# PRINCIPLES AND PRACTICE OF OBSTETRIC ANALGESIA AND ANESTHESIA

# PRINCIPLES AND PRACTICE OF OBSTETRIC ANALGESIA AND ANESTHESIA

JOHN J. BONICA, M.D.

*Chairman Emeritus and Professor*
*Department of Anesthesiology*
*University of Washington*
*Seattle, Washington*

JOHN S. McDONALD, M.D.

*Professor and Chairman*
*Department of Anesthesiology*
*The Ohio State University*
*Columbus, Ohio*

SECOND EDITION

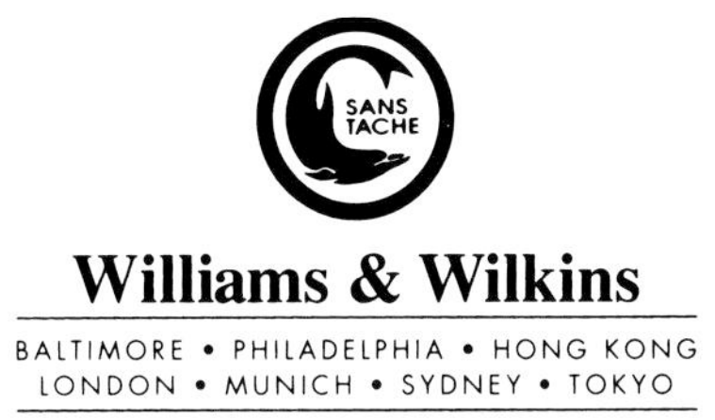


**Williams & Wilkins**

BALTIMORE • PHILADELPHIA • HONG KONG
LONDON • MUNICH • SYDNEY • TOKYO

A WAVERLY COMPANY
1995

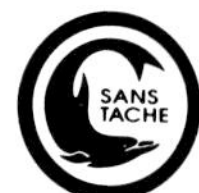


*Executive Editor:* Carroll C. Cann
*Developmental Editor:* Susan Hunsberger
*Production Coordinator:* Mary Clare Beaulieu
*Project Editor:* Robert D. Magee



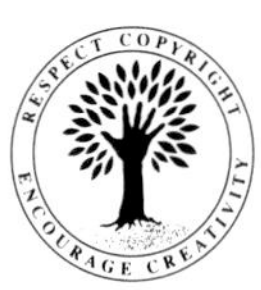




Accurate indications, adverse reactions, and dosage schedules for drugs are provided in this book, but it is possible they may change. The reader is urged to review the package information data of the manufacturers of the medications mentioned.

*Printed in the United States of America*

First Edition 1967

94 95 96 97 98
1 2 3 4 5 6 7 8 9 10

# IN MEMORIAM

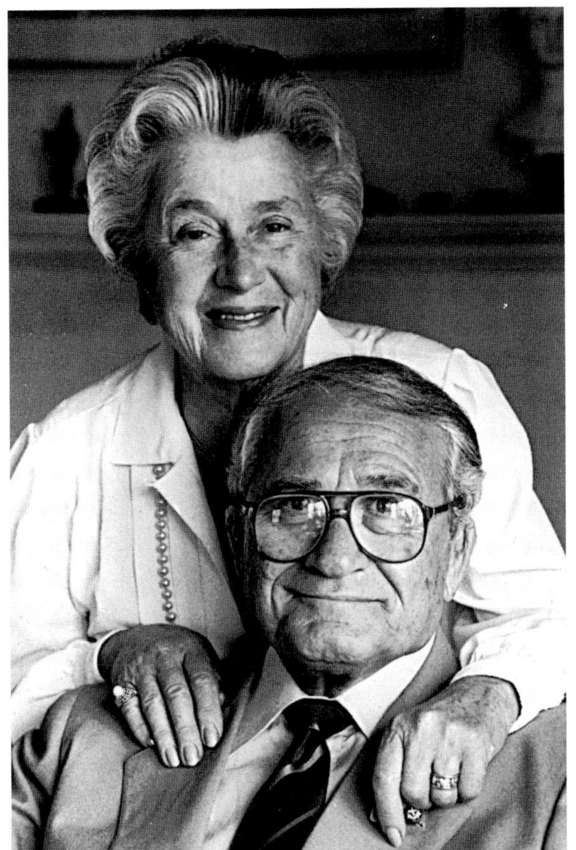



*Emma Bonica (1915–1994)*
*John Bonica (1917–1994)*

Dr. Bonica had three unmistakable passions in his life. The first, his beautiful family, consisting of his wife Emma, three daughters, Angela, Charlotte and Linda, and one son, John. The second, his work on pain, which culminated in his classic books of the first and second edition of *The Management of Pain.* The third, his work on obstetric anesthesiology, which culminated in a first edition of *The Principles and Practice of Obstetric Analgesia and Anesthesia* in 1968 and now in its second edition, this book, in 1994.

Dr. John J. Bonica championed the cause of obstetric anesthesia for over 50 years from 1940 until 1994. One dramatic but little known story is of his witness of near disaster during ether administration to his wife Emma during the birth of his first daughter, Angela. Dr. Bonica's speedy diagnosis of an airway problem and physical intervention prevented a catastrophe and prompted him to dedicate his life toward the improvement of care for the mother and her unborn baby. Dr. Bonica accomplished that during his life in providing us with the first comprehensive textbook on obstetric anesthesiology, the first edition of this book in 1968. Now, 26 years later, we are proud to present this revision of that original work. On a very personal note, after completion of this book this past June, Dr. Bonica expressed both his pride and pleasure with the work and hoped it would serve as an impetus for continued excellence in obstetric anesthesia management by anesthesiologists, obstetricians, neonatologists and other involved health care practitioners for many years to come.

John S. McDonald

# DEDICATION

This Volume is Dedicated to our families and foremost to our Wives:

Emma and Deborah

Man can ever be in awe of the unselfish love a woman gives over and over again in the best of times and in the worst of times. We were doubly blessed by the always present love and support of our wives. We thank them for the giving of our time to this important project.

And to our Children

Angela, Charlotte, Linda, and John

Douglas, Collin, Jeffrey, and Michelle

The writing of this book has deprived them of many hours and days of our time with them.

# PREFACE

The purpose of this text is to reconfirm the purpose of its predecessor, the first edition published in 1967. It is to offer an expansive, expressive, and exhaustive textbook of the many complex issues involved in providing the highest standard of care for the unborn baby and mother during the intrapartum challenge of labor and delivery. It is sighted toward all the many interactive disciplines of the field of perinatal medicine, including anesthesiology, obstetrics, neonatology, family medicine, nursing in all areas of perinatal medicine, and all physician assistants in these related fields so vital for the health and well being of the mother and her newborn baby.

Obstetric anesthesia is, today, finally, an established and even respected part of the delivery of anesthesia health care in today's environment. After so many years of attempting to be recognized as a valid entity and attempting to recruit interest from the speciality of anesthesiology, it now is fully accepted as one of the most vital and vivacious subinterest areas in the entire specialty. This has come about because of the persistence of so many dedicated physicians, including the senior author of this book, Dr. John J. Bonica. Dr. Bonica has spent the past 5 decades emphasizing that obstetric anesthesia deserves and even demands the highest of quality that anesthesiology can offer. He and many other of the early pioneers in the field did not stop the constant plea for improvement and involvement of anesthesiology in obstetrics. This book recognizes with profound appreciation the arduous and tiresome battles necessary to effect such a major change in attitude. Because of those who came before and laid this foundation for anesthesiology's involvement and because our fellow colleagues in obstetrics recognized that anesthesiology had not only much to offer for pain relief and humanitarian purposes but also in saving lives of both mothers and babies in many of the challenging complications of obstetrics, we do have that important acceptance in our country and many other countries today. Today's patients at tertiary care centers are being offered medical coverage consistent with other, similar levels of anesthesia care thoughout that hospital.

Research in the field of obstetric anesthesiology has come of age, evident by the increasing numbers of protocols and abstracts being submitted to hospitals, regional, national, and even international meetings in anesthesiology today. Regional analgesia, with the mother an active not passive participant, has become commonplace not extraordinary. Mothers now are able to take advantage of pain relief with reduced hazards to the fetus and newborn. Current methods of analgesia with combined therapy administered with small pumps at miniscule drip rates have revolutionalized this subspeciality and finally made the dream of labor and delivery with minimal pain and yet maximum safety for the mother and baby a realization.

The large number of illustrations will hopefully be appreciated by the readers as an expansion of the hidden textual material and as an easy method to quickly grasp the overview of a chapter. Naturally, some illustrations depict a method or technique of anesthesia, while others summarize in a visual fashion some of the complexity of issues in management. Certainly, one will agree that one picture can often crystallize a message that otherwise may be lost in detailed verbage. It is with these affirmations that we spent so many hours in search of the very best visuals to bring home a given point or descriptive.

This revision has been 5 years in the making. The involvement of busy, top-level academicians who are also solid practitioners has served to make it even more difficult. Busy schedules, lectures, travel, and clinical workloads made it an extremely abstruse task to adhere to schedules for the publisher. This book, like its first edition, has the unmistakable style of Dr. Bonica who has an uncanny way of distilling enormous amounts of literature into cohesive and coherent medical facts and doctrine. He offers the unparalled vision of the world's leading authority on pain in general, and his recent completion of his second edition of his monumental text on pain, *THE MANAGEMENT OF PAIN*, offers the readers a unique perspective not possible in any other textbook of obstetric anesthesiology. Thus, the leadership for this revision—from the individual chapter authors to the book's editors—brings the readers a comprehensive textbook for use by those in all levels of training and sophistication in the area of obstetric anesthesiology. In such a complex task there will be inevitable instances of repetition or at least of coverage of certain areas that are revisited due to the inescapable overlap that occurs. This overlapping sometimes acts as a benefit to the reader in helping to emphasize some difficult points of management or it sometimes prevents the "please refer to this subject on page x" scenarios, and thus allows the reader to maintain fluidity of thought on a given subject. We sincerely hope that readers will appreciate this aspect of the book's format. Special attention was paid to the last-minute update of literature for each chapter prior to publishing. Naturally, this up-to-dateness is vital to the solidarity of any contemporary textbook in a complex multidisciplinary area such as is encompassed by obstetrics, anesthesiology, and pediatrics-neonatology. This is a prodigious task and a time intensive one at that, but it must be done, again for the benefit of the reader and the references he or she may want to refer to at a later date. Finally, as mentioned, the enormity of the clinical experience of this group of authors is one for which the editors are very proud. Indeed, even the editors—one of whom (JSM) is still very active clinically—have enjoyed the privilege of either direct or indirect management of some 100,000 parturients between them over the past 5 decades.

The basic promise of this revision is based upon the same solid, simple credence of the first edition, i.e., the information in this text will hopefully give the reader the best and most up-to-date knowledge in regard to management of the many problems and challenges in the speciality of obstetric anesthesiology. It is our sincere wish that the many readers today, tomorrow, and in the distant future will appreciate the hundreds—even thousands—of hours necessary to bring this textbook to its final culmination.

Finally, no book can be brought to completion without the support and encouragement of a superb publisher. We found out the team responsible for the textbook with this country's oldest and one of the most respected publishers, Lea & Febiger. It has been a pleasure and a privilege to work with such a quality group of men and women throughout this effort. Their unremitting encouragement, understanding, patience, and direction have been most appreciated and important in the final, proud production of this book. If even one patient and/or her baby are helped by the fruits of this effort, then we can all rest well in the knowledge that something we have done may have contributed to the benefit of mankind in some small way.

It remains our fondest hope that this book will be both heralded and used as a definitive source of reference by the many practitioners of obstetric anesthesiology for the betterment and optimal management of the mother and her unborn baby.

John J. Bonica, M.D.
John S. McDonald, M.D.

# ACKNOWLEDGMENTS

This book, in its published form, as you see it, is the result of a major team effort. This acknowledgment is for the purpose of recognizing those many individuals who gave much time and effort to assure the final product. They are a talented and varied lot of specialists who form the infrastructure of that which is necessary to see a book of this complexity through to its completion and into its final published form.

We wish to acknowledge the authors of this book whose special qualifications made them authoritative and well versed for each particular chapter. We thank them for their many hours of research of the current literature and for combining that significant database with their own experience, as can be witnessed by their contribution. We are also grateful for their many hours spent in revising chapters in accordance with our numerous editorial suggestions.

We wish to acknowledge the immeasurable help of our in-house secretarial staff, including Julie Baker, Donna Rowe, Sue Naher, Cathy Chambers, Nancy Crawford, Jeri King, and Denise Ogden for their transcription, research, and organization of figures, tables, and references. Arlene Rogers was of superb help in regard to supervision of personnel and of immense support for helping to move the project along during its long evolution. The senior author also received significant research from the recent data supplied by Cliff Chadwick and Beth Glosten.

We wish to thank Mrs. Marjorie Domenowske for her untiring help and advice in regard to illustrations. She was able to redo and reformat many of the older figures from the first edition and make them pertinent for today's practice. She also did an excellent job of reviewing and redrawing many illustrations from other sources that were good but not quite clear enough to satisfy the standard we had established for this book.

Finally, we wish to thank the staff at Williams & Wilkins for their dedication and attention to detail in chapter editing, correcting, reformatting, clarifying, and substantiating of data. These include Carroll Cann, Susan Hunsberger, Bob Magee, and Mary Clare Beaulieu.

# CONTRIBUTORS

Alan J. Appley, MD
Neurological Surgery
Lake Mary, Florida

Sarah L. Artman, MD
Clinical Instructor
Obstetrics and Gynecology
Ohio State University
Columbus, Ohio

Eduardo Bancalari, MD
Professor of Pediatrics and Obstetrics/Gynecology
University of Miami School of Medicine
Miami, Florida

Costantino Benedetti, MD
Clinical Professor
Department of Anesthesiology
Ohio State University
Columbus, Ohio

Thomas J. Benedetti, MD
Professor, Department of Obstetrics and Gynecology
University of Washington
Seattle, Washington

John M. Bissonette, MD
Professor of Obstetrics/Gynecology
Obstetrical Research Laboratory
Oregon Health Sciences University
Portland, Oregon

John J. Bonica, MD, DSc, FRC Anaest.
Chairman Emeritus and Professor
Department of Anesthesiology
University of Washington
Seattle, Washington

Heathcliff S. Chadwick, MD
Associate Professor of Anesthesiology
Department of Anesthesiology
University of Washington
Seattle, Washington

Richard B. Clark, MD
Professor
Department of Anesthesiology
University of Arkansas for Medical Sciences
Little Rock, Arkansas

Barry C. Corke, MB, ChB, FFARCS
Director of Obstetrical Anesthesia
Department of Anesthesiology
Christiana Hospital
Newark, Delaware

Gabriel M. de Courten-Myers, MD
Associate Professor, Neuropathology
Department of Pathology and Laboratory Medicine
University of Cincinnati, College of Medicine
Cincinnati, Ohio

Richard Depp, MD
Professor and Chairman
Department of Obstetrics and Gynecology
Jefferson Medical College
Philadelphia, Pennsylvania

Cosmo A. DiFazio, MD, PhD
Professor of Anesthesiology
Department of Anesthesiology
University of Virginia, Health Sciences Center
Charlottesville, Virginia

Thomas R. Easterling, MD
Assistant Professor
Department of Obstetrics and Gynecology
University of Washington
Seattle, Washington

John P. Elliott, MD
Associate Director
Maternal-Fetal Medicine
Good Samaritan Medical Center
Phoenix, Arizona

Avroy Fanaroff, MB, FRCP, DCH
Professor and Vice Chairman
Department of Pediatrics
Case Western Reserve University
Cleveland, Ohio

John I. Fishburne, Jr, MD
Professor
Department of Obstetrics and Gynecology
University of Oklahoma Health Sciences Center
Oklahoma City, Oklahoma

Michael Foley, MD
Director, Obstetric Intensive Care Unit
Good Samaritan Regional Medical Center
Phoenix, Arizona

Roger K. Freeman, MD
Professor, Obstetrics and Gynecology
University of California
Irvine, California

Thomas M. Fuhrman, MD
Assistant Professor
Department of Anesthesiology
Ohio State University
Columbus, Ohio

Steven G. Gabbe, MD
Professor and Chairman
Department of Obstetrics and Gynecology
Ohio State University
Columbus, Ohio

Steven L. Giannotta, MD
Professor
Department of Neurological Surgery
University of Southern California School of Medicine
Los Angeles, California

Karen Hendricks-Muñoz, MD
Associate Professor
Department of Pediatrics
New York University Medical Center
New York, New York

L. Wayne Hess, MD
Assistant Professor/Director
Department of Obstetrics/Gynecology
Maternal-Fetal Medicine
University of Missouri Medical Center
Columbia, Missouri

Harold J. Hunter, Jr, Esq
Kirtland & Packard
Los Angeles, California

Jay Jacoby, MD, PhD
Professor and Chairman Emeritus
Department of Anesthesiology
Ohio State University
Columbus, Ohio

Kirk A. Keegan, MD
Assistant Professor
Department of Obstetrics/Gynecology
University of California, Irvine Medical Center
Orange, California

Robert R. Kirby, MD
Professor of Anesthesiology
Department of Anesthesiology, University of Florida
Gainesville, Florida

Mark B. Landon, MD
Assistant Professor
Department of Obstetrics and Gynecology
Division of Maternal-Fetal Medicine
Ohio State University
Columbus, Ohio

Jeff E. Mandel, MD, MS
Associate Professor of Anesthesiology
Department of Anesthesiology
Tulane University School of Medicine
New Orleans, Louisiana

John H. McAnulty, MD
Professor of Medicine
Division of Cardiology
Oregon Health Sciences University
Portland, Oregon

James McArthur, MD
Professor of Medicine
Division of Hematology
University of Washington
Seattle, Washington

James A. McGregor, MD, CM
Professor
Department of Obstetrics and Gynecology
University of Colorado Hospital, Health Sciences Center
Denver, Colorado

John S. McDonald, MD
Professor and Chairman
Department of Anesthesiology
Ohio State University
Columbus, Ohio

Frank C. Miller, MD
Professor and Chairman
Department of Obstetrics and Gynecology
University of Kentucky
Lexington, Kentucky

Houchang D. Modanlou, MD
Associate Professor, Pediatrics
University of California
Irvine, California

Mark A. Morgan, MD
Assistant Professor, Maternal Fetal Medicine
Department of Obstetrics and Gynecology
Division of Maternal-Fetal Medicine
University of California Irvine Medical Center
Orange, California

John C. Morrison, MD
Vice Chairman
Maternal-Fetal Medicine
University of Mississippi Medical Center
Jackson, Mississippi

Ronald E. Myers, MD, PhD
Associated Chief of Staff for Research
Department of Veterans Affairs Medical Center
Cincinnati, Ohio

J. Steven Naulty, MD
Director of Obstetric Anesthesia
George Washington University School of Medicine
Washington, D.C.

Richard W. O'Shaughnessy, MD
Professor
Department of Obstetrics and Gynecology
Maternal-Fetal Medicine
Ohio State University
Columbus, Ohio

Tim H. Parmley, MD
Professor of Obstetrics/Gynecology
Department of Obstetrics and Gynecology
University of Arkansas for Medical Sciences
Little Rock, Arkansas

Martin L. Pernoll, MD
Chairman Obstetrics/Gynecology
MacGregor Medical Association
Houston, Texas

Edward J. Quilligan, MD
Dean, School of Medicine
University of California Irvine Medical Center
Orange, California

James M. Roberts, MD
Professor and Vice-Chairman
Department of Obstetrics, Gynecology and Reproductive Sciences
Magee Women's Hospital
University of Pittsburgh
Pittsburgh, Pennsylvania

Patricia A. Robertson, MD
Assistant Professor
Department of Obstetrics, Gynecology and Reproductive Sciences
Universtity of California School of Medicine
San Francisco, California

Dan W. Rurak, D.Phil
Professor
Department of Obstetrics and Gynaecology
University of British Columbia
Vancouver, British Columbia, Canada

Merlin H. Sayers, MD, PhD
Medical and Laboratory Director
Puget Sound Blood Center and Program
Seattle, Washington

Jack Schneider, MD
Medical Director
Mary Birch Hospital for Women at Sharp Memorial Hospital, Women's Center
San Diego, California

John W. Seeds, MD
Professor and Director, Maternal and Fetal Medicine
Department of Obstetrics/Gynecology
University of Arizona Health Sciences Center
Tucson, Arizona

Penny Simkin, PT
Seattle, Washington

AnneMarie Sommer, MD
Associate Professor of Pediatrics
Genetics Section
Children's Hospital
Columbus, Ohio

Jon R. Sundin, MD
Clinical Assistant Professor
Department of Anesthesiology
University of Utah Health Sciences Center
Salt Lake City, Utah

Nikolai Tehin, Esq
Bostwick & Tehin
San Francisco, California

Kent Ueland, MD
Lahaina Maui, Hawaii

Robin J. Willcourt, MD
Director
Washoe Perinatal Services
Reno, Nevada

K. C. Wong, MD, PhD
Professor and Chairman of Anesthesiology
Professor of Pharmacology
University of Utah Health Sciences Center
Salt Lake City, Utah

Andrew M. Woods, MD
Associate Professor
Department of Anesthesiology
University of Virginia
Charlottesville, Virginia

# CONTENTS

## PART I. BASIC CONSIDERATIONS



## PART II: PHARMACOLOGY AND TECHNIQUES OF OBSTETRIC ANALGESIA AND ANESTHESIA

## Section D: Pharmacology and Techniques of General Analgesia and Anesthesia



## Section E: Nonpharmacologic Methods of Obstetric Analgesia and Anesthesia



# PART III: CLINICAL CONSIDERATIONS

## Section F: Analgesia and Anesthesia for Normal Labor and Vaginal Delivery



## Section G: Analgesia and Anesthesia for Major Obstetric Problems



## Section H: Nonobstetric Maternal Complications

## Section I: Obstetric Analgesia and Anesthesia for Fetal Complications

PART I

# BASIC CONSIDERATIONS

Section A

# HISTORIC CONSIDERATIONS

Chapter 1

# EVOLUTION AND CURRENT STATUS

JOHN J. BONICA

---

Understanding and controlling the pain associated with childbirth have concerned humankind since the beginning of time. While some authorities have suggested that childbirth pain is a product of human civilization (1–4), there is much evidence to suggest that women have suffered pain in childbirth for as long as humans have existed and continue to seek relief (5–18). In this chapter, a concise overview of the evolution and current status of obstetric analgesia and anesthesia is presented in three parts: (1) overview of the historic development of obstetric analgesia and anesthesia from prehistoric time to the mid-1950s; (2) the most important trends and advances made in this field from 1960 to 1994; and (3) the current status of obstetric analgesia and anesthesia in the United States, United Kingdom, Canada, and 31 other countries based on data acquired through two surveys made in 1984 and 1989. Because of space limitations, citation of the vast literature will be limited to key articles only, many of which can be consulted for more detailed accounts of specific issues.

## HISTORIC PERSPECTIVE

The concepts of pain associated with childbirth and its management throughout recorded history are some of the most interesting aspects in the evolution of medicine in general and in the development of the speciality of anesthesiology in particular. Indeed, the history of obstetric anesthesia has been the subject of discussion in books by Claye (7), Fulop-Miller (8), Sigerist (9), and Bellucci (10), and of extensive review articles by Dallenbach (11), Heaton (12), and Tainter (18). For some years I have categorized the evolution and development of obstetric analgesia and anesthesia into six periods or phases, *many of which overlap in time*:

1. The Preanesthesia Period, extending from prehistoric and ancient times to 1846;
2. The Period of the Great Discovery and promising beginning—the *naissance* (birth) of obstetric analgesia and anesthesia (1846 to 1860): (a) in the UK and (b) in the USA;
3. The Period of Technical Advances and the development of the speciality of anesthesiology (1900 to 1950);
4. The Period of Neglect, considered the "Dark Ages of obstetric analgesia and anesthesia" (1860–1940);
5. The "Renaissance of obstetric anesthesia," the transition from obstetrician to the anesthesiologist (1945-present, 1994);
6. The period of major growth and major advances (1960-present, 1994).

### The Preanesthesia Period

#### *Prehistoric Times*

There is evidence to suggest that the earliest attempts to control pain in childbirth consisted of psychologic, physical, and pharmacologic techniques or a combination of these (8,9,11,19,20). Primitive peoples considered pain an evil spirit and made many efforts to ward off, appease, or otherwise frighten away the pain demons by using various charms and incantations, conjurations, and spells made by the medicine man of the tribe, intent on putting the pain demons to flight. Obviously such combined distractions, suggestions, and subtle forms of hypnosis can be called collectively "psychologic analgesia."

Various physical maneuvers also were used by most primitive peoples to hasten labor and relieve pain. In his book, "Labor Among Primitive Peoples" (20), written over a century ago following intensive and extensive research, the American Engelmann discussed in detail the use of massage, external manipulation, and various forms of posture by primitive peoples from all parts of the world. Massage of the abdomen and back, Englemann found, while used primarily to help ameliorate pain, also stimulated uterine contractions and thus hastened labor. During uterine contractions among primitive people of the Pacific Islands, for example, Englemann found strong pressure applied to the abdomen, ribs, and low back (Figure 1–1). Recent research suggests that such massage and pressure relieves pain by stimulating large fiber input, as obtained with transcutaneous electrical nerve stimulation (TENS).

In some tribes the medicine man would encircle the parturient's abdomen by clasping his hands in front of the uterine fundus, thus forming a powerful compressor, while in other parturients, he would jump up and down upon the abdomen. Other physical measures included having the parturient tied to, or suspended from a tree, with arms tied over her head or with ropes secured under the armpits (20,21). In still others, parturients knelt with one or more assistants standing on her shoulders. Although all of these positions and maneuvers were used to hasten the delivery of the child, all had a most distracting effect and thus decreased the intensity of labor pain.

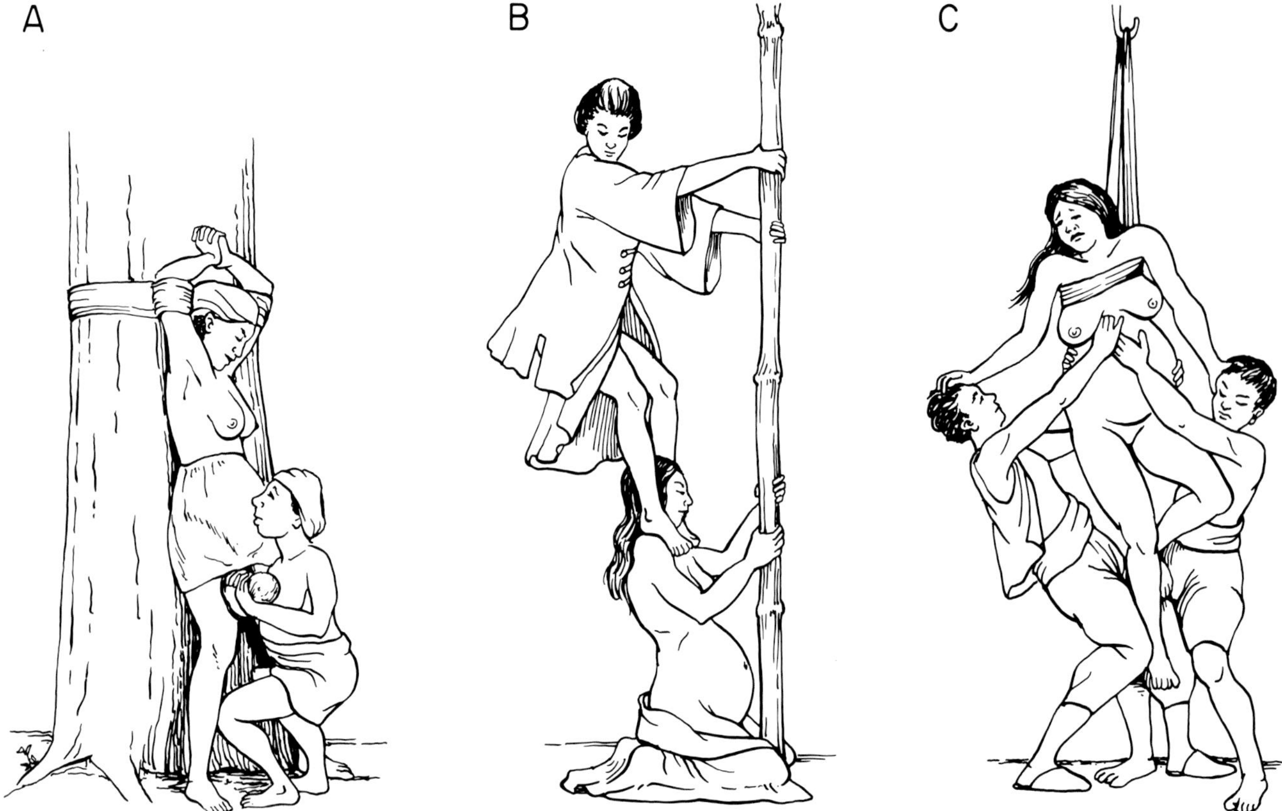


**Fig. 1–1.** Management of parturients among primitive people. **A,** Example of one form of a fixed, stressful position that may have helped to distract the mother's attention. Note that the arms are tied in place above the head, essentially lashing the patient to a tree. **B,** Example of kneeling position, with stress applied by an assistant standing on parturient's shoulders. Again, an obviously distractive maneuver. **C,** Another example of stress by which the parturient is suspended by both armpits from a pole, with added distraction from assistants rubbing the parturient's abdomen. (Modified from Englemann GL: Labor Among Primitive People. 2nd Ed. St. Louis, JH Chambers & Co., 1883.)

## *Ancient Cultures*

In addition to the psychologic and physical techniques, herbs were used by primitive and ancient peoples who, by experimenting with various plants as foods, discovered that some of these were efficacious in assuaging pain. The use of herbs was taken over gradually by the medicine man, who surrounded his knowledge of the mystic, herbal concoctions handed down to him by sorcerers and magicians with mystery, incantation, and ritual. Supplications and prayers for the relief of pain are found on Babylonian clay tablets and Egyptian papyri written in the days of the pyramid builders, in ancient Chinese writings and in the Hebrew books of the Old Testament that encompass 4,000 years of recorded history before Christ, on the parchment rolls from Troy, and in all ancient civilizations. All such writings entail the use of suggestions, distractions, and other psychologic forms of analgesia. The concentrated form of suggestions—which today we call hypnotism—was used by the Egyptians, Chinese, and other advanced cultures to relieve the pain of childbirth. Ellis (22) suggested that possibly the first recorded instance of hypnotism occurred with the proto-obstetric case found in Genesis 2:21 (Figure 1–2).

The concept of pain as punishment by the gods and its relief through prayer to these gods is found in the writings of ancient Greeks and Romans. There is reference to the Greek blonde goddess Agamede, who had exclusive power to relieve pain (9), and to the goddess Actemia, who having been terrified by her mother's suffering at her own birth, besought Zeus the favor of eternal virginity. Reference to the pain of childbirth and the need to relieve it is also found in the writings of Plato, Aristotle, and Theocritus, among others (4). The Greeks also recognized the importance of women who had special knowledge and powers to help women in labor. Theocritus (23) stated: "For then the daughter of Antigone, weighed down with throes, called out for Lucina, the friend of women in travail, and she with kind favor stood by her, and in sooth poured down her whole limbs an insensibility to pain, and so a lively boy, like his father, was born."

## *Judeo Hebraic and Christian Era*

The concept of pain related to sin and punishment was also prevalent in the Judeo-Hebraic civilization, which, of course, believed in only one God. Thus we find many references in the Old Testament to the pain of childbirth. In Genesis 3:16, it is found "unto the woman, I will greatly multiply thy sorrow and thy conception: in sorrow thou

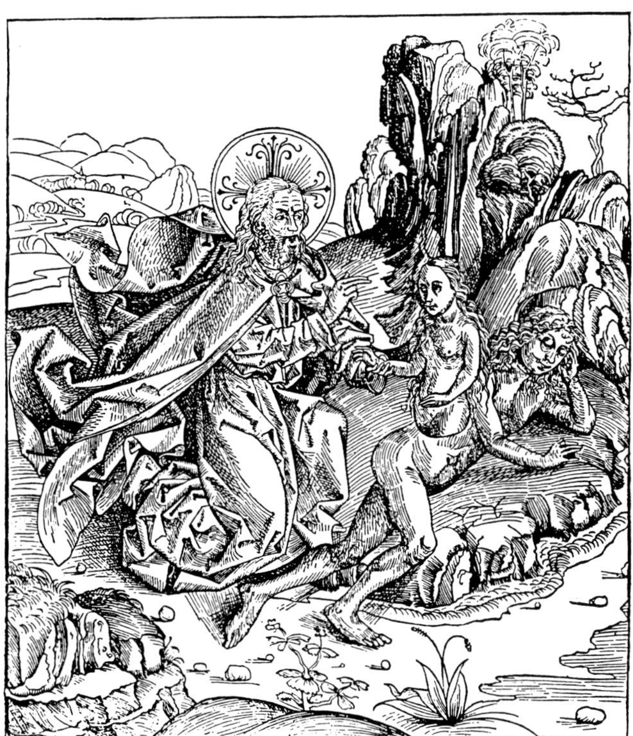

**Fig. 1–2.** "And the Lord God caused a deep sleep to fall upon Adam, and he slept; and He took one of his ribs, and closed up the flesh instead thereof." (Wood engraving attributed to Michael Wohlgemuth from the *Nuremberg Chronicle*, 1493. From Keys TE: The History of Surgical Anesthesia. New York, Shulman's, 1945.)

shalt bring forth children." The prophet Jeremiah (4:31) wrote, "for I have heard a voice as of a woman in travail and the anguish as of her that bringeth forth a first child, the voice of the daughter of Zion, that bewaileth herself that spreadeth her hands saying woe is me now."

The same concept of pain related to sin and punishment was adopted in the Christian ethic. The Apostle Paul probably reviewed all of the information on this subject in Romans 8:22 when he said, "For we know that the whole creation groaneth and travaileth in pain together until now." This concept of pain related to sin and punishment is emphasized by the origin of the word "pain," derived from the Latin "poena," meaning punishment and its relief through prayer. Consequently, pain became an important means of obtaining grace or a sacrament, and a woman in labor was expected to accept pain voluntarily without attempt to relieve it by other means. The same affirmation of pain was embraced by all Oriental as well as various Western religions.

Despite these religious principles and teachings, attempts to relieve childbirth pain continued. In addition to (or at times instead of) the psychologic analgesic action of prayer, concoctions and extracts of opium and other plants, alcohol, and various other techniques continued to be used for the relief of childbirth pain. In Europe during the Middle Ages, wine, beer, brandy, and other alcoholic beverages were kept beside the maternity bed for self-administration (9,18).

### *The Renaissance to the Nineteenth Century*

While the Renaissance fostered a great scientific spirit and effected remarkable advancements in chemistry, physics, physiology, and anatomy, it contributed little to the understanding and control of pain of childbirth. Thus we find that the same concepts and treatments of the ancients were used to control pain. Moreover, the religious opposition to efforts to relieve the pain of childbirth continued and was especially strong in some countries. As late as 1591, Eufame MacAlyane of Edinburgh was buried alive on Castle Hill for seeking the assistance of Agnes Sampsom for the relief of pain at the birth of her two sons (7). In those times many "witches" were persecuted for attempting to abolish the pains of labor. On the other hand, some physicians, realizing the needs of women suffering from labor pain, included prescriptions for their relief. Thus in 1660, Wecker (24) wrote a prescription titled "That a woman may be quickly delivered and without pain, an approved way," consisting of the following instructions: "Take clary a sufficient quantity, pound it well and press forth the juice; take half a cup full, mingle it with wine and give it to the woman to drink when she is in labour, then bind the herb that is pressed hot to her navel."

Six years later, Zerobabel Endecott (25), a physician of Salem, Massachusetts and the son of the governor, described a prescription titled "For sharpe and dificult travel in women with child," which, though hardly effective, revealed his conviction for the necessity of relieving pain in difficult labor.

> "Take a Lock of Vergins haire on any Part of ye head, of half the Age of ye Woman in trauill. Cut it very smale to fine Pouder than take 12 Ants Eggs dried in an ouen after ye bread is drawne or other wise make them dry & make them to pouder with the haire, giue this with a quarter of a pint of Red Cows milk or for want of it giue it in strong ale wort."

Such a prescription written by physician for the relief of pain continued for the next century and a half. In 1804 Peter Miller (26A) and two years later, William Dewees (26B), wrote theses for the Degree of Doctor of Medicine, in which they advocated the use of nauseating medicaments to distract a woman in labor, vigorous exercise, semistarvation, and copious bloodletting. A decade later Benajmin Rush, the great American physician, in his classic treatise, expressed the hope that a medicine would be discovered which "should suspend sensibility . . . and thereby destroy labor pains altogether (27)," without impairing uterine contractions.

## The Period of the Great Discovery

### *The* Naissance *of Obstetric Analgesia/Anesthesia*

Dr. Rush's hope was realized little over a quarter century later by Long, Morton, Simpson, Snow, and Channing, as each played a uniquely different role in making possible the conquest of surgical pain of which Sir William Osler later called "medicine's greatest gift to suffering humanity" (19). This milestone in the history of humankind was achieved through public demonstration of the effects of ether in producing surgical anesthesia and, subsequently, to relieve pain of childbirth—an event that can be called the *naissance* (birth) of obstetric analgesia/anesthesia.

The fact that Crawford Long, a physician in Georgia, did administer the first surgical anesthesia on March 30, 1842, some 4½ years before Morton's public demonstration in Boston (28), is well known. What is not widely appreciated is that Long had a special interest in obstetrics and used ether analgesia for vaginal delivery. Although Keys (19), based on a book on Long written later by his daughter (29), suggested that Long administered ether for childbirth at about the same time as Simpson, Raper (30) disputes this. In any case, because Long did not report his experience until 1849 (31), credit for the introduction of modern anesthesia in obstetrics rightly belongs to Sir James Y. Simpson of Edinburgh, Scotland, who used ether anesthesia in childbirth on January 19, 1847, to accomplish an internal version in a patient with fetopelvic disproportion due to a contracted pelvis. This took place 3 months after Morton's demonstration and 4 weeks after ether was first used in surgery in Britain (19). Simpson reported the event to the Edinburgh Obstetrical Society the next day and published the first paper a month later (32). A detailed account of Simpson's life and list of his publications relating to obstetric anesthesia is found in the book by Priestley & Stover (33), which contains his memoirs.

With subsequent experience Simpson became convinced that properly administered ether anesthesia eliminated the pain of childbirth without harm to the child and that it should be used not only in operative obstetrics but in the relief of the pain of normal labor. Simpson continued to improve the apparatus and began testing chloroform and finally used it for the first time as an obstetric anesthetic on November 8, 1847. In the ensuing months, Simpson's example was followed by many other obstetricians in Britain, Canada, France, Germany, Italy, the United States, and other countries throughout the world (7,12,19,34). It is of interest to note that in the same year the famous Russian surgeon Pirigoff reported the use of ether by rectum for surgical and obstetric anesthesia (19).

The use of anesthesia in childbirth aroused violent opposition from some physicians and from the public but aroused particularly the clergy, who labeled Simpson a heretic, a blasphemer, and an agent of the devil. Toward their cause, the clergy cited the Biblical admonition, "In sorrow thou shalt bring forth children." In rebuttal, Simpson, himself was an astute student of the Bible, cited the passage in Genesis 2:21 (i.e., anesthesia given to Adam), quoted in the Figure 1–2 legend. Simpson further added "What God, Himself did cannot be sinful," and argued, "But even if . . . we . . . were to admit that woman was, as the result of the primal curse, adjudged to the miseries of pure physical pain and agony in parturition, still, certainly, the Christian dispensation, the moral *necessity* of undergoing such anguish has ceased and terminated." Simpson also took on, as he had the religious leaders, British and American obstetricians and physicians who opposed obstetric anesthesia (33). His arguments were highly effective in neutralizing the opposition, and, within a short period, obstetric anesthesia was used worldwide. For a detailed and in-depth review of the controversy between Simpson and Meigs and others that makes interesting and, indeed, delightful reading, the reader should consult the article by Caton (35).

The incomparable contributions of John Snow to the early development of anesthesiology are too well known to repeat here. His precocious concepts, painstaking research, accurate and perspicacious writings, and clinical practice were among the most important factors for the initial development of anesthesia and accrued him a reputation as an outstanding practitioner of the art (36,37). It was logical, therefore, that, when in 1853 Queen Victoria requested she be given chloroform to relieve the pain that she anticipated with the birth of her eighth child Prince Leopold, Snow was called to administer it. On April 7, 1853, he gave his royal patient 15 minim doses intermittently on a handkerchief to achieve analgesia, a technique that became known as *anesthesie a la reine*. After the delivery the queen made the following note in her personal diary: "Dr. Snow gave that blessed chloroform and the effect was soothing, quieting and delightful beyond measure" (cited verbatim by Claye) (36). In a letter to Simpson dated April 19, 1853, Sir James Clark, the Queen's obstetrician, described the highly successful administration by stating, in part (35) ". . . the Queen had chloroform exhibited to her during her late confinement. It acted admirably. It was not at any time given so strongly as to render the Queen insensible. . . . Her Majesty was greatly pleased with the effect and she certainly never had a better recovery. . . . I know this information will please you and I have little doubt it will lead to a more general use of chloroform in midwifery practice in this quarter than hereto prevailed. . . ."

The epochal event was not publicized because of the great opposition by Mr. Thomas Wakley, editor of the *Lancet* (36). However, on April 18, 1857, the *Lancet* reported that Snow had administered with optimal results a 2½-hour chloroform analgesia to the Queen for delivery of Princess Beatrice. . . . This announcement was tantamount to moral, medical, and even religious sanction of the relief of pain of childbirth and must be considered one of the most important milestones in the history of obstetric anesthesia.

The last of Snow's many contributions to this field was his book "Chloroform and Other Anesthetics," published 2 months after his premature death in 1858 (38). The book contains detailed descriptions of the chemistry, pharmacology, side effects, complications, and clinical application of chloroform, ether, and amylene. The use of these agents for obstetric anesthesia was given special consideration, and his description of the technique of administering chloroform to parturients has never been improved.

> "The moment to begin is at the commencement of a pain; and the chloroform should be intermitted when the uterine contraction subsides, or sooner, if the patient is relieved of her suffering. It is desirable to give the chloroform very gently at first, increasing the quantity a little with each pain, if the patient is not relieved.

> The practitioner easily finds, with little attention, the quantity of vapour which it is desirable to give at any stage of the labour, and in each particular case; his object being to relieve the patient without diminishing the strength of uterine contractions and the auxiliary action of the respiratory muscles, or with diminishing it as little as possible. At first, it is generally necessary to repeat the chloroform at the beginning of each "pain"; but, after a little time, it commonly happens that sufficient effect has been produced to get the patient over one or two uterine contractions without suffering before it is resumed.... It may be remarked, that complete anesthesia is never induced in midwifery, unless in some cases of operative delivery" (38).

Throughout the book, Snow emphasized the importance of avoiding complications through careful and skillful administration and admonished the medical profession to limit the administration of these potent drugs to physicians with interest, scientific knowledge, and experience acquired first through preceptorship training.

### *Obstetric Anesthesia in America During the Initial Period*

The first recorded case of the use of ether for obstetrics in America was reported by N.C. Keep in the April 1847 issue of the *Boston Medical and Surgical Journal*, in an article entitled "Leoneon administered in a case of labor." In the article he described the intermittent administration of ether to a healthy parturient having a normal and uncomplicated but painful labor for her third child. As first pointed out by Thoms (39), Keep was apparently the first to use *analgesie a la reine*, because the parturients who were given ether did not lose consciousness. Although Simpson had used ether for obstetrics nearly 3 months earlier, it is obvious from his description of the case that he induced anesthesia with loss of consciousness.

A month later Walter Channing, Professor of Obstetrics at Harvard Medical School, reported in the same journal "A case of inhalation of ether in instrumental labor" and that summer published a pamphlet, making it the first independent publication on the subject in the United States. In September of the following year Channing, who by then had become the champion of obstetric analgesia in America, published the book "A Treatise on Etherization in Childbirth" (40). In this book, which in Channing's words "treats of a noble subject... the remedy of pain," he and some 20 physicians reported the use of ether in 581 cases. Throughout the book the author emphasized that his objective was to make ether "safe both to mother and to child."

At the second annual meeting of the American Medical Association held in Boston in 1849, the Committee on Obstetrics dealt chiefly with the consideration of anesthetics and their application in obstetric practice. It stated that the use of these agents "was not only justifiable for the purpose of alleviating the pain of labor, but also that in all *difficult and instrumental labors* their application *could not be rightfully withheld*" (41). On June 25, 1848, Dr. A.F. Holmes administered the first obstetric analgesia in Canada. That same year, analgesia/anesthesia was administered in Australia, New Zealand, and South Africa.

During those early years, the use of anesthesia in American obstetrics was strongly opposed by many medical and obstetric authorities as well as most of the clergy and some of the public. Outstanding among these was Professor Charles P. Meigs of Philadelphia, who had exchanged letters with Simpson. Like *some* present-day obstetricians, Meigs believed that anesthesia was neither necessary nor justifiable because childbirth pain was not sufficient to risk any possible complication and also because he "regarded labor pain as a most desirable, salutary, and conservative manifestation of life force" (42). In his authoritative textbook published in 1852 (43), Meigs calculated that because the average duration of labor was 4 hours and the number of contractions were about 50, each lasting 30 seconds, the woman experienced a total of 25 minutes of pain but not consecutively. He further stated that "it was improper at several points to contravene the operation of those natural and physiologic forces that the Divinity has ordained us to enjoy or to suffer."

### *The Latter Half of the 19th Century*

Despite the great achievements of the aforementioned preeminent physicians at mid-nineteenth century, development of obstetric analgesia and anesthesia was very slow and, as will be mentioned later, such development even regressed. The few advances related to this field made during the latter half of the 19th century include the following nine (5,10,12,19,44,45).

1. Introduction of the domette-covered wire frame mask by Skinner, a Liverpool obstetrician, in 1862;
2. Development of the needle and syringe during the period from 1845 to 1858;
3. Isolation of an alkaloid from the cocoa plant by Gaedeke in 1855 and its purification by Nieman, who called it cocaine 5 years later;
4. First use of nitrous oxide-oxygen for the relief of labor pains by Klikovich of St. Petersburg in 1881;
5. First clinical use of cocaine for local anesthesia by Karl Koller, a Viennese ophthalmologist, in 1884;
6. Invention of the first practical gas-oxygen machine and the use of nitrous oxide-oxygen for labor by Sir Frederick Hewit in 1887;
7. First description of the human pain pathways from the uterus by Henry Head in 1893 and the founding of the first society of physician anesthetists in London the same year;
8. First clinical use of spinal anesthesia for surgery by Bier in 1889;
9. Synthesis of a number of other local anesthetics during the last decade of the century.

Advances 2, 3, and 5 were important steps in the subsequent development of regional anesthesia (5,44).

## The Period of Technical Advances and the Development of the Specialty of Anesthesiology

During the first 5 decades of the twentieth century, various important developments took place related to anesthesiology in general, all of which may be referenced

**Table 1–1.** Period of Technical Advances in Obstetric Analgesia and Anesthesia

| | |
|---|---|
| 1900—*Kries, Doloris* | First use of spinal anesthesia in obstetrics |
| 1902—*Hopkins* | First use of spinal anesthesia for cesarean section in USA |
| 1905—*Einhorn* | Synthesized procaine for regional anesthesia |
| 1908—*Mueller* | First use of pudendal block for vaginal delivery |
| 1909—*Stoeckel* | First use of caudal anesthesia in obstetrics |
| 1923—*Labat* | Founded the American Society of Regional Anesthesia which was merged with the ASA in 1937 and reorganized in 1974 |
| 1925—*Miescher* | Synthesized dibucaine (Nupercaine) |
| 1926—*Gelert* | First paracervical block for labor pain |
| 1927—*Dellepiane* | First lumbar sympathetic block for labor pain |
| 1928—*Eisleb* | Synthetized tetracaine (Pontocaine) |
| 1928—*Cleland* | Animal experiments and paravertebral block in parturients to define uterine pain pathways |
| 1928—*Pitkin* | Controlled spinal (procaine/glucose) anesthesia in obstetrics |
| 1931—*Aburel* | Continuous paravertebral block for relief of labor pain |
| 1933—*Dogliotti* | Detailed study of lumbar and thoracic epidural anesthesia |
| 1934—*Cosgrove* | Extensive use of spinal anesthesia for labor, vaginal delivery, and cesarean section |
| 1935—*Graffignino* | First use of lumbar epidural block in obstetrics |
| 1940—*Lull & Ullery* | First use of continuous spinal for obstetric analgesia and anesthesia |
| 1942—*Hingson & Edwards* | First use of continuous caudal with malleable needle for obstetric analgesia/anesthesia |
| 1943—*Lundy et al.* | First use of catheter for continuous caudal block |
| 1943—*Lofgren* | Synthesized lidocaine (Xylocaine) |
| 1945—*Burton & Resnick* | Introduced modified "saddle" block in obstetrics |
| 1946—*Adriani et al.* | Standardized "saddle" block for obstetric analgesia and anesthesia |
| 1948—*Curbelo* | First continuous lumbar epidural block for surgery |
| 1949—*Flower et al.* | First continuous lumbar epidural block for obstetric analgesia and anesthesia |
| 1949—*Cleland* | Double catheter extradural obstetric analgesia and anesthesia |

in further detail (19,44,45) (Table 1–1). Interestingly, the direction of the development of anesthesia in Britain, the United States, Canada, and other English-speaking countries differed from the direction taken in continental Europe, Latin America, and Asia. In the latter countries, Bier's demonstration of spinal anesthesia for surgery initiated what I have called "The Golden Age of Regional Anesthesia" because during this period, virtually all of the techniques in current use were developed and applied widely. Moreover, a number of new and safer local anesthetics were synthesized and introduced into clinical practice. These developments were prompted by the conviction among most surgeons that properly applied, regional anesthesia afforded significant advantages over general anesthesia as then administered. Although these techniques were first developed to produce surgical anesthesia, most of them were promptly applied to obstetric patients. Table 1–1 lists the most important developments in the use of regional anesthesia for vaginal delivery and cesarean section. As noted, during the 1940s several Americans contributed significantly to the development of regional anesthetic techniques for obstetric patients.

During this period, European and some American obstetricians developed new techniques of systemic analgesia/anesthesia for obstetrics. In 1902, Von Steinbuchel (46) of Austria, and Gauss of Germany (47) began to use and advocate *Dammerschlaf*, or twilight sleep, which a year earlier had been used for surgical anesthesia. This technique entailed the injection of large doses of morphine for analgesia and scopolamine to produce amnesia, given at frequent intervals during labor and delivery. Soon after its introduction, it was given widespread publicity as a form of "painless childbirth" and thus caused many women to demand it, and in America a "Twilight Sleep Association" was formed. Although used subsequently in many obstetric centers throughout the world, many obstetricians became concerned about the severe neonatal depression inherent in this technique and resorted to less perinatal-depressing methods.

In 1911 Guedel (48) suggested the use of self-administration of nitrous oxide-air mixture during labor, and 2 years later Gwathmey (49) reported on the use of rectal ether-in-oil. In 1915, Webster (50), of Chicago, reported very favorable experience with nitrous oxide-oxygen administered during labor and delivery, while at about the same time Davis (51) published his book "Painless Childbirth: Eutocia and Nitrous Oxide-Oxygen Analgesia," which contained favorable statistics on over 500 parturients delivered in three Chicago hospitals. Despite its advantages, this method was not widely used for the first stage of labor, probably because it entailed the prolonged presence of the administrator. Consequently, during the ensuing quarter century, some obstetricians continued to rely on *Dammerschlaf* but many discarded this and used narcotics alone or combined narcotics with barbiturates or other sedatives to relieve the pain of the first stage.

During the late decades of the nineteenth century and into the early part of the twentieth century, in Britain, the United States, Canada, and other English-speaking countries, emphasis was placed on the development of physician anesthesia, reflected by the founding and growth of organized anesthesia societies (45), the development of new equipment, agents, and techniques for general anesthesia, and the publication of anesthesia journals and a number of textbooks. With the founding of organized societies, there was a steady, albeit slow, growth of physician anesthesia in the United States, Britain, Canada, and other English-speaking countries. Although exact figures for the first 2 decades are not available, it is estimated that by 1920 in the United States the number of physician-anesthetists had increased to 200; by 1930, there were about 350; by 1935, there were 500; and by 1940, there were about 1000. With the stimulus of World War II, there was a period of rapid growth of the specialty, so that by the end of the war, there were over 2000, and by 1950, there were 3400 trained physician-anesthetists (45). A somewhat similar pattern of growth of the specialty took place in the United Kingdom and Canada.

During this period, a number of technical and scientific advances were made, beginning with improved versions of machines for the administration of inhalation anesthesia and oxygen, the first introduced by Hewit in 1887. Advancements included better machines with flowmeters to measure the gas flow, which were developed by Teter, McKesson, Connell, Gwathmey, Forreger, and Boyle during the first 2 decades. The laryngoscope was introduced by Jackson in 1914 and was subsequently modified by Magill, Flagg, and Macintosh (45). In 1920, Magill and Rowbotham used endotracheal anesthesia for surgery, and 6 years later, Guedel and Waters introduced endotracheal tubes with inflatable cuffs. In 1923, Waters incorporated carbon dioxide absorption in inhalation anesthetic machines and later Guedel introduced controlled ventilation (52).

During this early period, some anesthesiologists suggested and some even administered various inhalation anesthetics for vaginal delivery. As already mentioned, Guedel suggested the self-administration of nitrous oxide-air mixture and in 1924 Heany reported on the first use of ethylene in obstetrics (19,45). A decade later Bourne, of Montreal, reported the first use of cyclopropane in obstetrics and a year later divenyl ether for vaginal deliveries. The use of cyclopropane was also reported by Griffith, of Montreal, in 1935 and Knight, of Minneapolis, in 1936. Trichlorethylene was first used in obstetrics in 1943 by Elam (45).

During this period, there was an increasing amount of new information derived from research by basic and some clinical scientists pertaining to the pharmacology and toxicology of various inhalation, intravenous, and local anesthetic drugs, along with a commensurate growth in the diffusion of scientific information about anesthesia through books and journals. Books on regional anesthesia were written by Braun, Allen, Pauchet, and Labat (5,6,44,53) while books written by Hewitt, Minnit, Boyle, Gwathmey, Flagg, Guedel, Dogliotti, and Beecher pertained to all aspects of anesthesia being used at the time (5,7,19,45).

Anesthesia journals that began publication during this period included "Current Researches in Anesthesia and Analgesia" in 1922, the "British Journal of Anaesthsia" in 1923, "Anesthesiology" in 1940, and "Anaesthesia" in 1946. Most of the regional anesthesia techniques and the sedatives, narcotics, and other drugs used for obstetric pain relief had been developed and introduced by obstetricians and were published in obstetric journals. Two such articles deserve special mention: first, the report by John Cleland (53), an Oregon surgeon who in 1933 published a summary of his extensive studies of the pathways of pain of childbirth carried out in animals and humans over a period of 6 years; second, the article by Moir (54) in which he discussed the various possible mechanisms of the pain of childbirth. Both studies were made during a period in which research in obstetrics was virtually non-existent. Both Cleland and Moir had an important impact on this field.

## The Period of Neglect (1860 to 1940)

### *"Dark Ages of Obstetric Analgesia and Anesthesia"*

Despite the obvious importance of obstetric analgesia/anesthesia and its very promising beginning affected by Simpson, Snow, Channing, and many others around the mid-nineteenth century, for the ensuing 9 decades, obstetric anesthesia went through its own Dark Ages. During the second half of the nineteenth century in America and most other countries, the administration of anesthesia was considered beneath the dignity of physicians; therefore, the task was relegated to such totally untrained personnel as orderlies, nurses, or medical students. Pleas by some American obstetricians and surgeons for only trained physicians to administer anesthetics fell on deaf ears. The lack of appreciation for the importance of obstetric anesthesia is reflected in part by the fact that a recent review of 10 obstetric textbooks published in English between 1860 and 1900 revealed that some did not mention analgesia at all and decried the use of anesthetics as too dangerous; while those who favored their use for vaginal delivery, particularly involving instrumentation, devoted two to four pages to the subject. Even in Britain the admonitions and teachings of Snow and Simpson were not fully effective, for although only physicians were permitted to administer anesthesia, many did so without the acquisition of available knowledge and the necessary preceptorship training. The same situation existed in Canada and other countries where physician anesthesia was being developed. Consequently, during this period (1860 to 1940), improperly administered anesthesia was one of the leading causes of death and complications among obstetric and surgical patients. Indeed, in some countries, particularly Britain and France, the problem developed into such magnitude as to become a major national issue.

During the first 5 decades of the twentieth century, when the aforementioned advances in anesthesiology were being made, obstetric anesthesia continued to be neglected. For one thing, of the textbooks on anesthesiology mentioned earlier, some did not include a discussion of obstetric anesthesia; and of those that did, none devoted more than a few pages. The same comment applies to various comprehensive textbooks in obstetrics published during this period. Only the textbook by DeLee (55), which was first published in 1913 and of which underwent nine revisions during this period, included a section on the practice of obstetric analgesia and anesthesia current at the time of each edition. Moreover, during this period, the number of articles on obstetric analgesia and anesthesia that appeared in the four English language journals of anesthesiology was very small—a fact which reflected that although there was a steady growth in the number of physician-anesthetists in the United States, Canada, Britain, and Australia, physician-anesthetists rarely, with few exceptions, became involved in obstetric analgesia/anesthesia because of the predominant demand for their services by surgeons. Exceptions included pioneers whose involvement in obstetric anesthesia was limited to the writing of articles on the basic principles of inhalation anesthesia or to the suggestion of applications for new techniques in inhalation anesthesia, and, as previously mentioned, to report the results of the newer inhalation anesthetics for vaginal delivery. During the 1920s, none of the few departments of anesthesia had an organized obstetric anesthesia service and, in the 1930s and early 1940s, less than a dozen such services existed in the United States and even fewer existed in Canada and Great Britain.

Because the proper application of inhalation anesthesia required training in anesthesiology, obstetricians were reluctant to use these techniques themselves, and, consequently, these were not widely employed. Moreover, although most of the regional analgesic techniques for pain relief during labor and anesthesia for vaginal delivery were first used and advocated by obstetricians, and although many obstetricians appreciated the advantages of regional anesthesia, these techniques did not become widely used. On the basis of my early observations, I suspect the reason for this was that many (if not most) obstetricians, believing that these techniques were simple to carry out, failed to acquire the necessary anatomic and pharmacologic knowledge, skill, and experience under a preceptor to carry them out effectively. Consequently, these obstetricians encountered failures and complications that prompted most of them to abandon these techniques. The serious complications with spinal analgesia in obstetrics during the first 4 decades, for example, prompted DeLee (55), Greenhill (56), and other obstetric authorities to decry its use.

Until the early 1940s most obstetricians relied on *Dammerschlaf* or other techniques of combining opioid analgesics with sedatives (e.g., barbiturates, chloral hydrate) in large doses to relieve pain and produce amnesia. Some used ether or chloroform for the actual delivery. These frequently produced perinatal depression and neonatal asphyxia, while the inhalation anesthetics, added to these effects, also produced maternal complications. For these reasons (deleterious effects), a significant number of obstetricians avoided any form of pharmacologic pain relief for labor and uncomplicated delivery. Information provided in a 1984 survey (see last section of this chapter) indicated that in Scandinavia, and in many of the Western and Eastern European countries, and in countries in the Near East and Asia, virtually all parturients had labor and delivery without any form of drug-induced pain relief. General anesthesia was used only for some operative vaginal deliveries.

During the 1920s, 1930s, and early 1940s, in the large- and medium-sized American hospitals nurse-anesthetists administered about 30% of the anesthesia for vaginal delivery and about 50% of the anesthesia for cesarean section. Notwithstanding their limited training and basic knowledge of obstetric anesthesia, they did a very credible job in filling the manpower needs. The remaining percentage of obstetric analgesia was administered by persons untrained in anesthesia, including interns, obstetric nurses, obstetric residents, or general practitioners. Unfortunately, it was the custom to assign the least trained nurse and the poorest type of anesthetic machine and other equipment to the obstetric suite. Untrained personnel played an even greater role in administering anesthesia for vaginal delivery in the small hospitals. Because these people had no training in the use of anesthetic machines, they relied on the use of open-drop ether or chloroform. Surprisingly, in the late 1930s and during the 1940s, the practice of relegating untrained personnel to administer anesthesia to obstetric patients was prevalent not only in small- or medium-sized hospitals, but also in outstanding medical centers in which surgical anesthesia was administered exclusively by anesthesiologists.

To emphasize these serious deficiencies that prompted my intense interest in obstetric anesthesia early in my career, I cite the following personal experience. My wife had her labor and delivery of our first child on July 18, 1943, at St. Vincent's Hospital in New York City, where I was chief anesthesiology resident. At the time, it was the custom at that hospital for all surgical anesthetics to be administered by anesthesiologists (there were no nurse anesthetists). The staff included such outstanding anesthesiologists of that time as Drs. Paul Wood, Paluel Flagg, James Gwathney, and Emory Rovenstine, who did their private cases there, but as anesthesiologists, they had absolutely no involvement in obstetrics. My wife's pregnancy, labor, and delivery were managed by a highly competent obstetrician who, having seen the severely depressed newborns from *Dammerschlaf* early in his career, did not give any medication to his patients during the first stage of labor. Consequently, my wife experienced moderately severe and eventually very severe pain during much of the active phase of labor. Moreover, although it had been planned that the chief obstetric resident, who had some anesthesia training, would administer the anesthetic to my wife, at the time of the imminent delivery he was busy doing a cesarean section and another obstetric resident with some training was also unavailable. Consequently, my wife was given open-drop ether by an intern who had started his internship 18 days earlier and who later admitted he had no training in anesthesia in medical school. Because of the archaic policy of not providing medical care to one's family members, I was restricted to the role of onlooker. After about a minute of open-drop ether, she developed laryngospasm that persisted for many seconds, during which time she became cyanotic. Had I not been there to take over and manage her, I would have lost my wife and baby. Later, while getting over the severe emotional stress, I fully realized and appreciated the great discrepancy in the quality of anesthetic care given to surgical and obstetric patients in one of the finest medical centers in the country. It was then that I made a firm commitment to help rectify these deficiencies.

These very serious deficiencies resulted in a high incidence of neonatal and maternal morbidity and sometimes death. Moreover, although obstetrics and pediatrics are two of the oldest clinical disciplines in the United States, Britain, and a number of other countries, surprisingly, during this period when scientific investigations were beginning in other medical clinical disciplines, research in obstetrics was virtually nonexistent. Thus continued "the Dark Ages of Obstetric Anesthesia" for nearly a century after the very promising beginning affected by Simpson, Snow, Channing, and others.

It should be noted that it was these deplorable conditions in obstetric anesthesia that, in 1923, prompted the English-trained physician, Grantly Dick-Read, to begin espousing "natural childbirth" (3). Similarly, it was the lack of any form of obstetric analgesia and anesthesia in the Commonwealth of Independent States (formerly the Soviet Union) that prompted Velvoski and associates (4) to begin espousing "psychoprophylaxis," which was later embraced and advocated throughout the world by the French obstetrician Lamaze (57) and his colleague Vellay. As noted in Chapter 21, both methods, although not very effective in relieving the pain of human parturition, have been widely embraced because they are far better than poor anesthesia and/or "no anesthesia."

## The Renaissance of Obstetric Anesthesia

### *The Transition from Obstetricians to Anesthesiologists*

This section focuses primarily on obstetric anesthesia in the United States and to a lesser extent in the United Kingdom because the involvement of anesthesiologists in this field began in these countries. Information on obstetric anesthesia in other countries is mentioned at the end of this chapter.

In the mid- and late 1940s and early 1950s a small nucleus of North American anesthesiologists, with the support of a few obstetricians with foresight and appreciation for good anesthesia, initiated what may be called "the Renaissance of obstetric anesthesia," characterized by a gradually increasing involvement of anesthesiologists in this field. The nucleus included Robert Hingson, Franklin Snyder, Bert Hershenson, and Virginia Apgar who devoted all of their time to this field and organized obstetric anesthesia services in their hospitals. In addition, Lull and Hingson (58), Snyder (59), and Hershenson (60) wrote the first textbooks on obstetric anesthesia, while Apgar (61) developed the Apgar Score—the first reproducible and reliable method for evaluating the newborn. They also wrote articles reporting the results of clinical studies done during the late 1940s and early 1950s.

In the United Kingdom, during this period, obstetric analgesia, primarily by the inhalation route, was given by midwives although a number of physicians were interested in administering the more complicated techniques of regional anesthesia. During this period, the literature on the subject was limited to articles appearing in anesthesia and obstetric journals, and small chapters in the major books on anesthesia. Beginning in 1947, J. Alfred Lee wrote the first edition of the classic book "A Synopsis of Anaesthesia," which contained a comprehensive, albeit concise, chapter on analgesia and anesthesia in obstetrics (62). This chapter provided an excellent summary of the history, development and the various agents and techniques used for the relief of pain of childbirth and anesthesia for cesarean section at the time (this section has been retained in all subsequent eleven editions) (63).

### *Obstetric Anesthesia Services*

In addition to the aforementioned individuals, there were a number of anesthesiologists in North America and the United Kingdom with interest in obstetric anesthesia who began to organize obstetric anesthesia services. Because of the aforementioned personal experience, in 1944 I organized an obstetric-anesthesia service at Madigan Army Hospital, Fort Lewis, Washington, and a year later administered the first continuous caudal analgesia given in the Northwest—the patient was my wife, whose almost painless labor was in great contrast to her 1943 experience. Moreover, promptly after I was appointed Chief of Anesthesia at Tacoma General Hospital, Tacoma, Washington, in February 1947, I organized an around-the-clock obstetric-anesthesia service that entailed the use of continuous caudal analgesia administered by myself and two residents, while the patient was monitored by nurse anesthetists who also administered inhalation analgesia. During the ensuing 4 years nurse anesthetists were replaced by anesthesiologists and anesthesia residents who also provided obstetric anesthesia on a 24-hour basis (64,65). My close friend, Daniel C. Moore, in 1948 also began to develop an obstetric-anesthesia service at the Virginia Mason Hospital, Seattle, Washington. Initially, the service involved nurses under his supervision, but later much of it was provided by anesthesiologists and anesthesia residents (66,67).

Other obstetric-anesthesia services initiated during the mid- and late 1940s included ones by Virginia Apgar in New York, Hingson and Edwards in Staten Island; Tovell and co-workers in Hartford; Volpitto and his group in Georgia; Pallin and associates, Green and associates, and Batten and associates in Brooklyn; Conroy in Chicago; Hugh Brown in Salt Lake; and Lundy and associates in Rochester, Minnesota. In addition to these known to me, it is likely that services were organized in other hospitals. During this early period the services were provided primarily by nurses under the supervision of physicians, but as more anesthesiologists were trained, these became involved.

Other related factors that contributed to the initial development of obstetric anesthesia included the publication of articles describing the practicality of 24-hour obstetric anesthesia service. These included the articles by Hingson and Hellman in 1952 (68), Webb and Leigh in 1953 (69), by Bonica and Mix in 1955 (64), by Bonica in 1957 (65), by Moore and associates in 1955 and 1957 (66,67), by Cull and Hingson in 1957 (70), by Nelson and associates in 1959 (71), by Papper in 1960 (72), and by Shnider in 1965 (73). Other factors that spurred the initial development of obstetric anesthesia included the publication of three surveys on obstetric anesthesia care in the United States that will be mentioned later. Moreover, studies on maternal mortality in the United States and the United Kingdom (74,75), which showed that anesthesia played a significant role in maternal deaths, did much to further generate concern and a sense of responsibility and interest among anesthesiologists and obstetricians in helping to develop obstetric anesthesia.

### Other Activities of the Early Pioneers

Through their persistent drum-beating in the form of publication of reports of new techniques or new aspects of obstetric anesthesia, editorials, personal presentation and personal involvement in obstetric anesthesia, these early "pioneers" of obstetric anesthesia began to get the attention of obstetricians. Special mention should be made of the techniques of continuous caudal by Hingson and Edwards (76) and the modified saddle block by Adriani and his associates (77) in the United States, and by Burton (78) and Resnick (79) in Britain. These were heralded as procedures that were highly effective in eliminating most of the pain of childbirth without depressing the mother or the fetus and newborn. Many obstetricians, who had experienced grave concern about the severely depressed infants delivered to mothers that had received *Dammerschlaff* and other forms of sedation and about the risks to the mother inherent in improperly administered inhalation anesthesia for the delivery, were ready to replace these methods with regional anesthesia.

During the first 5 decades of the present century, some obstetricians administered subarachnoid block, single-dose caudal, pudendal block, and local anesthesia themselves before the delivery. The aforementioned publications by Adriani and associates (77) and Hingson and associates, (76) and the widespread publicity that ensued, prompted some obstetricians to get training in these specialized techniques and administer them themselves. However, in those hospitals where anesthesiologists became involved in obstetric anesthesia, many obstetricians, realizing the risks inherent in both administering the anesthesia and giving obstetric care to the mother, were happy to relegate the task to their anesthesia colleagues.

### The Second and Subsequent Generations

In addition to provoking interest among obstetricians, these few early "pioneers" of obstetric anesthesia trained anesthesia residents and inculcated into them the importance of this aspect of the specialty. This, together with the aforementioned scientific and technical developments and other factors, provoked interest in a second generation of anesthesiologists who began to devote all or a major part of their professional time and efforts to obstetric anesthesia. By the mid-1950s, there were several dozens of such "second generation" obstetric anesthesiologists in the United States and a smaller but significant number in Canada and the United Kingdom. Another factor that helped to increase the interest of anesthesiologists in this field were the books on obstetric anesthesia by Hingson and Hellman (80), published in the USA, and the volume by J. Selwyn Crawford, who in 1959 published the first comprehensive book on obstetric anesthesia in Britain (81).

The second generation of obstetric anesthesiologists began their involvement during the 1950s and early 1960s and, in addition to providing services to parturients, they expanded the base of obstetric clinical care and training and thus produced a third generation of anesthesiologists. A number of these individuals collaborated with pediatricians and obstetricians in carrying out clinical research in perinatal medicine and in obstetrics. The opportunity to do research and the new knowledge acquired generated excitement and interest in the field in an increasing number of young anesthesiologists.

### Early Obstetric Anesthesia Services

#### Other Factors

#### Changes in Attitudes

Another important factor in the development of obstetric anesthesia during this period was the increasing interest in, and better appreciation of, the value of good anesthesiologic care by a modest percentage of obstetricians, gravidae, and anesthesiologists. In addition to the earlier unfavorable experiences and other factors mentioned above, obstetricians' increased interest in providing better anesthetic service was enhanced by the request and indeed by the demand of many expectant mothers not only in the United States and other English-speaking countries but also in a number of other countries throughout the world. This increased demand was provoked by information on the benefits of modern anesthesia by innumerable newspaper and magazine articles, radio and television programs, and by discussions with friends who had positive experiences with analgesia/anesthesia during childbirth.

This attitude among many expectant mothers was encouraged greatly by the approbation of methods to relieve childbirth pain by leaders of Christian and Hebraic-Judeo religions. In 1956 and 1957, Pope Pius XII, in response to the question posed by obstetricians regarding the obligation of women to accept suffering and refuse pain relief during their childbirth, stated "there is no obligation of this kind ... women retain the right of control over the forces of nature ... to suppress or avoid physical pain. The use of anesthesia gives no rise to moral or religious difficulties" (82).

By the late 1950s and early 1960s all of the aforementioned factors prompted an increasing number of American obstetricians to express strong desire for and indeed request (demand!) better obstetric analgesia and anesthesia through editorials published in major medical journals (83–86).

### Impact of Organized Medicine

One of the most important factors responsible for the gradual and further development of obstetric anesthesia in the United States in the 1950s and1960s was the cooperative and collaborative effort of the Committee on Maternal Welfare (CMW) (which in 1966 was renamed the Committee on Obstetric Anesthesia) of the American Society of Anesthesiologists (ASA/CMW) and the Committee on Obstetric Analgesia/Anesthesia of the American College of Obstetrics in Gynecology (ACOG/COAA). These two groups first joined forces in 1957 and became known as the "Combined Obstetric Anesthesia Liaison Committee on Maternal and Fetal Welfare" and included Apgar, Bonica, Hingson, Grossman, and Phillips representing the American Society of Anesthesiologists (ASA), and Randall, Douglas, Hellman, Pisani, Hendricks, and others representing the ACOG. At its 1957 meeting, this group discussed ways and means of improving obstetric anesthetic care in the United States, including presentations of scientific exhibits, panel discussions at national meetings of both organizations, and the publication of articles in their respective journals. As the Committee's co-chairman, I recommended that a survey of the then current status of obstetric anesthesia be made. This was approved unanimously by the combined group and Otto Phillips was given the responsibility of carrying it out.

## *Surveys of Obstetric Anesthesia Care*

In the years 1959 to 1981, three retrospective surveys on the status of obstetric anesthesia in varying percent of all hospitals in the United States were carried out. The first was by Otto Phillips on behalf of the Committee on Maternal Welfare (CMW) of the American Society of Anesthesiologists (ASA); the second was carried out by the Committee on Maternal Health of the American College of Obstetricians and Gynecologists (ACOG); and a third by Gibbs, et. al., on behalf of the Committee on Obstetric Analgesia (COA) of the ASA and Liasion Committee of the ACOG. The results of the surveys are summarized below and also in Tables 1–2 to 1–5.

### The First Survey

In 1960, Phillips retrospectively analyzed data on the status of obstetric anesthesia in 439 hospitals in the USA, which represented slightly less than 10% of those that had recorded live births in the previous year. A year later, Phillips, the Chairman of the ASA/CMW, distributed a summary of the data (87) to members of the committee; and in 1982, Phillips and Frazier published the results (88). These data revealed the startling fact that anesthesia for vaginal delivery was administered by: (1) anesthesiologists in 13.7% of the hospitals and 1.6% by anesthesia residents for a total of 15.3%; (2) nurse-anesthetists administered anesthesia in 31%; (3) obstetricians and obstetric residents gave a total of 26%; and (4) in the remaining 28%, anesthesia for vaginal delivery was administered by such wholly anesthesia-untrained personnel as medical and dental students, delivery room nurses, physicians untrained in anesthesia, and in some instances, even nonprofessional people. Table 1–2 shows these data as well as anesthesia for cesarean section, for which anesthesiologists and anesthesia residents administered anesthesia in about 40% of the cases.

Table 1–3 shows the degree of participation by anesthesiologists and anesthesia residents that increased from about 5% in hospitals with less than 300 births to about 38% in those hospitals with 2000 births. Moreover, anesthesiologists administered anesthesia for cesarean section in about 19% in hospitals with less than 300 deliveries; nearly 87% in hospitals that delivered between 1000 and 1500 parturients; and in 74% of hospitals with more than 2000 births. A very startling fact was that anesthesia residents provided no anesthesia for parturients in hospitals with less than 500 beds, and a total of 1.6% in hospitals that had between 500 and 2000-plus births per year. Another important point is that of this total only 15% of the hospitals had anesthesiology training programs.

This prompted the Committee to recommend the following resolution, which was approved by the ASA House of Delegates at the 1961 meeting (89).

> "Whereas anesthesia remains among the four leading causes of maternal mortality . . . whereas anesthesiologists assume the responsibility for anesthesia for only 13.7% and anesthesia residents for only 1.2% of vaginal deliveries, and 40% of cesarean section and whereas anesthesia residency programs evidently place minimal emphasis on the field of obstetric anesthesia; therefore be it resolved that the American Society of Anesthesiologists go on record as supporting an expanding program of participation by anesthesiologists recommends . . . to the Council on Postgraduate Education of the American Medical Association that greater emphasis be placed upon the training of anesthesia residents in the field of obstetric anesthesia."

### The Second Survey

A second survey of 3672 hospitals was carried out by the Committee on Maternal Welfare (CMW) of the American College of Obstetricians and Gynecologists (ACOG), which analyzed data for 1967 but published in 1970. This survey was carried out in the same manner as that done by Phillips (88). Hospitals were differentiated according to number of births. The survey revealed that analgesia for labor consisted mostly of systemic analgesics and sedatives and tranquilizers prescribed almost exclusively by the obstetrician (90). Analgesia/anesthesia for vaginal delivery in most instances was administered by (1) anesthesiologists in 12% of the hospitals; (2) certified registered nurse anesthetists (CRNA) in 25%; (3) obstetricians and obstetric residents in 33%; and (4) obstetric nurses, house staff, medical students, and "others" in 30%. The decreased participation of anesthesiologists compared to the 1959 survey was due to the fact that the 1967 survey included many more small hospitals in which anesthesiologists participated in only 5%, while in the larger hospitals they participated in 38%. For cesarean section, anesthesia was administered by (1) anesthesiologists or anesthesia residents in 74% of the hospitals; (2) nurse anesthetists in 19%; (3) obstetricians did not administer any anesthetic, while 7% was administered by other untrained personnel. As in the 1959 survey, anesthesiologists were involved much more frequently in administering anesthesia for both vaginal delivery and cesarean section in the larger hospitals than in the small units.

Comparison of the data in Table 1–2 shows virtually no improvement in the involvement of anesthesiologists or anesthesia residents in the care of parturients undergoing vaginal delivery, but there was significant improvement in the care of patients with cesarean section. There were many interrelated reasons responsible for this lack of progress in the care of parturients by anesthesiologists. These reasons involved anesthesiologists, obstetricians, hospital administrators, and health care agencies. Some obstetricians remained apathetic and, unlike other colleagues, failed to insist on the same high standards of an-

**Table 1–2.** Trends in Obstetric Analgesia/Anesthesia (OAA) in USA (Data Based on Survey of Various Percent of All Hospitals)

| Period of Survey | 1959 | 1967 | 1981 | | 1959 | 1967 | 1981 |
|---|---|---|---|---|---|---|---|
| **Author(s)** | **Phillips** | **OAC/AACOG** | **Gibbs et al.** | | **Phillips** | **OAC/ACOG** | **Gibbs et al.** |
| **Sponsoring Society** | **ASA/CMW** | **ACOG** | **ASA/ACOG** | | **ASA/CMW** | **ACOG** | **ASA/ACOG** |
| **No. of Hospitals Surveyed** | **439** | **3,672** | **617** | | **439** | **3,672** | **617** |
| **Personnel Administering Anesthesia (Figures in percent of total anesthesia administered)** | | | | **Type of Anesthesia Administered (In percent of total parturients managed)** | | | |
| | | | | **Analgesia/Anesthesia for Vaginal Delivery** | | | |
| Anesthesiologist | 13.7 | — | — | Subarachnoid Block | 8 | | 9 |
| Anesthesia Resident | 1.6 | — | — | Lumbar Epidural Block | 7 (a) | 0 | 14 |
| *Subtotal* | 15.3 | 12 (a) | 25 (b) | Caudal Epidural | | 6 | 0 |
| Nurse Anesthetist (CRNA) | 31 | 25 | 4 (c) | PCB/PNB/LI | 2 | 16 | 59 |
| | | | | Inhalation | | | |
| Obstetrician | 22 | | | Analgesia | 62* | 0 | 6 |
| Obstetric Resident | 4 | | | Anesthesia | | 36 | 3 |
| *Subtotal* | 26 | 33 | 54 | Other | 0 | 12 | 0 |
| Others (d) | 28 | 30 | 17 | None or Psychoprophylaxis | 21 | 22 | 15 |
| **Total** | 100 | 100 | 100 | Total | 100 | 100 | 100 |
| | | | | **Anesthesia for Cesarean Section** | | | |
| Anesthesiologist | 39.0 | | | Subarachnoid Block | 42 | 54 | 34 |
| Anesthesia Resident | 1.0 | | | Lumbar Epidural | 10* | 0 | 14 |
| *Subtotal* | 40.0 | 74 | 80 | Caudal Epidural | | 6 | 0 |
| Nurse Anesthetist (CRNA) | 33.0 | 19 | 16 | Local Infiltration | 1 | 1 | 0 |
| Obstetrician | 6.0 | | | General | 32 | 32 | 41 |
| Obstetric Resident | 1.0 | | | Combination | 15 | 10 | 10 |
| *Subtotal* | 7.0 | 0 | 4 | | | | |
| Other (c) | 20.0 | 7 | 0 | | | | |
| **Total** | 100 | 100 | 100 | Total | 100 | 100 | 96 (d) |

* Not differentiated in 1959 survey; (a) Anesthesiologist alone or with anesthesia resident; (b) Anesthesiologist or CRNA under supervision of anesthesiologist; (c) CRNA under supervision of Obstetrician; (d) values add to less than 100% because some respondents failed to answer all questions; ASA = American Society of Anesthesiologists; CMW = Committee on Maternal Welfare; OAC = Obstetric Anesthesia Committee; ACOG = American College of Obstetricians and Gynecologists; PCB = paracervical block; PNB = pudendal nerve block; GA = general anesthesia includes inhalation alone, or in combination with intravenous anesthesia, or others; RA = regional anesthesia.

**Table 1–3.** Persons Administering Obstetric Anesthesia According to Size of Hospital in U.S. (In Percent of Parturients Managed in Each Category of Hospital*)

| | | Vaginal Delivery | | | | | | Cesarean Section | | | | | |
|---|---|---|---|---|---|---|---|---|---|---|---|---|---|
| **Hospital Size by Number of Births per Year** | **No.** | **Anesthesiologist** | **Anesthesia Resident** | **Obstetrician** | **Obstetric Resident** | **Nurse Anesthetist** | **Other**** | **Anesthesiologist** | **Anesthesia Resident** | **Obstetrician** | **Obstetric Resident** | **Nurse Anesthetist** | **Other** |
| 1–149 | 90 | 4.4 | 0 | 20 | 1.0 | 26 | 56 | 15.6 | 0 | 8 | 0 | 36 | 41 |
| 150–299 | 82 | 6.1 | 0 | 22 | 0.4 | 31 | 37 | 17.1 | 0.2 | 1 | 0 | 43 | 28 |
| 300–499 | 71 | 12.7 | 0 | 22 | 1.0 | 24 | 34 | 28.2 | 0 | 4 | 2 | 38 | 27 |
| 500–999 | 87 | 16.1 | 0.2 | 25 | 0.2 | 38 | 20 | 44.8 | 0.5 | 5 | 0 | 39 | 1 |
| 1000–1499 | 37 | 24.3 | 0.7 | 24 | 0.2 | 35 | 6 | 86.5 | 0.2 | 0 | 0 | 11 | 0 |
| 1500–1999 | 30 | 13.3 | 0.2 | 27 | 0.2 | 43 | 10 | 76.7 | 0 | 0 | 3 | 20 | 0 |
| 2000+ | 42 | 35.7 | 0.5 | 18 | 1.0 | 23 | 10 | 73.8 | 0.2 | 5 | 3 | 20 | 0 |
| Total | 439 | | | | | | | | | | | | |
| Means | | 13.7 | 1.6 | 22 | 4.0 | 31 | 27 | 39.4 | 1.1 | 6 | 1 | 33 | 20 |

* Percentages for Anesthesiologist, Anesthesia Resident and Obstetric Resident are listed to nearest decimal; all others to the nearest unit. The total means for all categories of personnel administering anesthesia for vaginal delivery is less than 100, and those for cesarean section is slightly greater than 100 because numbers rounded to nearest unit. (Modified from Phillips, O.C. and Frazier, T.M., Obstetric anesthetic care in the United States. Obstet. Gynecol. 19:796–802, 1962.)
** Others—medical students, nurses or other persons untrained in obstetric anesthesia.

esthesiologic care for their obstetric patients as they did for their gynecologic patients. As aptly pointed out by Barnes (91), it was ironic that in some of the best hospitals in the United States, the removal of a brain tumor in a 70-year-old patient called for a large team, including an anesthesiologist and one assistant who would work 6 to 8 hours, to save someone whose life expectancy was 18 to 24 months at best, while a delivery at 4:00 a.m. was attended by one physician, one nurse, and inadequate or haphazard anesthesia coverage, thus risking the lives of two individuals whose combined life expectancy was more than 130 years. Even more serious was the outright opposition by some obstetricians who often gave as a reason the desire to have exclusive care of their patient and furthermore believed that sophisticated anesthesia was unnecessary. Some obstetricians had the paradoxical attitude that while they were agreeable to reasonable charges by an anesthesiologist for a 1½- to 2-hour gynecologic operation, they objected to a similar fee for a 4-hour analgesia/anesthesia provided to their obstetric patients. Table 1–2 includes a summary of the first two surveys and also the survey by Gibbs and associates carried out a decade after the second survey and described below.

With regard to anesthesiologists, a survey carried out independently by an ASA Committee chaired by Dr. Robert Dripps, during the period 1963 to 1965 when the number of anesthesiologists in the United States had increased to about 8000, revealed that all too many of them who had the time and opportunity to give obstetric anesthesia shunned this important responsibility (92). The survey revealed that this attitude hurt the anesthesiologist's status as a physician. The survey suggested that this neglect was due to several interrelated factors: (1) a predominant demand by surgeons that imposed a heavy clinical load on anesthesiologists in surgical anesthesia; (2) the emergency nature of obstetric anesthesia that would require night work; (3) lack of exposure and training in residency and consequent lack of appreciation of the importance of obstetric anesthesia; (4) lack of demonstrated interest by many directors of anesthesiology residency training programs; and (5) the aforementioned negative attitude of many obstetricians and the fact that fees for obstetric anesthesia were not commensurate with services rendered. Related to this issue was the deficiencies of health agencies that were at fault for allowing many hospitals to have small obstetric units that made it difficult, if not impossible, to support the services of anesthesiologists' work in obstetrics and to have ample resources for optimal obstetric and anesthetic care.

### *The Third Survey*

In 1982, Gibbs and associates (93), representing the Committee on Obstetric Anesthesia (COA) of the ASA and the Liasion Committee for Obstetrics and Gynecology (LCOG) of ACOG, carried out the third survey on the status of obstetric analgesia and anesthesia in the USA in 1981. The results were published in 1986 (93).

For this purpose, they divided the hospitals into three strata based on the number of births (as had been done for the 1961 survey): stratum I—more than 1,500 births; stratum II—between 500 and 1,499 births; and stratum III—less than 500 births. The survey consisted of two parts: (1) respondents agreed or disagreed with statements about why anesthesiologists were not more involved in obstetric anesthesia; and (2) respondents defined obstetric anesthesia practice in regard to both personnel and methods. The questionnaires were sent to 398 hospitals in stratum I, 396 in stratum II, and 377 in stratum III and responses were obtained from 272 (68%), 213 (54%), and 132 (35%) of the hospitals, respectively. Calculations for number of births indicated that nearly 30% of the total births in the United States in 1981 occurred in responding hospitals and because the largest number of responses came from stratum III hospitals, nearly 75% of the births among surveyed hospitals occurred in those with greater than 1,500 deliveries per year.

The data (expressed as means of the percent of parturients managed) pertaining to the anesthetic procedures used and the personnel performing them are summarized in Tables 1–4A, 1–4B, and 1–5. In these tables, percentages given to anesthesiologists (c) include staff anesthesiologists, anesthesia residents or a Certified Registered Nurse Anesthetist (CRNA) directed by an anesthesiologist; CRNA (d) indicates that the nurse anesthetists were directed by obstetricians, while "obstetricians" include obstetric staff or obstetric residents. As noted in Table 1–4B, a mean of 32% of all patients received no analgesia for labor, including nearly 45% of the patients in stratum III hospitals. Anesthesiologists or CRNAs supervised by an anesthesiologist administered 70% of the epidural blocks in stratum I and 61% in stratum II hospitals, but only 35% in stratum III units. The most frequently used form of pain relief in all strata were parenteral opioids, barbiturates, tranquilizers, or a combination of these.

For vaginal delivery (Table 1–4b), 15% of all patients received no anesthesia, and once again the percentages were higher in the smaller strata units. Local infiltration or pudendal block was used most frequently in all strata, and preexisting epidural block or subarachnoid block was used most frequently in larger stratum units and was administered by anesthesiologists or CRNA under their influence. General anesthesia was used infrequently.

For cesarean section (Table 1–5), regional anesthesia in the form of epidural or subarachnoid block were used in 55% and general anesthesia in 41% of all cases. Also note that in the larger stratum units regional anesthesia was used more frequently and general anesthesia less frequently than for the total population. Anesthesiologists or CRNA under their supervision administered 83% of the anesthetics, CRNA under the supervision of obstetricians administered 14%, and obstetricians/obstetric residents administered 3%.

The survey revealed that anesthesiologists were available in-house during the week in a significantly greater percentage of stratum I units than the other smaller stratum units. In 49% of the larger units, anesthesiologists were available nights and weekends, but they were also covering other anesthesia locations in those hospitals. Similarly, obstetricians were available full time for labor and delivery during the week in a significantly greater

**Table 1–4A.** Analgesia/Anesthesia Used for Labor and Personnel Performing Them (In Percent of Parturients Managed)

| Procedure | Hospitals: Stratum I (>1500 births) | Stratum II (500–1499 births) | Stratum III (<500 births) | All Strata |
|---|---|---|---|---|
| No analgesia/anesthesia | 27 | 33 | 45 | 32 |
| Intermittent inhalation (a) | 0 | 0 | 0 | 0 |
| Systemic Opioids (a) barbiturates tranquilizers | 52 | 53 | 37 | 49 |
| Paracervical Block (b) | 5 | 5 | 6 | 5 |
| Epidural Analgesia | 22 | 13 | 9 | 16 |
| Anesthesiologist or CRNA directed by one (c) | 70 | 61 | 35 | 62 |
| CRNA directed by an obstetrician (d) | 4 | 8 | 10 | 6 |
| Obstetrician or Obstetric resident | 26 | 31 | 46 | 30 |
| Other personnel | 0 | 0 | 10 | 1.3 |
| Total | 106* | 104* | 97† | 102* |

* Values add to greater than 100% because in some cases more than one procedure was used.
† Values add to less than 100% because some respondents failed to answer all questions.
(a) Prescribed by obstetrician and administered by obstetric nurse or Certified Registered Nurse Anesthetist (CRNA); (b) Carried out by obstetrician or obstetric resident; (c) Administered by anesthesiologist, anesthesia residents, or CRNA under direction of anesthesiologist; (d) Administered by CRNA under direction of obstetrician.
(Modified from Gibbs CP, et al. Obstetric anesthesia: a national survey. Anesthesiology, 1986;65:298, p. 301.)

percentage of the larger stratum units than in the medium-sized or smaller stratum units; indeed, obstetricians were available in-house more often in all stratum units than were anesthesiologists. In nearly 30% of the smaller stratum units, a family practitioner was the person available on a shared-time basis for obstetric care.

Table 1–2 compares the mean data of all strata revealed by this survey with the data provided by the two previous surveys and, as noted, there was some improvement in obstetric anesthesia care but it still remained far less than optimal. The reason for the insufficient coverage by anesthesiologists include some of the same reasons given in

**Table 1–4B.** Analgesia/Anesthesia Used for Vaginal Delivery and Personnel Performing Them (In Percent of Parturients Managed)

| Procedure | Hospitals: Stratum I (>1500 births) | Stratum II (500–1499 births) | Stratum III (<500 births) | All Strata |
|---|---|---|---|---|
| No analgesia | 11 | 13 | 27 | 15 |
| Local Infiltration or Pudendal Block | 54 | 68 | 59 | 59 |
| Inhalation Analgesia | 5 | 7 | 4 | 6 |
| Anesthesiologist or CRNA directed by one | 61 | 50 | 30 | 53 |
| CRNA directed by an obstetrician | 31 | 45 | 50 | 8 |
| Obstetrician or Obstetric resident | 5 | 4 | 11 | 6 |
| Other personnel | 3 | 2 | 8 | 3 |
| Preexisting Epidural Block | 20 | 11 | 7 | 14 |
| Subarachnoid Block | 11 | 7 | 5 | 9 |
| Anesthesiologist or CRNA directed by one | 63 | 45 | 17 | 51 |
| CRNA directed by an obstetrician | 5 | 3 | 11 | 5 |
| Obstetrician or Obstetric resident | 32 | 50 | 56 | 42 |
| Other personnel | 0 | 1 | 15 | 3 |
| General Anesthesia | 3 | 3 | 2 | 3 |
| Anesthesiologist or Anesthesia resident | 68 | 71 | 38 | 66 |
| CRNA directed by an obstetrician | 30 | 27 | 59 | 32 |
| Other personnel | 2 | 2 | 3 | 2 |
| Total | 104* | 109* | 104* | 106* |

* Values add to greater than 100% because in some cases more than one procedure was used.
(Modified from Gibbs CP, et al. Obstetric anesthesia: a national survey. Anesthesiology, 1986;65:298, p. 301.)

**Table 1–5.** Anesthetic Procedures Used for Cesarean Section and Personnel Performing Them (In Percent of Parturients Managed)

| Procedure | Hospitals | | | |
|---|---|---|---|---|
| | Stratum I (>1500 births) | Stratum II (500–1499 births) | Stratum III (<500 births) | All Strata |
| Epidural Block | 29 | 16 | 12 | 21 |
| Anesthesiologist (a), or CRNA directed by one | 89 | 83 | 61 | 84 |
| CRNA directed by an obstetrician | 4 | 11 | 15 | 7 |
| Obstetrician or Obstetric resident | 8 | 6 | 20 | 9 |
| Other personnel | 0 | 0 | 3 | 0.4 |
| Spinal Block | 33 | 35 | 37 | 34 |
| Anesthesiologist or CRNA directed by one | 94 | 86 | 49 | 83 |
| CRNA directed by an obstetrician | 4 | 8 | 39 | 12 |
| Obstetrician or Obstetric resident | 2 | 5 | 7 | 4 |
| Other personnel | 0 | 0 | 6 | 1 |
| General Anesthesia | 35 | 45 | 46 | 41 |
| Anesthesiologist or CRNA directed by one | 86 | 74 | 44 | 74 |
| CRNA directed by an obstetrician | 14 | 27 | 55 | 25 |
| Other personnel | 0.1 | 0.1 | 2 | 0.4 |
| Total | 97* | 96* | 95* | 96* |

* Values add to less than 100% because some respondents failed to answer all questions.
(a) Anesthesiologists include anesthesia residents as well as CRNAs.
(Modified from Gibbs CP, et al. Obstetric anesthesia: a national survey. Anesthesiology, 1986;65:298, p. 301.)

the Dripps report, as well as some new ones. These included: (1) the unpredictability of labor and delivery made scheduling difficult; (2) the fees for labor and vaginal delivery analgesia were not adequate; (3) obstetricians lacked sufficient background in anesthesia; (4) obstetricians tended to dictate the type and timing of anesthesia; (5) the risk of malpractice claims had increased for obstetric anesthesia; and (6) there was unanimity of opinion among obstetricians and anesthesiologists that the larger obstetric service would make it more practical to provide obstetric-anesthesia services. Obstetric units with less than 500 deliveries per year were considerably more understaffed than the larger units in most areas studied.

### *Corrective Measures*

During the 1960s and 1970s the aforementioned deficiencies and reasons for them were recognized by an increasing number of anesthesiologists and obstetricians interested and involved in obstetric anesthesia. Such deficiencies and their causes provided both groups with an impressive impetus to eliminate them. This was accomplished by continued drum beating, publication of an increasing number of articles in obstetric and anesthesiology journals, including an entire issue of *Anesthesiology* devoted solely to obstetric anesthesia (94), and a number of books (5,95–100), including the comprehensive two-volume, first edition of this book (5). Finally, and most important, was the founding of the Society of Obstetric Anesthesia and Perinatology (SOAP) in 1968 and the Obstetric Anaesthetists Association (OAA) in Britain a year later. Two other organizations, to which many of their members are involved in obstetric anesthesia care and research, are the American Society of Regional Anesthesia (ASRA), founded in 1974, and the European Society of Regional Anaesthesia (ESRA), founded in 1980.

It should be noted that this transition to the specialty of anesthesiology occurred at this time in the United States, Canada, Britain, Australia, and to a lesser extent in New Zealand and other English-speaking countries only. In other countries of Europe, Latin America, and Asia, where surgeons continued to dominate surgery and other aspects of medicine, the development of anesthesiology as a specialty was discouraged until after World War II. In the late 1940s and early 1950s, the advances in thoracic, cardiac, and neurosurgery prompted some leading surgeons in these countries to send some of their better assistants abroad to receive anesthesiology training. Consequently, the specialty of anesthesiology in Europe, Latin American, Japan, and other Asian countries did not develop until the mid-1950s; in what then existed as the Union of Soviet Socialist Republics (USSR) and in other Eastern European countries, this transition did not take place until the 1960s. Thus, in these countries, "the Dark Ages" of obstetric anesthesia continued and in all too many of these countries, most parturients continued to have childbirth without pharmacologic means of pain relief. The lack of anesthesiologists was and continues to be primarily responsible for the widespread and enthusiastic use of natural childbirth and, even more, psychoprophylaxis in most major obstetric centers of continental Europe and Latin America, where the claims by Lamaze of painless childbirth without the use of drugs replaced *Dammerschlaf* and improperly administered anesthesia.

## The Period of Growth and Major Advances

In the understanding and use of the principles of safe obstetric analgesia and anesthesia, more was accomplished from 1960 to the present (1994) than in the previous century. This achievement is attributable to continuation and marked expansion of those activities during the period of transition and other interrelated factors including: (1) remarkable advances in scientific knowledge in obstetrics, perinatal medicine, and anesthesiology in general, and obstetric anesthesia in particular; (2) further and impressive increase in the appreciation of the value of good obstetric anesthesia care by obstetricians, patients, anesthesiologists, hospital administrators, and some governmental agencies; (3) the increased number of obstetric anesthesia training programs, which resulted in an increased number of anesthesiologists who became interested and involved in obstetric anesthesia; (4) improvement in resources in obstetrics, anesthesiology, and perinatal medicine; and (5) the worldwide movement in childbirth education. These and other factors have effected a significant improvement in the care of many parturients and newborns. I will comment first on recent research and advances in knowledge, but because much of this will be discussed in subsequent chapters, only a concise overview will be given here. This will be followed by a summary of four surveys on obstetric anesthesia training programs.

## *Advances in Research, in Knowledge, and Practice*

During the past 30 to 35 years, there has been an increasing degree of collaboration among anesthesiologists, obstetricians, perinatologists, and basic scientists in perinatal research. As a result, there has been an unprecedented increase in our knowledge and understanding of the physiology, psychology, pharmacology, and pathophysiology of the gravida and the parturient; a vast amount of new knowledge of the physiology, pharmacology, and pathophysiology of the fetus and newborn; and of the placenta and the forces of labor. Three developments that must be considered milestones in the development of perinatal medicine and obstetric anesthesia are: (1) the advent of sophisticated electronic monitoring of fetal heart rate and uterine contractility; (2) serial measurements of the acid-base status of the fetus and newborn; and (3) the advent of neurobehavioral methods of assessing the newborn. These have sharpened our focus on the adverse effects of various agents and techniques used in obstetric anesthesia and has consequently refined the ability of the obstetric team to administer these procedures more precisely.

Another important area of research has concerned maternal pathophysiologic disorders including pregnancy-induced hypertension (toxemia), diabetes, heart disease, and a variety of other maternal disorders; such obstetric complications as placenta previa, rupture of the placenta, cephalopelvic disproportion and abnormal presentations; and such fetal complications as fetal distress, prematurity, postmaturity and multiple gestations. The new knowledge about these conditions has resulted in a marked increase in the use of cesarean sections, rather than traumatic vaginal deliveries. Moreover, this new knowledge and the advances in anesthesiology have enhanced the ability of the anesthesiologists to tailor various anesthetics of obstetric analgesia/anesthesia in such a fashion as to not only not aggravate the pathophysiology, but actually prove beneficial to the mother and infant.

During this same period, equally impressive advances have been made in anesthesiology in general and obstetric anesthesia in particular. As a result of intensive research, much new knowledge has been acquired concerning the pharmacology, pharmacokinetics, and pharmacodynamics of local, inhalation, and intravenous anesthetics and how they interact with the alteration produced by pregnancy, labor, and delivery. The advantages, disadvantages, limitations, and complications of paracervical and pudendal block administered by the obstetrician have been defined. Mechanisms of side effects and complications of various regional anesthetic techniques and how these can be prevented, and if they occur, how to effectively treat them, have been clarified and emphasized repeatedly. The refinement and widespread use of continuous lumbar analgesia for labor and vaginal delivery has demonstrated that *properly administered*, it produces almost complete pain relief with little or no adverse effects on the mother, fetus, and newborn. Moreover, as discussed in Chapter 9, this and other regional techniques, by blocking nociceptive impulses, prevent deleterious reflex responses consequent to labor and delivery.

These and many other advances in obstetric anesthesia have helped to improve the care of parturients and have effected the maturity of the subspecialty. This is reflected in part by the fact that during the past 20 years, there has been a large number of articles published in anesthesiology, obstetric, pediatric, and other types of journals, and by the fact that two entire issues of the *British Journal of Anaesthesia* (101,102), two issues of *Clinics in Obstetrics and Gynecology* (103,104), one issue of the *Clinical Anesthesia Series* (105), and one issue of *Clinics in Anesthesiology* (106) have been devoted to this field. Moreover, during this period, a total of nine new textbooks and monographs (107–115) were published in the United States and Britain alone: the second edition of "Anesthesia For Obstetrics" was published by Shnider and Levingson in 1987, and the third edition was published in 1993 (105); the second edition of Allbright, et al (109) was published in 1987, and the fifth edition of Jeff Crawford's book was published in 1984 before his tragic premature death (115). The fourth edition of the monograph by Moir has also been published (98b). In 1991 the *International Journal of Obstetric Anesthesia* began publication (by Churchill Livingstone, Edinburg, New York, London, Madrid, Barcelona, and Tokyo). Indicating the worldwide interest in this field, more than 110,000 copies of the first and second edition of the monograph of "Obstetric Analgesia and Anesthesia," which I wrote for the World Federation of Societies of Anaesthesiologists (WFSA), were distributed in 50 countries, and the book was translated into 5 languages (100,112). A new edition of the WFSA monograph, edited by McMorland and Marx, was published in 1992 (116).

## *Impact of Professional Organizations*

The American Society of Anesthesiology (ASA), through its Committee of Obstetric Anesthesia and members of the committee on maternal and fetal medicine of the American College of Obstetrics and Gynecology (ACOG), has continued to work closely to improve obstetric anesthesia care in the United States. Over the years this close cooperation, communication, and coordination between the two groups has resulted in the development of several important documents. One of these, *Guidelines for Obstetric Anesthesia*, was approved by the House of Delegates of the ASA in 1988 and amended in 1991. These guidelines deal primarily with regional anesthesia. The ACOG committee published guidelines for obstetric anesthesia in the Technical Bulletin 112, January 1988, and in 1992 the committee published an article on anesthesia for emergency deliveries. These documents, which are intended as educational aids for obstetricians, contain excellent summaries of the basic principles of obstetric anesthesia, discussions of various drugs and techniques used for labor and vaginal delivery and cesarean section. These have not only been informative, they have enhanced the relationship between the two major professional organizations responsible for obstetric anesthesia care in the United States.

In addition to the ASA and ACOG, the Society of Obstetric Anesthesia and Perinatology (SOAP) has played a critical role in the development and growth of obstetric anesthesia in the United States and reflects the maturity of this field. SOAP has increased its membership from a dozen in 1968 to nearly 800 active members (and an additional 600 who receive the newsletter) in 1992, comprising anesthesiologists, obstetricians, and neonatologists. In addition to enhancing collegiality, communication, and understanding among its members, SOAP's scientific meetings are devoted to the presentation of new data from basic and clinical research in the three fields, as well as presentations dealing with clinical problems. In addition to facilitating communication and transfer of information, these meetings also provoke questions that lead to new research directions. In 1992, SOAP adopted new articles of organization that require active and associate members to pay dues ($80.00), and consequently the number has decreased. However, many other anesthesiologists interested in obstetric anesthesia frequently attend the meetings. Moreover, during the past several years members of SOAP have worked closely with members of the Section of Obstetric Anesthesia of the American Society of Anesthesiologists (ASA), the American College of Obstetricians and Gynecologists (ACOG), and the American Academy of Pediatrics (AAP) to develop very important guidelines intended to improve obstetric anesthetic care in the USA These guidelines will be cited in the appropriate place in various chapters throughout this book.

The Obstetric Anaesthetists Association, with a membership of 1300 physicians in 1993, has had a similar impact in Britain and has influenced obstetric anesthesia in continental Europe. Consequently, a number of unofficial groups of obstetric anaesthesiologists exist in a number of continental European countries, where 20 years ago obstetric anesthesia administered by physicians was nonexistent. These groups collaborated with SOAP to have a European Congress on Obstetric Anesthesia. The section on Obstetric Anesthesia of the ASA, the American Society of Regional Anesthesia (ASRA), the American Society of Regional Anesthesia (ASRA) and the European Society of Regional Anesthesia (ESRA), as well as the World Federation of Societies of Anaesthesiologists (WFSA), have also played important parts in the development of obstetric anesthesia by devoting part of their scientific meetings to this subject.

## Obstetric Anesthesia Training Centers (OATC)

During the past 15 to 20 years, an impressively increasing number of physicians have become involved in obstetric anesthesia. In the United States, a small but important number have become trained and certified in both obstetrics and anesthesiology, and probably between 1200 and 1500 anesthesiologists are devoting all or much of their time to obstetric anesthesia. This favorable trend, which has resulted in the rapid growth of the subspecialty of Obstetric Anesthesia, has been provoked by a number of interrelated factors: (1) the earlier guidelines and regulations developed by the ASA and ACOG Committees which state that anesthesia residents should rotate on obstetric-anesthesia services to learn about principles and practices in obstetrics, and obstetric residents should rotate on anesthesia to learn management of the airway; (2) the impetus given by ASA, ACOG, SOAP, OAA, ASRA, and ESRA, and the acquisition of much new and relevant knowledge; (3) the increased importance given to obstetric anesthesia; and (4) the increased respect and prestige accorded obstetric anesthesiologists by obstetricians, perinatologists, and the rest of the medical profession. These factors have made possible greater interaction among anesthesiologists, obstetricians, and pediatricians and have improved somewhat the economic aspect of this field.

The improvement in the training of anesthesiologists and anesthesia residents in obstetric anesthesia is attested in part by comparing the results of the first survey of Obstetric Anesthesia Training Centers (OATC) carried out by Shnider (118) for the 2-year period (from July 1, 1961 to June 30, 1963) with those acquired by Hicks, et al (113) carried out a decade later; those acquired in the 1981 survey by Millar and Plumer (114); and the surveys I carried out in 1984 for inclusion in the first Gertie Marx Lecture and again in 1989 for inclusion in this chapter. Although the data derived from these surveys are not strictly comparable because of the nature of the questionnaires, they do show a rather impressive improvement in quantity and quality of training in obstetric anesthesia in the larger teaching centers and, consequently, improvement in the quality of anesthetic care to obstetric patients. The data are summarized in Table 1–6 included below.

### The First Survey on Obstetric Anesthesia Training Centers (OATCs)

Following the publication of the first survey of obstetric care in the USA by Phillips and Frazier (88), which revealed the virtual lack of involvement of the anesthesia resident in obstetric anesthesia, Shnider (117) was prompted to undertake the first survey on the status of training in obstetric anesthesia by anesthesiology residents in the United States. For this purpose he obtained data from the American Board of Anesthesiology (ABA)

**Table 1–6.** Surveys on Obstetric Anesthesia Training Centers (OATCs) in USA

| Period of Survey / Author(s) / Sponsoring Society / No. of Hospitals Surveyed | 1961–63 Shnider ABA/AMA 191/ATC* | 1974–75 Hicks et al. SOAP 39 OATC | 1981 Millar & Plummer SOAP 108 OATC | 1989 Bonica SOAP 40 (37) OATC |
|---|---|---|---|---|
| **Vaginal Delivery** | | | | |
| **Personnel Administering Anesthesia (Figures in percent rounded to nearest unit)** | | | | |
| Anesthesiologists: | | | | |
| Anesthesia Resident | 28/19 (a) | — | 67 | 21 |
| Staff Anesthesiologist | 2/23 (a) | — | 16 | 19 |
| Staff & Resident | 4/7 (a) | (b) | — | 42 |
| *Subtotal* | 34/49 (a) | 56 (61) | 83 | 82 |
| Certified Registered Nurse Anesthetist (CRNA) | 21/24 (a) | 10 (5) | 11 | 5 |
| Obstetrician or Obstetric Resident | 26/5 (a) | 32 (31) | 0 | 13 |
| Others (c) | 12/22 (a) | 2 (3) | 6 | 0 |
| **Total** | 100/100 | 100(100) | 100 | 100 |
| **Cesarean Section** | | | | |
| Anesthesiologists: | | | | |
| Anesthesia Resident | 71/24 (a) | (e) | (f) | 16 |
| Staff Anesthesiologist | 9/60 (a) | (e) | (f) | 13 |
| Staff & Resident | 12/14 (a) | (e) | (f) | (63) |
| *Subtotal* | 92/98 (a) | (e) | 83 | 92 |
| Certified Registered Nurse Anesthetist (CRNA) | 2/1 (a) | (e) | 11 | 8 |
| Obstetrician or Obstetric Resident | 0/0 (a) | (e) | 0 | 0 |
| Other (c) | 4/2 (a) | (e) | 6 | 0 |
| **Total** | 100/100 | (e) | 100 | 100 |

| Period of Survey / Author(s) / Sponsoring Society / No. of Hospitals Surveyed | 1974–75 Hicks et al. SOAP 39 OATC | 1981 Millar & Plumer SOAP 108 OATC | 1989 Bonica SOAP 40 (37) OATC |
|---|---|---|---|
| **Vaginal Delivery** | | | |
| **Type of Anesthesia Used (In percent rounded to nearest decimal)** | | | |
| Subarachnoid Block | 21 | 12 | 3.0 |
| Continuous LEB | 24 | 42 | 51 |
| Continuous CEB | 6 | 4 | 3.0 |
| Double Catheter | 0 | 1 | 2.0 |
| Local/PNB | 26 | 24 | 27 |
| Inhalation Analgesia | 13 | 7 | 2.0 |
| General Anesthesia | 6 | 0 | 1.0 |
| None or Psychoprophylaxis | 10 | 10 | 11 |
| **Total** | 106 (d) | 100 | 100 |
| **Cesarean Section** | | | |
| Subarachnoid Block | 24 | 18 | 19 |
| Continuous Lumbar Epidural Block | 32 | 48 | 62 |
| Continuous Caudal Epidural Block | 0 | 0 | 1.0 |
| Double Catheter Epidural Block | 0 | 0 | 1.0 |
| Local Infiltration | 1 | 0 | 0 |
| General Anesthesia | 43 | 34 | 18 |
| Other | 0 | 0 | 0 |
| Total | 100 | 100 | 100 |

ATC = anesthesiology training centers; OATC = obstetric anesthesia training center. (a) The first number is for non-private patients, and the second figure for private patients; (b) authors published two sets of numbers (see text); (c) Other = medical students, nurses or other doctors untrained in anesthesia; (d) the number is greater than 100% because more than one type of anesthetic was used in some patients; (e) Hicks et al. published only one set of numbers which applied to both vaginal delivery and cesarean section, and therefore cannot be cited under cesarean section; (f) percent for anesthesiologist, resident and combination of staff and resident were not differentiated. Cont. LEB = continuous lumbar epidural block analgesia; Cont. CEB = continuous caudal epidural block analgesia; PNB = bilateral pudendal nerve block.

regarding the number of obstetric cases performed during 24 months of residency training (1961 to 1963). In addition, he obtained information by means of a questionnaire sent to the chairmen of approved anesthesiology residency training programs in the United States.

The questionnaire included such items as hospital size according to number of births per year; the number of anesthesia residents; the presence of a staff anesthesiologist with major responsibility of training residents in obstetric anesthesia; whether a resident was assigned exclusively to obstetric anesthesia 24 hours per day, 7 days a week; whether a staff anesthesiologist was assigned exclusively to obstetric anesthesia for the same period; and various other important issues. Information was obtained on 387 residents during the 24-month training period, and this revealed that residents devoted between 6 to 10% of the total experience to anesthesia for vaginal delivery and 2% to anesthesia for cesarean section. Of 245 questionnaires sent to chairmen of anesthesiology departments, Shnider received 227 (93%) responses. Of those 227, obstetric services were not available at 31 institutions and five lacked residents. Therefore, complete data were obtained from 191 institutions with both active obstetric units and anesthesia residency training programs of which 40% were from departments of university hospitals.

The data concerning personnel who administered anesthesia for vaginal delivery and for cesarean section are listed in Table 1–6. As noted for vaginal delivery, anesthesia residents working alone administered 28% to patients in nonprivate hospitals and 19% to those in private hospitals; staff anesthesiologists administered 2% and 23%, respectively, while a combination of both staff and residents administered 4% and 7%, respectively, so that the subtotal for the category of "anesthesiologists" is 34/49. The involvement of CRNAs, obstetricians, obstetric residents, and other personnel is listed in the table as are the data for cesarean section. Unfortunately, no data was included in this early survey on the type of analgesia or anesthesia used, and consequently this information is missing in the right side of Table 1–6. Thus, the listings of types of anesthesia begin with the 1974–1975 survey.

The data also revealed that 40% of the residents in anesthesiology administered fewer than 50 anesthetics for vaginal delivery during a 2-year training period and almost 50% administered fewer than 20 anesthetics for cesarean section. Anesthesia residents administered anesthetics in only 28% of the hospitals where the majority of anesthetics were used for vaginal delivery for nonprivate patients. Anesthesia residents were assigned specifically for 24 hours per day, 7 days per week of obstetric anesthesia care in only 17% of the hospitals. Moreover, in 10% of the residencies, no instruction on obstetric anesthesia was given.

These very discouraging data and other factors prompted the ASA Committee on Obstetric Anesthesia to develop guidelines for training of obstetric anesthesiologists, and, subsequently, the ACOG/COAA made similar recommendations that obstetric residents be given training in anesthesia. These efforts led the Joint Commission on Accreditation of Healthcare Organizations (JCAHO, previously called JCAH) to develop similar guidelines.

### *The Second (1975) OATCs Survey*

The second OATC survey carried out in 1974 by Hicks, Levinson, and Shnider (118) was limited to 39 obstetric anesthesia training centers (OATCs) in the United States and revealed that these 39 centers were training 711 of the total 1376 anesthesia residents being trained that year. Because in all of these centers the residents rotated on anesthesia and were being taught by staff anesthesiologists, this permitted anesthesiologists and/or anesthesia residents to administer more anesthetics than CRNAs and obstetricians. In their report, authors presented two sets of figures of the personnel who administered anesthesia: under "Results" they indicated that anesthesiologists and anesthesia residents provided 56% of anesthetics; obstetricians 32%; CRNAs 10%; and others 2%. However, in another table in their report in which they compare the personnel administering anesthesia for vaginal delivery, the figures for "obstetrical anesthesia centers" was 61, 31, 5, and 3, respectively. In Table 1–6, the latter figures are presented in parentheses (Table 1–7).

On the right side of Table 1–6, the type of anesthesia used for vaginal delivery and cesarean section is listed. It is to be noted that 10% of the parturients studied by Hicks and associates (113) elected Lamaze or other psychoprophylactic techniques, but 60 to 70% of those who so elected required supplementation with pharmacologic analgesia. As may be noted in Table 1–6, some 77% of the patients who delivered vaginally received regional anesthesia including bilateral pudendal block or local block in about 26% of the cases; continuous lumbar epidural analgesia/anesthesia in 24%; continuous or single-dose caudal epidural analgesia in about 6%; inhalation analgesia in nearly 13%; and general anesthesia in a little more than 6%; and among these general anesthesia cases, an endotracheal tube was used in two-thirds of the parturients. For cesarean section, regional anesthesia was used in 56% of the cases; general anesthesia in 43%; and local block in 1%. Fifty-one percent of the programs with obstetric residents rotated through anesthesia; 21% of anesthesiology residents rotated on neonatology, while 33% of the programs trained nurse-anesthetists. In addition, these 39

**Table 1–7.** Trends in Obstetric Anesthesia in USA

| Personnel Administering OAA (Figures in percent of total) | | | | | | | |
|---|---|---|---|---|---|---|---|
| **Type of Hospitals** | **General Hospitals** | | | **Training Centers** | | | |
| Period of Survey | 1959 | 1967 | 1981 | 1963–64 | 1974–75 | 1981 | 1989 |
| Author | Phillips | OA Com | Gibbs | Shnider | Hicks et al. | Millar & Plumer | Bonica |
| Agency | ASA | ACOG | ASA/ACOG | ABA | SOAP | SOAP | SOAP |
| Number Hospital Surveyed | 439 | 3,672 | 617 | 191/ATC | 39/OATC | 108/ATC | 40 (37 OATC) |
| **Vaginal Delivery** | | | | | | | |
| Anesthesiologist; Anesthesia Resident | 15 | 12 | 28 (a) | 34/49 (c) | 56 (61) | 83 | 82 |
| Nurse Anesthetist | 31 | 25 | 4 (b) | 21/24 (c) | 10 (5) | 11 | 5 |
| Obstetrician; Obstetric Resident | 26 | 33 | 68 | 26/5 (c) | 32 (31) | 0 | 13 |
| Others (d) | 28 | 30 | 0 | 19/22 (c) | 2 (3) | 6 | 0 |
| Total | 100 | 100 | 100 | 100/100 | | 100 | 100 |
| **Cesarean Section** | | | | | | | |
| Anesthesiologist; Anesthesia Resident | 40 | 74 | 83 | 93/97 | (e) | 83 | 92 |
| Nurse Anesthetist | 33 | 19 | 14 | 2/1 | (e) | 11 | 8 |
| Obstetrician; Obstetric Resident | 7 | 0 | 3 | 0/0 | (e) | 0 | 0 |
| Others (d) | 20 | 7 | 6 | 5/2 | (e) | 6 | 0 |
| Total | 100 | 100 | 100 | 100/100 | | 100 | 100 |

(a) Anesthesiologist, anesthesia resident or CRNA under supervision of anesthesiologist; (b) CRNA under supervision of obstetrician; (c) the first number is for nonprivate patients and the second figure for private patients; (d) Other = medical students; (e) Hicks, et al. published only one set of numbers which applied to both vaginal delivery and cesarean section, and therefore cannot be cited under cesarean section; (f) percent for anesthesiologist, resident and combination of staff and resident were not differentiated. ATC = anesthesiology training centers; OATC = obstetric anesthesia training center.

centers had excellent facilities, provided a good education program for parturients and their spouses in a high percentage of cases, and more than half of patients had preanesthetic evaluation prior to arrival at the hospital.

### The Third (1981) OATCs Survey

The survey by Millar and Plumer (119), who acquired data on 108 training programs with more than 2,200 residents, revealed that 93% of the residents learned obstetric anesthesia on a specific rotation with an identified director for slightly less than 2 months. In most of the programs, an anesthesiologist was present at all times on the obstetric floor and the majority made daily obstetric anesthesia rounds. Half of the anesthesiology residents on obstetric anesthesia service were covered by faculty who were in the hospital at all times. Anesthesia was administered by a resident in 67% of cases and by the faculty in 16%, for a total of 83%, while CRNAs administered 11% and others (doctors and nurses untrained in anesthesia, medical students, etc.) administered only 6% of anesthesia. Anesthesia used for cesarean section consisted of spinal in 18%, lumbar epidural in 48%, and general anesthesia in 34% of parturients (data on the agents and techniques used for vaginal delivery were cited by Plumer in a personal communication in 1984).

### The Fourth (1984) and Fifth (1989) OATCs Surveys

As previously mentioned, in 1983 to 1984 I sent a questionnaire to members of SOAP and to leading anesthesiologists in 61 countries throughout the world. The questionnaire was simple and included data on the type of analgesia/anesthesia used for labor, vaginal delivery, and cesarean section. Responses were received from 41 members of SOAP and 37 from other countries. The 1989 survey consisted of a more detailed questionnaire and was sent to 50 members of SOAP who were known to have active obstetric anesthesia services and, through the courtesy of Dr. M. E. Tunstall, then president of the Obstetric Anaesthetists Association, to members in the United Kingdom. The questionnaire requested data on the following issues: (1) the type of analgesia/anesthesia used for labor, vaginal delivery, and for cesarean section; (2) the personnel administering the anesthesia for these various events; (3) whether the obstetric anesthesia program was a formal division of the department of anesthesiology; (4) data on training programs for anesthesia residents, obstetric anesthesia fellows, and obstetric residents and the duration of such training; and (5) information on psychoprophylaxis. Complete data was received from 40 members of SOAP, 37 of whom direct an obstetric anesthesia training center (OATC). A total of 45 responses were received from OATCs in the United Kingdom, but complete data for analysis were available from only 33 centers in England, Wales, and Ireland and five in Scotland.

### USA Data

The 40 American hospitals from which 1989 data were obtained had a total of 139,880 births; the mean was 3,497 per year, ranging from 1,560 to 16,000 per year. Obviously, all of these belong in the stratum III category, as defined by Gibbs, et al (93) in the survey of general hospitals. All of the 37 OATCs were directed by an obstetric anesthesiologist, i.e., a person who had special training and/or extensive experience in obstetric anesthesia and devoted most of the time to patient care, teaching, and research in this field. All of these programs had training for anesthesia residents for a mean of 1.6 months (range 1 to 4 months) and all but five had a fellowship that lasted a mean of 9 months (range 3 to 18 months). About half of the programs trained obstetric residents in obstetric anesthesia for a period of 1 month, while four trained for 2 months. Only one program also trained CRNAs in obstetric anesthesia.

Table 1–6 contains a concise summary of the data on the personnel administering anesthesia, the type of analgesia and anesthesia used in these programs, and the data acquired in the previous surveys presented for comparison and to indicate trends. In three hospitals without OATCs, analgesia/anesthesia for vaginal delivery was administered by a staff anesthesiologist in about 80% of the cases, and CRNAs in 20%. In the 37 OATC programs, anesthesia residents or obstetric anesthesia fellows administered a mean of 82% (range 65 to 100), invariably, with the help and/or supervision of an obstetric anesthesiologist in 42% (range 25 to 100) and by a staff anesthesiologist who provided night coverage in 35% of instances (range 5 to 60%). Analysis of the combined data of the administration by three types of anesthesiologists resulted in a mean of 82%. For cesarean section, the combined efforts resulted in a 92% coverage by anesthesiologists, staff, residents, and/or fellows. Nurse anesthetists were involved in administering obstetric anesthesia in only 11 of the hospitals, and they administered 5% of the analgesia/anesthesia for vaginal delivery and 8% of the anesthesia for cesarean section. Obstetricians or obstetric residents were involved in administering anesthesia for vaginal delivery in 13% and did not participate in the anesthetic care of patients undergoing cesarean section.

As part of the survey, data were acquired on the type of analgesia used for labor as well as analgesia and anesthesia used for vaginal delivery. Table 1–6 lists the summary of data acquired in the 1989 survey compared with those of two previous surveys of OATCs; as mentioned earlier, in the report of the first survey by Shnider (117) information on the type of anesthesia were not presented. The important points to be made about the data presented in Table 1–6 include the following: (1) there has been a progressive increase in parturients managed with continuous lumbar epidural alone or with continuous caudal epidural and a few with double catheter technique; and (2) the marked decrease in the use of spinal (saddle block) as well as inhalation analgesia and general anesthesia for vaginal delivery, which reflects current practice among most obstetric anesthesiologists. A similar trend obtains for anesthesia for cesarean section because over four-fifths of the patients received subarachnoid block or lumbar epidural block, while only 18% received general balanced anesthesia.

Tables 1–7 and 1–8 repeat the data from Tables 1–2

**Table 1–8.** Trends in Obstetric Anesthesia in USA

| | Type of OAA Administered (Figures in percent of total; rounded to nearest unit) | | | | | |
|---|---|---|---|---|---|---|
| **Type of Hospitals** | **General Hospitals** | | | **Training Centers** | | |
| Period of Survey | 1959 | 1967 | 1981 | 1974–75 | 1981 | 1989 |
| Author | Phillips | OA Com | Gibbs | Hicks et al. | Millar & Plumer | Bonica |
| Agency | ASA/OAC | ACOG | ASA/ACOG | SOAP | SOAP | SOAP |
| Number Hospital Surveyed | 439 | 3,672 | 617 | 39/OATC | 108/ATC | 40 (37 OATC) |
| | | | **Vaginal Delivery** | | | |
| Subarachnoid Block | 8 | 7 | 9 | 21 | 12 | 3 |
| Continuous LEB | 7* | 0 | 14 | 24 | 42 | 51 |
| Continuous CEB | — | 6 | 0 | 6 | 4 | 3 |
| Double Catheter | — | 0 | 0 | 0 | 1 | 2 |
| PNB/Local | 2 | 16 | 59 | 26 | 24 | 27 |
| Inhalation Analgesia | 62* | 0 | 6 | 13 | 7 | 2 |
| General Anesthesia | — | 36 | 3 | 6 | 0 | 1 |
| Type Not Specified | — | 22 | — | — | — | — |
| None or Psychoprophylaxis | 21 | (?) | 15 | 10 | 10 | 11 |
| Total | 100 | 100 | 106 (a) | 106 (b) | 100 | 100 |
| | | | **Cesarean Section** | | | |
| Subarachnoid Block | 42 | 54 | 34 | 24 | 18 | 19 |
| Lumbar Epidural Block | 10* | 0 | 21 | 32 | 48 | 62 |
| Caudal Epidural Block | | 3 | 0 | 0 | 0 | 1 |
| Local Infiltration | 1 | 1 | 0 | 1 | 0 | 0 |
| General (Balanced) | 32 | 32 | 41 | 43 | 34 | 18 |
| Combination (GA+RA) | 15 | 10 | 0 | 4 | 0 | 0 |
| Total | 100 | 100 | 96 (b) | 100 | 100 | 100 |

* Techniques not differentiated in 1959; (a) values greater than 100% because in some parturients more than one type was used; (b) values less than 100% because some respondents failed to answer all questions.

and 1–6 to show the trends in the United States in regard to the personnel administering anesthesia and the type of anesthesia used for vaginal delivery and cesarean section in general hospitals and OATCs over the course of the past 3 decades. In regard to personnel (Table 1–7), in general hospitals there was only a very modest and somewhat disappointing increase in the involvement of anesthesiologists/anesthesiology residents in the administration of anesthesia for vaginal delivery during the 22-year interval among the three surveys. As of this writing, the situation in general hospitals remains unknown, although Gibbs has initiated another survey similar to the one pertaining to 1981 that will be published probably in 1994. In contrast, from 1963 to 1989 there was an encouraging and indeed impressive increase in the number of anesthesiologists/anesthesiology residents or fellows involved in the administration of anesthesia for vaginal delivery in those hospitals that have large obstetric services and well organized and formalized obstetric anesthesia programs for patient care and training. Obviously, because the figures on OATCs represent the care of some 3 to 5% of all parturients that delivered in the United States during the periods of the surveys, these data *cannot reflect the national situation*. On the other hand, they do emphasize the *critical need* to discourage and indeed eliminate small and medium-sized obstetric units and concentrate obstetric care in hospitals that have a large obstetric service. This will facilitate the development and sustenance of high-quality obstetric anesthesia care and training and also facilitates better programs in perinatology and the acquisition of resources needed to permit optimal care of parturients and their babies.

It is important to recognize the role of the CRNA in the care of obstetric patients and to define the relationship with the anesthesiologist who, in many level 4 centers, has the prime medical responsibility of managing analgesia in the labor and delivery suite. It must be understood from the outset that often many CRNAs act in obstetric units without the supervision of the anesthesiologist because anesthesiologists are just not available in those units. In the latter case, it must be emphasized that the CRNAs are really dispatching their works under the license of the obstetrician responsible for the particular case involved. When the first edition of this book was published, some 25 years ago, the CRNA was often the chief person and power source for obstetric analgesia/anesthesia coverage. It has been estimated that nearly 50% of all obstetric anesthesia is still done primarily by the CRNA, while another undetermined percentage is performed by the CRNA under the direction of the anesthesiologist (120).

It is the opinion of the editors of this book that the CRNAs in the United States play a very important role in regard to obstetric anesthesia. It must be recognized that there are some small units across the country that are in need of the occasional anesthetic not covered by anesthesiologists, and they are administered by the CRNA. In such a scenario, although the administration of the anesthetic is by the CRNA, the sole physician responsible is the obstetrician, a practice which should be strongly discouraged, unless the obstetrician knows well the basic principles of obstetric anesthesia and is capable of helping the CRNA in treating serious anesthetic complications. It deserves emphasis that in urban areas this problem can and should be eliminated by closing down all small obstetric units in smaller hospitals and concentrate the care of patients in large obstetric units where a full staff of obstetric anesthesiologists are available.

In regard to the type of anesthesia, it is apparent that there has been a progressive increase in the use of regional anesthesia, both for vaginal delivery and cesarean section and an almost virtual elimination of the use of general anesthesia for vaginal delivery in both general hospitals and specialized centers. Lumbar epidural block, particularly, has emerged as the most frequently employed method in regional anesthesia, even for cesarean section.

## *Anesthesia in Obstetric Units in the USA/UK*

Table 1–9 contains comparative data on the type of analgesia used for labor and the type of analgesia and anesthesia used for vaginal delivery in the 30 hospitals in the United States and the 38 hospitals in the United Kingdom. Most striking is the similarity in the percentage of patients who received pharmacologic pain relief during labor and vaginal delivery. It is to be noted that for the purpose of computing the percentage of various types of analgesia and anesthesia used for labor and vaginal delivery, the groups that received no analgesia were omitted. Thus, the figures in the table represent the mean percentage of various types of analgesia and anesthesia given to all patients who received pharmacologic pain relief. Most striking are the similarities in percentage of parturients managed with systemic analgesia during labor and with local and/or pudendal block for vaginal delivery. Also of interest is the virtually discontinued use of paracervical block for pain relief during labor and of subarachnoid block for vaginal delivery. Differences in the two countries' practices pertain to inhalation analgesia during the first stage of labor and during vaginal delivery. This method is used in the UK in 29 of patients during labor and 24% during vaginal delivery, but only a few percent of parturients in the United States underwent such procedure. Indeed, many respondents in the UK indicated that nitrous oxide-oxygen in a 50/50 premixture contained in the Entonox was readily available in all obstetric suites and was used by many parturients in some instances to supplement other methods of analgesia. In contrast, in OATCs continuous epidural analgesia is being used twice as often in the United States than in the United Kingdom for both labor and vaginal delivery.

It is notable that in the USA the frequency of use of continuous epidural anesthesia during vaginal delivery was slightly lower than its use during labor. This is due probably to the fact that perineal analgesia was insufficient and consequently the patient received either a single-dose caudal analgesia or saddle block to provide perineal anes-

**Table 1–9.** Analgesia/Anesthesia for Labor and Vaginal Delivery (1989 Survey: Comparison between United States and United Kingdom)

| Analgesia for Labor | | | Analgesia/Anesthesia for Vaginal Delivery | | |
|---|---|---|---|---|---|
| **Procedure** | **USA (N = 30)** | **UK (N = 38)** | **Procedure** | **USA (N = 30)** | **UK (N = 38)** |
| Percent of All Labors | 85<br>(48–91) | 81<br>(25–100) | Percent of All Deliveries | 89<br>(47–98) | 80<br>(25–100) |
| Type* | | | Type* | | |
| Systemic Opioid Sedatives | 30.0<br>(44–90) | 42.0<br>(18–100) | Local or Pudendal Block | 30.0<br>(12–63) | 39.0<br>(5–100) |
| Continuous Epidural Analgesia | 62.0<br>(19–26) | 21.0<br>(7–70) | Continuous Lumbar Epidural Analgesia/ Anesthesia | 58<br>(30–89) | 21.0<br>(5–70) |
| Continuous Caudal Analgesia | 1.0<br>(0–11) | 0.0<br>— | Continuous or Single Caudal Anesthesia | 3.0<br>(0–17) | 1.0<br>(0–6) |
| Double Catheter Epidural | 3.0<br>(0–42) | 0.0<br>(10–27) | Double Catheter | 2.0<br>(0–42) | 0.0<br>(0–27) |
| Paracervical Block | 1.0<br>(0–19) | 0.0<br>— | Subarachnoid Block | 3.5<br>(0–23) | 3.0<br>(0–27) |
| Inhalation Analgesia | 3.0<br>(0–19) | 37.0<br>(10–58) | Inhalation Analgesia | 2.5<br>(0–10) | 34.0<br>(0–65) |
| | | | General Anesthesia | 1.0<br>(0–6) | 2.0<br>(0–18) |

* Shown in percent among those who received analgesia and anesthesia (does not include those who received psychoprophylaxis or no anesthesia). Figures in parentheses represent ranges recorded.

thesia or a perineal local block. Note should also be made of the percentage of patients who received no pharmacologic analgesia and managed with psychoprophylaxis decreased from 15 to 11%. Even though a larger percentage had planned initially not to have any pharmacologic analgesia or anesthesia, 4% of the patients among this group apparently requested and received anesthesia either because of very severe pain or to permit manipulation and instrumentation in difficult cases.

Among the 38 hospitals in the United Kingdom, *anesthesia for cesarean section* consisted of general anesthesia in 54% of the parturients, lumbar epidural anesthesia in 35%, and subarachnoid block in 11%. None of the patients were managed with local infiltration anesthesia. Comparison of the data in Table 1–9 with those in Tables 1–6 and 1–8 show that anaesthetists in the United Kingdom use general anesthesia about 2 to $2\frac{1}{2}$ times as frequently as their American counterparts. The data on cesarean section in the OTACs in the U.K. have been summarized above, and data for cesarean section for the general population is presented in Table 1–10.

## STATUS OF OBSTETRIC ANESTHESIA IN OTHER COUNTRIES

The 1984 questionnaire sent to anesthesiologists in 61 countries, of which 37 responded, consisted of three main sections: (1) date and person who gave the first anesthesia for vaginal delivery and cesarean section; (2) the evolution of obstetric anesthesia, the advent of the anesthesiologist in that country, and the factors responsible for it; (3) the current status regarding what percentage of patients received analgesia and anesthesia for labor, vaginal delivery, and cesarean section; and (4) of those receiving obstetric analgesia and anesthesia, what agents were being used for labor, vaginal delivery, and cesarean section. As previously mentioned, the early period was different for each country. In the United Kingdom, Canada, Australia, and New Zealand, the early period extended from the 1860s, while in most other countries, it did not begin until the early 1960s and 1970s. The 1989 survey was limited to the current status of obstetric analgesia and anesthesia of that year only. Because of space limitations, the evolutionary history of anesthesia in these various countries is omitted, while data on their current status is listed in Tables 1–10 through 1–13. It deserves emphasis here that many of the data reflect the current status in universities and major obstetric centers in each country, although some respondents have provided estimates for their overall population. Many respondents gave ranges for the use of various techniques, but for the sake of clarity in the tables that follow, in many instances, only the means are listed.

Because at the time of the publication of this book the data from Tables 1–10 to 1–13 are 9 and 4 years old, respectively, I hesitated to include them in this chapter. However, colleagues persuaded me to include them because they provide some information on the past trends of obstetric analgesia/anesthesia in various countries throughout the world. It deserves reemphasis that these data are not intended to provide precise information, but to give an idea of conditions in these countries. In view of the impressive growth of the World Federation of Societies of Anesthesiologists (WFSA) during the past decade, currently the status of obstetric analgesia and anesthesia should be better. The WFSA is in a good position to obtain more precise data on this and other aspects of anesthesiology.

### Canada, the United Kingdom, and Scandinavia

#### Canada

Table 1–10 contains data on Canada, the United Kingdom, and Scandinavia. For Canada, three sets of figures are listed. The first line of data was derived from a survey by McMorland and Jenkins (121) published in 1980, which revealed that the 13 Canadian University Departments of Anaesthesia that responded, representing 24 affiliated hospitals, delivered 17% of the total births in Canada. In their report, the authors did not provide data on percentage of parturients receiving analgesia for labor, but combined this together with "analgesia/anesthesia of vaginal deliveries" (in percentage of all deliveries). However, it may be reasonable to assume that continuous epidural analgesia, inhalation analgesia, and psychoprophylaxis were initiated during labor. The data are listed in the table as means above and ranges below. While epidural analgesia was widely used during labor, there were many hospitals where its use was limited, or it was not used at all. They reported that of 17% of parturients who started with "natural childbirth," 12% (70% of this group) eventually required some form of pharmacologic analgesia (range 0–100%). They reported that the majority of hospitals did not have adequate obstetrical anasthesia coverage, and that resident training in Obstetric Anasthesia was insufficient and that research programs on topics pertaining to it were rare.

The third line of the table contained 1989 data sent to me by Dr. Steve Rolbin of Toronto and reflected the situation in university and major general hospitals that had fairly large obstetric services throughout the country, and, as noted, epidural analgesia increased significantly for both vaginal delivery and cesarean section. The table also includes data on a survey carried out by McMorland, Jenkins, and Douglas in British Columbia that was initiated 1982 (122). They sent questionnaires to 78 hospitals and received responses from 42 (54%), three of which were affiliated with the University of British Columbia and annually had more than 2000 deliveries and 39 community hospitals of varying sizes. In their report, the authors did not provide information on the percent of parturients given analgesia for labor or analgesia/anesthesia for vaginal delivery, but like their first report, combined the data into "analgesia-anesthesia for vaginal delivery." Moreover, they did not compute means but published ranges that are listed in the second and third parts of the table.

#### United Kingdom

In 1984 Professor Michael Rosen provided me with mean figures for the majority of hospitals in England and Wales, and Dr. Bruce Scott, for most hospitals in Scotland. In Table 1–10 these figures are shown first and the 1989

**Table 1–10.** Status of Obstetric Analgesia/Anesthesia in Canada, United Kingdom, and Scandinavia

| Region | | Analgesia During Labor | | | |
|---|---|---|---|---|---|
| Country | Year* | Percent of All Labors† | IA / SA (1) | LEB | Other |
| **Canada** | | | | | |
| University Hospitals | 1980 | | | | |
| Mean | | N.R. | 22/21 | 40 cont. | PC-0.1, 17 PS |
| Range | | | 16–33 | 0–95 | 10–100 |
| University Hospitals | 1989 | 85 | 12 | 68 | 20 |
| **British Columbia** | | | | | |
| University Hospitals | 1986 | N.R. | 1–33/0 | 20–40 cont. | PCB 0–1 |
| Community Hospitals | | N.R. | 0–75/0 | 0–20 | 0–6 |
| **United Kingdom** | | | | | |
| England/Wales A | | 80 (81) | 80 (58) | 10 (22) | 10(20)PS |
| Scotland | | 90 (83) | 75 (55) | 15 (26) | 10 (19) PS |
| **Scandinavia** | | | | | |
| Sweden | | 75 | 60 | 25 | 15 PS |
| Finland | | 70 (75) | 75(68) | 12 (12) | 13 (16) PCB |
| Iceland | | 90 (99) | 72 (30/50) | 20 (33) | 8 (0) |

* Year of survey: †1984 cited first number; (without paranthesis) 1989 (numbers in parentheses). IA = inhalation analgesia; SA = systemic analgesics/sedatives/tranquilizers; LEB = lumbar epidural block; Cont. = continuous LEB; CEB = caudal epidural block; PNB = pudendal nerve block; LI = local infiltration; PCB = paracervical block; DCEB = double catheter epidural block; PS = psychoprophylaxis (Lamaze; natural childbirth); PS + S = psychoprophylaxis plus supplementary pharmacologic analgesia; GA = general anesthesia. (1) Single figures in the columns mean agents or techniques not differentiated in reports. (2) Figures that add more than 100% due to use of more than one procedure in the same patient. (3) Figures for British Columbia are presented in ranges of numbers published, N.R. = not reported.

**Table 1–11.** Status of Obstetric Analgesia/Anesthesia in Europe and the Near East

| Region | | Analgesia During Labor | | | |
|---|---|---|---|---|---|
| Country | Year* | Percent of All Labors | IA / SA (1) | LEB | Other |
| **Western Europe** | | | | | |
| West Germany | | 70 (90) | 70 (60) | 15 (30) | 15 (10) PS |
| France** | | 40 | 10 | 13 | 80 PS |
| Austria | (1984) | 65 | 60 | 10 | 30 PS |
| | (1989) | (5–95) | (2–98) | (5–98) | (10–60) |
| Italy | | 40 (60) | 50 (30) | 10 (25) | 40 (30) PS |
| Malta | | 80 (90) | 80 (75) | 20 (15) | 10 (10) AC |
| Spain | | 85 | 70 | 30 | — |
| **Eastern Europe** | | | | | |
| GDR (East Germany) | | 30 | 80 | 10 | 10 PS |
| Hungary | | 15 (20) | 3 (5) | 12 (15) | 85 (80) PS |
| Bulgaria | | 60 | 80 | 10 | 10 PS |
| Romania | | 10 | 95 | 1 | 4 |
| USSR | | 70+ | 95 | <5 | 95 PS |
| **Near East** | | | | | |
| Lebanon (AUH) | | 95 (80) | 25 (5) | 60 (80) | 15 (15) |
| Turkey | | 20 (25) | 90 (95) | 5 (3) | 5 (2) CEB |
| Egypt | | 2 | 80/20 | — | — |
| Kuwait | | 10 | 100 | — | — |

* Year of survey: 1984 cited first number; 1989 (numbers in parentheses). ** See text for explanation of the data on France. (1) Single figures in the columns means agents or techniques not differentiated in reports. (2) Figures that add up to more than 100% due to use of more than one procedure in the same patient. See Table 1–10 for abbreviations of anesthetic techniques.

| | Analgesia/Anesthesia for Vaginal Delivery | | | | Anesthesia for Cesarean Section | | |
|---|---|---|---|---|---|---|---|
| Percent of All Deliveries | PNB<br>LI (1) | LEB | IA<br>GA (1) | Other | GA | LEB | SAB |
| N.R. | 4.5/0<br>0–43 | 40 cont.<br>0–95 | 1.2/2<br>0–14 | SAB 0.5 PS<br>+S 12, 5 PS<br>alone | 21<br>2–10 | 28<br>0–98 | 1<br>0–10 |
| 85 | 20 | 70 | 10/0 | — | 5 | 95 | 0 |
| N.R. | 0–33/0 | 20–40 | 1–25 | — | 35–75 | 30–65 | 0–1 |
| N.R. | 0–80/0 | 0–20 | 1–15 | — | 20–100 | 0–50 | 0–42 |
| 95 (80) | 50/25 (10/39) | 10 (22) | 15 (27) | 7 PS (2 SAB) | 85 (54) | 14 (35) | 1 (11) |
| 90 (81) | 80 (0/38) | 16 (30) | 4 (26) | 8 PS (4 SAB) | 64 (55) | 31 (35) | 5 (10) |
| 90 | 70 | 25 | 0/5 | — | 25 | 70 | 5 |
| 80 (23) | 85 (80) | 10 (8) | 5 (12) | — | 35 (40) | 50 (35) | 15 (25) |
| 90 (99) | 21<br>5/15 | 2<br>35 | 40/0 | — | 10 (15) | 85 (81) | 5 (4) |

| | Analgesia/Anesthesia for Vaginal Delivery | | | | Anesthesia for Cesarean Section | | |
|---|---|---|---|---|---|---|---|
| Percent of All Deliveries | PNB<br>LI (1) | LEB | IA<br>GA (1) | Other | GA | LEB | SAB |
| 80 (90) | 55 (50) | 20 (30) | 15 (10) | 10 (10) PS | 80 (65) | 20 (30) | <1 (10) |
| 40 | 55 | 15 | 20 | 60 | 75 | 25 | — |
| 75 | 50 | 10 | 15 | 25 PS | 95 | 3 | 2 |
| (10–80) | (15–40) | (5–40) | (5–30) | (10–60) PS | (40–100) | (5–6) | (5–6) |
| 25 (35) | 80 (60) | 10 (35) | 7 (15) | 3 (9) SAB | 85 (75) | 15 (20) | 0 (5) |
| 90 (85) | 10 (45) | 85 (20) | 5 (15) | 0 (20) AC | 75 (90) | 15 (5) | 10 (5) |
| 75 | 10 | 75 | 0 | 15 SAB | 85 | 15 | — |
| 40 | 0/65 | 10 | 10/0 | 15 PS | 85 | 15 | — |
| 10 (20) | 55 (65) LI | 12 (15) | 5 (15) | 15 (10) PS | 85 (70) | 10 (20) | 5 (10) |
| 50 | 35/30 | — | 10/5 | 20 PS | 90 | 7 | 1 |
| 85 | 0/96 | 2 | 3 | — | 65 | 3 | 27 |
| 70+ | 1/5 | 3 | 96/0 | 95 PS | 89 | 10 | 1 |
| 95 (90) | 10 (8) | 90 (80) | 0 (12) | — | 90 (90) | 5 (2) | 5 (8) |
| 25 (30) | 75 (70) LI | 3 (5) | 22 (25) | — | 98 (95) | 1 (4) | 1 (1) |
| 20 | 0/10 | 2 | 85/3 | — | 98 | — | 2 |
| 75 | 0/100 | — | — | — | 99 | 0.5 | 0.5 |

**Table 1–12.** Status of Obstetric Analgesia/Anesthesia in Asia/Australasia

| Region | | Analgesia During Labor | | | |
|---|---|---|---|---|---|
| Country | Year* | Percent of All Labors | IA / SA (1) | LEB | Other |
| **Australia** | | 90+ | 70 | 30 | — |
| New Zealand | | 85 (60) | 40 (30) | 35 (40) | 25 (30) |
| Japan | | | | | |
| University Hospital | 1984 | 30 | 50 | 25 (20) | 25 CA/A |
| General Hospital | 1984 | 10 | 25 | 2 (5) | 5 PC |
| All Hospitals | 1989 | (10) | (40) | (20) | (20) DCEB |
| South Korea | | 70 | 60 | 35 | 5 CEB |
| Hong Kong | | 90–100 | 95 (75) | 5 (15) | 0 (10) |
| Malaysia | | 90 (80) | 90 (80) | 4 (10) | 6 (10) |
| Singapore | | 50 (100) | 90 (80) | 10 (20) | 0 (0) |
| Taiwan | | 5 | 15 | 85 | — |
| Philippines | | 92 (95) | 75 (70) | 10 (20) | 15 (10) CEB |
| Bangladesh | | 50 | 95 | 5 | — |

* Year of survey: 1984 cited first number; 1989 (numbers in parentheses). IA = inhalation analgesia; SA = systemic analgesics/sedatives/tranquilizers; LEB = lumbar epidural block; CEB = caudal epidural block; PNB = pudendal nerve block; LI = local infiltration; PCB = paracervical block; DCEB = double catheter epidural block; PS = psychoprophylaxis (Lamaze; natural childbirth). (1) Single figures in the columns means agents or techniques not differentiated in reports. (2) Figures that add up to more than 100% due to use of more than one procedure in the same patient.

**Table 1–13.** Status of Obstetric Analgesia/Anesthesia in Africa/Latin America

| Region | Analgesia During Labor | | | |
|---|---|---|---|---|
| Country | Percent of All Labors | IA / SA (1) | LEB | Other |
| **Africa** | | | | |
| South Africa | | | | |
| University Hospitals | 7 | 40 | 32 | 7 |
| Overall | 2 | 98 SA | 2 | — |
| Zimbabwe | 35 | 70 | 30 | — |
| Tanzania | 5 | 100 | — | — |
| Kenya | 50 | 95 | 3 | 2 |
| **Central Amer./Caribbean** | | | | |
| Guatemala | | | | |
| Major Hospitals | 10 (20) | 28 (20) | 60 (80) | 12 (9 CEB/3 DCEB) |
| Small Hospitals | (5–10) | (90) | (5) | (0/0) |
| Panama | 5 (15) | 80 (60) | 15 (40) | 5 (10) |
| Equador | (10) | (40) | (40) | (20 PS) |
| **South America** | | | | |
| Brazil | 70 | 980 | 2 | 8 PS |
| Colombia (UH) | 30 (25) | 53 (5) | 40 (80) | 5 (15) CEB |
| Venezuela (UH) | 80 | 60 | 35 | 5 |

Year of survey: 1984 cited first number; 1989 (numbers in parentheses). IA = inhalation analgesia; SA = systemic analgesics/sedatives/tranquilizers; LEB = lumbar epidural block; CEB = caudal epidural block; PNB = pudendal nerve block; LI = local infiltration; PCB = paracervical block; DCEB = double catheter epidural block; PS = psychoprophylaxis (Lamaze; natural childbirth). (1) Single figures in the columns means agents or techniques not differentiated in reports. (2) Figures that add up to more than 100% due to use of more than one procedure in the same patient.

| | Analgesia/Anesthesia for Vaginal Delivery | | | | Anesthesia for Cesarean Section | | |
|---|---|---|---|---|---|---|---|
| Percent of All Deliveries | PNB / LI (1) | LEB | IA / GA (1) | Other | GA | LEB | SAB |
| 100 | 10/40 | 30 | 10/0 | 10 | 60 | 35 | 5 |
| 90 (70) | 20 (30) | 25 (45) | 45 (15) | 10 (10) | 25 (50) | 70 (45) | 5 (5) |
| 44 | 10 | 40 | 45 | 5 | 5 | 45 | 50 |
| 33 (20) | 20 (20) | 25 (30) | 50 (30) | 5 | 3 | 35 | 60 |
| 20–35 | (20) | (35–40) | (25) | (15) CEB/SAB | (3) | (35) | (62) |
| 95 | 65/0 | 30 | 5 CEB | 5 CA | 80 | 8 | 12 |
| 90–100 | 90 (85) | 5 (15) | 0 (5) | — | 90 (85) | 5 (10) | 5 (5) |
| 90 (80) | 63 (55) | 12 (14) | 21 (26) | 4 (5) SAB | 93 (90) | 2 (5) | 5 (5) |
| 70 (100) | 75 (60) | 8 (20) | 2 (0) | 15 (20) SAB | 95 (80) | 4 (10) | 1 (10) |
| 10 | 10 | 85 | <1 | 15 | 95 | 5 | 0 |
| 90 (95) | 40 (50) | 20 (30) LEB<br>20 (15) CEB | 0 (0) | 10 (5) SAB | 5 (10) | 10 (35) | 85 (55) |
| 60 | 95 LI | 2 | 3 | — | 95 | 2 | 3 |

| | Analgesia/Anesthesia for Vaginal Delivery | | | | Anesthesia for Cesarean Section | | |
|---|---|---|---|---|---|---|---|
| Percent of All Deliveries | PNB / LI (1) | LEB | 1A / GA (1) | Other | GA | LEB | SAB |
| 7 | 80 | 18 | — | — | 90 | 10 | — |
| 2 | 18/80 | 2 | — | — | 94 | 5 | 1 |
| 30 | 60 | 30 | 10 | — | 80 | 15 | 5 |
| 5 | 100 | — | — | — | 90 | — | — |
| 20 | 95 | 1 | 4 | — | 98 | 1 | 1 |
| 30 (45) | 10 (5) | 50 (75) | 25 (10) | 15 SAB/CEB | 10 (3) | 80 (94) | 10 (3) |
| (10–15) | (75) | (10) | (5) GA | (5 SAB/5 CEB) | (40) | (10) | (50) |
| 10 (40) | 70 (30) | 15 (50) | 5 (10) | 10 (20) SAB | 4 | 90 | 1 |
| (10) | (80 LI) | 20 | — | — | (2) | (95) | (3) |
| 70 | 10/40 | 20 | — | 30 SAB | 17 | 3 | 80 |
| 70 (95) | 7 (10) | 70 (80) | 13 (5) | 10 (5) SAB | 15 | 55 | 30 |
| 90 | 10/15 | 65 | 5 | 10 SAB | 30 | 55 | 15 |

figures provided by the members of the Obstetric Anaesthesia Association are shown in parentheses. As previously mentioned, figures were derived from a survey that included 33 reports from hospitals in England, Wales, and Northern Ireland, while five reports involved hospitals in Scotland. Detailed data on analgesia during labor and analgesia and anesthesia for vaginal delivery are given in Table 1–9. It is obvious that in these hospitals one-third of the patients received continuous epidural analgesia for both vaginal delivery and cesarean section. It is also important to note that for a number of years in the United Kingdom the Royal College of Anaesthetists has required that all registrars receive training in epidural analgesia for obstetrics. In a survey by Hibbard and Scott (123) of 271 hospitals in the United Kingdom for the years 1982–1986, representing 3.4 million deliveries, lumbar epidural block was used in 17.4% of deliveries in England, 21.3% in Scotland, 6.7% in Wales, and 5.5% in Northern Ireland, with an overall mean of 17% for the entire United Kingdom. From the 38 hospitals that responded to the 1989 survey, the results are listed in Table 1–9 and indicate that obstetric anesthesia care had improved in major obstetric centers.

### Finland

Professor Arno Hollmen, of Finland, provided data in 1984 and again in 1989. The latter figures were gathered from 32 hospitals, including 14 local hospitals with one to three anesthesiologists, 14 central hospitals with five to 10 anesthesiologists, and four university obstetric units. The 1989 data, which are listed in parentheses, show that in Finland analgesia and anesthesia was used in 75% of the patients in labor but in only 23% of the patients during delivery. For labor, systemic analgesia meperidine was used in 68% (range 0 to 70%), epidural anesthesia in 12% (range 0 to 38%), paracervical block in 16% (0 to 75%), and nitrous oxide in 12% (0 to 95%). Among the 23% who received analgesia and anesthesia for vaginal delivery, local infiltration was used in 80% of the parturients, or pudendal block and epidural block in 8%. The decrease in the use of epidural block for vaginal delivery was apparently caused by the desire of obstetricians to have parturients deliver spontaneously. It is unfortunate that the double catheter technique is not used more widely because when properly performed, it permits spontaneous delivery in virtually every parturient. It is likely that other than 23% who received analgesia/anesthesia for vaginal delivery, many of the other patients still had the effects of systemic analgesics to care for their pain. Moreover, more recent personal discussion with Hollomen indicates that epidural analgesia for the second stage has increased in the past 4 years.

### Iceland

Professor T. Olafsson provided data for Iceland, which revealed significant improvement over the 1984 figures. Olafsson stated that during the early 1980s rapid progress was made in obstetric analgesia/anesthetic procedures with anesthesiologists supervising or administering virtually all of it. Currently, the field is in a steady state and no major changes are expected in the near future.

### Sweden

The data listed for Sweden are those provided by Professor Bertil Lofstrom in 1984; unfortunately, no response was received to the 1989 questionnaire. However, a recent report (124) contains the results of a survey on the use of analgesia in 99% of the 335,448 women in Sweden who had vaginal deliveries during the 4-year period, 1983–1986. This study revealed that lumbar epidural analgesia (LEA) was used in 16%, paracervical block (PCB) in 15%, pudendal block (PNB) in 82%, and meperdine or morphine in 49%. As expected, LEA was used in 27 to 35% of women delivered in major regional and central county hospitals, in 20 to 25% of women delivered in county hospitals specialized with obstetric services, but in only 5 to 8% in smaller nonspecialized county hospitals. Nulliparae were given LEA in 28%, PCB in 13%, opioids in 66%, and PNB in 70%, whereas the figures for multiparae were 7%, 11%, 38%, and 57%, respectively. Only 1.5% of parturients received no form of pharmacologic analgesia. These data, together with the fact that Nordic women (95% of the group) use regional analgesia slightly more often than the 5% non-Nordic women, prompted the authors to reemphasize that the current concept of Nordic women manifesting less pain behavior during labor than women of other ethnic origins is not correct.

## Western Europe

### Germany

Professor W. Dick provided data on the situation in Germany (see Table 1–11) that presumably represents the major obstetric centers in that country. Comparison of the data provided in 1989 with those of 1984 show that analgesia during labor increased from 70 to 90% of all labors and that analgesia/anesthesia for vaginal delivery increased from 80 to 90%.

### France

No response was received from France for the 1989 survey. The data shown in Table 1–11 reflects figures provided to me by several French colleagues during a tour in France and also the results of a study of the status of obstetric analgesia and anesthesia in France carried out by Professor G. Barrier and colleagues and submitted in the 1981 report to the French government (125). As noted, the Lamaze method of psychoprophylaxis was being used for labor and vaginal delivery in 60% of the parturients. In some university hospitals the use of epidural block was somewhat higher than that shown in the table. In that report (125), the authors pointed out deficiencies that existed at the time and made many recommendations to improve obstetric analgesia and anesthesia in France, especially the reorganization of obstetric units and the need for a greater financial support for optimal obstetric-anesthetic services carried out by anesthesiologists. In view of the fact that during the past decade regional anesthesia in France has been used at an increasing rate, it can be hoped that this has also been applied to obstetric patients.

### Austria

In 1984 Professor H. Bergmann sent data based on responses to questionnaires sent to 92 hospitals performing obstetrics in that country and received responses from 55% of these. Those data showed that 65% of all labors received some form of analgesia consisting of 60% opioids, 10% lumbar epidural block, and 30% psychoprophylaxis, while for vaginal delivery, 75% of parturients received anesthesia consisting of local or pudendal block in 50%, lumbar epidural block in 10%, general anesthesia in 10%, and psychoprophylaxis in 15. At the time, anesthesia for cesarean section consisted of of general anesthesia in 95%, lumbar epidural in 3%, and subarachnoid block in 2%. The 1989 figures were submitted by Dr. Heiblmayr of Professor Bergmann's department, who was unable to determine mean figures and therefore provided ranges. He commented that the mode of pain relief during labor and delivery varies widely and that psychoprophylaxis in the form of Lamaze technique is used frequently in many obstetric centers. For cesarean section, the majority of patients receive general anesthesia.

### Holland, Belgium, and Denmark

Although no responses were received from these countries, personal observations during several extensive teaching visits to these countries suggest that the current status of obstetric analgesia and anesthesia is similar to that of West Germany. Up to about 20 years ago, parturients received virtually little or no analgesia for labor and only a small percent received pharmacologic anesthesia for vaginal delivery. However, during the past 10 years, epidural analgesia/anesthesia has been used in an increasing number of parturients, and it is estimated that currently this form of analgesia is used in 10 to 15% of parturients undergoing vaginal delivery and in about 20 to 30% of parturients undergoing cesarean section. Of the remainder of parturients, the majority receive systemic analgesia for labor and local infiltration or pudendal block for delivery but a significant number deliver with psychoprophylaxis only.

### Italy

Professor E. Cosmi, Chairman of the Department of Obstetrics and Gynecology of the University of Perugia and Professor of Anesthesiology at the University of Rome, provided figures shown in Table 1–11. This is a significant improvement over the situation in earlier years, when parturients in Italy received little or no pharmacologic analgesia. In the major obstetric centers lumbar epidural analgesia is used in 25% during labor and vaginal delivery, whereas in general hospitals it is used in less than 10% of the cases. The use of psychoprophylaxis, which was very popular in the 1960s, has decreased to 30% during labor. For vaginal delivery, there has been a decrease of pudendal block and local infiltration from 80 to 60%, an increase in the use of inhalation analgesia, and a slight increase in subarachnoid block. For cesarean section, the majority of patients received general anesthesia; but based on personal observation during yearly visits to Italy, I have noted that in some university obstetric centers, epidural anesthesia is being used for 30–40% of the parturients.

### Malta

Dr. N. Azzoppardi provided information on obstetric analgesia and anesthesia in Malta. In the 1984 report, he indicated that that year an epidural service was initiated and at that time 80% of parturients received analgesia during labor and 90% received analgesia/anesthesia for vaginal delivery. For that period, cesarean section was done with general anesthesia in 75%, lumbar epidural in 15%, and subarachnoid block in 10%. The data for 1989, in parentheses, show a significant decrease in the use of epidural anesthesia because of the greater use of acupuncture for labor and vaginal delivery and also because of staffing problems.

### Spain

Professor M.A. Nalda, of Barcelona, provided figures for Spain that are shown in Table 1–11. It is likely that these figures reflect the practice in major university hospitals and other major obstetric centers, whereas in the smaller units regional analgesia in the form of epidural is used much less frequently.

## Eastern Europe

### German Democratic Republic

The figures in Table 1–11, reported from what was East Germany, were provided in 1984 by Professor Rose; unfortunately, no response was obtained from him in 1989 in that part of Germany. Based on personal discussion in 1990, it is likely that the figures presented reflect the current status of obstetric analgesia and anesthesia there. Although with reunification of the country, it is likely that some anesthesiologist from the West will attempt to improve the situation.

### Hungary

Professor J. Karovits provided information on obstetric analgesia and anesthesia in Hungary, both in 1984 and 1989, and a comparison of the data reveals that things have improved, as pharmacologic analgesia has increased from 15% to 20% and analgesia/anesthesia for vaginal delivery from 10 to 20%. The figures shown for systemic analgesia, epidural analgesia, and other forms of pharmacologic analgesia are the actual percent of the patients that received them, and although no other figures were reported, the majority of them had presumably either no analgesia or natural childbirth preparation. Karovits further reported that these are average values, reflecting a widely different anesthetic coverage of obstetric units. At some of the major university hospitals epidural pain relief during labor and delivery is used in 60 to 70% of parturients, but other units lack obstetric anesthesia completely. He further indicated there is no doubt that progressive developments in this field are on their way. It should be noted that the figures for local infiltration anesthesia includes patients who had an episiotomy, but no other method of pain relief for the delivery.

### *Bulgaria and Romania*

The figures for Bulgaria were provided by Professor E. Stonjanov in 1984 and, unfortunately, none were received for 1989. The figures for Romania were provided by Professor Z. Filipescu, who commented that in the past the anesthesiologist was rarely involved in the management of parturients and that the predominance of general anesthesia for cesarean section had been due to a recommendation of the "ancient" ministry of health and not of the Romanian Society of Anesthesiology and Critical Care Medicine, which should have liked to use more regional anesthesia. With the recent change in the governmental agencies related to health, regional anesthesia has increased significantly, especially for cesarean section.

### *USSR*

The figures for the Commonwealth of Independent States (formerly USSR), which is used as the heading in this report because the data were sent before the demise of Communism, were provided in 1984 by Professor E. Damir, then President of the Soviet Society of Anesthesiologists, who commented that there are no accurate statistics regarding obstetric anesthesia and that the figures presented reflect her own opinion based on observation throughout the country. It deserves reemphasis that the specialty of anesthesiology was not initiated until the late 1950s and early 1960s in the then Soviet Union. Although there has been an explosive increase in the number of specialists in those states, they have not been involved in obstetric anesthesia because of the wide use of psychoprophylaxis. In 1990 Damir commented to me personally that regional anesthesia is becoming more and more popular among anesthesiologists and, as a result of a significant increase in the percent of cesarean sections done by obstetricians during the past decade, has provided an opportunity to introduce the use of modern anesthesia to this group of patients.

## Near East

### *Lebanon*

Professor Anis Baraka of the American University Hospital (AUH) in Beirut provided information about conditions in Lebanon both in 1984 and in 1989 with data pertaining only to his own department. Comparison of the two sets of figures reveals that the percentage of parturients who received analgesia during labor has decreased from 95 to 80% and, among this latter group, 80% received lumbar epidural analgesia, about 5% received systemic analgesia, and apparently 15% received no analgesia. The percent of parturients who received anesthesia for the delivery has remained the same, but the use of lumbar epidural analgesia has decreased from 90% to 80%, while for cesarean section it decreased from 5 to 2%. I suspect that this trend is due to the situation in Lebanon, where few anesthesiologists are available. In the rest of the country, systemic analgesics or inhalation analgesia is used for a small percent of the patients, while the remainder receive no form of pharmacologic analgesia during childbirth.

### *Turkey*

Data was received in 1984 and again in 1989 on the situation in Turkey. Comparison of the two sets of figures reveals that the percentage of parturients who received analgesia during labor decreased from 25 to 15%, while analgesia and anesthesia for vaginal delivery increased from 25 to 81%. As may be noted, the majority of patients received systemic analgesia during labor and local infiltration for vaginal delivery; for cesarean section, 95% received general anesthesia, and the use of epidural anesthesia increased from less than 1 to 4%.

### *Egypt*

Professor Elshirbiny provided the data on the situation in Egypt in 1984, but no response was obtained to the 1989 survey. Although the number of anesthesiologists has increased significantly in the last decade, only a small percentage of patients received analgesia for labor, mostly in the form of nitrous oxide-oxygen, while 20% received anesthetic/analgesia for vaginal delivery, usually in the form of inhalation analgesia by mask. In 1984 Elshirbiny commented that despite the offer of services by some anesthesiologists, obstetricians in Egypt had not used their services because it added to the cost of the delivery.

### *Kuwait*

I received a response to the 1989 survey on the situation in that country before the invasion by Iraq. The data shown in Table 1–11 was computed from the actual files of about 50,000 parturients per year, and, as may be noted, both labor and vaginal delivery are managed with systemic analgesics and local infiltration, respectively. Anesthesia for cesarean section is administered by anesthesiologists.

## Asia/Australasia

### *Australia*

The data shown in Table 1–12 reflecting the situation in Australia were provided in 1984 by Dr. J. Paull, but, unfortunately, no information was received in 1989. In 1984, Paull had commented that in the course of the preceding 10 to 15 years, use of regional analgesia had increased in major hospitals. Based on personal observation in 1989, I speculate that regional anesthesia is being used in a higher percentage of parturients during labor and vaginal delivery in the major hospitals of Sydney, Melbourne, Adelaide, and Brisbane.

### *New Zealand*

Responses to the 1984 survey were made by Dr. C.H. Hoskins, of Auckland, while the 1989 figures were provided by Dr. David Sage, then president of the New Zealand Society of Anesthesiologists. The figures shown in Table 1–12 are those provided for 1984 and 1989. Comparison of the two sets of figures suggests that there has been a decrease in the use of analgesia during labor and for vaginal delivery, but an increase in the use of lumbar epidural block during labor, but, for some reason, a decrease for vaginal delivery. Dr. Sage commented that at the National Women's Hospital, the largest obstetric unit in New Zealand with 6,500 deliveries annually, the cesarean-section rate is 18%, the overall use of epidural 32%, with a rate of 28% among the general population and 50% for primiparae. Nitrous oxide-oxygen and meperidine are also used widely, often together or preceding epidural blockade. For all types of cesarean section (emergency and elective), general anesthesia was used in 50% of the patients, epidural anesthesia in 45%, and subarachnoid block in 5%. However, over 90% of elective cesarean sections were performed with regional anesthesia. A subsequent report indicated that epidural anesthesia was used in 76% of cesarean sections performed in 1990 at this same hospital (126).

### Japan

Information on obstetric analgesia and anesthesia in Japan was provided by Professor M. Fujimori both in 1984 and in 1989. The data listed in Table 1–12 pertaining to university hospitals were acquired from a survey by Fujimori (127) of 77 university hospitals and 102 general hospitals, and revealed that analgesia for labor was used in 30% of patients in university hospitals and 10% of patients in general hospitals, while anesthesia vaginally was used in 44% in university hospitals and in 33% in general hospitals, for an overall mean of 38%. Anesthesiologists administered 33% of the anesthetic given in university hospitals and only 20% of those given in general hospitals, for an overall mean of 25%. The data on the third line of figures for Japan represent the 1989 figures computed on the basis of 100%; thus, of the 10% of the patients who received analgesia for labor, 40% received systemic analgesics, 20% received lumbar epidural analgesia/anesthesia, 20% caudal analgesia, and an equal percentage received the double catheter technique (DCEB). Among the 20 to 35% of patients who received anesthesia for vaginal delivery, about 20% received either pudendal block or local infiltration, about 35 to 40% epidural analgesia, about 15% caudal or subarachnoid block, while the remainder received inhalation analgesia and 65% or less received no anesthesia for vaginal delivery. For cesarean section there is an obvious predominance of regional anesthesia, a significant portion of which was administered by the obstetrician. Fujimori (127) stated that the reason for the low figures for analgesia for normal labor is that the traditional concept of Japanese women in childbirth is that pain relief for delivery is unnatural, and they do not expect pain relief for the very severe pain. In addition, obstetricians are concerned for medical/legal problems. Should complications occur, they are likely to be attributed to anesthesia. Finally, there was a shortage of anesthesiologists to cover obstetric anesthesia and still meet the dominating demand of surgeons!

### Korea

Information on obstetric analgesia and anesthesia in Korea was provided by Dr. Ha In-Ho in 1984 but none was received for 1989. In 1984 he indicated that in university and major hospitals, 70% of the patients received analgesia for labor and nearly 100% received anesthesia for vaginal delivery and of course, for cesarean section. The great discrepancy between these data and those for Japan is difficult to understand in view of the fact that they involve somewhat similar Asian cultures.

### Hong Kong

Information on the status of obstetric analgesia and anesthesia in Hong Kong in 1989 was provided by Dr. J. Ronald, president of the Society of Anaesthetists of Hong Kong. Figures in Table 1–12 represent collected data from public hospitals and institutions in Hong Kong for which reliable information is available to the society. Data from private hospitals are not available, but they are not expected to be very different. Comparison of these figures with those of 1984 provided by Dr. J.M. Allison indicate a significant increase in the percentage of patients who received lumbar epidural block during labor from 5% to 15%. For vaginal delivery most of the patients received either pudendal block or local infiltration, while lumbar epidural block increased from 5% in 1984 to 15% in 1989. For cesarean section, general anesthesia was used in most of the patients.

### Malaysia

Information on the current status of obstetric analgesia and anesthesia in Malaysia was provided by Dr. Say Wan Lim, then executive secretary and currently president (1993) of the World Federation of Societies of Anaesthesiologists, who had also provided data in 1984. Comparison of the two sets of data suggests that there has been some decrease in the percentage of patients who received analgesia anesthesia for labor and vaginal delivery, from 90% to 80%, but the data suggest too that there has been an increase in the percentage of patients who received lumbar epidural block for both labor and vaginal delivery, from 12 to 14%. Type of anesthesia for cesarean section has not changed significantly.

### Singapore

Information on the status of obstetric analgesia and anesthesia in Singapore was provided for both 1984 and 1989 by Dr. Mun Kui Chin, then president of the Singapore Anesthetic Society. Comparison of these data revealed significant changes in the 5-year period. In 1984 only 50% of patients received analgesia during labor and only 70% for vaginal delivery, whereas in 1989 virtually every patient received analgesia for these events. Moreover, the use of lumbar epidural block during labor increased from 10 to 20%, and for vaginal delivery, it increased from 8 to 20%. Comment was made that the relatively low figure for epidural anesthesia for cesarean section is a reflection of a shortage of anaesthetists in Singapore. This is somewhat perplexing, because it takes more time to provide lumbar epidural analgesia for labor and vaginal delivery than for cesarean section.

### Taiwan

Information on the status of obstetric analgesia and anesthesia in Taiwan in 1984 was provided by Dr. Chin-Kai Tseng, but no data were sent for 1989. Dr. Tseng commented in 1984 that epidural anesthesia was fully developed in 1969 by anesthesiologists. In most major hospitals less than 5% of parturients receive analgesia for labor and less than 10% for vaginal delivery. However, based on this information and personal observation made during a week's practice in three major hospitals in Taipei, I suggest that most private patients received epidural block analgesia/anesthesia administered by anesthesiologists for labor and vaginal delivery, as reflected in the data on Table 1–12. In the smaller hospitals patients received systemic analgesic and local infiltration.

### Thailand

Although no responses were received from Thailand in both 1984 and 1989, observations made during a 6-day teaching visit to Bangkok suggest that the situation in that country is somewhat between those in Taiwan and Malaysia. In major hospitals, systemic analgesia, primarily with opioids, is used for the first stage and local infiltration or pudendal block for vaginal delivery. Cesarean sections are performed primarily with general anesthesia but subarachnoid block and occasionally epidural block are used in about 10% of the deliveries in major hospitals.

### The Philippines

Information on the Philippines was provided by Dr. M. V. Silao both in 1984 and in 1989. Comparison of two sets of data suggests that the percentage of patients who received analgesia during labor and vaginal delivery is essentially the same, but there was an increase in the use of epidural analgesia in labor from 10 to 20% and caudal epidural decreased from 15 to 10%. For vaginal delivery, the use of lumbar epidural increased from 20 to 30%, while caudal epidural anesthesia decreased from 10 to 15%, and the the use of subarachnoid block decreased from 10 to 5%. For cesarean section, there was an increase in lumbar epidural block from 10 to 35% but a significant decrease in the use of subarachnoid block from 85 to 55%.

### Bangladesh

Information on the current status of obstetric analgesia and anesthesia in Bangladesh was provided by Dr. S.N. Samad Choudhury, Chief of Anesthesiology at the major hospital in Dacca. During delivery virtually all patients receive systemic analgesia, while for vaginal delivery, pudendal block or local infiltration is used in most cases. Choudhury commented that his teaching hospital maintains good standard anesthetic technique for cesarean sections and that spinal/epidural analgesia was only recently introduced in teaching hospitals, but it is anticipated that there will be a slight increase in the use of these techniques in the future.

### People's Republic of China (PRC)

Although no information was received from PRC, my personal observation made in a 1973 visit and the observations of several colleagues who visited that country in 1983 and in 1987 suggest that less than 1% of parturients receive pharmacologic analgesia for labor and less than 5% receive it for vaginal delivery. For operative delivery, including cesarean section, regional anesthesia is used in 70% of the patients, general anesthesia in 25%, and acupuncture in less than 5%.

## Africa and Latin America

Data on the status of obstetric anesthesia in four South African countries was received in 1984 but none was obtained in 1989. Although the following information is now 9 years old, I will summarize the data found in Table 1–13 concisely.

### South Africa

Professor J.W. Downing, then Chairman of the Department of Anesthesiology at the University of Natal in Durban and currently in the United States, provided information on the Republic of South Africa derived from a survey of the eight university hospitals. This survey revealed that in those hospitals in which between 8,500 and 28,000 parturients were managed in 1982, analgesia during labor with meperidine alone or combined with a tranquilizer was received by 1.5 to 20% with an overall mean of 7% of parturients. Although all of the hospitals had an "epidural service" on a 24-hour basis, epidural analgesia for labor and delivery in these hospitals ranged from 2 to 20%, and most of these were peformed for cesarean section. In Downing's own department, therapeutic epidural-analgesia services were provided to 10% of over 16,000 deliveries per annum. For the entire country, he estimated that about 2% of patients received analgesia for labor and of these, 98% received systemic analgesia, while only 2% received epidural analgesia. Of the 2% who had anesthesia for delivery, local infiltration was used in 80%, pudendal block in 18%, and epidural block in 2%. For cesarean section, general anesthesia was used in 94%, epidural block in 5%, and subarachnoid block in 1%.

### Zimbabwe

In 1984, Dr. Daniel Goold provided information on the status of obstetric analgesia and anesthesia in Zimbabwe (formerly Rhodesia) and the data he provided us is summarized in Table 1–13.

### Tanzania

Dr. H. Lweno responded to the 1984 survey and provided the information about the conditions in Tanzania, East Africa, where only a few trained anesthesiologists and nurse-anesthetists provided service. The data submitted is summarized in Table 1–13.

### Kenya

In 1984 Professor E.N. Ayim of Nairobi University in Kenya provided information of obstetric analgesia and anesthesia in that country. The data are summarized in Table 1–13.

## Central America

### Guatemala

Information on the status of obstetric analgesia and anesthesia in Guatemala was provided in 1984 and again in 1989 by Dr. R. Samayoa de Leon. Comparison of the two sets of data suggests that analgesia for labor increased from 10 to 20% and for vaginal delivery from 20 to 30%. The techniques and agents used are summarized in Table 1–13. The majority of parturients received systemic analgesia for labor, but in those hospitals with anesthesiologists, the use of epidural analgesia increased from 60 to 80 percent. Nine percent of parturients were managed with caudal analgesia and 3% with double catheter caudal epidural block. For vaginal delivery, data for 1989 were obtained in five maternity hospitals, two federal, and three private institutions with large obstetric service. In these hospitals, epidural block for vaginal delivery was used in 50% of parturients in 1984, and this increased to 75% in 1989. However, the data for 1989 shows that in the smaller hospitals systemic analgesia was used for about 90% of patients during labor, and local infiltration or pudendal block was used in 75% of the patients, caudal analgesia in 5%, and subarachnoid block in 5%. The figures shown for anesthesia for cesarean section were derived from the five major hospitals. In the smaller obstetric units local infiltration, field block, and subarachnoid block were used more frequently.

### Panama

Information on the status of obstetric analgesia and anesthesia in Panama was provided in 1984 and in 1989 by Dr. S. Moscoso. Comparison of the two sets of data suggests that analgesia for labor has increased from 5 to 15% of the parturients and for vaginal delivery, from 10 to 40%. There has also been an increase of the use of lumbar epidural block for labor from 15 to 40%, vaginal delivery from 15 to 50%. This has caused a decrease of systemic analgesia from 80 to 60% during labor and for pudendal block and local infiltration from 70 to 30%, for vaginal delivery. The other techniques used are summarized in Table 1–13.

### Ecuador

Information on the status of obstetric analgesia and anesthesia in Ecuador for 1989 was received from Dr. Virgilio Paez, who indicated that as a result of small number of anesthesiologists, culture of the population, and the traditional practice of physicians who manage parturients, only about 10% of the women received pharmacologic analgesia for labor and vaginal delivery. In the university and private hospitals 40% receive epidural analgesia for labor, 20% for vaginal delivery, and an impressive 95% for cesarean section, all given by anesthesiologists. These data are shown in Table 1–13.

## South America

### Brazil

Information on the conditions in Brazil in 1984 was provided by Dr. Carlos Parsloe, then President of the World Federation of Societies of Anesthesiologists (WFSA), who obtained most of the data from Dr. R.S. Mathias, a prominent obstetric anesthesiologist in Brazil. They indicated that in the major university and general hospitals, 70% of parturients received analgesia during labor, consisting mostly of meperidine and benzodiazepines, and a similar percentage receive anesthesia for vaginal delivery, consisting of local infiltration in 40%, subarachnoid block in 30%, epidural in 20%, and pudendal block in 10%. In private hospitals, the incidence was even higher, and in those institutions cesarean section was performed with epidural anesthesia in 93%, subarachnoid block in 5%, and general anesthesia in 2% (Table 1–13). In the large governmental health service hospitals, general anesthesia was used in about 17% for cesarean sections, subarachnoid block in 80%, and epidural block in the remainder. Unfortunately, no data were received for 1989.

### Colombia

Information on obstetric analgesia and anesthesia in Colombia was provided by Dr. R. Sarmiento in both 1984 and 1989. Comparison of two sets of figures reveals a decrease in the percentage of parturients receiving analgesia during labor but not for vaginal delivery. In the university and major private hospitals an impressive 90 to 95% of the women received epidural analgesia administered by anesthesiologists. For cesarean section, most of the patients who received general anesthesia did so because of the emergency nature of the section. In the smaller cities and rural areas, the percentage of women who received pain relief during labor and vaginal delivery, consisting of systemic analgesia and local infiltration or pudendal block for vaginal delivery, is less than half of those percentages indicated in Table 1–13.

### Venezuela

Although no response was received from Venezuela, my many visits and extensive clinical teaching experiences at the university hospital and several private facilities in Caracas and Maracaibo suggest that the status of obstetric anesthesia there is similar to that of Colombia. In the university hospital and in private clinics, the majority of the parturients receive analgesia for labor and most receive anesthesia for vaginal delivery, as summarized in Table 1–13. Regional anesthesia in the form of epidural block and caudal block was used in the majority of patients undergoing vaginal delivery, especially when instrumentation was necessary. In private hospitals the percent of parturients who received analgesia/anesthesia for labor and vaginal delivery is higher.

## SUMMARY

An attempt has been made to provide a comprehensive overview of the history of pain relief for childbirth from prehistoric times to the present and of the evolution and current status of obstetric analgesia/anesthesia primarily in the United States. In addition, data from superficial surveys in various other countries have been presented. It deserves reemphasis that these data are very rough estimates of 5 to 10 years prior to publication of this chapter and are relevant primarily to major universities and general hospitals, and with few exceptions, do not even suggest the conditions throughout each country mentioned.

It is obvious that the development of obstetric analgesia and anesthesia was very slow during the 12 decades following its first use by Simpson, Snow, and other champions who practiced during the period of discovery of anesthesia. Although numerous anesthetic drugs and techniques were developed during the first 50 years of the present century, their application for the relief of childbirth pain lagged far behind that for surgical anesthesia. Fortunately, during the past 25 years various research efforts have produced much new data critically important to optimal anesthetic care. This, together with a gratifying trend of more anesthesiologists and nurse anesthetists becoming involved in this field, has made obstetric anesthesia safer in those institutions where such services are available.

These gains notwithstanding, there is still much to be done before we reach the long-sought goal of effective and safe pain relief of the parturient with pharmacologic means for the majority of women who desire or require it. This will require not only sustaining but increasing the efforts of the obstetric team as emphasized in the introduction of the first edition of this book.

Anesthesiologists must provide vigorous leadership and do everything possible to afford all parturients the best anesthesiologic care. Their contribution to this end will provide optimal pre-intra and post-anesthetic care to the parturient and child. Anesthesiologists must show interest and acquire the necessary knowledge of the physiology and pharmacology of various forms of anesthesia on the mother, fetus, and newborn. These are best done in hospitals that are large enough to have a formal obstetric service and active teaching programs in obstetrics and anesthesiology.

Anesthesiologists must play leading roles in informing and educating the rest of the medical profession and hospital administration about the need for the best anesthesiologic equipment and sufficient anesthesiologists to provide personal care and teaching related to obstetrics. The anesthesia staff should develop a training program for every anesthesia resident, not only to provide him/her with knowledge and skill, but also to stimulate the interest and sense of responsibility in this field. Because obstetricians and obstetric residents still provide a significant percentage of anesthesia in the United States, the anesthesiologic team should encourage the development of the training program for obstetric residents, obstetricians, child birth practitioners, and nurse anesthetists. Obstetricians should do whatever is necessary to encourage anesthesiologists to provide optimal care to obstetric patients. In their interaction, the anesthesiologist and obstetrician must adhere to the six cardinal *Cs* of medical practice: communication, cooperation, coordination, courtesy, and consideration and confidence.

Nurse anesthetists have played an important role in obstetric anesthesiology, and should continue to be involved. This is best done under the supervision of an anesthesiologist. Like the physician, they must acquire ample knowledge of the physiology and psychology of pregnancy and parturition, the physiology and pathophysiology of the placenta, fetus, and newborn, and again, the various drugs used in obstetric anesthesia.

In addition to the development and nurturing of optimal anesthesiologic care, anesthesiologists and other members of the obstetric team in the hospital should participate in research in this field. In addition to individual research projects, well-designed and well-executed collaborative and comprehensive research programs involving basic scientists, obstetricians, anesthesiologists, and pediatricians should be activated that will prove fruitful in providing new knowledge that will contribute to better care of the parturient and baby.

All members of obstetric teams should actively and aggressively collaborate with hospital administrators to influence the public and the national and state health agencies to encourage the closure of obstetric services in hospitals that have less than 500 deliveries per year. Data cited in this chapter makes it clear that obstetric units with less than that number of deliveries are not likely to have the personnel, the sophisticated equipment and other resources to provide high quality care in obstetrics, anesthesiology, perinatology, and related areas involved in this field. For smaller hospitals in rural areas, it is essential to develop training programs in obstetric anesthesia for nurse anesthetists, midwives, and family physicians. These programs, which should be of an appropriate period to teach the basic principles of obstetric anesthesia and the skill in administering drugs and techniques, should be implemented in all medical and nursing schools for those students who plan to practice in smaller communities in rural areas. Moreover, all small hospitals in such rural areas that are within reasonable driving distance should consolidate obstetric care in one institution in the region. This will not only be economically sound, but will permit personnel and resources to be consolidated and significantly improve the care of parturients and their neonates. The United States of America has the responsibility of providing very effective leadership in all aspects of health care, and there is no segment of the health care population as important for the optimal services of health care teams as the nearly 9 million partrurients and their newborn babies.

## REFERENCES


1. Lee R: Lectures on the Theory and Practice of Midwifery. Philadelphia, Barrington and Hoswell, 1844.
2. Behan RJ: Pain. New York, D. Appleton and Company, 1914.
3. Dick-Read G: Childbirth Without Fear. New York, Harper and Bros., 1953.
4. Velvovski IZ, et al: Psychoprophylactic. Leningrad, Medguiz, 1954.
5. Bonica JJ: Principles and Practice of Obstetric Analgesia

and Anesthesia. Philadelphia, F.A. Davis Company, Vol. 1, 1967; Vol. 2, 1969.
6. Bonica JJ: The Management of Pain. 2nd Ed. Lea & Febiger, Philadelphia, 1990, pp. 1283–1343.
7. Claye AM: The Evolution of Obstetric Analgesia. London, Oxford University Press, 1939.
8. Fulop-Miller R: Triumph Over Pain. E and G Paul (trans.). New York, Literary Guild of America, 1938.
9. Sigerist HE: A History of Medicine. Vol. 1. New York, Oxford University Press, 1951, pp. 274, 349.
10. Bellucci G: Storia Bella Anestesiologia. Padova, Piccin Editore, 1982, p.184.
11. Dallenbach KM: Pain: History and present status. Am. J. Psychol. 52:331, 1939.
12. Heaton CE: The history of anesthesia and analgesia in obstetrics. J. Hist. Med. 1:567, 1946.
13. Ford CS: A Comparative Study of Human Reproduction. Yale University Publications in Anthropology. New Haven, Yale University Press, 1945.
14. Freedman LZ, Ferguson VS: The question of "painless childbirth" in primitive cultures. Am. J. Orthopsychiatry 20: 363, 1950.
15. Levy-Strauss C: Sorciers et Psychanalyse. Geneva, Le Courier de l'Unesco, 1956, p. 808.
16. Riviere M, Chastrusse L: La douler en obstetrique. Rev. Franc. Gynec. Obstet. 49:247, 1954.
17. Preissman AB, Ogoulboston E: Some details of psychoprophylactic preparation for childbirth in the Turkomeaniam. Proceedings of the S.S.R. Kiev Congress of Psychiatry. Kiev, 1956, p. 66.
18. Tainter ML: Pain. Ann. N.Y. Acad. Sci. 51:3, 1948.
19. Keys TE: The History of Surgical Anesthesia. New York, Schuman's, 1945.
20. Engelmann GJ: Labor Among Primitive Peoples, 2nd Ed. St. Louis, J.H. Chambers and Company, 1883.
21. Ploss H, Bartels C: Dasweib in der Natur-und Volkerkund. Leipzig, T.H. Grieban's, 1902.
22. Ellis EH: Ancient Anodynes. Primitive Anesthesia and Allied Conditions. London, Wm. Heinemann Ltd., 1946, p.16.
23. Theocritus: Idylls, c. 3rd Century B.C. *In*: Ellis EH: Ancient Anodynes. Primitive Anesthesia and Allied Conditions. London, Wm. Heinemann Ltd., 1946, p. 17.
24. Wecker HJ: Eighteen Books of the Secrets of Art and Nature. London, 1660, p. 191.
25. Heaton CE: The history of anesthesia and analgesia in obstetrics. J. Hist. Med. 1:567, 1946.
26. Heaton CE: The history of anesthesia and analgesia in obstetrics. J. Hist. Med. 1:567, 1946.
26a. Miller P: An essay on the means of lessening pain of parturition. Thesis for the degree of doctor of medicine, University of Pennsylvania, 1804.
26b. Dewees WP: An essay on the means of lessening pain and facilitating certain cases of difficult parturition. Thesis for the degree of doctor of medicine, University of Pennsylvania, 1806.
27. Rush B: Medical Inquiries and Observations. 5th Ed. Philadelphia, 1818, p. 221.
28. Warren JC: Inhalation of aethereal vapor for the prevention of pain in surgical operation. Boston M.S. Jnl. 35:375, 1846.
29. Taylor FL: Crawford W. Long and the Discovery of Ether Anesthesia. New York, Paul B. Hoeber, Inc., 1928, p. 81.
30. Raper HR: A review of the Crawford Long Centennial Anniversary Celebration. Bull. Hist. Med. 13:340, 1943.
31. Long CW: An account of the first use of sulphuric ether by inhalation as an anesthetic in surgical operations. South Med. & Surg. J. 5:705, 1849.
32. Simpson JY: Notes on the inhalation of sulphuric ether in the practice of midwifery. Month. J. Med. & Sci. (London & Edinburgh). 1, 1946–47.
33. Priestley WO, Stover HR: The Obstetric Memoirs and Contributions of James Y. Simpson. Edinburgh, A. & C. Black, Vol. 2, 1856.
34. Snow J: On the Inhalation of the Vapour of Ether. London, John Churchill, 1847.
35. Caton D: Obstetric anesthesia: the first ten years. Anesthesiology 30:102–109, 1970.
36. Clark SJ: The Evolution of Obstetric Analgesia. Cited by AM Claye. London, Oxford University Press, 1939, pp. 15–16.
37. Sykes WS: Essays of the First One Hundred Years of Anaesthesia. Vol. 1. Edinburgh, E. & S. Livingston, Ltd., 1960, pp. 77–85.
38. Snow J: On Chloroform and Other Anesthetics: Their Action and Administration. Edited by BW Richardson. London, John Churchill, 1858, pp. 318–329.
39. Thoms H: "Anestesie a la Reine," a chapter in the history of anesthesia. Am. J. Obstet. Gynecol. 40:340, 1948.
40. Channing W: A Treatise on Etherization in Childbirth. Boston, W.D. Ticknor and Co., 1848.
41. Heaton CE: The history of anesthesia and analgesia in obstetrics. J. Hist. Med. 1:567, 1946.
42. Meigs CD: On the use of anesthesia in midwifery. Philadelphia, Med. Exam. Rec. of Medical Sciences, Nos. 4, 1848, pp. 145–53.
43. Meigs CD: Obstetrics: The Science and the Art. 2nd Ed. Philadelphia, Lea & Blanchard, 1852.
44. Fink BR: History of neural blockade. *In* Cousins MJ, Bridenbaugh OP (eds.): Neural Blockade in Clinical Anesthesia and Management of Pain. 2nd Ed. Philadelphia, J.B. Lippincott, 1988.
45. Betcher AM, Ciliberti BJ, Wood PM, Wright LH: The jubilee year of organized anesthesia. Anesthesiology 17:226, 1956.
46. Von Steinbuchel R: Vorlaufige mitteilung uber die anwendung von skopolamin-morphium-injectionen in der geburtschilfe. Zentralbl. Gynk. 26:1304, 1902.
47. Gauss CJ: Geburten in kunstlichen dammerschlaf. Arch. Gynk. 78:579, 1906.
48. Guedel AE: Nitrous oxide-air anesthesia self administered in obstetrics. Indianapolis Med. J. 14:476, 1911.
49. Gwathmey JP: Ether-oil rectal analgesia and obstetrics. N.Y. Med. J. 98:1101, 1913.
50. Webster JC: Nitrous oxide-oxygen analgesia in childbirth. J.A.M.A. 24:812, 1915.
51. Davis CH: Painless Childbirth: Eutocia and Nitrous Oxide-Oxygen Analagesia. 2nd Ed. Chicago, Forbes & Co., 1916.
52. Guedel AE: Inhalation Anesthesia. New York, The MacMillan Co., 1937.
53. Cleland JGP: Paravertebral anesthesia in obstetrics. Surg. Gynecol. Obstet. 57:51, 1933.
54. Moir C: The nature of the pain of labour. J. Obstet. Gynaec. Brit. Emp. 46:409, 1939.
55. DeLee JB: Obstetrics. 5th Ed. Philadelphia, W.B. Saunders, 1933.
56. Greenhill JP: Shall spinal anesthesia be used in obstetrics? Anesthesiology 11:283, 1950.
57. Lamaze F: Qu'est-ce que l'accouchement sans douleur par la methode psychoprophylactque? Ses principes, sa realisation, ses resultats. Paris, Savior et Connaitre, 1956.
58. Lull CB, Hingson RA: Control of Pain in Childbirth. Philadelphia, Lippincott, 1944.

59. Snyder FF: Obstetric Analgesia and Anesthesia. Philadelphia, W.B. Saunders Co., 1949.
60. Hershenson BB: Obstetrical Anesthesia: Its Principles and Practice. Springfield, IL, Charles C. Thomas, 1955.
61. Apgar V: A proposal for a new method of evaluation of the newborn infant. Curr. Res. Anesth. Analg. 32:260, 1953.
62. Lee JA: Synopsis of Anaesthesia. 1st Ed. Bristol, John Wright & Sons, 1947.
63. Atkinson RS, Rushman GB, Davies NJH, Lee JA: Lee's Synopsis of Anaesthesia, 11th Ed. Boston, Butter-Heinemann, 1993.
64. Bonica JJ, Mix G: Twenty-four hour medical anesthesia coverage for obstetric patients. J.A.M.A. 159:551, 1955.
65. Bonica JJ: Obstetric analgesia and anesthesia in general practice. JAMA 165:2146, 1957.
66. Moore DC, Bridenbaugh LD: Is it practical for medical anesthetists to supply 24 hour obstetric service? West. J. Surg. 63:382, 1955.
67. Lindstrom C, Morre DC: Trends in obstetrical anesthesia following the acceptance of a twenty-four hour physician anesthesia service. West J. Surg. 65:63, 1957.
68. Hingson RA, Hellman LM: Organization of obstetric anesthesia on 24 hour basis in large and small hospitals. Anesthesiology 12:745, 1951.
69. Webb E, Leigh MD: The private group practice of anesthesiology. Anesth. Analg. 32:199, 1953.
70. Cull WA, Hingson RA: Dedication, education and organization in the round-the-clock staffing of a modern obstetrical analgesia and anesthesia service. Bull. Mat. Welf. 4:17, 1957.
71. Nelson AT, Phillips OC, Savage JE: Obstetric anesthesia care—full-time coverage in a private hospital. Obstet. Gynecol. 13:426, 1959.
72. Papper EM: The organization of anesthesiology service for obstetrics. Bull. Sloane Hosp. Wom. 6:39, 1960.
73. Shnider SM: Organization of an obstetric anesthesia service. Anesthesiology 26:562, 1965.
74. Phillips OC, Hulka JF: Obstetric mortality. Anesthesiology 26:435, 1965.
75. Reports on Confidential Enquiries into Maternal Deaths in England and Wales, Her Majesty's Stationery Office, London (years studied, number of report, year published) a) 1955–57, #103, 1960; b) 1958–60, #108, 1963; c) 1961–63, #115, 1966; d) 1970–72, #11, 1975; e) 1979–81, #29, 1986 and f) 1982–84, #34, 1989.
76. Hingson RA, Edwards WB: An analysis of the first ten thousand confinements managed with continuous caudal analgesia with a report of the author's first one thousand cases. JAMA 123–538, 1943.
77. Adriani J, Roman-Vega D: Saddle block anesthesia. Am. J. Surg. 71:12, 1946.
78. Burton H: Low spinal anaesthesia during labour in cases of cardiac failure. Br. Med. J. 2:389, 1943.
79. Resnick L: Heavy nupercaine spinal analegesia in operative obstetrics with report on 394 cases. Br. Med. J. 2:722, 1945.
80. Hingson RA, Hellman LM: Anesthesia for Obstetrics. Philadelphia, J.B. Lippincott, 1956.
81. Crawford JS: Principles and Practice of Obstetric Anaesthesia. 1st Ed. Oxford, Blackwell Scientific Publications, 1959.
82. Address of His Holiness, Pope Pius XII, on February 24, 1957 in Reply to Three Questions Concerning Religious and Moral Aspects of Pain Prevention in Medical Practice. *In*: Anestesia e Persona Umana. Edited by L Gedda. Rome, Edizione dell Istituto Gregorio Mendel, 1957, p. 237.
83. Smith A: Editorial: obstetric analgesia and anesthesia. JAMA 165:2198, 1957.
84. Rhu HS: Editorial: obstetric anesthesia. Obstet. Gynecol. 1: 728, 1958.
85. Dumitru A: Editorial: anesthesia in obstetrics. Obstet. Gynecol. 16:634, 1960.
86. Phillips OC, Ott HA: Doctors call for better OB anesthesia. Mod. Hosp. January, 1964.
87. Phillips OC: Report of Committee on Maternal Welfare to the House of Delegates, American Society of Anesthesiologists, June 6, 1961. Proceedings the American Society of Anesthesiologists, Park Ridge, Iliinois, 1961.
88. Phillips OC, Frazier TM: Obstetric anesthetic care in the United States. Obstet. Gynecol. 19:796, 1962.
89. Phillips OC (Chairman): Maternal Welfare Committee Annual Report, Enclosure 2, Training in Obstetrical Anesthesia for Anesthesiology Residents. Proceedings of the American Society of Anesthesiologists, Park Ridge, Illinois, 1961.
90. National Study of Maternity Care: Survey of Obstetric Practice and Associated Services in Hospitals in the United States. Committee on Maternal Health, the American College of Obstetricians and Gynecologists, Chicago, 1970.
91. Barnes AC: Obstetric anesthesia today. Med. Tribune 4:24, 1963.
92. Dripps RD: The Anesthesia Survey: Proceedings of the House of Delegates of the American Society of Anesthesiologists, Park Ridge, Illinois, 1963–1965. The American Society of Anesthesiologists, 1963–1965.
93. Gibbs CP, Krischer J, Peckham BM, Sharp H, Kirschbaum TH: Obstetric anesthesia: a national survey. Anesthesiology 65:298, 1986.
94. Symposium on Maternal and Fetal Physiology in the Perinatal Period: Anesthesiology 26:377, 1965.
95. Moore DC: Anesthetic Techniques for Obstetrical Anesthesia and Analgesia. Springfield, IL, Charles C. Thomas, 1964.
96. Flowers CE, Jr: Obstetric Analgesia and Anesthesia. New York, Hoeber-Harper and Row, 1967.
97. Marx GF, Orkin LR: Physiology of Obstetric Anesthesia. Springfield, IL, Charles C. Thomas, 1969.
98. Moir C: Pain Relief in Labor. 1st Ed. Edinburgh, Churchill Livingstone, 1969.
99. Shnider SM: Obstetric Anesthesia, Current Concepts and Practice. Baltimore, Williams & Wilkins, 1970.
100. Bonica JJ: Obstetric Analgesia and Anesthesia, 1st Ed. Amsterdam, World Federation of Societies of Anesthesiologists, 1970.
101. Scott DB, Hunter AR : Symposium on obstetric anaethesia and analgesia. Br. J. Anaesth. 43:824, 1971.
102. Bush GH, Norman J: Symposium on the perinatal period. Br. J. Anaesth. 49:1, 1977.
103. Bonica JJ : Obstetric Analgesia and Anesthesia: Recent Advances and Current Status. Clinics in Obstetrics and Gynecology, Vol. 2. London, W.B. Saunders Co. Ltd., 1975.
104. Rosen M: Obstetric Anaesthesia and Analgesia: Safe Practice. Clinics in Obstetrics and Gynecology, Vol. 9:2. London, W.B. Saunders Co. Ltd., 1982.
105. Marx GF: Parturition and Perinatology, Clinical Anesthesia Series, 10/2. Philadelphia, F.A. Davis Co., 1973.
106. Ostheimer GW: Obstetric analgesia and anaesthesia. *In* Clinics in Anesthesiology 4:1 (Part 1); and 4:2, (Part II), 1986.
107. Abouleish E: Pain Control in Obstetrics. Philadelphia, J.B. Lippincott, 1977.
108. Shnider SM, Levinson G: Anesthesia for Obstetrics. 3rd Ed. Baltimore, Williams & Wilkins, 1993.

109. Allbright GA, Ferguson II JE, Joyce III TH, Stevenson DK: Anesthesia in Obstetrics. 2nd Ed. Menlo Park, CA, Madison-Wesley Publishers, 1987.
110. Marx GF: Clinical Management of Mother and Newborn. New York, Springer Verlag, 1979.
111. Marx GF, Bassell GM: Obstetric Analgesia and Anesthesia. Amesterdam, Elsevier-North Holland, 1980.
112. Bonica JJ: Obstetric Analgesia and Anesthesia, 2nd Ed. Amsterdam, World Federation of Societies of Anaesthesiologists, 1980.
113. Doughty A: Epidural Analgesia in Obstetrics. London, Loyd-Luke, 1980.
114. Cosmi EV: Obstetric Anesthesia and Perinatology. New York, Appleton-Century-Crofts, 1981.
115. Crawford JS: Principles and Practice of Obstetric Anaesthesia. 5th Ed. Oxford, Blackwell Scientific Publications, 1984.
116. McMorland GH, Marx GF: Handbook of Obstetric Analgesia and Anesthesia. Quala Lumpur, Malaysia, World Federation of Societies of Anesthesiologists, 1992.
117. Shnider SM: Training in obstetric anesthesia in the United States. Am. J. Obstet. Gynecol. 93:243, 1965.
118. Hicks JS, Levinson G, Shnider SM: Obstetric anesthesia training centers in the USA—1975. Anesthesia Analgesia. 55:845, 1976.
119. Millar WR, Plumer MH: Obstetric anesthesia teaching in the United States and anesthesia residencies. Anesthesiology 57:431, 1982.
120. American Hospital Association: Special AHA survey of hospitals. Chicago: AHA, 1981.
121. McMorland GH, Jenkins LC: A survey of obstetric anaesthesia practice, teaching and research in Canadian university departments of anaesthesia. Can. Anaesth. Sco. J. 27:417, 1980.
122. McMorland GH, Jenkins LC, Douglas MJ: A survey of obstetric anesthesia practice in British Columbia. Can. Anaesth. Soc. J. 33:1A85–94, 1986.
123. Hibbard BM, Scott DB: The availability of epidural anesthesia and analgesia. Br. J. Obstet. Gynecol. 92:402–405, 1990.
124. Gerdin E, Cnattingius S: The use of obstetric analgesia in Sweden 1983–1986. Br. J. Obstet. Gynaecol. 97:789, 1990.
125. Barrier G: Report Sur La Securite Maternelle Dans Les Services de Gynecologie-Obstetrique. Submitted to Commission de la Maternite Ministiere de la Sante, Paris, 1982.
126. Peskett WGH: The anaesthetic contribution to maternal mortality. New Zealand Int. J. Obstet. Anesth. 1:179, 1992.
127. Fujimori M: Present status of pain relief for normal labor in Japan. *In* Anesthesia: Anesthesiologists. Amsterdam, Excerpta Medica, 1984, p. 63.

Section B

# THE MOTHER, FETUS, AND NEWBORN

Chapter 2

# MATERNAL ANATOMIC AND PHYSIOLOGIC ALTERATIONS DURING PREGNANCY AND PARTURITION

JOHN J. BONICA

The process of pregnancy, labor, and parturition produces remarkable anatomic, physiologic, and biochemical alterations in the mother that invariably influence the fetus and newborn. Indeed, these changes that distinguish gravidae from nonpregnant females are so significant that Crawford categorized pregnant women collectively as the "third sex" (1). Physicians who participate in the management of obstetric patients need to be mindful of these changes, and to modify such management according to the individual needs of each patient. Evaluation of laboratory and clinical reports in light of these changes is especially important to the person who has the serious responsibility of providing anesthesiologic care.

From the viewpoint of optimal anesthesiologic care, the changes involving respiration, circulation, acid-base and electrolyte balance, metabolism, the function of the gastrointestinal, renal, hepatic, endocrine, and nervous systems are the most important. These changes, produced by placental hormones or mechanical effects of the growing uterus or both, develop to meet the increasing metabolic needs of the maternal-fetal-placental complex and also prepare the gravida for the stressses of parturition and the subsequent occlusion of the placental circulation. The purpose of this chapter is to present a summary of the most currently available data on the various processes. In contrast to the first edition of this book, in which the changes produced by pregnancy and those by labor and parturition were described in two different sections of the book, in this edition they are considered together in one chapter. Because there is a significant variation between different gravidae and parturients, alterations, in many instances, are expressed in percentages when in comparison to nonpregnant levels. Although the changes in the uterus are of primary interest to the obstetrician, these changes are briefly considered first because they have a major impact on the other changes in maternal anatomy and physiology. Following discussion of changes in each system, the clinical implications relevant to anesthesiologic management are summarized. As in the first edition, this chapter includes citation of the most relevant literature. More detailed discussion of most of the sections can be found in the books by Metcalfe and associates (2,3), Hytten and Chamberlain (4), Marx and associates (5,6), and Gabbe, et al. (7).

## CHANGES IN THE UTERUS

The uterus changes from a small, triangularly shaped, solid-like organ, weighing 30 to 60 g and measuring 6 cm long and 5 cm wide, into a thin-walled, globularly shaped, muscular sac, measuring about 30 cm long, 25 cm wide, and 20 cm deep, and weighing 700 to 1,000 g. This remarkable pregnancy metamorphosis results in a capacity increase of nearly 500 times over that of its nonpregnant state. A detailed discussion of the changes in the musculature and other structures of the uterus and cervix and uterine vasculature is found in Chapters 4 and 6.

Enlargement of the uterus during the first half of gestation is due primarily to hypertrophy of tissues. At about the twentieth week there is conversion of the conceptus from a spheroidal to a cylindrical shape and further uterine enlargement is accomplished by progressive stretching and thinning of the uterine wall. As a result, the thickness of the wall of the uterus is reduced from approximately 2 cm early in the pregnancy to 0.5 to 1.0 cm at term.

The uterus remains in the pelvis until the third month, but during the fourth month it ascends and partially fills the abdominal cavity, coming in contact with the anterior abdominal wall and gradually displaces the intestines to the sides and upward in the abdomen and finally rises to impinge upon the liver (Figure 2–1). The most notable consequence of this growth is an elevation of the diaphragm with a consequent decrease in expiratory reserve volume and residual volume, and a shift in the position of the heart as detailed below. In the latter part of pregnancy there is a tendency toward torsion of the uterus toward the right side. Acute torsion of the uterus may occur at any time during pregnancy and produce abdominal pain (6). Another cause of pain in and around the late first trimester and early second trimester is entrapment of the iliohypogastric nerve, likely produced by the rise of the uterus into the abdominal cavity. In the past this was often referred to, for lack of a better explanation, as round ligament pain. It was also often responsible for many emergency room visits and contemplation of appendicitis as a differential diagnosis. Local anesthetic injection of 1 to 2 ml at the correct junction will result in immediate and usually long-lasting pain relief. It will be noted that around

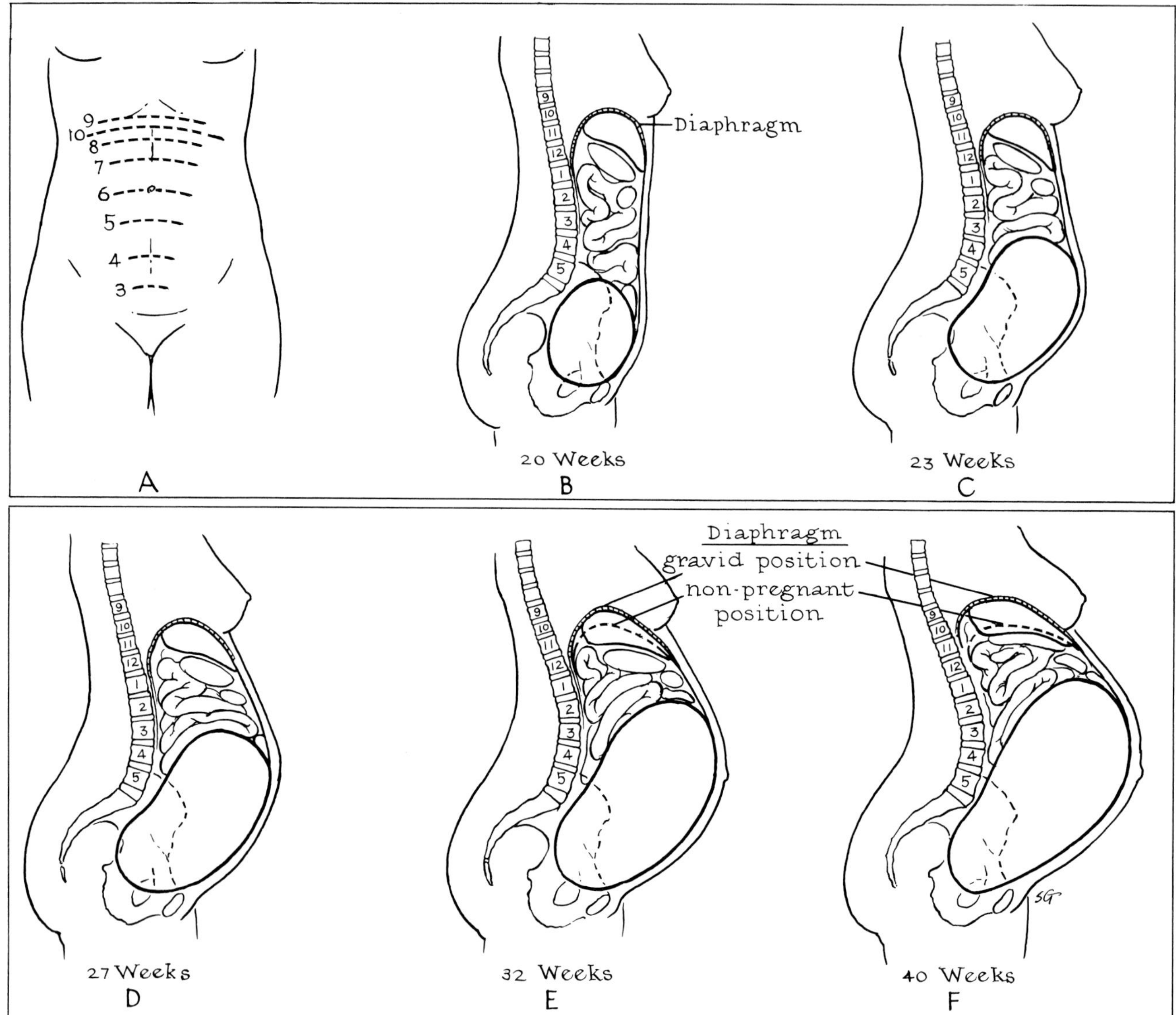


**Fig. 2–1.** Changes in shape and size of the uterus during pregnancy. **A,** Height of fundus at the end of each month of pregnancy according to Bartholomew's rule of fourths. **B** to **F,** Lateral views showing the changes in the size and shape of the uterus after the 20th week. These are modifications of Gillespie's original diagrams, which were drawn from actual x rays showing the relation of the uterus to the bony pelvis and spine. Note that the uterus, which is spheroid prior to the 20th week, becomes more and more elongated as the conceptus is converted from spheroid to cylindric form. Note also that the cephalad migration of the uterus pushes the abdominal contents cephalad, which in turn pushes the diaphragm upward to encroach on the lungs, causing the heart to be displaced.

the twentieth to twenty-fourth week the uterus is sufficiently large so that when the gravida is standing, it tends to fall forward and rests in great part on the anterior abdominal wall, but when the gravida assumes the supine position, it falls backward and comes to rest on the vertebral column and the large vessels anterior thereto. Consequently, it exerts pressure on these vessels resulting in diminution of blood flow through them. These phenomena are considered in detail in the section on circulation.

## CHANGES IN RESPIRATORY SYSTEM

The impressive anatomic and physiologic changes in the respiratory system are inter-related and involve the respiratory tract, the chest, lung volumes, and dynamics of breathing and ventilation, all of which have a significant relevance to anesthesiologic care (2–7).

### *Anatomic Changes*

#### Thoracic Cage

The upward pressure exerted by the growing uterus raises the diaphragm causing a decrease of as much as 4 cm in the vertical diameter of the chest (8,9). This is effectively counter-balanced, however, by an increase of 2 to 3 cm in the anteroposterior and transverse diameters and flaring out of the ribs so that the substernal angle is

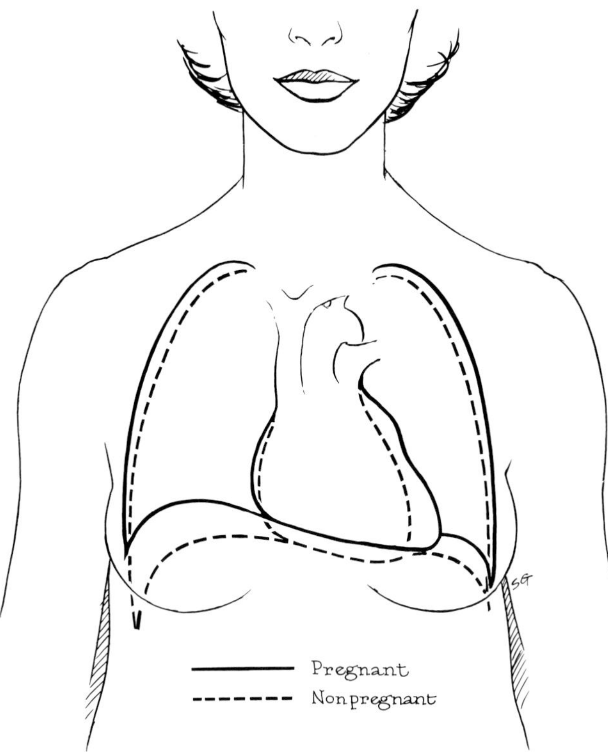


**Fig. 2–2.** Changes in the outline of the heart, lungs, and thoracic cage that occur in pregnancy. The gradual cephalad migration of the uterus causes the diaphragm to move upward and thus encroach on the lungs, and causes the heart to be displaced laterally and anteriorly. This is counterbalanced by an increase in the anterior-posterior and transverse diameters of the chest wall. (Modified from and courtesy of Klaften E, Palugyay H: Arch. Gynaek. 78:1, 1959.)

broadened from about 68° in the first trimester to 103° at term, an increase of about 50% (8,9). Consequently, the circumference of the thoracic cage is increased 5 to 7 cm (Figure 2–2). These changes are made possible in part by relaxation of the ligamentous attachment of the ribs (10), which is part of the hormonal changes on the musculoskeletal system. Despite its upward displacement, the diaphragm moves with greater excursions in gravidae than nonpregnant women, aided in part by the hormone-induced diminished tone of the abdominal muscles (11). Fluoroscopic studies have shown that during gestation breathing is primarily diaphragmatic because the thorax is limited in movement, whereas the movement of the diaphragm is unimpaired (8) and its descent increased compared to that of nonpregnant women. This allows the parturient to maintain adequate ventilation even during high levels of regional anesthesia, as evidenced by unchanged $PaO_2$ and $PaCO_2$ levels in parturients undergoing cesarean section with subarachnoid block (12).

### *Respiratory Tract*

In the majority of pregnant women, capillary engorgement takes place throughout the respiratory tract so that the nasopharynx, larynx, trachea, and bronchi, and particularly the false vocal cords and the arytenoid regions of the larynx, become swollen and reddened (2,3). These changes, together with the appearance of decidua-like cells in the submucosa, simulate histologic manifestations of inflammation. These histologic alterations may cause changes in the voice and make nose breathing difficult for some women at term. They are aggravated significantly in the presence of even minor upper respiratory infection or trauma and in pregnancy-induced hypertension.

One of the most important changes in the nasopharyngeal area is that of the engorgement of vessels and increase in vascularity associated with pregnancy. Because of the danger associated with placement of nasopharyngeal tubes of any kind, such engorgment and increase directly impacts on the anesthesiologic management. Increase in vascularity can and has been associated with dramatic nasopharyngeal hemorrhage of enormous proportions. This, of course, not only makes the airway difficult to isolate, but it also threatens oxygenation due to the aspiration of blood into the trachea.

The large airways are dilated, and this is associated with a 35% or more decrease in total pulmonary vascular resistance or an increase in reciprocal airway conductance (12–15). These changes in the large airways compensate for the increased resistance from the lower resting lung volumes and the decrease of the arterial partial pressure of carbon dioxide ($PaCO_2$). This change in the airways is also demonstrated by the lack of change of the forced expiratory volume at 1 minute ($FEV_1$), and no change in the ratio of this parameter to forced vital capacity ($FEV_1/FVC$), as well as an unaltered flow volume loop (15). The function of small airways remains unchanged, as shown by the flow characteristics of the flow volume loop, which are comparable in gravida and in nonpregnant women (see below).

### *Lungs*

Roentgenograms show increased lung markings (8) that simulate a picture of mild pulmonary edema, probably due to an increase of the blood volume in the pulmonary vessels (3). Comparison of roentgenograms in early and late pregnancy shows about a 4-cm elevation of the diaphragm, with a commensurate decrease in the length of the lungs and concomitant increase in the width. When observed under the fluoroscope, the excursions of the lungs appear normal (9).

Changes in lung volumes and capacities in pregnancy vary considerably among the various reports available. This is probably due to the equipment used and the position of the gravida at the time she is examined. Though values depicted in this chapter were derived from the data in Chapter 13 (references 13–23a), the primary source has been from the studies by Gudell, et al (16) and Foster and associates (23a).

## Lung Volumes and Capacities

### *Volumes*

The lung-volume profile begins to change early in pregnancy but significant deviations do not occur until the fifth or sixth month of gestation, after which the expiratory reserve volume (ERV) and residual volume (RV) gradually decrease as pregnancy advances, so that at near term the ERV is 150 to 175 ml (mean 150 ml or about 20%) less and the RV is 150 to 215 ml (mean 200 ml or about 20%) less than the nonpregnant state (13–15) (Figures 2–3 and 2–4). Consequently, the sum of these two, the functional residual capacity (FRC) decreases about 300 to 350 ml, or 18 to 20% (mean 20%) below the nonpregnant state (13–20). These effects are due to the progressive elevation of the diaphragm caused by the enlarged uterus and to a lesser extent by the increase in the pulmonary blood volume (6). During uterine contractions of labor, the increase in pulmonary blood volume reduces these lung volumes further. The decreases in FRC and RV are accentuated by the recumbent and lithotomy position (2,12,16). In the supine position, FRC falls to 70% of its value measured with the patient sitting (19) (Figures 2–3 and 2–4).

The closing volumes (CV), the closing capacity (CC), and the flow volume curves (FVC) remain unaltered during pregnancy. The CV is a lung volume at which terminal airways close during expiration. If a significant number of alveoli do not contribute to gas exchange, shunting of deoxygenated blood results in arterial hypoexmia. Whereas in normal young subjects, the tidal volume and FRC remain well above CV range so that airway closure does not occur in either the sitting or supine position, this may not be the case with gravidae in late pregnancy. Two studies carried out in gravidae in the sitting or semirecumbent position with a left lateral tip showed no airway closure and no physiologic shunting (19,21). On the other hand, studies of gravidae in the supine or lithotomy position showed airway closure in 25 to 50% of the subjects (21–24). Most of the evidence suggests that this is due primarily to reduction in FRC that leads to microatelectasis in the dependent portion of the lungs resulting in the lowering of Va/Q ratios and consequently lowered $PaO_2$ as is seen in some parturients at term in the supine or lithotomy position. Obviously, any further reduction in oxygenation that may happen during anesthesia may cause serious detrimental effects on both the mother and fetus.

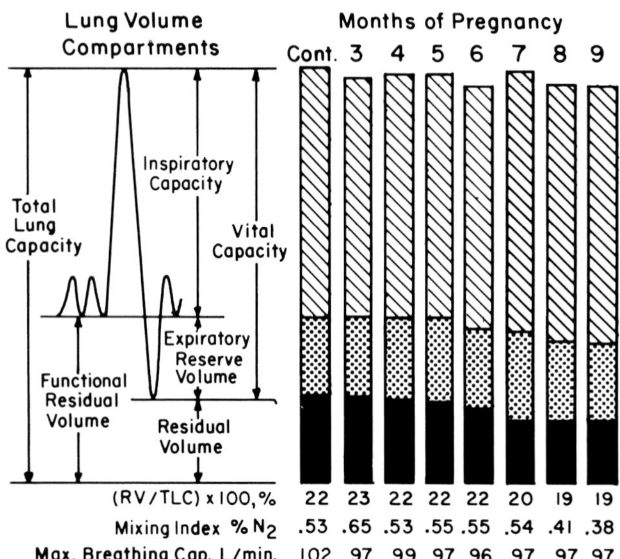


**Fig. 2–3.** Serial measurements of lung volume compartments, pulmonary mixing index, and maximum breathing capacity during normal pregnancy. Control values were obtained from the same women 4 to 9 months postpartum. The mean values were obtained in nine subjects by Cugell DW, et al.[13] Note that changes begin after the 5th month. Redrawn from Prowse CM, Gaensler EA: Respiratory and acid-base changes during pregnancy. Anesthesiology 26:381, 1965.)

### *Capacities*

The inspiratory capacity (IC) increases about 12 to 15% and is due to a 5% increase inspiratory reserve volume (IRV) and an increase in tidal volume (14,16b,18,22,23). In most instances, the increase is sufficient to compensate for the concomitant decrease in expiratory reserve volume and decrease in inspiratory capacity, so that the total lung volume remains within normal ranges or is decreased about 5% (16) (Table 2–1).

Vital capacity (VC) usually remains unaltered, but occasionally increases. A sustained decrease in vital capacity usually does not occur in normal gravidae, and when it is present it must be interpreted as pathologic (6,10,13). Because of the wide individual variations, a single measurement of vital capacity is of no clinical value—one must make serial measurements of vital capacity. Anatomic dead space is unaltered, but physiologic dead space is decreased due to a smaller alveolar dead space (24).

### *Dynamics*

The dynamics of respiration appear to be insignificantly affected by normal pregnancy. Cugell, et al (16) found that maximum breathing capacity was at a mean rate of 96 L/min in late pregnancy, as compared to 102 L/min some months after parturition. Timed vital capacity, peak flow rates, and velocity index, as well as intrapulmonary distribution of gas and diffusion capacity of the lungs, all remain within normal limits.

Lung compliance is also relatively unaffected by pregnancy, but chest wall compliance and thus total respiratory compliance are decreased significantly in late pregnancy in the supine position and even more so in the lithotomy position (14,25–29). Marx and associates (29) noted that total lung compliance increased by 25% after delivery of the infant compared with the value obtained immediately predelivery. In parturients in the supine-lithotomy position, the increase after delivery was 36%. Because there were only small and variable changes in lung compliance, the major contributing factor appeared to be an increase in chest wall compliance, which Marx and associates (29) attributed to a decrease in the degree of the elevation of the diaphragm by the enlarged uterus as soon as the infant was delivered. In most puerperae, the volume of FRC and RV recovers to its prepregnancy levels within 48 hours after delivery, but ERV may remain decreased for several months (18).

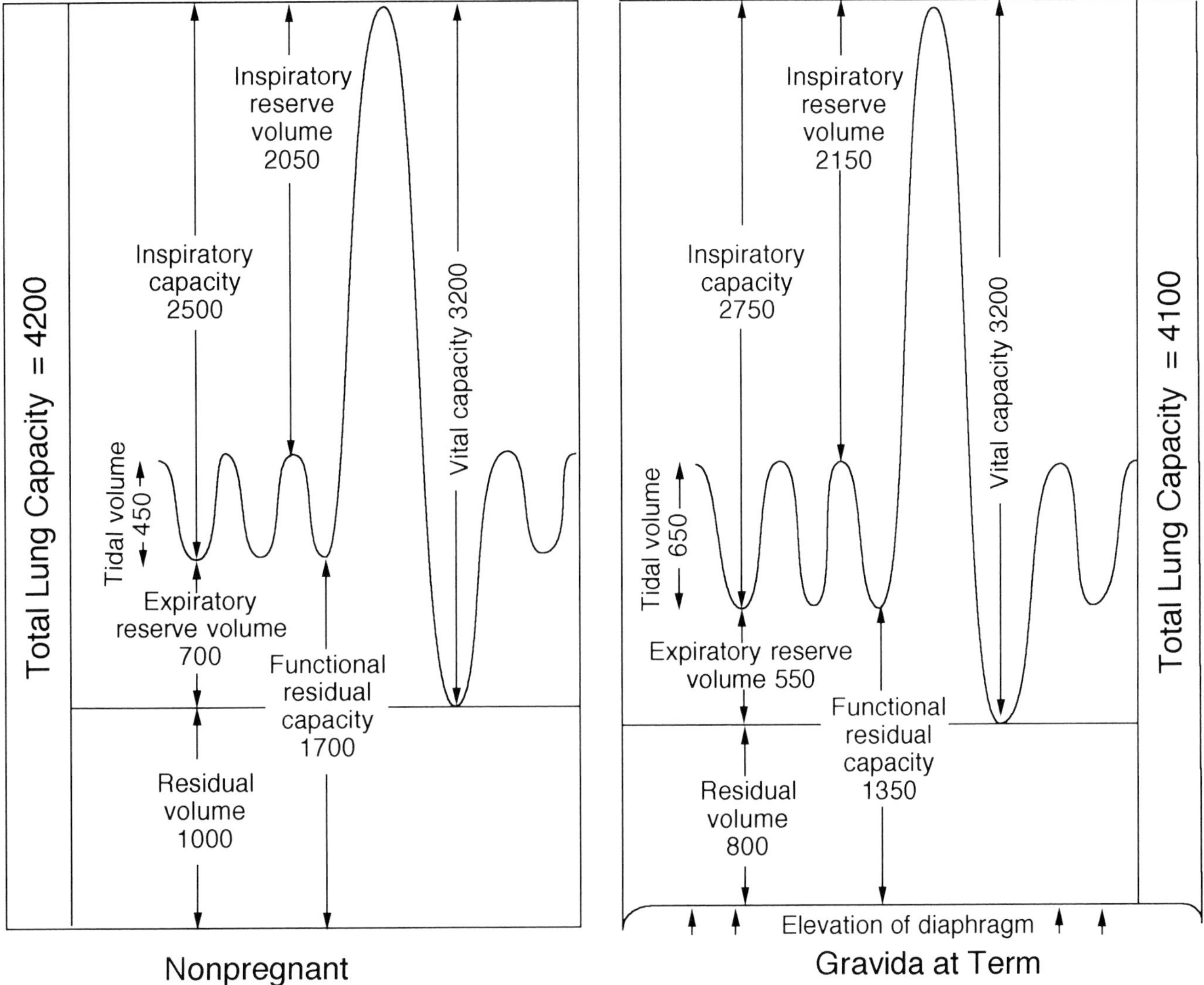


**Fig. 2–4.** Pulmonary volumes and capacities in the nonpregnant state and in the gravida at term.

## *Ventilation*

### *Ventilation During Pregnancy*

Ventilation during pregnancy is associated with an increase in minute ventilation, which begins during the early weeks of gestation and is 50% above normal at term (2,6,9,13–16,18,30). This change is effected by a 40 to 50% (mean 45%) increase in tidal volume and a 8 to 15% (mean 10%) increase in respiratory rate (Figure 2–5). Although some authors (16a), based apparently on only one study done at one interval in the third trimester of pregnancy (23), claim that there is no increase in respiratory rate, most investigators that have studied gravidae a number of times over the course of pregnancy have noted an increase of 10 to 15% (16,17,20,23,28). Earlier studies suggest that dead space remains normal during pregnancy, and, consequently, alveolar ventilation at term was higher (65 to 70% above nonpregnant levels) than minute ventilation. However, more recent studies (20,23) have shown that dead space increases about 45%, which is attributed to the larger conducting pathways (12,14). Moreover, the ratio of dead space to tidal volume (Vd/Vt) remains the same (20,24). Consequently, minute ventilation is 45 to 50% above nonpregnant level, and alveolar ventilation is the same as—or slightly higher than—minute ventilation (Table 2–1).

Earlier studies (9,12,16) suggested that the increase was progressive throughout the pregnancy, but more recent data (18,26,27,30) show that almost maximum hyperventilation occurs as early as the second or third month of gestation (Figure 2–6). In a study my colleagues and I carried out in women undergoing abortion at 8 to 10 weeks, minute ventilation was 30 to 35% above the values measured 2 weeks postoperatively (30). The hyperventilation is due to an increase in carbon dioxide production, a progesterone-induced increase in the slope of the ventilation response curve to arterial carbon dioxide and to stimulant effects of progesterone and estrogens (14,16a,28,31).

Changes in lung volumes and increased ventilation lead

**Table 2–1.** Summary of Ventilatory Changes during Pregnancy

| Parameters | Normal Nonpregnant Female | Gravida at Term | Change* |
|---|---|---|---|
| Tidal volume in ml. | 450 | 650 | +45% |
| Respiratory rate per minute | 15 | 16 | +10% |
| Minute ventilation in liters | 6.5 | 10 | +55% |
| Inspiratory capacity (IC) in liters | 2.5 | 2.75 | +10% |
| Expiratory reserve volume (ERV) in liters | 0.7 | 0.55 | −20% |
| Residual volume (RV) in liters | 1.0 | 0.8 | −20% |
| Functional residual capacity (FRC) in liters | 1.7 | 1.35 | −20% |
| Vital capacity (VC) in liters | 3.2 | 3.2 | None |
| Timed vital capacity | | | |
| a. 1 second | 82% | 80% | Insignificant |
| b. 2 seconds | 93% | 94% | Insignificant |
| c. 3 seconds | 98% | 98% | None |
| Maximum breathing capacity (MBC) in liters | 102 | 97 | −5% |
| Total lung volume in liters | 4.2 | 4.1 | −5% |
| Maximum air flows in liters per minute | | | |
| a. Inspiratory | 150 | 135 | −13% |
| b. Expiratory | 100 | 98 | −2% |
| Airway resistance in cm. $H_2O$/liter/second | 2.5 | 2.5 | None |
| Walking ventilation in liters per minute | 15 | 19 | +30% |
| Walking dyspnea index—% | 15 | 21 | +40% |

* Calculated in round figures.
(Based on data of Cugell DW, et al: Pulmonary function in pregnancy; serial observations in normal women. Am. Rev. Tuberc. 67:568, 1953.)

a reduction of arterial and alveolar carbon dioxide that begins at the end of the first trimester when it averages about 28 to 32 mm Hg, or a mean of about 30 mm Hg at term (26,30). The end-tidal carbon dioxide ($ETCO_2$) also decreases, and although there is a significant difference between $ETCO_2$ and $PaCO_2$ in nonpregnant subjects, there is no difference between the two parameters during the latter two-thirds of gestation, at term, and in the early puerperium (16,16a,25).

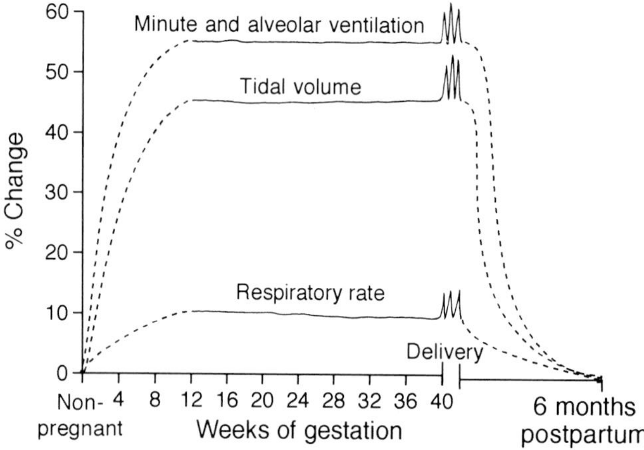


**Fig. 2–5.** Changes in ventilatory parameters during pregnancy. Note that almost maximum hyperventilation occurs as early as the second or third month of gestation. (Curves derived from data published by Bonica JJ: Maternal respiratory changes during pregnancy and parturition. *In* Parturition and Perinatology. Edited by GF Marx. Philadephia, FA Davis, 1972; and Bonica JJ, et al: Rev. Urug. Anethesiol. 5:45, 1971.)

Arterial oxygen tension ($PaO_2$) measured in the upright position is about 107 mm Hg at the end of the first trimester, 105 mm Hg at the second trimester, and 103 mm Hg at term compared to values of 95 mm Hg in the nonpregnant state (20,32). These increases are due to: 1) reduced $PaCO_2$; 2) slight decrease in physiologic shunt (20); and 3) reduced ateriovenous oxygen difference (A-$Vo_2$) (41). Reduced A-$Vo_2$ in the last trimester accounts for the slight reduction in $PaO_2$ at term. In the supine position, the $PaO_2$ at midgestation is frequently below 100 mm Hg, a fact that is due to: 1) a decrease in cardiac output consequent to aortocaval compression that increases the A-$Vo_2$ difference; and 2) the aforementioned further decrease in FRC in the supine position, whereas closing capacity does not change.

The respiratory alkalosis of pregnancy is compensated for by a significant increase in renal excretion of bicarbonate, which is reflected by decreases in milliequivalents per liter (mEq/L) in serum bicarbonate from 24–26 to 18–21, in buffer base from 47 to 42, in base excess from 0 to minus 2 to 3 (mean 1.5) mEq/L, lowering the total buffer base from 47 to 42. Because metabolic compensation does not fully offset the respiratory alkalosis, the pH increases from 7.40 to 7.44 (see section on acid base, metabolism, and nutrition later in the chapter, and the data listed in Table 2–3).

### *Metabolism and Oxygen Consumption*

Basal metabolic rate is slightly depressed during the first 14 to 16 weeks, then rises reaching a level 20% in 36 weeks, and then declines somewhat to 15% above nonpregnant levels at term (2,6,16a,33) (Figure 2–7). Components of the increased demand include the fetal-placen-

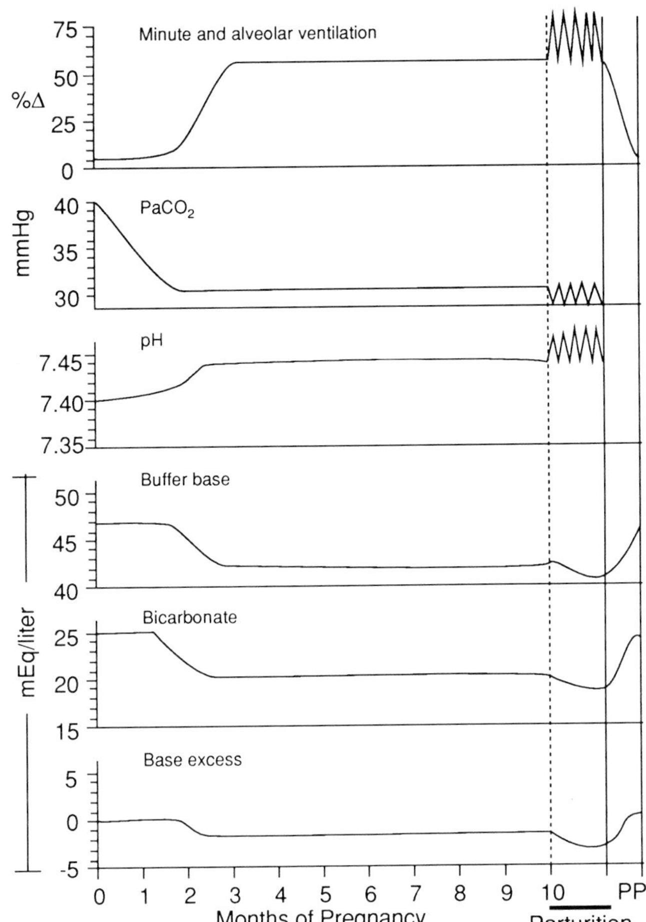


**Fig. 2–6.** Changes in alveolar ventilation, arterial carbon dioxide, pH, and acid-base changes during pregnancy, parturition, and the postpartum period. With the 50% increase in alveolar ventilation, the $PaCO_2$ decreases to levels of 30 mmHg at term, with concomitant changes in the acid-base. During parturition, especially during uterine contractions, further changes occur that increase ventilation and decrease $PaCO_2$. All of these variables return to normal 1 to 3 weeks after delivery. (From Bonica JJ: Maternal respiratory changes during pregnancy and parturition. *In* Parturition and Perinatology. Edited by GF Marx. Philadephia, FA Davis, 1972.)

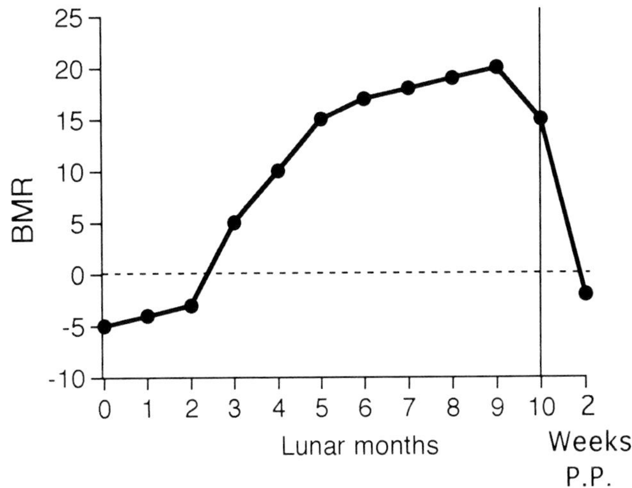


**Fig. 2–7.** Basal metabolic rate changes during pregnancy and puerperium. (From Russel KP: Basal metabolic rate changes during pregnancy and puerperium. Obstet. Gynecol. 8:207, 1956.)

tal complex, the hypertrophied maternal tissues, and increased cardiac rate and respiratory work (2,3). With ventilation rising about 50% and oxygen consumption only 20 to 25%, it becomes evident that there is considerable hyperventilation (5). Because of these two factors and because the basal metabolic rate increases about 10 to 15%, the ventilation equivalent for oxygen (ventilation in liters required for each 100 ml of oxygen consumption) is persistenly raised (13,30). During labor and vaginal delivery, oxygen consumption is increased an additional 60 to 75% primarily due to pain (30,30A,34,35) (Figure 2–7).

## Effects of Obesity

Because studies in nonpregnant subjects have shown that obesity is associated with a decrease of ERV, RV, FRC, tidal volume (TV) (36), mismatching of the ventilatory perfusion ratio (Va/Q) (37), and possibly in the sensitivity to $CO_2$ stimulation (38) and a concomitant increase in alveolar-arterial oxygen-tension difference ($AaDO_2$) (39), it has been assumed that these changes are accentuated significantly by pregnancy. This assumption is not substantiated by data derived from one study on obese gravidae. Eng, Butler, and Bonica (40), in a study of ten gravidae whose weight was 50 to 140% above the expected normal, found that such was not the case. Measurements or calculations of vital capacity, ERV, fraction of expired ventilation (FEV), FRC, $PaO_2$, $PaCO_2$, base excess, $AaDO_2$, and ventilatory response to $CO_2$ were made in the seated position during the last trimester and after the second postpartum month.

The data revealed that with the exception of FRC, the mean changes in lung volumes, blood gases, and other parameters were similar to those seen in nonobese gravidae. The FRC during pregnanacy was 2.06 liters and postpartum 2.14, a mean change smaller than that seen in nonobese gravidae. During pregnancy and postpartum, $PaO_2$ on room air was 86 and 86 mm Hg, respectively, while $PaO_2$ on 100% oxygen was 527 and 515, resulting in $AaDO_2$ of 62 and 167, respectively. These findings suggest that obesity of this magnitude does not exaggerate changes in ventilation induced by pregnancy as generally believed. Why in this obese population the decrease in FRC during pregnancy did not occur to the same degree as that seen in normal weight gravidae may be due in part to the fact that our studies were done with the gravidae in a sitting position, while many other data were obtained with the gravidae in the supine position.

## Dyspnea

During the last trimester, mild dyspnea is experienced by about 60 to 70% of normal gravidae (13,22), and this seems to be unrelated to either mechanics of respiration or exercise (14). Bader and coworkers (41) postulated that the high cost of breathing may contribute to the feeling of shortness of breath, while Gilbert and associates (42) suggested that this dyspnea is a sensation directly related to the unfamiliar low level of $PaCO_2$ during exercise and changes in perception of normal respiration. Cugell and coworkers (16) found that dyspnea did not correlate with the absolute level of ventilation nor the ratio of ventilation to maximum breathing capacity. On the other hand, a more recent and comprehensive study (23) demonstrated that increase in breathlessness is due to a normal awareness to the increase in minute ventilation. In any case, because hyperventilation results in more favorable conditions for gas exchange at the placenta, dyspnea can be considered a small price some women must pay for proper oxygenation and carbon dioxide elimination in the fetus.

## *Ventilation During Parturition*

During parturition, ventilation is further increased by the pain of labor, anxiety and apprehension, or by patients themselves trained voluntarily in natural childbirth or psychoprophylaxis (2,3,6,34,35,43–49). Moreover, during the second stage, the bearing-down effort, whether induced reflexively or carried out voluntarily consequent to coaching by a member of the obstetric team, also influences ventilation. The magnitude of hyperventiltion varies greatly, depending on the circumstances; respiratory rates as high as 60 to 174 during contraction; tidal volumes of up to 3042 ml; and maximum peak inspiratory flow rates of up to 340 L/min have been reported (30,43–45) (Figure 2–8).

Cole and Nainby-Luxmoore (43) measured respiratory volumes during labor in 25 patients and found a respiratory rate from 12 to 72 per minute and tidal volumes that varied from 350 ml to 2,250 ml, producing a range of respiratory minute volume from about 7 to 90 L/min. The higher values, which were close to the patients' maximum breathing capacity, were recorded in the second stage, while the lower figures were observed in parturients in the early first stage who had been given some sedation. Crawford and Tunstall (45) studied 20 parturients, 12 of whom were primigravidae. Measurements made during uterine contractions of the first stage and of the second stage showed wide patient-to-patient variations in ventilation. The values are listed in Table 2–2, which shows the great variation among parturients and the impressive values that are inspired during each contraction, and the values for the inspiratory flow rates during contractions as well as the inspiratory flow rates. Crawford and Tunstall noted that the values were greater in primigravidae than among multigravidae, and higher values were obtained from parturients nearing delivery (45).

In a study initiated in Caldeyro-Barcia's laboratory in Montevideo and completed in Seattle, Bonica and associates (30,30a) found that in primigravidae who had had no antepartal psychologic preparation and no sedation or analgesia during the first stage, ventilation was increased from a mean of 10.5 L/min between contractions to a mean of 22.4 L/min at the peak of contractions (Figure 2–7). In one patient, ventilation increased from 11 to 32 L/min, while in another it rose to 35 L/min—increases of more than 300% above prelabor ventilation and as much as a sixfold increase from nonpregnant values. Such significant hyperventilation caused a large, albeit transient, reduction of arterial carbon dioxide to 20 mm Hg. In the two patients who had ventilation above 30 L/min, $PaCO_2$ decreased to 15 and 11 mm Hg, respectively, while the pH rose to above 7.6. During the second stage, parturients without adequate analgesia hyperventilated to an even greater extent during contractions between bouts of involuntary bearing-down efforts causing even greater degrees of hypocapnia.

Similar results were recorded by Wulf and collaborators (35), who noted ventilation averaged 12 L/min before labor, but with the onset of labor noted its rapid rise to

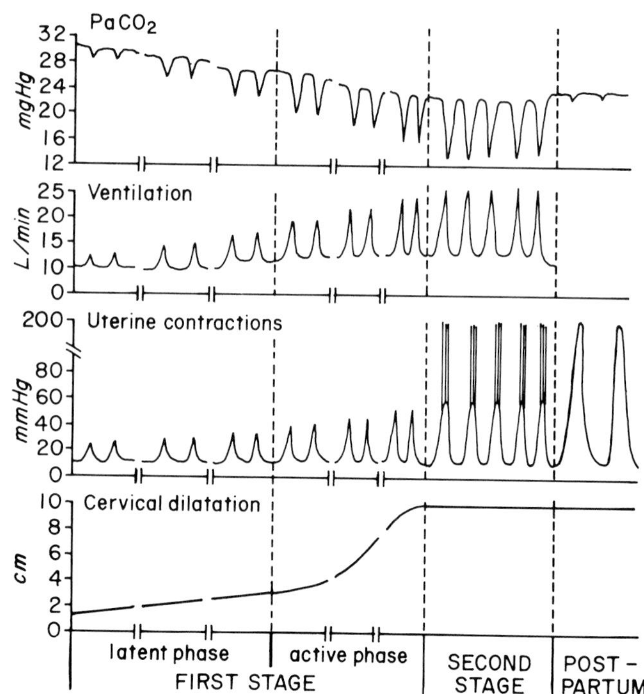


**Fig. 2–8.** Ventilatory changes during labor in unpremedicated gravida (schematic). Note correlation of the stage of labor as reflected by the Friedman's curve (lowermost tracing), the frequency and intensity of uterine contractions, minute ventilation, and arterial carbon dioxide tension (uppermost curve). Early in labor, uterine contractions are small and are associated with mild pain, causing only small increases in minute ventilation and decreases in $PaCO_2$, but, as labor progresses, the greater intensity of contractions causes greater changes in ventilation and $PaCO_2$. During the active phase, contractions with increased intrauterine pressure of 40 to 60 mmHg cause severe pain, that acts as an intense stimulus to ventilation with a consequent reduction of $PaCO_2$ to 18 to 20 mmHg. During the second stage, the reflex bearing-down efforts further increase intrauterine pressure and distend the perineum with consequent additional pain that prompts the parturient to ventilate at a rate almost twice that of early labor, causing a commensurate reduction in $PaCO_2$. (From Bonica JJ: Maternal respiratory changes during pregnancy and parturition. *In* Parturition and Perinatology (Clinical Anesthesia Series). Edited by GF Marx. Philadelphia, FA Davis Co., 1973.)

**Table 2–2.** Respiratory Performance During Labor (Numbers refer to mean of patients' means and ranges in parentheses*)

| Parameters | First Stage | Second Stage |
|---|---|---|
| No. of Contractions Observed | 11 (3–20) | 11 (1–24) |
| Duration of Contraction (seconds) | 33 (20–170) | 46 (20–120) |
| Number of Respirations During Each Contraction | 34 (2–124) | 45 (3–47) |
| Maximum Peak Inspiratory Flow Rate (liters per minute) | 112 (22–340) | 141 (30–300) |
| Volume of Inspired Air During Each Contraction (L/min) | 23 (2–95) | 12 (2–48) |
| Calculated Tidal Volume (in ml) | 750 (227–2,258) | 886 (104–3,024) |

* Figures rounded to nearest unit.
(Developed from data by Crawford JS, Tunstall MC: Notes on respiratory performance during labour. Br. J. Anaesth. 40:612–614, 1968.)

20 L/min and to 23 L/min at the time of delivery. Peak values of 40 L/min were observed in several instances. These investigators noted that oxygen uptake in ml/min$^{-1}$ $\times$ m$^{-2}$ was 140 before labor began and then rose steeply to 210 in early labor, and thereafter continued a progressive rise to 240 at 8 cm cervical dilation, 260 at full cervical dilation and during labor. During contractions, the oxygen uptake rose from 300 ml to 700 ml/min$^{-1}$ $\times$ m$^{-2}$. Moreover, the cardiac output increased from 6.4 liters per minute between contractions to over 14 liters (or 210%) during contractions. The metabolic rate in Kcal/(m$^2$ $\times$ min) in primiparae increased from 1.1 at the beginning of labor to 1.3 at 8 cm CxD, 1.5 at full dilation, and 1.4 during the second stage. For multiparae, the values during these time periods were from 0.75 to 1.0, 1.15, and 1.2, respectively. The metabolic rate for all of the patients studied were 0.7 just before the start of labor and rose steeply to 1.2 at 8 cm CxD, and 1.3 at 10 cm by the end of the second stage.

It is important to emphasize that with the end of painful contractions and the beginning of the relaxation phase, pain no longer stimulates respiration and that the hypocapnia causes a transient period of hypoventilation that can cause a decrease in $PaO_2$ to hypoxic levels (46–51). By using the noninvasive transcutaneous oxygen electrodes to monitor the mother and fetus, Huch, et al (47–50), Peabody (51), and many others (50) have shown that in parturients breathing air, the pain-induced hyperventilation and slight hyperoxia are followed by a transient period of hypoventilation and a decrease in $tcPO_2$ ranging from 5 to 50% or more, with a mean of 20 to 25% (Figures 2–9 and 2–10). They found administration of opiod analgesics such as 100 mg of meperidine intramuscularly to the mother or a sedative such as 5 mg of diazepam further depressed the ventilatory response to $CO_2$ causing even more severe hypoxemia between contractions. This can be remedied by instructing the mother to breathe in a normal fashion (Figures 2–9 and 2–10). When $PaO_2$ fell below 70 mm Hg, it frequently was reflected by a lowering of the fetal $tcPO_2$. Whether the transient periods of hypoventilation are dangerous to the fetus or not depends upon several factors, but mainly dependent upon the initial fetal $tcPO_2$. When it is high, a slight reduction will be without clinical significance, but when the fetus has a low intial $tcPO_2$ value, it is affected deleteriously by the superimposed transient lowering of $tcPO_2$ of the mother, resulting in a significant lowering of $tcPO_2$ and late decelerations (Figure 2–10). Huch, et al (49) also studied the efficacy of supplementary oxygen given to 40 parturients on a total of 64 occasions and found that in all but one instance fetal $PaO_2$ increased when the mother was given supplementary oxygen. The mean and $\pm$ standard deviation fetal $tcPO_2$ before and after maternal oxygen supplementation was $15 \pm 7.5$ and $21 \pm 7.9$ mm Hg, respectively. The beneficial effect of pain relief achieved with regional analgesia is discussed in detail in Chapter 13 (Figures 13–5 and 13–6).

## *Clinical Implications*

The anatomic changes are conducive to respiratory obstruction of the nasal passage, to an increased hazard of

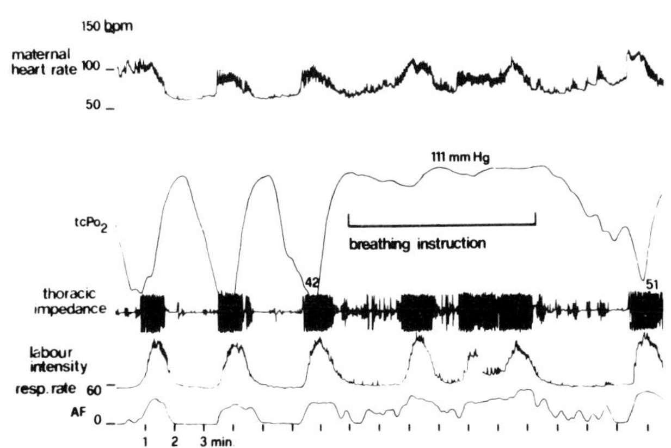


**Fig. 2–9.** Continuous recording of maternal heart rate, $tcPO_2$, thoracic impedance, uterine pressure, and respiratory rate after the parturient has been given 100 mg meperidine intramuscularly. With each uterine contraction, there was marked hyperventilation that caused $tcPO_2$ to increase to 110 mmHg but then fall to very low levels as a result of the marked respiratory alkalosis and the respiratory depressant effect of the meperidine. The large falls in $tcPO_2$ were avoided by giving the parturient breathing instructions during the relaxation period. (From Peabody JL: Transcutaneous oxygen measurement to evaluate drug effect. Clin. Perinatol. 6:109, 1979.)

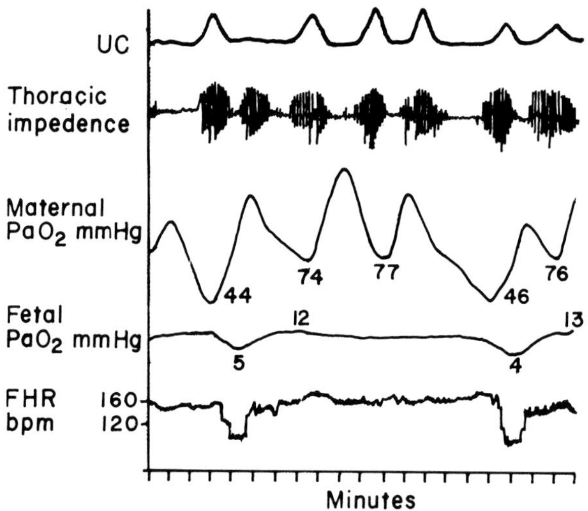


**Fig. 2–10.** Continuous recording of maternal transcutaneous oxygen tension ($tcPO_2$-mat), fetal oxygen tension ($tcPO_2$-fet), thoracic impedance, fetal heart rate (FHR), and uterine contractions (UC) in a primipara 120 minutes before spontaneous delivery of an infant with an Apgar 7. The same pattern was seen for 90 minutes, during which there were 22 contractions that provoked marked hyperventilation followed by hypoventilation or apnea between contractions. With the parturient breathing air, during and after the first and fourth periods of hyperventilation, the $tcPO_2$-mat fell to 44 and 46, with a consequent fall in fetal $tcPO_2$ and variable decelerations. Administration of oxygen to the mother prevents the maternal $tcPO_2$ from falling below 70 mm Hg and thus obviates decrease in fetal $tcPO_2$. [Modified from Huch A, et al: Continuous transcutaneous monitoring of fetal oxygen tension during labor. J. Obstet. Gynecol. 84(Suppl. 1):1, 1977.]

intubation, and to misinterpretation of physical findings. Special care must be taken in applying a face mask so that the patient is permitted to breathe through the mouth; nasopharyngeal tubes must be well lubricated and inserted carefully to avoid abrasion of the mucous membrane, and laryngoscopy and tracheal intubation must be performed skillfully and atraumatically. While the average nonpregnant female usually requires an 8 mm endotracheal tube, it is advisable to use a smaller (6 to 7 mm) tube in parturients to minimize the risk of injury to the larynx.

Changes in lung volumes, particularly the decrease in FRC, and ventilation increase the efficiency of gaseous transfer between maternal blood and alveolar air so that tension of $CO_2$ is decreased and that of oxygen increased. These changes, in turn, enhance the transfer of these gases between the mother and the fetus (52). On the other hand, these same changes and the increased oxygen consumption during labor make gravidae more susceptible to more rapid changes in respiratory blood-gas levels during respiratory complications than do they nonpregnant patients. Hypoventilation, breathholding, or respiratory obstruction will produce hypoxia, hypercarbia, and respiratory acidosis more readily in the gravida than in the nonpregnant woman. For example, even skillful tracheal intubation in a parturient breathing air frequently causes arterial oxygen tension to fall to 50 to 60 mm Hg after only 30 seconds of apnea (52). Archer and Marx (53) noted that even after adequate preoxygenation, the $PaO_2$ in apneic anesthetized gravidae fell by 81 mm Hg, more than in nonpregnant women (139 mm Hg in gravidae versus 58 mm Hg in nonpregnant women). Respiratory alkalosis may cause a leftward shift of the oxyhemoglobin curve causing oxygen to be tightly bound to a maternal hemoglobin, thus compromising its availability to the fetus (49). The tendency for rapid development of hypoxia is greatly enhanced by the high oxygen consumption during labor, the decreased functional residual capacity with less oxygen stored in the lungs, a decrease in cardiac output in the supine position, and airway closure.

Conversely, moderate-to-severe hyperventilation achieved spontaneously by the awake parturient or produced by the anesthesiologist through excessive positive-pressure ventilation during general anesthesia can quickly lead to severe respiratory alkalosis, which is often associated with a decrease in cerebral blood flow (54), a shift of the maternal oxygen-dissociation curve to the left, and possibly decreased uterine blood flow. Significant decrease in cerebral blood flow may produce a transient mental effect, and there is a transient analgesia and sometimes is manifested by carpopedal spasm and other signs of tetany. The shift of the maternal oxygen-dissociation curve produces fetal hypoxia and metabolic acidosis and consequent neonatal depression. The role of respiratory alkalosis and hypocapnia consequent to maternal hyperventilation in producing vasoconstriction of the uterine and umbilical vessels is controversial. While some older studies suggested that vasoconstriction was responsible for adverse effects on the fetus (55), later studies in parturients who voluntarily achieved severe hyperventilation showed that while maternal and fetal pH increased significantly, corresponding to changes in $PaCO_2$, fetal $PaO_2$ fell only 4 mm Hg and the condition of the newborn was good (56). Although progressive fetal acidosis does occur with excessive controlled hyperventilation during the course of general anesthesia, this is not likely to becaused by uterine vasoconstriction. In a study of mechanically hyperventilated pregnant ewes, Levinson and associates (57) found that added $CO_2$ did not restore uterine blood flow to normal. They concluded that decreases in venous return and cardiac output were more likely to be responsible for impaired uterine vasoconstriction.

As previously mentioned, the hypoventilation that can occur between contractions can cause maternal and fetal $PaO_2$ to fall and produce late deceleration in the fetus. This drop in $PaO_2$ can be prevented by giving the parturient instructions to breathe normally during the relaxation phase, or by giving her 100% oxygen through a tight-fitting face mask at flow rates of 8 to 20 L/min. Within a few minutes, maternal transcutaneous $PO_2$ rises to 175 to 260 mm Hg and fetal $PO_2$ rises about 8 mm Hg. If general anesthesia is to be used, 3 to 5 minutes of preanesthetic administration of 100% oxygen to the mother should be carried out to obviate any maternal and/or fetal hypoxia.

The respiratory changes during pregnancy and labor

also influence the induction of, and recovery from, inhalation anesthesia. With the increased alveolar concentration at the beginning of anesthesia and the decrease at the end, induction of, and emergence from, inhalation anesthesia is more rapid. This effect is less important with the less soluble gases such as nitrous oxide and cyclopropane than is it with the more soluble vapors such as diethyl ether, halothane, and enflurane. During general anesthesia, the minute ventilation with a normal pregnant $PaCO_2$ of 30 mm Hg in gravidae is 121 ml/Kg/min, a value significantly greater than the 77 ml/Kg/min required to maintain a comparable $PaCO_2$ in nonpregnant women (57a).

## CHANGES IN THE CIRCULATORY SYSTEM

### *Changes in the Blood*

#### Blood Volume

Next to the primary fetal and uterine development, the increase in blood volume is the greatest single physiologic alteration that occurs in pregnant women. While this augmentation is necessary to facilitate the interchange of gases and to better enable the parturient to withstand blood loss by holding blood in reserve, it imposes on the heart a burden of circulating a proportionately large quantity of blood per minute. This is an important factor in patients with heart disease.

These changes in blood volume begin at 4 to 8 weeks of pregnancy, and there is, subsequently, a progressive increase in total blood, plasma, and red cell volumes that reach maximum at 28 to 34 weeks and then remain constant until parturition (58–60). Earlier studies had suggested that these blood volumes were thought to decrease near term to obviate the additional stress of labor (6,61). However, recent data suggest that this fall in blood volumes during the latter part of pregnancy is an artifact resulting from measurements taken with the patient in the supine position and the consequent aortocaval compression (3). There is significant variation among gravidae, but one can estimate "average" values as listed in Table 2–3 and depicted in Figure 2–11.

*Plasma volume* is increased to 10 to 15% at 6 to 8

**Table 2–3.** Changes in Blood and Its Constituents During Pregnancy

| Variable | Nonpregnant | Average Values: Term Pregnancy | Average Values: Change |
|---|---|---|---|
| A. Volumes (ml) | | | |
| Total blood | 4000 | 5800 | 45% |
| Plasma 2700 | 2700 | 4200 | 55% |
| Red cell | 1400 | 2800 | +30% |
| B. Formed Elements | | | |
| RBC (million/mm³) | 4.6 | 4.3* | −0.3 |
| Hemoglobin (g/dl) | 14 | 12.8* | −1.2 |
| Hematocrit (%) | 41 | 36.5* | −4.5 |
| WBC | 6,000 | 9,000 | +3,000 |
| Platelets | 300,000 | 260,000 | −40,000 |
| C. Total Proteins | | | |
| Amount (gm) | 290 | 390 | ↑ |
| Concentration (gm/100 ml) | 7.3 | 6.5 | ↓ |
| D. Albumin | | | |
| Total (gm) | 127 | 144 | ↑ |
| Concentration (gm/100ml) | 5.5 | 4.4 | ↓ |
| E. Total Globulins | | Slight relative and absolute increase | |
| Alpha | | Slight increase | |
| Beta | | Slight increase | |
| Gamma | | Slight increase | |
| F. Electrolytes (mEq/L)** | | | |
| Total Base | 155 | 148 | ↓ |
| $Na^-$ | 143 | 138 | ↓ |
| $K^-$ | 4.3 | 4.1 | ↓ |
| $Ca^-$ | 4.4 | 4.6 | ↓ |
| $Cl^-$ | 105 | 103 | −2 |
| Mg** | 1.67 | 1.52 | −0.15 |
| $HPO^-$ | 1.96 | 1.15 | ↓ |
| $HCO^3$ | 26 | 21–23 | ↓ |
| G. Blood Gases and Acid-Base | | | |
| $PaO_2$ (mm Hg) | 95 | 105 | ↑ |
| $PaCO_2$ (mm Hg) | 40 | 30 | ↓ |
| Buffer base (mEq/L) | 47 | 42 | ↓ |
| Base excess (mEq/L) | 0.0 | −1.5 | ↓ |
| pH | 7.4 | 7.44 | slight ↑ |

* Values at term after iron and folic acid supplementation.
** Data on electrolytes. (From Newman RL: Serum electrolytes in pregnancy, parturition and puerperium. Obstet. Gynecol. 10:51, 1957.)

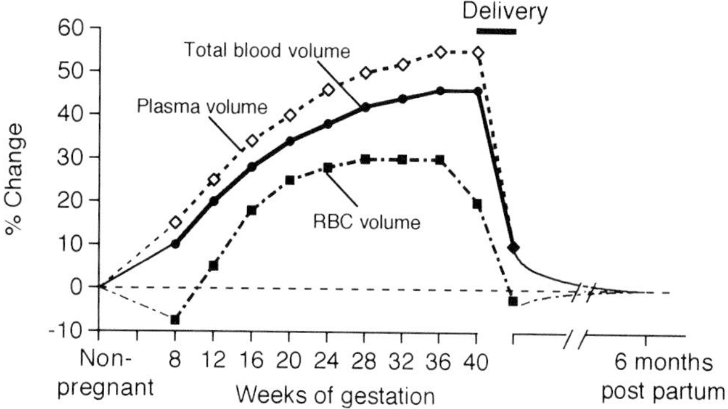


**Fig. 2–11.** Changes in blood volume, plasma volume, and red cell volume during pregnancy and in the puerperium. The curves were constructed from various reports in the literature and illustrate trends in percentage change rather than absolute values. Note that significant changes occur as early as 8 to 12 weeks. (From Bonica JJ: Obstetric Analgesia and Anesthesia. 2nd Ed. The World Federation of Societies of Anesthesiologists, Amsterdam, 1980, p. 2.)

weeks of gestation and then rises steeply until the twenty-eighth to thirty-fourth weeks of pregnancy, after which there is a subsequent, more gradual rise to levels of 50 to 55% above nonpregnant levels during the last several weeks of gestation. In primigravidae, the increase may be as high as 50% above the prepregnancy level. There is some evidence that in the normal multigravida the increase is even greater (up to 60% ) (62) and that an even larger increase occurs in case of multiple pregnancy (2–4). There is also good evidence that the degree to which plasma volume increases during pregnancy is directly correlated with the birth weight of the infant (62,63). This remarkable increase in plasma volume is due to elevation of aldosterone production, which is directly or indirectly caused by the estrogens, progesterone, and placental lactogen during gestation.

*The red cell volume* has an initial slight drop, but at 8 weeks it begins to rise and continues to do so in somewhat a more linear fashion than does the plasma volume, reaching 20 to 30% above the nonpregnant levels by the end of pregnancy (2–4,59–64). These effects on red blood cell volume are due to serum erythropoie, which does not increase its activity until the eighth to twelfth weeks of gestation, and is then increased to produce the elevation noted thereafter. The total blood volume increases from about 10% above nonpregnant levels at 8 weeks to about 40 to 50% (mean 45% ) at term. The specific gravities of whole blood and plasma are reduced and the relative blood viscosity declines about 12% (2,4).

This significant hypervolemia causes no evidence of circulatory overload in the healthy gravida, as most of the added volume is accommodated by the enlarged uterus and breasts and the increased blood flow to kidneys, skeletal muscles, and skin, and parallels the increased cardiac output and ventilation. These changes facilitate maternal/fetal exchange of blood gases, nutrients, and metabolites, and enable the gravida to tolerate the normal blood loss during parturition. The measured loss is 300 to 550 ml with vaginal delivery, and 600 to 1,000 ml with abdominal (cesarean) delivery (59,60). Crawford (1) noted that parturients who had spontaneous vaginal deliveries had a lower blood loss than those who had an episiotomy. It has also been shown that blood loss is less when the delivery is carried out with epidural blockade than when it is carried out with pudendal block or general anesthesia (12,65). At delivery, the autotransfusion of as much as 500 ml of blood into the maternal circulation from the uterus and placenta minimizes the impact of maternal hemorrhage. Moir (66) measured postpartum blood volume and found that although at 1 hour the decline was more severe following cesarean section than vaginal delivery, by 3 days postpartum, values had decreased by 16% in both groups of patients. Hematocrit rose by 5.2% after vaginal delivery because of hemoconcentration resulting from postpartum diuresis, whereas following cesarean section, hematocrit decreased by about 60%. By 8 weeks postpartum, the blood volume and its constituents have returned to nonpregnant values (59,60,63,64).

### *Hematologic Values*

#### Red Cells, Hemoglobin, Hematocrit

The red cell count, and the hemoglobin (grams/100 ml) and hematocrit values decrease during pregnancy, as depicted in Figure 2–12. However, there is an actual progressive increase in the total number of erythrocytes and in the hemoglobin content of the individual cells (Table 2–3), but this is obscured by the greater increase in plasma volume, resulting in hemodilution and an apparent decrease in erythrocytes and hemoglobin, producing what has long (and erroneously) been called the "physiologic anemia of pregnancy" (2–4,60–64). During the last 4 to 6 weeks of pregnancy, these values begin to increase toward normal levels. When hemopoiesis is stimulated by iron therapy, the fall in hemoglobin concentration and hematocrit is reduced significantly (2–4,60–64). With proper nutrition, iron and folic acid supplementation, the healthy gravida at term should have a red cell count of 3.7 to 3.8 million per mm$^3$, a hemoglobin concentration of about 12 to 13% ( 12.5% ) g/dL, and a hematocrit of 35% to 36% (mean 35.5% ) (1–3).

#### *Other Cellular Elements*

*The white cell count* in pregnancy usually is between 8000 and 9000 cells per mm$^3$, caused primarily by a significant increase in segmental neutrophils and monocytes, while the lymphocytes, the eosinophils, and basophils remain virtually unchanged (67,68) (Figure 2–13). Only leukocytosis in excess of 15,000 cu mm$^3$ should be regarded as indicating infection, and in such cases the count must be repeated to be significant.

*The platelet count*, reported in older studies, indicated an increase, decrease or no change during the course of pregnancy. However, most of these studies were cross-sectional in design and used visual techniques of cell counting. Pitkin and Witte (68a) used an automated technique of counting 10,000 cells in 23 women studied longitudinally throughout pregnancy and at 6 weeks after delivery. Figure 2–13b shows that the average platelet count

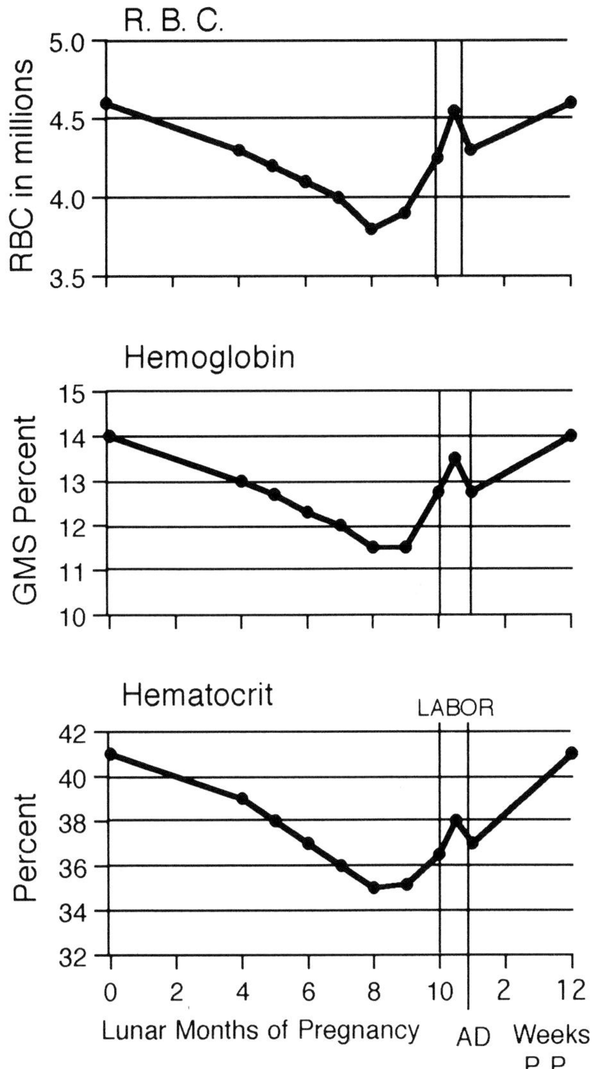


**Fig. 2–12.** Red blood cell, hemoglobin, and hematocrit values during pregnancy and the puerperium.

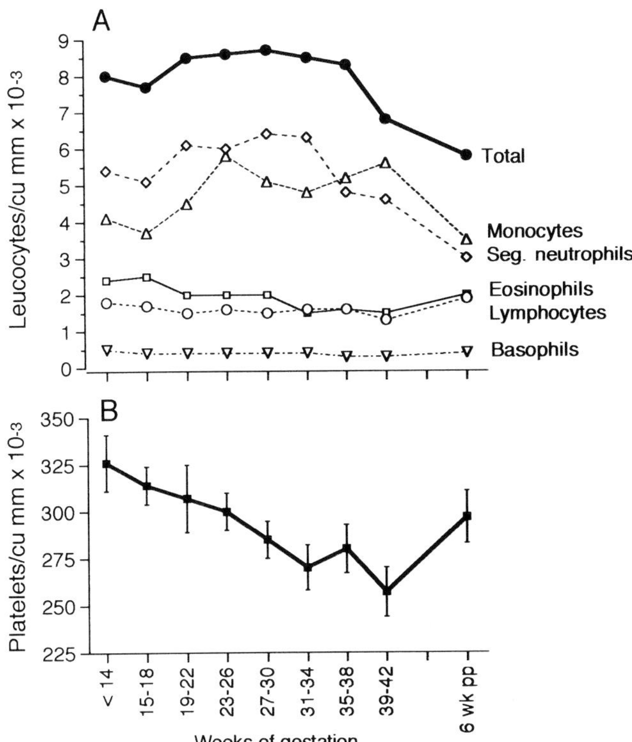


**Fig. 2–13.** The effect of pregnancy, labor and the puerperium on the white blood and platelet counts. (Modified from Pitkin RM, Witte DL: Platelet and leukocyte counts in pregnancy. JAMA 242:2696, 1979)

declined monotonically in a manner consistent with the gestational increase in blood volume. A progressive decline has also been reported by Sagi and associates (68b).

### Blood Composition

*Total circulating proteins* increase during pregnancy, but, because of the hemodilution, the concentration of the total proteins and the albumin fraction decreases, as do the specific gravity and viscosity of the blood (see Table 2–3). Because there is a concomitant relative, as well as absolute, increase in total globulins (with variation of different fractions (see Table 2–3), the albumin-globulin ratio declines from 1.5 in nonpregnant women to 1.1 at term but is not reversed. The globulin fractions differ in their trends; α-globulin and some β-globulins rise gradually, whereas some β-globulins and the γ-globulins decrease slightly (2–5). Maternal colloid oncotic pressure decreases from a nonpregnant level of 20.8 ± 1 mm Hg to 18.0 ± 1.5 mm Hg, a 15% reduction (13). Moreover, colloid oncotic pressure-pulmonary capillary wedge pressure gradient decreases from the nonpregnant value of 14.5 ± 2.5 mm Hg to 10.5 ± 2.7 mm Hg, or a 28% decline.

*Fibrinogen* is also increased significantly, both actually and relatively, from about 300 mg/dl to over 450 mg/dl in the third trimester (67). As a result of the increase in the fibrinogen level, the increase in erythrocyte sedimentation rising from a nonpregnant level of less than 10 mm$^3$ to a peak close to 80 mm$^3$ is of little diagnostic value in the pregnant patient.

*The total lipid concentration* of plasma increases from a mean of 650 to 700 mg/dl the first trimester to over 1,000 mg/dl at term, and all lipid factors are involved in this rise, including cholesterol, phospholipids, neutral fat, and nonesterized fatty acids (68).

*Serum cholinesterase activity* is reduced approximately 20% by the end of the first trimester, and 30% at midgestation at which level it remains until term (69,69a), but the enzyme remains unchanged qualitatively and the decreased amount is sufficient for normal hydrolysis of clinical doses of chloroprocaine, succinylcholine, and other drugs degraded by plasma. Some evidence suggests that the occasional case of prolonged neuromuscular blockade is not due to a decrease in cholinesterase, but rather potentiation by magnesium sulfate used in the treatment of obstetric complications (70).

### Blood Coagulation

During pregnancy, various components of the normal coagulation process are increased. In addition to the aforementioned rise in the amount of circulating fibrinogen (factor I), there is a significant increase in the concentrations of factors VII (proconvertin), VIII (antihemophilic factor), IX (Christmas factor), and X (Stuart-Prower factor), with other factors remaining unaltered (2–5,8). There is also a progressive increase in serum fibrin-fibrinogen degradation (71). These increases result in shortening, by approximately 20% of the prothrombin time and the partial thromboplastin time (68). Although these increased concentrations suggest that both fibrin formation and fibrinolysis increase as pregnancy progresses, gestation is associated with a hypocoagulative state that constitutes a double-edged sword; it protects the gravida against excessive blood loss during parturition, but also increases the risk of thromboembolism (2–5).

## Cardiac and Vascular Changes

### Changes in the Heart

#### Anatomic Changes

The aforementioned changes imposed on the diaphragm and thoracic cavity by the enlarging uterus cause a significant change in the position of the heart; it is lifted upward in toto, shifted to the left and anteriorly, and rotated toward a transverse position (Figure 2–2 and Figure 2–14). As a result, the apical impulse moves cephalad to the fourth intercostal space and laterally to, or beyond, the midclavicular line, and the transverse diameter of the heart increases as much as 1 cm. Radiographic studies have shown indentation of the esophagus by the left atrium and straightening of the left border of the heart (3,72). Although these changes simulate those of pathologic hypertrophy, they represent primarily a change in position (Figure 2–14).

#### Functional Changes

Functional changes involving the heart, as compared with normal values, include: a higher basal heart rate and louder heart sounds with an accentuated first apical and second pulmonic sounds; a faint hemic systolic murmur over the pulmonary and tricuspid areas; and a more forceful palpable apical beat (15,72). Moreover, there is a relative increase in the incidence of premature contractions, sinus tachycardia, and paroxysmal supraventricular tachycardia (62).

#### Electrocardiogram

The electrocardiogram may show a large Q-wave and inverted T-wave in lead III. In addition, there may also be a small Q in lead a Vf and inverted T-wave in leads $V_1$ $V_2$ and occasionally $V_3$, and a lowering of T in $V_4$. In many gravidae, there is a progressive tendency toward left axis deviation from the second to sixth month, but reversion to the right in the ninth month (13,72). Innocent depres-

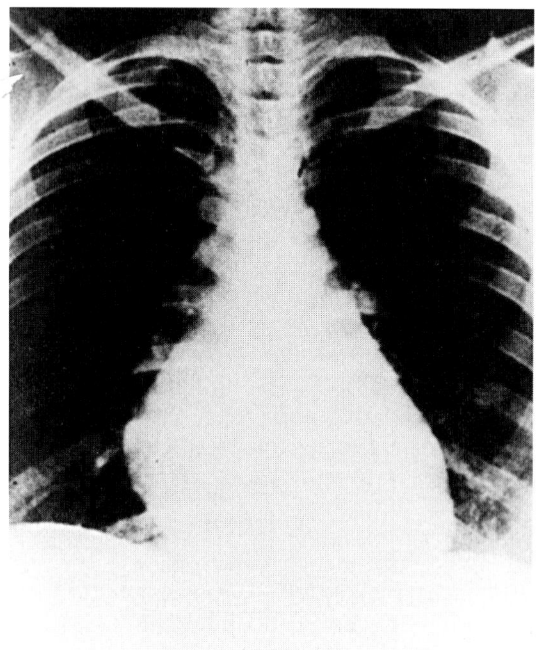

A

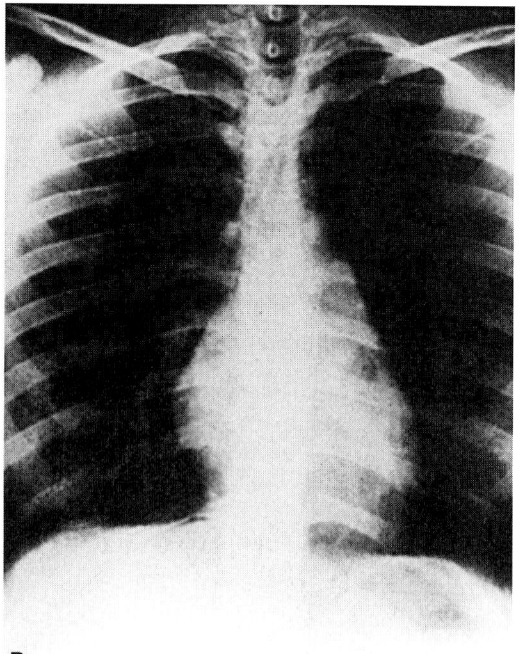

B

**Fig. 2–14.** Radiography of chest. Changes in heart size following delivery. These radiographs were taken at 7½ months of gestation **(A)** and 8 weeks following delivery **(B).** The patient was a 26-year-old woman who was asymptomatic throughout pregnancy and had no evidence of heart disease. The chest x-ray on the left, taken for tuberculosis screening (in 1964), was interpreted as showing "cardiac enlargement" and "increased vascular markings." The postpartum film on the right was taken to evaluate the previously suggested cardiomegaly and was read as "within normal limits." Note the difference in diaphragmatic height and of x-ray penetration as shown by the visibility of the spinal column in the postpartum film. (From Metcalf J, McAnulty JH, Ueland DK: Burwell and Metcalfe's Heart Disease and Pregnancy: Physiology and Management, 2nd Ed. Boston, Little, Brown, 1986, pp. 5–38.)

sion of the S-T segment and flattening of T-wave has been reported (73). None of these electrocardiographic changes is permanent.

## Hemodynamic Changes

### Changes During Pregnancy

### Cardiac Output

Cardiac output during pregnancy has been estimated or measured by a variety of techniques for nearly a century. In the first edition of this book, data published before 1966 that had been derived by measurement of pulse pressure, the application of direct Fick principle, by cardiac catheterization, and by the dye dilution technique were cited (74–78). Those data suggested that cardiac output began to increase about 10% by the twelfth week of gestation, reached a peak of 30 to 40% above a nonpregnant level at 28 to 32 weeks, and then fell to prepregnant levels by the thirty-eighth to fortieth week (75–78). The lowering of the heart's workload near the end of pregnancy was hypothesized as being a compensatory mechanism to obviate the added increase in myocardial work imposed by parturition.

In 1967, Lees and associates (79), who had previously defined the phenomena of the supine caval occlusion precisely, measured cardiac output in gravidae in the supine and lateral positions at three time periods: (1) 11 to 13 weeks; (2) 24 and 27 weeks; and (3) 34 to the 41st week. They found that cardiac output increased 30 to 40% above nonpregnant levels and that most of this increase had been established by the end of the first trimester. Moreover, measurements in the lateral position revealed that cardiac output during the last few weeks of pregnancy remained at the same high level as seen during the second trimester. In contrast, measurements in the supine position revealed a significant decrease during the third trimester. Lees and associates (79) concluded that because all previous studies had been done with the patient in the supine position, the decrease of cardiac output to nonpregnant levels near the end of pregnancy found by early investigators was due to compression of the inferior vena cava by the large uterus.

Soon thereafter, Ueland and associates (80) studied 11 gravidae serially during three periods and at 8 weeks postpartum when the values were considered to have returned to normal nonpregnant levels. The patients were measured in the supine, lateral, and sitting positions. Ueland and associates also studied the effects of mild and moderate exercise on a bicycle ergometer. Table 2–4 lists mean changes in actual values and in percentages. As noted, cardiac output had increased significantly by the 20 to 24 weeks of gestation and was maintained at these higher levels through 32 weeks. At 38 to 40 weeks, there was a decline somewhat toward normal in all three maternal positions (Figure 2–15). However, the greatest reduction did occur in the supine position; indeed, in the final weeks of pregnancy the cardiac output in the supine position was less than that found at 6 to 8 weeks postpartum (considered as the nonpregnant values). Mild exercise (100 kpm per minute) increased cardiac output about 75% throughout pregnancy. However, with moderate exercise (200 kpm per minute), the rise in cardiac output was progressively smaller as pregnancy advanced; the increases were 120% at 20 to 24 weeks; 83% at 28 to 32 weeks; and 71% at 38 to 40 weeks. This was due primarily to a decrease in stroke volume. These findings suggested to Ueland and associates (80) that there is a progressive decline in circulatory reserve as pregnancy advances.

During the past decade, noninvasive techniques have been used to carry out serial measurements of cardiac output at regular intervals during gestation (81–83). Atkins and associates (81) measured cardiac output by impedance cardiography in a total of 27 patients, 8 of whom were seen from before conception and throughout pregnancy, to several months postpartum, while the other 19 were measured at regular intervals from 8 to 11 weeks

**Table 2–4.** Cardiac Output, Stroke Volume and Heart Rate Related to Posture and Gestational Age (Expressed in Mean Values and Percent Change from Nonpregnant Values to Nearest Unit)

| | Gestational Age (weeks) | | | | | | |
|---|---|---|---|---|---|---|---|
| | 20–24 wk | | 28–32 wk | | 38–40 wk | | Postpartum (6–8 mos)!! |
| **Parameters** | **Actual** | **%** | **Actual** | **%** | **Actual** | **%** | **Value** |
| *Cardiac Output* (l/min) | | | | | | | |
| A. Supine | 6.4 | 28 | 6.0 | 22 | 4.5 | −12 | 5.1 |
| B. Lateral | 6.9 | 38 | 7.0 | 41 | 5.7 | 15 | 5.0 |
| C. Sitting | 5.9 | 29 | 6.4 | 39 | 5.2 | 13 | 4.6 |
| *Stroke Volume* (ml) | | | | | | | |
| A. Supine | 88 | 21 | 77 | 5 | 52 | −28 | 73 |
| B. Lateral | 95 | 33 | 88 | 23 | 69 | −2.8 | 71 |
| C. Sitting | 74 | 30 | 72 | 28 | 58 | −2.3 | 57 |
| *Heart Rate* (Beats/min) | | | | | | | |
| A. Supine | 74 | 7 | 83 | 20 | 8 | 23 | 70 |
| B. Lateral | 73 | 5 | 82 | 17 | 83 | 20 | 70 |
| C. Sitting | 83 | 3 | 92 | 13 | 89 | 10 | 81 |

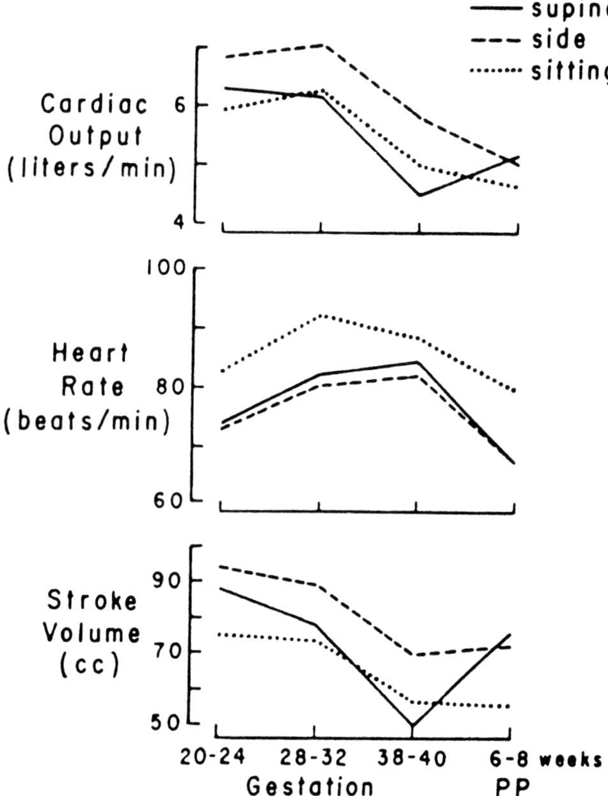


**Fig. 2–15.** Cardiac output, heart rate, and stroke volume in three positions. Resting cardiac output and its components. Maternal cardiac output was measured 3 times during pregnancy and once postpartum in 11 normal women. Measurements were made with the patient sitting, supine, and in the left lateral decubitus position at each study. As pregnancy nears term, assumption of the supine position causes a striking fall in cardiac output to levels below those found postpartum. Maternal heart rate increases slightly early in pregnancy and continues to rise as pregnancy advances. At term, the increments in cardiac output (above postpartum values) observed in the "sitting" and "side" positions are caused by a relative tachycardia. Stroke volume increases early in pregnancy and declines as pregnancy advances, particularly in the supine position. Most of the change in cardiac output at the twentieth week of pregnancy is caused by an increase in stroke volume. Near term, stroke volume is below the postpartum value with the patient supine. PP = postpartum. (From Ueland K, Novy MJ, Peterson EN, and Metcalf J: Material cardiovascular dynamics: VI. The influence of gestational age on maternal cardiovascular response to posture and exercise. Am. J. Obstet. Gynecol. 104:856, 1969.)

of pregnancy until 6 weeks postpartum. Although Atkins and associates made measurements in the supine, reclining, left and right lateral, and left and right tilt position, their first report contained data obtained in the left lateral position. They noted that from the eight to thirty-sixth week of pregnancy, the pulse rose from a prepregnant value of 68 to 76 to 80. Stroke volume and cardiac output began to rise shortly after conception and were significantly greater than the prepregnancy levels by the twelfth week. During the second half of pregnancy, these two values fell gradually and by term were lower than the prepregnancy levels. Subsequently, the method was criticized because it correlated poorly with cardiac output determined by thermal dilution and questioned because of the technique's validity during pregnancy (82).

As of this writing, Robson and associates (83) present the most comprehensive hemodynamic data throughout pregnancy. They carried out serial hemodynamic measurements in 13 women on two occasions before conception and then again at monthly intervals from the fifth to the thirty-eighth week of gestation. All measurements were made in the left semilateral position. Cardiac output was measured by Doppler and cross-sectional echocardiography at the aortic, pulmonary, and mitral valves, and the size of cardiac chambers and ventricular function investigated by M-mode echocardiography, both noninvasive techniques (Figure 2–16). Cardiac output increased a significant 10% by the fifth week, rose to 25% above nonpregnant levels at 8 weeks, 40 to 45% during the twelfth to the twenty-eighth week, then reached a peak of 50% during the thirty-second to the thirty-sixth weeks and decreased slightly (47% above prelabor values) at 38 weeks. Heart rate and left ventricular performance increased during the first trimester. Heart rate further in-

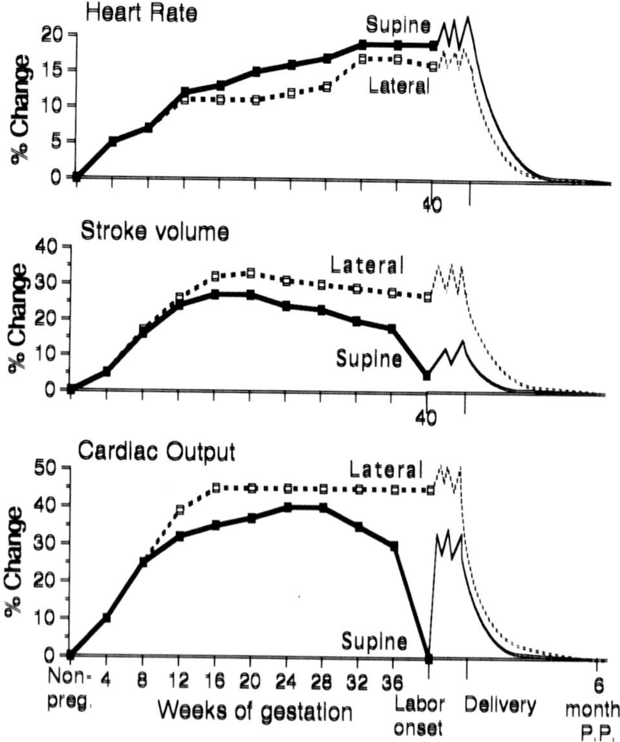


**Fig. 2–16.** Changes in maternal heart rate, stroke volume, and cardiac output during pregnancy with the gravida in supine and lateral positions. Note the significant changes that occur as early as 8 to 12 weeks. The curve in the lateral position was developed from Robson SC, et al: Cardiac output during labour. Br. Med. J. 295:1169, 1987. The curve in the supine position was developed from data published by Ueland DK, and Hansen JM: Maternal cardiovascular dynamics. II. Posture and uterine contractions. Am. J. Obstet. Gynecol. 103:1, 1969. The curve on cardiac output in the lateral position is leveled after the 20th week and does not show the decrease seen in the Figure 2–15.

**Table 2–5.** Effects of Position Change on Cardiac Output during Pregnancy

| Position | Percent Change* |
|---|---|
| Supine Horizontal | Control (0) |
| Lithotomy | −17 |
| Walcher | −8 |
| Trendelenburg Supine | −18 |
| Trendelenburg Left Side | +13 |
| Horizontal Left Side (Sims') | +13.5 |

* Approximate values.
From Vorys N, Ullery, Hanusek GE: The cardiac output changes in variable positions in pregnancy. Amer. Obstet. Gynec. 82:1312, 1961.

creased during the second and third trimester, during which time left atrial and left ventricular endiastolic dimensions increased suggesting an increase in venous return. Derived figures of total peripheral vascular resistance decreased 31% by the twelfth week, reached a low of 35% decrease by the twentieth week, and then remained at 30% below nonpregnant values. These changes were associated with a progressive increase in valve orifice area and left ventricular wall thickness during pregnancy. In contrast to the result in earlier reports (74–78) and those by Atkins and associates (81), these data suggest no significant changes in cardiac output or stroke volume during the later phases of pregnancy.

Table 2–5 lists effects of different positions on cardiac output during pregnancy based on data published by Vorys and associates (84) and Ueland and collaborators (80). Measurements of cardiac output in different positions by Vorys and associates (84) and Ueland and collaborators (80) revealed a rise of 14 to 20% in the lateral position as compared with the supine posture, but a further fall of 17% in the lithotomy position and of 18% in the steep Trendelenburg supine position. The increase that occurred when the gravida changed from supine to the left side was due to relief of vena cava compression (and probably the aortoiliac compression), whereas in the lithotomy and Trendelenburg position, it resulted in the uterus being pushed more posteriorly against the spine, thus compressing the inferior vena cava more than when the gravida is supine. Further detailed descriptions in regard to the maternal cardiovascular system can be found in Chapter 31.

Clark and 12 collaborators (13) carried out a comprehensive study of central hemodynamics in normal gravidae between 36 and 38 weeks of gestation who were carefully screened representing a uniform population. Selection was based on rigid criteria that included only primiparae of 26 years of age or less, a singleton fetus in vertex presentation, gestational age confirmed with ultrasonography, normal amniotic fluid volume, no fetal abnormalities, and the gravidae had no illnesses and did not use alcohol, tobacco or drugs. Various measurements were made during gestation and repeated between 11–13 weeks postpartum. The results are shown in Table 2–6 and, as noted, the group had a 43% increase in cardiac output, 17% increase in heart rate and 27% decrease in systemic vascular resistance, and a 34% decline in pulmonary vascular resistance reflecting the increased vascular reactivity in the pulmonary circulation. In contrast, they noted no significant difference in intrinsic left ventricular contractility as assessed by left ventricular stroke work index. Thus, normal pregnancies did not associate with hyperdynamic left ventricular function—a fact previously observed (87b). They noted no significant change in pulmonary capillary wedge pressure, central venous pressure or mean arterial pressure. The lack of increase in pulmonary capillary wedge pressure or central venous pressure, in the face of significant increases in vascular volume, reflects the significant decreases in systemic vascular resistance and pulmonary vascular resistance that allow both systemic and pulmonary vasculature to accommodate higher volumes than normal vascular pressures. They mentioned that their findings of significant fall in colloid osmotic pressure-pulmonary capillary wedge pressure gradient implies a greater propensity to pulmonary edema during pregnancy in the presence of any alteration in pulmonary capillary permeability or increase in cardiac load.

### Blood Pressures

Systolic and diastolic arterial blood pressures decrease slightly during early and mid-pregnancy because of the

**Table 2–6.** Central Hemodynamic Changes

| | Nonpregnant | Pregnant | Percent Change* |
|---|---|---|---|
| Cardiac output (L/min) | 4.3 ± 0.9 | 6.2 ± 1.0 | +43 |
| Heart rate (beats/min) | 71 ± 10.0 | 83 ± 1.0 | +17 |
| Systemic vascular resistance (dyne·cm·sec$^{-5}$) | 1530 ± 520 | 1210 ± 266 | −21 |
| Pulmonary vascular resistance (dyne·cm·sec$^{-5}$) | 119 ± 47.0 | 78 ± 22 | −34 |
| Colloid oncotic pressure (mm Hg) | 20.8 ± 1.0 | 18.0 ± 1.5 | −14 |
| Colloid oncotic pressure—pulmonary capillary wedge pressure (mm Hg) | 14.5 ± 2.5 | 10.5 ± 2.7 | −28 |
| Mean arterial pressure (mm Hg) | 86.4 ± 7.5 | 90.3 ± 5.8 | −NSC |
| Pulmonary capillary wedge pressure (mm Hg) | 6.3 ± 2.1 | 7.5 ± 1.8 | −NSC |
| Central venous pressure (mm Hg) | 3.7 ± 2.6 | 3.6 ± 2.5 | NSC |
| Left ventricular stroke work index (g·m·m$^{-2}$) | 41 ± 8 | 48 ± 6 | +NSC |

* NSC = no statistically significant change.
(From Clark SL, et al: Central hemodynamic assessment of normal term pregnancy. Am. J. Obstet. Gynecol. 161:1439, 1989.)

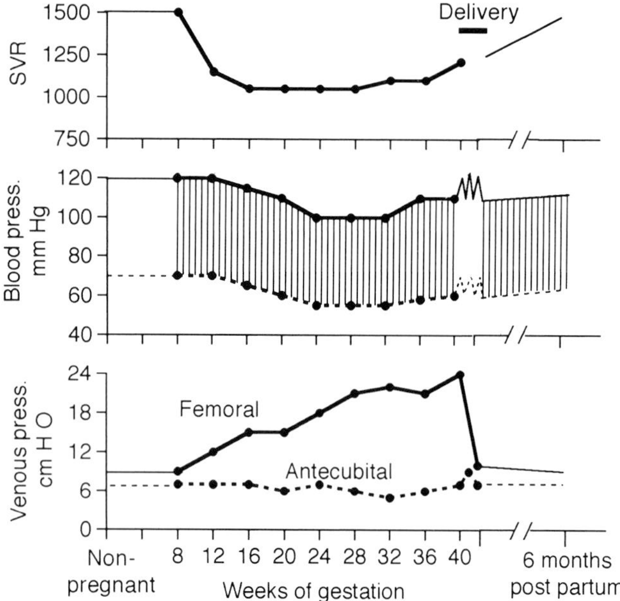


**Fig. 2–17.** Changes in arterial blood pressure, venous pressure, and total peripheral resistance during pregnancy. Note that the venous pressure in the upper limb remains level throughout pregnancy, whereas the pressure in the femoral vein rises progressively due to the progressive increase in encroachment of the inferior vena cava by the gravid uterus. (From Bonica JJ: Obstetric Analgesia and Anesthesia. 2nd Ed. Amsterdam. World Federation of Societies of Anesthesiologists. 1980, p. 2.)

concommitant 20% decrease in systemic peripheral resistance, which apparently more than offsets the increase in cardiac output noted during this period (74,75,77,80,83) (Figure 2–17). In the sitting or standing position, both systolic and diastolic pressures decreased significantly by 8 weeks gestation, and reached their lowest levels of 15 to 20 mm Hg at 15 to 25 weeks. During the last trimester, both systolic and diastolic pressure increased slightly to 8 to 10 mm Hg below the nonpregnant level at term. Both pressures were lower about 10 mm Hg in the lateral decubitus position than in the sitting position (13, 74,80,83).

Central and forearm venous pressures remain normal, but the femoral venous pressure increases progressively as pregnancy advances, and the uterus continues to enlarge and compress the inferior vena cava (and the aorta). This is compensated in part by the diversion of blood through the internal vertebral venous plexus and thence through the azygous venous system which empties into the superior vena cava.

## *Hemodynamic Changes During Parturition*

### Cardiac Output

During labor, cardiac output increases above prelabor, although this increase varies considerably, depending upon the prelabor value of cardiac output, the stage of labor, the intensity of pain, degree of anxiety and fear, and, most importantly, the position of the parturient in which cardiac output is measured. Several studies (84–87) in which measurements were made with patients in the *supine position*, suggest that between contractions, cardiac output is increased above prelabor as follows: during the early first stage (3 cm cervical dilatation, CxD), 10 to 15%; during mid-first stage (4–7 cm CxD) 15 to 20%; during the late first stage (8 cm CxD), 25 to 35%; during the second stage about 40 to 50%; in the third stage (immediately after delivery) 60 to 80% above prelabor; and 1 hour later, about 30 to 40% above prelabor.

Ueland and Hansen (87) studied maternal hemodynamic changes in 23 parturients who underwent induction of labor at term. Of these, 10 were managed with paracervical (PCB) and pudendal block (PB), and 13 were managed with continuous caudal analgesia. Measurements of cardiac output, continuous arterial, central venous, and intrauterine pressures were made before the onset of labor, which served as baseline values. Cardiac output was determined during and between contractions in early and late first stage of labor, in the second stage, immediately following delivery, and at 10 minutes and 1 hour postpartum. Measurements were made between contractions and during contractions with the parturient in the supine position during the first stage, in the lithomy position during the second stage and immediately 10 minutes after delivery, and in the supine position 60 minutes postpartum. Ueland and Hansen noted a progressive increase in cardiac output throughout labor.

Figure 2–18 shows increases of mean values of cardiac output between contractions in the 10 parturients managed with PCB/PB, which the authors called "local anesthesia," and they were as follows: early first stage about 13%; mid-first stage 26%; late first stage 40%; second stage 50%; immediately after delivery 80%; 10 minutes postpartum, 50%; and 1 hour postpartum, 40% above prelabor values. Because of a 22% increase in stroke volume and an 8% decrease in heart rate, contractions consistently increased cardiac output about 15% above values between contractions. This modest increase in cardiac

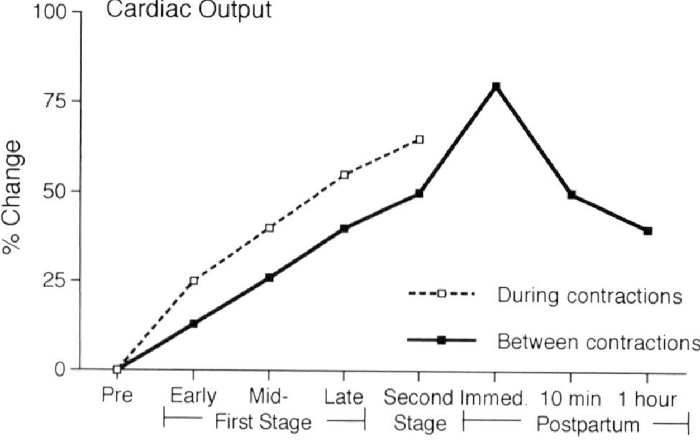


**Fig. 2–18.** Cardiac output during various phases of labor, between contractions, and during contractions measured in 10 parturients in the supine position managed with PCB and PB. Note a progesssive increase between contractions and a further 15 to 25% increase during contractions. (Developed from data of Hansen JM, Ueland K: The influence of caudal analgesia on cardiovascular dynamics during normal labor and delivery. Acta. Anaesthesiol. Scand. 23(Suppl.):49, 1966.)

**Table 2–7.** Effects of Posture on Maternal Cardiovascular Dynamics (Figures Represent Mean Values and 1 Standard Deviation (+) to Nearest Decimal or Unit)

| Position | Cardiac Output (l/min) | Stroke Volume (ml) | Heart Rate (Rate/min) |
|---|---|---|---|
| Supine | 5.15 (+1.3) | 59 (+14) | 90 (+14) |
| Lateral | 6.27 (+20) | 75 (+27) | 85 (+14) |
| Mean % Change | +22 | +27 | −6 |

* Before induction of labor. (From Ueland K, Hansen JM: Maternal cardiovascular dynamics: III. Labor and delivery under local and caudal analgesia. Am. J. Obstet. Gynecol. 103:8, 1969).

**Table 2–8.** Effects of Uterine Contractions on Maternal Cardiovascular Dynamics (Figures Represent Mean Values and 1 Standard Deviation (+) to Nearest Decimal or Unit)

| Condition | Cardiac Output (l/min) | Stroke Volume (ml) | Heart Rate (per min) |
|---|---|---|---|
| Between Contractions | 5.66 (+1.4) | 68 (+20) | 86 (+14) |
| During Contractions | 6.53 (+1.7) | 83 (+15) | 80 (+10) |
| Mean % Change | +15 | +22 | −8 |

output during uterine contractions is lower than that found by other investigators (35,85,88) whose studies suggested that uterine contractions increased cardiac output 20 to 30% above levels between contractions. The lower values obtained by Ueland and Hansen (86) were probably due to the fact that these patients had fairly good pain relief with paracervical and pudendal blocks. This is also suggested by the fact that among the 13 parturients managed with continuous caudal analgesia, the degree of increase in cardiac output between contractions and during contractions was significantly less, presumably due to a more effective degree of pain relief (see Chapter 9, Figure 9–20).

Ueland and Hansen (87) also studied the effects of maternal position and uterine contractions on cardiovascular dynamics in 23 patients who underwent induction of labor at term. Cardiac hemodynamics and pressures were measured before induction of labor and again once labor had been established and the cervix was 4 to 6 cm dilated. Table 2–7 shows the effects of posture on maternal hemodynamics in 20 gravidae before induction of labor was initiated. As noted, a change in the position from supine to lateral produced increases of 22% of cardiac output and 27% in stroke volume with a concomitant decrease of 6% in heart rate. This influence of position on cardiac output in gravidae has already been emphasized and is due to the fact that in the supine position there is obstruction of the inferior vena cava and other large veins in the lower part of the body causing a decrease in venous return and consequent lower cardiac output. When patients are turned on their side, the venous return is mostly relieved, and the pool of blood in the legs allowed to return to the general circulation, maintaining cardiac output at a higher resting level.

Table 2–8 contains data on the effects of uterine contractions on maternal cardiovascular dynamics in 23 parturients in early labor before analgesia was given and measurements made in the supine position. Thus, it is noted that uterine contractions caused a 15% increase in cardiac output produced by a 22% increase in stroke volume and 8% decrease in heart rate. Table 2–9 shows the effects of both posture and uterine contractions on maternal cardiovascular dynamics in nine parturients in early labor before sedation or analgesia was given. In this group, measurements of cardiac output, heart rate, and blood pressure were carried out in the supine position and then in the lateral position, both between contractions and during contractions. With patients in the supine position, uterine contractions caused increases of 25% in cardiac output, 33% in stroke volume, 18% in systolic blood pressure, 13% in diastolic pressure, 26% in pulse pressure, and a concomitant 15% decrease in heart rate. When the parturients were placed in the lateral position, uterine contractions produced significantly lower increases in the various parameters. Ueland and Hansen (86) explained these changes as follows: uterine contractions cause a significant amount (300 to 500 ml) of blood to be squeezed out from the uterus into the central circulation and, consequently, an increased venous return to the heart. This causes an increase in stroke volume and heart rate that results in an increase in cardiac output, followed by a rise in arterial pressure and reflex bradycardia.

In the supine position, uterine contractions also occlude the aorta, the volume redistribution is confined to the vascular tree above the obstruction and results in an augmented response in cardiac output. However, with the patient on her side, the vena caval obstruction is partially relieved and the pool of blood in the lower extremities allowed to return to the central circulation. A uterine contraction in this position does not cause obstruction of the aorta, and the volume redistribution encompasses the entire vascular tree and results in a much smaller change in maternal hemodynamics, thus explaining the smaller increase in cardiac output produced by uterine contractions in the lateral position.

Robson and associates (88), using the same noninvasive technique mentioned in the preceding section (Doppler and cross-sectional echocardiography), carried out serial measurements of cardiac output and mean arterial pressure in 15 women in the lateral position. Measurements were made first between the thirty-eighth and thirty-ninth weeks of gestation, during the first stage of labor, and at 1 and 24 hours after delivery. All parturients had an uncomplicated labor and a spontaneous vertex delivery and were given meperidine and nitrous oxide-oxygen for analgesia. Between contractions, cardiac output in L/min increased from a prelabor value of 6.99 to 7.49 at 4 cm CxD, and to 7.88 when the cervix was dilated at greater than 8 cm CxD. At 1 hour and 24 hours after delivery, it was 7.41 and 7.09, respectively. The highest value of 7.88 L/min reflects a 13% increase above prelabor. Over the same period, basal mean arterial pressure also increased. During uterine contractions there was a further increase in cardiac output as a result of increases in both stroke volume and heart rate. The increment in cardiac output during contractions became progressively greater as labor

**Table 2–9.** Effect of Posture & Uterine Contractions (UC) on Maternal Cardiovascular Dynamics (Figures Represent Mean Values and 1 Standard Deviation (+) to Nearest Decimal or Unit)

| Position | Cardiac Output (l/min) | Stroke Volume (ml) | Heart Rate (per min) | Systolic/Diastolic Blood Pressure (mm Hg) | Pulse Mean Pressure |
|---|---|---|---|---|---|
| **Supine** | | | | | |
| Between UC | 5.2(±1.4) | 59(±19) | 93(±17) | 112/70 | 42 |
| During UC | 6.5(±1.3) | 79(±14) | 79(±11) | 132/79 | 53 |
| Mean % Change | +25 | +33 | −15 | +18/+13 | +26 |
| **Lateral** | | | | | |
| Between UC | 6.3(±0.7) | 75(±10) | 80(±10) | 115/71 | 44 |
| During UC | 6.8(±0.9) | 81(±8) | 84(±10) | 126/80 | 46 |
| Mean % Change | +8 | +8 | +5 | +10/+13 | +5 |

(From Ueland K, Hansen JM: Maternal cardiovascular dynamics: II. Posture and uterine contractions. Am. J. Obstet. Gynecol. 103:1, 1969).

advanced; it increased 17% at less than 3 cm CxD, 23% at 4 to 7 cm CxD, and 34% at more than 8 cm CxD (Figure 2–19). There were also further increases in mean blood pressuring during contractions. One hour after delivery, heart rate and cardiac volume remained raised. By 24 hours after delivery, all hemodynamic variables had returned to prelabor values.

It is to be noted that the actual cardiac output values in L/min during prelabor and during the early part of the

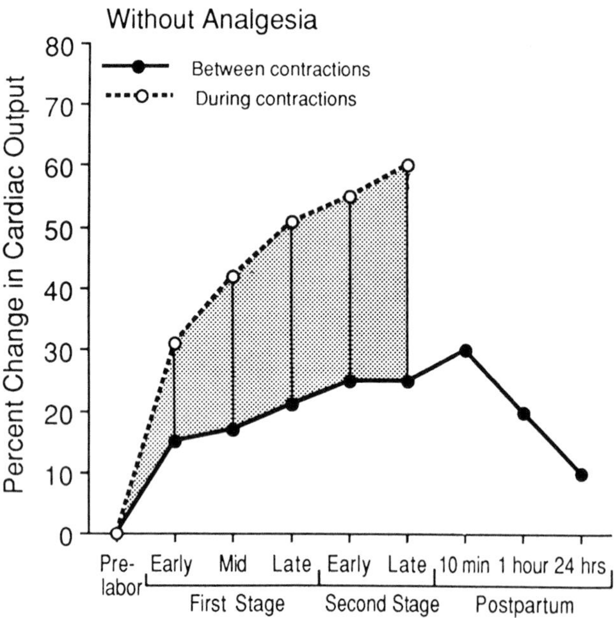


**Fig. 2–19.** Cardiac output during various phases of labor between contractions and during contractions measured in parturients in the lateral position. Note the difference between the increases shown in this graph and those in Figure 2–18. The increases between contractions are not as great as those seen in parturients in the supine position (Fig. 2–18), whereas the increases during contractions are much greater with the patient in the lateral position than in the patients in the supine position. This is due to the fact that there is less obstruction on the inferior vena cava and consequently more blood returns to the heart. (Developed from data by Robson SC, et al: Cardiac output during labour. Br. Med. J. 195:1169, 1987.)

active phase of the first stage were similar to those reported by Ueland and Hansen (87) when they measured cardiac output with the patient in the lateral position and between contractions. The progressively greater increase in cardiac output as labor advanced is not unexpected because during the latter part of the first stage and during the second stage, uterine contractions become progressively stronger and cause greater degress of pain. The fact that these values of cardiac output increase during contractions were greater than those reported by Ueland and Hansen (86) (50% increase) may be due to the parturients studied by Robson and associates (88) had insufficient pain relief produced by meperidine and nitrous oxide-oxygen, whereas those studied by Ueland and Hansen had better pain relief with paracervical and pudendal block (See Figure 9–20, Chapter 9).

## *Cardiovascular Responses During Each Contraction*

Ealier, Hendricks (85) reported on the hemodynamics of individual uterine contractions. Hendricks found that in most patients, cardiac output began to increase very early in the contraction, long before the patient could possibly be aware contractions were underway. Correlation with the amniotic fluid pressure showed that cardiac output began to increase when the pressure had risen by only about 3 mm Hg above the tonus level and reached an apex about 18 seconds before maximum amniotic fluid pressure was obtained. The pattern (Figure 2–20) was found to be identical whether the contractions were spontaneous or the result of intravenous oxytocin. Hendricks (85) further noted that the cardiac output was modified greatly by direct physical effort, anxiety, fright, or pain. In one patient Hendricks noted a prompt rise in cardiac output of nearly 500 ml when the parturient was startled by the noise caused by the dropping of a bedpan. Another patient in late labor, who was experiencing a combination of disturbing factors, had an increase in cardiac output during each contraction of as much as 2,500 ml. Hendricks (85) also noted a correlation between uterine contractions, blood pressure, heart rate, stroke volume, and venous pressure.

Figure 2–21 depicts the variation in heart rate and stroke volume during a uterine contraction. As may be noted, during each contraction there is first an increase

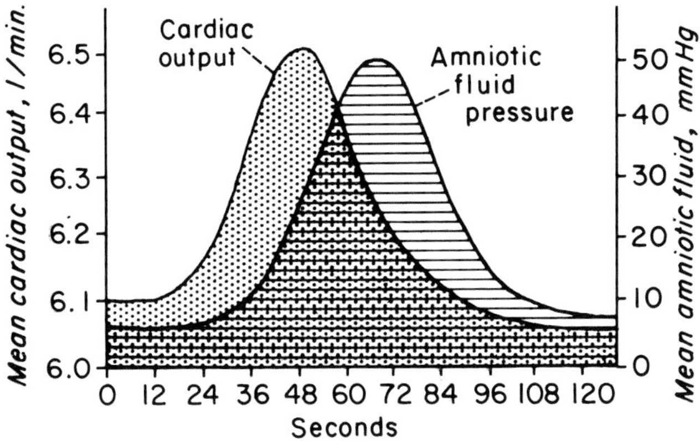


Fig. 2–20. Changes in cardiac output during uterine contraction. The mean cardiac output (as indicated by the pulse pressure method) for 20 complete contraction cycles shows a rise extremely early in the contraction and reaches an apex about 18 seconds before the maximum amniotic fluid pressure is reached. (Modified from Hendricks CH: Hemodynamics of Uterine Contractions. Am. J. Obstet. Gynecol. 76:969, 1958.)

in heart rate as the contraction develops, promptly followed by a decrease in rate which is now significantly (10 to 15%) lower than the rate between contractions, and, finally, as the uterus relaxes there is a gradual return to the original resting rate. During each contraction the stroke volume varies consistently in the opposite direction from variation in a cardiac rate, i.e., there is initially a small drop, but as the contraction develops there is a rise of 15 to 25% or more above the resting phase; finally, as the contraction subsides, the stroke volume decreases progressively toward the resting level. Figure 2–22 illustrates the mean variation in arterial blood pressure as found by Hendricks during 20 contraction cycles. Hansen and Ueland (89) noted that during contractions the systolic arterial pressure increased more than in diastolic pressure in all of their patients.

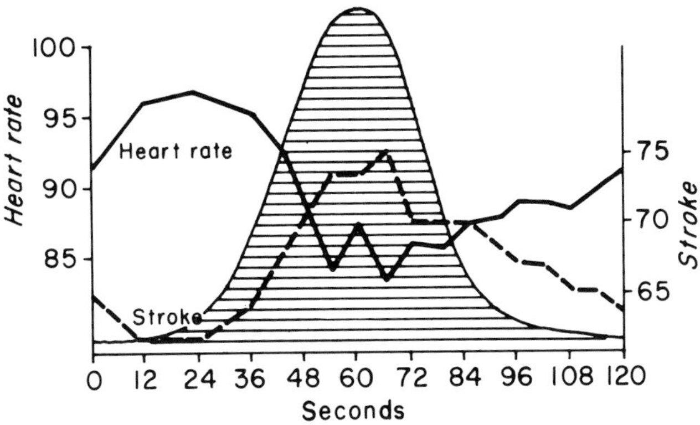


Fig. 2–21. Variations in heart rate and stroke volume during the uterine contraction (cross-hatched area). The mean values of the stroke (as indicated by the pulse pressure method) and of the heart rate were determined at 6-second intervals for 20 complete contraction cycles. There is a consistent reciprocal relation between these two parameters (see text). (Modified from Hendricks CH: Hemodynamics of uterine contractions. Am. J. Obstet. Gynecol. 76:969, 1958.)

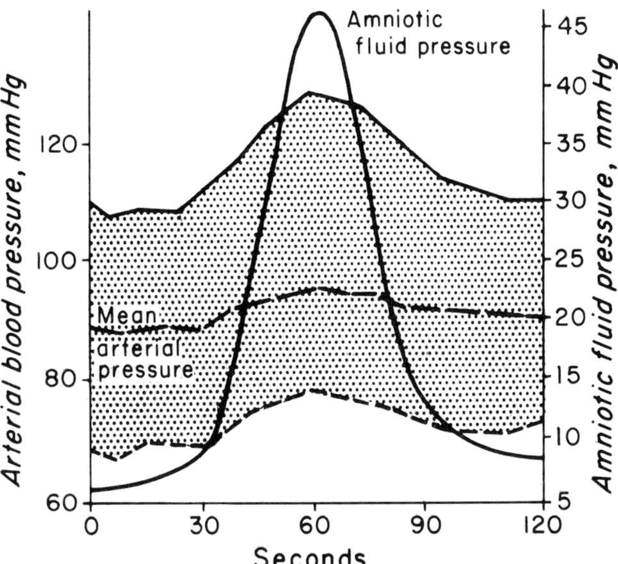


Fig. 2–22. Variation in arterial blood pressure during uterine contraction, indicated here by the amniotic fluid pressure. Although there is considerable variation in the magnitude of blood pressure response, there is a consistent tendency toward rise of pressure, with systolic rise substantially exceeding the diastolic rise. (Modified from Hendricks CH: Hemodynamics of uterine contractions. Am. J. Obstet. Gynecol. 76:969, 1958.)

## Blood Pressures

Arterial systolic and diastolic pressure, central venous pressure, femoral and intrathoracic venous pressure, also increase with each uterine contraction. Systolic arterial blood pressure increases 15 to 25%, diastolic, 10 to 15%

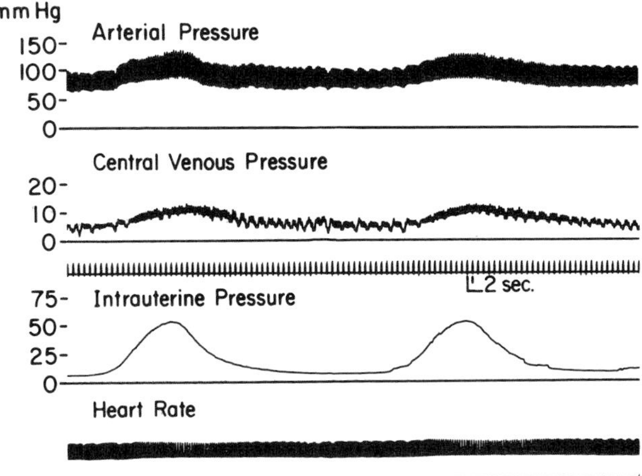


Fig. 2–23. Effect of uterine contractions on arterial and central venous pressure. Note that systolic pressure increases more than diastolic pressure, resulting in an increase in pulse pressure. Also note that the cardiac rate during peak of contractions is significantly decreased. (From Hansen JM, Ueland K: The influences of caudal analgesia on cardiovascular dynamics during normal labor and delivery. Acta Anaesth. Scand. 10(Suppl.)(23):449, 1966.)

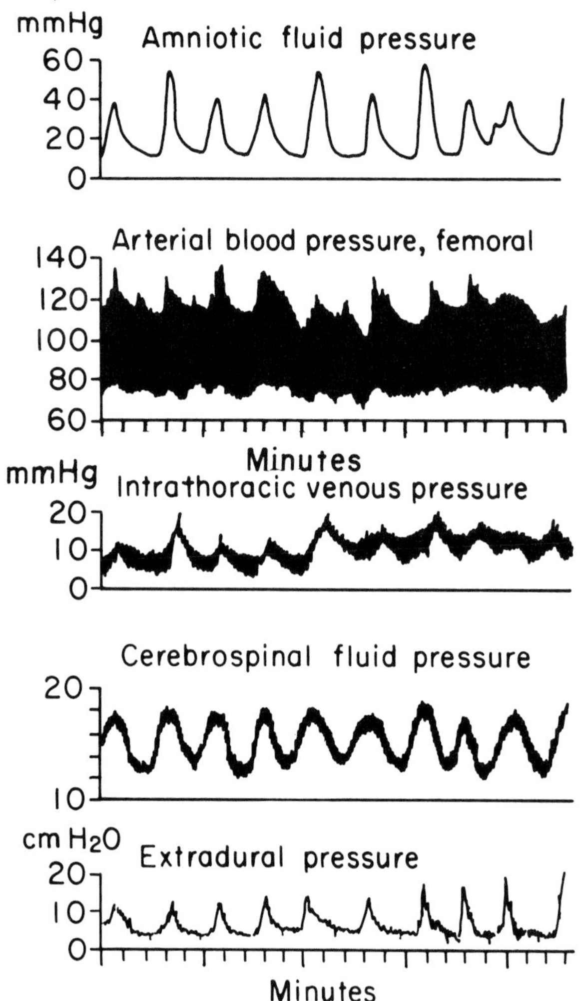


**Fig. 2–24.** Hemodynamic effects of uterine contractions. Note the increases in arterial blood pressure that are reflected in cerebrospinal fluid and extradural pressures.

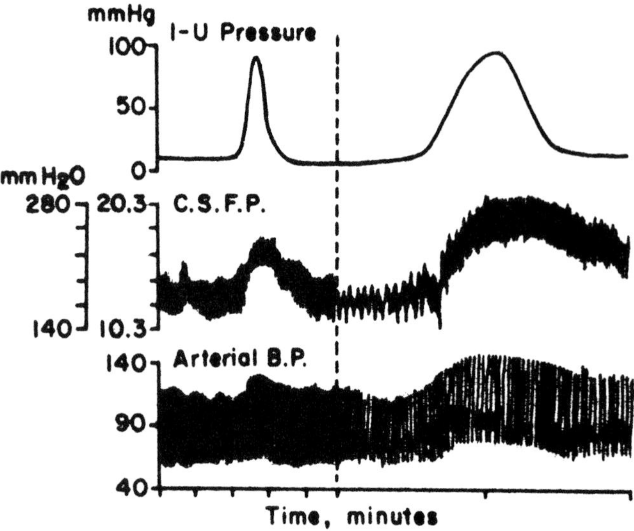


**Fig. 2–25.** Effect of typical uterine contractions on cerebrospinal fluid pressure and the arterial blood pressure. After the first 5 minutes, the recording speed was increased fourfold, so that the final 2 minutes of the record occupy more than half the area illustrated in order to better show time relations. A few seconds after the onset of uterine contractions, the arterial blood pressure began to rise to a maximum increase of about 20 mHg systolic and 10 mmHg diastolic about 35 seconds after the onset of the contractions. The peak in arterial pressure lasted 40 seconds, after which the arterial pressure dropped slowly. The changes in cerebrospinal fluid pressure mirrored those of arterial blood pressure: from an initial level of 167 $mmH_2O$ it began to rise a few seconds after the observed onset of blood pressure rise, attaining its peak of about 280 $mmH_2O$, about 10 seconds after the blood pressure had reached its maximum, remaining at that level for approximately 30 seconds and then subsiding slowly toward precontraction level. Blood pressure and spinal fluid pressure tended to reach their peak before the peak of the intrauterine pressure. (Modified from Hopkins EL, Hendricks CH, Cibils LA: Cerebrospinal fluid pressure in labor. Am. J Obstet. Gynecol. 93:907, 1965.)

(Figures 2–23 and 2–24). The magnitude of these changes varies and depends on the intensity of contractions and the associated pain, anxiety and apprehension, and the position of the parturient (see below). The changes in venous pressure are transmitted rapidly to the internal vertebral venous plexus, and thus cause a transient rise in extradural and cerebrospinal fluid pressure (Figure 2–25). During the second stage, the bearing-down efforts often alter blood pressure in a way similar to the Valsalva maneuver (Figure 2–26). For reasons mentioned above, these changes are greater in the supine than in the lateral position (Figures 2–24, 2–25, 2–26).

## *Aortocaval Compression*

Although the association of arterial hypotension in the supine position in late pregnant women was first recognized half a century ago (90), it was McRoberts (91) who, in 1951, suggested the correct etiology (Figure 2–27). Two years later, Howard, Goodson, and Mengert (92) reported that of 160 consecutive term pregnant women made to lie on their backs, 18 or 11.2% developed acute hypertension within 3 to 7 minutes associated with an increased pulse rate, increased femoral venous pressure, pallor and sweating—all of which disappeared when the women were turned on their sides or stood erect, a phenomenon which the investigators called "supine hypotensive syndrome." Experimental studies in dogs confirmed their hypothesis that the symptomatology was due to occlusion of the inferior cava. Within the decade, a number of investigators reported similar observations, and among other things, it was noted that the condition was aggravated by subarachnoid block (93). A decade after the report by Howard, et al (92), Scott and Kerr (94) used a catheter-transducer-recorder system for continuous measurement of the pressures in the inferior vena cava before and during cesarean section operation. They noted that while the gravida lay supine inferior vena cava (IVC) pressure was significantly higher than in the nonpregnant state, and the usual respiratory excursions were dampened. In the lateral posture, or with manual displacement of the uterus, there was an immediate fall in IVC pressure

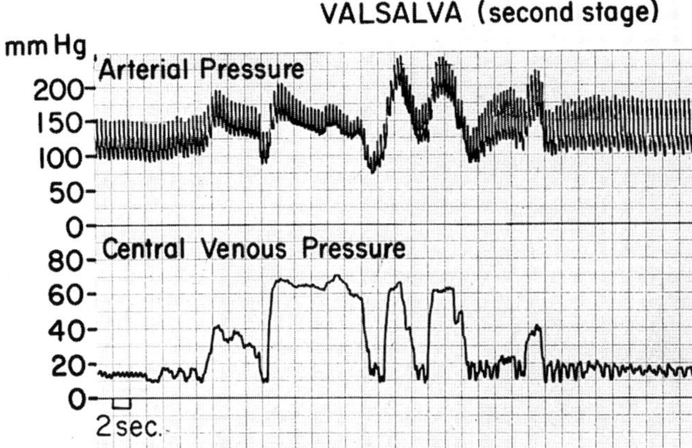


**Fig. 2–26.** Effects of bearing-down efforts on arterial pressure and central venous pressure. As a result of the Valsalva effect produced by each bearing-down effort, there is first a rise in the blood pressure. This is Phase I, or the "strain" phase of the Valsalva maneuver, which is thought to result from blood being forced out of the lungs into the left side of the heart. Since the Valsalva maneuver also impedes thoracic venous inflow, stroke output falls and consequently arterial, systolic, and pulse pressures decrease. Usually, this reduction in pressure (Phase II) begins within several seconds after onset of the acute rise in systemic arterial pressure. During Phase II, the systemic arterial pressure and pulse return toward normal levels. Phase III occurs as forced expiration is terminated and is characterized by a further and abrupt fall in systemic arterial pressure. Phase IV occurs after the release of forced expiration when vasoconstriction produces a characteristic rise in arterial systolic, diastolic, and pulse pressure to heights slightly in excess of normal levels. This phase, commonly called the "overshoot," occurs within 3 to 8 seconds after termination of positive pressure and is often followed by slight bradycardia. (From Hansen JM, Ueland K: The influence of caudal analgesia on cardiovascular dynamics during normal labor and delivery. Acta. Anaesth. Scand. 10(Suppl.)(23):449, 1966.)

concomitant with appearance of a normal respiratory fluctuation. Delivery of the fetus resulted in immediate reduction in IVC pressure with a further fall to the normal nonpregnant level consequent to lifting the empty uterus forward.

A year later, Kerr and a colleague (95) performed bilateral femoral venography with contrast medium (Urografin) in 12 healthy gravidae in the last trimester and noted that in 10 the inferior vena cava was almost completely occluded when examined in the supine position (Figure 2–28). They noted the venous return was redirected to the heart via the vertebral venous plexus and the paraspinal veins that empty into the azygous veins and the ovarian plexuses, which drain the uteroplacental vascular bed, and all enter the inferior vena cava proximal to the site of caval compression (95). In their study, Kerr and associates (94–96) noted that in the lateral position there was passage of some dye up the vena cava, although a significant degree of compression was still evident (Figure 2–28b). Venograms, taken right after the delivery of the infant, showed that the inferior vena cava had returned to normal size and permitted passage of the dye in a normal fashion (Figure 2–28c). It is of interest to note that half a century ago, McLennan (97) measured pressure in the antecubital and femoral veins and noted elevation in femoral venous pressure by 13 to 16 weeks of gestation—a finding that suggested that the hemodynamic consequences of caval compression begin early in pregnancy.

In 1935, Coutts and associates (98) first reported compression of the abdominal aorta and its branches was caused by the pregnant uterus. Some 3 decades later, Biarniz and associates (99), in Montevideo, began a systemic study of the problem by carrying out anteroposterior angiograms for direct visualization which showed significant aortoiliac compression by the uterus in late human pregnancy. They noticed that the uterus was displaced laterally and less densely opacified at the region of the lumbar lordosis (L3-L5) during relaxation; whereas during contraction or in the event of arterial hypotension, the aortic displacement was increased and the common iliac artery crossing the fourth and fifth lumbar vertebra was transiently occluded (Figure 2–29). Biarniz and associates (99) noted that the contracting uterus diminished its surface of support to a small fulcrum, whereas the relaxed uterus obstructed flow at hardly expected high cranial levels where its direct pressure could not reach. They attributed this to indirect effects consisting of kinking of the right renal artery over the convexity of the L1 vertebra due to displacement of the aorta and kidney each in an opposite direction (Figure 2–29). This aortoiliac compression was noted in gravidae between 27 weeks of pregnancy and term gestation. More recently, Marx and associates (100) measured the brachial and femoral arterial pressures in 202 unselected young primigravidae (198 teenagers) taken in both the supine and left lateral position at prenatal visits during the second and third trimester. They noted a decline of femoral pressure in the supine position as early as 19 weeks of gestation.

It has been previously mentioned that Ueland and associates (80,86,87) noted hemodynamic alterations when parturients changed from the lateral to the supine position and that this occurred as early as the twentieth to twenty-eighth weeks of gestation. As previously mentioned, the term pregnant subject in the lateral decubitus position exhibited a right ventricular filling pressure (central venous pressure), which is similar to that of the nonpregnant woman (13). These data suggest the venous return in this position is maintained by collateral circulation despite aortocaval compression. However, in the supine position, right atrial pressure falls substantially (94–96), indicating that the collateral circulation cannot compensate for almost complete obstruction of the inferior vena cava. Moving from the lateral decubitus to supine position, the cardiac filling pressure results in a decrease in stroke volume and cardiac output of about 25 to 30% (80,96,101). It is of interest to note that Milsom and Forssman (101) found that cardiac output in the supine, right lateral, and upright positions were all significantly lower than when the gravidae were in the lateral decubitus position.

In term gravidae, moving from the lateral to the supine position is usually associated with a significant elevation of blood pressure in the upper limb caused by an increase in the systemic vascular resistance consequent to in-

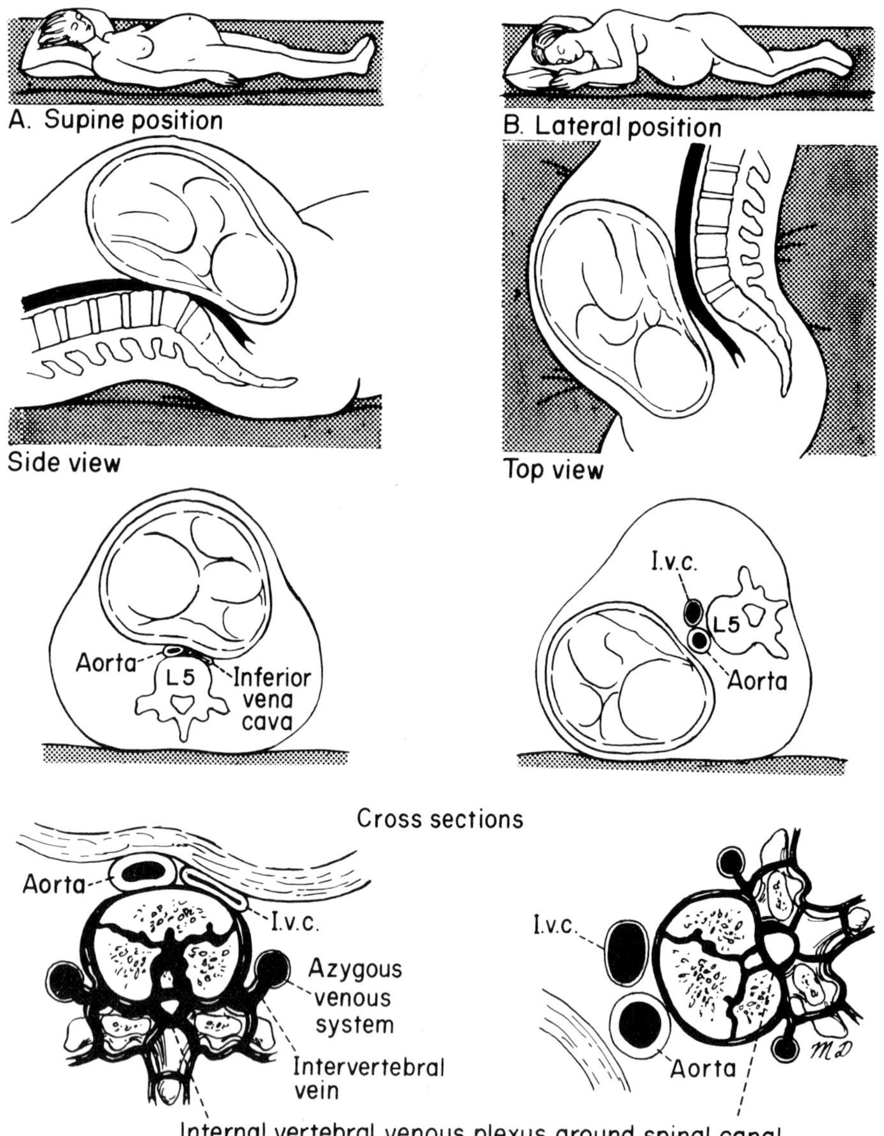


**Fig. 2–27.** The effects of the pregnant uterus on the inferior vena cava and the aorta in the supine position **(A)** and the lateral position **(B).** With the patient supine, the uterus is compressed almost completely against the vertebral column impairing the return of venous blood from the lower limb and pelvis to the heart. This results in diversion of the blood through the azygous system and the internal and external vertebral venous plexuses around the vertebral column and within the spinal canal, as depicted in the lowermost figure. This engorgement significantly decreases the size of the epidural and subarachnoid space in the lower thoracic and lumbar and sacral levels. With the parturient in the lateral position, the uterus falls away from the vertebral column and consequently the compression of the inferior vena cava and other large veins is decreased with consequent decrease in the engorgement of the vertebral venous plexus.

creased sympathetic nervous system outflow. However, in about 5 to 10% of gravidae, the obstruction of the vena cava is so low that despite the compensation of vasoconstriction and initial tachycardia (that is soon followed by bradycardia), blood pressure in the upper part of the body falls precipitously causing the supine hypotensive syndrome (SHS) (Figure 2–30). In one study of five parturients with subclinical supine hypotensive syndrome (SHS), there was a decrease in internal cartoid artery flow velocity of 37% (102). In two of the patients with symptomatic SHS, the internal cartoid flow velocities were below 10 cm/sec compared with control value of 30 cm/sec. In severe cases, this syndrome becomes evident within seconds, but, in moderate cases, hypotension does not develop for 3 to 5 minutes after the patient has assumed the supine position. "Supine hypotensive syndrome" can develop during the second trimester, become maximal at 36 to 38 weeks, and decrease with the descent of the fetal head into the pelvis.

The compression of the lower aorta leads to decreased blood flow to the kidneys, uterus, and lower extremities (96,99). As a result, maternal urine output and kidney function are significantly lower in the supine as compared with the lateral position, and fetal arrhythmia, indicative of fetal-placental insufficiency, may develop soon after the mother assumes a supine position. Compression is relieved when she changes to the left lateral position. In contrast to the caval compression, there is no compensation for the effects of the aortic compression. However, both are prevented or actively treated by left lateral uterine displacement achieved manually, or by a wedge under the right buttock and flank, or by tilting the table 15° to the left (103). In some parturients, right lateral uterine displacement is more effective than left lateral displacement. Which side is best should be determined prior to induction of regional analgesia.

Aortocaval compression also causes a 15 to 20% reduction in uterine blood flow with consequent decline in

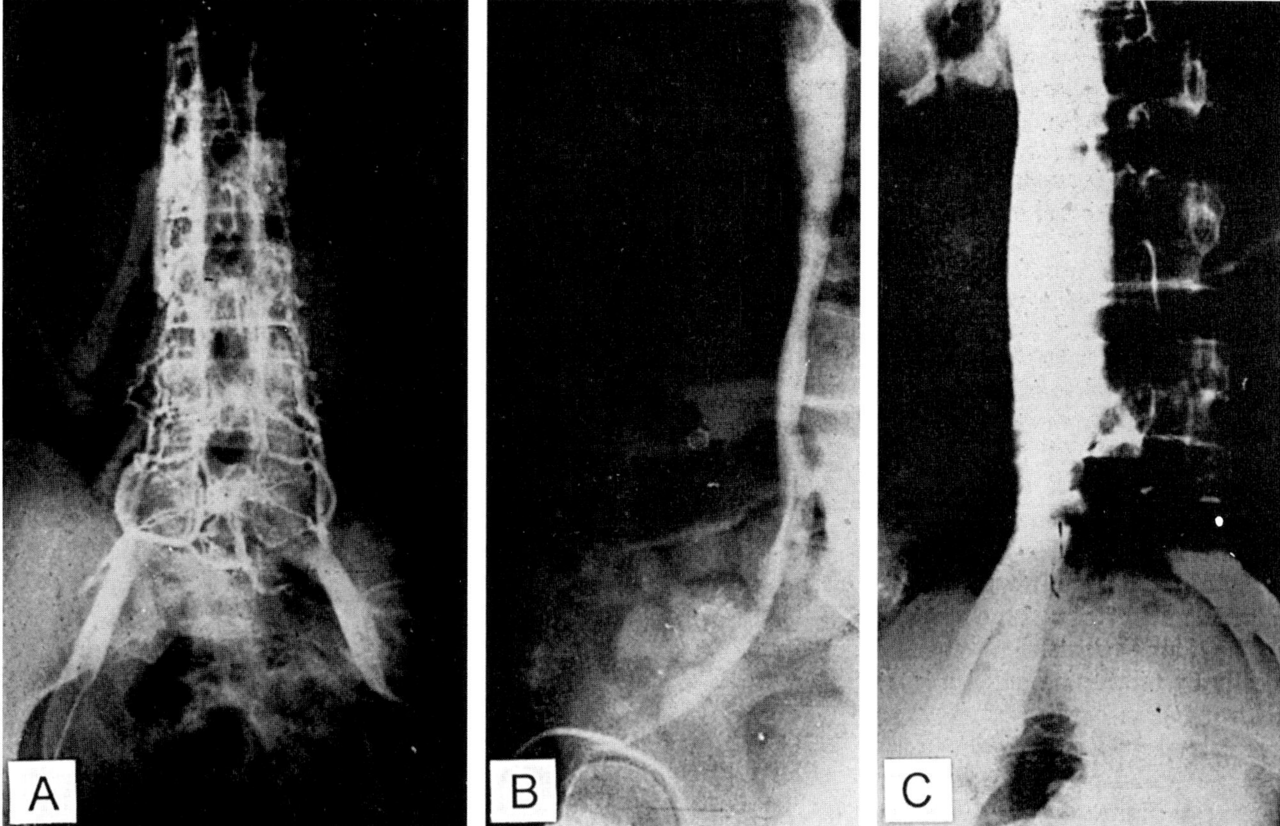


**Fig. 2–28.** Inferior vena cava grams during pregnancy and after delivery. **A)** The inferior vena cavagram in the supine position after injections of dye are made simultaneously into each femoral vein. Little or no dye enters the inferior vena cava. The collateral circulation via the paravertebral veins is clearly seen. **B)** The inferior vena cavagram in the lateral position in late pregnancy (lateral view). The dye is seen to pass through the vena cava, but there is considerable narrowing in the distal 5–10 cm of the vein. **C)** Inferior vena cava gram just after delivery of the fetus. Virtually all of the dye now travels cephalad through the inferior vena cava. (From Scott DB: Inferior vena caval occlusion in late pregnancy and its importance in anesthesia. Am. J. Anaesth. 40:120, 1968)

placental blood flow and perfusion of the placental fetal complex (104,105) (Figures 2–29, 2–30 and 2–31). This is because uterine perfusion pressure is the result of uterine artery pressure minus uterine venous pressure. Consequently, the placental and uterine perfusion pressures are decreased by: 1) compression of a lower aorta with consequent decrease in uterine arterial pressure; and 2) increase in uterine venous pressure due to compression of interior vena cava with consequent venous pooling in the pelvis and lower limbs. Thus, the fetus may be jeopardized by this double effect of aortocaval compression (Figure 2–30). In supine position, even without arterial hypotension, uterine perfusion pressure decreases as a result of increased uterine venous pressure.

Reed and associates (106) noted fetal bradycardia when the mother developed hypotension in the supine position. Hon (107) associated the arrhythmia with maternal hypotension and showed that late deceleration of fetal heart rate occurred while the mother was lying on her back, and that this could be reversed by turning her into a lateral position, regardless of whether or not there was concurrent maternal hypotension. Goodlin (108) noted that in about one-third of laboring parturients in the supine position, the femoral pulse decreased during a uterine contraction, and that this often was associated with subsequent fetal distress and/or maternal hypotension. Humphrey and his colleagues (109) studied the effects of maternal position on the infant in the course of vaginal delivery. Two groups were randomly assigned; one group of mothers delivering in the supine position; the other within 15° leftward tilt. In the offspring of the supine mothers, there was a time-related decrease in pH, whereas acid-base status was maintained within the normal range in the tilted group. Others have shown that a 10 to 15° left-sided downward tilt improves fetal oxygenation as compared to fetuses born of mothers in the supine position (100,109,110).

During labor, the compressive phenomena in the supine position are exaggerated by uterine contractions (Figures 2–29 and 2–31). As the uterus tenses, hardens, and increases its pressure on the major veins and arteries across the pelvic brim, there is often an apparent improvement in the mother's circulation but a hidden deterioration of the fetal environment. Each contraction tips the

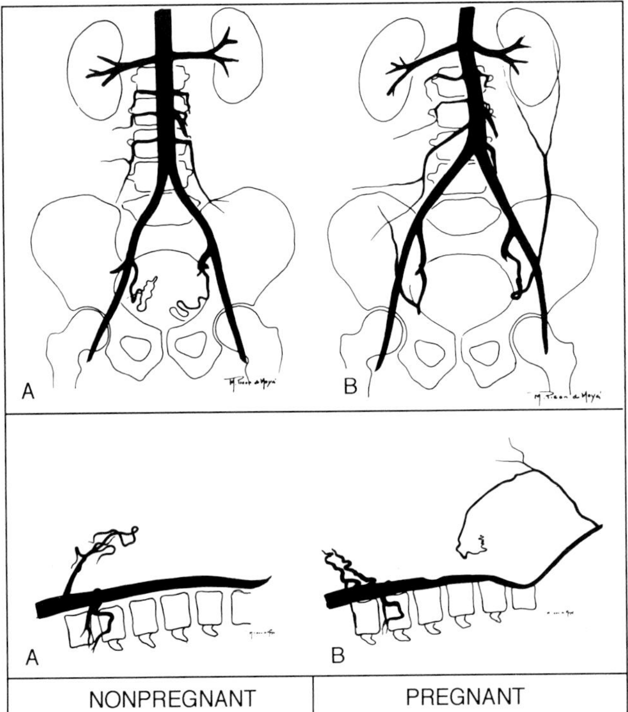


Fig. 2–29. Schematic diagram of the aorta and its branches based on angiograms taken in nonpregnant **(a)** and pregnant women near term **(b).** In the upper panel, the nonpregnant aorta is shown to be straight and uniformly wide, whereas in the pregnant state, it is displaced to the left and cranially as indicated by the more inclined curve of its branches, including the lumbar, renal and common iliac arteries. The latter is displaced in an outward direction so that the angles between them is increased. The lower panel shows the aorta and its branches based on an angiogram taken in the lateral and superior positions. In the nonpregnant state **(a),** there is a clear gap between the vertebral column and the aorta which is uniformly wide. During late pregnancy **(b),** the aorta is clearly displaced in the dorsal direction, encroaching on the shadow of the spine and is narrowed at the level of the lumbosacral region and its branches kinked. (From, and courtesy of, Biarniz J, et al: Aortocaval compression by the uterus in late human pregnancy. Am. J. Obstet. Gynecol. 100: 203, 1978)

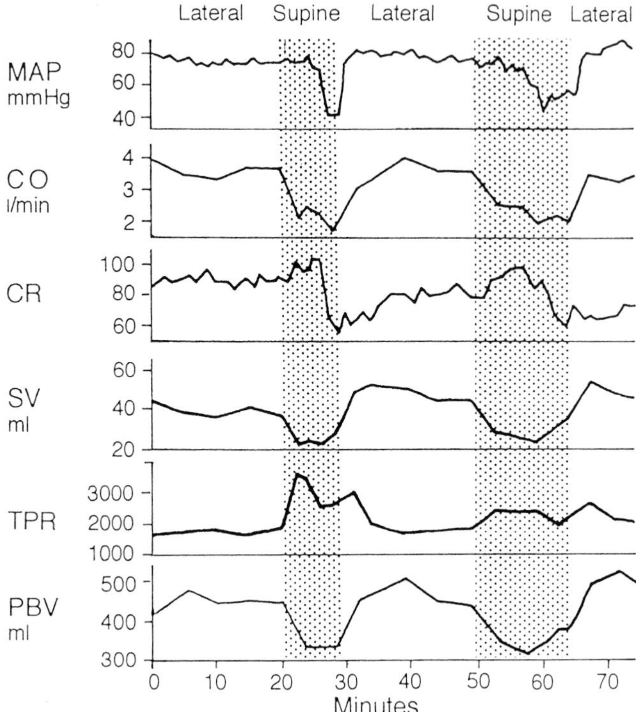


Fig. 2–30. The profound influence of the supine position on maternal hemodynamics in a parturient with the supine hypotensive syndrome. The impairment of venous return consequent to the pressure of the gravid uterus markedly decreased stroke volume (SV) and cardiac rate (CR), and consequently cardiac output (CO), and also reduced pulmonary blood volume (PBV). The compensatory increase in cardiac rate (CR) and total peripheral resistance (TPR) maintained blood pressure for about 5 minutes, but then the patient developed a marked reduction in mean arterial pressure (MAP). (Modified from and courtesy of Scott DB. Br. J. Anaesth. 40:120–128, 1968.)

uterus around a fulcrum formed by the lumbosacral vertebral prominence, and aortic compression is increased, leading to a hyperdynamic circulation above the compression but further deterioration below it. Consequently, there is a steep rise of maternal cardiac output and a hypertensive rise of blood pressure above the obstruction but a fall below it, as depicted in Figure 2–31. Figure 2–32 depicts the degree of compression of the lower aorta, iliac, and femoral arteries that can occur during uterine contractions in the supine position, with a consequent, significant decrease in uteroplacental blood flow. Figure 2–33 depicts the significant decrease in the pressure of the femoral arteries during each uterine contraction—called the Poseiro effect—with a concomitant increase in brachial artery pressure. As previously emphasized, the supine position will impair placental function with consequent deleterious impact on the fetus (Figure 2–34). Moreover, almost the entire 300 to 500 ml of blood squeezed out of the uterus are forced into the extradural and azygous systems during contractions, causing heightened peaks of extradural venous pressure (Figure 2–25).

## CLINICAL IMPLICATIONS

The above changes in blood volume, blood constituency, and hemodynamics produced by pregnancy, parturition, and puerperium are of great relevance to anesthetic care. The increase in blood volume increases cardiac preload, but this is compensated for by the significant reduction in the afterload consequent to the reduction of total peripheral resistance and blood viscosity. Although this hyperdynamic state increases cardiac workload and predisposes the development of functional murmurs, healthy gravidae have no impairment in the usual range (13,80). On the other hand, in gravidae with heart disease and consequent low myocradial reserve, the increase in work of the heart may constitute too great a strain and may precipitate pulmonary congestion. In such patients it is especially important to obviate further increase in the

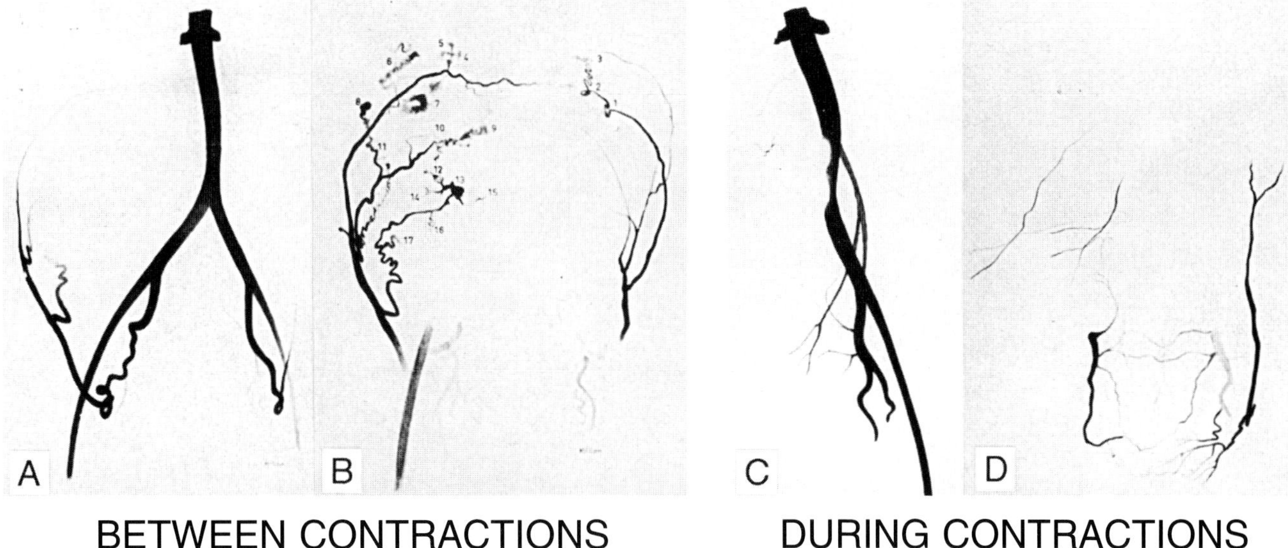


**Fig. 2–31.** Schematic illustration of the aorta and its branches based on anteroposterior angiograms taken between contractions (**a** and **b**) and during contractions (**c** and **d**). When the uterus was relaxed, the aorta was clearly displaced to the left, narrowed at L3–5 and less opacified here than proximally and distally to that region. Dye clearance was more rapid through the densely opacified internal iliac and uterine arteries than the through the external iliac, illustrating preferential flow toward the placenta. The overgrown uterine arteries coursed in an outward direction. In this gravida, the right uterine artery formed three wide arcuate branches, multiple spirals, and entries into the intervillous space, indicating good placental supply. The left uterine artery supplied only a small part of the placenta. The ovarian arteries are not visualized. During a contraction (**c** and **d**), the aorta was compressed, narrowed and displaced more than in the relaxed uterus, and completely occluded the right common iliac and uterine arteries. The only supply route through the left uterine artery was also obstructed, and its flow was retarded as compared with conditions between contractions. The intramural branches of the uterine artery were occluded at their entry into the contracting myometrium, markedly diminishing placental perfusion. (From, and courtesy of, Biarniz J, et al: Aortocaval compression by the uterus in late human pregnancy. Am. J. Obstet. Gynecol. 100:203, 1978.)

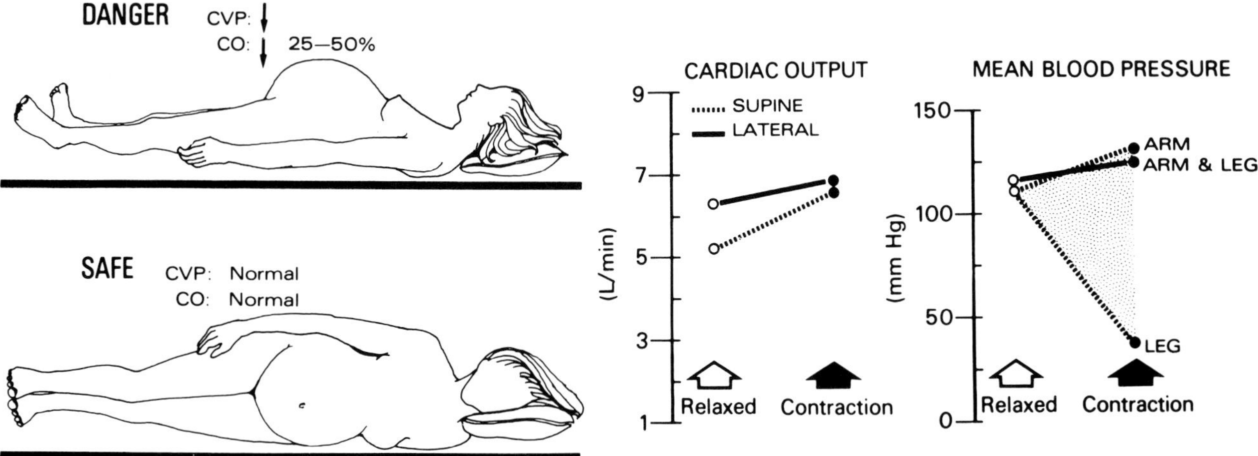


**Fig. 2–32.** Cardiovascular effects of posture and uterine contractions. The *left panel* shows the hazards of the supine position, which causes a decrease in central venous pressure and cardiac output; however, these promptly return to normal when the parturient assumes the lateral position. The *right panel* shows the changes in cardiac output and blood pressure during and between contractions. During contractions in the supine position, the cardiac output increases and pressure rises in the upper limb but falls in the lower limb because of partial aortic obstruction during uterine contractions. This effect is avoided by placing the parturient in the lateral position, which facilitates return of blood from the lower limbs to the general circulation so that cardiac output and blood pressure are maintained at a high resting level between contractions. Consequently, during contractions, the increase in cardiac output and blood pressure is less than in the supine position. (Courtesy of Bromage PR: Epidural Analgesia. Philadelphia, W.B. Saunders Co., 1978. Constructed from data of Ueland and Hansen, 1969; Galbert and Marx, 1974; and Bieniarz et al, 1968.)

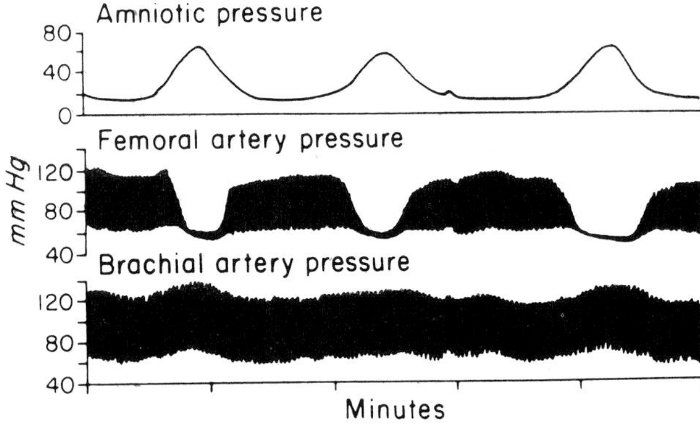


**Fig. 2–33.** Poseiro effect. In this patient each uterine contraction caused a marked fall in pressure in the femoral artery when she assumed the supine position. The systemic arterial pressure rose moderately during each contraction, indicating that the Poseiro effect is a local response caused by compression of the aorta and femoral arteries by the contracting uterus. (Modified from and courtesy of Bieniarz J, Crottogini JJ, Curuchet E, Romero-Salinas G, et al: Aortocaval compression by the uterus in late pregnancy. Am. J. Obstet. Gynecol. 100:203, 1968.)

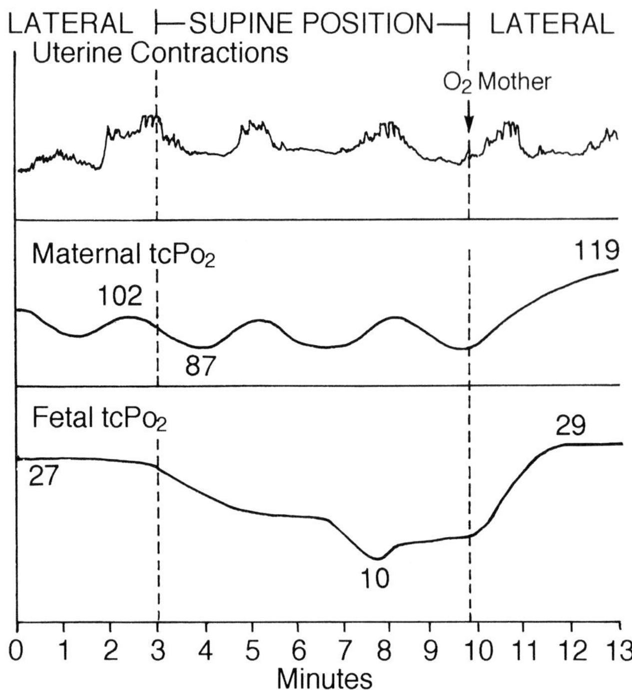


**Fig. 2–34.** The deleterious influence of the supine position on fetal oxygen tension. Continuous monitoring of uterine contractions and maternal and fetal oxygen tension obtained by the transcutaneous technique. Note that with each uterine contraction the maternal oxygen tension increases and between contractions it decreases due to maternal hypoventilation consequent to the respiratory alkalosis. However, this has little effect on fetal oxygen tension. When the mother assumed the supine position, uterine contraction and maternal oxygen tension continued to maintain the same profile, but the fetal $tcPO_2$ gradually decreased to 10 torr. When the mother was asked to turn to the lateral position and given oxygen by mask, the maternal oxygen tension steadily increased and the fetal oxygen tension turned to slightly above the level before positional changes. (Modified from Huch A, et al: Continuous transcutaneous monitoring of fetal oxygen tension during labour. Br. J. Obstet. Gynaecol. 84(Suppl 1):1, 1977.)

work of the heart during labor by providing effective analgesia, preferably with continuous epidural analgesia (see Chapters 9 and 13).

The diversion of blood consequent to the venous compression causes the internal vertebral venous plexus to become greatly engorged (45,111), and the capillary circulation of the meninges is slowed. These changes and some biochemical factors make it necessary to reduce the volume and amount of local anesthetic to achieve subarachnoid or epidural block for labor and vaginal delivery to a specific level, a reduction to about two-thirds of that used for nonpregnant women (111). The reduced need for local anesthetics is present regardless of the position of the gravida and despite the immediate effect of left uterine displacement. Moreover, the slowed capillary meningeal circulation delays the absorption of these drugs into the blood, leaving more for the target nerves, and thus decreases the latency (time of onset) and increases the duration of analgesia (5). Although some reports (112,113) dispute this effect, extensive clinical experience confirms this phenomenon. Recent evidence suggests that factors other than the engorgement of epidural veins, which reduces the volume of cerebrospinal fluid and enhances the cephalad spread of local anesthetics. These include: 1) increased neurosensitivity to local anesthetics (114–117); 2) reduced cerebrospinal fluid protein concentration (118), which increases local anesthetic effectiveness by reducing protein binding; and 3) elevated cerebrospinal fluid pH (119), which increases the proportion of un-ionized local anesthetic thus facilitating movement across neural membranes.

The local anesthetic dose required for segmental or standard lumbar epidural analgesia for labor and vaginal delivery requires 25 to 40% reduction of the dose compared with nonpregnant patients (111,113). In contrast, the administration of a large dose of local anesthetic as used for cesarean section produces the same spread of epidural anesthesia in term pregnant and nonpregnant patients (112,113). This issue is discussed in great detail in Chapter 13.

The fluctuation in cerebrospinal fluid (CSF) pressure produced by uterine contractions, bearing-down efforts, or straining, promotes turbulent current in the cerebrospinal fluid compartment. Consequently, injection of a local anesthetic into the subarachnoid space during such conditions may result in abnormally high spinal anesthesia. This may be accentuated by the exaggerated lumbar lordosis of pregnant women.

The postural hemodynamic changes make it mandatory that gravidae avoid the supine position during the second and third trimester of pregnancy and labor. Moreover, because induction of spinal or extradural anesthesia or other procedures that entail vasomotor blockade deprives gravidae of a compensatory vasoconstriction, they are likely to incur much greater falls in arterial blood pressure than nonpregnant patients (see Chapter 16). Unless prophylactic measures are carried out, severe hypotension may develop to a degree such as to threaten the life of the mother and fetus. Prophylactic measures include infusion of 800 to 1,000 ml of fluids before the block, placement of the parturient on her side during the duration of anesthesia and labor, and effective lateral displacement of the uterus during the delivery. Unilateral predominance of the block can be avoided by having the patient change sides every 2 to 3 minutes during the induction period. It is also desirable to ascertain the degree of compression and consequent supine hypotension before the induction of a block by measuring blood pressure with the patient on her side and measuring again at 2, 4, and 6 minutes after the patient has been in a supine position. This will permit diagnosis of supine hypotension in those gravidae who have delayed onset of the condition.

During the immediate postpartum period when the greatest increase in cardiac output occurs, the patient is able to maintain normal blood pressure by compensatory vasodilation. If the obstetric team deprives the mother of this compensatory vasodilation by administering the oxytoxic with such vasoconstrictor action as ergonovine maleate (Ergotrate) and/or such potent peripheral vasopressors as methoxamine (Vasoxyl) or phenylephrine (Neosynephrine), severe hypertension may develop which, in some patients, may cause a cerebrovascular accident. For this reason, it is preferable to use oxytocin and ephedrine to increase uterine contractility and blood pressure, respectively, during the delivery.

## CHANGES IN THE ALIMENTARY SYSTEM

### *Gastrointestinal Tract*

#### Stomach

During pregnancy, the stomach and intestines are progressively displaced cephalad by the enlarging uterus, the axis of the stomach is rotated to the right about 45° and is shifted from a vertical to a horizontal with the pylorus displaced upward and posteriorly, and the appendix is higher than the level of the iliac crest. This changes the angle of the gastroesophageal junction, impairs gastric emptying, and may even cause pocketing of gastric contents. There is usually slight diminution of gastric and intestinal tone and motility. Plasma motilin, the hormone that has a stimulative effect upon the smooth muscle of the lower esophageal sphincter and most of the gastrointestinal (GI) tract, is reduced during the latter two-thirds of pregnancy primarily due to increased progesterone, which has an inhibitory effect on the contractile activity of gastrointestinal tissue (120). Plasma motilin regains the prepregnancy level 1 week after delivery (120). The reduction of this hormone during pregnancy could contribute to the lowering of the lower esophageal sphincter pressure (LOSP) and the barrier pressure (BrP), particularly in gravidae who suffer from heartburn (121). Several studies (121,122) reveal that in the first trimester of pregnancy, lower esophageal sphincter pressure, barrier pressure, and gastric pressure (GP) were normal in the supine position, but that there was a significant reduction in lower esophageal sphincter pressure and barrier pressure in the lithotomy position unrelated to any change in intragastric pressure. These findings suggest that the lithotomy position is associated with increased risk or regurgitation even in early pregnancy.

Another factor that increases the risk of regurgitation is the presence of hiatal hernia, which is increased during pregnancy, especially in gravidae who are elderly or overweight or gravidae who have a particularly high intraabdominal pressure that may be related to multiple pregnancy, hydramnios, and other factors. Regurgitation of acid-stomach contents is common with hiatal hernia and is the cause of severe heartburn, esophagitis, and dysphagia, which is most likely due to an incompetent gastroesophageal sphincter. Lind and colleagues (121) measured mean intragastric pressure (MIP), maximum sphincter resistance (MSR), and pressure gradient (PG) in cm of water in 10 nonpregnant subjects and 20 gravidae in the final 2 months of pregnancy, resulting in the following: nonpregnant subjects—mean intragastric pressure 12; maximum sphincter resistance 35; pressure gradient 23; in gravidae without heartburn,17, 45, and 28, respectively; in gravidae with heartburn, the figures were 17, 24, and 7, respectively. Although it is obvious that sphincter pressure in those with heartburn was significantly lower than that measured in the other two groups, evidence of reflux, which suggests low barrier pressure, can be found even in pregnant patients who do not suffer from heartburn (123).

Gastric secretion of acid and pepsin is diminished during the first two trimesters of pregnancy, but during the final trimester it tends to increase and at term is above normal levels. Aspirates of gastric juice collected for 45 minutes from fasting gravidae yielded 79 ± 20 ml in the first trimester, 36 ± 12 ml in the second trimester, and 107 ± 28 ml in the last trimester, compared with 63 ± 8 ml in nonpregnant controls (124).

During pregnancy gastrin induces the secretion of water, electrolytic enzymes from within the upper gastrointestinal tract and by the pancreas, but it has no consistent effect upon gastric emptying time. This hormone is found to be increased in maternal blood throughout pregnancy and may play a role in increasing gastric residue noted in gravidae. Moreover, the concentration of gastrin in maternal blood has been found to rise during labor, to fall 30 minutes postdelivery, and to be higher in cord blood than in the maternal blood at delivery, suggesting that it was produced within the fetal-placental unit (124).

At about 15 weeks of gestation, over two-thirds of gravidae have a pH of 2.5 or less, about 50% have a volume of 25 ml or more, and, consequently, they are at risk of aspiration or regurgitation if a general anesthetic is given (124–127). Several studies (16a,124,125) have shown that at term 71% of parturients have a gastric pH of 2.5 or less compared with an instance of 87% among nonpregnant individuals. The volume in the stomach was found to be 25 ml or more in 59% of parturients, compared with 44% of nonpregnant subjects. Based on these data, Conklin (16a,124,125) concluded that the percentage of parturients at risk, i.e., those that have a pH of 2.5 or less and have a volume of 25 ml or more, was 49% at term versus 42% among nonpregnant subjects. He stated that "based on criteria of gastric volume and acidity, pregnant patients who have been without oral intake in preparation for elective cesarean section appear to be at little, if any, greater risk for aspiration pneumonitis than are nonpregnant individuals for elective surgery."

During labor the function of the gastrointestinal tract varies depending on circumstances. Radiographic studies in women who had no pain revealed that gastric performance was not altered (5). However, the pain of uterine contractions and any associated anxiety and stress produces segmental- and suprasegmental-reflex inhibition of gastrointestinal motility and function with consequent significant delay in gastric emptying (see Chapter 22). In a study of 52 term gravidae admitted to the hospital in active labor, the volume of gastric juice was greater than 40 ml in 36 (69%) compared to only 59% of those at term but not in labor, and the pH was below the critical level of 2.5 in 22 (52%) (126). Others have found that the mean gastric volume increases during labor (127–129). However, only 36% of patients in labor were found to have a gastric pH of 2.5 or less (126), and only 23% met the criteria of being "at risk" as defined by Conklin (16a).

Epidural analgesia achieved with local anesthetics has no effect on gastric volume or acidity and, indeed, may reverse the effects of the pain. However, if opioids are added to the local anesthetic, they may delay gastric emptying—an effect that has been shown in surgical patients (136) and in one study in obstetric patients in labor (137).

These reflex effects of nociception are aggravated in the recumbent position and by opioid analgesics and related drugs (127,131). In one study, the mean volume of a 750 ml test meal retained in the stomach of 8 women 30 minutes after ingestion was 221 ml during late pregnancy, but 339 ml during labor (130). Food may be retained for 24 to 36 hours during labor, and gastric juice and swallowed air may accumulate progressively (128,131). The delayed gastric emptying caused by opioid analgesia was shown by Holdsworth (128), who found the largest volume of gastric content among parturients who had received meperidine during labor and the smallest in those who had received either epidural or no analgesia. Similar findings were reported by Nimmo and associates (130), who used the acetaminophen absorption test as an indicator of the rate of gastric emptying. This effect is discussed further in Chapter 19. The issue of reducing the acidity of the gastric juice effectively by oral administration of antacid (126) is also discussed in Chapter 19.

### *Small Intestine*

The motility of the small bowel is reduced during pregnancy, and, consequently, transit time from the stomach to secum averages 58 ± 12 hours in the second trimester, compared with 52 ± 10 hours in the nonpregnant state (138). Absorption of nutrients from the small bowel, with the exception of enhancement of absorption of iron, is unchanged during pregnancy.

### *Large Intestine*

The tone and activity of the large intestines are reduced during pregnancy with a resulting tendency to constipation among gravidae—another effect of the reduced concentration of plasma motilin (120). Because the hormone does not regain its prepregnancy level until about 1 week postpartum, most puerperae do not have a bowel action until the third or possibly the fourth postpartum day, an effect that can be aggravated by the inhibiting effect of perineal pain. In addition to decrease in motilin, other factors that cause constipation include mechanical obstruction by the uterus and increased water absorption from the colon (138). Parry and associates (139) demonstrated a 59% increase in colonic water absorption and a 45% increase in sodium absorption during pregnancy, an effect which is said to be caused in part by increased alderstone levels. Crawford (1) also pointed out that hemorrhoids, induced in many instances by increased pressure within the pelvic veins and exacerbated or provoked by bearing-down efforts during the second stage and delivery, are a stressful complication in a significant proportion of puerperae and contribute to the incidence of constipation.

## *The Liver*

During pregnancy, the liver remains normal in size, hepatic blood flow is unaltered, and the histologic changes, which consist of mild fatty-swelling (140) lymphatic infiltration and evidence of mild glycogen deficiency, are not nonspecific and insignificant. Changes in hepatic metabolism are reflected in the aforementioned fall in plasma albumin and cholinesterase and rises in some of the globulin fraction. Fibrogen levels are increased 50% by the end of the second trimester, and the levels of ceruloplasmin and the binding proteins for corticosteroids, sex steroids, thyroid hormones, and vitamin D are also increased. Serum levels of bilirubin, aspartate aminotransferase (AST, formerly SGOT), allanine aminotransferase (ALT, formerly SGPT), and 5′-nucleotidase and prothrombin time are unchanged in normal pregnancy (7). Fibrogen levels are increased 50% by the end of the second trimester, while the level of ceruloplasmin and the binding proteins for corticosteroids, sex steroids, thyroid hormones, and vitamin D are also increased. There is an increase in serum alkaline phosphatase activity, as well. Serum cholesterol increases throughout pregnancy, often reaching 400 mg per 100 ml, but maternal and fetal cholesterol esterification remains normal.

Liver-function tests show minor impairment in the latter months of gestation, but this disappears soon after delivery (2,6,140). Bromsulphthalein blood levels decline more slowly in many gravidae than do they in nonpregnant women, but this is not indicative of impaired liver function because the reduced rate of clearance may result from delayed excretion of the dye into the bile or from increased binding of the dye to the plasma proteins (112). Thymol turbidity and cephalin floculation are elevated in 10 to 15% of normal gravidae. This is most likely because of extrahepatic obstruction rather than cellular damage (5).

### Gallbladder

Roentgenographic studies have shown a definite delay in the emptying of the gallbladder (141). This delay, which may be as long as 6 hours, appears to be caused by the widespread decrease in smooth muscle tone during pregnancy and to spasm of the sphincter of Oddi. The decrease in emptying time, together with increase of the cholesterol content of the blood, may be a factor in the causation of cholelithiasis. The gallbladder appears globular and distended in the majority of gravidae, and the bile is more viscid in the gravida than in the nonpregnant woman.

## CHANGES IN THE URINARY SYSTEM

### Kidneys

#### Anatomic Changes

In the second or third month of gestation there begins a progressive dilation of the renal pelvis and calyces and ureters (142). Because of the dextrorotation of the uterus, the right-sided structures are in general affected more frequently and more significantly than the left. That portion of each ureter that is below the pelvic brim appears not to be included in the process (142). This would suggest that these changes are caused primarily by the obstruction of flow due either to the enlarging uterus or to the dilatation of surrounding ovarian plexuses, which are more closely applied to the right ureter than the left. However, the fact that the process starts so early in pregnancy, before uterine enlarging is likely to be operative, also suggests that progesterone, which has a relaxing effect on all smooth muscle, produces a progressive decrease in muscular tone and rhythmic activity. At the end of the second trimester there is complete atony with absence of peristalsis (142). Consequently, the "urinary tract dead space" is enlarged and kidney drainage retarded. The mild hydroureter and hydronephrosis may also be a cause of pain referred to the 10th through 12th thoracic dermatome and can be relieved by having the patient lie on the contralateral side or in the Trendelenburg position. The process may be aggravated significantly during labor and be a source of severe discomfort. Moreover, if the process of damming back the urine is prolonged, as in protracted labor, the use of drugs, which are excreted by the kidneys, may be limited (6).

#### Renal Functional Changes

The effect of renal plasma flow (ERPF) and glomerular filtration rate (GFR) increased rapidly during the early part of gestation and thus increased urine formation (143–145). These changes reflect the larger expiratory load presented to the kidney by the augmented blood volume and cardiac output. As might be expected, the increases in renal function become evident as early as the tenth to twelfth week. Dunlop (145) documented an 80% increase in effective renal plasma flow during early pregnancy, which decreased during the third trimester, but the GFR remained elevated at 50% above nonpregnant levels. This indicated that the filtration fraction (GFR/ERPF) decreased during early pregnancy but increased during the third trimester. Similar results were shown by Ezimokhai and associates (146). Davison and Hytten (147) calculated a 24-hour creatinine clearance to be about 150 ml/min at 25 to 28 weeks of gestation, falling to 130 ml/min in late pregnancy. Renal function and urine formation are influenced significantly by the position of the gravida during the last trimester (Figure 2–35). Compression of the lower aorta and its branches in the supine position is associated with an average reduction of 20% in plasma flow and glomerular filtration, 60% in urine volume, and excretion of sodium and chloride.

The rise in glomerular filtration rate leads to a decrease in plasma levels of urea, nitrogen, and creatinine. Sims and Krantz (144) showed that the average plasma urea nitrogen (PUN) levels in $mg/dL^{-1}$ fell from 13 in the nonpregnant state to about 9 during the tenth to the twenty-ninth weeks of gestation to 8.5 during the last 7 weeks of gestation, and then rose to 13.6 $mg/dL^{-1}$ at 4 to 10 weeks postpartum. The plasma creatinine level in $mg/dL^{-1}$ fell from 0.67 in the nonpregnant state to about 0.46 at 10 to 20 weeks, 0.48 at 31 to 37 weeks, and 0.51 during the last 3 weeks of gestation, and then rose to 0.63 $mg/dL^{-1}$ at 4 to 10 weeks postpartum. Tubular reabsorptive function is modified so that the renal threshhold for certain substances is altered, a phenomenon that is demonstrated by the appearance in the urine of creatinine, glucose, histidine, uric acid, and other solutes normally absent or present in lesser amounts (142). Excretion of water and sodium is part of the pattern of changed homeostasis: progesterone increases the sodium excretion while aldosterone causes sodium retention. Consequently, there is neither excessive accumulation nor depletion of salt and water (5).

### The Urinary Bladder

#### Anatomic Changes

The bladder, like other pelvic organs, undergoes significant anatomic change in the form of hyperemia, hyperplasia of the muscular and connective tissue elements, and a significant deepening and widening of the trigone. In addition, the pressure of the presenting part impairs blood and lymph drainage of the base of the bladder so that this area is often edematous, easily traumatized, and more susceptible to infection than it is normally. This may be responsible for postpartum urinary difficulties, which may be wrongly attributed to regional anesthesia.

#### Functional Changes

*Lactosuria* and/or *glycosuria* occur as intermittent phenomenon in many healthy gravidae (2,6,144). Lactose, presumably formed by the mammary gland, is incom-

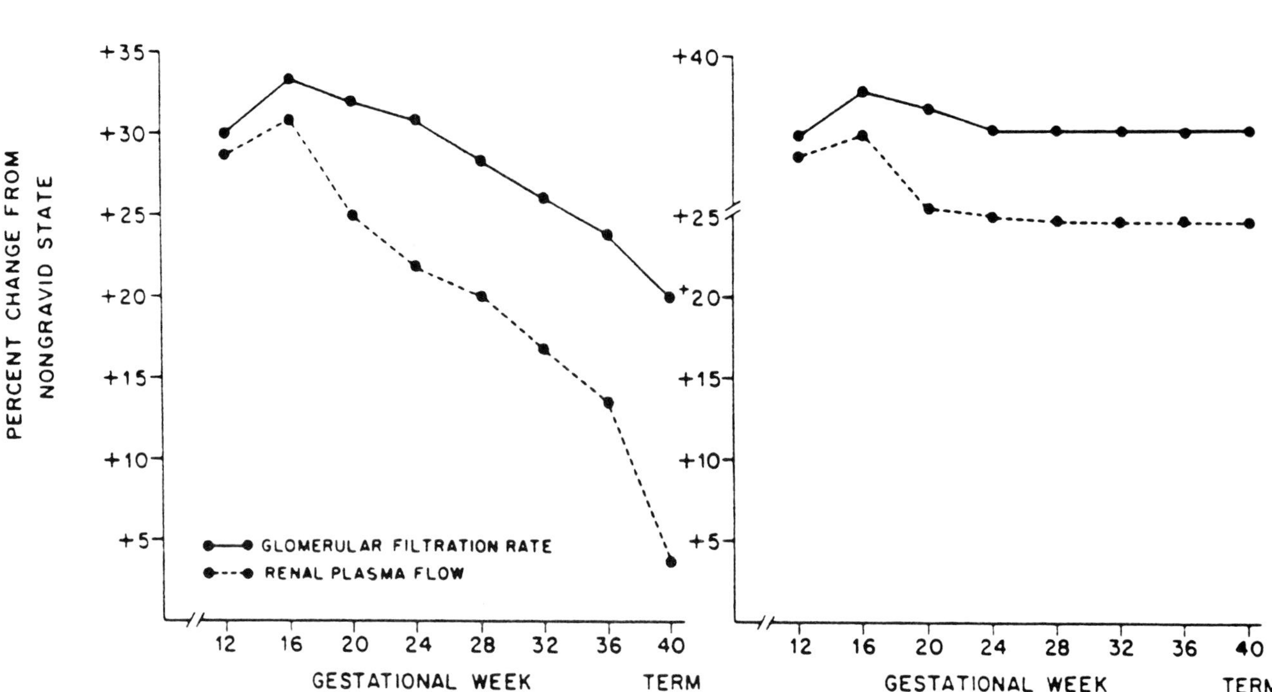


**Fig. 2–35.** Renal hemodynamics during pregnancy. The early increments in glomerular filtration rate and renal plasma flow are sustained until term when subjects are tested in lateral recumbency. Maintenance of the supine position causes each of these variables to fall substantially. (With permission from Lindheimer MD, Katz AI: Renal function in pregnancy. *In* Obstetrics and Gynecology Annual, 1972. Edited by RM Wynn. New York, Appleton-Century-Crofts, 1972.)

pletely reabsorbed in the tubules and appears in the urine from the third month on. Glycosuria is due to significant elevation in glomerular filtration rate for glucose with resultant predominance of filter load of a tubular reabsorptive capacity. The excretion of fructose also increases during pregnancy.

*Proteinuria* is present in about 20% of healthy gravidae, particularly those with accentuated lumbar lordosis. The condition appears to be related to increased venous pressure in one or both renal vessels. This can be ascertained by taking urine samples with the gravida in the upright or supine position and in the left lateral recumbent position, which reduces the uterine compression and thus decreases or eliminates the proteinuria.

## OTHER PHYSIOLOGIC CHANGES

### *Changes in the Acid-Base, Metabolism, and Nutrition*

#### Acid-base Balance

As has already been implied, changes in ventilation are associated with shifts of the balance between anionic and cationic constituents of the blood to a new equilibrium in pregnancy and labor. Total base decreases from the normal nonpregnant level of about 155 mEq/l to about 148 mEq/l with a corresponding decrease in sodium, potassium, calcium, and magnesium (148) (see Table 2–3). The total anions diminish commensurately, with the plasma bicarbonate decreasing from an average of 25 mEq/l to 21 to 22 mEq/l. The plasma buffer base (BB), which refers to the total available buffer and includes the bicarbonate, the protein, and the hemoglobin, decreases from a normal adult value of 47 mEq/l to 42 mEq/l and base excess decreases to −1.5 to −3.0 mEq/l (149). During normal pregnancy, gravidae have respiratory alkalosis and metabolic acidosis, both of which are accentuated during labor. As a response to the respiratory alkalosis, there is a fall in the level of concentration of plasma bicarbonate and its renal excretion. The metabolic acidosis, however, is not fully compensated so that a pH value of 7.44 is characteristic of maternal arterial blood during pregnancy, a condition that Sjostedt (149) defined "incompletely compensated respiratory alkalosis." The hyperventilation-induced hypocarbia has both maternal and fetal consequences: it accounts for the sensation of dyspnea, complained of by some gravidae, and it facilitates fetal disposition of carbon dioxide by providing a sizeable gradient across the placenta. The reduction of alkali reserve makes pregnant women more liable to development of metabolic acidosis while the decrease in plasma bicarbonate leads to a lowering of the plasma sodium level and thus the osmolality (6).

Labor and parturition are associated with a time-related progressive increase in metabolic acidosis, particularly during the second stage (150–154). There is now evidence that this metabolic acidosis is not due primarily to uterine work, but is caused mostly by the pain associated with uterine contractions and the neuroendocrine and metabolic responses consequent thereto. This is suggested by the observation that if pain relief is complete during the first stage, there is no change in the level of base excess (151–154). On the other hand, Marx and Greene (150) reported an increasing level of blood lactate concentration in patients undergoing labor in which pain was poorly relieved, and Maltau and associates (155) reported the occurrence of a steady rise in the level of concentration of free fatty acids in a similar group. In all three of these studies (150,151,155), relief of labor pain obviated these changes during the first stage of labor. As previously mentioned, hypoventilation between contractions can result in hypoxia and consequent deleterious effects on the fetus.

During the second stage, bearing-down efforts add to the metabolic acidosis caused by inadequate pain relief. Indeed, bearing-down efforts in themselves produce some of the metabolic acidosis—a fact impressively demonstrated by Pearson and Davies (151,152), who reported that among parturients who had total pain relief provided by epidural analgesia and did not bear down with contractions, there was no significant alteration in the value of either base excess or lactate concentration. However, patients who had total pain relief but who had also aided the expulsive efforts of the uterus by either voluntary or by the reflex bearing-down effort exhibited a slight time-dependent fall in base excess and rise in lactate (see Chapter 9, Figure 9–22). In contrast, in parturients who received only systemic analgesics during the first and second stage with consequent inadequate pain relief and who also had reflex-induced bearing-down efforts during the second stage, they developed a significantly greater incremental decrease in base excess and increase in lactate concentration and thus developed a significant degree of metabolic acidosis. This was reflected by an impressively greater degree of metabolic acidosis in the fetuses of these mothers than was noted in fetuses born of mothers who had received epidural analgesia (see Figure 9–22). As previously mentioned, hypoventilation between contractions can result in hypoxia and consequent deleterious effects on the fetus.

It has already been mentioned that basal metabolic rate and oxygen consumption rate increase progressively throughout gestation to peaks of 20% and 30%, respectively, at term and significantly more during labor.

*Protein metabolism* is enhanced to provide substrate for fetal as well as maternal anabolic pathways (2–4,6). Provided an adequate diet is ingested, there is an increased secretion of amino acids and greatly augmented retention of nitrogen that is most significant at mid-pregnancy, at which time the peak of phosphorus and sulfur retention occurs. This state of positive nitrogen balance is used not only for the growth of the fetus and the reproductive system, but also for the needs of lactation.

*Fat metabolism* also increases and includes a significant increase (double) in plasma neutral fats and a 25% increase in phospholipids and cholesterol. Total cholesterol may rise from 70 mg per 100 ml to 350 mg or more per 100 ml with a concomitant rise in free cholesterol so that the normal ratio between free and total serum cholesterol is maintained (2,4,6).

*Carbohydrate metabolism* is affected by the large amounts of human placental lactogen, which raise the free fatty acids and interfere with peripheral utilization of glucose (5). Because free fatty acids traverse the placenta only slowly, fetal energy needs are met by glucose transferral while maternal fasting glucose concentration becomes depressed. During labor, both aerobic and anaerobic carbohydrate metabolism undergo a steady rise as evidenced by progressively higher levels of lactate, pyruvate, and excess lactate with the latter indicating an oxygen debt (150).

### Water Balance

Increased water retention is a normal concomitant of pregnancy with water retained in all tissues, although the amount retained in vascular and extravascular spaces varies in each trimester. Intravascular retention of water increases only slightly during the first trimester, but thereafter the gradient steepens until just before the onset of labor when there is a sharp and significant fall. The increase in extravascular fluid in tissues, other than the uterus and breasts, begins about the thirtieth week and by term it amounts to 1.5 liters above nonpregnant levels (2–6). This fluid is distributed throughout the body as a general increase in the volume of "ground substance" which must of course be traversed by nutrients, metabolic products, and drugs. It is important to note, however, that much of the extravascular fluid is collected in the legs due to the combined effects of gravity and the impedance to venous return within the pelvis. Despite this local accumulation, edema is not necessarily present. The incremental increase in water retention continues during the final 10 weeks until just before spontaneous onset of labor when there is a sharp and significant fall. This generalized water retention is related closely to salt retention and both processes are probably related to the secretion of steroids by the placenta. During the postpartum period both water and salt retention are decreased through diuresis and diaphoresis.

### Nutrition

The requirement by the fetus for amino acids for protein synthesis, glucose for energy needs, and iron for erythropoiesis must be supplied by the mother. The total amount of iron required in pregnancy approximates 1.5 grams, which includes 500 mg incorporated into the expanded maternal red cell mass, 800 mg principally for fetal blood formation, and 200 mg for normal iron loss (in the absence of bleeding). The maternal body demand for folic acid also increases and with a marginal diet, deficiency will result. Daily supplementation with 30 to 60 mg of iron and with 200 to 400 mg of folic acid should be considered for most pregnant women. Needs for other vitamins and minerals are also higher, but these are usually met through diet (2,4–6).

## Changes in the Endocrine System

In addition to the persistence of corpus luteum and placental production of estrogen, progesterone, and chorionic gonadotropin, a number of endocrine changes take place. Because these are discussed in Chapter 32, only mention is made here.

### *Thyroid and Parathyroid Glands*

The thyroid gland undergoes a moderate degree of hyperplasia that is the result of the physiologic demand, as evidenced by an increase in the basal metabolic rate and the iodine content in the blood. The elevated level of estrogen in gestation causes increased production of $\alpha$-globulins and $\beta$-globulins by the liver, among which is thyroxin ($T_4$)-binding globulin (4–6,156). To maintain a euthyroid in the presence of higher levels of thyroxin-binding globulin and higher proportion of globulin($T_4$)-bound thyroxin, thyroid gland activity increases progressively (156). Thyroid uptake of radio-iodine is increased significantly, reflecting increased clearance of iodine by the thyroid, but not clinical hyperactivity. Moderate enlargement of the thyroid gland develops secondarily to glandular hypertrophy and increase of vascularity. Functionally, the gravida remains euthyroid and thyroid function tests must be interpreted with these physiologic alterations in mind (156). The hypothalmic-pituitary-thyroid relationships remain intact during pregnancy, the release of thyroid-stimulating hormone (TSH) in response to thyrotropin-releasing hormone (TRH) does not increase (157), and the thyroidal uptake if iodide also responds normally to thyroid hormone suppression and TSH stimulation during pregnancy (158). Serum TSH concentrations are decreased during the early weeks of gestation and then rise to prepregnancy levels by the end of the first trimester.

The parathyroid glands also undergo hyperplasia related to the increase in calcium and metabolism. Parathyroid hormone levels are elevated to meet the calcium needs of the infant while serum calcium levels are slightly lowered, probably secondary to the physiologic decreases in serum albumin concentration (160). As is well known, deficiency of the parathyroid contributes to the production of tetany.

#### The Pituitary Gland

The anterior lobe of the pituitary gland hypertrophies until it may be as large as twice its normal size (161). Both acidophilic and basophilic cells show evidence of increased activity, secreting more adenotropic and thyrotropic hormones to regulate metabolism processes and prolactin to effect lactation. The posterior infundibular portion of the pituitary, on the other hand, does not increase in size, but increases in activity, especially during labor. In addition to its well-known effects on blood pressure, it possesses the power of stimulating significantly uterine contractions through the excretion of oxytocin.

#### The Adrenal Glands

The adrenal glands enlarge during pregnancy and the activity of the adrenal cortex is significantly increased (162). This is manifested by elevated levels of free and bound plasma cortisol levels and a decrease in the circulating eosinophils. There is a progressive increase in 17-hydroxycorticosteroid levels with advancing pregnancy with a further rise during labor and delivery and a prompt decrease in the immediate postpartum period. There is also an increase in the androgen secretion and aldosterone secretion increases threefold after the third month.

#### The Endorphins

A number of recent studies have demonstrated a progressive increase in plasma beta endorphin, beta lipotrophin, and adrenocorticotropic hormone (ACTH), which are derived from a common precursor (163–165). Hormonal secretion from the adrenal cortex is similarly increased during labor. Because these will be discussed in detail in Chapter 9, no further comment is made here.

## Changes in the Nervous System

The organic changes that affect the nervous system are few. There is an increase in size of the pelvic plexuses. In the normal gravida, during pregnancy and during labor between uterine contractions, the cerebrospinal fluid pressure is within normal limits. During pregnancy, extradural pressures are higher than in nonpregnant subjects, whereas baseline pressures in the lumbar extradural space averaged $-1$ cm $H_2O$ in nonpregnant subjects; they were $+1$ cm $H_2O$ or above in gravidae. Cerebrospinal fluid, specific gravity, and total protein are insignificantly lower in healthy gravidae than in nonpregnant women, and the electrophoretic protein pattern remains unchanged (166). Resting cerebrospinal fluid pressures are within normal limits during uncomplicated gestation. Both extradural and cerebrospinal fluid pressures are changed significantly during labor (Figure 2–25). These are discussed in detail in Chapters 13 and 14.

## Changes in the Soft Parts of the Pelvis and Musculoskeletal System

The increased elasticity of the joints of the ribs and sternum consequent to widespread effects of progesterone and relaxin has been mentioned in the section on respiration. Similarly, the hormone-induced relaxation of abdominal muscles facilitates ventilation.

The increased vascularity and hypertrophy that occurs elsewhere also extend to a lesser degree to the various soft parts of the pelvis, including the skin and muscles. In addition, there is apparently an increase in the elastic tissue and softening of the other connective tissue elements, thus preparing the outlet for the strain of labor. This increased elasticity and flexibility of the joints make possible the increase in size of the outlet so necessary for the descent of the fetal head and eventual delivery of the baby at term. On the other hand, this elasticity and flexibility may be an indirect source of postpartum pain if the patient, under the influence of anesthesia, is improperly transported from the delivery table to the cart. During the latter part of pregnancy, there is a great exaggeration

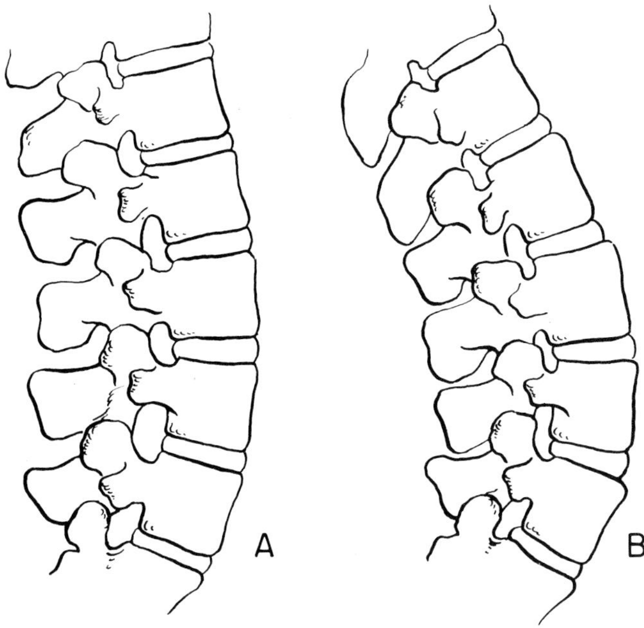


**Fig. 2–36.** Effect of pregnancy on posture and the lumbar lordotic curve: **A,** nonpregnant; **B,** pregnant. Note the marked increase in the lumbar lordosis and the consequent narrowing of the interspinous spaces.

of the lumbar dorsal curve of the spine producing the so-called lordosis of pregnancy (Figure 2–36). This may be a source of chronic backache and may increase the technical difficulty in carrying out puncture of the subarachnoid or epidural spaces when the mid-line entry method is used.

## REFERENCES

1. Crawford JS: Principles and Practice of Obstetric Anaesthesia, 5th Ed. Oxford, Blackwell Scientific Publications, 1984, pp. 1–100.
2. Metcalfe J, Stock MK, Barron DH: Maternal physiology during gestation. *In* The Physiology of Reproduction. Edited by K Knobil, L Ewing. New York, Raven Press, 1988, pp. 2145–2176.
3. Metcalfe J, McAnulty JH, Ueland K: Burwell and Metcalfe's Heart Disease and Pregnancy: Physiology and Management, 2nd edition. Boston, Little, Brown & Co, 1986, p. 25.
4. Hytten F, Chamberlain G: Clinical Physiology in Obstetrics. Oxford, Blackwell Scientific Publications, 1980.
5. Cruikshank DP, Hays PM: Maternal physiology in pregnancy. *In* Obstetrics: Normal and Problem Pregnancies. 2nd Ed. Edited by SG Gabbe, JR Niebyls, JL Simpson. New York, Churchill Livingstone, 1991, pp. 125–146.
6. Marx GF, Bassell GM: Physiologic consideration of the mother. *In* Obstetric Analgesia and Anesthesia. Amsterdam, Excerpta Medica, 1980, pp. 21–54.
7. Eastman NJ, Hellman LM: Williams Obstetrics, 12th Ed. New York, Appleton-Century-Crofts, 1961, pp. 221–266.
8. Thomson KH, Cohen ME: Studies on circulation in pregnancy; vital capacity observations in normal pregnant women. Surg. Gynecol. Obstet. 66:592, 1938.
9. Plass ED, Oberst FW: Respiration and pulmonary ventilation in normal nonpregnant, pregnant and puerperal women; with interpretation of acid-base balance during pregnancy. Am. J. Obstet. Gynecol. 35:441, 1938.
10. Campbell EJM, Agostini E, Newsome-Davis J: The Respiratory Muscles: Mechanics and Neuro Controlled. 2nd Ed. Philadelphia, WB Saunders Company, 1970, pp. 23–138.
11. McGinty AP: The comparative effects of pregnancy and phrenic nerve interruption on the diaphragm and their relation to pulmonary tuberculosis. Am. J. Obstet. Gynecol. 35:237, 1938.
12. Rubin A, Russo N, Goucher D: Effect of pregnancy upon pulmonary function in normal women. Am. J. Obstet. Gynecol. 72:963, 1956.
13. Clark S, Cotton DB, Lee W, et al: Central hemodynamic assessment of normal term pregnancy. Am. J. Gynecol. 161: 1439, 1989.
14. Gee JBL, Packer BS, Millen JE, Robin ED: Pulmonary mechanics during pregnancy. J. Clin. Invest. 46:945, 1967.
15. Milne JA, Mills RJ, Howie AD, Pack AI: Large airways function during normal pregnancy. Br. J. Obstet. Gynaecol. 84: 448, 1977.
16. Cugell DW, Frank NR, Gaensler EA, Badger TL: Pulmonary function in pregnancy; serial observations in normal women. Amer. Rev. Tuberc. 67:568, 1953.
16a. Conklin, KA: Maternal physiological adaptions during gestation, labor and the puerperium. Semin. Anesth. 4:221, 1991.
17. Leontic EA: Respiratory disease in pregnancy. Med. Clin. North. Am. 61:111–128, 1977.
18. Alaily AB, Carrol KB: Pulmonary ventilation in pregnancy. Br. J. Obstet. Gynaecol. 85:518, 1978.
19. Russell IF, Chambers WA: Closing volume in normal pregnancy. Br. J. Anaesth. 53:1043, 1981.
20. Templeton A, Kelman GT: Maternal blood gases ($PAO_2$)-$PaO_2$, physiological shunt and Vd/Vt in normal pregnancy. Br. J. Anaesth. 48:1001, 1976.
21. Baldwin GR, Moorthi DS, Whelton JA, MacDonnel KF: New lung functions and pregnancy. Am. J. Obstet. Gynecol. 127: 235, 1977.
22. Bevan DR, Holdcroft A, Loh L, MacGregor WG, et al: Closing volume and pregnancy. Br. Med. J. 1:13, 1974.
23. Holdcroft A, Bevan DR, O'Sullivan JC, Sykes MK, et al: Airway closure and pregnancy. Anaesthesia 32:517, 1977.
23A. Forster RE II, DuBois AB, Briscoe WA, Fisher AB: The Lung: Physiologic Basis of Pulmonary Function Tests. 3rd Ed. Chicago, Year Book Medical Publishers, Inc., 1986.
24. Weinberger SE: Pregnancy and the lung. Am. Rev. Respir. Dis. 121:559, 1980.
25. Prowse CM, Gaensler EA: Respiratory and acid-base changes during pregnancy. Anesthesiology 26:381, 1965.
26. Shankar KB, Mosely H, Vemula V, Kumar Y: Physiological dead space during general anesthesia for cesarean section. Can. J. Anaesth. 34:373, 1987.
27. Farman JV, Thorpe ME: Compliance changes during caesarean section. Br. J. Anaesth. 41:999, 1969.
28. Novy MJ, Edwards MJ: Respiratory problems in pregnancy. Am. J. Obstet. Gynecol. 99:1024, 1967.
29. Marx GF, Murthy PK, Orkin LR: Static compliance before and after vaginal delivery. Br. J. Anaesth. 42:1100, 1970.
30. Bonica JJ: Maternal respiratory changes during pregnancy and parturition. *In* Parturition and Perinatology (Clinical Anesthesia Series, Vol. 10/2). Philadelphia, FA Davis, 1973.
30a. Bonica JJ, Caldayro-Barcia R, Balitzky R, Grünwald I, Dalard G: Anesthesia peridural segmentaria en al periodo dilatacion del trabajo del parto. Revista Uruguaya de Anestesiologia 5:45, 1971.
31. Zwillich CW, Natalino MR, Sutton FD, Weil JV: Effects of

progesterone on chemosensitivity in normal man. J. Lab. Clin. Med. 92(2):262, 1978.
32. Andersen GJ, James GB, Mathers NP, Smith EL, et al: The maternal oxygen tension and acid-base status during pregnancy. J. Obstet. Gynaec. Br. Cwlth. 76:16, 1969.
33. Ang CK, Tan TH, Walters WAW, Wood C: Postural influence on maternal capillary oxygen and carbon dioxide tension. Br. Med. J. 4:201, 1969.
34. Hagerdal M, Morgan CW, Sumner AE, Gutsche BB: Minute ventilation and oxygen consumption during labor with epidural analgesia. Anesthesiology 59:425–427, 1983.
35. Wulf KH, Kunzel W, Lehmann V: Clinical aspects of placental gas exchange. *In* Respiratory Gas Exchange and Blood Flow in the Placenta. Edited by LD Longo and H Bartels. Bethesda, MD, U.S. Department of Health, Education and Welfare. DHEW publication no. (NIH) 73–361, 1972, pp. 505–521.
36. Tucker DH, Sieker HO: The effect of change in body position on lung volumes and intrapulmonary gas mixing in patients with obesity, heart failure and emphysema. Am. Rev. Resp. Dis. 82:6787, 1960.
37. Said SL: Abnormalities of pulmonary gas exchange in obesity. Ann. Intern. Med. 53:1121, 1960.
38. Bates DV, Macklem PT, Christie RV: Respiratory function in disease. 2nd Ed. Philadelphia, WB Saunders Company, 1971, pp. 100–101.
39. Barrera F, Reidenberg MM, Winters WL: Pulmonary function in the obese patient. Am. J. Med. Sci. 254:785, 1967.
40. Eng M, Butler J, Bonica JJ: Respiratory function in pregnant obese women. Am. J. Obstet. Gynecol. 123:241, 1975.
41. Bader RA, Bader ME, Rose DJ: The oxygen cost of breathing in dyspneic subjects as studied in normal pregnant women. Clin. Sci. 18:223, 1959.
42. Gilbert R, Epifano L, Auchincloss JH Jr: Dyspnea of pregnancy. JAMA 182:1073, 1962.
43. Cole PV, Nainby-Lusmoore RC: Respiratory volumes in labour. Br. Med. J. 1:1118, 1962.
44. Fisher A, Prys-Robergs C: Maternal pulmonary gas exchange. A study during normal labour and extradural blockade. Anaesthesia 23:350, 1968.
45. Crawford JS, Tunstall ME: Notes on respiratory performance during labour. Br. J. Anaesth. 40:612, 1968.
46. Gemzell CA, Robbe H, Stern B, Strom G: Observations on circulatory changes and muscular work in normal labour. Acta. Obstet. Gynecol. Scand. 36:75, 1957.
47. Huch A, Huch R, Lindmark G, Rooth G: Maternal hypoxaemia after pethidine. J. Obstet. Gynaecol. Br. Cwlth. 81:608, 1974.
48. Huch A, Huch R: Transcutaneous noninvasive monitoring of $PO_2$. Hosp. Pract. 11:43, 1976.
49. Huch A, Huch R, Schneider H, Rooth G: Continuous transcutaneous monitoring of fetal oxygen tension during labor. Br. J. Obstet. Gynaecol. 84S1:1, 1977.
50. Huch A, Huch R: Insight derived from perinatal monitoring. *In* Perinatal Medicine. Edited by Thalhammer O, Baumgarten K, and Pollak A. Sixth European Congress, Vienna, 1978. Stuttgart, Georg Thieme Publishers, 1979, pp. 284–293.
50a. Huch R, Huch A: Continuous Transcutaneous Blood Gas Monitoring. New York, Marcell Decker, 1983, pp. 495–647.
51. Peabody JL: Transcutaneous oxygen measurement to evaluate drug effect. Clin. Perinatol. 6:109–114, 1979.
52. Moya F: Consideration in maternal and placental physiology. Anesth. Analg. 42:661, 1963.
53. Archer GW, Marx GF: Arterial oxygen tensions during apnoea in parturient women. Br. J. Anaesth. 46:358, 1974.
54. Wollman H, Alexander SC, Cohen PHJ, Chase PE, et al: Cerebral circulation of man during halothane anesthesia. Anesthesiology 25:180, 1964.
55. Motoyama EK, Rivard G, Acheson F, Cook CD: Adverse effect of maternal hyperventilation on the foetus. Lancet 1:286–288, 1966.
56. Miller FC: Hyperventilation during labor. Am. J. Obstet. Gynecol. 120:489, 1974.
57. Levinson G, Shnider SM, deLorimier AA, Steffenson JL: Effects of maternal hyperventilation on uterine blood flow and fetal oxygenation and acid-base status. Anesthesiology 40:340, 1974.
57a. Rampton AJ, Mallaiah S, Garrett CPO: Increased ventilation requirements during obstetric general anaesthesia. Br. J. Anaesth. 61:730, 1988.
58. Assali NS, Brinkman III: Pathophysiology of Gestation. Vol. 1: Maternal Disorders. New York, Academic Press, 1972, p. 278–285.
59. Ueland K: Cardiorespiratory physiology of pregnancy. *In* Gynecology and Obstetrics, Vol 3. Baltimore, Harper and Row, 1979.
60. Pritchard JA: Changes in blood volume during pregnancy and delivery. Anesthesiology 26:393, 1965.
61. McLennan CE: Plasma volume late in pregnancy. Am. J. Obstet. Gynec. 59:662, 1950.
62. Campbell DM, MacGillivray I: Comparison of maternal response in first and second pregnancies in relation to baby weight. J. Obstet. Gynaecol. Br. Cwlth. 79:684, 1972.
63. Ueland K: Maternal cardiovascular dynamics. VII. Intrapartum blood volume changes. Am. J. Obstet. Gynecol. 126: 677, 1976.
64. Hytten FE, Lind T: Diagnostic indices in pregnancy. Basel, Ciba-Giegy, Ltd., 1973.
65. Moir DD, Wallace G: Blood loss at forceps delivery. J. Obstet. Gynaecol. Br. Cwlth. 74:424, 1967.
66. Moir DD: Anesthesia for cesarean section. Br. J. Anaesth. 42:136, 1970.
67. Pritchard JA, MacDonald PC: Maternal adaptation to pregnancy. *In* Williams Obstetrics. 15th Ed. Edited by JA Pritchard and PC MacDonald. New York, Appleton-Century-Crofts, 1976, pp. 171–203.
68. Talbert LM, Landgella RD: Normal values of certain factors in the blood clotting mechanism in pregnancy. Am. J. Obstet. Gynecol. 90:44, 1964.
68a. Sagi A, Creter D, Goldman J, et al: Platelet functions before, during and after labor. Acta. Haemat. 65:67, 1981.
68b. Pitkin RM, Witte DL: Platelet and leukocyte counts in pregnancy. JAMA 242:2696, 1979.
69. Shnider SM: Serum cholinesterase activity during pregnancy, labor and the puerperium. Anesthesiology 26:335, 1965.
69a. Leighton BL, Check TG, Gross JB, et al: Succinylcholine pharmacokinetics in peripartum patients. Anesthesiology 64:202,1986.
70. Morris A, Giesceke AH: Potentiation of muscle relaxants by magnesium sulfate therapy in toxemia of pregnancy. South. Med. J. 61:25, 1968.
71. Woodfield DG, Cole SK, Cash JD: Impaired fibrinolytic response to exercise stress in normal pregnancy. Am. J. Obstet. Gynecol. 102:440, 1968.
72. Mendelson CL: Cardiac Disease in Pregnancy. Philadelphia, FA Davis Co., 1960.
73. Oram S, Holt M: Innocent depression of the S-T segment and flattening of the T-wave during pregnancy. J. Obstet. Gynaecol. Brit. Cwlth. 68:765, 1961.
74. Adams JQ: Cardiovascular physiology in normal pregnancy: studies with dye dilution technique. Am. J. Obstet. Gynec. 67:741, 1954.
75. Bader RA, Bader ME, Rose DJ, Braunwald E: Hemody-

namics at rest and during exercise in normal pregnancy as studied by cardiac catheterization. J. Clin. Invest. 34: 1524, 1955.

76. Hamilton HFH: Cardiac output in normal pregnancy. J. Obstet. Gynaecol. Br. Cwlth. 56:548, 1949.

77. Palmer AJ, Walker AHC: Maternal circulation in normal pregnancy. J. Obstet. Gynaecol. Br. Cwlth. 56:537, 1949.

78. Rose DJ, Bader ME, Bader RA, Braunwald E: Catheterization studies of cardiac hemodynamics in normal pregnant women with reference to left ventricular work. Am. J. Obstet. Gynec. 72:233, 1956.

79. Lees MM, Taylor SH, Scott DB, Kerr MG: A study of cardiac output at rest throughout pregnancy. J. Obstet. Gynaecol. Br. Cwlth. 74:319, 1967.

80. Ueland K, Novy MJ, Peterson EN, Metcalfe J: Maternal cardiovascular dynamics. IV. The influence of testational age on the maternal cardiovascular response to posture and exercise. Am. J. Obstet. Gynecol. 104:856–864 1969.

81. Atkins AFJ, Watt JM, Milan P, Davies P, et al: A longitudinal study of cardiovascular dynamic changes throughout pregnancy. Eur. J. Obstet. Gynecol. Reprod. Biol. 12:215, 1981.

82. Easterling TR, Watts DH, Schmucker BC, Benedetti TJ: Measurement of cardiac output during pregnancy: validation of Doppler technique and clinical observations in preeclampsia. Obstet. Gynecol. 69:845, 1987.

83. Robson SC, Hunter S, Boys RJ, Dunlop W: Serial study of factors influencing changes in cardiac output during human pregnancy. Am. J. Physio. 256(4):H1060–1065, 1989.

84. Vorys N, Ullery JC, Hanusek GE: The cardiac output changes in various positions in pregnancy. Am. J. Obstet. Gynecol. 82:1312, 1961.

85. Hendricks CH: The hemodynamics of a uterine contraction. Am. J. Obstet. Gynecol. 76:969, 1958.

86. Ueland K, Hansen JM: Maternal cardiovascular dynamics: II. Posture and uterine contractions. Am. J. Obstet. Gynecol. 103:1, 1969.

87. Ueland K, Hansen JM: Maternal cardiovascular dynamics: III. Labor and delivery under local and caudal analgesia. Am. J. Obstet. Gynecol. 103:8, 1969.

87a. Katz R, Karliner J, Resnick R: Effects of a natural volume overload state (pregnancy) on left ventricular performance in normal human subjects. Circulation 58: 434–440, 1978.

88. Robson SC, Dunlop W, Boys RJ, Hunter S: Cardiac output during labour. Br. Med. J. 295:1169, 1987.

89. Kerr MG, Scott DB, Samuel E: Studies of the inferior vena cava in late pregnancy. Br. Med. J. 1:532, 1964.

90. Marx GF: Editorial. Aortal compression syndrome: its 50-year history. Int. J. Obstet. Anesth. 1:60, 1992.

91. Mc Roberts WA: Postural shock in pregnancy. Am. J. Obstet. Gynecol. 62:627, 1951.

92. Howard RK, Goodson JH, Mengert WF: Supine hypotensive syndrome in late pregnancy. Obstet. Gynecol. 1:371, 1953.

93. Kennedy RL, Friedman DL, Hatchka DM, et al: Hypotension during obstetrical anesthesia. Anesthesiology 20:153, 1959.

94. Scott DB: Inferior vena caval occlusion in late pregnancy and its importance in anaesthesia. Br. J. Anaesth. 40: 120–128, 1968.

95. Kerr MG, Scott DB, Samuel E: Studies of the inferior vena cava in late pregnancy. Br. Med. J. 1:532, 1964.

96. Lees MM, Scott DB, Kerr MG, et al: The circulatory effects of recumbent postural change in late pregnancy. Clin. Sci. 32:453,1967.

97. McLennan CE: Antecubital and femoral venous pressure in normal and toxemic pregnancy. Am. J. Obstet. Gynecol. 45:568, 1943.

98. Coutts WE, Opaga L, Banderas BT, Sanhueza DD: Abdominal circulation during late pregnancy as shown in aortogram. Am. J. Obstet. Gynecol. 29:566, 1935.

99. Biarniz J, Crottogini JJ, Curuchet E, et al: Aortocaval compression by the uterus in late human pregnancy. Am. J. Obstet. Gynecol. 100:203, 1968.

100. Marx GF, Husain FJ, Shiau HF: Brachial and femoral blood pressures during the prenatal period. Am. J. Obstet. Gynecol. 136:11, 1980.

101. Milsom I, Forssman L: Factors influencing aortocaval compression in late pregnancy. Am. J. Obstet. Gynecol. 148:764, 1984.

102. Ideda T, Ohbuchi H, Ikenoue T, Mori N: Physiology of pregnancy: maternal cerebral hemodynamics in the supine hypotensive syndrome. Obstet. Gynecol. 179:27–31, 1992.

103. Newman B, Derrington C, Dore C: Cardiac output and the recumbent position in late pregnancy. Anaesthesia 38: 332–335, 1983.

104. Arbitol MM: Aortic compression by pregnant uterus. NY. State. J. Med. 76:1470, 1976.

105. Kerr MG, Scott DB, Samuel E: Studies of the inferior vena cava in late pregnancy. Br. Med. J. 1:532, 1964.

106. Reed NE, Teteris NJ, Essig GF: Inferior vena caval obstruction syndrome with electrocardiographically documented fetal bradycardia. Obstet. Gynecol. 36:462–464, 1970.

107. Hon EH: An Introduction to Fetal Heart Rate Monitoring. New Haven, Harty Press, 1969, pp. 56–57.

108. Goodlin RC: Importance of the lateral position during labor. Obstet. Gynecol. 37:698, 1971.

109. Humphrey MD, Chang A, Wood EC, et al: A decrease in fetal pH during the second stage of labour, when conducted in the dorsal position. J. Obstet. Gynaecol Br. Commw. 81:600, 1974.

110. Ellington C, Katz VL, Watson WJ, et al: The effect of lateral tilt on materal and fetal hemodynamic variables. Obstet. Gynecol. 77:201–203, 1991.

111. Bromage P: Physiology and pharmacology of epidural analgesia. Anesthesiology 28:592–622, 1967.

112. Grundy EM, Zamora AM, Winnie AP: Comparison of spread of epidural anesthesia in pregnant and nonpregnant women. Anesth. Analg. 57:544–546, 1978.

113. Sharrock NE, Greenidge J: Epidural dose responses in pregnant and nonpregnant patients. Anesthesiology 51:S298, 1978.

114. Datta S, Lambert DH, Gregus J, et al: Differential sensitivities of mammalian nerve fibers during pregnancy. Anesth. Analg. 62:1070–1072, 1983.

115. Flanagan HL, Datta S, Lambert DH, Gissen AJ, et al: Effect of pregnancy on bupivacaine-induced conduction blockade in the isolated rabbit vagus nerve. Anesth. Analg. 66: 123–126, 1987.

116. Butterworth JF IV, Walker FO, Lysak SZ: Pregnancy increases median nerve susceptibility to lidocaine. Anesthesiology. 72:962–965, 1990.

117. Sevarino FB, Gilbertson LI, Gugino LD, Courtney MA, et al: The effect of pregnancy on the nervous system response to sensory stimulation. Anesthesiology 69:A695, 1988.

118. Sheth AP, Dautenhahn DL, Fagraeus L: Decreased CSF protein during pregnancy as a mechanism facilitating the spread of spinal anesthesia. Anesth. Analg. 64:280, 1985.

119. Dautenhahn DL, Fagraerus L: Acid-base changes of spinal fluid during pregnancy. Anesth. Analg. 63:204, 1984.

120. Chrisofides ND, et al: Decreased plasma motilin concentration in pregnancy. Br. Med. J. 284:1453, 1982.

121. Lind JF, Smith AM, McIver DK, Coopland AT, et al: Heartburn in pregnancy—a manometric study. Can. Med. Assoc. J. 98:571, 1968.
122. Hey VMF, Cowley DJ, Ganguli PC, Skinner LD, et al: Gastro-oesophageal reflux in late pregnancy. Anaesthesia 32:372, 1977.
123. Bainbridge ET, Nicholas SD, Newton JR, et al: Gastro-oesophageal reflux in pregnancy. Altered function of the barier to reflux in asymptomatic women during early pregnancy. Scand. J. Gastroenterol. 19:85, 1984.
124. Murray FA, Erskine JP, Fielding J: Gastric secretion in pregnancy. J. Obstet. Gynaecol. Brit. Emp. 64:373, 1957.
125. Wyner J, Cohen SE: Gastric volume in early pregnancy: Effect of metoclopramide. Anesthesiology 57:209, 1982.
126. Taylor G, Pryse-Davies J: The prophylactic use of antacids in the prevention of the acid-pulmonary-aspiration syndrom (Mendelson's syndrome). Lancet 1:288, 1966.
127. Dewan DM, Floyd HM, Thistlewood JM, et al: Sodium citrate pretreatment in elective cesarean section patients. Anesth. Analg. 64:34, 1985.
128. Holdsworth JD: Relationship between stomach contents and analgesia in labour. Br. J. Anaesth. 50:1145, 1978.
129. Wilson J: Gastric emptying in labour: some recent findings and their clinical significance. J. Int. Med. Res. 6(Suppl.): 54, 1978.
130. Nimmo WS, Wilson J, Prescott LF: Narcotic analgesics and delayed gastric emptying during labour. Lancet 1:890, 1975.
131. LaSalvia LA, Steffen EA: Delayed gastric emptying time in labor. Am. J. Obstet. Gynecol. 59:1075, 1950.
132. O'Sullivan GM, Sutton AJ, Thompson SA, et al: Non-invasive measurement of gastric emptying in obstetric patients. Anesth. Analg. 66:505–511, 1987.
133. Davidson JS, Davison MC, Hay DM: Gastric emptying time during pregnancy and labor. J. Obstet. Gynaecol. Br. Commw. 77:37, 1970.
134. Crawford JS: Some aspects of obstetric anaesthesia. Part III. Br. J. Anaesth. 28:201, 1956.
135. Carp H, Jayaram A, Stoll M: Ultrasound examination of the stomach contents of parturients. Anesth. Analg. 74:683, 1992.
136. Thorén T, Wattwil M: Effects on gastric emptying of thoracic epidural analgesia with morphine or bupivacaine. Anesth. Analg. 67:687, 1988.
137. Wright PM, Allen RW, Moore J, Donnelly JP: Gastric emptying during extradural analgesia in labor: Effect of fentanyl supplementation. Br. J. Anaesth. 68:248, 1992.
138. Parry E, Shields R, Turnbull AC: Transit time in the small intestine in pregnancy. J. Obstet. Gynaecol. Br. Commw. 77:900, 1970.
139. Parry E, Shields R, Turnbull AC: The effect of pregnancy on the colonic absorption of sodium, potassium, and water. J. Obstet. Gynaecol. Br. Commw. 77:616, 1970.
140. Combes B, Adams RH: Disorders of the liver in pregnancy. *In* Pathophysiology of Gestation. Edited by NS Assali. San Diego, 1971, p. 297.
141. Gerdes MM, Boyden EA: The rate of emptying of the human gall bladder in pregnancy. Surg. Gynecol. Obstet. 66:145, 1938.
142. Bellina JG, Dougherty CM, Mickal A: Pyeloureteral dilation and pregnancy. Am. J. Obstet. Gynecol. 89:108:356, 1970
143. Longo LD, Assali NS: Renal function in human pregnancy. Am. J. Obstet. Gynecol. 80:495, 1960.
144. Sims EAH, Krantz KE: Serial studies of renal function during pregnancy and the puerperium in normal women. J. Clin. Invest. 37:1764, 1958.
145. Dunlop W: Serial changes in renal hemodynamics during normal human pregnancy. Br. J. Obstet. Gynaecol. 88:1, 1981.
146. Ezimokhai M, et al: Non-postural serial changes in renal fucntion during the third trimester of normal human pregnancy. Br. J. Obstet. Gynaecol. 88:465, 1981.
147. Davison JM, Hytten FE: Glameral filtration during and after pregnancy. Br. J. Obstet. Gynaecol. 81:588, 1974.
148. Newman RL: Serum electrolytes in pregnancy, parturition and puerperium. Obstet. Gynecol. 10:51, 1957.
149. Sjostedt S: Acid-base balance of arterial blood during pregnancy, at delivery, and in the puerperium. Am. J. Obstet. Gynecol. 84:775, 1962.
150. Marx GF, Greene NM: Maternal lactate, pyruvate, and excess lactate production during labor and delivery. Am. J. Obstet. Gynecol. 90:786, 1964.
151. Pearson JF, Davies P: The effect of continuous lumbar epidural analgesia upon maternal acid-base status during the first and second stages of labour. Br. J. Obstet. Gynaecol. 80:218, 225, 1973.
152. Pearson JF, Davies P: The effect of continuous lumbar epidural analgesia upon fetal acid-base status of maternal arterial blood during the first and second stages of labour. Br. J. Obstet. Gynaecol. 81:971, 1979, 1974.
153. Thalme B, Belfrage P, Raabe N: Lumbar epidural analgesia in labour. Acta. Obstet. Gynaecol. Scand. 53:27, 1974.
154. Thalme B, Raabe N, Belfrage P: Lumbar epidural analgesia in labour. Acta. Obstet. Gynaecol. Scand. 53:113, 1974.
155. Maltau JM, Andersen HT, Skrede S: Obstetrical analgesia assessed by free fatty acid mobilization. Acta. Anaes. Scand. 19:245, 1975.
156. Nelson M, Wickus GC, Caplan RH, Beguin EA: Thyroid gland size in pregnancy: an ultrasound and clinical study. J. Reprod. Med. 32:888, 1987.
157. Burrow FN, Polackwich R, Donabedian R: The hypothalmic-pituitary-thyroid axis in normal pregnancy. *In* Perinatal Thyroid Physiology and Disease. Edited by DA Fisher, GN Burrow. New York, Raven Press, 1975, p.1
158. Kannan V, Sinha MD, Deri PK, Pastogi GK: Plasma thyrotropin and its response to thyrotropin releasing hormone in pregnancy. Obstet. Gynecol. 42:547, 1973.
159. Harada A, Hershman JM, Reed AW, et al: Comparison of thyroid stimulators and thyroid hormone concentrations in the sera of pregnant women. J. Clin. Endocrinol. Metab. 48:793, 1979.
160. Rovinsky JJ: Disease complicating pregnancy. *In* Gynecology and Obstetrics. The Health Care of Women. Edited by SL Romney, MJ Gray, AB Little, MA Merrill, et al. New York, McGraw Hill, 1975, pp. 777–866.
161. Gonzalez JG, Elizondo G, Saldivar D, et al: Pituitary gland growth during normal pregnancy: an in vivo study using magnetic resonance imaging. Am. J. Med. 85:217, 1988.
162. Jailer JW, Christy NP, Longson D, Wallace EZ, et al: Further observations on adrenal cortical function during pregnancy. Am. J. Obstet. Gynecol. 78:1, 1959.
163. Wardlaw SL, Frantz AG: Brain beta-endorphin during pregnancy, parturition and the post partum period. Endocrinology 113:164, 1983.
164. Genazzani AR, Facchinetti F, Nappi G, et al: Beta-lipotrophin and beta-endorphin plasma levels during pregnancy. Clin. Endocrinol. 14:409, 1981.
165. Genazzani AR, Petraglia N, Brilli G, Fabbri G, et al: Endogenous opioid peptides and pain disorders in humans. *In* Pain and Reproduction. Edited by AR Genazzani, G Nappi, F Facchinetti, E Martignoni. Casteron Holl, Carnfort, The Parthenon Publishing Group, 1988, pp. 15–22.
166. Marx GF, Orkin LR: Cerebrospinal fluid protein and spinal anesthesia on obstetrics. Anesthesiology 26:340, 1965.

Chapter 3

# PSYCHOLOGIC ASPECTS OF PREGNANCY, PARTURITION, AND ANESTHESIA

JOHN J. BONICA

Today in enlightened obstetric circles it is amply appreciated that to provide optimal care to parturients, understanding the psychologic and emotional impact that pregnancy, parturition, and anesthesia have on the parturient is as important as examining the urine and blood, measuring the pelvis, and recognizing physiologic deviations, as described in the preceding chapter. It is now well-established that negative psychologic reaction may deleteriously affect both the fetus in utero and the mother's later relations with her infant. It definitely can affect the course of labor and the incidence and intensity of pain during the entire parturition process and thus impact on the anesthesiologic management. Unfortunately, there are still some physicians who consider pregnancy and parturition as mere physiologic function and consequently do not award the psychologic aspects the attention that they deserve. This is especially true of some anesthesiologists who, because of the emergency nature of obstetric anesthesia, are frequently prompted to think mechanistically, in terms of a "case" rather than to think humanistically, in terms of a "person."

This chapter emphasizes that proper anesthesiologic management of the parturient requires consideration of the psychologic condition of the mother, not only to the method of pain relief, but also to the entire process of pregnancy and parturition. Although it may seem redundant to discuss parturient reactions that occur months before the actual time of anesthetic management, this is not the case because the entire life of a woman up to the time of childbearing may be regarded in a psychologic sense as in preparation for this event. Moreover, because significant numbers of gravidae undergo surgical operation during various phases of pregnancy, it is essential for the anesthesiologist to evaluate the psychologic as well as the physical condition of the patient. All concepts and attitudes that the gravida or parturient develops will influence her behavior at the time of her anesthesia.

## PSYCHOLOGY OF PREGNANCY

Numerous psychologic studies have revealed that pregnancy can provoke a variety of negative psychologic and emotional reactions (1–9). This is particularly true of primigravidae and many of those who have not been adequately informed and prepared. Earlier studies revealed that psychologic stress invariably accompanied a first pregnancy. Caplan (10) viewed the pregnancy period as a "biologically determined psychologic crisis." During pregnancy, both the interpersonal forces in the pregnant woman and the interpersonal forces in her family are in a state of disequilibrium. Bibring (11) also looked at pregnancy as a period of crisis and disequilibrium and postulated that, like puberty and the menopause, pregnancy is associated with significant somatic and psychologic changes. Bibring stated that "the crisis of pregnancy is basically a normal occurrence and indeed an essential part of growth which must precede and prepare maturational integration." During this period unsettled or partially resolved conflicts of earlier development stages are revived and other current problems may be present that can have deleterious effects on the mother, fetus and newborn, the process of labor, and the anesthetic management. Subsequently Grimm (12) stated, "in studies conducted over a number of years . . . it has been demonstrated that emotional disturbance and severe fatigue in the mother during the late stage of pregnancy were associated with an increase in activity of the fetus in utero and disturbances such as irritability, gastrointestinal disorders, higher than average heart rate, vasomotor irritability, or changes in respiratory patterns in the newborn."

Later studies (13–15) support this view of pregnancy as a period of crisis and the pregnancy itself as a causal agent in the onset of psychologic disorders. One study (15) indicated that depressive or anxiety neurosis occurred more in pregnant women than in the control group of nonpregnant, nonpuerperal women; however, the difference was significant for anxiety only (see Figure 3–1). In addition, as Figure 3–2 denotes, a dramatic increase of depression in the postpartum period occurs (16). Figure 3–3 depicts the proportion of women seeking professional help for emotional problems before and after pregnancy (16). In contrast, a number of recent studies dispute the view that pregnancy induces a "developmental crisis" and suggest that pregnancy is protective of women when they are less prone to the risk of psychologic disorders (17–19). More recently, Gottesman (19a) demonstrated the similarities and differences of the psychologic adaption during pregnancy among adult middle age and older gravidae.

Consideration of the general literature reveals that both views are correct. Normal women react to pregnancy in

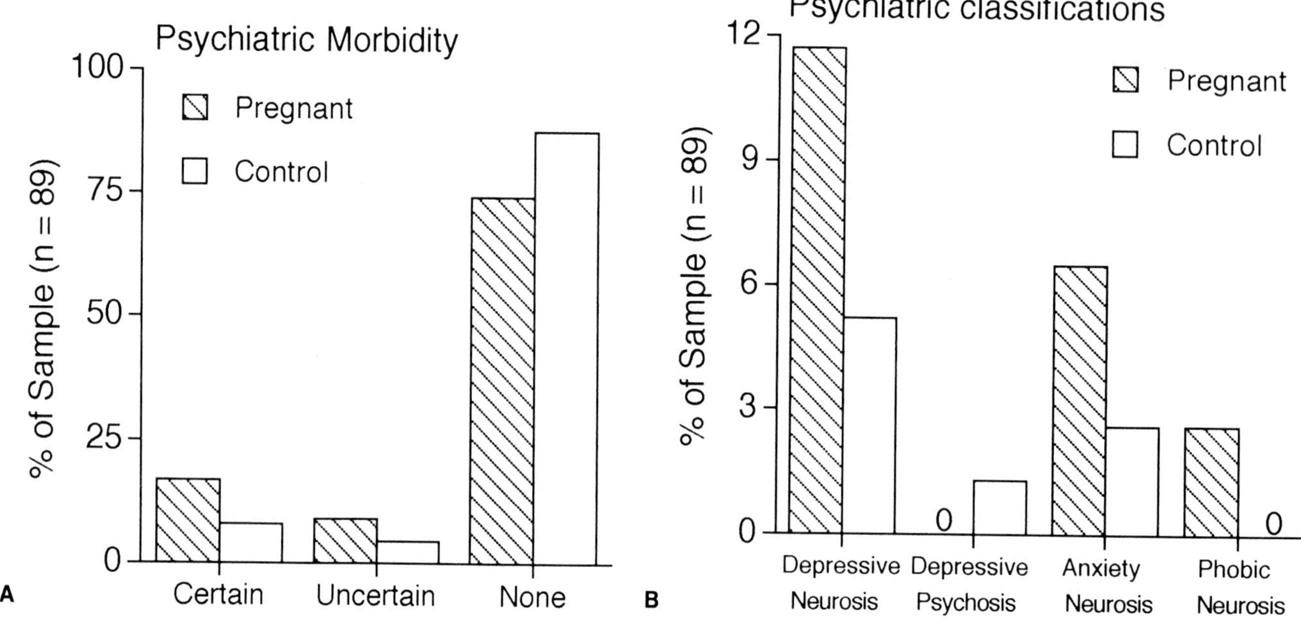


**Fig. 3–1A.** A comparison of the proportion of women with psychiatric morbidity in pregnant and controlled samples.
**Fig. 3–1B.** Psychiatric classification of women with certain psychiatric morbidity in control and pregnant samples.

a normal manner, just as they do to other situations in life, developing the ordinary, happy mental state in regard to their condition. The gravida anticipates and bears cheerfully the temporary discomforts, restrictions, and changes of appearance inherent in pregnancy, often with justifiable pride. Although she experiences certain anxieties, fears, and conflicts, these feelings are held in abeyance and effectively counterbalanced by the instinctive wish for and anticipated pleasure of having the baby; by the admiration, encouragement, and other gratifying reactions on the part of her husband, her parents, relatives and friends; by the confidence she develops in her physician; and by the knowledge of good health, and the satisfactory progress of pregnancy. However, women who were previously only marginally adjusted and in whom unresolved infantile and adolescent conflicts were previously repressed may develop psychologic, neurotic, and, very rarely, psychotic symptoms consequent to the psychologic stress of pregnancy.

## *Factors that Influence the Psychology of Pregnancy*

A variety of studies have suggested that a woman's psychologic response to pregnancy is conditioned by a complex series of interrelated influences, including five main groups of variables (1,5,20): (1) life history; (2) personality; (3) present life situation; (4) previous pregnancy experience; and (5) present pregnancy experience. In a comprehensive year-long study from the third month of pregnancy to 6 months postpartum of 60 healthy, young (18 to 28 years) primigravidae who were living with their husbands, members of middle-class families, had at least 4 years of high school education, and who lived in an urban setting, Shereshefsky, Yarrow, and others (1,20) studied the aforementioned variables other than (4). Because the high quality of their study of psychologically normal women, I selected their findings as representative of the normal American primigravidae.

### *Life History*

Based on the fact that psychoanalytic theory and contemporary research in human and animal psychology emphasize the significance of early mothering-influences on the emotional and behavioral pattern of the individual, Shereshefsky and Lockman (20), in studying the aforementioned 60 primigravidae, found that the mother/daughter relationship was one of the critical factors in assessing life history. They noted that women with good experience in being mothered are very likely to have adequate ego strength and be capable of handling the characteristic fears of pregnancy with minimal anxiety. The perception of experience in being mothered also appears to correlate with confidence in the maternal role, mother/infant adaptation, and husband/wife adaptation.

In contrast, women who were either temporarily or permanently separated from one or both parents during their childhood before the age of 12 had significantly more psychologic and mental problems, were more depressed and irritable, and had more and increasing problems in caring for the infant. Other less important factors that may influence the primigravidae include identification with one or both parents, experiences and adjustments at school and in work, peer relationship, and general health. In their study, Shereshefsky and Lockman (20) noted that among the 35 women who had suffered from a serious illness or accident before marriage gave evidence that pregnancy and especially labor and delivery

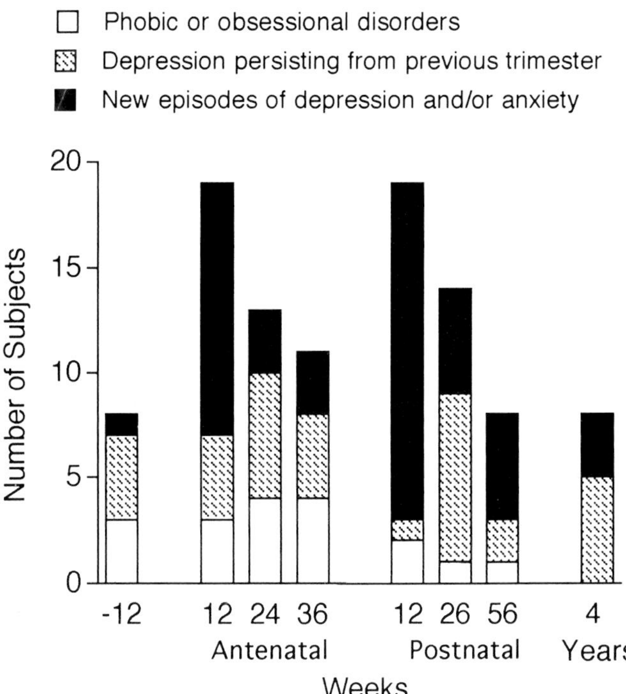


**Fig. 3–2.** The prevalence and incidence of neurotic disturbance in the main sample of first-time mothers is shown at different times of the longitudinal survey. The incidence of depression is significantly increased in the first trimester of pregnancy and also at 12 weeks postnatally. The numbers in parentheses refer to new cases. A subject is counted as a "new" case of depression only if she was not rated as depressed at the immediately previous occasion. Symptoms of anxiety mingled with depression in many subjects, but there were only two women with primary anxiety states, one in early pregnancy and the other 3 months after delivery. (Redrawn from Kumar R, Robson KM: A prospective study of emotional disorders in childbearing women. Br. J. Psychiatry 144:35, 1984.)

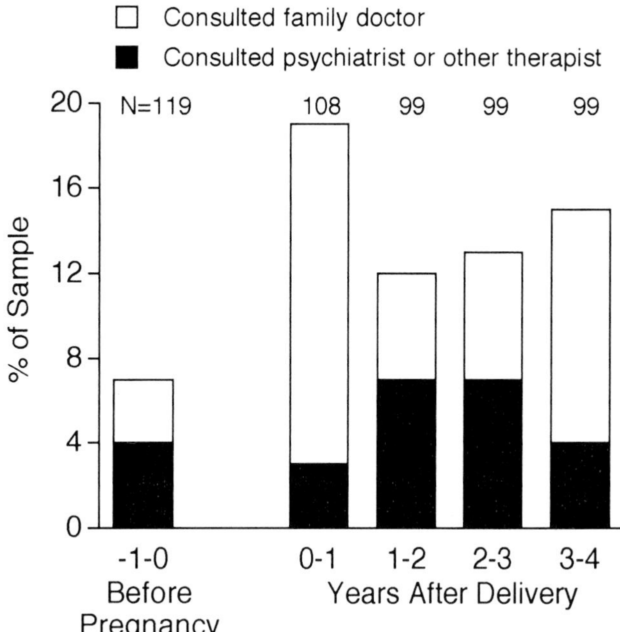


**Fig. 3–3.** The histograms show the proportion of women in the main sample (n = 119) who reported that they had consulted their family doctors or a specialist (e.g., psychiatrist, marriage guidance counsellor, lay psychotherapist) for emotional problems at various times during the survey. The data for the year before they conceived were obtained retrospectively at the first interview. Consultations between the first and fourth years after delivery were also measured retrospectively, when the women were interviewed at 4 years postnatally. (Redrawn from Kumar R, Robson KM: A prospective study of emotional disorders in childbearing women. Br. J. Psychiatry 144:35, 1984.)

often reactivated concern about body image and anxieties about doctors, medical procedures, and hospitalization.

## *Personality*

Of significant importance is the woman's personality, because this is clearly and closely related to her pregnancy experience. Among 28 items used in psychologic testing and psychiatric and social work interviews carried out at 3 months of gestation in evaluating the woman's personality, Shereshefsky and Lockman (20) reduced these items by factor analysis to factor scales, ego strength, and nurturing. Their collaborators, Saltzman and Schneidman (21), found these two factor scales to be very significant in the woman's adaptation to pregnancy. Ego strength includes: (1) degree to which a woman adapts emotionally; (2) level of general anxiety; (3) covert, underlying dependency pattern; (4) sense of human flexibility and ability to meet her own needs, including pleasure; (5) acceptance of her own identity; and (6) degree to which she has achieved an adult role and the overall adaptive behavior she exhibits. Nurturance involves the gratification in female sexuality, the responsiveness from her husband and others, the degree to which she is tender and affectionate and able to give help and support, and the responsiveness to her husband and to others.

Shereshefsky and collaborators (20,22) found that the characteristics of a well-developed ego strength and nurturance were closely related with the woman's ability to react not only to pregnancy, but also to the maternal period and, indeed, these characteristics could be used to predict a woman's response to pregnancy as well as to motherhood. In contrast, women with poorly defined ego strength and nurturance found it much more difficult to adapt to pregnancy and developed more symptoms.

## *Present Life Situation*

Current life situations including age, socioeconomic status, marital situation, and external stresses are other factors that influence the psychologic response to pregnancy. Age has been shown to influence the psychologic response to pregnancy and has also an important relationship to reproductive performance. The incidence of negative psychologic reactions is greater in primigravidae under 15 and over 35 years of age. Moreover, they have greater incidence of poor reproductive performance (5). Social class also has an important impact on psychologic reaction and reproduction. Studies in many countries have documented impressively the fact that gravidae in lower classes have greater psychologic reactions and poorer reproductive performance. Richardson (23) has suggested that the poorer reproductive performance among the financially poorer population is probably due to poor nutrition, stunting of physical growth, poor hygiene, inadequate education, prevalence of infectious disease, and close spacing of children, making this class a "population at risk."

### Marital Situation

The marital situation modifies significantly the gravida's psychologic reaction to pregnancy and motherhood. Shereshefsky and Lockman (20) found that the level of adjustment at first pregnancy, as well as the range in time of occurrence, showed wide variations. Well-adaptive marital relationships were characterized by such factors as an intense degree of affection, empathy, satisfying sexual adjustment, mutuality of goals, and flexibility of decision-making. Among this group there was much that was exciting and gratifying to counterbalance pregnancy-engendered anxieties. They noted that an emerging sense of common goals seemed to give new depth to the husband-wife relationship, which was expressed in many ways: shared preoccupation about what kind of parents they were likely to be and how they would meet crises and everyday issues, moments of wonder over the movements of the fetus and what they portended about the sex, and the future level of activity of the expected child. In many instances the men were able to sustain their wife with confidence, humor, affection, and reassurance.

In contrast, less adapted or poor husband-wife relationships showed such negative aspects as more conflict than mutuality, considerable hostility, more inhibition toward freedom in communication, and decisions arrived at with difficulty and further threat to mutuality. This group in conflict included two different patterns and processes: (1) those involved in differences that were essentially related to the earlier adjustment phase of the marriage—differences that were transitory; and (2) those involved in serious marital disharmony probably a long time in duration or predictive of eventual disruption of marriage (20). Among the first group were those who were caught up in the bewilderment of early marriage with its still surprising rewards and demands, and in the moments of discomforture of its disappointments and sharp encounters, but many of these issues were resolved with time. Serious marital disharmony, which was found in 21% of the families, had a negative impact on the woman's ability to adapt to pregnancy. Moreover, the pregnancy often became another source of discord for couples who were already in a conflict situation.

### External Stresses

External stresses consisting of a multitude of different life events also have a significant, negative impact on the psychologic reaction to pregnancy. Among the most important of these are financial concerns as it relates to the job satisfaction of the wife and husband, with the current economic crisis and effect of inflation and loss of earnings of the wife during the pregnancy and postpartum period. Moreover, housing problems, particularly in major cities, may contribute to family unhappiness and misery during pregnancy. In their study of this normal population, Shereshefsky and Lockman (20) found that about 30% of the families had concerns about finances.

Other factors that constitute specific stressors include an illness of the wife or husband during pregnancy or illness or death in the family, and isolation related to geographic distance from major family supports. Shereshefsky and Lockman (20) found that these, together with serious marital disharmony, occurred in 70% of their study population. Moreover, during the pregnancy 42% were involved with two or more stresses and 3% had a maximum of four. Naturally, unmarried women face a whole range of special problems that provoke negative psychologic reactions and make it more difficult for them to adapt to pregnancy (5).

### Previous Pregnancy Experience

A variety of problems that occurred during previous pregnancy can provoke a great deal of anxiety, fear, and apprehension and, consequently, have a negative influence on adaptation to pregnancy. These include miscarriage, abortion, or delivery of a preterm infant at risk, pregnancy-induced hypertension or any other severe complication during pregnancy, a painful vaginal delivery, an unpleasant forceps or cesarean section, or a number of other factors that are discussed below.

## Negative Psychologic Reactions During Pregnancy

### Resentment and Rejection

These are probably the earliest reactions to pregnancy. They usually develop as soon as the woman learns that she has conceived. Before the current era of planned parenthood, the majority of gestations were unplanned (3,6,9) and, consequently, the incidence of resentment and rejection was very high. In such patients, frustrations were frequent and at times anxiety reached an unreasonably high level. The majority of these patients gave reasons for rejection of the pregnancy that appeared partly unrealistic: economic insecurity or hardship; inadequate housing; or larger number of children. Some gravidae who experience these negative reactions may have such unconscious thoughts as the pregnancy's interference with social life or professional and economic pursuits, concern over the loss of physical attractiveness, and fear of discomfort or even death (3,6).

Rejection may even develop in planned pregnancies, which have been motivated by such illogical, immature or irrational reasons as pregnancies planned to obtain support, to prove femininity to domineering parents or a rival sister, or to reunite parents (3,5,6). Deutsch (3,4), Kanner (6), and Wengraff (9) reported the instances in which conception was planned by the woman as part of a scheme to induce her husband to assume proper responsibility for his family or to enhance the marital relationship or to allay his alcoholism, gambling or other bad habits. If the pregnancy resulted in accomplishment of the goal, it proved of great psychologic benefit to the mother. Unfortunately, in these circumstances all too frequently the gestation does very little to achieve the major purpose for which it was designated, and it is therefore resented as a bad investment (5).

### Ambivalence and Sense of Guilt

The aforementioned negative reactions to the coming child are in conflict with the female's basic inborn instinct to reproduce and thus provoke ambivalent reactions (3,4,25,26). Moreover, although society permits expression of pleasure and happiness at the prospect of having a child, it makes the gravida less free to express pleasure for negative feelings. Consequently, through shame or guilt she keeps these feelings to herself. As the suppressed or repressed negative feelings accumulate, they become magnified out of proportion to their significance and form the basis for some of the depression of pregnancy (4,25).

A sense of guilt may burden women who early in pregnancy experience resentment and rejection (3–6). Later when these women finally accept the pregnancy, they feel guilty for having resented the process. Some gravidae have a feeling of guilt and shame based on a background of biologic ignorance and unreasonable fears about the effects of intercourse during pregnancy (3–6).

## *Mood, Anxiety, Fear and Depression*

These are emotional reactions experienced by many pregnant women at one time or another during their gestation (1,3–6,24–29a).

### Mood

During pregnancy the mood varies according to different phases of gestation. During the first trimester, beginning with the discovery of conception, the mood changes are associated with hormonal changes with consequent increased emotional sensitivity (5,17). Consequently, women who are usually outgoing become edgy, nervous, tense, snappy, and tearful (5). They are often more demanding of their husband and, during the first trimester, have diminished vitality. Also, thought processes may become erratic, and hasty decisions sometimes made. Many women worry about becoming fat and unattractive, and the increasing fullness of a woman's breasts and changing curve of her abdomen is considered by some as threats to their self-esteem. Irrespective of her conscious attitude toward pregnancy, a woman's chief unconscious fantasy accompanying these changes is the sense of a foreign body jeopardizing her well-being, and not being in control of her body and mind may well create feelings of vulnerability. As previously mentioned, it is not uncommon for the gravida to experience vague misgivings or moderately angry feelings and resentment toward the developing baby (17). Shereshefsky and Lockman (20), based on their study, estimated that more than half the women in the first trimester experience and exhibit such reactions, but this usually falls to about one-third by the seventh month. On the other hand, there is usually a progressive increase in enhancement of their feeling of well-being as pregnancy continues: from 23% at 12 weeks to about 50% at 28 weeks (20). Moreover, by the end of the fourteenth week of pregnancy in most women, the nausea and fatigue have disappeared and the couple often enjoyed improved sexual relations. Also an increasing confidence in the woman's visualization of herself as a mother emerges as pregnancy advances, and, at the same time, there is usually a progressive improvement in the husband-wife relationship. The feeling of movement by the baby and the consequent reality that there is a separate, growing form within, tends to initiate and enhances strong feelings of protectiveness and a desire to nurture. Indeed, even unplanned, unwanted pregnancies may seem more acceptable at this time. A study on childbearing and maternal sexuality revealed there was clearly a fall in the frequency of sexual intercourse throughout pregnancy from the prepregnant state (8). In addition, the study revealed a slow but gradual return of frequency during the postpartum period (Table 3–1). Furthermore, sexual enjoyment was shown to have a similar fall throughout the antepartum period, and it too slowly returned in the postpartum period (Table 3–2). During pregnancy, most patients indicated that the decrease in frequency of sexual intercourse was due to fears, physical problems, discomfort, or lack of enjoyment (Figure 3–4). The overall prevailing effect on sexuality appears to be a decrease in both frequency and enjoyment of sexual intercourse throughout the antepartum period, and it persists well into the postpartum period (8).

### Anxiety and Fear

The gravida is usually beset by two types of fear that often run concurrently: fear for herself and fear for the

**Table 3–1.** Frequency of Sexual Intercourse

| Frequency per Week | Pre-pregnancy | Antepartum 12 wks | Antepartum 24 wks | Antepartum 36 wks | Postpartum 12 wks | Postpartum 26 wks | Postpartum 52 wks |
|---|---|---|---|---|---|---|---|
| ≥4 | 39.5% | 13.5% | 12.7% | 5.4% | 11.5% | 15.5% | 20.4% |
| 1–3 | 53.8 | 52.1 | 55.1 | 32.7 | 60.2 | 66.4 | 59.2 |
| <1 | 6.7 | 23.5 | 24.6 | 26.4 | 23.0 | 13.6 | 17.3 |
| 0 | | 10.9 | 7.6 | 35.5 | 5.3 | 4.5 | 3.1 |
| # of subjects | 119 | 119 | 118 | 110 | 113 | 110 | 98 |

(From Kumar R, Brant HA, Robson KM: Childbearing and maternal sexuality: a prospective survey of 119 primiparae. Psychosom. Res. 25:373, 1981.)

**Table 3–2.** Enjoyment of Sexual Intercourse

| Enjoyment | Pre-pregnancy | Antepartum 12 wks | Antepartum 24 wks | Antepartum 36 wks | Postpartum 12 wks | Postpartum 26 wks | Postpartum 52 wks |
|---|---|---|---|---|---|---|---|
| Pleasurable, no problems | 61.3% | 37.8% | 47.4% | 24.5% | 37.2% | 45.4% | 59.2% |
| Pleasurable, some problems | 17.6 | 21.0 | 27.9 | 16.4 | 31.9 | 31.8 | 22.4 |
| Very little or no pleasure | 21.1 | 30.3 | 17.1 | 23.6 | 25.6 | 18.2 | 15.3 |
| No sex | | 10.9 | 7.6 | 35.5 | 5.3 | 4.6 | 3.1 |

(From Kumar R, Brant HA, Robson KM: Childbearing and maternal sexuality: a prospective survey of 119 primiparae. Psychosom. Res. 25:373, 1981.)

baby (30). Recent studies have shown that the level of anxiety runs very high in the first trimester, is less in the second, but increases again in the last trimester (5,14,22). More than half of the patients studied by Shereshefsky and collaborators (22) revealed more anxiety and apprehension in these last periods than at previous periods of pregnancy (31). With labor and delivery imminent and physical awkwardness and discomfort more marked, they experienced more anxiety and expressed eagerness to have the pregnancy over with. Suggestive of mounting anxiety was the fact that approximately one-fourth of the women had some degree of false labor and several had to be admitted to the hospital for observation, sedation, and rest (30).

In a study of 220 women, 31 of whom were in the first trimester, 80 in the third trimester, and 60 in the postpartum period, Arizmendi and Alfonso (14) found that the anxiety level generated by most events varies across the gestation and delivery. Moreover, the events that were perceived to trigger the most anxiety were such internal events as fears or concerns regarding labor and delivery and the baby's welfare. They noted that the one category of external events that proved to be the most stressful was the gravida-spouse interaction, and that the intensity of stress was consistent across trimesters. They noted that the third trimester was associated with most acute stress. A woman's concern related to social feedback and self-image tended to peak during this period, as did stress related to emotional lability, a period of time when the woman's body is manifesting its greatest overt differences from the prepregnancy period. Thus, her body image becomes a central focus and feedback from others is likely to be more prevalent, influencing the gravida's self-image and level of self-esteem.

Arizmendi and Alfonso (14) and others have found that the woman's greatest stress is generated typically by anticipatory fears of complications involving herself or her baby. Apprehension and fear about herself affect her personal state of health during pregnancy and the possibility of complications during labor. Other "real" fears during pregnancy may be those of financial insecurity, fear of the new responsibility, fear that motherhood will ruin her

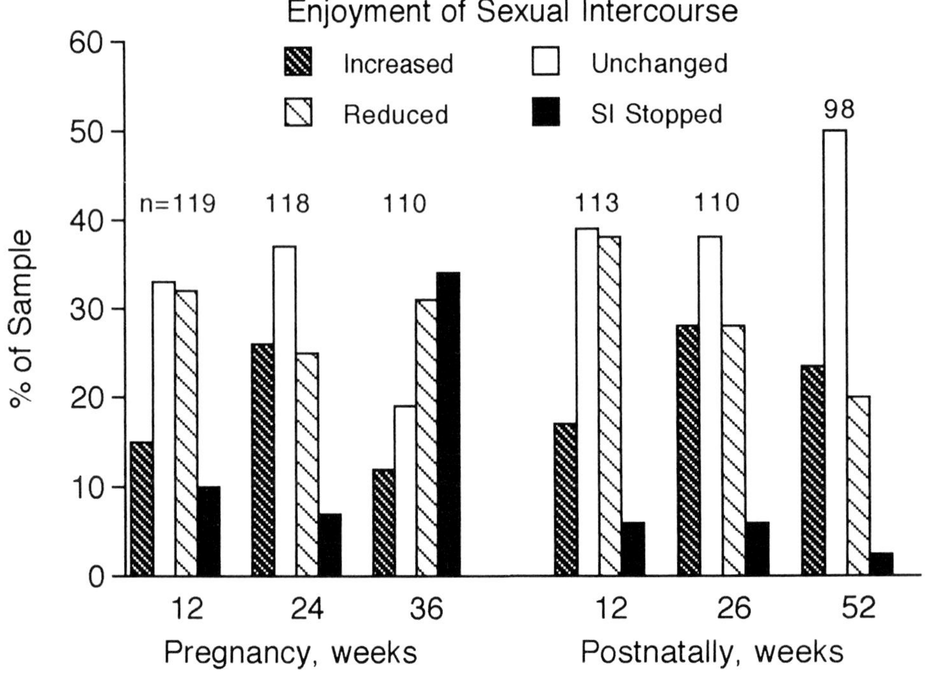


**Fig. 3–4.** Changes in subjects' enjoyment of sexual intercourse through pregnancy and after delivery are shown as differences from the ratings made of their reports of enjoyment in the month before conception. (Redrawn from Kumar R, Brant HA, Robson KM: Childbearing and maternal sexuality: A prospective survey of 119 primiparae. J. Psychosom. Res. 23:373, 1981.)

career and talents and frustrate her emotional goal (3,4). There is also evidence that the effects of pregnancy may be aggravated significantly in those who were afflicted previously with a crippling disease or had prior difficult pregnancies (1,3,4,26). Gravidae who have such medical complications as rheumatic disease or other conditions have even greater fears for themselves and their infant (26).

Concern for the health of the fetus is a frequent cause of anxiety and fear during pregnancy (1–6,26,32,33). The mother fears miscarriage, possible death of the fetus in utero or impairment of the child's mental capacity, and the possibility of having a complicated delivery with consequent harm to the infant. Some gravidae develop apprehension about the baby's gender, appearance, birthmarks, or deformities or even monstrosity (1,3–5,26). In a study of gravidae who experienced dreams during pregnancy, Gillman (34) found that 40% of these gravidae had anxiety-ridden dreams, compared with a group of nonpregnant college women, of whom only 10% had such dreams. Some 40% of the gravidae's dreams were about their babies, compared with 1% of the dreams of the college women who had dreamt about pregnancy or childbearing. A significant number of gravidae dreamt that the babies were crippled, deformed, or threatened. Similar findings had been reported 3 decades earlier by Deutsch (3), who also mentioned that some of the dreams concerned misfortunes, harm, or final threats to the mother: one gravida had dreamt she was surrounded, caught and in danger of being clawed by a wild beast (3).

### *Depression*

Like anxiety, depression is most common during the first 3 months, is usually not severe, and is probably related to the hormonal changes that are developing at the time. If depression occurs for the first time during the second or third trimester, it should receive urgent attention.

### ***Prophylaxis***

Proper psychologic preparation, information, and related care during the pregnancy are of inestimable value in helping the psychologically stable gravida to decrease or completely eliminate the impact of fear, anxiety, guilt feelings, and other negative emotional reactions (1,3,4, 5,10). These women are ready to seek and accept from their physician and other members of the obstetric team information and enlightenment regarding the physiology and psychologic reactions of pregnancy (1,10,24). Even most women with unplanned pregnancies are able to overcome the first shock of the discovery of conception and to adjust to the new situation without difficulty. Among the patients studied by Shereshefsky and associates (22), changes in terms of psychologic preparation for childbirth and maternity occurred in several major aspects. Among these involved clarification and confidence in visualizing herself as mother, on the feeling of well-being and improved husband-wife adaptation (except for the most acutely discordant families).

The story might be quite different in patients who have fundamental personality problems and are victims of powerful unconscious cross-currents that are reinforced by the aforementioned psychologic and emotional reactions (3,5,6). Unless the physician recognizes these problems very early and takes positive steps to effectively treat them, many of these patients will develop a variety of such somatic symptoms as headache, abdominal pain, low back pain, insomnia, and the usual symptoms of pregnancy such as nausea, vomiting, constipation, heart burn or indigestion, leg cramps and muscle pain, fatigue, and the preference or abhorrence for specific foods (3–6). Some of these patients manifest strong aggressiveness, and thus become dangerous for both fetus and mother and the pregnancy may suffer from spiteful neglect of antepartal care (3,5,6). In others the rejection of the pregnancy causes compulsive intake of liquor, tobacco, or food to the point of complicating the pregnancy by toxicity or marked obesity (6). In addition to the risk imposed on the pregnancy, these reactions may have deleterious effects on the nutrition of the fetus. Obviously, the emotional reactions may be severe enough to affect the parturient and thus complicate the anesthetic management.

## PSYCHOLOGIC ASPECTS OF PARTURITION

Labor and parturition reinforce many of the psychologic and emotional reactions mentioned previously and evoke certain others peculiar to these phases of the process of motherhood (35,36). It has already been mentioned that the mother's strong negative psychologic and emotional reactions may have a deleterious affect on fetal physiology and thus effect postnatal behavior and the mother's later relationship with her infant (10,28,29,32,37,38). Wengraff (9) depicted parturition, with all of its dangers and apprehensions, and its hopes and achievements, as a battle between strong opposing psychologic forces. On one side is fear, rejection, superstition, hostility and selfishness, and on the other, self-sacrifice, renunciation, and love. The childbirth process is particularly propitious for psychogenic influences (3).

The normal, well-adjusted, and properly prepared mother accepts the confinement as a hoped-for climax, at the end of which comes the coveted reward—the infant. The protective energies mobilized by the inborn instinct for reproduction are reinforced by education; by the mother's realization that parturition is a transition demanded by nature toward her ultimate goal which has been eagerly desired; and by her strong confidence in the physician whom she regards as an omniscient and omnipotent father-figure whose power and skill will be mobilized in her favor against the difficulties of her childbirth (5,6). In contrast, in emotionally unstable or psychologically unprepared women, parturition constitutes an intolerable psychologic stress that is conducive to abnormal behavior during labor and that may possibly produce prolonged and even permanent psychopathology. The devastating results of anxiety and fear on childbirth were effectively and dramatically emphasized by Dick-Read (39), who developed an entire philosophy of childbirth around this psychologic reaction.

### *Fear, Anxiety, and Apprehension*

The basic fear of death is the most important component of anxiety and apprehension because it provokes strong emotional reactions (3,4). Moreover, because the fear of death is a deep rooted, unconscious force that arises from the most primal source, its elimination by education and psychologic conditioning, as can be accomplished with other fears, is much more difficult if not impossible (3,40).

The fears of suffering, anesthesia, and of sustaining complications are very frequent and potent forces in disturbing emotional well-being during parturition. Primigravidae develop fears and anxiety as a result of extrapersonal influences while multigravidae usually have these reactions because of previous painful or complicated deliveries.

### *Causes of Fear and Anxiety During Labor*

#### Relatives and Friends

Formerly, from an early age on, girls were subjected to the fear-producing teachings that childbirth was a dangerous and painful process (3,38). Many grandmothers and even mothers of the present generation of gravidae, never having had the advantage of modern obstetric analgesia management, experienced suffering and sustained complications during their childbearing. As a result, they developed emotional tension and fearful attitudes which they have unintentionally imparted to their pregnant granddaughters and/or daughters (3,38). The influence of the husband is also particularly important: should he develop a state of anxiety or fear concerning the parturition, it will be communicated to the expectant wife and thus tends to reinforce her fears. It is unfortunate, and very strange indeed, to think that fears have been implanted frequently in the gravida by mature women, friends or acquaintances, who have delighted to an almost sadistic degree in recalling the dreadful experiences that they or someone they knew experienced during childbirth.

#### News Media

Apart from the more intimate source of information about childbirth, women cannot escape the influence of public opinions found in books, newspapers, radio, television, and motion pictures. Regrettably, in most instances, childbirth is depicted as an ordeal, essentially painful, and dangerous to the life of the mother. It is almost impossible for the expectant woman, especially if this is her first pregnancy, to see these representations without becoming acutely conscious of the possibility that they may attend her own confinement.

#### Attending Physician

The critical role played by the attending physician in offsetting these deleterious influences is stressed in Chapters 21 and 22. Here we will consider how physicians can unintentionally provoke these reactions by their behavior, attitude, admissions or comments. The use of such fear-provoking terminology as "labor pains," "lacerations," "hemorrhages," "stitches," "shots," and "mortality," is a not infrequent error. The physician may also cause fear by inadvertently stressing the importance of pain of childbirth. It is not uncommon for a young primigravida to receive such final instructions as "go to the hospital when your 'pains' are strong and regular." Unfortunately, even some outstanding authorities (41,42) have been unable to abandon the archaic custom of using the term "pains" for uterine contractions. Failure by the physician to see the patient soon after she enters the hospital may cause fear and anxiety in the parturient who has developed dependency upon the physician. Finally, if complications exist, physicians must suppress their own fears and anxieties about labor so that the patient will not sense this and become frightened. The same comments apply to the behavior of the house staff. The role played by the administrator of the anesthetic will be emphasized in the next section.

#### Hospitalization

In primigravidae and some multigravidae, apprehension, anxiety, fear, and mental anguish can be provoked by the trip to the hospital, of which institution the uninformed patient associates with illness, injury, surgery or accidents, and often considers it a strange and dangerous environment (43,44). Anxiety in going to the hospital produces anxiety and stress that correlate highly with the incidence and intensity of pain during childbirth (44,45). Volicer (45) showed that uninformed and unprepared patients who went to the hospital for a variety of conditions, who scored high in "hospital stress," and who had painful conditions experienced more pain and more morbidity than those who had low "hospital stress" scores. Some factors used to measure "hospital stress" included: lack of information before admission; separation from family; isolation from others; unfamiliar surroundings; and previous experience with inadequate pain treatment. Many of these factors are especially important in young primigravidae who have not experienced hospitalization before. On the other hand, multigravidae may develop anxiety and apprehension concerning the welfare of the children who may have to be left at home alone. These fears may remain throughout labor and may prove deleterious.

Fears and anxieties may be initiated or reinforced by the action, behavior or comments of the hospital personnel. A negative attitude or wrong comment by the admission clerk, elevator operator, nurse's aide, or any one of the many people with whom the parturient comes in contact with as she enters the hospital may precipitate fear and anxiety. Obstetric nurses, by the very nature of their work and close association with the patient, next to the attending physician, play the most important role in influencing the emotional status of the parturient. If, instead of managing the patient with a warm, sympathetic attitude, reassurance, and prompt response to requests, nurses treat the patient with an impersonal, rude, belligerent or otherwise unpleasant manner, they may cause the patient to promptly develop resentment and fear.

The patient's fears may be further reinforced and perhaps justified when she is placed in a community labor room with other women, some of whom may be crying out with each contraction. The uninformed primigravida entering such a room may become panic-stricken. Isolation in a single room may likewise produce fear if the patient is left unattended without words of explanation and with little or no instruction. An earlier study in Britain indicated that parturients considered insufficient companionship and attention as the most significant deficiency of the management of the first stage of labor within the hospital setting (46). Unless fully informed about the contractions, great fear, anxiety, and apprehension can be experienced at the height of a strong contraction, when, for example, the membranes rupture and a flow of blood or warm liquid is felt.

Many of these sources of anxiety and fear can be diminished or even eliminated by an active antepartal program of education and training, as discussed in detail in Chapter 21, and emphasized by many other authorities (46A,46B). In one study by Delke and associates (46C), it was shown that childbirth education and preparation significantly lowered plasma beta-endorphin immunoreactivity and reduced slightly the first stages of labor compared to a control group which did not receive adequate preparation. The authors hypothesized that this beneficial effect was due to the fact that childbirth preparation reduced fear, tension, and emotional stress of labor.

### *Role of the Pain of Labor*

In improperly prepared parturients, pain and suffering during labor invariably provoke or aggravate fear and anxiety. In the subconscious mind pain is allied with threat to life and impending disaster. Moreover, pain and fear are intimately interwoven into the fabric of life (47). Numerous studies have firmly established a direct relationship between pain and anxiety in childbirth (29,47–50). Figure 9–9 (see Figure 9–9, Chapter 9) demonstrates that labor pain in multiparae and primiparae exceeds the pain ascribed to common day-to-day pain syndromes (50). Table 9–1 demonstrates the severity of labor pain as interpreted after the fact by patients upon interview (50). Although early studies (51) suggested a curvilinear relation between anxiety and pain, most recent researchers now agree that there is a linear relationship between the two, i.e., increased anxiety is related to increased pain ( 51).

In a recent study, Wuitshik and associates (52) noted that anxiety, stress, and negative cognitive processes were associated with severe pain in the latent phase and that this was predictive of a longer latent phase and a long active phase of labor. Moreover, stress-related thoughts during the latent phase were predictive of a longer latent phase and longer second stage of labor and consequently in an increase in instrumental deliveries.

When fear, anxiety and apprehension, and pain are not significantly decreased or eliminated by proper antepartal preparation and the use of analgesia, they can cause havoc in an otherwise healthy parturient, and a normal labor can be converted into a horrible experience. While the memory of labor pain decreases over time (52a), in some puerperae the severe pain and suffering during labor may precipitate serious psychologic and emotional disturbances that can cause psychopathology and also influence the relationship between mother and child during their first few crucial days or weeks (52–56). Moreover, the parturient may develop intense fears of future pregnancies that seriously affect her sexual and emotional relationship with her husband (52,53). A number of studies have shown that many parturients who attempted natural childbirth without pharmacologic analgesia and experienced severe pain during labor and vaginal delivery developed serious negative emotional reactions (53–57). Stewart (57) reported that some of the patients in the postpartum period became miserable, depressed, and some even became suicidal, lost interest in sex and their marriage, and required psychotherapy. Indeed, in some cases the husbands who observed their wife experience severe pain and suffering also developed psychiatric symptoms and needed psychotherapy for impotence, phobias, and depression (57).

Stewart (57a) attributed the underlying causes to inadequate community-based childbirth preparation classes, which were inflexible and intolerant of medications and interventions. In 1981 and 1982, 18 of 125 patients attributed their postpartum psychologic problems to the birthing experience. In 1983, the hospital in which Stewart practiced initiated what was apparently better childbirth education programs with the result that only six of the 130 referrals with postpartum symptoms attributed them to the birthing experience. This emphasizes that fear, anxiety apprehension, and stress can be ameliorated by highly effective childbirth preparation classes.

## PSYCHOLOGIC ASPECTS OF ANESTHESIA

The psychologic and emotional reactions evoked by anesthesia are of serious concern to the entire obstetric team, but particularly to obstetric anesthesiologists who should mobilize their knowledge, skill, and all their attributes as physicians to obviate or counteract these reactions, and thus make the anesthesia not an unpleasant, but rather a pleasurable physical and emotional experience by relieving the pain and suffering. The reactions provoked by anesthesia are very similar to, and inextricably interrelated with, those that have been discussed in the preceding sections. They are discussed here separately to emphasize the role anesthesia plays in their development. In addition, certain other emotional phenomena peculiar to anesthesia need to be mentioned. These include the dreams that are experienced by the patient under general anesthesia and certain postanesthetic psychologic effects produced primarily by the anesthetic experience.

### *Emotional Reactions to the Preanesthetic Period*

The preanesthetic period begins when analgesia/anesthesia for labor and parturition is considered. Between this time and delivery the parturient may experience a variable degree of anxiety, apprehension, and fear about anesthesia. The most serious and most powerful is the basic fear of death which, as previously stated, is a potent, deep-rooted, unconscious force (3,4,47). Closely related to this is the fear of losing consciousness and coming into contact with the unknown (3,4). This is especially prone to develop in the uninformed or misinformed primigravida who has not had previous experience with anesthesia and who may think of unconsciousness and the loss of control of her body as a form of death (3,4). Some patients are able to ignore these fears by suppression.

The fear of possible anesthetic complications may disturb some gravidae. In this modern age of obstetric analgesia/anesthesia, there are many patients and, regrettably, even some physicians, who have serious misconceptions about the complications inherent in certain forms of anesthesia. In questioning the many patients who have expressed fears of paralysis due to spinal anesthesia, for example, among the over 8,000 parturients I have personally managed during the past 45 years of obstetric anesthesia practice I have not found a single authenticated case that could be used as a basis for such fears. In other instances the misconceptions are due to the complications or unpleasant experiences that occurred to their grandmother, mother or friends before the advent of modern anesthesia and the obstetric anesthesiologist (see Chapter 1). The disrepute that followed the over-enthusiastic and indiscriminate use of subarachnoid (spinal, caudal, and epidural) anesthesia in the early years of these techniques has been perpetuated in some quarters. This notwithstanding, the significant improvement in these procedures, when properly applied, is not only safe but has beneficial physical and psychologic effects on the mother and indirect beneficial effects on the fetus and newborn. Still another etiologic factor has been the unwarranted publicity given by newspapers on such rare occurrences of complication. Motion pictures and television, which often depict the administration of anesthesia as a dramatic between-life-and-death occasion, have also contributed to fear of anesthetics.

One of the most prevalent sources of fear is gross misrepresentations of the danger of anesthesia by well-meaning but misinformed authors. One of the greatest offenders in this respect was that outstanding crusader against fear of childbirth, Grantly Dick-Read (39), who committed the very sins for which he reprimanded others. In his books he called writers to task for instilling fear of what he considered a gross misrepresentation of the phenomenon of labor. In a similar fashion, Dr. Dick-Read misrepresented anesthetics as "poisons of the body" or "mutilating procedures." Throughout his book he exploited his extraordinary rhetorical talent in a very dramatic, often sarcastic, and fear-provoking manner, in arguing his belief that anesthesia is not necessary in 95% of parturients. However, in doing so he performed a great disservice because his writings have been widely read by prospective mothers who naturally may develop fear of anesthesia. Similar comments can be said of Lamaze (40) and other proponents of psychoprophylaxis and of LeBoyer (58) in extolling his concept of "birth without violence." Because a more detailed explanation of the subject is made in Chapter 21, nothing more will be said here except to note that the aversions of these writers to pharmacologic analgesia for parturients developed as a result of poor and at times disastrous experience with maladministered anesthetic agents and improper understanding of their action. In attempting to understand their viewpoints, we may perhaps attribute their negative anesthetic impressions on poor dedication to childbirth anesthesia during those times. Today, with the dedication of a large percentage of anesthesiologists to improving the delivery of obstetric anesthesia and improved coordination and education of obstetric anesthesiologists, pediatricians, gynecologists, and nurses, the situation has changed dramatically. These authors may have had quite different views entirely had they had the opportunity to interact with current practitioners in the area of obstetric anesthesia.

### *Prophylactic Measures*

Many of these negative psychologic and emotional reactions to anesthesia can be significantly minimized or even eliminated by having obstetric anesthesiologists participate in the antepartal preparation of the gravida during the latter part of pregnancy. During one of the prenatal visits, analgesia and anesthesia should be discussed in some detail, and the advantages, disadvantages, and limitations of each technique described. Although the obstetrician may indicate which technique he or she considers preferable, great caution should be exercised not to promise the patient either a specific method or painless labor. Rather, the patient should be assured that there are many means available for relieving pain and that all efforts compatible with safety will be made to lessen the discomfort.

In hospitals that have complete anesthesia services, it is essential for a member of the Obstetric Anesthesia Division to meet with groups of gravidae for periods of 60 to 90 minutes to present objectively the indication, advantages, disadvantages, and limitations of the various techniques used. Gravidae who are thus fully informed and are given an opportunity to ask questions about any aspect of the subject will accrue great benefits from a decrease in the anxiety and apprehension that they may be experiencing.

## *Emotional Reactions During the Intra-Anesthetic Period*

The most significant and affective emotional reactions concerning anesthesia occur just before the administration of the anesthetic. A frequent fear is that of being physically helpless and that something horrible will be done or that the obstetrician will start painful instrumentation before the onset of adequate analgesia (6,44,52,53,59). In some individuals inhalation anesthesia used for complicated deliveries or cesarean section symbolizes suffocation or strangulation and such persons develop great fears during the induction of the anesthetic (3,43,59,60). Subarachnoid or epidural block, on the other hand, may provoke fear of persistent low back pain or having the back damaged and fear even of permanent paralysis (44,59–62).

A relatively common fear is that general anesthesia will cause loss of sensation and inhibitions, that the patient will perform irresponsible acts or betray secrets (44, 57,60–62). Some patients express this fear before receiving the anesthetic, whereas others will manifest this fear postoperatively by avoiding their physician who, they believe, has learned their secrets or by asking such questions as: "Was I a bad patient during anesthesia?" (60,61).

Fear of the anesthesia can be instilled in the parturient by attitudes, behavior, comments or reactions from the obstetric team. I have seen reasonably calm parturients become agitated and fearful because of a nurse who manifested disdain or disapproval when the parturient told the nurse about the type of analgesia she was scheduled to receive. Similarly, enthusiastic approval of a certain type of anesthesia stated to one patient in the presence of another may cause the latter to fear the anesthetic she is to receive is not the best. Obviously, great care and discretion must be exercised by the nurse in making comments about a specific type of analgesia/anesthesia. Unless the gravida is prepared psychologically for a change in plans, fear is likely to develop should it become necessary to use a different form of anesthesia promised the patient.

The attitude of the anesthesiologist toward the parturient during the preanesthetic period, which includes preanesthetic evaluation of the patient and preparation of the parturient for the obstetric analgesia/anesthesia, is a potent force for either beneficial or deleterious psychologic reactions by the patients (44,59–61). During the preanesthetic visit when possible, the anesthesiologist establishes rapport with, and instills confidence in the parturient, becomes familiar with the patient's medical and anesthesia history, physical findings and obstetric conditions, and evaluates the physiologic and emotional status of the parturient. Once these tasks are completed, the anesthesiologist discusses plans with both the obstetrician and parturient, makes arrangements for analgesia and anesthesia, and participates in further psychologic preparation of the gravida.

During the immediate preanesthetic period the anesthesiologist can do much to decrease or eliminate the fears, anxieties, and apprehension by manifesting a sympathetic understanding, a willingness to participate in the management of the patient, and a reassurance to the parturient that everything will be done to help her through a comfortable and safe delivery. On the other hand, any manifestations of rudeness, frustration, aggressiveness, intolerance, or the slightest indication that the parturient's management has created an imposition on the anesthesiologist will cause the parturient to develop resentment, aggression, anxiety, and fear. Such terms used in anesthesia as "spinal" and "injection" may be fear-provoking and should be avoided.

During the period just before anesthesia, the anesthesiologist should be especially careful to avoid manifestation of frustrations, such as making vitriolic comments to the nurse assistant, being abrupt with the patient, or using such expressions as "now don't act foolish" because such manifestations may cause an unfavorable outcome on the part of the parturient during the initiation of the analgesia/anesthesia. Moreover, the anesthesiologist should avoid at all costs any manifestation of aggression in applying the mask to the parturient's face unnecessarily tight, or in not being gentle in positioning the patient for regional analgesia, or in inserting a needle roughly. Critically important to the emotional well-being of the parturient is to inform her of the various procedures to be carried out at the time of the preanesthetic visit and to repeat the information at the time of induction of anesthesia before each step is carried out. Should the anesthesiologist make the grave mistake of having the patient fit to the anesthesiologist's emotional needs rather than attempt to objectively conform to and satisfy the patient's, the anesthesiologist will create unfavorable psychologic reactions in the patient (60,61).

Fear and anxiety on the anesthesiologist's part may induce anxiety and apprehension in the patient (57,60). The anesthesiologist's fear and anxiety may be overt or concealed; such fear and anxiety are most commonly present in anesthesiologists who are concerned about their ability to cope with the needs of the patient. It is well to appreciate that to handle the patient's fear, one must have one's own fears well-resolved (59). Because the parturient is quick to sense these unfavorable attitudes and behaviors, the anesthesiologist should do everything possible to avoid or suppress them.

## *Dreams During Anesthesia*

Dreams during general anesthesia may evoke an immediate abnormal physical reaction or may produce deleterious psychologic effects in the postpartum period. Dreams are responses to external or internal stimuli that might disturb sleep (6). Through its biologic function to protect sleep, the successful dream belittles a danger, gratifies it, or substitutes one gratification for another. If, on the other hand, the dream is unsuccessful in performing its function, the sleeper awakens because the dream has been unable to cope with the situation. General anesthesia induces an artificial sleep that may be accompanied by dreams provoked by external sensory stimuli resulting from pharmacologic effects of the anesthetic.

Dreams can occur during induction of inhalation analgesia or anesthesia used for instrumental delivery or for manipulation necessary for vaginal delivery. Dreams rarely occur with modern balanced general anesthesia, which entails rapid induction with an intravenous agent, muscle relaxants, and followed by light inhalation anesthesia and muscle relaxant mixture, which is frequently used for cesarean section. Consequently, dreaming is not the problem it was at the time the first edition of this book was written. Nevertheless, it is important to emphasize that during induction of general anesthesia for either vaginal delivery or cesarean section, it is essential for the obstetrician and obstetric nurse to avoid premature auditory, visual or touch stimuli, which are grossly misinterpreted by the semiconscious patient and thus provoke dreams (60,61). I have seen patients react violently and awaken when a large instrument was dropped on the floor producing a sudden very loud noise during the early period of the induction of anesthesia. Upon questioning, some of them stated that they were dreaming of a bomb exploding. It was Freud (63) who first pointed out that in spontaneous dreams persons are represented in their normal size, whereas in dreams during anesthesia, the actors are gigantic, their power supernatural, the scenery cosmic, and plasticity unequaled by any spontaneous dream.

Premature preparation, manipulation, and placement of restraints by nurses during induction of inhalation anesthesia have caused patients to dream that they were being attacked or held incarcerated in chains (60,61). Premature examination or instrumentation by the obstetrician before the patient is adequately anesthetized are without doubt among the most grievous errors in obstetric practice. Such maneuvers not only interfere with smooth induction of general anesthesia, but may also provoke significant physical activity or cause abnormal sympathoadrenal response during the anesthesia and may cause severe postpartum emotional reaction. Kartchner (27) cites the case of a patient who, during the period between the birth of her first and that of her second child, was awakened frequently by nightmares filled with unremembered fear-ridden content. At the birth of the second child, while partially anesthetized, she screamed "there they are—the lights, the people, they said they wouldn't hurt me, but they did, they did." It was learned subsequently that as a primipara she had been subjected to pain for the duration of a forceps delivery.

Auditory sensation is the last sensation to disappear during induction of general anesthesia and the first to return (64–66). Indeed, Cheek (64,65) has presented convincing evidence that it is never eliminated completely with modern, balanced general anesthesia. Moreover, there have been a variety of instances of awareness under light, balanced anesthesia reported in the literature (66). These reports suggest that comments or suggestions made during light, balanced anesthesia may cause emotional reactions that are manifested in the postanesthetic period and may persist during the puerperium or lie deeply buried in the subconscious until reactivated, perhaps by a subsequent pregnancy.

### *Postanesthetic Reactions*

Psychologically impoverished women, as a result of culture, teaching or religious belief, may develop the misconception that pharmacologic pain relief is not necessary and should be avoided. These women may undergo negative postanesthetic reactions due to the administration of anesthetic agents while they are under the duress and stress of labor pains. If analgesia or anesthesia is used on a patient in this group, then the patient should participate in a discussion regarding how to avoid developing a sense of guilt, depression, or other psychiatric symptoms in the postpartum period. Enthusiastic proponents of natural childbirth, who inadvertently give the gravida the impression that failure with the method or the need for pharmacologic analgesia/anesthesia indicates psychologic and physiologic inadequacy, can be responsible for the patient's sense of guilt or other deleterious reactions following delivery. Mention has also been made of the number of reports of patients who develop psychiatric symptoms following failure with natural childbirth and the consequent need of pharmacologic analgesia/anesthesia.

Deutsch (4) suggested that abnormal reactions after general anesthesia in some women can be explained by the fact that the delivery took place during unconsciousness. The dynamism of the mother-child relationship is disturbed because the external child, psychologically, does not coincide with the being that was in the uterus and the mother has a feeling that it is not her child. In this respect Deutsch (4) supports the contention of Dick-Read (39) who belabored this point to an almost boresome and unjustifiable degree. Dick-Read (39) not only invoked his vitriolic condemnation on general anesthesia, but also on refined regional techniques currently available that should avoid such psychologic reactions because the mother remains conscious during the entire process of childbirth and can actively participate in the delivery. In discussing the use of spinal epidural block, subarachnoid (saddle) block, or caudal anesthesia, Dick-Read stated "women rarely know the joy of spontaneous delivery of a child. It is a painless sensationless birth without emotional rectitude. There is no sense of personal achievement. An offspring is produced by a magician from a paralyzed birth canal" (38).

This prompts comment. First, one should keep in mind the human trait to adapt to new situations. As pointed out many years ago by Van Dooren (67), it would be an insult to the emotionally healthy parturient to assume that she could not integrate the experience of pharmacologic analgesia, especially regional techniques, which are the most frequent method of providing pain relief during childbirth, into the process of childbirth and still come out with a feeling of accomplishment. Evidence obtained from postpartum observations, discussions, and evaluation of many thousands of patients who have delivered with various forms of pharmacologic analgesia and discussion with physicians who have followed up these patients for years, disputes impressively the contention that pharmacologic analgesia precludes the emotional fulfillment of childbirth. Second, the concept of the critical value of "early bonding" between the mother and the baby is being questioned, and according to Melzack (55) is "falling by the way side" (55A). Even admitting that it is important, it should not be interfered with in most parturients, who today receive pharmacologic analgesia in the form of epidural analgesia that permits immediate interaction between mother and baby. Melzack (55)—based on his very careful study—suggests that in many patients combining childbirth preparation and epidural analgesia affords the patient and the newborn the best of two worlds.

## PSYCHOPHYSIOLOGIC ASPECTS OF PARTURITION AND ANESTHESIA

In addition to the aforementioned psychologic effects, emotional reactions to labor and anesthesia invariably produce important physiologic and pathophysiologic responses. Although the magnitude of these responses varies according to the adaptive reactions characteristic of the individual parturient and the antepartal preparation, the general pattern is the same and involves neuroendocrine, metabolic, and biochemical responses, which have a major impact on the functions of the parturient (68). Because some of these have already been mentioned in the preceding chapter and are discussed in detail in Chapter 9, no further comments are made except to emphasize that anxiety, fear, and labor pain cause significant alterations in metabolism, cardiovascular, gastrointestinal, and respiratory function and influence the forces of labor (see Figure 9–14 for details).

## Psychologic and Emotional Reactions of the Puerperium

During the postpartum period the puerpera may develop emotional reactions that may or may not be related to anesthesia. She may become depressed because some of the physical burdens persist, or for some other reason. Some degree of depression is experienced by a significant portion of puerperae (68–71). This "blue period" usually appears 24 to 48 hours after delivery, lasts a few days and clears completely by the time the patient leaves the hospital.

During the immediate and long-term postpartum period, the puerpera's psychologic and emotional reactions vary depending on a variety of factors already mentioned in connection with the psychology of pregnancy. The majority of women who have had a favorable early experience in regard to their interest in children and experience with them, who have a good husband-wife relationship during the pregnancy, and who possess the personality characteristics of good ego strength and nurturance, were managed properly during labor and delivery, and had good pain relief, experienced few if any negative psychologic and emotional reactions. Moreover, the puerpera is able to develop a firm bond between herself and the infant, feels a great deal of pleasure, and manifests high qualities in her capacities as a mother, especially when birth occurred during effective regional analgesia that permits the mother to promptly hold and caress the newborn.

These comments notwithstanding, there are a significant number of puerperae who develop mild-to-moderate depression and/or other negative emotional reactions after delivery. They may become depressed because the physical burdens persist or for some other reason. Depression is experienced by a significant number of puerperae with some authors mentioning figures of 60 to 100% (68,69). Shereshefsky and coworkers (22) found that, among the 60 women studied, about one-third had special difficulty in the early postpartum period, particularly in taking care of their first-born infant. This difficulty was exhibited in such varied ways as an intense, sometimes disruptive, anxiety about the care of the infant or about adequacy in the mothering role, overreaction to such realistic problems as feeding adjustment and even hostile punitive acts toward the infant, as well as significant degrees of depression. It is to be reemphasized that this was a population of young, middle class, educated parturients of which the other two-thirds had no significant serious emotional problems.

In some puerperae the longing for the reunion with the child may be in conflict with the urge for liberation (4). As a result of this conflict, some young mothers are passive and demand loving care and attention. In others, apprehension and tension develop when they suddenly realize that with the new responsibilities the world has changed for them and that they must relinquish many former interests. The apprehension and tension are often manifested as backache, headache, fatigue, and many other conditions that may be wrongly attributed to the anesthesia. Fortunately, these emotional reactions usually subside and the mother assumes her proper responsibility, providing the infant with maternal affection that is now recognized undisputedly as an absolute need for the psychologic and emotional well-being of the child (6).

The highest incidence of negative psychologic and emotional reactions occurs in some women who have had a very unpleasant and stressful experience during labor and delivery. The role of severe unrelieved pain, particularly among those who have prepared for natural childbirth, in causing severe anxiety, depression, obsessive-compulsive behavior, other psychiatric symptoms, and sexual and marital problems has already been mentioned and is discussed in detail in Chapter 9.

Severe psychiatric disorders requiring hospitalization and intense psychotherapy occur in one or perhaps two of 1,000 women undergoing childbirth (70,71). An untold number of others suffer from incapacitating but less dramatic emotional disturbances that often go unrecognized. In the aforementioned study carried out by Shereshefsky and associates (1,70), seven women developed psychiatric symptoms within 6 months postpartum of their first or subsequent pregnancies. Of three women who were referred for psychiatric treatment following their first pregnancy, one was hospitalized. Moreover, during the 6 years following the initial study, four additional women were referred for psychiatric treatment after second pregnancies and two of these were hospitalized. Careful psychiatric evaluation revealed that of the seven, only two had disorders that were directly related to parturition and both had symptoms within days of the delivery. One women, who had appeared well-integrated during pregnancy, developed a profound schizophrenic disorder in the week following delivery, while the other, who had a tendency toward depressive mood-swings during pregnancy, developed a severe depressive disorder 4 days postpartum after two consecutive depressive mood-swings during pregnancy. Although each of the remaining five women had the onset of symptoms in what is usually designated as the postpartum period (6 months), it was clear to the investigators that childbirth itself had little to do with the onset of symptoms. They concluded that postpartum psychiatric disorders precipitated by childbirth can be distinguished from psychiatric disorders in the postpartum period, which is not critically related to the childbirth. In any case, it is essential for the obstetrician to monitor carefully women who manifest serious psychologic problems following parturition.

## REFERENCES

1. Shereshefsky, PM, Yarrow LJ: Psychological Aspects of a First Pregnancy and Early Postnatal Adaptation. New York, Raven Press, 1974.
2. Beck NC, Geden EA, Brouder GT: Preparation for Labor: a historical perspective. Psychos. Med. 41:243, 1979.
3. Deutsch H: Psychology of Women. Vol. II. New York, Grune & Stratton, 1945,
4. Deutsch H: Psychology of Pregnancy, Labor and Puerperium. *In* Obstetrics, Edited by JP Greenhill. 11th Ed. Philadelphia, W.B. Saunders, 1955.

5. Morris N: Psychologic problems during pregnancy. *In* Obstetric Anesthesia and Perinatology. Edited by E Cosmi. New York, Appleton-Century-Crofts, 1981, pp. 65–74.
6. Kanner L: Psychiatric aspects of pregnancy and childbirth. *In* Williams Obstetrics. 12th Ed. Edited by NJ Eastman, LM Hellman. New York, Appleton-Century-Crofts, 1961.
6A. Dobie SA, Walker EA: Deprerssion after childbirth. J. Am. Board Fam. Pract. 5(3), 1992, pp. 303–11.
7. Brockington IF, Winokur G, Dean C: Puerperal psychosis. *In* Motherhood and Mental Illness. Edited by IF Brockington, R Kumar. London, Academic Press, 1982, pp. 37–69.
8. Kumar R, Brant HA, Robson KM: Childbearing and maternal sexuality: a prospective survey of 119 primiparae. Psychosom. Res. 25:373, 1981.
9. Wengraff F: Psychosomatic approach to gynecology and obstetrics. Springfield, IL, C Thomas Publisher, 1953.
10. Caplan G: Concepts of mental health and consultation. United States Department of Health, Children's Bureau Publication No. 373. Washington, DC, 1959.
11. Bibring GL, Dwyer TF, Huntington DS, Valenstein AF: A study of the psychological processes in pregnancy and of the earliest mother-child relationship. Psychoanal. Study. Child. 16:9, 1961.
12. Grimm ET: Psychological and social factors in pregnancy, delivery and outcome. *In* Childbearing—Its Social and Psychological Aspects. Edited by SA Richardson, AF Guttmacher. Baltimore, Williams & Wilkins, 1967, p. 35.
13. Chalmers B: Psychological aspects of pregnancy: some thoughts for the eighties. Soc. Sci. Med. 16:323, 1982.
14. Arizmendi TG, Alfonso DD: Stressful events related to pregnancy and postpartum. J. Psychosom. Res. 31:743, 1987.
15. Cox JL: Psychiatric morbidity and pregnancy: a controlled study of 263 semi-rural Ugandan women. Br. J. Psychiatry. 134:401, 1979.
16. Kumar R, Robson KM: A prospective study of emotional disorders in childbearing women. Br. J. Psychiatry. 144:35, 1984.
17. Elliott SA, Rugg AJ, Watson JP, Brough DI: Mood changes during pregnancy and after the birth of a child. Br. J. Clin. Psychol. 22:295, 1983.
18. Knight RG, Thirkettle JA: Anxiety and depression in the immediate postpartum period: a controlled investigation of a primiparous sample. Aust. NZ. J. Psychiatry. 20:430, 1986.
19. Campbell EA: Neurotic disturbance in pregnancy—A review. Psychiatric Developments 4:311, 1988.
19A. Gottesman MM: Maternal adaption during pregnany among adult early, middle, and late childbearers: similarities and differences. Matern. Child Nurs. J. 20(2), 1992.
20. Shereshefsky PM, Lockman RF: Background variables. *In* Psychological Aspects of a First Pregnancy and Early Postnatal Adaptation. Edited by PM Shereshefsky, LJ Yarrow. New York, Raven Press, 1974, pp. 33–37.
21. Saltzman S, Schneidman T: Psychological study of the woman. *In* Psychological Aspects of a First Pregnancy and Early Postnatal Adaptation. Edited by PM Shereshefsky, LJ Yarrow. New York, Raven Press, 1974, pp. 37.
22. Shereshefsky PM, Plotsky H, Lockman RF: Pregnancy Adaptation. *In* Psychological Aspects of a First Pregnancy and Early Postnatal Adaptation. Edited by PM Shereshefsky, LJ Yarrow. New York, Raven Press, 1974, p. 67.
23. Richardson SA and Guttmacher AF. Childbearing—Its Social and Psychological Aspects. Baltimore, Williams & Wilkins, 1967.
24. Bernard VW: Needs of Unmarried Parents and Their Children as Seen by a Psychiatrist. Nat. Conference of Social Work, United States Department of Health and Welfare, NIH, Bethesda, MD, 1948.
25. Aldrich CK: Psychiatry for the Family Physician. New York, McGraw-Hill Book Co. Inc., 1955.
26. Rogers MP: Psychologic aspects of pregnancy in patients with rheumatic diseases. Rheumatic Disease Clinics of North America 15:361, 1989.
27. Kartchner FD: A study of the emotional reactions during labor. Am. J. Obstet. Gynecol. 60:19, 1950.
27A. Robson KM, Kumar R: Delayed onset of maternal affection after childbirth. Br. J. Psychiatry 4(136), 1980, pp. 347–53.
28. Davids A, DeVault S, Talmadge M: Anxiety, pregnancy and childbirth abnormalities. J. Consult. Psychol. 25:74, 1961.
28A. Levin JS: The factor structure of the pregnancy anxiety scale. J. Health Soc. Behav. 32(4), 1991, pp. 368–81.
29. Zuckerman M: Psychological correlates of somatic complaints in pregnancy and difficulty in childbirth. J. Consult. Psychol. 27:324, 1963.
29A. Marks MN, Wieck A, Checkley SA, Kumar R: Br. J. Psychiatry Suppl. May 1991.
30. Shereshefsky PM, Lockman RF: Comparison of counseled and non-counseled groups. *In* Psychological Aspects of a First Pregnancy and Early Postnatal Adaptation. Edited by PM Shereshefsky, LJ Yarrow. New York, Raven Press, 1974, pp. 151–163.
31. Liebenberg B: Techniques in prenatal counseling. *In* Psychological Aspects of a First Pregnancy and Early Postnatal Adaptation. Edited by PM Shereshefsky, LJ Yarrow. New York, Raven Press, 1974, pp. 123–151.
32. Magni G, Rizzardo R, Andreoli C: Psychosocial stress and obstetrical complications. Acta. Obstet. Gynecol. Scand. 65: 273, 1986.
33. Rizzardo R, Magni G, Cremonese C, Rossi RT: Variations in anxiety levels during pregnancy and psychosocial factors in relation to obstetric complications. Psychother. Psychosom. 49:10, 1988.
34. Gillman RD: The dreams of pregnant women and maternal adaptation. *In* Psychological Aspects of a First Pregnancy and Early Postnatal Adaptation. Edited by PM Shereshefsky, LJ Yarrow New York, Raven Press, 1974, p. 115.
35. Lee SR: Psychiatric disorders during pregnancy. Am. Fam. Physician. 28(3):187, 1983.
36. Carnes JW: Psychosocial disturbances during and after pregnancy. Postgrad. Med. 73(1):144, 1983.
37. Stott DH: Physical and mental handicaps following a disturbed pregnancy. Lancet 1:1006, 1957.
38. Thompson WR: Influence of prenatal maternal anxiety on motionality in young rats. Science 125:698, 1957.
39. Dick-Read G: Childbirth without Fear. New York, Harper & Brothers, 1944, pp. 152.
40. Lamaze F: L'experience francaise de l'accouchement sans douleur. Bull. Circle Claude Bernard 8:2, 1954.
41. Kubie LS: Discussion of H.B. Davidson's "The psychosomatic apects of educated childbirth." New York J. Med. 53:2508, 1953.
42. Greenhill JP: Obstetrics. 2nd Ed. Philadelphia, W.B. Saunders, 1965.
43. Davidson HB: The psychosomatic aspects of educated childbirth. New York J. Med. 53:2499, 1953.
44. Corman HH, Hornick EJ, Kritchman M, Terestman N: Emotional reactions of surgical patients to hospitalization, anesthesia and surgery. Am. J. Surg. 96:646, 1958.
45. Volicer BJ: Hospital stress and patient reports of pain and physical status. J. Human. Stress. 4:28, 1978.
46. Conrad K: Pain in childbirth: report of Subcommittee of Medical Women's Federation. Br. Med. J. 1:333, 1949.
46A. ICEA: The role of the childbirth educator and the scope of childbirth education. International Childbirth Education Association, Inc., Minneapolis, MN, 1986, p. 4.

46B. Beck NC, Siegel LJ: Preparation for childbirth and contemporary research on pain, anxiety, and stress reduction: a review and critique. Psychosom. Med. 42(4), 1980, pp. 429–47.
46C. Delkey I, Minkoff H, Grunebaum A: Effect of LaMaze childbirth preparation on maternal plasma beta-endorphin immunoreactivity in active labor. Am. J. Perinatol. 2:317–319, 1985.
47. Coleman LL: Freedom from Fear. New York, Hawthorn Books Inc, 1954.
48. Beck NC, Siegel LJ: Preparation for childbirth and contemporary research on pain, anxiety and stress reduction: a review of critique. Psychosom. Med. 42:429, 1980.
49. Klusman LE: Reduction in pain in childbirth by the alleviation of anxiety during pregnancy. J. Consult. Clin. Psychol. 213:162, 1975.
50. Melzack R, Taenzer P, Feldman P, Kinch RA: Labour is still painful after prepared childbirth training. Can. Med. Assoc. J. 125:357, 1981.
51. Peck CL: Psychological factors in acute pain management. *In* Acute Pain Management. Edited by MJ Cousins, GD Phillips. New York, Churchill Livingstone, 1986, pp. 251–274.
52. Wuitshik M, Bakal D, Lipshitz J: The clinical significance of pain and cognitive activity in latent labor. Obstet. Gynecol. 73:35–42, 1989.
52a. Norvell KT, Gaston-Johansson F, Fridh G: Remembrance of labor pain: how valued are retrospective pain measurements? Pain 31:77, 1987.
53. Hardy JD, Javert CT: Studies on pain; measurements of pain intensity in childbirth. J. Clin. Invest. 28:153, 1949.
54. Melzack R, Kinch R, Dobkin P, Lebrun M, et al: Severity of labour pain: Influence of physical as well as psychological variables. Can. Med. Assoc. J. 130:579, 1984.
55. Melzack R: The myth of painless childbirth (the John J Bonica Lecture). Pain 19:321, 1984.
55a Brody JE: Influential theory of birth "bonding" losing supporters. New York Times, reprinted in the Gazette, Montreal, April 2, 1983, pp.1–5.
56. Rogers FS: Dangers of the Read method in patients with major personality problems. Am. J. Obstet. Gynecol. 71: 1236, 1956.
57. Stewart DE: Psychiatric symptoms following attempted natural childbirth. Can. Med. Assoc. J. 127:713, 1982.
57A. Stewart D: Possible relationship of postpartum psychiatric symptoms to childbirth education programs. J. Psychosomatic Obstet. Gynecol. 4:295, 1985.
58. LeBoyer F: Birth Without Violence. Adelaide, Australia, Rigby, 1975.
59. Sheffer MB, Greifenstein FE: The emotional responses of patients to surgery and anesthesia. Anesthesiology 21:502, 1960.
60. Raginsky BB: Some psychosomatic aspects of general anesthesia. Anesthesiology 2:391, 1950.
61. Deutsch H: Some psychoanalytic observances in surgery. Psychosom. Med. 4:105, 1942.
62. Boverman M: Remarks on the psychologic aspects of anesthesia. Med. Ann. D. C. 24:179, 1955.
63. Freud S: The Problem of Anxiety. New York, W.W. Norton & Co, 1936.
64. Cheek DB: Surgical memory and reaction to careless conversation. Am. J. Clin. Hypn. 6:237, 1964.
65. Cheek DB: Further evidence of persistence of hearing under chemoanesthesia: Detailed case report. Am. J. Clin. Hypn. 7:55, 1964.
66. Guerra F: Awareness under general anesthesia. *In* Emotional and Psychological Responses to Anesthesia and Surgery. Edited by F Guerra, JA Aldrete. New York, Grune & Stratton, 1980, pp. 1–8.
67. Van Dooren H: Personal communication, 1967.
68. Asch SS, et al: Mental and emotional problems. *In* Medical, Surgical and Gynecological Complications of Pregnancy. 2nd Ed. Edited by JJ Rovinsky, AF Guttmacher. Baltimore, Williams & Wiklins Co., 1965.
69. Ploshette N, Asch SS, Chase J: A study of anxieties during pregnancy, labor, and the early and late puerperium. Bull. N. Y. Acad. Med. 32:436, 1956.
69A. Astbury J: Labor Pain: The role of childbirth education, information and expectaion. *In* Problems In Pain. Edited by C Peck, M Wallace. London, Pergamon, 1980.
70. Brown WA, Shereshefsky PM: Seven women: A prospective study of postpartum psychiatric disorders. Psychiatry 35: 139, 1972.
71. Normand, WC: Postpartum disorders. *In* Comprehensive Textbook of Psychiatry. Edited by AM Freedman, HI Kaplan Baltimore, Williams & Wilkins Co., 1967.

# Chapter 4

# ANATOMY AND PHYSIOLOGY OF THE FORCES OF PARTURITION

JOHN J. BONICA
FRANK C. MILLER
TIM H. PARMLEY

---

This chapter contains discussion of the anatomy and physiology of the forces of labor and how these may be affected by analgesia and anesthesia. As is well known, during the first stage, these forces consist of uterine contractions and the resistant forces offered by the cervix, while during the second stage these forces include uterine contractions that are aided by the auxiliary expulsive forces produced by reflex contraction of the diaphragm and abdominal muscles opposed by the resistance of the pelvic floor. During the third stage and the puerperium, uterine contractions are the primary forces involved.

The material includes detailed discussion of the anatomy of the uterus, physiology and biochemistry of uterine contractions and their characteristics during pregnancy and various stages of labor, the physiology of the auxiliary forces, the progress, pattern, and duration of labor and new advances in the clinical management. The material herein follows the same format and is an update of the subject found in the first edition of this book. It includes some of the older illustrations that remain relevant and others that are pertinent to new data. Miller and Parmley contributed material relevant to anatomy and changes in the uterus and cervix and to the section on biochemical factors that influence uterine contractility, especially the section on the contractile substance and the role of calcium. Omission errors or deficiencies in the rest of the chapter are the responsibility of the senior author.

Although the chapter deals with information that is primarily of interest to the obstetrician, it is the conviction of the senior author that this (and other chapters in Section II) contain fundamental information that the obstetric anesthesiologist must know well if he/she is to provide optimal anesthesiologic care to parturients. Although it may be omitted by experts in this field, no one on the obstetric team should manage parturients without this knowledge. More detailed discussion of the subject is found elsewhere (1–4).

## ANATOMY AND PHYSIOLOGY OF THE UTERUS

### *Uterine Structure*

Developmentally, the uterus and cervix are derived from the fusion of the paired müllerian ducts. These structures arise bilaterally, from the lateral surface to the urogenital ridge, migrate through the intermediate mesoderm into the pelvis where they meet in the midline and give rise to the upper vagina, the cervix, the uterus, and the fallopian tubes. Their fusion with each other occurs side-to-side so that the medial wall of each duct disappears. These embryologic details are apparently reflected in the structure that results.

#### *Anatomy of the Uterus*

The corpus of the uterus has three tissue layers: the endometrium or decidua, the myometrium, and the serosa. The cervix also consists of three layers: the innermost endocervical epithelia layer, the fibromuscular layer in the middle, and the outer squamous epithelial layer covering the vaginal portion. The myometrium is composed of smooth muscle cells in a matrix consisting mainly of collagen and glycosaminoglycans.

The uterine musculature appears to be arranged as fascicles that spiral around the lateral walls of the cavity, ending and meeting with similar fascicles from the other side in the midline of the organ (5). In addition, they tend to spiral from above, downward so that the result is that of two descending helices that have been joined in the middle by removing a portion of each. In addition, this structure has been described as being arranged in two or three layers (Figure 4–1). At least two layers clearly exist, divided by a prominent vascular layer. Beyond this, there is more muscle mass in the uterine fundus than in the lateral walls and during pregnancy the percentage of muscle in the uterine wall rises (6). This is in sharp contrast to the situation in the cervix where muscles taper off and constitute only 25% of the upper cervix, 16% of the middle part, and only 5% of the lower cervix, and there is no change with pregnancy (5–7). The two spiral halves of the uterine muscle may function as one or pathologically in an uncoordinated fashion. There is some proliferative growth in the uterine musculature in early pregnancy, but the greatest growth occurs in the form of cellular enlargement (6) (Figure 4–1).

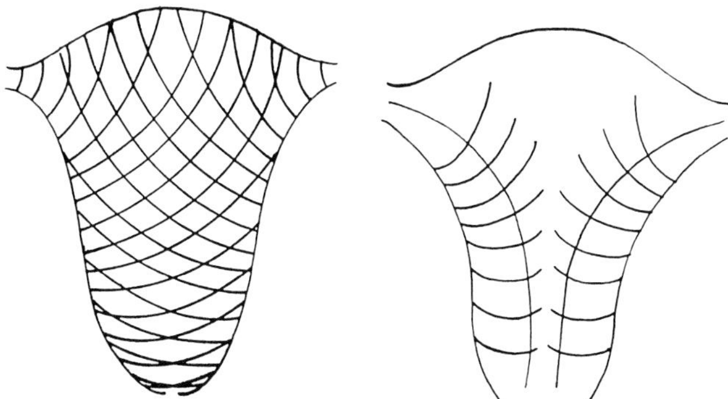

**Fig. 4–1.** Muscles of the uterus (see text for detail). Schematic arrangement of the muscular fibers of the external stratum of the uterine musculature. After penetrating the latter near the midline, the fibers are attached to deeper muscle stratum and, with their fellows from the opposite side, give rise to the upper vagina, the cervix, the uterus, and the fallopian tubes. (Modified from Beck AC, Rosenthal AH: Obstetrical Practice. 7th Ed. Baltimore, Williams & Wilkins, 1958, p. 133.)

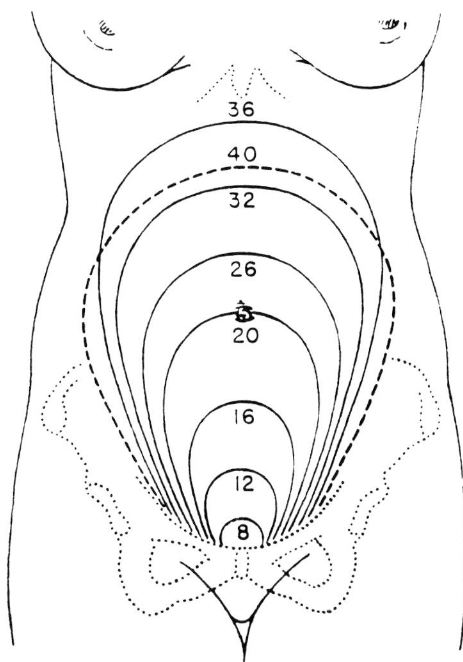


**Fig. 4–2.** Height of fundus at comparable gestational dates. There are usually significant variations between patients. Those shown in this illustration seem to be the most common. A convenient rule of thumb is that at 5-month gestation, the fundus is usually at or slightly above the umbilicus. (Modified from Beck AC, Rosenthal AH: Obstetrical Anesthesia. 7th Ed. Baltimore, Williams & Wilkins, 1958.)

### *Anatomy of the Cervix*

The majority of the cervix is composed of fibrous connective tissue (7–9). The predominant cells are fibroblasts, which are responsible for the production of large amounts of collagen and other ground substances including glycosaminoglycans, proteoglycans, and glycoproteins (6–10). The small amount of muscular fibers is continuous of the spiral bundles from the corpus. The glycosaminoglycan and hyaluronic acid possess an important structural feature in which each molecule expands in volume over 1000 times when hydrated. Proteoglycans are similar to glycosaminoglycans except that they bind to a core protein. They include dermatan sulfate, chondroitin sulfate, and heparin sulfate. Glycoproteins, of which fibronectin is an example, are believed to have a role in organizing the structure of the extracellular matrix.

## THE UTERUS AND CERVIX DURING PREGNANCY

### *Growth of the Uterus During Pregnancy*

During pregnancy, the uterus is converted from a small, almost solid organ weighing 30 to 60 g and 6 cm long and 4 cm wide, into a thin-walled muscular sac that at the time of labor is about 30 cm long, 25 cm wide, and 20 cm deep, weighing 700 to 1000 g (8,10). It increases approximately 500 times. During the first half of gestation, enlargement of the uterus is primarily due to hypertrophy of the tissues, but subsequently there is also cell division. The growth is induced not only by the pregnancy hormones estrogen and progesterone but also by stimulus of distention. At about the twentieth week, there is conversion of the conceptus from a spheroidal to a cylindrical shape, and further uterine enlargement is accomplished by progressive stretching and thinning of the uterine wall. As a result, the thickness of the wall of the uterus is reduced from approximately 2 cm early in pregnancy to 0.5 to 1.0 cm at term (1,6).

Until the third month, the uterus remains in the pelvis, but during the fourth month it ascends and partially fills the abdominal cavity, coming in contact with the anterior abdominal wall and gradually displacing the intestines to the sides and upward in the abdomen, and finally rising to impinge upon the liver (Figure 4–2, see also Figure 2–1, Chapter 2). This produces an elevation of the diaphragm with a consequent alteration in lung volume and a shift in the position of the heart, as discussed in Chapter 2.

The decidua, which is derived from the endometrium of the nonpregnant uterus, undergoes characteristic changes after implantation: the stromal cells enlarge and increase in number and the glands and blood vessels undergo increased growth. Subsequently, the decidua develops into three layers; the decidua basalis which is beneath the placenta, the decidua capsularis which covers the conceptus, and the decidua vera which is a parietal portion covering the inner surface of the myometrium.

### *Changes in the Cervix*

The development of cervical compliance is a process that begins early in pregnancy with softening of the cervix, but occurs much more rapidly in the hours immediately preceding and during labor (7). At this point the cervix is converted from a relatively firm, rigid structure to a very soft, flexible one that can be pulled up around the presenting part and dilated large enough to allow for the passage of the entire fetal body. Under normal circumstances, the development of myometrial contractility is coordinated with developing cervical compliance (7,10,11). In a primipara, the first clinical change, which may begin as early as the first part of the third trimester, is the flattening of the endocervical canal and the conversion of the cervix to become a portion of the lower uterine segment (Figure 4–3) (12). This process is referred to as "effacement." Dilatation of the cervical os continues at an accelerated pace and is oscillatory in character with some retraction after a contraction and loss of a dilating wedge (13). In multiparous individuals, however, these processes are less discrete: effacement may never appear to develop and dilation may begin significantly before the onset of labor. In apparent response to decreased cervical resistance, uterine activity may not need to be so strong as in primiparous women (14) (Figure 4–3).

These gross physical changes in the cervix are associated with even more dramatic cellular and biochemical events (10). As described above, there is little muscle in the cervix and most of that which is present is in the upper cervix. Even before definitive labor, this muscle thins with elongation of individual fibers. The fibrous connective tissue of the cervix contains morphologic fibroblasts that are probably many different cell types, each responsible for producing a component of the extracellular matrix (7). Prominent among these extracellular matrix molecules is collagen, which is found in the form of fibers. Collagen fibers in the cervical matrix are formed

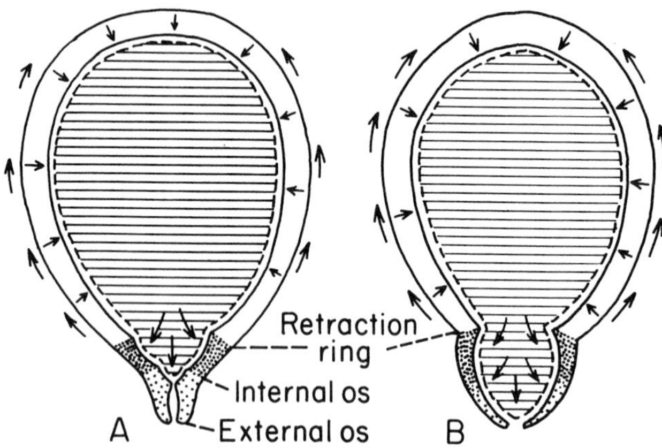


**Fig. 4–3.** The mechanism of cervical effacement. **A,** Muscles of the upper uterine segment contract, increasing the intrauterine pressure and causing a displacement of the amniotic fluid downward, which in turn causes distention of the weaker, lower part of the uterus. Simultaneously, the upper uterine segment retracts. All of these changes elevate the isthmus and dilate the internal os by pulling it upward around the presenting part, thus causing the beginning of cervical effacement. **B,** Effacement complete. The wall of the upper segment is shorter and thicker and the cervical canal is obliterated. As a result of this process, the upper part of the cervix becomes incorporated as part of the lower uterine segment, which also included the isthmus of the uterus. Note the rising of the physiologic retraction ring. This is the condition of the uterus at the onset of labor in the primigravida.

in extracellular sites from precursors produced in the fibroblasts and secreted. Early in pregnancy, collagen is dense and fills most of the extracellular space. Also present, however, are glycosaminoglycans, the most significant of which is hyaluronic acid. This unique molecule swells to greater than 1000 times its original volume when hydrated, and the hydration change in it may be the reason for the tremendous dispersion of collagen that occurs in the last part of pregnancy and during labor. Whether or not the collagen is actually degraded before the puerperium is less clear.

Proteoglycans such as elastin and glycoproteins such as fibronectin are also present. Their role is less clear but the former imparts some elasticity to the cervix. Fibronectin may help connect other structural proteins in the extracellular matrix. Estrogen tends to promote a decrease in collagen concentration as do the prostaglandins, among which the most effective is prostaglandin E. Direct mechanical stimulation also promotes cervical softening. Labor produces some undefined permanent change in cervical structure, as labors subsequent to the first are associated with more rapid cervical progress and a somewhat different cervical mechanism as described above.

## Uterine Contractility During Pregnancy, Labor, and Vaginal Delivery

### *Characteristics of Uterine Contractions*

A major advance in obstetric management made during the past 4 decades has been introduction and widespread use of tokodynamometry (TKD) to measure uterine contractility (1,15–22). Much of the work and publication have been produced by Alvarez, Caldeyro-Barcia, and Reynolds (1,15–23). Although the external tokodynamometry is useful for this purpose, the internal technique, entailing the insertion of a catheter into the amniotic space, provides more precise information about rhythmicity, coordination, intensity, frequency, and duration of uterine contractions (Figure 4–4). The parameters of uterine contractions include: 1) tonus which is the lowest pressure

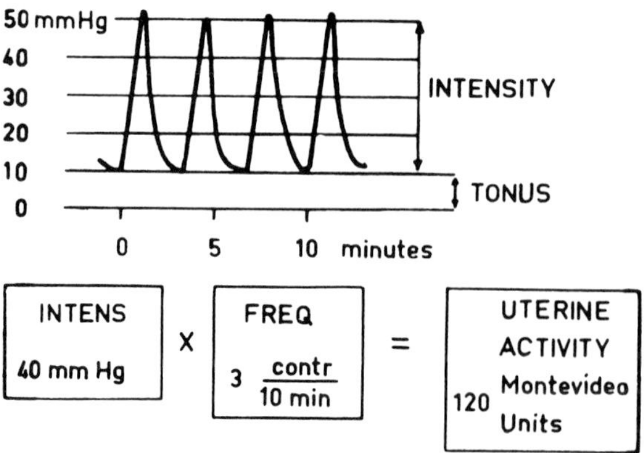


**Fig. 4–4.** Analysis of intra-amniotic fluid pressure tracing of uterine contractions. Several contractions are shown together with the parameters used for interpretation. (With permission from Sico-Blanco Y, Sala NL: Oxytocin. New York, Pergamon Press, 1960.)

recorded between contractions; 2) intensity (amplitude) of each contraction as measured by the rise in amniotic pressure in mm Hg above the tonus; 3) the frequency expressed as the number of contractions per 10 minutes; and 4) uterine activity defined as a product of intensity multiplied by the frequency, and expressed in mm Hg per 10 minutes, or Montevideo units (Mont.u.) (see Figure 4–4). To measure uterine activity, a large number of investigators use the area under the curve of each uterine contraction (23a,23b,23c). Figure 4–5, developed by Caldeyro-Barcia and his associates from analysis of over 500 different studies, depicts the evolution of spontaneous uterine activity throughout pregnancy and labor (22).

In 1977, Steer (23a) following the lead proposed originally by Caldeyro-Barcia, et al—who believed that the "active contraction area" (ACA) was the best measure of uterine activity, proposed the uterine activity integral (UAI), measured in kiloPascals × seconds and expressed as a 15-minute total (kPas per min), as the measure of uterine activity. Like Caldeyro-Barcia, et al (16), this method assumes that the baseline tone has little to do with the progress of labor. Steer and associates (23b), and others (23c), believe that by using modern electronic

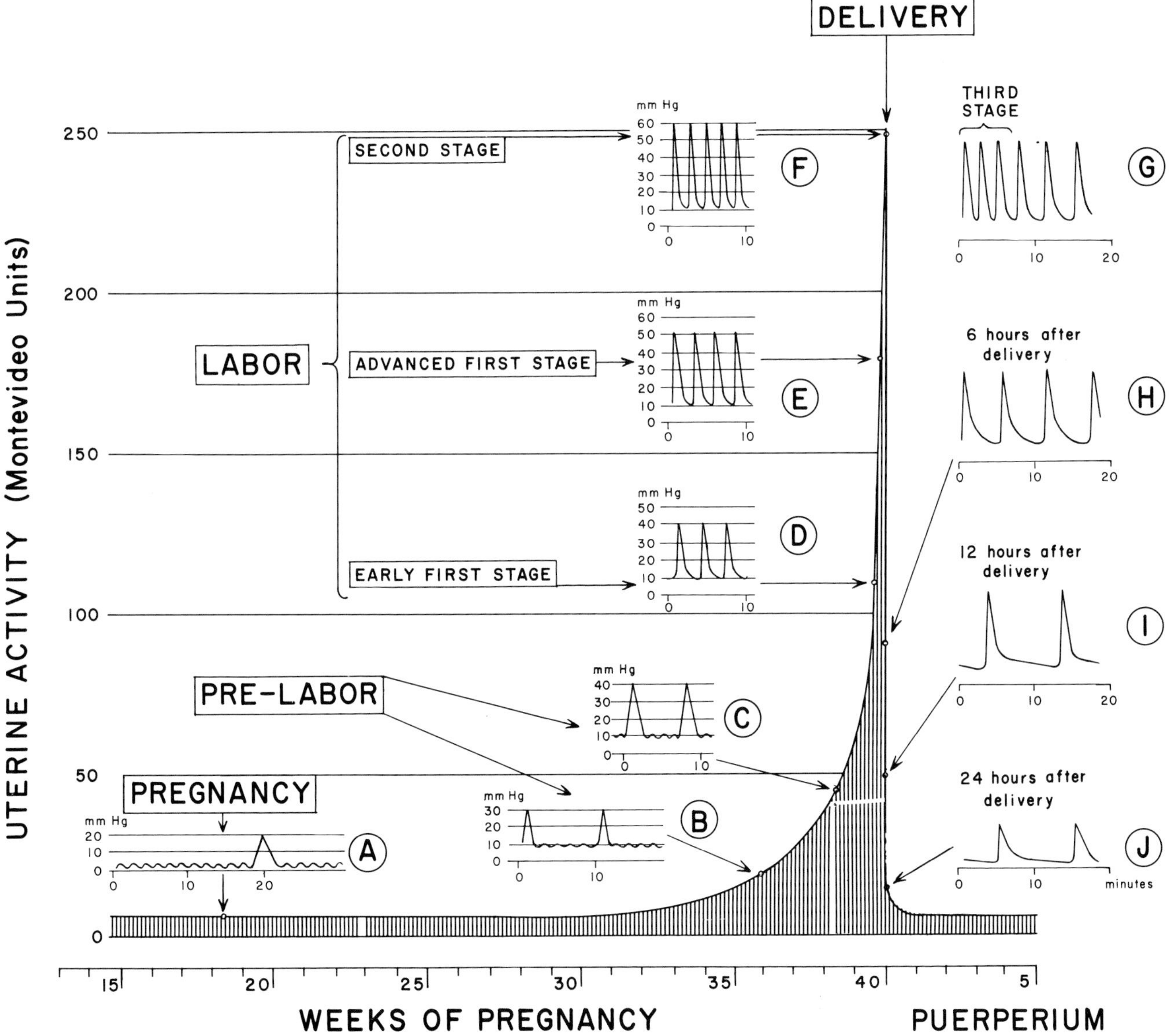


**Fig. 4–5.** Development, progression, and regression of spontaneous uterine contractility throughout pregnancy, labor, and early puerperium. The primary curve of uterine activity (shaded area) is the product of the intensity multiplied by the frequency expressed in mmHg/10 minutes and is referred to as Montevideo units. The curve shows the changes in magnitude of uterine activity in relation to the duration of pregnancy and to the successive stages of labor and puerperium, indicated by special points in the curve. Typical (schematic) tracings of uterine contractility are shown for each of these points. Contractions during the 24 hours after delivery are frequently more intense than shown. (Adapted from Caldeyro-Barcia R, Poseiro JJ: Oxytocin and contractility of the pregnant human uterus. Ann. N.Y. Acad. Sci. 75:813, 1959.)

technique, the active contact area is simpler to measure than in Mont.u. For an updated summary, the reader is referred to a recent publication by Allman and Steer (23c). Because the Montevideo unit measurements have been used much more frequently, especially in the United States, in this chapter much of the data is expressed in this measurement.

## Uterine Contractions During Pregnancy

The uterine musculature spontaneously contracts in the nonpregnant individual and may generate extremely high intrauterine pressures, particularly during the menses. However, when pregnancy ensues, the myometrium becomes almost quiescent (Figures 4–5A and 4–5B). During the first 30 weeks of gestation, uterine activity (Figure 4–5A: striped area) is less than 20 Mont.u. and consists of very slight contractions that remain localized to a small area of the uterus and occur at the rate of 1 per 10 minutes. Braxton Hicks contractions have a greater intensity (10 to 15 mm Hg) and spread to a larger area of the organ, and have a very low frequency (1 contraction per hour at 30 weeks) (Figures 4–5B and 4–6). The contractions are said to enhance the circulation in the intervillous space and thus to facilitate placental function (21,22). Assuming labor ensues at term, the last 10 weeks of pregnancy are characterized by gradually increasing uterine activity (Figure 4–5).

### Prelabor

During the last 3 to 4 weeks of pregnancy, uterine activity increases very rapidly and the small localized uncoordinated contractions are replaced by rhythmic coordinated contractions that increase progressively in frequency, intensity, and duration. The frequency is 1 to 2 per 10 minutes, and intensity is 25 to 40 mm Hg (Figures 4–5B, 4–5C, 4–6). These stronger and slow Braxton Hicks contractions of the prelabor period help demarcate the uterus into the upper segment, which is an active, thick, muscular contractile portion, and the lower segment, consisting of the lower part of the uterus and the cervix (11,17). These contractions also cause progressive ripening and effacement of the cervix (Figure 4–3).

At the onset of clinical labor, cervical effacement is usually complete in primigravidae but often is not in multiparae (1). Lightening also takes place, a phenomenon of special interest to the anesthesiologist because with the settling of the fetal head into the brim of the pelvis, the pressure against the diaphragm is relieved, maternal respirations become easier, and if dyspnea is present, it is relieved.

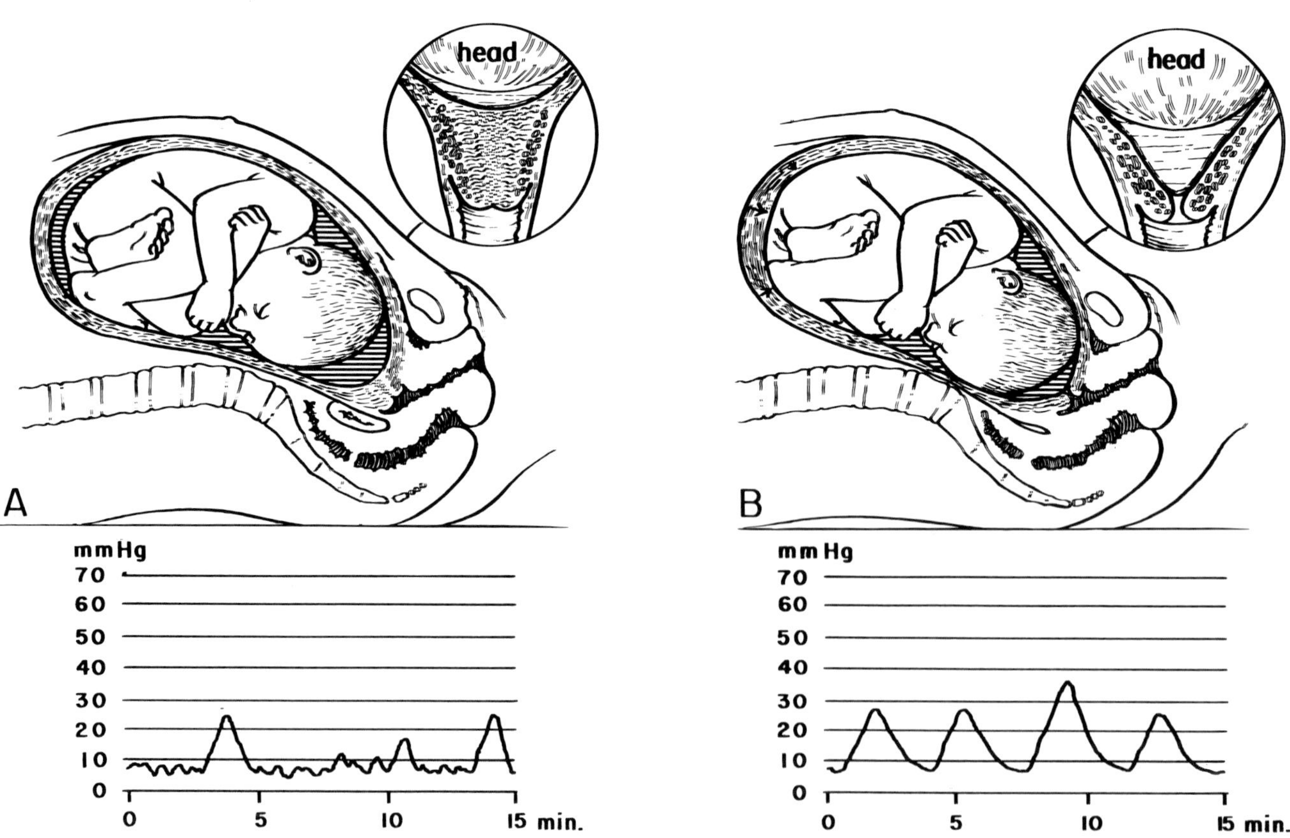


**Fig. 4–6.** Correlation between uterine contraction and changes in the cervix during pregnancy. **A,** Before prelabor. Note that the intensity of contractions is 20–25 mmHg and their frequency is one per 10 minutes. The cervix (insert) is thick, is very vascular and glandular, and contains mucus. **B,** At term, contractions are more frequent (typical of prelabor). The hydrostatic pressure of the forewaters exerts pressure in the direction of the lower segment and cervix. At first, this forces the blood out of the cavernous spaces in the cervical wall and later distends the lower uterine segment. Figures 4–7, 4–10, and 4–11 are continuations of this series.

### Definitions of Stages and Phases of Labor

From the standpoint of uterine contractility and cervical dilatation, there is no clear cut demarcation but a progressive transition between prelabor and labor (14). Traditionally, labor is divided into three stages, each of which is subdivided into phases.

*The first stage* consists of the latent phase that begins with the cervix dilated about 2 cm and is characterized by the onset of regular contractions that are mildly or moderately painful and ends when the cervix is 4 cm dilated. In the past, many of the labor curves, such as the Friedman curve, started at 0 cm dilatation, but current thought is that cervical dilatation is a minimum of 1 to 2 cm in the last few days before the onset of clinical labor. The latter is exemplified by the Hendricks curve, described at the end of the chapter. The active phase begins with the cervix dilating at a steady rate and ends with complete dilatation and retraction of the cervix.

*The second stage* of labor may be subdivided into a) descent phase, which begins with complete cervical dilatation and retraction and ends when the presenting part reaches the pelvic floor or 4+ station (approximately 4 cm below the plane of the ischial spines), and b) the pelvic floor phase.

*The third stage* of labor begins at delivery of the fetus and ends with delivery of the placenta.

In recent years, some clinicians have provided evidence that discrete signs between the latent and active phases of the first stage and the transition between the first and second stages are not so discrete and should be considered a continuous process. Moreover, some parturients experience the urge to bear down before complete cervical dilatation has occurred. Here we use the traditional classification because it is used by other contributors to this book.

## Contractions During Labor and Vaginal Delivery

### Contractions During the First Stage

During the latent phase of the first stage of labor, the uterine contractions usually have an intensity of 25 to 30 mm Hg and a frequency of about 2 to 3 contractions per 10 minutes (15–21). During the active phase, there is progressive increase in the intensity and frequency of contractions so that by the end of the active phase, the intensity is about 50 to 60 mm Hg, the frequency is 4 to 5 contractions per 10 minutes, and the tonus ranges from 8 to 12 mm Hg. The duration of normal contractions usually varies between 45 to 50 seconds during the early first stage, to 90 seconds during the end of the first stage. Generally, the more intense the contraction, the longer it lasts and hence as labor progresses, duration of the contraction tends to increase (Figures 4–5D, 4–5E, 4–6, 4–7, 4–8).

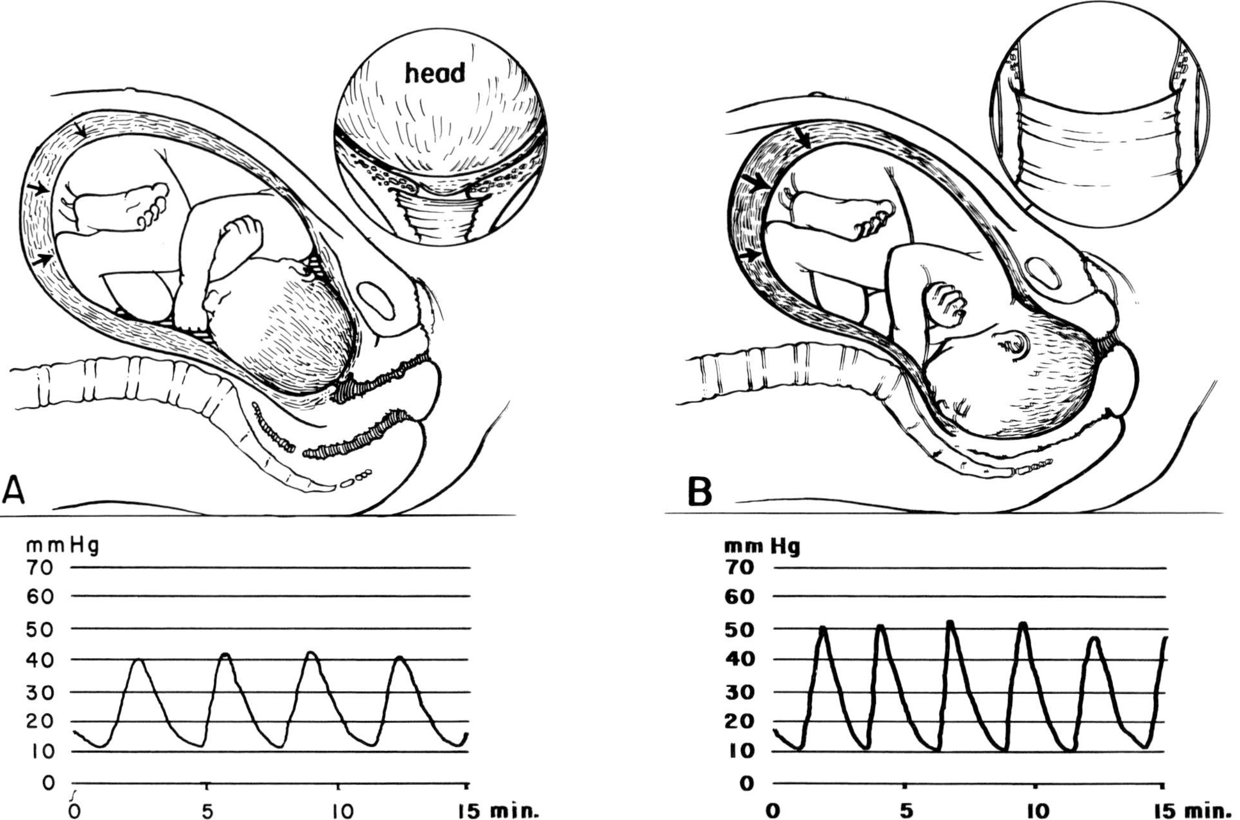


**Fig. 4–7.** Correlation between uterine activity and changes in the cervix and uterus during the first stage of labor (continuation of Fig. 4–6). **A,** At the onset of labor, uterine activity is 120 Montevideo units (40 mmHg × 3 contractions per 10 minutes). Cervix is effaced and 2 cm dilated. **B,** At the end of the first stage and entering second stage, the cervix is completely dilated and uterine activity is 200 Montevideo units.

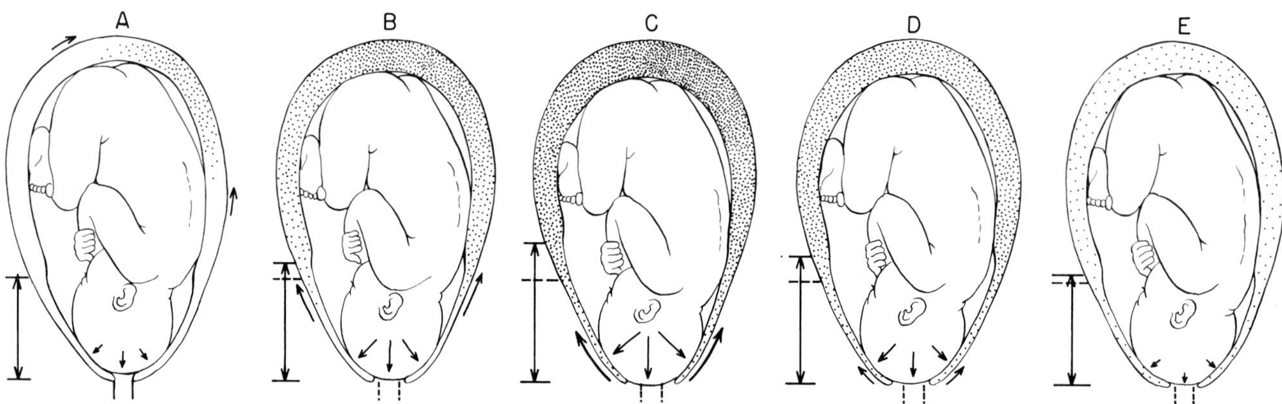


**Fig. 4–8.** Frontal sections of the uterus corresponding to successive stages from the beginning to the end of a uterine contraction. The dotted area indicates the part that is contracted, and the density of the dots represents the intensity of the contraction. The arrows at the head of the fetus show the pressure exerted by the head on the cervix. The arrows on the outside of the uterus indicate the traction exerted by the contracted parts, while the vertical arrows indicate the length of the lower uterine segment. (A) The beginning of the contraction at the site of initial impulse; (B) the contraction has spread throughout the uterus, is more intense and the length of the lower uterine segment is beginning to increase; (C) at the peak of contraction it is more intense, the length of the lower uterine segment is increased further and the cervix is more dilated; (D) with a regression of the contraction these changes regress but not to the original point. As a result, the upper segment remains shorter and thicker than before the contraction, while the cervix becomes more effaced and dilated and the lower uterine segment becomes thinner and longer. The upper segment shortens without losing its ability to contract (brachystasis) and the lower segment lengthens without changing its tension (mecystasis). (Modified from Alvarez H, Caldeyro-Barcia R: The normal and abnormal contractual wave of the uterus during labor. Gynaecologia 138:190, 1954.)

The function of these contractions during the latent phase is to efface and soften the cervix, while during the active phase, contractions complete effacement and effect progressive cervical dilatation. The mechanisms of these very important phenomena of labor are depicted in Figures 4–3, 4–6, 4–8 and 4–9. Although the hydrostatic dilator or wedging effect of the intact membranes contribute, it is not essential. The presenting part is just as effective as the membranes except in cases of cephalopelvic disproportion. During the height of the contraction, the pressure on the largest diameter fetal head is greater than 200 mm Hg (21–23). Effacement and dilation are accomplished solely by the uterine contractions of the first stage: contraction of the abdominal walls plays no role whatsoever in this process.

## *Contractions During the Second Stage*

The second stage is characterized by frequent, intense contractions of the uterus, aided by the reflex contraction of the intercostal and abdominal muscles and diaphragm (Figure 4–10). During this period, the intensity of contractions ranges between 50 to 60 mm Hg, and occasionally higher, and the frequency is 4 to 5 contractions per 10 minutes, so that the uterine activity ranges between 250 to 300 Mont.u (1,18–23). The pressure exerted by the auxiliary forces usually constitutes about 50% of the expulsive forces, and the pressure exerted by these reflex contractions superimposed on the pressure produced by uterine contractions increases the intrauterine pressure to about 100 to 120 mm Hg or higher (1,18,19,21–23).

The functions of these forces are further descent, flexion, internal rotation, and expulsion of the fetus. As shown in Figure 4–10, once cervical dilation is complete and

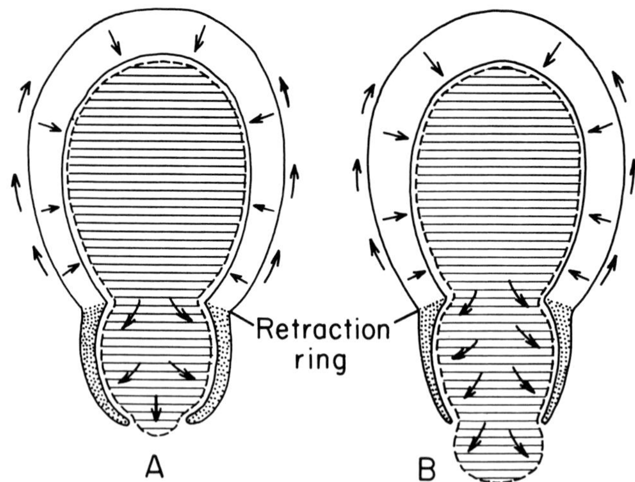


**Fig. 4–9.** Mechanism of dilatation of the cervix. **A,** During early labor. With each contraction, the presenting part is forced downward against the thinned-out cervix; at the same time, interaction of the muscle fibers in the upper segment pulls the lower segment and the cervix upward over the presenting part. Note the position of the retraction ring. **B,** Complete cervical dilatation. The physiologic retraction ring is now 7 to 10 cm above the external os. Note the increased thickness of the upper segment and the increased length and thinness of the lower segment. Descent can now take place without resistance from the cervix.

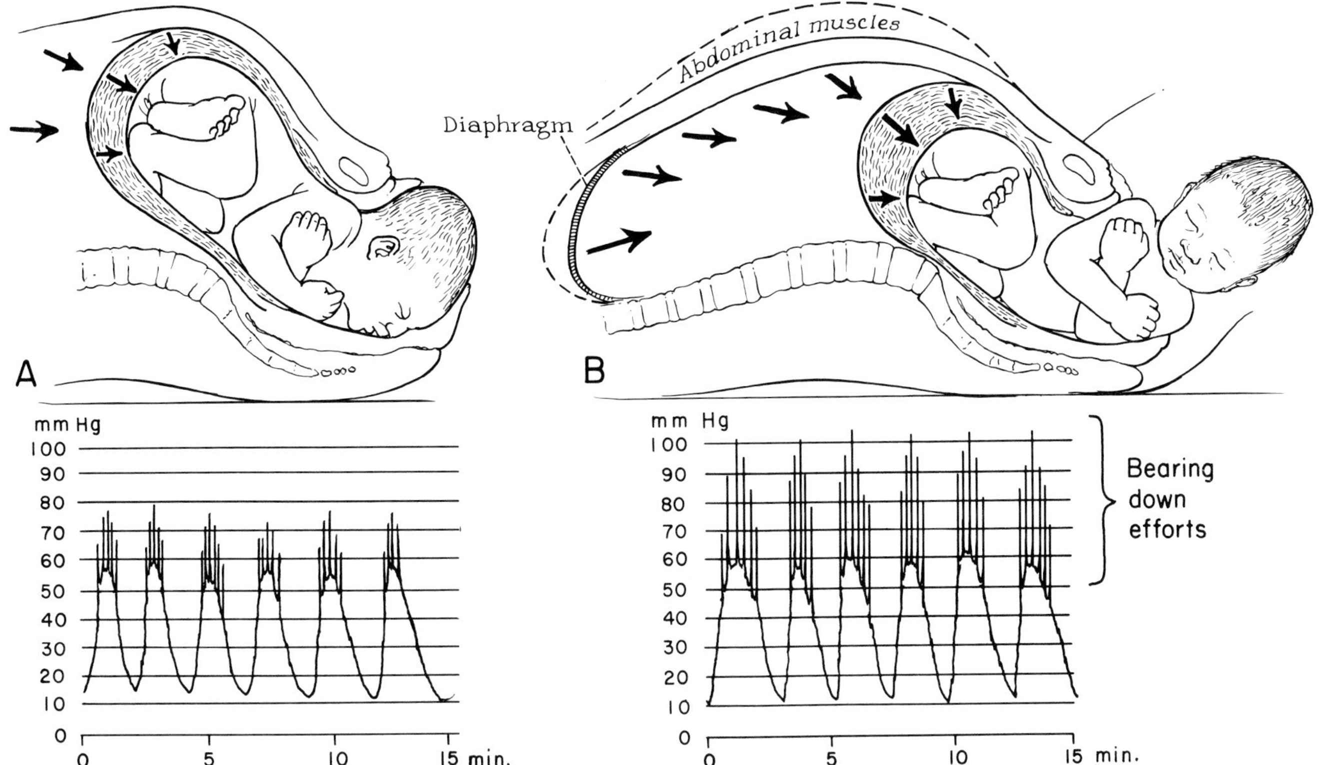


**Fig. 4–10.** The forces of the second stage of labor. **A,** Middle of the second stage. **B,** End of the second and beginning of the third stage. The intrauterine pressure caused by the uterine contraction is being reinforced by that produced by contraction of the diaphragm and the intercostal and abdominal muscles.

the second stage begins, the contracting uterus rapidly shortens and pushes the fetus downward. This mechanism is aided by action of the uterine ligaments: the uterosacrals and broad ligaments move the cervix to the pelvis while the contractions of the round ligaments that are simultaneous with those of the upper uterine segment tend to pull the uterus fundus anteriorly and bring its axis parallel to that of the inlet (1,24,25). As soon as the presenting part descends into the vagina and reaches the pelvic floor, it initiates the reflex urge to bear down and thus mobilizes the auxiliary forces to help the uterine contractions. In both nulliparae and multiparae, the descent phase is achieved normally with no more than 10 uterine contractions (22,23). Frequently, the presenting part is already on the pelvic floor at the time of complete cervical retraction, while at other times, only three or four contractions are required to achieve it (1,23). The pelvic floor phase is usually achieved in 10 contractions or less in nulliparae and three or four contractions in multiparae, with the assistance of normal bearing-down efforts.

## Contractions During the Third Stage

Immediately after the delivery of the fetus, the contractions continue rhythmically with continued high intensity, but with decreasing frequency (Figure 4–11). After delivery of the fetus, the uterine contraction compresses the placenta, causing rises in pressure of the fetal blood contained therein, and if the cord has not yet been clamped, it produces a transfusion of 60 to 100 ml of blood from the placenta to the fetus (22). At this time, the upper segment shortens markedly, and there is a very abrupt decrease in the size of the uterus and a concomitant decrease in the area of the placental site (Figure 4–11B). This marked shortening is the principal cause of separation of the placenta (23,25). Two or three contractions are sufficient to complete the separation of the placenta and to expel it (18). Thereafter, contractions, shortening, and tonus effect hemostasis of the placental site. The amount of blood lost in the average vaginal delivery is about 400 to 600 ml.

## The Early Puerperium (Fourth Stage of Labor)

During the immediate period after the delivery of the placenta, frequently referred to as the fourth stage of labor, uterine activity diminishes first in frequency and then intensity (Figures 4–5G, 4–5H, 4–5I). This phase is the most dangerous part of labor and requires constant attention to ascertain that the intensities of uterine contractions are maintained to obviate the risk of uterine relaxation and consequent increased risk of continuing blood loss. Continued vigorous manual massage of the uterus may be necessary with each contraction to avoid pushing the placenta deep in the pelvis with constant risk of losing control of excessive bleeding.

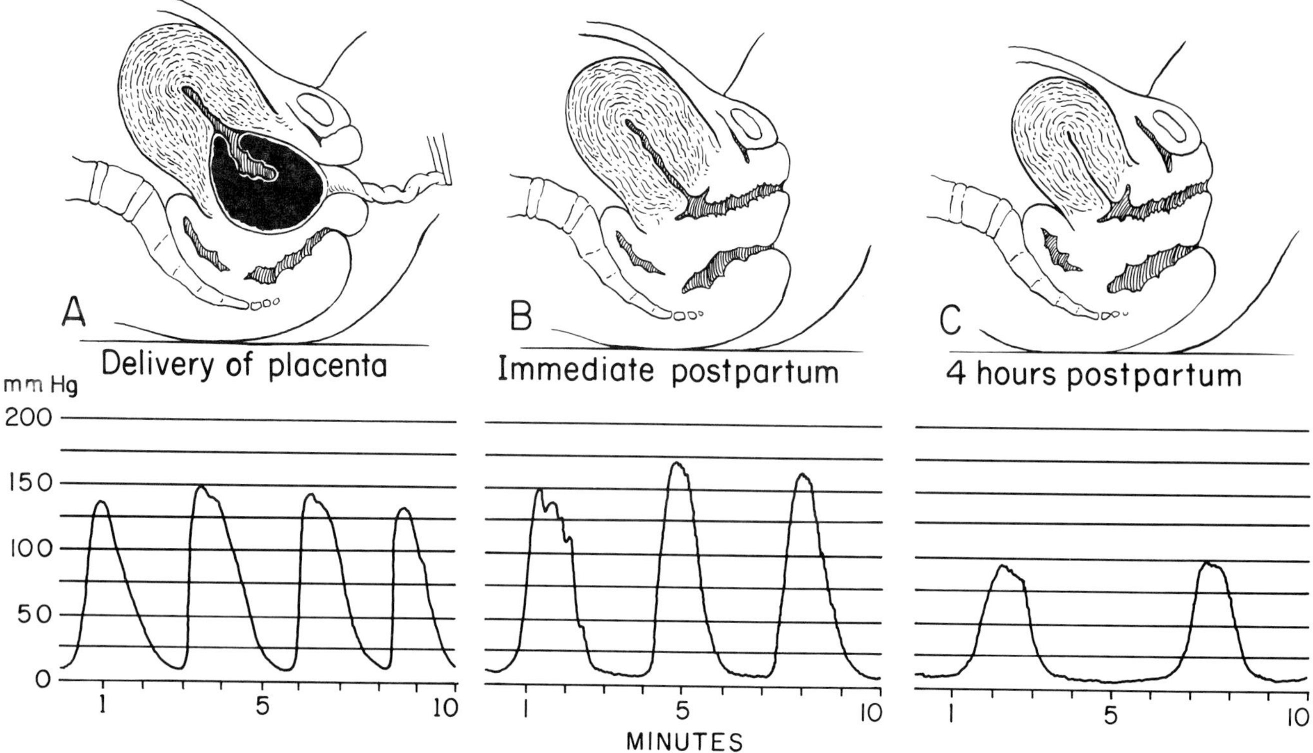


**Fig. 4–11.** Intrauterine pressures during the third stage of labor and early puerperium. **A,** The whole placenta is still inside the active upper segment. **B,** Immediately after the placenta has been delivered. **C,** Four hours after delivery. Uterine activity is markedly increased because delivery of the baby empties approximately seven-eighths of the contents of the uterus, which simply constricts around the remaining product of conception (the placenta). The high uterine activity persists for some time after delivery.

## Physiology of the Contractile Wave

Earlier teaching suggested that normal contractions originate near the uterine end of the fallopian tubes, which sites were referred to as "pacemakers" (16–18, 23,26), although Reynolds (23) long ago emphasized that there is no known morphologic entity in or about the uterus or tubes that may may be compared with the pacemaker of the heart. It was formerly believed that the stimulus for contractions started in these pacemakers and spread through the uterus at a speed of 2 cm per second, invading the whole organ within 15 seconds (16–18). However, recent evidence disputes the notion that there is any one pacemaker, but rather that uterine activity can commence in a variety of sites and only a group of highly excitable myometrial cells is required. Gap junctions, then, serve to propagate the impulse throughout the uterus. Normally, the spread of the impulses is from the upper part of the uterus downward—a phenomenon called the "contractile wave" (16–18, 22,23). Moreover, the contractions of the upper part of the uterus are stronger and of longer duration than those of the lower part that yield to and are distended by the contractions (Figure 4–12) (1,18,22,23). There is a gradient of contractility from above downward that is often called "gradient of activity," but more frequently called "fundal dominance."

In normal contractile waves, the activity of the different parts of the uterus is so well-coordinated that the acme of the contraction is attained almost simultaneously in all of them, despite the fact that the wave reaches them at different times. Consequently, the farther away the wave moves from the site of origin, the shorter is the duration of the "systolic" phase of the contraction. Moreover, the intensity of the contraction also diminishes from the upper to the lower segment. Because all parts of the uterus reach the acme of contraction almost simultaneously, the sum of their effects causes a significant increase in the amniotic pressure. The excellent coordination between all parts of the uterus is demonstrated by the regular form of the amniotic fluid pressure waves with its single peak. The synchronous relaxation of all parts of the uterus allows the amniotic pressure to fall to a minimum between contractions (tonus). The fact that the contraction begins earlier in the fundus and there is greater muscle mass results in a greater force of contraction in the upper uterus than in the lower segment (Figure 4–12.)

*Fundal dominance* is a term used to express the fact that in the fundus contractions begin earlier and are more intense and last longer. Fundal dominance plus developing cervical compliance result in the expulsive direction of the generated forces. In the upper uterus, myometrium tends to become thicker and muscle fibers become progressively shorter with each contraction as the fetus is pushed out of the fundus. However, in the lower uterine segment and in the cervix, the opposite occurs. The muscle wall thins and each fiber becomes slightly longer with

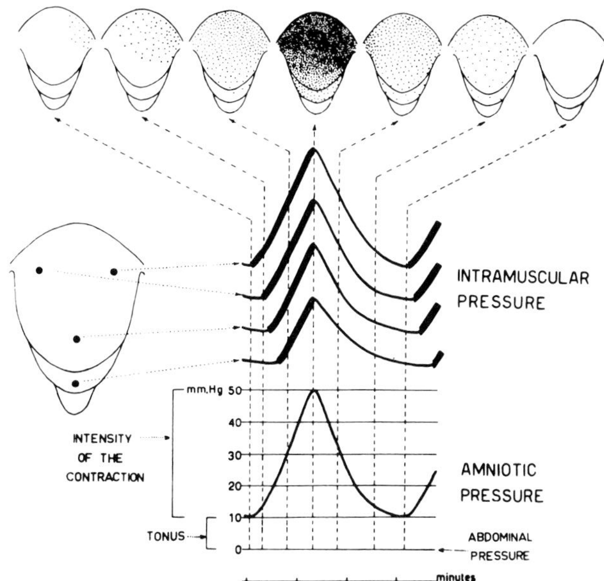


**Fig. 4–12.** Normal contractile wave of labor (schematic representation). The large uterus on the left shows the four points at which the intramyometrial pressure is recorded with a transabdominal plastic catheter. The four corresponding pressure tracings are shown in time relation to each other, to the amniotic pressure, and to the spread of the wave of contraction as indicated by the shading on the small uteri (above). The thick lines indicate the phase of contraction and thin lines denote the phase of relaxation. (From Caldeyro-Barcia R, Poseiro JJ: Physiology of uterine contraction. Clin. Obstet. Gynecol. 3:386, 1960.)

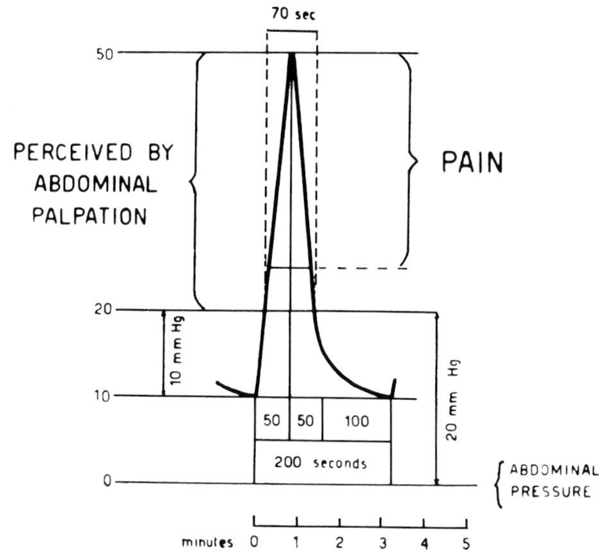


**Fig. 4–13.** Clinical aspects of the uterine contraction. The intrauterine pressure starts as 10 mmHg (tonus), increases another 10 mm before the uterus gets hard enough to be palpable through the abdominal wall, and increases to 25 mm before it starts to dilate the cervix and cause pain. Therefore, the lower part of the contraction is painless and is not perceived by abdominal palpation. The clinical duration of the contraction (the time it can be palpated and is painful) is 70 seconds—shorter than the actual duration revealed by the tracings (200 seconds). (From Caldeyro-Barcia R, Poseiro JJ: Physiology of uterine contraction. Clin. Obstet. Gynecol. 3:386, 1960.)

each contraction. The result is that the uterus not only forces the fetus down into the pelvis, but it also thins and then pulls the lower uterine segment and cervix upward. This is reflected in the process of effacement. It also produces a palpable ridge where the dense muscle mass of the upper portion of the organ meets the soft tissue of the compliant cervix. When delivery has been achieved, the muscle fibers of the lower segment and upper cervix also shorten.

These gradients in propagation, duration, and intensity of contraction were first noted by Reynolds and associates (1,16,23) who were the first to use the term "fundal dominance." These gradients, made possible by the difference in thickness of the myometrium and in the concentration of the contractile protein, actomyosin, in each part of the uterus, are essential for the efficiency of the contractions to dilate the cervix and to help expel the infant (18,19,22,23). Inversion of the gradient or incoordination of the various parts of the uterus impairs the efficiency of the contractions and thus produces abnormal labor (see below and Chapter 24).

## *Other Clinical Aspects of Uterine Contractions*

Several other important points about the intensity, duration, frequency, and coordination of uterine contractions need comment. There is a significant variation in each of these parameters, not only among different parturients, but also in the same patient at different times during labor; even in the same stage of labor, there may be a significant difference in the character of one contraction compared with the next. Figure 4–13 depicts schematically important clinical characteristics of a uterine contraction, summarized in the legend and the following text (15–19,22,23).

### *Intensity*

There is close correlation between the level of amniotic fluid pressure and the progress of labor: when the intensity is between 25 and 50 mm Hg labor progresses normally; when the intensity of uterine contraction is lower than 15 mm Hg labor does not start, or if it has started, it is delayed or even stopped (15–19,23). A minimum intensity of 15 mm Hg above tonus (or a total pressure of 25 mm Hg) is required to dilate the cervix. For the same reason, contractions do not become painful until their intensity exceeds 15 mm Hg above resting levels, i.e., the pressure totals 25 mm Hg (Figure 4–13). Occasionally, the intensity reaches 60 to 80 mm Hg and labor is extremely rapid and may end in precipitate delivery.

### *Frequency*

During the active phase of labor, contractions occur less frequently than 2 per 10 minutes, labor progresses very slowly; when contractions occur 2 to 5 per 10 minutes, labor progresses normally, and when contractions occur more frequently than 6 every 10 minutes they increase tonus, decrease the intensity and duration of the contractions, and thus frequently interfere with labor and cause fetal asphyxia.

### Duration

In normal labor, the contraction phase and rapid relaxation phase last approximately 40 to 60 seconds each, so that the total amount is approximately 80 to 120 seconds with an average of 100 seconds (Figure 4–13). The slow relaxation phase also averages about 100 seconds. Just using these means, each contraction and relaxation phase, totalling 200 seconds, would result in about three contractions per 10-minute period, which is the average rate at the time when the cervix is 3 to 4 cm dilated. During the latter part of the active phase (cervical dilation 7 to 10 cm), the duration of the first ascending phase of uterine contractility is faster and more intense, and, consequently, an average of four contractions occur per 10-minute period, resulting in uterine activity of approximately 160 to 170 Mont.u. During the second stage, the intensity, duration, and frequency are even greater, resulting in Mont.u. ranging between 175 to 225.

The duration of the "effective" contraction is shorter than the actual contraction, as is the duration of "clinical" contraction because uterine contractions are not perceived by abdominal palpation until the amniotic pressure increases at least 10 mm Hg above the tonus of the uterus (i.e., the amniotic pressure exceeds 20 mm Hg) (1,3, 15–23). This perception threshold is influenced by the thickness and tonus of the abdominal wall and by the experience of the obstetrician. Another important point: until the intensity of these contractions reaches 20 mm Hg, the uterine wall can readily be depressed by a finger, but above this pressure it becomes so hard that it resists depression.

## Some Factors That Affect Uterine Contractions

A number of physical and emotional factors influence intensity, frequency, and rhythmicity of uterine contraction. These include position of the parturient, circulatory alterations, parity, and strong emotional reactions.

### Position of Parturient

The effect of posture of the parturient of the forces of labor has been of great interest to physicians, midwives, and others since prehistoric times. A remarkable book published in 1883 by Engelmann (27) contains a comprehensive summary of the position assumed by parturients during labor among primitive people of all races. In a very extensive chapter, Engelmann described the postures used during labor and delivery, which among savages were determined by custom and tradition (Figure 1–1, Chapter 1). These included completely suspended, partially suspended, sitting erect, squatting, kneeling, and various horizontal or recumbent positions. Each position was used based on the degree of comfort, lack of risk, and the effect on labor. Many were also chosen based on the fact that the position enhanced uterine contractions, shortened labor, and was considered safe. The dorsal supine, or decubitus position, which was adopted with the advent of modern obstetrics, was considered very undesirable because it retarded labor, and increased the degree of discomfort and may have deleterious effect on the fetus.

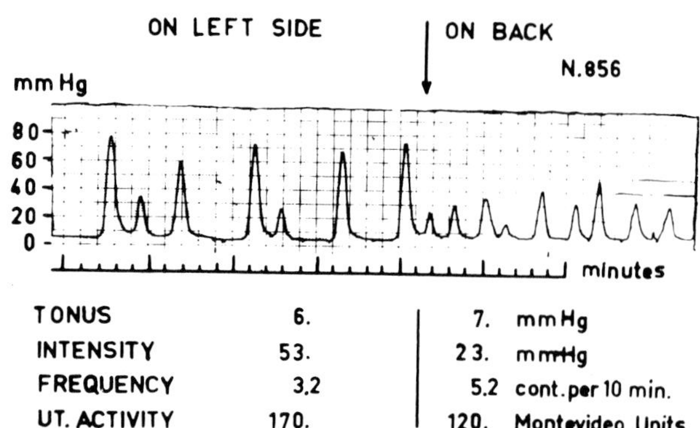


| | | | |
|---|---|---|---|
| TONUS | 6. | 7. | mm Hg |
| INTENSITY | 53. | 23. | mmHg |
| FREQUENCY | 3.2 | 5.2 | cont. per 10 min. |
| UT. ACTIVITY | 170. | 120. | Montevideo Units |

**Fig. 4–14.** The effect of position on uterine contractions. Contractions were more intense and less frequent when the patient was on her left side than when she was supine. (From Caldeyro-Barcia R, Poseiro JJ: Physiology of uterine contraction. Clin. Obstet. Gynecol. 3:386, 1960.)

The advent of new knowledge and the widespread use of the TKD, which measures intrauterine pressure precisely, has permitted acquisition of data that demonstrate the supine position is associated with a decrease in intensity, increase in frequency and higher tonus of uterine contractions, with consequent decrease in the progress of labor (Figure 4–14). This is undoubtedly due to the decrease in uterine blood flow in the supine position, compared to the lateral position. Many studies done during the past 2 decades have also shown that the vertical (sitting or standing) position is also associated with less pain during early labor (cervical dilatation 2 to 5 cm) but in late first stage and second stage, parturients have less pain in the lateral-horizontal position (28–34). It follows that uterine contractions with the parturient on her side or sitting or in Fowler's position are more efficient for the progress of labor than in the supine position. These effects appear immediately and last as long as the new position is maintained. They are more significant in spontaneous labor than in labor induced with oxytoxics, but neither the parity, the status of membranes, nor the positions of the fetus have an influence on this phenomenon (33).

### Circulatory Alterations

Systemic arterial hypotension frequently causes significant decrease in intensity and duration and impairs rhythmicity of uterine contractions (33,34). Hypertension, on the other hand, may cause an increase in intensity and frequency and in tonus (33,35). These effects are probably due to alterations (decrease or increase) in uterine blood flow (see Chapters 16 and 24 for more details).

### Parity

There is a definite correlation between the intensity, duration, and frequency of contractions and the parity of the gravida. During early labor the intensity of contrac-

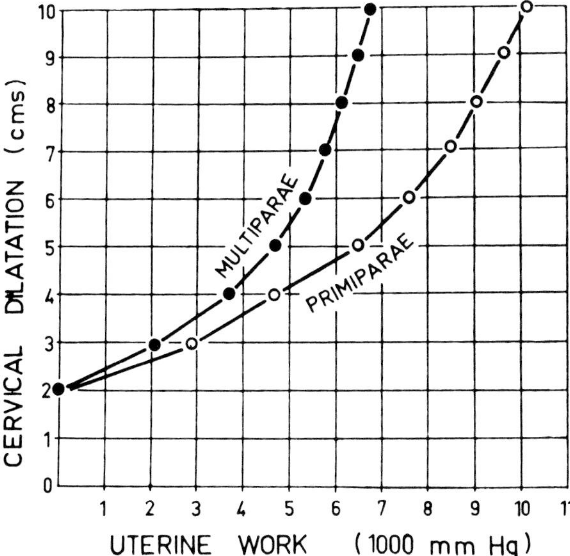


**Fig. 4–15.** Effect of the parity on uterine "work" required to dilate the cervix. The graph was developed from mean values obtained in 46 multiparae and 9 primiparae who were 38 to 40 weeks gestation. Labor was induced by oxytocin infusion. It is obvious that the uterus of a multipara is more efficient in dilating the cervix than the uterus of primigravida. Figure 4–33, shown later in this chapter, was developed using the same group of patients to show the duration of the first stage in multiparae and primiparae. (From Alvarez H, et al: *In* Oxytocin. Edited by R Caldeyro-Barcia, H Heller. New York, Pergamon Press, 1961.)

tions is greater in the primipara than in the multipara, whereas during the latter phase of the first stage of labor the reverse is true (1,14,22,23). The duration of uterine contractions in multiparae tends to exceed that in primiparae at all times during the first stage of labor. Reynolds, et al (23) suggest that it is primarily this factor that makes the multigravida uterus more efficient in dilating the cervix. Their data also show that in the early phase of the first stage of labor the weaker contraction in the multipara produces more cervical dilation in about one-third the time required by the nullipara. The greater efficiency of uterine contractions in multigravidae is effectively demonstrated by considering the hourly rate of work (intensity, frequency, and duration of contractions) (Figure 4–15).

### Other Factors

In the preceding chapter, ample evidence is presented that fear, anxiety, apprehension, and other negative emotional reactions and pain may alter uterine contractions. A recent study showed that parturients with severe pain in the latent phase, which is associated with anxiety, stress, and negative cognitive processes, causes a longer latent phase, a longer active phase of labor, and an increased incidence of instrumental deliveries (36). Other factors very relevant to this book are the use of analgesics and anesthetics that may directly or indirectly decreases uterine contractility. These are summarized briefly at the end of this chapter and considered in detail in Chapters 13, 14, 15 and 18.

## Abnormalities of Uterine Contractions

In Chapter 24, Ueland discusses the influence of hyperactivity and hypoactivity of uterine contractions and their treatment. *Hyperactivity* can occur with: 1) intensity higher than 50 mm Hg; or 2) a frequency greater than 5 contractions per 10 minutes (tachysystolia); or 3) a combination of both (21). Hyperactivity reduces placental blood flow and in the absence of mechanical obstruction produces a precipitate labor that may cause damage to both mother and infant.

*Hypoactivity* exists when the contractions have an abnormally low intensity (under 25 mm Hg) or abnormally low frequency (less than 2 contractions per 10 minutes.) In such cases, labor progresses much more slowly than normal or not at all (14,21,22).

*Hypertonicity* is present when the tonus is greater than 12 mm Hg. Caldeyro-Barcia and associates (17,18,22) classify it as weak (12 to 20 mm Hg), medium (20 to 30 mm Hg), or strong (greater than 30 mm Hg). Hypertonicity can be produced by: 1) overdistention of the myometrium as in polyhydramnios; 2) incoordination; 3) tachysystolia; and 4) abnormal augmentation of the tonic properties of uterine fibers (essential hypertonus). Hypertonicity impairs uterine function during labor.

*Inversion of gradient* occurs when the contractile waves start in the lower part of the uterus and spread upward (Figure 4–16). Although they may cause high ele-

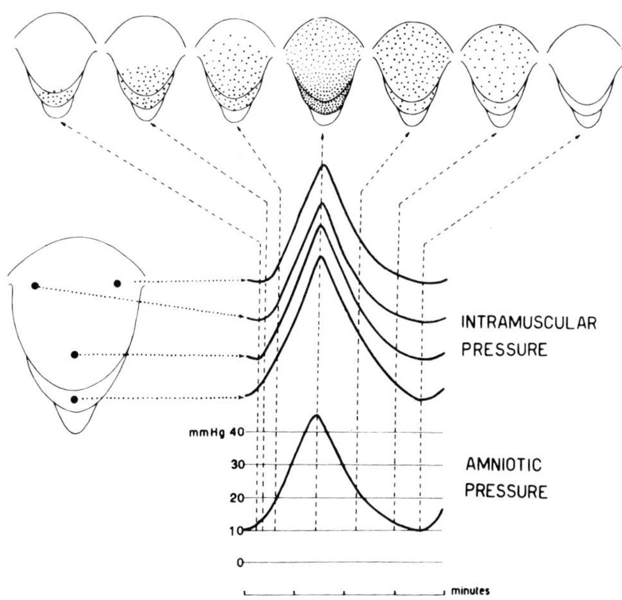


**Fig. 4–16.** Abnormal contractile wave with inverted gradients (schematic). The contraction starts in the lower uterine segment and spreads upward. It is stronger and lasts longer in the lower part than the upper part of the uterus (compare with Fig. 4–12). (From Caldeyro-Barcia R: Modern Trends in Gynaecology and Obstetrics. Vol. 1. Montreal, Librairie Beauchemin Limitee, 1959, p. 65.)

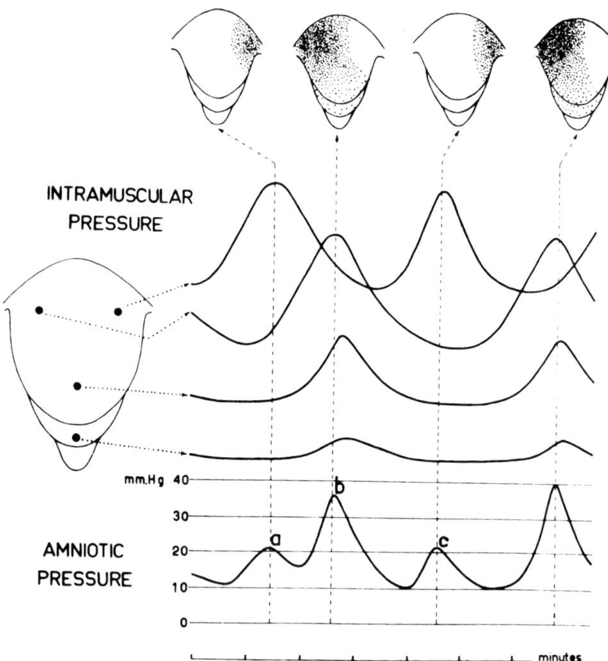


**Fig. 4–17.** First-degree incoordination (schematic). The contractile waves that originate in the left side remain localized in the area of the left horn. They cause only small elevations in the amniotic pressure and are ineffective in dilating the cervix. The wave that starts in the right side spreads over almost the whole of the uterus (except the left horn, which is still in the refractory period), causes a greater elevation in the amniotic pressure, and has some effect in dilating the cervix (compare with Fig. 4–12). (From Caldeyro-Barcia R, Poseiro JJ: Physiology of the uterine contraction. Clin. Obstet. Gynecol. 3:386, 1960.)

vation in intrauterine pressure, waves with inverted gradients are inefficient for dilating the cervix (1,15,22,23).

*Incoordination* occurs when the stimuli for the contraction initiate in different regions concomitantly and independently (first degree) (Figure 4–17) or when the uterus is divided functionally into numerous zones that contract asynchronously (second degree) (1,18,19,23). These either slow up labor or are totally ineffective in promoting cervical dilation (see Chapter 24 for details).

## BIOLOGY OF UTERINE ACTIVITY DURING LABOR

During the quarter century that has passed since the first edition of this book was published, we have acquired much information about the biological, biochemical, molecular, and cellular aspects of the function of the uterus during pregnancy and labor. However, despite the awesome scientific efforts worldwide, we still lack evidence about the precise mechanism responsible for the onset and progress of labor and delivery of the infant. Research in animals and humans suggests that these involve complex anatomic, structural, biochemical, endocrine, humoral, and circulatory factors which, at the critical time and adapted to the individual morphology, interact to initiate labor and eventually promote evacuation of the uterus. The following discussion summarizes briefly the most important of these factors. Additional details are found in Chapter 5, a recently published review (37), and books (2,38).

### Anatomic and Structural Factors

The widely accepted concept of considering labor in terms of smooth muscle function is no longer tenable. There are two distinct forces of labor that play a critical role: uterine contractions and the resistance of the cervix. It is the coordinated interplay of these two forces that produces the ultimate successful outcome—delivery of the infant. The anatomic and structural changes in the uterus and cervix during late pregnancy and labor have already been mentioned. These include the progressive increase in the thickness of the fundus, the consequent predominance of contractile power in it, and the concomitant progressive increase in the thinness and compliance of the cervix. The advantages of fundal dominance are further enhanced by favorable physical forces, including degree of stretching of uterine fibers (and consequently their length-tension relation) and the shape of the uterus that result in optimum radii for greatest efficiency (1,23). Changes in the uterine volume and uterine blood flow also have marked effects on uterine contractility. At term, uterine blood flow is about 700 to 800 ml per minute (39) and a decrease in blood flow impairs uterine contractility.

### Biochemical and Biophysical Factors

Contraction of uterine muscle, like other muscular contraction, involves the interaction of several systems: the contractile substance, a supply of energy, a stimulus brought about by electrical changes in muscle through ionic exchange across the cell membrane, particularly calcium, and a means of conducting the stimulus to the contractile element (37,38,40).

#### Contractile Substance

The contractile substance is a complex of two proteins, actin and myosin, neither of which is contractile, but when interacting they form "actomyosin" which is contractile. Each gram of human myometrium contains 1 to 5 mg of myosin and 16 to 60 mg of actin, which corresponds to the ratio of thin to thick filaments in myometrial cells.

Myosin forms the thick filaments, which are about 16 nm thick and 2.2 nm long and have a molecular weight (MW) of about 500,000. They consist of a helical tail and a globular head formed by two heavy chains (MW 200,000 each) (40). The head contains ATPase enzymatic activity and the site for combination with actin (Figure 4–18). Attached to each globular head are two pairs of light chains of myosin of 20,000 and 27,000 MW, respectively, which are sites of phosphorylation and calcium binding. Actin is the smaller molecule (42,000 MW) and in physiologic solution polymerizes to form thin filaments about 6 nm in diameter and longer than the thick filaments. Helically arranged strands of actin alternate with strands of tropomyosin. Actomyosin is formed when actin activates the magnesium-dependent myosin ATPase. The latter provides the energy for the attachment of the globular head

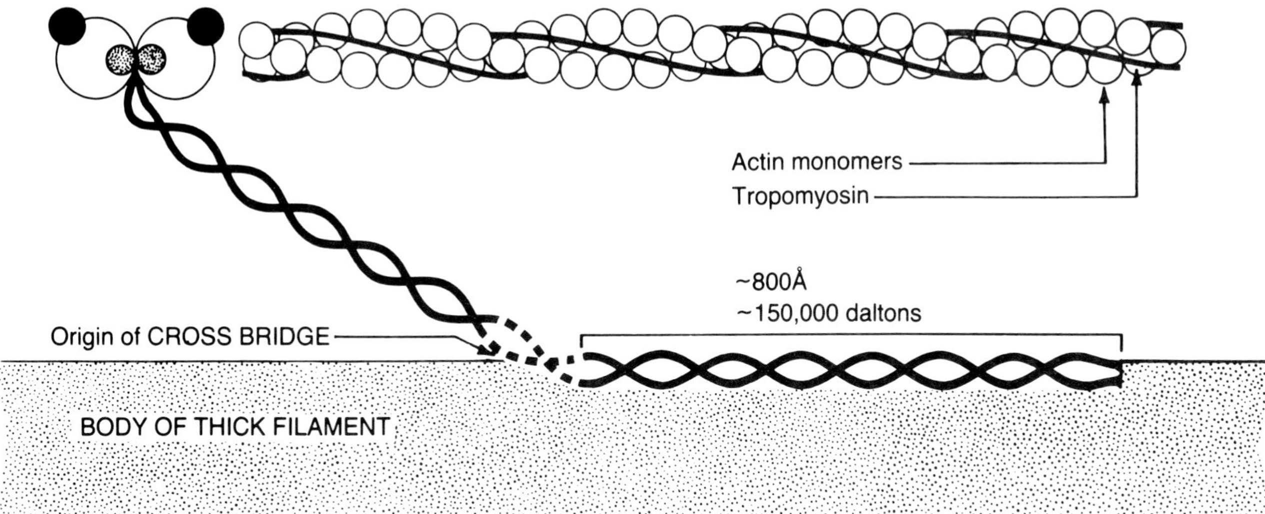


**Fig. 4–18.** Diagrammatic representation of the myosin molecule, which is a hexamer consisting of one pair of heavy chains and two pairs of light chains. The molecule is very asymmetric; the carboxyl-terminal portion of the heavy chain is a fibrous, almost completely α-helically coiled structure that forms the thick filaments (MW 20,000 each). The amino-terminal portion is globular in shape and is associated with the light chains, although their precise position is unknown. The globular head binds to actin and exhibits ATPase activity. The light chain of MW 20,000 contains the phosporylation site. The hinge region between head and tail is thought to be very flexible. (From Fuchs AR, Fuchs F: Physiology of parturition. *In* Obstetrics: Normal and Problem Pregnancies. 2nd Ed. Edited by SG Gabbe, JR Niebyl, JL Simpson. New York, Churchill Livingstone, Inc, 1986, pp 327.)

of myosin to the actin filament, forming cross bridges between thin and thick filaments. Once attached, the angle of the cross bridges changes, causing filaments to slide past each other, thereby generating contractile force (see Figure 5–3, next chapter). Relaxation occurs with detachment of the cross bridges.

Unlike striated muscle, the arrangement of actin and myosin filaments in smooth muscle cells is not parallel with the cell axis, but may be random, and the actin filaments connect through dense bodies with the cell membrane. This oblique arrangement allows actin and myosin to maintain contact and gives the smooth muscle cell the power to shorten by 50% or to lengthen by more than 100% of this resting length, and also gives it greater force and potential for lower velocity of contraction.

The contractile proteins are found in the small (10 μ) spindle-shaped cells that make up the larger (about 100 μ) myometrial bundles that compose the myometrium. These smooth muscle cells are much smaller than skeletal muscle cells: 1 mm of muscle contains 2.3 million smooth muscle cells, but only 17 skeletal muscle cells (37) (see Figure 5–5, next chapter). An important consequence of this difference is a much larger ratio of surface area to intracellular volume in smooth muscle. The surface area of smooth muscle is increased even more by the presence of surface invagination, caveolae, which are also present on about one-third of the cell surface. This accounts for the much greater influence of humoral agents acting on cell membrane on smooth muscle as opposed to skeletal muscles.

The contractile proteins are present in the gravid uterus in amounts that are about twice as much as those in the nonpregnant uterus, and its concentration in the fundus is more than double of that in the lowest part of the uterus (37,38,40). Because the work done by the myometrium is a factor of these contractile proteins, the biochemical makeup of the fundus and cervix is such that it favors fundal dominance—a condition essential for the onset and progress of labor and for the evacuation of the uterus.

## Role of Calcium

The stimulus that initiates the liberation of energy and thus causes the contraction of the uterus is brought about by ionic exchanges across the cell membrane, particularly calcium, which predominantly controls activation of the cells. For contractions to occur, the concentration of free $Ca^{++}$ ion within the cell must rise from $10^{-7}$M or $10^{-8}$M to $10^{-6}$M. This ion is derived from both extracellular and intracellular sources (Figure 4–19). The concentration of $Ca^{++}$ ion in the interstitial fluid is 10 to 3M. An action potential will cause it to enter the cell through calcium ion channels. These channels may be specifically blocked by so-called calcium channel blockers, and the usefulness of these agents in inhibiting uterine activity attests to the pertinence of this mechanism in uterine muscle contraction. However, extracellular calcium com-

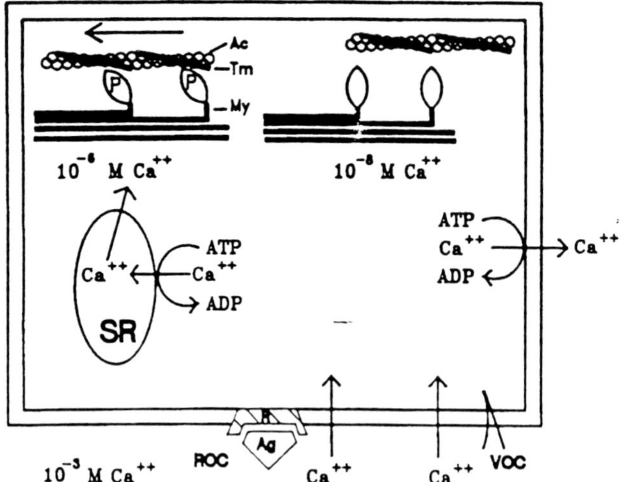


**Fig. 4–19.** Calcium sources for myometrial contraction. On top, sliding filament of muscle contraction (left) and relaxation (right). (Ac = actin; Tm = tropomyosin; My = myosin; P = phosphorylated; SR = sarcoplasmic reticulum; R = receptor; Ag = agonist; ROC = adenosine diphosphate; VOC = voltage-operated channel; ATP = adenosine triphosphate; ADP = adenosine diphosphate). (With permission from Carsten ME, Miller JD: A new look at uterine muscle contraction. Am. J. Obstet. Gynecol. 157:1303, 1987.)

ing through calcium ion channels appears to be a less important source of calcium ion than the intracellular stores that are contained with the sarcoplasmic reticulum.

These stores in the sacroplasmic reticulum are mobilized by another mechanism activated by hormones, rather than by an action potential (neural signals) (40,41). In this case, a hormone (oxytocin or prostaglandin) interacts with a specific receptor in the cell membrane. This interaction, mediated by a so-called G-protein, activates a cell membrane enzyme, phospholipase-C (PLC). This enzyme hydrolyzes a minor membrane component phosphatidylinositol 4,5 triphosphate (PIP2) to 1,4,5 inositol triphosphate (1,4,5, IP3) and diacylglycerol (DAG), both of which are second messengers. Inositol triphosphate acts on the sarcoplasmic reticulum to release Ca + + (Figure 4–20) from nonmitochondrial stores. The diacylglycerol activates protein kinase C, and possibly stimulates additional prostaglandin synthesis.

As the intracellular Ca + + level rises, the ion complexes with the protein calmodulin. This complex further interacts with the enzyme myosin-light-chain kinase (MLCK). The three molecules together then phosphorylate myosin at the site of the serine and threonine residues, and the phosphorylated myosin interacts with actin to produce contractions.

*Relaxation* occurs when this molecular sequence is reversed. Dephosphorylation of myosin occurs within smooth muscle cells at a steady rate by phosphatase. A protein kinase, which is cAMP-dependent, phosphorylates MLCK and inactivates it. Ca + + is lowered by sequestering it within the sarcoplasmic reticulum and by efflux across the cell membrane. The latter is achieved through Ca and Mg adenosine triphosphatase. Ca and Mg ATPases also facilitate the uptake of Ca + + by the sarcoplasmic reticulum. Calcium in the cytoplasm in the presence of ATP and the ATPase is transported across the membrane of the sarcoplasmic reticulum and stored. With a decrease in cytoplasmic concentration of Ca + +, calmodulin dissociates from MLCK, which becomes inactive (Figure 4–21).

## Gap Junctions

The remarkable coordination of uterine musculature that develops in association with the onset of labor is correlated with the development of gap junctions between individual muscle cells (42,43). These structures contain protein-linked channels that establish direct contact between the cytoplasm of one cell and that of another. Gap junctions are areas of specialized intimate contacts between cells of the same type and are sites of communication permitting rapid transmission of electrical impulses and chemical signals from one cell to the next.

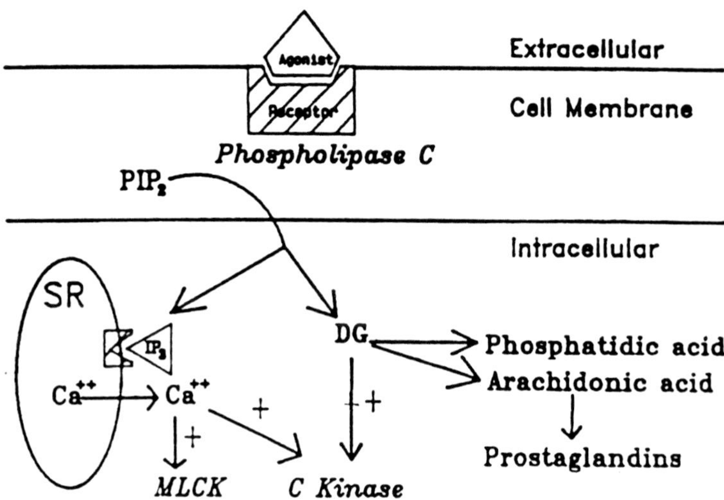


**Fig. 4–20.** Agonist-dependent second messengers: inositol triphosphate, calcium, and diacyglycerol. Agonist receptor-binding activates phospholipase C to hydrolyze phosphatidylinositol 4,5-bisphosphate ($PIP_2$) to 1,4, 5,inositol triphosphate (1,4,5$IP_3$) and diacylglycerol (DG). Myosin light-chain kinase (MLCK) and protein kinase C (C Kinase) phosphorylate various proteins, leading to biologic responses. (With permission from Carsten ME, Miller JD: A new look at uterine muscle contraction. Am. J. Obstet. Gynecol. 157:1303, 1987.)

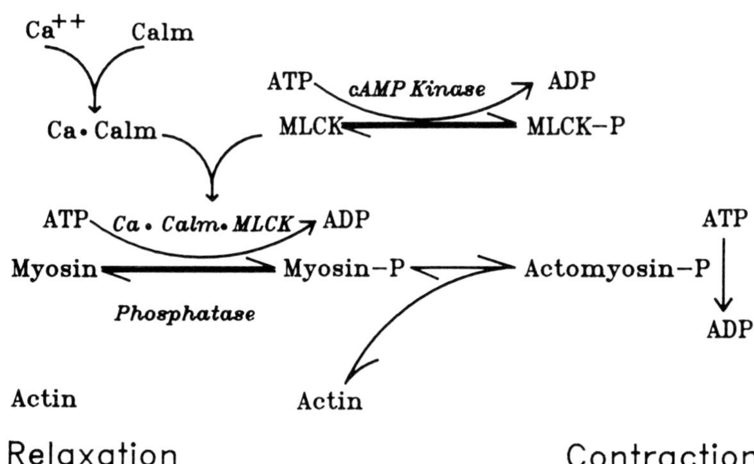


**Fig. 4–21.** Diagram of contraction-relaxation cycle of smooth muscle. (Calm = calmodulin; cAMP kinase = cAMP-dependent protein kinase; MLCK = myosin light-chain kinase; MLCK-P = phosphorylated myosin light-chain kinase; Myosin-P = phosphorylated myosin; Actomyosin-P = phosphorylated actomyosin; ADP = adenosinediphosphate; ATP = adenosine triphosphate.) (With permission from Carsten ME, Miller JD: A new look at uterine muscle contraction. Am. J. Obstet. Gynecol. 157:1303, 1987.)

This electrical coupling facilitates synchronization of the contraction of individual cells that is essential for the propagated activity of the organ (44). They permit electrical coupling of two adjacent cells as well as the passage of a variety of diffusible dyes. Thus, they permit coordinated activity. Exceedingly rare in the preterm uterus of humans and other species, they suddenly become extremely numerous just before labor, then as rapidly regress postpartum (43). Estrogen promotes their development and progesterone inhibits it. The production of gap junctions by estrogen requires protein synthesis. Some portion of the arachidonic acid cascade also seems to promote their development by mechanisms as yet unknown. In addition, both Ca ion and cAMP modulate their function. The concentration of free Ca + + in the cytoplasm of the smooth muscle cell is the type of biologic variable that is felt to be transferable via gap junctions.

## *Endocrine and Humoral Factors*

Humoral factors affecting myometrial function consist of (40): 1) steroid hormones estrogen and progesterone; 2) oxytocic hormones that include the α-adrenergic neurotransmitters, the neurohypophyseal hormones oxytocin and vasopressin, and prostaglandin F and E; and 3) relaxin hormones. Although the origin, synthesis, and most other aspects of the biochemistry of these various factors have been clarified, there remains controversies and differences of opinion about which of these play the dominant role in the initiation of labor.

There are four major hypotheses for the initiation of human labor: 1) progesterone withdrawal; 2) prostaglandin hypothesis; 3) oxytocin hypothesis; and 4) "fetal-maternal communication system proposition" (44,45). Let us briefly consider the first three.

### *Progesterone Withdrawal*

The oldest of the theories suggests that uterine quiescence during pregnancy is maintained by progesterone and that the uterus would contract spontaneously upon its withdrawal (46). However, the evidence for withdrawal of progesterone at the end of human pregnancy is not available (40). Recent studies, in which progesterone withdrawal without affecting the production of other steroids is possible, revealed that administration of progesterone antagonists to monkeys during late pregnancy produced spontaneous contractions and cervical effacement, but labor was not initiated unless oxytocin was administered (40).

### *Prostaglandins*

Studies by Casey and MacDonald (44,45) and many others (45a) suggest an increased release of $PGE_{2\alpha}$ from the amnion is the event that initiates human parturition and that prostaglandins are the sole force that drives the laboring uterus. Casey and MacDonald (45) have presented the proposition that the fetus is in control of its destiny with respect to the time of onset of parturition at term, and, it is the fetus that, after maturation of key organs and systems, is able to initiate a chain of events that culminate in labor.

Prostaglandins, both $PGF_2$ and $PGF_{2\alpha}$, are produced in the fetal membranes and the decidua vera and may be degraded by the chorion. Their production is enhanced by estrogen, which may increase in late pregnancy in response to rising fetal cortisol levels (44). Cortisol enhances the activity of the 17a-hydroxylase, the 17,20-desmolase, and the aromatase, that sequentially hydroxylate progesterone at the 17a position, remove the side chain, and aromatize the A ring, resulting in estrogen. Rising estrogen, with or without a decrease in progesterone, may increase prostaglandin levels. All of these changes tend to promote contraction of muscle, developing cervical compliance, and the appearance of gap junctions in the myometrium. Whether or not there is a drop in local progesterone production shortly before labor begins is debated (38,40). The sensitivity of the myometrium to oxytocin increases during labor, which also may be an effect of the prostaglandins.

$PGF_{2\alpha}$ is the main prostanoid released during labor and has similar action on the myometrium as oxytocin (40). $PGF_{2\alpha}$ raised intracellular-free calcium both by opening calcium channels and by release of calcium from intracellular vesicles. Equally, or more important, is the fact that $PGF_{2\alpha}$ increases the excitability of myometrium cells at concentrations lower than those required to produce contractions (40). This action enhances the properties of other oxytocics (47) and may explain the significant sensitization of oxytocin that occurs during labor (40) (Figure 4–21).

Figure 4–22 depicts levels of $PGF_{2\alpha}$ and its metabolite in amniotic fluid in late gestation and during labor. Figure 4–23 demonstrates the relationship of one of the plasma

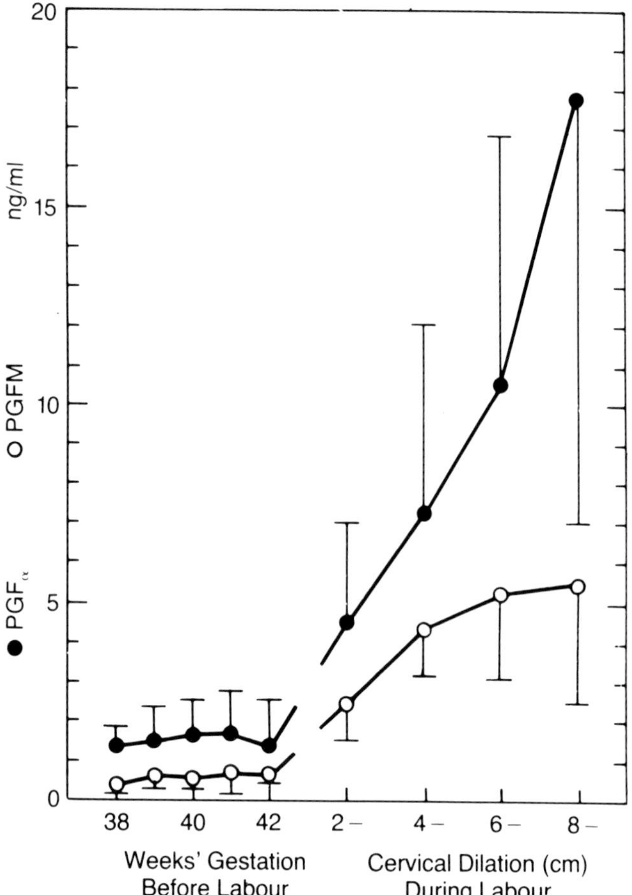


**Fig. 4–22.** Levels of $PGF_{2\alpha}$ (●) and its metabolite PGFM (○) in the amniotic fluid during late gestation and during labor. Values are for samples obtained at amniotomy in individual patients (not serial samples). The levels of the main metabolite in maternal plasma increased very slightly during pregnancy, reflecting growth of the uterus. With the onset of labor there is a rapid progressive rise from 4 to 5 cm cervical dilatation until after delivery of the baby, when maximum levels occur at the time of placental separation. The concentration of PGFM then falls rapidly, suggesting that the peak production during the third stage originates in the placenta or fetal membranes. However, levels remain increased at least 1 hour after delivery of the placenta and fetal membranes, indicating that they are a major source of uterine $PGF_{2\alpha}$ during labor. (From Keirse MJMC: Endogenous prostaglandins in human parturition. *In* Human Parturition. Edited by MFMC Keirse, ABM Anderson, JB Gravenhorst. Lyden, Lyden University Press, 1979, p. 101.)

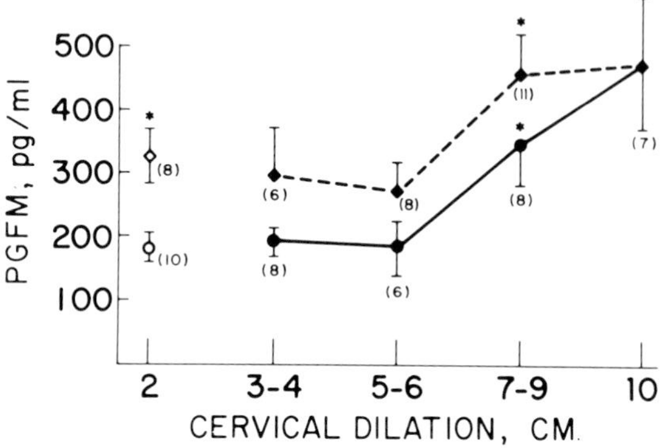


**Fig. 4–23.** Plasma prostaglandin F metabolite (PGFM) levels in parturients measured in serial samples taken during the first stage of labor and arranged according to cervical dilatation. Values for parturients with intact membranes (——) are shown separately from those with ruptured membranes (– – – –). Prelabor values are shown in women with premature ruptured membranes (◇) and intact membranes (○). It is obvious that no significant changes in PGFM occurred prior to labor; however, after cervical dilatation of 5 to 6 cm, there is a rapid progressive increase in the metabolite. Maximum levels occurred after the delivery of the baby and time of placental separation. (From Fuchs AR, et al: Oxytocin and the initiation of human parturition: III. Plasma concentration in 3,14-dihydro-15-ketoprostaglandin F2-α in spontaneous and oxytocin-induced labor at term. Am. J. Obstet. Gynecol. 147:497, 1983.)

prostaglandins (PGF) before the onset of labor and during labor, showing significant increase in plasma prostaglandin F metabolite during labor (48,49). It is this increased sensitivity that is pivotal in the susceptibility of the myometrium to the effect of oxytocin (40).

The increased production of prostaglandin during labor can result from: 1) withdrawal of inhibitory substances, such as lipocortins and the recently isolated protein, gravidin, which is active during pregnancy but loses activity in labor (40), or 2) increase in stimulatory synthesis of which oxytocin was the first endogenous compound shown to stimulate $PGE_2$ and $PGF_{2\alpha}$ synthesis in decidua and amnion. Oxytocin activates phospholipase C (PLC). The human decidua thereby increases $PGF_{2\alpha}$. Other stimulators include epidermal growth factor and platelet-activating factor found in amniotic fluid and thus constitutes the fetal signal that may also increase prostaglandin production (40). Another possibility is that prostanoid production is initiated by a shift in the balance of the inhibitory and stimulating substances. The shift need not be large, because once labor is in progress the production of prostanoid appears to be self-perpetuating. $PGF_{2\alpha}$ may stimulate its own release or due to contraction and intrauterine pressure changes may bring about sustained $PGF_{2\alpha}$ release (40).

## *Oxytocin Hypothesis*

Fuchs and associates (40,49) dispute the prostaglandin theory and present the following arguments to support their own hypothesis that it is oxytocin that is the critical factor. First is the fact that the levels of PGE and PGF in the amniotic fluid are not increased at the onset of labor over those noted in late pregnancy but only rise in the course of labor (45). In contrast, plasma oxytocin levels increase in early labor and precede the rise in levels of $PGF_{2\alpha}$ metabolite that occur in the course of active labor (49,50,51). Moreover, the responsiveness of oxytocin undergoes remarkable change during pregnancy and reaches a maximum at term, which is the optimal time for birth (51), whereas the uterine responsiveness to prostaglandins undergoes only minor alterations during the course of pregnancy (52). Finally, term labor can be induced with oxytocin in doses that result in plasma oxytocin levels in the physiologic range as shown long ago by Caldeyro-Barcia and his associates (51), and more recently by Fuchs and associates (49). In contrast, initiation of labor with prostaglandins results in plasma levels that far exceed the physiologic range regardless of the method of administration (49).

On the basis of these considerations, Fuchs and Fuchs (40) propose that initiation of labor depends on endogenous oxytocin as the maternal signal and on oxytocin, vasopressin, epidermal growth factor, platelet-activating factor, and perhaps other compounds as the fetal signal. These signals are integrated in the decidua parietalis and transmitted to the myometrium using prostaglandin as a second messenger. Notwithstanding these convincing arguments, many American obstetricians currently believe in the prostaglandins theory and use small doses of this agent to soften the cervix, which in many parturients initiates labor.

Endogenous oxytocin is created in the very special locale of the supraoptic and paraventricular area of the hypothalamus in the deep recesses of the endoplasmic reticulum. It is composed of the complex protein neurophysin, a glycine-lysine-arginine unit and the octapeptide oxytocin, which are then converted to secretory granules and transported to their storage depots in the posterior pituitary gland. The process of transportation is via neural pathways; subsequently, oxytocin and neurophysin are both released to magnocellular neurons. Impulses initiated by distention of the cervix and vagina reaching the hypothalamus caused a release of both hormones into the circulation. Oxytocin effects increase in uterine muscle tone. This remarkable physiological effect was first described by Dale as early as 1906 (53). Four decades later, Ferguson (54) described the reflex that bears his name, discovered in rabbits by elucidation of the fact that cervical dilatation produced uterine contractions.

It is now well-established that endogenous oxytocin is produced throughout pregnancy and it is the combined effect of increased receptivity of the target cells and the increased release of oxytocin that many investigators believe participates in the initiation and sustenance of the labor effort (51,55–57). The fetus also secretes oxytocin and studies have revealed that the concentration in the umbilical artery is about twice as high as in the umbilical vein, which is about the same concentration as maternal venous blood (55).

There is controversy as to whether or not the oxytocin levels change during pregnancy, with some studies suggesting an increase (51) while others indicating no change (40,55). Fuchs and Fuchs (40) state that mean plasma levels of oxytocin are relatively constant during pregnancy with individual fluctuations suggestive of sporadic release (55). During the first stage of labor, mean oxytocin levels in samples collected in 1- to 2-hour intervals were raised over values in nonlaboring women (49). During induction of labor, infusion rates of 1 to 6 Mont.u./min resulted in plasma levels of oxytocin that were similar to those observed during the first stage of spontaneous labor (58). Others have noted that with onset of labor there is significant increases of spikes of oxytocin, most frequently with maximum vaginal and cervical dilatation (20,59,60).

In one study in which plasma was collected at 1 minute intervals, a pulsatile oxytocin secretion pattern was confirmed (61). Fuchs, et al (61) noted that before the onset of labor the pulse frequency in 10 women was 1.3 per minute; in the first stage of labor, before cervical dilatation of 4 cm, the pulse frequency was 3 to 4 times greater; in the second stage, a further threefold increase was observed while in the third stage, the pulse frequency fell by about 60% but remained greater than before labor. Injections of 2 to 8 mU of oxytocin intravenously produced levels similar to the spontaneous pulses. This study, performed with a high specific and sensitive antibody, caused Fuchs and associates (61) to believe that it proved conclusively that oxytocin secretion in pregnant women occurs in a pulsative manner and is increased throughout the course of labor. This finding disputes data of an earlier study by Leake and associates (56) who found no evidence of pulsative secretions. Moreover, Fuch's group found that the pulsative administration of oxytocin was more effective than a continuous infusion in stimulating uterine contractions (62), and that this reduced significantly the amount of oxytocin required for the induction of labor or augmentation of dysfunctional labor (63).

The role of Ferguson's reflex, depicted in Figure 4–24, in provoking secretion of endogenous oxytocin remains a controversial issue. Some studies (40) failed to demonstrate the presence of the reflex in all species of animals, and Fuchs and Fuchs (40) doubt its existence in humans. On the other hand, a number of clinical studies have provided indirect evidence for its existence (55,59,60).

Vasicka and associates (59) found a significant increase of spikes of plasma oxytocin most frequently with maximum vaginal and cervical distention (vertex at 2+station). They reported that parturients in whom previous continuous epidural analgesia had worn off or had no analgesia had surges or spikes of oxytocin that they interpreted as a response to Ferguson's reflex, provoked by vaginal and cervical distention during the second stage of labor. They also noted that lumbar epidural anesthesia and subarachnoid block interrupted the final oxytocin surge that is peculiar to maximum cervical and vaginal distention.

Goodfellow and associates (60) noted an increase in the levels of oxytocin between cervical dilatation and the

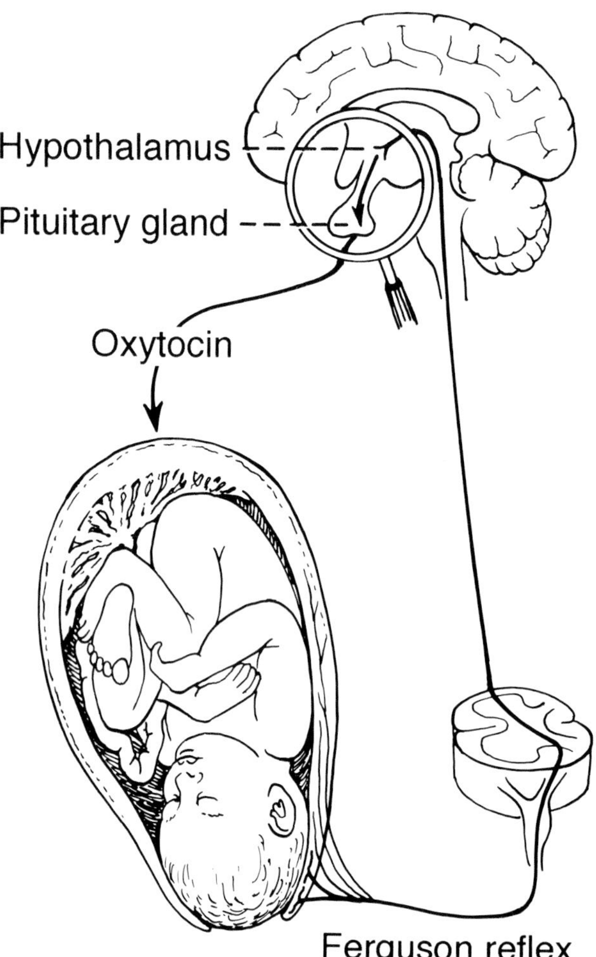


**Fig. 4–24.** The Ferguson reflex (schematic illustrations showing the probable pathways of the reflex). Distention of the lower uterine segment, cervix, and vagina (and perhaps other pelvic structures) provokes afferent impulses that pass into the spinal cord and proceed cephalad to reach the hypothalamus, where they provoke secretion of oxytocin. The oxytocin is then transported along the efferent hypothalamic-hypophyseal tract to the posterior pituitary, from which it passes into the circulation to eventually reach and stimulate uterine muscles. (Modified from Caldeyro-Barcia R, et al: Judicio critico sobre la induccion y conduccion del parto. Third Congr Lat Am Obstet Gynec, Mexico, 1:131, 1958.)

crowning of the fetal head, but this increase was not present in parturients given epidural anesthesia. Still another source of indirect evidence was provided by Dagwood and associates (55) who noted that oxytocin on maternal and fetal blood was high in parturients and their fetuses who had normal labor and spontaneous vaginal deliveries and in parturients and their fetuses who had cesarean section after the onset of labor, but not in a group of parturients who had elective cesarean section. The difference between the latter two groups was due to the fact that with the onset of labor there was cervical distention, while in those who had the elective cesarean section cervical distention had not occurred.

### *Oxytocin Receptors*

Many studies have also shown that low-affinity, low-capacity oxytocin receptors are present in both the myometrium and endometrium (40,64). During pregnancy the concentration of both rises dramatically; at 13 to 17 weeks they are about sixfold higher than nonpregnant levels, and at the end of pregnancy, they are about 80- to 100-fold higher (64,65). The highest concentration of receptors is found in early labor when levels are 2 to 3 times higher than those at term prior to labor (Figure 4–25). The distribution of oxytocin receptors in the fundus corpus and upper part of the lower uterine segment is rather uniform, but receptor concentration tapers off significantly in the lower part of the segment and is extremely low in the cervical tissue (Figure 4–26).

The rise in myometrial receptor concentration increases in response to oxytocin by two mechanisms (40): 1) the lowering the threshold for stimulation of contraction by oxytocin; and 2) by increasing the number of contractile units recruited to contract simultaneously, thereby causing the tension developed by a given oxytocin concentration to rise. The responsiveness to oxytocin

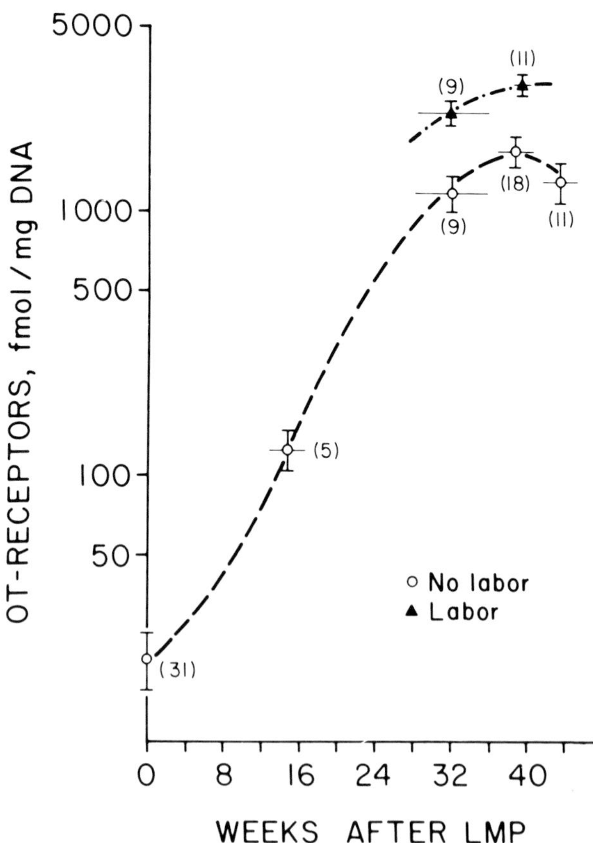


**Fig. 4–25.** Oxytocin receptors in human myometrium during pregnancy (○) and during preterm and term labor (▲). Note the logarithmic scale on the abscissa. Values are log-normal means; bars indicate SE. Note that the highest concentrations are found in early labor, when levels are 2 to 3 times higher than those at term prior to labor. (From Fuchs AR, Fuchs F, Husslein P, et al: Oxytocin receptors in the human uterus during pregnancy and parturition. Am. J. Obstet. Gynecol. 150:734, 1984.)

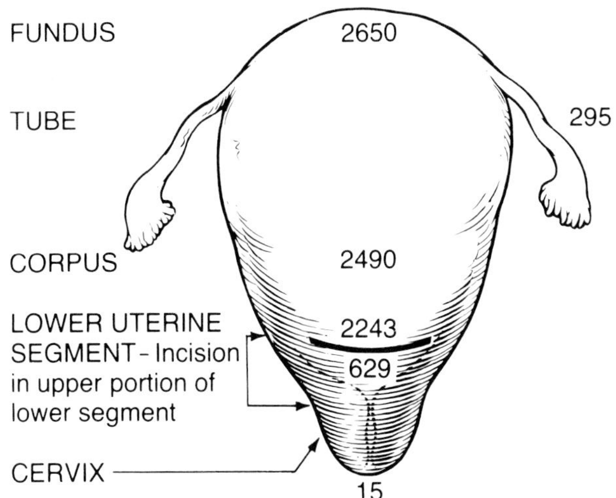


**Fig. 4–26.** Distribution of oxytocin receptors in a pregnant human uterus, removed from a preterm labor at 34 weeks. As stated in the text, the highest number is found in the top of the uterus; the receptors then gradually decrease in the lower uterine segment and cervix and are virtually absent in the vagina. (Adapted from Fuchs AR, Fuchs F, Husslein P, et al: Oxytocin receptors in the human uterus during pregnancy and parturition. Am. J. Obstet. Gynecol. 150:734, 1984.)

increases throughout pregnancy parallel to the receptor concentration (40,66). Results from serial daily measurements indicate that there is a significant rise in oxytocin sensitivity during the last 5 to 7 days before the onset of spontaneous labor (40).

The threshold level falls, reaching normally circulating oxytocin concentration when labor begins. These events are shown schematically in Figure 4–27. Although the factors that control oxytocin receptors concentrations are still not known precisely, there is experimental evidence that distention of the lower uterine segment acts synergistically with estrogen to increase oxytocin receptors density (40). Moreover, distention is probably responsible for the increase in oxytocin receptors during the last days of pregnancy, when the growth of the conceptus is faster than the myometrial growth, and consequently the uterine wall becomes increasingly distended by the growing fetus (40).

## *Neural Mechanisms*

The uterus, like all other viscera, is supplied by extrinsic autonomic sympathetic and parasympathetic nerves, and afferent (sensory) nerves associated with both types of autonomic nerves that supply the uterus, blood vessels, and glands. Moreover, the uterus and its adnexa, like other viscera, also have intrinsic nerves (67). Despite extensive studies, especially during the latter half of the nineteenth and early part of the twentieth centuries, the role of both sets of nerves in influencing uterine contractility during gestation and parturition remains unclear and controversial. We briefly summarize the available evidence here. The role of the sensory nerves that transmit pain during labor is discussed in detail in Chapter 9.

### *Extrinsic Innervation*

The uterus is supplied by sympathetic preganglionic neurons which originate in the anterolateral horn of the spinal cord of segments T-5 to L-2 (Figure 4–28A). They pass peripherally through the white rami communicantes and synapse with postganglionic neurons in the paravertebral chain and the prevertebral ganglia. Consequently, the

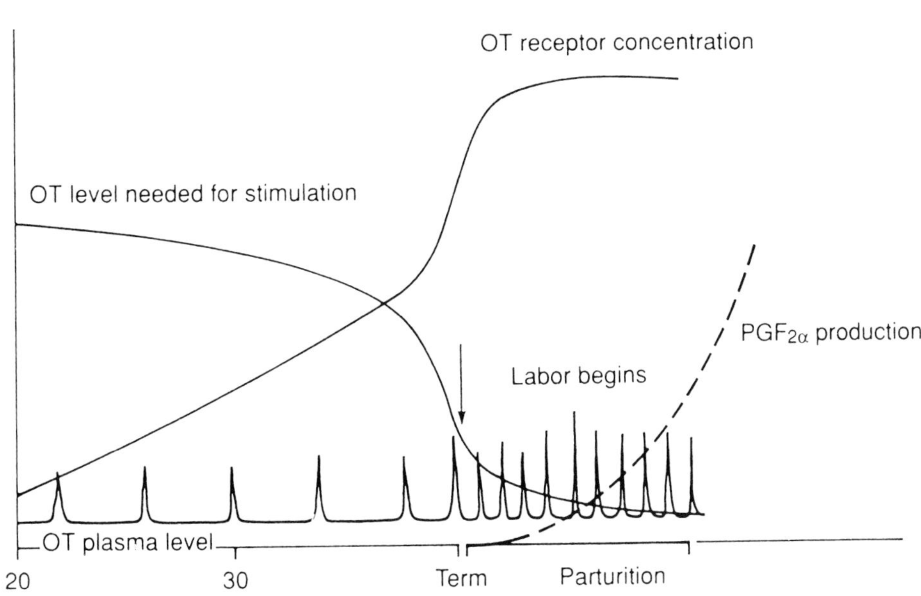


**Fig. 4–27.** Diagrammatic representation of the concentration of myometrial oxytocin, the level of oxytocin needed to elicit contractions, and the maternal plasma oxytocin levels at the end of gestation and during labor. Oxytocin is secreted in pulses of low frequency. During labor, pulse frequency increases. Fetal secretion of oxytocin can be considerable and may contribute to the oxytocin level reaching the myometrium. $PGF_{2\alpha}$ production does not increase significantly until labor is in progress and then increases progressively throughout the third stage of labor. OT = oxytocin. (From Fuchs AR, Fuchs F: Physiology of parturition. *In* Obstetrics: Normal and Problem Pregnancies. 2nd Ed. Edited by SG Gabbe, JR Niebyl, JL Simpson. New York, Churchill Livingstone, Inc, 1986, pp. 327–350.)

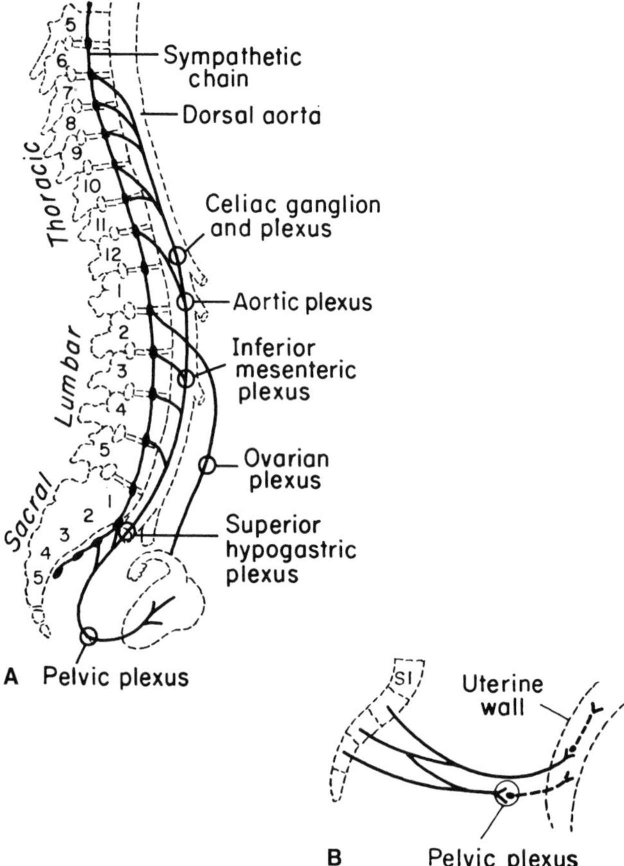


**Fig. 4–28.** The autonomic nerve supply to the uterus. Schematic diagram showing the sensory (pain) pathways (red) concerned with parturition, as well as the sympathetic nerves (white) and parasympathetic nerves (blue) to the uterus, and the somatic nerve (yellow) of the perineum. The sympathetic efferent nerves originate at T6 to L1 or L2 spinal cord segments and the afferent nerve supply enters the spinal cord at T10–L1 segments. The parasympathetic nerve supply to the uterus derives from S2, S3, S4 spinal cord segments and passes to the uterus near the pelvic plexus.

postganglionic neurons have a long course before they reach the uterus. Preganglionic parasympathetic neurons arise in the anterolateral horn of spinal segments S2, S3 and S4, pass peripherally in the pelvic nerve and without interruption they reach the wall of the uterus where they synapse with postganglionic neurons (Figure 4–28B). These postganglionic sympathetic and parasympathetic fibers supply the myometrium, blood vessels, and glands with an abundance of adrenergic and cholinergic nerve endings, respectively. In general, the action of these two sets of autonomic nerves is brought about by the neurohumoral transmitters, acetylcholine, and norepinephrine that are synthesized and stored at the cholinergic and adrenergic nerve endings, respectively. Epinephrine, the other catecholamine, is derived from the adrenal medulla and from the other chromaffin tissue which in the uterus is located in abundance along the periuterine nervous tissue, mainly the pelvic plexus (67).

Many older reports (67) and recent studies provide convincing evidence that the extrinsic autonomic nerves play no direct role in provoking uterine contractions, but are wholly under hormonal control (40). There is much indirect evidence showing that extrinsic nerves are not necessary for pregnancy or parturition (68–74). After complete denervation, the uterus of laboratory animals retains a high degree of autonomy, and the animal can deliver a full-term fetus (67). It has also been observed that pregnant patients with transection for the spinal cord at the upper thoracic or lower cervical region go into spontaneous labor (68,69) and that many parturients who have had presacral (sympathetic) neurectomy for dysmenorrhea subsequently had normal labor (70–72). Finally, it has been demonstrated that spinal anesthesia initiated after the onset of the active phase of labor had no effect, even when the level of the anesthetic was above the first thoracic segment (22,73–75). On the other hand, it has also been well-documented that interruption of the extrinsic nerve supply achieved with subarachnoid block, lumbar epidural block or caudal block initiated during the latent phase or very early active phase of labor frequently caused a weakening, and in some cases a complete cessation of uterine contractions. This suggests that the extrinsic nerves have some indirect influence in the initiation of labor, perhaps by interrupting neurohumoral reflexes.

### *Sensory (Afferent) Innervation*

In the discussion of oxytocin, it was implied that the sensory nerves that supply the uterus may play an important role in uterine contractions and, as will be noted in the next section, they play a major role in activating the auxiliary forces of labor. Distention of the lower uterine segment and vagina, produced by strong contractions and by the bearing-down efforts of the auxiliary forces, provokes various reflexes that in part cause secretion of oxytocin by the posterior pituitary.

The concomitant increase in oxytocin receptors and endogenous secretion of the hormone during the active phase is said to progressively increase the intensity of uterine contractions which, in turn, effect more dilatation of the cervix and distention of the pelvic structures (19–21). These in turn cause greater secretion of oxytocin, thus producing a sequence of events that Caldeyro-Barcia and his coworkers (19–21) called the "vicious circle" of parturition. This is said to explain why once parturition has started and cervical dilatation is sufficient, uterine contractility progressively increases until the fetus is expelled. Moreover, this would explain why interruption of the sensory pathways very early in labor, before an established pattern occurs, may result in a decrease of uterine contractility. Regardless as to whether the Ferguson reflex is present or not, there is ample evidence that distention and dilatation of the lower uterine segment and cervix and distention of the pelvic structures play an important role in the progress and termination of labor.

### *Intrinsic Adrenergic Innervation*

Intrinsic nerves play an important role in the function of most other hollow viscera, but there is difference of opinion as to whether such nerves exist in the uterus and what their function is. Krantz (76) cited a massive number of data from numerous studies by others and from his own work that showed the uterus to be supplied by a variety of myelinated and unmyelinated free nerve endings that appear to be terminations of extrinsic efferent fibers. The cervix and blood vessels receive the richest supply of these nerves. Adrenergic ganglion cells that make connection with adrenergic receptors richly supply the uterus, cervix, and vagina. Recent studies have clearly shown that the four types of adrenergic receptors, β-1 and β-2 and α-1 and α-2, are present in the myometrial tissues in a variety of species including humans (77–78A).

Diamond (77) has suggested that, generally speaking, the uterine relaxant's effect of catecholamines is exerted primarily through β-2 adrenoreceptors, whereas the uterine contractile effect of these agents is mediated via α-1 receptors (78). Ariens and Simons (79) have suggested that the α-1 and β-1 receptors are "innervated" receptors, i.e., they are located postsynaptically in close proximity to sympathetic nerve endings and preferentially activated by the sympathetic neurotransmitter norepinephrine, whereas the α-2 and β-2 receptors are "hormonal" receptors, located presynaptically and extrajunctionally and activated by the circulating hormone epinephrine.

The sympathetic adrenergic innervation of the uterus is not under the control of the extrinsic autonomic nerves, but under the control of ovarian hormones with estrogen increasing and progesterone decreasing the uterine content of norepinephrine. After an initial increase in early pregnancy, the histochemically demonstrable catecholamines virtually disappear from the body of the uterus, while the cervix and vagina retain their neurotransmitter content (80,81). Fuchs and Fuchs (40) have used this phenomenon to indicate that neural activity has no influence on myometrial function during parturition.

### Peptinergic Innervation

In addition to the classical cholinergic and adrenergic innervation of the uterus, recent studies have revealed there are nerves that can be classified as noncholinergic and noradrenergic and consist of peptinergic nervous elements (82). These include Substance P, vasoactive intestinal peptide (VIP), neuropeptide (NPY), gastrin releasing peptide (GRP), leucine-enkephalin, methionine-enkephalin, and such hypothalamic-releasing hormones as somastostatin and thyrotropin-releasing hormone (TH), and the neurohypophyseal hormones oxytocin, vasopressin and neurophysin, and calcitonin-gene-related peptide (CGRP) and relaxant among others. These peptides are localized to large vesicles and nerve terminals of afferent fibers or efferent nerves innervating blood vessels, nonvascular smooth muscle, lining epithelium, and glands (Figure 4–29). Some neuropeptides such as VIP and NPY participate in the local noncholinergic, nonadrenergic nervous control of myometrial smooth muscle activity and blood flow, and other peptides such as sP and GGRP appear to be sensory transmitters. It is of interest to note that VIP fibers, which are particularly numerous in the cervical region, vagina, and tube of isthmus have a strong relaxing effect on both the isthmus and cervical tissue. Moreover, like the adrenergic neurotransmitters, VIP fibers in the uterine body are significantly reduced during pregnancy, whereas the number in the cervix and vagina is less effective.

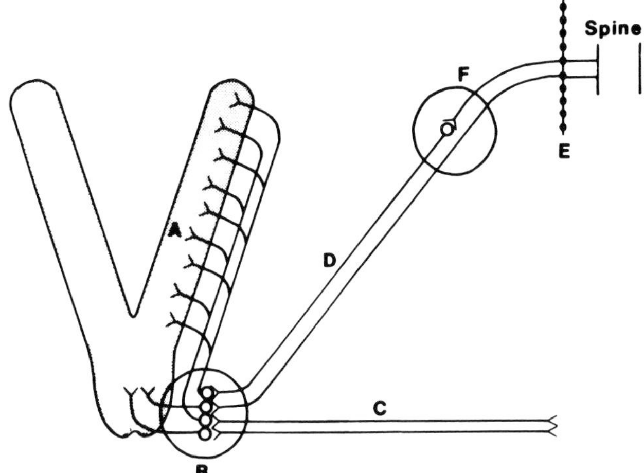


**Fig. 4–29.** Schematic drawing illustrating the relation between the uterine VIPnergic neurons in the hypogastric and pelvic nerves. VIPnergic neurons (**A**) have the cell body in the paracervical ganglia shown in **B.** These are activated via nicotinic receptors and preganglionic fibers that travel in the pelvic (**C**) and hypogastric nerves (**D**). The hypogastric fibers arise in either the lumbar chain (**E**) or the inferior mesenteric ganglion (**F**). Some fibers synapse in the inferior mesenteric ganglion, but the majority pass through to the spinal cord. (From Ottsen B, Fahrenkrug J: Regulatory peptides and uterine function. *In* Uterine Function: Molecular and Cellular Aspects. Edited by ME Carsten, JD Miller. New York, Plenum Press, 1990, p. 399.)

## Conclusion

What conclusions can be made from the aforementioned information on the role of various factors that leads to the initiation and maintenance of human parturition? At the outset it is permissible to emphasize that while we have acquired a vast amount of new information, the predominant factor(s) that initiate this process remains a controversial issue. The foregoing data suggest both prostaglandins and endogenous oxytocin, together with other factors, can initiate and maintain labor. However, none of the data provides conclusive evidence that either of these or both are the predominant factor responsible for the entire process. It is therefore necessary to repeat the statement made at the beginning of this chapter: The process of human parturition involves complex anatomic, structural, biochemical, endocrine, humoral and circulatory factors, and perhaps others that at the critical time and adapted to the individual morphology interact to initiate and eventually promote evacuation of the uterus. To determine the precise role that each of these factors plays requires much more productive research in this field.

## ANATOMY AND PHYSIOLOGY OF OTHER FORCES OF LABOR

### *The Auxiliary Expulsive Forces*

The progress of labor and expulsion of the fetus is affected by four factors: 1) uterine contractions; 2) resistant forces by the cervix during the first stage of labor; 3) auxiliary expulsive forces consisting of the reflex bearing-down efforts; and 4) resistance provided by the pelvic structure. Reynolds (1) calculated that the force necessary to expel the infant through the average pelvis varies between 80 to 100 pounds. The total force that the uterus exerts on the infant during normal labor is about 50 to 60 pounds. In other words, there is a deficit of some 30 to 50 pounds to be made up either by an auxiliary force or by the use of forceps (1). In spontaneous labor, the auxiliary force is contributed by the reflex contraction of the diaphragm, the abdominal and intercostal muscles, and by the action of accessory muscles of respiration. These muscles, acting together in a bearing-down effort, increase the intra-abdominal pressure sufficiently so as to make up the additional pressure on the uterus. The increase in intrauterine (amniotic fluid) pressure contributed by the Valsalva maneuver ranges between 25 and 60 mm Hg or higher (14,23). When this is combined with the pressure generated by uterine contraction, they produce a total intra-amniotic pressure of 100 to 120 mm Hg (1,15,21,22,83). The magnitude of this added pressure is variable and depends upon the quality of labor, physical status of the patient, the power of the muscles concerned, and the type and amount of analgesia and anesthesia being used. Although this effect usually plays an important role in the expulsive act, it is possible for uterine contractions alone to deliver an infant, as has been demonstrated in a variety of circumstances cited above.

Reynolds (1,23) reports that the contracting uterus at term can exert about 3.4 pounds per square inch. To rupture the membranes, a force of 0.25 to 3.0 (average 1.2) pounds per square inch is necessary and to rupture the normal uterus a force of 17 to 25 pounds per square inch (5 to 7 times that needed for labor) would be necessary. Of course, there are enormous individual variations depending on the blood supply, abnormalities of the uterine muscle, and the presence of disease, among other things.

Mobilization of the auxiliary forces is a reflex phenomenon initiated after cervical dilatation is complete and the head has reached the pelvic floor and creates pressure on the rectal ampulla and the pelvic muscle sling, thus stimulating sensitive pressure receptors that transduce the stimuli into impulses (Figure 4–30). The afferent path of the impulses is primarily through the pudendal nerve, although other sensory fibers in the sacral nerves are involved. The reflex is active only during uterine contractions that push the presenting part against the perineal floor. The process usually starts before the patient experiences pain: she develops an uncontrollable urge to bear down; she braces her feet in bed, while at the same time inhaling deeply, then closing her glottis, she contracts the intercostal and abdominal muscles and the diaphragm and bears down, thus producing a Valsalva effect. In a conscious parturient, this desire can be partially controlled voluntarily and either resisted or aided.

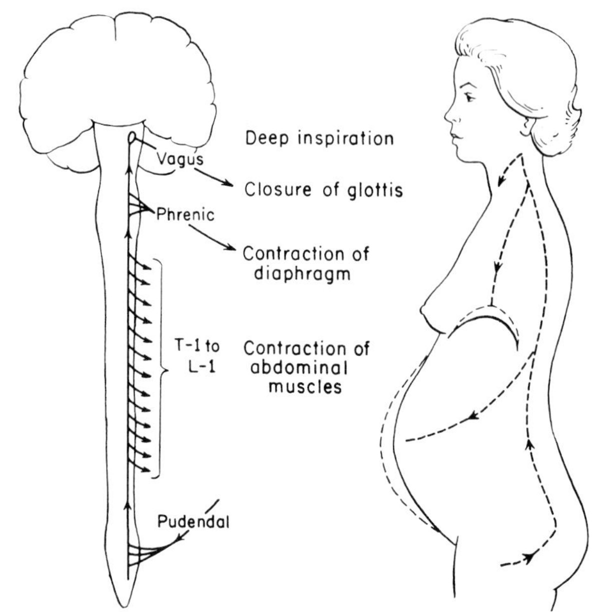


**Fig. 4–30.** Schematic diagram of nerves that supply the muscles that act as the auxiliary forces of labor and the pathways concerned with the bearing-down reflex.

The TKD of the second stage is characterized by pointed peaks on the crests of the uterine contractions (Figures 4–10, 4–31). There may be one or more of these sharp peaks on the contractions profile and the peaks may

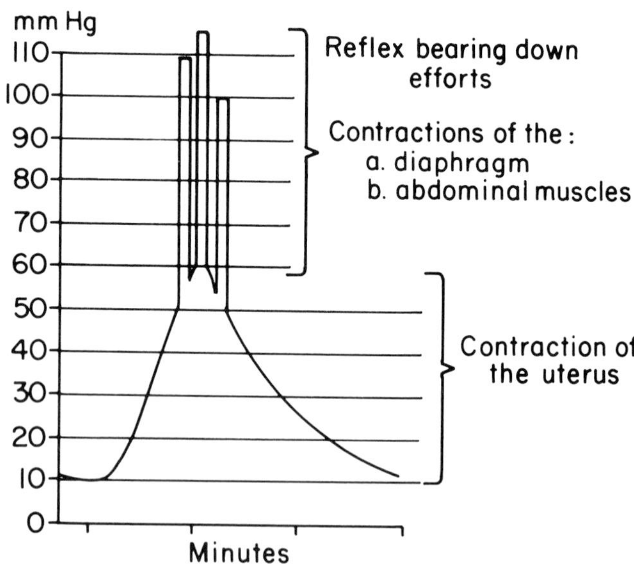


**Fig. 4–31.** The bearing-down efforts superimposed on a uterine contraction (schematic illustration of the effect on the record of amniotic pressure registered at a paper speed that is slower than in Fig. 4–10). Each reflex bearing-down effort causes an abrupt and short-lasting rise of intra-abdominal pressure that is fully transmitted in all directions. Voluntarily holding the bearing-down effort for several seconds produces a slower, smoother, and prolonged pressure-elevation period. The number of reflex bearing-down efforts often increases as the second stage advances.

add as much height to the contraction as that which the uterus itself exerts. The duration of these peaks is variable, but it is always much shorter than that of uterine contractions because frequently several of the efforts are exerted during each contraction (21,22). The longer the effort to bear down effected voluntarily by the parturient and the consequent augmented intra-abdominal pressure, the more effective the auxiliary forces. Moreover, parturients in semirecumbent position can exert greater pressure than those in supine position. Mengert and Murphy (83) found that females could effect an increase in intra-abdominal pressure of approximately 120 mm Hg in the lateral position, 125 mm Hg in the supine position, 135 mm Hg in the semirecumbent position, and 155 mm Hg in a sitting position.

To be effective, increase in intra-abdominal pressure must be superimposed upon a contracting uterus, so that the two forces produce enough increase in the intrauterine pressure to expel the infant and, subsequently, the placenta. Attempts at bearing down when the uterus is not contracting are not only futile, but also deplete the strength and energy of the parturient unnecessarily and may alter maternal hemodynamics. Because these auxiliary forces play no role whatsoever during the first stage, the patient should not be urged to bear down during this phase of labor.

Although many writers allude to these forces as "voluntary efforts," they are really mobilized by an involuntary reflex phenomenon similar to that set up during the act of defecation. Pudendal block, saddle block, caudal block, or epidural analgesia or any other technique that interrupts the afferent pathways of the reflex that involve S2, S3, and S4 spinal nerves will either impede or completely eliminate the reflex urge to bear down. Moreover, heavy sedation and confusion interfere with the coordination of the process and may prevent the patient from cooperating in bearing down at the correct time. In such instances, it is necessary to coach the patient to coordinate her efforts and to mobilize the auxiliary forces for the expulsion of the infant. Injury of the afferent pathways (e.g., in paraplegic parturients) also completely eliminates the reflex urge.

### Resisting Forces

The least studied force contributing to parturition is the resistance provided by the pelvic floor. The fusion of the müllerian ducts results in a slightly oval uterine cavity. The long axis of this oval is usually transverse with respect to the pelvic inlet, and the longest axis of the pelvic inlet is usually the transverse one (Figure 4–32a). Consequently, the fetal presenting part most commonly enters the pelvis with its longest axis transverse. In the pelvis, the presenting part is pushed against the pelvic floor, which consists of the levator ani group of muscles. These structures run from the anterior to the posterior walls of the pelvis, filling each side of it with a convex or bulging mass of muscle. Only in the midline is there an oval defect in this barrier, and the long axis of this defect is anteroposterior rather than transverse (Figure 4–32b). Consequently, to pass through this defect, the fetal presenting part must be rotated from the transverse diameter as it enters the pelvis, to the anteroposterior diameter of the pelvic outlet. This is accomplished when the expulsive forces push the fetal presenting part against the upwardly bulging side walls of the pelvic floor (Figure 4–32c). This forces the presenting part to rotate, and then it passes through the pelvic outlet.

A loss of tone in the pelvic floor muscles, caused by spinal block, lumbar epidural block, or caudal or pudendal block achieved with high concentration of a local anesthetics weakens or paralyzes the muscles. Consequently, the loss of muscle tone interferes with this mechanism as there is lessening of the resisting force to produce rotation. Ordinarily, the combined force exerted by uterine contractions and the auxiliary forces plus the continuous stretch and weakening of the pelvic muscles due to descent of the fetal head result in a successful completion of the second stage. As previously mentioned, weakening of the pelvic musculature caused by regional anesthesia

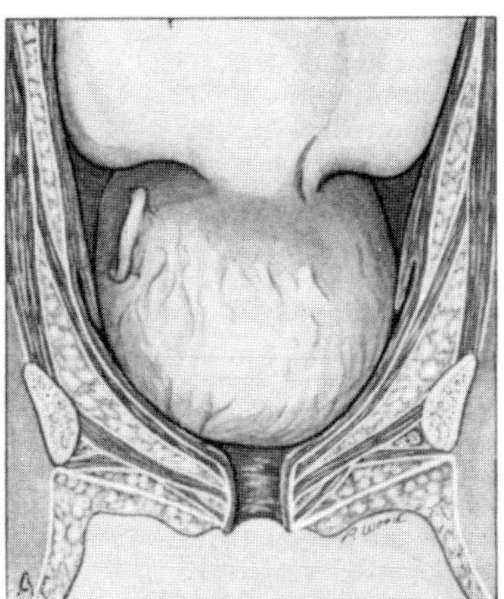


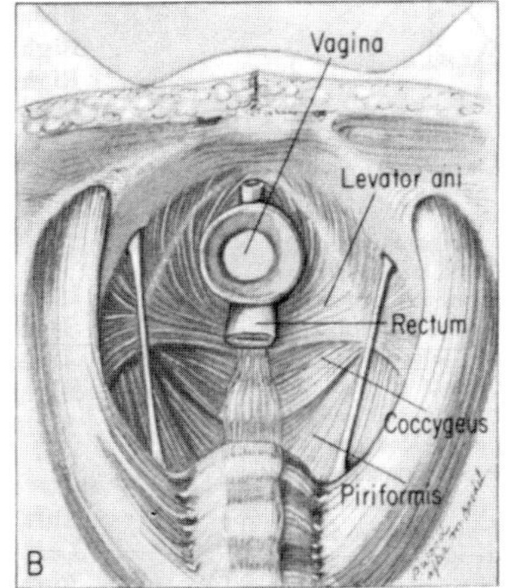


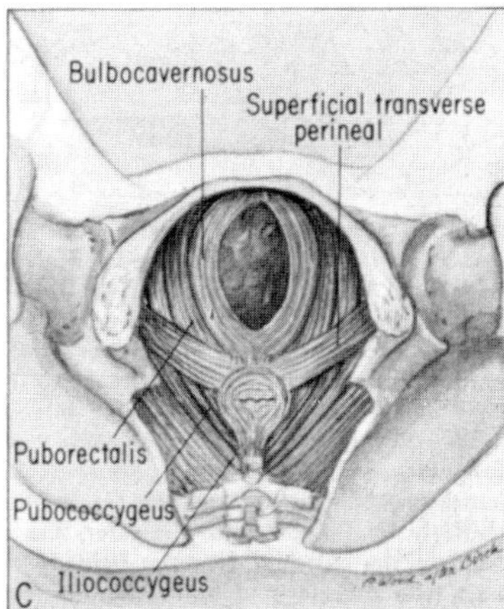


**Fig. 4–32.** The resisting forces in the pelvic floor. **A,** Coronal section showing the fetal head on the pelvic floor during early labor. **B,** Superior view showing the musculature through the pelvic floor that makes up the V-shaped sling that is so important in rotation of the head. **C,** Inferior view of the muscular pelvic floor just before birth.

will result in incomplete rotation of the fetal head and an increase in the length of the second stage of labor. Another important factor is the resistant forces offered by the vulvovaginal ring and contraction of the pelvic floor during the intervals between contraction in causing recession of the fetal head and thus facilitating temporary restoration of circulation.

## Progress, Pattern, and Duration of Labor

About mid-century, several groups of investigators provided vigorous leadership in applying advanced technology to study labor. Alvarez, Caldeyro-Barcia and associates (15–19) were among the first to use the internal TKD to measure uterine activity and to define the characteristics of uterine contractions in normal and abnormal labor as mentioned in the early part of this chapter. Reynolds and associates (1,23) also collaborated with Alvarez and Caldeyro-Barcia (16) to provide a comprehensive overview of the physiology and pathophysiology of labor that included description of the progress, pattern, and duration of normal and abnormal labor.

### *The Work of the Uterus and Duration of Labor*

Caldeyro-Barcia and his associates (15,21,22) estimated that the sum of the intensity of the successive contractions required for dilation of the cervix from 2 cm to full dilatation in multiparae was 4,000 to 8,000 mm Hg (average 7,000 mm Hg) (Figure 4–15). If the contractions had an average intensity of 40 mm Hg, about 175 contractions were required. If the frequency ranged from 4 to 5 contractions per 10 minutes, the duration of the first stage was 7 hours. Primiparae having the same type of contractions would require 10,000 mm Hg and a period of 10 hours to achieve full cervical dilatation. Figure 4–33 depicts the length of time required to achieve full cervical dilatation by both primiparae and multiparae by the same group of patients used to develop Figure 4–15. They also reported that if the membranes were ruptured when cervical dilatation was 2 cm, the uterine work required for dilating the cervix is reduced by 30 to 40%, suggesting that the intact membranes act as an obstacle opposing cervical dilatation.

As mentioned earlier in this chapter, an alternative in determining the work of labor is to measure the active contraction area that incorporates three variables: frequency, active pressure, and duration of contractions (40). With modern electronic equipment recording the active contraction area, it is easy to measure the work of labor by integrating the pressure above the baseline with time as expressed in units of kilo Pascal-seconds (kPas) (40). Steer, Carter and Beard (84) reported that the active contraction area correlates better than any other measure with the rate of cervical dilatation. The mean value for uterine activity over the whole first stage of labor was found to be 1100 kPas per 15 seconds, with an standard deviation of 333 kPas/15 min in 22 consecutive patients in spontaneous labor. During the period of dilatation from 4 to 10 cm, the active contraction area increased from about 800 to 1200 kPas/15 min, a 50% increase that occurred primarily between 7 and 9 cm of dilatation (Figure 4–34).

The rate of cervical dilatation achieved with a certain

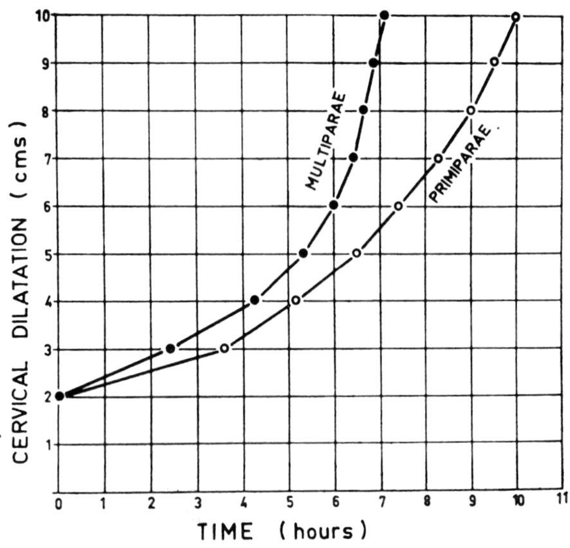


**Fig. 4–33.** Influence of parity on the time required for cervical dilatation. This is the same group of patients used in Figure 4–15. (From Alvarez H, et al: *In* Oxytocin. Edited by R Caldeyro-Barcia, H Heller. New York, Pergamon Press, 1961, p. 206.)

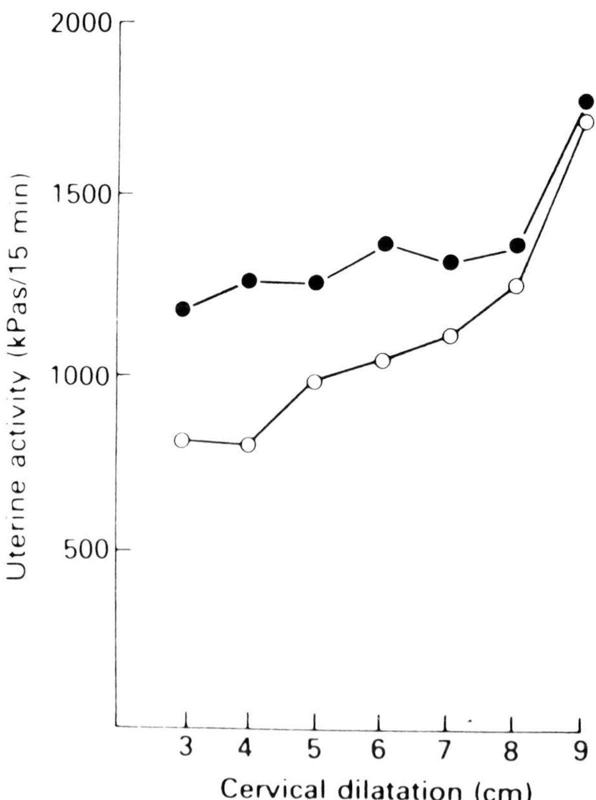


**Fig. 4–34.** Comparison of median uterine activity values on nulliparae (●) and multiparae (○) at each centimeter of cervical dilatation. (From Arulkumaran S: The effect of parity on uterine activity in labour. Br. J. Obstet. Gynaecol. 91:843, 1984.)

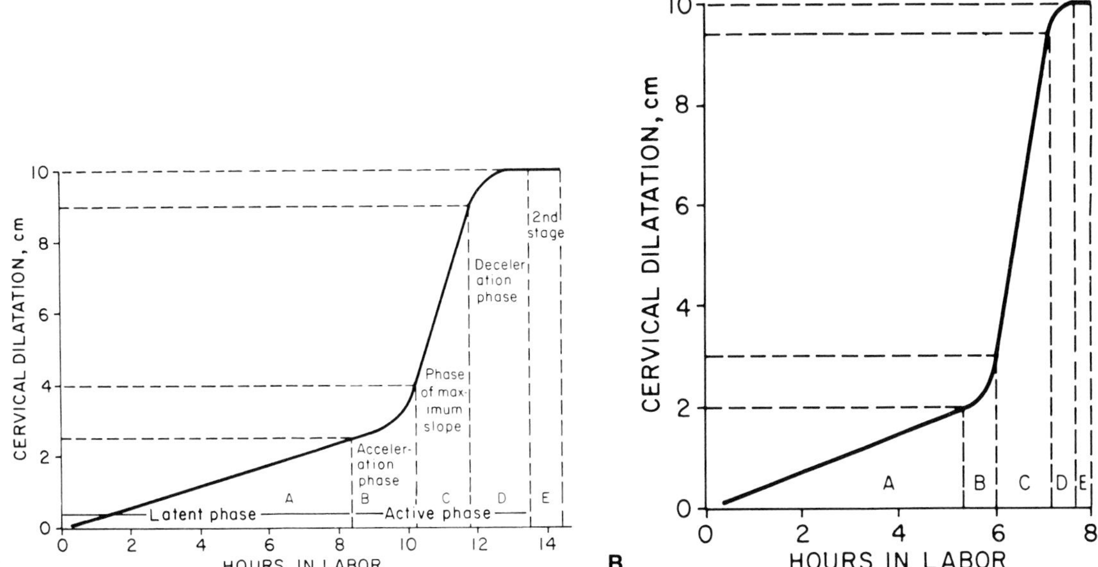


**Fig. 4–35.** **A,** The mean labor curve (cervical dilatation *vs.* time) based on a study of 500 primigravidae at term. The latent phase extends from the onset of labor, taken arbitrarily from the onset of regular uterine contractions to the beginning of the active phase. The onset of the active phase is apparent on the graph as that point at which dilatation (slope) begins to change and the curve becomes more steeply inclined. The active phase ends at full dilatation, giving way to the second stage of labor. Note that the active phase is divided into three phases. The middle of these is made up of that portion of the curve undergoing the most rapid change—the phase of maximum slope. The acceleration and deceleration phases precede and follow the latter, respectively. (Modified from Friedman EA: Primigravid labor. Obstet. Gynecol. 6:567, 1955.) **B,** The mean multiparous labor curve based on the study of cervical dilatation-time relation in 500 multiparae. **A,** Latent phase; **B,** Acceleration phase; **C,** Phase of maximum slope; **D,** Deceleration phase (**B** through **D** is the active phase); **E,** Second stage. (Redrawn from Friedman EA: Labor in multiparas. Obstet. Gynecol. 8:691, 1956.)

amount of uterine activity depends on the resistance of the cervix. Below 430 kPas/15 min, significant progress in labor is unlikely to occur, but even above 500 kPas/15 min some women will exhibit slow rates of cervical dilatation because of increased cervical resistance. Like Caldeyro-Barcia and associates (51), Arulkumaran, et al (13) noted that less uterine work is required to dilate the cervix in multiparae than in nulliparae.

Figure 4–33 emphasizes the point made earlier in the section on the "influence of parity on uterine contractions," i.e., during early labor the intensity of contractions (and consequently the work done by the uterus) is greater in primiparae than in multiparae. Fuchs and Fuchs (40) have pointed out the fact that uterine activity measured in kPas/15 min remains relatively stable at cervical dilatation up to 4 to 6 cm and then increases, suggesting that oxytocin is the main driving force in the early part of labor when mean levels of oxytocin remain rather constant. At cervical dilatation above 6 cm, PGF-generation increases rapidly potentiating oxytocin-induced activity and perhaps becoming the major myometrial stimulant (49,50,52).

### *Patterns of Cervical Dilatation*

In the early 1950s, Friedman (85,86) began to study the course of labor and eventually developed a graphico-statistical cervimetric technique that entailed plotting cervical dilatation on a time ordinate. A careful study of 500 primiparae and multiparae showed that normal labors followed a well-defined sigmoid curve, as shown in Figure 4–35. It should be noted that he divided the curve into five phases and that the latent phase began at 0 cervical dilatation and ended when cervical dilatation was 2 to 2.5 cm. Statistical limits for the various portions of the curve were obtained and these were utilized in depicting changes from the expected normal. By gleaning from the original series all those cases that presented no complications, he was able to list 200 cases of "ideal" labor. These patients had adequate pelves, the fetus was in vertex presentation and in occiput anterior position, and their labor progressed normally. Figure 4–36 depicts the mean "ideal" curve as compared to the mean curve for the entire series. Friedman's method also permitted statistical study of the abnormalities and definition of the responsible factors that are considered in detail in Chapter 23. Of particular importance are the effects of medication, potent inhalation anesthetics, and regional anesthesia, which will be summarized at the end of this chapter and in various chapters in Sections C & D.

Following their publication, these curves were used widely in many studies by a variety of individuals. Among this group were Hendricks and his associates (87,88) who studied 303 patients that were followed and delivered by Hendricks, beginning 4 weeks before labor and throughout various stages of labor. He carried out vaginal examination of cervical dilatation and noted a progressive increase in cervical dilatation from a little less than 1 cm at the fourth week before labor to a mean dilatation of 2.2 cm for multiparae and 1.8 cm for nulliparae within 3 days of labor (Figure 4–37). Their data and those of others indicated that the cervix dilated progressively in an orderly fashion during the last 4 weeks of gestation and that a completely closed cervix at the onset of labor was rare (10% in nulliparae and fewer in multiparae.) On admission to the hospital, cervical dilatation was about 2.5 cm multiparae and 3.5 nulliparae. They estimated that the progress of cervical dilatation from 2.5 cm, which they considered the beginning of the latent phase, to 4 cm, which is considered the beginning of active phase, was 108 minutes for nulliparae and 95 minutes for multiparae. These figures were shorter than what Friedman called the "acceleration phase" that began at 2.5 cm and ended at 4.0 cm dilatation. Hendricks and associates (88) concluded that in active normal labor, cervical dilatation tends to follow a pattern of constant acceleration rather than a linear progression, and that the mean rate of cervical dilatation during the active phase for nulliparae is just as fast as that for multiparae. They believed that the fact that the average nulliparae's labor is longer than that of the average multipara, is largely accounted for by the fact that the average multipara goes into labor with her cervix more dilated than that of nullipara. They also noted that the deceleration phase is rarely seen in otherwise perfectly normal labor. Finally, analysis revealed that 70% of the multiparae completed cervical dilatation in 3.8 hours, while 60% of the nulliparae had completed dilatation in less than 5 hours after the hospital admission.

Subsequently, many other clinicians tended to agree with some of the points made by Hendricks, particularly regarding the degree of cervical dilatation at the onset of labor. Indeed, in 1962, Friedman and Sachtleben (89) published additional observations that suggested the cervix was dilated to some degree before the onset of labor. Three years later (89), they published an amended dilatation curve based upon the observation of 591 nulliparae that indicated the latent phase started with the cervix dilated 1.8 to 2.0 cm and progressed to about 2.5 cm during the 6.4 hour latent period in nulliparae and 4.8 hours in multiparae. In his excellent textbook, first published in 1968 with a second edition published in 1978 (91), Friedman presented a comprehensive analysis of the course and pattern of normal labors and various forms of labor abnormalities based on intensive computer analysis of a series of over 10,000 gravidae selected for a study from a total of nearly 59,000 pregnant women (92).

Table 4–1 contains composite data on the course of labor in the general population while Table 4–2 contains data on the "ideal course of labor" gleaned from a group of nulliparae and multiparae with no complicating factors. Comparison of these data with those depicted in Figure 4–35 reveals that the only significant difference is in the mean duration of the latent phase that lasted 8.6 hours in the early group versus 6.4 in the later group. The cervical curve in nulliparae studies in this group is shown in Figure 4–38, which also shows the descent curve discussed below. One can speculate that the longer time in the duration of the latent phase noted in the initial group than the time in the later series was due to the fact that they began measuring the latent phase at zero cervical dilatation in the initial study, whereas in the later study they began to measure the latent phase when the cervix was 1.8 to 2.0 cm dilated.

Comparison of the data in Tables 4–1 and 4–2 indicates that nulliparae yielded data that differed significantly from those of the composite group of nulliparae at large. In contrast, the "ideal labor course," based on a series of uncomplicated multiparae, did not differ significantly from the average curve for multiparae in general. Friedman (91) attributed this to the very low complicating factors among nulliparae.

The large number of subjects studied confirmed the fact that both nulliparae and multiparae have the same type of sigmoid curve. Friedman (91) explained the differ-

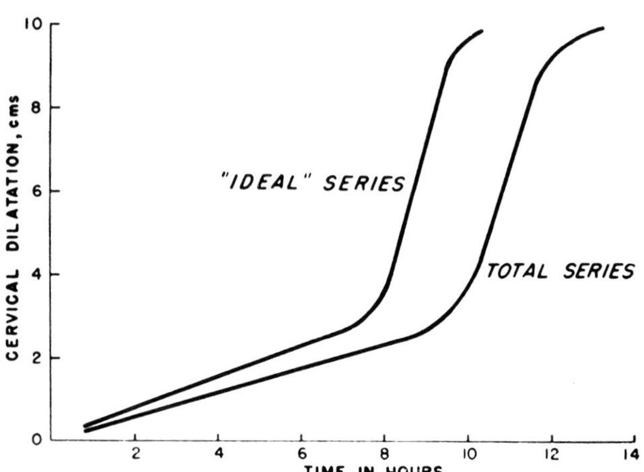


**Fig. 4–36.** The "ideal" labor curve based on the study of 200 uncomplicated labors contrasted with the overall mean labor curve in primiparae. (From Friedman EA: Primigravid labor. Obstet. Gynecol. 6:567, 1955.)

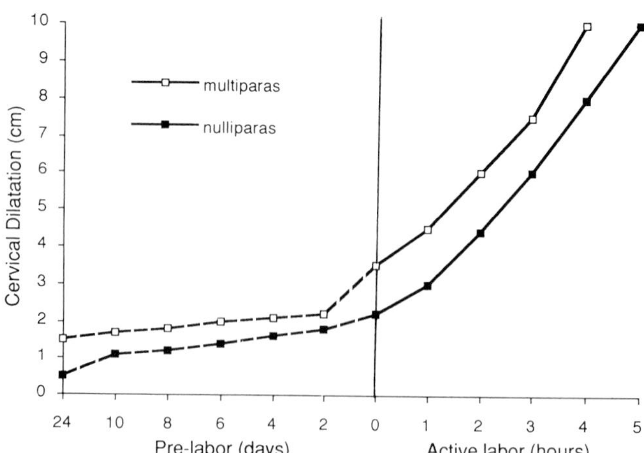


**Fig. 4–37.** Mean cervical dilatation by parity during the last 28 days of pregnancy and during labor among parturients with normal labors. Dashed lines are extensions of the lines that fit the known mean. (From Hendricks VH, et al: Normal cervical dilatation patterns in late pregnancy and labor. Am. J. Obstet. Gynecol. 106:1065, 1970.)

**Table 4–1.** Composite Data on Course of Labor

| Group | Latent Phase (hr) | Active Phase (hr) | Maximum Dilatation (cm/hr) | Deceleration Phase (hr) | Maximum Descent (cm/hr) | Second Stage (hr) |
|---|---|---|---|---|---|---|
| Nulliparas | | | | | | |
| Mean | 6.4 | 4.6 | 3.0 | 0.84 | 3.3 | 1.1 |
| SD* | 5.1 | 3.6 | 1.9 | 1.0 | 2.3 | 0.8 |
| Multiparas | | | | | | |
| Mean | 4.8 | 2.4 | 5.7 | 0.36 | 6.6 | 0.39 |
| SD* | 4.9 | 2.2 | 3.6 | 0.3 | 4.0 | 0.3 |

* Standard deviation.
(Modified from Friedman EA: Labor: Clinical Evaluation and Management. New York: Appleton-Century-Crofts, 1978.)

ences noted by Hendricks and others by the fact that the others took into consideration only the active phase of labor, whereas Friedman has insisted that the latent phase is important. This phase is the interval from the onset of regular uterine contractions, which are only mildly painful, to the active progressive dilatation phase, characterized by strong painful contractions that effect the acceleration phase and the phase of maximum slope. He emphasized that the acceleration phase is short and variable but is important in determining the outcome of labor: it leads from the phase of minimum slope of the latent phase to the maximum slope that follows (91,92). A slow acceleration phase generally presages a lower maximum slope and therefore a prolonged total labor, while a rapid change in the acceleration phase precedes a short residual labor. The phase of maximum slope is a good measure of the overall efficiency of the uterus because it gives a rather clear idea of how effective the motive force of the uterine contraction is in producing dilatation. The deceleration phase, which is the final phase of the first stage of labor, reflects a fetopelvic relationship that may be considered an artifactual phenomenon that Friedman admits may not be observed, or may not occur.

### *Pattern of the Descent Curve*

In 1970, Friedman and Sachtleben (93) published their results on patterns of descent and the reliably consistent relationship between the cervical dilatation curve and the pattern of descent curve. Figure 4–38 depicts the interrelationship between the descent curve and the concurrently developing dilatation curve shown in composite form representing the average labor curve for nulliparae. It is to be noted that contrary to previously held functional concepts, descent begins when the dilatation curve reaches its phase of maximum slope—well before the onset of the second stage (91). The earliest point of the acceleration of the descent curve in nulliparae coincides with that portion of labor in which the cervix is dilating at its most rapid rate, namely the phase of maximum slope. During this interval the speed of descent reaches to a maximum, just at the onset of the deceleration phase of dilatation and then rapidly continues in linear manner into the second stage of labor. Descent normally maintains this maximum rate until the perineal floor is reached. In multiparae, active descent may not begin until the dilatation curve reaches the beginning of the deceleration phase.

It is of interest to note that the expected pattern of descent in nulliparae is described in two parts analogous to the phase of cervical dilatation curve of the first stage. The latent period of the descent extends from the onset of labor to that point in time when active descent begins (90). This latter transition is concurrent with the time that the dilatation curve is entering its phase of maximum slope. The active period of descent comprises the remainder of the first and second stages. In their studies, Friedman and collaborators (93) studied the station of descent mostly by vaginal examination to define the position of the edge of the fetal presenting part as related to the interspinous plane.

Two years after Friedman's publication, Philpott and Castle (94) introduced the "partograph," which permitted plotting of the cervical dilatation and descent of the fetal presenting part through the maternal pelvis by reference to the proportion of the fetal skull that remained palpable abdominally. While this technique presents no

**Table 4–2.** Composite Ideal Labor Course

| Group | Latent Phase (hr) | Active Phase (hr) | Maximum Dilatation (cm/hr) | Deceleration Phase (hr) | Maximum Descent (cm/hr) | Second Stage (hr) |
|---|---|---|---|---|---|---|
| Nulliparas | | | | | | |
| Mean | 6.1 | 3.4 | 3.5 | 0.72 | 3.6 | 0.76 |
| SD* | 4.0 | 1.5 | 3.0 | 0.7 | 1.9 | 0.5 |
| Multiparas | | | | | | |
| Mean | 4.5 | 2.1 | 5.9 | 0.30 | 7.0 | 0.32 |
| SD* | 4.2 | 2.0 | 3.4 | 0.3 | 3.2 | 0.3 |

* Standard deviation.
(Modified from Friedman EA: Labor: Clinical Evaluation and Management. New York: Appleton-Century Crofts, 1978.)

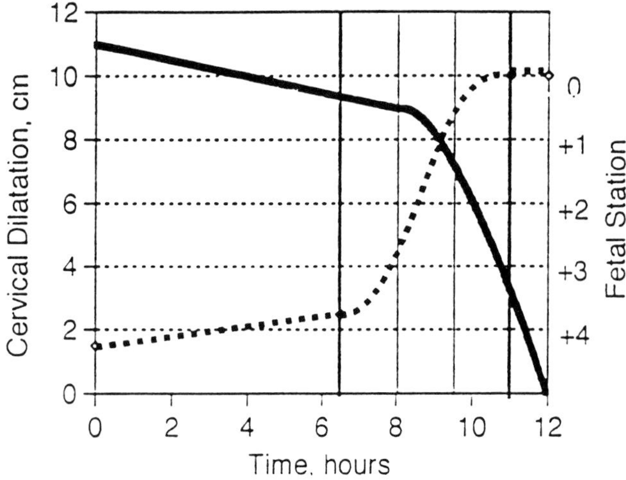


Fig. 4–38. Dilatation and descent curves (see text for details). (Modified from Friedman EA: Labor: Clinical Evaluation and Management. 2nd Ed. New York, Appleton-Century-Crofts, 1978, pp. 6–59.)

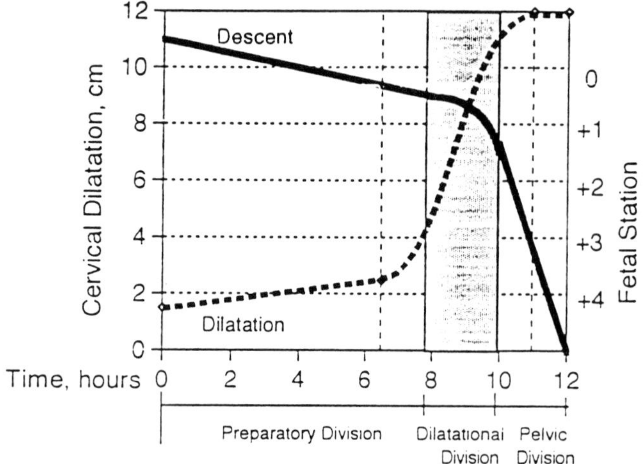


Fig. 4–39. The functional curve consisting of three phases depicted in the illustration. Inter-relationship between the descent curve (solid line) and the concurrently developing dilatation pattern (broken line) is shown in the composite form representing the average labor course for nulliparae. Active descent generally begins when the dilatation curve reaches its phase of maximum slope; the rate of descent reaches its maximum at the beginning of the deceleration phase of dilatation and continues in a linear manner until the perineum is reached. (Modified from Friedman EA: Labor: Clinical Evaluation and Management. 2nd Ed. New York, Appleton-Century-Crofts, 1978, pp. 6–59.)

problem in the normal gravida, it could be the cause of difficulty in precisely identifying the level of the skull in obese parturients.

In 1973, Studd (95) added to the partograph a part to include the fetal heart rate as well as the drugs given during labor. It is of interest to note that in the second volume of the first edition of this book, published 4 years earlier, Bonica presented an obstetric anesthesia chart that includes all of these factors plus an anesthesia chart that permitted recording the most important vital signs of the mother, the fetal heart rate of the infant, and the administration of various drugs and anesthetics (96).

## Pattern of the Functional Curve

Another important contribution by Friedman and his colleagues (90,97) was the development of "the functional curve" in which both the dilatation and descent curves were plotted in the same fashion as described above, but they also divided the entire period of the first stage into three functional divisions: 1) preparatory; 2) dilatational; and 3) pelvic divisions (Figure 4–39).

***The Preparatory Division.*** The preparatory division comprises that portion of labor from the onset of regular, perceived contractions to the end of the acceleration phase of dilatation. It ends when the labor enters that part of the active phase characterized by linear maximum slope of dilatation, during which time the descent curve is flat in its own latent period. The preparatory division is particularly sensitive to sedation and various types of analgesia and anesthesia, and their premature application of these agents impairs uterine contractility. Apparently, during this phase, myometrial function has not become sufficiently coordinated to withstand the inhibitory effects of such exogenous influences. The changes that occur in the cervix during this interval are both overt and subtle. Some apparent transformation is seen with softening, effacement, and the beginning of dilatation. More subtle variations occur in the subcellular alteration of ground substance, collagen, reticulum, and other fibrillar connective tissue components.

***The Dilatational Division.*** The dilatational division occupies the time interval during which cervical dilatation is proceeding at its most rapid pace. In addition to the dilatation that has occurred before labor begins {as mentioned by Hendricks (88)} and the negligible additional amount that takes place during the preparatory division (i.e., during the latent and acceleration phases combined), all of dilatation except the terminal retraction aspects of deceleration phase take place during the relatively short interval of the phase of maximum slope (91,97). It is during this important, albeit brief, span of time that the results of all the driving forces of uterine contractions become manifest in effecting cervical dilatation. The steeply inclined slope of dilatation is the result of a favorable combination of factors regardless of the particular clinical picture of labor in terms of contractility pattern.

In contrast to the preparatory division, the dilatational division of labor is essentially unaffected by sedation or anesthesia administered to provide maternal pain relief. The inhibitory pharmacologic effects of various exogenous agents, so readily demonstrated in the latent phase, are rarely seen here. It is only in the presence of a preexisting, disordered state of myometrial function or with some major intrinsic impedance or obstruction, that any potentially deleterious influences of extraneous factors become manifest during this phase. When the phase of maximum slope is progressing slowly or abnormally, the effects of inhibitory factors become apparent. Under such circumstances, excessive sedation or administration of a potent inhalation anesthetic in high concentration can readily

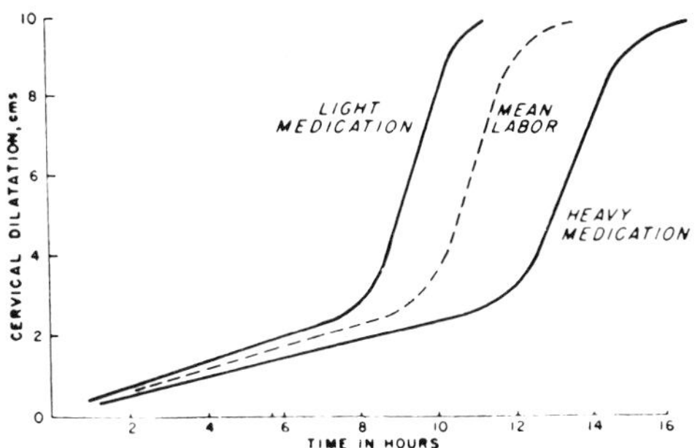


**Fig. 4–40.** The effects of sedatives on the labor curve. Note that light medication produced a shorter labor than the mean curve, suggesting that it was beneficial to the group of gravidae. In contrast, heavy medication prolonged the latent phase. (From Friedman EA: Primigravid labor. Obstet. Gynecol. 6:567, 1955.)

diminish or even stop further progress (see Figure 4–40, showing the effects of deep halothane anesthesia).

***The Pelvic Division.*** The pelvic division includes the deceleration phase and the second stage, and this is characterized by a linear descent of the presenting part that in normal labor proceeds without interruption until the perineum is reached (91). The classic mechanisms of labor, describing the cardinal movements of the fetus as it adjusts to the various pelvic dimensions during its descent, take place almost exclusively during this division. The linear descent pattern constitutes a fine measure of the overall efficiency of the labor process, analogous in value to that of the linear active dilatation curve. Its inclination provides a measure of the effectiveness of the motive force in producing the work required of it, i.e., descent of the fetus through the birth canal.

Friedman (91) justified this type of classification of the functional divisions of labor because of the clear-cut distinctions between them as to function, technique of assessment, manifestation of disorders, management regimen, and prognosis. The essential characteristic must be recognized so that appropriate diagnostic, evaluative, and therapeutic approaches will be available in the methodology of the practitioner. This simple view provides a meaningful and practical framework for understanding the complex process of labor.

## Other Important Advances

Another important advance pertaining to the forces of labor in the management of parturients is the use of what O'Driscoll and Meagerd (98) advocated as "active management of labor." This entails the infusion of exogenous oxytocin in those parturients where no complications are obvious but where uterine activity remains insufficient. This concept is being practiced in most countries where obstetricians and other health professionals have full knowledge of the pharmacology and complications of exogenous oxytocin and administer the drug in physiologic doses to avoid these.

Still another advance has been the demonstration that delaying the bearing-down efforts during the second stage is associated with a normal rotation of the presenting part, an increase in the incidence of spontaneous delivery, and a concurrent decrease in forceps delivery (99–101). This is contrary to the traditional concept and practice that neonatal mortality increases with longer labors (102). The old obstetric preaching dictated delivery of the fetus if the second stage persisted more than 1 hour in multiparae and 2 hours in primiparae. The advent and widespread use of electronic fetal heart rate (FHR) monitoring and widespread use of continuous epidural analgesia have provided impressive evidence that as long the FHR remains normal, it is not necessary to terminate the delivery by rotational forceps because an arbitrary amount of time has elapsed. Several studies have shown that delaying maternal expulsive efforts until the fetal head is below the ischial spines (99), or is visible at the introitus or until 1 hour has passed since full cervical rotation was achieved, reduced the incidence of forceps delivery. Indeed Maresh, Choong and Beard (100) demonstrated that the second stage of labor could be allowed to continue for as long as 4 hours without risk of harm to the fetus or mother, provided continuous monitoring shows no serious complications. As a result of these and other data, the American College of Obstetricians and Gynecologists (ACOG) in 1988 defined a prolonged second stage as more than 3 hours in nulliparous patients managed with regional anesthesia, as compared with 2 hours in those managed without regional anesthesia (103). For multiparae, the figures were more than 2 hours with regional analgesia and more than 1 hour without regional analgesia (Table 4–3). Because most of the recent studies pertain to the influence of continuous lumbar epidural analgesia, this topic will be discussed in much more detail in Chapter 13.

**Table 4–3.** ACOG Definitions for Prolonged Second Stage of Labor*

| |
|---|
| *Primigravidas:* |
| A) More than 2 hours without regional analgesia |
| B) More than 3 hours with regional analgesia |
| *Multigravidas:* |
| A) More than 1 hour without regional analgesia |
| B) More than 2 hours with regional analgesia |

* Based on a study by the Committee on Obstetrics: Maternal and fetal medicine: Obstetric forceps ACOG. Committee opinion #59, 1988.

## Effects of Analgesia and Anesthesia on the Forces of Labor

The effects of analgesia and anesthesia on the progress of labor and vaginal delivery and on the newborn depend on: 1) prevailing obstetric conditions; 2) technique or method of providing analgesia/anesthesia; 3) most importantly, the knowledge, skills, and experience of the administrator. Numerous studies provide evidence that uterine contractility and the progress and total length of labor may or may not be influenced by sedatives, opioids, and various forms of analgesia and anesthesia. In the early 1990s, we have continued to develop drugs and techniques that provide effective pain relief with minimum amount of side effects on the mother and fetus, including undesirable effects on the forces of labor. This type of analgesia minimizes or eliminates the pain-induced deleterious effects on the mother and fetus discussed Chapter

9 and enhances their well-being, while at the same time provides the mother with a pleasurable labor experience. Because the effects of various analgesic/anesthetic agents/techniques are discussed in detail in each chapter of Section C & D, only brief comments are made here. A comprehensive review of the subject has been published by Conklin (104).

## Systemic Sedatives and Analgesics

Given in optimal doses at the proper time these agents have little or no effect on the forces of labor. On the other hand, given prematurely during the latent phase or the preparatory phase of the functional curve, sedatives and opioid analgesics contribute to the failure of organizing urine activity to develop. Figure 4–40 shows the effect of light and heavy medication on the mean labor curve of nulliparae. If sedation or analgesia improves the quality of uterine activity in labor, then it is believed that this is due to a decrease in maternal anxiety and apprehension and a consequent increased secretion of catecholamines. The curve showing "heavy sedation" of a consequent prolongation of the first stage by particularly the latent phase may be due to either premature administration of the drugs or very large doses of both. Later sedation and systemic analgesia are likely to produce a minor impairment of uterine contractility but very frequently it produces confusion in the parturient, thus interfering with coordination of bearing-down efforts during the second stage.

A small percentage of parturients will experience very severe pain in the latent phase and recent studies have shown this phase to be associated with anxiety, stress, and negative cognitive processes, all of which portend a longer latent phase and longer active phase of labor and increased incidence of instrumental delivery (36). In such parturients it is essential to relieve the pain completely, thus minimizing the risk of prolonged labor with an ample dose of morphine given intravenously or 0.25 mg injected into the subarachnoid space.

## Regional Analgesia and Anesthesia

Administering regional analgesia or anesthesia in the latent phase may contribute to failure of organizing uterine activity to develop and labor to progress normally. For this reason most clinicians wait until labor is well within the active phase (4 to 5 cm cervical dilatation) before initiating the analgesia (the catheters should be put in place early in labor when the parturient is not very uncomfortable and to abstain from injecting analgesic solution until proper conditions are present). On the other hand, for parturients who are being induced with exogenous oxytocin or other oxytoxics early in labor, it is appropriate and indeed humanitarian to begin the analgesia as soon as the patient starts to have moderate-to-severe pain. Carried out in a well-planned, coordinated fashion, this method of managing patients during the induction of labor obviates needless suffering.

In well-established spontaneous labor, administration of new techniques of regional analgesia may have slight transient inhibition of uterine contractility but it has no effect on the progress of labor during the first stage (Figure 4–41). Indeed, patients with incoordinate uterine ac-

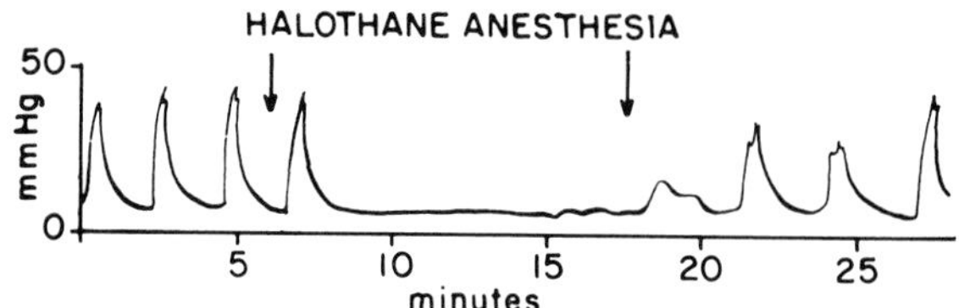


**Fig. 4–41.** Effect of halothane on uterine contractions (first arrow). A mixture containing 4% halothane, 65% nitrous oxide, and 31% oxygen was administered using controlled ventilation. Note the rapid and complete depression of myometrial activity and prompt recovery when the halothane was discontinued (second arrow). During this period, the patient's blood pressure decreased from 122/76 to 88/60. (Modified from Vasicka A, Kretchmer H: Effect of conduction and inhalation anesthesia on uterine contractions. Am. J. Obstet. Gynecol. 82:600, 1961.)

tivity that persists for a few hours without improvement should have the benefit of continuous lumbar epidural analgesia or other regional technique. Frequently, this will cause improvement in the intensity, frequency, and duration of uterine contractions and eventually lead to a normal labor and vaginal delivery. In these and all other cases, improvement is felt to result from decreased maternal catecholamine levels consequent to the relief of pain. Temporary decrease of uterine activity when it occurs is not consistent and has been attributed to the supine position or large doses of epinephrine in the local anesthetic, or to arterial hypotension and other factors previously discussed.

Older techniques of regional anesthesia that weaken the intercostal and abdominal muscles, decrease the efficacy of the auxiliary forces and thus prolong the second stage and increase the incidence of instrumental delivery. The same result may occur if regional anesthesia of the perineum develops thus eliminating the afferent limb of the reflex urge to bear down. However, in such circumstances most parturients can push effectively if instructed correctly during the antepartal period and encouraged to bear down forcefully when the presenting part is at the level of the ischial spines or lower. Coaching of a cooperative, alert patient during the second stage can substitute effectively for the perineoabdominal reflex that provokes the bearing-down efforts.

Older techniques of subarachnoid block often produced analgesia from T-5 to S-5, or the older techniques of continuous lumbar epidural and continuous caudal block achieved with large doses of local anesthetics administered before internal rotation had taken place, caused premature relaxation of the pelvic floor and thus prolonged the second stage. This increased the incidence of instrumental deliveries, and often caused transverse arrest of the presenting part. This fact was emphasized by Bonica in the first edition of this book, at which time he suggested modification of the technique such as using the double-catheter technique. The recent widespread use of continuous lumbar epidural analgesia achieved with continuous infusion of low concentration of local anesthetics and opioids can decrease or completely obviate this problem. This and many other aspects of epidural anesthesia are discussed in detail in Chapter 13.

Bilateral paracervical block or bilateral lumbar sympathetic block used to provide relief of pain due to uterine contractions and the use of local infiltration of the perineum during the second stage have no effect on uterine activity unless excessive doses of local anesthetics are used and cause direct depression of the myometrium. Administration of bilateral pudendal block with local anesthetics in concentrations that are relatively high for such small nerves (e.g., 1% lidocaine or 0.25% bupivacaine with 1:200,000 epinephrine) before internal rotation has taken place will relax the perineum sufficiently to interfere with the bearing-down efforts and thus prolong the second stage and increase the incidence of instrumental delivery (105). The problem may be obviated by using an analgesic concentration of local anesthetics (e.g., 0.5% lidocaine or 0.125 bupivacaine) that provides relief of pain but produces less perineal muscle relaxation. These issues are discussed further in Chapter 15.

In the late 1960s, the obstetric anesthesia and obstetric groups of the University of Washington Medical Center initiated a study of the effects of various techniques on uterine contractions (UC) and the bearing-down efforts (BDE) during the second stage of labor. In 1972, the results of the study in 42 parturients were published by the late Dr. Wayne Johnson (106). Patients who were selected were alert and cooperative, and all were having a normal spontaneous or induced labor with vertex presentation and an anticipated vaginal delivery. After the anesthetic and study procedures were explained to the patient, intrauterine pressure measurements (in mm Hg) were initiated. When the cervix was completely dilated and the second stage of labor was starting, the patients were coached in voluntary bearing-down efforts to coincide with the peak of uterine contractions. After two or more of these contractions with superimposed bearing efforts were recorded, the regional anesthetic was given. The study included: a) a control group of 6 parturients who had local or no anesthesia; b) 12 parturients managed with bilateral pudendal block achieved with 10 ml of 1% lidocaine on each side; c) subarachnoid block achieved with 6 to 8 mg of tetracaine; and d) standard continuous epidural anesthesia achieved with 15 to 18 ml of 1% lidocaine without epinephrine in 8 and 1% lidocaine with 1:200,000 epinephrine in 4 (the latter containing a total of 75 to 90 μg epinephrine). Measurements taken of both parameters before the administration of anesthesia were then compared to the contractions after stabilization of anesthesia, thereby using each patient as her control. In 4 of the 12 parturients given standard epidural block, measurements were made at the time the block was at T9-T12, and a second set of measurements was made when the block finally stablilized at T3-T7. Table 4–4 contains the data published by Johnson and associates (106), containing mean values and standard deviation of the various parameters. In the six patients who received local or no anesthesia, measurements were made in the first half and again during the last half of the second stage of labor. As noted, there was no difference in the intensity of uterine contraction, but the bearing-down effort increased significantly. In the 12 patients given pudendal block, there was no change in the intensity of uterine contraction, but the bearing-down effort increased significantly similar to that seen in patients with local or no anesthesia. With subarachnoid block, at T9-T12, there was no significant change in intensity of uterine contraction, but a significant decrease in bearing-down effort. In the two patients who had subarachnoid block at T3, the decrease of bearing-down effort was much higher than in the other 10 patients. With epidural anesthesia at the level of T9-T12, there were decreases in intensity of uterine contractions and bearing-down efforts, but the difference was not significant. In the four patients whose block eventually reached T3-T7, intensity of uterine contraction was not significantly different but the mean bearing-down efforts were significantly diminished when compared with the blockade at higher levels. The addition of epinephrine to lidocaine in the 12 patients had only mild greater depressant effects on uterine contraction, as compared to those who received plain lidocaine.

Subsequently, additional studies were carried out by Bonica and associates using these three techniques, and, additionally, they evaluated the effects of: e) segmental epidural anesthesia during the first stage that extended to the sacral segments during the second and third stages,

**Table 4–4.** Effects of Regional Anesthesia on the Forces of Labor and Vaginal Delivery

| Technique | Number of Patients | Uterine Contractions (UC) (mmHg) | | Bearing Down Efforts (BDE) (mmHg) | |
|---|---|---|---|---|---|
| | | Before Block | After Block | Before Block | After Block |
| Local or No Analgesia/Anesthesia | 6 | | | | |
| a) 1st half of 2nd stage | | 48 ± 20 | — | 58 ± 24 | — |
| b) 2nd half of 2nd stage | | 48 ± 18 | — | 72 ± 27 | — |
| Bilateral Pudendal Block | 12 | 32 ± 12 | 33 ± 13 | 53 ± 24 | 70 ± 23 |
| Subarachnoid Block Upper Levels | 12 | | | | |
| a) T9–T12 | 10 | 35 ± 13 | 32 ± 15 | 63 ± 28 | 46 ± 18 |
| b) T3 | 2 | 28 ± 14 | 28 ± 10 | 55 ± 30 | 31 ± 24 |
| Standard Epidural Block Upper Levels | 12 | | | | |
| a) T10–T12 | 12 | 34 ± 19 | 28 ± 10 | 57 ± 32 | 55 ± 22 |
| b) T3–T7* | 4* | 33 ± 18 | 25 ± 20 | 59 ± 14 | 46 ± 19 |

* Final cephalad extension of blockade in 4 of the 12 parturients.

achieved with 0.125% bupivacaine; and, f) the double-catheter technique, as described in detail in Chapter 13. In group (e), segmental (T10-L1) analgesia was initiated when the cervix was 4 to 5 cm dilated and carried out throughout the first and second stages so that by the time of the delivery nearly half of them had analgesia of the perineum, while the rest had perineal pain and required a bolus injection of 1% lidocaine with the patient sitting. In group (f), the segmental (T9-T10 to L1-L2) analgesia was also initiated at the beginning of the active phase of the first stage and maintained, limited to these segments throughout the second and third stages of labor. With the onset of perineal pain, an injection of 4 ml of analgesic concentration of local anesthetics (e.g., 0.125% bupivacaine) was given through the caudal catheter, and 15 minutes before the anticipated delivery another bolus of 3 to 4 ml of a high concentration of local anesthetics (e.g., 1.5% lidocaine or 1% etidocaine) was given. Measurements in most patients of groups (a), (b), and (c) were taken with the patient supine; whereas in groups (e) and (f), measurements were made with the patient in the lateral position during the first and early second stages. When the patient started to bear down, she was placed supine with a lift under the buttocks on one side so that the uterus would be displaced laterally to avoid compression of the inferior vena cava and aorta.

Table 4–5 contains a summary of the results of the expanded study, and these data can be compared with those in Table 4–4. As may be noted from review of the two tables, pudendal block achieved with 6 to 10 ml of 1% lidocaine or 0.25% bupivacaine injected in each side produced no significant effect on uterine contractions; but the relief of perineal pain and vigorous coaching of the patient resulted in a significant increase in bearing-down efforts in 14 parturients, a slight decrease in two, and one remained the same, so that the mean intensity of bearing-down efforts increased from 55 ± 19 to 72 ± 21.

Of the 18 patients who received subarachnoid block, 12 had a stabilized upper level of T9-T12, and this was associated with no significant change in uterine contractility, but the bearing-down efforts decreased from a mean of 60 ± 26 mm Hg to 48 ± 21 (20 %), which was of some significance. In the six patients with the upper level of block extending to T3-T7, decrease in uterine contractions was insignificant (15%), but bearing-down efforts decreased profoundly (46%). The decrease in uterine contractions was probably related to interruption of Ferguson's reflex, and in some instances was due to transient maternal hypotension, while the profound decrease in bearing-down efforts was due to the loss of the reflex to bear down and, more importantly, due to the weakness of the abdominal and lower thoracic muscles. The group given subarachnoid block required elective (outlet), or indicated low forceps in 55% and mid-forceps in 3% of the patients.

The standard continuous epidural block was achieved with 1% plain lidocaine in nine and 1% lidocaine and 1:200,000 epinephrine in the other nine (total 75 to 90 μg). In parturients in whom the upper level of standard epidural block was at T9–12, there was a mild (12%), insignificant decrease in the intensity of uterine contractions and no significant effect on bearing-down efforts. In the five patients who had the upper level at T3-T7, the intensity of uterine contractions decreased significantly (27%), probably due to the fact that it interrupted the Ferguson's reflex, which plays an important role during the second

**Table 4–5.** Effects of Regional Analgesia/Anesthesia on the Forces of Labor and Vaginal Delivery

| Technique | Number of Patients | Uterine Contractions (UC) (mmHg) | | Bearing Down Efforts (BDE) (mmHg) | |
|---|---|---|---|---|---|
| | | Before Block | After Block | Before Block | After Block |
| Local or No Analgesia/Anesthesia | 10 | | | | |
| a) 1st half of 2nd stage | | 46 ± 20 | — | 56 ± 21 | — |
| b) 2nd half of 2nd stage | | 48 ± 18 | — | 71 ± 26 | — |
| Bilateral Pudendal Block | 16 | 34 ± 14 | 38 ± 16 | 55 ± 19 | 72 ± 21 |
| Subarachnoid Block Upper Level | 18 | | | | |
| a) T9–T12 | 12 | 35 ± 12 | 33 ± 15 | 60 ± 26 | 48 ± 21 |
| b) T3–T6 | 6 | 35 ± 10 | 30 ± 16 | 63 ± 14 | 34 ± 19 |
| Standard Epidural Block Upper Levels | 18 | | | | |
| a) T9–T12 | 18 | 33 ± 19 | 28 ± 16 | 57 ± 28 | 58 ± 21 |
| b) T3–T7 | 6* | 34 ± 19 | 25 ± 13 | 58 ± 11 | 44 ± 17 |
| Continuous Intermittent Segmental Epidural Analgesia | 15 | | | | |
| a) First Stage | | 35 ± 17 | 38 ± 21 | — | — |
| b) Second Stage | | | | | |
| i) No perineal analgesia | 8 | 40 ± 14** | 43 ± 18** | 55 ± 23 | 61 ± 18 |
| ii) Perineal analgesia | 7 | 39 ± 16** | 36 ± 12** | — | 54 ± 12 |
| Double Catheter Technique | 20 | | | | |
| a) First Stage (T9–L2) | | 36 ± 16 | 38 ± 18 | — | — |
| b) Second Stage (S2–S5) | | 35 ± 19** | 41 ± 17** | 56 ± 16 | 76 ± 21 |

* Final cephalad extension of 6 of the 18 parturients.

** These figures represent the intensity of uterine contractions during the second stage before and after perineal analgesia was produced.

stage. Moreover, the intensity of uterine contractions among the nine parturients who had lidocaine-epinephrine decreased 16%, whereas in those who received plain lidocaine uterine contractions decreased 8%. High epidural block also decreased the bearing-down efforts about 24%. It is of interest to note that standard epidural block had greater effects on uterine contractions than subarachnoid block, probably due to a combination of the high concentration of local anesthetic with direct myometrial effects and mild effects of epinephrine. Among this group, 53% required elective or indicated outlet forceps, and one parturient required mid-forceps.

Continuous epidural analgesia by intermittent injection was used in 15 parturients achieved with 0.125% bupivacaine during the first and early second stages. As internal rotation took place, a 10 ml bolus of either 1.5% lidocaine or 0.5% bupivacaine was injected. As previously mentioned, the analgesia was initiated early in the active phase of the first stage of labor. The measurements of uterine contractions were made at 5 to 8 cm cervical dilatation, and, as noted, there was no significant change after the block. This difference between the standard and the segmental epidural analgesia is probably due to the fact that the latter did not interfere with Ferguson's reflex, and also that there was a concomitant decrease in catecholamine release with pain relief. During the early second stage, eight patients had no perineal analgesia, and these were associated with only a slight increase in uterine contractions to nearly the level that is expected in the second stage. In these patients, the intensity of bearing-down efforts increased slightly. On the other hand, in seven patients who had perineal analgesia throughout the second stage, bearing-down efforts were of slightly lower intensity, possibly because the stimulus for the bearing-down effort was eliminated. Of this group about 35% of the patients were delivered with elective or indicated low forceps.

Among the 20 parturients who had double-catheter technique during the first stage, analgesia was achieved with 4 to 5 ml of 0.25% bupivacaine during the first stage, and the levels were maintained from between T9-T10 and L1–2 throughout the entire first stage and early second stage, thus obviating interference with Ferguson's reflex and, concurrently, probably decreasing catecholamine release. With onset of perineal pain during the beginning of the second stage, 4 to 5 ml of 0.125% bupivacaine were injected into the sacral catheter to provide pain relief without motor block of the perineal sling. Once internal rotation had taken place, injection of 3 to 4 ml of 0.5% bupivacaine or 1% were given through the sacral catheter. As may be noted, during the second stage before the onset of sacral analgesia the intensity of uterine contractions is slightly lower than that during the first stage, probably due to increased secretion of catecholamines. With the onset of analgesia of the perineum, there was a significant increase in the intensity of uterine contractions. The most important effect, however, was on the bearing-down efforts, which increased from a mean of 56 ± 16 mm Hg to 76 ± 21 mm Hg. Figure 13–20 (Chapter 13) illustrates the efficacy of this technique in increasing the ability of parturients to bear down forcefully. Of this group, three (15%) required elective outlet forceps. In view of the trend among some obstetricians not to have the parturient push, there is a decrease in need for this technique. However, in the experience of the senior author the double catheter is the best regional anesthetic technique for all parturients and particularly for those who are at risk.

### *Inhalation and Intravenous Anesthesia*

Inhalation anesthetics administered in analgesic concentration for the relief of pain of uterine contractions and delivery have no effect on uterine contractility, or the course and progress of labor, nor do they effect the reflex urge to bear down. Indeed the analgesia may improve uterine contractility if the parturient is having severe pain that is usually associated with increased secretion of catecholamines. Many older studies in which analgesic concentrations of nitrous oxide, ethylene, cyclopropane, chloroform, or ether produced complete pain relief in about 25% of the patients, very good relief in another 45%, mild-to-moderate relief in 20% and no relief in 10%. In the United Kingdom, the Entonox inhaler, which delivers 50% oxygen and 50% nitrous oxide, is used frequently for self-administration by the patient or administered by a midwife. This type of mixture has no significant effect on the forces of labor.

In contrast, virtually all potent inhalation anesthetics have a depressant effect on uterine contractility that is dose dependent. In very light concentrations, used as part of balanced anesthesia that includes the concomitant administration of a muscle relaxant, uterine contractility is depressed only slightly. On the other hand, administering these agents in concentration that is twice the minimum alveolar concentration (MAC) produces profound myometrial depression and relaxation (Figure 4–42). For these and other reasons, potent inhalation agents—even in light concentrations—are rarely used for vaginal deliv-

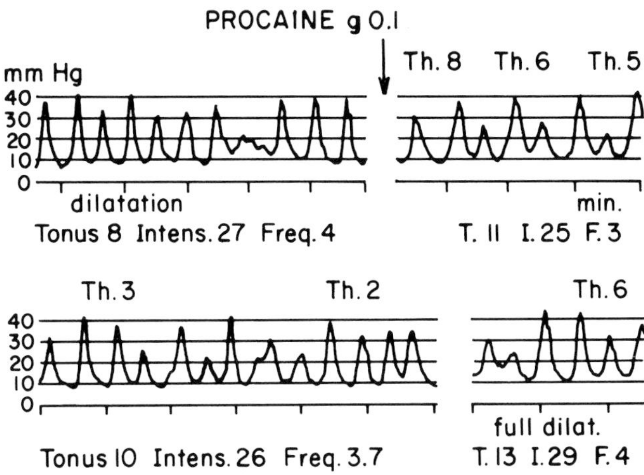


**Fig. 4–42.** Lack of effect of subarachnoid block produced with 100 mg of procaine on uterine contractions. Note that the block was extended to the second thoracic dermatome without producing changes in intensity or frequency of contractions. (Modified from Caldeyro-Barcia R: Modern Trends in Gynaecology and Obstetrics. Montreal, Librairie Beauchemin Limitee, 1959.)

ery because of the high risks of regurgitation and pulmonary aspiration and difficulty in tracheal intubation. Potent inhalation anesthetics such as halothane are the method "par excellence" to rapidly relax the uterus to facilitate manipulation of the fetus or terminate tetanic contractions. Other drugs that have been used to achieve myometrial relaxation include magnesium sulfate, terbutaline sulfate, ritodrine, indomethacin, and aspirin. The advantages of the use of a potent inhalation agent over these other uterine relaxants are that once the intrauterine or extrauterine maneuver of the fetus has been completed or the tetanic contraction has stopped, the drug can be rapidly eliminated so that within a few minutes the uterus regains its normal tone.

## REFERENCES


1. Reynolds SRM: Physiology of the uterus. New York, Hafner Publishing Company, 1965.
2. Huszar G: The Physiology and Biochemistry of the Uterus in Pregnancy and Labor. Boca Raton, FL, CRC Press, 1986.
3. Friedman EA: Labor: Clinical Evaluation and Management. New York, Appleton Century-Crofts, 1978.
4. Gabbe SG, Neibyl JR, Simpson JL: Obstetrics: Normal and Problem Pregnancies. 2nd Ed. New York, Churchill Livingstone, 1991.
5. Schwalm H, Dubrauszky V: Structure of the musculature of the human uterus-muscle and connective tissue. Am. J. Obstet. Gynecol. 94:391, 1966.
6. Hytten FE, Cheyne GA: The size and composition of the human pregnant uterus. J. Obstet. Gynecol. Br. Commonw. 76:400, 1969.
7. Danforth DN: The fibrous nature of the human cervix, and its relation to the isthmic segment in gravid and nongravid uteri. Am. J. Obstet. Gynecol. 53:431, 1947.
8. Danforth DN, Buckingham JC, Roddick JW Jr: Connective tissue changes incident to cervical effacement. Am. J. Obstet. Gynecol. 80:1960, 1960.
9. Danforth DN. The morphology of the human cervix. Clin. Obstet. Gynecol. 26:7, 1983.
10. Golichowski AM: Biochemical basis of cervical maturation. *In* The Physiology and Biochemistry of the Uterus in Pregnancy and Labor. Edited by G Huszar. Boca Raton, FL, CRC Press, 1986.
11. Huszar G, Cabrol D, Naftolin F: The relationship between myometrial contractility and cervical maturation in pregnancy and labor. *In* The Physiology and Biochemistry of the Uterus in Pregnancy and Labor. Edited by G. Huszar. Boca Raton, FL, CRC Press, 1986.
12. Richardson JA, et al: The development of an instrument for monitoring dilatation of the cervix during labor. Biomed. Eng. 11:311, 1976.
13. Kok FT, Wallenburg HCS, Wladimiroff JW: Ultrasonic measurement of cervical dilatation during labor. Am. J. Obstet. Gynecol. 126:288, 1976.
14. Arulkumaran S, et al: The effect of parity on uterine activity in labor. Br. J. Obstet. Gynecol. 91:843, 1984.
15. Alvarez H, Caldeyro-Barcia R: Studies of the contractility of the human uterus recorded by new methods. Surg. Gynecol. Obstet. 91:1, 1950.
16. Caldeyro-Barcia R, Alvarez H, Reynolds SRM: A better understanding of uterine contractility through simultaneous recording with an internal and a seven-channel external method. Surg. Gynecol. Obstet. 91:641, 1950.
17. Caldeyro-Barcia R, Alvarez H: Abnormal uterine action in labor. J. Obstet. Gynecol. Br. Emp. 59:646, 1952.
18. Alvarez H, Caldeyro-Barcia R: The normal and abnormal contractile waves of the uterus during labor. Gynaecologia 138:190, 1954.
19. Caldeyro-Barcia R, Alvarez H, Poseiro JJ: Normal and abnormal uterine contractility in labour. Triangle 2:41, 1955.
20. Caldeyro-Barcia R, Poseiro JJ: Oxytocin and contractility of the pregnant human uterus. Ann. NY. Acad. Sci. 75:813, 1959.
21. Caldeyro-Barcia R: Uterine contractility in obstetrics. Main Lecture II World Congr. In. Fed. Obstet. Gynaecol., 1960.
22. Caldeyro-Barcia R, Poseiro JJ: Physiology of the uterine contraction. Clin. Obstet. Gynecol. 3:386, 1960.
23. Reynolds SRM, Harris JS, Kaiser IH: Clinical Measurement of Uterine Forces in Pregnancy and Labor. Springfield, IL, Charles C. Thomas, 1954.
23A. Steer PJ: The measurement and control of uterine contractions. *In* The Current Status of Fetal Heart Rate Monitoring and Ultrasound In Obstetrics. Edited by RW Beard, S Campbell. London, Royal College of Obstetricians and Gynaecologists, 1977, pp. 48–68.
23B. Allman ACJ, Steer PJ: Monitoring uterine activity. Br. J. Hosp. Med. 49:649, 1993.
23C. Gibb DM: Measurement of uterine activity in labour—clinical aspects. Br. J. Obstet. Gynaecol. 100(Suppl.9): 28, 1993.
23D. Steer PJ: Standards in fetal monitoring—practical requirements for uterine activity measurement and recording. Br. J. Obstet. Gynaecol. 100(Suppl.9):32, 1993.
24. Danforth DN, Graham RJ, Ivy AD: The functional anatomy of labor as revealed by frozen sagittal sections in the Macacus Rhesus monkey. Surg. Gynecol. Obstet. 74:188, 1942.
25. Jeffcoate TNA: Physiology and mechanisms of labour. *In* British Obstetrics and Gynaecological Practice. Edited by J Holland. London, William Heinemann, Ltd, 1955.
26. Larks SD: Electrohysterography: The Electrical Activities of the Human Uterus in Pregnancy and Labor. Springfield, IL, Charles C Thomas, 1960.
27. Engelmann GJ: Labor Among Primitive Peoples. 2nd Ed. St. Louis. JH Chambers & Co, 1983, pp 51–151.
28. Melzack R, Schaffelberg D: Low-back pain during labor. Am. J. Obstet. Gynecol. 156:901–905, 1987.
29. Roberts JE, Wodell DA: The effects of maternal position on uterine contractility and efficiency. Birth 10:243–249, 1983.
30. Roberts J, Asanos L, Mendez-Bauer C: Maternal positions in labor: analysis in relation to comfort and efficiency. Birth Defects (Original Article Series) 17:97–128, 1981.
31. Mendez-Bauer C, et al: Effects of standing position on spontaneous uterine contractility and other aspects of labor. J. Perinat. Med. 3:89–100, 1975.
31A. Roberts JE, Mendez-Bauer C, Wodell DA: The effects of maternal position on uterine contractility and efficiency. Birth 10:243, 1983.
31B. Chen SZ, Aisaka K, Mori H, Kigawa T: Effects of sitting position on uterine activity during labor. Obstet. Gynecol. 69:67, 1987.
32. Caldeyro-Barcia R, et al: The influence of maternal position on time of spontaneous rupture of the membranes, progress of labor, and fetal head compression. Birth Fam. J. 6:7–16, 1979.
33. Caldeyro-Barcia R, et al: Effect of position changes on the intensity and frequency of uterine contractions during labor. Am. J. Obstet. Gynecol. 80:284, 1960.
34. Steward T, Calder AA: Posture in Labor: Patients' choice and its effect on performance. Br. J. Obstet. Gynaecol. 91: 1091–1095, 1984.

35. Vasicka A, Kretchmer HE: Uterine dynamics. Clin. Obstet. Gynecol. 4:17, 1961.
36. Wuitshik M, Bakal D, Lipshitz J: Clinical significance of pain and cognitive activity in latent labor. Obstet. Gynaecol. 73:35–42, 1989.
37. Carsten ME, Miller JD: A new look at uterine muscle contraction. Am. J. Obstet. Gynecol. 157:1303–1315, 1987.
38. Carsten ME, Miller JD: Uterine Function: Molecular and Cellular Aspects. New York, Plenum Press, 1990, a) pp. 361–392; b) pp. 501–518.
39. Thailer I, Manor D Itskovitz J, Rottem S, Levit N, et al: Changes in uterine blood flow during human pregnancy. Am. J. Obstet. Gynecol. 162:121–125, 1990.
40. Fuchs AR, Fuchs F: Physiology of parturition. *In* Obstetrics: Normal and Problem Pregnancies. 2nd Ed. Edited by SG Gabbe, JR Niebyl, JL Simpson. New York, Churchill Livingstone, Inc, 1986, pp 327–350.
41. Kao CY: Electrophysical properties of the uterine smooth muscle. *In* Biology of the Uterus. Edited by RR Wynn. New York, Plenum Press, 1977, p 423.
42. Verhoeff A, Garfield RE: Ultrastructure of the myometrium and the role of gap junctions in myometrial function. *In* The Physiology and Biochemistry of the Uterus in Pregnancy and Labor. Edited by G Huszar. Boca Raton, FL, CRC Press, 1986.
43. Daniel EE: Gap junctions in smooth muscle. *In* Gap Junctions. Edited by MLV Bennett, DC Spray. New York, Cold Spring Harbor, 1985.
44. Casey ML, McDonald PC: Initiation of labor in women. *In* The Physiology and Biochemistry of the Uterus in Pregnancy and Labor. Edited by G Huszar. Boca Raton, FL, CRC Press, 1986.
45A. Wiquist N, Bryman I, Lindblom B, Norstrom A, Wikland M: The role of prostaglandins for the coordination of myometrial forces during labour. Acta. Physiol. Hung. 65:313, 1985.
45. Casey ML, MacDonald PC: Endocrinology of pregnancy and parturition. *In* Uterine Function: Molecular and Cellular Aspects. Edited by ME Carsten, JD Miller. New York: Plenum Press, 1990, pp. 501–517.
46. Csapo A: Function and regulation of the myometrium. Ann. NY. Acad. Sci. 75:790, 1962.
47. Coleman HA, Parkington H: Indication of prolonged excitability in myometrium of pregnant guinea pigs by $PGF_{2\alpha}$. J. Physiol. (Lond) 399:33, 1988.
48. Keirse MJNC: Endogenous prostaglandins in human parturition. *In* Human Parturition, Boehave Series for Postgraduate Medical Education, Vol. 15. Edited by MJNC Keirse, ABM Anderson, JB Gravenhorst. Leiden, Leiden University Press, 1979, pp 101.
49. Fuchs AR, Goeschen K, Husslein P, et al: Oxytocin and the initiation of human parturition. III. Plasma concentrations of oxytocin and 13,14-dihydro-15-keto-prostaglandin $F_{2-\alpha}$ in spontaneous and oxytocin-induced labor at term. Am. J. Obstet. Gynecol. 147:497, 1983.
50. Ghodganokar RB, Dubin NH, Blake DA, King TM: The 13,14-dihydro-15-keto-prostaglandin concentrations in human plasma and amniotic fluid. Am. J. Obstet. Gynecol. 134:265, 1979.
51. Caldeyro-Barcia R, Sereno JA: The response of human uterus to oxytocin throughout pregnancy. *In* Oxytocin. Edited by R Caldeyro-Barcia, H Heller. London: Pergamon Press, 1959, p. 177.
52. Dubin NH, Johnson JWC, Calhouin S, et al: Plasma prostaglandin in pregnant women with term and preterm deliveries. Obstet. Gynecol. 57:203, 1981.
53. Dale HH: On some physiological actions of ergot. J. Physiol. 34:163, 1906.
54. Ferguson JKW: A study of motility of the intact uterus at term. Surg. Gynecol. Obstet. 73:359, 1941.
55. Dagwood MY, Raghavan KS, Pociask C, Fuchs F: Oxytocin in human pregnancy and parturition. Obstet. Gynecol. 51: 138, 1978.
56. Leake RD, Weitzman RE, Glatz PH, Fisher DA: Plasma oxytocin concentrations in men, nonpregnant women and pregnant women before and during spontaneous labor. J. Clin. Endocrinol. Metab. 53:730, 1981.
57. Dagwood MY, Wang CF, Gupta R, Fuchs F: Fetal contribution to oxytocin in human labor. Obstet. Gynecol. 52:205, 1978.
58. Fuchs AR. The Role of Oxytocin and Parturition Biochemistry of the Human Uterus. Boca Raton, FL, CRC Press, 1986, pp. 163–170.
59. Vasicka A, Kumaresan P, Han GS, Kumaresan M: Plasma oxytocin in initiation of labor. Am. J. Obstet. Gynecol. 130: 263–273, 1978.
60. Goodfellow CF, Hull MG, Swaab DF, Dogterom J, Buijs RM: Oxytocin deficiency at delivery with epidural analgesia. Br. J. Obstet. Gynaecol 90:214, 1983.
61. Fuchs AR, Romero R, ParraM, et al: Pulsatile release of oxytocin: significant increase in spontaneous labor. Am. J. Obstet. Gynecol. 1990.
62. Randolph GW, Fuchs AR: Pulsatile administration enhances the effect and reduced the dose of oxytocin required for induction of labor. Am. J. Perinatol.
63. Dagwood MY: Evolving concepts of oxytocin for induction of labor. Am. J. Perinatol. 6:167, 1989.
64. Fuchs AR, Fuchs F, Husslein P, et al: Oxytocin receptors in the human uterus during pregnancy and parturition: a dual role for oxytocin in the initiation of labor. Science 215:1396, 1982.
65. Fuchs AR, Fuchs F, Husslein P, et al: Oxytocin receptors in the human uterus during pregnancy and parturition. Am. J. Obstet. Gynecol. 150:734, 1984.
66. Fuchs AR, Fuchs F: Endocrinology of human parturition: a review. Br. J. Obstet. Gynaecol. 91:948, 1984.
67. Kuntz A: The Autonomic Nervous System. 4th Ed. Philadelphia, Lea & Febiger, 1953, pp. 297–307.
68. Mulla N: Vaginal delivery in a paraplegic patient. Am. J. Obstet. Gynecol. 73:1346, 1957.
69. Robertson DNS, Guttman L: Paraplegic patient in pregnancy and labor. Proc. Roy. Soc. Med. 56:381, 1963.
69A. Greenspoon JS, Paul RH: Paraplegia and quadriplegia: special considerations during pregnancy and labor and delivery. Am. J. Obstet. Gynecol. 155:738, 1986.
69B. Kulkami S, Morgan OS: Pregnancy outcome in paraplegic women. West Indian Med. J. 41:99, 1992.
70. Blinick G: Painless labors following presacral neurectomy. Am. J. Obstet. Gynecol. 54:148, 1947.
71. Dumond M: Etude de l'accouchement chez les primipares operees avec success de resection dur nerf presacre pour dysmenorrhea. Gynecol. Obstet. 50:35, 1951.
72. Rysanek WJJr, Cavanagh D: Presacral neurectomy and its effect on subsequent pregnancies. Am. Surg. 24:335, 1958.
73. Alvarez H, et al: Effects of the anesthetic blockage of the spinal cord on the contractility of the pregnant uterus. XXI Int. Congr. Physiol. Sci. Buenos Aires, Communications 14, 1959.
74. Caldeyro-Barcia R, et al: Jucio critico sobre la induccion y conduccion del parto. III Congr. Lat. Am. Obstet. y Ginec. 1: 131, 1958.
75. Cibils LA, et al: Uterine work during labor. XXI Int. Congr. Physiol. Sci. Buenos Aires, Communications 65, 1959.

76. Krantz KE: Innervation of the human uterus. Ann. NY. Acad. Sci. 75:770, 1959.
77. Diamond J: Beta adrenoceptors, cyclic AMP, and cyclic GMP in control of uterine motility. *In* Uterine Function: Molecular and Cellular Aspects. Edited by ME Carsten, JD Miller. New York: Plenum Press, 1990, pp. 249–275.
78. Bottari SP, Vokaer A, Kaivez E, Lescrainier JP, Vanquelin G: Regulation of alpha- and beta-adrenergic receptor subclasses by gonadal steroids in human myometrium. Acta. Physiol. Hungarica. 65:335–346, 1985.
78A. Berg G, Andersson RG, Ryden G: Alpha-adrenergic receptors in human myometrium during pregnancy. Am. J. Obstet. Gynecol. 154:601, 1986.
79. Ariens EJ, Simonis AM: Physiological and pharmacological aspects of adrenergic receptor classification. Biochem. Pharmacol. 32:1539–1545, 1983.
80. Owman CH, Rosengren E, Sjoberg NO: Adrenergic innervation of the human female reproductive organs: a histochemical and chemical investigation. Obstet. Gynecol. 30: 763, 1967.
81. Sjoberg NO: Considerations of the cause for the disappearance of adrenergic transmitter in uterine nerves during pregnancy. Acta. Physiol. Scand. 72:510, 1968.
82. Ottesen B, Fahrenkrug J: Regulatory peptides and uterine function. *In* Uterine Function: Molecular and Cellular Aspects. Edited by ME Carsten, JD Miller. New York, Plenum Press, 1990, pp. 393–422.
83. Mengert WF, Murphy DP: Intra-abdominal pressures created by voluntary muscular effort. Surg. Gynecol. Obstet. 57:745, 1933.
84. Steer PG, Carter MC, Beard RW: Normal levels of active contraction area in spontaneous labor. Br. J. Obstet. Gynaceol. 91:211, 1984.
85. Friedman EA: Primigravid labor: A graphicostatistical analysis. Obstet. Gynecol. 6:567, 1955.
86. Friedman EA: Labor in multiparas: A graphicostatistical analysis. Obstet. Gynecol. 8:691, 1956.
87. Hendricks CH, Eskes TK, Saameli K: Uterine contractility at delivery and in the peurperium. Am. J. Obstet. Gynecol. 83:890, 1962.
88. Hendricks VH, Brenner WE, Kraus G: Normal cervical dilatation patterns in late pregnancy and labor. Am. J. Obstet. Gynecol. 106:1065–1082, 1970.
89. Friedman EA, Sachtleben NR: The determinant role of initial cervical dilatation on the course of labor. Am. J. Obstet. Gynecol. 84:930, 1962.
90. Friedman EA, Sachtleben NR: Station of the fetal presenting. Part I. Pattern of descent. Am. J. Obstet. Gynecol. 93: 522, 1965.
91. Friedman EA: Labor: Clinical Evaluation and Management. 2nd Ed. New York, Appleton-Century-Croft, 1978, pp. 6–59.
92. Friedman EA, Kroll DH: Computer analysis of labor progression. II. Distribution of data and limits of normal. J. Reprod. Med. 6:20, 1971.
93. Friedman EA, Sachtleben NR: Station of the fetal presenting part. IV. Slope of descent. Am. J. Obstet. Gynecol. 107: 1031, 1970.
94. Philpott RM, Castle WM: Cervical graphs in the management of labor in primigravidae. J. Obstet. Gynaecol. Br. Commonw. 79:599, 1972.
95. Studd JWW: Partogram and normalgrams of cervical dilatation in the management of primigravid labour. Br. Med. J. 4:451, 1973.
96. Bonica JJ: Analgesia during normal labor. *In* Bonica JJ: Principles and Practices of Obstetric Analgesia & Anesthesia.Vol. 2. Edited by JJ Bonica. Philadelphia: FA Davis, 1969, p. 866.
97. Friedman EA: Functional division of labor. Am. J. Obstet. Gynaecol. 109:274, 1971.
98. O'Driscoll K, Meagher D: Active Management of Labor. London, WB Saunders, 1981.
99. Phillips KC, Thomas TA: Second stage of labor with or without extradural analgesia. Anaesthesia 38:972–976, 1983.
100. Maresh M, Choong KH, Beard RW: Delayed pushing with lumbar epidural analgesia in labor. Br. J. Obstet. Gynaecol. 90:623–627, 1983.
101. Goodfellow CF, Studd C: The reduction of forceps in primigravidas with epidural analgesia: control trial. Br. J. Clin. Pract. 33:287–288, 1979.
102. Niswander KR, Gordon M: Safety of the low-forceps operation. Am. J. Obstet. Gynaecol. 117:619–629, 1973.
103. Committee on Obstetrics: Maternal and fetal medicine: Obstetric forceps ACOG. Committee opinion #59, 1988.
104. Conklin KA: Effects of obstetric analgesia and anesthesia on uterine activity and uteroplacental blood flow. *In* Uterine Function: Molecular and Cellular Aspects. Edited by ME Carsten, JD Miller. New York, Plenum Press, 1990, pp. 539–575.
105. Zador G, Lindmark G, Nilsson, BA: Pudendal block in normal vaginal delivery. Acta. Obstet. Gynecol. Scand. Supplement 34:51–64, 1974.
106. Johnson WL: Effect of pudendal spinal epidural block anesthesia on the second stage of labor. Am. J. Obstet. Gynecol. 113:166–175, 1972.

# Chapter 5

# THERAPEUTIC PHARMACOLOGY OF UTERINE CONTRACTILITY

PATRICIA A. ROBERTSON
JAMES M. ROBERTS

---

Current concepts of the mechanisms and control of uterine contractility permit rational therapy usage with drugs that modify uterine contractions (1). The expansive use of agents that stimulate or inhibit myometrial contractions mandates that clinicians who manage the anesthetic care of the pregnant woman and her fetus be familiar with the mechanism of action of these drugs and their side effects as well as interactions with other drugs.

In this chapter we will first review briefly the current understanding of the control of uterine contractility. Although this subject is discussed in Chapter 4, we will discuss the several classes of agents used clinically to modify myometrial contractions. In addition to discussion of the mechanisms of action of tocolytics and oxytocics, we will also consider indications and contraindications for their usage; maternal, fetal, and neonatal effects, and their interaction with other agents, with special emphasis on anesthetic drugs. More detailed information on these various drugs can be found elsewhere (2,3,4,5).

## BASIC CONSIDERATIONS

### *Myometrial Structure and Function*

The pregnant uterus is a remarkable organ. It expands from a nonpregnant volume of 10 cc to 3.5 liters in late pregnancy, maintaining its ability to contract forcefully despite striking changes in the length of muscle fibers. Myometrial changes resulting in the increased uterine size are determined by circulating hormones. This responsiveness to not only neural but also humoral influences provides for exquisite "fine tuning" of structural and contractile responses. The ability of the uterus to sustain contractions with a minimum of energy expenditure ideally suits it for the arduous process of labor. These adaptive characteristics are a function of the unique features of smooth muscle exemplified by the uterine smooth muscle, myometrium. Because skeletal muscle has formed the basis for much of our knowledge about muscle structure and function, we will consider these features of smooth muscle as contrasted to this more familiar tissue.

### The Mechanism of Smooth Muscle Contraction

#### *Contractile Proteins*

As in skeletal muscle, the primary contractile proteins of smooth muscle are actin and myosin. Actin is a globular protein that is arranged as a helical polymer to form the thin filaments (Figure 5–1). Myosin is an asymmetric protein, consisting of a globular head that contains myosin light chains and an actin activatable ATPase. The remainder of the protein is linear (Figure 5–2a). The thick filaments are made up of myosin molecules arranged with the linear portion toward the interior and the heads projecting outward as potential contact points with actin (Figure 5–2b).

In both skeletal and smooth muscle, the transduction of biochemical to mechanical energy is accomplished by an energy-dependent conformational change in the relationship of the myosin head to the remainder of the protein. This is stimulated by actin myosin interaction and causes the myosin head to become acutely angulated with its tail (Figure 5–3). As this is repeated, the thin filaments slide across the thick filaments and the muscle contracts. For both types of muscle this is a calcium-dependent event. The major effect of this ion, however, is quite different in the two muscles.

### *The Role of Calcium in Smooth Muscle Contraction*

Skeletal muscle contains a high concentration of troponin, a globular protein which in association with tropomyosin is present in the groove of the α-helix of actin. These proteins effectively occlude the binding site for myosin at resting intracellular calcium concentration. With increased intracellular free calcium concentration, troponin undergoes a conformational change, the myosin binding site is exposed and the muscle contracts. In smooth muscle, very little troponin and tropomyosin are present, and this mechanism is probably of minor importance. In contrast to skeletal muscle where myosin appears to be activated in the resting state needing only access to the actin binding site for contraction to occur, in smooth muscle, the activation step is the predominant control for contraction. This activation is under control of calcium, acting through the intracellular transducer calmodulin (Figure 5–4). With increased intracellular free calcium, the calcium-calmodulin complex binds to and activates the enzyme, myosin light chain kinase (MLK). This enzyme, when activated, catalyzes the phosphorylation of myosin light chains that results in the activation of myosin and

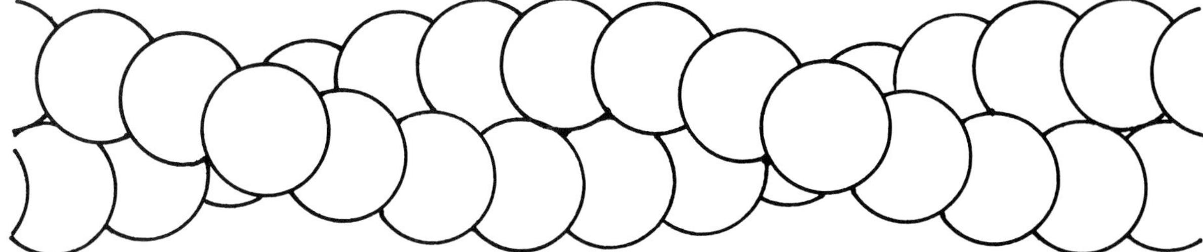

**Fig. 5–1.** Actin polymers. Actin is a globular protein that is present intracellularly as a pair of polymers coiled in an alpha felix. (Redrawn from Lenniger AL: Biochemistry. 2nd Ed. New York, Worth, 1975, p. 760.)

its binding to actin and subsequent contraction of the smooth muscle (6).

Although little information is available on myometrium specifically, it is evident from work in other smooth muscles that there are other important calcium-sensitive regulators. In tracheal smooth muscle, while the initiation of contraction correlates quite well with increased intracellular calcium and myosin light chain phosphorylation, contraction is maintained when calcium concentrations have returned to nearly resting levels and there is no longer an increase in light chain phosphorylation (7). This has stimulated interest in other calcium-sensitive proteins one of which, kinase-C, is discussed below.

### The Structure of Smooth Muscle

Several important structural contrasts between smooth and skeletal muscle contribute to functional differences. Smooth muscle cells are much smaller than skeletal muscle cells. As indicated in Figure 5–5, one cubic millimeter of muscle contains 17 skeletal muscle cells but 2.3 million smooth muscle cells (8). An important consequence of this difference is a much larger ratio of surface area to intracellular volume in smooth muscle. The surface area of smooth muscle is increased even more by the presence of surface invaginations, caveolae, which are present on about one-third of the cell surface. This accounts for the much greater influence of humoral agents acting at the cell surface on smooth as opposed to skeletal muscle.

On electron microscopy the arrangement of the contractile proteins is quite orderly in skeletal muscle (Figure 5–6a) but appears almost random in smooth muscle (Figure 5–6b). On closer examination (Figure 5–7) it is evident that the arrangement is not random but that the fibers are oriented obliquely with the fibers anchored to the plasma membrane and dense bodies within the cytoskeleton. This oblique arrangement allows actin and myosin to maintain contact and gives the capacity to cause contractions at much greater stretch than skeletal muscle. This arrangement also permits smooth muscle to shorten to 25% of its resting length, a considerably greater reduction in length than is possible for skeletal muscle.

## Modulation of Smooth Muscle Contraction

### Stimulation of Contraction

In both skeletal and smooth muscle, modification of intracellular free calcium concentration is the primary determinant of muscle contraction or relaxation. However, in addition to the mechanisms by which calcium acts, striking differences exist in the manner in which this changing calcium concentration is achieved in these muscles. In skeletal muscle this is almost exclusively by neural signals, while in smooth muscle, agents acting at surface receptors are at least as important. Calcium concentration can be influenced by alteration of entry or egress of calcium or release of calcium from intracellular stores (Figure 5–8). The entry of calcium is through voltage sensitive or independent channels, while several calcium egress pumps have been described (9).

### Receptor Mediated Phosphatidylinositol Hydrolysis

Most agents that act through receptor interactions to increase calcium intracellularly use the receptor-mediated activation of a specific, membrane bound, phospholipase-C (10). This phospholipase has as its preferred substrate a phospholipid that makes up only about 1% of membrane phospholipids, phosphatidylinositol 4,5 bisphosphate (PIP2). The products of PIP2 hydrolysis are the polyphosphorylated sugar, 1,4,5 inositol trisphosphate (1,4,5 IP3) and diacylglycerols (DAG) (Figure 5–9). Both of these products are second messages. Inositol trisphosphate releases calcium from nonmitochondrial stores and initiates smooth muscle contraction. Diacylglycerols activate a membrane-associated kinase, kinase-C, which is implicated in the maintenance of smooth muscle contraction (11). Diacylglycerols are also important potential precursors for arachidonic acid. About 65% of phosphatidylinositol molecules contain arachidonate in the 2 position that can be released by specific diacylglycerol lipases present intracellularly. Thus, it is possible for receptors activating phospholipase-C to generate not only the 2-second messages described but also to provide substrate for other messages, the eicosanoids.

### Inhibition of Contraction

The relaxation of smooth muscle is characterized by a return of intracellular calcium to resting levels. Thus, agents that inhibit contraction can have as their targets reduced entry of calcium, enhanced egress of calcium or intracellular sequestration of this ion. Other potential targets are steps in contraction beyond calcium, inhibition of calmodulin or myosin light chain kinase, for example.

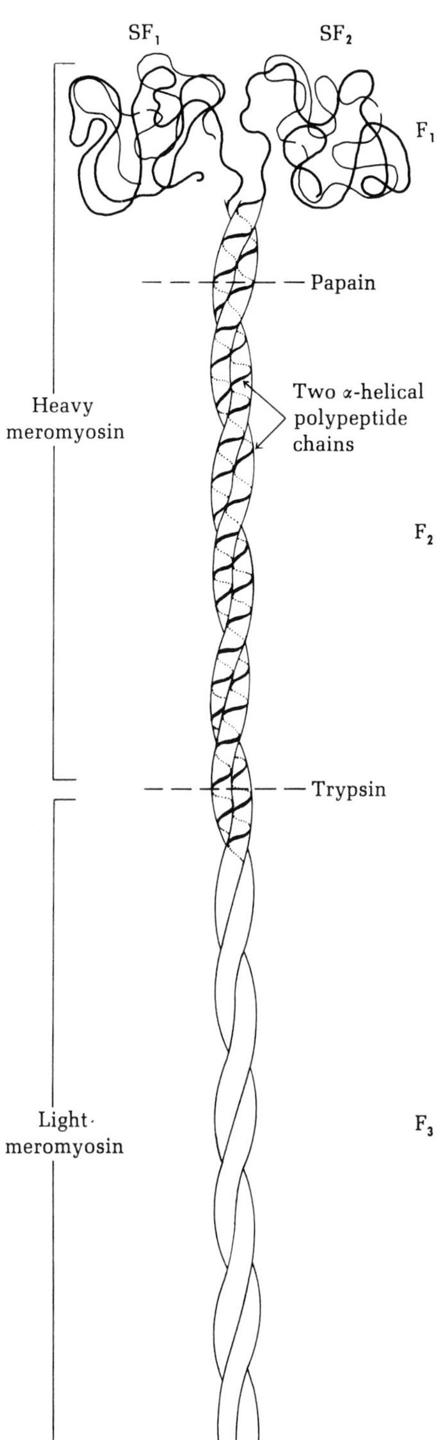


**Fig. 5–2.** **A,** Myosin. Myosin consists of heavy and light chains, the light chains are included in the head portion of myosin. (Also indicated are the sites of proteolytic cleavage, which have been useful in defining the function of the different portions of the molecule.) (Redrawn from Lenniger AL: Biochemistry. 2nd Ed. New York, Worth, 1975, p. 755.) **B,** The thick filaments. In the thick filaments, monomers of myosin are precisely arranged with the myosin heads projecting outward and oriented to the active sites of actin. (Redrawn from Lenniger AL: Biochemistry. 2nd Ed. New York, Worth, 1975, p. 752.)

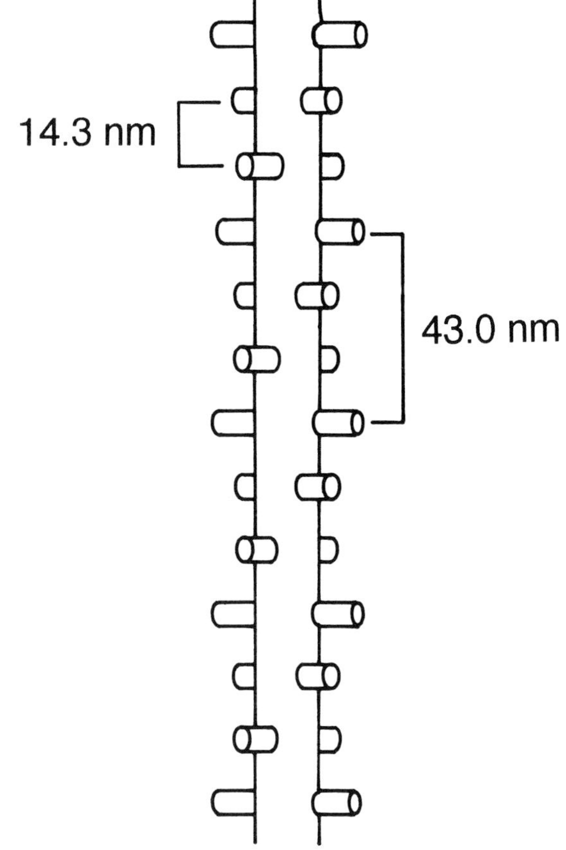


**Fig. 5–2.** *(Continued)*

At present, the best characterized inhibitory pathway is that mediated by cAMP. Cyclic AMP inhibits contractions by at least three mechanisms (12): (1) increased cAMP acting through its protein kinase, kinase-A, phosphorylates ML (Figure 5–4), and intracellular calcium-binding proteins; (2) phosphorylation of ML reduces its affinity for calcium calmodulin and prevents the activation of myosin light chains; and (3) phosphorylated calcium-binding proteins have a greater affinity for calcium, bind more of this ion, and reduce intracellular free calcium concentration. A less well-characterized mechanism is cAMP stimulation of calcium egress (13).

The mechanism by which receptor activation results in the formation of cAMP is the prototype for receptor-mediated responses that utilize similar receptor transducer systems (14). The components of the receptor adenylyl response cascade (Figure 5–10) are the receptor, a guanylyl nucleotide-sensitive transducing-protein complex, Gs, and the component that catalyzes the conversion of ATP to cAMP. Occupancy of the receptor by an agonist stimulates a conformational change facilitating receptor Gs interaction. Gs is a heterotrimer of α, β, and γ subunits. Receptor Gs interaction reduces the affinity of Gsa for GDP, which dissociates from its binding site and is replaced by GTP, present in excess intracellularly. The agonist receptor Gs complex dissociates as does the Gs heterotrimer. This allows Gsa to interact with the catalytic component and cAMP is generated. The system is recy-

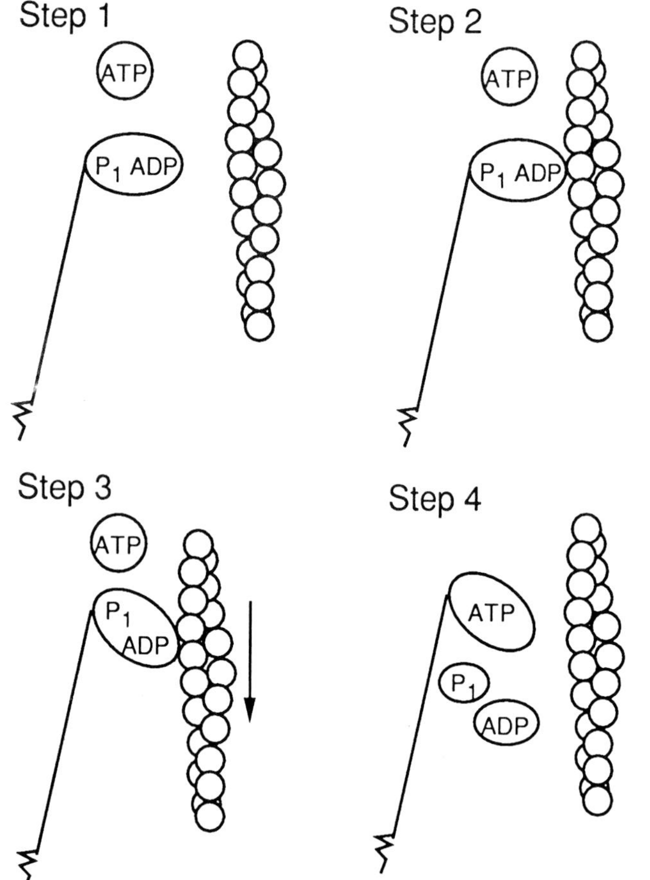


**Fig. 5–3.** Transduction of biochemical to mechanical energy. The energized myosin head binds to the active site of actin (Step 2), which induces conformational change as the myosin head assumes a 45° angle with the tail (Step 3). ADP and inorganic phosphorus ($P_1$) are exchanged for ATP and the interaction is terminated (Step 4). The head–tail configuration changes to a 90° angle with subsequent hydrolysis of ATP (Step 1). (Redrawn from Lenniger AL: Biochemistry. 2nd Ed. New York, Worth, 1975, p. 763.)

cled by the hydrolysis of GTP to GDP by a specific GTPase present on Gsa. The concentration of cAMP is further modified by the degradatory enzymes (phosphodiesterases) present intracellularly.

## Modification of Contractile Responses by Sex Steroids

A unique feature of myometrium is the modification of its structural and response characteristics by sex steroids. Progesterone and estrogen dramatically affect the contractility of the uterus by several mechanisms. In general, progesterone "quiets" the uterus, while estrogen facilitates the uterine response to contractile agents.

Progesterone uncouples the excitation-contraction potential of the cell membranes, suppresses the production of prostaglandins, and reduces the intracellular concentration of free calcium by causing this ion to be more tightly bound to cell membranes and intracellular organelles (15). Estrogen increases membrane potential (hyperpolarization) facilitating spontaneous depolarization by pacemaker cells, and promotes the formation of gap junctions, which aids the transmission of contractile stimuli. Estrogen also stimulates the production of contractile proteins and increases the generation of prostaglandins. In addition it can modify the response to specific contractile agonists, acting to increase the concentration of specific receptors or modifying transduction steps beyond the receptor to augment contractile responses (16).

## Uterine Relaxants

Preterm birth (birth before 37 completed weeks of gestation) remains a significant public health problem, accounting for approximately 80% of all deaths of otherwise healthy neonates. Approximately 9% of all births in the United States occur prematurely (17). In the majority of cases, preterm labor precedes preterm birth. If preterm labor (the presence of regular uterine contractions with progressive cervical effacement or dilation) can be diagnosed early, tocolytic therapy may decrease or obliterate uterine activity, prolonging gestation and avoiding the serious sequelae of a preterm birth. The number of available

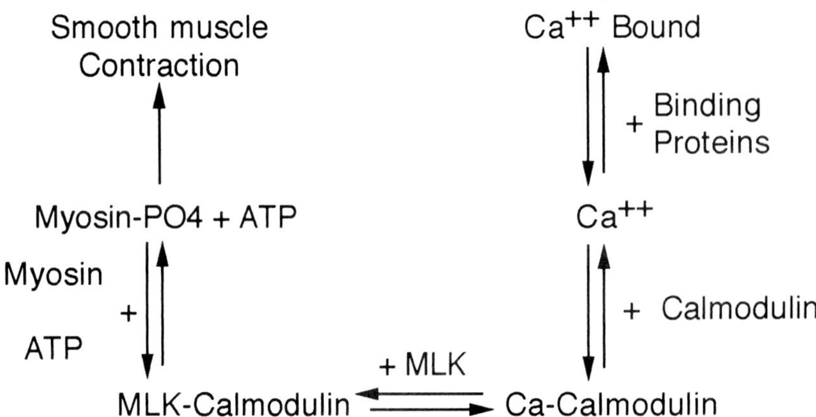


**Fig. 5–4.** Calcium calmodulin activation of myosin light chain kinase (MLK). Increased intracytoplasmic free calcium facilitates the binding of calcium to calmodulin. Calcium-calmodulin then binds to MLK, activating this enzyme that subsequently phosphorylates and activates myosin light chains leading to smooth muscle contraction.

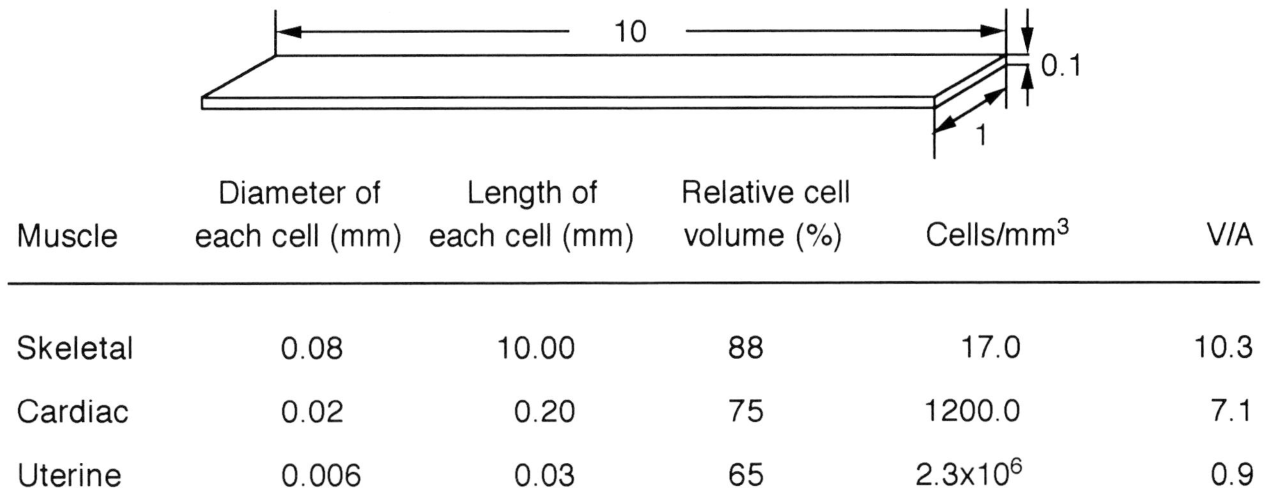


| Muscle | Diameter of each cell (mm) | Length of each cell (mm) | Relative cell volume (%) | Cells/mm$^3$ | V/A |
|---|---|---|---|---|---|
| Skeletal | 0.08 | 10.00 | 88 | 17.0 | 10.3 |
| Cardiac | 0.02 | 0.20 | 75 | 1200.0 | 7.1 |
| Uterine | 0.006 | 0.03 | 65 | $2.3 \times 10^6$ | 0.9 |

**Fig. 5–5.** Comparison of skeletal, cardiac, and uterine muscle. Based on a hypothetical preparation of 10 by 1 by 0.1 mm with a volume of 1 mm. (Redrawn from Kao CY: Electrophysiological properties of the uterine smooth muscle. *In* Biology of the Uterus. Edited by RM Wynn. New York, Plenum Press, 1977, p. 423.)

tocolytic medications has increased greatly in the past decade. Each of these drugs has side effects and anesthetic implications. The following descriptions of the different tocolytic medications will familiarize the anesthetist with the medications and address specific anesthetic issues.

## BETA ADRENERGIC AGENTS

### *History*

Betamimetic tocolytic agents are the most widely used class of tocolytic medications. Early pharmacological studies indicated that adrenergic agonists acting through beta adrenoreceptors could inhibit myometrial contractions in vitro. However, interactions of these agents with beta adrenoreceptors in other organ systems, primarily the cardiovascular system, made their clinical use impractical. The recognition of subtypes of beta receptors, with beta-1 adrenoreceptors primarily in the heart and beta-2 receptors in the uterus and other organs, encouraged the development of subtype selective beta adrenergic drugs. The use of beta agonists for the treatment of preterm labor began in the 1960s with the availability of the modestly selective beta-2 agonist, isoxsuprine (Vasodilan). Isoxsuprine was replaced in the 1970s by the more specific beta-2 agonist, ritodrine. This agent remains the only tocolytic that has been extensively tested for its efficacy and side effects and which is approved by the FDA (18,19,20). However, primarily because of lower cost, the beta-2 agonist, terbutaline, is used extensively by many practitioners. Although no beta adrenergic tocolytic has been as thoroughly tested as ritodrine, a large body of information indicates similar efficacy and side effects for both of these agents, as well as other beta agonists used outside of the USA, such as hexoprenaline, fenoterol, orciprenaline, and salbutamol (21). Ritodrine can be administered intravenously or orally; terbutaline intravenously, orally, or by subcutaneous infusion pump (22).

### *Mechanism of Action*

The tocolytic action of beta adrenergic agents can be largely explained by its activation of adenylyl cyclase leading to an increase in cAMP intracellularly (see Figure 5–10). An important consideration in the use of these agents is the propensity of beta adrenergic agonists to induce tachyphylaxis or desensitization (23). With continued exposure of beta receptors to beta agonists, the effectiveness of the drug decreases strikingly. Biochemically, this can be caused by a decrease in the number of receptors and a reduction in the ability of the remaining receptors to activate adenylyl cyclase (24).

### *Pharmacokinetics*

The synthetic betamimetic drugs are excreted in urine unaltered or as conjugates. Ritodrine has been most thoroughly studied. The initial rapid half-life of an intravenous injection of ritodrine is 5 to 10 minutes, followed by a second phase half-life of 1.5 to 2.5 hours. With oral medication, the bioavailability is about 30% of the intravenous route. The maximum serum concentration with this route is at 30 to 60 minutes with an initial half-life of 1 to 2 hours and a second phase decrease of 10 to 12 hours (25).

### *Indications and Efficacy*

The primary indication for these drugs is the treatment of preterm labor. They are also used prophylactically for fetal surgery or cervical cerclage, or to relax the uterus before external maneuvers to turn the fetus from the breech to vertex position. The anesthesiologist may also be faced with managing the woman who has been acutely medicated with beta agonists in an attempt to relieve fetal asphyxia secondary to uterine contractions before cesarean section (26). Another setting in which the anesthesiologist may have to deal with the acute effects of beta agonists is with acute uterine inversion. In this setting

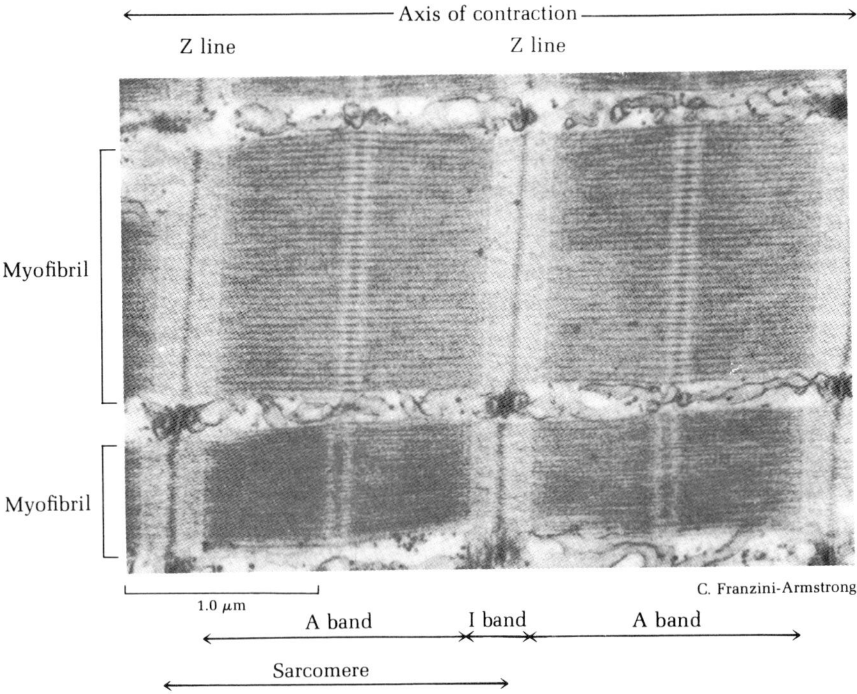


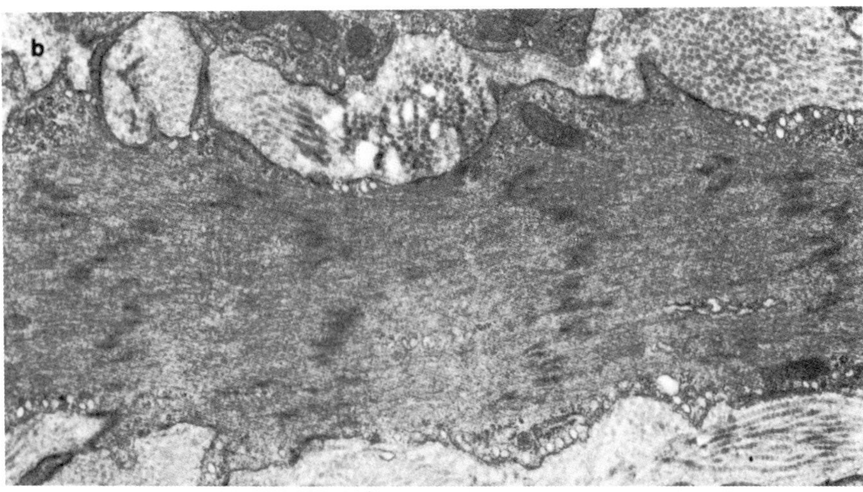


**Fig. 5–6.** Ultrastructure of skeletal and smooth muscles. Electron micrographs of frog skeletal muscle **(A)** and mouse myometrium **(B).** (**A** from Lenniger AL: Biochemistry. 2nd Ed. New York, Worth, 1975, p. 750; **B** from Schoenberg CF: The contractile mechanism and ultrastructure of the myometrium. *In* Biology of the Uterus. 2nd Ed. Edited by RM Wynn. New York, Plenum, 1977, p. 497.)

intravenous tocolytics are used to relax the uterus to allow manual restitution of normal uterine position.

Contraindications to the use of beta agonists include pulmonary hypertension, cardiac disease, hyperthyroidism, myasthenia gravis (27) or myotonia (28), and uncontrolled diabetes (29). With controlled placebo studies, the betamimetic medications can delay delivery for a minimum of several days, and in some studies, for weeks (30).

### Side Effects

The betamimetic drugs are derivatives of epinephrine, and many of their side effects can be understood from this perspective. Ideally, beta-2 adrenergic effects on the uterus are maximized and beta-1 effects minimized with these medications. However, the drugs available are selective, not specific, and at the doses used affect many responses mediated by beta-1 adrenoreceptors (Table 5–1).

The heart is a primary target for these effects, with stimulation of myocardial responses both by direct actions of the drug and by reflex responses to the vasodilatation secondary to activation of beta-2 receptors on vascular smooth muscle. The maternal heart rate increases by about 19 to 40 beats/minute and cardiac output is increased by 50%. The pulse pressure widens, with an increase in the systolic pressure of 12%, and a decrease in the diastolic pressure of 10% (31).

Serious cardiovascular complications can occur, including myocardial ischemia and arrhythmias. The most common cardiovascular complication is pulmonary edema, which occurs in 1 to 5% of women receiving these agents intravenously. This prevalence increases to as much as 50% with twin gestations. Pulmonary edema typically develops 36 to 72 hours after the initiation of therapy. This complication is caused by cardiac effects of the drug, so-

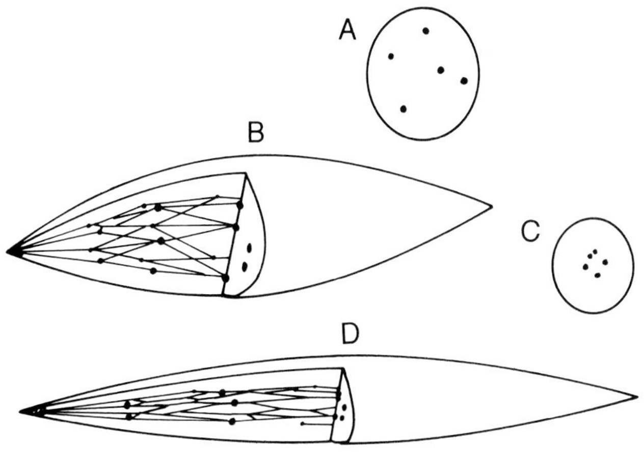


**Fig. 5–7.** Orientation of smooth muscle fibers (schematic representation of the orientation of myofibrils in resting (A, B = stretched muscle; C, D = smooth muscle). (Redrawn from Schoenberg CF: The contractile mechanism and ultrastructure of the myometrium. *In* Biology of the Uterus. 2nd Ed. Edited by RM Wynn. New York, Plenum, 1977, p. 497.)

dium and water retention secondary to beta-2 adrenergic stimulation of renin release, increased arginine vasopressin, and perhaps direct effects on endothelial permeability. It is often associated with iatrogenic fluid overload, maternal anemia, and the presence of amnionitis (32,33,34).

Stimulation of beta-2 adrenoreceptors leads to increased glycogenolysis, hyperglycemia, and hyperinsulinemia with secondary hypokalemia, as activation of the $K^+ - Na^+$ pump increases the entry of potassium into cells. The effects on serum potassium are usually limited to intravenous treatment and return to normal within 30 minutes of discontinuing therapy (35). Incomplete glycogenolysis, secondary to activation of this process in skeletal muscle, results in increased circulating lactate and occasionally lactic acidosis. Increased adrenergically stimulated lipolysis increases circulating free fatty acids. The summation of several of these effects is hypocalcemia, decreased pH, reduced colloid osmotic pressure, and dilutional anemia. Other frequent maternal side effects are tremor, headaches, nausea, vomiting, anxiety, and ileus (36).

Fetal effects include a slight tachycardia at high doses. Neonatally, hypoglycemia, hypocalcemia, ileus, and hypotension have been reported with the use of intravenous ritodrine (37).

To reduce the serious cardiovascular complications, careful maintenance of fluid balance (restricting total fluid intake to 2,400 cc/24 hours), monitoring of electrolytes (although not replacing $K^+$ unless the level is less than 2.5) and not allowing the maternal heart rate to exceed 130 beats/minute is mandatory. Betamimetic therapy must be immediately discontinued if the patient develops shortness of breath, chest pain or arrhythmia.

### *Anesthetic Considerations*

Before administering anesthetics to the patient being treated with betamimetics, specific issues must be addressed. Fluid balance must be carefully assessed, especially if major regional anesthesia (epidural or subarachnoid) is contemplated. The usual infusion of intravenous fluids prior to the use of regional anesthesia may contribute to pulmonary edema. See Figure 5–11. Also, vasodilatation secondary to the sympatholysis of the procedure itself may be additive to the cardiovascular effects of the beta agonists and can contribute to uteroplacental insufficiency. Electrolytes, CBC, and glucose should be mea-

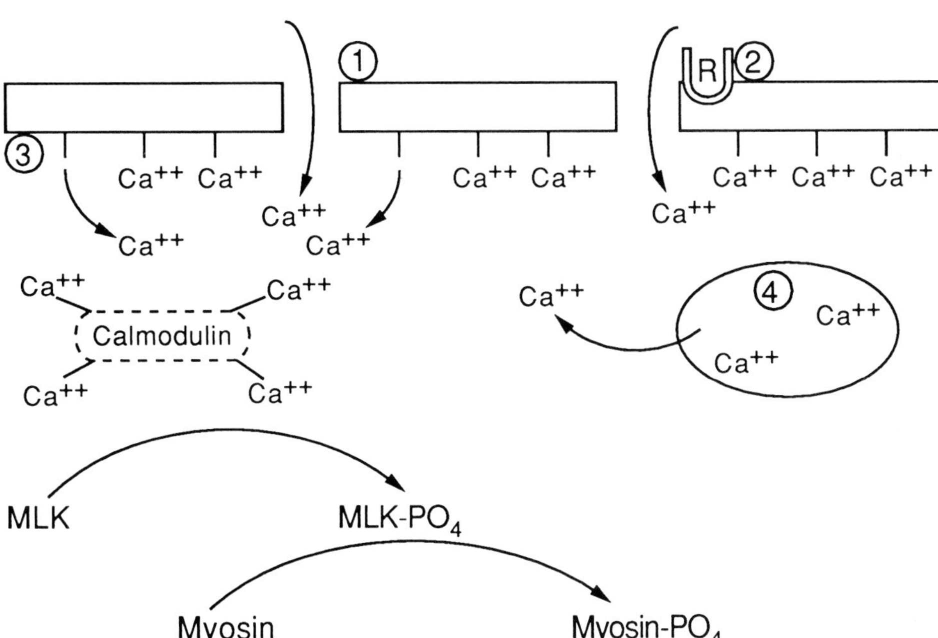


**Fig. 5–8.** Methods by which free calcium ($Ca^{++}$) concentration can be increased intracellularly. Calcium entry into the cell can be potentiated by either receptor-mediated (1) or voltage-dependent (2) calcium channels. Calcium can also be released from stores bound intracellularly, either on the plasma membrane (3) or in intracellular organelles (4). Calcium homeostasis is maintained by pumps that reduce intracellular concentration to resting levels (5). Reduction of the activity of such pumps also increases free calcium concentration.

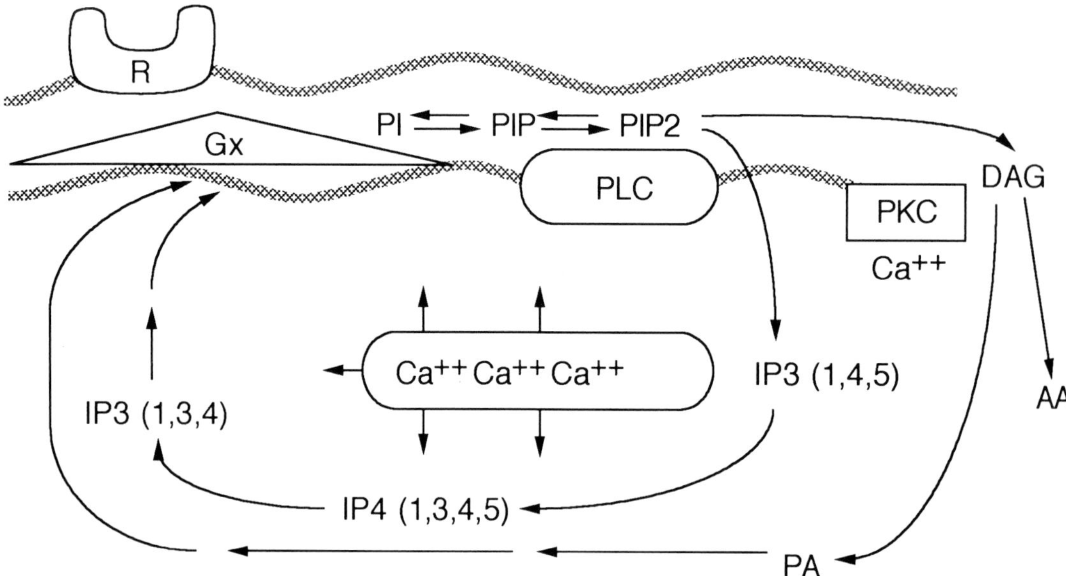


**Fig. 5–9.** Receptor-activated phosphatidylinositol 4,5-bisphosphate (PIP2) hydrolysis. Occupancy of the receptor (R) activates a PIP2-specific phospholipase-C (PLC), an effect mediated by a guanyl-nucleotide-sensitive transducing protein (Gx). The results of this hydrolysis are the generation of diacylglycerols (DAG) and inositol 1,4,5-triphosphate (IP3 1,4,5). IP3 1,4,5 stimulates the release of calcium ($Ca^{++}$) from nonmitochondrial intracellular stores. This phosphorylated sugar is metabolized to 1,3,4,5-tetraphosphate (IP4 1,3,4,5). Further metabolism generates 1,3,4-inositol triphosphate and, with sequential removal of the remaining phosphates, inositol is regenerated and reincorporated into phosphatidyl inositol (PI). The relative concentration of the phosphorylated forms of phosphatidylinositol (PI, PIP, PIP2) in the membrane is determined by the activity of specific kinases. The other product of PIP2 hydrolysis, diacylglycerol, interacts with protein kinase C (PKC), increasing its sensitivity to $Ca^{++}$. In addition, diacylglycerols can be further metabolized by lipases to release arachadonic acid (AA), which is contained in a high proportion of diacylglycerols in phosphatidylinositol.

sured preoperatively. A preoperative EKG in the woman receiving betamimetics may reveal the following: sinus tachycardia (96%), depression of S-T segment (70%), T-wave flattening or inversion (55%), and prolongation of QT interval (35%) (38,39).

Halothane anesthesia sensitizes the myocardium to the arrhythmogenic effects of the beta agonists medication and is contraindicated in these patients (40). Atropine and glycopyrrolate should be avoided as premedications, as they may increase the preexisting maternal tachycardia or arrhythmias, and pancuronium should be used with caution. Dextrose-free intravenous solutions are used to avoid increasing the hyperglycemia associated with betamimetic agents. Close attention should be directed to the volume of fluids administered so as not to increase the risks of pulmonary edema secondary to betamimetics. Magnesium sulfate, diazoxide, morphine, and meperidine may also potentiate the hypotensive effects of betamimetics.

## MAGNESIUM SULFATE

### History

Magnesium sulfate has been used extensively, for many years, to prevent seizures in the management of preeclampsia. Recently, a side effect of its use in this condition, the inhibition of uterine contractions, has been exploited and the drug used as treatment for preterm labor (41). In some institutions, because of familiarity with this common obstetrical medication and the undesirable side effects of betamimetic medications, magnesium sulfate has become the first line intravenous tocolytic.

### Mechanism of Action

Magnesium sulfate decreases smooth muscle activity by several mechanisms. In in vitro studies of vascular smooth muscle, elevated magnesium concentrations (about 9.6 mEq/liter) reduced resting vascular tone and contractile responses to several agonists. This phenomenon occurred in association with decreased entry of calcium into cells and enhanced egress of calcium out of cells. This is postulated to be secondary to increased magnesium binding to membranes, which interferes with calcium uptake, or perhaps competition with calcium for entry through calcium channels. In broken-cell preparations, magnesium also inhibits the calcium-sensitive ATPase involved in calcium egress (42). Although no such information has been generated for other tissues, similar mechanisms are postulated for myometrial cells and the cardiac conduction system. Magnesium also has a central depressant effect; it alters nerve transmission by decreasing acetylcholine release and reduces sensitivity at the motor endplate of skeletal muscle.

### Pharmacokinetics

The volume of distribution of magnesium is greater than extracellular fluid because magnesium also enters

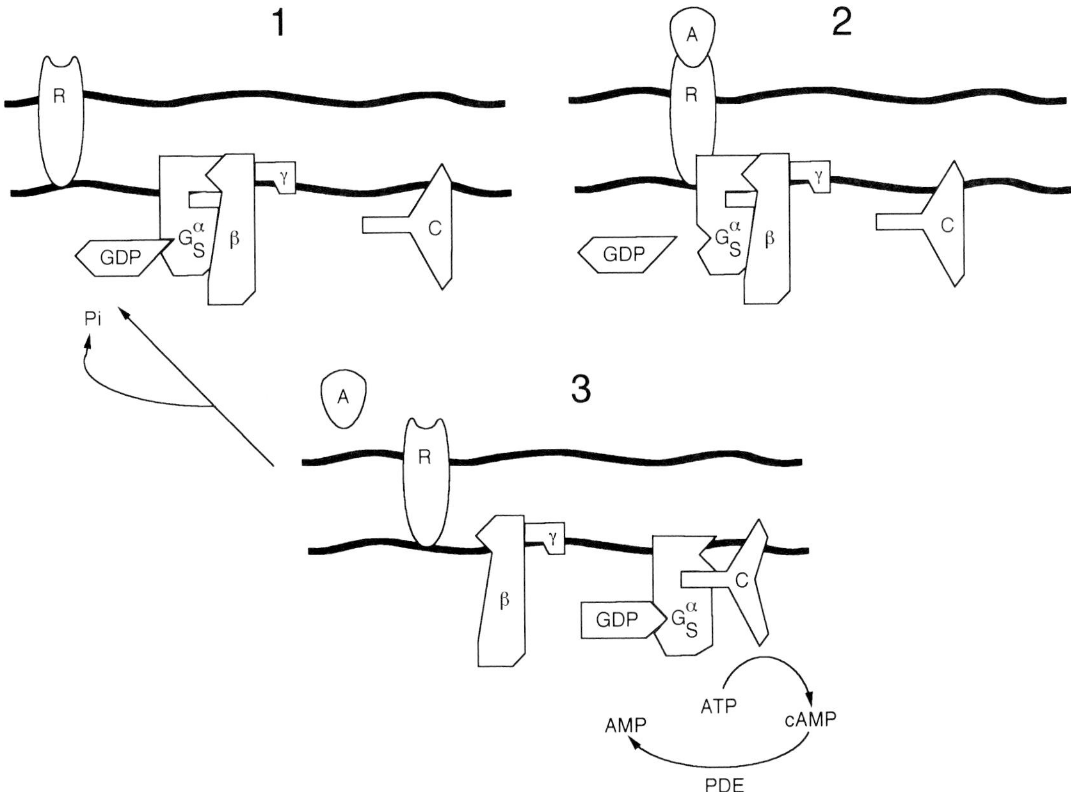


**Fig. 5–10.** Receptor-mediated activation of adenylate cyclase. In the unstimulated state (1), there is minimal interaction between the receptor (R) and the guanyl nucleotide-sensitive regulatory heterotrimer ($Gs_{\alpha,\beta,\gamma}$). In the heterotrimeric state, GDP (guanosine diphosphate) is bound to $Gs_\alpha$, and there is minimal interaction with the catalytic component of adenylate cyclase (C). With the binding of an agonist to the receptor (2), the interaction between R and the heterotrimer is facilitated. As a result of the interaction of R and $Gs_{\alpha,\beta,\gamma}$, the affinity of GDP is reduced and GDP dissociates. This form of Gs is very transient because GDP is rapidly replaced by GTP (Guanosine Triphosphate), which is present at high concentrations intracellularly (3). GTP reduces the affinity of $Gs_\alpha$ for $Gs_{\beta,\gamma}$ and the heterotrimer dissociates, allowing the interaction of $Gs_\alpha$ with C. This activates C, which catalyzes the conversion of ATP to cAMP, which is then subject to degradation by phosphodiesterases (PDE). Note that GTP reduces the affinity of R for Gs and the agonist for the receptor. The system is recycled by the hydrolysis of GTP to GDP and inorganic phosphorus (Pi).

bones and cells. Magnesium is minimally bound to protein and is almost exclusively excreted in urine. It is reabsorbed in the proximal tubule by a process limited by transport maximum ($T_{max}$). Its excretion increases as the filtered load exceeds $T_{max}$ (43). In patients with normal renal function the half-time for excretion is 4 hours. Because excretion is determined by the filtered load of magnesium, the time for excretion is prolonged in women with reduced glomerular filtration rate.

**Table 5–1.** Side Effects of Betamimetic Agents

| Beta-1 | Beta-2 |
|---|---|
| Cardiac | Smooth muscle relaxation |
| Inotropic | Gut (adynamic ileus) |
| Chronotropic | Blood vessels (hypotension) |
| Arrhythmogenic | Renal |
| Lipolytic | Increased renin release |
| Increased free fatty acid | Hepatic glycogenolysis |
| | Hyperglycemia |
| | Hyperinsulinemia |
| | Hypokalemia |
| | Skeletal muscle glycogenolysis |
| | Lactic acidosis |

With the administration of the usual 4 g loading dose, the resulting blood level is 3.5 mg/dl with a range of 1.6 to 4.8 mg/dl, determined largely by the volume of distribution and not renal function. Thus, the initial loading dose may be administered without knowledge of renal status. However, subsequent blood levels are determined by glomerular filtration and must be guided by the woman's renal function. This should be determined by an assessment of serum creatinine before therapy and adequate urine output (greater than 50 ml/hour) during therapy. Because the effect of magnesium upon neuromuscular transmission occurs at concentrations lower than those resulting in serious cardiac or respiratory problems (Table 5–2), the presence of deep tendon reflexes is a valuable marker of the approximate upper limit of serum magnesium concentration.

## *Indications and Efficacy*

In clinical trials, magnesium sulfate is as efficacious in treating preterm labor as betamimetic medications (44).

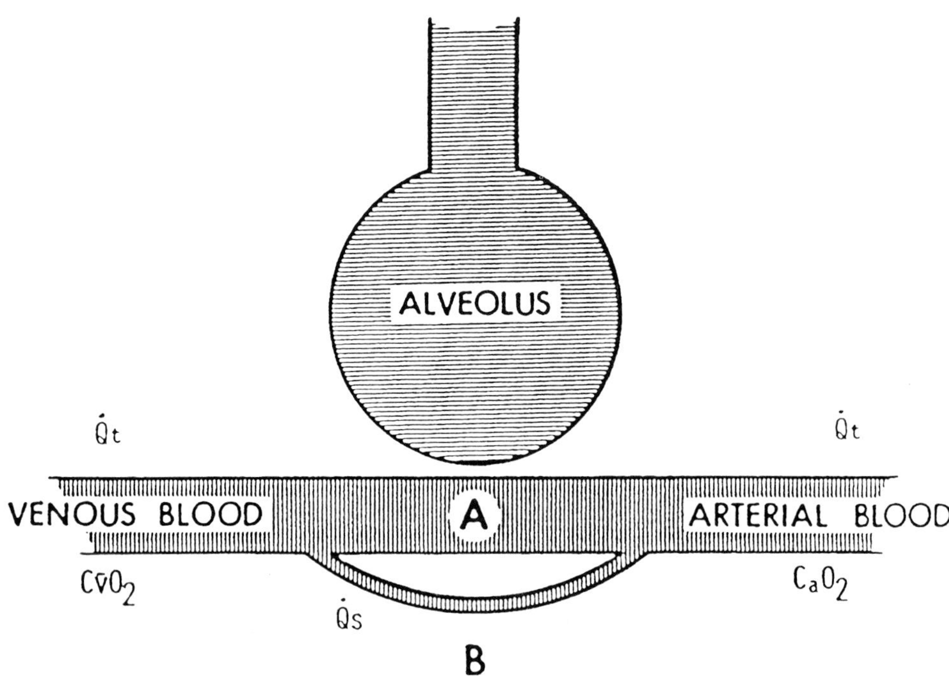


**Fig. 5–11.** Venous blood in the pulmonary circulation may pass through well-ventilated areas (A) or areas of low or absent ventilation (B). If cardiac output is reduced and/or systemic oxygen extraction increases, the venous oxygen content ($CvO_2$) will be less than normal. Any blood passing through B will reduce arterial oxygen content ($CaO_2$) below its normal value and $PaO_2$ will decrease. (Qs = shunted blood; Qt = cardiac output.) (With permission from Kirby RR: An overview of anesthesia and critical care medicine. *In* Anesthesia. 2nd Ed. Edited by RD Miller. New York, Churchill Livingstone, 1986, p. 2161.)

It is the drug of choice for tocolysis in women who have contraindications to betamimetic therapy, e.g., women with diabetes, or hyperthyroidism. Contraindications to magnesium sulfate treatment are heart block, myasthenia gravis, or myocardial damage (21,45). The drug must be used at lower doses and with frequent determination of blood levels in women with impaired renal function.

### Side Effects

The side effects of magnesium are caused by central actions and effects on the neuromuscular junction. The complications and corresponding serum levels of the drug are well established from the years of usage in the management of preeclampsia (Table 5–2). The most serious side effects of magnesium sulfate treatment are respiratory depression and cardiac arrest. Pulmonary edema has also been reported. As with the betamimetics, judicious management of fluid balance (i.e., less than 2,400 cc in 24 hours) may play an important role in avoiding pulmonary edema. Common side effects, especially with the loading dose, are due to vasodilatation by magnesium (flushing, transient decrease in blood pressure, sweating) and nausea. Other annoying side effects are vomiting, headache, and palpitations. Ileus can occur with prolonged administration. Serum calcium concentration is decreased by 25%, with an associated increase of parathyroid hormone (46). It is imperative that women treated with magnesium sulfate have serum magnesium levels determined serially, to avoid the serious complications of respiratory depression and cardiac arrest. Complications of elevated serum magnesium concentration can usually be reversed with calcium gluconate. One gram (10 ml of a 10% solution) injected over 5 to 10 minutes intravenously is usually effective. If this is unsuccessful renal dialysis may be necessary.

Hypocalcemia is also a potential neonatal problem, although not to the extent present in the mother (47). Despite concerns about the depressant effects of magnesium on neonatal respiration, this rarely occurs (48).

**Table 5–2.** Serum Magnesium Concentrations and Clinical Responses

| Clinical Response | Magnesium Concentration (mEq/L) |
|---|---|
| EKG changes | 5 to 10 |
| Areflexia | 10 to 12 |
| Respiratory arrest | 12 to 15 |
| Cardiac arrest | 25 |

### Anesthetic Considerations

Because of the effects of magnesium on smooth muscle, the neuromuscular junction, and central responses there are important considerations when administering anesthetics to women receiving this therapy. Increased serum levels of magnesium (7 to 11 mg/dl) can reduce anesthetic requirement by 20% (Figures 5–12 and 5–13) (49). Barbiturates and narcotics must be used cautiously because of additive effects of these agents and magnesium on respiratory depression. Magnesium also potentiates the response to depolarizing and nondepolarizing agents. Precurarization with nondepolarizing neuromuscular blockers before succinylcholine is **not recommended** as it may result in profound muscle weakness, loss of airway protective reflexes, and aspiration (49). Monitoring of neuromuscular blockade with a nerve stimulator is recommended during general anesthesia. Full reversal of the

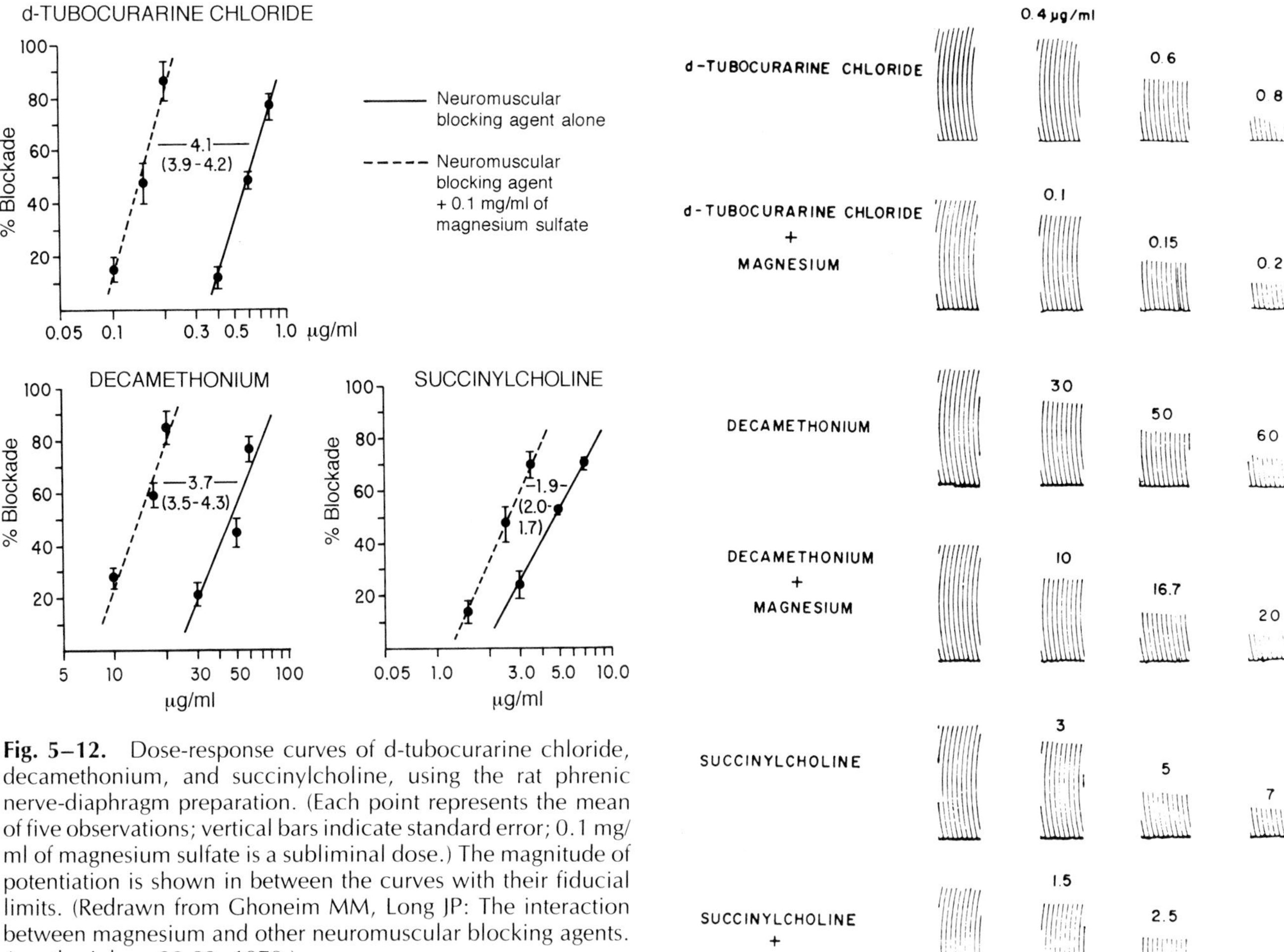


**Fig. 5–12.** Dose-response curves of d-tubocurarine chloride, decamethonium, and succinylcholine, using the rat phrenic nerve-diaphragm preparation. (Each point represents the mean of five observations; vertical bars indicate standard error; 0.1 mg/ml of magnesium sulfate is a subliminal dose.) The magnitude of potentiation is shown in between the curves with their fiducial limits. (Redrawn from Ghoneim MM, Long JP: The interaction between magnesium and other neuromuscular blocking agents. Anesthesiology 32:23, 1970.)

**Fig. 5–13.** Effects of magnesium on degrees of neuromuscular blockade produced by d-tubocurarine chloride, decamethonium, and succinylcholine. When a subliminal dose of magnesium (0.1 mg/ml) is added, the reduction in dosage of the other drugs required to produce a comparable degree of blockade is apparent. (From Ghoneim MM, Long JP: The interaction between magnesium and other neuromuscular blocking agents. Anesthesiology 32:23, 1970.)

neuromuscular blockade must be documented prior to extubation. Preoperatively, electrolytes, serum calcium, and fluid status should be carefully assessed. When interpreting EKG findings, it is important to take into account the effects of magnesium, including prolongation of the P-R interval, increased duration of the QRS complex, and increased height of the T-waves.

## CALCIUM CHANNEL BLOCKERS

### *History*

Calcium channel blockers have been used for many years to manage cardiac arrhythmias, ischemic myocardial disease, and hypertension. In the 1970s, calcium channel blockers were first used in Europe to treat preterm labor. Verapamil was the calcium channel blocker first used for this indication but was an ineffective tocolytic at tolerable doses (50). More recently, studies from Britain, Sweden, and the United States examined the calcium channel blocker nifedipine as a treatment for preterm labor (51).

### *Mechanism of Action*

Nifedipine blocks transmembrane calcium movement through voltage-sensitive calcium channels to reduce intracytoplasmic free calcium concentration. This blockade of transmembrane movement of calcium may also inhibit release of calcium from intracellular stores. This effect is, in theory, exerted on all tissues. Thus, the relaxation of vascular smooth muscle may lower blood pressure, and effects on the cardiac conduction system and inotropic responses could depress cardiac function. The likelihood of this response varies with the particular class of agent (Table 5–3). In practice, the depressant cardiac effects of nifedipine are countered by the reflex beta adrenergic response to vasodilatation, although in certain settings (valvular heart disease) myocardial depression may be evident (52). In addition, the combination of beta blockers and nifedipine is reported to be associated with hypotension, angina, and pulmonary edema (53), although this combination is used extensively in the treatment of hypertension without problems.

**Table 5–3.** Cardiovascular Effects of Calcium Channel Blockers

| | Diltiazem | Nifedipine | Verapamil |
|---|---|---|---|
| Arterial vasodilation | + + | + + + + | + + |
| Atrioventricular block | + + | 0 | + + + |
| Negative inotropic effect | + | + | + + |

### *Pharmacokinetics*

The absorption of nifedipine orally is 90%, with 65% bioavailability. It is metabolized by the liver, with 70 to 80% excreted by the kidneys as inactive metabolites. The peak concentration after oral administration is at 30 minutes, with a half-life for elimination of 2.5 hours (54). There is currently no parenteral preparation of nifedipine.

### *Indications and Efficacy*

There are not, as yet, a large number of clinical trials published on the use of nifedipine as a tocolytic. Preliminary studies suggest that nifedipine may be as effective as the betamimetics in treating preterm labor (55). On the basis of its known pharmacological effects, it might be a safe alternative in women with cardiovascular contraindications to betamimetics.

### *Side Effects*

The most common side effects are from arteriolar vasodilatation and decreased vascular resistance, which result in flushing, headache, nausea, reduced diastolic blood pressure, and occasionally dizziness (56). Significant hypotension has not been reported when the drug is used to treat preterm labor. Theoretically, there is an increased risk of postpartum hemorrhage, although this has not been reported. Elevated digoxin levels have been reported with concomitant digoxin nifedipine therapy (57). Nifedipine also interacts with cimetadine causing central nervous side effects. The combined use of magnesium and nifedipine has been associated with hypotension (58).

### *Anesthetic Considerations*

The effects of arteriolar dilation with decreased peripheral vascular resistance must be considered when administering anesthesia to women treated with nifedipine. Especially with regional anesthesia, accentuation of the decreased peripheral vascular resistance may lead to hypotension that might decrease uterine blood flow and adversely affect the fetus.

## PROSTAGLANDIN SYNTHESIS INHIBITORS

### *History*

The administration of prostaglandin synthetase inhibitors (PGSI) to inhibit preterm labor has recently been reevaluated for efficacy and safety, especially fetal side effects. In the 1970s, several case reports raised concerns about the possible role of the prostaglandin synthetase inhibitors, indomethacin, which caused premature closure of the fetal ductus arteriosus, resulting in persistent fetal circulation at birth. The results in these case reports were confounded by concurrent chorioamnionitis, fetal asphyxia from the birth process, and other fetal and neonatal problems (59). Recently, randomized trials and careful follow up of infants exposed to indomethacin confirm that this is a very effective tocolytic agent, used alone or in conjunction with another tocolytic agent, and is safe for the fetus in acute follow up (60,61,62). Nonetheless, there remain specific concerns. These include the possible constriction of the ductus arteriosus in utero and decreased fetal urine output (63,64). In most clinical trials, only a 48 to 72 hour course of indomethacin was undertaken, although in smaller studies, prolonged courses resulted in a benign outcome for the neonate (65).

### *Mechanism of Action*

Prostaglandins are produced by all tissues and in most cases act in a paracrine fashion on adjacent tissues. They are produced by a series of enzymatic reactions (Figure 5–14) from precursor arachidonic acid, either circulating or supplied by the activity of phospholipase-A2 and phospholipase-C upon endogenous phospholipids. Prostaglandin synthetase inhibitors affect the biochemical cascade of prostaglandin synthesis, at the prostaglandin synthase step. Thus, the agents currently used as tocolytics prevent the synthesis of all prostaglandins. They cross the placenta, and similar effects are exerted on the synthesis of fetal prostaglandins.

### *Pharmacokinetics*

Indomethacin is administered either by rectal suppository or orally for the treatment of preterm labor. Bioavail-

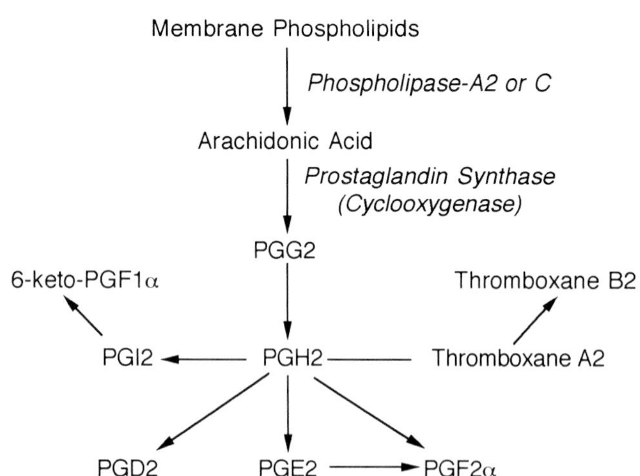


**Fig. 5–14.** Synthesis and metabolism of prostaglandins. The prostaglandin precursors, the major source of arachidonates, are from membrane phospholipids, either directly by the action of phospholipase A or indirectly by the formation of diacylglycerols by phospholipase C. The cyclo-oxygenase enzyme converts arachidonate to PGG2, which is subsequently converted to PGG and then to the specific prostaglandins by specific synthetic enzymes. (PG = prostaglandin; PGI = prostacycline.)

ability is complete with either route, with no evidence of first pass metabolism. The peak serum concentration with oral administration occurs between 30 minutes and 2 hours, and later and to lower peak concentration with rectal dosing. The range of plasma half-life is between 3.1 and 9.8 hours. There is no evidence of dose-dependent elimination. The fecal recovery of indomethacin has been reported to be 21 to 61%, from enterohepatic circulation. The remainder is eliminated by the kidneys (66).

### *Indications and Efficacy*

In view of concerns about the effect of prostaglandin synthetase inhibitors on fetal homeostatic functions, these agents are rarely the first line medication for the treatment of premature uterine contractions. When used, they are preferably restricted to a short course (1 to 3 days), either alone or supplementary to another tocolytic. If the preterm labor is refractory to more conventional therapy, prostaglandin synthetase inhibitors may be considered for long-term treatment, carefully weighing the known effects of delivery at the gestational age of the fetus in question against the largely unknown fetal effects of these agents. Prolonged administration must be accompanied by careful follow up of both maternal and fetal status, including renal function. In certain settings, the drugs are especially useful, probably reflecting their effect on the specific stimulant of uterine contraction. Thus, prophylactic treatment, shortly preoperatively and postoperatively for perturbations known to increase uterine prostaglandin production such as cervical cerclage placement or fetal surgery, is particularly effective. Some practitioners limit the use of prostaglandin synthetase inhibitors to gestations less than 32 weeks, because after this gestational age, the ductus may be most sensitive to the constricting effects of the drug (67).

### *Side Effects*

The most commonly reported side effects in pregnant women treated with prostaglandin synthetase inhibitors are nausea, vomiting, dyspepsia, occasional epistaxis, and maculo-papular skin eruption. Hyperkalemia and hypernatremia have been reported in nonpregnant adults treated with prostaglandin synthetase inhibitors, attributed to the effect of the drug on the proximal and distal tubule of the kidney (68), as have effects on GFR, as reflected by increased serum creatinine (69). Other side effects reported in nonpregnant patients chronically exposed to prostaglandin synthetase inhibitors include abdominal pain, anorexia, aplastic anemia, diarrhea, frontal headaches, mental confusion, hepatitis, neutropenia, fluid retention, thrombocytopenia, and ulcerative lesions of the bowel (70). Nonetheless, of major concern are the recognized side effects upon the fetus (oliguria and constriction of the ductus arteriosus) (71) and the unknown consequences of disrupting components of fetal homeostasis dependent on fetal or maternal prostaglandin synthesis.

### *Anesthetic Considerations*

The pregnant woman treated with prostaglandin synthetase inhibitors, who requires an anesthetic, should

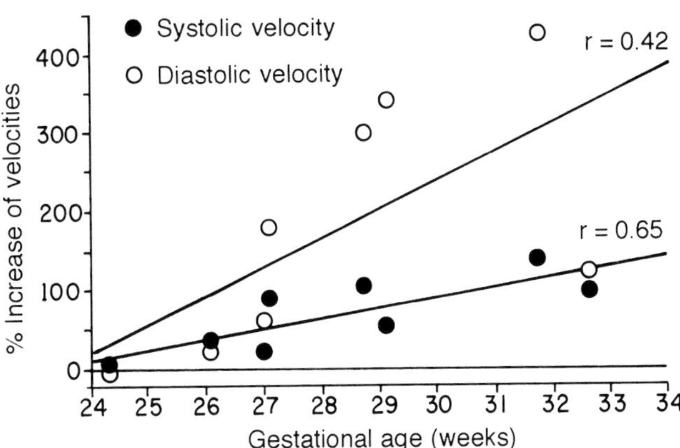


**Fig. 5–15.** Percentage increases of systolic and diastolic velocities in fetal ductus during maternal indomethacin treatment. (Redrawn from Eronen M, Pesonen E, Kurki T, Ylikorkala O, and Hallman M: The effects of indomethacin and a sympathomimetic agent on the fetal ductus arteriosus during treatment of premature labor. A randomized double-blind study. Am. J. Obstet. Gynecol. 164:141, 1991.)

have a thorough a preoperative evaluation based on the recognized effects of prostaglandin synthetase inhibitors. Laboratory assessment includes a CBC with platelet count, (in light of the known alterations of platelet function it is important to exclude coexistent thrombocytopenia), liver function tests, electrolytes, and serum creatinine. A baseline neurological exam should be done to rule out any existing altered mental status caused by the drug. Prophylactic antacids are especially important because gastritis may be associated with the drug. Careful monitoring of fluids is necessary because of the effects of prostaglandin synthetase inhibitors on renal function. Figure 5–15 demonstrates the effect of maternal indomethacin treatment on the systolic and diastolic velocities in fetal ductus.

## LESS COMMONLY USED TOCOLYTIC AGENTS

### *Phosphodiesterase Inhibitors*

Phosphodiesterase inhibitors (e.g. aminophylline) are occasionally used as tocolytic agents. These agents slow the degradation of cAMP, thus increasing cAMP with attendant uterine relaxation. They potentiate the effects of beta adrenergic agonists.

Potential maternal side effects are nausea and restlessness. Serious toxicity can occur (convulsions, ventricular arrhythmias) at high serum concentrations of the drug, indicating the importance of monitoring serum levels. Halothane anesthesia in conjunction with aminophylline can induce sinus tachycardia or arrhythmia. Toxic potentiation of the effects of ephedrine or betamimetic agents may also occur. Caution should be used when aminophylline is administered to patients with impaired liver function. Maternal contraindications include severe cardiac disease, hypertension, hyperthyroidism, and a history of peptic ulcer disease.

### *Combined Tocolytic Agents*

Single agent tocolytic therapy fails in approximately 20 to 40% of patients. One approach to this problem is to use multiple tocolytic agents either sequentially or concurrently. The latter approach is especially pertinent to the anesthesiologist because of additive or synergistic accentuation of side effects of these drugs.

Clinical trials have tested the simultaneous administration of beta agonists and magnesium sulfate (72,73), nifedipine and terbutaline (74), and ritodrine and indomethacin (75). Although some of the trials suggest a greater efficacy than single agents, this is at the price of substantially increased side effects (76).

Another approach is to replace the failed tocolytic with a tocolytic with a different mechanism of action (e.g., substituting magnesium for a beta agonist). It appears that this approach can safely prolong gestation longer than the use a single agent (77).

## OXYTOCICS

Oxytocic drugs have been used for many centuries, beginning with ergotate, continuing with the development of synthetic oxytocin, and now broadening with the prostaglandins $E_2$ and $F_{2\alpha}$. It is important that the anesthetist be familiar with each category so that the indications for the use of the drug will result in more benefit than risk to the pregnant patient and her fetus. The following section will discuss each category and the anesthetic implications.

### Oxytocin

#### *History*

The use of oxytocin in obstetrics is based on observations from the early twentieth century. In 1906, Dale recognized the contractile effects of pituitary extracts on myometrium (78). The "hormone" that Bell named "Pituitrin" (79) contained both oxytocin and vasopressin and certain properties were inappropriately attributed to oxytocin. Many of these misconceptions persist in clinical folklore to the present. Thus, women receiving synthetic oxytocin continue to have blood pressure frequently monitored because of the mistaken concept that oxytocin has a hypertensive effect. In 1953, du Vigneaud (80) determined the biochemical structure of oxytocin and the pure synthetic substance (Syntocinon) was manufactured.

#### *Mechanism of Action*

Oxytocin acts both directly and indirectly to cause uterine contractions. Activation of myometrial oxytocin receptors stimulates contraction and similar receptors in the uterine mucosa (decidua) release prostaglandins with contractile activity (81). Although the mechanism by which this is accomplished is not completely established, it appears that an important part of oxytocin action is mediated by the activation of receptor-linked phospholipase-C (see Figure 5–9). In myometrial cells the active second message is 1,4,5, IP3, which releases calcium from intracellular stores, while in decidual cells the diacylglycerols produced serve as a source of arachidonic acid for the generation of prostaglandins (82). Another reported mechanism is the inhibition of calcium egress from myometrial cells (83).

An important component determining oxytocin response is the modulation of oxytocin-receptors concentration by estrogen and progesterone. Estrogen increases the concentration of receptors increasing oxytocin sensitivity, while progesterone has the opposite effect (84). In humans, the recognized increase in oxytocin sensitivity with advancing gestation is accompanied by a twelvefold increase in oxytocin-receptors concentration between the second trimester and 36 weeks of gestation. Because the concentration of oxytocin does not increase before labor, this increased oxytocin-receptors concentration in late gestation has rekindled interest in oxytocin as a potential signal for the onset of parturition.

Previous studies have documented increased oxytocin concentration only in the second stage of labor (85). This increase, which appears to be neurally mediated as it can be blunted by epidural anesthesia, is of unknown significance in labor (85). The clinical impact (if any) of blockade of increased oxytocin secretion with regional anesthesia is probably minimal compared to the effects of such anesthesia on reflex voluntary expulsive efforts.

#### *Pharmacokinetics*

Oxytocin is rapidly degraded by a peptidase present in high concentration in the blood of pregnant women (86). The half-life of oxytocin in maternal blood is 10 minutes. This rapid degradation is the predominant factor determining the time to steady state, which, by both theoretical predictions (circa 4 half-lives) and actual measurement, is 40 minutes (87).

#### *Indications and Efficacy*

Oxytocin is used for the induction or augmentation of labor and for treatment of postpartum hemorrhage. It is also used as a stimulator of uterine contractions to assess fetal well-being (contraction stress test) and to stimulate milk "let down" for breast feeding. Oxytocin has been used for labor induction since the early twentieth century. During the early years of use, oxytocin was delivered by several different routes (intramuscularly, intranasally, and as buccal tablets). The significant variation in uterine sensitivity to oxytocin makes potential overdose by these routes both likely and difficult to reverse. The short half-life of intravenous oxytocin (about 10 minutes) and the development of accurate, controlled methods of delivery of the intravenous medication makes the use of other routes for the induction or augmentation of labor obsolete. When used appropriately (see Side Effects) virtually all women will achieve adequate uterine activity with intravenous oxytocin. The rare exceptions are probably explained by cervical factors (failure of the cervix to undergo biochemical changes necessary for dilatation) or fetopelvic disproportion. Oxytocin used as prophylaxis or therapy for postpartum hemorrhage is also usually administered intravenously; however, intramuscular administration is also safe in this setting. On some occasions, women have difficulty establishing the milk "let down" factor in the cascade of events necessary for successful breast feeding. Intranasal oxytocin can be used to facilitate this series of reactions. Contraindications to oxytocin relate to its use to induce or augment labor and include evidence of fetal distress or the presence of a contracted pelvis (absolute fetopelvic disproportion).

## Side Effects

The side effects of oxytocin relate primarily to its activity to increase the frequency and amplitude of uterine contractions. In the past, oxytocin was used frequently at dosages 5 to 50 times higher than the currently recommended dose. At these dosages uterine rupture was a reported complication. In current practice this is an extremely rare complication. Similarly, fetal trauma indicated by hyperbilirubinemia is a previously reported complication that is not reported with current usage. The major current complication is fetal asphyxic distress related to uterine hyperstimulation. With uterine contractions, the blood supply to the intervillus space is transiently interrupted. With normal contraction frequency (about 3/10 minutes) and with the return of uterine tonus to resting levels between contractions, this does not result in significant hypoxemia in the healthy fetus. However, if contractions are more frequent than every 2 minutes, even normal fetuses will display fetal heart rate evidence of distress. Similarly, if uterine tonus remains elevated between contractions, fetal asphyxic distress can occur in normal fetuses. The former anomaly can be detected simply by palpation or external tocodynanometry to determine contraction frequency. The return of uterine tonus to resting levels is impossible to detect with these techniques and difficult to diagnose with conventional intrauterine pressure monitoring methods.

With oxytocin delivery rates of greater than 8 mU/minute, precise measurement of intrauterine pressure will frequently reveal increased uterine tonus. However, with conventional equipment, which may not accurately determine uterine tonus, it is mandatory to monitor fetal heart rate continuously with oxytocin doses higher than 8 mU/minute. Many of the problems of uterine hyperstimulation can be avoided with oxytocin dosing based on the established pharmacokinetics of the drug. Oxytocin should be started at low delivery rates (1 mU/minute) and increased only when sufficient time has elapsed to achieve steady-state concentration (40 minutes) (88).

Another important oxytocin side effect is caused by activation of renal vasopressin receptors leading to the retention of free water. At 16 mU/minute of oxytocin the antidiuretic effect is equivalent to the maximal effect of arginine vasopressin. Thus, the pregnant woman receiving oxytocin is at risk for water intoxication (89). This complication is easily avoided by either limiting fluid input or even more simply avoiding the use of hypotonic fluids.

The affinity of oxytocin for vascular vasopressin receptors is substantially lower than its affinity for the renal receptors, and synthetic oxytocin does not increase blood pressure. In fact, the major cardiovascular complication of oxytocin is hypotension resulting from myocardial depression with extremely high doses (e.g. 10 units administered as an intravenous bolus!) of oxytocin (90,91). Rapid intravenous injections of synthetic oxytocin are shown to cause an increase in the heart rate and a decrease in blood pressure, as shown in Table 5–4 (91). There is no significant difference between the responses in patients receiving repeated injections of synthetic oxytocin, as shown in Table 5–5. Figure 5–16 shows the typical response to rapid injection of oxytocin. Anaphylactoid reaction to oxytocin has been described, hypotension being a major issue (treated with epinephrine) (Figure 5–17) (92). A patient whose blood pressure approaches shock is in possible danger when given large IV doses of oxytocin, as shown in Figure 5–18.

## Anesthetic Considerations

Prior to a cesarean section it is important to assess the fluid volume and electrolyte status of the woman who has undergone extended oxytocin induction or augmentation.

In addition, oxytocin should usually not be administered postpartum until after the placenta has delivered, as

**Table 5–4.** Mean Effects of Synthetic Oxytocin in 22 Patients

| Time | Systolic Blood Pressure (mm Hg) | | Diastolic Blood Pressure (mm Hg) | | Heart Rate (beats/min) | |
|---|---|---|---|---|---|---|
| | | Mean difference | | Mean difference | | Mean difference |
| Before oxytocin | 121 | | 69 | | 95 | |
| | | −41* | | −28* | | +14* |
| 30 seconds following oxytocin | 80 | | 41 | | 109 | |
| | | +34* | | +23* | | −11** |
| 2 minutes, 36 seconds following oxytocin | 114 | | 64 | | 98 | |

The means of the maximal changes in systolic and diastolic blood pressures and in heart rate after rapid intravenous injection of 10 units synthetic oxytocin in 22 patients following delivery by cesarean section. The time of onset of the maximal effects varied between 18 and 52 seconds (average 36 seconds), and the duration of the effects varied from 1 to 6 minutes (average 2 minutes, 36 seconds).

* $P < 0.001$

** $P < 0.01$

(From Andersen TW, De Padua CB, Stenger V, Prystowsky H: Cardiovascular effects of rapid intravenous injection of synthetic oxytocin during elective cesarean section. Clin. Pharm. Ther. 6:345, 1965.)

**Table 5–5.** Comparison of Mean Effects of Repeated Oxytocin Injections in 5 Patients

| | Mean Arterial Pressure (mm Hg) | Mean difference | Heart Rate (beats/min) | Mean difference | Cardiac Output (L/min) | Mean difference | Stroke Volume (ml) | Mean difference | Total Peripheral Resistance (MAP/CO/sec) | Mean difference |
|---|---|---|---|---|---|---|---|---|---|---|
| First injection | −21* | | +2 | | 1.26** | | +13 | | −0.412*** | |
| | | 7 | | 5 | | 0.08 | | 5 | | 0.103 |
| Second injection | −14*** | | +7 | | 1.18** | | +8 | | −0.309*** | |

The mean effects of the initial and a repeat intravenous injection of 10 units synthetic oxytocin on mean arterial pressure (MAP), heart rate, cardiac output (CO), stroke volume, and total peripheral resistance (TPR) are shown. Both oxytocin injections caused significant changes in MAP, CO, and TPR. There were no significant differences in responses to the two injections. The time interval between the two injections varied from 4 to 32 minutes (average 18 minutes).
* $0.02 > P > 0.01$
** $P < 0.001$
*** $0.05 > P > 0.02$
(From Anderson T, et al: Clin. Pharm. Ther. 6:345, 1965.)

the uterus may contract prematurely leading to retained placenta.

## PROSTAGLANDINS

### *History*

In the 1930s a gynecologist, Rafael Kuzrock, discovered an agent in semen that stimulated uterine contractions. Because this material was eventually isolated from prostatic secretions it was termed prostaglandin. It was soon evident that there were many prostaglandins and that these ubiquitous substances were found in virtually all tissues. The activities of prostaglandins include not only contraction or relaxation of smooth muscle, but also secretion, platelet activation, and inflammation. With the availability of synthetic prostaglandins, the role of prostaglandin therapy has expanded in obstetrics, including pregnancy termination, cervical ripening (preinduction cervical shortening, softening, and dilation), and treatment for uterine atony with postpartum hemorrhage.

### *Mechanism of Action*

The two important prostaglandins in obstetrics are prostaglandin $F_{2\alpha}$ ($PGF_{2\alpha}$) and prostaglandin $E_2$ ($PGE_2$)

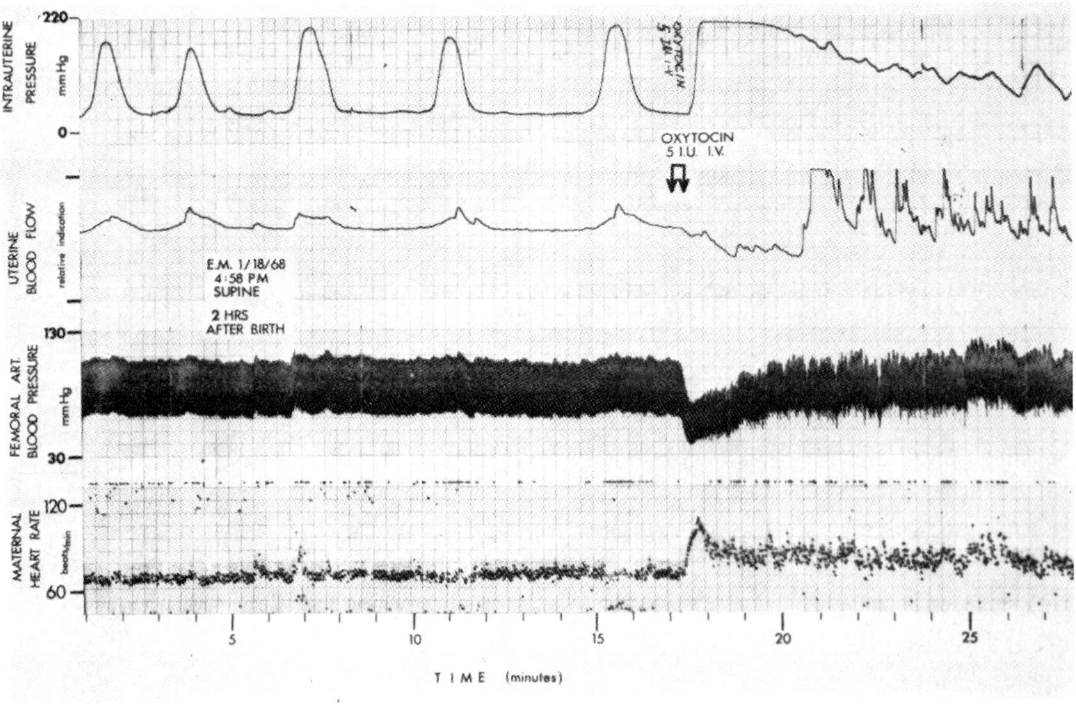


**Fig. 5–16.** The rapid injection of 5 IU of oxytocin intravenously was followed promptly by a tetanic type of uterine contraction (top line), a significant alteration in relative uterine blood flow (second line), a dramatic fall in the arterial blood pressure from 115/60 to 72/38 (third line), and an equally pronounced transient increase in the fetal heart rate (bottom line). (From Hendricks CH, Brenner WE: Cardiovascular effects of oxytocic drugs used postpartum. Am. J. Obstet. Gynecol. 108:751, 1970.)

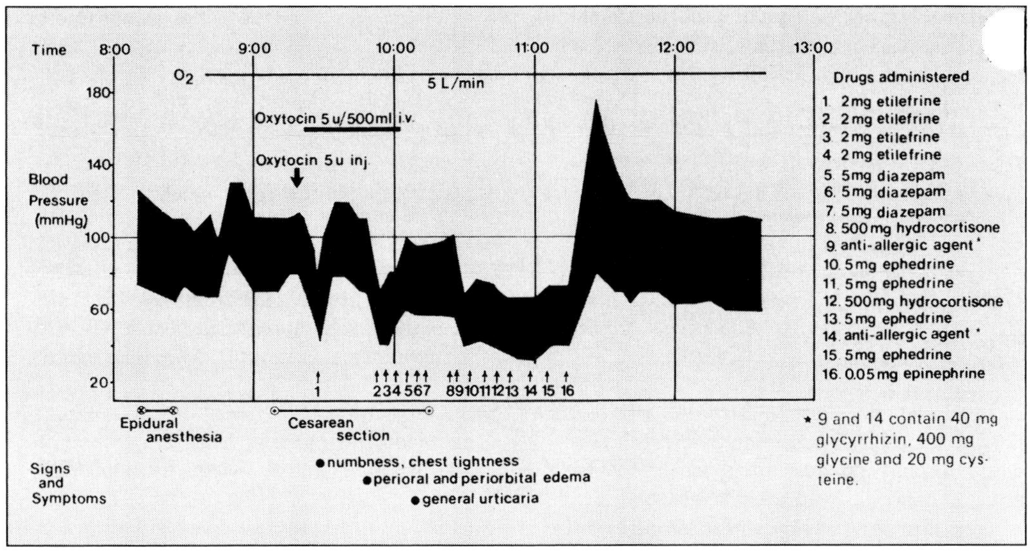


**Fig. 5–17.** Summarized clinical course in the patient. (From Kawarabayashi T, Narisawa Y, Nakamura K, Sugimori H, et al: Anaphylactoid reaction to oxytocin during cesarean section. Gynecol. Obstet. Invest. 24:277, 1988.)

(see Figure 5–14). $PGF_{2\alpha}$ causes the uterus to contract and also constricts the smooth muscle of blood vessels, the gastrointestinal tract, and bronchioles. By contrast, $PGE_2$ also causes contraction of the uterus and gastrointestinal tract, but relaxes smooth muscle of the bronchial tree and has minimal effects on vascular smooth muscle (93). $PGE_2$ has an important additional effect for obstetric purposes. It has a direct effect (independent of its contractile activity) on cervical collagen, increasing ground substance and separating collagen bundles to "ripen" the cervix, making it more easily distensible (94). Interestingly in spite of its long usage and ubiquitous activities, the biochemical mechanism by which prostaglandins establish these responses is not clearly established. Preliminary findings suggest that many of these responses may be mediated by activation of phospholipase-C (see Figure 5–9).

### Pharmacokinetics

Native prostaglandins are rapidly metabolized by enzymes in the lung and liver. These enzymes metabolize about 90% of the compounds in one circulation (95). The substitution of the 15 methyl group, e.g., 15 methyl $PG_{2\alpha}$, inhibits the first, most rapid, degradation step by inactivating the enzymatic oxidation of the C 15 hydroxyl group, yielding longer-acting compounds.

### Indications and Efficacy

Indication for the use of $PGE_2$ and $PGF_{2\alpha}$ is primarily pregnancy termination. Most trials of labor induction with these agents indicate they are no more efficacious than oxytocin and have substantially more side effects (96). Their use is currently reserved for preterm pregnancy termination or as induction after fetal demise. In this setting they offer an advantage over oxytocin, because the uterus is responsive to prostaglandins throughout gestation. $PGE_2$, as a low-dose intravaginally administered gel, is also useful before oxytocin induction, taking advantage of the ability of $PGE_2$ at low doses to preferentially effect cervical ripening rather than smooth muscle contractions. Either of these agents can be used as treatment of postpar-

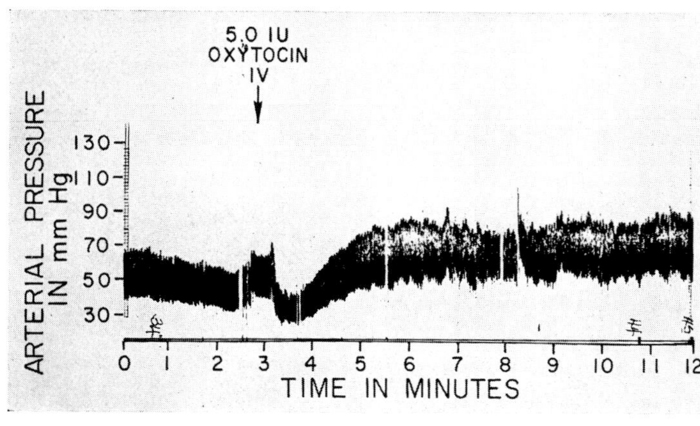


**Fig. 5–18.** Effect of oxytocin in postpartum hemorrhage. In one patient (18 minutes postpartum) already hemorrhaging and with blood pressure approaching shock levels, the administration of 5 IU of oxytocin in a single intravenous dose brought about a brief but significant additional further depression of the blood pressure to a level of 44/26. (From Hendricks CH, Brenner WE: Cardiovascular effects of oxytocic drugs used postpartum. Am. J. Obstet. Gynecol. 108:751, 1970.)

tum uterine atony. In view of their short circulatory half-life and ability to be absorbed and act locally, they are usually administered vaginally or directly into myometrium (97). The methyl ester of PGF with prolonged half-life in the circulation can be administered by intramuscular injection (98). Contraindications to the use of prostaglandins include known hypersensitivity to the agents, active cardiac, pulmonary or hepatic disease, or a fundal uterine scar. $PGF_{2\alpha}$ but not $PGE_2$ is contraindicated in women with a history of asthma. If $PGE_2$ is to be used for cervical ripening in a setting in which fetal compromise is suspected, the ability of the fetus to tolerate contractions must be determined before its administration. This is most safely accomplished by controlled oxytocin infusion.

### Side Effects

As with any uterotonic agent, uterine rupture has been reported with the use of prostaglandins. However, $PGE_2$ has been used to safely terminate pregnancy in a large series of women with prior low-segment uterine incisions (99). In the doses used to stimulate uterine contractions, all have significant side effects. These include fever, nausea, vomiting, diarrhea, hypertension, and with $PGF_{2\alpha}$ bronchospasm. Many of these problems can be reduced by predosing with antiemetic and antipyretic agents.

### Anesthetic Considerations

Administration of the prostaglandin $F_{2\alpha}$ has anesthetic implications, both respiratory and cardiovascular. $PGF_{2\alpha}$ decreases vital capacity, forced expiratory volume, and expiratory flow rates in both nonasthmatic and asthmatic patients (100). Acute hypertension has been reported with the intramyometrial administration of $PGF_{2\alpha}$ for uterine atony at the time of cesarean section (101).

## ERGOT ALKALOIDS

### History

For over 2000 years, ergots have been recognized as potent stimulators of uterine activity. Ergot is a product of the fungus *Claviceps purpurea*, which grows on rye and other grain. Currently, three preparations of ergots are used in obstetrics for the treatment of uterine atony: methylsergide maleate (oral), ergonovine maleate (injectable and oral), and methylergonovine maleate (injectable and oral). Figure 5–19 shows the uterine and cardiovascular response to a 0.2 mg injection of ergonovine.

### Mechanism of Action

The ergot alkaloids are α-adrenergic agonists and stimulate the contraction of smooth muscle through the receptor specific phospholipase-C (see Figure 5–9). They increase the force and frequency of uterine contractions, often causing a sustained contraction (102).

### Pharmacokinetics

The peak effect of orally administered ergot preparations is at 2 hours. The rate of clearance of ergot from the plasma corresponds to hepatic blood flow, as 90% of these drugs are excreted in bile. The clinical response to intramuscular administration is at approximately 5 minutes and to an oral dose, 20 minutes. Ergot alkaloids should never be administered intravenously, because of complications secondary to acute vascular constriction.

### Indications and Efficacy

Ergot alkaloids are commonly used for the prevention and treatment of postpartum hemorrhage. Currently the preventive use of ergots has been largely abandoned because of their potent side effects (103,104). They are commonly the second line drug (after oxytocin) to treat postpartum hemorrhage. Ergot alkaloids are never used before the delivery of the fetus, because sustained uterine contractions compromise placental perfusion. Similarly, ergots administered before the delivery of the placenta substantially increase the risk of placental entrapment. These agents are contraindicated in women with hypertension or a history of hypertension, and who are especially susceptible to increased vascular constriction by activation of vascular α-adrenergic receptors (105). This phenomenon reduces tissue perfusion and increases blood pressure with the attendant risk of myocardial or cerebral ischemia, or intracranial bleeding. Women with Raynaud's phenomenon also may have profound digital

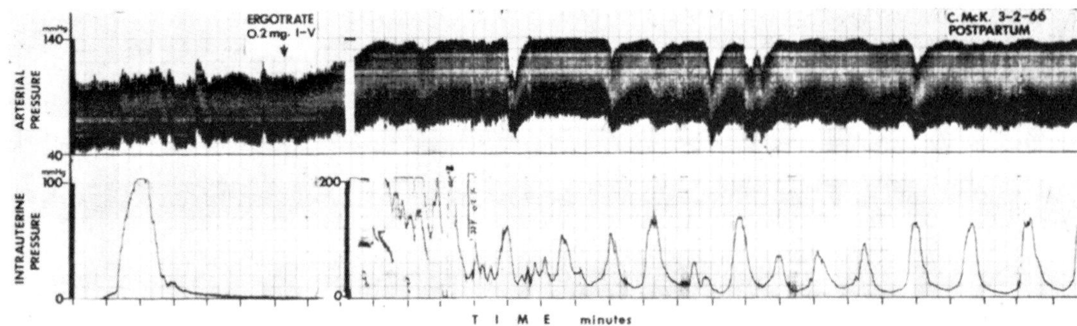


**Fig. 5–19.** The administration of 0.2 mg of ergonovine maleate intravenously was followed by a substantial rise in the blood pressure within 3 minutes after injection (top line) and an enormous increase in uterine contractility (bottom line). (From Hendricks CH, Brenner WE: Cardiovascular effects of oxytocic drugs used postpartum. Am. J. Obstet. Gynecol. 108:751, 1970.)

ischemia and necrosis. Other contraindications to ergot alkaloids include obliterative vascular disease and hepatic or renal disease (106).

### Side Effects

The major side effects of ergot alkaloids are caused by the stimulation of α-adrenergic receptors on gut and vascular smooth muscle. Complications include myocardial infarction, hypertensive crisis, and convulsions (107,108,109). In addition to the severe side effects, when the drugs are administered to women in whom the drug is contraindicated, common and less serious problems are headache, nausea, vomiting, diarrhea, dizziness, weakness, pruritus, and cold skin (110).

### Anesthetic Considerations

The anesthetist is commonly called upon to administer ergot alkaloids in the acute situation of uterine atony. It is imperative that the patient be assessed to determine the safety of the administration of these agents. This includes not only a review for the patient characteristics discussed under contraindications, but also knowledge of medicines received in labor. If the woman has received ephedrine during the course of regional anesthesia, ergots must be used with caution, if at all. Combined effects of ephedrine and the ergot alkaloid can produce an acute hypertensive crisis (111). It is also imperative to remember that regardless of the urgency of the situation, the risks of intravenous ergots usually outweigh any potential advantage.

## Conclusion

Increased knowledge of contractile physiology and the control of uterine contractions should lead to less empiric and more selective use of uterotonic and tocolytic medications. The increasing array of agents being used to treat pregnant women with preterm labor who may require anesthetic intervention, mandates that the anesthetist be familiar with recognized side effects of these agents and drug interactions and also be cognizant of their mechanisms to predict other potential interactions and effects.

## REFERENCES


1. Riemer RK, Roberts JM: Activation of uterine smooth muscle contraction: Implications for eicosanoid action and interaction. Semin. Perinatol. 1:276, 1986.
2. Besinger R, Niebyl J: The safety and efficacy of tocolytic agents for the treatment of preterm labor. Ob. Gyn. Survey. 45(7):415–40, 1990.
3. Creasy R, Resnik R: Maternal fetal medicine: maternal-fetal medicine. *In*: Principles and Practice. Philadelphia, W.B. Saunders, 1989.
4. Pritchard J, MacDonald P, Gant N: Williams Obstetrics. 17th Ed. New York, Appleton-Century-Crofts, 1985.
5. Gilman AG, Goodman LS, et al : Goodman and Gilman's Pharmacological Basis of Therapeutics. 7th Ed. New York, Macmillan, 1985.
6. Kamm KE, Stull JT: The function of myosin and myosin light chain kinase phosphorylation in smooth muscle. Ann. Rev. Pharmacol. Toxicol. 25:539, 1985.
7. Rasmussen H, Takuwa Y, Park S: Protein kinase C in the regulation of smooth muscle contraction. FASEB 1:177, 1987.
8. Kao CY: Electrophysiological properties of the uterine smooth muscle. *In* Wynn RM (ed): Biology of the Uterus. Edited by RM Wynn. New York, Plenum Press, 1977, p. 423.

8A. Hamon G, Worcel M: Electrophysiological study of the action of angiotensin II on the rat myometrium. Circ. Res. 45(2), 1979, pp. 234–43.

9. Carafoli E: Intracellular calcium regulation, with special attention to the role of the plasma membrane calcium pump. J. Cardiovasc. Pharmacol. 12:S77, 1988.
10. Putney JW Jr, Takemura H, Hughes AR, Horstman DA, et al: How do inositol phosphates regulate calcium signaling? FASEB J. 3:1899, 1989.
11. Housey GM, Johnson MD, O'Brian CA, Weinstein IB, et al: Structural and functional studies of protein kinase C. Adv. Exp. Med. Biol. 234:127, 1988.
12. Roberts JM, Reimer JM, Bottari SP, Wu YY, et al: Hormonal regulation of myometrial adrenergic responses: the receptor and beyond. J. Dev. Psychol. 11(3):123–134, 1989.
13. Meisheri KD, van Breemen C: Effects of β-adrenergic stimulation on calcium movements in rabbit aortic smooth muscle: relationship with cAMP. J. Physiol. 331:429, 1982.
14. Stryer L, Bourne HR: G proteins: A family of signal transducers. Ann. Rev. Cell. Biol. 2:391, 1986.
15. Riemer RK, Roberts JM: Endocrine modulation of myometrial response. *In* The Physiology and Biochemistry of the Uterus in Pregnancy and Labor. Edited by G Huszer. Boca Raton, FL, CRC Press, 1986, p. 53.
16. Roberts JM, Reimer RK, Bottari SP, Wu YY, et al: Myometrial postreceptor responses: Targets for steroidal regulation. *In* The Onset of Labor: Cellular and Intergrative Mechanisms. Edited by D McNellis, JRG Challis, PC McDonald, Nathanielsz P, et al. Ithaca, NY, Perinatolog Press, 1988, pp. 37–50.
17. Main DM, Main EK: Preterm birth. *In* Obstetrics Normal and Problem Pregnancies. Edited by SG Gabbe, JR Niebyl, JL Simpson. New York, Churchill Livingstone, 1991.
18. Barden TP, Peter JB, Merkatz IR: Ritodrine hydrochloride: a betamimetic agent for use in preterm labor, part 1. Pharmacology, clinical history, administration, side effects and safety. Obstet. Gynecol. 56:1, 1980.
19. Merkatz IR, Peter JB, Barden TP: Ritodrine hydrochloride: a betamimetic agent for use in preterm labor, part 2. Evidence of efficacy. Obstet. Gynecol. 56:7, 1980.
20. Wesselius-de Casparis A, Thiery M, Yo Le Sian A, Baumgarten K, et al: Results of double-blind multicenter study with ritodrine in premature labor. Br. Med. J. 3:144, 1971.

20A. Lauersen NH, Merkatz IR, Tejani N, Wilson KH, et al: Inhibition of premature labor: a multicenter comparison of ritodrine and ethanol. Am. J. Obstet. Gynecol. 127(8), 1977, pp. 837–45.

20B. Comments: Treatment of preterm labor with the beta-adrenergic agonist ritodrine. The Canadian Preterm Labor Investigators Group. N. Engl. J. Med. 327(5), 1992, pp. 308–12.

21. Caritas SN, Darby MJ, Chan L: Pharmacologic treatment of preterm labor. Clin. Obstet. Gynecol. 31:635, 1988.
22. Lam F, Gill P, Smith M, Kitzmiller J, Katz M: Use of the subcutaneous terbutaline pump for long term tocolysis. Obstet. Gynecol. 72:810–813, 1988.
23. Berg G, Andersson RRG, Ryden G: Beta-adrenergic receptors in human myometrium during pregnancy; changes in the number of receptors after beta-mimetic treatment. Am. J. Obstet. Gynecol. 151:392, 1985.

24. Harden TK: Agonist-induced desensitization of the beta-adrenergic receptor-linked adenylate cyclase. Pharmacol. Rev. 35:5, 1983.
25. Caritis SN, Lin LS, Toig G, Wong LK: Pharmacodynamics of ritodrine in pregnant women during preterm labor. Am. J. Obstet. Gynecol. 147:752, 1983.
26. Ingemarrson I, Arulkumaran S, Ratnam SS: Single injection of terbutaline in term labor. Am. J. Obstet. Gynecol. 153: 865, 1985.
27. Catanzarite VA, McHargue AM, Sandberg EC, Dyson DC: Respiratory arrest during therapy for premature labor in a patient with myasthenia gravis. Obstet. Gynecol. 64:819, 1984.
28. Sholl JS, Hughey MJ, Hirshmann RA: Myotonic muscular dystrophy associated with ritodrine tocolysis. Am. J. Obstet. Gynecol. 151:83, 1985.
29. Mordes D, Kreutner K, Metzger W, Colwell JA: Dangers of intravenous ritodrine in diabetic patient. JAMA 248:973, 1982.
30. Larsen JF, Eldon K, Lange AP, Leegaard M, et al: Ritodrine in the treatment of preterm labor. Second Danish Multicenter Study. Obstet. Gynecol. 67:607, 1986.
31. Bieniarz J, Ivankovich A, Scommegna A: Cardiac output during ritodrine treatment in preterm labor. Am. J. Obstet. Gynecol. 118:919, 1974.
31A. Bieniarz J, Ivankovich A, Scommegna A: Cardiac output during ritodrine treatment in premature labor. Am J. Obstet. Gynecol. 118(7), 1974, pp. 910–20.
32. Katz M, Roberson PA, Creasy RK: Cardiovascular complications associated with terbutaline treatment for preterm labor. Am. J. Obstet. Gynecol. 135:605, 1981.
33. Benedetti T: Maternal complications of parenteral beta-sympathomimetic tocolytic therapy. Am. J. Obstet. 145:1, 1983.
34. Pisani RJ, Rosenow EC: Pulmonary edema associated with tocolytic therapy. Ann. Intern. Med. 110:714, 1989.
35. Moravee MA, Hurlburt BJ: Hypokalemia associated with terbutaline administration on obstetrical patients. Anesth. Analg. 59:917, 1980.
36. Robertson PA, Herron M, Katz M, Creasy RK: Maternal morbidity associated with isoxsuprine and terbutaline tocolysis. Eur. J. Obstet. Gynaecol. Reprod. Biol. 11:371, 1981.
37. Epstein MF, Nicholls E, Stubblefield PG: Neonatal hypoglycemia after beta-sympathomimetic tocolytic therapy. J. Pediatr. 94:449, 1979.
38. Mulders LGM, Boers GHJ, Prickartz-Wijdeveld MMJF, Hein PR: A study of maternal ECG characteristics before and during intravenous tocolysis with β-sympathomimetics. Acta. Obstet. Gynaecol. Scand. 66:417, 1987.
39. Hendricks SK, Keroes J, Katz M: Electrocardiographic changes associated with ritodrine-induced maternal tachycardia and hypokalemia. Am. J. Obstet. Gynecol. 154:921, 1986.
40. Ravindran R, Viegas OJ, Padilla LM, LaBlonde P: Anesthetic considerations in pregnant patients receiving tocolytic therapy. Anesth. Analg. 59:391, 1980.
41. Spisso KR, Herbert GM, Thiajarajah S: The use of magnesium sulfate as the primary tocolytic agent to prevent premature delivery. Am. J. Obstet. Gynecol. 142:840, 1982.
42. Altura BM, Altura BT: Magnesium ions and contraction of vascular smooth muscles: relationship to some vascular diseases. Fed. Proc. 40:2672, 1981.
43. Massey SG: Pharmacology of magnesium. Ann. Rev. Pharmacol. Toxicol. 17:67, 1977.
44. Hollander DI, Nagey DA, Pupkin MJ: Magnesium sulfate and ritodrine hydrochloride: a randomized comparison. Am. J. Obstet. Gynecol. 156:631, 1987.
45. Gambling DR, Birmingham CL, Jenkins LC: Magnesium and anesthesiology. Can. J. Anaesth. 35:644, 1988.
46. Cruikshank DP, Pitkin RM, Donnelly E, Reynolds WA: Urinary magnesium, calcium and phosphate excretion during magnesium infusion. Obstet. Gynecol. 58:430, 1981.
47. Cruikshank DP, Pitkin RM, Reynolds WA, Williams GA, et al: Effects of magnesium sulfate treatment on perinatal calcium metabolism. Am. J. Obstet. Gynecol. 134(3):243–249, 1979.
48. Pruett KM, Kirshon B, Cotton DB, Adam K, et al: The effects of magnesium sulfate therapy on Apgar scores. Am. J. Obstet. Gynecol. 159:1047, 1988.
49. Ghoneim MM, Long JP: The interaction between magnesium and other neuromuscular blocking agents. Anesthesiology. 32:23, 1970.
49A. Bradley RJ: Calcium or magnesium concentration affects the severity of organophosphate-induced neuromuscular block. Eur. J. Pharmacol. 127(3), 1986, pp. 275–8.
49B. Tsai SK, Liao KT, Lee CM: Modification by ketamine on the neuromuscular actions of magnesium, vecuronium, pancuronium and alpha-bungarotoxin in the primate. Can. J. Anaesth. 39(1), 1992, pp. 79–82.
50. Strigl R, Pfieffer U, Erhardt W, Krieglsteiner P, et al: Does the administration of the calcium-antagonist verapamil in tocolysis with beta-sympathicomimetics still make sense? J. Perinat. Med. 9:235, 1981.
51. Ulmsten U: Treatment of normotensive and hypertensive patients with preterm labor using oral nifedipine a calcium antagonist. Arch. Gynecol. 236:69, 1984.
52. Staffurth JS, Emery P: Adverse interaction between nifedipine and beta-blockade. Br. Med. J. 282:225, 1981.
53. Gillmer DJ, Kark P: Pulmonary edema precipitated by nifedipine. Br. Med. J. 280:1420, 1980.
54. Pueh P, Krebs R: Nifedipine pharmacokinetics. 4th International Adalat Symposium. Excepta Medical, Amsterdam, 1980, p. 14.
55. Ferguson JE II, Dyson DC, Schutz T, Stevenson DK: A comparison of tocolysis with nifedipine or ritodrine analysis of efficacy, maternal, fetal and neonatal outcome. Am. J. Obstet. Gynecol. 63(1, Part 1):105–111, 1990.
56. Lewis JG: Adverse reactions to calcium antagonists. Drugs. 25:196, 1983.
57. Belz GG: Digozin plasma concentration and nifedipine. Lancet. 1(8223):844–845, 1981.
58. Waisman GD, Mayorga LM, Cmera MI, Vignolo CA, et al: Magnesium plus nifedipine: potentiation of hypotensive effect in preeclampsia? Am. J. Obstet. Gynecol. 159:308, 1988.
59. Manchester D, Margolis A, Sheldon R: Possible association between maternal indomethacin therapy and primary pulmonary hypertension of the newborn. Am. J. Obstet. Gynecol. 126:467, 1976.
60. Dudley D, Hardia M: Fetal and neonatal effects of indomethacin used as a tocolytic agent. Am. J. Obstet. Gynecol. 151:181, 1985.
61. Niebyl J, Blake DA, White RD, Kumor KM, et al: The inhibition of premature labor with indomethacin. Am. J. Obstet. Gynecol. 136:1014, 1980.
62. Zuckerman H, Shalev E, Gilad G, Katzuni E: Further study of the inhibition of preterm labor by indocin. J. Perinatal. Med. 12:19, 1984.
63. Kirshon B, Moise KJ Jr, Wasserstrum N, Ou C-N, et al: The influence of short-term indomethacin therapy on fetal urine output. Obstet. Gynecol. 72:51, 1988.
64. Moise KJ Jr, Huhta JC, Sharif DS, Ou C-N, et al: Indomethacin treatment of preterm labor: effects on the fetal ductus arteriosus. N. Engl. J. Med. 319:327, 1988.

65. Edersheim T, et al: Prolonged indomethacin use in intractable premature labor. Proc. Soc. Perinat. Obstet. February 1988.
66. Alván G, Orme M, Bertilsson L, Ekstrand R, et al: Pharmacokinetics of indomethacin. Clin. Pharmacol. Ther. 18:364, 1975.
67. Repke JT, Kiebyl J: Role of prostaglandin synthesis inhibitors in treatment of preterm labor. Semin. Endocrinol. 3: 259, 1985.
68. de Jong PL: Incidence of hyperkalemia induced by Indocin. Br. Med. J. 12:19, 1984.
69. Orme MLE: Nonsteroidal antiinflammatory agents and the kidney. Br. Med. J. 292:1621, 1986.
70. Gilman AG, Goodman LS, Rall TW, Murad F: Goodman and Gilman's Pharmacological Basis of Therapeutics. 7th Ed. New York, Macmillan, 1985.
71. Eronen M, Pesonen E, Kurki T, Ylikorkala O, Hallman M: The effects of indomethacin and a sympathomimetic agent on the fetal ductus arteriosus during treatment of premature labor. A randomized double-blind study. Am. J. Obstet. Gynecol. 164:141–146, 1991.
72. Ferguson JE, Hensleigh PA, Kredenster D: Adjunctive use of magnesium sulfate with ritodrine for preterm labor tocolysis. Am. J. Obstet. Gynecol. 148:166, 1984.
73. Hatjis CG, Swain M, Nelson LH, Meis PJ, et al: Efficacy of combined administration of magnesium sulfate and ritodrine in the treatment of preterm labor. Obstet. Gynecol. 69:317, 1987.
74. Kaul AF, Osathanondh R, Safon L, Frigoletto F, et al: The management of preterm labor with the calcium channel-blocking agent nifedipine combined with the beta-mimetic terbutaline. Drug. Intell. Clin. Pharm. 19:369, 1985.
75. Katz Z, Lancet M, Yemini M: Treatment of premature labor contractions with combined ritodrine and indomethacin. Int. J. Gynaecol. Obstet. 21:337, 1983.
76. Thiagarajah S, Harbert G, Bourgeois FJ: Magnesium sulfate and ritodrine hydrochloride: systemic and uterine hemodynamic effects. Am. J. Obstet. Gynecol. 153:666, 1985.
77. Valenzuela G, Cline S: Use of magnesium sulfate in premature labor that fails to respond to beta-mimetic drugs. Am. J. Obstet. Gynecol. 143:718, 1982.
78. Dale HH: On some physiological actions of ergot. J. Physiol. 34:163, 1906.
79. Bell WB: The pituitary body and the therapeutic value of the infundibular extract in shock uterine atony and intestinal paresis. Br. Med. J. 2:1609, 1909.
80. DuVigneaud V, Ressler C, Swan JM, Roberts CW: Synthesis of an octapeptide amide with hormonal activity of oxytocin. J. Am. Chem. Soc. 75:79–80, 1953.
81. Wilson T, Liggins GC, Whittaker DJ: Oxytocin stimulates the release of arachidonic acid and prostaglandin $F_{2\alpha}$ from human decidual cells. Prostaglandins 35:771, 1988.
82. Flint APF, Leat WMF, Sheldrick EL, Stewart HJ: Stimulation of phosphoinositide hydrolysis by oxytocin and the mechanism by which oxytocin controls prostaglandin synthesis in the ovine endometrium. Biochem. J. 237:797, 1986.
83. Batra S: Effect of oxytocin on calcium influx and efflux in the rat myometrium. Eur. J. Pharmacol. 120:57, 1986.
84. Jacobson L, Riemer RK, Goldfin AC, Lykins D, et al: Rabbit myometrial oxytocin and alpha 2-adrenergic receptors are increased by estrogen but are differentially regulated by progesterone. Endocrinology 120:1184, 1987.
85. Goodfellow CF, Hull MGR, Swaab DF, Dogterom J, Buij RM: Oxytocin deficiency at delivery with epidural anesthesia. Br. J. Ob. Gyn. 90:214–219, 1983.
86. Fuchs AR, Fuchs F, Husslein P, Soloff MS: Oxytocin receptors in the human uterus during pregnancy and parturition. Am. J. Obstet. Gynecol. 150:734, 1984.
87. James NT: Histochemical demonstration of oxytocinase in the human placenta. Nature. 210:1276, 1976.
88. Seitchik J, Amico JA, Castillo M: Oxytocin augmentation of dysfunctional labor. V. An alternative oxytocin regimen. Am. J. Obstet. Gynecol. 151:757, 1985.
89. Eggers TR, Fliegner JR: Water intoxication and syntocinon infusion. Aust. NZ. J. Obstet. Gynaecol. 19:59, 1979.
90. Hendricks CH, Brenner WE: Cardiovascular effects of oxytocic drugs used postpartum. Am. J. Obstet. Gynecol. 108: 751–760, 1970.
91. Andersen TW, De Padua CB, Stenger V, Prystowsky H: Cardiovascular effects of rapid intravenous injection of synthetic oxytocin during elective cesarean section. Clin. Pharm. Ther. 6:345, 1965.
91A. Sorbe B: Active pharmacologic management of the third stage of labor. A comparison of oxytocin and ergometrine. Obstet. Gynecol. 52(6), 1978, pp. 694–697.
92. Kawarabayashi T, Narisawa Y, Nakamura K, Sugimori H, et al: Anaphylactoid reaction to oxytocin during cesarean section. Gynecol. Obstet. Invest. 24:277–279, 1988.
93. Secher NJ, Thayssen P, Arnsbo P: Effect of prostaglandin $E_2$ and $F_{2\alpha}$ on the systemic and pulmonary circulation in pregnant anesthetized women. Acta. Obstet. Gynaecol. Scand. 61:213, 1982.
94. Jagani N, Schulman H, Fleischer A, Mitchell J, et al: Role of prostaglandin-induced cervical changes in labor induction. Obstet. Gynecol. 63:225, 1984.
95. Lands WEM: The biosynthesis and metabolism of prostaglandins. Ann Rev. Physiol. 41:633, 1979.
96. Calder AA, Embrey MP: Comparison of intravenous oxytocin and prostaglandin $E_2$ for induction of labour using automatic and non-automatic infusion techniques. Br. J. Obstet. Gynecol. 82:728, 1975.
97. Herz RH, Sokol RJ, Dierker LJ: Treatment of postpartum uterine atony with prostaglandin $E_2$ vaginal suppositories. Obstet. Gynecol. 56:129, 1980.
98. Hayashi RH, Castillo MS, Noah M: Management of severe postpartum hemorrhage with prostaglandin $F_{2\alpha}$ analogue. Obstet. Gynecol. 63:806, 1984.
99. MacKenzie IZ, Bradley S, Embrey MP: Vaginal prostaglandins and labour induction for patients previously delivered by cesarean section. Br. J. Obstet. Gynaecol. 91:7, 1984.
100. Brown R, Ingram RH, McFadden ER: Effects of prostaglandin $F_{2\alpha}$ on lung mechanics in nonasthmatic and asthmatic subjects. J. Appl. Physiol. 44:150, 1978.
101. Silva DA, Singh PP, Bauman J, Miller R: Acute hypertensive response to prostaglandin F2α during anesthesia administration. J. Reprod. Med. 32:700, 1987.
102. Fitzgerald WJ: The use of a semisynthetic oxytocic (Methergine) in the third stage of labor. Am. J. Obstet. Gynecol. 63:865, 1952.
103. Prediville W, Elbourne D, Chalmers I: The effects of routine oxytocic administration in the management of third stage of labour: an overview of the evidence from controlled trials. Br. J. Obstet. Gynaecol. 95:3, 1988.
104. Dumoulin JG: A reappraisal of the use of ergotamine. J. Obstet. Gynaecol. 1:178, 1981.
105. Hendricks CH, Brenner WE: Cardiovascular effects of oxytocic drugs used postpartum. Am. J. Obstet. Gynecol. 108: 751–760, 1970.
106. Ringroses CAD: The obstetrical use of ergot. Can. Med. Assoc. J. 87:712, 1962.
106A. Hansen JM, Ueland K: Maternal cardiovascular dynamics during pregnancy and parturition. Clin. Anesth. 10(2), 1974, pp. 21–36.

107. Valentine BH, Martin MA, Philips NV: Collapse during operation following intravenous ergometrine. Br. J. Anaesth. 49:81, 1977.

108. Taylor GJ, Cohen B: Ergonovine-induced coronary artery spasm and myocardial infarction after normal delivery. Obstet. Gynecol. 66:821, 1985.

109. Abouleish E: Postpartum hypertension and convulsion after oxytocic drugs. Anesth. Analg. 55:813, 1976.

110. Browning DJ: Serious side effects of ergometrine and its use in routine obstetric practice. Med. J. Aust. 1:957, 1974.

110A. Secher NJ, Arnsbo P, Wallin L: Haemodynamic effects of oxytocin (syntocinon) and methyl ergometrine (methergin) on the systemic and pulmonary circulations of pregnant anaesthetized woman. Acta. Obstet. Gynecol. Scand. 57(2), 1978, pp. 97–103.

110B. Gilbert L, Porter W, Brown VA: Postpartum haemorrhage—a continuing problem. Br. J. Obstet. Gynaecol. 94(1), 1987, pp. 67–71.

111. Cassady GN, Moore DC, Bridenbaugh LD: Postpartum hypertension after use of vasoconstrictor and oxytocic drugs. JAMA 172:1011, 1960.

111A. Abouleish E: Postpartum hypertension and convulsion after oxytocic drugs. Anesth. Analg. 55(6), 1976, pp. 813–815.

Chapter 6

# ANATOMY AND PHYSIOLOGY OF THE PLACENTA

DAN W. RURAK

The placenta is a remarkable, multi-functional organ that is essential for normal embryonic and fetal development. It provides protection for the fetus from the maternal immune system, but allows the transfer of the substrates necessary for maintenance and growth of the conceptus, as well as for the transfer of fetal waste products to the mother. The placenta also is a important endocrine organ, producing large amounts of steroid and protein hormones that are released into the maternal and fetal circulations. And because of this synthetic activity as well as other metabolic processes, the placenta has a very high metabolic rate, and for most of pregnancy consumes more of the nutrients supplied to the uterus than does the fetus. It grows rapidly, and by the end of pregnancy is receiving significant fractions of maternal and fetal cardiac output. Yet at birth it is normally expelled from the mother with minimal blood loss. Although placental functions remain important, much of the interest to the obstetric anesthesiologist liesin those areas relating to the maternal-fetal transfer of the anesthetics and other drugs administered to pregnant women and knowledge of the factors affecting the transfer of oxygen and other nutrients under normal and pathological conditions. Moreover, there is increasing evidence that abnormalities in implantation and placentation in the first trimester can ultimately lead to the development of problems, such as preeclampsia, later in pregnancy. This chapter will discuss briefly: (1) the development, anatomy, and maturation of the placenta; (2) uteroplacental and umbilical circulations; and (3) transfer functions of the placenta, with particular reference to respiratory gases. The transfer of sedatives, analgesics, anesthetics, and other drugs used in obstetric anesthesia are discussed in Chapter 9.

## DEVELOPMENTAL ANATOMY OF THE PLACENTA

Our knowledge of the morphologic aspects of implantation and placental development in the human has largely come from carefully dated in situ specimens, collected over decades at several centers, as well as punch biopsy specimens of the placental bed obtained at cesarean section; these are described extensively by Boyd and Hamilton (1). However, some stages of implantation and placentation are not represented in these specimens; for example, penetration of the uterine epithelium by the blastocyst. Data from animal species, particularly the monkey, in part make up for these deficits, but it is important to note that there are several features of the development of the human placenta, which taken together, make it almost unique among mammals (2,3). In addition to the morphologic information that has been accumulated over many years, there has been study more recently of the functional aspects of placentation, particularly of the characteristics of the embryonic trophoblast and maternal endometrial cells that are intimately involved in the formation of the placenta (4).

### Implantation and Early Trophoblast Expansion

During the process of implantation there is the attachment of the blastocyst to the uterine wall and the subsequent burrowing of the blastocyst into the uterine stroma (Figure 6–1a). This is a critical period of development, because it is then that most of the genetically abnormal embryos are likely lost (5). At the time of implantation the blastocyst consists of an inner cell mass, which will give rise to the embryo proper, and an outer sphere of trophoblast cells, which will be involved primarily in formation of the placenta. At the interface between the conceptus and uterine wall, the trophoblast consists of an outer syncytial layer and an inner layer of cytotrophoblast cells. It appears that the syncytial layer is involved in the initial invasion of maternal tissues, but there is not universal agreement on this point (6).

In the human, implantation likely occurs 6 to 7 days after conception, most frequently on the upper portion of the posterior uterine wall (1). However, no in situ human specimen has yet been obtained that shows the initial stages of the process; in the earliest specimens, at 7.5 and 8 days, the blastocyst is partially or completely embedded in the endometrium. Thus, the precise mechanism by which the human blastocyst penetrates the uterine epithelium is not clear. In the various other species studies, three different modes of penetration have been described (7): displacement of uterine epithelial cells by the trophoblast, fusion of trophoblast and uterine epithelial cells, and intrusion or infiltration of trophoblast between adjacent uterine epithelial cells. There is evidence for the fusion mode from in situ human specimens and for an intrusive process with implantation in vitro of a blastocyst on a monolayer of uterine epithelial cells (8). Also, in vitro studies of cytotrophoblast cells from first term pregnancies suggest that infiltration of trophoblast cellular processes could also be important (9). Denker (10) has pointed out that whatever the mode of trophoblast pene-

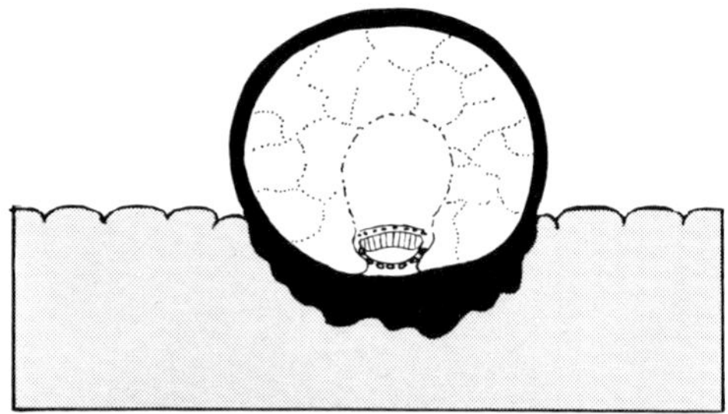

Fig. 6–1. Diagrammatic representations of various stages of early placentation. **A,** Implantation; **B,** Expansion of the syncytiotrophoblast and formation of the lacunar spaces; **C,** Development of primary chorionic villi; **D,** Formation of the cytotrophoblast shell. (From Boyd JD, Hamilton WJ: The Human Placenta. Cambridge, W. Heffer & Sons, 1970.

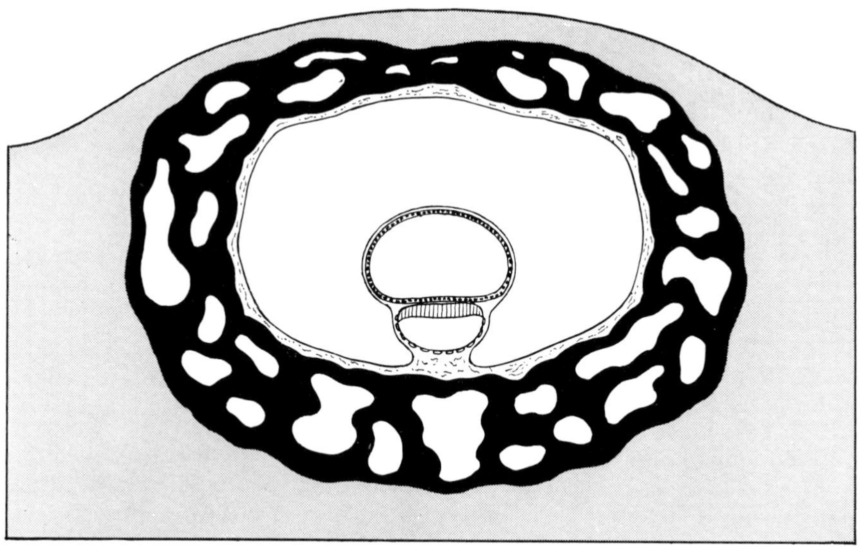

tration of the uterine epithelium, the first event is the physical attachment of the two cell types via their apical membranes, whereas in other epithelial systems, it is only the basal membrane that exhibits adhesive properties. Thus, implantation must involve alteration of the cell surface properties of the trophoblast and uterine epithelial cells, and with the latter cells, some degree of loss of apico-basal polarity may also be involved. Changes in various properties (cell surface charge, lectin binding, glycoprotein constituents) of both cell types occur around the time of implantation, and there is evidence that factors from both the blastocyst (histamine, estrogen, prostaglandins) and mother (ovarian steroids) mediate this process (11,12,13). However, our understanding of the precise mechanisms of implantation is far from complete.

Following implantation, there is expansion of the syncytiotrophoblast layer into the uterine stroma, with destruction of maternal cells. By day 8 to 9, there is the formation of lacunar spaces in the syncytium, some of which extends to the underlying cytotrophoblast layer (Figure 6–1b). These spaces, which ultimately form the intervillous space, become filled with maternal blood that eventually comes to circulate through the spaces, although as discussed below, there are different opinions as to the time at which this occurs. This process continues until about day 12, by which time the conceptus as a whole has become completely embedded in the uterine wall, with the regrowth of uterine epithelium over it. Thus, the provision of a rudimentary maternal blood supply to the trophoblast at this time is likely important for nutrient supply to the embryo, because access to uterine fluids is lost. Also by day 12, the syncytiotrophoblast has come to extend completely around the conceptus.

## Formation of the Definitive Placenta

### *Villus Formation*

A key process in placentation begins on about day 13 postconception: formation of primary villi, the elements that will ultimately form the fetal component of the exchange system in the placenta (14) (Figure 6–1c). The process begins with finger-like projections of cytotrophoblast cells into the syncytial layer. Initially, these outgrowths are covered with a syncytial layer, which lines the lacunar spaces and the maternal/fetal interface. Branching of the cytotrophoblast columns begins to form additional anchoring columns, as well as floating villi that project into the intervillous space. The primary villi develop a mesenchymal core and become secondary villi and tertiary villi, resulting from the formation of vascular elements within the villus mesenchyme, a process that begins on about day 18 (1).

### *Formation of the Cytotrophoblast Shell*

When the outgrowing cytotrophoblast villi reach the outer limits of the syncytial layer, the tips of the villi expand laterally to link up with cytotrophoblast cells from adjacent villi (Figure 6–1d). By this process, a complete layer of cytotrophoblast cells, the cytotrophoblast shell,

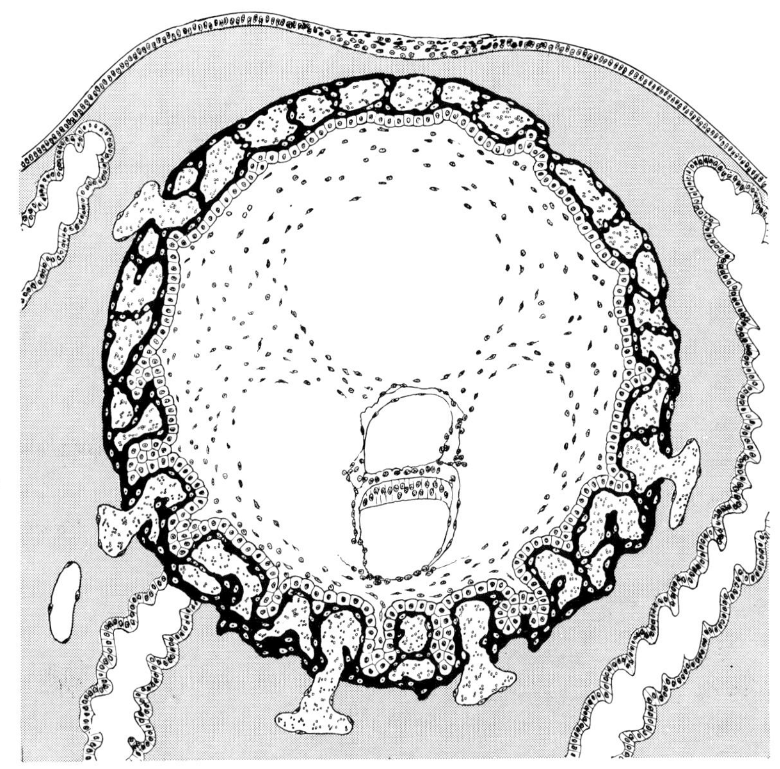

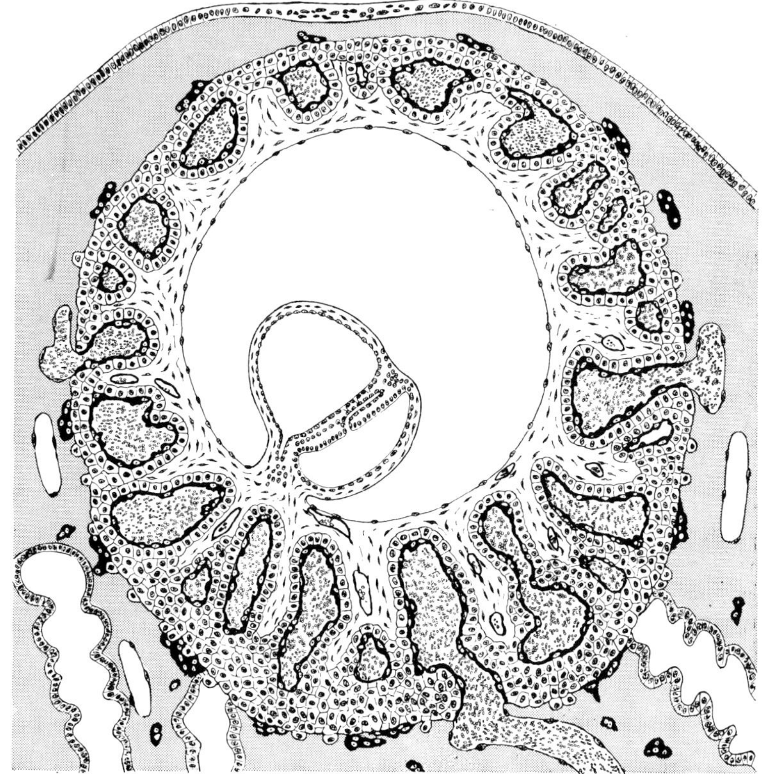

**Fig. 6–1.** *(Continued)*

comes to surround the conceptus, splitting the syncytial layer into the lining of the lacunar spaces and that in contact with maternal tissue. The process appears complete by about day 20. Boyd and Hamilton (1) feel that the cytotrophoblast shell allows for rapid expansion of the implantation area. And although the cytotrophoblast shell regresses to some extent later in pregnancy (6) with its initial formation, we have the definitive elements of the placenta: a chorionic plate of cytotrophoblast from which the vascularized villi arise, a basal plate to which the villi are anchored distally, and an intervillous space through which maternal blood can flow. While these changes in the trophoblast are occurring, there are significant changes in the surrounding endometrial tissue, the decidua, with destruction of uterine glands and the walls of the spiral arteries, a process discussed in more detail below. There is also the appearance of large venous sinusoids adjacent to the implantation site.

## *Extravillous Trophoblast*

Aside from the cytotrophoblast cells that make up the villi (Langhans cells) and the cytotrophoblast shell, there are others, termed nonvillous or extravillous trophoblast. These cells, which appear to arise from the ends of the anchoring villi and from the cytotrophoblast shell, invade further into the decidua and the myometrium, largely, as individual cells (1,6,15,16,17) (Figure 6–2). In the myometrium, the greatest numbers of trophoblast cells are found toward the center of the placental bed and in the superficial myometrial layers, with the numbers peaking at 11 to 12 weeks gestation (16). There are also multinuclear giant cells, whose numbers increase progressively between 8 and at least 18 weeks gestation; they may result from fusion of cytotrophoblast cells. Beyond 18 weeks, mononuclear trophoblast cells are not found in the myometrium, whereas giant cells are. The functional consequences of trophoblast invasion of the myometrium are not clear, but it has been suggested that it may alter myometrial contractile properties or be involved in human chorionic hormone production (16).

In the decidua, the most obvious location of the extravillous cytotrophoblasts is in the vicinity of the spiral arteries where they are located both perivascularly and within the lumen of the vessels in large numbers. Although the precise timing of events is as yet unclear, it is now generally accepted that these cells are involved in what are termed the "physiological changes" in the spiral arteries (18,19). These comprise loss of the endothelial layer and the muscular and elastic components of the vessel wall, which are replaced by fibrinoid material and fibrous tissue. There also appears to be incorporation of cytotrophoblasts into the vessel wall. These changes in wall structure appear to occur in two phases, with alteration of the decidual segments in the first trimester and then in the myometrial segments in the second trimester, likely the result of a second wave of trophoblast migration. They result in the thick-walled muscular spiral arteries being transformed into flaccid, presumably, noncontractile channels that can accommodate the tremendous increase in maternal placental blood flow that occurs later

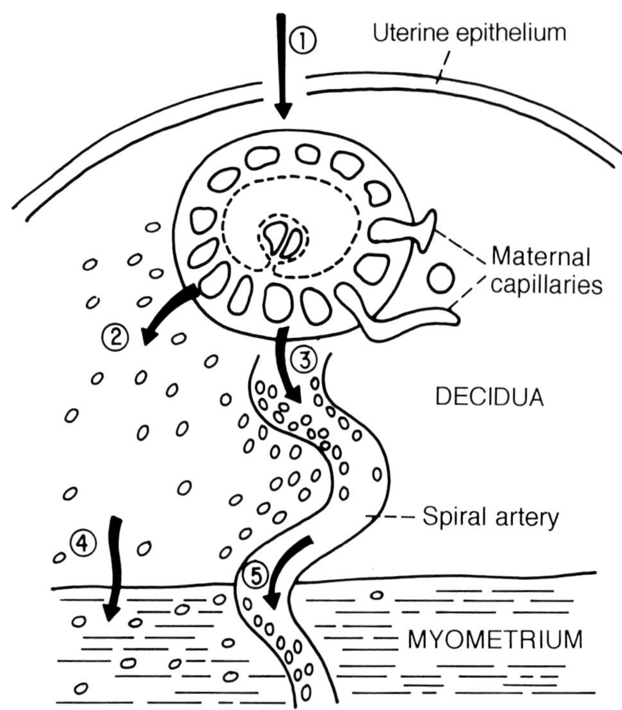


**Fig. 6–2.** Diagram illustrating successive steps in trophoblast invasion during human placentation. Key: 1) Implantation (epithelial penetration); 2) Interstitial cytotrophoblast in decidua (*first month*); 3) Tapping of spiral arteries and first wave of endovascular trophoblast invasion (*first month*); 4) Interstitial cytotrophoblast in myometrium (*8 weeks*); 5) Second wave of endovascular trophoblast invasion (*from 14 to 15 weeks*). (Redrawn from Pijnenborg R: Trophoblast invasion and placentation in the human morphological aspects. *In* Trophoblast Invasion and Endometrial Receptivity. Trophoblast Research, Vol. 4. Edited by H-W Denker, JD Aplin. New York, Plenum, 1990, pp. 33–47.)

in pregnancy (Figure 6–3a). Of great clinical significance are the observations that this process does not appear to go to completion in pregnancies associated with hypertension and/or fetal growth restriction, in that the physiological changes are restricted to the decidual segments of the arteries and, in some vessels, they are absent along the entire length (20,21,22,23) (Figure 6–3b). And, as will be discussed below, these pregnancies also exhibit evidence in increased uterine vascular resistance later in gestation.

As yet, the factors regulating the expansion and invasion of cytotrophoblast are unknown. Recently, however, exciting information on the cellular properties that permit cytotrophoblast cells to invade maternal tissues has been obtained, largely through the work of Fisher and colleagues (9,24,25). In vitro studies of cytotrophoblasts isolated from first trimester placentas indicate that they have the ability to degrade and pass through a basement membrane-like extracellular matrix; this activity is absent from cytotrophoblasts obtained from second and third trimester placentas. The matrix degrading properties of first trimester cytotrophoblasts correlated with the expression of metalloproteinases, in particular a 92 kD type IV colla-

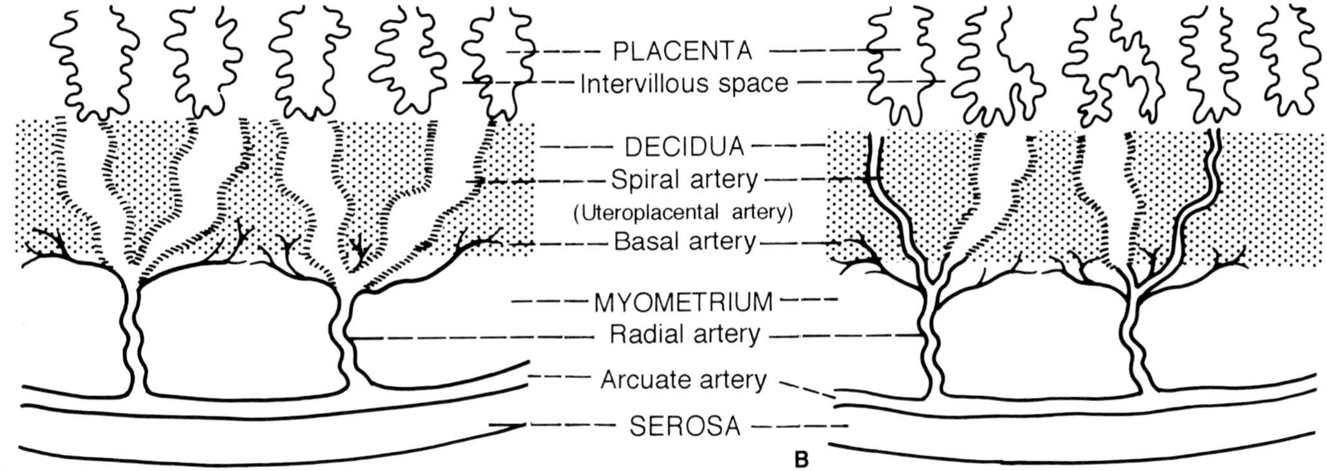


**Fig. 6–3.** Diagram of the maternal blood supply to the human placenta. **A,** Normal situation, **B,** Situation with preeclampsia. (Redrawn from Khong TY, De Wolf F, Robertson WB, Brosens I: Inadequate maternal vascular response to placentation in pregnancies complicated by pre-eclampsia and by small-for-gestational age infants. Br. J. Obstet. Gynaecol. 93:1049–1059, 1986.)

genase. Inhibition of this enzyme with a specific antibody abolishes trophoblast invasiveness. More recently, in situ immunohistochemical studies of first trimester cytotrophoblast in floating and anchoring villi and in the decidua have demonstrated differences in the cell surface adhesion (extracellular matrix) receptors of the cytotrophoblasts and in the extracellular matrix components of these regions. And there also appear to be differences in the types of cell surface receptors found on villi at different stages of pregnancy (26). These data suggest that changes in cytotrophoblast adhesion receptors and decidual extracellular matrix components could be involved in the development of invasiveness in the cytotrophoblasts at the terminal end of the anchoring villi and in the cytotrophoblast shell, as has been shown for differentiation in other systems (24). The factors regulating these components remain to be identified. In the golden hamster, which also has invasive, extravillous trophoblast, estrogen and progesterone are required for endovascular trophoblast migration (27), and it seems possible that the permissive effects of the steroids could be mediated in part via alterations in decidual extracellular matrix components. As indicated above, inadequate endotrophoblast migration in human pregnancy appears to be involved in the development of preeclampsia and other pregnancy-induced hypertensive disorders and of fetal growth restriction. It may also result in spontaneous first trimester abortion (21,28). In contrast, excessive trophoblast invasion is associated with placental accreta (21). With the recent development of in vitro and in vivo methods to study the cellular characteristics of trophoblast cells (9,24,25) and of model systems for maternal-fetal interactions (4), it is likely that significant advances will soon be made in our understanding of the pathogenesis of these conditions, and perhaps in better methods to diagnose and treat them.

## Placental Growth and Maturation

As was discussed above, by about day 20 of gestation, the essential elements of the placenta have formed. Development beyond this time involves elaboration of these elements as well as physical growth of the placenta. Initially, when the conceptus remains entirely embedded within the uterine wall, it is completely surrounded by chorionic villi and decidua. But with growth, the conceptus first projects into and then fills the lumen of the uterus, and the villi and decidua (decidua capsularis) cover the exposed portions degenerate, leaving the definitive, discoid placenta at the maternal/fetal interface (Figure 6–4). The placenta appears to grow throughout pregnancy, and roughly at the same rate as the fetus, so that fetal/placental weight ratio (~6) is constant through gestation (1,29). Initially, the increase in placental size and weight occurs largely via an increase in diameter, but later in pregnancy, it occurs via an increase in placental thickness (1). At term, the placenta is 15 to 20 cm in diameter, 2 to 3 cm in thickness, and weighs 500 to 600 grams.

There are three main processes that occur in the morphologic maturation of the placenta from its initial formation in the first weeks of pregnancy. These are growth and expansion of the cytotrophoblast sheet/basal plate into the uterine stroma to tap the spiral arteries (see below), continued branching of the fetal villi, and formation of partial septa arising from the basal plate and projecting into the intervillous space. The branching of the villi that occurs results in increases in both anchoring and floating villi. At term there are 50 to 60 fetal villi, with a fairly complex structure (Figure 6–4). Each arises from the chorionic plate via a main stem (truncus chori) that then divides into successive orders of branches (ramuli), ultimately ending in terminal villi. Kaufmann and his colleagues have classified villi into four types depending on their position in the villous tree and histologic appearance (30,31,32,33) (Figure 6–5). Stem villi occupy central positions in the villous tree, with few fetal capillaries, centrally located arteries and veins, and a fibrous connective tissue stroma; their main function would appear to be support. The stem villi branch into intermediate villi, which are of two types: immature and mature intermedi-

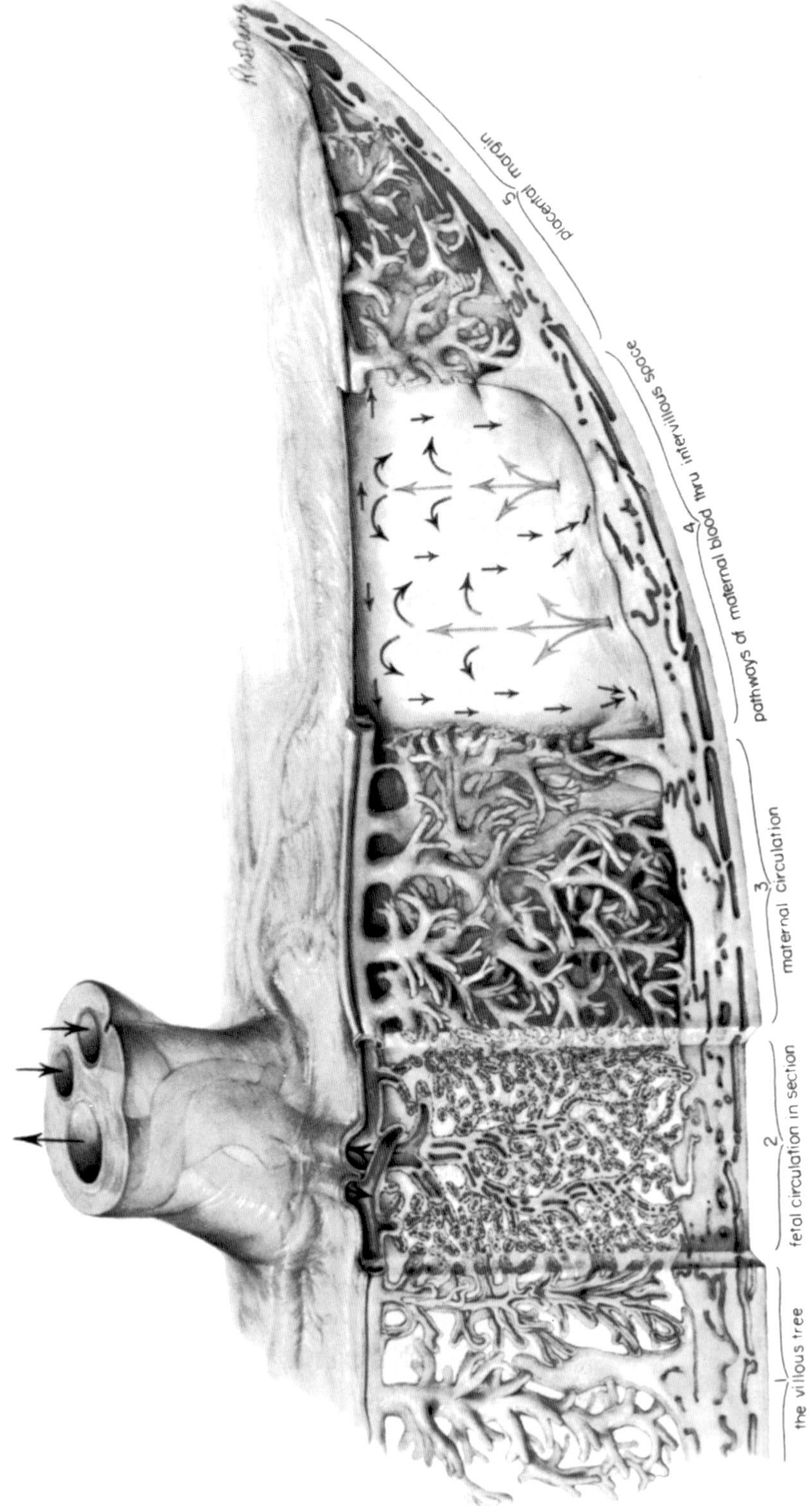


**Fig. 6–4.** Composite drawing of placenta showing its structure and circulation. 1, villus tree; 2, cross section of the fetal circulation; 3 and 4, hemodynamics of maternal circulation according to the concepts of Ramsey and associates (see text). (From Ramsey EM, the Carnegie Institution of Washington. In Obstetrics, 13th Ed. Edited by JP Greenhill. Philadelphia, WB Saunders Co., 1965.)

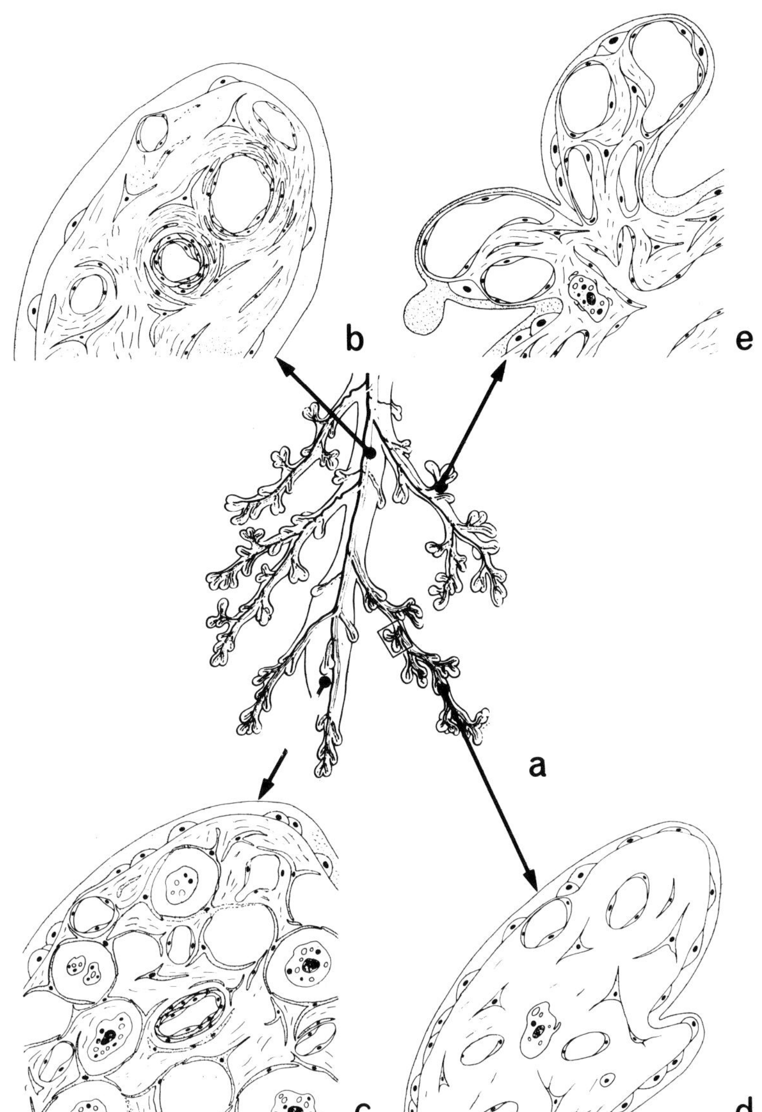


**Fig. 6–5.** **A,** Highly simplified drawing of a peripheral part of a villous tree. The surrounding cross-sections represent the characteristic structure of the different segments: **B,** Stem villus, **C,** Immature intermediate villus, **D,** Mature intermediate villus, eterminal villus. (From Kaufmann P: Basic morphology of the fetal and maternal circuits in the human placenta. Contr. Gynecol. Obstet. 13:5–17, 1985.)

ate villi. The immature type are few in number in mature placenta; however, they are the first type to appear, at about 8 weeks of pregnancy and are the dominant type until midpregnancy. They appear to be important for growth of the villous tree and differentiate into both stem and mature intermediate villi (30,34). They have arterioles and venules and a large component of connective tissue and give off few terminal villi. The mature type, in contrast, gives rise to about 95% of the terminal villi, and possesses capillaries as well as arteries and venules, and a large volume of loose connective tissue. The terminal villi, which are the final branches of villous tree, contain capillaries that are dilated in the bulbous peripheral parts of the terminal villi and usually separated from maternal blood by only the basal lamina and syncytiotrophoblast layer; the average diffusion distance is 4.25 [micrometer]. In the mature placenta, the terminal villi comprise about 40% of the total villous volume and 47% of the villous surface area, and are undoubtedly the most important site of maternal/fetal exchange (32,33). The mechanisms that regulate branching and maturation of the villous system are as yet unknown. However, Castellucci and colleagues (34,35) have described characteristic differences in the connective tissue stroma for the various villous types, suggesting that changes in extracellular matrix components and perhaps cell surface adhesion receptors could be involved.

The interlobar septa first arise from the cytotrophoblast shell in the third month of pregnancy (1). Initially, they appear to consist solely of cytotrophoblast cells, but by the fourth month also contain maternal decidual tissue. In the mature placenta, the septa are of varying width and depth, but in no case do they extend to the chorionic plate (Figure 6–4). The effect, then, of the septa is to partially subdivide the intervillous space into a number of compartments, and they result in the maternal surface of the placenta being divided into 10 to 40 lobules or cotyledons (1). By injecting contrast media into the fetal vessels and then comparing radiologic and visual observations of the placenta, Boyd and Hamilton (1) determined that each of these maternal cotyledons is occupied by several fetal villous trees. The maternal vascular supply to the intervillous space and cotyledons will be discussed below.

## UTEROPLACENTAL CIRCULATION

### *Vascular Anatomy of the Placenta*

#### *Maternal Placental Vascular Anatomy*

Blood is supplied to the uterus via the uterine and ovarian arteries (1). These vessels anastomose and send 9 to 14 branches to each of the lateral margins of the uterus. These penetrate about one-third of the myometrial thickness and divide to form the arcuate arteries, which pass circumferentially to the anterior and posterior uterine walls, there to meet with the arcuate vessels from the other side. From the arcuate system arise radial arteries that pass deeper into the myometrium. Each radial artery then divides to form several spiral arteries, which supply the intervillous space and basal arteries that supply the myometrium and decidua (36) (Figure 6–3). There are varying estimates of the number of spiral arteries that enter the intervillous space, but the most common estimate is around 100 (1,37). Also in dispute is the location of the openings of the spiral arteries into the intervillous space, with one view being that the openings are predominantly located below the center of the fetal villi (31), while the other is that they are located in the interlobar septa, at the periphery of the villi (37,38). With the former situation, maternal blood would presumably enter the intervillous space in the center of the villi and then flow toward the periphery, whereas with the latter situation, the direction of blood movement would be reversed, from periphery to center. Radioangiographic studies of rhesus monkey and human placenta appear to support a central location of the openings. Maternal blood was observed to enter the intervillous space in discreet spurts or jets and to travel upward toward the chorionic plate before dispersing laterally (31,39) (Figure 6–6). The maternal veins that drain the intervillous space number 50 to 100 and are situated around the periphery of the villous trees (1,38). The veins frequently unite beneath the basal plate to form venous lakes (1,37).

#### *Fetal Placental Vascular Anatomy*

Fetal blood is supplied to the placental villi via the paired umbilical arteries (although rarely a single artery is present), which contact the chorionic surface of the placental disk usually at the center (Figure 6–4), but sometimes at the periphery. The arteries then divide to send ~20 branches (chorionic arteries) over the surface of the placenta, and these in turn give off vertical branches to the stem villi, with each stem villi being supplied with one artery (1). A similar pattern of branching occurs for the umbilical vein, with the result that each stem villi is supplied with one artery and vein. These pass down the stem villi into the immature and mature intermediate villi, giving off branches to supply the villous branches (32,40) (Figure 6–7). At the level of the intermediate villi, the vessels are transformed into arterioles and venules, with a reduction in the muscle cell layers. Also present in the stem and intermediate villi is a perivascular capillary net (14,41). This receives its blood supply from branches from the arterioles and drains into the venules. The capillaries of the net are generally straight and tend to run parallel to the long axis of the villi and thus with the arterial and venous vessels. They extend into the proximal portions of the mature intermediate villi. When terminal villi arise directly from stem villi, they can be supplied

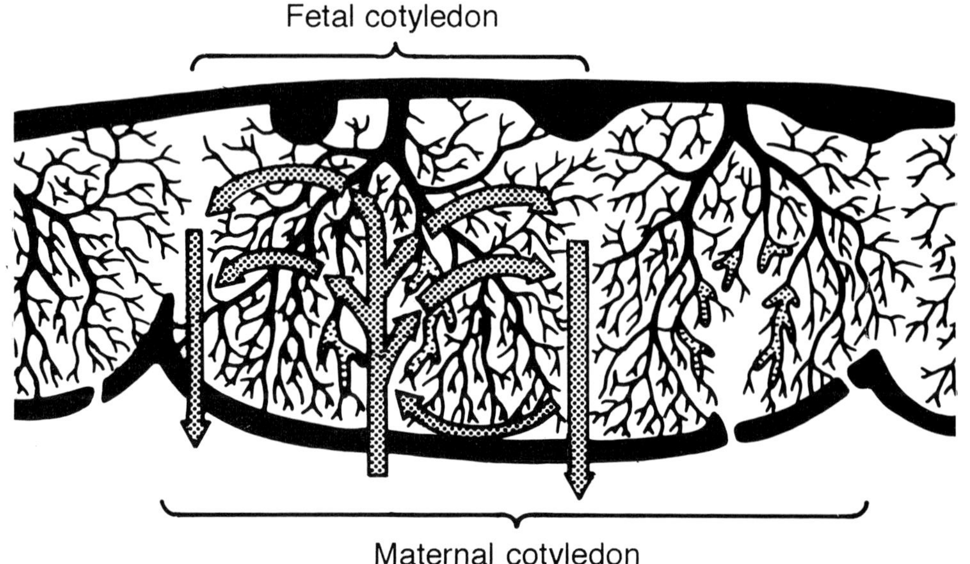


**Fig. 6–6.** Diagram of one postulated pattern of maternal blood flow through the intervillous space. A vertical section of one maternal cotyledon, with two villous trees, is shown. (Redrawn from Kaufmann P: Basic morphology of the fetal and maternal circuits in the human placenta. Contr. Gynecol. Obstet. 13:5–17, 1985.)

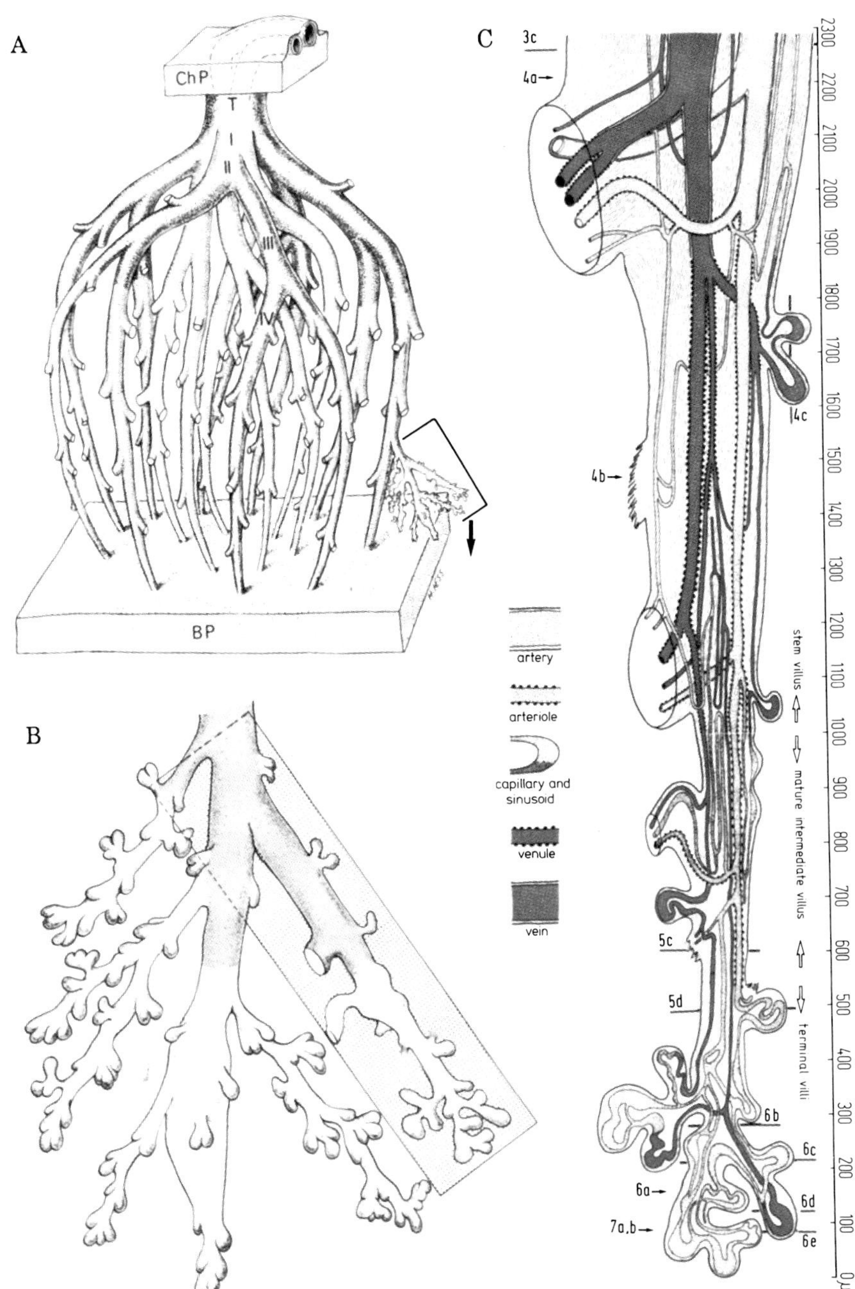


**Fig. 6–7.** Diagrammatic representation of the villous circulation. **A,** Main branches of a villous, **B,** Magnified view of the branch indicated in A, **C,** Magnified section of the branch indicated in B, showing the villous vasculature, Ch. P = chorionic plate, BP = basal plate, T = truncus, I, II, III, IV = rami chorii of the 1st to the 4th order, the number and letter in C refer to histologic sections discussed in the original publication. (From Kaufmann P, Luckhard M, Leiser R: Three-dimensional representation of the fetal vessel system in the human placenta. *In* Placental Vascularization and Blood Flow, Basic Research and Clinical Application. Trophoblast Research, Vol. 3. Edited by P Kaufmann, RK Miller. New York, Plenum, 1988, pp. 113–137.)

from this perivascular net. But for the bulk of the terminal villi that originate from mature intermediate villi, the capillaries are supplied from arterioles and venules of the main villous vascular trunk. As was mentioned previously, the capillaries in the terminal villi exhibit sinus-like dilations; these may serve to reduce blood flow velocity in the terminal villi and promote maternal/fetal exchange, or they may function to reduce vascular resistance by increasing mean capillary diameter. In the classic description of the villous circulation by Arts (41), each terminal villus was described as having its own arterial supply, so that the terminal villi were supplied in parallel. However, more recent studies (31) have indicated a series arrangement, with blood from an arteriole flowing through the capillary loops of several terminal villi before reaching a venule (Figure 6–7).

### Relative Orientation of Maternal and Fetal Placental Blood Flows

Numerous theoretical and animal studies indicate that the relative directions of maternal and fetal placental blood flows have a major effect on the efficiency of transplacental transfer of lipid soluble molecules, including respiratory gases. Species such as the horse, in which there is a countercurrent flow arrangement, exhibit a more efficient placenta in terms of transfer, and this is reflected in a higher fetal vascular $Po_2$ when compared to species, such as the sheep, where there appears to be a crosscurrent arrangement (42,43). In the human placenta, there are of course no actual maternal vascular channels in the placenta, although the dimensions of the spaces between villous branches through which maternal blood flows are similar to capillary diameters (44). However, it is unlikely only one type of maternal/fetal flow arrangement exists; rather there is likely to be a heterogeneous situation, with maternal and fetal blood flowing in the same and opposite directions or at varying angles to each other in different regions of the intervillous space. It is now generally accepted that there is a multivillous arrangement of maternal/fetal flow in the human placenta (Figure 6–8), in which a given volume of maternal blood passes and exchanges with the capillaries of a large number of villous branches (12,45). As is discussed below, this arrangement is consistent with the maternal/fetal oxygen relationship now known to exist in the human.

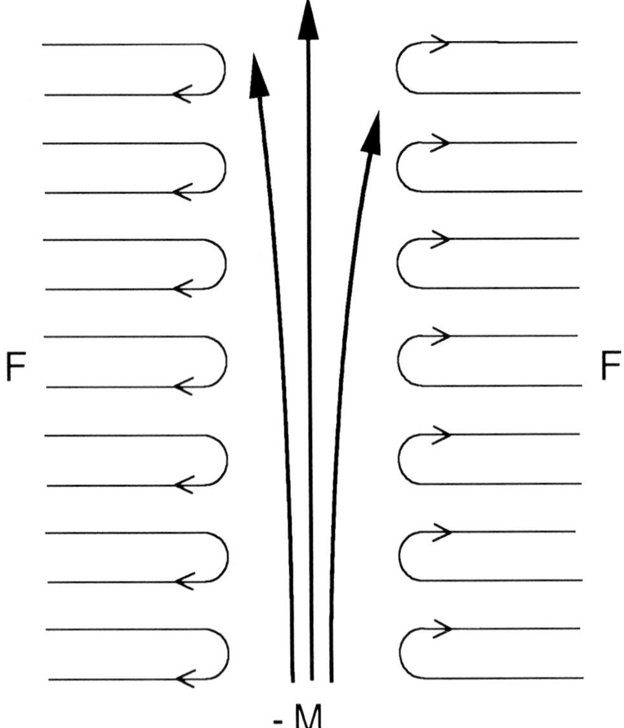


**Fig. 6–8.** A schematic diagram of a multivillous pattern of maternal (M) and fetal (F) blood flow in the placenta. (Redrawn from Bartels H, Moll W, Metcalfe J: Physiology of gas exchange in the human placenta. Am. J. Obstet. Gynecol. 84:1714–1730, 1962.)

## MATERNAL AND FETAL PLACENTAL BLOOD FLOW

### Methods of Measurement

A number of methods have been developed to measure uterine and umbilical blood flows in human and animal pregnancies. But before discussing these, the terms uterine and umbilical flows should be distinguished from maternal and fetal placental blood flows. Only a portion of the former flows actually supplies the maternal and fetal components of the placenta. A portion of uterine blood flow supplies the myometrium and nonplacental endometrium, and in various species, the fraction of total uterine blood flow going to these tissues ranges from 7 to 29% (46,47,48,49), with the only primate species that has been studied (rhesus monkey) having a value of about 19% (48). The proportion of nonplacental umbilical blood flow appears to have been estimated only in sheep, and averages 6% (47). Specific knowledge of the maternal and fetal placental blood flows is of particular importance when considering maternal/fetal flow relationships. Also, our attempts to understand the control of maternal and fetal placental blood flows have been confounded by the fact that most of the methods to estimate flow actually measure total and uterine and umbilical flows.

Measurement of uterine and umbilical blood flows in the human is obviously more difficult than in animals because of ethical constraints. The first estimates of uterine blood flow in humans were obtained at pregnancy termination or delivery using electromagnetic flow transducers on the uterine artery or by nitrous oxide equilibration (29). As these estimates were obtained under acute conditions, at a single point in time, there are of limited value. An indirect method of estimating maternal placental blood flow involves measuring the metabolic clearance rate of dehydroisoandrosterone sulfate (DS) in the mother following bolus intravenous injection of a small amount of (14C-labelled DS (50). DS is a precursor for placental estradiol synthesis, and there is evidence that its clearance from the maternal circulation, particularly its specific conversion to estradiol, is directly related to maternal placental blood flow. The method has been used primarily to assess placental flow in preeclamptic patients in comparison to normal, and to examine the effect of thiazide diuretics (50). More recently, several methods have been described that involve the monitoring of placental uptake or disappearance rates of gamma ray emitting radionuclides (xenon-133, indium-113m, technecium-99) following injection intravenously or locally into the intervillous space (51,52). These methods give only relative values for maternal placental blood flow, not absolute values in ml/min. They have been used primarily to estimate blood flows in pregnancies with various pregnancy complications (52,52A) or before and after specific interventions (53,54,55). Although it has been proposed that compartmental analysis of the placental uptake curves of the isotopes allows separate determination of intervillous, myometrial and umbilical blood flows (52,54), studies of xenon-133 washout from isolated, perfused guinea pig placentas suggest that this is not the case (56).

By far the most commonly employed, current methods of assessing the uterine and umbilical circulations in

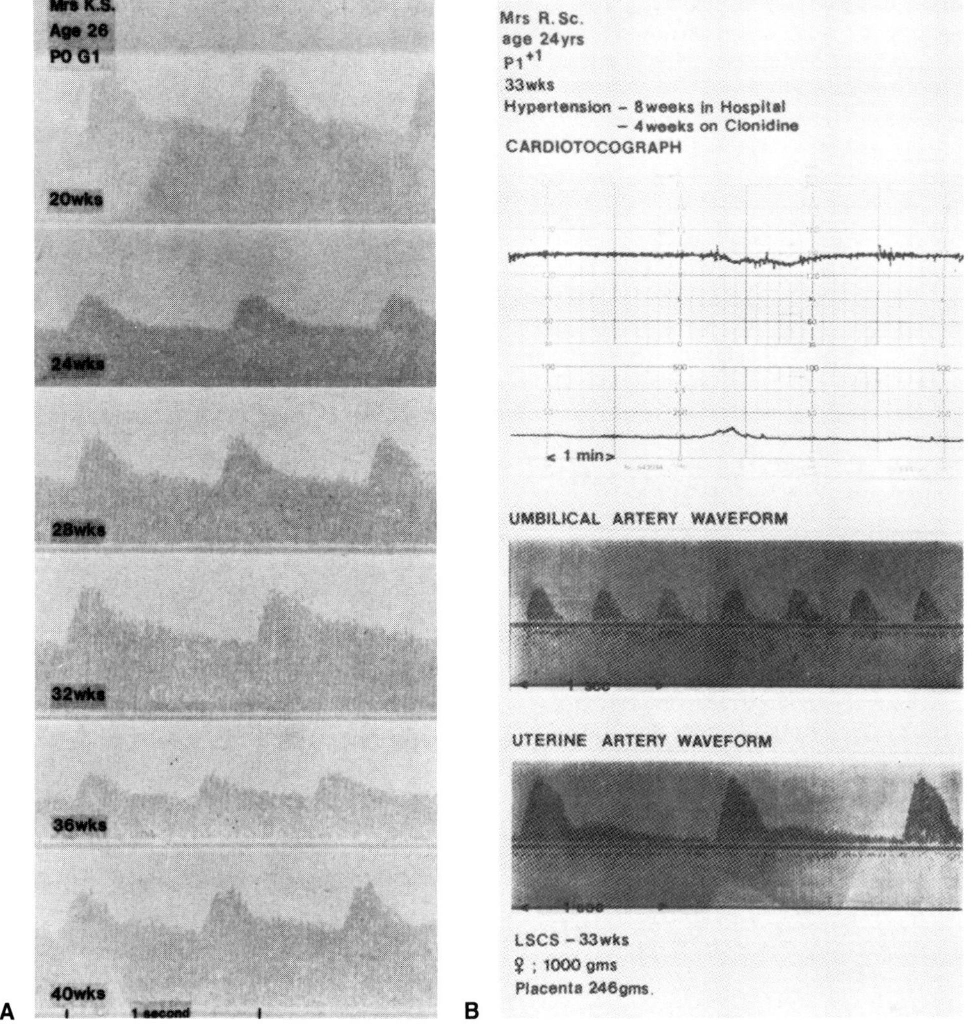


**Fig. 6–9.** Serial studies of Doppler flow velocity waveforms in the umbilical (A) and uterine (B) arteries. (From Trudinger BJ, Giles WB, Cook CM: Flow velocity waveforms in the maternal uteroplacental and fetal umbilical placental circulations. Am. J. Obstet. Gynecol. 152:155–163, 1985.)

human pregnancy are those based upon noninvasive Doppler ultrasound monitoring of blood velocity waveforms (57,58). The method exploits the fact that when an ultrasound beam transects a blood vessel, some of the beam will be reflected (backscattered) by the cellular elements of the moving blood and the frequency of that reflected ultrasound will be shifted from that of the initial beam. With appropriate processing of the backscattered signal, the velocity profile of the blood in the vessel can be estimated and displayed (Figure 6–9). The magnitude of the Doppler frequency shift is determined by several factors, as indicated by the Doppler equation:

$$f_d = [2f_i \cdot v \cdot cos\theta]/c$$

where: $f_d$ = Doppler shift frequency
$f_i$ = initial frequency
$v$ = blood flow velocity
$\theta$ = angle between the incident ultrasound beam and the axis of blood flow
$c$ = velocity of sound in tissue

It can be seen that the determination of absolute blood flow velocity requires knowledge of θ, the angle between the initial ultrasound beam, and the axis of blood flow. This can be achieved with a pulsed wave Doppler system, which transmits short pulses of ultrasound. This allows for depth selection of the target vessel and for combined use with a real-time ultrasound scanner as a duplex system to permit visualization of the vessel and thus determination of θ. In addition, the diameter of the vessel can be measured, so that the vessel cross sectional area and blood volume flow can be estimated. This technique has been primarily utilized to measure fetal umbilical venous blood flow (59,60,61,62,63), although recently the development of transvaginal duplex scanners has allowed for measurement of volume flow in the main uterine arteries (64).

The other main Doppler method used to assess the umbilical and uterine circulations employs continuous wave systems of the type used for fetal heart rate monitoring. In this case, the observations are done "blind," in that the specific vessel being isonated is not visualized, nor is depth selection possible. However, the method works well for the umbilical artery, which lies in the amniotic fluid compartment, relatively removed from other blood vessels or moving tissue interfaces and which also has a characteristic blood velocity profile. And although absolute blood velocity cannot be determined because θ is unknown, qualitative assessment of the velocity curves is possible, because the degree of pulsatility of the Doppler shift waveform is independent of θ (65). The primary use of continuous wave systems has been to assess umbilical arterial blood velocity pulsatility using the various measures noted in Figure 6–10, measures that give an indication of downstream vascular resistance in the villous circulation of the placenta (57). These indices relate diastolic flow velocity to systolic or mean velocity, as it is the diastolic component that is mainly affected by changes in downstream resistance, with decreasing, absent or reversed diastolic velocities with increasing resistance. The approach has also been used to assess vascular resistance in the maternal uterine circulation (65,66,67). But here the situation is complicated by the fact that different elements of the uterine arterial vasculature have different velocity profiles, and these in turn are different from nonuterine arteries in the pelvic region. This likely explains the variability in flow velocity waveforms obtained using continuous wave methods, but the situation is improved when duplex or color Doppler systems are employed to allow identification of the specific vessel being examined (51,68,69,70,71). Because continuous wave systems are cheaper than pulsed Doppler duplex equipment and more readily available, they are much more widely used for assessment of the umbilical and uterine perfusion. However, it must be borne in mind that, while they are providing some information on downstream vascular resistance, flow is determined by both vascular resistance and the arteriovenous perfusion pressure gradient. Doppler velocity waveform analysis provides no information on the latter variable. This likely explains the relatively weak correlation between umbilical arterial pulsatility and umbilical volume flow under normal conditions in both human and animal studies (63,72). Moreover, recent work in pregnant sheep has indicated that it is changes in the resistance of the microvascular placental circulation rather than in the umbilical arteries that primarily affect umbilical waveform pulsatility (73,74). The methods are thus of limited value in assessing the effects of vasoactive drugs on the umbilical circulation, as these primarily affect the umbilical arteries (72,73).

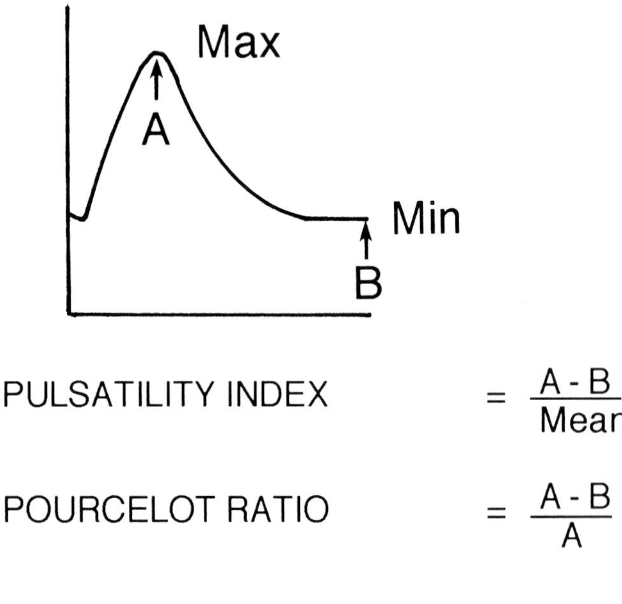


**Fig. 6–10.** Three indices of down-stream resistance used in the analysis of Doppler flow velocity waveforms. (Redrawn from Cook CM, Connelly AJ, Trudinger BJ: Doppler assessment of the umbilical circulation. Sem. Ultrasound. CT. MR. 10:417–427, 1989.)

Although the use of noninvasive Doppler techniques has added greatly to our knowledge of uterine and umbilical blood flow in the human, much of the information on the regulation of these circulations continues to come from animal studies. A number of methods have been used to estimate uterine and umbilical blood flow in animals (75). Three methods are primarily used today. The radioactive microsphere method employs 15 to 50 μ diameter plastic spheres which contain gamma ray emitting radionuclides (76). When these are injected as a bolus into the vascular system via a route that results in their presence in systemic arterial blood, they are distributed to tissues in proportion to tissue blood flow. If a reference arterial blood sample is withdrawn at a constant, known rate in conjunction with the microsphere injection, tissue blood flows can be calculated from the tissue and reference radioactive counts and the withdrawal rate. The method obviously gives flow estimates at a single point in time, but with separate injections of microspheres labelled with different radioisotopes, multiple flow measurements can be obtained in the same animal. Advantages of the method are that the different components of uterine and umbilical blood flow can be measured (47) and that maternal and fetal blood flows can be estimated in different regions of the placenta, thereby allowing examination of maternal/fetal placental flow relationships (77). A disadvantage of the technique is that continuous or long term flow measurements are not possible. These can be achieved with electromagnetic or ultrasound transit-time blood flow transducers (78,79). Both techniques require the implantation of a perivascular probe on the vessel of interest. With the electromagnetic transducer, the movement of blood through an electromagnetic field created by the probe generates a voltage whose amplitude is in part determined by the blood flow velocity. As the probe must fit tightly around the vessel for the generated voltage to be detected, the vessel cross sectional area can be determined from the internal diameter of the probe thereby allowing volume flow estimates to be obtained. The transit-time flow transducer compares the time taken for a ultrasound signal to travel in upstream and downstream directions between a pair of transmitting/receiving crystals. The difference in upstream and downstream transit times is proportional to volume flow. One advantage of the transit-time flowmeter over the electromagnetic type is that a tight fit of the transducer around the vessel is not necessary, thereby allowing for the increase in uterine and umbilical vessel diameters that occurs during pregnancy. Also, the transit-time estimates are not affected by the precise alignment of the probe, whereas the electromagnetic flow measurements are.

## *Flow Changes in Normal Pregnancy*

Before discussing the changes in uterine and umbilical blood flow that occur during normal pregnancy, the time at which maternal blood flow through the intervillous space first occurs should be considered. Until recently it has been generally assumed that an effective maternal intervillous circulation (i.e. from the spiral arteries) occurs early in the first trimester, with the latest estimate being the seventh week (80). However, Hustin and his colleagues (80,81) have presented several lines of evidence that suggest that this does not occur until week 12. Before this the distal ends of the spiral appear to be occluded by trophoblastic plugs that are contiguous with the cytotrophoblast shell, thereby preventing the entry of normally constituted maternal blood into the intervillous space, although plasma flow and entry of some red cells may occur. Moreover, when contrast material was injected into the uterine arteries following hysterectomy before 12 weeks gestation, it appeared in the uterine vein, but the not intervillous space, suggesting the existence of uterine arteriovenous shunts proximal to the intervillous space. Hustin, et al have suggested that until ~12 weeks gestation the number and effectiveness of anchoring villi are insufficient to prevent disruption of the placenta if there were unimpeded entry of maternal blood into the intervillous space, and that failure of this mechanism may be responsible for some cases of first trimester pregnancy loss. They also hypothesize that because of the apparent lack of true maternal placental blood flow (i.e. whole blood) in early pregnancy, embryonic development may occur at low oxygen levels.

The changes in uterine blood flow in human pregnancy, determined using duplex Doppler ultrasonography, are illustrated in Figure 6–11. There is more or less a linear increase in flow from 6 to 8 weeks gestation until term. The values are for the left uterine artery only, so that if there is the same flow in the right artery, total flow at term is ~700 ml/min or ~12% of maternal cardiac output (64). Other methods of estimating intervillous blood flow in late pregnancy suggest a value of ~500 ml/min (50). Thus, the myometrium and nonplacental endometrium could receive ~25% of total uterine blood flow, although firmer data are warranted. In pregnant sheep, the proportion of uterine flow going to the placenta increases progressively during gestation, while the fractions going to the endometrium and myometrium decrease (82). The gestational rise in uterine blood flow is associated with increases in uterine arterial diameter and peak systolic blood velocity and decreases in the indices of the flow velocity waveform that reflect vascular resistance, largely as a result of increases in diastolic flow velocity (64,68,71,83,84). Some studies report discrepancies in the flow velocity characteristics of the left and right uterine arteries, at least in the first and second trimesters, but there is not universal agreement on this point.

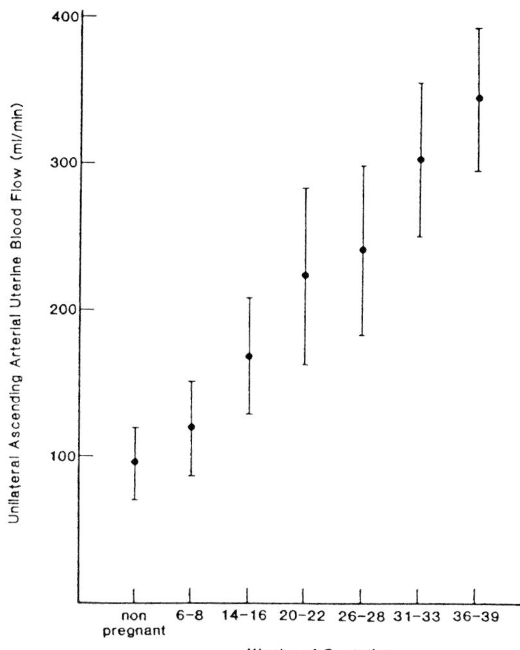


**Fig. 6–11.** Changes in blood flow in one uterine artery during human pregnancy. (From Thaler I, Manor D, Itskovitz J, Rottem S, et al: Changes in uterine blood flow during normal human pregnancy. Am. J. Obstet. Gynecol. 162:121–125, 1990.)

The changes in human fetal umbilical venous flow during gestation have been measured in several studies (60,63,85,86), and a representative example of the findings is given in Figure 6–12. Absolute flow increases exponentially, but this is not quite sufficient to keep up with fetal growth, so that flow/kg estimated fetal weight declines as gestation proceeds. The increase in flow is associated with decreases in the measures of downstream vascular resistance, as a consequence of an increase in the diastolic flow component (87,88,89,90) (Figure 6–9). The average value for umbilical flow/kg fetal weight ranges from 100 to 130 ml/min kg, and this is about one-third of fetal combined ventricular output (91). Some studies have reported a decrease in flow/kg in near or after normal term (85), whereas others have not, and it was not observed in the one study in which patients were studied longitudinally (60).

## *Control and Matching of Maternal and Fetal Flows*

There has been a very large number of studies on the control of maternal and fetal placental blood flows in recent years, primarily in animal species, and the reader is referred to reviews for a comprehensive discussion of this subject (75,92,93,94). However, several general points can be made here.

In considering the regulation of maternal and fetal placental blood flows, it is convenient to divide the topic into three parts: factors that affect the flows over the short

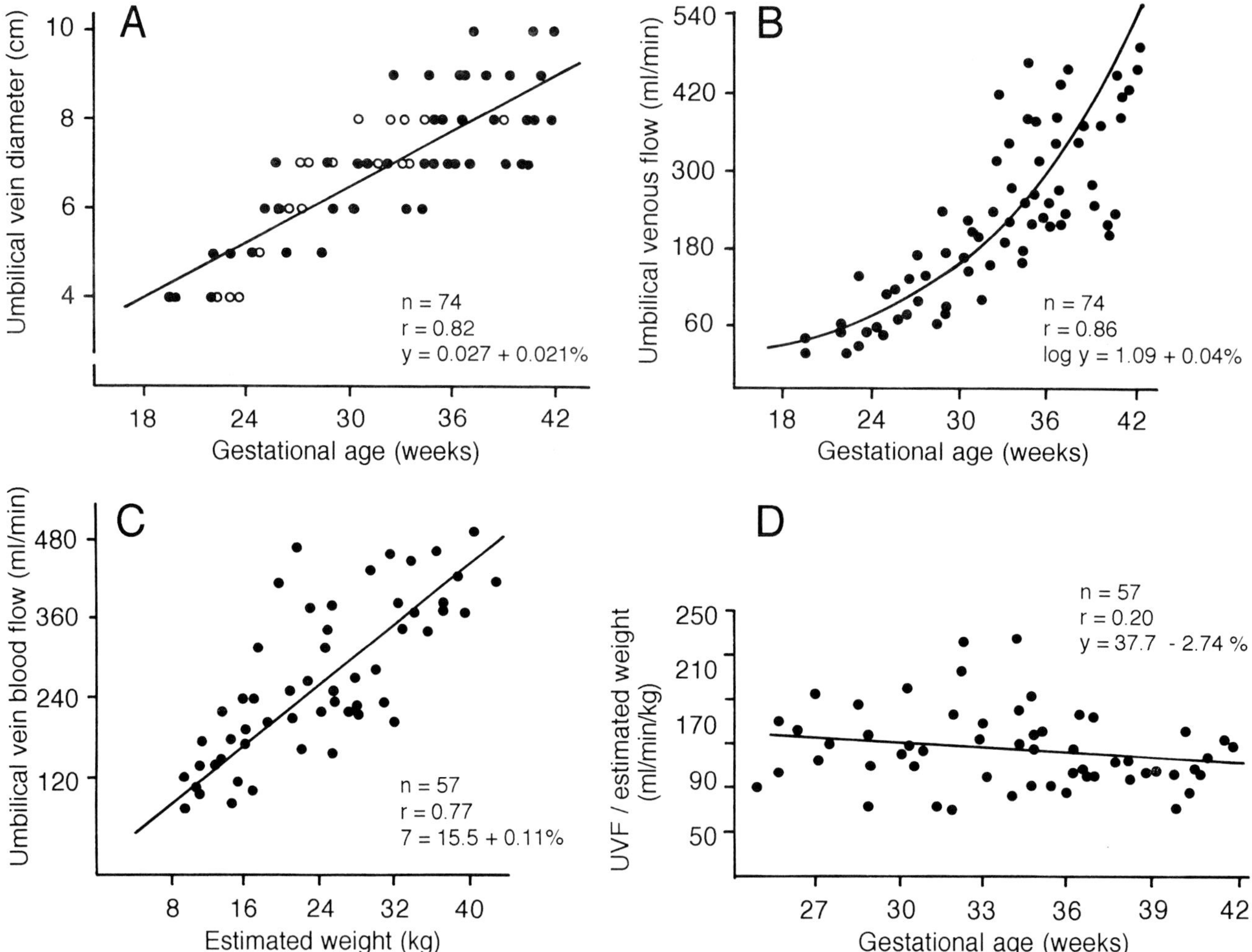


**Fig. 6–12.** Umbilical venous blood flow in human pregnancy measured with Doppler and real-time ultrasound. **A,** Umbilical vein diameter during gestation, **B,** Umbilical venous flow in relation to gestational age, **C,** Umbilical venous flow in relation to estimated fetal weight, **D,** Umbilical venous flow/kg estimated fetal weight in relation to gestational age. (Redrawn from St. John Sutton M, Theard MA, Bhatia SJS, Plappert T, et al: Changes in placental blood flow in the normal human fetus with gestational age. Pediatr. Res. 28:383–387, 1990.)

term, long term control through gestation, and whether and how there is control of the matching of maternal and fetal placental flows, both for the whole placenta and for localized regions. It is also useful to recall that the flow is determined by vascular resistance and the hydrostatic driving pressure, so that any factor affecting or controlling flow has to influence one or both of these variables, usually the former. With hemochorial placentae, it appears that the main site of resistance in the maternal placental circulation, and hence the most effective site for regulation, is in the main arteries outside of the uterus. Moll and Kunzel (95) found that the pressure in the arteries entering the placenta in guinea pigs, rabbits, and rats was only 18%, 8%, and 11% of central arterial pressure, respectively. The situation appears similar in rhesus monkeys, where hydrostatic pressures measured at various sites within the intervillous space average ~5 to 15 mm Hg, with maternal arterial pressures of 75 to 85 mm Hg (96). And given the above described changes in the vascular wall of the spiral arteries that occurs in the human, a similar situation is likely in this species as well. In contrast, in the sheep epitheliochorial placenta, "preplacental" arterial pressure is 79% of central arterial pressure, indicating that in this species, the main site of resistance is within the placenta (29). The hydrostatic pressure drop across the fetal umbilical circulation appears to have been measured only in sheep (29). In this species, 85% of the total vascular resistance lies between the umbilical arteries and the liver, and the bulk of this is in the villous circulation. If a similar situation exists in species with a hemochorial placenta, then it seems that the regulation of the uterine and umbilical circulations occurs at different sites. Also, it appears possible that the regulation of uterine blood flow in sheep, which is the most widely studied animal species, could differ from the species, including the human, which possess a hemochorial placenta. Finally, there is no evidence for neural regulation of the uterine and umbilical circulations (75); any control that does occur appears mediated by the chemical and physical mechanisms discussed below.

### *Short Term Regulation of Uterine and Umbilical Flows*

Most of the studies that have examined short term changes in uterine and umbilical flows have been conducted with pregnant sheep. Under normal circumstances, the main factors affecting uterine blood flow are prelabor uterine contractions (also termed contractures) and postural changes (Figure 6–13, Harding, et al, 1984). Prelabor uterine contractions occur at fairly regular intervals of ~30 to 90 minutes in pregnant sheep, are associated with intrauterine pressure increases of ~5 mm Hg, and last ~5 minutes; they may be analogous to Braxton-Hicks contractions in human pregnancy (97). Uterine flow decreases by 7 to 16% during contractions and by 6 to 12% with the change from lying to standing (98,99,100). Umbilical blood flow is not consistently changed during these contractions (101) nor with changes in maternal posture. However, there are periodic increases in umbilical flow associated with the transient fetal heart accelerations and hypertension (Figure 6–14), which in turn are associated with fetal movement (102). And there are transient decreases in umbilical blood flow with changes in fetal behaviorial state from rapid eye movement to quiet sleep (91,103). Both uterine and umbilical blood flows exhibit reciprocal diurnal variations in pregnant sheep, with uterine perfusion being ~9% higher than average flow during the day, while umbilical flow is ~3% higher during the night (104). A similar diurnal variation in uterine blood flow is observed in the rhesus monkey. However, the amplitude of the variation of about twofold is greater than in the sheep, and the nocturnal decrease in flow is associated with increased uterine activity (105). In contrast, there are no rhythms in intrauterine pressure, nor in maternal or fetal arterial pressures in pregnant ewes (104,106). Alterations in uterine or umbilical perfusion pressures result in corresponding changes in uterine and umbilical flows, respectively, in sheep (Figure 6–15), i.e., there is no evidence for autoregulation in these vascular beds (107). But the situation with the hemochorial placenta of the rabbit appears different, because uterine blood flow, at least, is well maintained with decreases of maternal arterial pressure down to ~70% of normal (108) (Figure 6–15). One other mechanism has been postulated to affect umbilical flow acutely. This is the effect of the pressure in the tissue surrounding the fetal placental capillary beds (i.e. the intervillous space in a human placenta). Experiments performed with perfused placental cotyledons in pregnant sheep suggested that it was the difference between fetal arterial pressure and the surrounding pressure that determined the hydrostatic pressure gradient, and that, further, the surrounding pressure was high enough to affect fetal placental blood flow by a "sluice" or "waterfall" phenomenon (109,110). However, subsequent studies of chronically instrumented fetal lambs in utero have failed to confirm these observations, suggesting that in this species, at least, the mechanism does not operate (101,111).

A number of vasoactive agents have been shown to affect either uterine and/or umbilical blood flow acutely. However, a functional role for any of the agents in regulating the flows has yet to be conclusively demonstrated (75,92,94). In terms of uterine and maternal placental flow, the substances most widely studied are angiotensin II, epinephrine, and norepinephrine. The numerous studies of angiotensin II effects in several species have reported both increases and decreases in uterine perfusion (112). A possible explanation for these discrepant results is provided by studies in pregnant sheep, which indicate that the uterine circulation has a lower responsiveness to angiotensin than does the systemic circulation, and thus with lower doses of the hormone, the systemic vasoconstriction leads to hypertension, which in turn leads to increased uterine blood flow (113). With higher angiotensin doses, uterine vasoconstriction overrides the increase in pressure, resulting in reduced uterine blood flow. Similar findings have been made on pregnant rabbits (114); however, other studies in rabbits and in monkeys report much greater percentage increases in uterine blood flow than in arterial pressure with angiotensin administration,

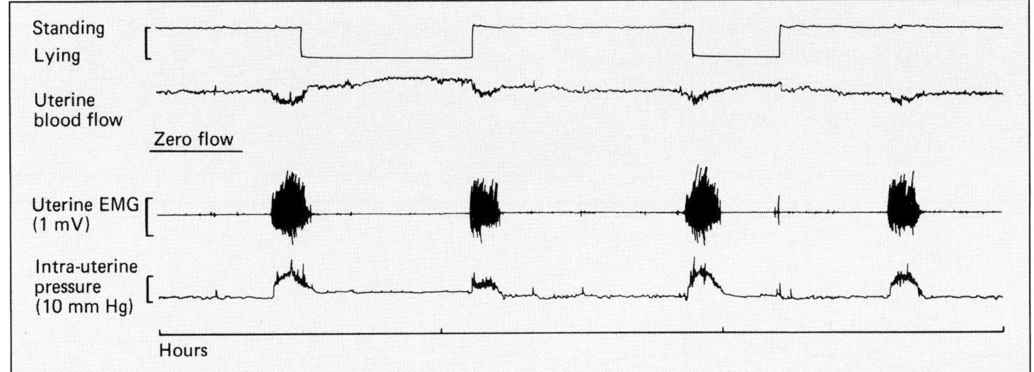


**Fig. 6–13.** The relationship between nonlabor uterine contractions and uterine blood flow in a pregnant sheep. The influence of maternal posture on uterine blood flow is also evident. (From Harding R, Poore ER: The effects of myometrial activity on fetal thoracic dimensions and uterine blood flow during late gestation in the sheep. Biol. Neonate. 45:244–251, 1984.)

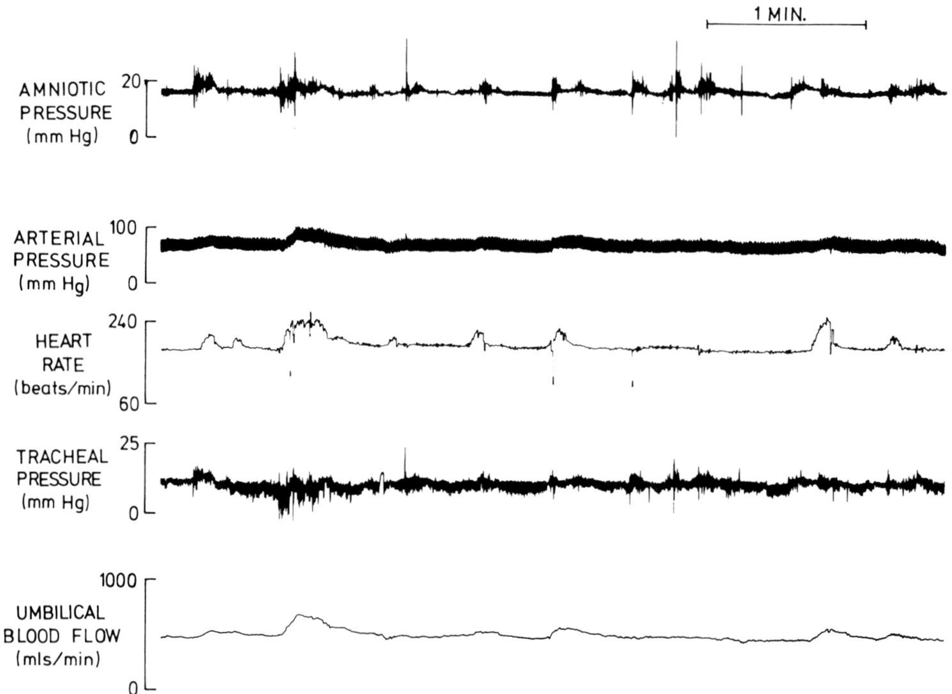


**Fig. 6–14.** Amniotic pressure, and fetal arterial pressure, heart rate, tracheal pressure and umbilical blood flow in a chronically instrumented pregnant sheep. The transient increase in umbilical blood flow in association with heart rate accelerations is evident. (From Dan Rurak, M.D., unpublished observations.)

suggesting uterine vasodilation (115,116). In pregnant sheep, the relative refractoriness of the uterine circulation to angiotensin is due to a limited responsiveness of the maternal placental circulation; angiotensin-induced vasoconstriction in the myometrium and endometrium is similar to that in systemic tissues (117). Because of this limited responsiveness, it is unlikely that maternal endogenous angiotensin II levels could increase to levels high enough to reduce uterine perfusion. Treatment of pregnant sheep and rabbits with sarlasin, a competitive inhibitor of angiotensin II, leads to hypotension and reduced uterine and maternal placental blood flow (118,119), and similar results have been reported in rabbits and sheep following treatment with the angiotensin converting enzyme inhibitor, captopril (117,120,121). With both saralasin and captopril treatment in these species, placental blood flow was reduced to a greater extent than myometrial flow. Also, the decrease in flow tended to be greater than the decrease in arterial pressure, i.e. there was apparent placental vasoconstriction. However, because captopril or saralasin-induced vasodilation in other vascular beds is likely greater than the changes in resistance in the maternal placental circulation, it may be that there was diversion of blood from the placenta to these other beds, rather than actual placental vasoconstriction (121). Although these results suggest that the renin-angiotensin system may sustain uterine blood flow via the maintenance of maternal arterial pressure, Ferris and Weib (117) found than when arterial pressure in pregnant rabbits was reduced with magnesium sulfate to a similar extent as with saralasin and captopril, uterine blood flow was unchanged. There may well be species differences in the role of the renin-angiotensin system in the regulation of uterine blood flow, because in species such as the rabbit and human, there appears to be a synthesis and release of renin by the uterus, whereas in others, such as sheep, there is not (114,122). Moreover, studies in pregnant rabbits have shown that when uterine perfusion is reduced experimentally, uterine renin secretion is increased (114).

In contrast to the relative insensitivity of the uterine vasculature to angiotensin II, there is a significant responsiveness to catecholamines in several species, a response mediated by α-adrenergic mechanisms (79,112, 123,124,125). In pregnant sheep, the degree of α agonist-induced vasconstriction is greater in the uterine circulation than in systemic vascular beds (124,126). However, the vasoconstriction in the placenta is less than in myometrium and endometrium (125). In spite of the sensitivity of the uterine vasculature to catecholamines, it is unlikely that endogenous α-adrenergic tone plays a role in the regulation of uterine blood flow, because treatment of pregnant sheep with α receptor antagonists does not affect uterine blood flow or vascular resistance (112,127). However, very significant reductions in uterine perfusion can be achieved with elevated catecholamine levels, either via exogenous administration or as a result of psychological stress, and this can lead to significant fetal hypoxemia and acidemia (79,124,128,129). And similar reductions in uterine blood flow, although to varying degrees with different agents, are observed with sympathomimetic agents (ephedrine, metarminol, mephentermine, methoxamine) used as vasopressors (130). In contrast, the β2-adrenergic agonists, such as ritodrine, used for treatment of premature labor, have no effects on uterine or umbilical blood flows, except as very high concentrations, when modest vasodilation occurs (112,131).

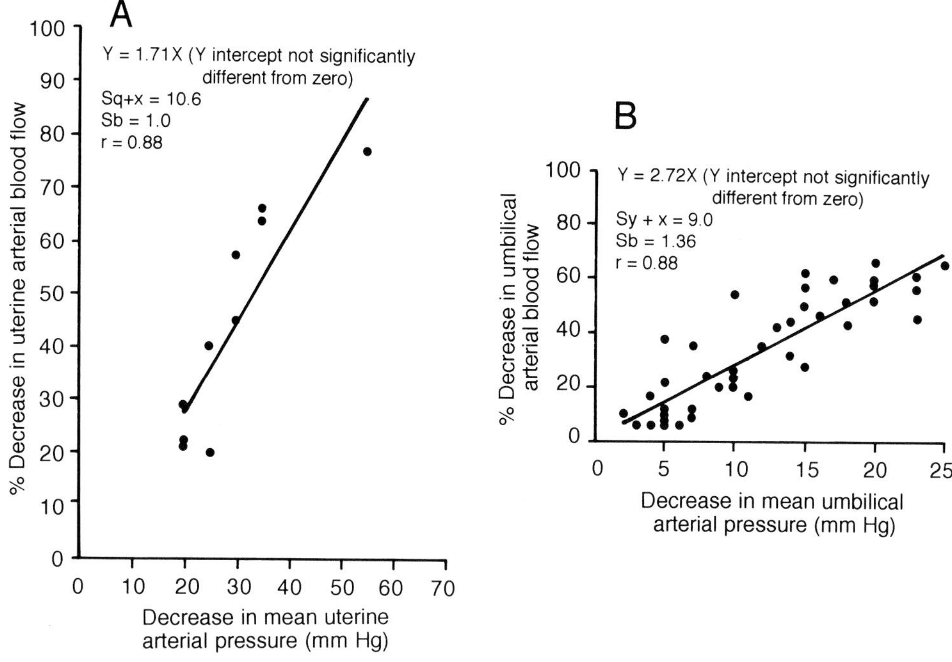


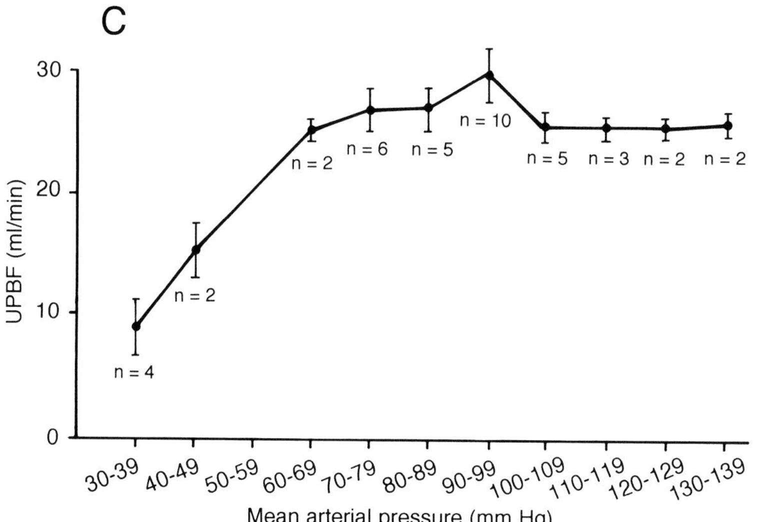


**Fig. 6–15.** Relationship between arterial pressure and (A) uterine and (B) umbilical in pregnant sheep and (C) uterine blood flow in pregnant rabbits. (A and B redrawn from Berman W Jr, Goodlin RC, Heymann MA, Rudolph AM: Relationships between pressure and flow in the umbilical and uterine circulations of the sheep. Circ. Res. 38:264–266, 1976.) (C redrawn from Venuto RC, Cox JW, Stein JH, Ferris TF: The effect of changes in perfusion pressure on uteroplacental blood flow in the pregnant rabbit. J. Clin. Invest. 57: 938–944, 1976.)

Angiotensin II also causes umbilical vasoconstriction and reduced flow in fetal lambs (79,132,133,134). Administration of angiotensin antagonists has no effect on fetal placental blood flow or vascular resistance (135,136), suggesting that the hormone is unlikely to affect umbilical vascular resistance under normal conditions. However, the angiotensin-converting enzyme inhibitor, captopril, results in hypotension, decreased umbilical blood flow, and an apparent increase in placental vascular resistance in the fetal lamb (120). But as was discussed above for captopril effects on uterine blood flow, the apparent increase in fetal placental resistance may actually reflect diversion of blood from the placenta to other fetal vascular beds that vasodilate in response to captopril. The fetal umbilical circulation is generally unresponsive to norepinephrine in sheep (79,127,132,133,137). Thus, the relative potencies of angiotensin II and norepinephrine in increasing umbilical vascular resistance are reversed from that observed in the uterine circulation. Arginine vasopressin in another endogenous vasoconstrictor increases placental vascular resistance in the fetal lamb (138), and it may play a role in the umbilical vascular responses to hypoxemia. Fetal plasma levels of the hormone increase during hypoxemia (139,140), and when a vasopressin $V_1$ antagonist is administered, there is a significant rise in fetal placental blood flow and decrease in vascular resistance (141). Overall then, although some of these vasoconstrictors may be involved in the uterine or umbilical responses to stress, they do not appear to contribute to the regulation of these circulations under normal conditions.

## *Long Term Regulation of Uterine and Umbilical Blood Flows*

So far, the discussion of the control of uterine and umbilical blood flow has dealt with short term regulation in late pregnancy. What remains to be considered are possible mechanisms responsible for the dramatic increases in maternal and fetal placental blood flow during the course of gestation. Also, because in sheep at least, there appears to be relatively equal rates of maternal and fetal perfusion to localized areas of the placenta both under control conditions and when umbilical blood flow is altered (77,110), the possibility that there is some form of local regulation to achieve matching of maternal and fetal flows will also be discussed.

There is considerable evidence to suggest that estrogens are responsible, in part at least, for the increase in uterine blood flow during pregnancy (142). Bolus administration of exogenous estrogens has been shown to increase uterine blood flow in numerous species, including the human (143). The effect is most striking in nonpregnant, ovariectomized animals and when given locally to the uterus by intra-arterial injection (144,145). However, increased flow is also observed with acute estrogen administration to pregnant ewes, with increased perfusion occurring for all elements of the uterus (myometrium, endometrium, placenta). In absolute terms, the flow increase is similar in nonpregnant and pregnant animals, but because of the large increase in basal flow in pregnancy, the percentage rise following estrogen is less than in the nonpregnant ewes (142) (Figure 6–16). Chronic systemic administration of estrogen to ovariectomized nonpregnant ewes does not result in a sustained increase in uterine blood flow; rather tachyphylaxis develops (146). However, when estradiol is administered into the uterine lumen in nonpregnant sows, uterine blood flow was dramatically increased for up to 6 days (147), suggesting that local estrogen production by the placenta could be involved in the increase in uterine blood flow during gestation. Further evidence for a role of estrogens in the long term regulation of uterine blood flow is provided by the studies that demonstrate correlations between plasma estrogen and progesterone levels and uterine blood flow in sheep during the estrus cycle, early and late pregnancy, and immediately following parturition (148,149).

Our understanding of the long term control of umbilical blood flow is far from complete (95). However, it seems likely that the progressive increase in umbilical blood flow during gestation is due in large part to the elaboration of new fetal placental vessels that occurs as a component of villous growth and branching, and thus may be regulated locally by angiogenic factors. Certainly, no endocrine regulator has been identified. Faber, et al (150) have demonstrated that fetal blood volume is a major determinant of umbilical blood flow in sheep, suggesting that transplacental fluid acquisition by the fetus during growth, and hence transplacental hydrostatic, osmotic and oncotic gradients, could be a long term modulator of fetal placental perfusion (92,151). However, when umbilical blood flow in fetal lambs was reduced by ~30% for an average of 14 days, via an adjustable occluder placed on the descending aorta to reduce placental perfusion pressure, fetal arterial pressure did not increase nor did fetal placental vascular resistance decrease (152). Thus, the negative feed-back mechanisms via which umbilical blood flow could be restored did not operate; rather estimated fetal daily growth rate fell to about 50% of normal, presumably due to decreased umbilical delivery of oxygen and nutrients (153). In addition, when the occlusion was momentarily released each day and unrestricted flow observed, the flow immediately returned to the level appropriate for that gestational age (Figure 6–17). The findings reinforce the view that the increase in umbilical flow during gestation is "programmed" by placental villous

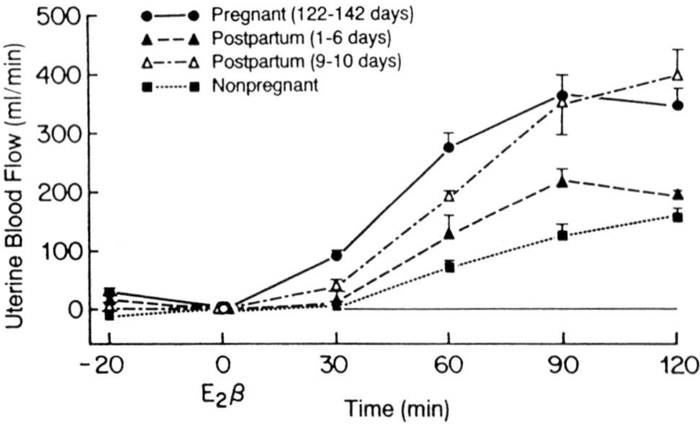


**Fig. 6–16.** Effects of intravenous estradiol-17β on the absolute change in uterine blood flow from baseline in ovariectomized nonpregnant, intact postpartum (days 1–6 and 9–10) and late pregnant (days 122–142) sheep. (From Magness RR, Rosenfeld CR: The role of steroid hormones in the control of uterine blood flow. *In* The Uterine Circulation. Edited by CR Rosenfeld. Ithaca, Perinatology Press, 1989, pp. 239–271.)

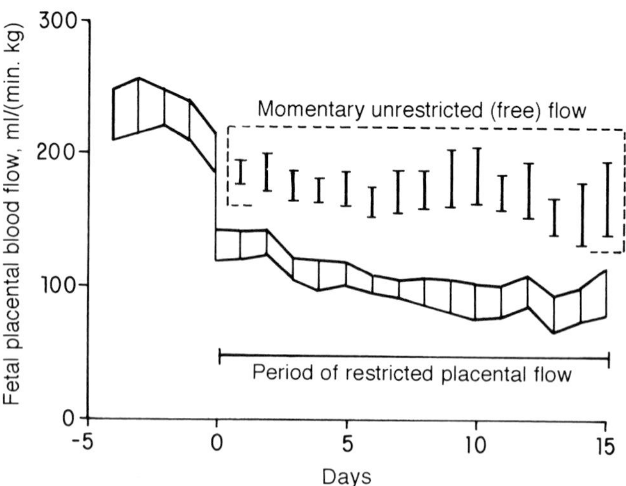


**Fig. 6–17.** Fetal placental blood flow in a control period and for 15 days after restricting flow. During each of the latter days, the restriction was momentarily relieved and the unrestricted flow was observed. (Redrawn from Anderson DF, Faber JJ: Regulation of fetal placental blood flow in the lamb. Am. J. Physiol. 247:R567–R574, 1984.)

growth and maturation and is not subject to regulation by fetal homeostatic mechanisms.

There is another class of vasoactive substances that might affect maternal and fetal placental blood flows on a short or long term basis. These are the prostaglandins, thromboxanes, and other products of arachidonic acid. There are several lines of evidence to suggest that these compounds could regulate placental perfusion. They are produced by the decidua, placenta and fetal membranes, and some prostaglandins and/or their metabolites are released into the maternal and fetal circulations (117,154,155,156). As a group, prostaglandins exhibit both vasoconstrictor and vasodilator actions on the placental vasculature in vitro and in vivo (157). However, clear elucidation of their role has been hindered by the fact that while prostanoids and thromboxane are produced and act locally within the placenta, and the study of their effects on placental perfusion in vivo has involved systemic administration, leading to the potential confounding influences of systemic or oxytocic effects. Thus, when exogenous prostanglandin $E_2$ is administered to pregnant sheep there is a fall in uteroplacental blood flow and increase in vascular resistance, but this is associated with a uterine contraction (158). And although prostacyclin is a vasodilator of the uterine and umbilical vasculature in vitro (103), administration of the agent to fetal lambs in utero generally results in a fall of umbilical blood flow, with no change in calculated vascular resistance, but this is due to a significant fetal hypotension, this in turn being the result of systemic vasodilation (159). Thus, there may be diversion of blood flow from the umbilical circulation to the vasodilated beds, resulting in an apparent increase in umbilical resistance. In vitro studies indicate that thromboxane, prostaglandins $F_2\alpha$, $E_2$, $D_2$ elicit placental vasoconstriction, while prostacyclin (prostaglandin $I_2$) is a vasodilator (157). However, in pregnant sheep $PGE_2$ causes uterine vasodilation, at least when given via the fetus, so as to avoid the confounding effect of $PGE_2$-elicited uterine contractions (158). And, $PGE_2$ has also been implicated as the mediator of angiotensin II-induced uterine vasodilation in pregnant rabbits (117), and as at least one of the mechanisms for the attenuated responsiveness of the pregnant uterus to angiotensin (156). And as will be discussed below, prostaglandin $E_2$ has been suggested as a mediator in the matching of maternal and fetal blood flows in the sheep placenta. Prostaglandins have also been proposed to be involved in the alterations in uterine and umbilical flows that occur with some pregnancy complications. Decreased placental production of prostacyclin and increased production of thromboxane occurs in pregnancies associated with preeclampsia and diabetes (160), and the changes in the ratio of this vasodilator and vasoconstrictor have been postulated to cause the alterations in umbilical arterial hemodynamics that occur with the former condition (159,161). However, exogenous prostacyclin does not improve uterine or umbilical blood flows in preeclamptic pregnancies (162). Finally, studies involving inhibition of prostaglandin synthesis with indomethacin or antipyrine have not provided evidence for the involvement of prostaglandins in the regulation of uterine or umbilical blood flow. While bolus indomethacin injection in pregnant sheep leads to uterine and umbilical vasoconstriction, the responses are transient and do not follow the time course of prostaglandin synthesis (163,164). And infusion of antipyrine in pregnant sheep, at a dose that significantly reduces uterine venous but not fetal arterial prostaglandin levels, has no effect on either uterine or umbilical blood flow (165). Similarly, indomethacin therapy for premature labor or polyhydramnios in pregnant women is not associated with any change in umbilical arterial pulsatility index, although a reduction in fetal prostaglandin levels was indicated by constriction of the ductus arteriosus (166). It may be that these studies did not achieve a sufficient enough degree of local placental prostaglandin synthesis inhibition to affect perfusion. It is also possible that there could have been synthesis inhibition of both a vasodilatory and vasoconstrictive prostaglandins, with no resultant change in placental perfusion. Clearly, further work is needed to establish the role of prostaglandins in the control of uterine and umbilical blood flow under both normal conditions and in disease states.

As noted above, studies in pregnant sheep have indicated that maternal and fetal perfusion to localized areas of the placenta is generally closely matched, a phenomenon similar to the matching of ventilation and perfusion in different regions of the lung (77,167,168,169). Moreover, when maternal blood flow is reduced to portions of the sheep placenta, there is a reduction in fetal flow to these same areas over the next 24 hours, and a similar change occurs in maternal placental flow when fetal placental flow is experimentally decreased to a limited area of the placenta (77,170,171). These findings suggest the presence of a local mechanism in the placenta to match maternal and fetal blood flows, and which acts to shunt either maternal or fetal blood away from regions that are underperfused from the other side (169), a view also supported by recent studies of the matching of maternal and fetal perfusion to individual placental cotyledons before and after maternal captopril administration (120). There are also data suggesting that maternal and fetal placental flows in toto respond to long term flow alterations on the other side of the placenta. In pregnant sheep and rabbits, experimental death of the fetus in utero is followed by a progressive reduction uterine blood flow over the next 24 hours (170,172), and when uterine vascular resistance is increased by embolization of the uterine circulation, there is also a rise in umbilical vascular resistance, but only in those fetuses that subsequently demonstrate evidence of growth restriction (173). Rankin (174) suggested that placental prostaglandin E2 was the mediator of this matching of maternal and fetal placental blood flows. This was based upon observations that prostaglandin E2 elicits vasoconstriction of the umbilical circulation and vasodilation of the uterine vasculature (158,175). Thus, when maternal blood flow to one portion of the placenta fell, prostaglandin E2 would be produced locally to elicit maternal vasodilation to increase maternal flow, while at the same time cause fetal placental vasoconstriction to reduce fetal blood flow, thereby moving the maternal/fetal perfusion ratio back to unity. This is the situation that has been examined to date in the experimental studies of flow matching, i.e. one or other flows have been decreased. What has not been studied is the situation where flow on one side is increased. Nor has there been examination of the effect of inhibition of placental prostaglandin synthesis on the degree of matching of maternal and fetal placental blood flows. Also, this mechanism appears most plausible for the type of placenta present in sheep, where there are both maternal and fetal vessels whose vascular tone could be altered to achieve localized regulation of flow. In the human, however, localized regulation of maternal blood flow within the intervillous space seems unlikely.

### *Maternal and Fetal Flows in Compromised Pregnancies*

As was outlined earlier, there is increasing evidence that in pregnancies that ultimately develop preeclampsia and fetal growth restriction, there is a failure of the process of spiral artery wall alteration to go to completion. It has also been well-demonstrated that later in gestation, these pregnancies exhibit alterations in the Doppler velocity waveforms obtained from the umbilical and uterine arteries (65,176). The characteristic alteration in the fetal placental vasculature is a reduced diastolic velocity for gestational age (67,177,178,179) (Figure 6–18a). In the most extreme cases, there can be absent or reversed diastolic velocity (180,181,182) (Figure 6–18b). Several lines of evidence indicate that the cause of these alterations appears to be an increase in downstream umbilical vascular resistance or impedance. The abnormal waveforms are associated with a reduction in number of small arterial vessels in the tertiary stem villi, which may be due to obliteration of vessels (183,184). Moreover, measurement of umbilical volume flow in preeclamptic pregnancies and in other conditions associated with fetal hypoxia indicates lower than normal flows (61,185). In pregnant sheep, similar alterations in umbilical arterial velocity waveforms can be achieved by embolization of the umbilical circulation with microspheres, and this is associated with an increase in umbilical vascular resistance and decreased umbilical blood flow (186,187,188). However, waveform alterations precede decreased flow and increased resistance. Animal studies have also demonstrated that umbilical arterial waveforms are not altered by other features of preeclamptic pregnancies, such as fetal hypoxia, hyperviscosity and maternal hypertension, nor by elevated fetal catecholamine levels or reductions or embolization of the uterine circulation (189,190,191,192). The embolization experiments in sheep also are associated with fetal hypoxemia and acidemia, which worsen as the degree of embolization and waveform alteration increase. Sampling of human fetal blood by cordocentesis has also indicated hypoxemia and acidemia with reduced umbilical arterial diastolic velocity, and the degree of blood gas deterioration appears greatest with absent end-diastolic velocity (193,194,195). But it is important to emphasize that abnormal umbilical velocity waveforms are primarily an indication of placental pathology, rather than of fetal hypoxia. In fact, fetal hypoxia is better correlated with alterations in fetal carotid arterial and aortic Doppler velocity waveforms that likely reflect hypoxia-induced changes in the distribution of cardiac output (196). The umbilical arterial waveform can also be altered in twin and diabetic pregnancies and in association with placental abruption (197,198,199,200, 201,202). Reduced diastolic velocity has also been observed in the uterine vasculature associated with preeclampsia and fetal growth restriction (67,203). This is consistent with the reports of reduced uterine perfusion in such pregnancies, estimated from the metabolic clearance rate of dehydroisoandrosterone sulfate (50) and from placental uptake of radioisotopes (204,205,206). However, the problem of precisely identifying the uterine vessels being examined that was mentioned earlier in relation to examining the uterine circulation in normal pregnancies likely explains, in part at least, the low correlation between this measure and clinical outcome (176,207,208).

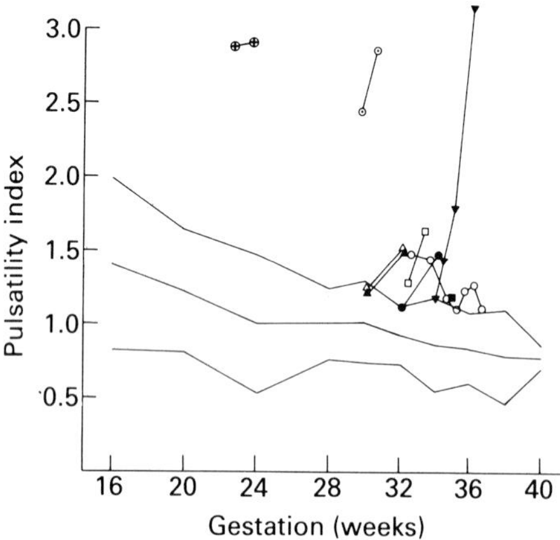


**Fig. 6–18.** Abnormal umbilical arterial flow velocity waveforms. **A,** Normal range of pulsatility index during gestation (mean ± 2SD) compared to individual values from nine growth-retarded fetuses. (From Erskine RLA, Ritchie JWK: Umbilical artery blood flow characteristics in normal and growth-retarded fetuses. Br. J. Obstet. Gynaecol. 92:605–610, 1985.) **B,** Serial waveforms from one patient at 25, 26, 27 weeks showing the reduction then loss of the diastolic velocity component. (From Woo JSK, Liang ST, Lo RLS: Significance of an absent or reversed end diastolic flow in Doppler umbilical artery waveforms. J. Ultrasound. Med. 6:291–297, 1987.)

## PLACENTAL TRANSFER FUNCTIONS

### *Methods of Transfer*

As is the case with other biologic membrane systems, a number of different transfer mechanisms are utilized by the placenta (93,209). By far the most common method is simple diffusion down a physicochemical gradient. It is the mechanism of transfer for respiratory gases, some electrolytes (e.g. sodium), fatty acids, steroids and other lipid soluble compounds, and most therapeutic agents. The permeability values for a number of hydrophilic compounds have been determined for the human placenta in vitro and in vivo, and these are similar to estimates obtained in other species (e.g. rabbit, guinea pig) that also possess a hemochorial placenta (93,210, 211, 212, 213). Not surprisingly, permeability decreases progressively

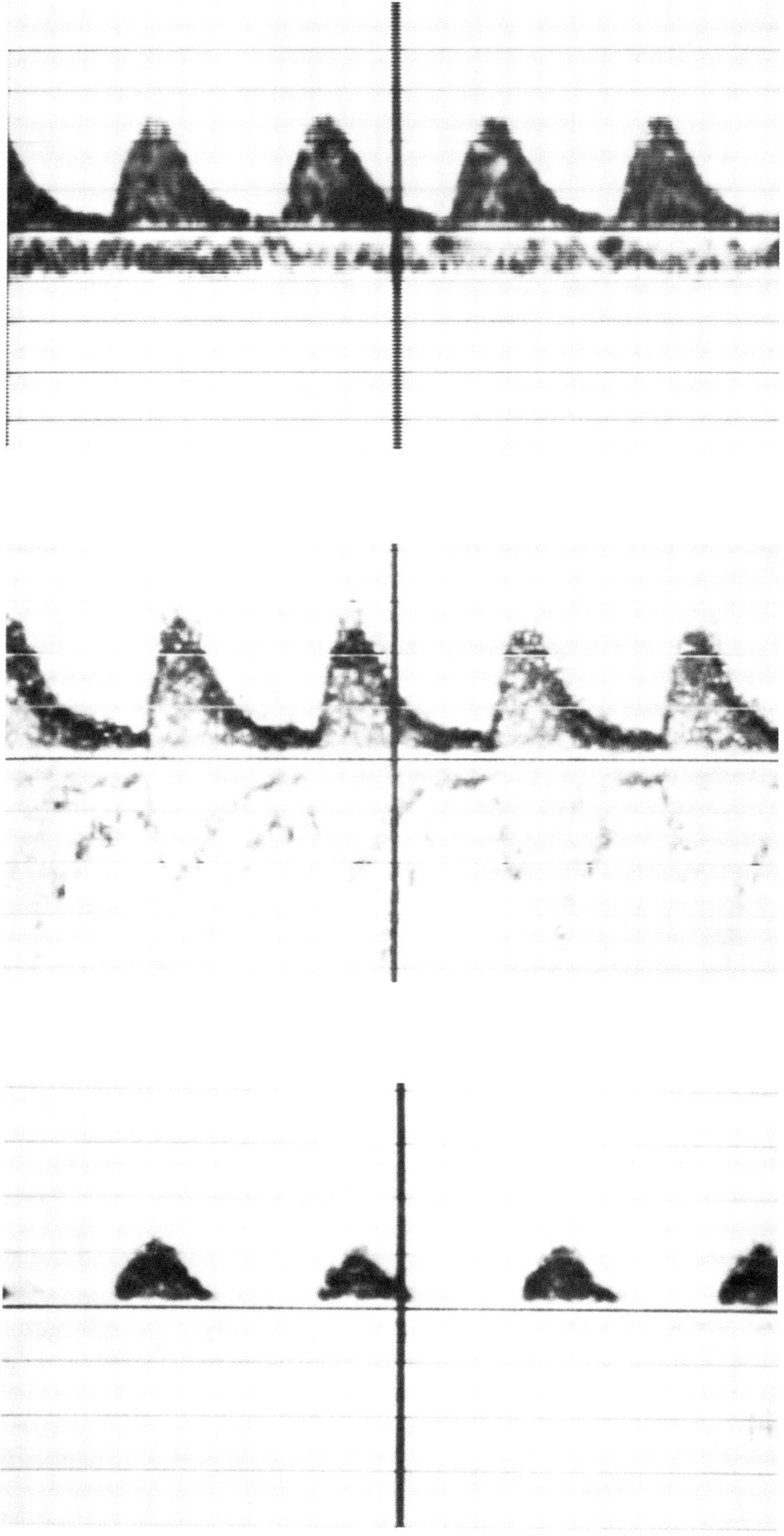

Fig. 6–18. (*Continued*)

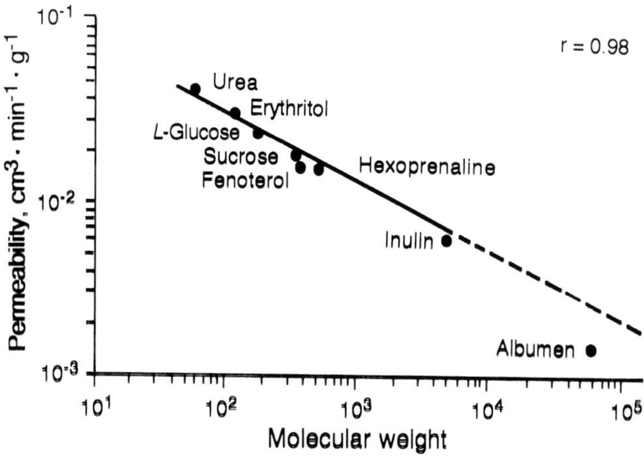


**Fig. 6–19.** Plot of the logarithm of permeability against molecular weight for several substances in perfused human placentae. (Redrawn from Schneider H, Sodha RJ, Progler M, Young MPA: Permeability of the human placenta for hydrophilic substances studied in the isolated dually in vitro perfused lobe. Contr. Gynecol. Obstet. 13:98–103, 1985.)

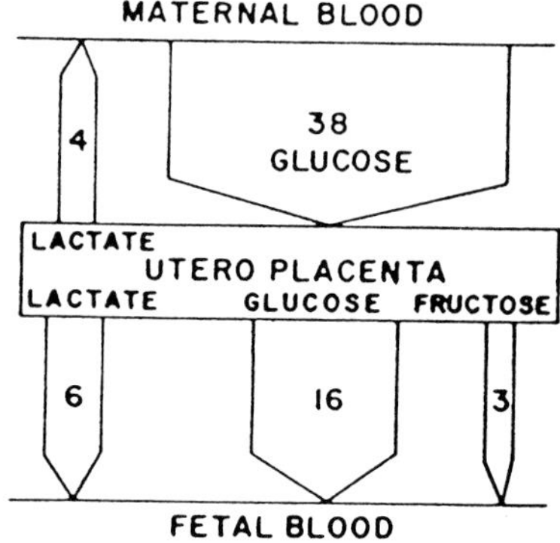


**Fig. 6–20.** Representative normal values for net fluxes (mg/min) of glucose, lactate, and fructose between maternal blood, uteroplacenta, and fetal blood in a pregnant ewe carrying a 3 kg fetus. (From Battaglia FC, Meschia G: Fetal nutrition. Ann. Rev. Nutr. 8:43–61, 1988.)

with increased molecular weight (Figure 6–19). For lipid soluble drugs, transfer occurs relatively unimpeded up to molecular weights of ~600, while for hydrophilic drugs the limit is ~100 (214).

Placental transfer of glucose and some other carbohydrates occurs via facilitated diffusion, i.e., transfer via a membrane-bound carrier at rates significantly greater than would occur via simple diffusion (93). Membrane vesicle preparations have been obtained from human trophoblast cells, which allow study of the kinetics of this membrane-bound exchanger (215). In vivo, transfer is still down a physicochemical gradient, so that fetal plasma glucose levels are lower than in the mother. Moreover, if fetal glucose levels rise as a result of endogenous glucose mobilization to reduce the maternal-fetal glucose concentration gradient, net fetal uptake of glucose from the placenta can cease or reverse (131). Conversely, infusion of glucose to the mother will increase placental glucose transfer and fetal glucose concentration, although to a lesser extent than in the mother (216). Fetal plasma concentrations of most amino acids are higher than those in the mother, suggesting active placental transport of these molecules (217,218). There are energy requiring amino acid transporters coupled to $Na+$-$K+$ ATPase-driven $NA+$ and $H+$ exchange that transfer amino acids from maternal plasma into the intracellular space of the trophoblast, where amino acid concentrations are much higher than in maternal or fetal plasma (219,220,221). It is then thought that the compounds diffuse from the trophoblast into fetal plasma, down a concentration gradient, although it does not appear that the presence of active processes in trophoblast to fetal transfer have been investigated. Active maternal-to-fetal transport appears to occur for calcium and phosphorus (209). An active process also appears to be involved in the placental transport of iron, via transferrin uptake from maternal blood by the trophoblast, followed by removal of the iron and its active transport into fetal plasma (93,222,223). Pinocytosis is important for the maternal-to-fetal transport of proteins, particularly immunoglobulins. In species with a functional yolk sac placenta (e.g. rat, guinea pig), the transfer occurs specifically via this organ and not via the hemochorial placenta, whereas in humans and other species that lack a functional yolk sac placenta, the same functions appear to be carried out by the hemochorial placenta (93,224,225).

It is important to note that with maternal/fetal exchange of nutrient molecules (e.g carbohydrates, lipids, amino acids), the placenta is not functioning simply as an organ of transfer, but rather also is a significant consumer and/or converter of these compounds (226). In pregnant sheep, uteroplacental consumption of glucose accounts for more than half of the glucose taken up from the uterine circulation, although the bulk of this does not come directly from maternal blood but rather from the fetal umbilical circulation (227,228). A portion of the glucose taken up by the uteroplacental is converted to lactate which is released in the maternal and fetal circulations (227)(1988). The fetus, then, is a net consumer of lactate (Figure 6–20). And there is also placental processing of amino acids and lipids, and in the case of the former compounds, cycling of amino acids between the placenta and fetal liver (226,227,229).

## Placental Gas Transfer

### *Factors Affecting Placental Oxygen Transfer*

It is the respiratory gases, particularly oxygen, that have been most intensively studied in terms of placental transfer, undoubtedly because of the critical importance of oxygen in prenatal development. One of the earliest observations made on maternal/fetal oxygen relationships was the low value of fetal vascular $Po_2$, which led to the view that the placenta presented a barrier to oxygen transfer and that the fetus developed in an hypoxic environment (230). However, subsequent investigations, which have employed a variety of techniques such as measurement of placental CO diffusing capacity (231), fetal oxygen consumption (232,233), and observing the effects of maternal hyperoxia on fetal oxygen consumption (234) have indicated that the placenta is not a barrier to oxygen in the sense of limiting fetal oxygen utilization, although as discussed below in some species it may contribute to the difference between maternal and fetal $Po_2$. Moreover, in fetal lambs in late gestation, oxygen consumption can be increased by ~25% above the resting level by various factors including fetal activity, hyperglycemia, hyperinsulinemia, norepinephrine, triiodothyrinine, and ritodrine, suggesting that, in this species at least, there is a modest reserve in the capacity of the placenta to transfer oxygen to the fetus (131,235,236,237,238). These studies have also identified a number of factors that can affect fetal oxygen supply and blood oxygen tension, and these are discussed briefly below. More comprehensive discussion is found in several excellent reviews (93,239,240,241).

The factors that affect transplacental oxygen transfer include the oxygen capacities and dissolved oxygen concentrations of maternal and fetal blood, the permeability of the placenta to oxygen, the area of the exchange surface, the rate of oxygen consumption by placental tissues, and the relative orientations and matching of maternal and fetal placental blood flows. Much of the research that has investigated these factors has been done on pregnant sheep. This species has an epitheliochorial placenta that differs significantly in structure and permeability characteristics from the hemochorial placenta present in the human (93). There appears to be a crosscurrent arrangement between maternal and fetal vessels in the placenta, and, for highly diffusible molecules, the sheep placenta appears to behave as a venous equilibrator, i.e. there is equilibration in the concentrations of such substances between maternal and fetal blood leaving the placental exchange areas (42).

Thus, one would expect that uterine and umbilical venous $Po_2$'s would be equal. However, in sheep uterine venous $Po_2$ is in fact ~18 mm Hg greater than that in the umbilical vein (43). Two separate, but not mutually exclusive, hypotheses have been postulated to explain this phenomenon (241). They both involve the concept of the placental diffusing capacity for oxygen, which is the rate of transplacental oxygen diffusion per units of time and partial pressure difference between maternal and fetal blood (239). It is determined by many of the factors listed above that affect maternal/fetal $O_2$ transfer, including placental $O_2$ permeability, area of exchange, and the properties of maternal and fetal placental blood. As with placental $O_2$ diffusing capacity in the lung, the placental variable is estimated from measurements of the diffusing capacity for CO (231). One hypothesis is that placental $O_2$ diffusing capacity is low relative to the rate of blood transport capacity (blood flow x $O_2$ capacity) on the fetal side of the placental, thereby requiring a large maternal-fetal oxygen gradient to sustain an adequate rate of fetal $O_2$ supply and resulting in a lack of equilibration between maternal and fetal blood within the placenta. The second hypothesis is that placental diffusing capacity is adequate in relation to fetal blood transport capacity, and thus that there is complete equilibration of maternal and fetal blood within the placenta. The ~18 mm Hg $Po_2$ difference between uterine and umbilical venous blood is explained by the high rate of placental $O_2$ consumption, which is similar to that of metabolically active tissues like renal cortex and brain (241), and by unequal distribution of maternal and fetal blood flows in localized areas of the placenta. The latter phenomenon is equivalent to ventilation/perfusion inequalities in the lung. The second hypothesis is supported by measurements of placental CO diffusing capacity coupled with a mathematical model of placental $O_2$ transfer, which suggests that there is ~99% equilibration of maternal and fetal $Po_2$ in the placental exchange areas, with a difference in maternal/fetal placental end-capillary $Po_2$ of ~0.5 mm Hg, in contrast to the ~18 mm Hg difference between uterine and umbilical $Po_2$'s (242,243). The second hypothesis is also supported by assessment of the degree of local inequalities in maternal and fetal placental blood flows, which suggests that this could account for up to 50% of the maternal/fetal $Po_2$ difference in sheep (168). However, reexamination of the data of Hill, et al (242) and Longo, et al (243) led Faber and Thornburg (93) to conclude that the equilibration is nearer to 90 to 95% complete, with placental end-capillary $Po_2$ difference being ~3 mm Hg. And recently, experiments involving transient occlusion of one umbilical artery in fetal lambs (244) also support the hypothesis that there is incomplete equilibration of maternal and fetal blood, and thus that placental $O_2$ diffusing capacity is a limiting factor in placental $O_2$ transport in sheep.

Overall, the data from pregnant sheep suggest that limited placental $O_2$ diffusing capacity, high placental $O_2$ consumption, and unequal distribution of maternal and fetal placental blood flows are all important factors in placental oxygen transfer, and that together they are responsible for the large maternal-fetal $O_2$ gradient in this species. Whether the same situation exists in other species is not yet clear. In some animal species, the maternal/fetal $O_2$ gradient is much lower that in the sheep. Thus, in the horse, another species with an epitheliochorial placenta, the difference between uterine and umbilical venous $Po_2$ is only ~2 mm Hg (43). The explanation for this difference between the sheep and the horse appears to relate to differences in the geometry of the maternal and fetal placental circulations, as in the latter species there is good evidence for a countercurrent flow arrangement. As was discussed earlier, this system is more efficient for the transfer of highly diffusible substances (Figure 6–21). In theory, with a countercurrent system, umbilical venous $Po_2$ could equal maternal arterial $Po_2$. That it does not in the horse could be due to the same factors as in the sheep: low placental $O_2$ diffusing capacity, placental $O_2$ consumption, and unequal placental flow distribution. However, experiments to assess the relative importance of these factors in the horse have not been carried out. A similar situation exists in the human (Table 6–1). Blood gas values from fetal and maternal intervillous space blood obtained via cordocentesis indicate the $Po_2$ difference between maternal blood in the intervillous space and fetal umbilical venous blood is ~7 mm Hg, i.e. about one-half the value in sheep (245). At least two factors could be responsible for this species difference. First, placental CO diffusing capacity appears to be higher in the human (246) (2.7 ml/min mm Hg kg fetal weight) than in the sheep (231) (0.55 ml/min mm Hg kg fetal weight) as is

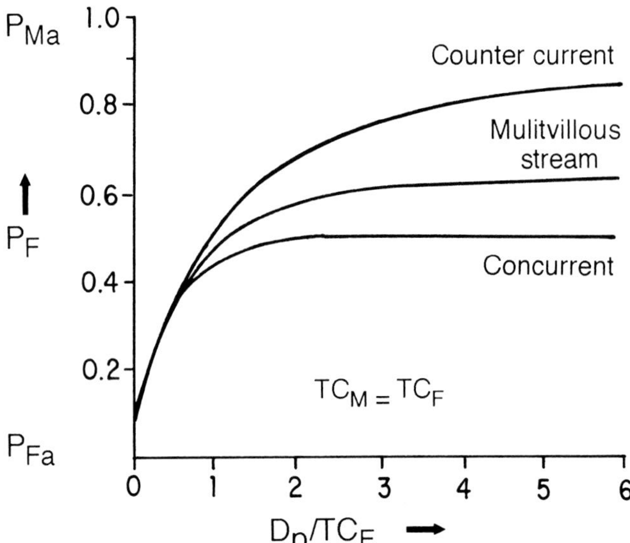


**Fig. 6–21.** Comparison of the $O_2$ transfer efficiency of the countercurrent, concurrent, and multivillous systems. The transport capacities of the mother ($TC_M$) and fetus ($TC_F$) are assumed equal. The abscissa plots the diffusion capacity of the placenta in relation to the transport capacity of the fetus. The ordinate plots umbilical venous $Po_2$ in relation to the maximum difference in oxygen tension between maternal arterial and umbilical arterial bloods. (Redrawn from Bartels H, Moll W, Metcalfe J: Physiology of gas exchange in the human placenta. Am. J. Obstet. Gynecol. 84:1714–1730, 1962.)

the case with the rabbit (247) and guinea pig (248) species which, like the human, possess an epitheliochorial type of placenta. Second, there appears to be a multivillous arrangement of maternal/fetal flow in the human placenta (45) (Figure 6–8), and this flow pattern is predicted to result in lower uterine-umbilical vein $Po_2$ difference than with the crosscurrent flow geometry found in the sheep placenta (Figure 6–21).

There are several other factors that may be important in maternal/fetal oxygen transfer, in terms of promoting fetal oxygenation. These include the $O_2$ affinity and capacity of fetal compared to maternal blood, and transplacental Bohr effects. The first two factors act to compensate for the low fetal vascular $Po_2$ and result in values of blood $O_2$ saturation and content that are not much different from the adult range (Table 6–1). It has been well-demonstrated in many species that fetal hematocrit and hemoglobin concentrations are higher than the values in the mother (e.g. Table 6–1). This of course increases the $O_2$ carrying capacity of fetal blood. Also present in most species is a higher oxygen affinity of fetal blood; the $O_2$ dissociation curve for fetal blood is shifted to the left in relation to the adult (249) (Figure 6–22). The magnitude of the fetal-adult difference in hemoglobin $O_2$ affinity, which can be expressed by the adult-fetal difference in $P_{50}$, varies considerably in the species that have been examined, from a high value of 17 mm Hg in the sheep to no difference at all in the cat (93). The maternal-fetal $P_{50}$ difference in the human is 4 mm Hg. Thus, even with the low $Po_2$ values, fetal blood has a relatively high saturation and total $O_2$ content. The high $O_2$ affinity could limit the unloading of oxygen from blood to fetal tissues. But this is minimized by the steepness of that portion of the dissociation curve over which the fetus normally operates. Even with the relatively small drop in $Po_2$ that occurs between arterial and systemic venous bloods, there is a large fall in $O_2$ saturation. However, the importance of this mechanism to fetal survival seems limited, because with intrauterine blood transfusion to treat erythroblastosis in the human fetus, almost complete replacement of fetal red cells by adult cells is apparently well-tolerated (249). It may be that mechanism is most important in species such as the sheep, which have a large maternal/fetal $Po_2$ gradient and maternal-fetal difference in $P_{50}$, and a relatively low fetal vascular $Po_2$. However, even in this species, studies involving acute replacement of fetal blood with mater-

**Table 6–1.** Representative Blood Gas, pH, Hemoglobin (Hb), and Lactate Values in Maternal Arterial (MA), Intervillous Space (IS), and Umbilical Arterial (UA) and Venous (UV) Blood in Human Pregnancy in the Third Trimester

| | MA | IV | UV | UA |
|---|---|---|---|---|
| $Po_2$ (mm Hg) | 96 | 50 | 43 | 28 |
| $Pco_2$ (mm Hg) | 28 | 33 | 35 | 42 |
| pH | 7.45 | 7.41 | 7.41 | 7.37 |
| (lactate) (mM) | 0.87* | — | 0.99 | 0.92 |
| $O_2$ saturation (%) | 97 | — | 83 | 46 |
| (Hb)(g%) | 12.5 | — | 16 | 16 |
| $O_2$ content (vol. %) | 15.9 | — | 17.1 | 13.6 |

Values obtained from Ramanathan S, et al (1982), Soothill PW, et. al. (1986), and Nicolaides KH, et al (1989). * maternal venous value, — data not available.

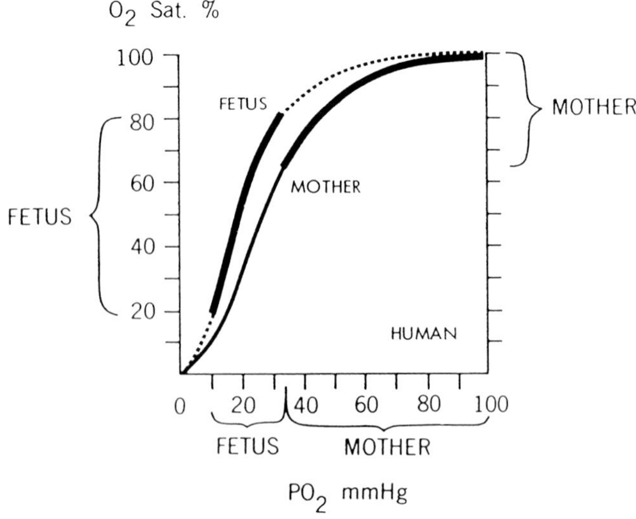


**Fig. 6–22.** Oxygen dissociation curves for human maternal and fetal blood, indicating the physiologic range of $Po_2$ and $O_2$ for mother and fetus. (From Towell ME: Fetal respiratory physiology. *In* Perinatal Medicine. Edited by JW Goodwin, GW Chance. Toronto, Canada, Longman, 1976, pp. 171–186.)

nal blood have not consistently observed adverse effects on fetal oxygenation and acid-base status (28,250,251).

Transplacental Bohr effects result from the reciprocal changes in acid-base status that occur in maternal and fetal blood in transit through the placenta. Thus, with fetal blood there is loss of $CO_2$, a rise in pH, and a leftward shift of the hemoglobin-oxygen dissociation curve to increase $O_2$ affinity, whereas in the mother there is gain of $CO_2$, a fall in pH, and a leftward shift of the curve to decrease $O_2$ affinity. Bartels, et al (45) estimated that this mechanism results in fetal $O_2$ saturation being 13% higher than it would otherwise be. However, the magnitude of the effect is dependent upon the maternal and fetal placental arteriovenous change in $P_{CO_2}$ and pH. The estimate of Bartels, et al (45) was based upon maternal and fetal blood gas measurements at delivery. As discussed below, there is a deterioration in fetal and likely intervillous blood gases during delivery. The maternal (0.09) and fetal (0.08) arteriovenous pH differences used by Bartels, et al are larger than those present in utero (Table 6–1). Thus, the transplacental Bohr effect may be more important during delivery than in the antenatal period. However, there is another aspect of the Bohr effect that is relevant to maternal-fetal $O_2$ relationships. This is the effect of maternal hypercapnia or hypocapnia of fetal vascular $P_{O_2}$. The former situation will increase fetal oxygenation (237), while maternal hypocapnia will result in a fall in fetal $P_{O_2}$ (252). In both cases, the mechanism is a Bohr shift in the maternal hemoglobin-oxygen dissociation curve, to the left with hypercapnia and to the right with hypocapnia. Maternal hypocapnia, due to hyperventilation, is most likely during labor, and this is at a time when fetal oxygenation is already likely to be reduced.

### *Oxygen Tensions in Fetal Blood*

***In utero.*** A major advance in our understanding of human fetal oxygenation has resulted from the development of cordocentesis procedures, which permit sampling of blood from the fetus in utero from the first trimester to the end of pregnancy (253,254). Table 6–1 gives representative fetal (and maternal) blood gas values from the third trimester, while Figure 6–23 illustrates the average changes in intervillous, umbilical venous, and umbilical arterial $P_{O_2}$'s from ~16 to 36 weeks gestation. Two features are obvious from these data. First, at any stage of pregnancy fetal vascular $P_{O_2}$ is higher than it is at delivery, either vaginally or via cesarean section (see below). Second, fetal vascular $P_{O_2}$ decreases during gestation. A similar situation may exist in the fetal lamb (255), but the data are much more scanty. Because, in the human, intervillous $P_{O_2}$ also declines with gestation, the transplacental maternal-fetal $O_2$ gradient does not change. Thus, the fall in intervillous and fetal vascular $P_{O_2}$'s likely reflects a failure of uterine blood flow and hence uterine oxygen delivery to keep pace with the increase in fetal oxygen requirements resulting from growth.

The 95% confidence limits of the data in Figure 6–23 indicate considerable variability in human fetal $P_{O_2}$ at any stage of gestation. In fetal lambs, vascular $P_{O_2}$ fluctuates almost continuously, with frequent, transient drops of 3 to 4 mm Hg (97,101,238,256,257). This is due to prelabor uterine contractions and periods of increased skeletal muscle activity in the form of breathing and body movements. Harding, et al (257) have elegantly shown that when contractures and fetal skeletal muscle activity are temporarily abolished with a $\beta_2$ adrenergic tocolytic and a neuromuscular blocking agent, respectively, the variability in fetal vascular $P_{O_2}$ and $O_2$ saturation is virtually eliminated (Figure 6–24). With contractures, $P_{O_2}$ falls because of the transient decrease in uterine blood flow that was mentioned earlier, while the fall in $P_{O_2}$ with increased skeletal muscle activity is associated with a 15 to 30% increase in fetal $O_2$ consumption, at least during episodes of fetal breathing (237,238). Conversely, when fetal activity is abolished by a neuromuscular blocking agent or general anesthesia, $O_2$ consumption falls by 8 to 23% associated with a rise in vascular $P_{O_2}$ (258,259,260). Thus, in the fetus there is an inverse relationship between $O_2$ con-

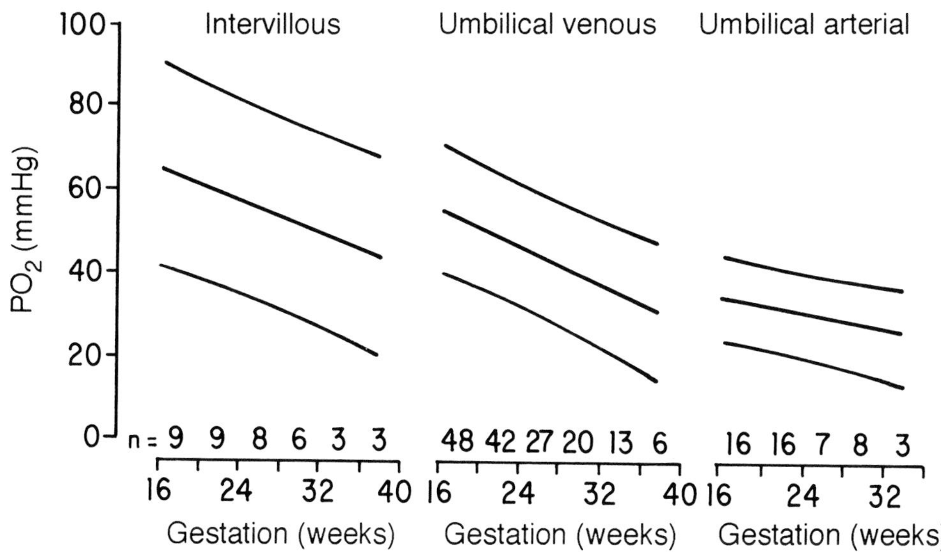


**Fig. 6–23.** $P_{O_2}$ values (mean ± 95% confidence intervals) during gestation in human intervillous, umbilical venous, and umbilical arterial blood. (Redrawn from Soothill PW, Nicolaides KH, Rodeck CH, Campbell S: Effect of gestational age on fetal and intervillous blood gas and acid-base values in human pregnancy. Fetal. Therapy. 1:168–175, 1986.)

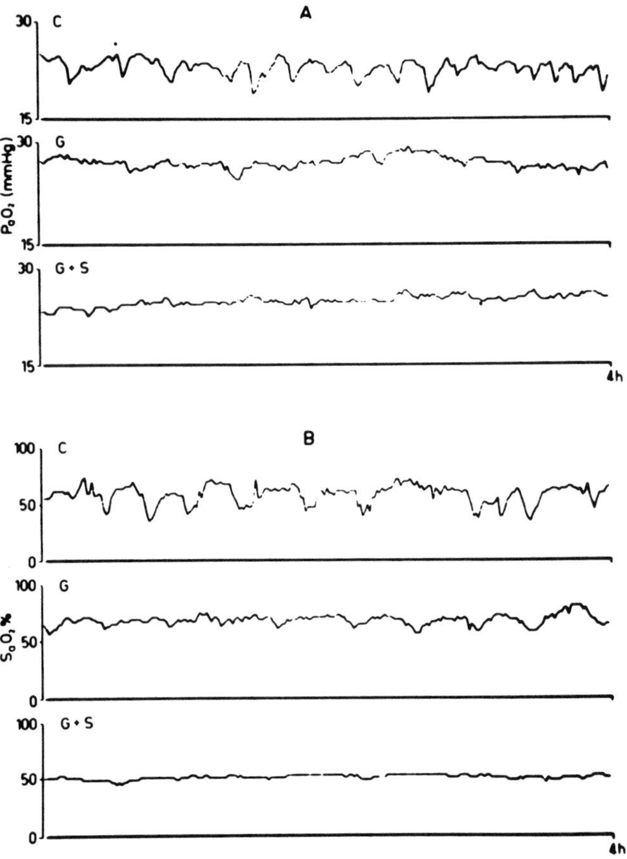


**Fig. 6–24.** Reconstruction of 4-hour periods of control and experimental arterial $Po_2$ and $O_2$ saturation from two chronically instrumented pregnant fetal lambs, one of which was fitted with an intravascular $Po_2$ electrode (A) and one with a fibre optic catheter oximeter (B). C = control data, G = fetus paralyzed with gallamine, G+S = fetus paralyzed with gallamine and uterine activity abolished with salbutamol. (From Harding R, Sigger JN, Wickham PJD: Fetal and maternal influences on arterial oxygen levels in the sheep fetus. J. Dev. Physiol. 5:267–276, 1983.)

sumption and arterial blood oxygen levels, a situation not normally present in the adult. However, after birth, increases in tissue $O_2$ demands are matched by elevations in cardiac output, ventilation, and pulmonary $O_2$ uptake. The equivalent responses in the fetus would require that uterine blood flow fluctuate to match transient changes in fetal oxygen uptake and this does not occur. It is likely that similar fluctuations in $Po_2$ occur in the human fetus in association with Braxton-Hicks contractions (261) and with episodic fetal breathing and body movements (262,263).

***During Labor and Delivery.*** Labor and delivery are times when the fetus would seem to be most at risk from reductions in oxygen delivery leading to hypoxemia and/or hypoxia as a result of decreased uterine and/or umbilical blood flows or placental separation. However, as with the fetus before birth, its relative inaccessibility during labor until fairly recently prevented assessment of fetal oxygenation and acid-base balance. With the development of fetal scalp sampling, such data became available and indicate that in healthy human fetuses $Po_2$, $Pco_2$, and pH are reasonably well-maintained until the late second stage of labor, when there are falls in $Po_2$, $O_2$ saturation, pH and base excess and an increase in $Pco_2$ (264,265) (Figure 6–25). The acidemia is thus of a mixed respiratory and metabolic nature, and in normal pregnancies the changes are slight and innocuous. Similar changes are observed with intravascular blood gases and pH in fetal lambs during labor and delivery (266). More recently there has been the use of methods for the continuous measurement of fetal oxygenation and acid-base status during labor. Transcutaneous $Po_2$ and $Pco_2$ electrodes utilize localized heating of the fetal scalp to increase scalp blood flow and provide for "arterialized" estimates of $Po_2$ and $Pco_2$ (267,268). Pulse oximeters, which are widely used in anesthesia, intensive care, and neonatal care have also been applied to the measurement of $O_2$ saturation of the fetal scalp or breech during labor (269,270), and there has also been use of a miniature pH electrode to measure fetal scalp tissue pH (271,272). Although these methods have various limitations (269,273,274,275), they have provided useful information on the changes in fetal blood gas and acid-bases status that occur with uterine contractions during labor (276). There is sometimes but not always transient hypoxemia and hypercarbia during a contraction and pH may also decrease slightly (268,269,276,277,278,279). The magnitude of the hypoxemia depends on the strength and frequency of the uterine contractions; with a normal contraction, the decrease in $Po_2$ is 2 to 3 mm Hg (268,278). This is similar to the transient hypoxemia observed in fetal lambs associated with contractures (see above) and the mechanism is the same in both situations: a transient fall in uterine blood flow that in human patients during labor has been demonstrated by measurement of uterine artery blood velocity and the Doppler velocity waveform (280) (Figure 6–26). Moreover, the magnitude in the alteration of uterine artery Doppler indices is related to the strength of the uterine contraction, suggesting that greater reductions in uterine perfusion occur with stronger contractions (36,281), and this is consistent with the greater decrease in fetal scalp transcutaneous $Po_2$ in this situation (268). Similar observations of contraction-related uterine hypoperfusion have been made in animal species during labor (282,283). Monitoring of umbilical arterial Doppler velocity waveforms suggests that in uncomplicated labors umbilical blood flow is not altered during uterine contractions (36,281,284,285). However, when fetal heart rate decelerations are associated with a uterine contraction, there is also an increase in umbilical pulsatility index, suggesting reduced umbilical blood flow (284). These data indicate that in uncomplicated deliveries the deteriorations in fetal oxygenation and acid-base balance are minimal and pose no risk to the fetus. However, in pregnancies with maternal or obstetric complications, prolonged labor or with delays in induction-delivery time, there can be much more severe fetal hypoxemia and acidemia (286,287,288,289) (Figure 6–27).

***In Compromised Pregnancies.*** Until fairly recently, the occurrence of hypoxemia and acidemia in the

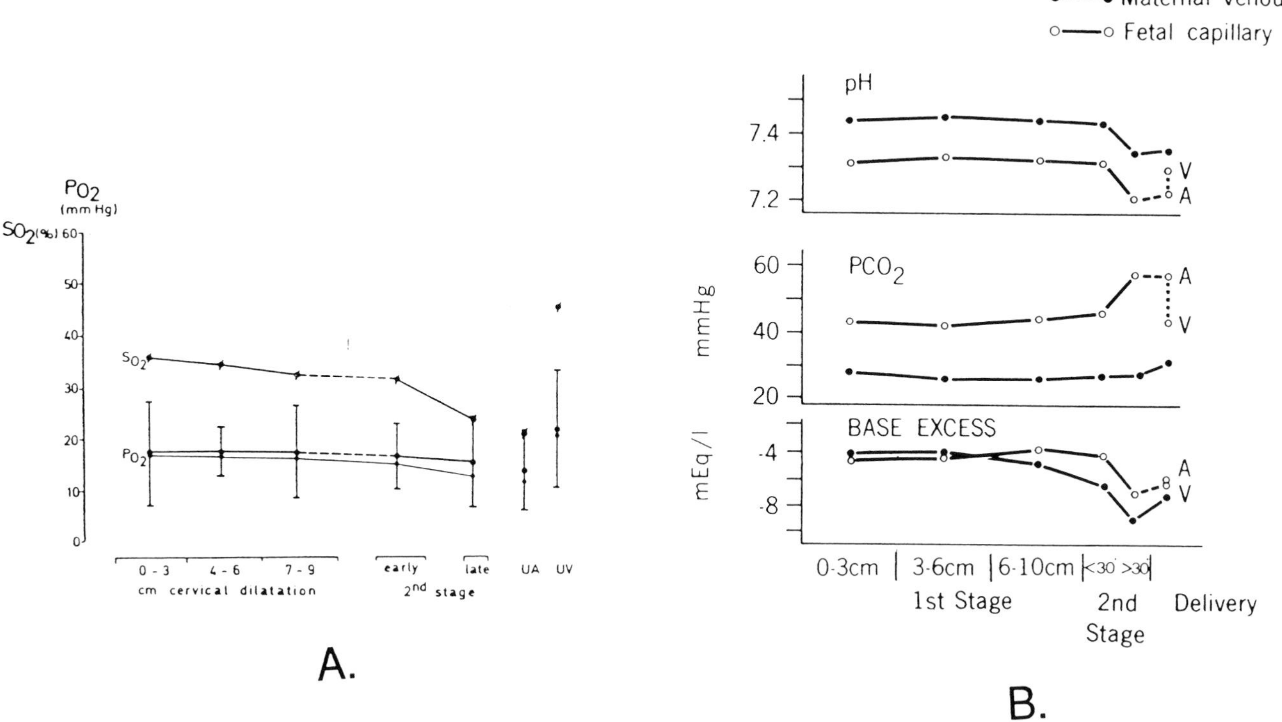


**Fig. 6–25.** Blood gas values from fetal scalp blood during labor and from umbilical artery and vein at delivery. A $Po_2$ and $O_2$ saturation, the thin line for $Po_2$ gives values corrected to pH = 7.4, UA = umbilical artery, UV = umbilical vein. (From Berg D, Saling E: The oxygen partial pressures in the human fetus during labor and delivery. *In* Respiratory Gas Exchange and Blood Flow in the Placenta. Edited by HD Longo, H Bartels. Bethesda, Dept. of Health, Education, and Welfare, 1972, pp. 441–457.) B. pH, $Pco_2$, and base excess, A = umbilical artery, V = umbilical vein. (From Towell ME: Fetal acid-base physiology. *In* Goodwin JW, Godden JO, Chance GW (eds.): Perinatal Medicine. Edited by JW Goodwin, JO Godden, GW Chance. Toronto, Canada, Longman, 1976, pp. 187–208.)

human fetus was diagnosed unequivocally only after delivery, on the basis of cord blood gas and acid-base status (290). It is now clear, however, that in pregnancies with various complications, particularly fetal growth restriction or premature labor, the occurrence of fetal hypoxemia and acidemia at birth is a reflection of a similar situation in the antenatal period and not just the result of the birth process itself. Information in support of this view has come from a number of sources. There are retrospective analyses of human stillbirths that indicate that fetal hypoxia accounts for a significant proportion of the deaths (291). Also, there are studies of perinatal deaths or surviv-

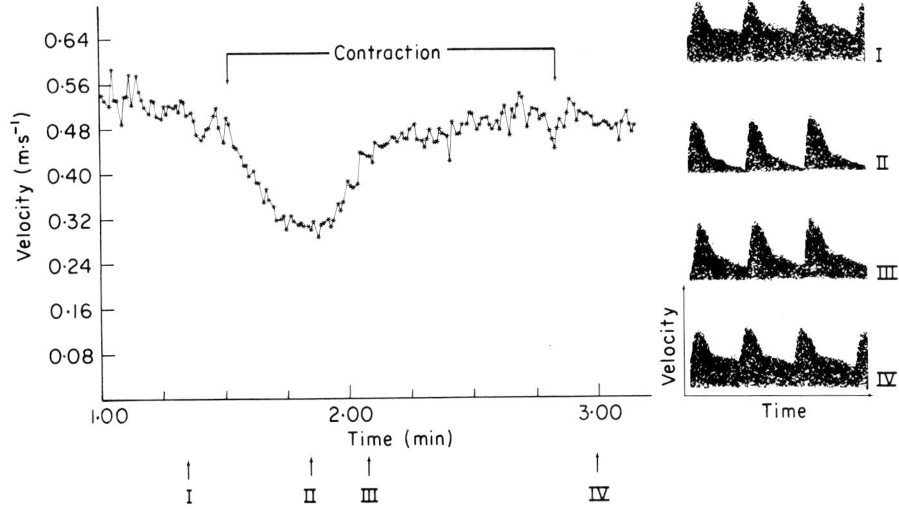


**Fig. 6–26.** Doppler ultrasound estimated of uterine blood flow in a patient during labor. **A,** Mean flow velocity before, during, and after a uterine contraction, **B,** Flow velocity waveforms at the times indicated by the roman numerals in A. (From Janbu T, Koss KS, Nesheim B-I, Wesche J: Blood velocities in the uterine artery in humans during labour. Acta. Physiol. Scand. 124:153–161, 1985.)

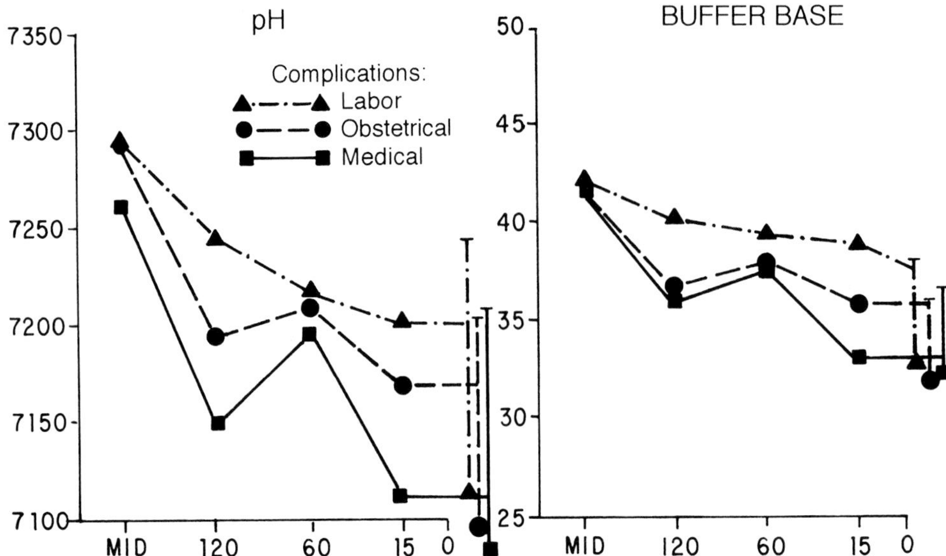


Fig. 6–27. pH and buffer base in fetal scalp blood during labor and in umbilical artery and vein in patients with maternal medical, obstetric or labor complications. (Redrawn from Low JA, Pangham SR, Worthington D, Boston RW: Clinical characteristics of pregnancies complicated by intrapartum asphyxia. Am. J. Obstet. Gynecol. 121: 452–456, 1975.)

ing infants that indicate that, in a proportion of the cases with neuropathologic lesions characteristic of asphyxia, the asphyxial insult occurred in the antenatal period (292,293). Then, there are the many studies involving the commonly employed diagnostic tests of fetal health that have demonstrated an association between an abnormal test result and evidence of fetal hypoxemia and/or acidemia at delivery. This applies to fetal heart rate monitoring (294,295), fetal activity, and the biophysical profile score (296) and, as noted above, Doppler ultrasound measurements of blood velocity profiles in the umbilical and fetal systemic circulations. Moreover, the alterations in fetal functions that have been revealed or suggested by these tests (e.g. reduced fetal heart rate variability and skeletal muscle activity, redistributed fetal cardiac output) are similar to the changes that have been observed in studies of pregnant animals where fetal hypoxemia has been imposed experimentally or occurred spontaneously (297,298,299). However, the most recent and compelling evidence has resulted from the development of cordocentesis techniques. Application of such techniques to pregnancies complicated by preeclampsia and/or fetal growth retardation has demonstrated that in a proportion of such cases, there is fetal hypoxemia, hypoglycemia, reduced concentrations of essential amino acids, and, in fewer cases, metabolic acidemia (195,217,300,301, 302,303,304,305) (Figure 6–28a). Also, in fetuses that are anemic as a result of Rh isoimmunization, there is increasing lactic acidemia with decreasing fetal hemoglobin concentration (306). In such compromised cases, comparison of fetal blood gases and pH with fetal biophysical variables and heart rate patterns indicates that the most severe deteriorations in blood gas and acid-base status (hypoxemia, associated with hypercapnia and acidemia) tend to be associated with the most abnormal fetal monitoring results, i.e. no fetal movements or tone in the case of biophysical activities and repetitive decelerations or a terminal pattern in the case of fetal heart rate (307,308,309) (Figure 6–28b). Moreover, it is clear that when fetal metabolic deterioration of the fetus has reached the point of hypoxic acidemia associated with prolonged fetal quiescence and a terminal heart rate pattern, continued fetal survival is measured in days at most (310).

***Fetal Oxygen Therapy.*** Maternal oxygen administration is commonly employed during cesarean section, with the aim being to increase fetal $Po_2$. Numerous studies have demonstrated that this is indeed the case, and that fetal cord arterial and venous $Po_2$, $O_2$ saturation, and $O_2$ content values increase in proportion to maternal inspired oxygen concentrations (311) (Figure 6–29). However, the degree of rise in fetal $Po_2$ is much less than the increase in maternal arterial oxygen tension. This due to the fact that maternal arterial blood is nearly fully saturated under normal circumstances, so that maternal $O_2$ content increases only slightly, even with 100% $O_2$. Moreover, while fetal oxygenation can be improved if maternal oxygen administration is employed throughout the entire operative procedure, no such effect is observed if maternal inspired oxygen concentration is only increased for the period between hysterotomy and birth (312). In the antenatal period, maternal oxygen administration (50%) for 30 to 120 min is associated with increased fetal breathing activity in growth retarded, but not normally grown fetuses; however, fetal gross body movements, fetal heart rate accelerations, and fetal heart rate variability are not affected (313,314). Recently, there have also been reports of prolonged maternal oxygen administration (55%) in the antenatal period, in situations involving fetal growth retardation, abnormal Doppler flow velocity waveforms, and hypoxemia/acidemia (315,316). Improvements in fetal Doppler waveform patterns and fetal blood gas status occurred with maternal oxygen administration. The effect of chronic maternal oxygen administration on fetal growth and perinatal outcome is not yet clear, because of the small patient numbers and uncontrolled study design of the investigations conducted to date.

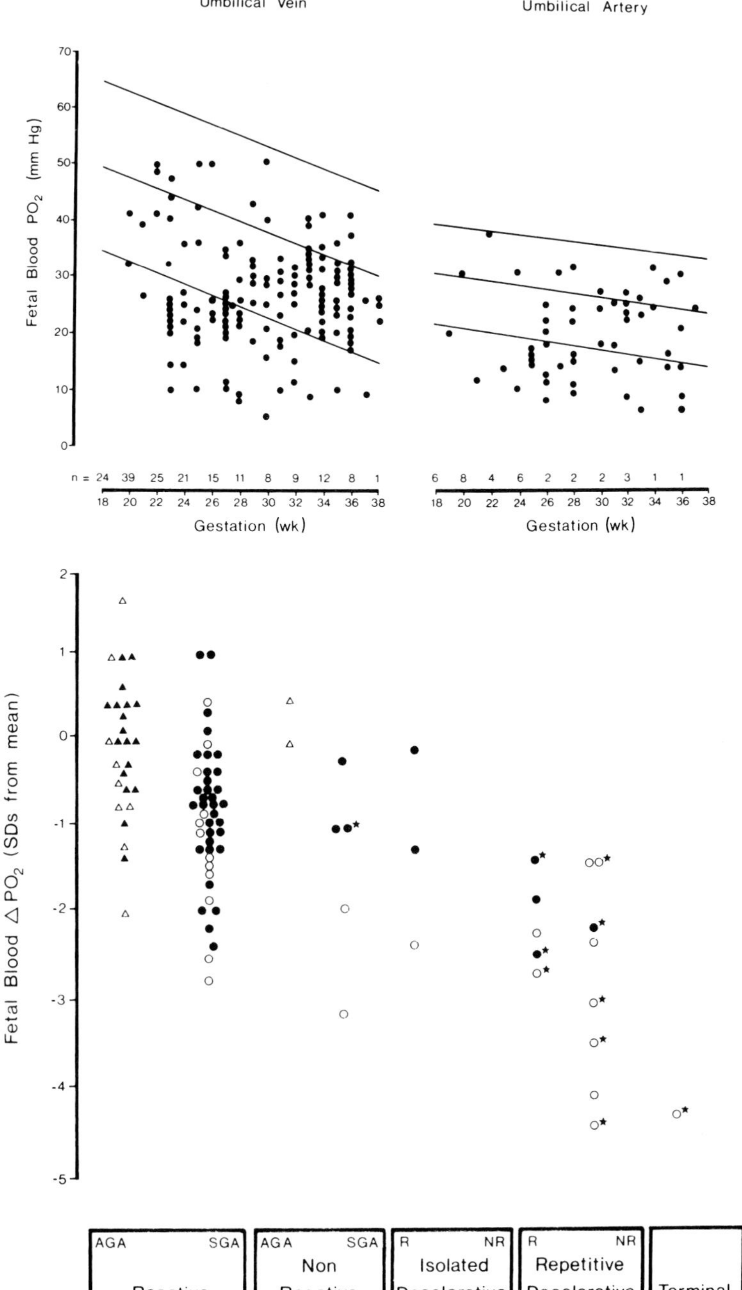


**Fig. 6–28.** Fetal $Po_2$ in compromised pregnancies. **A,** $Po_2$ in individual small-for-gestational-age fetuses (closed circles) in relation to the normal range (mean ± 95% confidence intervals). (From Nicolaides KH, Economides DL, Soothill PW: Blood gases, pH and lactate in appropriate- and small-for-gestational-age fetuses. Am. J. Obstet. Gynecol. 161:996–1001, 1989.) **B,** Relationship between fetal heart rate patterns and the deviation in fetal $Po_2$ from the normal range. AGA = appropriate-for-gestational-age, SGA = small-for-gestational-age, R = reactive, NR = non-reactive AGA and SGA fetuses indicated by △ and ○, respectively. Open symbols denote to pregnancies of 27–32 weeks gestation, closed symbols to pregnancies of 33–38 weeks, asterisks denote cases with fetal acidemia. (From Visser GHA, Sadovsky G, Nicolaides KH: Antepartum heart rate patterns in small-for-gestational third-trimester fetuses: Correlations with blood gas values obtained at cordocentesis. Am. J. Obstet. Gynecol. 162:698–703, 1990.)

## *Carbon Dioxide Transfer*

$CO_2$ is produced by fetal tissues at about the same rate as oxygen is consumed, and, to maintain $CO_2$ balance, the rate of fetal $CO_2$ production must equal the rate of $CO_2$ loss to the mother. Carbon dioxide in blood is hydrated in a reaction catalyzed by carbonic anhydrase to form carbonic acid that spontaneously dissociates to bicarbonate and a proton:

$$CO_2 + H_2O \rightarrow H_2CO_3 \rightarrow H^+ + HCO_3^-$$

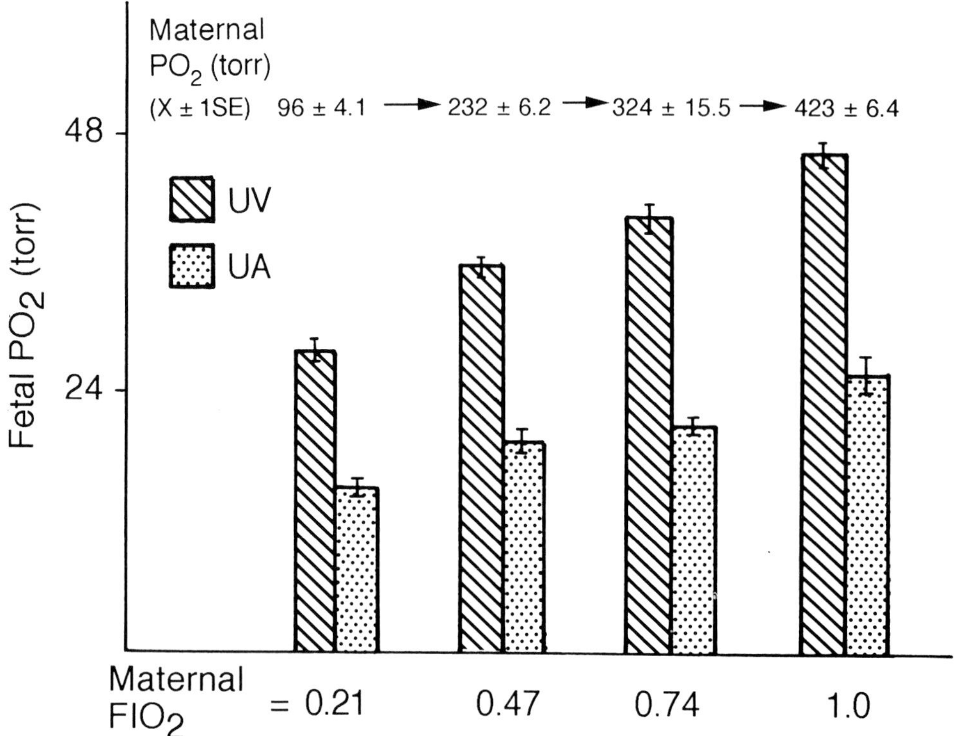


**Fig. 6–29.** Histograms showing umbilical vein (UV) and umbilical artery (UA) $Po_2$ values obtained at delivery in relation to maternal fractional inspired $O_2$ concentration ($FIO_2$). (Redrawn from Ramanathan S, Gandhi S, Arismendy J, Chalon J, et al: Oxygen transfer from mother to fetus during cesarean section under epidural anesthesia. Anesth. Analg. 61:56–81, 1982.)

Carbonic acid levels in the blood are very low, so $CO_2$ and $HCO_3$- are the dominant species, with the latter ion accounting for most of the carbon dioxide in blood; there is also $CO_2$ reversibly bound to hemoglobin.

Table 6–1 gives representative values for maternal and fetal blood $Pco_2$ and pH values. As with fetal $Po_2$, there are changes in fetal $Pco_2$ values during gestation, in this case with a progressive increase (245). Data from pregnant sheep suggest that the bulk of fetal-maternal carbon dioxide transfer occurs via diffusion of dissolved $CO_2$ (317), and the apparent limited permeability of the human placenta to bicarbonate suggests the same situation in humans (1). As with oxygen, the permeability of the placenta to $CO_2$ is high, and equilibration between maternal and fetal placental venous bloods would be expected. However, as indicated in Table 6–1, umbilical venous $Pco_2$ is about 2 mm Hg higher than in intervillous blood. This difference is likely due to the same factors that are responsible for the maternal-fetal $Po_2$ differences discussed earlier, namely local inequalities in maternal and fetal placental blood flows and placental $CO_2$ production. The umbilical-intervillous $Pco_2$ gradient is lower than the maternal-fetal $Po_2$ gradient (Table 6–1). Fetal $Pco_2$ is affected by maternal arterial $Pco_2$ and thus is altered by maternal hypo- and hyper-ventilation, which increase and decrease fetal $Pco_2$, respectively. In pregnant sheep fetal $Pco_2$ can also be increased acutely by decreases in uterine and umbilical blood flows (318,319) and, as noted above, hypercapnia can occur in the human fetus during labor and in pregnancies complicated by fetal growth retardation. In both pregnant sheep and humans, the effects of fetal hypercapnia have been most commonly studied by increasing maternal inspired $CO_2$ for ~1 hour (237,298,320,321). The resulting fetal hypercapnia elicits effects similar to those in adults: respiratory stimulation and an increase in cerebral blood flow. And as was noted above, there is also a rise in fetal vascular $Po_2$, apparently due to Bohr shifts in the oxygen dissociation curves of maternal and fetal blood. Overall, the effects of raised fetal $CO_2$ levels appear to be relatively benign.

## REFERENCES


1. Boyd JD, Hamilton WJ: The Human Placenta. Cambridge, W Heffer & Sons, 1970.
2. Ramsey EM, Houston ML, Harris JWS: Interactions of the trophoblast and maternal tissues in three closely related primate species. Am. J. Obstet. Gynecol. 124:647–652, 1976.
3. Steven DH: Interspecies differences in the structure and function of the trophoblast. *In* Biology of the Trophoblast. Edited by Locke and Whyte. New York, Elsvier, 1983.
4. Denker H-W, Aplin JD: Trophoblast invasion and endometrial receptivity. Trophoblast Research, Vol. 4. New York, Plenum, 1990.
5. Short RV: When a conception fails to become a pregnancy. *In* Maternal Recognition of Pregnancy. Edited by J Whelan. Ciba Foundation Symposium 64 (New Series), Amsterdam, Excerpta Medica, 1979.
6. Pijnenborg R: Trophoblast invasion and placentation in the human: morphological aspects. *In* Trophoblast Invasion and Endometrial Receptivity. Edited by H-W Denker, JD Aplin. Trophoblast Research, Vol. 4. New York, Plenum, 1990, pp. 33–47.
7. Schlafke S, Enders AC: Cellular basis of interaction between trophoblast and uterus at implantation. Biol. Reprod. 12: 41–65, 1975.

8. Lindberg S, Hyttel P, Lenz S, Holmes PV: Ultrastructure of the early implantation in vitro. Human Reproduction. 1: 533–538.
9. Librach CL, Werb Z, Fitzgerald ML, Chiu K, et al: 92-kD type IV collagenase mediates invasion of human cytotrophoblasts. J. Cell. Biol. 113:437–449, 1991.
10. Denker H-W: Trophoblast-endometrial interactions at embryo implantation: a cell biological paradox. *In* Trophoblast Invasion and Endometrial Receptivity. Edited by H-W Denker, JD Aplin. Trophoblast Research, Vol. 4. New York, Plenum, 1990, pp. 3–29.
11. Glasser SR: Biochemical and structural changes in uterine endometrial cell types following natural or artificial deciduogenic stimuli. *In* Trophoblast Invasion and Endometrial Receptivity. Edited by H-W Denker, JD Aplin. Trophoblast Research, Vol. 4. New York, Plenum, 1990, pp. 377–416.
12. Kennedy TG: Embryonic signals and the initiation of blastocyst implantation. Aust. J. Biol. Sci 36:531–543, 1983.
13. Psychoyos A: Endocrine control of egg implantation. *In* Handbook of Physiology, Section 7, Endocrinology Vol. II, Part II. Edited by RO Greep, EB Astwood, SR Geiger. Washington, D.C., American Physiological Society, 1973, pp. 187–215.
14. Boe F: Studies on the vascularization of the human placenta. Acta. Obstet. Gynecol. Scand. 32, Suppl. 5:1–92, 1953.
15. Harris CH, Ramsay EM: The morphology of the human uteroplacental vasculature. Contrib. Embryol. 38:43–58, 1966.
16. Pijnenborg R, Bland JM, Robertson WB, Dixon G, et al: The pattern of interstitial trophoblast invasion of the myometrium in early human pregnancy. Placenta 2:303–316, 1981.
17. Pijnenborg R, Dixon G, Robertson WB, Brosens I. Trophoblast invasion of human decidua for 8 to 18 weeks of pregnancy. Placenta 1:3–19, 1980.
18. Brosens I, Robertson WB, Dixon HG: The physiological response of the vessels of the placental bed to normal pregnancy. J. Path. Bact. 93:569–579, 1967.
19. Pijnenborg R, Bland JM, Robertson WB, Brosens I: Uteroplacental arterial changes related to interstitial trophoblast migration in early human pregnancy. Placenta 4:387–414, 1983.
20. Khong TY, De Wolf F, Robertson WB, Brosens I: Inadequate maternal vascular response to placentation in pregnancies complicated by pre-eclampsia and by small-for-gestational age infants. Br. J. Obstet. Gynaecol. 93: 1049–1059, 1986.
21. Khong TY, Sawyer IH: The human placental bed in health and disease. Reprod. Fertil. Dev. 3:373–377, 1991.
22. Pijnenborg R, Anthony J, Davey DA, Rees A, et al: Placental bed arteries in the hypertensive disorders of pregnancy. Br. J. Obstet. Gynaecol. 98:648–655, 1991.
23. Robertson WB, Brosens I, Dixon HG: The pathological response of the vessels of the placental bed to hypertensive pregnancy. J. Path. Bact. 93:581–592, 1967.
24. Damsky CH, Fitzgerald ML, Fisher SJ: Distribution patterns of extracellular matrix components and adhesion receptors are intricately modulated during first trimester cytotrophoblast differentiation along the invasive pathway, in vivo. J. Clin. Invest. 89:21–222, 1992.
25. Fisher SJ, Cui T-Y, Zhang L, Hartman L, et al: Adhesive and degradative properties of human placental cytotrophoblast in vitro. J. Cell. Biol. 109:891–902, 1989.
26. Korhonen M, Ylanne J, Laitinen L, Cooper HM, et al: Distribution of the $\alpha 1$-$\alpha 6$ integrin subunits in human developing, term placenta. Lab. Invest. 65:347–356, 1991.
27. Pijnenborg R, Robertson WB, Brosens I: The role of ovarian steroids in placental development and endovascular trophoblast migration in golden hamster. J. Reprod. Fert. 44:43–51, 1975.
28. Itskovitz J, Goetzman BW, Roman C, Rudolph AM: Effects of fetal-maternal exchange transfusion on fetal oxygenation and blood flow distribution. Am. J. Physiol. 247: H655–H660, 1984.
29. Dawes GS: Foetal and Neonatal Physiology. Year Book Medical Publishers, Chicago, 1968.
30. Kaufmann P: Development and differentiation of the human placental villous tree. *In* Structural and Functional Organization of the Placenta. Edited by P Kaufmann, BF King. Basel, Karger, Biblthca. Anat. 22:29–39, 1982.
31. Kaufmann P: Basic morphology of the fetal and maternal circuits in the human placenta. Contr. Gynecol. Obstet. 13:5–17, 1985.
32. Kaufmann P, Sen DK, Schweikhart G: Classification of human placental villi, I. Histology. Cell. Tiss. Res. 200: 409–423, 1979.
33. Sen DK, Kaufmann P, Schweikhart G: Classification of human placental villi, II. Morphometry. Cell. Tiss. Res. 200: 425–434, 1979.
34. Castellucci M, Kaufmann P: Evolution of the stroma in human chorionic villi throughout pregnancy. *In* Structural and Functional Organization of the Placenta. Edited by P Kaufmann, BF King. Basel, Karger, Bibl Anat 22:40–45, 1982.
35. Castellucci M, Schweikhart G, Kaufmann P, Zaccheo D: The stromal architecture of the intermediate villous of the human placenta. Gynecol. Obstet. Invest. 18:95–99, 1984.
36. Brar H, Platt LD, DeVore GR, Horenstein J, Medaris L: Qualitative assessment of maternal uterine and fetal umbilical artery blood flow and resistance in laboring patients by Doppler velocimetry. Am. J. Obstet. Gynecol. 158: 952–956, 1988.
37. Brosens I, Dixon HG: The anatomy of the maternal side of the placenta. J. Obstet. Gynaecol. Commonw. 73:357–363, 1966.
38. Gruenwald P: Lobular architecture of primate placentas. *In* The placenta and its maternal supply line. Edited by P Gruenwald. Lancaster, MTP, 1975, pp. 35–55.
39. Ramsey EM: Maternal and foetal circulation of the placenta. Ir. J. Med. Sci. 140:151–168, 1971.
40. Kaufmann P, Luckhard M, Leiser R: Three-dimensional representation of the fetal vessel system in the human placenta. *In* Placental Vascularization and Blood Flow, Basic Research and Clinical Application. Trophoblast Research, Vol 3. Edited by P. Kaufmann, RK Miller. New York, Plenum, 1988, pp. 113–137.
41. Arts NFT: Investigations of the vascular system of the placenta. Am. J. Obstet. Gynecol. 82:147–158, 1961.
42. Battaglia FC, Meschia G: An Introduction to Fetal Physiology. New York, Academic Press, 1986.
43. Comline RM, Silver M: Placental transfer of blood gases. Br. Med. Bull. 31(1), 1975, pp. 25–31.
44. Crawford JM: Vascular anatomy of the human placenta. Am. J. Obstet. Gynecol. 84:1543–1567, 1962.
45. Bartels H, Moll W, Metcalfe J: Physiology of gas exchange in the human placenta. Am. J. Obstet. Gynecol. 84: 1714–1730, 1962.
46. Johnson RL, Gilbert M, Meschia G, Battaglia FC: Cardiac output distribution and uteroplacental blood flow in the pregnant rabbit: a comparative study. Am. J. Obstet. Gynecol. 151:682–696, 1985.

47. Makowski EL, Meschia G, Croegemueller W, Battaglia FC: Distribution of uterine blood flow in the pregnant sheep. Am. J. Obstet. Gynecol. 101:409–412, 1968.
48. Novy MJ, Thomas CL, Lees MH: Uterine contractility and regional blood flow responses to oxytocin and prostaglandin $E_2$ in pregnant monkeys. Am. J. Obstet. Gynecol. 122: 419–433, 1975.
49. Peeters LLH, Sparks JW, Grutters G, Girard J, et al: Uteroplacental blood flow during pregnancy in chronically catheterized guinea pigs. Pediatr. Res. 16:716–720, 1982.
50. Gant NF, Worley RJ: Measurement of uteroplacental blood flow in the human. *In* The Uterine Circulation. Reproductive and Perinatal Medicine (X). Edited by NF Gant, RJ Worley. Ithaca, Perinatology Press, 1989, pp. 53–73.
51. Anderson KV, Hermann N: Placenta flow reduction in pregnant smokers. Acta. Obstet. Gynecol. Scand. 63:707–709, 1984.
52. Lunell NO, Sarby B, Lewander R, Nylund L: Comparison of uteroplacental blood flow in normal and intrauterine growth-retarded pregnancy. Gynecol. Obstet. Invest. 10: 106–118, 1979.
52A. Karr K, Jouppila P, Kuikka J, Luotola H, et al: Intervillous blood flow in normal and complicated late pregnancy measured by means of an intravenous 133Xe method. Acta. Obstet. Gynecol. Scand. 59:7–10, 1980.
53. Leodolter S, Phillip K: Estimation of the uteroplacental perfusion by use of ¹13m In-Tranferrin and an iterative regression method. Gynecol. Obstet. Invest. 16:172–179, 1983.
54. Jouppila P, Jouppila R, Barinoff T, Koivula A: Placental blood flow during caesarean section performed under subarachnoid blockade. Br. J. Anaesth. 56:1379–1383, 1984.
55. Kauppila A, Koskinen M, Puolakka J, Tuimala R, et al: Decreased intervillous and unchanged myometrial blood flow in supine recumbency. Obstet. Gynecol. 55:203–205, 1980.
56. Lehtovirta P, Forss M: The acute effect of smoking on intervillous blood flow of the placenta. Br. J. Obstet. Gynaecol. 85:729–731, 1978.
57. Schroder H, Voss G, Leichtweiss HP: Washout of xenon-133 from isolated perfused guinea-pig placenta. Gynecol. Obstet. Invest. 17:25–35, 1984.
58. Cook CM, Connelly AJ, Trudinger BJ: Doppler assessment of the umbilical circulation. Sem. Ultrasound. CT. MR. 10: 417–427, 1989.
59. Maulik D: Doppler for clinical management: what is its place? Obstet. Gynecol. Clin. NA. 18:853–874, 1991.
60. Eik-Nes SH, Brubakk AO, Ulstein MK: Measurement of human fetal blood flow. Br. Med. J. 280:283–284, 1980.
61. Erskine RLA, Ritchie JWK: Quantitative measurement of fetal blood flow using Doppler ultrasound. Br. J. Obstet. Gynaecol. 92:600–604, 1985.
62. Gill R, Kossoff G, Warren PS, Garrett WJ: Umbilical venous flow in normal and complicated pregnancy. Ultrasound. Med. Biol. 10:349–363, 1984.
63. Krujak A, Rajhvajn B Jr: Ultrasonic measurements of umbilical blood flow in normal and complicated pregnancies. J. Perinat. Med. 10:3–16, 1982.
64. St. John Sutton M, Theard MA, Bhatia SJS, Plappert T, et al: Changes in placental blood flow in the normal human fetus with gestational age. Pediatr. Res. 28:383–387, 1990.
65. Thaler I, Manor D, Itskovitz J, Rottem S, et al: Changes in uterine blood flow during normal human pregnancy. Am. J. Obstet. Gynecol. 162:121–125, 1990.
66. Cohen-Overbeek TE, Campbell S: Doppler ultrasound techniques for the measurement of uterine and umbilical blood flow. *In* The Uterine Circulation. Ithaca, Perinatology Press, 1989, pp.75–112.
67. Trudinger BJ, Giles WB, Cook CM: Flow velocity waveforms in the maternal uteroplacental and fetal umbilical placental circulations. Am. J. Obstet. Gynecol. 152: 155–163, 1985.
68. Trudinger BJ, Giles WB, Cook CM: Uteroplacental blood velocity-time waveforms in normal and complicated pregnancy. Br. J. Obstet. Gynaecol. 92:39–45, 1985.
69. Bewley S, Campbell S, Cooper D: Uteroplacental Doppler flow velocity waveforms in the second trimester A complex circulation. Br. J. Obstet. Gynaecol. 96:1040–1046.
70. Gudmundsson S, Fairlie F, Lingman G, Marsal K: Recording of blood flow velocity waveforms in the uteroplacental and umbilical circulation: reproducibility study and comparison of pulsed and continuous wave Doppler ultrasonography. J. Clin. Ultrasound. 18:97–101, 1990.
71. Jauniaux E, Jurkovic D, Campbell S, Kurjak A, et al: Investigation of placental circulations by color Doppler ultrasonography Am. J. Obstet. Gynecol. 164:486–488, 1991.
72. Jurkovic D, Jauniaux E, Kurjak A, Hustin J, et al: Transvaginal color Doppler assessment of the uteroplacental circulation in early pregnancy. Obstet. Gynecol. 77:365–369, 1991.
73. Irion GL, Clark KE: Relationship between ovine fetal umbilical artery blood flow waveform and umbilical vascular resistance. Am. J. Obstet. Gynecol. 163:222–229, 1990.
74. Adamson SL, Morrow RJ, Langille BL, Bull SB, et al: Site-dependent effects of increases in placental vascular resistance on the umbilical arterial velocity waveform in fetal sheep. Ultrasound. Med. Biol. 16:19–27, 1990.
75. Schmidt KG, Di Tommaso M, Silverman NH, Rudolph AM: Evaluation of changes in umbilical blood flow in the fetal lamb by Doppler waveform analysis. Am. J. Obstet. Gynecol. 164:1118–1126, 1991.
76. Rankin JHG, McLaughlin MK: The regulation of placental blood flows. J. Dev. Physiol. 1:3–30, 1979.
77. Heymann MA, Payne BD, Hoffman JIE, Rudolph AM: Blood flow measurement with radionuclide labelled particles. Progr. Cardiovasc. Dis. 20:55–79, 1977.
78. Stock MK, Reid DL, Phernetton TM, Rankin JHG: Matching of maternal and fetal flow ratios in the sheep. J. Dev. Physiol. 11:20–35, 1989.
79. Berman W Jr, Goodlin RC, Heymann MA, Rudolph AM: The measurement of umbilical blood flow in fetal lambs in utero. J. Appl. Physiol. 39:1056–1059, 1975.
80. Clark KE, Irion GL, Mack CE: Differential responses of uterine and umbilical vasculatures to angiotensin II and norepinephrine. Am. J. Physiol. 259:H197-H203, 1990.
81. Hustin J, Schaaps J-P, Lambotte R: Anatomic studies of the utero-placental vascularization in the first trimester of pregnancy. *In* Placental Vascularization and Blood Flow, Basic Research and Clinical Application. Trophoblast Research, Vol. 3. Edited by P. Kaufmann, RK Miller. New York, Plenum, 1988, pp. 49–60.
82. Hustin J, Schaaps J-P: Echocardiographic and anatomic studies of the maternotrophoblastic border during the first trimester of pregnancy. Am. J. Obstet. Gynecol. 157: 162–168, 1987.
83. Rosenfeld CR: Considerations of the uteroplacental circulation in intrauterine growth. Sem. Perinatol. 8:42–51, 1984.
84. Deutinger J, Rudelstorfer R, Bernaschek G: Vaginosonographic velocimetry of both main uterine arteries by visual recognition and pulsed Doppler method during pregnancy. Am. J. Obstet. Gynecol. 159:1072–1076, 1988.
85. Schulman H, Fleischer A, Farmakides G, Bracero L, et al: Development of uterine artery compliance in pregnancy

as detected by Doppler ultrasound. Am. J. Obstet. Gynecol. 155:1031–1036, 1986.

86. Gill RW, Trudinger BJ, Garrett WJ, Kossoff G, et al: Fetal umbilical venous flow measured in utero by pulsed Doppler and B-mode ultrasound. I. Normal pregnancies. Am. J. Obstet. Gynecol. 139:720–725, 1981.
87. Lingman G, Marsal K: Fetal central blood circulation in the third trimester of normal pregnancy—a longitudinal study. I. Aortic and umbilical blood flow. Early. Human. Dev. 13:137–150, 1986.
88. Arstrom K, Eliasson A, Hariede JH, Marsal K: Fetal blood velocity waveforms in normal pregnancies: a longitudinal study. Acta. Obstet. Gynecol. Scand. 68:171–178, 1989.
89. Schulman H, Fleischer A, Stern W, Farmakides G, et al: Umbilical velocity wave ratios in human pregnancy. Am. J. Obstet. Gynecol. 149:985–990, 1984.
90. Stuart B, Drumm J, Fitzgerald D, Duigan NM: Fetal blood velocity waveforms in normal pregnancy. Br. J. Obstet. Gynaecol. 87:780–785, 1980.
91. Thompson RS, Trudinger BJ, Cook CM: Doppler ultrasound waveform indices: AB ratio, pulsatility index and Pourcelot ratio. Br. J. Obstet. Gynaecol. 95:581–588, 1988.
92. Slotten P, Phernetton TM, Rankin JM: Relationship between fetal electrocorticographic changes and umbilical blood flow in the near-term sheep fetus. J. Dev. Physiol. 11:19–23, 1989.
93. Anderson DF: Regulation of umbilical blood flow. *In* Fetal and Neonatal Physiology, Vol. 1. Edited by RA Polin, WA Fox. W.B. Philadelphia, Saunders, 1992, pp. 694–701.
94. Faber JJ, Thornburg KL: Placental Physiology. New York, Raven Press, 1983.
95. Moll W, Kunzel W: The blood pressure in the arteries entering the placentae of guinea-pigs, rats, rabbits and sheep. Pflugers. Arch. 338:125–131, 1975.
96. Rosenfeld CR: The Uterine Circulation. Perinatology Press, Ithaca, 1989.
97. Reynolds SRM, Freese UE, Bieniarz J, Caldeyro-Barcia R, et al: Multiple simultaneous intervillous space pressures recorded in several regions of the hemochorial placenta in relation to the functional anatomy of the fetal cotyledon. Am. J. Obstet. Gynecol. 102:1128–1134, 1968.
98. Jansen CAM, Krane AL, Beck NFG, Lowe KC, et al: Continuous variability of fetal $Po_2$ in the chronically catheterized fetal sheep. Am. J. Obstet. Gynecol. 134:776–783, 1979.
99. Harding R, Poore ER: The effects of myometrial activity on fetal thoracic dimensions and uterine blood flow during late gestation in the sheep. Biol. Neonate. 45:244–251, 1984.
100. Longo LD, Dale PS, Gilbert RD: Uteroplacental $O_2$ uptake: continuous measurements during uterine quiescence and contractions. Am. J. Physiol. 250:R1099–R1107, 1986.
101. Sunderji SG, El Badry A, Poore ER, Figueroa JP, et al: The effect of myometrial contractures on uterine blood flow in the pregnant sheep at 114–140 days' gestation measured by the 4-aminoantipyrine equilibrium diffusion technique. Am. J. Obstet. Gynecol. 149:408–412, 1984.
102. Llanos AJ, Block BSB, Court DJ, Germain AM, et al: Fetal oxygen uptake during contractures. J. Dev. Physiol. 10: 525–529, 1988.
103. Bocking AD, Harding R, Wickham JD: Relationship between accelerations and decelerations in heart rate and skeletal muscle activity in fetal sheep. J. Dev. Physiol. 7: 47–54, 1985.
104. Walker AM, Fleming J, Smolich J, Stunden R: Fetal oxygen consumption, umbilical circulation and electrocortical activity in fetal lambs. J. Dev. Physiol. 6:267–274 1984.
105. Walker AM, Oakes GK, McLaughlin MK, Ehrenkranz RA, et al: 24-hour rhythms in uterine and umbilical blood flows of conscious pregnant sheep. Gynecol. Invest. 8:288–298, 1977.
106. Harbert GM: Biorhythms of the pregnant uterus (Macaca mulatto). Am. J. Obstet. Gynecol. 129:401–407, 1977.
107. Lawler FH, Brace RA: Fetal and maternal arterial pressures and heart rates: histograms, correlations, and rhythms. Am. J. Physiol. 243:R433-R444, 1982.
108. Berman W Jr, Goodlin RC, Heymann MA, Rudolph AM: Relationships between pressure and flow in the umbilical and uterine circulations of the sheep. Circ. Res. 38: 264–266, 1976.
109. Venuto RC, Cox JW, Stein JH, Ferris TF: The effect of changes in perfusion pressure on uteroplacental blood flow in the pregnant rabbit. J. Clin. Invest. 57:938–944, 1976.
110. Bissonnette JM, Farrell RC: Pressure-flow and pressure-volume relationships in the fetal placental circulation. J. Appl. Physiol. 35:355–360, 1973.
111. Power GG, Longo LD: Sluice flow in the placenta: maternal vascular pressure effects on fetal circulation. Am. J. Physiol. 225:1490–1496, 1973.
112. Thornburg KL, Bissonnette JM, Faber JJ: Absence of fetal placental waterfall phenomenon in chronically prepared fetal lambs in utero. Am. J. Physiol. 230:886–892, 1976.
113. Naden RP, Rosenfeld CR: Uteroplacental circulation: renin-angiotensin and adrenergic systems. *In* The Uterine Circulation. Edited by CR Rosenfield. Ithaca, NY, Perinatology Press, 1989, pp. 207–238.
114. Albertini R, Seino M, Scili G, Carretero OA: Uteroplacental renin in regulation of blood pressure in the pregnant rabbit. Am. J. Physiol. 239:H266–H271, 1980.
115. Naden RP, Gant NF, Rosenfeld CR: The pressor response to angiotensin II: the roles of peripheral and cardiac responses in pregnant and nonpregnant sheep. Am. J. Obstet. Gynecol. 148:450–457, 1984.
116. Ferris TF, Stein JH, Kauffman J: Uterine blood flow and uterine renin secretion. J. Clin. Invest. 51:2827–2833, 1972.
117. Ferris TF, Weir EK: Effect of captopril on uterine blood flow and prostaglandin E synthesis in the pregnant rabbit. J. Clin. Invest. 71:809–815, 1983.
118. Rosenfeld CR, Naden RP: Uterine and nonuterine vascular responses to angiotensin II in ovine pregnancy. Am. J. Physiol. 257:H17-H24, 1989.
119. Speroff L, Haning RV, Levin RM: The effect of angiotensin II and indomethacin on uterine blood flow in pregnant monkeys. Obstet. Gynecol. 50:611–614, 1977.
120. McLaughlin MK, Chez RA: The effect of $Sar^1$ $ala^8$ AII on ovine uterine and umbilical blood flow. Clin. Exper. Hypertens. 2:851–863.
121. Binder ND, Faber JJ: Effects of captopril on blood pressure, placental blood flow and uterine oxygen consumption in pregnant rabbits. J. Pharmacol. Exp. Ther. 260:294–299, 1992.
122. Lumbers ER, Kingsford NM, Menzies RI, Stevens AD: Acute effects of captopril, an angiotensin-converting enzyme inhibitor, on the pregnant ewe and fetus. Am. J. Physiol. 262: R754-R760, 1991.
123. Brar HS, Do Y-S, Tam HB, Valenzuela G, et al: Uteroplacental unit as a source of elevated circulating prorenin levels in normal pregnancy. Am. J. Obstet. Gynecol. 155: 1223–1226, 1986.
124. Chestnut DH, Weiner C, Martin JG, Herrig JE, et al: Effect of intravenous epinephrine on uterine artery blood flow velocity in the pregnant guinea pig. Anesthesiology 65: 633–636.
125. Magness RR, Rosenfeld CR: Systemic and uterine responses

to α-adrenergic stimulation in pregnant and nonpregnant ewes. Am. J. Obstet. Gynecol. 155:897–904, 1986.
126. Rosenfeld CR, West JA: Circulatory responses to systemic infusions of norepinephrine in the pregnant ewe. Am. J. Obstet. Gynecol. 127:376–383, 1977.
127. Magness RR, Rosenfeld CR: Mechanisms for attenuated pressor responses to α-agonists in ovine pregnancy. Am. J. Obstet. Gynecol. 159:252–261, 1988.
128. Oakes GK, Ehrenkranz RA, Walker AM, McLaughlin MG, et al: Effect of α-adrenergic agonist and antagonist infusion on the umbilical, uterine circulations of pregnant sheep. Biol. Neonate. 38:229–237, 1980.
129. Gu W, Jones CT: The effects of elevation of maternal plasma catecholamines on the fetus and placenta of pregnant sheep. J. Dev. Physiol. 8:173–186, 1986.
130. Shnider SM, Wright RG, Levinson G, Roizen MF, et al: Uterine blood flow and plasma norepinephrine changes during maternal stress in the pregnant ewe. Anesthesiology 50: 524–527, 1979.
131. Ralston DH, Shnider SM, deLorimier AA: Effects of quipotent ephedrine, metaraminol, mephentermine and methoxamine on uterine blood flow in the pregnant ewe. Anesthesiology 40:354–370, 1974.
132. van der Weyde MP, Wright MR, Taylor SM, Axelson JE, et al: Metabolic effects of ritodrine in the fetal lamb. J. Pharmcol. Exp. Ther. 262:48–59, 1992.
133. Adamson SL, Morrow RJ, Bull SB, Langille BL: Vasomotor responses of the umbilical circulation in fetal sheep. Am. J. Physiol. 256:R1056–R1062, 1989.
134. Berman W Jr, Goodlin RC, Heymann MA, Rudolph AM: Effects of pharmacologic agents on umbilical blood flow in fetal lambs in utero. Biol. Neonate. 33:225–235, 1978.
135. Iwamoto H, Rudolph AM: Effects of angiotensin II on the blood flow and its distribution in fetal lambs. Circ. Res. 48:183–189, 1981.
136. Iwamoto H, Rudolph AM: Effects of endogenous angiotensin II on the fetal circulation. J. Dev. Physiol. 1:283–287, 1979.
137. Rankin JHG, Phernetton TM: Alpha and angiotensin receptor tone in the near-term sheep fetus. Proc. Soc. Exp. Biol. Med. 158:166–170, 1978.
138. Rankin JHG, Phernetton TM: Effect of norepinephrine on the ovine umbilical circulation. Proc. Soc. Exp. Biol. Med. 152:312–317, 1976.
139. Iwamoto H, Rudolph AM: Hemodynamic responses of the sheep fetus to vasopressin infusion. Circ. Res. 44:430–436, 1979.
140. Daniel SS, Stark RI, Zubrow AB, Fox H, et al: Factors in the release of vasopressin in the hypoxic fetus. Endocrinology 113:1623–1628, 1983.
141. Rurak DW: Plasma vasopressin levels during hypoxaemia and the cardiovascular effects of exogenous vasopressin in foetal and adult sheep. J. Physiol. Lond. 277:341–357, 1978.
142. Perez R, Espinoza M, Riquelme R, Parer JT, et al: Arginine vasopressin mediates cardiovascular responses to hypoxemia in fetal sheep. Am. J. Physiol. 256:R1011-R1018, 1989.
143. Magness RR, Rosenfeld CR: The role of steroid hormones in the control of uterine blood flow. *In* The Uterine Circulation. Edited by CR Rosenfeld. Ithaca, NY, Perinatology Press, 1989, pp. 239–271.
144. Prill HJ: Blood flow in the myometrium and endometrium of the uterus. Am. J. Obstet. Gynecol. 82:102–108, 1961.
145. Killam AP, Rosenfeld CR, Battaglia FC, Makowski EI, et al: Effect of estrogens on the uterine blood flow of oophorectomized ewes. Am. J. Obstet. Gynecol. 115:1045–1052, 1973.
146. Magness RR, Rosenfeld CR: Local and systemic estradiol-17β: effects on uterine and systemic vasodilation. Am. J. Physiol. 256:E536–E542, 1989b.
147. Clewell WH, Stys S, Meschia G: Stimulation summation and tachyphylaxis in estrogen response in sheep. Am. J. Obstet. Gynecol. 138:485–493, 1980.
148. Ford SP, Magness RR, Farley DB, Van Orden DE: Local and systemic effects of intrauterine estradiol-17β on luteal function in nonpregnant sows. J. Anim. Sci. 55:657–664, 1982.
149. Caton D, Karla PS: Endogenous hormones and the regulation of uterine blood flow during pregnancy. Am. J. Physiol. 250:R365–R369, 1986.
150. Faber JJ, Gault CF, Green TJ, Thornburg KL: Fetal blood volume and fetal placental blood flow in lambs. Proc. Soc. Exp. Biol. Med. 142:340–344, 1973.
151. Caton D, Wilcox CJ, Karla PS: Correlation of the rate of uterine blood flow and plasma steroid concentrations at parturition in sheep. J. Reprod. Fert. 58:329–337, 1980.
152. Faber JJ: Regulation of fetal placental blood flow. *In* Respiratory Gas Exchange and Blood Flow in the Placenta. Edited by LD Longo, H Bartels. Washington, DC, U.S. Government Printing Office, 1972, pp. 157–173.
153. Anderson DF, Faber JJ: Regulation of fetal placental blood flow in the lamb. Am. J. Physiol. 247:R567–R574, 1984.
154. Anderson DF, Parks CM, Faber JJ: Fetal $O_2$ consumption in sheep during controlled long-term reductions in umbilical blood flow. Am. J. Physiol. 250:H1037–H1042, 1986.
155. Laifer SA, Ghodgaonkar R, Caritis SN, Dubin NH: Changes in uterine venous prostaglandin F metabolites following intravenous infusion of ritodrine in sheep. Obstet. Gynecol. 78:753–756, 1991.
156. Magness RR, Mitchell MD, Rosenfeld CR: Uteroplacental production of eicosanoids in ovine pregnancy. Prostaglandins 39:75–88, 1990.
157. Magness Rosenfeld, CR Faucher, DJ Mitchell MD: Uterine prostaglandin production in ovine pregnancy: effects of angiotensin II and indomethacin. Am. J. Physiol. 263:H188-H197, 1992.
158. Walsh SW, Parisi VM: The role of prostanoids and thromboxane in the regulation of placental blood flow. *In* The Uterine Circulation. Edited by CR Rosenfeld. Ithaca, NY, Perinatology Press, 1989, pp. 237–310.
159. Rankin JHG, Phernetton TM: Effect of prostaglandin $E_2$ on ovine maternal placental blood flow. Am. J. Physiol. 231: 754–759, 1976.
160. Trudinger BJ, Connelly AJ, Giles WB, Hales JR, et al: The effects of prostacyclin and thromboxane analogue (U46619) on the fetal circulation and umbilical flow velocity waveforms. J. Dev. Physiol. 11:179–184, 1989.
161. Walsh SW: Physiology of low dose aspirin therapy for the prevention of preeclampsia. Semin. Perinatol. 14:152–170, 1990.
162. Makila U-M, Jouppila P, Kirkinen P, Viinikka L, et al: Placental thromboxane and prostacyclin in the regulation of placental blood flow. Obstet. Gynecol. 68:537–540, 1986.
163. Jouppila P, Kirkenen P, Koivula A, Ylikorkala O: Failure of exogenous prostacyclin to change placental and fetal blood flow in preeclampsia. Am. J. Obstet. Gynecol. 151: 661–665, 1985.
164. Naden RP, Iliya CA, Arant BS, Gant NF Jr, et al: Hemodynamic effects of indomethacin in chronically instrumented pregnant sheep. Am. J. Obstet. Gynecol. 151:484–493, 1985.
165. Rankin JHG, Berssenbrugge A, Anderson D, Phernetton T:

Ovine placental vascular responses to indomethacin. Am. J. Physiol. 236:H61–H64, 1979.
166. Cashner KA, Skillman CA, Brockman D, Mack C, et al: Effect of antipyrine on prostaglandin levels and uterine and umbilical blood flow. Am. J. Obstet. Gynecol. 155: 1305–1310, 1986.
167. Moise KJ, Mari G, Kirshon B, Huhta JC, et al: The effect of indomethacin on the pulsatility index of the umbilical artery in human fetuses. Am. J. Obstet. Gynecol. 162: 199–202, 1990.
168. Lumbers ER, Kingsford NM, Menzies RM: The relationship between fetal and maternal placental blood flows. J. Dev. Physiol. 16:125–132, 1991.
169. Power GG, Dale PS, Nelson PS: Distribution of maternal and fetal blood flow within cotyledons of the sheep placenta. Am. J. Physiol. 241:H486–H496, 1981.
170. Rankin JHG: Interaction between the maternal and fetal placental blood flows. *In* The Uterine Circulation. Edited by CR Rosenfeld. Ithaca, NY, Perinatology Press, 1989, pp. 175–190.
171. Rankin JHG, Goodman A, Phernetton T: Local regulation of uterine blood flow by the umbilical circulation. Proc. Soc. Exp. Biol. Med. 150:690–694, 1975.
172. Stock MK, Anderson DF, Phernetton TM, McLaughlin MK, et al: Vascular responses of the fetal placenta to local occlusion of the maternal placental vasculature. J. Dev. Physiol. 2:339–346, 1980.
173. Raye JR, Killam AP, Battaglia FC, Makowski EL: Uterine blood flow and $O_2$ consumption following fetal death in sheep. Am. J. Obstet. Gynecol. 111:917–924, 1971.
174. Rankin JHG: A role for prostaglandins in the regulation of the placental blood flows. Prostaglandins 11:343–353, 1976.
175. Clapp JF III, Szeto HH, Larrow R, Hewitt J, et al: Umbilical blood flow response to embolization of the uterine circulation. Am. J. Obstet. Gynecol. 138:60–67, 1980.
176. Rankin JHG, Phernetton TM: Circulatory responses of the near-term sheep fetus to prostalgandin $E_2$. Am. J. Physiol. 231:760–765, 1976.
177. Ritchie JWK: Use of Doppler technology in assessing fetal health. J. Dev. Physiol. 15:121–123, 1991.
178. Erskine RLA, Ritchie JWK: Umbilical artery blood flow characteristics in normal and growth-retarded fetuses. Br. J. Obstet. Gynaecol. 92:605–610, 1985.
179. Fleischer A, Schulman H, Farmakides G, Bracero L, et al: Umbilical artery velocity waveforms and intrauterine growth retardation. Am. J. Obstet. Gynecol. 151:502–505, 1985.
180. Trudinger BJ, Giles WB, Cook CM, Bombardieri J, et al: Fetal umbilical artery flow velocity waveforms and placental resistance: clinical significance. Br. J. Obstet. Gynaecol. 92:22–30, 1985.
181. Brar H, Platt LD: Reverse end-diastolic flow velocity on umbilical artery velocimetry in high-risk pregnancies: an ominous finding with adverse pregnancy outcome. Am. J. Obstet. Gynecol. 159:559–561, 1988.
182. Divon MY, Girz BA, Leiblich R, Langer O: Clinical management of the fetus with markedly diminished umbilical artery end-diastolic flow. Am. J. Obstet. Gynecol. 161: 1523–1527, 1989.
183. Woo JSK, Liang ST, Lo RLS: Significance of an absent or reversed end diastolic flow in Doppler umbilical artery waveforms. J. Ultrasound. Med. 6:291–297, 1987.
184. Giles WB, Trudinger BJ, Baird PJ: Fetal umbilical artery flow velocity waveforms and placental resistance: pathological correlation. Br. J. Obstet. Gynaecol. 192:31–38, 1985.
185. McCowan LM, Mullen BM, Ritchie K: Umbilical artery flow velocity waveforms and the placental vascular bed. Am. J. Obstet. Gynecol. 157:900–902, 1987.
186. Jouppila P, Kirkenen P: Umbilical vein flow as an indicator of fetal hypoxia. Br. J. Obstet. Gynaecol. 91:107–110, 1984.
187. Morrow RJ, Adamson L, Bull SB, Ritchie JWK: Effect of placental embolization on the umbilical arterial velocity waveform in fetal sheep. Am. J. Obstet. Gynecol. 161: 1055–1060, 1989.
188. Muijsers GJJM, van Huisseling H, Hasaart THM: The effect of selective umbilical embolization on the common umbilical artery pulsatility index and umbilical vascular resistance in fetal sheep. J. Dev. Physiol. 15:259–267, 1991.
189. Trudinger BJ, Stevens D, Connelly A, Hales JRS, et al: Umbilical artery flow velocity waveforms and placental resistance: The effects of embolization of the umbilical circulation. Am. J. Obstet. Gynecol. 157:1443–1448, 1987.
190. Morrow RJ, Adamson L, Bull SB, Ritchie JWK: Hypoxic acidemia, hyperviscosity, and maternal hypertension do not affect the umbilical arterial velocity waveform in fetal sheep. Am. J. Obstet. Gynecol. 163:1313–1320, 1990.
191. Muijsers GJJM, Hasaart THM, Ruissen CJ, van Huisseling H, et al: The responses of the umbilical and femoral artery pulsatility indices in fetal sheep to progressively reduced uteroplacental blood flow. J. Dev. Physiol. 13:215–221, 1990.
192. Muijsers GJJM, Hasaart THM, van Huisseling H, de Haan J: The response of the umbilical artery pulsatility index in fetal sheep to acute and prolonged hypoxaemia and acidaemia induced by embolization of the uterine microcirculation. J. Dev. Physiol. 13:231–236, 1990.
193. van Huisseling H, Muijsers GJJM, de Haan J, Hassart THM: Fetal hypertension induced by norepinephrine infusion and umbilical artery flow velocity waveforms in fetal sheep. Am. J. Obstet. Gynecol. 165:450–455, 1991.
194. Nicolaides KH, Bilardo CM, Soothill PW, Campbell S: Absence of end diastolic frequencies in umbilical artery: a sign of fetal hypoxia and acidosis. Br. Med. J. 297: 1026–1027, 1988.
195. Okamura K, Watanabe T, Tanigawara S, Shintaku Y: Biochemical evaluation of fetus with hypoxia caused by severe preeclampsia using cordocentesis. J. Perinat. Med. 18: 441–447, 1990.
196. Soothill PW, Nicolaides KH, Bilardo CM, Hackett GA, et al: Utero-placental blood velocity resistance index and umbilical venous pO2, pCO2, pH, lactate and erythroblast count in growth-retarded fetuses. Fetal Therapy 1: 176–179, 1986.
197. Bilardo CM, Nicolaides KH, Campbell S: Doppler measurements of fetal and uteroplacental circulations: relationship with umbilical blood gases measured at cordocentesis. Am. J. Obstet. Gynecol. 162:115–120, 1990.
198. Bracero L, Schulman H, Fleischer A, Farmakides G, et al: Umbilical artery velocimetry in diabetes and pregnancy. Obstet. Gynecol. 68:654–658, 1986.
199. Degani S, Lewinsky R, Shapiro I, Sharf M: Fetal and uteroplacental flow velocity waveforms in the expectant management of placental abruption. Gynecol. Obstet. Invest. 30: 59–60, 1990.
200. Farmakides G, Schulman H, Saldana LR, Bracero LA, et al: Surveillance of twin pregnancy with umbilical arterial velocimetry. Am. J. Obstet. Gynecol. 153:789–792, 1985.
201. Giles WB, Trudinger BJ, Cook CM: Fetal umbilical artery flow velocity-time waveforms in twin pregnancies. Br. J. Obstet. Gynecol. 92:490–497, 1985.
202. Morrow RJ, Ritchie JWK: Uteroplacental and umbilical ar-

tery blood velocity waveforms in placental abruption assessed by Doppler ultrasound case report. Br. J. Obstet. Gynaecol. 95:723–724, 1988.

203. Nimrod C, Davies D, Harder J, Dempster C, et al: Doppler ultrasound prediction of fetal outcome in twin pregnancies. Am. J. Obstet. Gynecol. 156:402–406, 1987.
204. Saldena LR, Eads MC, Schaefer TR: Umbilical blood waveforms in fetal surveillance of twins. Am. J. Obstet. Gynecol. 157:712–715, 1987.
205. Fleischer A, Schulman H, Farmakides G, Bracero L, et al: Uterine artery Doppler velocimetry in pregnant women with hypertension. Am. J. Obstet. Gynecol. 154:806–813, 1986.
206. Karr K, Jouppila P, Kuikka J, Luotola H, et al: Intervillous blood flow in normal and complicated late pregnancy measured by means of an intravenous 133Xe method. Acta. Obstet. Gynecol. Scand. 59:7–10, 1980.
207. Lunell NO, Nylund L, Lewander R, Sarby B: Uteroplacental blood flow in pre-eclampsia measurements with indium-113m and a computer-linked gamma camera. Clin. Exp. Hypertens. In. Pregnancy. B1(1), 1982, pp. 105–117.
208. Nylund L, Lunell N-O, Lewander R, Sarby B: Uteroplacental blood flow index in intrauterine growth retardation of fetal or maternal origin. Br. J. Obstet. Gynaecol. 90:16–20, 1983.
209. Jacobsen S-L, Imhof R, Manning N, Mannion V, et al: The value of Doppler assessment of the uteroplacental circulation in predicting preeclampsia or intrauterine growth retardation. Am. J. Obstet. Gynecol. 162:110–114, 1990.
210. McCowan LM, Ritchie K, Mo LY, Bascom PA, et al: Uterine artery flow velocity waveforms in normal and growth-retarded pregnancies. Am. J. Obstet. Gynecol. 158:599–504, 1988.
211. Sibley CP, Boyd RDH: Control of transfer across the mature placenta. Oxford. Rev. Repr. Biol. 10:382–435, 1988.
212. Bain MD, Copas DK, Landon MJ, Stacey TE: In vivo permeability of the human placenta to inulin and mannitol. J. Physiol. (Lond.) 399:313–319, 1988.
213. Schneider H, Sodha RJ, Progler M, Young MPA: Permeability of the human placenta for hydrophilic substances studied in the isolated dually in vitro perfused lobe. Contr. Gynecol. Obstet. 13:98–103, 1985.
214. Thornburg KL, Burry KJ, Adas AK, Kirk EP, et al: Permeability of placenta to inulin. Am. J. Obstet. Gynecol. 158: 1165–1169, 1988.
215. Willis DM, O'Grady JP, Faber JJ, Thornburg KL: Diffusion permeability of cyanacobalamin in human placenta. Am. J. Physiol. 250:R459–R464, 1986.
216. Reynolds F, Knott C: Pharmacokinetics in pregnancy and placental drug transfer. Ox. Rev. Reprod. Biol. 11: 389–449, 1989.
217. Bissonnette JM: Membrane vesicles from trophoblast cells as models for placental exchange studies. Placenta 3: 99–106, 1982.
218. Cordero L, Yeh SY, Grunt JA, Anderson GG: Hypertonic glucose infusion in labor. Am. J. Obstet. Gynecol. 107: 295–302, 1970.
219. Cetin I, Corbetta C, Serini LP, Marconni AM, et al: Umbilical amino acid concentrations in normal and growth-retarded fetuses sampled in utero by cordocentesis. Am. J. Obstet. Gynecol. 162:253–261, 1990.
220. Yudilevich DL, Swiery JH: Transport of amino acids in the placenta. Biochem. Biophys. Acta. 822:169–201, 1985.
221. Balkovetz DF, Leibach FG, Mahesh VB, Devoe LD, et al: Characterization of tryptophan transport in human placental brush-border membrane vesicles. Biochem. J. 238: 201–208, 1986.
222. Hill PMM, Young M: Net placental transfer of free amino acids against varying concentrations. J. Physiol. (Lond.) 235:409–422, 1973.
223. Lemmons JA: Fetal-placental nitrogen metabolism. Sem. Perinatol. 3:177–190, 1979.
224. van Dijk JP, van Kreel BK, Heeren JWA: A study of the relationship between placental non-haem iron and iron transfer in the guinea pig: the maturation of the transfer process. J. Dev. Physiol. 8:347–354, 1986.
225. Wong CT, Morgan EA: Placental transfer of iron in the guinea pig Quart. J. Exp. Physiol. 58:47–48, 1973.
226. McArdle HJ, Priscott PK: Uptake and metabolism of transferrin and albumin by rat yolk sac placenta. Am. J. Physiol. 247:C409–C414, 1984.
227. Thornburg KL, Faber JJ: Transfer of hydrophilic molecules by placenta and yolk sac of the guinea pig. Am. J. Physiol. 233:C111–C124, 1977.
228. Hay WW Jr: The placenta: not just a conduit for maternal fuels. Diabetes 40(suppl.2):44–50, 1991.
229. Battaglia FC, Meschia G: Fetal nutrition. Ann. Rev. Nutr. 8: 43–61, 1988.
230. Hay WW Jr, Molina R, DiGiacomo JE, Meschia G: Model of placental glucose consumption and glucose transfer. Am. J. Physiol. 258:R569–R577, 1990.
231. Coleman RA: Placental metabolism and transport of lipid. Fed. Proc. 45:2519–2523, 1986.
232. Hellegers AE: Some developments in opinions about the placenta as a barrier to oxygen. Yale. J. Biol. Med. 42: 180–190, 1969.
233. Longo LD, Ching KS: Placental diffusing capacity for carbon monoxide and oxygen in unanesthetized sheep. J. Appl. Physiol. 43:885–893, 1977.
234. Battaglia FC, Meschia G: Principle substrates of fetal metabolism. Physiol. Rev. 58:499–527, 1978.
235. Bonds DR, Crosby LO, Cheek TG, Hagerdal M, et al: Estimation of human fetal-placental unit metabolic rate by application of the Bohr principle. J. Dev. Physiol. 8:49–54, 1986.
236. Battaglia FC, Meschia G, Makowski EL, Bowes W: The effect of maternal oxygen administration upon fetal oxygenation. J. Clin. Invest. 47:548–555, 1968.
237. Hay WW Jr, DiGiacomo JE, Meznarich HK, Hirst K, et al: Effects of glucose and insulin on fetal glucose oxidation and oxygen consumption. Am. J. Physiol. 256:E704–E713, 1989.
238. Lorijn RHW, Longo LD: Clinical and physiologic implications of increased fetal oxygen consumption. Am. J. Obstet. Gynecol. 136:451–457, 1980.
239. Rurak DW, Cooper CC, Taylor SM: Fetal oxygen consumption and $PO_2$ during hypercapnia in sheep. J. Dev. Physiol. 8:447–459, 1986.
240. Rurak DW, Gruber NC: Increased oxygen consumption associated with breathing activity in fetal lambs. J. Appl. Physiol. 54:701–707, 1983.
241. Carter AM: Factors affecting gas transfer across the placenta and oxygen supply to the fetus. J. Dev. Physiol. 12: 305–322, 1989.
242. Longo LD: Respiratory gas exchange in the placenta. *In* Handbook of Physiology, Section 3, The Respiratory System, Volume IV, Gas Exchange. Bethesda, MD, American Physiological Society, 1987, pp. 351–401.
243. Wilkening RB, Meschia G: Current topic: comparative physiology of placental oxygen transport. Placenta 13: 1–15, 1992.
244. Hill EP, Power GG, Longo LD: A mathematical model of placental $O_2$ transfer with consideration of hemoglobin reactions rates. Am. J. Physiol. 222:721–729, 1972.

245. Longo LD, Hill EP, Power GG: Theoretical analysis of placental $O_2$ transfer. Am. J. Physiol. 222:730–739, 1972.
246. Wilkening RB, Meschia G: Effect of occluding one umbilical artery on placental oxygen transport. Am. J. Physiol. 260:H1319–H1325, 1991.
247. Soothill PW, Nicolaides KH, Rodeck CH, Campbell S: Effect of gestational age on fetal and intervillous blood gas and acid-base values in human pregnancy. Fetal Therapy 1: 168–175, 1986.
248. Delivoria-Papadopoulus M, Coburn RF, Forster RE II: The placental diffusing capacity for carbon dioxide at term. *In* Respiratory Gas Exchange and Blood Flow in the Placenta. Edited by HD Longo, H Bartels. Bethesda, MD, Dept. of Health, Education, and Welfare, 1972, pp. 259–265.
249. Rocco E, Bennett TR, Power GG: Placental diffusing capacity in unanesthetized rabbits. Am. J. Physiol. 228:465–469, 1975.
250. Nelson PS, Gilbert RD, Longo LD: Fetal growth and placental diffusing capacity in guinea pigs following long-term maternal exercise. J. Dev. Physiol. 5:1–10, 1983.
251. Towell ME: Fetal respiratory physiology. *In* Perinatal Medicine. Edited by JW Goodwin, JO Godden GW Chance. Toronto, Canada, Longman, 1976, pp. 171–186.
252. Battaglia FC, Bowes W, Mcgaughey HR, Makowski EL, et al: The effect of fetal exchange transfusions with adult blood upon fetal oxygenation. Pediatr. Res. 3:60–65, 1969.
253. Edelstone DI, Darby MJ, Bass K, Miller K: Effect of reductions in hemoglobin-oxygen affinity and hematocrit level on oxygen consumption and acid-base state in fetal lambs. Am. J. Obstet. Gynecol. 160:820–828, 1989.
254. Carter AM, Gronlund J: Contribution of the Bohr effect to the fall in fetal $Po_2$ caused by maternal alkalosis. J. Perinat. Med. 13:185–193, 1985.
255. Meizner I, Glezerman M: Cordocentesis in the evaluation of the growth-retarded fetus. Clin. Obstet. Gynecol. 35: 126–137, 1992.
256. Nicolaides KH, Soothill PW, Rodeck CH, Campbell S: Ultrasound-guided sampling of umbilical cord and placental blood to assess fetal well-being. Lancet I 1065–1067, 1986.
257. Bell AW, Kennaugh JM, Battaglia FC, Makowski EL, et al: Metabolic and circulatory studies of fetal lambs at midgestation. Am. J. Physiol. 250:E538–E544, 1986.
258. Harding R, Poore ER, Cohen GL: The effect of brief episodes of diminished uterine blood flow on breathing movements, sleep state and heart rate in fetal sheep. J. Dev. Physiol. 3:231–243, 1981.
259. Harding R, Sigger JN, Wickham PJD: Fetal and maternal influences on arterial oxygen levels in the sheep fetus. J. Dev. Physiol. 5:267–276, 1983.
260. Rurak DW, Gruber NC: The effect of neuromuscular blockade on oxygen consumption and blood gases in the fetal lamb. Am. J. Obstet. Gynecol. 145:258–262, 1983.
261. Rurak DW, Taylor SM: Oxygen consumption in the fetal lamb after maternal administration of sodium pentobarbital. Am. J. Obstet. Gynecol. 154:674–678, 1986.
262. Wilkening RB, Boyle DW, Meschia G: Fetal neuromuscular blockade: effect on oxygen demand and placental transport. Am. J. Physiol. 257:H734-H738, 1989.
263. Mulder EJH, Visser GHA: Braxton Hicks contractions and motor behavior in the near-term human fetus. Am. J. Obstet. Gynecol. 156:543–549, 1987.
264. Patrick J, Campbell K, Carmichael L , Natale R: Patterns of human fetal breathing during the last 10 weeks of pregnancy. Obstet. Gynecol. 54:24–30, 1980.
265. Patrick J, Campbell K, Carmichael L , Natale R: Patterns of gross fetal body movements over 24-hour observation periods during the last 10 weeks of pregnancy. Am. J. Obstet. Gynecol. 142:363–371, 1982.
266. Berg D, Saling E: The oxygen partial pressures in the human fetus during labor and delivery. *In* Respiratory Gas Exchange and Blood Flow in the Placenta. Edited by HD Longo, H Bartels. Bethesda, MD, Dept. of Health, Education, and Welfare, 1972, pp. 441–457.
267. Towell ME: Fetal acid-base physiology. *In* Perinatal Medicine. Edited by JW Goodwin, JO Godden GW Chance. Toronto, Canada, Longman, 1976, pp. 187–208.
268. Comline RM, Silver M: The composition of foetal and maternal blood during parturition in the ewe. J. Physiol. (Lond.) 222:233–256, 1972.
269. Nickelson C: Monitoring of fetal carbon dioxide tension during labour. Dan. Med. Bull. 36:537–551, 1989.
270. Rooth G, Fall O, Huch A, Huch R: Integrated interpretation of fetal heart rate, intrauterine pressure and transcutaneous $Po_2$. Gynecol. Obstet. Invest. 10:265–280, 1979.
271. Gardosi JO, Schram CM, Symonds EM: Adaptation of pulse oximetry for fetal monitoring during labour. Lancet 337: 1265–12167, 1991.
272. Johnson N, Johnson VA, Fisher J, Jobbings B, et al: Fetal monitoring with pulse oximetry. Br. J. Obstet. Gynaecol. 98:36–41, 1991.
273. Uzan S Sturbois, G Salat-Baroux, J Sureau C: Application technique of tissue pH electrode on human fetuses. Arch. Gynaekol. 226:61–667, 1978.
274. Young BK, Noumoff J, Klein SA, Katz M: Continuous fetal tissue pH measurement in labor. Obstet. Gynecol. 52: 533–538, 1978.
275. Jansen CAM, Bass FG, Lowe KC, Nathanielsz PW: Comparison of continuous transcutaneous and continuous intravascular $Po_2$ measurement in fetal sheep. Am. J. Obstet. 138: 670–676, 1980.
276. Smits TM, Aarnoudse JG: Variability of fetal scalp blood flow during labour: continuous transcutaneous measurement by the laser Doppler technique. Br. J. Obstet. Gynaecol. 91:524–531, 1984.
277. Wallenburg HCS, Verhoeff A Jansen, TC van der Wiel, AR: Effects of experimental head compression on transcutaneous scalp $Po_2$ in fetal lambs. Obstet. Gynecol. 64:239–243, 1984.
278. Okane M, Shigemitsu S, Inaba J, Koresawa M, et al: Noninvasive continuous transcutaneous $Po_2$ and $Pco_2$ monitoring during labor. J. Perinat. Med. 17:399–410, 1989.
279. Hansen PK, Thomsen SG, Secher NJ, Weber T: Transcutaneous carbon dioxide measurements in the fetus during labor. Am. J. Obstet. Gynecol. 150:47–51, 1984.
280. Klink F, Grosspeitzsch R, Klitzing LV, Oberheuser F: Uterine contraction intervals and transcutaneous levels of fetal oxygen pressure. Obstet. Gynecol. 57:437–440, 1981.
281. Thomsen SG, Weber T: Fetal transcutaneous carbon dioxide tension during the second stage of labour. Br. J. Obstet. Gynaecol. 91:1103–1106, 1984.
282. Janbu T, Koss KS, Nesheim B-I, Wesche J: Blood velocities in the uterine artery in humans during labour. Acta. Physiol. Scand. 124:153–161, 1985.
283. Fleischer A, Anyaegbunam AA, Schulman H, Farmakides G, et al: Uterine and umbilical artery velocimetry during normal labor. Am. J. Obstet. Gynecol. 157:40–43, 1987.
284. Assali NS, Dasgupta K, Kolin A, Holmes L: Measurement of uterine blood flow and uterine metabolism. V. Changes during spontaneous and induced labor in unanesthetized pregnant sheep and dogs. Am. J. Physiol. 195:614–620, 1958.
285. Greis FC: Effect of labor on uterine blood flow. Am. J. Obstet. Gynecol. 93:917–923, 1965.

286. Fairlie FM, Lang GD, Sheldon CD: Umbilical artery flow velocity waveforms in labour. Br. J. Obstet. Gynaecol. 96: 151–157, 1989.
287. Stuart B, Drumm J, Fitzgerald D, Duigan NM: Fetal blood velocity waveforms in uncomplicated labour. Br. J. Obstet. Gynaecol. 88:865–869.
288. Low JA, Pangham SR, Worthington D, Boston RW: Clinical characteristics of pregnancies complicated by intrapartum asphyxia. Am. J. Obstet. Gynecol. 121:452–456, 1975.
289. Wood C, Ng KH, Hounslow D, Benning H: The influence of differences of birth times upon fetal condition in normal deliveries. J. Obstet. Gynaecol. Br. Commonw. 80: 289–294, 1973.
290. Wood C, Ng KH, Hounslow D, Benning H: Time—an important variable in normal delivery. J. Obstet. Gynaecol. Br. Commonw. 80:295–300, 1973.
291. Yudkin PL, Johnson P, Redman CWG: Obstetric factors associated with cord blood gas values at birth. Eur. J. Obstet. Gynecol. Reprod Biol 24:167–176, 1987.
292. Towell ME: The rationale for biochemical monitoring of the fetus. J. Perinat. Med. 16 (suppl 1):55–70, 1988.
293. Morrison IB, Olsen J: Weight-specific stillbirths and associated causes of death: an analysis of 765 stillbirths. Am. J. Obstet. Gynecol. 152:975–980, 1985.
294. Bejar R, Wozniak P, Allard M, Bernischke K, et al: Antenatal origin of neurologic damage in newborn infants. I. Preterm infants. Am. J. Obstet. Gynecol. 159:357–363, 1988.
295. Low JA, Robertson DM, Simpson LL: Temporal relationships of neuropathologic conditions caused by perinatal asphyxia. Am. J. Obstet. Gynecol. 160:608–614, 1989.
296. Brown R, Patrick J: The nonstress test: how long is enough. Am. J. Obstet. Gynecol. 141:646–651, 1981.
297. Smith JH, An KJS, Cotes PM, Dawes GS, et al: Antenatal fetal heart rate variation in relation to the respiratory and metabolic status of the compromised human fetus. Br. J. Obstet. Gynaecol. 95:980–989, 1988.
298. Manning FA, Morrison I, Lange IR, Harman CR, et al: Fetal assessment based on fetal biophysical profile scoring: experience in 12,620 referred high-risk pregnancies. Am. J. Obstet. Gynecol. 151:343–350, 1985.
299. Bocking AD, Harding R, Wickham PJD: Effects of reduced uterine blood flow on accelerations and decelerations in heart rate of fetal sheep. Am. J. Obstet. Gynecol. 154: 329–335, 1986.
300. Boddy K, Dawes GS, Fisher R, Pinter S, et al: Foetal respiratory movements, electrocortical, and cardiovascular responses to hypoxemia and hypercapnia in sheep. J. Physiol. (Lond.) 243:599–618, 1974.
301. Cohn HE, Sacks EJ, Heymann MA, Rudolph AM: Cardiovascular responses to hypoxemia and acidemia in fetal lambs. Am. J. Obstet. Gynecol. 120:817–824, 1974.
302. Bernardini I, Evans MI, Nicolaides KH, Economides DL, et al: The fetal concentrating index as a gestational age-independent measure of placental dysfunction in intrauterine growth retardation. Am. J. Obstet. Gynecol. 164: 1481–1490, 1991.
303. Economides DL, Nicolaides KH: Blood glucose and oxygen tension levels in small-for-gestational-age fetuses. Am J Obstet. Gynecol. 160:385–389, 1989.
304. Economides DL, Nicolaides KH, Gahl WA, Bernardini I, et al: Plasma amino acids in appropriate- and small-for-gestational-age fetuses. Am. J. Obstet. Gynecol. 161: 1219–1227, 1989.
305. Nicolaides KH, Economides DL, Soothill PW: Blood gases, pH and lactate in appropriate- and small-for-gestational-age fetuses. Am. J. Obstet. Gynecol. 161:996–1001, 1989.
306. Pearce JM, Chamberlain GVP: Ultrasonically guided percutaneous umbilical blood sampling in the management of intrauterine growth retardation. Br. J. Obstet. Gynaecol. 94:318–321, 1987.
307. Soothill PW, Nicolaides KH, Campbell S: Prenatal asphyxia, hyperlacticaemia, hypoglycaemia, and erythroblastosis in growth retarded fetuses. Br. Med. J. 294:1051–1053, 1987.
308. Soothill PW, Nicolaides KH, Rodeck CH, Clewell WH, et al: Relationship of fetal hemoglobin and oxygen content to lactate concentrations in Rh isoimmunized pregnancies. Obstet. Gynecol. 69:268–270, 1987.
309. Nicolaides KH, Sadovsky G, Visser GHA: Heart rate patterns in normoxemic, hypoxemic and anemic second-trimester fetuses. Am. J. Obstet. Gynecol. 160:1034–1037, 1989.
310. Vintzileos AM, Fleming AD, Scorza WE, Wolf EJ, et al: Relationship between fetal biophysical activities and umbilical cord blood gas values. Am. J. Obstet. Gynecol. 165: 707–713, 1991.
311. Visser GHA, Sadovsky G, Nicolaides KH: Antepartum heart rate patterns in small-for-gestational third-trimester fetuses: Correlations with blood gas values obtained at cordocentesis. Am. J. Obstet. Gynecol. 162:698–703, 1990.
312. Visser GHA, Redman CWG, Huijes HJ, Turnbull AC: Nonstressed antepartum heart rate monitoring: implications of decelerations after spontaneous contractions. Am. J. Obstet. Gynecol. 138:429–435, 1980.
313. Ramanathan S, Gandhi S, Arismendy J, Chalon J, et al: Oxygen transfer from mother to fetus during cesarean section under epidural anesthesia. Anesth. Analg. 61:56–81, 1982.
314. Perreault C, Blaise GA, Meloche R: Maternal inspired oxygen concentration and fetal oxygenation during Caesarean section. Can. J. Anesth. 39:155–157, 1992.
315. Dornan JC, Ritchie JWK.: Fetal breathing movements and maternal hyperoxia in the growth retarded fetus. Br. J. Obstet. Gynaecol. 90:210–213, 1983.
316. Gagnon R, Hunse C, Vijan S: The effect of maternal hyperoxia on behavioral activity in growth-retarded human fetuses. Am. J. Obstet. Gynecol. 163:1894–1899, 1990.
317. Battaglia C, Artini PG, D'Ambrogio G, Galli PA, et al: Maternal hyperoxygenation in the treatment of intrauterine growth retardation. Am. J. Obstet. Gynecol. 167:430–435, 1992.
318. Nicolaides KH, Bradley RJ, Soothill PW, Campbell S, et al: Maternal oxygen therapy for intrauterine growth retardation. Lancet I (#8539):942–945, 1987.
319. Longo LD, Delivoria-Papadopoulus M, Forster RE II: Placental $CO_2$ transfer after fetal carbonic anhydrase inhibition. Am. J. Physiol. 226:703–710, 1974.
320. Aarnoudse JG, Illsley NP, Penfold P, Bardsley S, et al: Permeability of the human placenta to bicarbonate: in-vitro perfusion studies. Br. J. Obstet. Gynaecol. 91:1096–1102, 1984.
321. Yaffe H, Parer JT, Block BS, Llanos AJ: Cardiorespiratory responses to graded reductions of uterine blood flow in the sheep fetus. J. Dev. Physiol. 9:325–336, 1987.

# Chapter 7

# PHYSIOLOGY OF THE FETUS AND NEWBORN

EDUARDO BANCALARI
KAREN HENDRICKS-MUÑOZ

Knowledge of fetal and newborn physiology is essential in the provision of excellent obstetric anesthesia and care to the neonate in the delivery room. This knowledge must encompass normal development and physiology as well as the adaptational responses of the fetus and newborn to physiologic alterations, particularly as they relate to the birth process and to pharmacologic interventions in the mother. Knowledge of the development and function of the different fetal organ systems is becoming more critical as the survival of infants delivered at very low gestations increases rapidly.

Growth and development of different organs during fetal life occur at different rates. The brain, the kidneys, and the liver develop relatively early during gestation, and at 20 to 24 weeks past conception they are proportionately much larger in the fetus than in the adult. The brain at 20 to 24 weeks, for example, accounts for approximately 13% of the total fetal weight, while in the adult it accounts for only 2% of the body weight. On the other hand, development of the skeletal muscles occurs mainly postnatally, and while in the adult skeletal muscle constitutes 40% of the body weight, in the newborn at term it only accounts for 25% of the weight.

For the obstetric anesthesiologist, it is important to have a basic understanding of each fetal and neonatal organ system and especially the cardiovascular and respiratory systems. These systems have different functions during fetal life than do they during extrauterine life, and therefore undergo dramatic changes at birth. Consequently, most of the pathologic conditions in the immediate neonatal period are related to problems of the cardiovascular and respiratory systems.

The viability of the fetus in the extrauterine environment depends mainly on the stage of development at birth. The limit of viability is not static, and has been moving upward in gestation as a result of new developments in the management of the small preterm infants. For example, the survival of infants with birth weights between 500 g and 1500 g at the University of Miami/Jackson Memorial Medical Center has increased from 48% in 1970 to 68% in 1980, and 88% in 1990. The mortality of infants with birth weights above 1500 g is very low today, and it is mostly due to severe congenital malformations. Intrauterine growth and development occur at a very fast rate during the last trimester, and therefore even a few weeks of difference in gestation can determine a large difference in birth weight and survival rate for the infant. At 24 weeks of gestation, for example, the fetus weighs approximately 700 g, while at 28 weeks the weight is 1100 g; at 32 weeks 1700 g; and at 40 weeks approximately 3500 g (Figure 7–1). The smaller the infant at birth, the greater the risk for developing some of the complications that account for most of the neonatal morbidity and mortality. Among these complications, the most prominent include hypothermia, hypoglycemia, respiratory distress, apnea, intracranial hemorrhage, patent ductus arteriosus, and infections. It is for this reason that strict attention be paid to the prevention of these complications from the first minutes of extrauterine life. The care that these infants receive in the delivery room and in the immediate neonatal period is crucial, and many times that care is the main determinant of the survival and subsequent outcome of the infant.

This chapter discusses the most important physiologic changes that occur during the stages of embryonic and fetal development and during perinatal transition, with an emphasis on cardiorespiratory function. It also discusses the effects that pharmacologic interventions may have on fetal well-being during these periods. A more detailed description of fetal and neonatal physiology is found elsewhere (1–7).

## CARDIOVASCULAR DEVELOPMENT AND PHYSIOLOGY

### *Embryology of the Heart*

The human heart originates from a tubular structure that is formed during the first month of gestation of the embryonic period (Figure 7–2) (8–10). The cardiac tube is composed of four segments: the truncus arteriosus, the bulbus cordis, the ventricle, and the sinoatrium, arranged in series (Figure 7–2A). Differential growth of the cardiac cells causes the tubular structure to bend to the right (Figure 7–2B) (11). The bulbus and ventricle then take on a U-shape and the two ventricles, initially in series, loop to eventually lie side-by-side (Figure 7–2C and Figure 7–2D). The atrioventricular canal then migrates toward the right so that it lies over both ventricles (Figure 7–2D). The sinoatrial chamber is divided by the endocardial cushions to become the right and left atrium (12). The tricuspid and mitral atrioventricular valves develop dividing the atrioventricular canal and, in connecting the

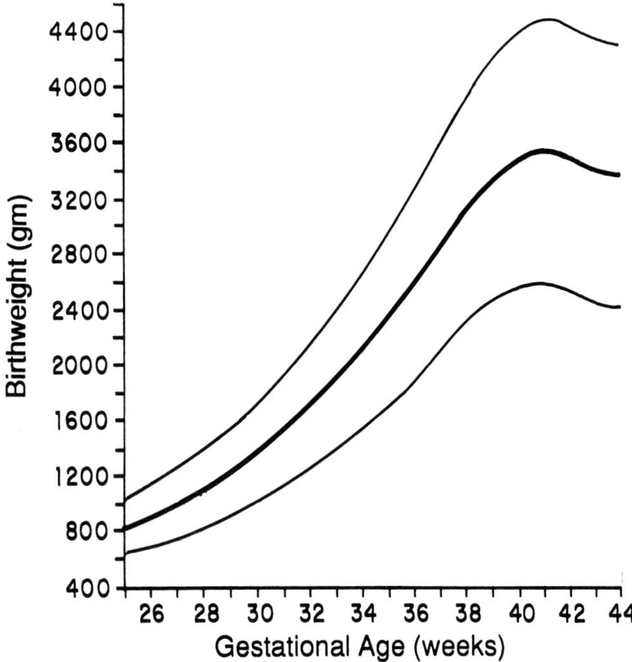


**Fig. 7–1.** Smoothed curve values for the mean ±2 standard deviations of birth weight against gestational age. (Redrawn from Usher and McLean. J. Pediatr. 74:901, 1969.)

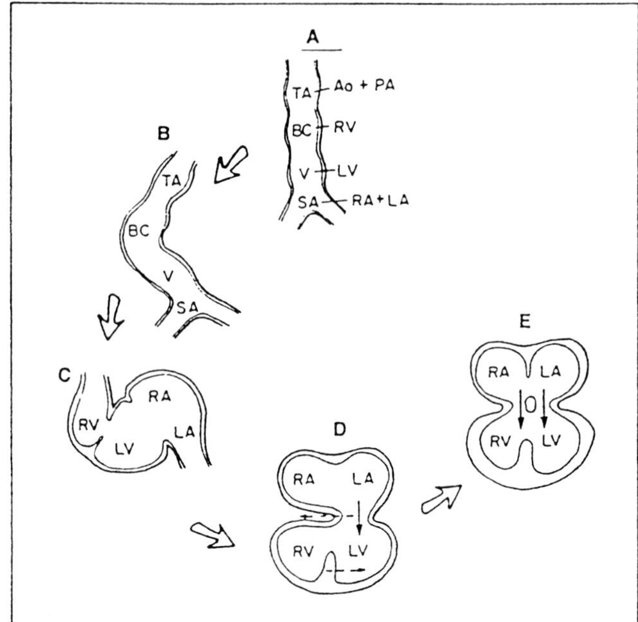


**Fig. 7–2.** The transition of the embryonic cardiac tube to four-chamber heart. **A,** Straight cardiac tube. The four segments are in series: sinoatrium (SA) destined to become the right and left atria (RA, LA); the ventricle (V) precursor to the left ventricle (LV); the bulbus cordis (BC) precursor to the right ventricle (RV); and the truncus arteriosus (TA) precursor of the aorta (Ao) and main pulmonary artery (PA). **B,** The cardiac tube is fixed at the proximal and distal ends, causing the tube to bend to the right in response to differential growth. **C,** The ventricular portion doubles over on itself so that the right and left ventricles once in series lie side by side. **D,** The atrioventricular (AV) canal migrates toward the right to overlie both ventricles. **E,** The endocardial cushions meet dividing the AV canal into mitral and tricuspid openings. (From Abraham Rudolpf Textbook of Pediatrics. 17th Ed. East Norwalk, Appleton-Century-Crofts Publishers, 1982.)

primitive ventricles, permit forward flow of blood entering through the sinoatrium and leaving via the truncus arteriosus (13).

These embryonic changes lead to a heart composed of four chambers with two outflow great vessels and two pumping systems in parallel (Figure 7–2E).

## *Development of the Great Vessels*

The fetal truncus arteriosus is destined to become the great vessels while the distal end of the bulbus cordis divides into two muscular portions becoming the subaortic and the subpulmonic conus. The subpulmonic conus increases in length, but the subaortic conus resorbs as the aorta migrates posteriorly to connect with the left ventricle (14,15).

Failure of reabsorption of the subaortic conus may cause truncus arteriosus. In addition, abnormalities of great artery connection to the ventricles may produce such anomalies as double-outlet right ventricle, or transposition of the great vessels (16,17).

Blood flow patterns are important to the embryonic development of the heart. Changes in blood flow patterns may cause such anomalies as endocardial cushion defects, large ventricular septal defects, and double-outlet right ventricle (13,17,18). Furthermore, any subaortic obstruction can produce aortic hypoplasia (18).

The pulmonary veins develop from the common pulmonary vein. The veins develop initially as a small bud from the posterior left atrium that enlarges and connects with the splanchnic plexus attached to the lung buds (Figure 7–3) (19). Abnormal communication of the pulmonary veins can result in total anomalous pulmonary venous return or cor triatriatum (20).

The tenth week of gestation signals the end of the embryonic period. The subsequent fetal period is a time of growth and maturation of the established major structures.

## *The Fetal Circulation*

In the preceding chapter, the function of the placenta as the organ of exchange of gases and nutrients is discussed in detail. Here we will briefly discuss the fetal circulation, which has four features that distinguish it from the adult circulation. These include: (1) umbilical vessels; (2) ductus venosus; (3) foramen ovale; and (4) ductus arteriosus. The umbilical vein carries blood saturated with oxygen and nutrients from the placenta to the fetus, while the umbilical arteries carry the oxygen desaturated blood, carbon dioxide, and catabolic products from the fetus to the placenta (Figure 7–4).

The umbilical vein in the fetus is as large as the descending aorta, which divides into two branches just below the liver. The larger branch becomes the ductus venosus, a

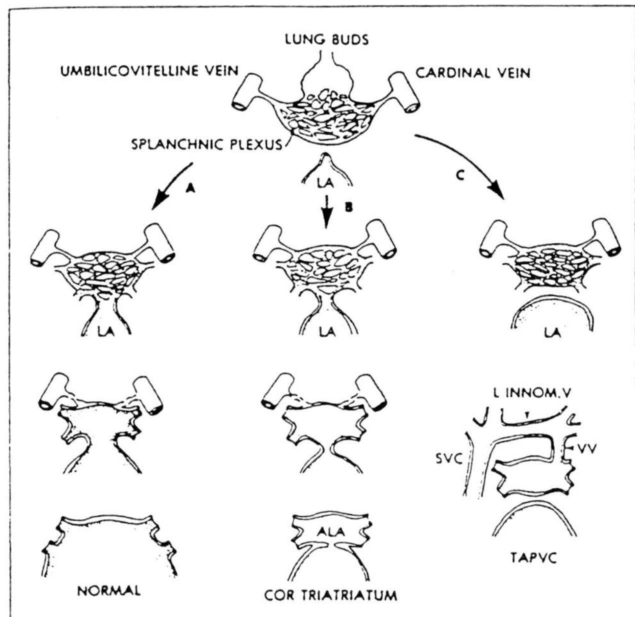


**Fig. 7–3.** The development of the normal pulmonary veins, cor triatriatum, and total anomalous pulmonary venous connection. **A,** Normal pulmonary vein development. **B,** Cor triatriatum development caused by a narrowed common pulmonary vein and left atrial junction, which creates a membrane producing an accessory chamber (ALA = accessory left chamber) that receives the pulmonary veins. **C,** Total anomalous pulmonary venous return connection (TAPVC). (VV = vertical veins; L INNON V = innominate vein; SVC = superior vena cava.) (From Abraham Rudolpf Textbook of Pediatrics. 17th Ed. East Norwalk, Appleton-Century-Crofts Publishers, 1982.)

low resistance bypass (21) that carries about 50% of the umbilical blood flow to the inferior vena cava, while the slightly smaller branch unites with the portal vein to carry the remainder of the umbilical venous blood and venous blood in the portal vein to empty into the liver. After the latter blood circulates through the liver, it enters the inferior vena cava through the hepatic vein. The blood from the ductus venosus is thus joined by venous return from the lower extremities and the abdominal organs. However, the two streams of blood from the abdominal and inferior vena cava and the ductus venosus do not mix; preferentially, the blood from the ductus venosus enters the left atrium through the foramen ovale and then into the left ventricle, which pumps it into the ascending aorta, bypassing the lungs (22–24). Through this preferential streaming, high-oxygen-saturated umbilical venous blood supplies the brain and myocardium via the brachiocephalic and coronary arteries, respectively. The remaining inferior vena cava blood is mixed with superior vena caval and coronary sinus blood from the upper body and heart and enters the right atrium that is then directed through the tricuspid valve into the right ventricle and thence to the pulmonary trunk. This desaturated blood enters the descending aorta through the ductus arteriosus, joining the oxygenated blood from the ascending aorta. A small percentage (7%) of this desaturated blood, however, passes through the pulmonary arteries into the high resistance lung vascular bed (25,26). The high pulmonary vascular resistance in the fetal lung is due to the presence of thick medial smooth muscle layer in the fetal small precapillary pulmonary arterioles and the constriction of this muscle in response to the intrauterine environment (27).

The foramen ovale and ductus arteriosus thus affect hemodynamics and the course of fetal blood in such a way that most of the oxygenated blood from the placenta returning to the fetus, via the inferior vena cava, bypasses the lungs and goes directly to the left ventricle, while most of the desaturated blood from the upper part of the fetus and the lower limbs and abdominal organs bypasses the left ventricle and passes through the ductus arteriosus to the descending aorta. In this way the two ventricles of the fetal heart work parallel to pump blood simultaneously from the great veins to the aorta.

The foramen ovale lies between the inferior vena cava and atrium but does not join the two atria. The valve is composed of cardiac muscle and contracts during atrial systole. The stream of blood from the inferior vena cava bifurcates on a protruding fold of endocardial tissue, the crista dividens, into a larger stream that passes through the foramen ovale into the left atrium and a smaller stream that remains in the right atrium to become mixed with blood entering by way of the superior vena cava.

The ductus arteriosus is a wide channel whose internal diameter is the same as that of the pulmonary artery and aorta—a characteristic of this structure that permits it to serve as a channel from the pulmonary trunk to the descending aorta, delivering right ventricular blood to the placenta and lower part of the body. Although the media of the great vessels are composed of elastic tissue, the media of the ductus arteriosus consist of muscular fibers that encircle the ductal channel. Because, as previously mentioned, the pressure in the branch of the pulmonary artery is much higher than the aortic pressure, about 90% of the right ventricular output passes (right-to-left) through the ductus arteriosus into the aorta where it joins blood from the left ventricle (see below).

## *Fetal Oxygen Tension and Cardiac Output*

The fetal arterial blood oxygen tension is lower than the neonatal or adult oxygen tension (24,25). Umbilical venous blood has an oxygen tension of about 30 to 35 mm Hg. The oxygen tension of the inferior vena caval blood entering the heart after mixing with portal venous and inferior vena caval blood is about 26 to 28 mm Hg. This decreases slightly, due to admixture, to 23 to 25 mm Hg in the ascending aorta. Therefore, the brain and coronaries are supplied with the most oxygenated blood via the ascending aorta. Venous blood returning from the superior vena cavae has an oxygen tension of about 12 to 14 mm Hg. When this mixes with inferior vena caval blood, the oxygen tension of right ventricular and pulmonary arterial blood is about 18 to 19 mm Hg before flowing into the descending aorta.

It has already been mentioned that during fetal life the two ventricles work in parallel. Although measurements

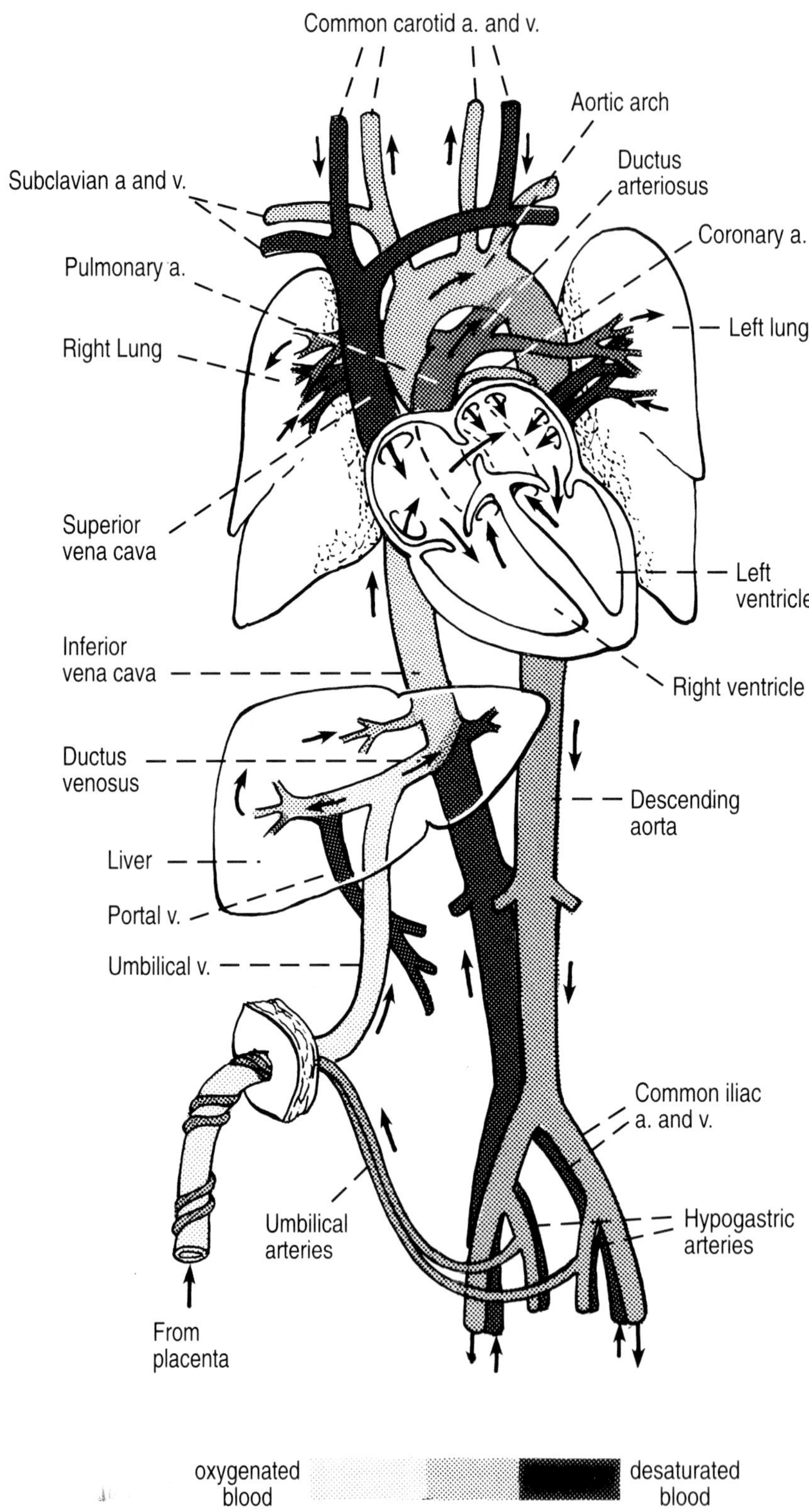


**Fig. 7–4.** The directional flow of venous and arterial systems from and to the placenta; specific oriented intracardiac patterns are shown. (Courtesy of Ross Laboratories.)

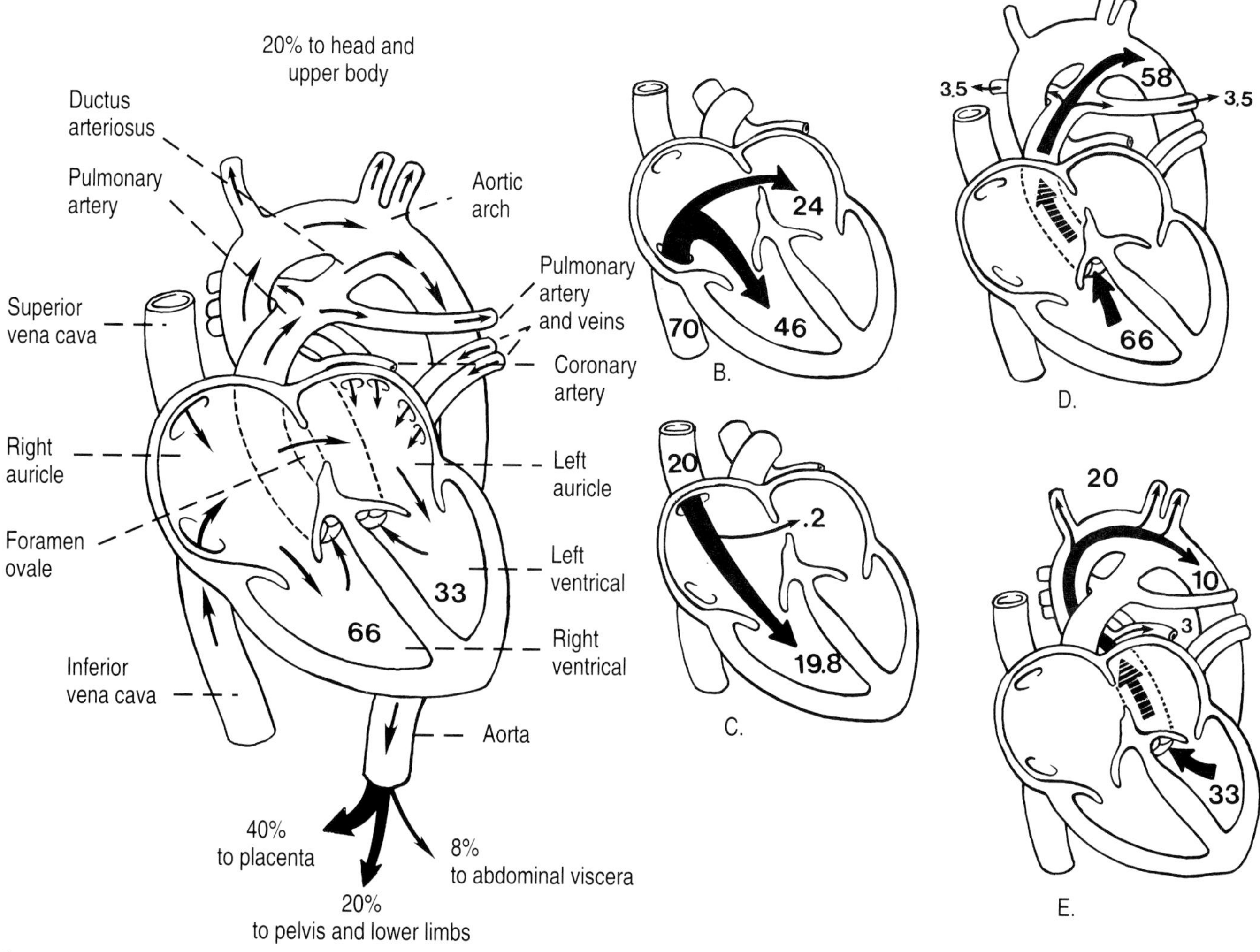


**Fig. 7–5.** The percentage return of blood from inflow and outflow patterns on directional orientation.

of blood flow have not been done in humans, echographic studies have suggested that circulatory changes in the human are similar to those described in the lamb (28) (Figure 7–5). The combined ventricular output (CVO) during the last half of gestation is 450 to 500 ml/kg fetal body weight per minute (29). Of this amount, about 70% returns to the heart via the inferior vena cava, 20% via the superior vena cava, 3% from pulmonary veins, and 3% from coronary veins. With the circulation in parallel, the right ventricle serves and develops as a systemically dominant ventricle. Of the 70% of the cardiac output (CO) that returns to the heart via the inferior vena cava, about one-third (24% of CO) passes through the foramen ovale to the left atrium and thence to the left ventricle, while the other two-thirds (46% of CO) pass to the right atrium and right ventricle (Figure 7–5B). Of the 20% of the CO returning to the heart via the superior vena cava, virtually all is directed toward the tricuspid valve, and in normal fetuses an insignificant volume of superior vena caval blood passes through the foramen ovale (Figures 7–5A and 7–5C). Thus, the right ventricle receives and ejects about 66% of CO, of which 58% is ejected into the pulmonary trunk and thence through the ductus arteriosus to the descending aorta, and 7% is distributed to the pulmonary circulation (Figure 7–5D). In addition to the blood that passes into the left atrium via the foramen ovale (26% of CO), it also receives 7% from the lungs so that the left ventricle receives and ejects about 34% of CO (Figure 7–5D). Of this amount, about 3% enters the coronary arteries, about 20% supplies the head, brain, neck, and upper body and arms, while the remaining 10% is ejected by the left ventricle into the descending aorta (Figure 7–5E).

Cardiovascular output as determined by fetal echographic studies demonstrates that about 40% supplies the placenta, 20% supplies the head, brain, and neck, upper body and arms (including the brain, which receives about 4%), 3 to 5% supplies the myocardium, 7 to 8% supplies the lungs, 5 to 6% supplies the gastrointestinal tract, 2 to 3% the kidneys, while the remainder supplies the rest of the lower part of the body. Blood flow to the human brain appears to be a larger proportion of cardiac output than

**Table 7–1.** Cardiac Rate of Fetus and Newborn

| | Fetus | | | Newly Born (Minutes after Birth) | | | Newborn (Days after Birth) | | | |
|---|---|---|---|---|---|---|---|---|---|---|
| **Rate at:** | **20 Weeks** | **30 Weeks** | **40 Weeks** | **Birth** | **10 Min.** | **60 Min.** | **1** | **2** | **4** | **6** |
| Mean | 160 | 150 | 140 | 170 | 160 | 140 | 112 | 114 | 116 | 120 |
| Range | 150–200 | 140–180 | 130–160 | 130–200 | 130–180 | 120–160 | 95–130 | 90–140 | 100–134 | 100–140 |

in animals. Although the data are limited, cerebral blood flow in previable human fetuses as measured by radionuclide-labeled microspheres may be as high as 31% of the combined ventricular output (30). Additionally, in infants from 29 to 38 weeks gestation, cerebral blood flow measurements made by venous occlusion plethysmography were similar to measurements of adult cerebral flow (31).

### *Fetal Myocardial Function*

Although cardiac output is determined by preload (ventricular filling) and afterload (the resistance to ventricular ejection), myocardial contractility (inotropic capacity of the heart muscle) and heart rate are contributing factors (32). Fetal myocardial studies demonstrate immaturity of myocardial sympathetic innervation, as well as immature structure and myocardial performance (33,34). Fetal muscle cells are smaller than the adult and contain approximately 50% less myofibrils. This immaturity results in a myocardium that normally functions at the top of its cardiac performance curve. Development of myocardial sympathetic innervation is incomplete and fetal cardiac tissue is more sensitive to the inotropic effects of norepinephrine due to a lower response threshold (35).

### *Control of the Fetal Cardiovascular System*

The cardiovascular system appears to be controlled by a complex interaction of local and reflex vascular responses, the central and autonomic nervous system, and hormonal influences (35,36). Blood flow to the fetus over a wide range of perfusion pressures is maintained by autoregulation. Although local responses to changes in oxygen content are not found for all fetal organs, autoregulation is in effect in the fetal brain, heart, and adrenal gland where blood flow increases in response to a fall in oxygen content (37,38). Umbilical placental circulation does not display autoregulation, and changes in blood flow can affect arterial perfusion (39). Fetal baroreceptors are present but are poorly developed and may not be involved in normal cardiovascular control in utero (40). In the fetus, central and carotid chemoreceptors are less sensitive than the aortic chemoreceptors (41,42). However, abnormal aortic chemoreceptors appear to be responsible for the bradycardia and hypotension resulting from fetal exposure to hypoxia, for this response is abolished with sinoaortic denervation (43).

Fetal sympathetic innervation is not complete until term. Cholinergic innervation, as evidenced by the presence of acetyl cholinesterase, is fully developed during fetal life (44). Adrenergic receptors are present in fewer number in the fetal myocardium and response to agonist is blunted compared to the adult (45,46).

The renin-angiotensin system is important in regulating the fetal circulation and its response to hemorrhage (47,48,49). Plasma renin and circulatory angiotensin II are present in fetal plasma during early gestation. In fetal sheep moderate hemorrhage (15 to 20%) causes hypertension, increased heart rate, increased combined ventricular output, as well as increased blood flow to the lungs and myocardium. Although these changes occur, the effects of fetal stress caused by small hemorrhages on the angiotensin system are controversial. In general the response to hemorrhage is peripheral vascular constriction to maintain systemic arterial blood pressure.

## Other Aspects of the Fetal Circulation

### *Cardiac Rate*

By 20 weeks gestation, the cardiac rate is about 160 per minute, and gradually decreases to about 140 per minute at term (Table 7–1). Following birth, the heart rate declines to an average of 110 to 115, with a minimum rate of 95 and a maximum rate of 130 (50,51). This decline results from changes in cardiac output, vascular re-

**Table 7–2.** Blood Pressure of Fetus and Newborn

| | Fetus* (Months of Gestation) | | | | | Newborn** (Days after Birth) | | | | |
|---|---|---|---|---|---|---|---|---|---|---|
| | **5** | **6½** | **7** | **8** | **9** | **Birth** | **1st Hour** | **2nd Day** | **4th Day** | **10th Day** |
| Systolic | 39 | 55 | 70 | 85 | 80 | 90 | 70 | 90 | 90 | 95 |
| Diastolic | 21 | 25 | 35 | 45 | 40 | 50 | 40 | 50 | 50 | 55 |

* Recorded in the umbilical artery at premature birth by Woodbury et al.
** From James et al.
(From Woodbury et al and James, et al: J. Pediatr. 51:5, 1957.)

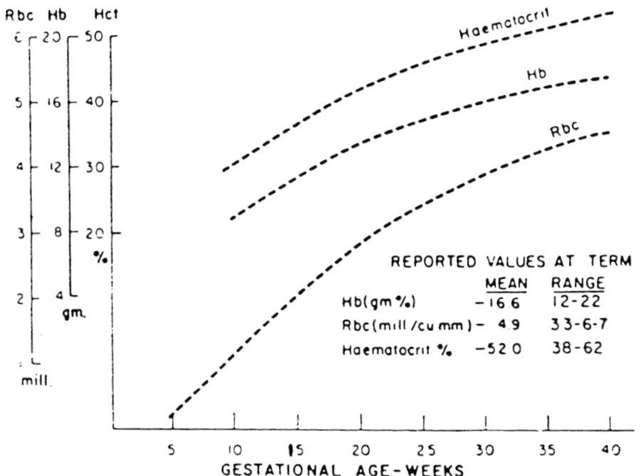


**Fig. 7–6.** Changes in hemoglobin concentration, red cell count, and hematocrit during fetal life. (From Schulman I: Characteristics of the blood in fetal life. *In* Oxygen Supply of the Human Foetus. Edited by J Walker, AC Turnbull. Philadelphia, Blackwell Scientific Publications, 1959.)

sistance, and other factors of circulatory dynamics, rather than alteration in neurogenic control (2).

## Blood Pressure

In contrast to the fetal heart rate, the fetal arterial blood pressure follows a steady increase as gestation advances (Table 7–2) (52). The difference in pressure between the umbilical arteries and umbilical vein represents the perfusion gradient that maintains fetal circulation in the placenta (53).

## Blood Volume

Total blood volume in relation to fetal weight is practically uniform throughout most of fetal life, being 8% of the combined weight of the fetus and placenta in the first half of gestation and about 10% at term (2). At the beginning of the last trimester, the blood volume is divided equally between the placenta and the fetus, while at term approximately one-fourth is in the placenta and three-fourths in the infant (54).

## Hematologic Values

There is progressive increase in erythrocyte, hemoglobin, and hematocrit values of the fetus as gestation advances and in the newborn (55,56) (Figure 7–6 and Table 7–3). The erythrocytes of the immature fetus are nucleated and much larger than those of the adult. As gestation advances, there is progressive decrease in the number and size of nucleated cells, but even at term they are still larger than those in postnatal life, so that the hemoglobin content at this time is higher than that of the adult.

Fetal hemoglobin (HbF) is similar to adult hemoglobin (HbA) in molecular weight, but differs in chemical and physical properties (57). The erythrocytes during early gestation contain only fetal-type hemoglobin, but by the fifth or sixth month, the adult form appears (58,59). Thereafter, the percentage of fetal hemoglobin gradually decreases with a corresponding increase in the percentage of adult hemoglobin. At birth, term infants have about 85% HbF, premature infants about 90%, and "postmature" infants about 65% (60,61).

## Effects of Labor on Fetal Cardiovascular Function

During early labor, when the membranes are still intact, uterine contractions lead to increased fetal blood pressure concomitant with the rise in amniotic fluid pressure, thus keeping constant the pressure gradient between the fetus and that part of his environment. During this time, there is an equivalent rise in the pressure in the intervillous space. Mild hypoxia in animals produces an increase in blood pressure that increases fetal blood flow and placental oxygen extraction leading to improved oxygenation to the fetal tissues (62,63). This compensatory mechanism is affected by an increase in cardiac rate and stroke volume, presumably mediated by the fetal autonomic nervous system and is lacking in immature fetuses before midpregnancy. The mechanism has its limit, however, for with more severe anoxia, umbilical vascular resistance rises, presumably from the effects of catecholamines released from the fetal adrenals (64,65). Eventually, a point is reached when the blood pressure and cardiac output fall, thus accentuating the hypoxia and producing deepening fetal distress (66). Similar responses probably occur in the human fetus (64,65).

## Fetal Heart Rate

Alterations in fetal heart rate occur frequently during labor. Bradycardia is the most frequent alteration of fetal heart rate (67–69). Early decelerations, a decrease in fetal heart rate (FHR) not associated with fetal compromise, produce a FHR tracing that resembles a mirror image of the contraction. They are mild in nature, never more than 20 beats/min below baseline. These heart rate changes

**Table 7–3.** Hemotologic Values of Fetus and Newborn

| | Fetus | | | | Newborn | | |
|---|---|---|---|---|---|---|---|
| | 12 Weeks | 24 Weeks | 36 Weeks | 38 Weeks | Birth | 1st Day | 7th Day |
| Weight (grams) | 15 | 600 | 2,000 | 3,000 | 3,200 | 32,000 | 3,200 |
| Erythrocytes (RBC) in millions | 1.5 | 3.5 | 4.4 | 5 | 5.0 | 5.0 | 4.0 |
| Hematocrit (Ht) | 25 | 43 | 48 | 50 | 52 | 53.5 | 43 |
| Hemoglobin (Hb) grams/100 ml. | 8 | 13 | 15 | 15.5 | 16.5 | 17.0 | 15.0 |

Developed from data of Walker and Turnbull and Wintrobe and Schumacher.
(Walker and Turnbull: Lancet 2:312, 1953; Arch. Dis. Child. 30:111, 1955; Wintrob and Schumacher: Am. J. Anat. 58:313, 1936.)

are due to vagal reflexive responses to mild hypoxia and can be reproduced by fetal head compression. Late decelerations, also a mirror image of contractions, differ from early deceleration in that their onset, peak, and recovery are delayed 10 to 30 seconds after the onset, peak, and termination of the contraction. Late decelerations can result from maternal hypotension or may result from fetal myocardial hypoxia. The latter is associated with prolonged asphyxia and is associated with loss of fetal heart rate variability. Variable decelerations differ in conformation from contraction to contraction, and can occur in response to umbilical cord compression or head compression. Some of these episodes occur frequently during normal labor. The rapidity of onset, magnitude, and duration of bradycardia and its relation to the uterine contraction and to the phase of labor may vary considerably.

Occasionally, uterine contractions are associated with fetal heart rate accelerations. Transient tachycardia may be associated with a loose cord around the neck or trunk. Sustained tachycardia suggests fetal distress or may be a response to maternal hyperthermia. Transient fetal cardiac arrhythmias may also occur during normal labor, but when they exist are indicative of fetal hypoxia.

## Transition From Fetal to Neonatal Circulation

Immediately following birth, major circulatory changes occur that comprise the neonatal period of cardiorespiratory adaptation (Figure 7–7) (70). With the separation of the umbilical placental unit, the lungs now assume the role of the organ of gas exchange. When umbilical-placental circulation is disrupted, inferior vena caval blood flow is decreased, reducing right atrial blood flow and pressure. Pulmonary vascular resistance falls associated with a rapid increase in pulmonary blood flow (Figure 7–8). The observed fall in pulmonary vascular resistance is due to vasodilation of the pulmonary vascular bed in response to lung expansion, increased oxygen tension, and synthesis or release of prostaglandins and other vasoactive substances such as bradykinin (46–49). Prostaglandins, the products of arachidonic acid metabolism, appear to be released with lung distension (71,72). Of the various prostaglandins, $PGI_2$ seems to be the most powerful dilator of the fetal lamb pulmonary circulation, followed by $PGE_1$ and $PGE_2$. Recently, another prostaglandin, $PGD_2$, has been shown to be a pulmonary vasodilator in perfused fetal lungs and may have a physiologic role in the production of pulmonary vascular resistance during the transitional period (73).

The increase in pulmonary blood flow and increased venous return to the left atrium raises left atrial pressure above right atrial pressure, resulting in functional closure of the foramen ovale. Closure of the ductus arteriosus in response to increased oxygen tension and decreased levels of circulating prostaglandins completes the separation of the pulmonary and systemic circulation (74–76). Postnatally, pulmonary vascular resistance continues to fall, changing the circulation from the "parallel" flow pattern of fetal life to the adult "series" flow pattern.

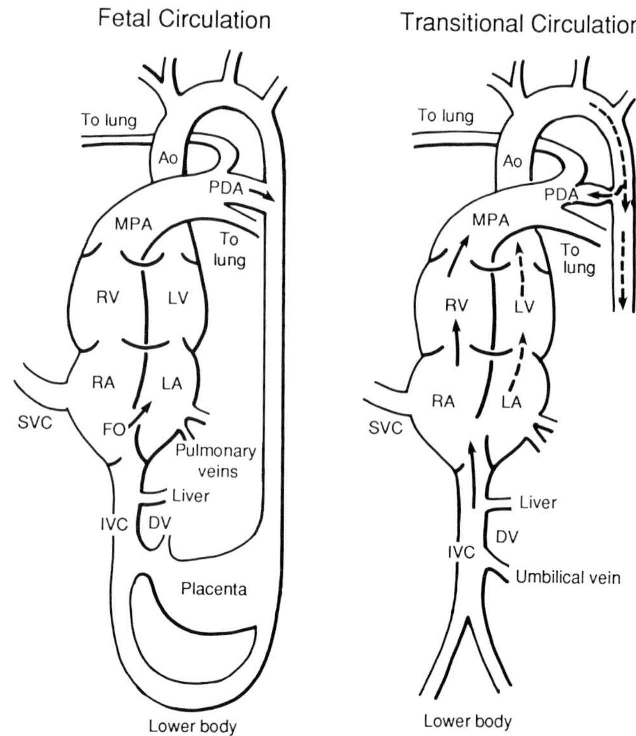


**Fig. 7–7.** Cardiovascular circulatory patterns of the fetal, transitional, and neonatal periods. During the fetal period, desaturated blood bypasses the lungs by way of the ductus arteriosus. During the transitional period, the series pattern is established with the lungs becoming the organ of oxygenation. During the neonatal period and adult life, the ductus arteriosus is closed. (PDA = patent ductus arteriosus; FO = foramen ovale; RV = right ventricle; RA = right atrium; DV = ductus venosus; LV = left ventricle; LA = left atrium; Ao = aorta; MPA = main pulmonary artery; SVC = superior vena cava; IVC = inferior vena cava.) Solid arrows indicate desaturated blood; broken arrows indicate flow of oxygenated blood. (Redrawn from Pollin RA, Burg FD: Workbook in Practical Neonatology. Philadelphia, WB Saunders Co., 1983.)

### *Closure of Fetal Shunt Pathways*

#### Ductus Arteriosus

In most full-term infants, the ductus arteriosus remains partially patent until about 15 hours of age (74). The tone and patency of the ductus arteriosus are reactive to oxygen as well as many vasoactive agents such as prostaglandins, kinins, catecholamines, and angiotensin. Persistence of the ductus arteriosus is common in the prematurely born infant who has a decreased response to a rise in $PO_2$ and has an age-dependent increase in sensitivity of the immature ductus to endogenous prostaglandins (75,76). This effect is reduced by glucocorticoids, which underlies the lower incidence of prolonged patency of the ductus in premature infants treated with steroids prenatally to accelerate lung maturation (77,78). Functional closure of the ductus arteriosus occurs between 24 and 96 hours of life, with bidirectional shunts occurring during the first few hours of life, which indicates that pulmonary vascular resistance levels are near those of the systemic circulation

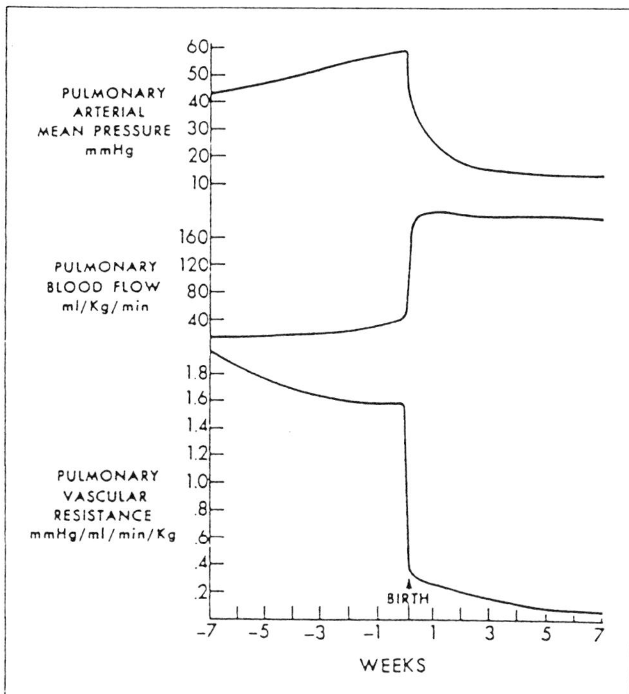


**Fig. 7–8.** The cardiovascular changes that occur during neonatal transition. Fetal pulmonary arterial pressure and vascular resistance decrease dramatically at birth and are associated with a large increase in pulmonary blood flow. (From Abraham Rudolpf Textbook of Pediatrics. 17th Ed. East Norwalk, Appleton-Century-Crofts Publishers, 1982.)

(79,80). During this early transitional neonatal period, because of the small differences between systemic and pulmonary vascular resistance, lung pathology such as sepsis, asphyxia, and meconium aspiration potentially can increase pulmonary vascular resistance, raising right atrial pressure over left atrial pressure, causing right-to-left shunting through a reopened foramen ovale and the development of persistent fetal circulation (81).

### *Foramen Ovale*

With the separation of the umbilical-placental unit and resultant increased pulmonary blood flow, the left atrial pressure rises above that of the right atrial pressure, functionally closing the foramen ovale (82). Anatomic closure of the foramen ovale generally occurs about 2 to 3 months postnatally, on average, but in some cases can be as late as the end of the first year or even later.

### *Ductus Venosus*

After birth, when the umbilical venous blood flow ceases, the portal venous and sinus pressures fall. The ductus venosus narrows and retracts from the portal sinus. With portal pressure gradually decreasing, the ductus venosus closes. Although it is functionally closed, the ductus venosus is usually patent 3 to 5 days after birth with anatomic closure occurring between 2 to 3 weeks postnatally. Closure of the ductus venosus, unlike the ductus arteriosus, is not dependent on changes in oxygen tension nor physiologic levels of catecholamines or vasoactive agents (83).

## Neonatal Cardiovascular Function

### *Cardiac Output*

After the transitional period, neonatal cardiac output represents the volume of blood ejected by each ventricle in series. While right ventricular output increases little compared to fetal cardiac output, left ventricular output increases 2- to 2.5-fold (24,70). The combined ventricular output therefore increases to 600 to 850 ml/kg/min, which represents a small rise over fetal combined ventricular output of 500 ml/kg fetal body weight/min (84).

Over the first 8 to 10 weeks after birth, the cardiac output falls rapidly to about 150 ml/kg/min whereupon it falls more slowly to the adult level of about 70 to 80 ml/kg/min (85). Oxygen consumption appears to parallel the changes that occur in cardiac output during neonatal transition (86).

### *Fetal Hemoglobin and Neonatal Oxygen Consumption*

The rapid fall in cardiac output over the first 8 weeks after neonatal transition is thought to be related to replacement of fetal hemoglobin by adult hemoglobin in circulating erythrocytes (Figure 7–9) (87). The leftward shift of the curve is advantageous during fetal life because it facilitates oxygen uptake in the placenta. However, after birth when $PaO_2$ is approximately 90 mm Hg and venous $PaO_2$ is 40 mm Hg, a rightward shift increases the amount of oxygen released to tissues allowing a smaller blood flow to provide the same amount of tissue $O_2$ delivery.

Although fetal oxygen consumption is about 7 ml/min/kg, it rises initially to 15 to 20 ml/min/kg in the newborn but falls again to 8 to 10 ml/min/kg by the eighth week of life (87). The rise in oxygen consumption during the neonatal transitional period is related to the increased metabolic and oxygen consumption needs of the newborn to maintain body temperature independently.

### *Neonatal Heart Rate and Arterial Blood Pressure*

The resting fetal heart rate of 160 to 180 beats/min decreases to 140 to 160 beats/min postnatally in the awake infant, but may vary from 90 to 120 beats/min during sleep (Table 7–1) (88). Eventually, the heart rate gradually decreases with advancing age. Systemic arterial blood pressure varies with gestational and birth weight, and postnatal age (Figure 7–10A and Figure 7–10B) (89).

### *Effects of Blood Volume on Neonatal Circulation*

### *Umbilical Vessels*

Changes in neonatal blood volume can alter the process of cardiorespiratory adaptation to extrauterine life (90–92). After placental separation, umbilical circulation stops within the first minute. In normal-term infants, blood flow through the umbilical arteries ends within 30

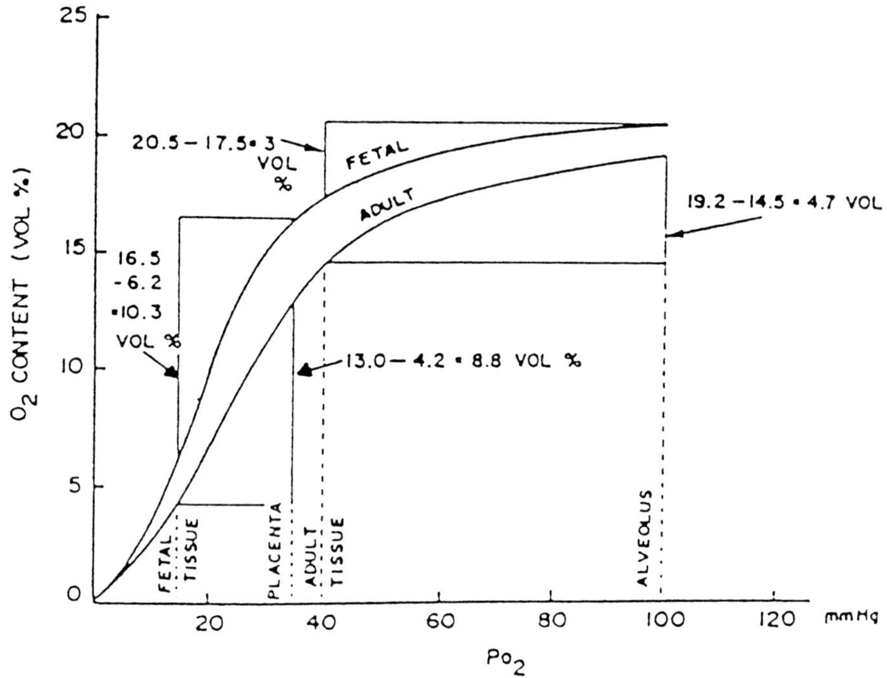


**Fig. 7–9.** Oxygen-unloading capabilities of fetal and adult hemoglobin. Each respective curve demonstrates the Hb-$O_2$ dissociation; the ordinate indicates ml $O_2$/100 ml blood. The fetal Hb-$O_2$ unloading capacity of 10.3 ml $O_2$/100 ml blood is greater than the adult Hb-$O_2$ unloading capacity of 8.8 ml $O_2$/100 ml blood at $PO_2$ in the fetal range. Conversely, $PO_2$ in the adult range, adult Hb has a greater unloading capacity then the fetus (4.7 vs 3.0 ml $O_2$/100 ml blood). (From Scarpelli EM, Moss IR: Transition from fetal to neonatal breathing in perinatal cardiovascular function. Edited by N Gootman, PM Gootman. New York, Marcel Dekker, Inc., 1983.)

seconds and umbilical vein blood gases and pH are unchanged during the first 6 to 8 minutes. Uterine contractions compress the placenta, and these contractions, which can occur after the first minute and up to 6 minutes in the term infant, produce blood flow through the umbilical vein into the infant. Placental blood flow to the infant is favored as long as the umbilical cord is left intact and the infant kept at or below the level of the placenta.

Drugs used at delivery including anesthetics, oxytocic agents, sedatives and analgesics, may either hasten or delay closure of the umbilical arteries after birth thereby affecting blood volume transfusion (90). Acetylcholine, for example, has a mildly constrictive effect on the vessels that is enhanced by oxytocin, while meperidine can dilate the vessels by depressing the intense vasoconstrictive effect of 5-hydroxytryptamine.

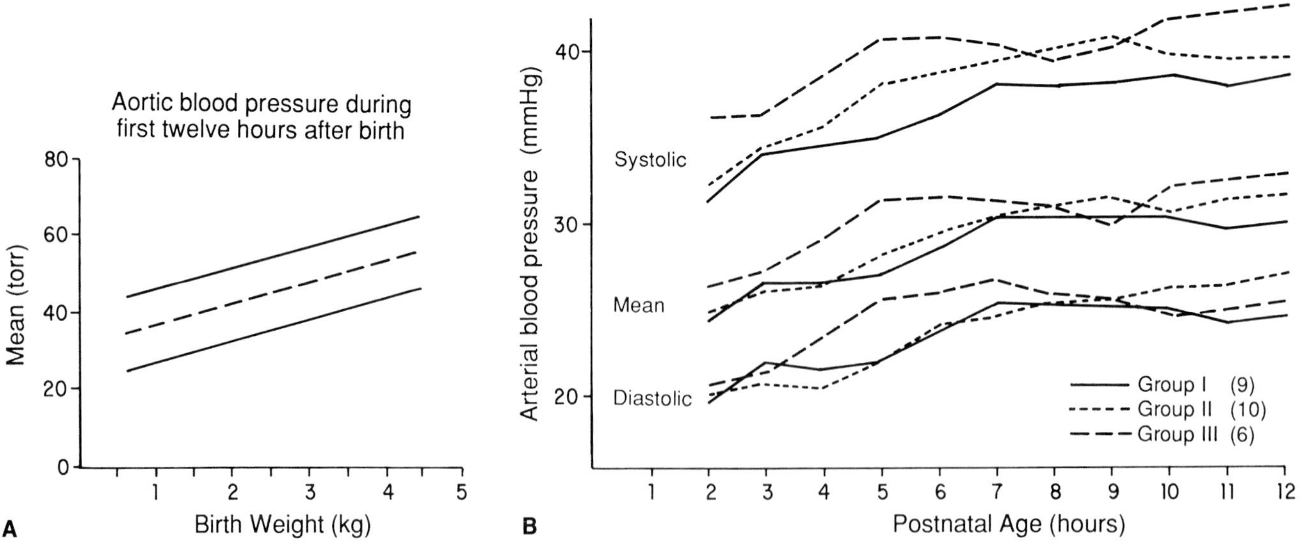


**Fig. 7–10.** **A,** Mean arterial blood pressure obtained from umbilical artery catheter measurements at varying birth weights during the first 12 hours of postnatal life. Dotted lines indicate the average mean; solid lines indicate the highest and lowest corresponding arterial pressures at 95% confidence intervals. (Redrawn from Avery G: Neonatology Pathophysiology and Management of the Newborn. 3rd Ed. Philadelphia, JB Lippincott Co. 1987.) **B,** Systolic, mean, and diastolic arterial blood pressures of very low birth weight infants from birth to 12 hours of postnatal age. (Redrawn from Moscoso P, Goldberg R, Jamieson J, Bancalari E: Spontaneous elevation in arterial blood pressure during the first hours of life in the very-low-birth-weight infant. J. Pediatr. 103:114, 1983.)

### Effects of Placental Transfusion on Neonatal Circulation

A full placental transfusion occurring with late cord clamping (greater than 3 minutes) can increase the circulating blood volume of the term infant from 65 to 70 ml/kg body weight to 110 to 120 ml/kg body weight (91). During cesarean section blood drainage from the infant to the placenta is especially favored, potentially placing these infants at risk of hypovolemia when cord clamping is delayed (Figure 7–11) (92–94).

Small-for-gestational-age (SGA) infants generally have an increased hematocrit due to enhanced erythropoiesis regardless of cord clamping time. Premature infants receive placental transfusions at a slower rate than term infants receiving a full transfusion in 5 minutes (95). The consequences of a high initial blood volume due to late cord clamping are the development of hemoconcentration. Infants normally contract their blood volume rapidly to about 100 ml/kg at 30 min and 80 to 90 ml/kg at 4 hours postnatally (96). With additional blood volume the development of hyperviscosity could potentially increase right and left ventricular afterload adding to myocardial work load. Furthermore, a full placental transfusion may be associated with a prolonged period of pulmonary hypertension associated with lower lung compliance and functional residual capacity (FRC) due to pooling of blood and plasma fluid extravasation in the lungs (97).

## Abnormalities of the Cardiovascular System

### Fetal Myocardial Response to Loading

The fetal heart has a limited ability to increase stroke volume in response to an increased volume load by a rapid intravenous infusion or in response to increased outflow resistance. The myocardium does improve its performance with increasing gestation presumably due to the increased sympathetic innervation.

Because of the cardiovascular and myocardial characteristics during fetal development, volume loading may adversely affect cardiac output. The fetal myocardium has a limited ability to increase stroke volume or cardiac output depending on gestational age. After birth, however, cardiovascular output can increase in response to volume loading by 35% during the first week and by 65% by 6 to 8 weeks of postnatal age (98).

### Cardiovascular Response to Stress

Hypoxic insults that occur during fetal development are associated with increasing cardiac output and heart

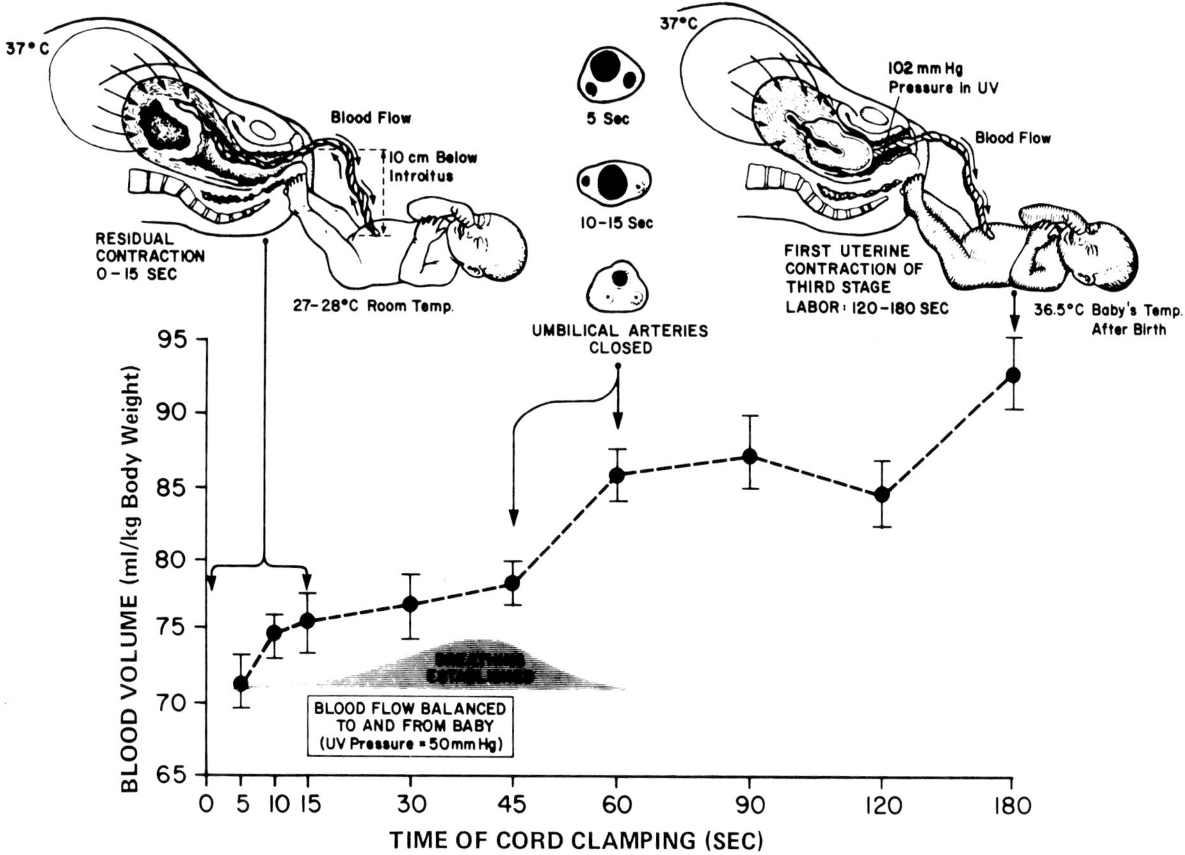


**Fig. 7–11.** Effect of delayed cord clamping on neonatal blood volume. The mean full–term neonatal blood volume at 30 minutes of age plotted against the time of cord clamping after birth indicating a stepwise transfer of blood to the infant occurring at 10, 60, and 180 seconds after cord sampling. (From Gootman N, Gootman PM: Perinatal Cardiovascular Function. New York, Marcel Dekker, Inc., 1983.)

rate due to chemoreceptor or autonomic activity that tends to preserve brain blood flow (99,100). During fetal hypoxemia the major circulatory changes are a redistribution of fetal cardiac output. Umbilical-placental blood flow is maintained but flow to the fetal body falls. During this time, blood flow to the fetal myocardium, cerebrum, and adrenals increases while blood flow to the gut, spleen, kidney, skin, muscle, and bone falls (62). The overall effect is the maintenance of blood flow and oxygen delivery to the heart and brain, as well as maintenance of systemic arterial blood pressure for placental perfusion. This fetal response to hypoxia is dependent on gestational age.

When the organ of gas exchange, the placenta or the lungs, fails, fetal or neonatal asphyxia occurs. Tissues continue to consume oxygen leading to tissue hypoxia and the need for anaerobic metabolism. When blood flow to some tissues is reduced, acidemic blood can be pooled in the vasculature of some tissues rather than returning to the central circulation, and arterial blood gas values may fail to reflect the full extent of the asphyxia.

Normal labor itself is associated with a transient hypoxemia that occurs with uterine contractions. However, healthy infants can withstand this mild hypoxemia. Additional episodes of asphyxia can occur when umbilical blood flow is interrupted by cord compression, when there is failure of placental exchange due to placental separation and abruption, or when there is inadequate maternal perfusion.

Although mild asphyxia associated with normal labor and delivery reverses spontaneously, severe asphyxia may be lethal and spontaneous reversal is unlikely because of irreversible circulatory and neurologic changes (101). Perfusion of vital organs during asphyxia is maintained by redistribution of blood flow as a result of regional vasoconstriction in less vital tissues such as the gut, kidneys, muscle, and skin (102). Total body oxygen consumption decreases and blood flow to vital organs including brain, myocardium, and adrenals is maintained or increased to deliver adequate oxygen even though arterial blood oxygen content is reduced (103). The newborn respiratory center responds to asphyxia with increased respiratory rate and gasping. If asphyxia becomes more severe, the respiratory center may be suppressed and spontaneous ventilation decrease (104). As myocardial glycogen stores for energy are exhausted, the myocardium is exposed to low oxygen and acidosis leading to myocardial failure and additional decreased blood flow to organs (105). Endocrine responses to asphyxia include elevations in plasma concentrations of catecholamines, renin, vasopressin, and glucocorticoids (106–108).

### *Persistent Fetal Circulation*

During the early neonatal transitional period hypoxia and acidosis from any cause may produce increased pulmonary vascular resistance with accompanying decreased pulmonary blood flow. The fetal pattern of circulation with right-to-left shunting through the ductus arteriosus and foramen ovale is reestablished causing persistence of the fetal circulation or persistent pulmonary hypertension (PPHN) (109). Without a functioning placenta this leads to progressive acidosis and hypoxia with increasing pulmonary vasoconstriction and a fatal condition unless pulmonary vasoconstriction is reversed. Therapy of this disorder has included a combination of hyperventilation and pharmacotherapy aimed at producing pulmonary vasodilatation and improved pulmonary blood flow. Hyperventilation produces respiratory alkalosis that has been associated with pulmonary vasodilation (110). No specific pulmonary vasodilator drugs have currently been used successfully with infants with PPHN. Tolazoline (priscoline), an alpha adrenergic antagonist with a histamine-like action, has been used to treat this disorder but results in both systemic as well as pulmonary vasodilation. Results with tolazoline are variable but must still be considered unproven. Drugs such as prostaglandins $D_2$ and $E_1$ aimed at selectively dilating the pulmonary circulation are being investigated (73,111). Supportive care for these infants also includes maintenance of systemic circulation by volume expansion and/or inotropic agents, such as dopamine.

### *Persistent Patent Ductus Arteriosus*

Delayed closure or persistence of ductus arteriosus occurs frequently in disorders associated with hypoxemia such as neonatal respiratory distress, prematurity, and infants born at high altitude. Ductal closure is dependent on oxygen content, and prostaglandin levels and constriction can be reversed potentially by decreased oxygen content. Premature infants with respiratory distress syndrome are known to have delayed ductal closure presumably due to immaturity of the muscle tissue's response to oxygen (112,113). Studies using isolated ductal tissue and studies of the fetal lamb indicate that prostaglandins play a central role in maintaining fetal ductal relaxation and patency. Indomethacin and inhibitors of prostaglandin synthesis have been used successfully for ductal closure (113,114). Other stimuli that may cause ductal constriction include: kinins, adrenaline, noradrenalin, and angiotensin. The effect of prostaglandin on the ductus appears to be reduced by glucocorticoids and may account for the lower incidence of patent ductus in premature infants who were treated with prenatal steroids to accelerate lung maturation (77,78). Persistence of the ductus arteriosus can lead to pulmonary edema when associated with a left-to-right shunt, which occurs when pulmonary vascular resistance falls.

Factors that prevent ductal closure include hypoxemia as well as atropine and prostaglandin $E_1$ ($PGE_1$) (111). $PGE_1$ has been successfully used to dilate a closed ductus to maintain patency in congenital heart disease in which infant survival is dependent on the persistence of an open ductus.

## Maternal Drugs that May Affect the Fetal or Neonatal Cardiovascular System

Maternal aspirin intake or prostaglandin antagonist ingestion late during pregnancy can result in delivery of hydropic infants presumably from premature closure of the ductus arteriosus and development of neonatal pulmonary arterial hypertension (115). Maternal therapy of pregnancy-induced hypertension as well as treatment for preterm labor recently encompasses the use of low-dose aspirin (60 to 100 mg) or indomethacin, respectively. When used before 32 weeks gestation and in low doses, aspirin and indomethacin have not been associated with ductal closure and the development of persistent pulmonary hypertension (116,117).

Maternal anesthetic treatment may cause fetal cardiovascular depression (118). All inhalation agents, such as methoxyflurane, isoflurane, and halothane, if given in large enough concentrations, can lead to maternal cardiac depression leading to fetal compromise (119,120). Given in routine concentrations, however, these agents usually do not affect the fetal cardiovascular system. In laboring women, large or excessive dosage of local anesthetics can decrease fetal heart rate variability and produce fetal bradycardia and acidosis (121,122). Furthermore, local anesthetics inserted near the uterine artery may produce uterine vascular spasm leading to severe fetal bradycardia (123). Atropine can depress fetal heart rate, while halothane and scopolamine can lead to fetal tachycardia and lethargy. Obstetrical use of magnesium sulfate to suppress labor or treat maternal preeclampsia is associated with neonatal respiratory depression, hypotonia, intestinal ileus, and hypocalcemia because it freely crosses the placenta (124). Maternal treatment with cardiovascular agents may have a variety of effects on the fetal cardiovascular system (125,126). Aldomet may cause neonatal systolic hypotension while propranolol and nadolol are associated with neonatal bradycardia, hypoglycemia, and respiratory depression (122). Quinidine sulfate may lead to the development of infants who are thrombocytopenic, smaller for gestational age and more susceptible to asphyxia at birth (127). Maternal treatment with β-sympathomimetic agents for premature labor is based on the agents' ability to increase intracellular cAMP, which is responsible for uterine smooth muscle relaxation. Ritodrine, terbutaline, isoxsuprine, and salbutamol have been used for inhibition of premature labor (125,126). β-agonists increase heart rate, cardiac output, and pulmonary artery pressure, and lower the arterial pressure and systemic and pulmonary vascular resistances. β-sympathomimetics are known to cross the placental barrier and their concentration in fetal blood is equal to that of the mother producing similar short-term effects as those seen with maternal treatment. About 1 to 5% of pregnant women receiving intravenous β-sympathomimetic agents for inhibition of premature labor develop pulmonary edema within 24 to 36 hours after treatment. The development of maternal pulmonary edema can potentially result in neonatal asphyxia (126).

## RESPIRATORY DEVELOPMENT AND PHYSIOLOGY

### *Development of the Fetal Lung*

With the viability of infants being shifted progressively into shorter gestational ages, understanding the morphological and functional development of the respiratory system becomes very important. The survival of prematurely born infants is closely related to the maturation of their respiratory system and the possibility of gas exchange. Although development of the respiratory system follows a relatively predictable pattern, a number of circumstances may accelerate or retard the maturation process, both structural and functional. The structural development of the lung has been divided into five stages. In the first stage, the embryonic period that spans from 0 to 7 weeks, marks the beginning of the lung development from a diverticulum of the endodermal foregut that results in the formation of the first 20 to 24 branches of the airways. By the seventh week there are rudimentary bronchopulmonary segments and the left and right pulmonary arteries have formed plexuses. Interaction with the intrathoracic mesenchyme give rise to the pulmonary interstitium, smooth muscle, blood vessels, and cartilage. The next stage is the pseudoglandular, from 8 to 16 weeks, and is characterized by rapid proliferation and branching of the airways (128,129). This is followed by the canalicular stage from 17 to 27 weeks, characterized by the appearance of vascular channels that approximate the potential air spaces (130,131). It is only in this stage that effective gas exchange becomes possible. This is also the time when surfactant appears and provides stability to the air spaces. Acinar units are formed during this period and there is also thinning of the extracellular matrix. By 20 to 22 weeks Type I and Type II epithelial cells can be identified. The sacular stage follows, between the 28 to 35 weeks of gestation. In this stage, most of the peripheral air spaces are formed with further thinning of the interstitial spaces. Septation of air spaces with small capillaries divides the saccules increasing the gas exchange surface area. The final alveolar stage, from 36 weeks to term, is characterized by the rapid increase in the number of alveoli, thinning of septal walls, and attenuation of cuboidal epithelium. Type I and II cells are well-differentiated. This process of alveolarization continues after birth and 80 to 85% of the adult 300 million alveoli will form during the first 2 years of life and continue to later childhood (132–135).

### *Fetal Breathing Movements*

It is well-established that the fetus has breathing movements from early in pregnancy (136–143). These movements do not play a functional role in gas exchange but may be important for the growth and development of the fetal respiratory system. Fetal breathing occurs intermittently and mainly during low voltage electrocortical activity. It is usually irregular and generates a negative tracheal pressure of 2 to 5 mm Hg. The fetus is capable of responding with increased breathing activity to increased $PaCO_2$ (140,144) and $PaO_2$ (145). Hypoxia, on the other hand, decreases fetal breathing activity (140,146). Pharmacologic agents such as morphine and indomethacin induce continuous fetal breathing movements probably through central stimulation (147–149).

### *Fetal Gas Exchange*

The oxygenation of fetal blood in the placenta is accomplished by passive diffusion of oxygen from maternal to the fetal blood stream across the placental membrane. The rate of diffusion depends on the gradient of gas tensions between the two circulations, the diffusibility of the membrane, and the type of vascularization of the placenta (150).

The type of vascular geometry in the human placenta has not been clearly defined. The fact that gas exchange occurs between two circulatory systems has some advantages in that the Bohr and Haldane effects work simultaneously but in opposite directions on both sides of the placenta, facilitating gas exchange. As the fetal blood approaches the capillaries in the intervillous spaces and $CO_2$ diffuses from fetal to the maternal side, the resultant increase in fetal blood pH increases oxygen affinity of the fetal hemoglobin. The opposite occurs in the maternal side facilitating the release of oxygen from the maternal to the fetal blood (Bohr effect) (Figure 7–12A). At the same time, the increased oxygen content of the fetal hemoglobin decreases its affinity for $CO_2$ facilitating the diffusion of $CO_2$ into the maternal circulation and the opposite occurs on the maternal side (Haldane effect) (Figure 7–12B) (151). The oxygenated blood returning from the placenta into the fetus through the umbilical vein has a $PO_2$ of approximately 30 to 35 mm Hg that is lower than the maternal venous $PO_2$ (152,153). This gradient between maternal and fetal $PO_2$ results from arteriovenous connections in both the uterine and the umbilical circulations, from the oxygen consumption of the placenta, from the actual gas tension gradient across the placental membrane, and more importantly from inhomogeneities of blood flow in the fetal and maternal sides of the placenta (154–157).

Reduction in blood flow in either the maternal or fetal side of the placenta may result in a reduction in gas exchange and fetal hypoxia. The same occurs with inflammation or edema of the placenta that results in an impairment of gas diffusion.

Despite the relatively low oxygen tension in the fetal blood there is no evidence that under normal conditions the fetus is under hypoxic conditions. This is mainly due to the relatively low oxygen consumption of the fetus, the distribution of the blood flow with preferential flow of the more oxygenated blood to brain and heart, and to the higher oxygen affinity of the fetal hemoglobin.

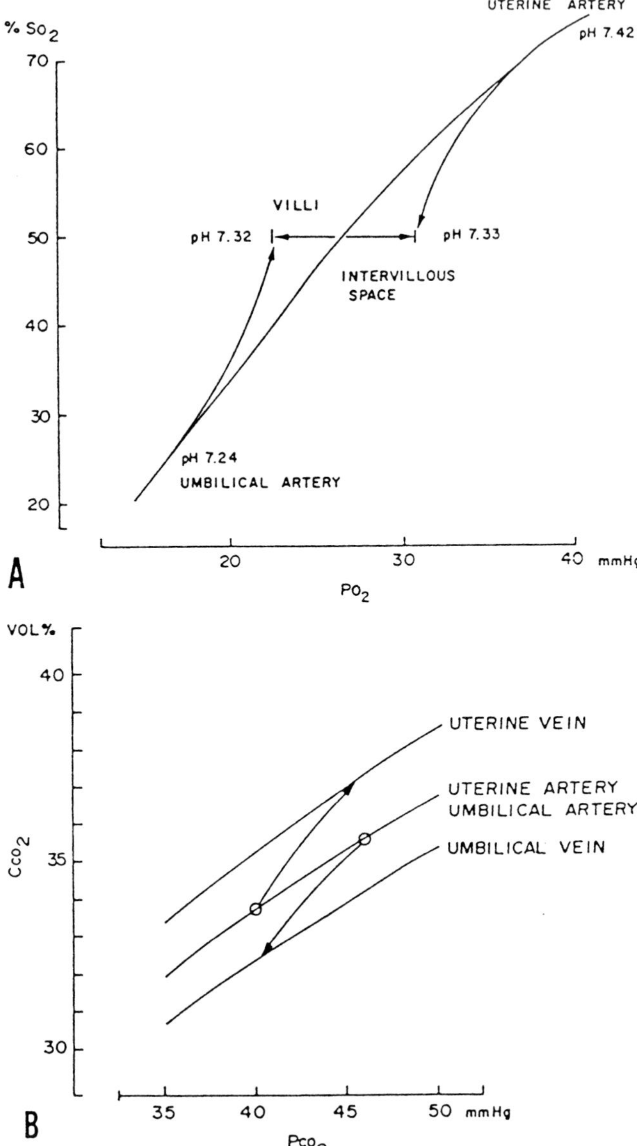


**Fig. 7–12. A,** Bohr effect in the placenta. As maternal blood flows into the placenta and gains $CO_2$, its pH decreases shifting the oxygen dissociation curve to the right and releasing more oxygen at a gastrointestinalven $PO_2$. The opposite occurs with the fetal blood. **B,** Haldane effect in the placenta. As fetal blood gains oxygen in the placenta its capacity to carry $CO_2$ decreases. The reverse is true for maternal blood flowing into the placenta. (From Smith and Nelson. The Physiology of the Newborn Infant. 4th Ed. Springfield, IL. Charles C. Thomas, 1976.)

## *Effects of Labor on Oxygenation and Acid Base Status*

During labor, the uterine contractions frequently interfere with placental gas exchange, resulting in variable decreases in fetal $PO_2$ and also increase in $PCO_2$ (158–161). This effect is due to a decrease in uterine and placental blood flow and in some situations can also be related to compression of the umbilical cord and reduction of umbilical blood flow. These changes in fetal oxygenation are frequently associated with variations in fetal heart rate that also decrease during uterine contractions. The decrease in uterine oxygen uptake is more significant during contractions induced by oxytocin, and after the contractions oxygen uptake increases above baseline for a short period of time (161). Animal work has demonstrated that the fetus has a large reserve in terms of oxygen availability. Fetal $O_2$ uptake did not change significantly until uterine blood flow was reduced to approximately 50% of control by arterial embolization (162).

Fetal acid base balance can also be influenced by several actors during labor. As mentioned before, during uterine contractions, there may be an increase in fetal $PCO_2$ that produces an acute reduction in pH. This change reverses rapidly after the contraction ceases and gas exchange is restored. Prolonged fetal hypoxemia, when sufficiently severe to produce tissue hypoxia, leads to anaerobic metabolism with increased lactic acid production and metabolic

**Table 7–4.** Effects of Labor on Oxygenation and Acid-Base Status of Fetus and Newborn

| | First Stage Cervical Dilation (cm.) | | | Second Stage | | After Birth | |
|---|---|---|---|---|---|---|---|
| | 1–3 | 6–8 | 10–12 | Early | Late | Umbilical Vein | Umbilical Artery |
| Oxygen saturation (%) | | | | | | | |
| a. mean | 42.3 | 35.9 | 36.1 | 34.9 | 30.4 | 50.3 | 20.2 |
| b. range | (23–62) | (18–54) | (14–59) | (12–58) | (12–49) | (17–83) | (0–45) |
| Carbon dioxide tension (mm Hg) | | | | | | | |
| a. mean | 44.5 | 45.3 | 49.1 | 48.8 | 51.1 | 43.4 | 56.8 |
| b. range | (27–62) | (28–63) | (30–68) | (35–63) | (30–72) | (30–57) | (33–80) |
| pH | | | | | | | |
| a. mean | 7.31 | 7.33 | 7.31 | 7.30 | 7.28 | 7.30 | 7.25 |
| b. range | (7.23–7.40) | (7.19–7.46) | (7.21–7.42) | (7.21–7.40) | (7.14–7.42) | (7.15–7.45) | (7.09–7.40) |
| Buffer base (mEq/L) | | | | | | | |
| a. mean | 41.16 | 42.42 | 40.96 | 30.84 | 36.96 | 37.23 | |
| b. range | (35.3–47.0) | (34.1–50.7) | (35.4–46.5) | (34.4–45.3) | (32.4–41.5) | (30.8–43.7) | |
| Standard bicarbonate (mEq/L) | | | | | | | |
| a. mean | 18.92 | 20.27 | 18.90 | 18.01 | 16.48 | 16.62 | |
| b. range | (15–22.9) | (14.2–26.4) | (16–21.8) | (15.6–20.4) | (13.1–19.8) | (11.8–21.4) | |
| Base excess (mEq/L) | | | | | | | |
| a. mean | 5.63 | 4.19 | 5.65 | 6.92 | 10.13 | 9.54 | |
| b. range | (−11.4 to +0.1) | (−12.2 to +3.8) | (−11.4 to +0.1) | (−12.8 to −1.1) | (−17.28 to −2.4) | (−16.6 to −2.5) | |

Effects of labor on oxygenation and acid-base status of fetus and newborn. (From Saling and Schneider: Z. Geburtsh. Gynak. 161:262, 1963; J. Obstet. Gynaec. Br. Commw. 74:799, 1967.)

acidemia. This has been the base for the use of scalp blood pH measurements as an indirect way of evaluating fetal oxygenation (163–166). Even during normal labor there is a gradual decrease in buffer base3 and pH (163) (Table 7–4 and Figure 7–13).

Because scalp blood sampling only provides information for the particular instant in which the sample is obtained, a number of investigators have described different methods to measure pH, $PCO_2$, and $PO_2$ continuously in the fetal scalp. These methods include pH and $PO_2$ electrodes (167–169) and mass spectrometry (159). Although these methods have great potential for early detection of problems in fetal gas exchange, they have not yet been sufficiently developed to gain widespread clinical application.

It has been long debated whether administration of oxygen to the mother is beneficial to the fetus or not. Most evidence, both in animals and humans, suggests that an increase in maternal $PaO_2$ results in a small but significant increase in umbilical venous $PO_2$ and fetal arterial $PO_2$ (169–174). Even when the increase in $PO_2$ may be only a few mm Hg, this increase can have a striking effect on blood $O_2$ saturation and content and improve tissue oxygenation because at the low fetal $PO_2$ levels the hemoglobin oxygen dissociation curve is very steep.

## Initiation of Regular Breathing after Birth

As discussed before, the fetus has rhythmic respiratory activity in utero, but this is not constant. After delivery, this pattern of intermittent breathing movements must change to an uninterrupted breathing pattern to assure normal gas exchange in the lungs. The exact mechanism that determines this change from fetal to neonatal respiration is not fully understood but a number of factors seem to play a role. The sudden changes in physical environment, with changes in temperature, sound, and tactile stimulation are all known to stimulate the respiratory center. The increase in $PCO_2$ and decrease in pH that occurs during labor may also stimulate breathing. During the minutes that follow birth, a number of dramatic circulatory changes occur and under normal conditions the arterial $PO_2$ increases from fetal levels to values above 50 to 70 mm Hg during the first hour. This increase in arterial oxygen tension may also contribute to the establishment of regular breathing because low $PaO_2$ in the fetus and neonate is a strong respiratory depressant (175,176).

### *The First Breath and the Establishment of a Functional Residual Capacity*

During the passage through the birth canal, the chest is significantly compressed to a lower volume (Figure 7–14). When the head is delivered, the airway is exposed to a lower pressure and this determines the flow of lung fluid out of the airways. When the trunk is delivered, there is some expansion due to elastic recoil that produces the passive inspiration of the tidal volume (177–180). Nevertheless, most of the gas inspired during the first breath is moved by the active contraction of the respiratory muscles. Karlberg, et al (179,180) measured tidal volume and esophageal pressure change during the first breath in normal neonates and found that the change in volume followed a decrease in esophageal pressure (Figure 7–15). They recorded negative esophageal pressures that ranged from 30 to 100 cm $H_2O$ and tidal volumes between 35

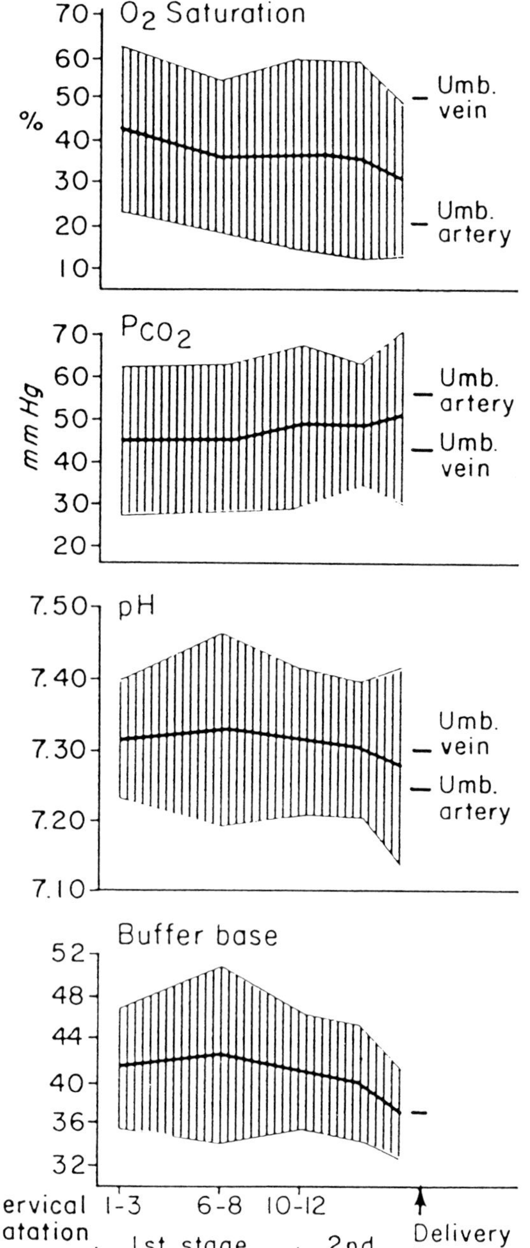


**Fig. 7–13.** Oxygen saturation, carbon dioxide tension, pH, and buffer base of arterial blood in the cephalic circulation of the fetus during labor. (From Saling E: Z. Gerburtsh. Gynaek. 161:262, 1963.)

to 45 ml, both several times higher than the values observed later during normal breathing. During expiration they also recorded large positive pressure swings, but in spite of this, the exhaled volume was smaller and a substantial amount of the inspired volume was retained in the lungs at the end of the first expiration (Figure 7–16). This contributes to the rapid establishment of the functional residual capacity.

The large negative intrathoracic pressure during the first breaths is required mainly to overcome the elastic recoil of the lung tissue and the frictional resistance to the movement of fluid and air through the airways. As air starts filling the air spaces, surface tension forces also become an important factor that opposes lung expansion, especially in the immature infant with insufficient surfactant.

The expiration that follows the first inspiration is prolonged by active closure of the upper airway and is often accompanied by active expiration that results in positive airway and intrathoracic pressures (see Figure 7–16) (180–183). This may favor reabsorption of lung fluid and can improve the distribution of the inspired gas promoting a more even lung expansion.

After the first expiration, a volume of 11 to 19 ml of gas remains in the lungs and this initiates the establishment of FRC (Figure 7–17)(180–184). The amount of gas that remains at the end of each expiration is mainly determined by the elastic recoil of the chest wall and the lung, each acting in opposite directions, and also by the duration of the expiration and the time constant of the respiratory system. Increased surface tension in the alveolar surface decreases alveolar stability at low lung volumes and therefore the presence of surfactant to lower surface tension in the alveolar surface is an important factor for the establishment of a normal FRC (185). Insufficient synthesis of surfactant in the preterm infant results in Respiratory Distress Syndrome, one of the major causes of respiratory failure in the neonatal period. This condition is characterized by alveolar collapse and inability to establish or maintain a normal FRC (186–188). The capacity to produce surfactant is primarily related to the gestational age of the infant and under normal circumstances becomes sufficient between the 30 to 32 weeks of gestation (189).

### *Subsequent Breaths*

The changes that follow the initiation of breathing after birth are characterized by the reabsorption of the lung fluid and by the establishment of a normal FRC (Figure 7–17 and Figure 7–18). During the hours that follow birth, the respiratory rate is increased and varies between 60 to 90 breaths/min. These high rates are due to the low lung compliance observed during the first hours after birth and to the activation of irritant receptors (190–192). Partial closure of the glottis during expiration, "grunting," is characteristic of the first hours of extrauterine life and plays an important role in the establishment of the FRC. It improves the distribution of the alveolar gas and also favors the reabsorption of the lung fluid into the pulmonary circulation and lymphatics (189–195).

## *Lung Liquid Reabsorption after Birth*

In the fetus the lung is filled with fluid that is continuously secreted at the alveolar surface. Fetal lung growth depends on the balance between production and elimination of this fluid from the airways into the amniotic cavity. After birth, the rapid elimination of the lung fluid becomes essential for the establishment of pulmonary gas exchange. The secretion of fluid into the alveolar space is due to active chloride secretion at the fetal pulmonary epithelium (196). The fluid production in the fetal lamb

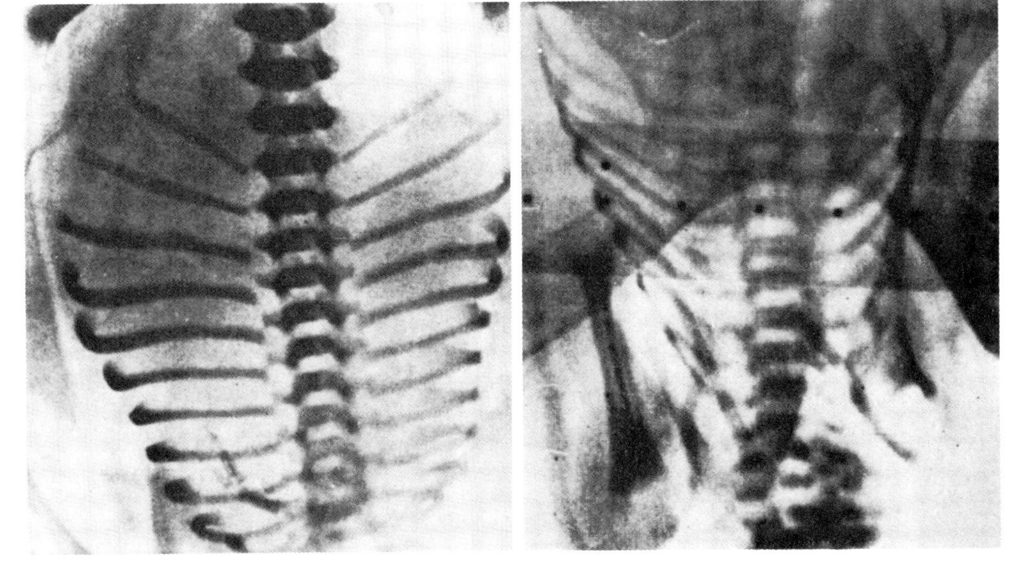


**Fig. 7–14.** Roentgenograms showing configuration of thorax of fetus taken in frontal planes. **A,** within the uterus before labor **B,** during passage through the birth canal. (From Karlberg P: P. J. Pediatr. 56:585, 1960.)

increases throughout gestation reaching approximately 5 ml/kg at term (197). Liquid secretion is influenced by hormonal changes, especially catecholamines. β-adrenergic agonists, epinephrine, and isoproterenol reduce lung water in rabbit pups and in fetal lambs (198,199). Arginine vasopressin has been shown to reduce lung liquid secretion in fetal goats (200) and infusion of prostaglandin $E^2$ reduces lung liquid in fetal lambs (201).

The reduction in fetal lung liquid that is observed in response to hypoxia is most likely related to the increase of catecholamine and prostaglandin levels that occur during the hypoxic stress. Interestingly, lung liquid production starts to decline a few days before spontaneous delivery (202,203). This may also be related to the increase in plasma epinephrine concentration observed at this time and explains the increased lung liquid that is present in animals that are delivered operatively before initiation of labor (202,204).

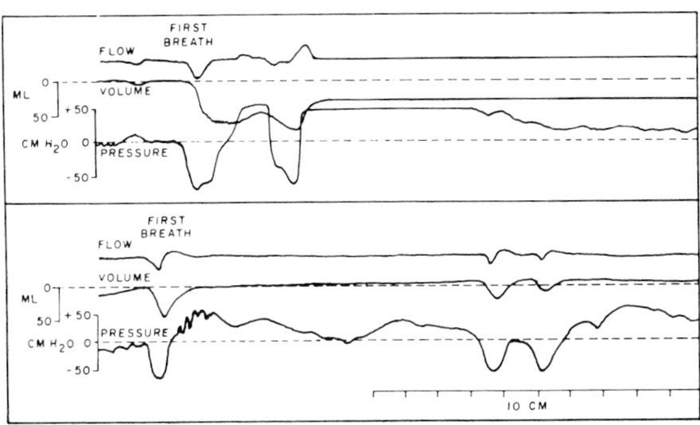


**Fig. 7–15.** Two records of simultaneously recorded volume and changes in intraesophageal pressure before, during, and after first breath. In upper tracing, there is residual volume from first breath. In lower one, there is none. (Modified from Karlberg P: P. J. Pediatr. 56:585, 1960.)

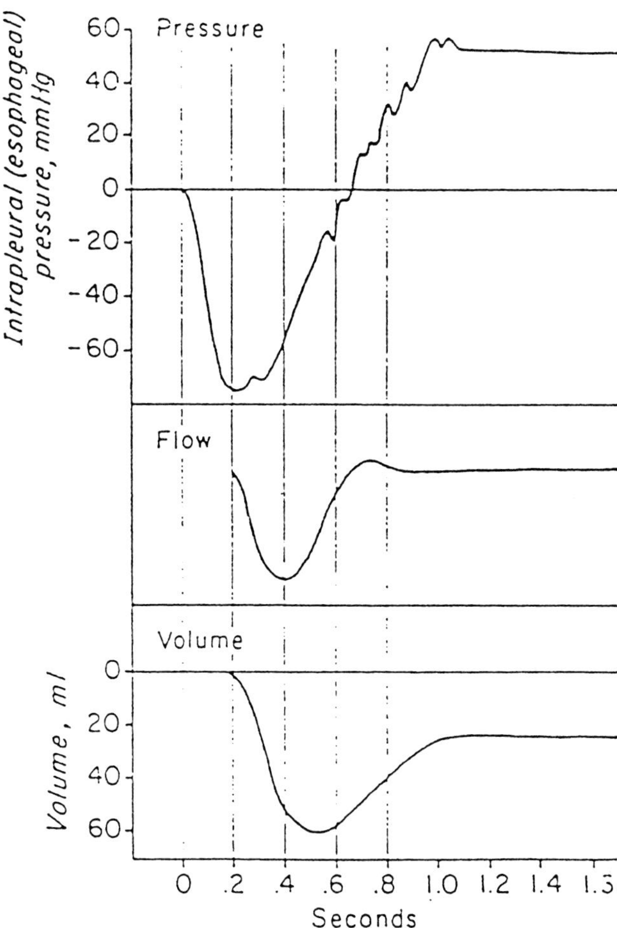


**Fig. 7–16.** Characteristics of first breath. Note time lag between negative intrathoracic pressure and flow and volume changes. Also note slow expiratory phase consisting of a series of short expiratory efforts and relatively small inspiratory efforts.

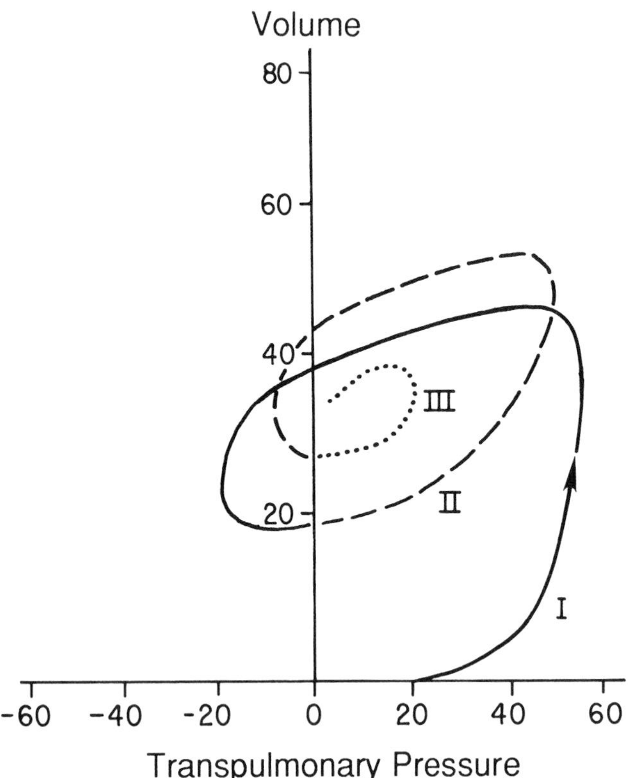


**Fig. 7–17.** The first breaths. Each successive breath requires less pressure and more residual gas remains in the lung at end of expiration. (Redrawn from Smith and Nelson. The Physiology of the Newborn Infant. 4th Ed. Springfield, IL. Charles C. Thomas, 1976.)

A prenatal increase in the concentration of plasma proteins may also facilitate the reabsorption of fluid into the pulmonary circulation. The removal of all the fluid from the air spaces after birth takes several hours. The liquid is first absorbed into the interstitial space and from this into the small blood vessels and lymphatics. The pulmonary circulation is the most important route of liquid clearance and in normal mature lambs all the fluid is absorbed by 6 hours of birth (204,205). The absorption of lung liquid into the interstitium is secondary to active sodium transport across the pulmonary epithelium. This active transport can be blocked by amiloride and this produces a delay in liquid reabsorption (206). The decrease in pulmonary vascular pressure and the increase in pulmonary blood flow also contributes to the rapid fluid reabsorption after birth.

## *Control of Breathing in the Newborn*

The exact mechanisms that explain the change from the intermittent breathing in the fetus to the continuous regular breathing after birth are not known. As mentioned earlier the increase in afferent input to the respiratory neurons generated from the multiple sensory stimulation to which the neonate is exposed after birth is one possible mechanism that explains this change. Increased sensitivity of the peripheral chemoreceptors to arterial oxygen tension may also play a role. The fetus and young neonate respond to hypoxia with a depression of respiratory activity and therefore the increase in arterial oxygen tension that occurs immediately after birth may stimulate the respiratory activity of the newborn.

Perinatal asphyxia, depressant drugs administered to the mother, fetal infection, and prematurity are conditions that may interfere with the normal initiation of breathing and may lead to neonatal apnea requiring resuscitation shortly after birth (207,208). The ventilatory response to hypoxia in the neonate is characterized by a transient hyperventilation followed by a fall in minute ventilation to levels close or even below baseline (175). This paradoxical response persists for several days after birth in the fullterm and may last weeks to months in the premature infant. The exact mechanism for this hypoxic depression is not known but it appears to be of central origin and can be mediated by an increase in concentration of depressant neuromodulators such as dopamine and adenosine (209). The ventilatory response to carbon dioxide is normal in the full-term infant but may be depressed in the premature, especially in those with apnea of prematur-

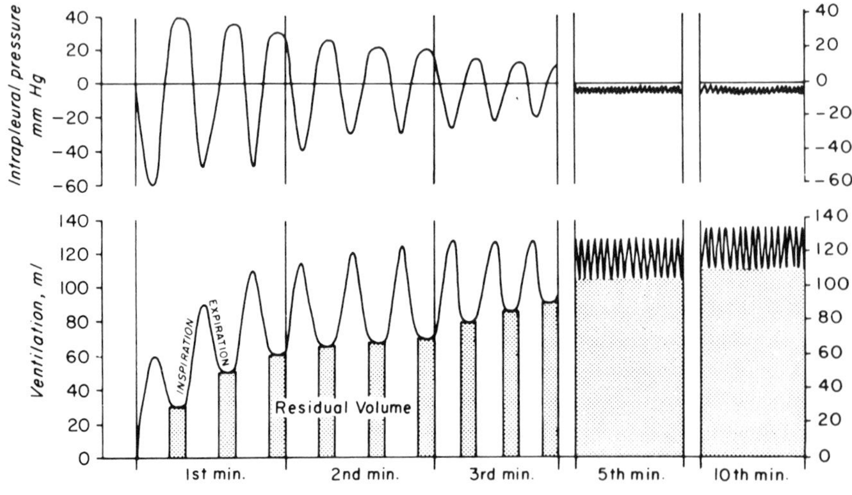


**Fig. 7–18.** Ventilation during first minutes after birth. During the first several breaths pressure changes and tidal volume are smaller, and residual volume, functional residual capacity, and lung aeration increase progressively. Thereafter a progressively smaller negative pressure is exerted and smaller volumes are respired. After a few minutes, respiration becomes quiet and the mechanics of breathing are similar to those found later in the neonatal period when pressure changes are -2 mmHg during expiration and -7 mmHg during inspiration, and tidal volume is 15 to 20 ml.

ity (210). The ventilatory response to $CO_2$ in the preterm infant is further depressed by hypoxemia (211).

### *Respiratory Reflexes*

In the neonate there are some respiratory reflexes that are different from the adult and may be responsible for some of the specific patterns of breathing observed in this age group.

### *Hering Breuer Inflation Reflex*

This reflex can be elicited in the fetus and in the neonate by inflating the lung, which results in inspiratory inhibition. It may also be triggered by occluding the airway at end expiration. Because there is no volume change the duration of the following inspiratory effort is prolonged (212–214). This reflex is more active in the full term but may also remain active for several weeks in the premature infant (Figure 7–19). The active Hering Breuer reflex can explain the higher respiratory rate observed during the neonatal period. This higher respiratory rate may be important in maintaining a larger functional residual capacity because inspiration begins before total relaxation of the respiratory system has occurred. This prevents the lung from emptying to its lower passive resting volume and allows the infant to maintain a higher dynamic FRC.

### *Head's Reflex*

This reflex consists of an increased inspiratory effort in response to a rapid lung inflation. This reflex is also present during the first few days of postnatal life and then disappears (212). This reflex may explain the biphasic sigh pattern of breathing observed in some neonates. This reflex may also be important in promoting lung inflation in the early postnatal period.

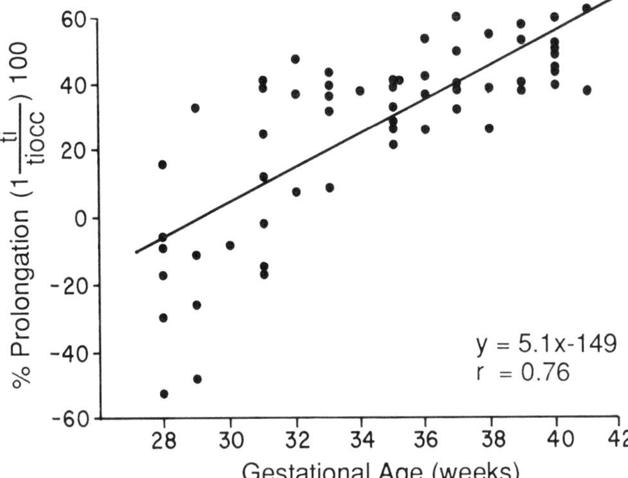


**Fig. 7–19.** Percent prolongation of inspiratory effort during airway occlusion in infants of different gestational ages. More mature infants have longer inspiratory efforts. (Redrawn from Gerhardt T, Bancalari E: Maturation changes of reflexes influencing inspiratory timing in newborns. J. Appl. Physiol. 50:1282, 1981.)

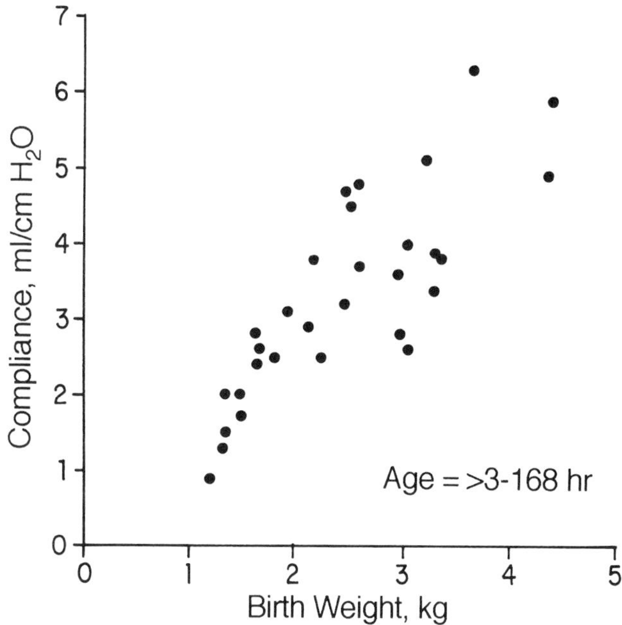


**Fig. 7–20.** Pulmonary compliance of normal infants during first week after birth. Note that compliance changes little with neonatal age after first hour, but is related to volume of lungs, and, therefore, to body size. (Redrawn from Smith CA: Physiology of the Newborn. 3rd Ed. Springfield, IL. Charles C. Thomas, 1959.)

## *Ventilation and Mechanics of Breathing*

The fluid reabsorption and increase in gas lung volume after birth produce a gradual increase in lung compliance from about 2.5 ml/cm $H_2O$ a few minutes after birth to 4 ml/cm $H_2O$ at 1 hour and 5.6 ml/cm $H_2O$ at 1 week of life (1.5 to 2 ml/cm $H_2O$/kg body weight) (Figure 7–20) (180,215). Specific compliance (CL/1 liter FRC) in the neonate is around 50 to 60 ml/cm $H_2O$/liter FRC, a value similar to that observed in the normal adult. Lung volume and compliance are lower in the premature infant, and this is more striking in infants with Respiratory Distress Syndrome. The compliance of the chest wall is increased in the neonate especially in the premature infant (216). This explains the significant distortion of the chest wall that occurs with the increased inspiratory effort that is generated by some infants with respiratory failure. The increased compliance of the chest wall is an additional factor that contributes to the propensity to lose lung volume, a characteristic of the preterm infant.

Airway and total pulmonary resistance is high during the neonatal period with values that range from 30 to 130 cm $H_2O$/liter/sec (217). These values are also higher in the premature than in the full-term infant and decrease with increasing postnatal age as the diameter of the airways becomes larger. Nearly half of the total pulmonary resistance is given by the upper airways. Because of the very small diameter, even a slight reduction in the lumen of the airway may produce a very substantial increase in resistance.

## *Lung Volume*

The functional residual capacity increases very rapidly after birth as lung fluid is reabsorbed from the alveolar spaces. Within a few hours of postnatal life the FRC is between 20 to 30 ml/kg body weight, and this relationship is maintained relatively constant during the first years of life. Because of the relatively low lung compliance and high chest wall compliance in the preterm infant, FRC tends to decrease leading to alveolar collapse and hypoxemia. There are mechanisms that compensate for this tendency, such as shorter expiratory time that prevent passive relaxation of the respiratory system. Under certain pathologic conditions there is partial closure of the airway during expiration ("grunting") and this maintains a positive airway pressure for a longer time during expiration, also preventing alveolar collapse and loss of FRC.

### *Respiratory Rate, Tidal Volume, and Minute Ventilation*

The respiratory rate varies significantly during the first days after birth. During the first hours it is not uncommon to observe rates of 60 to 80/breaths min that decrease gradually as lung fluid is reabsorbed to stabilize at rates of 30 to 40 after the first day. The premature infant frequently remains with higher rates than the fullterm. Tidal volume in the normal neonate ranges from 5 to 7 ml/kg body weight, and is similar in infants of different gestational ages (Figure 7–21). Minute ventilation is also related to body weight and ranges from 150 to 250 ml/kg/min (Figure 7–22) (218). Minute ventilation per body weight is higher in smaller infants because of the higher metabolic rate in proportion to body weight and the proportionally higher dead space ventilation. Figure 7–23 illustrates the changes in lung mechanics, lung volume, and ventilation that occur in the newborn during the first day after birth.

## Neonatal Gas Exchange

During the process of labor and delivery fetal gas exchange is frequently compromised by a reduction in the uterine and placental blood flows produced by the uterine contractions, by cord compression or by partial separation of the placenta. Because of this, most infants are born with some degree of hypoxemia and hypercapnia. In most cases the hypoxemia is not sufficiently severe to produce anaerobic metabolism and severe metabolic acidemia. As soon as the infant initiates regular breathing, the oxygenation improves and within minutes of birth the arterial $PO_2$ is over 50 mm Hg and the $PCO_2$ is less than 50 mm Hg (Figures 7–24 and 7–25). By 2 to 3 hours of age the $PaO_2$ in the normal full-term infant is around 70 mm Hg with $O_2$ saturations over 90% and the $PaCO_2$ is within normal limits (219).

In premature infants, specially those under 30 weeks of gestation, $PaO_2$ normally remains at lower values, between 50 to 70 mm Hg and their $PaCO_2$ is frequently

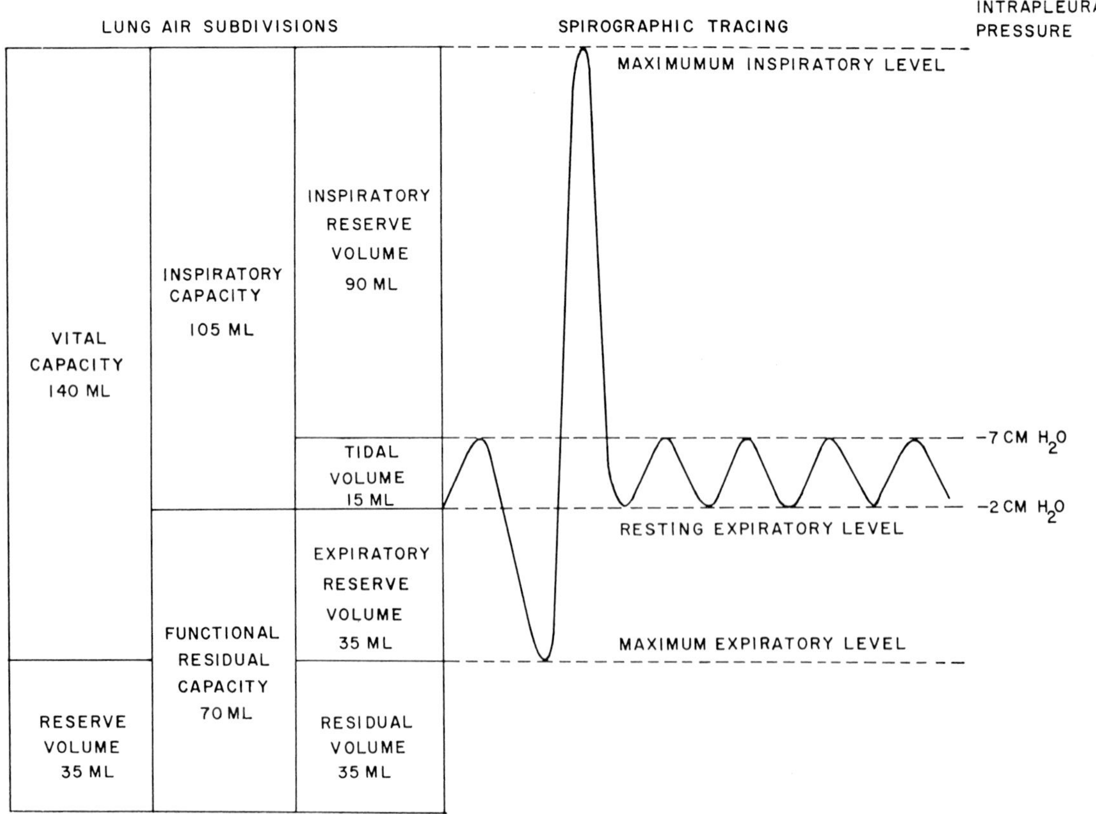


**Fig. 7–21.** Lung volumes and intrathoracic pressures in the normal, 2.5 kg infant. In the term newborn weighing 3.2 kg these volumes are larger. (Modified from Cook CD, et al: N. Engl. J. Med. 254:562, 1956.)

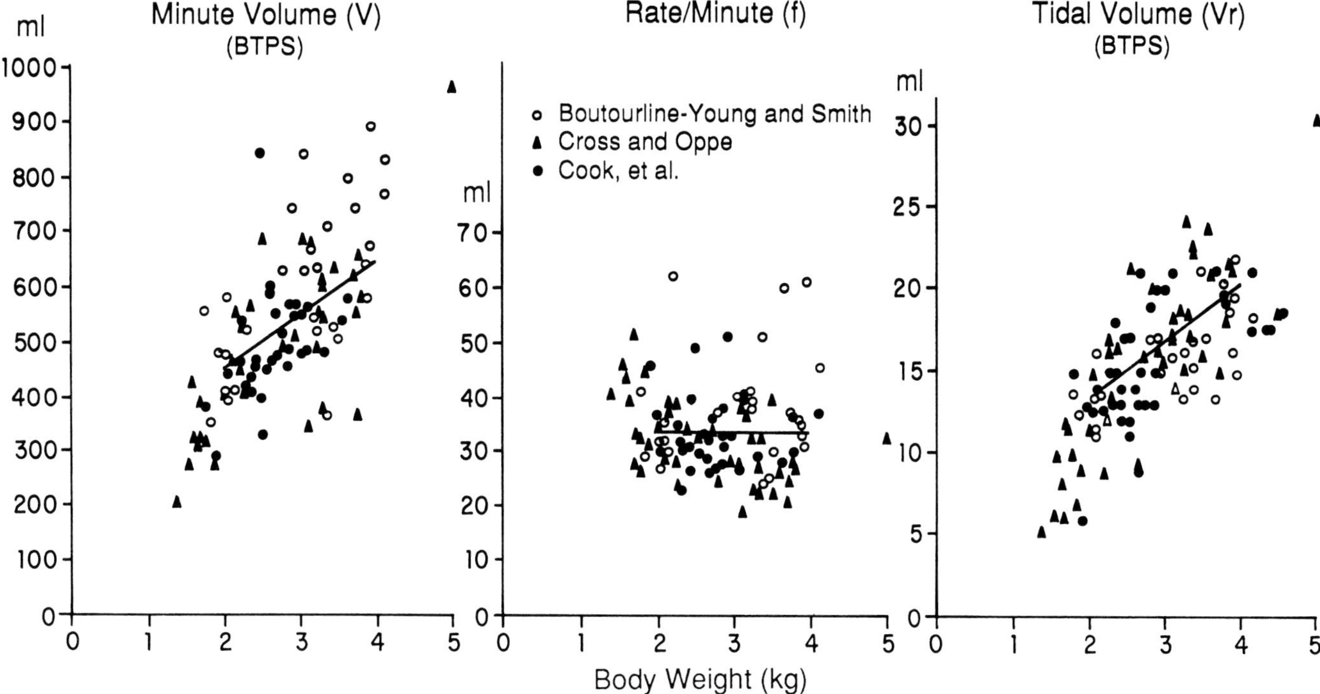


**Fig. 7–22.** Minute volume, rate, and tidal volume of 107 normal infants. BTPS signifies at body temperature and pressure, saturated with water vapor. Note correlation between weight and volumes, but not between weight and rate. (Redrawn from Cook CD, et al: J. Clin. Invest. 34:975, 1955.)

higher than 40 mm Hg. The lower $PaO_2$ in these infants is due to low VA/Q secondary to alveolar collapse and to lower diffusion capacity (220). Very immature infants also have variable degrees of alveolar hypoventilation due to decreased respiratory effort. This may be secondary to central depression and relative insensitivity to $CO_2$ and to chest wall instability. This can be aggravated by the relatively low lung compliance and high airway resistance characteristic of very small preterm infants.

## FETAL AND NEONATAL METABOLISM

The metabolic needs of the human fetus are similar in magnitude to those of the adult when adjusted for body weight. In the human fetus, oxygen consumption varies between 2.9 to 10.3 ml/kg/min with an average of 5.0 ml (221). In the newborn the needs are higher averaging 6.2 ml/kg/min during the first days of life (222). This increase is partly due to the energy required for temperature control. The high energy requirements of the fetus and newborn are necessary to support the rapid organ growth and differentiation. While glucose is the major energy substrate during fetal life, after birth the infant has the capacity to utilize fatty acids, ketone bodies, and amino acids. While the 7-month-old fetus has only 3.5% of body weight as fat at birth, this is approximately 16%. Therefore, most of the fat accumulation occurs during the last 6 to 8 weeks of gestation (223). This means that the prematurely born infant has considerably less fat reserves to meet metabolic needs than the full-term infant.

In the immediate postnatal period, a number of changes must occur to adapt the infant to the different substrates available. There is a sudden cessation of placental glucose transfer and therefore the newborn must mobilize stored glycogen to meet its metabolic needs. The newborn also is capable of oxidizing long chain fatty acids and ketone bodies. Fatty acid oxydation becomes a source for about 40% of the energy requirements of the neonate.

The fetal liver also accumulates glycogen during later stages of gestation (224,225). This glycogen serves as substrate for energy until gluconeogenesis, fatty acid oxidation, and exogenous caloric intake are established. These glycogen deposits are rapidly depleted during the first 24 hours after birth (226). This explains the propensity of the newborn to develop hypoglycemia if proper supply is not provided soon after birth. The risk for developing hypoglycemia is much higher in premature infants because of their lower glycogen deposits.

After birth, there is a dramatic increase in serum fatty acids levels that peak at 24 hours and decrease gradually over the next 6 to 12 months (227). This active lipolysis may be triggered by the very high catecholamine levels that are present at birth. The capacity to oxidize fatty acids after birth appears to be related to the increase of the enzyme carnitine palmitoyl tranferase (228,229). Carnitine derived from breast milk also seems to play a key role in the capacity for fatty acid oxidation of the newborn (230,231). Ketone bodies also increase significantly after birth and become an important energy substrate for the newborn (232).

The plasma amino acid pattern also suffers a striking change after birth. While levels of glycine and glutamine increase after birth the other amino acids decrease (233).

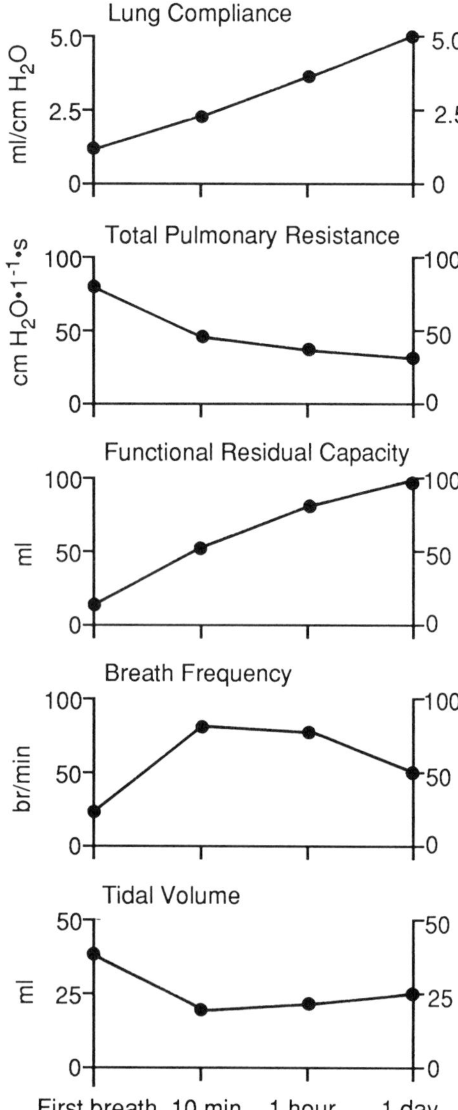


**Fig. 7–23.** This figure shows dynamic changes in five lung parameters that occur in the neonate from delivery through the first 24 hours of life. (Modified from Mortola J: Physiol. Reviews. 67: 202, 1987.)

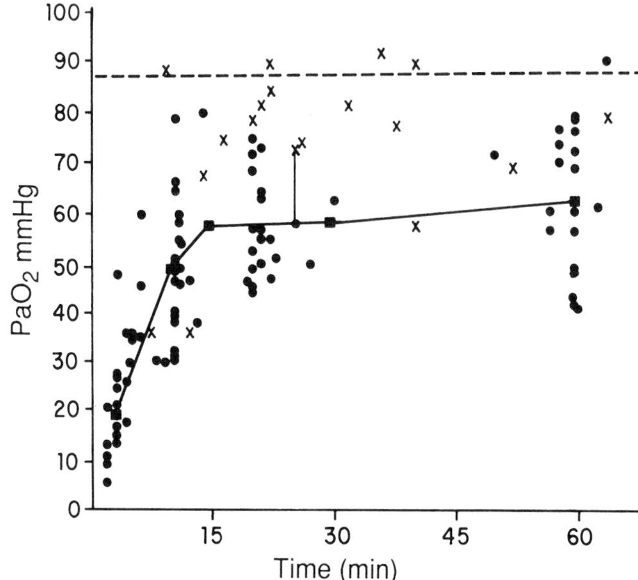


**Fig. 7–24.** Postnatal adjustments of oxygen tension in arterial blood. Figures are the means of the five time periods. Dots indicate arterial samples, and crosses, left atrial samples. Dashed line is the lower limit of normal $PaO_2$ for older children and adults (88 mmHg). Note that the largest increment of change in mean values occurred in the 6 to 10 minute period when the $PaO_2$ rose from a mean of 19.5 mmHg to a mean of 48.7 mmHg; during the next 10 minutes the $PaO_2$ rose to 56.3 mmHg with only very slight changes thereafter. (Redrawn from Oliver TJ Jr, Demis JA, Bates GD: Acta. Paediatr. 50:346, 1961.)

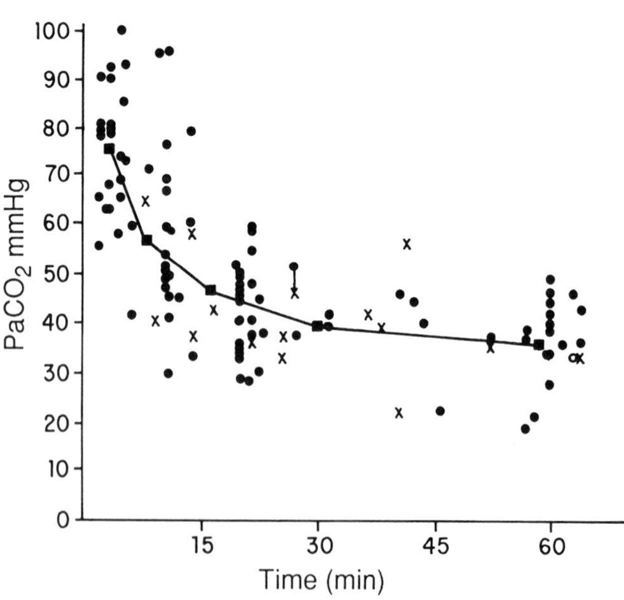


**Fig. 7–25.** Postnatal changes in arterial $CO_2$ tension. Dots indicate arterial sample, and crosses, left atrial sample. Note that during the first 10 minutes of life the $PaCO_2$ fell from a mean of 76.4 mmHg to 57.2 mmHg; during the next 10 minutes it fell further, to 46.3 mmHg, but during the remainder of the first hour there were only slight changes. (Redrawn from Oliver TJ Jr, Demis JA, Bates GD: Acta. Paedriatr. 50:346, 1961.)

These changes are closely linked with the alterations in carbohydrate and fat metabolism that occur after birth. Amino acids are mobilized from muscle to liver where they can be utilized for hepatic glucose synthesis. Amino acids therefore are also utilized as energy sources in the neonate and Alanine plays a major role in hepatic glucose synthesis (234). This is especially important in infants who suffer hypogylcemia, perinatal asphyxia or intrauterine growth retardation.

Metabolic rate per body weight is much higher in the newborn than in the adult. This is because of the larger surface area in relation to body weight of the newborn and because of the additional energy required for growth. Neonatal oxygen consumption varies with maturity, age, and environmental temperature but averages around 7 ml/kg body weight (222,234).

An important characteristic of the neonatal metabolism is that during hypoxia the newborn infant is capable of reducing oxygen consumption (235). This reduction in metabolism occurs before there is any evidence of anaerobic metabolism and may offer some degree of protection to the infant during the first days of life when episodes of hypoxia are more likely to occur.

## Neonatal Temperature Control

The fetal temperature is slightly above maternal temperature and is closely influenced by the latter. Because of this gradient there is normally transfer of heat from the fetus to the mother. The heat produced by the fetus is transferred to the mother who eliminates it through her heat control mechanisms.

After birth, the infant is exposed to a new environment in which heat losses may increase several fold (236). The environment is cooler, dryer, and the skin comes in contact with objects that are below body temperature. Therefore, the infant can loose heat by conduction, convection, radiation, and evaporation. This results in a rapid drop in temperature in most neonates that is influenced by the environmental conditions of the delivery room. Heat losses are greatly influenced by the temperature gradient between skin and the environment, and this gradient will determine the metabolic response of the infant. The larger the gradient, the more striking is the increase in oxygen consumption that the infant will have in an attempt to maintain body temperature relatively constant. The infant also responds with a reduction in skin blood flow to decrease heat loss.

The capacity of the newborn to thermoregulate is influenced by gestational and postnatal age and is reduced by factors such as perinatal asphyxia, hypoxia, hypoglycemia, and infections. For the normal full-term infant, during the first 8 to 24 hours of life, an environmental temperature of 28 to 34 degrees with a relative humidity of 40 to 60% provides a thermoneutral environment with minimal energy consumption (236). In the premature infant, this temperature is higher and varies depending on the gestational and postnatal age from 28° Celsius in an 1800 g infant, to 36° Celsius in extremely low birth weight infants (237).

The newborn is homeotherm, but is capable of increasing heat production by nonshivering mechanisms only. The maximal rate of thermogenesis is around 15 ml/kg/min, about double the resting metabolic rate. Nonshivering thermogenesis seems to occur mainly in brown adipose tissue, liver, and muscle (237).

The newborn's thermal stability is less efficient than in the adult, and it is especially limited in the preterm infant. This is mainly due to the large body surface area in relation to mass that increases the potential for heat loss. The increase in oxygen consumption in response to cold is predominantly a function of the gradient between body surface area and environmental temperature, rather than rectal, skin or environmental temperatures alone (238,239). The thermoregulatory response can also be impaired by hypoxia, arterial hypotension, CNS depression, by sedatives or analgesics given to the mother, and by infection. At birth the evaporation of the amniotic fluid in the infant's skin produces a rapid fall in skin temperature. This can be prevented by drying the skin and by placing the infant in a neutral thermal environment as rapidly as possible (238).

# RENAL DEVELOPMENT AND FUNCTION

Renal tubular function is present in the human metanephric kidney between the tenth and twelfth week of gestation when the loop of Henle is functional and there is tubular reabsorption of water. New nephrons are formed up to the thirty-sixth week of gestation (240). While the fetal kidney receives only 2 to 4% of the cardiac output in the last trimester, in the newborn this increases to 15 to 18%. After birth, there is a rapid increase in glomerular filtration rate due to an increase in arterial blood pressure and a decrease in renal vascular resistance. Both the fetus during the last trimester and the neonate have the capacity to autoregulate glomerular filtration rate within a certain range of fluctuations in arterial blood pressure.

During fetal life the reabsorption of Na is comparatively low. For this reason, the preterm infant excretes a larger fraction of sodium than the term infant. This may be related to a relative insensitivity of the tubular cells to aldosterone (241,242).

Fetal urine is hypo-osmotic with respect to plasma, but the fetus is capable of producing more concentrated urine in face of water deprivation but the ability to concentrate urine to adult levels is not reached until 6 to 12 months after birth (241–243). This may be due in part to a lower sensitivity of the fetal nephron to arginine vasopressin (AVP) and aldosterone. The ability of the newborn to excrete sodium loads is also limited and therefore they are more susceptible to develop hypernatremia (244).

Although hydrogen ion excretion increases in the fetal kidney during metabolic academia, the neonatal kidney is unable to excrete an acid load as efficiently as an adult. Both ammonium and tritatable acidity are limited in the newborn kidney. This predisposes the newborn to metabolic acidosis in situations when acid load is increased (245).

# GASTROINTESTINAL DEVELOPMENT AND FUNCTION

The gastrointestinal tract develops from the endodermal and mesodermal layers. By 4 weeks of gestation, there is already a simple tube that protrudes into the umbilical cord. By 6 to 8 weeks, the small intestine rotates around the axis of the superior mesenteric vessels inside the umbilical cord. At 10 weeks, the intestine re-enters the abdominal cavity and continues to elongate at a rapid rate. Enzyme activity is present from the seventh to eighth week, and increases rapidly so by 24 to 26 weeks infants are usually able to tolerate small feedings (246).

In very immature infants proteolytic enzyme activity is diminished, and these infants can present with protein malabsorption. Although bile acid concentration is also low in preterm infants, they are able to absorb most vegetable fat and fats contained in breast milk.

Other than some lactose intolerance in the preterm infant (247), the newborn can absorb most carbohydrates unless there is intestinal damage produced by hypoxia or ischemia.

Motility develops in the gastrointestinal tract in a craniocaudal progression. Muscle layers in the gut are present by 12 weeks of gestation, and ganglion cells are found in a normal distribution by the twenty-fourth week.

Swallowing is already present at 16 to 18 weeks of gestation, but the coordination between sucking and swallowing is not well-developed until the thirty-fourth week of gestation. The transit time is prolonged in the preterm infant, due to poor coordination of peristalsis and possibly decreased hormonal secretions (248,249).

## REFERENCES


1. Polin R, Fox W: Fetal and Neonatal Physiology. Edited by R Polin, W Fox. Orlando, FL, W.B. Saunders, Co., 1992.
2. Smith CA, Nelson NM: The Physiology of the Newborn Infant. 4th Ed. Springfield, IL, Charles C. Thomas, 1976.

2A. Yecco GJ: Neurobehaviorial development support of premature infants. J. Perinat. Neonatal. Nurs. (United States). 7(1), 1993, pp. 56–65.

3. Longo LD, Reneau DD: Fetal and newborn cardiovascular physiology. Fetal and Newborn Circulation. Vol. 2. Edited by LD Longo, DD Reneau. Bryn Mawr, PA, Garland Publishing, Inc., 1978.
4. Stave U: Physiology of the perinatal period. Functional and Biochemical Development in Mammals. Vol. 2. Edited by U Stave. New York, Appleton-Century-Crofts, Educational Division, Meredith Corp., 1970.

4A. Richardson BS: The effect of behaviorial state on fetal metabolism and blood flow circulation. Semin. Perinatol. 16(4), 1992, pp. 227–233.

4B. Ramer JC, Mowrey PN, Robins DB, Ligato S, et al: Five children with del (2)(q31q33) and one individual with dup (2)(q31q33) from a single family: review of brain, cardiac, and limb malformations. Am. J. Med. Genet. 37(3), 1990, pp. 392–400.

5. Strang LB: Neonatal respiration. Physiological and Clinical Studies. Edited by LB Strang. London, Blackwell Scientific Publications, 1977.
6. Sinclair JC: Temperature Regulation and Energy Metabolism in the Newborn. Edited by JC Sinclair. New York, Grune & Stratton, Inc., 1978.
7. Cowett RM: Principles of Perinatal-neonatal Metabolism. Edited by RM Cowett. New York, Springer-Verlag New York, Inc., 1991.
8. Davis CL: Development of the human heart from its first appearance to the stage found in embryos of twenty paired somites, Carnegie Inst. Wash. Contrib. Embryol. 23:252, 1932.
9. Dische MR: Observations on the morphological changes of the developing heart. Cardiovasc. Clin. 4:175, 1972.
10. Krediet P, Klein HW: Synopsis of normal cardiac development. *In* Mechanism of Cardiac Morphogenesis and Teratogenesis: Perspectives in Cardiovascular Research. Vol. 5. Edited by T Pexeider. New York, Raven Press, 1981, p. 7.
11. Manasek FJ, Burnside MB, Waterman RE: Myocardial cell shape change as a mechanism of embryonic heart looping. Dev. Biol. 29:349, 1972.
12. O'Rahilly R: The timing and sequence of events in human cardiogenesis. Acta. Anat. 79:70, 1971.
13. Grant RP: The embryology of the ventricular flow pathways in man. Circulation 25:756, 1962.
14. Van Praagh R, Van Praagh S: The anatomy of common aorticopulmonary trunk (truncus arteriosus communis) and its embryologi implications. A study of 57 necropsy cases. Am. J. Cardiol. 16:406, 1965.
15. Van Praagh R, Ongley PA, Swan HJC: Anatomic types of single or common ventricle in man. Morphologic and geometric aspects of 60 necropsied cases. Am. J. Cardiol. 13:367, 1964.
16. Van Mierop LH, Alley RD, Kausel HW, Stranahan A, et al: Pathogenesis of transposition complexes. I. Embryology of the ventricles and great arteries. Am. J. Cardiol. 12:216, 1963.
17. De Vries PA, deSaunders JB: Development of the ventricles and spiral outflow tract in the human heart. Contributions to Embryology 37:87, 1962.
18. Rupolph AM, Heymann MA, Spitznas Y: Hemodynamic considerations in the development of narrowing of the aorta. Am. J. Cardiol. 30:514, 1972.
19. Neill CA: Development of the pulmonary veins, with reference to the embryology of anomalies of pulmonary venous return. Pediatrics 18:880, 1956.
20. Lucas RV Jr, Anderson RD, Amplatz K, Adams P Jr, Edwards JE: Congenital causes of pulmonary venous obstruction. Pediatr. Clin. North. Am. 10:781, 1983.
21. Meyer WW, Lind J: The ductus venosus and the mechanism of its closure. Arch. Dis. Child. 41:597, 1966.

21A. Friedman AH, Fahey JT: The transition from fetal to neonatal circulation: normal reponses and implications for infants with heart disease. Semin. Perinatol. (United States). 17(2), 1993, pp. 106–121.

21B. Loberant N, Barak M, Gaitini D, Hersovits M, et al: Closure of the ductus venosus in neonates: findings on real-time gray-scale, color-flow Doppler, and duplex Doppler sonography. AJR. 159(5), 1992, pp. 1083–1085.

22. Lind J: Human fetal and neonatal circulation: some structural and functional aspects. Eur. J. Cardiol. 5:265, 1977.
23. Edelstone DI, Rudolph AM: Preferential streaming of ductus venosus blood to the brain and heart in fetal lambs. Am. J. Physiol. 237:H724, 1979.
24. Rudolph AM, Heymann MA: Fetal and neonatal circulation and respiration. Ann. Rev. Physiol. 36:187, 1974.

24A. Friedman AH, Fahey JT: The transition from fetal to neonatal circulation: normal responses and implications for infants with heart disease. Semin. Perinatol. (United States). 17(2), 1993, pp. 106–121.

25. Rudolph AM, Heymann MA, Lewis AB: Physiology and pharmacology of the pulmonary circulation in the fetus and newborn. *In* Lung Biology in Health and Disease, The Development of the Lung. Edited by WA Hodson. New York, Marcel Dekker, Inc., 1977, p. 497.
26. Reid L: The pulmonary circulation: remodeling in growth and disease. Am. Rev. Respir. Dis. 119:531, 1979.
27. Rudolph AM, Yaun S: Response of the pulmonary vasculature to hypoxia and Hp+ ion concentration changes. J. Clin. Invest. 45:399, 1966.

27A. McMurty IF, Rodman DM, Yamaguchi T, O'Brien RF: Pulmonary vascular reactivity. Chest 93(3 Suppl.), 1988, pp. 88S–93S.

28. Barclay AE, Barcroft J, Barron DH, Franklin, KJ: Radiographic demonstration of circulation through heart in adult and in foetus, and identification of ductus arteriosus. Br. J. Radiol. 12:505, 1939.

28A. Edwards DK, Higgins CB: Radiology of neonatal heart disease. Radiol. Clin. North Am. 18(3), 1980, pp. 369–85.

29. Rudolph AM, Heymann MA: Circulatory changes with growth in the fetal lamb. Circ. Res. 26:289, 1970.
30. Rudolph AM, Heymann MA, Teramo KA, Barrett CT, et al:

Studies on the circulation of the previable human fetus. Pediatr. Res. 5:452, 1971.

31. Leahy FAN, Sankaran K, Cates D, MacCallum M, et al: Quantitative noninvasive method to measure cerebral blood flow in newborn infants. Pediatrics 64:277, 1979.
32. Friedman WF: The intrinsic physiologic properties of the developing heart. Prog. Cardiovasc. Dis. 15:87, 1972.
33. Lebowitz EA, Norwick JS, Rudolph AM: Development of myocardial sympathetic nerve innervation in the fetal lamb. Pediatr. Res. 6:887, 1972.
34. McPherson RA, Kramer MF, Covell JW, Friedman WF, et al: A comparison of active stiffness of fetal and adult cardiac muscle. Pediatr. Res. 10:660, 1976.
35. Gennser G, Nilsson E: Response to adrenaline, acetylcholine and changes of contraction frequency in early human fetal hearts. Experientia 26:1105, 1970.
36. Eckberg DL: Parasympathetic cardiovascular control in human disease: a critical review of methods and results. Am. J. Physiol. 239:H581, 1980.
37. Papile L, Rudolph AM, Heymann MA: Autoregulation of cerebral blood flow in the preterm fetal lamb. Pediatr. Res. 19:159, 1985.
38. Peeters LLH, Sheldon RE, Jones MD Jr, Makowski EL, et al: Blood flow to fetal organs as a function of arterial oxygen content. Am. J. Obstet. Gynecol. 135:637, 1979.
39. Berman W Jr, Goodlin RC, Heymann MA, Rudolph AM: Relationships between pressure and flow in the umbilical and uterine circulation of the sheep. Circ. Res. 38:262, 1976.
40. Dawes GS, Johnston BM, Walker DW: Relationship of arterial pressure and heart rate in fetal, newborn, and adult sheep. J. Physiol. (Lond). 309:405, 1980.
41. Dawes GS, Duncan SLB, Lewis BV, Merlet CL, et al: Cyanide stimulation of the systemic arterial chemoreceptors in foetal lambs. J. Physiol. (Lond). 281:117, 1969.
42. Goodlin RC, Rudolph AM: Factors associated with initiation of breathing. *In* Proceedings of the International Symposium of Physiologi Biochemistry of the Fetus. Edited by AA Hodari, FG Mariona. Springfield, IL, Charles C. Thomas, 1972, p. 294.
43. Daly M, Angell-James JE, Elsner R: Role of carotid-body chemoreceptors and their reflex interaction in bradycardia and cardiac arrest. Lancet 1:764, 1979.
44. Wildenthal K: Maturation of responsiveness to cardioactive drugs. Differential effects of acetylcholine, norepinephrine, theophylline, tyramine, glucagon and dibutyryl cyclic AMP on atrial rate in hearts of fetal mice. J. Clin. Invest. 52:2250, 1973.
44A. Hondeghem LM, Mouton E, Stassen T, De Geest H: Additive effects of acetylcholine released by vagal nerve stimulation on atrial rate. J. Appl. Physiol. 38(1), 1975, pp. 108–113.
45. Friedman WF, Pool PE, Jacobowitz D, Seagren SC, et al: Sympathetic innervation of the developing rabbit heart. Biochemical and histochemical comparisons of fetal, neonatal and adult myocardium. Circ. Res. 23:25, 1968.
45A. Kast A, Hermer M: Beta-adrenocepter tocolysis and effects on the heart of fetus and neonate. A review. J. Perinat. Med. (Germany). 21(2), 1993, pp. 97–106.
45B. Watanabe T, Matsuhashi K, Takayama S, Morita H: Study on the functional development of the sympathetic nervous system of fetal heart in rats. Nippon Yakurigaku Zasshi. 84(2), 1984, pp. 229–241.
46. Wyse DG, Van Petten GR, and Harris WH: Responses to electrical stimulation, noradrenaline, serotonin, and vasopressin in the isolated ear artery of the developing lamb and ewe. Can. J. Physiol. Pharmacol. 55:1001, 1977.
47. Niarchos AP, Pickering TG, Case DB, Sullivan P, et al: Role of the renin-angiotesin system in blood pressure regulation. The cardiovascular effects of converting enzyme inhibition in normotensive subjects. Circ. Res. 45:829, 1979.
48. Heymann MA, Rudolph AM, Nies AS, Melmn KL, et al: Bradykinin production associated with oxygenation of the fetal lamb. Circ. Res. 25:521, 1969.
48A. Stalcup SA, Lipset JS, Odya CE, Goodfriend TL: Angiotensin-converting enzyme activity and its modulation by oxygen tension in the guinea pig fetal-placental unit. Circ. Res. 57(4):646, 1985.
49. Mott JC: The place of the renin-angiotensin system before and after birth. Br. Med. Bull. 31:44, 1975.
50. Bowes WA, Gabbe SB, Bowes C: Fetal heart rate monitoring in premature infants weighing 1500 grams or less. Am. J. Obstet. Gynecol. 137:791, 1980.
51. Benedict FG, Talbot FB: Physiology of newborn infant; character and amount of catabolism. Carnegie Inst., Carnegie Inst. Publ. #233, 1915.
52. Woodbury RA, Robinov M, Hamilton WF: Blood pressure studies on infants. Am. J. Physiol. 122:472, 1938.
52A. Rasoulpour M, Marinelli KA: Systemic hypertension. Clin. Perinatol. 19(1), 1992, pp. 121–137.
53. Reynolds SRM: Hemodynamic characteristics of the fetal circulation. Am. J. Obstet. Gynecol. 68:69, 1954.
53A. Vetter K, Favre Y, Suter T, Huch R, Huch A: Doppler sonographic determination of specific hemodynamic changes in fetal circulation during the last four weeks before birth. Z. Geburtshilfe Perinatol. 193(5), 1989, pp. 215–218.
54. Yao AC, Lind Tiisala, R Michellson, K: Placental transfusion in the premature infant with observation on clinical course and outcome. Acta. Paediatr. Scand. 58A:561, 1969a.
54A. Betke K: The effect of intra-partum and intra-uterine asphyxia on placental transfusion in premature and full-term infants. Eur. J. Pediatr. 127(2), 1978, pp. 91–99.
55. Bloom W, Bartelmez BW: Hematopoises in young human embryos. Am. J. Anat. 67:21, 1940.
56. Gilmour JR: Normal haemopoises in intrauterine and neonatal life. J. Path. Bact. 52:25, 1941.
57. Walker JL, Turnbull EPN: Haemoglobin and red cells in the human foetus, III. Foetal and adult haemoglobin. Arch. Dis. Child. 30:111, 1955.
58. Armstrong DH, Schroeder WA, Fennigre WD: A comparison of the percentage of fetal hemoglobin in human umbilical cord blood as determined by chromatography and by alkali denaturation. Blood 22:554, 1963.
58A. Huisman TH, Schroeder WA: The chemical heterogeneity of the chain from human fetal hemoglobin. Crit. Rev. Clin. Lab. Sci. 1(3), 1970, pp. 514–526.
59. Beuzard Y, Vainchenker W, Testa U, Dubart A, et al: Fetal to adult hemoglobin switch in cultures of early erythroid precursors from human fetus and neonates. Am. J. Hematol. 7:207, 1979.
60. Wood WG, Weatherall DJ: Haemoglobin synthesis during human foetal development. Nature 244: 162, 1973.
61. Bard H, Makowski EL, Meschia G, Battaglia FC: The relative rates of synthesis of hemoglobins A and F in immature red cells on newborn infants. Pediatrics 45:766, 1970.
61A. Forestier F, Daffos F, Galacteros F, Bardakjian, et al: Hematalogical values of 163 normal fetuses between 18 and 30 weeks of gestation. Pediatr. Res. 20(4), 1986, pp. 342–346.
61B. Stamatoyannopoulos G, Papayannopoulou T: The switching from hemoglobin F to hemoglobin A formation in man: parallels between the observations in vivo and the findings in erythroid cultures. Prog. Clin. Biol. Res. 55, 1981, pp. 665–678.
62. Cohn HE, Sacks EJ, Heymann MA, Rudolph AM: Cardiovas-

cular responses to hypoxemia and acidemia in fetal lambs. Am. J. Obstet. Gynecol. 120:817, 1974.

63. Eaton JW, Skelton TD, Berger E: Survival at extreme altitude: protective effect of increased hemoglobin-oxygen affinity. Science 183:743, 1974.

64. Delprado WJ, Baird PJ: The fetal adrenal gland: lipid distribution with associated intrauterine hypoxia. Pathology 16: 25, 1984.

65. Fenton AN, Steer CH: Fetal distress. Am. J. Obstet. Gynecol. 83:354, 1962.

65A. Parer JT, Livingston EG: What is fetal stress. Am. J. Obstet. Gynecol. 162(6), 1990, pp. 1421–1425.

66. Fleischyer A, Schulman H, Jagani N, Mitchell J, Randolph G: The development of fetal acidosis in the presence of an abnormal heart rate tracing. Am. J. Obstet. Gynecol. 144: 55, 1982.

67. Creasy RK, Resnik R, Saunders WB: Maternal Fetal Medicine. 2nd Ed. Philadelphia, The Curtis Institute, 1989.

68. Martin CB: Regulation of the fetal heart rate and genesis of FHR patterns. Semin. Perinatol. 2:131, 1978.

69. Thaler I, Timor-Tritsch IE, Blumenfeld Z: Effect of acute hypoxia on human fetal heart rate. Acta. Obstet. Gynecol. Scand. 64:46, 1986.

70. Yao AC: Cardiovascular changes during the transition from fetal to neonatal life. *In* Perinatal Cardiovascular Function. Edited by PM Gootman, Gootman N. New York, Marcel Dekker, Inc., 1983, p. 4,

71. Edmonds JF, Berry E, Wyllie JH: Release of prostaglandins caused by distension of the lungs. Br. J. Surg. 56:622, 1969.

72. Leffler CW, Hessler JR, Terragno NA: Ventilation-induced release of prostaglandin-like material from fetal lungs. Am. J. Physiol. 238:H282, 1980.

73. Soifer SJ, Morin FC, Kaslow DC, Heymann MA: The developmental effects of prostaglandin D2 on the pulmonary and systemic circulations in the newborn lamb. J. Dev. Physiol. 5:237, 1983.

74. Moss AJ, Emmanouoilides G, Duffie ER: Closure of the ductus arteriosus in the newborn infant. Pediatrics 3: 225,1963.

74A. Friedman AH, Fahey JT: The transition from fetal to neonatal circulation: normal responses and implications for infants with heart disease. Semin. Perinatol. (United States). 17(2), 1993, pp. 106–121.

74B. Barst RJ, Gersony WM: The pharmacological treatment of patent ductus arteriosus. A review of the evidence. Drugs. 38(2), 1989, pp. 249–266.

75. Heymann MA, Rudolph AM: Control of the ductus arteriosus. Physiol. Rev. 55:62, 1975.

76. McMurphy DM, Heymann MA, Rudolph AM, Melmon KL: Developmental change in constriction of the ductus arteriosus: responses to oxygen and vasoactive substances in the isolated ductus arteriosus of the fetal lamb. Pediatr. Res. 6:231, 1972.

77. Clyman RI, Mauray F, Roman C, Rudolph AM, et al: Glucocorticoids alter the sensitivity of the lamb ductus arteriosus to prostaglandin E2. J. Pediatr. 98:126, 1981.

78. Clyman RI, Ballard PL, Sniderman S, Ballaard RA, et al: Prenatal administration of betamethasone for prevention of paten ductus ateriosus. J. Pediatr. 98:123, 1981.

79. Christie A: Normal closing time of foramen ovale and ductus arteriosus, anatomic and statistical study. Am. J. Dis. Child. 40:323, 1930.

80. McMurphy DM, Boreus LO: Studies on the pharmacology of the perfused human fetal ductus arteriosus. Am. J. Obstet. Gynecol. 109:937, 1971.

81. Lind J, Wegelius CE: Human fetal circulation: changes in the cardiovascular system at birth and disturbances in the postnatal closure of the foramen ovale and ductus arteriosus. Cold Spring Harbor, Symp. Quant. Biol. 19:109, 1954.

82. Kobayashi K: The foramen ovale cordis in man. Mem. Anthropol. Hum. Constit. 37:25, 1960.

83. Ehinger R, Gennser B, Owman C, Sjoberg N-O: Histochemical and pharmacological studies on amine mechanisms in the umbilical cord, umbilical vein and ductus venosus of the human fetus. Acta. Physiol. Scand. 72:15, 1968.

84. Klopfenstein HS, Rudolph AM: Postnatal changes in the circulation and response to volume loading in sheep. Circ. Res. 42:839, 1978.

85. Lister G, Walter TK, Versmold HT, Dallman PR, et al: $O_2$ delivery in lambs: cardiovascular and hematologic development. Am. J. Physiol. 236:H668, 1979.

86. Rudolph AM: Physiologic Events occurring during the transitional circulation. *In* Cardiovascular sequelae of asphyxia in the newborn. 83rd Ross Conference on Pediatric Research. Edited by GJ Pevkham, MA Heymann. Columbus, OH, Ross Laboratories, 1982, p. 30.

87. Heymann MA: Fetal and neonatal circulation. *In* Moss' Heart Diseases in Infants, Children, and Adolescents. Edited by FH Adams, GC Emmauouillded, TA Riemenschneider. Baltimore, Williams and Wilkins Publishers, 1989, p. 30.

88. Hastreiter AR, Abella JB: The electrocardiogram in the newborn period: I. The normal infant. J. Pediatr. 78:146, 1971.

89. Moscoso P, Goldberg RN, Jamieson J, Bancalari E: Spontaneous elevation in arterial blood pressure during the first hours of life in the very-low-weight infant. J. Pediatr. 103: 114, 1983.

90. Yao AC, Lind J: Effect of early and late cord clamping on the systolic time intervals of the newborn infant. Acta. Paediatr. Scand. 66:489, 1977.

91. Usher RH, Shepard M, Lind J: The blood volume of the newborn infant and placental transfusion. Acta. Paediatr. Scand. 52:497, 1963.

92. Yao AC, Wist A, Lind J: The blood volume of the newborn infant delivery by caesarean section. Acta. Paediatr. Scand. 56:585, 1967.

93. Yao AC, Hirvensalo M, Lind J: Placental transfusion-rate and uterine contraction. Lancet 1:380, 1968.

94. Yao AC, Nergardh AM, Boreus LO: Influence of oxytocin and meperidine on the isolated human umbilical artery. Biol. Neonate 29:333, 1976.

95. Saigal S, O'Neill A, Surainder Y, Chua L, et al: Placental transfusion and hyperbilirubinemia in the premature. Pediatrics 49:406, 1972.

96. Oh W, Lind J, Gessner IH: Circulatory and respiratory adaptation to early and late cord clamping in newborn infants. Acta. Paediatr. Scand. 55:17, 1966.

96A. Iso H, Yuge K, Hirayama T: Spatial and quantitative analysis of the QRS and T waves by Frank-lead orthogonal electocardiography in normal children. Comparative study in an early and late cord-clamping groups in newborns. Nippon Ika Daigaku Zasshi. 59(5), 1992, pp. 409–417.

96B. Linderkamp O, Nelle M, Kraus M, Zilow EP: The effect of early and late cord-clamping on blood viscosity and other hemorheological parameters in full-term neonates. Acta. Paediatr (Norway). 81(10), 1992, pp. 745–750.

97. Oh W, Wallgren G, Hanson JS, Lind J: The effects of placental transfusion on respiratory mechanics of normal term infants. Pediatrics 40:6, 1967.

98. Downing SE, Talner NS, Gardner TH: Ventricular function in the newborn lamb. Am. J. Physiol. 208:931, 1965.

98A. Downing SE, Lee JC: Cardiac function and metabolism

following hemorrhage in the newborn lamb. Ann. Surg. 184(6), 1976, pp. 743–751.
99. Gootman PM, Buckley NM, Gootman N: Postnatal maturation of neural control of circulation. *In* Review in Perinatal Medicine, Vol. 3. Edited by EM Scarpelli EM, EV Cosmi. New York, Raven Press, 1979, p. 1.
100. Hirsch EF: Embryologic and fetal development of cardiac innervation in the human heart. *In* Innervation of the Vertebrate Heart. Springfield, IL, Charles C. Thomas, 1970, p. 125.
101. Parer JT, Krueger TR, Harris JL: Fetal oxygen consumption and mechanisms of heart rate response during artificially produced late decelerations of fetal heart rate in sheep. Am. J. Obstet. Gynecol. 136:4781, 1980.
102. Behrman RE, Lees MH, Peterson EN, DeLannoy CW, et al: Distribution of the circulation in the normal and asphyxiated fetal primate. Am. J. Obstet. Gynecol. 108:956, 1970.
103. Burnard ED, James LS: Failure of the heart after cardiac asphyxia at birth. Pediatrics 28:545, 1961.
104. Rudolph AM, Itskovitz J, Iwamoto H, Reuss ML, et al: Fetal cardiovascular responses to stress. Semin. Perinatol. 5:109, 1981.
105. Bucciarelli R, Nelson RM, Egan EA, Eitzman DV, et al: Transient tricuspid insufficiency of the newborn: A form of myocardial dysfunction in stressed newborns. Pediatrics 59:330, 1977.
106. Drummond WH, Rudolph AM, Keil LC, Gluckman PD, et al: Arginine vasopressin and prolactin after hemorrhage in the fetal lamb. Am. J. Physiol. 238:E214, 1980.
107. Comline RS, Silver IA, Silver M: Factors responsible for the stimulation of the adrenal medulla during asphyxia in the foetal lamb. J. Physiol. (Lond). 178:211, 1965.
108. Lewis AB, Evans WN, Sischo W: Plasma catecholamine responses to hypoxemia in fetal lambs. Biol. Neonate 41:115, 1982.
109. Fox WW, Duara S: Persistent pulmonary hypertension of the neonate: diagnosis and clinical management. J. Pediatr. 103:505, 1983.
110. Drummond WH, Gregory GA, Heymann MA, Phibbs RA: The independent effects of hyperventilation, tolazoline and dopamine on infants with persistent pulmonary hypertension. J. Pediatr. 98:603, 1981.
111. Haworth SG, Suer U, Buhlmeyer K: Effect of prostaglandin E1 on pulmonary circulation in pulmonary atresia. Br. Heart. J. 43:306, 1980.
112. Siassi B, Blanco C, Cabal LA, Coran AG: Incidence and clinical features of patent ductus arteriosus in low-birth weight infants. A prospective analysis of 150 consecutively born infants. Pediatrics 57:347, 1976.
113. Clyman RI: Ontogeny of the ductus arteriosus response to prostaglandins and inhibitors of their synthesis. Semin. Perinatol. 4:115, 1980.
114. Clyman RI, Mauray F, Rudolph AM, Heymann MA: Age dependent sensitivity of the lamb ductus arteriosus to indomethacin and prostaglandins. Journal of Pediatrics 96:94, 1980.
115. Csaba IF, Sulyok E, Ertl T: Relationship of maternal treatment with indomethacin to persistence of fetal circulation syndrome. J. Pediatr. 92:484, 1978.
116. Sibai BM, Mirro R, Chesney CM, Leffler C: Low-dose aspirin in pregnancy. Obstet. Gynecol. 74:551, 1989.
117. Morales WJ, Smith SG, Angel JL, O'Brien WF, et al: Efficacy and safety of indomethacin versus ritodrine in the management of preterm labor. A randomized study. Obstet. Gynecol. 74:567, 1989.
118. Datta S, Alper MH: Anesthesia for cesarean section. Anesthesiology 53:142, 1980.
119. Kryc JJ: Management of pain during labor. *In* Drug Therapy in Obstetrics and Gynecology. 2nd Ed. Rayburn WF, Zuspan FP (eds). Norwalk, CT, Appleton-Century-Crofts, 1986, p. 205.
120. Ralston DH, Shnider SM: The fetal and neonatal effects of regional anesthesia in obstetrics. Anesthesiology 48:34, 1978.
121. Lavin JP: Effects of bupivicaine and chloroprocaine as local anesthetics for epidural anesthesia. Am. J. Obstet. Gynecol. 141:717, 1981.
122. Petrie RH: Effects of drugs and anesthetics on the fetal heart rate. Semin. Perinatol. 2:147, 1978.
123. Petrie RH, Yeh SY, Murata Y, Paul RH, et al: The effect of drugs on fetal heart rate variability. Am. J. Obstet. Gynecol. 130:294, 1978.
124. Green KW, Key TC, Coen R, Resnik R: The effects of maternally administered magnesium sulfate on the neonate. Am. J. Obstet. Gynecol. 146:29, 1983.
125. Gross TL, Kuhnert BR, Kuhnert PM, Rosen MG, et al: Maternal and fetal plasma concentration of ritodrine. Obstet. Gynecol. 65:793, 1985.
126. Katz M, Robertson P, Creasy RK: Cardiovascular complication associated with terbutaline treatment for preterm labor. Am. J. Obstet. Gynecol. 139:605, 1981.
127. Hill LM, Malkasian GD Jr: The use of Quinidine sulfate throughout pregnancy. Obstet. Gynecol. 54:366, 1979.
128. Boyden EA: Development and growth of the airways. *In* Developments of the Lung. Edited by WA Hodson. New York, Marcel Dekker, 1977, p. 3.
129. Boyden EA, Tompsett DH: The changing patterns in the developing lungs of infants. Acta. Anat. (Basel) 61:164, 1965.
130. Boyden EA: Development of the human lung. *In* Practice of Pediatrics. New York, Harper and Row Publishers, Chapt. 64:1, 1975.
131. Boyden EA: The programming of canalization in fetal lungs of man and monkey. Am. J. Anat. 145:125, 1976.
132. Dunnill MS: Postnatal growth of the lung. Thorax. 17:329, 1962.
133. Zeltner TB, Caduff JH, Gehr P, Pfenninger J, et al: The postnatal development and growth of the human lung. I. Morphometry. Respir. Physiol. 67:247, 1987.
134. Zeltner TB, Burri PH: The postnatal development and growth of the human lung. II. Morphology. Respir. Physiol. 67:269, 1987.
135. Loosli CG, Potter EL: Pre-and postnatal development of the respiratory portion of the lung. Am. Rev. Resp. Dis. 80:5, 1959.
136. Snyder FF: Fetal respiratory movement. Clin. Obstet. Gynecol. 3:874, 1960.
137. Snyder FF, Rosenfeld M: Direct observation of intrauterine respiratory movements of the fetus and the role of carbon dioxide and oxygen in their regulation. Am. J. Physiol. 119: 153, 1937.
138. Barcroft J: The onset of respiratory movement. *In*: Researchers on PreNatal Life. Oxford, Blackwell Scientific Publications, 1977, p. 260.
139. Boddy K, Dawes GS: Fetal breathing. Br. Med. Bull. 31:3, 1975.
140. Boddy K, Dawes GS, Fisher R, Pinter S, Robinson JS: Fetal respiratory movements, electrocortical and cardiovascular responses to hypoxaemia and hypercapnia in sheep. J. Physiol. (Lond). 243:599, 1974.
141. Dawes GS: Breathing before birth in animals and man. N. Engl. J. Med. 290:557, 1974.
142. Moloney JE, Bowes G, Wilikinson M: "Fetal breathing" and

the development of patterns of respiration before birth. Sleep 3:299, 1980.

143. Patrick J, Campbell K, Carmichael L, Natale R, et al: Patterns of human fetal breathing during the last 10 weeks of pregnancy. Am. J. Obstet. Gynecol. 56:24, 1980.

144. Rigatto H, Lee D, Davi M, Moore M, et al: Effect of increased arterial $CO_2$ on fetal breathing and behavior in sheep. J. Appl. Physiol. 64:982, 1988.

145. Baier RJ, et al: The effects of continuous distending airway pressure under various background concentrations of oxygen, high frequency oscillatory ventilation, and umbilical cord occlusion on fetal breathing and behavior in sheep. Proceedings of the Society for the Study of Fetal Physiology, Cairns, Australia, 1988, p. 26.

146. Clewlow F, Dawes GS, Johnston BM, Walker DW: Changes in breathing, electrocortical and muscle activity in unanesthetized fetal lambs with age. J. Physiol. (Lond). 341:463, 1983.

147. Hansan SU, Lee DS, Gibson DA, Nowaczyk BJ, et al: Effect of morphine on breathing and behavior in fetal sheep. J. Appl. Physiol. 64:2058, 1988.

148. Kitterman JA, Liggins GC, Clements JA, Tooley WH: Stimulation of breathing movements in fetal sheep by inhibitors of prostaglandin synthesis. J. Dev. Physiol. 1:453, 1979.

149. Olsen GD, Dawes GS: Morphine effects on fetal lambs. Fed. Proc. 42:1251, 1983.

150. Carter AM: Factors affecting gas transfer across the placenta and the oxygen supply to the fetus. J. Dev. Physiol. 12:305, 1989.

151. Metcalfe J, Bartels H, Moll W: Gas exchange in the pregnant uterus. Physiol. Rev. 47:782, 1967.

152. Wulf H: The oxygen and carbon dioxide tension gradients in the human placenta at term. Am. J. Obstet. Gynecol. 88: 38, 1964.

153. Parker HR, Purves MJ: Some effects of maternal hyperoxia and hypoxia on the blood gas tensions and vascular pressures in the foetal sheep. Quart. J. Exp. Physiol. 52:205, 1967.

154. Friedman EA, Little WA, Sachtleben MR: Placental oxygen consumption in vitro. II. Total uptake as an index of placental function. Am. J. Obstet. Gynecol. 84:561, 1962.

155. Campbell AGM, Dawes GS, Fishman AP, Hyman AI, et al: Oxygen consumption of the placenta and foetal membranes in the sheep. J. Physiol. 182:439, 1966.

156. Power GG, Longo LD, Wagner HN Jr, Kuhl DE, et al: Uneven distribution of maternal and fetal placental blood flow, as demonstrated using macroaggregates, and its response to hypoxia. J. Clin. Invest. 46:2053, 1967.

157. Longo LD, Schwarz RH, Forster RE II: $O_2$ tensions of blood from uterine wall venules, maternal placental venules, and uterine vein. J. Appl. Physiol. 24:787, 1968.

158. Jansen CAM, Krane EJ, Thomas AL, Beck NFG, et al: Continuous variability of fetal $PO_2$ in the chronically catheterized fetal sheep. Am. J. Obstet. Gynecol. 134:776, 1979.

159. Sykes GS, Molloy PM, Wollner JC, Burton PJ, et al: Continuous, noninvasive measurement of fetal oxygen and carbon dioxide levels in labor by use of mass spectrometry. Am. J. Obstet. Gynecol. 150:847, 1984.

160. Lye SJ, Wlodek ME, Challis JRG: Relation between fetal arterial $PO_2$ and oxytocin-induced uterine contractions in pregnant sheep. Can. J. Physiol. Pharmacol. 62:1337, 1984.

161. Longo LD, Dale PS, Gilbert RD: Uteroplacental $O_2$ uptake: continuous measurements during uterine quiescence and contractions. Am. J. Physiol. 250:R1099, 1986.

162. Boyle JW, Lotgering FK, Longo LD: Acute embolization of the placental circulation: uterine blood flow and placental CO diffusing capacity. J. Dev. Physiol. 6:377, 1984.

163. Saling E: Micro blood pH determinations from fetal scalp. Z. Gerburtsh. Gynak. 161:262, 1963.

164. Saling E, Schneider D: Biochemical supervision of the foetus during labour. J. Obstet. Gynaec. Br. Commonw. 74: 799, 1967.

165. Beard RW, Morris ED, Clayton SG: pH of foetal capillary blood as an indicator of the condition of the foetus. J. Obstet. Gynaec. Br. Commonw. 74:812, 1967.

166. Parer JT: The current role of intrapartum fetal blood sampling. Clin. Obstet. Gynec. 23:565, 1980.

167. Antoine C, Silverman F, Young BK: Current status of continuous fetal pH monitoring. Clin. Perinatol. 9:409, 1982.

168. Lauersen NH, Miller FC, Paul RH: Continuous intrapartum monitoring of fetal scalp pH. Am. J. Obstet. Gynecol. 133: 44, 1979.

169. Huch A, Huch R, Schneider H, Rooth G: Continuous transcutaneous monitoring of fetal oxygen tension during labour. Br. J. Obstet. Gynaecol. 84 (Suppl1):4, 1977.

170. Althabe Jr O, Schwarcz RL, Pose SV, Escarcena L, et al: Effects on fetal heart rate and fetal $PO_2$ of oxygen administration to the mother. Am. J. Obstet. Gynecol. 98:858, 1967.

171. Battaglia FC, Meschia G, Makowski EL, Bowes W: The effect of maternal oxygen inhalation upon fetal oxygenation. J. Clin. Invest. 47:548, 1968.

172. Young DC, Popat R, Luther ER, Scott KE, et al: Influence of maternal oxygen administration on the term fetus before labor. Am. J. Obstet. Gynecol. 136:321, 1980.

173. Morishima HO, Daniel SS, Richards RT, James LS: The effect of increased maternal $PaO_2$ upon the fetus during labor. Am. J. Obstet. Gynecol. 123:257, 1975.

174. Khazin AF, Hon EH, Hehre FW: Effects of maternal hyperoxia on the fetus. I. Oxygen tension. Am. J. Obstet. Gynecol. 109:628, 1971.

175. Brady JP, Ceruti E: Chemoreceptor reflexes in the newborn infant: effect of varying degrees of hypoxia on heart rate and ventilation in a warm environment. J. Physiol. 184: 631, 1966.

176. Cross KS, Oppe TW: The effect of inhalation of high and low concentrations of oxygen on the respiration of the premature infant. J. Physiol. 117:38, 1952.

177. Karlberg P: The adaptive changes in the immediate postnatal period, with particular reference to respiration. J. Pediatr. 56:585, 1960.

178. Karlberg P, Adams FH, Geubelle F, Wallgren G: Alterations of the infant's thorax during vaginal delivery. Acta. Obstet. Gynecol. Scand. 41:223, 1962.

179. Karlberg P, Escardo F, Cherry RB, Lind J, et al: I. Studies on the respiration of the newborn in the first minutes of life. Acta. Paediatr. 46:396, 1957.

180. Karlberg P, Cherry RB, Escardo FE, Koch G: Respiratory studies in newborn infants. II. Pulmonary ventilation and mechanics of breathing in the first minutes of life, including the onset of respiration. Acta. Paediatr. 51:121, 1962.

181. Milner AD, Saunders RA: Pressure and volume changes during the first breath of human neonates. Arch. Dis. Child. 52:918, 1977.

182. Saunders RA, Milner AD: Pulmonary pressure/volume relationships during the last phase of delivery and the first postnatal breaths in human subjects. J. Pediatr. 93:667, 1978.

183. Vyas H, Milner AD, Hopkin IE: Intrathoracic pressure and volume changes during the spontaneous onset of respiration in babies born by cesarean section and by vaginal delivery. J. Pediatr. 99:787, 1981.

184. Mortola JP, Fisher JT, Smith JB, Fox GA, et al: Onset of

respiration in infants delivered by caesarean section. J. Appl. Physiol. 52:716, 1982.
185. Scarpelli EM, Agasso EJ, Kikkawa Y: Demonstration of the significance of pulmonary surfactants at birth. Respir. Physiol. 12:110, 1971.
186. Avery ME, Mead J: Surface properties in relation to atelectasis and hyaline membrane disease. Am. J. Dis. Child. 97: 517, 1959.
187. Brumley GW, Chernick V, Hodson WA, Normand C, et al: Correlations of mechanical stability, morphology, pulmonary surfactant, and phospholipid content in the developing lamb lung. J. Clin. Invest. 46:863, 1967.
188. Gribetz L, Frank NR, Avery ME: Static volume-pressure relations of excised lungs of infants with hyaline membrane disease newborn and stillborn infants. J. Clin. Invest. 38: 2168, 1959.
189. Gluck L, Kulovich MV, Eidelmar A, Cordero L, et al: Biochemical development of surface activity in mammalian lung. Pediatr. Res. 6:81, 1972.
190. Paintal AS: Vagal sensory receptors and their reflex effects. Physiol. Rev. 53:159, 1973.
191. Sellick H, Widdicombe JD: The activity of lung irritant receptors during pneumothorax, hyperpnia and pulmonary vascular congestion. J. Physiol. (Lond). 203:359, 1969.
192. Widdicombe JG: Respiratory reflexes: *In*: Handbook of Physiology. Respiration. Washington, DC, Am. Physiol. Soc., Sect. 3, Vol. I, Chapt. 24, 1964, p. 585.
193. Milner AD, Saunders RA, Hopkin IE: Tidal pressure/volume and flow/volume respiratory loop patterns in human neonates. Clin. Sci. Mol. Med. 54:257, 1978.
194. Mortola JP, Fisher JT, Smith B, Fox G, et al: Dynamics of breathing in infants. J. Appl. Physiol. 52:1209, 1982.
195. Radvanyi-Bouvet MF, Monset-Couchard M, Morel-Kahn F, Vincente G, et al: Expiratory patterns during sleep in normal full-term and premature neonates. Biol. Neonate 41: 74, 1982.
196. Olver RE, Strang LB: Ion fluxes across the pulmonary epithelium and the secretion of lung liquid in the foetal lamb. J. Physiol. 241:327, 1974.
197. Adamson TM, Brodecky V, Lambert TF, Maloney JE, et al: Lung liquid production and composition in the "in utero" foetal lamb. Aust. J. Exp. Biol. Med. Sci. 53:65, 1975.
198. Enhorning G, Chamberlain D, Contreras C, Burgoyne R, et al: Isoxsuprine-induced release of pulmonary surfactant in the rabbit fetus. Am. J. Obstet. Gynecol. 129:197, 1977.
199. Walters DW, Olver RE: The role of catecholamines in lung liquid absorption at birth. Pediatr. Res. 12:239, 1978.
200. Perks AM, Cassin S: The effects of arginine vasopressin and other factors on the production of lung liquid in fetal goats. Chest 81 (Suppl):63S, 1982.
201. Kitterman JA: Fetal lung development. J. Dev. Physiol. 6: 67, 1984.
202. Kitterman JA, Ballard PL, Clements JA, Mescher EJ, et al: Tracheal fluid in fetal lambs: spontaneous decrease prior to birth. J. Appl. Physiol. 47:985, 1979.
203. Bland RD, Bressack MA, McMillan DD: Labor decreases the lung water content of newborn rabbits. Am. J. Obstet. Gynecol. 135:364, 1979.
204. Bland RD, Hansen TN, Haberkeren CM, Bressack MA, et al: Lung fluid balance in lambs before and after birth. J. Appl. Physiol. 53:992, 1982.
205. Raj JU, Bland RD: Lung luminal liquid clearance in newborn lambs. Effect of pulmonary microvascular pressure elevation. Am. Rev. Resp. Dis. 134:305, 1986.
206. O'Brodovich H, Hannam V, Seear M, Mullen JBM: Amiloride impairs lung liquid clearance in newborn guinea pigs. J. Appl. Physiol. 68:1758, 1990
207. James LS: Physiologi adjustments at birth: effects of labor, delivery, and anesthesia on the newborn. Anesthesiology 26:501, 1965.
208. James LS, Adamsons K Jr: Respiratory physiology of the fetus and newborn infant. N. Engl. J. Med. 271:1352; 1403, 1964.
209. Mueller RA, Lundberg DBA, Breese GR, Hedner J, et al: The neuropharmacology of respiratory control. Pharmacol. Rev. 34:255, 1982.
210. Gerhardt T, Bancalari E: Apnea of prematurity: I. Lung function and regulation of breathing. Pediatrics 74:58, 1984.
211. Rigatto H, de la Torre Verduzco R, Cates DB: Effects of $O_2$ on the ventilatory response to $CO_2$ in preterm infants. J. Appl. Physiol. 39:896, 1975.
212. Cross KW, Klaus M, Tooley WH, Weisser K: The response of the newborn baby to inflation of the lungs. J. Physiol. 151:551, 1960.
213. Olinsky A, Bryan MH, Brayan AC: Influence of lung inflation on respiratory control in neonates. J. Appl. Physiol. 36: 426, 1974.
214. Gerhardt T, Bancalari E: Maturational changes of reflexes influencing respiratory timing in newborns. J. Appl. Physiol. 50:1282, 1981.
215. Drorbaugh JE, Segal S, Sutherland JM, Oppe TE, et al: Compliance of lung during first week of life. Am. J. Dis. Child. 105:63, 1963.
216. Gerhardt T, Bancalari E: Chestwall compliance in full-term and premature infants. Acta. Paediatr. Scand. 69:359, 1980.
217. Cook CD, Sutherland JM, Segal S, Cherry RB, et al: Studies of respiratory physiology in the newborn infant. III. Measurements of mechanics of respiration. J. Clin. Invest. 36: 440, 1957.
218. Cook CD, Cherry RB, O'Brien D, Karlberg P, et al: Studies of respiratory physiology in the newborn infant. I. Observation on normal premature and full-term infants. J. Clin. Invest. 34:975, 1955.
219. Oliver TK Jr, Demis JA, Bates GD: Serial blood-gas tensions and acid-base balance during the first hour in human infants. Acta. Paediatr. 50:346, 1961.
220. Nelson NM, Prod'hom S, Cherry RB, Lipsitz PJ, et al: Pulmonary function in the newborn: The alveolar-arterial oxygen gradient. J. Appl. Physiol. 18:534, 1963.
221. Romney SL, Reid DE, Metcalfe J, Burwell CS: Oxygen utilization by the human fetus in utero. Am. J. Obstet. Gynecol. 70:791, 1955.
222. Oliver TK Jr, Karlberg P: Gaseous metabolism in newly born human infants. Am. J. Dis. Child. 105:427, 1963.
223. Widdowson E: Chemical composition of newly born mammals. Nature 166:626, 1950.
224. Shelly HJ, Neligan GA: Neonatal hypoglycaemia. Br. Med. Bull. 22:34, 1966.
225. Devos P, Hers H: Glycogen metabolism in the liver of the fetal rat. Biochem. J. 140:331, 1974.
226. Allen D, Kornhauser D, Schwartz R: Glucose homeostasis in the newborn puppy. Am. J. Dis. Child. 112:343, 1966.
227. Novak M, Melichar V, Hahn P, Koldovsky O: Release of free fatty acids from adipose tissue obtained from newborn infants. J. Lipid. Res. 6:91, 1965.
228. Warshaw JB: Cellular energy metabolism during fetal development. IV. Fatty acid activation, acetyl transfer and fatty acid oxidation during development of the chick and rat. Dev. Biol. 28:537, 1972.
229. Foster P, Bailey E: Changes in the activities of the enzymes of hepatic fatty acid oxidation during fetal development of the rat. Biochem. J. 154:49, 1976.
230. McGarry JD, Robles-Valdes C, Foster DW: Role of carnitine

in hepatic ketogenesis. Proc. Natl. Acad. Sci. U.S.A. 72:4385, 1975.

231. Robles-Valdes C, McGarry D, Foster D: Maternal-fetal carnitine relationships and neonatal ketosis in the rat. J. Biol. Chem. 251:6007, 1976.

232. Tildon JT, Cone AL, Cornblath M: Coenzyme transferase activity in rat brain. Biochem. Biophys. Res. Commun. 43: 225, 1971.

233. Lindblad BS, Baldesten A: Time studies on free amino acid levels of venous plasma during the neonatal period. Acta. Paediatr. 58:252, 1969.

234. Karlberg P: Determination of standard energy metabolism (basal metabolism) in normal infants. Acta. Paediat. (Supp. 89) 41:1, 1952.

235. Cross KW, Tizard JPM, Trythall DAH: The gaseous metabolism of the newborn infant breathing 15% oxygen. Acta. Paediatr. Scand. 47:217, 1958.

236. Swyer PR: Heat loss after birth. *In* Temperature Regulation and Energy Metabolism in the Newborn. Edited by JS Sinclair. New York, Grune & Stratton, Inc., 1978, p. 91.

237. Hull D, Smales ORC: Heat loss after birth. *In* Temperature Regulation and Energy Metabolism in the Newborn. Edited by JS Sinclair. New York, Grune & Stratton, Inc., 1978, p.129.

238. Dahm LS, James LS: Newborn temperature: heat loss in the delivery room. Pediatrics 49:504, 1972.

239. Adamsons K Jr, Towell ME: Thermal homeostasis in the fetus and newborn. Anesthesiology 26:531, 1965.

240. Smith F, Robillard JE: Functional development of the fetal kidney. *In* Pediatric Nephrology: From Old to New Frontiers. Current Concepts in Diagnosis and Management. Edited by J Strauss, L Strauss. Coral Gables, FL, University of Miami Press, 1991, p. 15.

241. Kleinman LI: Developmental renal physiology. Physiologist 25:104, 1982.

242. Spitzer A: The developing kidney and the process of growth. *In* The kidney: Physiology and Pathophysiology Edited by. DW Seldin Gilbisch G. New York, Raven Press, 1985, p. 1979.

243. Rees L, Brook CGD, Forsling ML: Continuous urine collection in the study of vasopressin in the newborn. Hormone Res. 17:134, 1983.

244. Aperia A, Broberger O, Thodenius K, Zetterstrom R: Developmental study of the renal response to an oral salt load in preterm infants. Acta. Paediatr. Scand. 63:517, 1974.

245. Sulyok E, Heiem T, Soltesz G, Jaszai V: The influence of maturity on renal control of acidosis in newborn infants. Biol. Neonate 21:418, 1972.

246. Grand RJ, Watkins JB, Torti FM: Development of the human gastrointestinal tract: a review. Gastroenterology 70:790, 1976.

247. MacLean WC Jr, Fink BB: Lactose malabsorption by premature infants: magnitude and clinical significance. J. Pediatr. 97:458, 1980.

248. Sunshine P, Herbst JJ, Koldovsky O, Kretchmer N: Adaptation of the gastrointestinal tract to extrauterine life. Ann. NY. Acad. Sci. 176:16, 1971.

249. Deren JJ: Development of intestinal structure and function. *In* Handbook of Physiology. Vol. 3. Edited by CF Code. Baltimore, Waverly Press, Inc., 1968.

Chapter 8

# PLACENTAL TRANSFER OF ANESTHETICS AND RELATED DRUGS AND EFFECTS

JOHN M. BISSONNETTE

## INTRODUCTION

This chapter outlines the physiological principles that govern the transport of nutrients and other solutes between mother and fetus. Based on these principles, the transport of an individual solute can then be predicted from its known physical properties such as molecular size, lipid solubility, and ionic charge. More detailed discussion of placental physiology can be found in the monograph by Faber and Thornburg (1) and in recent reviews by Longo (2) and by Sibley and Boyd (3).

## DEFINITIONS

The term permeability is used to denote the number of molecules of a given solute that cross a defined area of a membrane during a defined time period under the conditions of a known concentration difference across the membrane. Permeability coefficients have the dimensions of a velocity and if the concentration of the solute is given in moles/ml, the area of the membrane in $cm^2$, and the time of transfer in seconds, then the unit of permeability would be cm/sec.

When dealing with a whole organ such as the placenta, the unit area available for transport is usually not known. Therefore, the term permeability is derived from the number of molecules that transfer per unit time per unit concentration difference, and it has the dimensions of ml/sec. It is often referred to as the permeability surface area product or P·S. In measurements of solute concentrations across complex organs such as the placenta it is difficult to estimate the true concentration difference because only inflow (arterial) and outflow (venous) samples are available for measurement. In many studies the term placental clearance (4) has been used to define the number of molecules that are transferred per unit time divided by the concentration difference between the maternal uterine artery and the fetal umbilical artery. The units for clearance are the same as those for the permeability surface area product.

A deviation from the above definitions takes place when the solute in question is a respiratory gas. Instead of moles/ml the concentration differences across the placenta are expressed as partial pressure, with units of mmHg and the amount transferred per unit time, given as ml/min. The resultant expression of permeability of a respiratory gas is the diffusing capacity of the placenta and its units are ml/min/mm Hg. It is customary to express the volume of respiratory gas that crosses the placenta in terms of standard temperature and pressure dry (STPD).

Two other terms have gained common usage in discussions of relative permeability of the placenta: flow-limited and diffusion-limited. The term "flow-limited" really means "not limited by diffusion" (1) and is applied to solutes whose permeability across the placenta is such that there is complete equilibration in concentration between the maternal and fetal blood. An increase in permeability for such a solute would result in equilibration at an earlier time during transit, but would not lead to any increase in the concentration in the fetal blood. Thus, the arteriovenous difference would not be altered by an increase in permeability for the solute in question. Because the amount transferred to the fetus is the product of umbilical blood flow and arteriovenous difference between the umbilical vessels, any increase in permeability would not result in a change in the amount transferred. However, an increase in flow would result in an increase in the amount of solute transferred.

At the other end of the spectrum of solute permeabilities is that there is very little decrease in concentration in the maternal blood, producing a small arteriovenous difference. In this situation any change in blood flow would not result in a change in the amount of solute transferred across the placenta. This situation has been termed "diffusion-limited" although it really means "not limited by flow" (1).

### Methodologies in the Study of Placental Transport

#### *In Vivo Methodologies*

In large animal studies the amount of solute transferred can be measured by application of the Fick principle, found in Figure 8–1. The major potential limitation of this approach is that not all uterine blood flow is placental blood flow; the latter can be determined using labeled microspheres. In addition, one must be reasonably assured that the concentration of the solute in question measured in the uterine vein represents that leaving the placenta, that is, that there is no significant admixture from venous blood representative of nonplacental uterine tissues. The Fick principle applied to placental transport also assumes that the solute under study is not metabolized or otherwise sequestered in the placenta itself. For

$$\frac{Q}{t} = K\frac{A(Cm - Cf)}{D}$$

**Fig. 8–1.** Fick's Law of Diffusion. *Q/t* is the rate of diffusion (quantity per unit time), *A* is the surface area, *Cm* is the maternal blood concentration, *Cf* is the fetal blood circulation, *D* is the thickness of the membrane, and K the diffusion constant of the drug.

nutrients such as glucose this is a significant fraction (5,6). To determine the amount of metabolized solutes transferred to the fetus, the Fick principle must be applied to the concentration difference between the umbilical vein and artery and umbilical blood flow.

In smaller animals, placental transport can be estimated by introducing a labeled solute into the maternal circulation and then obtaining serial samples in the mother's arterial blood. A single sample is obtained in fetal blood. The amount transferred to the fetus is the product of the concentration in fetal blood and the volume of distribution in the fetus. The permeability surface area product can then be calculated from the amount transported divided by the concentration differences between mother and fetus, integrated over time. This method can only be used for solutes in which a wide maternal-to-fetal gradient scan is maintained over the period of time the study is performed. The method has been used to study transport in the human (7,8).

An attempt is often made to estimate placental transport from single samples taken from the mother and from cord blood. The results are then expressed as a percentage of the maternal level and inferences made concerning the effectiveness of transfer across the placenta. Substances in which the fetal concentration is a significant percentage of the maternal are considered to be transferred efficiently. However, as shown in Figure 8–2, the time at which the two samples are taken with respect to the time at which the test solute is introduced in the maternal circulation is very critical. Very different conclusions with respect to placental transfer will be obtained from data gathered at different sampling times.

## In Vitro Methodologies

Perfusion of the human placenta in vitro has been used for some time to study transport mechanisms (9,10). The current studies employ circulations both through the fetal umbilical vessels, often to only one cotyledon, and also through the maternal intervillous space (11,12). These type of studies can shed information on transfer across the entire placenta. In an effort to gain insight into basic membrane transport at a cellular and molecular level investigations have recently turned to isolated plasma membrane vesicles from human placenta. Methods have been described for the isolation of both the maternal or microvillous plasma membrane (13) and also the fetal or basal (14) membrane of the human trophoblast. Studies with these membrane vesicles can precisely control the solute composition on either side of the membrane to examine the specificity of uptake for a given solute. Knowledge of basic mechanisms gained from the study of isolated plasma membranes can then be used to reconstruct the picture of transport across the intact trophoblast cell as it occurs in vivo (15).

Certain questions of placental transport such as the effect of hormone regulation on transfer of a particular nutrient may require the entire trophoblast cell rather than its isolated plasma membrane. Methods have been developed for the isolation of intact sealed human trophoblasts (16). It would be a significant advance if these isolated trophoblast cells could become confluent in cell culture such that they could be studied in plastic chambers and transport monitored from one side to the other. A preliminary report has indicated that this may be possible (17). In the past much effort was devoted to the study of human chorioamniotic membranes mounted in plastic chambers. However, it is now recognized that while transport across this tissue has some significance with respect to the regulation of amniotic fluid volume, it contributes little information with respect to transport across the trophoblast.

## Transport of Specific Solutes

### *Respiratory Gases*

#### Oxygen

As outlined above, the volume of oxygen transferred into the umbilical circulation can be obtained in animal studies from measured oxygen content values in the umbilical vein and that in the umbilical artery and then multiplying this value by the umbilical blood flow. Such studies are obviously not possible in man. However, an estimate of the oxygen taken up by the fetus has been made in humans. These studies consist of determining oxygen consumption of the pregnant women at term, usually under anesthesia just before cesarean section. After the infant is delivered, the maternal oxygen consumption measurement, made from the subjects' expired air, is repeated. The difference represents the oxygen consumption of the fetus. Care must be taken to make the repeat measurement rapidly so that placental oxygen consumption is still intact. Such studies reveal that fetal oxygen consumption is about 8 ml/kg fetal weight per minute or about 24 ml/min for a 3.0 kg fetus (2). Dividing this value for oxygen transferred across the placenta by the mean partial pressure gradient across the organ will yield the diffusing capacity of the placenta. However, because there is approximately a 55 mm Hg fall in $PO_2$ from uterine artery to uterine vein (2,18,19) and a 8 to 10 mm Hg rise from umbilical artery to umbilical vein, the mean gradient will differ depending on the conceptual model one assumes from these changes in oxygen tension. The gradient will be large (resulting in a relatively smaller diffusing capacity) if a linear change in $PO_2$ is used, and it will be small (resulting in a relatively larger diffusing capacity) if an exponential change in $PO_2$ is assumed. Because of the ambiguity of these attempts in defining the diffusing capacity of the placenta from oxygen measurements studies have been performed using carbon monoxide (20,21). Carbon monoxide has an affinity for the erythrocyte,

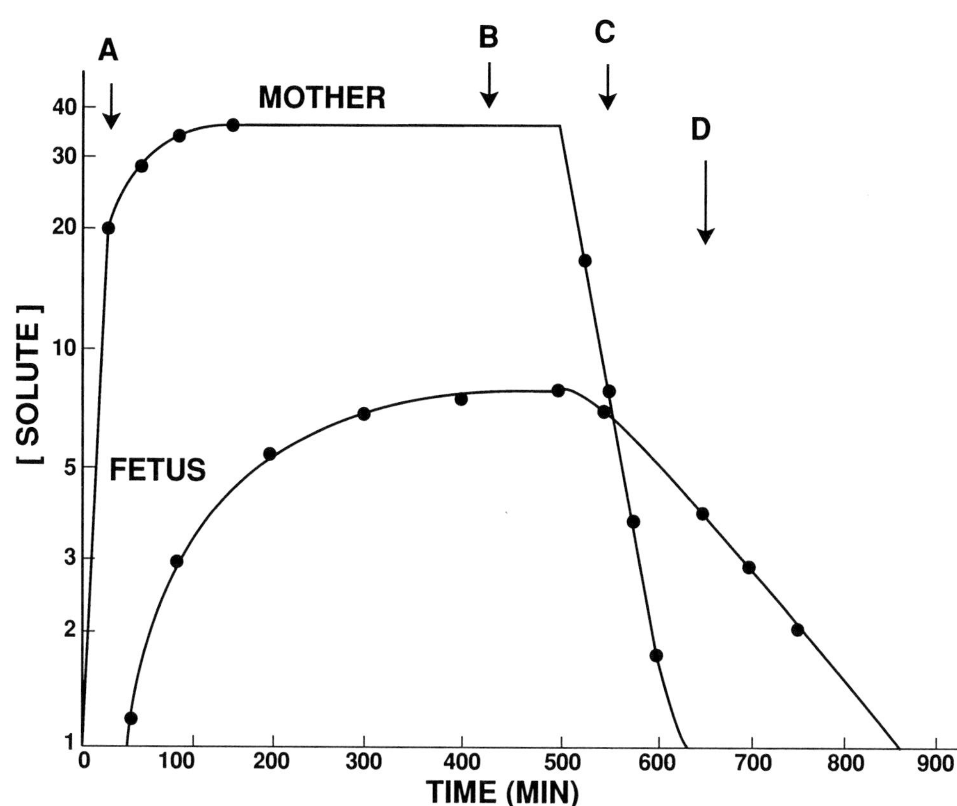


**Fig. 8–2.** Relationship of sampling time to interpretation of maternal-fetal transport across the placenta. Hypothetical data shown for a solute which in the steady state has a relatively low placental transport. Single samples at time A in maternal and fetal blood (umbilical cord blood at delivery) would lead to the conclusion that the placenta is impermeable to this solute. Sampling at point B would lead to the proper interpretation that the solute is relatively permeable and fetal levels are about one-fourth of those in the mother at steady state conditions (note log scale of the Y-axis). Blood obtained at point C would lead to the conclusion that the placenta is freely permeable to the solute, and sampling at point D would be interpreted as evidence for active transport from mother to fetus. (Adapted from Anderson DF, Phernetton TM and Rankin JHG: Prediction of fetal drug concentrations. Am. J. Obstet. Gynecol. 137:735, 1980.)

which is in excess of two-hundred-fold that of oxygen. Because it is so tightly bound there is very little change in carbon monoxide tension from artery to vein on the maternal side or from vein to artery on the fetal side of the placenta. Thus, the partial pressure gradient is little influenced by choice of models for carbon monoxide tension changes as blood passes through the placenta.

Diffusing capacity of the placenta measured with carbon monoxide can then be used to estimate how close blood in the fetal villus comes to being in equilibrium with the tension of maternal blood in the intervillous space. These estimates predict that the two bloods should have an identical partial pressure. Despite these calculations, actual measurements either between the uterine vein or the maternal intervillous space and the umbilical vein show an 8 to 10 mm Hg gradient for oxygen (18,19,22). Factors other than a diffusional limitation for oxygen account for this measured gradient. These include oxygen consumption by the placenta that may account for one-half the total oxygen that leaves the maternal circulation across the uterus (23), shunting in both the uterine and umbilical circulations and, most importantly, uneven maternal relative to fetal flow ratios analogous to uneven ventilation perfusion in the lung (24). Because oxygen comes either to complete equilibrium or nearly so between maternal and fetal blood, uterine blood flow is an important factor in regulating oxygen supply to the fetus. Situations that result in a fall in uterine blood flow will cause a fall in oxygen delivery to the fetus. However, it has been suggested that uterine blood flow must fall significantly before fetal oxygen consumption is affected (25).

### *Carbon Dioxide*

Despite its greater solubility in both blood and lipids compared to oxygen, there also exists a measured $PCO_2$ gradient between fetal blood and that in the intervillous space (26). The reasons for this are similar to those listed above for oxygen, especially carbon dioxide production by the trophoblast itself. Carbon dioxide could in theory be transferred from fetus to mother as bicarbonate as well as dissolved $CO_2$. However, experiments in which carbonic anhydrase was used to block $CO_2$ release from $HCO_3$ showed that it is physically dissolved $CO_2$, which accounts for the exchange across the placenta with little contribution from bicarbonate (27). However, in the perfused human placenta it has been shown that over a short time period (30 minutes) of maternal metabolic acidosis, bicarbonate derived from the placental tissues can buffer the fetus against changes in pH (28).

## ***Nutrients***

### *Glucose*

As with most lipid insoluble nutrients, glucose gains entrance to syncytiotrophoblast from the maternal intervillous space by means of plasma membrane spanning or integral membrane proteins. These proteins, termed glucose transporters, have recently been characterized to a considerable extent. They are thought to form a water-filled channel that has a certain specificity for various carbohydrates. Thus D-glucose, 2-deoxy-D-glucose, and 3-0-methyl-D-glucose are transported well, D-galactose less so, and D-fructose, L-glucose and L-xylose virtually not transported by these proteins (29,30).

The molecular nature of the glucose transporter is understood to a certain extent. In its glycosylated form it has a molecular weight of approximately 52,000 (16,29). There are 12 membrane spanning domains that together form the channel through which the sugars are transported (31). There is a family of genes that encode these glucose transporters, two of which, located on chromosomes 1 and 12, are abundantly expressed in the human placenta (32,33). In human fibroblasts, insulin increases the transcription of the glucose transporter gene (34) and in rat glial cells the gene is repressed by hyperglycemia and stimulated by hypoglycemia at physiological concentrations (35). It is not known whether insulin or plasma glucose levels influence the expression of the glucose transporter gene in the placenta.

The glucose transporter in the placenta enables sugar to be translocated across this organ at least 50 times what would be seen if transport were based on the physical characteristics of glucose alone (29,30,36). The transporter is half-saturated at glucose levels of about 100 mg/dl (37), thus during hypertonic infusions of glucose into the mother the fetus does not reach the same elevated glucose levels as seen in the maternal circulation (38). The presence of integral membrane proteins within the trophoblast on both its maternal surface and also on the fetal surface (39) results in a mechanism with potential for regulation of sugar transport from mother to fetus. In contrast to amino acids (see below) the entry of glucose into the trophoblast cell is not coupled to sodium so that there is no mechanism whereby glucose can be concentrated in the placenta (29,30). In a number of tissues, including human fat cells, insulin causes a significant increase in the rate of glucose uptake (40). This stimulation, which occurs within minutes at physiological temperature, is due to the translocation of intracellular vesicles, which contain glucose transporter, to the plasma membrane where they can increase glucose entry. It is to be distinguished from the longer term (hours) effect of insulin on the genes that encode the glucose transporter referred to above. In human placenta, however, insulin does not result in a stimulation of glucose transport on a short term basis (16,29).

### *Lactate*

In contrast to glucose less is known about the mechanisms of membrane transport for the three carbon solute lactate. However, carrier mechanisms that distinguish L-lactate from D-lactate are present at both the maternal and fetal surfaces of the trophoblast (41,42). L-lactate is transferred to a greater extent than D-lactate although the magnitude of this facilitated diffusion is much less than that seen for D-glucose, indicating that passive diffusion accounts for a considerable portion of lactate transport (42). In addition to the net transfer of lactate from mother to fetus or fetus to mother, there is also a considerable contribution of lactate that originates in the trophoblast and is then secreted into the maternal and fetal circulations (6,28,43). Despite the demonstration that when lactate transfer is measured from maternal-to-fetal circulations or in the opposite direction the rates are similar, lactate secretion by the trophoblast itself is predominantly in the maternal direction (6,28,43). The maternal-facing trophoblast plasma membrane has an $H^+$-lactate cotransporter that under the usual conditions of intracellular pH lower than extracellular would function to eliminate lactate into the maternal circulation (44). The secretion of lactate by the trophoblast is not an index of anaerobic metabolism, as the oxygen uptake of the placenta is quite high in fact, comparable to that of the brain (23).

### *Amino Acids*

The concentration of many amino acids is higher in fetal than in maternal plasma under steady state conditions (45,46). This is accomplished by plasma membrane transporters in which the transport of the amino acid is coupled to sodium (Figure 8–3). Because sodium levels in the trophoblast are much lower than in the maternal intervillous space due to the presence of $Na^+$-$K^+$-ATPase on the basal or fetal side of the cell (47), sodium runs down its concentration gradient into the placental cells. This sodium-dependent uptake of amino acids allows the intracellular concentration to rise above that in the maternal circulation. The amino acids then move from this concentrated intracellular level to the lower concentration present in fetal plasma. There are at least three separate transport systems for amino acids in the placenta. Among the 20 amino acids some use more than one transport system. Although there are regulatory factors that influ-

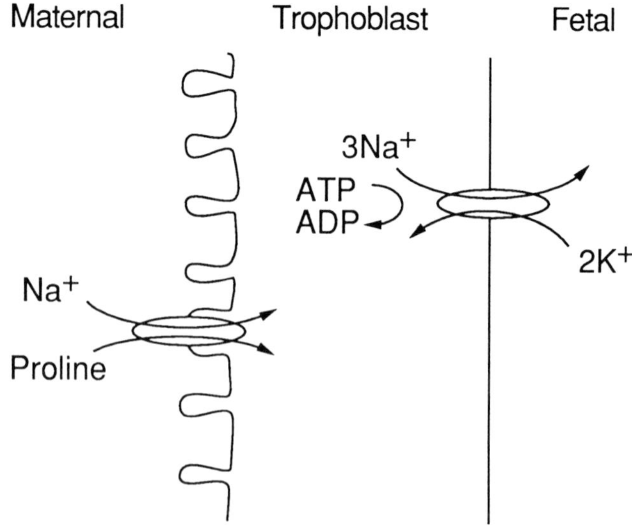


**Fig. 8–3.** Placental transfer of amino acids. A sodium-driven amino acid co-transporter drives proline such that trophoblast concentrations exceed those of the maternal blood. The low intracellular sodium concentration is maintained by $Na^+$-$K^+$ ATPase on the basal side of the trophoblast.

ence some of the amino acid systems, they are not influenced by insulin (48).

Alanine, proline, serine, and glycine are transported by the sodium-dependent alanine (A) system (49). This system at the interface with maternal blood accounts for two-thirds of the total transport of alanine. The remainder is divided between the leucine (L) system and diffusion with a negligible contribution from the alanine, sernine, and cysteine (ASC) system (48,50). The alanine system is regulated such that it is enhanced by preincubation of placental slices in vitro by a mechanism that requires the synthesis of protein (51,52). In addition, the presence of elevated intracellular concentrations of the amino acids which use system alanine inhibits transport (49). In combination these two methods in vivo probably result in a stable level of amino acid concentration within the trophoblast and buffer the fetus against fluctuating levels in maternal plasma.

The L amino acid uptake system is used by leucine, phenylalanine, valine, and isoleucine (49). It is not sodium dependent and does not have regulatory control as seen for the alanine system. In the microvillous plasma membrane of the trophoblast that is in contact with the maternal intervillous space, there is both a high-affinity and low-affinity component to this system (50). The high-affinity transport system is used by amino acids with hydrophobic side chains, while the low-affinity system is used by serine and alanine.

The third amino acid transport system, termed alanine, serine, and cysteine, is used by alanine, serine, cysteine, and threonine. It is sodium dependent but not regulated by intracellular amino acid concentrations (49). This system is localized to the basal or fetal side of the trophoblast (50).

## *Cholesterol, Triglycerides, and Free Fatty Acids*

The placenta requires a considerable amount of cholesterol for the synthesis of progesterone and other steroids. In addition, cholesterol is also transported to the fetus (53). The maternal-facing microvillous membrane of placental trophoblast has binding sites for both low-density (LDL) and very-low-density lipoproteins (VLDL). However, there is preferential binding due to a much higher affinity constant for very-low-density lipoproteins (54), thus, cholesterol associated with apoliproprotein E entry via receptor-mediated endocytosis (55) may be the major route into the placenta. Subsequent steps in transport to the fetus at the molecular level are not completely understood.

The relative contribution of the very-low-density lipoproteins receptor and entry as triglyceride compared to transport across the lipid bilayer of the cell membrane for free fatty acids are unknown. With respect to free fatty acids, placental transfer is strongly influenced by the length of the fatty acid carbon chain (Figure 8–4). Placental transfer is sharply increased with a shortening of carbon chain length for fatty acids between 8 and 16 carbons (56,57). This is due to a decrease in binding to albumin over this range. Although protein binding continues to decrease for fatty acids of 6 and 4 carbons, the rate of

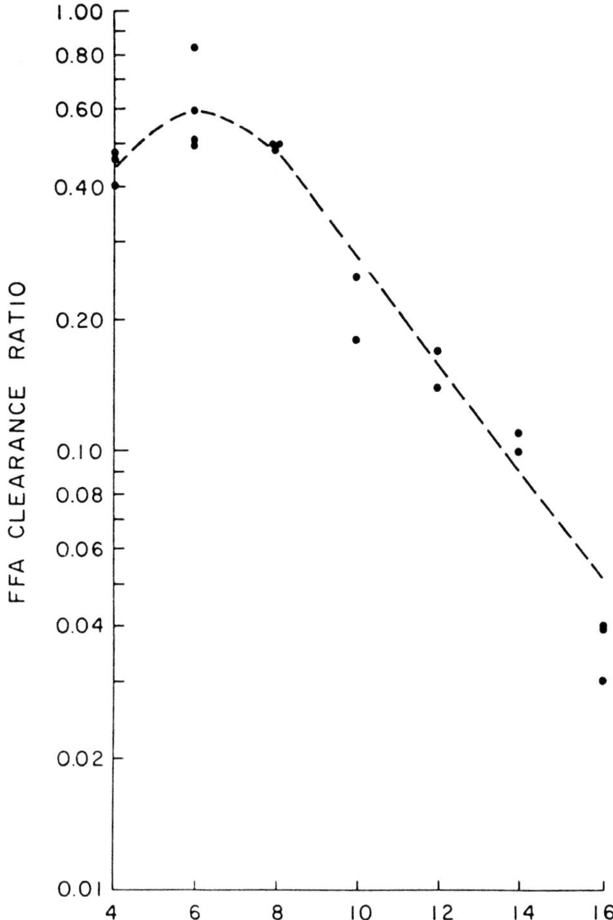


**Fig. 8–4.** This figure shows that placental transfer is affected by the FFA chain length. This placenta was perfused with FFA and antipyrine. Note the significantly increased clearance ratio of the small chain lengths as opposed to the long chain lengths, especially in lieu of fact that the vertical ordinate is a logarithmic scale. (From Dancis J, Jansen V, Levitz M: Transfer across perfused human placenta. IV. Effect of protein binding on free fatty acids. Pediatr. Res. 10:5, 1976.

placental transfer decreases. This is due to the fact that although they are more easily released from albumin they are less lipid soluble, which retards their movement through the lipid bilayer (56,57). These principles of protein binding and relative hydrophilic nature may well govern the placental transfer of other solutes.

## *Nonelectrolytes*

The placental transport of solutes, which do not have specialized systems such as exist for ions or nutrients, is governed by their lipid solubility and molecular size. In using only these two criteria, it is understood that the solute in question is not bound to any plasma protein, does not have a protein or other binding site in the trophoblast cell, and is not metabolized by the trophoblast. For solutes that are insoluble in lipids, placental transport over the molecular weight range from 180 to 5200 daltons appears to be directly proportional to the free diffusion of these molecules in water (Figure 8–5) (7,8,58).

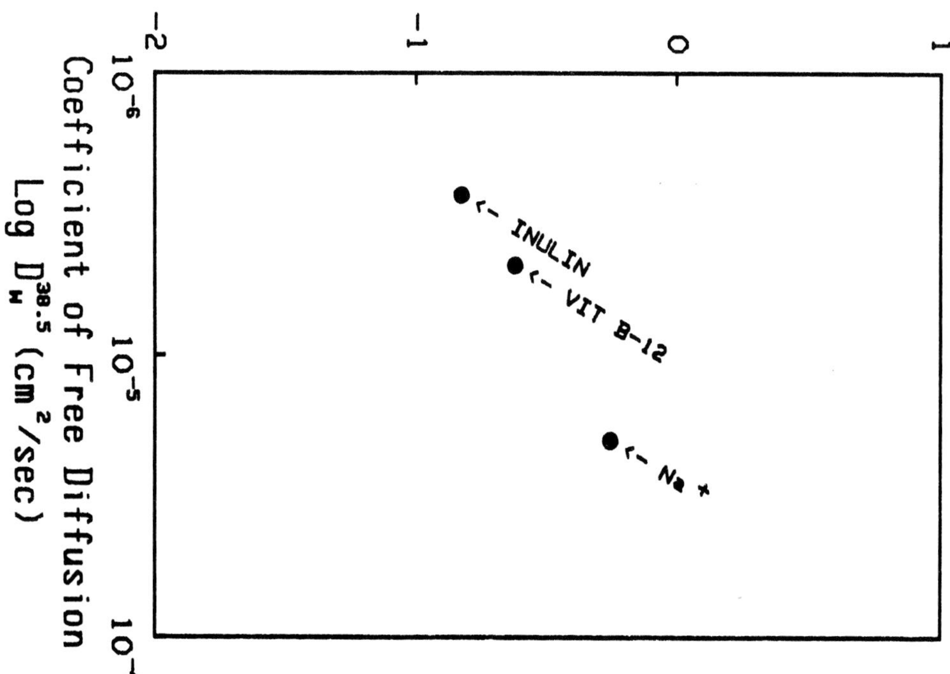


**Fig. 8–5.** Permeability across the human placenta as a function of the coefficient of free diffusion in water. Note log scale for both axes of this figure. Molecular weights range from 23 to 5,000 daltons. (From Willis DM, O'Grady JP, Faber JJ, Thornburg KL: Diffusion permeability of cyanocobalamin in human placenta. Am. J Physiol. 250:R459, 1986; and Thornburg KL, Burry KJ, Adams AK, Kirk EP, et al: Permeability of placenta to inulin. Am. J. Obstet. Gynecol. 158:1165, 1988.)

That is, there is no physiological evidence for pores or channels that would hinder transport over this size range. However, there is preliminary evidence that the rate of transport across the microvillous membrane vesicles of the human placenta is much restricted compared to the in vivo measurements across the intact placenta (59). This would imply that there is considerable transport by means of a paracellular route. Because the trophoblast forms a syncytium, the anatomic nature of this route remains to be established.

Lipid solubility is an important factor for the placental transport of many solutes. Ethanol is transferred almost 10 times the rate of urea (60) due to its considerable lipid solubility in spite of the fact that their molecular weights are similar.

### *Ions*

Ion transport across the placenta may take place by a number of routes. In addition to simple diffusion across cell membranes or especially by paracellular routes, there are a variety of specific mechanisms attributable to transcellular membrane proteins. These consist of cotransport systems such as described above for sodium and certain amino acids, in which the ion moves across the membrane coupled to its cotransported solute, which may be another ion. These are sometimes termed symports. An alternate system involves the exchange of one ion for another such that one moves out of the cell at the same time as its exchange ion is moving in. These systems are termed antiports. In addition to these types of carriers there are also ion-specific channels for sodium, chloride, potassium, and calcium. These channels can now be studied using single cell patch pipette methods (61). To date only a preliminary description of the potassium and chloride channels in first trimester placental cells is available (62). However, because in their open state these channels can pass at least $6 \times 10^6$ monovalent ions/sec (61), their contribution to intracellular ion composition of the trophoblast is very important. In contrast the turnover number for the ion carrier $Na^+$-$K^+$-ATPase is $5 \times 10^2$/sec (61).

Under steady state conditions, if the sum of all carriers and channels for ions is such that an excess of either cations or anions were present on the fetal side of the trophoblast with respect to the maternal, a transplacental membrane potential would exist. This membrane potential would then serve to either attract or repel charged solutes depending on their net charge. The question of the magnitude and even the sign of a transplacental potential difference in human placenta is at present unsettled (3). There is more agreement with respect to the existence of a potential difference between the interior of the trophoblast and the bath solution in vitro, which would correspond to the maternal intervillous space. This potential difference appears to be about 30 mV, the interior of the cell being negative (63). The potential difference is maintained to a considerable extent by $Na^+$-$K^+$-ATPase but not exclusively by this ion pump. Extracellular potassium is more important than sodium for the maintenance of the transcellular potential difference in trophoblast (63).

### *Sodium*

In vitro studies of whole placentas show a small net movement of sodium toward the fetus. This net sodium uptake by the fetal compartment is enhanced by β-adrenergics and inhibited by blocking $Na^+$-$K^+$-ATPase (64). The placental β-adrenergic receptors are localized on the fetal facing or basal side of the trophoblast (65). In addition to $Na^+$-$K^+$-ATPase, which exchanges three intracellular $Na^+$ ions for two extracellular $K^+$ and is predominantly localized on the basal aspect of the trophoblast (47), there are at least three $Na^+$ carriers on the microvillous or maternal-facing side of the cell. One of these is the sodium amino acid cotransport system described above. The microvilli also contain a sodium-phosphate cotransporter that translocates two sodium ions for each phosphate radical, resulting in a positively charged complex (66). Because the inside of the cell is negative (see above) the uptake of sodium and phosphate by this carrier is enhanced. In addition, there is a sodium-proton antiport in trophoblast microvilli in which one $Na^+$ enters for each $H^+$ that leaves the microvillous cytosol. Inhibition of this $Na^+$-$H^+$ exchanger in the absence of amino acids eliminates the majority of sodium transport across the maternal-facing side of the trophoblast (67).

### *Chloride*

In addition to the presence of chloride channels mentioned above the placenta has at least one chloride carrier. This is a chloride-anion exchanger that is present in the microvillous membrane and accounts for approximately half of the chloride flux into the placenta from the maternal intervillous space (68). The mechanisms involved in chloride transport on the fetal side of the cell have not been studied.

### *Potassium*

As noted by Sibley and Boyd, there is evidence that fetal plasma potassium levels are maintained in the presence of maternal hypokalemia, though the mechanism is unclear (3). The basal side of the trophoblast does contain $Na^+$-$K^+$-ATPase (47) and potassium channels with high conductances have been demonstrated in human placental cells (62). However, an integrated picture of transmembrane or transplacental potassium homeostasis is not available at present.

### *Calcium*

Fetal plasma calcium levels exceed those of the mother (69). In addition, the level of free calcium within the trophoblast must be kept at nanomolar concentrations, in contrast to the millimolar levels in fetal and maternal blood. At least two mechanisms are involved with these processes. The placenta contains a specific calcium binding protein composed of 70,000 molecular weight dimers (69). This enables sequestration of calcium that enters at the maternal face. The fetal or basal membrane of the trophoblast contains an ATP-dependent calcium pump, which has a high affinity (100 nM) for free calcium. This calcium pump is magnesium dependent up to concentrations of 5 mM. At higher magnesium concentrations, activity of the pump is suppressed (70). The calcium-dependent regulatory protein calmodulin enhances the activity

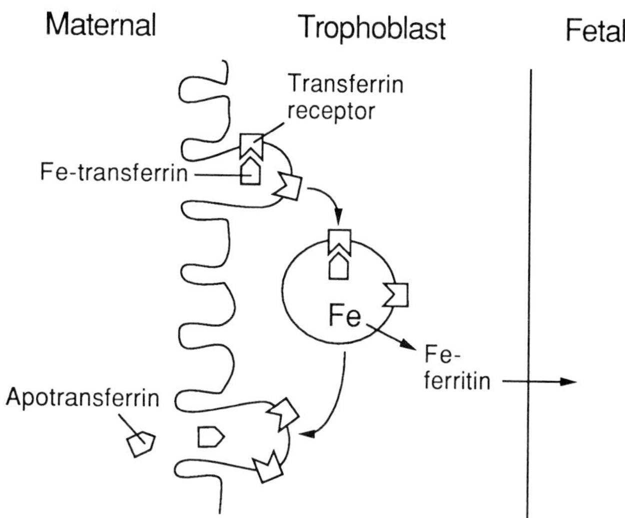


**Fig. 8–6.** Placental transfer of iron. Iron coupled to transferrin is internalized after binding to the transferrin receptor. In the endosome it dissociates from transferrin and is coupled to ferritin. Apotransferrin is recycled to the maternal surface. (Modified from Douglas GC, King BF: Uptake and processing of 125I-labeled transferrin and 59Fe-labeled transferrin by isolated human trophoblast cells. Placenta. 11:41, 1990.)

of this calcium ATPase at physiological concentrations (70). The basal location of this calcium transporter is in keeping with the observed high levels of calcium in fetal blood.

### *Iron*

Unlike the ions discussed above, iron is carried in plasma bound to the protein transferrin. Because iron is a major essential fetal nutrient, mechanisms must be available for its transport across the placenta (Figure 8–6). Transferrin receptors are present on the maternal face of the placenta (71). After binding transferrin, the receptor ligand complex is internalized where, influenced by the hydrogen ion environment of the cell, transferrin is released and returned to the maternal surface of the cell as apotransferrin, that is, without divalent iron (72,73). Although the basal or fetal aspect of the trophoblast contains transferrin, its affinity for apotransferrin, like the receptor at the maternal face, is much less than that for transferrin. Thus, basal receptors are not likely to internalize apotransferrin, which could in turn pick up cytosolic iron for delivery to the fetus (73)

## FETAL DRUG DISTRIBUTION, TISSUE UPTAKE, AND EXCRETION

When a drug is administered to the mother, a certain amount of it is transmitted to the fetus; the response of the fetus is dependent upon the amount of the drug that reaches it. Since the fetus is completely sustained physiologically by the mother via the uteroplacental unit, there is no real jeopardy in regard to oxygenation and ventilation unless the fetal cardiac output is reduced enough to cause respiratory embarrassment with resultant hypoxia, hypercarbia, and acidosis. The latter may follow fetal cardiac depression or rhythm disturbances, both of which reduce fetal output from the heart. In fact, the only two organ systems that experience major impact are the central nervous system, which at low drug levels experiences depression, and at higher levels experiences stimulation or seizure activity, and the heart, which at low plasma levels exhibits bradycardia, and at higher levels exhibits heart block and electromechanical dissociation. The global impact upon the fetus due to either stimulation or depression of the central nervous system is minimal; however, the same is not true of the impact on the myocardium. Because the fetal heart serves as the only generator for exchange of blood at the uteroplacental interface, significant changes in its effectiveness can have major global impact. Specifically, as noted above, a reduction in fetal cardiac output for extended periods can result in both hypoxia, due to ineffective oxygenation, and hypercarbia, due to poor ventilation. These alterations can lead first to respiratory acidosis, and then to metabolic acidosis.

Naturally, the neonatal response to a particular drug must also be considered. The neonatal response will be similar to that of the mother, and depends chiefly on the concentration of the drug in the plasma, the regional blood flow, the tissue solubility of the drug, and the effective excretory rate of the drug. The added physiologic embarrassment to the neonate is, once again, depression of the respiratory system, with possible resultant hypoxia and hypercarbia, and depression of the myocardium.

### Fetal Circulation

Once a drug traverses the placenta and arrives at the fetus, a complex array of mixing of blood from various fetal compartments occurs. A familiar illustration, Figure 8–7 from the first edition, is still applicable today and should be referred to in order to understand two important dilutional pathways that go into play immediately. One is that the large majority of blood, nearly 85%, funnels directly into the liver and its drug concentration is thus immediately reduced due to some hepatic absorption. The second is that the remainder of the blood, some 15%, bypasses the liver and enters the inferior vena cava directly by way of the ductus venosus. This blood is immediately diluted with blood coming from both lower extremities of the fetus and regional blood flow from the viscera.

The total amount of drug reaching a fetal organ or tissue during a given period is directly related to the organ's blood supply. Because the brain is a highly vascular organ, initially it receives a larger amount than most other tissues. The heart is also a highly vascularized organ, thus it also receives a larger proportion of drug after initial exposure. Because of the distribution phase, these high drug levels in the fetal brain and heart decrease over time as redistribution to other fetal organs occurs. It is important to keep in mind that drug pharmacokinetics in the fetus are the same as in the adult organism in that they are governed by the four basic principles of uptake, distribution, biotransformation, and excretion. In the distribution phase drug levels will change over time according to the following priority: (1) highest vascularized group; (2) muscle rich group; (3) vessel poor group; and (4) fat.

### Absorption

To present an effective rate of absorption a drug must first reach the target system in substantial amounts. In the case of the fetus this is accomplished by the fact that the four most prioritized organs for distribution are the brain, the heart, the kidney, and the liver/placenta. The actual entry rate of that drug, however, is governed by other important pharmacokinetic mechanisms, such as those listed in Table 8–1. Because the brain acts essentially as a lipid barrier, the drug entry rate is determined by its lipid solubility and unionization ratio; there is an increase in the blood-brain barrier permeability in neonates. Protein binding also decreases a drug's permeability to the blood-brain barrier because the large protein molecules do not pass readily. Last, but not least, permeability to drugs is also increased with conditions of hypoxia and/or hypercarbia.

### Excretion

Both fetal and neonatal drug excretion are important in relation to the overall drug impact. Fetal excretion is by both the kidneys and the placenta, the latter of which serves as the fetal liver in utero. The placenta serves as the most important fetal excretory pathway because large volumes of blood turn over in a rapid fashion. Furthermore, this pathway is naturally time-dependent because as the mother's drug concentration decreases, the fetal transfer to the mother is enhanced, and it is clear that redistribution back to the mother occurs, as depicted in period D of Figure 8–2. If fetal myocardial compromise occurs this important excretory pathway can be limited due to the reduced flow of blood volume to the placenta; such compromise can also reduce renal blood flow and thus impede excretion by this route.

Neonatal drug excretion is primarily by the renal route. Pulmonary excretion can also occur, but is important only in instances of volatile anesthetics, such as $N_2O$ and enflurane, isoflurane, or desflurane. If minute ventilation is depressed after birth, this method of excretion can be significantly affected and thus result in continued and prolonged respiratory embarrassment with reduced $O_2$ and elevated $CO_2$ levels.

### Drug Metabolism

Drug metabolism by the fetus is the key method of its limiting the effect and duration of a given drug. There has been some question as to the effectiveness of the fetal biotransformation process because certain catabolic enzymes may be deficient. It would appear from recent studies that preterm fetuses, as opposed to term fetuses, have different cardiovascular adaptive capacities when challenged with local anesthetics in conditions of threatened asphyxia (74,75). Metabolic enzyme system activity is present shortly after birth and it equals adult enzyme activity around 8 weeks after delivery. The immaturity of

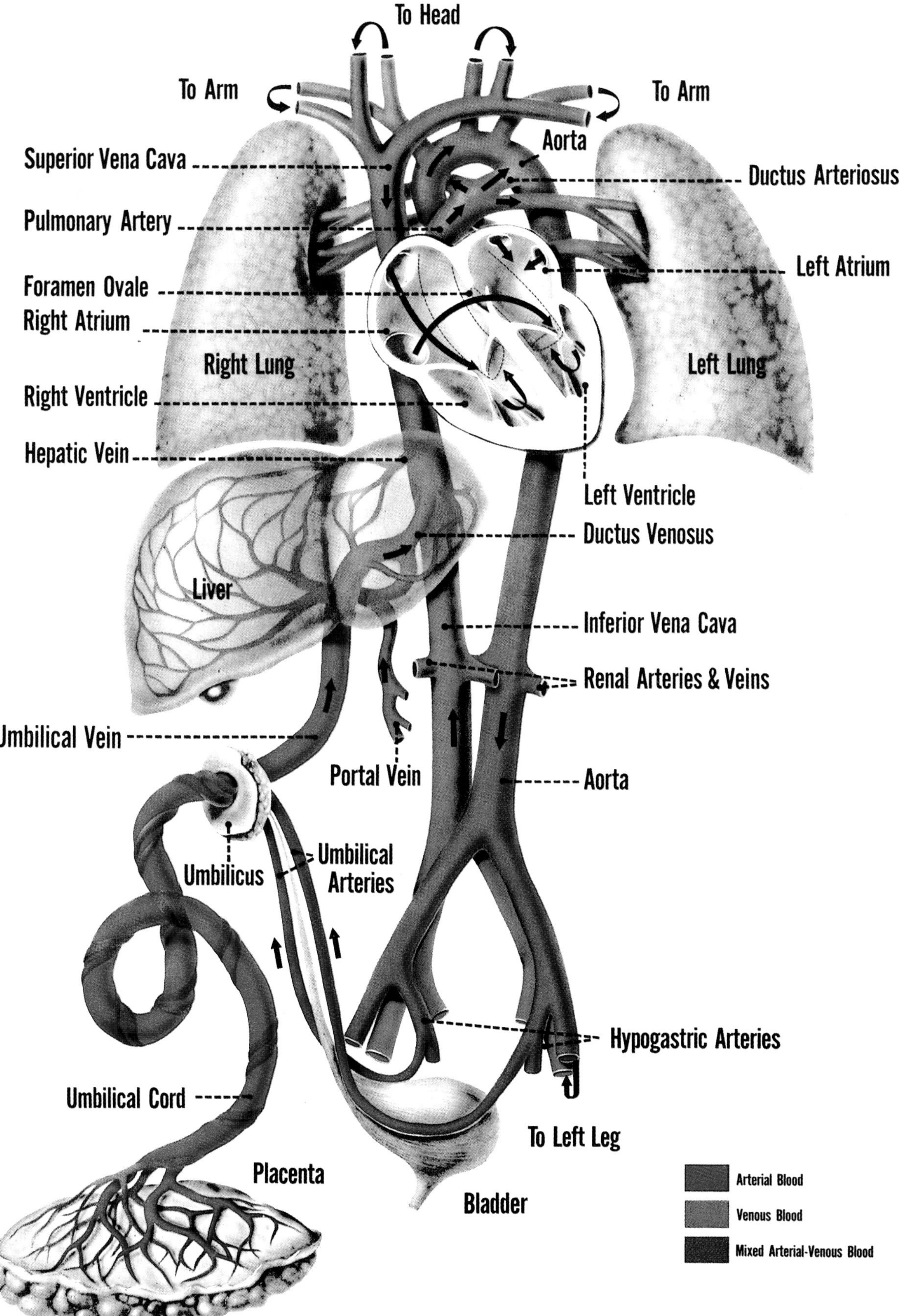


**Fig. 8–7.** Fetal circulation. Arrows indicate course of blood. Oxygen saturation is highest in the umbilical vein and progressively lower in the vessels to the head and neck, the aorta, and finally the inferior vena cava below the liver, which has the most desaturated blood. (Courtesy Ross Laboratories.)

**Table 8–1.** Pharmacokinetic Mechanisms that Affect Entry Rate of Drugs

| |
|---|
| (1) lipid solubility; |
| (2) degree of unionization; |
| (3) degree of protein binding; |
| (4) hypoxia and hypercarbia. |

these metabolic enzyme systems may be the reason for the increased neonatal susceptibility. Earlier studies have shown that the newborn animal is many times more susceptible to the effects of depressant drugs than is the adult (76). Stechler (77) has shown in human newborns that the depressant effects of narcotics, barbiturates, and promethazine (Phenergan) persist for from 2 to 4 days after birth. In contrast to this, it should be noted that at least one agent, thiopental, has been shown to have an elimination half-life of about 8 hours in neonates, roughly the same as in adults (78).

## PLACENTAL TRANSFER AND CLINICAL EFFECTS OF SPECIFIC DRUGS

### *Barbiturates*

The barbiturates, once very popular and used extensively by colleague obstetricians to maintain the calm on the delivery floor, are still used occasionally as sedatives during the first stage of labor, but only for providing a good night's sleep for the mother diagnosed as having false labor (79). Formerly, the barbiturates were used in rather large dosages to produce complete pain relief and amnesia during the first stage. Such misuse resulted in significant neonatal depression, maternal confusion, and labor prolongation (80). Today, fortunately, barbiturate use as sedatives during the early stages of labor is rare. For false labor, overnight sedation, and hypnosis, the shorter-acting barbiturates, such as pentobarbital and secobarbital, are used. Certainly, by far the most important current contribution of barbiturates to obstetric anesthesiology is the short-acting hypnotic, thiopental, which is still used universally for induction of general anesthesia for cesarean section.

Local anesthetics are the most frequently used anesthetic agent for obstetric anesthesia. This is true because of the fact that many more anesthetics are administered for labor and delivery than for cesarean section alone. Agents used for cesarean section alone are barbiturates, tranquilizers, other hypnotics and sedatives, narcotics, and inhalation anesthetics. We will turn our attention to these latter drugs later in the chapter. For now, we must turn our attention to one of the most important aspects of placental transfer of which the clinician must be aware. In fact, clinicians have the ultimate control over how much local anesthetic gets to the fetus by placental transfer, because they control the sub-m (maternal concentration of the drug, which is local anesthesia in this case) administered to the mother.

According to the Fick equation in Figure 8–1, it is readily apparent that the primary determinant of the numerator, other than surface area of membranes for diffusion, is concentration of the drug in the maternal compartment. This concentration is directly controlled by the anesthesiologist, who determines both the amount of drug given and the rate at which that given amount is administered. In other words, anesthesiologists, by their own hands, can somewhat govern placental transfer of local anesthetics by administering the smallest amount of drug over the longest period of time. The clinical application of this is readily apparent, and today it is practiced by use of a low dosage continuous administration method by some method of pump delivery. What the editors wish to emphasize is that clinicians must not be placed into a clinical situation when the patient has poor analgesia, and clinicians must quickly "block" the patient. These situations encourage administration of large doses of drugs in short time quadrants, and maximize both maternal and placental drug delivery. In such situations, the clinician may consider alternative analgesic methods, such as a combination of nitrous oxide and oxygen for analgesia during unexpected, emergent second stage analgesic situations. The final admonishment is to administer drugs slowly in obstetric anesthesia, just as is practiced in anesthetic management of other patients.

### *Placental Transfer*

The placenta acts as an interface between maternal and fetal circulations. It transmits biological substances essential for fetal growth and development.

Drugs cross the placenta by diffusion at varying rates depending on their physical and chemical properties. Nonionized particles cross more rapidly than ions, and small molecules cross more rapidly than large ones. The amount of a drug that actually reaches the fetus depends upon: (1) dose and route of administration to the mother; (2) amount of protein binding; (3) amount of free drug in the mother's serum; (4) lipid solubility; (5) concentration of nonionized free drug (Figure 8–8); and (6) uterine blood flow.

The placenta readily transmits most anesthetic drugs to the fetus, because most have low molecular weights, low ionization, and high lipid solubility. The muscle-paralyzing drugs, however, are not transferred across the placenta easily, because they are highly ionized and poorly lipid soluble. For this reason, the newborn rarely exhibits any effect even though the mother may have complete muscle paralysis.

Early speculation on the speed and completeness of placental transfer of barbiturates was confusing. Some reports related slow maternal-to-fetal transfer, while other reports related the transfer was rapid. This confusing picture has its greatest confounding effect clinically upon the timing of delivery of the fetus after general anesthesia induction. There emerged the slow-delivery school and the fast-delivery school, both with the same idea—to deliver the fetus at its lowest drug concentration after induction. Finally, the definitive work of a study from Japan confirmed that barbiturate transfer was almost instantaneous (81) and, in fact, that barbiturate levels peaked by 3 to 5 minutes and were low again by 6 to 8 minutes.

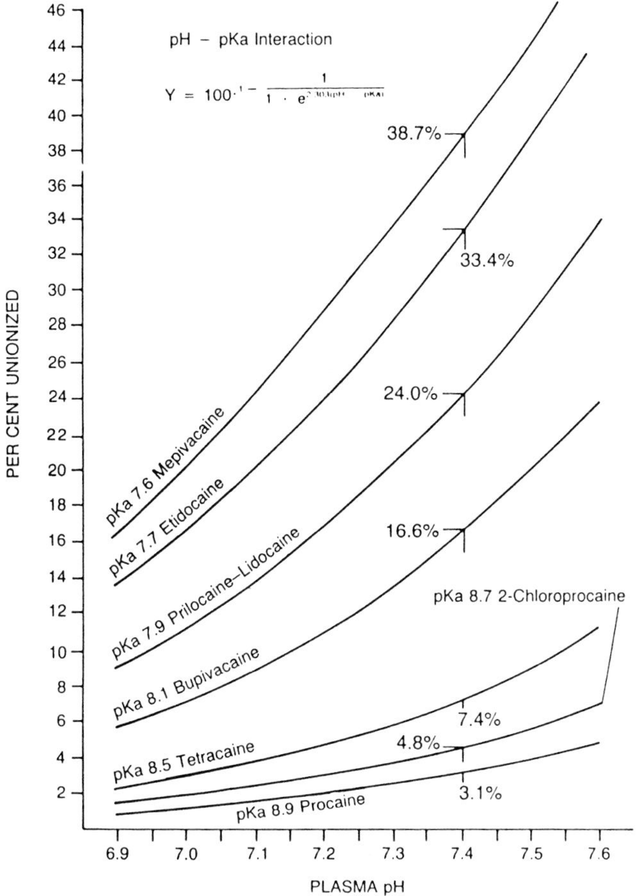


**Fig. 8–8.** This figure shows that the proportion of local anesthetic that remains in the nonionized state ranges from as low as 3.1% for procaine to as high as 38.7% for mepivacaine. Naturally, the nonionized fraction is free to achieve equilibrium between the maternal and fetal sides by diffusion. It is also easy to see from this figure that as the mother's blood becomes more alkaline, the nonionized proportion will increase. (From Yurth DA: Placental transfer of local anesthetics. Clinics in Perinatology. 9:13–28, 1982.)

Because induction-to-delivery times usually were in the 6 to 10 minute range, this correlated well with the fetal peak and decay curve as demonstrated in Figure 8–9.

For historical completeness, the following section reviews the excellent summary found in the first edition of this book. It may be recalled that in earlier days, there were statements about delays or blockage of barbiturates at the placental barrier. Subsequent work has disproved this, of course, and now it is a well-known fact that this class of drugs traverses the placenta immediately. This work began with Fabre (82) and Dille (83) in the early 1930s and continued 2 decades later with Flowers (84) and Martland (85). Within a short period of time, phenobarbital, pentobarbital, and secobarbital (Figure 8–10) were all shown to cross the placenta freely and rapidly. McKechnie and Converse (86) were among the first to show that thiopental also crossed the placental immediately (Figure 8–11), and subsequent work by Kosaka (81) revealed the maternal uptake, fetal transfer, and redistribution of thiopental at the time of induction of anesthesia for cesarean section. Although many of the suggested theories of why there was little fetal/neonatal depression after use of thiopental doses that caused maternal sleep had to do with maternal/fetal dilution patterns and variances in placental barrier, the most reasonable cause became the small quantity used for maternal hypnosis and the rapid redistribution back to the mother, thus resulting in minimal fetal levels. The general anesthetic regimen described in 1974 by McDonald, et al (87) laid the groundwork for the application of safe tenets for cesarean section anesthesia for nearly the next 2 decades (Table 8–2).

The rapid sequence induction regimen has withstood the test of time with few criticisms from the "too light side" with recall to the "too deep side" with depressed neonates. In 1000 cesarean section cases at the University of Southern California in the early 1970s, there was not a statistically significant difference between Apgars and umbilical artery pHs with the general versus regional anesthesia such as the lumbar epidural or spinal method (JS McDonald, personal communication, 1974).

***Thiamylal (Surital sodium).*** The placental transfer of thiamylal was first demonstrated by Kahn and coworkers (88) and later by Flowers (89), and Kosaka, Takahashi, and Mark (81), who found that the drug passed to the fetus as rapidly as thiopental (Figure 8–12). Thiamylal's chief advantage over thiopental is a slightly more rapid induction. This benefit is more than offset by the tendency of thiamylal to cause hiccoughs; it is unlikely, therefore, that thiamylal will ever supplant thiopental as the preferred standard induction agent. Table 8–3 shows the Apgar scores of infants of mothers receiving thiamylal injections, per Figures 8–9 and 8–12.

## Tranquilizers

Benzodiazepines are readily transferred to the fetus, and the practitioner must bear in mind the slow elimination rate due to slow metabolism of these agents. As such, in late pregnancy and parturition, benzodiazepines should be used in their lowest effective dose to prevent fetal and neonatal depression. In the last 2 decades, diazepam was clearly the drug of choice, but in the 1990s, midazolam is by far the most popular drug. In fact there is really the question, "Should this class of drug ever be used in labor and delivery?" It has its primary effect upon the hypocampus and amygdala and effects a tranquil state effectively, but does the mother require such a drug? The authors believe not, because the primary problem associated with the pain of labor should be countered with adequate analgesia effected by analgesic agents and the problems associated with anxiety best countered by effective education and training early in the gestation. Such a pharmacologic solution for maternal anxiety is a poor solution at best, and one with fetal consequences due to the poor metabolism of the fetus. Much, if not all, of the original interest in use of the tranquilizer class of drugs was due to the conception that there was a substantial enhancement of the narcotic effect when these two drugs were combined. Today, there is more a tendency to use the analgesics alone for their singular effect and not to worry about

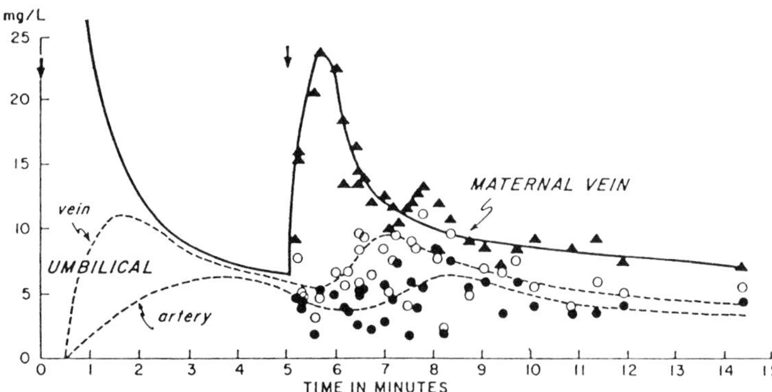


**Fig. 8–9.** Cesarean section Group II. Supplementary method: two injections (4 mg/kg and 1 1/3 mg/kg). Thiamylal concentrations in maternal vein (▲—▲), umbilical vein (O---O), umbilical artery (---). Curves drawn by inspection. (From Kosaka Y, Takahashi T, Mark LC: Intravenous thiobarbiturate anesthesia for cesarean section. Anesthesiology. 31:489, 1981.)

potentiation. It should also be noted that all agents are present in small, usually pharmacologically insignificant, amounts in breast milk.

## *Other Hypnotics and Sedatives*

Ethyl alcohol was first shown to cross the placental membrane by Nicloux (90). Later studies have confirmed this (91,92). Cord blood levels of alcohol were found to be approximately 20% below those in the maternal blood following slow intravenous administration, but no neonatal respiratory depression was noted in 95% of the infants (87).

Magnesium sulfate, often used in obstetrics for its sedative action, has been shown to pass the placental barrier. Pritchard (93) found that in 16 parturients given magnesium sulfate, 4 gm every 4 hours, the maternal and fetal plasma level had reached equilibrium by the time of delivery. A recent study (94) suggested that magnesium sulfate reduced the vascular resistance of the umbilical and placental vascular beds in addition to having the usual sedative and therapeutic effect in regard to treatment of the pregnancy-induced hypertensive state.

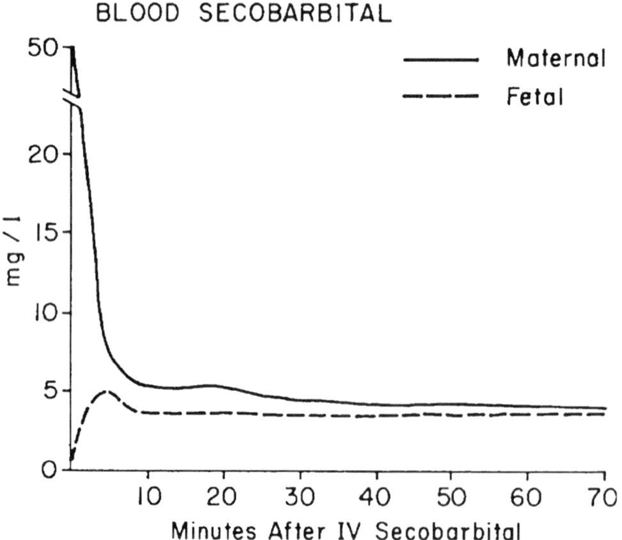


**Fig. 8–10.** Secobarbital (Seconal) blood levels of mother and newborn. The drug crossed the placenta rapidly and obtained early equilibrium. Blood level in the infant was approximately 70% of that of the mother. (Modified from Root B, Eichner E, Sunshine I: Blood and secobarbital levels and their clinical correlation in mothers and newborn infants. Am. J. Obstet. Gynecol. 81:948, 1961.)

Still another study (95) looked at the effects of magnesium sulfate and ritodrine hydrochloride on cardiovascular physiology in 70 human subjects treated for preterm labor. Though systolic blood pressure was affected minimally by either agent, diastolic pressure, unaffected by magnesium sulfate, decreased 26.3% during ritodrine therapy. As anticipated, the heart rates were affected minimally by magnesium sulfate, but, as no surprise, ritodrine increased both maternal and fetal heart rates significantly. This same study also had an animal study of magnesium sulfate and ritodrine effect on uterine and placental blood flows. While magnesium sulphate increased both uterine and placental flows, ritodrine decreased placental flow by an average of 27.6%. Ritodrine would therefore seem contraindicated with a compromised fetal environment.

An interesting bench study by Altura and Altura (96) revealed that umbilical vessels sustained in an in vitro environment had magnesium deficiency induced spasms, and further, that a reduced magnesium concentration potentiated the contractile response to bradykinin, angiotensin II, serotonin, and prostaglandin $F_2$ alpha.

## Narcotics

A drug that has gained enormously popularity over the past decade is fentanyl. It is now a popular drug in the obstetric management of the first stage of labor. A rabbit study of placental transfer of fentanyl revealed that it was intermediate between meperidine and bupivacaine (97). A sheep study noted that fentanyl was detected in 1 minute after maternal injection and levels peaked at 5 minutes. Maternal levels remained 2.5 times greater than fetal levels and both drug levels declined similarly during the degradation phase (98). In an alfentanil study for elective cesarean section, 10 μg/kg resulted in a maternal plasma concentration of 23.5 mg/ml and a neonatal umbilical alfentanil plasma level of 7.5 mg/ml (99).

In earlier days narcotic antagonists such as nalorphine

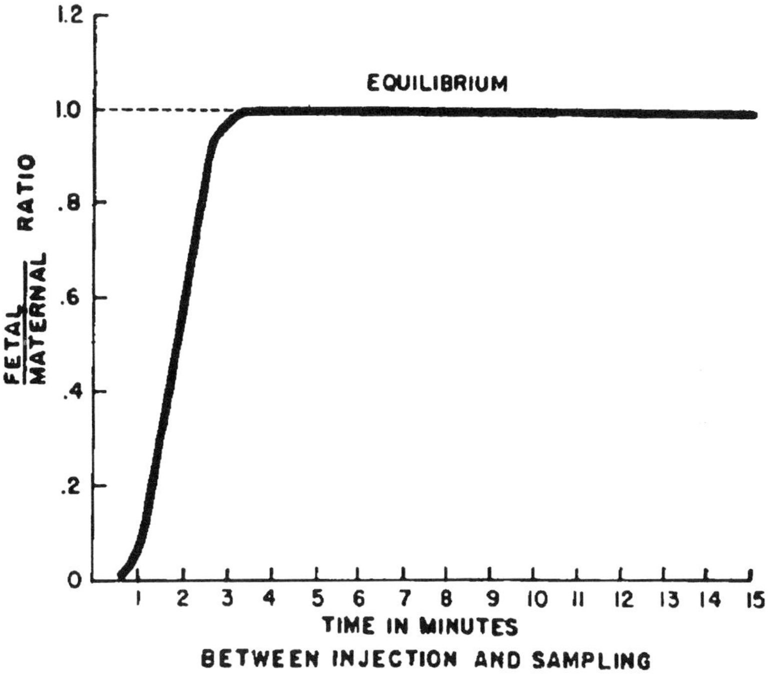


**Fig. 8–11.** Concentrations of thiopental (Pentothal) in the material and fetal blood reach equilibrium within 3 minutes. Diagram based on data of McKechnie and Converse. (From Moya F, Thorndike V: Passage of drugs across the placenta. Am. J. Obstet. Gynecol. 84:1778, 1962.)

(Nalline) and levallorphan (Lorfan) were the mainstays of treatment; current use is now almost entirely with naloxone. This compound represents only slight modification of the molecular structure of morphine, levorphan, and oxymorphone, respectively. Although no data are available, they most likely cross the placental membrane readily. This is supported by reports of their efficacy in preventing narcotic depression in the newborn by administration to the mother shortly before labor (100,101). Since their introduction, many attempts have been made to combine their use with narcotics to provide optimum maternal pain relief without neonatal depression. Telford and Keats (102), after reviewing the literature, concluded that none of the studies satisfactorily demonstrated any decrease in the degree of neonatal depression. It has also been well-demonstrated that the narcotic antagonists potentiate depression produced by agents other than narcotics. Therefore, extreme care has been exercised in using them in obstetrics in the past. Today, they are rarely used because of the trend toward almost exclusive use of naloxone.

**Table 8–2.** General Anesthetic Regimen for Cesarean Section Anesthesia

(1) rapid nitrogen wash-out of functional reserve capacity by oxygen;
(2) cricoid pressure;
(3) the use of a small hypnotic dose of thiopental, 2.5 to 3.0 mg/kg;
(4) immediate followup injection of succinylcholine 100 mg right after thiopental;
(5) laryngoscopy and intubation and inflation of tracheal cuff;
(6) $N_2O/O_2$ at 50% concentration.

(Modified from McDonald JS, Mateo CV, Reed EC: Modified nitrous oxide or ketamine hydrochloride for cesarean section. Anesth. Analg. 51:975, 1972.)

One study of naloxone revealed that maternal-to-fetal transfer occurred in 1 to 2 minutes after intravenous administration and was variable following intramuscular administration (103).

Finally, a new induction drug, propofol, has also been studied. Neonatal effects and placental transfer of propofol were investigated in elective cesarean section under general anesthesia (104). Women were induced with an intravenous bolus of 2.5 mg/kg of propofol. Propofol crossed the placenta, as demonstrated by concentrations found in umbilical venous blood (0.13 to 0.75 μg/ml) in phase 1, where anesthesia was maintained with 50% nitrous oxide in oxygen and halothane; and 0.78 to 1.37 μg/ml in phase 2, where a continuous infusion of propofol at a rate of 5 mg/kg/hr was started after the induction dose. The ratio of the drug concentration in umbilical venous blood to that in maternal blood was $0.70 \pm 0.06$ for phase 1 and $0.76 \pm 0.10$ for phase 2 (104).

Some mention should be made of the effect on the fetus of recreational drugs. One recent study outlined the many problems associated with maternal cocaine use (105). Intravenous (44%) and freebasing (31%) were the main routes of exposure. Abnormal labors were found in nearly 64% and meconium in another 21%. Birth weights were significantly lower than the general hospital population; for example, less than 2500 g occurred in 37% and small for gestational age 32%. In addition, Burkett's study found

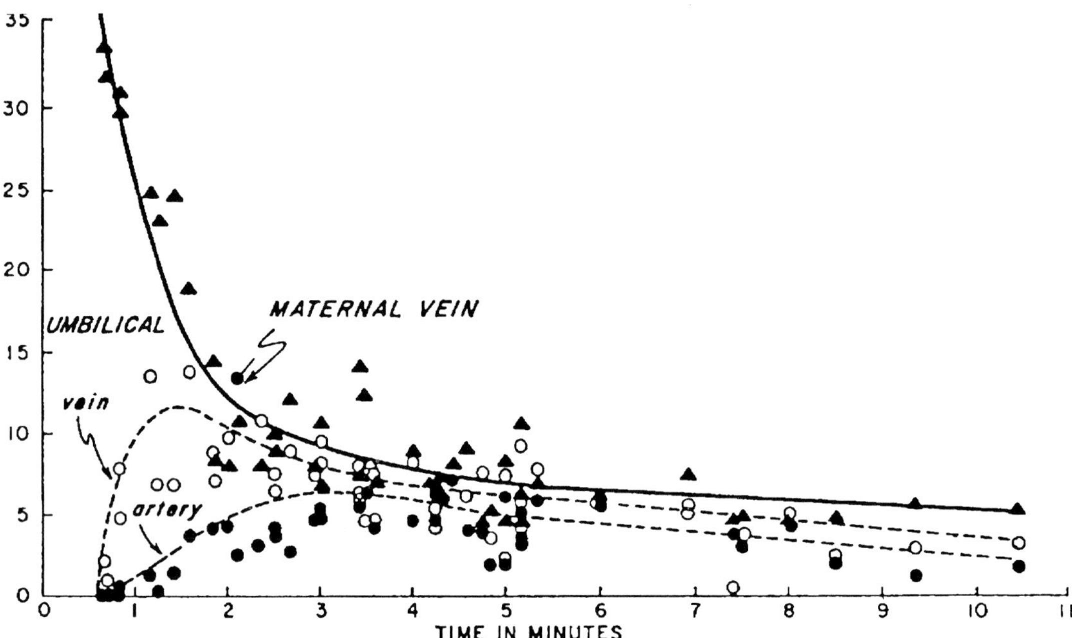


**Fig. 8–12.** Cesarean section Group 1. Single injection method (4 mg/kg). Thiamylal concentrations in maternal vein (▲—▲), umbilical vein (○---○), unbilical artery (---). Curves drawn by inspection. (From Kosaka Y, Takahashi T, Mark LC: Intravenous thiobarbiturate anesthesia for cesarean section. Anesthesiology. 31:489, 1981.)

neurologic problems in 31%, congenital problems in 17%, and syphilis in 15%.

## Inhalation Anesthetics

All inhalation anesthetics traverse the placental barrier with ease. The transfer is due to their diffusion capability, their high fat solubility, and their low molecular weight. It is, however, rare to have fetal depression due to inhalation anesthetics today because the concentrations of anesthetics used currently are so minimal and used so briefly as to have little or no clinical effect on the newborn. The practice of administration of analgesic concentrations of inhalation anesthetics to mothers during vaginal delivery is no longer in vogue, so that again it is not a concern in regard to fetal depression.

**Table 8–3.** Technique of Administration and Apgar Score

| | Group I | | | | Group II | |
|---|---|---|---|---|---|---|
| | 4 mg/kg | | 6 mg/kg | | | |
| No. of cases | 140 | | 10 | | 34 | |
| No. of babies | 143 | | 10 | | 34 | |
| | No. | Percent | No. | Percent | No. | Percent |
| Apgar Score | | | | | | |
| 7–10 | 130 | 90.9 | 8 | 80 | 25 | 73.5 |
| 4–6 | 9 | 6.3 | 2 | 20 | 7 | 20.6 |
| 0–3 | 4 | 2.8 | | | 2 | 5.9 |

(Modified from Kosaka Y, Takahashi T, Mark LC: Intravenous thiobarbiturate anesthesia for cesarean section. Anesthesiology 31:489, 1981.)

At the time of the first edition of this book, it was common to have nitrous oxide administered for the delivery phase of vaginal birth. It is still a common practice today to use $N_2O/O_2$ analgesia at the time of delivery. In some areas, it was also the practice to have nitrous oxide analgesia self-administered during the first stage of labor for periodic relief of uterine contraction pain. This is *not* common practice nor recommended today.

One study revealed transfer of $N_2O$ in the fetal vascular system of the guinea pig placenta (106). It was found that the effectiveness of the $N_2O$ transfer was about 90% (SD = 6%) when the maternofetal flow ratio was 2 and about 75% (SD = 13%) when the ratio was 1. The placenta has the properties of a countercurrent system in which the effectiveness of gas transfer is decreased by about 25% at a flow ratio of 1 and by 10% at a flow ratio of 2 by inhomogeneity of the maternofetal flow ratio.

Another interesting study looked at the use of higher doses of enflurane and isoflurane in 100% oxygen so as to avoid the awareness problem in lieu of no nitrous oxide (107). This feasibility was studied in 113 cesarean sections. Isoflurane 1.25% was compared with 1.5% enflurane. Criteria for a satisfactory general anesthetic technique for cesarean section were fulfilled: there was no maternal awareness, no undue depression of the fetus, and no adverse effect on uterine contractility. Isoflurane and enflurane by themselves appear to be suitable anesthetic agents for facilitating hyperoxygenation during cesarean section.

In consideration of an asphyxiated situation or one in which the maternal or fetal stress is identified but not certain, a recent study (108) would confirm that isoflurane-oxygen anesthesia would be a good choice because

**Table 8–4.** Acid Base and Blood Gas Data.* No Significant Differences Between Groups Using Analyses of Variance Test

| | Isoflurane 0.5% (n = 20) | Isoflurane 1.0% (n = 20) | Halothane 0.5% (n = 20) |
|---|---|---|---|
| Umbilical vein | | | |
| pH | 7.36 ± 0.01 | 7.36 ± 0.01 | 7.36 ± 0.01 |
| $PO_2$ (kPa) | 4.80 ± 0.53 | 4.53 ± 0.27 | 4.93 ± 0.27 |
| $PCO_2$ (kPa) | 5.60 ± 0.13 | 5.87 ± 0.13 | 5.73 ± 0.13 |
| BE (mmol/l) | −1.15 ± 0.53 | −0.46 ± 0.44 | −0.65 ± 0.66 |
| Umbilical artery | | | |
| pH | 7.30 ± 0.01 | 7.30 ± 0.01 | 7.31 ± 0.01 |
| $PO_2$ (kPa) | 2.40 ± 0.13 | 2.40 ± 0.13 | 2.53 ± 0.13 |
| $PCO_2$ (kPa) | 7.20 ± 0.27 | 7.33 ± 0.13 | 7.20 ± 0.13 |
| BE (mmol/l) | 0.68 ± 0.60 | 2.10 ± 0.59 | 0.85 ± 0.47 |

* Values are mean ± S.E. mean.
(From Abboud TK, D'Onofrio L, Reyes A, Mosaad P, et al: Isoflurane or halothane for cesarean section: comparative maternal and neonatal effects. Acta. Anesthesiol. Scand. 33:578, 1989, p. 580.)

the fetal lamb model demonstrated that acidosis was increased, that cardiac output was redistributed to vital organs, and that the cerebral oxygen supply-demand was maintained.

***Halothane and Isoflurane.*** In a recent clinical study, Abboud, et al (109) compared the concentration of isoflurane and halothane in maternal and fetal blood (Tables 8–4 and 8–5). Both isoflurane and halothane were present in the earliest blood samples drawn, indicating rapid placental passage. Maternal fluoride levels were not substantially altered from preanesthetic values. Furthermore, newborn fluoride levels were barely detectable. Acid-base values for both the mother and baby were within acceptable values of norm. The authors concluded that either isoflurane or halothane, in small doses, could safely be used to supplement the accepted general anesthetic technique of $N_2O/O_2$ (104). They noted that isoflurane does not enhance the arrhythmogenic effects of epinephrine as halothane does, and that in some cases, isoflurane might be preferred to halothane (104).

**Table 8–5.** Fluoride Level (μMol/l)

| | Isoflurane 0.5% (n = 20) | Isoflurane 1.0% (n = 20) | Halothane 0.5% (n = 20) |
|---|---|---|---|
| Maternal serum | | | |
| Antepartum | 5.60 ± 0.00 | 5.88 ± 0.27 | 5.88 ± 0.27 |
| Postpartum | 5.59 ± 0.01 | 5.60 ± 0.00 | 5.60 ± 0.00 |
| Maternal urine | | | |
| Antepartum | 37.94 ± 3.53 | 37.49 ± 4.79 | 30.00 ± 6.95 |
| Postpartum | 39.72 ± 4.64 | 41.94 ± 4.85 | *27.22 ± 3.14 |
| Baby urine | | | |
| First voided | 6.52 ± 0.90 | 6.47 ± 0.62 | 5.60 ± 0.00 |

* $P < 0.05$ compared to 0.5% or 1% isoflurane using analyses of variance test.
** Values are mean ± S.E. mean.
(From Abboud TK, D'Onofrio L, Reyes A, Mosaad P, et al: Isoflurane or halothane for cesarean section: comparative maternal and neonatal effects. Acta. Anesthesiol. Scand. 33:578, 1989, p. 580.)

***Other Inhalation Anesthetics.*** Desflurane is a new methyl ethyl ether that is halogenated solely with fluorine. Its low blood/gas (0.42) and oil/gas (18.7) partition coefficients indicate it will function basically as fast as nitrous oxide with rapid wash-in and wash-out characteristics. Its minimum anesthetic concentration (MAC) value is about 5%. It has at this time not been used in obstetrics, but early work on volunteers reveals that they responded to verbal commands on an average of 2.7 minutes after discontinuing the anesthetic. It could, therefore, be an especially beneficial agent for use in obstetrics.

## REFERENCES


1. Faber JJ, Thornburg KL: Placental Physiology. New York, Raven Press, 1983.
2. Longo LD: Respiratory gas exchange in the placenta. *In* Handbook of Physiology, Section 3: The Respiratory System, Vol. IV. Gas Exchange. Edited by LE Farhi, SM Tenney. Bethesda, American Physiological Society, 1987, p. 351.
3. Sibley CP, Boyd RDH: Control of transfer across the mature placenta. *In* Oxford Reviews Reprod Biol Vol. 10. Edited by JR Clarke. Oxford, Oxford University Press, 1988, p. 382.
4. Meschia G, Battaglia FC, Bruns PD: Theoretical and experimental study of transplacental diffusion. J. Appl. Physiol. 22:1171, 1967.
5. Holzman I, Philipps AF, Battaglia FC: Glucose metabolism, lactate and ammonia production by the human placenta in vitro. Pediatr. Res. 13:117, 1979.
6. Hauguel S, Challier J-C, Cedard L, Olive G: Metabolism of the human placenta perfused in vitro: glucose transfer and utilization, $O_2$ consumption, lactate and ammonia production. Pediatr. Res. 17:729, 1983.
7. Willis DM, O'Grady JP, Faber JJ, Thornburg KL: Diffusion permeability of cyanocobalamin in human placenta. Am. J. Physiol. 250:R459, 1986.
8. Thornburg KL, Burry KJ, Adams AK, Kirk EP, et al: Permeability of placenta to inulin. Am. J. Obstet. Gynecol. 158: 1165, 1988.
9. V Euler US: Action of adrenaline, acetylcholine and other substances on nerve-free vessels (human placenta). J. Physiol. 93:129, 1938.

9A. Paci A, Cocci F, Piras F, Niedermeyer HP, et al: Demonstration of beta 1-adrenergic receptors in human placenta by 125-iodocyanopindolol binding. J. Nucl. Med. Allied Sci. 33(1), 1989, pp. 15–21.

10. Panigel M: Placental perfusion experiments. Am. J. Obstet. Gynecol. 84:1664, 1962.
11. Schneider H, Panigel M, Dancis J: Transfer across the perfused human placenta of antipyrine, sodium, and leucine. Am. J. Obstet. Gynecol. 114:822, 1972.
12. Krantz KE, Panos TC: Apparatus for establishment of separate extracorporeal fetal and maternal circulations in the human placenta. Am. J. Dis. Child. 98:674, 1959.
13. Smith NC, Brush MG, Luckett S: Preparation of human placental villous surface membrane. Nature 252:302, 1974.
14. Kelly LK, Smith CH, King BF: Isolation and partial characterization of the basal cell membrane of human placental trophoblast. Biochem. Biophys. Acta. 734:91, 1983.
15. Bissonnette JM: Membrane vesicles from trophoblast cells as models for placental exchange studies. Placenta 3:99, 1982.
16. Bissonnette JM, Ingermann RL, Thornburg KL: Placental sugar transport. *In* Carrier-mediated Transport of Solutes

from Blood to Tissue. Edited by DL Yudilevich, GE Mann. London, Pitman, 1985, p. 65.

17. Bullen B, Bloxam D: Human placental trophoblast cultured on amnion basement membranes: a model for transport studies. 11th Rochester Trophoblast Conference, Abstract 131, 1988.
18. Rooth G, Sjostedt S: The placental transfer of gases and fixed acids. Arch. Dis. Child. 37:366, 1962.

18A. Blechner JN: Placental gas transfer. Clin. Obstet. Gynecol. 11(4), 1968, pp. 1165–1181.

19. Stenger V, Eitzman D, Anderson T, et al: Observations on the placental exchange of the respiratory gases in pregnant women in cesarean section. Am. J. Obstet. Gynecol. 88: 45, 1964.

19A. Longo LD: Transplacental gas exchange. Rev. Mal. Respir. 5(3), 1988, pp. 197–206.

20. Longo LD, Power GG, Forster RE, II: Respiratory function of the placenta as determined with carbon monoxide in sheep and dogs. J. Clin. Invest. 46:812, 1967.
21. Delivoria-Papadopoulos M, Coburn RF, Forster RE II: The placental diffusing capacity for carbon monoxide in pregnant women at term. *In* Respiratory Gas Exchange and Blood Flow in the Placenta. Edited by LD Longo, H Bartles. Bethesda, Department of Health, Education and Welfare, 1972, p. 259.
22. Sjostedt S, Rooth G, Caligara F: The oxygen tension of the blood in the umbilical cord and intervillous space. Arch. Dis. Child. 35:529, 1960.
23. Meschia G, Battaglia FC, Hay WW Jr, Sparks JW: Utilization of substrates by the ovine placenta in vivo. Fed. Proc. 39: 245, 1980.
24. Power GG, Dale PS, Nelson PS: Distribution of maternal and fetal blood flow within cotyledons of the sheep placenta. Am. J. Physiol. 241:H486, 1981.
25. Meschia G: Safety margin of fetal oxygenation. J. Reprod. Med. 30:308, 1985.
26. Wulf H: Der gasaustausch in der reifen plazenta des menschen. Geburtsh. Gynak. 158:117, 1962.
27. Longo LD, Delivoria-Papadolpoulos M, Foster RE II: Placental $CO_2$ transfer after fetal carbonic anhydrase inhibition. Am. J. Physiol. 226:703, 1974.
28. Aarnoudse JG, Illsey NP, Penfold P, Bardsley SE: Permeability of the human placenta to bicarbonate: In-vitro perfusion studies. Br. J. Obstet. Gynaecol. 91:1096, 1984.
29. Johnson LW, Smith CH: Monosaccharide transport across microvillous membrane of human placenta. Am. J. Physiol. 238:C160, 1980.
30. Bissonnette JM, Black JA, Wickham WK, Acott KM: Glucose uptake into plasma membrane vesicles from the maternal surface of human placenta. J. Membr. Biol. 58:75, 1981.
31. Mueckler M, Caruso C, Baldwin SA, Panico M, et al: Sequence and structure of a human glucose transporter. Science 229:941, 1985.
32. Fukumoto H, Seino S, Imura Y, Bell GI: Characterization and expression of human HepG2/erythrocyte glucose-transporter gene. Diabetes 37:657, 1988.
33. Kayano T, Fukomoto H, Eddy RL, Fan Y-S, et al: Evidence for a family of human glucose transporter-like proteins. J. Biol. Chem. 263:15245, 1988.
34. Kosaki A, Kuzuha H, Yosimasa Y, et al: Regulation of glucose transporter gene expression by insulin in cultured human fibroblasts. Diabetes 37:1583, 1988.
35. Walker PS, Donovan JA, VanNess BG, Fellows RE, et al: Glucose-dependent regulation of glucose transport activity, protein and mRNA in primary cultures of rat brain glial cells. J. Biol. Chem. 263:15594, 1988.
36. Bissonnette JM: Studies of in vivo of glucose transfer across the guinea-pig placenta. *In* Placental Transfer: Methods and Interpretations. Edited by M Young, RDH Boyd, LD Longo, G Telegdy. Philadelphia, W.B. Saunders, 1981, p. 155.
37. Ingermann RL, Bissonnette JM: Effect of temperature on kinetics of hexose uptake by human placental plasma membrane vesicles. Biochem. Biophys. Acta. 734:329, 1983.
38. Cordero L Jr Yeh S-Y, Grunt JA, Anderson GG: Hypertonic glucose infusion during labor. Am. J. Obstet. Gynecol. 407: 295, 1970.
39. Johnson LW, Smith CH: Glucose transport across the basal plasma membrane of human placental syncytiotrophoblast. Biochem. Biophys. Acta. 815:44, 1985.
40. Ciaraldi TP, Kolterman OE, Siegel JA, Olefsky JM: Insulin-stimulated glucose transport in human adipocytes. Am. J. Physiol. 236 (Endocrinol. Metab. Gastrointest. Physiol. 5): E621, 1979.
41. Carstensen MH, Leichtweiss HP, Schröder H: Lactate carriers in the artificially perfused human term placenta. Placenta 4:165, 1983.
42. Illsley NP, Wooten NP, Penfold P, Hall S, et al: Lactate transfer across the perfused human placenta. Placenta 7: 209, 1986.
43. Schneider H, Challier J-C, Dancis J: Transfer and metabolism of glucose and lactate in the human placenta studied by a perfusion system in vitro. Placenta (Suppl.2):129, 1981.
44. Balkovetz DF, Leibach FH, Mahesh UB, Ganapathy V: A proton gradient is the driving force for uphill transport of lactate in human placental brush border membrane vesicles. J. Biol. Chem. 263:13823, 1988.
45. Hayashi S, Sanada K, Sagawa N: Umbilical vein-artery differences of plasma amino acids in the last trimester of human pregnancy. Biol. Neonate. 34:11, 1978.
46. Philipps AF, Holzman IR, Teng C, Battaglia FC: Tissue concentrations of free amino acids in term human placentas. Am. J. Obstet. Gynecol. 131:881, 1978.
47. Whitsett JA, Wallick ET: [3H] Oubain binding and Na+ −K-ATPase activity in human placenta. Am. J. Physiol. 238 (Endocrinol. Metab. 1) E38, 1980.
48. Steel RB, Mosley JD, Smith CH: Insulin and placenta: degradation and stabilization, binding to microvillous membrane receptors, and amino acid uptake. Am. J. Obstet. Gynecol. 135:522, 1979.
49. Smith CH: Mechanisms and regulation of placental amino acid transport. Fed. Proc. 45:2443, 1986.
50. Johnson LW, Smith CH: Neutral amino acid transport systems of microvillous membrane of human placenta. Am. J. Physiol. 254:C773, 1988.
51. Longo LD, Yuen P, Gusseck DJ: Anaerobic glycogen-dependent transport of amino acids by the placenta. Nature 243: 531, 1973.
52. Smith CH, Depper R: Placental amino acid uptake. II. Tissue preincubation, fluid distribution and mechanisms of regulation. Pediatr. Res. 8:697, 1974.
53. Lin DS, Pitkin RM, Connor WE: Placental transfer of cholesterol into the human fetus. Am. J. Obstet. Gynecol. 128: 735, 1977.
54. Naoum HG, DeChazal RCS, Eaton BM, Contractor SF: Characterization and specificity of lipoprotein binding to term human placental membrane. Biochem. Biophys. Acta. 902: 193, 1987.
55. Brown MS, Anderson RGW, Goldstein JL: Recycling receptors: the round trip itinerary of migrant membrane proteins. Cell 32:663, 1983.
56. Dancis J, Jansen V, Kayden JH: Transfer across perfused human placenta. III. Effect of chain length on transfer of free fatty acids. Pediatr. Res. 8:796, 1974.

57. Dancis J, Jansen V, Levitz M: Transfer across perfused human placenta. IV. Effect of protein binding on free fatty acids. Pediatr. Res. 10:5, 1976.
58. Bain MD, Copar DK, Landon MJ, Stacey TE: In vivo permeability of the human placenta to inulin and mannitol. J. Physiol. 399:313, 1988.
59. Illsley NP: Non-electrolyte permeability of the human placental microvillous membrane. 11th Rochester Trophoblast Conference, Abstract 130, 1988.
60. Bissonnette JM, Cronan JZ, Richards LL, Wickman WK: Placental transfer of water and nonelectrolytes during a single circulatory passage. Am. J. Physiol. 236 (Cell Physiol. 5): C47, 1979.
61. Hille B: Ionic channels of excitable membranes. Sunderland, MA, Sinauer Assoc Inc., 1984, p. 181.
62. Bissonnette JM, Maylie J: Abnormal chloride channel activity in human placental cells in cystic fibrosis. FASEB J. 2: A1723, 1988.
63. Bara M, Challies JC, Guiet-Bara A: Membrane potential and input resistance in syncytiotrophoblast of human term placenta. Placenta 9:139, 1988.
64. Sibley CP, Ward BS, Glasier JD, Moore WMO, et al: Electrical activity and sodium transfer across in vitro pig placenta. Am. J. Physiol. 250:R474, 1986.
65. Bahouth SW, Kelly LK, Smith CH, Arbabian MA, et al: Identification of a novel Mr = 76-kDa form of beta-adrenergic receptors. Biochem. Biophys. Res. Commun. 141:411, 1986.
66. Lajeunesse D, Brunette MG: Sodium gradient-dependent phosphate transport in placental brush border membrane vesicles. Placenta 9:117, 1988.
67. Balkovetz DF, Leibach FH, Mahesh VB, Devoe LD, et al: $Na^+$-$H^+$ exchanges of human placental brush-border membrane: identification and characterization. Am. J. Physiol. 251:C852, 1986.
68. Shennan DB, Davis B, Boyd CAR: Chloride transport in human placental microvillous membrane vesicles I. Evidence for anion exchange. Pflugers. Arch. 406:60, 1986.
69. Tran RS: Identification and characterization of a calcium-binding protein from human placenta. Placenta 3:145, 1982.
70. Fisher GJ, Kelly LK, Smith CH: ATP-dependent calcium transport across basal plasma membranes of human placenta. Am. J. Physiol. 252:C38, 1987.
71. Wada HG, Hass PE, Sussman HH: Transferrin receptor in human placental brush border membranes. J. Biol. Chem. 254:12629, 1979.
72. Douglas GC, King BF: Receptormediated endocytosis of 125I-labeled transferrin by human choriocarcinoma (JAR) cells. Placenta 9:253, 1988.
73. Vanderpuye OA, Kelly LK, Smith CH: Transferrin receptors in the basal plasma membrane of the human placental syncytiotrophoblast. Placenta 7:391, 1986.
73A. Kennedy ML, Douglas GC, King BF: Expression of transferrin receptors during differentiation of human placental trophoblast cells in vitro. Placenta 13(1), 1992, pp. 165–197.
74. Morishima HO, Santos AC, Pedersen H, Finster M, et al: Effect of lidocaine on the asphyxial responses in the mature fetal lamb. Anesthesiology 66:502, 1987.
75. Morishima HO, Pedersen H, Santos AC, Schapiro HM, et al: Adverse effects of maternally-administered lidocaine on asphyxiated fetal lambs. Anesthesiology 71:110, 1989.
76. Burkhalter A: Drug Metabolism—General Concepts. *In* Perinatal Pharmacology. Report of the Forty-First Ross Conference on Pediatric Research. Edited by CD May. Columbus, OH, Ross Laboratories, 1962, p. 43.
77. Stechler G: Newborn attention as affected by medication during labor. Science 144:315, 1964.
77A. Clark RB, Seifen AB: Systemic medication during labor and delivery. Obstet. Gynecol. Annu. 12, 1983, pp. 165–197.
78. Morgan DJ, Beamiss CG, Blackman GL, Paull JD: Urinary excretion of placentally transferred thiopentone by the human neonate. Dev. Pharmacol. Ther. 5:136, 1982.
79. Clark RB, Seifen AB: Systemic medication during labor. Obstet. Gynecol. Annu. 12:165, 1983.
80. Shnider S, Levinson G: Anesthesia for Obstetrics. Baltimore, Williams & Wilkins, 1979.
81. Kosaka Y, Takahashi T, Mark LC: Intravenous thiobarbiturate anesthesia for cesarean section. Anesthesiology 31:489, 1981.
82. Fabre R: De la Permeabilité Placentaire auxdérivés barbituriques. C.R. Soc. Seances. Soc. Biol. Fil. 113:1380, 1933.
83. Dille JM: Studies on barbiturates; placental transmission of non-anesthetic doses of barbital. Am. J. Obstet. Gynecol. 32:328, 1936.
84. Flowers CE Jr: Placental transmission of sodium barbital. Obstet. Gynecol. 9:332, 1957.
85. Martland HS, Martland HS Jr: Placental barrier in carbon monoxide, barbiturate and radium poisoning (some original observations in humans). Amer. J. Surg. 80:270, 1950.
86. McKechnie FB, Converse JG: Placental transmission of thiopental. Am. J. Obstet. Gynecol. 70:639, 1955.
86A. Celleno D, Capogna G, Emanuelli M, Varrassi G, et al: Which induction drug for cesarean section? A comparison of thiopental sodium, propofol, and midazolam. J. Clin. Anesth. 5(4), 1993, pp. 284–288.
86B. Teviotdale BM: Vecuronium-thiopentone induction for emergency caesarean section under general anesthaesia. Anaesth. Intensive Care (Australia). 21(3), 1993, pp.288–291.
87. McDonald JS, Mateo CV, Reed EC: Modified nitrous oxide or ketamine hydrochloride for cesarean section. Anesth. Analg. 51:975, 1972.
88. Kahn JB, Nicholson DB, Assali NS: Placental transmission of thiobarbiturate in parturient women. Obstet. Gynecol. 1:663, 1953.
88A. Celardo A, Passerini F, Bonati M: Placental transfer and tissue distribution of thiopental in the pregnant rat. J. Pharmacokinet. Biopharm. 17(4), 1989, pp. 425–440.
89. Flowers CE Jr: The placental transmission of barbiturates and thiobarbiturates and their pharmacological action on mother and infant. Am. J. Obstet. Gynecol. 78:730, 1959.
90. Nicloux M: Passage de l'alcohol ingere de la niere au foetus et passage de l'alcohol ingere dans le lait en particulier chez la femme. Obstetrique 5:97, 1900.
91. Belinkoff S, Hall OW: Intravenous alcohol during labor. Am. J. Obstet. Gynecol. 59:429, 1950.
92. Chapman ER, Williams PT: Intravenous alcohol as an obstetrical analgesia. Am. J. Obstet. Gynecol. 61:676, 1951.
93. Pritchard JA: The use of the magnesium ion in the management of eclamptogenic toxemia. Surg. Gynecol. Obstet. 100:131, 1955.
94. Kovac R, Gaborikova V, Stencl J: Functional reserve of umbilico-placental circulation. Cesk. Gynekol. 54:581, 1989.
95. Thiagarajah S, Harbert Jr GM Bourgeois FJ: Magnesium sulfate and ritodrine hydrochloride: systemic and uterine hemodynamic effects. Am. J. Obstet. Gynecol. 153:666, 1985.
96. Altura BM, Altura BT, Carellac A: Magnesium deficiency-induced spasms of umbilical vessels: relation to preeclampsia, hypertension, growth retardation. Science 221:376, 1983.
97. Vella LM, Knott C, Reynolds F: Transfer of fentanyl across

the rabbit placenta. Effect of umbilical flow and concurrent drug administration. Br. J. Anaesth. 58:49, 1986.
98. Craft JB Jr, Coaldrake LA, Bolan JC, Mondino M, et al: Placental passage and uterine effects of fentanyl. Anesth. Analg. 62:894, 1983.
99. Cartwright DP, Dann WL, Hutchinson A: Placental transfer of alfentanil at caesarean section. Eur. J. Anaesthesiol. 6: 103, 1989.
100. Eckenhoff JE, Hoffman GL, Funderburg LW: N-allylnormorphine: antagonists to neonatal narcosis produced by sedation of the parturient. Am. J. Obstet. Gynecol. 65:1269, 1953.
101. Eckenhoff JE, Oech SR: The effects of narcotics and antagonists upon respiration and circulation in man. Clin. Pharmacol. Ther. 1:483, 1960.
102. Telford J, Keats JS: Narcotic-narcotic antagonist mixtures. Anesthesiology 22:465, 1961.
103. Hibbard BM, Rosen M, Davies D: Placental transfer of naloxone. Br. J. Anaesth. 58:45, 1986.
104. Dailland P, Cockshott ID, Didier Lirzin J, Jacquinot P, et al: Intravenous propofol during cesarean section: placental transfer, concentrations in breast milk, and neonatal effects. Anesthesiology 71:827, 1989.
105. Burkett G, Yasin S, Palow D: Perinatal implications of cocaine exposure. J. Reprod. Med. 35:35, 1990.
106. Moll W, Kastendieck E: Transfer of $N_2O$, CO and HTO in the artificially perfused guinea-pig placenta. Respir. Physiol. 29:283, 1977.
107. Tunstall ME, Sheikh A: Comparison of 1.5% enflurane with 1.25% isoflurane in oxygen for caesarean section: avoidance of awareness without nitrous oxide. Br. J. Anaesth. 62:138, 1989.
108. Baker BW, Hughes SC, Shnider SM, Field DR, et al: Maternal anesthesia and the stressed fetus: effects of isoflurane on the asphyxiated fetal lamb. Anesthesiology 72:65, 1990.
109. Abboud TK, D'Onofrio L, Reyes A, Mosaad PA, et al: Isoflurane or halothane for cesarean section: comparative maternal and neonatal effects. Acta. Anesthesiol. Scand. 33:578, 1989.

Chapter 9

# THE NATURE OF THE PAIN OF PARTURITION

JOHN J. BONICA

A thorough understanding of all aspects of the nature of pain of childbirth is a *sine qua non* for optimal obstetric anesthesiologic care. As emphasized in Chapter 1, effective relief of the pain of childbirth has long been and today remains an important health and sociologic issue worldwide. The importance stems from several interrelated reasons. For one thing, contrary to the claims of proponents of "natural childbirth" and "psychoprophylaxis" that this physiologic process should be painless, it has long been appreciated that labor and vaginal delivery are painful events for most women. For another, misconceptions exist among the public, some physicians, nurses, midwives, and other health professionals about its nature, function, and effects and about methods for its control. Many believe that pain has an important biologic function and should not be relieved, while others believe that pharmacologic methods of pain relief have deleterious effects on the mother and fetus and should be avoided.

As emphasized later, while pain has the important biologic function of indicating to the gravida that labor is imminent, it should be effectively relieved once it has served this function because persistent, severe pain has harmful effects on the mother and might also have harmful effects on the fetus and newborn. Although improperly administered analgesia/anesthesia can entail the risk of complications and can contribute to maternal and perinatal morbidity and even mortality, there is now an impressive body of evidence that suggests that properly administered analgesia/anesthesia does not contribute to maternal and perinatal morbidity or mortality but may help to reduce them, especially in high-risk pregnancies. Finally, many gravidae in developed countries have been informed of the benefits of modern pharmacologic analgesia by the news media and other sources and many expect effective pain relief during childbirth.

In this chapter I present a comprehensive overview of all aspects of the pain of childbirth. The terms labor pain, parturition pain, and childbirth pain are used interchangeably for the pain experienced by parturients during their three stages of labor and vaginal delivery.

The material is presented in three major sections: (1) a brief overview of the current concepts of acute pain in general, including its neurophysiologic and biochemical substrates, its modulation, and its function; (2) the nature of the pain of childbirth, including discussion of the incidence, intensity, and quality of labor pain; detailed description of the intrinsic mechanisms and other factors that influence it; the peripheral pathways and the central nociceptive mechanisms; and (3) the effects of parturition pain and their modification by properly administered analgesia/anesthesia. This chapter represents an updated summary of the subject as presented in the first edition of this book (1), two recent review articles (2,3), and chapters recently published in major textbooks on pain (4,5).

## CURRENT CONCEPTS OF PAIN

In this chapter only a brief review of some of the new facts will be given under the following headings: (1) neurophysiology and biochemistry of acute pain, including the peripheral system; central mechanisms and spinal cord; ascending afferent systems, brain stem and cerebral cortex; (2) modulating systems; and (3) psychologic aspects. Comprehensive review of the historical evolution of pain concept and many of these aspects appears in recently published books and articles (14–17).

### *Neurophysiology and Biochemistry of Acute Pain*

#### Peripheral System

The peripheral system consists of afferent neurons of spinal and cranial nerves; their distal axonal branches, which end as, or into, receptors in body tissues; their cell bodies in sensory ganglia; and their proximal axonal branches, which make contact with second-order neurons in the neuraxis (Figure 9–1a). Many recent electrophysiologic studies have shown an impressive degree of specialization among receptor-afferent units (14–17). Several types of receptors have been identified: mechanoreceptors, thermoreceptors, and nociceptors or pain receptors. Nociceptors are characterized by high threshold, small receptive fields, persistent discharge for a suprathreshold stimulus, and are terminals of small A delta and C afferent fibers. Some A delta afferents are activated only by very strong mechanical stimulation, and thus are known as mechanical nociceptors (high-threshold mechanoreceptors or HTMs). Other A delta afferents respond to both noxious heat stimuli (greater than 45° C) and to intense mechanical stimuli and are thus known as myelinated mechanothermal nociceptors (MMTNs). Most (95% in human skin) of C afferent fibers are activated by intense mechanical (greater than 1 g), thermal (maximal firing range 45 to 53° C), and chemical stimuli and are therefore known as polymodal nociceptors (CPNs).

Studies have also indicated that repeated stimulation

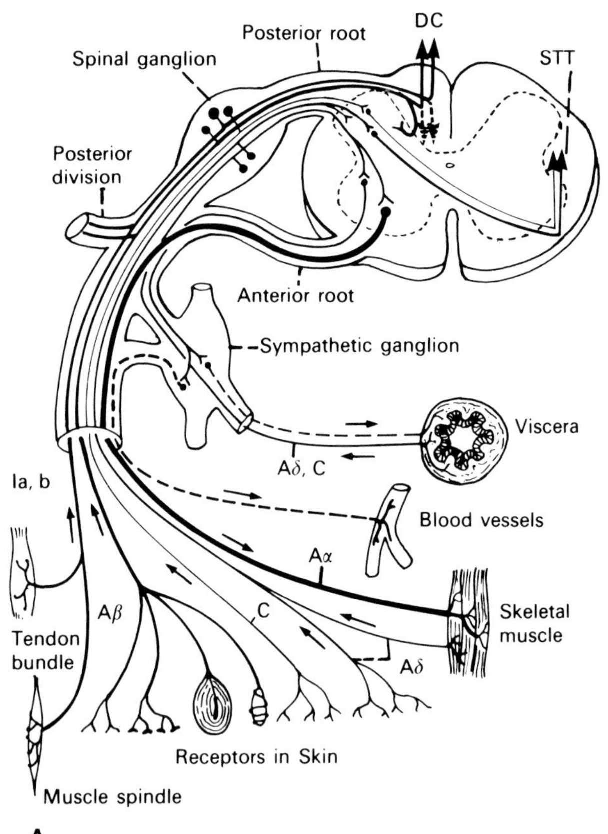


**Fig. 9–1.** A very simplified schema of the components of a peripheral nerve **(A)** and a cross section of the input and output of the dorsal horn of the spinal cord as well as the interneurons and axonal terminals of the descending control systems **(B).** Many of the small, thinly myelinated Aδ and unmyelinated C fibers transmit innocuous mechanical and thermal information, but a significant number transmit nociceptive impulses. These Aδ and C fibers supply skin, deep somatic structures, and viscera. They synapse primarily in laminae I, II°, and V, although they make synoptic contact through interneurons with cells in other laminae. Cutaneous nociceptive afferents project to laminae I, II°, and V, whereas visceral and muscle nociceptive afferents project to laminae I and V but not to lamina II. Note the convergence of cutaneous and visceral afferents on viscerosomatic neurons in laminae I and V [C cells, which are wide-dynamic range (WDR) neurons] the axons of which pass to the anterolateral fasciculus (ALF) of the opposite side and project to the brain. Similarly, Aδ and C muscle nociceptive afferents and cutaneous afferents also converge on neurons in laminae I and V, including some with long ascending axons that make part of the anterolateral fasciculus. Although most of the axons ascend in the contralateral anterolateral fasciculus, some ascend ipsilaterally. The collaterals from Aβ fibers, which course along the medial side of the dorsal horn, take a retroflex course at the level of lamina V, ascend dorsally, and then branch out to make contact with interneurons and output neurons. In this way they modulate dorsal horn output. Note the interneurons in laminae II and III and an "antenna" cell in lamina IV (cells B) that may project rostrally as dorsal column postsynaptic fibers or as spinocervical fibers. Raphespinal and reticulospinal fibers (from n. reticularis magnocellularis) descend in the lateral fasciculus to make contact with cells in laminae I, II, and V, and deeper laminae to exert modulating influences on dorsal horn function (see Figure 9–4) S = stalk cell, I = islet cell. The dorsolateral funiculus (DLF) contains descending axons of cells in the brain stem that are inhibitory (off-cells) of perhaps facilitatory (on-cells).

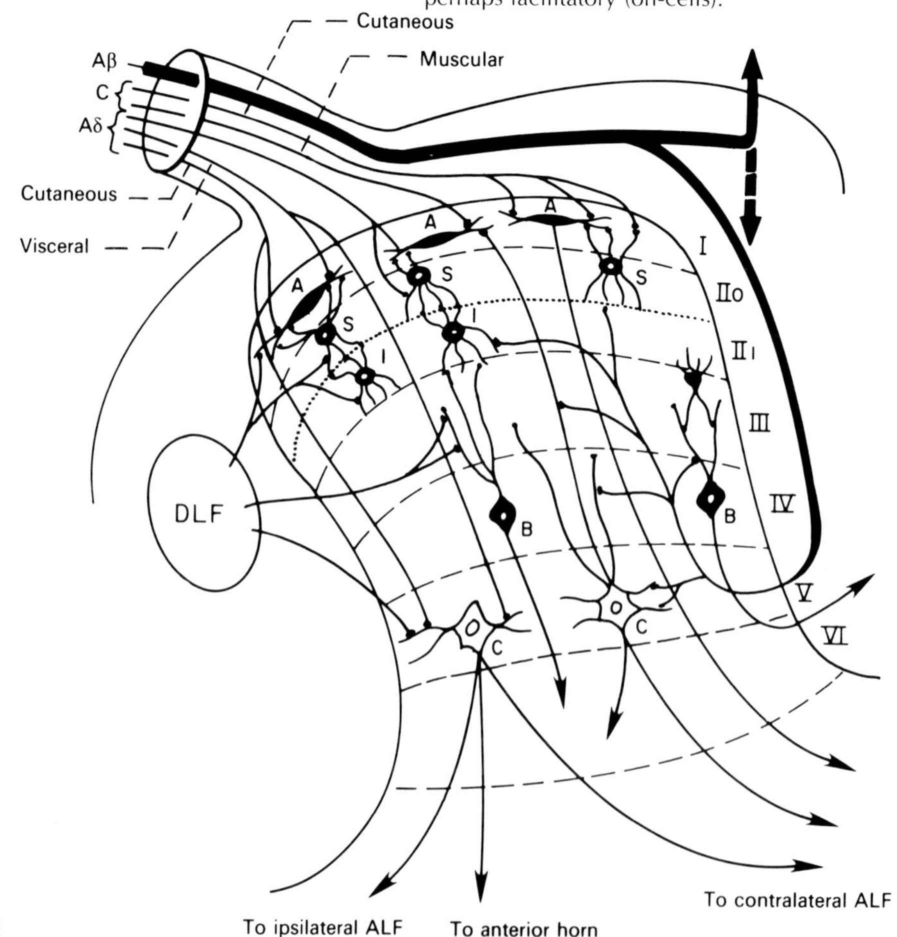

produces sensitization consisting of a decrease in threshold, an augmented responsiveness to suprathreshold stimuli, and spontaneous activity. Sensitization is also produced directly or indirectly by biochemical agents liberated with tissue damage or inflammation, such as bradykinin, histamine, substance P, the leukotrines, prostaglandins, and other arachidonic acid metabolites. There is evidence that the terminals of postganglionic sympathetic efferents are also involved, possibly by the release of a neuropeptide or of ATP. Data from single-fiber and multiple-fiber studies in animals and in man support earlier observation that these A delta and C fibers are essential for pain sensation (17,20). These nociceptor-afferent fibers supply not only the skin and subcutaneous tissue, but also the muscle, fascia, periosteum, and other deep structures (Figure 9–1). Viscera are also supplied by afferent fibers that under certain circumstances [inflammation, spasm of hollow viscera, contraction of hollow viscera under isometric conditions (contraction against obstruction), sudden abnormal distension, stretching or tearing of these structures], act as nociceptive afferents (16).

From the peripheral spinal nerves, the sensory information from below the head is transmitted to dorsal horn cells of the spinal cord while the sensory information from the head is carried via the cranial nerves to the nucleus caudalis of the trigeminal nuclear complex, also called the "medullary dorsal horn." It is then transmitted to higher parts of the neuraxis via ascending neural systems. In contrast to the idea of the straight-through transmission without modification, it is now clear that there is a great degree of modulation all along the course of transmission of impulses: at the first synapse in the spinal dorsal horn or medullary dorsal horn and at every level of the neuraxis (12,13,17,21–23). Within the somatosensory system there are mechanisms that permit distinction between mechanical, thermal, and chemical events in spatial, temporal, and intensity domains.

### *Spinal and Medullary Dorsal Horn*

On reaching the dorsal horn of the spinal cord or the nucleus caudalis, some primary peripheral nociceptive afferents terminate and make direct or indirect contact with cells in the superficial part of these structures (laminae I and II°) and send collaterals that terminate in deeper laminae (V), while others terminate more medially (laminae VII and VIII) (Figure 9–1b) (15,16). Some of the cells in laminae I and II of the dorsal horn are known as nociceptive-specific (NS) neurons because they receive input exclusively from high-threshold peripheral afferents. Those in laminae V (and perhaps IV and VI) are known as "wide dynamic range" (WDR) neurons because they receive input from low-threshold fibers concerned with touch sensation and also from nociceptive afferents so that they are able to respond with increasingly higher frequency of impulse discharge to touch, pressure, and noxious stimuli. The convergence of visceral high-threshold afferents and low-threshold afferents from the skin, supplied by the same spinal cord segments on laminae V neurons, is said to provide the neural basis for the phenomenon of referred pain associated with visceral deep and somatic disorders (16).

In addition to making synaptic contact and receiving input from primary nociceptive afferents, these dorsal horn neurons also receive input from the large myelinated peripheral afferents, from short axon interneurons of the substantia gelatinosa and from the terminals of supraspinal descending neural control systems. Thus, it is obvious that the dorsal horn and nucleus caudalis, which were traditionally considered simple relay stations, are very complex structures containing a large number and many varieties of neurons and synaptic arrangements that permit not only reception and transmission, but a high degree of sensory processing, including local abstraction, integration, selection, and appropriate dispersion of sensory impulses. This complex form of local processing is achieved through the phenomena of central convergence, central summation, excitation, and inhibition coming from the periphery, from local and segmental interneurons, and from the brain and brain stem. These processes involve the liberation of putative excitatory neurotransmitters, including substance P and somatostatin, and the liberation of the endogenous opioid peptide enkephalin and other inhibitory neurotransmitters including norepinephrine and 5-hydroxytriptamine. These very complex interactions determine the modulation, transmission, and dispersion of nociceptive information.

After being subjected to these modulating influences in the dorsal horn, some of the nociceptive impulses pass through internuncial neurons to the anterior and anterolateral horn cells where they stimulate somatomotor neurons that supply skeletal muscles and sympathetic neurons, which supply blood vessels, viscera, and sweat glands. These are involved in segmental reflex (autonomic) responses that are described later. Other nociceptive impulses are transmitted to neurons, the axons of which make up the spinothalamic tract and other ascending systems and are thus conveyed to the brain stem and the brain to provoke suprasegmental reflex responses and cortical responses.

### *Ascending Pathways*

It has long been known that the spinothalamic tract transmits pain messages from below the head and that the trigeminothalamic tract transmits impulses from the head (17,24). However, evidence acquired during the past 2 decades indicates that this system also transmits other sensory information and is composed of two parts that have different anatomical, physiologic, and functional characteristics: the neospinothalamic tract and the paleospinothalamic tracts (Figure 9–2). More recent evidence also suggests that several other ascending systems participate in transmission of pain signals; on the basis of their anatomical and functional characteristics, these and the spinothalamic tracts have been grouped into two major systems: the lateral system and the medial system (Figure 9–3) (25).

### *The Lateral System*

The lateral system includes the neospinothalamic and neotrigeminothalamic tracts, the spinocervical tract, and the dorsal column postsynaptic system (16). This group is composed of long, thick fibers that conduct rapidly, have a discrete somatotopic organization, and make con-

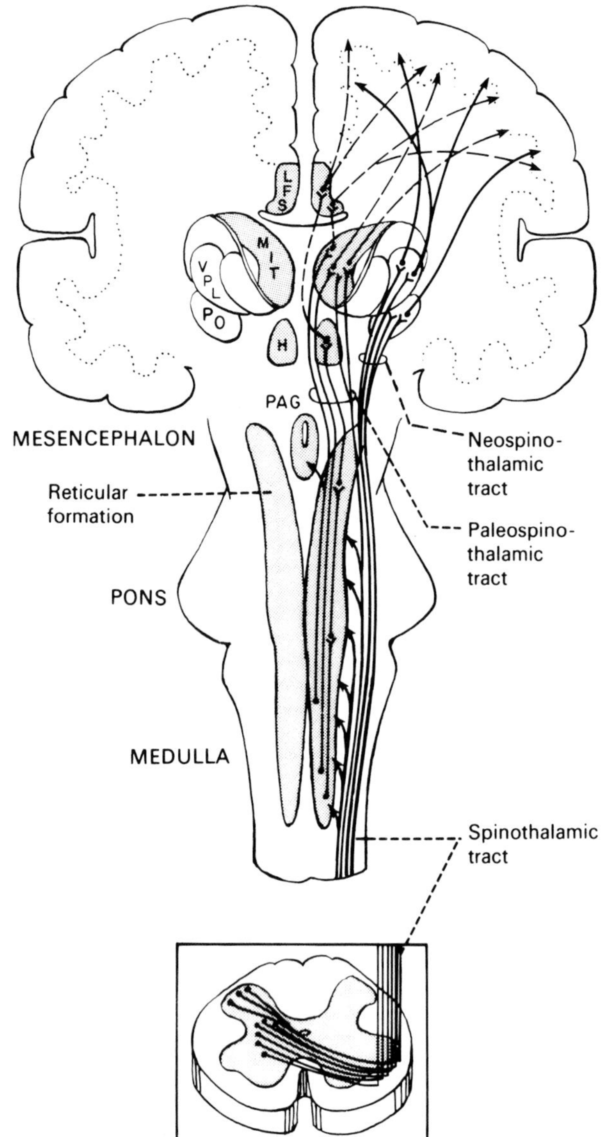


**Fig. 9–2.** Simple diagram of the course and termination of the spinothalamic tract. Most of the fibers cross to the opposite side and ascend to the brain stem and brain, although some ascend ipsilaterally. The neospinothalamic (nSTT) part of the tract has cell bodies located primarily in laminae I and V of the dorsal horn, whereas the paleospinothalamic tract (pSTT) has its cell bodies in deeper laminae. The neospinothalamic fibers ascend in a more superficial part of the tract and project without interruption to the caudal part of the ventroposterolateral thalamic nucleus (VPLc) the oral part of this nucleus (VPLo), the medial part of the posterior thalamus (POm). In these structures they synapse with a third relay of neurons, which project to the somatosensory cortex (SI, SII, and retroinsular cortex) [solid lines]. Some of the fibers of the paleospinothalamic pass directly to the medial/intralaminar thalamic nuclei (MIT), and others project to the nuclei and the reticular formation of the brain stem and thence to the periaqueductal gray (PAG), hypothalamus (H), nucleus submedius, and medial/intralaminar thalamic nuclei. In these structures these axons synapse with neurons that connect with the limbic forebrain structure (LFS) via complex circuits and also send diffuse projection to various parts of the brain [dashed lines].

nection with the ventrobasal thalamus and posterior thalamic nuclei where they synapse with another relay of fibers that project to the somatosensory cortex. The evidence suggests that the lateral system is concerned with rapid transmission of phasic discriminatory information about the onset of injury, its precise location, its intensity and duration, and can quickly bring about responses that prevent further damage.

### The Medial System

The medial system is composed of the paleospinothalamic, paleotrigeminothalamic, spinoreticular, and propriospinal systems (16,25). The paleospinothalamic, paleotrigeminothalamic, and spinoreticular fibers consist of a few long and many short, thin fibers that are not somatically organized and that pass medially to project to the reticular formation, the periaqueductal grey matter (PAG), the hypothalamus, and the medial and intrathalamic nuclei where they synapse with neurons that connect with the limbic forebrain structures and with diffuse projections to many other parts of the brain. The multisynaptic propriospinal system also consists of very short, thin fibers that ascend through the cord in the grey matter (in contrast to the ventrolateral tracts which lie in the white matter) and project to unknown destinations in the brain. Because of the thinness of the fibers, their multi-synaptic nature, and the lack of somatotopic organization, impulses passing through this system are said to transmit tonic information about the state of the organism. As previously mentioned, these impulses also provoke the suprasegmental reflex responses, the powerful motivational drive, and the unpleasant effect characteristic of pain, and some stimulate cells in the PAG and thus activate descending control systems.

### Brain Stem

The reticular formation serves an integrative function and from the midbrain level an ascending activating system of fibers maintains both tonic and phasic stimulation of an overlying diffuse thalamic projection system, which in turn modulates the level of arousal of widespread areas of cerebral cortex, particularly the association cortex (16,17,26–31). The hypothalamus integrates and regulates autonomic nervous system functions and the neuroendocrine response to stress, and organizes visceral and somatic reaction patterns (16,28,29). The limbic system does not have primary control of behavioral processes, but rather has a complex modulatory suppressor influence upon attention, mood, and motivation, as well as upon processes underlying the performance of certain types of behavior (16,30,31).

### Cerebral Cortex

The somatosensory cortex serves a discriminatory function and may regulate subcortical activity related to pain through highly complex reflexes, but is not essential to pain perception (12,13,16,32). The frontal cortex probably plays a significant role in mediating between cognitive activities and motivational and affective features of pain because it receives information via intracortical fiber sys-

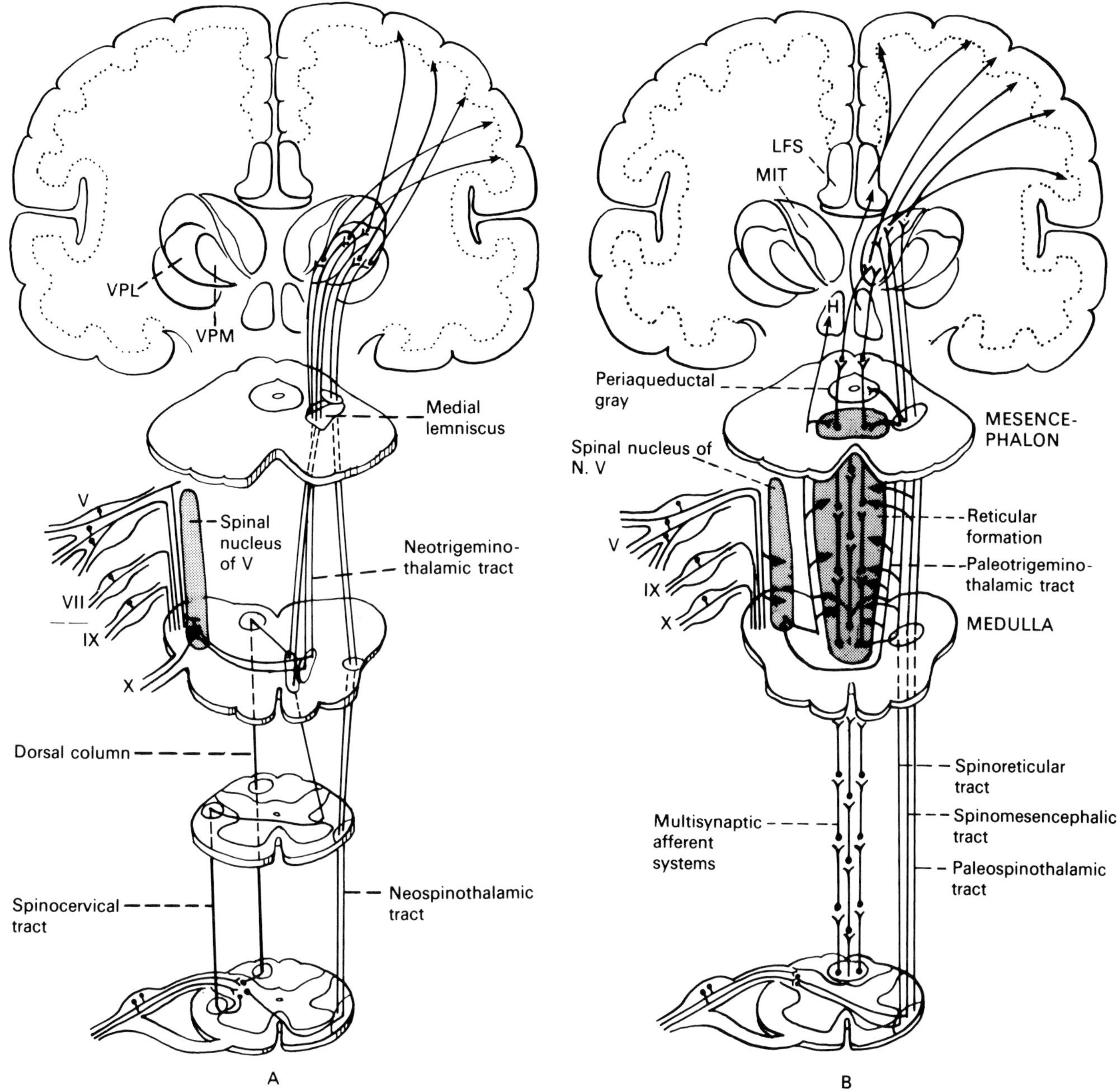


**Fig. 9–3.** Diagrams illustrating the origin, course, and projection of the lateral system **(A)** and the medial system **(B).** See text for details.

tems from virtually all sensory and associated cortical areas and projects strongly to reticular and limbic structures (13–16). These make possible mobilization of all sorts of associations based upon past experience, judgements, and emotions, and is involved in the evaluation of the sensation. It appears essential in maintaining a negative affect and aversive motivational dimension of pain. Neocortical processes subserve cognitive and psychologic factors, including early experience, prior conditioning anxiety, attention, suggestion, cultural background, and evaluation of the meaning of the pain-producing situation. Through the neocortical processes and corticifugal impulses, these factors may affect both sensory, affective, and motivational dimensions of pain or they may modify primarily the affective and motivational and leave the sensory discriminatory dimensions relatively undisturbed (13–16).

## *Modulation of Nociception and Pain*

One of the most exciting areas in recent research concerns the various neural, biochemical, and psychophysiologic mechanisms that participate in the modulation of nociceptive information from tissues to the brain (22–24). In the peripheral system, injury or inflammation causes the liberation of pain-producing substances and/or damages nerves and thus lowers the threshold of the nociceptive afferent units so that innocuous stimulation

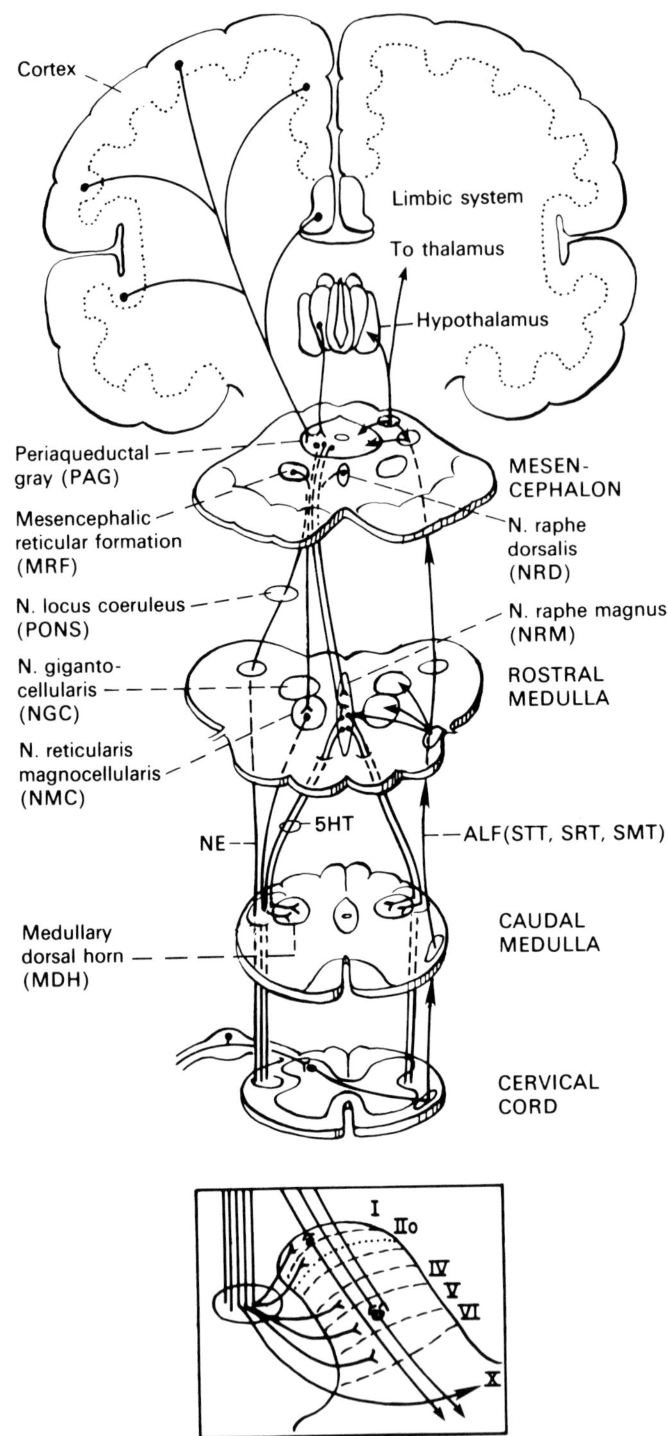


**Fig. 9–4.** Schema of the most extensively studied and probably the most important descending control system, composed of four tiered parts. The ascending anterolateral fasciculus (anterolateral fasciculus), composed of the spinothalamic, spinoreticular, and spinomesencephalic tracts, has important inputs into the nucleus raphe magnus (NRM), nucleus magnocellularis (NMC), nucleus reticularis gigantocellularis (NGC), and the periaqueductal gray (PAG) via the nucleus cuneiformis. The anterolateral fasciculus also has input to the medullary/pontine reticular formation, the nucleus raphe dorsalis (NRD), and the mesencephalic reticular formation (MRF). The periaqueductal gray receives important input from such rostral structures as the frontal and insular cortex and other parts of the cerebrum involved in cognition, and from the limbic system, the thalamus, and, most importantly, the hypothalamus, which sends beta endorphin axons to the periaqueductal gray. The locus coeruleus in the pons is a major source of noradrenergic input to the periaqueductal gray and dorsal horn. These mesencephalic structures (periaqueductal gray, nucleus raphe dorsalis, mesencephalic reticular formation) contain enkephalin (ENK), dynorphin (DYN), serotonin (5HT), and neurotensin (NT) neurons, but only the latter two send axons that project to nucleus raphe magnus and nucleus reticularis gigantocellularis. Here they make synapse with neurons that are primarily serotonergic, whose axons project to the medullary dorsal horn and descend in the dorsolateral funiculus to send

(light touch) produces pain. On the other hand, innocuous stimulation of the skin by rubbing, by application of cold or by transcutaneous electrical stimulation in some way impairs the transmission of nociceptive impulses from the periphery to the dorsal horn. Nociceptive transmission in the dorsal horn is affected by the activity and interactions of local interneurons and supraspinal descending systems (Figure 9–3).

In 1969 Reynolds (33) reported that electrical stimulation of the lateral periaqueductal grey (PAG) and periventricular grey (PVG) matter of the midbrain produced a profound analgesia without apparently interfering with motor function or with the animal's response to other sensory stimuli. A series of brilliant experiments by Liebeskind and coworkers (34–36) and many others (21,37) done during the ensuing decade have shown that: (1) this phenomenon, known as stimulation-produced analgesia or SPA, often outlasts stimulation by many seconds or minutes; (2) stimulation-produced analgesia inhibits the activity of dorsal horn neurons involved in nociception but not those concerned with other sensations; (3) the effects of stimulation-produced analgesia are partly or wholly diminished by administration of naloxone, a morphine antagonist; and (4) injection of very small amounts of morphine directly into PAG produces analgesia indicating that a major effect of morphine is to activate descending inhibitory neurons in the brain stem. The anatomical and biochemical characteristics of this descending pathway have been elucidated (21–23) (Figure 9–4).

These studies were paralleled by the discovery of opiate receptors on nerve cells that led to the quest and identification of endogenously produced substances, which were named endorphins (endogenous morphine-like substances) and enkephalins (opioid substances in the brain). As a result of these and other studies, it was found that stimulation-produced analgesia produced impulses that descend in the dorsolateral funiculus and make contact with and stimulate a variety of short axon interneurons in the substantia gelatinosa at every level of the spinal cord. Some of these interneurons contain enkephalin, which inhibits transmission of nociceptive information by preventing the release of substance P, the neurotransmitter, and permits the transfer of nociceptive impulses from one nerve to another. This descending modulating system has input from the brain, limbic system, and other structures that are known to be involved in the psychologic dimensions of pain.

More recent studies have suggested that there are other descending inhibitory systems that do not involve opioids (21,38,39). The data acquired to date make it perfectly clear that there are a number of mechanisms of pain inhibition, some involving spinal mechanisms; others involving supraspinal mechanisms; some involving opioids and some not; and some involving contrifugal control on spinal nociceptive systems and some not. In addition to drastically changing our conceptualization of pain mechanisms, the new data have had a major impact on the development of new modalities for relief of pain.

Even more recent electrophysiologic experiments in animals revealed that stimulation of the rostral ventromedial medulla (RVM) can also exert facilitatory effects on spinal nociceptive neurons. Fields and associates (40) used a tail-flick reflex (TF) response in lightly anesthetized rats to study the characteristics of cells in the rostral ventromedial medulla and found a class of tail-flick reflex-related bulbospinal neurons in this region that they called "on-cells." Pharmacologic evidence supports the thesis that on-cells have an enhancing effect on nociception. The activity of these on-cells is completely suppressed by morphine given in doses sufficient to block tail-flick reflex—a response that is due to stimulation of "off-cells." When the "spontaneous" activity of on-cells and off-cells is studied simultaneously, they are found to have a reciprocal period of activity. When on-cells are active, tail-flick reflex response latency is short and the threshold is lower, whereas when off-cells are active, tail-flick reflex response latency is longer. Given the extensive independent support for the role of rostral ventromedial medulla neurons and modulation of spinal nociception, these observations that tail-flick reflex response latency is inversely related to on-cell firing and is directly related to off-cell firing, are consistent with bidirectional modulation or control of nociception by these two populations of rostral ventromedial medulla neurons: on-cells that enhance nociceptive transmission and off-cells that suppress it.

### *Psychologic and Emotional Factors*

During the past quarter-century much new scientific data have been acquired that impressively emphasize the importance of the motivational, affective, cognitive, emotional, and other psychological factors on the individual's total pain experience (41–46). Moreover, it has put into sharper focus the influence of perceptual factors, learning, personality, ethnic and cultural factors, and the environment, and has helped to clarify the psychodynamics of anxiety, anticipation of pain, the meaning or significance of the pain-producing sensation, attention, motivation, suggestion, and placebos—factors well-known to influence the pain experience. Early experience, perceptual factors, personality, ethnic and cultural patterns play varying roles in the individual's pain behavior. In some cultures tolerating pain without expression of suffering is required, while in others overt expression of suffering is encouraged.

Anxiety is a particularly powerful factor in reducing pain tolerance or, in other worlds, producing greater pain behavior (45,46). Conversely, pain tolerance can be increased by reducing anxiety with information or attention to another task. Attention, the selective orientation of the receptor system to one source or pattern of stimulation to the exclusion of others, can either enhance or diminish

terminals to all laminae of the spinal gray (the densest populations are found in laminae I, II°, and V of the dorsal horn and the motor neuron pools of lamina IX). The projection from nucleus raphe magnus is bilateral, whereas the projection from nucleus reticularis gigantocellularis is ipsilateral. Noradrenergic fibers descend and project to the medullary dorsal horn and then descend in the dorsolateral funiculus of the spinal cord to send terminals to laminae I, II°, IV–VI, and X.

the painful experience. It is, of course, well-known that athletes injured during play and soldiers injured in battle often do not experience pain at the moment of injury. In contrast, the same individuals often manifest overt pain behavior consequent to minimal noxious stimulation induced by hypodermic needles in the emergency room. Under such conditions, attention and anxiety both decrease tolerance to pain.

Motivation is another psychodynamic mechanism that can have significant influence on the physiologic, behavioral, and affective aspects of pain experience (10,44). In some instances motivation is so strong as to permit the individual to sustain severe injury without any of the pain responses. In such cases, psychophysiologic mechanisms probably inhibit transmission of impulses in the dorsal horn as well as other parts of the nervous system. In others, the mechanism is not sufficient to block reflex responses but is sufficient to suppress overt pain behavior.

How do these psychologic factors influence pain? In view of the recent data, it is not taking an unreasonable degree of scientific license to suggest that various emotional, motivational, and affective factors can stimulate parts of the brain that, when activated, exert powerful inhibition. These send descending impulses, which have the capability of preventing transmission of noxious impulses in the dorsal horn and at different levels of the neuraxis. On the other hand, under appropriate conditions psychologic factors through action of the limbic system and descending pathways can stimulate "on-cells" and thus enhance transmission of noxious impulses to the brain with consequent greater pain experience.

## Biology and Pathophysiology of Acute Pain

Transient acute pain occurs when an individual touches a hot stove or steps on a sharp object that promptly alerts the individual and causes him or her to immediately withdraw the limb and thus avoid further damage. Acute pain associated with severe injuries involving deep somatic structures, such as fractures or sprains, imposes limitation of action and therefore tends to prevent further damage or aggravation of pathophysiology. The biologic function of acute pain under these circumstances is widely accepted and appreciated. Similarly, acute pain of visceral disease has the biologic function of warning the individual that something is wrong and prompting him or her to consult a physician, and is used by the physician as an aid in making the diagnosis. Moreover, acute pain caused by injury or disease is often associated with certain segmental and suprasegmental reflex responses that help the organism maintain homeostasis (see below).

Although the biologic function of acute pain is widely and universally accepted, what is not generally realized or appreciated, even by some physicians, is that some types of pain, such as that which occurs after an operation, has no biologic function, but instead produces abnormal physiologic and psychologic reactions that often cause complications. Similar deleterious effects result if the severe pain of injury or of such diseases as myocardial infarction and acute pancreatitis is not effectively relieved after it has served its biologic function. Indeed, as will be duly emphasized later, even severe pain associated with certain physiologic processes such as parturition, if allowed to persist, will produce deleterious effects. These detrimental effects are consequent to progression of the segmental and suprasegmental reflex responses and cortical responses to an abnormal state. To fully appreciate this thesis, a brief discussion of the responses to tissue injury is presented.

### Responses to Tissue Injury

Tissue destruction, whether from crush injury, fracture, operation, internal disease or the injury inherent in parturition, results in local biochemical changes and autonomic reflex responses that are intended to maintain body integrity (47,48). The local biochemical changes produced by liberation of intracellular chemical substances into the extracellular fluids surrounding nerve endings to induce local pain, tenderness, and hyperalgesia have been discussed earlier. In addition to sensitizing the nerve endings, these algogenic substances also act indirectly by altering the microenvironment consisting of smooth muscles, capillaries, and efferent sympathetic fibers. The nociceptors, thus activated, transduce the noxious stimuli into impulses that are transmitted to the neuraxis. As previously mentioned, upon reaching the spinal or medullary dorsal horn, these impulses are promptly subjected to peripheral, local, segmental and supraspinal descending modulating influences which, together with other factors, determine their further transmission throughout the neuraxis. Some stimulate somatomotor and sympathetic preganglionic fibers of the same and adjacent segments to produce segmental (spinal) reflex responses. Other nociceptive impulses stimulate dorsal horn neurons, the axons of which make up ascending afferent systems and thus provoke suprasegmental reflex responses and cortical responses (Figure 9–14).

### Segmental (Spinal) Reflexes

Segmental (spinal) reflexes may, and often do, enhance nociception and produce alteration of ventilation, circulation, and gastrointestinal and urinary function. Thus, stimulation of somatomotor cells results in increased skeletal muscle tension or spasm, which decreases chest wall compliance and initiates positive feedback loops that generate nociceptive impulses from the muscle (47,48).

Stimulation of sympathetic preganglionic neurons in the anterolateral horn of the spinal cord causes an increase in heart rate, stroke volume, and, consequently, cardiac work, and myocardial oxygen consumption. Moreover, severe pain may cause cardiac arrhythmia, which may become serious. In addition, sympathetic hyperactivity causes decrease of gastrointestinal tone that may progress to ileus and a decrease in urinary function that reduces urinary output. Because these responses to noxious stimuli occur in animals who have had vagotomy and C1 spinal section, they are produced by truly spinal segmental reflexes.

Recent studies in animals and clinical observations in man suggest that intense nociceptive stimulation as occurs during the latter part of the active phase of the first stage and during the second stage of labor, not only sensitizes peripheral nociceptor afferents and perhaps sympathetic efferents but also produces a nociceptor barrage that is likely to sensitize both the dorsal horn neurons, interneurons, preganglionic sympathetic neurons, and anterior motor neurons (20). This produces a long-latency, long duration facilitation that effects cells in lamina I and in deeper laminae, and thus triggers very prolonged increase in excitability of cells in these regions. Massive nociceptive input also produces a large expansion of the cutaneous fields. The input can convert spinal cord nociceptive specific cells to cells that respond to light as well as to intense stimulation (wide dynamic range, WDR). Although the facilitation is triggered by the arrival of impulses in afferent fibers from deep tissues, it is sustained by an intrinsic spinal cord process (20,21). This prolonged increase of excitability of central cells is probably the basis for widespread prolonged tenderness, hyperalgesia, and spasm of the low back muscles that cause low back pain hypoalgesia that many puerperae experience postoperatively.

### Suprasegmental Reflex Responses

Suprasegmental reflex responses result from nociceptive-induced stimulation of medullary centers of ventilation and circulation, of hypothalamic (predominantly sympathetic) centers of neuroendocrine function, and of some limbic structures (47). These responses consist of hyperventilation, increased hypothalamic neural sympathetic tone, and increased secretion of catecholamines and other endocrines. The increased neural sympathetic tone and catecholamine secretion add to the effects of spinal reflexes and further increase cardiac output, peripheral resistance, blood pressure, cardiac workload, and myocardial oxygen consumption (48). In addition to catecholamine release, there is an increased secretion of cortisol, ACTH, glucagon, cAMP, ADH, growth hormone (GH), renin, and other catabolically acting hormones, with a concomitant decrease in the anabolically acting hormones insulin and testosterone (47–50). This type of endocrine secretion, characteristic of the stress response, produces widespread metabolic effects, including increased blood glucose, free fatty acids, blood lactate, and ketones, as well as generalized increased metabolism and oxygen consumption. The endocrine and metabolic changes result in substrate utilization from storage to central organs and injured tissue and lead to a catabolic state with a negative nitrogen balance. The degree and duration of these endocrine and metabolic changes are related to degree and duration of tissue damage, and many of these biochemical changes last for days (50) see Figure 9–14 in section on).

### Cortical Responses

The intense anxiety and fear that invariably develops in patients who experience severe acute pain consequent to an unexpected severe injury or acute myocardial infarction greatly enhance the hypothalamic responses characteristic of stress through cortical stimulation. Indeed, cortisol and catecholamine responses to anxiety may exceed the hypothalamic responses provoked directly by nociceptive impulses reaching the hypothalamus (47). Moreover, anxiety causes cortically mediated increased blood viscosity, clotting time, fibrinolysis, and platelet aggregation (see 47 for references). Recent advances in medicine, surgery, and anesthesia, together with much new information about the metabolic and biochemical responses to injury, now suggest that these reflex responses might have become maladaptive because the persistent pain and associated reflex responses may cause a variety of complications. In the next section I will present impressive evidence that blocking the afferent and efferent pathways involved in these responses proves beneficial.

## THE NATURE OF PARTURITION PAIN

### *Magnitude of the Problems*

Mention has been made of the misconceptions and confusion about the nature of the pain of childbirth and its treatment. This has been and continues to be a result of inadequate dissemination of information to the public about advances in knowledge and current therapeutic procedures. Many proponents of natural childbirth have compounded the problem by insisting that pain need not occur during normal labor and that when it occurs it is the product of modern cultural and environmental factors. The origin of this notion is not known, but Lee in 1844 mentioned parturition as a painless process, and 70 years later Behan (51) stated in his classic book that "like menstruation, childbirth naturally should be a painless process. It is only as culture advances that the labor becomes painful, for in women of primitive races pain is absent. Savages of a low degree of civilization are generally little troubled by parturiency." Nineteen years later the same argument was put forth by Dick-Read (52), who for the ensuing 25 years traveled worldwide espousing this thesis, strongly condemning pharmacologic analgesia, and encouraging the use of his method of "natural childbirth." In 1950, in the then called USSR, Velvovski and associates (53) began to use the technique of "psychoprophylaxis," which they had developed and which was a modification of the Dick-Read method. Psychoprophylaxis was subsequently embraced by Lamaze (54) of France, who did much to popularize it in Europe and the Western hemisphere. The claim by these clinicians and their followers that childbirth among primitive peoples is painless has been disputed by many studies (55–59).

Ford (55), who studied this and other problems of reproduction in 64 primitive societies, wrote that "the popular impression of childbirth in primitive society as painless and easy is definitely contradicted by our cases. As a matter of fact, it is often prolonged and painful." After studying 80 primitive groups, Freedman and Ferguson (56) reported that the pain response in these groups during childbirth was similar to that observed in American and European parturients. Similar views have been expressed by others who studied the problem of labor pain in primitive societies (57). I observed over 24 parturients in primitive societies in Australia and Africa, most of whom manifested severe pain behavior (unpublished data). Mention of the prevalence of pain during childbirth and its importance is found in the writings of the ancient Babylonians, Egyptians, Chinese, Hebrews, and Greeks, and in the writings of many subsequent cultures and civilizations (58). Finally, a recent study by Lefebvre and Carli (59) of parturition of 88 individuals of 29 species of captive and wild nonhuman primates, revealed that 69 (78%) manifested moderate to very severe pain characterized by straining, stretching, arching, grimacing, writhing, shaking, doubling-up, restlessness, and vocalizations. This article provides impressive evidence that while the behavior of the monkeys varied upon the circumstances of the environment, the process of parturition in these animals provoked what in humans we call pain of varying degrees.

### *Incidence, Intensity, and Quality of Parturition Pain*

Although it is a common observation in obstetrics that parturients vary in the amount of suffering associated with labor and vaginal delivery, few well-designed studies on the prevalence, intensity, and quality of labor pain have been performed. Lundh (60) published a survey of several Swedish investigations, which included both primiparae and multiparae; these revealed that the incidence of intolerable severe pain ranged from 35 to 58%, with the remainder having moderate pain. Bundsen (61) found that 77% of primiparae reported that their pain during childbirth was severe or intolerable. In a study of 78 Swedish randomly selected primiparae, Nettelbladt and colleagues (62) found that 35% reported intolerable pain, 37% had severe pain, and 28% had moderate pain during labor and delivery. Records on 2700 parturients observed (and many interviewed) by Bonica while visiting or working (demonstrating obstetric anesthetic techniques) in 121 obstetric centers (with some having 100 to 150 deliveries daily) in 35 countries on 6 continents indicated that the frequency and intensity of labor pain was as follows: 15% had little or no pain, 35% had moderate pain, 30% had severe pain, and 20% had extremely severe pain. The data are similar to those noted among over 8000 American parturients to whom I have administered personally or directly supervised residents providing anesthetic care during a period of 40 years (Bonica, unpublished data). Obviously, these surveys and observations were based on simple numeric or verbal descriptions of pain, and thus lack quantification. One of the first attempts to quantify the intensity of labor pain was made by Javert and Hardy (63), who used the Hardy-Wolff-Goodell dolorimeter to induce experimental pain and asked the parturients to compare it to the pain of their labor. The method entails the application of thermal heat, measured in millicalories (mc), to 3.5 cm of skin for 3 seconds. The stimulus was increased in intensity stepwise until perceptible pain (pain threshold) and eventually the greatest perceivable pain (ceiling or maximum pain) were induced. They used a pain scale that ranged from 1 pain unit ("dol"), assigned to pain threshold, to 10½ dol, denoting maximum pain, which was produced by a stimulus of sufficient intensity to produce a third-degree burn. They studied 26 primiparae and 6 multiparae during the course of normal labor and delivery and found that the intensity of pain in the early part (latent phase) of the first stage was 2 to 3 dol (very mild), increasing progressively to 3 to 4 dol at about 4 cm cervical dilatation, 5 to 7 dol at 6 to 8 cm, and 8 to 9 dol at full dilatation, and ranging from 9 to 10½ dol (maximum pain) as the head of the baby dilated and stretched the perineum during the second stage of labor.

The incidence, intensity, quality, and other aspects of labor pain have been elucidated more precisely by Melzack and associates (64–67,68), who have carried out a series of studies using the McGill Pain Questionnaire (MPQ) (69), the most extensively tested multidimensional scale of pain measurements available. The McGill Pain Questionnaire consists of 20 sets of words describing the sensory, affective, and evaluative dimension of the pain experience. The first 10 sets represent sensory quality, the next 5 affective, 16 are evaluative, and the last 4 are miscellaneous words (Figure 9–5). Two major indices can be obtained from the questionnaire: first is a pain rating index (PRI), which is the sum of the rank values of the words chosen based on the position of the words in each category of subclass; second is an index of present pain intensity (PPI), a measure of the overall pain intensity on a scale of 0 to 5 with 0 representing no pain, 1 mild, 2 discomforting, 3 distressing, 4 horrible, and 5 excruciating.

In their first study (64), labor pain was measured with the McGill Pain Questionnaire in 87 primiparae and 54 multiparae, all of whom had cervical dilatation of at least 2 to 3 cm and contractions at intervals of 5 minutes or less. Of the 141 parturients, 61 primiparae and 31 multiparae had received prepared childbirth training in special-

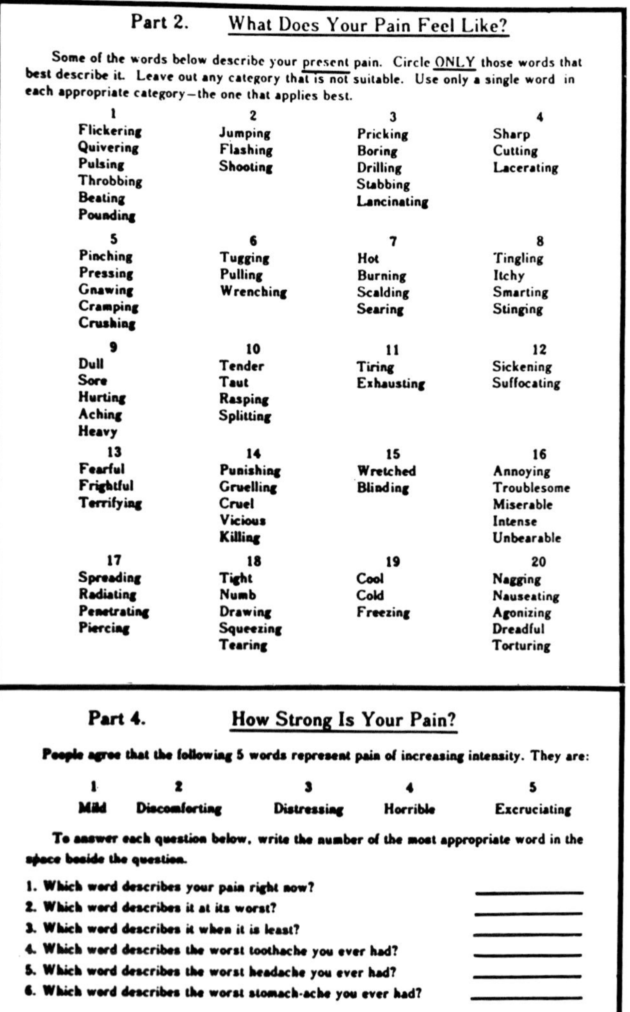

Part 2. What Does Your Pain Feel Like?

Some of the words below describe your present pain. Circle ONLY those words that best describe it. Leave out any category that is not suitable. Use only a single word in each appropriate category—the one that applies best.

| 1 | 2 | 3 | 4 |
|---|---|---|---|
| Flickering<br>Quivering<br>Pulsing<br>Throbbing<br>Beating<br>Pounding | Jumping<br>Flashing<br>Shooting | Pricking<br>Boring<br>Drilling<br>Stabbing<br>Lancinating | Sharp<br>Cutting<br>Lacerating |
| **5** | **6** | **7** | **8** |
| Pinching<br>Pressing<br>Gnawing<br>Cramping<br>Crushing | Tugging<br>Pulling<br>Wrenching | Hot<br>Burning<br>Scalding<br>Searing | Tingling<br>Itchy<br>Smarting<br>Stinging |
| **9** | **10** | **11** | **12** |
| Dull<br>Sore<br>Hurting<br>Aching<br>Heavy | Tender<br>Taut<br>Rasping<br>Splitting | Tiring<br>Exhausting | Sickening<br>Suffocating |
| **13** | **14** | **15** | **16** |
| Fearful<br>Frightful<br>Terrifying | Punishing<br>Gruelling<br>Cruel<br>Vicious<br>Killing | Wretched<br>Blinding | Annoying<br>Troublesome<br>Miserable<br>Intense<br>Unbearable |
| **17** | **18** | **19** | **20** |
| Spreading<br>Radiating<br>Penetrating<br>Piercing | Tight<br>Numb<br>Drawing<br>Squeezing<br>Tearing | Cool<br>Cold<br>Freezing | Nagging<br>Nauseating<br>Agonizing<br>Dreadful<br>Torturing |

Part 4. How Strong Is Your Pain?

People agree that the following 5 words represent pain of increasing intensity. They are:

| 1 | 2 | 3 | 4 | 5 |
|---|---|---|---|---|
| Mild | Discomforting | Distressing | Horrible | Excruciating |

To answer each question below, write the number of the most appropriate word in the space beside the question.

1. Which word describes your pain right now? ______
2. Which word describes it at its worst? ______
3. Which word describes it when it is least? ______
4. Which word describes the worst toothache you ever had? ______
5. Which word describes the worst headache you ever had? ______
6. Which word describes the worst stomach-ache you ever had? ______

**Fig. 9–5.** The McGill Pain Questionnaire. (From Melzack R: The McGill Pain Questionnaire: Major properties and scoring methods. Pain. 1:277, 1975.)

ized training units in hospitals or private clinics, while 26 primiparae and 23 multiparae had received no training. Although the McGill Pain Questionnaire was completed between contractions, the patients were asked to measure the amount of pain they felt during contractions. They found that the mean total PRI was 34 for primiparae and 30 for multiparae, thus confirming the widely held view that labor is significantly more painful for the first birth than for later births. Significant differences were also found between primiparae and multiparae for each of the four classes of words describing their pain. The sensory qualities of the pain were described as sharp, cramping, aching, throbbing, stabbing, hot, shooting, or heavy; the affective qualities were described as tiring by 50% and exhausting by more than a 33%. The evaluative word *intense* was chosen by 52% and the miscellaneous word *tight* by 44% (Table 9–1). Subsequently, Melzack (68) compared the mean total PRI scores for several pain syndromes obtained in earlier studies (69,70) with those of labor and noted that the scores for labor pain were some 8 to 10 points higher than those associated with back pain, cancer pain, phantom limb pain or postherpetic neuralgia and even greater than acute pain that occurs after accidents (Figure 9–6).

As might be expected, although the average intensity of labor pain was extremely high, a wide range in pain scores was observed, which Melzack (68) divided into six groups within the range of the PRI scores recorded (ranging from 2 to 62) (Figure 9–7). Assigning verbal descriptors of pain intensity to these data suggests that about 10% of primiparae and about 24% of multiparae experienced mild to moderate pain, about 30% of both groups rated their pain as severe, about 38% of primiparae and 35% of multiparae felt very severe pain, and 23% of primiparae and 11% of multiparae experienced horrible or excruciating pain. The mean PRI scores of 61 primiparae who received prepared childbirth training were 33 and, for the 26 primiparae who received no training, it was 37 (Figure 9–8). On the other hand, no significant difference was noted in any of the PRI measures of the 30 multiparae who had received training and 24 who received no training. Of the 28 parturients who were given successful epidural analgesia, the PRI score decreased from a mean of 28 before the block to a mean of 8 and 7.6 at 30 and 60 minutes, respectively, after induction of analgesia. These scores were based on the use of such words as numbness, pressing, and tingling.

In the second study (65) involving 79 parturients (42 primiparae and 37 multiparae), parturients were given several successive questionnaires at hourly intervals until they entered the delivery room, or had an epidural block,

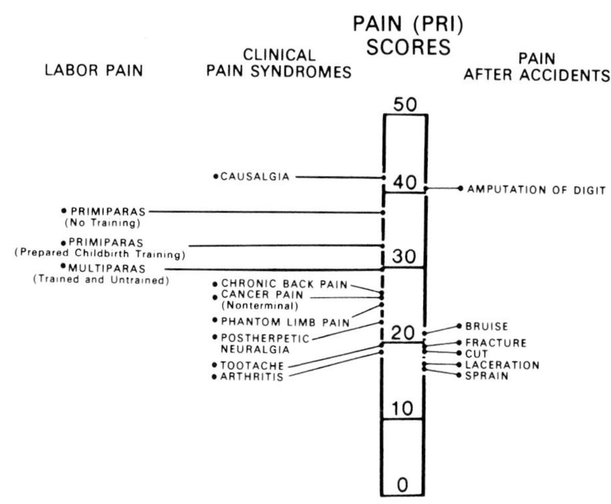


**Fig. 9–6.** Comparison of pain scores using the McGill Pain Questionnaire obtained from women during labor and from patients in general hospital clinics, and an emergency department. The Pain Rating Index represents the sum of the rank values for ll words chosen from 20 sets of pain descriptions. (From Melzack R: The myth of painless childbirth (The John J. Bonica Lecture) Pain. 19:321, 1984.)

**Table 9–1.** Qualities of Labor Pain

| Class | % of Women |
|---|---|
| Sensory | |
| Sharp | 62 |
| Cramping | 54 |
| Aching | 45 |
| Throbbing | 43 |
| Stabbing | 40 |
| Hot | 36 |
| Shooting | 33 |
| Heavy | 33 |
| Affective | |
| Tiring | 49 |
| Exhaustive | 36 |
| Evaluative | |
| Intense | 52 |
| Miscellaneous | |
| Tight | 44 |

(From Melzack R, et al: Labour is still painful after prepared childbirth training. Can. Med. Assoc. J. 125:357, 1981.)

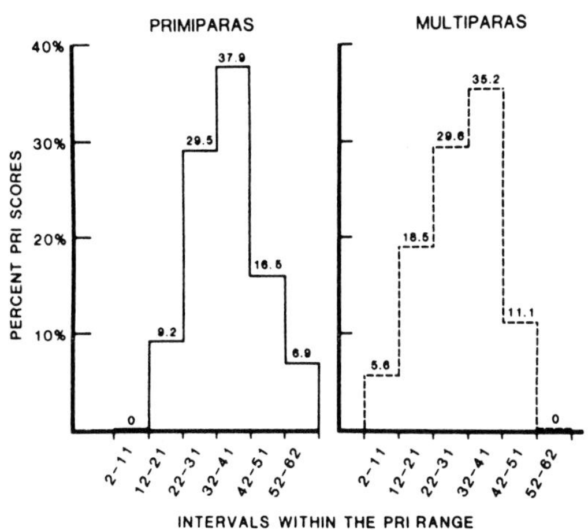


**Fig. 9–7.** Distribution of Pain Rating Index scores for primiparae and multiparae in six intervals of the total Pain Rating Index range. (From Melzack R: The myths of painless childbirth (The John J. Bonica Lecture) Pain. 19:321, 1984.)

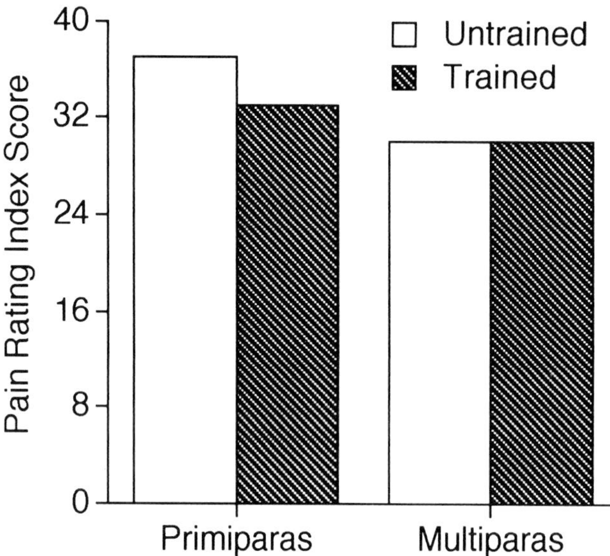


**Fig. 9–8.** The mean Pain Rating Index scores of pain by untrained and trained primiparas and multiparas. Untrained primiparas had a pain-rating-index score of 37, while the trained primiparas had a score of 33, but both untrained and trained multiparas had a similar score of 30. (Modified from Melzack R: The myth of painless childbirth (The John J. Bonica Lecture) Pain. 19:321, 1984, and Melzack R, et al: Labour is still painful after prepared childbirth training. Can. Med. Assoc. J. 125:357, 1981.)

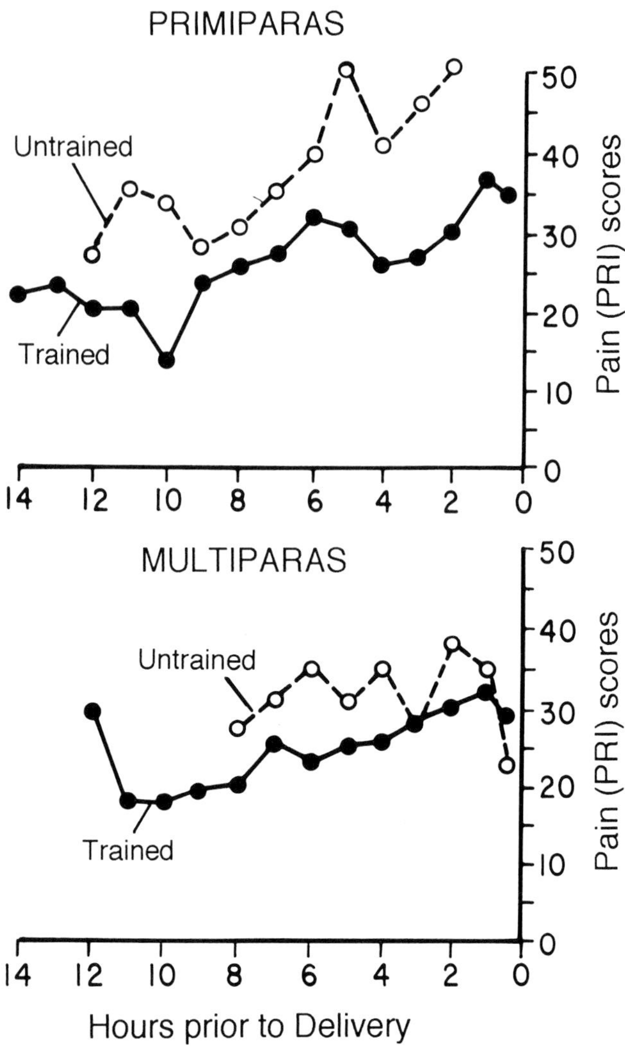


**Fig. 9–9.** Average Pain Rating Index (PRI) scores reported by primiparas and multiparas at successive hours before delivery. Pain scores, shown separately for trained and untrained women, were assigned to the nearest hour for purposes of calculation. (Modified from Melzack R: The myths of painless childbirth (The John J. Bonica Lecture) Pain. 19:321, 1984.)

or asked the experimenter to stop. Figure 9–9 shows the average pain curves for trained and untrained women. Although these curves indicate a gradual, rising pain intensity, graphs of pain scores obtained from individual parturients revealed a high level of variability as labor progressed. Instead of the idealized rising curve usually seen in obstetric textbooks, Figure 9–9 shows its group scores depicting a remarkable variety of patterns. Some parturients showed the expected rising curve, while others showed rises and falls in pain level. Some women had extremely high levels of pain early in labor, while others, up to the time of delivery, showed fairly low, constant pain scores.

In both studies, Melzack and associates (64,65) noted that the high level of individual variability was also reflected in the spatial distribution of the pain. Some women had widespread pain of a large part of the abdomen and back, while others had discrete painful areas. Spatial variability prompted Melzack and Schaffelberg (66) to carry out another study involving 46 parturients (29 primiparae and 17 multiparae) to define more precisely the location of the pain during contractions and between contractions. All 46 women had abdominal pain and 44 (96%) rated the contraction pain as the worst. In contrast, 34 parturients (74% of the subjects) had low back pain with 19 having the pain only during contraction, while 15 (33% of the whole group) had continuous low back pain that was rated worse than the abdominal and back pain associated with contractions. The parturients found this type of pain as intense and as difficult to bear and described it as "unrelenting" and "exhausting." The mechanisms of back pain are discussed in the next section.

Gaston-Johansson and associates (71) carried out a study similar to that of Melzack, et al in 138 Swedish women (50 primiparae, 88 multiparae) using the Johansson Pain-O-Meter and Visual Analog Scale (VAS) when the cervix was dilated 2 to 4 cm (stage I), 5 to 7 cm (stage II), and 8 to 10 cm (stage III). The Pain-O-Meter is made of a hard plastic and is 8 inches long by 2 inches wide and 1 inch thick with one side having 11 affective and 12 sensory pain word descriptors and the other side having the VAS scale. Two major indices obtained from the sensory and affective components of pain are: (1) the number of words chosen (NWC); and (2) the pain rating index rank (PRIR), based on accumulation of numerical values assigned to the chosen words. Among the 138 women, 80% of the primiparae and 20% of the multiparae had received prepared childbirth training. Moreover, 72% of primiparae and 27% of multiparae received meperidine, while epidural anesthesia was administered to 30% and 7%, respectively, and nitrous oxide oxygen was administered to 70% and 57%, respectively. Table 9–2 shows the mean value of pain intensity scores during three stages of labor. As may be noted, the intensity scores for the sensory component of pain were highest during stage I of labor, rather than stage II or III, while pain intensity scores for the affective component reached the highest peak during stage III of labor and delivery. Primiparae reported more intense sensory pain in stage I and III and more intense affective pain in all three stages of labor than multiparae, even though they consumed significantly more pain medication than did the multiparae. It is of interest to note that subjects who had participated in prepared childbirth training reported significantly higher in-labor pain scores during stage I and stage III than those who did not. The authors commented that prepared childbirth, while providing much information, may lead to unrealistic expectations about in-labor pain. In another study, Fridh and Gaston-Johansson (72) found that neither primiparae nor multiparae had realistic expectations of in-labor pain and experienced much more pain than they had anticipated. More detailed discussion about the effect of prepared childbirth on labor pain is presented in Chapter 21. The findings reported in this study are in agreement with earlier reports by Javert and Hardy (63), Cogan, et al (73), and Scott-Palmer and Skevington (74).

**Table 9–2.** Correlation between Postpartum Information and Scores in Subclasses of the Pain Rating Index (PRI) Obtained during Labor for the 141 Women

| Subclass and Variable | Pearson Correlation Coefficient | P Value |
|---|---|---|
| Primiparae | | |
| Sensory | | |
| Prepared childbirth practice | −0.30 | 0.008 |
| Complications (this pregnancy) | −0.20 | 0.05 |
| Prepared childbirth training | −0.19 | 0.04 |
| Affective | | |
| Complications (this pregnancy) | −0.21 | 0.04 |
| Intend to breast-feed | −0.20 | 0.05 |
| Prepared childbirth training | −0.18 | 0.04 |
| Menstrual difficulties | +0.28 | 0.009 |
| Religious | +0.22 | 0.03 |
| Evaluative | | |
| Cervical dilation | −0.18 | 0.052 |
| Miscellaneous | | |
| Socioeconomic status | −0.45 | 0.002 |
| Age | −0.31 | 0.002 |
| Prepared childbirth practice | −0.24 | 0.03 |
| Total | | |
| Prepared childbirth practice | −0.32 | 0.005 |
| Socioeconomic status | −0.29 | 0.04 |
| Complications (this pregnancy) | −0.23 | 0.02 |
| Age | −0.22 | 0.02 |
| Prepared childbirth training | −0.19 | 0.04 |
| Multiparae | | |
| Sensory | | |
| Socioeconomic status | −0.42 | 0.02 |
| Felt prepared by childbirth training | −0.37 | 0.02 |
| Affective | | |
| Contraction frequency | −0.37 | 0.04 |
| Evaluative | | |
| Felt prepared by childbirth training | −0.32 | 0.03 |
| Miscellaneous | | |
| Complications (previous pregnancy) | −0.27 | 0.05 |
| Menstrual difficulties | +0.38 | 0.009 |
| Total | | |
| Socioeconomic status | −0.42 | 0.02 |
| Felt prepared by childbirth training | −0.34 | 0.03 |
| Menstrual difficulties | +0.29 | 0.04 |

## *Mechanisms of the Pain of Parturition*

To provide optimal pain relief with regional analgesia, it is essential for the obstetric team to understand the peripheral mechanisms and pathways of the pain of parturition and the factors that influence its intensity, duration, and quality. Most of these factors vary during the different phases and stages of labor and are therapeutically significant, so they are considered separately.

### *Pain of the First Stage of Labor*

During the first stage, labor pain initially is entirely in the uterus and its adnexa during contractions. Earlier, it was proposed that labor pain was caused by the following: (1) pressure on nerve endings between the muscle fibers of the body and fundus of the uterus (75); (2) contraction of the ischemic myometrium and cervix consequent to expulsion of blood from the uterus during the contraction (76) or as a result of vasoconstriction consequent to sympathetic hyperactivity (52); (3) inflammatory changes of uterine muscles (75); (4) contraction of the cervix and lower uterine segment consequent to fear-induced hyperactivity of the sympathetic nervous system (52); and (5) dilatation of the cervix and lower uterine segment (76). Most data support the concept that the pain of the first stage of labor is predominantly a result of dilatation of the cervix (CX) and lower uterine segment (LUS) and of the consequent distension, stretching, and tearing of these structures during contractions. Contractions of the uterus under isometric conditions—that is, against the obstruction presented by the cervix and perineum—also probably contribute to the pain of uterine contractions. These hypotheses are based on the following considerations:

1. Stretching of smooth muscle of a hollow viscus is an adequate stimulus for visceral pain (77).
2. The degree of cervix and lower uterine segment dilatation is correlated with the rapidity with which it occurs on the one hand and with the intensity of the pain on the other (1).
3. The time of onset of uterine contractions is related to the time of onset of the pain. This lag, which is longest in the early stages of labor and lessens as labor progresses, occurs because uterine contractions need time to increase the amniotic fluid pres-

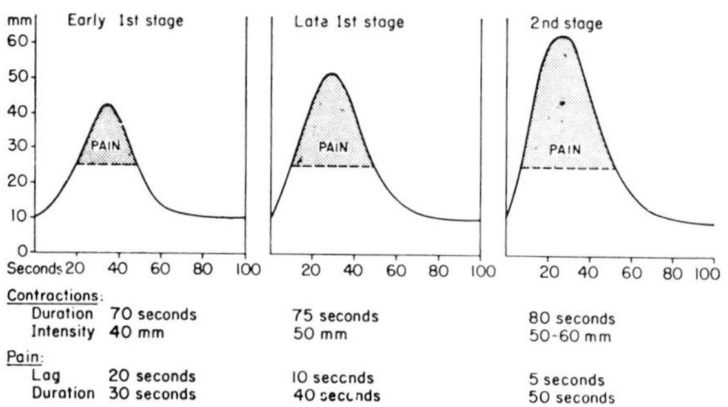


**Fig. 9–10.** Relation between duration of uterine contraction and duration of pain associated with the contraction. Because intensity of contraction must reach 25 mm Hg before pain is provoked, there is a lag of 20 seconds during early phase of first stage when the buildup of the contraction is slower. As labor progresses the contraction reaches its peak more rapidly and the lag is shortened.

sure to 15 mm Hg above tonus (Figure 9–10). This has been determined to be the minimum pressure required to initiate distension of the cervix and lower uterine segment (78).

4. In the parturient undergoing cesarean section with abdominal field block, the exposed but unanesthetized uterus can be incised and gently palpated without discomfort to the conscious parturient (63,76), while forceful palpation and stretching of the cervix and lower uterine segment produce pain similar in quality and location to that experienced during labor (78).
5. When the cervix is suddenly and widely dilated in parturients or in gynecologic patients, they feel pain similar in quality, distribution, and intensity to that experienced during uterine contractions (63,76,79).

The evidence that contractions of the body of the uterus contribute to the pain of labor is somewhat puzzling. Braxton-Hicks contractions of prelabor are frequently painless, even though they can attain a high intensity of labor contractions, and this detracts from this hypothesis. Moreover, during the immediate postpartum period, the intensity of uterine contractions of the empty uterus might be 2 to 3 times stronger than the contractions of active labor but are associated either with much less intense pain or with no pain at all. On the other hand, strong contractions are associated with severe pain in most parturients with mechanical distortion caused by abnormal fetal positions and in those in whom the cervix dilates slowly. Because in such situations the uterine muscle is contracting under isometric conditions (i.e., its exit, the cervix and perineum, present an obstruction), the strong contractions are probably also a source of pain.

The validity of various other hypotheses is also disputed. The suggestion that pain is a result of ischemia during uterine contractions is disputed by monkey studies that showed that, although placental (intervillous) perfusion decreased to nearly 50% of control values, myometrial blood flow increased significantly during contractions (80) and increased to an even greater degree during a sustained (8-minute) contraction (81). Moreover, no evidence of an inflammatory process in the uterine muscles has been found (1,3). Dick-Read's (52) hypothesis that contraction of the cervix brought about by fear-induced hyperactivity of the sympathetic nervous system as the cause of pain is unwarranted in view of the fact that the cervix is composed mostly of connective tissue, with little muscle and elastic tissue (82). Moreover, during uncomplicated childbirth, the lower uterine segment and cervix manifest only a small contractile force, which becomes even weaker as labor progresses (78).

### *Second and Third Stages of Labor*

Once the cervix is fully dilated, the amount of nociceptive stimulation arising in this structure decreases, but the contractions of the body of the uterus and distension of the lower uterine segment continue to cause pain in the same areas of reference as in the first stage of labor. In addition, the progressively greater pressure of the presenting part on pain-sensitive structures in the pelvis and distension of the outlet and perineum becomes a new source of pain. Progressively greater distension causes intense stretching and actual tearing of fascia and subcutaneous tissues and pressure on the skeletal muscles of the perineum.

## *Other Factors that Influence the Pain of Childbirth*

In addition to the role played by such intrinsic factors as the intensity, duration, and pattern of contractions and related physiologic and biochemical mechanisms, the amount or degree of pain and suffering associated with childbirth is influenced by physical, physiologic, biochemical, psychologic, emotional, and motivational factors (60–62,64–66,74,83–87). Although different investigators found differences in the role played by each of the various factors mentioned below, there is consensus that many of these play an important role in determining the incidence, intensity, and quality of pain in the general parturient population.

### *Physical Factors*

Physical factors that influence the incidence, severity, and duration of the pain of childbirth include the age, parity, and physical condition of the parturient, the condition of the cervix at the onset of labor, and the relationship of the size of the infant to the size of the birth canal. Many of these factors are interrelated. Generally, an uninformed unmarried teenage gravida may experience more anxiety-induced pain. Moreover, older (greater than 40 years old) primiparae experience a longer, more painful labor than a young primipara. The cervix of the multipara begins to soften even before the onset of labor and is less sensitive than that of the primipara. In general, the intensity of uterine contractions in early labor tends to be higher in primiparae than in multiparae, whereas in the latter phase of labor the reverse is true (64–66,71).

In the presence of dystocia caused by a contracted pelvis, a large baby, or abnormal presentation, the parturient experiences more pain than under normal conditions. Melzack and associates (65) found that the heavier the primipara per unit of height, the higher the pain scores. The same variable contributed to the pain scores of multiparae and, in addition, heavier mothers and those with heavier babies had higher pain scores. There are also a number of reports cited by Kohenen (86) that women who labor and deliver in the vertical position (sitting, standing or squatting) experience less pain and have a shorter second stage of labor. However, in a recent study by Melzack and Belanger (67) in which they used part of the McGill Pain Questionnaire and Visual Analog Scale to measure pain intensity, they found that in the latent and early first stage of labor, parturients had less pain in the vertical position, but in the late first stage and second stage they experienced less pain in the lateral horizontal position. This confirms results reported by others.

Melzack and associates (64,66) found that high pain scores were associated with menstrual difficulties. They also noted that menstrual pain felt in the back, but not in the front, was correlated with increasing levels of pain in the abdomen and back, during contractions and with continuous low back pain previously mentioned. Similar relationships between menstrual pain and higher pain scores were reported by Fridh and associates (72) who noted that primiparae had more pain in late first stage, whereas multiparae had more pain in the early first stage. Marx (87) has presented strong evidence that women who have dysmenorrhea produce excessive amounts of prostaglandins that trigger uterine contractions and that drugs that inhibit prostaglandin synthesis also diminish menstrual pain. Melzack (68) has suggested that because of the positive correlation between menstrual pain and the pain during childbirth, it is conceivable that parturients who suffer severe labor pain may also produce excessive prostaglandins during labor. Fatigue, loss of sleep, and general debility influence a parturient's tolerance of the painful experience and increase the pain behavior. This is particularly significant in parturients with prolonged labor.

## *Physiologic and Biochemical Factors*

A number of studies have demonstrated a progressive increase in plasma beta-endorphin, beta-lipotropin, and ACTH levels, all of which are derived from a common precursor (88–93). These values have been found to peak at delivery or in the immediate postpartum period at 4 to 10 times the prelabor and nonpregnant values. These findings have led to the speculation that plasma beta-endorphin might have an intrinsic analgesic role during parturition (93). The fact that plasma beta-endorphin levels, which are considerably higher than those observed in these studies do not appear to cross the blood-brain barrier or have analgesic effects on nonpregnant humans (94), has questioned the efficacy of beta-endorphin as an analgesic during parturition.

On the other hand, other opioid systems may play a role in increasing the pain-tolerance threshold. This suggestion is based on the findings of Gintzler (95) who in 1980 noted in rats that pain threshold rises at the end of pregnancy, peaks around delivery, and returns to normal nonpregnant levels within 12 hours of delivery. This "pregnancy-induced analgesia" or more properly "hypalgesia" is blocked by the opioid antagonists naloxone and naltrexone. This phenomenon has been observed using several noxious modalities including response threshold to electric foot shock and tail withdrawal latencies (96,97). Similar increases in pain threshold have been noted in studies involving humans during late pregnancy in which responses to radiant heat to dermatomes C1 or S1 or intense pressure applied to the forearm were used as aversive (noxious) stimuli (98,99). Gintzler, et al (97) have identified the pregnancy-induced hypalgesia as resulting from action of spinal dynorphin/kappa opioid receptor systems. These data suggest that in parturients who experience low levels of pain, the activation of this system may be sufficient to lower the intensity and perhaps modify the quality of the pain of parturition.

Related to this issue are the recent studies carried out by Kristal and associates (100–103) that show that ingestion of amniotic fluid or the placenta by rats enhanced several types of opioid-mediated analgesia: that induced by morphine, by foot shock, by vaginal/cervical stimulation and that of late pregnancy, but not analgesia produced by aspirin injection. In the absence of opioid-mediated analgesia, however, ingestion of placenta and amniotic fluid do not produce the enhancing effects. Opioid antagonists such as naloxone and naltrexone not only block the opioid mediated analgesia, but also render placental ingestion and amniotic fluid ingestion ineffective. Kristal and associates (101–103) have named the active substance in placenta and amniotic fluid, Placental Opioid-Enhancing Factor or POEF. They have also shown that placental opioid-enhancing factor enhances the central effects of opioid analgesia but not its peripheral effects, perhaps by stimulating "off-cells" in the periaqueductal gray.

Because most nonaquatic, nonhuman mammalian mothers engage in ingestion of the afterbirth termed *placentophagia* or at least lick amniotic fluid from themselves or the newborn infant, and in view of the measurable increase in pain threshold produced by elevated endogenous opioids present before delivery, Kristal and associates (103) have explored in rats the possibility that a significant benefit of parturitional placentophagia is an enhancement of the pregnancy-mediated analgesia during labor and delivery. Their studies have revealed that 1 ml placenta or 0.25 ml amniotic fluid, which is the amount available during the delivery of one rat pup, is the optimum dose for enhancement of morphine-induced analgesia. Moreover, the enhancement produced by 0.25 ml amniotic fluid by orogastric tube is detectable within 5 minutes and lasts for about 30 minutes, the approximate duration of the interpup interval during delivery. Because amniotic fluid is available to the mother before the emergence of the first neonate and the placenta is not available until after delivery of each pup, amniotic fluid is probably the more important substance in enhancement of pregnancy-mediated analgesia.

The importance of these findings is twofold: first, it demonstrates that nonaquatic nonhuman mammalian mothers have two factors that tend to diminish nociception and pain behavior, pregnancy-induced hypalgesia and the hypalgesic effect of amniotic fluid and placenta; second, it demonstrates the possibility of isolating the active substance in human placenta and, on the basis of the findings, it may be possible to develop new and different analgesic agents.

### Psychologic Factors

Psychologic factors that can and frequently do affect the incidence and intensity of parturition pain include the mentation, attitude, and mood of the parturient at the time of labor, and other emotional factors. Fear, apprehension, and anxiety probably enhance pain perception and pain behavior (85,104–108). One of the most frequent causes of fear and anxiety is ignorance of or misinformation about the process of pregnancy and parturition, and what the onset of labor signifies. An uninformed parturient, especially a primipara, can be disturbed by fear of the unknown, death, suffering, mutilation, possible complications, and concern for her condition or that of her fetus (71,85,107). Parturients who have had an unplanned or illegitimate pregnancy or have an ambivalent or negative reaction to gestation report more pain than those who do not (see Chapter 3 for details regarding the psychologic aspects of pregnancy, labor, and analgesia) (62,77).

In a relatively recent study, Wuitshik and associates (108) noted that anxiety, stress, and negative cognitive processess were often associated with severe pain in the latent phase and that the latter was predictive of a longer latent phase and a long active phase of labor. Moreover, stress-related thoughts during the latent phase were predictive of a longer latent phase, a longer second stage of labor, and, consequently, in an increase in instrumental deliveries.

The relationship between the parturient and her spouse plays an important role in the degree of pain she experiences. Melzack (68) reported that the affective pain scores were higher when the husband was in the labor room than when he was absent. He suggested that this may reflect genuinely higher affective pain scores or may be due to a deliberate choice of descriptors in the attempt to impress the husband or express anger at him, but in any case, the finding was not spurious. Melzack (68) cited that H. Wallach found a similar effect in an independent study (unpublished thesis). In contrast, Nettelbladt and associates (62), Norr, et al (84), and Fridh, et al (85) found that positive feelings of the expectant father toward the pregnancy seemed to be an important factor in decreasing the mother's feelings of apprehension during pregnancy. When fathers were more supportive of their mates during pregnancy and labor, women experienced less pain during parturition. Fridh, et al (85) emphasized the need to include supportive fathers in prenatal training.

In contrast, other emotional factors such as intensive motivation and cultural influences can affect modulation of sensory transmissions and certainly can influence the affective and behavioral dimensions of pain. Moreover, cognitive intervention such as giving the parturient preparatory information about labor, thus reducing uncertainty while focusing attention or producing distraction and dissociation from pain (all parts of an "educated" childbirth program) reduces pain behavior. In a study of 134 low-risk parturients at term, Lowe (109) found that confidence in ability to handle labor was the most significant predictor of all components of pain during active labor. The greater the confidence the parturient had, the lesser the pain and vice versa.

### Cultural and Ethnic Factors

Racial, cultural, and ethnic factors have long been considered to be important in influencing pain tolerance and pain behavior. Persons of Italian and other Latin cultures or of Jewish or Mediterranean background are said to express pain in an emotive fashion and to exaggerate their verbal report, whereas those of Anglo-Saxon origin (e.g., English, third-generation Americans, Irish), as well as Scandinavians, Asians, American Indians, and Eskimos, are said to be more stoic and to manifest less pain behavior (110). Experimental data and clinical observations, however, suggest that, although racial, cultural, and ethnic differences do exist, there appears to be differences in expressiveness consequent to underlying attitudes toward the pain rather than differences in the sensory experience or pain perception.

Pesce (110a) studied 22 Australian-born gravidae, 10 Italian-born gravidae, and 8 graviadae born in Australia of Italian parents. The three groups were tested using the Present Pain Index (PPI), the Pain Rating Index (PRI) (ranking), and the Number of Words Chosen Index (NWCI) from the McGill Pain Questionnaire (MPQ). Mann-Whitney U Test (one failed) were performed between the three groups on the PPI, the PPR (R), and the NWC. All of the results proved to be statistically insignificant at the stated level. Among the three groups regarding the PRI, PPI, and NWC Scale, all were all statistically insignificant. Contrary to data produced by prior studies, the data obtained by Pesce suggest that the Italian groups could not be said to exaggerate the intensity of the reported pain as measured on the PPI or the PRI (R) Scale. Results with the NW Scale were also statistically insignificant at the 0.01 level. The author concluded that the absence of statistically significant results in this comparison of Australian mothers and those of Italian origin on measures of childbirth pain suggests that the ascription of a lower pain threshold to people with an Italian background is not appropriate. Therefore, it cannot be said that this group is any more likely to talk about pain, to exaggerate it or to be diffuse in describing it. Pesce (110a) concluded, by paraphrasing Pasquarelli (110b), that in the reporting of childbirth pain, the screams of the Australian and the Italian women are equally loud, equally frequent, and equally exaggerated.

True (111) reported that Mohave Indian women experienced a great deal of pain during childbirth but avoided expressing their suffering for fear of ridicule. In an experimental study, Meehan and colleagues (112) found no significant differences between pain tolerance of American Indians, Eskimos, and Caucasions. In a study of Turkomenian women, Preissman and Ogoulbostan-Essenova (113) noted that they behaved calmly during childbirth and manifested no pain behavior but inquiry revealed that the process was very painful. Nettelbladt and associates (62), in a study of 78 women, noted that 56% of parturients who reported intolerable pain were not rated by the midwives as having very painful deliveries. This discrepancy probably occurred because the parturients manifested less overt pain behavior than they actually felt, which is a characteristic of Scandinavian culture. Winsberg and Greenlick (114) examined pain behavior in Negro and Caucasion parturients who were matched on such parameters as age, social class, and education and found no differences in pain responses or estimated degrees of pain.

The thesis that cultural and racial differences can have some influence on pain behavior but probably not on the pain felt by parturients is supported by my own studies (unpublished data) of 2700 parturients in other countries and of 8000 parturients in the United States (see previous: Incidence and Intensity of Labor Pain). In Western and Eastern Europe, Latin America, Africa, Asia-Australia, the Near East, and North America parturients who were not "educated" and who were psychologically unprepared for childbirth manifested a similar incidence of pain behavior, although the patterns of behavior varied. During the contractions some women moaned, others screamed, others writhed and had facial expression of suffering with little or no verbal expression, while still others used incantations (said to be specific for labor pain in that particular country). Contrary to traditional belief, Asian women (including Japanese, Chinese, Malaysians, Indians, Cambodians, and Thais) did not remain stoic but manifested as much pain behavior as American and European parturients.

Moreover, the large Oriental population of Seattle and the recent influx of refugees from Indochina afforded the opportunity to observe and interview several hundred parturients from various countries in Southeast Asia. These studies revealed that the frequency and intensity of labor pain and the request for analgesia was the same as for Occidental parturients living in Asia, and the pain behavior was similar to that observed among parturients in their native countries (Bonica, unpublished data).

The influence of education and psychologic conditioning inherent in psychoprophylaxis and natural childbirth in modifying pain behavior without significantly affecting pain behavior is now widely appreciated. During 5-day to 10-day visits to obstetric centers that practice psychoprophylaxis or natural childbirth in the Soviet Union, France, Germany, Italy, The Netherlands, Sweden, and the United States, made over a 5-month period in 1959, Bonica observed about 700 parturients (and interviewed many) who had received training in one of these methods, and over 85% of them manifested little or no pain behavior during labor and delivery. When questioned the next day, however, most of them indicated that the process had been painful but many quickly added that they were pleased to cooperate with their instructor and obstetric team. Especially impressive was the significant change in behavior of Italian parturients in a large obstetric center in Turin noted during two visits made 5 years apart. During the first visit, in 1954, the labor ward was a scene of cacophony caused by the screaming, pleading, and praying of the nearly 50 laboring women in the same ward. In contrast, 5 years later, one heard only an occasional moan from a similar number of parturients who had undergone an intensive course of psychoprophylaxis. Most went through the entire labor and delivery with minimal pain behavior but later stated that they had had moderate to severe pain.

### *Summary*

It is obvious that the pain-associated responses to noxious stimulation provoked by uterine contractions and other tissue-damaging factors during labor and vaginal delivery are the net effects of highly complex interactions of various neural systems, modulating influences, and psychologic and cultural factors. Through the interaction of the afferent system and neocortical processes, the parturient receives perceptual and discriminate information that is analyzed and that usually activates motivational and cognitive processes. These, in turn, act on the motor system and initiate psychodynamic mechanisms of anxiety and apprehension that produce the complex physiologic, behavioral, and affective responses that characterize acute pain.

## NEURAL PATHWAYS OF PARTURITION PAIN

Although the extrinsic nerve supply to the uterus was well described during the seventeenth and eighteenth centuries, it was not until 1893 that Henry Head (115) published the first description of the specific nociceptive pathways of the uterus and cervix. Based on his studies of the segments of hyperalgesia associated with various uterine disorders, as well as of hyperalgesia during the second stage of labor, Head (115) concluded that the sensory nerve supply of the uterus always involved the T11, often the T12, and not infrequently the T10 and L1 and sometimes L2 segments, and that the cervix was supplied by the S2, S3, and S4. During the ensuing 4 decades, much confusing and conflicting evidence and difference of opinion existed in textbooks concerning this issue. It remained for John Cleland (116) to clarify the issue by extensive animal experiments and studies on parturients. Cleland used the visceromotor reflex to determine the critical sensory pathways from the uterus and subsequently carried out paravertebral somatic nerve block in parturients to eliminate the pain of the first stage of labor. Based on these studies, Cleland concluded that in humans the sensory supply of the uterus is through the T11 and T12 spinal segments and that pain caused by stretch of the birth canal was transmitted through "undetermined sacral segments." The latter finding was interpreted to mean that the cervix and vagina are supplied by the sacral segments. As a result of these two studies it became widely taught that nociceptive impulses from the body of the uterus are transmitted through the T11 and T12 nerves, and that pain from the lower uterine segment and cervix is transmitted through the pelvic nerves to the S2, S3, and S4 spinal segments.

Because my clinical observations were at variance with this concept, in collaboration with my colleagues Akamatsu, Kohl, and others, I carried out a study that involved 305 parturients and 41 gynecologic patients investigated

**Table 9-3A.** Influence of Various Nerve Blocks on Different Aspects of Pain Parturition

| Technique | Spinal Segments Blocked | Number of Observations | Effects on Pain of Parturition: Uterine Pain, Early | Uterine Pain, Late | Perineal Pain | Other Pain |
|---|---|---|---|---|---|---|
| A. *Paravertebral somatic nerve block* | $T_{11,12}$ | 10 | + + + + | + + | 0 | 0 |
| | $T_{10-12}$ | 10 | + + + + | + + + | 0 | 0 |
| | $T_{11,12}$, $L_1$ | 10 | + + + + | + + + | 0 | 0 |
| | $T_{10}$-$L_1$ | 10 | | | | |
| B. *Extradural block* | | | | | | |
| a) 1 catheter ($T_{12}$) | $T_{11-12}$ | 10 | + + + + | + + | 0 | 0 |
| b) 2 catheters ($T_{12}$, $S_3$) | $T_{10}$-$L_1$ | 10 | + + + + | + + + + | 0 | 0 |
| c) 3 catheters ($T_{12}$, $L_4$, $S_3$) | $T_{10}$-$L_1$<br>$S_2$-$S_5$ | 15 | + + + + | + + + + | + + + + | 0 |
| | $T_{10}$-$L_1$<br>$L_2$-$S_1$<br>$S_2$-$S_5$ | 15 | + + + + | + + + + | + + + + | + + + + |

0, no relief; + +, + + + +, increasing levels of pain relief.
(From Bonica, JJ: Mechanisms and pathways of parturition pain. *In* Pain and Reproduction. Edited by AR Genazzani, G Nappi, F Facchinetti, E Martignoni. Casterton Holl, Carnfort, The Parthenon Publishing Group, 1988, pp. 182–191.)

**Table 9–3B.** Influence of Continuous Caudal and Transsacral Block on Different Aspects of the Pain of Parturition

| Technique | Spinal Segments Blocked | Number of Observations | Uterine Pain | Perineal Pain | Other Pain |
|---|---|---|---|---|---|
| *Continuous caudal* | $S_{2-5}$ | 10 | 0 | + + + + | 0 |
| | $L_5$-$S_5$ | 10 | 0 | + + + + | + |
| | $L_3$-$S_5$ | 10 | 0 | + + + + | + + + |
| | $L_1$-$S_5$ | 10 | + | + + + + | + + + + |
| | $T_{10}$-$S_5$ | 22 | + + + + | + + + + | + + + + |
| *Transsacral nerve block* | $S_2$ | 10 | 0 | + + | 0 |
| | $S_3$ | 10 | 0 | + | 0 |
| | $S_4$ | 10 | 0 | + | 0 |
| | $S_{2,3}$ | 10 | 0 | + + + | 0 |
| | $S_{3,4}$ | 10 | 0 | + + | 0 |
| | $S_{2,3,4}$ | 12 | 0 | + + + + | 0 |
| *Lumbar sympathetic block* | | 20 | + + + + | 0 | 0 |
| *Paracervical block* | | 20 | + + + + | 0 | 0 |
| *Pudendal block* | | 20 | 0 | + + + + | 0 |
| *Paracervical/pudendal block* | | 30 | + + + | + + + | 0 |

0, no relief; + + +, + + + +, increasing levels of pain relief.
(From Bonica, JJ: Mechanisms and pathways of parturition pain. *In* Pain and Reproduction. Edited by AR Genazzani, G Nappi, F Facchinetti, E Martignoni. Casterton Holl, Carnfort, The Parthenon Publishing Group, 1988, pp. 182–191.)

over a period of 22 years (117). The study entailed the use of discrete blocks of various nociceptive pathways by paravertebral block, segmental epidural block, caudal block, and trans-sacral block of various segments (Table 9–3). Their results demonstrated conclusively that the upper part of the cervix and the lower uterine segment are not supplied by sensory fibers that accompany the pelvic nerves (nervi erigentes) as stated in almost every modern anatomy and obstetric textbook. Rather, these structures are supplied by afferents that, like those that supply the body of the uterus, accompany the sympathetic nerves in the following sequence: the uterine and cervical plexus; the pelvic (inferior hypogastric) plexus; the middle hypogastric plexus or nerve; and the superior hypogastric and aortic plexuses. The nociceptive afferents then pass to the lumbar sympathetic chain and course cephalad through the lower thoracic sympathetic chain, which they leave by way of the rami communicantes associated with the T10, T11, T12, and L1 spinal nerves. Finally, they pass through the posterior roots of these nerves to make synaptic contact with interneurons in the dorsal horn (Figures 9–11 and 9–12).

These findings have been recently confirmed in animal experiments carried out by a number of investigators (118–122). Berkeley and her associates (118–120) have carried out a series of systematic comprehensive experiments using in vitro and in vivo electrophysiologic studies and behavioral studies of the nerve supply of the uterus and other pelvic organs. These investigators have used mechanical and chemical stimuli of the uterine cavity including the cervix and vagina. The results can be summarized as follows:

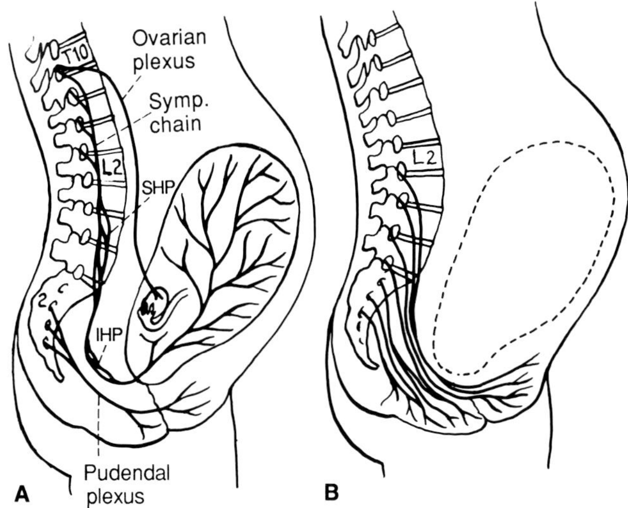


**Fig. 9–11.** Schematic depiction of the peripheral nociceptive pathways involved in the pain of childbirth. **(A)** the uterus, including the cervix and lower uterine segments, is supplied by afferents that pass from the uterus to the spinal cord by accompanying sympathetic nerves through the inferior hypogastric plexus (IHP), the hypogastric nerve, the superior hypogastric plexus (SHP), the lumbar and lower thoracic sympathetic chain, and the nerves at T10, T11, T12, and L1. **(B)** the nerves involved in transmission of nociceptive impulses are provoked by noxious stimulation of other pelvic structures.

1. Afferent fibers in the hypogastric nerve have receptive fields confined to the uterus and cervix with most fibers located in the lower portion of the cervix and that they respond primarily to noxious stimuli. Effective mechanical stimuli included steady pressure, stretching, squeezing and probing in intensities greater than 5 g, which produced transient ischemia around the probe (118–119). Using in-vitro preparations, the fibers responded to injection into the uterine artery of high doses of algesic substances such as bradykinin, 5 hydroxytriptamine, and KCl and they also responded to high doses of $CO_2$ in saline and sodium cyanide (NaCN) but rarely to lower doses. Afferent fibers in the hypogastric nerve also responded to uterine contractions after sensitization by prior manipulations.
2. Afferent fibers in the pelvic nerve (nervi erigentes) have receptive fields located mostly in the upper part of the vaginal canal and the cervix (120). Effective stimuli that activated these fibers were much less intense, rarely producing ischemia and responded to much lower doses of algesic substances.
3. Gentle distension of the vaginal canal of anesthetized rats showed response of sensory fibers in the pelvic nerve and the responses increased as distension increased into the noxious range. Berkeley, et al (119) also examined the relation between this neural response and sensation caused by vaginal distension in rats that had previously been trained to perform an operant escape response to terminate in noxious somatic stimulus (tail pinch). At the gentle level of distension, rats oriented toward the stimulus, but failed to make the escape responses but as the levels of stimulation were gradually increased into the noxious range, the probability of the rats making an escape response gradually increased to 100%. Although this would suggest that both pain and nonpainful stimulation arising from mechanical stimulation of the vaginal canal is subserved at least in part by activity in afferent fibers of pelvic nerve, this apparently is not the case because bilateral pelvic neurectomies had no significant effect on the animals' response to noxious stimulation of the vagina (119,120).

The above findings led Berkeley and associates (118–120) to conclude that afferent fibers in the hypogastric nerves are concerned with the transmission of nociceptive information. In contrast, the uterine pelvic nerve afferent fibers are capable of conveying information regarding more physiologic innocuous events that are likely to subserve a wide range of reproductive functions. These afferent fibers differ considerably from, but must somehow be coordinated with, those of the hypogastric nerve fibers during the lifetime course of reproductive events.

### *Patterns of Pain of Parturition*

Typical of pain arising from viscera, the pain of the first stage of labor is referred to the dermatomes supplied by the same spinal cord segments that receive nociceptive input from the uterus and cervix. During the latent (very early) phase of the first stage, the pain is felt as an ache or moderate cramp and is limited to the T11 and T12 dermatomes (Figure 9–13a). As labor progresses to the active phase of the first stage (usually 3 to 4 cm cervical dilatation) and the uterine contractions become more intense, the pain in the T11 and T12 dermatomes becomes more severe, is described as sharp and cramping, and spreads to the two adjacent (T10 and L1) dermatomes (Figure 9–13b).

The distribution of the T10, T11, T12, and L1 dermatomes in the back overlies the lower three lumbar vertebrae and the upper half of the sacrum. This distribution of pain during the first stage of labor has been misinterpreted by some as being transmitted by the lower lumbar and sacral spinal segments. Proof that the low back pain is the result of nociceptive transmission in the T10-L1 segments is derived from the fact that epidural block limited to these four segments produces relief of the low back pain until descent of the presenting part causes pressure on the pelvic structures that are supplied by lower lumbar and the sacral segments (see below). As previously mentioned, often the pain is not referred to the entire dermatome, but can be more severe in one or more patches of varying size within a territory of one or more dermatomes. However, one can demonstrate hyperalgesia in the entire extent of the involved dermatomes.

In the late first stage and second stages of labor, the pain is felt most sharply in the perineum, in the lower part of the sacrum, anus, and frequently in the thighs (Figures

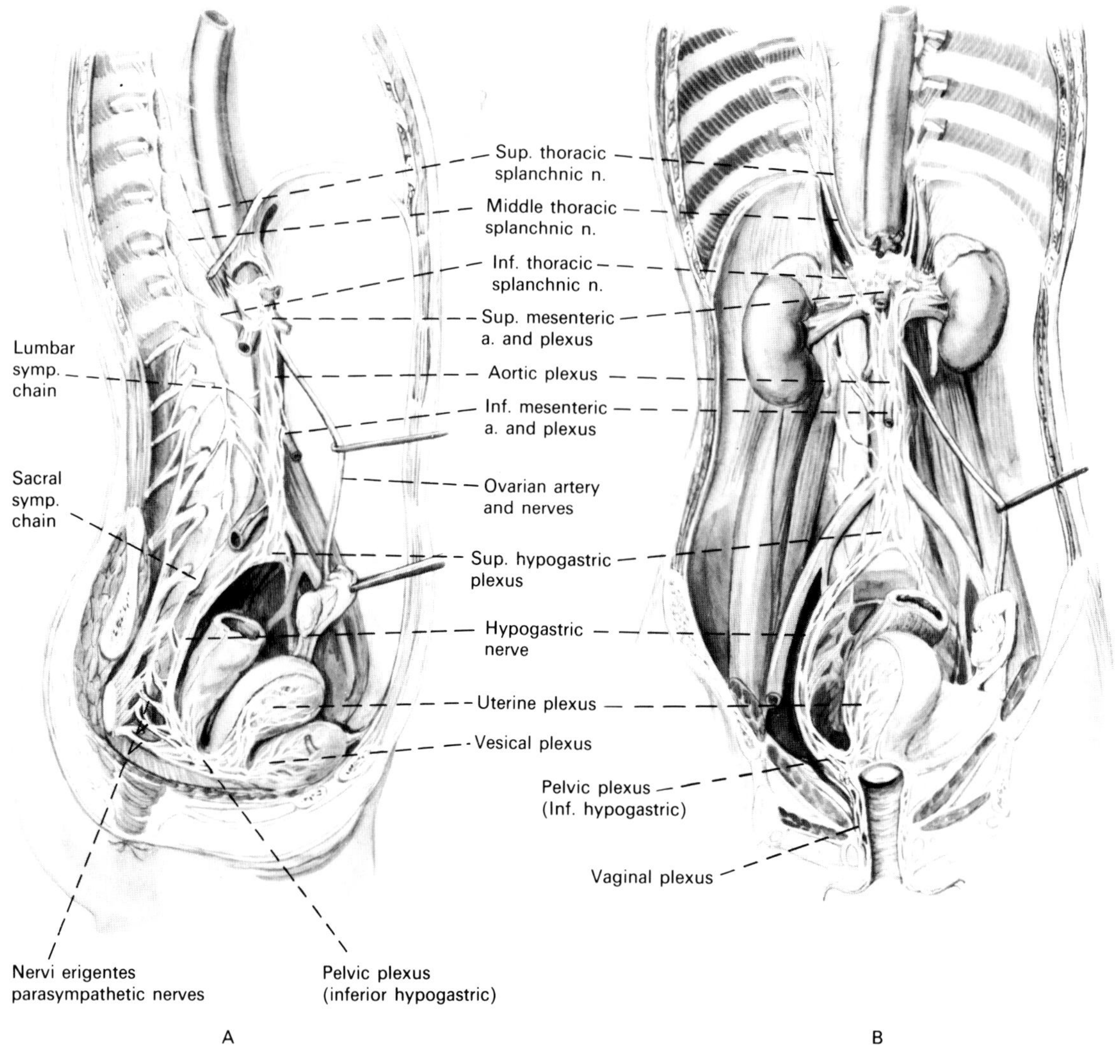


**Fig. 9–12.** Gross anatomy of the nerve supply to the uterus. **(A)** lateral view, **(B)** anterior view. The uterus is shown in the nonpregnant state to permit the various nerves that supply it to be depicted. Note that the uterine and cervical plexuses are derived from the pelvic plexus, which contains parasympathetic and sympathetic efferents. The parasympathetic efferents have their cell bodies in the middle three sacral segments, and the parasympathetic afferents pass through these segments and progress cephalad through the neuraxis. The sympathetic efferents and afferents pass through the hypogastric nerve, which in turn is a continuation of the superior hypogastric and aortic plexuses. Note that fibers from the latter two plexuses pass on to the lumbar sympathetic chain, the afferents of which mediate nociceptive impulses and accompany the sympathetic fibers through these structures. From the lumbar and lower thoracic sympathetic chain the nociceptive afferents pass to the T10, T11, T12, and L1 spinal nerves and reach the spinal cord via their posterior roots and rootlets.

9–13b and 9–13c). Like other pain caused by stimulation of superficial somatic structures, the perineal pain is sharp and well-localized, predominantly in the region supplied by the pudendal nerves and can be eliminated by block of these nerves. Moreover, in the late part of the first stage, and during the second stage a number of parturients develop aching, burning or cramping discomfort in the thigh and less frequently in the legs (Figures 9–13c and 9–13d). This is presumably a result of stimulation of pain-sensitive structures in the pelvic cavity, including the following: (1) traction on the pelvic parietal peritoneum and on the structures it envelops, including the uterine ligaments; (2) stretching and tension of the bladder, urethra, and rectum; (3) stretching and tension of ligaments, fascia, and muscles in the pelvic cavity; and (4) undue pressure on one or more roots of the lumbosacral plexus. These factors usually produce mild pain referred to the lower lumbar and sacral segments (Figure 9–12b); but, if the fetus is in an abnormal position, with undue pressure by the presenting part, the referred pain can become moderate or severe (Figures 9–13c and 9–13d).

The transmission of the nociceptive information that arises from these various structures to the dorsal horn and then to other parts of the spinal cord and to the ascending systems to the brain is presumably similar to that of other types of acute pain. Because this was discussed in the first section of this chapter, nothing more will be said except to reemphasize that the tissue damage in the cervix and

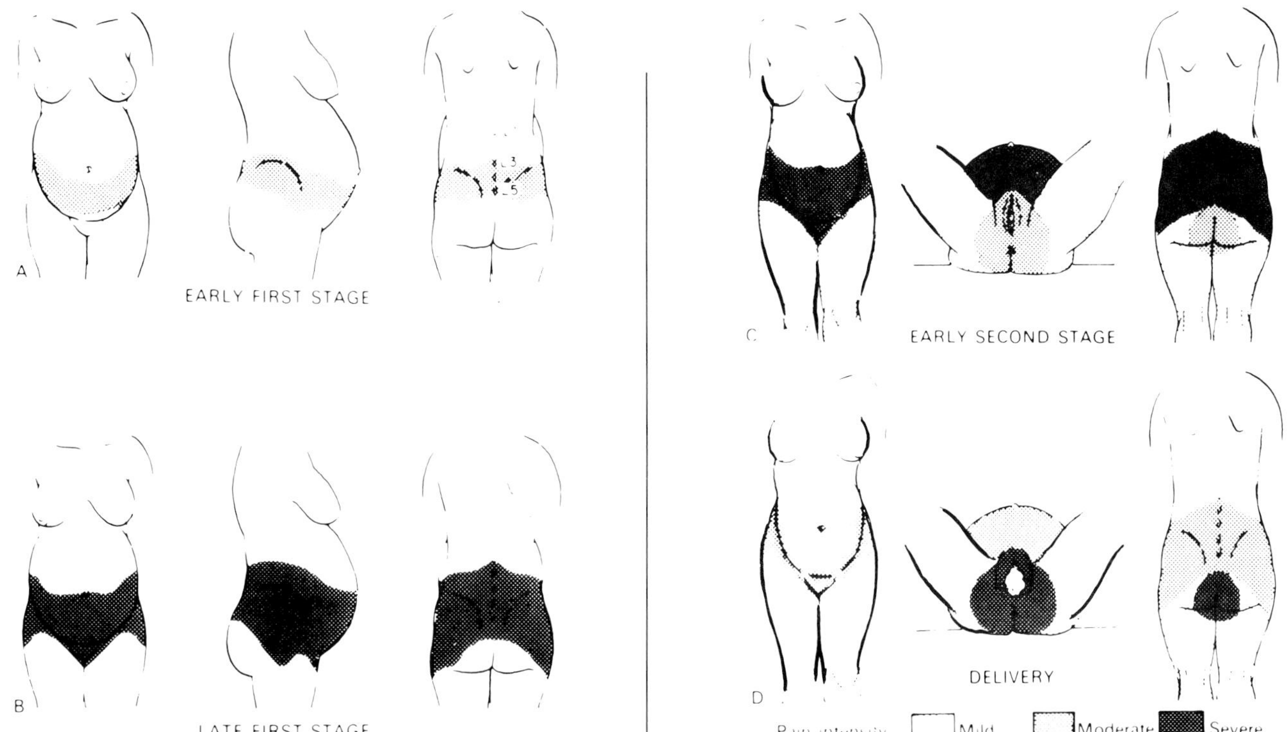


**Fig. 9–13.** The intensity and distribution of parturition pain during the various phases of labor and delivery. **(A)** in the early first stage the pain is referred to the T11 and T12 dermatomes. **(B)** in the late mid and first stage, however, the severe pain is also referred to the T10 to L1 dermatomes. **(C)** in the early second stage uterine contractions remain intense and produce severe pain in the T10 to L1 dermatomes. At the same time the presenting part exerts pressure on pelvic structures and thus causes moderate pain in the very low back and perineum and often produces mild pain in the thighs and legs. **(D)** intensity and distribution of pain during the latter phase of the second stage and during actual delivery. The perineal component is the primary cause of pain whereas uterine contractions produce moderate pain.

perineum causes the responses to injury mentioned in the section on pathophysiology of the pain of parturition.

## EFFECTS OF PARTURITION PAIN AND THEIR MODIFICATION WITH ANALGESIA

This last section is devoted to discussion of the effects of parturition pain on the mother, fetus, and newborn and how these can be modified and, in many instances, completely eliminated. This will require repetition of some of the information contained in Chapter 2, which presents data on the effects of the forces of labor and that superimposed by the associated pain on ventilation, circulation, and other body functions. In addition, I will stress the effects of labor pain on uterine contractility and forces of labor and on the fetus and newborn. Figure 9–14 depicts the nociceptive output from the uterus and the responses provoked by tissue damage and pain during uterine contractions.

### *Effects of Childbirth Pain*

#### Changes in Ventilation

In Chapter 2 the remarkable changes in ventilation are described in detail. Because the pain of childbirth is a powerful respiratory stimulus, it causes significant increases in tidal volume and minute ventilation and even greater increases in alveolar ventilation, causing a fall of $PaCO_2$ from a normal pregnant level at term of 30 mm Hg (4.27 kPa) to a value of 16 to 20 mm Hg (2.13 to 2.67 kPa), with some as low as 10 to 15 mm Hg (1.33 to 2.00 kPa), and a concomitant increase in pH to 7.55 to 7.60 (Figure 9–15). With the onset of the relaxation phase, pain no longer stimulates respiration, so that hypocapnia causes a transient period of hypoventilation that decreases the maternal $PaO_2$ by 10 to 50%, with a mean of 25 to 30%. In parturients who received an opioid the depressant effects of the respiratory alkalosis are enhanced by the action of the opioid. When the maternal $PaO_2$ falls below 70 mm Hg (9.33 kPa), it has a significant effect on the fetus, consisting of a decrease in the fetal $PaO_2$ and late decelerations (Figure 9–16).

#### *Effects of Analgesia*

Partial relief of pain with opioids decreases hyperventilation somewhat so that the $PaCO_2$ is in the 22 to 25 mm Hg (3.0 to 3.3 kPa) range and oxygenation improves (123). However, between contractions the respiratory alkalosis combined with the depressant effects of the opioid may cause hypoventilation and hypoxemia (Figure 9–17). Complete pain relief achieved with extradural analgesia

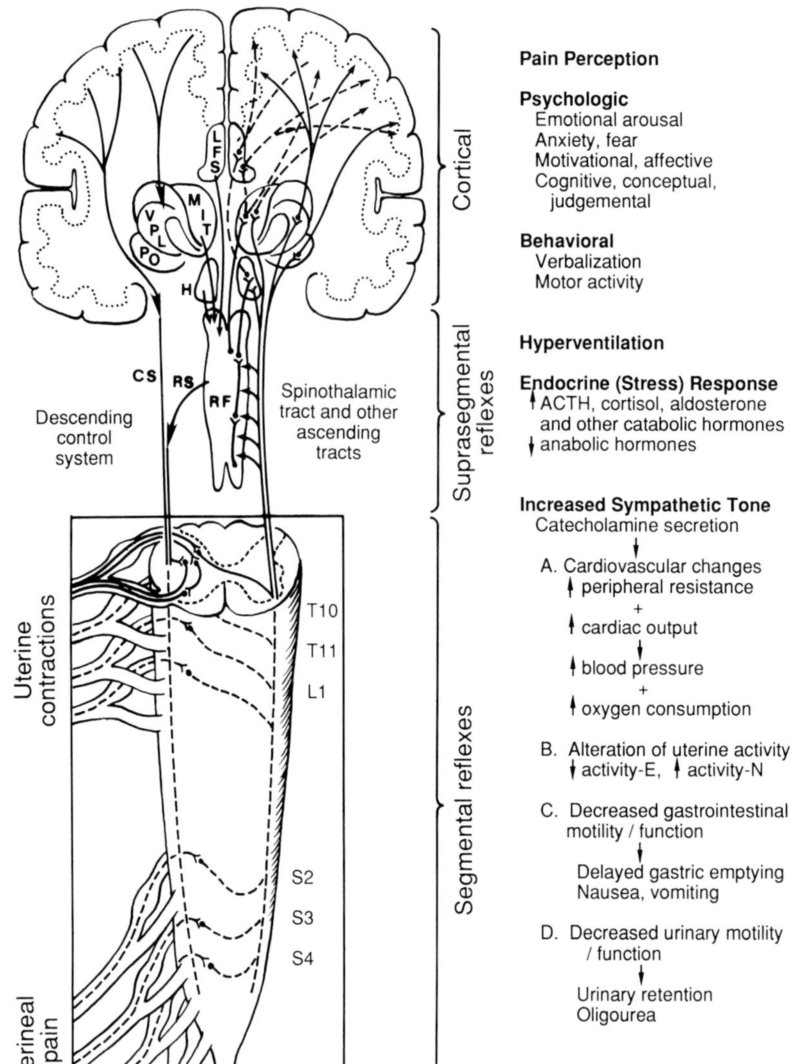


**Fig. 9–14.** Schematic depiction of the nociceptive input to the spinal cord provoked by uterine contractions throughout labor and simulation of the perineum during the second and third stages of labor. The spinothalamic tract and other ascending tracts in the neuraxis are primarily involved in central transmission of nociceptive information to the anterior and anterolateral horn cells of the spinal cord which provoke segmental reflex responses and impulses that reach the brain stem that provoke suprasegmental responses listed on the right. The nociceptive impulses that reach the brain provoke the cortical responses that include perception of pain, initiation of psychologic mechanisms and behavioral responses. On the reader's left shows a simple schematic illustration of descending pathways that convey modulating influence from the brain to the spinal cord. RF = reticular formation; RS = reticulospinal; CS = corticospinal; H = hypothalamus; PO = posterior thalamus; VPL = ventral posterolateral thalamus; MIT = medial and intralaminar thalamic nuclei; LFS = limbic forebrain structures.

prevents the transient period of hyperventilation during a contraction and prevents hypoventilation during relaxation, so that the $PaCO_2$ remains in the range of 28 to 32 mm Hg (mean 30 mm Hg) (3.73 to 4.27 kPa) and the $PaO_2$ increases to about 100 mm Hg (13.3 kPa) Figures 9–15 and 9–16).

## *Neuroendocrine Effects*

Animal studies have shown that acute pain caused by noxious stimulation produces a significant (20 to 40%) increase in catecholamine levels, particularly norepinephrine, with a consequent 35 to 70% decrease in uterine blood flow (Figures 9–18 and 9–19) (124,125). Human studies have shown that severe pain and anxiety during active labor cause a 300 to 600% increase in the epinephrine (E) level, a 200 to 400% increase in the norepinephrine (NE) level, a 200 to 300% increase in the cortisol level, and significant increases in corticosteroid and ACTH levels during the course of labor; these reach peak values at or after delivery (126–128). Lederman and associates (126,127) noted that, during the period of active labor, the epinephrine level increased by nearly 300%, the norepinephrine level by 150%, and the cortisol level by 200%. They noted that the higher epinephrine levels

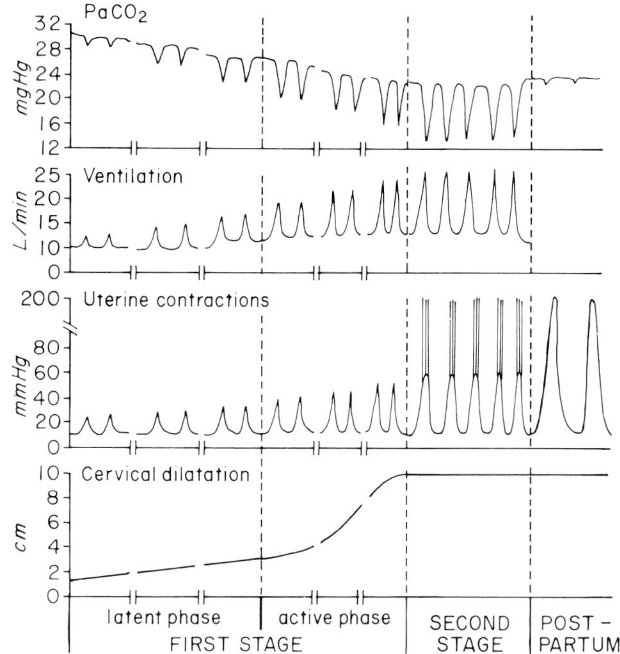


**Fig. 9–15.** Schematic representations of ventilatory changes during labor in an unpremedicated gravida. Note the correlation of the stages of labor as reflected by the Friedman's curves *(bottom tracing)*, the frequency and intensity of uterine contractions, minute ventilation, and arterial carbon dioxide tension *(top tracing)*. Early in labor uterine contractions are mild and are associated with mild pain, causing only small increases in minute ventilation and decreases in the $PaCO_2$. As labor progresses, however, the greater intensity of contractions causes greater changes in ventilation and $PaCO_2$. During the active phase, contractions with an increased intrauterine pressure of 40 to 60 mm Hg cause severe pain, which acts as an intense stimulus to ventilation with a consequent reduction of the $PaCO_2$ to 18 to 22 mm Hg. During the second stage the reflex bearing-down efforts further increase intrauterine pressure and distend the perineum, producing consequent additional pain that prompts the parturient to ventilate at a rate almost twice that of early labor and causing a commensurate reduction in the $PaCO_2$.

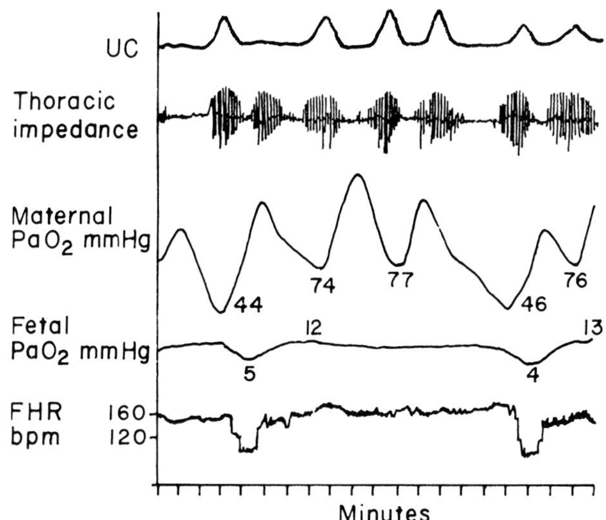


**Fig. 9–16.** Continuous recording of uterine contractions (UC), maternal thoracic impedance, maternal transcutaneous oxygen tension ($PaO_2$), fetal oxygen tension, and fetal heart rate (FHR) in a primipara 120 minutes before spontaneous delivery of an infant with an Apgar of 7. Marked hyperventilation during uterine contraction was followed by hypoventilation or apnea between contractions. With the parturient breathing air during and after the first and fourth periods of hyperventilation, the maternal $PaO_2$ fell to 44 and 46 mm Hg, with a consequent decrease in fetal $PaO_2$ and variable decelerations, which reflected fetal hypoxia. (Modified from Huch A, et al: Continuous transcutaneous monitoring of foetal oxygen tension during labour. J. Obstet. Gynecol. 84(Suppl. 1):1, 1977.)

were significantly associated with uterine contractile activity at the onset of active labor (3 cm cervical dilatation) and with longer labor during the active phase (3 to 10 cm cervical dilatation). Increased epinephrine and cortisol levels were correlated significantly with anxiety and pain.

Ohno and associates (129) carried out a comprehensive study of catecholamines and cyclic nucleotides during labor and following delivery and noted a nearly twofold increase in the dopamine level, a threefold increase in the epinephrine level, and a twofold increase in the norepinephrine, as well as a small increase in the cAMP level. They noted a positive correlation between epinephrine on the one hand and heart rate and systolic blood pressure on the other, as well as a correlation between norepinephrine and cAMP during labor. The greater increase in epinephrine than in norepinephrine was contrasted with the findings of a previous study, which showed that norepinephrine was much greater than epinephrine during physical exercise. This led them to con-

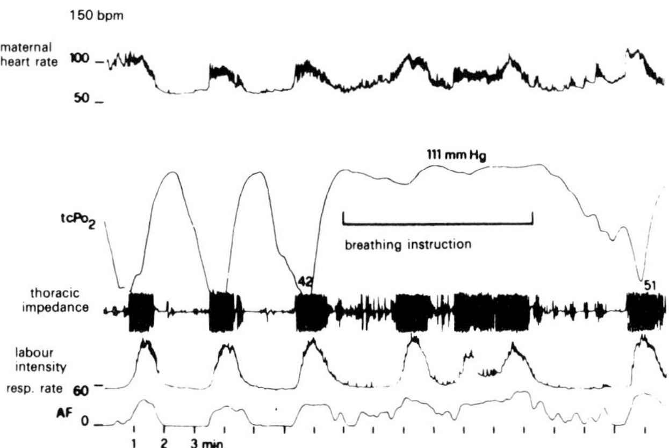


**Fig. 9–17.** Continuous recording of maternal heart rate, transcutaneous (tc) $PO_2$, thoracic impedance, uterine pressure (labor intensity), and respiratory rate after the parturient was given 100 mg meperidine IM. With each uterine contraction marked hyperventilation caused the $tcPO_2$ to increase to 110 mm Hg but then to fall to low levels as a result of the marked respiratory alkalosis and of the respiratory depressant effect of the meperidine. The large decreases in $tcPO_2$ were avoided by giving the parturient breathing instructions during the relaxation period. (From Peabody JL: Transcutaneous oxygen measurement to evaluate drug effect. Clin. Perinatol. 6:109, 1979.)

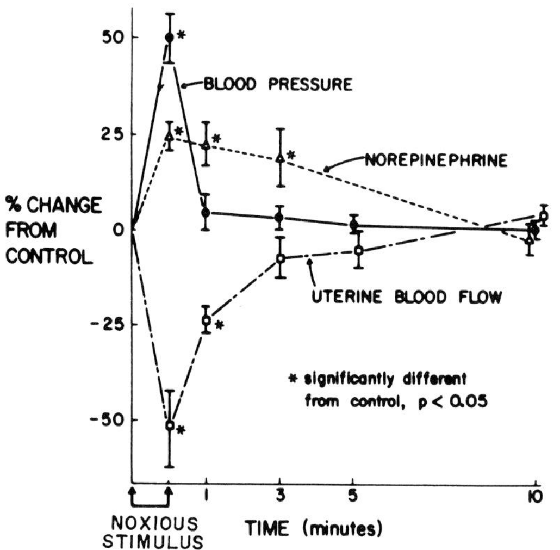


**Fig. 9–18.** Effects of noxious stimulus on maternal arterial blood pressure, norepinephrine blood level, and uterine blood flow. The stress was induced by application of an electric current onto the skin of an ewe at term. The increase in arterial pressure is transient but the decay in norepinephrine level is more protracted, and is reflected by a mirror image decrease in uterine blood flow. (From Shnider SM, et al: Uterine blood flow and plasma norepinephrine changes during maternal stress in the pregnant ewe. Anesthesiology. 50:524, 1979.)

clude that elevated sympathoadrenal activity during labor is a result of pain and anxiety rather than of physical effort. Other data, however, show that although pain is a major factor in the elevation of catecholamine levels, physical effort during the second stage does contribute to the increase in catecholamine levels.

### Effective Analgesia

Recent studies have provided impressive evidence that epidural analgesia, by blocking nociceptive input and sympathetic efferents, reduces the release of catecholamines, beta-endorphins, ACTH, and cortisol (130–137). This neuroendocrine-lowering effect is primarily a result of relief of pain during labor and was demonstrated by Abboud and associates (138), who noted that spinal anesthesia at the T4-dermatomal level decreased catecholamine levels in women in labor, but did not do so in women who were not in labor. This selectivity suggests that the mechanism by which catecholamine release is decreased is relief of maternal pain.

Epidural analgesia during labor and delivery does not decrease catecholamine and beta-endorphin release in the fetus and newborn (92,131,135–138), and norepinephrine predominates over epinephrine (138). This response indicates that, even during completely uncomplicated deliveries with adequate maternal analgesia, the infant is considerably distressed by the process of birth by vaginal delivery. A number of studies have suggested that catecholamines have an important role for neonatal adaptation to the extrauterine environment, including surfactant synthesis and release, lung liquid resorption, nonshivering thermogenesis, glucose homeostasis, cardiovascular changes, and water metabolism (138).

### Cardiovascular Changes

During labor the progressive increase in cardiac output is about 40 to 50% higher than the prelabor value during

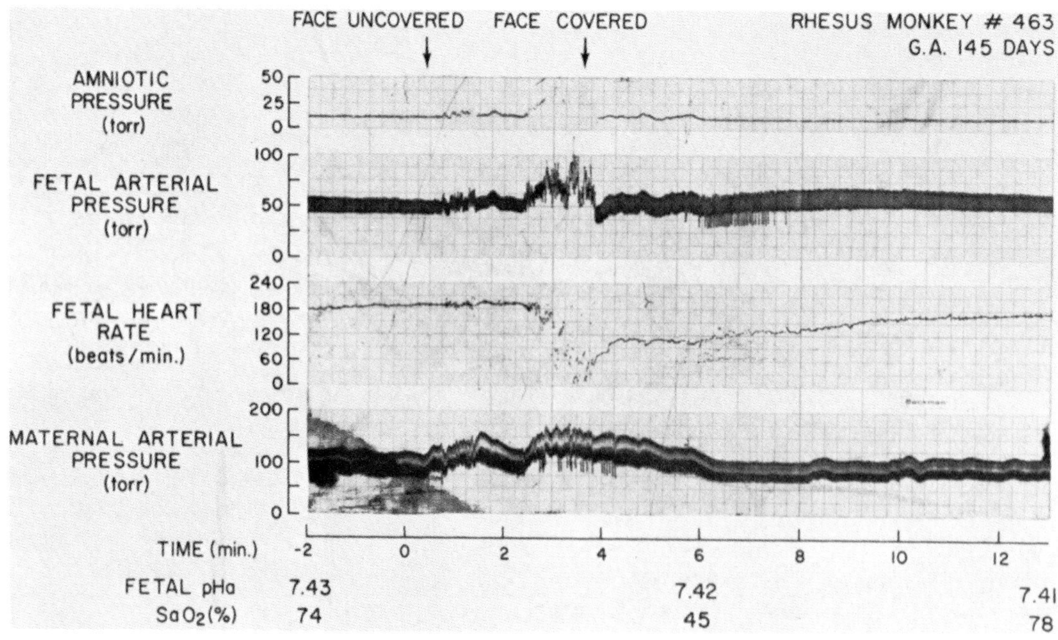


**Fig. 9–19.** Effects of pain-induced stress on maternal arterial pressure, intrauterine pressure, and fetal heart rate in a pregnant monkey. Note the adverse effect of the stress on fetal heart rate and oxygenation. (Modified from Morishima et al: Am. J. Obstet. Gynecol. 131:286, 1978.)

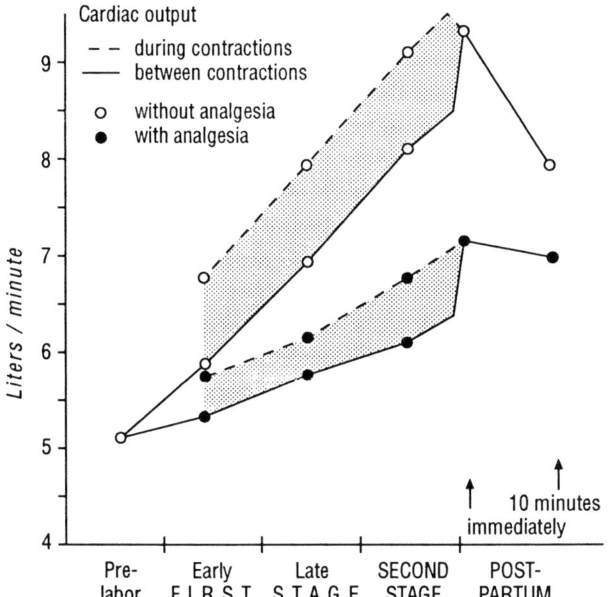


**Fig. 9–20.** Cardiac output during various phases of labor between contraction and during contractions. In a group of patients laboring without analgesia, the progressive increases between contractions and the further increases during each contraction were much greater than corresponding changes in a group of patients who received continuous epidural analgesia.

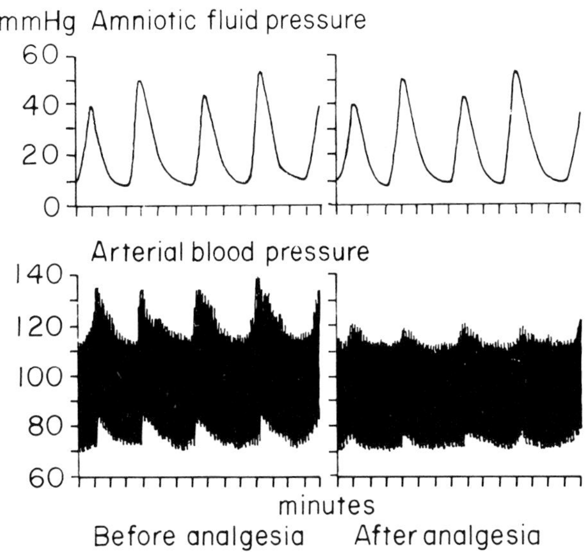


**Fig. 9–21.** Fluctuations in blood pressure produced by uterine contractions before and after induction of continuous epidural analgesia. Like the cardiac output changes (Figure 9–20), complete relief of pain resulted in decreasing the contraction-induced fluctuations to nearly 50% of the values measured before analgesia.

the late first and second stages, and some parturients have an increase of nearly 100% with a further increase of 20 to 30% during each painful uterine contraction (Figure 9–20) (139–143). Available data suggest that 40 to 50% of the increase during the contraction is caused by the extrusion of 250 to 300 ml of blood from the uterus and by increased venous return from the pelvis and lower limbs into the maternal central circulation (139,142). The rest is caused by an increase in sympathetic activity provoked by pain, anxiety, apprehension, and the physical effort of labor, which contribute to the progressive rise in cardiac output as labor advances (140,141). Uterine contractions in the absence of analgesia also cause increases of 20 to 30 mm Hg (2.6 to 6.4 kPa) in the systolic and diastolic blood pressures. The increases in cardiac output and systolic blood pressure lead to a significant increase in left ventricular work that is tolerated by healthy parturients but can prove deleterious if the parturients have heart disease, pregnancy-induced hypertension (preeclampsia), essential hypertension, pulmonary hypertension, or severe anemia.

## *Effective Analgesia*

By decreasing the pain-induced sympathetic hyperactivity and neuroendocrine response, epidural analgesia eliminates that portion of the increase in cardiac output and blood pressure caused by pain. Figure 9–21 shows that epidural analgesia decreases the progressive increase in cardiac output and its further increase during uterine contractions to about 50% of that without analgesia. A similar decrease in periodic increase in blood pressure is depicted in Figure 9–20. Several studies have proven the value of epidural analgesia in dampening the increase in cardiac output, cardiac work, and blood pressure in laboring parturients with heart disease, pregnancy-induced hypertension (preeclampsia), and pulmonary hypertension, provided, of course, that maternal hypotension is avoided (143,144).

## *Metabolic Effects*

During the first and second stages of labor, free fatty acids and lactate levels increase significantly, apparently as a result of the pain-induced release of catecholamines and the consequent sympathetic-induced lipolytic metabolism (133). This assumption is based on the fact that, with complete blockade of nociceptive (afferent) and efferent pathways achieved with epidural or other forms of regional analgesia, only slight increases in maternal free fatty acid and lactate levels and acidosis are seen. During the second stage of labor, maternal acidosis is a result of the pain and physical exertion inherent in the active bearing-down (pushing) effort during contractions.

Increased sympathetic activity caused by labor pain and anxiety also increases metabolism and oxygen consumption and decreases gastrointestinal and urinary bladder motility. The increased oxygen consumption, plus that inherent in the work of labor, together with the loss of bicarbonate from the kidney as compensation for the pain-induced respiratory alkalosis and often reduced carbohydrate intake, produce a progressive metabolic acidosis that is transferred to the fetus. The maternal pyruvate level increases, along with an even greater increase in the lactate level and a progressive accumulation of excess lactate, which is reflected by a progressive increase in base excess (145–147).

### Effects of Analgesia

The relief of pain and associated anxiety with continuous epidural analgesia decreases the total work of labor, maternal metabolism, and oxygen consumption. Buchan (133) showed that, during labor, epidural analgesia reduced internal stress by abolishing pain, thus eliminating the progressive increase in the 11-hydroxycorticosteroid levels normally seen throughout labor. Consequently, epidural analgesia significantly reduces maternal and fetal metabolic acidosis. The superiority of epidural analgesia over opioids and other systemic drugs in decreasing maternal work, oxygen consumption, and maternal and fetal metabolic acidosis has been impressively demonstrated by a number of investigators (130,145–152). Because active pushing during the second stage of labor contributes to metabolic acidosis, epidural analgesia does not completely eliminate metabolic and fetal acidosis. Figure 9–22 demonstrates that epidural analgesia and elimination of the bearing-down effort (pushing) during the second stage almost eliminates maternal metabolic acidosis. Moreover, under these conditions it decreases but does not eliminate the degree of fetal acidosis. Undoubtedly, this is a result of the physical stress on the fetus inherent in the process of birth.

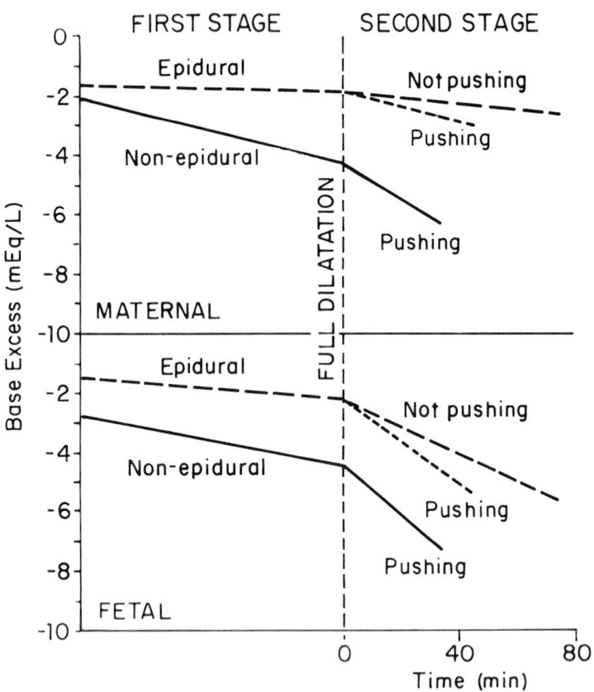


**Fig. 9–22.** Mean changes in extent of maternal (top) and fetal (bottom) metabolic acidosis during the first and second stages of labor in a group of parturients managed without lumbar epidural analgesia and in two similar groups managed with epidural analgesia, one of which retained the bearing-down reflex while the other did not. The parturients were delivered by outlet forceps. Significant metabolic acidosis was experienced by those in the nonepidural group of parturients whereas those given epidural analgesia experienced little or no changes in their acid-base status. Fetuses born of mothers managed without epidural also developed metabolic acidosis during the first stage, and to an even greater degree, during the second stage. In contrast, fetuses of mothers given epidural had no change in acid-base status during the first stage but showed a time-dependent increase in metabolic acidosis during the second stage.

### Changes in Gastrointestinal Function

The pain of labor affects the function of the gastrointestinal tract. Gastrin release is stimulated during painful labor and results in an increase in gastric acid secretion (153). Moreover, the pain and associated anxiety and emotional stress produce segmental and suprasegmental reflex inhibition of gastrointestinal motility and function, and consequently a significant delay in gastric emptying. These reflex effects of nociception are aggravated by the recumbent position and by the use of opioids and other depressant drugs (153–155). The combined effect of pain and depressant drugs can cause food and fluids other than water to be retained for as long as 36 hours or more, and during this period swallowed air and gastric juices accumulate progressively, with the pH of the stomach contents decreasing below the critical value of 2.5 in most parturients. Delayed gastric emptying of acidic gastric contents increases the risk of regurgitation and pulmonary aspiration, especially during the induction of general anesthesia.

### Effect of Analgesia

Epidural analgesia by completely blocking the nociceptor input obviates the reflex inhibition of gastrointestinal function and unlike opioids, have no effect on gastrointestinal function. Consequently, the parturient does not incur the delay in gastric emptying and other changes mentioned above in gastrointestinal function (155).

### Psychologic Effects

Severe labor pain can produce serious long-term emotional disturbances that might impair the parturient's mental health, negatively influence her relationship with her baby during the first few crucial days, and cause fears of future pregnancies that could affect her sexual relationship with her husband (62–65,148–151). Kartchner (156), Rogers (157), Melzack, et al (64,65,68), Gaston-Johansson and associates (71,72) and others (74,158) reported a significant number of women who had participated in natural childbirth developed or had aggravation of prelabor depression and other deleterious emotional reactions in the postpartum period, consequent to the pain experienced during their childbirth without analgesia. Cheetam and Rzadkowolski (157) reported that nearly two-thirds of parturients experienced some type of emotional upset characterized predominantly by a decrease in mental acuity and in social interests, and an increase in their feelings of dysphoria, depression, and anxiety. They pointed out that psychologic aspects of labor are accentuated by the well-cited triad of "fear-tension-pain," which might in turn decrease uterine activity and thus prolong labor. In addition, Melzack, et al (68) noted that some women might experience an added burden of guilt, anger, and failure when they anticipate "natural, painless childbirth" and are then confronted with such severe pain that they require epidural analgesia. Stewart (159) reported that some women who failed to achieve "painless" childbirth and experienced such severe pain as to require epidural analgesia subsequently became miserable, depressed, and even suicidal, and lost interest in sex. In some cases, the husbands of women who anticipated "natural" childbirth had to undergo psychotherapy for serious reactions after seeing their wives experience such severe pain that they developed feelings of guilt and subsequent impotence, and phobias. Melzack (68) also mentioned other reports of similar reactions by parturients who failed to achieve painless childbirth.

### *Effects of Analgesia*

Properly administered epidural analgesia will relieve most of the pain and thus obviate many of the psychologic and emotional reactions to the severe pain mentioned above. Melzack (68) summarized the data from the studies mentioned earlier in this chapter in a review article titled "The myth of painless childbirth." As previously mentioned, epidural analgesia decreased the PRI scores from a mean of 28 before the block to a mean of about 8 at 30 and 60 minutes after induction of analgesia, and these scores were based on the use of such words as numbness, pressing, and tingling. Indeed, by using the double-catheter technique described in Chapter 13, virtually all the discomfort of the parturient can be eliminated. Based on his studies and data from other sources, Melzack (68) pleaded for a well-developed and well-balanced approach, whereby all prospective parturients are given education and training for childbirth and if they experience more than mild pain, to have skillfully administered epidural analgesia, because these are compatible and complementary procedures that allow the recognition of the individuality of each woman.

### *Effects on Uterine Activity and Labor*

Through increased secretion of catecholamines and cortisol, pain and emotional stress can either increase or decrease uterine contractility and thus influence the duration of labor. Norepinephrine increases uterine activity, whereas epinephrine and cortisol decrease it (126,127). Morishima and colleagues (124,160) reported that, in pregnant baboons and Rhesus monkeys, nociceptive stimulation increased uterine activity about 60 to 65%, and was associated with a decrease in fetal heart rate and oxygenation. In contrast, severe pain and anxiety in some parturients caused such an increase in epinephrine and cortisol levels that uterine activity was consequently decreased and labor was prolonged (126,127). In a small number of parturients, pain and anxiety produce "incoordinate uterine contractions" manifested by a decrease in intensity coupled with an increase in frequency and uterine tonus (161).

### *Effects of Analgesia*

By decreasing the sympathetic-induced hyperactivity, sedation and complete analgesia can reduce or eliminate uterine hyperactivity or hypoactivity and can change incoordinate uterine contractions to a normal labor pattern (161,162). Equally important is the efficacy of analgesia in reducing placental hypoperfusion and any existing deterioration in uterine blood flow, thus decreasing or even eliminating any impairment of blood gas transfer that might be a result of increased catecholamines or uterine hyperactivity (122).

### *Effects on the Fetus*

During labor the intermittent reduction of intervillous blood flow during the peak of a contraction leads to a temporary decrease in placental gas exchange. This impairment is often further increased by pain-induced severe hyperventilation, which causes severe respiratory alkalosis (see above) and results in the following: (1) shift (to the left) in the maternal oxygen dissociation curve, which diminishes the transfer of oxygen from mother to fetus; (2) maternal hypoxemia during uterine relaxation; and (3) reduction in uterine blood flow, which is provoked by an increase in norepinephrine and cortisol release (Figures 2–34 and 9–22). These deleterious effects on the fetus have been demonstrated in several species of animals and in humans (118,119,130,132,160). Figure 9–17 depicts the deleterious effects on fetal heart rate that are caused by significant hyperventilation during a contraction and by hypoventilation between contractions. Lederman and associates (127) also noted that parturients who were anxious and had pain had a higher incidence of abnormal fetal heart rate patterns, and that their infants had lower 1-minute and 5-minute Apgar scores.

Under the conditions of normal labor, such series of transient and intermittent impairments of blood gas exchange are tolerated by the normal fetus because oxygen is stored in the fetal circulation and intervillous space, and is sufficient to maintain adequate fetal oxygenation during the brief period of placental hypoperfusion. Moreover, the fetus can compensate by increasing the proportion of cardiac output that is distributed to the myocardium and brain (163,164). If the above factors are combined with an excessive increase in uterine activity, however, fetal hypoxia, hypercapnea, and acidosis develop that might still be tolerated by the normal fetus, although its ability to withstand oxygen deprivation is limited. It the fetus is already at risk because of obstetric or maternal complications (e.g., preeclampsia, heart disease, diabetes), the pain-induced reductions of oxygen and carbon dioxide transfer can be the critical factors that produce perinatal morbidity, and could even contribute to mortality (124,125,160). The maternal metabolic acidosis is transferred to the fetus, making it more vulnerable to the effects of intrauterine asphyxia caused by cord compression, prolapse, or other obstetric complications (160,165).

### *Effects of Analgesia*

These benefits of pain relief, best achieved with regional analgesia, are likely to be of value to many infants, but they are especially important to the fetus at risk (1,130,145–152,155,166,167). It has been found to be the best method of analgesia for breech delivery and for multiple pregnancies (1,155,166,167). It has been shown that epidural analgesia, through its vasomotor blocking effect, increases intervillous blood flow in parturients with severe preeclampsia and probably also in those with hypertension, diabetes, and other conditions that decrease placental blood flow and function (1,155,166,167). Janisch and coworkers (168) found that continuous epidural analgesia administered to preeclamptics during their last few weeks of gestation produced a 100% increase in placental blood flow. Jouppila and colleagues (169) studied the influence of lumbar epidural analgesia that was limited to a few segments and the effect of a more extensive type of lumbar epidural block on parturients with severe preeclampsia. They found that the limited block increased intervillous blood flow by 34%, whereas the more extensive block increased it by a mean of 77%. They attributed this effect to the relief of severe vasoconstriction by the vasomotor block. Maternal hypotension must be strictly avoided by appropriate prophylactic measures (e.g., intravenous infusion of fluids, lateral displacement of the uterus) to achieve these benefits.

## REFERENCES


1. Bonica JJ: Principles and Practice of Obstetric Analgesia and Anesthesia, Vol. 1 and 2. Philadelphia, FA Davis, 1969.
2. Bonica JJ: The nature of pain of parturition. Clin. Obstet. Gynecol. 2:499, 1975.
3. Bonica JJ: Pain of parturition. Clin. Anesthesiol. 4:1, 1986.
4. Bonica JJ, Chadwick HS: Labour Pain. *In* Textbook of Pain. 2nd Ed. Edited by PD Wall, R Melzack. New York, Churchill Livingstone, 1989, pp. 482–499.
5. Bonica JJ: The pain of childbirth. *In*, JJ:The Management of Pain, ed 2. Philadelphia, Lea & Febiger, 1990 pp. 1313–1343.
6. Bonica JJ: History of pain concepts and therapies. *In* The Management of Pain. 2nd Ed. Edited by JJ Bonica. Philadelphia, Lea & Febiger, 1990, pp. 2–17
7. Wolff HG, Wolf S: Pain. Springfield, IL, Charles C. Thomas Publisher, 1948.
8. Hardy JC, Wolff HG, Goodell H: Pain Sensations and Reactions. Baltimore, The Williams & Wilkins Co., 1952.
9. Hardy JC: The nature of pain. J. Chron. Dis. 4:22, 1956.
10. Beecher HK: Measurement of Subjective Responses. New York, Oxford University Press, 1959.
11. Szasz TS: Pain and Pleasure. New York, Basic Books,Inc., 1957.
12. Melzack R, Wall PD: Pain mechanisms: a new theory. Science 150:971, 1965.
13. Melzack R, Casey KL: Sensory, motivational, and central control determinants of pain: a new conceptual model. *In* International Symposium on the Skin Senses. Edited by D Kenshalo. Springfield, IL, Charles C. Thomas Publisher, 1967.
14. Bonica JJ: Presidential address. *In* Advances in Pain Research and Therapy, Vol. 5. Edited by JJ Bonica, U Lindblom, A Iggo New York, Raven Press, 1983.
15. Wall PD, Melzack R: Textbook of Pain. 2nd Ed. New York, Churchill Livingstone, 1989.
16. Bonica JJ: Anatomic and physiologic basis of nociception and pain. *In* The Management of Pain. 2nd Ed. Philadelphia, Lea & Febiger, 1990. Edited by JJ Bonica 1990, pp. 28–94.
17. Dubner R, Bennett GJ: Spinal and trigeminal mechanisms of nociception. Ann. Rev. Neurosci. 6:381, 1983.
18. Perl ER: Pain and nociception. *In* Handbook of Physiology. Section I, The Nervous System, Vol. 3. Bethesda, American Physiologic Society, 1984, pp. 915–975.
19. Lynn B: The detection of injury and tissue damage. *In* Textbook of Pain. Edited by PD Wall, R Melzack. New York, Churchill Livingstone, 1984, pp. 19–31.
20. Woolf CJ: Long-term alterations in the excitability of deflection reflex produced by peripheral tissue injury in the chronic decerebrate rat. Pain 18:325, 1984.
21. Woolf CJ: Recent advances in the pathophysiology of acute pain. Br. J. Anaesth. 63:139, 1989.
22. Fields HL, Basbaum AI: Brain stem control of spinal pain transmission neurons. Ann. Rev. Physiol. 40:193, 1978.
23. Basbaum AI, Fields HL: Endogenous pain control systems: brain stem spinal pathways and endorphin circuitry. Ann. Rev. Neurosci. 7:309, 1984.
24. Willis WD: The pain system: the neural basis of nociceptive transmission in the mammalian nervous system. Basel, Karger, 1985.
25. Dennis SG, Melzack R: Pain signalling systems in dorsal and ventral spinal cord. Pain 4:97, 1977.
26. Casey KL: Reticular formation and pain: toward a unifying concept. *In* Pain. Edited by JJ Bonica. New York, Raven Press, 1980, pp. 93–105.
27. Brodal A: The Reticular Formation of the Brain Stem. Anatomical Aspects and Functional Correlations. Springfield, IL, Charles C. Thomas, 1957.
28. Jänig W: The autonomic nervous system. *In* Human Physiology. Edited by RF Schmidt, G Thews. New York, Springer-Verlag, 1983, pp. 111–144.
29. Haymaker W, Anderson E, Nauta WJH: The Hypothalamus. Springfield, IL, Charles C. Thomas, 1969.
30. Isaacson RL: The Limbic System. New York, Plenum Press, 1974.
31. MacLean PD: Contrasting functions of limbic and neocortical systems of the brain and their relevance to psychophysiological aspects of medicine. Am. J. Med. 25:611, 1958.
32. Kenshalo DR Jr, Isensee O: Responses of primate SI cortical neurons to noxious stimuli. J. Neurophysiol. 50:1479, 1983.
33. Reynolds DV: Surgery in the rat during electrical analgesia induced by focal brain stimulation. Science 164:444, 1969.
34. Mayer DJ, et al: Analgesia from electrical stimulation in the brain stem of the rat. Science 174:1351, 1971.
35. Liebeskind JC: Pain modulation by central nervous system stimulation. *In* Advances in Pain Research and Therapy, Vol. 1. Edited by JJ Bonica, D Albe-Fessard. New York, Raven Press, 1976, pp. 445–453.
36. Liebeskind JC, Paul LA: Psychological and physiological mechanisms of pain. Annu. Rev. Psychol. 28:41–60, 1977.
37. Besson JMR: Supraspinal modulation of the segmental transmission of pain. *In* Pain and Society. Edited by HW Kosterlitz, LY Terenius Weinheim, Verlag Chemie, 1980, pp. 161–181.
38. Lewis JW, et al: Neural, neurochemical, and hormonal bases of stress-induced analgesia. *In* Advances in Pain Research and Therapy, Vol. 6. Edited by JJ Bonica, L Kruger, JC Liebeskind New York, Raven Press, 1984, pp. 277–288.
39. Mayer DJ, Watkins LR: Multiple endogenous opiate and nonopiate analgesia systems. *In* Advances in Pain Research and Therapy, Vol. 6. Edited by JJ Bonica, L Kruger, JC Liebeskind New York, Raven Press, 1984, pp. 253–276.
40. Fields HL, et al: The activity of neurons in the rostral medulla of the rat during withdrawal from noxious heat. J. Neurosci. 3:2545, 1983.

41. Merskey H, Spear FG: Pain: Psychological and Psychiatric Aspects. London, Bailliere, Tindall and Cassell, 1967.
42. Fordyce WE: Behavioral Methods of Chronic Pain and Illness. St. Louis, C.V. Mosby, 1976.
43. Sternbach RA: The Psychology of Pain. New York, Raven Press, 1978.
44. Pilowsky I: Abnormal illness behavior and sociocultural aspects of pain. *In* Pain and Society. Edited by HW Kosterlitz, LY Terenius. Weinheim, Verlag Chemie, 1980, pp. 445–460.
45. Chapman CR, Turner JA: Psychologic and psychosocial aspects of acute pain. *In* The Management of Pain. 2nd Ed. Edited by JJ Bonica. Philadelphia, Lea & Febiger, 1990, pp. 122–132.
46. Chapman CR: Psychological factors in postoperative pain and their treatment. *In* Acute Pain, Vol. 1. Edited by G Smith, B Covino. London, Butterworths International Medical Review, 1985.
47. Bonica JJ: General considerations of acute pain. *In* The Management of Pain. 2nd Ed. Edited by JJ Bonica. Philadelphia, Lea & Febiger, 1990, pp. 159–179.
48. Kehlet H: Influence of epidural analgesia on the endocrine-metabolic response to surgery. Acta. Anesthesiol. Scand. 70:39, 1978.
49. Kehlet H: Pain relief and modification of the stress response. *In* Acute Pain Management. Edited by MJ Cousins, GD Philips, New York, Churchill Livingstone, 1986, pp. 49–75.
50. Wilmore DW, et al: Stress in surgical patients as a neurophysiologic reflex response. Surg. Gynecol. Obstet. 142: 257, 1976.
51. Behan RJ: Pain. New York, D. Appleton and Company, 1914.
52. Dick-Read G: Childbirth Without Fear. New York, Harper & Bros., 1953.
53. Velvovski IZ, Chougom EA, and Plotitcher VA: The psychoprophylactic and psychotherapeutic method in painless childbirth. Pediatriya, Akusherstvo ta Ginekologiya 1:32, 1950.
54. Lamaze F: Qu'est-ce que l'accouchement sans douleur par la methode psychoprophylactique? Ses principes, sa realisation, ses resultats. Paris, Savouret Connaitre, 1956.
55. Ford CS: A Comparative Study of Human Reproduction. Yale University Publications in Anthropology. New Haven, Yale University Press, 1945.
56. Freedman LZ, Ferguson VS: The question of "painless childbirth" in primitive cultures. Am. J. Orthopsychiatry 20: 363, 1950.
57. Jochelson W: The Yukaghir and the Youkaghirized Tungus: Vol. XIII of the Memoirs of American Museum of Natural History which constitutes at the same time Vol. IX, Part I, of the Jesup North Pacific expedition. Am. Museum of Natural History, New York and Leiden, 1910.
58. Levy-Strauss C: Sorciers et psychanalyse. Geneva, LeCourier de l'Unesco, 1956, pp. 808–810.
59. Lefebvre L, Carli G: Parturition pain in non-human primates: pain and auditory concealment. Pain 21:315, 1985.
60. Lundh W: Modraundervisning, Forlossningstraning eller foraldrakunskap? Ph.D. Dissertation, Pedagogiska Institutionen, Stockholms Universitet, 1974.
61. Bundsen P: Subjectiva resultat av smartlindring under forlossning-En enkatundersokning. Lakartidningen 3:129, 1975.
62. Nettelbladt P, Fagerstrom CF, Uddenberg N: The significance of reported childbirth pain. J. Psychol. Res. 20:215, 1976.
63. Javert CT, Hardy JD: Measurement of pain intensity in labour and its physiologic, neurologic and pharmacologic implications. Am. J. Obstet. Gynecol. 60:552, 1950.
64. Melzack R, et al: Labour is still painful after prepared childbirth training. Can. Med. Assoc. J. 125:357, 1981.
65. Melzack R, et al: Severity of labour pain: influence of physical as well as psychological variables. Can. Med. Assoc. J. 130:579, 1984.
66. Melzack R, Schaffelberg D: Low-back pain during labor. Am. J. Obstet. Gynecol. 156:901, 1987.
67. Melzack R, Belanger E: Labour pain: correlations with menstrual pain and acute low-back pain before and during pregnancy. Pain 36:225, 1989.
68. Melzack R: The myth of painless childbirth. The John J. Bonica Lecture. Pain 19:321, 1984 b.
69. Melzack R: The McGill Pain Questionnaire: major properties and scoring methods. Pain 1:277, 1975.
70. Melzack R, Wall PD, Ty TC: Acute pain in an emergency clinic: latency of onset and descriptor patterns related to different injuries. Pain 14:33, 1982.
71. Gaston-Johansson F, Fridh G, Turner-Norvell K: Progression of labor pain in primiparas and multiparas. Nurs. Res. 37:86, 1988.
72. Fridh G, Gaston-Johansson F: Expectations of labor pain held by primiparas and multiparas. Manuscript under review, 1988, unpublished.
73. Cogan R, Henneborn W, Klopper F: Predictors of pain during prepared childbirth. J. Psychosom. Res. 20:523, 1976.
74. Scott-Palmer J, Skevington SM: Pain during childbirth and menstruation: a study of locus of control. J. Psychosom. Res. 25:151, 1981.
75. Reynolds SRM: Physiology of the Uterus. 2nd Ed. New York, Paul B Hoeber, 1949.
76. Moir C: The nature of the pain of labour. Br. J. Obstet. Gynaecol. 46:409, 1939.
77. Hurst AF: The Sensibility of the Alimentary Canal. Oxford, Oxford University Press, 1911.
78. Caldeyro-Barcia R, Poseiro JJ: Physiology of the uterine contraction. Clin. Obstet. Gynaecol. 3:386, 1960.
79. Paul WM, et al: Clinical tone and pain threshold. Am. J. Obstet. Gynecol. 7:SlQ 1956.
80. Lees MH, et al: Maternal placental and myometrial blood flow of the rhesus monkey during uterine contractions. Am. J. Obstet. Gynecol. 110:68, 1971.
81. Novey MJ: The effect of sustained uterine contractions on myometrial and placental blood flow in the rhesus monkey. *In* Respiratory Gas Exchange and Blood Flow in the Placenta. Edited by LD Longo, H Bartels. Bethesda, Department of Health, Education and Welfare, Publ. No. (NIH) 7–361, 1972, pp. 143–152.
82. Danforth DN: Distribution and functional significance of the cervical musculature. Am. J. Obstet. Gynecol. 68:1261, 1954.
83. Eustace TD: Cognitive, attitudinal, and socioeconomic factors influencing parents' choice of childbirth procedure. Dissertation Abstracts International 39:1474B, 1978.
84. Norr KL, et al: Explaining pain and enjoyment in childbirth. J. Health. Soc. Behav. 18:260, 1977.
85. Fridh G, et al: Factors associated with more intense labor pain. Res. Nurs. Health 11:117, 1988.
86. Kohnen N: "Natural" childbirth among the Kankanaly-Igorot. Bull. NY. Acad. Med. 62:768, 1986.
87. Marx JL: Dysmenorrhea: basic research leads to a rational therapy. Science 205:175, 1979.
88. Csontos K, Rust M, Hollt V: The role of endorphins during parturition. Rockville, MD, National Institute of Drug Abuse Research, Monograph Series, 1980, pp. 264–271.
89. Goland RS, et al: Human plasma beta-endorphin during

pregnancy, labour and delivery. J. Clin. Endocrinol. Metabol. 52:74, 1981.
90. Abbound TK, et al: Effects of epidural anesthesia during labor on maternal plasma beta-endorphin levels. Anesthesiology 59:1, 1983.
91. Fettes I, et al: Plasma levels of immunoreactive beta-endorphin and adrenocorticotropic hormone during labor and delivery. Obstet. Gynecol. 64:359, 1984.
92. Goebelsmann U, et al: Beta-endorphin in pregnancy. Eur. J. Obstet. Gynecol. Reprod. Biol. 17:77, 1984.
93. Facchinetti F, et al: Opioid plasma levels during labour. Gynecol. Obstet. Invest. 13:155, 1982.
94. Foley KM, et al: B-endorphin: analgesic and hormonal effects in humans. Proc. Natl. Acad. Sci. U.S.A. 76:5377, 1979.
95. Gintzler AR: Endorphin-mediated increases in pain threshold during pregnancy. Science 210:913, 1980.
96. Gintzler AR, Peters LC, Komisaruk BR: Attenuation of pregnancy-induced analgesia by hypogastric neurectomy in rats. Brain Research 277:186, 1983.
97. Sander HW, Portoghese PS, Gintzler AR: Spinal k-opiate receptor involvement in the analgesia of pregnancy: effects of intrathecal nor-binaltorphimine, a k-selective antagonist. Brain Research 474:343, 1988.
98. Cogan R Spinnato JA: Pain and discomfort thresholds in late pregnancy. Pain 27:63, 1986.
99. Rust M, et al: Verminderte Schmerzempfindung wahrend Schwangerschaft und Geburt. Arch. Gynecol. 235:676, 1983.
100. Kristal MB, Thompson AC, Grishkat HL: Placenta ingestion enhances opiate analgesia in rats. Physiol. Behav. 35:481, 1985.
101. Kristal MB, et al: Modification of periparturitional pain threshold by ingestion of amniotic fluid in the rat. Soc. Neurosci. Abstr. 14(Part 2):1158, 1988.
102. Kristal MB, Tarapacki JA, Barton D: Amniotic fluid ingestion enhances opioid-mediated but not nonopioid-mediated analgesia. Physiol. Behav. 47:79, 1990.
103. Kristal MB, et al: Amniotic-fluid ingestion by parturient rats enhances pregnancy-mediated analgesia. Life Sci. 46: 693, 1990.
104. Reading AE Cox DN: Psychosocial predictors of labor pain. Pain 22:309, 1985.
105. Brown WA, Manning T, Grodin J: The relationship of antenatal and perinatal psychologic variables to the use of drugs in labor. Psychosom. Med. 34:119, 1972.
106. Zuckerman M, et al: Psychological correlates of somatic complaints in pregnancy and difficulty in childbirth. J. Consult. Psychol. 27:324, 1963.
107. Deutsch H: Psychology of Pregnancy, Labour and Puerperium. *In* Obstetrics. llth Ed. Edited by JP Greenhill JP. Philadelphia, W.B. Saunders, 1955, pp. 349–360.
108. Wuitshik M, Bakal D, Lipshitz J: The clinical significance of pain and cognitive activity in latent labor. Obstet. Gynecol. 73:35–42, 1989.
109. Lowe NK: Explaining the pain of active labor: the importance of maternal confidence. Res. Nurs. Health. 12:237, 1989.
110. Wolff BB, Langley S: Cultural factors and the response to pain: a review. *In* Pain: Clinical and Experimental Perspectives. Edited by M Weisenberg. St. Louis, C.V. Mosby, 1975, pp. 144–151.
110A. Pesce G: Measurement of reported pain of childbirth: a comparison between the Australian and Italian subjects. Pain 31:87, 1987.
110B. Pasquarelli G: The general medical associated problems of the Italian migrant family. Med. J. Aust. 1:65, 1966.
111. True RM: Obstetrical hypnoanalgesia. Am. J. Obstet. Gynecol. 67:373, 1953.
112. Meehan JP, Stoll AM, Hardy JD: Cutaneous pain threshold in Native Alaskan Indians and Eskimos. J. Appl. Physiol. 6: 397, 1954.
113. Preissman AB, Ogoulbostan E: Some details of psychoprophylactic preparation for childbirth in the Turkomenian. S.S.R. Kieve Congress 90:66, 1956.
114. Winsberg B, Greenlick M: Pain response in Negro and white obstetrical patients. J. Health. Soc. Behav. 8:222, 1967.
115. Head H: On disturbances of sensation with special reference to the pain of visceral disease. Brain 16:1, 1893.
116. Cleland JGP: Paravertebral anaesthesia in obstetrics. Surg. Gynaecol. Obstet. 57:51, 1933.
117. Bonica JJ: Mechanisms and pathways of parturition pain. *In* Pain and Reproduction. Edited by AR Genazzani, G Nappi, F Facchinetti, E Martignoni. Casterton Holl, Carnfort, The Parthenon Publishing Group, 1988, pp. 182–191.
118. Berkley KJ, Robbins A, Sato Y: Afferent fibers supplying the uterus in the rat. J. Neurophysiol. 59:142, 1988.
119. Berkley KJ, Wood E: Responses to varying intensities of vaginal distension in the awake rat. Soc. Neurosci. Abstr. 15:979, 1989.
120. Berkley KJ: The role of various peripheral afferent fibers in pain sensation produced by distension of the vaginal canal in rats. Pain (Suppl. 5):S239, 1990.
120A. Berkley KJ, Scofield S, Wood E: Uterine pain: the role of ischemia and the hypogastric nerve. Society for Neuroscience Abstracts 16:416, 1990.
120B. Berkley KJ, Robbins A, Sato Y: Functional differences between afferent fibers in the hypogastric and pelvic nerves innervating female reproductive organs in the rat. J. Neurophysiol. 69:533, 1993.
121. Peters LC, Kristal MB, Komisaruk BR: Sensory innervation of the external and internal genitalia of the female rat. Brain Res. 408:199, 1987.
122. Kawatani M, et al: An analysis of the afferent and efferent pathways to the uterus of the cat using axonal tracing techniques. Soc. Neurosci. Abstr. 12:1055, 1988.
123. Bonica JJ: Maternal respiratory changes during pregnancy and parturition. *In* Parturition and Perinatology. Clinical Anesthesia Series, Vol. 10, No. 2. Edited by GF Marx Philadelphia, FA Davis, 1973, pp. 9–21.
124. Morishima HO, Pedersen H, Finster M: The influence of maternal psychological stress on the fetus. Am. J. Obstet. Gynecol. 134:286, 1978.
125. Shnider SM, et al: Uterine blood flow and plasma norepinephrine changes during maternal stress in the pregnant ewe. Anesthesiology 50:524, 1979.
126. Lederman RP, et al: Endogenous plasma epinephrine and norepinephrine in last-trimester pregnancy and labour. Am. J. Obstet. Gynecol. 129:5, 1977.
127. Lederman RP, et al: The relationship of maternal anxiety, plasma catecholamines, and plasma cortisol to progress in labor. Am. J. Obstet. Gynecol. 132:495, 1978.
128. Falconer AD Powles AB: Plasma noradrenaline levels during labour. Anaesthesia 37:416, 1982.
129. Ohno H, et al: Maternal plasma concentrations of catecholamines and cyclic nucleotides during labor and following delivery. Res. Commun. Chem. Pathol. Pharmacol. 51:183, 1986.
130. Joupplila R, Hollmen A: The effect of segmental epidural analgesia on maternal and foetal acid-base balance, lactate, serum potassium and creatine phosphokinase during labour. Acta. Anaesthesiol. Scand. 20:259, 1976.
131. Abboud TK, et al: Effects of epidural anesthesia during

labor on maternal plasma beta-endorphin levels. Anesthesiology 59:1, 1983.
132. Motoyama EK, et al: The effects of changes in maternal pH and $PCO_2$ on the $Po_2$ of fetal lambs. Anesthesiology 28: 891, 1967.
133. Buchan PC: Emotional stress in childbirth and its modification by variations in obstetric management—epidural analgesia and stress in labor. Acta. Obstet. Gynecol. Scand. 59:319, 1980.
134. Shnider SM, et al: Maternal catecholamines decrease during labor after lumbar epidural anesthesia. Am. J. Obstet. Gynecol. 147:13, 1983.
135. Raisanen I, et al: Beta-endorphin in maternal and umbilical cord plasma at elective cesarean section and in spontaneous labor. Obstet. Gynecol. 67:384, 1986.
136. Westgren M, Lindahl SGE, Norden NE: Maternal and fetal endocrine stress response at vaginal delivery with and without an epidural block. J. Perinat. Med. 14:235, 1986.
137. Neumark J, Hammerle AF, Biegelmayer C: Effects of epidural analgesia on plasma catecholamines and cortisol in parturition. Acta. Anaesthesiol. Scand. 29:555, 1985.
138. Abboud TK, et al: Effects of spinal anesthesia on maternal circulating catecholamines. Am. J. Obstet. Gynecol. 142: 252, 1982.
139. Adams JQ, Alexander AM: Alterations in cardiovascular physiology during labor. Obstet. Gynecol. 12:542, 1958.
140. Hansen JM and Ueland K: The influence of caudal analgesia on cardiovascular dynamics during normal labor and delivery. Acta. Anaesthesiol. Scand. 23(Suppl 10):449, 1966.
141. Lees MM, Scott DB, Kerr MG: Haemodynamic changes associated with labour. Br. J. Obstet. Gynaecol. 77:29, 1970.
142. Hendricks CH, Quilligan EJ: Cardiac output during labour. Am. J. Obstet. Gynecol. 71:953, 1956.
143. Bonica JJ, Ueland K: Heart disease. *In* Principles and Practice of Obstetric Analgesia and Anesthesia, Vol. 2. Edited by JJ Bonica Philadelphia, FA Davis, 1969, pp. 941–977.
144. Sorenson MB, et al: The use of epidural analgesia for delivery in a patient with pulmonary hypertension. Acta. Anaesthesiol. Scand. 26:180, 1982.
145. Pearson JF, Davies P: The effect of continuous lumbar epidural analgesia on maternal acid-base balance and arterial lactate concentration during the second stage of labour. Br. J. Obstet. Gynaecol. 80:225, 1973.
146. Marx GF, et al: Effect of pain relief on arterial blood gas values during labor. NY. J. Med. 69:819, 1969.
147. Marx GF, Greene NM: Maternal lactate, pyruvate and excess lactate production during labour and delivery. Am. J. Obstet. Gynecol. 90:786, 1964.
148. Pearson JF, Davies P: The effect of continuous lumbar epidural analgesia upon fetal acid-base status during the first stage of labour. Br. J. Obstet. Gynaecol. 81:971, 1974.
149. Pearson JF, Davies P: The effect of continuous lumbar epidural analgesia upon fetal acid-base status of maternal arterial blood during the first stage of labour. Br. J. Obstet. Gynaecol. 81:975, 1974.
150. Thalme B, Belfrage P, Raabe N: Lumbar epidural analgesia in labour. Acta. Obstet. Gynaecol. Scand. 53:27, 1974.
151. Thalme B, Raabe N, Belfrage P: Lumbar epidural analgesia in labour. Acta. Obstet. Gynaecol. Scand. 53:113, 1974.
152. Zador G, et al: Low dose intermittent epidural anaesthesia with lidocaine for vaginal delivery. Acta. Obstet. Gynaecol. Scand. 34(Suppl):17, 1974.
153. Hayes JR, et al: Stimulation of gastrin release by catecholamines. Lancet 1:1, 1972.
154. Nimmo WS, Wilson J, Prescott LF: Narcotic analgesics and delayed gastric emptying during labour. Lancet 1:890, 1975.
155. Crawford JS: Principles and Practice of Obstetric Anesthesia. 5th Ed. Oxford, Blackwell Scientific, 1984.
156. Kartchner FD: A study of the emotional reactions during labour. Am. J. Obstet. Gynecol. 60:19, 1950.
157. Rogers FS: Dangers of the Read method in patients with major personality problems. Am. J. Obstet. Gynecol. 71: 1236, 1956.
158. Cheetam RW, Rzadkowolski A: Psychiatric aspects of labour and the puerperium. S. Afr. Med. J. 58:814, 1980.
159. Stewart DE: Psychiatric symptoms following attempted natural childbirth. Can. Med. Assoc. J. 127:713, 1982.
160. Morishima HO, Pedersen H, Finster M: Effects of pain on mother, labour and fetus. *In* Obstetric Analgesia and Anaesthesia. Edited by GF Marx, GM Bassell Amsterdam, Elsevier North Holland, 1980, pp. 197–210.
161. Bonica JJ, Hunter CA Jr: Management in dysfunction of the forces of labor. *In* Principles and Practice of Obstetric Analgesia and Anesthesia, Vol. 2. Edited by JJ Bonica. Philadelphia, FA Davis, 1969, pp. 1188–1208.
162. Moir DD, Willocks J: Management of incoordinate uterine action under continuous epidural analgesia. Br. Med. J. 3: 396, 1967.
163. Assali NS, Holm IW, and Sehgal N: Hemodynamic changes in foetal lamb in utero in response to asphyxia, hypoxia and hypercanpia. Circ. Res. 11:423, 1962.
164. Cohn HE, et al: Cardiovascular responses to hypoxemia and acidemia in foetal lambs. Am. J. Obstet. Gynecol. 120: 817, 1974.
165. Beard RW, Morris ED, Clayton SG: pH of foetal capillary blood as an indication of the conditions of foetus. Br. J. Obstet. Gynaecol. 74:812, 1967.
166. Shnider SM, Levinson G: Anesthesia for Obstetrics. Baltimore, Williams & Wilkins, 1984.
167. Albright GA: Anesthesia and Obstetrics: Maternal, Fetal and Neonatal Aspects. 2nd ed. Boston, Butterworths, 1986.
168. Janisch H, et al: Der Einfluss der kontinuierlichen Epiduralanaesthesia auf die uteroplazentare Durchblutung. Z. Gerburtshilfe. Perinatol. 182:343, 1978.
169. Jouppila P, et al: Lumbar epidural analgesia to improve intervillous blood flow during labour in severe preeclampsia. Obstet. Gynecol. 59:158 1982.

# Chapter 10

# ASSOCIATED PAIN MANAGEMENT PROBLEMS OF PARTURITION

JOHN S. McDONALD

This chapter deals with those many mysterious pain conditions of pregnancy that are a constant source of discomfort and irritation to the pregnant mother. It is necessary to establish an understanding of certain neuroanatomic features that are involved with the pain processes. It is also necessary to discuss pertinent physiologic changes of pregnancy as they relate to these conditions. After these foundation points follows a brief discussion of the important elements of the clinical evaluation of the pregnant patient who has pain. The remainder of the chapter will be consumed by discussions of various pain disorders, including the main categories of pregnancy disorders, medical disorders, joint instability disorders, neuropathies, and myopathies. A discussion of the signs and symptoms and the prevention and diagnosis of these main categories will complete the chapter. It is hoped that this chapter will bring attention to and aid the physician who is confronted with and confounded by some of these painful conditions associated with pregnancy.

## BASIC CONSIDERATIONS

Pain associated with the first, second, and third trimesters of pregnancy is unusual and often associated with pathology of the gestation, such as threatened abortion in the first trimester, incompetent cervix with dilatation in the second trimester, and abruptio placenta in the third trimester. Otherwise, there are some painful disorders of pregnancy that become apparent in the second and third trimesters not associated with fetal jeopardy but due directly to pathologic conditions that develop in the mother sometimes secondary to the pregnancy itself. These will be stressed in this chapter so as to alert the primary physician and the specialist of their existence and signs and symptoms to diminish hopefully the frustration of the diagnostician and to improve the health care of the pregnant women in pain due to such disorders.

The pelvis contains viscera made up of the uterus, tubes, ovaries, broad ligaments, round ligaments, cardinal ligaments, uterosacral ligaments, cervix, vagina, bladder, ureters, urethra, sigmoid colon, rectum, lymph vessels, and nodes. It also contains many nerve structures that will be mentioned in the next section on neuroanatomy. The peritoneum of the female pelvis acts as a completely investing layer anteriorly covering the bladder and the uterus and forming the vesicouterine pouch, and posteriorly covering the back of the uterus, tubes, and ovaries and extending downward over the rectum to form the rectouterine pouch. It also spreads entirely lateral to both side walls to complete the investature of all the pelvic organs.

The following section lays the foundation for an understanding of the neuroanatomic aspects associated with assorted neuropathies, is basic to understanding the causative factors, and instrumental in the diagnosis of many of the disorders. A thorough knowledge of the anatomy of the most common entrapment areas will be indispensable to the clinician presented with the parturient in pain. In each of the five pain sections to follow, the appropriate innervation will be discussed and the innervation pathways identified in a figure to reinforce the visualization of the problem. This knowledge will help the reader to understand the signs and symptoms of the various disease processes and will aid in the selection of the optimum treatment and prevention decisions.

### Neuroanatomy

#### *First Order Nerve Plexus*

The entire pelvic viscera are heavily innervated by two sets of efferent and afferent nerve networks, the sympathetic and the parasympathetic nerves. There are really two main sympathetic control centers to the pelvis, and these are the superior and inferior hypogastric plexuses. There is anatomically one other, referred to as the middle hypogastric plexus, which is really made up of the right and left hypogastric nerves that connect the superior and inferior plexuses.

#### *Second Order Nerve Plexus*

Second order plexuses connect to the two primary ones, namely the superior and inferior hypogastric plexuses. They include: (1) uterovaginal plexus, which lies at the base of the broad ligament and makes connections to the cervix, the body of the uterus, and fallopian tubes; (2) vesicle plexus, which arises in the inferior hypogastric plexus and passes to the bladder proper; and (3) middle rectal plexus, which also arises in the inferior hypogastric plexus and passes to the rectum proper.

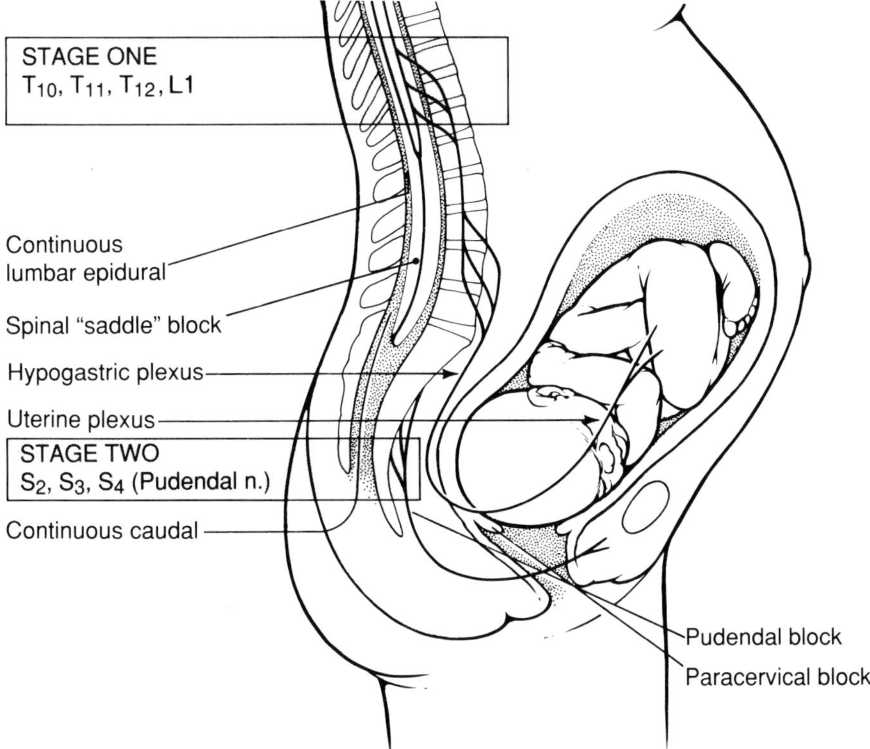


**Fig. 10–1.** Representation of the completely separate pain fibers responsible for transmission of pain in the first stage of labor, T10, T11, T12, and L1, as opposed to the second stage (S2, S3, and S4). (Modified from Chestnut DH, Gibbs CP: Obstetric anesthesia. *In* Obstetrics: Normal & Problem Pregnancies. 2nd Ed. Edited by SG Gabbe, JR Niebyl, JL Simpson. New York, Churchill Livingstone Inc., 1991.)

### *Other Innervations*

The rectum and anal canal innervation is from the superior, middle, and inferior rectal plexus. The latter is derived from the pudendal nerves. The vagina is innervated from nerve fibers from the uterovaginal plexus (Figure 10–1). Table 10–1 lists the pelvic viscera and nerve structures.

## Pertinent Physiologic Changes of Pregnancy

### *Cardiac*

The enlarged uterus effects an anatomic shift in the heart of the parturient. The heart is thus elevated and slightly rotated toward the upward portion of the fourth rib. In so doing, it is also shifted lateralward with the apex pointed to the midclavicular line instead of the usual anterior clavicular line. This causes the left ventricle to move outward from between the sternum anteriorly and the vertebral bodies posteriorly and has great significance in regard to the ineffective use of external cardiac massage during cardiac arrest in the parturient. In the latter situation, internal cardiac massage should be used immediately if inadequate carotid pulsations are noted. Of course the most important item in the treatment of a maternal arrest is to immediately empty the uterus so that fresh blood can enter the ventricle via the vena cava once the uterus is emptied.

Early work on the cardiac dynamics of pregnancy before 1966 suggested cardiac output increased initially by some 10% at the end of the first trimester but then rose to a maximum of 40% by the end of the second trimester (1–5). By the end of the third trimester, the cardiac output was said to return to nonpregnant levels. However, these studies were repeated by Lees and associates (6) and later Ueland and associates (7) who did measurements of cardiac output in the lateral and supine positions and discovered the increase topped-out by the end of the first trimester near 30 to 40% and then did not fall substantially near term unless measurements were taken in the supine position with vena caval compression artifactually giving lowered values. The most recent work by Robson and associates (8) with Doppler and echocardiography reveals a very early trend in increased cardiac output with 10% by 5 weeks, 25% by 8 weeks, and finally to 45% thereafter and during the rest of the gestation. This detail of cardiac changes is repeated here to emphasize to the reader that there is significant increase in the workload of the heart during pregnancy.

### *Liver*

As is well appreciated, many of the liver function tests become elevated toward the end of pregnancy, including the sulfobromophthalein test, thymol turbidity, and cephalin flocculation tests. These changes are believed to be

**Table 10–1.** Innervation of Pelvic Viscera

| Pelvic Viscera | Nerve Structures |
|---|---|
| Uterus: | Motor fibers from parasympathetic pelvic nerves from S2, S3, S4, and sympathetic sensory fibers via the hypogastric plexus from T12, L1 |
| Tubes/Ovaries: | Motor fibers from parasympathetic pelvic nerves from S2, S3, S4, and sympathetic sensory fibers via the ovarian plexus from T12, L1 |
| Broad ligament: | Motor fibers from parasympathetic pelvic nerves from S2, S3, S4, and sympathetic sensory fibers via the hypogastric plexus from T12, L1 |
| Cervix: | Motor fibers from parasympathetic pelvic nerves from S2, S3, S4 and sympathetic sensory fibers via the hypogastric plexus from T12, L1 |
| Vagina: | Motor fibers from parasympathetic pelvic nerves from S2, S3, S4 and sympathetic sensory fibers via the hypogastric plexus from T12, L1 |
| Vestibule/Hymen: | Erectile vasodilator fibers from parasympathetic pelvic nerves from S2, S3, S4 |
| Labia: | Posterior labial nerve S2, S3 and perineal branch of the posterior femoral cutaneous nerve S1, S2, S3 |
| Clitoris: | Erectile vasodilator fibers from parasympathetic pelvic nerves from S2, S3, S4 |
| Perineum: | Motor and sensory innervation from the pudendal nerve arising from S2, S3, S4 |
| Bladder: | Sympathetic fibers from T11, T12, L1, L2 via the superior/inferior hypogastric plexuses control the sphincter and parasympathetic fibers from S2, S3, S4 control filling/emptying of the bladder |
| Anus: | Motor and sensory innervation from the pudendal nerve arising from S2, S3, S4 |

due to obstruction of the extrahepatic pathways and not evidence of actual cellular changes that might belie impaired liver function. When this author was a resident at the University of Iowa, one particularly difficult case to diagnose was illustrated by the young parturient who presented near term with severe abdominal pain in the location of the right upper quadrant. All liver function tests were abnormal as noted above but not out of the ordinary for the gestational date. All gallbladder tests were normal, as were radiographic studies that were done to rule out the possibility of a subhepatic hematoma. The differential diagnosis became liver hepatoma with subcapsular stretching, old gallbladder disease with adhesions to the liver capsule, pancreatic disease, and duodenal ulceration. The patient had to be hospitalized due to the severity of the pain, and premature labor at 36 weeks resulted in such severe right upper quadrant pain with contractions that a decision was made to perform a cesarean section. At laparotomy a long pedunculated fibroid was found to be imbedded into the inferior capsule of the liver just lateral to the gallbladder bed. Evidently, with the onset of contraction and further movement of the liver, there was augmentation of the pain due to the attached fibroid from the dome of the uterus.

### Gallbladder

The sluggish activity of the gallbladder is due to the decreased smooth muscular effect, and emptying is delayed accordingly. There is some distension in most pregnant patients that may be due to a triad of events, the smooth muscle effect, the added effect of some spasm of the sphincter of Oddi, and the increased viscosity of the bile.

### Kidney

As early as the first trimester there is dilatation of the kidney's pelvis, calyces, and ureters. The greatest ureteral effect is noted above the pelvic brim, which suggests it is secondary to uterine compression and relative obstruction. The obstructive factor, however, could not be effective at such an early date, thus it is likely that some of the effect early on is due to progesterone's effect on relaxing smooth muscle tension in a progressive course so that by the beginning of the third trimester there is nearly complete atony with poor peristalsis. This naturally results in the development of hydroureter and further up hydronephrosis. In addition, there is an increase in the glomerular filtration rate, renal plasma flow, rate of filtration, and tubular reabsorption that all eventually results in a decrease in the blood urea nitrogen level.

### Uterus

Naturally, the uterus undergoes the most dramatic changes of any internal organ during pregnancy. It is transposed into an organ that is enlarged nearly 10 to 20 times its normal dimensions. Its nonpregnant weight is some 60 grams, its pregnant weight, nearly 1000 grams. Its nonpregnant length is 6 cm, its pregnant length 60 cm. Early increases in dimensions are due to tissue hypertrophy, while later increases are due to stretching. The most demonstrative effects on the nervous system are due to the latter phases of pregnancy when the uterus becomes an abdominal organ and rests upon the vertebral column posteriorly compressing the vena cava and aorta; additionally, the fetal presenting part exerts pressure upon the vasculature and the nerves of the pelvis during descent in labor. This latter point will become important in regard to the possible stretching of some of these pelvic nerves during prolonged second stages with large babies.

### Muscles

The general effect of relaxin upon the musculoskeletal system is to effect muscular softening and relaxation. This effect is notable in the muscles of the pelvis, abdomen, and lower back. This effect can work to the benefit of the mother by allowing room for expansion of the abdomen anteriorly due to the anatomic effect on the rectus abdominal muscles during the third trimester and by allowing compensation in the pelvis for the descent of the presenting fetal part during labor.

### Joints

The effect of the hormone-stimulated general relaxation by relaxin has been alluded to in previous portions of this section on changes in physiology during pregnancy. Nevertheless, the most demonstrative effect is due to its effect on the target organ it was made for—the joints. It is natural that this hormone increases late in the third trimester to assure flexibility of the joints of the pelvis, including, most dramatically, the symphysis pubis.

### Nervous System

To date, there are no published documented effects upon the nervous system. There are many possible stretch effects on peripheral nerves that may be fixed at various points within the pelvis and near the pelvic brim. This results in stretch due to the descent of the fetal presenting part during late second stage and delivery itself.

### Clinical Evaluation

The first order of business in the clinical evaluation consists of determining a complete history of the pain, its onset, characteristics, intensity, and factors that bring it on and alleviate it. It is important to be a good listener and to take careful notes so that the patient is not asked to repeatedly answer the same question. Few things are more irritating to the patient than having to state her history over and over. Next must follow a comprehensive review of all the past studies and laboratory tests performed on the patient. This is important so that studies are not repeated and costly bills incurred without reason. Every patient will appreciate a genuine interest in her welfare and planning, holding expensive tests to a minimum. Discuss these items with the patient and involve her in the decision-making process. It will help the patient to feel in some control and help her to develop respect for your openness. Discuss the patient's pain to develop a pain score based upon *her* personal evaluation and past pain experience. The comparison of different pain scores is shown in Figure 10–2.

The second order of business in the clinical evaluation is the careful physical examination of the patient. Be thorough and complete, but do not spend inordinate lengths of time on minutia that has little to do with the patient's primary complaint. A complete neurologic examination is a must and should be performed in one sitting.

The third order of business is the examination of the muscles in the area affected by the pain. Care must be taken to be gentle yet persistent to elicit discomfort, tension or injury. This can be done with the tips of the fingers or with the probe of a blunt object, such as the blunt end of a pen with gradually increasing pressure to elicit tender points in the muscle tissue.

The fourth order of business is the examination of the dermatomes in the area of pain so that some insight may be developed in regard to the sensory cord level of the transmission. This is best performed with cotton for the light touch evaluation and then the finger for gradually increasing levels of sensory discrimination.

The fifth order of business is a careful examination and manipulation of the joints located in the area of the pain complaint. This can give many hints as to what role the joint or joint space may have upon the genesis of the pain condition. This examination includes the full range of motion of both the upper and lower extremities to detect any abnormalities.

The sixth order of business is the pelvic examination.

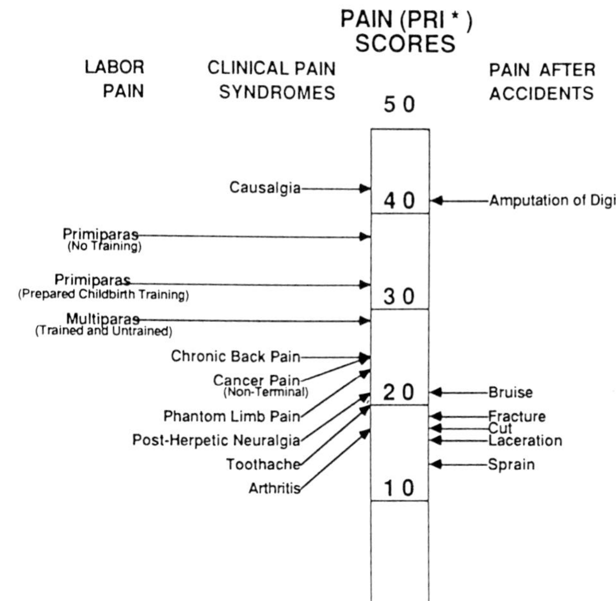


**Fig. 10–2.** Representation of pain-score column, with the lowest pain of 10 with regular graduations to the highest pain of 50. It is quite evident that the pain of labor is interpreted by parturients as significant, as primiparae and multiparae are spread through the 30 and 40 index marks. Other typical pain, i.e., toothache, arthritis, fractures, lacerations, etc., are included for comparison. (From Melzack R: The myth of painless childbirth (The John J. Bonica Lecture). Pain 19:321–327, 1984.)

This exam must be performed by someone who is schooled in the complexity of the exam, its sensitivity, its completeness, and its salient pathologic points. This must include evaluation of the external genitalia, the outlet, the vagina, cervix, the uterus, tubes, parametria, and ovaries. In addition to the usual bimanual exam for detection of any abnormalities in size, configuration or pain, the vaginal area, outlet, and immediate parametrial area must be probed with a small instrument or small padded sponge stick to detect any signs of pain. The pelvic exam may be supplemented with the use of the vaginal ultrasound.

## PAIN DISORDERS—SIGNS, SYMPTOMS, DIAGNOSIS, AND TREATMENT

### Pregnancy Disorders

#### Parovarian Cysts

Parovarian cysts originate from the broad ligament and are derived from mesothelium, mesonephric, and paramesonephric elements. Various torsion accidents of pelvic adnexa occur and precipitate acute pain. These can include the ovary and other cystic masses, such as corpus luteum cysts, in addition to parovarian cysts. Parovarian cysts comprise between 10 to 20% of all adnexal masses (Figure 10–3) (9–11). In a case in which a parovarian cyst grows during pregnancy, it can present as acute back or flank pain (12). Two cases are presented for examples of the clinical course during pregnancy.

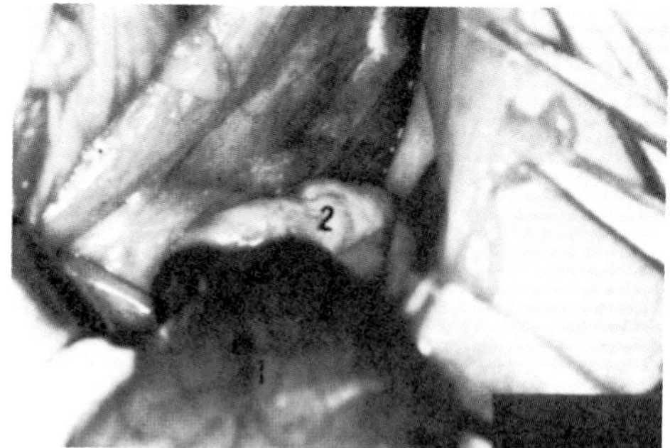

**Fig. 10–3.** The shell of a ruptured parovarian cyst with the darkened center core representing the middle of the cyst. (From Hasuo Y, Higashijima T, Mitamura T: Torsion of parovarian cyst. Kurume. Med. J. 38:39–43, 1991.)

Case #1: 35-year-old primipara admitted with sudden severe flank pain at 32 weeks. All vital signs were within normal limits on admission. The patient's heart rate was 82 and the fetal heart rate was 146. Pelvic exam revealed a closed firm cervix without bleeding. The abdomen was soft but had tenderness in the right lower quadrant. Complete blood count (CBC) and white blood cells (WBC) were normal. Pelvic sonograms revealed a 40 × 47-mm cystic mass on the right side of the uterus. Ultrasound performed five times during the first and second trimesters revealed no cystic masses. At laparotomy a right black cyst 40 × 50 mm with a tense capsule was found.

Case #2: 32-year-old woman experienced dull lower abdominal pain. Exam on admission revealed normal vital signs and a tender lower abdomen with rebound localized to the right lower quadrant. Red blood cells (RBC) and white blood cells were normal. A pelvic conogram revealed a small cyst. Admission diagnosis was acute appendicitis. Laparotomy was performed at which time a normal appendix was found with a small parovarian cyst, which was blue-black and twisted.

These two cases illustrate that clinical symptoms are due to torsion of the cyst and compromise of its blood supply after it has grown sufficiently to undergo torsion. The most common symptom is mild-to-moderate lower abdominal pain that can become severe if torsion and greater compromise of blood supply or stretching of the overlying peritoneum occur. Many parovarian cysts are found during the course of other surgical procedures. In pregnancy it is suggested that they should be removed in the first-half of pregnancy if diagnosed because they often tend to enlarge and undergo torsion later. In one of the presented cases illustrated here, five ultrasounds did not reveal a parovarian cyst, thus it must have grown rapidly in the third trimester (13).

### *Hydronephrosis*

Almost all pregnant patients have anatomic dilatation of the upper collecting system, including the calyces, pelves of the kidney, and ureters (Figure 10–4). One of the symptoms of hydronephrosis of pregnancy can be acute pain secondary to symptomatic infections, refractory infections, and, in some cases, even renal failure. The following case illustrates this condition. The patient was a 19-year-old women at 26 weeks. She presented at the emergency room with acute right flank pain, nausea, and vomiting. She had no history of fever nor urinary tract symptoms. Urine culture was negative. Ultrasound revealed right hydronephrosis. On the second hospital day the pain became localized to the right lower quadrant with guarding and rebound tenderness. A laparotomy was performed with a working diagnosis of appendicitis. The appendix was normal. The patient was discharged from the hospital but returned 2 weeks subsequently with a recurrence of the same pain. An excretory urographic study revealed significant dilatation of the right collecting system with evident extravasation of contrast into the retroperitoneum. The patient was treated with a cutaneous nephrostomy and antibiotics and underwent delivery by cesarean section without incident. In summary, hydronephrosis detected by renal ultrasonographic studies is a normal finding unless it is associated with acute flank pain such as illustrated by the aforementioned case. Such a severe case of hydronephrosis of pregnancy with extravasation of urine is rare with only one other case noted in the literature (14), but it must be kept in mind should all the signs and symptoms fit (15).

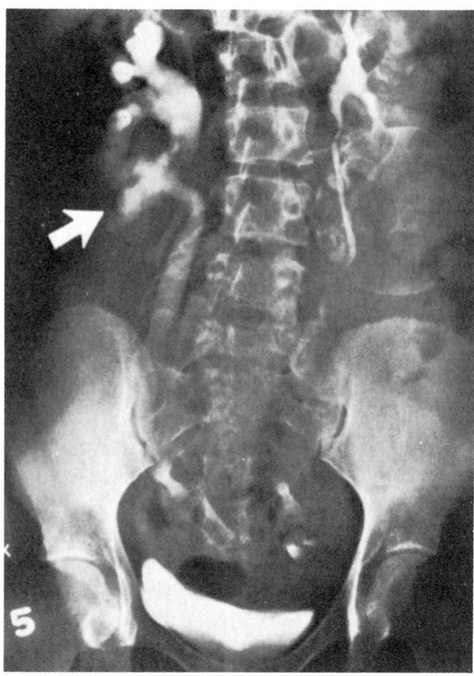


**Fig. 10–4.** Excretory urogram which reveals right-sided hydronephrosis and extravation of contrast material. (From Ferguson T, Bechtel W: Hydronephrosis of pregnancy. American Family Physician 43:2135–2137, 1991.)

### *Appendicitis and Abruptio Placenta*

The combined occurrence of an appendicitis and abruptio placenta may pose as a diagnostic problem. The following case illustrates such an occurrence. The patient was a 26-year-old woman who complained of sudden abdominal pain and vomiting. An ultrasound study performed before admission to the hospital indicated a normal pregnancy. The patient had uterine tenderness and normal uterine size for dates. Biophysical profile was normal and the placenta showed no signs of abruption. The patient went into labor with passage of clots through the cervix precipitating cesarean section. At the time of delivery purulent peritoneal fluid was encountered. A near 2500-gm fetus was delivered with good Apgar scores. The placenta immediately followed delivery of the fetus with numerous blood clots on over 30% of its surface. Exploration of the abdomen revealed a ruptured appendix, which was removed. The peritoneal cavity was rinsed several times and the patient recovered uneventfully. It is suggested that leakage of bacteria into the peritoneum may stimulate prostaglandin synthesis and precipitate placental disruption, and thus the occurrence of these two pathologic conditions may be more than coincidental (16).

### Inguinal Endometriosis

Six patients out of 958 patients with endometriosis were found to have inguinal endometriosis (Table 10–2) (17). The signs were tenderness, small bulge in inguinal area, hard inguinal nodule, tender inguinal mass, 3-cm inguinal mass, 1-cm nodule at inguinal ring, and tender 2-cm mass at superficial inguinal ring. The symptoms were swelling, pain, fever, and pain with menses. Most patients were diagnosed as having inguinal hernia and some with incarceration; some patients were correctly diagnosed with inguinal endometriosis. Surgical treatments included excision of the inguinal masses and in some instances excision of ovarian endometriomas, adnexal resections, and, in one case, a hysterectomy with bilateral salpingo-oophorectomy. Followup revealed only one patient subsequently had recurrence of the local inguinal endometriosis. A few patients underwent later endometrioma resection for recurrent pelvic endometriosis. This is an important diagnosis to keep in mind as a differential of pain and swelling in the inguinal region. There is one other study of inguinal endometriosis reported to date in the world literature (18).

### Pelvic Inflammatory Disease

Pelvic inflammatory disease during pregnancy is not common (19). It occurs during the first trimester of gestation unlike pelvic abscess, which can occur at any trimester. The diagnosis is many times made incidental to operative intervention for other conditions, such as appendicitis. It is important to diagnose this condition because it is amenable to antibiotic therapy if treated early. It is also important to realize that pregnancy is not a barrier to salpingitis because the uterine cavity is not totally occluded before 12 weeks and thus the pathway of infection can still be effective. The most consistent symptoms in pregnancy are acute lower abdominal pain, anorexia, nausea, vomiting, and low grade fever. Some of the other causes of acute abdominal pain in pregnancy include, appendicitis, adnexal torsion, abortion, ectopic pregnancy, abruption, bowel obstruction, pancreatitis, and renal stone.

## Medical Disorders

### Budd-Chiari Syndrome

The Budd-Chiari Syndrome complicating preeclampsia is illustrated by a case of a 25-year-old preeclamptic woman who had third-trimester right upper quadrant pain of a severe degree, an elevation of serum aminotransferase, and disseminated intravascular coagulation associated with a cesarean delivery (20). This patient had a liver CT scan that revealed a specific hepatic abnormality located on the patient's right side. A subsequent magnetic resonance image was suggestive that this hepatic mass looked hemorrhagic. Also noted on magnetic resonance imaging (MRI) was a partial thrombosis of the right hepatic vein that appeared to extend into the inferior vena cava (Figure 10–5). The patient completely recovered after anticoagulation, and followup magnetic resonance imaging at 8 months was normal. This case is suggestive that Budd-Chiari Syndrome can occur in association with preeclampsia and that venous obstruction can be traced to disseminated intravascular coagulation. One of the differential diagnoses that such a condition can be confused with is hepatic hemorrhage with or without capsular tear, the latter being related to sever symptoms of pain in the right upper quadrant. This is an example in which the use of magnetic resonance can be absolutely diagnostic. Certainly, liver disorders in pregnancy promote concern. The Budd-Chiari Syndrome is basically hepatic venous outflow obstruction.

### Ehlers-Danlos Syndrome Type III

Ehlers-Danlos Syndrome Type III during pregnancy is another unusual disorder, a truly rare disorder of connective tissue. In association with pregnancy it can be responsible for complications varying from major to minor degrees. A typical sign of this syndrome is the patient's ability to dislocate joints either walking or even standing. The joints include both the knees and the hips. The patient in this report had severe knee dislocation and nerve root pain from a prolapse of an intervertebral disc (21). The patient was placed in the hospital at 27 weeks, placed at bed rest, given analgesics, and given pelvic traction after being placed on prophylactic heparin. Worsening pain resulted in a cesarean section at 35 weeks due to uncontrollable pain.

### Partial Absence of the Left Pericardium

Partial absence of the left pericardium during pregnancy is another rare congenital entity that can cause chest pain during parturition. It carries a high risk of death due to herniation of the left atrial appendage through the pericardial remnant with eventual strangulation. One case report of the first known condition to be followed throughout pregnancy involved a 22-year-old Malaysian woman (22). Her initial referral was for chest pain. The patient's condition was previously diagnosed by chest

**Table 10–2.** Endometriosis of the Round Ligament

| | Patient 1 | Patient 2 | Patient 3 |
|---|---|---|---|
| Age at diagnosis | 23 | 30 | 46 |
| Gravidity and parity | Nulligravid | Nulligravid | 2–0–0–2 |
| Presenting symptoms | Right inguinal swelling for 10 mo, painful during menses | Right inguinal nodule for 6 mo, painful during menses | Bilateral inguinal mass with catamenial pain for 1 y |
| Physical findings | Tender 3-cm bulge at right superficial inguinal ring, 6-cm right adnexal mass | Hard 2-cm right inguinal nodule | Tender 3-cm left inguinal mass, nontender 2-cm right inguinal nodule, uterine leiomyomas |
| Tentative diagnosis | Right inguinal hernia and ovarian cyst | Right inguinal hernia | Incarcerated left inguinal hernia |
| Surgical diagnosis and treatment | Endometriosis of right round ligament: excision; right ovarian endometrioma: right adnexectomy | Endometriosis of right round ligament: excision | Bilateral round ligament endometriosis: excision; ovarian endometriomas: TAH-BSO |
| Follow-up | Pregnancy not attempted, right-thigh endometriosis recurrence after 14 y | Pregnancy not attempted, TAH-BSO for ruptured right ovarian endometrioma 19 y later, no inguinal recurrence | No recurrence after 18 y |

TAH-BSO = total abdominal hysterectomy and bilateral salpingo-oophorectomy.
(From Candiani GB, Vercellini P, Fedele L, Vendola N, et al: Inguinal endometriosis: pathogenetic and clinical implications. Obstet. Gynecol. 78: 191, 1991.)

x ray that revealed a prominent left atrial appendage. The patient refused surgical repair. One physician recommended a cesarean delivery to avoid possible herniation of the atrial appendage with a Valsalva maneuver. Nevertheless, a vaginal delivery was recommended and performed under local anesthesia without incident. This is an example of how many different techniques can be effective treatment for given conditions. In this case, the patient did not require a Valsalva maneuver and thus avoided one of the apparent risks of promotion of atrial herniation. Another recommendation would be for first stage analgesia via a continuous epidural with dilute solutions of local anesthetic; opioid for the first stage of labor; and use of a caudal or saddle block anesthetic for the second stage with shortening of the latter by forceps extraction (22).

## *Sickle Cell Syndrome*

Sickle Cell Syndrome also causes pain in pregnancy (Table 10–3). Clinical variation is the hallmark of this disease process. Patients not in threat nor in the throes of a crises may function entirely normal. Other patients may experience repeated hospitalizations with repeated complications. The perinatal complications include intrauterine growth retardation, stillbirths, and perinatal deaths. Sickle cell anemia maternal-related complications include hypoxic-based injury, such as painful crises with associated fever and leukocytosis (23), seizures, splenic sequestration, anemia, pyelonephritis, and cholecystitis. Special attention must be given to the patient in regard to counseling, strict antepartum care with frequent visits emphasizing blood pressure, complete blood count, reticulocyte count, urine analysis (UA), fetal monitoring with the biophysical profile, and contraction stress or the nonstress test. Labor management should be directed toward reduction of cardiac work, providing extra oxygen, epi-

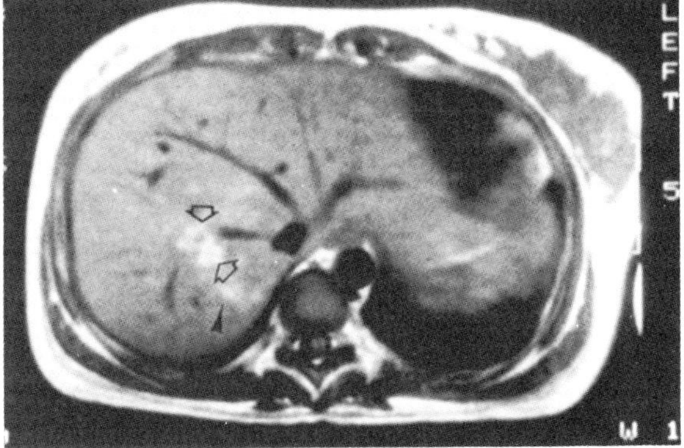


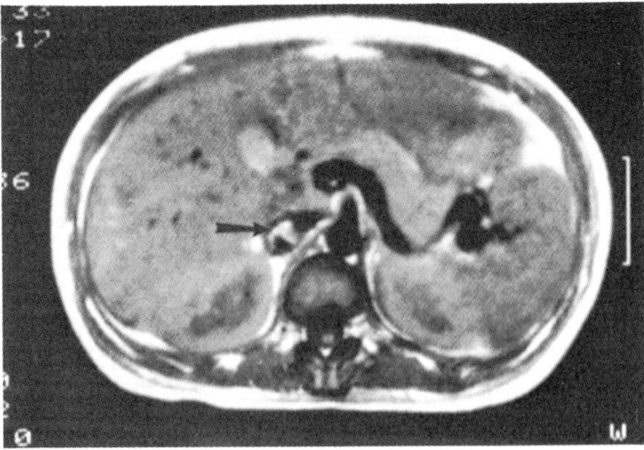

**Fig. 10–5.** Magnetic resonance images showing clot in inferior venal cava. (From Gordon SC, Polson DJ, Shirkhoda A: Budd-Chiari syndrome complicating pre-eclampsia: diagnosis by magnetic resonance imaging. J. Clin. Gastroenterol. 13:460–2, 1991.)

| Patient 4 | Patient 5 | Patient 6 |
|---|---|---|
| 38 | 29 | 22 |
| 2–0–0–2 | Nulligravid | Nulligravid |
| Severe dysmenorrhea, mild fever and catamenial right inguinal pain for 1 y | Infertility, right inguinal nodule with catamenial pain for 18 mo | Right inguinal nodule, painful during menses, mild fever for 1 y |
| Tender 3-cm right inguinal mass, 5-cm right adnexal cyst | 1-cm nodule at right superficial inguinal ring, nodular uterosacral ligaments | Tender 2-cm mass at right superficial inguinal ring |
| Right inguinal hernia and ovarian cyst | Pelvic and inguinal endometriosis | Inguinal endometriosis |
| Endometriosis of right round ligament: excision; right ovarian endometrioma enucleation | Endometriosis of right round ligament: excision | Endometriosis of right round ligament: excision |
| Pregnancy not attempted, TAH-BSO for ovarian endometrioma recurrence after 2 y, no inguinal recurrence | Pelvic endometriosis at laparoscopy 2 y later for persistent infertility, no inguinal recurrence | Pregnancy not attempted, pelvic endometriosis diagnosed at laparoscopy 1 y later for chronic pelvic pain, no inguinal recurrence |

dural analgesia to reduce stress of labor, shortening of the second stage of labor with forceps delivery with good sacral analgesia with a caudal or saddle block anesthetic, and careful fetal monitoring. In the postpartum period, anemia must be avoided and good oxygenation maintained, and the avoidance of thromboembolism by exercise and ambulation of the patient (24).

### *Pseudotrochanteric Bursitis*

Pseudotrochanteric bursitis and the differential diagnosis of lateral hip pain can be another problem in the pain syndromes of pregnancy. A group of patients who were classified as refractory trochanteric bursitis patients was deemed to have pseudotrochanteric bursitis (25). The most common causes were found to be lumbar radiculopathy involving L2 and L3, lumbar facet syndrome, and entrapment neuropathies of the subcostal or iliohypogastric nerves. Pseudotrochanteric bursitis can be of somatic origin from various branches of sciatic, femoral, and obturator nerves; of neuropathic origin due to inflammatory, compression or ischemia of the iliohypogastric, subcostal or lumbar rootlets; or of referred origin from facet joints and paraspinous ligaments. Diagnosis can be made by injection of local anesthetic into the peritrochanteric area or specific local injection into the involved nerves noted above should neuropathy be the etiology.

**Table 10–3.** Sickle Cell Complications

| | Randomized SS | | Not Randomized | | |
|---|---|---|---|---|---|
| | Transfusion (Group A) | Control (Group B) | SS | SC | SB Thal |
| Pain crisis* | 14 | 50 | 29 | 25 | 30 |
| Seizure disorder | 3 | 3 | 11 | 2 | 0 |
| Headaches | 3 | 3 | 0 | 0 | 0 |
| Splenic sequestration | 0 | 3 | 0 | 3 | 9 |
| Acute chest syndrome | 6 | 8 | 11 | 3 | 9 |
| Congestive heart failure | 3 | 3 | 7 | 0 | 4 |
| Severe anemia | 3 | 8 | 11 | 3 | 13 |
| Pyelonephritis | 3 | 3 | 7 | 2 | 0 |
| Urinary tract infection | 6 | 17 | 11 | 9 | 4 |
| Nephrotic syndrome | 3 | 3 | 0 | 0 | 0 |
| Chronic renal failure | 0 | 3 | 4 | 0 | 0 |
| Cholecystitis | 0 | 6 | 0 | 0 | 0 |

* $P = <0.01$
(From Koshy M, Burd L: Management of pregnancy in sickle cell syndromes. Hematology/Oncology Clin. of North America 5:585–96, 1991.)

### *Endometrioma*

Endometrioma and pain in the pubis and the hip, though unusual in early pregnancy, can be considered in refractory pain problems of the area. The original descriptive of endometriosis was by Sampson in 1921 (26). Aberrant cellular rests can occur in locales distant from the pelvic cavity and are responsive to cyclic stimulation (27). Endometriomas of the sciatic nerve are responsible for pain in the thigh and buttock area. Similarly, small endometrial implants in and around the round ligament can be responsible for causing pain in the groin and subpubic area (28). The original descriptive of adenomyoma of the round ligament was made in 1896 (29). It is a possible consideration in patients with refractory groin pain who may present with a small nodule or mass that appears to be cyclic in nature.

### *Rapidly Progressive Glomerulonephritis (RPGN)*

Pregnancy associated with rapidly progressive glomerulonephritis (RPGN) and arthralgia is an unusual condition that causes painful joints. At 28 weeks gestation, a 35-year-old woman was eventually diagnosed as rapidly progressive glomerulonephritis (RPGN) (30). The final diagnosis after renal and skin biopsies was polyarteritis nodosa. Prednisolone was administered with good relief. Labor was induced at 36 weeks with successful delivery of a female infant in good condition.

## Joint Disorders

### Sacroiliac Subluxation

The documentation of sacroiliac subluxation during pregnancy as a cause of low-back pain was determined in a retrospective review between June 1986 and June 1989 (31). Approximately two-thirds of all patients with severe low-back pain met the criteria for sacroiliac subluxation. The incidence of sacroiliac subluxation was 11% compared to 14% reported by Golighty (32) and 6% by Berg (33). Pain onset was before the twenty-sixth week of gestation in 55% of the cases compared to 66% of cases described by Berg. Sacroiliac subluxation and its associated pain affect many women during the second trimester of pregnancy, as work and household responsibilities were often interrupted for a significant part of the pregnancy. Manipulation relieved pain in 10 of 11 women (91%) in this uncontrolled study. Other accepted methods of treatment include use of a trochanteric belt (33) and physical therapy (34,35). No study has shown any risk to the fetus from rotational pelvic manipulations. Even though early descriptions of sacroiliac subluxation in pregnancy came from the United States (31), the condition is largely unrecognized in this country. There are several reasons sacroiliac subluxation is not more commonly diagnosed and treated: (1) medical practitioners are skeptical about manipulative therapy in general and associate it only with chiropractic diagnosis; and (2) the orthopedic literature has traditionally taught that the sacroiliac joint does not move (36) and that it should not be considered a source of low-back pain (37). Most obstetricians are not schooled in this disease process and are not taught corrective manipulative techniques (31).

### Sacroiliac Joint Infection

Pregnancy and the association of sacroiliac joint infection were the source of another paper on the cause of pain in pregnancy (38). The article stressed that magnetic resonance imaging will be used more and more frequently as a diagnostic tool in pregnancy because of its complete safety to the mother and fetus (Figure 10–6). A case of such a use in a 24-year-old woman at 26 weeks gestation illustrates the applicability of this substitute for radiographic study of medical or surgical conditions. The patient presented with right-sided back pain, an old history of rheumatic fever, and four recent episodes of fever. A differential diagnosis included infection in a pelvic kidney, herniated disc, and sacroiliac or hip joint disease. Bacterial endocarditis was diagnosed by echocardiography, which revealed a ventricular septal defect (VSD) with vegetation attached to the tricuspid valve. The patient was treated with antibiotic therapy and became afebrile. She continued to have pain in the right iliac and thigh areas that increased with walking. A magnetic resonance imaging of the right hip and sacroiliac joint was performed and revealed right sacroiliac joint irregularity and widening consistent with septic arthritis. The patient's antibiotic therapy was increased and the patient became asymptomatic. Magnetic resonance imaging can also be effective as a diagnostic tool in pregnancy with suspected herniated lumbar disc disease (39). Figure 10–7 shows the complex anatomic relationship of the sacrum at the iliac articulation and demonstrates the protective massive architecture of this boney process.

### Impact of Low-Back Pain and Pelvic Pain

Another study looked at the impact of low-back and pelvic pain in pregnancy (40). Pregnancy and back pain are often considered to go hand-in-hand. Several studies show that nearly one-half of pregnant patients have back pain (see Figure 10–8) (33,41–43). Part of the blame is given to hormonal changes from relaxin, which promotes necessary tissue changes in the cervix and ligaments of the pelvis. The latter allows for the necessary joint flexibility in the symphysis, lumbosacral and sacroiliac joints so that the fetal head can traverse the pelvic inlet during labor (44–47). This study analyzed 855 pregnant women in regard to back pain and found that those with precedent back pain had more intense pain during gestation, that back pain resulted in a higher rate of induction and cesarean deliveries, and that back pain disappeared in the first 6 months postpartum except in those women with the aforementioned precedent pain (Figure 10–9) (40). Eighty-two percent of those still had pain at 18 months.

### Protecting the Back

Protecting the back during pregnancy was the source of another study (48). Back pain occurs in about 50% of all pregnant patients (49). The important physiologic changes responsible for this include: (1) the hormones progesterone and relaxin, which relax and soften pelvic joints and ligaments; (2) the instability of the pelvis due to this relaxation; (3) uterine enlargement and tipping, which shifts the center of gravity forward and the resultant lumbar strain; (4) weakening of the rectus abdominal muscles due to stretch; (5) back muscles and buttock muscles, which overcompensate to offset the weak abdominals; and (6) the exaggerated lumbar curve, which compensates for the shifted center of gravity. Several important considerations can help the pregnant patient combat these changes, including: (1) maintenance of good posture by keeping the pelvis tilted backward by using the anterior muscle group to lift the pelvis upward and by use of the posterior muscle group to pull the posterior pelvis downward; (2) use of the pelvic tilt exercise to relieve stress and back strain and at the same time strengthen the abdominal muscles (Figures 10–10 and 10–11); (3) use of a good shoe that has a thick but moderate heel to decrease the lumbar curve; and (4) development of strong abdominal muscles, which provides the

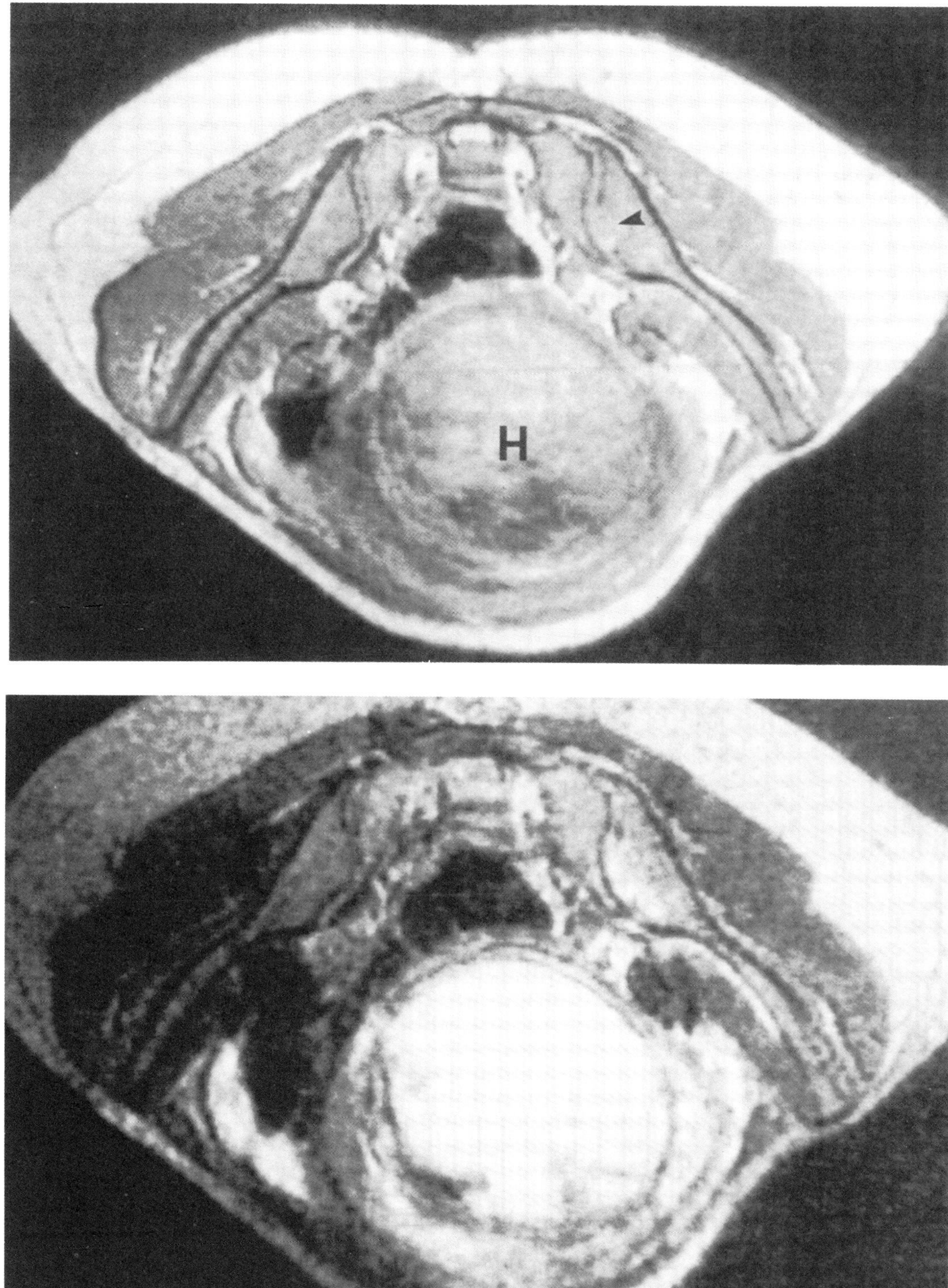


**Fig. 10–6.** Magnetic resonance images being used in pregnancy in lieu of radiographic studies. Images are of lower sacroiliac joint through the plane of the fetal head. (From Wilbur AC, Langer BG, Spigos DG: Diagnosis of sacroiliac joint infection in pregnancy by magnetic resonance imaging. Mag. Reson. Imaging. 6:341–343, 1988.)

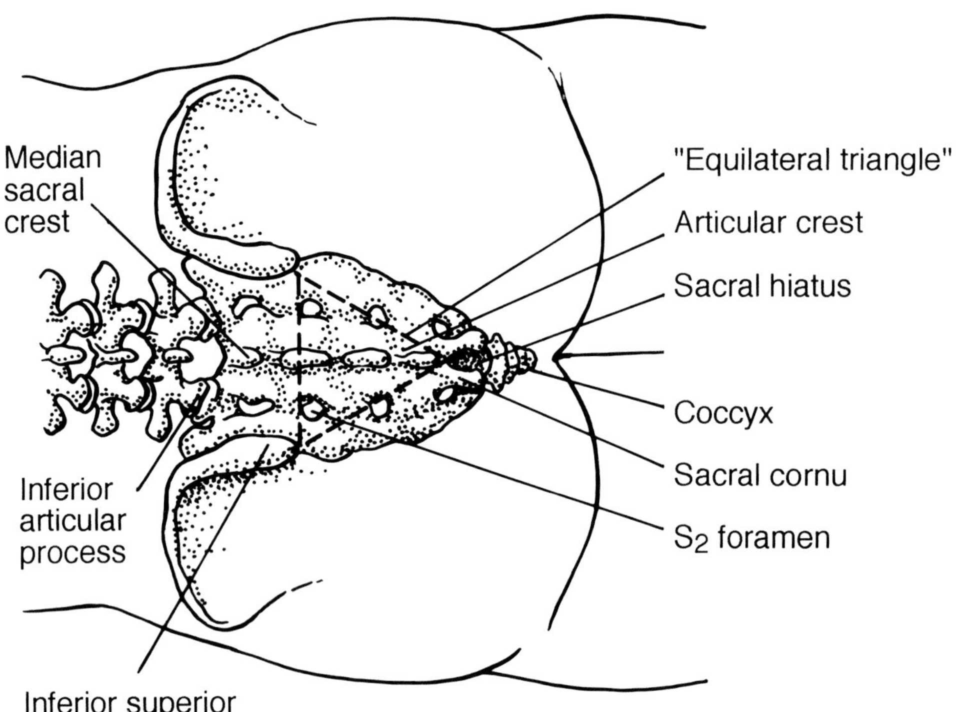


**Fig. 10–7.** This figure demonstrates the equilateral triangle that can be drawn conceptually from the sacral hiatus to the iliac spines. This helps define the sacral area for caudal block.

key to support of the pregnant pelvis (40). Figure 10–8 illustrates the difference in pain threshhold of pregnant versus nonpregnant patients and the obvious increase in discomfort due to the physiologic stress imposed upon the musculoskeletal systems.

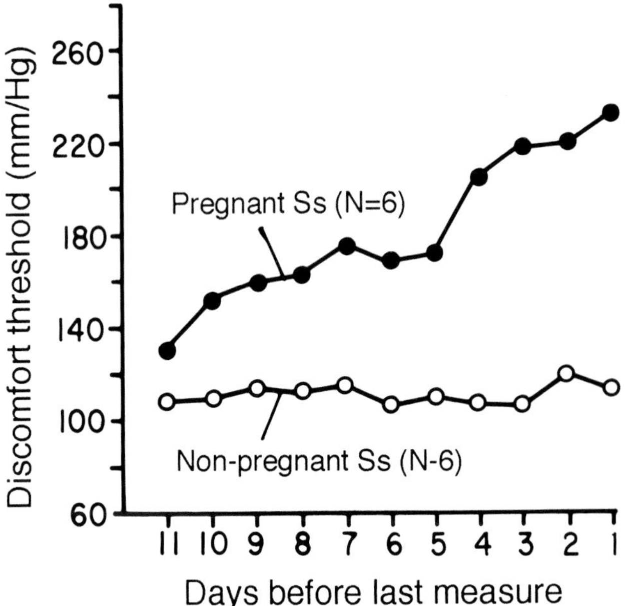


**Fig. 10–8.** Discomfort threshold of non-pregnant and pregnant patients in the last 11 days of pregnancy. It is obvious that pregnant patients have a significant increase in pain index during the last 4 days.

*Low-Back Pain During Pregnancy*

The well-known problem of low-back pain during pregnancy was the source of an interesting study (33). In this study of 862 pregnant women, it was discovered that sacroiliac joint pain was the most common dysfunction that caused common low-back pain, i.e., in 43% of the women (Table 10–4). The increased biomechanical stress on ligaments, muscles, and the skeletal structure is the underlying reason for such low-back pain of pregnancy. In this

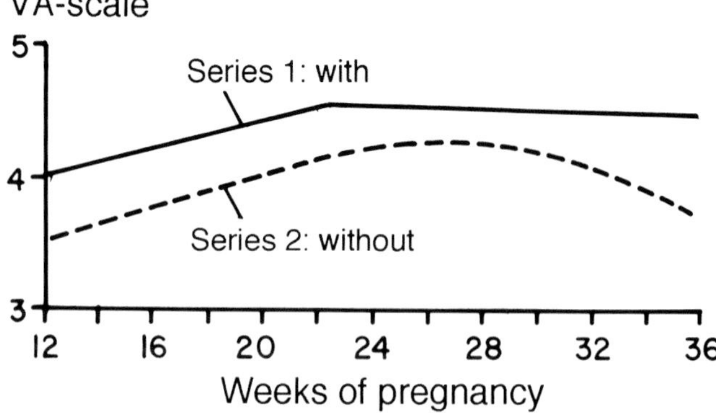


**Fig. 10–9.** Graph of two groups of patients, one with history of back pain, and the other without. There is both a higher scale of pain in women with prior back pain, and a higher plateau reached, regardless of the week of pregnancy when comparing the two groups.

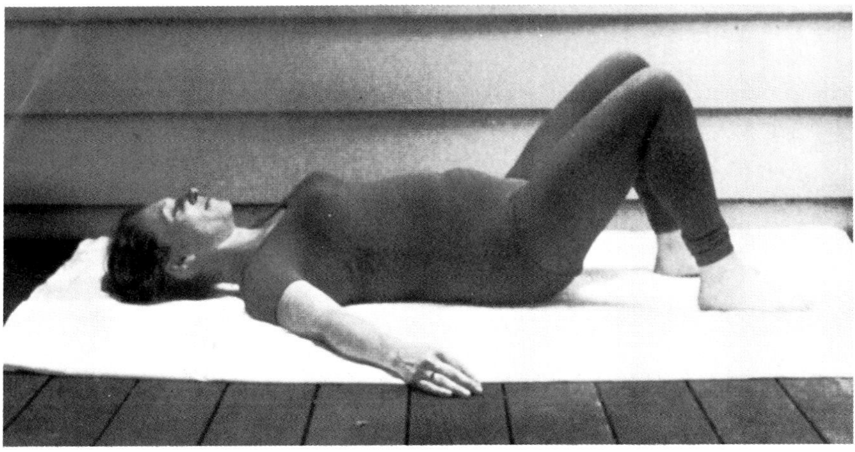

A

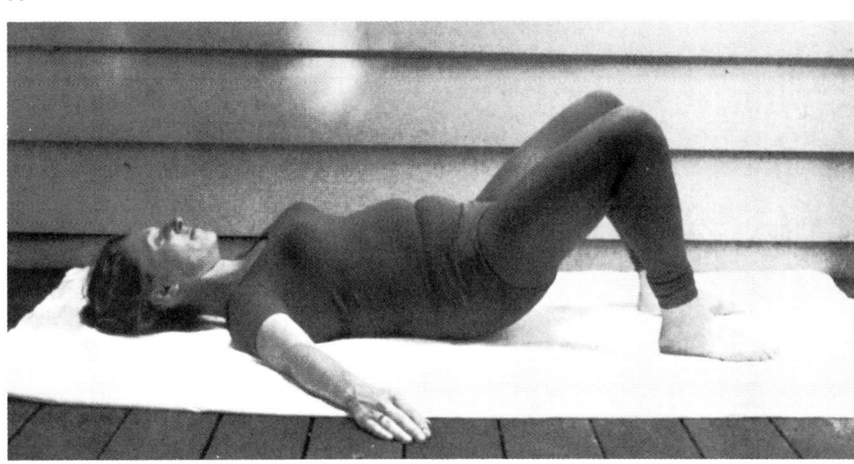

B

**Fig. 10–10.** The correct position for pelvic tilt exercise. The left photograph **(A)** is the standard position before changes, and the right photograph **(B)** is with the pelvic tilt in effect. (From Jacobson H: Protecting the back during pregnancy. AAOHN. J. 39:286–291, 1991.)

study, low backache was also a problem, which persisted well after delivery in some instances for a year after delivery (Table 10–4). Seven of the 10 patients were treated with sacroiliac mobilization.

### *Low-Back Pain in Pregnancy*

Another study of low-back pain in pregnancy sought to view the effect of pregnancy on the abdominal muscles and how that effect relates to low-back pain of pregnancy (50). Pregnancy results in a biomechanical strain on muscles, ligaments, and the skeletal system. The progressive weakening of abdominal muscles has been implicated in the genesis of the low-back pain of pregnancy (Figure 10–12). The study design included 164 women in two groups, pregnant and nonpregnant that were paired for race, age, height, weight, parity, profession, abdominal length, and physical fitness. Results revealed abdominal muscle length is longer in pregnancy due to overstretch by the uterus, eventual abdominal muscle insufficiency, and inability to perform the hook lying setup 86% of the time. Twelve percent of the pregnant patients complained of severe back pain located in the sacroiliac joint. Another study revealed higher relaxin levels in pregnant patients with back pain during the third trimester and higher relaxin levels in incapacitated patients (44).

**Table 10–4.** Pain Syndromes

| Diagnosis | Total Number of Patients | Patients With Pain after Delivery |
|---|---|---|
| SI joint infection | 52 | 34 |
| Muscular insufficiency | 10 | 9 |
| Thoracic pain | 9 | 8 |
| Symphysiolysis | 3 | 2 |
| Sciatic nerve involvement | 3 | 2 |
| Lumbago | 2 | 2 |
| Total | 79 | 57 |

SI = Sacroiliac
(Modified from Berg G, Hammar M, Möller-Nielsen J, Linden U, et al: Low back pain during pregnancy. Obstet. Gynecol. 71:71–4, 1988.)

## NEUROPATHIES

### *The Role of the Saphenous Nerve in Insomnia*

A most interesting study of the role of the saphenous nerve in insomnia proposed that the "Restless Legs Syndrome" played a role. Ekbom, in 1960, first described Restless Legs Syndrome (RLS) in pregnancy to have an incidence of 11% (51). Goodman at a later date described

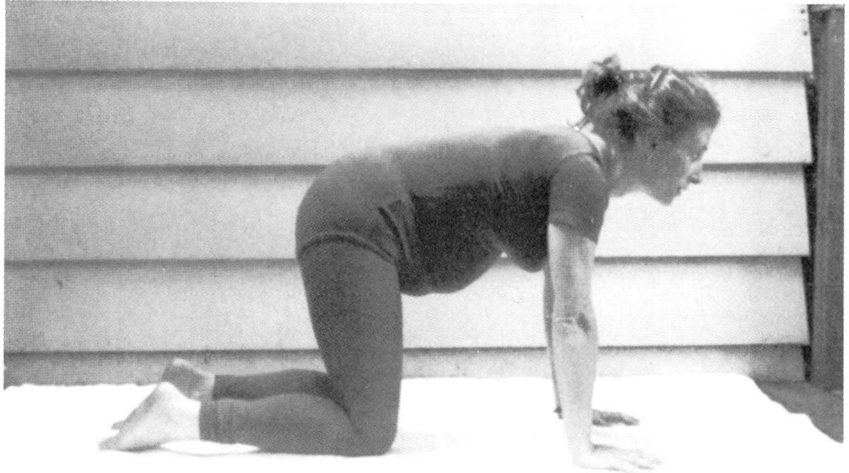

A

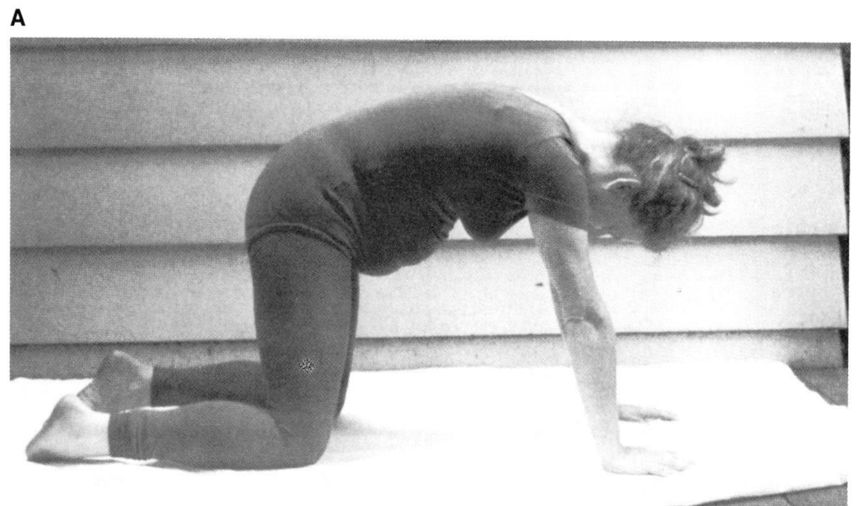

B

Fig. 10–11. A different approach to performance of the pelvic tilt, with patient in the "all fours position." The top (A) photograph is prior to the tilt, and the bottom (B) is the performance of the tilt with extension and curvature of the spine. (From Jacobson H: Protecting the back during pregnancy. AAOHN. J. 39: 286–291, 1991.)

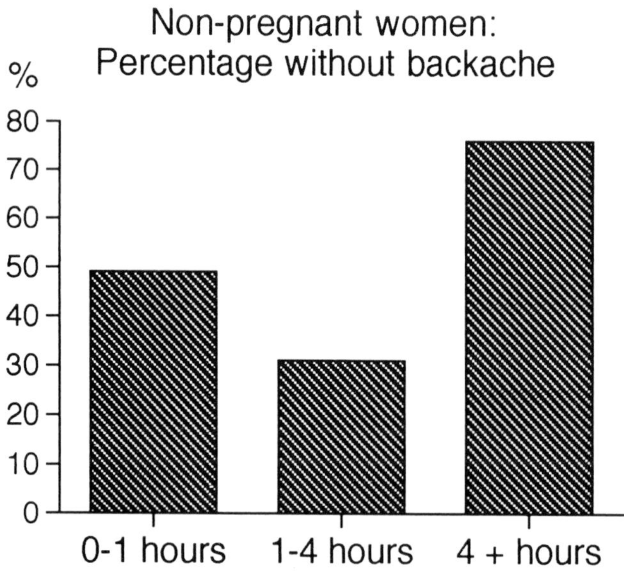


Fig. 10–12. This figure reveals that women with over 4 hours of exercise have a significantly smaller incidence of backache.

the same syndrome and said it occurred in 19% of pregnant women (52). Two of the associated pregnancy changes, venous obstruction and anemia, have been implicated as possible etiologies in RLS. Additional physiologic changes associated with effects on emerging nerves, include fetal head pressure on the lumbosacral plexus, which in turn may cause referred pain into the hips and down the lower limbs (53). Meralgia Paresthetica is an entrapment syndrome of the lateral femoral cutaneous nerve in the region of the anterior superior iliac spine; it may be caused at times by an intra-abdominal or pelvic mass (i.e., pregnancy) (54). The compressed nerve of RLS would have to be pure sensory to account for the absence of motor function impairment and innervation of the area of the calf in RLS, as this is the area of chief complaint. The only nerve that fits both criterion is the saphenous nerve. Pressure on the median nerve at the wrist (carpal tunnel syndrome) usually causes sensory symptoms with paraesthesia and pain in the median nerve distribution. Here the patient often wakes at night with the pain and almost involuntarily shakes the hand about to gain relief (55). The shaking about of the hand to gain relief is analogous to the moving of the legs for relieving sensations in RLS (56).

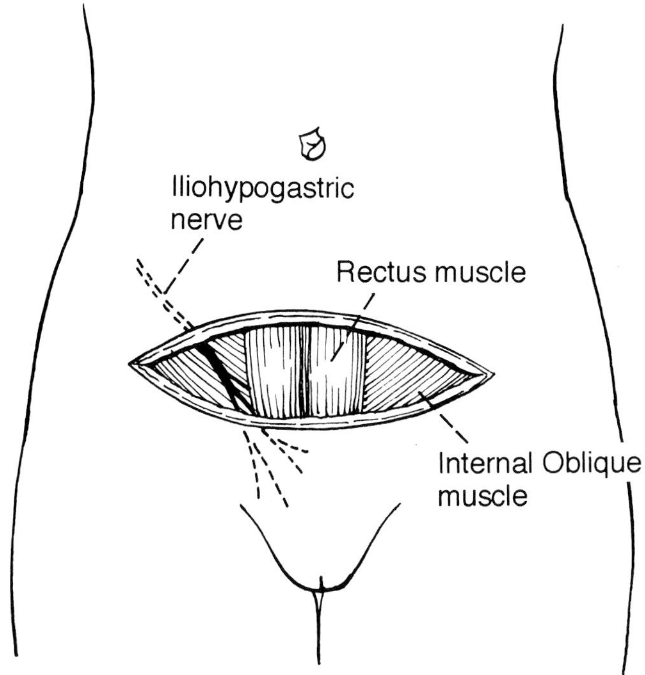


**Fig. 10–13.** The position of the iliohypogastric nerve lies just lateral to the abdominal rectus muscle.

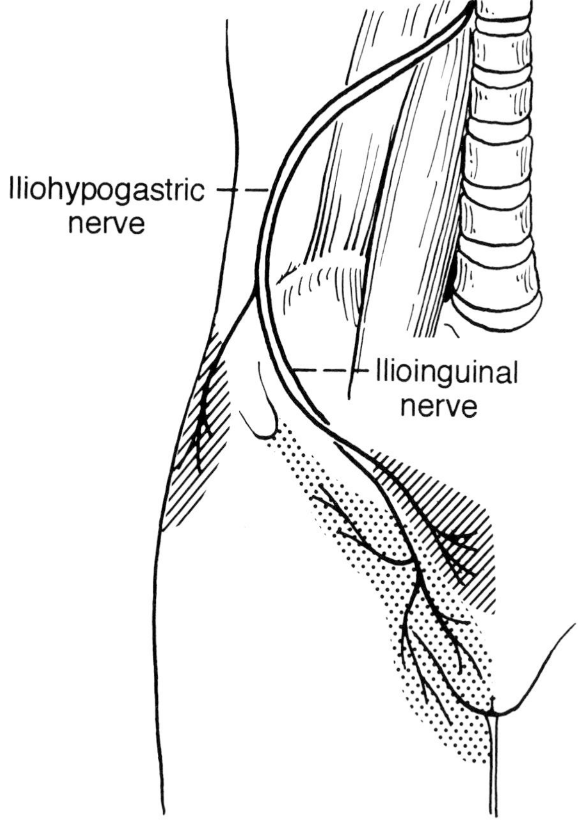


**Fig. 10–14.** Anatomic cutaneous list of pain from the ilioinguinal (dotted area) and iliohypogastric (lined area) nerves.

### *Iliohypogastric Nerve Injury*

Iliohypogastric nerve injury is a frequent cause of abdominal or "pelvic" pain. The transverse abdominal incision was described first by Baudelocque in 1823 (57), but it was not popularized until the 1900s by Pfannenstiel (58). This incision often involves the iliohypogastric nerve either by direct nerve injury or by stretching due to the use of retractors. This report summarizes the injury sustained by four patients' postPfannenstiel incision, three by hysterectomies, and one by an appendectomy (59). All patients had a small painful nodule in their well-healed incision line that became pain free with injection of a local anesthetic. Subsequent surgical exploration revealed entrapment or neuroma of the iliohypogastric nerve. This nerve, the highest branch of the first lumbar nerve, runs across the psoas major muscle over to the quadratus lumborum then forward into the transversalis muscle where it penetrates the internal oblique before surfacing just above the superficial inguinal ring in the external oblique muscle (Figure 10–13) (59).

### *Peripheral Nerve Injuries*

Another article reviewed peripheral nerve injuries as a result of common surgery in the lower abdomen (60). Twenty-three patients had painful nerve entrapments of the ilioinguinal and/or iliohypogastric nerves (Figure 10–14) after lower abdominal surgery (Table 10–5). A diagnostic triad discovery included burning pain with radiation to the skin dermatome, impaired nerve function by sensory tests, and relief of pain by local anesthetic injection. Treatment modalities included administration of anti-inflammatory agents, local anesthetic injection, 5% phenol injection, physiotherapy or surgical repair of the scar with neurectomy. The former treatment methods were found to be temporary, but surgery resulted in cures for 16 patients. Seven of the patients still suffer from chronic pain.

### *Genitofemoral Neuralgia*

The diagnosis and management of genitofemoral neuralgia are other concerns to keep in mind. This type of

**Table 10–5.** Peripheral Nerve Injuries

| Operation | Asymptomatic | Persistent Pain | Total |
|---|---|---|---|
| Neurotomy | | | |
| Ilioinguinal nerve | 5 | 0 | 5 |
| Iliohypogastric nerve | 9 | 5 | 14 |
| Both | 2 | 1 | 3 |
| Neurolysis of iliohypogastric nerve | 0 | 1 | 1 |
| Total | 16 | 7 | 23 |

(From Stulz P, Pfeiffer KM: Peripheral nerve injuries resulting from common surgical procedures in the lower portion of the abdomen. Arch. Surg. 117:324–327, 1982.)

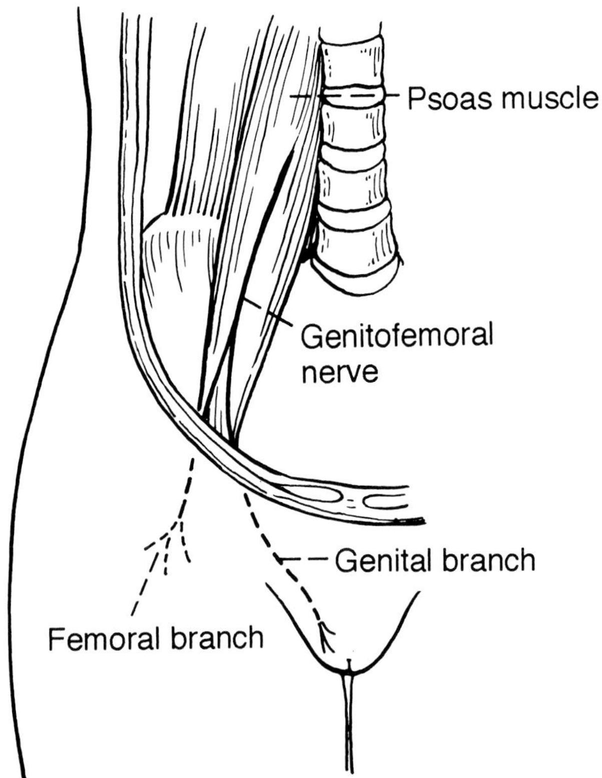


**Fig. 10–15.** The course of genitofemoral nerves from exit at L3 area and its course down through the abdomen to its point of exit on anterior abdominal wall. Note its close association with the psoas muscle.

neuralgia has been described after inguinal hernia repair, appendectomy, and cesarean section. Genitofemoral entrapment must be distinguished from ilioinguinal nerve entrapment by local anesthetic nerve blocks of the ilioinguinal nerve and the genitofemoral nerve. Magee first described genitofemoral neuralgia in 1942 (61). Typical pain is located in the inguinal region and/or the medial aspect of the upper thigh (Figure 10–15). It increases with hip extension, walking or even pressure from sitting. The pain may begin shortly after a surgical procedure responsible for the injury or it may be delayed for several months. Extraperitoneal surgical excision of the genitofemoral nerve was found to be the treatment of choice. The sensory loss was small with loss of cremasteric reflex also (62).

### *Ilioinguinal Nerve Entrapment and Results of Operative Treatment*

Forty-six women who complained of lower abdominal and pelvic pain had hyperasthesia and pain located at the nerve exit point as major symptoms. (63). Hypoasthesia was rarely found. The cause for the entrapment may be previous surgery or contraction of the transversalis, internal oblique, and external oblique muscular layers (64). The symptoms are sudden, stabbing, colicky pain in an area located close to the inguinal ligament on the low medial aspect of the abdomen that is elicited by exercise and relieved by rest. Many patients can no longer exercise and obtain relief by curling up into the fetal position. Often, the gynecologist is the physician who examines the patient due to the complaint of pelvic pain. Slocumb described a referred pelvic pain treatable by trigger point injections (65). He had a 90% success rate in 131 patients. Others' experience is that local injections are short-lived. Applegate described a similar treatment in 1972 that was a similarly short-lived success. (66). Howe suggested that nerve damage either by external trauma or entrapment can result in regeneration of new nerve endings or sprouts that can establish the generation of pain impulses locally (67).

### *Ilioinguinal-Iliohypogastric Nerve Entrapment*

Another instance of nerve entrapment was illustrated by the combined ilioinguinal-iliohypogastric nerve entrapment as described by Stulz and Pfeiffer in 1982 (60). One patient complained of a pain that radiated from her right inguinal region into her labia (68). This was a pain similar to what she had experienced in her recent pregnancy for which she had a cesarean section. The patient had also had inguinal hernia repairs at 8 months, another at 23 years of age, and one other cesarean section. All were by Pfannenstiel incision. After local anesthetic injection, the patient experienced nearly complete relief of symptoms. Resection of the ilioinguinal-iliohypogastric nerve was performed and a pathology report confirmed connective tissue trapping of multiple nerves (Figure 10–16). The entrapment is most likely a pressure phenomena due to chronic compression factors from surrounding anatomic structures.

### *Thoracic Lateral Cutaneous Nerve Entrapment*

An associated problem is the thoracic lateral cutaneous nerve entrapment (Figure 10–17). The case presented was of a patient who suffered the problem without previous surgery (69). Examples of widespread anatomic problems with nerves, compression and entrapment, are from the top of the head, as in occipital neuralgia, to the tip of the toe, as in interdigital neuromas. Patients who suffer from nerve entrapment syndromes can be labeled as somatizers with suggestions for psychology or psychiatric evaluations due to the fact that many times practitioners are not familiar with these maladies and are ill-trained and ill-equipped to handle the diagnosis and treatment of these problems. This case report is of a 36-year-old woman who complained of left lower abdominal pain activated by exercise and described as dull and superficial in nature. She related the problem had begun when she was in her seventh month of her last pregnancy and experienced a sudden excruciating pain in her left upper abdomen. Studies at the time were negative. A local anesthetic nerve block of the cutaneous branches of the tenth and eleventh thoracic nerves was performed with complete success. The patient's pain did not return. The slipping rib syndrome is another problem of upper abdominal irritation that elicits a neuropathy (70). Most neuropathies

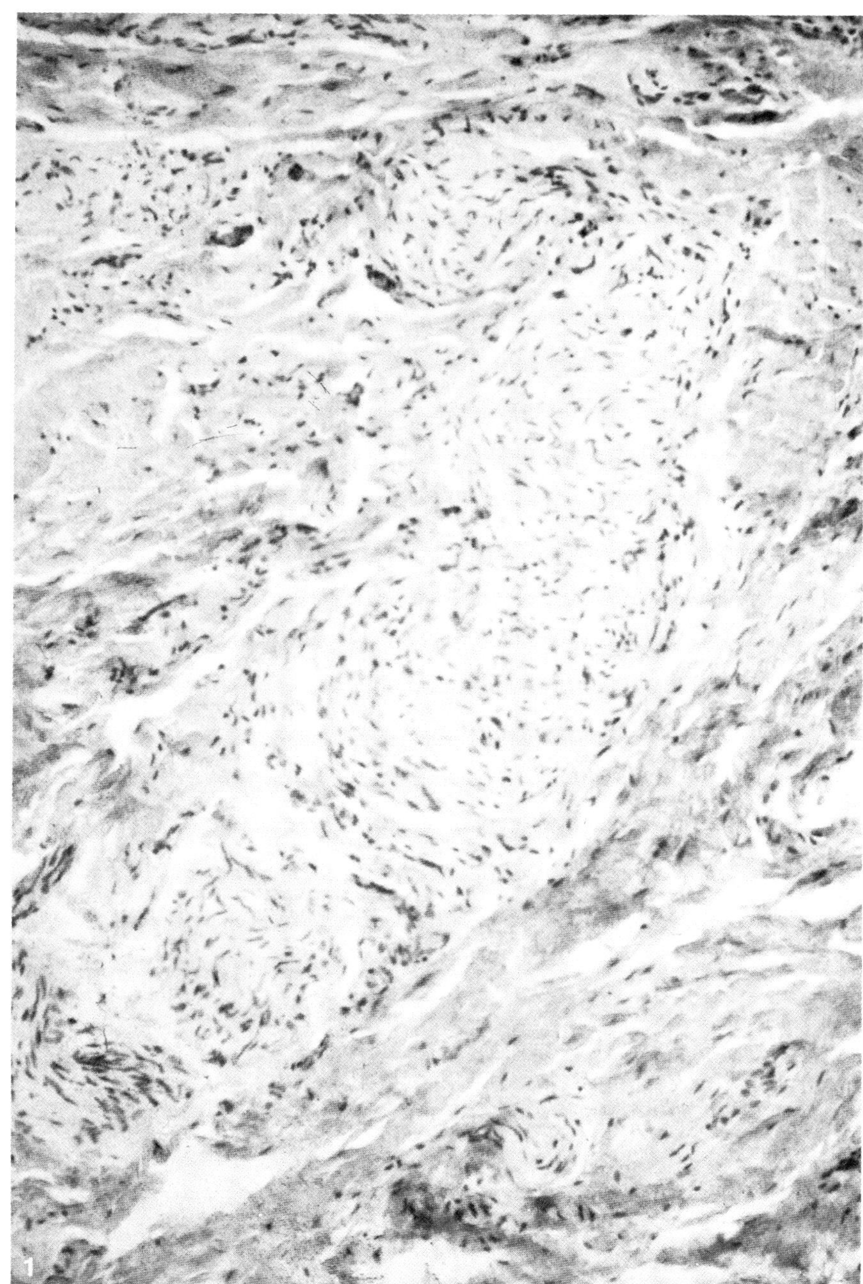

**Fig. 10–16.** Nerve filaments that are dispersed throughout with connective tissue. (From Melville K, Schultz EA, Dougherty JM: Ilioinguinal-iliohypogastric nerve entrapment. Ann. Emerg. Med. 19:925–29, 1990.)

of the abdomen are following surgery, but this case is an exception.

### *Iliac Bone Grafting*

Afflictions of nerves can follow iliac bone grafting, as illustrated by a case of ilioinguinal neuralgia (71). Two case histories are presented of pain associated with the ilioinguinal nerve following bone grafting (Figure 10–18). One was in a 35-year-old woman who had undergone a bone graft from the anterior iliac crest. The pain, characterized as burning in the inguinal area on the side of the operation, was increased by walking or coughing. The ilioinguinal nerve was blocked with complete relief noted for 12 hours. With no further treatment the pain subsided over several days and did not return. A second woman was 57-years-old and had a bone graft taken from her right iliac crest for cervical fusion. Six months later the patient had abdominal pain on the affected side described as sharp in nature. After ilioinguinal nerve block, the patient got good pain relief. This is the first known report of ilioinguinal neuralgia after bone grafting, but the genesis of the injury is no doubt retraction of the nerve during exposure of the anterior iliac crest. The diagnosis may be confused with thrombophlebitis, hip pathology including trochanteric bursitis, and inguinal hernia. This nerve is particularly sensitive to traction and compression

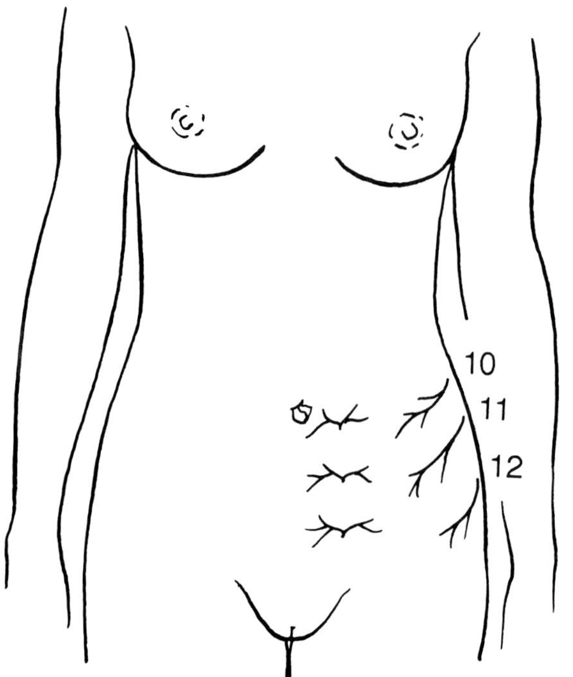


Fig. 10–17. Distribution of pain in mid-abdominal area from T10, T11, and T12. Treatment can be directed at local infiltration in skin area.

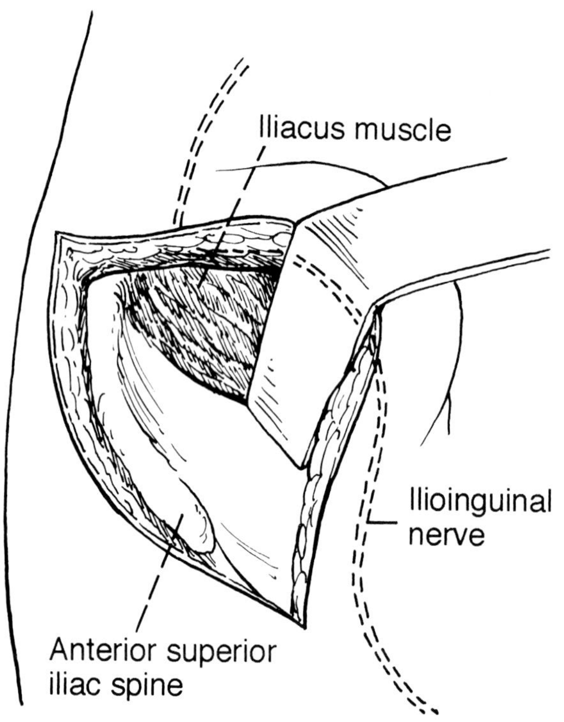


Fig. 10–18. Demonstration of neuropathy generated by pressure exerted by the retractor on the ilioinguinal nerve.

injury because of its stair-like path through the muscles of the abdominal wall.

### Cryoanalgesia

Cryoanalgesia for pain following herniorrhaphy can be effective for pain control. This was a study of postoperative pain relief by freezing the ilioinguinal nerve in a double blind study of 36 patients (72). An experimental group had nerve freezing while the control group did not. Pain relief was assessed over a 48-hour period of time by three methods of pain evaluation. The conclusion was that cryoanalgesia of the ilioinguinal nerve did not offer adequate posthernia repair pain relief. Perhaps one of the lessons learned from the study was not that the method of cryoanalgesia was not effective but that the freezing of a single nerve is ineffective in pain relief for a procedure that necessitates the blockade of three individual nerves, namely, the ilioinguinal, the iliohypogastric, and the genitofemoral.

## MYOPATHIES

### Unusual Clinical Variants of the Pubic Pain Syndrome

Unusual clinical variants of the pubic pain syndrome can occur in women. One specific case occurred in a woman athlete after vigorous exercise (73). Gynecologic pain in vigorous exercise and in sportswomen can be traumatic due to bony, muscular or cartilaginous tissue injury in the pubic area. This case description is of vaginal pain due to abductor tendonitis in the hip in a long-distance walker. Some of the disease processes that can be considered in the differential diagnosis are instability of symphysis of the pubis, muscular lesions of the abdominal group, hip abductors, and iliopsoas muscles. In addition, stress fractures of the pubic rami and subsequent inflammation of the symphysis due to stress and osteomyelitis can also occur.

### Postpartum Cervical Myofascial Pain Syndrome

The postpartum cervical myofascial pain syndrome can be the cause of postpartum headaches in patients who have had epidural anesthesia (74). These patients are usually assumed to suffer pain due to an inadvertent dural puncture with loss of spinal fluid. However, there are other considerations to keep in mind, including withdrawal from caffeine or nicotine and subarachnoid hemorrhage due to strenuous pushing efforts of the second stage. Another possibility might be cervical myofascial pain, which is an associated headache in the occipital region down to the neck and shoulder girdle. It is associated with significant muscular tenderness, but is not positional in nature. Most of the patients presented complained of constant, dull, aching pain of an intense nature in the neck, upper back, and both shoulders that was also associated with an intense throbbing occipitofrontal headache. Treatment consisted of heat, massage, and exercises that stretch the involved muscle groups. If this treatment was not effective, then cold packs and ethyl chloride spray with stretching of the muscles was used along with nonsteroidal anti-inflammatory agents. The problem of myofascial pain is quite common but is not commonly known to obstetricians and gynecologists, while they are quite familiar with the concept of postdural puncture headache.

## Summary

The aforementioned pain disorders will hopefully alert physicians to many of the problems they may be faced with in handling the pregnant patient with a pain complaint. The iliohypogastric entrapment is a perfect example of a condition that does perpetually perplex the physician when the patient and husband call in with complaints of right or left lower quadrant acute and severe pain. The first reflex thought is the appendix. But remember from the foregoing discussions how the iliohypogastric nerves can be compressed and pushed laterally by the growing and descending pelvic mass, the fetus. This was referred to earlier, for lack of understanding, by many practitioners as "round ligament syndrome." It can save the physician and the patient precious time and money if it is considered, a local anesthetic block of the iliohypogastric nerve performed for diagnosis, and the outcome carefully observed. Should the patient suddenly become painfree, then you instantly become very sage; should it do nothing, the differential diagnosis is continued with the appropriate laboratory exam and surgical consultation.

The key suggestion is for physicians to be in the listening, learning, probing, and exploring mode so that nothing will escape them.

## REFERENCES

1. Burwell CS, Metcalfe JA: Heart Disease and Pregnancy. Boston, Little, Brown, & Co., 1958.
2. Bader RA, Bader ME, Rose DJ, Braunwald E: Hemodynamics at rest and during exercise in normal pregnancy as studied by cardiac catheterization. J. Clin. Invest. 34:1524, 1955.
3. Hamilton HFH: Cardiac output in normal pregnancy. J. Obstet. Gynaecol. Br. Commnw. 56:548, 1949.
4. Palmer AJ, Walker AHC: Maternal circulation in normal pregnancy. J. Obstet. Gynaecol. Br. Commnw. 56:537, 1949.
5. Rose DJ, Bader ME, Bader RA, Braunwald E: Catheterization studies of cardiac hemodynamics in normal pregnant women with reference to left ventricular work. Am. J. Obstet. Gynecol. 72:233, 1956.
6. Lees MM, Taylor SH, Scott DB, Kerr MG: A study of cardiac output at rest throughout pregnancy. J. Obstet. Gynaecol. Br. Commnw. 74:319, 1967.
7. Ueland K, Novy MJ, Peterson EN, Metcalfe J: Maternal cardiovascular dynamics. IV. The influence of gestational age on the maternal cardiovascular response to posture and exercise. Am. J. Obstet. Gynecol. 104:856, 1969.
8. Robson SC, Hunter S, Boys RJ, Dunlop W: Serial study of factors influencing changes in cardiac output during human pregnancy. Am. J. Physiol. 256(4):H1060–1065, 1989.
9. Stenback F, Kauppila A: Development and classification of parovarian cysts. An ultrasound study. Gynecol. Obstet. Invest. 12:1–10, 1981.
10. Alpern MB, Sandler MA, Madrazo BL: Sonographic features of parovarian cysts and their complication. AJR 143: 157–160, 1984.
11. Athey PA, Cooper NB: Sonographic features of parovarian cysts. AJR 144:83–86, 1985.
12. Inoue H, Fukushima Y: Twisted parovarian cysts. Jpn. J. Med. Ultrasonics 14:626–630, 1987.
13. Hasuo Y, Higashijima T, Mitamura T: Torsion of parovarian cyst. Kurume. Med. J. 38:39–43, 1991.
14. Quinn AD, Kusuda L, Amar AD, Das S: Percutaneous nephrostomy for treatment of hydronephrosis of pregnancy. J. Urol. 139:1037–8, 1988.
15. Ferguson T, Bechtel W: Hydronephrosis of pregnancy. American Family Physician 43:2135–2137, 1991.
16. Yaron Y, Lessing JB, Peyser MR: Abruptio placentae associated with perforated appendicitis and generalized peritonitis. Am. J. Obstet. Gynecol. 166:14–15, 1992.
17. Candiani GB, Vercellini P, Fedele L Vendola N, et al: Inguinal endometriosis: pathogenetic and clinical implications. Obstet. Gynecol. 78:191, 1991.
18. Clausen I, Nielsen KI: Endometriosis in the groin. Int. J. Gynaecol. Obstet. 25:469–71, 1987.
19. Blanchard AC, Pastorek JG II, Weeks T: Pelvic inflammatory disease during pregnancy. South. Med. J. 80:1363–65, 1987.
20. Gordon, SC, Polson DJ, Shirkhoda A: Budd-Chiari syndrome complicating pre-eclampsia: diagnosis by magnetic resonance imaging. J. Clin. Gastroenterol. 13:460–2, 1991.
21. Sakala EP, Harding MD: Ehlers-Danlos syndrome type III and pregnancy. J. Reprod. Med. 36:622–4, 1991.
22. Savage RW, Nolan TE: Pregnancy in a woman with partial absence of the left pericardium. J. Reprod. Med. 33:385–6, 1985.
23. Charache S, Lubin B, Reid CD (eds): Cooperative study of the clinical course of sickle cell disease: management and therapy of sickle cell disease: NIH Publication No. 89:2117. Bethesda, U.S. Dept Health Human Services, Public Health Service, Revised September 1989.
24. Koshy M, Burd L: Management of pregnancy in sickle cell syndromes. Hematology/Oncology Clin. of North America 5:585–96, 1991.
25. Traycoff RB: "Pseudotrochanteric bursitis": the differential diagnosis of lateral hip pain. J. Rheumatol. 18:1810–2, 1991.
26. Pellegrini VD, Pasternak HS, Macaulay WP: Endometrioma of the pubis: a differential in the diagnosis of hip pain. J. Bone. Joint. Surg. 63:1333–4, 1981.
27. Forrest JS, Brooks DL: Cyclic sciatica of endometriosis. J. Am. Med. Assn. 222:1177–1178, 1972.
28. Novak ER, Woodruff JD: Gynecologic and Obstetric Pathology, with Clinical and Endocrine Relations. 8th Ed, Philadelphia, WB Saunders, pp. 561–584, 1979.
29. Cullen TS: Adeno-myoma of the round ligament. Bull. Johns Hopkins Hosp. 7:112–114, 1896.
30. Ishii K, Kobayashi M, Koyama A, Narita M: Pregnancy associated RPGN (rapidly progressive glomerulonephritis) with repeated attacks of purpura and arthralgia. Jap. J. Nephrol. 31:71–75, 1989.
31. Daly JM, Frame PS, Rapoza PA: Sacroiliac subluxation: a common, treatable cause of low-back pain in pregnancy. Fam. Pract. Res. J. 11:149–59, 1991.
32. Golighty R: Pelvic arthropathy in pregnancy and puerperium. Phys. Ther. 68:216–20, 1982.
33. Berg G, Hammar M, Möller-Nielsen J, Linden U, et al: Low back pain during pregnancy. Obstet. Gynecol. 71:71–4, 1988.
34. Greive GP: Modern Manual Therapy of the Vertebral Column. New York, Churchill Livingston, 1986. pp. 805–14.
35. Greive GP: Common Problems of the Vertebral Column. New York, Churchill Livingston, 1981. pp. 418–9.
36. Cyriax JH: Textbook of Orthopedic Medicine. Baltimore, Williams & Wilkins, 1971, p. 292.
37. Abramson D, Roberts SM, Wilson PD: Relaxation of pelvic

joints in pregnancy. Surg. Gynecol. Obstet. 58:595–613, 1934.
38. Wilbur AC, Langer BG, Spigos DG: Diagnosis of sacroiliac joint infection in pregnancy by magnetic resonance imaging. Mag. Reson. Imaging. 6:341–343, 1988.
39. McCarthy S: Magnetic resonance imaging in obstetrics and gynecology. Mag. Reson. Imaging. 4:59–66, 1986.
40. Östgaard HC, Andersson GBJ, Wennergren M: The impact of low back and pelvic pain in pregnancy on the pregnancy outcome. Acta. Obstet. Gynecol. Scand. 70:21–24, 1991.
41. Mantle MJ, Greenwood RM, Curry HLF: Backache in pregnancy. Rheumatol. Rehab. 16:95–101, 1977.
42. Fast A, Shapiro D, Ducommun EJ, Friedmann LW, et al: Low back pain in pregnancy. Spine 12:4:368–71, 1987.
43. Melzack R, Berlanger E: Labour pain: correlations with menstrual pain and acute low-back pain before and during pregnancy. Pain 36:225–9, 1989.
44. MacLennan AH, Nicholson R, Green RC, Bath M: Serum relaxin and pelvic pain of pregnancy. Lancet 2:243–5, 1986.
45. MacLennan AH, Nicholson R, Green RC: Serum relaxin in pregnancy. Lancet 2:241–3, 1986.
46. Kroc RL, Steinetz BG, Beach VL: The effects of estrogens, progestagens, and relaxin in pregnant and non-pregnant laboratory rodents. Ann. NY. Acad. Sci. 75:942–80, 1959.
47. Fridh G, Kopare T, Gaston-Johansson F, Norvell KT: Factors associated with more intense labor pain. Research in Nursing and Health 11:117–24, 1988.
48. Jacobson H: Protecting the back during pregnancy. AAOHN J. 39:286–291, 1991.
49. Scott J (Ed): Danforth's obstetrics. Philadelphia, J.B. Lippincott, 1990.
50. Fast A, Weiss L, Ducommun EJ, Medina E, et al: Low-back pain in pregnancy—abdominal muscles, sit-up performance, and back pain. Spine 15:28–30, 1990.
51. Ekbom KA: Restless legs syndrome. Neurology 10:868–73, 1960.
52. Goodman DS, Brodie C, Ayida GA: Restless leg syndrome in pregnancy. BMJ 297:1101–2, 1988.
53. Boshes B: The nervous system in pregnancy. *In* Gynecology and Obstetrics. Edited by C Davis, Hagerstown, Harper & Row, 1965.
54. Jones RK: Meralgia paresthetica as a cause of leg discomfort. CMA Journal, Vol. III, 1974.
55. Schott GD: Peripheral neuropathies. The Practitioner 227: 401–10, 1983.
56. Lewis F: The role of the saphenous nerve in insomnia: a proposed etiology of restless legs syndrome. Medical Hypothesis 34:331–333, 1991.
57. Baudelocque CA: Nouveau Procédé Pour Pratiquer l'Operation Césarienne. Paris, Théses d L'Ecole de Medecine, 1823, p.132.
58. Pfannensteil J: Sammlung klinischer vortage. Leipzig, Gynakologie, No. 268 (Gynak No. 97), 1900:1735–56.
59. Grosz CR: Iliohypogastric nerve injury. Am. J. Surg. 142: 628, 1981.
60. Stulz P, Pfeiffer KM: Peripheral nerve injuries resulting from common surgical procedures in the lower portion of the abdomen. Arch. Surg. 117:324–327, 1982.
61. Magee RK: Genito-femoral causalgia. Can. Med. Assoc. J. 46: 326–329, 1942.
62. Harms BA, DeHaas DR Jr, Starling JR: Diagnosis and management of genitofemoral neuralgia. Arch. Surg. 119:339–41, 1984.
63. Hahn L: Clinical findings and results of operative treatment in ilioinguinal nerve entrapment syndrome. Brit. J. Obstet. Gynaecol. 96:1080–83, 1989.
64. Kopell HP, Thompson WAL, Postel A: Entrapment neuropathy of the ilioinguinal nerve. N. Engl. J. Med. 161:16–19, 1962.
65. Slocumb JC: Neurological factors in chronic pelvic pain: trigger points and the abdominal pelvic pain syndrome. Am. J. Obstet. Gynecol. 71:118–24, 1984.
66. Applegate WV: Abdominal cutaneous nerve entrapment syndrome. Surgery 71:118–24, 1972.
67. Howe JF, Loeser JD, Calvin WH: Mechanosensitivity of dorsal root ganglia and chronically injured axons: a physiological basis for the redicular pain of nerve root compression. Pain 3:25–40, 1977.
68. Melville K, Schultz EA, Dougherty JM: Ilioinguinal–iliohypogastric nerve entrapment. Ann. Emerg. Med. 19:925–29, 1990.
69. Sharf M, Shvartzman P, Farkash E, Horvitz J: Thoracic lateral cutaneous nerve entrapment syndrome without previous lower abdominal surgery. J. Fam. Prac. 30:211–214, 1990.
70. Wright JT: Slipping-rib syndrome. Lancet 2:632–3, 1987.
71. Smith SE, DeLee JC, Ramamurthy S: Ilioinguinal neuralgia following iliac bone-grafting. J. Bone Joint Surg. 66-A: 1306–8, 1984.
72. Khiroya RC, Davenport HT, Jones JG: Forum: cryoanalgesia for pain after herniorrhaphy. Anaesthesia 41:73–76, 1986.
73. Baeyens L: An unusual clinical variant of the pubic pain syndrome in a woman: the case of an athelete. J. Gynecol. Obstet. Biol. Reprod. 16:339–341, 1987.
74. Hubbell SL, Thomas M: Postpartum cervical myofascial pain syndrome: review of four patients. Obstet. Gynecol. 65:56S 1985.

# PART II

# PHARMACOLOGY AND TECHNIQUES OF OBSTETRIC ANALGESIA AND ANESTHESIA

Section C

# REGIONAL ANALGESIA/ANESTHESIA

Chapter 11

# PHARMACOLOGY OF LOCAL ANESTHETICS AND RELATED DRUGS

ANDREW M. WOODS
COSMO A. DIFAZIO

This chapter discusses the pharmacology of local anesthetics and other closely related drugs. The mechanisms of anesthetic action, including the effect on the nerve membrane itself, set the foundation of the chapter toward understanding the basics of local anesthetic effect. This is followed by presentation of physiochemical properties of the present day, commonly used local anesthetics. For an overview and detailed view of local anesthetics prominent in years past, we refer the reader to the first edition of "Principles and Practices of Obstetric Analgesia and Anesthesia." The important aspects of placental transfer and final disposition of drugs, including fetal and neonatal effects, are discussed and followed by further discussion of the clinical considerations, and, the most valuable section, on the important clinical properties of drugs. A section is included on the modification of local anesthetic action by various means, and the concern for complications attendant to the use of local anesthetics is presented.

Such a chapter is required for all those using local anesthetics in the treatment of mothers during labor. These patients form fundamental considerations for understanding the use of such potent analgesics to obtain the desired effect of pain relief. But far more important than the pain relief itself is the element of safety for both the mother and her unborn baby. Many complications alluded to in that section of the chapter are due to a poor understanding of these basics. As pointed out in the first edition of this book, the practitioner who uses regional anesthesia must have an essential knowledge base consisting of at least an understanding of anatomy, dose and administration, pharmacology, and physiologic alterations of the mother that may create potential hazards inherent in these drugs. It is still true today throughout the world that many practitioners who use such local anesthetics for either local or regional anesthesia are practitioners other than anesthesiologists. A basic knowledge base must be obtained by these individuals before using these potent drugs. The most effective and safest practitioner will be one who has such an aforementioned knowledge base and who keeps current throughout his/her lifetime.

The pharmacology of local anesthetic agents used in obstetric patients became a focus of concern following a number of maternal deaths attributed to intravascular injections of drugs intended for epidural administration for cesarean section (1). Since that time, our knowledge of the mechanisms of action of local anesthetics, both therapeutic and toxic, has been greatly expanded. The authors believe that fetal and maternal mortality and morbidity as a complication of local anesthetic agents most frequently result from improper technique or inadequate knowledge of local anesthetic activity on the part of the practitioner. This chapter, then, reviews the basic pharmacology of local anesthetic agents and addresses specifically special concerns arising from the pregnant state and the presence of a fetus inside the primary patient.

## BASIC CONSIDERATIONS

### *Mechanisms of Anesthetic Action*

#### Nerve Membrane as Site of Action

The desired action of all clinically useful local anesthetics is the reversible blockade of nerve conduction at the level of the axonal membrane (2). Nerve conduction involves propagation of an electrical signal that is generated by the rapid movement of several ionic species across the nerve cell membrane. The ionic concentration of sodium ($Na^+$) is high extracellularly and low intracellularly, while that of potassium ($K^+$) is high intracellularly and low extracellularly. This ionic gradient for sodium and potassium across the cell membrane is maintained by an ion-translocating sodium-potassium ATPase pump mechanism within the nerve (3). In the resting state, the nerve membrane is much more permeable to potassium ions than to sodium ions, and there is a continual leakage of potassium ions from the interior of the nerve cell to the exterior. This leakage of a cation, with its positive charge, leaves the interior of the nerve negatively charged relative to the exterior. In humans, this results in an electrical potential of $-60$ to $-70$ mV across the resting nerve membrane.

Sensory nerves have receptors at one end that are, in effect, transducers, and convert various energy inputs (mechanical, chemical, thermal) into tiny electrical currents. For example, a surgical incision causes the release of chemical mediators resulting from tissue injury, and these chemicals interact with receptors in the nerve terminal to generate minuscule electrical currents. This current alters the electrical potential across the portion of the nerve membrane that is nearest to the receptor, making it slightly less negative. If a level of approximately $-55$ mV (the threshold potential) is reached, a sudden increase in

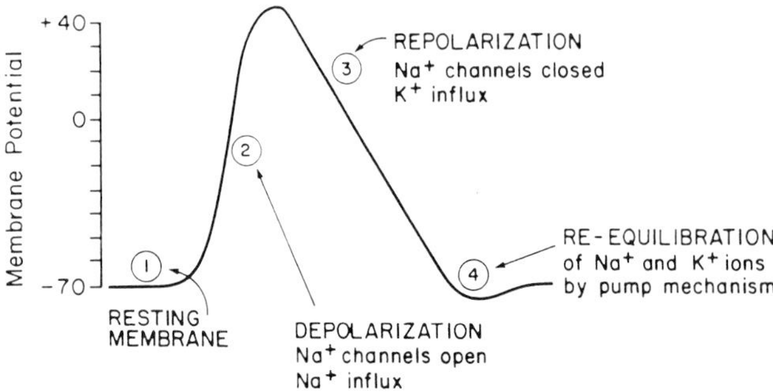


**Fig. 11–1.** Sodium and potassium ion movement during course of an action potential in a nerve.

the permeability of the nerve membrane to sodium ions occurs and, in a very narrow segment of the nerve fiber, the inside becomes positive relative to the outside due to the rapid influx of positively charged sodium cations. This transient reversal of charge, or depolarization, is followed by repolarization as the sodium permeability abruptly decreases; an increase in potassium permeability occurs and allows for a large efflux of potassium from the cell, restoring the negative intracellular charge. Both ions are subsequently restored to their initial intra- and extracellular concentrations by the $Na^+/K^+$-ATPase-dependent pump mechanism. This sequence of localized depolarization and repolarization is referred to as an action potential (Figure 11–1). Just as the initial electrical signal from the receptor initiated an action potential in its immediate vicinity, this depolarization generates a current that, if of sufficient magnitude, depolarizes the next adjacent segment of nerve, thus allowing the action potential to be propagated along the entire length of the nerve.

The rapid influx of sodium ions, which produces the initial upswing of an action potential, occurs through specific sodium channels in the cell membrane. The sodium channel is a protein structure, part of which has been sequenced, that penetrates the full depth of the membrane bilayer. The opening of the sodium channel is voltage-dependent, and has been postulated to result from a conformational change in the channel structure induced by the action potential (4).

In the case of myelinated nerves, the depolarization occurs at nodes of Ranvier where there is no encircling myelin and where there is a high density of sodium channels. The adjacent nerve is surrounded by myelin, which is an effective insulator, and the underlying nerve contains very few sodium channels. The absence of myelin at the nodes allows this area to be in close contact with extracellular fluid, which can conduct an electrical current, and the depolarizing currents spread, not to adjacent nerve, but to the next adjacent node of Ranvier. This process greatly facilitates conduction velocity and also decreases the energy required to restore the resting membrane potential, as $Na^+/K^+$-ATPase activity occurs in very limited regions of the nerve, rather than along the entire length.

## *Mechanism of Local Anesthetic Blockade of Nerve Conduction*

Local anesthetic drugs prevent the development of an action potential in a nerve by preventing sodium ions from moving intracellularly through sodium channels (2). While the exact mechanism by which this occurs is unknown, one widely held theory is that local anesthetic binding to the sodium channel causes a change in the conformation of the channel that prevents it from assuming an open (ion conducting) state (4). The impediment to ion movement may be a function of the radius of the channel pore or, alternatively, could be due to electrostatic forces; i.e., the interaction between the local anesthetic molecule and the sodium channel might produce an area of positive charge within the channel that repels the like-charged sodium ions.

The sodium channel progresses through a series of conformational changes in response to an action potential, going from a resting closed state to a series of preopen, open, and inactivated states; each of these states binds local anesthetic more avidly than the resting closed state (5). Repetitive stimulation of a nerve results in more channels being in open or inactivated conformations, thus facilitating anesthetic binding. This results in conduction blockade at a lower anesthetic concentration than when the nerve is not repetitively stimulated, and most channels are predominantly in the resting closed position. This action potential reduction during a train of impulses is referred to as a "use-dependent" or "phasic" block.

Local anesthetics can produce conduction blockade by interacting with sodium channels that are in the resting state. This is referred to as a "tonic block," and is much weaker than a phasic block in terms of impeding sodium flux. Our current understanding is that the variable states of the sodium channel with its associated local anesthetic receptors determine the strength of the interaction with the local anesthetic molecule, and excitable membranes with a higher depolarization frequency are more sensitive to the blocking effects of local anesthetics.

Factors that favor the presence of open or inactivated channels will enhance local anesthetic phasic block. Because most neurons depend upon an outward current mediated through voltage-gated $K^+$ channels, agents that block these channels slow repolarization. $K^+$ channel blockers have been shown to enhance the efficacy of local anesthetics (6).

Almost all clinically relevant local anesthetics exist in both charged and uncharged forms and it appears that both species interact with the active site on the sodium channel. However, the un-ionized form rapidly dissociates from the receptor, while the cationic (protonated) form remains bound for a longer period of time; the protonated form is thus believed to play the major role in channel blockade for most local anesthetics (7).

The current state of knowledge postulates that local anesthetic molecules predominantly interact with sodium channel active sites in the following manner: a portion of the drug that is in an uncharged state crosses the lipid membrane of the axon and enters the cell cytoplasm, where it then reequilibrates into a predominantly charged form that readily dissolves in water, and that is able to reach the active site on the sodium channel when the channel is open (Figure 11–2). Thus, the ability of local anesthetics to assume two forms, charged and uncharged, with vastly different solubilities in lipids versus water, is fundamental to their mechanism of action.

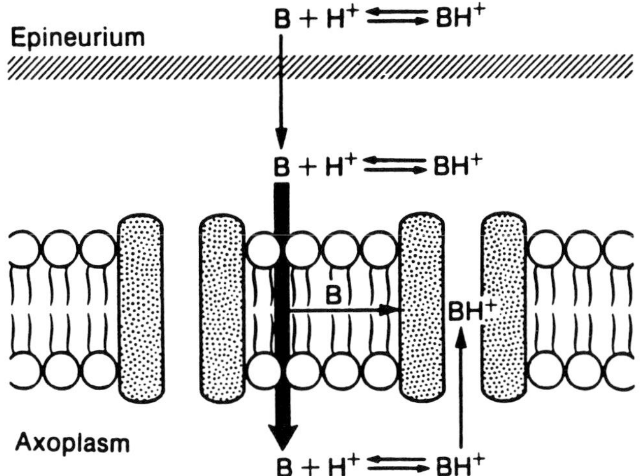


**Fig. 11–2.** Schematic of nerve membrane and surrounding epineurium depicting interaction of local anesthetics. The base (B) form of the drug crosses the epineurium; the drug then reequilibrates with the cationic form ($BH^+$); the base is free to traverse the lipid bilayer (circles with squiggly tails) of the nerve membrane. While a portion of the drug may interact with the sodium channel (stippled column) via the hydrophobic domain of the nerve membrane, the majority of the drug enters the aqueous axoplasm where it reequilibrates with the cationic form, which is believed to reach the local anesthetic receptor site on the sodium channel by traversing the channel pore while it is in an open state. (From Carpenter RL, Mackey DC: Local anesthetics. *In* Clinical Anesthesia. Edited by PG Baras, BF Cullen, RK Stoelting. JB Lippincott Company, Philadelphia, 1992.)

One exception to this postulated mechanism (interaction of the cationic form with the sodium channel receptor) is benzocaine, which has local anesthetic activity and is permanently uncharged. Benzocaine is believed to affect the sodium channel in a different manner than ionized local anesthetics. The fact that permanently uncharged benzocaine is effective in blocking sodium currents indicates that forms other than cations can effect channel blockade. In fact, interference with sodium conductance by local anesthetics is fairly nonspecific, and local anesthetic activity is displayed by a wide range of dissimilar compounds, including volatile general anesthetics, barbiturates, opiates, alcohols, adrenergic blocking compounds, and numerous naturally occurring toxins.

The mechanism of epidural and subarachnoid blockade may be more complex than just simple blockade of sodium channels, as local anesthetics affect other membrane-associated enzymes and second messenger systems, such as adenylate cyclase, (guanylate cyclase, ion pumping enzymes such as $Na^+/K^+$-ATPase, $Ca^{++}/Mg^{++}$-ATPase, (and phospholipase A2 and C (4). Also, synoptic transmission can be inhibited by local anesthetic modification of postsynaptic receptors (8) or presynaptic calcium channel blockade (9).

## Structure-Activity Relationships and Physiochemical Properties

### *Chemical Structure*

A number of aspects of the chemical structure of local anesthetics are similar for a large number of different agents, and it is this common basic structure that accounts for similar effects upon nerves, i.e., the reversible blockade of sodium channels. Superimposed upon this generic structure are other chemical variations that account for the differences between the various local anesthetics in such properties as anesthetic potency, duration of anesthesia, and methods of metabolism and elimination. Figure 11–3 presents the chemical structure of the local anesthetic agents in current clinical use. All are characterized by an aromatic moiety (benzene ring) at one end of the local anesthetic molecule. This ring structure is a major contributor to the lipophilic nature, i.e., lipid solubility, of the drug. At the other end of the molecule, one finds a hydrophilic (water soluble) amino group that usually has three organic groups attached (tertiary amine). The ability of this amino group to accept a hydrogen ion accounts for the polar nature of the molecule and its interaction with the charged sodium channel. Joining the aromatic ring to the amino group is a chemical linkage that is usually either an ester or an amide. This structural difference is fundamental and determines the metabolic fate of the molecule in the body; aminoesters are rapidly metabolized in plasma by plasma cholinesterase, while aminoamides undergo oxidative metabolism in the liver. This linkage is also important in that partial ionization in the area of the double bond (C = O) of the amide or ester results in a partial negative ionic charge that may facilitate local anesthetic binding within the sodium channel. Ester-linked anesthetics also tend to be more hydrophobic and more ionized at body pH than structurally similar compounds with amide linkages (10).

Structural modifications produce physiochemical changes in the compounds and major changes result from modest structural modifications; addition of a propyl (3 carbon) moiety to the cyclic amino group of mepivacaine (Figure 11–3) converts the compound to bupivacaine; the latter compound is 30 times more lipid soluble.

### *Chiral Forms*

Carbon atoms with four different substituents attached can be configured in two different patterns of spatial arrangement of the substituents around the carbon atom; such carbon atoms are referred to as asymmetric, and the compounds in which they reside display stereoisomerism. That is, the compound exits in two forms, referred to as enantiomers, that are mirror images of each other and are not superimposable. These compounds are also referred to as chiral forms. A number of local anesthetics have symmetric carbon atoms and thus exist in chiral forms that contain identical atoms and identical linkages. However, differences in the arrangement of the four substituent groups around the asymmetric carbon atoms result in compounds with a slight difference in chemical structure that is, in many cases, sufficient to produce differences in the physiochemistry and the clinical pharmacology of the compounds.

Originally, enantiomers were described as D and L on the basis of the arrangement of the substituents attached to the carbon atom; in more recent literature this nomenclature has been changed to R and S, respectively. These compounds are also optically active, meaning that they

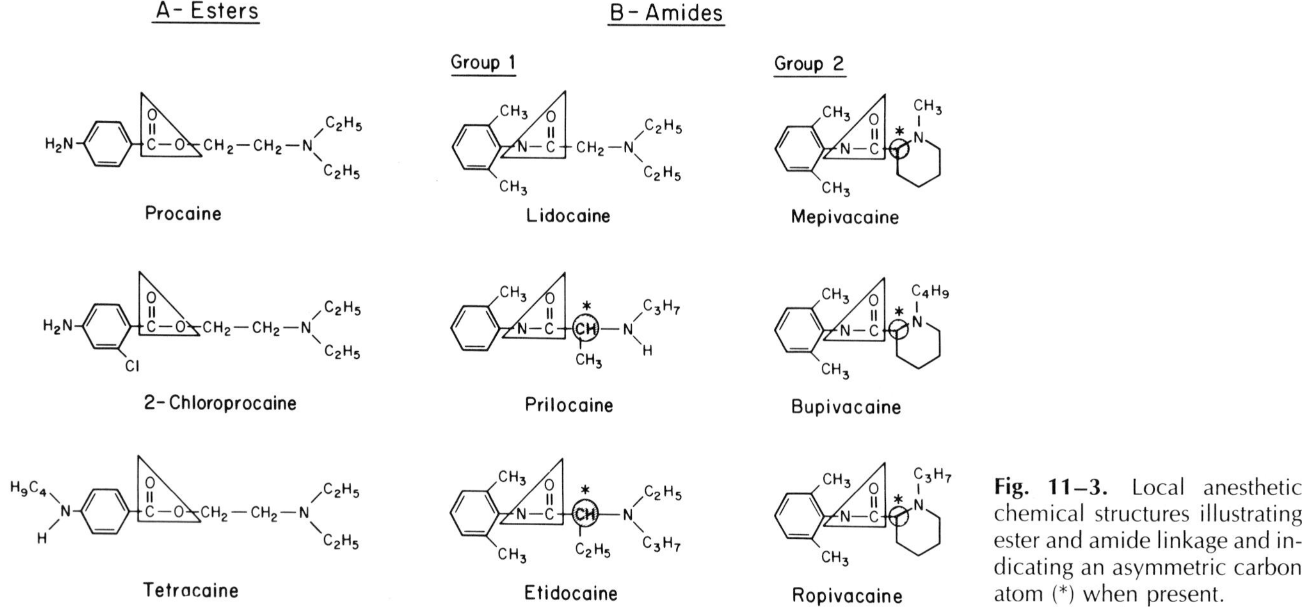


**Fig. 11–3.** Local anesthetic chemical structures illustrating ester and amide linkage and indicating an asymmetric carbon atom (*) when present.

rotate the plane of polarization of plane-polarized light. The direction of this rotation is indicated by ( + ) or ( − ) signs following the R or S designation.

Local anesthetics that display stereoisomerism exhibit varying degrees of differences in activity and toxicity for the enantiomers. In the case of bupivacaine, the S − enantiomer has been noted to have a slightly longer duration of action yet lower systemic toxicity when compared to its R − enantiomer or to the racemic mixture of both enantiomers (11,12). However, this less toxic compound is not commercially available, as bupivacaine is marketed as the racemic mixture.

Ropivacaine is structurally very similar to bupivacaine, differentiated only by a single methyl ( $-CH_3$) group; ropivacaine has a 3-carbon propyl group attached to the amino terminus, whereas bupivacaine has a 4-carbon butyl group. As shown in the table of physiochemical properties (Table 11–1), this results in very little difference between the two drugs, although ropivacaine is less lipid soluble. The S − enantiomers of both ropivacaine and bupivacaine appear to be less cardiotoxic than their R − forms or their racemic preparations (13). More relevant clinically is the fact that S − ropivacaine (the commercial preparation) appears to be less cardiotoxic than the commercial preparation of bupivacaine, which is the racemic mixture. In animal studies, ropivacaine, at equipotent doses, appears to have a safety margin that is almost twice that of racemic bupivacaine in terms of cardiac electrophysiologic toxicity (14). For peripheral nerve blocks (sciatic nerve, brachial plexus, etc.), the duration of action of ropivacaine and bupivacaine is similar; ropivacaine has a slightly shorter duration of action than bupivacaine when used for central blocks (epidural and spinal), (but is distinctly longer acting than bupivacaine when used for infiltration (13), possibly due to vasoconstrictive properties at clinical concentrations (15), as well as the fact that the S − form of ropivacaine has slower absorption than the racemic bupivacaine compound). Ropivacaine is only about half as lipid soluble as bupivacaine (16). For bupivacaine, the S − form is also absorbed much more slowly than the R − form. These differences may be explained by slight differences in the shape of the molecule: the angle between the two ring systems in the bupivacaine molecule is slightly different for the R and the S forms (17). These two drugs clearly illustrate the clinical significance of slight differences in molecular structure, both in terms of the single methyl group differentiating bupivacaine from ropivacaine and, for ropivacaine, the difference in the arrangement of substituent groups around the asymmetric carbon that allows preparation of the less toxic S − form.

For mepivacaine, there appears to be no difference between the R − and the S − forms after rapid intravenous injection. However, after slow intravenous or subcutaneous injection, the S − form was less toxic than the R − form (11,12). Following slow infusion, lung concentration of the S − form is over twice that of the R − form, while brain levels were higher for the R − form. Thus, differential binding to lung tissue may account for differences in toxicity between the enantiomers of mepivacaine (12).

A recent study found that, following combined psoas compartment/sciatic nerve block with mepivacaine, plasma concentrations of the S − form were consistently higher than the R − form. The authors explained these differences on the basis of a larger volume of distribution and a higher rate of total body clearance of the R − form (18).

In addition to clinical utility, as illustrated in the case of ropivacaine, stereoisomers have been useful in laboratory investigations probing the topology of local anesthetic binding sites on sodium channels. Because optical isomers have identical physicochemical properties and have identical uptake into nerve and other biologic membranes

**Table 11–1.** Physiochemical Characteristics of Local Anesthetics

| Generic Name<br>Proprietary Name | Procaine<br>(Novocaine) | 2-Chloroprocaine<br>(Nesacaine) | Lidocaine<br>(Xylocaine) | Mepivacaine<br>(Carbocaine) | Tetracaine<br>(Pontocaine) | Bupivacaine<br>(Marcaine) | Etidocaine<br>(Duranest) | Ropivacaine |
|---|---|---|---|---|---|---|---|---|
| Molecular weight | 236 | 271 | 234 | 246 | 264 | 288 | 276 | 274 |
| Potency** ratio | 1 | 2 | 3 | 3 | 15 | 15 | 15 | — |
| Toxicity ratio | 1 | 0.5 | 2 | 2.5 | 10 | 10 | 10 | — |
| Anesthetic index | 1 | 2 | 1.5 | 1.25 | 1.5 | 1.5 | 1.5 | — |
| pKa (25° C) | 9.05 | 8.97 | 7.9 | 7.16 | 8.46 | 8.16 | 7.7 | 8.0 |
| Lipid solubility | 1 | — | 4 | — | — | 30 | 140 | 2.8 |
| Protein binding | | | | | | | | |
| Maternal | 66 | — | 64 | 77 | 75 | 95 | 94 | 90–95 |
| Fetal | — | — | 25 | — | — | 66 | — | — |
| % Nonionized at | | | | | | | | |
| pH 7.4 | 3 | 4.8 | 24 | 39 | 7.4 | 17 | 33 | — |
| pH 7.2 | 2 | 3.1 | 17 | 28 | 48 | 11 | 24 | — |
| Partition coefficient (n-Heptane 7.4) | 0.02 | 0.14 | 2.9 | 0.8 | 4.1 | 27.5 | 141 | g* |
| Maternal Arterial Concentration | — | — | 1.2–3.5 | 2.0–7.0 | — | 0.26 | 0.25–1.3 | — |
| Umbilical Vein Concentration | — | — | 0.8–1.8 | 2.0–5.0 | — | 0.08–0.1 | >0.07–0.45 | — |
| UV/M ratio | — | — | 0.5–0.7 | 0.7–0.72 | — | 0.3–0.44 | 0.14–0.35 | |
| Half-life | | | | | | | | |
| Adult | — | 21 sec | 1.6 hr | 1.9 hr | — | 9.4 hr | 2.6 hr | — |
| Newborn | — | 43 sec | 3.0 hr | 9.0 hr | — | 8.1 hr | — | — |
| Equipotent concentration % | — | — | 2.0 | 1.5 | — | 0.5 | 1.0 | 0.75 |

* Estimated from data by Rosenberg PH: Absorption of bupivacaine, etiducaine, lignocaine, and ropivacaine into n-heptane, rat sciatic nerve, and human extradural and subcutaneous fat. Br. J. Anaesth. 58:310, 1986.
** Procaine used as standard of reference = 1. Ratios vary according to technique of regional anesthesia used.

(19), differences in potency for these isomers appear to reflect differences in binding to the receptor (17).

## *Physicochemical Properties*

While the basic chemical structure of local anesthetics is similar, specific structural differences account for the differences in physicochemical properties and anesthetic actions. The physicochemical properties determine the nature of interactions between local anesthetic molecules and body tissues, and affect such factors as rates of diffusion and vascular uptake. The physicochemical properties of the local anesthetics in common clinical use are presented in Table 11–1. The clinical significance of these properties is discussed in detail below.

### Molecular Weight

Molecular weights of clinically useful local anesthetics vary from 234 for lidocaine to 307 for 2-chloroprocaine. Benzocaine, which probably has a different mechanism of action than the ionizable local anesthetics in Table 11–1, has a molecular weight of 166. Molecular weight is one of the physicochemical factors that influence the rate of diffusion for all compounds. The relative uniformity of size of the different local anesthetics accounts more for their similarity in being able to cross biologic membranes such as the placenta, blood vessels, and nerves than for any clinical differences. However, there is some evidence to suggest that molecular weight might be a factor in the diffusion of local anesthetics within the sodium channels of the nerve membrane (6,20). Molecular weight has been shown to be the principle determinant of drug (narcotic) flux through dura mater (21), but to have no influence on the movement of narcotics and local anesthetic through the arachnoid mater (22). Decreases in local anesthetic activity appear to occur when molecular weight exceeds 500 and molecules above this size do not diffuse freely across the placental membranes.

### Ionization

Ionization, the capacity for an uncharged species to assume a charged form, is an essential aspect of the physicochemical properties of almost all clinically applicable local anesthetics, as it is the charged form that is believed to interact with the sodium channel receptor. However, local anesthetics in the charged form do not appear to have ready access to this active site on the channel from the exterior of the nerve. Small, permanently charged local anesthetics do not block sodium currents when applied outside the nerve cell membrane, whereas these same compounds strongly block sodium currents when applied on the cytoplasmic side of the same membrane (23). These charged compounds are relatively lipid insoluble and membrane impermeable. Thus, for most local anesthetics, it appears that ionization is an essential feature of its interaction with the nerve membrane, allowing it to alternate between a neutral, lipid soluble phase for

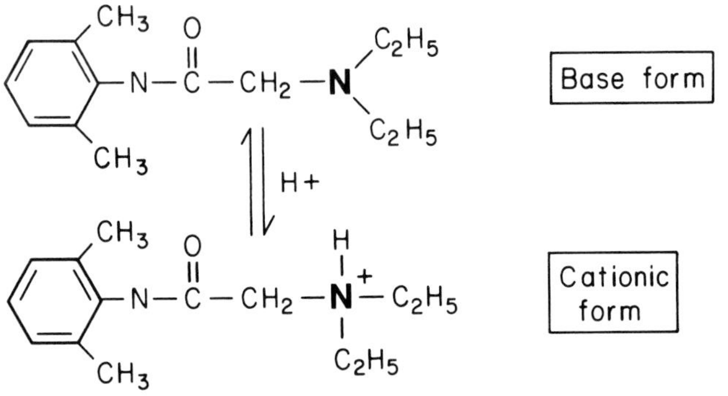

**Fig. 11–4.** The equilibration of lidocaine into base and cationic forms. The amount of available hydrogen ion (pH) will determine the equilibrium concentration of the two forms.

nerve membrane penetration and a charged hydrophilic phase for activity on the sodium channel.

Local anesthetics are usually hydrochloride salts produced by the combination of a weak base and a strong acid. In solution at physiologic pH, the salt dissociates and the local anesthetic exists in one of two forms, either an uncharged base or a positively charged cation (Figure 11–4). The base form is soluble in lipids, and is thus able to penetrate the lipid bilayer of the nerve membrane much more rapidly than the protonated form. Once across the nerve membrane, the drug reequilibrates in the axoplasm between the charged cationic and the uncharged base form.

The structural basis for ionization resides in the amino portion of the local anesthetic molecule; the addition of a hydrogen ion to the uncharged amino group converts the un-ionized base form into the ionized cationic form of the drug (Figure 11–4). The pKa, which is defined as the pH at which 50% of a drug is ionized and 50% is present as base, falls within a narrow range (7.6 to 8.9) for all of the clinically used local anesthetic drugs. The relationship between pH and pKa and the concentration of cation and base forms of the local anesthetic is described by the Henderson-Hasselbach equation:

$$\mathrm{pKa} = \mathrm{pH}^{+}\log\,[\mathrm{cation/base}]. \qquad (1)$$

With rearrangement this equation can also be expressed as:

$$\mathrm{pH} = \mathrm{pKa}^{+}\log\,[\mathrm{base/cation}]. \qquad (2)$$

Because each of the local anesthetics has a pKa greater than 7.6, these drugs will exist at equilibrium at normal body pH predominantly in the cationic (charged) form. The closer the pKa of a drug is to 7.4 (body pH), the greater will be the fraction of drug present in its base form as it equilibrates in body fluids, thereby increasing the concentration of the membrane-crossing form surrounding the axon. Conversely, the further from body pH (local anesthetics with a very high pKa), the greater will be the proportion of drug existing in the ionized form at body pH. This has implications for clinical utility. For example, tetracaine has a relatively high pKa (8.9 at 36° C), resulting in an ionized fraction of 97% at normal body pH. Compared to local anesthetics with lower pKa's and less ionization, tetracaine does not readily diffuse through tissues, which accounts in part for the lower efficacy of this agent when used for nerve blocks in which extensive tissue penetration is required. However, when placed in the subarachnoid space in immediate contact with nerve roots, tetracaine is quite efficacious.

For any local anesthetic with a given pKa, changes in pH will affect the degree of ionization and movement into and out of tissue (24). As a general principle, lowering the pH will increase the fraction of ionized drug, a form that does not readily cross biologic membranes. This may impair neural blockade, as seen when a local anesthetic is injected into acidotic tissue for peripheral nerve block (i.e., an ankle block in a diabetic with an ischemic, acidotic foot). It also has implications for toxicity in that once a local anesthetic is in a tissue, such as the heart or brain, an intracellular decrease in pH may increase the concentration of the active (ionized) form intracellularly while concomitantly retarding the ability of the drug to leave the tissue, a condition referred to as "ion trapping." This concept will be discussed more fully below, as pH effects upon drug transfer to the fetus are considered.

The addition by practitioners of bicarbonate to solutions of local anesthetic marketed in an acidic medium represents an attempt to use our knowledge of the physicochemistry of these agents to improve their efficacy; elevation of the pH of the local anesthetic solution shifts the equilibrium toward the un-ionized form and thus may shorten the onset time for anesthesia (25). This effect is limited, however, and an excess amount of bicarbonate results in precipitation of the local anesthetic from solution.

### *Lipid Solubility and Hydrophobicity*

Because local anesthetics must traverse lipid membranes to reach the sodium channel active site, lipid solubility is an essential aspect of the physiochemical properties of clinically applicable local anesthetics. The interaction of local anesthetics with nerve membranes is described by several terms that are commonly used interchangeably. "Lipophilic" (attracted to lipids) on the one hand and "hydrophobic" (water avoiding) on the other, both refer to the degree to which molecules are excluded from aqueous domains (e.g., extracellular and intracellular fluid) or solubilized in lipid solutions. There are technical differences between the terms (4,26), but for practical purposes, lipid solubility and hydrophobicity refer to the same property, one that is important because it correlates in a nonlinear manner with anesthetic potency; thus, the more hydrophobic the drug, indicative of greater lipid solubility, the greater the potency (11).

Clinically, there is a limit on the additional potency achieved by further increases in lipid solubility. One explanation for this is that local anesthetics with very high lipid solubilities have enhanced uptake into non-neural tissues, including perineural fat and blood vessels. Such uptake effectively decreases the concentration that remains in the vicinity of the nerve.

Another explanation for the limitation on potency with increases in lipid solubility is that as lipid solubility increases, aqueous solubility decreases. However, both water solubility and lipid solubility are necessary for drug diffusion from the injection site to the nerve membrane. For example, drug deposited in the epidural space must traverse the dura, the arachnoid, and the pia mater to reach the subarachnoid space and hence the spinal cord or nerve roots (27). Because these three tissues consist of multiple layers of overlapping cells, this cellular barrier contains both hydrophilic domains (extracellular and intracellular fluid) and hydrophobic domains (cell membrane lipids). The consequence of this hydrophobic/hydrophilic barrier has been demonstrated in studies of the diffusion of various drug molecules through the spinal meninges of animals in in vitro models (21,28). The permeability coefficients for the various drugs were found to be related in a biphasic manner to lipid solubility as assessed by octanol:buffer distribution coefficients. Hydrophobic drugs, those with low octanol:buffer coefficients, such as morphine, and those with high octanol:buffer coefficients, the hydrophilic drugs fentanyl and sufentanil, were found to cross the meningeal barrier less readily than drugs of intermediate hydrophobicity, such as lidocaine, bupivacaine, and alfentanil. This suggests that there is an optimal hydrophobicity that will result in maximal meningeal permeability. Of course, the model in the study just cited is an in vitro model, and in the in vivo situation there will be other factors that will also influence meningeal permeability, such as vascular uptake from the epidural space and local tissue binding.

The aromatic ring present at one end of the local anesthetic molecule is the major contributor to the lipophilic nature of the drug. When the drug exists in its uncharged base form, this lipophilicity allows the molecule to rapidly enter and pass through the lipid-containing nerve membrane into the axoplasm of the nerve, from whence it appears to enter the sodium channel, albeit most likely in a protonated, less lipid-soluble form (5). Alterations in chemical structure may alter lipid solubility. As an example, the addition of chlorine to the 2-position of the aromatic ring in procaine yields 2-chloroprocaine and an eightfold increase in lipid solubility.

Lipid solubility is approximated in vitro by measuring the concentration of a drug in an immiscible mixture, such as an organic solvent (heptane, octanol) and an aqueous buffer that resembles extracellular fluid in terms of pH, ionic strength, temperature, etc. Organic solvent: buffer partition coefficients may differ from membrane: buffer partition coefficients by several orders of magnitude for the same drug, indicating that the complexity of biologic membranes is not easily approximated with a single organic compound. Rosenberg, et al have demonstrated the lack of correlation between in vitro solubilities in a pure organic solvent (n-heptane) and uptake into biologic tissues (nerve, subcutaneous fat, epidural fat) (16). The relative n-heptane partitioning (37°) of etidocaine: bupivacaine: ropivacaine: lidocaine was approximately 40:10:3:1. Thus, etidocaine was found to be 40 times more lipid soluble than lidocaine, and four times more lipid soluble than bupivacaine, in an organic solvent. However, when uptake into rat sciatic nerve was measured for these same local anesthetics, the comparable ratios were 4:3.3:1.8:1. There was much less variation between drugs in biologic tissue (nerve) than in an organic solvent. There was also much less difference among the various local anesthetics in comparable solubilities in epidural and subcutaneous fat as opposed to n-heptane. Thus, while in vitro organic solvent measurements allow a ranking of local anesthetics based upon lipid solubilities, they do not provide a sound basis for predicting the in vivo behavior of different local anesthetics. Thus, the greater in vitro lipid solubility of bupivacaine compared to lidocaine does not result in a faster onset of nerve blockade during, for example, epidural anesthesia, presumably due to differences in uptake by non-neuronal tissues such as epidural fat.

In summary, increases in lipid solubility correlate with increases in drug potency, indicating greater access to, or affinity for, the site of action. Lipid solubility is associated primarily with the neutral form of local anesthetics and appears to determine the rate at which a local anesthetic reaches its binding site. Drug charge (protonation) appears to determine whether it will stay there (4).

### Protein Binding

In the body, varying proportions of all local anesthetics are bound to proteins in plasma and in tissues. Protein binding has major implications for the activities, toxicities, and metabolic fates of these drugs, because drugs are not pharmacologically active or readily metabolized while in the bound form (28). It is the free drug that is able to penetrate into tissues such as heart and brain, and thus it is the concentration of free drug that has implications for toxicity. Lidocaine entry into brain and cerebrospinal fluid is highly correlated with the fraction of free (unbound) drug, which is inversely correlated with the concentration of binding proteins (29,30). Thus, particularly for drugs that are highly protein bound, either qualitative or quantitative changes in protein binding may have important consequences for potential systemic toxicity. Protein binding is also a major factor influencing placental transfer of local anesthetic; bound drug does not cross the placental membranes.

Protein binding is an equilibrium phenomenon. It is not a case of local anesthetic filling up all the binding sites and then accumulating as unbound drug. At all local anesthetic concentrations, there is a continual binding and release of local anesthetic-protein complexes so that, at any given moment, there are unoccupied binding sites on proteins, and, at any given moment, there are also unbound local anesthetic molecules, no matter how many unoccupied protein binding sites are available. However, the fraction of protein bound drug decreases in a curvilinear manner as the local anesthetic concentration in the plasma is increased (Figure 11–5) (31).

Thus, when one speaks of the degree of protein binding of a particular local anesthetic, one must also specify the serum concentration at which that binding was measured.

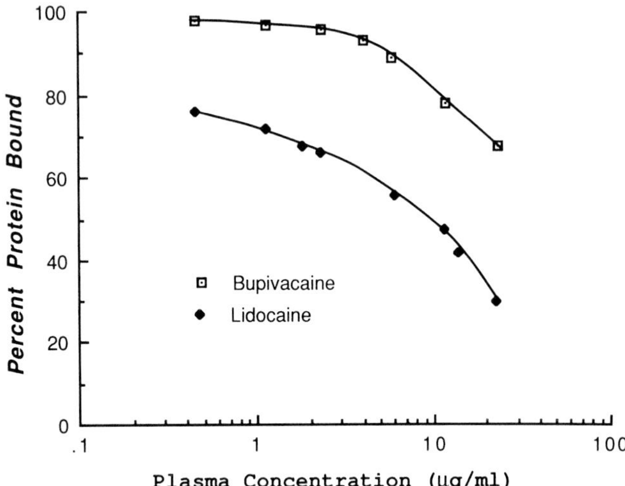


**Fig. 11–5.** The effect of increasing plasma drug concentration on the protein binding of bupivacaine and lidocaine. Note that the concentration is a log scale. Increasing drug concentration is associated with decreased protein binding and hence a greater fraction of free, biologically active drug. (From Tucker GT, Mather LE: Pharmacology of local anesthetic agents. Brit. J. Anaesth. 47:213, 1975.)

The commonly used value for the degree of protein binding for lidocaine of 65% assumes a serum level in the 1 to 2 µg/ml range. With increasing concentrations, i.e., 5 to 10 µg/ml, the portion of protein bound lidocaine is 50 to 55%. Decreased protein binding at increasing serum concentrations of local anesthetic has implications for toxicity. For example, the serum level of lidocaine in adults following a typical epidural anesthetic is in the range of 2 to 4 µg/ml (unless stated otherwise, reported serum levels for local anesthetics refer to the total amount of drug in plasma, and include both bound and unbound drug). In this concentration range, 65% of this amount will be protein bound, leaving a free fraction of 35% (Figure 11–5). However, at a serum level of 20 µg/ml, a level that might be achieved following an accidental intravascular injection, the bound fraction decreases to 30% and the free fraction increases to 70%. Thus, the amount of free, biologically active lidocaine at a serum level of 3 µg/ml is approximately 1 µg/ml; at 20 µg/ml, this free amount increases to 14 µg/ml. In this example, a sevenfold increase in total drug concentration results in a fourteenfold increase in the active form of the drug.

The most important binding proteins for local anesthetics in plasma are albumin and alpha-1-acid glycoprotein (AAG). Alpha-1-acid glycoprotein is an acute phase reactant and circulating levels of alpha-1-acid glycoprotein increase to a variable degree in response to tissue injury. Thus, surgery, trauma, infection, inflammation, and malignancy are all associated with increased serum levels of alpha-1-acid glycoprotein (26,32). Epidural anesthesia does not block the increase in alpha-1-acid glycoprotein in response to surgery (33). In addition to quantitative changes, the binding affinity of alpha-1-acid glycoprotein may be altered in disease states; such qualitative changes are reflected in a patient with cancer in whom a doubling of alpha-1-acid glycoprotein concentration was associated with a sixfold increase in bupivacaine binding (34). This accounts for reports of asymptomatic patients who have measured plasma levels of bupivacaine that are in the range normally associated with toxic reactions.

Fortunately, there appear to be few clinical situations in which low plasma concentrations of alpha-1-acid glycoprotein are encountered, with the major exceptions being the fetus and newborn and the parturient at term. These special cases are discussed more fully below.

Albumin levels vary with nutritional status and certain disease states. Nephrotic syndrome is associated with decreased albumin levels. However, alpha-1-acid glycoprotein is an acute phase reactant and may be normal, elevated or decreased in nephrotic syndrome. Because, as will be discussed, alpha-1-acid glycoprotein is the principle binding protein at usual anesthetic blood levels, one cannot predict that hypoalbuminemia will result in a greater local anesthetic free fraction without knowing the status of alpha-1-acid glycoprotein levels.

The binding to alpha-1-acid glycoprotein has been characterized as high-affinity, low-capacity binding, while binding to albumin is best described as low-affinity, high-capacity binding (35). At plasma concentrations below 10 µg/ml, local anesthetics preferentially bind to alpha-1-acid glycoprotein; above this level, alpha-1-acid glycoprotein becomes progressively saturated and albumin plays the major role in binding local anesthetics. The binding capacity of albumin for local anesthetics is very large; albumin is able to bind these drugs without saturation up to an order of magnitude greater than blood levels clinically achieved. The clinical significance of the differential binding affinities of alpha-1-acid glycoprotein and albumin for local anesthetics is that alterations in albumin binding, either qualitative or quantitative, have very little impact on free drug levels at plasma levels associated with routine clinical procedures, e.g., epidural, intercostal, or axillary block. However, at these same levels, alterations in alpha-1-acid glycoprotein binding can result in major changes in the levels of free drug. At very high plasma drug concentrations, such as occur following accidental intravascular injections of intermediate-potency local anesthetics such as lidocaine or mepivacaine, the affinity and capacity of albumin binding are the primary determinants of the amount of free and potentially toxic drug; alterations in alpha-1-acid glycoprotein binding assume less significance, because, in such cases, saturation occurs.

The effects of alterations in the binding proteins are illustrated in Figures 11–6 and 11–7. In Figure 11–6, it can be seen that below a total bupivacaine serum level of 10 µg/ml, moderate hypoalbuminemia has almost no effect on the amount of free drug. This is because drug binding over this range is primarily related to the affinity and capacity of alpha-1-acid glycoprotein. Once the high-affinity, low-capacity sites on alpha-1-acid glycoprotein are saturated (above 10 µg/ml), free levels of anesthetic progressively increase in low-albumin sera compared to control. However, even following accidental intravascular injection of high-potency local anesthetics such as bupivacaine, ropivacaine or etidocaine, one would not expect

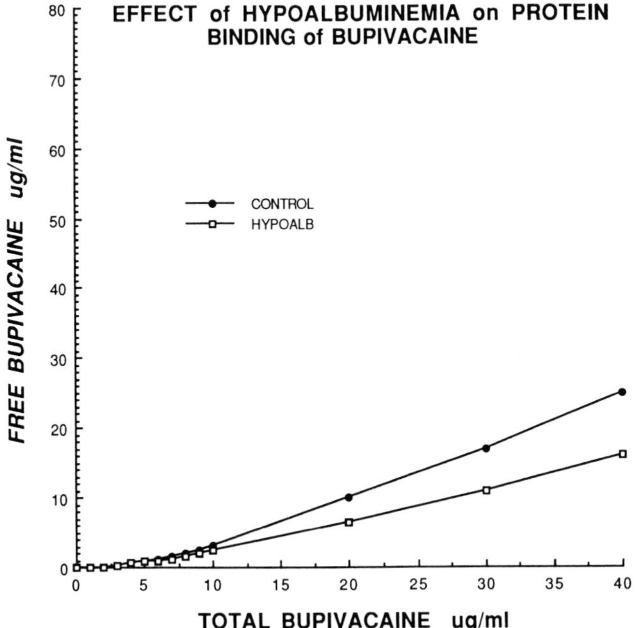


**Fig. 11–6.** The effect of hypoalbuminemia on the plasma protein binding of bupivacaine. At drug concentrations below 10 μg/ml no effect is seen because it is the major binding protein over this range. About 10 μg/ml, while there is a significant increase in the amount of free drug with hypoalbuminemia, these levels of bupivacaine are above those that would be achieved clinically, even following an accidental intravenous injection of an intended epidural dose of bupivacaine. (From Denson DD, Mazoit JX: Physiology, pharmacology, and toxicity of local anesthetics: adult and pediatric considerations. *In* Clinical Practice of Regional Anesthesia. Edited by PP Raj. New York, Churchill Livingstone, 1991.)

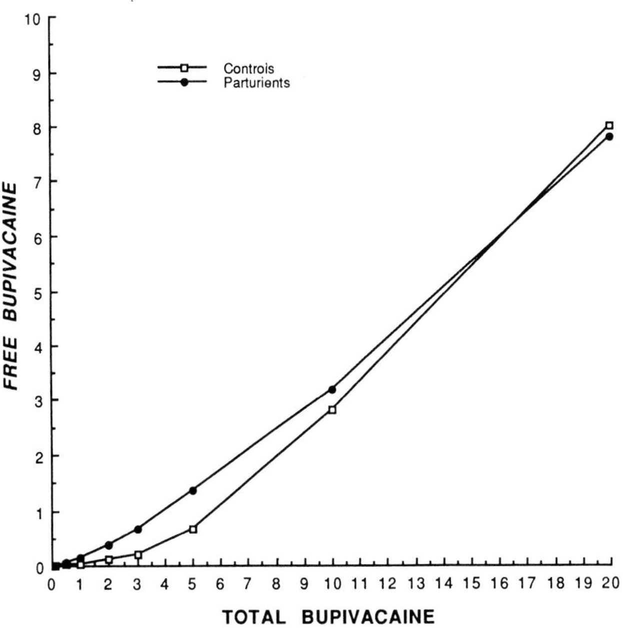


**Fig. 11–7.** The effect of pregnancy on the protein binding of bupivacaine. Pregnancy is associated with a decrease in binding to AAG, which is the predominant binding protein at plasma levels below 10 μg/ml. Above this level, albumin becomes increasingly important, and the pregnancy related differences disappear. While the differences seem rather small, note that the concentration of free bupivacaine at a total level of 5 μg/ml is increased two-fold. (From Denson D, Coyle D, Thompson G, Santos D, et al: Bupivacaine protein binding in the term parturient: effects of lactic acidosis. Clin. Pharmacol. Ther. 35:702, 1984.)

to achieve blood levels significantly above the 10 μg/ml range, and this represents a highly toxic level. Thus, for the high-potency agents, alterations in albumin binding are unlikely to be of clinical consequence.

Figure 11–7 illustrates the effects of moderate decreases in the binding capacity of alpha-1-acid glycoprotein as occurs during pregnancy. At the levels associated with central nervous system (CNS) toxicity (4 to 6 μg/ml), pregnancy results in approximately 50% more free drug. In animal studies, pregnancy enhances the toxicity of bupivacaine, presumably due to decreased binding by alpha-1-acid glycoprotein (36). In pregnant ewes, cardiovascular collapse occurred at a blood concentration of bupivacaine of 5.5 μg/ml, while nonpregnant ewes had significantly higher blood levels (8 μg/ml) at this end point. The concentration of drug in the myocardium at toxicity was not significantly different between the two groups. Thus, for a given dose, decreased plasma protein binding results in higher tissue levels of bupivacaine and lowers the threshold for toxic reactions.

For mepivacaine, circulatory collapse does not occur until quite high serum levels are achieved (~50 μg/ml). Thus, even though decreased alpha-1-acid glycoprotein binding in pregnancy results in almost twice as much free drug (at a mepivacaine serum concentration of 8.5 μg/ml), these levels are not associated with toxicity and the decrease in binding is not clinically significant (Figure 11–8) (37). At the cardiotoxic doses, there is no difference in drug binding when pregnant ewes are compared to nonpregnant ewes. This is because binding at these drug levels is a function of albumin, not alpha-1-acid glycoprotein, and albumin binding is not decreased during pregnancy. These studies illustrate the clinical importance of protein binding, with major differences existing among different drugs and at different drug concentrations.

Protein binding is influenced by pH in that the percentage of bound drug decreases as pH decreases. Thus, with the development of an acidic environment, an increase in the amount of free drug occurs (Figure 11–9). For example, in the adult, lidocaine at pH 7.4 at a 5 to 10 μg/ml blood concentration is 50% protein bound; with a decrease in pH to 7.0, the drug is 35% bound at the same total concentration (38,39).

While acidosis results in a greater fraction of unbound drug, the significance of decreased protein binding with acidosis is unclear. Because acidosis also increases the protonated form, which does not readily cross biologic membranes, the increase in free fraction during combined metabolic/respiratory acidosis (as might occur during local anesthetic induced seizures) does not result in greater movement of drug into myocardium or brain in

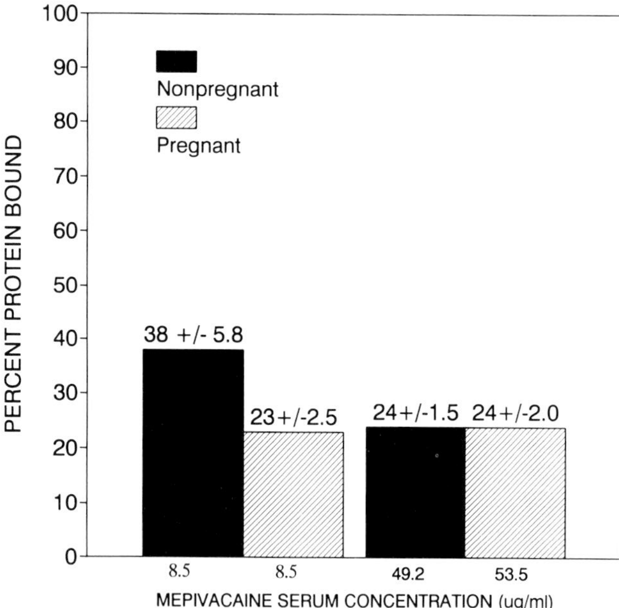


**Fig. 11–8.** Effects of pregnancy upon mepivacaine protein binding at low (8.5 μg/ml) and high (~50 μg/ml) plasma concentrations. Decreased binding, and hence increased amounts of free mepivacaine, is seen at the low range of drug at which there is no clinical toxicity. At the levels at which cardiac toxicity occurs (50 μg/ml) there is no difference in protein binding and hence no increased toxicity related to the pregnant state. (From Santos AC, Pedersen H, Harmon TW, Morishima HO, et al: Does pregnancy alter the systemic toxicity of local anesthetics? Anesthesiology. 70:991, 1989.)

sheep (40). It appears that if acidosis potentiates local anesthetic toxicity, it does so by mechanisms other than decreased protein binding, possibly by increasing the concentration of ionized local anesthetic at the active site on the sodium channel.

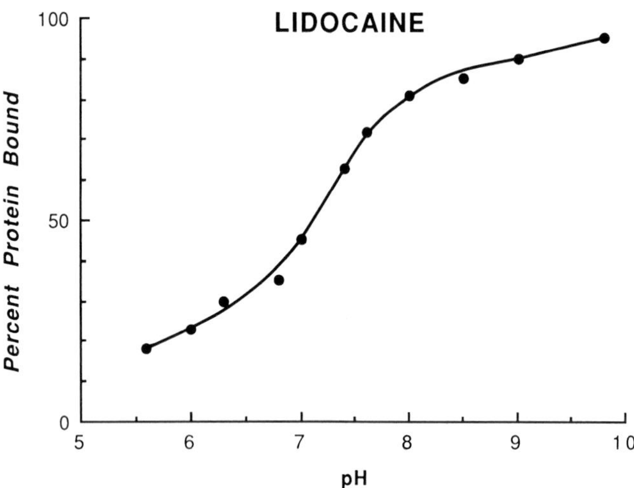


**Fig. 11–9.** pH of plasma and protein binding of lidocaine. Acidosis is associated with decreased binding and a greater fraction of free drug.

The fraction of drug bound to protein in plasma correlates with duration of local anesthetic activity, i.e., bupivacaine/ropivacaine/etidocaine ≥ mepivacaine ≥ lidocaine ≥ procaine/2-chloroprocaine. This suggests that binding between the local anesthetic molecule and the amino acids of the receptor proteins on the sodium channel may be similar to that between the local anesthetic molecule and plasma proteins, i.e., electrostatic and/or hydrogen binding.

***Effects of Pregnancy on Protein Binding.*** As already alluded to, protein binding appears to change with pregnancy. Although the plasma concentration of albumin decreases in parturients (41,42), this is offset by an increase in the total amount of albumin due to the expansion in total blood volume associated with pregnancy. Also, Denson, et al have reported an approximate doubling of binding sites per molecule of albumin, resulting in an increased capacity at the low-affinity, high-capacity site (albumin) (42). However, as explained above, alpha-1-acid glycoprotein, not albumin, is the predominate binding protein when local anesthetic blood levels are in the normal clinical range, and in both normal and preeclamptic pregnant subjects, variations in albumin levels do not affect the free fraction of lidocaine in maternal blood (43).

The concentration of alpha-1-acid glycoprotein in maternal plasma has been reported to be decreased as much as 50% in pregnancy at term (44), while other investigators have found no differences between pregnant and nonpregnant subjects in alpha-1-acid glycoprotein concentration (42,45). However, in both of these latter studies, the free fraction of local anesthetic [lidocaine (45) bupivacaine (42)] was increased despite lack of major changes in alpha-1-acid glycoprotein levels, suggesting a decrease in binding capacity. Denson, et al reported a 50% decrease in the number of available binding sites per molecule of alpha-1-acid glycoprotein in pregnant subjects. The decrease in binding capacity is not due to increased progesterone or nonesterified fatty acids, two substances that are increased in pregnancy and are bound by the same proteins that bind local anesthetics, i.e., alpha-1-acid glycoprotein and albumin, but could theoretically displace the local anesthetics from protein binding sites (46).

As a consequence of qualitative and possibly quantitative changes in alpha-1-acid glycoprotein, the free fraction of bupivacaine is increased in pregnancy. Thus, for a given serum level, there will be a larger proportion of the drug that is biologically active and potentially toxic in pregnant patients (Table 11–2). To illustrate, at blood levels resulting from proper epidural anesthesia with bupivacaine (~1 μg/ml), the concentration of free bupivacaine is 0.155 μg/ml in pregnant subjects compared to 0.042 μg/ml in nonpregnant subjects, almost a fourfold increase. Note that, in nonpregnant subjects, a serum level of 5 μg/ml (a concentration at which seizures would be expected), is associated with a concentration of free bupivacaine of 0.675 μg/ml. Because of decreased protein binding (primarily to alpha-1-acid glycoprotein) the same amount of free drug (0.675 μg/ml) is found in pregnant patients at a lower total serum concentration, 3 μg/ml. Clearly, for drugs in which toxicity occurs at plasma levels below 10

**Table 11–2.** Effect of Pregnancy on Protein Binding of Bupivacaine

| Total Plasma Concentration (μg/ml) | Free Bupivacaine Concentration μg/ml | |
|---|---|---|
| | Nonpregnant | Pregnant |
| 0.1 | 0.004 | 0.012 |
| 0.5 | 0.019 | 0.068 |
| 1.0 | 0.042 | 0.155 |
| 2.0 | 0.107 | 0.384 |
| 3.0 | 0.214 | 0.677 |
| 5.0 | 0.675 | 1.37 |
| 10.0 | 2.8 | 3.2 |
| 20.0 | 8.0 | 7.8 |

(From Denson D, Coyle D, Thompson G, Santos D, et al: Bupivacaine protein binding in the term parturient: effects of lactic acidosis. Clin. Pharmacol. Ther. 35:702, 1984.)

μg/ml (bupivacaine, ropivacaine, etidocaine), the decrease in the binding capacity of alpha-1-acid glycoprotein during pregnancy can be of major significance.

Because toxicity with lidocaine and mepivacaine occurs at much higher blood levels compared to bupivacaine, ropivacaine or etidocaine, the alterations in alpha-1-acid glycoprotein binding with pregnancy have much less implications for toxicity in the case of excessively high plasma levels. This was discussed in the preceding section, and is well illustrated in Figure 11–7.

To summarize, for high-potency local anesthetics such as bupivacaine, ropivacaine or etidocaine, in which cardiotoxic plasma levels are in the range of 4 to 10 μg/ml, pregnancy results in a greater free fraction of drug due to decreased protein binding and hence potentiates toxicity. In the case of intermediate-potency drugs such as lidocaine and mepivacaine, cardiac toxicity is associated with much higher plasma levels (30 to 50 μg/ml); at these levels alpha-1-acid glycoprotein sites are saturated in both pregnant and nonpregnant subjects, and decreases in alpha-1-acid glycoprotein binding are offset by increases in albumin binding. For the intermediate agents, the effects of pregnancy upon protein binding do not appear to result in any increase risk of cardiac toxicity.

## PHARMACOKINETICS

In clinical practice, when local anesthetics are administered for neural blockade, the anesthesiologist is chiefly concerned with the onset, spread, quality, and duration of the block, as well as potential local anesthetic toxicity. However, the variation in these clinical phenomena is ultimately determined by pharmacokinetic principles affecting the local disposition, absorption, distribution, metabolism, and elimination of these drugs. The pharmacokinetic characteristics of local anesthetics have great clinical significance, as both the therapeutic activity and the toxicity of local anesthetic depend upon a balance among these various factors.

### *Local Disposition*

For regional anesthesia, factors relating to local disposition tend to be the most important determinants of successful neural blockade. Because direct injection of local anesthetic into a nerve is painful and injurious, neural blockade using local anesthetics of necessity involves placing the drug at some distance from the nerve to be blocked. The drug must then move from the site of injection to the interior of the nerve cell, a journey that always requires traversing tissue barriers such as fat, interstitial fluid or connective tissue surrounding the nerve. There are three basic mechanisms associated with the movement of local anesthetic molecules in the body and these mechanisms influence drug movement into the nerve, as well as drug movement away from the nerve:

1. Bulk flow of the injected solution at the site of injection;
2. Diffusion into and through aqueous and lipoprotein barriers;
3. Vascular transport either free in solution in the blood or bound to circulating plasma proteins.

### *Bulk Flow*

Bulk flow can be thought of as movement of a substance on the basis of energy supplied from a source external to the substance. For example, the mixing of isobaric lidocaine with spinal fluid injected into the subarachnoid space is primarily by bulk flow. The energy is supplied by the force applied to the barrel of the syringe and this kinetic energy is transferred to the lidocaine molecules. Energy for dispersal of the lidocaine within the spinal fluid also is supplied by kinetic energy within the spinal fluid itself, which is in circulatory motion. The energy is supplied by the heart; as blood is pumped into the brain, a certain amount of spinal fluid is displaced from the cranial vault and pushed into the spinal canal. During diastole, as blood leaves the brain, this process is reversed. This repetitious process sets up currents of spinal fluid that can affect the dispersal of drugs within the subarachnoid space. This is true for local anesthetics as well as other drugs. For example, when epidural morphine is administered, a certain portion of the opiate reaches the spinal fluid, presumably by diffusing through the dura, and is then carried by bulk flow to the brain. The energy is supplied by the moving currents of spinal fluid. The slowness of this process is seen clinically by a delay of several hours in the onset of brain-related symptoms (itching, nausea, somnolence and, on rare occasion, respiratory depression) following epidural administration.

Bulk flow may be affected by a number of variables, including the volume of solution injected; the force (speed) with which it is injected (47) although this is of minimal importance in the epidural space (48); the size of the injected space; physical resistance offered by tissues and fluids; and gravity and patient position during and after injection.

### *Diffusion*

Diffusion is the property whereby a substance spreads through a given space based upon random molecular motion. In pharmacological terms, it most often is used to describe the movement of a substance across a membrane or porous barrier. The rate of such diffusion is described by the equation:

$$Q/t = A(C_1 - C_2)kD\text{-}1 \qquad (3)$$

where the quantity diffusing per unit of time (Q/t) depends upon the thickness (D) and surface area (A) of the membrane, the concentration gradient of the substance (free, unbound drug in the case of local anesthetics) from one side to the other ($C_1 - C_2$), and a diffusion constant k for each substance that is related to the physicochemical properties of the drug (molecular weight, lipid solubility, and degree of ionization).

Any anesthesiologist who has waited for 30 minutes for an axillary or epidural block to set up has had a demonstration of the fact that diffusion is a very slow process. For any given drug targeted at a specific nerve, the rate of diffusion can be accelerated by increasing the concentration of drug surrounding the nerve (thus initially altering $C_1 - C_2$). Altering the pH of the injectate may in some cases increase the concentration of un-ionized local anesthetic molecules, a form that more readily diffuses through lipid membranes. The variables A (surface area) and D (membrane thickness) are also subject to change; for example, the thickness of the trophoblastic epithelium decreases from 26 μm during early pregnancy to 2 μm at term.

The concentration of drug available to diffuse across the nerve membrane is also affected by local tissue binding. For example, perineural fat will absorb drugs in accordance with their lipid solubilities (16) and will effectively decrease the concentration gradient tending to move drug into the nerve.

### Vascular Transport

Local anesthetics also move through the body via vascular transport. This can have grave clinical consequences, as when an accidental intravascular injection of local anesthetic during regional nerve blockade allows high blood concentrations to be carried to the brain and heart and cause seizures and potentially lethal cardiac arrhythmias. Vascular transport is important even when the drug is properly placed, as a portion of the local anesthetic is absorbed into the bloodstream and removed from the injected area, thus lowering the effective concentration at the nerve site. The use of local vasoconstrictors such as epinephrine to prolong duration of action represents an attempt to impair local vascular transport. Vascular transport also plays an essential role in drug metabolism, as all amide local anesthetics (i.e., lidocaine, bupivacaine, ropivacaine, mepivacaine, etidocaine) must be transported from the site of injection to the liver to be biotransformed.

### Absorption

Absorption of local anesthetic refers to the movement of drug from the site of injection into the bloodstream. The resultant blood levels of local anesthetic are important in that systemic toxicity affecting the heart and/or central nervous system is directly related to peak blood concentration ($C_{max}$) of the drug, and specifically the concentration of free drug (30).

Absorption of local anesthetic produces blood levels that are directly related to: amount of drug injected; vascularity of the site injected; and tissue binding of local anesthetic at the injection site. The larger the total dose of anesthetic injected, the higher the $C_{max}$ that can be expected. For example, epidural doses of ropivacaine of 100, 150, and 200 mg produced mean peak plasma concentrations of 0.53, 1.07, and 1.53 μg/ml, respectively (49), confirming the linear relationship between dose and $C_{max}$ reported earlier for other amide anesthetics (50).

Injection into areas of high vascularity tends to result in higher blood levels compared to less vascular areas. With a given dose of drug, the blood levels seen are highest with intercostal and intrapleural blocks, lowest for subcutaneous infiltration of skin and axillary blocks, and intermediate for epidural and caudal blocks (51). For lidocaine or mepivacaine, the general range of blood levels to be expected for each 100 mg of drug injected in the average adult will vary from 0.5 μg/ml following subcutaneous administration or axillary blockade to 1.0 μg/ml for epidural and caudal injections to 1.5 μg/ml for intercostal blocks (Figure 11–10). Vascularity also affects the rate of absorption; equal doses of lidocaine injected into the epidural and subarachnoid spaces appear in the blood much more rapidly following epidural administration (52).

Local tissue binding also influences anesthetic absorption. Partitioning into the various tissue compartments at the site of injection (fat, muscle, interstitial fluid, nerve) is a function of the physical properties of the various local anesthetic agents. The more potent agents tend to have high lipid solubilities and to readily partition into fat (16). Thus, one would predict that highly potent agents such as bupivacaine, ropivacaine, and etidocaine would display high binding to epidural fat and would hence produce a lower $C_{max}$ than the less potent and less lipid soluble agents such as lidocaine and mepivacaine, which are less bound to fat and more free to diffuse into the vascular space. This has been demonstrated by the epidural injection of a mixture of equal milligram doses of three agents (bupivacaine, lidocaine, and mepivacaine), thus controlling for any differences in local anesthetic-induced vasodilatation (53). The $C_{max}$ for bupivacaine was lower than that for either mepivacaine or lidocaine.

The addition of a vasoconstrictor to the local anesthetic also affects absorption and hence peak blood levels. Vasoconstrictors such as epinephrine have the greatest effect in terms of decreasing peak plasma levels when the injection site is a highly vascular area. For example, plasma levels of lidocaine following paracervical (a highly vascular area) injection are decreased 50% by the addition of epinephrine 1:200,000 to the anesthetic solution, whereas epinephrine decreases lidocaine plasma levels by only 33% when the injection site is the comparatively less vascular epidural space (51). Likewise, epinephrine will have a greater effect in terms of decreasing peak plasma levels when the local anesthetic is a low-potency agent (e.g., lidocaine) as opposed to a high-potency drug such as bupivacaine or etidocaine, because tissue binding

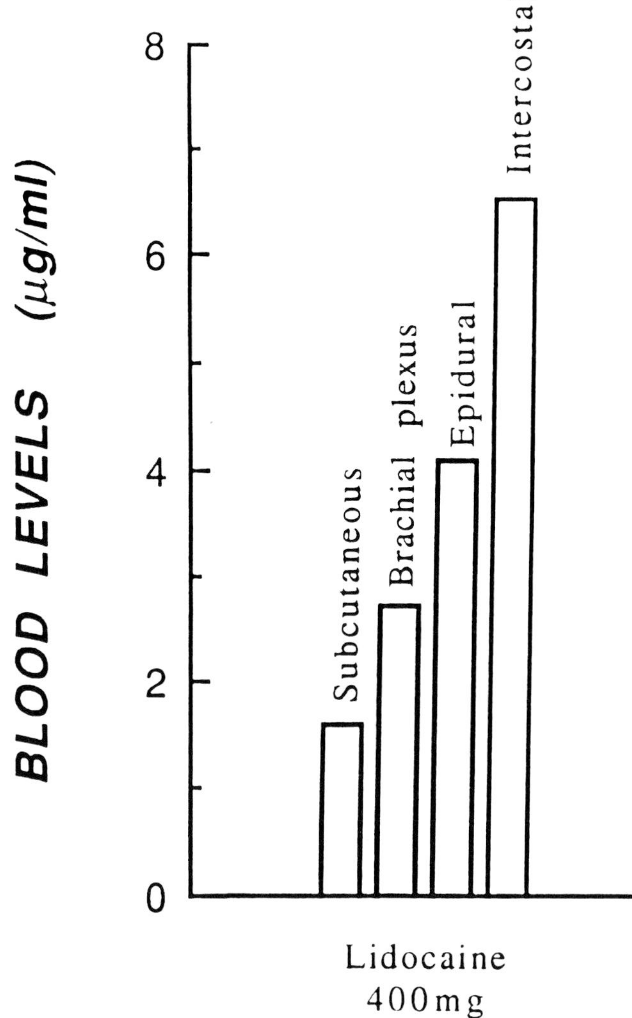


**Fig. 11–10.** Plasma concentration after a 400 mg dose of lidocaine at different sites. (From Covino BG, Vassallo HG: Local Anesthetics: Mechanisms of Action and Clinical Use. New York, Grune & Stratton, 1976.)

(to epidural fat and neural tissue) is more important than tissue blood flow in determining peak blood levels for these agents, and the addition of epinephrine to epidural solutions of etidocaine, for example, has no significant effect on peak plasma levels (54).

### Distribution

Distribution refers to the delivery of absorbed drug to various tissues in the body. Distribution of local anesthetic has special emphasis in the pregnant patient, because one of the organs that will be exposed to absorbed drug is the fetoplacental unit. Because of importance of drug transfer to the fetus, this aspect of distribution will be discussed in a subsequent section.

The time course and tissue distribution of amide-linked local anesthetics is influenced by multiple factors, including: cardiac output and tissue blood flow; the solubility of the drug in various body tissues and organs: the physicochemical properties of the drug (pKa, protein binding) and the physicochemical state of the body (temperature, pH); and ongoing metabolism and elimination.

#### Tissue Blood Flow, Tissue Solubility, and Cardiac Output

Amide-linked local anesthetics are distributed first to the lungs once the drug is in the blood. Local anesthetics are highly soluble in lung tissue, and there is a large uptake of drug into the lung (55). This initially results in a lower concentration of drug on the left side of the heart and the coronary circulation than is present in the venous blood reaching the right heart. This rapid uptake by the lung is transitory, however, lasting only about 10 seconds in the case of lidocaine, after which the drug appears in the arterial circulation. Eventually, all drug taken up by the lung is released back into the systemic circulation, there being no significant pulmonary metabolism of local anesthetics. For the more lipid soluble agents, the ability of the lung to serve as a sink following a rapid intravenous injection, followed by a slower release into the arterial circulation, may be of clinical significance. For example, in a study comparing the toxicities of bupivacaine and ropivacaine following intravenous infusion, it was noted that for both drugs the venous blood levels in the arm opposite the injection site were higher 5 minutes after the infusion ended than at the moment the infusion was stopped (56). Thus, passage through the pulmonary circulation appears to provide some degree of protection in the event of excessive blood levels of long-acting local anesthetics; conversely, individuals with right-to-left cardiac lesions may be at greater risk from cardiac and CNS toxicity in the event of accidental intravascular injection of such agents.

After traversing the lungs, local anesthetic is then distributed primarily to those organs with the highest tissue blood flow; heart, brain, liver, kidney, and, in the case of a pregnant subject, the uterus and placenta. In this regard the distribution of local anesthetics is similar to inhalational anesthetics. Also, uptake into these organs is a function of the blood:tissue solubility of the drug, and this will vary for different agents and different body tissues (16). Lesser amounts of local anesthetic are simultaneously distributed to organs with less relative blood flow, such as muscle and fat, as well as to organs with very poor perfusion, such as connective tissue.

Pregnancy is associated with major changes in cardiac output, with a normal increase in the range of 40%. Cardiac output affects not only the rate of local anesthetic delivery to various tissue beds but also the rate of clearance by the liver.

#### Physicochemical Factors (protein binding, pKa, pH, ionization, lipid solubility)

All of these factors are discussed in detail elsewhere. As a general rule, increased protein binding results in less free drug that can redistribute to body organs. The converse is also true. pKa, pH, and ionization primarily determine the electrochemical nature of the drug (charged versus uncharged) that greatly affects movement through aqueous and nonaqueous tissues, and may also affect protein binding. Lipid solubility influences not only what tissues a drug penetrates but how long it remains there.

### Biodegradation and Elimination

An ester or amide linkage is present between the lipophilic and the amide end of the drug molecule. The type of link present determines the site of metabolic inactivation of the drug: ester-linked local anesthetics are inactivated predominantly in plasma, while amide-linked drugs undergo inactivation in the liver.

Ester-linked local anesthetics are hydrolyzed in plasma by plasma pseudocholinesterase. In addition to the ester-linked local anesthetics, this plasma enzyme also hydrolyzes natural choline esters and succinylcholine. The rate of hydrolysis of ester-linked local anesthetics depends on the substitutions present in the aromatic ring structure, with 2-chloroprocaine being hydrolyzed about four times faster than procaine, which in turn is hydrolyzed about four times faster than tetracaine. In the case of 2-chloroprocaine, the half-life in the normal adult is approximately 30 seconds. Thus, distribution pharmacokinetics as discussed for amide-linked drugs are not clinically relevant in the case of drugs such as 2-chloroprocaine. Assuming adequate levels of plasma pseudocholinesterase, metabolism occurs in the bloodstream before significant tissue uptake can occur.

In individuals with atypical plasma pseudocholinesterase, the rate of hydrolysis of the ester-linked local anesthetic is markedly decreased and a prolonged half-life of these drugs results. Therefore, while the potential for toxicity from accumulation of the ester linked local anesthetics such as 2-chloroprocaine in plasma is extremely remote in normal individuals, this likelihood should be considered in the administration of large or repeated doses of this drug to individuals with atypical pseudocholinesterase (57). In the pregnant patient, there is a 25% decrease in plasma pseudocholinesterase activity. However, this appears to be of no clinical significance, given the short plasma half-lives of the commonly used ester-linked local anesthetics.

In contrast, the amide-linked local anesthetics need to be transported by the circulation to the liver before hepatic biotransformation can take place. The two major factors controlling the clearance of the amide-linked local anesthetics by the liver are hepatic blood flow (delivery of drug to the liver) and hepatic function (drug extraction by the liver). Factors or drugs that decrease hepatic blood flow or hepatic drug extraction will result in an increase in the elimination half-life ($T_{1/2}b$) of these local anesthetics. Drugs such as general anesthetics, norepinephrine, histamine $H_2$ receptor blockers, beta blockers, and calcium channel blockers all can decrease hepatic blood flow and increase the elimination half-life of amide local anesthetics. Severe hemodynamic derangements must be present for hepatic blood flow to be affected enough to have a significant affect on local anesthetic blood levels.

Decreases in hepatic function caused by a lowering of body temperature, immaturity of the hepatic enzyme system, or liver damage such as in cirrhosis can lead to a decrease in the rate of hepatic metabolism of amide local anesthetics. The hepatic extraction ratio, clearance, and elimination half-life of amide local anesthetics in the normal adult are presented in Table 11–3.

**Table 11–3.** Pharmacokinetic Parameters of Local Anesthetics in Adults

| | Elimination half-life ($T_{1/2b}$) (min) | Volume Distribution $(V_D)_{ss}$ (liters) | Clearance (Cl) (liters/min) | Hepatic Extraction |
|---|---|---|---|---|
| Lidocaine | 96 | 91 | 1.0 | 0.7 |
| Bupivacaine | 162 | 73 | 0.6 | 0.4 |
| Mepivacaine | 114 | 84 | 0.8 | 0.5 |
| Etidocaine | 162 | 73 | 0.6 | 0.4 |

(Modified from Tucker GT: Pharmacokinetics of local anesthetics. Br. J. Anaesth. 58:717, 1986.)

Only a small fraction of local anesthetic is cleared by the kidney. Thus, renal failure has minimal impact upon the metabolism and clearance of these drugs.

## PLACENTAL TRANSFER AND FETAL/NEONATAL DISPOSITION

All local anesthetics readily cross the placenta. Thus, it becomes critically important to understand the factors that influence the amount and rate of drug transferred from the maternal circulation to the fetus. Although this topic is discussed in detail in Chapter 8 and a number of maternal factors affecting transfer have been discussed above, this subject is briefly reviewed here for the sake of emphasis and summarized in Table 11–4.

The transfer of drug from the mother to the fetus via the placenta is influenced by factors specific to each, and these will be considered in turn. However, it should be noted that there are routes other than placental transfer whereby excessive doses of local anesthetic may reach the fetus. There have been tragic cases of direct injection into the fetal brain due to misguided needle placement during attempted caudal analgesia. There have also been fetal deaths associated with paracervical blocks, possibly due to uptake by uterine blood vessels and rapid transfer to the fetus, even when the maternal doses were in a safe range (58).

### Maternal Factors

The maternal factors all have as a common endpoint the amount of local anesthetic delivered to the intervillous space of the placenta. This is determined by the absorption, distribution, metabolism, and elimination of the local anesthetic by the mother. There are some aspects of these pharmacokinetic factors that are particularly relevant to the pregnant patient, and these will be reviewed.

For any given injection site, maternal blood levels of local anesthetic are a direct consequence of the total dose of drug administered. The larger the dose, the higher will be the resulting maternal blood levels. Direct intravenous injection bypasses all absorption barriers and produces the highest maternal blood levels for a given dose of local

**Table 11–4.** Factors that Influence Placental Transfer and Fetal Disposition of Local Anesthetics

I. Maternal Factors
  A. Absorption
    1. Total amount of drug administered
    2. Vascularity of site of injection
    3. Addition of epinephrine
  B. Distribution
    1. Characteristics of drug (Ionization, lipid solubility, protein binding, etc)
    2. pH of maternal blood
    3. Distribution of cardiac output to different organs
  C. Metabolism and Elimination
  D. Uteroplacental Blood Flow
II. Placental Factors
  A. Characteristics of Placenta (Normal, pathologic)
  B. Characteristics of Local Anesthetic
    1. Molecular weight
    2. Degree of ionization
    3. Lipid solubility
    4. Spatial configuration
  C. Maternal-Fetal Concentration Gradient
III. Fetal Disposition
  A. Fetal Uptake
    1. Solubility of drug in fetal blood
    2. Quantity and distribution of fetal blood in intervillous space
    3. Concentration of drug in fetal blood returning to placenta
    4. pH of fetal blood
  B. Fetal Distribution
    1. Difference between adult and fetal circulation (see Chapter 6)
    2. Concentration of drug returning to placenta influenced by fetal circulation, fetal tissue uptake, fetal pH, protein binding, and nonplacental routes of fetal elimination
    3. Protein binding in the fetus and newborn
  C. Fetal Metabolism and Elimination

anesthetic; maternal blood levels are considerably lower following epidural, caudal, paracervical or pudendal block, and are a function of site vascularity and local tissue binding characteristics for the specific agent administered.

Vasoconstrictors such as epinephrine and phenylephrine can be used to alter the absorption profile from various injection sites for some local anesthetics. Local vasoconstriction impedes systemic absorption of lidocaine and mepivacaine, resulting in lower maternal peak blood levels and hence lower fetal levels (59). For the more lipid soluble drugs such as bupivacaine and etidocaine, tissue binding, particularly to epidural fat, is a much more significant determinant of maternal absorption than local blood flow, and hence vasoconstrictors do not appreciably alter maternal epidural absorption profiles for these drugs.

In terms of distribution, 10% of maternal cardiac output is diverted to the low-resistance uteroplacental unit during pregnancy. Intervillous blood flow is normally pressure dependent, so that maternal hypotension can affect fetal blood drug levels by decreasing uterine blood flow. Uterine vascular resistance also affects uterine blood flow. Amide local anesthetics have been shown in vitro to produce uterine artery vasoconstriction at concentrations in excess of those normally obtained clinically, but do not appear to have a significant effect upon uterine blood flow at clinically useful concentrations; in pregnant sheep, lidocaine, bupivacaine, and ropivacaine have been shown to have no significant effects on uterine blood flow or fetal condition (60,61). Epinephrine is also a known vasoconstrictor of the uterine vasculature and is frequently used with local anesthetics; however, when used in doses of less than 100 μg for epidural anesthesia, no significant effects upon uterine blood flow are noted (62).

## Placental Factors

Once the drug reaches the intervillous space, the quantity of local anesthetic transferred per unit of time is given by equation 3, which describes the diffusion of drug across, in this case, the placental membranes. The rate and amount of drug transfer depend upon the surface area of the maternal/fetal interface; the concentration of free drug on each side of the interface; the thickness of the biological membranes separating maternal and fetal blood; and a number of physicochemical properties of the drug, including molecular weight, extent of ionization, and lipid solubility.

## Fetal Disposition

The same general patterns of uptake, distribution, and elimination of local anesthetic occur in the fetus as in the mother. However, differences arise due to differences in pH, protein binding, circulation, and maturity of metabolic pathways.

## Fetal Uptake

***Ionization.*** The free fraction of local anesthetic rapidly equilibrates across the placenta, presumably crossing in the base (uncharged) form (Figure 11–11). At equilibrium, the base form will be equal in concentration on both sides of the placenta, because it can freely cross as long as there is a concentration gradient. In Figure 11–11, note that the concentration of the base form is 0.5 μg/ml in both maternal and fetal blood. However, differences in pH between maternal and fetal blood will result in differences in the amount of ionized drug in equilibrium with the base form in the mother as compared to the fetus. Because the charged species does not cross the placenta, it is possible for the free local anesthetic concentration to be higher in the fetus than that in the mother, with the degree of difference due to the degree of difference in pH. According to the Henderson-Hasselbach equation (equation 1), local anesthetics will increasingly exist in the cationic form as the environment becomes more acidic. The fetus, with a normal pH range of 7.30 to 7.35, is slightly acidotic relative to the mother and the amount of cation associated with the 0.5 μg/ml of base is 1.5 μg/ml in the fetus compared to 1.2 μg/ml in the mother. Thus, the total concentration of free lidocaine (base plus cation) in the example is 2.0 μg/ml in the fetus compared to 1.7 μg/ml in the mother.

This increased free fraction in the fetus compared to the mother will increase even further as the difference between fetal and maternal pH increases. This is illustrated in Figure 11–11 in which, as the fetus becomes more acidotic and the pH decreases to 7.0, the cationic

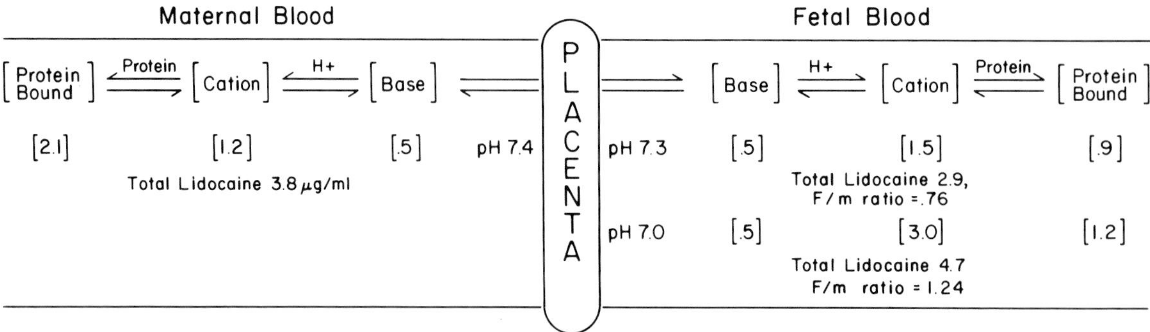


**Fig. 11–11.** Schematic of maternal/fetal transfer of lidocaine across the placenta at varying pH.

concentration in the fetus increases to 3.0 μg/ml and, even though the concentration of base remains the same, the total free drug concentration increases.

This phenomenon whereby a lower fetal pH than that in the mother increases the amount of ionized drug on the fetal side of the placenta is referred to as "ion trapping" and has been confirmed in animal studies in which direct infusions of acidic solutions into the fetus caused increases in fetal local anesthetic concentration (63). Likewise, the acidosis associated with fetal asphyxia has been shown to increase the tissue concentration (brain, heart, liver, lungs, kidneys) of lidocaine in baboons compared to values measured in nonasphyxiated fetuses (64).

***Protein Binding.*** Fetal uptake is also influenced by protein binding. Protein binding of local anesthetics is decreased in the fetus and newborn. This is due to decreased levels of alpha-1-acid glycoprotein and is age related. Alpha-1-acid glycoprotein levels in the premature infant (less than 30 weeks gestation) are half those seen in term newborns, and newborn levels are still decreased three to four times in comparison to adults (46,65). As with adults, acidosis can further decrease the fraction of protein bound drug (Figure 11–9).

***Fetal/maternal Ratios.*** The term "fetal/maternal ratio" is commonly used to describe the differential distribution of drug between the fetus and the mother. However, this term includes both free drug as well as that which is protein bound, and hence not biologically active. Protein binding is greatly decreased in the fetus. Thus, referring to Figure 11–11, when the amount of free drug is added to the amount that is protein bound in both the mother and the fetus, there is more total drug in the mother (3.8 μg/ml) than the fetus (2.9 μg/ml) at normal pH levels, resulting in a fetal/maternal ratio of 0.76 for lidocaine. With fetal acidosis (pH 7.0) the ratio shifts considerably to 1.24, as the total amount of drug in the fetus increases due to an increase in the amount of ionized drug as well as the total amount bound to protein.

For drugs that are highly protein bound, such as bupivacaine, the fetal/maternal ratios appear even more favorable than those for lidocaine in terms of large differences between maternal and fetal blood levels. However, it must be stressed that these numbers have very little clinical significance, because it is the amount of free drug that is of consequence. Maternal:fetal ratios refer to amount of total drug that equilibrates between the mother and the fetus and includes protein bound drug. However, it is the unbound form that rapidly equilibrates across the placenta and with other compartments in the fetus and, if the maternal levels of free drug are dangerously high, then the fetus will be exposed to a similar concentration.

### Fetal Distribution

The fetal circulation is unique in several respects that serve to modify drug distribution and these are discussed more fully in Chapter 7. Fetal blood from the placenta is carried by the umbilical vein; a variable portion of this blood may bypass the liver by traversing the ductus venosus, thus avoiding liver extraction before reaching the heart. The umbilical vessels empty into the inferior vena cava and blood from this vessel tends to be shunted across the foramen ovale, thus bypassing the fetal lung in reaching the left atrium. The output from the left heart goes preferentially to the fetal brain, which gets a proportionately larger share of cardiac output compared to an adult. Blood draining the brain returns to the right heart and again bypasses the lung by traversing the ductus arteriosus. This blood then is preferentially returned to the placenta via the umbilical arteries. To the extent that local anesthetic is taken up, it will be distributed in accordance with this pattern of blood flow and based upon physicochemical considerations already covered.

During acidosis, the fetus makes circulatory adjustments to maintain cerebral and myocardial blood flow at the expense of other tissues. Thus, local anesthetic delivered via the placenta will tend to be preferentially delivered to the heart and brain in situations such as asphyxia that produce fetal acidosis.

### Fetal Metabolism and Elimination

In the newborn there is typically a two- to threefold prolongation of the elimination half-life of local anesthetics (66,67). This is primarily a reflection of hepatic immaturity and a larger volume of distribution in neonates as compared to adults. For the amides, there is marked variation in elimination half-lives between agents based upon differences in the metabolic pathways used and differences in maturation of enzymes systems that make up these pathways. For example, the principal metabolic re-

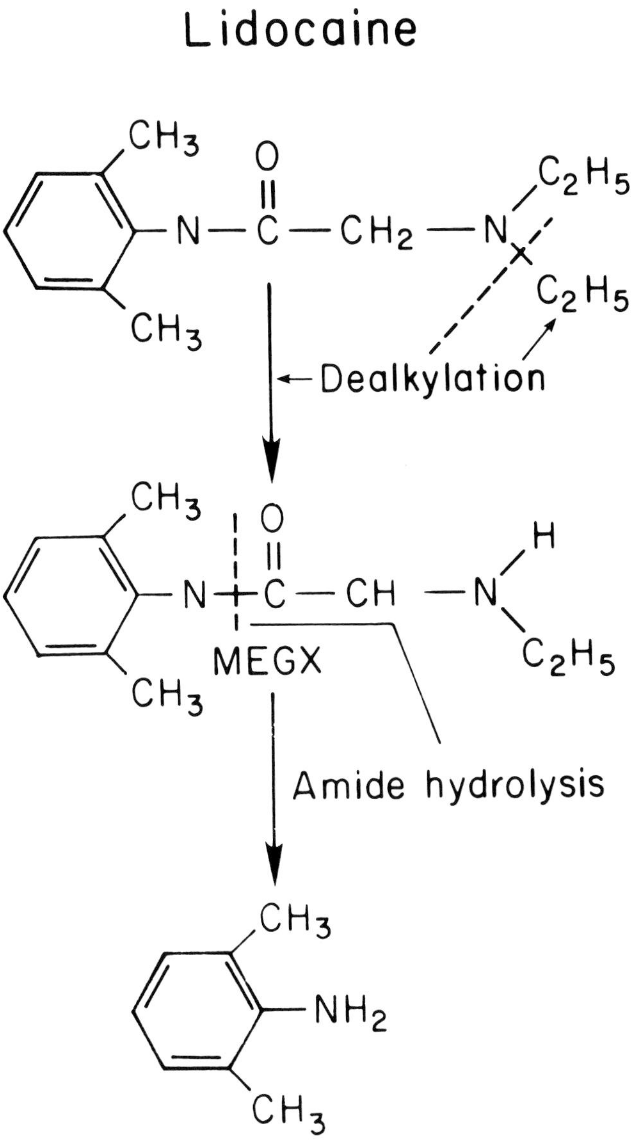

**Fig. 11–12.** Metabolism of lidocaine illustrating a dealkylating reaction.

action used for metabolism of lidocaine is dealkylation (Figure 11–12). This primary step in the biotransformation of lidocaine appears to be only slightly slower in the newborn than the adult, indicating functional maturity of this particular enzyme system. Thus, the twofold increase in the elimination half-life of lidocaine in the newborn in comparison to the adult is not due to enzymatic immaturity but rather reflects the larger volume of distribution for lidocaine in the newborn. A larger volume of distribution means that a given dose of drug will have a lower plasma concentration and thus less drug will be delivered per unit time to the liver for metabolism and to the kidney for excretion. Thus, it will take longer to clear the drug from the body.

Renal clearance of lidocaine in the adult is small (3 to 5% of the total dose administered). In contrast, in the newborn, because of decreased tubular reabsorption, approximately 20% of a lidocaine dose is excreted unchanged in the urine.

Biotransformation of bupivacaine, as with lidocaine, progresses via a dealkylation reaction as the primary step. (Figure 11–13) Because of an increased volume of distribution, a somewhat longer half-life is to be anticipated in the newborn in comparison to the adult (68).

Other hepatic enzyme systems in the newborn are not as well developed as those subserving dealkylation. Specifically, oxidative pathways involving ring oxidation or hydroxylation are characterized by slow rates of enzymatic activity in the newborn. Thus, local anesthetics that require such oxidative pathways for biotransformation can be expected to have a prolonged elimination half-life. This is seen in the case of mepivacaine, which, in the adult, is metabolized primarily by way of ring hydroxylation (Figure 11–14). The immaturity of this enzymatic mechanism in the neonate results in an elimination half-life that is five times that of an adult (69). This occurs despite a marked increase in renal clearance of unchanged mepivacaine. Repeated mepivacaine administration has been associated with poor neonatal neurobehavioral scores following delivery.

Initially, following local anesthetic administration to the mother, drug concentrations on the maternal side of

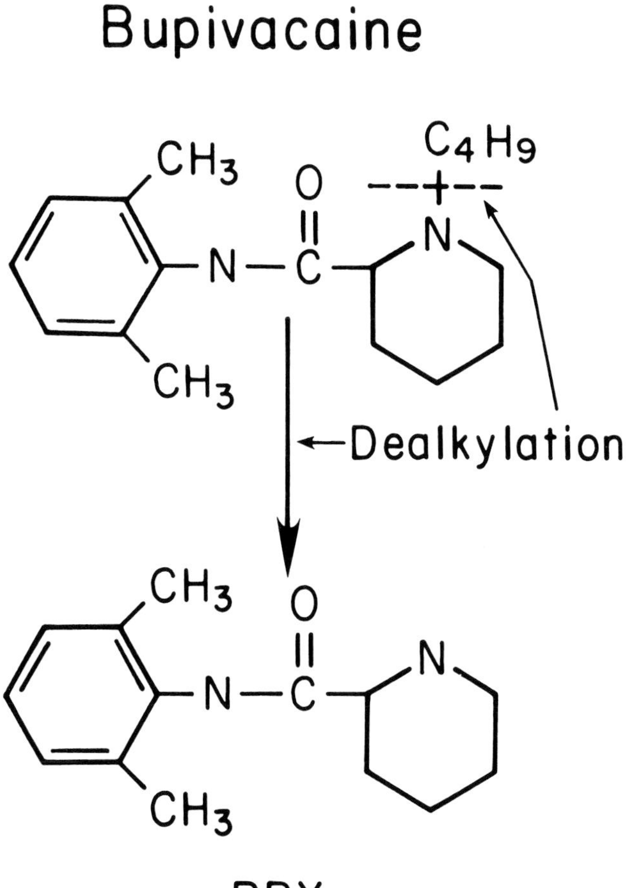

**Fig. 11–13.** Metabolism of bupivacaine.

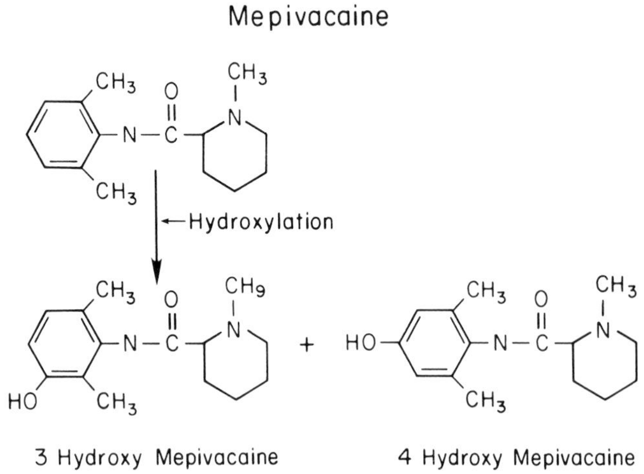

Mepivacaine

Hydroxylation

3 Hydroxy Mepivacaine 4 Hydroxy Mepivacaine

**Fig. 11–14.** Metabolism of mepivacaine illustrating the hydroxylation reaction required.

the placenta will be much higher than on the fetal side. With time, however, as the maternal levels decrease (due to further redistribution, metabolism, and elimination) drug concentration on the fetal side of the placenta may be higher, and drug will then move from the fetus to the mother. Thus, as long as the fetus is in utero, differences in biotransformation of local anesthetic are of no consequence, because, if needed, the fetus has access to the more efficient metabolic pathways of the mother. This maternal assistance is ended the moment the umbilical cord is cut.

Decreased plasma pseudocholinesterase activity in the fetus results in a twofold increase in the elimination half-life for 2-chloroprocaine. Yet, the clinical significance of this change is negligible because the elimination half-life for the newborn is still only 1 minute.

## CLINICAL CONSIDERATIONS

### *Modification of Local Anesthetic Action*

#### *Addition of Epinephrine*

In general, the addition of epinephrine increases intensity and duration of local anesthetic action (70). This effect of epinephrine has been postulated as being caused by decreased local tissue blood flow and hence decreased absorption of the local anesthetic from the site injected. This results in increased availability of the drug for diffusion into the nerve. With infiltration, this decreased absorption and increased duration occur with all local anesthetics when epinephrine is added to the local anesthetic solutions. All local anesthetics are not the same, however, when given for epidural anesthesia. Little to no change in duration of anesthesia or in the resultant blood levels is seen following epidural administration of bupivacaine or etidocaine (54) with and without epinephrine. In contrast, when lidocaine and mepivacaine are used for epidural anesthesia, the addition of epinephrine does result in increased duration and decreased blood levels in both the pregnant and the nonpregnant patient.

The usual concentration of epinephrine used in the local anesthetic solutions is 1:200,000 (5 μg/ml). Many concentrations of epinephrine have been tried; however, little difference is seen following the epidural administration of 1:200,000, 1:400,000, or 1:600,000 epinephrine solutions of lidocaine solutions (71). As even the 1; 200,000 concentration of epinephrine may not consistently identify an intravascular injection based upon increases in heart rate when used in a 3 ml test dose, use of the more dilute solutions would be even less reliable in this regard.

#### *Reducing Latency Time*

Producing an adequate level of neural blockade with a fixed dose of local anesthetic in an acceptable period of time is of concern to the clinician. To achieve this goal, various approaches have been made to manipulate the factors involved in producing anesthesia of nerves with local anesthetics. Recall that local anesthetic drugs need to be able to: (1) pass through the nerve membrane as un-ionized lipid soluble drugs, and then (2) once in the nerve axoplasm, reequilibrate into an ionic form (Figure 11–2). The rate-limiting step in this cascade is step (1) because the commercially available local anesthetic solutions contain very little drug as un-ionized base. The fraction of un-ionized base and of cationic forms present is determined by the pKa of the drug and the pH of the drug solution ($pKa = pH^{+} \log [cation/base]$). All local anesthetic solutions commercially available are acidic (low pH) (72) and exist predominantly in the cationic form, which is much more soluble and more stable than the base form. Yet, this cationic form will not cross biologic membranes readily. Thus, to increase the amount of drug in the base form, one can either alter the pH or the pKa of the solution to be injected.

***pH Adjustment.*** pH adjustment is an old technique, first reported in 1910, and more recently repopularized (25). Reports of marked decreases in onset time have been achieved when major pH changes in the local anesthetic solution injected are accomplished. This is more likely to occur when commercially available epinephrine-containing local anesthetic solutions are used, because the epinephrine requires an acidic environment for stability, and these solutions are pH adjusted to make them more acidic. DiFazio and colleagues demonstrated that a greater than 50% decrease in onset time for epidural anesthesia took place when the pH of commercially available lidocaine with epinephrine was raised from pH 4.5 to an adjusted pH level of 7.2 (66). Similarly, Hilgier reported a marked improvement in onset time for brachioplexus anesthesia when bupivacaine with epinephrine (pH 3.9) was alkalized to pH 6.4 (73). These relatively large changes in pH resulted in major increases in the amount of free base available in solution.

Plain lidocaine to which epinephrine has been freshly added has a pH of 6.5, in contrast to the 4.5 value seen in commercially available epinephrine-containing solutions. Therefore, only a small change in pH can be achieved by the addition of bicarbonate to plain lidocaine solutions, and decreases in onset time will be approximately 20%, compared to a 50% decrease when commercially available lidocaine with epinephrine is pH adjusted (65). Similarly, adjusting the pH of bupivacaine from 5.5 to the maximal level permitted by its solubility produces small changes in the fraction of free base and hence decreases in onset time are modest at best (74,75).

Increases in the amount of free base in solution achieved by increases in pH are limited by the solubility of the free base in solution. For each local anesthetic, there is a pH at which the amount of free base in solution is maximal (saturated solution). Further increases in pH will result in precipitation of the drug.

***Carbonation of Local Anesthetics.*** Another approach to shortening onset time for surgical anesthesia has been through the use of carbonated local anesthetic solutions, which at the present time are not available in the United States. In two clinical studies, Bromage found that spread of anesthesia was more extensive, and a better quality of neural blockade occurred when the carbonated rather than an uncarbonated lidocaine solution was used (76,77). Numerous animal studies using carbonated lidocaine have also shown shortened onset time and improved blockade. Clinically, a recent study by Sukhani and Winnie (78) similarly observed that when using a carbonated lidocaine with epinephrine solution, more rapid and more complete anesthesia occurred than when a comparable uncarbonated solution was used. Several explanations have been put forth to define the role of carbonation: (1) carbon dioxide may cause some degree of direct neural blockade, and (2) the increased $CO_2$ that results in the axoplasm can cause an increase in ion trapping of the local anesthetic in the axoplasm. A further contribution may result from mechanisms operational in the pH adjustment of local anesthetics, as discussed above. Solutions of carbonated lidocaine have a pH of 6.5 with a $pCO_2$ of 700 mm Hg. As the $CO_2$ is lost on opening of the vial, the pH of the solutions increases toward 7, thus modestly increasing the fraction of free base available for nerve penetration.

However, studies using carbonated bupivacaine epidurally have failed to demonstrate similar improvements. It would appear that carbonation of the local anesthetic solutions produces more pronounced effects when lidocaine is the agent compared with bupivacaine.

***Warming Local Anesthetic Solutions.*** Yet another technique that has been demonstrated to modify latency is the warming of the local anesthetic solution. Although the exact mechanism for this result is not totally clear, it would appear that it is due to the increase in the pKa of the local anesthetic that occurs with increases in temperature (Table 11–5). Again, referring to the Henderson-Hasselbach equation, an increase in pKa at a constant pH will result in an increase in the fraction of free base available. A consistently faster onset of action was seen in women having vaginal deliveries and cesarean sections when bupivacaine was warmed to 37.7° before injection (79). The duration of the anesthetic was the same, as was the degree of motor blockade and the incidence of hypotension requiring treatment when compared with patients who received bupivacaine at room temperature.

**Table 11–5.** Relationships between Temperature and pKa

| | Temperature | | |
|---|---|---|---|
| | 10° C | 25° C | 38° C |
| Lidocaine | 8.24 | 7.91 | 7.57 |
| Bupivacaine | 8.49 | 8.16 | 7.92 |
| Mepivacaine | 8.02 | 7.76 | 7.55 |
| Chloroprocaine | 9.37 | 8.97 | 8.77 |
| Procaine | 9.38 | 9.05 | 8.66 |

(From Kamaya H, Hayes JJ and Ueda, I: Dissociation constants of local anesthetics and their temperature dependence. Anesth. Analg. 62:1025, 1983.)

***Opiate Addition.*** Recently, there has been a great deal of interest in the area of intensification of regional anesthesia by the combined use of local anesthetics and opiates such as fentanyl. The original observations by Justins, et al (80,81) and of subsequent studies were that onset is more rapid and anesthesia is more complete and more prolonged when fentanyl is added to bupivacaine solutions for epidural use. Other studies have subsequently shown that very dilute solutions of local anesthetic combined with an opiate produce anesthesia that is comparable to that produced by a more concentrated solution of the same local anesthetic alone, yet with much less motor blockade. For instance, Chestnut demonstrated that a 0.0625% bupivacaine solution combined with fentanyl produced good analgesia with minimal motor blockade during labor (82).

At present labor epidural analgesia with local anesthetic alone in many institutes is being replaced with the above described dilute local anesthetic-opiate combination. Pharmacologically, opiates do not have local anesthetic activity in the concentrations administered clinically, with the exception of meperidine and methadone. The action of opiates at spinal cord receptors mediating pain in the dorsal horn of the spinal cord has been well documented. It would appear that the observed interaction of opiate and local anesthetic may be the result of a combined action in which the epidurally administered local anesthetic acts to decrease or obtund sensory input somewhere along the nerve root before it enters the spinal cord, while the opiate acts at the next synoptic region in the neural pathway for transmission of the pain stimulus, the dorsal horn of the spinal cord. The final result of improved labor analgesia and a more mobile patient with this pharmacologic combination deserves careful, further evaluation.

## COMPLICATIONS OF LOCAL ANESTHETICS

### *Central Nervous System Toxicity*

#### *Maternal Effects*

Major complications associated with the use of local anesthetics are related to the systemic effects of high blood levels of drug that may be achieved. Potentially toxic blood levels can occur whenever a drug is injected intravenously, intra-arterially, or whenever a large dose of drug is injected into a highly vascular area. The blood levels of local anesthetic are important in that they are predictive of the systemic effects that may be seen. Systemic toxicity of local anesthetic drugs occurs when certain critical levels are acutely achieved in the heart and brain. Using lidocaine as an example, blood levels of 1 to 5 μg/ml are in the therapeutic range and are sought for the treatment of arrhythmias and for supplementation of general anesthesia. At blood levels of 3 to 5 μg/ml, systemic symptoms with this drug include a metallic taste in the mouth, ringing in the ears, and circumoral numbness. In humans, serum concentrations of 10 to 12 μg/ml for lidocaine or 4 to 6 μg/ml for bupivacaine are associated with clinically evident seizure activity, assuming normal protein binding. At these levels, there is selective blockade of inhibitory pathways in the brain, allowing facilitatory neurons to function unopposed. The seizures appear to originate in the amygdala and hypocampus and then spread to the cortex (83). The signs and symptoms that precede the onset of seizures usually include slow speech, jerky movements, tremors, and hallucinations. These warning signs and symptoms of high blood levels are most commonly seen with lidocaine and less frequently seen when bupivacaine or etidocaine is the offending agent.

The effect of lidocaine and most local anesthetics on the brain is triphasic: at low blood levels the drugs have an anticonvulsant action; as the concentration of the drug increases in blood and brain, seizures will occur, and at very high blood levels, there is global CNS depression and seizures will be suppressed (84). However, at these high levels one can expect cardiotoxicity, and the detrimental effects on the brain will be a function of the inadequacy of cardiac output and cerebral blood flow.

Pregnancy does not appear to confer an increased risk of central nervous system toxicity in association with high plasma levels of lidocaine or mepivacaine. No differences in blood or brain concentrations of lidocaine were found when seizures were induced using this drug in pregnant and nonpregnant rats (85), and no differences in plasma lidocaine (86) or mepivacaine (37) levels were reported when pregnant versus nonpregnant sheep were given doses of local anesthetic sufficient to cause seizures. This is consistent with the earlier discussion of changes in protein binding in pregnancy (Figures 11–6, 11–7, and 11–8). At the plasma levels at which central nervous system toxicity with lidocaine or mepivacaine occurs (greater than 10 to 15 μg/ml), albumin is the major binding protein and the capacity of albumin is apparently increased in pregnancy (41).

When highly protein-bound drugs such as bupivacaine are used in pregnancy, the risk for CNS toxicity may be increased. Pregnancy is associated with a 30% decrease in protein binding of bupivacaine in sheep; (an almost identical decrease was noted in the dose of intravenous bupivacaine necessary to produce convulsions in sheep when nonpregnant sheep (2.7 mg/kg) were compared to pregnant sheep (1.9 mg/kg) (37). It would appear that decreased protein binding during pregnancy allows for higher brain levels of bupivacaine for a given dose of drug.

Somewhat surprisingly, this does not appear to be true for ropivacaine, a drug that is similar to bupivacaine in terms of potency. In sheep, pregnancy is not associated with changes in the protein binding of this drug as it is for bupivacaine, and there is no difference in the dose of ropivacaine necessary to produce seizures in pregnant animals versus nonpregnant ones (87). Ropivacaine is around 50% less lipid soluble than bupivacaine, and its protein binding in sheep more closely resembles that of intermediate-potency agents such as lidocaine in humans. For example, at a serum concentration of 1.7 μg/ml, ropivacaine is 65% protein bound in both pregnant and nonpregnant sheep; at a serum concentration of 9.0 μg/ml, ropivacaine is approximately 50% protein bound in sheep regardless of pregnancy. Referring to Figure 11–5, it can be seen that the protein binding of lidocaine in humans is almost identical to that of ropivacaine in sheep. Thus, in both nonpregnant humans (88) and sheep (87), ropivacaine appears to have less central nervous system toxicity than equipotent doses of bupivacaine, and pregnancy does not seem to enhance the brain toxicity of ropivacaine as it does for bupivacaine.

### Fetal Effects

Sensitivity of the fetal central nervous system to local anesthetics was evaluated by Teramo, et al by infusing lidocaine directly into fetal lambs of varying gestational ages (89). A negative correlation for age and blood concentration at the onset of seizures was observed with the least mature fetal lambs requiring the highest concentration to produce seizures and the lowest seizure-inducing concentration being seen in the full-term lamb. The blood concentration in the full term lamb was also found to be somewhat higher than that required in adult sheep to produce seizures. This would suggest that the risk in the fetus for local anesthetic induced seizures is no greater than that in the mother, and may be less.

### Treatment

Treatment of local anesthetic seizures consists primarily of preventing the detrimental effects of hypoxia. Therefore, adequate ventilation with 100% oxygen must be first established (90) and the airway protected with cricoid pressure, at a minimum; then, suppression of seizures can be achieved by raising the seizure threshold with a CNS sedating drug such as thiopental (50 to 100 mg), diazepam (5 to 10 mg), or midazolam (1 to 2 mg). Cardiac output and cerebral blood flow normally increase during seizure activity, so that high maternal brain levels of local anesthetic resulting from an intravenous injection will decrease rapidly due to redistribution. However, if the local anesthetic levels are high enough to cause significant cardiac toxicity, and cardiac output is greatly diminished, then this redistribution will not occur. The use of thiopental to treat seizures in the situation of concurrent cardiac toxicity is of concern because this drug can further depress myocardial function and, hence, should be administered judiciously, if at all. Patients with severe toxicity warrant tracheal intubation, and succinylcholine used for this purpose provides the additional benefit of terminating the tonic-clonic muscle activity. Failure to stop seizure activity at the earliest possible moment will lead to progressive acidosis, a condition that may further potentiate toxicity by increasing the intracellular fraction of ionized drug, as discussed earlier. Succinylcholine does not stop neuronal seizure activity. This may be clinically significant in cases in which cardiac output and oxygen delivery are impaired during a time of increased metabolic activity (and increased oxygen need) in the central nervous system. In this circumstance, it is important to treat the CNS seizure activity in a paralyzed patient.

### Cardiovascular Toxicity

Concern for the cardiac toxicity of the long acting local anesthetics, particularly bupivacaine and etidocaine, developed following numerous reports of maternal cardiac arrest followed by difficult and often unsuccessful resuscitations (1). In all cases, the patients apparently had excessively high serum levels of local anesthetic, either due to an unintended intravascular injection of a large amount of drug or premature release of a tourniquet following intravenous regional anesthesia. Numerous animal studies have subsequently provided further insight into the cardiac toxicity of different local anesthetic drugs.

### Mechanism of Action

All local anesthetics cause a dose-dependent depression of contractility in cardiac tissue (91,92). This cardiodepressant effect on contractility of cardiac muscle parallels anesthetic potency in blocking peripheral nerves (93). Thus, bupivacaine, which is four times more potent than lidocaine, is also four times more cardiodepressant (94,95). However, human death in cases of bupivacaine overdose is usually characterized by progressive prolongation of ventricular conduction time (widened QRS complex) followed by the sudden onset of ventricular fibrillation. It is theorized that the delay in ventricular conduction predisposes to reentrant phenomena. Experimental studies have shown that all local anesthetics cause a dose-dependent depression of conduction velocity (intra-atrial, A-V nodal, His-Purkinje, intraventricular) in cardiac tissue. When this potential for electrophysiologic toxicity (reentrant arrhythmias, as opposed to cardiodepressant toxicity) has been studied, bupivacaine has been shown to be, on average, 16 times more toxic than lidocaine and approximate two times more toxic than ropivacaine (95).

In vitro studies have demonstrated that local anesthetics block cardiac sodium channels as well as cardiac calcium channels, and that blockade of these channels is better tolerated for lidocaine than for bupivacaine. The best current explanation for the differences seen in the toxicity of these agents has been put forth by Clarkson and Hondeghem (96). They theorize that during systole (depolarization of cardiac tissue) lidocaine rapidly enters the sodium channel; during diastole, lidocaine rapidly dissociates from the sodium channel and there is no accumulation of block at normal heart rates. This pattern of movement is referred to as fast in/fast out and produces minimal cardiac blocking effects, as long as the heart rate is not so fast as to allow insufficient time for the drug to dissociate from the sodium channel during diastole. In contrast, bupivacaine (in high concentration) also rapidly enters sodium channels during systole but, most likely due to differences in binding, it is slow to leave during diastole (fast in/slow out) and thus strongly blocks inactivated open channels and does not allow for recovery during diastole. This in turn leads to susceptibility to reentrant arrhythmias and can lead to fibrillation.

Some investigators have speculated that the cardiac dysrhythmias associated with local anesthetics may be mediated by local anesthetic effects on the CNS, based upon animal studies in which local anesthetic infused into the ventricles of the brain produced cardiac tachyarrhythmias, with bupivacaine having a much greater tendency to do so than lidocaine (97,98). While direct CNS effects cannot be excluded, an animal model in which local anesthetics are injected directly into the left anterior descending coronary artery (LAD) has allowed study of the direct effects upon the left ventricle (95). Independent of CNS effects, local anesthetics administered into the left anterior descending coronary artery cause slowing of ventricular conduction and, at sufficient doses, ventricular fibrillation.

### Effects of Acidosis and Hypoxia

Increases in the cardiac toxicity of local anesthetics may be further enhanced when acidosis, hypoxia, hypercarbia or hyperkalemia is present (99–101). In addition to membrane effects, acidosis may enhance toxicity by affecting ionization and protein binding. As discussed earlier, acidosis decreases the protein binding of local anesthetics, thus increasing the free, active fraction; at the same time, acidosis shifts the equilibrium toward the ionized form, which tends to prevent transmembrane passage. Thus, in the case of high serum levels following an accidental intravascular injection, there is rapid movement of local anesthetic into neural cells and cardiac cells. If the brain levels are high enough, seizures will occur. The resultant combined metabolic and respiratory acidosis leads to a rapid decrease in pH (from normal to 7.0 in less than two minutes) (102). The fall in intracellular pH increases the amount of ionized, biologically active drug relative to the base form, so there is more potential for interaction with the sodium channel.

Overdoses of bupivacaine have resulted in a clinical picture of cardiovascular collapse, in which drug-induced myocardial depression is accompanied by acidosis and hypoxia, which in turn leads to vasodilatation and extreme hypotension. It is unlikely that the vasodilatation is the result of circulating local anesthetic, because animal studies have shown that these agents actually produce vasoconstriction at the levels associated with clinical toxicity, and that vasodilatation does not occur until levels several orders of magnitude higher are achieved (103).

### Effects of Pregnancy

Cardiac toxicity of the long acting agents may be further enhanced in the pregnant patient. Significantly lower doses of bupivacaine are required to produce cardiovascular collapse in pregnant ewes compared to nonpregnant sheep (36). The free fraction of bupivacaine has been found to be 50% in pregnant sheep at serum concentrations associated with cardiovascular collapse, compared to a free fraction of 33% in nonpregnant animals at this high concentration. Tissue levels of bupivacaine in sheep were essentially the same for pregnant and nonpregnant animals given a dose sufficient to cause circulatory collapse, even though the mean dose required was 5.1 mg/kg in the pregnant animals and 8.9 mg/kg in the nonpregnant ones. The increased sensitivity of pregnant patients to local anesthetic toxicity may be a function of decreased protein binding with an increased fraction of free drug, as discussed earlier. Other factors, such as possible hormonally induced alterations in neural sensitivity (104), membrane permeability (105) or progesterone-increased cardiac sensitivity (106) may also contribute to toxicity. Again, it should be noted that these factors do not appear to influence the toxicity of ropivacaine.

If collapse does occur in a pregnant patient therapy should be directed toward reestablishing gas exchange and circulation by cardiopulmonary resuscitation. The airway should be protected by a cuffed endotracheal tube at the earliest possible moment. This should be done while chest compressions are initiated and epinephrine is administered. Attention to restoration of circulation must not be delayed, because to do so will allow progression of the acidosis and a worsening of toxicity. Resuscitation of the parturient is complicated by the problem of inferior vena cava obstruction caused by the uterus in the supine position. To overcome this problem, either the fetus should be delivered immediately or the legs should be lifted to a near vertical position, and the uterus manually displaced to the left. Vigorous volume therapy may be necessary to restore cardiac output in the vasodilated state produced by local anesthetic toxicity. Successful animal resuscitations following massive bupivacaine overdose have required multiple doses of epinephrine and atropine when indicated for bradycardia. It is desirous to administer epinephrine into the central circulation, if possible. Bretylium has been suggested as an alternative to lidocaine in the treatment of serious ventricular arrhythmias arising from local anesthetic overdose (107).

## *Administration and Safety*

Systemic toxicity is directly related to blood levels of local anesthetics. The potential for producing systemic toxicity can be significantly reduced in the clinical situation by careful attention to the following details:

1. Select a dose that should be associated with a clinically safe blood level based on the site of injection. As a general rule, the maximum drug dose administered should be selected so that the peak blood concentration that is achieved does not exceed ½ to ⅔ of the convulsant blood level. Suggested maximum doses for epidural administration are indicated in Table 11–6.
2. Administer the dose of drug in a manner that will identify an unintended intravascular injection and minimize the volume of drug injected. This is achieved by adhering to the practice of fractionating the dose of local anesthetic, aspirating frequently during injection, and maintaining verbal contact with the patient. The latter is essential in identify early subjective sensations such as circumoral tingling and ringing in the ears that are associated with an unintentional intravascular injection of local anesthetic. The addition of epinephrine in a 1:200,000 concentration to a small first dose—test dose—also has been advocated to allow for the more rapid recognition of intravascular injections. An alternative agent that has been proposed is isoproteranol. The advantages it potentially offers, compared to epinephrine, are more specific chronotropic effects (Beta-1) and the absence of alpha adrenergic activity, thus eliminating concerns for uterine artery constriction.

**Table 11–6.** Recommended Epidural Doses of Local Anesthetics for Cesarean Section

| | Suggested** Initial Dose (mg) | Approx Peak Blood Level (μg/ml) | Recommended Maximum Initial Dose (μg/Kg) | Approx Peak Blood (μg/ml) |
|---|---|---|---|---|
| 2-chloroprocaine (3%) | 600 | — | 20 | — |
| Lidocaine (2% with 1 : 200,000 Epi) | 400 | 3–4 | 7 | 5–6 |
| Bupivacaine | 100 | 1.8–1.0 | 2 | 1.5–2.0 |

Average heights in pregnant females is 62–68 inches. Dose may be increased 20% for patients above 68 inches in height.
** Initial dose should be administered incrementally, checking frequently for signs and symptoms of toxicity or subarachnoid block.

In the obstetrical patient there is good documentation that a reduced dose of epidural local anesthetic drug is indicated. Past observations by Crawford (108) and later by Bromage (109) have demonstrated that a 30 to 35% greater spread occurs in obstetrical patients receiving either a caudal or an epidural anesthetic with a fixed volume/dose in comparison to a nonpregnant adult. For many years, the prevailing explanation for this increased spread theorized that obstruction to venous return by the enlarging uterus increased blood flow through alternate venous pathways, including the azygous and intravertebral plexi, which pass through the epidural space. Because the epidural space is a semi-rigid one, it was postulated that venous engorgement in this space should decrease the remaining potential epidural volume and favor an exaggerated spread from a fixed dose of local anesthetic. This theory, however, fails to account for the fact that these engorged veins may actually potentiate systemic uptake of local anesthetic from the epidural space, an effect that would tend to limit spread. This theory also fails to explain the fact that increased spread of epidural analgesia after a fixed dose is seen in the first trimester of pregnancy, before significant venous engorgement in the epidural space (110).

Thus, factors other than venous engorgement must be considered, and an alternative hypothesis has been put forward by Datta, et al (105,106). Using a rabbit vagus nerve model, bupivacaine was observed to produce a much more rapid onset of anesthesia in the vagus nerve of the pregnant animal in comparison to those animals that were not pregnant. They postulated that increases in the hormones of pregnancy, and most likely progesterone, increase the transneuronal diffusion of the local anesthetic and therefore increase neuronal sensitivity. This increased sensitivity probably also accounts for the decreased dosage requirements for spinal anesthetics in the pregnant patient.

All of the above support the initial statement that the dose required and that which should be used for epidural analgesia is significantly less in the pregnant patient than in other comparable patients.

## CLINICAL APPLICATION

### *Vaginal Delivery*

The maternal and fetal effects of local anesthetics have already been discussed and certainly the complications mentioned for each are to be avoided. The clinical use of the local anesthetics must meet the conditions of safety for the fetus and the mother before they are used at all. There is no question that complications can occur despite the best intentions by the physician due to unexpected idiosyncratic reactions of the mother or even due to an unexpected vascular uptake. The fact that complications can and will occur must be accepted by the physicians practicing in this area, and those facts must also be mentioned to the mother to fulfill a legitimate informed consent before a local anesthetic is administered. The anesthesiologist may quote the statistics for complications from the literature, or he/she may mention what the complications have been locally in his/her center over the years of practice. What is important is that the physician administering such anesthetics be alert to the detection, diagnosis, and immediate treatment of any and all complications as they arise. With the exception of the cardiac arrests with bupivacaine, other local anesthetic complications, if diagnosed and treated early, have been able to be reversed successfully. And when taken in the light of today's practice of small dosage delivery, this provides even a greater degree of safety for the mother and fetus. As mentioned, the use of the epidural method in labor today has undergone dramatic changes over just the last decade such that very small amounts of drug are now used and the effect on both the fetus and the mother are negligible. Thus, the preferred method is the lumbar epidural with small doses given via the pump on a continuous delivery system. For the most part, this is on a preset delivery amount somewhere in the range of 8 to 10 ml per hour. However, there have been some who have advocated the pump as a patient-controlled epidural by allowing the patient to over-ride the continuous delivery with a bolus amount as desired.

The local anesthetic agents used today are classified in one of two groups: (1) the ester-linked agents, and (2) the amide-linked agents. The esters are metabolized in the bloodstream by the enzyme pseudocholinesterase. They have lower molecular weights, higher lipid solubility, higher ionization, moderate protein binding,and pass the placental barrier with less ease. The common ester-ype derivatives include tetracaine and chloroprocaine. Tetracaine has been the most popular drug used for spinal blocks and still maintains high popularity even today. Chloroprocaine was very popular in the 1970s but after reports of nerve damage with the drug implicated in spinal spillage and animal documentation of nerve damage, the drug fell into disfavor. It is only now being used once again after production without the preservative metabisulfite. The amides are metabolized by the liver and have more complex radicals so as to prolong their biological effect. They have higher molecular weights, lower lipid solubility, lesser ionization, higher protein binding,and pass the placental barrier with lesser ease. The common amide-ype derivatives include bupivacaine and lidocaine. They are today, by far, the most popular local anesthetics used in labor for the first and second stages. Today,these local anesthetic agents are mixed with other potent agents such as opioids or vasoconstrictors and often administered over time via some type of pump mechanism.

The pharmacokinetics of the local anesthetic agents mentioned above are important to summarize for the clinician. Molecular weight, lipid solubility, ionization, and protein binding are all important because of their varying degree of placental solubility. Protein binding does not effect the placental transference of local anesthetics; however, the greater uptake of the highly bound agents will have lower fetal blood levels due to the fact that they have bound to fetal tissues and are thus not available for blood level results. Refer to Table 11–7 for a comparison of these pharmacokinetic features.

### *Cesarean Section*

The anesthetic technique and the agents used for cesarean section are for the most part the same as the ones mentioned for labor and delivery. What is different is the concentration of the drug. For the analgesic effect and for the muscle relaxant effect, lidocaine is used in the 2% form and bupivacaine in the 0.5% form for epidurals; for spinal block, tetracaine in the 1% concentration or bupivacaine in the 0.75% concentration is used. Since the first edition of this book, there have been many articles written to extoll the salient features of the epidural technique or the spinal technique for use in cesarean section. In those earlier days, often the epidural technique was performed by injection of the entire amount of local anesthetic into the epidural space after administration of the test dose. Likewise, the spinal technique was performed by injection of the entire amount of local anesthetic into the subarachnoid space at the time of spinal puncture. Now both techniques have been modified so that the epidural is always done with a catheter with slow injection of the local anesthetic over time until the desired level is attained; further, the spinal is now sometimes done with a catheter with fractionated levels administered over time until the de-

**Table 11–7.** Clinical Characteristics and Concentrations of Local Anesthetics

| Generic Name Proprietary Name | Procaine (Novocaine) | 2-Chloroprocaine (Nesacaine) | Lidocaine (Xylocaine) | Mepivacaine (Carbocaine) | Tetracaine (Pontocaine) | Bupivacaine (Marcaine) | Etidocaine (Duranest) |
|---|---|---|---|---|---|---|---|
| Anesthetic Potency Ratio | 1 | 2 | 3 | 3 | 15 | 15 | 15 |
| Latency | Moderate | Fast | Fast | Moderate | Very Slow | Fast | Very Fast |
| Penetrance | Moderate | Marked | Marked | Moderate | Poor | Moderate | Moderate |
| Duration | Short | Very Short | Moderate | Moderate | Long | Long | Long |
| (Ratio) | 1 | 0.75 | 2 | 2 | 6–8 | 6–8 | 6–8 |
| Infiltration | 0.5 | 0.5 | 0.25 | 0.25 | 0.05 | 0.05 | 0.1 |
| Field Block | 0.75 | 0.75 | 0.5 | 0.5 | 0.1 | 0.1 | 0.2 |
| Pudendal/ Paracervical | 1.5 | 1.5 | 0.75–1.0 | 0.75–1.0 | 0.15 | 0.125 | 0.37 |
| Extradural Block | | | | | | | |
| Analgesia | 1.0 | 1.0 | 0.5–1.0 | 0.5–1.0 | 0.1–0.2 | 0.125–0.25 | 0.5–0.75 |
| Motor Block | 3 | 3 | 2 | 2 | 0.4 | 0.5–0.75 | 1.0–1.5 |
| Maximum Amount (mg/kg) | 12 | 15 | 6 | — | 2 | 2 | 2 |

sired level is attained. These modifications have diminished the incidence of the complication of hypotension in both techniques. It is even difficult today to say one technique is beneficial over the other. Certainly, if the epidural is now compared to the single-shot spinal, one could predict a higher proportion of patients with hypotension with the latter due to the more rapid onset of the sympathetic block. In addition, some mothers prefer to have less of a profound sensory block of their legs, which is more common with the spinal technique. Finally, with the addition of fentanyl 50 μg per 10 ml of local anesthetic in the epidural technique, the intensity of the sensory block is equal to that found with the spinal technique with regard to intra-abdominal manipulation, so the epidural can be viewed as being on an equal par with spinals as far as analgesia potency.

## REFERENCES


1. Albright GA: Cardiac arrest following regional anesthesia with etidocaine or bupivacaine. Anesthesiology (Editorial) 51:285, 1978.

1A. Skou JC: The identification of the sodium-pump as the membrane-bound Na + /K + -ATPase: a commentary on 'The Influence of Some Cations on an Adenosine Triphosphatase from Peripheral Nerves.' Biochim. Biophys. Acta. 1000, 1989, pp. 435–8.

2. Hille B: Common mode of action of three agents that decrease the transient change in sodium permeability in nerves. Nature 210:1220, 1966.
3. Rang HP, Ritchie JM: On the electrogenic sodium pump in mammalian non-myelinated nerve fibers and its activation by various cations. J. Physiol. 196:183, 1968.
4. Butterworth JF, Strichartz GR: Molecular mechanisms of local anesthesia: a review. Anesthesiology 72:711, 1990.
5. Hille B: Local anesthetics: hydrophilic and hydrophobic pathways for the drug-receptor reaction. J. Gen. Physiol. 69:497, 1977.
6. Drachman D, Strichartz G: Potassium channel blockers potentiate impulse inhibition by local anesthetics. Anesthesiology 75:1051, 1991.
7. Chernoff DM, Strichartz GR: Kinetics of local anesthetic inhibition of neuronal sodium currents. pH and hydrophobicity dependence. Biophys. J. 58:69, 1990.
8. Ruff RL: The kinetics of local anesthetic blockade of endplate channels. Biophys. J. 37:625, 1982.
9. Frelin C, Vigne P, Pazdunski M: Biochemical evidence for pharmacological similarities between a-adrenoreceptors and voltage-dependent $Na^+$ and $Ca^{++}$ channels. Biochem. Biophys. Res. Commun. 106:967, 1982.
10. Strichartz GR, Sanchez V, Arthur R, Chafetz R, et al: Fundamental properties of local anesthetics. II. Measured octanol: buffer partition coefficients and pKa values of clinically used drugs. Anesth. Analg. 71:158, 1990.
11. Luduena FP, Bogado EF, Tullar BF: Optical isomers of mepivacaine and bupivacaine. Arch. Int. Pharmacodyn. Ther. 200:359, 1972.
12. Aberg G: Toxicological and local anesthetic effects of optically active isomers of two local anaesthetic compounds. Acta. Pharmacol. Toxicol. 31:273, 1972.
13. Akerman B, Hellberg IB, Trossvik C: Primary evaluation of the local anesthetic properties of the amino amide agent ropivacaine (LEA 103). Acta. Anaesthesiol. Scand. 32:571, 1988.
14. Reiz S, Haggmark S, Johansson G, Nath S: Cardiotoxicity of ropivacaine-a new amide local anaesthetic agent. Acta. Anaesthesiol. Scand. 33:93, 1989.
15. Kopacz DJ, Carpenter RL, Mackey DC: Effect of ropivacaine on cutaneous capillary blood flow in pigs. Anesthesiology 71:69,1989.
16. Rosenberg PH, Kytta J, Alila A: Absorption of bupivacaine, etidocaine, lignocaine, and ropivacaine into n-heptane, rat sciatic nerve, and human extradural and subcutaneous fat. Br. J. Anaesth. 58:310, 1986.
17. Lee-Son S, Wang GK, Concus A, Crill E, et al: Stereoselective inhibition of neuronal sodium channels by local anesthetics. Anesthesiology 77:324, 1992.
18. Vree TB, Beumer EMC, Lagerwerf AJ, Simon MAM: Clinical pharmacokinetics of R(+) and S(−)-mepivacaine after high doses of racemic mepivacaine with epinephrine in the combined psoas compartment/sciatic nerve block. Anesth. Analg. 75:75, 1992.
19. Ackerman B: Uptake and retention of the enantiomers of a local anesthetic in isolated nerve in relation to different degrees of blocking of nervous conduction. Acta. Pharmacol. et Toxicol. 32:225, 1973.

20. Courtney KR: Size-dependent kinetics associated with drug block of sodium currents. Biophys. J. 45:422, 1984.
21. Moore RA, Bullingham RES, McQuay HJ, Hand CW, et al: Dural permeability to narcotics:in vitro determination and application to extradural administration. Br. J. Anaesth. 54: 1117, 1982.
22. Bernards CM, Hill HF: Physical and chemical properties of drug molecules governing their diffusion through the spinal meninges. Anesthesiology 77:750, 1992.
23. Strichartz GR: The inhibition of sodium currents in myelinated nerve by quaternary derivatives of lidocaine. J. Gen. Physiol. 62:37, 1973.
24. Hille B: The pH-dependent rate of action of local anesthetics on the node of Ranvier. J. Gen. Physiol. 69:475, 1977.
25. DiFazio CA, Carron H, Grosslight KR, Moscicki JC, et al: Comparison of pH-adjusted lidocaine solutions for epidural anesthesia. Anesth. Analg. 65:760, 1986.
26. Van de Waterbeemd H, Testa B: The parametrization of lipophilicity and other structural properties in drug design. Adv. in Drug Res. 6:85,1987.
27. Bernards CM, Hill HF: Morphine and alfentanil permeability through the spinal dura, arachnoid and pia mater of dogs and monkeys. Anesthesiology 73:1214, 1990.
28. Wood M: Plasma drug binding: implications for anesthesiologists. Anesth. Analg. 65:786, 1986.
29. Marathe PH, Shen DD, Artru AA, Bowdle A: Effect of serum protein binding on the entry of lidocaine into brain and cerebrospinal fluid in dogs. Anesthesiology 75:804, 1991.
30. Wood M: Plasma binding and limitation of drug access to site of action (editorial). Anesthesiology 75:721, 1991.
31. Tucker GT, Mather LE: Pharmacokinetics of local anesthetic agents. Brit J Anaesth 47:213, 1975.
31A. Berde CB: Toxicity of local anesthetics in infants and children. J. Pediatr. 122(5), 1993, pp. S14–20.
32. Kremer JMH, Wilting J, Janssen LHM: Drug binding to human alpha-1-acid glycoprotein in health and disease. Pharmacol. Rev. 41:1, 1988.
33. Wulf H, Winckler K, Denzer D: Plasma concentrations of alpha-1-acid glycoprotein following operations and its effect on the plasma protein binding of bupivacaine. Prog. Clin. Biol. Res. 300:457, 1989.
34. Denson DD, Mazoit JX: Physiology, pharmacology, and toxicity of local anesthetics: adult and pediatric considerations. *In* Clinical Practice of Regional Anesthesia. Edited by PP Raj. New York, Churchill Livingstone, 1991, p. 83.
35. Denson D, Coyle D, Thompson G, Myers J: Alpha-1-acid glycoprotein and albumin in human serum bupivacaine binding. Clin. Pharmacol. Ther. 35:409, 1984.
36. Morishima HO, Pedersen H, Finster M, Hiraoka H, et al: Bupivacaine toxicity in pregnant and nonpregnant ewes. Anesthesiology 63:134, 1985.
37. Santos AC, Pedersen H, Harmon TW, Morishima HO, et al: Does pregnancy alter the systemic toxicity of local anesthetics? Anesthesiology 70:991, 1989.
38. Burney RG, DiFazio CA, Foster JA: Effects of pH on protein binding of lidocaine. Anesth Analg 57:478, 1978.
39. McNamara PJ, Slaughter RL, Pieper JA, Wyman MG, et al: Factors influencing serum protein binding of lidocaine in humans. Anesth. Analg. 60:395, 1981.
40. Nancarrow C, Runciman WB, Mather LE, Upton RN, et al: The influence of acidosis on the distribution of lidocaine and bupivacaine into the myocardium and brain of the sheep. Anesth. Analg. 66:925,1987.
41. Denson D, Coyle D, Thompson G, Santos D, et al: Bupivacaine protein binding in the term parturient: effects of lactic acidosis. Clin. Pharmacol. Ther. 35:702, 1984.
42. Ganrot PO: Variation of the concentration of some plasma proteins in normal adults, in pregnant women, and in newborns. Scand. J. Clin. Lab. Invest. 29(suppl. 124):83, 1972.
43. Bottorf MB, Pieper JA, Boucher BA, Hoon TJ, et al: Lidocaine protein binding in preeclampsia. Eur. J. Clin. Pharmacol. 31:719, 1987.
44. Hinnerk W, Munstedt P, Maier C: Alpha-1-acid glycoprotein and protein binding of bupivacaine in the plasma of pregnant women at term. Prog. Clin. Biol. Res. 300:461, 1989.
45. Wood M, Wood AJJ: Changes in plasma drug binding and alpha-1-acid glycoprotein in mother and newborn infant. Clin. Pharmacol. Ther. 29:522, 1981.
46. Coyle DE, Denson DD, Essell SK, Santos DJ: The effect of nonesterified fatty acids and progesterone on bupivacaine protein binding. Clin. Pharmacol. Ther. 39:559, 1986.
47. Rigler ML, Drasner K: Distribution of catheter-injected local anesthetic in a model of the subarachnoid space. Anesthesiology 75:684, 1991.
48. Burn JM, Guyer PB, Langdon L: The spread of solutions injected into the epidural space. Brit. J. Anaesth. 45:338, 1973.
49. Katz JA, Bridenbaugh PO, Knarr DC, Helton SH, et al: Pharmacodynamics and pharmacokinetics of epidural ropivacaine in humans. Anesth. Analg. 70:16, 1990.
50. Scott DB, Jepson PJ, Braid DP, Ortengren B, et al: Factors affecting plasma levels of lidocaine and prilocaine. Brit. J. Anaesth. 44:1040, 1972.
51. Covino BG, Vassallo HG: Local Anesthetics: Mechanisms of Action and Clinical Use. New York, Grune & Stratton, 1976, p. 97.
52. Giasi RM, D'Agostino E, Covino BG: Absorption of lidocaine following subarachnoid and epidural administration. Anesth. Analg. 58:360,1979.
53. Reynolds F: A comparison of the potential toxicity of bupivacaine, lidocaine, and mepivacaine during epidural blockade for surgery. Brit. J. Anaesth. 43:567–571, 1971.
54. Lund PC, Bush DF, Covino BG: Determinants of etidocaine concentration in the blood. Anesthesiology 42:497, 1975.
55. Jorfeldt L, Lewis DH, Lofstrom JB, Post C: Lung uptake of lidocaine in healthy volunteers. Acta. Anaesthesiol. Scand. 23:567, 1979.
56. Scott DB, Lee A, Fagan D, Bowler GMR, et al: Acute toxicity of ropivacaine compared with that of bupivacaine. Anesth. Analg. 69:563, 1989.
57. Smith AR, Hur D, Resano F: Grand mal seizures after 2-chloroprocaine epidural anesthesia in a patient with plasma cholinesterase deficiency. Anesth. Analg. 66:677, 1987.
58. Rosefsky JB, Petersiel ME: Perinatal deaths associated with mepivacaine paracervical block anesthesia in labor. New Eng. J. Med. 278:530, 1968.
58A. Phillipson EH, Kuhnert BR, Syracuse CB, Reese AL, Rosen MG: Intrapartum paracervical block anesthesia with 2-chloroprocaine. Am. J. Obstet. Gynecol. 146(1), 1983, pp. 16–22.
59. Abboud TK, David S, Nagappala S, Constandi J, et al: Maternal, fetal and neonatal effects of lidocaine with and without epinephrine for epidural anesthesia in obstetrics. Anesth. Analg. 63:973, 1984.
60. Biehl D, Schnider SM, Levinson G, Callender K: The direct effects of circulating lidocaine on uterine blood flow and foetal well-being in the pregnant ewe. Can. Anaesth. Soc. J. 24:445, 1977.
61. Santos AC, Arthur GR, Roberts DJ, Wlody D, et al: Effect of ropivacaine and bupivacaine on uterine blood flow in pregnant ewes. Anesth. Analg. 74: 62, 1992.

62. Albright GA, Jouppila R, Hollmen AL, Jouppila P, et al: Epinephrine does not alter human intervillous blood flow during epidural anesthesia. Anesthesiology 54:131, 1981.
63. Diehl D, Shnider SM, Levinson G, Callender K: Placental transfer for lidocaine: effects of fetal acidosis. Anesthesiology 48:409, 1978.
64. Morishima HO, Covino BG: Toxicity and distribution of lidocaine in nonasphyxiated baboon fetuses. Anesthesiology 54:182, 1981.
65. Lerman J, Strong HA, LeDez KM, Swartz J, et al.: Effects of age on the serum concentration of alpha-1-acid glycoprotein and the binding of lidocaine in pediatric patients. Clin. Pharmacol. Ther. 46: 219, 1989.
66. DiFazio CA: Metabolism of local anaesthetics in the fetus, newborn and adult. Br. J. Anaesth. Vol. 51, Supp. 1:295, 1979.
67. Mihaly GW, Moore RG, Thomas J, Triggs EJ, et al: The pharmacokinetics and metabolism of the anilide local anaesthetics in neonates. Europ. J. Clin. Pharmacol. 13:143, 1978.
68. Bricker SRW, Telford RJ, Booker PD: Pharmacokinetics of bupivacaine following intraoperative intercostal nerve block in neonates and in infants aged less than 6 months. Anesthesiology 70:942, 1989.
69. Meffin P, Long GJ, Thomas: Clearance and metabolism of mepivacaine in the human neonate. Clin Pharmacol Ther. 14:218, 1973.
69A. Boyes RN: A review of the metabolism of amide local anaesthetic agents. Br. J. Anaesth. 47(Suppl.), 1975, pp. 225–30.
70. Fink BR, Aasheim GM, Levy BA: Neural pharmacokinetics of epinephrine. Anesthesiology 48:263, 1978.
71. Hiroshi O, Watanabe M, Saitoh J, Saegusa Y, et al: Effect of epinephrine concentration on lidocaine disposition during epidural anesthesia. Anesthesiology 68:625, 1988.
72. Moore DC: The pH of local anesthetic solutions. Anesth. Analg. 60:833, 1981.
73. Hilgier M: Alkalinization of bupivacaine for brachial plexus block. Reg. Anaesth. 10:59, 1985.
74. McMorland GH, Douglas MJ, Jeffery WK, Ross PLE, et al: Effect of pH-adjustment of bupivacaine on onset and duration of epidural analgesia in parturients. Can. Anaesth. Soc. J. 33:537, 1986.
75. Bedder MD, Kozody R, Craig DB: Comparison of bupivacaine and alkalinized bupivacaine in brachial plexus anesthesia. Anesth. Analg. 67:48, 1988.
76. Bromage PR: A comparison of the hydrochloride and carbon dioxide salts of lidocaine and prilocaine in epidural analgesia. Acta. Anaesth. Scand. Suppl XVI:55, 1965.
77. Bromage PR, Burfoot MF, Crowell DE, Truant AP: Quality of epidural blockade III: carbonated local anaesthetic solutions. Br. J. Anaesth. 39:197, 1967.
77A. Sukhani R, Winnie AP: Clinical pharmacokinetics of carbonated local anesthetics. Anesth. Analg. 66(8), 1987, pp. 739–45.
78. Sukhani R, Winnie AP: Clinical pharmacokinetics of carbonated local anesthetics II: interscalene brachial block model. Anesth. Analg. 66:1245, 1987.
79. Mehta PM, Theriot E, Mehrotra D, Patel K, et al: A simple technique to make bupivacaine a rapid-acting epidural anesthetic. Reg. Anesth. 12:135, 1987.
80. Justins DM, Francis D, Houlton PG, Reynolds F: A controlled trial of extradural fentanyl in labour. Br. J. Anaesth. 54:409, 1982.
81. Justins DM, Knott C, Luthman J, Reynolds F: Epidural versus intramuscular fentanyl: analgesia and pharmacokinetics in labour. Anaesthesia 38:937, 1983.
82. Chestnut DH, Owen CL, Bates JN, Ostman LG, et al: Continuous infusion epidural analgesia during labor: a randomized double-blind comparison of 0.0625% bupivacaine/0.0002% fentanyl versus − 0.125% bupivacaine. Anesthesiology 68:754, 1988.
83. Wagman IH, deJong RH, Prince DA: Effect of lidocaine on the central nervous system. Anesthesiology 28:155, 1967.
83A. Bishop D, Johnstone RE: Lidocaine toxicity treated with low-dose propofol. Anesthesiology. 78(4), 1993, pp. 788–9.
84. Modica PA, Templehoff R, White PF: Pro- and anticonvulsant effects of anesthetics (part II). Anesth. Analg. 70:433, 1990.
85. Bucklin BA, Warner DS, Choi WW, Todd MA, et al: Pregnancy does not alter the threshold for lidocaine-induced seizures in the rat. Anesth. Analg. 74:57, 1992.
86. Morishima HO, Finster M, Arthur GR, Covino BG: Pregnancy does not alter lidocaine toxicity. Am. J. Obstet. Gynecol. 162:1320, 1990.
87. Santos AC, Arthur GR, Pedersen H, Morishima HO, et al: Systemic toxicity of ropivacaine during ovine pregnancy. Anesthesiology 75:137, 1991.
88. Scott DB, Lee A, Fagan D, Bowler GMR, et al: Acute toxicity of ropivacaine compared to that of bupivacaine. Anesth. Analg. 689:563, 1989.
89. Teramo K, Benowitz N, Heymann MA, Rudolph AM: Gestational differences in lidocaine toxicity in the fetal lamb. Anesthesiology 44:133, 1976.
90. Moore DC: Administer oxygen first in the treatment of local anesthetic-induced convulsions. Anesthesiology 53: 346, 1980.
91. Block A, Covino BG: Effect of local anesthetic agents in cardiac conduction and contractility. Reg. Anesth. 6:55, 1981.
92. Lynch C III: Depression of myocardial contractility in vitro by bupivacaine, etidocaine, and lidocaine. Anesth. Analg. 65:551, 1986
93. Feldman HS, Covino BG, Sage DJ: Direct chronotropic and ionotropic effects of local anesthetic agents in isolated guinea pig atria. Reg. Anesth. 7:149, 1982.
94. Liu P, Feldman HS, Covino BM, Giasi R, et al: Acute cardiovascular toxicity of intravenous amide local anesthetics in anesthetized ventilated dogs. Anesth. Analg. 61:317, 1982.
95. Nath S, Haggmark S, Johansson G, Reiz S: Differential depressant and electrophysiologic cardiotoxicity of local anesthetics: an experimental study with special reference to lidocaine and bupivacaine. Anesth. Analg. 65:1263, 1986.
96. Clarkson DW, Hondegham LM: Mechanism for bupivacaine depression of cardiac conduction: fast block of sodium channels during the action potential with slow recovery from block during diastole. Anesthesiology 62:396, 1985.
97. Heavner JE: Cardiac dysrhythmias induced by infusion of local anesthetics into the lateral cerebral ventricle of cats. Anesth. Analg. 65:113, 1986.
98. Thomas RD, Behbehani MM, Coyle DE, Denson DD: Cardiovascular toxicity of local anesthetics: an alternative hypothesis. Anesth. Analg. 65:444, 1986.
99. Avery P, Redon D, Schaenzer G, Rusy B: The influence of serum potassium on the cerebral and cardiac toxicity of bupivacaine and lidocaine. Anesthesiology 61:134, 1985.
100. Sage DJ, Feldman HS, Arthur GR, Datta S, et al: Influence of bupivacaine and lidocaine on isolated guinea pig atria in the presence of acidosis and hypoxia. Anesth. Analg. 63: 1, 1984.
101. Reiz S, Nath S: Cardiotoxicity of local anaesthetic agents. Br. J. Anaesth. 58:736, 1986.

102. Moore DC, Crawford RD, Scurlock JE: Severe hypoxia and acidosis following local anesthetic-induced convulsions. Anesthesiology 53:259, 1980.
103. Johns RA, Seyde WC, DiFazio CA, Longnecker DE: Dose-dependent effects of bupivacaine on rat muscle arterioles. Anesthesiology 65:186, 1986.
104. Datta S, Lambert D, Gregus J, Gissen AJ, et al: Differential sensitivity of mammalian nerve fibers during pregnancy. Anesth. Analg. 62:1070, 1983.
105. Flanagan H, Datta S, Lambert D, Gissen AJ, et al: Effect of pregnancy on bupivacaine-induced conduction blockade in the isolated rabbit vagus nerve. Anesth. Analg. 66:123, 1987.
106. Moller RA, Datta S, Fox J, Johnson M, et al: Progesterone-induced increase in cardiac sensitivity to bupivacaine. Anesthesiology 76:604, 1992.
107. Kasten GW, Martin ST: Bupivacaine cardiovascular toxicity: comparison of treatment with bretylium and lidocaine. Anesth. Analg. 64:911, 1985.
108. Crawford OB, Chester RV: Caudal anesthesia in obstetrics: a combined procaine-Pontocaine single injection technique. Anesthesiology 10:473, 1949
108A. Dennerstein G: Caudal analgesia by the obstetrician. Aust. N.Z. J. Obstet. Gynaecol. 30(3), 1990, pp. 203–5.
109. Bromage PR: Spread of analgesic solutions in the epidural space and their site of action: a statistical study. Br. J. Anaesth. 24:161, 1962.
110. Fagraeus L, Urban BJ, Bromage PR: Spread of epidural analgesia in early pregnancy. Anesthesiology 58:184, 1983.

# Chapter 12

# VASOPRESSORS AND VASOCONSTRICTORS

RICHARD B. CLARK

This chapter is devoted to the pharmacology and uses in obstetric anesthetic practices of vasoconstrictors and vasopressors, including epinephrine, norepinephrine, ephedrine, and several other vasoactive agents. The obstetric team frequently uses these agents as vasoconstrictors to delay the absorption of local anesthetics and as vasopressors to treat hypotension that may follow the use of regional analgesia anesthesia. Epinephrine and some of its relatives have also been used as myometrial relaxants. Moreover, endogenous epinephrine and norepinephrine play a major role in the body's adaptation to pain and emotional reactions during labor. These drugs have diverse actions; therefore, for optimal use it is essential to know not only the direct effects on body functions, but also how they interact with other drugs used during labor. This review is especially desirable in view of the vast amount of new data on these drugs acquired during recent years that have clarified their action and modified their clinical use.

The chapter from the first edition serves as a basis of this discussion, retaining information that has not changed in the past decade, (1) adding modifications and a significant amount of new material where necessary, and updating references. More extensive reviews can be found elsewhere (2–7).

Epinephrine and norepinephrine are discussed first and are used as a standard of reference for evaluation of other agents mentioned in the last part of the chapter.

## EPINEPHRINE AND NOREPINEPHRINE

### Basic Pharmacology

Epinephrine and norepinephrine are naturally occurring catecholamines (compounds with a catechol nucleus) and have similar structural formulas. The absence of a methyl group in norepinephrine indicated by the prefix *nor*, derived by the elision of the German phrase Nitrogen Ohne Radikal (nitrogen without radical), results in significant differences in pharmacologic activity. The primary function of norepinephrine appears to be the maintenance of normal sympathetic tone, whereas epinephrine is the great emergency hormone that stimulates metabolism and promotes blood flow to skeletal muscles, thus preparing the individual for fight or flight (7). Epinephrine, norepinephrine, and dopamine are naturally occurring catecholamines. Some useful synthetic catecholamines are isoproterenol and dobutamine.

#### *Norepinephrine*

Norepinephrine carries out its primary function by being the adrenergic transmitter. It is synthesized and stored at nerve endings, ready to be mobilized by the passage of an impulse. Once released, it interacts with the receptor. Synthesis of norepinephrine begins with the amino acid tyrosine, which enters the neuron by active transport. Tyrosine hydroxylase catalyzes the conversion of tyrosine to dihydroxyphenylalanine (DOPA); dopamine is formed from dihydroxyphenylalanine by dihydroxyphenylalanine decarboxylase. Dopamine then enters the storage vesicles. Dopamine is converted to norepinephrine by dopamine-beta-hydroxylase. Norepinephrine is the neurotransmitter at postganglionic nerve endings, and is released from the storage vesicles upon the arrival of an action potential, crossing the synoptic cleft to the receptors of the postjunctional membrane of the receptor cell (Figure 12–1) (5). In the adrenal medulla, the additional step of conversion of norepinephrine to epinephrine is accomplished by a transferase. Norepinephrine is inactivated at the synoptic cleft by three mechanisms: (1) reuptake into the presynaptic terminals; (2) extraneuronal uptake; and (3) diffusion. Termination of norepinephrine at the effector site is almost entirely by reuptake of norepinephrine into the terminals of the presynaptic neuron. Furthermore, the conversion of tyrosine to dihydroxyphenylalanine by tyrosine hydroxylase is inhibited by increased norepinephrine synthesis.

To summarize, junctional transmission involves the following steps: (1) synthesis of the transmitter; (2) storage of the transmitter; (3) release of the transmitter by a nerve action potential; (4) interaction of the released transmitter with receptors on the effector cell membrane and the associated change in the effector cell; (5) rapid removal of the transmitter from the vicinity of the receptors; and (6) recovery of the effector cell to the state that preceded transmitter action (4). Epinephrine is inactivated by catechol-o-methyl-transferase. The final metabolic product of the catecholamines is vanillylmandelic acid.

Norepinephrine activates the receptors on the postjunctional membrane. It is, therefore, the first messenger of the adrenergic nervous system. Cyclic adenosine monophosphate (CAMP) serves as the intracellular moderator of the catecholamine, and is termed the second messenger. The third messenger is calcium (for a thorough discussion, see Durrett and Lawson (5)).

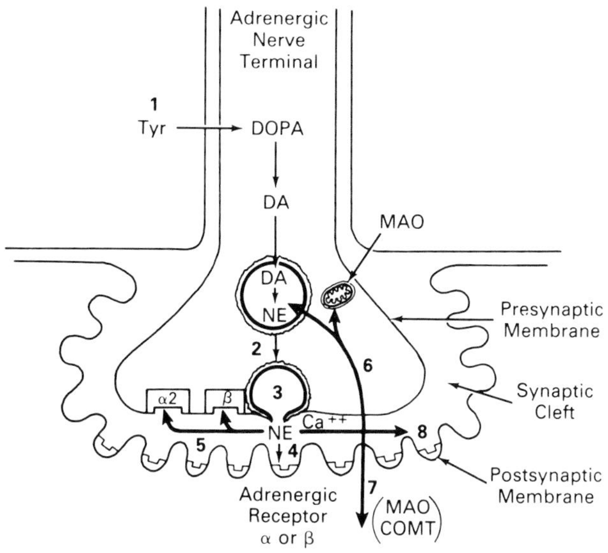


**Fig. 12–1.** Schematic diagram of sympathetic end organ synapse, showing presynaptic and postsynaptic membranes, synaptic cleft, and pre- and postsynaptic receptors. Norepinephrine (NE) stimulation of postsynaptic receptors produce classic beta and alpha effects. Note that stimulation of alpha-2 receptors by norepinephrine released into the synaptic cleft inhibits further release of norepinephrine. Presynaptic beta stimulation increases norepinephrine uptake, augmenting its availability. Other receptors, such as muscarinic receptors (MUSC) exist but are not pertinent to this discussion. (From Durrett LR, Lawson NW: Autonomic nervous system, physiology and pharmacology. *In* Clinical Anesthesia. Edited by P. Barash, BF Cullen, RK Stoelting. Philadelphia, JB Lippincott, 1989.)

### *Epinephrine*

Epinephrine, on the other hand, is synthesized and stored in granules of the adrenal medulla and in scattered chromaffin cells located in various tissues such as the myocardium, carotid body, walls of peripheral vessels, and ganglia of the pelvic plexus. Here it is accompanied by high concentrations of adenosine triphosphate (ATP), a substance that seems to play a role in the binding or concentrating mechanisms for various biologically active amines (8,9). The amount of epinephrine released when sympathetic nerves are stimulated is usually less than 10% of the total catecholamines (10).

However, epinephrine constitutes 80% of the catecholamines in the adrenal medulla (11,12), while norepinephrine comprises 20%. Bilateral adrenalectomy in humans produces a more than 80% reduction in the amount of epinephrine normally excreted in the urine, reducing the ratio of epinephrine to norepinephrine from about 20% to 3% to 5% (13). The normal plasma level of epinephrine ranges from 0.10 to 0.12 μg/l, while norepinephrine ranges 0.2 to 0.5 μg/l. Sympathetic denervation affects the norepinephrine content of an organ without producing any significant decrease in epinephrine content. Reserpine depletes the norepinephrine stores in tissues (as much as 95% in the heart) (14).

## *Receptors*

In 1941 Dale (15) proposed the terms cholinergic and adrenergic (from adrenal) to describe neurons that liberated acetylcholine and norepinephrine, respectively (7). Cannon and Uridil (16) reported that stimulation of hepatic sympathetic nerves released a substance that increased blood pressure and heart rate (16). They called this sympathin, which was revealed to be norepinephrine. Von Euler (17) differentiated the physiologic effects of epinephrine and norepinephrine. Ahlquist (18), on the basis of the observed selectivity of action of the agonists and antagonists, proposed two types of adrenoreceptors. These were designated as alpha and beta receptors. Receptors that responded with an order of potency of norepinephrine ≥ epinephrine ≥ isoproterenol were called alpha receptors. Those responding with an order of potency of isoproterenol ≥ epinephrine ≥ norepinephrine were called beta receptors. The development of new agonists and antagonists with relatively selective activity allowed Lands (19) to subdivide the beta receptors into beta-1 and beta-2 in 1967. In 1974, Langer (20) subdivided alpha receptors into the alpha-1 and alpha-2 receptors.

The alpha-1 receptors are located at postjunctional (postsynaptic) sites on tissues innervated by adrenergic neurons. Originally, alpha-2 receptors were thought to have only a presynaptic (i.e., neuronal) location and to be involved in the feedback inhibition of norepinephrine release from nerve terminals (see Figure 12–1). It now appears that alpha-2 receptors also can occur postjunctionally (21). The beta-1 receptors are found chiefly in the heart and in adipose tissue, while beta-2 receptors are located in several sites, including bronchial smooth muscle, skeletal muscle, blood vessels, and uterus (5,22,23).

The existence of other receptors responsible for dilatation of mesenteric and renal vessels with the administration of dopamine has been suspected since 1979 (24). These dopaminergic receptors (DA) are a matter of controversy, as no peripheral dopaminergic neurons have been identified. They are, however, very important to this discussion.

Stimulation of alpha-1 receptors in smooth muscle of blood vessels leads to vasoconstriction, while activation of beta-2 receptors in blood vessels of skeletal muscle produces vasodilation. Stimulation of beta-1 receptors in cardiac tissue produces an increase in heart rate and contractile force. Table 12–1 describes the action of vasopressors on adrenergic receptors. Stimulation of beta-2 receptors also results in relaxation of the smooth muscles of the bronchi and of the uterus. Alpha adrenergic activity can change with pregnancy (25).

Norepinephrine and epinephrine are potent alpha receptor agonists, but isoproterenol is not similarly active in usual therapeutic doses. Norepinephrine and epinephrine are thus potent vasoconstrictors of those vascular beds that contain alpha receptors, while isoproterenol has little effect on those vessels. Isoproterenol and epinephrine are potent beta-2 receptor agonists; norepinephrine is a relatively weak beta-2 receptor agonist. Isoproterenol and

**Table 12–1.** Classification, Mechanism of Action, and Dose of Vasopressor Drugs

| Drug | Receptors Stimulated | | | Mechanism of Action | Single IV Dose (70 kg adult) | Continuous Infusion Dose (70 kg adult) |
|---|---|---|---|---|---|---|
| | Alpha | Beta-1 | Beta-2 | | | |
| Methoxamine | + + + | 0 | 0 | direct | 5–10 mg | not used |
| Phenylephrine | + + + | ? ± | ? | direct | 50–100 mg | 20–50 μg/min |
| Metaraminol | + + | + | + | direct & indirect | 1.5–5.0 mg | 40–500 μg/min |
| Epinephrine | + | + + | + + | direct | 200–350 μg | 2–20 μg/min |
| Norepinephrine | + + + | + + | 0 | direct | not used | 4–16 μg/min |
| Ephedrine | + + | + | + | indirect, some direct | 10–25 mg | not used |
| Mephentermine | + + | + | + | indirect | 10–25 mg | not used |
| Dopamine | + + | + + | + | direct | not used | 2–20 μg/kg/min |
| Dobutamine | + | + + + | 0 | direct | not used | 2–10 μg/kg/min |
| Isoproterenol | 0 | + + + | + + + | direct | 1–4 μg | 1–5 μg/min |
| Amrinone | | | | direct | 0.75 mg | 5–10 μg/kg/min |
| Angiotensin | | | | direct | | |

(Compiled from Stoelting R: Sympathomimetics. *In* Pharmacology and Physiology in Anesthetic Practice. Edited by R Stoelting: J.B. Lippincott, Philadelphia, 1987, p. 251; Lawson NW, Wallfisch HK: Cardiovascular pharmacology: a new look at the "pressors." *In* Advances in Anesthesia. Edited by R Stoelting: Yearbook Medical Publishers, Chicago, 1986, p. 195; and Kaplan JA: How can the heart be treated by treating the peripheral circulation? ASA Refresher Courses 116:1–7, 1980.)

epinephrine produce vasodilatation in skeletal muscle, but norepinephrine does not. Low doses of dopamine have dopaminergic effects and result in increased renal blood flow.

Isoproterenol, epinephrine, and norepinephrine are potent beta-1 receptor agonists; all three can stimulate the heart. Epinephrine is the most potent stimulator of alpha receptors, being 2 to 10 times more active than norepinephrine and more than 100 times more potent than isoproterenol. Isoproterenol is the most potent stimulator of beta receptors because it is 2 to 10 times more active than epinephrine, and 100 or more times more active than norepinephrine. Thus, epinephrine has a strong effect on both alpha and beta receptors; norepinephrine is much more active on alpha than beta receptors; and isoproterenol acts primarily on the beta receptors.

### *Antagonists*

Various compounds have been developed that block the effects of adrenergic agonists. Phentolamine (Regitine), phenoxybenzamine (Dibenzyline), tolazoline (Priscoline), and prazosin (Minipress) block alpha responses, while propranolol (Inderal) and nadolol (Corgard) block beta responses (26). Esmolol (Brevibloc), metoprolol (Lopressor), and atenolol (Tenormin) are cardioselective (beta-1) adrenergic blocking agents. Labetalol (Trandate) is both an alpha and a nonselective beta blocking agent.

#### *Classification*

These drugs may thus be classified by the cardiovascular responses that effect vasoconstriction or vasopressor. Some cause solely peripheral vasoconstriction (alpha effect), others predominantly cardiac stimulation (beta effect), and still others have multiple actions. This is the basis of their classification in Table 12–1, which contains a summary of dose and pharmacologic effects. Like epinephrine and norepinephrine, the vasopressor effectiveness of these agents is decreased in the presence of acidosis, electrolyte imbalance, and hypovolemia.

## PHARMACODYNAMICS

Exogenous epinephrine and norepinephrine administered for therapeutic purposes have diverse effects on the mother and certain specific effects on the uterus, and thus may affect the fetus. These effects have importance for the obstetric team.

### Effects on the Mother

#### Cardiovascular Effects

The cardiovascular effects of epinephrine and norepinephrine are similar in many respects and different in others. Moreover, each drug produces variable cardiovascular responses under different conditions. The variability depends primarily upon: (1) amount of drug injected; (2) route of administration; and (3) potentiation by other drugs or inhibition by metabolic disorders. The greatest difference between the two drugs is seen when small amounts are used. With very large unphysiologic doses, the difference between the two agents is slight. These effects are listed in Table 12–2.

***Epinephrine.*** Epinephrine evokes three distinct responses of the heart: (1) cardioacceleration through the sino-auricular node (chronotropic effect); (2) increased force of ventricular contraction (inotropic effect); and (3) altered arrhythmic function (dromotropic) of the ventricle (12,27). These are distinct responses, each of which can be checked separately by different agents. The effects of epinephrine on the peripheral vascular bed include vasoconstriction (increased resistance), vasodilation (decreased resistance) or both, depending on the vascular bed involved and the dose of the drug used. The use of epinephrine in small subcutaneous doses, as when it is used as a vasoconstrictor with local anesthetics at the

**Table 12–2.** Comparative Effects of Epinephrine and Norepinephrine on the Human Cardiovascular System

| Response | Epinephrine Minimum Dose IV | Epinephrine Large Dose IV | Norepinephrine Minimum Dose IV | Norepinephrine Large Dose IV |
|---|---|---|---|---|
| Blood pressure, mean | No change* | ↑ ↑ | ↑ | ↑ ↑ ↑ |
| Systolic | Slight ↑ | ↑ ↑ ↑ | ↑ | ↑ ↑ ↑ |
| Diastolic | Slight ↓ | ↑ | ↑ | ↑ ↑ ↑ |
| Cardiac output | ↑ | ↑ ↑ | No change | No change or ↓ |
| Pulse rate | No change or ↑ | ↑ ↑ | No change | No change or ↓ |
| Peripheral resistance | ↓ | ↑ ↑ | ↑ | ↑ ↑ |

↑ = increase
↓ = decrease
* These responses can result from a moderate to large dose given subcutaneously, or a very small dose given intravenously.

proper concentration (see below), is followed by a slight increase in cardiac rate and stoke volume, resulting in an increase in cardiac output, and a concomitant and somewhat commensurate decrease in total peripheral resistance. Consequently, the blood pressure remains normal. With larger subcutaneous or intramuscular injections (e.g., 0.5 to 1.0 mg) in normal adults, the cardiac rate is increased by about 20 to 25%, cardiac output and left ventricular work by about 40 to 50%, and stroke volume by about 20 to 25%. At the same time, there is a fall of 10 to 15% in diastolic pressure and of 30 to 40% in peripheral resistance (7,12,28).

Intravenous infusion at rates of 0.5 to 10 μg/min produces similar responses, although the degree of response is influenced by the dose. The decrease in blood pressure may be due in part to exaggeration of the beta response and consequent greater decrease in peripheral resistance and blood pressure that is usually seen in subjects with elevated vascular tone given minute doses of epinephrine intravenously. Under such circumstances, the increase in cardiac output is not sufficient to overcome the intense vasodilation.

It is apparent that following subcutaneous or intramuscular injection of even large doses and following intravenous infusion of small to moderate doses of epinephrine, the intense vasoconstriction (alpha effect) produced in the skin and certain viscera is overshadowed by an equally intense vasodilation (beta effect) in skeletal muscles and elsewhere. However, with relatively large intravenous doses generalized vasoconstriction and subsequent increase in total peripheral resistance are seen, resulting in a significant increase in systolic and diastolic blood pressure. Rises in blood pressure from 120/80 to 170/120 within 20 seconds of the injection of 3 ml of local anesthetic containing epinephrine in a 1:200,000 concentration (i.e., containing 15 μg of epinephrine) that was inadvertently injected into an epidural vein in the course of epidural anesthesia have been noted (1). Blood pressures of 400/300 mm Hg following accidental administration of therapeutic doses intended for subcutaneous injection have been reported (7). In such excessive doses, the very intense vasoconstriction predominates so that there is increased peripheral resistance and reduction in blood flow through skeletal muscles (7,12).

***Norepinephrine.*** Norepinephrine increases systolic, diastolic, mean blood pressure, and total peripheral resistance, usually diminishes cardiac rate, and has either no effect or decreases cardiac output (Figure 12–2). Although norepinephrine is capable of stimulating the ventricular force, the hypertension initiates reflex bradycardia, which offsets or masks the myocardial effect with the net result of either no change or reduction in cardiac output (29). This indicates that the pressor response is entirely due to vasoconstriction, unless reflex pathways are blocked either by atropine or ganglionic blocking agents. In the latter instance, there is an increase in cardiac output that contributes to the rise in blood pressure. The difference between norepinephrine and epinephrine in humans appears to be that the reflex bradycardia caused by the former is more intense, whereas cardiac stimulation caused by the latter is more prominent. Zuspan and his associates (30) found in parturients that norepinephrine intravenous infusion rates of 2 μg/min had an insignificant effect on blood pressure, but that rates of 5 to 10 μg/min had a significant effect.

***Cardiac Arrhythmias.*** It is well-known that exogenous epinephrine produces ventricular extrasystoles, multifocal ventricular tachycardia, and may even lead to ventricular fibrillation in subjects with a diseased heart or other pathologic conditions, including hypercarbia. This effect is related to the dose because intravenous infusion rate of epinephrine must exceed 10 μg/min to precipitate ventricular arrhythmia (31). The incidence and severity of the ventricular arrhythmias are increased by certain inhalation anesthetics such as halothane. Johnson, et al (32) calculated the $ED_{50}$ of three anesthetics when epinephrine was utilized. They found that 2.1 μg/kg epinephrine with halothane, 10.9 μg/kg with enflurane, and 6.7 μg/kg with isoflurane were the $ED_{50}$s, indicating the relative safety of these agents. Norepinephrine is thought to produce a smaller incidence of ventricular arrhythmia.

### *Effects on Regional Blood Flow*

All adrenergic drugs have direct and indirect effects on blood flow to the brain, heart, kidney, liver, and other

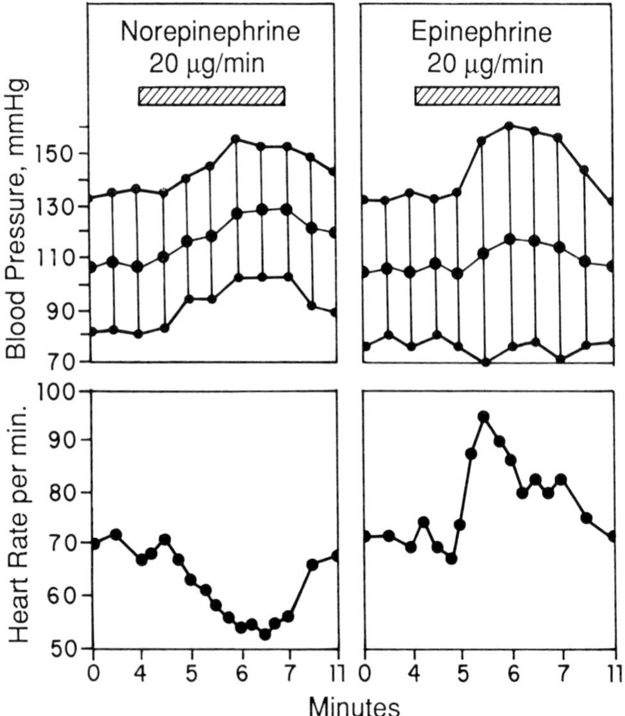


**Fig. 12–2.** Effect of norepinephrine and epinephrine infusion on blood pressure and heart rate in man. Note that following infusion of norepinephrine there is an increase in systolic, diastolic, and mean pressure and a concomitant decrease in heart rate; whereas following infusion of epinephrine the systolic pressure increases, and the diastolic and mean pressures remain essentially unchanged, with a consequent increase in pulse pressure and tachycardia. (Redrawn from Barcroft H, Konzett H: On actions of noradrenaline, adrenalin and isopropyl noradrenalin on arterial blood pressure, heart rate and muscle blood flow in man. J. Physiol. 110:194, 1949.)

body organs, and thus influence their function. The effects vary depending on (1) infusion rate and dose; (2) preinfusion blood pressure; and (3) preinfusion vascular resistance of the organ.

***Coronary Circulation.*** The coronary circulation, as part of the central circulation, has certain unusual features: (1) it supplies blood to a contracting hollow viscus; (2) the flood flow is phasic, because most of it occurs during diastole; (3) it is little influenced by sympathetic nervous system activity, but is primarily under the influence of local metabolites (carbon dioxide, lactic acid, etc.); and (4) the extraction of oxygen, and consequently the A-V oxygen difference (12 volumes per cent) is larger than any other vascular bed. Therefore, any decrease in perfusion pressure or fall in arterial tension cannot be compensated by further oxygen extraction, as occurs in other organs, because this is almost maximum, but must be countered by vasodilation. Compensatory vasodilation occurs with normovolemic hypotension, so that the proportion of the total cardiac output diverted to the coronary circulation is increased from 4.5% to as much as 12%. (33). This continues until the blood pressure reaches a low level of 60 mm Hg, below which vasodilation can no longer compensate for the decreased blood flow and ischemia follows.

Reduction of blood pressure by hemorrhage causes a progressive increase in coronary resistance and decrease in coronary blood flow (34). When the blood pressure is restored by blood transfusion, the coronary flow and resistance return to normal. Infusion of exogenous epinephrine or norepinephrine increases coronary blood flow by decreasing coronary vascular resistance and increasing systemic pressure. The coronary flow increases linearly as the pressure is raised (34).

***Cerebral Circulation.*** The cerebral circulation is under the influence of many of the same factors as the coronary circulation. In normal subjects, the primary determinant of cerebral blood flow is cerebral autoregulation, which maintains a constant flow between cerebral perfusion pressures of approximately 50 to 150 mm Hg. When the perfusion pressure falls below 50 mm Hg, the brain is unable to compensate with further vasodilation and blood flow decreases in linear relation to the perfusion pressure. When cerebral blood flow falls below the threshold for ischemia, symptoms such as mental disturbance, agitation, apprehension, syncope, unconsciousness, and focal neurologic deficits may appear. Other factors such as cerebral metabolic rate, arterial $CO_2$, and arterial $O_2$ can also influence cerebral blood flow.

Systemically administered vasopressors have little effect on cerebral blood flow in normal subjects. The blood-brain barrier normally excludes many circulating compounds from the brain. The blood-brain barrier is composed of both a physical barrier (tight endothelial cell junctions) and an enzymatic barrier (monoamine oxidase and catechol O-methyltransferase) (35). Intracarotid infusion of epinephrine, angiotensin or norepinephrine have little effect on cerebral blood flow in humans (36). When evaluating the effects of vasopressors on cerebral blood flow, it is important to separate direct effects from indirect effects. Systemic administration of epinephrine with resultant hypertension will lead to an increase in cerebral vascular resistance. This increase in cerebral vascular resistance is not due to direct effects of the epinephrine, however, but is due to cerebral autoregulation that causes the vasoconstriction to maintain cerebral blood flow constant in the face of an increase in mean arterial pressure. When these agents are infused into hypotensive individuals, they cause a consistent increase in cerebral blood flow and disappearance of any symptoms of cerebrovascular insufficiency that might have existed before infusion (34).

***Renal Circulation.*** The renal circulation is unique in that there is a large blood flow (20 to 25% of total cardiac output) with very little oxygen extraction or A-V oxygen difference (37). This suggests that there is a considerable latitude in the alteration of blood flow without production of ischemia. Although the renal circulation is directly related to blood pressure, the resistance to blood flow in the kidney is directly under control of the sympathetic nervous system. The renal circulation, like that of the splanchnic bed and skin, participates in compensatory adjustment to changes in central blood pressure, and thus plays a major role in circulatory homeostasis. Vasoconstriction is usually associated with decrease in secretion of urine and renal ischemia, which can be tolerated for much longer periods of time than occurs with the heart and brain. Even a slight decrease in blood volume due to hemorrhage is followed by renal vasoconstriction (34,37).

The effects of exogenous epinephrine and norepinephrine on renal function will vary according to: (1) dose and route of administration of the drug; and (2) preinfusion blood pressure and blood volume. In normotensive individuals, these drugs cause a significant decrease in renal blood flow, diuresis, and filtration rate (37,38). Administered in small doses to patients with normovolemic hypotension, these drugs cause an increase in renal blood flow, diuresis, and filtration rate, indicating that the rise in blood pressure overcompensates for the vasoconstriction produced (38). Large doses of either epinephrine or norepinephrine cause a decrease in blood flow, diuresis, and filtration rate, and decrease in excretion of sodium and potassium, with epinephrine having a stronger vasoconstrictive effect than norepinephrine (10). Apparently, such large doses produce vasoconstriction of both afferent and efferent arterioles and closure of some nephrons. Epinephrine may also produce antidiuresis by a central effect mediated by the posterior pituitary (12).

When either drug is used to restore the blood pressure in patients with hypovolemic hypotension associated with hemorrhagic, renal blood flow decreases further, and at the same time renal vascular resistance increases significantly (34). This decrease in renal blood flow occurs despite the rise in blood pressure. Excessive doses that raise the blood pressure of hypovolemic, hypotensive patients to hypertensive levels are associated with cessation of renal blood flow. Restoration of the blood volume in hypovolemic subjects restores the renal blood flow to normal levels (34).

***Hepatic Blood Flow.*** The hepatic circulation and the major portion of the splanchnic circulation are involved in the autonomic response to changes in central circulation with resultant vasoconstriction and vasodilation. Total hepatic blood flow is usually considered to contribute approximately 40% of venous return to the heart (39). A fall in blood pressure, either due to decreased peripheral resistance or decreased blood volume, is associated with vasoconstriction in the entire splanchnic region, including the hepatic and mesenteric arteries. Administration of very small doses of epinephrine (0.1 μg/kg/min) increases hepatic blood flow and decreases splanchnic vascular resistance (12). This is due to action on beta receptors and is abolished by propranolol (40). However, larger doses of epinephrine or norepinephrine (or any other vasopressor) are associated with a decrease in hepatic blood flow. Although there is an increase in hepatic blood flow, this is not sufficient to compensate for the decrease in portal vein flow, with a result of net decrease in total hepatic flow (34).

***Mesenteric Blood Flow.*** It is known that the vasopressor drugs decrease blood flow to the intestines and other abdominal viscera supplied by the mesenteric vessels (41). This apparently includes uterine blood flow which, because of its importance, will be discussed in detail under "Effects on the Uterus." The decrease in visceral blood flow is commensurate with the dose of the vasopressor agent: the greater the dose, the greater the decrease. Epinephrine and norepinephrine (and other vasopressors) have been shown to aggravate the ischemia of the intestines produced by hemorrhagic and endotoxic shock (41).

***Skeletal Muscles.*** Epinephrine produces dilation of the blood vessels of the skeletal muscles through its beta effect, as does isoproterenol. As previously mentioned, following subcutaneous or intramuscular injection, or infusion at low flow rates, epinephrine produces a vasodilation in skeletal muscles that is so intense that it more than offsets the vasoconstriction that occurs in cutaneous and visceral vessels, so that the net effect is a significant decrease in total peripheral resistance. Usual doses of norepinephrine produce vasoconstriction, as do excessive intravenous doses of epinephrine.

## Other Effects

The central nervous system is stimulated by the usual therapeutic doses of epinephrine, so that patients frequently experience anxiety and apprehension when epinephrine is used with local anesthetics, of which the dosage should never exceed 0.2 mg (200 μg). Norepinephrine is much less active in this respect.

***Respiration.*** Respiration is usually stimulated and bronchodilation produced with the usual therapeutic doses of epinephrine or norepinephrine, or during continuous intravenous infusion. Large doses produce apnea, probably due in part by direct action on the respiratory center and in part by reflex action.

***Gastrointestinal Tract.*** The gastrointestinal tract is relaxed and peristalsis is reduced, while the muscles of the pyloric and the iliocecal sphincters may contract or relax, depending upon their state at the time of injection. Epinephrine also has a stimulating effect on the gallbladder. In dogs and cats, the smooth muscle in the capsule of the spleen is contracted by the drug with a consequent increase in the volume and number of erythrocytes in the circulatory blood, but this effect has not been demonstrated in humans (12). The detrusor muscle of the urinary bladder is relaxed and the trigone and sphincter are contracted, whereas the amplitude and frequency of ureteral peristaltic waves are increased. Norepinephrine has much less effect on the gastrointestinal and urinary tract.

***Metabolic Effects.*** Metabolic effects of epinephrine include: (1) glycogenolysis with consequent elevation of the blood sugar and lactic acid and decrease of glycogen content of the liver and skeletal muscles; and (2) increased metabolic rate and heat production. Epinephrine also stimulates the anterior pituitary to increase the release of ACTH and consequent secretion of adrenocortical hormones. It also causes a significant decrease in the number of circulating eosinophils. In therapeutic doses, norepinephrine causes much less hyperglycemia and other metabolic and central nervous system effects than epinephrine.

## Effects on the Uterus

The effects of epinephrine on the pregnant uterus have been the subject of studies since 1907 when Neu (42) observed that the administration of what is now considered a large dose of adrenal extract to patients undergoing cesarean section produced a powerful uterine contraction. In 1925, Rucker (43), in the course of studies of the effect of caudal anesthesia on the uterus in labor, noted diminution of uterine activity when the anesthetic mixture contained epinephrine. He extended these studies, and two years later advocated its use as a uterine depressant (44). During the ensuing years, many clinical reports attested to the efficacy of epinephrine in treatment of constriction ring and premature labor (45).

In the first edition of this book, numerous studies were cited on the effects of epinephrine and norepinephrine on uterine blood flow and uterine contractility. In most of these pioneering studies, these drugs were administered intravenously and occasionally intramuscularly in very large doses that showed a significant reduction of uterine blood flow and also a significant decrease in uterine contractility. For example, in studying the effects of epinephrine on uterine blood flow, Greiss (46) used doses of epinephrine of 1 μg/kg per minute (or 50 μg/min for the average parturient) and, as expected, produced a significant decrease in uterine blood flow (shown in Figure 12–3). Similarly, Stroup found that epinephrine given at the rates of 4.2 μg/min produced a depression of intense contractions but had no effect on frequency (47). While these studies were relevant at the time when epinephrine was being used as a uterine relaxant, they are not applicable today because in most instances epinephrine is used as a vasoconstrictor added to local anesthetic solution that produces regional anesthesia, particularly epidural analgesia and anesthesia. Therefore, in this section we will focus on recent studies pertaining to the use of epinephrine as a vasoconstrictor added to a local anesthetic used for regional anesthesia or as part of the test dose. For the sake of clarity, the effect of uterine blood flow and uterine blood contractions is considered separately. Before proceeding with reports, we cite some background data.

In a series of studies carried out in the 1960s and early 1970s (48–50), Bonica and coworkers showed that epinephrine added to local anesthetics and doses ranging from 20 μg to 400 μg injected into the epidural space or around major nerves, consistently produced a beta adrenergic action, which produced alterations in cardiovascular function consisting of increases in stroke volume and heart rate and, consequently, cardiac output and left ventricular stroke work in a concomitant decrease in total peripheral resistance and mean arterial pressure. These beta adrenergic effects of epinephrine were first noted at 5 minutes and reached their peak at 15 minutes, remained at this level for 15 to 20 minutes, and subsequently returned to normal levels. The duration of the peak and the time for the decay were dose dependent. The least and shortest was with a 20-μg dose, and the highest and longest was with the 400-μg dose. They also noted that injection of as little as 15 to 20 μg of epinephrine as a bolus produced a transient (15 to 30 seconds) alpha adrenergic action consisting of increase in stroke volume and heart rate and, consequently, increase in blood pressure and peripheral resistance resulting in an increase in blood pressure. This led them to suggest that for the first time that such doses of epinephrine be included as a test dose to help predict the accidental intravenous injection. These studies are cited to help explain the conflicting results obtained in recent studies.

### *Uterine Blood Flow*

In one of the earlier studies on uterine blood flow, Barton and associates noted that the injection of epinephrine in doses of 0.10 to 1.00 μg/kg/min caused maternal blood

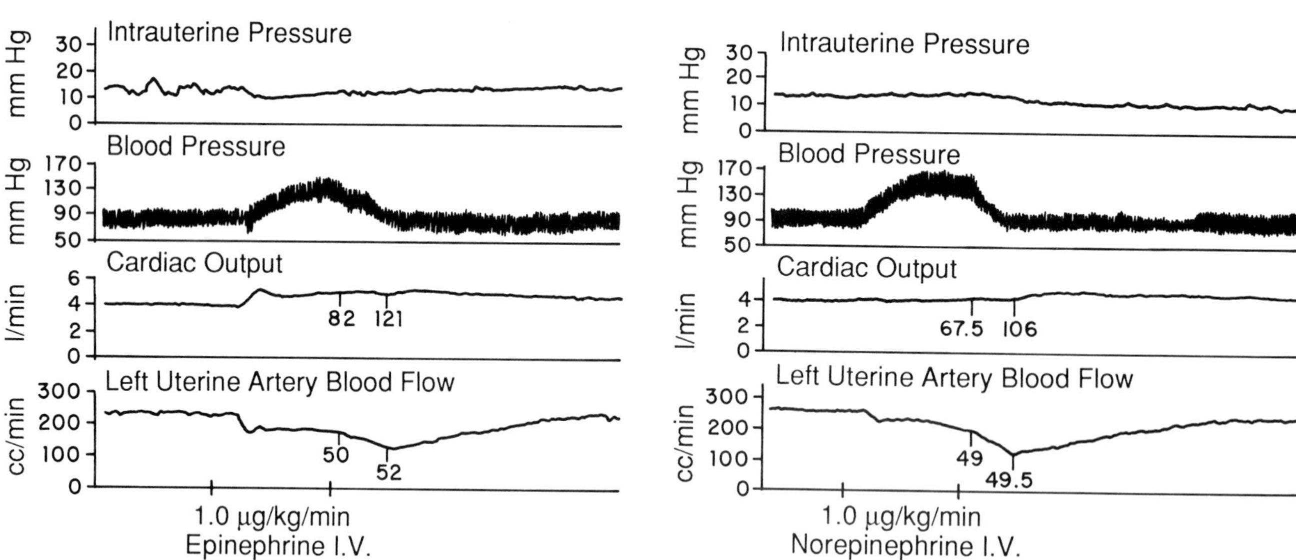


**Fig. 12–3.** Effects of intravenous epinephrine and norepinephrine on blood pressure and myometrial tonus as reflected in intrauterine pressure, integrated uterine blood flow, and cardiac output in pregnant ewes at term. The numbers show the maximum calculated changes in control conductance, the reciprocal of resistance (flow in ml/min divided by perfusion pressure in mm Hg). (Redrawn from Greiss FC Jr: The uterine vascular bed: Effect of adrenergic stimulation. Obstet. Gynecol. 21:295, 1963.)

pressure to rise 65% and uterine blood flow to fall 55 to 75% (51). Obviously, these investigators used infusion rates that produced blood levels that could cause predominantly alpha adrenergic action. Similarly, they infused 50 to 100 μg of epinephrine intravenously over a 5-minute period into pregnant ewes and produced what they believed to have been a generalized beta adrenergic effect consisting of tachycardia and an increase in cardiac output, decreased peripheral resistance, and no change in blood pressure with a 50% decrease in uterine blood flow. They postulated that the uterine artery in pregnant ewes may be more sensitive to the alpha adrenergic effects of epinephrine, while the vessels of skeletal muscles, viscera, and adipose tissue may be more sensitive to beta adrenergic effects. Wallis and associates (52) measured uterine blood flow and percentage of uterine blood flow distributed to the placenta of pregnant ewes during lumbar epidural anesthesia achieving 1.5% chloroprocaine of the same drug with 60 to 80 μg of epinephrine. They noted transient 14% decrease in uterine blood flow in the ewes receiving chloroprocaine epinephrine solution but uterine blood was sufficient at all times and maintained stable fetal acid-base and blood gas values. The percentage of uterine blood flow distributed to the placenta in the absence of uterine contractions was not altered by epidural anesthesia achieved by chloroprocaine epinephrine solution. Skjoldebrand and associates (53) noted that the addition of epinephrine to the local anesthetic to produce epidural anesthesia for cesarean section resulted in a decrease in placental blood flow. A disturbing finding in this study was the decrease in total maternal placental blood flow of 34% with a p value of less than 0.01. This methodology may be questioned because it is a human study using computer-linked gamma camera, and it may be that the camera positioning may affect the total read-out and slight variations in camera angle may affect the results.

Nonetheless, the authors have validated their technique in pregnant monkeys against radioactive microspheres as a referenced method and indeed found them to be valid. Furthermore, it should be realized that 2.5 μg/ml is equivalent to 1:400,000 solution of epinephrine, which is a very dilute solution as most of the solutions currently in use are 1:200,000, and certainly in epidural use. 1:200,000 solution is equivalent to 5 μg/ml compared to the 2.5 μg/ml referred to in the study, which is a 1:400,000 solution.

A number of other studies have shown little or no effect on uterine blood flow. Thus, de Rosayo and associates (54) studied the effects of 100 μg of epinephrine added to the epidural local anesthetic solution on cardiovascular system of anesthetized pregnant ewes and noticed that except for slight tachycardia there were no significant cardiovascular changes and uterine blood flow remained stable. Albright and associates (55) studied the effects of epidural anesthesia achieved with 10 ml of chloroprocaine and 1:200,000 epinephrine in humans and noted that despite a slight reduction in mean arterial pressure, there was no alteration in intervillous blood flow. This was corroborated by a Abboud and his coworkers (56) who compared 2% lidocaine alone to 2% lidocaine with 1:200,000 epinephrine administered for epidural anesthesia for cesarean section and found no adverse effects of epinephrine on the mother or neonate as assessed by the incidence of hypotension, low Apgar scores or abnormal fetal acid-base status.

In view of the current practice of using continuous infusions of dilute solutions of local anesthetics and opioids for epidural analgesia and anesthesia for labor and delivery, the problem of epinephrine effect on uterine blood flow no longer exists. On the other hand, we and many other clinicians often add epinephrine 1:200,000 to the local anesthetics for cesarean section because this does decrease the level of the local anesthetic in maternal blood and does decrease the risk of maternal and fetal toxicity. Although there may be transient fluctuation in uterine blood flow with such epinephrine containing solutions, there has been little or no effect on the fetus except the mothers who are very anxious and apprehensive and are secreting increased amounts of exogenous epinephrine. Under such circumstances, there was high instance of abnormal fetal heart rate patterns compared to those fetuses born to mothers who were less anxious (57).

## *Effects on Uterine Contractions*

Following Rucker's publication (45), the effects of exogenously administered epinephrine on uterine contractility were studied by many who used large intravenous doses to produce inhibition of uterine activity. As previously mentioned, because epinephrine is no longer used as a uterine relaxant, these studies are no longer relevant to the current issues. However, the series of studies by Zuspan and associates (30) deserve brief mention. Zuspan and associates measured uterine activity by internal tocodynamometry technique to study the effects of l-epinephrine and norepinephrine on the uterus and correlated those with plasma levels for catecholamines. They noted that l-epinephrine infused at rates of 0.5 and 0.25 μg/min had little effect on uterine contractility, but when the infusion was increased to 5 μg/min a decrease in uterine activity occurred within 3 minutes and lasted for the duration of infusion and for 20 minutes thereafter. Further increases in infusion rates increased inhibitory effects. Norepinephrine produced a definite increase in uterine activity (tonus, intensity, and frequency of contraction) in all patients and with higher doses it produced incoordinate uterine activity. The plasma level of the catecholamines was related to the infusion rates. The studies demonstrated that low blood levels of epinephrine have little or no effect on uterine contractility.

During the past 2 decades, numerous clinical studies have evaluated the effect of epinephrine added to the local anesthetic to achieve continuous epidural analgesia and anesthesia for labor and vaginal delivery. These studies are detailed in Chapter 11. To briefly recapitulate here, we cite first the study by Gunther and associates (58) who carried out double-blind, randomized investigations that totalled 1946 parturients managed with continuous caudal analgesia. They noted the addition of epinephrine increased the duration of the first stage of labor 30 to 40 minutes for nulliparae and about 26 minutes in multiparae. That such occurred is not surprising in view of the fact that total dose of 175 to 250 μg of epinephrine was used during periods ranging from 2 to 2½ hours from the time the block was initiated to complete cervical dilatation. The influence of epinephrine added to the local anesthetic solution for epidural analgesia on uterine contractility was evaluated by a number of investigators. Zador and Nilsson (59,60) evaluated the effects of epinephrine in two studies. In one, epidural analgesia was achieved by repeated injections of 10 to 15 ml of 0.5% lidocaine with 1:200,000 epinephrine, while in the second study they used continuous infusion of 1.2 mg of lidocaine per minute with solutions containing epinephrine. In most instances, there was a decrease in intensity in uterine contractions and of uterine activity, which lasted about 15 to 30 minutes and returned to normal. Matadial and Cibils (61) noted that when lidocaine with epinephrine 1: 200,000 was administered as initial dose of 3 to 4 ml and as a therapeutic dose of 6 to 10 ml, a transient decrease in uterine activity followed. Lowensohn and associates (62) also found a significant reduction in uterine activity lasting 30 minutes after lidocaine epinephrine injection. The latter two studies only provided information up to 60 minutes after the study was initiated. A similar transient decrease in uterine activity followed injection of lidocaine with epinephrine 1:200,000, as was noted by Craft and associates (63), who compared the effects of 1.5% lidocaine 1:200,000 when 1.5% plain lidocaine for continuous lumbar epidural analgesia was used. They noted that while there was transient decrease in uterine activity, there was no significant difference on the rate of cervical dilatation and duration of the first stage of labor between the two groups, nor was there any demonstrable difference of uterine response to oxytocin in both groups of patients. In view of this and because currently continuous infusion of dilute solutions of local anesthetics combined with opioids are being used for labor and vaginal delivery, the effects of epinephrine on uterine contractility are no longer an important issue.

### *Endogenous Epinephrine and Norepinephrine in Relation to Uterine Contractility*

It has long been known that emotional or physical distress provokes sympathetic hyperactivity with a consequent increase in the secretion of catecholamines from various body stores and the adrenal medulla. The presence of such stimuli in pregnancy, and particularly in labor, suggested the possibility that changes in the blood levels of the catecholamines may be related to the onset and maintenance of labor, problems of uterine dysfunction, and some complications of pregnancy, such as toxemia. Among the first to consider this possibility were Hardy and Javert (64), and Kaiser and Harris (65), who suggested that there may be a relationship between emotionally provoked increase in endogenous catecholamines and uterine inertia. In an attempt to substantiate this hypothesis, Garcia and Garcia (66) measured blood levels of epinephrine in: (1) patients with normally progressing labor; (2) apprehensive patients with moderately painful labor; and (3) patients with slow (inertial) labor. From these results, they concluded that there is a definite correlation between the blood levels of epinephrine and uterine inertia.

Animal studies have shown that acute pain caused by noxious stimulation produces a significant (20 to 40%) increase in catecholamine levels, particularly norepinephrine, with a consequent 35 to 70% decrease in uterine blood flow (67–69). Human studies have shown that severe pain and anxiety during active labor cause a 300 to 600% increase in the epinephrine level, a 200 to 400% increase in the norepinephrine level, a 200 to 300% increase in the cortisol level, and significant increases in corticosteroid and ACTH levels during the course of labor; these reach peak values at or after delivery (1). Lederman and associates (70,71) noted that, during the period of active labor, the epinephrine level increased by nearly 300%, the norepinephrine level by 150%, and the cortisol level by 200%. They noted that the higher epinephrine levels were significantly associated with uterine contractile activity at the onset of active labor (3 cm cervical dilatation) and with longer labor during the active phase (3 to 10 cm cervical dilatation). Increased epinephrine and cortisol levels were correlated significantly with anxiety and pain.

Ohno and associates (72) carried out a comprehensive study of catecholamines and cyclic nucleotides during labor and following delivery, and noted a nearly twofold increase in the dopamine level, a threefold increase in the epinephrine level, and a twofold increase in the norepinephrine level, as well as a small increase in the CAMP level. They noted a positive correlation between epinephrine on the one hand and heart rate and systolic blood pressure on the other, as well as a correlation between norepinephrine and CAMP during labor. The greater increase in epinephrine than in norepinephrine was contrasted with the findings of a previous study, which showed that norepinephrine was much greater than epinephrine during physical exercise. This led these investigators to conclude that elevated sympathoadrenal activity during labor is a result of pain and anxiety rather than of physical effort. In a small, albeit significant percentage of parturients, pain and anxiety produce "incoordinate uterine contractions" manifested by decrease in uterine intensity, coupled with an increase in frequency and uterine tonus (72).

### Effect on the Fetus

Epinephrine and norepinephrine administered to the mother may influence the fetus directly or indirectly, or both. As long ago as 1932, G.A. Clark (73) noted in animals that injection of epinephrine into the mother affected the fetal heart rate, an action that he ascribed to minute amounts of catecholamines crossing the placental barrier and reaching the fetal heart. His interpretation was subsequently doubted by Martin and Young (74), whose experiments led them to conclude that changes in the fetal heart rate, following administration of catecholamines to the mother, were secondary to hypoxia caused by uterine arterial constriction. It was then generally believed that catecholamines were destroyed by placental monoamine oxidate, so that none ever reached the fetus. However,

Sandler and associates (75) have shown in humans that norepinephrine labeled with radioactive carbon crosses the placental barrier in significant amounts. They were able to detect the agent in afferent cord blood, whereas efferent blood showed very little radioactivity, which presumably had been bound or inactivated during its passage through fetal tissues. These findings, together with clinical observation, indicate that exogenous catecholamines administered to the mother do cross the placental barrier and provoke a cardiovascular response in the fetus.

Mothers who are very anxious during labor have increased circulating epinephrine blood levels and a higher incidence of abnormal fetal heart patterns compared to those less anxious. As previously mentioned, the pain of uterine contraction frequently causes anxiety and apprehension with consequent increase in catecholamines resulting in decreasing uterine blood flow. Morishima and colleagues (68) reported that in pregnant baboons and rhesus monkeys nociceptive stimulation increased catecholamines and uterine activity about 60 to 65% and was associated with decreased fetal heart rate and oxygenation. Similar results were reported by Shnider, et al (69) and Martin and Gingerick (76). Lederman and associates (71) also noted that parturients who were anxious and had pain had a higher incidence of abnormal fetal heart rate patterns, and that their infants had lower 1- and 5-minute Apgar scores.

## Therapeutic Use

### *Use as Vasoconstrictor*

It has already been mentioned that the use of epinephrine in obstetric practice is limited to produce vasoconstriction and as a test dose. This drug is no longer used as a myometrial relaxant because of its serious side effects and also because better and more effective agents have been produced, as discussed in Chapter 5.

Epinephrine can be used to retard the absorption of local anesthetic and thus: (1) increase intensity and the duration of analgesia; and (2) decrease the incidence of toxic reaction, provided that not more than 100 μg are used, the fetus is not already compromised, and the mother does not have a disease (e.g., thyrotoxicosis, mitral valve disease or heart failure, and contraindicating cardiac stimulants). For optimum effect, the best concentration of epinephrine is 1:200,000 (5 μg/ml).

Although for optimum effect the best concentration of epinephrine is 1:200,000 (5 μg/ml), lower concentrations (1:400,000) are used in patients with pregnancy-induced hypertension. The use of epinephrine to retard the absorption of local anesthetics used for labor and vaginal delivery has decreased and in some centers it has been eliminated altogether. On the other hand, this author adds epinephrine 1:200,000 to the local anesthetic for epidural anesthesia used for cesarean section.

One of the most frequent and grievous errors in regional anesthesia practice is to measure the amount of epinephrine or other vasoconstrictor crudely and inaccurately by the drop method. For accurate measurement, it is best to use a 1.0 ml tuberculin syringe. A basic rule for this purpose is to use 0.1 ml of 1:1,000 epinephrine (i.e., 100 μg) for each 20 ml of local anesthetic solution. Because the regional anesthetic methods described and recommended in this book usually entail the use of 10 to 20 ml of local anesthetic, and never more than 30 ml, amounts greater than 150 μg of epinephrine need never be given at any one time. Every precaution should be taken to avoid accidental intravenous injection of the solution, so that the patient will not develop a toxic reaction to the local anesthetic and epinephrine with resultant severe hypertension.

### *Use of Test Dose*

Controversy also exists as to the components of the test dose for epidural anesthesia. Traditionally, the test dose consists of a small amount of local anesthetic and epinephrine. The former reveals if the test dose is injected into the subarachnoid space, and the latter shows an intravascular injection. Moore and Batra (77) state that the components of a test dose must contain 15 μg epinephrine and 1 mg of the local anesthetic drug, which rapidly results in evidence of spinal anesthesia. Albright (78) believes that epinephrine should be used with the therapeutic dose of bupivacaine in obstetrics. On the other hand, Leighton and colleagues (79) have shown that epinephrine produces only a transient tachycardia in laboring women. They have studied isoproterenol as a marker for a test dose (80). Epinephrine in the test dose also has been criticized because it may produce a significant reduction in uterine blood flow if given intravenously. Indeed, Hood, et al (81) found that intravenous injection of 10 to 30 μg of epinephrine decreased uterine blood flow for more than 3 minutes. However, because the total reduction over time in uterine blood flow was not greater than that associated with a normal uterine contraction, only fetuses so compromised in which immediate cesarean section is indicated would demonstrate any adverse effects (82). These authors commonly use a test dose of lidocaine 1.5%, 3 ml, with epinephrine 1:200,000.

### *Norepinephrine*

The use of norepinephrine, either to stimulate the uterus or to raise the blood pressure in the gravida, is potentially dangerous to the mother and fetus. Because it produces incoordinate uterine activity and increased tonus, it is a poor oxytoxic agent and likely will compromise the fetus. Its administration is particularly dangerous for the treatment of hypovolemic hypotension, because it will further decrease placental circulation and may initiate premature separation of the placenta, and thus prove disastrous to the infant and the mother.

## PHARMACOLOGY AND CLINICAL EFFICACY

Vasopressors produce an increase in blood pressure by: (1) direct action on smooth muscle; (2) indirect action through the release of endogenous stores of catecholamines; or (3) mixed action, i.e., they have both direct and indirect effects (see Table 12–1). Phenylephrine, like epinephrine, angiotensin, and norepinephrine, has a direct effect on smooth muscle. It is, therefore, a drug that might be considered if catecholamine stores have been depleted. Methoxamine also has a direct effect (2,5). Mephentermine has an indirect effect. Ephedrine and metaraminol have a mixed effect, and thus might not be as effective as the aforementioned drugs in subjects whose catecholamines have been depleted. However, for reasons that become apparent below, ephedrine is the most frequently used drug in raising maternal blood pressure in obstetric anesthesia.

In obstetric practice, the most important vasopressors are ephedrine, mephentermine (Wyamine), dopamine (Intropin), and, under certain circumstances, phenylephrine (Neo-Synephrine). Other agents that have been developed and used include methoxamine (Vasoxyl), metaraminol (Aramine), dobutamine (Dobutrex), isoproterenol (Isuprel), Aamrinone (Inocor), milrinohe (Primacor), and angiotensin (Hypertensin).

### *Ephedrine*

Ephedrine is the vasopressor of choice in obstetrics. Ephedrine acts both directly and indirectly, releasing stores of catecholamines, and increases arterial pressure by both peripheral vasoconstriction and by cardiac stimulation. There is an increase in heart rate, stroke volume, and blood pressure. The hemodynamic picture is similar to epinephrine except that ephedrine does not dilate blood vessels. Ephedrine possesses both beta and alpha properties (83), but increases rather than decreases uterine blood flow (see Figure 12–4) (84). The alpha effects may be exerted mostly on capacitance vessels (5,6,85). Ramanathan and Grant (86) found that both ephedrine and phenylephrine increase cardiac preload by constricting venous capacitance vessels (alpha effect). Perhaps the resistance vessels are spared. Ephedrine stimulates the central venous system, produces tachyphylaxis, and its duration of action is much longer than that of epinephrine or levarterenol. It passes the placenta (87). Ephedrine finds its greatest usefulness when given intravenously (5 to 10 mg) for the treatment of maternal hypotension (88) after more physiologic measures (fluid loading, left uterine displacement) have not been successful (88–90). Fetal acidosis is improved by ephedrine (91). The treatment by ephedrine of spinal or epidural anesthesia hypotensions, if preceded by generous infusion of crystalloid and left uterine displacement, has been known by many investigators not to be associated with fetal or neonatal acidemia (92–96).

Much of the information that we have on vasopressors in obstetrics has been generated from animal work. One should be skeptical in extrapolating animal blood flow data to human placental blood flow (97). Although controversial, human uterine vessels (unlike those of the ewe) do dilate with beta-adrenergic stimulation, making the interpretation of uterine blood flow data in sheep studies questionable (55) Marx, et al (98) clearly demonstrated that ephedrine prophylaxis or treatment of spinal hypotension in the human have adverse effect on the clinical or biochemical status.

Ephedrine may be given intramuscularly (50 mg) for attempted prophylaxis of maternal hypotension. Gutsche (99) found a 100% hypotension rate in nine patients (placebo group) given spinal anesthesia for cesarean section; this was reduced to 25% (two of eight patients) when prophylactic ephedrine was utilized. This method could be criticized because it is not 100% effective and, in certain patients, could produce undesirable hypertension. Rolbin, et al (100) using 25 or 50 mg of intramuscular ephedrine prophylactically did find that 50 mg caused a persistent hypertension in 8 of 12 patients. The incidence of hypotension was 8 to 12% in all three groups. Thus, prophylactic intramuscular ephedrine is of dubious value.

Ephedrine may be given as soon as any fall in maternal blood pressure is detected to offset a longer period of hypotension and thus a possible decrease in uteroplacental blood flow. Datta, et al (101) found this quite effective, giving increments of ephedrine 10 mg intravenously until

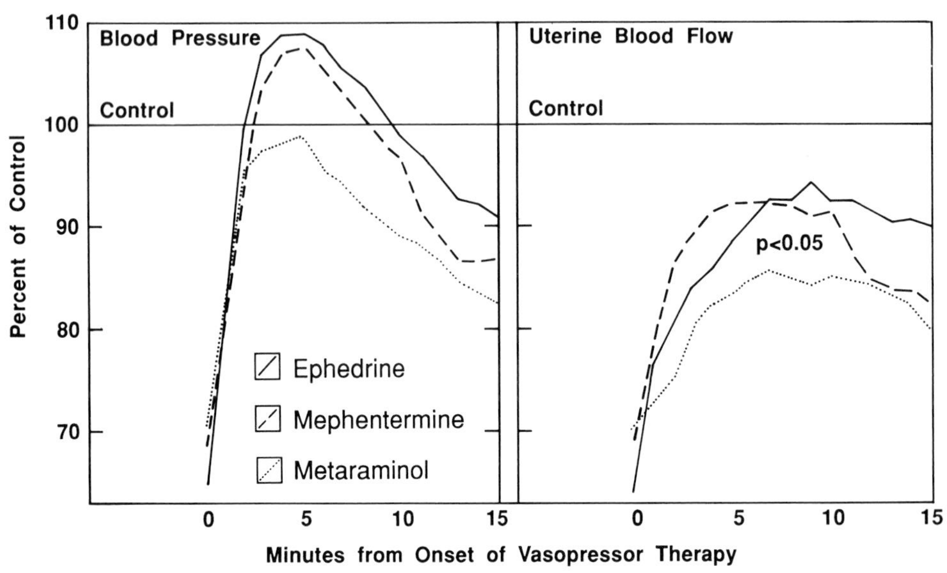


**Fig. 12–4.** Pooled average response patterns to ephedrine, mephentermine, and metaraminol given at varying rates with and without atropine in sheep. After 1 and 2 minutes with ephedrine and mephentermine, respectively, uterine blood flow was significantly higher than with metaraminol. (From James FM III, Greiss FC, Kemp RA: An evaluation of vasopressor therapy for maternal hypotension during spinal anesthesia. Anesthesiology. 33: 25, 1970.)

the blood pressure was restored. Kang, et al (90), Hollmën (102), and Jouppila, et al (103) used a prophylactic intravenous ephedrine infusion, also with good results. Marx, et al (98) gave prophylactic ephedrine and found good acid-base status in the infants.

Many authors have demonstrated excellent acid-base condition of infants whose mothers became hypotensive, and then treated with ephedrine (86,90,104,105). The optimal approach now seems to be to displace the uterus to the left, load the patient with 1500 to 2000 ml crystalloid before the spinal or epidural anesthetic takes effect, then to administer a small dose of ephedrine if the systolic blood pressure drops at all, giving further increments in an attempt to keep the blood pressure close to baseline. Ephedrine crosses the placenta, increases fetal heart rate, but does not affect fetal outcome (106). Ephedrine also does not affect the neurobehavioral status of the newborn infant, but does influence the power and the frequency of the spectral electroencephalogram (EEG) (107).

## *Mephentermine*

This sympathomimetic amine has an indirect action, mediated through release of catecholamines (see Table 12–1). As with ephedrine, tachyphylaxis occurs readily (5). Senties and coworkers (92) studied the effect of mephentermine on uterine contractility in pregnant women at term. Results were quantitatively similar to norepinephrine. Intravenous infusion increased intensity and frequency of uterine contractions as well as resting uterine tone. Increase in blood pressure is due mostly to cardiac stimulation (7); its alpha activity is relatively weak. Of considerable interest was the finding in 1970 by James and colleagues (84) that mephentermine raises uterine blood flow after spinal hypotension, as does ephedrine (see Figure 12–4)).

## *Dopamine*

This precursor of norepinephrine, unlike other vasopressors, has an effect on receptors that is dose dependent. At low doses (2 μg/kg/min) it has dopamine effects, resulting in an increase in renal blood flow (108). Higher doses (3 to 12 μg/kg/min) cause primarily beta stimulation and with more than 12 μg/kg/min, alpha effects may predominate. For these reasons, infusions of low dose dopamine might seem to be an effective treatment of hypotension in obstetrics. Animal studies are conflicting on this point. Blanchard and Cabalum (109,110), using an electromagnetic flow probe on the common internal iliac artery in pregnant ewes, demonstrated significant increases in uterine blood flow in response to dopamine at increasing concentrations (Figure 12–5). Callender and associates (111,112), on the other hand, applied an electromagnetic flow probe to a branch of the uterine artery and recorded decreased uterine blood flow, particularly at the higher concentrations of 20 to 40 μg/kg/min (Figure 12–6). The work of Fishburne (113) supports the latter view. The difference may be one of methodology. The ewe possesses a common internal iliac artery (Figure 12–7) (94), essentially a trifurcation of the aorta. It is suggested that a flow probe on the common internal iliac

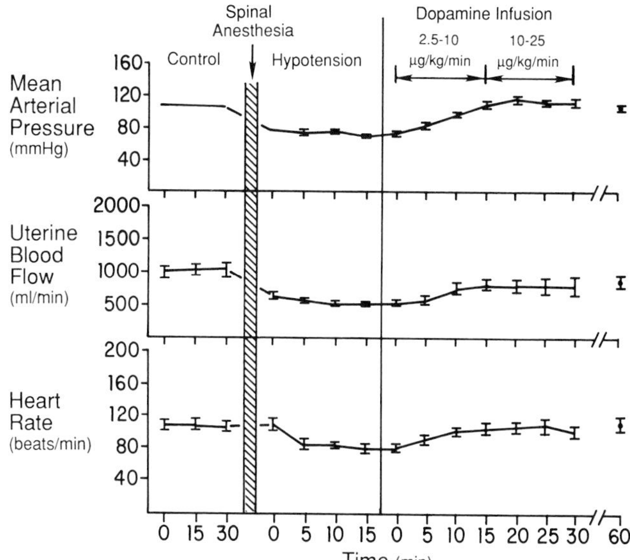


**Fig. 12–5.** Effect of dopamine on uterine blood flow in sheep made hypotensive with spinal anesthesia. Average values (+1 SE) for systemic arterial pressure, uterine blood flow, and heart rate during control, spinal anesthesia, and dopamine-infusion periods. Average values obtained 30 minutes after interruption of dopamine infusion are represented by one datum to avoid expansion of the graph. Note that in this report uterine blood flow returned to normal. (Redrawn from Cabalum T, Zugaib M, Lieb S, Nuwayhid B, et al: Effect of dopamine on hypotension induced by spinal anesthesia. Am. J. Obstet. Gynecol. 133:630, 1979.)

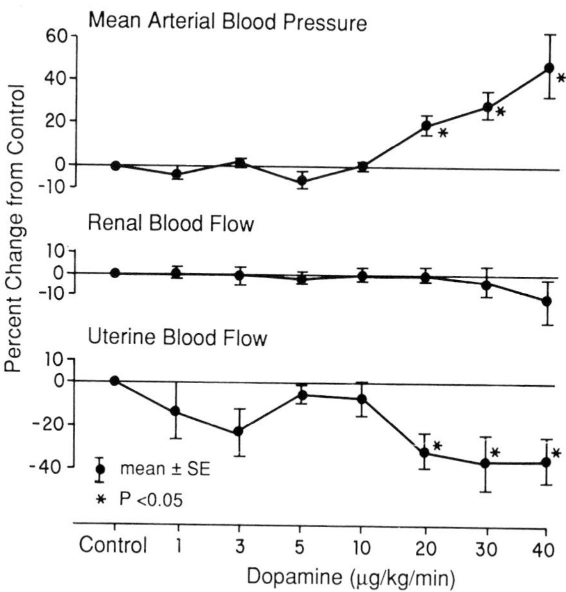


**Fig. 12–6.** Changes in mean arterial pressure, renal blood flow, and uterine blood flow from control with administration of varying dopamine dosages. Note there is minimal, if any, effect on renal blood flow but some reduction in uterine blood flow even at lower dose ranges of dopamine in the pregnant ewe. (Redrawn from Callender K, Levinson G, Shnider SM, Feduska NJ, et al: Dopamine administration in the normotensive pregnant ewe. Obstet. Gynecol. 51:586, 1978.)

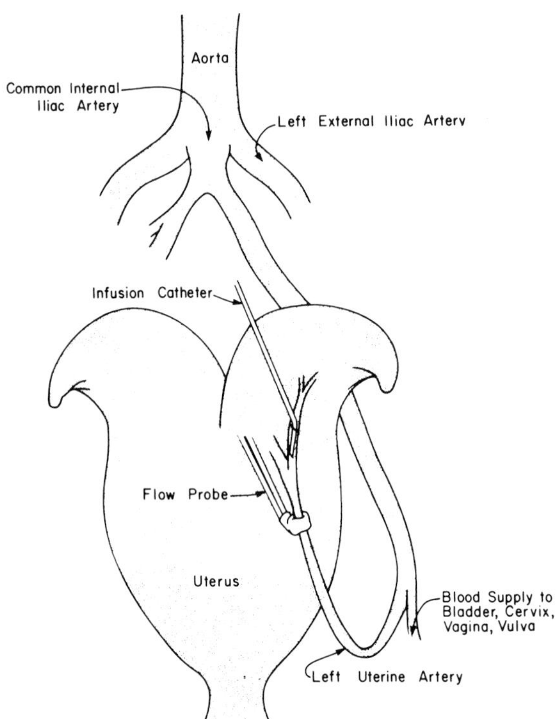


**Fig. 12–7.** Schematic diagram of the uterine vasculature in the ewe. Note presence of common internal iliac artery, which does not appear in humans. (From Miodovnik M, Lavin JP, Harrington DJ, Leung LS, et al: Effect of maternal ketoacidemia on the pregnant ewe and fetus. Am. J. Obstet. Gynecol. 144:585, 1982.)

artery measures more than the uterine vascular bed. One may therefore conclude that the correct values are recorded from the middle uterine artery and that the true dopamine response is one of decreased uterine blood flow. Dopamine was studied in human pregnant patients using spinal anesthesia (108). Umbilical cord acid-base studies and Apgar scores were evaluated, rather than uterine blood flow. Of the total study group of 68 patients, 15 did not become hypotensive. Of those who did become hypotensive, 27 received ephedrine and 26 received dopamine. There were only two depressed infants, (Apgar less than 7), one in the control group, and one in the dopamine group. Acid-base values are shown in Table 12–3. It can be noted that the only significant differences occurred in the $PO_2$ values not the pH values. These differences can be interpreted several ways.

First, one might say that there is a great deal of placental and fetal reserve, and our methodology was not sensitive enough to detect harm from dopamine. Second, one could argue that $pO_2$ was significantly lower in both dopamine and ephedrine groups; hypotension, even when it is treated promptly with vasopressors, is deleterious to the fetus. Third, it could be said that only $pO_2$ was affected (more so in the ephedrine than in the dopamine group). It is only when pH is affected that harm to the fetus can result. Therefore, dopamine has a beneficial effect.

Dopamine may have a place in obstetrics. However, the studies in the literature are in regard to the animal model,

**Table 12–3.** Umbilical Artery and Umbilical Vein Blood Gas Values at Delivery in Humans (Mean ± SE)

| | Control | Ephedrine | Dopamine |
|---|---|---|---|
| Umbilical artery | | | |
| pH | 7.26 ± 0.03 | 7.24 ± 0.01 | 7.26 ± 0.02 |
| $PO_2$ (mm Hg) | 23.3 ± 4.1 | 16.4 ± 1.1* | 14.6 ± 1.0* |
| $PCO_2$ (mm Hg) | 46.9 ± 4.0 | 48.5 ± 2.7 | 49.8 ± 2.9 |
| Base excess (mEq/l) | −5.4 ± 1.1 | −5.9 ± 0.9 | −6.2 ± 1.0 |
| Umbilical vein | | | |
| pH | 7.33 ± 0.03 | 7.33 ± 0.01 | 7.32 ± 0.02 |
| $PO_2$ (mm Hg) | 32.1 ± 3.4 | 26.4 ± 2.1 | 23.5 ± 1.2* |
| $PCO_2$ (mm Hg) | 44.5 ± 3.6 | 42.8 ± 2.4 | 42.9 ± 2.4 |
| Base excess (mEq/l) | −3.0 ± 1.5 | −4.4 ± 0.7 | −4.3 ± 0.7 |

* Significantly different from control, $P < 0.05$.
(From Clark RB, Brunner JA: Dopamine as a vasopressor for the treatment of spinal hypotension during cesarean section. Anesthesiology 53:514, 1980.)

not the human model. Furthermore, dopamine is currently not a popular drug in obstetrics, and most likely will not be in the future. In other words, adequate results have been obtained with the aforementioned drugs, such as ephedrine, and it is unlikely that dopamine will replace this time-tried agent. Occasionally, when spinal anesthesia is given for cesarean section, hypotension still occurs, despite aggressive prespinal fluid loading and left uterine displacement. Intravenous ephedrine in doses of 10 to 15 mg usually treats the hypotension satisfactorily. Rarely, extremely large doses of ephedrine (greater than 60 mg total) with spinal anesthesia have been inadequate to sustain an acceptable blood pressure (author's experience). These instances are quite unusual now that it is routine to administer over 1000 ml crystalloid or more before the block takes effect. In these instances, dopamine 10 μg/kg/min as an intravenous infusion resolved the hypotension, with no apparent harm.

## *Phenylephrine*

This potent alpha agonist has been used as a vasopressor in obstetrics. In this writer's experience, phenylephrine appears to be without deleterious clinical effect on the human infant when given by intravenous infusion to the mother, although studies have demonstrated an increase followed by a decrease in uterine blood flow (Figure 12–8)(23,94,95). Greiss and Crandell, when studying the drug, used fairly high doses (2.5 μg/kg/min) (95). The dose may explain this action. The effect of phenylephrine on the uterus independently has not been studied, but one would expect the uterus to contract, a response similar to methoxamine. It has a direct action on blood vessels (see Table 12–1). Phenylephrine is primarily an alpha agonist; some believe it exhibits slight beta activity (see Table 12–1). Reflex bradycardia can occur. Because of its alpha activity and decrease in uterine blood flow in animal models, it would presumably have detrimental fetal effects. However, Ramanathan and colleagues (86,96) studied ephedrine and phenylephrine in human subjects undergoing cesarean section under epidural anesthesia.

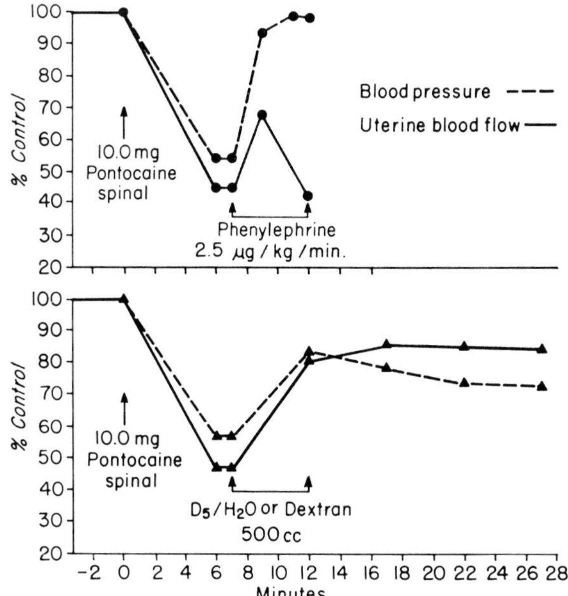


**Fig. 12–8.** Average blood pressure and uterine blood flow response to rapid infusion of dextrose and water or to dextran in sheep made hypotensive by spinal anesthesia (lower figure). The upper figure illustrates the response to phenylephrine. Note that uterine blood flow increases initially, then decreases when phenylephrine is used, but returns to near normal when dextrose and water, or dextrose is used. (Adapted from Greiss FC, Crandell DL: Therapy for hypotension induced by spinal anesthesia during pregnancy. JAMA. 191:793, 1965.)

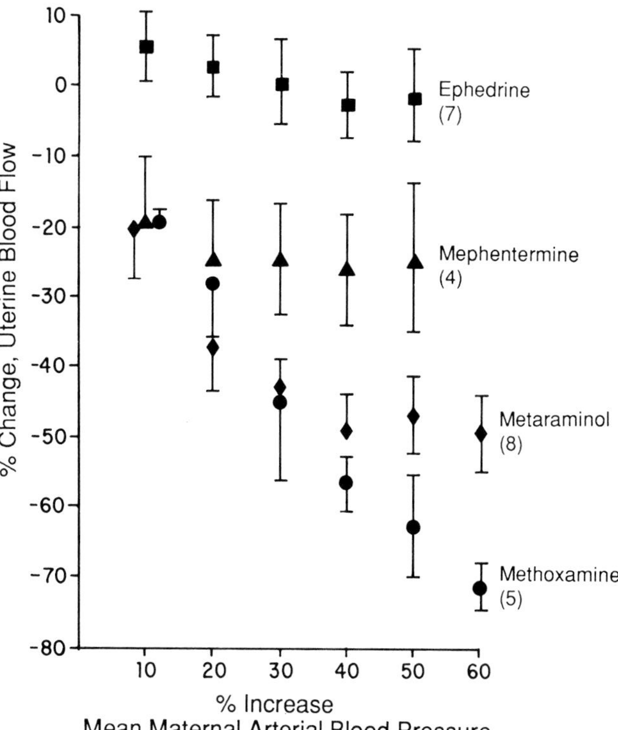


**Fig. 12–9.** Mean changes in uterine blood flow at equal elevations of mean arterial blood pressure following vasopressor administration in sheep. (Redrawn from Ralston DH, Shnider SM, deLorimier AA: Effects of equipotent ephedrine, metaraminol, mephentermine, and methoxamine on uterine blood flow in the pregnant ewe. Anesthesiology. 40:354, 1974.)

The patients were prehydrated with 1200 ml lactated Ringer's solution. Hypotension, if it occurred, was treated either with ephedrine (5-mg increments) or phenylephrine, 100-μg doses. The patients that did not become hypotensive were used as controls. Neonatal Apgar scores and acid-base profiles were not significantly different among the three groups of neonates.

Moran and colleagues (114), in well-hydrated pregnant humans undergoing elective cesarean section, found that phenylephrine in small doses (20 to 40 μg) to be as effective as ephedrine in restoring maternal blood pressure, with little difference in maternal or fetal acid-base parameters. Neurobehavioral scores were similar in both groups. One explanation is that when these small doses are employed, phenylephrine may constrict only venous capacitance vessels. If these findings are confirmed by further studies, phenylephrine in small doses may well be acceptable in well-hydrated patients. Of course, acid-base studies may not demonstrate deleterious effects, as there may be substantial placental reserve, and the decrease in blood flow may not be evidenced by fetal acidosis. Direct measurements of uterine blood flow (Figures 12–9 and 12–4) are superior to indirect studies, which depend on acid-base changes.

Demonstration of the vasoconstrictive aspects of phenylephrine in the pregnant ewe (115) opened the door to studies of the other commonly used vasopressors.

Etilefrine, a homologue of phenylephrine, also increases the vascular resistance of human maternal arteries (116).

## *Methoxamine*

This amphetamine is a pure alpha agonist (5). It raises blood pressure by vasoconstriction (117). There may be a reflex bradycardia. Vasicka and associates (118) reported that methoxamine, given intravenously in single doses of 3 mg for the treatment of hypotension caused by epidural block, consistently produced increased uterine tone and tetanic contractions. Uterine blood flow is decreased (Figure 12–9) (119,120). In the pregnant-ewe preparation, maternal blood pressure is restored by methoxamine, but fetal asphyxia is worsened (120).

## *Metaraminol*

This sympathomimetic amine has been characterized as a "weak levophed" (see Table 12–1). Indeed, it shares the alpha and beta effects of norepinephrine, although it is not as potent an alpha agonist as is norepinephrine. Blood flow to brain, kidneys, and splanchnic organs is decreased in both normotensive and hypotensive patients. Uterine effects and placental transfer do not appear to have been studied. Lucas, et al (121) demonstrated in the pregnant ewe an increase in maternal arterial pressure, uterine blood flow, and uterine vascular resistance when metaraminol was infused during spinal hypotension. Because of this apparent increase in uterine blood flow, this drug was recommended in the past for the treatment of obstetric hypotension. Shnider, et al (122) found that metaraminol improved uterine blood flow, but did not stop progressive metabolic acidosis. More recent studies have indicated that it tends to restore uterine blood flow, but not to normal, and not as well as ephedrine or mephentermine (Figure 12–9) (84,116).

### *Dobutamine*

This synthetic catecholamine acts primarily on beta-1 receptors (see Table 12–1) (2). It is an analog of dopamine and in contrast to dopamine, which produces a significant proportion of its cardiac effects through the release of norepinephrine from adrenergic nerves, dobutamine acts directly on beta-1 adrenoreceptors in the heart (4). It is recommended for cardiogenic shock. Heart rate does not increase to the extent that it does with dopamine. Fishburne and colleagues (113) studied both dopamine and dobutamine in pregnant ewes and found a decrease in uterine blood flow with both drugs. Dopamine use resulted in an increase in mean arterial pressure and uterine tone while the heart rate response was variable. Dobutamine administration resulted in a significant increase in heart rate (as it also does in humans), while mean arterial pressure and uterine tone remained essentially unchanged. Smith and Hess (123) administered dobutamine to pregnant ewes and found a decrease in uterine artery blood flow (Figure 12–10).

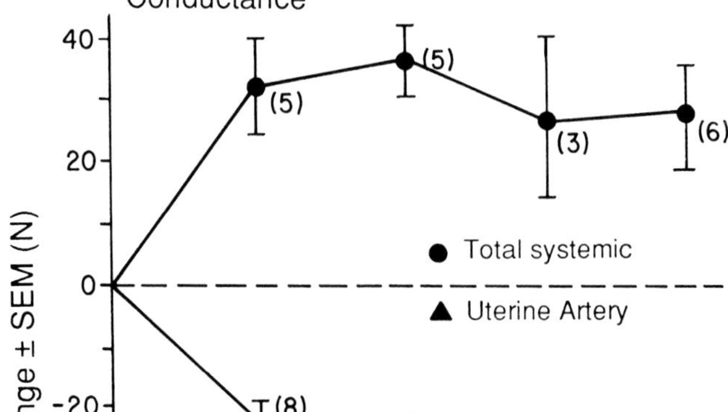


**Fig. 12–10.** The effect of dobutamine on uterine blood flow in sheep. Note decreased flow with increasing doses of dobutamine. The ewes were undergoing nitrous oxide, halothane, and curare anesthesia. (Redrawn from Smith BE, Hess DG: Effects of dobutamine infusion on uterine artery conductance and blood flow in the pregnant ewe. Presented at the annual meeting, Society for Obstetric Anesthesia and Perinatology, Cambridge, MA, May 9, 1980. SOAP Abstract, p. 14.)

### *Isoproterenol*

This classic synthetic catecholamine has almost no alpha activity. Because of vasodilatation, blood pressure would tend to fall, rather than rise, when administered. Isoproterenol causes a decrease in mean blood pressure and uterine blood flow (23). No direct vasodilatation of gravid uterine vessels has been demonstrated (124). Uterine contractions are inhibited by approximately 50% when doses of 2 to 8 µg/min are administered (57,125).

### *Amrinone*

Amrinone is not a sympathomimetic amine, but rather a bipyridine derivative that produces strong inotropic activity and weak vasodilatory effects (3). It increases cellular cyclic AMP by inhibition of phosphodiesterase (126). In gravid baboons, Fishburne, et al (126) found that an infusion of 40 µg/kg/min produced a slight increase in iliac artery blood flow, but did not significantly alter mean arterial pressure, heart rate or uterine artery blood flow. Regional infusion produced a significant increase in iliac artery blood flow without changing uterine artery blood flow or mean arterial pressure (127). Amrinone has no place as a vasopressor in obstetrics. Baumann and colleagues (127) studied milrinone, a relative of amrinone in pregnant sheep, and contrasted it with dopamine. Milrinone treatment resulted in an increase in uterine blood flow, in which there was a decrease in uterine blood flow with dopamine.

### *Angiotensin*

Angiotensin is an octapeptide formed in the body to promote the secretion of the mineralocorticoid aldosterone from the adrenal cortex (1). It is a potent vasoconstrictor. Symonds and associates (128) found lower levels in patients receiving epidural anesthesia during labor and after elective cesarean section, indicating it is produced partially by stress. Greiss and Van Wilkes (94), and Greiss and Gobble (129) studied angiotensin in ewe preparations and found that it caused an increase in blood pressure, an increase in vascular resistance, and a decrease in uterine blood flow.

## Relation of Vasopressors to Physiologic Measure in Restoring Maternal Blood Pressure

It has long been known that compression of the inferior vena cava by the pregnant uterus occurs when the patient assumes the supine position (130). It has long been less well-appreciated that the aorta is also compressed in this situation (131). Bieniarz demonstrated with arteriography that the arterial, as well as the venous system, is com-

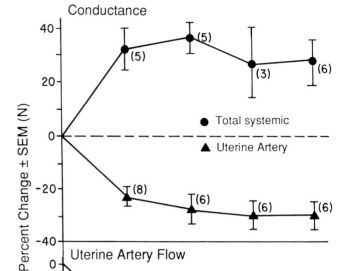

**Table 12–4.** Spinal Anesthesia for Cesarean Section and Incidence of Hypotension

| | Patients Not in Labor (Elective Section) | | | Patients in Early Labor (Primary or Repeat Section) | | |
|---|---|---|---|---|---|---|
| | No Prevention | Fluid Loading | Fluid Loading + SLUDER** | No Prevention | Fluid Loading | Fluid Loading + SLUDER** |
| # patients | 27 | 76 | 53 | 18 | 39 | 34 |
| Hypotension incidence (systolic pressure < 100 mm Hg) | 25/27 (92%) | 43/76 (57%) P ≤ 0.005* | 28/53 (52.8%) NS* | 9/18 (50%) | 18/39 (46.1%) NS* | 5/34 (14.7%) P ≤ 0.005* |
| # patients receiving ephedrine IV | 13/25 (52%) | 32/43 (74%) | 23/28 (82%) | 4/9 (44%) | 13/18 (72%) | 5/5 (100%) |
| Mean total dose of ephedrine in those who received ephedrine | 21.8 mg | 20.1 mg | 26.2 mg | 27 mg | 27 mg | 22.5 mg |
| Mean induction-delivery interval | 27.5 min | 23.5 min | 25.6 min | 28.1 min | 27.9 min | 24.0 min |
| # infants with 1-minute Apgars of 1–6 | 0/27 (0%) | 3/76 (3.9%) | 1/53 (1.9%) | 2/18 (11.1%) | 0/39 (0%) | 0/34 (0%) |

Note that the incidence of hypotension was much greater in the patients not in labor than for those in labor. The incidence of ruptured membranes was higher in the patients in labor, presumably resulting in a smaller uterine volume and less caval compression. Also note the progression of decreasing incidence of hypotension as fluid loading, and then fluid loading plus uterine displacement were employed.

* Statistical significance compared with preceding group by Chi-square test.

** Sustained left uterine displacer.

(Modified from Clark RB, Thompson DS, Thompson CH: Prevention of spinal hypotension associated with cesarean section. Anesthesiology 45: 670, 1976.)

promised (132). As stated throughout this book, parturients should labor while in the lateral position, and deliver with some sort of uterine displacement to prevent these complications. If this is done, pharmacologic treatment of maternal hypotension is often unnecessary. The use of vasopressors is also often unnecessary when the blood volume of the parturient is expanded with 1000- to 2000-ml crystalloid before institution of an epidural or spinal block. Wollman and Marx (133) were the first to call our attention to this modality; their recommendation of 1 liter of fluid given prophylactically has been extended, until now, as many anesthesiologists administer double that amount to prevent hypotension.

The incidence of hypotension when spinal or epidural anesthesia depends not only upon uterine displacement and preloading, but also on whether or not the patient is in labor.

Spinal anesthesia for elective cesarean section in the nonlaboring patient without uterine displacement or fluid loading was reported in 1970 to be 82% (134). We found it to be 92% (88). If fluid loading only is performed, the hypotension rate is 57%; if both fluid loading and uterine displacement are attended to, the rate is 53% (Table 12–4). These rates are lower when the patient is in labor; the corresponding figures are 50%, 46%, and 15% (see Table 12–4). Antoine and Young (135) also observed the differences between patients in labor and not in labor, in patients receiving epidural anesthesia, saying "only 38% of the elective cesarean section patients had stable blood pressure with epidural anesthesia, compared with 65% in the labor" (135). Brizgys, et al (136) also found a difference—with epidural anesthesia—"Non laboring mothers had a significantly higher incidence of hypotension than laboring mothers, 36% versus 24%" (136).

How does one account for these differences? We originally explained the differences by noting the autotransfusion of 300 ml of blood into the general circulation by each uterine contraction. This would periodically increase the effective blood volume. Dr. J.S. Crawford, in a personal communication, inquired if most of the patients in labor had ruptured membranes. He replied in the affirmative. It was his opinion, then, that the patients in labor had smaller uterine volumes, resulting in less caval compression (137). This seemed like a very rational explanation. Both Antione and Young, and Brizgys, et al, believed their patients who were in labor were better hydrated than those sectioned electively, and this was their explanation for the difference. We are currently studying patients who are to have elective cesarean section with epidural anesthesia and are vigorously hydrated, comparing them with section patients who have been in labor, to ascertain if it is the difference in hydration that makes elective section patients more prone to hypotension. It could be that all three mechanisms are operative; autotransfusion, a greater incidence of uterine size and less caval compression in laboring patients, and better hydration in laboring patients.

The primary message, however, remains clear. The infusion of 1000- to 2000-ml balanced salt solution and uterine displacement results in a much decreased number of patients who require vasopressor therapy. If this fluid infusion does not prevent hypotension, the uterus should be moved manually to the left and the legs of the patient elevated so that the patient forms a reverse L; in other words, the legs are straight up in the air. This results in an autotransfusion of some 500 or more ml that results in an increase in both systolic and diastolic pressure within seconds of the maneuver. This rarely fails in treatment of hypotension secondary to sympathectomy of regional analgesia. If hypotension does occur despite these measures, the vasopressor of choice is ephedrine.

## REFERENCES


1. Bonica JJ: Principles and Practice of Obstetric Analgesia and Anesthesia. Philadelphia, F.A. Davis, 1967, p. 289.
2. Stoelting R: Sympathomimetics. *In* Pharmacology and Physiology in Anesthetic Practice. Edited by RK Stoelting. Philadelphia, J.B. Lippincott, 1987, p. 251.
3. Lawson NW, Wallfisch HK: Cardiovascular pharmacology: a new look at the "pressors." *In* Advances in Anesthesia. Edited by RK Stoelting. Chicago, Yearbook Medical Publishers, 1986, p. 195.
4. Craig CR, Stitzel RF: Modern Pharmacology. 2nd Ed. Boston, Little Brown, 1986, p. 158.
5. Durrett LR, Lawson NW: Autonomic nervous system, physiology and pharmacology. *In* Clinical Anesthesia. Edited by P Barash, BF Cullen, RK Stoelting. Philadelphia, J.B. Lippincott, 1989, p. 165.
6. Smith NT, Corbasicio AN: The use and misuse of pressor agents. Anesthesiology 33:58, 1970.
7. Hoffman BB, Lefkowitz RJ: Catecholamines and sympathomimetic drugs. *In* The Pharmacological Basis of Therapeutics. 8th Ed. Edited by L Goodman, A Gilman., New York, Macmillan, 1990, p. 187.
8. Carllson A: The occurrence, distribution and physiological role of catecholamines in the nervous system. Pharmacol. Rev. 11:490, 1959.
9. Hillarp NA, Hokfelt B, Nilson BP: The cytology of the adrenal medullary cells with special reference to the storage and secretion of the sympathomimetic amines. Acta. Anat. 21:155, 1954.
10. Von Euler US: Epinephrine and norepinephrine: actions and use in man. Clin. Pharmacol. Ther. 1:65, 1960.
11. Ahlquist RP and Woodbury RA: Influence of drugs and uterine activity upon uterine blood flow. Fed. Proc. 6:305, 1947.
12. Ahlquist RP: Adrenergic drugs. *In* Pharmacology In Medicine. Edited VA Drill. New York, McGraw-Hill, 1971, p. 627.
13. Von Euler US, Franksson C, Hellstrom J: Adrenaline and noradrenaline output in urine after unilateral and bilateral adrenalectomy in man. Acta. Physiol. Scand. 31:1, 1954.
14. Morrow DH, Gaffney TE, Chidsey CA: The effect of norepinephrine infusion in reserpine induced myocardial catecholamine depletion: implications in anesthesiology. Anesth. Analg. 42:21, 1963.
15. Dale HH: The action of certain esters and ethers of choline and their relation to muscarine. J. Pharmacol. Exp. Ther. 6:147, 1941.
16. Cannon WG, Uridil JE: Studies on the conditions of activity in endocrine glands. VIII. Some effects on the denervated heart of stimulating the nerves of the liver. Am. J. Physiol. 58:353, 1921.
17. Von Euler US: A specific sympathomimetic ergone in adrenergic nerve fibers (sympathin) and its relation to adrenaline and noradrenaline. Acta. Physiol. Scand. 12:73, 1946.
18. Ahlquist RP: A study of the adrenotropic receptors. Amer. J. Physiol. 153:586, 1948.
19. Lands AM, Arnold A, McAuliff JP, Luduena FP, et al: Differentiation of receptor system activated by sympathomimetic amines. Nature 214:597, 1967.
20. Langer SZ: Presynaptic regulation of catecholamine release. Biochem. Pharmacol. 23:1793, 1974.
21. Ariens EJ, Simons AM: Physiologic and pharmacological aspects of adrenergic receptor classification. Biochem. Pharmacol. 32:1539, 1983.
22. Stander RW, Barden TP: Adrenergic receptor activity of catecholamines in human gestational myometrium. J. Obstet. Gynecol. 28:768, 1966.
23. Greiss FC, Pick JF: The uterine vascular bed: adrenergic receptors. Obstet. Gynecol. 23:209, 1964.
24. Kebabian JW, Calne DB: Multiple receptors for dopamine. Nature 277:93, 1979.
25. McLaughlin MK, Keve TM, Cooke R: Vascular catecholamine sensitivity during pregnancy in the ewe. Am. J. Obstet. Gynecol. 160:47, 1989.
26. Datta S, Kitzmiller JL, Ostheimer GW, Scoenbaum SC: Propranolol and parturition. Obstet. Gynecol. 51:577, 1978.
27. Cotten M, Moran NC: Cardiovascular pharmacology. Ann. Rev. Pharmacol. 1:261, 1961.
28. Kennedy WF, Bonica JJ, Ward RJ: Cardiorespiratory effects of epinephrine when used in regional anesthesia. Acta. Anaesth. Scand. Suppl. 23:320, 1966.
29. Barcroft H, Konzett H: On actions of noradrenaline, adrenalin and isopropyl noradrenalin on arterial blood pressure, heart rate and muscle blood flow in man. J. Physiol. 110: 194, 1949.
30. Zuspan FP, Cibils LA, Pose SV: Myometrial and cardiovascular responses to alterations in plasma epinephrine and norepinephrine. Am. J. Obstet. Gynecol. 84:841, 1962.
31. Price HL, Lurie AA, Jones RE, Price ML, et al: Cyclopropane anesthesia. II. Epinephrine and norepinephrine in initiation of ventricular arrhythmias by carbon dioxide inhalation. Anesthesiology 19:619, 1958.
32. Johnson RR, Eger EI, Wilson C: A comparative interaction of epinephrine with enflurane, isoflurane and halothane in man. Anesth. Analg. 55:709, 1976.
33. Eckenhoff JE: Physiology of coronary circulation. Anesthesiology 11:168, 1950.
34. Corday E, Williams JH Jr: Effect of shock and of vasopressor drugs on the regional circulation of the brain, heart, kidney and liver. Amer. J. Med. 29:228, 1960.
35. Oldendorf WH: Brain uptake of radiolabeled amino acids, amines and hexoses after arterial injection. Am. J. Physiol. 221:1629, 1971.
36. Olesen J: The effect of intracarotid epinephrine, norepinephrine, and angiotensin on the regional cerebral blood flow in man. Neurology 22:978, 1972.
37. Moyer JH and Handley CA: Norepinephrine and epinephrine effect on renal hemodynamics. Circulation 5:91, 1952.
38. Smythe CM, Nickel J, Bradley SE: The effect of epinephrine (U.S.P.) 1-epinephrine and l-norepinephrine on glomerular filtration rate, renal plasma flow, and the urinary excretion of sodium, potassium and water in normal man. J. Clin. Invest. 31:449, 1952.
39. Coleridge JCG, Hemingway A: Partition of the venous return of the heart. J. Physiol. 142:366, 1958.
40. Greenway CV, Lawson AE: The effects of adrenalin and noradrenalin on venous return and regional blood flows in the anaesthetized cat with special reference to intestinal blood flow. J. Physiol. (Lond.) 1986:579–595, 1966.
41. Lillehi RC: The modern treatment of shock based on physiological principles. Clin. Pharmacol. Ther. 5:63, 1964.
42. Neu M: Untersuchungen uber die bedeutung des suprarenins fur diei geburtshulfe. Eine experimentelle and klinische studie. Berlin, L Schumacher, 1908.
43. Rucker MP: The action of adrenalin on the human pregnant uterus. Southern Med. J. 18:412, 1925.
44. Rucker MP: Treatment of contraction ring dystocia with adrenalin. Am. J. Obstet. Gynecol. 14:609, 1927.
45. Rucker MP: Adrenalin in treatment of contraction ring with note on action of adrenalin upon tubal contractions. Southern Med. J. 24:258, 1931.

46. Greiss FC Jr: The uterine vascular bed: effect of adrenergic stimulation. Obstet. Gynecol. 21:295, 1963.
47. Stroup PE: The influence of epinephrine on uterine contractility. Am. J. Obstet. Gynecol. 84:595, 1962.
48. Ward RJ, Bonica JJ, Freund FG, Akamatsu T, et al: Epidural and subarachnoid anesthesia: cardiovascular and respiratory effects. JAMA 191:275–278, 1965.
49. Bonica JJ, Berges PU, Morikawa K: Circulatory effects of peridural block: I. Effects of level of analgesia and dose of lidocaine. Anesthesiology 33:619–626, 1970.
50. Bonica JJ, Akamatsu TJ, Berges PU, Morikawa K, et al: Circulatory effects of peridural block. II. Effects of epinephrine. Anesthesiology 34:514–522, 1971.
51. Barton MD, Kilam AP, Meschia G: Response of ovine uterine blood flow to epinephrine and norepinephrine. Proc. Soc. Exp. Biol. Med. 145:996–1003, 1974.
52. Wallis KL, Shnider SM, Hicks JS, Spivey HT: Epidural anesthesia in the normotensive pregnant ewe: effects on uterine blood flow and fetal acid-base status. Anesthesiology 44:481, 1976.
53. Skjoldebrand A, Eklund J, Lunell N-O, Nylund L, et al: The effects on uteroplacental blood flow of epidural anaesthesia containing adrenaline for cesarean section. Acta. Anaesthesiol. Scand. 34:85, 1990.
54. de Rosayo AM, Nahrwold ML, Hill AB: Cardiovascular effects of epidural epinephrine in the pregnant sheep. Reg. Anesth. 6:4, 1981.
55. Albright GA, Jouppila R, Hollmën AI, Jouppila P, et al: Epinephrine does not alter human intervillous blood flow during epidural anesthesia. Anesthesiology 54:131, 1981.
56. Abboud TK, Sheik-ol-Eslam A, Yanagi T, Murakawa K, et al: Safety and efficiency of epinephrine added to bupivacaine for lumbar epidural analgesia in obstetrics. Anesth. Analg. 64:585, 1985.
57. Shnider SM, Levinson G: Anesthesia for Obstetrics. 2nd Ed. Baltimore, Williams & Wilkins, 1987, p. 32.
58. Gunther RE, Baumann AL: Obstetrical caudal anesthesia. I. A randomized study comparing 1% mepivacaine with 1% lidocaine plus epinephrine Anesthesiology 31:5, 1969.
59. Zador G, Nilsson BA: Low dose intermittent epidural anesthesia with lidocaine for vaginal delivery. II. Influence of labour and foetal acid-base status. Acta. Obstet. Gynecol. Scand. (Suppl) 34:17, 1974.
60. Zador G, Nilsson BA: Continuous drip lumbar epidural anaesthesia with lidocaine for vaginal delivery. II. Influence on labour and foetal acid-base status. Acta. Obstet. Gynecol. Scand. (Suppl) 34:41, 1974.
61. Matadial L, Cibils LA: The effect of epidural anesthesia on uterine activity and blood pressure. Am. J. Obstet. Gynecol. 125:846, 1976.
62. Lowensohn RI, Paul RH, Fales S, Yeh S-Y, et al: Intrapartum epidural anesthesia. Obstet. Gynecol. 44:388, 1974.
63. Craft JB, Epstein BS, Coakley CS: Effect of lidocaine with epinephrine vs. lidocaine (plain) on induced labor. Anesth. Analg. 51:243–246, 1972.
64. Hardy JD, Javert CT: Studies on pain: measurements of pain intensity in childbirth. J. Clin. Invest. 28:153, 1949.
65. Kaiser IH, Harris JS: The effect of adrenalin on the pregnant human uterus. Am. J. Obstet. Gynecol. 59:775, 1950.
66. Garcia CR, Garcia E: Epinephrine-like substances in the blood and their relation to uterine inertia. Am. J. Obstet. Gynecol. 69:812, 1955.
67. Myers RE: Maternal psychological stress and fetal asphyxia: a study in the monkey. Am. J. Obstet. Gynecol. 122:47–59, 1975.
68. Morishima HO, Pedersen H, Finster M: The influence of maternal psychological stress on the fetus. Am. J. Obstet. Gynecol. 131:2868–290, 1978.
69. Shnider SM, Wright RG, Levinson G, Roizen MF, et al: Uterine blood flow and plasma norepinephrine changes during maternal stress in the pregnant ewe. Anesthesiology 50: 524–527, 1979.
70. Lederman RP, Lederman E, Work BA Jr, McCann DS: The relationship of maternal anxiety, plasma catecholamines and plasma cortisol to progress in labor. Am. J. Obstet. Gynecol. 132:495–500, 1978.
71. Lederman RP, Lederman E, Work Jr B, McCann DS: Anxiety and epinephrine in multiparous labor: relationship to duration of labor and fetal heart rate pattern. Am. J. Obstet. Gynecol. 153:870–877, 1985.
72. Ohno H, Yamashita K, Yahata T, Doi R, et al: Maternal plasma concentrations of catecholamines and cyclic nucleotides during labor and following delivery. Res. Commun. Chem. Pathol. Pharmacol. 51:183, 1986.
73. Clark GA: Some Foetal blood pressure reactions. J. Physiol 74:391, 1932.
74. Martin JD, Young IM: Influence of gestational age and hormones on experimental foetal bradycardia. J. Physiol. 152 1, 1960.
75. Sandler M, Ruthven CRJ, Contractor SF, Wood C, et al Transmission of noradrenaline across the human placenta Nature 197:598, 1963.
76. Martin CG Jr, Gingerick B: Uteroplacental physiology JOGN Nurs. (Suppl) 5:16–25, 1976.
77. Moore DC, Batra MS: The components of an effective test dose prior to epidural block. Anesthesiology 55:693, 1981
78. Albright GA: Epinephrine should be used with the therapeutic dose of bupivacaine in obstetrics. Anesthesiology 61:217, 1984.
79. Leighton BL, Norris MC, Sosis M, Epstein R, et al: Limitations of epinephrine as a marker of intravascular injection in laboring women. Anesthesiology 66:688, 1987.
80. Leighton BL, Desimore CA, Norris MC, Chayen B: Isoproterenol is an effective marker of intravenous injection in laboring women. Anesthesiology 71:206, 1989.
81. Hood DD, Dewan DM, James FM III: Maternal and fetal effects of epinephrine on gravid ewes. Anesthesiology 64 610, 1986.
82. Albright G, Ferguson JE, Joyce TH III, Stevenson DK: Anesthesia in Obstetrics: Maternal, Fetal and Neonatal Aspects Boston, Butterworths, 1986, p. 67.
83. Butterworth JF, Piccione W Jr, Berrizbeitia LD, Dance G, et al: Augmentation of venous return by adrenergic agonists during spinal anesthesia. Anesth. Anal.g 65:612, 1986.
84. James FM III, Greiss FC, Kemp RA: An evaluation of vasopressor therapy for maternal hypotension during spinal anesthesia. Anesthesiology 33:25, 1970.
85. Ramanathan S, Grant G, Turndorf H: Cardiac pre-load changes with ephedrine therapy for hypotension in obstetrical patients. Anesth. Analg. 65:S125, 1986.
86. Ramanathan S, Grant GJ: Vasopressor therapy for hypotension due to epidural anesthesia for cesarean section. Acta Anaesthesiol. Scand. 32:559, 1988.
87. Wright RG, Shnider SM, Levinson G, Rolbin SH, et al: The effect of maternal administration of ephedrine on fetal heart rate and variability. Obstet. Gynecol. 57:734, 1981
88. Clark RB, Thompson DS, Thompson CH: Prevention of spinal hypotension associated with cesarean section. Anesthesiology 45:670, 1976.
89. Datta S, Alper MH: Anesthesia for cesarean section. Anesthesiology 53:142, 1980.
90. Kang YG, Abouleish E, Caritas S: Prophylactic intravenou

ephedrine infusion during spinal anesthesia for cesarean section. Anesth. Analg. 61:839, 1982.

91. Shnider SM, de Lorimier AA, Holl JW, Chapler FK, et al: Vasopressors in obstetrics. I. Correction of fetal acidosis with ephedrine during spinal hypotension. Am. J. Obstet. Gynecol. 102:911, 1968.
92. Senties LG, Arellano G, Casellas AF, Ontiveros E, et al: Effects of some vasopressor drugs upon uterine contractility in pregnant women. Am. J. Obstet. Gynecol. 107:892, 1970.
93. Miodovnik M, Lavin JP, Harrington DJ, Leung LS, et al: Effect of maternal ketoacidemia on the pregnant ewe and fetus. Am. J. Obstet. Gynecol. 144:585, 1982.
94. Greiss FC, Van Wilkes D: Effects of sympathomimetic drugs and angiotensin on the uterine vascular bed. Obstet. Gynecol. 23:925, 1964.
95. Greiss FC, Crandell DL: Therapy for hypotension induced by spinal anesthesia during pregnancy. JAMA 191:793, 1965.
96. Ramanathan S, Friedman S, Moss P, Arismendy J, et al: Phenylephrine for the treatment of maternal hypotension due to epidural anesthesia. Anesth. Analg. 63:S262, 1984.
97. Albright GA: Effects of anesthesia on the fetus and neonate. *In* Fetal and Neonatal Brain Injury. Edited by DR Stevenson. Toronto, BC Decker, 1989, p. 46.
98. Marx GF, Cosmi EV, Wollman SB: Biochemical status and clinical condition of mother and infant at cesarean section. Anesth. Analg. 48:986, 1969.
99. Gutsche BB: Prophylactic ephedrine preceding spinal anesthesia for cesarean section. Anesthesiology 45:462, 1976.
100. Rolbin SH, Cole AFD, Hew EM, Pollard A, et al: Prophylactic intramuscular ephedrine before epidural anesthesia for cesarean section: efficacy and actions on the fetus and newborn. Can. Anaesth. Soc. J. 29:148, 1982.
101. Datta S, Brown WU Jr: Acid-base status in diabetic mothers and their infants following general or spinal anesthesia for cesarean section. Anesthesiology 47:272, 1977.
102. Hollmën AI, Jouppila R, Albright GA, Jouppila P, et al: Intervillous blood flow during cesarean section with prophylactic ephedrine and epidural anesthesia. Acta. Anaesth. Scand. 28:396, 1984.
103. Jouppila P, Jouppila R, Barinoff T, Koivula A: Placental blood flow during cesarean section performed under spinal blockade. Br. J. Anaesth. 56:1379, 1984.
104. Caritis SN, Abouleish E, Edelstone DI, Mueller-Heubach E: Fetal acid-base state following spinal or epidural anesthesia for cesarean section. Obstet. Gynecol. 56:610, 1980.
105. Norris M: Hypotension during spinal anesthesia for cesarean section: does it affect neonatal outcome? Reg. Anesth. 12:191, 1987.
106. Hughes SC, Ward MG, Levinson G, Shnider SM, et al: Placental transfer of ephedrine does not affect neonatal outcome. Anesthesiology 63:217, 1985.
107. Kangas-Saarela T, Hollmën AI, Eskelinen P, Alahuhta S, et al: Does ephedrine influence newborn neurobehavioral responses and spectral EEG when used to prevent maternal hypotension during cesarean section? Acta. Anaesthesiol. Scan. 34:8, 1990.
108. Clark RB, Brunner JA: Dopamine as a vasopressor for the treatment of spinal hypotension during cesarean section. Anesthesiology 53:514, 1980.
109. Blanchard K, Dandavino A, Nuwayhid B, Brinkman CR III, et al: Systemic and uterine hemodynamic responses to dopamine in pregnant and nonpregnant sheep. Am. J. Obstet. Gynecol. 130:669, 1978.
110. Cabalum T, Zugaib M, Lieb S, Nuwayhid B, et al: Effect of dopamine on hypotension induced by spinal anesthesia. Am. J. Obstet. Gynecol. 133:630, 1979.
111. Callender K, Levinson G, Shnider SM, Feduska NJ, et al: Dopamine administration in the normotensive pregnant ewe. Obstet. Gynecol. 51:586, 1978.
112. Rolbin SH, Levinson G, Shnider SM, Biehl DR, et al: Dopamine treatment of spinal hypotension decreases uterine blood flow in the pregnant ewe. Anesthesiology 51:36, 1979.
113. Fishburne JI, Meis PJ, Urban RB, Greiss FC, et al: Vascular and uterine responses to dobutamine and dopamine in the gravid ewe. Am. J. Obstet. Gynecol. 137:944, 1980.
114. Moran DG, Perillo M, Bader AM, Datta S: Phenylephrine in treating maternal hypotension secondary to spinal anesthesia. Anesthesiology 71:A857, 1989.
115. Ralston DH, Shnider SM, deLorimier AA: Effects of equipotent ephedrine, metaraminol, mephentermine, and methoxamine on uterine blood flow in the pregnant ewe. Anesthesiology 40:354, 1974.
116. Rasanen J, Alaahuhta S, Kangas-Saarela T, Jouppila, R, et al: The effects of ephedrine and etilefrine on uterine and fetal blood flow and on fetal myocardial function during spinal anesthesia for cesarean section. Int. J. Obst. Anes. 1:1, 1991.
117. Moya F, Smith B: Spinal anesthesia for cesarean section: clinical and biochemical studies of effects on maternal physiology. JAMA 179–609, 1962.
118. Vasicka A, Hutchinson HT, Eng M, Allen CR: Spinal and epidural anesthesia, fetal and uterine response to acute hypo- and hypertension. Amer. J. Obstet. Gynecol. 90:800, 1964.
119. Eng M, Berges PU, Ueland K, Bonica JJ, et al: The effects of methoxamine and ephedrine in normotensive pregnant primates. Anesthesiology 35:354, 1971.
120. Shnider SM, de Lorimier AA, Asling JH, Morishima HO: Vasopressors in obstetrics, II. Fetal hazards of methoxamine administration during obstetric spinal anesthesia. Am. J. Obstet. Gynecol. 106:680, 1970.
121. Lucas WE, Kirschbaum TH, Assali NS: Effects of autonomic blockade with spinal anesthesia on uterine and fetal hemodynamics and oxygen consumption in the sheep. Biol. Neonat. 10:166, 1966.
122. Shnider SM, deLorimer AA, Steffenson JL: Vasopressors in obstetrics. III. Fetal effects of metaraminol infusion during obstetric spinal hypotension. Am. J. Obstet. Gynecol. 108: 1017, 1970.
123. Smith BE, Hess DG: Effects of dobutamine infusion on uterine artery conductance and blood flow in the pregnant ewe. Presented at the annual meeting, Society for Obstetric Anesthesia and Perinatology, Cambridge, MA, May 9, 1980. SOAP Abstract, p. 14.
124. Krasnow N, Rolett EL, Yurchak PM, Hood WB Jr, et al: Isoproterenol and cardiovascular performance. Am. J. Med. 37:514, 1964.
125. Mahon WA, Reid DWJ, Day RA: The in vivo effects of beta adrenergic stimulation and blockade on the human uterus at term. J. Pharmacol. Exp. Ther. 156:178, 1967.
126. Fishburne JI, Dormer KJ, Payne GG, Gill PS, et al: Effects of amrinone and dopamine on uterine blood flow and vascular responses in the gravid baboon. Am. J. Obstet. Gynecol. 158:829, 1988.
127. Baumann AL, Santos AC, Wlody D, Pedersen H, et al: Maternal and fetal effects of milrinone and dopamine. Anesthesiology 71:A855, 1989.
128. Symonds EM, Pipkin FB: Factors affecting plasma angiotensin II concentration in labour. Br. J. Obstet. Gynecol. 87: 869, 1980.

129. Greiss FC Jr, Gobble FL Jr: Effect of sympathetic nerve stimulation on the uterine vascular bed. Am. J. Obstet. Gynecol. 97:962, 1967.
130. Howard BK, Goodson JH, Mengert WF: Supine hypotensive syndrome in late pregnancy. Obstet. Gynecol. 1:371, 1953.
131. Clark RB: Prevention and treatment of aortocaval compression in the pregnant patient. Anesthesiology Review 7:13, 1980.
132. Bieniarz J, Yoshida T, Romero-Salinas G, Curuchet E, et al: Aortocaval compression by the uterus in late human pregnancy. IV. Circulatory homeostasis by preferential perfusion of the placenta. Am. J. Obstet. Gynecol. 103:19, 1969.
133. Wollman SB, Marx GF: Acute hydration for prevention of hypotension of spinal anesthesia in parturients. Anesthesiology 29:374, 1968.
134. Shnider SM: Obstetrical Anesthesia: Current Concepts and Practice. Baltimore, Williams and Wilkins, 1970, p. 8.
135. Antoine C, Young BK: Fetal lactic acidosis with epidural anesthesia. Am. J. Obstet. Gynecol. 142:55, 1982.
136. Brizgys RV, Dailey PA, Shnider SM, Kotelko DM, et al: The incidence and neonatal effects of maternal hypotension during epidural anesthesia for cesarean section. Anesthesiology 67:782, 1987.
137. Crawford JS: Principles and Practice of Obstetric Anaesthesia. 4th Ed.. Cambridge, MA, Blackwell Scientific Publications, 1978, p. 266.

## SUGGESTED READINGS

* Rout CC, Rocke DA, Levin J, et al: A reevaluation of the role of crystalloid preload in the prevention of hypotension associated with spinal anesthesia for elective cesarean section. Anesthesiology 79:262–9, 1993

Despite prophylactic measures, such as plasma volume expansion and uterine displacement, mild hypotension is a fairly frequent occurrence during obstetric epidural (or spinal) anesthesia.

* Zakowski M, Otto T, Baratta J, et al: Phenylephrine for hypotension in risk paturients during cesarean section. Anesthesiology 77:A973, 1992

Phenylephine is effective in restoring maternal blood pressure, without adversely affecting indices of well being, such as Apgar score and biochemical status.

* Alahuhta S, Rasanen J, Jouppila P, et al: Ephedrine and phenylephrine for avoiding maternal hypotension due to spinal anaesthesia for cesarean section. Effects on uteroplacental and fetal hemodynamics. International Journal Obstetric Anesthesia 1:129–34, 1992

Phenylephrine and methoxamine are effective in restoring maternal blood pressure, without adversely affecting Apgar score or biochemical status.

* Santos AC, Pedersen H: Current controversies in OB anesthesia. Anesthesia & Analgesia 78:752–60, 1994

A good review, includes "Alpha Agonists in the Treatment of Maternal Hypotention".

* Corke BC, Datta S, Ostheimer GW, Weiss JB, Alper MH: Spinal anesthesia for caesarean section: the influence of hypotention and neonatal outcome. Anaesthesia 37:658–62, 1982

Short periods of maternal hypotension (less than 2 minutes) are not harmful to the neonate.

* (Mentioned in Santos & Pedersen's Review)

# Chapter 13

# EPIDURAL ANALGESIA AND ANESTHESIA

JOHN J. BONICA
JOHN S. McDONALD

## A. CLINICAL CONSIDERATIONS

### INTRODUCTION

Epidural analgesia/anesthesia is one of the most frequently used techniques for the relief of pain of childbirth. Indeed, in most hospitals that have an obstetric anesthesia service, it is the most prominently used technique for labor and vaginal delivery and for cesarean section (see Table 1–6, Chapter 1). It is well known that this technique entails the injection of a local anesthetic or an opioid or a combination of these into the epidural (extradural, peridural) space.*

This can be achieved by injection of a solution into the lumbar or lowermost part of the thoracic epidural space and most frequently referred to as lumbar epidural block or into the sacral canal through the sacrococcygeal hiatus, referred to as caudal epidural block. Although the single bolus injection technique can be used, in most instances, the administration of the solution is made through an indwelling epidural catheter that permits either single bolus injections repeated at appropriate intervals or a continuous infusion or a combination of these. The advantages of the catheter technique over single injection, are that it provides far better control of the intensity, extent, and duration of neural blockade. In some institutions, a catheter is placed in the lumbar epidural space and the second catheter in the sacral canal—the so-called Double-Catheter Epidural block, which, in the opinion of the authors, provides greater flexibility and advantages not obtained with other techniques. The quantity of analgesic solution varies depending on the stage of labor and the spinal nerve segments that need to be blocked for pain relief. The different techniques are described and depicted in Part B of this chapter.

In the first edition of this book, lumbar epidural block and caudal epidural block were discussed in separate chapters. In this present edition, they are considered together for the following reasons: First, the site of action of both techniques in blocking nociceptive (pain) and other sensory and motor fibers is the same (i.e., the epidural space). Second, placement of the catheter in the epidural space, though dissimilar methodologically, does entail insertion and placement of the catheter into the same body space, i.e., the potential epidural space. Third, pharmacodynamic effects on the mother and fetus are the same regardless of whether lumbar epidural or caudal epidural technique is used. As a consequence, the mechanism of analgesia and the side effects of the blockade on maternal function, on the forces of labor, and on the fetus and newborn are similar. Any differences between the two techniques are due to the volume and concentration (i.e., the total amount) of drug used and the extent of analgesia and the number of vasomotor and somatomotor segments blocked. Therefore, the two techniques will be considered together for both lumbar epidural block and caudal epidural block, and, where clinically relevant, the differences pointed out. This approach is intended to obviate repetition of similar information. On the other hand, the section and subsections that deal with epidural puncture, and insertion of the catheter and complications with each technique are sufficiently different to require separate consideration. Similarly, the historical perspectives are somewhat different and will be considered separately.

Our discussion of epidural analgesia and anesthesia is presented in two major parts: Chapter 13-A contains a comprehensive discussion of the clinical aspects of these techniques, including: 1) evaluation of the analgesic efficacy; 2) the adverse and beneficial effects on the mother; 3) the effects on the forces of labor; 4) the effects on the fetus and newborn; and 5) based on the preceding information, a summary of the indications, contraindications, advantages and disadvantages of lumbar epidural, caudal epidural, and double-catheter epidural technique block, and a comparison with other methods in current use—primarily with respect to the United States, the United Kingdom, and other countries in which the art and science of anesthesiology has advanced sufficiently enough to permit provision of optimal relief of pain associated with labor and vaginal delivery and anesthesia for cesarean section. Chapter 13-B is devoted to the technical aspects of these procedures, including: 1) the anatomic and pharmacologic bases; 2) general principles of techniques that must be adhered to achieve optimal results; 3) description of each specific technique: lumbar epidural block, caudal epidural block, and double-catheter epidural block using local anesthetics alone and the combined use of these agents and opioids; and 4) description of the technique of carrying out epidural anesthesia for cesarean section. The last part of 13-B is devoted to a

* The terms epidural, peridural and extradural are synonymous and can be used interchangeably.

discussion of general principles in management of the mother and newborn during the intrapartrum and postpartum period. Because this last topic is discussed in detail in Chapter 23, only those points relevant to epidural analgesia/anesthesia will be covered. In discussing all aspects, save the historical perspectives, we consider lumbar epidural block before caudal epidural block because it is used much more frequently and because the use of lumbar epidural block has major advantages over the use of caudal epidural block. Finally, it should be noted that all references can be found at the end of Part B.

## Historical Perspectives

Epidural injection of therapeutic drugs was first achieved accidentally in 1884 by Corning (1), a New York neurologist who administered cocaine via a needle inserted between T11 and T12 vertebrae to a patient for the treatment of a medical disorder. It was not until 1901, however, that caudal epidural anesthesia was reported by Cathelin (2) of France, and another 2 decades elapsed before spinal epidural anesthesia was reported by Pages (3) and Dogliotti (4). These reports, which pertained to the use of these procedures for surgical operations, prompted the use of both the techniques in many surgical centers. Their application to obstetric patients lagged behind about a decade for each technique.

## *Caudal Epidural Blockade*

Caudal (sacral) anesthesia was first used in obstetrics by the Germans, by Stoeckel (5) in 1909 and by Schlimpert and Schneider (6) a year later. Meeker and Bonar (7), and Rucker (8) were the first Americans to report its use in obstetrics during the period 1923–1925. In 1928, Pickles and Jones (9) reviewed the literature on the use of caudal epidural anesthesia published to date and reported its successful use for the second stage of labor. In the subsequent 2 decades, many reports appeared in the literature attesting to the value of single injection caudal anesthesia for vaginal delivery (9–12). In 1932, Cleland (12), while studying the pathways of pain associated with uterine contractions by using paravertebral block of T11 and T12 (see Chapter 1), complemented this procedure with caudal block to provide relief of perineal pain. This was the prelude to the development and use of the double-catheter technique a decade later.

The application of the "continuous" technique to caudal block for obstetrics, first reported in 1942 by Edwards and Hingson (13), must be considered one of the most important advances in obstetric analgesia and anesthesia up to that time. Their technique entailed the insertion of a malleable needle into the sacral canal connected to a tubing through which repeated doses of local anesthetic could be injected. A year later Adams, Lundy and Seldon (14) replaced the malleable-needle technique with vinyl plastic catheter introduced into the sacral canal via an 18-gauge thin-walled needle. These advances helped to popularize continuous caudal analgesia, and by 1948 a total of 264 papers had been published recording results in more than 600,000 parturients and emphasized the fact that in addition to effective relief for the mother with this technique, a reduction in neonatal morbidity and mortality was realized (15). By the early 1960s, published reports indicated that continuous caudal analgesia had been used in over 3 million parturients in the United States alone during the preceding 2 decades (16–28), thus attesting to its growing popularity, which spread from the United States to Britain (29–33) and Australia (34,35), and other parts of the world (36). In addition to providing analgesia, continuous caudal analgesia became to be used as a therapeutic measure in the treatment of disorders of uterine function, prolonged labor, and of primary cervical dystoci (29–34).

Up to the early 1960s, continuous caudal analgesia was considered the best all-around method of providing pain relief during childbirth, and, indeed, it was heralded as the ultimate form of obstetric anesthesia, permitting "painless childbirth." This popularity can be attributed to obstetricians having learned the technique themselves and then teaching it to their trainees. This trend was motivated by lack of obstetric anesthesia services by anesthesiologists and by the fact that the use of systemic analgesia for the first stage and pudendal block for the second and third stages of labor provided less satisfactory degrees of pain relief. Moreover, reports of deaths from aspiration of gastric contents with general anesthesia and from "spinal shock" associated with spinal anesthesia helped the efforts of Hingson and others to popularize continuous caudal anesthesia.

With the increasing popularity of lumbar and thoracic epidural anesthesia for surgery, young anesthesiologists became highly skilled in performing lumbar epidural puncture, but acquired little or no experience with the technically more difficult needle puncture through the sacrococcygeal hiatus into the sacral canal necessary to achieve caudal block. These and other disadvantages of caudal analgesia in comparison with spinal epidural analgesia, especially during the first stage of labor, prompted a gradual shift to the latter technique. Consequently, since the first edition of this book, caudal analgesia has sharply declined in popularity (see Table 1–6). Indeed, today with the exception of a few hospitals in which caudal analgesia was entrenched as the predominant form of regional analgesia for childbirth, continuous caudal is rarely used for labor. In some institutions, its use is limited to supplement lumbar epidural analgesia in cases in which the latter does not produce adequate perineal analgesia and relaxation, but even in such circumstances, in most instances, low subarachnoid (saddle) block is used for the delivery.

Today, the greatest usefulness of low caudal blockade is in combination with segmental lumbar epidural analgesia to effect the double-catheter technique, which offers the ultimate in the precise control of pain of the first and second Stages of labor (see below). Moreover, single-dose caudal block can be used to provide perineal analgesia and anesthesia for the delivery, and a high caudal technique with blockade of T4-S5 can be used for cesarean section in the very rare instances in which lumbar epidural, subarachnoid block, and general anesthesia are contraindicated or unsuccessful. Therefore, obstetric anesthesiologists should learn and acquire sufficient skill with caudal anesthesia to be able to carry it out as easily as spinal epidural blockade.

### Lumbar Epidural Blockade

The first use of lumbar epidural analgesia in obstetrics is somewhat uncertain. In 1935, Graffagnino and Seyler (37) published the first reports in the American literature on the use of epidural analgesia in obstetrics. Despite these and other sporadic reports, its use in obstetrics remained limited for another 2 decades. During the 1940s and 1950s, two important developments took place that later contributed to the popularity of spinal epidural block. One of these events was the advent of lidocaine, chloroprocaine, and other more penetrating and fast-acting local anesthetics; the other was the introduction of the "continuous" technique.

Soon after Lemmon's description of continuous spinal anesthesia (38), Hingson and Southworth (39) considered the use of the same equipment for spinal epidural block, but because of technical difficulties in keeping the needle in place, they abandoned the idea in favor of continuous caudal analgesia. In January, 1947, the technical problem was solved by Manuel Curbelo of Cuba, who used a 3.5 ureteral catheter introduced through a Tuohy needle to produce continuous epidural anesthesia for surgery and who described the technique in September of the same year at the 22nd Annual Congress of Anesthetists (40). Soon after hearing Curbelo's presentation, Umstead and Dufresne (41) began to apply the technique to obstetric patients and a year later published a description of the technique and its successful use in 26 parturients. This was the year before Curbelo's report was published (42), and the year that Flowers, Hellman, and Hingson (43), reported on the use of vinyl plastic tubing for continuous lumbar epidural block in obstetric patients.

In 1949, Cleland (44) described the double-catheter technique, which was a refinement of the paravertebral-caudal block he had used during the 1930s and 1940s. This technique represented a beautiful example of integrating sound anatomic knowledge and the desire to use the least amount of local anesthetic to achieve more precise analgesia during various stages of labor and vaginal delivery. During the ensuing 3 decades Dr. John Cleland, Sr., used the double-catheter technique very successfully in several thousand private patients in his practice in Oregon City. In the 1970s, he was joined by his son, Dr. John Cleland, Jr., who has continued this practice and achieved the same high degree of analgesia with great safety to the mother and the fetus in nearly 4000 parturients during the course of 49 years (personal communication, 1994). In the same year, Bonica implemented one of the first round-the-clock obstetric anesthesia services in the United States, using first continuous caudal analgesia, but later applying lumbar epidural and the double-catheter techniques.

During the period 1943–1960, for reasons previously mentioned, continuous caudal analgesia was used much more frequently than was the lumbar epidural approach, but in the mid-1950s a number of factors converged to initiate a shift in this trend toward favor of continuous lumbar epidural block. Among the most important of these factors was the large amount of new information on the physical, biochemical, and pharmacologic bases and other clinical aspects of lumbar epidural analgesia acquired from extensive studies by Bromage and associates (45–49), Bonica and associates (50–52), Lund (53), and many others, (cf. 53 for references) and the increasing recognition of the advantages of the lumbar approach over the sacral technique, particularly in obstetrics. Also very important was the widespread use of the Apgar score in evaluating the newborn (54), and several technologic advances that permitted precise measurements of the forces of labor (55–57); continuous monitoring of the fetal heart rate (58); of the acid-base status of the fetus in utero and after birth (59); the measurements of blood concentration of local anesthetics in the mother, fetus, and newborn; and, finally, the introduction of neurobehavioral methods of evaluating the newborn (60).

During the ensuing decade (1960–1970), the method became increasingly popular among anesthesiologists and obstetricians as attested by the numerous publications on its use in obstetrics. Thus, Eisen, Hellman and their associates (61,62) published favorable results on its use in nearly 37,000 parturients who underwent labor and vaginal delivery or cesarean section. Reports on its use in large obstetric series were also published by Shnider (63), Chaplin and Renwick (64), Hehre and Sayig (65), Lund et al (53), Bromage (66), Nielsen and associates (67), Crawford and associates (67–70), and Moir (71), among others. Most of these reports in the 1960s and early 1970s pertained to its use in obstetrics in North America and the United Kingdom (68–72). Subsequently, the technique became increasingly popular in Australia (73,74), Scandinavia (75–85), Germany (86) and other Western European countries (87,88), and Japan (89).

With increasing clinical experience during the 1970s and 1980s, a number of modifications of continuous lumbar epidural analgesia/anesthesia were made to minimize some of its adverse side effects on the mother, on the forces of labor, and on the fetus and newborn. These adverse effects include maternal hypotension and the risk of systemic toxic reactions from large amounts of local anesthetic used with the standard epidural technique that produced blockade from T10 to S5 neurotomes that had been in widespread use. Moreover, obstetricians, particularly those in the United Kingdom and Scandinavia, while appreciating the value of epidural analgesia in relieving parturition pain and in the treatment of incoordinate uterine contractions and other pathophysiologic conditions, expressed concern about the increased incidence of nonrotation of the presenting part and the consequent need for instrumental delivery—also associated with the standard technique. These and other concerns led to the development of a sequential series of modifications: 1) use of lower concentrations of local anesthetics; 2) limiting the analgesia to spinal segments extending from T10 to L1 neurotome during the first stage, and then extending it to the sacral segments during the second and third stages; 3) evaluation of the effects of epinephrine in the epidural solutions; 4) use of continuous infusions of low concentrations of local anesthetics; and 5) combined use of dilute solutions of local anesthetic with opioids to enhance the analgesic efficacy of continuous epidural analgesia. These techniques have been shown to produce a more stable level of analgesia, less incidence and smaller degree of maternal hypotension, and significantly decrease the risk of systemic toxic reaction or accidental high or total spinal anesthesia. The last two modifications have also decreased the incidence of motor block, especially during the second stage, so that the occurrence of lack of rotation of the presenting part is decreased, and the mother can voluntarily mobilize the expulsive forces of labor to achieve spontaneous delivery, if this is desired. After discussing relevant clinical considerations, including efficacy and effects on the mother, each of these modifications is briefly considered and supporting references given.

## Clinical Considerations

Proper and effective application of epidural analgesia and anesthesia in its various forms, like the use of other techniques of obstetric anesthesia, requires knowledge and evaluation of the therapeutic (analgesic) efficacy and their effect on the mother, on the forces of labor and delivery, and on the fetus and newborn. This, in turn, requires thorough knowledge of the information contained in Chapters 2 through 9, inclusive, in which the maternal physiologic and psychologic alterations produced by pregnancy and parturition, the anatomy and physiology of the forces of labor, the physiology and pharmacology of the maternal/fetal/placental complex, and the mechanism and effects of pain of parturition are considered in detail. Some of the material that follows below is a repetition of information contained in these various chapters, including duplication of a number of the illustrations. This is done purposely to duly emphasize the importance and interrelationship of the information that is clinically relevant to the proper application of continuous lumbar epidural analgesia/anesthesia.

The discussion that follows reflects: 1) the two authors' combined total 60 years of clinical experience in personally administering or directly supervising trainees in the application of these various forms of epidural analgesia in over 30,000 parturients; 2) the experience of all of their colleagues in the six departments with which they have been affiliated and in which these techniques have been used in well over 60,000 deliveries; and 3) on the publications of authors who have published reports based on its use in large series of cases.

Before discussing the clinical aspects of the various epidural analgesia/anesthesia techniques, Figures 13–1 and 13–2, and Table 13–1, are presented to provide the reader with a very brief overview of each of these techniques, including the procedures involved in achieving the technique and in managing the first and second stages of labor, as well as brief mention of its advantages and disadvantages. Detailed description of each of these procedures is presented in Part B.

### *Efficacy of Epidural Analgesia/Anesthesia for Labor and Vaginal Delivery*

When properly carried out and the block develops as intended, epidural analgesia provides complete relief of

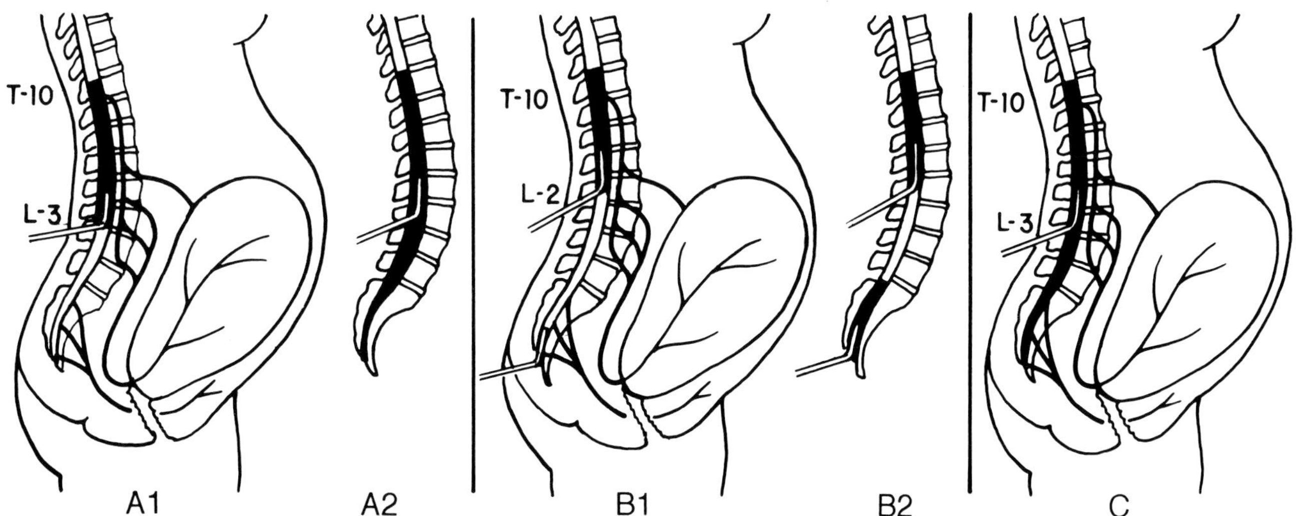


**Fig. 13–1.** Various techniques of epidural block used in obstetrics. White tube indicates level of catheter; black area in spinal canal indicates extent of diffusion of the local anesthetic. **A**: 1) depicts the extent of analgesia after the initial injection of continuous segmental epidural block during the early part of the active phase of labor; 2) shows the extent of analgesia during the latter part of the first stage. The caudad extension results from repeated injections through the lumbar epidural catheter or continuous infusion of local anesthetic and opioids. **B**: 1) and 2) depict the extent of analgesia/anesthesia achieved with the double-catheter technique. 1) shows the extent of segmental (T10-L1) analgesia during the first and throughout the second stage. At the onset of perineal pain, an injection is given through the caudal catheter to produce analgesia of the perineum (S2-S5). **C**: Standard lumbar epidural block for labor and vaginal delivery. The catheter is inserted through the L3-L4 interlaminar space, and its tip is advanced to the middle of the second lumbar vertebra. Injection of 12 to 15 ml of analgesic solutions of a local anesthetic produces analgesia extending from T10-S5.

**Table 13–1.** Summary of Various Techniques of Epidural Analgesia/Anesthesia for Labor and Vaginal Delivery*

| Techniques | Initial Procedure | Management During First Stage of Labor |
|---|---|---|
| I. CONT. SEGMENTAL LUMBAR EPIDURAL → SACRAL BLOCK | | |
| A. Intermittent Technique | 1) Procedure done during latent phase<br>2) Needle puncture L3–L4<br>3) Advance catheter 3 cm → L2<br>4) Withhold injections until onset of moderate labor pain<br>5) Inject test dose | 1) After neg. test dose → inject 5–7 ml LAnalS (1) → Extent of analgesia T10–L1<br>2) Closely monitor patient and fetus<br>3) Top-up injections every 40–70 min (2)<br>4) Titrate dose to maintain T10–L1 analgesia<br>5) Gradual caudad extention and analgesia |
| B. Continuous Infusion LAnalS alone or with opioids | (Same as above) | 1) After steps 1 and 2 in IA., connect to infusion pump<br>2) Infuse at rate of solution to provide effective analgesia at T10–L1 initially<br>3) After 3–4 hrs, analgesia extends to lumbar and sacral segments |
| II. DOUBLE CATHETER TECHNIQUE | 1) Needle puncture at L2–3 → catheter advanced 5 cm to T12<br>2) Needle puncture thru SCH (5) → advance catheter 2 cm in sacral canal to S3 vertebra<br>3) Both catheters inserted at same time during latent phase | 1) After neg. test dose → inject 4–5 ml LAnalS thru *upper* catheter → segmental (T10–L1) analgesia<br>2) Top-up and titrate doses as required to maintain T10–L1 analgesia<br>———<br>3) Alternatively connect to infusion pump and deliver at rate to maintain T10–L1 analgesia |
| III. STANDARD LUMBAR EPIDURAL BLOCK (T10–S5) | 1) Needle puncture at L4–5<br>2) Advance catheter 3 cm<br>3) Site of injection at L3<br>4) Catheter inserted during latent phase | 1) Same as IA, except inject boluses of 12–15 ml of LAnalS<br>2) Top-up and titrate as necessary to maintain T10–S5 analgesia |
| IV. CAUDAL BLOCK (T10–S5): | | |
| A. Continuous Caudal | 1) Needle puncture thru SCH →<br>2) Advance catheter 2 cm to S3<br>3) An alternate is to advance catheter 8 cm to S1–L5<br>4) Puncture done during latent phase | 1) After neg. test dose → inject 18–20 ml of LAnalS if catheter tip at S2–3<br>2) Inject 12–15 ml of LAnalS if catheter tip at S1–L5<br>3) Analgesia extends T10–S5<br>4) Top-up and titrate as necessary |
| B. Low Caudal Block (S1–S5) | 1) Not used during 1st stage<br>2) Used as terminal perineal anesthesia<br>3) Injection of 5–8 ml thru caudal needle → analgesia/anesthesia S1–S5 | (Not used) |

* Includes lumbar epidural and caudal block; (1) LAnalS = Local Analgesic Solution; (2) Interval depends on local anesthetic used; (3) LAntS = Local Anesthetic Solution; (4) BDE = Bearing down efforts (Push during latter part of second stage); (5) SCH = Sacrococcygeal hiatus

pain due to uterine contractions to 75 to 85% of parturients and incomplete, but sufficient, relief in another 10 to 15% so that a combined total of 90 to 95% of parturients are highly satisfied with the procedure whether achieved with intermittent injections or by continuous infusions (61–70,74–85,90–94). In this regard, it is important to differentiate failure to technically achieve a successful epidural block and the perception of the patient of the degree of pain before the block and the overall evaluation of the efficacy of the procedure in providing relief of pain and meeting her expectations.

In regard to the former, the degree of technical success depends on the knowledge or skill and experience of the administrator. Unfortunately, most of the reports published in the past 2 decades do not include data on the incidence of technical failure, but the older data suggest the following: Foldes (95) reported an overall technical failure rate of about 5%, Bromage (49) 1.5%, Hehre & Sayig (65) 2.3%, Nielsen and coworkers (67) 4%, Crawford (82) 3%, and Hellman, Eisen and associates (61,62) who reported their experience in nearly 37,000 parturients, experienced technical failure of less than 3%. In the

| Management During Second and Third Stages | Advantages | Disadvantages |
|---|---|---|
| 1) Onset of pain in legs/perineum → inject 10–12 ml LAnalS → Analgesia T10–S5<br>2) Repeat & titrate LAnalS to maintain analgesia<br>3) After flexion/internal rotation → inject 10–12 ml LAntS (3) with patient sitting | 1) Provides effective 1st stage analgesia<br>2) Segmental block →<br>a) No effect on Ferguson's Reflex<br>b) No premature block of perineum<br>c) Little/no numbness of legs in 1st stage | 1) Patient may experience pain between injections<br>2) Less stable analgesic level<br>3) Many patients experience pain in perineum during 2nd & 3rd stages<br>4) Prolonged 2nd stage → increased instrumental delivery |
| 1) Increase infusion rate at beginning of 2nd stage<br>2) Test for perineal analgesia<br>3) 15 min pre-delivery inject 10 ml LAntS with patient sitting | 1) Effective analgesia during 1st stage<br>2) Little or no motor block<br>3) Effective BDE (4) → spontaneous delivery | 1) 20–50% feel perineal pain during 2nd and 3rd stages<br>2) Inadequate perineal relaxation for delivery |
| 1) If pain in lower limbs/back, inject 5 ml SAnalS thru upper catheter<br>2) With onset of perineal pain, inject 3–4 ml LAnalS thru lower catheter → perineal analgesia<br>3) 15 min pre-delivery inject 3–4 LAntS → perineal relaxation | 1) Most specific technique of LEB "Rolls Royce" of obstetric A/A<br>2) Requires less drug than other Epidural techniques<br>3) Least effect on mother, labor, fetus, and newborn<br>4) No premature numbness or weakness of limbs<br>5) No premature perineal relaxation → no interference of flexion/internal rotation<br>6) Little or no impairment of BDE → spontaneous delivery | 1) Two catheters are required → theoretically greater risk of complications or failures (These obviated by skilled anesthesiologists) |
| 1) Continue analgesia to 15 min pre-delivery →<br>2) Inject 10 ml of LAntS with patient sitting | 1) Puncture done in lower lumbar area<br>a) Larger space → easier puncture<br>b) Less risk of damage to spinal cord | 1) Premature numbness of lower limbs during 1st stage<br>2) Use of much larger amt of local anesthetic → risk of toxicity to mother, fetus and newborn<br>3) For above reasons, no longer used |
| 1) Continue injection of LAnalS as necessary<br>2) After 2nd or 3rd dose, perineal relaxation present | 1) None over above techniques | 1) Premature analgesia/anesthesia of perineum and lower limbs<br>2) Premature relaxation of perineum → impairs flexion/internal rotation → instrumental delivery necessary<br>3) Risk of injection or puncture of rectum<br>4) For above reasons, no longer used |
| 1) Used as complementary to analgesia for labor<br>2) Injection made after flexion and internal rotation | 1) Useful as perineal analgesia/anesthesia as supplementary to other analgesia (PCB or inhalation or opioid analgesia) | 1) Does not provide relief of labor pain<br>2) Risk of infection or puncture of rectum<br>3) Risk of accidental puncture of fetal scalp |

four series reported by Zador and associates (76–78), there are no specific data on the incidence of technical failure, but based on the data of evaluation of the efficacy by an anesthetic nurse and midwife, suggest that they experienced technical failure rates in about 3%. In our own departments, technical failure rate among trainees has been 3 to 5%, and among attending staff 1 to 2%.

The technical failure rate with caudal block is higher than that with lumbar epidural analgesia performed by the same individuals. This is due to the fact that anatomic anomalies of the sacrum are present in some persons and these make puncture through the sacrococcygeal hiatus difficult. In others, if it is difficult to achieve analgesia after successful penetration of the sacrococcygeal hiatus, it is due to the lack of fusion of some of the laminae of the sacral vertebrae so that some of the local anesthetics are lost into the soft tissue posterior to the sacrum (see anatomic considerations in Part B). In a survey of the first 10,000 parturients managed with continuous caudal analgesia/anesthesia, Hingson and Edwards (16) reported an 8% failure rate. A number of other papers, published during the first decade of continuous caudal analgesia usage,

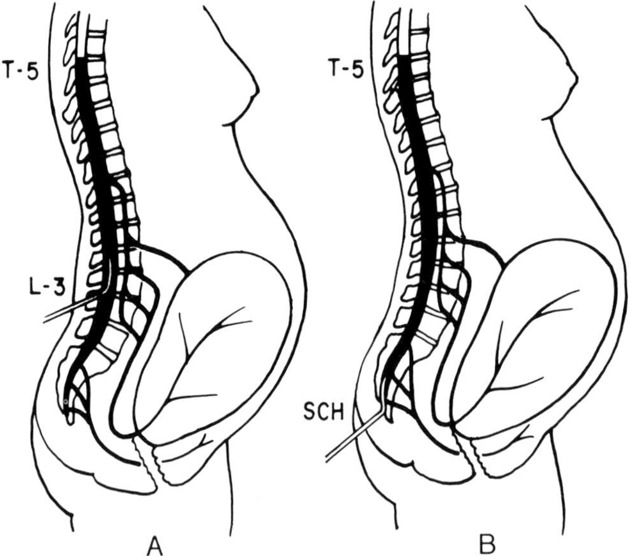


**Fig. 13–2.** Schematic illustration of continuous lumbar epidural block for cesarean section. **A:** The catheter is inserted through a needle that has been passed through the L3-L4 interlaminar space, and its tip advanced to the level of the upper part of L2 vertebra. Injection of increments of 5 ml every 2 to 3 minutes until the upper level of analgesia is at T4-T5 dermatome. The total dose of 18 to 22 ml of local anesthetic can be injected as a single dose very slowly, so that it takes 3 to 4 minutes to complete the injection. **B:** Continuous caudal anesthesia for cesarean section. The catheter is inserted through the sacrococcygeal hiatus and advanced 10 to 12 cm so that its tip is at the level of L5 or S1 vertebra. The injection of 18 to 22 ml of local anesthetic produces analgesia from T4-T5 to S5, and motor block extends from T8-T9 to S5.

reported failure rates ranging from 10 to 15% (14,22). However, subsequent reports of larger series indicated a failure rate of between 3 to 6% in those departments in which the procedure was used extensively. Chapter 35 in the first edition of this book, devoted to caudal block, contains Table 35–1 which lists the results of 10 reports that present more than half the total number of over 101,000 patients with a mean failure rate of about 6%. One of these studies included 16,000 parturients managed by Bonica and associates, working in Tacoma General Hospital, Tacoma, Washington, during the late 1940's to 1955, reported an overall failure rate of 6%. Further analysis revealed that the failure rate with continuous anesthesia occurred in about 1% when the procedure was done by senior attending staff with 10 years' experience, 2.5% among staff with 2 to 5 years experience, 12% when the procedure was done by first-year residents, and 4% when performed by the second-year residents. Although in the early 1950s Bonica began to use lumbar epidural block and the double-catheter technique, many of the staff continued to use continuous caudal analgesia for labor and vaginal delivery in 85% of the parturients. Even today most of the staff in that hospital manage parturients with this procedure—primarily due to its long tradition of a high (96% + ) success rate. The significant improvement in results during the first decade was due not to only generally improved technical skill in its use, but also to the advent of better (more penetrating) local anesthetic drugs, better equipment, and refinement of techniques. As previously mentioned, during the last several decades, caudal blockade has been virtually abandoned and consequently most anesthesiologists have not acquired the skill necessary for success with this technique. This is unfortunate because, as will be emphasized later in this chapter, the double-catheter technique eliminates many of the major problems encountered during the second stage of labor.

Notwithstanding the high technical success rate with lumbar epidural analgesia, about 15 to 25%, or more, of patients fail to enjoy *total* pain relief during the entire labor and vaginal delivery. This may be due to one or more of the following factors: 1) a "missed segment," i.e., some pain is felt in a single segment either unilaterally or bilaterally; 2) analgesia on one side is only partial or totally unilateral; 3) among parturients in whom lumbar epidural analgesia is achieved with a single catheter using either intermittent injections or continuous infusions, a significant percentage will not have sufficient perineal analgesia/anesthesia and will experience pain of varying severity during the latter part of the second stage, during the delivery, or both, especially if instrumental delivery is necessary; 4) about 5 to 8% of parturients will have varying degrees of discomfort in the back, flanks, or abdomen, with each uterine contraction or continuous back pain even between contractions (see Chapter 9). These latter types of pain and discomfort are more frequent among parturients with persistent posterior position or abnormal presentations. In these patients, it is probable that the concentration of the local anesthetics is not sufficient to block very intense nociceptive impulses produced by very strong uterine contractions. In Part B, which details the techniques, suggestions are given to prevent or to promptly correct these problems.

In addition to these technical problems that prevent parturients from enjoying a completely painless and pleasurable experience with their childbirth, there is another issue that has gained the attention of the public, particularly in the United Kingdom; and it's importance is somewhat exaggerated by the proponents of natural childbirth. This refers to an emotional experience of "deprivation," which Crawford (69,70,90) considered as a "complication," or "disadvantage," of epidural anesthesia. The condition is one in which the mother states that although she was grateful and appreciative for the pain relief provided by the epidural analgesia, in the postpartum period she experiences a feeling of disappointment that she was deprived or, to use Crawford's word, "cheated" of the anticipated pleasure of "natural" labor and delivery, or that she had not fulfilled her proper role in the process. Crawford reported that this was experienced by 1.4% of puerpera interviewed within 6 days of the delivery. Subsequently, Billewicz-Driemel and Milne (96) interviewed 99 mothers who had received epidural anesthesia 18 to 24 months before the interview and noted an incidence of 4%, though only occurring in primigravidae. After considering additional factors (included in their report) that might have contributed to this experience, the authors concluded that the "absence of long-term ill effects associated with deprivation leads us to suggest that the small incidence of 'deprivation' is of little significance and should not influence the decision to perform extradural blockade." Subsequently, a number of other investigators studied the incidence of this phenomenon which occurred in 4 to 7%. (97–105).

The most recent report, published in 1993 by MacArthur and associates (98), involved an extensive questionnaire sent to 11,701 women 13 months to 9 years after giving birth in the same maternity unit in which Crawford had worked. The opinion sought from the respondees related to both levels of satisfaction with the particular form of pain relief used and the presence of any feelings of deprivation of the birth process. Among the 3484 women who had received epidural analgesia for vaginal delivery and responded to this specific issue, 7% reported feelings of deprivation of the full pleasure of childbirth—a figure much higher than that reported by Crawford, but still only representing a minority of women. It is of interest to note that women who had spontaneous deliveries and shorter labors were least satisfied with the epidural anesthesia, while the opposite was generally true for the other forms of pain relief. Moreover, after an emergency cesarean section carried out under epidural anesthesia, feelings of deprivation were expressed by 5.1%, but by only 1.7% after an elective cesarean section. In the women who had had inhalation analgesia, pethidine (meperidine), or relaxation techniques, the incidence of deprivation was less than 1%. Moreover, the various studies also revealed that among women who had experienced deprivation, two-thirds to three-quarters indicated they would have epidural analgesia for subsequent labor and delivery—an indication that freedom from pain is more important than the effects of deprivation.

These and other data contained in the various reports suggest that a feeling of deprivation with epidural anesthesia reflected, in part, inadequate antepartal preparation, which should have included comprehensive information on the physiologic and psychologic aspects of pregnancy and labor and vaginal delivery and the possible problems that may be encountered that require forceps delivery and other active interventions. Moreover, many uninformed primigravidae without previous experience have fears and anxiety about epidural and other forms of regional anesthesia, as discussed in detail in Chapter 3. Some reports also suggest that lack of emotional and psychologic support by the spouse, and one or more members of the obstetric team, contributes to this experience. Obviously, this is a very important issue, but one that can be virtually eliminated by providing gravidae and parturients with optimal care that includes, among other things, strong physiologic and psychologic support and other tactics that counteract negative reactions.

## Conclusion

The aforementioned problems and issues notwithstanding, many published reports cited above under "efficacy" and a significant number in which various forms of analgesia have been compared, make clear the fact that continuous epidural analgesia, *properly administered*, is the most effective form of pain relief during labor and vaginal delivery currently available (76–79,98–106). Of the numerous controlled trials comparing epidural analgesia with other methods and control groups, we will cite the data of only a few.

In the four studies of Zador and associates (76–79) already cited, the efficacy of epidural analgesia was evaluated independently by an anesthetic nurse, a midwife, and patients using a detailed scoring system. Among the 190 patients managed with intermittent injection of lidocaine alone (100 patients) or lidocaine/epinephrine, very good (complete) pain relief was achieved by 70 to 86% (mean 77%) of the parturients and good (almost complete) pain relief was experienced by 14 to 28% (mean 20%) of the subjects for a total of 97%. Results were better among the 90 patients who were given lidocaine with 1:200,000 epinephrine than were the results with 100 patients who had plain lidocaine. In the two control groups with the same demographic characteristics (except that the study group had had a more prolonged and painful labor and were more tired before induction of block than was the control group), the control groups experienced less than 50% satisfactory pain relief. In the 22 parturients in whom lidocaine alone, or lidocaine-epinephrine, was administered as a continuous-drip infusion, clinically satisfactory analgesia was achieved by nearly all (96%) of the patients, though the results were somewhat better when epinephrine was added to the local anesthetic solution. Additional information from these studies will be presented in subsequent sections.

The study by MacArthur and associates (98) revealed that, among the 3484 parturients who had had epidural anesthesia and responded positively to the questionnaire, 74% were fully satisfied (complete pain relief), 12% felt that epidural analgesia helped, while only 7% stated "it was no good." Among the 3825 women who received inhalation analgesia, the figures for pain relief were 37%, 47%, and 15%, respectively; among the 1139 women who had been managed with meperidine, the figures were 28%, 29%, and 28%, respectively; while of the 2709 women who had used relaxation techniques, the figures were 34%, 48%, and 13%, respectively. Philipsen and Jensen (103) carried out a prospective randomized study to evaluate the opinion of 97 parturients on the efficacy of segmental epidural analgesia, compared with parental meperidine. Using the visual analog scale that extended from 0 to 100, they noted that of the 51 patients who received epidural analgesia for labor and delivery, those patients had a mean VAS score of 11, in contrast to the score of 65 among women who were managed with pethidine. Moreover, 59% of the women in the epidural group, compared to the 20% in the pethidine group, had a painless labor and delivery. Philipsen and Jensen also reported that for subsequent deliveries, 73% of the epidural group stated that they would request epidural blockade compared to 30% in the pethidine group. The other reports cited in the reference list had similar incidents of pain relief with epidural analgesia as compared with other methods used, which included nitrous oxide-oxygen, opioids, pudendal nerve block, spinal anesthesia, and a combination of different techniques (96–103,105,106).

A summary of these and other prospectively controlled clinical trials comparing epidural analgesia with nonepidural forms of pain relief during labor has been recently published by Howell and Chalmers (105). This report has reviews of numerous publications on epidural analgesia and is highly recommended to the reader. It should also be mentioned that in the mid-1980s Chalmers and his associates developed the Oxford Data Base of Perinatal Trials, and, in 1991, a large amount of data was published by the Oxford University Press (106). This promises to become an unparalleled source of information about epidural analgesia as well as other forms of obstetric pain relief.

## *Other Clinical Aspects*

### Optimal Time for Starting Analgesia

The optimal time to start analgesia depends on several factors, including: 1) whether epidural analgesia is being used for spontaneous or induced labor; 2) severity of the pain; 3) the obstetric conditions; 4) preference of the obstetrician regarding use of oxytocics, manual rotation of the presenting part, and outlet forceps; and 5) the presence of special indications for the procedure.

### Induced Labor

In induced labor, the catheter should be introduced and a test dose given before starting the induction. Continuous lumbar epidural (or even continuous caudal block) is the ideal analgesia during induction of labor because it provides continuous pain relief without significantly altering the response of the uterus to physiologic doses of oxytocin (16,17,24,25,65,69,90). By administering the oxytocin at physiologic rates, labor progresses at a normal rate, even when standard epidural or caudal block analgesia is used that may interfere with Ferguson's reflex. Properly applied and rigidly supervised, the combined use of elective induction of labor and early continuous epidural is especially useful in cases in which there are maternal or obstetric indications for induction.

### Spontaneous Labor

In spontaneous labor that is uncomplicated by maternal disease or obstetric difficulty, the conditions listed in Table 13–2 should exist before block is started. Usually, it is not necessary to start epidural analgesia earlier because during the latent phase most parturients can be managed adequately with psychologic support and small doses of sedatives. On the other hand, there is a small, albeit significant, percentage of parturients who experience severe pain during the latent phase that requires effective therapy. As discussed in detail in Chapters 3 and 9, recent studies have shown that parturients with severe pain in the latent phase have longer latent phases and active phases of labor and increased incidence of instrumental delivery (57,68,72–74). These may be related to the presence of anxiety, stress, and negative, cognitive processes that may precipitate marked increase in catecholamines and cortisol and thus predispose the parturient to inefficient labor pattern that could continue through the second stage (107). By effectively relieving the pain during the latent phase, this chain of events might be obviated or at least minimized.

**Table 13–2.** Conditions Essential to Initiation of Epidural Analgesia/Anesthesia

1) The parturient should be in active phase of labor and experiencing moderate to severe pain during uterine contractions.
2) The contractions should be regular, of good intensity, and occurring at intervals of 3 minutes or less and lasting 35 to 40 seconds or longer.
3) The presenting part should be engaged in the pelvis.
4) The cervix should be dilated 3 to 4 cm in multiparas and 4 to 5 cm in primiparas.

Other indications for an early initiation of epidural block include parturients with heart disease or other disorders, which require that the adverse hemodynamic and metabolic effects of labor be reduced. It can also be started early if the infant is premature or if there are other obstetric complications that preclude the use of intramuscular or intravenous opioids during early labor. At the University of Washington Medical Center, parturients who experience severe pain during the latent phase are given a subarachnoid injection of 0.2 to 0.3 mg morphine. This technique provides partial or complete relief of the pain without any adverse side effects on the mother, fetus, or labor. After the onset of active phase, they are managed with continuous epidural infusion of dilute local anesthetic solution alone or in combination with opioids.

It is highly desirable to insert and fix the catheter in place early in labor before there is need for analgesia even in patients whose labor is not induced. The injection of the local anesthetic is withheld until the parturient experiences moderate pain. Such early insertion of the catheter affords certain advantages. For one thing, the procedure is carried out when the patient is not having as much discomfort and therefore can cooperate better. Moreover, it decreases the chance of inadequate analgesia in case labor progresses very rapidly. This is especially important in multiparae who are often deprived of the benefit of epidural analgesia because the procedure is postponed until it is too late, in which there is just not enough time to do the puncture, insert the catheter, and allow time for effective analgesia to develop. In patients managed with continuous caudal analgesia, early insertion decreases the risk of the most serious complication—puncture of the fetal head. Theoretical disadvantage of early insertion is risk of infection, but with proper technique this risk is virtually eliminated.

## *Epidural Anesthesia for Cesarean Section*

Lumbar epidural anesthesia that extends from T4–5 to S5 is adequately suited for cesarean section. Indeed, in major obstetric centers where obstetric anesthesia is available, it is currently the most frequently used technique for this purpose (see Table 1–6 in Chapter 1). The technique itself is discussed in detail later in this chapter.

Although anesthesia can be achieved with a single injection, the use of the continuous technique provides much better control of the extent, intensity, and duration of the anesthesia. Moreover, it permits injection of several small volumes, and thus decreases the frequency and magnitude of maternal arterial hypotension (see Chapter 16).

Since the writing of the first edition, one of the most significant improvements in patient care has been the addition of an opioid to the usual drugs used for cesarean section. The drugs most commonly used today are 0.5% bupivacaine, 2% lidocaine, or 3% chloroprocaine; although some physicians combine lidocaine or chloroprocaine with bupivacaine. Currently, most clinicians also add fentanyl to the local anesthetic to enhance the analgesic action. The usual dose of solution is 20 ml of local anesthetic combined with 100 μg of fentanyl given in divided 5 ml aliquots every 2 minutes four times. Others use injections of the entire 20 ml of solution in slowly taking 3 to 4 minutes to inject the entire solution. All of these steps in the technique prolong the onset of the analgesia but decrease the incidence and magnitude of maternal hypotension. This small amount of opioid eliminates most of the previous "bladder flap" discomfort, and helps most all epidurals convert the cesarean section experience into a pleasant one for the parturient. McDonald and associates at The Ohio State University have been using this modification since early in 1990 with impressive clinical results.

## Effects of Epidural Analgesia/Anesthesia on the Mother

### *Respiration*

Uncomplicated epidural analgesia/anesthesia, whether achieved via the lumbar or sacral route, has no direct effect on the respiratory center, and the changes in pulmonary function caused by it are clinically insignificant. When the uppermost level of analgesia is at the ninth or tenth thoracic segment, there is no weakness of the intercostal or abdominal muscles because the concentration of the local anesthetic is usually insufficient to affect the large thickly myelinated motor fibers in the four or five uppermost segments involved in the block. Even when sensory block extends to the fourth or fifth thoracic segment as required for cesarean section, it is likely that motor block does not extend above T8–9 (108). Although no electromyographic data in obstetric patients are available, studies in surgical patients and human volunteer subjects showed that the level of motor block following extradural analgesia was usually 4 to 5 segments below the level of analgesia (108) (Figure 13–3). Even if the lower intercostal and abdominal muscles are weakened or paralyzed, there is no decrease in pulmonary ventilation because the diaphragm and the unaffected intercostal muscles are able to compensate (Figure 13–4). Moreover, a study of 19 parturients undergoing cesarean section in whom serial measurements of peak expiratory flow rates were recorded revealed that all except one had adequate expiratory reserve volume and residual abdominal muscle power consistent with an effective cough (109). On the other hand, if complete motor block extends much above

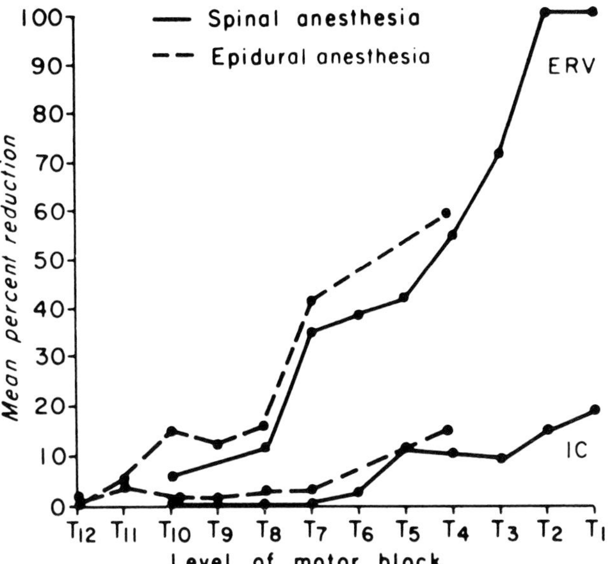


**Fig. 13–3.** The effect of spinal and epidural anesthesia on inspiratory capacity (IC) and expiratory reserve volume (ERV). Solid analgesia to T9-T10 results in motor block of L1, producing no significant effects on IC and ERV. However, epidural analgesia extending to T4 results in motor block up to T8 that results in insignificant change in IC and 15 percent decrease in ERV. Because the level of sensory block is usually about four spinal segments above motor blockade, excessively high blockade to T1 results in motor block up to T4 with consequent 12 to 14% decrease in IC, but a profound (60%) reduction in ERV. This usually results in fall of end-tidal ventilation below the pulmonary closing volume with consequent atelectasis and arterial desaturation. (From Freund FG, et al: Ventilatory reserve and level of motor block during high spinal and epidural anesthesia. Anesthesiology 28:834–837, 1967).

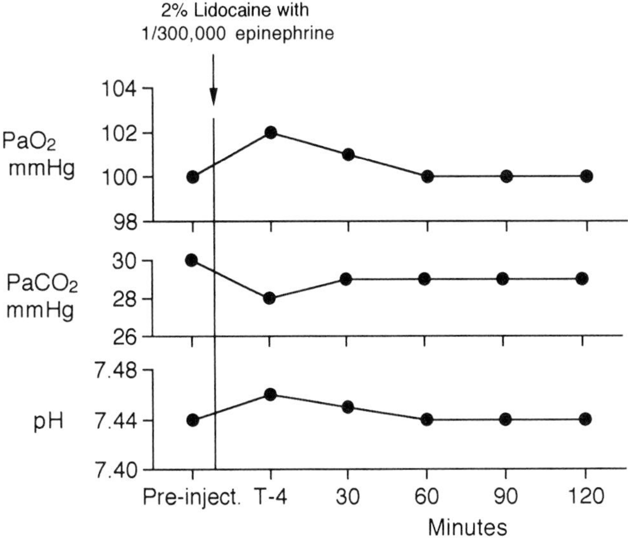


**Fig. 13–4.** Effect of high (T4-T5) epidural block on ventilation. Mean values obtained in 15 parturients who received epidural block with 2% lidocaine and 1:200,000 epinephrine. Notice the slight rise in $PaCO_2$ and decrease in $PCO_2$ within 15 minutes of the injection, probably due to hyperventilation consequent to anxiety and apprehension caused by the execution of the block.

T7, there is significant reduction of the expiratory reserve volume that results in end-tidal ventilation falling below pulmonary closing volume with consequent atelectasis and hypoxemia. This condition is most likely to occur in parturients undergoing cesarean section with an unduly high epidural block. To obviate the risk of hypoxemia, patients should be given 100% oxygen by mask.

Inadequate alveolar ventilation can occur with epidural anesthesia when: 1) there is marked maternal hypotension with consequent medullary ischemia and impairment of respiratory center function; 2) there is impediment to diaphragmatic movement caused by an abnormally large uterus, by suprafundic pressure, or by extreme lithotomy or Trendelenburg position; 3) there is concomitant respiratory depression from parenteral opioids; or, 4) toxic reaction or accidental total spinal anesthesia complicates the epidural block. As discussed in detail in Chapter 16, which discusses complications of regional anesthesia, all of these can be obviated or minimized with proper technique and effective management of the parturient.

## The Beneficial Effects on Ventilation

The beneficial effects of complete pain relief achieved with lumbar epidural analgesia on ventilation are summarized in Chapter 9 and depicted in Figures 13–5 and 13–6. As may be noted, the pain-induced hyperventilation during uterine contractions that produces respiratory alkalosis and the hypoventilation between contractions consequent to the respiratory alkalosis that produces hypoventilation and frequently hypoxemia are eliminated with significant benefit to the mother and the fetus.

### *Cardiovascular Function*

The effects of epidural analgesia on cardiovascular function depend on: 1) the physical condition of the parturient, especially the degree of hydration and her blood volume; 2) the influence of compression of the inferior vena cava and other veins by the gravid uterus; 3) the lability of the cardiovascular system; 4) the number of vasomotor segments that are interrupted with each of the various

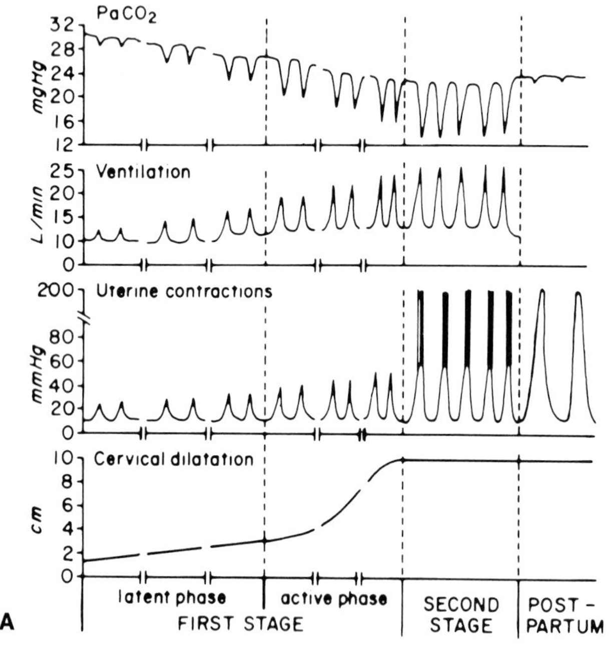


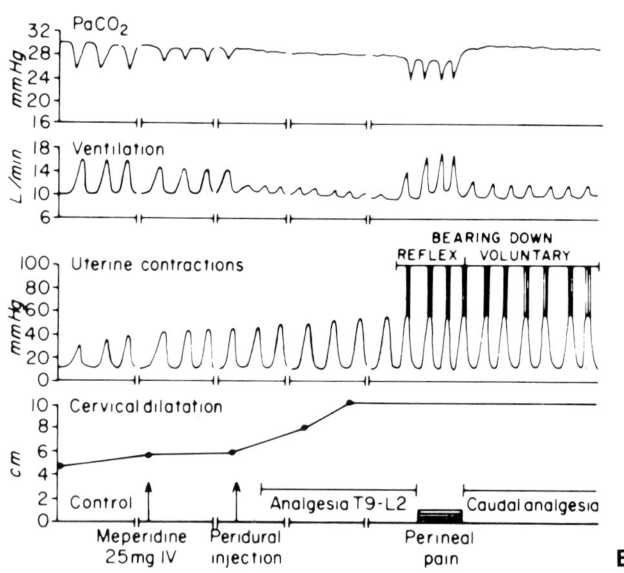


**Fig. 13–5.** The beneficial effects of continuous double-catheter epidural analgesia on the parturient. **A**: Schematic representation of ventilatory changes during labor in an unpremedicated gravida. Note the correlation of the stages of labor as reflected by the Friedman's curve (bottom tracing), the frequency and intensity of uterine contractions, minute ventilation, and arterial carbon dioxide tension (top tracing). During the latent phase, uterine contractions are mild and cause little discomfort with consequent minimal changes in ventilation and $PaCO_2$. As labor progresses, however, the greater intensity of contractions causes greater changes in ventilation and $PaCO_2$. During the active phase of the first stage, contractions cause an increase in intrauterine pressure of 50 to 60 mm Hg, or more, cause moderate to severe pain that acts as an intense stimulus to ventilation with a consequent reduction of $PaCO_2$ as low as 20 mm Hg or lower (see text). During the second stage, the reflex bearing-down efforts further increase intrauterine pressure and distend the perineum producing additional pain that prompts the parturient to ventilate at a rate that is about twice that of early labor and causing a commensurate reduction in $PaCO_2$ as low as 15 to 20 mm Hg. **B**: The effects of epidural analgesia achieved with a double-catheter on ventilation based on measurements in a primipara. At 5 cm cervical dilatation, 25 mg of meperidine, given intravenously, result in partial relief of pain and consequently produced smaller changes in ventilation and $PaCO_2$. Subsequent induction of segmental epidural analgesia produced complete relief of pain caused by uterine contractions, and consequently virtually eliminated maternal hyperventilation and $PaCO_2$ changes without affecting uterine contractions. During the second stage, the onset of perineal pain and initiation of reflex bearing-down efforts caused concomitant increase in ventilation and a slight decrease in $PaCO_2$, which were eliminated with the induction of low caudal (S2-S5) analgesia. (From Bonica JJ: Obstetric Analgesia and Anesthesia, 2nd Ed. Seattle, University of Washington Press, 1980, p. 114).

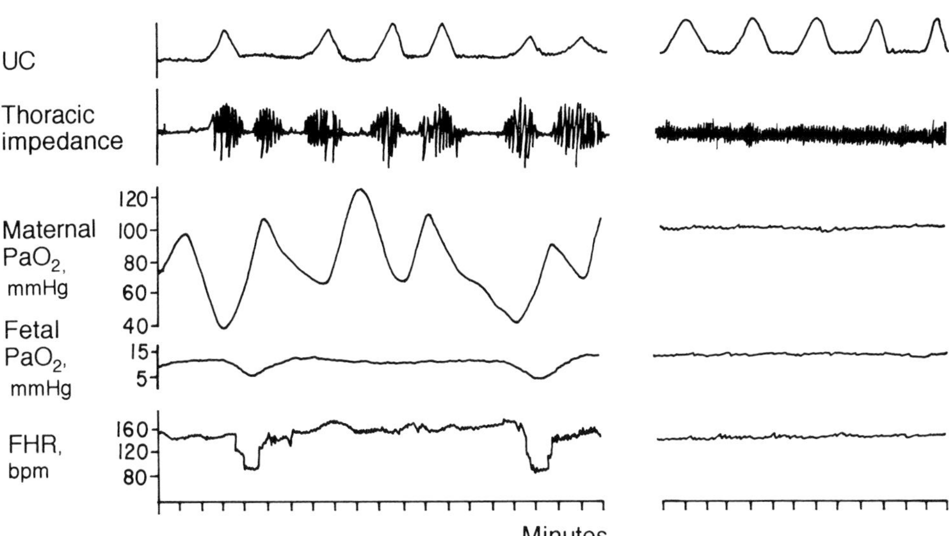


**Fig. 13–6.** Polygraph recording of maternal heart rate, transcutaneous oxygen tension ($tcPO_2$), thoracic impedance, and respiratory rate during labor. Before the induction of epidural analgesia, the pain of uterine contractions caused marked hyperventilation and a consequent increase in $tcPO_2$ to 100 to 105 mm Hg and concomitant decrease in $PaO_2$. When the uterus relaxed, the respiratory alkalosis produced hypoventilation with consequent fall of $PaO_2$ to low levels that in turn caused a fall in fetal $PaO_2$ and a late and variable deceleration reflecting the fetal hypoxia. After initiating and maintaining epidural analgesia, all curves became more regular and the maternal and fetal $PcPO_2$ was maintained at a stable 100 mm Hg. (From Huch A, et al: Continuous transcutaneous monitoring of fetal oxygenation during labor. J. Obstet. Gynecol. 84(Suppl 1): 1977; and Peabody JL: Transcutaneous oxygen measurement to evaluate drug effect. Clin. Perinatol. 6:109, 1979).

techniques; and 5) the total amount of local anesthetic used alone or in combination with epinephrine.

### *Effects of T10 Block*

With the uppermost level of analgesia at T10, as needed for labor and vaginal delivery, the five lowermost vasomotor segments, which control the blood vessels that supply the pelvis, lower trunk, and lower limbs are interrupted with a consequent decrease in total peripheral resistance, venous return, and cardiac output, all of which combine to produce a reduction of arterial pressure. In normal nonmedicated parturients lying on their side, a reduction in blood pressure provokes compensatory reflex cardiovascular mechanisms that counteract these effects and thus maintain blood pressure near normal levels (Figure 13–7). Because the efficacy of these mechanisms cannot be predicted, it is essential to carry out prophylactic measures to minimize the degree of arterial hypotension by: 1) preload intravenous infusion of 800 to 1000 ml of solution prior to initiation of the block; 2) having the parturient lie on her side after analgesia is achieved; and 3) avoiding large or excessive doses of the local anesthetic because these can have a direct depressant effect on the myocardium and peripheral vessels (see Chapter 16 for detailed discussion).

Standard criteria that defines treatable maternal hypotension include a decrease of systolic pressure below 100 mm Hg or decreases in mean arterial pressure of 30% from control. With proper management of parturients in good physical condition lying on their side, analgesia extending to T9–10 used for labor and vaginal delivery achieved with single boluses will be associated with a reduction of systolic pressure of 5 to 10 mm Hg in 40 to 50% of parturients, 10 to 20% with drops of 10 to 15 mm Hg, while in the remainder the pressure remains within normal limits. With continuous infusion of local anesthetics alone or continuous infusion of local anesthetic combined with opioids, the decrease in blood pressure is less than that which occurs with the intermittent injection technique. Crawford (71,72) reported a fall below 100 mm Hg that occurred within 20 minutes of the injection of a therapeutic dose as a single bolus in 1.4% of almost 6000 top-up doses given to 1035 parturients. In properly managed parturients in good physical condition, a fall of systolic pressure below 100 mm Hg occurs in less than 2 to 4%, while a fall below 90 mm Hg is even less frequent (49,53,61–70,72–85,90–94,98–104). When these degrees of hypotension occur, one should suspect low blood volume and/or venous compression of the inferior vena cava, which can occur even in the lateral position.

The higher incidence and magnitude of hypotension reported in the literature and published before the 1960s was probably due to several factors, which include: 1) most parturients did not receive preloading with intravenous infusion of fluids prior to starting of the block; 2) following achievement of the analgesia, parturients were made to lie in the supine position with consequent compression of the inferior vena cava; and 3) in using caudal analgesia achieved with the usual technique of injecting the local anesthetic at S3 level, larger amounts of local anesthetic were needed to extend the analgesia to T10. This, together with the fact that in former years higher concentrations of LA were used, may have been

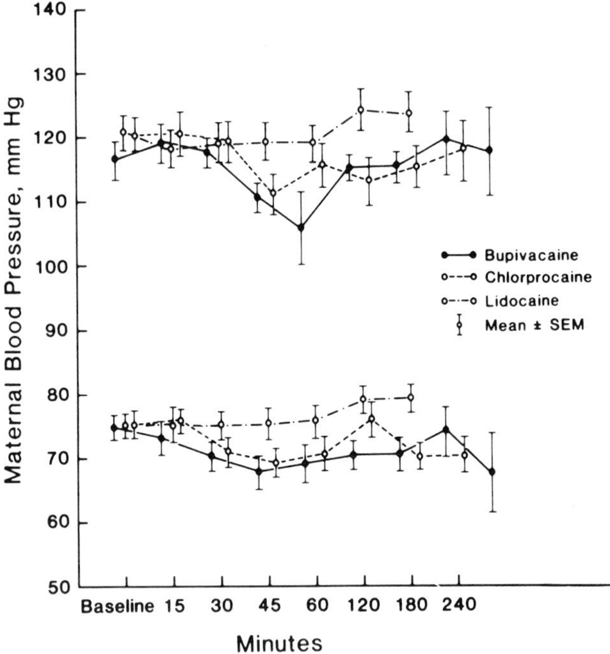


**Fig. 13–7.** Effects of continuous infusion epidural analgesia with three different local anesthetics on maternal systolic and diastolic pressure. (mean ± SEM). After the initial injection of 6 ml of each of the solutions, maternal hypotension developed in 13% of the group that received 0.5% bupivacaine, in 21% of the group that received 2% chloroprocaine, and 15% of the group that received 1.5% lidocaine. Blood pressure was promptly restored with injection of ephedrine. None of the parturients in any of the three groups developed hypotension during the period of infusion, which was started after analgesia was established with initial injection. There were no significant changes in blood pressure compared to baseline value, as determined by Student's t-test. (From Abboud TK, et al: Continuous infusion epidural analgesia in parturients receiving bupivacaine, chloroprocaine or lidocaine—maternal, fetal, and neonatal effects. Anesth. Analg. 63:421–428, 1984).

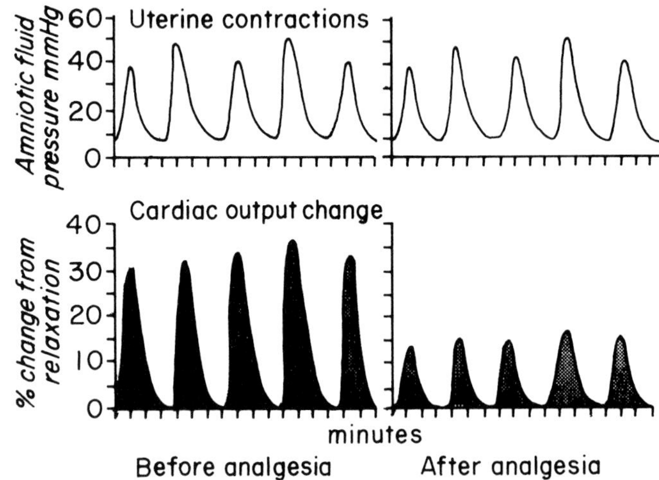


**Fig. 13–8.** Increases in cardiac output during each uterine contraction before and after induction of continuous epidural analgesia in a primipara. With pain relief, the increases in cardiac output during contractions were about 40 to 50% of those before induction of analgesia. (From Bonica JJ: Labor pain. *In* Textbook of Pain. Edited by PD Wall, R Melzack. Edinburgh, Churchill Livingstone, 1984, pp. 327–392).

responsible for some direct depression of the myocardium and the blood vessels. These and other important aspects of hypotension are discussed in detail in Chapter 16.

## The Beneficial Effects on Cardiovascular Function

The beneficial effects of the pain relief produced by epidural analgesia and anesthesia on cardiovascular function are discussed in detail in Chapter 9 and shown in Figures 13–8, 13–9, and 13–10. By decreasing the pain-induced neuroendocrine stress response and the consequent increase in catabolic hormones and other effects directly, it reduces the degree of the progressive increase in cardiac output that occurs during labor without pain relief. This, in turn, decreases myocardial work and oxygen consumption and the repeated increases in arterial blood pressure (Figure 13–11) and venous pressure seen during contractions (see Chapter 9 for details). As emphasized in Chapters 2 and 9, this is beneficial to all parturients, but is especially important in those with cardiovascular disease, essential hypertension, pulmonary hypertension, pregnancy-induced hypertension, kidney disease, and other maternal disorders in which the repeated increases in cardiac output and blood pressure might prove critical to the condition of the parturient.

### *High Epidural Anesthesia (T4-S5)*

Epidural anesthesia that extends from T4 to S5 spinal segments inclusive as needed for cesarean section is associated with a significant incidence and magnitude of hypotension. This is not unexpected because of the 15 vasomotor preganglionic axons contained within the spinal canal that control blood pressure throughout the body, high epidural block interrupts 12 or 13 of these segments as compared to 5 to 6 segments with block extending to T10. However, parturients in good physical condition and lying on their side are able to compensate so that the degree of hypotension is not as great as would otherwise be expected. Another factor that undoubtedly plays an important role is compression of the inferior vena cava and the veins draining the lower limbs and pelvis when the patient is supine. In seven parturients given high epidural block with 2% lidocaine and 1:200,000 epinephrine studied in the supine position by Stenger and associates (110), the fall in systolic pressure averaged 34% and diastolic pressure about 40%.

Ueland, Bonica, and associates (111) studied the cardiovascular dynamics in 16 parturients undergoing cesarean section with lumbar epidural anesthesia achieved with 16 ml of 2% plain mepivacaine. They noted a mean reduction of 13% in systolic pressure and 10% diastolic pressure soon after the onset of epidural anesthesia to T2–5. Left lateral uterine displacement was used in all of the patients. Figure 13–12 depicts the course of cardiovascular dynam-

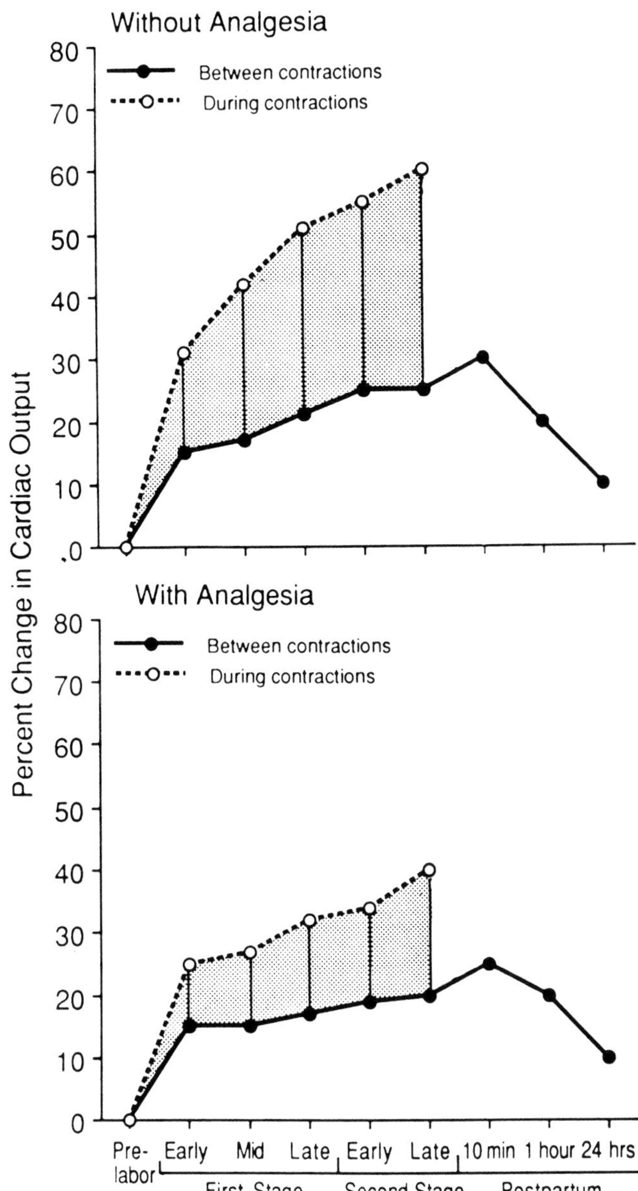


**Fig. 13–9.** Cardiac output during various phases of labor between contractions and during contractions measured in parturients in the lateral position. In parturients laboring without analgesia (upper) the progressive increase between contractions and the further increase during each contraction were much greater than the corresponding changes in a group of parturients who received continuous epidural analgesia (lower). The curve on the left was derived in part from data from Robson SC, et al: Cardiac output during labor. Br. Med. J. 295:1169, 1987 (confirmed by unpublished data at the University of Washington). The curve on the right was developed from data obtained in gravidae laboring on the side with continuous epidural analgesia/anesthesia.

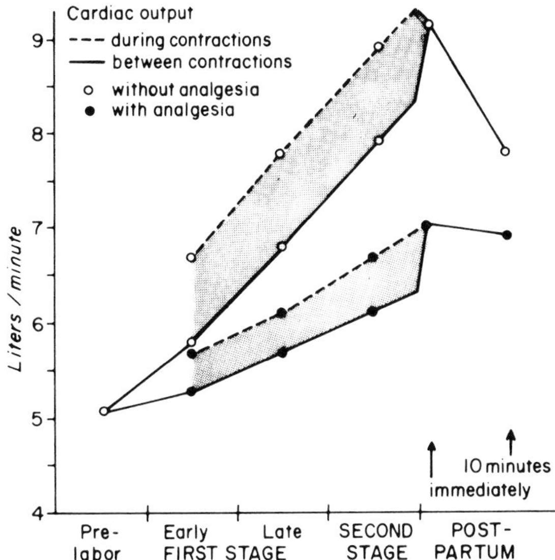


**Fig. 13–10.** Cardiac output during various phases of labor between contractions and during contractions in a group of parturients laboring without analgesia, the progressive increase between contractions and the further increase during each contraction were much greater than the corresponding changes in a group of patients who received continuous epidural analgesia. In this group of patients, cardiac output was measured in the supine position. (Based on data from Hendricks CH: Cardiac output during labor. Am. J. Obstet. Gynecol. 71:953, 1956; and Hansen JM, Ueland K: The influence of caudal analgesia on cardiovascular dynamics during normal labor and delivery. Acta. Anaesthesiol. Scand. 23(Suppl. 10):449, 1966).

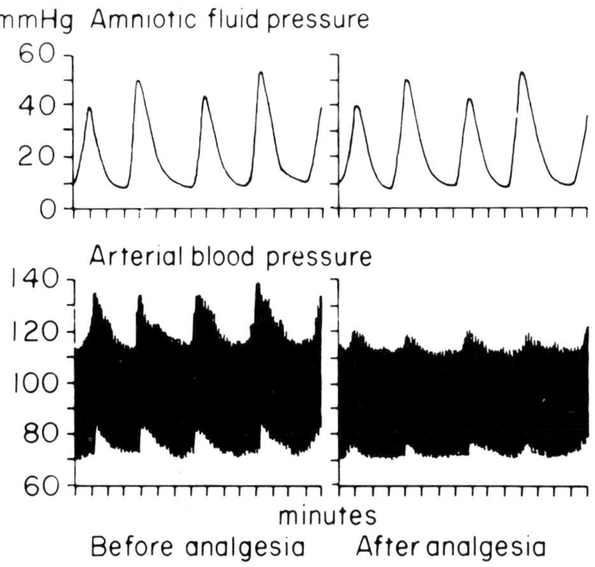


**Fig. 13–11.** Arterial blood pressure before induction of analgesia (left) and during continuous epidural analgesia (right).

ics and, as noted, the blood pressure declined from 116/72 to 101/65 promptly after the onset of anesthesia, but upon opening the abdomen there was an increase in cardiac output due primarily to increase in stroke volume with consequent slight increase in blood pressure. Imme-

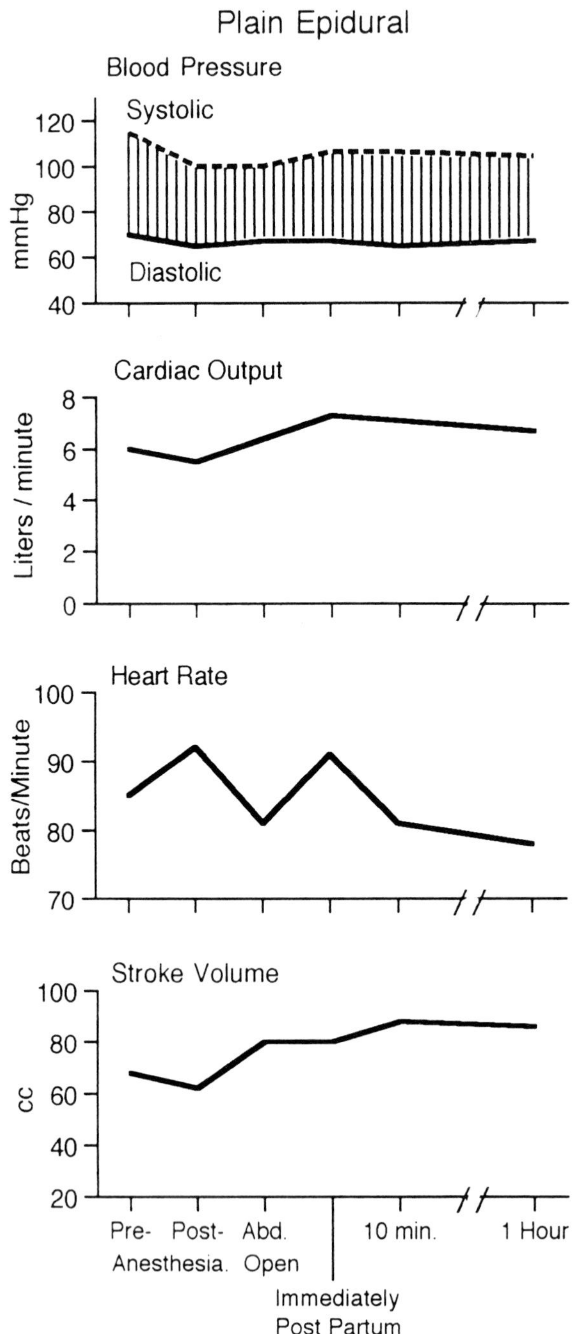


**Fig. 13–12.** Cardiovascular parameters in patients undergoing cesarean section with lumbar epidural anesthesia achieved with 16 ml of 2% plain mepivacaine. Measurements were made with the patient supine and left lateral uterine displacement. Blood pressure declined at the onset of anesthesia, but upon opening the abdomen there was an increase of cardiac output and stroke volume, resulting in restoration of the blood pressure after delivery of the infant (see text for details). (Based on data from Ueland K, et al: Maternal cardiovascular dynamics. VI. Cesarean section under epidural anesthesia without epinephrine. Am. J. Obstet. Gynecol. 114:775–780, 1972).

diately after delivery of the infant, there was a further and marked increase in cardiac output, with consequent restoration of the blood pressure. This strongly suggests that much of the decrease of the blood pressure was due to compression of the inferior vena cava and other veins in the lower part of the body. The study emphasizes the critical need of not only giving a preload infusion of fluid, but effectively displacing the uterus laterally, either with a wedge under the buttocks, or manually, or with a mechanical instrument. Although displacement to the left is used most frequently, in some patients it is not as effective in displacement to the right so that measurement of blood pressure should be made with displacement of the uterus to one side and then to the other. Another point that needs to be made is that even with correct lateral uterine displacement, there remains some venous compression (see Figure 2–28), which added to the extensive vasomotor blockade is responsible for the greater incidence and magnitude of hypotension noted in patients given epidural anesthesia for cesarean section. It is, therefore, essential to monitor the parturient closely and, as soon as maternal hypotension as defined above develops, to promptly give increments of 10 to 15 mg of ephedrine intravenously and repeat these as necessary to maintain the maternal blood pressure above the aforementioned levels.

Because ways to deal with this and other problems regarding hypotension are discussed in detail in Chapter 16, only two other comments are made here. First, the fall in arterial pressure following epidural anesthesia to a specific level is greater in parturients than in nonparturients (see Figure 16–5, Chapter 16). Second, both the frequency and the degree of hypotension with epidural anesthesia are lower than with subarachnoid block extending to similar levels (107,111–115). This is probably due to several interrelated factors, which include: 1) the slow onset of extradural anesthesia, which allows sufficient time for cardiovascular homeostatic mechanisms to become effective; and 2) the area of differential block between sensory and vasomotor interruption, which is wider with the subarachnoid technique than with the extradural method. (50,107)

## Other Cardiovascular Effects

S-T segment changes, nausea and vomiting, tachycardia and chest wall pain have been noted in a number of patients undergoing cesarean section with continuous lumbar epidural anesthesia (116). One study was done to assess if the electrocardiographic changes were associated with echocardiographic evidence of myocardial wall motion abnormality or change in the CPK-NB fraction changes, postoperatively, that might be indicative of myocardial ischemia (117). Of 26 patients given epidural anesthesia achieved with 2% lidocaine and 1:200,000 epinephrine undergoing cesarean section, 6 (23%) had S-T segment depression but no wall motion abnormalities or elevation of CPK-NB. Tachycardia (more than 130), nausea and vomiting, or chest pain occurred in 7, 12, and 10 of the patients, respectively, without wall motion abnormality. However, 3 patients (11%) developed septal wall motion abnormality without ECG changes or symptoms. Left atrial and ventricular dimensions were not significantly different at any time, and all patients had normal posterior and septal wall systolic/diastolic thickness. Ejection fraction significantly decreased during episodes of tachycardia, and all CPK-NB results and ECG changes were normal.

Another study done to detect myocardial ischemia during cesarean section entailed monitoring 111 parturients with continuous ambulatory electrocardiogram (Holter) during and after cesarean section (118). Twenty-two parturients undergoing vaginal delivery were similarly monitored. S-T segment depression was present in 25% of the patients undergoing cesarean delivery, but was not found in those patients delivering vaginally. S-T segment elevation was not detected in either group. The incidence of S-T segment depression during cesarean delivery was similar with epidural (29%), spinal (17%), and general (18%) anesthesia—occurring most commonly in the 30 minutes following delivery. Transthoracic echocardiographic imaging was performed in 23 patients undergoing cesarean section, and of this group 5 had seven episodes of intraoperative S-T segment depression, but wall motion abnormality did not occur in any of the patients.

### Effects on Neuroendocrine Stress Response

In Chapters 2 and 9, many data are presented that reflect marked increases in epinephrine, norepinephrine, dopamine, ACTH, cortisol, glucagon, and other catabolic hormones depicted in Figure 9–14 (Chapter 9). These, in turn, produce some of the cardiovascular changes that impose stress on the mother, may impair uterine contractility, cause dysfunction of labor (discussed later), and increased metabolism and oxygen consumption (see Chapter 9 for references). Equally or more important is that catecholamines and other hormones decrease uteroplacental blood flow with consequent deleterious effects on the fetus (119–123). Morishima (122), Lederman (124), Abboud and associates (125), and Ohno and associates (126), among others, have shown that these effects in parturients during labor and vaginal delivery are caused predominantly by the pain and the associated nociceptive barrage that impacts the neuraxis and the pain-induced anxiety and psychologic stress; and, in part, it is due to the physical stress during the second stage and delivery of the infant when there is marked increase in metabolic demands on the maternal organisms. A number of studies have provided impressive evidence that epidural analgesia, by blocking all nociceptive input and some of the sympathetic efferents, significantly reduces the release of catecholamines, beta endorphins, ACTH, cortisol, and other aforementioned catabolic hormones (125, 127–135).

Epidural analgesia during labor and delivery does not decrease catecholamines and beta endorphin release in the fetus and newborn (125,127,132–138), and norepinephrine predominates over epinephrine (125). This response indicates that, even during completely uncomplicated deliveries with adequate maternal analgesia, the infant is considerably distressed by the process of birth by vaginal delivery. A number of studies have suggested that catecholamines have an important role for neonatal adaptation to the extrauterine environment, including surfactant synthesis and release, lung liquid resorption, nonshivering, thermogenesis, glucose homeostasis, cardiovascular changes, and water metabolism (130–138).

The beneficial effects of continuous epidural analgesia, regarding the neuroendocrine stress response, are even greater among parturients undergoing cesarean section than during labor and delivery because all afferent nociceptive barrage provoked by intra-abdominal manipulation that is transmitted above the T-10 epidural eliminates all sensory input that provokes the endocrine stress response and block of all the sympathetic efferents of the adrenal medulla. Consequently, there is not only dampening but virtual elimination of the increased secretion of catecholamines and other catabolic response (139–145). Hollmen, Jouppila and associates (130–142), and others (143–145) have shown that uteroplacental blood flow is increased *provided* that maternal blood pressure is maintained within normal limits, with vasopressor if necessary. These effects of blocking of the neuroendocrine stress response are beneficial to the well-being of the normal gravida, but are critically important to the gravida with pregnancy-induced hypertension and, as previously mentioned, those that have severe heart disease and other medical or obstetric problems that compromise the wide margin of tolerance necessary to undergo cesarean section. The influence on uteroplacental blood flow and intervillous perfusion on the fetus is discussed in Section 4.

The value of continuous epidural anesthesia, in managing patients with severe preeclampsia undergoing cesarean section, has been demonstrated by several studies. Hodgkinson and associates (146) were among the first to show that in patients, managed with continuous epidural anesthesia, mean arterial pressure, pulmonary capillary wedge pressure, and pulmonary artery pressure remain unchanged, whereas those managed with general anesthesia incurred significant increases in these important parameters. Subsequently, Abboud and associates (147) showed that in women with severe preeclampsia, epidural anesthesia was associated with decreases in catecholamine levels and, as already mentioned, Jouppila and associates (140–142) and others (143–145) have shown that epidural anesthesia significantly improved uteroplacental and intervillous blood flow. Others have used continuous epidural blockade in these patients (148,149). Most recently, Ramanathan and associates (150) demonstrated the superiority of epidural anesthesia in maintaining hemodynamic and neuroendocrine stress responses to cesarean section near normal, whereas general anesthesia was associated with marked increases provoked by the nociceptive input associated with the abdominal incision and delivery of the infant. A more detailed discussion of the management of pregnancy-induced hypertension is presented in Chapter 28.

### Effects on Metabolism and Oxygen Consumption

In Chapters 2 and 9 evidence is presented that pain-induced increase in catecholamines and other catabolic hormones and the physical effort inherent in labor, especially during the second stage, significantly increases metabolism and oxygen consumption (141–158). In one older study, Gemzell and associates (156) noted that oxygen consumption in 19 parturients averaged about 300 ml/min during the early active phase of the first stage, 350 ml/min during the latter part of the active phase, and then rose to 470 ml/min during the second stage. A more recent (Wulf and collaborators (157) study presented data that metabolism measured in Kcal/($m^2$ × min) increased from 0.7 before labor began to 1.2 at 4–6 cm dilatation to 13 during the second stage and delivery, and the figure was doubled during uterine contractions. Oxygen uptake and consumption, measured in ml/($m^{-1}$ × $m^2$), increased from 140 before labor, then rose steeply to 210 during early labor, to 240 at 8 cm dilation, to 260 at full cervical dilatation, and about 300 during the second stage. Moreover, uterine contractions increased oxygen uptake from 300 to 700 ml/($m^{-1}$ × $m^2$). As a result, there is marked increase of free fatty acids from the sympathetically induced increased lipolytic metabolism (81), an increase in hydroxycorticosteroid levels (155), and a steady rise in both aerobic and anaerobic carbohydrate metabolism as evidenced by higher levels of lactates, pyruvates, and excess lactate, which is reflected by a progressive rise in base excess (158). These changes, plus increase in metabolism and oxygen consumption inherent in the work of labor, together with the loss of bicarbonate from the kidneys, produce a progressive maternal metabolic acidosis, which is transferred promptly to the fetus (151–154,158,159).

A number of studies have demonstrated that providing parturients with effective analgesia achieved with continuous lumbar epidural block not only relieves the pain but decreases or completely eliminates many of these deleterious metabolic consequences during the first stage of labor (77–79,81–84,90,91,147–153). Moreover, the superiority of epidural analgesia over opioids and other systemic drugs in decreasing maternal work oxygen consumption, and maternal and fetal metabolic acidosis has been impressively demonstrated by a number of investigators. Figure 13–13, developed from the comprehensive studies by Pearson and Davis (151–154), shows the efficacy of continuous epidural analgesia and the elimination of bearing-down efforts during the second stage in almost eliminating maternal metabolic acidosis. Moreover, under these conditions, it decreases but does not eliminate degree of fetal acidosis. Undoubtedly, this is the result of physical stress on the fetus inherent in the delivery process.

In regard to oxygen consumption, Sangoul and associates (160) were among the first to show the efficacy of lumbar epidural analgesia on decreasing oxygen consumption during the first stage of labor from 317 ± 7.5 ml/min to 274.2 ± 6.4. They concluded that the 15% decrease in oxygen consumption was not only due to decrease in catecholamines but also due to a decrease or elimination of hyperventilation. The oxygen cost of ventilation is 1% of total oxygen consumption in normal subjects (161,162), but increases disproportionately as minute ventilation increases because of the low efficiency of

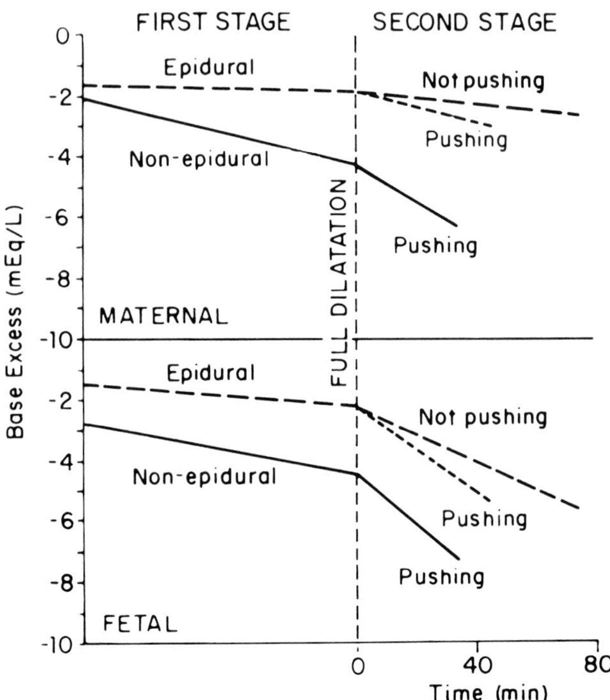


**Fig. 13–13.** Mean changes in extent of maternal (above) and fetal (below) metabolic acidosis during the first and second stages of labor in a group of parturients managed without lumbar epidural analgesia, one of which retained the bearing-down reflex while the other did not. The parturients were delivered by outlet forceps. Significant metabolic acidosis was experienced by those in the nonepidural group of parturients, whereas those given epidural analgesia experienced little or no change in their acid-base status. Fetuses born of mothers managed without epidural also developed metabolic acidosis during the first stage, and to an even greater degree during the second stage. In contrast, fetuses of mothers given epidural had no change in acid-base status during the first stage but showed a time-dependent increase in metabolic acidosis during the second stage. [Based on data from Pearson JF, Davis P: The effect of continuous lumbar epidural analgesia on the acid-base status of maternal and fetal blood during the first and second stages of labor. J. Obstet. Gynaecol. Br. Commonw. 80:218–229 and 81:371–379, 1974. (From Bonica JJ: Obstetric Analgesia and Anesthesia, 2nd Ed. Seattle, University of Washington Press, 1980, p. 115)].

the respiratory muscles (161,162). Moreover, elimination of the purposeless muscle movements and apprehension associated with labor pain contributes to the decrease of oxygen demand after efficient neural blockade. Marx and Greene (158) showed that maternal analgesia is followed by a significant decrease in lactate and excessive lactate.

Reduction of oxygen consumption is especially useful in parturients with acute respiratory distress syndrome. Ackerman and associates (163) reported the successful use of continuous epidural analgesia for labor and epidural anesthesia for subsequent cesarean delivery in a parturient with respiratory distress. This involved a 28-year-old woman (gravida II, para I) admitted to the hospital at 32 weeks gestation because of tachypnea, dyspnea, vomiting, and syncopal episodes that had developed 24 hours after a severe upper respiratory infection. On admission, she had a normal blood pressure but a pulse rate of 140 per minute and respiratory rate of 44 per minute, pH 7.47, $PaCO_2$ 26 mm Hg, $PaO_2$ 61 mm Hg, and base excess −41 mEq/L. A chest examination revealed bilateral expiratory wheezes, and a radiograph showed diffuse pulmonary infiltrate bilaterally. The patient was admitted to the intensive care unit wherein a tracheal intubation was carried out, and ventilation begun with a volume limited ventilator using a tidal volume of 800 ml, and intermittent mandatory ventilation rate of 12 per minute and forced expiratory oxygen of 60% with positive end-expiratory pressure (PEEP) of 5 $cmH_2O$. She improved her oxygenation slightly, but there were no acute changes in the patient's respiratory status after 48 hours except that the PEEP was increased to 10 $cmH_2O$ to maintain a $PaO_2$ above 65–70 mm Hg. On the third day after admission, the patient went into active labor, and it was noted that after nearly each uterine contraction, the patient's mixed venous oxygen saturation ($SvO_2$) decreased. Because the patient became progressively uncomfortable during labor, epidural analgesia with 0.25% bupivacaine without epinephrine was initiated. As analgesia was established, the $SvO_2$ remained relatively constant during and immediately after each uterine contraction. After about 3 hours of labor when it was noted that she had not progressed, a decision was made to do a cesarean section. This was carried out after four 3-ml incremental doses of 2% lidocaine produced a bilateral T4 blockade. A female infant with Apgar score of 7 and 9 at one and 5 minutes, respectively, was delivered. The cord pH at the time of delivery was normal. No significant change in the patient's hemodynamic or pulmonary pressure was noted intraoperatively; and the postpartum course was unremarkable. After removal of the pulmonary artery catheter and endotracheal tube on the second postoperative day, there was no clinical significant decreases in $SvO_2$ in the acute postoperative period. The case demonstrates that decrease in sympathetic tone after establishing epidural analgesia/anesthesia probably improved regional tissue perfusion due to increased blood flow that together with a concomitant increase in oxygen delivery played a role in improving $SvO_2$ during epidural analgesia/anesthesia. Ackerman and associates concluded that the absence of venous desaturation, with contractions after the onset of analgesia, confirmed that pain was the major cause of increased oxygen consumption in this critically ill parturient.

### *Effects on Alimentary Function*

The effects of pregnancy and labor on gastric intestinal function, and the liver and gallbladder, are discussed in detail in Chapter 2, and the effects of pain during labor and vaginal delivery are considered in Chapter 9. To briefly recapitulate, gastric emptying and decrease in the lower esophageal sphincter (LES) tone and other functions are altered during the last 4 to 6 weeks of pregnancy, and are markedly enhanced during labor. The pain, anxiety, and stress associated with uterine contractions in vaginal delivery, and the consequent increased nociceptive barrage to the neuraxis produce segmental and suprasegmental reflex stimulation of the sympathetic nervous system with a consequent inhibition of gastrointestinal motility and function. These reflex effects of nociception are aggravated by the recumbent position and markedly so by the use of opioids (164,165) (see Chapter 9 for other references).

Some studies have shown that continuous epidural anesthesia with local anesthetics, by interrupting the nociceptive barrage and some of the sympathetic efferents to the gastrointestinal tract, decreases the magnitude of the gastrointestinal inhibition and tends to increase the LES tone (166–170). This, together with the fact that the parturient remains awake and alert and retains the pharyngeal/laryngeal reflexes, greatly minimizes the risk of regurgitation and aspiration of gastric contents that in the past have been a leading cause of maternal deaths. From this viewpoint, continuous lumbar epidural analgesia, properly carried out, imposes much less risk to the parturient and her baby.

The above comments do not strictly apply to the current practice of achieving continuous epidural analgesia with low concentrations of local anesthetics and opioids because recently it has been shown that epidural opioids delay gastric emptying. Thoren (170) noted that epidural injected opioid delayed gastric emptying and, indeed, he and coworkers (171) noted that the epidural injection of morphine produced a greater degree of delay in gastric emptying than if the same amount had been given intramuscularly. Subsequently, Wright and associates (172) studied the problem in 30 women in labor in whom they measured gastric emptying by paracetamol absorption and the duration of analgesia in 30 women, 15 of whom received an epidural injection of 10 ml of 0.375% bupivacaine alone, while the other 15 received a combination of the local anesthetic with fentanyl 100 mg. Treatment was administered double-blind and by random allocation. The median time to maximum serum concentration of paracetamol was 60 minutes in the control group and 75 minutes in the fentanyl group, respectively. The correspondent mean maximal concentration of paracetamol was 27.3 $\mu g/ml^{-1}$ and 18.0 $\mu g/ml^{-1}$, respectively. Mean duration of analgesia in those given bupivacaine alone was 113 minutes, while it was 154 minutes when fentanyl was added to the local anesthetic. These results showed that while the fentanyl prolonged the analgesia, it also enhanced the delayed gastric emptying. The fact that in this study the investigators injected a relatively large dose of fentanyl, together with the fact that there are significant advantages of the combination of local anesthetic and opioids regarding latency and duration of analgesia, suggests that for labor and vaginal delivery, these data should not cause discontinued use of the combined solutions. On the other hand, in patients in whom epidural anesthesia is used for emergency cesarean section in parturients who have been in active labor associated with painful contractions, it may be wise to be cautious in using opioids in combination with local anesthetic because there is risk of regurgitation and aspiration of stomach contents should the parturient require supplementation with general anesthesia.

## *Other Effects of Epidural Analgesia*

### *Effects on the Liver and Gallbladder*

Although we know of no studies done on the effects of continuous epidural analgesia and anesthesia used for labor and vaginal delivery on the function of the liver and gallbladder, indirect evidence suggests that it should have no adverse effects. Indeed, it may prove beneficial by decreasing the pain-induced sympathetic hyperactivity and increase in catecholamine secretion, which have been shown to reduce hepatic blood flow and deplete oxygen in the liver. Because hepatic blood flow is largely dependent on mean systemic blood pressure, high epidural block to T4–5 achieved with 2% lidocaine carried out in human volunteers by Kennedy and associates (173), caused a 25% decrease in hepatic blood flow block in mean arterial pressure. In those volunteers in whom the epidural was achieved with local anesthetic and epinephrine 1:200,000, there was little change of splanchnic resistance, suggesting that epidural blockade with epinephrine 1:200,000 provides very stable hepatic hemodynamic conditions (49,173), provided, of course, that cardiac output and systemic blood pressure are maintained near normal levels. Continuous epidural analgesia does not seem to affect the function of the gallbladder, except perhaps by increasing the emptying time due to blockade of the sympathetics to the organ.

### *Urinary System*

Epidural analgesia/anesthesia has no effect on renal blood flow or function, provided normal arterial pressure is maintained. In this regard, it proves beneficial because sympathetic hyperstimulation tends to reduce total renal blood flow and urine output, which are also aggravated by distension of the bladder and ureters (49). Neural blockade of the nerve supply to the kidney and bladder eliminates the reductions of renal blood flow caused by pain-induced sympathetic stimulation.

The effects of epidural analgesia on urinary bladder control depend on the segments that are interrupted. Segmental epidural analgesia produces very little disturbance of bladder function, but blockade that involves the sacral segments produces an analgesic bladder with distension, usually accompanied by functional obstruction. Therefore, during prolonged epidural analgesia caused by a prolonged labor, it is necessary to observe the height of the bladder fundus by palpation and to drain the bladder by catheterization should distension become severe. Post-block urinary retention, which is often attributed to the anesthesia, very frequently is the result of reflex-induced inhibition of the muscles of the ureters and urinary bladder caused by postoperative pain.

## *Complications*

In addition to arterial hypotension, which occurs even with meticulous technique, certain maternal complications can occur as a result of technical error. These include: 1) systemic toxic reactions from the use of excessive doses of the local anesthetic or accidental intravenous injection or both; 2) perforation of the dura, with consequent risk of postpuncture headache; 3) total spinal anesthesia due to accidental subarachnoid injection of the larger local anesthetic dose intended for epidural use; 4) shearing of the catheter; 5) local or epidural infection or possible abscess; 6) shivering; and 7) serious neurologic sequelae. In addition to these, the risks of caudal technique include perforation of the rectum with consequent infection and the risk of accidental injection of the local anesthetic into the fetal scalp. Horner's syndrome associated with either caudal or lumbar epidural anesthesia can also occur. The problem of the "sense of deprivation," already discussed in detail, can be diminished or eliminated by proper information and psychologic preparation for labor and delivery, as discussed earlier in this chapter. Prevention and effective management of the other complications are discussed in Chapter 16.

## Effects on the Course of Labor and Vaginal Delivery

The effect of epidural analgesia and anesthesia on the progress of labor and on the type of delivery of the infant was formerly (and in some quarters still is) a source of controversy among obstetricians, anesthesiologists, and midwives. In their report of 1000 cases, Edwards and Hingson (13) stated that the first and third stage of labor were definitely shortened but that the terminal part of the second stage was greatly prolonged unless outlet forceps were used. Subsequently, other writers (15,16,26) reported that cervical dilatation was enhanced and labor was shortened; others (16,23) reported that labor was slowed; and still others (24–28) claimed that caudal analgesia properly administered had no effect on the progress of labor.

With the increasing use of lumbar epidural block to provide analgesia for labor and vaginal delivery during the past 3 decades, similar discrepant results regarding its effects on the forces of parturition have been published. Thus, some clinicians have reported that lumbar epidural block has no significant inhibitory effects on uterine contractions or the progress of cervical dilatation and, if properly managed, does not significantly influence the resistant forces and the auxiliary forces of labor so that it has little or no effect on the incidence of spontaneous delivery (74,80,85,88,91–94,174–190). Others reported that lumbar epidural block caused a decrease in intensity and frequency of uterine contraction so that cervical dilatation was slowed and the second stage prolonged (77,79,90,115,184–191). Still others reported that epidural analgesia did not effect the progress of cervical dilatation but markedly increased the incidence of the lack of adequate rotation (i.e., malrotation) of the presenting part and the need for instrumental delivery (68,76,90,190–197). Bonica (112) reported that these adverse effects can be obviated with the double-catheter technique.

These and various other reports suggest that the discrepant results can be attributed to: 1) different obstetric conditions existing at the time the block was initiated, as many parturients who have received the lumbar epidural analgesia arrive at the hospital at an earlier stage of labor and already had had prolonged labors before the block was begun (76–79,114,191–194); 2) in many instances, epidural block was reserved for patients with dysfunctional labor that by its nature is longer and often requires stimulation of uterine contractions and applications of forceps delivery (76–79,191,192); 3) Floberg, Belfrage and Ohlsen (197) reported that patients who requested epidural analgesia were more likely to have small pelvic outlet capacity; (4) the posture of the parturient during labor differed; in the past, most parturients having epidural analgesia were kept supine during labor with consequent aortocaval compression and decrease in uterine blood flow with consequent impairment of uterine activity (179,181, 182,185,186); 5) differences in the obstetrician's preference concerning the use of oxytocics and outlet forceps; and 6) the technique of epidural block used, but particularly the extent of the block, the amount of local anesthetic used, and whether or not epinephrine was incorporated in the local anesthetic solution. To help reduce the confusion and clarify a number of these issues, below we summarize some of the most important studies on the effects of various epidural techniques on the three major forces of parturition:

1. Uterine contractions during the first stage of labor, which are the critical factors for effacement and dilatation of the cervix and that help in the descent of the presenting part during the second stage;
2. The effect on resistant forces produced by the perineal muscle sling, which is essential for the cardinal movements of flexion, internal rotation, and extension of the presenting part;
3. The effects on the auxiliary expulsive forces produced by a reflex contraction of the diaphragm and the abdominal muscles, which increase intra-abdominal and intrauterine pressures and thus help the uterus to achieve further descent of the presenting part and finally expulsion of the fetus.

## Effects on Uterine Contractility

The advent of the internal tokodynamometer (TKD) permitted a number of clinicians to study the effects of various techniques of epidural analgesia (as well as other types of regional anesthesia, systemic analgesia, and general anesthetics) on uterine contractions. During the 1950s and early 1960s, TKD studies were carried out by Alvarez, Caldeyro-Barcia and associates (55), Reynolds, et al. (56), Cibils and Spackman (187), Vasicka and associates (115,188,189), Alfonsi and Massi (190), Bonica in collaboration with Caldeyro-Barcia and associates (178), and subsequently with Johnson, Ueland and associates at the University of Washington (112,183,196). These studies were carried out in parturients receiving the older methods of caudal or epidural analgesia/anesthesia that entailed the use of high concentrations and large volumes. With the modifications that occurred in the ensuing 2 decades, TKD and well-controlled clinical studies were carried out that demonstrated the superiority of these procedures over the older techniques, particularly in regard to uterine contractility, progress of labor, and the effects on auxiliary forces of labor during the second and third stages (74–85,91–94,182–186). Below, we summarize the results of these studies on the: A) the effects of the local anesthetic per se; B) the influence of epinephrine incorporated into the local anesthetic; and C) the effects of continuous infusion techniques using low concentration local anesthetics and/or in combination with opioids.

### *Effects of the Local Anesthetic*

Among the first who used TKD studies to evaluate the influence of regional analgesia were Alvarez, Caldeyro-Barcia and their associates (55,56) who noted no significant alteration of the pattern of uterine contractions of the progress of labor in parturients receiving either continuous caudal or continuous epidural analgesia. Cibils and Spackman (187) studied the effects of continuous caudal block in 56 term or near term gravidae and noted that uterine contractility pattern, uterine activity, the efficiency of cervical dilatation, and the total progress of labor were not influenced by the procedure in two-thirds of the patients, were enhanced in 25%, and decreased in 10%. From their results, they concluded that overall first stage of labor was not influenced by continuous caudal analgesia.

The influence of lumbar epidural analgesia/anesthesia was subsequently studied by Henry and associates (176), Sala and coworkers (177), Bonica and associates, (112,178,196), Matadial and Cibils (181), and Craft and associates (182), most of whom used 1% lidocaine to achieve either segmental or mid-epidural analgesia. Similar negative TKD studies were subsequently reported by Schellenberg (179) and Tyack and associates (180) who used intermittent injections of 0.25% bupivacaine. The lack of deleterious effects of continuous lumbar epidural analgesia used for labor and vaginal delivery on uterine contractions and the progress of cervical dilatation have also been demonstrated by a number of well-designed clinical studies, including those of Potter and MacDonald (74), who used 1% lidocaine and those of Matouskova and associates (85), Maltau and Andersen (174), Phillips and associates (175), Studd and collaborators (193,195), Hollmen, Jouppila and coworkers (75,184,185), and Gal and associates (186), all of whom used bupivacaine to achieve lumbar epidural block in concentrations of 0.125% (175), 0.25% (85,174,186), and 0.5% (184,185).

Earlier, Friedman and Sachtleben (198) studied the effects of continuous caudal anesthesia in 500 multiparae and 500 primiparae and compared these with 118 primiparae and 215 multiparae from the general obstetric population that served as control. They noted that caudal anesthesia per se produced an essentially normal cervimetric pattern in primiparae with slight lengthening of the latent and active phases and a pattern in multigravidae characterized by prolongation of the deceleration phase.

In recent years, Abboud and her associates (91–93) have carried among the most comprehensive studies of the effects of lumbar epidural analgesia achieved with various local anesthetic drugs on the mother, uterine activity, fetus, and newborn. They have shown that the use of dilute solution of local anesthetics, including lidocaine, bup-

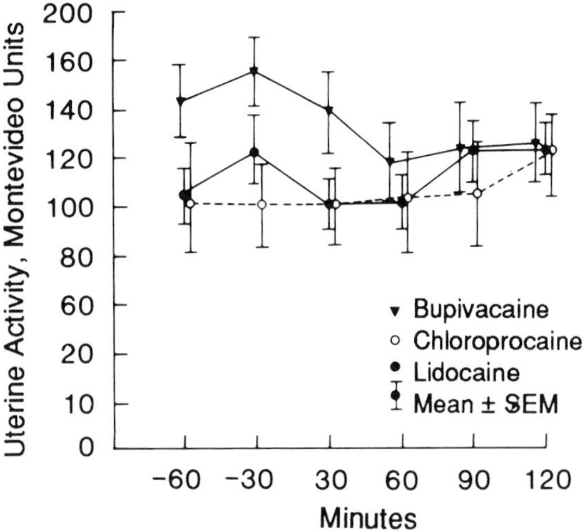


**Fig. 13–14.** Uterine activity measured in Montevideo units 30 minutes before and 120 minutes after induction of continuous infusion epidural analgesia with three different local anesthetics. Although there was a decrease in uterine activity with bupivacaine and lidocaine after induction of epidural analgesia, the analysis using Student's t-test revealed no statistically significant changes during the 120 minutes after the block was initiated. (From Abboud TK, et al: Continuous infusion epidural analgesia in parturients receiving bupivacaine, chloroprocaine or lidocaine—maternal, fetal, and neonatal effects. Anesth. Analg. 63: 421–428, 1984).

ivacaine, and chloroprocaine, produced no statistically significant changes in uterine activity measured in Montevideo units during 120 minutes of the active phase of the first stage of labor (91) (Figure 13–14).

In contrast, a number of other investigators have reported that following the injection of the local anesthetic, they noted transient decreases in the intensity of uterine contractions (76–79,115,188–195). This phenomenon was first reported by Vasicka and Kretchmer (188,189) who noted that soon after the injection of a test dose and a therapeutic dose of lidocaine, the intensity of uterine contractions was reduced by 10 to 20 mm Hg and lasted 10 to 30 minutes, after which contractions resumed their preanesthetic intensity. Similar observations were noted by Alfonsi and Massi (190) in 10 parturients given lumbar epidural analgesia who manifested a slight decrease in the intensity of uterine contractions that occurred about 10 minutes after the injection and lasted 20 to 30 minutes after which contractions returned to normal. Cervical dilatation progressed as expected, and, in some instances, it was accelerated so that the duration of the first stage of labor was shortened. A similar pattern was noted by Craft and associates (182) who used a total of 8 to 10 ml of 1.5% lidocaine to produce segmental lumbar epidural analgesia.

Also using the TKD technique, Zador and Nilsson (76) studied 100 parturients and observed a similar type of transitory decrease in the intensity (but not the frequency) of uterine contractions and uterine activity in Montevideo units after injecting each bolus. This consisted of 10 ml of 0.5% plain lidocaine injected with the patient in the supine position during the first stage and 10 ml of 1% lidocaine injected for the second stage. On the average, the interval between top-up doses was only 38 minutes (range 15 to 60 minutes) during the first stage and 48 minutes (range 20 to 90 minutes) during the second stage. The reduction of the intensity of uterine contractions and uterine activity was less with each subsequent injection (Figure 13–15). The results of various parameters obtained in these groups were compared with those in control groups of equal size of primiparae and multiparae who had been managed with occasional doses of meperidine and nitrous oxide-oxygen analgesia. They noted that the active phase of the first stage was shorter in multiparae who received epidural analgesia than it was in the control group, whereas in primiparae it was longer as was the duration of the second stage in both primiparae and multiparae. Similar results were reported by Willdeck-Lund (109).

Because others had not noted this effect with bupivacaine (70,90) or with propitocaine (199), the transitory uterine depression was attributed to the lidocaine. However, subsequent TKD studies by Willdeck-Lund, et al (192) noted a similar transitory decrease in uterine activity whether bupivacaine or lidocaine was used. Unfortunately, they only measured uterine activity for 30 minutes, so it is difficult to know if it caused prolongation of the first stage of labor. Tyack and associates (180) studied the effects of plain bupivacaine in 10 parturients who were given caudal epidural analgesia. They noted a slight reduction in uterine activity 5 to 15 minutes after injection and then noted an increase above preblock level for a period of 15 minutes and, thereafter, a plateau to preblock level. They concluded that the study failed to show any significant change in uterine activity during the active phase of labor following caudal epidural analgesia as compared

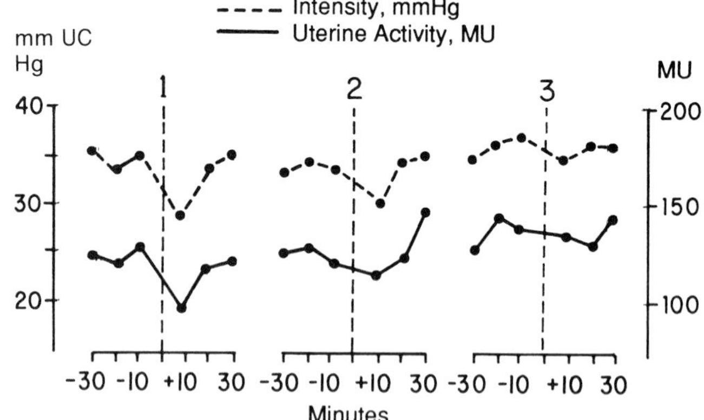


**Fig. 13–15.** The mean intensity of uterine contractions (UC) in mm Hg, and the mean uterine activity (UA) expressed in Montevideo units in 10 patients following three subsequent epidural injections of 10 ml of 0.5% lidocaine (50 mg). Values are given for three 10-minute periods before and after each dose. Note that the intensity of uterine contractions and uterine activity was less with each subsequent injection. (From Zador G, Nilsson BA: Low dose intermittent epidural anaesthesia with lidocaine for vaginal delivery. II. Influence on labour and foetal acid-base status. Acta. Obstet. Gynecol. Scand. (Suppl.) 34:17–30, 1974).

with a control period of uterine activity before block was initiated. No correlation was noted between uterine activity and the bupivacaine blood levels.

## Mechanisms of Decrease in Uterine Activity

The precise mechanism of the transient decrease in uterine activity following injection of local anesthetics is not known. The time sequence of the myometrial depression parallels that of the concentration of the local anesthetic, suggesting that these agents produced myometrial depression. This may have played a part when older techniques of caudal or epidural block were used. However, because the dose of local anesthetic used for segmental epidural block is small, the blood level of local anesthetic from epidural absorption is far lower than needed to produce myometrial depression (200). Moreover, because uterine inhibitory effects of continuous infusions of low concentrations of local anesthetics, alone or with opioids, are much less marked than with the intermittent injections, it is possible that the bolus injection may initiate a reflex inhibition of uterine contractility.

Based on the result of his own study in which the patients were managed on the side and in view of the fact that virtually all of the other studies that reported transient decreases in uterine activity were done on patients in the supine position, Schellenberg (179) attributed transient effects on uterine hypoperfusion caused by aortocaval compression when the parturient is supine. This issue is discussed in more detail later in this chapter.

In addition, it is important to mention that Zador and Nilsson (77,78) and other Scandinavian authors (80,184, 185,191,192) emphasized that prolongation of labor in their parturients was due in part to the fact that parturients who requested epidural analgesia had had more prolonged and painful labor and were more tired before induction of the lumbar epidural analgesia and were more sensitive to pain than the parturients in the control groups that had not requested epidural analgesia. These same etiologic factors contributing to prolonged labor and increased instrumental delivery were also noted by a number of British authors (69–72,193,195). As already mentioned, the study by Wuitchik and associates (106) revealed that in women without epidural analgesia, the presence of severe pain in the latent phase of labor was predictive of longer latent and active phase of labor while distress-related thoughts during latent phase were predictable of longer latent and second stages of labor. These were probably present in many of the patients who received epidural analgesia.

### *Effects of Epinephrine in Epidural Solutions*

There has long been and continues to be a controversy about whether or not epinephrine should or should not be added to the epidural solution given to obstetric patients. There is ample evidence that epinephrine reduces vascular absorption from the epidural space by 15 to 30%, and this has beneficial effects to the mother and infant (49,51,201–205). Reduction in absorption leaves more drug for the target nerves and, consequently, analgesia is more intense and lasts longer, both of which prove beneficial to the mother (203–205). There is also evidence that improved analgesia may be due to alpha-adrenergic antinociceptive effect operating at the level of the spinal cord (206). Moreover, with a lower blood concentration of the local anesthetic, less of the drug is usually transferred to the fetus and thus decreases risk of perinatal depression. On the other hand, there is concern that epinephrine absorption leads to decrease in uterine contractility and prolonged labor.

The results of various studies demonstrate that the myometrial depressant action of epinephrine is a dose-dependent effect. Thus, the incorporation of 1:200,000 of epinephrine into the local anesthetic solution in volumes of 8 ml currently used for segmental epidural block includes 25 to 40 μg epinephrine, while incorporation of epinephrine 1:300,000 in each injection includes about 19 to 30 μg epinephrine. The use of epinephrine in infusion solution delivers even a lower concentration of the vasoconstrictor. A number of studies have shown that this amount does not impair uterine contractility (203–205). Similarly, incorporation of epinephrine in continuous infusion solution during labor has little or no effect on uterine contractility. In contrast, some of the older techniques of continuous lumbar epidural block, which usually entailed the injection of 10 to 15 ml of solution, would include 50 to 75 μg of epinephrine in a 1:200,000 concentration and about 40 to 60 μg if the 1:300,000 concentration was used. These amounts are likely to enhance the transient decrease of uterine contractions and uterine activity mentioned earlier in connection with local anesthetics (77,79,90,183,187,188,190,196,199). With continuous caudal block used for pain relief in labor and vaginal delivery, epinephrine in amounts of 100 to 250 μg incorporated in the local anesthetic solution produced even greater degree of depression in uterine contractility and thus prolonged the first and second stages of labor significantly (202).

In their comprehensive studies, Zador and Nilsson (76–79) evaluated the effects of 1:200,000 epinephrine included in the local anesthetic solution given either intermittently or by continuous infusion. They evaluated the effects of lidocaine-epinephrine in 90 parturients who remained in the supine position and who were managed with 10 ml of 0.5% lidocaine with epinephrine 1:200,000 (50 μg) during the first stage of labor. At the beginning of the second stage, 10 ml of 1% lidocaine with 1:200,000 epinephrine (50 μg) was given in the sitting position. The total dose of lidocaine for the entire procedure was 258 ± 117 mg, whereas in Series I (lidocaine alone) the total dose was 409 ± 245 mg—a significantly greater amount of the drug required when epinephrine was not included in the solution. The quality of analgesia evaluated by the patient, by the anesthetic nurse, and midwife was rated as very good (excellent) or good in 95 to 97% of the parturients. Figure 13–16 depicts the effects on uterine activity in this series of patients (compare with Figure 13–15). Figure 13–17 shows the effect of continuous epidural infusion of lidocaine plain and lidocaine with 1: 200,000 epinephrine.

Matadial and Cibils (181) noted that lidocaine with epinephrine 1:200,000 administered as initial dose of 3 to 4 ml and a therapeutic dose of 6 to 10 ml were followed

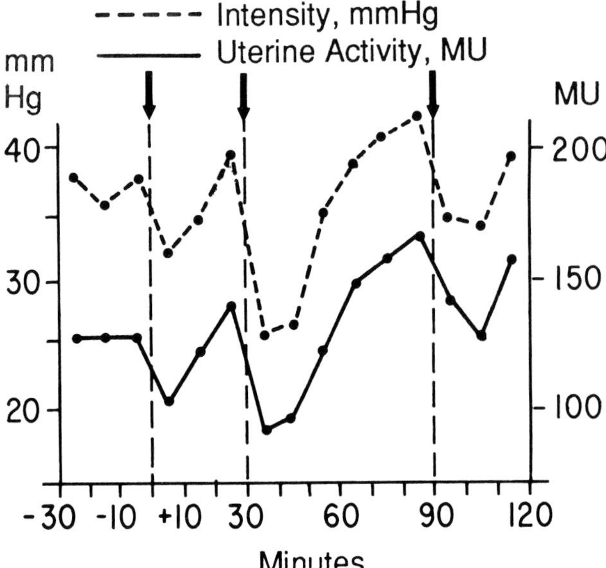


**Fig. 13–16.** The mean intensity of uterine contractions in mm Hg and the mean uterine activity expressed in Montevideo units in 12 patients after injection of 10 ml of 0.5% lidocaine (15 mg) given as test dose into the epidural space, followed by two subsequent injections of 10 ml of 0.5% lidocaine with epinephrine 1:200,000 (as indicated by the arrows). In comparison with Figure 13–14, it shows that lidocaine-epinephrine was followed by a significantly more marked reduction than the first injection, which was given with plain lidocaine. The third injection, however, caused less reduction than the second one in this series. (From Zador G, Nilsson BA: Low dose intermittent epidural anaesthesia with lidocaine for vaginal delivery. II. Influence on labour and foetal acid-base status. Acta. Obstet. Gynecol. Scand. (Suppl.) 34:17–30, 1974).

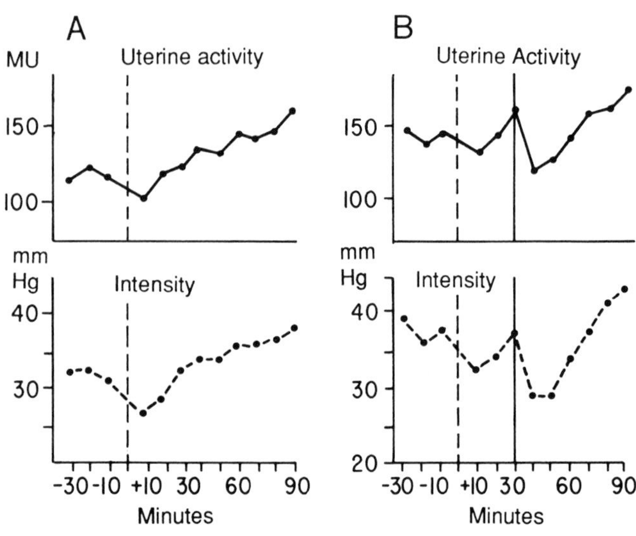


**Fig. 13–17.** The mean intensity of uterine contractions (UC) in mm Hg, and the mean uterine activity (UA) expressed in Montevideo units in two series of continuous drip lumbar epidural anesthesia achieved with plain lidocaine (**A**) and lidocaine-epinephrine (**B**), measured at three 10-minute periods prior to and nine 10-minute periods after epidural block. The broken vertical line in **A** indicates the onset of analgesia with 50 mg of lidocaine as a test dose, which was followed by a slight decrease in mean intensity of uterine contractions and mean uterine activity after which it rapidly returned to normal and continued to increase as labor advanced. In **B**, the broken vertical line indicates the injection of 50 mg of plain lidocaine, which caused a similar decrease in uterine activity as in **A**. The solid vertical lines indicate the injection of 50 mg of lidocaine with 1:200,000 epinephrine immediately before the start of the drip infusion. This caused a substantial decline after the second injection; and that after the fifth 10-minute period, there was a gradual restoration of both parameters toward normal, and as in **A** continued to increase above the preblock level as labor advanced. (From Zador G, Nilsson BA: Continuous drip lumbar epidural anaesthesia with lidocaine for vaginal delivery. II. Influence on labour and foetal acid-base status. Acta. Obstet. Gynecol. Scand. (Suppl.) 34:41–49, 1974).

by a significant decrease in uterine activity. Computation suggests that they used epinephrine in doses of 45 to 60 μg. Unfortunately, they did not provide data beyond the 60 minutes and, therefore, one is not able to determine to what degree it slowed cervical dilatation. Lowensohn and associates (199) also found impairment of uterine contractility with lidocaine epinephrine 1:200,000 but not with propitocaine (Citanest). Like the study by Matadial and Cibils (181), mentioned above, unfortunately, no information is given beyond a 60-minute period. Therefore, one is not able to determine whether or not analgesia slowed cervical dilatation and, if so, to what degree.

The importance of evaluating the entire course of labor to determine the precise influence of the local anesthetic solution and epinephrine is emphasized by the study by Craft and associates (182). A total of 55 healthy parturients with normal obstetric conditions and ample cervical dilatation (4 to 6 cm) were randomly assigned to receive either 1.5% lidocaine with 1:200,000 epinephrine ($L_E$) or 1.5% plain lidocaine ($L_O$) for continuous lumbar epidural analgesia. Following injection of 2 ml test dose, 6 to 8 ml of solution were injected to raise the level of the sensory block to T10. They measured uterine activity in Montevideo units using TKD, and cervical dilatation was estimated in centimeters noted during the next 2- to 20-minute periods. Time from the first injections of the epidural until complete cervical dilatation was also measured. Statistical analysis revealed no significant difference in duration of labor between the two groups, nor was there any demonstrable difference of uterine response to oxytocin in both groups of patients. This study demonstrated that while the addition of epinephrine to even small volumes of lidocaine used for segmental lumbar epidural analgesia caused a slight decrease in uterine activity, the cervix continued to dilate and efface, and labor progressed normally. A similar conclusion had been reported earlier by Vasicka and Kretchmer (115,189) and is supported by the clinical studies mentioned earlier (74,174–178).

Abboud and associates studied the effects of the addition of epinephrine to lidocaine (203), to bupivacaine (204), and to chloroprocaine (205) administered by single injection of the local anesthetic after a negative test dose. They found that the addition of epinephrine produced no statistically significant changes in uterine activity. In the first study, they evaluated the maternal, fetal, and neonatal effects of lidocaine with and without epinephrine for epidural analgesia during labor (203). Sixteen parturients (Group I) received 1.5% lidocaine with 1:300,000 epinephrine ($L_E$), while another 14 parturients received epidural analgesia with 1.5% lidocaine alone ($L_O$). Table 13–3 contains the clinical data on this study, and, as noted, the duration of analgesia achieved with lidocaine epinephrine was 62% longer than that produced with plain lidocaine. Figure 13–18, depicting the effects of epidural analgesia on uterine activity, shows no statistically significant change between the two groups. The duration of analgesia was a mean of 107 minutes with $L_E$ and 66 minutes with plain lidocaine. Epidural analgesia with $L_O$ or $L_E$ had no significant adverse effects on Apgar scores, neonatal acid-base status, and neurobehavioral status of the infant. Similar results were noted in the groups of patients who received epidural analgesia with plain bupivacaine ($B_O$) and bupivacaine epinephrine ($B_E$) (204). The duration of analgesia in minutes was significantly longer in the $B_E$ group than in the $B_O$ group (187 ± 12 versus 85 ± 6. Uterine activity, as measured in Montevideo units, did not change significantly in any of the patients in either group, nor did it differ significantly in the two groups (Figure 13–19). Plasma concentration of bupivacaine in maternal and neonatal blood was significantly lower in the $B_E$ than in the $B_O$ group. In another study, Abboud and associates (205) evaluated the maternal, fetal, and neonatal effects of chloroprocaine with and without epinephrine, they noted that the addition of 1:200,000 epinephrine to 2% chloroprocaine ($CH_E$), as compared to the group that received the 2% chloroprocaine alone ($CH_O$). The duration of analgesia in the $CH_E$ group was 78% longer than in the $CH_O$ group. Again, the effects of epidural analgesia on uterine activity showed no statistically significant difference between the two groups as measured by the Student t-test. There was no significant difference in the duration of the second stage in both groups. Moreover, epinephrine showed no adverse effects in the mother, fetus, or neonate.

**Table 13–3.** Data on Clinical Conditions, Blood Concentrations, Blood Gases and Acid-Base Status of Parturients Given Continuous Epidural Infusion of Lidocaine Alone and Lidocaine-Epinephrine

| | Group I ($n$ = 16) Lidocaine with Epinephrine | Group II ($n$ = 14) Lidocaine Alone |
|---|---|---|
| Clinical Data | | |
| Total amount of drug (mg) | 350.8 ± 51.4 | 464.3 ± 53 |
| No. patients: | | |
| Hypotension | 7 | 2 |
| Tachyphylaxis | 1 | 5 |
| Duration (min): | | |
| Analgesia | 106.9 ± 6.6* | 66.2 ± 4.4 |
| 1st stage (≥4–10cm) | 270.4 ± 44.3 | 230.8 ± 30.5 |
| 2nd stage | 74.0 ± 15.2 | 100.2 ± 35.3 |
| Last dose-delivery | 123.8 ± 19 | 76.5 ± 24 |
| Mode of delivery: | | |
| Spontaneous | 14 | 12 |
| Forceps | 1 | 2 |
| Cesarean | 1 | 0 |
| Plasma Concentrations of Lidocaine (μg/ml): | | |
| Maternal vein | 1.32 ± 0.17 | 1.84 ± 0.18 |
| Umbilical vein | 0.56 ± 0.08† | 1.23 ± 0.26 |
| Umbilical artery | 0.61 ± 0.14 | 1.20 ± 0.28 |
| Umbilical vein/maternal vein ratio | 0.42 ± 0.03† | 0.67 ± 0.08 |
| Acid-Base and Blood Gas Data‡ | | |
| Umbilical vein: | | |
| No. | 10 | 12 |
| pH | 7.32 ± 0.01 | 7.30 ± 0.01 |
| $P_{O2}$ (mm Hg) | 27.1 ± 1.8 | 25.3 ± 2.2 |
| $P_{CO_2}$ (mm Hg) | 37.5 ± 1.0 | 39.1 ± 1.6 |
| Base excess (mEq/L) | −5.2 ± 2.9 | −5.4 ± 1 |
| Umbilical artery: | | |
| No. | 10 | 12 |
| pH | 7.27 ± 0.02 | 7.23 ± 0.01 |
| $P_{O_2}$ (mm Hg) | 20.1 ± 2.8 | 20.3 ± 1.7 |
| $P_{CO_2}$ (mm Hg) | 38.7 ± 3.8 | 43.5 ± 1.6 |
| Base excess (mEq/L0 | −6.9 ± 1.5 | −5.3 ± 0.7 |

Values are ± SEM; * = $P < 0.001$; † = $P < 0.05$ compared to group II patients as determined by Student's *t*-test; ‡ = No significant differences between groups as determined by Student's *t*-test.
[Modified from Abboud, TK, et al, Anesth. Analg. 63:973, 1984]

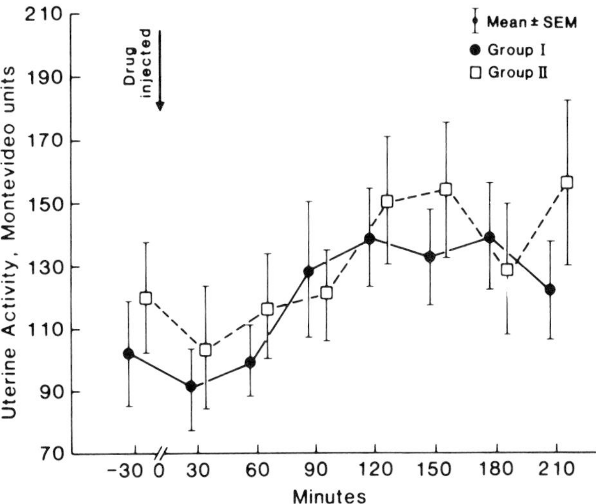


**Fig. 13–18.** Uterine activity measured in Montevideo units for 30 minutes before and 120 minutes after induction of epidural analgesia using 1.5% lidocaine with 1:300,000 epinephrine in 16 parturients (group I), and 1.5% lidocaine alone in 14 parturients (group II). Statistical analysis using Student's t-test revealed no statistically significant change in any of the two groups of parturients, nor did it differ significantly in the two groups. (From Abboud TK, et al: Maternal, fetal and neonatal effects of lidocaine with and without epinephrine for epidural anesthesia in obstetrics. Anesth. Analg. 63:973–979, 1984).

## *Continuous Infusion of Local Anesthetics*

In the late 1960's, continuous infusion of dilute solution of local anesthetics was introduced first using the drip technique (207–209) and later precise infusion pumps to provide analgesia for labor and vaginal delivery (93,94,210–225). The earlier techniques entailed placement of a catheter with its tip in the upper lumbar epidural space and injection of a bolus of 3 to 5 ml as a test

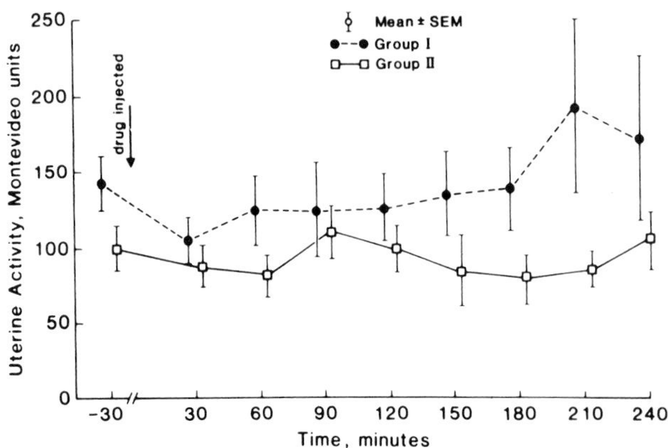


**Fig. 13–19.** Uterine activity measured in Montevideo units 30 minutes before and for 240 minutes after induction of epidural anesthesia achieved with 0.5% bupivacaine with 1:300,000 epinephrine in 16 parturients (group I) and 14 parturients who received 0.5% bupivacaine alone (group II). Statistical analysis using the Student t-test showed no significant change in any of the patients in either group, nor did it differ significantly in the two groups. (From Abboud TK, Eslam AS, Yanagi T, et al: Safety and efficacy of epinephrine added to bupivacaine for lumbar epidural analgesia in obstetrics. Anesth. Analg. 64:585–591, 1985).

dose and 5 to 10 ml as therapeutic doses of low concentrations of local anesthetics (e.g., 0.5 to 1.0 lidocaine or 0.125 or 0.25% bupivacaine, or 2% chloroprocaine). Once effective analgesia was established, the continuous infusion was initiated at flow rates to produce T10-L1 analgesia in the first stage and gradually extending to the analgesic level caudad during the second and third stages.

The advantages purported for this technique included the following (215–226): 1) continuous infusion produced a more stable level of analgesia because of the elimination of the return of painful contractions, which some writers call "roller-coaster" analgesia (224), which is the usual indication for a repeat injection of local anesthetics with the intermittent injection technique. With the intermittent technique, delays between the request for reinjection and the onset of analgesia are not infrequently inevitable. Infusions overcome this to a large degree and the infusion rate can be adjusted to introduce an element of fine tuning and provide a level of analgesic block that suits the patient (223,224); 2) significant reduction in the incidence of maternal hypotension and fluctuations of the blood pressure, which usually occur soon after a bolus injection; and although this is most pronounced after the initial dose, it also occurs with subsequent reinjections (93,212,221); 3) continuous infusions tend to provide a more steady blood level, and, consequently, reduce the incidence of transient decrease in uterine contractions, which is noted in some patients given intermittent injections of the local anesthetics mentioned previously; 4) continuous infusion theoretically should decrease the risk of systemic toxicity provided the total dose is well below 300 to 320 mg of bupivacaine over a 12- to 14-hour period, and the blood concentration is significantly less than 1.6 μg/ml$^{-1}$ that Reynolds and associates found to be related with mild toxic reactions (211,224). A number of studies have shown that epidural infusion, with which plasma bupivacaine concentration was measured, was well below the 1.6 μg/ml (93,209,212). Moreover, while a number of studies have shown an increase in total dose with infusion when compared with the intermittent injection, the total dose falls well below 320 mg (211, 222–223). Still another advantage of continuous infusion is that it reduces relaxation of the perineal muscle sling, and may reduce the incidence of malrotation and the need for instrumental delivery (222). Moreover, infusion regimens properly administered have shown to produce little or no adverse effects on the fetus (93,212). Finally, it has been shown that once stable analgesia is achieved with the infusion, the parturient and fetus remain stable, and the amount of time that is required of physicians and nurses to properly care for them is significantly reduced (209,215,222,225).

Zador and Nilsson (78,79) were among the first to study the effects of continuous infusion of local anesthetics on uterine activity as measured by TKD. They studied a total of 22 parturients with uncomplicated pregnancies who were given continuous epidural infusion using a 0.4% lidocaine drip solution. In two series of patients, one consisting of 10 patients managed with lidocaine without epinephrine ($L_O$), while another 12 patients received lidocaine with epinephrine ($L_E$). Figure 13–17A depicts uterine contractility response in the series with plain lidocaine, and, as may be noted, with the slight decrease caused by the test dose, there was a rapid return to normal and this continued to increase as labor advanced. Consequently, the first stage of labor was not prolonged because the cervix dilated in a normal fashion of about 2 cm/hr. Physical conditions of the mother and fetus, including blood gases and acid-base status, were similar to those of the control group. Figure 13–17B depicts the effect of 15 ml of 0.5% lidocaine containing 50 μg of epinephrine injected at the third 10-minute period, causing a substantial decline in the mean intensity of uterine contractions and the mean uterine activity. Immediately thereafter, a drip infusion was started at a rate of 6 to 7 drops per minute (1.2 to 1.4 mg lidocaine and 0.036 to 0.04 μg of epinephrine). Note that the recovery of the parameters after the lidocaine-epinephrine was injected worked more slowly than after the first, which did not contain epinephrine. In view of the fact that in both series the duration of the first and second stages was similar (10.7 hours in Series I, 10.9 hours in Series II), it is of interest to note that the duration of analgesia in Series I was 258 ± 91 minutes while in Series II it was 188 ± 90 minutes, suggesting that despite the initial myometrial depression caused by lidocaine-epinephrine, the subsequent continuous administration of the drug did not interfere with uterine activity. Figure 13–16B shows that the intensity of uterine contractions and uterine activity declined substantially from the end of the third 10-minute period, when an epidural dose of 50 mg of lidocaine containing 50 μg of epinephrine was injected as a test dose prior to the start of the drip infusion at a rate of 6 to 7 drops per minute (1.2 to 1.4 mg lidocaine and 0.036 to 0.042 μg per ml). It is apparent from the figure that the recovery after the second dose, which contained epinephrine, worked more slowly than after the first dose, which did not contain epinephrine.

Lowensohn and associates (199) also noted no significant effect on the progress of cervical dilatation and the duration of the first stage of labor in 97 parturients who received 0.25% plain bupivacaine by an infusion pump at a rate of 10 ml/hr (25 mg/hr). Abboud and associates (93) also used TKD measurements in 61 parturients at term who received continuous infusion epidural analgesia achieved with three different local anesthetics. Figure 13–16 shows no statistically significant effect on the uterine activity in Montevideo units produced by continuous epidural infusion of 0.125% bupivacaine at a rate of 14 ml/hr, 0.75% chloroprocaine at a rate of 27 ml/hr, and 0.75% lidocaine at a rate of 14 ml/hr. Consequently, the progress of cervical dilatation and duration of the first stage of labor was not influenced by the continuous infusion of the three local anesthetics.

### *Effects of Local Anesthetic and Opioids*

In view of the use of the utility of epidural opioids for the management of acute and chronic pain, a number of workers attempted to provide analgesia for labor and vaginal delivery with epidural opioid injected alone, but these proved to be ineffective-especially during the second stage and for instrumental delivery (226–229). This prompted a number of anesthesiologists to carry out clinical trials combining various concentrations of bupivacaine or lidocaine with one of the opioids, including fentanyl (230–238), sufentanil, (233,234,236,239,240), alfentanil (241), meperidine (242), and butorphanol (231,240,243,244). All of these studies, performed with the intermittent injection technique, showed that the combination of local anesthetic and opioid produced an analgesia that was faster at onset, more intense and longer lasting, and provided excellent analgesia during the first stage without interfering with uterine contractility. Indeed, in some instances, there was a tendency to decrease the duration of the active phase of the first stage, e.g., Bazin and associates (238) studied 40 parturients given segmental epidural block with 0.375% bupivacaine who were then assigned to three groups: group I received 75 to 100 μg of fentanyl in 10 ml saline through the epidural catheter; group II received the same amount of fentanyl intravenously; and group III received plain saline through the epidural catheter. Tokodynamometer studies were used to measure basal tone and the frequency, intensity, and duration of uterine contractions and uterine activity determined by the area under the contraction curve before and after the injections. There were no changes produced in groups II and III, but in group I there was a significant increase in the intensity of uterine contractions and uterine activity, while the basal tone remained normal.

Skerman and associates (242) published one of the first reports on the use of continuous epidural infusion of a local anesthetic and opioids. In their study, they noted that a continuous epidural infusion of 0.125% bupivacaine and 0.00025% fentanyl produced more profound analgesia than a continuous epidural infusion of 0.125% bupivacaine alone. Subsequently, many studies were carried out to evaluate the effects of low concentrations of local anesthetics and of various opioids administered by continuous infusion, which now has become almost the established technique in many centers. Phillips (243) evaluated the efficacy of continuous infusion epidural analgesia achieved with bupivacaine alone and bupivacaine-sufentanil in 40 healthy parturients. Group I consisted of 20 parturients who were given epidural analgesia instituted with a bolus injection of 10 to 15 ml of 0.125 bupivacaine containing sufentanil 2 μg/ml followed 30 minutes later by starting an epidural infusion of 0.125% bupivacaine containing sufentanil 1 μg/ml at a rate of 10 ml per hour. In group II, the epidural analgesia was started with 10 or 15 ml of 0.25% bupivacaine with an epidural infusion of 0.125% bupivacaine begun 30 minutes later at the rate of 10 ml/hr. Infusion rates were altered as required to maintain analgesic level to the tenth thoracic dermatome. Parturients given bupivacaine-sufentanil had significantly better analgesia during labor as determined by a visual analog pain score before epidural and at 10, 20, and 30 minutes after epidural injection. The level of analgesia was checked hourly and was maintained at the level of tenth thoracic dermatome by increasing or decreasing the infusion rate by 2 ml/hr. Group I experienced 95% decrease in initial pain score, while in group II the reduction was 80%. Complete analgesia for delivery occurred in 80% of group I but in only 35% of group II. Jones and associates (245) obtained similar results with bupivacaine-fentanyl compared with bupivacaine alone, administered in a randomized double-blind study of 39 parturients. The fentanyl produced more consistently sustained analgesic levels, and the duration of analgesia was extended significantly. Surprisingly, 20% of the bupivacaine-fentanyl group had a systolic arterial pressure of less than 95, compared with 10% in the bupivacaine group. Other side effects included pruritis, but otherwise the course of labor was similar. They concluded that the addition of fentanyl significantly reduced the amount of local anesthetic required, as compared to bupivacaine alone.

Chestnut and associates (94) have also reported that a continuous infusion of 0.0625% bupivacaine-0.0002% fentanyl given to primiparae did not prolong, but rather, tended to decrease the duration of the active phase of the first stage of labor compared to the general obstetric population. As noted in the next section, it also did not prolong the second stage of labor and was associated with a high incidence of spontaneous delivery. Abboud and associates (246,247), Huckaby, et al (248), and Rodriguez (249), studied the efficacy of pain relief in the maternal and neonatal effects of continuous epidural infusion of 0.0625% bupivacaine/0.02% butorphanol compared with the infusion of 0.125% bupivacaine alone in a randomized double-blind study of 32 parturients. A test dose of 2 ml of 0.5% bupivacaine was given to every patient and followed by two epidural regimens in a randomized double-blind manner. Group bupivacaine/butorphanol (BB) patients received 7.5 ml of 0.125 bupivacaine plus 1 mg of butorphanol followed by an infusion of 0.0625% bupivacaine/0.002% butorphanol at the rate of 12/ml/hr, in which group B (bupivacaine alone) patients received 8 ml of 0.25% bupivacaine followed by an infusion of 0.125 bupivacaine at a rate of 12 ml/hr. In the event of additional pain, a bolus of 5 ml of 0.125 bupivacaine or 0.0625 bupivacaine was given to group B. Total dose use of bupivacaine for the entire group was 71 ± 14 in group BB versus 99 ± 13 in group B. Both groups had excellent pain relief reducing the visual analog pain score from 9 to 1 within 30 minutes, and remained stable for the ensuing 270 minutes. All of the patients rated their analgesia as good to excellent. There was no significant difference regarding onset of analgesia, dermatome level of block, or the number of spinal segments blocked. Progress of labor and mode of delivery did not differ significantly between the two groups. All infants were vigorous and had normal acid-base status and NACS evaluation.

In another study, Abboud and associates (247) evaluated the effects of epidural bupivacaine/butorphanol with and without 1:300,000 epinephrine in 33 parturients during labor and delivery. Group I received 0.25 bupivacaine plus 1 mg butorphanol plus 1:300,000 epinephrine, and those in group II received the same agent without the epinephrine. The incidence of maternal hypotension episode did not differ significantly between the two groups. Apgar score, neonatal base status, and the NACS were equally good and did not differ significantly between the two groups. The duration of analgesia was 176 minutes ± 11 in group I versus 132 ± 10 in group II that received the bupivacaine-butorphanol alone. They concluded that the addition of epinephrine to bupivacaine-butorphanol during epidural anesthesia in all parturients had no adverse effects on the mother, fetus of neonate, or on the progress of labor, and it significantly prolonged the duration of analgesia, thus replicating the results previously mentioned regarding the addition of epinephrine to bupivacaine, lidocaine, and chloroprocaine.

Vertommen and 10 other anesthesiologists (250), representing five hospitals in Belgium, carried out a double-blinded, randomized, prospective multicenter study of 695 parturients to evaluate the influence of sufentanil to 0.125% bupivacaine with epinephrine 1:800,000 $B_E$ given to 347 parturients that constituted the control group. Of the parturients who received sufentanil, 94 experienced no pain or short periods of pain during the first stage of labor, whereas of those who did not received sufentanil, only 76% had no or only short periods of pain. The spread of analgesia was comparable between the two groups with a mean cephalad dermatome level for sensory anesthesia of T10. The mean total dose of bupivacaine in the $BS_E$ group was 34 ± 17 mg compared to 42 ± 19 in the control group. The duration of labor after epidural was 3.6 ± 2.6 hours in the control group and 3.7 ± 2.7 hours in the BSF group. As will be discussed in the next section, the sufentanil group had a lower incidence of instrumental deliveries in cesarean section than the control group. The studies by Chestnut and others and an editorial by Chestnut (251) discussed some of the problems in the study by Vertommen, et al (250) and are summarized in the section dealing with the second and third stages of labor.

A recent analysis of data of the first 1000 parturients managed by McDonald and associates (unpublished data) at Ohio State University Medical Center, Columbus, given a combination of 0.0625% bupivacaine, 0.0005% sufentanil, and epinephrine 1.6 μg/ml at a flow rate of 8 to 10 ml/hr, revealed that 88% of patients achieved complete pain relief during the first stage and 83% during the second stage. The maternal blood pressure was reduced 3% and there were no other adverse maternal effects, and the mean Apgar scores were 8 to 9 at 1 minute and 9 at 5 minutes.

### *Effects of Maternal Position and Arterial Pressure*

It has been long known, but not fully appreciated, that when the parturient lies supine, uterine contractions have a lower intensity, faster frequency, and higher tonus than when she lies on her side or sits (253). Figure 4–14 (Chapter 4), derived from a study by Caldeyro-Barcia and associates (253,254), shows that having the parturient change from her side to the supine position significantly decreased the intensity and increased the frequency of contractions with a consequent decrease in uterine activity. It follows that uterine contractions with the parturient on her side or sitting or in the Fowler's position are more efficient for the progress of labor than in the supine position. These effects appear immediately and last as long as the supine position is maintained, and are more marked in spontaneous labor than in labor induced with oxytocics but neither the parity, the status of the membrane, nor the position of the fetus has an influence on this effect of the supine position on uterine contractility (253). Based on current evidence, this phenomenon is probably caused by aortocaval compression when the parturient is supine with consequent decrease in uterine blood flow and myometrial (and possibly fetal) depression. As previously mentioned, Schellenberg (179), based on the results of his own study and comparison with others, believes that the transient myometrial depression noted by many investigators who used small volumes of local anesthetics for segmental lumbar epidural analgesia was due primarily to the fact that they studied their parturients in the supine position, which was associated with a decrease in uterine perfusion.

The supine position is also important because it decreases maternal arterial pressure and this is related to myometrial depression. Vasicka and associates (115) used the TKD technique in a study of 30 parturients and noted that immediately following the injection of the local anesthetic, there was suppression of intensity of uterine contractions that lasted 10, 15, or at most 30 minutes and that this was associated with reduction of maternal arterial blood pressure ranging from 20 to 30 mm Hg. Because they studied their patients in the supine position, the decrease in blood pressure was the combined effect of sympathetic blockade and the hemodynamic alterations consequent to the supine position, i.e., decrease in venous return with consequent decrease in cardiac output. A close correlation between decrease in uterine blood flow and uterine activity was reported by Brotanek and associates (145).

Schellenberg (179) has emphasized that even in parturients who do not develop arterial hypotension, there may be decrease in uterine blood flow consequent to aortocaval compression that occurs in the supine position. He cited the work of Weaver and associates (255) who noted that when pregnant women at term with epidural block were turned on their back, the fall in mean arterial pressure in the upper limbs was only marginally significant when compared to pre-epidural measurements, whereas the decrease in blood flow in the legs was highly significant. This suggests that systemic blood pressure may be a poor criterion for blood flow in the lower limbs and probably also in the uterus and that the absence of measurable systemic blood pressure changes in the upper limb does not exclude the possibility of changes in uterine blood flow. These and various other data reemphasize the importance of having the parturient with epidural analgesia labor on her side and to displace the uterus laterally when she is placed in the lithotomy position for delivery.

### *Other Factors that Effect Uterine Contractility*

Other factors that can impair uterine contractility include maternal metabolic acidosis, the use of excessive amounts of local anesthetics, and systemic toxic reactions from accidental intravenous injection of large therapeutic doses of local anesthetics. Parturients who have very painful, prolonged, and exhaustive labor are likely to develop metabolic acidosis (256,257). Experiments have shown that drop in maternal pH impedes uterine contractility and depresses the sensitivity to oxytocin of the pregnant human uterus (258). The beneficial effects of effective pain relief in such patients are discussed in detail below.

Large doses of local anesthetics, as required for continuous caudal anesthesia or for extensive lumbar epidural anesthesia, are likely to cause mild depression of uterine contractility. In a study by Johnson and associates (196), continuous caudal anesthesia achieved with 20 ml of 1% (200 mg) lidocaine and lumbar epidural anesthesia achieved with 15 to 18 ml of 1% (150 to 180 mg) mepivacaine administered at the beginning of the second stage of labor caused the intensity of uterine contractions to decrease from 34 ± 19 before the block to 25 ± 16 after the block. As will be noted later, this study, carried out in the late 1960s, led Bonica and associates to abandon the use of continuous caudal block (T10-S5) and standard lumbar epidural analgesia (T5-S5) and to use either the segmental epidural block or the double-catheter technique frequently.

## *Effect on Progress of First Stage of Labor*

The results of the foregoing reports and personal observation provide convincing evidence that the refined techniques of continuous epidural analgesia that are in current use have little or no effect on the progress of cervical dilatation and the duration of the first stage of "normal" (uncomplicated) labor. As previously emphasized, this requires that: 1) the analgesia is initiated at the appropriate time under the conditions previously mentioned; 2) a preload infusion of fluid is given to minimize the incidence and degree of maternal hypotension; 3) the procedure is properly carried out and should the intermittent injection of boluses be used, these be given with the uterus laterally displaced; 4) the parturient is made to lie on her side during labor; and 5) maternal blood pressure is maintained. Factors that tend to decrease uterine activity for transient (10 to 20 minutes) periods include: 1) bolus injection with the parturient in a supine position with consequent aortocaval compression; 2) bolus injection of solutions containing large doses of epinephrine; and 3) maternal arterial hypotension among others. It is important to note, however, that while epinephrine produces a transient decrease in uterine contractile forces, used in amounts included in solutions that are employed for current techniques, it has little or no effect on the progress of the first stage of labor. The majority of studies that showed a prolonged first stage also provided evidence that the patients were already experiencing protracted labor prior to initiation of the epidural analgesia. Properly executed, continuous epidural analgesia is likely to enhance the progress of the first and second stage of labor in parturients with incoordinate uterine contractions and in those, who because of insufficient pain relief, are in distress, exhausted, and have metabolic acidosis. In the latter circumstances, effective epidural analgesia reverses the situation and the progress of labor reverts to normal pattern.

## Effects on Auxiliary Forces of Parturition and the Second Stage of Labor

Consideration of the effects of various techniques of epidural analgesia/anesthesia on the auxiliary forces of parturition, which are important during the second stage and for the delivery of the infant, requires a thorough understanding of their anatomy, physiology, and mechanical effect as discussed in Chapter 4. To briefly recapitulate, in addition to the uterine contractions, essential for dilatation and effacement of the cervix and descent of the presenting part, during the second stage, the cardinal mechanisms of labor with vertex presentation include internal flexion, internal rotation, and extension of the fetal head, and promptly after its delivery restitution, which is followed in sequence by delivery of the shoulder, external rotation of the head and finally delivery of the infant. Of particular importance to the anesthesiologic management is the influence of epidural analgesia on internal flexion, internal rotation, and extension of the presenting part, which are dependent on the resistant forces and the expulsive forces (see Chapter 4 for details.)

The resistant forces consist primarily of the firm tone of the perineal muscles, especially the levator ani and their fascia, other soft tissues, and the bony configuration of the pelvis, upon which impinge the fetal head in a vertex presentation. With continued descent of the fetal head, it flexes and rotates and finally extends the presenting part. For maximum efficiency of the resistant forces, the perineal muscles must retain their tone and strength, which, of course, are predominantly dependent on the motor fibers supplied by the two pudendal nerves and the muscular fibers of S2, S3, S4, and the anococcygeal nerve. The auxiliary expulsive forces consist of the reflex forceful contraction of the diaphragm, the abdominal and intercostal muscles, and the accessory muscles of respiration that produce marked increases in intra-abdominal and intrauterine pressures to help the uterus in effecting progressive descent of the presenting part, thus enhancing the effects of the resistant forces and finally expelling the fetus (259). The physiology of this reflex is described in Chapter 4.

Regional analgesia achieved with low concentrations of local anesthetics alone or combined with opioids does not significantly influence the tone of the perineal muscle sling, but regional anesthesia achieved with high concentrations of local anesthetic produces motor block, and thus interferes with these basic mechanisms. While regional analgesia blocks the afferent limb of the reflex urge to bear down, with proper coaching, a cooperative and motivated parturient can mobilize the expulsive forces voluntarily. Moreover, while the two sets of auxiliary forces of labor are important during the second stage in the majority of parturients, they are not absolutely essential, as attested to by the fact that spontaneous labor and spontaneous vaginal delivery can eventually occur without their active participation—a fact that was emphasized over 12 decades ago by Simpson (260), the patriarch of obstetric anesthesia, and by the reports of parturients with transsection of the spinal cord at the upper thoracic or lower cervical levels who have proceeded into spontaneous labor and can deliver the infant (261,262).

### *Effects of Older Techniques of Epidural Anesthesia on the Second Stage*

During the time period that continuous caudal analgesia was the predominant form of regional anesthesia used for labor and vaginal delivery, the incidence of persistent occiput posterior and persistent occiput transverse of the presenting part, and the need to use forceps delivery, were high (11,13,16,18,20–24). This is not unexpected because, as previously mentioned, this type of regional anesthesia reverses the logical sequence of blockade, producing perineal analgesia/anesthesia and frequently perineal relaxation too early in labor at the time when the former is unnecessary and the latter is contraindicated.

The increase in forceps delivery was due in part to the fact that in the United States, episiotomy and outlet (prophylactic) forceps delivery, considered the hallmark of American optimal obstetric practice since it was first proposed by DeLee (263) in 1920, was widely used to shorten the second stage. This widespread use of episiotomy and outlet forceps, done *only* after the fetal head was on the pelvic floor with complete anterior rotation and showing through a parted introitus, was based on DeLee's conviction that such interference in the normal process of labor was justified in order to: 1) reduce the physical strain on the mother incident to expulsive efforts; 2) preserve the integrity of the supporting tissue of the pelvis and avoid cervical tears; 3) decrease the amount of blood lost incident to delivery; and 4) decrease the adverse effect of continued pressure on the fetal head during the second stage. It was firmly believed and taught that properly carried out, outlet forceps decreased maternal and fetal morbidity and perhaps mortality (264).

Continuous caudal anesthesia also increased the rate of indicated low forceps and mid-forceps deliveries. Many experienced American clinicians believed that these adverse effects of continuous caudal anesthesia (increased incidence of lack of internal rotation and forceps delivery) were offset by the fact that a relaxed perineum facilitated manual rotation and also delivery of the infant. This was in contrast to the obstetric practice in the United Kingdom, continental Europe, and other parts of the world where the use of forceps delivery was equated with increased risk to the mother and infant. This was due to the fact that in Europe outlet (prophylactic) forceps were not used, but low, mid, and high forceps were used for obstetric complications in which the newborn was frequently depressed by the preexisting pathophysiology and the forceps delivery. The greater appreciation of these unwanted side effects of continuous caudal anesthesia by obstetricians and anesthesiologists played an important role in discontinuing its clinical application and replacing it with continuous lumbar epidural analgesia/anesthesia.

During the 1950s and early 1960s the decreases in these undesirable effects were not as great as they should have been. In the United States this was due to two major factors: the concept of the beneficial effects of outlet forceps and the use of fairly large volumes and relatively high concentrations of local anesthetics to produce midepidural anesthesia. Thus, the standard technique during this period was to initiate continuous epidural analgesia with a test dose of 3 to 5 ml and a therapeutic dose of 14 to 18 ml of 1 to 1.5% lidocaine or equivalent concentrations of other local anesthetics. This so-called "standard epidural" anesthesia resulted in intense anesthesia extending from S5 to T9–10 and frequently as high as T6 or higher with consequent paralysis of the resistant forces and not infrequently weakness of the lower abdominal muscles. Thus, flexion and internal rotation were impaired and the mother not only lost the afferent limb of the reflex urge to bear down, but voluntarily was unable to contract the abdominal muscles forcibly enough to be effective.

In the study by Johnson and associates (196) (discussed in detail in the last section of Chapter 4), the intrauterine pressure was measured by TKD in mm Hg to evaluate the force of uterine contractions and the superimposed expulsive force before and after anesthesia achieved with pudendal block or subarachnoid block or lumbar epidural block. Among 42 parturients who were studied, 6 preferred no anesthesia or only local infiltration, and the values for the intensity of uterine contractions and the expulsive forces were considered as "normal" controls. Here we will limit the discussion to lumbar epidural block, which was initiated after the onset of the second stage, and two or more baseline measurements made after which 5 ml of 1% lidocaine were injected as test dose and 5 minutes later 15 to 18 ml were injected as therapeutic doses. These produced anesthesia extending from S5 to T9–12 when measurements were made, and these were repeated subsequently when the level of analgesia became stable at upper levels extending from T8 to T3. The results are summarized in Table 13–4. These data emphasize two important points. In parturients with T10 block, the majority were able to increase their expulsive force almost as much as patients who received no analgesia, while in

**Table 13–4.** Effects of Epidural Anesthesia on the Forces of Labor and Vaginal Delivery Using the Standard Epidural Technique

| Technique | Number of Patients | Uterine Contractions (UC) (mmHg) | | Bearing Down Efforts (BDE) (mmHg) | |
|---|---|---|---|---|---|
| Local or No Analgesia/Anesthesia | 6 | *Before Block* | *After Block* | *Before Block* | *After Block* |
| a) 1st half of 2nd stage | | 48 ± 20 | — | 58 ± 24 | — |
| b) 2nd half of 2nd stage | | 48 ± 18 | — | 72 ± 27 | — |
| Standard Epidural Block Upper Levels | 12 | | | | |
| a) T10–T12 | 12 | 34 ± 19 | 28 ± 10 | 57 ± 32 | 55 ± 22 |
| b) T3–T7* | 4* | 33 ± 18 | 25 ± 20 | 59 ± 14 | 46 ± 19 |

* Final cephalad extension of blockade in 4 of the 12 parturients.
(Modified from Johnson WL, et al, Am. J. Obstet. Gynecol. 113:116, 1972)

the minority there was a significant decrease either because of inadequate instruction of how to bear down and/or excessive sedation and consequent confusion, improper coaching during the second stage, or because of the lack of motivation on the part of the parturient. The second point is that with peridural block to T4 or above, it is likely that motor block extends as high as T8 or 9 or even as high as T6 causing weakness or paralysis of the abdominal and intercostal muscles and peripheral part of the diaphragm supplied by motor fibers of the lowermost 5 to 7 thoracic spinal segments. Moreover, as many of these patients would incur a significant degree of hypotension and, as we shall see in the next section, it invariably produced varying degrees of perinatal depression.

During the mid-1960s, these adverse side effects, together with the advent of various factors already mentioned, merged to provoke modifications of lumbar epidural analgesia. The most frequently used and most practical technique of lumbar epidural analgesia used for labor and vaginal delivery has already been summarized in Table 13–1. Despite these improvements in the technique of lumbar epidural analgesia, the rate of malrotation or lack of rotation and the consequent need for forceps delivery remained high in the United States. Malrotation resulted from the fact that in an attempt to provide the mother with ample perineal anesthesia, there was relaxation of the perineal sling with consequent impairment of the cardinal mechanisms of flexion and internal rotation, and the fact that with the loss of the reflex urge to bear down, many parturients were not properly instructed and coached to forcefully do so voluntarily.

Up to several years ago, these undesirable effects of lumbar epidural analgesia were accepted by most American obstetricians who, appreciating the beneficial effects of analgesia, compensated for them by continuing to use manual or instrumental rotation and outlet forceps delivery. In contrast, until the mid-1970s, most obstetricians in the United Kingdom, Scandinavia, and many other countries in Europe and elsewhere, concerned about the increased incidence of malrotation and the need for instrumental deliveries, deterred them from using continuous lumbar epidural anesthesia in "normal labor," while in a few centers it was limited to parturients with dysfunctional labor (71,73,80–83,90). With the advent of more refined techniques of producing "selective" continuous epidural analgesia, many obstetricians in Britain, and other European countries, realizing the value of the technique in providing effective pain relief and as a therapeutic modality in treatment of incoordinate uterine contraction in very prolonged and painful labor, in breech and multiple deliveries, in preeclampsia and in a number of other obstetric and maternal complications, prompted them to progressively increase the use of lumbar epidural analgesia in normal labor as well as for the aforementioned pathophysiologic conditions (69–72,75–85,88,102,184, 185,191–195).

While most obstetricians appreciated the value of lumbar epidural analgesia, they repeatedly expressed concern that its use increased the number of instrumental deliveries and malpositions. Hoult and associates (194) reported a five-fold increase in instrumental deliveries and a three-fold increase in fetal malrotation (persistent occiput posterior and persistent occiput transverse) in parturients given epidural analgesia compared with those given meperidine or no anesthesia. Of note in this study was a self-imposed time limit of 1 hour for the second stage and the use of high concentrations (0.5%) of bupivacaine. Others in the United Kingdom reporting high incidence of instrumental deliveries included Crawford (69,70,90), Studd, et al (193,195), Morgan and associates (265), Thornburn and Moir (266), and Read and colleagues (267). In Scandinavia, a high incidence of instrumental deliveries was reported by Zador and associates (76–79), Willdeck-Lund and colleagues (191), Hollmen, et al (75,184), and others. Shnider (63), Johnson and associates (196), and Cowles (268) in the United States, also reported a significant increase in the use of forceps delivery with epidural anesthesia over that seen in the general obstetric population managed with mild systemic and/or inhalation analgesia, or no anesthesia at all. Many of these were older reports involving the use of larger doses of local anesthetics, more extensive epidural block, and significant motor nerve involvement that impaired the mechanisms of the second stage of labor. It is also of interest to note that many of those authors who used the newer, refined techniques of lumbar epidural analgesia reported that increased malrotations and instrumental deliveries did not have any deleterious effects on the fetus and newborn, and that in many instances, the condition of the newborn of mothers who had received epidural analgesia was better than was the condition of infants born of mothers in the control group (62,70,74,75,77,79,82–85,184,185,188,191–193, 195).

In Britain, the notion that lumbar epidural analgesia increased the incidence of malrotation and forceps delivery was challenged by Doughty (72) who reported on a series of 800 parturients he managed personally from 1957 to 1969 during which period epidural analgesia in the hospitals he worked in increased from 1% during the first 3-year period to 26% during the second 3-year period, and 78% during the last 3-year period. He reported that among those given lumbar epidural anesthesia during these three periods, the percent of parturients delivered by forceps were 100, 75, and 24, respectively, suggesting that with increase in the use of lumbar epidural anesthesia, there was a decrease in forceps delivery. Analysis of the data for the last period revealed that of 151 primiparae given epidural analgesia, 63 (42%) were delivered by forceps; while among the 197 multiparae, forceps were used in 21 (11%), for an overall rate of 24% among both groups. In a subsequent report, Doughty (269) emphasized that in addition to the special indications for epidural analgesia in patients with a variety of pathophysiologic problems, a significant number of obstetricians used outlet forceps to avoid the progressive maternal and fetal acidemia during a prolonged second stage. Doughty (269) admitted that by using segmental epidural analgesia during the first stage and analgesic concentrations during the second stage, the mother is frequently deprived of the reflex desire to bear down in the second stage. However, he argued that labor can be managed in anticipation of a spontaneous delivery despite the use of regional analgesia by improving the strength of uterine contractions with oxytocin, digital assistance of the rotation of the fetal head, and judicial application of fundal pressure once the head is in the perineum and by encouraging the mother to push in concert with the contractions.

This position that properly administered epidural analgesia did not increase significantly the incidence of forceps delivery was subsequently supported by Bailey and associates (270), who stated that the increased use of forceps delivery is not a direct consequence of epidural analgesia, but, in part, a reflection of the fact that epidural analgesia is used more frequently in complicated deliveries, which commonly require forceps or surgical intervention. To support their contention, Bailey and associates (270) carried out a study and compared all deliveries at their medical center, the Doncanster Royal Infirmary, that occurred during a 2-year period (1976 and 1977) before the use of epidural anesthesia was adopted, with deliveries carried out during 1978, 1979, and 1980 when epidural analgesia was used in 27%, 37%, and 43%, respectively, of all deliveries. The incidence of instrumental deliveries among primiparae was a mean of 24% during the 1976 and 1977 period, compared with 28% during the period when epidural analgesia was used. The figures for multiparae were means of 7.7% and 8.5%, respectively. The combined incidence for both multiparae and primiparae were 14% during the pre-epidural analgesia period compared with 15.5% during the 3-year period when epidural analgesia was used. Cesarean section was done in about 8% before the advent of epidural and between 8.5 and 9.6% during the 3-year period of epidural. In a more recent report, Bailey (271) presented yearly data from 1977 up to the end of 1988 and reported that of all deliveries done in that hospital: 1) epidural anesthesia has continued to be used between 40 to 45% of the cases; 2) spontaneous delivery has been between 70 to 80%; 3) forceps delivery between 12 to 15%; and 4) cesarean section between 10 to 15%.

Similar findings were reported by Maltau and Anderson (80), who used continuous lumbar epidural analgesia/anesthesia in 204 parturients including 133 primiparae and 71 multiparae. These were managed with intermittent injections of 5 ml of either 0.25% bupivacaine or 1% lidocaine that produced complete pain relief in 93% of parturients. The incidence of instrumental deliveries (vacuum extraction or forceps delivery) occurred in a mean of 7.6% of primiparae and 1.3% multiparae during a 19-month period before epidural analgesia was introduced, compared with means of 7.7% and 1.3%, respectively, during a similar period when epidural analgesia was employed. The incidence of emergency cesarean section was reduced to half of that seen prior to the introduction of epidural analgesia. Apgar scores and the condition of the newborn were the same in both the epidural and control groups. Many other studies showed that nulliparae who received epidural analgesia are more likely to require instrumental delivery than multiparae (69,70,72,76–80, 191–195,269–273).

During the late 1970s and 1980s, the controversy regarding high incidence of malrotation and forceps delivery among obstetricians and anesthetists, especially in the United Kingdom and Scandinavia, continued unabated. This prompted obstetric anesthesiologists and some obstetricians to modify the technique and to also modify the obstetric management in order to decrease the incidence of the undesirable side effects on the forces of the second stage of labor. These modifications included: 1) the use of "selective" lumbar epidural analgesia in the first and second stage of labor and the avoidance of perineal analgesia/anesthesia altogether; 2) in patients who had developed perineal analgesia during the latter part of the first stage, some obstetricians let the blockade in the perineum wear off during the second stage so that the parturient could bear down forcibly; 3) the progressive increase and refinement of continuous lumbar epidural infusion analgesia achieved with very low concentration of local anesthetics alone or combined with opioids; 4) some obstetricians had parturients delay the bearing-down efforts until the fetal head was in the introitus, discarding the concept that the second stage should be limited to less than 1 hour and allowing the parturient to continue the second stage until spontaneous delivery occurred; and, 5) the emphasis on "active management of labor," as an integrated program that includes augmentation of uterine contractions with oxytocin during the second stage of labor. All of these are briefly discussed below.

## Segmental Analgesia During the Second Stage

Concern about the problem of increased malrotation and the need for forceps delivery prompted Hollmen, Jouppila and associates (184,185) of the University of Oulu, Finland, who are among the most experienced and authoritative obstetric anesthesiologists in Europe, to adopt the practice of using segmental epidural analgesia limited to the lower three thoracic and the upper two lumbar segments without producing any perineal analgesia during the second or third stages. In one of their reports, they state that "Most of the mothers consider the first stage of labor the most painful and want effective pain relief precisely during this stage." They further state that although the parturients experience pain in the perineum during the second stage, this is compensated by the fact that they have a good bearing-down reflex and can actively take part in the delivery. They further justified this method by stating that this observation and the common obstetric practice in Scandinavia, which in the past has strictly avoided instrumental deliveries in normal labor, was the reason why selective segmental epidural analgesia instead of caudal or standard lumbar epidural analgesia has been used as the routine obstetric technique in their obstetric service with "good results."

They reported a study of 100 parturients (77 primiparae and 23 multiparae) given segmental epidural analgesia and 100 parturients with the same demographic characteristics given none or conventional analgesia considered the control group. They initiated analgesia when the cervix was about 3.5 cm dilated, at which time 4 ml of 0.5% bupivacaine was given and repeated as needed, and this was continued until after delivery. The results showed that in the primiparae epidural group, the progress of labor before analgesia was induced was significantly slower than in the control group, but after the block was initiated, the subsequent course of labor was of equal duration in both groups. Moreover, the duration of the second stage of labor did not differ significantly between the groups, nor did the incidence of malposition or the rate of vacuum extraction, nor was there any significant difference in the condition of the newborn. They concluded that the results signify a normal progress and outcome of labor after low dose segmental epidural analgesia.

To achieve the same objective, some practitioners allow the epidural block involving the sacral segments to wear off as cervical dilatation nears completion or use top-up doses of insufficient volume or concentration near the end of the first stage and beginning of the second stage to avoid block of the sacral segments (191,192,266). This permits the parturient to retain the reflex urge to bear down forcibly. We agree with Crawford (82) that having parturients experience severe pain during the second stage is not only cruel to the mother, but is actually counterproductive because it may be associated with a higher incidence of forceps delivery, probably because of the imposed maternal distress. That this may be the case was demonstrated by a study by Phillips and Thomas (272) who carried out a randomized study on a total of 56 parturients, all of whom were given segmental epidural analgesia for the first stage, achieved with 4 ml of 0.5% bupivacaine injected as the first dose and subsequent "top-up" doses of 6 ml of 0.25% bupivacaine. Just prior to the start of the reflex urge to bear down during the second stage, the extent of epidural analgesia was assessed and subsequent management differed between those in group A and those in group B. In group A, parturients, when the fetal head was below the ischial spine, received no further top-up doses, the epidural analgesia was allowed to wear off, and the mother started to push when she felt the urge to bear down. In group B parturients' analgesia was maintained throughout the second stage and when the fetal head was below the ischial spine, the parturient was asked to begin bearing down. Parturients in group A experienced considerable pain and distress, whereas parturients in group B were relatively pain free throughout the second and third stages of labor; the second stage was not prolonged, the incidence of forceps delivery was lower than in group A, and there were fewer persistent malrotations without increasing dosage of bupivacaine.

In a more recent study, Philipsen and Jensen (275) carried out a randomized study to evaluate epidural analgesia with 0.375% bupivacaine with intramuscular meperidine. There was no significant difference between the two groups in incidence of instrumental deliveries, but the investigators gave no additional bupivacaine after 8-cm cervical dilatation; and in the second stage, 85% of each group received bilateral pudendal block for delivery. Although the bilateral block was effective, neither group consistently had satisfactorily analgesia during the second stage except for the pudendal block during the mid-second stage. In a previous section of this chapter, this group of patients was mentioned regarding the degree of analgesia and patient's satisfaction.

## Low Concentrations of Local Anesthetics

In attempts to reduce the adverse effects on the forces of the second stage and also to eliminate fetal depression, a number of investigators used low concentrations of local anesthetics administered by either the intermittent or infusion technique. Vanderick, Steenberg, and their associates (88) published a report on the use of 0.125% bupivacaine with 1:800,000 epinephrine for labor and vaginal delivery and 5 years later the group published a second report on its successful use in about 1500 primiparae and 1500 multiparae (273). They reported good to excellent analgesia in 92% of parturients who developed minimal motor block and who had short second stages of labor. Spontaneous delivery occurred in 39% of primiparae and 73% of multiparae, forceps delivery was used in 1%, and vacuum extraction used in the remainder of the patients. One subsequent study in a small group of parturients indicated that 0.125% concentration produced a high failure rate in achieving analgesia (274). In contrast, Phillips and associates (175) used 0.125% bupivacaine with epinephrine 1:200,000 given in a total of 598 parturients who received, following a negative test dose, 6 to 10 ml of solution with the patient placed in 20° lateral position. Effective pain relief was achieved by 97% of the parturients. The rate of forceps delivery was no greater than the general obstetric population in that institution.

### Continuous Epidural Infusion with Local Anesthetic

In a previous section it was mentioned that, with the advent of precise infusion pumps in the mid-1970s and early 1980s, an increasing number of anesthesiologists began to use this method for labor and vaginal delivery (209–225). Among the advantages mentioned earlier included the fact that with this technique, it was intended to reduce or eliminate relaxation of the perineal muscle sling and the abdominal muscles and thus reduce the incidence of malrotation and the need for instrumental delivery.

Those published reports in which parturients received low concentration of bupivacaine or lidocaine were said to produce effective analgesia in 80 to 90% of parturients during the first stage, did not prolong the first or second stage, and thus did not increase the frequency of malrotation or instrumental delivery, but produced much lower rates (40 to 60%) of effective analgesia during the second and third stage of labor (68,69,85,88,209,210,218,219, 220,222,223). Those investigations that had entailed the use of higher concentrations (e.g., 0.25 to 0.375 bupivacaine or 1 to 1.5% lidocaine) and fast infusion rates (>15 ml/hr) or both and used top-up doses before delivery, provided good perineal pain relief, but prolonged significantly the second stage and consequently increased the incidence of malrotation and instrumental delivery (215–217, 221,221).

### Continuous Infusion of Local Anesthetics and/or Opioids

To solve the problem of high instrumental delivery during the second stage, Chestnut and colleagues began to carry out several randomized, double blind, placebo-controlled studies to evaluate the analgesic efficacy and the effect on the second stage of labor (94,219,220,244). The first study, a continuous infusion of 0.75% lidocaine administered beyond 8 cm of cervical dilatation, did not prolong the second stage nor increase the incidence of forceps delivery in primiparae, but it also did not reliably provide second stage analgesia (219). In contrast, continuous infusion of 0.125% bupivacaine provided excellent intrapartum analgesia but it also prolonged the second stage and increased the incidence of instrumental delivery (220). In a third study (244), they noted that continuous epidural infusion of 0.0625% bupivacaine with 0.0002% fentanyl (2 μg/ml) (group BF) produced first stage analgesia similar to that produced by continuous infusion of 0.125% bupivacaine (group B). At complete cervical dilatation, the known continuous infusions were stopped and, if the parturient did not have perineal analgesia during the second stage, one or two boluses of 0.0625% bupivacaine were given to the BF group and 0.125% bupivacaine given to the B group. Although the BF infusion produced less intense motor block than the B solution, parturients did not have a significantly shorter second stage nor lower incidence of instrumental delivery than parturients who received B alone.

In still another study, Chestnut and colleagues evaluated a continuous epidural infusion of 0.0625% bupivacaine-0.0002% fentanyl (94). Each patient received a sequence of: 1) 3 ml of 1.5% lidocaine with 1:200,000 epinephrine as a test dose and 5 minutes later 6 ml of 0.125% bupivacaine-0.008% fentanyl as therapeutic dose; and 2) at 10 minutes a continuous epidural infusion of 0.0625% bupivacaine-0.002% fentanyl at a rate of 12.5 ml/hr was given by infusion pump to all patients. When the cervix was fully dilated, the known infusion combination was stopped and one of two coded study solutions was given: one group of 29 parturients was given the coded solution containing bupivacaine-fentanyl in the same concentration as used during the first stage (group BF), while the second group of 34 parturients were given saline placebo (group SP). If near the time of delivery patients had no perineal analgesia, two 5-ml boluses of the study solution were given. The two groups had similar degrees of pain relief during the first stage of labor, but during the second stage only 70% of the BF group and only 48% of the SP group had good to excellent analgesia. Table 13–5 contains the pertinent data of the results. Chestnut and colleagues concluded that maintenance of epidural infusion of the BF solution until delivery provided better second stage analgesia than did the SP group and that, further, it did not significantly increase the incidence of instrumental delivery. Thus, the objective of decrease in the duration of the second stage and the high incidence of spontaneous delivery were achieved but at the price of ineffective analgesia during the second stage, which occurred in 30% of the BF group.

Several other groups have carried out double-blind randomized studies in an attempt to decrease the incidence of instrumental deliveries, most of which were mentioned in the previous section (216,230,234,235,245,246a,246b, 249,250). The study by Vertommen and colleagues (250) deserves special mention not only because it is a multicenter study involving a large group of patients, but that it was also done in a randomized double-blind fashion, and also because the authors observed a decrease in instrumental deliveries. In the group of patients who received bupivacaine, sufentanil, and epinephrine (BSE), required instrumental deliveries were 24% versus a 36% incidence in the group managed with bupivacaine-epinephrine. The authors attribute this reduction to the decreased dose of bupivacaine (34 ± 17 versus 42 ± 19, $p < 0.001$) and a decreased intensity of motor block in the BSE group. Moreover, they noted no adverse effect of epidural sufentanil on the mother or the neonates. Chestnut (251) wrote an editorial in which he mentioned some of the deficiencies of the study. For example, they did not prohibit elective instrumental deliveries, and they did not distinguish between elective and indicated deliveries. Because Belgium obstetricians usually terminate the second stage at 1 hour, Chestnut pointed out that had the obstetrician allowed the second stage to progress beyond 1 hour, it is possible that there would have been no difference between groups in the incidence of instrumental deliveries. Moreover, patients expectations, perception of labor pain, and epidural anesthetic requirements differ significantly between Belgium women and women in other

**Table 13–5.** Data on Continuous Infusion of Epidural Analgesia Bupivacaine/Placebo

| | **Bupivacaine-Fentanyl (*n* = 29)** | **Saline-Placebo (*n* = 34)** |
|---|---|---|
| Conduct of Labor: | | |
| Duration of active phase of first stage (min)* | 316 ± 188 | 317 ± 199 |
| Duration of known bupivacaine-fentanyl infusion (min)* | 227 ± 159 | 215 ± 164 |
| Bupivacaine dosage before start of study solution (mg)* | 47 ± 30 | 44 ± 29 |
| Bupivacaine dosage after start of study solution (mg)* | 16 ± 13 | 0 |
| Fentanyl dosage before start of study solution (μg)* | 169 ± 80 | 161 ± 84 |
| Fentanyl dosage after start of study solution (μg)* | 50 ± 41 | 0 |
| Duration of second stage (min)† | 53 (5–283) | 63 (16–181) |
| Position of vertex immediately before delivery: | | |
| Occiput anterior | 27 (93%) | 31 (91%) |
| Occiput posterior | 1 (3%) | 3 (9%) |
| Occiput transverse | 1 (3%) | 0 (0%) |
| Method of Vaginal Delivery: | | |
| Spontaneous | 22 (79%) | 29 (85%) |
| Outlet forceps | 0 (0%) | 0 (0%) |
| Low forceps | 2 (7%) | 4 (12%) |
| Midforceps | 2 (7%) | 1 (3%) |
| Midvacuum followed by low forceps | 2 (7%) | 0 (0%) |
| Newborn Assessment: | | |
| Infant weight (g)* | 3258 ± 528 | 3314 ± 390 |
| Meconium-stained amniotic fluid | 2 (7%) | 5 (15%) |
| 1-min Apgar ≥7 | 25 (86%) | 31 (91%) |
| 5-min Apgar ≥7 | 29 (100%) | 34 (100%) |
| Umibilical venous blood analysis:* | | |
| pH | 7.33 ± 0.08 | 7.32 ± 0.06 |
| $P_{O_2}$ (mmHg) | 27 ± 7 | 25 ± 6 |
| $P_{CO_2}$ (mmHg) | 37 ± 7 | 39 ± 5 |
| Base excess (mEq/l) | −4.8 ± 2.7 | −4.9 ± 2.4 |
| Umbilical arterial blood analysis:* | | |
| pH | 7.26 ± 0.07 | 7.27 ± 0.06 |
| $P_{O_2}$ (mmHg) | 18 ± 7 | 18 ± 5 |
| $P_{CO_2}$ (mmHg) | 46 ± 6 | 45 ± 7 |
| Base excess (mEq/l) | −5.7 ± 3.3 | −5.7 ± 2.8 |

*P* was not significant; * = Mean ± SD; † = Median (range) (excluding one woman in the bupivacaine-fentanyl group who underwent cesarean section after full cervical dilation).
(Modified from Chestnut DH, et al, Anesthesiology 72:613, 1990)

countries such as the United States. Finally, Chestnut pointed out that an important limitation to the study was that the authors did not specifically evaluate and report the quality of analgesia during the second stage or the quality of perineal anesthesia during delivery. After raising a number of other problems, he states "to date no published study has been shown that one can consistently provide effective analgesia throughout the second stage of labor without risk of the instrumental delivery."

## *Problem with Analgesia During Second Stage and Delivery*

It is to be noted that many reports of the use of either intermittent injection or continuous infusion of local anesthetics given alone or in combination with opioids through a single lumbar epidural catheter indicate that significant percentages (20 to 50%) of parturients did not have adequate perineal analgesia during part of the second stage and/or for the delivery (68–70,85,88,90,186,209, 218–220,). In a few instances, this was done purposely so that the parturient would retain perineal muscle tone and reflex urge to bear down in order to minimize the incidence of malrotation and instrumental delivery (75,184–186,191,192). In other instances, insufficient perineal analgesia resulted from the fact that diffusion of the local anesthetics to the sacral segment was inadequate. In any case, it is most unfortunate that parturients were deprived of effective pain relief during the second stage and delivery. Although many of the them had good analgesia during the first stage, the lack of sufficient analgesia during the second stage caused them to consider the entire experience as very unpleasant. Certain anesthesiologists and surgeons would not tolerate having a patient with only partial analgesia for the surgical procedure; nor would a dental patient tolerate only partial anesthesia during an otherwise painful procedure.

This serious problem can be eliminated in one of several ways. In parturients receiving intermittent injection for epidural analgesia, at the time they complain of perineal pain, one or two boluses of the local anesthetics are injected in the sitting position. If perineal pain is experienced during the early part of the second stage, before flexion and internal rotation have taken place, 10 ml of an analgesic concentration of the local anesthetic and/or opioid is injected in the sitting position with the expectation that this will cause diffusion of the local anesthetic to the sacral segments. In such cases, it is suggested that

15 minutes before the expected delivery another bolus of an high concentration of local anesthetics/opioid be injected to produce perineal relaxation for the delivery. Occasionally, injections with a patient sitting do not cause diffusion of the solution to the sacral segments.

In parturients receiving continuous infusions of local anesthetics alone or with opioids, the infusion is continued throughout labor with the parturient lying on either the left or right side with the upper part of the body raised about 15 to 20°. Provided that the infusion rate is titrated to the needs of the patient (i.e., increased or decreased) to maintain analgesia with an upper level of T10, with each subsequent hour, the extent of the cephalad level of analgesia usually remains constant at T9–10, but the caudal level tends to extend after about the fourth or fifth hour to the lumbar and sacral segments. This technique is used by Chadwick, Ross, Glosten and other colleagues of the senior author who work in the Division of Obstetric Anesthesia at the University of Washington. They have noted that most patients will have ample perineal analgesia, and, in some instances, there is eventually some motor block. For those who do not have sufficient perineal analgesia, about 15 minutes before the anticipated delivery, they are given 10 ml of 1% lidocaine in a sitting position. If these measures are not effective, a saddle block or bilateral pudendal block can be used to provide some perineal analgesia. Again, in a small percentage of women, the injections during the second stage fail to provide total perineal pain relief.

The third and the most effective alternative to obviate the problem of inadequate perineal analgesia/anesthesia is to use the double-catheter technique, which is summarized in Table 13–1 and described in detail in Part B of this chapter. This is the technique that assures obtaining the objective mentioned by Chestnut in the editorial cited above. Properly done, the double-catheter technique assures effective perineal analgesia without risk of instrumental delivery unless maternal anatomic problems exist. Anesthesiologists who have the technical knowledge and skill to carry out a continuous caudal, inserting the catheter soon after carrying out the insertion of the lumbar epidural catheter, is simpler than doing bilateral pudendal block on a patient who is having severe perineal pain during the second stage when the presenting part fills the pelvis. Using either the intermittent boluses injection or continuous infusion titrated to produce T10-L1 analgesia throughout the first stage, an injection of an analgesic concentration through the lower (sacral) catheter at the time that perineal pain is experienced, the parturient can remain pain free throughout the first and second stages and still retain good perineal muscle tone to permit flexion and internal rotation of the presenting part. This obviates the need for the parturient to sit up at a time when the fetal head is on the perineum. Moreover, provided parturients have been thoroughly informed in advance of the procedure, are not confused by heavy sedation, are cooperative and motivated, and properly coached to bear down forcefully during each contraction in late second stage, they are able to mobilize sufficient increases in intra-abdominal and intrauterine pressures to achieve spontaneous delivery. Indeed, the majority of patients who are pain free are able to not only muster greater pressure, but control also their expiratory efforts for a longer period of time than is the case among parturients who are experiencing severe pain with contractions.

Figure 13–20 shows one of many typical tracings obtained by the senior author from dozens of patients managed with the double-catheter technique (DCEB). Table 13–6 also lists the mean data (and range) in 20 parturients managed with double-catheter technique. Comparison of these data with those obtained by Johnson et al (196) when standard epidural block with large doses of local anesthetic was being used in the Division of Anesthesia at the University of Washington, shows the advantage of DCEB. Another advantage of this technique is that once flexion and internal rotation have taken place, very small amount (3 ml) of high concentration of the local anesthetic is injected through the lower catheter to produce maximal perineal relaxation and to facilitate delivery either spontaneously or with outlet forceps, if this is indicated. Although some authorities (49,63,252) consider the technique as "a complicated procedure" and some

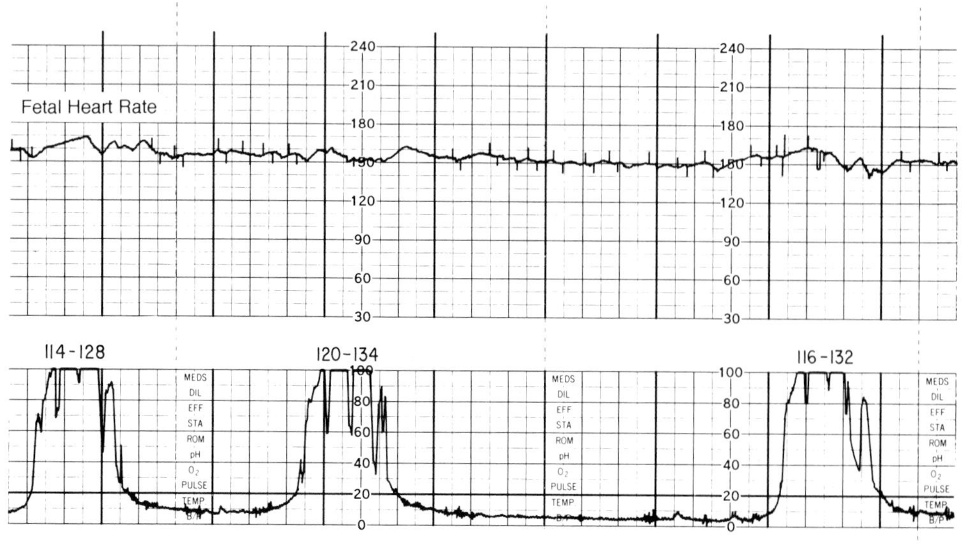


**Fig. 13–20.** Tracing of uterine contractions and the superimposed bearing-down efforts in a parturient managed with double-catheter technique. Through cooperation and motivation of the patient and coaching by the anesthesiologist bearing-down efforts resulted, which were maintained for several seconds causing the intrauterine pressure to reach values between 115 and 135 mm Hg.

**Table 13–6.** The Effects of Standard Epidural Block, Segmental Epidural Analgesia/Anesthesia that Eventually Diffuses to the Sacral Segments, and the Double-Catheter Technique (Note the significant difference on the bearing-down efforts between the first and the last technique.)

| Technique | Number of Patients | Uterine Contractions (UC) (mmHg) | | Bearing Down Efforts (BDE) (mmHg) | |
|---|---|---|---|---|---|
| Local or No Analgesia/Anesthesia | 10 | *Before Block* | *After Block* | *Before Block* | *After Block* |
| a) 1st half of 2nd stage | | 46 ± 20 | — | 56 ± 21 | — |
| b) 2nd half of 2nd stage | | 48 ± 18 | — | 71 ± 26 | — |
| Standard Epidural Block Upper Levels | 18 | | | | |
| a) T9–T12 | 18 | 33 ± 19 | 28 ± 16 | 57 ± 28 | 58 ± 21 |
| b) T3–T7 | 6* | 34 ± 19 | 25 ± 13 | 58 ± 11 | 44 ± 17 |
| "Continuous" Intermittent Segmental Epidural Analgesia | 15 | | | | |
| a) First Stage | | 35 ± 17 | 38 ± 21 | — | — |
| b) Second Stage | | | | | |
| i) No perineal analgesia | 8 | 40 ± 14** | 43 ± 18** | 55 ± 23 | 61 ± 18 |
| ii) Perineal analgesia | 7 | 39 ± 16** | 36 ± 12** | — | 54 ± 12 |
| Double Catheter Technique | 20 | | | | |
| (a) First Stage (T9–L2) | | 34 ± 16 | 37 ± 18 | — | — |
| b) Second Stage (S2–S5) | | 39 ± 19** | 41 ± 17** | 56 ± 16 | 76 ± 21 |

* Final cephalad extension of 6 of the 18 parturients.
** These figures represent the intensity of uterine contractions during the second stage before and after perineal analgesia was produced.
(Modified from Bonica JJ, Abstracts of the Fifth World Congress of Anaesthesiologists, Amsterdam, September 19–23, 1973, p. 331)

also suggest that it causes more pain for the parturient and increases the risks of complications, these are not the experiences of the present authors or other clinicians who have used the procedure extensively (44,178,183,251a). As mentioned earlier, Doctors Cleland, Sr., and Cleland, Jr., have carried out the procedure in private practice in Oregon City. In the course of 39 years, they have performed over 3950 procedures with a success rate exceeding 95%. The issue of inserting an epidural catheter virtually pain free is discussed in Chapter 13-B.

## *Other Therapeutic Measures for the Second Stage*

### *Delaying the Bearing-Down Efforts*

It has long been standard obstetric teaching and practice to encourage the parturient to bear down soon after complete cervical dilatation occurs, and that the second stage must not be allowed to continue for longer than 60 minutes in primiparae and 30 minutes in multiparae (276). It was believed that exceeding these periods might jeopardize the infant and cause greater degrees of maternal and fetal acidemia and increase the incidence of neonatal death (277). However, there is recent evidence that suggests in parturients with effective epidural analgesia a second stage that is prolonged, even up to 3 hours, is not detrimental to the mother or fetus provided there is continuous electronic monitoring of the fetal heart rate and the mothers are well hydrated and not fatigued by a very long and painful first stage (74). In addition to adequate epidural analgesia, this requires that the parturient not expend energy unnecessarily with premature bearing-down efforts that are likely to cause exhaustion and metabolic acidosis. There is now evidence that postponing the bearing-down efforts until the fetal head is seen in the parted introitus will result in not only more effective bearing-down efforts when they are needed, but will also result in spontaneous deliveries (74,278–280).

Potter and McDonald (74) were among the first to propose that delaying the bearing-down efforts until the fetal head was visible upon parting the labia resulted in a spontaneous delivery in 72% of their Australian-born parturients. Subsequently, several others suggested that bearing-down efforts be delayed until the presenting part is visible (278–280). Maresh and associates (281) investigated this problem by studying 76 primiparae with epidural analgesia and who were randomly assigned to one of two groups that were well matched for maternal, obstetric, and fetal characteristics, including position and level of the presenting part at full dilatation and fetal scalp blood pH. Once full dilatation of the cervix was reached, the parturients in group I (early pushing) were encouraged to bear down as soon as they had the desire. The parturients in group II (late pushing) continued to lie on their side and if they had the desire to bear down and the head was not visible on parting the labia, one epidural top-up dose was given and the vulva inspected every 15 minutes to see whether the fetal head was visible. If after 2 hours the fetal head was not visible, the vagina was visualized every 15 minutes to assess the level of the vertex, and if no further descent occurred after two subsequent inspections, the parturients were instructed to bear down as soon as they felt the urge. All had continuous fetal heart monitoring throughout the course of labor, and maternal and fetal pH and Apgar scores were recorded. Although the total duration of the second stage was significantly increased in group II, for those who delivered spontaneously, the actual pushing time was almost identical with that of group I. The delay was not associated with an increase in fetal heart rate abnormalities nor any decrease in umbilical cord pH nor Apgar scores. In contrast, the delay was associated with an increase in spontaneous delivery and a concomitant decrease in forceps delivery. They further demonstrated that the second stage of labor could be allowed to continue as long as 4 hours without risk of harm to the fetus or mother.

The data prompted the conclusion that it is necessary to redefine the management of the second stage of labor with epidural analgesia to include delayed pushing. This concept was espoused by Crawford (82) and others. As a result of these and other favorable data, the American College of Obstetricians and Gynecologists in 1988 defined a prolonged second stage as greater than 3 hours in nulliparous patients with a regional anesthesia as compared with greater than 2 hours in nulliparous patients without regional anesthesia, and greater than 2 hours of multiparae with regional anesthesia as compared with 1 hour without regional anesthesia (282) (see Table 4–4).

### Active Management of Labor

Another modification in the management of labor in parturients receiving continuous epidural analgesia in whom decrease in uterine activity is noted is to administer exogenous oxytocin by continuous infusion at physiologic rates. This technique has been practiced in the United States for over half a century and especially with the increasing popularity of continuous caudal and continuous lumbar epidural analgesia. In Britain, O'Driscoll and associates (283), in 1973, proposed the concept of "active management of labour," which included, as part of the integrated program, stimulation of inefficient uterine activity with continuous infusion of oxytocin, including its use in parturients with subnormal uterine contractility associated with lumbar epidural analgesia. According to Crawford (82), this concept now dominates the philosophy of management of labor in probably the great majority of obstetric units in Great Britain and Ireland, and is described in detail in the monograph by O'Driscoll and Meaghe (284).

More recently, Goodfellow and his associates (285) reported a decrease in the incidence of forceps delivery rate in primiparae with the routine use of oxytocin infusion during the second stage. The routine use of oxytocin was based on the premise that epidural analgesia interfered with Ferguson's reflex and the consequent increase in oxytocin released from the posterior pituitary in response to stretching of the birth canal. Measuring oxytocin levels in parturients, Goodfellow and his associates (285) found a significant increase in the levels between complete cervical dilatation and the crowning of the fetal head but this increase was not present in parturients given epidural analgesia. Similar findings had been previously reported by Vasicka and associates (286) (see Chapter 4 for more details).

## Summary

The foregoing review of the effects of continuous epidural analgesia/anesthesia on the resistant and expulsive forces, on the duration of the second stage, and on the delivery of the infant, reveals that these effects vary considerably depending on the technique used and the obstetric management. With continuous caudal analgesia or mid lumbar epidural anesthesia, the resistance by the pelvic muscles is diminished, usually resulting in delayed and slower rotation of the advancing fetal head and, in some instances, rotation may not take place. Moreover, the afferent limb of the reflex urge to bear down is eliminated and in some patients there is weakness of the lower abdominal muscles, especially if high concentration of local anesthetics is used. All of these factors contribute to prolonging the second stage of labor and to increasing the incidence of nonrotation and the need for instrumental delivery.

The use of segmental epidural anesthesia for the first stage and its extension to the sacral segments for the second stage and delivery achieved with concentration of 0.25% bupivacaine or 1% lidocaine decreases the incidence of these adverse side effects, but the majority of studies still shows a longer duration of the second stage (by 15 to 45 minutes) and increase in instrumental delivery.

The recent development and increasing clinical application of continuous infusion of a low concentration of local anesthetics (e.g., 0.0625% bupivacaine or 0.25% lidocaine) administered alone or in combination with opioids (e.g., 0.0002% fentanyl) have shown to produce little or no perineal muscle weakness and, in most instances, the duration of the second stage was not increased, nor was the incidence of nonrotation and instrumental delivery. Unfortunately, a significant percentage of these patients experienced moderate to severe perineal pain during the delivery because the analgesia was not sufficiently intense to block nociceptive impulses from the perineum. The application of the double-catheter technique virtually obviates the latter problem because it permits injection of dilute solutions of local anesthetics as soon as perineal pain occurs. Moreover, although the afferent limb of the reflex urge is blocked, parturients can bear down forcibly and thus increase the intra-abdominal and intrauterine pressures sufficiently to deliver the infant spontaneously.

Delay in the bearing-down efforts until the presenting part is visible in the parted introitus is likely to prolong the second stage; but as long as the electronic monitoring of the fetal heart rate shows no distress, it will decrease significantly the incidence of nonrotation and increase the incidence of spontaneous delivery. Obviously, optimal care of parturients during the first and second stage of labor requires maximum communication and cooperation, exquisite coordination and, whenever necessary, compromise among all members of the obstetric team and between this group and the parturient. The overall plan of the management of the patient during the second stage should be made in advance and should be based on the physical and emotional condition of the patient, her motivation, and her wishes and desires of the type of delivery she wishes to experience, and the amount or degree of pain relief she desires and/or needs.

## Beneficial Effects on Abnormal Forces of Labor

It has already been mentioned that continuous epidural analgesia has been used in the management of patients with prolonged labor due to incoordinate uterine contractions and certain other types of uterine and cervical dystocias. Prolonged painful labor produces a great deal of anxiety and apprehension that causes liberation of catecholamines, resulting in incoordinate or weak uterine contractions, which are usually associated with maternal fatigue and acidosis and perinatal depression. Indeed, a century ago one in six mothers who had excessively prolonged labor (more than 30 hours) died (287). Moreover, such excessively prolonged labor is associated with an increased perinatal morbidity and even mortality (288). Providing such parturients with effective pain relief achieved with continuous epidural analgesia not only accrues beneficial humanitarian effects on the mother, but has beneficial effects on uterine contractility and, most importantly, on the fetus and newborn. Some of the important studies are summarized below.

Galley (29) was among the first to report the successful use of continuous caudal analgesia in patients with prolonged labor due to incoordinate uterine contractions. Subsequently, Johnson and coworkers (31–33) published several reports in which they presented convincing data that continuous caudal analgesia does in fact enhance contractions in parturients with abnormal contractile patterns and improve placental function. The last published report contained data derived from a controlled clinical trial involving 44 patients with prolonged labor (over 48 hours) caused by subnormal or incoordinate uterine contractions (33). The patients were assigned, according to a random table, to either the test group (caudal) or to the control group managed with morphine and fluids. Vaginal delivery was achieved by 87% of the parturients given caudal analgesia compared to 62% of the control group. Moreover, despite the fact that twice as many infants in the caudal group as in the control group were in distress before therapy was instituted, the condition of newborns immediately after birth in the caudal group was far better than in the control group.

Climie (73) reported similar results in 65 parturients with abnormally prolonged labor managed with continuous lumbar epidural block. He noted that very commonly, contractions ceased for 10 to 15 minutes after the first injection of analgesic solution, but then returned spontaneously. Although the quality varied from patient to patient, in no patient were uterine contractions poorer than before the block, and in about 25% the contractions were considerably improved, as indicated by internal uterine pressure recordings. Tokodynamometer studies showed a change to stronger, shorter contractions with a longer resting time than before.

Moir and Willocks (71,289) studied the effects of continuous epidural analgesia on severe incoordinate uterine contraction. In the first report (71), they gave details concerning the first 75 patients in whom they used the Friedman method of cervimetric graphic analysis to measure the progress of labor and in eight patients they also used the tokodynamometry. Definite cephalopelvic disproportion was present in 25% of these patients, but a relative disproportion was probably present in many others. Almost all of the patients were primiparae, had postmature large babies in occiputoposterior position, ruptured membranes, ketonuria, and many had vomited. When continuous epidural analgesia was started, the patients had been in labor for an average of 20 hours and had severe pain despite very large doses of narcotics and other depressant drugs. Graphic analysis of labor showed an increased rate of cervical dilatation in 78% of patients who had no cephalopelvic disproportion and in 67% of those with definite disproportion. In the remainder, the progress of labor was either unaltered or slowed. Moir and Willocks concluded that in addition to providing much needed relief and improving the progress of labor, epidural analgesia allows time for a correct diagnosis to be made and precludes the need to terminate labor solely because of maternal discomfort. A year later, the second report (289) included an additional 25 parturients treated with continuous epidural block with similar results.

In the first edition of this book, Bonica and Hunter (290) reported their own results in the treatment of incoordinate uterine contraction with segmental epidural analgesia or with lumbar sympathetic blockade as an effective method of pain relief and in successfully treating abnormal uterine contractile patterns (Figure 13–21). They also provided a comprehensive overview in the overall management of parturients with various dysfunctions of the forces of labor, not only with regional analgesia but also with other measures. Hunter (291) used bilateral lumbar sympathetic block successfully for correction of abnormal contractile pattern. Monitoring uterine activity continuously by TKD, he noted that in approximately 75% of patients treated with this technique, the abnormal contractile pattern was converted to normal contractions, i.e., a midsegment dominance changed to a fundal dominance with good progress of labor ensuing.

Subsequently, Maltau and Andersen (80) reported the

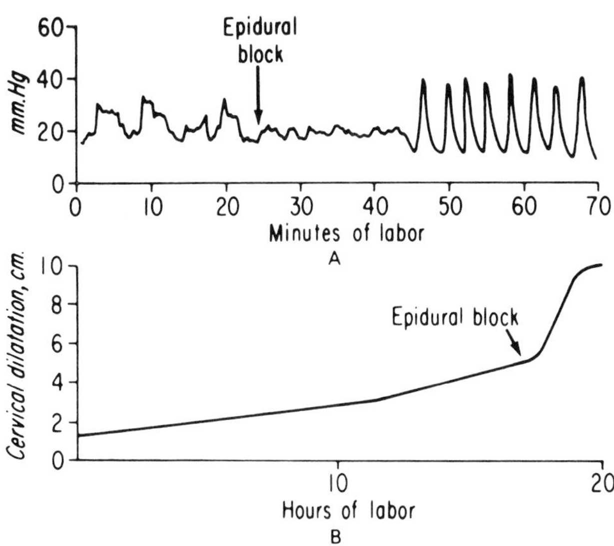


**Fig. 13–21.** Effect of epidural analgesia on incoordinate uterine activity. **A**. Intrauterine pressure tracings. Note the temporary decrease in uterine contractions and the subsequent normalization of the previously irregular contractions. **B**. Cervimetric curve showing the rapid cervical dilation that followed start of the epidural block.

successful use of epidural analgesia in the treatment of very prolonged, exhaustive labor consequent to weak or incoordinate uterine contractions in nine parturients who had been considered candidates for delivery by cesarean section. Among 88 parturients managed with lumbar epidural analgesia during a 6-month period, eight primigravidae and one multipara, 19 to 34 years of age, and a gestational age from 39 to 41 weeks were selected for a study of the therapeutic efficacy of lumbar epidural analgesia. All nine had been admitted to the hospital with severe painful labor that could not be relieved with intramuscular doses of 100 mg meperidine and 10 mg diazepam and nitrous oxide-oxygen inhalation analgesia. Despite oxytocin infusion, uterine contractions were weak or incoordinate and consequently cervical dilatation was slow and the fetus did not descend. Several hours after admission, the parturients presented a picture of maternal distress due to prolonged, very painful and exhaustive labor and had severe maternal metabolic acidosis. At this point, satisfactory pain relief with systemic and inhalation analgesics could not be obtained and further attempt to stimulate uterine contractions was no longer feasible. Under such circumstances, parturients normally would be considered candidates for emergency cesarean section. Instead of surgical intervention, the parturients were given segmental epidural analgesia, which provided complete relief of pain associated with contractions. Once labor pains were relieved, regular uterine contractions were often reestablished spontaneously, and the uterus responded to moderate doses of oxytocin given by infusion at rates of from 5 to 30 Mu/min with the guidance of continuous monitoring of fetal heart rate and intrauterine pressure. Cervical dilatation and descent of the presenting part progressed satisfactorily and consequently seven delivered spontaneously, one with outlet forceps and another with a vacuum extractor to terminate the second stage within 1 hour (Figure 13–22). In view of the fact that regular uterine contractions were frequently evoked by pain relief alone, Maltau and Andersen attributed the beneficial effects of epidural analgesia to minimizing or eliminating the increased release of epinephrine, the consequent severe sympathetically-induced lipolysis, and the very high concentration of circulating free fatty acids (81). Moreover, because the response of the uterus to oxytocin was prompt and predictable when pain had been relieved, they suggested that epidural analgesia may reduce or reverse metabolic acidosis, which, as previously mentioned, impedes uterine contractility and decreases the sensitivity to oxytocin (256–258).

### *Effects of Epidural Analgesia/Anesthesia on the Fetus and Newborn*

In considering the effects of epidural analgesia/anesthesia (and other anesthetics) on the newborn, it is important to recall that before the introduction of the Apgar score (54), the condition of neonates was evaluated by the time interval between birth and the first gasp, the first cry and the time for sustained respiration, the heart rate, skeletal muscle tone, and the skin color, while some clinicians also used mortality rate to evaluate long-term results. To the early pioneers who introduced and advocated the use of various forms of regional anesthesia for parturients, it was promptly obvious that newborns of mothers managed with properly administered epidural analgesia did not manifest the neonatal depression noted in infants whose mother had received Dammerschlaff or large doses of opioids and barbiturates, inhalation anesthesia, or other central nervous system depressants that were in wide use during the first 4 decades of the present century (see Chapter 1). In this section, we first very briefly mention the effects of older techniques of regional anesthesia on the fetus and newborn, and then focus on the influence of the more refined methods that were introduced during the past 3 decades.

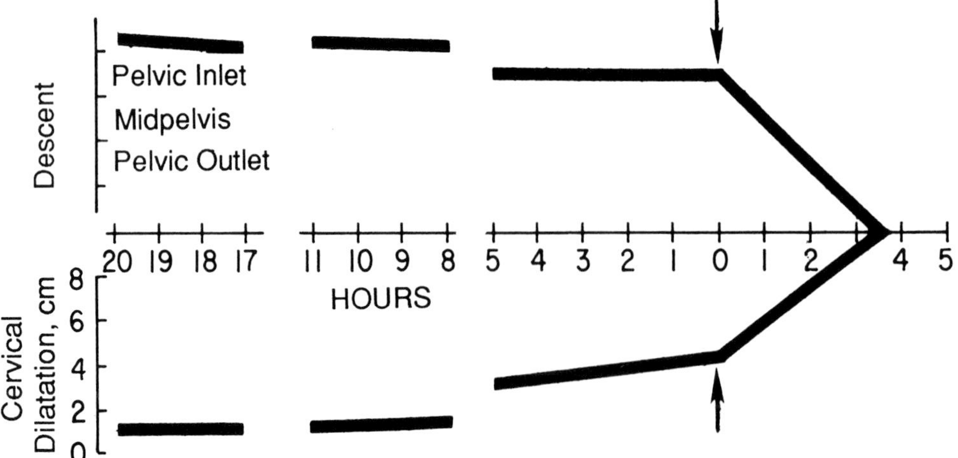


**Fig. 13–22.** Schema of the mean Partogram of 7 parturients who had had prolonged, painful, and exhaustive labor and were considered candidates for delivery by cesarean section, but upon initiation of continuous epidural analgesia at time zero hours, or indicated by arrows, the labors progressed rapidly with cervical dilitation and fetal descent, as diagrammatically illustrated. Because effective pain relief occurred, regular uterine contractions became spontaneously re-established and the uterus responded to moderate doses of oxytocin to effect spontaneous delivery. (Modified from Maltau JM, Andersen HT: Epidural anaesthesia as an alternative to caesarean section in the treatment of prolonged, exhaustive labour. Acta. Anaesthesiol. Scand. 19:349–354, 1975).

The widespread use of continuous caudal analgesia and saddle block for nearly 2 decades after they were introduced was due to a large part to the apparent lack of neonatal depression noted among infants delivered of mothers managed with these techniques. Thus, it is noted that after analyzing the first 10,000 continuous caudal analgesia cases used in obstetrics, Hingson and Edwards (16) concluded that newborns delivered of mothers managed with caudal anesthesia were as wide awake as those delivered of mothers given no sedation or anesthesia. Later, Hingson and associates (26) reported that neonatal death rates and delayed onset of respiration in full term and premature infants were statistically diminished with continued caudal anesthesia as compared with control groups. Bush (24) found the neonatal death rate among normal infants and those weighing between 1 to 2 kg to be significantly lower with caudal analgesia than with general anesthesia, and markedly lower than with minor analgesia (self-administered inhalation, or local infiltration or pudendal block), or no anesthesia (patients managed using the Dick-Read technique of natural childbirth). The overall death rate per 1000 live births was as follows: regional analgesia (most of which were continuous caudal blocks), 9.6; general anesthesia, 15.9; and minimal or no anesthesia, 24. Many others reported diminished neonatal mortality in normal births (20,23,25–26), in premature births (16,18,20,23,25,26,28), and among infants delivered by breech and other abnormal presentations (15,16,18,20,24,26). Because mortality rates involve complex issues, and other criteria used were not systematically observed and recorded, the validity of these data might be questioned. Nevertheless, the reports published in the late 1940s and 1950s comparing systemic opioids and other depressant agents including general anesthesia with properly administered continuous caudal analgesia/anesthesia provided convincing evidence that the latter technique was superior from the viewpoint of the fetus and newborn. The comparison of the results obtained with continuous caudal analgesia with the results obtained in nonmedicated group of parturients was less convincing but even here in parturients with high risk pregnancies continuous caudal epidural anesthesia was still better for the fetus and newborn.

The introduction of the Apgar score (54) is considered one of the milestones in the history of obstetric anesthesia because it provided a more systematic and reproducible measurement of the condition of the newborn that became widely used not only in the United States but in many hospitals throughout the world. Many data were published that confirmed the advantages of continuous caudal analgesia and standard continuous epidural analgesia/anesthesia over general anesthesia used for vaginal delivery (23–36,43,44,61–70,74,76,83–85,174,191–194, 272,273). As a consequence of these data, many believed that local anesthetic had no direct effects on the fetus or newborn and that barring maternal systemic complication, regional anesthesia provided "optimal conditions for the neonate" (292).

Subsequently, the widespread use of segmental epidural analgesia/anesthesia, entailing the use of smaller doses of local anesthetics than with the standard technique, showed that most neonates were given Apgar scores of 7 to 10 at 1 minute and 8 to 10 at 5 minutes, demonstrating minimal or no adverse effects on the parameters that constitute the Apgar score. It is essential to keep in mind that many obstetric factors also contribute to the condition of the fetus and newborn, and, therefore, local anesthetics and regional techniques usually play a variable, albeit usually minor role, in affecting the condition of the mother and her offspring.

Obviously, if the execution of the technique and the management of the parturient and the fetus were not carried out correctly, complications occurred. These are mentioned at the end of this section.

### *Advances in Methods of Evaluating the Fetus and Newborn*

In the early part of this chapter, mention was made that during the past 3 decades remarkable advances have been made in developing new methods of assessing the effects of epidural analgesia/anesthesia (as well as other obstetric anesthetic techniques) on the fetus and newborn that have been widely used together with the Apgar score. These include: 1) serial measurements during the course of labor and delivery, and in some cases, during the postpartum period, of the concentration of local anesthetics in the mother, fetus, and newborn; 2) similar serial measurements of blood gases and acid-base status of the mother and offspring; 3) intrauterine continuous electronic monitoring of the fetal heart rate (FHR) and the beat-to-beat variability and other sophisticated measurements; 4) uteroplacental blood flow and blood flow in the fetus; and 5) neurobehavioral assessments of the newborn. These newer measurements, which are described in detail in Chapter 40, frequently confirm data acquired with the Apgar score, but also demonstrate subtle changes in the newborn not always evident from the use of the Apgar score. We will not attempt to review the mass amount of data that have been published, but will summarize below some of the important reports on each of these methods.

#### Evaluation by Measurements of Blood Levels of Local Anesthetics

The misconception about the lack of direct effects on neonates whose mothers had been managed with continuous caudal or continuous epidural anesthesia prevailed throughout the 1960s despite the fact that in 1961 Bromage and Robson (293) reported that lidocaine administered to the parturient appeared in measurable quantities in umbilical cord blood. Many subsequent studies verified their findings and documented the rapid placental transfer of every local anesthetic in clinical use (see 294 for references). Thus, it became evident that regional anesthesia of any type administered to parturients may effect their fetuses and newborn in one or three ways: 1) directly through placental transfer and fetal uptake of the local anesthetic used with possible fetal central nervous system and cardiovascular depression; 2) indirectly through changes in maternal homeostasis that secondarily alter the fetal environment; and 3) a combination of these. The direct effects of local anesthetics on the fetus and newborn are dependent on: 1) the total dose of the local anesthetic, route of administration, and presence of epinephrine in solution; 2) maternal metabolism and maternal protein binding; 3) intervillous blood flow and fetal to maternal concentration ratio; 4) the uptake and distribution of the local anesthetic by the fetus; and 5) biotransformation or excretion of local anesthetic by the fetus and neonate. Indirect effects of these agents on the fetus and neonate are due to a decrease in uterine blood flow consequent to maternal hypotension or systemic toxic reactions, local anesthetic-induced uterine vasoconstriction, adrenergic stimulation of uterine vasculature, and uterine hypertonus plus maternal hypoxia caused by any factor, as well as changes in duration of labor and rate of forceps delivery.

The pharmacology, pharmacokinetics and placental transfer and how these drugs affect the fetus are discussed in detail in Chapter 11. A comprehensive review of almost all reports published up to 1978 on the effects of various local anesthetics and regional techniques on the fetus and newborn was published by Ralston and Shnider (294). Table 13–7 (page 388) contains a summary of the concentration of local anesthetics in the mother, fetus, and newborn that is representative of data acquired with standard epidural block using intermittent injections of local anesthetics, with continuous infusion of dilute solution of local anesthetics alone or combined with opioids, and with the double-catheter technique, achieved with the three primary local anesthetics in current use, employed alone, and with the addition of epinephrine. (295–318). As expected, the concentrations found in mother, fetus, and newborn were greater with the older technique that entailed large amounts of local anesthetics than were they with the segmental intermittent injections and continuous infusion techniques. Figure 13–23 depicts the maternal/fetal scalp concentration in a patient receiving continuous epidural analgesia to whom hourly epidural injections of 50 to 60 mg of lidocaine to 1:200,000 epinephrine were given for five doses. Just before delivery, the parturient received 100 to 120 mg of lidocaine-epinephrine (302).

Figure 13–24 depicts the data published by Zador and associates (76) showing the means and standard deviation in maternal venous blood, fetal capillary blood, and the umbilical cord blood following intermittent injections of 0.5% and 1% lidocaine, while Figure 13–25 depicts the data obtained by Zador, et al in groups of parturients managed by continuous drip lumbar epidural analgesia. Figure 13–26 depicts the concentrations of lidocaine in the mother's venous blood, fetal scalp blood, umbilical vein blood, and umbilical artery blood published by Brown and associates (304) compared with the data published by Zador and associates (76) and data obtained in 20 parturients managed with the double-catheter technique by Bonica and associates (112,178). The data by Brown and associates did not include a figure for fetal scalp blood. Note the significant difference between the older standard epidural technique used by Brown, et al (304) and the segmental epidural analgesia used by Zador and associates, and the very low figures obtained with the double-catheter technique (Bonica, unpublished data).

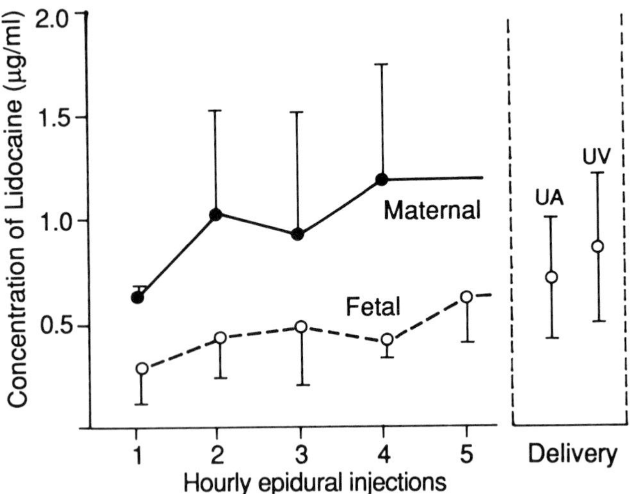


**Fig. 13–23.** Maternal and fetal scalp blood concentrations of lidocaine during labor and delivery after hourly epidural injection of 50 to 60 mg lidocaine with 1:200,000 epinephrine over the course of 5 hours. Before delivery, the parturient received 100 to 120 mg lidocaine. After delivery, the values in the umbilical vein and umbilical artery were 0.84 ± 0.35 and 0.72 ± 0.30, respectively. (From Fox GS, et al: Intrauterine fetal lidocaine concentrations given continuous epidural anesthesia. Am. J. Obstet. Gynecol. 110:896–899, 1971).

These data are of some use, but do not reflect the condition of the fetus and newborn because there are many other factors pertaining to the pharmacokinetics, placental transfer, and fetal tissue update that influence the condition of the fetus and neonate that are discussed in detail in Chapter 11. To recapitulate some of the essential points, it is important to note that because the free unchanged base is that portion of the local anesthetics that penetrates membranes, the amount transferred across the placenta and taken up by fetal tissues is influenced by the pKa of the drug and pH of tissues. Figure 13–27 (page 386) depicts that the calculated percentage of free base available for placental transfer is 18% for bupivacaine, 26% for lidocaine, and 36% for mepivacaine (49). These data suggest that bupivacaine is the best choice and mepivacaine the least favorable from the viewpoint of the fetus, but there are other factors to consider. One is that bupivacaine has profound effect in the amount of free base across the placenta and is available in the fetal circulation, is the degree of protein binding in maternal and fetal blood. Figure 13–28 shows the relative degrees of protein binding of bupivacaine and lidocaine in maternal and fetal blood and, as noted, little amount of bupivacaine is available for placental transfer (321). However, once in the fetal blood, the local anesthetic becomes less protein bound and therefore relatively more toxic than in the maternal circulation as shown in Figure 13–29 (page 386). There are two reasons for this effect: 1) there are quantitative and possibly qualitative differences in the protein fractions because there are greater amounts of globulin, especially β-2 globulin in maternal blood (321);

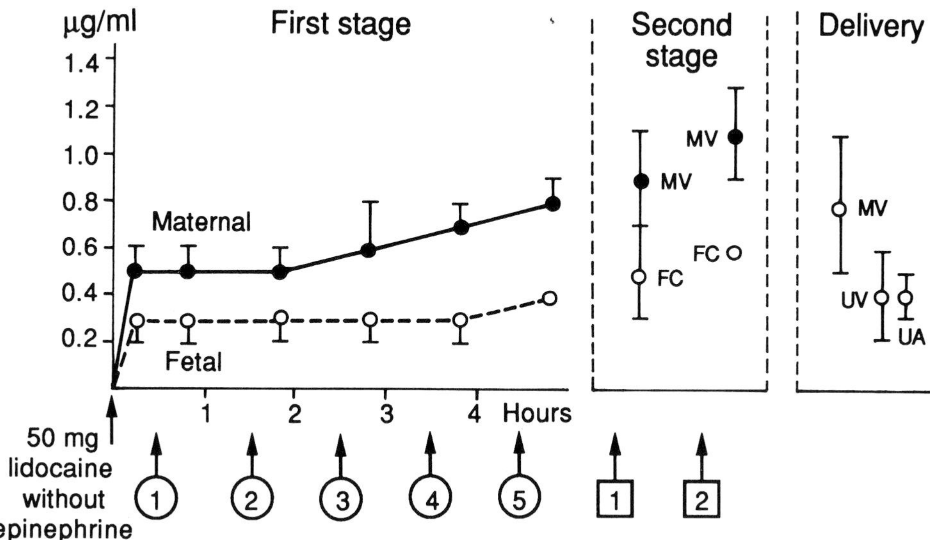


**Fig. 13–24.** Mean and standard deviation of lidocaine concentration in the maternal venous blood (MV), fetal capillary blood (FC), umbilical vein blood (UV), and umbilical artery blood (UA) following intermittent administration of 0.5% and 1% lidocaine with epinephrine 1:200,000 in doses as indicated in the figure. Figure in circle: 50 mg doses. Figure in square: 100 mg doses. (From Zador G, Englesson S, Nilsson BA: Low-dose intermittent epidural anaesthesia with lodicaine for vaginal delivery. Acta. Obstet. Gynaecol. Scand. (Suppl.) 34:3–16, 1974).

and 2) the number of binding sites in fetal plasma is reduced by competition from bilirubin, which exists in higher concentrations in the fetus than in the mother (322). As Bromage (49), among others, has pointed out, ultimately the toxic effects of a local anesthetic are not due to concentration of blood, but rather in tissue which depends on the partition coefficient of the drug between blood and tissue and on the rate of tissue perfusion which is greatest in highly perfused organs as the heart and brain. Thus, measurements of blood concentration give little indication of the tissue concentrations, some of which are 3 to 4 times higher than in the blood level. Fetal-tissue uptake of local anesthetic will rise in increasing degrees of fetal acidosis; hence, the importance of the acid-base status of the fetus and newborn.

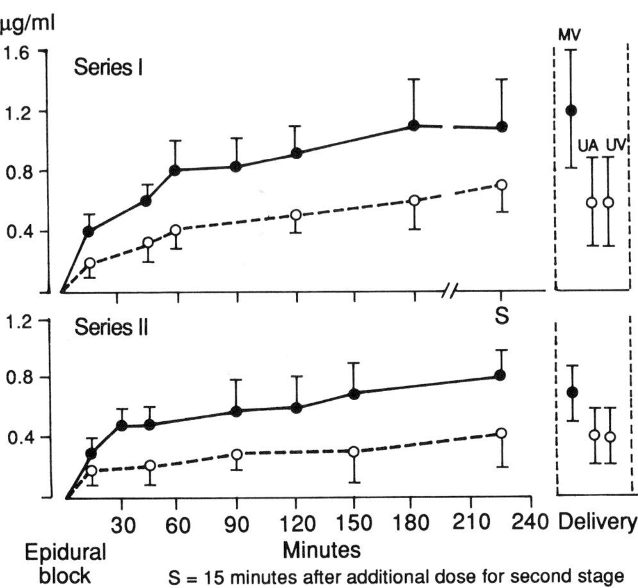


**Fig. 13–25.** Mean and standard deviation of lidocaine concentration in maternal venous blood (MV), fetal capillary blood (FC), umbilical vein blood (UV), and umbilical artery blood (UA) following lidocaine infusion into the epidural space. Series I 120 mg lidocaine without epinephrine per hour, series II 60 mg lidocaine with epinephrine 1:200,000 per hour. (From Zador G, Willdeck-Lund G, Nilsson BA.: Continuous drip lumbar epidural anaesthesia with lidocaine for vaginal delivery. Acta. Obstet. Gynecol. Scand. (Suppl.) 34:31–40, 1974).

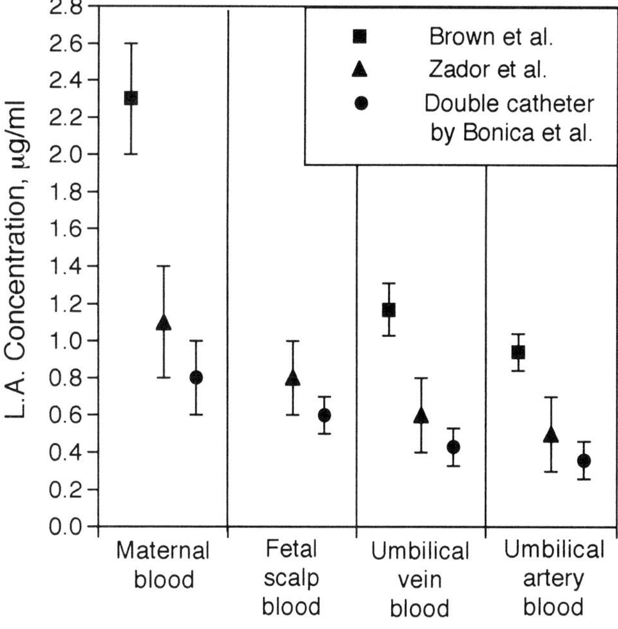


**Fig. 13–26.** Blood levels in maternal venous blood, fetal scalp blood, and blood in the umbilical vein and umbilical artery derived from three studies pertaining to lumbar epidural analgesia for labor and vaginal delivery. The data pertain to lidocaine alone and is included in Table 13–7. Brown, et al (304) used standard lumbar epidural (T10-S5); Zorab, et al (78) used semisegmental block with 10 ml of 0.5 to 1% lidocaine; while Bonica and associates (112,178) used the double-catheter technique injecting 4 to 6 ml in the lumbar catheter and 3 to 5 ml in the caudal catheter (see text for details).

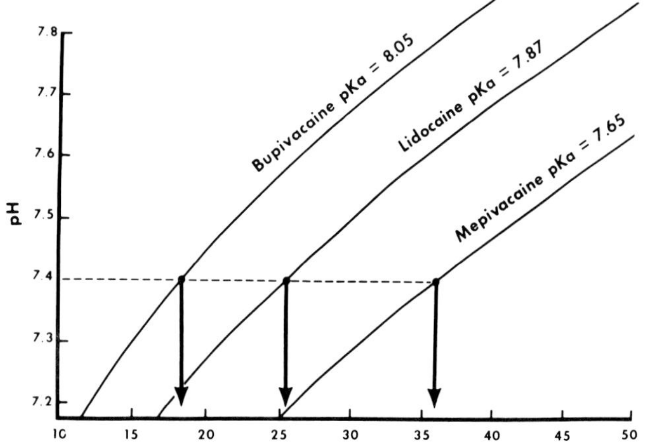


**Fig. 13–27.** Placental transfer of local anesthetics related to pKa, ionization, and pH. Comparison of bupivacaine, lidocaine, and mepivacaine showing relative proportions of free base available for diffusion across the placenta at pH 7.4. (From Bromage PR: Epidural Analgesia. Philadelphia, W.B. Saunders, 1978, p. 531).

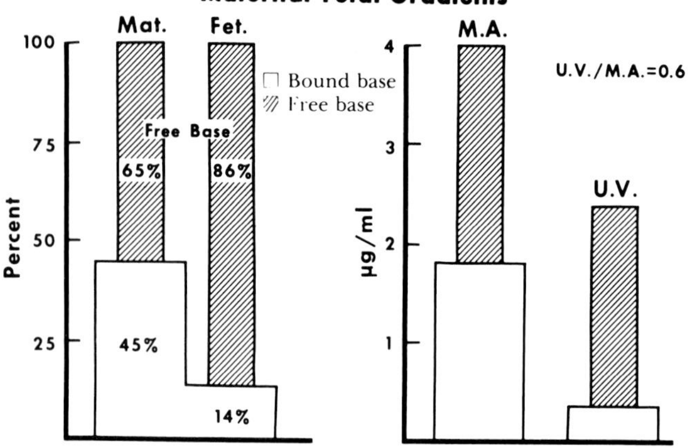


**Fig. 13–29.** Relative toxicity of local anesthetics in maternal and fetal blood. Approximate distribution of bound and free lidocaine in adults and fetal plasma assuming an umbilical/maternal artery ratio of 0.6. Although the total concentration of lidocaine is less in the umbilical vein than in the maternal artery, the smaller degree of protein binding in fetal plasma leaves relatively more free unbound and pharmacologically active base available in the fetus, and the drug can accrue in the mother and fetus. (From Bromage PR: Epidural Analgesia. Philadelphia, W.B. Saunders, 1978, p. 532. Developed from data from Tucker, et al.: Binding of anilide type local anesthetics in human plasma. Anesthesiology 33:304, 1970).

Finally, it deserves reemphasis that the addition of epinephrine in concentrations of 1:200,000 to 1:400,000 has been shown to reduce the concentration of lidocaine and mepivacaine in maternal blood by 25 to 35%, and in fetal or neonatal blood by 15 to 20%. In regard to the effects of epinephrine on the placental transfer of bupivacaine, there are contradictory data. Abboud and associates (204) and Reynolds and coworkers (308) showed a decrease in the placental transfer with consequent decrease in plasma concentration in the mother and fetus. However, others, including Reynolds and associates (323–325), have shown that epinephrine caused a slight but insignificant rise in total and free levels of bupivacaine (see Table 13–7). In their latest report, Fletcher, Reynolds and associates (325) showed that the F/M ratio of bupivacaine was significantly increased in the presence of epinephrine—a phenomenon that was not associated with protein binding in mother or baby, nor with an increase in placental transfer rate or ion trapping, but probably can be accounted for by more rapid equilibrium of bupivacaine within the fetal compartment. Nevertheless, we and many others add epinephrine to bupivacaine to enhance its efficacy of the analgesia/anesthesia for both vaginal delivery and cesarean section (204,318,326).

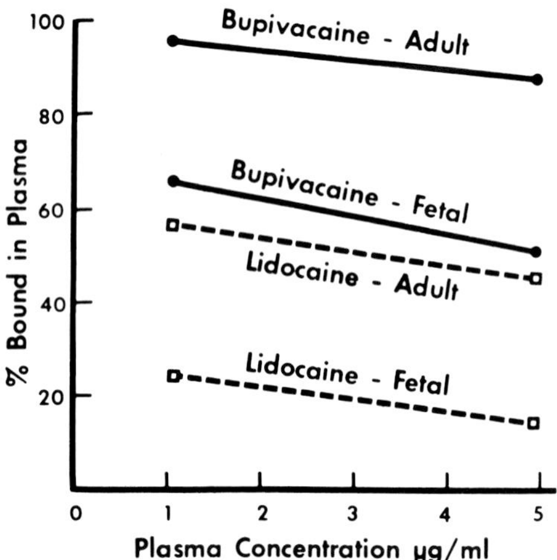


**Fig. 13–28.** Placental transfer of local anesthetics. Relative proportions of bupivacaine and lidocaine bound to plasma proteins in adult and fetal blood at concentrations between 1 and 5 μg/ml. (From Bromage PR: Epidural Analgesia. Philadelphia, W.B. Saunders, 1978, p. 532. (Developed from data from Tucker, et al.: Binding of anilide type local anesthetics in human plasma. Anesthesiology 33:304, 1970).

## *Blood Gases and Acid-Base Status*

In the preceding section on the "Second Stage of Labor," it was mentioned that many of the authors who reported an increased prolongation of the second stage and increased incidence of instrumental deliveries with continuous epidural analgesia noted no deleterious effects on the fetus and newborn (74,75,77,93,95,112). Indeed, in many instances, the condition of the newborns of mothers who had received continuous epidural analgesia was better than that of newborns delivered of mothers in the control group consisting of either minimal systemic analgesia with opioids, sedatives and nitrous oxide-oxygen inhalation analgesia, and in some no analgesia at all (63,72,75,76,91–94,203–205,272,273). Table 13–8 lists the data on blood gases and acid-base status of the fetus as reported by representative studies and, as may be noted, these parameters were normal.

The results obtained by Pearson and Davis (151–154) are depicted in Figure 13–13 and show the markedly greater increase in metabolic acidosis in both the mother, fetus, and newborn when the mother was managed with systemic opioid (meperidine) compared to those managed with continuous epidural analgesia. Belfrage and associates (82) reported that during continuous epidural analgesia, fetal scalp blood pH was within normal limits and no pathologic fetal heart rate tracings were elicited by the analgesia. Thalme and associates (83,84) found less maternal and fetal metabolic acidosis during the lumbar epidural analgesia with bupivacaine than in a control group who received conventional analgesia (meperidine and inhalation analgesia for the first stage and pudendal block for the second stage). Zador and his associates (77,79) noted that fetal and neonatal acid blood gases and acid-base status during either low dose intermittent or continuous lumbar epidural analgesia was not significantly different from a control group of parturients who received no analgesia. Abnormal fetal heart rate patterns indicating hypoxia were rare and occurred almost exclusively in association with transient maternal hypotension. Similar results on the effects of epidural analgesia/anesthesia on blood gases and acid-base status have been reported by Abboud and associates in the many studies they have carried out (Figures 13–30 to 13–32) (91–93,246,249, 303–305,317), by Chestnut and associates (94,219, 220,244), Shnider (83,119,128,252), and many others (191,210,245,246,249,266,294,314).

Another way that continuous epidural analgesia improves the blood gases of the fetus is by eliminating the hyperventilation so that maternal $PaCO_2$ returns to prelabor levels; and although this reduces transplacental carbon dioxide gradient, it also has the effect of reducing the affinity of maternal hemoglobin for oxygen thereby potentially enhancing oxygen transfer to the fetus. Swanström and Bratteby (327) showed that the $PaO_2$ values in newborns whose mothers had received epidural lidocaine analgesia during labor were higher than in controls, but unlike the results reported by Thalme and associates (83,84), they found no difference in the acid-base status between the groups.

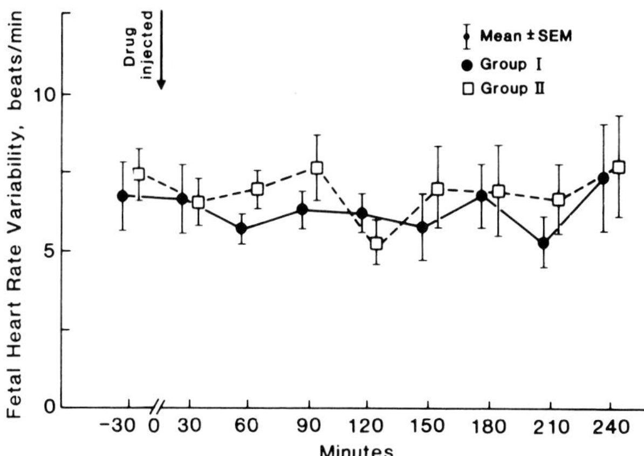


**Fig. 13–31.** Effects of epidural anesthesia on fetal heart rate variability (mean ± SEM) in fetuses of 16 parturients in whom anesthesia was achieved with lidocaine-epinephrine (group I) and 14 parturients given plain lidocaine (group II). Statistical analysis by Student's t-test showed there was no statistically significant change between the two groups. (From Abboud TK, et al: Maternal, fetal and neonatal effects of lidocaine with and without epinephrine for epidural anesthesia in obstetrics. Anesth. Analg. 63:973, 1984).

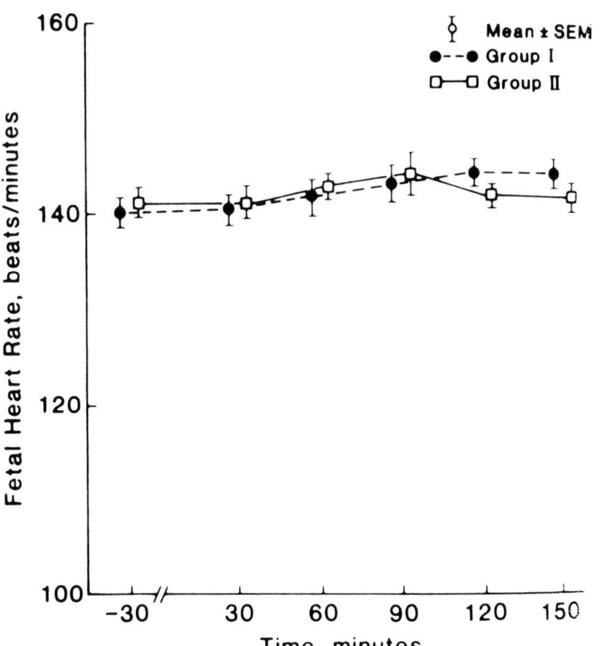


**Fig. 13–30.** Effects of epidural anesthesia on beat-to-beat variability (mean ± SEM) in fetuses of mothers given bupivacaine plain (group II) and bupivacaine with epinephrine 1:300,000 (group I). (From Abboud TK, et al: Safety and efficacy of epinephrine added to bupivacaine for lumbar epidural analgesia in obstetrics. Anesth. Analg. 64:585, 1985).

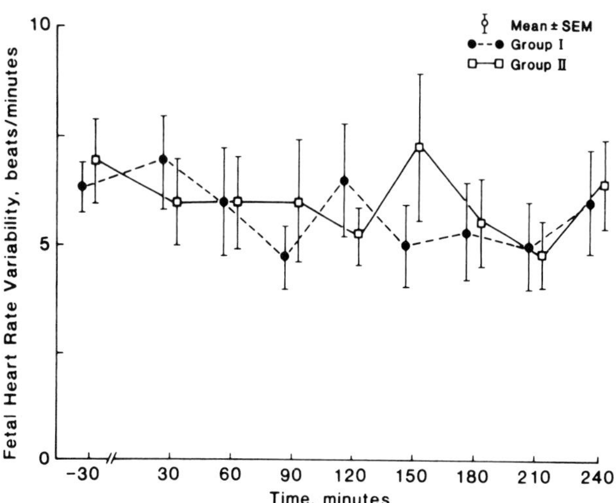


**Fig. 13–32.** Effects of epidural anesthesia on fetal heart rate (mean ± SEM) in a group of parturients given bupivacaine-epinephrine (group I), and another group given bupivacaine alone (group II). Statistical analysis by Student's t-test revealed changes were not statistically significant. (From Abboud TK, et al: Safety and efficacy of epinephrine added to bupivacaine for lumbar epidural analgesia in obstetrics. Anesth. Analg. 64:585, 1985).

**Table 13–7.** Placental Transfer of Local Anesthetics Achieved with Various Epidural Techniques Used for Labor, Vaginal Delivery, and Cesarean Section

| Authors Year Ref. # | Epidural Technique[1] | Injection Technique[2] | Number of Patients (Position)[3] | Anesthetic Agent[4] P = Plain E = Epinephrine |
|---|---|---|---|---|
| A. Labor and Vaginal Delivery | | | | |
| *Lidocaine:* | | | | |
| Shnider & Way 1968 (303) | St. LEB | Rep./Interm. | 27 S | 1.5% LE |
| Thomas, et al. 1968 (295) | St. LEB | Rep./Interm. | 18 S | 2% LP |
| | | | 24 S | 2% LE |
| Thomas, et al. 1969 (296) | St. LEB | Single dose | 12 S | 1.5% LP |
| | | Rep./Interm. | 7 S | 1.5% LE |
| Epstein, et al. 1968 (297) | St. LEB | Rep./Interm. | 46 S | 2% LP |
| | | | 46 S | 2% LE |
| Hehre, et al. 1969 (298) | Seg. LEB →Sacral | Rep./Interm. | 3 S | 2% LE |
| Fox & Houle 1969 (299) | Seg. LEB →Sacral | Rep./Interm. | 19 S | 2% LE |
| Lurie & Weiss 1970 (300) | St. LEB | Rep./Interm. | 13 S | 1.5–2% LE |
| Houle, et al. 1971 (301) | Seg. LEB →Sacral | Rep./Interm. | 25 SL | 1% LE |
| | | Rep./Interm. | 25 SL | 1% $LCO_2E$ |
| Fox, et al. 1971 (302) | Seg. LEB →Sacral | Rep./Interm. | 22 S | 1% LE |
| Brown, et al. 1975 (304) | St. LEB | Rep./Interm. | 11 S | 1.5–2% LP |
| | | | 30 S | 1.5–2% LE |
| Zador, et al. 1974 (76) | Seg. LEB →Sacral | Rep./Interm. | 100 SL | 0.5–1% LP |
| Zador & Nilsson 1974 (76) | Seg. LEB →Sacral | Rep./Interm. | 90 SL | 0.5–1% LE |
| Zador, et al. 1974 (78) | Seg. LEB →Sacral | Cont. Infusion | 10 SL | 0.4% LP |
| Zador & Nilsson 1974 (78) | Seg. LEB →Sacral | Cont. Infusion | 11 SL | 0.4% LE |
| | **DCEB** | | | |
| Bonica, et al. 1974 (178) | Seg. LEB | Rep./Interm. | 12 L | 1.5% LP |
| | Caudal | Rep./Interm. | 12 L | 1.5% LE |
| Abboud, et al. 1982 (91) | Seg. LEB →Sacral | Rep./Interm. | 50 L | 1.5% LP |
| Abboud, et al. 1984 (203) | Seg. LEB →Sacral | Rep./Interm. | 14 L | 1.5% LP |
| | | | 16 L | 1.5% LE |
| Abboud, et al. 1984 (94) | Seg. LEB →Sacral | Cont. Infusion | 19 L | 1.5% LP |
| Scanlon, et al. 1974 (60) | St. LEB | Rep./Interm. | 11 S | 2% LP |
| Milaszkiewicz, et al. 1992 (314a) | St. LEB | Cont. Infusion | 42 L | 0.75% LP |
| *Mepivacaine* | | | | |
| Morishima, et al. 1966 (305) | Caudal | Single dose | 32 S | 1.5% MP |
| | St. LEB | Rep./Interm. | 24 S | 1.5% MP |
| Lurie & Weiss 1970 (300) | St. LEB | Rep./Interm. | 19 S | 1.5–2.0% MP |
| Brown, et al. 1975 (304) | St. LEB | Rep./Interm. | 11 S | 1.5–2.0% MP |
| | | Rep./Interm. | 30 S | 1.5–2.0% ME |
| Scanlon 1974 (60) | St. LEB | Rep./Interm. | 42 S | 1.5% MP |
| *Bupivacaine* | | | | |
| Thomas, et al. 1969 (301) | St. LEB | Single dose | 18 S | 0.5% BE |
| | | Repeat 1 × | 2 S | |
| Reynolds & Taylor 1971 (308) | Seg. LEB →Sacral | Rep./Interm. | 9 S | 0.5 BP |
| | | Rep./Interm. | 9 S | 0.5 BE |
| Hyman & Shnider 1979 (309) | St. LEB | Single dose | 11 S | 0.25–0.5% BP |
| | St. LEB | Single dose | 21 S | 0.25–0.5% BE |
| | St. LEB | Rep./Interm. (multiple doses) | 32 S | 0.25–0.5% BE |
| Reynolds, et al. 1973 (211) | Seg. LEB →Sacral | Rep./Interm. | 35 S | 0.5% BP |
| | | | 35 S | 0.5% BE |
| Scanlon, et al. 1976 (310) | St. LEB | Rep./Interm. | 20 S | 0.5% BP |

*(continued)*

| Total Anesthetic Administered (mg) mean (± SD or range)[5] | Maternal Concentration at Delivery (μg/ml) mean (± SD or range)[5] | Umbilical Vein Concentration (μg/ml) mean (± SD or range) | Umbilical Vein / Maternal Blood Ratio |
|---|---|---|---|
| N.G. | 2.7 (0.2–5.5) | 1.3 (0.4–3.4) | 0.5 |
| 540 (100–900) | 2.53 (1.5–4.5) | 1.25 (0.6–0.21) | 0.5 |
| 490 (300–1070) | 2.75 (1.1–4.7) | 1.65 (1.0–4.3) | 0.6 |
| 400 ± 218 | 3.43 (1.3–6.0) | 1.56 (1.1–2.9) | 0.45 |
| 400 ± 169 | 2.62 (1.5–4.0) | 1.33 (0.7–2.5) | 0.5 |
| 502 ± 218 | 2.6 (0–6.7) | 1.8 (0–3.6) | 0.7 |
| 424 ± 169 | 1.23 ± 0.1 | 0.8 ± 0.06 | 0.65 |
| 130 ± 5.8 | 1.23 ± 0.09 | 0.8 ± 0.06 | 0.65 |
| 315 ± 36 | 1.39 (0.5–2.4) | 0.83 (0.4–1.4) | 0.6 |
| 567 (135–930) | 2.2 (0.95–3.34) | 1.55 (0.7–2.6) | 0.7 |
| 326 ± 141 | 1.3 ± 0.5 | 0.73 ± 0.4 | 0.5 |
| 251 ± 97 | 1.1 ± 0.5 | 0.64 ± 0.4 | 0.6 |
| 318 ± 132 | 0.99 ± 0.58 | 0.84 ± 0.35 | 0.8 |
| 423 ± 40 | 2.3 ± 0.29 | 2.27 ± 0.14 | 0.52 |
| 414 ± 36 | 1.5 ± 0.12 | 0.89 ± 0.07 | 0.59 |
| 409 ± 245 | 1.08 ± 0.34 | 0.63 ± 0.22 | 0.58 |
| 258 ± 117 | 0.79 ± 0.25 | 0.42 ± 0.17 | 0.53 |
| 591 ± 203 | 1.22 ± 0.42 | 0.65 ± 0.32 | 0.57 |
| 258 ± 117 | 0.79 ± 0.25 | 0.42 ± 0.17 | 0.53 |
| 325 ± 87 | 0.67 ± 0.18 | 0.38 ± 0.06 | 0.56 |
| 266 ± 61 | 0.48 ± 0.8 | 0.26 ± 0.03 | 0.54 |
| No data | 1.22 ± 0.11 | 0.80 ± 0.07 | 0.66 |
| 464 ± 53 | 1.84 ± 0.18 | 1.23 ± 0.26 | 0.67 |
| 351 ± 51 | 1.32 ± 0.17 | 0.56 ± 0.08 | 0.42 |
| 623 ± 50 | 2.4 ± 0.1 | 1.27 ± 0.09 | 0.53 |
| 423 ± 40 | 2.3 ± 0.3 | 1.17 ± 0.14 | 0.52 |
| 762 ± 264 | 3 ± 1.2 | 1.4 ± 6 | 0.57 |
| No data | 2.91 ± 0.28 (SEM) | 1.90 ± 16 (SEM) | 0.65 |
| No data | 3.9 ± 0.39 | 2.68 ± 0.22 | 0.69 |
| 396 | 2.2 (1.3–3.6) | 1.6 | 0.7 |
| 374 ± 21 | 2.89 ± 0.16 | 1.84 ± 0.12 | 0.64 |
| 349 ± 31 | 2.26 ± 0.22 | 1.54 ± 0.15 | 0.69 |
| 374 ± 21 | 2.89 ± 0.16 | 1.84 ± 0.12 | 0.64 |
| 62.5 | 0.22 (0.12–0.4) | 0.11 | 2 |
| 128 ± 20 | 0.67 ± 0.12 | 0.16 ± 0.04 | 0.24 |
| 116 ± 17 | 0.49 ± 0.08 | 0.18 ± 0.03 | 0.37 |
| 57 ± 7 | 0.22 ± 0.03 | 0.082 ± 0.02 | 0.26 |
| 83 ± 7 | 0.39 ± 0.08 | 0.098 ± 0.02 | 0.20 |
| 96 ± 6 | 0.24 ± 0.02 | 0.082 ± 0.01 | 0.38 |
| 147 ± 13 | 0.54 ± 0.65 | 0.14 ± 0.02 | 0.26 |
| 126 ± 12 | 0.36 ± 0.69 | 0.09 ± 0.01 | |
| 112 ± 7 mg | 0.41 ± 0.05 | 0.11 ± 0.02 | 0.27 |

*(continued)*

**Table 13–7.** Placental Transfer of Local Anesthetics Achieved with Various Epidural Techniques Used for Labor, Vaginal Delivery, and Cesarean Section—*(continued)*

| Authors Year Ref. # | Epidural Technique[1] | Injection Technique[2] | Number of Patients (Position)[3] | Anesthetic Agent[4] P = Plain E = Epinephrine |
|---|---|---|---|---|
| Belfrade, et al. 1975 (81a) | Seg. LEB →Sacral | Rep./Interm. | 33 L | 0.25% BE 0.5% × 4 |
| Belfrage, et al. 1975 (82) | Seg. LEB →Sacral | Rep./Interm. | 37 L | 0.25% BP |
| Bonica 1977 (unpubl.) | Seg. LEB | Rep./Intem. | 20 L | 0.25% BP |
| | Caudal | Rep./Interm. | | 0.5% BP |
| Abboud, et al. 1982 (91) | Seg. LEB →Sacral | Rep./Interm. | 50 L | 0.5% BP |
| Abboud, et al. 1984 (93) | Seg. LEB →Sacral | Rep./Interm. | 23 L | 0.125% BP |
| Abboud, et al. 1985 (204) | Seg. LEB →Sacral | Rep./Interm. | 16 L | 0.5% BP |
| | | | 16 L | 0.5% BE |
| Li, et al. 1985 (216) | Seg. LEB →Sacral | Cont. Infusion | 20 L | 0.125% BP |
| | | Cont. Infusion | 20 L | 0.065% BP |
| | | Cont. Infusion | 15 L | 0.125% BP |
| | | Cont. Infusion | 16 L | 0.125% BP |
| *Continuous Caudal:* | | | | |
| Morishima 1961 (305) | Caudal | Continuous | 24 S | 1.5% MP |
| | Caudal | Single dose | 32 S | 1.5% MP |
| Moore, et al. 1971 (312) | Caudal St. LEB | Continuous | 57 S | 1.5% MP |
| *B. Cesarean Section* | | | | |
| Fox & Houle 1969 (313) | St. LEB | Single dose | 19 SL | 2% L/E |
| Houle, et al. 1971 (313a.) | St. LEB | Single dose | 18 SL | 2% $LC_{O_2}$/E |
| Magno, et al. 1976 (316) | St. LEB | Single dose | 14 SL | 0.75% BP |
| Reynolds, et al. 1989 (323) | St. LEB | Single ractionated | | |
| | | a. Elective CS | 20 SL | 0.5 BP |
| | | | 20 SL | 0.5 BE |
| | | b. Emergency CS | 20 SL | 0.5 BP |
| | | | 20 SL | 0.5 BE |
| McIntic, et al. 1991 (314) | St. LEB | Single dose | 10 SL | 2% LP |
| | | | 9 SL | 2% LE |
| Loftus, et al. 1991 (323a) | St. LEB | Single dose | 30 SL | 0.5%$BC_{O_2}$/E |
| | | | 30 SL | 2% LE |

(1) Epidural Techniques: a) St. LEB = Standard (T10–S5) Lumbar epidural block; b) Seg. LEB = Segmental (T9–10 to L1–2) epidural block; c) Seg. LEB/→Sacral = Segmental (T10–L1) block that gradually diffuses to sacral segments; DCEB = Double catheter epidural block. St. LEB for cesarean section usually extends to T4 or higher.
(2) Injection Techniques: All techniques used to achieve continuous blockade, except for S.D. = Single dose; Rep/Interm. = Repeated intermittent injection to provide continuous analgesia; c) Cont. Infusion = Continuous infusion
(3) Position: S = supine; L = lateral; SL = supine with lateral uterine displacement.
(4) Local Anesthetic: LP = Lidocaine plain; LE = Lidocaine/epinephrine; MP = Mepivacaine plain; ME = Mepivacaine/epinephrine; BP = Bupivacaine plain, BE = Bupivacaine epinephrine
(5) Dosage: Rounded to nearest unit or decimal; mg/ml = milligram per milliliter; μg/ml = microgram per milliliter; pt/ml = picogram per milliliter; ng/ml = nanogram per milliliter. Blood concentrations are listed in μg/ml except where otherwise indicated.

### *Uteroplacental Blood Flow and Intervillous Perfusion*

An important means by which continuous lumbar epidural blockade may affect respiratory gas exchange is by altering placental blood flow because respiratory gases are flow-dependent in their placental transfer rates (328). Many studies have shown that well-conducted epidural analgesia/anesthesia, in the absence of hypotension or having the patient in the supine position, does not have a detrimental effect on uterine blood flow (130,131, 140–145), fetal heart rate (82–84,91–93,329–331), or acid base or blood gas status (82–84,91–93,103–105, 329–331). In fact, many studies document an increase in uterine blood flow and improvement in fetal acid-base status following epidural analgesia, especially in parturients with pregnancy-induced hypertension (144–150,332,333). The improvement noted in these studies have been attributed to relief of the vasospasm of uteroplacental circulation, but more likely it is an indirect effect of eliminating the sympathetic hyperactivity conse-

| Total Anesthetic Administered (mg) mean (± SD or range)[5] | Maternal Concentration at Delivery (μg/ml) mean (± SD or range)[5] | Umbilical Vein Concentration (μg/ml) mean (± SD or range) | Umbilical Vein / Maternal Blood Ratio |
|---|---|---|---|
| 62 ± 31 | 185 ± 1.04 μg/ml | 51 ± 29 μg/ml | 0.26 |
| 50 mg | 257 ± 58 ng/ml | 27 ± 11 ng/ml | 0.2 |
| 60 ± 28 | 0.21 ± 0.22 | 0.034 ± 0.015 | 0.25 |
| No data | 0.3 ± 0.05 | 0.10 ± 0.02 | 0.3 |
| 182 ± 36 | 0.54 ± 0.11 | 0.18 ± 0.04 | 0.33 |
| No data | 0.57 ± 0.17 | 0.19 ± 0.1 | 0.27 |
| No data | 0.45 ± 0.12 | 0.15 ± 0.04 | 0.31 |
| 135 ± 52 | 0.24 ± 0.9 | 0.16 ± 0.08 | 0.67 |
| 165 ± 67 | 0.33 ± 0.9 | 0.15 ± 0.12 | 0.44 |
| 171 ± 65 | 0.44 ± 0.2 | 0.16 ± 0.05 | 0.41 |
| 198 ± 64 | 0.33 ± 0.15 | 0.11 ± 0.04 | 0.37 |
| No data | 2.9 (2.0–5.0) | 1.9 (0.5–3.6) | 0.7 |
| No data | 3.9 (1.0–8.6) | 2.68 (0.8–4.5) | 0.7 |
| 900–1400 | 6.9 (3.9–8.6) | 4.9 (2.5–7.9) | 0.7 |
| 315 ± 36 | 1.39 ± 0.83 | 0.83 ± 0.35 | 0.6 |
| 297 ± 31 | 1.93 ± 0.54 | 0.91 ± 0.66 (UV) | 0.48 |
| | 0.64 ± 0.48 (UA) | | 0.33 |
| 103 ± 35 EM | 494 ± 21 ng/ml | 2.14 ± 24 | 0.41 |
| | | UV UA | |
| 100 | 0.64 ± 0.38 | 1.59 ± 0.08 0.14 ± 0.06 | 0.31 |
| 100 | 0.51 ± 0.12 | 0.17 ± 0.74 0.18 ± 0.11 | 0.32 |
| 100 | 0.92 ± 0.27 | 0.33 ± 0.15 0.27 ± 0.15 | 0.37 |
| 100 | 0.88 ± 0.22 | 0.32 ± 0.15 0.29 ± 0.15 | 0.39 |
| 493 ± 64 | 2.22 ± 0.66 | 1.4 ± 0.52 | 0.6 |
| 400 ± 108 | 1.32 ± 0.57 | 0.8 ± 0.37 | 0.6 |
| | | UV UA | |
| 120 ± 33 | 1.04 ± 0.09 | 0.27 ± 0.6 0.15 ± 0.01 | 0.29 |
| 418 ± 34 | 2.61 ± 0.09 | 1.17 ± 0.06 0.8 ± 0.1 | 0.48 |

quent to the relief of pain. Because the uteroplacental vascular bed does not appear to be innervated by the sympathetic nervous system, reduction of intrinsic vascular resistance would have to be accounted for by the reduction of epinephrine and norepinephrine blood levels that occur with regional analgesia mentioned earlier (168).

During epidural analgesia for cesarean section, changes in intervillous blood flow may be inconsistent, depending on the status of the maternal arterial pressure. The reduced blood flow usually coincides with a fall in maternal arterial pressure, but this can be minimized by the effects of preload, maintaining the gravida in the lateral position and admnistering ephedrine to maintain the maternal pressure within normal limits. On the other hand, if the maternal hypotension is not promptly treated, there is a significant decrease in uterine blood flow as a consequence of decrease in uterine perfusion pressure. This is usually associated with the impaired fetal or neonatal well-being, as evidenced by deterioration of the fetal heart rate pattern, fetal blood gas status, and umbilical blood gas status measurement at the time of delivery (334–337).

Doppler ultrasound has been used to measure flow-velocity wave forms in both maternal and fetal circulation by a number of investigators, including Marx and associates (338), Giles and associates (339), and Long, et al (340)—all of whom used continuous wave Doppler ultrasound systems to record uteroplacental wave forms. Marx and associates (338) used the system to measure the umbilical blood velocity waves in the fetuses of healthy partu-

**Table 13–8.** Effects of "Continuous" Epidural Analgesia/Anesthesia on Blood Gases and Acid-Base Status in the Mother,

| Authors Year (Ref. #) | Epidural Technique Used[1] | Number of Patients and Position[2] | Local Anesthetic Used[3] | Total Dose[4] (mg) | Maternal | | | |
|---|---|---|---|---|---|---|---|---|
| | | | | | $P_{O_2}$ mm Hg | $P_{CO_2}$ mmHg | pH | Base Defic. |
| Fox & Houle 1971 (299) | St. LEB for CS | 13 S $O_2$<br>13 S air | 2% $L_O$<br>2% $L_E$ | 310 ± 32<br>316 ± 25 | 340 ± 10<br>75 ± 12 | 29 ± 5<br>28 ± 5 | 7.42<br>7.43 | −4.05<br>−4.23<br>$BD_{ECF}$[6] |
| Zador, et al. 1974 (76) | Intermittent Seg. LEB | 100 S<br>90 S | 0.5–1% $L_O$<br>0.5–1% $L_E$ | 409 ± 245<br>258 ± 117 | —<br>— | 31 ± 2<br>31 ± 2 | 7.36<br>7.37 | 7.3<br>8.5 |
| Zador & Nilsson 1974 (77) | Control | 100 S | — | — | — | 31 | 7.36 | 7.4 |
| Zador, et al. 1974 (78) | Continuous LEB | 10 S<br>11 S | 2 mg/min<br>1.2–1.4 ml/min | 591 ± 203<br>293 ± 108 | —<br>— | 28.5<br>28.6 | 7.39<br>7.40 | −7.2<br>−6.6 |
| Zador, et al. 1974 (79) | Control | 71 S | — | — | — | 23.0 | 7.36 | 7.4 |
| Thalme, et al. 1974 (83) | Intermittent Seg. LEB | 23 S<br>12 S | 0.5 $B_O$<br>0.5 $B_E$ | NP<br>NP | —<br>— | —<br>— | —<br>— | —<br>— |
| Abboud, et al. 1982 (91) | Intermittent Seg. LEB | 50 L<br>50 L<br>50 L | 0.5 $B_O$<br>2% $Chlor_O$<br>1.5% $L_O$ | NP<br>NP<br>NP | —<br>—<br>— | —<br>—<br>— | —<br>—<br>— | —<br>—<br>— |
| Abboud, et al. 1983 (92) | Continuous LEB | 25 L<br>19 L<br>19 L | 0.125 $B_O$<br>0.75 $Chlor_O$<br>0.25 $L_O$ | NP<br>NP<br>NP | —<br>—<br>— | —<br>—<br>— | —<br>—<br>— | —<br>—<br>— |
| Abboud, et al. 1985 (204) | Seg. LEB<br>→Sacral Bl. | 16 L<br>16 L | 0.5% $B_E$<br>0.5 $B_O$ | NP<br>NP | —<br>— | —<br>— | —<br>— | —<br>— |
| Chestnut, et al. 1988 (244) | Cont. LEB<br>→Sacral Bl. | 41 L | 0.0625% $B_O$<br>Fen. 0.0002% | 67 ± 32<br>Fen. 132 ± 23 µg | — | — | — | — |
| | | 39 L | 0.125% $B_O$ | 99 ± 49 | — | — | — | — |
| Abboud, et al. 1989 (246b) | Seg. LEB<br>2 ml Test Dose<br>8 ml Ther. Dose | 17 L | 0.5% $B_O$<br>1 mg Buto.<br>1:300,000 E. | 64 ± 7<br>2.1 ± 0.2<br>55 ± 6 µg | — | — | | — |
| | | 16 L | 0.5% $B_O$<br>1 mg Buto.<br>Epin. | 62.5 ± 9<br>1.8 ± 0.2<br>0 | — | — | — | — |
| Abboud, et al. 1984 (203 | | (See Table 13–3 for detailed data on blood gases.) | | | | | | |
| Chestnut, 1990 (94) | | (See Table 13–5 for detailed data on blood gases.) | | | | | | |

(1) Epidural Techniques: St. LEB = Standard (T10–S5) Lumbar epidural block; Inter. LEB = Segmental (T10–L1) Lumbar epidural block; Inter. LEB →Sacral Bl. = Intermittent injection of local anesthetic initiated with segmental block, then gradually diffusing to lower lumbar and sacral segments
(2) Number of patients and Position: S = supine; L = lateral, during labor
(3) Local Anesthetic Used: $L_O$ = lidocaine alone; $L_E$ = lidocaine-epinephrine; $B_O$ = bupivacaine alone; $B_E$ = bupivacaine-epinephrine; $Chlor_O$ = Chloroprocaine alone; Fen. = fentanyl; Buto. = butorphanol
(4) Total Dose: Most given in milligrams (mg), but some given in micrograms (µg); NP = not published
(5) Numbers listed to nearest unit or decimal
(6) $BD_{ECF}$ = Base deficit extracellular fluid

rients in early active labor to assess the influence of different maternal positions in 16 and the effects of epidural anesthesia in another 16. The ratio of systolic peak to diastolic trough (S/D) of the umbilical blood flow velocity (UBFV) wave is reflective of vascular resistance distal to the point of measurement on the fetal side of the placenta. In 16 parturients, the S/D ratio was significantly lower in the lateral position than in the supine position, indicating that the umbilical artery vascular resistance (UAVR) was lower when the mother lies lateral. After epidural blockade (T9–10 to L1–2), the S/D ratio remained unchanged in three and decreased in 13 parturients, indicating that relief of labor pain beneficially affects the UAVR.

Giles and his associates (339) demonstrated a fall in the systolic/diastolic ratio following infusion of Hartmann's solution and continuous epidural analgesia with plain lidocaine, which they attributed to reduced resistance to blood flow and therefore beneficial. On the other hand, Long and associates (340) detected no significant change in the uteroplacental pulsatility index following fluid loading and epidural anesthesia for cesarean section. Reynolds (341) has pointed out that more accurate estimates of maternal flow in the lower part of the body can be made from measuring the dorsalis pedis artery using pulsed Doppler. Following positional changes in parturients with epidural blockade, changes in this artery are likely to reflect those in the uterine vessels. Janbu (342) measured changes in dorsalis pedis blood velocity that occurred consequent to labor pain and in the presence and absence of epidural analgesia. In the nonepidural group of parturients, there were marked fluctuations in velocity, while with epidural analgesia, flow was consistent and well maintained.

Others have used real-time ultrasound and a pulsed Doppler technique to measure fetal aortic or umbilical blood flow. Lindblad and associates (343) found that preloading, followed by continuous epidural analgesia/anesthesia with bupivacaine or etidicaine for cesarean section, had no significant effect on these parameters. Giles and associates (339), using continuous-wave Doppler, sug-

Fetus, and Newborn

| Blood Gases and Acid-Base Status[5] | | | | | | | | | | | | | |
|---|---|---|---|---|---|---|---|---|---|---|---|---|---|
| Fetal | | | | Umbilical Vein | | | | Umbilical Artery | | | | APGAR Score | |
| $Pa_{O_2}$ mmHg | $Pa_{CO_2}$ mmHg | pH | Base Defic. | $Pa_{O_2}$ mmHg | $Pa_{CO_2}$ mmHg | pH | Base Defic. | $Pa_{O_2}$ mmHg | $Pa_{CO_2}$ mmHg | pH | Base Defic. | 1 min ≥ 7 | 5 min ≥ 7 |
| — | — | — | — | 35 ± 6 | 38 ± 2 | 7.33 | −5.29 | 19 ± 6 | 45 ± 6 | 7.28 | −6.6 | 8.1 | 9.6 |
| — | — | — | — | 29 ± 6 | 37 ± 6 | 7.32 | −6.55 | 16 ± 6 | 49 ± 9 | 7.27 | −8.9 | 8.2 | 9.5 |
| | | | $BD_{ECF}$ | | | | $BD_{ECF}$ | | | | $BD_{ECF}$ | | |
| — | 46 | 7.27 | 4.4 | — | 43 | 7.30 | 5.8 | — | 52 | 7.23 | 4.8 | 97% | 98% |
| — | 44 | 7.29 | 4.8 | — | 44 | 7.29 | 5. + 8 | — | 53 | 7.24 | 4.8 | 86% | 99% |
| — | 52 | 7.20 | 7.0 | — | 42 | 7.32 | 6.0 | — | 52 | 7.25 | 6.0 | 95% | 97% |
| — | 45 | 7.32 | 2.6 | — | 42 | 7.29 | −6.1 | — | 51 | 7.24 | 5.3 | 8.5 | 9.7 |
| — | 46 | 7.32 | 2.2 | — | 44 | 7.29 | 5.1 | — | 52 | 7.25 | 6.1 | 8.5 | 9.8 |
| — | 52 | 7.20 | 7.0 | — | 42 | 7.32 | 6.0 | — | 52 | 7.32 | 6.0 | 8.5 | 9.4 |
| — | 42 | 7.34 | 4.7 | — | 38 | 7.26 | 11.6 | — | — | — | — | 8 | 8 |
| — | 32 | 7.33 | 5.7 | — | 45 | 7.17 | 11.6 | — | — | — | — | 100% | 100% |
| — | — | — | — | 31 | 36 | 7.34 | −6.5 | 20 | 42 | 7.26 | −7.0 | 79% | 100% |
| — | — | — | — | 29 | 36 | 7.32 | −6.6 | 19 | 47 | 7.23 | −7.0 | 78% | 100% |
| — | — | — | — | 29 | 37 | 7.33 | −7.9 | 20 | 47 | 7.25 | −8.0 | 88% | 100% |
| — | — | — | — | 30 | 37 | 7.32 | −5.5 | 25 | 41 | 7.6 | −5.9 | 7–81% | 100% |
| — | — | — | — | 32 | 33 | 7.35 | −6.3 | 25 | 40 | 7.3 | −6.9 | 7–89% | 100% |
| — | — | — | — | 28 | 36 | 7.35 | −4.3 | 22 | 35 | 7.3 | −6.4 | 7–89% | 100% |
| — | — | — | — | 26 ± 2 | 39 ± 2 | 7.3 ± 0.02 | −5 ± 0.7 | 18 ± 2 | 47 ± 2 | 7.25 ± 0.1 | −5.6 ± 0.6 | 7–88% | 100% |
| — | — | — | — | 27 ± 2 | 38 ± 1 | 7.32 ± 0.001 | −5 ± 0.5 | 17 ± 0.9 | 49 ± 1.5 | 7.26 ± 0.02 | −2.9 ± 1.2 | 88% | 95% |
| — | — | — | — | 28 ± 6 | 36 ± 5 | 7.33 ± 0.05 | −5.5 ± 2 | 16 ± 6 | 46 ± 6 | 7.3 ± 0.05 | −6 ± 2 | 83% | 100% |
| — | — | — | — | 27 ± 8 | 46 ± 6 | 7.32 ± 0.07 | −5.5 ± 2 | 16 ± 9 | 47 ± 8 | 7.22 ± 0.08 | −7.4 ± 4.3 | 82% | 100% |
| — | — | — | — | 26 ± 2 | 45 ± 1 | 7.34 ± 0.01 | −1 ± 0.4 | 20 ± 2.8 | 57 ± 3.4 | 7.26 ± 0.02 | −0.8 ± 1 | 76% | 95% |
| — | — | — | — | 30 ± 2 | 42 ± 2 | 7.33 ± 0.01 | −3 ± 0.9 | 21 ± 3.4 | 53 ± 4.3 | 7.25 ± 0.02 | −2.7 ± 0.8 | 88% | 95% |

gested that umbilical resistance was reduced by epidural analgesia achieved with plain bupivacaine, whereas, Veille, et al (344), recorded negative findings with chloroprocaine-epinephrine solution. Lindblad and associates (345) found that fetal aortic flow increased following epidural analgesia achieved with bupivacaine-epinephrine and with plain bupivacaine, but not following block with etidocaine-epinephrine prior to cesarean section. They also found that epidural analgesia during labor was associated with small increase in fetal aortic flow (346). A similar increase was seen in the control group but not in the group whose mother received meperidine, which obviously did not relieve labor pain effectively.

### *Effect on Cardiotocography*

For many years, changes in fetal heart rate and beat-to-beat variability have been used as an index of fetal well-being, but currently it is considered not such an important criterion of the condition of the fetus (341). Lavin and associates (347) found changes in fetal heart rate in 34 low-risk parturients receiving continuous epidural analgesia with bupivacaine or chloroprocaine and reported some increased beat-to-beat variability following bupivacaine, whereas the same group subsequently found that epidural analgesia with lidocaine was associated with tachycardia or loss of variability. Rickford and Reynolds (348) studied the fetal heart tracing in a series of 70 women before and for 30 minutes after epidural analgesia was established with bupivacaine, and found no change or improvement in 63 and loss of variability and advent of decelerations in seven, and in only two of whom was it found associated with maternal hypotension. Abboud and associates (93) reported occasional decelerations in the fetuses of 61 parturients receiving bupivacaine, chloroprocaine or lidocaine, most frequently with the former. Figures 13–27 to 13–29 depict the fetal heart rate and beat-to-beat variability noted by Abboud and associates (203,204). Nel (349) reported abnormalities, usually loss of variability, in the fetal heart tracing in 13 of 58 women given epidural analgesia achieved with bupivacaine. Reynolds (341) has come to the conclusion that, with the exception of the occasional dip apparently provoked by the initial injection of the local anesthetic into the epidural space, changes with bupivacaine are probably random and unimportant.

## *Neurobehavioral Evaluation*

### *Labor and Vaginal Delivery*

In the early 1970s, Brazelton (353) described a scale that could be used to evaluate neonatal changes in a standardized way within the first few days of life and subsequently used this to evaluate the effects of analgesics on the newborn that became known as the Brazelton Neonatal Neurobehavioral Assessment Scale (BNNAS). Soon thereafter Scanlon developed a neurobehavioral examination that combines standard neurologic testing and evaluation of the newborn response to repeated external stimuli and is considered a measurement of sophisticated central nervous system functioning (60), which he called the Early Neonatal Neurobehavioral Scale (ENNS). Later Amiel-Tison and associates (354) developed a Neurologic and Adaptive Capacity Scoring (NACS) system as another refined neurobehavioral assessment of the newborn.

Scanlon and associates (60) used the ENNS technique in evaluating the effects of local anesthetic on infants born of mothers who had received continuous lumbar epidural anesthesia achieved with lidocaine or mepivacaine. One group of nine parturients was given continuous lumbar epidural anesthesia with 1.5 to 2.5% lidocaine administered in four intermittent doses that totaled 423 ± 40 mg over a period of 3 hours, while a second group of 19 parturients were given 1.5 to 2.5% mepivacaine in three divided doses that totaled 374 ± 21 mg given over a 2½-hour period. They also used the ENNS technique in assessing the infants of 13 parturients, seven of whom received low spinal anesthesia while six did not receive any analgesia or anesthesia and were considered as the "control group." The ENNS assessment revealed that infants born of mothers given continuous lumbar epidural anesthesia had lower scores in attentiveness, greater muscular hypotonia, less vigorous motor and rooting responses, and altered decremental responses to pin prick than did the neonates born of mothers in the control group. A subsequent study published by Scanlon and collaborators (311), published in 1976, indicated that mothers managed with continuous lumbar epidural anesthesia achieved with 0.5% bupivacaine in two intermittent doses that totaled 112 ±7 mg over a 3-hour period revealed no neurobehavioral changes as compared to the control group.

The following year Hodgkinson, Marx and associates (355) used the Scanlon ENNS technique to evaluate effects on the newborn of analgesia and anesthesia given for labor and vaginal delivery in three groups: 1) thiopental-nitrous oxide in 45 parturients; 2) ketamine-nitrous oxide in 45 patients; and 3) lumbar epidural analgesia produced with 2% chloroprocaine in 127 mothers. Analysis of the results revealed that all infants weighing over 2500 grams had Apgar scores of at least 8 at 1 minute and 10 at 5 minutes. However, infants delivered of mothers who received chloroprocaine epidural analgesia had ENNS scores of 79 at day one and 88 at day two, compared with 71 and 74 among infants whose mothers had been given ketamine-nitrous oxide, and 50 and 64 among infants whose mothers had been given thiopental-nitrous oxide anesthesia. The difference between the group of infants born of mother given epidural analgesia and those of mothers who had been given ketamine or thiopental with nitrous oxide was highly significant ($p < 0.001$). In discussing the report by Hodgkinson, Marx and associates (355) and Brown (356), a member of the same group as Scanlon, also reported that 69 infants born of mothers who had been given chloroprocaine epidural analgesia had high ENNS scores in about 97% of infants compared to the same figures for 20 infants born of mothers given bupivacaine epidural analgesia, and scores of about 98% given no analgesia, which constituted the control that had been used by Scanlon, and also the data on lidocaine-bupivacaine used in Scanlon's report that showed that only half of the neonates had high scores.

Tronick, Brazelton and associates (357) used the Brazelton BNNAS system to evaluate neonatal neurobehavioral performance for as long as 10 days postnatally following maternal regional anesthesia with lidocaine and mepivacaine. Although changes in neonatal tone were demonstrated, they were transient and led them to conclude that they were of little or no clinical significance. Corke (358) used the Scanlon ENNS technique to evaluate infants of epidural analgesia achieved with 0.25 to 0.5% bupivacaine in 15 parturients and compared these with the effects of repeated doses of 100 mg of meperidine and 25 mg of promazine in 22 parturients and the results obtained in 14 parturients who received no analgesia or anesthesia during labor and delivery. They noted that the overall total for six tests, which would give a maximum score of 42, was 24 in the meperidine/promazine group, 30 in the no analgesia group, and 31 in the epidural group, again showing that bupivacaine had less effect on neurobehavioral scores than meperidine.

In another study, Wiener, Hogg and Rosen (359) compared the effects of continuous lumbar epidural anesthesia achieved with 0.5% bupivacaine, using a total dose of 130 mg for the entire labor and delivery given to 11 parturients with the results noted in 18 parturients given meperidine in doses of 100 to 300 mg (mean 183 mg) and those in 15 other parturients who were given a mean dose of 157 mg of meperidine and 200 μg of naloxone, which was given to the neonates intramuscularly at birth. They noted that bupivacaine had less effect on neonatal ventilation ($PaCO_2$) than meperidine, but had somewhat similar effects to the opioid on feeding behavior, general and elicited reflexes, and was associated with lesser muscle tone than the meperidine group only. Infants in the meperidine-naloxone group had at all times lower $PaCO_2$ and higher $V_{CO_2}$ indicating more metabolic activity than both the bupivacaine- and meperidine-only groups. Interestingly, there were no important differences between the two groups and in the values of umbilical venous pH at delivery and the Apgar scores at 1 or 5 minutes. On the hand, Rosenblatt and associates (360), using large doses of bupivacaine to achieve continuous epidural analgesia without preload, demonstrated rather variable and inconsistent decrement in attention and responsiveness scores, but an increase in muscle tone a few days after birth, suggesting that low doses of bupivacaine had some protective effect on the babies. It is to be noted that in most of these neurobehavioral studies carried out during the 1970s, lumbar epidural anesthesia was achieved with moderately large amounts of local anesthetics.

The reports by Scanlon and collaborators (60,311) that continuous lumbar epidural analgesia with lidocaine or with mepivacaine produced lower ENNS scores than with bupivacaine caused many obstetric anesthesiologists to avoid lidocaine for both labor and vaginal delivery for cesarean section. Because of the many advantages of lidocaine proven over many years of its use, this prompted Abboud and associates (91) to evaluate 1.5 to 2% lidocaine, 2% chloroprocaine, and 0.5% bupivacaine used for intermittent continuous lumbar epidural analgesia done in a very comprehensive study that included measurements of fetal heart rate, fetal heart variability, uterine activity, maternal blood pressure, newborn Apgar scores, neonatal acid-base status, and the ENNS. They found that none of the three local anesthetics used had any significant effect on either baseline fetal heart rate, beat-to-beat variability, or uterine activity but noted late or delayed deceleration patterns in 8 of 42 infants whose mother received intermittent bupivacaine, 0 of 34 who received intermittent chloroprocaine, and 3 of 47 of the fetuses that received intermittent lidocaine. These changes in fetal heart rate disappeared after repositioning the patient and administering oxygen and intravenous fluids, suggesting they were due to inadequate uterine blood flow. The ENNS did not differ among the three groups of neonates, nor did any of the neonates in the three groups score lower than a control group of 20 neonates whose mothers did not receive any analgesia or medication for labor and delivery. In the three studies, Abboud and associates evaluated the effects of the local anesthetic alone and the local anesthetic with additions of epinephrine (203–205). In these studies, they evaluated the condition of the fetus by using the NACS that had been proposed by Amiel-Tison and associates (354) and noted that the behavioral score was the same in the plain solution and the solution containing epinephrine 1:300,000.

Because in the first study (93) the total amount of lidocaine given was 240 ± 17 mg while in the Scanlon study it was 423 ± 40 mg, Abboud and associates (361) carried out a similar study on 22 parturients who received continuous lumbar epidural block with 1.5% lidocaine without epinephrine given frequently enough so that the total dose given was 446 ± 22 mg, and this produced mean plasma levels similar to those reported by Scanlon. Despite the fact that in this study by Abboud, et al the research produced doses that were comparable to those by Scanlon, et al, they found the status of the newborns delivered of these mothers to be the same as 17 neonates whose mothers did not receive analgesia, medication, or local anesthetic for labor and delivery. There was no significant difference in ENNS in the two groups of neonates. Abboud, et al concluded that lidocaine, even in larger doses, has no adverse effects on early neurobehavioral status of the newborn.

Kangas-Saarela, Jouppila and associates (362) studied neonatal effects for the first 4 to 5 days after birth in infants whose mothers had been managed with segmental epidural anesthesia achieved with bupivacaine and compared these with a group of neonates born of mothers who had not received medication. They found that the only significant difference was on day one when the babies born of mothers given epidural analgesia habituated and oriented better than controls.

The increasing use of the continuous infusion technique of low-dose local anesthetics and opioid has provided both direct and indirect benefits to the fetus and newborn. Hoyt and Youngstrom (363) showed that the combination of a dilute solution of bupivacaine and opioid had no effect on the neurobehavioral responses of the newborn while Mokriski et al (364) showed that epidural opioids had no effect on the variability of the fetal heart rate pattern. Because, as previously mentioned, the continuous technique provides more consistent and more stable analgesia and hemodynamic responses and consequently more stable maternal blood pressure, continuous infusion techniques should prove even more beneficial to the fetus and newborn than the intermittent technique. That such is the case was shown by Abboud and associates (93) who studied the effects of continuous epidural analgesia for labor and delivery using a continuous infusion technique on fetal heart rate, uterine activity, maternal blood pressure, Apgar scores, neonatal acid-base status, and NACS scores. None of the three local anesthetics used had any significant effect on baseline fetal heart rate or uterine activity, although bupivacaine had a higher incidence of variable and late decelerations in fetal heart rate that agrees with the previous study in which bupivacaine was administered intermittently (Figure 13–32). The neonatal outcome was invariably good as evaluated by the Apgar score, acid-base status, and the NACS system. Capogna and associates (365) found that the addition of fentanyl with bupivacaine did not affect neurobehavioral performance. The lack of any deleterious depressant effects on the fetus and newborn as measured by the Apgar score and acid-base status was also reported by Chestnut and associates (84) who used continuous epidural analgesia as previously described.

### *Elective Cesarean Section*

A number of studies of the neurobehavioral effects of epidural anesthesia used for elective cesarean section have been reported. Hollmen and his associates (366) examined infants of mothers who had received either standard general anesthesia or epidural anesthesia achieved with lidocaine epinephrine after colloid preload. As expected, they found that in the presece of maternal hypotension, during epidural anesthesia, infants had impaired rooting and sucking responses, muscle tone, and reflexes. Abboud and associates (317) compared epidural anesthesia with lidocaine or with chloroprocaine, with tetracaine subarachnoid block, and with general anesthesia. They found that adaptive capacity, tone, primary reflexes, and total NACS were worse after general anesthesia at 15 minutes and at 2 hours, but by 24 hours there was no difference among the four groups.

A number of other workers have also looked at the effect of different local anesthetics for epidural anesthesia. Kuhnert and her associates (367) claimed that the use of chloroprocaine provided the nearest thing to a drug-free control group because chloroprocaine is generally unmeasurable in newborns, and using the BNNAS cluster, compared this agent with lidocaine for both vaginal delivery and cesarean section. The changes they recorded were variable and lacked consistency, and they concluded that prenatal factors were more important than the choice of the local anesthetic. In a subsequent study, however, the same team (269) compared bupivacaine for cesarean section with chloroprocaine historical controls. They noted that bupivacaine babies performed better or improved their performance more rapidly than did the controls. Scores were not related to bupivacaine cord levels and were lower with prolonged dose-delivery intervals, confirming the extreme unlikelihood that these scores relate to any pharmacologic effect of the drug in the newborn (341). This was confirmed by the findings of Jani and associates (370) in a 1989 study in which they noted no difference in responses between babies born under subarachnoid block and epidural bupivacaine.

Kileff and associates (371) compared plain lidocaine with bupivacaine, and despite the use of large doses of lidocaine (which Reynolds (341) considered toxic amounts because several mothers reported dizziness and dyspnea), analgesia was inadequate in 6 of 23 patients given lidocaine, but hypotension was more frequent. Kileff, et al (371) reported that there was no difference in neurobehavioral scores between groups, but because this was after excluding 13 babies in the lidocaine group with low Apgar scores, need for special care as well as inadequate block, Reynolds (341) cast doubt on the results.

Marx, et al (350) noted that the time to onset of sustained respiration was shorter with regional anesthesia than with general anesthesia. While in a study of nearly 4000 neonates, Ong, et al (351) noted that following both elective and nonelective cesarean section (urgent delivery for dystocia and fetal distress), the Apgar scores of both at 1 minute and 5 minutes were lower with general anesthesia than with regional anesthesia. In addition, in instances of general anesthesia, there were greater requirements for intubation and artificial ventilation.

Evans, et al (352) underscored this in a 5-year study of 139 cesarean patients with epidural block compared to 471 cesarean patients with general anesthesia. Their findings concluded that no babies in the epidural group were depressed with Apgar scores less than 4 while 6.2% of babies in the general anesthesia group were depressed. Furthermore, only 4.3% of the epidural babies had Apgars in the 4 to 6 range compared to 15.4% of the babies of the general anesthesia group. It may be that general anesthesia by itself may be responsible for some percentage of the depressed infants born at cesarean section. Marx et al (350) in an early study found that neonatal depression appeared to be associated with the time of administration of general anesthesia and speculated that it was the time of greater saturation of the nitrous oxide that may be responsible. McDonald, in unpublished data of over 1000 cases from USC, found that by using a reduced nitrous oxide regimen, i.e., 50% nitrous oxide, and more rapid reduction to delivery times, that the percentage of depression could be reduced some. Nevertheless, it would seem prudent in light of all the aforementioned studies to urge greater use of epidural anesthesia for all types of cesarean section deliveries, i.e., elective and otherwise.

### *Indirect Benefit of Lumbar Epidural Analgesia*

The indirect benefits of continuous epidural analgesia by infusion to the fetus and newborn consist of providing the mother with more stable and more even relief of the pain and more stable blood pressure. The beneficial effects of relieving maternal pain are derived from elimination of hyperventilation during contractions and hypoventilation between contractions, as well as diminishing or eliminating the increase in catecholamines and other neuroendocrine stress responses to pain in the mother. Consequently, epidural analgesia obviates or minimizes the adverse maternal effects that otherwise might have an adverse impact on the fetus and newborn. By decreasing the intensity of the bearing-down efforts during the second stage of labor, it is not only beneficial to the mother by conserving her energy, but also epidural analgesia has been shown to decrease the incidence of retinal hemorrhages in the newborn. In a study of the incidence of retinal hemorrhages in the newborn, Maltau and Egge (372) assessed three groups of newborn infants within the first 72 hours of life. It was found that infants delivered by vacuum extraction had an incidence of retinal hemorrhages of 50%, among those delivered by forceps the incidence was 16%, and among those delivered spontaneously, retinal hemorrhages occurred in 41% of the cases.

Egge and associates (373) studied the influence of epidural analgesia on perinatal retinal hemorrhages in 100 cases, 50 of whom received epidural analgesia while the other 50 received conventional analgesia consisting of occasional dose of meperidine and nitrous oxide-oxygen analgesia. Although the second stage of labor was longer in the epidural group (which contained a higher number of primiparae than did the controls), they found that 81% of the epidural group had no retinal hemorrhage compared with 64% of the control group. Moreover, whereas among neonates born of mothers managed with epidural analgesia, only 5% had grade II and 1% had grade III retinal hemorrhages, while among neonates in the control group, the figures were 16% and 9%, respectively. They attributed the lower incidence in the epidural group to the fact that this type of anesthesia reduces the intensity of the bearing-down effort and produces adequate relaxation of the pelvic musculature.

Another important advantage is the fact that the fetuses and newborns benefit by epidural analgesia because it permits a more predictable and orderly delivery in a quiet and respectable environment in the birthing area. The dangers associated with forceps delivery are markedly diminished and less intracranial pressure differentials occur which decrease the degree of birth asphyxia. For these reasons, continuous epidural analgesia preferably combined with low caudal block (the double-catheter technique) is especially useful in cases of prematurity, postmaturity, and whenever maternal or obstetric complications are present and are likely to decrease placental efficiency or increase birth asphyxia. Forceps delivery when indicated result in less trauma to the neonate in a cooperative mother with a relaxed perineum. The use of such a sophisticated technique in consultation with the obstetrician who is managing the labor and delivery and the fetal monitoring and in consultation with the neonatologist who will be responsible for the important minutes and hours of that patient in the postnatal period is a fine example of cooperation among members of the obstetric team.

The value of continuous epidural analgesia to the fetus and newborn is further emphasized by a Canadian study of 10 university teaching hospitals in which the perinatal death rate in babies delivered without maternal anesthesia was 8.2% per 1000 compared with 4.9 per 1000 among those whose mothers were managed by various forms of regional anesthesia (374). In premature infants, the difference was even more striking: the perinatal mortality rate was 440 per 1000 when no anesthesia was administered compared 140 per 1000 when regional anesthesia was administered. These differences probably reflect a large number of precipitous or poorly controlled deliveries with subsequent fetal head injury when no anesthesia was used.

## *Fetal/Neonatal Complications of Epidural Analgesia/Anesthesia*

With the techniques currently used and the mother and fetus properly monitored, epidural analgesia/anesthesia has little or no adverse effects on the fetus and newborn. Indeed, in the presence of preeclampsia and other maternal or obstetric complication, epidural analgesia provides beneficial effects. In the past, the most frequent causes of maternal/fetal/neonatal complications included: 1) persistent untreated maternal hypotension, regardless of its cause; 2) uterine hyperactivity associated with poorly relieved severe pain; 3) oxytocin-induced uterine hypertonus and hyperactivity; 4) excessive doses of local anesthetics that may cause maternal systemic toxic reaction, or may rapidly transfer through the placenta to produce fetal depression; and 5) rarely accidental injection of the local anesthetic in the fetal scalp in the course of carrying out caudal block. Because most of these have already been mentioned and are discussed in detail in Chapter 16, only a few important points will be made here.

### Maternal Hypotension

It is well known that healthy parturients will tolerate systolic blood pressure of 80 to 90 mm Hg without ill effects to the brain, heart, and kidneys. The fetus, however, is highly sensitive to decrease in maternal blood pressure because there is no autoregulation of the uteroplacental circulation and intervillous perfusion, so that when maternal hypotension occurs, uterine blood flow falls linearly with blood pressure. The consequences of reduced uteroplacental blood flow depend on the degree and duration of the hypotension and the preexisting status of uteroplacental circulation in the fetus. When uteroplacental blood flow becomes inadequate, fetal asphyxia associated with consequent late decelerations and deterioration of the blood gases and acid base balance will develop (331,334–337).

The precise degree and duration of hypotension necessary to cause fetal distress seems to be variable. Hon, et al (334) and Bonica and Hon (375) found that, with maternal systolic pressure, less than 100 for about 5 minutes abnormal fetal heart rate patterns developed. Zilianti et al (376) reported that a systolic pressure of less than 100 mm Hg for 10 to 15 minutes usually leads to fetal acidosis and bradycardia. Moya and Smith (371) reported an increased incidence of low Apgar scores when maternal systolic pressure fell to between 90 to 100 mm Hg for longer than 15 minutes. Women who have had even greater falls in pressure, but were promptly treated, delivered vigorous neonates.

Because maternal hypotension is more likely to occur with the parturient in the supine position after receiving the epidural anesthesia (115,333–337,348,375–379), prompt treatment that includes changing the parturient to the lateral position, increasing IV fluids, and frequently giving the mother small intravenous doses of ephedrine will not only increase the maternal pressure but reverse the alteration of fetal heart rates. Many authors have shown that, promptly applied, this form of treatment obviates any deleterious effects on the infant, and that newborns will have high Apgar scores, normal acid base, and pH, and high neurobehavioral scores (115,140–145, 329–335,366,371). Decrease in uteroplacental blood flow with consequent deleterious effects on the fetus and newborn can occur even when maternal blood pressure in the upper limbs is normal. In such cases, compression of the lower aorta, iliac vessels, and uterine artery decrease uterine blood flow without affecting blood pressure in the upper limb. In such cases, one should suspect aortocaval compression and measure the blood pressure in a lower extremity and, if available, use a pulsed Doppler on the dorsalis pedis artery, mentioned previously. The etiology, pathophysiology, and therapy of these complications are discussed in greater detail in Chapter 16.

### Effects of Uterine Hyperactivity and Maternal Posture

Bromage (49) has emphasized the impact of severe pain associated with intense uterine contractions by comparing the results of a study in Lund, Sweden, where normal labor was hard and the pain unrelieved, with those of a study in Edmonton, Alberta, where labor pain was managed with regional anesthesia. In Lund, maternal pH was 7.36 and fetal pH 7.26 compared with figures in Edmonton of 7.45 and 7.39. Figure 13–33 depicts: 1) maternal and fetal pH values in a group of parturients given epidural analgesia for complete relief of pain in which pH was not depressed; 2) a group in whom severe pain associated with intense uterine contraction depressed maternal and fetal pH as secondary events: and 3) worst of all, the presence of severe pain, together with uterine hyperactivity in parturients in the supine position with partial aortocaval compression, showing that these affected primarily fetal pH. Bromage (49, p. 558) took this occasion to remind the reader that a great deal of past research on anesthesia and fetal acid base balance was published without this basic information, and, consequently, it is impossible to know what role the epidural (or other regional anesthetic) played in the development of profound fetal acidosis.

### Oxytocin Infusion and Uterine Hypertonus

In Chapter 4, mention was made that uterine hypertonus, occurring either naturally or more frequently by infusion of oxytocin in excessive amounts, is another nonan-

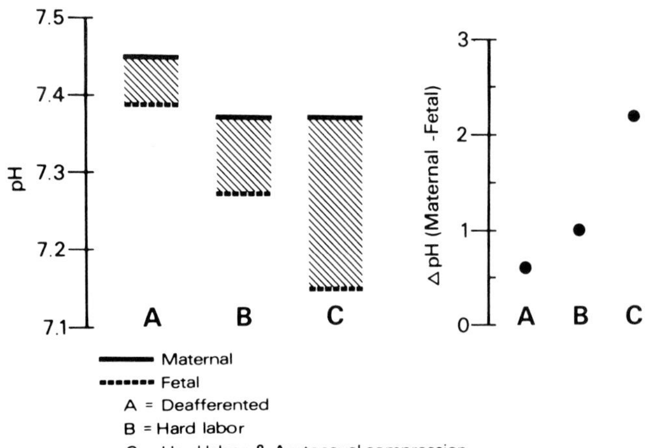


**Fig. 13–33.** Effects of muscular effort and supine posture on maternal and fetal acidosis. **A**). Labor with complete pain relief by epidural blockade with the patient in the lateral position does not depress pH in either mother or fetus. **B**. Hard labor depresses maternal pH and fetal pH falls as a secondary event. **C**. Intense uterine contractions (hard labor) and supine posture with partial aortocaval compression. Fetal and maternal pH fall in a time-dependent manner. (From Bromage PR: Epidural Analgesia. Philadelphia, W.B. Saunders, 1978, p. 569).

esthetic variable that may affect the fetus adversely. This problem is aggravated if the parturient is lying supine. Schifrin (378) examined the influence of oxytocin combined with epidural analgesia or general anesthesia in the supine position in a series of 360 parturients. Of this group, 119 parturients (group I) received neither analgesia/anesthesia nor oxytocin infusion; 135 parturients received epidural analgesia without oxytocin (group II); 65 parturients received epidural anesthesia combined with oxytocin (group III); and 41 parturients received oxytocin and systemic analgesics (group IV). The frequency of uteroplacental insufficiency (UPI) manifested by late decelerations in the fetuses, occurred in 16.8% in group I, 24.4% in group II, 40% in group III, and 27% in group IV. He noted that, in the supine position, when the fall in maternal systolic pressure was greater than 20 mm Hg during epidural anesthesia, 72% of fetuses developed late deceleration characteristic of UPI. Moreover, when uterine hypertonus developed during oxytocin infusion alone administered from a crude and rather unprecise manually controlled intravenous drip given at 10 mU/ml with rates of up to 20 mU/min, in these patients 50% of the fetuses, including 5 of 7 fetuses subjected to tetanic contraction, developed late decelerations. Prompt correction of oxytocin infusion and of the maternal hypotension by hydration and avoidance of the supine position caused prompt improvement of the fetal heart rate patterns. Fetuses of parturients in the supine position who had no analgesia nor oxytocin infusion had an abnormal fetal heart of 17%, whereas in fetuses whose mothers in the supine position received oxytocin and systemic analgesics, late decelerations occurred in 27%. In a subsequent unpublished study sent to Bromage (49), Schifrin reported that he had studied another group of parturients in labor on their side and administered oxytocin with a precise infusion pump. Fetuses in parturients who received epidural analgesia without oxytocin had late deceleration in less than 2% of the group, whereas in those whose mothers had received epidural analgesia and oxytocin, abnormal FHR occurred in less than 5%. In the other two groups, late deceleration did not occur.

## Excessive Amounts of Local Anesthetic

Excessive amounts of local anesthetic may adversely affect the fetus, either by producing maternal systemic toxic reactions alone or combined with transfer of excessive amounts into the fetus with consequent central nervous system and cardiovascular depression. Maternal convulsions, which may occur from accidental injection of the local anesthetic into a vein, impairs maternal respiration and circulation and invariably produces fetal asphyxia with resultant marked perinatal depression manifested by late deceleration and variable deceleration of fetal heart rate and fetal acidosis.

## Inadequate Obstetric Management

Birth asphyxia with consequent residual neonatal depression can occur if obstetric management is not diligent. For example, lack of spontaneous rotation due to a paralyzed perineal sling consequent to caudal or lumbar epidural anesthesia may prolong the second stage excessively and thus may cause an increase in degree of metabolic acidosis in the fetus. This is particularly important as when after the fetal head is on the perineum for a prolonged period of time without progress, the fetus is subjected to repeated compression during the uterine contractions. Because it has been estimated that one-third of fetuses have umbilical cord compression during the last phase of the second stage, this is likely to produce variable decelerations. In such cases of signs of UPI, the obstetrician should use the perineal relaxation to advantage and rotate the infant manually, and perhaps use outlet forceps to terminate the prolonged second stage, and, thus, this complication can be minimized or avoided. This is another nonanesthetic type of complication that is often attributed to the epidural analgesia/anesthesia.

## Accidental Fetal Local Anesthetic Intoxification

Finally, a rare complication of caudal analgesia is accidental fetal injection of the local anesthetic (see Figure 13–88, page 457). In 1965, Finster, et al (380) and Sinclair and associates (381) reported four such accidents. In each instance, the mothers were given epidural anesthesia administered by nonanesthesiologists who gave a total of 20 to 25 ml of 1.5% (300 to 375 mg) mepivacaine yet failed to produce pain relief. In three patients, fetal bradycardia occurred shortly after the first injection. All infants were delivered either spontaneously or with low forceps. Three of the babies were profoundly depressed at birth, with 1-minute Apgar scores being 1, 2, and 1, respectively. These infants were limp and unresponsive, had severe bradycardia, markedly dilated pupils, and did not breathe spontaneously. The fourth infant, more vigorous initially with a 1-minute Apgar score of 6, soon became apneic and manifested bradycardia within minutes. Immediately after artificial ventilation, the infants became pink but they remained apneic and unresponsive, and severe bradycardia continued. Convulsions occurred soon after the infants were oxygenated and continued intermittently for several hours. Visible puncture marks in the scalps of all four infants indicated that indeed an accidental injection of the local anesthetic directly into the fetuses had occurred. The first two infants died at 12 and 31 hours of age. Postmortem examination revealed needle tracks in the head and significant drug levels in the brain and blood. The third infant underwent a two blood-volume exchange transfusion; 24 hours later, the plasma drug level fell markedly, pupillary reactivity to light returned, heart rate increased to 140 beats per minute, and seizures stopped. The fourth infant underwent two exchange transfusions and three gastric lavages during the first 19 hours of life. Drug measurements in the wasted blood from the exchange transfusions and in the return from the gastric lavages contained significant amounts of local anesthetic. The third and fourth infants recovered fully: neurologic and electroencephalographic examinations 3 months later displayed no disorders and normal motor development in both infants. These cases emphasize two major points: First, major regional anesthesia should not be administered by obstetricians or other physicians without having been trained in these techniques under the supervision of an expert. Second, if a caudal block is used alone or as part of the double-catheter technique, the needle and catheter should be inserted early in labor when the fetal head is high. If severe perineal pain cannot be relieved with an already placed continuous lumbar epidural block, it is best to use a true (S2-S5) saddle (spinal) block by injection of 3 to 4 mg of tetracaine or 25 to 30 mg of lidocaine with the patient sitting for 45 to 50 seconds and then having her lie in a semi-Fowler's position with a lateral tilt for the delivery.

## *Conclusions about Clinical Applications*

### *Indications*

Properly carried out, continuous lumbar epidural block provides most parturients with continuous and complete intrapartum analgesia with little or no significant side effects or complications. In the early years, continuous caudal analgesia was used in some centers for 80 to 90% of parturients, while in others it was reserved for special cases. Today, continuous caudal is used in only a few centers for reasons given in the earlier part of this chapter. Therefore, much of the discussion about clinical application will deal with continuous lumbar epidural analgesia using modern techniques described in preceding pages. In some centers, the double-catheter technique is used to assure solid perineal analgesia during the second stage in a significant percent of the parturients, while in most centers, it is reserved for very special cases.

It is now the general consensus among obstetric anesthesiologists that continuous epidural analgesia properly carried out with correct monitoring of the mother and fetus is the best all around method of pain relief during childbirth. In addition to its use in normal labor, it is especially indicated whenever certain maternal, obstetric, or fetal complications exist. Because these are discussed in other chapters of this book, only reference to the most important reports will be made here.

### *Maternal Complications*

The absence of pain and the consequent reduction in anxiety and apprehension (without having to resort to opioids or sedatives) makes it particularly useful in the following maternal complications:

1. Congenital or acquired heart disease in which epidural analgesia reduces the load imposed on the cardiovascular system by pain and neuroendocrine stress response (This topic is discussed in detail in Chapter 31).
2. Pregnancy induced hypertension (PIH). Epidural analgesia/anesthesia is useful not only because it provides superior analgesia but dampens or attenuates the hypertensive response to pain, control of the hypertension is facilitated, intervillous blood flow is improved, renal blood flow is improved, excellent analgesia is provided for elective forceps delivery if this is indicated, and the fatigue associated with maternal expulsive efforts in the second stage can be obviated. This subject is discussed in detail in Chapter 25.
3. Essential hypertension and pulmonary hypertension are also indications for continuous epidural analgesia for labor and vaginal delivery because they dampen the aggravation of the hypertension by blocking the pain-induced catecholamine release. This is further discussed in Chapters 25 and 31.
4. Endocrine disorders: Diabetes is a common medical problem during pregnancy that requires optimal obstetric and anesthesiologic care. The aim is to optimize placental blood flow and blood glucose levels during labor and delivery and avoid hypotension to minimize fetal acidosis. These and other issues are discussed in detail in Chapter 32.
5. Renal or hepatic disease in parturients is another indication for continuous epidural analgesia provided their overall management takes account of both the renal disease and the obstetric welfare. Fluid balance must be managed carefully during labor and hypotension avoided, especially the hypertensive patient with renal transplant. Similarly, parturients with hepatic disease derive benefit from continuous epidural analgesia, provided that maternal blood pressure is maintained near normal limits. These subjects are discussed further in Chapter 34.
6. Pulmonary disease, of which asthma is the most commonly encountered in obstetric patients, is another indication for epidural analgesia by infusion, which is probably better than intermittent technique because avoidance of episodes of pain prevent periods of hyperventilation that can precipitate wheezing. Most other respiratory disorders, such as bronchitis, bronchiectasis, and common cold are best managed with epidural blockade for labor or

operative delivery. These and other pulmonary disorders are discussed in Chapter 33.

7. Neuromuscular disease: Epidural blockade is especially indicated in any condition in which a rise in intracranial pressure during labor and delivery would be dangerous. Management of the analgesia must be meticulous, and continuous infusion is preferable to avoid episodes of pain-induced rise in intracranial pressure. Patients who are paraplegic or quadraplegic may not require analgesia for labor, but if pain is present it is the procedure of choice because it will prevent or minimize the incidence of reflex muscle spasms. Management of the blood pressure may prove difficult due to autonomic dysfunction, but close monitoring and the appropriate use of drugs will minimize this problem. Controversy may still surround the use of epidural blockade in patients with multiple sclerosis, but provided they are properly informed preoperatively, there is no reason to deprive them of this superior quality of pain relief achieved with epidural analgesia. Epidural blockade is indicated in most patients with neuromuscular disorder unless there is an associated severe cardiomyopathy or respiratory insufficiency. Epileptic patients benefit from epidural blockade, but opioid analgesia is best avoided to minimize the likelihood of attacks during labor and to allow continued use of anticonvulsants. These subjects are discussed in more detail in Chapter 36.

In those with the necessary experience and expertise, the double-catheter technique is particularly suitable in managing parturients with any of these disorders and the following fetal conditions (349).

### *Fetal Conditions*

Epidural analgesia is indicated in breech deliveries and in multiple pregnancies, whether these are done by the vaginal route or cesarean section. These are discussed in detail in Chapters 41 and 42.

Continuous epidural analgesia/anesthesia with a single or, better still, a double-catheter technique has special indication in cases of prematurity, postmaturity, multiple births, fetal distress from depressant factors, or any other situation that requires that opioids, sedatives, and general anesthetics be avoided. See Chapter 28 for detailed discussion.

### *Obstetric Complications*

Continuous lumbar epidural block, using the double-catheter technique, if the anesthesiologist has the necessary skill and experience is especially indicated in: (1) prolonged labor due to primary cervical dystocia or abnormal uterine contractions as already mentioned; (2) induction of labor; (3) forceps delivery; (4) breech delivery; (5) any other obstetric complications that place great stress on the mother and thus may impact deleteriously on the fetus and newborn. It has already been mentioned that continuous lumbar epidural analgesia is especially

**Table 13–9.** Contraindications to Lumbar Epidural Analgesia/Anesthesia

1) Parturients who refuse the block or have great fear of puncture of the spine. In our experience, many patients who are concerned initially about epidual block will consent to be managed with this technique provided they are properly informed. However, if they still refuse, it is an absolute contraindication to the technique.
2) Lack of skill by the administrator, not only in carrying out the procedure, but in the management of the parturient and in the prompt treatment of complications.
3) Infection at the puncture site or in the epidural space.
4) Severe hypovolemia from hemorrhage, dehydration, or malnutrition.
5) Coagulopathies.
6) Lack of resuscitation equipment in the immediate area ready for *prompt* use.
7) In addition to the above, absolute contraindication to continuous caudal epidural anesthesia are infection or cyst in the area of the sacrococcygeal region and having the presenting part close to the perineum.

*Relative Contraindications Include:*

8) Lack of appreciation by the obstetrician as to how the procedure influences the management of labor.
9) A very rapid or precipited labor, or in any case which requires immediate anesthesia. On the other hand for the anesthesiologist who is very skilled and has had extensive experience, extension of the epidural block in patients who have had the catheter in place during labor can be done as rapidly as getting things ready for anesthesia (172).
10) Cephalopelvic disproportion unless the block is used for a trial of labor prior to cesarean section.

**Table 13–10.** Advantages and Disadvantages of Regional Analgesia/Anesthesia

*Advantages:*

1) In contrast to opoids, regional analgesia produces complete relief of pain in most parturients.
2) The hazards of pulmonary aspiration of gastric contents that is inherent in general anesthesia is diminished and can be even eliminated.
3) *Provided it is properly administered* and no complications occur, regional analgesia/anesthesia causes no serious maternal or neonatal complications.
4) Administered at the proper time, it does not impede the progress of labor at the first stage.
5) Continuous techniques can be extended for delivery and may even be modified for cecarean section if this becomes necessary.
6) Regional analgesia permits the mother to remain awake during labor and delivery so that she can experience the pleasure of actively participating in the birth of her child.
7) Regional anesthesia for cesarean section also permits the mother to be awake and immediately develop bonding with the newborn.
8) Provided the mother is doing well, the anesthesiologist can leave her and resuscitate the newborn if this is necessary.

*Disadvantages:*

1) Regional techniques require greater skill to administer than do administration of systemic drugs or inhalation agents.
2) Technical failures occur even in experienced hands.
3) Certain techniques produce side effects (e.g., maternal hypotension) that if not promptly and properly treated can progress to complications in the mother and fetus.
4) Techniques that produce perineal muscle paralysis interfere with the mechanism of internal rotation and increase the incidence of posterior positions and thus require instrumental deliveries.
5) These procedures can only be carried out in the hospital.

**Table 13–11.** Requisites for Optimal Results with Regional Anesthesia

1) Anesthesiologists must know well the pain pathways of labor, the pharmacology of local anesthetics and must have acquired sufficient skill and experience with the technique and know how to manage the patient after regional analgesia has been established.
2) Anesthesiologists must know the possible complications, their prevention and their prompt therapy.
3) *None of the regional techniques should be begun without an intravenous infusion running, giving a preload amount of fluids and having all monitoring equipment in functioning order.*
4) *None of the regional procedures should be begun without having equipment for treatment of complications and for resuscitation immediately available and ready for prompt use.*
5) Each regional technique has contraindications which must be observed.
6) Except in circumstances in which the use of regional technique is especially indicated and provides significant advantages over all other methods, it should not be used against the wishes of the parturient.
7) Regional analgesia should not be started until the cervix is 3 to 4 cm in multiparae and 4 to 5 cm in primiparae, contractions are strong—last 35 to 40 seconds or more and occur at an interval of 3 minutes or less. The only exception to this rule are with patients who have experienced extreme pain during the latent phase of labor or with patients in whom labor has been induced and maintained with oxytocin.
8) During and following administration of analgesia, the parturient should be given attention continuously and must be carefully observed, and her blood pressure, pulse, respiration measured every ½ minute during the first 15 to 20 minutes and every 5 minutes thereafter.
9) Continuous monitoring of the fetal heart rate must be available.
10) All patients should be given psychological support by every member of the obstetric team, but particularly the anesthesiologist and spouse if present.
11) In patients who are unusually nervous and anxious, a mild sedative should be given intravenously, whereas if the patient experiences pain the regional anesthesia should be supplemented with either inhalation analgesia or intravenous opioids in small doses.
12) The anesthesiologist must have time, skill and willingness to supervise the patient properly. If it is necessary to have a nurse anesthetist supervise the patient, he/she must have the knowledge and skill to fulfill all of these requisites.

indicated in patients who have impairment of uterine placental blood flow or the placental circulation.

## *Contraindications*

The absolute and relative contraindications are listed in Table 13–9.

## *Advantages And Disadvantages*

Because this is the first chapter on regional anesthetic techniques, we first summarize the advantages of the major regional anesthetic procedures and compare these to systemic opioid and adjunctive drugs, inhalation analgesia/anesthesia, and general balanced anesthesia (Table 13–10). To achieve the advantages and stated objectives, i.e., effective maternal pain relief with little or no risk to her or the infant, it is essential for the physician to fulfill the requisites listed in Table 13–11. Table 13–12 compares lumbar epidural analgesia with subarachnoid block. Table 13–13 then compares lumbar epidural block with caudal block in general terms. Comparison among the various techniques of epidural anesthesia will be presented in Chapter 13 to B.

**Table 13–12.** Comparison Between Lumbar Epidural Block with Subarachnoid Block

ADVANTAGES OF EPIDURAL ANALGESIA/ANESTHESIA

1. Incidence of magnitude of maternal hypotension less because slower onset of vasomotor block → more time to mobilize compensatory mechanisms.
2. No postpuncture headache unless dura perforated accidentally.
3. Theoretically less risk of neurologic sequelae (rare even when subarachnoid block).
4. Theoretically less risk from continuous catheter in extradural space than in subarachnoid space.
5. Continuous epidural block technique permits use of analgesic concentration during the first and early second stage:
   a) Less or no effect on perineal sling → less interference with internal rotation.
   b) Better bearing–down efforts.

DISADVANTAGES OF EXTRADURAL ANALGESIA/ANESTHESIA:

1. Technique more difficult than subarachnoid block, requires more skill, precision, and experience to insert needle bevel into the extradural space and to insert a catheter.
2. It carries the risk of accidental intravenous injection with consequent systemic reaction, or accidental high subarachnoid block if the amount is injected into the subarachnoid space.
3. Onset of analgesia/anesthesia slower, and therefore cannot be initiated for emergency cesarean section or in a patient who is ready to deliver.
4. With the older technique more (3 to 4 times) local anesthetic injected:
   a) Fetal/neonatal depression may occur.
   b) Greater risk of maternal systemic toxicity.
   c) Greater risk of accidental total spinal anesthesia.
5. With the current methods of continuous epidural analgesia disadvantage #4 is obviated.

**Table 13–13.** Comparison of Lumbar Epidural Block and Caudal Block

ADVANTAGES OF LUMBAR EPIDURAL BLOCK:

1. Less local anesthetic required.
2. Onset of uterine pain relief faster because injection site nearer to uterine sensory fibers.
3. Less risk of infection: more difficult to keep skin clean over sacral hiatus than skin over lumbar region.
4. No risk of puncturing rectum or fetal head.
5. Less anatomic anomalies in lumbar spine than sacrum.

DISADVANTAGES OF LUMBAR EPIDURAL BLOCK:

1. Greater risk of dural puncture → more risk of postpuncture headache.
2. Greater risk of accidental subarachnoid injection → total spinal.
3. Occasional inadequate diffusion to sacral segments → deficient perineal analgesia/relaxation (decrease risk by injecting final dose in Fowler's or sitting position).

# B. TECHNICAL CONSIDERATIONS OF EPIDURAL ANALGESIA/ANESTHESIA

## INTRODUCTION

This section constitutes the second part of the discussion of epidural analgesia/anesthesia for obstetrics and can be considered the sequence of the preceding Chapter 13-A. The material is divided into four major sections: (1) lumbar epidural block; (2) caudal epidural block; (3) double-catheter technique; and, (4) management of the mother and newborn. Sections one and two contain discussion of the following subjects: 1) the anatomic, physicochemical, and pharmacologic bases of epidural block; 2) general principles in the preparation of the gravida for the analgesia/anesthesia; 3) general principles of regional anesthetic techniques that must be adhered to achieve optimal results; 4) description of each specific technique of lumbar epidural block, caudal epidural block, and the double-catheter epidural block using local anesthetics alone or the combined use of these agents with opioids; 5) description of the technique of epidural anesthesia for cesarean section considered under section one; and 6) monitoring of the mother, fetus, and newborn during labor and vaginal delivery, and the postpartum care of the mother. Because this last topic is discussed in detail in Chapter 23, only those points relevant to epidural analgesia/anesthesia will be made here.

With the exception of the first edition of this book and the book by Aboulesh (382) and Albright (383), other textbooks on obstetric anesthesia omit discussion of these basic aspects. And because this material should be well known to obstetric anesthesiologists and to anesthesia residents rotating in obstetric anesthesia, these aspects are included here for those members of the obstetric team who have not been exposed to this information. Moreover, because during the past decade there has been a great surge of interest in carrying out laboratory and clinical research on the anatomic bases of lumbar epidural neural blockade that is critically important to the success of the technique, they are presented in this chapter in detail. Another reason for presenting basic information is that our experience reveals that technical errors are committed even by some well-trained anesthesiologists who have not learned such critically important details such as the anatomy of the epidural space, and this ignorance has led to failures and complications. Finally, due to the trend in the mid-1960s to discontinue the use of continuous caudal and replace it with lumbar epidural blockade, many anesthesiologists trained during the past quarter century have not been taught and, consequently, have not acquired the skill and experience essential to carry out a successful caudal blockade. This is unfortunate because it precludes consideration of the use of the double-catheter technique that some other authors (49,63,90,252) consider to be "very difficult" trauma, "impractical," as "inserting the needle into the sacral canal is very painful," " associated with a high failure rate" and "high risk of complications." However, as mentioned in the preceding chapter, a number of problems with single-catheter lumbar epidural block, of which inadequate perineal pain is the most frequent, can be obviated by using the double-catheter technique. It is hoped that in this chapter we describe the technique that minimizes all of the "disadvantages" mentioned above so that the technique will be used more frequently.

## Lumbar Epidural Block

### *Anatomic Bases*

#### Vertebral Column

The vertebral column is composed of 33 tightly packed vertebra, held together with a number of ligaments, which in the standing erect position, presents four curves: the cervical, thoracic, lumbar, and sacral. In the supine position, the region of the fourth and fifth lumbar vertebra is the highest part, and the sixth thoracic and second sacral vertebra the lowest parts of the column. The curves of the spinal column play an important role in the spread of the local anesthetic in the subarachnoid space, but play little or no role in epidural bloc (384). Here we focus our attention to the anatomic aspects of the lower thoracic and lumbosacral vertebral column as depicted in Plate A (Figure 13–34) and in Figures 13–35 and 13–36 that, together with the legend, provide detailed description of the most important points related to epidural analgesia. As may be noted in both Plate A (Figure 13–34) and Figure 13–35, the spinous processes of the lower thoracic vertebrae are somewhat rounded, whereas those of the lumbar vertebrae are thick, broad, somewhat quadrilateral, 3 to 4 cm long and projecting posteriorly and slightly anteriorly making an angle of about 70 to 80° with a longitudinal axis on the caudad side. The free posterior edge of the spinous process of the lumbar vertebra is a rough, uneven rectilinear prominence about 3 cm high and thickest below where not infrequently it is notched (Figure 13–45A and C). The laminae are broad, flat, and thinner than the pedicles, and the posterior surface of each limina slants so that its upper portion is considerably deeper from the skin than its lower portion, a fact of clinical importance.

Between adjacent spinous processes, there are the interspinous spaces, and between the two (pair) of laminae of adjacent vertebrae there are the interlaminar spaces (Figure 13–36). These spaces provide the most practical avenues of entrance into the spinal canal with a needle to achieve epidural or subarachnoid block. In the normal (upright) position, these spaces are somewhat pear-shaped, being wider below and apical above.

### *Ligaments*

Figures 13–37 and 13–38 provide an overview of all of the ligaments of the lumbosacral part of the vertebral column. The most important ligaments related to epidural anesthesia are the supraspinous and interspinous ligaments, the ligamenta flava, and the posterior longitudinal ligament.

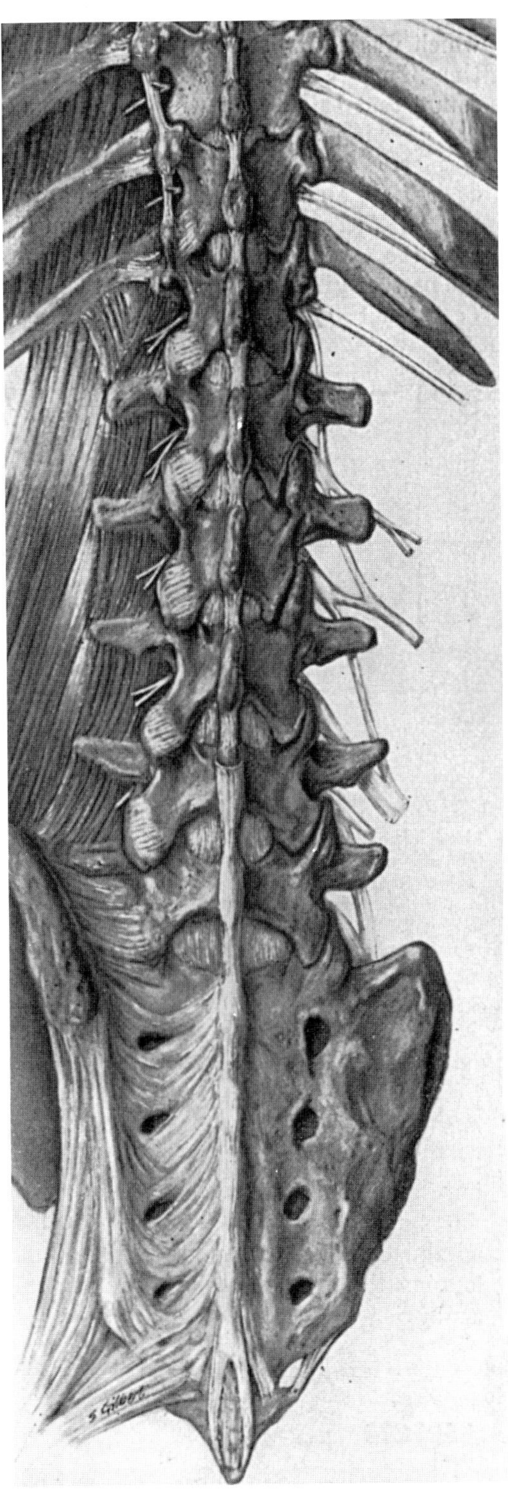

**Fig. 13–34.** Posterior view of the lower thoracic and lumbosacral parts of the vertebral column showing ligamentous structures that must be traversed by a needle inserted into the spinal canal that contains the epidural space. Note the shape of the posterior end of the spinous processes, which are quadrilateral with their lower posterior edge being thick (1 to 1.5 cm). The supraspinous ligament is shown connecting the spinous process of the fourth and fifth lumbar vertebrae with the midline crest of the sacrum. The interlaminar space is shown deep to the spinous processes and is covered by the ligamentum flavum. The midline approach to the epidural space entails penetration of the skin, supraspinous ligament, interspinous ligament, and ligamentum flavum, whereas the paramedian approach is just lateral to the spinous process through the paraspinal muscles, which have been removed in the specimen. The illustration also depicts the relationship of the transverse processes of the lumbar spine to the lumbar plexus and lumbosacral trunk. Note also the posterior sacral foramina through which the posterior division of the sacral nerves pass posteriorly to supply bones, ligaments, and muscles of the low back. This is a first of four illustrations of the lower part of the vertebral column noted in subsequent pages.

### *The Supraspinous Ligament*

The supraspinous ligament is a strong fibrous cord that connects the apices of the spinous processes of all of the vertebrae from the lower most portion, which covers the sacrococcygeal hiatus, to the tip of the seventh cervical vertebra where it continues cephalad to the external occipital protuberant as a ligamentum nucha (384). This ligament is thicker and broader (1 to 1.5 cm wide) in the lumbar area than in the thoracic region and is composed of three layers of fibers: the most superficial fibers extend over three or four vertebrae, those coursing more deeply pass between two or three vertabrae, and the deepest ones connect the spinous processes of neighboring vertebrae and become continuous with the interspinous ligament (385).

### *The Interspinous Ligament*

The interspinous ligament runs obliquely between adjoining spinous processes, attached to the lower border of the spinous process above, through the upper border of its caudad neighbor, and is continuous posteriorly with the tough supraspinous ligamen (384–387). A study of the transverse section from the mid-lumbar region shows that it is narrower posteriorly and in much of its course, but as it approaches its anterior part, it splays out anterolaterally in the sagittal plane to become continuous with the posterior fibers of the two parts of the ligamentum flavum forming the vertex of the midline sulcus.

### *The Ligamenta Flava*

The yellow ligament is composed of two halves, each of which is attached to a lower half or lower third of the anterior surface and the lower border of the lamina above and passes caudad to be attached to the posterior surface and upper border of the lamina below (Figures 13–37, 13–38, 13–39). The anterolateral border extends from the intervertebral foramen where it blends with the capsule of the joint between the articular process and then proceeds posteromedially to end where the two laminae join. In most individuals, the two bands of ligamenta lie at an angle of less than 90° to each other with a discreet gap between the medial borders that allows passage of small veins and otherwise filled with fat (386–388). Although this vertical slit between the medial border of the two bands has been known for nearly a century and emphasized in the 1920s by Bertocchi (388), it has been ignored by virtually every textbook, including some ana-

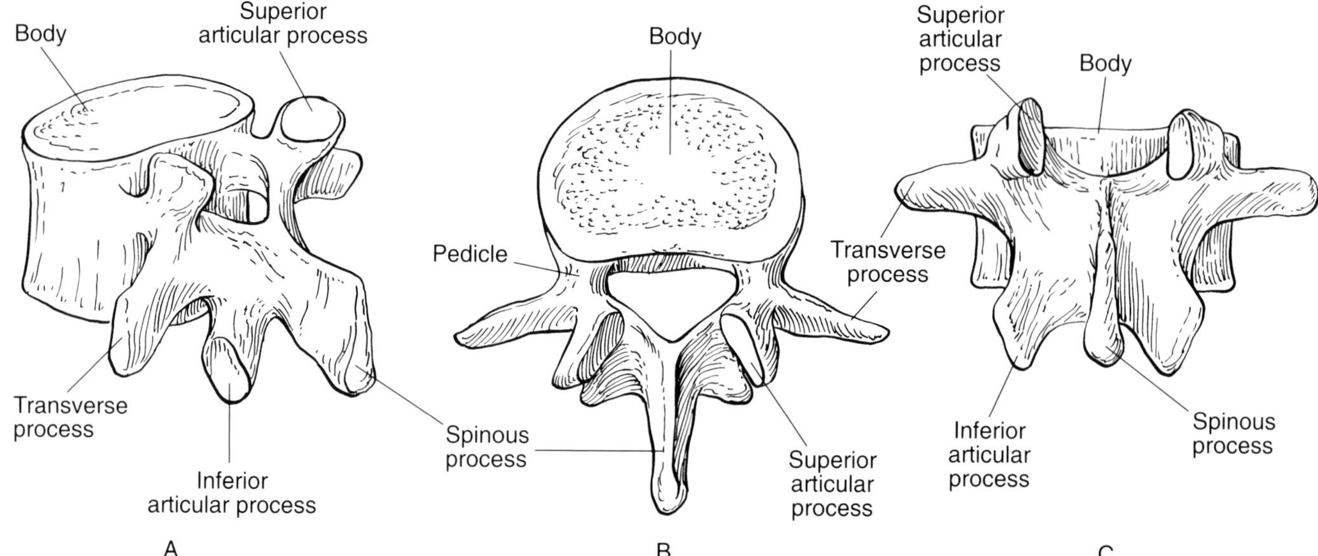


**Fig. 13–35.** Anatomy of the lumbar vertebra. **A**: Lateral view. **B**: Superior inferior view. **C**: Superior (cranial) aspect. The body is wider transversely than anteroposteriorly. The cranial (superior) and caudal (inferior) surfaces are flat or slightly concave, while the sides of the centrum are definitely concave. It is of interest to note the quadrilateral shape of the spinous processes which are thick, broad, and ending posteriorly in an uneven border that is thickest caudally where it is occasionally notched. **B** shows the shape of the laminae which are broad, short, and strong, and the vertebral canal is triangular in shape and larger than in the thoracic spine. **B** and **C** show the thick, broad spinous processes, which are about 2.5 to 3 cm long, about 1 to 1.5 cm thick, and 2 to 2.5 cm high. (From Bonica JJ: The Management of Pain, 2nd ed. Philadelphia, Lea & Febiger, 1992, p. 1396).

tomic treatises (394,395), which consider the ligamentum flavum as a continuous structure running the entire length of the interlaminar space.

The presence of this vertical slit is of significant importance to epidural anesthesia. Anatomic, radiologic, magnetic resonance imaging, epiduroscopy, and computerized tomography studies during the past decade have provided more precise descriptions of the anatomy of these two bands of ligamentum flavum (386,387). Each of the two bands is rectangular in shape, about 20 mm in width (with a range of 12 to 22 mm), 17 mm high (with a range 13 to 20 mm), and 3 mm thick (with a range of

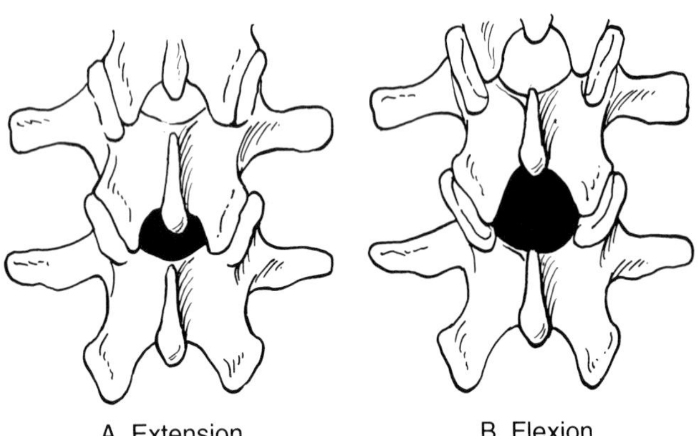


**Fig. 13–36.** Simple schematic view of lumbar vertebrae showing the shape of the interlaminar space with the lumbar spine in normal position **(A)** and in a flexed position **(B)** which significantly increases the size of the space.

2.5 to 5 mm) (386,387,389,392,393). The angle formed between the internal surfaces of the two nearly contiguous ligamenta flava is about 70° with a range of 60° to 85° (389,390,392,393)

## *The Posterior Longitudinal Ligament*

The posterior longitudinal ligament (PLL) extends along the posterior surface of the body of the vertebra from the axis to the sacrum and contributes to the anterior wall of the vertebral (spinal) canal. This ligament is intact and broad throughout the length of the vertebral column until it reaches the first lumbar vertebra where it begins to narrow progressively, so that on reaching the last lumbar and first sacral interspace, it is only one-half of its original width.

## *Nerve and Blood Supply of the Lumbar Spine*

The lumbar spine and the contents of the spinal canal are supplied by the meningeal (recurrent) nerves, which are derived from the spinal nerves, and by the articular and ligamentous branches, which are derived from the posterior primary division (384,385). These nerves are shown in Figure 13–40, which contains a description of the articular and meningeal nerves in the legend.

***Blood supply.*** Each lumbar vertebra is supplied by a pair of segmental lumbar arteries that arise from the aorta and are accompanied by the venous system (384,385) as shown in Figure 13–41 and described in the legend. Figure 13–42 depicts the connections between the internal and external plexuses and the inferior vena cava, and pos-

Ligamentum flavum
Intervertebral disk
Supraspinous ligament
Post. longitudinal ligament
Interspinous ligament
Anterior longitudinal ligament
A
B
Pedicle (cut)
D
Ligamentum flavum
Synovial joint
Posterior longitudinal ligament
Intervertebral disk
Anterior longitudinal ligament
C

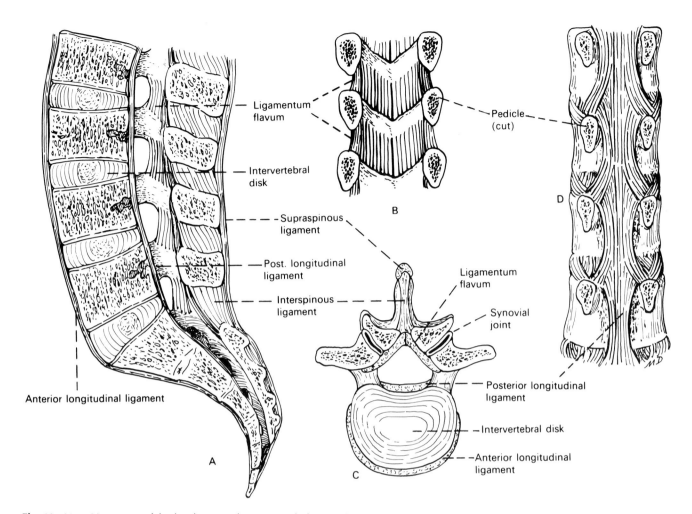

**Fig. 13–37.** Ligaments of the lumbar vertebra. **A**: Medial sagittal section of three lumbar vertebra and their ligaments. The supraspinous ligament is a strong fibrous cord that connects the apices of the spinous processes of the vertabrae. The interspinous ligaments are thin and membraneous and interconnect the adjoining spinous processes with their attachment extending from the root to the apex of each spinous process. **B**: Anteroposterior view from the inside of the spinal canal showing the ligamenta flava and their attachment to adjacent laminae. Note the slit between the two halves of the ligament for passage of small veins and arteries and often occupied by fat. **C**: Superior view of the lumbar vertebrae showing the position of the various ligaments in the lumbar region, including the anterior longitudinal ligament, which covers the anterior surface. **D**: The posterior longitudinal ligament, which covers the posterior surface of the vertebra and the ligamentum flavum (see text for additional information). (From Bonica JJ: The Management of Pain, 2nd ed. Philadelphia, Lea & Febiger, 1992, p. 1398).

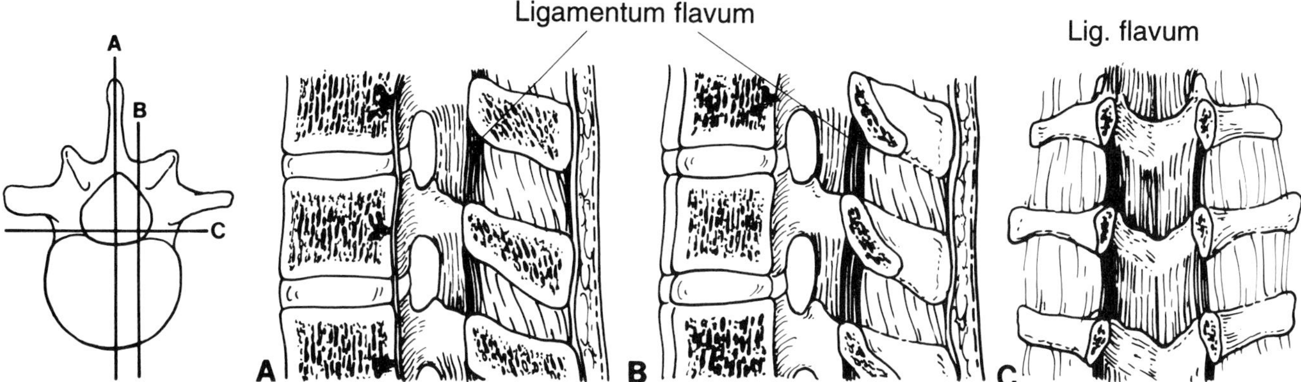


**Fig. 13–38.** Anatomy of the ligamenta flava. **A** and **B** show sagittal sections to demonstrate the attachment of the ligamentum flavum to the anterior surface and lower border of the lamina above and the superior border of the lamina below. **C**: Anteroposterior view of the spinal canal showing the attachments of the ligamenta flava.

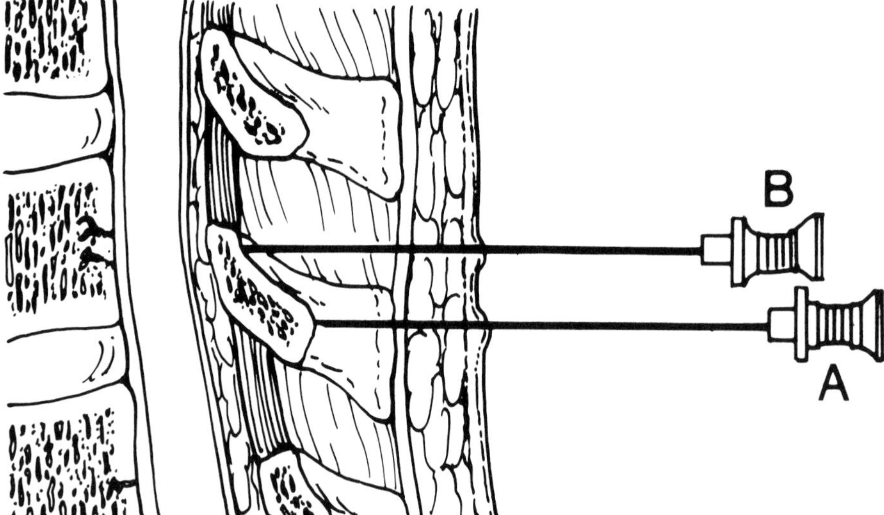


**Fig. 13–39.** Sagittal section of the spinal column with tips of needles contacting the superior part of the lamina **(A)** which is deeper than the inferior part **(B)**. [Modified from MacIntosh RR: Lumbar Puncture and Spinal Anesthesia. Edinburgh. E.S. Livingstone, 1957).

sible sites of obstruction of the latter, which cause engorgement of the internal vertebral venous plexus as occurs in pregnancy.

### *Vertebral (Spinal) Canal*

The vertebral (spinal) canal extends from the foramen magnum to the sacrococcygeal hiatus where it is covered by sacrococcygeal ligament. It is bounded anteriorly by the posterior surface of the vertebral body, intervertebral disk, and overlying posterior longitudinal ligament, laterally by the pedicles, laminae, ligamenta flava, and the lateral vertebral ligaments, and posteriorly by the anterior surfaces of the vertebral arches, liminae, and the ligamenta flava. Its shape and size vary in different parts of the vertebral column to conform to the shape of the spinal cord: it is oval and large in the cervical region, round and cylindrical in the thoracic region, triangular prismatic in the lumbar region, and prismatic and semilunar in shape in the sacral region (389,394–396). In the cervical, thoracic, and first lumbar vertebral level, it accommodates the two enlargements of the spinal cord. The diameters of the canal in the thoracic region are 17 mm transversally and 17 mm anteroposteriorly, while in the lumbar region they are 23 and 18 mm, respectively. The size of the canal is about twice the size of the spinal cord (384).

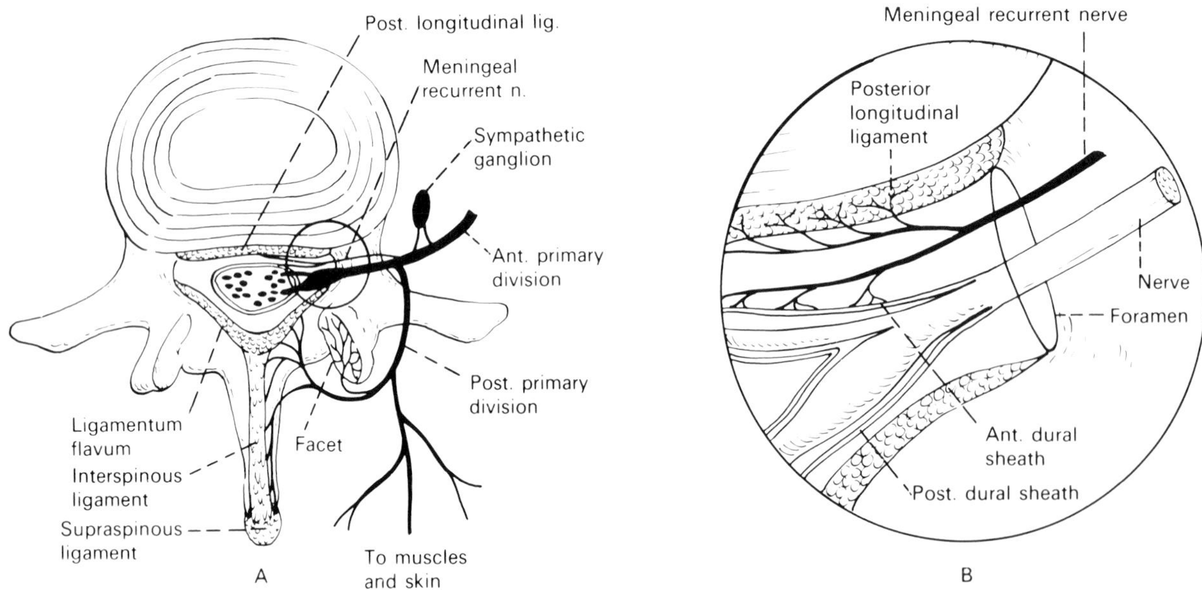


**Fig. 13–40.** Nerve supply to the lumbar vertebrae, consisting of the meningeal branch of the spinal nerve and the articular branch of the posterior primary division. **B**: Enlargement of the part circled in **A** showing details of the distribution of the meningeal recurrent nerve, also called the recurrent nerves of Luschka, which supply many structures within the spinal canal and also the longitudinal ligaments. These nerves arise from the spinal nerves close to, or in common with, the rami communicantes and consist of both somatic afferent and sympathetic fibers.

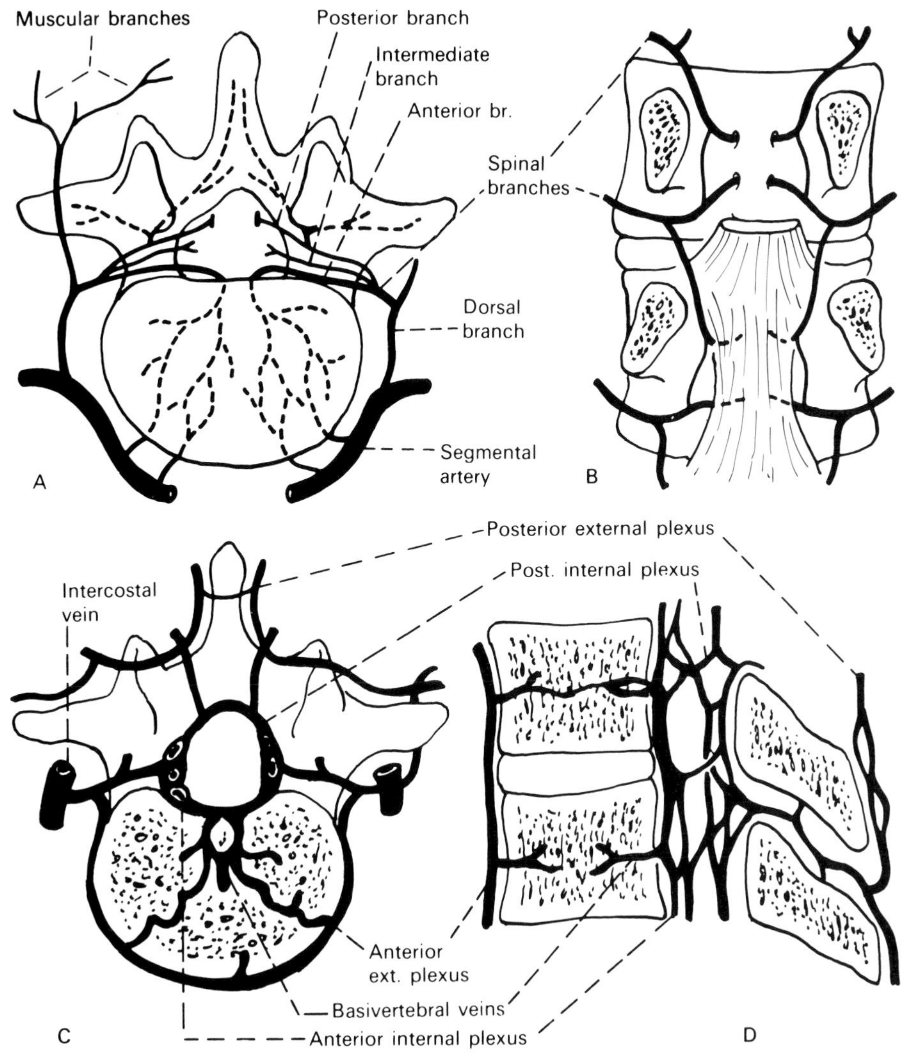


**Fig. 13–41.** Blood supply to a lumbar vertebra. **A**: Inferior view of a lumbar vertebra surrounded by the two segmental arteries derived from the aorta. These contribute branches that pass through the anterior surface of the body and, importantly, provide the spinal branch, which breaks up into three branches that supply the body of the vertebra, the contents of the spinal canal, and the ipsilateral lamina and spinous process. The posterior branch also gives off branches that supply the paravertebral muscles and cutaneous tissue. **B**: Posteroanterior view of the body of the vertebra showing arterial branches to the vertebral bodies. The cut surfaces of the pedicles are recognizable, and part of the posterior longitudinal ligament has been removed. **C**, **D**: Venous drainage of the vertebrae by the external and internal vertebral venous plexuses. Note the complex drainage within the spinal canal and the body of the vertebra.

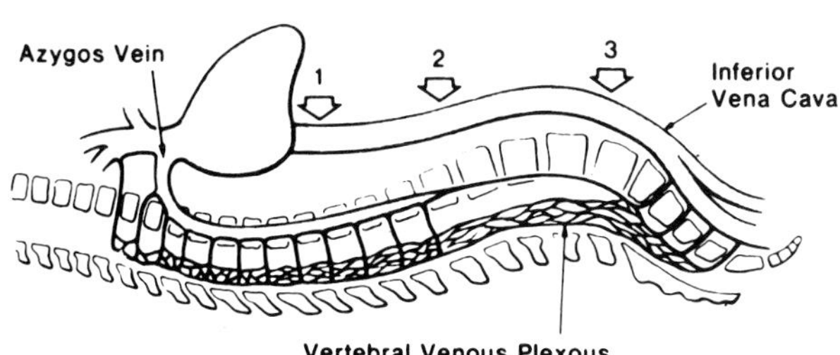


**Fig. 13–42.** Epidural veins (vertebral venous plexus) and their connections with inferior vena cava (IVC) and azygos vein. Epidural veins are protected from compression by the vertebral canal; thus, obstruction to IVC results in rerouting of venous return by way of epidural veins, and thence to the azygos vein above the level of obstruction. Some common sites of IVC obstruction are shown: 1) below the liver (e.g., severe ascites); 2) thoracolumbar junction (e.g., abdominal pressure) in prone position; 3) pelvic brim (e.g., pregnancy). (Modified from Bromage P.R.: Epidural Analgesia. Philadelphia, W.B. Saunders, 1978. Reproduced from Cousins MJ, Bromage PR: Epidural neural blockade, in: Neural Blockade in Clinical Anesthesia and Management of Pain, 2nd ed., edited by MJ Cousins, PO Bridenbaugh. Philadelphia, J.B. Lippincott, 1988, p. 271).

## *Spinal Cord*

The spinal cord in the adult occupies the upper two-thirds of the vertebral canal, being continuous above with the brain stem and ending below in a conical extremity, the conus medullaris, usually at the level of the lower border of the L1 vertebra (Figures 13–43 and 13–44). Because the cord is a great deal shorter than the vertebral column in adult life, the spinal cord segments do not lie exactly opposite the correspondingly named vertebrae. As a result of this unequal growth between the spinal cord and spinal column, the spinal nerve rootlets and roots course laterally in the upper two or three cervical vertebral levels, but course more and more obliquely in a caudad direction from their points of origin in the spinal cord to the same intervertebral foramina through which they made their exits in the fetus before the vertebral column lengthened. Thus, the lumbar, sacral, and coccygeal nerves descend vertically, occupying the subarachnoid space below the conus medullaris in a voluminous group of fibers, the cauda equina (Figure 13–44).

The spinal cord presents two fusiform enlargements: an upper or cervical enlargement, which extends from the C3 to the T2 vertebrae and corresponds to the attach-

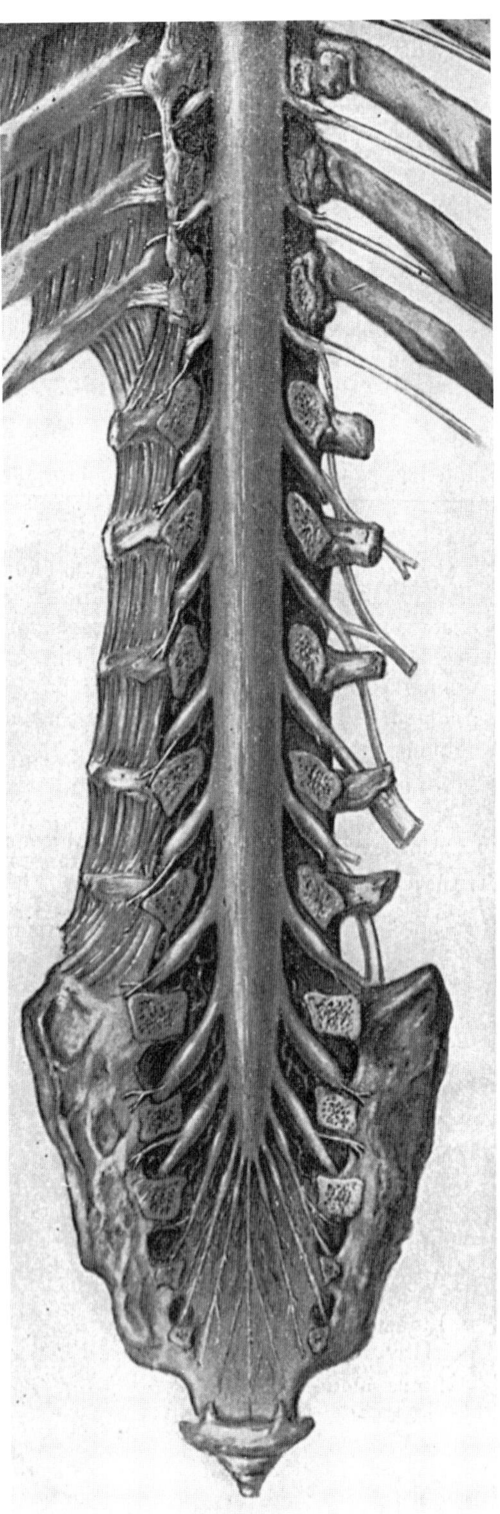

**Fig. 13–43.** View of the dural sac after removal of all structures contained in the epidural space (see Figure 13–47).

The sac ends at the level of S2. Each nerve root passes peripherally and is contained in its own dura-arachnoid cuff (see text for details).

ments of the nerves that supply the upper extremities, and a lower, lumbar enlargement, which extends from the T9 to the upper border of the L1 vertebrae and corresponds to the attachments of the nerves that make up the lumbar and lumbosacral plexuses and their branches that supply the lower extremities. Below the lower enlargement, the spinal cord tapers rapidly into the conus medullaris from whose apex a fibrous cord, the filum terminalae, arises. The latter descends first inside the dura and then extradurally in the sacral canal to become attached to the posterior surface of the first coccygeal vertebra.

## The Spinal Meninges

***The Pia Mater.*** The pia mater is a thin, delicate vascular membrane intimately adherent to the spinal cord, dipping into all its depressions, carrying with it the numerous blood vessels that nourish the cord, and forming their adventitial tissue. The pia ensheaths the spinal nerve roots, forming a sleeve-like investment that extends as far as the intervertebral foramen. In addition, it sends out prolongations laterally, anteriorly, posteriorly, and inferiorly, all of which reach and become attached to the arachnoid dura.

***The Arachnoid Mater.*** The arachnoid mater is a thin, delicate membrane that loosely invests the spinal cord, each of the spinal nerve roots, and the accompanying blood vessels as far as the intervertebral foramen. It also invests the denticulate ligaments and the septum posticum. The spinal arachnoid is continuous with the arachnoid membrane of the brain, and below it, it widens out and invests the cauda equina. It is on the inner surface of the dura mater with a potential space between the two coverings known as the subdural space, which contains serous fluid between the surfaces of the opposed membranes. The spinal arachnoid does not communicate directly with the subarachnoid space but continues a short distance along the nerve roots, possibly communicating with lymph spaces and venous channels (Figure 13–45). The subarachnoid space, which exists between the arachnoid and pia mater, is filled with cerebrospinal fluid. Crossing the space and connecting the two membranes are many trabecullae, which form a sponge-like mass in the subarachnoid space that results in the formation of innumerable channels that are lined by mesothelial cells and that aid mixing of any fluid injected into the subarachnoid space. The subarachnoid space and its fluid contents encircle the spinal cord along its length, being continuous below the conus medullaris as the cisterna terminale and continuous above with the cranial subarachnoid space.

***The Dura Mater.*** The dura mater, covering the spinal cord, is a tough fibroelastic tube cylindrical in shape that forms a loose sheath around the spinal cord. It is composed principally of longitudinal connective tissue fibers with a proportionately small amount of circular, yellow elastic tissue fibers. The spinal dura mater extends from the foramen magnum to which it is closely adherent by its outer surface to the S2 vertebra where it ends in a cul-de-sac (Figure 13–43). Below this level, the dura mater closely invests the filum terminale and descends to the back of the base of coccyx where it fuses with the perio-

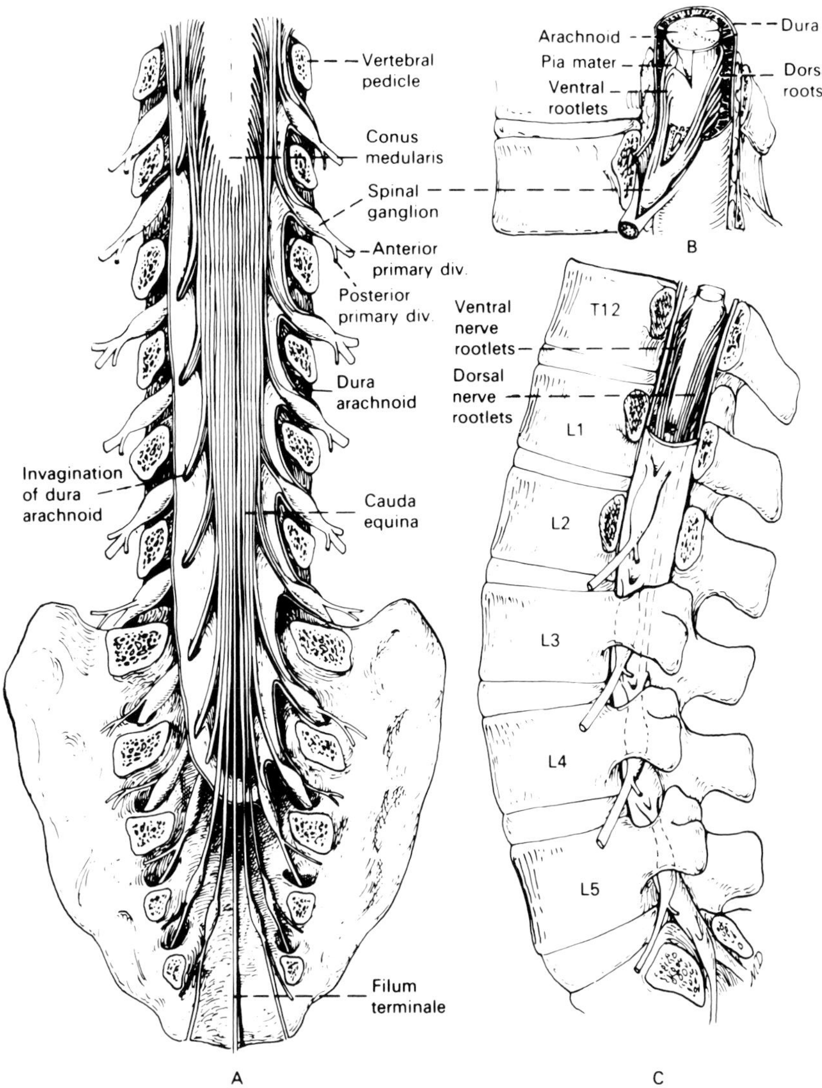


**Fig. 13–44.** Anatomy of the lower part of the spinal cord. Detailed anatomy of the nerve rootlets and roots of the lumbar, sacral, and coccygeal nerves. **A** Posterior view. **B.** Lateral view at midthoracic vertebral level. **C.** Lateral view of the lumbar spine. The rootlets and roots of the lumbar, sacral, and coccygeal nerves course some distance before they leave the spinal canal. Gathered from their respective rootlets, they proceed caudad toward their respective interver-tebral foramina and traverse the subarachnoid space within the dura-arachnoid sac in their own separate dura-arachnoid sleeves. As the nerve roots of the lumbar nerves descend in the spinal canal they cross the disk immediately above the foramina through which they exit and then enter the foramina beneath the pedicles. After entry into the foramina on their extravertebral course each root invaginates the dura-arachnoid and carries the sheath of each into the foramen, so that each of the two roots has its own separate investment of dura-arachnoid as far as lateral to the spinal root ganglion where the roots unite. At this point the two separate sheaths likewise merge so that the formed spinal nerve is invested by a single sheath, which continues for a short distance before it fuses with the epineurium of the spinal nerves. Within the foramen part of the dura fuses with connective tissue and thus anchors the dural sleeve to protect the nerve root from being stretched during movements of the spine. **C.** Within the foramen the smaller anterior (motor) root is located anteriorly and inferiorly near the intervertebral disk. After leaving the foramina the lumbar nerves incline caudad, laterally and slightly anteriorly. The roots and dorsal ganglia of the S1, S2 and S3 nerves lie in sheaths immediately external to the arachnoid-dura cisterna or cul de sac, while the roots and ganglia of the S4, S5, and coccygeal nerves lie within their sheaths in the bony sacral canal at a considerable distance from the dural cul de sac. (From Bonica, JJ, The Management of Pain, 2nd Ed, Philadelphia, Lea & Febiger, 1990, p. 1413.)

steum. The thickness of the spinal dura mater is between 1.5 and 2 mm in the cervical region, is about 1 mm thick in the thoracic region and thinner as it proceeds to and in the lumbosacral region (397). However, throughout its entire length, the dura mater is thicker in its posterior aspect than the anterior aspect, and this is especially true in the posterior midline. Moreover, the dura surrounds anterior and posterior roots, becoming progressively thinner as it proceeds through the intervertebral foramina, and becomes continuous with the epineural and perineu-

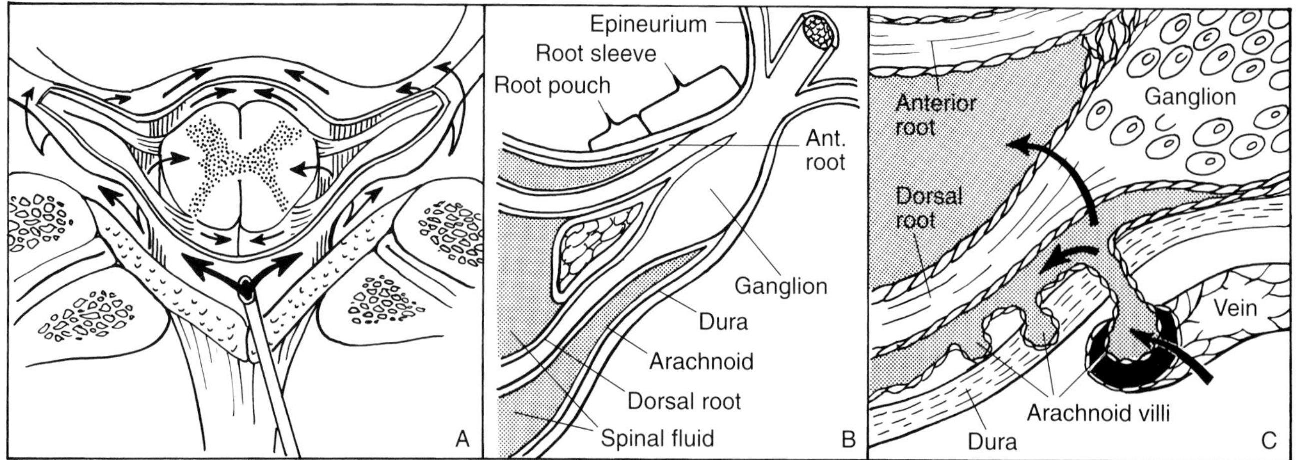


**Fig. 13–45.** Spread of local anesthetic solution following epidural injection, shown in **A**. The arrows indicate the horizontal spread of the anesthetic. Major spread posteriorly to the region of the root sleeve or "dural cuff," which is soon followed with entry to the cerebrospinal fluid (CSF) and spinal cord, as well as into the anterior epidural space. **B**: Detailed anatomy of the root sleeve and root pouch as well as the anterior and posterior roots invested in their own dura arachnoid until they fuse to become the peripheral nerve at the distal end of the root sleeve. **C**: Enlarged view of the dural cuff region showing rapid entry of the local anesthetic into CSF by way of arachnoid granulations (villi), many of which protrude through the dura and contact the epidural veins. (Modified from Cousins MJ, Bromage PR: Epidural neural blockade. *In*: Neural Blockade in Clinical Anesthesia and Management of Pain, 2nd ed. Edited by MJ Cousins, PO Bridenbaugh. Philadelphia, J.B. Lippincott, 1988, p. 256).

ral connective tissue of the formed nerve. The dura mater, like the arachnoid and pia mater, sends out sleeve-like prolongations that surround each posterior and anterior spinal nerve roots (Figures 13–44, 13–45).

Each spinal nerve root receives a special, separate investment of dura-arachnoid and pia mater (Figure 13–45). Thus, the anterior and posterior roots, as they approach each other, are encased in separate sheaths as far as the lateral extremity of the spinal root ganglion where the two roots unite. At this point the three separate sheaths (pia, arachnoid, and dura) likewise merge, so that the formed spinal nerve is invested by a single sheath that continues for a short distance before it fuses with the epineurium of the nerve. These prolongations occasionally extend beyond the intervertebral foramina. The arachnoid covering of each root has a special feature consisting of proliferation of arachnoid cells forming villus structures of different types (shown in Figure 13–45).

The meningeal prolongations around the roots and formed nerves are usually short in the upper part of the vertebral column but gradually become longer and longer below, enclosing the roots of the lower spinal nerves. The roots and dorsal ganglia of the S1, S2, and S3 nerves lie in sheaths immediately external to the cul-de-sac, while part of the roots and ganglia of the S4, S5, and the coccygeal nerves lie within their sheaths in the bony sacral canal at a considerable distance caudad to the lower end of the cisterna terminalis (Figure 13–44).

The dura mater is connected to the walls of the spinal canal by fibrous connective tissue strands, which are shorter and stronger anteriorly, and thinner, weaker, and longer posteriorly. Blomberg (398,399) and Blomberg and Olson (400) have used a 2.2-mm epiduroscope to study the epidural space and noted the presence of a strong midline fibrous band. Blomberg found the structure, which he called the dorsomedian connective tissue band, in 96% of autopsy subjects (398) and 8 of 10 live humans prior to partial laminectomy for herniated lumbar disc. This dorsomedian connective tissue band is a strong posterior midline band that attaches the midline dura to the ligamentum flavum (Figure 13–46).

***Special Features of the Spinal Dura.*** In 1963, Luyendyjk (401) described what he called "plica mediana dorsalis durae matris" in the lumbar region for the median translucency seen on a postero-antero projection in periduragraphy consisting of radiologic examination following injection of contrast material into the epidural space which was interpreted as a middle fold of the dura mater. Subsequently, various methods have been used to identify this anatomic feature, including studies on cadavers in which ink or resin have been injected into the epidural space (402–405) by Blomberg (398–400) with the use of the aforementioned 2.2-mm diameter epiduroscope into the epidural region to visualize the various structures, and by the use of computerized tomography after epidural injection of a contrast medium (405,406). Although all of these techniques succeeded in demonstrating the presence of such structures as the fold of dura mater and dorsomedian connective tissue band, all of these techniques require distortion of the anatomy by the injection of a substance into the epidural space regardless of the material. Gaynor (387) and Westbrook, et al (406) point out that these have not been described in anatomic studies, nor by unenhanced computerized tomography or MRI, so that a definite conclusion cannot be made.

In this regard, it is important to differentiate between Luyendyjk's (401,403) plica of the dura, which is apparently an artifact, and fibrous bands that extend posteriorly between the dura and the ligamentum flavum. These are different structures and should not be confused with each

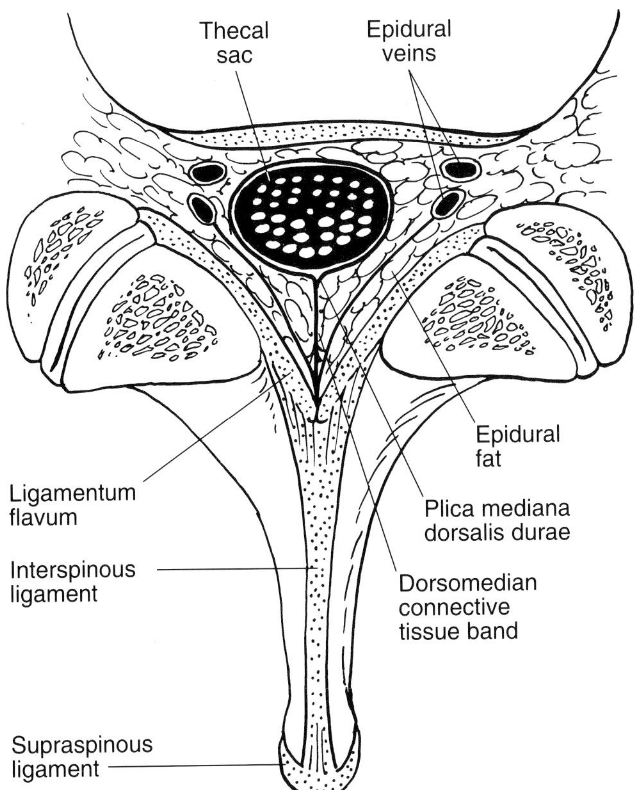


**Fig. 13–46.** Cross section of lumbar vertebra depicting various structures, noted by Savolaine and associates who used CT extradurography in 40 subjects. Note the thecal sac containing the nerves that make up the cauda equina. He also noted the dorsomedian fibrous band and mistakenly called this the plica medianus dorsalis durae. Note also fibers that separate the fat in the epidural space and communicate with epidural veins. The interspinous ligament is thin and splays on the ligamentum flavum anteriorly and posteriorly contacts the supraspinous ligament. [Modified from Savolaine BR, et al: Anatomy of the human epidural space: new insights using CT epidurography. Anesthesiology 68:217–220, 1988).

other. Such bands can be strong enough to impede the cephalad progress of epidural catheters. Although Savolaine (405) using CT extraduragraphy in 40 subjects described the plica medialis dorsalis as being present in 38 of the specimens, they were inappropriately using the term to describe the posterior midline fibrous band and not a true fold of dura (Figure 13–46). As with other studies that did not involve the injection of fluid into the extradural space, this study showed no evidence of a true plica medialis dorsalis durae. Westbrook, et al (406) have concluded that previous descriptions of the plica by a number of workers have been the result of partial collapse of dura by injected contrast of polyester resin or on opening the extradural space at surgery. Under these circumstances, the fibrous bands support the mid-portion of the dura giving the impression of a dural fold.

### The Cerebrospinal Fluid

The cerebrospinal fluid (CSF) is a colorless, transparent, watery fluid, a form of lymph, that is found in the arachnoid space surrounding the entire central nervous system and in the ventricles of the brain. It has a specific gravity of about 1.0065 and is mildly alkaline in reaction (pH 7.6). Of the total volume of 120 to 150 ml of fluid in the average adult, 20 to 35 ml of CSF is in the spinal portion of the subarachnoid space. Because the makeup of CSF is discussed in detail in the next chapter, it is omitted here.

### Subdural Space

The subdural space, between the dura and arachnoid, is a potential space containing a film of serous fluid between the surfaces of the opposing membranes. It does not communicate directly with the subarachnoid space but continues a short distance along the nerve roots, possibly communicating with lymph spaces and venous channel (391,408). In former years, it was thought that the two membranes were so close together that it would be impossible to penetrate the dura without also penetrating the arachnoid. However, in the course of diagnostic myelography, a number of workers noted sometime ago that some of the contrast media would be located in the subdural extra-arachnoid space. Anesthesiologists began to hypothesize that partial subdural injection might be the cause of failure in subarachnoid anesthesia or epidural anesthesia. Indeed, in 1977 Mehta (408) reported a series of epidural anesthetic blocks performed by trained anesthetists and showed with the radiologic technique that the position of the Tuohy needle was partially subdural in seven cases. More recently, Blomberg (407) carried out a study using spinaloscopy in 15 autopsy subjects and found that in 10 of the cases the space opened up with ease, and that the bevel of an 18-gauge Tuohy needle introduced into the subdural space could be visualized in 8 of 13 cases. Whether this is applicable to parturients is unknown, but it should be considered as a cause of inadequate epidural analgesia.

## Anatomy of the Epidural Region (Space)

The epidural space is the interval between the periosteum lining the vertebral canal and the dura mater surrounding the canal in its extension from the foramen magnum to the lower end of the dural sac (Figure 13–47). Superiorly, it does not extend beyond the foramen magnum, where the dura attaches to the entire circumference of the foramen, and thus forms a coarse barrier to any fluid moving cephalad. The epidural space is bound anteriorly by the posterior longitudinal ligament of the vertebral bodies; laterally, by the pedicles and the 48 intervertebral foramina which permit it to communicate with the paravertebral spaces and which contain the anterior and posterior roots and the formed nerve; posteriorly, by the laminae and ligamenta flava; and inferiorly, by its continuation with the sacral canal (Figure 13–48) (discussed in the next section).

### Size of the Epidural Space

The size of the epidural space varies greatly. The anterior portion is very narrow (1 mm) throughout the length of the canal because the dural tube tends to hug the ante-

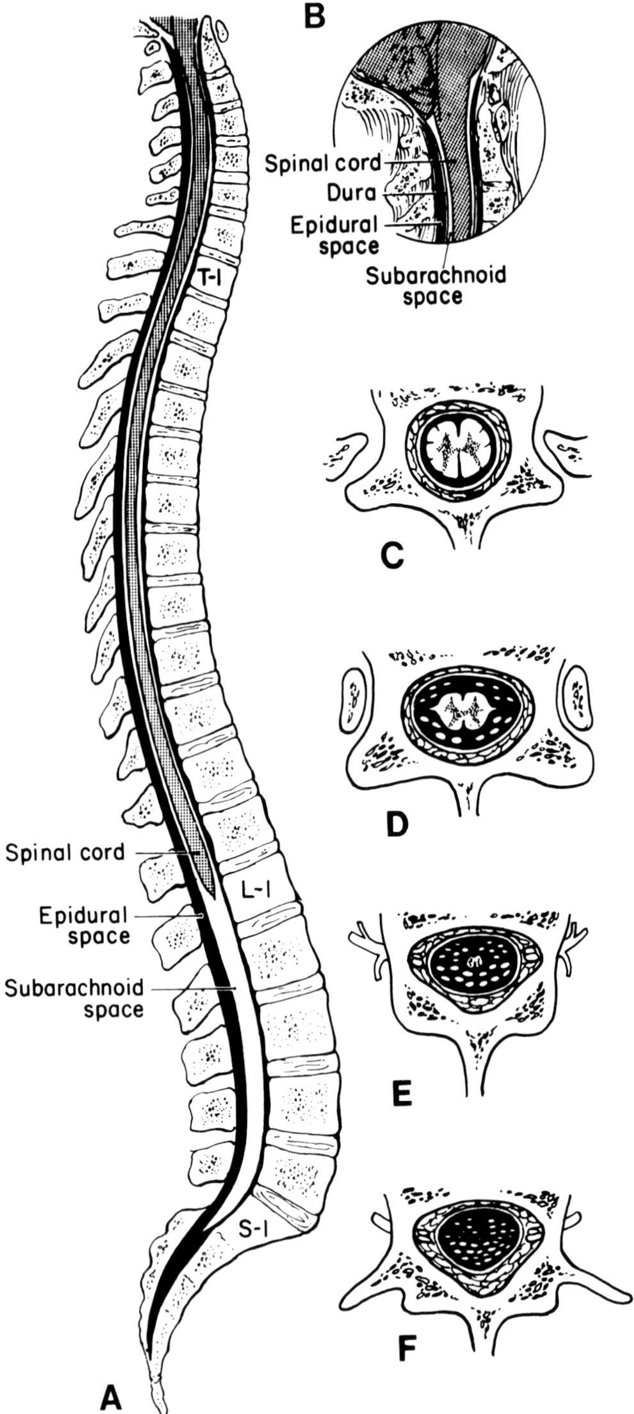


**Fig. 13–47.** Schema depicting the epidural space in the sagittal plane, **A**. Its cephalad termination is around the foramen magnum where the dura-arachnoid fuses with the dura-arachnoid of the cranial cavity **(B)**. **C**: A cross section of the spinal canal at T8, D at T10, E at the first lumbar, and F in the sacral region. [Section C-F modified from MacIntosh RR: Lumbar Puncture and Spinal Anesthesia. Edinburgh. E.S. Livingstone, 1957).

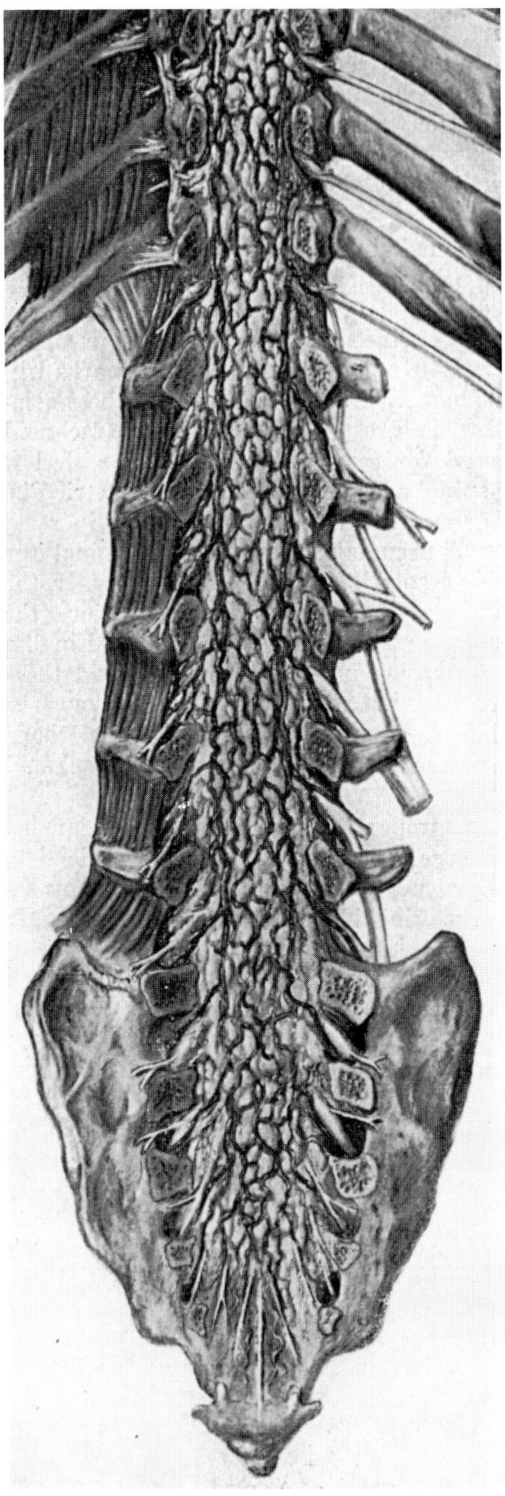

**Fig. 13–48.** Posteroanterior view of the epidural space and its contents which consists mostly of the internal vertebral venous plexus, arteries, solid and liquid fat, and lymphatics. This view is after the root of the laminae have been sawn so that the posterior part of the vertebral canal has been removed. Injection of the local anesthetic into the canal will diffuse easily through the various structures noted in this illustration.

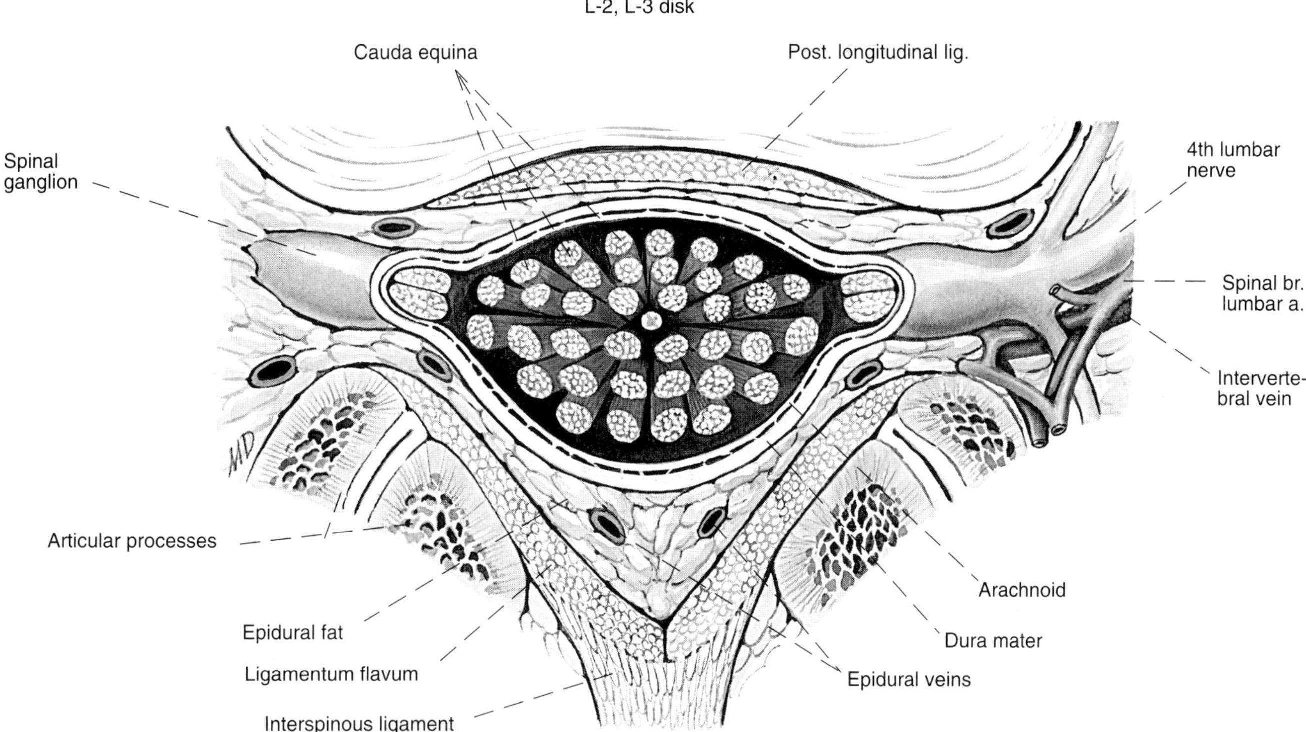


**Fig. 13–49.** Cross section of the spinal canal and surrounding structures in the third lumbar region showing 18 posterior and 18 anterior roots that make up the caudad equina. Each root contains fibers destined to structures below this level. Note also the triangular configuration of the epidural space that besides the nerve roots is filled with fat, the internal venous plexus, and other structures already mentioned. The size of the epidural space, anteriorly, that is between the posterior longitudinal ligament and the dura-arachnoid, is very narrow. Two halves of the ligamentum flavum that approximate each other in the midline, posteriorly, containing a slit for passage of small vessels and occupied with some fat.

rior wall of the canal, being separated by a few fibrous tissue strands and epidural veins. The fibrous strands pass from the posterior longitudinal ligament to the anterior aspect of the dura, anchoring it in place and tending to divide the anterior epidural space into longitudinal compartments. The posterolateral portion, existing between the dura and the laminae and the ligamenta flava (Figure 13–49), is wider, ranging from 1.5 to 2 mm in the cervical region, from 3 to 5 mm in the mid-thoracic region, and from 4 to 6 mm in the lumbar region (39,390,399). Measurements with MRI show that the distance is 6 mm with a range of 4–9 mm in the cranial two-thirds of the interlaminar space and is 4 mm with a range of 2 to 7 mm in the caudal part of the space (406). At the second lumbar interspace, the distance between the posterior surface of the dural sac and the ligamentum flavum ranges from 4 to 9 mm. At the level of the anterior portion of the laminae, the dura sac is closely applied to the periosteum producing a "saw tooth" shape of the epidural region, as seen in MRI scans (Figure 13–50).

## The Contents of the Epidural Space

Figures 13–47 to 13–50 depict the contents of the epidural space, which include fat and loose areolar tissue through which run the internal vertebral venous plexus, lymphatics, arteries, and the dural projections that surround the spinal nerves.

***Epidural Fat.*** The epidural fat is mainly localized in the posterior sulcus between the ligamentum flavum and dura and also in the anterolateral space and in the intervertebral foramina. It is usually described as semi-fluid and lobulated with pads of solid fat intermingled in the vessels that pass through it. Observations of patients undergoing laminectomy show the fat to be enclosed within loose areolar tissue that varies in appearance from a diaphanous layer to a pseudomembrane (389). The fat is highly vascular with many capillary walls appearing in serial microscopic sections. The greater part of the fat lies free and unattached in the spinal canal, but collagen bundles become increasingly numerous in the region of the nerve roots as a considerable amount of connective tissue is intermingled with the fat within the intervertebral foramina (39).

The fat itself does not hinder the identification of the epidural space nor the spread of local anesthetic solution nor contrast media injected in it. It constitutes an important "pharmacologic space" and depot for the injected local anesthetic agent, and it is one of the three main competitors for the share of the drug, the other two being nervous tissue of the spinal roots and spinal cord and blood vessels within the spinal canal. Drugs with high

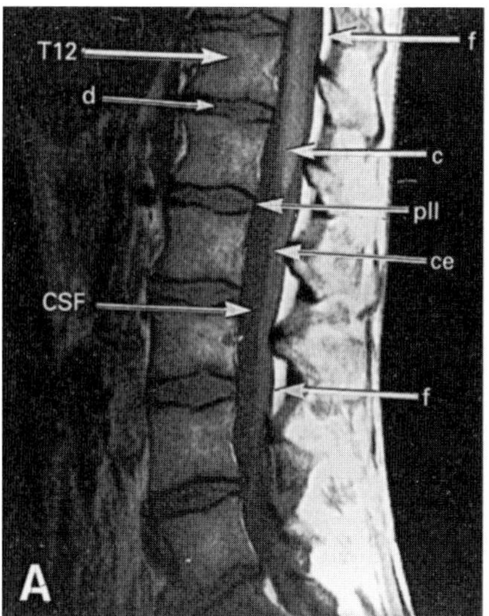


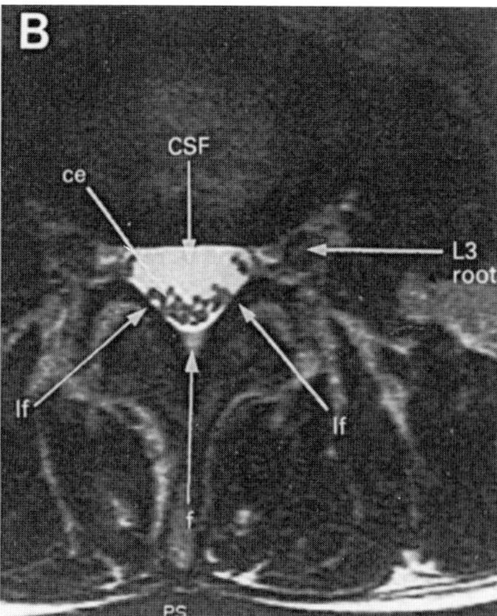


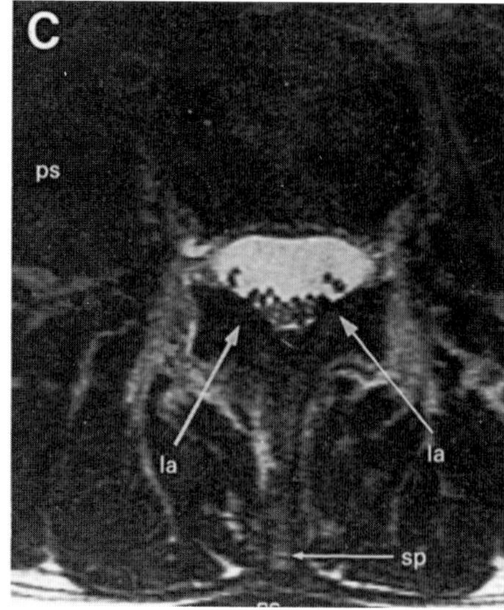


**Fig. 13–50.** Anatomy of the extradural region using magnetic resonant imaging. **A**: T1W sagittal midline MR image showing vertebrae T11-S2, the intervening discs (d), and the overlying posterior longitudinal ligament (pll). The dural sac lies within the spinal canal. The CSF is of low signal (dark) and the conus (c), of higher signal, is located at L1. The nerve roots of the cauda equina (ce) are demonstrated to lie posteriorly. Posterior to the dural sac, extradural fat (f), which is of high signal (white) on TlW images, is demonstrated at levels T11–12 to L3–4, giving a "saw toothed" pattern to the extradural region. The fat is divided into segments by the interposing laminae. The extradural space is deeper at the cranial end than at the caudal end. **B**: T2W axial MR image at L3–4, between the two laminae. On 2W sequences CSF is of high signal (white) and the nerve roots of the cauda equina (ce) are well demonstrated within the dural sac. Fat is of intermediate signal; posterior to the dura is a triangle of extradural fat (f), bordered posterolaterally by the ligamentum flavum (lf). Laterally, the confines of the extradural space are less defined. **C**: T2W axial image at the level of the L3 lamina. The dural sac is located adjacent to the anterior surface of the lamina (la). There is no intervening extradural fat. wp = Spinous process of L3; ps = psoas muscle. [Reproduced with permission from Westbrook JL, Renowden SA, Carrie LES: Study of the anatomy of the extradural region using magnetic resonance imaging. Br. J. Anaesth. 71, 1993, p. 496).

lipid solubility and lipoprotein binding characteristics will tend to enter the fat phase and remain there for periods of time depending on their pharmacodynamics and on the briskness of the blood flow competing for uptake (409).

***The Internal Vertebral Venous Plexus.*** The internal vertebral venous plexus that drains both the spinal cord and canal lies mainly in the anterolateral parts of the epidural space (Figure 13–42B). In the valveless plexus is a double anterior system of large veins, the anterointernal and antero-external veins, which run together at the anterolateral border of the vertebral canal, except at the intervertebral foramina where they divide to allow the nerve root to pass through (410). The internal vertebral venous plexus connects to the systemic venous circulation through the internal iliac veins, the intercostal and azygous veins, and through the vertebral veins to the cerebral sinuses (Figure 13–43). In gravidae and individuals with an increase in intra-abdominal pressure, which compresses the inferior vena cava, such pressure forms important alternate routes of venous drainage; indeed, through this venous network increase intra-abdominal and intravascular pressure such as coughing and straining. The engorged veins during pregnancy displace the dura mater locally away from the walls of the vertebral canal.

***Spinal Arteries.*** The endings of the spinal arteries in the epidural space are depicted in Figure 13–41 and described in the legend (384).

***Lymphatics.*** Lymphatic networks surrounding and draining the neural cul-de-sacs of the dural root sleeves run anteriorly from each intervertebral foramina and empty into the longitudinal channels in front of the vertebral column (411). These networks share a vital role with the arachnoid villi in eliminating debris from the subarachnoid space.

## Distances and Measurements

In a recent study using magnetic resonance imaging, Westbrook, Renowden and Carrie (406) have clarified many important issues about the anatomy and contents of the epidural space that in previous studies caused confusion and presented contradictions. Table 13–14 lists the measurements that are of critical importance in carrying

**Table 13–14.** Measurements Taken from MR Images at the $L_{2-3}$ Level (mean ± SD [range] in millimeters)*

| | |
|---|---|
| —Skin-ligamentum flavum | 47.7 ± 11.75 (30–85) |
| —Ligamentum flavum-dura mater: | |
| Cranial | 4.97 ± 1.35 (4–9) |
| Mid-point | 6.15 ± 1.31 (4–9) |
| Caudal | 3.95 ± 1.1 (2–7) |
| —Interlaminar distance | 21.44 ± 2.79 (15–27) |
| —Angle of spinous process to | 70.7 ± 5.1 (63–83) |

(Modified from Westbrook JL, et al.: Study the anatomy of the extradural region using magnetic resonance imaging. Br. J. Anaesth. 71:496, 1993.)

**Table 13–15.** Frequency of Distribution (in Percent) of Distances from the Skin to the Epidural Space Just Inside the Ligamentum Flavum at Different Lumbar Interspaces

| Distance Skin to Ligament | Lumbar Interspace L1–2 | L2–3 | L3–4 | L4–5 | % of Total |
|---|---|---|---|---|---|
| 3–4 | 43 | 17 | 49 | 20 | 14 |
| 4–5 | 33 | 38 | 44 | 39 | 41 |
| 5–6 | 18 | 26 | 24 | 29 | 25 |
| 6–7 | 3 | 12 | 14 | 10 | 13 |
| >7 | 3 | 7 | 9 | 2 | 7 |
| Total | 100 | 100 | 100 | 100 | 100 |

out the epidural puncture, and Figure 13–50 shows important features. As may be noted, in the midline the distance between the skin and inner surface of the ligamentum flavum, which constitutes the epidural space, is a mean of less than 5 cm with a range between 3 and 8.5 cm. In a more detailed study, in 1000 parturients, Harrison and Cowles (412) measured the distance of the skin and the epidural space at various lumbar interspaces. They measured the distance in the first lumbar interspace in 33 parturients; at L2–3 in 344, at L3–4 in 543, and at L4–5 in 80. Table 13–15 lists the percentage of gravidae's skin/epidural space (S-ES) distance at each lumbar interspace, while Table 13–16 lists the median and the 5th and 95th percentiles of the S-ES distance. The results, taken as whole, indicate that the median distance from the skin to the lumbar epidural space is 4.7 cm and in only 5.4% of subjects is it greater. These findings are in agreement with the data derived from the old study by Gutierriez (413) who measured the distance in the mid lumbar space in 3200 subjects and similar also to the more recent findings by Palmer, et al (414) who measured the distance in 125 obstetric patients (Table 13–17). Palmer, et al (414) found no relationship between the S-ES measurement and height of the parturient, but as expected, the distance varied directly with the weight (obesity) of the subject ($p < 0.0001$). They concluded that the fat in the subcutaneous tissue accounted for most of the variation in distance from skin to the epidural space, others (414a,414b) have confirmed these data.

**Table 13–16.** The Median, 5th and 95th Percentiles of the Distance from the Skin to Epidural Space at Each Interspace

| Lumbar Interspace | Distance from Skin to Epidural Space (in centimeters) Median | Percentile 5th | 95th |
|---|---|---|---|
| L1–2 | 4.23 | 3.12 | 6.33 |
| L2–3 | 4.66 | 3.29 | 7.32 |
| L3–4 | 4.93 | 3.57 | 7.44 |
| L4–5 | 4.78 | 3.25 | 6.75 |

**Table 13–17.** Distribution of Frequencies of Distances from Skin to Epidural Space*

| Depth (centimeters) | Frequency (in % of patients) |
|---|---|
| 3–3.5 | 3.0 |
| 3.5–4.0 | 11.0 |
| 4.0–4.5 | 21.0 |
| 4.5–5.0 | 21.4 |
| 5.0–5.5 | 16.0 |
| 5.5–6.0 | 13.6 |
| 6.0–6.5 | 9.0 |
| 6.5–7.0 | 3.0 |
| > 7 | 2.0 |
| | 100 |

* (Modified from Palmer SK, et al: Distance from the skin to the lumbar epidural space in an obstetric population. Anesth. Analg. 62:944–946, 1983.)

Soon after introducing the paramedian (paraspinous) approach to the epidural space, Bonica (415) measured the distance between the skin and the point at which there was loss of resistance to injection of saline with both the midline and paramedian approach. The distance in the midline was found to be a mean of 4.9 cm (range 4.6 to 5.1 cm); whereas with the paramedian approach, as precisely described by Bonica (cephalad angle with longitudinal axis 135° and with cross-sectional angle of 15° (see Figure 13B-62), the S-ES distance was 6.1 cm (range 5.4 to 8.6 cm), i.e., the paramedian needle was passed 1.2 cm deeper than the midline needle. Very similar figures were reported by Blomberg (416) in his comprehensive study of various aspects of the epidural space, on 14 cadavers, carried out 3 decades later. For this purpose, he used insertion of a Tuohy needle at L3–4 interspace in the midline and a rigid needle arthroscope (Olympus Selfoscope 2211S) with an external diameter of 2.2 mm and with the lens directed 90° to the length of the endoscope, introduced percutaneously into the epidural space at the L2–3 interspace. The Tuohy needle was then advanced so that its orifice was directed cephalad and was seen to lie entirely in the space. Then it was further advanced to contact the dura mater. The distances from the point of loss of resistance to these two points were measured, and the risk of puncture of the dura mater with further advancement of the needle was judged by the appearance of the dura mater as the needle pressed against it and was determined as imminent (+ +), possible (+), or none (−). The midline needle was then retracted toward the ligamentum flavum and then another Tuohy needle was introduced by way of the paramedian approach, about 1.5-cm lateral to the caudal part of the spinous process of L4 and directed toward the midline of the epidural space in L3–4. The distance from the skin to the point of loss of resistance was measured and the needle then

**Table 13–18.** Other Distances: Midline *versus* Paramedian Approach (measurements in millimeters)

| Measurements | Midline | Paramedian |
|---|---|---|
| — Skin to dura mater | 48.6 (42–56) | 57.9 (52–67) |
| — Loss of resistance to point needle orifice entirely in epidural space | 2.4 (0–5) | 3.4 (0–9) |
| — Loss of resistance to contact with dura | 3.9 (1–7) | 7.6 (5–13) |
| — Cephalad angle of needle with dorsal plane of skin | 90°–100° | 120°–135° |
| — Angle of needle with cross-sectional plane | 0 | 15–25 |
| — Risk of dural puncture* | + + | none |
| — Tenting of dura* | + + | none |

* Risk puncture of dura mater: ** imminent; + possible; – no risk; Tenting of dura mater: + + great; + moderate; – no tenting. [Modified from Blomberg RG: Technical advantages of the paramedian approach for lumbar epidural puncture and catheter introduction. Anaesthesia 43: 839, 1988]

advanced so that its orifice, again directed cephalad, was seen to be entirely in the space and then further to contact the dura mater. The distances from the point of loss of resistance to these two positions were measured and the risk of puncture of the dura mater with further advancement of the needle was judged by the appearance of the dura in the same manner as with the midline needle. Both needles were then placed just inside the ligamentum flavum with the orifice directed cephalad, and an epidural catheter was inserted first through the midline needle and subsequently through the paramedian needle. The results were as follows: the S-ES distance in the midline averaged 48.6 mm (range 42 to 56 mm) with the midline needle and 57.9 mm (range 52 to 67 mm) for the paramedian needle, i.e., the paramedian needle was passed an average of 9.3 mm (range 5 to 18 mm) further than the midline needle to reach the epidural space (note that measurements are listed in millimeters not centimeters). The distance from the point of loss of resistance to the point when the orifice could be seen to lie entirely in the epidural space was 2.4 mm (range 0 to 5 mm) with the midline needle and 3.4 mm (range 0 to 9 mm) for the paramedian needle. The cephalad angle of the midline needle to the dorsal plane of the skin varied from 90° and 100° in the sagittal plane. The cephalad angle of the paramedian needle varied between 120° and 135°, while its angle to the cross-sectional plane was between 15° and 25° (see Table 13–18). The midline needle presented an imminent risk of perforating the dura mater in all 14 subjects if advanced further from the point of contact, whereas the paramedian needle presented an imminent risk of perforation of the dura mater in only 2 of the 14 subjects. The tip of the catheter introduced into the midline needle caused considerable tenting of the dura in 10 subjects and moderate tenting in 4; whereas the tip of the paramedian catheter did not cause tenting in any case. The midline catheter took a varying course, whereas the paramedian catheter was passed easily on a straight cephalad course without any resistance in all 14 subjects.

### *The Distance Between the Ligamentum Flavum and the Dura Mater*

Another point to focus on is the distance between the center of the posterior sulcus and the intervening ligamentum flavum and the dura, which is wider in the upper two-thirds of the space (about 6 mm with a range of 4 to 9 mm) than in the lower third (4 mm with a range or 2 to 7 mm) (see Table 13–14). This is due to the fact that the upper edge of the lamina below is more anteriorly than the lower edge of the lamina above (Figure 13–51). Blomberg (416,417), using the aforementioned technique, found that the distance from the point of loss of resistance to contact with the dura by the needle was an average of 3.9 mm (range 1 to 7 mm) for the midline needle and 7.6 mm (range 5 to 13 mm) for the paramedian needle at the initial CSF pressure. Thus, the paramedian needle was advanced an average of 3.7 mm (range 1 to 10 mm) deeper than the midline needle in the epidural space to reach the dura mater. This was probably due to angulation of the trajectory of the needle with the paramedian approach (see Figures 13B-63 and 13B-64), which is discussed later in this chapter.

Figure 13–50 is an MRI image of the sagittal midline showing the twelfth thoracic to the second sacral vertebra and, as noted, the segmental shape of the posterior extradural space caused by the fact that the posterolateral part of the laminae is in direct contact with the dura and that fat is in the posterior recess between the adjacent laminae. Some researchers have called it "saw-toothed" shape.

### *Other Important Features*

It is also important to note that the epidural space narrows abruptly at its cranial end as the lamina becomes adjacent to the dura. This is critically important in introducing an epidural needle because should its bevel touch the upper end of the space, introduction of the catheter would be impeded by the inferior surface of the lamina above.

In discussing the paramedian approach, we emphasize that the shape of the spinous processes is such ("trough-like") that it will direct the needle toward the midline to pass through the anterior portion of the interspinous ligament and then "walk off" the back of the Huber point of the Tuohy needle with the opening cephalad off the upper edge of the lamina through the medial part of the ligamentum flavum, midway between the cranial and caudad end. This precludes the problems mentioned above and almost always causes the bevel to enter the epidural space at its midpoint from the cranial and caudad end where the distance between the ligamentum flavum and dura is widest. This is in contrast with the midline approach, which would cause the point of the needle to penetrate the ligamentum flavum at its lower end. Because of the angle the needle makes with the longitudinal axis with the paramedian approach, the bevel of the Tuohy needle traverses obliquely the epidural space, and, thus, the back of the bevel will contact the dura in the upper third of the space. Moreover, the oblique passage of the needle through the space provides the greatest distance between the ligamentum flavum and the posterior portion of the dura mater so that the back part of the Huber point comes to lie against the dura (see Figure 13–67). Most importantly, the oblique passage causes the catheter to be in line, longitudinal with the long axis, and thus proceeds straight cephalad parallel to the dura.

## *Epidural Pressures*

### Negative Epidural Pressure

The presence of a negative pressure registered when the epidural space in the lumbar region is penetrated with a needle has been the subject of controversy. Some writers believe that it exists normally, while the majority of evidence suggests that the original observation of Jansen (418) in 1926, those of Eaton (419) 13 years later, and the data of many others published subsequently (420–422) provide overwhelming evidence that it is an artifact produced by "tenting" of the dura mater by the point of the needl (39). This occurence has been demonstrated by the fact that the negative pressure increases as the needle advances across the epidural space toward the dura, that blunt needles with side openings produce the greatest negative pressure: blunt needles (421,422) produce a good "coning" effect on the dura without puncturing or transmitting the negative pressure well because of their side opening. Moreover, slow introduction of a needle produces the greatest negative pressure. Even if the needle is halted and the pressure equalized, further advance of the needle will continue to produce a negative pressure until the dura is eventually punctured.

Eaton (419) provided the critical data when he showed that tenting of the dura with a blunt stylet in the third lumbar interspace and having placed an epidural needle in the second lumbar interspace caused negative pressures of up to $-14$ cm$H_2O$, which were recorded via means of the epidural needle in the second interspace. The pressure could be returned to zero by withdrawing the stylet from the dura, and then the same level of negative pressure could be obtained by advancing the stylet again. These data and data by Usubiaga and collaborators (421,422) showed that the negative pressure may last for a few seconds in 60% of the subjects. Usubiaga, et al (421,422) suggested that the use of the "hanging drop" negative pressure test in the lumbar region is not as certain as the "loss of the resistance" test.

In the thoracic region, a negative pressure of $-1$ to $-9$ is present at the point of needle entrance into the epidural space in virtually all individuals. This negative pressure is the transmission of the mean negative intrapleural pressure of $-7$ cm$H_2O$ (range $-5$ to $-10$ cm$H_2O$) and, therefore, can be used in the thoracic region, but we prefer the loss of resistance test even at these higher levels.

### Epidural Pressures During Pregnancy

The epidural pressure during pregnancy and labor has been studied by Bromage (49), Usubiaga and associates (421,422), Gabbert and Marx (423), and Messich (424), among others. Gabbert and Marx (423) showed that the extradural pressures during pregnancy and labor were more pronounced than those of the cerebrospinal fluid pressure, which had been demonstrated to remain within the usual range throughout pregnancy and labor. In contrast, the extradural pressures in early pregnancy were higher (+1 cm$H_2O$ or above) than those of nonpregnant patients ($-1$ cm$H_2O$ or below), and the baseline pressures increased gradually during the course of labor. These findings indicate progressed venous engorgement. Figure 13–51 shows tracings of the extradural pressure during contractions with bearing-down efforts in the supine position with those of contractions with bearing-down efforts with left uterine displacement. Obviously, these pressures are likely to interfere with the "hanging drop" technique for identifying the extradural space. The decrease in the pressure during uterine contraction following lateral uterine displacement demonstrates a more efficient venous return of the blood expelled from the uterus during a contraction to the right heart, both with and without bearing-down efforts.

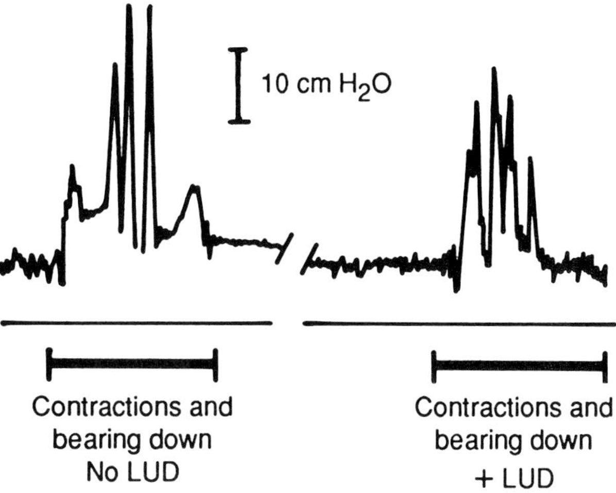


**Fig. 13–51.** Extradural pressure during labor, which was more pronounced than those of cerebrospinal fluid pressure that remains within the usual range throughout pregnancy and labor. The left tracing shows the pressure during contractions and bearing down without left uterine displacement (LUD), whereas on the right the pressure is caused by contractions and bearing-down efforts with the left uterine displacement in place. The lower pressure with uterine displacement is due to the more efficient venous return to the right heart of the blood expelled from the uterus during contraction. (Modified from Galbert MW, Marx GF: Extradural pressures in the parturient patient. Anesthesiology 40:499, 1974).

Messich (424) carried out a very extensive study on 21 full-term pregnant patients before and during labor and 6 to 12 hours postpartum in different positions. He found that prior to induction of labor or prior to cesarean section the pressures in 18 parturients each with a singleton fetus when placed in the lateral position had an epidural pressure of 4.8 ± 1.5 mm Hg, in the supine position; without lateral tilt the pressure was 29 ± 5 mm Hg; whereas in the supine position with a lateral tilt, it dropped to 11.6 ± 3. Figure 13–52 shows: 1) a synchronous rise in the epidural space pressure with a rise of intrauterine pressure with parturients aware of uterine con-

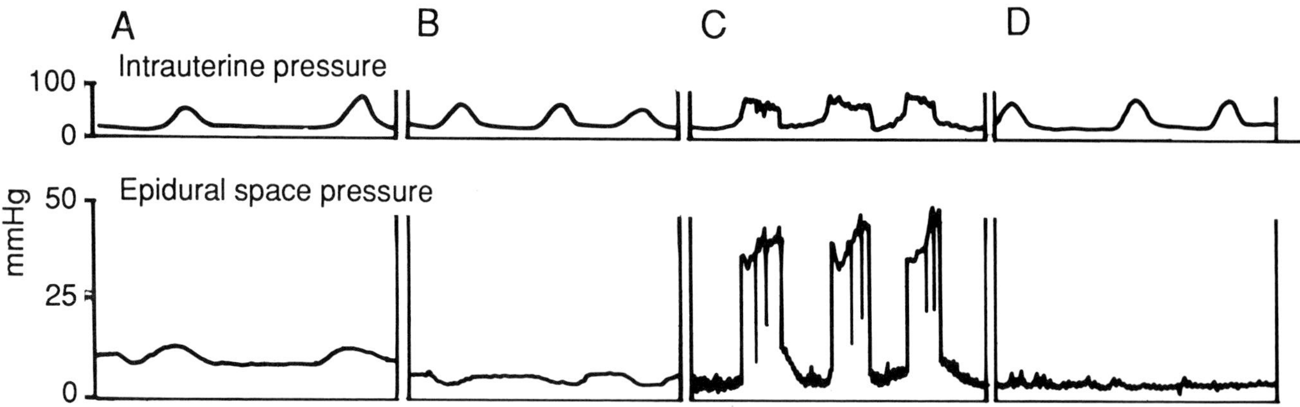


**Fig. 13–52.** Extradural pressures recorded in 21 full-term gravida before and during labor and 6 to 12 hours postpartum in different positions. In **A**, synchronous rise in the epidural space pressure with a rise in intrauterine pressure, with the parturient aware of uterine contractions during the active phase of labor. **B**: Fall in the epidural space pressure synchronous with uterine contractions in single fetus pregnant patients with motor loss as a result of epidural block in the lateral position. **C**: Rise in epidural pressure with the patient "bearing down" during the second stage of labor. **D**: Absence of rise in the epidural space pressure with uterine contractions during the active phase of labor with established epidural block, with the parturient unaware of the contraction. (Modified with permission from Messih MN: Epidural space pressures during pregnancy. Anaesthesia 36, 1981, 775–782).

tractions during the active phase of labor (first group); 2) the fall in epidural pressure synchronous with uterine contractions in single fetus pregnant patients with motor loss as a result of epidural block in the lateral position; 3) rise in epidural pressure with the patient bearing down during the second stage of labor; and, 4) the absence of rise in epidural pressure with uterine contractions during the active phase of labor with established epidural block, but with the patients unaware of the contractions. These data show that the epidural space pressure in the full-term pregnant patient is closely related to the degree of inferior vena caval obstruction imposed by the gravid uterus. These data also suggest that when the patient is aware of uterine contractions, the synchronizing of epidural space pressure with the contraction is a result of reflex increase in abdominal muscle tone. With established epidural block and the parturient unaware of the contraction, such a rise is minimal and is replaced by a drop in pressure in patients with single fetuses who develop loss of motor muscle power. In all patients, 6 to 12 hours postpartum, the mean epidural pressures were between −5.7 mm Hg and −6.8 mm Hg in the lateral position—pressures that are much lower than those of nonpregnant patients. This suggests that the lumbar subarachnoid space capacity 6 to 12 hours in parturients postdelivery is still smaller than in the normal nonpregnant woman.

In a more recent study, Zarzur and Gonzalves (425) used a sharp spinal needle with a long (2 mm) bevel and measured the distance the dura could be indented and the negative pressure produced before penetration of the dura-arachnoid occurred. They noted that the indentation of the dura was a mean of 4.06 ± 1.33 mm (range 2 to 6), and that the pressure was a mean of −12.9 ± 6.3 $cmH_2O$.

In a somewhat related anatomic study intended to determine if an epidural catheter could penetrate the dura mater and pia mater, Hardy (426) tested three different catheters in common use on specimens removed from the midline theca from the cervical, thoracic, and lumbar regions. The dura was peeled off the arachnoid and the outer surface wiped dry before each experiment. Hardy's specimens were pinned to a workbench by one end and held taut. The catheters were supported to within 5 mm of their tips using the epidural needle with the tip removed. Each catheter was held in turn, and attempts were made to perforate the dura-arachnoid using as much force as possible with the catheter tip held perpendicular to the tissue. Of the 30 specimens of dura, none were perforated, whereas perforation of the arachnoid occurred in every specimen. It is obvious that the dura is tough and difficult to penetrate with a catheter, and when penetration occurs, it is likely that the dura has already been damaged by the needle, resulting in a subdural puncture (407).

## Spread of the Local Anesthetic Solution

Following injection of fluid into the epidural space, there is spread of the solution in all directions away from the point of the needle: cephalad, caudad, and laterally, and within a few seconds, the solution passes through the intervertebral foramina and into the paravertebral spaces (4,46–49,427). [In the thoracic region, colored solution has been found as far distal as the angle of the ribs (4,46,427). At the same time, some of the solution is absorbed by the contents of the epidural space (especially the fat in which it is retained as a depot), while in some, it is removed by the venous plexus.]

Early in the history of epidural anesthesia, it was believed that the segmental spread of the local anesthetic in the epidural space depended almost entirely on the volume injected: the larger the volume, the greater the spread (Figure 13–53). However, the painstaking and meticulous studies of Bromage and associates of 3 decades ago (46–49,430–431) and of many others (53,65,95, 427–429,432–437) suggest other factors may play some role in the spread of epidural analgesia. These include: 1)

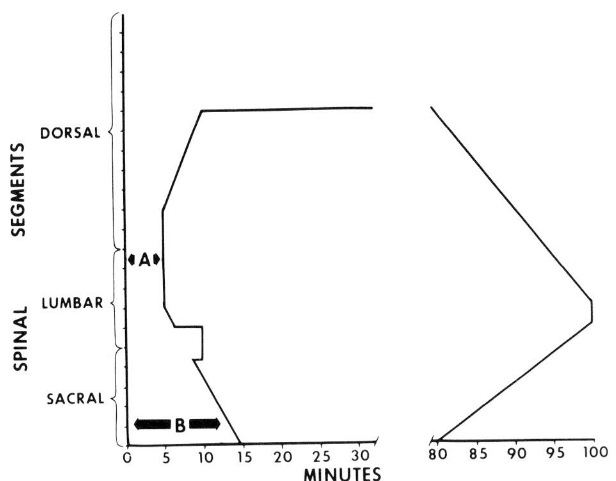


**Fig. 13–53.** Segment-time diagram of spread and regression of epidural analgesia after injection at the second lumbar interspace. **A**: Latency of initial onset; **B**: latency of complete spread of analgesia. Note the delay in block of L5 and S1. [Reprinted with permission from Bromage PR: Mechanism of action. [In] Epidural Analgesia, W.B. Saunders 1978, p. 132).

site of injection and nerve root size; 2) age, weight, and height of the patient; 3) size of the epidural space as affected by pregnancy, large abdominal tumor, or obesity; 4) posture of the patient and the effects of gravity; 5) speed of injection of the local anesthetic; 6) epidural pressure at the time of injection; and 7) the concentration, latency, and penetrance of the local anesthetic injected. Let us now briefly consider each of these.

***Site of Injection and Nerve Root Size.*** It can be readily seen from the time segment diagram in Figure 13–53 that blockade tends to be most intense and has the most rapid onset close to site of injection. The subsequent spread of analgesia depends to some extent on whether the injection is made in a thoracic or lumbar region. In this diagram, which pertains to lumbar epidural injection, analgesia spreads more in a cranial than caudal direction, and there may be a delay in L5-S1 root due to the large size of these nerve root (39,428).

***Age, Weight, and Height.*** In adults there appears to be no correlation between spread of analgesia with weight of the subject. However, Bromage (48,49) found a correlation between age and dose requirements when more than 2000 patients between ages 4 and 102 years were assessed by a standard technique. There was an increase in dose requirements from ages 4 to 18 and then a gradual decrease in dose requirements from ages 19 to 102. However, if one examines the data of dose requirements in subjects between ages 20 and 40, the age groups in which most parturients fall under, there is a variation of 1 to 1.6 ml of 2% lidocaine per segment. The larger volume in the younger age group as opposed to the older group is due to the fact that there is probably a greater loss of local anesthetic through the two escape routes: the intervertebral formina are free from occlusion by fibrous tissues as is the case in older people, and blood runs faster in the veins of younger people, flushing epidural drugs into the general circulation faster than in older people.

Bromage (46) reported a trend to increase dose requirements with increases in height, although the correlation is weak when injections are made in the lumbar region. A dose of 1 ml of lidocaine per segment is adequate for most patients 5 feet tall (150 cm), whereas a dose of 1.6 ml per segment is sufficient for most subjects 6 feet tall (160 cm). A simple rule of thumb, suggested by Bromage (431), is to use 1 ml per segment for 5 feet of height and then add 0.1 ml per segment for each additional 2 inches (5 cm). Similar negative findings regarding height and dosage were reported by Sharrock, et al (434)

***Size of the Epidural Space.*** Although there remains some confusion and controversy, it is generally agreed that gravidae at term need about one-third less epidural local anesthetic dosage than women in the nonpregnant state. This phenomenon was first described in 1949 by Oral B. Crawford and R. V. Chester (438) who were using caudal analgesia for labor, and showed that the dermatomal level for caudal injections with a mixture of 1.5% procaine and 0.125% tetracaine rose as high as eighth or ninth thoracic segment in women in labor, whereas such injections seldom rose above the first to second lumbar segment in nonpregnant patients. In the subsequent decade, this phenomenon was confirmed in studies carried by Bromage and associates (66) who showed that the lumbar dose requirements in parturients was one-third less than in nonpregnant women (depicted in Figure 13–53). Similar findings were reported by Nielsen and associates (439), Kandel and coworkers (440), and others in Canada, while Hehre and his group (429) at Yale found even greater reduction in segmental dose requirements. Bromage and others (66) attributed the phenomenon to the fact that during the last trimester of pregnancy, engorgement of the internal vertebral venous plexus consequent to obstruction of the inferior vena cava by the uterus decreases size of epidural (and subarachnoid) spaces.

Additional mechanical factors that have been suggested that enhance the spread of epidural analgesia include the exaggerated lumbar lordosis at term and an increased epidural pressure during pregnancy, with pressures being higher in the supine than in the lateral position (423). Epidural space pressures also rise during uterine contractions (66), although this effect is lessened after epidural analgesia (424). Uterine contractions per se, however, have little influence on the physical spread of local anesthetic in the epidural space (441). Bromage (47,49,66) and others (437) believe that hormonal influences contribute to the increased spread of epidural anesthetics in gravidae.

The role of mechanical factors in facilitating epidural spread of local anesthetics has been questioned by the findings of Fagraeus and associates (437) who observed the increased spread of epidural analgesia, even in early pregnancy when mechanical factors related to the gravid uterus are unlikely to be significant. They proposed a biochemical explanation that goes as follows: the hyperventilation that occurs early in the first trimester produces respiratory alkalosis, which is compensated by lowered

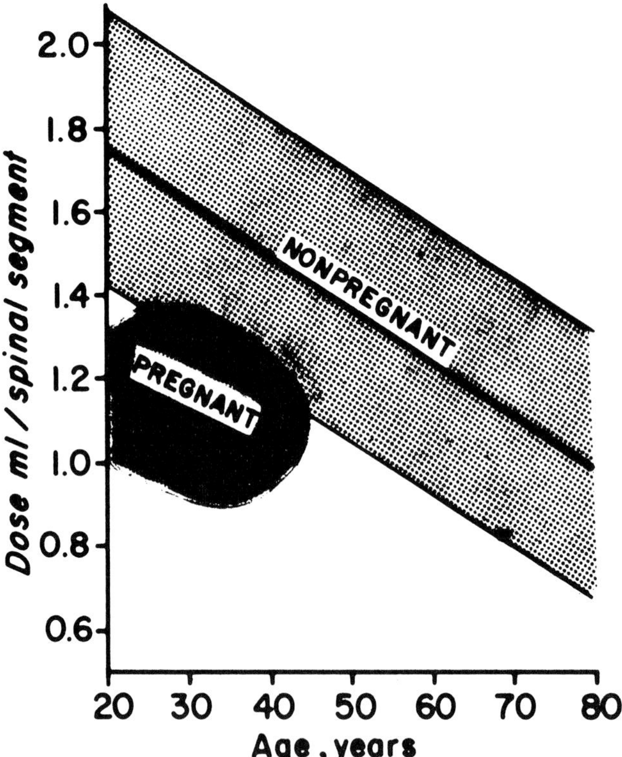


**Fig. 13–54.** Regression lines for dose of epidural solution and age in nonpregnant women, and in pregnant women at term. As may be noted, the gravida requires about two-thirds of the dose of the nonpregnant woman. [Modified from Bromage PR: Continuous lumbar epidural analgesia for obstetrics. Can. Med. Assoc. J. 85:1136, 1961).

bicarbonate levels. Because local anesthetics are salts that need buffer to convert to the base for transport across membranes into the central nervous system and circulation, a decreased buffer capacity allows the local anesthetic to remain as a salt for a longer period and, therefore, stay longer in the area of injection (epidural space). This increased time to complete analgesia and the local anesthetic will have time to spread further within anatomic tissue planes and further increase dermatomal spread.

Other factors that may contribute to the enhanced spread of local anesthetics include: 1) increased sensitivity of nerve fibers to local anesthetic caused by increased levels of progesterone during pregnancy (442–446); 2) reduced cerebrospinal fluid protein concentration (447), which increases local anesthetic effectiveness by reducing protein binding; and 3) elevated cerebrospinal fluid pH, which increases the proportion of non-ionized local anesthetics and thus facilitates movement across neural membrane (448).

The traditional concept that during pregnancy there is facilitated spread of local anesthetic has been challenged by the findings of Sharrock (434) and Sharrock and Greenridge (443) and by those of Grundy and associates (435,436). Grundy, et al (436) reported that the volumes of local anesthetic solution (either 15 ml or 20 ml of 0.25% bupivacaine without epinephrine) administered to 61 nonpregnant women scheduled to undergo surgical procedures were the same with 45 gravidae who were given the local anesthetic for cesarean section. They did not note any statistically significant difference in sensory levels in these groups. Based on this and in view of the fact that lower volumes of local anesthetics have been required to manage the pain of labor and vaginal delivery, some writers suggested that the use of small volumes for labor and vaginal delivery is associated with enhanced spread, whereas the administration of a large dose of local anesthetic as used for cesarean section produces the same spread of epidural anesthesia in term pregnant and nonpregnant patients (449). In view of the fact that currently many parturients receive infusion of local anesthetic and opioids for the management of pain of labor and vaginal delivery, it has now become an almost moot issue.

***Posture.*** Several studies have shown that having parturients in the sitting position for 5 minutes or longer after standard epidural injection in labor does not influence the caudad spread of the local anesthetic as presumed by many clinicians who use this technique to produce perineal analgesia for the delivery (450–453). Indeed, Merry and associates (451) showed that a significant shift of the mean lower limit occurred in 35 patients who were kept in the sitting position for 5 minutes, but contrary to what might be expected, this spread was in a cephalad direction. Comparing the results of this group with those of 54 patients who were kept in the left lateral horizontal position showed that the lower level of block was 5.6 ± 3.5 spinal segments above S5 in the sitting group and 4.1 ± 3.1 spinal segments in the horizontal group. It was noted that there was no difference in the cephalad level of the block, being T10 in both groups. Thus, group I had analgesia from T10 to L5, while group II had block from T10 to S2, i.e., the group who remained in the sitting position had a narrower analgesia band. The investigators concluded that the sitting position conferred no clinical advantage to patients receiving epidural analgesia in labor, and, indeed, they pointed out that placing the patient in the sitting position during late labor when contractions are strong may be a cause of discomfort and distress. Therefore, the only possible indication to place the parturient in the sitting position is to limit the cephalad spread of the local anesthetic in very obese patients (452). Somewhat similar results were reported by Grundy, et al (450).

In a study of 250 term parturients, Hodgkinson and Husain (452) found that the sitting position for 5 minutes after injection of 20 ml of 0.75% bupivacaine in increments of 5 ml every 4 to 5 minutes. The results were compared with those obtained in a previous study in which the parturients were kept on the left horizontal at all times. The data showed that the sitting position limited the cephalad spread of anesthesia only in obese patients, and that the decrease in spread was proportional to the degree of obesity. The results confirmed the previous findings: cephalad spread is positively correlated to body mass index (BMI) (weight in kilograms divided by height in meters squared). Roldin and associates (453) have shown that maintenance of the lateral position after induction of epidural anesthesia produces highly satisfactory analgesia for labor. They and others have noted that maintaining the patient in the lateral position the extent of epidural analgesia is increased by about two spinal segments on the dependent side. Turning the patient to the contralateral position after injection of 12 ml of 0.25% bupivacaine improved the quality of analgesia. They concluded that it is not necessary to have the patient in the supine position to produce bilateral analgesia or blockade.

***Speed of Injection.*** Increase in the speed of injection through a needle has little or no effect on bulk flow of the solution in the epidural space, and the spread of analgesia is only minimally influenced (554,555). On the other hand, rapid injection through a large needle of large volumes of solution may increase CSF pressure, decrease spinal cord blood flow, increase intracranial pressure, and pose risk of spinal and cerebral complications. Fortunately, with continuous epidural analgesia the speed of injection has a minimal role in determining the spread of analgesia, although a slow injection will cause more drug to be deposited in each segment and consequently increase the intensity and duration of the analgesia.

***Concentration, Latency and Penetrance of Local Anesthetic.*** Early extensive studies by Bromage (456) suggested that the dose of drug (concentration x volume) determines the spread of analgesia, at least between the concentration of 2% and 5% lidocaine and 0.2% and 0.5% tetracaine. However, data were not obtained to compare 0.5% lidocaine within a range of 1 to 2%, which is the typical clinical range of concentration for the clinical use of this drug. Data from Bromage (456) suggested that dose requirements diminished from about 30 mg per segment to 20 mg per segment when concentrations were reduced from 2% to 1%. Erdemir and colleagues (457) showed that 30 ml of 1% lidocaine produced a higher sensory level than 10 ml of 3% solution.

In regard to motor blockade, it is well established that below the concentration of 1% lidocaine, motor block is minimal regardless of the dose unless the injections are repeated at frequent intervals—a mechanism that is critically important in obstetric analgesia when using dilute solutions of 0.125% or 0.0625% bupivacaine. Increasing dosage results in a linear increase in degree of sensory block and duration of epidural block, while increase in concentration results in reduction in onset time and intensity of motor block. Clinically, the degree of motor block is estimated by the method of Bromage (49) and the RAM test of abdominal muscles (Table 13–19).

**Table 13–19.** Methods for Testing Motor Block

| | |
|---|---|
| *Bromage Scale** | |
| No block (0%) | Full flexion of knees and feet possible |
| Partial (33%) | Just able to flex knees, still full flexion of feet possible |
| Almost complete (66%) | Unable to flex knees, Still flexion of feet |
| Complete 100% | Unable to move legs or feet |
| *"RAM" Test of Abdominal Muscles** | |
| 100% | Able to rise from supine to sitting position with hands behind head |
| 80% power | Can sit only with arms extended |
| 60% power | Can lift only head and scapulae off bed |
| 40% power | Can lift only shoulders off bed |
| 20% | An increase in abdominal muscle tension can be felt during effort. No other response. |

* (Modified with permission from: Cousins MJ, Bromage PR: Epidural neural blockade, *In* Cousins MJ, Bridenbaugh PO: Neural Blockade, 2nd ed. Philadelphia, J.B. Lippincott Co., 1988, pp. 309, 310.)

## *Mechanism (Site) of Action of Epidural Analgesia*

The exact site where block is effected following injection of local anesthetic agents into the epidural space remains a controversial issue. Early studies by Sicard and Forestier (458) and Cathelin (2) indicated that the solution injected into the epidural space did not penetrate the dura; consequently, it was believed that the site of action of epidural block was outside the subarachnoid space. Improved methods for determining the quantity of local anesthetics in tissues have demonstrated that following epidural injection these drugs do penetrate the dura. Studies by Bromage and coworkers (459) using [$^{14}$C] labeled lidocaine injected into the epidural space of dogs and then carrying out autoradiographic and tissue essays, showed that rapid diffusion of local anesthetic into the CSF epidural cuff region is the most important determinant of onset of epidural blockade: peak local anesthetic concentrations in CSF were reached within 10 to 20 minutes of epidural injection when concentrations were high enough to produce blockade of the spinal nerve roots and rootlets. The same study also showed that by 30 minutes after the injection the Cm for lidocaine (0.28 μg/mg) had been exceeded in the peripheral spinal cord (1.38 μg/mg) as well as in spinal nerves in the paravertebral space (1 μg/mg). Data from other studies, in which local anesthetics were injected directly into the CSF, indicated that Cm is not exceeded in the dorsal root ganglion or in the more central part of the spinal cord (460–463).

Bromage (39) suggests that diffusion into intradural spinal nerve root most likely plays a major role during the early stage of disease, which is in keeping with the rapid onset of the segmental pattern of blockade. Subsequently, local anesthetic seepage through the intervertebral foramina and the arachnoid villi may contribute by producing multiple paravertebral block (464). After long epidural block, diffusion through the CSF to the spinal cord is probably a secondary phenomenon, although it may occur more rapidly when local anesthetic is injected closer to the spinal cord in the thoracic region.

Somewhat different results about the primary site of action of epidural (as well as subarachnoid) block have been published by Frumin, et al (463) and Galindo and associates (465,466). Galindo and coworkers confirmed the earlier work of Frumin, et al (463) by a study, which, in part, involved supportive neurophysiologic and anatomic evidence that the dorsal root ganglion is a structure more vulnerable to local anesthetics in the afferent system. Galindo and Witcher (466) stated that Cohen (461) and Bromage (459), from their aforementioned autoradiographic studies in dogs, have not been given due importance to their findings in locating a site of action for

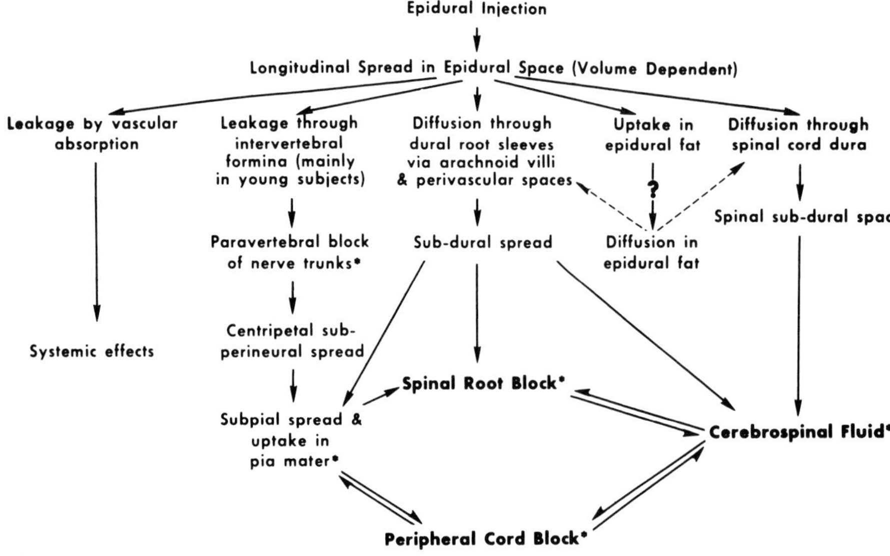


**Fig. 13–55.** Mechanism of action of epidurally injected local anesthetic solution in producing analgesia/anesthesia (see text for details). [Reprinted with permission from Bromage PR: Mechanism of action of extradural analgesia. Br. J. Anaesth. 47:199, 1975).

local anesthetics during epidural (and spinal) anesthesia because of relatively low concentrations of local anesthetics were found on the ganglion when compared to the roots in the spinal cord. However, their findings demonstrated that the ganglion is much more vulnerable to the frequency-dependent block than the nerve roots and therefore require a lesser concentration to cause a functional blockade.

On the other hand, other evidence supports Bromage's hypothesis. Urban (467) reported that the regression of analgesia after epidural block follows a circumferential pattern in the sagittal plane rather than follow the classic segmental pattern seen during the onset of epidural analgesia. This finding is consistent with the persistent action of local anesthetics on the peripheral spinal cord after the initial effect on the spinal nerve roots has abated. Moreover, Bromage (462) has shown reflex changes in the lower limbs during thoracic epidural blockade that spares the lumbar segments. Penetration of the spinal cord depends on the local anesthetic used and its concentration. Various important effects of local anesthetic on the spinal cord may follow initial action on dorsal roots and explain differences in sensory and motor blockade. Bromage's data (462) indicate that all local anesthetic reaches the spinal cord with significant blocking concentrations, and that penetration to different structures in the cord then depends on the physical, chemical, and perhaps other properties of the local anesthetic. Thus, drugs with low lipid solubility, such as lidocaine, penetrate predominantly to the superficial areas of the spinal cord, such as the spinothalamic tract and sympathetic excitatory tract.

Evidence from pharmacokinetic and analgesic efficacy studies of epidural opioids gives further insights because molecular weight, and physical and chemical properties of opioids are similar to those of local anesthetics. Epidural opioids have their predominant site of action in the superficial layer of the dorsal horn (substantia gelatenosa), and lipid soluble drugs such as sufentanil have an almost immediate onset of action in animal studies (468) and an onset time of 5 to 15 minutes in humans (469). This suggests that the drug reaches the laminae II regions of the dorsal horn almost immediately. Diffusion across the dural cuff into the CSF and then the spinal cord may be rapid for highly soluble opioids or local anesthetics. Another possibility is that the fine posterior reticular arteries convey drug by way of branches that penetrate directly into the dorsal horn. On the basis of these findings, Bromage suggests the schema shown in Figure 13–59.

## *Sequence of Block*

The sequence of epidural block is like that of subarachnoid block, except its onset is more delayed, probably because of the greater distance the drug must travel to reach its primary site of action. As Bromage (39) so aptly described it: "This initial spread through the epidural space is just a prelude for the drug's more difficult journey through the connective tissue barriers of nerve and cord, across the waters of the cerebrospinal fluid, either by free diffusion or along the root bridges leading to the cord and perhaps the brain itself." The first effect is slight relief of uterine pain, which occurs in 4 to 8 minutes, depends on the latency of the local anesthetic. Subsequently, there is evidence of sympathetic block, loss of temperature sense, and hypalgesia. Then, there is progressive total loss of sense of pain and light touch, and, if the concentration of the local anesthetic is high, proprioception, deep touch, and motor functions are lost. These effects occur first and are most profound near the site of injection; the farther away from the site, the longer the time for their onset and the less their effect.

Brull and Greene (470) found that during epidural anesthesia achieved with 2% lidocaine there were differential levels among light touch (LT), pinprick (PP), and cold temperature discrimination (TE). The median thoracic dermatomal levels were 4.5 for LT, 2.0 for PP, and 2.0 for TE. Zones of differential sensory block developed within 5 minutes of the epidural injection of the local anesthetic and persisted for the next 55 minutes. In all instances, PP extended more cephalad than LT, and TE extended above PP levels. Thus, during epidural anesthesia, sympathetic denervation extended 1 to 2 segments above sensory levels of LT and PP. They noted that age affected neither the cephalad extent nor the width of zone of differential block, and that pinprick levels of analgesia were closer to presumed levels of sympathetic block and those to light touch. Stevens and associates (471) also showed zones of differential block with epidural anesthesia and noted that the more extensive the block, the greater the band of differential block for analgesia (pain), anesthesia (touch), and cold. Thus, with the first injection, temperature sense and analgesia were at the same level, but anesthesia was almost two spinal segments below. With a second injection, achieved with larger volumes, analgesia extended at T4, temperature sense loss extended at T5, and anesthesia at T8. Following a third and fourth injection, the level of analgesia was at T7, temperature sense loss at T2, and anesthesia at T4.

## Clinical Aspects

### *Preparation of the Gravida*

The antepartal, intrapartal, and postpartum management of the gravida are discussed in detail in Chapter 22. Because this is the first chapter on regional anesthesia, we feel compelled to recapitulate some of the information there.

#### *Antepartal Preparation*

One of the most basic considerations in obstetric analgesia and anesthesia is the proper mental, psychologic, and physiologic preparation of the gravida. It is generally acknowledged that the pregnant patient of today deserves and will reap great benefits from the time and effort spent by her physician in informing her (and the child's father) about the course of pregnancy. This can be accomplished during the prenatal visits to the office, or it can be done by having monthly group-information periods. During these periods, information is disseminated verbally and with such aides as slides, video tapes, motion pictures, manikins, and charts.

A discussion of the physiology and clinical course of labor will similarly provide the mother with useful information and will help her to cooperate during labor. The procedures she is to follow during labor and delivery should be explained in detail, with the emphasis placed on the importance of properly bearing down during the second stage (to provide the uterus with the assistance of the auxiliary powers of labor) and of relaxing between contractions. This form of education and information is of inestimable value in freeing the expectant mother from misconceptions, superstitions, false beliefs, and fears that may have been instilled in her by misinformed relatives and friends or by improper teachings. Most important in the mental preparation of the gravida is the physician's or midwife's manifestation of friendship and sympathetic understanding, his or her kindness and reassurance, and those other human qualities that comprise the "art" of medicine and enhance the development of rapport. An optimal relationship between health worker and patient is a potent force in relieving pain and enhancing the action of analgesics.

During one of these prenatal visits, analgesia and anesthesia should be discussed in some detail and the advantages, disadvantages, and limitations of each technique should be briefly discussed. Although the obstetrician may indicate which technique he or she considers preferable, great caution should be exercised not to promise the patient either a specific method or painless labor. Rather, the patient should be reassured that there are many means available for relieving pain and that all efforts compatible with safety will be made to lessen the discomfort. In hospitals that have complete anesthesia service, it is useful for a member of the obstetric anesthesia service to meet with groups of gravidae for periods of 60 to 90 minutes to discuss analgesia/anesthesia in some detail.

The gravida should be specifically instructed to refrain from eating solid foods after labor begins. It will prove profitable to explain to her that labor and medication markedly interfere with digestion and absorption and delay gastric emptying to such an extent that partially digested food my remain in the stomach for as long as 24 hours. Aspiration of gastric contents is currently the second most frequent cause of anesthesia-related maternal deaths in most parts of the world. The importance of lying on her side to avoid aortocaval compression during the last 12 weeks of pregnancy and during labor should be emphasized.

#### *Preanesthetic Care*

Ideally, the anesthesiologist should meet and visit with the gravida during the prenatal period. This preanesthetic visit by the anesthesiologist is as important, if not more important, for obstetric patients than it is for surgical patients. During such a visit, the anesthesiologist, the nurse anesthetist, or midwife: 1) establishes rapport with and instills confidence in the parturient; 2) becomes familiar with the patient's medical and anesthesia history, physical findings, and obstetric conditions; 3) evaluates the physiologic and emotional status of the parturient at the time she enters the hospital; 4) discusses the plans with both the obstetrician and the parturient and makes arrangements for analgesia and anesthesia; and 5) participates actively in the psychologic preparation of the gravida. The gravida should be asked what drugs she has taken during pregnancy and if she has had any drug reactions, allergy, or other abnormal response to previous therapy. The anesthesia history should include details about her previous experience with anesthetics and how she feels about them. Because most patients have a subconscious fear of death, the anesthetist should make a point of emphasizing the safety of modern anesthesia.

A physical examination should be performed by the anesthetist not only to obtain additional information, but also to enhance rapport, for it manifests interest and concern for the patient's welfare. In gravidae who are beyond the thirty-fourth week of gestation, the blood pressure and pulse must be measured with the patient in the lateral position and again at 1, 2, and 5 minutes in the supine position, to ascertain the degree of compression of the inferior vena cava and aorta by the uterus. The maneuver will help detect severe aortocaval compression. The patient should again be impressed with the importance of lying on her side during the entire labor. If the decision has been made that the patient will receive epidural or other regional technique, the technical aspects of the procedure should be described in great detail using illustrations, if deemed advisable. For instance, most individuals have a fear of needles and it is essential for the anesthesiologist to emphasize that once an intracutaneous anesthetic wheal is made, the remainder of the procedure can be totally painless by appropriate use of dilute solution of local anesthetics as described below, to make penetration of the epidural needle and insertion of the catheter as well as other parts of the procedure virtually painless. The patient should be assured that everything will be done to keep her as comfortable as possible.

Once the patient is admitted and all preliminary steps accomplished, the obstetric nurse can arrange to have the patient taken to a comfortable labor room or ward. Once she is comfortable, all of the monitoring equipment, including an automatic blood pressure cuff, electrocardiogram, and continuous monitoring of fetal heart should be applied and observed for a number of minutes to be sure that all equipment is functioning properly. Equally important is having all of the equipment to carry out the epidural blockade (discussed below and as emphasized in preceding chapters) and equipment for the prevention and treatment of possible complications placed in the room, tested for proper functioning and ready for immediate use to effectively treat possible complications should they occur.

During the immediate preanesthetic period, the patient is reassured, informed once again of each detail of what procedures are to be done, and given psychological support in every other way. The maternal blood pressure, pulse, respiration, and other vital signs are measured and recorded while the fetal heart rate and uterine activity are measured continuously. In patients in whom epidural anesthesia is planned, there should be an electrocardiogram that provides continuous monitoring of the heart. In high-risk patients, central venous pressure should be used to measure the load on the right atrium, and in patients with cardiovascular disease, a Swan-Ganz catheter should be employed.

Details of the management of the mother, fetus, and newborn during analgesia/anesthesia will be presented after description of the various epidural block techniques.

## Techniques of Lumbar Epidural Block

### *Preliminary Tasks*

Following completion of the aforementioned preparation of the gravida, including detailed discussion of the procedure, the anesthesiologist together with the obstetric nurse initiate certain preliminary procedures. Once the patient is comfortable in bed, an intravenous infusion should be initiated and given at the normal flow rate until 20 to 25 minutes before the injection of the therapeutic dose of the local anesthetic. At this point the flow is speeded so that 800 to 1000 ml of fluid has been given by the time the block is initiated. It is highly desirable to carry out the various procedures to achieve proper placement of the catheter in the latter part of the latent phase, or the early part of the active phase when the pain caused by uterine contraction is mild and the parturient can cooperate fully with the obstetric team. Postponing these procedures until the patient has severe uterine contraction pain is likely to cause the patient trauma no matter her motivation to keep still as instructed and is likely to cause her to "squirm" and move during contractions making it difficult if not impossible to carry out these various technically precise steps in placing the catheter.

Moreover, placing the catheter early affords the obstetric team control of the situation should the patient suddenly begin to have strong contractions, which are likely to hasten labor and delivery. This is particularly important in multiparae, many of whom are likely to have a transition from the mild uterine activity of the latent phase and early active phase to very frequent and intense contractions that hasten labor. In any case, the test and therapeutic dose should not be injected until the uterine conditions mentioned in Chapter 13-A are present. If induction of labor is contemplated, the placement of an epidural catheter should be carried out before starting the oxytocin administration to again provide full control of the management of uterine activity.

The placement of the catheter is usually done in the parturient's own labor bed, provided there is enough room for the anesthetic equipment and the equipment for monitoring the mother and fetus, and equipment and drugs for prompt resuscitation in the event that an adverse effect or complication occurs. It deserves re-emphasis here that all equipment should be tested and proven to be fully functional just before beginning the anesthetic procedure, and that the drugs and equipment for the treatment of side effects and complications be within reach of an arm's length of the anesthetist. In all instances of these procedures, it is essential to have an obstetric nurse, nurse anesthetist, or other qualified person to assist the anesthesiologist, and equally important to provide the parturient with psychologic support and to help the anesthesiologist expedite prompt treatment of any adverse reaction. Obviously, the anesthesiologist should continue to provide psychologic support and reassurance before, during, and after placement of the catheter. At the risk of belaboring the point, it is also essential that the physician again describe the procedure before initiating it to refreshen the patient's memory. Then, once the catheter is in place, the parturient should be monitored continuously by a nurse, and analgesia and anesthesia initiated at the appropriate time.

### *Anesthetic Equipment*

Regional anesthesia, because of its complex nature, is not easy to achieve even by the expert, but it is impossible to successfully complete with poor or insufficient anesthetic equipment. Up to 2 decades or so ago, permanent equipment was used in the sense that the syringes and most other equipment was re-usable. Figure 13–56 depicts a tray used by the senior author that contains all of

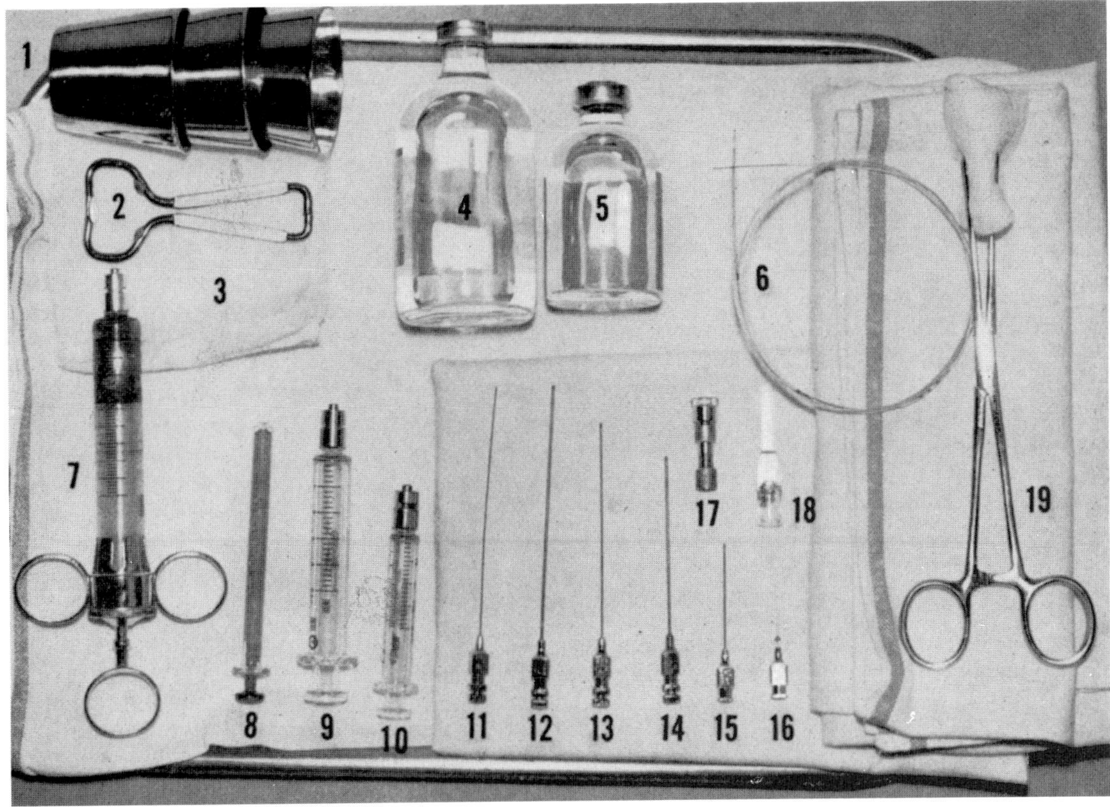


**Fig. 13–56.** Tray that may be used for lumbar epidural or caudal epidural block: (1) three medicine glasses; (2) bottle opener to remove caps of items: 4 and 5. (3) Sponges; (4) saline used to dilute the anesthetic (5); (6) vinyl plastic catheter with steel stylet; (7) 10-ml Luer-Lok control syringe; (8) tuberculin syringe to measure epinephrine; (9) 5-ml syringe; (10) 2-ml syringe; (11) 22-gauge spinal needle used for infiltration of subcutaneous tissue and muscle, and to explore the paravertebral structures; (12) 18-gauge thin-walled needle with short bevel for continuous lumbar epidural block; (13) 20-gauge, short-bevel needle for single-dose epidural block; (14) 18-gauge thin-walled, 5 cm needle for continuous caudal block; (15) 25-gauge, 3-cm needle for exploration of the sacrococcygeal hiatus; (16) 30-gauge needle for intracutaneous injection; (17) Tuohy-Borsch adaptor; (18) epinephrine ampule; (19) sponge forceps and towels for draping.

the items necessary to successfully achieve placement of the catheter and initiating and managing epidural analgesia/anesthesia. Currently, most anesthesiologists use disposable trays (Figure 13–57). Although these trays possess all the advantages of disposability, together with sharp needles and catheters constructed of the best material, it is obvious that the tray requires many additional items to carry out epidural analgesia. Table 13–20 lists the items necessary in the tray to carry out epidural analgesia.

### Local Anesthetic Agents

The pharmacology, including pharmacokinetics, and clinical characteristics of the various local anesthetics currently available are discussed in Chapter 11. Some of these characteristics are mentioned in Chapter 13-A also. No further comments are made here. Although any of the commonly available local anesthetic solutions may be used, the authors prefer lidocaine because of its short latency, penetrance, and intermediate duration, and bupivacaine because of its prolonged duration and, in dilute solution, its ability to produce minimal or no perineal muscle relaxation. Chapter 13-A stresses that if intermittent injections are used, low concentrations or in combination with opioids are preferable during labor because risk of toxicity is less and lower analgesic concentrations do not produce perineal muscle relaxation likely to interfere with flexion and internal rotation of the presenting part after it has descended on the perineum. Once this is accomplished, relaxation may be desirable and a higher concentration may be used.

Currently, most obstetric anesthesiologists are using dilute solutions administered by continuous infusion alone or in combination with opioids, and some also add epinephrine to the infusion. Many modifications of epidural blockade have been described using different agents or combination of agents and different techniques of injecting the analgesic/anesthetic solution, such as patient-controlled epidural analgesia versus physician controlled, and many others. None has enjoyed as much widespread use as the two agents and techniques recommended by the present authors that are presented later in this chapter.

### Epinephrine

The addition of epinephrine or other vasoconstrictors reduces venous absorption of local anesthetic so that a

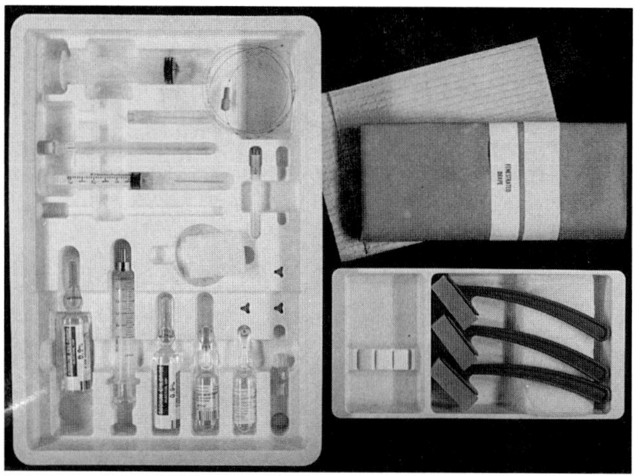

**Fig. 13–57.** This modern disposable tray offers many advantages. It is clean, has all needed equipment in one spot, and is very convenient because it mimics the utility of reusable equipment.

greater amount of the solution is left in the epidural space. This, in turn, increases the spread slightly and decreases the time of onset of block and increases the intensity and duration of analgesia by 30 to 40% (46,49,51). Although this applies to lidocaine and mepivacaine, it does not apply strictly to bupivacaine: addition of epinephrine to bupivacaine increases the percent of placental absorption of the drug. Some investigators have reported that adding epinephrine to bupivacaine not only significantly enhances the analgesic efficacy (shortening the onset and producing more intense block) but that the addition also increases the duration of blockade (204,246b,472,473), while others (211,308) have noted no effect on duration

**Table 13–20.** Equipment Required for Epidural Blockade

| | |
|---|---|
| A satisfactory preparation of the tray includes: | |
| 4 | swabs, a swab holder, sterile towels |
| 1 | 1 inch, 30-gauge needle for skin analgesia |
| 1 | 4 cm, 25-gauge needle for subcutaneous infiltration |
| 1 | 8 cm, spinal needle for deep infiltration |
| 1 | 18 gauge, needle for drawing up epidural solutions |
| Epidural needle (Tuohy or Crawford) | |
| Epidural catheter | |
| 1 | 2 ml, glass syringe for aspiration, syringe mount |
| 2 | 10 ml, Luer-Lok control syringes for loss of resistance tests and drawing up local anesthetic |
| 2 | Local anesthetic mixing cups |
| 1 | cup for antiseptic |
| Normal saline | |
| Local anesthetic(s) | |
| Filters and caps for epidural catheter | |
| Sterility indicator | |

of analgesia. As will be noted in the description of the technique we use, epinephrine is included in the local anesthetic solution unless it is contraindicated by systemic disease. We continue to employ a dilute solution of epinephrine to enhance analgesia, particularly anesthesia for cesarean section.

Ever since Braun (474), in 1905, began to use and recommend epinephrine in concentration of 1:200,000—a recommendation confirmed by many others, but particularly by Bieter (475) two decades later—it has been the tradition to use epinephrine in this concentration. However, some recent studies have shown that lower concentrations of the vasoconstrictor are just as effective in decreasing the placental transfer so that maternal and fetal concentrations are lower and the duration of blockade very similar to when a 1:200,000 concentration is used. Brose and Cohen (476) studied the problem in 40 healthy parturients with similar characteristics who were scheduled to undergo cesarean section with epidural anesthesia. They segregated the 40 patients into four groups of 10, all of whom received 20 ml of 2% lidocaine, with group I receiving no epinephrine, group II receiving the lidocaine with 1:400,000 epinephrine, group III 1:300,000, and group IV 1:200,000. The transplacental concentrations are listed in Table 13–7, while the condition of the fetus, particularly the blood gas and Apgar scores, are listed in Table 13–8. Here we can state that epinephrine decreases the blood levels of lidocaine concentrations 7%, 26%, and 50%, respectively. The onset of analgesia occurred in about 5 to 6 minutes, and the peak lidocaine concentrations in groups II, III, and IV decreased 7%, 26%, and 50%, respectively, which are not significantly different either from each other or from controls. The condition of the newborn, as measured by blood gases, pH and base deficit, and the neurologic and adaptive capacity scores were all normal.

Ohno and associates (477) studied the problem in 40 women scheduled to undergo pelvic operations and divided them into four groups of 10. All received 15 ml of 2% lidocaine with: no epinephrine in group I; epinephrine 1:200,000 in group II; 1:400,000 in group III; and 1:600,000 in group IV. Figure 13–56 is a graph depicting the mean arterial serum concentration of lidocaine following epidural group injections. As may be noted, group I developed arterial serum concentrations of about 4 μg/ml, whereas the other three groups developed very similar decreases in the concentrations of lidocaine. An important point is that in concentrations of 1:200,000 added to 20 ml of local anesthetic to achieve anesthesia for cesarean section, it amounts to 100 μg of epinephrine. In studies by Bonica and associates (51) mentioned in Chapter 16, this amount produced significant cardiovascular effects consisting of increase in stroke volume and heart rate and consequently cardiac output and a concomitant but greater decrease in total peripheral resistance, resulting in significant decrease in mean arterial pressure. As in another study by Bonica's group (478) it was shown that the cardiovascular effects of epinephrine are dose dependent, the study by Ohno, et al (477) is persuasive in its use of concentrations of 1:300,000 or 1:400,000 added to 20 ml of local anesthetic solution for cesarean sec-

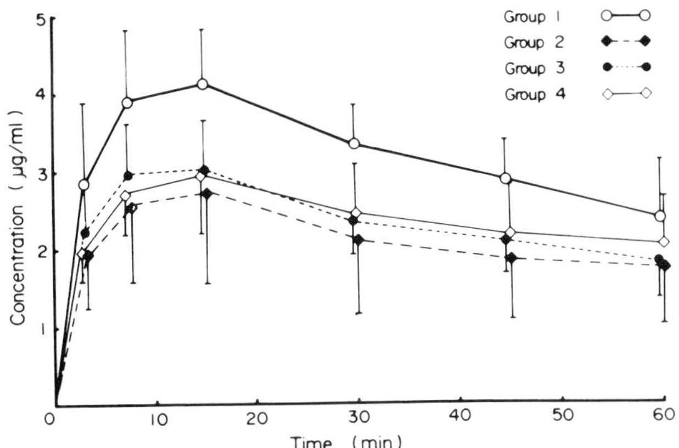


**Fig. 13–58.** Mean arterial serum concentration of lidocaine following epidural injection. Group 1 received 15 ml of 2% lidocaine plain solution, while , groups 2, 3, and 4 contained epinephrine with: 1:200,000, 1:400,000, and 1:600,000 epinephrine, respectively. Patients number 10 in all groups except group I at 60 min (n = 3) and groups 2 and 3 at 60 min (n = 9, respectively). Each bar represents the standard deviation (SD). [Reprinted with permission from: Ohno H, et al: Effect of epinephrine concentration on lidocaine disposition during epidural anesthesia. Anesthesiology 68, 1988, p. 626).

tion—concentrations that would total 75 μg and 50 μg of epinephrine, respectively. In addition to these considerations, it is important to recall the discussion in 13-A concerning the influence of large doses of epinephrine on uterine activity during labor. Fortunately, with the current techniques the amounts of epinephrine used produce very low blood levels and consequently have little or no effect on uterine contractility and should produce no significant cardiovascular changes—a fact that has been shown by many, as discussed in chapter 12.

### *Position of the Parturient*

Penetration of the epidural space and injection of the local anesthetic solution can be achieved with the patient in the lateral position or in the sitting position. The lateral position is much more comfortable and safer for the parturient than is the sitting position because in some instances the parturient may develop syncope should she have had any premedication or for some other reason. Moreover, the cerebrospinal fluid pressure in the lumbar region is higher than when she is in the lateral position causing the dura to bulge posteriorly and thus decrease the size of the epidural space and increase the risk of perforating the dura with the point of the advancing needle. The only exception to the preference for the lateral position is in an obese individual in whom the lateral position causes shift of the midline of the skin lower than the spinous processes. Indeed, in some excessively obese individuals, it is difficult to palpate the spinous processes in the lateral position, but this is more feasible with the patient in the sitting position and able to flex as much as possible.

It is essential that the patient be attended by a nurse assistant who should continuously encourage the patient and prevent her from changing position. As in spinal anesthesia, flexion of the thoracolumbar spine increases the width of the interspinous and interlaminar space and thus facilitates introduction of the needle.

## *General Principles*

### *Identification of Landmarks and Check of Equipment*

The anatomic landmarks necessary for performance of the block should be identified before the physician puts on sterile gloves and the antiseptic solution applied. This step has the advantage of permitting the operator to get a good perspective and to palpate the area without fear of contaminating it.

No needle should be inserted until it has been tested for sharpness, "hooks," and patency by injecting saline through it. Although currently available equipment is disposable and theoretically without hooks and is sharp, it is essential to test them before they are inserted into the patient. The anesthetic solution should be prepared just before the block is carried out with freshly added epinephrine from the 1 mg dose vial. In regard to sterility of the local anesthetic solution, stock solutions manufactured by reputable pharmaceutical firms can be used, provided the container has been sterilized with heat (autoclave) or gas, and is not opened until just before the block. Solutions that have been exposed to air, heat, or light might be decomposed or concentrated and should be discarded. This preliminary check of equipment and preparation of solution should be done out of sight of the patient.

### *Asepsis*

It is hardly necessary to emphasize the importance of carrying out the block procedure under strictly aseptic conditions. This is, of course, especially important when the block procedure entails invasion of the subarachnoid space, paravertebral region, sacral canal, epidural space, or any other region of the body in which an infection might be a serious problem. After the injection site has been adequately prepared, towels should be placed so that they do not obscure the landmarks or distort the perspective of the field.

## *Initial Steps of Epidural Block*

### *Preparation of the Skin*

The skin is sterilized with an antiseptic solution and the field is properly draped using strictly aseptic technique. After wiping the skin with a dry sponge to remove excess antiseptic solution, the landmarks are again identified. For obstetric analgesia, the second, third, or fourth lumbar interspace is chosen, because at these levels the epidural space is largest. Which of these interspaces is used depends on the contemplated technique (Table 13–1 and Figure 13–1). The senior author usually prefers to pass the epidural needle through the second lumbar interspace whenever rather unusual circumstances cause him to use a single catheter. In most instances, he uses the double catheter, and for this the needle is passed through the first lumbar or the twelfth thoracic interspace (L1–2, T12-L1).

The reason for use of such high interspaces is to place the tip of the catheter as near as the middle of the T10-L1 segments of the epidural area so that the local anesthetic is deposited very near the segments involved in the pain of uterine contractions.

In the early publication of "The Management of Pain" in 1953 (479) and in a number of subsequent publications (480–483) Bonica and associates reported that placing the tip of the epidural catheter at the T11 or T12 vertebral level through a needle introduced in the T11-L1 or L1–2 intervertebral spaces produced adequate segmental blockade extending from T9–10 to L1–2 by injecting a mean of 4 ml (range 3 to 6) of local anesthetics. This is part of a double-catheter technique that consistently produced complete pain relief during labor and reduced the total amount of local anesthetic to two-thirds or one-half of that used by others (see Table 13–7). Recently, Ackerman and associates (484) completed a study involving four groups of patients, the results of which are summarized in Table 13–21. As noted in Table 13–21, the duration of the first stage of labor from initiation of the epidural analgesia was similar in all four groups, but the initial volume of bupivacaine needed to provide complete pain relief during the first stage was less than one-half when the tip of the catheter was at T12-L1 or L1–2, as was the total amount of bupivacaine to sustain analgesia during the entire first stage.

Tables 13–15 (p 415) and 13–21 list the frequency of distribution (in percentages) of distances from the skin to the epidural space just inside the ligamentum flavum. Obviously, insertion of the needle above the L2 interspace is inherent in the risk of damaging the conus medullaris when the procedure is carried by a person not experienced with epidural puncture above L1. Over the course of 4½ decades, 14,000 epidural blocks in the thoracic and cervical cord have been carried out by Bonica and associates with only one transient neurologic injury due to needle-induced trauma of the thoracic cord. During this period, he taught over 700 residents who within a few months mastered punctures at such high levels in both surgical and obstetric patients, and patients requiring blocks for acute or chronic pain. The one case of neurologic damage, which occurred when an anesthesia fellow ignored the instructions to proceed very slowly in traversing the ligamentum flavum, was published in 1953 (479)

### Methods of Identifying the Epidural Space

Accurate identification of the epidural space with the needle is the most important requisite for success. It is essential that the operator recognize immediately when the point of the needle penetrates the ligamentum flavum and enters the space, and that the advance be halted instantly, so that the dura-arachnoid is not perforated. After having given ample trial in several dozens of patients to all of the procedures that have been suggested for this purpose, including, the Ikle spring loaded syringe (86), the MacIntosh balloon (485), and the "sign of the drop" espoused particularly by Gutierriez (413) (Figure 13–59), the authors prefer the "loss of resistance" technique (Figures 13–60 and 13–61) with saline as first used by Sicard and Forestier (458) and later popularized by Dogliotti (3). Others use air to promptly detect the "lack of resistance." The reason for the preference of saline is that, early on, the senior author gave ample trial to both techniques and noted that saline was the most reliable method of identifying the epidural space. In contrast with air, saline permits the use of tactile as well as visual sensation, and provides additional confirmatory evidence other than visual signs perceived from insensate apparatus (45,432) Saline is a rigid, incompressible liquid filled system and is ideal for providing an unequivocal, crisp endpoint to the loss of resistance so that the transition from complete resistance to total loss of resistance is immediate and convincing. Moreover, as first pointed out by Sicard (486), the sudden forceful ejection of saline from

**Table 13–21.** Influence of Site of Tip of Catheter on the Doses Needed for First Sage of Labor*

| | Group | | | |
|---|---|---|---|---|
| | I | II | III | IV |
| Interspace for Needle Placement | (L3–4) | (L2–3) | (L1–2) | L12–L1) |
| Initial vol (ml) of 0.5% bupivacaine to obtain analgesia | 9.4 (1.02) | 8.4 (1.96) | 4.1 (1.41)** | 3.4 (0.05)** |
| Time to achieve relief from total initial dose (min) | 11.8 (1.32) | 10.6 (2.15) | 3.77 (3.0)** | 2.05 (2.31)** |
| Time to first redose (min) | 78 (28.67) | 85.33 (29.41) | 81.33 (29.28) | 81.67 (37.01) |
| Total mg of bupivacaine for initial pain relief | 47 (5.09) | 42 (9.79) | 20 (7.07)** | 17 (5.10)** |
| Pain score pre-block | 9.73 (0.77) | 8.47 (0.72) | 8.4 (0.61) | 8.46 (0.12) |
| Total mg of bupivacaine for first stage of labor | 65.75 (3.31) | 60.75 (3.56) | 38.75 (7.07)** | 35.75 (5.10)** |
| Incidence of hypotension with initial injection (N/%) | 4/26.7%** | 3/20%** | 0/0% | 0/0% |
| Incidence of hypotension with delivery dose (N/%) | 1/6.7% | 2/3.3% | 2/3.3% | 1/67% |
| Motor score after analgesia established | 0.133 (0.38) | 0.33 (0.47) | 1.6 (0.88) | 1.93 (0.68) |
| Time until first dose (min) | 68 (18.68) | 75.33 (19.41) | 71.33 (19.29) | 77.67 (23.01) |
| Number of reinjections for 1st stage of labor | 1.8 (0.04) | 1.73 (0.068) | 1.67 (0.47) | 1.64 (0.38) |
| Incidence of pudendal block supplementation required (N/%) | 4/26.7% | 5/33.3% | 4/26.7% | 4/26.7% |

* Values are mean (± S.D) unless otherwise stated.
** $P < 0.05$.
(Modified from Ackerman WE, et al: Mid-East J. Anesthesiol. 10;181, 1989.)

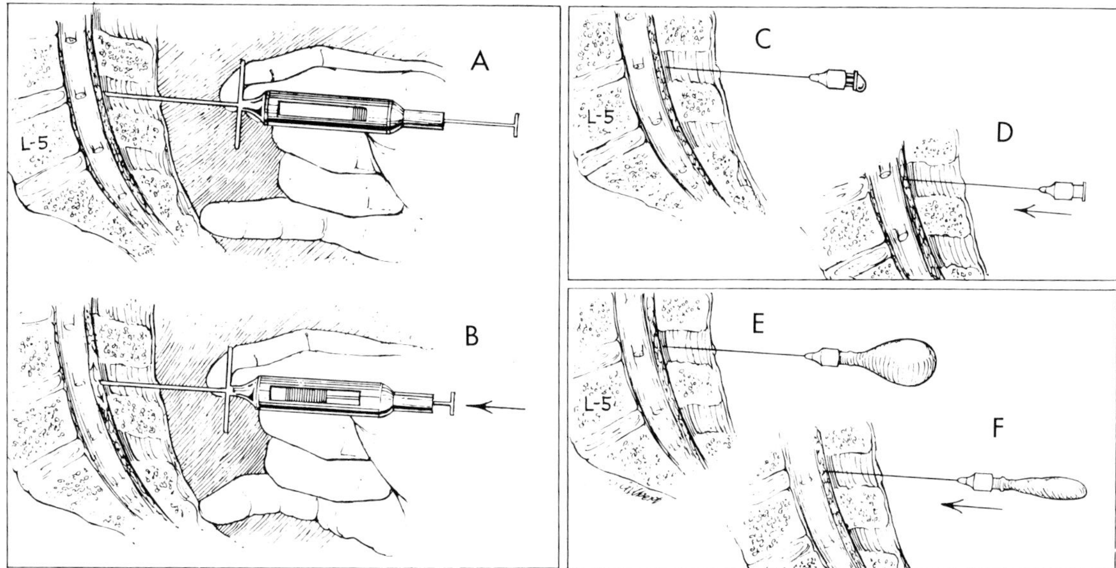


**Fig. 13–59.** Techniques of identifying epidural space. **A** and **B** show use of the Ikle syringe. Syringe has a spring which can be loaded before introducing the needle into the patient. When the point of the needle is in the ligamentum flavum the spring is released, but because of the resistance offered by the ligament the solution remains in the syringe under pressure **(A).** As soon as the point of the needle enteres the epidural space **(B),** lack of resistance permits the solution under pressure to pass easily into the epidural space. **C** and **D,** Use of "sign of the drop" (*signa de gota*) of Gutierrez. When the point of the needle is in the ligamentum favum a drop of fluid is placed so that it will overhang the hub. As soon as the point of the needle enters the epidural space, the negative pressure created sucks the fluid into the epidual space and the drop promptly disappears. **E** and **F,** Use of the Macintosh balloon. The balloon with glass adaptor at its opening and a ring of hard rubber at its base is inflated by injecting 2 ml. of air when the point of the needle has been placed into the ligamentum flavum. As the needle is advanced its point enteres the epidural space, air diffuses into the space and collapses the balloon. Occasionally, deflation of the balloon does not occur promptly as soon as the needle point enters the epidural space, but is gradual, thus misleading the operator. This may be the result of a piece of tissue in the distal lumen of the needle which was "punched out" as the needle, without stylet, was advanced through the ligament. Because of disadvantages inherent in each of these procedures, the lack-of-resistance test if preferred.

the needle adds to the safety of the procedure by pushing the dura-arachnoid away from the needle point (Figures 13–61 and 13–62). Bonica demonstrated this phenomenon by means of forcefully injecting contrast media into the epidural space and taking radiographs at 30 seconds, 1 minute, 2 minutes, and 3 minutes (487). The fact that this dural indentation occurs, despite the dural-anchorling effect of the dorsomedian fiberous band, casts doubt about its existence and/or its function.

Distention of the epidural space with saline not only decreases the risk of dural puncture, but should the catheter be inserted within 2 to 3 minutes of the saline injection the distention may help its cephalad passage. The concern expressed by some that the injection of saline before injection of the local anesthetic dilutes the latter and consequently causes inadequate intensity of block is not valid. Bonica has shown conclusively that saline injected into the epidural space is removed within 3 to 5 minutes, which is a much shorter time than that required to insert the catheter and carry out two or three aspiration tests, inject the test dose, and wait 3 to 5 minutes to evaluate its effects before the injection of the therapeutic dose (487).

A significant reduction in the accidental dural puncture rate using saline has been reported by Doughty (488), MacDonald (489), Galea (490), and Reynolds (491). In contrast, testing with air may result in the formation of air bubbles with irregular spread of local anesthetic solution and subsequent uneven analgesia (492), and pain in the neck and shoulder (493). Naulty, et al (494) also emphasized the risk of venous air embolism with the use of air. The problem of break up of air bubbles with consequent inadequate analgesia was reported by Valentine and his associates (495) who studied 50 parturients, half of whom had saline and half air, to ascertain the loss of resistance in performing epidural analgesia. Once the lack of resistance was demonstrated, each patient received two increments of 4 ml of 0.5% bupivacaine given 5 minutes apart and then the resulting analgesia was followed for 30 minutes. The first segment blocked, the time of onset, the number of blocked segments, and the height of block were comparable on both sides. At 30 minutes, unblocked segments were present in eight parturients (32%) in the air group compared with two (8%) in the saline group ($p < 0.01$). Subsequently, all unblocked subjects were blocked by injecting further doses of bupivacaine. The authors concluded that air is much more likely than saline to produce unblocked segments in the initiation of extradural analgesia in labor. In view of the aforementioned evidence, the development and use by Candido and Winnie (496) of a dual-chambered syringe that allow identification of the epidural space with the loss of resistance with air and with saline seems to us a step that will tend

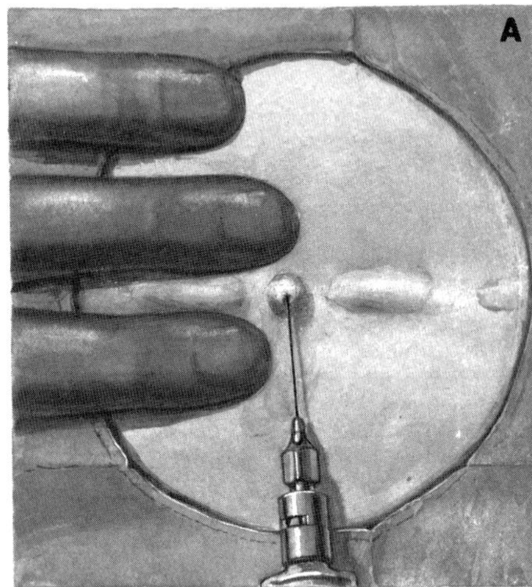


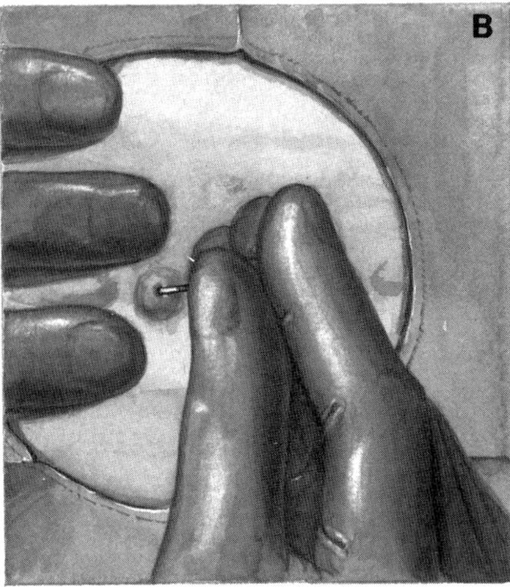


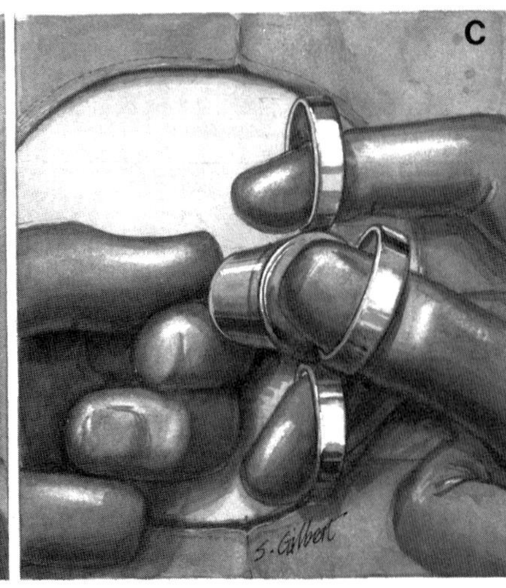


**Fig. 13–60A.** Technique of midline approach. **A,** Following the aforementioned preparation, a skin wheal is made at the midpoint between the second and third lumbar spinous processes with 0.5% lidocaine. The 30-gauge needle is then replaced with a 22-gauge 8-cm disposable spinal needle with a sharp point that is inserted through the opening in the skin made by the small needle. As the point of the needle passes into the subcutaneous tissue, a small amount (0.5 ml) of solution is injected. Great care must be exercised to maintain this 22-gauge needle in the midsagittal plane with its shaft at an angle of 105° (on the cephalad side) with the long axis of the spine. As soon as the needle point reaches the supraspinous ligament, significant resistance is encountered in injecting a small amount of solution because of the density of the ligament. The needle is then advanced 2½ to 3 cm through the loose interspinous ligament, which offers less resistance, and a small amount of solution is injected there. When the point of the needle engages the ligamentum flavum, more resistance is encountered. An attempt should be made to inject while advancing the needle slowly. As soon as the point of the needle passes through the ligamentum flavum, a loss of resistance is felt. The needle is then withdrawn slowly while injecting small amounts of local anesthetic to create a track of analgesia for the larger 18- or 17-gauge epidural needle. After waiting about 15 seconds, the epidural needle is inserted through the same opening in the skin. As noted in **B**, the right hand of a right handed operator is used to control movement of the needle by grasping the hub of the needle firmly between the thumb and third finger while the second finger is placed over the stylet to prevent its retrenchment that would result in punching out a piece of tissue as the needle advances. **C,** The relative positions of the fascial structures should be maintained by having the second and third finger of the left hand straddling the midline and holding it firmly. When the bevel of the needle is 2 to 2½ cm deep, the stylet is removed and the 10 ml Luer-Lok control syringe filled with saline is carefully adapted to the needle. Again, if the operator is right handed, it is easier to manage the syringe with the right hand while the needle is grasped firmly between the thumb and index finger of the left hand and the other fingers and the back of the left hand resting against the patient's back, as depicted in **C**. An attempt is then made to inject the saline. If the point of the needle is still in the interspinous ligament, only moderate resistance to the injection is encountered, but if it is in the tough, dense ligamentum flavum, attempts to inject are met with considerable resistance (see also **A** and **B** of Figure 13–60B).

to make a simple technique (loss of resistance with saline) more complicated and, we believe, unwarranted.

### *Analgesia for the Puncture Site*

From the patient's viewpoint, complete anesthezation of all of the structures to be traversed by the large epidural needle is among the most important obligations of the anesthesiologist. All of the "minor" procedures prior to insertion of the large epidural needle should be made completely painless. This requires the operator to know all of the structures that are to be traversed and their degree of nociception, and to use ample amount of injection of the local anesthetic and to wait sufficient time for analgesia to develop. In making rounds with residents and staff, the senior author often asked the patient to evaluate the procedure, and in all patients in which the block was successful they expressed pleasure and delight about analgesia during uterine contractions, but many commented that the introduction and placement of the epidural needle was a painful experience that detracted from the overall value of the anesthetic. Although this unpleasant experience occurred infrequently, it was usually due to not allowing enough time for analgesia of the various structures to develop; or due to the fact that the step was omitted. Both authors of this chapter feel so strongly about this issue as to repeat description of the analgesia for the puncture site with both the midline and paramedian approach.

## ***Techniques of Epidural Puncture***

To place the bevel of the needle in the posterior midline sulcus of the epidural space, the patient is made to lie on her left side, her spine well flexed so as to increase the size of the interlaminar spaces, and thus facilitate the entrance of the needle into the spinal canal. Following the aforementioned preparation, the epidural needle is introduced and made to follow a course in the exact midsagittal plane—the so-called midline or median approach; or the needle is introduced by the Bonica paramedian technique.

### *Midline Approach*

The midline approach to penetrate and identify the epidural space was first described by Sicard (458), popular-

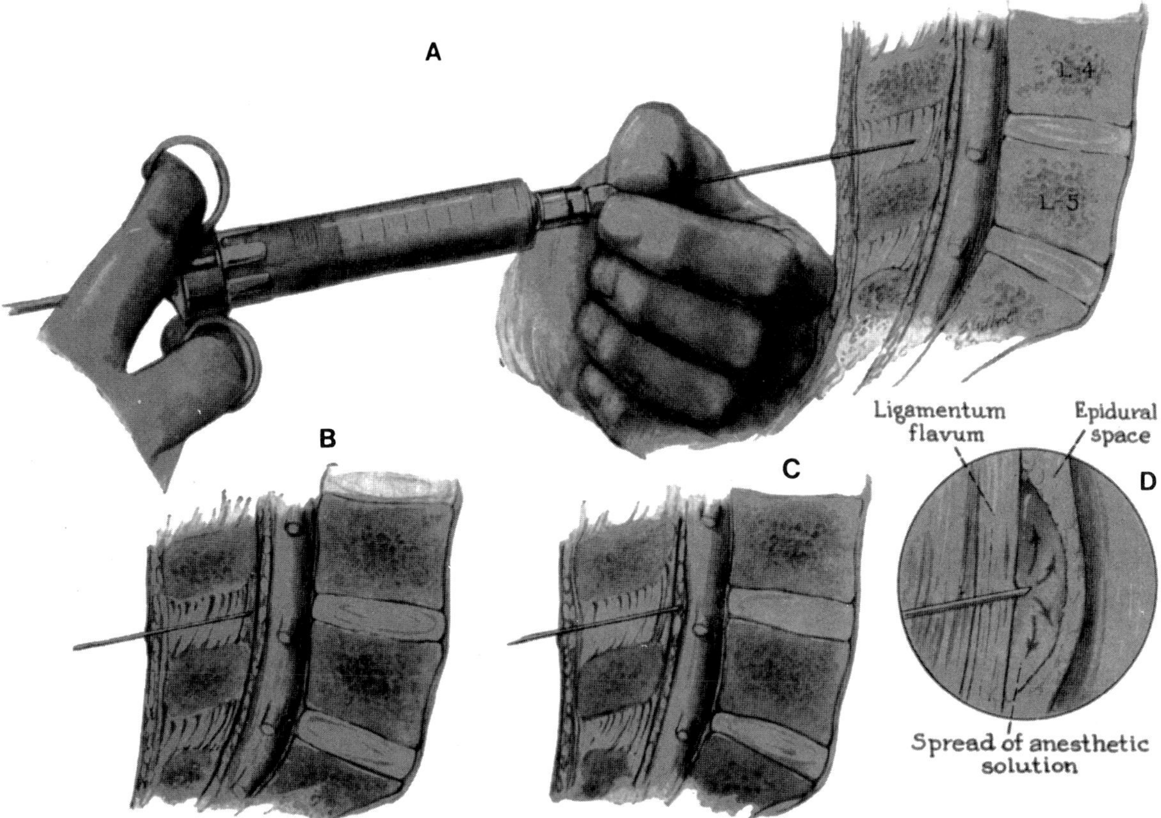


**Fig. 13–60B.** Technique of epidural puncture using the midline approach (continued). Showing side view of the hand and syringe and the sagittal view of the spinal column. **A** shows the back of the left hand of a right handed operator is held against the patient's back with the thumb and index finger grasping the hub of the needle so as to act as a fine control of the advance of the needle while it is pushed anteriorly with the right hand, which controls the syringe by having the second and third fingers in the rings of the syringe and the thumb in the ring of the distal part of the plunger. In **A**, an attempt to inject saline solution while the point of the needle is in the interspinous ligament meets with some resistance; but as soon as the point of the needle enters the ligamentum flavum **(B)**, there is marked resistance that makes injection of the solution virtually impossible. The point of the needle must be advanced very slowly through the ligamentum flavum while the thumb of the right hand exerts constant, unremitting pressure on the plunger of the syringe. Some physicians prefer to advance the needle intermittently 2 mm and then stop and apply pressure on the plunger; the maneuver is repeated several times until the point of the needle enters the space. In any case, it is essential to advance the needle through the ligamentum flavum very slowly; 20 to 25 seconds should be allowed to advance the needle through the 3 to 4 mm thickness of the ligament. As soon as the bevel of the needle enters the epidural space, there is a sudden lack of resistance and the liquid, which up to this point has encountered obstruction, now escapes rapidly and freely **(C)**. The advance of the needle is stopped instantly and the 6 to 8 ml of saline solution discharged forcefully pushing the dura-arachnoid away from the point of the needle **(D)**. When the bevel of the needle is wholly within the epidural space, it is possible to inject saline with little or no resistance: the feeling is the same as injecting fluid into the subarachnoid space. If the operator experiences the sudden marked decrease in resistance, indicating passage of the point of the needle through the ligament but still feels the injection is not free or there is reflux of the fluid, the point of the needle is either not entirely within the epidural space or contains a particle of tissue which was "punched out" by the bevel. To eliminate this possibility, the stylet is replaced into the needle and the needle slowly advanced 1 to 2 mm and injection again attempted. If resistance is still encountered or if there is still reflux, the needle has missed its target and should be withdrawn and another attempt made.

ized by Dogliotti (4), and today remains the most frequently used technique despite the drawbacks inherent in it, which will be discussed later. As already mentioned, it is essential to anesthetize the skin, subcutaneous tissue, and supraspinous and interspinous ligaments with dilute solutions of a local anesthetic (e.g., 0.5% lidocaine or 0.125% bupivacaine). After a lapse of 20 to 30 seconds, a special 18-gauge thin-walled epidural needle is introduced. For ease of introduction and penetration of the tissues, the bevel of the Tuohy needle should face cephalad from the start of the procedure; whereas with the Crawford needle, the bevel faces caudad as depicted in Figures 13–63 and 13–64. Because of its density and toughness, the supraspinous ligament is difficult to penetrate and unless the tissues are held in the midline firmly with two fingers on each side of the interspace, there is a tendency for the needle to slip lateral to the ligament. Therefore, great care must be exercised to maintain the epidural needle in the midsagittal plane. At this point, the 10 ml Leur-Lok control syringe filled with saline is adapted

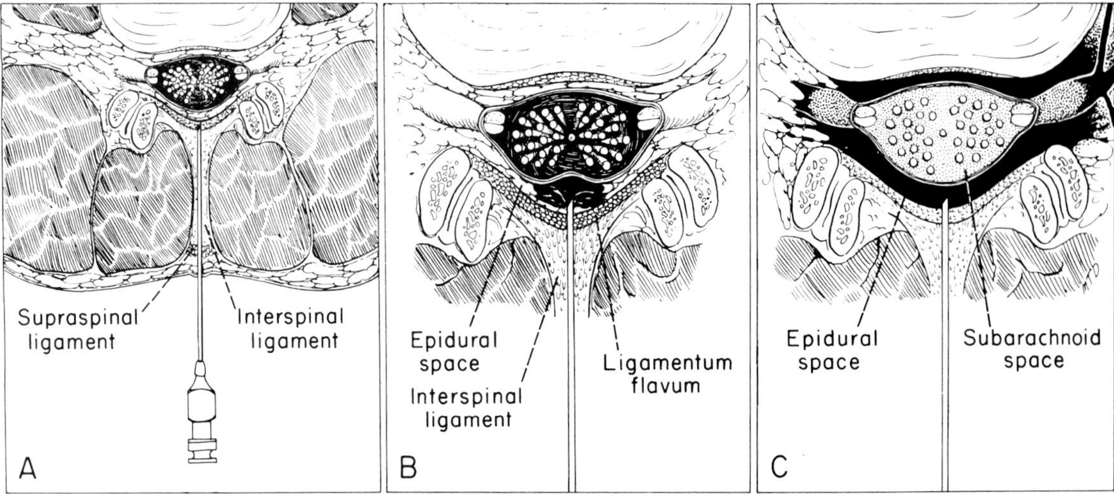


**Fig. 13–61.** Cross section of the lumbar region depicting technique of epidural puncture using the midline approach (continued). In **A**, the point of the needle is in the ligamentum flavum so that injection of saline solution is met with great resistance. In **B**, entrance of the bevel of the needle into the epidural space, while forceful pressure is being applied to the plunger of the syringe, causes complete loss of resistance, and efflux of the 6 to 8 ml of saline causes the dura to be pushed anteriorly away from the point of the needle. Following injection of large volumes of saline into the epidural space, there is a temporary buildup of local epidural pressure causing the solution to reflux briskly through the hub of the needle. The refluxing solution may be mistaken for cerebrospinal fluid. Distinction between the two can be made by: 1) using saline at room temperature for injection: if suspicion of the reflux occurs, 1 or 2 drops are allowed to fall on the bare arm of the operator (without contaminating the field!). Saline is felt much colder than cerebrospinal fluid (at room temperature); 2) observing the reflux for a minute: if the needle is in the epidural space, the dripping ceases within 30 to 60 seconds, but if the point of the needle is in the subarachnoid space, the dripping persists; and 3) attempting to aspirate gently in 4 planes with a dry 2 ml syringe, care being taken not to displace the needle. **C**: Depicts the solution in the epidural space and eventual diffusion into the subarachnoid space.

to the needle. Advance of the needle proceeds through the ligamentum flavum with constant unremitted pressure exerted on the plunger of the syringe. Upon entering the epidural space, there is sudden lack of resistance and rapid eflux of the saline into the epidural space causing the dura-arachnoid to be pushed anteriorly from the point of the needle (Figure 13–60B).

Following injection of the large volume of saline into the epidural space, there is a temporary buildup of local epidural pressure causing the solution to reflux briskly through the hub of the needle. The refluxing solution may be mistaken for cerebrospinal fluid, but distinction between the two can be made by several maneuvers. One is using saline at room temperature for injection so that if there is suspicion of the reflux, one or two drops are allowed to fall on the bare arm of the operator (without contaminating the field!); saline is felt colder than cerebrospinal fluid pressure, which, of course, is at body temperature. A second technique is to observe the reflux for a minute or so: if the needle is in the epidural space, the dripping ceases within 30 to 60 seconds; but if the point is in the subarachnoid space, the dripping persists. A third technique is to attempt to aspirate gently in four planes with a dry 2-ml syringe with care being taken not to displace the needle. If these signs indicate that the point of the needle is in the subarachnoid space, some clinicians prefer to proceed with subarachnoid block while others remove the needle and reinsert it through an adjacent interspace. If blood-tinged fluid is aspirated, 2 ml of saline are injected, the stylet replaced within the needle, and then a minute is allowed to elapse before other steps are taken. If after this interval bloody fluid is aspirated freely, the needle should be withdrawn and reinserted into an adjacent interspace. Should blood again be aspirated, it is best to abandon the procedure because it indicates that a blood vessel has been lacerated and this increases the risk of systemic toxic reaction.

There are three other problems particular to the midline approach that deserve comment. For one thing, this penetration of the supraspinous and interspinous ligaments, because of their structural makeup, make it difficult for the needle to be maintained in a precise, midsagittal plane, and, consequently, the point of the needle may deviate laterally slightly so that the bevel of the needle not infrequently does not reach the midline of the epidural space. Second, penetration of the needle through the supraspinous and interspinous ligaments is associated with more trauma to nociceptive-rich structures, and consequently a percentage of patients will have postpuncture backache (442,497–499). Third, and most important, is the fact that once the catheter passes beyond the bevel of the Crawford needle it is directed almost perpendicular to the long axis of the dura making it difficult to go through the almost right angle curve necessary to proceed cephalad (Figure 13–63). Even with the Tuohy needle, the trajectory of the epidural catheter passing from the bevel is not at right angles to the long axis of the epidural space as some clinicians believe but usually makes an angle of 130° to 140° cephalad to the long axis of the epidural space, and consequently the tip of the catheter is

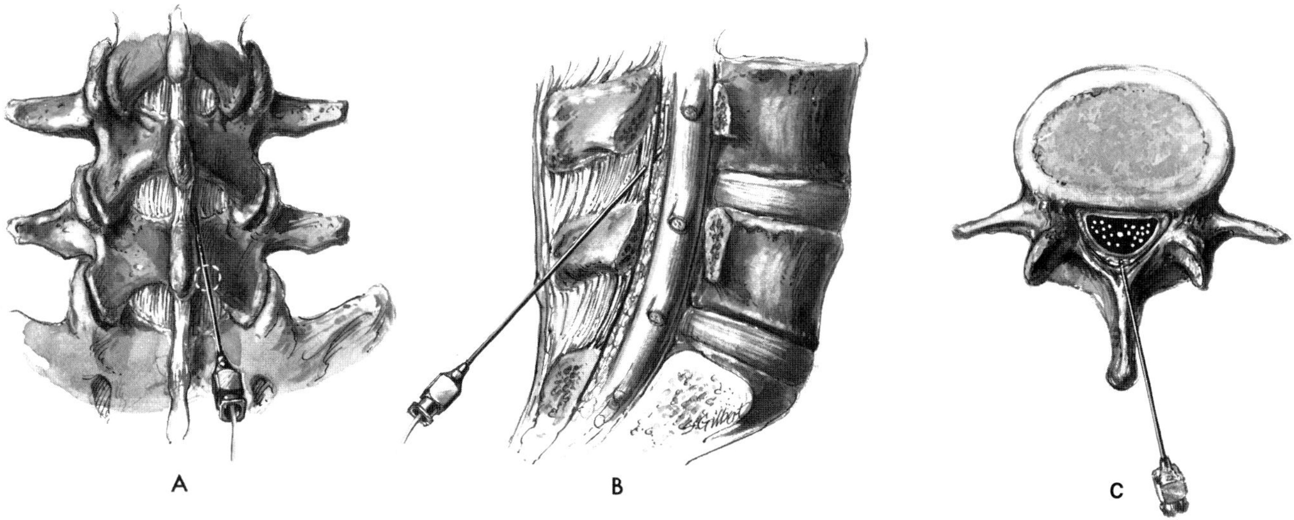


**Fig. 13–62.** Technique of continuous epidural block in the lumbar region using the Bonica paramedian approach. **A**: Posterior view; **B**: side view; and **C**: superior view to show the relationship of the site of puncture, direction of the needle in relationship to the spinous process. **A** shows that the anesthetic wheal is made 1.5 cm from the precise midsagittal plane at the same cross-sectional level as the lower tip of the spinous process of the vertebra below the site of puncture of the ligamentum flavum and final position with the bevel of the needle in the epidural space. Because the spinous process at its lower end is about 1 cm wide, the wheal is about 0.5 to 1 cm lateral to the process. The anesthetic intracutaneous wheal is produced with a 30-gauge, 1-cm needle and injection made of 0.5 ml of 0.5% lidocaine or 0.125% bupivacaine. Next, a 22-gauge 8-cm disposable spinal needle is used to produce a track of anesthesia that will permit penetration with the special 18-gauge epidural needle painlessly and also permit exploration of the deeper structures. As soon as the 22-gauge needle penetrates the skin, 0.5 ml of local anesthetic is injected into the subcutaneous tissue and then the needle directed superiorly and medially so as to make an angle of 15° with the midsagittal plane and 135° cephalad to the long axis of the body. Advancing in this trajectory while at the same time injecting small amounts of local anesthetic as the needle is advanced slowly. At a depth of 3 to 3.5 cm, the bevel of the needle is likely to make contact with the lateral aspect of the proximal portion of the spinous process whose topography at this point is such that it will direct the needle toward the medial aspect of the ipsilateral lamina. The needle is maneuvered to pass superior to the superior edge of the lamina where it usually makes contact with the medial part of the ligamentum flavum. An attempt is made to inject at this point, and if the needle is still outside of the ligamentum flavum, the injection is made without resistance; whereas, if the point of the needle has engaged the ligamentum flavum, significant resistance to injection is encountered. The needle is advanced *very slowly* until sudden lack of resistance is experienced, indicating that the point of the needle has entered the epidural space. Once this is achieved with the 22-gauge needle, it is withdrawn slowly, and the remaining amount of local anesthetic (about 3 to 4 ml) is injected continuously until the point of the needle is out of the skin. (Because of the dilute nature of the local anesthetic and the fact that the needle is moved and the region has only small vessels, the danger of injecting any more than 0.1 to 0.2 ml of solution intravenously is rare.) Within 30 seconds a track of anesthesia that is about 1 to 1.5 cm in diameter is present to permit the penetration with the larger epidural needle painlessly. In **B**, depicting the relationship and position of the needle with the epidural catheter in it shows that, after penetration of the epidural space, the long access of the needle makes a cephalad angle with the long access of the body of about 135° while the caudad angle is 45°. Also note that the bevel of the needle is in the upper part of the epidural space, which is usually wider than its lower portion. **C**: The superior view showing the relationship of the needle to the midsagittal plane and the position of the needle point in the epidural space with the bevel of the needle facing cephalad. For reasons presented in previous pages, with the paramedian technique, the advance of the catheter is invariably cephalad and being adjacent to the dura is straight in the midline sulcus of the epidural space.

directed against the dura. Not infrequently, as the catheter advances beyond the bevel of the needle, its tip is buried into a fat pad or between an epidural vein and other contents of the epidural space. If the tip of the catheter is against a vein and its advancement beyond the bevel of the needle requires some force, it is likely to tear and/or lacerate the vein. As already mentioned, Blomberg (416) studied the insertion of a lumbar epidural catheter in the 14 autopsy subjects already cited and noted that midline approach to the epidural space caused tenting of the dura in all 14 cases and that the direction of the midline catheter took varying courses. In contrast, none of these problems occurred with the paramedian approach as described below.

## *The Paramedian Approach*

### *Development of the Parmedian Approach*

Soon after the report by Curbelo (42) and the one by Flowers, et al (43) on the use of continuous lumbar epidural anesthesia for surgery and obstetrics using the midline approach, the senior author began to use the technique and continued at an increased rate and often in place of continuous caudal. He soon noted that in contrast to continuous caudal, in which the catheter could be advanced without much difficulty, problems were encountered with advancement of the catheter inserted in the lumbar epidural space. This prompted him to take the problem to his anatomy laboratory at the University of

Washington where he began to systematically study the configuration of the lumbar vertebra and the relationship of the Crawford needle that was being widely used for this purpose. At the time, Bonica was aware that the paraspinous technique for spinal (subarachnoid) block had been described by Sicard, Forestier, Dogliotti, MacIntosh, and many others—all of whom introduced the needle and catheter at the same horizontal cross-sectional level as the interlaminar space and dural sac intended to be penetrated. Because this approach was inherent in the same problem of requiring that the catheter make a 90 to 105° angle cephalad to the long axis of the epidural space, not infrequently the catheter would impinge on the posterior wall of the epidural space and become caught in a fat pad or a vessel making it impossible to advance further. This made it obvious that to minimize or overcome this problem, it would be necessary to introduce the needle in a paramedian (or as some prefer, "paraspinous") angle so that on entering the epidural space the bevel (opening) of the needle would be at an angle that would facilitate the catheter advance cephalad.

To determine the optimal angle in which to introduce the needle, Bonica carried out a comprehensive, systematic study in 25 cadavers and 125 patients in whom he introduced the epidural needle at different angles in relation to both the long axis and the cross-sectional aspects of the epidural space. Analysis of the data revealed that the optimal angles in the average individual would place the needle with its axis making an angle of 15° with the cross-sectional plane and a cephalad angle of 135° with the long axis of the spinal canal. In some of the volunteer subjects, as well as in patients, it was noted that introduction of the needle more lateral than 1.5 cm from the midsagittal plane caused the needle to reach and enter the contralateral ligamentum flavum and advance within this ligament until its point reached the intervertebral foramen and elicited paresthesia caused by stimulation of the nerve as it comes out of the intervertebral foramen (Figure 13–63A). On the other hand, using an angle of less than 15°, the needle will pass through the ligamentum flavum lateral to the midline and enter the lateral aspect of the very thin epidural space and enter the subarachnoid space (Figure 13–63B).

By 1955, sufficient experience had been gained, not only by Bonica but also the faculty and residents, to adapt the final modification depicted in Figures 13–62 and 13–65, and a year later, it was published (415). Figures 13–64 and 13–65 are enlarged schematic depictions that show more clearly the differences between the midline and paramedian approaches. Over the 4 decades the technique has been used in the departments in which Bonica and McDonald have worked, in over 100,000 obstetric and surgical patients and in those requiring pain therapy, with a success rate of 90 to 95%, or even higher among those with long experience. On the basis of the findings in the literature, 15 years elapsed between the first publication by Bonica and the first reference to its clinical use, published by Carrie in 1971 (497) and 4 years later by

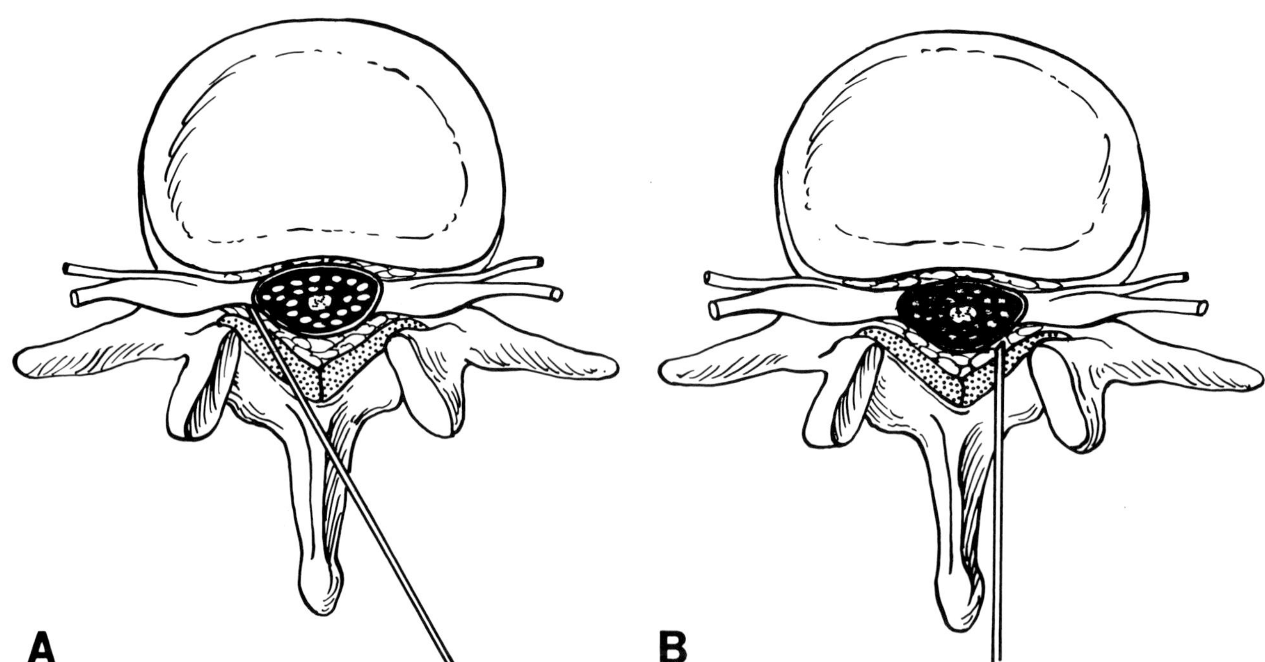


**Fig. 13–63.** Misdirection of the needle introduced by the paramedian approach. **A**: The angle the needle makes with coronal plane is greater than 15° so that its point will advance to the contralateral ligamentum flavum and then proceed anteriorly within the ligament for 2 to 3 cm without encountering loss of resistance and until its point is in the intervertebral foramen. At this juncture it may contact the nerve and cause lancinating paresthesia. **B**: Introduction of the needle intended for the paramedian approach is misdirected to the lateral aspect of the ipsilateral ligamentum flavum. Because the ligament is much thinner than in the midline and the epidural space at this point of needle penetration is very narrow, it is likely that it will pass into the subarachnoid space without experiencing loss of resistance.

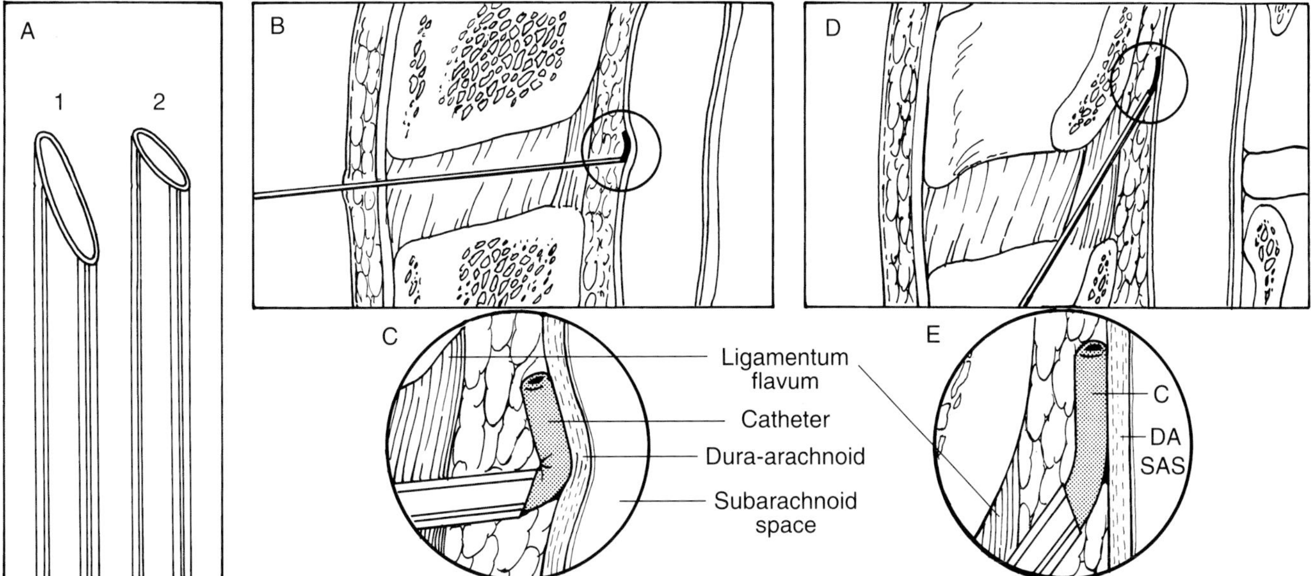


**Fig. 13–64.** Enlarged schema of midline puncture of the epidural space using the Crawford needle. Insert A shows the bevel (1) of the regular 18 gauge thin-walled needle, while 2 depicts the shorter Crawford bevel. B shows the midline approach to the epidural space. In this case the needle is advanced until the bevel is near the dura, at which point the catheter is introduced. Because of the toughness of the dura mater the bevel of the Crawford needle, being short and facing the dura, does not penetrate the structure but causes bulging inward until finally the catheter passes through the bevel and advances usually cephalad, although this is not always the case: It may deviate laterally into one of the intervertebral foramen or may even proceed cephalad. In D, the Crawford needle has been introduced via the paramedian approach to facilitate the advance of the catheter cephalad. In either case, the needle is introduced with the bevel (opening) facing the dura, and with the paramedian approach the catheter will impinge on the dura and slide cephalad. C = catheter; DA = dura mater; SAS = subarachnoid space.

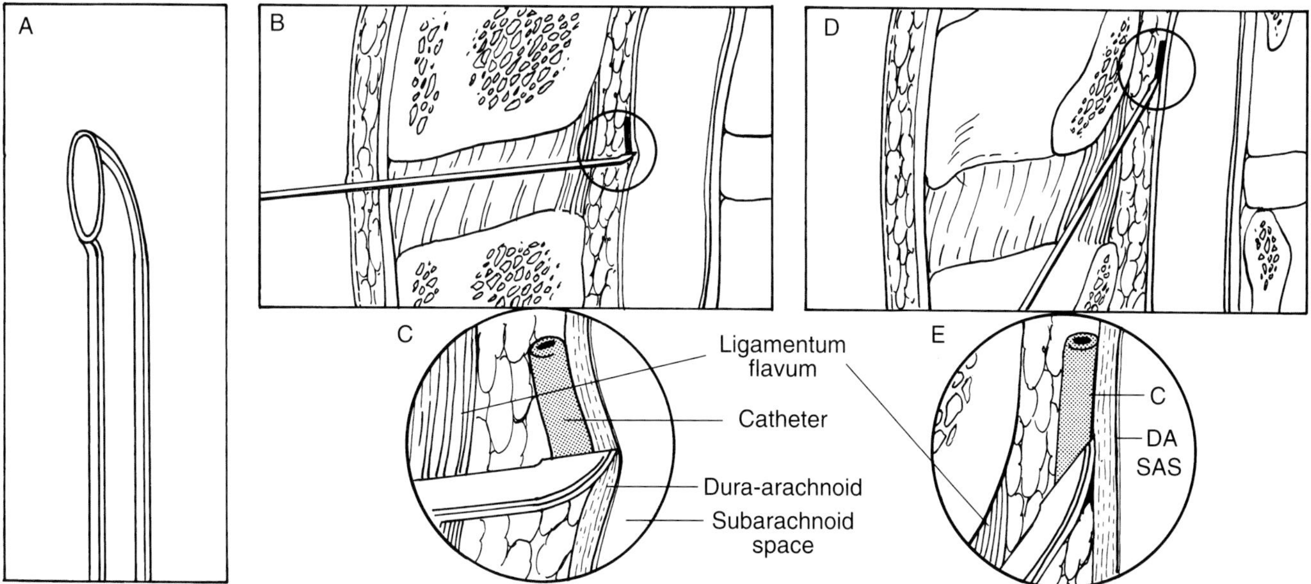


**Fig. 13–65.** Schema of the penetration of the Tuohy needle and the course of the catheter cephalad. A Tuohy needle is introduced through the midline and advanced sufficiently so that its entire bevel is within the epidural space. Because the needle makes a cephalad angle of about 100° with the long axis of the epidural space, the trajectory of the epidural catheter will usually make about 140° cephalad to the long axis of the epidural space causing its tip to impinge on the dura mater. Consequently, to advance further it is necessary to exert enough pressure to indent significantly the dura, after which the tip of the catheter will slip and pass cephalad. If the epidural space is narrow or if the needle is advanced too far, the very sharp point of the Tuohy needle may cause a nick (or a small hole) into the dura that permits loss of fluid during the postpartum period with consequent postpartum headache. **B**: With the Bonica paramedian approach, the angle of the needle is such that the back of the bevel comes to be flush against the dura, the orifice faces cephalad, and the advance of the catheter is straight cephalad within the epidural space. Because the point of the needle is directly cephalad, the possibility of puncturing the dura is small (see text for more details).

Armitage (498) who spent part of his postgraduate studies with Bonica and associates in Seattle.

In the 1980s and early 1990s, a number of very informative experimental and clinical studies related to epidural anesthesia, but especially to the paramedian technique, were published and most of which have been cited in various sections of preceding pages of this chapter. Of particular value have been the studies of Blomberg (398–400,407,416,427), Gaynor (397), Harrison and coworkers (392–394,412), Parkin and Harrison (389), Westbrook and associates (406), and Zurzur (390), among others and a number of clinical studies (498–501). Jacout (499) reported on the largest published retrospective study involving 1010 parturients, which were used to compare the midline and paramedian approach. Although some of the authors made slight changes in Bonica's technique, all of these reports confirm the advantages of the paramedian over the midline (median) technique that have been claimed by Bonica in the many writings published on this subject.

### Technique of the Paramedian Approach

As in the midline approach, the paramedian approach is carried out with the patient on her left side and after proper preparation in carrying out all of the aforementioned tasks, including discussion with the patient, analgesia of the skin, subcutaneous tissue, muscle, and periosteum of the spinous process, and lamina with dilute local anesthetic solution achieved. Using dilute solutions, one can inject a total of 15 ml of lidocaine (75 mg) to produce a track of anesthesia that will make introduction of the 18-gauge epidural needle painless. In addition, the maneuver serves to explore the region before inserting the larger needle. Although this extra step of injecting these structures with the 22-gauge needle consumes more time, it is well worthwhile from the viewpoint of making the procedure painless for the patient. The senior author has had continuous epidural analgesia for both surgery and postoperative pain on 14 occasions, in all except one done with prepuncture analgesia carried out to determine the difference between analgesia and no analgesia. In one instance without analgesia, puncture with a large Tuohy needle caused acute pain superficially and referred acute pain when the periosteum of the lamina was contacted. It is important to wait about 20 to 30 seconds between the formation of the track of analgesia and the penetration of the tissues with the large needle to allow sufficient time for the lidocaine to block the small nociceptive afferent terminals. Once this is accomplished, the 18-gauge epidural needle is introduced through the track of anesthesia and it is maneuvered so that its bevel faces caudad and is flush with the superior surface of the lamina. It is then slowly advanced to engage and then traverse the ligamentum flavum. When this is achieved, the stylet is removed and a 10 ml Leur-Lok control syringe filled with saline is carefully adapted to the needle and attempt made to inject it. If the point of the needle is still within the paraspinal muscle, the saline can be injected with ease; but if it is within the tough yellow ligament, marked resistance is encountered. It is important to note in Figures 13–62, 13–63, and 13–64 that when the opening of the Crawford needle is fully within the epidural space, it faces anteriorly, while with the bevel of the Tuohy needle, the opening faces cephalad and its back is against the dura (as shown in Figures 13–67 and 13–68).

### Comparison Between Midline and Paramedian Approach

A comparison between the midline and paramedian approach suggests the following differences and advantages, most of which have been cited by Bonica (415), Armitage (498), Blomberg (399,400,498), Carrie (497), Gaynor (442), Jacout (500), and Barretta (501).

1. With the paramedian technique, penetration of the epidural space is easier and provides more definitive landmarks—factors that in the hands of anesthesiologists experienced with the technique account for the high (95 to 99%) success. Once the bevel of the epidural needle penetrates the skin, about 1.5 cm to the precise mid-sagittal plane and angled posteriorly and rostrally, it is made to contact the superficial surface of the spinous process, the topography of which is such as to direct the bevel of the needle to the medial edge of the ipsilateral ligamentum flavum.
2. In the midline, the resistance to injection of saline provided by the interspinous ligament varies and may be a factor in confusion as to where the point of the needle is; whereas with the paramedian approach, the penetration of the muscles offers virtually no resistance. Consequently, contact with the lamina provides a much better deep landmark that is an excellent osseous indication of the depth of the ligamentum flavum.
3. Injection with the bevel of the needle above the lamina provides no resistance, but upon entering the yellow ligament there is a marked increase in resistance that leaves no doubt in the mind of operator to which structure the bevel of needle is in.
4. The angle by which the back of the bevel of the Tuohy needle approaches the dura is so acute as to virtually eliminate risk of piercing the dura mater—a factor that some consider the most important advantage of the paramedian approach. This is in contrast to the midline technique in which the bevel of the needle approaches the dura mater at a 100 to 110° angle cephalad to the long axis. Although it has been shown that the dura mater is resistant to needle penetration (425,426,500), not infrequently the point of the epidural needle is advanced more than 6 cm from the skin. On such occasions, it is likely to make a very small hole in the dura that in the postpartum period causes leakage of cerebrospinal fluid with consequent postpartum headache (see Figure 13–64).
5. Intravenous cannulation with the point of the needle occurs much less frequently with the paramedian approach than with the midline approach. Indeed, if the point of entry of the needle into the skin is paraspinal, entrance of the epidural space is made

through the medial edge of the ligamentum flavum, and the subsequent insertion of the catheter causes it to run into the space between the venous plexuses that lies on each side of the midline.

6. With the paramedian technique, the opening of the bevel of the Tuohy needle faces directly cephalad (Figure 13–64B) and facilitates the advance of the catheter in a straight rostral direction. This was impressively demonstrated by Blomberg and associates in their studies, but particularly in the study of 14 cadavers (417). In this study, one Tuohy needle was inserted in the midline, another paramedian using Bonica's angles for the introduction of the paramedian needle and epidural visualization with the 2.2 mm Olympus Selfoscope 2211S. The cephalad angle of the midline needle to the dorsal plane of the skin varied between 90° and 100°, whereas the cephalad angle of the paramedian needle varied between 120° and 135°. In its angle to the cross-sectional (coronal) plane, it was between 15° and 20°. They noted that with the midline catheter there was significant tenting of the dura that did not occur with the paramedian needle. The course of the midline catheter was unpredictable because contact with the dura caused variable deviations. Strands of connective tissue that restricted movement of the dura mater in the region of catheter contact contributed to this behavior. A loop of catheter was seen to be formed when the tip caught on connective tissue strands as the catheter was being advanced, but a normal CSF pressure with catheter changed to a straight cephalad course in only two instances while a straight course was changed into a deviated one in two other cases. In contrast, the paramedian catheter was advanced easily in a straight cephalad direction without any resistance in all 14 cases, and even in the subjects with a dense dorsomedian connective tissue band no obstacle was presented to the paramedian catheter that passed through the strands and advanced parallel to the dorsomedian aspect of the dura mater. A number of studies have demonstrated a great variation in the course of epidural catheters introduced via a midline approach, whereas Barretta, et al (501) noted that in 13 patients in whom catheters were introduced by the paramedian approach, all of them assumed a straight cephalad direction.

   In another study by Blomberg and associates (417), 49 live patients scheduled for transurethral resection of the prostate or resection of bladder neoplasm on 50 occasions were allocated randomly into two groups of epidural puncture-midline or paramedian. Technical difficulties and the occurrence of complications as well as extents of sensory and motor blockade were compared. The paramedian approach was associated with a significantly lower frequency of technical problems compared to the midline approach. Statistically significant differences were demonstrated between the two techniques for the following factors: 1) repeated attempts at needle insertion; 2) difficulty in identification of the epidural space; 3) resistance to introduction of the catheter into the epidural space; 4) resistance to injection through the epidural catheter; and, 5) production of paresthesia which occurred in 18% of patients in the midline group and only 2% in the paramedian group.

7. Another advantage of the paramedian approach is that passage through muscle and the ligamentum flavum present much less trauma from the large epidural needle and, consequently, there has been a lesser incidence of residual backache among patients who have received epidural anesthesia achieved by the paramedian technique compared to those achieved with the midline approach (442,499).
8. For parturients who have difficulty in flexing their back, the ligamentum flavum is easier to reach with the paramedian than with the midline technique, thus providing an important advantage.
9. Finally, a simple clinical issue: Because the catheter makes an acute angle with the skin, its placement and adjustment allows the parturient to lie on it with less or no risk of being kinked.

The technique of the paramedian approach to the epidural space is depicted in Figure 13–64 and described in detail in the legend with the hope that those clinicians who have not employed it might be encouraged to do so and use it more widely to afford the patient and the anesthesiologist the aforementioned advantages over the midline technique.

### *Placement of the Catheter*

Currently, very few obstetric anesthesiologists use single-dose epidural block for labor and vaginal delivery, and even for cesarean section, which in the hands of an experienced surgeon should be carried out within the time of anesthesia produced with the appropriate doses of bupivacaine. The authors believe, even in circumstances in which operative delivery can be accomplished within the period of the duration of block following a single dose, it is best to have a catheter in place because it provides control of extent and intensity of blockade. The technique of placing and fixing the catheter is depicted in Figure 13–66. The following comments are intended to supplement and/or emphasize certain points.

Once the point of the catheter is beyond the bevel of the needle, it is advanced 3 to 4 cm. If it is introduced less than this distance, there is the possibility that the tip may be withdrawn from the space during manipulation and taping of the catheter. However, if the catheter is advanced too far, there is the possibility of: (1) laceration of veins; (2) tying a true knot within the epidural space; and (3) migration of its point through an intervertebral foramen to the paravertebral space.

Occasionally, the catheter cannot be advanced beyond the point of the needle. This may be because: (1) the bevel of the needle is totally outside of the epidural space; or (2) the bevel of the needle is only partially within the epidural space, so that the catheter does not have an opening large enough to permit its exit from the needle.

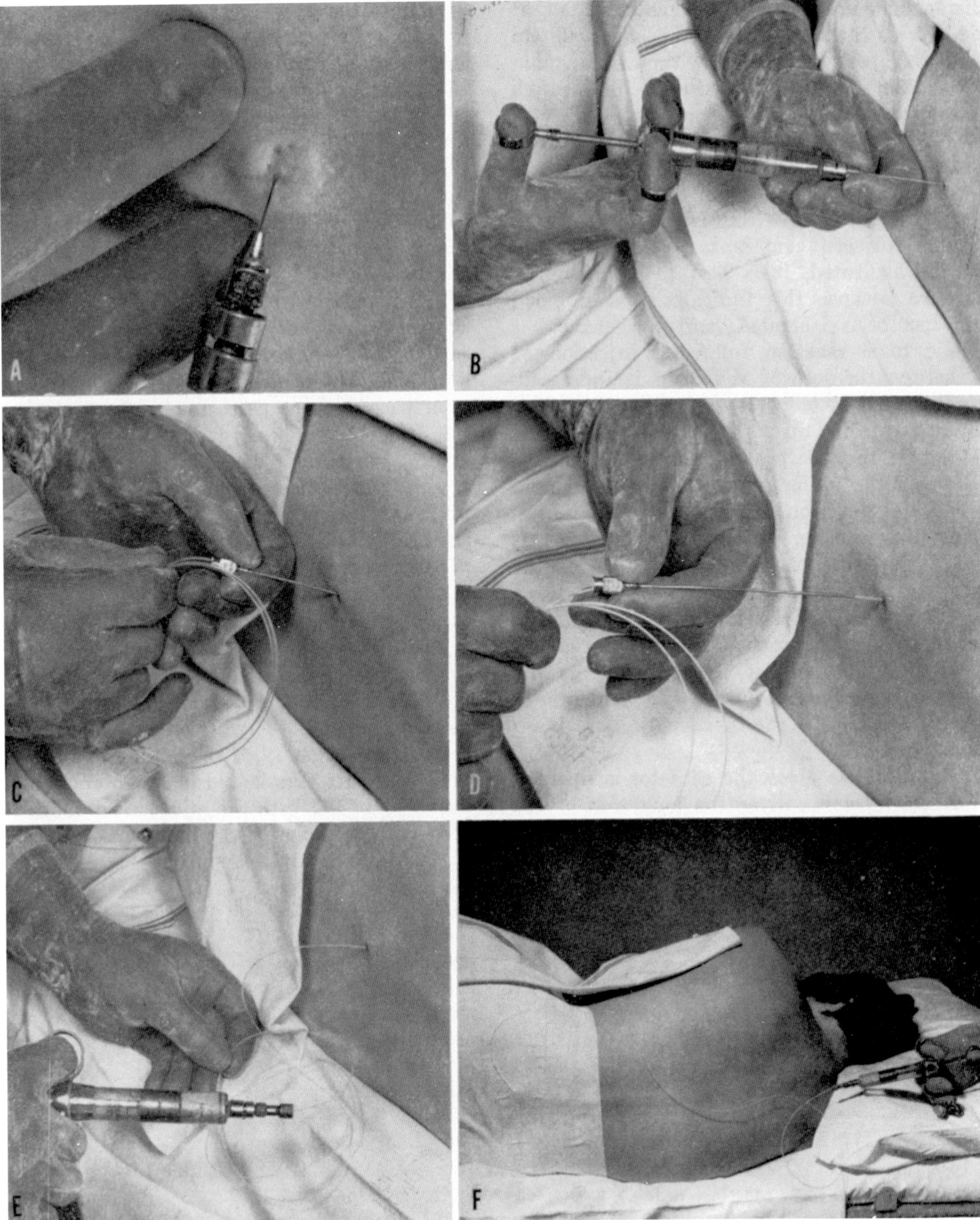


**Fig. 13–66.** Technique of continuous epidural block using paramedian approach. **A**: Formation of intracutaneous wheal just lateral to lower portion of spinous process of third lumbar vertebra. **B**: Advance of needle through ligamentum flavum of the second lumbar interspace. Note that puncture is just lateral to the crest made by the spinous processes. Needle is controlled by grasping its hub with the thumb and index finger of the left hand while the right hand is exerting constant, unremitting pressure on the plunger of the syringe filled with saline. **C**: Introduction of catheter through needle. Note that hub of needle is pulled caudad toward the patient, increasing the angle its shaft makes with the epidural space. Also note technique of holding the tubing: it is wound around the right hand. **D**: Withdrawal of needle over the tubing which is held steady with the right hand. **E**: Injection of test dose after needle has been withdrawn. Tuohy-Borsch adaptor is placed at the end of catheter and adapted to a syringe filled with local anesthetic. **F**: Catheter is immobilized with adhesive tape. Note the large circle made by the catheter to decrease risk of kinking at its point of exit from the skin.

The latter condition may result from not advancing the needle sufficiently, so that the proximal portion of the bevel is still within the ligamentum flavum, or because it has been advanced too far, so that its distal portion is buried in the posterior longitudinal ligament. To find out which is the case, an attempt should be made to advance the needle an additional 2 or 3 mm and then to advance the catheter. If part of the bevel was in the yellow ligament, this step will solve the problem. However, if the bevel was already against the anterior wall of the spinal canal, the needle cannot be advanced. Obviously, in this case the needle must be withdrawn before attempting to pass the catheter again. Occasionally, the catheter is advanced 1 or 2 cm only to meet an obstruction. This may be because its tip is impinged on a fat pad or vessel, or the pedicle of vertebra above the site of injection. In such cases, gently twisting the catheter on its axis will often change the position of its point so that it can be further advanced without difficulty. During such maneuver, extreme care must be exercised not to withdraw the catheter through the needle once its tip has passed into the epidural space; otherwise, it is likely to be sheared off and cannot be retrieved without laminectomy.

When the catheter is properly placed, the needle is withdrawn from the patient's back over the plastic tubing (Figure 13–66C). After removal of the needle, the tubing is withdrawn 1 cm just in case its tip has been pushed into a foramen or into fat. A Tuohy-Borsch adaptor (Becton, Dickinson Company, Rutherford, NJ) is then attached to the end of the tubing and aspiration attempted with a dry 2-ml syringe. If blood or blood-tinged fluid is aspirated, the tubing should be withdrawn an additional 5 mm and aspiration repeated. If no blood or cerebrospinal fluid can be aspirated, the syringe is disconnected and 1 ml of saline is injected to dislodge any tissue that may be against the tip of the plastic tubing. Then another attempt is made at aspiration. If again nothing is aspirated, a further precaution is taken: the syringe is detached and the end of the tubing is placed about 2 feet below the level of the spinal column. If the tubing is within the subarachnoid space, CSF fluid will drip out. In such a case, 0.5 ml of CSF should be aspirated and injected on the bare forearm of the anesthesiologist or another person to confirm the suspicion as to whether or not the catheter tip is in the CSF, which, of course, is warmer (body temperature) than the local anesthetic at room temperature. If this further attempt confirms the position of the catheter inside the subarachnoid space, one can either withdraw the catheter and reintroduce the needle and catheter one or two segments above or below the original site of the needle penetration. Many anesthesiologists proceed in this manner and are usually successful in carrying epidural anesthesia without any serious complications from subarachnoid injection. Many prefer, on the other hand, to abandon epidural anesthesia and proceed with subarachnoid block.

### *Injection of Test Dose*

The introduction by Moore and Batra (502) of the epidural test dose (ETD) has been an important advance in obstetric anesthesia. It consists of injection of a: 1) combination of epinephrine intended to indicate whether or not the tip of the catheter is in the vein, in which case it will cause increase in maternal heart rate and blood pressure; and 2) small amount (45 to 60 mg) of lidocaine, which will produce a definite subarachnoid block extending to T10–12 if the catheter is in the subarachnoid space. Prior to injection, the patient should be encouraged to relax and all monitoring equipment shown to be functional, including: the electrocardiograph and automatic blood pressure cuff that measures blood pressure every 3 minutes; a pulse oximeter to continuously monitor pulse rate, continuous monitoring of fetal heart rate (FHR) and uterine activity (UA) either by external or internal TKD. After observation of the various parameters for 1 minute, the injection is made about 15 seconds after termination of uterine contraction and the associated pain. A number of studies have shown that continuous observation of all of the parameters for 1 minute will cause maximal changes in maternal heart rate (MHR) due to the injection of intravenous epinephrine occur within 30 to 45 seconds (502). In addition, limiting the MHR observation time to 1 minute after the intravenous injection reduces the possible number of pain-induced MHR variations due to uterine contractions, and this, in turn, improves the sensitivity and specificity of this technique. The importance of limiting the observation time to 1 minute is also supported by findings of Leighton, et al (503) who noted that intravenous administration of 15 μg epinephrine cause significant increases in MHR at 45 seconds after the injection, but not at 60 or 90 seconds.

While the recommendations by Batra and Moore (502) were widely applied, a number of negative studies (504–508) cast doubt and challenged the validity of this method and discouraged the use of the test, especially in parturients because of several concerns: 1) the specificity and sensitivity of the test as a marker for accidental intravenous injection were not high enough; 2) the fact that in animals intravenous injection of epinephrine doses reduced uterine blood flow (UBF) for a transient period but without changes in FHR pattern, and this effect was dose dependent. In gravid ewes, intravenous epinephrine in doses of 10 and 20 μg reduced UBF by 30% and 50%, respectively. Supporters of the EDT have pointed out that these reductions in UBF were significantly lower than the 100% decrease noted in humans when contraction-induced increase in intrauterine pressure reaches 30 to 40 mm Hg (509–513).

In one recently published study, Colonna-Romano and associates (511) carried out a well-designed study to determine the sensitivity and specificity and lowest effective dose of epinephrine for ETD. Fifty-nine parturients were assigned randomly to receive an intravenous injection of either normal saline solution (NS group I or 1% lidocaine with epinephrine 1:200,000 in which the 3 ml contained 5 μg epinephrine; a second group in which the solution contained 10 μg; and a third group in which the solution contained 15 μg, all diluted to 3 ml. Based on their comprehensive study, they came to the following conclusion: 1) epinephrine is a 100% sensitive marker of intravascular injection in laboring women; 2) within 1 minute after injection, the baseline-to-peak criterion was a reliable in-

**TABLE 13–22.** Technique and Characteristics of Single Catheter Continuous Lumbar Segmental Block

| Technique | Comparison with Other Extradural Techniques |
|---|---|
| —Needle puncture at $L_3 \rightarrow$ catheter advanced 3 cm ($L_2$) | Advantages |
| —Aspiration test and injection of test dose | 1. Requires less drug than the standard technique |
| —If negative at 5 min, inject 5–6 ml of dilute (analgesic) solution of local anesthetic $\rightarrow$ analgesia $T_{10}$–$L_1$ | 2. No effect on uterine contractions |
| —Continuous oxygen and frequent monitoring | 3. No premature numbness of the limbs |
| —Top-up analgesic dose as soon as slight pain returns | 4. No premature perineal relaxation $\rightarrow$ no interference with flexion or rotation |
| —When pain in limbs and perineum inject 10–12 ml of analgesic concentration with patient in Fowler's position | 5. Less effect of local anesthetic on mother and fetus |
| —After internal rotation inject higher concentration to relax perineum | Disadvantages |
| | 1. May produce incomplete analgesia/relaxation of perineum |
| | 2. Requires Fowler's or sitting up position |

(From Bonica JJ: Obstetric Analgesia and Anesthesia, 2nd Ed., University of Washington Press, Seattle, 1980, p. 106.)

dicator of intravenous injection; 3) 10 μg epinephrine is as effective as 15 μg; 4) the pattern of epinephrine induced tachycardia could be clinically differentiated from tachycardia from other sources. Gieraerts and associates (513) reported a double blind study that entailed the injection of 12.5 mg of bupivacaine and 12.5 μg of epinephrine with a highly reliable epidural test dose to detect accidental intravascular injection in obstetric patients with a 99% specificity and 97.5% sensitivity.

The positive position of Bonica's colleagues of the Division of Obstetric Anesthesia at the University of Washington was published by Chadwick and associates in 1987 (512). The test dose (3 ml of 0.25% bupivacaine containing a total of 7.5 mg of bupivacaine) is an indicator of intrathecal injection and 15 μg of epinephrine is a reliable indicator of accidental intravenous injection. At the time, Chadwick and associates reported that in the preceding 6 years, during which time they had carried out 7000 continuous epidural blocks in the obstetric service, they had no instance of accidental intravascular injection following the use of an epinephrine-containing test dose. Since then, about an equal number of epidurals have been performed with the same results. The same degree of efficacy has been observed at the University Medical Center of Ohio State University with the obstetric service under the leadership of McDonald. In view of our own results and those of many others, we recommend the routine use of the EDT and feel that further discussion of the many articles reporting discrepant techniques and discrepant results would be useless and wasteful consumption of the reader's time.

## Specific Techniques of Lumbar Epidural Obstetric Analgesia/Anesthesia

The specific techniques of epidural analgesia/anesthesia used for labor and vaginal delivery are summarized in Tables 13–21, 13–22, 13–23, and depicted in Figures 13–67, 13–68 and 13–69.

### *Continuous Segmental Epidural Block*

#### *Intermittent Injection Technique*

Continuous segmental epidural block achieved with a single catheter placed in the lumbar epidural space is the most frequently used technique. Many obstetric anesthesiologists still use the intermittent injection technique, while others use the continuous infusion technique (Figure 13–67). Although the number of studies comparing one method with the other by the same group is small,

**Table 13–23.** Technique and Characteristics of Double Catheter Technique

| Technique | Comparison with Other Extradural Techniques |
|---|---|
| —Needle puncture at $L_1 \rightarrow$ catheter advanced 3 cm ($T_{11}$) | Advantages |
| —Needle puncture in sacrum at $S_4 \rightarrow$ advance catheter to $S_3$ | 1. Requires less drug than standard or single catheter techniques |
| —Aspiration test and injection of test dose | 2. The most specific technique for labor and delivery |
| —If negative at 5 min, inject 4–5 ml analgesic solution of local anesthetic in upper catheter $\rightarrow$ analgesia $T_{10}$–$L_1$ | 3. Least effect on mother and fetus |
| —Continuous oxygen and frequent monitoring | 4. No effects on newborn |
| —Top-up analgesic dose in the upper catheter as soon as uterine pain returns | 5. No premature numbness or weakness of limbs |
| —With onset of pain in limbs and perineum inject 5–7 ml of analgesic solution through caudal catheter $\rightarrow$ analgesia in limbs and perineum | 6. No premature perineal relaxation $\rightarrow$ no interference with flexion and internal rotation |
| —Continue analgesia until after internal rotation $\rightarrow$5–7 ml 0.75% bupivacaine or 1.5% etidocaine via lower catheter $\rightarrow$ profound perineal muscle relaxation | 7. "Rolls-Royce" of obstetric analgesia |
| | Disadvantages |
| | 1. Two catheters are required $\rightarrow$ greater risk of complication and failure (Obviated by skilled anesthetist) |

(From Bonica JJ: Obstetric Analgesia and Anesthesia, 2nd Ed., University of Washington Press, Seattle, 1980, p. 112.)

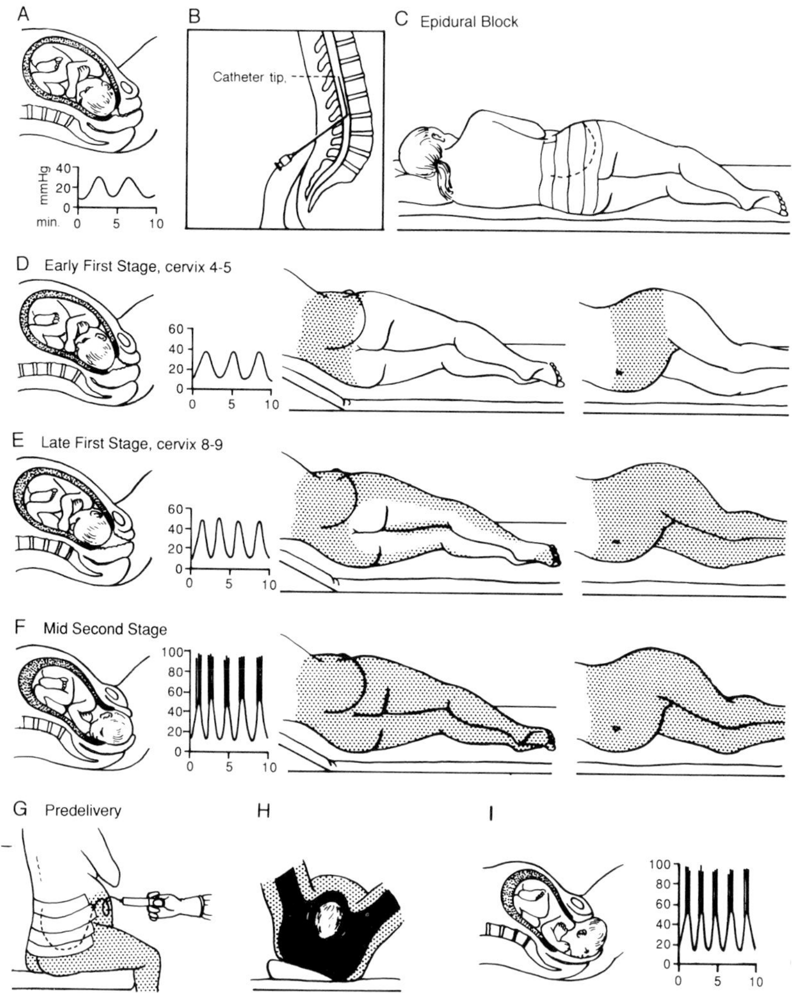


**Fig. 13–67.** Lumbar epidural analgesia using a single catheter to produce "continuous" analgesia, for the first, second, and third stages of labor, using the intermittent, "top-up" technique. This illustration shows a schematic correlation between the intensity of uterine contractions, the phase of the first and second stages of labor (shown on the left column), and the pattern of analgesia that is produced at different stages of labor using the intermittent injection technique. Because the sacral segments are not blocked, it is unlikely to interfere with uterine contractions caused by interruption of Ferguson's reflex, and therefore the injections can be started earlier if the parturient is experiencing severe pain during the latent phase or if there is another special indication to start the procedure before 4 cm cervical dilatation. The analgesia can be achieved with intermittent injections of a local anesthetic alone or combined with an opioid or by continuous infusion of these agents. Here we will consider the technique of repeated intermittent injections. When the parturient begins to experience moderate to severe pain, a test dose of 3 ml of solution is given, and after waiting 5 minutes if there is no evidence of subarachnoid block or intravascular injection, a bolus of 5 to 7 ml of local anesthetic (e.g., 0.125% to 0.25% bupivacaine or 0.75% to 1% lidocaine) to produce segmental analgesia limited to T10-L1 and perhaps one adjacent to each side **(D)**. Once established, intermittent injections or top-up doses are given to maintain effective analgesia during the first stage of labor. The patient is placed with a 15° to 20° head up position, to presumably cause diffusion of the analgesia caudad. In a number of cases, by the second or third injection, analgesia extends to all of the lumbar and the upper sacral segments, and by mid-second stage analgesia has diffused to involve all of the sacral segments producing blockade from T10 to S5. Unfortunately, however, in many instances the lower sacral segments are not blocked and it is therefore necessary during the second stage, when the parturient is experiencing moderate to severe perineal pain to inject 10 to 12 ml of analgesic concentration of the local anesthetic (0.125% bupivacaine or 1% lidocaine) with the patient in the 30° to 45° semi-Fowler position and this is maintained for the duration of labor. Once flexion and internal rotation have taken place, perineal relaxation is desirable to facilitate delivery so that the final injection should consist of a higher concentration of the local anesthetic (0.5% bupivacaine or 1.5% lidocaine) carried out.

those that have been published (514–518) suggest that, provided each method is administered in an optimal fashion, there is little or no difference regarding different aspects of the procedure: in the degree of pain relief using the VAS Scores; the patient's degree of satisfaction of pain relief; duration of the first and second stages of labor; the amount of drug used; the incidence of hypertension and other side effects; the height of sensory blockade; and the degree of motor dysfunction, among other aspects. The one difference between the two methods may be the amount of time required of the personnel monitoring and administering the drug.

On the other hand, if the response from the patient's request for "top-up" doses is delayed, the overall degree of

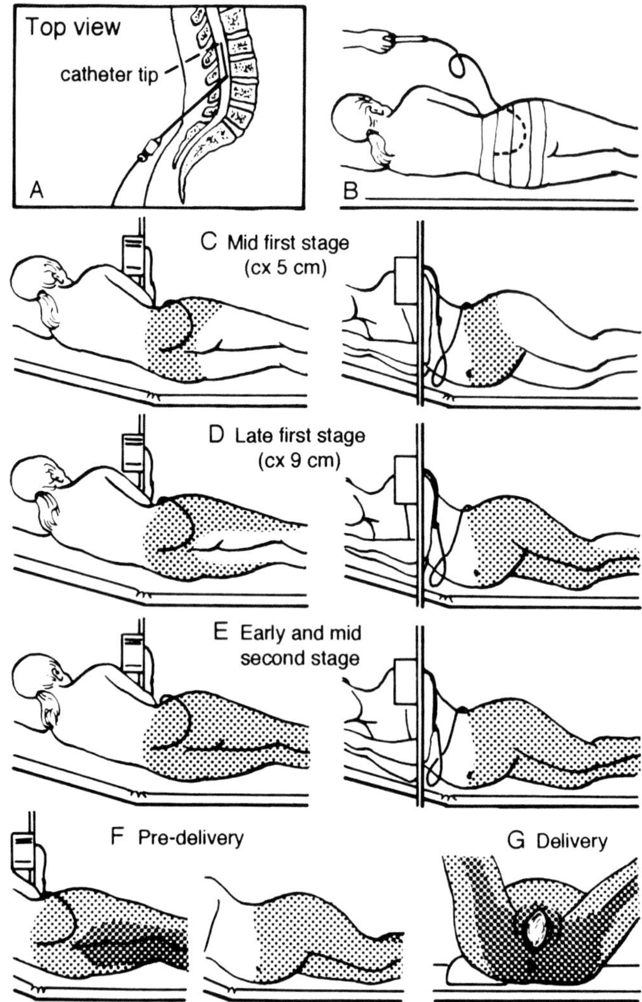


**Fig. 13–68.** Continuous epidural analgesia using the continuous infusion technique. When the parturient begins to experience moderate to severe pain, a test dose of 3 ml of solution is given; and after waiting 5 minutes if there is no evidence of subarachnoid block or intravascular injection, a bolus of 5 to 7 ml of local anesthetic to produce segmental analgesia, limited to T10-L1 and perhaps one adjacent to each other, is carried out as described for Figure 13–67. Once segmental epidural analgesia is established with the test dose and the first therapeutic dose, a continuous infusion is initiated using a volumetric infusion pump that delivers low concentration of local anesthetic alone (e.g., 0.125% bupivacaine or 0.75% lidocaine), or a combination such as that used by McDonald and collegues at The Ohio State University since 1989, of 0.0625% bupivacaine and 0.0002% sufentanyl with 1: 200,000 epinephrine infused at a rate of 8 to 12 ml/hr. With this approach, there is a progressive caudad spread of analgesia so that by the third or fourth hour the level of blockade extends to the lower lumbar and even the upper sacral segments. By the early second stage, analgesia extends to all of the sacral segments **(E)**. With this technique, motor block is usually minimal so that flexion and internal rotation progress normally and the parturient is able to voluntarily mobilize her expulsive force to achieve spontaneous delivery. On the other hand, with such dilute solutions in about one-third to one-fifth of the parturients, the perineal blockade is insufficient to provide good pain relief for the latter part of the second stage and for the delivery. In such instances, 10 ml of 1% lidocaine or 2% chloroprocaine is injected slowly while the patient is in the sitting or semirecumbent position about 10 to 15 minutes before the delivery of the infant. This results in more intense analgesia and some motor block depicted by the heavier stippling in **F**. **G** shows the patient ready for the vaginal delivery.

pain relief will be lower with the intermittent technique. Similarly, if the amount of local anesthetic administered by intravenous infusion is markedly higher than with the "top-up" technique, the blood concentration effects on the mother, fetus, and newborn will be greater. Several studies (517–519) have suggested that patient-controlled epidural analgesia (PCEA) is as good if not better than continuous infusion epidural analgesia and superior to intermittent injection of epidural analgesia on a p.r.n. basis. It has been suggested that the patients appreciate control over their own pain relief and less reliance on the medical staff. However, this patient-controlled analgesia is not being used as widely as one might expect.

### *Continuous Infusion Technique*

In well-organized obstetric anesthesia services, protocols are eventually evolved and applied as to have little or no difference between the techniques. Notwithstanding these data, the fact remains that in many departments continuous infusion technique has steadily increased over the past several years to the point that it is currently being used in some two-thirds to three-quarters of the parturients (Figure 13–68). A recent survey by Plumer (518) of members of the Society of Obstetric Anesthesiology and Perinatology (SOAP), for example, revealed that: continuous infusion for labor was used routinely by 85% of the respondents; that bupivacaine was used for the infusion in 98%; that an opioid was used by between 25% and 73%, with fentanyl most popular (85%) and sufentanil second (12%). Obviously, the technique used is determined by the experience, results, and a variety of other factors that influence the obstetric anesthesia staff.

### *The Double-Catheter Technique*

Throughout this chapter it has been mentioned repeatedly that in the opinion of the authors the double-catheter technique properly performed is the ultimate in analgesia/anesthesia for labor and vaginal delivery, and is often referred to by anesthesiologists as the "Rolls-Royce" of OAA (Figure 13–69). In our opinion, it provides all of the advantages of regional analgesia/anesthesia without most of its disadvantages. The technique permits exquisitely specific analgesia for the first and second stage and anesthesia for the delivery. The process is accomplished with smaller individual and total doses so that: 1) hypotension and other side effects and the risk of systemic toxic reaction in the mother are minimized; 2) it causes little or no effect on uterine contractions (because of the small doses of local anesthetic); 3) it permits the voluntary use of the abdominal muscles because the analgesic concentrations do not produce motor block; 4) although the caudal analgesia interrupts the afferent limb of the reflex urge to bear down, the parturient voluntarily can exert almost as much increase in intra-abdominal pressure as she does reflexively; and 5) most important, with this technique the fetus receives less local anesthetic than with any of the other extradural techniques and, therefore, incurs no cardiovascular and central nervous system depression (see Table 13–22). In experienced hands, the only disadvantage of the technique is that it requires two catheters so that,

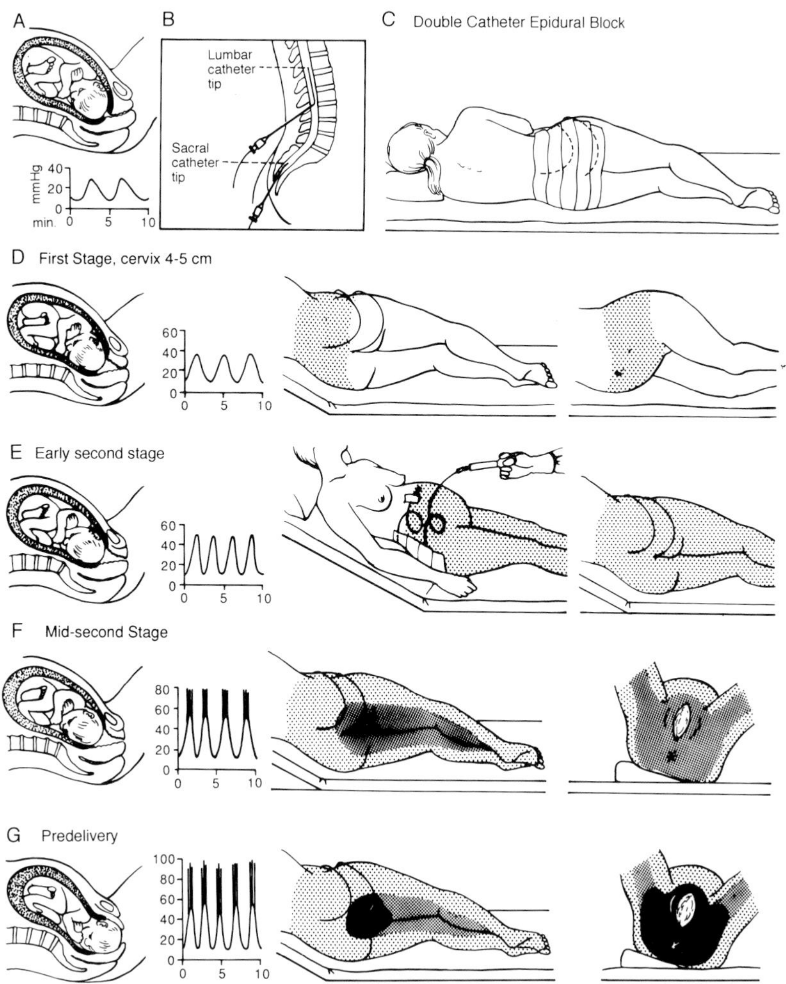


**Fig. 13–69.** Schematic depiction of the double-catheter technique. This entails the insertion of one catheter into the first lumbar interspace and it is advanced until its tip is at the level of T11 or T12 vertebra; and a second catheter is placed into the sacral canal with its tip at the level of the third sacral vertebra (**A**, **B**, and **C**). Both catheters should be inserted and fixed in place early in labor before the parturient becomes uncomfortable with painful contractions. The lumbar epidural block is initiated as described with a single-catheter technique except that following the test dose, the initial therapeutic dose consists of 4 to 5 ml of analgesic concentration of local anesthetic (e.g., 0.25% bupivacaine) to establish a truly segmental (T10-L1) analgesia and these are repeated as often as necessary to maintain continuous pain relief during the first stage of labor. An alternative technique that can be used once the segmental epidural block is established is to adapt the upper catheter to an infusion pump and administer a continuous infusion of 0.25% bupivacaine alone at a rate of 5 ml/hr or a combination of 0.0625% bupivacaine, 0.0002% sufentanil, and epinephrine administered at rates of 7 to 10 ml/hr. The fact that the tip of the catheter is at T12 permits the use of lower volumes or lower infusion rates to consistently achieve segmental block and provide effective pain relief during the first stage. Because during the latter part of the first stage or during the second stage about one-third of the parturients experience moderate to severe pain in the low back and anterior thighs and legs, it is essential to block all of the lumbar and the first sacral segment. This is achieved by injecting through the upper catheter either a bolus of 5 to 7 ml of 0.25% bupivacaine or increasing the infusion rate to 8 to 10 ml/hr. The aforementioned problem of inadequate perineal pain relief that occurs with single-catheter epidural block is definitely obviated by having the second catheter into the sacral canal. When the parturient develops moderate to severe pain in the perineum, 4 to 5 ml of local *analgesic* solution (e.g., 0.125% bupivacaine) is injected through the caudal catheter. This is usually sufficient to produce pain relief without causing significant motor block, and the perineal muscles retain sufficient muscle tone, so that flexion and internal rotation of the presenting part progresses normally and be completed near the end of the second stage. Usually analgesia will last until delivery, but if it does not, a second dose of the same concentration of the local anesthetic is injected. About 15 to 20 minutes before delivery, a caudal injection of 4 ml of 1.5% lidocaine or 3% chloroprocaine is injected through the caudal catheter to produce profound perineal muscle relaxation and thus facilitate delivery of the fetus whether this occurs spontaneously or with the aid of outlet forceps. If the parturient has had an extensive episiotomy and/or other tissue damage that is likely to produce moderate to severe postoperative pain, an injection of a bolus of 3 ml of 0.125% bupivacaine and of 5 μg of fentanyl is injected and the catheter removed, or if it is anticipated that postoperative pain will persist for the next day or two, the catheter is left in place and a reinjection of the local anesthetic opioid is given at 8-hour intervals.

theoretically, there is greater risk of complications and failure, but this can and should be obviated by the skilled anesthesiologist.

Obviously, proper application of the procedure requires the administrator to have acquired experience and skill in introducing a needle and catheter into the sacral canal, but as previously emphasized, every obstetric anesthesiologist should possess skill with this technique. As previously mentioned, although some authorities consider this technique a "complicated procedure" while some also suggest that it causes more pain for the parturient and increases the risk of complications, they are not the experiences of the present author or other clinicians who have used the procedure extensively. Some authorities believe that this technique should be reserved only for parturients who have obstetric or maternal and/or fetal complications. However, with the exception of tertiary obstetric care facilities that care for a large number of complicated cases, in other obstetric units where complicated cases are not seen as frequently, most will not provide the opportunity to carry out the procedure often enough to acquire a high degree of skill so that it can be executed effectively when the parturients who really need this type of anesthesia present themselves. Moreover, we believe that parturients with normal labor should be afforded the advantage of this technique.

### *Standard Lumbar Epidural Block (T10-S5)*

In the 1960s and early 1970s, the standard lumbar epidural technique, which as previously mentioned entails the use of injection of sufficient quantities (12 to 15 ml or more) of dilute solution of local anesthetic at L3 or L2 spinal level, was the most frequent technique employed (Figure 13–70). Because the injection of such amounts often interrupt the sacral segments early, it impairs the function of Ferguson's reflex which plays an important role in the liberation of endogenous oxytocin during labor (see Chapter 4), and thus may prolong the latent and early active phase of the first stage. Moreover, block of the sacral segments early in labor causes unnecessarily premature numbness and often weakness of the lower limbs, which annoys most patients and disables many of them. Another major disadvantage of standard epidural analgesia is that it will result in an injection of a larger amount of local anesthetic during the first stage than is necessary. Moreover, premature weakness or paralysis of the perineal muscle sling is likely to develop and potentially interfere with flexion and internal rotation. For these reasons, this technique is no longer used in most obstetric centers.

## Technical Aspects of Caudal Epidural Analgesia

To carry out caudal block properly, it is essential to know the anatomy of the sacrum and coccyx, the sacral canal and its contents, and the possible sacral anomalies. In addition, knowledge of certain physical, physiologic, and pharmacologic facts is necessary. Each is presented below, with a description of the technique of caudal block following.

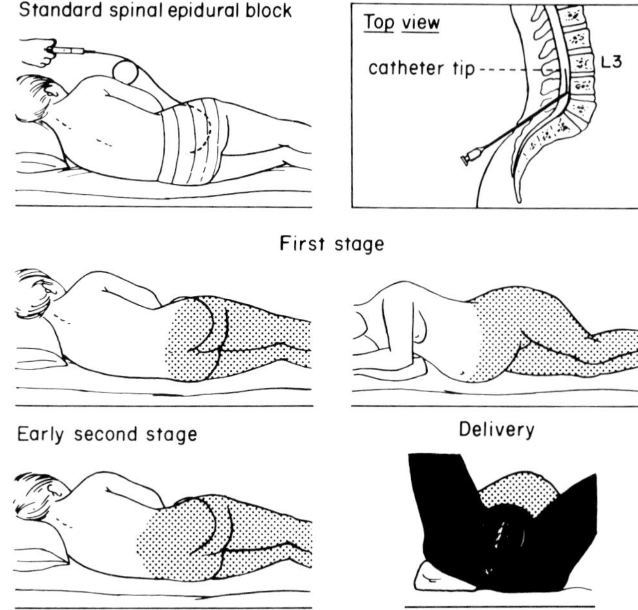


**Fig. 13–70.** Technique for standard epidural analgesia for labor and vaginal delivery. A continuous catheter is inserted through a needle placed in the fourth interlaminar space and advanced so that its tip is at the level of the third lumbar vertebra. In the first stage, analgesia extending from T10 to S5 is achieved with low concentrations of local anesthetics. This is continued until just before delivery, when a higher concentration is injected, with the patient in the semirecumbent position, to produce perineal relaxation and anesthesia as depicted in the lower right figure. The wedge under the right buttock causes the uterus to displace toward the left side. This technique is inherent in a number of disadvantages, which include the injection of large dose and premature weakness or paralysis of the perineal muscle sling that interferes with flexion and internal rotation and is associated with marked increase in instrumental deliveries.

## *Anatomy of the Sacrum and Coccyx*

The sacrum is a large, triangle-shaped bone composed of the five fused sacral vertebrae and located as a wedge between the two iliac bones to which it is connected by an intricate network of ligaments (Figures 13–71 and 13–72). Its long axis is curved, with the convexity facing posteriorly and parallel to the axis of the pelvic cavity. Compared with the male sacrum, the female sacrum is shorter, wider, with the upper portion making a greater angle with the lower portion and inclined more obliquely posteriorly. This formation increases the size of the pelvic cavity and renders the lumbosacral angle more prominent.

### *The Coccyx*

The coccyx is also a triangle-shaped structure formed of rudimentary vertebrae, which are destitute of pedicles, laminae, and spinous processes. The first vetebra is the largest and often exists as a separate structure. It resembles the lowest sacral vertebra with which it articulates. The other three diminish in size from cephalad downward and are usually fused to one another. The anterior surface

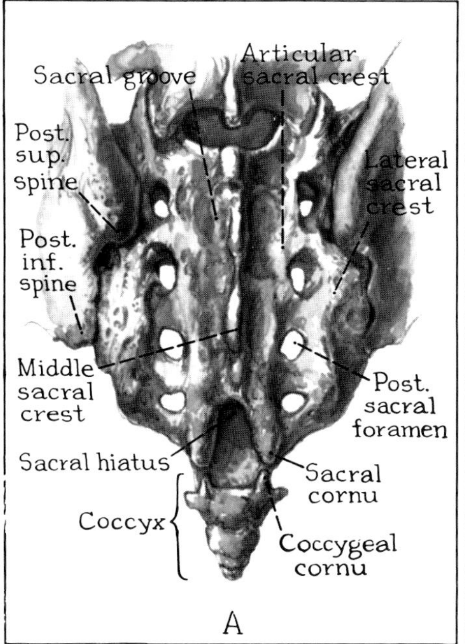


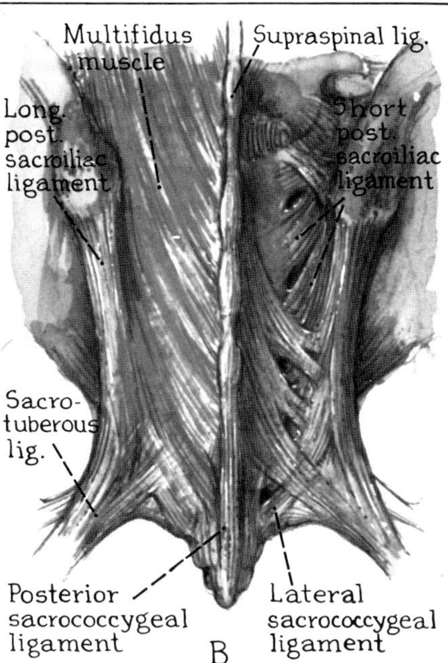


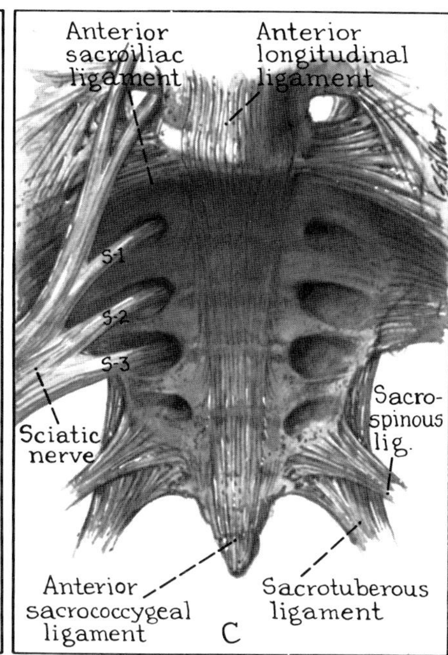


**Fig. 13–71.** Some anatomic aspects of the sacrum and coccyx. **A**: Shows the anterior aspect of the sacrum which is a smooth, concave, triangular surface that constitutes the posterior wall of the true pelvis. It is important to note that the anterior foramina are not obstructed by muscles or ligaments, as happens posteriorly, and that each foramen is very large: the nerve passing through it and the loose areolar tissue, fat, and blood vessels around it, take up only a small (one-third) portion of the opening. The posterior surface of the sacrum is rough, irregular, and convex, facing superiorly and posteriorly. In the midline is the middle sacral crest, surmounted by 3 or 4 tubercles, the rudimentary spinous processes of the upper 3 or 4 sacral vertebrae. These serve as important landmarks in carrying out caudal block. The spinous process and laminae of the fifth sacral vertebra are usually absent, giving rise to the sacral hiatus. The lowest part of the intermediate sacral crest, representing the inferior articular process of the fifth sacral vertebra, is prominent and prolonged downward as a rounded process known as the sacral cornu. The cornu on each side is connected with the ipsilateral coccygeal cornu by the lateral sacrococcygeal ligament. Lateral to the articular processes are located the posterior sacral foramina, through which the posterior primary divisions of the sacral nerves make their exit. The posterior surface of the sacrum gives attachments to dense ligamentous bands that bridge the foramina and to the multifidus and erector spinae muscles. These ligaments and muscles are tightly packed and effectively seal the underlying posterior sacral foramina and thus hinder the escape of fluid injected into the sacral canal.

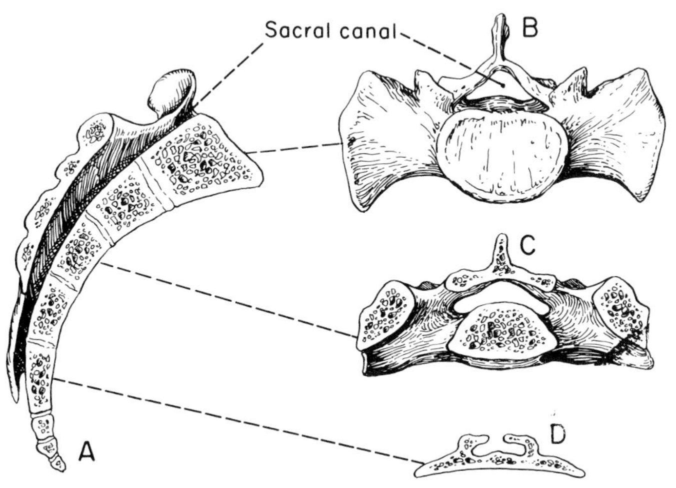


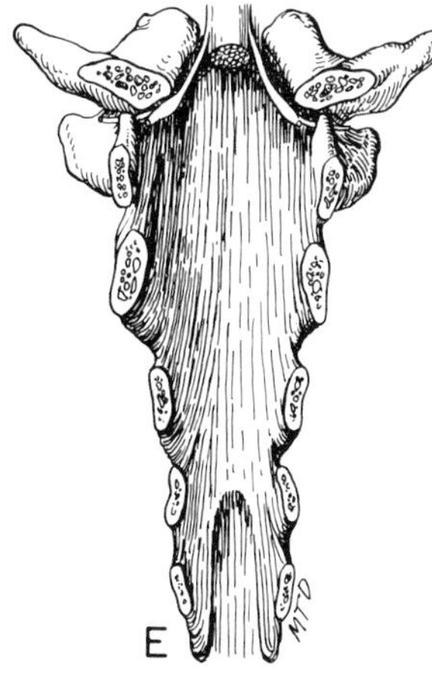


**Fig. 13–72.** The sacral canal: **A**: sagittal view; **B**: super view; **C**: horizontal cross section of the level of the second sacral vertebra. Note that the longitudinal axis of the canal is curved like the sacrum, with its convexity backward. The angle made by the axis of the lumbar portion of the vertebral canal (as represented by the direction of the upper 3 lumbar vertebrae) and the axis of the upper portion of the sacral canal, called the lumbosacral angle, is 50 to 70° in the female, and even greater in the parturient. On cross section, the sacral canal is triangular at the cephalad end and flattened at the lower end. In its cephalad portion, the transverse diameter is about 2.5 cm and the anteroposterior diameter about 1 cm, whereas at its lower end the transverse diameter is 1 cm and the anteroposterior diameter 2 to 3 mm. Its length in the female is 8 to 10 cm. On cross section, the intervertebral foramina appear as lateral extensions of the canal. Each foramen, containing the short, mixed spinal nerve, opens into the medial wall of its homologous transsacral canal. These funnel-shaped canals connect the large anterior foramina with their homologous posterior foramina.

of the coccyx is smooth and concave, whereas the posterior surface is convex, has transverse grooves, and presents on either side a linear row of tubercles, the rudimentary articular processes. The superior pair are large and are called the coccygeal cornua, and constitute important landmarks in caudal block.

The sacrococcygeal articulation is an amphiarthroidal joint with a disc of fibrocartilage interposed between contiguous surfaces of the sacrum and coccyx and surrounded by the anterior, posterior, and lateral sacrococcygeal ligaments. In the young female, the joint has sufficient motion to permit backward movement of the coccyx of 2.5 cm or more if forced by the presenting part of the fetus as it advances during labor.

## *The Sacral Canal*

The sacral canal is a prismatic cavity extending the length of the sacrum. It is the continuation of the vertebral canal, and may be considered as the sacral prolongation of the epidural (peridural) space. The canal is bounded anteriorly by the posterior surface of the fused vertebral bodies and the overlying posterior longitudinal ligament; laterally by the pedicles and the sacral intervertebral foramina; posteriorly by the fused laminae, and caudad by the posterior sacrococcygeal ligament. The anterior wall is rough, due to the transverse ridges found between the fused vertebrae. These transverse ridges are sometimes so prominent that they obstruct the advance of a caudal block needle. In addition, the canal may present lateral deviations and other variations of its usual curves, anteroposterior narrowing, or it may be divided into loculi by connective tissue septa. All of these anomalies represent unfavorable conditions for the insertion of the needle and the homogeneous dispersion of an anesthetic solution injected into the canal. The posterior wall of the canal is smooth and is a rather deep and narrow groove in the midline where the two laminae of each of the fused vertebrae meet. This groove facilitates the cephalad advance of the catheter.

## *Contents of the Sacral Canal*

Contents of the sacral canal, depicted in Figure 13–73A, include: 1) the dura-arachnoid cul-de-sac; 2) the menin-

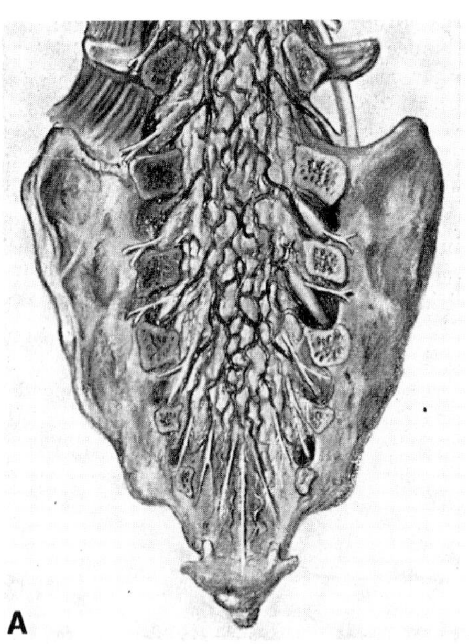


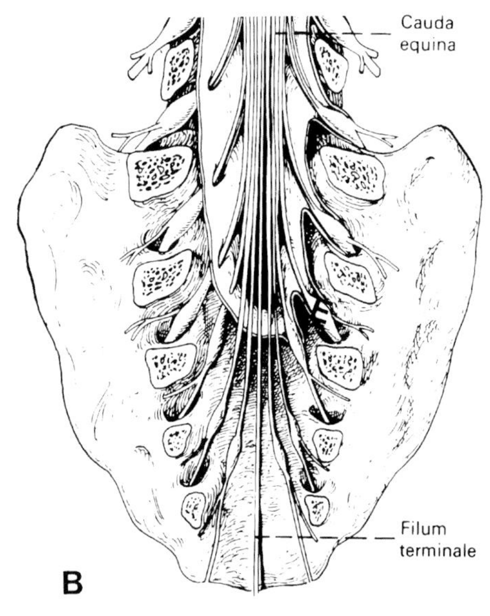


**Fig. 13–73.** **A**: The anatomy of the sacral canal with its contents. The solid fat fills the entire canal, being particularly thick posteriorly, where it appears as a pad separating the nerves and cul-de-sac (above) from the posterior wall of the canal. The fat and loose areolar tissue also surround the blood vessels and each nerve, not only it its position in the canal, but also in the foramen where they act as a substantial protective pad. The fat is very loosely attached to the walls of the canal and to the nerves and their coverings by delicate strands, but it can be easily stripped out and permits seepage of solutions injected into the canal. The liquid fat surrounds and is interspersed with the solid fat and appears to act as a lubricant. **B**: The sacral canal with all but the nerves removed. The roots and dorsal ganglia and the dura-arachnoid covering of the first and second sacral nerves lie immediately lateral to the cul-de-sac. Below the level of the second sacral vertebra, the dura-arachnoid extensions surround each pair of the third, fourth, and fifth sacral spinal nerve roots and the coccygeal spinal nerve roots. These coverings extend to the point where the anterior and posterior roots meet just distal to the dorsal root ganglion. Each ganglion is located 1 to 3 cm below the termination of the dural sac. The third, fourth, and fifth formed sacral spinal nerves and the coccygeal nerve traverse the sacral canal for a short distance before they divide into a larger anterior division and much smaller posterior division. These two divisions proceed caudad together until they reach their respective foramina, where they separate and make their exit. The anterior divisions pass through the anterior foramina and make up the sacral, pudendal, and coccygeal plexuses. The posterior divisions pass through the posterior foramina and then to the fascia, muscles, and skin of the low back. The fact that the lower sacral spinal nerves are situated within the sacral canal for some distance is of clinical importance in caudal block because in this situation the nerves become exposed to the anesthetic solution to a greater degree than if this was not the case.

geal prolongations investing the nerve roots; 3) the beginning of the sacral nerves; 4) loose areolar tissue; and 5) solid and liquid fat, lymphatics, and blood vessels. The vessels consist mostly of veins representing the lower end of the internal vertebral venous plexus. These veins, which are thin-walled and large in parturients (because of increased venous pressure in the lower part of the body), lie at the periphery of the canal, being most numerous anteriorly and laterally.

The dural cul-de-sac tapers off as a cone-shaped structure and usually ends at the level of the second sacral vertebra. The dura-arachnoid then contracts around the internal filum terminale to become the external filum terminale, which passes caudad to become fused to the periosteum of the dorsal surface of the coccyx. The point of termination of the dural sac may vary from the level of the middle of the first sacral vertebra to the level of the middle of the third sacral vertebra. Lanier, McKnight, and Trotter (519–521) found the level of termination to be above the middle of the second sacral vertebra in one-third the specimens, and below this level in nearly one-half of the specimens examined. Figure 13–73B shows the contents of the sacral canal with all but the nerves removed.

## The Sacral Hiatus

The sacral hiatus is an aperture shaped like an inverted V or U, resulting from the failure of fusion of the laminae of the lower sacral vertebrae. The cephalad end of the hiatus is usually considered to be at the level of the middle of the fourth sacral vertebra, but this is variable (Figures 13–74 and 13–75). The hiatus is bound above by the fused laminae, inferiorly by the posterior surface of the body of the fifth sacral vertebra, and laterally by the edges of the deficient laminae of the fifth and sometimes fourth sacral vertebrae. At the lower end of the lateral boundaries is the two prominent sacral cornua, which are valuable topographic landmarks in performing caudal block. Figure 13–74 depicts a detailed anatomy of the sacral hiatus viewed from behind and a sagittal view showing the superficial and deep part of the posterior segmental coccygeal ligament, the supraspinous ligament, and the sacral canal with the felum terminale traversing it and its attachment to the posterior surface of the coccygeal vertebra.

In addition to the fibrous sacrococcygeal ligament, the sacral hiatus is covered by subcutaneous tissue and skin. The subcutaneous tissue is composed primarily of fat, the amount of which varies considerably, being greater in the obese individual and in the female. Frequently, parturients have a particularly thick, edematous layer over the hiatus, making its identification difficult.

## Physical and Dynamic Aspects

### Spread of Anesthetic Solution

Local anesthetic solutions injected into the sacral canal spread in all directions, up and down the canal, and laterally to the transsacral canals, and then through the sacral foramina. If a sufficient quantity is injected, the solution will spread cephalad along the epidural space of the lumbar and thoracic space, and with large quantities even to the cervical region. From the epidural space it escapes through the intervertebral foramina to the paravertebral

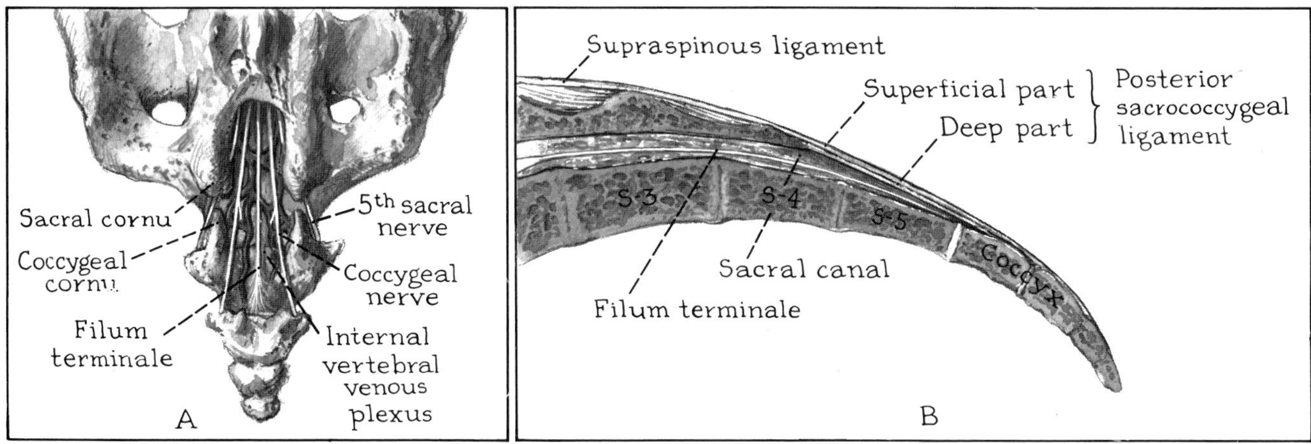


**Fig. 13–74.** Dimensions of the sacral hiatus. In the average parturient the hiatus is 1.5 cm wide and 2 cm long. Rarely, the hiatus is very small (2 to 3 mm in diameter) (Figure 13–75B) because of the presence of the laminae of all the sacral vertebrae, making introduction of a caudal needle almost impossible. The center of the hiatus, where the caudal needle is inserted, is cephalad to the sacrococcygeal joint, about 5 cm above the tip of the coccyx and directly beneath the upper limit of the intergluteal crease of the skin. The distance between this point of insertion of the needle and the lower end of the dural sac is about 6 cm, but this varies depending on the level of the termination of the dural sac and the upper extent of the hiatus. Lanier and Trotter (520) found the distance between the apex of the hiatus (which is usually about 1 cm above the point of insertion) and the termination of the dural sac to range between 2 and 7.5 cm, with a mean of about 5 cm. About 42% of the specimens were less than the mean, and 36% greater than the mean. The posterior (dorsal) sacrococcygeal ligament forms the roof of the sacral hiatus. It consists of a short, deep layer that extends from the lower margin of the sacral canal to the upper posterior surface of the coccyx, and a thin, superficial layer that is much longer and blends superiorly with the supraspinous ligament and is attached inferiorly to the lower posterior surface of the coccyx. This ligament usually has a cleft in the midline where the caudal needle is inserted and through which pass the coccygeal and fifth sacral nerve and the filum terminale.

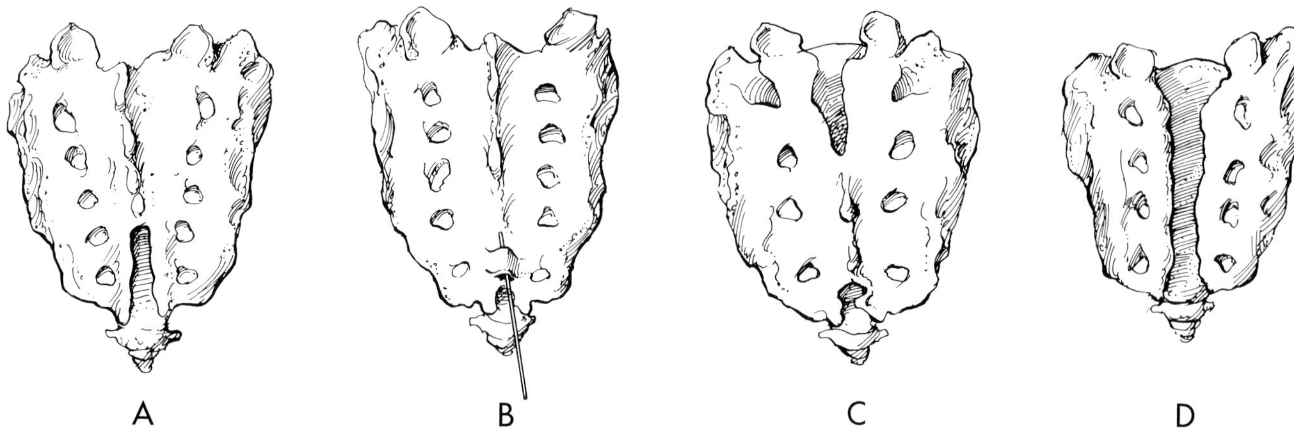


**Fig. 13–75.** Anomalies of the sacrum. In addition to the sacrococcygeal ligament, the sacral hiatus is covered by subcutaneous tissue and skin. The subcutaneous tissue is composed primarily of fat, the amount of which varies considerably, being greater in obese individuals and in the female. Frequently, parturients have a particularly thick, edematous layer over the hiatus making its identification difficult. In a series of 1227 sacra, Trotter and Letterman (521) found it to be at the level of the lower part of the fourth sacral vertebra in about 33% of the specimens, below this level in about 20%, and above this level in nearly 50%, with some of the latter being as high as the upper third of the laminae of the second sacral vertebra. In a few (2 to 3%) it extended to the fifth lumbar vertebra because of the failure of the laminae of all the sacral vertebrae to fuse (Figure 13–74).

spaces. Of course, the solution must seep through the fat, loose areolar tissue, and blood vessels to reach the formed spinal nerve where it exerts its primary anesthetic action. The spread of the local anesthetic solution is influenced by various factors, including: 1) total dose of the anesthetic; 2) volume of solution injected; 3) capacity of the sacral canal and the epidural space; 4) patency of the sacral foramina and the intervertebral foramina; 5) gravity; and 6) site of injection in the sacral canal. These factors are all, of course, interrelated and, except for the third and fourth, are under the control of the anesthetist.

## Dose

Bromage (49,55) has shown that the actual dose of the analgesic solution itself is the most important factor in determining the segmental spread of caudal extradural block. With caudal anesthesia, the dose assumes greater importance if the site of injection is high, and lesser importance if injection is made in the lower sacral canal, because much of the solution escapes before it has an opportunity to come in contact with nerve tissue.

***Volume of Solution and Capacity of Sacral Canal.*** All other factors being equal, the greater the volume of solution, the greater its spread and the higher the level of block. Also involved with this is the capacity of the sacral canal with its normal contents to contain injected fluid. In the average female, this capacity is about 4 to 6 ml, but is significantly reduced in the parturient, probably because of the engorgement of the internal venous plexuses. Consequently, a parturient requires approximately two-thirds the volume she requires when not pregnant.

***Foramina.*** The patency of the foramina, the exits, or escape routes for solutions injected into the epidural space, is important with all extradural techniques. The large anterior sacral foramina are by far the most important of these exits. Unlike other foramina, these are unobstructed by ligaments or muscles, so that the solution passes through them and to the retrorectal space unhindered. In some instances, the leak through the anterior foramina is so great that it is virtually impossible to effect anesthesia above the sacral segments. However, the posterior sacral foramina are sealed effectively by the overlying ligaments and muscles and permit very little solution to escape from the sacral canal.

***Gravity and Site of Injection.*** Gravity is more important in the spread of the anesthetic solution in caudal anesthesia than in lumbar epidural block, though not as important as in subarachnoid block. If the patient is kept in the lateral position during and after injection, more intense analgesia of the lower side results. If the patient remains prone during and after injection, gravity causes most of the solution to spread toward the upper sacral and lumbar epidural space (Figure 13–76).

With the parturient supine and the injection of the anesthetic made in the lower part of the sacral canal (through a continuous catheter), the spread of the solution is influenced by gravity, leakage through the anterior sacral foramina, and also by the lumbosacral angle. Under such conditions, the solution must first fill the lower sacral canal and then the upper part before it overflows to the lumbar epidural space. As the canal is being filled, much of the solution escapes through the anterior foramina which, in this position, act as holes on the side of the column of fluid being developed. Bryce-Smith (521) has emphasized that occasionally it is impossible to inject the anesthetic solution fast enough to keep pace with the leakage through the anterior sacral foramina and at the same time to build up the required column of solution within the sacral canal. Consequently, the level of analgesia de-

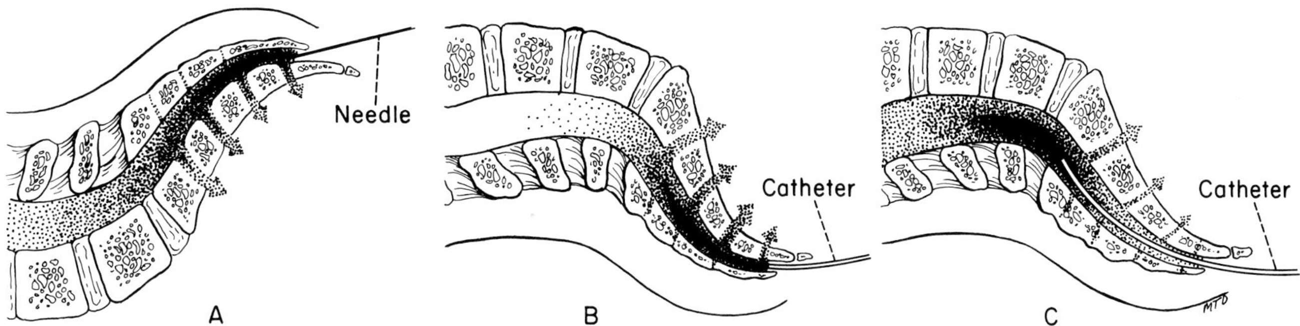


**Fig. 13–76.** Effects of gravity, site of injection, and size of anterior sacral foramina on the spread of local anesthetic introduced into sacral canal. Thickness of arrows indicates degree of diffusion. **A,** Patient prone with a roll under the hips. Injection through a needle with the point at the level of the fourth sacral vertebra causes most of the solution to diffuse cephalad, toward upper sacral and lumbar canal. Only moderate amounts diffuse through the anterior sacral foramina. **B,** Patient supine and point of injection at the level of the fourth sacral vertebra. As the canal is being filled, much of the solution escapes through the anterior sacral foramina, which act as holes on the side of the column of fluid being developed. **C,** Patient supine but point of injection is at the first sacral vertebral level. The drug tends to diffuse toward the posterior aspect of the sacral canal because of gravity and because the catheter is usually placed against the posterior surface. Moreover, solution diffusing cephalad has less distance to travel to reach the lumbar and lower thoracic level. Because of gravity, much less solution diffuses through the anterior sacral foramina than in **B.**

veloped will be lower than anticipated, although the intensity will be greater. Theoretically, this difficulty can be overcome by bringing the sacral canal into the horizontal plane by tilting the patient's head down. However, because 30° is the maximum tilt that can be obtained on most delivery tables and because the lumbosacral angle in most parturients is greater than 30°, it is practically impossible to bring the sacral canal into the horizontal plane, even while disregarding the comfort of the patient. These effects of gravity are even greater if the patient is sitting or in Fowler's position.

The higher the site of injection, the less important are leakage and gravity to the spread of solution. If the injection is made at the level of the first sacral or fifth lumbar vertebra, that part of the solution spreading cephalad will have less distance to travel to reach the lumbar and lower thoracic nerve. And so, less anesthetic is required for a given level. For example, to produce analgesia to the tenth thoracic segment, 20 to 25 ml of lidocaine are needed if the injection is made low (S3), and only 12 to 14 ml if the injection is made at the first sacral or fifth lumbar segment. For this reason, in our obstetric patients the continuous caudal catheter is advanced to the upper segment.

### *Pharmacodynamics*

The site of anesthetic action following caudal injection is similar to that following lumbar epidural block (Figure 13–53). Consequently, the anesthetic effects of the block are the same as those of spinal epidural block, and the effects of both are similar to those of subarachnoid block. However, onset is slower probably because the extradural solution must penetrate the connective tissue coverings before it comes in contact with individual axons. In 4 to 8 minutes (depending on the latency of the local anesthetic), the parturient experiences subjective warmth of the extremities and relief of pain. Objectively, there is evidence of sympathetic block, decrease in temperature sense, and hypalgesia. Subsequently, there is progressive loss of pain, light touch, deep touch, motor function, and proprioception. These effects occur first and are most profound near the point of injection, and the further away from this point, the longer the time of onset and the less the effects. Because conditions are such that the sacral nerves come in contact with a greater amount of solution, the intensity and duration of block are significantly greater in the sacral segments than in the lumbar and lower thoracic segments.

## Technique of Caudal Epidural Block

Preparation of the parturient is the same as any other form of regional anesthesia. It is essential to explain the procedure to the patient and to reassure her to allay apprehension and fear and to obtain her cooperation.

### *Drugs and Equipment*

The equipment and drugs are similar to those for lumbar epidural block except that the 18-gauge thin-walled caudal needle is only 5 cm long and its bevel is of normal length. If a single injection is contemplated, a 20-gauge spinal needle replaces the larger thin-walled needle. Any of the commonly available local anesthetics may be used. In our programs, the following are preferred: 1) 1 to 3% 2-chloroprocaine for blocks of short duration; 2) 0.5 to 2% lidocaine or mepivacaine for blocks of intermediate duration; and 3) 0.125 to 0.25% bupivacaine for blocks of longer duration. Because it is necessary to use larger volumes to achieve a certain level of epidural block, the lowest effective concentration should be used. During labor, the lowest possible concentrations should be used because the amount of drug is considerably less and therefore the risk of toxicity is diminished. Equally important, analgesic concentrations will not produce perineal muscle relaxation, and are therefore less likely to interfere with flexion and internal rotation and descent of the presenting part. Moreover, after these cardinal movements

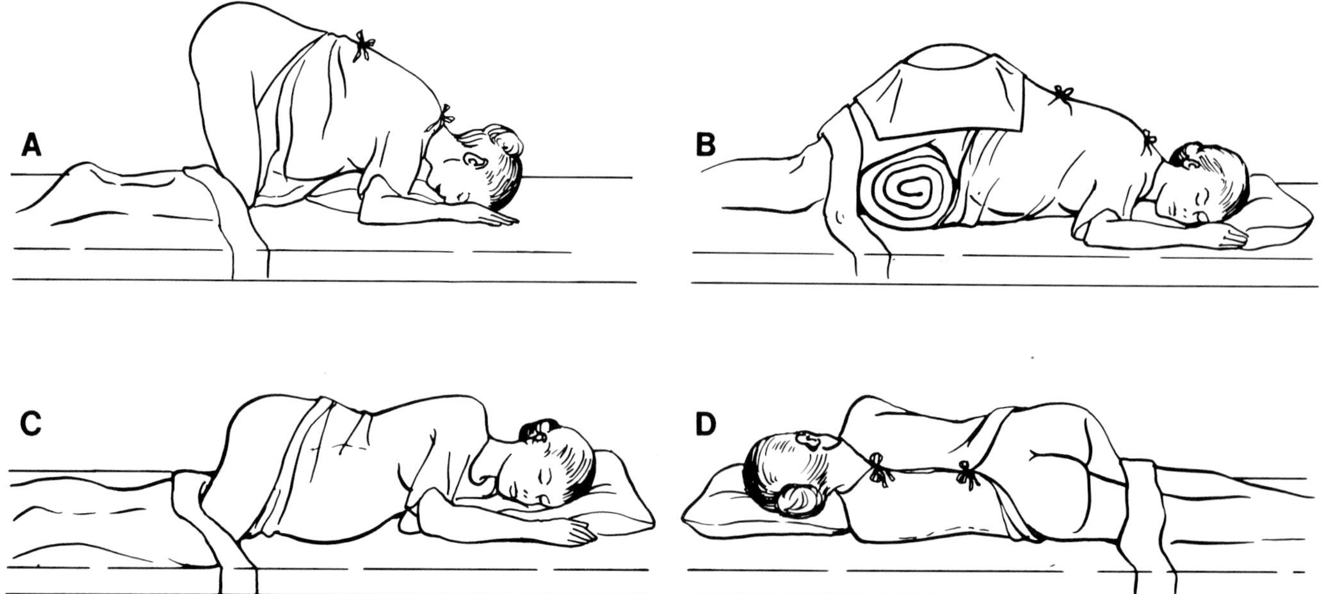


**Fig. 13–77.** Different positions of the patient for performing caudal block: **A**: knee-chest; **B**: prone with a roll 10 inches in diameter under upper part; **C**: lateral position, view from the front; **D**: lateral position, view from the back.

are completed, relaxation may be considered desirable so that higher concentrations are used, such as 1% lidocaine or 0.25% bupivacaine.

Epinephrine 1:300,000 or preferably 1:400,000 concentration should be used to delay and decrease absorption, which, in turn, results in an increase in the intensity and duration of blockade and decreases the risk of systemic toxicity. This is particularly important in the unusual circumstance in which continuous caudal anesthesia (with the tip of catheter at L5) for cesarean section is contemplated. If carefully measured with a tuberculin syringe, the amount of epinephrine contained in 18 to 22 ml of solution required for cesarean section with an anesthesia level to T4 will total 45 to 50 μg when used in 1:400,000 concentration, and between 67 and 75 μg if the 1:300,000 concentration is used.

## *Position of the Patient*

Caudal block in obstetrics may be carried out with the patient in the lateral, prone, knee-elbow, or knee-chest position. The knee-elbow or knee-chest position (Figure 13–77A) is best for inexperienced operators because it makes the lower portion of the sacrum prominent and facilitates identification of landmarks. However, this is a very uncomfortable position for the patient and is disliked by most parturients. The prone position can be used by placing a roll about 10 inches in diameter under the upper part of the thighs to avoid pressure on the abdomen (Figure 13–77B). This position also makes it easier to identify landmarks and, from the patient's standpoint, is slightly better than the knee-elbow posture, though still uncomfortable.

The lateral-semiprone posture, shown in Figure 13–77C and D, which is actually a modification of the Sims' position, is preferred by the authors and their colleagues because most frequently the continuous caudal catheter is inserted and taped in the lying-in room with the patient in her own bed; and because some of these beds have a sag in the center, the parturient can roll forward sufficiently, so that the surface of the back makes a 45° angle or less with the horizontal plane instead of the 90° angle as in the true lateral position. For the physician who is right-handed, the patient is requested to lie on her left side at the very edge of the bed. She is then rolled forward as much as she can without feeling pressure on her abdomen, and her legs placed in a modified Sims' position (Figure 13–77D). For left-handed physicians, the patient lies on her right side.

## *Identification of Landmarks*

With the patient in the lateral-prone position, the physician palpates the midline crest of the sacrum and adjusts the skin so that the midline of the skin is over the middle sacral crest and the midpoint of the sacral hiatus. In obese patients in whom the shift of the skin is marked, it is advisable to have the nurse assistant retract the lateral aspect of the upper buttock so as to place the midline of the skin over the middle sacral crest.

To identify the sacral hiatus, it is best to first palpate the middle sacral (spinous) crest and then proceed caudad with the palpating finger. At about the intergluteal crease of the skin (anal fold), there is felt a semisolid depression with the shape of an inverted V or U. This is the sacral hiatus. The location of the hiatus is confirmed by palpating the movable coccyx, whose tip is easily identified, and then proceeding cephalad with the palpating finger. The hiatus is located about 5 cm above the tip of the coccyx where the same semisolid depression was previously identified. Palpation of its lateral edges and prominent sacral cornua on each side helps to confirm the identity of the opening. If identification of the sacral hiatus is difficult because the parturient is obese or because of edema, the knee-elbow position is used.

### *Procedures Before Puncture*

Because of the nearness of the puncture site to the anus, it is especially important to cleanse the skin thoroughly with Phisohex and ether before applying antiseptic solution. The perianal and anal mucosa and perineum should be protected against the irritating action of the antiseptic by holding a sterile towel or sponge firmly against the skin of the anal fold. After putting on sterile gloves and using aseptic technique, the area is draped with a double-thickness drape (with a window in it), and the skin is wiped with a dry sponge to remove any excess antiseptic. The position of the hiatus is then reaffirmed and anesthetization of the region should be initiated. Because the skin, the sacrococcygeal ligament, and periosteum of the lower sacrum and coccyx are among the most nociceptive sensitive areas of the body, the preblock anesthetization should be done slowly using several different-sized needles to minimize the discomfort inherent in needle penetration. Moreover, 0.5% lidocaine is used because of the short latency, and at least 25 to 30 seconds should be allowed after each injection before the larger needles are inserted. Prior to the procedure, each step is again described to the parturient in a slow, reassuring, confidence-inducing manner and she is further informed to promptly indicate to the physician if any discomfort occurs. The physician should do everything he or she can to have the patient as relaxed as possible. A basic principle is to allow 25 to 30 seconds between injections to have the local anesthetic anesthetize the very small nerve endings in these structures. Figures 13–78 and 13–79 depict the major steps required to eventually place the caudal needle in the canal. Additional details may be found in the legends for these illustrations.

### *Difficulties*

The two most frequent difficulties encountered during puncture are in locating the puncture site and in advancing the needle within the sacral canal. In the first instance, the needle is systematically inserted several times along the midline at intervals of 0.5 cm (Figure 13–80). Because the coccyx is easier to identify, the first of these punctures is made at the level of the first coccygeal vertebra and subsequent ones cephalad thereto. For each of these "exploratory punctures," the point of the needle is withdrawn to the subcutaneous tissue, the skin is moved cephalad 0.5 cm, and the needle then advanced. The angle of the needle in its relation to the skin should be maintained. The skin is sufficiently movable to permit exploration along the length for about 3 cm.

In some instances advance of the needle is obstructed at a short distance (0.5 to 1 cm) from its point of entrance by an abnormally high transverse ridge between the fourth and fifth vertebrae (Figure 13–81). In this case, more pressure should be applied on the shaft of the needle to cause its point to move posteriorly and thus glide over the ridge. This is further facilitated by having the bevel of the needle facing anteriorly. If this maneuver is not successful, the needle is inserted through the ligament more caudad, or an attempt is made to inject the solution without advancing the needle further. As long as the entire bevel of the needle is within the sacral canal, a successful block can be effected with a little larger volume of solution.

### *Tests to Ascertain Position of Needle*

When the needle is in its proper place, the stylet is removed, 1 ml of saline is injected to displace any tissue away from the needle point, and the aspiration test is performed in four different planes by rotating the needle 90° on its axis each time. During each attempt at aspiration, the plunger must be kept withdrawn for at least 10 seconds to allow sufficient time for viscid blood-liquid fat to pass through the length of the needle (Figure 13–80A). If cerebrospinal fluid is obtained, the needle should be withdrawn and the block abandoned, so that massive subarachnoid block does not develop following injection of the therapeutic dose. If blood is obtained, the needle is moved 0.5 cm and a few minutes allowed for the blood to clot before going ahead with the injection.

The next step is to inject rapidly 3 to 5 ml of air while the palm of the free hand rests firmly on the skin of the lower part of the sacrum (Figure 13–82), and as soon as the injection is completed, the finger on the plunger removed. This maneuver helps to detect misplacement of the point of the needle into the subcutaneous tissue posterior to the sacrum because in such instances air produces crepitation and saline causes tumefaction (Figure 13–82). If the needle point is not in the canal, there will be reflux of 0.5 ml or more of air or solution as soon as pressure on the plunger is removed. Should the needle be misplaced subperiosteally, resistance to injection is almost absolute and requires the needle to be withdrawn 5 mm. (Figure 13–83C).

The caudal needle is considered to be properly placed in the sacral canal when: 1) no blood or cerebrospinal fluid is obtained; 2) no tumefaction is palpated during injection of the solution or there is no crepitation during injection of air; 3) no resistance to injection is evident; and 4) no rebound of air nor reflux of fluid is present.

Some authors have advocated a rectal exam to rule out penetration of the rectum by the caudal needle. The present authors maintain that careful attention to minute details in performing the caudal technique as outlined previously will prevent such an unusual accident. Furthermore, if the administrator is so unsure and unskilled in regard to such placement without adequate supervision, then the technique should not be attempted, and the lumbar epidural technique substituted.

## ***Injection of Local Anesthetic***

### *Injection of Single-Dose Block*

When the needle is judged to be properly placed, a test dose of 3 ml of anesthetic solution with epinephrine is injected through the needle. The needle is then left in place for 5 minutes before the full therapeutic dose is

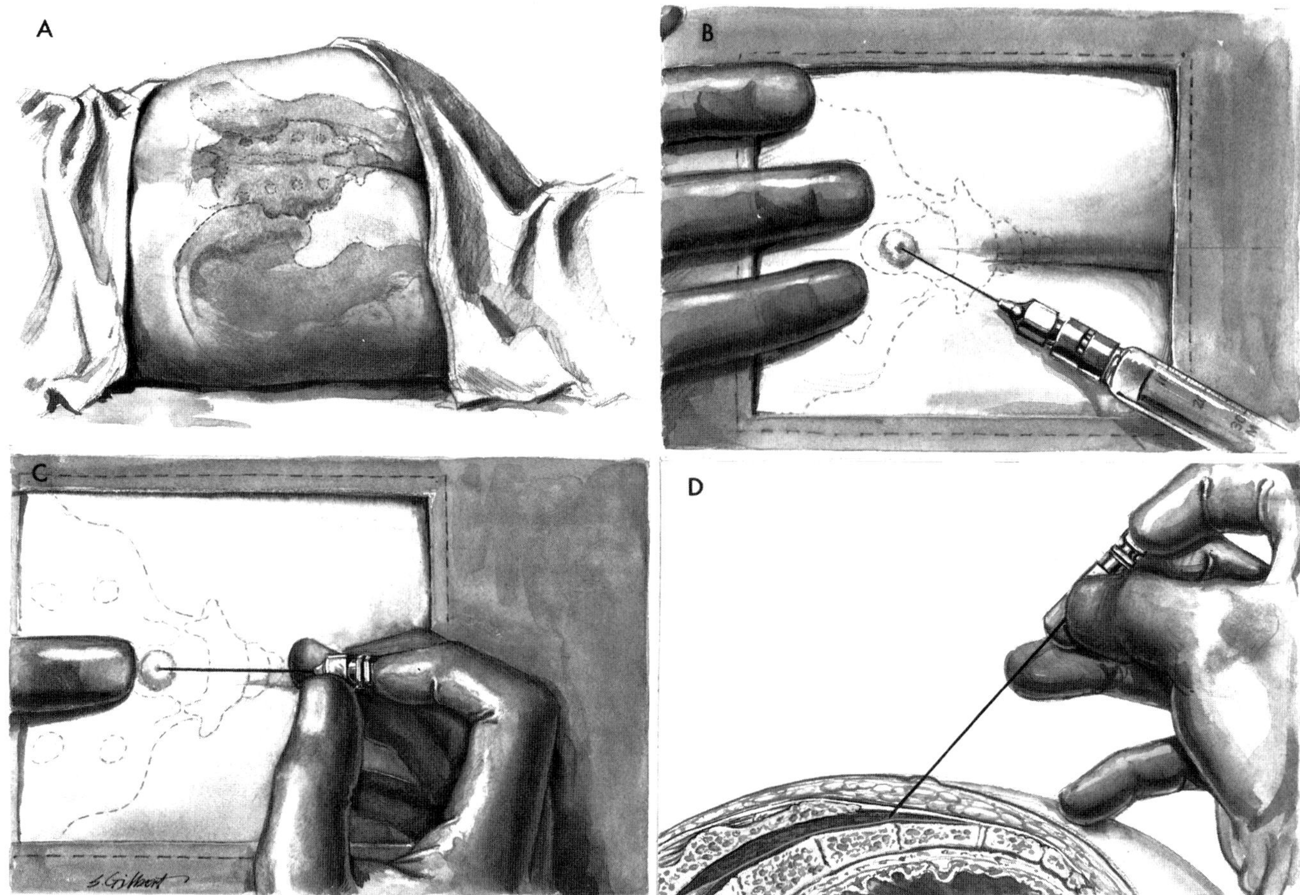


**Fig. 13–78.** Technique of puncture of the sacral canal. **A** shows sacrum in phantom to indicate landmarks. The initial step is to reaffirm the position of the hiatus and then produce good analgesia of the different steps in carrying out the procedures. **B**: Formation of an anesthetic wheal at the center of the hiatus using a 30-gauge, 1-cm needle and approaching the skin with the bevel of the needle facing the skin and its shaft being parallel to the skin. This initial preparation should be the only painful phase of the procedure if the subsequent steps are carried out effectively. A total of 0.5 ml of solution is injected into the skin slowly because rapid injection produces great discomfort. Next, the 30-gauge needle is replaced with a 25-gauge, 3½-cm needle, which is inserted through the same hole in the skin. In following injection of a few centimeters in the subcutaneous tissue, the direction of the needle is changed so that its axis is almost perpendicular to the plane of the posterior sacrococcygeal hiatus. This usually makes a caudal angle of 40 to 50° with the skin. Injection of 1 to 1.5 ml of 0.5% lidocaine into the subcutaneous tissue and sacrococcygeal ligament. The needle is advanced through the ligament and one can sense passing through the ligament and touching the posterior surface of the fourth sacral vertebra, whereupon another increment is injected into the periosteum to anesthetize this very sensitive structure. **C**: The next step is to grasp the 18-gauge, 5-cm long, thin-walled caudal needle between the first and third fingers, while the tip of the second finger is held over the top of the stylet so that it will not be displaced during insertion. While the skin immediately cephalad to the anesthetic wheal is held firm by the second finger of the opposite hand (right-handed physicians should use the right hand to hold the needle and syringe and the left hand to immobilize the skin, and vice versa for the left-handed physician), the point of the caudal needle, with its bevel facing posterosuperiorly, is inserted through the same wound made by the smaller needle. **D**: Sagittal view showing direction of the needle. Index finger of the left hand that holds the skin just cephalad to point of puncture that immobilizes the skin has been omitted. The shaft of the caudal needle should make angles with the skin of 125° cephalad to it and 90° laterally. In this direction it is advanced through the subcutaneous tissue and posterior sacrococcygeal ligament. If absolute resistance is encountered before the ligament is engaged, it indicates that the needle has impinged on bone and should be withdrawn before reinserting it. Extreme care must be exercised to avoid inserting the needle lateral to the lateral edge of the coccyx or lower portion of the sacrum, because this may result in invasion of the retrorectal space and perhaps the rectum and even the fetal head. This can be avoided by repeatedly checking the position of the coccyx and making certain that the needle remains in the midline.

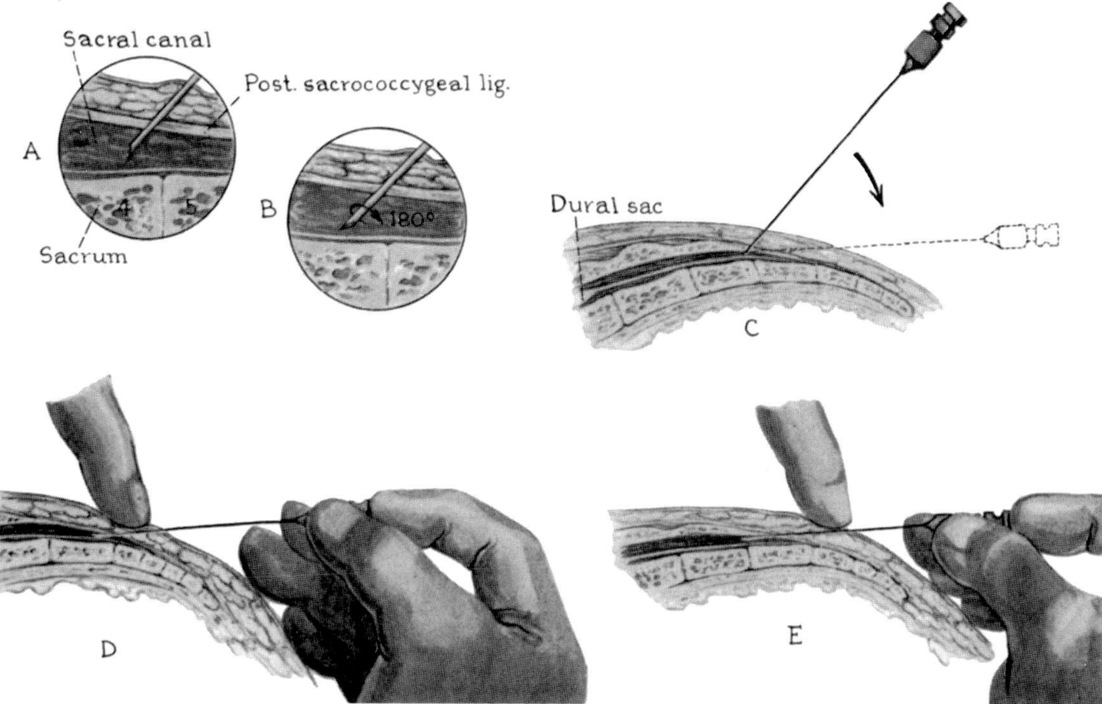


**Fig. 13–79.** Technique of puncture of the sacral canal (continued). **A**: Penetration of the ligament and entrance of the needle point into the sacral canal are indicated by a sudden lack of resistance and a snap. The point of the needle usually impinges on the posterior aspect of the body of the fourth sacral vertebra, as shown in the enlargement of the structures at site of puncture. The needle has already been advanced to the posterior surface of the fourth sacral vertebra and withdrawn so that its bevel is halfway between the anterior and posterior surface of the canal. **B**: The needle is then rotated 180° so that the bevel faces the anterior surface of the sacral canal. **C**: Change in direction of the needle is necessary before it is advanced cephalad so that the long axis of the needle is in the same plane as the sacral canal. This movement is facilitated by simultaneously depressing the hub of the needle with the right hand and applying pressure with the second finger of the left hand on the shaft of the needle at its point of entrance into the skin, as shown in **D** and **E**. Unless this is done, an attempt to press on the hub will merely cause that part of the needle outside the skin to bow without altering the direction of that part within the ligament and canal. The needle is then advanced 2 cm to the level of the lower border of the third vertebra, always keeping it in the midline. The concavity of the long axis of the canal is such that when the point of the needle is advanced to the lower part of the third sacral vertebra, it will be near the posterior wall and away from the anterior part of the canal which contains important structures.

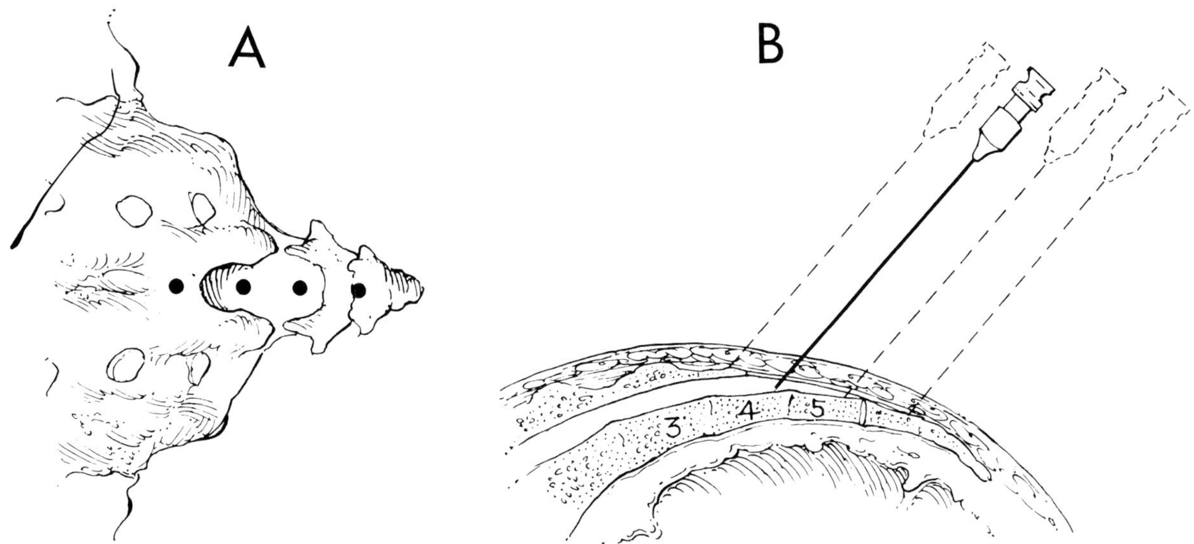


**Fig. 13–80.** Technique of making exploratory punctures to locate center of sacral hiatus. **A**: Posterior view. Dots indicate sites of insertion. **B**: Sagittal view.

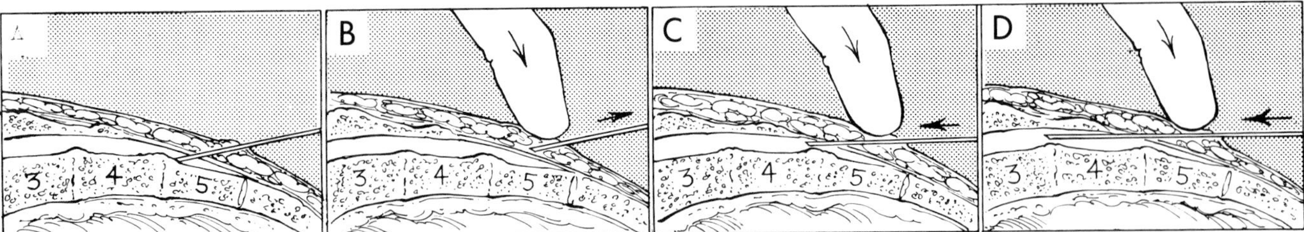


**Fig. 13–81.** Technique of overcoming bony obstructions to advance needle in sacral canal. **A**: Point of needle against obstruction. **B**: Needle has been withdrawn and is reinserted through the sacrococcygeal ligament at a point more cephalad and in a direction more parallel to the sacral canal. The finger exerts more pressure to facilitate this change in direction. **C**: Point of needle is just over obstruction. **D**: Final position of needle.

injected. During this period, the patient is reassured, cautioned not to move, her blood pressure and pulse measured, and mental condition evaluated. When 5 minutes have elapsed (accurately measured with a watch), skin sensation and muscle function are tested. If there is no evidence of subarachnoid block, the therapeutic dose is injected while the palm of the free hand is held against the skin to detect tumefaction. The amount injected depends on the purpose of the block and the concentration of the local anesthetic. Injection is made slowly because rapid injection may cause discomfort to the patient, including vertigo, headache, and a sense of fullness or actual pain in the legs, particularly the posterior aspect of the thigh. This latter sign is fairly constant and is another sign that the needle is properly placed. Immediately after the injection is completed, the needle is withdrawn, drapes removed, and the parturient requested to assume the supine position. Thereafter, she is managed as described below.

## *Continuous Caudal Block*

Continuous caudal analgesia is usually effected by use of a catheter introduced into the sacral canal and maintained in this position during labor and for vaginal delivery or for cesarean section. Preliminary preparations are the same as discussed above. Special equipment consists of:

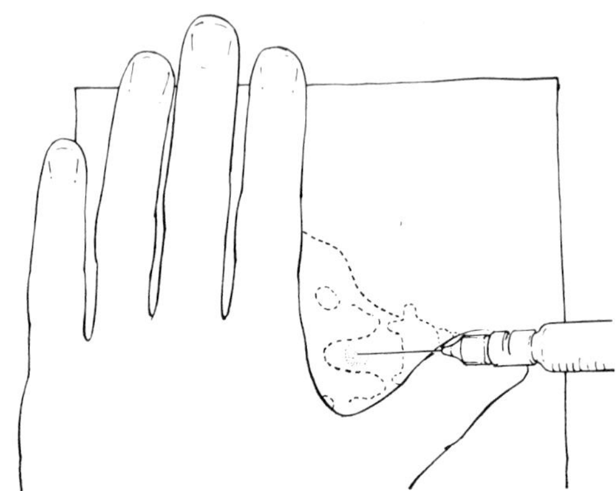

**Fig. 13–82.** Technique of palpating for subcutaneous displacement of needle point. The palm of the free hand resting firmly against skin over the sacrum will easily detect tumefaction, indicating injection of solution outside of sacral canal.

1) a special 18-gauge, thin-walled, 5-cm needle with well-fitting stylet (Becton, Dickinson Company, Rutherford, NJ); 2) vinyl plastic catheter, 100 cm long with the distal 20 cm marked at 5-cm intervals, and a wire stylet sufficiently stiff to prevent buckling or curling of the catheter within the sacral canal (Cobe Laboratories, Los Angeles, CA); 3) a Tuohy-Borsch adaptor to connect the tubing to the syringe; and, 4) a three-way stopcock and assembly. The vinyl plastic catheter is preferred because it is cheaper and can be discarded after use, and also because it permits the use of the 18-gauge, thin-walled needle.

The procedures before puncture and the technique of inserting the caudal needle are exactly the same as already described. The special 18-gauge needle is introduced as described in Figure 13–84. After it penetrates the posterior sacrococcygeal ligament, the needle is rotated 180° so that its bevel faces anteriorly, and the shaft of the needle is depressed through an arc of approximately 45°. Because this needle is stouter than that used for the single-dose technique, it is less likely to bow, and, consequently, it is easier to change its direction. Following this maneuver, the needle is advanced approximately 1 cm and then rotated 180° on its axis so that its bevel again faces posteriorly. This positioning helps guide the plastic tubing toward the posterior wall (roof) of the sacral canal, which is usually smooth, with a groove that facilitates the advance of the catheter. However, if the point of the needle is too near the anterior wall, the tip of the catheter will more likely contact one of the structures in the sacral canal and its cephalad advance will be obstructed.

The various maneuvers (described previously) to ascertain if the needle is in the proper place are carried out. The next step is to measure the length of the needle on the catheter by placing the needle stylet alongside the distal part of the catheter. The hub of the needle stylet should be at the 6-cm mark on the catheter. The stylet of the catheter is then withdrawn 1 cm so that its distal 1 cm does not contain stylet and is less rigid. If the caudal is intended to be used as part of the double-catheter technique, the catheter is advanced 1 to 1.5 cm within the sacral canal so that its tip is at the level of the third sacral vertebra. This is followed by a test for patency by injecting 2 ml of saline. The catheter is then fixed in place and ready for the test dose and the subsequent therapeutic dose at the appropriate time (second stage).

If the caudal is to be used for continuous extradural

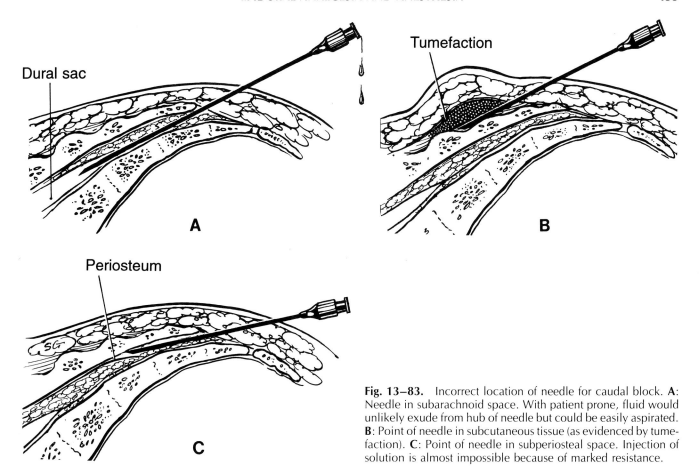

**Fig. 13–83.** Incorrect location of needle for caudal block. **A**: Needle in subarachnoid space. With patient prone, fluid would unlikely exude from hub of needle but could be easily aspirated. **B**: Point of needle in subcutaneous tissue (as evidenced by tumefaction). **C**: Point of needle in subperiosteal space. Injection of solution is almost impossible because of marked resistance.

analgesia for labor and vaginal delivery or for cesarean section, it is best to advance the catheter cephalad so that its tip is at L5 or S1 (Figure 13–85). As previously mentioned, this will permit to achieve the same cephalad extent of blockade with smaller doses than if the tip of the catheter is lower. If the needle is properly placed, the tip of the catheter will proceed cephalad along the smooth posterior wall (roof) of the sacral canal without difficulty. The trough-like deep groove in the middle part of the posterior wall helps maintain the catheter in the midline.

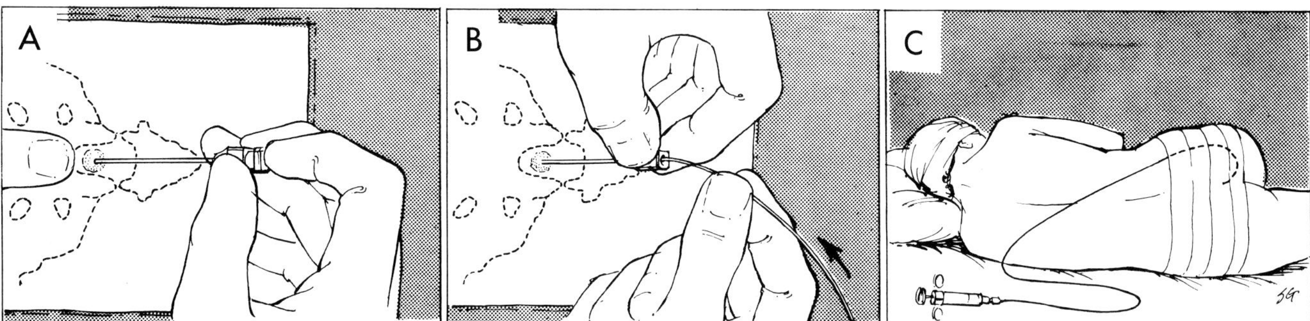

**Fig. 13–84.** Technique of continuous caudal block. **A**: Insertion of special 18-gauge, thin-walled caudal needle through posterior sacrococcygeal ligament. **B**: Needle has already been advanced 1 to 2 cm, and its shaft rotated 180° so that its bevel faces the roof of the sacral canal. The catheter is then introduced through the needle as shown. For clarity, the left hand has been displaced. Usually, it is held so that ulnar surface is against the low back. If the caudal is being used as part of the double-catheter technique, the point of the catheter is placed so that it is at the level of the third lumbar vertebra, i.e., it is advanced 0.5 cm beyond the bevel of the needle. If the caudal is being used for cesarean section, the catheter needs to be advanced in the midline to the level of the first sacral or fifth lumbar vertebral. For the latter purpose, it is essential that the needle with its bevel facing posteriorly is in the exact midline and its shaft depressed with the fingers of the left hand so that the needle opening is within the groove that exists in a "roof" of the canal. Advance of the catheter in the groove will cause it to proceed cephalad without difficulty and without deviation. **C**: Needle has been removed, catheter taped in place and connected to a syringe.

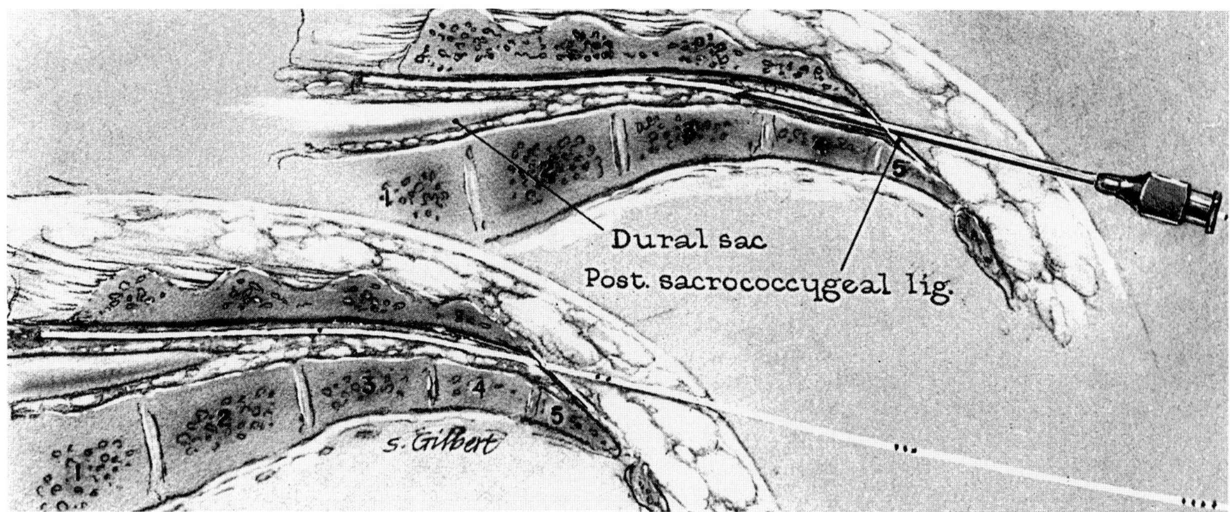


**Fig. 13–85.** Placement of the epidural catheter in the sacral canal advanced to the level of the first sacral vertebra procedure which is facilitated by the presence of the groove in the "roof" of the sacral canal. The lower figure shows the catheter in place after the needle has been withdrawn.

If the tubing does not pass beyond the point of the needle, the point of the needle is probably misplaced in subcutaneous, muscular, or subperiosteal tissue. However, if the point of the catheter passes for 1 or 2 cm beyond the point of the needle and then becomes obstructed, it is likely that the needle is in the sacral canal, and that the tip of the catheter is buried in the fat pad overlying the nerve structure or is against one of the lower sacral nerves, or it may even be in a blood vessel. If the patient experiences paresthesia in the perianal region, contact with nerves should be suspected. Occasionally, the tip of the catheter may become trapped anterior to one or more nerves, and when attempt is made to force its advance, the catheter may migrate into one of the anterior sacral foramina and then to the retrorectal space. If any of these problems is expected, the needle and catheter are withdrawn about 0.5 cm (without disturbing the relation of one to the other!) to remove the catheter tip from the obstructing structure, and then an attempt is again made to advance the catheter.

A very important point that requires strong emphasisis this: The plastic tubing must never be withdrawn from the needle, otherwise it is likely to be sheared off by the sharp bevel and the sheared section left in the sacral canal and cannot be retrieved without surgical access to it. Nor should the needle be advanced after part of the catheter is beyond the bevel of the needle, because the catheter tip may be trapped and advancing the needle will only force it to bend and even shear off. If repeated difficulties are encountered, it is best to remove the needle first and then to withdraw the catheter before repeating the entire procedure.

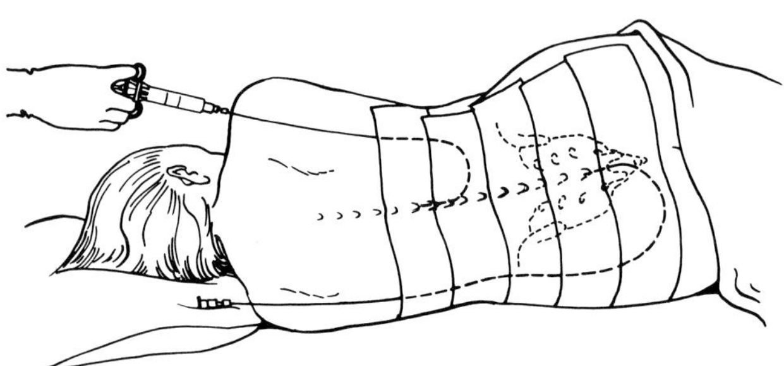

**Fig. 13–86.** Double-catheter technique of continuous epidural analgesia. The upper catheter is placed with its tip at T11 and the lower catheter is placed with the tip at S3.

When the catheter is judged to be properly placed, the needle is withdrawn from the patient's back over the plastic tubing. This should be done carefully to avoid accidental withdrawal of the catheter out of the sacral canal. After removing the needle, the catheter is withdrawn 1 cm in case its tip had been pushed against fat or has migrated into a foramen. A Tuohy-Borsch adaptor is then attached to the end of the catheter and aspiration is attempted with a dry, 2-ml syringe. If blood or blood-tinged fluid is aspirated, the tubing should be withdrawn an additional 1 cm and aspiration repeated. If either blood or cerebrospinal fluid can not be aspirated, 1 ml of saline is injected to dislodge any tissue that may be against the tip of the tubing and then another aspiration attempt made. If this also proves negative, a further precaution is taken; the syringe is detached and the end of the tubing with the adaptor is placed about two feet below the level of the sacral canal. The difference in the level of the tip and the end of the catheter facilitates flow of cerebrospinal fluid even when its pressure is low, or when the tip of the catheter is against the arachnoid or a nerve root.

When all of these maneuvers indicate that the tip of the catheter is properly placed, a test dose of 3 ml of anesthetic solution is injected. The syringe is disconnected and a cap is placed on the Tuohy-Borsch adaptor, which is wrapped in sterile gauze or the adaptor connected to a closed system. The plastic catheter is then firmly fas-

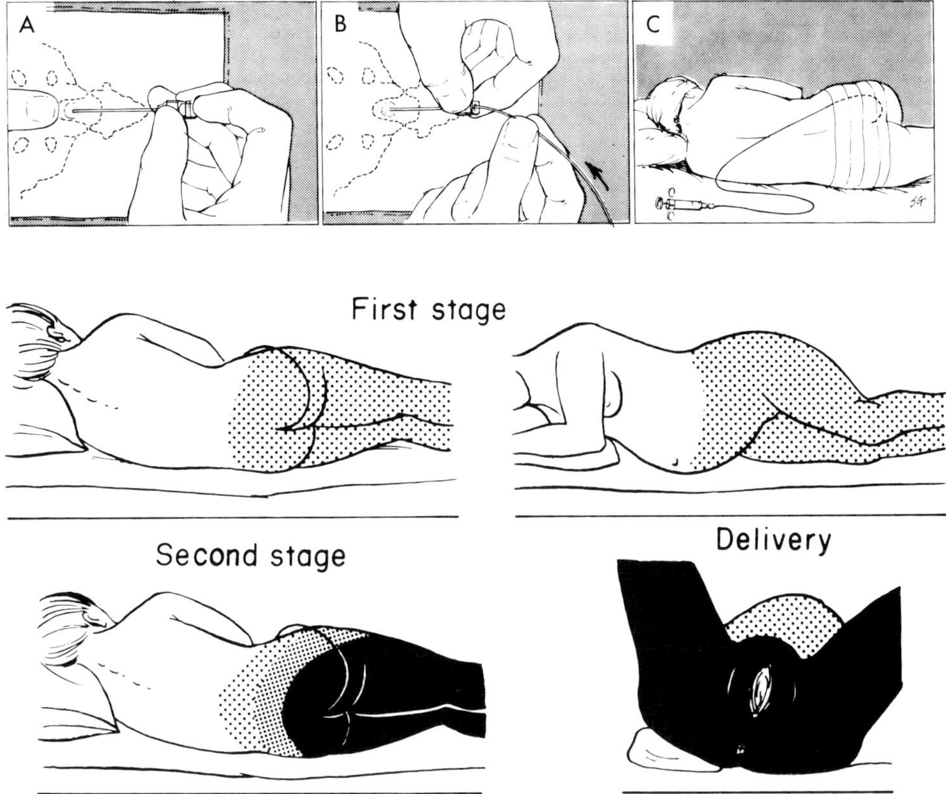


**Fig. 13–87.** Technique of continuous caudal analgesia. The uppermost figure, **A**, shows insertion of a special 18-gauge, thin-walled 5-cm needle through posterior sacrococcygeal ligament. **B**: The needle has already been advanced 2 cm and its shaft turned 180° so that its bevel faces the roof of the sacral canal, and the plastic catheter is being introduced and advanced 8 to 10 cm to place its tip at the level of the first sacral-fifth lumbar vertebrae, as depicted in Figure 13–85. For the first stage and early second stage, low concentrations of anesthetics are used to produce only analgesia. After internal rotation of the presenting part, a higher concentration is injected to achieve motor block and perineal relaxation (black) and differential block T10–12 (light stippling) and lumbar segments (heavy stippling). (**A** From Bonica JJ: Obstetric Anesthesia and Analgesia. WFSA , Seattle, University of Washington Press, 1980, p. 110)

tened to the skin with adhesive tape, and the patient requested to turn on her side (Figure 13–86). Figures 13–87 and 13–88 depict the technique of continuous caudal analgesia/anesthesia for labor and vaginal delivery.

### *Intrapartal and Intra-Anesthetic Care*

During labor, uterine contractions, cervical dilatation, and advance of the presenting part should be monitored. The cervicographic method of following the progress of labor is recommended. In home deliveries and in hospital deliveries where modern equipment is not available, the fetal heart rate (FHR) is followed by auscultation. The limitations of this method and of palpating uterine contractions are generally recognized and emphasize the need for the clinical use of more sophisticated systems, especially in monitoring the labor of women with high-risk pregnancies. Combined with these is a measurement of cervical dilatation in advance of the presenting part. These are recorded in a partograph that also has space for recorded maternal blood pressure, respiration, the administration of oxytocin, sedatives or other drugs used during labor and delivery. In many centers, facilities are also available for assessment of pH and other biochemical parameters of the fetal blood obtained from the scalp or the buttocks.

During labor, the patient is made to lie on her side and only assume the supine position for brief periods (seconds) during which the left lateral tilt or left uterine displacement is used. In the event there is concern about having predominantly a unilateral analgesia, it may be desirable to have the parturient change sides 3 to 4 minutes after the initial injection.

With 0.5 to 1% lidocaine or chloroprocaine, or 0.125% bupivacaine, subjective relief of pain due to contractions develops 3 to 5 minutes of the injection of the therapeutic dose, and objective analgesia (as evidenced by pinprick test) is present in 8 to 15 minutes. The spread of analgesia/anesthesia is complete in 15 to 20 minutes after the injection. If 10 minutes after injection of the therapeutic dose there is no subjective or objective evidence of block, it is likely that the solution was injected outside of the epidural space because the catheter has migrated, or it may have been absorbed too rapidly through lacerated veins to effect block.

If analgesia is present, but not at a sufficiently high level,

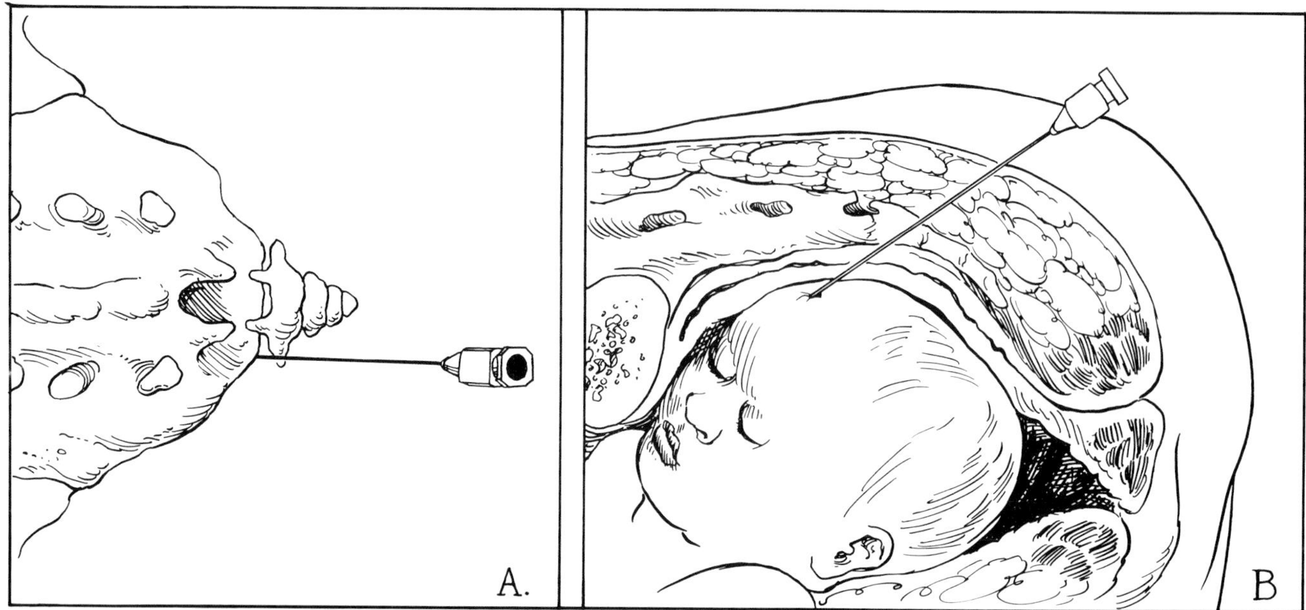


**Fig. 13–88.** Improper placement of needle lateral to edge of sacrum **(A)** and into rectum and fetal head **(B)**. In the reported cases of this complication, the scalp lesions were situated over or adjacent to the anterior fontonelle as would be anticipated from the spatial relations in occipito-anterior position.

reinjection may be carried out with a larger dose; or if an infusion is being used, the infusion rate increased. The ability to control the height, extent, and intensity is one of the major advantages of the continuous technique of achieving lumbar epidural or caudal block. As previously mentioned, occasionally, some patients may have one or more unblocked segments, or may have only limited block on one side. In such instances, the patient should be turned to the poorly anesthetized or unblocked side and an additional dose of the drug injected.

## EXTRADURAL ANESTHESIA FOR CESAREAN SECTION

Extradural anesthesia for cesarean section is best accomplished with continuous lumbar epidural block—a technique that has evolved as the most frequently used procedure to carry out abdominal operative delivery in many major obstetric centers. Steps of preparation of the patient, the site of field, the administration of 1000 to 1500 ml of fluids intravenously, and of epidural puncture with a special Tuohy needle are similar to that described earlier in this chapter. The procedure is carried out with the patient in the left lateral position, which is inherent with more rapid cephalad spread of the solution. As previously mentioned, injection of the solution with the patient in the sitting position is associated with a less caudal spread and more céphalad spread. The Tuohy needle is introduced into the second or third lumbar interspace and the catheter inserted through it and advanced 3 cm beyond the point of the needle. Following a negative test dose, a total of 18 to 22 ml of 0.5% bupivacaine with 1: 300,000 epinephrine or 2% bupivacaine with the same concentration of epinephrine is injected. The entire volume of the solution can be injected slowly or injected in four increments at intervals of 2 to 3 minutes between injections. The use of the slow, single-bolus injection ensures a rapid and reliable onset of block as speed is essential, whereas the use of an incremental technique has a slower incidence of hypotension but is unquestionably slower in onset and may require a slightly larger dose of local anesthetic (521,522).

Once the placement of the catheter has been accomplished, the patient is made to lie in the supine semilateral position with a wedge under the buttock and left lateral uterine displacement to minimize the aortocaval compression. The patient is then observed constantly and her blood pressure, pulse, and respiration measured and recorded every 2 minutes following the injection of the therapeutic dose. Pleasant conversation should be encouraged, not only for its distracting effect, but also to permit the physician to note promptly any cerebral dysfunction (manifestation of systemic toxic reaction or hypotension). Hypotension, if it occurs, develops more gradually than with subarachnoid block. If the systolic blood pressure drops more than 20% of normal for the parturient or drops below 100 mm Hg systolic, prompt therapy is instituted, including: 1) administration of 100% oxygen; 2) administration of an additional 500 ml of fluids very rapidly; and 3) intravenous administration of small increments (5 to 10 mg) of ephedrine until the blood pressure is stabilized. More detailed discussion of the use of epidural anesthesia for cesarean section is contained in Chapter 29.

## REFERENCES

1. Corning JL: Spinal anaesthesia and local medication of the cord. N.Y. J. Med. 42:483, 1885.

2. Cathelin MF: A new route of spinal injection: a method for epidural injections by way of the sacral canal; application to man. Compt. Rend. Soc. Biol. 53:452, 1901.
3. Pages F: Metameric anesthesia. Rez. Sanid. Milit. 11:351, 1921.
4. Dogliotti AM: A new method of block anesthesia: segmental peridural spinal anesthesia. Am. J. Surg. 20:107, 1933.
5. Stoeckel D: Sakrale anesthesia. Z. Gynaek. 33:3, 1909.
6. Schlimpert H, Schneider K: Sacral anesthesia in gynecology and obstetrics. Munchen Med. Wschr. 57:2561, 1910.
7. Meeker WR, Bonar BE: Regional anesthesia in gynecology and obstetrics. Surg. Gynecol. Obstet. 37:816, 1923.
8. Rucker MP: The use of novacaine in obstetrics. Am. J. Obstet. Gynecol. 9:35, 1925.
9. Pickles W, Jones SS: Regional anesthesia in obstetrics with a report of twenty-eight deliveries under epidural block. N. Engl. J. Med. 199:988, 1928.
10. Baptisti A Jr: Caudal anesthesia in obstetrics. Am. J. Obstet. Gynecol. 38:642, 1939.
11. Lahmann AH, Mietus AC: Caudal anesthesia: its use in obstetrics. Surg. Gynecol. Obstet. 74:63, 1942.
12. Cleland JGP: Paravertebral anesthesia in obstetrics. Surg. Gynecol. Obstet. 57:51, 1933.
13. Edwards WB, Hingson RA: Continuous caudal anesthesia in obstetrics. Am. J. Surg. 57:459, 1942.
14. Adams RC, Lundy JS, Seldon TH: Continuous caudal anesthesia or analgesia: a consideration of the technic, various uses and some possible dangers. JAMA 122:152, 1943.
15. Hingson RA, Edwards WB, Lull CB, Whitacre FE, et al: Newborn mortality and morbidity with continuous caudal analgesia. JAMA 136–229:221, 1948.
16. Hingson RA, Edwards WB: An analysis of the first ten thousand confinements managed with continuous caudal analgesia with a report of the authors' first one thousand cases. JAMA 123:538, 1943.
17. Siever JM, Mousel LH: Continuous caudal anesthesia in three hundred unselected obstetric cases. JAMA 122:424, 1943.
18. Lull CB: Some observations in use of continuous caudal analgesia. Am. J. Obstet. Gynecol. 47:312, 1944.
19. Brown HO, Thomson JM, Fitzgerald JE: An analysis of 500 obstetrical cases with continuous caudal anesthesia using Pontocaine. Anesthesiology 7:355, 1946.
20. Lusk HA: Continuous caudal analgesia in obstetrics. Am. J. Obstet. Gynecol. 59:437, 1950.
21. Lewis MS, Austin RB: Continuous caudal versus saddle-block anesthesia in obstetrics. Am. J. Obstet. Gynecol. 59: 1146, 1950.
22. Downing GC: Caudal anesthesia in private obstetric practice: Review of 2139 cases. West. J. Surg. 59:19, 1951.
23. Ritmiller LF, Rippman ET: Caudal analgesia in obstetrics: report of thirteen years' experience. Obstet. Gynecol. 9: 25, 1957.
24. Bush RC: Caudal analgesia for vaginal delivery. Anesthesiology 20:31, 186, 1959.
25. Friedman A, Schantz S, Page HR: Continuous caudal analgesia and anesthesia in obstetrics. A critical evaluation of 510 consecutive cases. Am. J. Obstet. Gynecol. 80:1181, 1960.
26. Hingson RA, Cull WA, Benzinger M: Continuous caudal analgesia in obstetrics. Curr. Res. Anesth. Analg. 40:119, 1961.
27. Evans TN, Morley GW, Helder L: Caudal anesthesia in obstetrics. Obstet. Gynecol. 20:726, 1962.
28. Moore DC, Bridenbaugh LD: Physician anesthesia, regional block and father participation: the ultimate in care for vaginal delivery. West. J. Surg. 72:73, 1964.
29. Galley AH: Continuous caudal analgesia in obstetrics. Anaesthesia 4:154, 1949.
30. Ostlere B: Epidural analgesia in the treatment of hypertension due to toxemia of pregnancy. Anaesthesia 7:169, 1952.
31. Johnson GT: Continuous caudal analgesia: Experiences in the management of disordered uterine function in labour. Br. Med. J. 1:627, 1954.
32. Johnson T, Clayton CG: Studies in placental action during prolonged and dysfunctional labours using radioactive sodium. J. Obstet. Gynaecol. Br. Commonw. 62:513, 1955.
33. Johnson GT: Prolonged labour (a clinical trial of continuous caudal analgesia). Br. Med. J. 2:386, 1957.
34. Ball HCJ, Chambers JSW: Primary cervical dystocia treated with caudal analgesia. Br. Med. J. 1:1275, 1956.
35. Solomon HJ: Caudal anesthesia and analgesia in obstetrics: A preliminary report. Med. J. Aust. 2:215, 1963.
36. McCaul K: Regional anesthesia for vaginal delivery. Abstracts of the Fifth World Congress of Anaesthesiologists, Kyoto, Japan, September 19–23. Excerpta Medica, Amsterdam, 1973, p 329.
37. Graffagnino P, Seyler LW: Epidural anesthesia in obstetrics. Am. J. Obstet. Gynecol. 35:597, 1938.
38. Lemmon WT: A method for continuous spinal anesthesia. Ann. Surg. 111:141, 1940.
39. Hingson RA, Southworth JL: Continuous peridural anesthesia. Curr. Res. Anesth. Analg. 23:215, 1944.
40. Curbelo MM: Continuous peridural segmental anesthesia by means of a ureteral catheter. Presented before the 22nd Annual Congress of Anaesthetists, New York, September 8–11, 1947.
41. Umstead HW, Dufresne WJ: Continuous lumbar peridural anesthesia in obstetrics. R.I. Med. J. 31:489, 1948.
42. Curbelo MM: Continuous peridural segmental anesthesia by means of ureteral catheter. Curr. Res. Anesth. Analg. 28:1, 1949.
43. Flowers CE Jr, Hellman LM, Hingson RA: Continuous peridural anesthesia/analgesia for labor, delivery and cesarean section. Curr. Res. Anesth. Analg. 28:181, 1949.
44. Cleland JGP: Continuous peridural and caudal analgesia in obstetrics. Curr. Res. Anesth. Analg. 28:61, 1949.
45. Bromage PR: Spinal Epidural Analgesia. Baltimore, The Williams & Wilkins Co., 1954.
46. Bromage PR: Spread of analgesic solutions in the epidural space and their site of action: a statistical study. Br. J. Anaesth. 34:161, 1962.
47. Bromage PR: Spread and site of action of epidural analgesia. Int. Anesthesiol. Clin. 1:547, 1963.
48. Bromage PR, Burfoot MF, Crowell DE, Pettigrew RT: Quality of epidural blockade. I. Influence of physical factors. Br. J. Anaesth. 36:342, 1964.
49. Bromage PR: Epidural Analgesia. Philadelphia, W.B. Saunders, 1978, pp. 513–600.
50. Bonica JJ, Berges PU, Morikawa K: Circulatory effects of peridural block. I. Effects of levels of analgesia and doses of lidocaine. Anesthesiology 33:619, 1970.
51. Bonica JJ, Akamatsu TJ, Berges PU, Morikawa K, et al: Circulatory effects of peridural block. II. Effects of epinephrine. Anesthesiology 34:514, 1971.
52. Bonica JJ, Kennedy WF Jr, Akamatsu TJ, Gerbershagen HU: Circulatory effects of peridural block. III: Effects of acute blood loss. Anesthesiology 36:219, 1972.
53. Lund PC, Cwik JC, Quinn JR: Experiences with epidural anesthesia, 7730 cases. Analg. Anesth. 40:153, 1961.
54. Apgar V: A proposal for a new method of evaluation of the newborn infant. Curr. Res. Anesth. Analg. 32:260, 1953.
55. Caldeyro-Barcia R, y Alvarez H, Reynolds SRM: A better

understanding of uterine contractility through simultaneous recording with an internal and a seven-channel external method. Surg. Gynecol. Obstet. 91:641, 1950.
56. Reynolds SRM, Harris JS, Kaiser IH: Clinical Measurement of Uterine Forces in Pregnancy and Labor. Springfield, Charles C. Thomas Publisher, 1954.
57. Friedman EA: a) Primigravid labor: A graphicostatistical analysis. Obstet. Gynecol. 6:567, 1955; b) Labor in multiparas: A graphicostatistical analysis. Obstet. Gynecol. 8:691, 1956.
58. Hon EH: The diagnosis of fetal distress. Clin. Obstet. Gynecol. 3:860, 1960.
59. Saling E: Die amnioskopie, ein neues verfahren zum Erkennen von Gefahrenzustanden des feten bei noch stehender fruchtblase. Geburtsh Frauenheilk 22:830, 1962.
60. Scanlon JW, Brown WU, Weiss M, Alpert MH: Neurobehavioral responses of newborn infants after maternal epidural anesthesia. Anesthesiology 40:121–128, 1974.
61. Eisen SM, Rosen N, Winesander H, Hellmann K: The routine use of lumbar epidural anesthesia in obstetrics: Clinical review of 9532 cases. Can. Anaesth. Soc. J. 7:280, 1960.
62. Hellmann K: Epidural anaesthesia in obstetrics: A second look at 26,127 cases. Can. Anaesth. Soc. J. 12:398 1965.
63. Shnider S: Experience with regional anesthesia for vaginal delivery. *In* The Anesthesiologist, Mother and Newborn. Edited by SM Shnider, SM Moya. Baltimore, Williams & Wilkins, 1974, pp. 38–46.
64. Chaplin RA, Renwick WA: Lumbar epidural anaesthesia for vaginal delivery. Can. Anaesth. Soc. J. 5:414, 1958.
65. Hehre FW, Sayig JM: Continuous lumbar peridural anesthesia in obstetrics. Am. J. Obstet. Gynecol. 80:1173, 1960.
66. Bromage PR: Continuous lumbar epidural analgesia for obstetrics. Can. Med. Assoc. J. 85:1136, 1961.
67. Nielsen JS, Spoercl WE, Keenleyside HB, Slater PE, et al: Continuous epidural analgesia for labour and delivery. Can. Anaesth. Soc. J. 9:143, 1962.
68. Crawford JS: Principles and Practice of Obstetric Anaesthesia, 2nd edition. London, Blackwell Scientific Publications, 1965.
69. Crawford JS: Lumbar epidural block in labour: A clinical analysis. Br. J. Anaesth. 44:66, 1972.
70. Crawford JS: The second thousand epidural blocks in an obstetric hospital's practice. Br. J. Anaesth. 44:1277–1286, 1972.
71. Moir DD, Willocks J: Continuous epidural analgesia in incoordinate uterine action. Acta. Anaesthesiol. Scand. Suppl. 23:144, 1966.
72. Doughty A: Selective epidural analgesia and the forceps rate. Br. J. Anaesth. 41:1058, 1969.
73. Climie CR: The place of continuous lumbar epidural analgesia in the management of abnormally prolonged labour. Med. J. Aust. 2:447, 1964.
74. Potter N, MacDonald RD: Obstetric consequences of epidural analgesia in nulliparous patients. Lancet 1:1031, 1971.
75. Hollmen A: Lumbar epidural analgesia as an obstetric analgesic method. Acta. Anaesthesiol. Scand. Suppl. 37:251, 1970.
76. Zador G, Englesson S, Nilsson BA: Low-dose intermittent epidural anaesthesia with lidocaine for vaginal delivery. I. Clinical efficacy and lidocaine concentration in maternal, foetal and umbilical cord blood. Acta. Obstet. Gynaecol. Scand. Suppl. 34:3–16, 1974.
77. Zador G, Nilsson BA: Low dose intermittent epidural anaesthesia with lidocaine for vaginal delivery. II. Influence on labour and foetal acid-base status. Acta. Obstet. Gynecol. Scand. (Suppl) 34:17–30, 1974.
78. Zador G, Willdeck-Lund G, Nilsson BA: Continuous drip lumbar epidural anaesthesia with lidocaine for vaginal delivery. I. Clinical efficacy in lidocaine concentration in maternal, foetal and umbilical cord blood. Acta Obstet. Gynecol. Scand (Suppl) 34:31–40, 1974.
79. Zador G, Nilsson BA: Continuous drip lumbar epidural anaesthesia with lidocaine for vaginal delivery. II. Influence on labour and foetal acid-base status. Acta Obstet. Gynecol. Scand. (Suppl) 34:41–49, 1974.
80. Maltau JM, Andersen HT: Epidural anaesthesia as an alternative to caesarean section in the treatment of prolonged, exhaustive labour. Acta. Anaesthesiol. Scand. 19:349–354, 1975.
81. Maltau JM, Andersen HT: Obstetrical analgesia assessed by free fatty acid mobilization. Acta. Anaesthesiol. Scand. 19: 245, 1975.
82. Belfrage P, Raabe N, Thalme B: Lumbar epidural analgesia with bupivacaine in labor. Determinations of drug concentrations and pH in fetal scalp blood and continuous fetal heart rate monitoring. Am. J. Obstet. Gynecol. 121:365, 1975.
83. Thalme B, Raabe N, Belfrage P: Lumbar epidural analgesia in labour. I. Acid-base balance and clinical condition of mother, fetus, and newborn child. Acta. Obstet. Gynecol. Scand. 53:27, 1974.
84. Thalme B, Raabe N, Belfrage P: Lumbar epidural analgesia in labour. II. Effects on glucose, lactate, sodium, chloride, total protein, haematocrit and haemoglobin in maternal, fetal, and neonatal blood. Acta. Obstet. Gynecol. Scand. 53: 113, 1974.
85. Matouskova A, Dottori O, Forssman L, Victorin L: An improved method of epidural analgesia with reduced instrumental delivery rate. Acta. Obstet. Gynecol. Scand. 54: 231–235, 1975.
86. Ikle A: Die Periduralanaesthesie in der Geburtshilfe. Anaesthesist 2:29, 1953.
87. Schaudig H: On problems and current technic of peridural anaesthesia in obstetrics and gynecology. Anaesthesist 10: 152, 1961.
88. Vanderick G, Doud TK, Khoo SS, et al: Bupivacaine 0.125% in epidural block analgesia during childbirth: clinical evaluation. Br. J. Anaesth. 46:838, 1974.
89. Fujimori M: Present status of pain relief for normal labor in Japan. *In*: Anesthesia: Safety for All. Edited by QJ Gomez, LM Egay, MF Cruz-Odi. Proceedings of the 8th World Congress of Anesthesiologists, Excerpta Medica, Amsterdam, 1984, p. 63.
90. Crawford JS: Principles and Practice of Obstetric Anaesthesia, 5th edition. London, Blackwell Scientific Publications, 1984, p. 239.
91. Abboud TK, Khoo SS, Miller F, et al: Maternal, fetal and neonatal epidural anesthesia with bupivacaine, 2-chloroprocaine, or lidocaine. Anesth. Analg. 61:638, 1982.
92. Abboud TK, Kim KC, Noueihed R, et al: Epidural bupivacaine chloroprocaine, or lidocaine for cesarean section: maternal and neonatal effects. Anesth. Analg. 62:914, 1983.
93. Abboud TK, Afrasiabi A, Sarkis F, Daftaria N, et al: Continuous infusion epidural analgesia in parturients receiving bupivacaine, chloroprocaine, or lidocaine: Maternal, fetal, and neonatal effects. Anesth. Analg. 63:421–428, 1984.
94. Chestnut DH, Laszewski LJ, Pollack KL, Bates JN, et al: Continuous epidural infusion of 0.0625% bupivacaine—0.0002% Fentanyl during the second stage of labor. Anesthesiology 72:613–618, 1990.
95. Foldes FF, Colavincenzo JW, Birch JH: Epidural anesthesia: A reappraisal. Anesth. Analg. 35:33, 1956.
96. Billewicz-Driemel AM, Milne MD: Long-term assessment

of extradural analgesia for the relief of pain in labour: Sense of "deprivation" after analgesia in labour, relevant or not. Br. J. Anaesth. 48:139–144, 1976.
97. Robinson JO, Rosen M, Evans JM, Revill SI, et al: Maternal opinion about analgesia for labour. A controlled trial between epidural block and intramuscular pethidine combined with inhalation. Anaesthesia 35:1173, 1980.
98. MacArthur C, Lewis M, Knox EG: Evaluation of obstetric analgesia and anaesthesia: long-term maternal recollections. Int. J. Obstet. Anesth. 2:3, 1993.
99. Morgan BM, Bulpitt CJ, Clifton P, Lewis PJ: Effectiveness of pain relief in labour: survey of 1000 mothers. BMJ 285: 689, 1982a.
100. Morgan BM, Bulpitt CJ, Clifton P, Lewis PJ: Analgesia and satisfaction in childbirth. (The Queen Charlotte's 1000 mother survey). Lancet ii:808, 1982.
101. Morgan BM: Mothers' views of epidural practices. *In* Epidural and Spinal Blockade in Obstetrics. Edited by F Reynolds. London: Bailliere Tindall, 1990, pp. 219–228.
102. Reynolds F.: Epidural and Spinal Blockade in Obstetrics. London: Bailliere-Tindall, 1990.
103. Philipsen T, Jensen NH: Maternal opinion about analgesia in labour and delivery. A comparison of epidural blockade and intramuscular pethidine. Eur. J. Obstet. Gynecol. Reprod. Biol. 34:205, 1990.
104. Kitzinger S: Some women's experience of epidurals—a descriptive study. London: National Childbirth Trust, 1987.
105. Howell CJ, Chalmers I: A review of prospectively controlled comparisons of epidural with nonepidural forms of pain relief during labour. Int. J. Obstet. Anaesth. 1:93, 1992.
106. Chalmers I: Oxford database of perinatal trials, version 1.2 disk issue 6. Oxford: Oxford University Press, Autumn 1991.
107. Wuitshik M, Bakal J, Lipshitz JM: Clinical significance of pain and cognitive activity in latent labor. Obstet. Gynecol. 73:35–42, 1989.
108. Freund FG, Bonica JJ, Ward RJ, Akamatsu TJ, et al: Ventilatory reserve and level of motor block during high spinal and epidural anesthesia. Anesthesiology 28:834, 1967.
109. Gamil M: Serial peak expiratory flow rates in mothers during cesarean section under extradural anaesthesia. Br. J. Anaesth. 62:415, 1989.
110. Stenger V, Andersen T, Eitzman D, Prystowski H: Extradural anesthesia for cesarean section. Obstet. Gynecol. 25: 802, 1965.
111. Ueland K, Akamatsu TJ, Eng M, Bonica JJ, et al: Maternal cardiovascular dynamics. VI. Cesarean section under epidural anesthesia without epinephrine. Am. J. Obstet. Gynecol. 114:775–780, 1972.
112. Bonica JJ: Effects of double-catheter epidural analagesia on the mother, labor, fetus and newborn. Abstracts of the Fifth World Congress of Anaesthesiologists, Kyoto, Japan, September 19–23. Excerpta Medica, Amsterdam, 1973, pp. 331–350.
113. Bonica JJ, Kennedy WF Jr, Ward RJ, Tolas AG: A comparison of the effects of high subarachnoid and epidural anesthesia. Acta. Anaesthesiol. Scand. (Suppl.) 23:429, 1966.
114. Ueland K, Gills RE, Hansen JM: Maternal cardiovascular dynamics: I. Cesarean section under subarachnoid block anesthesia. Am. J. Obstet. Gynecol. 100:42, 1968.
115. Vasicka A, Hutchinson HT, Eng M, Allen CR: Spinal and epidural anesthesia, fetal and uterine response to acute hypo- and hypertension. Am. J. Obstet. Gynecol. 90:800, 1964.
116. Palmer CM, Norris MC, Giudici MC, Leighton BL, et al: Incidence of electrocardiographic changes during cesarean delivery under regional anesthesia. Anesth. Analg. 70: 36, 1990.
117. Baratta J, Czinier D, Zakowski M, Kromzon I, et al: Echocardiographic changes during cesarean section. Anesthesiology 77:A1043, 1992.
118. Mathew JP, Fleisher LA, Rinehouse JA, Sevarino FB, et al: ST segment depression during labor and delivery. Anesthesiology 77:635, 1992.
119. Shnider SM, Wright RG, Levinson G, Roizen MF: Uterine blood flow and plasma norepinephrine changes during maternal stress in the pregnant ewe. Anesthesiology 50:524, 1979.
120. Rosenfeld CR, Barton MD, Meschia G: Effects of epinephrine on distribution of blood flow in the pregnant ewe. Am. J. Obstet. Gynecol. 124:156, 1976.
121. Adamsons K, Mueller-Heubach E, Myers RE: Production of fetal aphyxia in the rhesus monkey by administration of catecholamines to the mother. Am. J. Obstet. Gynecol. 109: 248, 1971.
122. Morishima HO, Pedersen H, Finster M: The influence of maternal psychological stress on the fetus. Am. J. Obstet. Gynecol. 131:286, 1978.
123. Myers RE: Maternal psychological stress and fetal asphyxia: A study in the monkey. Am. J. Obstet. Gynecol. 122:47, 1975.
124. Lederman RP, Lederman E, Work BA Jr, McCann DS: The relationship of maternal anxiety, plasma catecholamines, and plasma cortisol to progress in labor. Am. J. Obstet. Gynecol. 132:495, 1978.
125. Abboud TK, Artal R, Henriksen EH, Earl S, et al: Effects of spinal anesthesia on maternal circulating catecholamines. Am. J. Obstet. Gynecol. 142:252, 1982.
126. Ohno H, et al: Maternal plasma concentrations of catecholamines and cyclic nucleotides during labor and following delivery. Res. Commun. Chem. Pathol. Pharmacol. 51:183, 1986.
127. Abboud TK, Sarkis F, Goebelsmann U, Hunt TT, et al: Effects of epidural anesthesia during labor on maternal plasma β-endorphin levels. Anesthesiology 57:A382, 1982.
128. Shnider SM, Abboud MD, Artal Raul, A, et al: Maternal catecholamines decrease during labor after lumbar epidural anesthesia. Am. J. Obstet. Gynecol. 147:13, 1983.
129. Falconer AD, Powles AB: Plasma noradrenaline levels during labour: Influence of elective lumbar epidural blockade. Anaesthesia 37:417, 1982.
130. Jouppila R, Jouppila P, Hollmen A, Kuikka J: Effect of segmental extradural analgesia on placental blood flow during normal labour. Br. J. Anaesth. 50:563, 1978.
131. Hollman AI, Jouppila R, Jouppila P, Koivula A, et al: Effect of extradural analgesia using bupivacaine and 2-chloroprocaine on intervillous blood flow during normal labour. Br. J. Anaesth. 54837, 1982.
132. Goebelsmann U, et al: Beta-endorphin in pregnancy. Eur. J. Obstet. Gynecol. Reprod. Biol. 2777, 1984.
133. Raisanen I, et al: Beta-endorphin in maternal and umbilical cord plasma at elective cesarean section and in spontaneous labor. Obstet. Gynecol. 67:384, 1986.
134. Westgren M, Lindahl SGE, Norden NE: Maternal and fetal endocrine stress response at vaginal delivery with and without an epidural block. J. Perinat. Med. 14:235, 1986.
135. Neumark J, Hammerle AF, Biegelmayer C: Effects of epidural analgesia on plasma catecholamines and cortisol in parturition. Acta Anaesthesiol. Scand. 29:555, 1985.
136. Irestedt L: How does anaesthesia influence fetal and neonatal stress? Abstr. Eur. Soc. Reg. Anaesth., Oulu, Finland p. 27, 1989.
137. Haberer JP, Monteillard C: Effets de l'anesthesie peridurale

obstetricale sur le foetus et le nouveau ne. Ann. Francaises Anesth. Reanimation 5:381, 1986.
138. Hagnevik K, Irestedt L, Lundell B, Skolderfors E: Cardiac function and sympathoadrenal activity in the newborn after caesarean section under spinal and epidural anaesthesia. Acta. Anaesthesiol. Scand. 32:234, 1988.
139. Loughran PG, Moore J, Dundee JW: Maternal stress response associated with caesarean delivery under general and epidural anaesthesia. Br. J. Obstet. Gynaecol. 93:943, 1986.
140. Hollmen AI, Jouppila R, Jouppila P, Koivula A, et al: Effect of extradural analgesia using bupivacaine and 2-chloroprocaine on intervillous blood flow during normal labour. Br. J. Anaesth. 54:837, 1982.
141. Jouppila R, Jouppila P, Karinen JM, Hollmen A: Segmental epidural analgesia in labour: Related to the progress of labour, fetal malposition and instrumental delivery. Acta. Obstet. Gynecol. Scand. 58:135, 1979.
142. Jouppila R, Puolakka J, Kauppila A, Vuori J: Maternal and umbilical cord plasma noradrenaline concentrations during labour with and without segmental extradural analgesia and during caesarean section. Br. J. Anaesth. 56:251, 1984.
143. Huovinen K, Lehtovirta P, Forss M, Kivalo I, et al: Changes in placental intervillous blood flow measured by the 133 xenon method during lumbar epidural block for elective caesarean section. Acta. Anaesth. Scand. 23:529, 1979.
144. Janisch H, Leodolter S, Neumark J, Philipp K: Der Einfluss der Kontinuierlichen Epiduralanaesthesie auf die uteroplazentare Durchbluntung. Z. Geburtshife u Perinatol. 182: 343, 1978.
145. Brotanek V, Vasicka A, Santiago A, Brotanek JD: The influence of epidural anesthesia on uterine blood flow. Obstet. Gynecol. 42:276, 1973.
146. Hodgkinson R, Marx GF, Kim SS, Miclat NM: Neonatal tests following vaginal delivery under ketamine, thiopental, and extradural anesthesia. Anesth. Analg. 56:548–552, 1977.
147. Abboud T, Artal R, Sarkis F, Kenriksen EH, et al: Sympathoadrenal activity, maternal, fetal and neonatal responses after epidural anesthesia in the pre-eclamptic patient. Am. J. Obstet. Gynecol. 144:915, 1982.
148. Newsome LR, Bramwell RS, Curling PE: Severe preeclampsia: hemodynamic effects of lumbar epidural anesthesia. Anesth. Analg. 65:31, 1986.
149. Benedetti TJ, Benedetti JK, Stenchever MA: Preeclampsia—maternal and fetal outcome. Part B. Hypertension in pregnancy. Clin. Exp. Hypertens. 2/3:401–416, 1982.
150. Ramanathan J, Coleman P, Sibai B: Anesthetic modification of hemodynamic and neuroendocrine stress response to cesarean delivery in women with severe preeclampsia. Anesth. Analg. 73:772–779, 1991.
151. Pearson JF, Davies P: The effect of continuous lumbar epidural analgesia on the acid-base status of maternal arterial blood during the first stage of labour. J. Obstet. Gynaecol. Br. Commonw. 80:218–224, 1973.
152. Pearson JF, Davies P: The effect of continuous lumbar epidural analgesia on maternal acid-base balance and arterial lactate concentration during the second stage of labour. J. Obstet. Gynaecol. Br. Commonw. 80:225–229, 1973.
153. Pearson JF, Davies P: The effect of continuous lumbar epidural analgesia upon fetal acid-base status during the first stage of labour. J. Obstet. Gynaecol. Br. Commonw. 81: 971–974, 1974.
154. Pearson JF, Davies L: The effect of continuous lumbar epidural analgesia upon fetal acid-base status during the second stage of labour. J. Obstet. Gynaecol. Br. Commonw. 81:975–979, 1974.
155. Buchan PC, Milne MK, Browning MCK: The effect of continuous epidural blockade on plasma 11-hydroxycorticosteroid concentrations in labour. J. Obset. Gynaecol. Br. Commonw. 80:974–977, 1973.
156. Gemzell CA, Robbe H, Stern B, Strom G: Observations on circulatory changes and muscular work in normal labour. Acta. Obstet. Gynecol. Scand. 36:75, 1957.
157. Wulf KH, Kunzel W, Lehmann V: Clinical aspects of placental gas exchange in respiratory gas exchange and blood flow in the placenta. Edited by LD Longo, H Bartels. Bethesda, Maryland, U.S. Department of Health, Education and Welfare, DHEW Publication No. (NIH 73–61), 1972, p. 505–521.
158. Marx GF, Greene NM: Maternal lactate, pyruvate, and excess lactate production during labor and delivery. Am. J. Obstet. Gynecol. 90:786, 1964.
159. Jouppila R, Hollmen AI: The effects of segmental epidural analgesia on maternal and fetal acid-base balance, lactate, serum potassium and creatine phosphokinase during labour. Acta. Anaesthesiol. Scand. 20:259–266, 1976.
160. Sangoul F, Fox GS, Houle GL: Effect of regional analgesia on maternal oxygen consumption during the first stage of labor. Am. J. Obstet. Gynecol. 121:1080, 1975.
161. Best CH, Taylor NB: The Physiological Basis of Medical Practice, 8th ed. Baltimore, the Williams & Wilkins Company, 1966, p1002.
162. Otis AB: *In* Handbook of Physiology, Section 3. Respiration, volume I. Washington, American Physiological Society, 1964, p. 463.
163. Ackerman WE III, Molnar JM, Juneja MM: Beneficial effect of epidural anesthesia on oxygen consumption in a parturient with adult respiratory distress syndrome. South. Med. J. 86:361–364, 1993.
164. Holdsworth JD: Relationship between stomach contents and analgesia in labour. Br. J. Anaesth. 15:1145, 1978.
165. Nimmo WS, Wilson J, Prescott LF: Narcotic analgesics and delayed gastric emptying during labor. Lancet i:890:1975.
166. Conklin KA: Maternal physiologic adaptation during gestation, labor and the puerperium. Sem. Anaesth. 10:221, 1991.
167. O'Sullivan GM, Sutton AG, Thompson SA, et al: Noninvasive measurement of gastric emptying in obstetric patients. Anesth. Analg. 66:505, 1976.
168. Conklin KA: The effects of anesthesia and analgesia. *In* Uterine Function: Molecular and Cellular Aspects. Edited by ME Carsten, JD Miller. New York, Plenum Press, 1990, pp. 531–574.
169. Thoren T, Tangho J, Wattwill M: Epidural morphine delays gastric emptying in small intestinal tract in volunteers. Acta. Anaesthesiol. Scand. 33:174, 1989.
170. Thoren T, Wattwill M: Effects on gastric emptying of thoracic epidural analgesia with morphine or bupivacaine. Anesth. Analg. 67:687, 1988.
171. Wright PM, Allen RW, Moore J, Donnelly J: Gastric emptying during extradural analgesia in labor: Effect of fentanyl supplementation. Br. J. Anaesth. 68:248, 1992.
172. Reynolds F: Epidural analgesia in obstetrics: Pros and cons from mother and baby. Br. Med. J. 229:751, 1989.
173. Kennedy WF, Everett GB, Cobb LA, Allen GD: Simultaneous systemic and hepatic hemodynamic measurements during high peridural anesthesia in normal man. Anesth. Analg. 50:1016, 971.
174. Maltau JM, Andersen HT: Continuous epidural anaesthesia with a low frequency of instrumental deliveries. Acta. Obstet. Gynecol. Scand. 54:401–406, 1975.
175. Phillips JC, Hochberg CJ, Petrakis JK, Van Winkle JD: Epi-

dural analgesia and its effects on "normal" progress of labor. Am. J. Obstet. Gynecol. 129:316–323, 1977.

176. Henry JS Jr, Kingston MB, Maughan GB: The effect of epidural anesthesia on oxytocin-induced labor. Am. J. Obstet. Gynecol. 97:350–359, 1967.

177. Sala NL, Schwarcz RL, Altabe O: Effect of epidural anesthesia upon uterine contractility induced by artificial cervical dilatation in human pregnancy. Am. J. Obstet. Gynecol. 106:26–31, 1970.

178. Bonica JJ, Caldeyro-Barcia R, Belitzky R, Grunwald I, et al: Anesthesia peridural segmentaria en el periodo de dilatacion del trabajo del parto. Revista Uruguaya de Anestesiologia 5:45–52, 1971.

179. Schellenberg JC: Uterine activity during lumbar epidural analgesia with bupivacaine. Am. J. Obstet. Gynecol. 127: 26–31, 1977.

180. Tyack AJ, Parsons RJ, Millar DR, Nicholas ADG: Uterine activity and plasma bupivacaine levels after caudal epidural analgesia. J. Obstet. Gynaecol. Br. Comm. 80:896–901, 1973.

181. Matadial L, Cibils LA: The effect of epidural anesthesia on uterine activity and blood pressure. Am. J. Obstet. Gynecol. 125:846–854, 1976.

182. Craft JB, Epstein BS, Coakley CS: Effect of lidocaine with epinephrine versus lidocaine (plain) on induced labor. Anesth. Analg. 51:243–246, 1972.

183. Bonica JJ: Effects of analgesia and anesthesia on the mother, fetus, and newborn. *In* Advances in Obstetrics and Gynecology. Edited by SL Marcus, C Marcus. Baltimore, The Williams and Wilkins Company, 1978, pp. 293–312.

184. Hollmen A, Jouppila R, Pihlajaniemi R, Karvonen P, et al: Selective lumbar epidural block in labour: A clinical analysis. Acta. Anaesthesiol. Scand. 21:174–186, 1977.

185. Jouppila R, Jouppila P, Karinen J-M, Holmen A: Segmental epidural analgesia in labour: Related to the progress of labour, fetal malposition and instrumental delivery. Acta. Obstet. Gynecol. Scand. 58:135–139, 1979.

186. Gal D, Choudhy R, Ung K-A, Abadir A, Tancer ML: Segmental epidural analgesia for labor and delivery. Acta. Obstet. Gynecol. 58:429–431, 1979.

187. Cibils LA, Spackman TJ: Caudal analgesia in first-stage labor: Effect on uterine activity and the cardiovascular system. Am. J. Obstet. Gynecol. 84:1042–1050, 1962.

188. Vasicka A, Kretchmer H: Effect of conduction and inhalation anesthesia on uterine contractions. Am. J. Obstet. Gynecol. 82:600–607, 1961.

189. Vasicka A, Kretchmer HE: Uterine hemodynamics. Clin. Obstet. Gynecol. 4: 17–23, 1961.

190. Alfonsi PL, Massi GB: Effetti degli anesthetici sulla contrattilita uterina. Riv. Ostet. Ginec. 18:37, 1963.

191. Willdeck-Lund G, Lindmark G, Nilsson BA: The effect of segmental epidural block upon the course of labour and the condition of the infant during the neonatal period. Acta. Anaesthesiol. Scand. 23:301–311, 1979.

192. Willdeck-Lund G, Lindmark G, Nilsson BA: Effect of segmental epidural analgesia upon the uterine activity with special reference to the use of different local anaesthetic agents. Acta. Anaesthesiol. Scand. 23:519–528, 1979.

193. Studd JWW: Epidural anaesthesia in labour. *In* Management of Labour. Edited by R Beard. London, Royal College of Obstetricians and Gynaecologists, 1975, p. 179.

194. Hoult IJ, MacLennan AH, Carrie LES: Lumbar epidural analgesia in labour: relation to fetal malposition and instrumental delivery. Br. Med. J. 1:14–16, 1977.

195. Studd JWW, Crawford S, Duignan HW, et al: The effect of lumbar epidural analgesia on the rate of cervical dilatation and the outcome of labour of spontaneous onset. Br. J. Obstet. Gynaecol. 87:1015–1021, 1980.

196. Johnson WL, Winter WW, Eng M, Bonica JJ, Hunter CA: Effect of pudendal, spinal, and peridural block anesthesia on the second stage of labor. Am J Obstet. Gynecol. 113: 166–175, 1972.

197. Floberg J, Belfrage P, Ohlsen H: Influence of the pelvic outlet capacity on fetal head presentation at delivery. Acta. Obstet. Gynecol. Scand. 66:127–130, 1987.

198. Friedman EA, Sachtleben MR: Caudal anesthesia. The factors that influence its effect on labor. Obstet. Gynecol. 13: 442–448, 1959.

199. Lowensohn RI, Paul RS, Fales F, Yeh S, Hon EH: Intrapartum epidural anesthesia. Obstet. Gynecol. 44:388–393, 1974.

200. McCaughey HS Jr, Corey EL, Eastwood D, Thornton WN: The effect of anesthetics on the spontaneous motility of human uterine muscle in vitro. Obstet. Gynecol. 19:233, 1962.

201. Mather LE, Tucker GT, Murphy TM, et al: The effects of adding adrenaline to etidocaine and lignocaine in extradural anesthesia. II. Pharmacokinetics. Br. J. Anaesth. 48: 989–994, 1976.

202. Gunther RE, Bellville JW: Obstetrical caudal anesthesia. II. A randomized study comparing 1% mepivacaine with 1% mepivacaine plus epinephrine. Anesthesiology 37: 288–298, 1972.

203. Abboud TK, David S, Shakuntala N, et al: Maternal, fetal and neonatal effects of lidocaine with and without epinephrine for epidural anesthesia in obstetrics. Anesth. Analg. 63:973–979, 1984.

204. Abboud TK, Eslam AS, Yanagi T, et al: Safety and efficacy of epinephrine added to bupivacaine for lumbar epidural analgesia in obstetrics. Anesth. Analg. 64:585–591, 1985.

205. Abboud TK, Sarkissian LD, Terrasi J, et al: Comparative maternal, fetal and neonatal effects of chloroprocaine with and without epinephrine for epidural anesthesia and obstetrics. Anesth. Analg. 66:71–75, 1987.

206. Kozody R, Swartz J, Palahniuk RJ, et al: Spinal cord blood flow following subarachnoid lidocaine. Can. Anaesth. Soc. J. 32:472–478, 1985.

207. Scott DB, Walker LR: Administration of continuous epidural analgesia. Anaesthesia 18:82–83, 1963.

208. Dawkins M: Relief of postoperative pain by continuous epidural drip. Survey Anesthesiol. 1:616–617, 1957.

209. Glover DJ: Continuous epidural analgesia in the obstetric patient: A feasibility study using a mechanical infusion pump. Anaesthesia 32:499, 1977.

210. Evans KRL, Carrie LES: Continuous epidural infusion of bupivacaine in labour: A simple method. Anaesthesia 34: 310, 1979.

211. Reynolds F, Hardgrove RL, Wyman JB: Maternal and foetal plasma concentrations of bupivacaine after epidural block. Br. J. Anaesth 45:341–344, 1973.

212. Clark MJ: Continuous mini-infusion of 0.125% bupivacaine into the epidural space during labour. J. Am. Obstet. Assoc. 81:484–491, 1982.

213. Taylor HJC: Clinical experience with continuous epidural infusion of bupivacaine at 6 ml per hour in obstetrics. Can. Anaesth. Soc. J. 30:277, 1983.

214. Kenepp NB, Cheek TG, Gutsche BB: Bupivacaine: Continuous infusion epidural analgesia for labor. Anesthesiology 59:A407, 1983.

215. Morison DH, Smedstad KG: Continuous infusion epidurals for obstetric analgesia (Editorial). Can. Anaesth. Soc. J. 32: 101, 1985.

216. Li DF, Rees GAD, Rosen M: Continuous extradural infusion

of 0.0625% or 0.125% bupivacaine for pain relief in primigravid labour. Br. J. Anaesth. 57:264, 1985.
217. Rosenblatt R, Wright R, Benson D, Raj T: Continuous epidural infusion for obstetric analgesia. Reg. Anesth. 8: 10–14, 1983.
218. Nadeau S, Elliott RD: Continuous bupivacaine infusion during labour: Effects on analgesia and delivery. Can. Anaesth. Soc. J. 32:S70, 1985.
219. Chestnut DH, Bates JN, Choi WW: Continuous infusion epidural analgesia with lidocaine: Efficacy and influence during the second stage of labor. Obstet. Gynecol. 69: 323–327, 1987.
220. Chestnut DH, Vandewalker GE, Owen CL, Bates JN, Choi WW: The influence of continuous epidural bupivacaine analgesia on the second stage of labor and method of delivery in nulliparous women. Anesthesiology 66:774–780, 1987.
221. Ewen A, McLeod DD, MacLeod DM, Campbell A, et al: Continuous infusion epidural analgesia in obstetrics: a comparison of 0.08% and 0.25% bupivacaine. Anaesthesia 42:143–147, 1986.
222. Gaylard DG, Wilson IH, Balmer HGR: Forum. An epidural infusion technique for labour. Anaesthesia 42:1098–1101, 1987.
223. Hicks JA, Jenkins JG,Newton MC, Findley IL: Continuous epidural infusion of 0.075% bupivacaine for pain relief in labour. Anaesthesia 43:289, 1988.
224. Gaylard D: Epidural analgesia by continuous infusion. *In* Epidural and Spinal Blockade in Obstetrics, edited by F Reynolds. London, Bailliere Tindall, 1990, pp. 49–58.
225. Caldwell JE, Bradwood JM: Epidural analgesia by infusion. Anaesthesia 39:493–494, 1984.
226. Husemeyer RP, O'Connor MC, Davenport HT, Thayer F: Failure of epidural morphine to relieve pain in labour. Anaesthesia 35:161, 1980.
227. Carrie LES, O'Sullivan GM, Seegobin R: Epidural fentanyl in labour. Anaesthesia 36:965, 1981.
228. Justins DM, Francis D, Houlton PG, Reynolds F: A controlled trial of extradural fentanyl in labour. Br. J. Anaesth. 54:409, 1982.
229. Heytens L, Cammu H, Camu F: Extradural analgesia during labour using alfentanil. Br. J. Anaesth. 59:331–337, 1987.
230. Youngstrom P, Eastwood D, Patel H, Bhatia R, et al: Epidural fentanyl and bupivacaine in labor: Double-blind study. Anesthesiology 61:A414, 1984.
231. Naulty JS, Malinow A, Hunt CD, Haushoer J, et al: Epidural butorphanol-bupivacaine for analgesia during labor and delivery. Anesthesiology 65:A369, 1986.
232. Cohen SE, Tan S, Albright GA, Halpern J: Epidural fentanyl/bupivacaine mixtures for obstetric analgesia. Anesthesiology 67:403–407, 1987.
233. Little MS, McNitt JD, Choi HG, Tremper KK: Low dose sufentanil and bupivacaine for labor anesthesia. Anesthesiology 67:A444, 1987.
234. Van Steenberge A, Debroux HC, Noorduin H: Extradural bupivacaine with sufentanil for vaginal delivery. A double-blind trial. Br. J. Anaesth. 59:1518, 1987.
235. Celleno D, Capogna G: Epidural fentanyl plus bupivacaine 0.125% or labor: Analgesic effects. Can. J. Anaesth. 35: 375–378, 1988.
236. Naulty JS, Ross R, Bergen W: Epidural sufentanil-bupivacaine for analgesia during labor and delivery. Anesthesiology 71:A842, 1989.
237. Reynolds F, O'Sullivan G: Forum. Epidural fentanyl and perineal pain in labour. Anaesthesia 44:341–344, 1989.
238. Bazin JE, et al: Variations in uterine activity related to epidural fentanyl during labor. Anesthesiology 71:A849, 1989.
239. Williams B, Kwan W, Chen B, Wu Y: Comparison of 0.0312% bupivacaine plus sufenta and 0.0625 bupivacaine plus sufenta for epidural anesthesia during labor and delivery. Anesthesiology 73:A950, 1990.
240. Zhu J, Abboud TK, Afrasiabi A, et al: Epidural butorphanol augments lidocaine analgesia during labor. Anesthesiology 73:A979, 1990.
241. Kavuri S, Janandhan Y, Fernando E, et al: A comparative study of epidural alfentanil and fentanyl for labor pain relief. Anesthesiology 71:A846, 1989.
242. Skerman JH, Thompson BA, Goldstein MT, Jacobs MA, et al: Combined continuous epidural fentanyl and bupivacaine in labor: A randomized study. Anesthesiology 63: A450, 1985.
243. Phillips G: Continuous infusion epidural analgesia and labor: The effect of adding sufentanil to 0.125% bupivacaine. Anesth. Analg. 87:462–465, 1988.
244. Chestnut DH, Owen CL, Bates JN, et al: Continuous infusion epidural analgesia during labor: A randomized double-blind comparison of 0.0625% bupivacaine/0.0002% fentanyl versus 0.125% bupivacaine. Anesthesiology 68: 754–759, 1988.
245. Jones G, Paul DL, Elton RA, McClure JH, et al: Comparison of bupivacaine and bupivacaine with fentanyl in continuous extradural analgesia during labor. Br. J. Anaesth. 63: 254, 1989.
246a. Abboud TK, Afrasiabi A, Zhu J, Mantilla M, et al: Epidural morphine or butorphanol augments bupivacaine analgesia during labor. Reg. Anesth. 14:115–120, 1989.
246b. Abboud TK, Afrasiabi A, Zhu J, Mantilla M, et al: Bupivacaine/butorphanol/epinephrine for epidural anesthesia in obstetrics: Maternal and neonatal effects. Reg. Anesth. 14: 219–224, 1989.
247. Huckaby T, Gerard K, Scheidlinger J, et al: Continuous epidural infusion of alfentanil-bupivacaine versus bupivacaine for labor and delivery. Anesthesiology 71:A847, 1989.
248. Hoyt M, Youngstrom P: Neonatal neurobehavioral effects of continuous epidural infusion of fentanil/bupivacaine/epinephrine in labor. Anesthesiology 73:A984, 1990.
249. Rodriguez J, Payne M, Afrasiabi A, Abboud PK, et al: Continuous infusion epidural anesthesia during labor: A randomized, double-blind comparison of 0.0625% bupivacaine/0.002% butorphanol and 0.125% bupivacaine. Reg. Anesth. 15:300–302, 1990.
250. Vertommen JD, Vandermeulen E, Van Aken H, et al: The effects of the addition of sufentanil to 0.125% bupivacaine on the quality of analgesia during labor and on the incidence of instrumental deliveries. Anesthesiology 74: 809–814, 1991.
251. Chestnut DH: Epidural anesthesia and instrumental vaginal delivery (Editorial). Anesthesiology 74:805–808, 1991.
252. Shnider SM, Levinson G, Ralston DH: Regional anesthesia in labor and vaginal delivery. *In* Anesthesia for Obstetrics. 3rd Ed. Edited by SM Shnider, G Levinson. Baltimore, Williams & Wilkins, 1993, pp. 135–153.
253. Caldeyro-Barcia R, et al: Effect of position changes on the intensity and frequency of uterine contractions during labor. Am. J. Obstet. Gynecol. 80:284, 1960.
254. Caldeyro-Barcia R, Poseiro JJ: Physiology of the uterine contraction. Clin. Obstet. Gynecol. 3:386, 1960.
255. Weaver JB, Pearson JF, Rosen M: Posture and epidural block in pregnant women at term. Anaesthesia 30:752, 1975.
256. Fadl ET, Utting JE: Acid-base disturbance in obstetrics. Proc. R. Soc. Med. 68:77, 1970.

257. Rooth G, McBride R, Ivy BJ: Fetal and maternal pH measurements. Acta. Obstet. Gynecol. Scand. 52:47, 1973.
258. Mark RF: The dependence of uterine muscle contraction on pH with reference to prolonged labor. J. Obstet. Gynaecol. Br. Comm. 68:584, 1961.
259. Reynolds SRM: Physiology of the Uterus, 2nd edition. New York, Paul B Hoeber, 1949.
260. Simpson Sir JY: Selected Obstetrical Works. Edinburgh, Adams & Charles Black, 1871, p. 150.
261. Mulla N: Vaginal delivery in a paraplegic patient. Am. J. Obstet. Gynecol. 73:1346, 1957.
262. Robertson DNS, Guttman L: The paraplegic patient in pregnancy and labor. Proc. R. Soc. Med. 56:381, 1963.
263. DeLee JB: The prophylactic forceps operation. Am. J. Obstet. Gynecol. 1:34, 1920.
264. Dennen EH: Forceps Deliveries, 2nd edition. Philadelphia, F.A. Davis, 1964.
265. Morgan BM, Rehar S, Lewis PJ: Epidural analgesia for uneventful labour. Anaesthesia 5:57, 1980.
266. Thornburn J, Moir DD: Extradural analgesia: The influence of volume and concentration of bupivacaine on the mode of delivery, analgesic efficacy and motor block. Br. J. Anaesth. 53:933, 1981.
267. Read M, Hunt LP, Anderson AM, Lieberman BA: Epidural block and the progress and outcome of labour. J Obstet. Gynecol. 4:35 1983.
268. Cowles GT: Experiences with lumbar epidural block. Obstet. Gynecol. 26:734, 1965.
269. Doughty A: Epidural analgesia in labour: the past, the present and the future. J R Soc Med 71:879, 1978.
270. Bailey PW, Howard FA: Epidural analgesia and forceps delivery: laying a bogey. Anaesthesia 38:282, 1983.
271. Bailey PW: Epidural analgesia in the management of the second stage of labor: A failure to progress. *In* Epidural and Spinal Blockade in Obstetrics. Edited by F Reynolds. London, Bailliere Tindall, 1990, pp. 59–72.
272. Phillips KC, Thomas TA: Second stage of labour with and without extradural analgesia. Anaesthesia 38:972, 1983.
273. Bleyaert A, Soetens M, Vaes L, Van Steenberge AL, Van der Donk A: Bupivacaine 0.125 percent in obstetric epidural analgesia. Anesthesiology 51:435, 1979.
274. Stainthorp SF, et al: 0.125 percent bupivacaine for obstetric analgesia? Anaesthesia 33:3, 1978.
275. Phillipsen T, Jensen NH: Epidural block or parental pethidine as an analgesic in labor: A randomized study concerning progress in labor and instrumental deliveries. Eur. J. Obstet. Gynecol. Reprod. Biol. 30:27–33, 1989.
276. Calkins LA: Normal Labor. Springfield, Charles C. Thomas, 1955.
277. Goodwin JW, Reid DE: Risk to the fetus in prolonged and trial labor. Am J Obstet. Gynecol. 85:209, 1963.
278. Hibbard B, et al: Lumbar epidural analgesia in labour (letter). Br. Med. J. i:286, 1977.
279. Bakhoum S, Lewis BV, Tipton RH: Lumbar epidural analgesia in labor (letter). Br. Med. J. i:641, 1977.
280. McQueen J, Mylrea L: Lumbar epidural analgesia in labour (letter). Br. Med. J. i:640, 1977.
281. Maresh M, Choong KH, Beard RW: Delayed pushing with lumbar epidural analgesia in labour. Br. J. Obstet. Gynaecol. 90:623, 1983.
282. Committee on Obstetrics: Maternal and fetal medicine: Obstetric forceps. ACOG Committee Opinion No. 59, 1988.
283. O'Driscoll K, Strong JM, Minogue M: Active management of labor. Lancet 2:135, 1973.
284. O'Driscoll K, Meaghe RD: Active Management of Labor. Saunders, London, 1981.
285. Goodfellow CF, Hull MGR, Swaab DF, et al: Oxytocin deficiency at delivery with epidural analgesia. Br. J. Obstet. Gynaecol. 90:214, 1983.
286. Vasicka A, Kumaresan DV, Han GS, Kumaresan M: Plasma oxytocin in initiation of labor. Am. J. Obstet. Gynecol. 130: 263, 1978.
287. Sturrock J, Brown R: Prolonged first stage of labour. J. Obstet. Gynaecol. Br. Emp. 63:83, 1956.
288. Keettel WC, Pettis GS: Prolonged labor: Review of 891 cases with special reference to perinatal mortality. Obstet. Gynecol. 7:15, 1956.
289. Moir DD, Willocks J: Management of incoordinate uterine action under continuous epidural analgesia. Br. Med. J. 3: 396, 1967.
290. Bonica JJ, Hunter CA Jr: Management in Dysfunction of the Forces of Labor. *In* Principles and Practice of Obstetric Analgesia and Anesthesia, Vol. 2. Edited by JJ Bonica. Philadelphia, F.A. Davis, 1969, p. 1188.
291. Hunter CA Jr: Uterine motility studies during labor. Am. J. Obstet. Gynecol. 85:681, 1963.
292. Snyder FF: Obstetric Analgesia and Anesthesia: Their Effects upon Labor and the Child. Philadelphia, W.B. Saunders, 1949, p. 383.
293. Bromage PR, Robson JG: Concentrations of lignocaine in the blood after intravenous, intramuscular, epidural and endotracheal administration. Anaesthesia 16:461, 1961.
294. Ralston DH, Shnider SM: The fetal and neonatal effects of regional anesthesia in obstetrics. Anesthesiology 48:34, 1978.
295. Thomas J, Climie CR, Mather LE: Placental transfer of lignocaine following lumbar epidural administration. Br. J. Anaesth. 40:965, 1968.
296. Thomas J, Climie CR, Long G, Nighjoy LE: The influence of adrenaline on the maternal plasma levels and placental transfer of lignocaine following lumbar epidural administration. Br. J. Anaesth. 41:1029, 1969b.
297. Epstein BS, Banerjee SG, Coakley CS: Passage of lidocaine and prilocaine across the placenta. Anesth. Analg. 47:223, 1968.
298. Hehre FW, Hook R, Hon EH: Continuous lumbar peridural anesthesia in obstetrics. VI. The fetal effects of transplacental passage of local anesthetic agents. Anesth. Analg. 48: 909, 1969.
299. Fox GS, Houle GL: Transmission of lidocaine hydrochloride across the placenta during caeserean section. Can. Anaesth. Soc. J. 16:135, 1969.
300. Lurie AO, Weiss JB: Blood concentrations of mepivacaine and lidocaine in mother and baby after epidural anesthesia. Am. J. Obstet. Gynecol. 106:850, 1970.
301. Houle GL, Fox GS, Torkington IMG: A comparison between lignocaine hydrochloride and lignocaine carbon dioxide base for epidural analgesia during vaginal delivery. Br. J. Anaesth. 43:1145, 1971.
302. Fox GS, Houle GL, Desjardins PD, Mercier G. Intrauterine fetal lidocaine concentrations during continuous epidural anesthesia. Am. J. Obstet. Gynecol. 110:896, 1971.
303. Shnider SM, Way EL: Plasma levels of lidocaine (Xylocaine™) in mother and newborn following obstetrical conduction anesthesia: Clinical applications. Anesthesiology 29:951–958, 1968.
304. Brown WU Jr, Bell GC, Lurie AO, Weiss JB, et al: Newborn blood levels of lidocaine and mepivacaine in the first postnatal day following maternal epidural anesthesia. Anesthesiology 42:698–707, 1975.
305. Morishima HO, Daniel SS, Finster M, Poppers PJ: Transmission of mepivacaine hydrochloride (Carbocaine) across the human placenta. Anesthesiology 27:147, 1966.

306. Scanlon JW, Hollenbeck AR: Neonatal behavioral effects of the anesthetic exposure during pregnancy. *In* Advances in Perinatal Medicine, Vol. III. Edited by EA Friedman, A Milunsky, A Gluck. New York, Plenum Press, 1983.
307. Thomas J, Climie CR, Mather LE: The maternal plasma levels and placental transfer of bupivacaine following epidural analgesia. Br. J. Anaesth. 41:1035, 1969.
308. Reynolds F, Taylor G: Plasma concentrations of bupivacaine during continuous epidural analgesia in labour: The effect of adrenaline. Br. J. Anaesth. 43:436–440, 1971.
309. Hyman MD, Shnider SM: Maternal and neonatal blood concentration of bupivacaine associated with obstetrical conduction anesthesia. Anesthesiology 34:81–86, 1971.
310. Reynolds F, Hargrove RL, Wyman JB: Maternal and foetal plasma concentrations of bupivacaine after epidural block. Br. J. Anaesth. 45:1049, 1973.
311. Scanlon JW, Ostheimer GW, Lurie AO, Brown WU, et al: Neurobehavioral responses and drug concentrations in newborns after maternal epidural anesthesia with bupivacaine. Anesthesiology 45:400–405, 1976.
312. Moore DC, Bridenbaugh LD, Bridenbaugh PO, Tucker GT: Caudal and epidural blocks with bupivacaine for childbirth. Report of 657 parturients. Obstet. Gynecol. 37:667, 1971.
313. Fox GS, Houle GL: Acid-base studies in elective caesarean sections during epidural and general anaesthesia. Can. Anaesth. Soc. J. 18:60, 1971.
314. McLintic AJ, Danskin SH, Reid JA, Thorburn J: Effects of adrenaline on extradural anesthesia, plasma lignocaine concentrations and feto-placental unit during elective caesarean section. Br. J. Anaesth. 67:683–689, 1991.
315. Eddleston JM, Maresh M, Horsman EL, Young H: Comparison of maternal and fetal effects associated with intermittent or continuous infusion of extradural analgesia. Br. J. Anaesth. 69:154–158, 1992.
316. Magno R, Berlin A, Karlsson K, Kjellmer I: Anesthesia for cesarean section. IV. Placental transfer and neonatal elimination of bupivacaine following epidural analgesia for elective cesarean section. Acta Anaesth. Scand. 20:141, 1976.
317. Abboud TK, Naggappala S, Murakawa K, et al: Comparison of the effects of general and regional anesthesia for cesarean section on neonatal neurologic and adapative capacity scores. Anesth. Analg. 64:996–1000, 1985.
318. Laishley RS, Morgan BM: A single dose epidural technique for caesarean section. Anaesthesia 50:275–279, 1978.
319. Tucker GT, Boyes RN, Bridenbaugh PO, Moore DC: Binding of anilide-type local anesthetics in human plasma. II. Implications in vivo, with special reference to transplacental distribution. Anesthesiology 33:304, 1970b.
320. Brownridge P, Obst D: Epidural bupivacaine-pethidine mixture: Clinical experience using a low dose combination labor. Aust. N. Z. J. Obstet. Gynaecol. 28:17–24, 1988.
321. Mather LE, Long GJ, Thomas J: The binding of bupivacaine to maternal and foetal plasma proteins. J. Pharm. Pharmacol. 23:359, 1971.
322. Chignell CF, Vesell ES, Starkweather DK, Berlin CM: The binding of sulfaphenazole to fetal, neonatal and adult plasma albumin. Clin. Pharmacol. Ther. 12:897, 1971.
323. Reynolds F, Laishley R, Morgan B, Lee A: Effect of time and adrenaline on the feto-maternal distribution of bupivacaine. Br. J. Anaesth. 62:509–514, 1989.
324. Laishley RS, Carson RJ, Reynolds F: Effect of adrenaline on the distribution of bupivacaine in the rabbit fetus. Br. J. Anaesth. 63:721–725, 1989.
325. Fletcher S, Carson R, Reynolds F, Howell P, et al: Plasmal total and free concentrations of bupivacaine and lignocaine in mother and fetus following epidural administration, singly or together. Int. J. Obstet. Anesth. 1:135–140, 1992.
326. Laishley RS, Morgan BM, Reynolds F: Effect of adrenaline on extradural anaesthesia and plasma bupivacaine concentrations during casesarean section. Br. J. Anaesth. 60: 180–186, 1988.
327. Swanstrom S, Bratteby LE: Metabolic effects of obstetric regional analgesia and of asphyxia in the newborn infant during the first 2 hours after birth. III. Adjustment of arterial blood gases and acid-base balance. Acta. Paediatr. Scand. 70:811–818, 1981.
328. Reynolds F: Placental Transfer: In Foundation of Obstetric Anaesthesia. London, Farrand Press, 1987, pp. 137–157.
329. Raabe N, Belfrage P: Epidural analgesia in labour. IV. Influence on uterine activity and fetal heart rate. Acta. Obstet. Gynecol. Scand. 55:305–310, 1976.
330. Maltau JM: The frequency of fetal bradycardia during selective epidural anaesthesia. Acta Obstet. Gynaecol. Scand. 54:357–361, 1975.
331. Noble AD, Craft IL, Bootes JAH, Edwards PA, et al: Continuous lumbar epidural analgesia using bupivacaine: A study of the fetus and newborn child. J. Obstet. Gynaecol. Br. Commonw. 78:559–563, 1971.
332. Phillipp K, Leodolter S, Neumark J: The influence of continuous epidural block on uteroplacental blood-flow. *In* Pregnancy Hypertension. Edited by J Bonnar, I MacGillivray, M Symonds. Lancaster, MTP Press, 1980, pp. 539–542.
333. Jouppila P, Jouppila R, Hollmen A, Koivula A: Lumbar epidural analgesia to improve intervillous blood flow during labor in severe preeclampsia. Obstet. Gynecol. 59: 158–161, 1982.
334. Hon EH, Reid BL, Hehre FW: The electronic evaluation of fetal heart rate: II. Changes with maternal hypotension. Am. J. Obset. Gynecol. 79:209–215, 1960.
335. Jouppila P, Jouppila R, Kaar K, Merila M: Fetal heart rate patterns and uterine activity after segmental epidural analgesia. Br. J. Obstet. Gynaecol. 84:481–486, 1977.
336. Kandel PF, Spoerel WE, Kinch RAH: Continuous epidural analgesia for labour and delivery: Review of 1000 cases. Can. Med. Assoc. J. 95:947–953, 1966.
337. Thomas G: The aetiology, characteristics and diagnostic relevance of late deceleration patterns in routine obstetric practice. Br. J. Obstet. Gynaecol. 82:121–125, 1975.
338. Marx GE, Patel S, Berman JA, et al: Umbilical blood flow velocity waveforms in different maternal positions and epidural analgesia. Obstet. Gynecol. 68:61–64, 1986.
339. Giles WB, Lah FX, Trudinger BJ: The effect of epidural anaesthesia for caesarean section on maternal uterine and fetal umbilical artery blood flow velocity waveforms. Br. J. Obstet. Gynaecol. 94:55–59, 1987.
340. Long MG, Price M, Spencer JAD: Uteroplacental perfusion after epidural analgesia for elective caesarean section. Br. J. Obstet. Gynaecol. 95:1081–1082, 1988.
341. Reynolds F: Effects on the baby of conduction blockade in obstetrics. *In* Epidural and Spinal Blockade in Obstetrics. Edited by F Reynolds. London, Billiere Tindall, 1990, pp. 205–218.
342. Janbu T: Blood velocities in the dorsal pedis and radial arteries during labour. Br. J. Obstet. Gynaecol. 96:70–79, 1989.
343. Lindblad A, Marsal K, Vernersson E, Renck H: Fetal circulation during epidural analgesia for caesarean section. Br. Med. J. 2881329–1330, 1984.
344. Veille JC, Youngstrom P, Kanaan C, Wilson B: Human umbilical artery flow velocity waveforms before and after regional anesthesia for cesarean section. Obstet. Gynecol. 72:890–893, 1988.

345. Lindblad A, Bernow J, Marsal K: Obstetric analgesia and fetal aortic blood flow during labour. Br. J. Obstet. Gynecol. 94:306–311, 1987.
346. Lindblad A, Bernow J, Vernersson E, Marsal K: Effects of extradural anaesthesia on human fetal blood flow in utero. Comparison of three local anaesthetic solutions. Br. J. Anaesth. 59:1265–1272, 1987.
347. Lavin JP, Samuels SV, Miodovnik M, et al: The effects of bupivacaine and chloroprocaine as local anesthetics for epidural anesthesia on fetal heart rate monitoring parameters. Am. J. Obstet. Gynecol. 141:717–722, 1981.
348. Rickford WJK, Reynolds F: Epidural analgesia in labour and maternal posture. Anaesthesia 38:1169–1174, 1983.
349. Nel JT: Clinical effects of epidural block during labour. A prospective study. S. Afr. Med. J. 63:371–374, 1985.
350. Marx GF, Luykx WM, Cohen S: Fetoneonatal status following caesarean section for fetal distress. Br. J. Anaesth. 56: 1009–1013, 1984.
351. Ong BY, Cohen MM, Palahniuk RJ: Anesthesia for cesaean section—effects on neonates. Anesth. Analg. 68:270–275, 1989.
352. Evans CM, Murphy JF, Gray OP, Rosen M: Epidural versus general anaesthesia for elective caesarean section. Effect on Apgar score and acid-base status of the newborn. Anaesthesia 44:778–782, 1989.
353. Brazelton TB: Neonatal Behavioral Assessment Scale. 2nd Ed. Philadelphia, J.B. Lippincott, 1984
354. Amiel-Tison C, Barrier G, Shnider SM: A new neurologic and adaptive capacity scoring system for evaluating obstetric medication in full term newborns. Anesthesiology 56: 340, 1982.
355. Hodgkinson R, Marx GF, Kim SS, Miclat NM: Neonatal neurobehavioral tests following vaginal delivery under ketamine, thiopental and extradural anesthesia. Anesth. Analg. Curr. Res. 56:548–552, 1977.
356. Brown WU: Discussion of paper by Hodgkinson, et al. Anesth. Analg. Curr. Res. 56:552–553, 1977.
357. Tronick E, Wise S, Als H, Adamson L: Regional obstetric anesthesia and newborn behavior: Effect over the first ten days of life. Pediatrics 58:94, 1976.
358. Corke BC: Neurobehavioral responses of the newborn: The effect of different forms of maternal analgesia. Anaesthesia 32:539, 1977.
359. Wiener PC, Hogg MJ, Rosen M: Neonatal respiration, feeding, and neurobehavioral state. Anaesthesia 34:996, 1979.
360. Rosenblatt B, Belsey EM, Lieberman BA, et al: The influence of maternal analgesia on neonatal behaviour. II. Epidural bupivacaine. Br. J. Obstet. Gynaecol. 88:407–413, 1981.
361. Abboud TK, Sarkis F, Blikian A, Varakian L, et al: Lack of adverse neonatal effects of lidocaine. Anesth. Analg. 62: 473–475, 1983.
362. Kangas-Saarela T, Jouppila R, Jouppila P, et al: The effect of segmental epidural analgesia on the neurobehavioral responses of newborn infants. Acta. Anaesth. Scand. 31: 347–351, 1987.
363. Hoyt M, Youngstrom P: Neonatal neurobehavioral effects of continuous epidural infusion of fentanyl/bupivacaine/ epinephrine in labor. Anesthesiology 73:A984, 1990.
364. Mokriski BLK: Epidural narcotic analgesia for labor and fetal heart rate variability. Anesthesiology 71:A856, 1989.
365. Capogna G, Celleno D, McGannon P, Richardson G, et al: Neonatal neurobehavioral effects following maternal administration of epidural fentanyl during labor. Anesthesiology 67:A461, 1987.
366. Hollmen AI, Jouppila R, Albright GA, et al: Intervillous blood flow during caesarean section with prohylactic ephedrine and epidural anaesthesia. Acta. Anaesth. Scand. 28:396–400, 1984.
367. Kuhnert BR, Harrison MJ, Linn PL, Kuhnert PM: Effects of maternal epidural anesthesia on neonatal behavior. Anesth. Analg. 63:301–308, 1984.
368. Kuhnert BR, Linn PL, Kuhnert PM: Obstetric medical and neonatal behavior. Current controversies. Clin. Perinatol. 12:423–440, 1985.
369. Kuhnert BR, Kennard MJ, Linn PL: Neonatal neurobehavior after epidural anesthesia for cesarean section: A comparison of bupivacaine and chloroprocaine. Anesth. Analg. 67: 64 1988.
370. Jani K, McEvedy B, Harris S, Samaan A: Maternal and neonatal bupivacaine concentrations after spinal and extradural anaesthesia for caesarean section. Br. J. Anaesth. 62: 226P-227P, 1989.
371. Kileff ME, James FM, Dewan DM, Floyd HM: Neonatal neurobehavioral responses after epidural anesthesia for cesarean section using lidocaine and bupivacaine. Anesth. Analg. 63:413–417, 1984.
372. Maltau JM, Egge K: Epidural analgesia and perinatal retinal hemorrhages. Acta. Anaesthesiol. Scand. 24:99, 1980.
373. Egge K, Lyng G, Maltau JM: Effect of instrumental delivery on the frequency and severity of retinal haemorrhages in the newborn. Acta. Obstet. Gynecol. Scand. 60:153, 1981.
374. Ontario Perinatal Mortality Study Committee: Second Report of the Perinatal Mortality Study in Ten University Teaching Hospitals. Three Reports, Toronto, Ontario, Department of Health, 1967. Section I, 1961, Supplement to Second Report, pp. 108–124, 1967.
375. Bonica JJ, Hon EH: Fetal distress. *In* Principles and Practice of Obstetric Analgesia & Anesthesia, Vol. 2. 1st Ed. Edited by JJ Bonica. Philadelphia, F.A. Davis, 1969, pp. 1245–1262.
376. Zalianti M, Salazar JR, Aller J, Aguero O.: Fetal heart rate and pH of fetal capillary blood during epidural analgesia in labor. Obstet. Gynecol. 36:881–886.
377. Moya F, Smith B.: Spinal anesthesia for cesarean section. Clinical and biochemical studies of effects on maternal physiology. JAMA 179:609–614, 1962.
378. Schifrin BS: Fetal heart rate patterns following epidural anaesthesia and oxytocin infusion during labour. J. Obstet. Gynaecol. Br. Commonw. 79:332–339, 1972.
379. Antoine C, Young BK: Fetal lactic acidosis with epidural anesthesia. Am. J. Obstet. Gynecol. 142:55–59, 1982.
380. Finster M, Poppers PJ, Sinclair JC, et al: Accidental intoxification of the fetus with local anesthetic drug during caudal anesthesia. Am. J. Obstet. Gynecol. 92:922, 1965.
381. Sinclair JC, Fox HA, Lentz JS, et al: Intoxification of the fetus by a local anesthetic. N. Engl. J. Med. 273:1173, 1965.
382. Aboulesh E: Pain Control in Obstetrics. Philadelphia: J.B. Lippincott Co., 1977.
383. Albright GA, Ferguson JE, Joyce TH, Stevenson D: Anesthesia in Obstetrics: Maternal, Fetal and Neonatal Aspects, 2nd edition. Boston: Butterworths, 1986.
384. Clemente CD: Gray's Anatomy of the Human Body. 30th Ed. Philadelphia, Lea & Febiger, 1985.
385. Hollingshead WH: The Back and Limbs. *In* Anatomy for Surgeons, Vol. 3. 3rd Ed. Philadelphia: Harper & Rowe, 1982.
386. Harrison GR: The anatomy of the epidural space. Jacksonian Prize Essay. London, Royal College of Surgeons, 1984.
387. Gaynor PA: The applied anatomy of lumbar epidural anaesthesia. May & Baker Prize Essay. London, Royal Society of Medicine, 1986.
388. Bertocchi L: Cited by Dogliotti AM: Trattato di anestesia:

Narcosi, anestesie locali, regionali spinali. Unione Tipografico Editrice Torinese, 1935, p. 433.
389. Parkin IG, Harrison GR: The topographical anatomy of the lumbar epidural space. J. Anat. 141:211–217, 1985.
390. Zarzur E: Anatomic studies of the human ligamentum flavum. Anesth. Analg. 63:499–502, 1984.
391. Williams PL, Warwick R: Gray's Anatomy. 37th Ed. Edinburgh, Churchill Livingstone, 1989.
392. Harrison GR, Parkin IG, Shah JL: Resin injection studies of the lumbar extradural space. Br. J. Anaesth. 57:333–336, 1985.
393. Harrison GR: The topographical anatomy of the lumbar epidural region: a study using computerised tomography. Ann. Roy. Coll. Surg. (England) 68:110, 1986.
394. Snell RS, Katz J: Clinical Anatomy for Anesthesiolgists. Norwalk, CT: Appleton & Lange, 1988.
395. Ellis H, Feldman S: Anatomy for Anaesthetists, 3rd edition. Oxford: Blackwell Scientific Publications, 1979, pp. 138–143.
396. Elsenstein S: The trefoil configuration of the lumbar vertebral canal. J. Bone Joint Surg. 62B:73–77, 1980.
397. Cheng PA: The anatomical and clinical aspects of epidural anesthesia. Anesth. Analg. 42:398–415, 1963.
398. Blomberg RA: A method for epiduroscopy and spinaloscopy. Acta. Anaesthesiol. Scand. 29:1113–1116, 1985.
399. Blomberg RG: The dorsomedian connective tissue band in the lumbar epidural space of humans: An anatomical study using epiduroscopy in autopsy cases. Anesth. Analg. 65:747–752, 1986.
400. Blomberg RG, Olsson SS: The lumbar epidural space in patients examined with epiduroscopy. Anesth. Analg. 68: 157–160, 1989.
401. Luyendijk W: Canalography. J. Belge Radiol. 46:236–254, 1963.
402. Lewit K, Sereghy T: Lumbar peridurography with special regard to the anatomy of the lumbar peridural space. Neuroradiology 8:233–240, 1975.
403. Luyendyjk W: The plica mediana dorsalis of the dura mater and its relation to lumbar peridurography (canalography). Neuroragiology 11:147–149, 1976.
404. Husemeyer RP, White DC: Topography of the lumbar epidural space. Anaesthesia 35:7–11, 1980.
405. Savolaine ER, Pandya JB, Greenblatt SH, Conover SR: Anatomy of the human lumbar epidural space: New insights using CT-epidurography. Anesthesiology 68:217–220, 1988.
406. Westbrook JL, Renowden FA, Carrie LEF: Study of the anatomy of the extradural region using magnetic resonance imaging. Br. J. Anaesth. 71:795–798, 1993.
407. Blomberg RG: The lumbar subdural extra-rachnoid space of humans: Anatomical study using spinaloscopy in autopsy cases. Anesth. Analg. 66:177–180, 1987.
408. Mehta M, Maher R: Injection into the extra-arachnoid subdural space. Anaesthesia 32:760–766, 1977.
409. Morikawa KI, Bonica JJ, Tucker GT, Murphey TM: The effect of acute hypovolaemia on lignocaine absorption and cardiovascular response following epidural block in dogs. Br. J. Anaesth. 46:431, 1974.
410. Renard M, Larde D, Masson JP, Roland J: Anatomical and radio-anatomical study of the lumbo-sacral intervertebral venous plexuses. Anatomica Clin. 2:21–28, 1980.
411. Field EJ, Brierley JB: The lympatic connexions of the subarachnoid space. Br. Med. J. 1:1167, 1948.
412. Harrison GR, Cowles NWB: The depth of the lumbar epidural space from the skin. Anaesthesia 40:685–687, 1985.
413. Gutierrez A: Anesthesia extradural. Rev. Cerug. (Buenos Aires), 1939.
414. Palmer SK, Abram SE, Maitra AM, von Colditz JH: Distance from the skin to the lumbar epidural space in an obstetric population. Anesth. Analg. 62:944–946, 1983.
414a. Meiklejohn BH: Distance from the skin to the lumbar epidural space in an obstetric population. Reg. Anesth. 3: 134–136, 1990.
414b. Sutton DN, Linter SPK: Depth of extradural space and dural puncture. Anesthesia 46:97–98, 1991.
414c. Upton PM, Carrie LES, Reynolds K: Epidural insertion: how far should the epidural needle be inserted before testing for loss of resistance? Int. J. Obstet. Anesth. 1:71–73, 1992.
414d. Crosby ET: Epidural catheter migration during labour and hypothesis for inadequate analgesia. Can. J. Anesth. 37: 789–793, 1990.
415. Bonica JJ: Continuous peridural block. Anesthesiology 17: 626–630 1956.
416. Blomberg RG: Technical advantages of the paramedian approach for lumbar epidural puncture and catheter introduction: A study using epiduroscopy in autopsy subjects. Anaesthesia 43:837–843, 1988.
417. Blomberg RG, Jaanivald A, Walther S: Advantages of the paramedian approach for lumbar epidural analgesia with catheter techniques: A clinical comparison of midline and paramedian approaches. Anaesthesia 44:742–746, 1989.
418. Jansen E: Der negative Vorschlag bei Lumbalpunktion. Deutsche Zeitschrift für Nervenheilkunde 94:280, 1926.
419. Eaton LM: Observations on the negative pressure in the epidural space. Proc. Mayo Clin. 14:566, 1939.
420. Heldt TJ, Moloney JC: Negative pressure in epidural space. Amer. J. Med. Sci. 175:371, 1928.
421. Usubiaga JE, Moya F, Usubiaga LE: A note on the recording of epidural negative pressure. Can. Anaesth. Soc. J. 14:119, 1967.
422. Usubiaga JE, Wijinski JA, Usubiaga LE: Epidural pressure and its relation to spread of local anesthetic solutions in epidural space. Anesth. Analg. 46:440, 1967.
423. Galbert MW, Marx GF: Extradural pressures in the parturient patient. Anesthesiology 40:499–502, 1974.
424. Messich MNA: Epidural space pressures during pregnancy. Anaesthesia 36:775–782, 1981.
425. Zarzur E, Gonzalves JJ: The resistance of the human dura mater to needle penetration. Reg. Anesth. 17:216–218, 1992.
426. Hardy PAJ: Can epidural catheters penetrate dura mater? An anatomical study. Anaesthesia 41:1146–1147, 1986.
427. Moore DC, Bridenbaugh D, Van Ackerman EG, Belda FB, Cole FV: Spread of radiopaque solutions in the epidural space of the human adult corpse. Anesthesiology 19: 377–385, 1958.
428. Galindo A, Hernandez J, Benavides O, Ortegon de Munoz S, Bonica JJ: Quality of spinal extradural anaesthesia: The influence of spinal nerve root diameter. Br. J. Anaesth. 47: 41, 1975.
429. Hehre FW, Moyes AZ, Senfield RM, Lilly EJ: Continuous lumbar peridural anesthesia in obstetrics. II. Use of minimal amounts of local anesthetics during labor. Anesth. Analg. 44:89, 1965.
430. Bromage PR: Exaggerated spread of epidural analgesia in arteriosclerotic patients. Dosage in relation to biological and chronological ageing. Br. Med. J. 2:1634, 1962.
431. Bromage PR: Spread of analgesic solution in the epidural space and their site of action. Br. J. Anaesth. 34:161, 1962.
432. Bonica JJ, Backup PH, Anderson CE, Hadfield B, et al: Peridural block: Analysis of 3637 cases in a review. Anesthesiology 18:723–784, 1957.
433. Dawkins DJM: The relief of pain in labour by mean of con-

tinuous-drip epidural block. Acta. Anaesthesiol. Scand. 37 (Suppl.):248, 1970.
434. Sharrock NE: Lack of exaggerated spread of epidural anesthesia in patients with arteriosclerosis. Anesthesiology 47: 307–308, 1977.
435. Grundy EM, Ramamurthy S, Patel KP, Mani M, Winnie AP: Extradulral analgesia revisited. A statistical study. Br. J. Anaesth. 50:805–809, 1978.
436. Grundy EM, Zamora AM, Winnie AP: Comparison of spread of epidural anesthesia in pregnant and non-pregnant women. Anesth. Analg. (Cleve.), 57:544, 1978.
437. Fagraeus L, Urban BJ, Bromage PR: Spread of epidural analgesia in early pregnancy. Anesthesiology 58:184–187, 1983.
438. Crawford OB, Chester RV: Caudal anesthesia in obstetrics: A combination of procaine and pontocaine single injection technique. Anesthesiology 10:473, 1949.
439. Nielsen JS, Spoerel WE, Keenleyside HB, Slater PE, Clancy PR: Continuous epidural analgesia for labor and delivery. Can. Anaesth. Sod. J. 9:143, 1962.
440. Kandel PF, Spoerel WE, Kinch RA: Continuous epidural analgesia for labor and delivery: A review of 1000 cases. Can. Med. Assoc. J. 95:947, 1956.
441. Sivakumaran C, Ramanathan S, Chalon J, Turndorf H: Uterine contractions and the spread of local anesthetics in the epidural space. Anesth. Analg. 61:127–129, 1982.
442. Gaynor A: The lumbar epidural region: anatomy and approach. *In* Epidural and Spinal Blockade in Obstetrics. Edited by F Reynolds. London, Bailliere Tindall, 1990, pp. 3–18.
443. Sharrock NE, Greenridge J: Epidural dose responses in pregnant and nonpregnant patients. Anesthesiology 51: S298.
444. Datta S, Lambert DH, Gregus J, et al: Differential sensitivities of mammalian nerve fibers during pregnancy. Anesth. Analg. 62:1070–1072, 1983.
445. Butterworth JF IV, Walker FO, Lysak SZ: Pregnancy increases median nerve susceptibility to lidocaine. Anesthesiology 72:962–965, 1990.
446. Sevarino FB, Gilbertson LI, Gugino LD, Courtney MA, et al: The effect of pregnancy on the nervous system response to sensory stimulation. Anesthesiology 69:A695, 1988.
447. Seth AP, Dautenhahn DL, Fagraeus L: Decreased CSF protein during pregnancy as a mechanism facilitating the spread of spinal anesthesia. Anesth. Analg. 64:280, 1985.
448. Dautenhahn DN, Fagraeus DC: Acid base changes of spinal fluid during pregnancy. Anesth. Analg. 63:204, 1984.
449. Conklin KA: Maternal, physiological adaptations during gestation, labor and puerperium. Semin. Anesth. 4:221, 1991.
450. Grundy EM, Rao LN, Winnie AP: Epidural anesthesia and the lateral position. Anesth. Analg. (Cleve.), 57:95, 1978.
451. Merry AF, Cross JA, Mayaded SV, Wild CJ: Posture and spread of extradural analgesia in labour. Br. J. Anaesth. 53: 303, 1983.
452. Hodgkinson R, Husain FJ: Obesity, gravity, and spread of epidural anesthesia. Anesth. Analg. 60:421–424, 1981.
453. Roldin SH, Cole AFD, Hew EM, Virgin TS: Effect of lateral position and volume on the spread of epidural anesthesia in the parturient. Can. Anaesth. Soc. J. 28:431–435, 1981.
454. Nishimura N, Kitahara T, Kusakabe T: The spread of lidocaine and I-131 solution in the epidural space. Anesthesiology 20:785, 1959.
455. Husemeyer RP White DC: Lumbar extradural injection pressure in pregnant women. An investigation of relationships between rate of injection, injection pressures and extent of analgesia. Br. J. Anaesth. 52:55, 1980.
456. Bromage PR: Mechanism of action of extradural analgesia. Br. J. Anaesth. 47:199, 1975.
457. Erdemir HA, Soper LE, Sweet RB: Studies of factors affecting peridural anesthesia. Anesth. Analg. (Cleve.) 44:400, 1965.
458. Sicard JA, Forestier J: Radiographic method for exploration of the extradural space using lipiodol. Rev. Neurol. (Paris) 28:1264, 1921.
459. Bromage PR, Joyal AC, Binney JC: Local anesthetic drugs: Penetration from the spinal extradural space into the neuraxis. Science 140:392, 1963.
460. Cohen EN: Distribution of local anesthetic agents in the neuraxis of the dog. Anesthesiology 29:1002, 1968.
461. Howarth, F: Studies with a radioactive spinal anesthetic. Br. J. Pharmacol. 4:333, 1949.
462. Bromage PR: Lower limb reflex changes in segmental epidural analgesia. Br. J. Anaesth. 46:504, 1974.
463. Frumin MJ, Schwartz H, Burns JJ, Brodie BB, Papper EM: Sites of sensory blockade during segmental spinal and segmental peridural anesthesia in man. Anesthesiology 14: 576, 1953.
464. Shantha TR, Evans JA: The relationship of epidural anesthesia to neural memberanes and arachnoid villi. Anesthesiology 37543, 1972.
465. DeCampo T Macias-Loza M, Cohen H Galindo A: Lumbar epidural anaesthesia and sensory profiles in term pregnant patients. Can. Anaesth. Soc. J. 27:274–278, 1980.
466. Galindo A, Witcher T: Blockade of sensory and motor pathways by bupivacaine, etidocaine and lidocaine: Clinical significance of spinal ganglion vulnerability. Reg. Anesth. 7: 7–13, 1982.
467. Urban BJ: Clinical observations suggesting a changing site of action during induction and recession of spinal and epidural anesthesia. Anesthesiology 39:496, 1973.
468. Cousins MJ, Mather LE: Intrathecal and epidural administration of opioids. Anesthesiology 61:276, 1984.
469. Klepper ID, Sherril DL, Boetger CL, Bromage PR: The analgesic and respiratory effects of epidural sufantanil in volunteers and the influence of adrenaline as an adjunct. Br. J. Anaesth. (in press).
470. Brull SJ, Greene NM: Zones of differential sensory block during extradural anesthesia. Br. J. Anaesth. 66:651–655, 1991.
471. Stevens RA, Bray JG, Artuso JD, et al: Differential epidural block. Reg. Anesth. 17:222–225, 1992.
472. Eisenbach JC, Grice SC, Dewan DM: Epinephrine enhances analgesia produced by epidural bupivacaine during labor. Anesth. Analg. 66:447–451, 1967.
473. Grice SC, Eisenbach JC, Dewan DM: Labor analgesia with epidural bupivacaine plus fentanyl: Enhancement with epinephrine inhibition with 2-chloroprocaine. Anesthesiology 72:623–628, 1990.
474. Braun, H: Local anesthesia. 3rd Ed, Translated by P. Shields, Philadelphia, Lea & Febiger, 1914.
475. Bieter RN: Applied Pharmacology of Local Anesthetics. Am. J. Surg., 35:500, 1936.
476. Brose WG, Cohen SE: Epidural lidocaine for cesarean section: Effect of varying epinephrine concentration. Anesthesiology 69:936–938, 1988.
477. Ohno H, Watanabe M, Saitoh J, Saegusa Y, et al: Effect of epinephrine concentration on lidocaine disposition during epidural anesthesia. Anesthesiology 68:625–628, 1988.
478. Martin WE, Kennedy WF Jr, Bonica JJ, Stegall F, Ward RJ: Effect of epinephrine on arteriolar vasodilation produced by brachial plexus block. Acta. Anaesth. Scand. Suppl. 23: 313–319, 1966.

479. Bonica JJ: Management of Pain. Philadelphia, Lea & Febiger, 1953.
480. Bonica JJ: Clinical Applications of Diagnostic and Therapeutic Nerve Block. Springfield, Charles C. Thomas, 1955, 354 p.
481. Bonica JJ: Principles and Practice of Obstetric Analgesia and Anesthesia. Philadelphia, F.A. Davis Company, 1967.
482. Bonica JJ: Obstetric Analgesia and Anesthesia. Amsterdam, World Federation of Societies of Anaesthesiologists, 1980.
483. Bonica JJ: The Management of Pain. 2nd Ed. Philadelphia, Lea & Febiger, 1990.
484. Ackerman WE et al: The deposition of epidural bupivacaine in approximation to T10–11 decreases the onset time and the dose needed to establish labor analgesia. Mid. East. J. Anesthesiol. 10:177–183, 1989.
485. MacIntosh RR: Lumber puncture and spinal analgesia, 2nd. Ed. Baltimore, Williams & Wilkins, 1957.
486. Sicard JA and Forestier J: Radiographic method for exploration of the extradural space using Lipiodol. Rev. Neural. 37:1264, 1921.
487. Bonica JJ: The Management of Pain. 2nd edition. Philadelphia, Lea & Febiger, 1990, p. 1954.
488. Doughty A: A precise method of cannulating the lumbar epidural space. Anaesthesia 29:63–65, 1974.
489. MacDonald R: Dr. Doughty's technique for the location of the epidural space. Anaesthesia 38:71–72, 1983.
490. Galea PJ: Avoiding accidental dural puncture (letter). Br. J. Anaesth. 60:347, 1988.
491. Reynolds F: Avoiding accidental dural puncture (letter). Br. J. Anaesth. 61:515–516, 1988.
492. Dalens B, Bazin JE, Harberer JP: Epidural bubbles as a cause of incomplete analgesia during epidural anesthesia. Anesth. Analg. 66:679–683, 1987.
493. Heggie NM: Unexplained pain during epidural anaesthesia (letter). Anaesthesia 39:609–610, 1984.
494. Naulty JS, Ostheimer GW, Datta S, et al: Incidence of venous air embolism during epidural catheter insertion. Anesthesiology 57:410–412, 1982.
495. Valentine SJ, Jarvis AP, Shutt LE: Comparative study of the effects of air or saline to identify the extradural space. Br. J. Anaesth. 66:224–227, 1991.
496. Candido KD, Winnie AP: A dual-chambered syringe that allows identification of the epidural space using the loss of resistance technique with air and with saline. Reg. Anesth. 17:163–165, 1992.
497. Carrie LES: The approach to the extradural space (letter). Anaesthesia 26:252–253, 1971.
498. Armitage EN: The paramedian approach to lumbar epidural analgesia. Anaesthesia 31:1287–1288, 1976.
499. Jacout J: Paramedian approach of the peridural space in obstetrics. Acta Anaesthesiol. Belgica 37:187–192, 1986.
500. Reference deleted.
501. Barretta C, Hook R, Seah CH: Use of the Tuohy needle in paramedian approach for peridural block. Anesth. Analg. 56:582–584, 1977.
502. Moore DC, Batra MS: The components of an effective test dose prior to epidural block. Anesthesiology 55:693–696, 1981.
503. Chestnut DH, Owen CL, Brown CK, Vanderwalker GE, Weiner CP: Does labor affect the variability of maternal heart rate during induction of epidural anesthesia? Anesthesiology 68:622–625, 1988.
504. Hood DD, Dewan DM, James FM: Maternal and fetal effect of epinephrine in gravid ewes. Anesthesiology 64: 610–613, 1986.
505. Leighton BL, Norris MG, Sosis M, Epstein R, et al: Limitations of epinephrine as a marker of intravenous epinephrine upon uterine blood flow velocity. Anesthesiology 66: 688–691, 1987.
506. Dain SL, Rolbin SH, Hew EM: The epidural test dose in Obstetrics: is it necessary? Can. J. Anaesth. 34:601–605, 1987.
507. Cartwright PD, McCarroll SM, Antzoka C: Maternal heart rate change with plain epidural test dose. Anesthesiology 65:226–228, 1986.
508. Scott DB: Test doses in extradural blockade. Br. J. Anaesth. 61:129–130, 1988.
509. Sosis A: Limitations of adrenaline test doses in obstetric patients undergoing extradural anaesthesia. Br. J. Anaesth. 62:578–581, 1989.
510. Shnider SM, Levinson G: Anesthesia for Obstetrics. 2nd Ed. Baltimore, Williams & Wilkins, 1987.
511. Colonna-Romano P, Lingaraju N, Godfrey SD, Braitman LE: Epidural test dose and intravascular injection in obstetrics: Sensitivity, specificity, and lowest effective dose. Anesth. Analt. 75:372–376, 1992.
512. Chadwick HS, Benedetti C, Ready LB, Williams V: Epinephrine-containing test doses-don't throw the baby out with the bath water. Anesthesiology 66:571, 1987.
513. Gieraerts R, Van Zundert A, De Wolf A, Vaes L: Ten ml bupivacaine 0.125% with 12.5μ epinephrine is a reliable epidural test dose to detect inadvertent intravascular injection in obstetric patients. A double-blind study. Acta. Anaesthesiol. Scand. 36:656–659, 1992.
514. Smedstad KG, Morison DH: A comparative study of continuous and intermittent epidural analgesia for labour and delivery. Can. J. Anaesth. 35:234–241, 1988.
515. Gambling DR, McMorland GH, Yu P, Laszlo C: Comparison of patient-controlled epidural analgesia and conventional intermittent "top-up" injections during labor. Anesth. Analg. 70:256–261, 1990.
516. Gambling DR, Yu P, McMorland GH, Palmer L: A comparative study of patient controlled epidural analgesia (PCEA) and continuous infusion epidural analgesia (CIEA) during labour. Can. J. Anaesth. 35:249–254, 1988.
517. Ferrante FM, Lu L, Jamison SB, Datta S: Patient-controlled epidural analgesia: Demand dosing. Anesth. Analg. 73: 547–552, 1991.
518. Plumer M: How anesthesiologists practice obstetric anesthesia. II. A limited survey of routine practice. The SOAP Newsletter 25 (Summer):8–21, 1993.
518a. Ducrow M: The occurrence of unblocked segments during continuous lumbar epidural analgesia for pain relief in labour. Br. J. Anaesth. 43:1172–1173, 1971.
519. Lanier VS, McKnight HE, Trotter M: Caudal analgesia: An experiment and anatomical study. Am. J. Obstet. Gynecol. 47:633, 1944.
520. Lanier P, Trotter M: Volume of sacral canal. Am. J. Phys. Anthrop. 4:227, 1946.
521. Trotter M, Letterman GS: Variations of the female sacrum: Their significance in continuous caudal anesthesia. Surg. Gynecol. Obstet. 78:419, 1944.
522. Bryce-Smith BR: The spread of solutions in the extradural space. Anaesthesia 9:201, 1954.

Chapter 14

# SUBARACHNOID BLOCK

JOHN S. McDONALD
DOMINIC A. MANDALFINO

When Corning first performed a spinal anesthetic in 1885 it is doubtful that he had any conception of the tremendous impact this regional anesthetic technique would have. It was introduced into surgical practice by Bier in 1898. The application to obstetrics was championed by numerous clinicians over the ensuing decade. Yet, it was not until Pitkin's (1928) (1) and Cosgrove's (1937) (2) reports that subarachnoid anesthesia became popular.

Two obstetricians, DeLee (3) and Greenhill (4), condemned the technique because of parturient complications. These complications were undoubtedly due to a lack of appreciation for the altered physiology of a woman at term, especially the reduced size of the subarachnoid space and the impaired venous return. The renewal of its popularity in obstetrics had to wait until the restricted "saddle block" method was introduced to clinical anesthesia by Adriani in the late 1940s (5–9). Since that time, innumerable reports have solidly entrenched the saddle block as the premier late second stage analgesic. This is due to its simplicity of performance, reliability, low complication rate, and overwhelming acceptance by patients. After enduring a painful period of first and early second stage labor, patients had the miracle of sudden pain relief and tranquility presented to them in the form of the "saddle block," usually performed by obstetricians before they performed the delivery. Throughout the 1930s and 1960s, this method was the most popular anesthetic technique used in obstetric anesthesia. It has only been since the later years of the 1970s that the lumbar epidural technique has become popular as a suitable method of pain relief for both first and second stage of labor. Lumbar epidural as a second stage anesthetic has only recently gained solid popularity due to the use of an opioid addition to the local anesthetic in providing a more reliable and intense sacral block.

## CLINICAL EVALUATION

Advantages of spinal anesthesia that are responsible for its current popularity include: relative simplicity, rapidity, certainty, duration, low failure rate, and minimal side effects. There is no question that the spinal technique is far easier to master than any of the other regional methods. The spinal technique also offers exposure to the lowest anesthetic drug concentrations and therefore the least exposure to systemic toxic reactions. This is, of course, due to the fact that a minimal amount of anesthetic is injected into an area where the nerve fibers are vulnerable, and the area is compartmentalized, allowing minimal systemic uptake of drugs.

The primary disadvantages to the use of spinal anesthesia and the contraindications to spinal anesthesia as listed in the first edition are listed in Table 14–1. It was mentioned in the first edition that only the first and the last two contraindications were absolute, and that the others were relative. However, in today's climate of the practice of medicine we would have to say that numbers (2), (3), (5), and (6) would also be absolute contraindications if they were of a serious nature. It has been well understood for years that pain relief for the second stage can be obtained by administration of $N_2O$ in conjunction with pudendal anesthesia. The obstetrician and anesthesiologist work together in harmony for the benefit of the patient.

In today's practice, there are three important uses of spinal anesthetics in obstetrics: (1) very low spinal block, i.e., the true "saddle" block limited to the sacral segments, for delivery only; (2) low spinal block, in which analgesia extends to the tenth thoracic dermatome to give relief for painful contractions and delivery; and (3) high spinal block, in which analgesia extends to T-2 or T-4 dermatome, for cesarean section.

### *Analgesia-Anesthesia*

The saddle block, affecting only sacral segments, provides complete relief of pain caused by perineal distention. If the block is the low spinal variant, extending from S-5 up to T-10, then significant pain relief from contractions will be noted. The primary use today is for primiparae for delivery or completion of the second stage. Naturally, it is sometimes used also for multiparae for the same effect, but the timing can be tricky, because the time between complete dilatation and actual delivery can be quite short. High subarachnoid block in the region of T-2 to T-4 provides satisfactory anesthesia for cesarean section. Many patients previously experienced discomfort during manipulation within the peritoneal cavity. This is now avoided by the addition of morphine or fentanyl to the local anesthetic agents used for the spinal block.

While it is true that the success rate varies with the skill of the operator, the overwhelming advantage of the spinal method is its simplicity. Thus, the statement was made in the previous edition that "any physician properly

**Table 14–1.** The Primary Disadvantages of the Use of Spinal Anesthesia and the Contraindications as Listed in the First Edition

| Primary Disadvantages |
|---|
| (1) frequency of hypotension |
| (2) postdural puncture headaches |
| **Contraindications** |
| (1) infection at the site of puncture |
| (2) disease of the central nervous system |
| (3) severe hypovolemia due to hemorrhage, dehydration or malnutrition |
| (4) fetopelvic disproportion unless the block is used for a trial of labor prior to cesarean section |
| (5) parturient refusal or fear of the procedure, or emotional unsuitability for regional anesthesia |
| (6) severe hypotension or hypertension |
| (7) lack of skilled physicians |
| (8) lack of resuscitation equipment in the immediate area |

trained in the technique can produce subarachnoid block in over 95% of parturients." This is probably still valid, because failures are almost always due to technical errors. When successful, spinal block provides complete relief of perineal pain and relief of pain associated with operative deliveries. The latter, plus the excellent motor relaxation obtained, makes spinal anesthesia the favorite for obstetricians who plan a forceps delivery to shorten the second stage. When they have a level at T-10, perhaps 10% of patients experience some discomfort in the back, flanks or abdomen during uterine contractions, and a dragging, uncomfortable sensation during traction by forceps. This is more likely to occur with a persistent fetal occiput posterior position. With occiput posterior positions, it may be that transmission of pain may be via sensory nerves that enter the spinal cord through segments higher than the tenth thoracic dermatome.

## *Effects on the Mother*

### Cardiovascular

The saddle (S-2 to S-5) or low subarachnoid block (T-10 to S-5) has no harmful effects on the mother or infant, and does not interfere with labor. These outstanding advantages make this the technique of choice in parturients who are in poor physical condition due to preexisting conditions or pregnancy-related disorders. However, mid- or high subarachnoid block may alter maternal cardiovascular function because of the more extensive chemical sympathectomy, and, therefore, greater reduction in vascular resistance.

### Respiratory

A major advantage of low spinal anesthesia is the minimal effect on the patient's pulmonary physiology. With a T-10 level there is no weakness of the intercostal muscles. However, a high spinal block can have a significant effect upon pulmonary physiology because of weakness, or even paralysis, of the abdominal muscles and many intercostal muscles. This causes an increase in respiratory dead space but a decrease in functions listed in Table 14–2. Alveolar ventilatory insufficiency in the parturient does occur when any of the conditions in Table 14–3 exist.

**Table 14–2.** Decreases in Pulmonary Physiology Due to High Spinal Block

| |
|---|
| (1) total lung volume |
| (2) expiratory reserve volume |
| (3) vital capacity |
| (4) functional reserve capacity |
| (5) peak expiratory flow rate |
| (6) ability to cough |

The author has experienced personally the effect of items (2) and (4) from Table 14–3 in a 24-year-old patient who had an excessively high spinal with resultant respiratory and cardiovascular impairment. This patient first developed hypotension and then developed alveolar ventilatory insufficiency within 3 to 5 minutes of receiving a high spinal for cesarean section. The intended level was T-2 to T-4 but the eventual level was high cervical. The patient was noted to be in extremis, and resuscitative measures were immediately instituted, including intubation, controlled ventilation with oxygen, external cardiac massage, and additional intravenous vasopressor administration. Despite these efforts, the patient did not have an effective carotid pulsation. A decision was made to proceed with immediate delivery and concomitant open chest cardiac massage. These resulted in the delivery of a depressed infant who recovered well, and a mother who also recovered because of prompt and effective therapy.

It must be emphasized that whenever respiratory depression follows subarachnoid block, it is essential to assist or control respiration promptly, so that the patient does not develop hypoxia and hypercarbia. This patient undoubtedly survived because of the swift action to: (1) obtain an airway and supply oxygen; and (2) enhance cardiovascular dynamics in the mother by delivery of the fetus and elimination of aortic and vena caval compression. Subsequent papers touching on this issue now suggest just such a maneuver, i.e., rapid delivery of the baby while continuing cardiac resuscitation (10,11).

### Cardiovascular Function

Subarachnoid block has a significant effect on the cardiac and systemic systems of the mother, as demonstrated by the case illustration above. This is indirectly by effect upon blood flow and reduction in peripheral vascular resistance. This is due to interruption of preganglionic vaso-

**Table 14–3.** Conditions Associated With Alveolar Ventilatory Insufficiency

| |
|---|
| (1) depression of the respiratory center by drugs |
| (2) impairment of respiratory center by medullary ischemia |
| (3) hindrance of diaphragm movement by an abnormally large uterus |
| (4) paralysis of respiration by block of the intercostal and phrenic nerves. |

motor fibers resulting in peripheral vasodilation. The low block or "saddle block" used strictly for perineal effect has no significant vasomotor impact, and thus, little or no effect on cardiovascular function. However, the higher block used for cesarean section interrupts a large number of vasomotor segments and decreases all three important cardiovascular parameters—peripheral resistance, venous return, and cardiac output. Such a scenario can cause maternal arterial hypotension in a very short period of time. The degree of hypotension depends on the rapidity of onset of the block and the preexisting state of the mother's cardiovascular system, i.e., whether the volume depleted at the time of the spinal block. In addition, the degree of hypotension will depend on the speed of detection, diagnosis, and definitive therapy. The latter are very important and worthy of emphasis here because one cannot reduce vigilance after a block is successfully performed and be lulled into inactivity. The blood pressure must be taken every minute for the first 5 to 8 minutes, and if a rapid and steep fall in pressure is detected, one must institute immediate treatment. Two additional important points were made in the first edition:

1. following block to a specific level, the fall in arterial pressure is greater in parturients than in nonpregnant patients; and
2. following subarachnoid block, both the frequency and severity of hypotension are greater than after either caudal or epidural block.

There is still the same concern today, as there was 20 years ago at the time of the publishing of the first edition of this book, to respect, understand, and be prepared to detect, diagnose, and treat all of the significant cardiovascular complications associated with spinal anesthesia in obstetrics.

## Effects on Hepatic Function

The primary innervation of the blood supply of the visceral organs is controlled by the sympathetic side of the autonomic nervous system. The blood vessels of the liver, kidney, adrenal gland, small bowel, and uterus are controlled via the superior mesenteric plexus. Thus, a reduction in neuronal input would cause an increase in blood flow, not a decrease, assuming that the maternal systemic blood pressure was maintained at a normal level. All previous studies of these major visceral organs basically concluded that during pregnancy they are not any more susceptible to the effects of anesthesia than in the nonpregnant state. During pregnancy total proteins and the albumin-globulin ratio are decreased (12,13). There is also a decrease in the cholinesterase activity of plasma during pregnancy, down to 70% of normal (14). The latter, of course, should alert the anesthesiologist to carefully monitor recovery from the effects of succinylcholine after cesarean section or elective surgery in the second or third trimester. In one study of nearly 1000 patients there were, in fact, instances of delayed recovery from succinylcholine (15). There are mild elevations in many liver-associated laboratory values in the third trimester such as SGOT, LDH, alkaline phosphatase, cholesterol, and bilirubin. However, a recent study of hyperemesis gravidarum revealed that all liver function tests during pregnancy were actually normal. Serum levels of total bilirubin and gamma-glutamyl-transferase were significantly decreased and those of total serum bile acids were increased in emesis-prone women. Finally, a recent study of the clearance of BSP as a measure of hepatic function in pregnancy concluded that alterations in liver function are physiologic rather than pathologic in nature (16).

## Renal Function

During pregnancy, renal blood flow increases consistent with the increase in cardiac output. By the second trimester, renal blood flow is increased by nearly 40% (17). This causes a parallel increase in glomerular filtration rate, which results in lowered values for BUN and creatinine during pregnancy. Mild glycosuria and proteinuria are common findings in normal pregnancy (17). In recent studies of the effect of pregnancy upon chronic renal disease, it was discovered that a few women experienced deterioration of renal function during gestation, but it was deemed unlikely to be due to the pregnancy itself. Furthermore, serial clearances in creatinine did not increase in half of the patients who had compromised renal function, and did not increase at all in those with severe dysfunction (18). Last, but not least, pregnancy did not seem to alter the rate of progression of neuropathy in diabetic patients. All the patients in this latter study had hypertension and proteinuria with pregnancy, but their mean serum creatinine before conception and after delivery were not significantly different (19).

### *Other Maternal Effects*

The clear advantage of the subarachnoid block for vaginal delivery or for cesarean section is its maternal compartmentalization, and its lack of effect upon other maternal organ systems such as the heart, brain, liver, kidney, and the uteroplacental complex. There is no appreciable effect upon the endocrine system, carbohydrate and protein metabolism or acid-base balance. Because there is no effect upon respiration or ventilation in the saddle block or low spinal technique, oxygen consumption is either unaffected or decreased. The only global effect occurs in instances of extensive sympathetic blockade, when it causes blood pressure drops secondary to a reduction in peripheral vascular resistance. The severity of the blood pressure drop is proportional to the speed of onset and the height of the block.

There are two side effects of high spinal for cesarean section that are important clinically. One side effect is the denervation of sympathetic segments. The primary side effect here that is a threat to the mother is a decrease in peripheral vascular resistance that results in hypotension, a condition which can be severe at times. This can be severe enough to result in ineffective circulatory volume of blood to the heart and brain. This, in turn, results in either cardiac arrest or syncopy. In addition, the overwhelming sympathetic denervation results in leaving the parasympathetic system in control. This results in increased gastric motility and contraction of the entire bowel. This improves surgical exposure. However, the unopposed vagal effect on the bowel, with the added stimulation of the emesis center produced by medullary ischemia and hypoxia that result from arterial hypotension, is sufficient to cause a high incidence of nausea and vomiting. The second side effect is denervation of the motor fibers of the respiratory system. This is even more important. A high spinal may cause impairment of normal ventilation, elevation of $paCO_2$, and reduction of $paO_2$. It is a threat to maternal and fetal viability if not recognized and treated early and aggressively with ventilation and oxygenation. The best way to make sure that a tragedy does not develop is to examine blood pressure by use of a continuous or recycling monitor set at 1 minute, along with a pulse oximeter, in every case of high spinal for cesarean section.

Neurologic complications of spinal anesthesia have had a high degree of visibility in the past. Many of the problems were probably caused by inadequate sterilization of needles or by improper technique. The use of disposable needles and the standardization of technique has done much to reduce the frequency and severity of neurologic complications. The post dural puncture headache is the most frequent but minor complication of spinal anesthesia for obstetrics. The incidence over the years has really not varied appreciably in spite of diligent efforts by many people. Variation in needle design and angle of penetration has little effect. The incidence of headache is still highly dependent upon the size of the needle used, with small 25- or 26-gauge needles resulting in about a 0.5 frequency. It has been reported that both the drug and vehicle influence the frequency of headache. There is a higher incidence when dextrose is used, and it is highest with lidocaine, and lowest with tetracaine (20).

Postpartum neuropathy was reported in a series of 143,000 births to include four cases of femoral neuropathy, five cases of footdrop, and two cases of meralgia paresthetica (21). The incidence of obstetrical neuropathies is reduced because cesarean sections reduce the mother's time in lithotomy position and reduce the traumatic use of forceps. Prolonged paralysis of the lower extremities associated with spinal anesthesia has become very rare. One incident occurred in association with placenta accreta and postpartum curettage, which required that the patient remain in the lithotomy position for some time. The lower extremity paralysis lasted three days, with subsequent recovery (22). Finally, two ophthalmic complications should be mentioned: optic nerve palsy after spinal anesthesia was reported, involving the third, fourth or sixth cervical nerves, and bilateral scotoma was reported in two patients after spinal anesthesia for cesarean section; both patients had hypotension and moderate blood loss, which may have resulted in transient macular ischemia (23,24).

### Auxiliary Forces of Labor

Spinal anesthesia for management of the second stage obtunds the bearing-down reflex because of the intense analgesic block of the perineum. Expulsion is either assisted with the mother's Valsalva maneuver or assisted with outlet forceps. The low spinal "saddle block" does not interfere with the diaphragm or the upper abdominal musculature, so that adequate generation of a Valsalva can be effected. In the past, some patients have simply just "run out of energy" because of the exhaustion of a long first stage labor with minimal analgesia and sleep. Naturally, their response was to relax and to hope that delivery could be effected by forceps. Some obstetric colleagues probably blamed the spinal for having forced them to use forceps, when it was really just due to lack of maternal motivation and spirit after an arduous labor. It is undoubtedly true that some women, due to lack of instruction, improper coaching or sheer exhaustion, could not spontaneously expel the fetus to end the second stage.

## Conclusions

All in all, spinal block for obstetrics still today has a definite place in certain circumstances. Although there may be some disagreement about the role of spinal for second stage, there is probably little argument about its role in anesthesia for cesarean section. In the latter circumstance, it has two chief advantages over the epidural method: its rapidity of onset and its tendency to be compartmentalized in the subarachnoid space with little spread into the maternal compartment and fetal compartment. There are several recent papers that attest to the fact that this method of anesthesia is acceptable and successful for deployment in obstetrics today (25–27). Yet there are still those today who question the usefulness of the spinal method of anesthesia compared to epidural for cesarean section. Crawford's summary of his review of his Birmingham experience was that the spinal method was too unreliable and too fraught with dangerous complications compared to his favorite method of epidural anesthesia (28). On the other hand, there are those who believe that in the hands of experienced obstetric anesthesiologists spinal anesthesia for cesarean section still has an important part to play today (29).

### Effects on Fetus and Newborn

As mentioned above, subarachnoid block has the distinct advantage of compartmentalization and thus by itself has no direct fetal effect. The epidural method demands far more local anesthetic usage than the small quantity used for spinal anesthesia; thus, not only is the drug injected a barrier away from the maternal systemic compartment, but it is present in such minute quantities that by the time it does reach the fetal circulation, its presence is in quantities that do not threaten depression of the fetus/newborn. One study revealed maternal plasma levels only 5% of that with epidural (30). The lack of direct fetal and neonatal depression is the prime advantage of spinal anesthesia over narcotics/general anesthesia, and epidural anesthesia whose drugs pass the placental barrier in sufficient quantities do sometimes result in neonatal depression. In the first edition of this book, there was mention of the fact that the induction to delivery times may have an impact on the condition of the newborn at birth and immediately thereafter. In the early 1970s, this author noted that the more extended the delivery of the fetus was after uterine incision, the more depressed the neonate seemed to be regardless of whether the anesthetic was regional or general. In the intervening years, we have verified that the uterine incision to delivery time is the more important of the two time intervals and that the prolonged delivery times after uterine incision result in depression due to malfunction of the placenta, and oxygenation and ventilation at the intervillous space interface. In one study in which the uterine incision-to-delivery interval was prolonged, there was a definite higher incidence of lower pH values in the umbilical arterial samples and a higher incidence of elevated norepinephrine levels. In another study, uterine incision-to-delivery interval times greater than 90 and 150 seconds were associated with more acidotic umbilical cord values than those with times shorter than 90 seconds (31,32).

## Technical Aspects

Because spinal anesthesia is established by performance of a lumbar puncture, often it is viewed as a technique anyone can do because lumbar punctures are one of the earliest procedures learned in medical school training. It seems simple to insert a needle into the spine posteriorly and obtain spinal fluid, and indeed often it is; nevertheless, the actual administration of an anesthetic and the resultant physiologic and nonphysiologic consequences can cause serious harm and injury to both the mother and unborn baby. It must be taken seriously and it must be emphasized that strict attention to detail, technique, and complete knowledge of drugs and their effects in the parturient are prerequisites to such a procedure. Many of the tragic complications of the past were due to lack of thorough knowledge of both anatomy and physiology; often these were combined with inaccurate preparation in management of complications due to lack of understanding the involved pharmacology. This is totally unacceptable today. Some of the material on technical aspects from the first edition will be repeated here because it was so well done in the first edition.

Figure 14–1 shows some important anatomic aspects concerned with subarachnoid, caudal, and spinal epidural block.

### *Vertebral Column*

The following points are noteworthy in studying the lumbar vertebrae. The spinous process is a thick, broad, somewhat quadrilateral structure, 3 to 4 cm long and projecting almost directly posteriorly. The free posterior edge of each spinous process is a rough uneven rectilinear prominence about 3 cm high and thickest below where it is occasionally notched. The laminae are broad, flat, and thinner than the pedicel, and the posterior surface of each slants so that its upper portion is considerably deeper from the skin than its lower portion, a fact of clinical importance. The spinal canal is in the shape of a triangle (Figure 14–2).

Between adjacent spinous processes there is an interspinous space, and between the laminae of adjacent vertebra there is an interlaminar space. These provide the most practical avenue of entrance into the spinal canal with a needle. In the normal (upright) position, these spaces are somewhat pear-shaped, being wider below and apical above, but during extreme spinal flexion the inferior articular process slides upward and the interlaminar foramina enlarge and become somewhat diamond-shaped (33). Each spinous process identifies the interspinous space and interlaminar foramen below.

### *Ligaments*

The supraspinous ligament is a ribbon-like band passing longitudinally over the posterior tips of the spinous processes, and is the first ligament traversed by the spinal needle when inserted at the midline. The interspinous ligament is a fibroelastic band binding adjacent spinous processes by attachment to the inferior surface of the process above and the superior surface of the one below. The ligamentum flavum is a tough, dense ligament composed almost entirely of elastic fibers. Each is attached to the anterior and inferior aspect of the lamina above and the superior and posterior aspect of the lamina below. It extends from the articular process, and its associated capsular ligaments, posteromedially to meet in the midline with the ligament of the opposite side, and these become continuous with the deep fibers of the interspinous ligament. The anterior and posterior longitudinal ligaments extend the length of the vertebral column. They are firmly attached to the intervertebral discs, but very loosely connected to the bodies of the vertebrae.

### *Curves*

The curves of the spinal column play an important role in the spread of spinal anesthetic. With the parturient supine, the region of the fourth lumbar vertebra is the highest part and the sixth thoracic and second sacral the lowest part of the column (Figure 14–3).

### *Spinal Cord*

The spinal cord occupies the upper two-thirds of the vertebral canal, ending as the conus medullaris at the level of the first lumbar vertebra (Figure 14–4). This level of termination of the cord is, however, subject to some variability (34). Because the spinal cord is a great deal shorter than the vertebral column, spinal cord segments do not lie opposite the corresponding named vertebrae. Laterally, the spinal cord is fixed by a series of nerve roots and the dentate ligaments, and below, by the filum terminale.

### *Spinal Nerves*

Each of the 31 pairs of symmetrically arranged spinal nerves (Figure 14–5) is attached to the spinal cord by two roots. The smaller anterior root emerges from the anterior surface of the cord as three or four filaments, which converge into a single compact root extending toward its intervertebral foramen wherein it meets and fuses with the posterior root. The larger, dorsal (posterior) root is composed of 6 to 10 rootlets attached to the spinal cord. These converge peripherally into two bundles that, in turn, unite near the dorsal root ganglion into the single

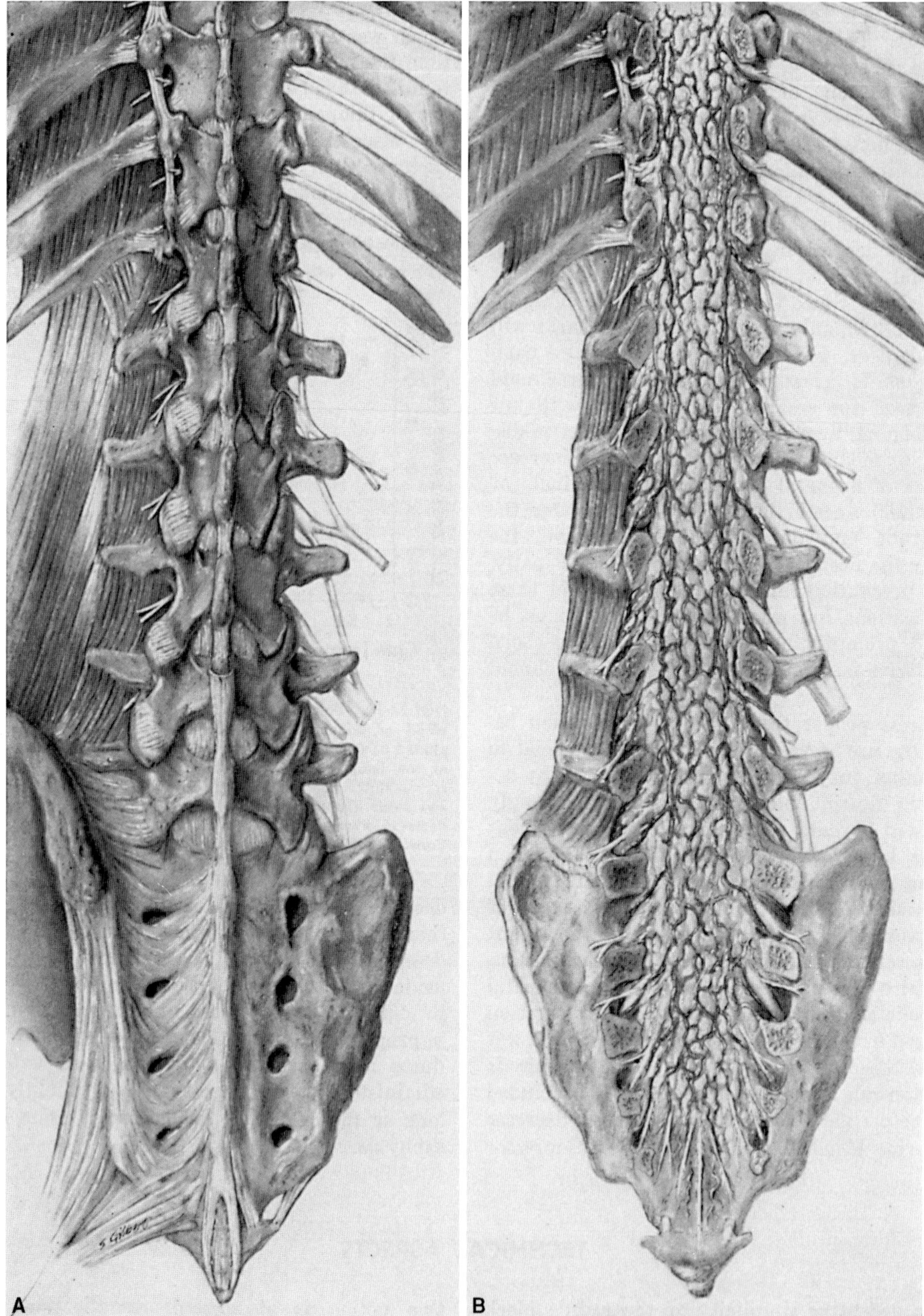


**Fig. 14–1.** Important aspects of subarachnoid, caudal, and spinal epidural block. **A,** vertebral column showing the ligamentous structures that must be traversed by a needle inserted into the spinal canal or sacral canal. **B,** spinous processes and lamina have been removed to show contents of the epidural space—the internal vertebral venous plexus and accompanying arteries, loose areolar tissue, and fat.

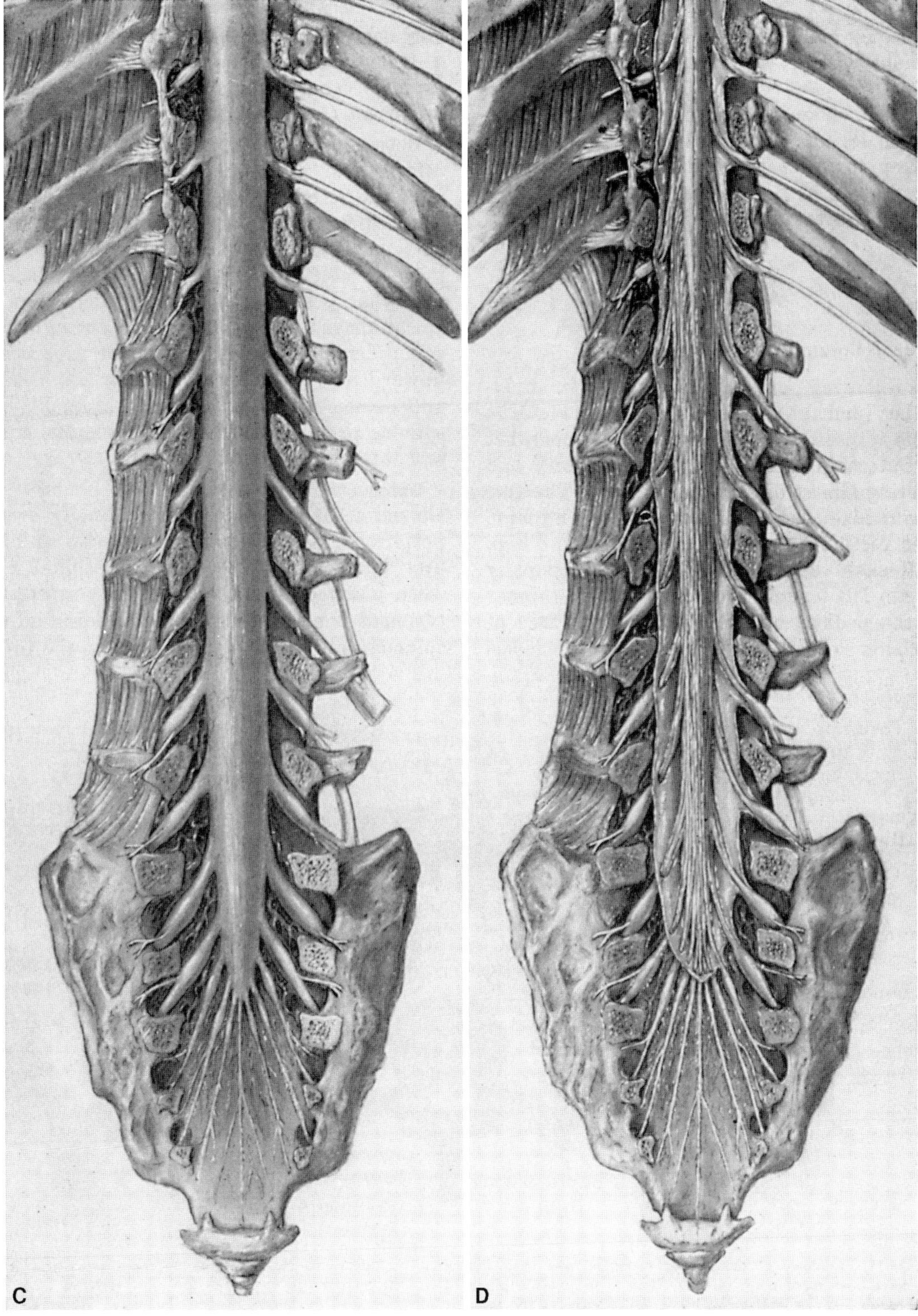


**Fig. 14–1.** **C,** deeper dissection. Contents of the epidural space have been removed to show position of the dural sac. **D,** dura-arachnoid has been opened and cerebrospinal fluid removed to show conus medullaris and caudal equina. In this subject the spinal cord ended at the level of the first vertebra. On the right, the dural cuffs have been opened to show their fusion with the epineurium of the formed nerves.

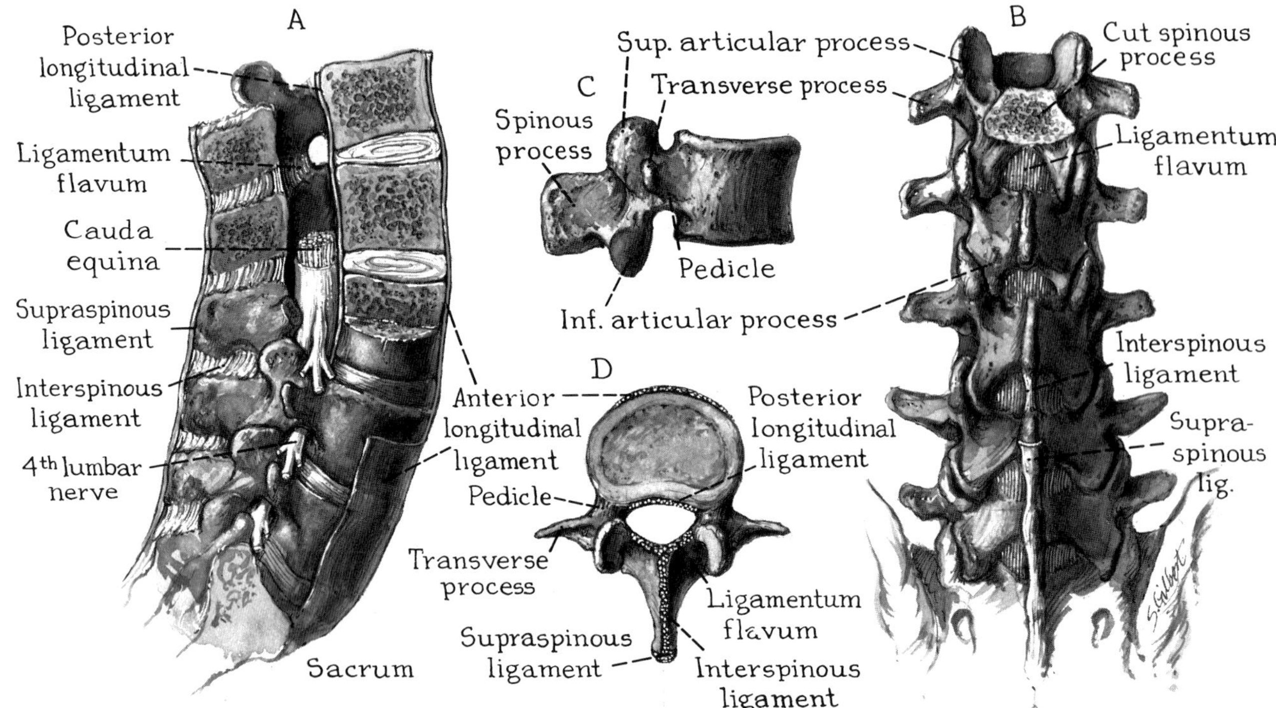


**Fig. 14–2.** Lumbar vertebral anatomy. **A,** side view of vertebral column with midline cuts through lumbar vertebrae 1, 2, and a portion of 3. This shows the relationship of the vertebral bodies to the intervertebral discs, the fact that the anterior and posterior longitudinal ligaments are actually a continuum, that the ligamentum flavum forms the lateral wall of the spinal canal, and that the relationship between the interspinous ligament and supraspinous ligament is very intimate. **B,** posterior view showing that ligamentum flavum forms also the posterior wall of the spinal canal and attaches intimately with both the leading edge and trailing edge of the laminar processes. It also demonstrates from above again the close relationship of the supraspinous and interspinous ligaments. **C** and **D,** side view and top view of an individual lumbar vertebra with important anatomical parts identified.

posterior root. The rootlets consist of many individual fibers, which are nearly devoid of the external fibrous tissue covering characteristic of peripheral nerves.

The roots of the lumbar and sacral nerves are the largest and the longest, extending the height of 5 to 10 vertebrae, and their filaments are the most numerous of all the spinal nerves. Consequently, they provide a greater surface area to be exposed to the action of local anesthetics. This and the lack of fibrous tissue covering allow for rapid onset of anesthesia. The voluminous group of the lumbar and

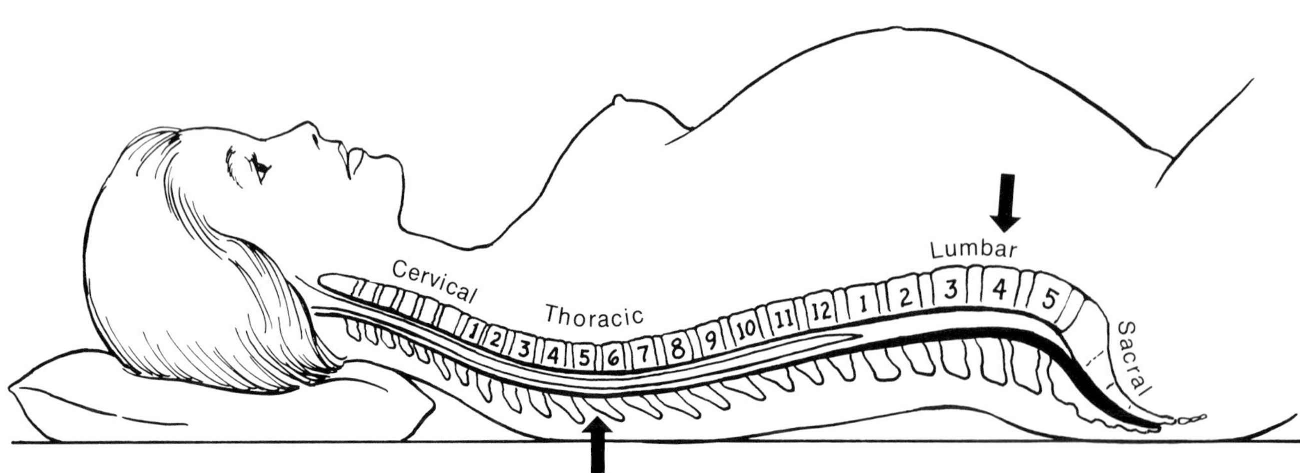


**Fig. 14–3.** The intrinsic curves of the spine of a female in the supine position, such as is assumed just after successful spinal anesthesia. Note that the level could ascend easily to T-3 level by natural gravity effect and that the lowest point of the thoracic curve is T-5, while the highest point caudally is L-4. This shows how important it is to adjust the table with a head-up tilt early on in the spinal anesthetic to assure that the anesthetic stays at a lower level.

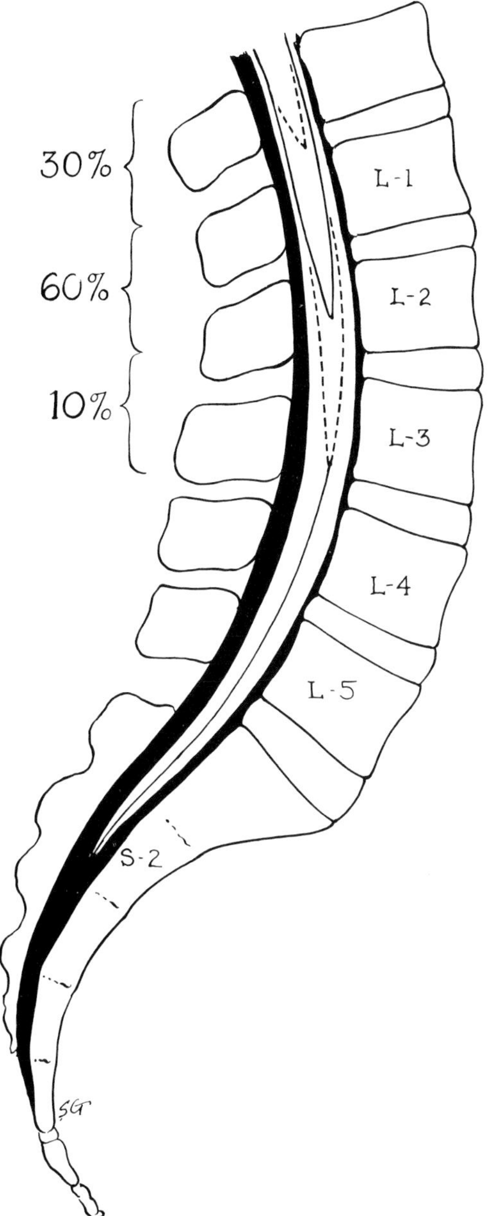


**Fig. 14–4.** The percentage of cord terminations relative to the lumbar spine. It must be recalled that where the cord ends, the caudal equina begins, filling the space with its dangling spinal nerve roots.

sacral roots, known as the caudal equina, occupies the dural sac between the end of the spinal cord and the end of the dura at the level of the second sacral vertebra. In the supine position, the nerve bundles of the caudal equina are displaced posteriorly; when the patient is acutely flexed in the lateral position for spinal puncture, they are displaced anteriorly (35).

## Meninges of Spinal Cord

The spinal dura mater is a tough fibroelastic tube that forms a loose sheath around the spinal cord. It is composed principally of longitudinal connective tissue fibers and some circular yellow elastic fibers (33). The spinal dura mater extends from the foramen magnum, to which it is closely adherent by its outer surface, to the second sacral vertebra where it ends in a cul-de-sac. Below this level, the dura mater closely invests the filum terminale, which descends to the back of the base of the coccyx, where it fuses with the periosteum.

The arachnoid is a thin, delicate membrane closely applied to the dura mater, and with it forms the cul-de-sac containing the caudal equina. Although there is a capillary interval between the dura and arachnoid (the subdural space), the two membranes are in such close contact that it is almost impossible to pierce the dura mater without piercing the arachnoid.

The pia mater is a thin, delicate vascular membrane intimately adherent to the spinal cord, dipping into all its depressions, carrying with it the numerous blood vessels that nourish the cord, and forming their adventitial tissue. The pia ensheathes the spinal nerve roots, forming a sleeve-like investment that extends as far as the intervertebral foramen. In addition, it sends out lateral branches called the dentate ligaments.

The dura and the arachnoid also send out sleeve-like branches that surround the spinal nerve roots. Usually, this dural cuff extends just beyond the dorsal root ganglion where the two roots fuse to form the mixed spinal nerve and where the meninges become adherent with the epineurium. Occasionally, the dural cuff and its subarachnoid space extend laterally as far as the paravertebral space—a point of considerable importance in paravertebral block (35). These branches of dura-arachnoid around the emergent nerve roots form pockets into which anesthetic solution injected subarachnoidally tends to become "trapped" if the patient remains in the lateral position or sitting position.

## Subarachnoid Space

The subarachnoid space exists between the dura and pia mater and is filled with cerebrospinal fluid. Crossing this space are numerous trabeculae, which form a sponge-like mass in the subarachnoid space, resulting in innumerable channels lined by mesothelial cells and harboring the cerebrospinal fluid. These trabeculae act as baffle bars, which aid in the mixing of any fluid injected into the subarachnoid space. The subarachnoid space and its fluid encircle the spinal cord for its entire length, being continuous below the conus medullaris, as the so-called cisterna terminale, and above as the cranial subarachnoid space. Engorgement of the internal vertebral venous plexus, which occurs during the late stages of pregnancy, as well as during large intra-abdominal tumors, causes a decrease in the capacity of the lower portion of the spinal subarachnoid space—a fact of great importance in spinal anesthesia.

## Cerebrospinal Fluid

Cerebrospinal fluid is colorless, transparent, and is formed at the rate of 400 ml/day (36). Its constituents and characteristics are listed in Table 14–4 (37). The average adult has a total of 120 to 150 ml of fluid, of which only

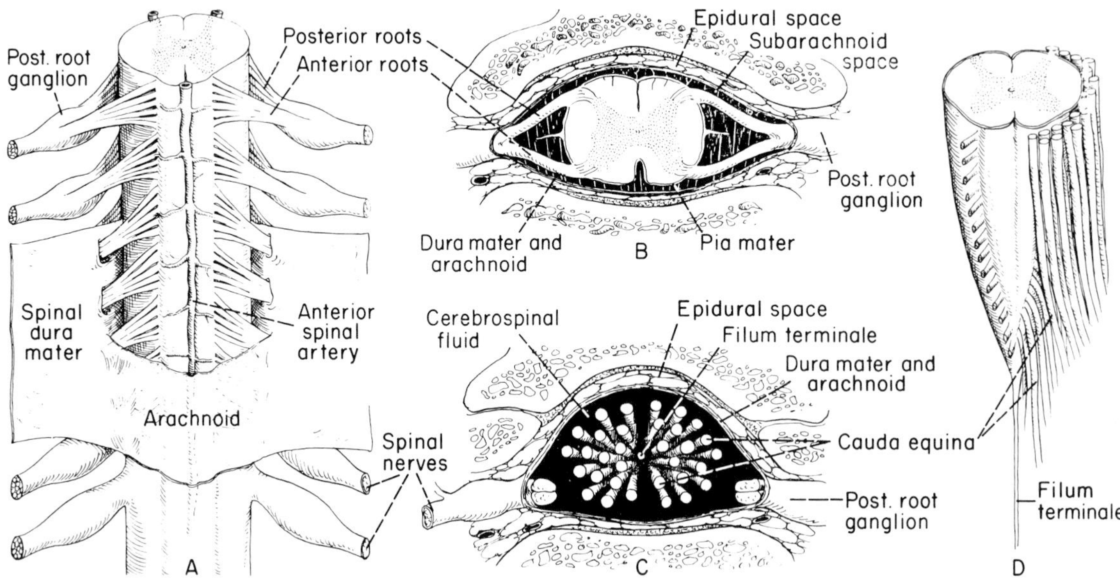


**Fig. 14–5.** Anatomy of the spinal cord and nerves. **A,** Anterior view of cord showing details of attachment of spinal nerve roots. Dura mater is reflected, showing the delicate arachnoid. **B,** Cross section of spinal canal and its contents at the midthoracic level. **C,** Schematic drawing giving three dimensional view of the subarachnoid space at the level of the third lumbar vertebra. The spinal nerve roots, which make up the caudal equina, are proceeding caudad. **D,** Anterior view of lower portion of spinal cord with the spinal nerve roots (present on left, removed on right).

20 to 35 ml are in the spinal portion of the subarachnoid space. In parturients, this volume in the spinal canal is decreased. Following uneventful spinal anesthesia, changes in cerebrospinal fluid protein content are directly related to similar changes in the blood. There is an increase in the number of red cells, but no change in white cell count (38). In gravidae suffering from toxemia and in normal puerperae who develop postpuncture headache or other neurologic complaints, the protein content is higher (39).

Cerebrospinal fluid pressure in the lumbar region is usually 150 to 300 mm $H_2O$ of water when the subject is supine and 200 mm higher in the sitting position. Cerebrospinal fluid pressure is increased slightly with each uterine contraction and respiratory movements and augmented to a greater extent by pain and movements of the body or any other activity that increases arterial and central venous pressure. It is significantly increased by bearing-down efforts (Figure 14–6). As mentioned, subarachnoid block to T-10 or above eliminates all these increases except the primary one due to increase in cardiac output.

**Table 14–4.** Characteristics and Constituents of Cerebrospinal Fluid

| | |
|---|---|
| Specific gravity | 1.007* (1.001–1.010) |
| pH | 7.4–7.6 |
| Proteins (60% albumin, 40% globulin) | 25–30 mg/100 ml |
| Sugar | 50 mg/100 ml |
| Sodium | 325 mg/100 ml |
| Chloride | 425 mg/100 ml |
| Urea | 15 mg/100 ml |
| Potassium | 10 mg/100 ml |
| Calcium | 5 mg/100 ml |
| Bicarbonate | 65 mg/100 ml |
| Lymphocytes | 2–3 $mm^3$ |
| Other cells | None |
| Phosphates, uric acid, cholesterol amino acids, solids | Traces only |

* This figure is at body temperature (37° C) relative to water at the same temperature. Relative to water at 4° C (the proper standard of reference), specific gravity is 1.003.37

## Spread of Spinal Anesthetics

The spread of local anesthetics within the subarachnoid space and the consequent level of analgesia is influenced by gravity, volume, and amount of anesthetic, speed of injection, site of injection, and size of needle (40). Table 14–5 lists the various sized needles used today.

### *Gravity*

With the techniques currently used, the most important factor is gravity as determined by: (1) difference between the specific gravity of the injected solution and that of the spinal fluid; and (2) position of the patient during and immediately after injection. A hyperbaric solution (specific gravity greater than spinal fluid) injected into a patient who remains in the sitting position will gravitate to the lower part of the dural sac, whereas if the patient is placed in the Trendelenburg position immediately after injection, it will gravitate cephalad. Hypobaric solutions will disperse in the opposite direction. The spread of isobaric solutions (the same specific gravity as spinal fluid) is unaffected by gravity.

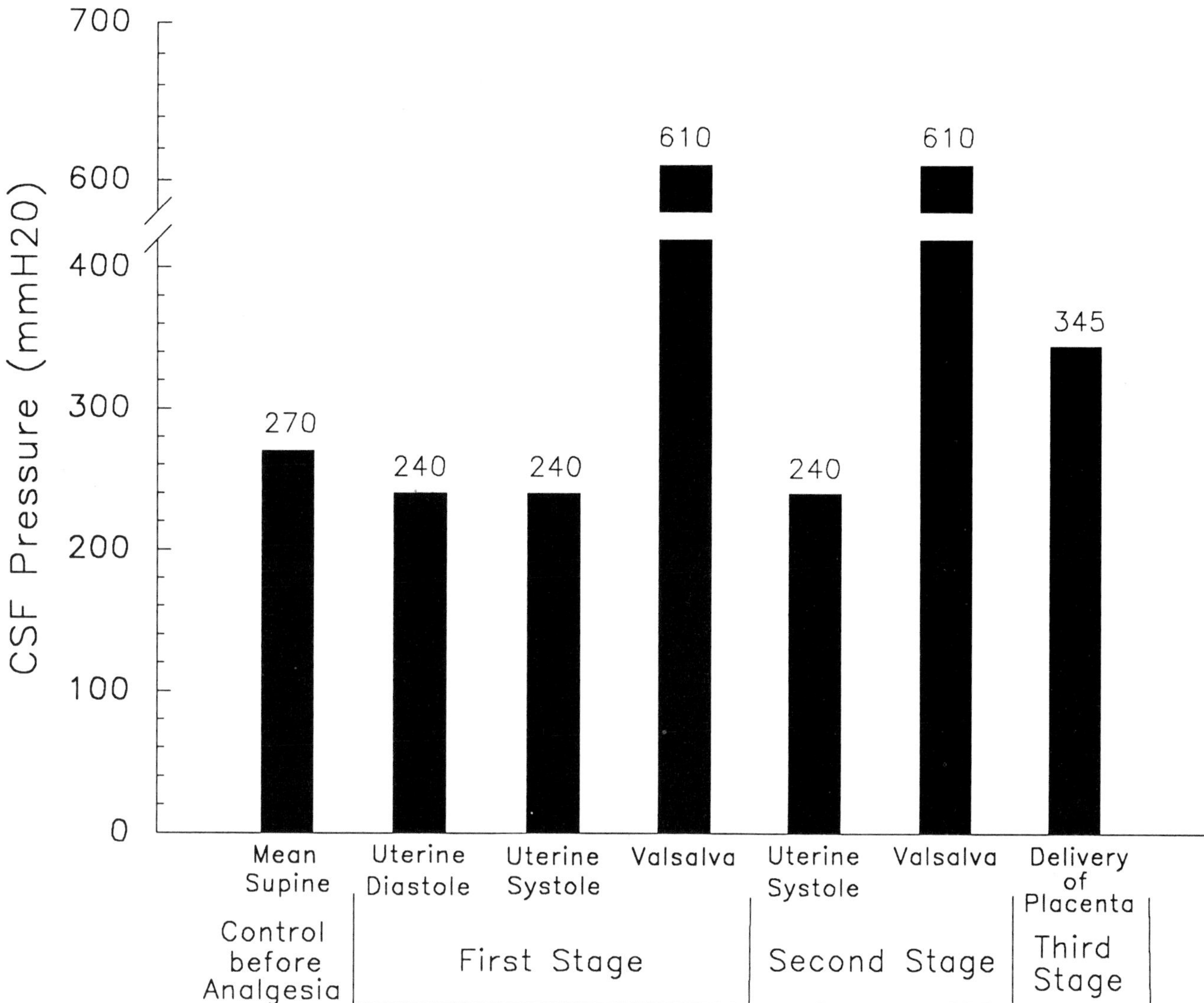


**Fig. 14–6.** Variation in cerebrospinal fluid pressures throughout labor. Note the baseline resting pressures around 240 mm $H_2O$ with the significant increase during Valsalva. Note also the increase in pressure during termination of the third stage that is often associated with either Valsalva or manual expression, which increases abdominal pressure. (From Marx GF, Saifer A, Orkin LR: Cerebrospinal fluid cells and proteins following spinal anesthesia. Anesthesiology. 24:305, 1963.)

### *Volume and Total Dose of Local Anesthetic*

The larger the volume, the greater the displacement of spinal fluid and the greater the extent of the anesthetic. Similarly, the greater the total dose, the more drug that will be available to spread away from the site of injection (Table 14–6).

### *Speed of Injection and Size of Needle*

When using large needles, the faster the injection, the greater the spread (40). At slow rates of injection, the spread is greater with small needles than it is with larger needles (velocity of solution varies inversely with the cross section area of the needle).

### *Other Factors*

The site of injection may also influence the level of the block, but in obstetric practice this must be considered of little significance because the site of injection is usually in the lower lumbar spinal area. Although the direction of the bevel of the needle at the time of injection, the pressure of the cerebrospinal fluid, its churning action caused by pulsation of the arteries, and diffusion are often mentioned as affecting spread of local anesthetic, they probably play an insignificant role.

### *Effect of Pregnancy*

The spread of spinal anesthetics is significantly influenced by pregnancy. The same dose (volume and

**Table 14–5.** Various Spinal Needles

| Manufacturer | Needle Size | Comments |
|---|---|---|
| Becton Dickinson Division | 1) Quincke Tip, 18 to 29 gauge, 1½ to 3½ inches | |
| | 2) Long Length Spinal, 18 to 29 gauge, 4¹¹⁄₁₆ to 7 inch | |
| | 3) Pediatric Needle, 25 gauge, 1–2 inch | |
| | 4) Whittaker Needles, 22 to 27 gauge, 3½ to 4¹¹⁄₁₆ inch | Pencil Point |
| Popper and Sons, Inc. | 1) Quincke Standard Sizes, 17 to 26 gauge, 1½ to 6 inch | |
| | 2) Pitkin Spinal Needle, 20 to 22 gauge, 3 to 4 inch | 45° angle |
| | 3) Thinwall Needles, 12 to 21 gauge, 1½ to 7 inch | Custom needles available |
| Sherwood Medical Co. | 1) Diamond Point Spinal Needles with metal HVB 18 to 26 gauge, 1½ to 3½ inches | Autoclavable |
| | 2) Sensitouch Spinal Needle with plastic HVB 18 to 26 gauge, ½ to 4½ inch | |
| | 3) Whittaker Type Pencil Point with metal HVB 22 gauge, 3½ inch | |
| Pajunk | 1) Sprotte Needle, 22 to 24 gauge, 3½ inch | Rounded tip |

amount) of drug produces a considerably higher spinal block in parturients than in nonpregnant women. We now know that in the intrapartum period, one-third to one-fourth the amount of drug was needed to obtain the same level of sensory block as that required after delivery. This is due to a decreased subarachnoid space produced by engorgement of epidural vein. The slight increase in the maternal lumbar lordotic curve may also contribute to the greater spread following injection of hyperbaric solutions. Sudden increase in intra-abdominal pressure during bearing down, active effort to change position or phonation may cause alteration in cerebrospinal fluid pressure, which produces waves or eddies that may enhance the spread of solution. Uterine contractions in themselves do not significantly effect spread of spinal anesthetics.

## Concentration of Anesthetic in Cerebrospinal Fluid

The injection of a local anesthetic into the subarachnoid space mimics the injection of one liquid into another of varying density and other properties. Naturally, there is a dispersion that is dictated by the various physical parameters of the two liquids. These include density, volume, and concentration differentials at the least. The concentration of the local anesthetic is maximum at the point of injection, but there is a rapid decline from that point in the spinal fluid in all directions from the point of injection. We know this from the earlier work of Helrich and associates, who measured concentrations of procaine at various distances from the site of injection (41). In time this concentration gradient continues to change with ever-increasing dilution as the local anesthetic disperses in all directions. This change is one of a continuing dilution as more and more area of the spinal canal is involved. Moreover, with this type of spread, the concentration finally reaches its minimum at the most remote points from initial injection. Thus, the concentration minimum necessary to block various nerve complexes is varied and depends on the site of injection, the concentration of the local anesthetic injected, and the amount injected. Most always, with the concentrations used today, the anesthetic in the subarachnoid space is sufficient to block both motor and large A sensory fibers. At some point, however, enough dilution occurs so that only the smaller C and A-delta fibers responsible for pain, touch, temperature, and sympathetic function are blocked. Finally, with further dilution there is only blockade of vasoconstriction and temperature perception. Usually, this so-called "differential block" between the level of analgesia and vasomotor block is only two spinal segments; sometimes, however, it can cover as many as four to six spinal segments.

## Technique of Subarachnoid Block

### *Preparations*

#### *Equipment*

Today most all equipment used for spinal blocks in modern centers is disposable (Figure 14–7). There are

**Table 14–6.** Dose-Volume of Hyperbaric Local Anesthetics for Spinal Anesthesia in Obstetrics

| | Vaginal Delivery | | | | Cesarean Section | | |
|---|---|---|---|---|---|---|---|
| | Low Block ($S_1$–$S_5$) (Saddle Block) | | Modified Saddle Block ($T_{10}$–$S_5$) | | $T_4$–$T_8$ Level | | |
| **Drug (Proprietary Name)** | **Dose (mg)** | **Vol (ml)** | **Dose (mg)** | **Vol (ml)** | **Dose (mg)** | **Vol (ml)** | **Approx Duration** |
| Lidocaine 5% with Dextrose (Xylocaine) | 35 | 0.7* | 50 | 1.0 | 50–80 | 1–1.6 | 45–75 min |
| Bupivacaine 0.75% with 8.25% Dextrose (Marcaine, Sensorcaine) | 3 | 0.4* | 5 | 0.7* | 8–12 | 1–1.6 | 120–180 min |
| Tetracaine 1% with 10% Dextrose (Portocaine) | 5 | 0.5* | 7 | 0.7* | 7–10 | 0.7–1.0 | 120–180 min |

* additional dilution may be added to simplify handling and administration
** addition of epinephrine 100–200 mg will increase duration by approximately 50%

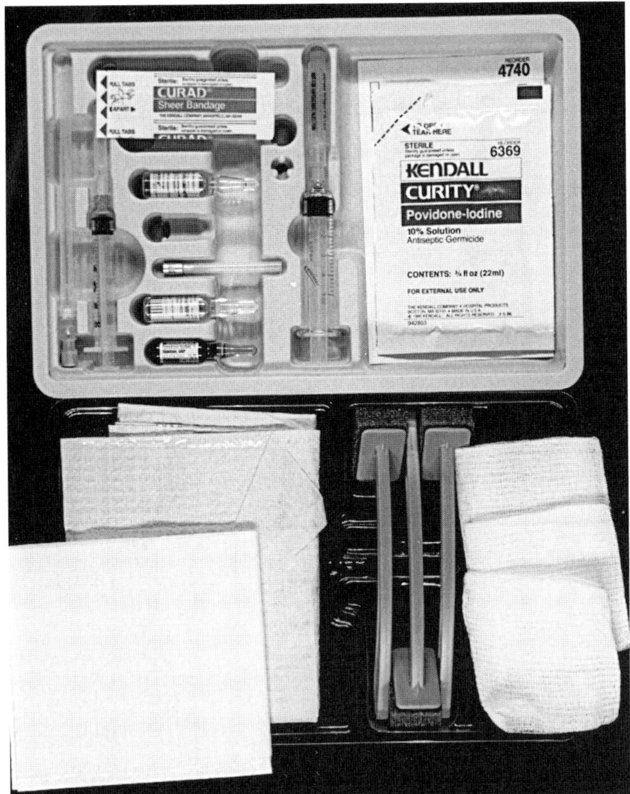


**Fig. 14–7.** An example of one of the currently available disposable spinal anesthetic kits. The use of these kits has eradicated the worry of subarachnoid contamination from incompletely sterilized reusable needles. (Photo courtesy of Ohio State University)

many different manufacturers of disposable trays with various needles and drug combinations ready-made. Some of these are listed in Table 14–7. One very nice spinal needle is a small gauge, pencil-point needle, which is now a 25-gauge size but the needle puncture is purportedly equivalent to the dural damage done by a much smaller 29-gauge needle because of the way the rounded nose of the needle spreads the dural fibers rather than cutting them.

## *Patient*

The entire procedure is explained to the patient; it is necessary to give informed consent that includes a mention of all the hazards associated with the technique. The patient may wish not to hear all of these and if so can be requested to sign a form stating such and giving the physician permission for performance of the spinal. Naturally, the ideal time to take care of all of these housekeeping matters is before labor and/or immediate cesarean section. This can be accomplished on an outpatient basis during one of the patient's visits to the doctor's office or hospital for initial workup. Before performance of the actual technique of spinal block, there are certain patient preparatory measures that must be taken. Blood pressure, pulse, respiration, and color are noted and recorded frequently, and an intravenous infusion is started by inserting

**Table 14–7.** Anesthesia Spinal Kits

| Manufacturer | Needle Size | Comments |
|---|---|---|
| Abbot Laboratories/ Hospital Products | 22, 25, 26, 27 gauge Quincke 3½ inch<br>22 gauge Whittaker needle 3½"<br>Tetracaine HCl 1% 2 ml<br>Lyophilized Tetracaine 1% 2 ml<br>Lidocaine 5% 2 ml<br>Bupivacaine 0.75% 2 ml | Multiple combinations of kit components i.e., epinephrine, ephedrine |
| Baxter Health Care Corp, Hospital Supply (Pharmaseal) | 22 to 25 gauge Quincke Tip needle, 3½ inch<br>Tetracaine, 1% 2 ml<br>Tetracaine lyophilized 20 mg–5 ml<br>Lidocaine 5% 2 ml | Complete kit |
| Kendall Health Care | 24 gauge Sprotte needle<br>22, 25, 26 gauge Quincke Tip needle<br>Tetracaine 1% 2 ml<br>Lidocaine 5% 2 ml<br>Tetracaine lyophilized 20 mg<br>Bupivacaine 0.75% 2 ml | Complete kit |

an 18-gauge plastic catheter into one of the veins in the middle of the forearm or hand.

## *Position*

### *Sitting*

Some anesthesiologists may prefer the patient in a sitting position. This position is reasonably comfortable for the patient. Positioned with her legs over the side of the delivery table with support from her arms planted firmly at both her sides, she may also be assisted by a nurse who stands in front of her and instructs her to "arch her back" by flexing her head and resting it on the nurses shoulder (Figure 14–8).

This position is popular because: (1) it is often the first exposure to spinal block taught by another house staff in training; (2) it is comfortable for the doctor who easily approaches the patient from the back; (3) it may seem to make flexion of the spine more prominent; and (4) perhaps most importantly it helps to present a more definable midline view or straight line up of the spinous processes for the operator. This position is often most appreciated in the morbidly obese parturients. Of course this position is preferred for the saddle block technique to prevent spread of the anesthetic above the tenth thoracic dermatome.

### *Lateral*

Others prefer the lateral position because: (1) there is definitely more comfort for the mother; (2) the hazard

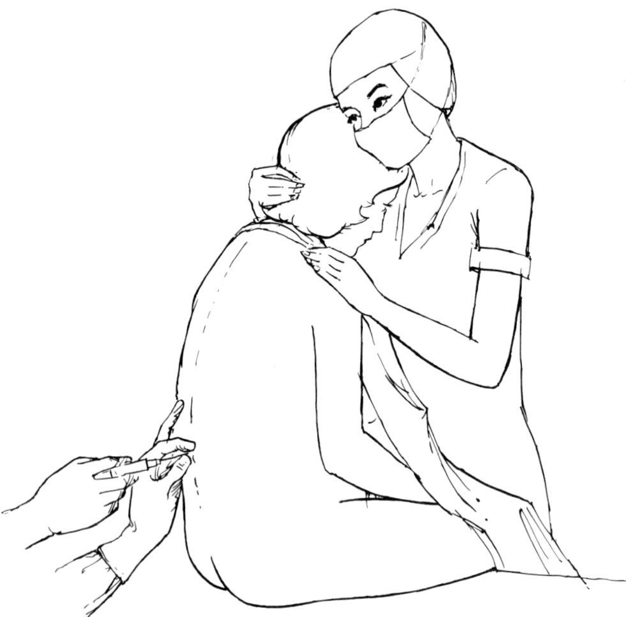

**Fig. 14–8.** A common and helpful positioning of the patient by a nurse assistant. From her position in front of the patient, the nurse is able to both support the patient and help allay the patient's anxiety during the procedure.

of eminent delivery with the fetus being trapped because of the sitting position is obviated; (3) postural hypotension is not an issue; and (4) there is more comfort and control seemingly from the operator's viewpoint because he/she can sit comfortably adjusted behind the patient and have the back immediately next to the edge of the bed along the long axis of the bed.

## Puncture

In obstetric patients, the best site of puncture is the space that can be most easily palpated in the area of the third or fourth lumbar interspace. Punctures above the second lumbar space are potentially hazardous because of the danger of trauma in an area where the spinal cord terminates. One may wish to examine the patient and draw several spinous interspaces and spinous processes to feel comfortable with the patient's anatomy.

### Procedures before Puncture

The tray containing equipment for the puncture is placed in a suitable and comfortable position for the operator on some type of mayo stand or an acceptable substitute. An operating room trash receptacle is not an acceptable substitute although it is tempting because often it is the first stand of reasonable height available. The technique of spinal block must carry rigid requisites for sterility, and this is inclusive of: (1) the location and opening of the spinal tray; (2) skin preparation; (3) glove donning; (4) drug handling; and (5) needle insertion. The tray should be opened before donning gloves and careful attention must be paid to making sure the inside of the tray is not contaminated with the bare hands. Next, the patient's skin is prepared by use of several betadine swabs with circular motions with each swab assuring the center is protected by gradually enlarging circles (Figure 14–9). A circular area the size of 8 to 10 inches in all directions is adequate preparation with the disposable betadine swabs. If the latter are used, the operator then dons gloves and prepares the medication and needles on the tray. If the prep tray from the disposable tray is used and betadine poured for skin prep, then of course the gloves are donned first. Lighting is a personal preference and varies tremendously, so suffice it to say that it should be something the operator feels comfortable with and intense enough to be pleasant and provide sufficient illumination. It is important for the physician to maintain close verbal reassuring contact with the patient all during the performance of the procedure to allay anxiety and to prevent sudden unexpected moves by the patient. The skin is first wiped with 4 × 4-inch sterile gauze so that any excess betadine is removed (Figure 14–10). Then the analgesic for the puncture is made with care and consideration for the patient's feelings. What is meant by this is that often one may be so engrossed in his/her technique that no communication is made with the patient until she feels a sharp needle. This is best avoided by warning the patient in advance that she will feel various sensations during the procedure and that the operator will give her advance warning before proceeding to actual needle puncture. In fact, it is best to develop a continuous dialogue with the patient so that she may become comfortable with your style and assured that you will not do anything without telling her first. The only area in need of analgesia is the skin and that can be accomplished by injection of only 1 ml of local anesthetic. This is often the most painful part of the procedure and it can be reduced by: (1) addition of bicar-

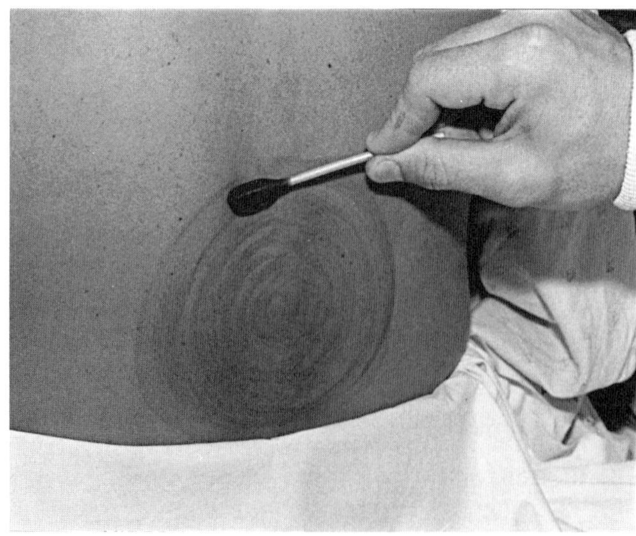

**Fig. 14–9.** The betadine prep of the patient begins at the center of where the actual puncture will be made and continues in ever-increasing circles until an approximate 6-inch diameter is attained. Then the routine is repeated two more times, each time starting at the center and ending at the outermost ring. (Photo courtesy of Ohio State University)

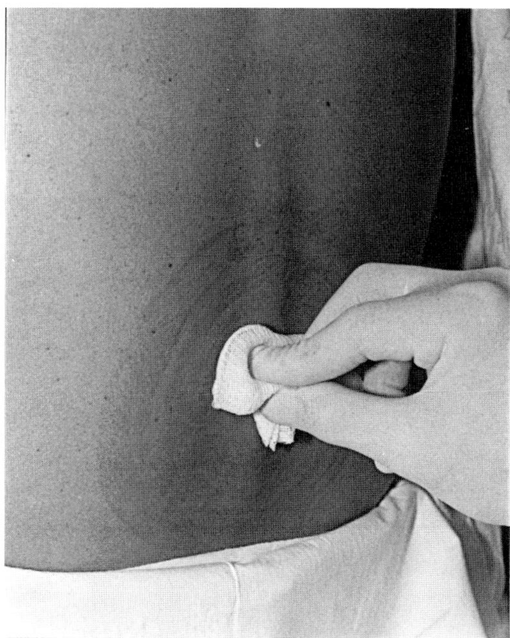

**Fig. 14–10.** Before puncture, the center of the prep area is wiped dry with 4″ × 4″ gauze so that no excess betadine will be carried into the deeper tissues.

bonate to the local anesthetic, whose normal pH is extremely acidotic, and (2) firm pressure with the first two fingers of the operator's left hand so that the patient will sense primarily deep pressure just at the time of skin needle penetration. As the local anesthetic is injected, a small papular area is developed, which is often referred to as an orange peel effect (Figure 14–11). Now the operator has a few moments to go back over the drugs, the solution for intraspinal injection, a final check of the patient's vital signs, and the fetal heart tones, before picking up the chosen needle for performing the puncture.

## *Technique of Puncture*

### *Midline Approach*

The midline puncture method is shown in Figures 14–12 and 14–13 and described in detail in the accompanying legends. This is still the most popular approach because it is thought to be the easiest to learn, it is often the first method taught to the medical student in reference to spinal puncture, and often older residents teach younger residents the method they were introduced to first and have found most comfortable. Because the needle passes in the midsagittal plane, it would appear that there would be less chance for error in directing it to the spinal space. However, occasionally it is difficult to advance the needle in the midline, either because the needle is directed onto a bony process, the upper or lower margin of the spinous process, the left or right side of the lamina at that level or, if widely misdirected, it can impinge near the foramina and even produce a paresthesia. The spinal procedure is notorious for ego reduction in instances where the above problems are repeatedly encountered on a "bad" day and any one individual is prone to such a problem, because regardless of how many and how well or fast one has become at needle placement, there is always a chance that repeated errors may occur, which can frustrate tremendously even the most calm and most level-headed anesthesiologist. In such instances, it is best to go back to the basics and "think anatomical." First, take a close look at the patient's position, for she may be slightly rotated in one direction or another that will cause the

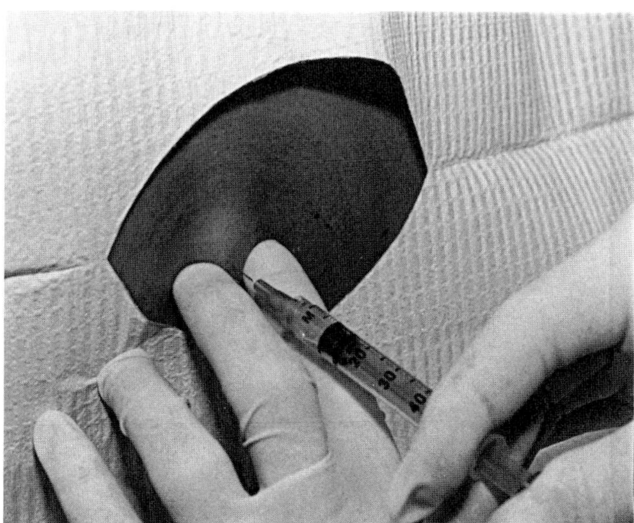

**Fig. 14–11.** A 25-gauge short needle is used to make the superficial skin wheal, which provides really the bulk of the anesthetic effect for the procedure. A 1-cm rounded orange-peel effect is created by a slow injection of lidocaine into the dermis. The slow injection is most important because it helps to minimize the pain of injection. (Photo courtesy of Ohio State University)

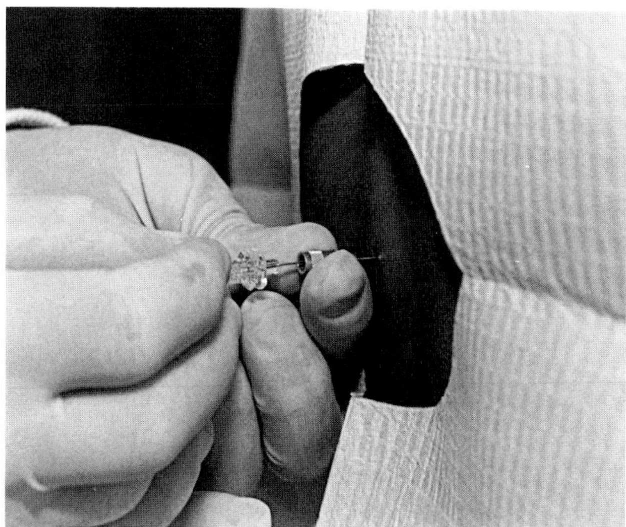

**Fig. 14–12.** Demonstration of the midline spinal puncture with use of the 25-gauge spinal needle and the short introducer needle, which helps get through the tough epidermis/dermis layers and the superficial layer of the superficial fascia. (Photo courtesy of Ohio State University)

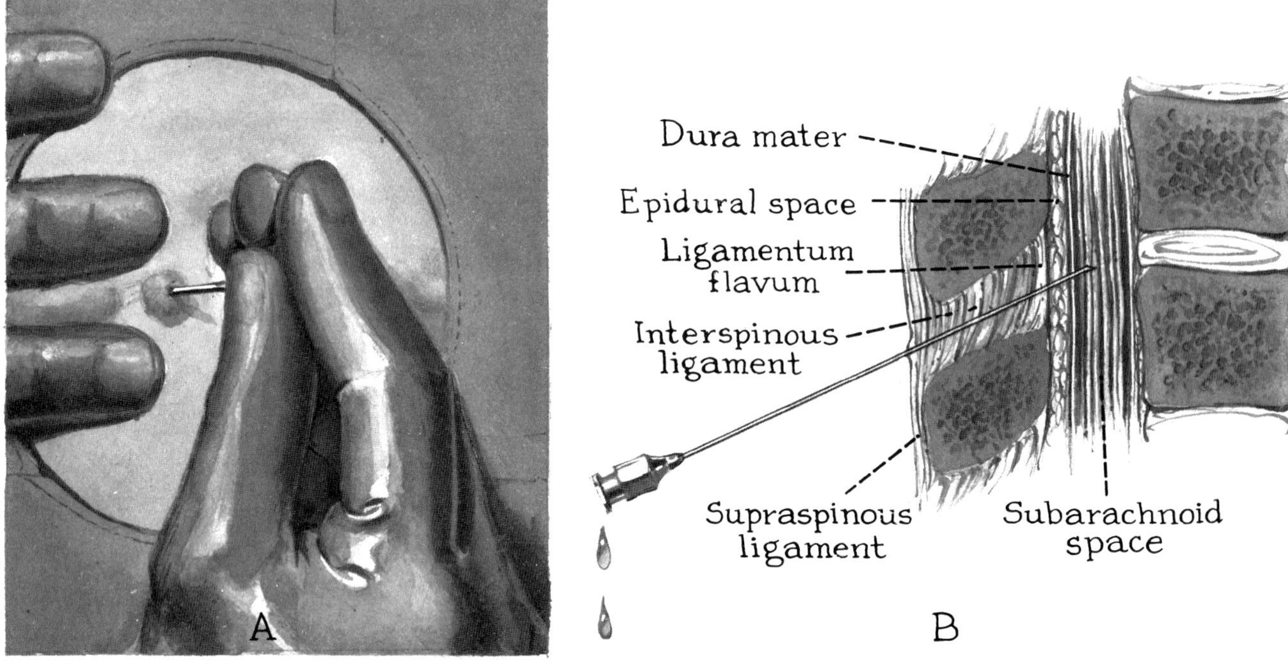


**Fig. 14–13.** Demonstration of the midline technique showing finger positioning (*A*) and needle path (*B*). **A,** The index and second finger of the left hand are placed on either side of the posterior aspect of the spinous process and the right hand then directs the needle puncture into the midline and the middle of the interspace. **B,** The needle course is directed slightly at an angle with the tip of the needle inclined ever so slightly in the cranial direction. The needle penetrates the supraspinous ligament, the interspinous ligament, and finally the ligamentum flavum before it punctures the dura and enters the subarachnoid space.

needle to miss the entire spinal canal due to the augmentation of the offset as the distance to the spinal space increases. Second, examine the spinal vertebral process you are working with and see if it is perhaps not misaligned somewhat with the vertebral processes above and below (Figure 14–14). This can cause the needle to "just miss" the spinal space because of a regional misalignment of the vertebrae (Figure 14–15). This error in alignment and the increased deviation of the tip of the needle as it drives deeper into the tissue is one of the most frustrating elements of performing spinal anesthesia. The spinal space is missed over and over again until the anesthesiologist is quite frustrated. In the latter instance, one may decide it best to select a space immediately above or below the original one selected; this may just be the solution, and result in immediate success. Finally, it just may not be that given individual's day! Don't press the issue, ask another colleague to do the honors for you. He or she may be successful the first time. In such a case, be grateful and

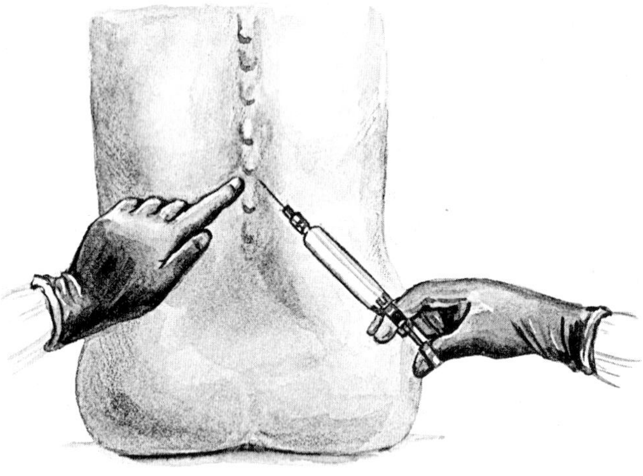

**Fig. 14–14.** This shows palpation of the spinous process at the interspace of the puncture, while careful visual examination assures that the spinous process above and below are in line with one another.

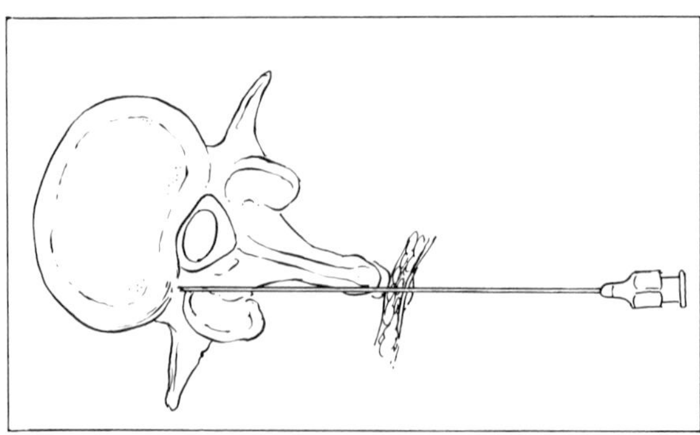

**Fig. 14–15.** A misalignment of a spinous process due to patient tilt can cause the needle direction to be directed away from the midline and result in the needle tip to just miss the spinal space, resulting in repeated "dry taps."

thankful that "there will be another day" and your honor will once again be vindicated.

## *Paramedian Approach*

The paramedian puncture method is shown in Figures 14–16 and 14–17, and described in the accompanying legends. In this method, the operator has a definite anatomical plan in mind and it is based upon visualizing the three-dimensional relationship of the ipsilateral lamina of the space selected and the pathway of the needle as it penetrates the skin, superficial fascial layers, superior muscle fascia, multifidus muscle belly, inferior muscle fascia, and, finally, the ligamentum flavum itself as it attaches just in front of the leading edge of the lamina. In this method, the needle avoids completely the supraspinous and interspinous ligaments. If a bony process is encountered in this approach, it is most likely the front edge of the ispilateral lamina (Figure 14–18). This is in direct contrast to the midline method in which one can never be sure of what bony anatomical landmark is involved. Once the lamina is encountered, it becomes relatively simple to "walk off" the lamina with successive needle movements cephalad and medial until ligamentum flavum is met. This method is extremely useful in obese patients where the exact midline is in question, but where a spinous process can be palpated. See the figures on method of subarachnoid block in obese individuals and the accompanying legends. The authors prefer the paramedian approach because it is more "anatomical" in its concept, because it obviates the question of which ligamentous structure the needle is in because, in the midline method, the posterior spinous ligament, the interspinous ligament, and the ligamentum flavum are traversed, and because it removes the need for excessive flexion of the lumbar spine and thus avoids the discomfort associated with such positioning. When the fully flexed position is necessary parturients can become uncomfortable because the thighs are pushed up against the abdomen, which, in turn, pushes up the diaphragm and impairs ventilation.

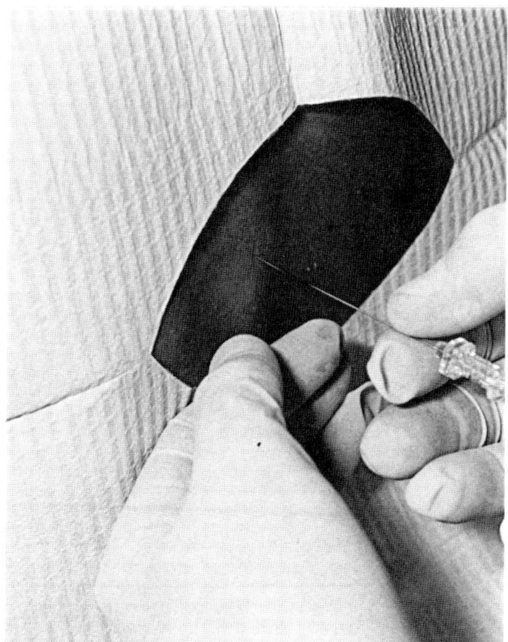

**Fig. 14–17.** In the paramedian approach the idea is to identify the lamina of the identified spinous process. This is done by driving the needle all the way down to the lamina at the midline offset point shown in Figure 14–16. The point of the puncture is the midpoint of the spinous process so that the direction of the needle is inclined gradually toward the cephalad direction, "walking" off the superior border of the lamina. (Photo courtesy of Ohio State University)

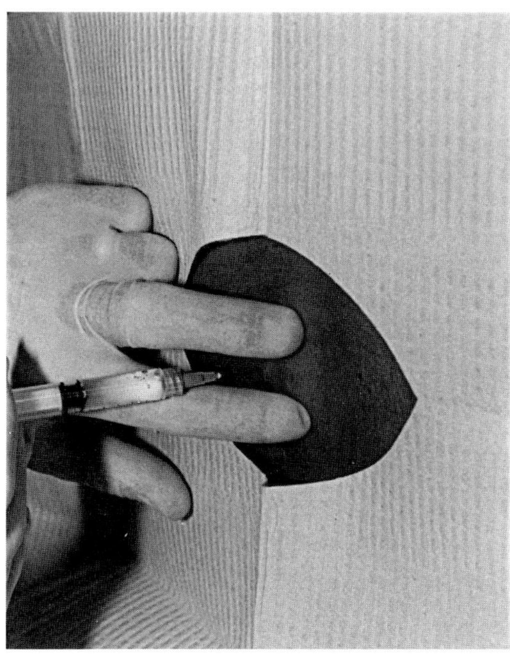

**Fig. 14–16.** The fingers of the operator are in the midline on either side of a spinous process. The skin wheal is being made off the midline in the area of the middle of the spinous process. (Photo courtesy of Ohio State University)

One more approach should be mentioned for completeness, although it is not taught vigorously today and this is the **Taylor approach**. This special technique (Figure 14–19) of paramedian puncture is performed through the fifth lumbar interlaminar space (42). Anatomically, this is the largest spinal space available and usually the last to be closed by arthritic processes; it is especially useful in patients with disease of the spine and may be useful in other situations where spinal surgeries have been previously performed or even in instances where bone is repeatedly encountered and the operator is becoming frustrated.

## *Double Needle*

The double-needle technique can be quite helpful in difficult cases where the small-gauge needle is bending. It is performed basically by use of an epidural guide needle first, so that a larger 21- or 20-gauge spinal needle is placed and serves as an introducer for a 26- or 25-gauge needle, which is used for the actual dural puncture. Occasionally, the use of small-gauge slanted sharp needle point

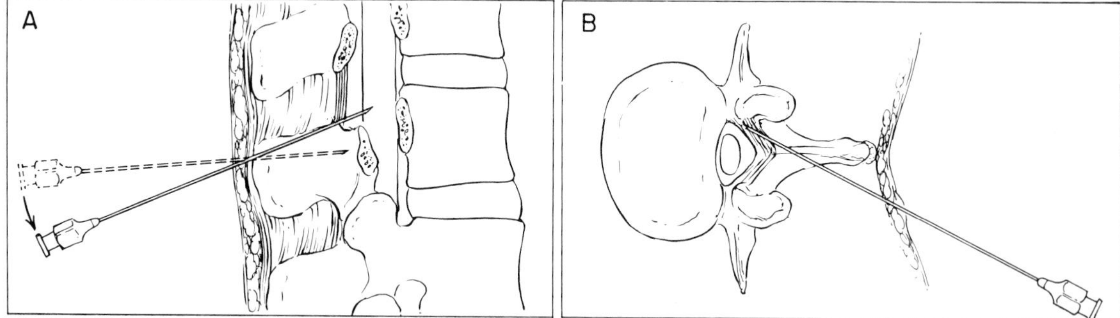


**Fig. 14–18.** The lamina "walking" technique. The ligamentum flavum attaches to the leading edge of the lamina, and the epidural space and dural barrier lie just below this anatomical point. This method of anatomical entry is especially advantageous for catheter placement in the continuous spinal technique because of the slanted direction of the needle.

will result in the needle following a "cutting" path through the muscle belly wall. This may cause a curve in direction that the operator just cannot counteract. The use of the "over needle" of a larger bore obviates this (43). This situation may also be avoided by use of a rounded pencil-point needle—perhaps another advantage of this type of needle (Figure 14–20). Puncture of the dura-arachnoid with these small needles is followed by a much lower incidence of headache—a consideration of great importance. The outside needle also avoids contact of the skin with the needle used for dural puncture and thus decreases contamination. This technique can also be performed with a shorter needle used as the guide with placement through the skin, superficial fascial layers, superior muscle fascia and muscle belly wall in the paramedial method, or the posterior longitudinal ligament and the interspinous ligament in the midline method thus serving as an aid in directing the point of the small-gauge needle to its target.

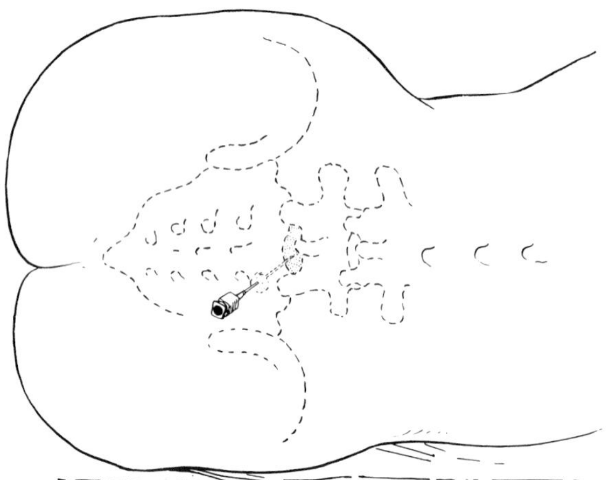

**Fig. 14–19.** With repeated frustrations in obtaining spinal fluid at the midlumbar space, it may be worthwhile to consider entry just above the rim of the sacrum. This area is said to be open and unaffected by some of the problems that affect the spaces above. The needle is introduced 1 cm cephalad and medial to posterior-superior iliac spine with a slight bias toward both the medial and cephalic directions.

## *Subarachnoid Tap*

One of the major advantages of the spinal method of analgesia is the free flow of spinal fluid, which serves as the immediate evidence of success. When the larger 22-gauge needle is used, the appearance of spinal fluid is almost immediate, but when the smaller 25- or 26-gauge needle is used, one must be patient for a few seconds before appearance of spinal fluid. If no fluid appears, the needle can be rotated on its axis to avoid the possibility of the end of the needle being occluded by a nerve root (Figure 14–21) or too deep a penetration to the posterior longitudinal ligament (Figure 14–22). It is usually not advisable to take time to aspirate fluid because fluid should return if the needle is correctly positioned. In the

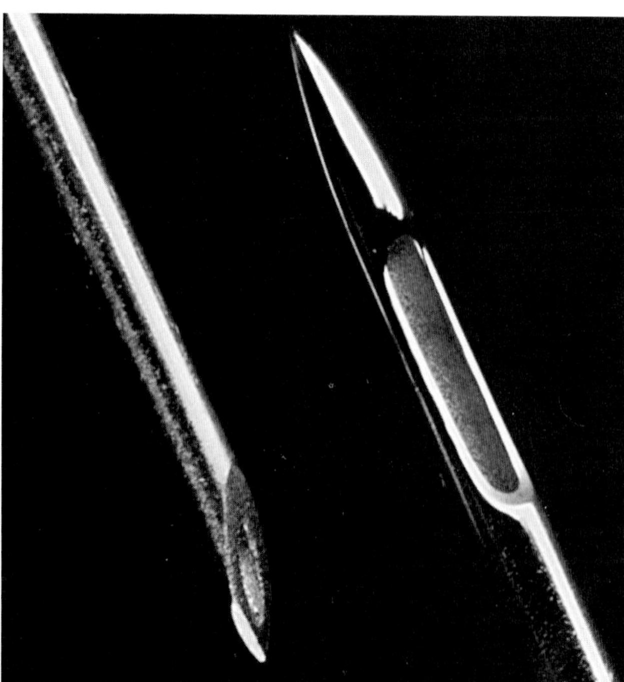

**Fig. 14–20.** Comparison of the points of two 25-gauge needles, the slanted needle (left) and the "pencil point" needle (right). (Photo courtesy of Ohio State University)

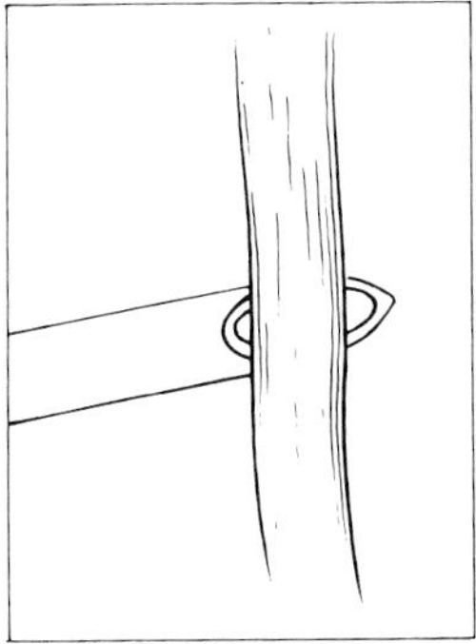

Fig. 14–21. One of the frustrations of subarachnoid block. A portion of the needle bevel is in the spinal fluid space, so that fluid is aspirated, but upon injection of the anesthetic, much of it is distributed outside the spinal space through the portion of the needle that rests outside the space.

case where a couple of punctures have not been successful, operators should take a moment with observation of the patient's position, needle direction, and depth of penetration so that they can reposition the needle more successfully the next time. The cerebrospinal fluid should be clear and if it is blood tinged, it should be allowed to flow until it does clear. If it does not clear, the stylet should be replaced and the needle slightly withdrawn, presumably out of a blood vessel. If difficulty is repeatedly encountered, the needle should be withdrawn completely, the position of the patient carefully checked, and a visual, anatomical three-dimensional picture created to help the operator understand what is causing the failures to occur. While it is permissible to make two or three attempts at one interspace, promiscuous probing should be strictly avoided. Choose another interspace. Finally, if difficulty is encountered in the subsequent interspace, the lateral or paramedian approach should be attempted or the Taylor technique tried.

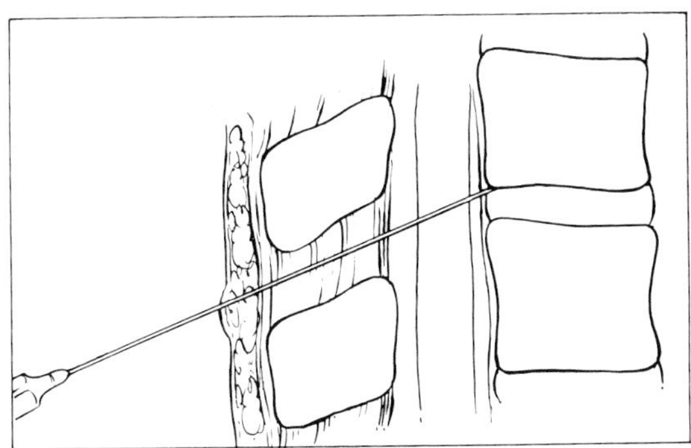

Fig. 14–22. Another reason for spinal block failure. **A,** The needle is within the spinal space, but the tip is at the very front part of the space. **B,** The operator has noted free flow of fluid, attached the anesthetic-filled syringe to the needle, and, without his knowledge, simultaneously allowed the needle tip to move forward ever so slightly. The tip now rests *outside* the spinal fluid space in the area of the posterior longitudinal ligament.

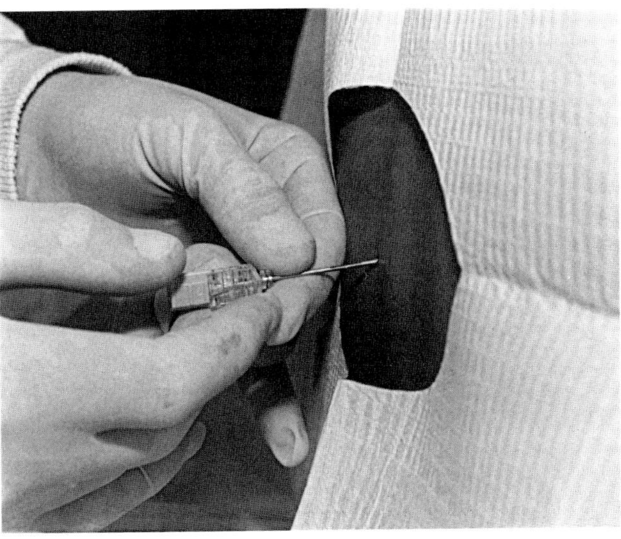

Fig. 14–23. Movement of the needle can be reduced by placement of the hand against the patient's back and *locking* the thumb and forefinger tightly onto the needle hub. In this way, when the syringe is placed onto the hub, minimal forward movement can be assured. (Photo courtesy of Ohio State University)

## *Injection of Analgesic Agent*

In adapting the syringe to the needle, the hub of the needle is grasped between the index finger and thumb of the left hand, with the operator's hand resting against the skin of the patient's back to steady it (Figure 14–23). The syringe is adapted to the needle by rotating the shaft around the needle's long axis, instead of trying to push two individual pieces together. Once this is completed, a small amount (0.1 ml) of cerebrospinal fluid is aspirated to again ascertain the proper position of the needle, and then the local anesthetic solution injected at a rate of 1 ml/3 to 5 seconds. During injection, one may wish to aspirate to ensure free flow and to be certain that the point of the needle remains within the subarachnoid space throughout injection. When the needle is withdrawn, it is important to take time to place the fingers just at the skin surface and pull the needle out observing its direction and depth so that the next time on a patient of similar build, you can better gauge the depth and direction of needle placement; in essence, each puncture should be a learning process for the operator regardless of how many times he has performed the procedure.

## *Position of Patient after Injection*

After injection is completed in the preferred position, i.e., sitting for a classical saddle block, lateral decubitus for a low spinal or high spinal for cesarean section, it is important to carefully position the patient yourself. First of all, before the procedure is completed you should make the patient aware of the necessity of letting you handle all the aspects of positioning with your assistant. Admonish the patient not to cough, Valsalva, grunt or attempt to move herself in the few moments just after drug placement. It is during this time that careful positioning can make the difference between success and failure of the level of analgesia and attendant complications such as hypotension. In all cases, first make sure the head of the patient is above the spinal level so that an extremely high level does not occur by mistake (Figure 14–24). Second, begin to take blood pressures every minute for the next 10 to 15 minutes so that you can be warned early of a fall in systemic pressure. Third, at the same time begin to evaluate the level of the spinal block by use of either a blunted needle with pin prick or ethyl chloride for temperature definition. In this way, you can adjust the table accordingly at an early stage in an attempt to have some effect on final level. Ordinarily, the table is placed in a slightly head-up position just after supine positioning of the patient, and this is changed over the next 10 minutes or so based upon feedback of the analgesic skin level. The saddle block and low spinal methods are simple because you simply keep the head of the table substantially elevated to assure the level stays low; it is the high spinal at T-4 that is complicated and that necessitates careful attention to detail in the first few minutes after injection of the drug. The goal of course is to make sure the level is not too low and at the same time make sure it does not ascend above the T-4 level to avoid severe problems with hypotension. In any event, as mentioned earlier in this chapter, one can quickly counteract hypotension with left uterine displacement and elevation of the patient's legs straight into the air, with the patient assuming the "reverse L" position (Figure 14–25). This is followed by use of small amounts of ephedrine to assure continued blood pressure stability.

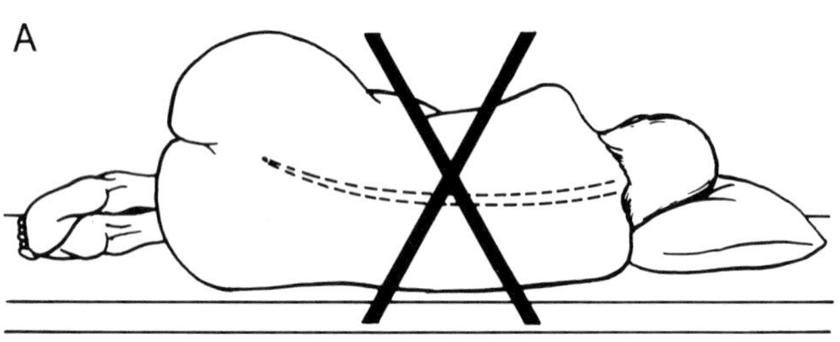


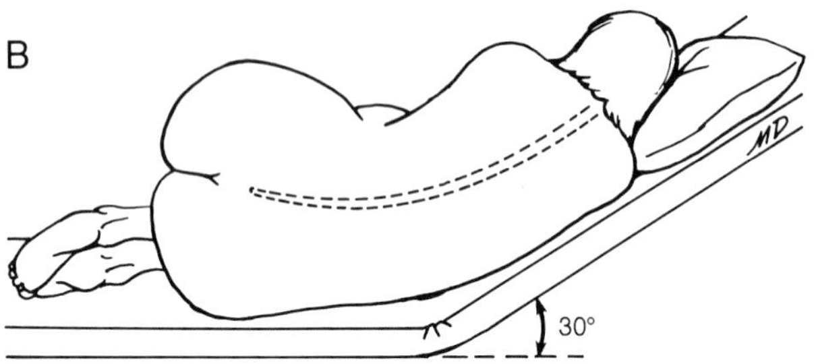


**Fig. 14–24.** It is most important to remember that the spinal level after injection can be influenced greatly by patient positioning. This figure shows why it is important to immediately place the patient in a slight head-up position just after turning and why not to leave the patient in the lateral neutral position very long. The block will become elevated because of the lateral curvature of the spinal canal due to the greater hip width over the shoulder width and, of course, the block will tend to be higher on the downside of the patient with standard hyperbaric solutions. (Photo courtesy of Ohio State University)

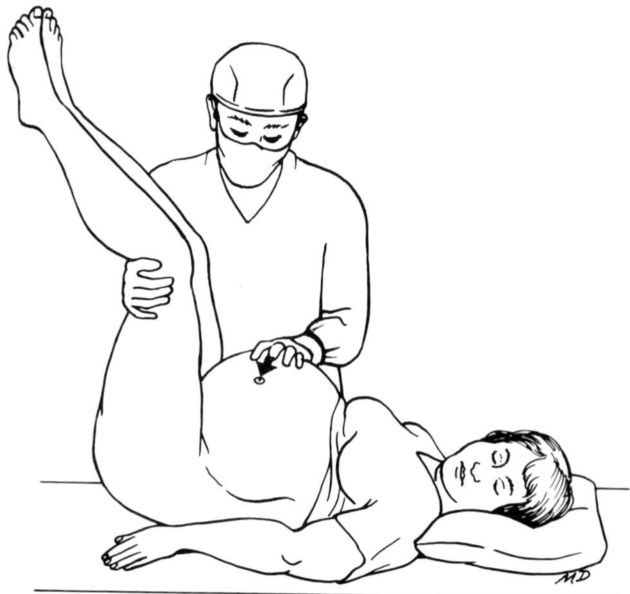

**Fig. 14–25.** Obese patient in "reverse L" position with sustained left uterine displacement to prevent maternal hypotension. The leg elevation provides extra intraveolar fluid volume almost instantaneously.

## Specific Technique for Vaginal Delivery

### *Original "Saddle Block" Technique*

The standard technique originally described by Adriani and associates, (5–9) is shown in Figure 14–26 and described in detail in the legend. This technique is duplicated here similar to as it was presented in the first edition of this book because of its importance still today. There is no question that this method of analgesia has been the mainstay of primigravidae pain relief for second stage delivery for nearly 5 decades since its popularization in 1943. There are tales of anesthesiologists at lying-in hospitals becoming so adept at this technique that they were able to perform the procedure in remarkably brief times. Some claim they could perform the spinal and obtain a block in less than 60 seconds, others claimed and have records to prove that they performed over 32 spinals in a 28-hour period. (Ray T. Smith, Jr., MD, written communication, February 1991).

The subarachnoid injection is usually made at lumbar interspace number three or four. Today, the preferential drugs are 5% lidocaine or 0.5% bupivacaine, rather than 1% tetracaine. The patient is kept in the sitting position after drug administration for 30 to 60 seconds. After this she is placed in typical lithotomy position for delivery with a pillow under her head for comfort. The delivery table is also positioned so that it is in a 30° head up tilt to make sure the level remains low. Just as is the case after any drug injection into the subarachnoid space, the

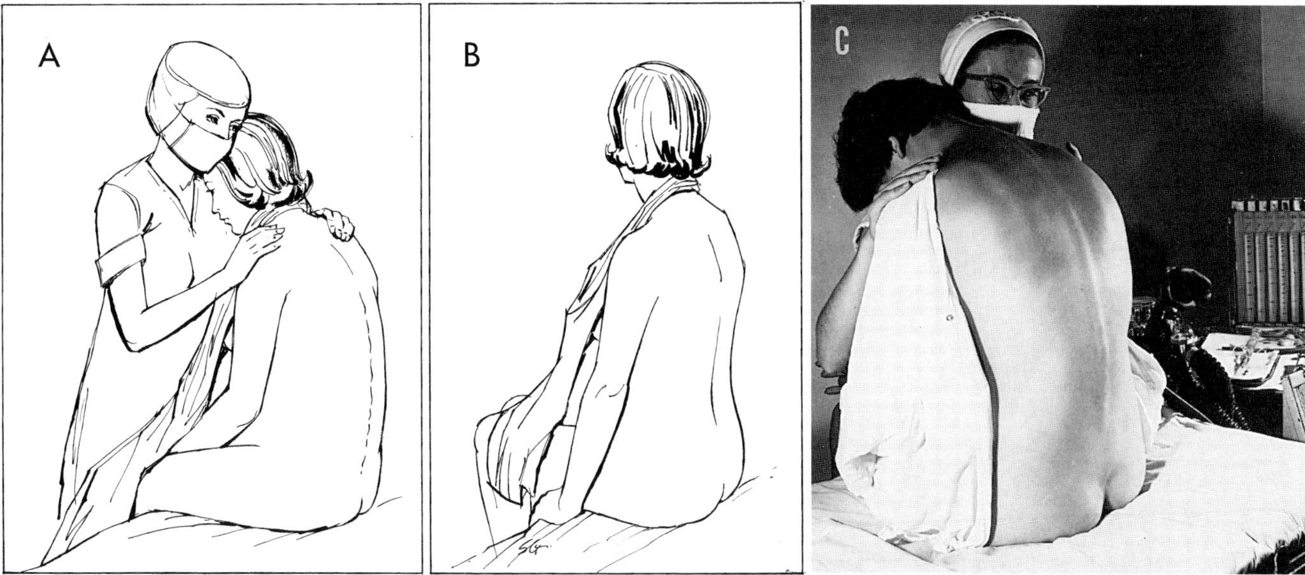


Fig. 14–26. The classic sitting position that helped popularize the "saddle block" technique in the early 1940s.

parturient is asked to refrain from coughing or using the Valsalva maneuver for 5 or so minutes after injection.

### *Mid-Subarachnoid Block*

To produce analgesia for a mid-subarachnoid block the authors prefer use of the lateral decubitus position because of comfort for the mother. Often at this time, the fetal head is right on the perineum so it is certainly more comfortable and most likely more protective for the fetus also. The same drugs are preferred in these cases as mentioned above for saddle block because of their rapid setup. The injection is made slowly, and directly after the needle is withdrawn, the patient is gently turned to the supine position. Immediately after assumption of the supine position, the table is placed in the 30° head up position and sensory levels tested every minute until a satisfactory T-10 level is reached. It is important to remember that the level can be shifted during this early time after injection of the drug and that the safety is assured by careful attention to detail in positioning immediately after the block and adjustments instituted thereafter accordingly.

## Technique of Subarachnoid Block for Cesarean Section

For cesarean section subarachnoid analgesia should extend to the upper thoracic levels but not beyond the fourth thoracic dermatome. This level is adequate for the abdominal incision, manipulation of the uterus, and the discomfort inherent in manipulation of various visceral mesentery and upper intra-abdominal structures. Puncture and injection are carried out in the usual manner as noted previously in this chapter with the patient in the more comfortable lateral decubitus position, with the table adjusted so that the plane of the subarachnoid space is in a slight head up position with horizontal plane. Otherwise, the mechanics of the puncture are identical to what has already been described earlier. After injection, the patient is placed in the supine position with left uterine displacement, the head of the table elevated so that there is nearly a 20 to 30° plane with the horizontal, and the sensory level checked every minute over the next 5 minutes. A pillow is placed under the patient's head for comfort, and the table position can be changed frequently depending upon the level of the block so that a sensory level of near T-4 can be achieved. Particular care should be taken in moving the patient from the lateral to the supine position, as this maneuver can result in a significant increase in intra-abdominal pressure, with consequent sudden change in cerebrospinal fluid pressure, which, in turn, can produce turbulence and increase the spread of the local anesthetic and, in turn, the analgesic level.

## Technique of Continuous Subarachnoid Block

Continuous subarachnoid block for cesarean section, and even for labor, surprisingly came into use in some hospitals as early as 1940 for about a decade after Lemmon first described the technique. (44,45). The technique soon fell into disuse because of a combination of factors, including the concerns over sterility, headaches with the use of a large 16-gauge needle, possible injury to exposed nerve roots, and the fact that the need for a continuous method was less popular due to the introduction of new, longer-acting agents. Despite Bizzarri's introduction in 1964 of a special 20- or 21-gauge thin-walled needle through which a soft radiopaque catheter could be introduced, there was not a revitalization of the continuous technique. Now some thirty years later, there seems to be a rekindled interest based soundly upon its solid application to the special problem of managing the morbidly obese parturient. There is also new technology available in the form of new continuous disposable equipment for the procedure (Figure 14–27). There is little question that this type of pregnant patient has presented many seri-

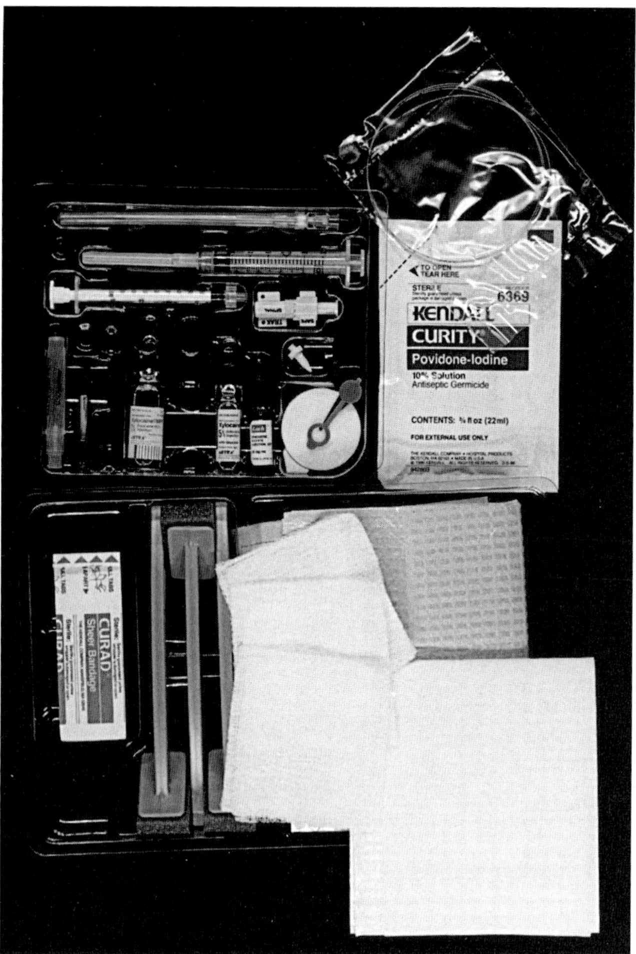


**Fig. 14–27.** A typical disposable *continuous* spinal-block kit. The use of the 22-gauge needle and the 25-gauge catheter has helped improve the success of the continuous technique greatly. (Photo courtesy of Ohio State University)

ous challenges to management over the past years and may be one of the chief causes of maternal morbidity and mortality of recent years (46–49). Certainly, many of the complications of past years associated with mismanagement of regional anesthetics, lack of anesthesiologists for obstetric anesthesiology, and lack of organization of obstetric anesthesia units in maternity centers has been largely overcome by recent commitment by scores of anesthesiologists all over the country who have answered the call to improve this area of our speciality of anesthesiology. In recent years, there have been reports of the concern about the security of the airway of the morbidly obese patient, and now there are those who believe the continuous subarachnoid block is the answer to this problem. The authors presented a solution to management of such a problem at a perinatal conference in the summer of 1990 and suggested at that time that the continuous spinal should be administered to all morbidly obese patients so that it could be used for labor with first stage narcotic injections, and, should a cesarean section subsequently be indicated, then small aliquots of 5% lidocaine could be substituted for development of a rapid, adequate analgesic level (50,51). Naturally, even the successful lumbar puncture may be difficult in a morbidly obese patient, and the passage of a small spinal catheter only compounds that problem, but the use of the paramedian technique and careful attention to passing of the catheter can often overcome these obstacles (Figure 14–28). It is important to recall that often the sitting position will aid the success here because of the superficial skin folds occluding the anatomy in the lateral decubitis position (Figure 14–29). There are also several different-sized disposable needles available today that greatly enhance success (Table 14–7). The ideal point about use of this method is that it also answers the question about what to do in cases of declaration of emergency cesarean section for fetal distress. In as few as only 2 to 3 minutes after the injection of the hyperbaric 5% lidocaine, the extent of skin hypalgesia and analgesia can be determined by the usual pinprick test. If the spread of anesthetic is closely followed by repeated testing, spread of the anesthetic above the desired level can be promptly detected and diffusion of the drug reversed by adjusting the patient's position. Changes in the parturient's position to reverse drug diffusion should be made within the first 5 minutes after injection.

Because small aliquots of the drug can be injected slowly and the eventual level more gradually developed in most cases except those declared emergency, the usual fall in systemic pressure of nearly 20% of patients usually does not occur. However, if the blood pressure should drop more than 20 mm Hg, active treatment must be instituted. In addition to administering oxygen, the patient is placed in the previously mentioned "reverse L" position with the uterus displaced to the left for 1 to 2 minutes and then placed flat again. If these maneuvers are not effective within 30 seconds, and the pressure still remains down, a vasopressor is used. The vasopressor of choice

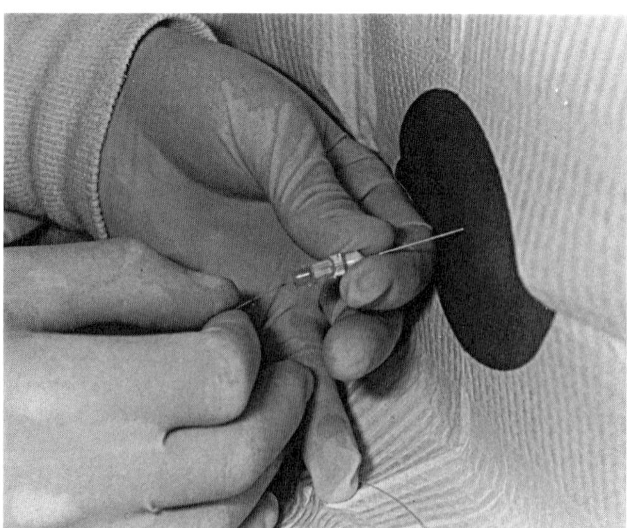

**Fig. 14–28.** Because the needle angle is augmented, passage of the catheter will be aided occasionally by the use of the paramedian technique, allowing for easier catheterization into the subarachnoid space.

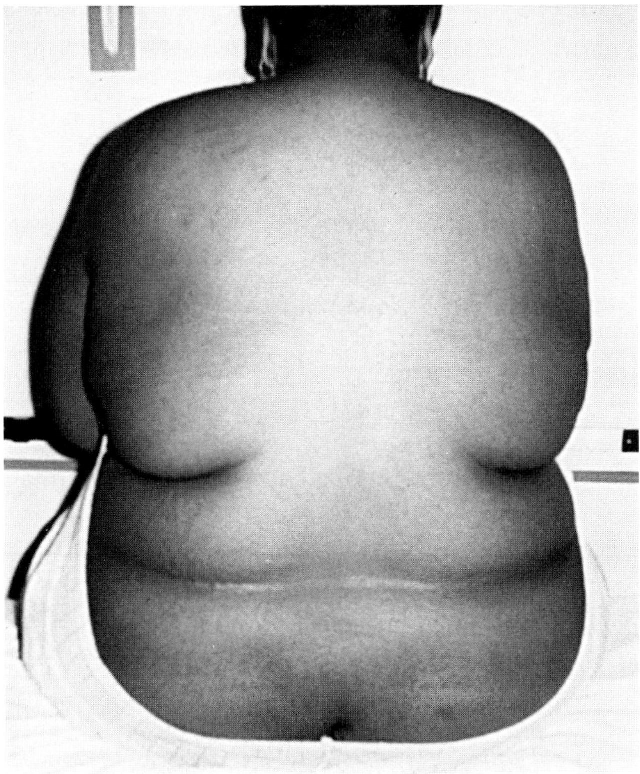

**Fig. 14–29.** Demonstration of how spinous process location by a standard 3½ in. 25-gauge spinal needle can help visualize the midline and location of the laminar processes. The longer 5 or 7 in. 22-gauge spinal needle is used to "walk" off the lamina in the paramedian approach or to penetrate the three ligamentous layers in the midline technique.

is, of course, ephedrine in intermittent aliquots of 10 mg injected intravenously.

An important question that must be asked is: Can the anesthetic-associated causes of maternal mortality in obese parturients be lessened by use of regional anesthetics for all or nearly all cesarean sections? If it is true that the majority of deaths of mothers are due to failed intubation and patient airway, then it is probably time that we made our colleague obstetricians aware of this sobering fact and encouraged their support for regional anesthesia for all of these obese pregnant patients.

Finally, to belabor the point, and to once and for all discourage the use of general anesthesia in the morbidly obese parturient who may present an airway problem, let us review that these obese pregnant patients are at great risk because of those reasons listed in Table 14–8. All of these reasons spell potential disaster for the unsuspecting anesthesiologist who is not well-acquainted with the multiplicity of these hazards and the patient and her unborn baby.

One of the very early discussions that must be aired with the anesthesiologists and the obstetricians is the question of regional anesthesia, even in light of the declared cesarean section. In past years, it has always been assumed and, in fact, practiced that these would be done under general anesthesia because it was faster. This is not necessarily so, and where the life of the mother may hang in the balance, it certainly makes sense to reevaluate this past practice, especially because often the subarachnoid block may really not take much longer than the complete process of induction of general anesthesia with laryngoscopy and intubation (52–54).

**Table 14–8.** Risk Factors in the Morbidly Obese Pregnant Patient

(1) elevated diaphragm
(2) incompetent gastroesophageal sphincter
(3) higher incidence of low pH
(4) higher gastric volume
(5) excessively heavy breasts
(6) reduced functional reserve capacity

## Causes of Failure

No one likes to be thought of as a failure. In medicine, two of the most common failures on an everyday basis are inability to start an IV and inability to do a spinal. Both of these experiences are tremendously ego-reducing. But everyone now and then will have a problem with a spinal. The spinal failure may be that no fluid is obtained or that no block is obtained.

The causes of the failure are different for the two different failures noted. The failure to obtain spinal fluid is usually due to misalignment of the needle, which causes the reactions listed in Table 14–9.

The failure to obtain a block after injection of anesthetic may be due to reasons listed in Table 14–10. Failure of the block is mostly due to reasons (1) and (2), which are both really technique failures due to misplacement of the anesthetic outside the subarachnoid space (55). Sometimes injection through a very long beveled needle can

**Table 14–9.** Reactions to Misalignment of Spinal Needle

(1) the needle to veer off center and miss the centrally located spinal space
(2) the needle to be advanced too far into tissues beyond the spinal space
(3) the needle to not be advanced far enough, so that it does not reach the spinal space

**Table 14–10.** Causes of Failure to Obtain Block After Anesthetic Injection

(1) needle movement out of the spinal space during anesthetic injection
(2) injection of the anesthetic into a loculated spinal space, i.e., subdural space, etc.
(3) a high spinal fluid pH
(4) an inactive anesthetic agent
(5) patient resistance to the anesthetic

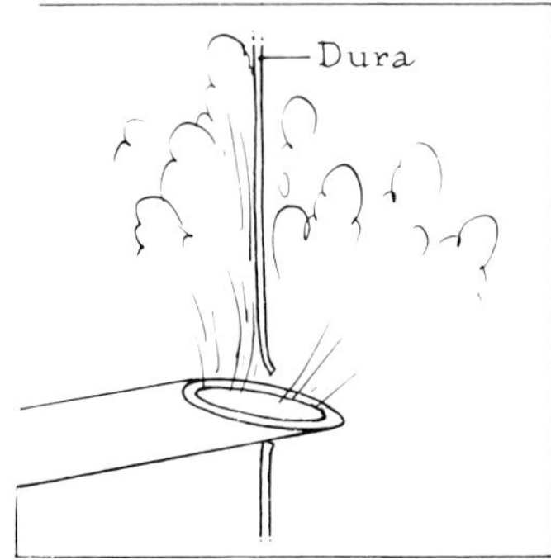


**Fig. 14–30.** Loss of anesthetic potency because of injection partly outside the spinal space, due to slight needle movement during injection.

be a problem in this regard (Figure 14–30). In such a case, fluid aspiration can be accomplished but upon injection a large portion of the anesthetic may be misplaced. Last, but not least, some of the newer, longer, very small-gauge needles may have such high resistance that no fluid is aspirated despite the needle tip being accurately placed within the subarachnoid space (56).

## *Complications*

The various complications of subarachnoid block include: (1) physiologic complications, such as the cardiac problems of bradycardia, and even arrest; (2) nonphysiologic complications, including the total anesthetic block with respiratory arrest and toxic reactions; and (3) neurologic complications, including paraplegia, arachnoiditis, and the enigmatic post dural puncture headache.

## *Post Dural Puncture Headache*

The post dural puncture headache is such a notoriously noted complication of the spinal method of anesthesia that it will be mentioned briefly here. When the first edition of this book was written, its incidence and diagnosis was similar to that of today, but its treatment was radically different. Its primary treatment in the late 1960s was bed rest, medication and hydration, plus a tincture of time. It was and still is a devastating complication because the mother so wants to be with, take care of, and bond with her newborn baby, and, at the same time she is responsible for receiving and greeting various visitors and relatives—hardly a time when she wants to be restricted to a supine position suffering from a horrendous headache. The treatment in the early 1970s shifted to a more aggressive epidural blood patch. Early reports were favorable and complications from the treatment few, although a large fraction of physicians were concerned about later repercussions in the form of epidural band formation and obliteration of the epidural space altogether. Most important, there were no neurologic sequelae and by the late 1970s, it was accepted as the primary method for relief of the post dural puncture headache syndrome. Other effective methods, including caffeine injections, are detailed along with the results of the epidural blood patch method in Chapter 16, Complications of Regional Anesthesia.

There is little question that the smaller gauge needle is less liable to cause a post dural puncture headache. Perhaps the recent work on fluid dynamics through dural puncture sites offers the best insight into this question. This study revealed that cerebrospinal fluid leakage stopped in a 5-minute time period in only 10% of instances of 22-gauge needle use, 28% of instances of 26-gauge needle use, and 65% of instances of 29-gauge needle use (57).

Recent innovations with needles have produced a new type of graduated or rounded tip known as the "Sprotte" needle. Another innovation, the Quincke needle of small caliber, also has sparing effects on the dura at the entry point. Such needles have encouraged renewed interest in the dream of minimal CSF loss and thus reduction in postpuncture headache sequelae. Current research focuses on comparative statistics between the two needles and ease of use in the pregnant patient (36A,58,59,60,61).

## REFERENCES

1. Pitkin GP, McCormack FC: Controllable spinal anesthesia in obstetrics. Surg. Gynecol. Obstet. 47:713, 1928.
1A. Russell IF, Holmquist EL: Subarachnoid analgesia for caesarean section. A double-blind comparison of plain and hyperbaric 0.5% bupivacaine. Br. J. Anaesth. 59(3), 1987, pp. 347–53.
2. Cosgrove SA, Hall PO, Gleeson WJ: Spinal anesthesia with particular reference to its use in obstetrics. Curr. Res. Anesth. Analg. 16:234, 1937.
2A. Mets B, Broccoli E, Brown AR: Is spinal anesthesia after failed epidural anesthesia contraindicated for ceasaren section? Anesth. Analg. 77(3), 1993, pp. 629–31.
3. DeLee JP: Obstetrics. 6th Ed. Philadelphia, W.B. Saunders Co., 1933.
4. Greenhill JP: Shall spinal anesthesia be used in obstetrics? Anesthesiology 11:283, 1950.
4A. Juhani TP, Hannele H: Complications during spinal anesthesia for cesarean delivery: a clinical report of one year's experience. Reg. Anesth. 18(2), 1993, pp. 128–31.
5. Adriani J, Roman-Vega D: Saddle block anesthesia. Amer. J. Surg. 71:12, 1946.
6. Burton H: Low spinal anesthesia during labour in cases of cardiac failure. Brit. Med. J. 2:389, 1943.
6A. Pflug AE, Halter JB: Effect of spinal anesthesia on adrenergic tone and the neuroendocrine responses to surgical stress in humans. Anesthesiology. 55(2), 1981, pp. 120–6.
7. Parmley RT, Adriani J: Saddle block anesthesia with Nupercaine in obstetrics. Am. J. Obstet. Gynecol. 52:636, 1946.
7A. Sivarajan M, Amory DW, Lindbloom LE, Schwettmann RS: Systemic and regional blood-flow changes during spinal anesthesia in the rhesus monkey. Anesthesiology. 43(1), 1975, pp. 78–88.
8. Resnick L: Heaby Nupercaine spinal analgesia in operative obstetrics with report on 394 cases. Brit. Med. J. 2:722, 1945.
9. Roman-Vega DA, Adriani J: A simplified technique for spinal anesthesia using Nupercaine. Anesth. Analg. 25:79, 1946.
10. Katz VL, Dotters DJ, Droegemeuller W: Perimortem cesarean delivery. Obstet. Gynecol. 68:571, 1986.
11. Lindsay SL, Hanson GC: Cardiac arrest in near term pregnancy. Anaesthesia 42:1074, 1987.
12. Seymour CA, Chadwick VS: Liver and gastrointestinal function in pregnancy. Postgrad. Med. J. 55:343, 1979.
13. Tindall VR: The liver in pregnancy. Clin. Obstet. Gynaecol. 2:441, 1975.

13A. Fisk NM, Storey GN: Fetal outcome in obstetric cholestasis. Br. J. Obstet. Gynaecol. 95(11), 1988, pp. 1137–43.
14. Shnider SM: Serum cholinesterase activity during pregnancy, labour and puerperium. Anesthesiology 26:335, 1965.
14A. Satyanarayana M: Maternal serum cholinesterase levels in pregnant women in healthy and diseased states. Asia Oceania J. Obstet. Gynaecol. 12(3), 1986 pp. 425–31.
15. Evans RJ, Wroe JM: Plasma cholinesterase changes during pregnancy. Anaesthesia 35:651, 1982.
15A. Evans RT, O'Callaghan J, Norman A: A longitudinal study of cholinesterase changes in pregnancy. Clin. Chem. 34(11), 1988, pp.2249–52.
16. West HJ: The clearance of bromosulphthalein from plasma as a measure of the changes in hepatic function during pregnancy and lactation in ewes. Br. Vet. J. 145:506, 1989.
17. Dunlop W: Renal physiology in pregnancy. Postgrad. Med. J. 56:642, 1979.
18. Cunningham FG, Cox SM, Harstad TW, Mason RA, et al: Chronic renal disease and pregnancy outcome. Am. J. Obstet. Gynecol. 163:453, 1990.
19. Reece EA, Winn HN, Hayslett JP, Coulehan J, et al: Does pregnancy alter the rate of progression of diabetic nephropathy? Am. J. Perinatol. 7:193, 1990.
20. Naulty JS, Hertwig L, Hunt CO, Datta S, et al: Influence of local anesthetic solution on postdural puncture headache. Anesthesiology 72:450, 1990.
21. Vargo MM, Robinson LR, Nicholas JJ, Rulin MC: Postpartum femoral neuropathy: relic of an earlier era? Arch. Phys. Med. Rehabil. 71:591, 1990.
22. Bachmann MB, Michaelis G, Biscoping J, Kleinstein J: Neurologic complication following spinal anesthesia for manual detachment of the placenta [in German]. Geburtshilfe Frauenheikd 50:231, 1990.
23. Stilma JS, de Lange JJ, Crezee FC: Bilateral central scotoma with preservation of central vision in 2 patients following caesarean section under spinal anesthesia. Doc. Ophthalmol. 67:59, 1987.
24. Haruta M, Funato T, Naka Y, Saeki N, et al: Neonatal effects of the delivery interval during cesarean section under spinal anesthesia [in Japanese]. Nippon Sanka Fujinka Gakkai Zasshi 38:2207, 1986.
25. Mincheva-Saeva M, Smilov I, Traikova V, Mlechkova L, et al: Our experience with spinal anesthesia in cesarean section [in Bulgarian]. Akush Ginekol 29:40, 1990.
26. Eckstein KL, Vicente-Eckstein A: A clinical report of 11 years' experience of anesthesia for cesarean section (n = 721)—particularly spinal anesthesia (n = 648)—in a hospital outpatient clinic (in German). Reg. Anaesth. 13:47, 1990.
27. Dmyterko W: Subarachnoid anesthesia in cesarean section (in Polish). Ginekol. Pol. 60:283, 1989.
28. Crawford JS: There is only a limited place for spinals in obstetrics. Acta. Anaesthesiol. Belg. 39:181, 1988.
29. Carrie LE: Debate on use of spinal anesthesia in obstetrics: spinal anesthesia has definite indications in obstetrics. Acta. Anaesthesiol. Belg. 39:177, 1988.
30. Kuhnert BR, Zuspan KJ, Kuhnert PM, Syracuse CD, et al: Bupivacaine disposition in mother, fetus, and neonate after spinal anesthesia for cesarean section. Anesth. Analg. 66: 407, 1987.
31. Bader AM, Datta S, Arthur GR, Benvenuti E, et al: Maternal and fetal catecholamines and uterine incision-to-delivery interval during elective cesarean. Obstet. Gynecol. 75:600, 1990.
32. Haruta M, Funato T, Naka Y, Saeki N, et al: Neonatal effects of the delivery interval during cesarean section under spinal anesthesia [in Japanese]. Nippon Sanka Fujinka Gakkai Zasshi 38:2207, 1986.
33. Macintosh RR: Lumbar Puncture and Spinal Anesthesia. 2nd Ed. Baltimore, Williams and Wilkins, 1957.
34. Nikolenko UN: Length of spinal dural sac, sex differences and correlations with the length of the spinal cord in adults. Arkh. Anat. Gistol. Embriol. 88:23, 1985.
35. Bonica JJ: The Management of Pain. 2nd Ed. Philadelphia, Lea & Febiger, 1990.
36. Frankson C, Gordh R: Headache after spinal anesthesia and a technic for lessening its frequency. Acta. Chir. Scand. 94: 443, 1946.
36A. Ross BK, Chadwick HS, Mancuso JJ, Benedetti C: Sprotte needle for obstetric anesthesia: decreased incidence of post-dural puncture headache. 17(1), 1992, pp.29–33.
37. Davis H, King WR: Densities of cerebrospinal fluid of human beings. Anesthesiology 15:666, 1954.
37A. Thornberry EA, Thomas TA: Posture and post-spinal headache. A controlled trial in 80 obstetric patients. Br. J. Anaesth. 60(2), 1988, pp. 195–7.
38. Marx GF, Saifer A, Orkin LR: Cerebrospinal fluid cells and proteins following spinal anesthesia. Anesthesiology 24:305, 1963.
39. Marx GF, Oka Y, Orkin LR: Cerebrospinal fluid proteins and spinal anesthesia in obstetrics. Anesthesiology 26:340, 1965.
39A. Davis LE: Normal laboratory values of CSF during pregnancy. Arch. Neurol. 36(7), 1979, p. 443.
40. Schwagmeier R, Schmidt A, Nolte H: The effect of injection speed and needle gauge on spinal anesthesia (in German). Reg. Anaesth. 13:148, 1990.
41. Helrich M, Papper EM, Brodie BB, Fink M, et al: The fate of intrathecal procaine and the spinal fluid level required for surgical anesthesia. J. Pharmacol. Exp. Ther. 100:78, 1950.
42. Taylor JA: Lumbosacral subarachnoid tap. J. Urol. 43:561, 1940.
43. McLeskey CH: Introducers for 25-gauge spinal needles (letter). Anesth. Analg. 62:1046, 1983.
44. Carpenter SL, Cervolo AJ, Foldes FF: Continuous-drop subarachnoid block with dilute procaine solution for labor and delivery. Amer. J. Obstet. Gynecol. 61:1277, 1951.
44A. Moran DH, Johnson MD: Continuous spinal anesthesia with combined hyperbaric and isobaric bupivacaine in a patient with scoliosis. Anesth. Analg. 70(4), 1990, pp.445–7.
45. Lemmon WT: A method for continuous spinal anesthesia. Ann. Surg. 111:141, 1940.
45A. Giuffrida JG, Bizzarri DV, Masi R, Bondoc R: Continuous procaine spinal anesthesia for cesarean section. Anesth. Analg. 51(1), 1972, pp. 117–24.
46. Endler GC, Mariona FG, Sokol RJ, Stevenson LB: Anesthesia related maternal mortality in Michigan 1972–1984. Am. J. Obstet. Gynecol. 159:187, 1988.
47. Hofmeister EJJ: Mothers are still mortal. South. Med. J. 71: 1193, 1978.
48. Stratmann D: Choice of anesthesia procedure in cesarean section. Reg. Anaesth. 9:94, 1986.
49. Green RA: Changes in obstetric anesthesia in the last twenty-five years. J. Int. Med. Res. 6:33, 1978.
49A. Kopacz DJ, Bridenbaugh LD: Maternal serum cholinesterase levels in pregnant women in healthy and diseased states. Reg. Anesth. 18(2), 1993, pp. 84–7.
50. Moran DH, Johnson MD: Continuous spinal anesthesia with combined hyperbaric and isobaric bupivacaine in a patient with scoliosis. Anesth. Analg. 70:445, 1990.
51. Malan TP Jr, Johnson MD: The difficult airway in obstetric

anesthesia: techniques for airway management and the role of regional anesthesia. J. Clin. Anesth. 1:104, 1988.
52. Marx GF, Luykx WM, Cohen S: Fetal-neonatal status following caesarean section for fetal distress. Br. J. Anaesth. 56: 1009, 1984.
53. Gale R, Zalkinder-Luboshitz I, Slater PE: Increased neonatal risk from the use of general anesthesia in emergency cesarean section. A retrospective analysis of 374 cases. J. Reprod. Med. 27:715, 1982.
54. Ramanathan J, Ricca DM, Sibai BM, Angel JJ: Epidural vs general anesthesia in fetal distress with various abnormal fetal heart rate patterns. Anesth. Analg. 67:S180, 1988.
55. Levy JH, Islas JA, Ghia JN, Turnbull C: A retrospective study of the incidences and causes of failed spinal anesthetics in a university hospital. Anesth. Analg. 64:705, 1985.
56. Toomey PJ: Resistance to fluid flow through two spinal needles. Anaesthesia 45:751, 1990.
57. Cruikshank RH, Hopkinson JM: Fluid flow through dural puncture sites. Anaesthesia 44:415:1989.
58. Lewis IH: Headache after spinal anesthesia for cesarean section: a comparison of the 27-gauge Quincke and 24-gauge Sprotte needles [letter]. Anesth. Analg. 76(6), 1993, p. 1377.
59. Mayer DC, Quance D, Weeks SK: Headache after spinal anesthesia for cesarean section: a comparison of the 27-gauge Quincke and 24-gauge Sprotte needles. Anesth. Analg. 75(3), 1992, pp. 377–80.
60. Pollock JE, Neal JM: Postdural puncture headache with a Sprotte needle [letter]. Reg. Anesth. 17(1), 1992, pp. 54–55.

# Chapter 15

# OTHER REGIONAL ANALGESIC/ANESTHETIC TECHNIQUES

JOHN J. BONICA
JOHN S. McDONALD

This chapter is devoted to discussion of regional analgesic/anesthetic techniques not considered in the two preceding chapters. These techniques are presented in order of importance, based on frequency of use, efficacy, simplicity of the technique, and the incidence and degree of side effects and complications. Five techniques are included: 1) bilateral pudendal block; 2) local anesthesia of the perineum to provide analgesia/anesthesia for the second and third stages of labor; 3) paracervical block; 4) lumbar sympathetic block to provide analgesia for the relief of general labor pain due primarily to uterine contractions; and 5) local infiltration and field block for cesarean section. Four miscellaneous regional techniques—thoracic paravertebral block, transsacral block, presacral block, and intracutaneous infiltration of the lower abdomen—discussed in the first edition of this book, are not considered because they are rarely, if ever, used in modern obstetric practice.

Each of the five techniques discussed affords the following advantages: 1) they can be carried out by the obstetrician and are especially useful in hospitals where expert obstetric anesthesia service provided by anesthesiologists is not available; 2) properly carried out, they provide effective analgesia/anesthesia for the specific indication; 3) generally, they are inherent in not producing serious harmful effects on the mother or the fetus, nor do they cause deleterious action on labor. Unfortunately, these very desirable advantages have caused many obstetricians and generalists doing obstetrics to be misled into thinking that: 1) these techniques are simple to carry out; 2) they require little or no knowledge of their anatomic basis or the clinical pharmacology of local anesthetics; 3) many obstetricians have used these without proper instructions in regional anesthesia; and 4) most importantly, they have had no knowledge or clinical experience in the prevention and treatment of side effects and complications of regional anesthesia. Although these methods are always mentioned as the most useful analgesic procedures for nonanesthesiologists, little space is devoted to a description of these techniques or those aspects mentioned above in the average obstetric textbook. Indeed, in the most recent two-volume edition of Williams' classic textbook on obstetrics (1), only three-fourths of a page is devoted to a description of pudendal block (although two illustrations are included), one paragraph to paracervical block, while other techniques are not mentioned at all. Consequently, this has resulted in a disappointingly high incidence of failures and complications. It is for these reasons that they are considered here in great detail for physicians practicing obstetrics.

In discussing each of these five techniques, the format used in the two preceding chapters is followed. The material is presented in three subsections: 1) a brief historical overview of its development and clinical use; 2) clinical evaluation, including assessment of its efficacy for analgesia/anesthesia and effects on the mother, on labor, and on the fetus and newborn; and 3) technical considerations, including: anatomic basis for the procedure; agent and equipment required; c) detailed description of the techniques; and mention of complications and how to prevent them. (A more detailed discussion of these complications is presented in the next chapter.) This chapter is an update of the chapters in the first edition of the book and a summary of the most important studies carried out after the publication of the first edition. An important difference in format between this and the first edition is that the description of the technique is presented as the legend under the illustration, and thus precludes the often-encountered annoyance and frustration of having to turn pages when the text and the illustrations are presented in pages that are separate and apart.

## BILATERAL PUDENDAL NERVE BLOCK

Bilateral pudendal nerve block in obstetric practice was first described in 1908 by Mueller (2) in Germany and was widely advocated by Ilman and Sellheim (3), and Ilmer (4) two years later. In 1916, King (5) published the first American article, an excellent dissertation on the subject. Since that time, many techniques and modifications of techniques have been described. Most of these involve not only block of the two pudendal nerves, but also multiple, almost indiscriminate infiltration of the perineum, which, because it is richly vascular, usually resulted in numerous small hemorrhages with a consequent increase in postpartum morbidity. The scholarly presentation by Klink (6) contained a refinement of the transperineal approach. His studies demonstrated that if each nerve is properly blocked in its position near the ischial spine, the resultant analgesia is sufficient and additional infiltration of the perineum not necessary. This has proved to be one of the most significant advances in obstetric anesthesia.

Another extremely important refinement in pudendal block has been the widespread use of the transvaginal approach. Although this technique was said to have been first used by Dugger (7) and Sheares (8) in 1948 and by Kobak (9) in 1950, it was my late colleague, Dr. Gerald Kohl of Tacoma, Washington, who, in 1954, published the first article advocating this approach (10). Dugger and Kobak published their first reports two years later, and Sheares never published his account but was cited by Apgar (11). During the ensuing decades, numerous articles have been published proclaiming its ease, reliability, and safety over the transperineal approach (12–23). The popularity of this technique has remained fairly steady, especially in the United States, Scandinavia, western European countries, the United Kingdom, Australia, and South Africa, as indicated in Table 1–4 and Table 1–8 (see end of Chapter 1). In the obstetric survey of the United States, carried out by Gibbs and associates in 1981–1982 and published in 1986 (24), pudendal block and local infiltration were not differentiated, but both techniques were carried out by obstetricians in 54% of the parturients delivered in obstetric units that had more than 1,500 births; in 68% in units that had 500 to 1499 births; and 59% in units that had less than 500 births for an overall mean of 59%. Surveys of major obstetric units that have obstetric anesthesia training programs indicate that pudendal block is being used less frequently consequent to the increase in the use of continuous epidural analgesia, but even in these units it is being used for vaginal delivery in about one-third of the parturients who receive pharmacologic analgesia (see Table 1–9). In countries other than those mentioned above, it is used less frequently than local infiltration of the perineum, a procedure that is used in some 30 to 80% of the vaginal deliveries (see Table 1–10 to 1–13 in Chapter 1).

The transvaginal approach is simpler to carry out, and there is less risk of infection or hemorrhage than in the transperineal approach and less discomfort to the parturient. However, it must be done before the presenting part completely fills the vagina. If the block is done late in labor, it is better to use the transperineal approach rather than to push the presenting part out of the way (and possibly provoke undue pressure on it) in order to do the transvaginal technique.

During the 1950s and 1960s, the widespread use of paracervical block became another important development in contributing to the usefulness of pudendal block in obstetrics. Because pudendal block does not relieve pain of uterine contractions, the combined use of paracervical and pudendal block should provide the obstetrician or generalist peforming obstetrics with a method of regional anesthesia that affords the parturient good pain relief during the latter phase of the first stage and during the entire second and third stages of labor. As discussed later, in recent years the use of paracervical block has decreased significantly in most institutions because of side effects on the fetus, but it is still being used for labor in some parturients and even more widely to provide analgesia for therapeutic abortion, for artificial insemination, and other painful procedures inherent in manipulation of the cervix.

## Clinical Evaluation

Of a small number of well-planned and controlled studies on bilateral pudendal block (BPB), two provide among the most comprehensive overview on its effect on the mother, labor, and on the fetus (18,19). The study by Zador and associates (19) provides comprehensive data on 24 randomly selected healthy parturients with uncomplicated pregnancies, in spontaneous labor, and with the fetus in the vertex position. In this study, BPB was achieved with injection of 10 ml of 1% lidocaine on each side of which 14 parturients (group I) received plain lidocaine, ($L_o$) and in 10 parturients epinephrine 1/200,000 was added to the solution ($L_E$) (group II). A control series of 24 parturients (group III) fulfilling the same criteria of normality as the other two groups was used. Analgesia during the first stage of labor was achieved with 50% nitrous oxide-50% oxygen, and in a few 10 mg diazepam was given early in the first stage. The second study, carried out by our group at the University of Washington (18), provides comprehensive data on the effects of BPB on the forces of labor and will be described under that section. Additional studies with pertinent information on one or more aspects of obstetric analgesia and anesthesia are cited.

### *Analgesia/Anesthesia*

Properly executed BPB alone is sufficient to produce highly effective perineal analgesia/anesthesia for spontaneous delivery, low forceps delivery, episiotomy, and repair (7–19b). As shown by Klink (6), and subsequently confirmed by many other clinicians, it is not necessary to block the ilioinguinal nerve, the genital branch of the genitofemoral nerve, and the perineal branch of the posterior femoral cutaneous nerve to provide almost complete pain relief during the second and third stages of labor. By using dilute solutions of local anesthetics (e.g., 0.5 to 0.75% lidocaine or 0.125 to 0.25% bupivacaine) analgesia with minimal muscle relaxation is achieved, whereas higher concentrations (e.g., 1.5 to 2.0% lidocaine or 0.375 to 0.5 bupivacaine) produce paralysis of the perineal muscles.

In their study, Zador and associates (19) assessed the efficacy of the block by three methods: 1) the area of dermal anesthesia by pinprick testing 10 minutes after the injection; 2) patients were asked to evaluate the degree of pain relief during the first part of the second stage (S), during expulsion of the fetus (D), and repair of episiotomy or lacerations (R) using a scale of 0 to 3, with 0 indicating complete pain relief and a total of 9 as no relief during any of the three periods; 3) assessment by the midwife using audible or visible reactions to pain during the same three time periods. The total score could range from 0, indicating total absence of reaction to pain, to 27, indicating no relief. The results were summarized in two tables that indicated that in two parturients analgesia on the right side was inadequate and that one of these had the highest pain score. The table indicates that the $L_E$ group had a cumulative score from the six subcategories (three from the patient and three from the midwife) of 36, out of a total score of 348 or 10.3%, while the $L_o$ group had a cumulative score of 91 out of a possible 420 total, or 21.6%. Because the lower the score the better the pain relief, parturients who received $L_E$ solution had much better pain relief than those who received plain lidocaine. The authors point out that the higher pain scores with $L_o$ can be explained in part by the fact that after a period of acceptable analgesia, the pain returned toward the end of the second stage of rather long duration (50 to 100 minutes). With $L_E$, low pain scores were recorded even in parturients who delivered 85 to 115 minutes after the administration of the block. Also, the belief was expressed by the authors that the addition of epinephrine to the local anesthetic improved the quality of the block.

Finally, epinephrine decreased the maternal and fetal blood level of lidocaine. As with other regional techniques, significant amounts of local anesthetic are found 5 to 8 minutes after the injection, attaining peak levels 10 to 30 minutes later, and then gradually decaying to lower levels. In group I ($L_o$), mean lidocaine concentration in μg/ml increases from 0.8 at 5 minutes after the injection to a peak level of about 1.1 within 10 to 20 minutes, and then declines continuously to 0.6 at 90 minutes after the block, and was 1.0 at delivery. In fetal scalp blood, the mean concentration in μg/ml increased from 0.4 at 5 minutes after the injection to a level of about 0.6 at 20 minutes, and this was maintained for about 30 minutes. The mean values for lidocaine concentration in the umbilical vein and artery were 0.4 and 0.3, respectively. In group II ($L_E$), the mean lidocaine concentration in μg/ml in maternal blood was 0.5 at 5 minutes after injection (0.3 μg/ml lower than the corresponding level in group I), then reached a peak level of 0.8 during the period 10 to 20 minutes after injection, and then declined gradually to 0.5 at 90 minutes, and was 0.8 at delivery. In fetal scalp blood, the mean concentration in μg/ml was 0.4 at 5 minutes, then rose to 0.5 at 10 to 20 minutes, and declined to 0.3 at 50 minutes. The umbilical vein and umbilical artery values were 0.4 and 0.3, respectively. Zador and associates (19) mentioned that the maternal blood levels appear lower after BPB than after epidural or paracervical block, but definitive data from comparative control studies are lacking. In any event, using a total of 20 ml of local anesthetic, either without or with epinephrine, produces maternal and fetal blood levels that are significantly lower than even minimal toxic levels of local anesthetics.

### *Effects on the Mother*

Properly executed pudendal block does not have deleterious effects on respiratory, cardiovascular, gastrointestinal, hepatic or other maternal bodily functions. In their comprehensive study of BPB, Zador and associates (19) found no statistically significant differences between the pH, $PCO_2$, and $BD_{ECF}$ (base deficit in extracellular fluid). Inadequate pain relief from improper block may provoke or aggravate apprehension, anxiety, fear, and cause tachycardia, hypertension, and may even cause uterine inertia due to increase of catecholamines and other hormones involved in the neuroendocrine stress response.

Possible complications include: 1) systemic toxic reactions from accidental intravenous injection; 2) trauma to the sciatic nerve resulting in anesthesia of the legs; 3) hematoma; 4) puncture of the rectum; and 5) hip pain and femoral head abscess (25). The use of very large volumes of local anesthetics (e.g., 20 to 30 ml injected into each side) to compensate for lack of anatomic knowledge and technical skill may result in systemic local anesthetic reactions with consequent convulsions that unless properly treated may cause death of the mother and fetus. A case in which pure epinephrine solution was mistakenly injected instead of the local anesthetic causing the death of the mother and fetus was reported in the older literature (26). Detailed discussion of the prevention and treatment of these complications is discussed in the next chapter.

### *Effects on the Forces of Labor*

As already mentioned, two studies are summarized here to reflect the effects of BPB on the forces of labor. The first of these carried out at the University of Washington Medical Center, Seattle, by my colleagues and I, entailed tokodynamometri (TKD) studies carried out in 42 parturients, some of whom received BPB, subarachnoid block, or continuous epidural block. The results of the first phase involving the 42 parturients were published in 1972 by the late Dr. Wayne Johnson as first author (18). Subsequently, my colleagues and I continued the study and increased the total number to 97 parturients, including studies on the effects of continuous double-catheter epidural analgesia and the use of different local anesthetic agents. Because the protocol and results are presented in detail in Chapter 4, here we summarize only the study of BPB. It is suggested that the reader review the protocol and the data in the control group in that chapter to better appreciate the results obtained with BPB.

Table 15–1 contains the results obtained in 15 parturients who received local or no anesthesia and 16 parturients given bilateral pudendal block. Data on the intensity of uterine contraction show no consistent differences. This is not surprising in view of the fact that the afferent fibers in the pudendal nerves constitute the primary limb of the reflex urge (see Figure 4–31). However, because other sacral nerves contain afferents that supply the periphery of the perineum and other pelvic structures, some parturients retain the reflex urge to bear down. Even if the reflex is eliminated, the parturient can bear down as effectively as she can without the block (sometimes even more effectively because the block relieves the perineal pain), so that she is able to deliver spontaneously. This requires imparting the parturient with ample information about the physiology of this process during the prenatal period, and then reinforcing it repeatedly during the second stage. The efficacy of voluntary bearing down is impressively down in Figure 13–20, which is the record obtained in a well-informed, highly motivated parturient working in close collaboration with an effective coach during the entire second stage.

**Table 15–1.** Intensity of Uterine Contraction (UC) and Bearing-Down Efforts (BDE) in Parturients with Local or No Anesthesia (mean mm Hg ± SD)

| Number of Patients | Parity* P | Parity* M | 1st Half of Second Stage UC | 1st Half of Second Stage BDE | 2nd Half of Second Stage UC | 2nd Half of Second Stage BDE |
|---|---|---|---|---|---|---|
| 15 | 8 | 7 | 42 ± 18 | 56 ± 22 | 46 ± 20 | 69 ± 31 |

| Number of Patients | Parity* P | Parity* M | No Coaching UC | No Coaching BDE | Coaching Before Block UC | Coaching Before Block BDE | Coaching After Block UC | Coaching After Block BDE |
|---|---|---|---|---|---|---|---|---|
| 16 | 7 | 7 | 35 ± 14 | 58 ± 19 | 38 ± 16 | 68 ± 21 | 41 ± 15 | 76 ± 21 |

* P = primipara; M = multipara

***Further comment.*** In regard to the effects of BPB on the auxiliary forces of labor, two additional issues need to be addressed. First is the necessity to have the cardinal mechanism of internal rotation take place. Dilute solutions of local anesthetics (e.g., 0.5 to 0.75 percent lidocaine or 0.125 to 0.25% bupivacaine) produce minimal depressant effect on the nerve supply to the pelvic muscle sling, so they retain some tone and thus provide the resistant forces essential for the presenting part to rotate, so that the occiput is anterior or anterolateral. This, of course, makes manipulation of the perineum more difficult for the application of forceps. On the other hand, if perineal relaxation is essential to facilitate fetal manipulation, the block is carried out with a higher concentration of LA (e.g., 1.5 to 2% lidocaine or 0.375 to 0.5% bupivacaine).

The second issue is the effect of BPB on the perineoabdominal reflex, which is involved in initiating and sustaining the bearing-down effort effectively and thus increasing the intra-abdominal and intra-amniotic pressure sufficiently to help the uterus expel the fetus. Clinical studies suggest that 35 to 45% of parturients who have BPB with high concentration lose the reflex urge to bear down (23), and in many the urge is significantly weakened for reasons given above. It deserves re-emphasis that even in such patients, with proper coaching, a well-informed and highly motivated parturient can mobilize the bearing-down efforts so that she can generate an increase in intra-abdominal and intra-amniotic pressure equal to or even higher than that generated by parturients who have no perineal anesthesia.

The importance of "voluntary" bearing-down efforts was emphasized by Zador and associates (19) in explaining the fact that duration of the second stage in primiparae who received BPB lasted 60 minutes in group I and 65 minutes in group II, whereas in the control group it lasted 45 minutes. Obviously, the control group retained the reflex urge to bear down, but in their report Zador, et al (19) imply that in the groups that received the block, the reflex urge was either absent or weakened. This is suggested by their statement that "The tendency to a prolongation of the second stage can, in our experience, be considerably reduced by liberal use of the episiotomy, proper coaching, and active assistance during the bearing-down efforts," and cite our report as one in which these procedures were practiced. They further stated that "Such an act of conduct of the second stage is often necessary in order to achieve successful, spontaneous deliveries without unnecessary delay after pudendal block." It is of interest to note that in the six multiparae in group I, the second stage lasted 25 minutes, while in the four parturients in the control group it lasted 20 minutes (no multiparae were included in group II). The significant lack of prolongation of the second stage in multiparae is undoubtedly due to condition of the perineum, which facilities more rapid delivery.

## *Effects on the Fetus and Newborn*

Properly executed BPB has no clinically significant effects on the fetus and newborn as measured by the Apgar score, acid-base values, and neurobehavioral studies (18,19,21,23). In the study by Zador and associates (19), the Apgar score in 1 minute in 14 newborns in group I was 9–10 in 12 and 7–8 in 2; in 10 newborns of group II, 9 had scores of 9–10 and one had a score of 7–8; while in 24 newborns in the control group, 22 had scores of 9–10 and two had scores of 7–8. None of the newborns in the study had scores lower than 7.

As in the mothers, no statistically significant difference could be demonstrated between the pH, $pCO_2$, and $BD_{ECF}$ values among the newborns whose mothers received BPB and those of the control group at corresponding sampling times. They did note that significant prolongation of the second stage was associated with a small, increasing tendency to fetal acidosis in both the anesthetized and the control groups. A few studies have shown that bilateral pudendal block does not have clinically significant neurobehavioral effects on the newborn.

Merkow and associates (21) studied the neurobehavioral effects of BPB achieved with 30 ml of one of three local anesthetics used in random sequence: 15 parturients had 0.5% bupivacaine, 21 received 1% mepivacaine and 18 had 3% 2-chloroprocaine. Except for a significant difference in the responses to pinprick, there was no significant effect of any of these local anesthetics on infant neurobehavior, and no differences were found among the agents themselves. Neonates in the mepivacaine-treated group had the ability to modify or abolish their response to a repeated nonmeaningful stimulus sooner than neonates in the bupivacaine- and chloroprocaine-treated groups. This difference existed only at 4 hours of age and had disappeared by 24 hours. The bupivacaine-treated group was not significantly different from the chloroprocaine-treated group. Other neurobehavioral variables in which differences might have been expected, such as muscle tone and alertness, showed no significant difference among the three local anesthetic groups. Mean mepivacaine levels in neonatal capillary blood at 4 hours of age were low (0.10 ± 0.02 l/ml) compared with those in previous studies because of the short interval between maternal injection and delivery (13 ± 3 min). Bupivacaine gave higher neonatal capillary blood levels (0.15 μg/ml at 4 hours of age) than previously reported, but the drug still produced no detectable neonatal neurobehavioral effects.

## Technical Considerations

### *Anatomic Bases*

#### Nerve Supply of the Female External Genitalia

Figures 15–1 and 15–2 illustrate the anatomy and the nerve supply of the external genitalia and perineum. The labia majora and labia minora are supplied primarily by posterior labial branches of the perineal nerve (a branch of the pudendal nerve). In addition, the lateral edge of each labium receives terminations of the perineal branches of the posterior femoral cutaneous nerve, while a small anterior portion is supplied by terminations of the anterior labial branches of the ilioinguinal and genitofemoral nerve. The extremely sensitive labia minora are abundantly supplied with vasomotor and sensory fibers by the same nerves that supply the labia majora. The mons pubis is supplied by terminal branches of the ilioinguinal and genitofemoral nerve.

The clitoris, consisting of the two corpora cavernosa and comprised primarily of erectile tissue, is richly supplied with nerve endings derived primarily from the dorsal nerve of the clitoris, which is a major branch of the pudendal nerve. The vagina is supplied primarily by the perineal branch of the pudendal nerve, although the upper part also receives afferent fibers through the nervi erigentes (pelvic nerve). The bulb of the vestibule, consisting of elongated masses of erectile tissue on either side of the vaginal orifice, contains afferent and efferent fibers supplied by both sympathetic and parasympathetic nerves.

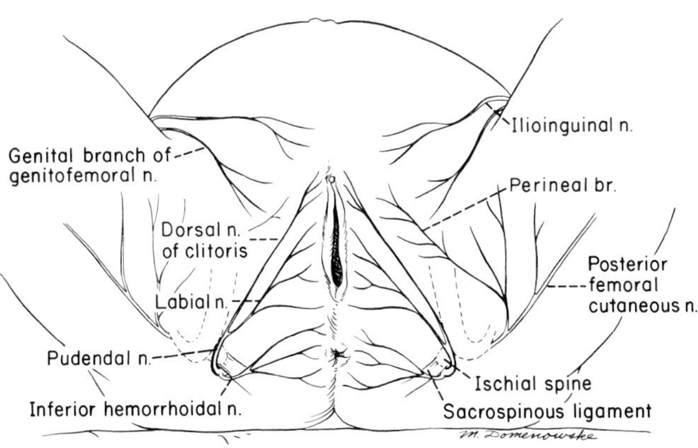


**Fig. 15–1.** The cutaneous nerve supply of the perineum. The major supply is provided by branches of the pudendal nerve, including the inferior hemorrhoidal nerve that supply the posterior portion, the superficial branch of the perineal nerve that divides into a medial and lateral parts known as the posterior labial nerves, and the dorsal nerve of the clitoris. The perineal branch of the posterior femoral cutaneous nerve, the genital of the genitofemoral nerve, and the ilioinguinal nerve supply the periphery of the perineum and are not primarily involved in transmission of pain during labor.

### *Neurology of the Perineum*

The perineum derives its nerve supply primarily from various branches of the pudendal nerve. It also receives some fibers from the anterior labial branches of the ilioinguinal, the genital branch of the genitofemoral, the perforating cutaneous and muscular branches of the second, third, and fourth sacral nerve, and the anococcygeal nerve. Because the branches of the ilioinguinal and genitofemoral need not be blocked, they are not described.

#### Pudendal Plexus

The pudendal plexus is formed by the union of the anterior divisions of the second and third sacral nerve and all of the fourth sacral nerve (Figure 14–3). This structure lies in the lower part of the posterior wall of the pelvic cavity and the anterior surface of the piriformis muscle, where it divides into the pudendal nerve, the perforating cutaneous nerve, visceral branches, and muscular branches. The visceral branches make up the pelvic nerve, which leaves the pudendal plexus and proceeds anteriorly to join the pelvic plexuses to contribute parasympathetic fibers.

The muscular branches of the pudendal plexus are provided mainly by the fourth sacral nerve to supply the levator ani, coccygeus, and sphincter ani externus muscles. The nerves to the levator ani and coccygeus muscles enter these structures on their pelvic surface. The nerve to the sphincter ani externus, generally known as the perineal branch of the fourth sacral nerve, pierces the sacrotuberous ligament and the coccygeus muscle, and enters the ischiorectal fossa to supply muscular branches to the sphincter and cutaneous branches to the skin between the anus and coccyx. The perforating cutaneous branches of the second and third sacral nerves descend in front of the coccygeus muscle and pass through it, then perforate the sacrotuberous ligament, turn around the inferior border of the gluteous maximus muscle to supply the skin of the buttocks. Some of the fibers, however, run anteriorly to the perineum. The anococcygeal nerve, derived from the fourth and fifth sacral and the coccygeal nerve, also penetrates the sacrotuberous ligaments to supply the skin behind the anus in the anococcygeal area.

### *Anatomy of the Pudendal Nerve*

The pudendal, or pubic nerve, the largest and most important branch of the pudendal plexus, is composed of somatic sensory, somatic motor, and autonomic (vasomotor) fibers. The anatomy of the nerve is shown in Figures 15–3, 15–4, and 15–5, which should be studied with the description that follows. The somatic fibers are derived

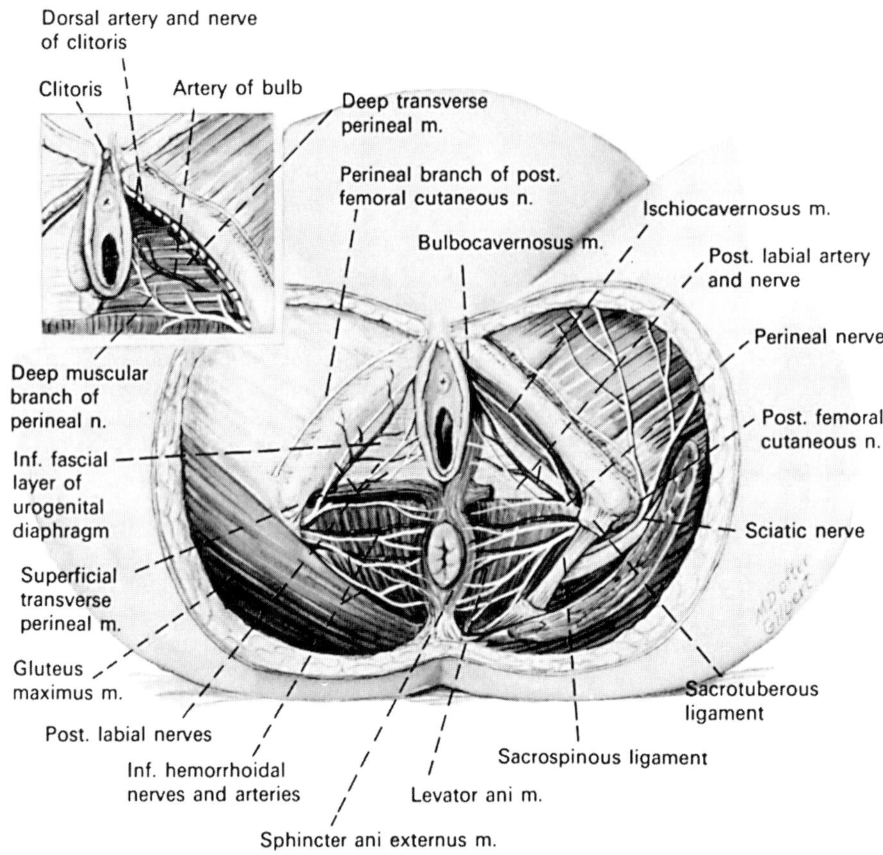


**Fig. 15–2.** Nerve supply of the perineum of a gravida showing the principal branches of the pudendal nerve, as well as the posterior femoral cutaneous nerve and other nerves that supply sensory fibers to the skin, subcutaneous tissue, external genitalia, and muscular fibers to the various muscles. The superficial transverse perineal muscles have been cut to show the course of the perineal nerve. *Inset:* Deeper dissection after inferior (superficial) fascia of the urogenital diaphragm has been removed shows the course of the dorsal nerve of the clitoris. The posterior two-thirds of the nerve passes through the thickness of the muscle.

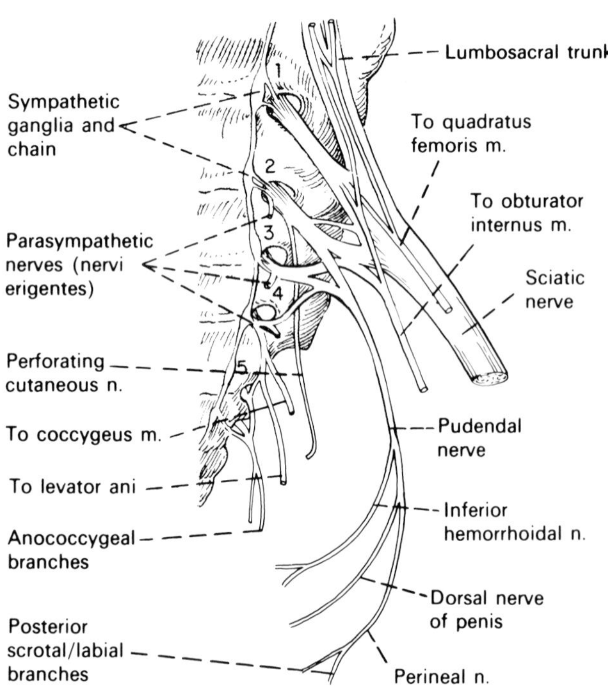


**Fig. 15–3.** **A)** Anatomy of the pudendal plexus and its branches and their relation to the large sciatic nerve and the nerves to the obturator internus and quadratus femoris muscles. The plexus is formed by the union of the anterior divisions of the second and third sacral nerve and all of the fourth sacral nerve, all of which lie in the lower part of the posterior wall of the pelvic cavity and the anterior surface of the piriformis muscle where it divides into the pudendal nerve, perforating cutaneous nerve, and in visceral and muscular branches that supply the levator ani, coccygeus, and the sphincter ani externus muscles. The pudendal nerve, after leaving the pelvic cavity, divides into the inferior hemorrhoidal, the perineal and the dorsal nerve of the clitoris. **B)** Anatomy of pudendal plexus and particularly three branches of the pudendal nerve, which are discussed further in Figure 15–4.

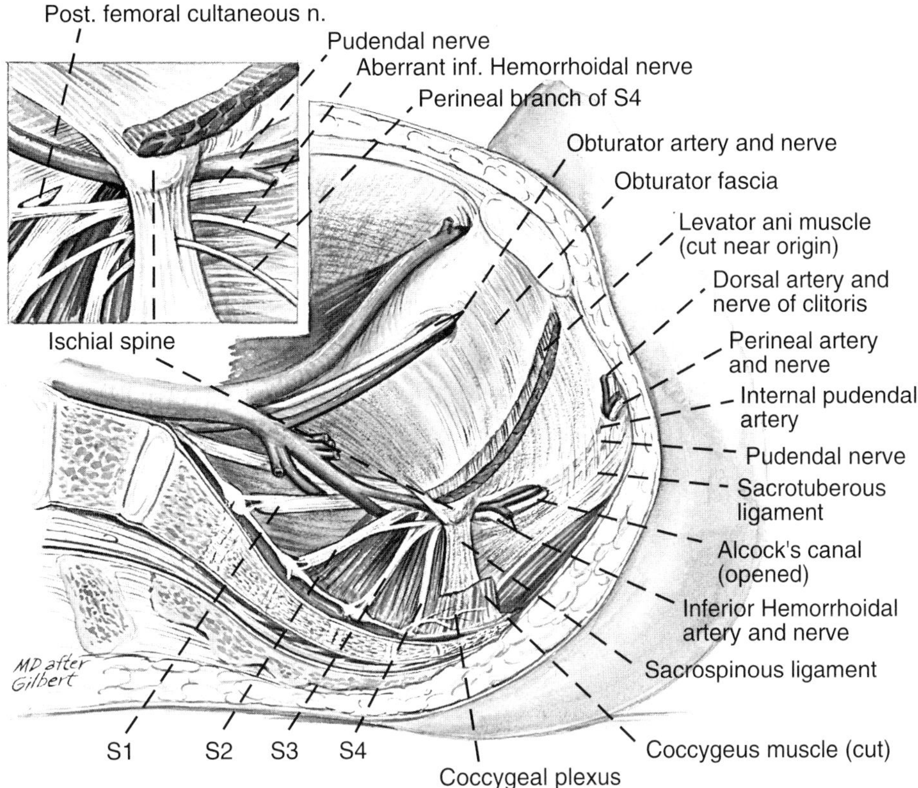


**Fig. 15–4.** Sagittal section of the perineum showing the origin and course of the pudendal nerve. Its three roots derive from the second, third, and fourth sacral nerves, unite about 1-cm proximal (cephalad) to the ischial spine, then leave the pelvic cavity by passing through the greater sciatic foramen. The formed nerve then passes posterior to the junction between the ischial spine and the sacrospinous ligament, then re-enters the pelvic cavity through the lesser sciatic foramen and proceeds anteriorly through Alcock's (pudendal) canal. In half of the individual, the inferior hemorrhoidal branch leaves the parent nerve in the posterior part of the canal while in the other half, this branch arises directly from the third and fourth sacral nerves as shown in the inset. In the former instance, it branches off from the parent nerve about 1-cm distal to the sacrospinous ligament and then accompanies the pudendal nerve within the posterior part of Alcock's canal. The inferior hemorrhoidal nerve then pierces the medial wall of Alcock's canal and crosses the ischiorectal fossa and proceeds medially and anteriorly across the ischiorectal fossa accompanied by the inferior hemorrhoidal vessels to reach the perianal region. When it arises separately, it does not pass through Alcock's canal but proceeds anteriorly from its origin, lying significantly more medial than the pudendal nerve. Upon emerging from Alcock's canal more distally, the pudendal nerve breaks into two major branches, the perineal nerve and the dorsal nerve of the clitoris (cut). All branches proceed medially to supply the perineum as depicted in Figure 15–2.

from the anterior primary division of the second, third, and fourth sacral nerve, while the sympathetic fibers are contributed by the sacral portion of the sympathetic chain. All of these fibers combine to form a single trunk, about 1-cm proximal (cephalad) to the ischial spine. The formed nerve is directed anteriorly and inferiorly and leaves the pelvic cavity by passing through the greater sciatic foramen (Figure 15–5) inferior to the piriformis muscle, between it and the coccygeal muscle. It then re-enters the pelvic cavity through the lesser sciatic foramen and proceeds anteriorly through Alcock's (pudendal) canal. Because the nerve is best blocked in its position posterior to the sacrospinous ligament, it may be profitable to focus our attention on the details of the relation of the nerve in this region.

The nerve passes posterior to the junction between the ischial spine and the sacrospinous ligament and anterior to the sacrotuberous ligament (Figures 15–4 and 15–5). Except when the ischial spine is unusually long and prominent, the nerve does not pass behind the spine, but rather diagonally across the posterior surface of the sacrospinous ligament, just as it attaches to the spine. At this point, it is medial to the internal pudendal vessels that separate it from the nerve to the obturator internus muscle (see inset in Figure 15–4). The posterior femoral cutaneous nerve lies lateral and posterior to the pudendal nerve but close to it, thus explaining the frequent involvement of the posterior femoral cutaneous nerve during pudendal block (Figure 15–3A). The sciatic nerve is much more lateral and at some distance from the pudendal nerve, and is infrequently involved in the block. In addition to the pudendal vessels, the inferior gluteal vessels are near the pudendal nerve and are liable to injury during performance of the block. Moreover, the proximity of these vessels to the point of injection increases the risk of accidental intravenous injection of local anesthetic.

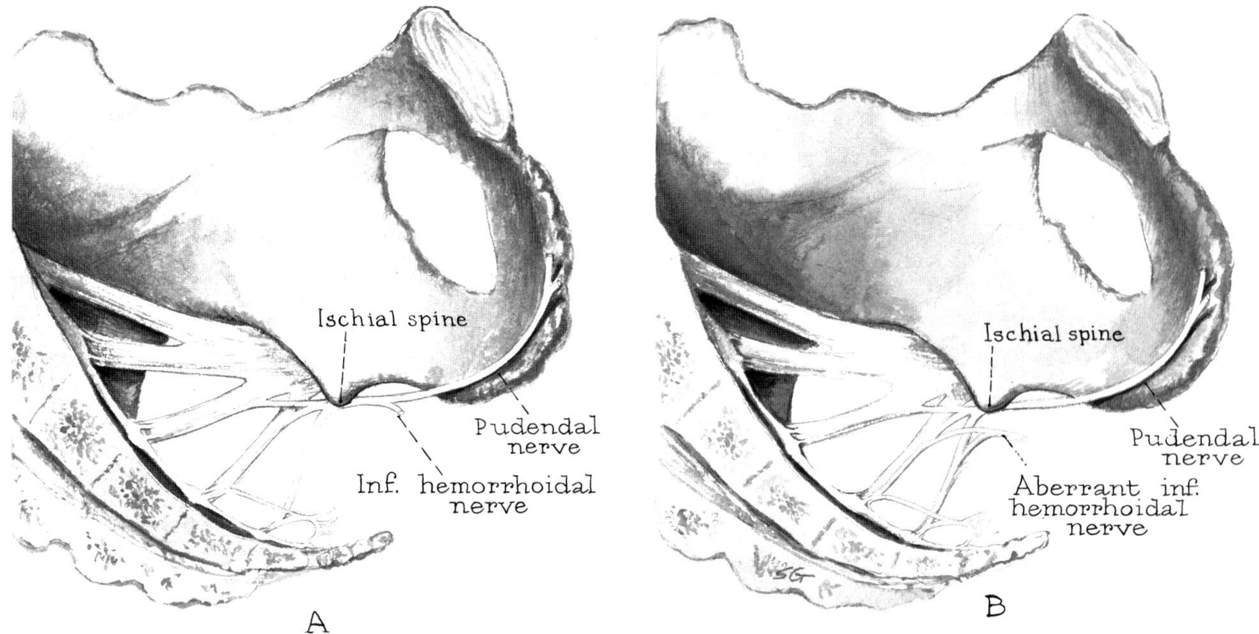


**Fig. 15–5.** Sagittal view of the pelvis showing the relationship of the pudendal nerve to the ischial spine and the bones of the pelvis. **A)** Shows the anatomy of the nerve in half of patients. **B)** Shows the anatomy of the nerve in the aberrant inferior hemorrhoidal nerve arising separately that does not pass through Alcock's canal but proceeds anteriorly from its origin.

The pudendal nerve trunk divides into three main branches: the inferior hemorrhoidal nerve, the perineal nerve, and the dorsal nerve to the clitoris. All make an important contribution to the sensory nerve supply of the perineum (Figures 15–1, 15–2, 15–3).

***Inferior hemorrhoidal nerve.*** In approximately half the individuals, the inferior hemorrhoidal nerve arises directly from the third and fourth sacral nerves, while in the other half it arises from the pudendal nerve. In the latter instance, it branches off from the parent nerve just distal to the sacrospinous ligament and then accompanies the pudendal nerve within the posterior part of Alcock's canal. The inferior hemorrhoidal nerve then pierces the medial wall of Alcock's canal and crosses the ischiorectal fossa and proceeds medially and anteriorly across the ischiorectal fossa accompanied by the inferior hemorrhoidal vessels to reach the perineal region. Midway in its course to the anus it divides into: 1) muscular branches for the sphincter ani externus; 2) cutaneous filaments that supply the skin around the anus; and 3) branches that communicate with other nerves of the perineum. When the inferior hemorrhoidal arises separately, it does not pass through Alcock's canal, but proceeds anteriorly from its origin, lying significantly more medial than the pudendal nerve.

***The perineal nerve.*** This is the largest of the three branches of the pudendal nerve. It arises near the base of the urogenital diaphragm, approximately 3 cm above the inferior border of the ischial tuberosity, and divides almost immediately into the superficial cutaneous and deep muscular branch. The superficial part of the perineal nerve is purely cutaneous, consisting of two nerves, medial and lateral, and often known as the posterior labial nerves. These supply the skin of the perineum and the major portion of the ipsilateral labia majora and minora. They also communicate with the interior hemorrhoidal nerves and with the perineal branch of the posterior femoral cutaneous nerve.

The deep branch of the perineal nerve arises at the anterior end of the ischiorectal fossa and proceeds anteriorly by passing between the superior and inferior layers of the urogenital diaphragm to reach the urethra. Its branches supply the following muscles: the transversus perinei superficialis, bulbocavernosus, ischiocavernosus, transverus perinei profundus, the sphincter urethrae, and the anterior part of the levator ani and sphincter ani externus muscles. It also supplies sensory fibers to the fascia of these muscles, all of which are very much involved in the pain of the second stage of labor. The deep branch of the perineal nerve terminates in the urethra and supplies the erectile tissue of the bulb of the vestibule, urethra, and the mucous membrane of the urethra with vasomotor nerves.

***The dorsal nerve of the clitoris.*** The third branch of the pudendal nerve, the dorsal nerve of the clitoris, emerges from the anterior end of Alcock's canal and passes through the urogenital diaphragm and proceeds anteriorly, lying between the two layers of fascia of the diaphragm. Near the apex of the urogenital diaphragm it pierces the lower (superficial) fascial layer and proceeds anteriorly on the side of the dorsal artery of the clitoris to reach the dorsum of the clitoris, which it supplies. This nerve also supplies a small branch to the corpus cavernosum clitoridis and carries sympathetic fibers, which supply the erectile tissue in this structure.

## Technique of Pudendal Nerve Block

### *Agents and Equipment*

Any of the local anesthetic agents may be used. If it is desirable to produce very prompt but brief anesthesia, 1% chloroprocaine (Nesacaine) offers the advantage of low toxicity. Lidocaine (Xylocaine) provides the advantage of prompt effect and intermediate action and is a very penetrant drug. Bupivacaine (Marcaine) and tetracaine (Pontocaine) produce prolonged analgesia. Some clinicians combine a fast, short-acting agent like chloroprocaine or lidocaine and bupivacaine to obtain rapid onset and prolonged effect. Table 15–2 indicates the concentrations and amounts of various local anesthetics that may be used for this purpose. The lower concentration should be used in patients in whom it is desirable to retain some tone in the pelvic muscle sling and in those who are in poor physical condition. The higher concentration produces anesthesia that is more prompt, more intense, and of longer duration, and is used in patients in whom paralysis of pelvic muscle is desirable. If epinephrine is used, it should be carefully measured with a 0.25-ml tuberculin syringe, adding 0.25 ml of the vasoconstrictor to 50 ml of the local anesthetic solution to make a 1:200,000 concentration.

Equipment for pudendal block includes a disposable kit (Figure 15–6) with all the necessary items for either the pudendal or paracervical block or both. In carrying out the transvaginal approach, some obstetricians use the second and third finger of the opposite hand to position the needle guide into the vagina and advance it to its target. Usually, using only the fingers to guide the needle is unsatisfactory because: 1) the needle point frequently catches the vaginal mucosa; 2) the depth of penetration cannot be controlled accurately; and 3) there is hazard of losing complete control of the needle in a restless patient with consequent injury to the fetal presenting part. These problems prompted a number of clinicians to devise various types of guides, such as the one advocated by Kobak and the Iowa Trumpet. Figure 15–6 depicts a simple guide currently available in disposable pudendal block sets.

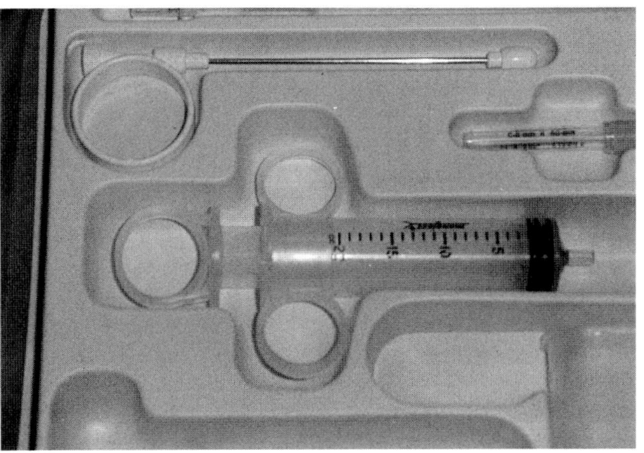

**Fig. 15–6.** Equipment for pudendal nerve block consisting of 10-ml syringe containing the local anesthetic solution, a 20-gauge 12-cm needle, and a guide used for insertion of the needle into the vagina.

### *Transvaginal Approach*

Figure 15–7 depicts the site of pudendal nerve block and, as noted, nerves from the uterus are not involved with this technique. As previously mentioned, the nerve at this site can be blocked by the transvaginal or by the transperineal approach. The transvaginal approach is easier and less painful to the patient, but it can only be carried out in the last part of the first stage before the presenting part is on the perineum and when it is possible to insert the second and third fingers (or at least the second finger) into the vagina without causing undue pressure on the fetal head (Figures 15–8 and 15–9). This technique is similar to the transperineal technique and is carried out with the patient in the lithotomy position with the uterus displaced laterally. After adequate preparation of the perineum and vagina (using gloves), the status of the presenting part and the location of the ischial spine is determined by insertion of one or two fingers. In most parturients, a 12-cm 22-gauge needle, adapted to a 10-ml syringe, filled

**Table 15–2.** Clinical Characteristics and Concentrations of Local Anesthetics

| | Procaine (Novocaine) | 2-Chloroprocaine (Nesacaine) | Lidocaine (Xylocaine) | Mepivacaine (Carbocaine) | Tetracaine (Pontocaine) | Bupivacaine (Marcaine) |
|---|---|---|---|---|---|---|
| Anesthetic Potency Ratio | 1 | 2 | 3 | 3 | 15 | 15 |
| Latency | Moderate | Fast | Fast | Moderate | Very Slow | Fast |
| Penetrance | Moderate | Marked | Marked | Moderate | Poor | Moderate |
| Duration | Short | Very Short | Moderate | Moderate | Long | Long |
| (Ratio) | 1 | 0.75 | 2 | 2 | 6–8 | 6–8 |
| Infiltration | 0.5 | 0.5 | 0.25 | 0.25 | 0.06 | 0.06 |
| Field Block | 0.75 | 0.75 | 0.5 | 0.5 | 0.1 | 0.125 |
| Pudendal/ Paracervical | 1.5 | 1.5 | 0.75–1.0 | 0.75–1.0 | 0.15 | 0.125 |
| Maximum Amount (mg/kg) | 12 | 15 | 6 | 6 | 2 | 2 |

From Bonica, JJ: Obstetric Analgesia and Anesthesia. 2nd Ed. Amsterdam, 1980. World Federation of Societies of Anaesthesiologists.

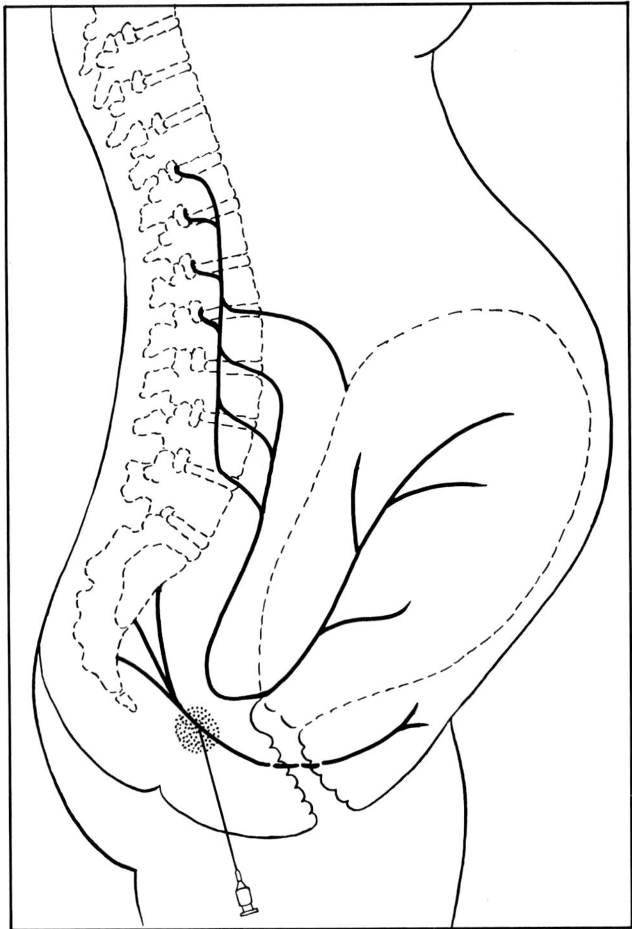

**Fig. 15–7.** Schematic illustration showing the site of pudendal nerve block. The nerves to the uterus are not involved with the use of this technique.

with anesthetic solution is used. If a special needle guide is not available, the needle is held so that its shaft is in the groove formed by the opposition of the second and third fingers of the left hand for a left pudendal nerve block and between those of the right hand for right pudendal nerve block. Some obstetricians prefer to hold the needle so that its tip is pressed against the pad of the second finger. The steps of the technique are depicted in Figures 15–8 and 15–9 and described in detail in the legend.

### *Transperineal Approach*

The transperineal approach, though rarely used today, is an option when the fetal presenting part on the perineum prohibits insertion of the operator's fingers into the vagina without causing undue pressure on the fetal head. The technique is carried out also with the patient in the lithotomy position while an assistant displaces the uterus laterally to decrease or obviate aortocaval compression. Because the guiding finger is usually inserted through the rectum, special care should be taken to prepare the perineum with antiseptic solution and proper draping and having available two pairs of gloves. The technique is de-

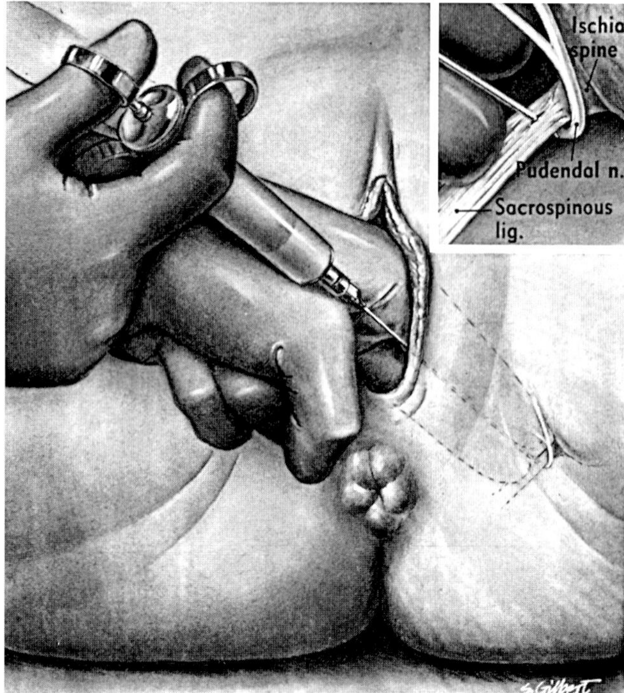


**Fig. 15–8.** Technique of pudendal nerve block using the transvaginal approach. With the patient in the lithotomy position, a 20-gauge 12-cm needle inserted into the outer guide is adapted to a syringe filled with local anesthetic solution. The guide and needle are passed into the vagina with the shaft being held in the groove formed by the apposition of the second and third finger of the left hand for a left pudendal nerve block as shown here. For a right pudendal nerve block, the guide and needle are held between the second and third finger of the right hand. If a guide is not available, the needle is held between the two fingers as it is advanced into the vagina. Some clinicians prefer to hold the shaft of the needle so that its tip is pressed against the pad of the second finger. Protected and guided by the fingers, the needle is carried into the vagina, directly laterally and posteriorly until the tip of the ischial spine is palpated by the tip of the third finger. The point of the needle is then cautiously advanced into the vaginal mucosa overlying the sacrospinous ligament just anterior and medial to the tip of the ischial spine. One or 2 ml of solution is injected into the mucosa and the submucosa to anesthetize these structures. The needle is then advanced slowly through the sacrospinous ligament very near its attachment to the spine, while at the same time an attempt is made to inject the anesthetic solution. As long as the short beveled tip of the needle is within the ligament, there is considerable resistance to the injection. With constant pressure on the plunger of the syringe, the needle is then very slowly and cautiously advanced through the ligament until there is a sudden lack of resistance. This indicates the needle point has emerged from the posterior surface of the ligament and entered the space where the pudendal nerve and associated vessels are located. (The sudden lack of resistance aids in proper placement of the needle point in the same way as it does in epidural anesthesia depicted in Chapter 13.) After attempts at aspiration in two planes to make sure that the needle is not in a blood vessel, 3 to 5 ml of the solution are injected. The needle is then advanced another 5 to 7 mm (no more!), attempts at aspiration are made, and, if negative, the remainder of the solution is injected. Not infrequently, once the bevel of the needle passes through the sacrospinous ligament, it contacts the nerve causing paresthesia throughout its branches. If the needle is advanced too far, the solution will be injected into the gluteal muscle or may even contact the sciatic nerve, causing paresthesia along its course. In such circumstances, the needle should be promptly withdrawn until its bevel is again into the sacrospinous ligament and the procedure is repeated.

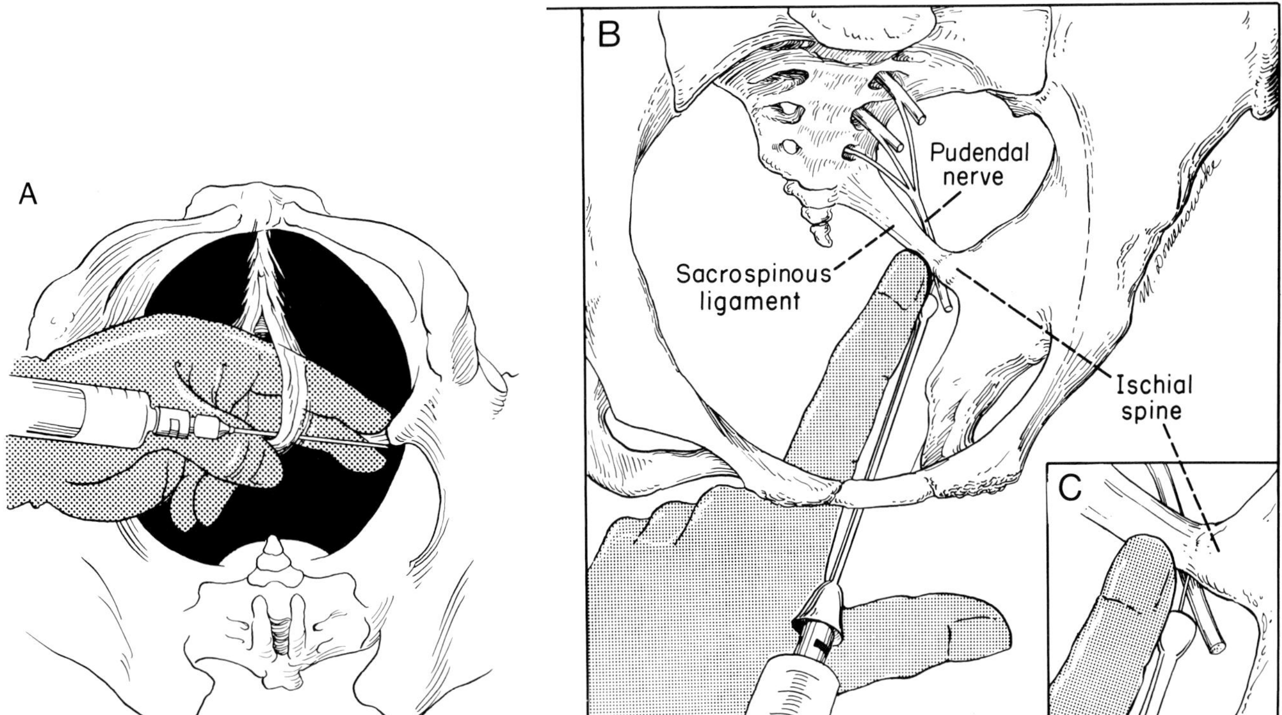


**Fig. 15–9.** Schematic views showing the technique of transvaginal approach to pudendal nerve block, with the point of the needle passed behind the sacrospinous ligament instead of through the ligament as depicted in Figure 15–8. **A)** inferior view of the pelvis showing the needle having passed through the vagina and advanced until its bevel is just posterior to the junction of the ischial spine and sacrospinous ligament and is in contact with the pudendal nerve. **B)** superior view of the pelvis showing how the second finger is used to direct the guide containing a needle with its final position for injection of the pudendal nerve. Note that the needle is longer than the guide so that its distal 1.0 cm protrudes beyond the end of the guide and thus permits passing the needle through the sacrospinous ligament or posterior to it. **C)** is an enlargement that shows the distal part of the guide is 1 cm from the ligament so that the bevel of the needle is just posterior to the junction of the spine and ligament next to the pudendal nerve.

picted in Figures 15–10, 15–11, and 15–12 and described in detail in the legends below these figures. In contrast to the transvaginal approach, with this technique a skin wheal is made with a 30-gauge needle about 2.5 cm posteromedial to the tuberosity of ischium. Once this is done, a 8-cm 22-gauge disposable spinal needle is used for infiltration of the subcutaneous tissue and fascia to produce a tract of anesthesia. Several points made in the legend deserve re-emphasis. First, it is much easier to insert and advance the needle without the syringe attached. Second, because of its length and the resistance of the skin, the needle is likely to buckle unless its shaft is supported by the left hand. Third, the second finger of the hand not holding the needle should be inserted into the rectum to guide the needle to its target. Fourth, most obstetricians inject one-third of the solution at each of three points depicted in the inset in Figure 15–12.

Usually, one who is right handed prefers using this hand to guide the needle. There are other obstetricians who change hands using the left second finger in the rectum for block of the patient's right pudendal nerve and the right second finger for block of the parturient's left pudendal nerve. This, of course, requires a change of gloves. Some clinicians prefer placing the guiding second finger into the vagina instead of the rectum, even with the transperineal technique, to avoid contamination. However, when the presenting part is bulging on the perineum and the transperineal technique is especially indicated, transvaginal palpation is difficult if not impossible.

### *Resultant Analgesia-Anesthesia*

The parturient experiences relief of perineal pain within 3 to 5 minutes after block is completed, and anesthesia develops within 5 to 10 minutes. The area of analgesia that usually develops is shown in Figure 15–13. Many parturients lose the urge to bear down because the afferent limb of the reflex has been eliminated.

## Local Anesthesia and Field Block of the Perineum

Analgesia of the perineum can also be effected with local infiltration or field block. Local infiltration is achieved by injecting dilute solutions of local anesthetics into tissues for the purpose of blocking or interrupting nerve endings that supply these tissues. Field block is injection of the solution at some distance from nerve endings to systematically block small nerves that supply specific structures.

## Clinical Evaluation

### *Analgesic Efficacy*

Local infiltration or field block of the perineum for vaginal delivery has been used and advocated for many years,

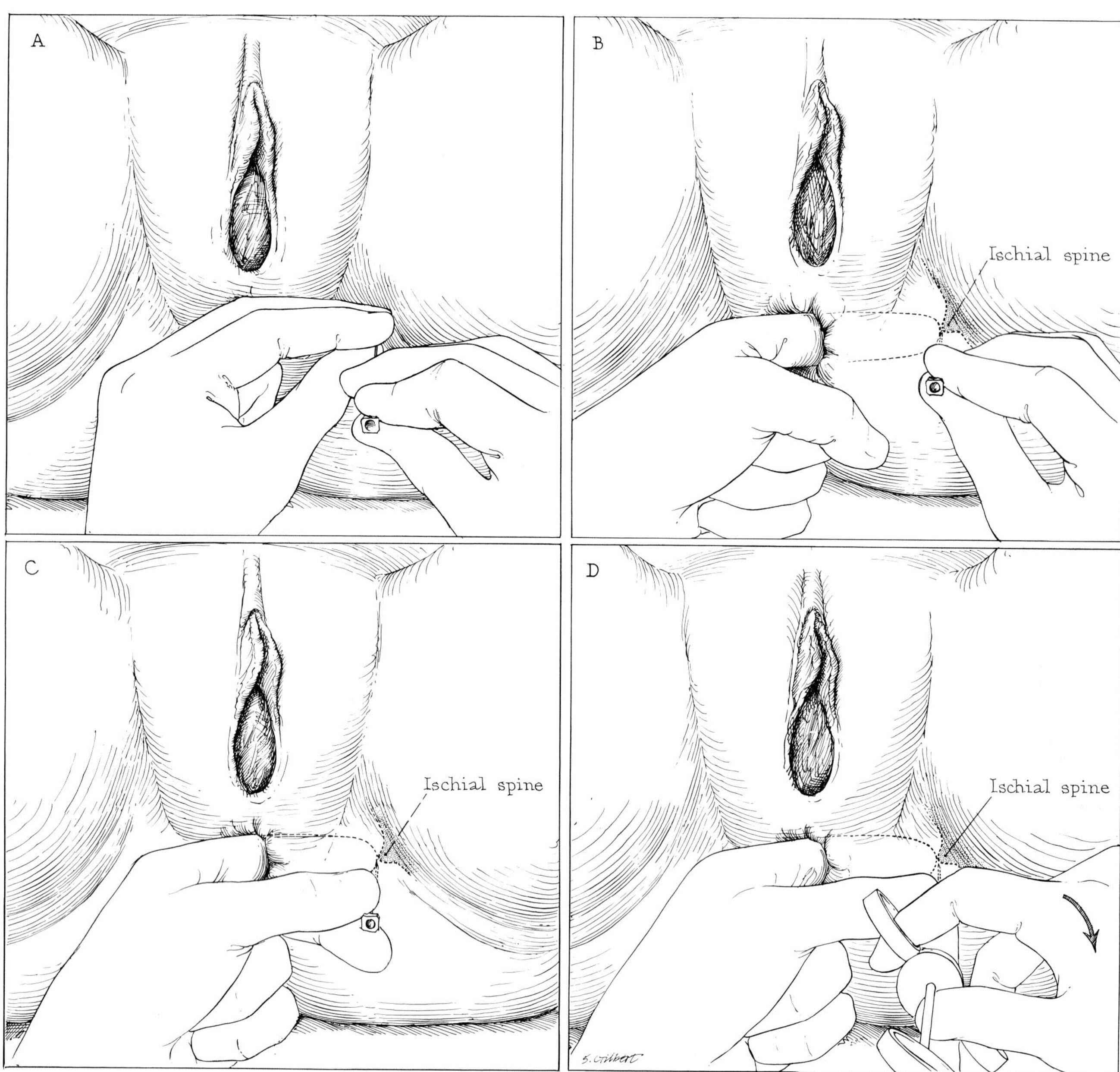


**Fig. 15–10.** Pudendal nerve block using the transperineal approach. With the patient in the lithotomy position, the perineum is prepared with antiseptic and draped. A skin wheal is made with a fine, 30-gauge needle about 2.5-cm posteromedial to the tuberosity of the ischium. A 25-gauge 8-cm disposable spinal needle is attached to the 10-ml Luer-Lok control syringe containing 0.5% lidocaine solution. Needle is then inserted through the wheal and the solution injected as the needle is advanced through the subcutaneous tissue as far as the fascia. Infiltration with 5 ml of this solution will produce a tract of analgesia that will permit passage of the larger pudendal block needle painlessly. Once this is done, the 20-gauge 12-cm pudendal block needle is introduced perpendicular to the skin. It is much easier to maneuver and insert and advance the larger needle without the syringe attached. Because of its length and the resistance of the skin, the needle is likely to buckle unless its shaft is supported by the left hand (as shown in **A**), until its point passes through the skin and into the subcutaneous tissue. At this point, the second finger of the left hand is inserted into the rectum to guide the needle to its target and also to minimize the chance of puncturing the rectum (as shown in **B**). The needle is slowly advanced in the ischiorectal fossa toward the ischial spine by having it pass behind the urogenital diaphragm and levator ani muscle. As the needle approaches the ischial spine, it is pushed posterior to it by the guiding finger as shown in ***C.*** This usually places the bevel of the needle into the beginning of Alcock's canal. Frequently, the patient experiences paresthesia in the ipsilateral half of the perineum—a sure sign that the point of the needle has contacted the nerve and its advance should be promptly stopped. Moreover, if the bevel of the needle is in the canal, it can be moved back and forth without resistance, whereas if it is in muscle or ligament, resistance is felt. Once the needle is thought to be properly placed, the 10-ml syringe filled with the local anesthetic solution is adapted to the needle, attempts to aspirate in two planes are made to make sure that the point of the needle is not in a blood vessel, and 3 to 4 ml of solutions are injected posterior to the tip of the spine. The needle is then advanced an additional 5 mm into the canal and another 3 ml of solution are injected. The needle is then advanced a second time another 5 mm, and the remaining 3 to 4 ml of solution are injected. The last step assures block of the aberrant inferior hemorrhoidal nerve in parturients in whom it arises as a separate nerve, but also invariably blocks other branches of the pudendal plexus and the posterior femoral cutaneous nerve.

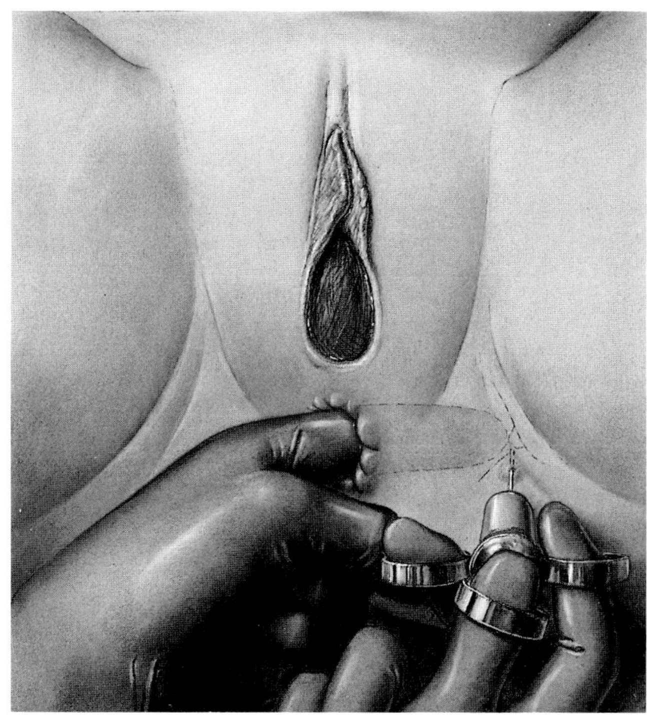

**Fig. 15–11.** A larger view than seen in Figure 15–10 depicting the transperineal approach to pudendal nerve block. The spine and ligament are palpated by the tip of the left index finger, which is inserted into the rectum to guide the point of the needle.

especially by Greenhill (25). He firmly believed that these procedures are not only simple and effective, but also are practically free of complications either to the mother or infant. Although theoretically such is the case, practically it is difficult to produce complete relief of perineal pain unless large (and sometimes toxic) amounts of local drugs are used. This is because the nerves supplying the perineum are widely scattered in many fascial and muscular compartments. Field block is effective for episiotomy, but does not eliminate spontaneous pain from perineal distension completely. Thus, for analgesia, these techniques are inferior to pudendal, subarachnoid, caudal or epidural block.

### Effects on the Mother

Properly executed local infiltration and field block do not alter respiratory, cardiovascular, gastrointestinal or other maternal bodily functions. However, improper technique that results in inadequate pain relief may provoke or aggravate apprehension, anxiety and fear, and cause tachycardia, hypertension, and uterine inertia. Systemic toxic reactions produce significant alteration of bodily functions. This complication, discussed in detail in the next chapter, is clearly due to errors in technique and can be avoided.

### Effects on Labor

Local infiltration and field block, properly carried out, have no effect on uterine contractility or the auxiliary forces, and thus do not alter the progress or duration of labor. However, an overdose of a local anesthetic may alter uterine contractility either directly or indirectly by producing maternal hypoxemia and hypercapnea. Even more important is the inhibiting action of epinephrine if used with the local anesthetic. Epinephrine, in excess of 0.20 mg (200 μg) and injected into vascular tissue, produces temporary inhibition of uterine contractions.

### Effects on the Infant

The most important advantage of local infiltration and field block is the lack of depressant effect on the infant, provided they are properly executed. However, systemic toxic reactions, if they occur, impair maternal ventilation and circulation and have a harmful effect on the fetus and newborn. Moreover, because these drugs pass the placental membrane, a high fetal blood level also may be produced, with consequent depression of the cardiovascular and central nervous system of the fetus and newborn. Because of the large volumes of solutions used, the risk of these complications is greater with local blocks than with most other regional techniques.

## Technical Considerations

To obviate the disadvantages of these techniques, it is essential to know well the fascial compartments that contain the nerves that supply the perineum. Knowledge of the anatomy of the perineum and pelvic diaphragm is also important because these trough-like structures participate in normal internal rotation and flexion of the head, and their resistance must be overcome by the forces of labor before birth can take place. Detailed description of the anatomy of the perineum—including description of the superficial and deep fascia, the urogenital diaphragm, superficial and deep perineal pouches, and the anal region—is beyond the scope of this book. Figures 15–14 and 15–15 are included for the sake of completeness.

## *Technique of Infiltration*

The technique of infiltrating the various fascial planes of the perineum to produce anesthesia is depicted in Figure 15–16. The concentrations of the various local anesthetic drugs that may be used for this purpose are indicated in Table 15–2. Note that 0.5% lidocaine or chloroprocaine or 0.25% of mepivacaine and 0.125% of bupivacaine are effective in producing analgesia. Because of its prolonged action, bupivacaine is preferable, not only to produce anesthesia for the delivery, but also for postoperative pain relief. Greater concentrations are neither necessary nor desirable because they increase the risk of systemic toxic reactions. Because lidocaine is more penetrant and thus likely to diffuse more widely than bupivacaine, some clinicians use a combination of these to take advantage of the more rapid and penetrant action of the lidocaine and the prolonged effect of bupivacaine. However, if this is done, it is essential that the final concentrations of both solutions do not exceed those cited above. Hyaluronidase is useful in carrying out infiltration of the perineum or regional block because it not only enhances anesthesia but also may help to minimize hematomas.

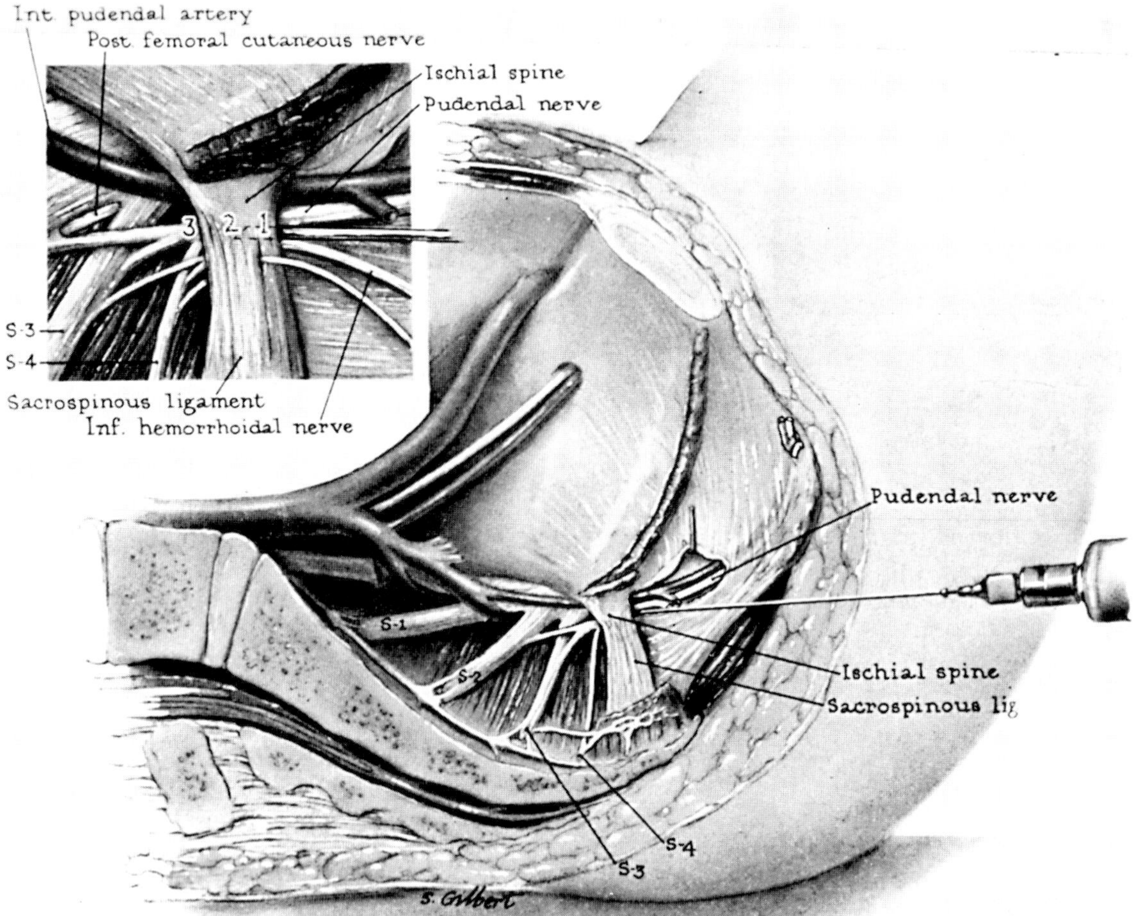


**Fig. 15–12.** Sagittal view of the perineum showing the needle having passed through the pelvic structures until its point is just posterior to the junction of the ischial spine and the sacrospinous ligament in the proper position for injection of the local anesthetic to block the pudendal nerve. Inset enlargement of the area of the ischial spine showing the numbers that indicate the position of the bevel of the needle for three separate injections. After attempt at aspiration in two planes to make sure that the point of the needle is not in a blood vessel, 3 to 4 ml of solution are injected with the bevel of the needle in position 1, which is just posterior to the anterior part of junction of the ischial spine and sacrospinous ligament. The needle is then advanced an additional 5 mm into the canal, placing its bevel in position 2, and another 3 ml of solution are injected. The point of the needle is advanced to beyond the spine into the greater sciatic notch, and after negative aspirations the remaining 3 to 4 ml of solution are injected. The last step should assure block of the inferior hemorrhoidal nerve in those parturients in whom it arises as a separate trunk. This technique also invariably involves other branches of the pudendal plexus and the posterior femoral cutaneous nerve. Again, if the needle is advanced too far, it may contact the sciatic nerve itself.

A 10-cm (4 inch) 22-gauge (no larger!) needle with a short, sharp bevel should be used for infiltration. Care must be taken to avoid punctures of the bulb of the vestibule, Bartholin's gland, and other important paralabial structures. Because the anesthetic requires sufficient time to penetrate the various structures and block the nerves, effective analgesia requires 10 to 15 minutes to develop.

### *Technique of Field Block of the Perineum*

Field block of the perineum is carried out by forming a wheal with a 30-gauge needle at a point medial and slightly posterior to the tuberosity of the ischium. A 10-cm 22-gauge needle is then substituted for the skin-wheal needle and subcutaneous infiltration is performed anteriorly (Figure 15–17). Then infiltration is carried into the ischiorectal fossa to create a wall of anesthesia through which the deeper branches of the perineal and hemorrhoidal nerves pass. It is advisable to insert the left index finger into the rectum to avoid puncture of the rectum through a misguided needle into it.

In the usual case, field block of the branches of the pudendal nerve suffices. In the unusual case, when the patient experiences discomfort in the parts supplied by branches of the ilioinguinal and genitofemoral nerve, these can be blocked by making subcutaneous infiltration. The comment about a latency of 10 to 15 minutes for the development of effective analgesia/anesthesia applies to this technique.

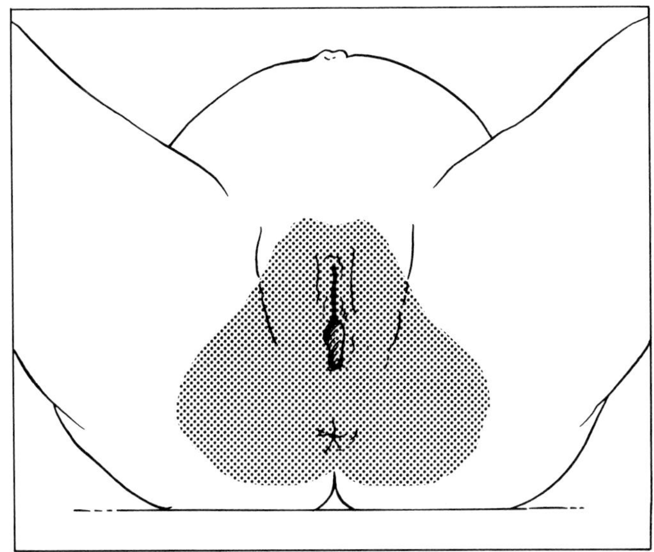

**Fig. 15–13.** The stippled area shows the extent of analgesia/anesthesia with pudendal nerve block. This is usually sufficient to relieve pain of the second and third stage of labor and for episiotomy.

## *Field Block for Episiotomy*

The technique of local infiltration for episiotomy and repair is shown in Figure 15–18. Because this is usually carried out when the skin is partially anesthetized due to stretching and pressure, it can be performed without a preliminary wheal. Note that several fanwise injections are made in two planes to block the nerve endings. It is absolutely essential that the obstetrician awaits sufficient time to permit effective analgesia to develop before making the incision. This author has observed many obstetricians who have carried out the infiltration and promptly thereafter attempted to do the episiotomy before the onset of analgesia, causing significant amount of pain and suffering, and thus provoking a great deal of anxiety and apprehension.

***Supplemental analgesia.*** In view of the fact that local infiltration of field block of the perineum may not provide complete relief of pain during the second stage, it is important for the obstetrician to be prepared to complement the procedure with either inhalation analgesia or an intravenous opioid. If the additional analgesia is needed for the delivery of the infant as well as for the postdelivery period for repair of episiotomy or laceration, continuous inhalation analgesia is preferred because when properly administered, it has no effect on the mother or on the fetus and newborn. Nitrous oxide, in concentrations of 50 to 60% in oxygen, administered continuously, provides sufficient additional analgesia to result in a pain free experience by the parturient. As discussed in Chapter 19, it can be self-administered by the patient, by a nurse anesthetist or by an anesthesiologist. Data on its use as a complement to bilateral pudendal block are not available, but it is likely that it is frequently used in centers where major regional analgesia/anesthesia (epi-

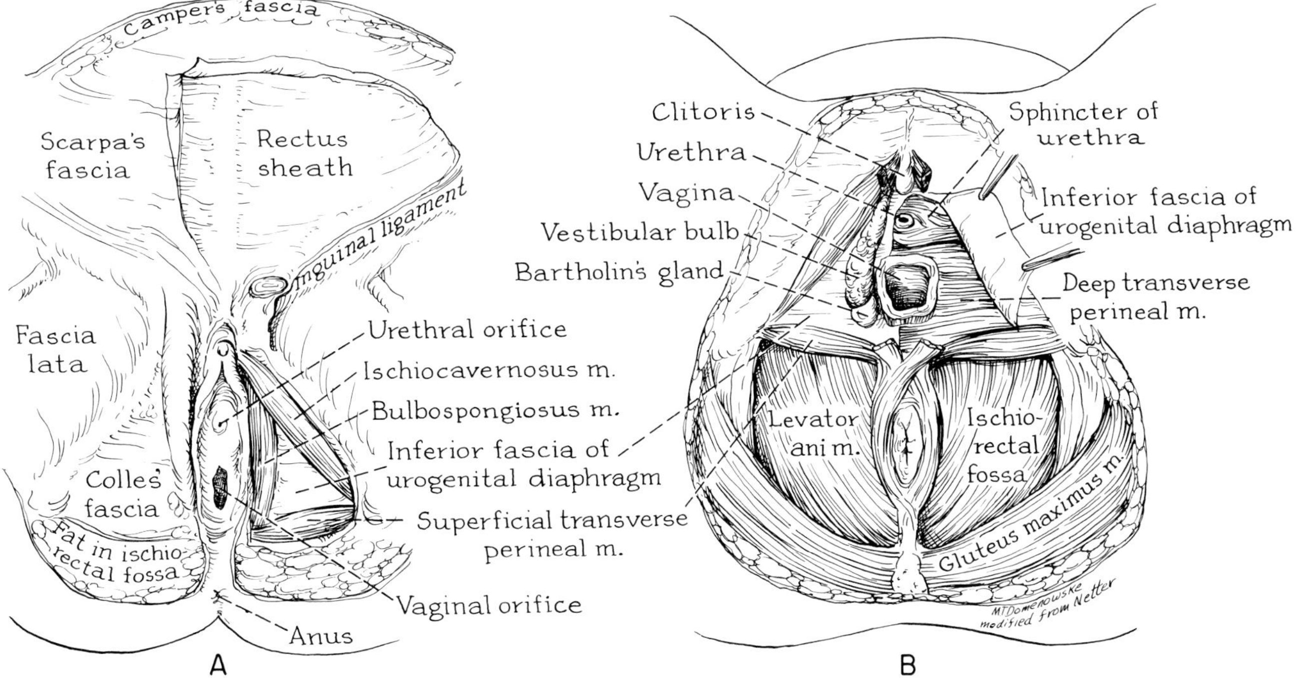


**Fig. 15–14.** Structures of the perineum. **A)** and **B)** inferior superior view and **C)** sagittal section. In **A)** the outer layer of the superficial fascia has been removed showing on the right of the specimen the deeper layer (Colles' fascia), while on the left side this has been removed to show the muscle. The vessels and nerves are omitted but these are shown in Figure 15–4. **B)** deeper section to show the urogenital diaphragm and the ischiorectal fossa, which contain important nerves involved in the pain of the second stage of labor (also not shown here but shown in Figure 15–2). **C)** is schematic diagram of the sagittal section of the perineum showing that the bladder and rectum are compressed by the advancing head. The nerves and blood vessels are omitted.

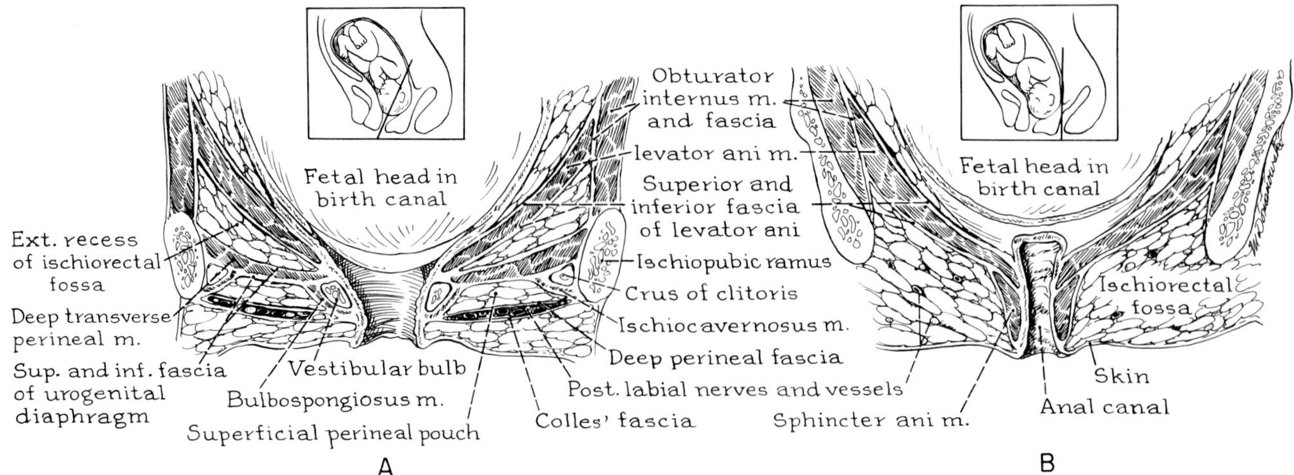


**Fig. 15–15.** Schematic diagram of coronal sections of perineum. **A)** section through the vagina (indicated by line in inset). Note location of posterior labial nerves and vessels. **B)** section through the anal canal (indicated by line in the inset, and also showing position of posterior labial nerves).

dural or subarachnoid block) is not available. In parturients who experience pain after delivery of the infant, a long-acting opioid can be given intravenously that will provide additional relief during the surgical procedure and for several hours postpartum.

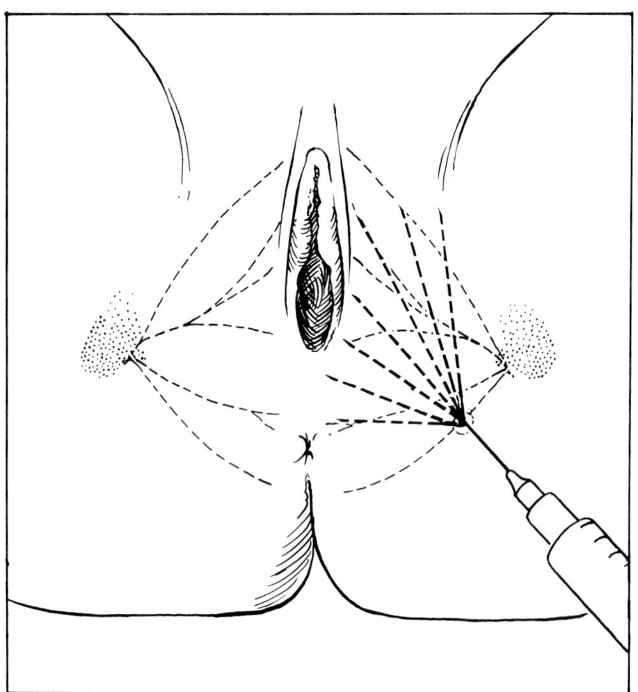

**Fig. 15–16.** Technique of infiltrating the perineum. The light solid lines indicate the nerves, while the heavy dashed lines indicate directions of the needle from the point of entrance. Note the fanwise infiltration that must be made subcutaneously and through the various fascial planes and muscles containing the nerves. In addition to the fact that it requires multiple punctures that may be painful, it may also cause damage to vessels and other structures and produce postoperative pain and morbidity.

## Paracervical Block

In the 1950s and 1960s, paracervical and uterosacral block were widely applied for the relief of pain of uterine contractions. The first publications on the subject were published in 1926 by Gellert (27) in Germany who reported a series of 50 cases. In the next 2 decades, a number of articles appeared in the European literature (28,29). The first American article was published in 1945 by Rosenfeld (30) who reported that all 100 patients in whom the procedure was used experienced relief of pain during the first stage of labor. Subsequently, Freeman and his associates (31–34) published several reports with very favorable results, and later many other reports were published, all attesting to the simplicity, safety, and usefulness of paracervical block (PCB) (17,35–40). In 1959, Spanos and Steele (41) published a description of a modification of the paracervical technique, which they called uterosacral block.

Although the earlier reports included observation of fetal bradycardia, the procedure continued to be used widely until the late 1960s when an increasing number of published reports of fetal morbidity, and even mortality, associated with fetal bradycardia began to question the usefulness of the procedure. Because of the aforementioned advantages of PCB, in the 1970s two important trends were followed: one was the numerous studies in an attempt to determine the incidence and mechanism of fetal bradycardia and the associated fetal morbidity; while the other was the progressive decrease in the use of this procedure for the relief of pain caused by uterine contractions (42). An admirably valiant effort in 1972 by Thiery and Vroman (42) was made by publishing a comprehensive review of the literature, which cited 179 articles involving over 70,000 cases and summarized virtually every aspect of the procedure reported up to that time. A year later, Freeman and Schifrin (43) published another, though smaller but still impressively "balanced," review of paracervical with a detailed discussion of the incidence

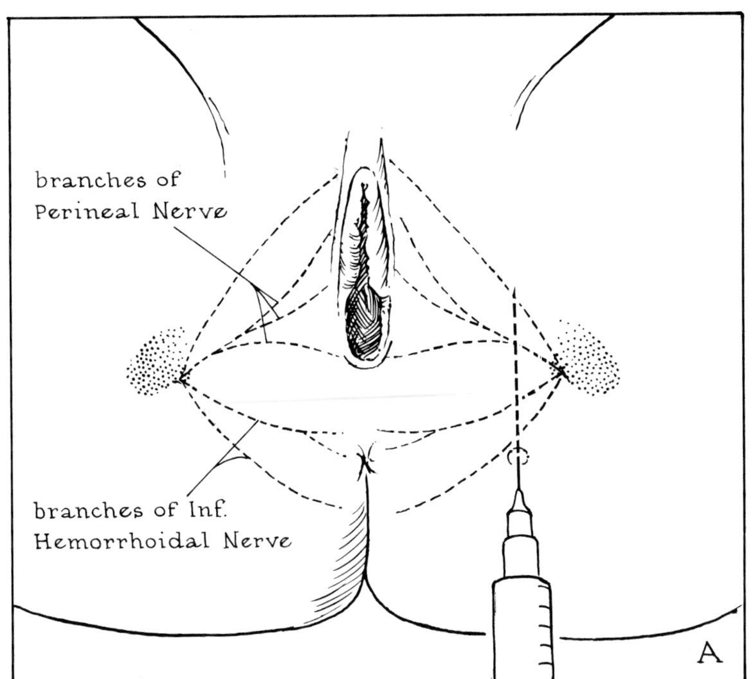


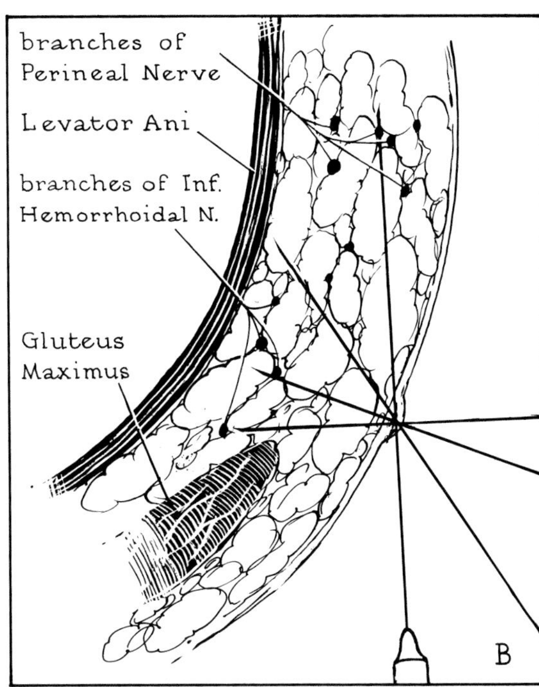


**Fig. 15–17.** Technique of field block of the perineum. **A)** inferior superior view showing the distribution of the branches of the pudendal nerve and the direction of the needle attached to the syringe. **B)** sagittal view showing fanwise technique of infiltrating in various directions. The dilution solution is injected while the needle is being advanced and withdrawn rapidly. The rapid movement of the needle with steady injection virtually eliminates accidental intravascular injection of any more than 0.5 ml of solution.

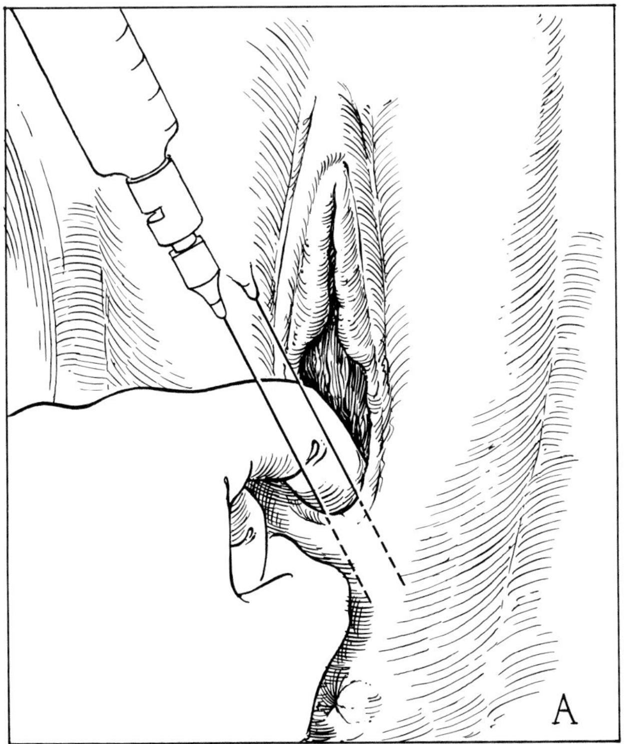


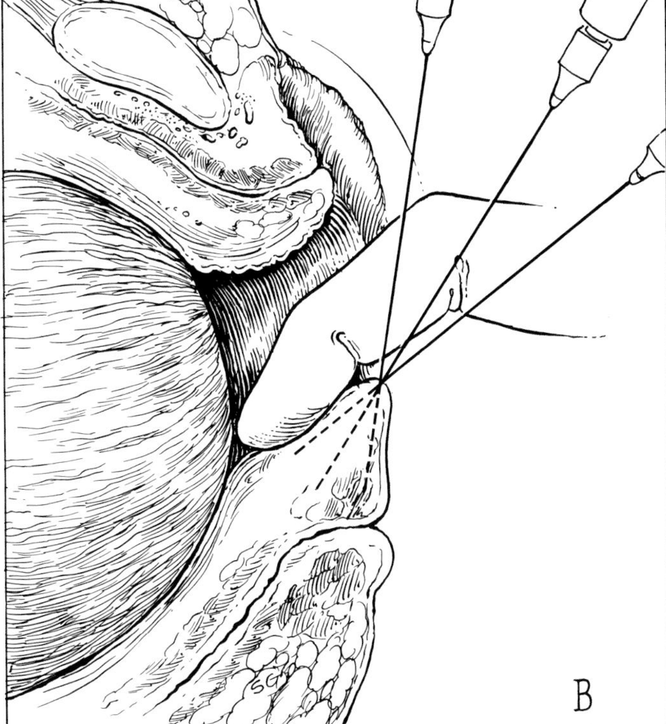


**Fig. 15–18.** Technique of local infiltration for episiotomy and repair. **A)** anterior view showing the directions of the needle insertion on each side of the proposed incision. **B)** sagittal view showing fanwise pattern of the three injections that must be made on each side of the proposed episiotomy to ascertain that all superficial and deeper structures are anesthetized.

and mechanisms of fetal bradycardia and the effects of PCB on the course of labor and neonatal outcome based on their own personal experience. A third important review published in 1978 by Cibils and Santonja-Lucas (44) focused on the incidence of heart rate pattern changes in parturients given PCB during labor. They reviewed 28 reports involving over 12,000 parturients and discussed various hypotheses of fetal bradycardia and other alteration of FHR patterns. These and other reports form the basis of the discussion that follows.

Currently, paracervical block (PCB) is being used much less frequently than formerly. Table 1–3 (Chapter 1) indicates that in the national survey carried out by Gibbs and associates (24) in 1981 (but published in 1986), paracervical block was used in 5 to 6% of the parturients undergoing vaginal delivery. In many of the major obstetric centers in the United States, PCB has been abandoned and is not used at all based on the admonition of some obstetricians and obstetric anesthesia authorities (45–47) who believe that the procedure is contraindicated in vaginal delivery because of the high risk to the fetus. On the other hand, a number of obstetricians still use PCB, especially in general community hospitals with small obstetric units where the services of obstetric anesthesiology are not available. In a relatively recent report, Day (48), of the Department of Family Medicine and Community Health of the University of Minnesota, reported that PCB was used in 63% of 883 obstetric patients delivered in a community hospital. About 65% of the patients obtained good pain relief and another 20% had partial relief. Infants delivered after PCB were compared with infants whose mothers did not receive PCB, and they were found to have similar Apgar scores and only 6% had alteration of fetal heart rate. Day (48) concluded that PCB properly done remains an effective and low risk form of obstetric anesthesia in most parturients that deliver in a community hospital. Other recent reports have suggested that with proper technique, PCB is safe and has been used in a significant percentage of parturients undergoing vaginal delivery (49–52). This technique apparently remains an important procedure in some Scandinavian hospitals (50–52). Cibils and Santonja-Lucas (44), after analyzing the data in their extensive review in addition to an analysis of 401 of their own patients, also consider the procedure safe and stated that it can be used. In their report, Freeman and Schifrin (43) indicate that the procedure can be used provided certain guidelines are followed, discussed later in this chapter.

In 1992, Goins (52a) reported the use of bilateral paracervical block in a private practice group of 182 parturients during a 3-year period with excellent results. The block, which was achieved with 10 ml of plain 1% mepivacaine injected bilaterally into the lateral fornices (total drug dose 200 mg ) through a needle that was inserted 5 mm or less, was successful in 94% of the parturients. The incidence of fetal bradycardia (fetal heart rate dropped below 100 beats per minute and lasted more than 30 seconds) was 13.2%, occurred within an injection-bradycardia interval of 8 minutes and lasting a mean of 4.5 minutes. Apgar scores of less than 7 occurred in 10.4% of fetuses at 1 minute and 2.2% at 5 minutes, compared with 7% and 1.2%, respectively, among the control group of 343 parturients managed by the author during the same period.

## Clinical Evaluation

### *Analgesic Efficacy*

Paracervical block interrupts uterine nociceptive pathways as they pass through the uterovaginal plexus in the parametrium, whereas uterosacral block interrupts them as they pass in, and below, and between the uterosacral ligament. Either procedure effects complete relief of pain of the first stage of labor, but does not relieve perineal pain of the second and third stages. The block is usually begun when the patient begins to experience moderate to severe pain with each uterine contraction. Most parturients require this after the onset of the active phase of the first stage, usually at the phase of maximum slope (acceleration phase), when the cervix is 4 cm dilated, the presenting part is above 2+ station, and the contractions have an intensity of 35 to 40 mm Hg, a frequency of at least 3 per minute, and a duration of 45 to 60 seconds. Some clinicians disregard this degree of cervical dilatation and administer the procedure when the parturient is experiencing moderate to severe pain (42). When administered too late (i.e., with cervical dilatation too far advanced, greater than 8 cm) and the head well-engaged, paracervical block is inherent in three disadvantages: 1) the procedure is more difficult to carry out, 2) the block is less effective, and 3) fetal hazard is increased.

Analgesia develops rather dramatically within 3 to 5 minutes and lasts 1 to 2 hours, depending on the local anesthetic used. With 2% chloroprocaine alone it lasts about 40 to 55 minutes; whereas when dextran is added to the local anesthetic, the analgesia lasts about 75 minutes (53,54). With 1% lidocaine (Xylocaine) or 1% mepivacaine (Carbocaine), the block lasts 50 to 75 minutes; with 0.125% bupivacaine, it lasts 60 to 90 minutes; whereas with 0.25% bupivacaine, without epinephrine, it lasts 90 to 120 minutes (39). The addition of epinephrine in concentration of 1:200,000 to 1:300,000 increases the duration of analgesia, with 1% lidocaine or 1% mepivacaine, by 30 to 50 percent; whereas with bupivacaine, opinions are somewhat contradictory. However, some agree that at least the maximal duration of effect is higher with than without epinephrine (39). Based on a controlled study, Freeman, Bellville and Barno (32) stated that epinephrine substantially increased the duration of analgesia produced by PCB. When the block "wears off" pain returns rather abruptly. Therefore, to relieve discomfort, the procedure is repeated as soon as the parturient begins to sense any discomfort.

The success rate with paracervical block depends primarily on the skill and experience of the operator. Many writers (16,32–40,48–55) have reported that they were able to provide complete relief of uterine pain to about 70% of parturients, and partial relief to another 15 to 20%. The latter group usually experienced some residual backache or unilateral suprapubic pain. Failure to produce relief with the initial injection occurs in 10 to 15% of cases and is due to technical error. Using the technique discussed below, Jagerhorn (52) achieved effective analgesia in 95% of the parturients. Thiery and Vroman (42) cited over a dozen reports that stated success (complete or good relief of pain) occurred in virtually 100% and failure rate under 1%. In one study, the success rate of 71% and complete failure in 4% was obtained in patients who were unaware of the aim of the procedure (56).

When the parturient begins to experience perineal pain, either a bilateral pudendal block or low (S1-S5) caudal, or even a true "saddle" block can be done. This supplementary perineal analgesia is usually required at the end of the first stage. If the effect of the paracervical block has worn off at that time, the patient is ready for delivery and pudendal block has been done for perineal pain. The pain of uterine contraction can be relieved with inhalation analgesia as discussed above.

### *Effects on the Mother*

Properly carried out, neither technique alters respiratory, cardiovascular, gastrointestinal or other bodily functions of the mother. Sangoul, Fox, and Houle (57) reported that following the administration of paracervical block, oxygen consumption, tidal volume, and minute volume decreased during the first stage of labor. Effective analgesia with PCB was associated with a decrease in tidal and minute volumes, and in apprehension, and, consequently, there was a decreased metabolic rate that contributed to a decrease in maternal lactic acidosis during labor. Grenman and associates (58) studied the effects of paracervical block in 39 parturients on catecholamines, arginine, and vasopressin and noted that analgesia decreased the plasma levels of epinephrine significantly during the period of analgesia, suggesting that PCB is effective in diminishing the neuroendocrine stress response.

Maternal complications that can occur include: 1) possible damage to the uterine vessels, 2) hematoma, 3) infections, 4) systemic toxic reactions, 5) transient rectal sphincter relaxation, and 6) possibly sensory disturbances from involvement of the sciatic or other nerves in the pelvis. The incidence of systemic toxic reaction is said to be 3.5 per 10,000 cases (59). Thiery and Vroman (42) reported that only five cases of hematoma of the broad ligament due to laceration of major uterine vessel had been reported. Infection is rare (42). The overall incidence of adverse effects is less than 1% (36,37,48–53). Severe convulsions, vascular collapse, and even death were reported by Davis, et al (38). Albright (59) cited two deaths that had occurred with PCB used for therapeutic abortion. These complications are usually caused by technical error and can be avoided by using thin, sharp needles, avoiding accidental intravenous injection, and using a proper dose of the local anesthetic. Although the paracervical veins are very large and dilated at this stage of labor, they are drawn upward to a much higher level and therefore can be avoided. Rarely, the sacral nerves become involved in the block, with consequent anesthesia of the affected leg.

### *Effects on Labor*

The effects of PCB on the factors that determine the progress of labor are often contradictory and inconclusive. Thiery and Vroman (42) cite numerous reports in which the rate of cervical dilatation was said to be increased and others that reported it is unaffected. Uterine contractility, measured by abdominal palpation, external tacography, and continuous measurements of amniotic fluid pressure (internal TKD) produces contradictory conclusions. Many studies have shown that PCB produces a small transient decrease in contractility (15,32–34,37,39,44), as has been reported with epidural analgesia (see Chapter 13). Fewer reports indicated that uterine contractility was augmented by PCB.

Miller, Schifrin and his coworkers (62) assessed the effects of PCB with 200 mg of lidocaine on sequential changes in uterine activity. Statistically significant diminution in uterine activity over preblock levels was demonstrated in patients receiving the block during the latent phase of labor and those receiving oxytocin stimulation. Patients in the normal active phase of labor showed progressive increases in uterine activity before the block, but this increase was not seen after the block was administered, although it returned to preblock levels in about 40 to 50 minutes. Thiery and Vroman (42) cited many reports in which paracervical block interferes with uterine contractility pattern for a transient period but then returns to normal levels so as to not effect the progress of labor. Most of the published data suggest that the progress of labor is unaffected if the procedure is started at the proper time (phase of maximum slope when uterine contractions are strong and frequent). However, if the block is started during the latent phase of the first stage, it is likely to slow or even arrest labor, probably as a result of interrupting the afferent limb of the so-called Ferguson's reflex. Some writers (15,17,33,38,50) claim that paracervical block hastens labor due to softening of the cervix and relaxation of the lower uterine segment, but proof of this claim is lacking. In a TKD study of 43 parturients, Zourlas and Kumar (61) found that paracervical block diminished uterine activity in about half the patients. The inhibitory effect was minor (an average of 50 Mont. u.) and resulted from a diminution of either frequency or intensity of contraction (Figure 15–19). It occurred within 5 to 10 minutes of the injection and lasted for about 30 minutes. The rate of cervical dilation was unaffected.

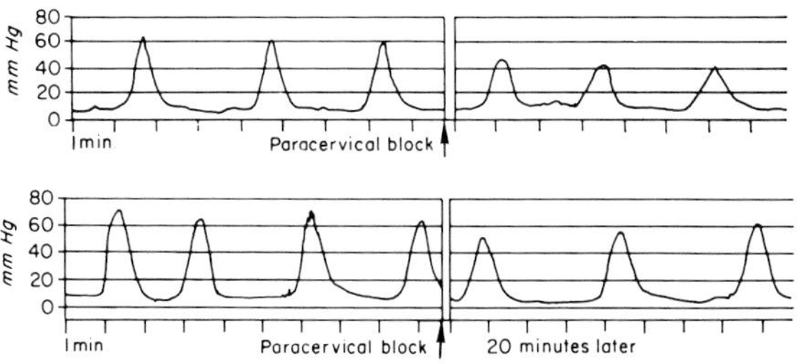


**Fig. 15–19.** Tracing of uterine contractions that indicate mild inhibitory effects of paracervical block. **A)** intensity of uterine contractions decreased about 20 mm Hg. **B)** in this patient, frequency of contractions decreased from 4 per 10 minutes to 3 per 10 minutes. (After Zourlas TA, Kumar D: Am. J. Obstet. Gynecol. 91:217, 1965.)

Notwithstanding the effects on uterine contractility, the cause and progress of labor are unaffected by paracervical block. In a study by Schifrin and associates (62), they divided patients according to parity and compared them to Friedman's ideal curves for nulliparae and multiparae (63). Despite the observed changes in contractility, no significant differences could be demonstrated in the mean durations of the latent phase, active phase, deceleration phase, and second stage of labor nor the maximum slope of cervical dilatation. These studies served to illustrate the limited correlation between transient changes in contractility and longterm changes in cervical dilatation and the progress of labor.

The mechanism for the temporary impairment of uterine contractility following injection of various drugs for regional anesthesia remains unknown. Early studies indicate that perhaps this was caused by interruption of the sympathetic and parasympathetic influence on the uterus, and if epinephrine is used, it may be caused by this agent or by both. Although the influence of the autonomic nerves on uterine contractility remains uncertain, it is known that their interruption is usually followed by transient inhibition of uterine contractility. This interval is short when the uterus is very active (during the active phase of the first stage and in the second stage of labor), but may be prolonged during the latent phase. Because this transient inhibitory effect is seen with all local anesthetic agents used for various regional techniques in obstetrics, one is left with the conclusion that the sudden interruption of the extrinsic neurogenic influences produces inhibition as occurs with interruption of the autonomic nerve to other viscera. This varying period of quiescence is followed by spontaneous resumption of contractility, which then continues uninfluenced by extrinsic nerve activity.

The effect of a given dose of epinephrine is probably greater with paracervical block than with other regional techniques because the drug is injected in the vicinity of the uterine vessels. Because of this and the uterine inhibitory effect, and the possibility of diminished uterine blood flow, generally I do not recommend the use of a vasoconstrictor with the local anesthetic in carrying out paracervical block. In a clinical study using the double-blind technique, Pitkin and Goddard (55) found the incidence of diminished frequency and intensity of uterine contractions to be 41% of 27 cases in which local anesthetic contained epinephrine, and only 7% of 56 cases in which epinephrine was omitted. Freeman and his associates (31,33,34) reported that it was common for contractions to cease for 10 to 15 minutes following block with solutions containing 1:100,000 epinephrine. To avoid this transient inhibitory effect, many clinicians (15,17,35,36) omitted the use of epinephrine.

The auxiliary forces of labor are not affected because paracervical block, unlike pudendal block, does not interrupt the reflex urge to bear down. Even when pudendal block is combined with paracervical block, the patient is able to deliver spontaneously, provided she is properly coached when to bear down. The incidence of spontaneous delivery ranges from 70 to 80% (17,32,33,38–40).

### *Effects on the Fetus and Newborn*

Theoretically, properly carried out, paracervical block should have no direct effect on the infant. However, fetal bradycardia (fetal heart rate less than 100) has been reported by almost every writer, with an incidence ranging from 0 to 70% (17,32,33,35–37,42,44,55,64–71). Others have also noted little or no fetal bradycardia with the use of 2-chloroprocaine (53,54).

Read and Miller (49) used 5 ml of 0.25% bupivacaine on each side (total dose 25 mg) in 32 parturients and noted no adverse effects on the fetus as reflected by baseline fetal heart rate (FHR), beat-to-beat variability, and Apgar scores, and no adverse effects on the mother (81% of whom obtained excellent to good analgesia). Jagerhorn (52), using the refined technique mentioned below in which he achieved PCB with 5 ml of 0.25% bupivacaine with 1/400,000 epinephrine on each side, not only produced effective analgesia in 94% of the parturients, but noted only "extremely slight" changes in fetal heart rate, Apgar scores at 1 minute of 8–10 in 87%, and scores at 10 minutes of 8–10 in all of the infants, and acid-base status similar to the control group. Bradycardia, associated with PCB, occurred in only one case, although slow FHR caused by other factors was encountered in several other cases.

Freeman and Schifrin (43,62), in their extensive studies, evaluated 100 paracervical block-induced fetal bradycardias in parturients whose fetuses previously had benign heart rate patterns. Under these circumstances, the incidence of fetal bradycardia or neonatal depression was not increased even in high-risk pregnancy compared with the control group. Their findings show that in the majority of instances, there is no discernible change in FHR pattern, uterine activity or acid-base balance following PCB when 20 ml of 1% lidocaine or mepivacaine was used. Characteristic bradycardia was encountered in 15% of parturients in which PCB was performed with mepivacaine and 7% with those who had lidocaine. The bradycardia was heralded by an abrupt increase in baseline irregularity beginning 2 to 10 minutes following PCB (Figure 15–20). FHR drops suddenly, usually during a uterine contraction or in association with uterine hypertonus, and it may fall as low as 70 beats per minute and remain depressed for up to 30 minutes. During the bradycardia, the baseline variability of the heart rate is diminished, and episodes of beat-to-beat arrhythmia may occur.

Bradycardia is often followed by a brief period of tachycardia, and as the rate recovers, late deceleration patterns may be observed. Freeman and Schifrin (43) and others have noted that the development of fetal bradycardia coincides with appearance of an increased frequency of uterine contractions and elevated baseline tone (Figure 15–20). With the development of fetal bradycardia, the P-R interval diminishes, and as FHR decreases further, the P-wave becomes biphasic and then disappears (15–21), suggesting vagal suppression of the sinoatrial node followed by ventricular or nodal escape. During this period, beat-to-beat arrhythmias are common but no change in intraventricular conduction is noted as evidenced by the QRS complex (Figure 15–21).

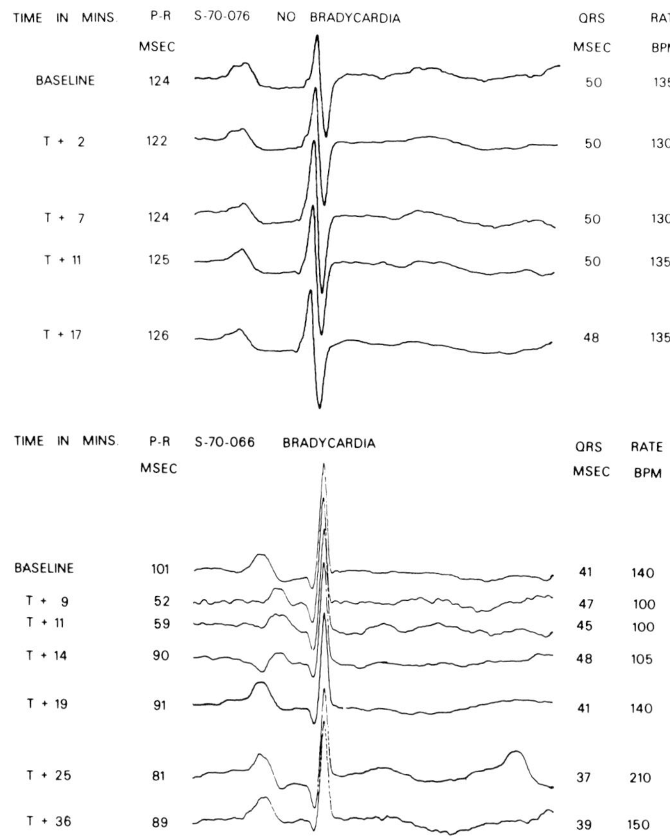


**Fig. 15–20.** Fetal bradycardia following bilateral paracervical block. Note the association of the slowing of the fetal heart rate with uterine hypertonus. (From Freeman RK, Schifrin BS: Whither paracervical block? Int. Anesthesiol. Clin. 11:69–91, 1973.)

Severe fetal bradycardia is followed by fetal acidosis, which recovers slowly and is preceded by a recovery of FHR and, as noted above, rebound tachycardia (74). Bradycardia occurs more frequently with high doses of local anesthetics in which there are FHR abnormalities before PCB, in premature or postmature fetuses, and in association with high-risk pregnancies (42,64,65,68–71,74). In the absence of fetal bradycardia, there is little or no alteration in fetal acid-base status. When fetal bradycardia is corrected 30 to 50 minutes before delivery, neonates have a normal range of Apgar scores; but if it is severe and persists, it may result in fetal death or a severely depressed infant at birth.

Murphy and associates (71) reported two perinatal deaths that resulted from using bupivacaine with epinephrine. Rosefsky and Petersiel (72) reported the perinatal death of two fetuses after fetal bradycardia for 40 to 80 minutes following paracervical blocks with 240 and 300 mg of bupivacaine. Taw (73) reported a perinatal death from direct fetal scalp injection during a paracervical block. Thiery and Vroman (42), in their extensive review, reported 50 fetal mortalities, many of which were associated with serious complications of pregnancy. They stated that local anesthetics, in achieving paracervical block, probably do not cause death in a healthy fetus, but in a fetus already compromised death may occur. Albright (59) cited the case of a death in a lower risk parturient, and also the fact that the FDA was aware of about 17 fetal or neonatal deaths before 1971 (principally from the foreign literature) that followed the paracervical block with bupivacaine. In 11 of these cases, there were obvious other causes of death, including intrafetal injection in three cases. It is the firm belief of this author that all of these deaths were due to technical error, including the use of excessive amounts of local anesthetic, and could have been prevented.

***Mechanisms of bradycardia.*** Despite a number of animal and human studies, the mechanisms for the bradycardia remain controversial. Nyirjesy and his associates (75) attributed fetal bradycardia and acidosis, as well as one intrapartal fetal death, to rapid lidocaine absorption. Fetal intoxication by local anesthetic drugs and their metabolites results from direct flow of a high concentration of the drug to the intervillous space (42–44,55,64,68–71,75). This can be achieved by diffusion of the drug across the uterine wall or by direct injection into the artery (64,68,75). Others have suggested that fetal arrhythmias are the result of acute fetal asphyxia caused by transient uterine artery spasm that in turn is provoked by high concentration of the local anesthetic agent in the paracervical region (64,68,71,75). Still others have attributed this complication to the effects of high concentration of epinephrine (75). The larger the dose of local anesthetic and epinephrine, the more serious the fetal heart rate changes. Accidental intra-arterial injection has also been reported and results in the rapid development of high fetal blood level of the local anesthetic with the consequent depression of the cardiovascular and central nervous system of the fetus, resulting in fetal and neonatal depression and even death. Perinatal depression and

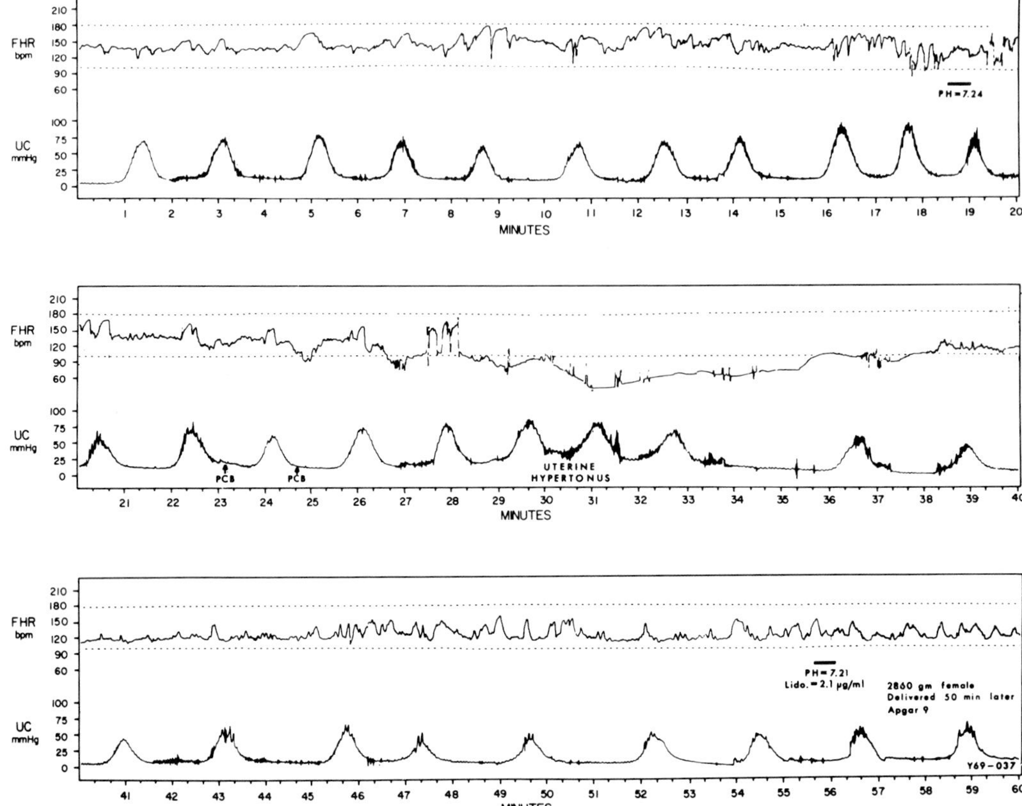


**Fig. 15–21.** The fetal electrocardiogram (FECG) using averaging techniques of the signal-to-noise ratio. **A)** The FECG pattern in the absence of fetal bradycardia. **B)** Changes in group-averaged FECG during fetal bradycardia following bilateral paracervical block. Note the progressive decreases in PR integral gradually diminishes, and as the heart rate decreases further, the P-wave becomes biphasic and then disappears (see text for details). (From Freeman RK, Schifrin BS: Whither paracervical block? Int. Anesthesiol. Clin. 11:69–91, 1973.)

even death may also occur as a result of maternal complications (convulsions, severe hypotension consequent to systemic reactions) and impairment of the forces of labor (prolonged contraction or contracture). For a comprehensive review of mechanisms of fetal bradycardia, the reader is referred to articles by Thiery and Vroman (42), and Cibils and Santonja-Lucas (44).

***Comment.*** Despite the considerable controversy and speculation regarding the mechanisms of PCB-induced bradycardia, there is little doubt that it reflects fetal compromise. Freeman and Schifrin (43) suggest the following guidelines for the use of paracervical block:

1. PCB should be avoided in fetuses with demonstrable asphyxial FHR patterns or acidosis.
2. Because bradycardia appears to be related to dosage and concentration, or total amount of local anesthetic used, it is essential to use the least amount of drug that would be effective. It is best to limit the dosage to 5 ml of 1% lidocaine or 0.25% bupivacaine for each side; and if expertly administered, this should provide sufficient analgesia.
3. Despite the aforementioned precautions, fetal bradycardia is encountered. Because the bradycardia is associated with acidosis and accumulation of local anesthetic in the fetus, it is better to avoid immediate delivery to give the fetus time to recover. The intact placenta undoubtedly can remove the local anesthetic from the fetus quicker and with greater safety than man-made apparatus can remove it from a depressed neonate. When bradycardia is diagnosed, attempts should be made to maximize fetal-maternal exchange. Obviously, the parturient should be turned on her side after the block is administered because the supine position itself may cause fetal bradycardia. She should be given 100% oxygen by tight face mask. If delivery cannot be delayed, resuscitation of the depressed newborn should include usual measures and gastric lavage.

## Technical Considerations

### *Anatomic Basis*

To properly understand and perform paracervical block, it is essential to know the anatomy of the pelvic plexus (also known as the hypergastric plexus) and its various related structures. These include: the uterine vessels and the cardinal and uterosacral ligaments. In addition to Figures 15–22 and 15–23, the reader is invited to study

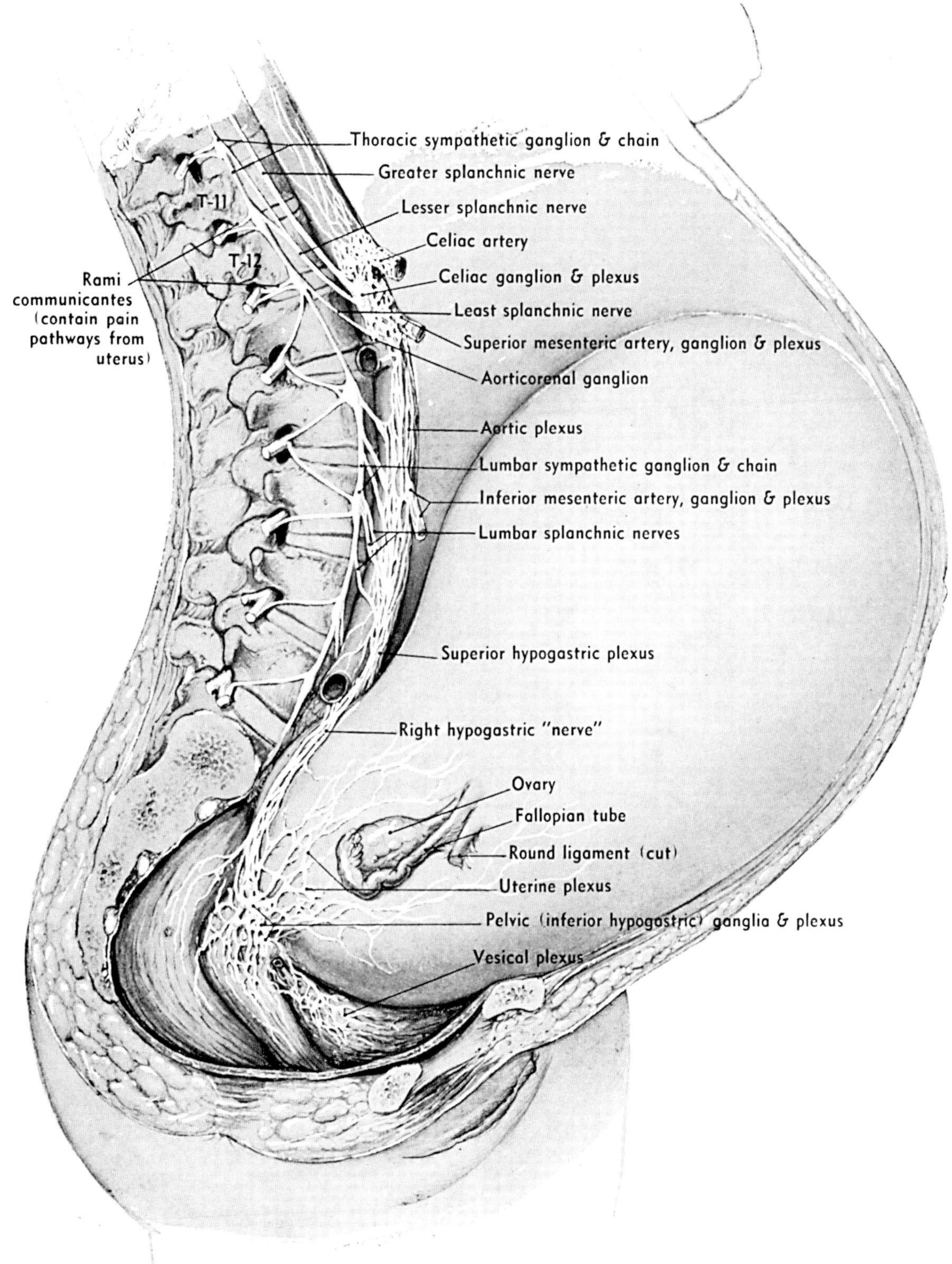


**Fig. 15–22.** Schematic parasagittal section view showing the nerves that supply the uterus and that are involved in lumbar sympathetic and paracervical block. Note relation of the lumbar sympathetic chain to the aortic plexus, superior hypogastric plexus, and the pelvic plexus. The latter breaks up into the rectal, uterovaginal, and vesical plexus. Pain from the uterus and cervix can be relieved by injecting the pelvic plexus on both sides as achieved with bilateral paracervical block or lumbar sympathetic chain as discussed in Figure 15–30 and 15–31.

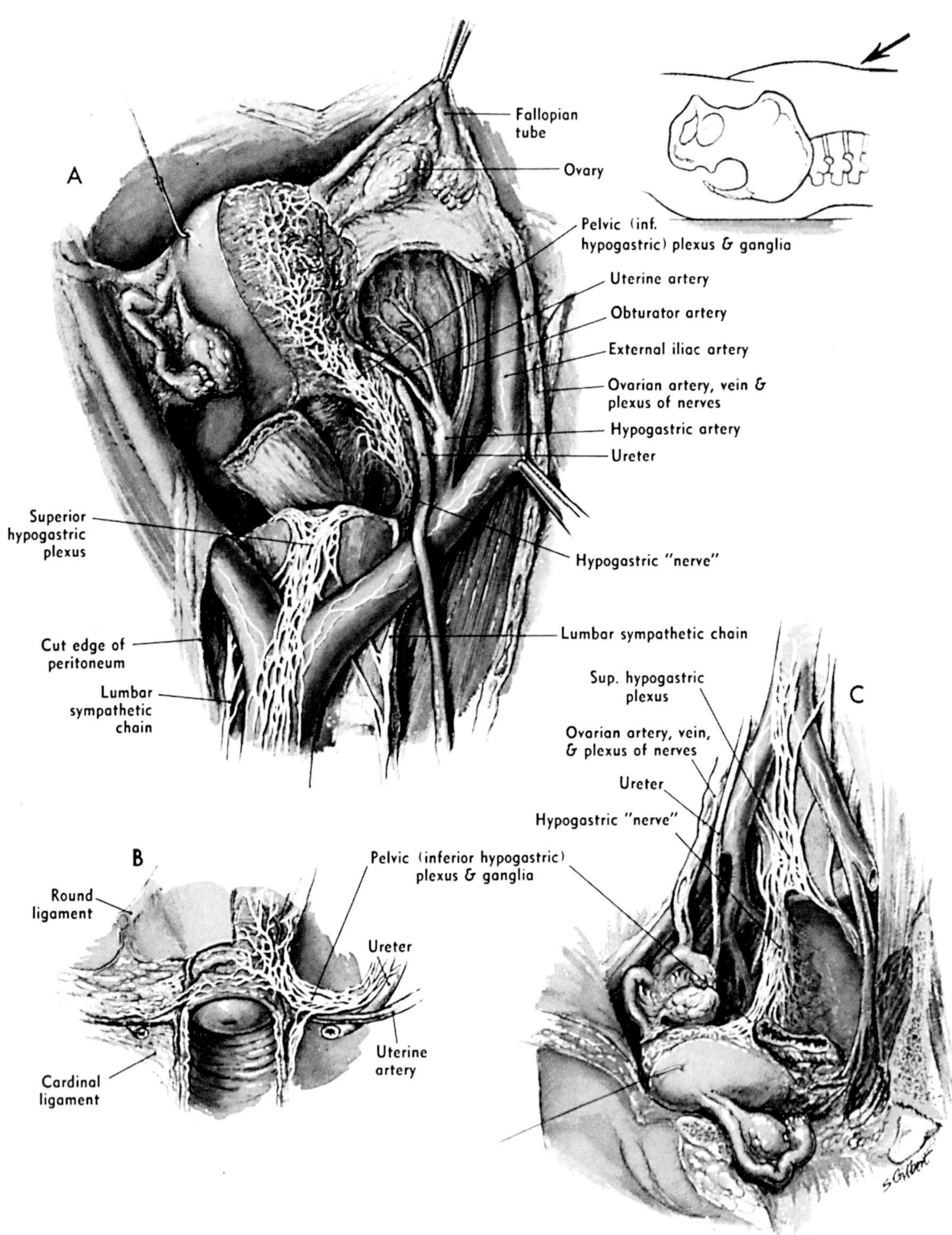


**Fig. 15–23.** Nerve supply of the uterus. **A)** Superior view of pelvis (indicated by arrow in inset). The peritoneum has been removed to show the distribution of the lower portion of the aortic plexus, the superior hypogastric plexus, and the pelvic plexus. Note the relation of the nerve supply to the uterus; this forms the anatomic basis for paracervical block. **B)** Coronal section of the cervix and vagina showing distribution of the pelvic plexus in the paracervical region. Note the relation of the plexus to the uterine artery and the ureter. **C)** Sagittal section of pelvis with a view of its right lateral wall showing course and relation of some of the nerves to the uterus.

the Figure 9–12, as this also provides a good perspective of the relevant anatomy.

### Pelvic Plexus

The pelvic plexus represents the focal point of distribution for sympathetic, sensory, and parasympathetic nerves to the uterus, vagina, bladder, and rectum. It gives rise to subordinate plexuses of which the uterovaginal plexus is one of the larger and most important subdivisions. Figure 15–23 shows the relation of these structures to the uterine artery and veins. During labor these vessels are drawn cephalad to a higher level. The pelvic plexus reaches the parametrial region by passing medial to these structures. In this region, the inferior hypogastric plexus passes downward and laterally near the sacral end of each uterosacral ligament, and then passes forward over the lateral aspect of the rectal ampulla and to the vagina. The nerve fibers then course through this focal anatomic area in, under, and between the terminal 2.5 cm of the uterosacral ligaments. In the immediate vicinity of the cervix, the nerve fibers leave the uterosacral ligament and proceed anteriorly and pass, along with the uterovaginal vessels, to the uterus and vagina.

Figure 35–24 depicts the site of paracervical block to interrupt the afferent nociceptive pathways from the cervix and uterus, and thus relieves pain caused by uterine contractions. At the site of injection in the lateral vaginal fornices, the plexus lies just beneath the stratified squamous epithelium, which is about 2 mm thick. At a depth of about 3 to 4 mm, lie the paracervical venous, arterial plexuses, and loose intervascular connective tissue, and deeper to this, the cervical substance, which is very thin during labor.

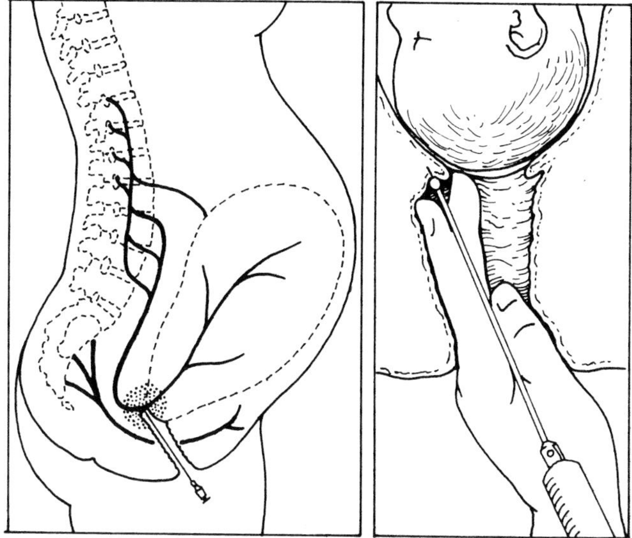

**Fig. 15–24.** Technique of bilateral paracervical block. **A)** Schematic diagram showing sensory (pain) pathways concerned with parturition and the site of interruption when using paracervical block. The pathways from the uterus, including the cervix, are interrupted, thus relieving the pain caused by uterine contraction during the first and second stages of labor. **B)** Schematic coronal section of the vagina and lower part of the uterus showing proper handling of the guide and needle. The injections are made into the lateral fornices of the vagina on each side. Many obstetricians inject at 3 and 9 o'clock, but this writer prefers to inject between 4 and 5 o'clock on the right, and between 7 and 8 o'clock on the left. These injections are made at sites where the pelvic plexus lie, whereas injection at 3 and 9 o'clock are at risk of involving the uterine arteries and ureters (see Figure 15–28). The technique of block is as follows: Following vaginal examination to determine the position of the presenting part, these points of injections are palpated and identified. The distal end of the guide is then carried up to the junction of the cervix and vagina by passing it between the index and middle finger, and then the needle that has already been adapted to the syringe, is passed through the proximal end of the guide. Some obstetricians insert the guide with the needle within it in one step. In any case, as soon as the point of the needle begins its penetration of vaginal mucosa, it is advanced 2 to 3 mm. Whether the guide is used or not, it is very important to avoid inserting the needle more than 4 mm. If the point of the needle is inserted 4 to 6 mm, the solution will be injected in or close to the venous plexus causing rapid absorption of the local anesthetic. Older techniques, in which the point of the needle protruded 1.5 cm beyond the end of the beaded metal tube, advance of the needle to this depth is likely to cause its bevel to enter the peritoneal cavity so that the injected solution would not involve the paracervical plexus. (From Bonica JJ: Obstetric Analgesia and Anesthesia. World Federation of Societies of Anaesthesiologists, Amsterdam, 1980, p. 135.)

## *Preliminary Considerations*

### Agents and Equipment

The concentration and volume of the various analgesic agents that can be used are shown in Table 15–2 and are the same as those used for bilateral pudendal nerve block. Although procaine was used and advocated by the early writers, lidocaine or mepivacaine is far more effective because of their penetrating action, while bupivacaine provides longer analgesia. The penetrating action of lidocaine and bupivacaine is particularly advantageous because the nerves lie among loose areolar tissue, uterosacral ligament, blood vessels, and other tissues. Although epinephrine 1:200,000 can be added to the local anesthetic to delay its absorption and thus decrease the risk of local anesthetic toxicity and increase the intensity and duration of the block, most clinicians no longer use it because the addition of the vasoconstrictor tends to increase the severity of the fetal heart rate changes. For this reason, it is advisable to rely on either 0.25% bupivacaine alone or a mixture of equal parts of 1% lidocaine and 0.375% bupivacaine to achieve more rapid and longer lasting analgesia. Other clinicians (52) add lesser amounts of epinephrine so that the final concentration is 1:300,000 or 1:400,000 (i.e., the amount of epinephrine is 3.75 μg or 2.5 μg per ml of solution).

The equipment required for the procedure is contained in the disposable kit, as noted in Figure 15–6. Currently, most obstetricians use disposable sets that include a 10-ml plastic syringe, preferably with a Luer-Lok, a 15-cm 20-gauge needle with 0.5-cm spacer, an Iowa Trumpet needle guide, a 3.5-cm 22-gauge needle to aspirate the local anesthetic from a container, sponges, and plastic drape to appropriately prepare the field. With the spacer in place, the needle protrudes about 1 cm beyond the end of the guide. Although the manufacturer suggests that the spacer be removed to permit a greater length of needle to protrude beyond the guide, this should not be done for reasons given below.

### *Preliminary Guidelines*

To minimize the aforementioned maternal and perinatal complications, the following guidelines should be adhered to: 1) the procedure should not be started until optimal obstetric conditions prevail; 2) an infusion of fluid should be initiated before the induction of the block, not only to provide fluid, but also to provide a means of immediate injection of appropriate drugs to treat possible complications; 3) it is essential to use low concentrations of local anesthetics, e.g., 0.125 to 0.25% bupivacaine, 2% 2-chloroprocaine and 1% lidocaine or mepivacaine in volumes ranging from 5 to 10 ml, injected into one or two sites of each side; 4) the bevel of the needle should not be deeper than 2 to 3 mm beyond the surface of the vaginal mucosa; 5) adherence to basic principles of regional anesthesia, including aspiration before injection; 6) the maternal and fetal heart rate should be monitored continuously after injection; and 7) this technique should not be used in parturients with chronic uteroplacental insufficiency or in the presence of preexisting fetal distress.

#### Technique of Paracervical Block

Blocks are usually performed in the delivery room using the usual technique for vaginal examination with the patient in the lithotomy position, whereas Jagerhorn (52) prefers to carry out the procedure with the patient in the supine position, relaxed, with the thighs and legs spread apart as much as possible. In either case, it is essential that the uterus be displaced to one side to avoid or minimize aortocaval compression. Obviously, it is necessary to prepare the perineum and vagina and drape the patient as for vaginal examination. The block is best carried out when the cervix is at least 3 to 4 cm dilated, and the presenting part is at 0 to 2+ station. Although most authors believe that the procedure becomes more difficult when the cervix is more than 7 to 8 cm dilated or the presenting part is lower, some clinicians repeat PCB once, twice or even three times (52). The actual technique of blocking the paracervical plexus is depicted in Figures 15–24 to 15–26 and described in the legends. It is important not to penetrate more than 2 to 3 mm into the fornices for the injection of the local anesthetic.

Jagerhorn (52) carried out a study in women who were to undergo legal abortion at the fourteenth to nineteenth week of pregnancy and injected a mixture of contrast medium and local anesthetic into various sites and at various depths to ascertain the best site for the absorption from the paracervical space. Jagerhorn concluded that the injection should be made 2 to 3 mm at which point a slow diffusion of the local anesthetic into the loose intervascular connective tissue occurs. He noted that a depth of 4 mm at each injection site venous absorption occurred, although it was not as significant as at greater depths of injection. With injection at a depth of 6 mm, the risk of vascular absorption is very high. He emphasized the importance of placing the needle strictly tangential to the descending fetal part. If the needle is directed more medially at a slight angle, injection may be made into the cervical substance that—although it produces analgesia—may cause rapid absorption of the local anesthetic. More importantly, having the needle at an angle instead of tangentially is inherent in the risk of injecting the anesthetic directly into the fetus, which has serious consequences as discussed above. By using this technique in administering 204 paracervical blocks to 134 parturients, Jagerhorn was able to produce good to excellent analgesia in 94% of parturients with no adverse effects on the mother and only minimal adverse fetal effects. He used 0.25% bupivacaine with 1:400,000 epinephrine and injected 3 ml at 4 and 8 o'clock and 2 ml at 5 and 7 o'clock on each side. He repeated the procedure a second time in 43% of parturients, a third injection in 7%, and a fourth or more injections in 3% of the patients. The mean duration of each block was 95 ± 32 minutes.

The fact that the procedure described by Jagerhorn (52) produced analgesia that was 10 to 20% better than others using bupivacaine, and that a total of only 10 ml of 0.25% bupivacaine with epinephrine 1:400,000 was used, is an impressive accomplishment. Based on these results, the technique described by Jagerhorn is recommended to obstetricians. However, this writer believes that a single injection of 5 to 7 ml of solution at a site between 3 and 4 o'clock on the patient's left side, and between 7 and 8 o'clock on the patient's right side should produce equally effective results. If the bevel of the needle is in the submucosal space, the solution is likely to diffuse anteriorly and posteriorly as depicted in Figure 15–26.

#### Continuous Techniques of PCB and BPB

In the mid-1960s, continuous techniques of paracervical block were described by Burchell and Sadove (77) and a year later by Tafeen, Freedman and Harris (78), but they never achieved widespread use for several reasons. The technique of Burchell and Sadove required a large 13-gauge needle guide, was passed through the perineum into the vagina and thus was more traumatic. The same could be said for the technique of Tafeen and associates (78) who initially used also a 13-gauge needle to introduce the 20-gauge precurved Teflon catheter. Two years later, they published an article describing a combined continuous paracervical and continuous pudendal nerve block for labor using the same type of instrument except that the needle had been reduced to a 17 gauge, and that the precurved catheter was a 23 gauge. They used continuous paracervical block in 525 patients, and, of these, 284 had combined techniques with continuous paracervical and continuous pudendal catheters being used. Although they reported that gratifying analgesic effects occurred in over 90% of the patients, 68% of those with the combined technique required inhalation anesthesia for about 45 seconds to complete delivery. With their technique, they reported low instances of fetal bradycardia and virtually no complications in the mother. Despite these favorable results, the procedure did not gain widespread use; indeed,

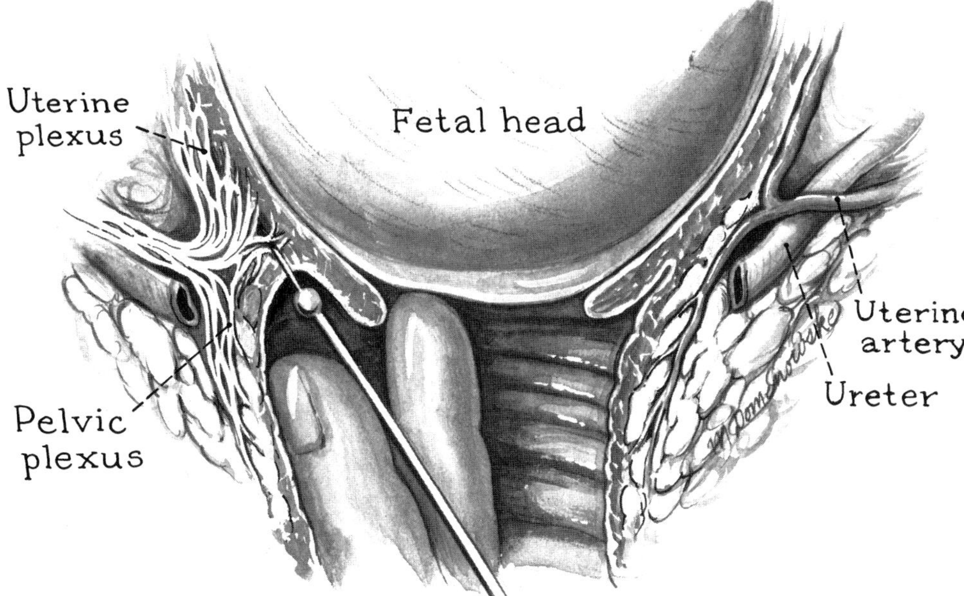


**Fig. 15–25.** Technique of paracervical block. Schematic coronal section (enlarged) of the lower portion of the cervix and upper portion of the vagina showing the end of the needle projecting beyond the beaded end of the guide within the paracervical plexus. Note the thinness of the vaginal mucosa and the fact that the needle projects only about 3 mm beyond the beaded end of the guide.

a brief survey at the time of this writing revealed that the procedure is not used by any obstetrician, except perhaps by the group associated with the original authors. Therefore, it will not be included in this chapter. The interested reader may wish to review the technique in the first edition of this book (pp. 514–518) or the authors' original article (79).

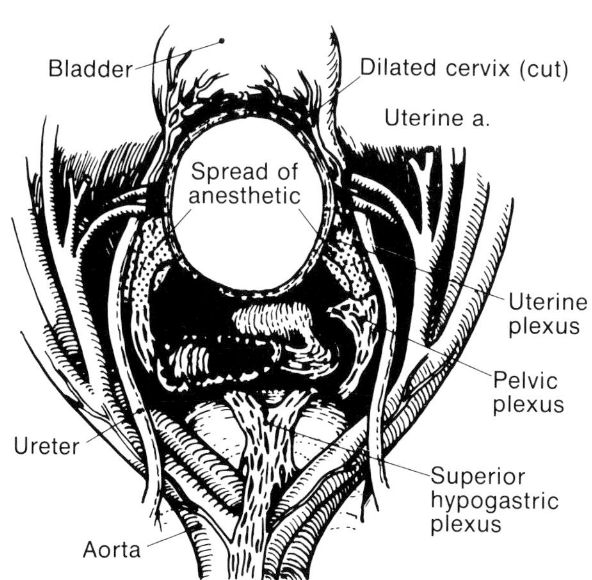


**Fig. 15–26.** Superior view of the pelvis depicting the relative positions of the pelvic plexus and uterine arteries and ureter and the area of diffusion of the local anesthetic. Note that the pelvic plexus is located at 4 and 8 o'clock, whereas the uterine arteries and ureter are located at 3 and 9 o'clock. This indicates that the optimal sites of injection are as described in the text and Figure 15–25. (From Bonica JJ: Obstetric Analgesia and Anesthesia. World Federation of Societies of Anesthesiologists, Amsterdam, 1980, p. 135)

### Management of the Patient

Following each injection, the patient is observed closely for signs of systemic toxicity or other complications. Blood pressure, pulse and respiration, and fetal heart rate are measured frequently and recorded every 3 to 5 minutes. Uterine contractions are also monitored. As soon as the pain of uterine contractions returns, the paracervical injections are repeated. If at the time the patient is made ready for delivery and 60 to 75 minutes have elapsed since the last injection, the block is repeated—if this is possible without having to exert too much pressure on the presenting part. When the parturient begins to experience perineal pain, bilateral pudendal block or saddle block is carried out.

## Bilateral Lumbar Sympathetic Block

Bilateral lumbar sympathetic block (BLSB), like bilateral paracervical block, interrupts the sensory pathways from the uterus, including the cervix, and thus relieves the pain caused by uterine contractions. It was first used for this purpose in 1927 by Dellepiane and Badino (80) who reported good relief of pain in 20 to 25 parturients following infiltration of the sympathetic chain at the level of the third lumbar vertebra. They noted no deleterious effects on uterine contractility or on the newborn. The report also contained a detailed discussion of the nerve supply to the uterus and the conclusion that pain of the first stage of labor is carried by sensory nerves incorporated into the lumbar sympathetic chain, a fact that was overlooked for over 30 years. Despite this favorable report, the technique was not adapted to obstetric practice until nearly 2 decades later. In 1943, Schumaker, Hellman, and Manahan (81) published the first American report; they were unimpressed with the procedure and abandoned its use. A year later, Jarvis (82) reported its use on 70 patients with excellent results. In the same year, Cleland (83) used a combination of lumbar sympathetic block for the first stage of labor and continuous caudal analgesia for the second stage. He noted best results using block at the level of the second lumbar vertebra. In 1951, Reich (84) reported on a continuous lumbar paravertebral block technique he had used in 700 patients. Subsequently, Byrd and associates (85,86) reported its successful use in several thousand cases. Hunter (87) reported the therapeutic value of lumbar sympathetic block in patients with uterine inertia. Despite its simplicity of administration, relative safety, and effectiveness, bilateral lumbar sympathetic block (BLSB) has not achieved widespread acceptance because most obstetricians consider it too complicated and perhaps inherent in the high risk of complications. Nevertheless, in patients in whom PCB is contraindicated, BLSB is highly effective and does not carry the risk of fetal bradycardia associated PCB. In such circumstances, the obstetrician should require the services of an anesthesiologist who has expertise with this technique (usually for pain therapy) to carry it out in selected parturients. With knowledge of the anatomy and technique, this procedure is as simple as bilateral PCB.

## Clinical Evaluation

### *Analgesic Efficacy*

Lumbar sympathetic block is usually initiated when the parturient begins to experience moderate to severe pain during the active phase of the first stage of labor. The conditions that should be present are the same as those present for paracervical block, i.e., cervical dilatation of at least 3 to 4 cm and uterine contractions occurring every 3 minutes, lasting 30 to 45 seconds, and having an intensity of 35 to 40 mm Hg. The best site for injection is the level of the second lumbar vertebra (Figures 15–26 and 15–27).

The success rate with the initial injection should be over 90% of the parturients. In a series of 1200 cases, Byrd (85) noted adequate relief of labor pain in all but three cases. Duration of analgesia was 1 hour with 1% procaine, 1 1/2 hours with 1% lidocaine without epinephrine, and 2 hours with 1% lidocaine with epinephrine 1:300,000. In 65 parturients, the block had to be repeated once, and in eight of them it had to be repeated twice. With 0.25% plain bupivacaine block and consequent analgesia lasting 2 1/2 to 3 hours, the addition of 1:300,000 epinephrine will extend the block to 3 to 4 hours—sufficient for providing pain relief for most of the active phase of the first stage of labor. Although a continuous technique has been described and reported to be effective by Riekse (86), this writer has experienced discouraging results because after the first injection the catheter moved and inadequate analgesia resulted. Because of this and because of the advent of bupivacaine, a single injection technique with 0.25% bupivacaine and 1:300,000 epinephrine is preferred. Because the procedure has no effect on the perineal pain, it is necessary to supplement it with bilateral pudendal block, low saddle block or low caudal for the second and third stages of labor.

#### *Effects on the Mother*

Properly carried out, BLSB should not cause alteration of maternal function except mild hypotension. This occurs in 10 to 15% of parturients if the patient is made to lie supine after the block or as a result of the spread of an excessive volume of local anesthetic solution with consequent spread to the celiac plexus and splanchnic nerves. The more solution used above that recommended (5 to 7 ml for each side), the more likely the spread and the greater the incidence and magnitude of hypotension. Alteration in maternal function may also result from systemic toxic reaction or accidental injection of the drug into the epidural or subarachnoid space. In her series of 1200 cases, Byrd (85) encountered generalized convulsions in three patients, minor systemic reactions in four, accidental subarachnoid block in two, and accidental epidural anesthesia (extending to levels ranging from T9 to T6 dermatomes) in five patients. All of these patients were successfully treated without consequences either to the patient or to the infant. Other possible complications include accidental involvement of some lumbar somatic nerves with consequent analgesia/anesthesia of the anterior thigh. All of these complications, except mild hypotension, can be prevented with proper technique and having the patient lie on her side after the block.

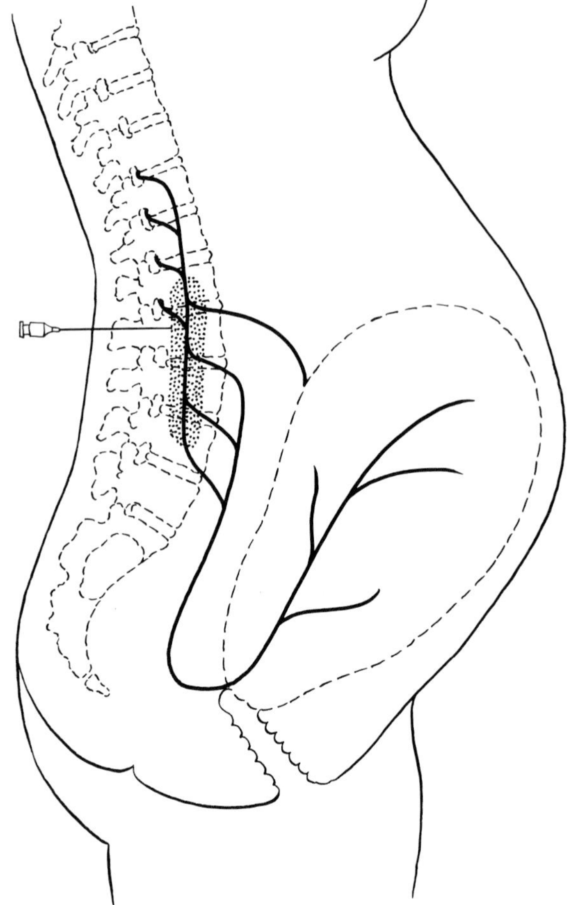

**Fig. 15–27.** Schematic diagram showing site of lumbar sympathetic block. Note that this technique interrupts pain pathways from the uterus and cervix, but it has no effect on those from the perineum, which is supplied by the pudendal nerves.

### Effects on Labor

Normal labor is usually not affected by BLSB. Among 39 parturients studied by Hunter (87) using the TKD technique, 20 exhibited acceleration of the first stage of labor, following temporary (5 to 15 minutes) uterine hypertonus. The remaining 19 subjects exhibited no change in uterine contractions following block. This technique should be slightly better than paracervical block in this regard because it interrupts sympathetic pathways. Hunter (87) found that sympathetic block converts abnormal (midsegment dominance) uterine contractions to normal contractions in three-fourths of the patients in whom this procedure was used. He attributed the beneficial effect to release of the uterus from an inhibitory effect of the sympathetic nervous system. Unlike subarachnoid or epidural blocks, or pudendal block, this procedure does not involve the nerves to the perineum so that spontaneous internal rotation and the reflex urge to bear down are not interfered with.

### Effects on the Infant

Lumbar sympathetic block has no direct effect on the fetus, and the newborn sustains no depression except in those cases in which maternal complications develop or excessive amounts of local anesthetics are used.

## Technical Considerations

### *Anatomic Bases*

The pertinent anatomy for lumbar sympathetic block is illustrated in Figures 15–26 and Figure 15–27, which should be studied together with Figure 15–22 in the preceding section and with Figure 9–12 in Chapter 9, as these give better perspective.

The lumbar portion of the sympathetic trunk consists of two ganglionated cords that extend from the first to the fifth lumbar vertebra and which are continuous above with the thoracic portion and below with the pelvic portion of the trunk. Each chain lies on the anterolateral surface of the vertebral column. The chain on each side is situated anterior to the lumbar vessels that separate it from the vertebral column and medial to the origin of the psoas muscle and its fascia. On the right side, the trunk lies posterior to the lateral edge of the vena cava, which in most cases completely covers the trunk. However, on the left side, the chain is rarely covered by the aorta, being 2 to 10 mm lateral to the lateral edge of the vessel. Inferiorly, the cords pass posteriorly to the iliac vessels to become continuous with the sacral trunk.

The lumbar sympathetic chain is the most variable portion of the sympathetic system, particularly in regard to the number of ganglia and the general forms of the two chains. Although there are usually 3 or 4 ganglia, this number varies. Moreover, one only rarely finds a chain on one side that is the same shape, size, and position as the one on the other. In some instances, the ganglia are segmentally located, while others are closely grouped and lie over particular segments—the most common location being between the second lumbar and the inferior border of the fourth lumbar vertebra. The ganglia may be situated on the body of the vertebra or next to aponeurotic arcades giving origin to the psoas muscle, or they may lie anterolateral to an intervertebral disc—one portion of the ganglion in front of the vertebra above and the other in front of the vertebra below.

The above description makes apparent two important points. First, the inconsistency of the location and number of the sympathetic ganglia makes any attempt to anesthetize a particular ganglion impractical. Regardless of the indication for the block, the operator should strive to place the point of the needle near the chain at the level of the second lumbar vertebra. Because the chain is contained within fascial planes that act as "pouches," the local anesthetic solution injected into the "pouch" will spread along the length of the chain (88). The second point is the close proximity of the sympathetic chain to the aortic (intermesenteric) plexus, the celiac plexus, and the superior hypogastric plexus. If large volumes of solution are used, all of these preaortic sympathetic nerves will likely be involved with consequent block of the motor fibers to the uterus, and the vasomotor fibers to the splanchnic region. The latter effect is likely to produce arterial hypotension.

### *Agents and Equipment*

The concentrations and volumes of the various anesthetic agents that may be used for lumbar sympathetic block are shown in Table 15–2. As previously mentioned, I prefer the use of 5 to 8 ml of 0.25% bupivacaine with epinephrine 1:300,000.

The equipment needed for the single-dose technique includes the usual block tray and two 10-cm 22-gauge needles with long, sharp bevels. Resuscitation equipment should be in the room ready for immediate use.

### Technique of Block

The best position for the patient is dependent upon at which phase of the first stage of labor the block is to be started. If it is started before the head of the fetus is on the perineum, it is best to have the patient in a sitting position with her legs over the edge of the bed or delivery table, and her spine flexed as much as possible (Figure 15–28). It is essential that an attempt be in front of the patient to encourage her constantly and also to detect any reactions. Because some parturients who have received narcotics develop postural hypotension, it is especially important to have the attendant keep a close watch on the patient's color, pulse rate, and respiration. Later on in labor, the lateral position is probably more comfortable.

Maximum flexion of the lumbar spine facilitates identification of the spinous process of the lumbar vertebrae which are found as rectilinear prominences about 2 cm in length and about 0.5 cm thick. The mid portion of the spinous process is marked with a thumbnail impression or indelible pencil because this is at the same cross section level as the site of injection. After this, the skin is prepared with an antiseptic solution, and the procedure is carried out as depicted in Figure 15–28 and described in the legend.

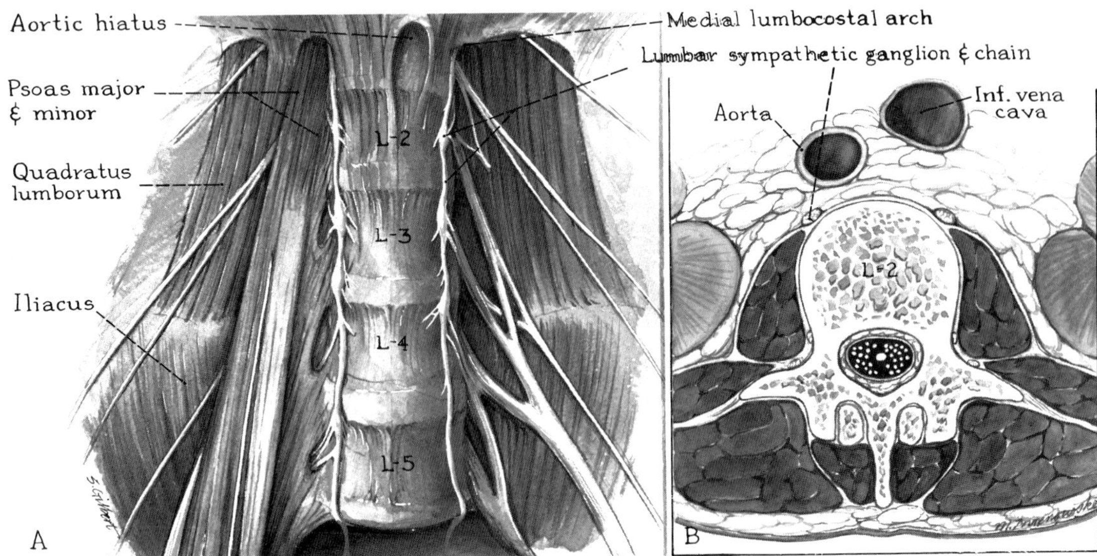


**Fig. 15–28.** Lumbar sympathetic chain. **A)** Anterior view showing its position on the anterolateral surface of the vertebral bodies. **B)** Cross sectional level showing the relation of the chain to the vertebrae and to the iliopsoas muscle and its fascia. The superior vena cava and aorta are closer to the spinal column than shown here and overlie the sympathetic chains with the aorta just anterior to the left chain and the inferior vena cava anterior to the right chain.

### *Management of the Patient*

The parturient should be monitored closely for signs of systemic toxicity, accidental subarachnoid block or other complications during and after the block. Promptly after the block is completed, the patient is made to lie on her side. Blood pressure, pulse, and respiration are measured frequently and recorded every 3 to 5 minutes. If pain returns before the patient is positioned for the delivery, the procedure is repeated. When the patient begins to have perineal pain, bilateral pudendal block, low caudal block or a low saddle block is performed.

## Local Analgesia and Field Block of the Abdomen

Local analgesic techniques for cesarean section are intended to anesthetize the abdominal wall and parietal peritoneum (89). Usually no attempt is made to interrupt the visceral sensory pathways initially because the gravid uterus makes these inaccessible until it has been exposed. The abdominal wall may be anesthetized by local infiltration techniques and rectus block.

## Clinical Evaluation

Properly executed, these techniques provide adequate analgesia of the abdominal wall. They do not usually anesthetize the visceral peritoneum, uterus or other viscera; but because the "adequate stimulus" for pain in viscera is stretching, sudden distention, contraction, tearing or ischemia, incision of the uterus will not produce pain. (90) Therefore, abdominal delivery can be carried out without discomfort provided analgesia of the abdominal wall is complete and the surgeon is gentle in exposing the uterus. If extensive intra-abdominal exploration and manipulation are required, it will be necessary to supplement regional analgesia/anesthesia with systemic analgesic achieved with opioids or inhalation analgesia with 60 to 70% nitrous oxide in oxygen or balanced general endotracheal anesthesia given after the infant has been delivered.

The deceptive simplicity of the infiltration field block techniques has misled many obstetricians and surgeons into thinking that there is no need to learn the technique or the pharmacology of the local anesthetic drug. As a result, the incidence of partial failure and complications is relatively high. In some instances, the parturient experiences moderate to severe pain because the operator does not wait long enough for the local anesthetic to produce its effects. In others, it is because the injection has not been made in the proper fascial compartments.

### *Effects on the Mother*

Side effects on the mother occur only as a result of improper technique. In addition to inadequate pain relief—with consequent apprehension, anxiety and fear, tachycardia—systemic toxic reactions may develop. I have observed operators who used 2% procaine and, in some instances, even 2% lidocaine for infiltration. Because of the large volume required, the total dose injected was naturally excessive. These patients frequently developed tremors that in some progressed to convulsions, and some suffered cardiovascular collapse that required prompt aggressive resuscitative measures.

### *Effects on the Fetus and Newborn*

The fetus and newborn are usually not affected—a most important advantage of these techniques. However, if the mother sustains a systemic toxic reaction with convulsions, the fetus will suffer asphyxia. Moreover, because these drugs pass the placental membrane, a high fetal blood level also may be produced with consequent direct depression of the cardiovascular and central nervous system of the fetus and newborn. Because of the larger volume used, the risk of these complications is greater with this technique than with extradural or subarachnoid block.

## Technical Considerations

### *Anatomy of the Abdominal Wall*

Like all other regional techniques, success with these procedures requires thorough knowledge of the topographic landmarks of the abdominal wall and the fasciae muscles, and most important, the course and location of the nerves that supply these structures. Because these techniques are usually done by obstetricians who know these anatomic facts, only a very brief description, supplemented with illustrations, is presented.

Figures 15–29 and 15–30 depict the topographic landmarks and muscles of the abdominal with a brief description of each given in the legend. Figures 15–31 and 15–32 depict the nerve supply, which is described briefly in the legend. As noted in the first two figures, the musculature of the abdominal wall consists of four pairs of muscles and their aponeuroses: 1) the rectus; 2) external oblique; 3) internal oblique; and 4) transversus abdominis. These

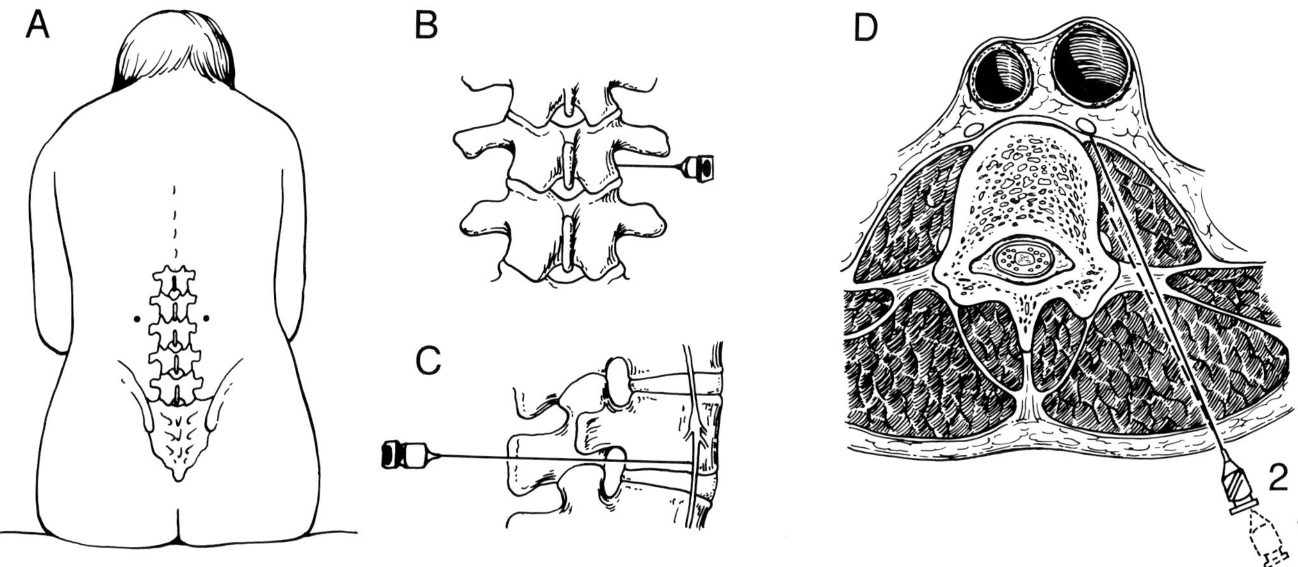


**Fig. 15–29.** Technique of lumbar sympathetic block to provide relief of pain during the first stage of labor. **A)** Patient is sitting with the lumbar spine flexed. Note that two skin wheals are opposite the midportion of the spinous process of the second lumbar vertebra about 7-cm lateral to the spinous process. **B)** Enlarged posterior view of the vertebral column depicting the relation of the needle to the vertebra and its spinous process. **C)** Parasagittal view of the vertebral with the needle in place in contact with the sympathetic chain, showing its position just below the transverse process and its relation to the midportion of the spinous process. **D)** Cross section showing the steps in carrying out the block. A 22-gauge 10-cm needle is threaded with a depth marker and inserted through the skin wheal with its point directed anteriorly and medially. In step 1, the shaft of the needle should make an angle of about 25° to 30° with the midsagittal plane or 70° to 75° with the skin lateral to it. The needle is advanced until the lateral aspect of the lumbar vertebra is contacted, usually at a depth of 6 to 8 cm from the skin in normal individuals but possibly as deep as 10 cm from the skin in obese parturients. The depth marker is placed 2 cm from the skin, and the needle is withdrawn until its point is subcutaneous and then redirected more laterally so that it will pass through the psoas major muscle (step 2) and the lateral aspect of the vertebra. When the point of the needle is 1-cm anterior to the site of contact with the lateral aspect of the vertebra, it is useful to adapt a 2- or 5-ml syringe filled with air or saline solution. As the needle traverses the psoas muscle, steady pressure on the plunger of the syringe encounters some resistance to injection. The needle is further advanced while gentle pressure is applied to the plunger of the syringe. As the point of the needle passes through the thick medial junction of the psoas fascia, significant resistance is encountered, but as soon as the bevel pierces the fascia, a sudden lack of resistance can be felt and the air or saline can be injected easily indicating that the needle point is in the retroperitoneal space, on the anterolateral surface of the vertebra, and is near the sympathetic chain. The procedure is repeated on the opposite side and attempt at aspiration is made in two planes to detect blood or cerebrospinal fluid. If cerebrospinal fluid is aspirated, it is best to abandon the procedure. If blood is aspirated, the position of the needle should be changed and then one must wait at least 5 minutes to permit clot formation. When both needles are considered to be properly placed, 3 ml of solution containing 1/200,000 (15 μg) of epinephrine is injected and the patient is observed for 2 minutes. If, despite the negative aspiration, the solution is injected accidentally into a vein, the patient will develop increase in heart rate and blood pressure due to the epinephrine. If the point of the needle was accidentally in cerebrospinal fluid, the 3 ml of solution will produce a midsubarachnoid block. If neither complication occurs, the remaining 7 ml of solution are injected through each needle. This is sufficient to spread and involve the chain for the length of 3 vertebrae. Larger volumes will likely result in widespread diffusion and involvement of the prevertebral sympathetic plexuses (celiac, aortic, and mesenteric plexuses) with consequent hypotension. Because the procedure does not interrupt the pudendal nerve and the perineal pain pathways contained therein, it needs to be combined with bilateral pudendal block or low caudal or low subarachnoid block initiated when the patient begins to have perineal pain at the end of the first stage and beginning of the second stage.

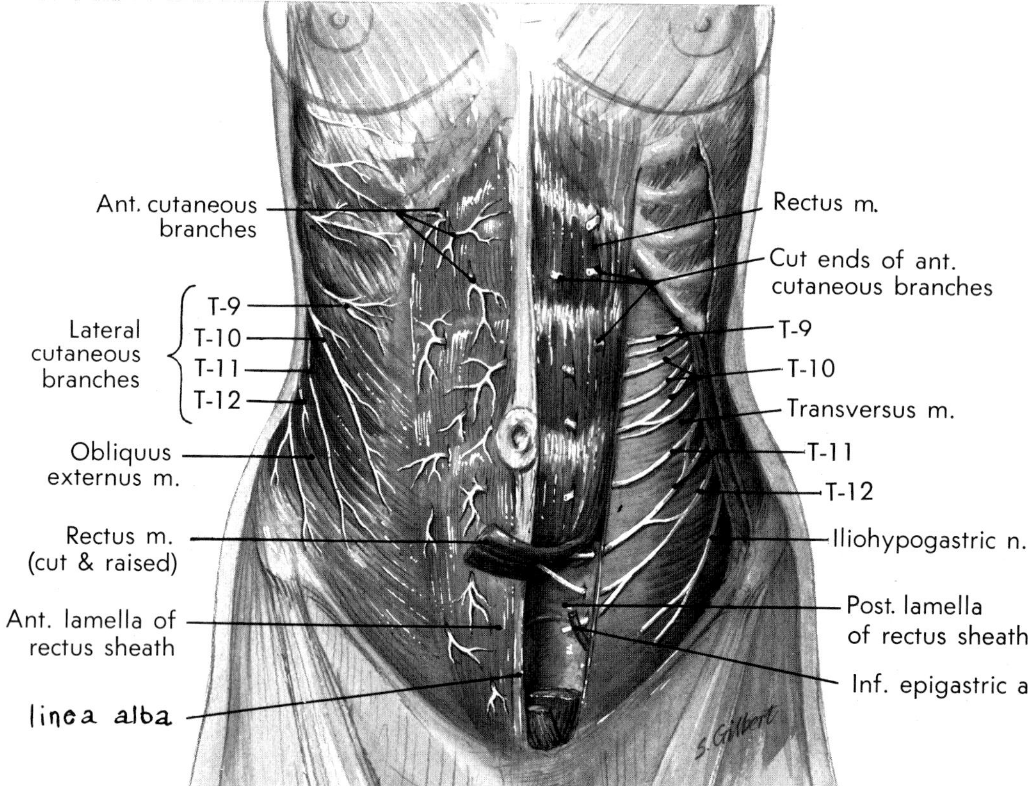


**Fig. 15–30.** Anterior view of abdominal wall with skin removed to show nerve supply and muscles. Note that the important landmarks of the abdominal wall include: a) the umbilicus, b) the linea alba, which extends in the midline from the xiphoid process to the symphysis pubis, and represents a line of union between the aponeurosis of the sides of the abdominal wall; c) the linea semilunaris, which indicates the lateral margin of each rectus muscle; and d) the three linea transversae, which have shallow grooves extending across the upper part of each rectus muscle. These landmarks are vague in obese individuals and in gravidae at term because of the significant stretching of the abdominal wall and consequent thinning of its components. Moreover, there is rupture of the elastic fibers of the reticular stratum of the skin and formation of the striae of pregnancy. Note that various muscles that include: a) the rectus; b) the external oblique; c) the internal oblique; and d) the transversus abdominis. In the figure's left side, the external and internal oblique muscles have been cut to show the course of some of the intercostal nerves between the internal oblique and the transversus. The endings of these nerves that pass through the rectus abdominis are the anterior cutaneous branches. Note also the lateral cutaneous branches of the nerves (compare with Figure 15–34).

are attached above and laterally to the sternum and ribs, and below to the bones of the pelvis. The important functions of these muscles in the bearing-down effort during the second stage of labor have been emphasized in Chapter 4. Here, we are primarily concerned with the fascial compartments and the course of the nerves within them. Three pertinent points to field block or local infiltration should be made.

First is that the greater part of the rectus sheath is formed by the splitting at the linea semilunaris of the aponeurosis of the internal oblique muscle into two layers that envelop the rectus muscle. Each of these lamellae is thickened and strengthened by: 1) the aponeurosis of the external oblique, which blends with the anterior layer; and 2) the aponeurosis of the transverse abdominis, which blends with the posterior layer (Figure 15–30). In the lower portion of the abdominal wall below the semicircular line of Douglas, the posterior rectus sheath is missing. This is because the aponeuroses of the three flat muscles pass to the linea alba in front of the rectus, so that the posterior surface of the rectus muscle is in direct contact with the fascia transversalis and extraperitoneal fat.

Second, the rectus muscle is crossed by three fibrous bands, the inscriptiones tendineae. One is usually situated opposite the umbilicus, one at the level of the lower tip of xiphoid process, and the third about midway between the xiphoid and the umbilicus (Figure 15–29). Occasionally, another one or two incomplete ones are present below the umbilicus. These inscriptions pass transversely or obliquely and are intimately and firmly adherent to the anterior wall of the rectus sheath but do not involve the posterior portion of the muscle. Injection of local anesthetic solution between the anterior sheath and the anterior aspect of the muscle is limited by these inscriptions, whereas when injected posterior to the muscle it is free to spread cephalad and caudad.

The third important point is that in the gravida at full term the rectus muscle is stretched and thinned, and the anterior and posterior layers of the sheath are less than 5 mm apart. The abdominal wall between the medial bor-

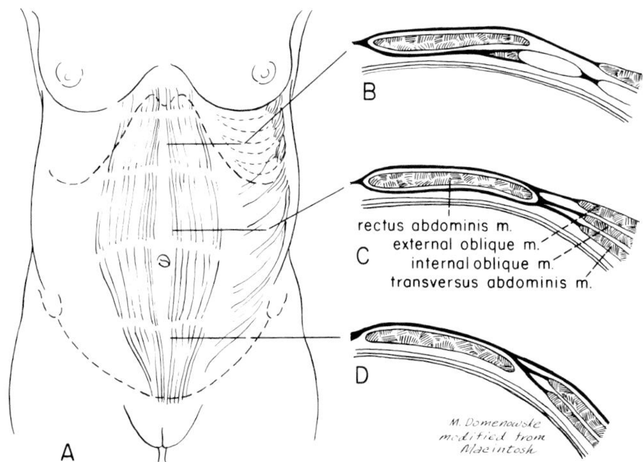


**Fig. 15–31.** Muscles and fascia of abdominal wall. **A)** the rectus muscles become stretched and thinned as the abdomen enlarges. Above the costal margin, the muscles lie directly on the costal cartilages and intercostal spaces. **B)** cross section showing the fibers of the transversus abdominous fused with the aponeurosis of the internal oblique in the posterior wall of the sheath. **C)** typical formation of the rectus sheath. **D)** below the arcuate line, the rectus muscle is separated from peritoneum only by the transversalis fascia and extraperitoneal fat.

ders of these two rectus muscles consists merely of the skin, the fascia, and the peritoneum. Moreover, under the strain of the enlarged abdomen, the two rectus muscles often separate permitting the uterus to fall forward and thus giving rise to diastasis. These effects (which occur to a much greater degree in multiparae than in primiparae) significantly increase the difficulty in carrying out local anesthesia.

The nerve supply of the abdominal wall consists of the anterior division of the lower six thoracic nerves and by the ilioinguinal and iliohypogastric nerves (Figures 15–31 and 15–32). The anterior primary division of the seventh to eleventh nerves, called the thoracoabdominal intercostal nerves, enters the abdominal wall by passing behind the costal cartilages and entering the interval between the transversus abdominis and internal oblique muscle. The course within this muscle is shown in Figure 15–32. As noted, these nerves end as the anterior cutaneous nerves of the abdominal wall. The anterior primary division of the twelfth thoracic nerve, known as the subcostal nerve, is much larger than the others. After emerging from its intervertebral foramen, it proceeds anterolaterally in front of the quadratus lumborum, then perforates the transversus abdominis to gain the interval between this muscle and the internal oblique. Therefore, its course and distribution are the same as the intercostal nerves.

The iliohypogastric and the ilioinguinal nerves arise from the anterior primary division of the first lumbar nerve. Their course is similar to and parallel with that of the twelfth thoracic nerve. After leaving the intervertebral foramen, these nerves pass in front of the quadratus lumborum and course between the transversus abdominis and the internal oblique. The iliohypogastric nerve continues this course as far as 2 cm anterior to the anterior-superior iliac spine where it gains the interval between the internal oblique and external oblique muscle. In this position, it proceeds medially as far as 3 cm above the subcutaneous

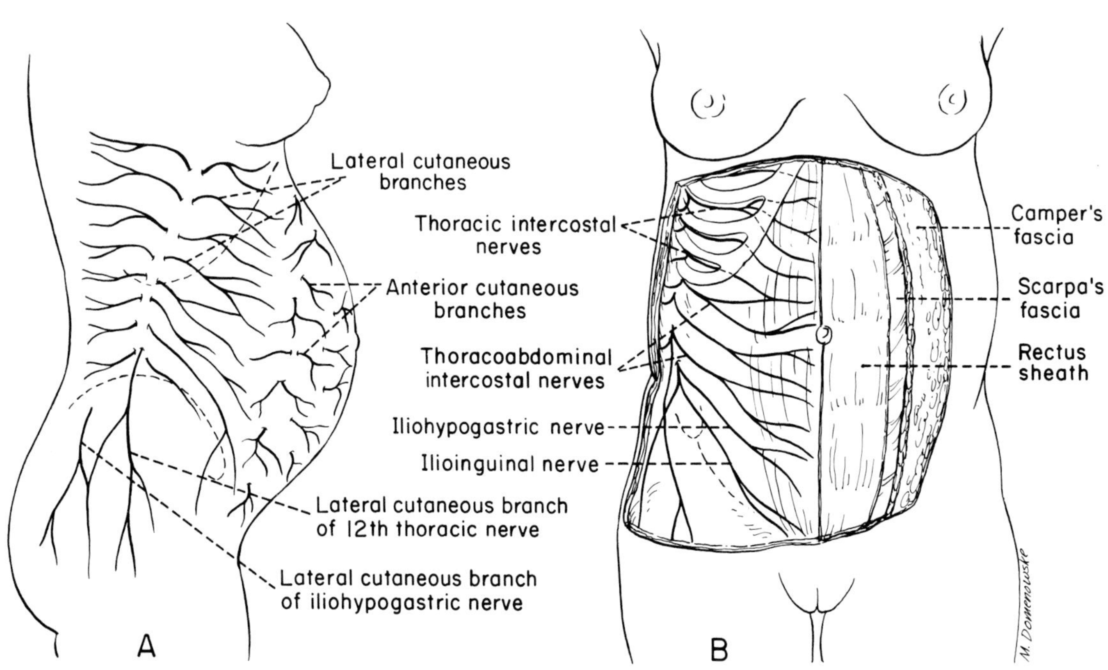


**Fig. 15–32.** Schematic diagram of the nerve supply of the abdominal wall. **A)** side view showing the distribution of the lateral and anterior cutaneous branches of the lower seven intercostal and the first lumbar nerves. **B)** anterior view showing the various layers of the fascia (patient's left side), and a deeper dissection (patient's right side), showing the course of the lower seven thoracic and first lumbar nerve.

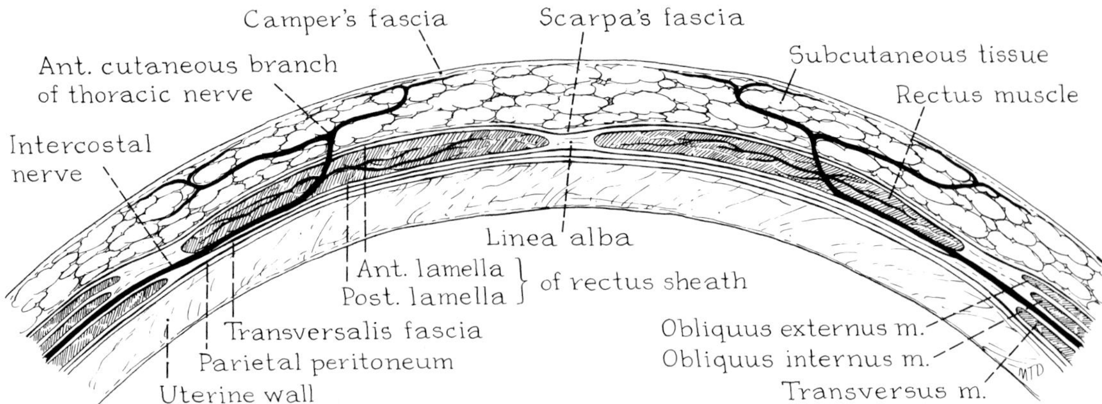


**Fig. 15–33.** Cross section of the anterior abdominal wall showing details of the nerve supply. After passing behind the costal cartilages, the intercostal nerves enter the interval between the transversus abdominis and internal oblique muscle. They run medially within this interval as far as the semilunar line, where they perforate the posterior sheath of the rectus abdominis near its lateral margin. They then course between the posterior aspect of the muscle and its posterior sheath as far as the middle of the muscle, where they abruptly turn anteriorly, pass through the substance of the muscle, and perforate its anterior sheath to become the anterior cutaneous nerves of the abdominal wall. While within the rectus sheath, they give off branches to the rectus muscle.

inguinal ring where it becomes superficial to supply sensory fibers to the abdominal wall just above the pubic bone. The ilioinguinal nerve perforates the internal oblique muscle at the anterior part of the iliac crest and then descends within the inguinal canal. At the external inguinal ring it becomes superficial to terminate as cutaneous branches that supply the skin overlying the symphysis pubis and a very small portion of the labium majus, as well as the upper medial part of the thigh. Neither the iliohypogastric nor ilioinguinal enters the rectus sheath.

In general, the anterior cutaneous branch of the seventh thoracoabdominal intercostal nerve supplies primarily the skin over the xiphoid process; that of the eighth and ninth, the skin between the xiphoid process and the umbilicus; that of the tenth, the skin around the umbilicus; that of the eleventh, the skin just below the umbilicus; and that of the twelfth thoracic and first lumbar nerve, the skin above and over the pubis. Each nerve, except the ilioinguinal, also gives off a lateral cutaneous branch at approximately the midaxillary line. The lateral cutaneous branch of the seventh to eleventh nerves, inclusive, divides into a short posterior and long anterior branches that run anteromedially to supply the skin of the abdominal wall as far as the linea semilunaris. The lateral cutaneous branches of the twelfth thoracic and iliohypogastric do not divide but pass downward over the iliac crest to supply the skin of the gluteal region (Figure 15–31).

The relative distribution of sensory nerve endings in various layers of the abdominal wall is suggested by the diagram in Figure 15–33. The skin is the most sensitive, with the fasciae next in order; the muscles and fat are almost insensitive.

## Local Infiltration and Field Block

### *Anesthetic Agents and Equipment*

Although earlier writers advocated the use of procaine, it is best to use a combination of 0.5% lidocaine to obtain rapid onset, and 0.125% bupivacaine to achieve prolonged action. Because about 125 ml of solution is required to carry out the whole procedure, it is advisable to mix 65 ml of 1% lidocaine and an equal amount of 0.25% bupivacaine to obtain the aforementioned concentrations (Table 15–3). The first step requires 10 ml of the plain solution to achieve intracutaneous analgesia. The epinephrine is omitted for this step to avoid possible slough of the skin. For subsequent steps, it is essential to decrease the total amount of the vasoconstrictor for a final concentration of 1:400,000. Thus, a total of about 290 μg of epinephrine is added to the remainder of the solution (i.e., 0.3 ml of the 1:1,000 epinephrine contained in the standard ampule, and this results in a dose of 2.5 μg/ml of the anesthetic solution). Because the technique requires 12 to 15 minutes to complete, the cardiovascular effects of epinephrine are not as great as when the injection is completed within a few minutes. The sterile tray containing the equipment for local infiltration is similar to that used for other regional techniques, and the size of various needles are mentioned in the legends.

### *Technique of Infiltration*

The procedure should be done with the uterus displaced laterally, achieved with a wedge under the right buttock for displacement to the left or vice versa. The technique of producing analgesia of the abdominal wall entails six separate steps of injections: 1) intracutaneous, 2) subcutaneous, 3) intrarectus, 4) parietal peritoneal, 5) visceral peritoneal, and 6) paracervical. These steps are shown and described individually in Figures 15–34 to 15–37, inclusive. To carry out these procedures, the right-handed operator stands at the left side of the table and begins at the upper part of the proposed incision. If circumstances warrant, block can be carried out on both sides simultaneously by the operator and his or her assistant. To avoid getting in each other's way, it is best that

**Table 15–3.** Doses of Various Local Anesthetics for Abdominal Wall Analgesia

| Procedure | Total Volume Required (ml) | Procaine 2-Chloroprocaine Conc. (%) | Procaine 2-Chloroprocaine Total Dose (mg) | Lidocaine Mepivacaine Conc. (%) | Lidocaine Mepivacaine Total Dose (mg) | Bupivacaine Tetracaine Conc. (%) | Bupivacaine Tetracaine Total Dose (mg) |
|---|---|---|---|---|---|---|---|
| 1. Intracutaneous Infiltration (no epinephrine) | 10 | 0.5 | 50 | 0.4 | 40 | 0.06 | 6 |
| 2. Subcutaneous Injection (epinephrine) | 20 | 0.5 | 100 | 0.4 | 80 | 0.06 | 6 |
| 3. Intrarectus (epinephrine) | 25 | 1.0 | 250 | 0.6 | 125 | 0.125 | 31.5 |
| 4. Parietal Peritoneal Injection (epinephrine) | 10 | 0.5 | 50 | 0.4 | 40 | 0.06 | 6 |
| 5. Visceral Peritoneal (Vesicouterine) Injection (epinephrine) | 15 | 0.5 | 75 | 0.4 | 60 | 0.06 | 9 |
| 6. Paracervical Injection (epinephrine) | 20 | 1.0 | 200 | 0.6 | 120 | 0.125 | 25 |
| TOTAL | 100 | | 725 | | 465 | | 83.5 |

the operator on the right side of the table begins injections in the lower part of the incision, while his or her assistant on the opposite side of the table begins in the upper part of the incision.

### *Complications*

Systemic toxic reaction from an overdose of local anesthetic solution has been the most frequent complication with this technique. This is more likely to occur if the maximum therapeutic dose is exceeded. It also occurs from accidental intravenous injection. This can be avoided by carrying out the aspiration test each time the needle is moved when its point is near a large vessel. Accidental invasion of the uterus can be avoided by observing the precaution mentioned above.

## Rectus Block

Injection of the anterior portion of the thoracic nerves within the rectus sheath may be used to produce anesthesia of the anterior abdominal wall. In this technique, the local anesthetic solution is deposited between the rectus muscle and the posterior layer of its sheath, thus blocking the nerves before they enter the substance of the muscle. The technique is shown in Figure 15–38 and described in the legend. This procedure has the advantage over the infiltration technique in permitting the use of smaller amounts. However, this advantage is offset by the danger of invading the peritoneal cavity and even the uterus. It should only be used by those who have had experience with this technique in nonpregnant patients.

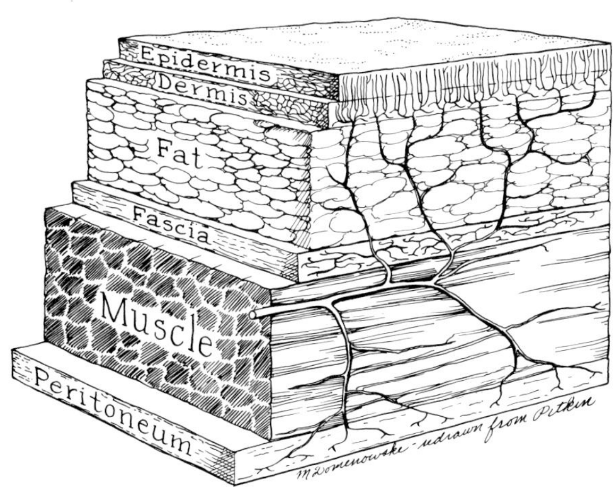


**Fig. 15–34.** Distribution of nerves in the skin. Note the large number of nerve endings in the epidermis and outer layer of the dermis that are the most sensitive parts of the abdominal wall (and the skin in other parts of the body). The fascia and peritoneum are also supplied by numerous nociceptive fibers.

### *Technique*

The concentrations of various local anesthetics that may be used for this procedure are the same as suggested in Table 15–3 for Step 3 (intrarectus block). Skin wheals are formed with a 30-gauge needle at the appropriate intervals (as indicated in Figure 15–39a), and the procedure is carried out as described in the legend.

It is advisable to wait approximately 5 minutes following injection of lidocaine, chloroprocaine, or mepivacaine, and even longer following injection of other drugs, to permit maximum effect. In the immediate suprapubic region, the injections must be carried out not only perpendicularly but also tangentially in an inferior direction to block endings of the iliohypogastric and ilioinguinal nerve. This produces analgesia of the abdominal wall for about 5 cm from the midline (Figure 15–39f).

### *Management of the Patient*

The management of the patient is the same as described with other regional techniques, and requires continuous monitoring of the parturient and the fetus. It deserves reemphasis that during the procedure, and after the block is completed, the uterus be displaced onto one side and for the operator to wait sufficient time to have maximum analgesia/anesthesia before the skin incision is made. If the parturient becomes unduly apprehensive, injection of 100 mg of thiopental intravenously may be given at any time during the procedure. This is usually sufficient to decrease apprehension, anxiety, and also to have a slight decrease in the cardiovascular effects of epinephrine without producing any clinically significant fetal or neonatal depression.

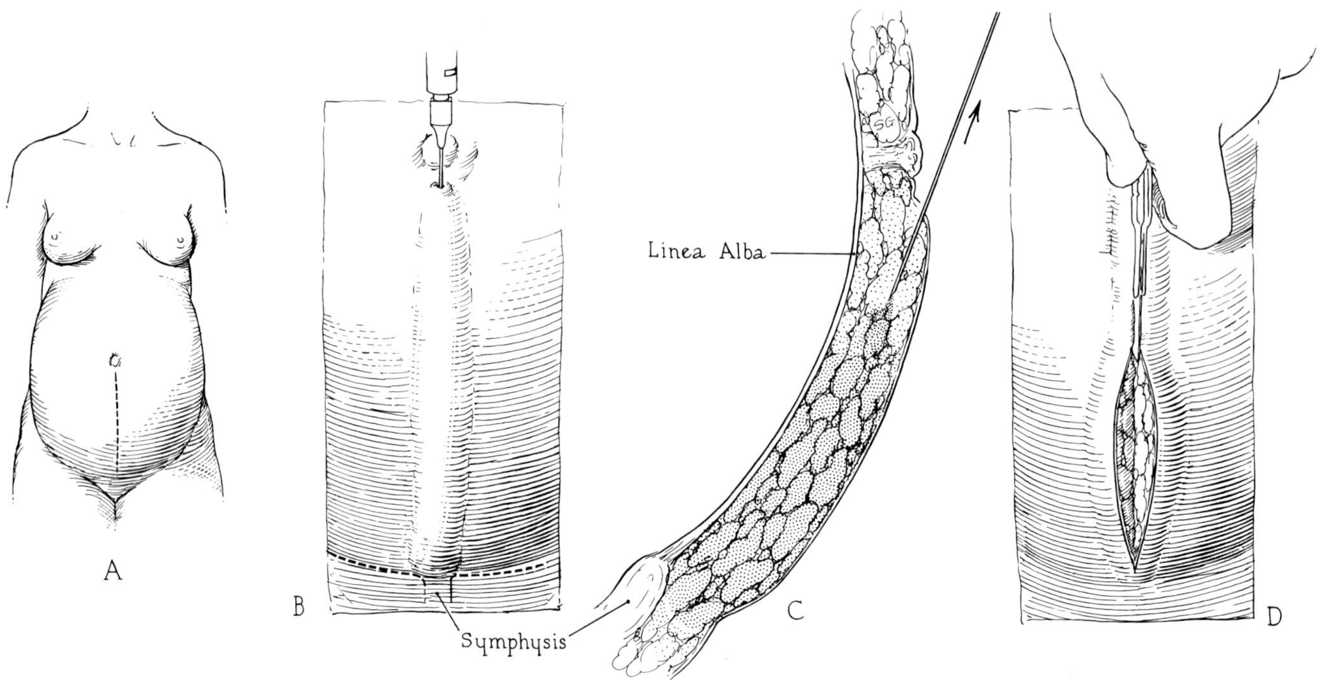


**Fig. 15–35.** Technique of abdominal anesthesia. Steps 1 and 2. Intracutaneous and subcutaneous injection. **A)** site of the proposed intracutaneous and subcutaneous injection. **B)** anterior view showing tumefaction, produced by the subcutaneous infiltration. **C)** sagittal view showing distribution of the anesthetic agent (stippled area). **D)** incision carried out. The intracutaneous injection is initiated by an intracutaneous wheal raised with a 30-gauge 2-cm needle just below the umbilicus. A 25-gauge 5-cm needle is then thrust through the skin wheal with its shaft almost parallel to the skin and its point directed toward the pubis and 0.5 ml of solution (Table 15–3) is injected. The needle is then advanced intracutaneously for about 1 cm and injection repeated. With a 25-gauge 5-cm needle, four such injections can be carried out without removing the point of the needle from the skin. This produces less discomfort for the patient and avoids repeated skin punctures, as would be the case if the needle were removed after each wheal. The point of the fine needle can be guided by digital pressure to avoid piercing the skin or deflecting its point into the subcutaneous structures. There is no need to carry out an aspiration test before injecting because the blood vessels are so small that there is absolutely no danger of intravascular injection. If properly carried out, 10 ml of dilute solution are sufficient to produce instantaneous analgesia of the skin (Table 15–3). For the subcutaneous injection (Step 2), a 22-gauge 10-cm needle is used. The syringe is held in the right hand so that the shaft of the needle makes a 45° angle with the surface of the skin. Then, the point of the needle is deliberately thrust through the uppermost intracutaneous wheal, and advanced 0.5 cm until it is in the subcutaneous tissue. Because of its length, the needle is likely to buckle unless its shaft is held with the fingers of the left hand. To decrease the risk of inserting the needle too far into the patient with a very thin abdominal wall and diastasis, it is advisable to grasp the skin of the abdomen near the site of injection between the thumb and the index finger of the left hand and to insert the needle with its axis parallel to the surface of the skin. Once the needle point is in the subcutaneous tissue, the needle is advanced toward the pubis while the solution is being injected continuously. As long as the injection is carried out while the needle is in motion, there is very little chance of intravenous injection. The convexity of the abdominal wall requires that the point of the needle be guided by digital pressure. In this manner, the shaft of the needle follows the same plane as the abdominal wall, otherwise the needle point is likely to protrude through the skin. The needle is advanced for about 8 cm and then rapidly withdrawn while the injection is continued to produce a linear tumefaction as shown in ***B.*** About 6 to 8 ml of solution are injected during this maneuver. The point of the needle is then reinserted through the intracutaneous wheal at a point overlying the lowermost part of the subcutaneous injection and the procedure repeated. The needle is advanced until its point impinges on the pubic bone. Because the area just above the symphysis pubis is especially sensitive, it should be well infiltrated. About 3 to 4 minutes are allowed to elapse for analgesia to develop (stippled area in **C**). With the described technique using the more penetrant drugs (lidocaine), the analgesic area usually extends for 2 cm beyond the midline. This is more than adequate to carry out the cutaneous and subcutaneous incision **(D)** and retract the skin sufficiently to expose the medial border of the rectus sheath to carry out the step 3 (next figure). For the surgeon who is rough or who requires wider retraction, it will be necessary to carry out the subcutaneous infiltration laterally. However, this entails the use of larger volumes of solution, which increases the risk of toxic reactions. After analgesia develops, the incision is carried down to the fascia (Figure 35–38) and the skin gently retracted to expose the medial portion of the rectus fascia in preparation for step three.

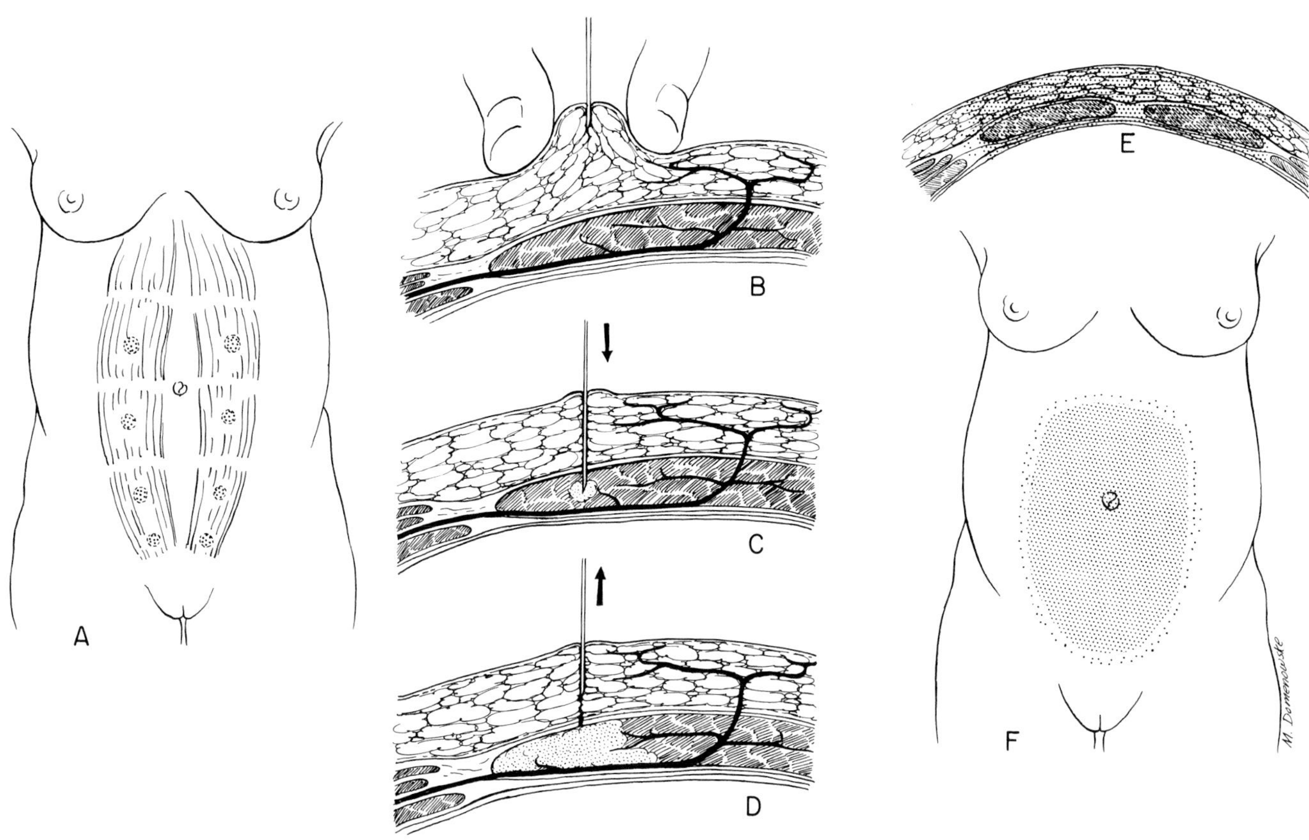


**Fig. 15–36.** Technique of abdominal wall analgesia/anesthesia (step 3), intrarectus injection. **A)** anterior view showing insertion of needle through the medial part of the anterior lamella of the rectus muscle. **B)** the two edges of the incisions are already anesthetized from the subcutaneous infiltration (step 2). The needle point is in the lateral edge of the rectus sheath where the injection (stippling) is begun. **C)** completion of the intrarectus injection as the needle is withdrawn, resulting in block of the anterior cutaneous branch of the nerves. Stippled area indicates distribution of analgesia. To carry out each of these injections, the wound edges are gently separated. At each selected site, the bevel of the 8-cm 22-gauge needle, which already attached to a syringe filled with the local anesthetic solution, is inserted through the medial part of the anterior lamella of the rectus sheath **(B).** It should be noted that the axis of the needle makes an angle of not more than 10° to 15° with the abdominal fascial layers. As the needle point passes through the sheath of the rectus, a distinct snap is felt. It is then advanced laterally and slightly posteriorly for approximately 3 to 5 cm until its point is thought to be at the lateral and posterior edges of the muscle, but still within the rectus sheath **(B).** After aspiration indicates that the needle is not within a blood vessel, 2 ml of solution are injected without moving the needle and another 2 ml is injected as the needle is being withdrawn **(C).** Because the sheath is not attached to the muscle posteriorly this technique permits free spread of fluid upward and downward, so that if injections are carried out at intervals of 3 cm, a continuous layer of anesthetic solution is produced between the posterior surface of the muscle and the posterior layer of the rectus sheath where the nerves are situated. This step should result in analgesia of the abdominal wall between the lateral edges of the 2 recti muscles **(C)** and also relaxation of the recti muscles, as well as analgesia of the underlying peritoneum. To be certain that the area of analgesia extends beyond the limits of the incision, one or two oblique injections should be made at the upper and lower ends of the incision. It is especially important to infiltrate extensively the suprapubic area to block terminations of the iliohypogastric nerve. No more than the prescribed volume of solution listed in Table 15–3 should be injected. For best results it is best to wait 3 to 5 minutes after injections are completed. The fascia is then incised the entire length of the incision and the peritoneum is exposed.

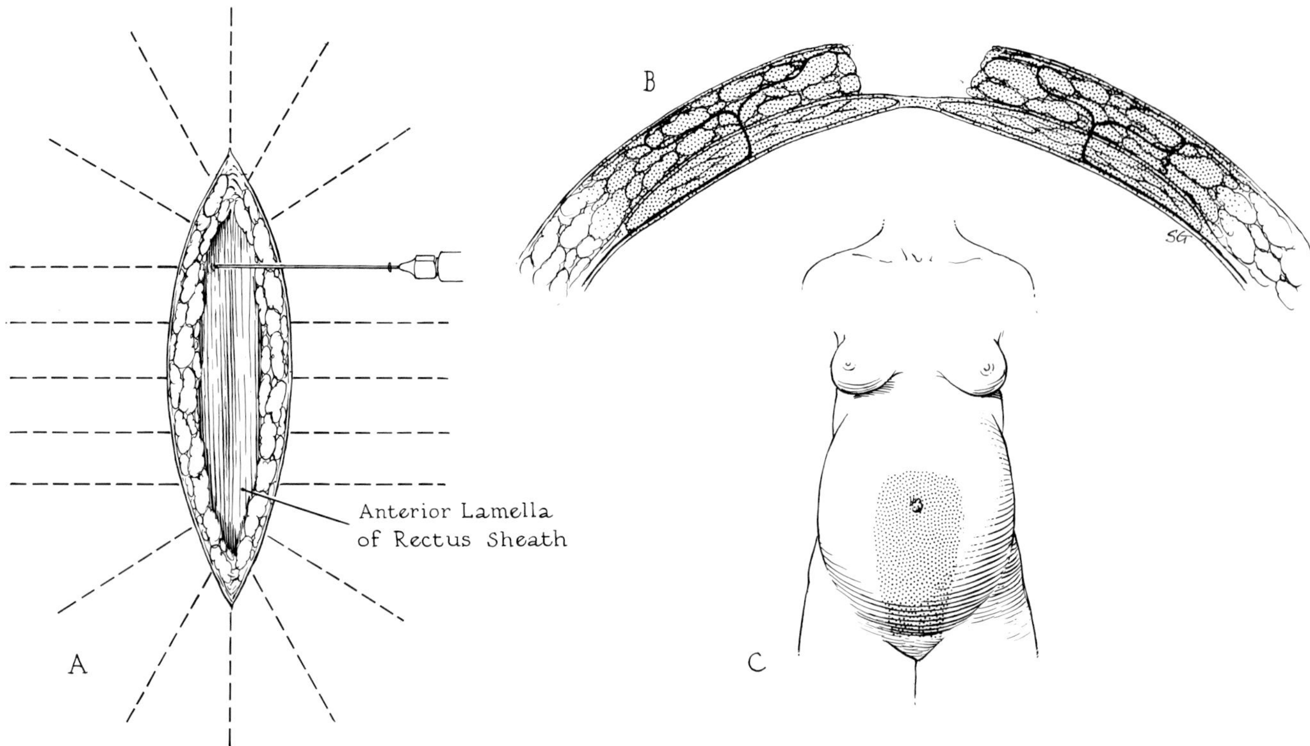


**Fig. 15–37.** Technique of abdominal wall anesthesia. Step 3. intrarectus injection (continued). **A)** sites of various intrarectus injections (dashed lines). **B)** cross section, and **C)** anterior view showing distribution of anesthesia (stippled area). (See legend of Figure 15–36 for details)

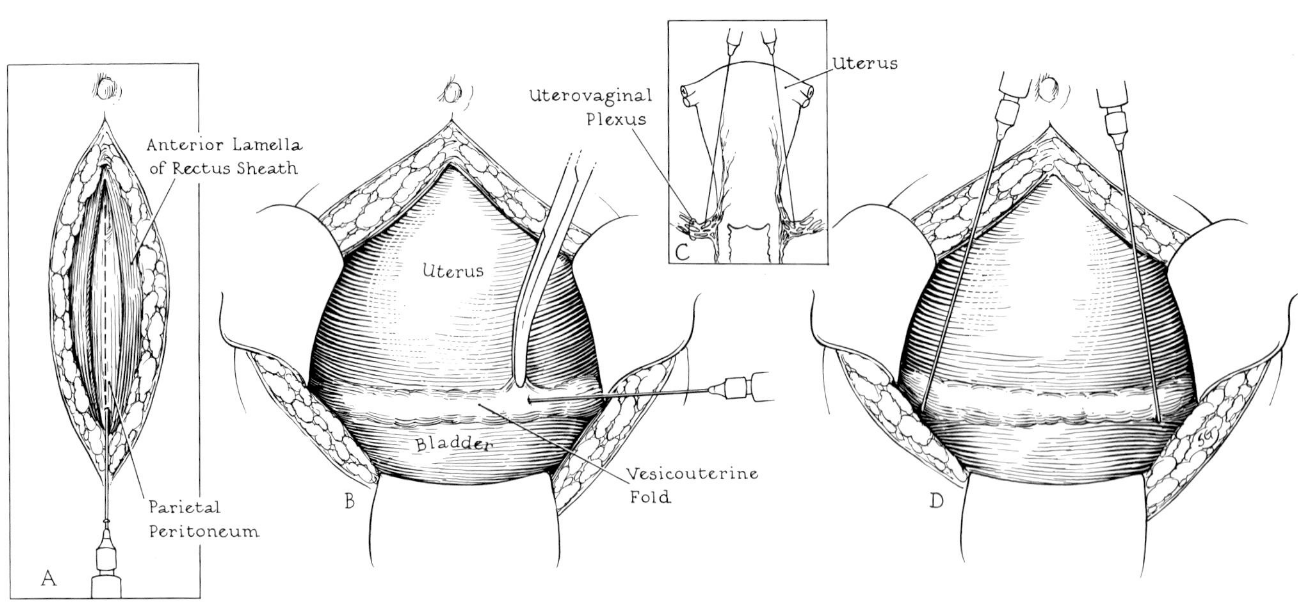

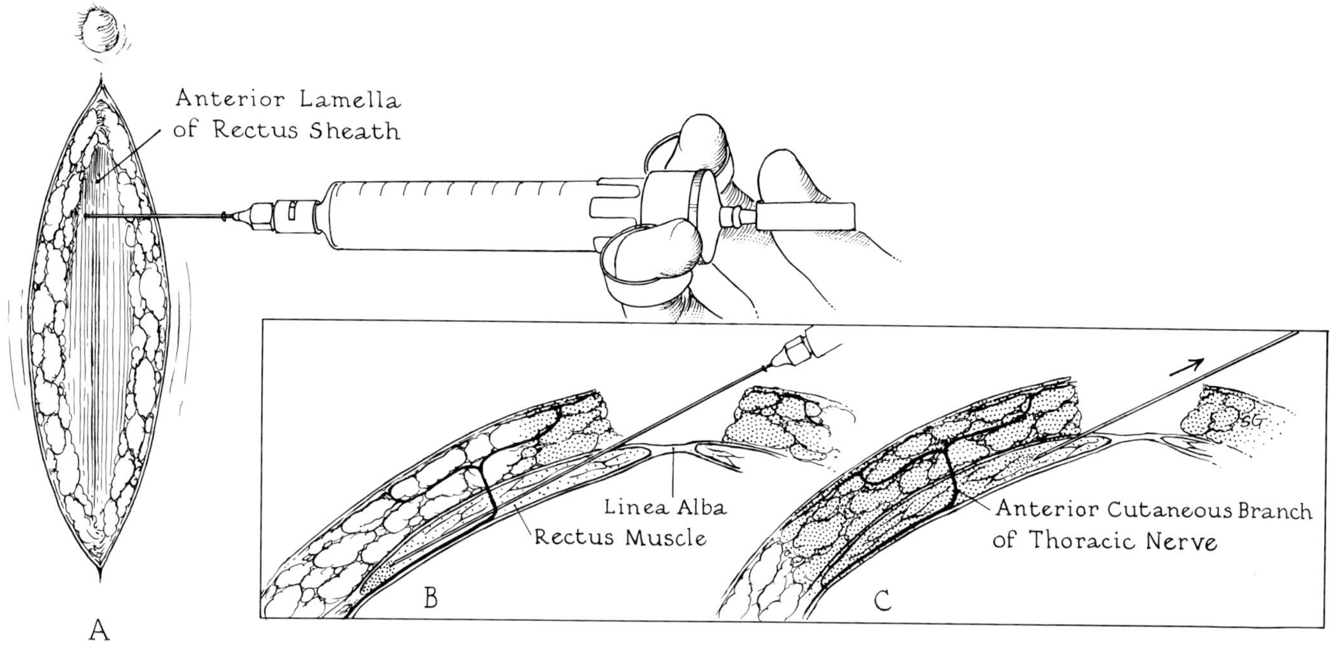


**Fig. 15–39.** Technique of rectus block. **A)** anterior view showing location of intracutaneous wheals and injection sites (stippled area). The transverse lines may be difficult to make out in the gravida. The skin wheals are made over the lateral part of the rectus muscle. In patients with marked diastasis, the skin wheals are formed at a greater distance from midline than shown. **B)** the skin is picked up before the point of the needle is passed through it. This is done to decrease the risk of accidental passage of the needle through the thinned abdominal wall and into the abdominal cavity. **C)** the point of the needle has passed through the anterior lamella of the rectus sheath and is in the rectus compartment, where 5 ml of solution (stippled area) are injected. **D)** the needle is withdrawn after the injection of the solution within the sheath of the muscle. The terminal part of the thoracoabdominal and intercostal nerves are thus blocked before they course anteriorly to reach the subcutaneous and cutaneous structures. **E)** cross section, and **F)** anterior view of the abdominal wall showing the area of anesthesia produced by the block (stippled area).

←

**Fig. 15–38.** Technique of abdominal wall anesthesia. Steps 4, 5, and 6. **A)** injection of the parietal peritoneum. **B)** injection of the vesicouterine fold. **C** and **D)** technique of paracervical injection to anesthetize the "pain" nerves supplying the uterus. If the intrarectus injections have been properly carried out and sufficient time permitted for the nerve block to be complete, the peritoneum can be grasped with clamps and incised painlessly without further injection. If the clamps cause discomfort, either more time is allowed, or the peritoneum can be injected. Peritoneal injection is carried out by gently lifting the peritoneum and inserting the point of the 22-gauge 10-cm needle (already attached to a syringe) through the uppermost or lowermost part of the incision **(A)**. A total of 10 ml is injected. Another way of producing analgesia of the parietal peritoneum is to apply topically one of the more penetrant local anesthetics (e.g., 0.5% lidocaine with 0.125% bupivacaine) and then wait 2 to 3 minutes. The anesthetic is rapidly absorbed and desensitizes the peritoneum. The peritoneum is then gently grasped with forceps and cut the entire length of the incision. If a classic cesarean section is to be carried out, an attempt is made to inject the visceral peritoneum overlying the uterus, whereas in the case of low cesarean section, the solution is injected into the vesicouterine reflection of the peritoneum **(B)**. To carry out a paracervical injection depicted in C and D, 10 ml of solution is infiltrated into the paracervical region. This will produce interruption of nociceptive fibers from the uterus so that it may be manipulated without discomfort. First, gently palpate and identify the paracervical region. Identification can be facilitated by incising the peritoneum and reflecting that portion over the bladder and over the lower uterine segment. Injection is then carried out with a 22-gauge 10-cm needle. Not more than 10 ml of solution are needed for each site. Great care should be exercised to avoid intravascular injection.

## REFERENCES


1. Cunningham FG, MacDonald PC, Gant NF: Williams' Obstetrics. 18th Ed. Norwalk, CT, Appleton & Lange, 1989.
2. Mueller B: Narcologie. 88 Berlin Trenkel, Volume 11, 1908.
3. Ilman and Sellheim: Cited by de Alvarez RR, Gray EW: Influence of hyaluronidase and epinephrine on pudendal block anesthesia. Obstet. Gynecol. 4:635: 1954.
4. Ilmer W: Ueber nervus pudendus anasthesie, Zentralbl. f.d. ges. Gynak U Geburtsh 34:699, 1910.
5. King R: Perineal anesthesia in labor. Surg Gynec Obstet 23: 615, 1916.
6. Klink EW: Perineal nerve block: an anatomic and clinical study in the female. Obstet. Gynecol. 1:137, 1953.
7. Dugger JH, Kegel EE, Buckley JJ: Transvaginal pudendal block: the safe anesthesia in obstetrics. Obstet. Gynecol. 8: 393, 1956.
8. Sheares BH: Cited by Apgar V. Pudendal block. Anesth. Analg. 36:77–78, 1957.
9. Kobak AJ, Evans EF, Johnson GR: Transvaginal pudendal nerve block. Am. J. Obstet. Gynecol. 71:981, 1956.
10. Kohl GC: New method of pudendal nerve block. Northwest. Med. 53:1012, 1954.
11. Apgar V: Pudendal block. Anesth. Analg. 36:77–78, 1957.
12. Wilds PL: Transvaginal pudendal nerve block. Obstet. Gynecol. 8:385, 1956.
13. Kohl GC: Transvaginal pudendal nerve block with an improved instrument. Obstet. Gynecol. 11:314, 1958.
14. Sahay PA: Pudendal nerve block. Brit. Med. J. 1:759, 1959.
15. Kobak AJ, Sadove MS: Transvaginal regional anesthesia simplified by a new instrument. Obstet. Gynecol. 15:387, 1960.
16. Egbert DS, Keettel WC, Lee JG: "Iowa trumpet," pudendal needle guide. J. Iowa. Med. Soc. 50:499, 1960.
17. Kobak AJ, Sadove MS, Kobak AJ Jr: Childbirth pain relieved by combined paracervical and pudendal nerve blocks. JAMA 183:931, 1963.
18. Johnson WL, Bonica JJ, et al: Effect of pudendal spinal and peridural block anesthesia on the second stage of labor. Am. J. Obstet. Gynecol. 113:166–175, 1972.
19. Zador G, Lindmark G, Nilsson BA: Pudendal block in normal vaginal deliveries. Acta. Obstet. Gynecol. Scand. Suppl. 34: 51, 1974.
19A. Schierup L, Schmidt JF, Torp Jensen A, Rye BAO: Pudendal block in vaginal deliveries: mepivacaine with and without epinephrine. Acta. Obstet. Gynecol. Scand. 67:195, 1988.
19B. Langhoff-Roos J, Lindmark G: Analgesia and maternal side effects of pudendal block at delivery. Acta. Obstet. Gynecol. Scand. 64:269, 1985.
20. Marin RD: A review of the use of Barton's forceps for the rotation of the fetal head from the transverse position. Aust. N. Z. J. Obstet. Gynaecol. 18:234–237, 1978.
21. Merkow AJ, McGuinness GA, Erenberg A, Kennedy RL: The neonatal neurobehavioral effects of bupivacaine, mepivacaine, and 2-chloroprocaine used for pudendal block. Anesthesiology 52:309–312, 1980.
22. Schierup L, Schmidt JF, Torp Jensen A, Rye BA: Pudendal block in vaginal deliveries. Mepivacaine with and without epinephrine. Acta. Obstet. Gynecol. Scand. 67:195–197, 1988.
23. Langhoff-Roose J, Lindmark G: Analgesia and maternal side effects of pudendal block at delivery. A comparison of three local anesthetics. Acta. Obstet. Gynecol. Scand. 64: 269–672, 1985.
24. Gibbs CP, et al: Obstetric anesthesia: a national survey. Anesthesiology 65:298, 1986.
25. Greenhill JP: Analgesia and Anesthesia in Obstetrics. 2nd Ed. Springfield, IL, Charles C. Thomas, 1962, pp. 54–60.
26. Stevenson CS: Obstetric analgesia and anesthesia—current problems. J. Michigan Med. Soc. 53:857, 1954.
27. Gellert P: Aufhebung der Wehenschmerzen and Wehenuberdruck. Monatschr. f. Geburtsh u Gynak 73:143, 1926.
28. Henriet J: Les bases anatomo-physiologiques et technique personnelle de l'infiltration du plexus pelvi-perinatal. Strasbourg Med. 97:623, 1937.
29. Pribam E: Die schmerzlose geburtsleitung in lokal-anestesie. Klin Wschr 6:1282, 1927.
30. Rosenfeld SS: Paracervical anesthesia for the relief of labor pains. Am. J. Obstet. Gynecol. 50:527, 1945.
31. Gillam JS, Freeman DW: Paracervical block anesthesia during labor. Lancet 70:206: 1950.
32. Freeman DW, Bellville TP, Barno A: Paracervical block anesthesia in labor. Obstet. Gynecol. 8:270, 1956.
33. Baken MP, Freeman WD, Barno A: Transvaginal regional blocks. Surg. Gynecol. Obstet. 114:375, 1962.
34. Freeman DW: Paracervical block anesthesia. Am. J. Obstet. Gynecol. 89:554, 1964.
35. Page EP, Kamm ML, Chappel CC: Usefulness of paracervical block in obstetrics. Am. J. Obstet. Gynecol. 81:1094, 1961.
36. Seeds E, Stein-Messinger P, Dorsey JH: Paracervical block: results of a double-blind evaluation. Obstet. Gynecol. 21: 462, 1962.
37. Davis JE, et al: Paracervical block for pain relief in labor. Obstet. Gynecol. 19:195, 1962.
38. Davis JE, Frudenfeld JC, Frudenfeld K, Frudenfeld KH, Webb AN: The combined paracervical and pudendal block anesthesia for labor and delivery. A review of 2,100 private cases. Am. J. Obstet. Gynecol. 89:366–376, 1964.
39. Sandmire HF, Stephen DA: Paracervical block anesthesia in obstetrics. JAMA 187:775 1965.
40. White CA, Pitkin RM: Paracervical block anesthesia in obstetrics. Postgrad. Med. 33:585, 1963.
41. Spanos WJ, Steele JC: Uterosacral block. Obstet. Gynecol. 13:129, 1959.
42. Thiery M, Vroman S: Paracervical block analgesia during labor. Am. J. Obstet. Gynecol. 113:988–1336, 1972.
43. Freeman RF, Schifrin BS: Whither paracervical block? Int. Anesthesiol. Clin. 11:69–91, 1973.
44. Cibils LA, Santonja-Lucas JJ: Clinical significance of fetal heart rate patterns during labor. Am. J. Obstet. Gynecol. 130:73–100, 1978.
45. Ostheimer GW: Anesthesia in childbirth. Fam. Pract. Annu., 1985, pp. 61–75.
46. LeCron L: L'anesthesie loco-regionale. Complications en obstetrique. Anesth. Analg. (Paris) 38:141–145, 1981.
47. Ueland K: Comment on paracervical block. *In* Anesthesia and Obstetrics: Maternal, Fetal and Neonatal Aspects. 2nd Ed. Edited by GA Albright, et al. Boston, Butterworths, 1986, pp. 229–221.
48. Day TW: Community use of paracervical block in labor. J. Fam. Pract. 28:545–550, 1989.
49. Read JA, Miller FC: The bupivacaine paracervical block in labor and its effect on quantitative uterine activity. Obstet. Gynecol. 53:166–170, 1979.
50. Jenssen H: The effect of paracervical block on cervical dilatation and uterine activity. Acta. Obstet. Gynecol. Scand. 52: 13–22, 1973.
51. Jenssen H: Fetal systolic time intervals after paracervical block during labor. Acta. Obstet. Gynecol. Scand. 59: 115–121, 1980.
52. Jagerhorn M: Paracervical block in obstetrics. An improved injection method. A clinical and radiologic study. Acta. Obstet. Gynecol. Scand. 54:9–27, 1975.
52A. Goins, JR: Experience with mepivacaine paracervical

block in an obstetric private practice. Am. J. Obstet. Gynecol. 167:342–345, 1992.
53. Weiss RR, Nathanson HG, Tehrani MR, Rejani NA, et al: Paracervical block with 2-chloroprocaine. Anesth. Analg. 56: 709–716, 1977.
54. Strauss RG, Dase D, Doering PL: Prolonging block anesthesia: addition of dextran to 2-chloroprocaine. Am. J. Obstet. Gynecol. 133:891–893, 1979.
55. Pitkin RM, Goddard WB: Paracervical and uterosacral block in obstetrics—a controlled, double blind study. Obstet. Gynecol. 21:737, 1963.
56. Cooper K, Moir JC: Paracervical nerve block: a simple method of pain relief in labour. Br. Med. J. 5342:1372–1374, 1963
57. Sangoul F, Fox GS, Houle GL: Effect of regional analgesia on maternal oxygen consumption during the first stage of labor. Am. J. Obstet. Gynecol. 121:1080–1083, 1975.
58. Grenman S, et al: Epidural and paracervical blockades in obstetrics. Catecholamines arginine vasopressin and analgesic effect. Acta. Obstet. Gynecol. Scand. 65:699–704, 1986.
59. Albright GA: Paracervical block. *In* Anesthesia in Obstetrics: Maternal, Fetal, And Neonatal Aspects. 2nd ED. Edited by GA Albright, et al. Boston, Butterworths, 1980, pp. 212–222.
60. Jenssen H: The shape of the amniotic pressure curve before and after paracervical block during labour. Acta. Obstet. Gynecol. Scand. Suppl. 42:1–29, 1975.
61. Zourlas PA, Kumar D: An objective evaluation of paracervical block on human uterine contractility. Am. J. Obstet. Gynecol. 91:217, 1965.
62. Miller FC, Yeh SY, Schifrin BS, Paul RH, et al: Quantitation of uterine activity in 100 primiparous patients. Am. J. Obstet. Gynecol. 124:398–405.
63. Friedman EA: Labor: Clinical Evaluation and Management. New York, Appleton-Century-Crofts, 1967.
64. Shnider SM, et al: Paracervical block in obstetrics. I. Fetal complications and neonatal morbidity. Am. J. Obstet. Gynecol. 107:619, 1970.
65. Rogers RE: Fetal bradycardia associated with paracervical block anesthesia in labor. Am. J. Obstet. Gynecol. 106: 913, 1970.
66. Gabert HA, Stenchever MA: Electronic fetal monitoring in association with paracervical blocks. Am. J. Obstet. Gynecol. 116:1143, 1973.
67. Santonja-Lucas JJ, Bonilla-Musoles F: Anestesia paracervical en obstetricia: efectos sobre la dinamica uterina y frecuencia cardiaca fetal. Rev. Espanola Obstet. Gynecol. 33:87, 1974.
68. Shnider SM, et al: High fetal blood levels of mepivacaine and fetal bradycardia. N. Eng. J. Med. 279:947, 1968.
69. Ralston DH, Shnider SM: The fetal and neonatal effects of regional anesthesia in obstetrics. Anesthesiology 48:34–64, 1978.
70. Asling JH, Shnider SM, Margolis AJ, Wilkinson GL, et al: Paracervical block anesthesia and obstetrics. II. Etiology of fetal bradycardia following paracervical block anesthesia. Am. J. Obstet. Gynecol. 107:626–634, 1970.
71. Murphy PJ, Wright JD, Fitzgerald TB: Assessment of paracervical nerve block anesthesia during labor. Br. Med. J. 1:526, 1970.
72. Rosefsky JB, Petersiel ME: Perinatal deaths associated with mepivacaine paracervical anesthesia in labor. N. Engl. J. Med. 278:530–533, 1968.
73. Taw R: In discussion of the report of Davis JE, et al: The combined paracervical and pudendal block anesthesia for labor and delivery; a review of 2,100 private cases. Am. J. Obstet. Gynecol. 89:366–376, 1964.
74. Teramo K, et al: Effects of lidocaine on heart rate, blood pressure, electrocardiogram in fetal sheep. Am. J. Obstet. Gynecol. 118:935, 1974.
75. Nyirjesy I, et al: Hazards of the use of paracervical block anesthesia in obstetrics. Am. J. Obstet. Gynecol. 87:231, 1963.
76. Shnider SM, Way EL: The kinetics of transfer of lidocaine across the human placenta. Anesthesiology 29:944, 1968.
77. Burchell RC, Sadove MS: Continuous paracervical block in obstetrics. Obstet. Gynecol. 23:112, 1964.
78. Tafeen CH, Freedman HL, Harris H: A system of continuous paracervical block anesthesia. Am. J. Obstet. Gynecol. 94: 854, 1966.
79. Tafeen CH, Freedman HL, Harris H: Combined continuous paracervical and continuous pudendal nerve block anesthesia in labor. Am. J. Obstet. Gynecol. 100:55–62, 1968.
80. Dellepiane G, Badino P: L'anestesie paravertebrale in ostetricia e ginecologia. Clin. Obstet. 29:537, 1927.
81. Schumaker HB, Hellman LM, Manahan CP: Sympathetic anesthesia in labor. Am. J. Obstet. Gynecol. 45:129, 1943.
82. Jarvis SM: Paravertebral sympathetic nerve block, a method for the safe and painless conduct of labor. Am. J. Obstet. Gynecol. 47:335, 1944.
83. Cleland JCP: Continuous peridural and caudal anesthesia in obstetrics. Curr. Res. Anesth. Analg. 28:61–76, 1949.
84. Reich AM: Paravertebral lumbar sympathetic block in labor. Am. J. Obstet. Gynecol. 61:1263, 1951.
85. Byrd ML: Lumbar sympathetic block for obstetrical analgesia; preliminary report of over 1,200 cases, 1959. Unpublished data.
86. Riekse JM: Terminal obstetric anesthesia by means of lumbar sympathetic paravertebral block. Am. J. Obstet. Gynecol. 78:411, 1959.
87. Hunter CA: Uterine motility studies during labor. Observations on bilateral sympathetic nerve block in the normal and abnormal first stage of labor. Am. J. Obstet. Gynecol. 85:681, 1963.
88. Bonica JJ: Clinical Application of Diagnostic and Therapeutic Nerve Blocks. Springfield, IL, Charles C. Thomas Publisher, 1959, pp. 142–148.
89. Busby T: Local anesthesia for cesarean section. Am. J. Obstet. Gynecol. 87:399, 1963.
90. Bonica JJ: The mechanisms of referred pain. *In* The Management of Pain. 2nd Ed. Edited by JJ Bonica. Malvern, PA, Lea & Febiger, 1990, pp. 171–173.

Chapter 16

# COMPLICATIONS OF REGIONAL ANESTHESIA

H.S. CHADWICK
JOHN J. BONICA

This chapter contains a comprehensive, albeit concise, discussion of the complications mentioned in the three preceding chapters pertaining to various regional anesthetic techniques that can occur as a direct or indirect effect of carrying out the procedure and/or managing the patient. Complications that are associated with general anesthesia are considered in Chapter 20. The complications considered here are based on the primary pathophysiology involved. For example, because arterial hypotension can occur with lumbar epidural, caudal epidural or subarachnoid block, it is discussed not in relation to the technique, but in relation to the primary pathophysiologic process.

The material is presented in four major sections: 1) cardiovascular complications including arterial hypotension and cardiac arrest; 2) systemic toxic reactions to the local anesthetic that involve primarily dysfunction of the cardiovascular and neurologic systems, or other systemic reactions not related to the local anesthetic; 3) neurologic complications; and 4) a heterogeneous grouping, which includes complications that do not fit in any of the other categories and that may have deleterious effects on several organs/functions. In discussing the same complication caused by different techniques, we point out differences and similarities in the characteristics of the complication. Portions of this chapter have been taken from the first edition of this book (1) and from a chapter written by Chadwick and Ross (2)

## CARDIOVASCULAR COMPLICATIONS

Cardiovascular dysfunction, but specifically arterial hypotension, has been and continues to be the most frequent complication associated with subarachnoid block, lumbar epidural block, and caudal epidural block administered to parturients. In the past, death consequent to profound hypotension that ended in cardiac arrest was not an infrequent cause of maternal mortality (1,2) and a major contributing factor to perinatal morbidity and perhaps mortality. In the first edition of this book, Bonica presented detailed analysis of data published between 1940 and 1965 that revealed that among the causes of maternal mortality due to anesthesia, cardiovascular complications were the most frequent cause of death associated with regional anesthesia (1). The analysis revealed that cardiovascular complications accounted for about 30% of the maternal deaths associated with anesthesia. These deaths caused by cardiovascular complications were only second to deaths caused by aspiration of gastric contents during the course of general anesthesia.

Fortunately, during the past 25 to 30 years, advances have been made in the fields of obstetrics, perinatology, and anesthesiology, and these have converged to greatly improve obstetric anesthesia services and to drastically reduce maternal and perinatal mortality. We have acquired a great amount of new information about the physiology and pathophysiology of the mother, fetus and newborn, and placental function. These have been followed by improvement in the prevention and treatment of complicating disorders. Moreover, in the United States there has been a significant increase in the number of physicians who are currently devoting their time and effort to obstetric anesthesia and many of who have continually modified and improved the various techniques of regional anesthesia so that they can be applied safely. Still another very important factor that has helped the care of parturients subjected to regional anesthesia has been the large number of studies on human volunteers and low-risk obstetric and surgical patients. The results of these studies have greatly helped to define the action of various techniques of lumbar epidural, caudal epidural, and subarachnoid block on the mother, fetus and newborn, and on the forces of labor. These have led to the development and application of prophylactic measures to avoid or minimize complications. We will briefly review recently published data relevant to each issue.

### *Arterial Hypotension*

#### *Basic Considerations*

In gravidae and parturients who are otherwise "normal" and do not have complicating disorders, arterial hypotension is defined as a 20 to 30% reduction in baseline systolic pressure or a reduction of mean arterial pressure below 100 mm Hg. Because data on the frequency and magnitude of arterial hypotension consequent to the older techniques of subarachnoid block and epidural block and its incidence with the modifications currently practiced are presented in Chapters 13, 14 and 15, they are only briefly mentioned here. We will focus much of the discussion on the pathophysiologic factors that underlie its occurrence.

Until the early 1960s, it was believed and taught that the degree of arterial hypotension consequent to neuraxial blocks was directly related to the number of vasomotor segments interrupted, a concept that Bonica discussed in the first edition of this book (1). Although he mentioned or briefly discussed other causes that contribute to hypotension, the extent of the vasomotor block was considered the most influential factor. However, data derived from the aforementioned clinical observations and controlled studies published subsequently, suggested that the condition of the patient and the presence of complicating disorders are the most important etiologic factors that determine the frequency and degree of arterial hypotension. These include: 1) degree of sympathetic vasomotor tone before the block (especially if a high tone is present, provoked by anxiety and apprehension or by injury or disease); 2) blood volume and nutrition of the patient; 3) presence or absence of cardiovascular disease; and 4) efficiency of circulatory homeostatic mechanisms that may be impaired by depressant drugs or by pathophysiologic factors. In otherwise normal parturients, the degree of a aortocaval compression by the gravid uterus is by far the most important factor that determines the degree of hypotension consequent to subarachnoid or extradural blockade. In addition to these and the extent of sympathetic blockade produced, other factors that may play a role in determining the magnitude of arterial hypotension include the total amount of local anesthetic used and whether or not epinephrine is included in the solution injected.

To duly emphasize the relevance of all of these findings from recent studies toward the prevention and treatment of arterial hypotension in obstetric patients, we first discuss very briefly the physiology of circulatory homeostasis and then briefly summarize some of the data derived from controlled studies.

### *Physiology of Circulatory Homeostasis*

It has long been known that circulatory homeostasis is maintained primarily by intrinsic and extrinsic mechanisms and the volume of blood, all working in concert and with exquisite interaction, integration, and coordination, which continuously detect and compensate for any deviation in the blood pressure (3–5). The intrinsic mechanisms include the vasomotor tone of the blood vessels, the Frank-Starling mechanisms of the heart, and the blood volume, which frequently shifts from one vascular bed to another in response to the needs of different body tissues. The extrinsic mechanisms are comprised of the vagal parasympathetic function, which when stimulated decreases chronotropic and inotropic action of the heart, and the sympathetic system, which when stimulated increases inotropic and chronotropic activity and constricts blood vessels. Normally, tonic sympathetic outflow partly controls the tone of vessels of both the arterial and venous system. Blockade of sympathetic outflow results in dilatation of arterial resistance vessels and the venous capacitance vessels. Vasoconstrictive tone of blood vessels is composed of an extrinsic part provided by continuous sympathetic vasoconstrictor impulses and an intrinsic vasomotor tone. Sympathetic blockade eliminates the former, but not the latter, i.e., during sympathetic blockade associated with subarachnoid, epidural or peripheral nerve block, decrease in vascular resistance is rarely maximal because the intrinsic vasomotor tone is autonomously maintained. Intrinsic vasomotor tone can be decreased or eliminated by drugs that directly depress the smooth muscle of the vessels. Factors that decrease or eliminate intrinsic vasomotor tone include histamine, halothane, thiopental, hypoxemia, and severe acidosis, among others. The clinical implication of these effects is that administration of such drugs or development of asphyxia will increase the degree of hypotension in a patient already under the influence of sympathetic blockade.

The exquisitely sensitive extrinsic neurogenic influences involve reflexes that are activated by stimulation of baroreceptors and chemoreceptors in the carotid sinus and aortic arch, and by atrial and ventricular stretch receptors and the receptors in the low pressure vessels of the thorax as depicted in Figure 16–1. The afferent pathways are contained in the glossopharyngeal and vagus nerves, which convey afferent impulses to the vasomotor and cardiac centers where they are integrated and interpreted, and thence provoke efferent impulses that reach the target organs—the heart and blood vessels—via the vagus and sympathetic efferent fibers. The vagi act as the parasympathetic mediators to the cardiovascular system and carry impulses to the sinoatrial and the atrioventricular nodes and the atrial myocardium, while the sympathetic nerves innervate all of the tissues of the cardiovascular system. In healthy individuals with normal blood volume, these two fundamental regulatory mechanisms—the intrinsic and extrinsic controls—continue to be operative, acting in concert and in exquisite coordination to maintain circulatory homeostasis. Impairment of one factor results in increase in the effect of the other. Thus, if the extrinsic sympathetic nervous system control is decreased, the Frank-Starling mechanism assumes a more prominent role. Conversely, in patients with impaired myocardial function, there is increased sympathetic activity and concomitant decrease in parasympathetic influence.

### *Response to Neural Blockade in Healthy Humans*

In this section we briefly review data derived from the aforementioned controlled studies in human volunteers and low-risk surgical and obstetric patients on the cardiovascular effects of: 1) the different levels of neural blockade; 2) rapidity with which high blockade is produced; 3) influence of the local anesthetics on the heart and blood vessels; 4) effects of epinephrine included in the local anesthetic solution; and 5) influence of hypovolemia and of agents and conditions that impair circulatory homeostatic mechanisms. The data cited were published by many workers including, Greene (3), Bromage (6,7), Defalque (8), Shimosato and Etsten (9), Otton and colleagues (10,11), and by Bonica and associates, who, during the course of a decade and a half, carried out 43 different studies involving 700 human subjects (12–27). These subjects were healthy, unmedicated volunteers who were used to determine the influence of vasomotor block. In addition, the studies included patients undergoing surgical operations, and gravidae who underwent vagi-

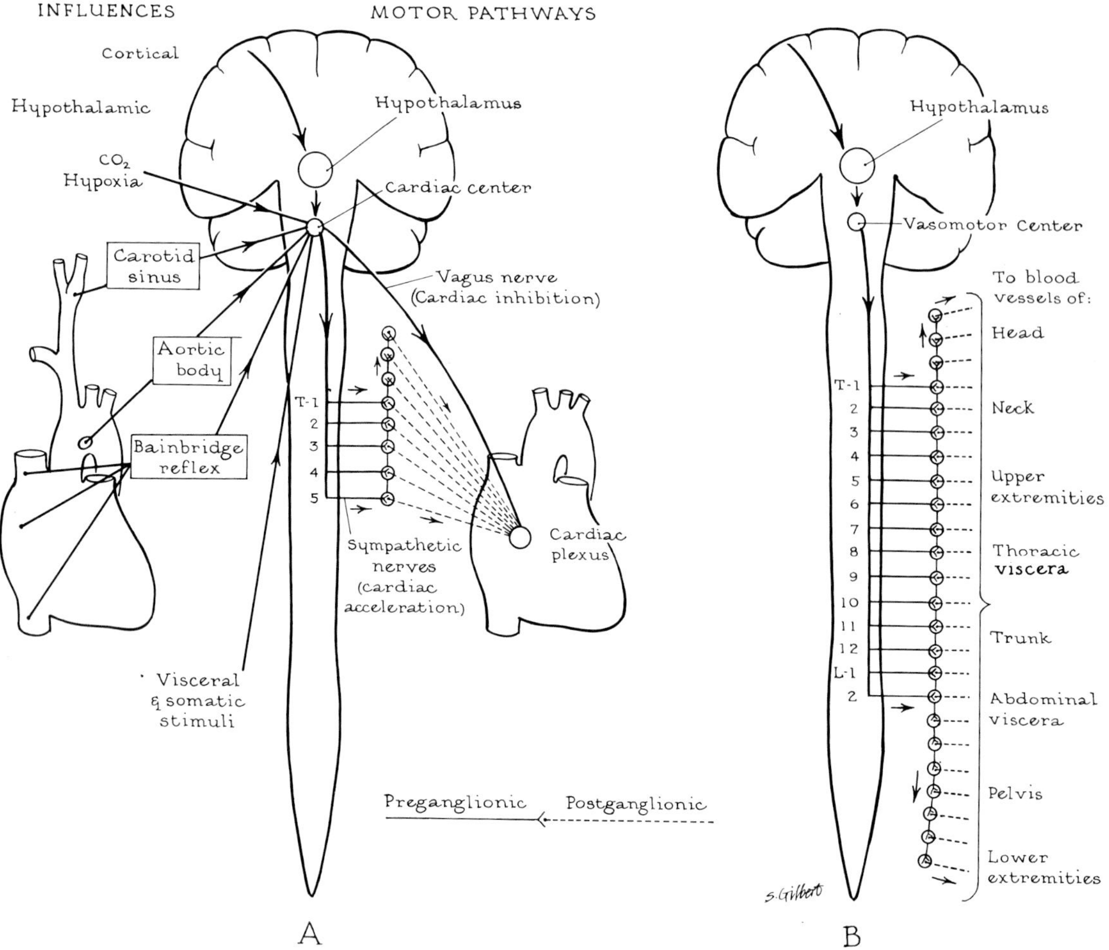


**Fig. 16–1.** Neural pathways involved in the control of circulation. **A,** Afferent fibers from the heart and great vessels, which provide information about alteration and blood pressure, cardiac function, and biochemical factors to the cardiac and vasomotor centers on the reader's left, and the neural pathways, which control cardiac function. **B,** Pathways for neural control of blood vessels. Note the efferents from the cortex hypothalamus and biochemical environment that influence cardiac function as well as the peripheral vessels. The preganglionic sympathetic fibers, which have their cell bodies in the spinal cord, pass along the anterior root of the spinal nerves and enter the paravertebral chain where they make connection with postganglionic fibers.

nal delivery or cesarean section (20–22,25,26). Here we cite only those relevant to this present subject (12–34).

Effects of Levels of Neural Blockade

1. In several studies in which cutaneous analgesia to T10 was achieved with either subarachnoid or epidural block in healthy unmedicated volunteers, no significant changes in any of the hemodynamic parameters were found (13,14,19).
2. Comparison of the effects of T4–5 continuous epidural analgesia (CEA) with T4–5 subarachnoid block (SAB) carried out in the same group at different times showed that SAB produced a much greater degree of hypotension than did epidural analgesia (12,13).
3. Studies were done to determine the hemodynamic effects of high epidural and high subarachnoid block achieved by injecting the drug in small, incremental doses to produce a step-wise analgesia to T10, T8, T6, T4. Figure 16–2 shows that with SAB below T6 there were minimal, clinically insignificant changes in mean arterial pressure (MAP), cardiac output (CO), and total peripheral resistance (TPR), but block above T1 was associated with a significant decrease in CO and TPR resulting in a 20% decrease in MAP. Figure 16–3 shows the results obtained with CEA, achieved with 2% lidocaine injected in a similar step-wise fashion (21).

The much greater degree of hypotension seen with a single dose of the local anesthetic, than which occurred with several small, incremental doses, was attributable to the fact that the onset of sympathetic blockade was much faster with a single dose than with several small, incremental doses. These data strongly suggest that, ideally, epidural anesthesia for cesarean section should be achieved by giving incremental doses over a period of 15 to 20 minutes or more.

4. Another important issue relevant to obstetric anesthesia brought out by a study of progressively higher levels of continuous epidural blockade was the cardiac stimulating effect of lidocaine. Figure 16–3 shows that blockade to the T4-T5 segments produced only small changes in the various hemodynamic parameters. Even more important is the fact that with analgesia block at T2-T3 level, which was achieved after the fourth or fifth injection entailing the use of a total of 1000 to 1200 mg of lidocaine given over a 4-hour period (17) and resulting in arterial blood lidocaine levels ranging between 4 and 6 μg/ml, there was a significant increase in CO due solely to increase in cardiac rate. On the basis of these data and the experimental results reported by Kao and Jalar (28) and Jorfeldt and associates (29), we speculated that this chronotropic effect represented a predominance of lidocaine-induced stimulation of cardiovascular centers in the brain stem with consequent increase in sympathetic nervous system stimulation and some direct peripheral vasoconstriction. In a subsequent study, this hypothesis was confirmed (16) in subjects who were given intravenous infusions of lidocaine that produced a similar increase in CO and cardiac rate, and this was eliminated by producing a segmental SAB with 2 to 3 mg tetracaine injected at T2 interspace to produce sympathetic blockade of the heart.

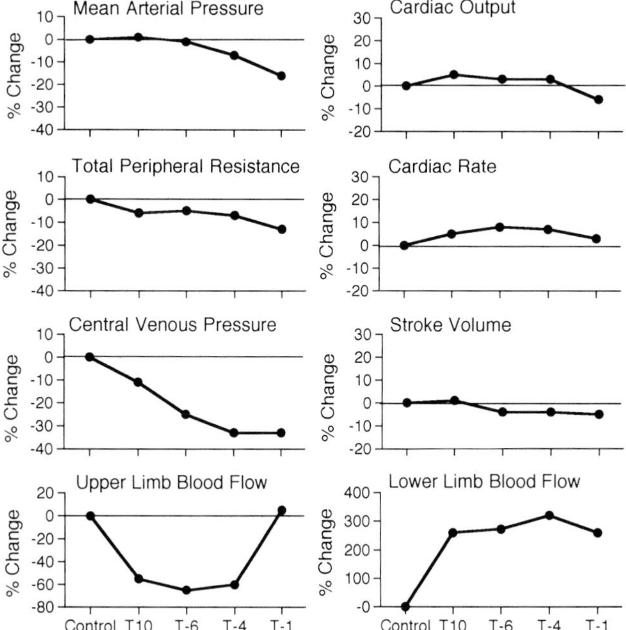


**Fig. 16–2.** Hemodynamic changes in healthy volunteers subjected to progressively higher levels of subarachnoid block. Note that mean arterial pressure (MAP) decreased only about 4% with block as high as T4. The decrease in total peripheral resistance (TPR) and central venous pressure (CVP) were offset by an increased cardiac output (CO), which was primarily due to an increase in heart rate. Note that with T10 block there was a 350% increase in lower limb blood flow due to block of T10, L2 vasomotor segments that control blood flow to the lower limbs. Concomitantly, there was a 60% decrease in upper limb blood flow produced by compensatory vasoconstriction of the vessels in the upper limb. In parturients in the supine position, the increase of blood volume in the lower limbs is trapped by the compression of the inferior vena cava, and because the large volume in the limbs does not return to the heart, it will cause maternal hypotension. (Based on data from Berges PU, Morikawa K, Bonica JJ: Proceedings of the ASA Annual Meeting, 1970, pp 50–59.)

Because blood levels of 4 μg/ml of lidocaine usually develop following single epidural injection of 400 mg or following several injections of 200 to 300 mg of lidocaine (27), these findings have obvious clinical implications in obstetric patients who require continuous epidural anesthesia for prolonged labor for which repeated injections are usually given hourly. Because adult humans require considerably longer than 1 hour to metabolize and eliminate lidocaine, the drug will accumulate to significant levels in blood plasma and body tissues (30).

## Effects of Epinephrine

Many studies have also shown that epidural block achieved with lidocaine containing epinephrine in total doses ranging from 40 to 250 μg produces a predominant beta-adrenergic action consisting of increases in heart rate (HR), stroke volume (SV) and CO and a significant decrease in TPR resulting in a decrease in MAP (2,13,18). Apparently, absorption of these amounts of epinephrine is so slow as to produce almost a pure beta-adrenergic action that affects the peripheral portion of the circulation to a slightly greater degree and slightly longer time than its action on the heart.

The remarkably small alterations usually seen in normovolemic unmedicated subjects given high epidural or subarachnoid block are in contrast with significant cardiovascular depression seen among surgical patients, particularly those given high block for upper abdominal surgery. The most important factors contributing to cardiovascular depression seen in these patients include: 1) high degree of sympathetic tone before the block, provoked by anxiety and apprehension, injury, or by disease; 2) acute or chronic hypovolemia from any cause; 3) cardiovascular disease; 4) impairment of homeostatic circulatory mechanisms; and 5) mechanical obstruction of venous return to the heart.

## Effects of Acute Blood Loss

Studies were carried out to determine the influence of acute blood loss in healthy human volunteer subjects given: 1) high (T4–5) subarachnoid block achieved with 40 to 50 mg of lidocaine and dextrose; 2) the influence of high epidural block achieved with 18 to 22 ml of 2% lidocaine containing 1:200,000 epinephrine; and 3) high epidural achieved with 2% lidocaine alone. The general protocol included usual rest periods and measurements of all hemodynamic and respiratory parameters, before and during the duration of the block in the normovolemic state. This was followed by another rest period and a second group of control measurements, after which 10 ml/kg of whole blood was withdrawn within a fixed period

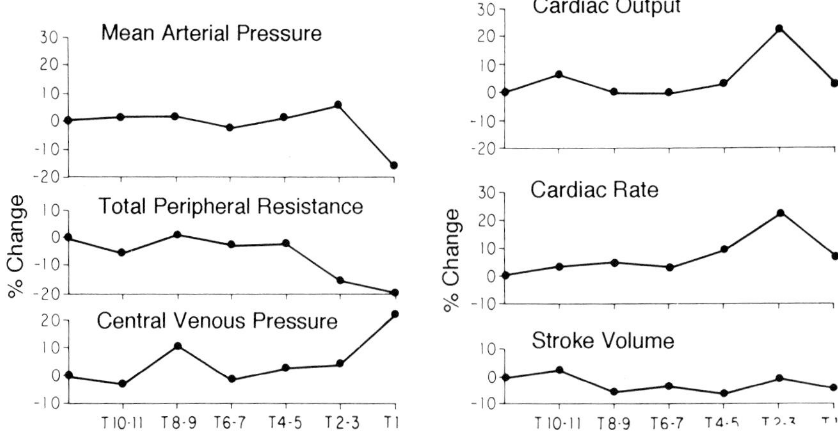


**Fig. 16–3.** Hemodynamic changes in healthy human subjects produced by progressively higher levels of epidural analgesia achieved by injection of small but progressively larger doses of local anesthetic. Note there is virtually no change in MAP and CO with block below T4-5. With block at T2-3, there was a moderate increase in MAP due primarily to an increase in CO caused exclusively by an increase in heart rate. A subsequent study demonstrated these increases were due to stimulation of the cardiac and vasomotor centers in the midbrain by the moderate levels (4 to 6 μg/ml) of lidocaine in arterial blood. The increase in CO was more than adequate to offset the decrease in TPR, resulting in moderate increase in arterial blood pressure. When the block was extended above T1 (involving all sympathetic outflow to the body), heart rate, CO, and MAP decreased to below control levels due to elimination of sympathetic innervation to the heart. (From Bonica JJ, Akamatsu TJ, Berges PU, Morikawa K, et al: Circulatory effects of peridural block: I. Effects of level of analgesia and dose of lidocaine. Anesthesiology 33:619–626, 1970.)

of 15 to 20 minutes which, according to the studies of Moore and associates (31), represents 13% of the total blood volume and simulates moderate hemorrhage. Measurements were repeated at 10 and 30 minutes after blood withdrawal, followed by a 10-minute rest period, and a second injection of the same amount of local anesthetic. Measurements were repeated when T5 block was established and every 30 minutes thereafter until all signs of blockade disappeared. After completion of the study, the blood was reinfused into the subject.

Figure 16–4 summarizes the results obtained in one study in which the effects of high epidural block were measured in the normovolemic state (not shown) and after acute blood loss (19). Part A shows the response to T5 epidural block achieved with 2% lidocaine and 1:200,000 epinephrine in 15 subjects after they had been made hypovolemic. Apparently, the epinephrine produced a positive inotropic and chronotropic effect increasing CO to about 18%, which offset the 30% decrease in TPR, resulting in a 22% decrease in MAP. It had been planned that the study would be repeated in 15 subjects using similar volumes of 2% lidocaine without epinephrine. However, because five of the first seven subjects had a precipitous fall in MAP to profound levels and 2 had an asystole lasting about 10 seconds, the study was terminated (Figure 16–4B). The five subjects who developed severe cardiovascular depression were immediately given 15 to 25 mg ephedrine via the superior vena cava catheter to restore arterial blood pressure to near normal levels.

In the latter group, MAP decreased to a mean of 41% of control, central venous pressure (CVP) from 2 to -0.7 cm$H_2O$, and HR to 70% of control (Figure 16–4B). The difference between the results of the two epidural solutions is the fact that the epinephrine-containing lidocaine had some beneficial cardiac-stimulating effect to prevent the profound cardiovascular depression seen with lidocaine alone. This profound depression was probably due to the rapid absorption of lidocaine producing arterial blood levels in excess of 11 μg/ml (27), which together with the metabolic acidosis consequent to the hypotension produced severe myocardial depression. A similar study with high subarachnoid block was carried out before and after acute blood loss. In this group, MAP was reduced 30% below control value; cardiac output was reduced 15%; stroke volume had decreased nearly 22%, and central venous pressure was 66% below the control values.

It is apparent that loss of moderate quantities of blood in young healthy unmedicated persons significantly increased the deleterious effects of high SAB or epidural anesthesia. The clinical implications of these studies are obvious. High subarachnoid or epidural block should be avoided in parturients who have moderate to severe hypovolemia. In very rare and special circumstances in which the patient's conditions contraindicate general anesthesia or present even greater risks, subarachnoid or epidural block can be used provided a T4-T5 analgesia can be used, but only after the blood volume is increased with whole blood or colloid solutions and other prophylactic measures are taken, as mentioned later. Moreover, the analgesia should be achieved with several incremental doses, and the parturient's hemodynamics should be monitored continually with techniques that provide second-to-second information.

### Effects of Pregnancy

Fall in arterial blood pressure following subarachnoid or epidural block to a specific level is greater and more

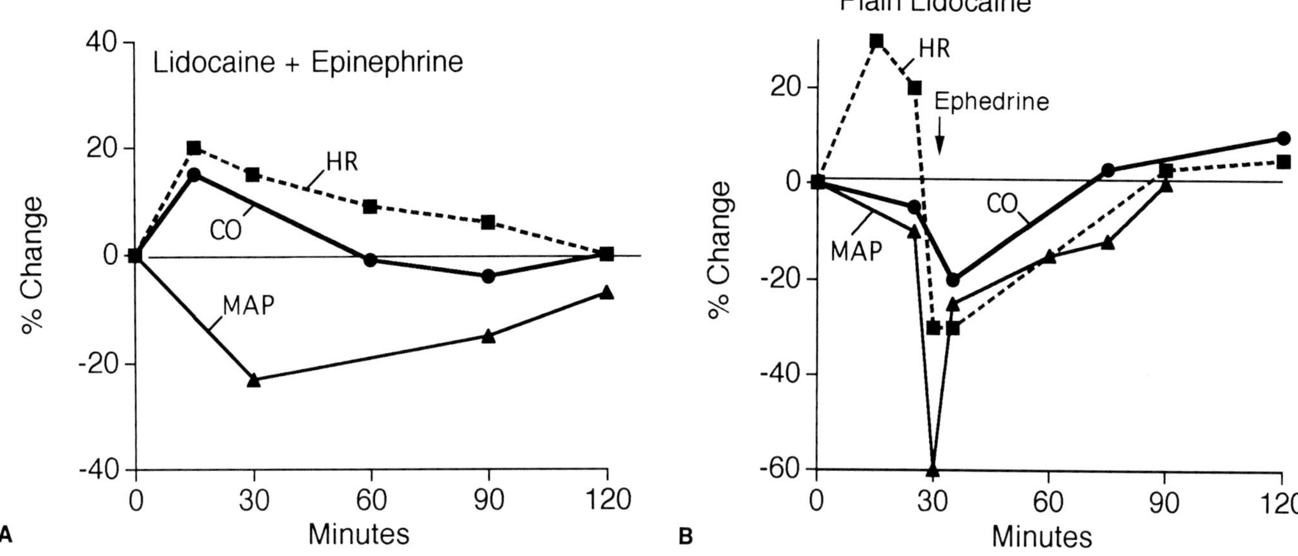


**Fig. 16–4.** Effects of epidural blockade to T5 in healthy human subjects after the administration of either plain lidocaine or lidocaine containing epinephrine 1:200,000 after 13% of blood volume was withdrawn to simulate moderate hypovolemia. The effects of blockade in the normovolemic state are not shown. **A)** Blockade with lidocaine/epinephrine produced a beta-adrenergic effect consisting of an increase in heart rate and CO, which partially offset the decrease in TPR to produce a 22% decrease in MAP. **B)** Blockade without epinephrine given during hypovolemia led to severe cardiovascular depression probably due to direct depression of the myocardium by the lidocaine. This required immediate therapy with intravenous ephedrine and very rapid infusion of fluid. In this case, the lack of epinephrine precluded the beta-adrenergic stimulating action on the heart. (Modified from Bonica JJ, Kennedy WF Jr, Akamatsu TJ, Gerbershagen HU: Circulatory effects of peridural block. II. Effects of acute blood loss. Anesthesiology 36: 219–227, 1972.)

rapid in pregnant than in nonpregnant women. This has been demonstrated in a number of studies during the past 3 decades. One of the first studies was carried out by Assali and Prystowsky (32), who noted a "negligible fall" in arterial pressure in normotensive, nonpregnant women during high subarachnoid block, compared to normotensive term pregnant women. When anesthetic block was repeated 35 to 48 hours after delivery, the average fall in systolic pressure was similar to that of nonpregnant level (Figure 16–5). In otherwise healthy gravidae, the primary reason for the greater degree of hypotension is decreased venous return to the heart due to occlusion of the inferior vena cava and other large veins by the gravid uterus. The effect of caval compression by the uterus was clearly demonstrated in half a dozen studies carried out by Ueland, Hansen, and Bonica and associates at The University of Washington.

In each of the studies pertaining to obstetrics, term gravidae were used and cardiovascular and respiratory parameters measured before and after induction of the block with the patient in the supine position, and then repeated in the lateral position before surgery was initiated. Because studies were carried out to evaluate the influence of these various types of anesthesia, the usual prophylactic measures of a given infusion of fluids and/or administration of vasopressors were omitted. The measurements were then repeated during the operation in the supine position: 1) at the moment the abdomen was opened; 2) immediately after delivery of the infant; and 3) at 10 minutes and 1 hour postpartum. Measurements of blood volume and arterial hematocrit were obtained before delivery and at 10 minutes and 1 hour postpartum, and on postpartum days 1, 3, and 5. Table 16–1 contains a summary of the maximum changes in maternal hemodynamics, noted with three types of regional anesthesia and with balanced general anesthesia.

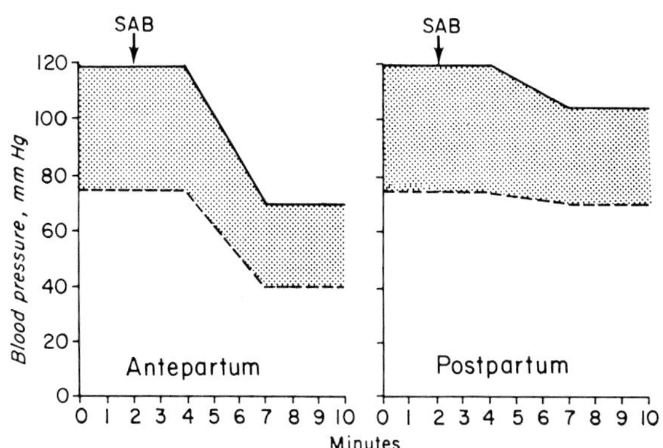


**Fig. 16–5.** Response of ten gravidas to high vasomotor block produced by T1 differential spinal block during pregnancy, and 36 to 48 hours after delivery. In the antepartum period, blood pressure was measured with the patient in the supine position, which caused compression of the inferior vena cava and consequent profound hypotension. In the postpartum period, hypotension was much less because there was no longer obstruction of venous return to the heart by the gravid uterus. (Developed from data of Assali NS, Prystowsky H: J. Clin. Invest. 29:1367, 1950.)

**Table 16–1.** Comparison of Hemodynamic Changes During Cesarean Section Carried Out With 4 Different Methods of Anesthesia

(Percent Changes from Control)

| Anesthetic Phases of Operation | Cardiac Output (L/min) | Cardiac Rate (per minute) | Stroke Volume (ml) | Total Peripheral Resistance (dynes/sec/cm$^{-5}$) | Mean Arterial Pressure (mmHg) |
|---|---|---|---|---|---|
| Postanesthesia Preoperative Supine Position | | | | | |
| SAB | −35 | +21 | −15 | −12 | −46 |
| Epidural LA | −6 | +8 | −10 | −1 | −11 |
| Epid LA & Epi | −17 | +5 | −16 | −16 | −37 |
| General | +7 | +7 | N/C | +21 | +13 |
| Abdomen Open | | | | | |
| SAB | +2 | +6 | N/C | −19 | −20 |
| Epidural LA | +12 | −5 | +17 | −18 | −11 |
| Epid LA & Epi | N/C | −10 | +5 | −24 | −14 |
| General | +25 | −5 | +32 | +4 | +18 |
| Immediate Post-Delivery | | | | | |
| SAB | +56 | −6 | +71 | −38 | −7 |
| Epidural LA | +25 | +7 | +17 | −26 | −7 |
| Epid LA & Epi | +32 | +19 | +26 | −31 | −12 |
| General | +32 | −11 | +46 | −9 | +12 |
| 10 minutes After Delivery | | | | | |
| SAB | +56 | +6 | +52 | −40 | −16 |
| Epidural LA | +20 | −6 | +28 | −23 | −10 |
| Epid LA & Epi | +22 | +19 | +20 | −24 | −15 |
| General | +40 | −11 | +57 | −5 | +10 |
| 60 minutes After Delivery | | | | | |
| SAB | +35 | −5 | +37 | −25 | −10 |
| Epidural LA | +14 | +2 | +26 | −16 | −8 |
| Epid LA & Epi | +22 | +2 | +17 | −29 | −3 |
| General | +24 | −16 | +49 | −2 | +8 |
| Effect of Tracheal Intubation/Extubation | | | | | |
| Intubation | +25 | +15 | +4 | −15 | +18 |
| Extubation | +15 | +7 | +14 | −27 | +16 |

N/C = no change
(Table developed from data published by: Ueland K, Gills RE, Hansen JM: Maternal cardiovascular dynamics: I. Cesarean section under subarachnoid block anesthesia. Am J. Obstet. Gynecol. 100:42, 1968; Ueland K, Akamatsu TJ, Eng M, Bonica JJ, et al: Maternal cardiovascular dynamics: VI. Cesarean section under epidural anesthesia without epinephrine. Am. J. Obstet. Gynecol. 114:775–780, 1972; and Akamatsu TJ, DerYuen D, Ueland K, Bonica JJ: Cardiovascular effects of epidural anesthesia with epinephrine for cesarean section. Obstet. Gynec. News. 9:3, 1974.)

In the first study, subarachnoid block achieved with 7 to 10 mg tetracaine and 200 μg epinephrine was used (20). The levels of analgesia were below T5 in three of the parturients. Moreover, these patients had lateral uterine displacement, but no vasopressors for the treatment of hypotension to assess the magnitude of the hemodynamic changes. In another 14 patients who underwent cesarean section with SAB, hypotension was treated promptly with vasopressors. Figure 16–6, developed from data of the first group, shows the significant difference in various cardiovascular parameters when the patient was supine and when the patient was in the lateral position. This illustration, which shows mean values, clearly demonstrates that the compression of the inferior vena cava was the sole etiologic factor responsible for the cardiovascular changes. Thus, it is noted that merely opening the abdomen resulted in some restoration of MAP toward normal levels, a result of improved SV and HR, and, consequently, CO and MAP. This restoration effect probably resulted from a decrease of intra-abdominal pressure and in turn decrease of the pressure exerted on the inferior vena cava and consequent increase in venous return. This beneficial effect was further enhanced after delivery of the infant, when these various parameters return to normal or slightly above normal. Because the level of sympathetic blockade at the latter two points and at the point marked postpartum remained at the same level as before the delivery of the infant, the only conclusion that can be considered is that the compression of the veins was the primary etiologic factor in producing hypotension. That the level of vasomotor block played little or no role in these changes is suggested by the fact that in this study group and in the other 14 patients who had cesarean section with subarachnoid block, patients with T8 or T9 block before the opening of the abdomen had the same degree of cardiovascular depression as those who had T4 or T5 block. The authors concluded that there was a lack of correlation between the level and dose of anesthesia and

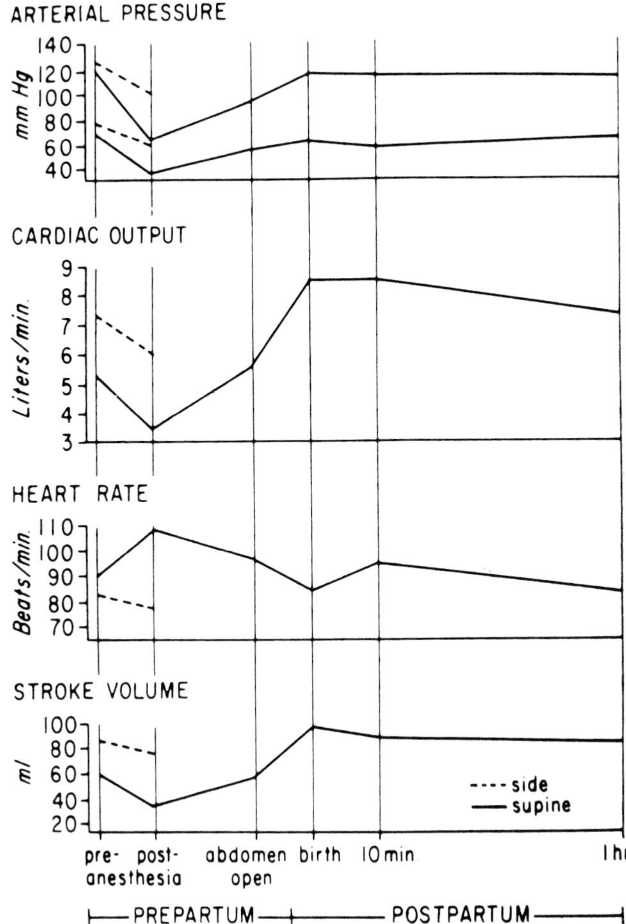


**Fig. 16–6.** Hemodynamic changes in gravidas undergoing cesarean section with subarachnoid block. Measurements were made in both the lateral and supine position before and after induction of anesthesia. Note the greater effect in the supine position, the block had on all hemodynamic variables as compared with the lateral position. With the onset of the operation, with the patient in the supine position, merely opening the abdomen increased blood pressure due primarily to increases in stroke volume and cardiac output. Following delivery of the infant, blood pressure increased to preanesthetic levels, while stroke volume and cardiac output increased even further above preanesthetic levels. The fact that at this point the parturients still had about the same level of vasomotor block provides evidence that the hypotensive episodes were due primarily to compression of the inferior vena cava and consequent decrease in venous return by the gravid uterus. In the postpartum period elimination of the venous obstruction and extrusion of blood from the uterus into the central circulation caused further significant increases in the various parameters. (Developed from data of Ueland K, Gills RE, Hansen JM: Maternal cardiovascular dynamics: I. Cesarean section under subarachnoid block anesthesia. Am. J. Obstet. Gynecol. 100:42, 1968.)

severity of maternal cardiovascular depression. Measurement of blood gases and pH revealed that some of the patients hyperventilated with a consequent increase in $PaO_2$, decrease in $PaCO_2$, and increase in pH. In this group, the hypotension did not appear to have any consistent deleterious effects on newborn infants whose blood gases were within normal limits, and the Apgar rating ranged from 6 to 9, with a mean score of 8 for the group. It was also noted that the administration of oxytocin injected intravenously after the delivery produced a transient (3 to 4 minutes) decrease in systolic and diastolic pressure and increase in HR. The mean blood volume decreased 16% (1004 ml), with a range of 400 to 1650 ml.

In a second study, the group evaluated the effects of a continuous epidural block achieved with 12–16 ml of 2% mepivacaine (Carbocaine) without epinephrine (21). In several patients, the level of anesthesia was inadequate and required supplementation with 50% $N_2O$ and oxygen by mask before delivery. In two patients, increments of 3 mg of morphine sulfate were given intravenously for relief of discomfort encountered during closure of the uterine incision. This study showed the same trend in cardiovascular and respiratory parameters as with subarachnoid block except that the degree of hypotension was significantly less. Table 16–1 shows that the block before the operation caused a decrease of about 6% in CO and 11% in MAP. Upon opening the abdomen, CO increased 12%, which together with an 18% decrease in TPR consequent to the vasomotor block resulted in an 11% decrease in MAP. Following delivery of the infant, CO increased 25%, which together with a 26% decrease in TPR resulted in an 11% decrease in MAP. Subsequently, these parameters remained the same, indicating stabilization of the hemodynamics. None of the patients required vasopressors as had been the case with subarachnoid block. It is apparent that continuous epidural block without epinephrine caused less hemodynamic alteration than did subarachnoid block. Maternal and fetal blood gases and Apgar scores were within normal limits, and the amount of blood loss was similar to the group that received subarachnoid block.

A third study was carried out with epidural anesthesia achieved with 12 to 16 ml of mepivacaine with 1:200,000 epinephrine injected as a single bolus (22). To the surprise of the investigators, the parturients manifested a decrease of 16% in SV, which resulted in a 17% decrease in CO. These, together with a 16% decrease in TPR, resulted in a 37% decrease in MAP, which was somewhat smaller than the effects with subarachnoid block but significantly greater than the effects of epidural achieved with plain mepivacaine. Because of the rapid onset of hypotension, 10 of the 12 parturients required therapy soon after the onset of block, consisting of left uterine displacement, rapid intravenous infusion, pressure booted inflation of the legs, and intravenous injection of ephedrine. The reason for the greater alterations in this group of patients as compared to the group receiving epidural with mepivacaine alone was primarily due to a decrease in stroke volume and a much greater decrease in TPR from the epinephrine-induced vasodilation. Following opening of the abdomen, SV and CO were restored to preanesthetic levels and were due to lessening of the compression of the inferior vena cava and the consequent decrease in venous return. The effects on peripheral resistance remained until 1 hour after the operation. Notwithstanding the significant differences between the two groups, maternal and fetal blood gases and pH and Apgar scores were within normal limits and were very similar to those noted in the group receiving mepivacaine alone.

To recapitulate, from these and other data it is obvious that the primary reason for the hypotension with subarachnoid block and epidural block achieved with a local anesthetic without epinephrine is due to compression of the inferior vena cava by the gravid uterus. The addition of epinephrine may exaggerate the hypotension by additional peripheral vasodilation. The significant increase in stroke volume and cardiac output immediately after delivery of the infant and 10 minutes later is primarily due to removal of the compression on the inferior vena cava and extrusion of about 500 ml of blood from the contracting uterus into the central blood volume. Ueland and associates (20–22) suggested that, together with the removal of the vena cava compression, the blood that had pooled into the lower limbs during the compression increased the venous return to the heart of about 1000 ml. This is reflected by the significant increase in SV and CO after delivery of the infant, and it was just sufficient to offset the decrease in TPR caused by the vasomotor block resulting in a parallel increase in blood pressure.

## Supine Hypotensive Syndrome

At this point mention is made of the "supine hypotension syndrome" discussed in detail in Chapter 2. This term, first used in 1953 by Howard and associates (33), applies to 10 to 15% of gravidae who develop hypotension in the supine position, and is due to impeded venous blood return from the pelvis and lower limbs to the heart. The other 85 to 90% maintain their blood pressure by compensatory vasoconstriction and an increase in HR, but despite these compensations, most gravidae have a decrease in CO (34,35). Moreover, because there is concomitant compression of the lower aorta, blood pressure is decreased below the obstruction, with consequent reduction of perfusion to the placenta and lower limbs (36). This is reflected by the fact that maintaining parturients in the supine position during labor for even a short period is associated with a progressive decrease in fetal pH (37). As noted in these and other studies, having the gravida on her side relieves more (but not all!) of the compression resulting in a 35 to 40% increase of SV and CO and consequent restoration of blood pressure toward normal (see Figures 2–28 and 2–30 from Chapter 2).

Other factors that aggravate the degree of hypotension in a parturient receiving subarachnoid or epidural block include: 1) hypertension; 2) hypovolemia; 3) severe anemia; 4) severe electrolyte imbalance or acidosis; 5) depression or elimination of intrinsic vasomotor tone; 6) depression of catecholamines from prolonged antihypertensive therapy; and 7) adrenocortical depression from prolonged cortisone administration.

In patients with hypovolemia, peripheral vasodilation results in a greater proportion of the blood being pooled at the periphery than is the case in normal individuals, and, consequently, there is a disproportionately greater reduction in venous return to the heart. For example, in a patient with a normal blood volume of 5 liters, the volume of blood in the legs during spinal blockade is approximately 800 to 1000 ml, or about 16 to 20% of the total blood volume (38). In a patient with a blood volume of only 3 liters, the same area of vasodilation may contain 25 to 30% of the circulating blood volume. Many patients with chronic hypovolemia are able to compensate sufficiently to maintain normal blood pressure, but when spinal block is given, even if it is limited to low spinal levels, it may eliminate enough vasomotor segments to disturb the delicate balance that exists, and the patient develops disproportionately severe hypotension.

Depression of intrinsic vasomotor tone may also play an important role. Normally, dilation of the arteries, arterioles, and metarterioles that follows sympathetic interruption is rarely maximum because of a residual intrinsic tone inherent in all smooth muscle, including that of the arterial tree. The degree of effectiveness of this residual intrinsic tone varies from organ to organ, being most effective in cerebral, cardiac, and renal vessels, less so in splanchnic vessels, still less in vessels of striated muscle, and least effective in skin vessels. This intrinsic tone is diminished or even eliminated by hypercarbia and depressant drugs due to direct effects on the smooth muscle of the vessels.

Patients with pregnancy induced hypertension (PIH) are at particular risk of becoming hypotensive with regional anesthesia. Intravascular volume, which may be less than 80% of normal pregnant values (39), predisposes these patients to significant hypotension with the onset of even midthoracic sympathetic block. The risk of fetal distress is further compounded by the fact that these patients often have abnormal placental vasculature and uteroplacental insufficiency. Any intervention that may lower maternal blood pressure, such as antihypertensive therapy or regional block, must be initiated in a slow, controlled fashion with close attention to intravascular volume status (40). Fetal heart rate monitoring, when available, should be used by the anesthesiologist in conjunction with more routine monitors to gauge the effects of anesthetic intervention.

## Effects of Hypotension on the Mother

### Cardiac Effects

Although it is widely believed that bradycardia is often seen in association with spinal hypotension, this was never seen in any of the studies carried out by Ueland and associates (20–22). It occurred in a group of healthy human volunteers who developed severe hypotension, bradycardia, and eventually asystole in two instances (19). Usually, this slowing of the heart can be attributed to paralysis of the cardiac accelerator fibers with high segmental block (T1-T4). However, bradycardia can be seen with spinal hypotension in the absence of total sympathetic blockade. A number of studies indicate that decreased venous return to the heart causes a rapid decrease in ventricular volume and provokes the Bezold-Jarish reflex characterized by vagal predominance, which may be even more important in causing bradycardia with arterial hypotension. In some patients, severe hypotension will produce medullary ischemia with consequent depression of respiration that results in hypercapnea, which further aggravates hypotension by its vasodilating effect. Bradycardia can usually be reversed by giving atropine and oxygen. It is important to emphasize that if hypotension and bradycardia are not quickly diagnosed and treated, they can rapidly progress to cardiac arrest in otherwise normal patients having spinal anesthesia (41–44). In many reports, the subjects had anesthesia to T4 or above and very likely developed total sympathetic blockade.

## Coronary Blood Flow (CF)

Coronary blood flow is decreased during spinal hypotension. However, the ability of the coronary circulation to autoregulate combined with the reduced metabolic demand on the heart during spinal hypotension results in the heart being able to tolerate considerable hypotension without developing myocardial ischemia (45–47). At some poorly defined critical level of hypotension, myocardial ischemia will begin to occur. The degree of hypotension that can be tolerated will be less in patients with coronary artery disease, ventricular hypertrophy, or in patients whose heart is required to perform a greater amount of work, e.g., women in active labor. Recently Palmer, et al (48) reported electrocardiographic (ECG) changes characteristic of myocardial ischemia in 35 out of 93 healthy parturients undergoing cesarean section under regional anesthesia. Although it is not clear if these ECG changes were due to myocardial ischemia, the authors postulated that ventricular distention due to rapid fluid administration combined with decreased diastolic blood pressure might lead to myocardial ischemia in this setting.

## Central Nervous System Effects

Cerebral blood flow is governed largely by mean arterial blood pressure and local metabolic factors. A decrease in blood pressure is followed by compensatory cerebral vasodilation resulting in a stable level of blood flow. However, at some critical degree of hypotension the cerebral vasculature will be unable to further compensate; any additional fall in blood pressure will result in decreased cerebral blood flow and eventually signs and symptoms of cerebral ischemia. In healthy normotensive men, cerebral ischemia will occur when mean arterial pressure falls to 35 to 40 mm Hg (3,49). Because of considerable individual variation it is best to assume that the critical mean arterial pressure is about 55 mm Hg in healthy patients and considerably higher in those with chronic hypertension, PIH, or other vascular disease (3). One of the most serious effects of hypotension on the central nervous system is medullary ischemia, which can cause autonomic instability and depression of respiratory centers. If not diagnosed and treated quickly, the result can be respiratory arrest and cardiovascular collapse. The most common cause of central nervous system (CNS) ischemia during spinal anesthesia is the head up position (3).

## Effects on Other Organ Systems and Metabolism

Reports from the literature indicate that as mean arterial pressure decreases below 80 to 85 mm Hg during spinal anesthesia, renal blood flow, glomerular filtration, and urinary output decrease in a linear fashion (49–51). The kidney is able to tolerate hypotension quite well and when perfusion pressure is returned to normal, renal function also returns. Precise data are lacking on how low blood pressure may go with high spinal anesthesia before irreversible damage becomes apparent. However, it should be assumed that below a mean pressure of 35 mm Hg renal ischemia and permanent renal damage will occur (3). In patients with renal vascular disease, this critical level of hypotension may be much higher. Hepatic blood flow is reduced during spinal hypotension (49–51). Whether this is due to a reduction in cardiac output or to a redistribution of blood flow away from the liver is not clear. However, there is no correlation between reduction in hepatic blood flow and development of postoperative hepatic dysfunction. Greene, et al (49) found that hepatic function following spinal hypotension with systolic pressures of 60 mm Hg or lower was similar to that found among patients who had received spinal anesthesia and maintained normal blood pressure. He concluded that the reduction in hepatic blood flow produced by moderate hypotension for a moderate period of time during spinal anesthesia does not contribute to postoperative changes in liver function (3).

Hypotension associated with spinal block is usually not followed by significant changes in electrolytes and hematological values. Metabolism and oxygen consumption are decreased, and the $pO_2$, $pCO_2$, pH, and other biochemical parameters remain normal, except when severe hypotension persists (3,52). In a study of parturients who had received subarachnoid block for cesarean section, Stenger and his associates (52) found that oxygen capacity, oxygen saturation, and oxygen tension of those in whom severe hypotension remained uncorrected were the same as those in whom the hypotension had been corrected. This lack of serious metabolic alteration contrasts with the significant biochemical changes associated with hypovolemic hypotension (shock). In hypovolemic shock, there is elevation of serum lactate, pyruvate, and potassium due to tissue hypoxia and consequent abnormal capillary permeability and anaerobic metabolism. This difference in biochemical effects is caused by the different effects on the peripheral vascular bed produced by the two hypotensive conditions.

### *Effects on Labor*

Mild to moderate hypotension has little or no effect on the intensity or frequency of uterine contractions; however, severe hypotension has been associated with decreased uterine activity. Vasicka and associates (53) found a consistent correlation between maternal hypotension and decrease in uterine contractility. Although this observation has not been uniformly reported, it stands to reason that if sufficient hypoperfusion is allowed to occur, the uterus will be deprived of sufficient substrate to meet the metabolic demands of the contracting uterus. Schellenberg (54) has proposed that supine positioning with decreased uterine perfusion accompanying aorto-caval compression may have been a confounding factor resulting in decreased uterine activity in a number of studies assessing the effect of epidural anesthesia on the outcome of labor.

### *Effects on the Fetus and Newborn*

Maternal organ systems will tolerate moderate degrees of hypotension quite well; however, because the uterus is essentially a nonautoregulating organ (55), uterine blood flow will decrease linearly with decreased perfusion pressure. Because of this, the placenta may be inadequately perfused while the parturient remains asymptomatic. It is difficult to predict at what maternal blood pressure level fetal asphyxia will develop. It appears that the uteroplacental anatomy, the normal maternal blood pressure, and the duration of hypoperfusion are all critical. Ebner, et al (56) studied the influence of degree and duration of spinal hypotension on the fetal heart rate. They observed a progressively greater incidence of fetal bradycardia when the maternal systolic blood pressure was less than 70 mm Hg. Even when maternal blood pressure was between 70 and 80 mm Hg for longer than 4 minutes, there was a progressive increase in the incidence of fetal bradycardia. Hon and associates (57), using electronic fetal heart rate assessment, found that maternal hypotension of less than 100 mm Hg systolic for longer than about 5 minutes resulted in signs of fetal distress. Others have reported a decrease in fetal scalp pH (37) and low Apgar scores (58) with maternal systolic blood pressures of less than 100 mm Hg for periods as short as 5 to 15 minutes. From these data one can conclude that a systolic blood pressure of less than 100 mm Hg in a previously normotensive parturient should be treated promptly. In such instances, if the hypotension is promptly corrected, it has no effect on the clinical condition of the newborn as assessed by the Apgar score at 1 and 5 minutes and the Neurologic Adaptive Capacity Score (NACS) at 15 minutes, 2 hours, and 24 hours of age (59). On the other hand, in patients who are hypertensive, signs of fetal distress often occur at systolic blood pressures greater than 100 mm Hg. Conversely, fetuses of mothers who normally have systolic blood pressures of less than 100 mm Hg seem to tolerate this without difficulty.

### *Prevention*

Some decrease in blood pressure is to be expected with spinal or epidural anesthesia in obstetric patients. However, a number of measures can be taken to minimize the incidence and severity of hypotension. All forms of neuraxial anesthesia are contraindicated in the presence of moderate or severe hypovolemia. This, however, may not always be apparent. Blood loss can be chronic or occult, and dehydration or maternal disease can result in nonhemorrhagic intravascular volume depletion. If there is any doubt about maternal intravascular volume status, hematocrit and urine output should be checked. Orthostatic blood pressure determinations may provide an indication of intravascular volume status. In some patients, central hemodynamic monitoring may be necessary to help assess a patient's volume status.

### Intravenous Infusions

The single best measure in preventing hypotension before induction of spinal or epidural anesthesia is the rapid infusion of balanced nondextrose containing fluid. Experience has shown that 1500 to 2000 ml of balanced nondextrose containing solution should be infused within 30 minutes of a high spinal or epidural anesthetic in the uncomplicated healthy parturient. Before a low segmental block, such as may be used for labor analgesia, 500 to 1000 ml of solution is usually adequate. The safety of rapid fluid preloading with crystalloid solutions in this setting has been well established (59,60). Although some recommend the inclusion of colloid solution to increase the time the fluid load remains in the vascular compartment (61), they are more expensive and can have other disadvantages, including anaphylactoid reactions. Dextrose-containing solutions are best avoided because of such adverse side effects as maternal hyperglycemia, fetal hyperglycemia, and subsequent neonatal hyperinsulinemia and hypoglycemia (62). There is also some evidence that such solutions increase the brain's susceptibility to anoxic injury (63).

### Lateral Uterine Displacement

The importance of maintaining continuous left lateral uterine (LUD) displacement cannot be overemphasized. Simply placing a wedge under the hip provides no guarantee of avoiding aorto-caval compression. Fifteen to 30° of tilt and/or manual displacement of the uterus may be necessary to avoid signs of vascular obstruction. Some patients appear to have a more satisfactory result with right uterine displacement. The importance of attention to uterine displacement during cesarean sections has been demonstrated by improved fetal acid base status and Apgar scores (64).

### Vasopressors

Some authors have recommended the use of prophylactic intramuscular (65) or intravenous (66) ephedrine administration before spinal anesthesia for cesarean section. But in one study, which included a large series of parturients (583) having cesarean sections performed under epidural anesthesia following prehydration and left uterine displacement, prophylactic intramuscular ephedrine did not seem to provide additional protection against hypotension (67). On the other hand, others have reported that prophylactic ephedrine administration is associated with better newborn outcomes when hypotension was prevented rather than treated (68,69). In addition to the other prophylactic measures mentioned, we recommend giving ephedrine intravenously as soon as a significant downward trend in blood pressure becomes apparent or as soon as the patient complains of symptoms associated with hypotension, e.g., nausea, vomiting, or pallor. Because of the low incidence of hypotension with current methods of continuous epidural analgesia used for labor and delivery, prophylactic ephedrine is not recommended.

### *Treatment*

The preventative measures outlined above are often sufficient to prevent moderate or severe hypotension with the induction of subarachnoid or epidural anesthesia. However, if the parturient becomes hypotensive or manifests symptoms associated with hypotension, then the following steps should be taken: 1) place the patient in the full lateral position or further displace the uterus laterally; 2) in parturients ready to undergo cesarean section, place them in a modified Trendelenberg position consisting of lowering the head of the table 5° and raising the legs 30° (70); 3) rapidly administer additional intravenous fluids; 4) administer oxygen; and 5) administer increments of 10 mg ephedrine intravenously as needed.

Ephedrine has been shown to have the least detrimental effect on uterine perfusion and is considered to be the vasopressor of choice in obstetric patients (71). As a rule of thumb, a systolic blood pressure of 100 mm Hg should be used as a lower limit in previously normotensive patients. In the hypertensive patient, any sudden decrease in blood pressure of greater than 20% should be treated. A recent clinical study in which low-risk parturients were treated in accordance with this usual rule of thumb, demonstrated that changes in maternal blood pressure were not correlated with any signs of fetal distress (72).

## Systemic Toxic Reactions to Local Anesthetics and Related Drugs

A number of systemic reactions can occur during regional anesthesia, including: 1) toxic reaction to local anesthetics; 2) accidental overdose of epinephrine or other vasopressors; 3) psychogenic reaction to the procedure rather than reaction to the drug; and 4) allergic/hypersensitivity reactions to the local anesthetic.

### *Toxic Reactions to the Local Anesthetic*

Systemic toxic reactions to local anesthetics are among the most dramatic and distressing complications in obstetric anesthesia and represent one of the main causes of maternal mortality associated with epidural anesthesia (73). Central nervous system and cardiovascular toxic reactions have long been recognized as complications of local anesthetic overdose or, more commonly, unintentional intravascular injection. However, before the widespread use of long-acting amide local anesthetics such as bupivacaine, these reactions rarely lead to fatal cardiac arrest. In 1979, Albright (74) reported six cases of cardiac arrest following bupivacaine or etidocaine injections. Albright speculated that the long-acting amide local anesthetics may be more cardiotoxic and that resuscitation from cardiac arrest induced by these agents may be more difficult. Since then, he has collected at least 44 cases of maternal cardiac arrests, 30 of which have been fatal (75). Data from the ASA Closed Malpractice Claims Study indicate that convulsion was the single most common critical event that led to serious complications among the obstetric-related claims (76). Of 19 convulsions in the obstetric group of claims, 17 were likely due to local anesthetic toxic reactions with epidural anesthesia. Bupivacaine was the local anesthetic used in 15 of the 17 cases. In the remaining two cases, the anesthetic was not specified. Eighty-three % of the convulsions resulted in neurologic injury or death to the mother, newborn, or both.

#### *Etiology*

Although systemic local anesthetic toxicity can result from overdose, rapid absorption, or abnormally slow elimination of the local anesthetic, the most common cause is unintentional intravenous injection. Epidural veins become engorged in gravidae because these veins serve as an alternate route for blood return to the heart when the inferior vena cava is obstructed by the gravid uterus. It is not rare for an epidural catheter to enter an epidural vein while the catheter is being advanced into the epidural space. Local anesthetic injected into an epidural vein under these conditions may travel to the heart via the azygos vein at a rate many times greater than when the inferior vena cava is not obstructed (77). It has been suggested that cannulation of epidural veins may be more common with the use of end hole catheters than with blunt tipped multiple side hole catheters. However, the positioning of multiple side hole catheters may be ambiguous because one or more of the side holes may be properly placed while others may be intravascular, subarachnoid, or in some other undesired location. In our experience, as many as 5 to 10% of end hole epidural catheters may enter an epidural vein (in the laboring patient) as judged by the ability to aspirate blood or by repeated test doses positive for intravascular injection.

#### *Pathophysiology*

Many factors influence the toxicity of local anesthetics. One important factor is the relative potency of the anesthetic. A number of studies have indicated that the seizure-producing potential of a local anesthetic is directly related to its anesthetic potency (78,79). The relationship between anesthetic potency and cardiovascular toxicity is less clear. Liu, et al, (80) using cumulative doses of lidocaine or bupivacaine in anesthetized and ventilated dogs, concluded that the cardiotoxicity was similar to the intrinsic potency of the drugs when hypotension and asystole were used as the endpoint. Since then, a number of other studies using a variety of animal models have demonstrated that bupivacaine has a greater potential for causing cardiac arrhythmias (81–85). In large or excessive doses, all local anesthetics have direct myocardial depressing properties. Typically, increasing local anesthetic plasma concentrations produce progressive conduction block with widened QRS complexes and eventually result in asystole. Bupivacaine, however, differs from other local anesthetics (such as lidocaine) in that it can induce cardiac tachyarrhythmias such as ventricular tachycardia and fibrillation. Research has been directed toward explaining these observations, but the answers are not conclusive. Clarkson and Hondegham (86) have postulated that differential binding properties of local anesthetic at the sodium channel may explain the greater dysrhythmia potential of bupivacaine. Other investigators have emphasized the potential role of the central nervous system in explaining the potential for bupivacaine, but not lidocaine, to induce cardiac dysrhythmias (87,88).

## Effects of Pregnancy

Many maternal deaths have been associated with the unintentional intravascular injection of local anesthetics during attempted epidural anesthesia in the obstetric patient (75). Part of the reason for this may be the greater epidural blood flow in the pregnant patient. Bromage (89) has postulated that this increased blood flow would result in a more rapid delivery of injected local anesthetic to the heart. Bupivacaine in particular has been associated with many of the maternal deaths from local anesthetic toxicity. Animal studies have shown that many factors may lower the cardiotoxic threshold for bupivacaine including, hyperkalemia (90), hypoxia and acidosis (91), as well as pregnancy itself (92). Morishima, et al (84) showed that the pregnant sheep is more sensitive to the cardiotoxic effects of bupivacaine than the nonpregnant sheep. This appears to be due to decreased plasma protein binding for bupivacaine in the pregnant animal as compared to the nonpregnant animal (92). In addition, it may be more difficult to resuscitate the pregnant patient than the nonpregnant patient because of partial occlusion of the inferior vena cava by the gravid uterus (93).

## Effects on the Mother

If local anesthetic blood levels increase relatively slowly such as in the case of an anesthetic overdose, rapid absorption, or slow elimination, a predictable series of signs and symptoms may be observed. The patient may first complain of numbness around the mouth, altered taste, tinnitus, and manifest excitement or confusion with slurred speech. The patient may then demonstrate muscular twitches and become unresponsive. This is quickly followed by generalized clonic seizure activity. Typically, seizures are brief although repeated, with interspersed periods of flaccidity. In the case of an accidental intravenous injection, there may be no warning signs, and the patient may immediately demonstrate seizure activity. If the patient has been given an anticonvulsant drug such as a benzodiazepine, barbiturate or a general anesthetic, seizure activity may never occur. The first signs of local anesthetic toxicity may be cardiovascular collapse. When ventilation is supported during experimental infusions of local anesthetics, the margin of safety between CNS toxicity and cardiovascular collapse is much wider than when ventilation is not supported. Moore, et al (94,95) have demonstrated profound acidosis and hypoxia within 30 seconds following the onset of local anesthetic induced convulsions in humans. This is thought to be due to impaired ventilation during seizure activity combined with the increased oxygen consumption and metabolic work associated with CNS and motor seizure activity. These metabolic changes greatly increase the cardiotoxicity of local anesthetics (91,96).

## Effects on Labor

Local anesthetics appear to have little direct effect on uterine activity at typical blood concentrations reached

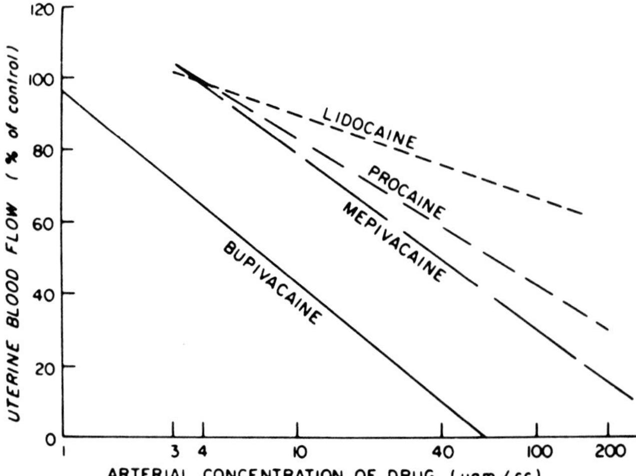


**Fig. 16–7.** Dose-response curves for four local anesthetics in nonpregnant ewes, illustrating the relationship between the arterial concentration of the drug and their effects in reducing uterine blood flow. (From Greiss FC Jr, Still JG, Anderson FG: Effects of local anesthetic agents on the uterine vasculature and myometrium. Am. J. Obstet. Gynecol. 124:889–899, 1976.)

with epidural anesthesia (54,97). However, at much higher concentrations that are reached during toxic reactions, direct effects of the local anesthetic may become apparent. At high blood concentrations, local anesthetics cause vasoconstriction and increased uterine tone resulting in decreased placental perfusion (Figure 16–7) (98). Unintentional intravenous injections of local anesthetic may result in tetanic uterine contractions and fetal bradycardia (Figure 16–8).

## Effects on the Fetus and Newborn

Fetal distress usually occurs rapidly in the face of overt maternal local anesthetic toxicity. There are a number of reasons for this. Maternal hypoxia and acidosis, which occur within seconds of a convulsion, rapidly result in fetal hypoxia and acidosis. Tetanic uterine contractions, which may result from the direct action of high local anesthetic blood concentrations, are poorly tolerated by the fetus because of impaired uterine and placental perfusion. Even if a convulsion is avoided and uterine perfusion is not adversely affected, high local anesthetic blood levels will be transferred to the fetus resulting in potential neonatal depression. Finally, neonatal depression may be made worse as a result of benzodiazepine or barbiturate therapy used to treat maternal convulsions.

## Prevention

Obviously, local anesthetic systemic toxic reactions are better avoided than treated. Since the editorial by Albright (74), the anesthesia community has become more aware of the potential problems with local anesthetic toxicity in general and bupivacaine cardiotoxicity in particular. Since 1983, the year that the Food and Drug Administration and the manufacturers of bupivacaine recommended

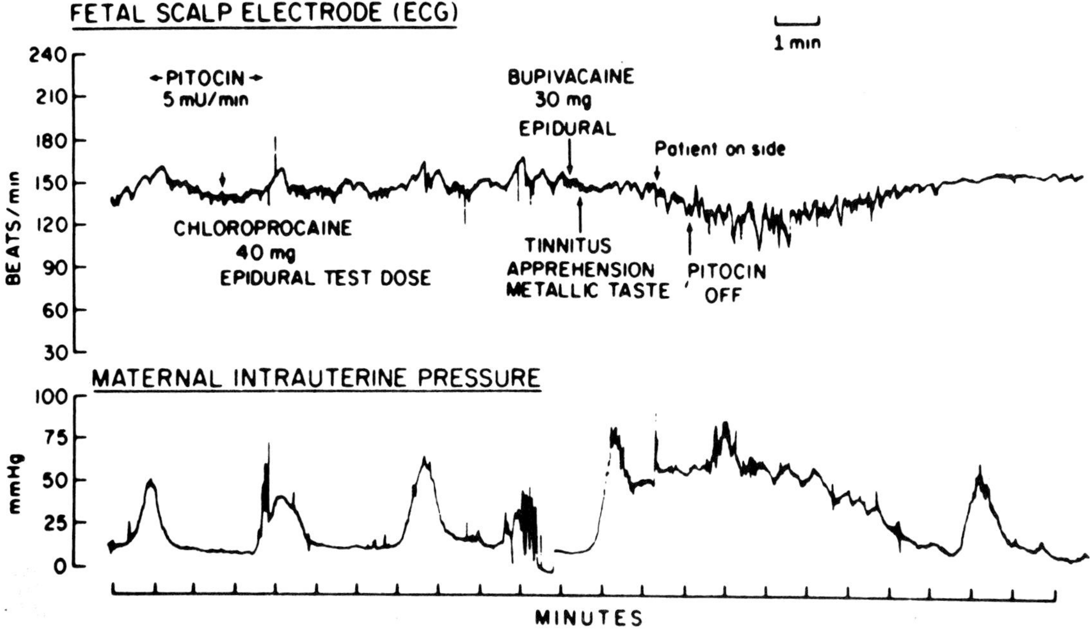


**Fig. 16–8.** Tetanic uterine contraction occurring after accidental intravenous injection of bupivacaine. Upper tracing shows fetal heart rate per minute, and indicates symptoms of mild toxicity following accidental injection of 30 ml of bupivacaine apparently into a vein. This caused disappearance of the uterine contraction curve and marked increase in uterine tone. (From Greiss FC Jr, Still JG, Anderson SG: Effects of local anesthetic agents on uterine vasculature and myometrium. Am. J. Obstet. Gynecol. 124: 889–899, 1976.)

that 0.75% bupivacaine should not be used in obstetrics because of cardiotoxic potential, there have been very few deaths associated with bupivacaine toxic reactions (Albright, personal communication, 1990). A number of steps can be taken to eliminate the risks of serious systemic toxic reactions to local anesthetics. At this point, it is appropriate to reemphasize points made in various chapters of this section of the book: no regional anesthetic procedure should be attempted without having a person to assist, and all equipment and drugs needed to treat various complications must be available for immediate use. Intravenous infusion should have been initiated and running with a large enough catheter to deliver fluids rapidly. Obstetric patients should be monitored with ECG and blood pressure cuff as one would any surgical patient in the operating room. Before initiating a regional anesthetic have all necessary resuscitation drugs and equipment at hand and ready for immediate use. We discourage the use of single dose epidurals injected through the epidural needle. Epidural catheters limit the rate at which anesthetic drugs can be injected and facilitate incremental injection of local anesthetics. We advocate the use of single end hole catheters to avoid the potential for some of the drug to be injected into an unintended area. A test dose should be used to rule out intravascular placement. Inject epidural local anesthetics in an incremental fashion, i.e., do not inject more than 5 ml of anesthetic solution at one time. Use the minimum effective dose and avoid exceeding the maximum recommended dose.

Before injecting local anesthetic, the catheter should be carefully aspirated; however, the inability to aspirate blood does not rule out intravascular placement. To minimize the chances of unintentional intravascular injection, an effective test dose should be used. In 1970, Bonica and associates (21) demonstrated that the intravenous injection of 15 to 20 μg of epinephrine produced a beta-adrenergic effect consisting of an increase in SV and HR with a consequent increase in CO that, together with the vasoconstriction, produced hypertension. On the basis of this, it is suggested that epinephrine together with a small amount of local anesthetic be injected as a test dose before injecting a full therapeutic dose of local anesthetic. Moore and Batra (99) carried out a much larger study that showed that 15 μg of epinephrine, when injected intravenously, resulted in a predictable increase in heart rate within 20 to 45 seconds. Since then, epinephrine has become the most commonly used marker for detecting intravenous injection. Data from the ASA Closed Claims Study shows that in none of the claims involving local anesthetic-induced convulsions was an epinephrine containing test dose documented (76,100).

Some have suggested that epinephrine, given intravenously, might have deleterious effects on uterine blood flow and fetal well-being (101,102). In addition, heart rate changes seen with intravenous epinephrine might be difficult to distinguish from the normal variation in maternal heart rate that may occur with uterine contractions (103,104). While these concerns may be valid, there are few case reports in the literature linking epinephrine test doses with adverse outcomes, while the advantages of the epinephrine test dose have been repeatedly documented (105). Hood and James (101) point out that the reduction in uterine blood flow caused by intravenous boluses of epinephrine were of the same magnitude and duration as those which occur with uterine contractions. Moreover, the concomitant use of 5 to 10 mg of bupivacaine or an equal anesthetic dose of another local anesthetic in the test dose is very useful to detect unintentional subarachnoid injection and consequently decrease the risk of total spinal anesthesia.

Epinephrine test doses should be used with caution, or perhaps not at all, in patients with uteroplacental insufficiency or in those who have a potential for an exaggerated response to intravenous epinephrine (e.g., PIH) (106). Some patients, e.g., those being treated with beta-blockers, may respond with hypertension and bradycardia (not tachycardia) when epinephrine is injected intravenously (107,108). Complications can be avoided by identifying these patients before an epinephrine test dose is administered. Recently, alternatives to the epinephrine test dose have been proposed, including: a bolus of plain local anesthetic solution (109,110), isoproterenol (111), or injecting a small volume of air and using a precordial Doppler for detection (112). However, more validation of these techniques is necessary before one can recommend replacing the epinephrine in local anesthetic solution as test dose. Regardless of the type of test dose chosen, there is no substitute for close observation of the patient by someone trained to detect adverse signs and symptoms of local anesthetic toxicity.

### Treatment

Early symptoms of local anesthetic toxicity should be treated with oxygen administration and preparation for intubation. The occurrence of local anesthetic induced convulsions constitutes an emergency condition and must result in immediate action. The patient must be ventilated with oxygen without delay; the trachea should be intubated to protect the airway from aspiration and to facilitate hyperventilation with 100% oxygen thereby counteracting respiratory and metabolic acidosis. Succinylcholine (80to100 mg) will facilitate intubation and stop the motor activity associated with convulsions thereby reducing metabolic work and the progression of acidosis. Conservative doses of a benzodiazepine or a barbiturate can be given to suppress CNS seizure activity; large doses, however, may further depress myocardial function. Animal studies have indicated that when ventilation is supported during experimental infusions of local anesthetics, the margin of safety between CNS toxicity and cardiovascular collapse is much wider than when ventilation is not supported.

Early and effective intervention may prevent the progression to cardiovascular collapse. If a nonperfusing cardiac rhythm has established itself, CPR must be initiated. Studies have shown that it is possible to resuscitate animals after massive bupivacaine infusions (82,113) and that it may not be more difficult to resuscitate animals following bupivacaine-induced, than it is following lidocaine-induced, cardiac arrest (82). It may, however, be much more difficult to resuscitate a pregnant patient than a nonpregnant patient because of impaired venous return to the heart due to partial occlusion of the inferior vena cava by the gravid uterus (93). For this reason, emergent delivery should be performed if resuscitation efforts are not quickly successful (114,115).

There is little information regarding the optimum resuscitation protocols for obstetric patients suffering cardiotoxic events due to local anesthetic. Animal studies would suggest that the most important factor is establishing effective circulation to redistribute the local anesthetic. Toxic blood levels of local anesthetic decline rapidly with effective CPR (82). General recommendations include facilitating blood return to the heart by elevating the legs, infusing fluids rapidly, and maintaining left uterine displacement during CPR. In some case reports resuscitation was not accomplished until after emergent delivery of the infant (114,115). Large doses of epinephrine and correction of acidosis may be required to establish adequate diastolic coronary perfusion pressure. Atropine and large doses of epinephrine may be particularly important in resuscitation from asystole. The optimum treatment of bupivacaine-induced arrhythmias may be different. Based on animal studies, some have recommended treating bupivacaine-induced tachyarrhythmias with lidocaine (116) or with bretylium (117); both drugs, however, may cause further hemodynamic depression. Resuscitation efforts should not be abandoned early and, if necessary, cardiopulmonary bypass should be considered (118).

## Other Systemic Reactions

### *Reaction to Vasoconstrictors*

Rapid uptake of epinephrine is a common cause of systemic reactions during or following regional anesthesia. The patient experiences palpitation, dyspnea, tachycardia, dizziness, perspiration, pallor, and tremor. Although these reactions simulate mild local anesthetic toxic reactions, epinephrine rarely causes convulsions or disorientation. Treatment consists of a small intravenous dose of a benzodiazapine or fast-acting barbiturate to allay apprehension. If hypertension is severe, an anti-hypertensive drug should be injected intravenously and titrated to control hypertension.

### Psychogenic Reactions

Some parturients who are scheduled for regional anesthesia and who have not been prepared psychologically by the anesthesiologist become apprehensive and fearful of the procedure per se. As a result, some develop dizziness, faintness, tinnitus, tachypnea, tachycardia, and pallor. This psychogenic reaction frequently occurs as soon as the procedure is started, and in some instances, even before the anesthetic is injected. Some of these patients develop hypotension, particularly if they are sitting, with consequent dizziness and faintness. In parturients with cardiac disease, the hypotensive episode may precipitate cardiac arrythmia. Treatment consists of reassurance, immediately placing the patient in a lateral recumbent position, administration of oxygen, and atropine, if necessary.

### *Allergic/Hypersensitive Reactions*

Not uncommonly, patients will be seen by an anesthesiologist claiming "allergy" to local anesthetics. Often this is based on some type of systemic reaction that the patient experienced during a dental procedure. Usually, these responses are due to psychogenically induced vasovagal episodes or due to subjective symptoms from intravenous injections of local anesthetic, often containing high concentrations of epinephrine. A detailed history should be taken to determine the probable cause of the reaction. Often the classic symptoms of allergic or anaphylactoid reaction will not be present. On the other hand, a history of urticaria, angioedema, bronchospasm or airway compromise must be taken seriously.

True allergic reactions to local anesthetics are rare. Most of the reported cases have involved amino ester local anesthetics such as procaine, chloroprocaine, and tetracaine (119). This is not surprising as these drugs are derivatives of para-aminobenzoic acid (PABA), which can act as a hapten and is known to be allergenic in nature. Allergic reactions to the amino amides such as lidocaine, bupivacaine, and mepivacaine are extremely rare but have been reported (120). Some cases of suspected amide local anesthetic allergy have been found to be a result of immunologic reaction to methylparaben, which is sometimes added to local anesthetics as a preservative. The structure of methylparaben is similar to PABA and can cause anaphylactic reactions. Cross-sensitivity does not occur with the two classes of local anesthetic agents. Consequently, if a patient is known to be sensitized to one class of local anesthetic it may be safe to administer a drug of the other class. Intradermal skin testing has been recommended to rule out hypersensitivity reactions (121). Skin testing, however, is associated with a number of problems. False positive reactions are very common, especially with ester local anesthetics. Patients who are truly allergic may develop anaphylactic reactions even from very small doses injected intradermally. For this reason, skin testing should only be carried out with full resuscitation equipment and drugs at hand.

## Cardiac Arrest

Cardiac arrest in the pregnant patient is without doubt the most dramatic and frightening complication that can occur in obstetric anesthesia. Cardiac arrest occurs when the heart ceases to function as an effective pump. This can be due to cardiac dysrhythmia, asystole, or electromechanical dissociation. The incidence of cardiac arrest in the parturient is not known. Some older reports suggested that it may have occurred once in every 8000 to 10,000 deliveries (122,123). More recent data from the Confidential Inquiries into Maternal Deaths in England and Wales estimate the incidence of cardiac arrest in late pregnancy at once in every 30,000 pregnancies (124,125). However, it has been suggested that advances in modern medicine and surgery have allowed more women with pre-existing serious medical conditions to become pregnant and thus has increased the likelihood of events that may require cardiopulmonary resuscitation (126).

**Table 16–2.** Predisposing Factors in Cardiac Arrest

| |
|---|
| Preexisting Conditions |
| Heart disease |
| anatomic disease, e.g., valvular disease |
| idiopathic dysrhythmias |
| myocardial infarction |
| cardiomyopathy |
| Cerebrovascular disease |
| Pulmonary disease, reactive airway disease |
| Hypertensive disease |
| Allergy |
| Other serious systemic diseases |
| Physiologic Changes Associated with Pregnancy |
| Hypercoagulation |
| Gastric reflux |
| Compression of the inferior vena cava and the aorta |
| Increased metabolic rate and oxygen consumption |
| Anemia |
| Obstetric Diseases and Complications |
| Preeclampsia |
| Hyperemesis |
| Hepatic necrosis |
| Disseminated Intravascular Coagulation |

### *Etiology*

Cardiac arrest can occur in the pregnant woman with or without obvious predisposing risk factors. Some of the normal physiological changes associated with pregnancy may increase the risk of cardiopulmonary arrest. In addition to the pregnant state itself, a variety of pathologic conditions and complications of pregnancy may further increase the risk to the parturient. These risks can be compounded by a variety of pre-existing medical conditions that the patient may have. Some predisposing risk factors are listed in Table 16–2. Cardiac arrest is usually preceded by an identifiable event that leads to the cardiac arrest. A number of such events are outlined in Table 16–3.

**Table 16–3.** Causes of Cardiac Arrest

| |
|---|
| Accidental |
| Drowning |
| Electrocution, lightning |
| Trauma |
| Obstetric and Medical Complications |
| Paradoxical embolism to brain or coronary circulation |
| thromboembolism |
| amniotic fluid embolism |
| air embolism |
| Intracranial hemorrhage |
| Massive hemorrhage |
| Myocardial infarction |
| Septic shock |
| Anesthetic Interventions |
| Hypoxia due to inability to secure airway, aspiration |
| Spinal shock |
| Anesthetic overdose |
| Systemic local anesthetic toxicity |
| Respiratory insufficiency |
| Drug Induced |
| Magnesium toxicity |
| Anaphylactoid, anaphylactic reactions |
| Miscellaneous |
| Reflex induced, e.g., mesentery traction, intubation, laryngospasm |

## Prevention

Although it is not always possible to prevent cardiac arrest in the obstetric patient, careful planning, good judgment, and technical expertise can prevent many of the causes of cardiac arrest. This is facilitated by a cooperative, coordinated effort on the part of all members of the obstetric team. Special emphasis should be given to the following issues:

1. Evaluation of the history and physiologic status of the parturient. Particular attention should be given to pre-existing medical conditions, including allergy to drugs, cardiac and pulmonary disease, and history of problems with prior pregnancies and anesthetics. Current obstetrical problems should be evaluated, including any history of bleeding, signs of preeclampsia, and labor pattern. Medications that the patient has been taking, recreational drug use, and recent oral intake should be reviewed. Available laboratory data should be checked and the need for additional laboratory studies ascertained. Physical examination must be guided by the history but a careful airway examination and cardiac and chest auscultation should always be performed before any anesthetic intervention.
2. The optimum analgesic or anesthetic plan should be chosen for each patient. This will be guided by the physical status and obstetric requirements of the patient, as well as the experience of the anesthesiologist.
3. Constant vigilance. ECG monitoring and frequent blood pressure monitoring should be employed for patients having regional anesthesia for labor analgesia, as well as for patients undergoing surgical procedures. Patients having operative deliveries should also be monitored with pulse oximetry and with capnography if a general anesthetic is employed.
4. It deserves re-emphasis that resuscitation equipment must be immediately available to treat any complication including cardiac arrest. Resuscitation drugs and airway equipment must be in the room when starting any regional anesthetic or general anesthetic. A "code cart" with defibrillator should be available on every labor and delivery unit.

## Treatment

Cardiopulmonary resuscitation (CPR) must be initiated immediately once the diagnosis of cardiac arrest has been made. The American Heart Association has developed algorithms to guide the physician in both basic life support and advanced cardiac life support (ACLS) techniques. These guidelines and algorithms are reviewed and revised periodically to incorporate advances in medical science. All physicians should be familiar with the current ACLS recommendations.

The current life support recommendations for pregnant women are similar to those for any adult patient and emphasize the ABC approach to resuscitation, i.e., airway, breathing, and circulation. Table 16–4 outlines basic CPR guidelines for pregnant women. For effective CPR, it is important that the patient be placed supine on a hard, flat surface. In this position, however, the gravid uterus may completely occlude the inferior vena cava. The adverse effect of partial occlusion of the inferior vena cava on CPR has been demonstrated in animal studies (93). Tilting the patient to the side improves venous return but makes effective cardiac compression more difficult. For this reason, CPR in late pregnancy must involve some degree of compromise in patient positioning. Recent studies indicate that effective compression forces can be generated with appropriate training when the patient is inclined laterally at angles of 30° or less (127). Advanced therapeutic interventions such as electrical and pharmacologic therapy must be guided by examination of the patient and electrocardiography. A discussion of the relevant ACLS protocols for various cardiac arrest conditions is beyond the scope of this text. For current standards and guidelines, the reader is encouraged to consult appropriate publications (128).

**Table 16–4.** Basic Life Support for Pregnant Women

Airway
- Determine unresponsiveness
- Call for help
- Position patient on firm flat surface
- Displace uterus to the left either manually or with wedge
- Open the airway with head-tilt and chin-lift or jaw-thrust maneuver

Breathing
- Look, listen and feel for air movement
- If breathing is absent, deliver two slow breaths (1.5 to 2.0 seconds each)

Circulation
- Feel for presence of carotid pulse
- If pulse is absent, begin external chest compression at a rate of 80 to 100 per minute
- Alternate 15 chest compressions with two slow breaths
- Reassess patient after four complete cycles
- If breathing and pulse are absent, continue CPR

Two-Rescuer CPR
- Same as above, except five compressions are followed by a pause to allow delivery of one slow breath

(Based on the recommendations of the American Heart Association Emergency Cardiac Care Committee and Subcommittees: Guidelines for cardiopulmonary resuscitation and emergency cardiac care, 1992.)

Some authors have recommended considering fetal status and viability when making resuscitation decisions in pregnant women (126,129). Before fetal viability (approximately the twenty-fourth week of gestation) all efforts should be directed toward saving the mother's life. The fetus may be able to tolerate the stresses of maternal cardiac arrest and full CPR without ill effect. Complete recovery of mother and fetus has been documented after 22 minutes of CPR following massive lidocaine overdose in a pregnant women at 15 weeks gestation (130). Resuscitation included epinephrine and electrical defibrillation. The patient went on to deliver a healthy neurologically normal infant at 40 weeks gestation.

It has been suggested that because many ACLS interventions may be harmful to the fetus, such interventions should be carefully considered or not used at all in pregnancies with a potentially viable fetus (129). Cardioversion or defibrillation can potentially result in fetal fibrillation, although this seems to be a very remote concern (131,132). Lidocaine and most other antiarrhythmic drugs cross the placenta and can potentially have adverse effects. However, when used in standard doses, there appears to be little adverse effect on the fetus from lidocaine and many other antiarrhythmic drugs (133). Epinephrine and other vasopressors with potent alpha-adrenergic activity cause uterine vasoconstriction. Administration of these drugs can result in severe fetal distress. It is our opinion, however, that, except in very unusual circumstances, all necessary resuscitative interventions should be made available to the mother even if fetal well-being may be compromised.

Although some have advocated attempting to assess fetal well-being during maternal CPR using external Doppler monitoring or real-time ultrasound (in an effort to guide decision making) (126,129), we feel that such efforts are misdirected and interfere with the primary objective, which is to resuscitate the mother. If CPR is not effective in generating a palpable pulse or adequate perfusion pressure or if resuscitation is not successful in 5 minutes, then emergent surgical delivery of the fetus should be considered while CPR is continued. The primary purpose of delivery is to improve blood return to the heart and facilitate resuscitation. Numerous cases have been reported in which resuscitation of the mother was not accomplished until after delivery of the fetus (114,115,134,135). An added benefit of early delivery is the possibility of salvaging a viable infant. Prolonged CPR may only worsen the prognosis of a good outcome for both mother and infant. Delivery should not be delayed even if the infant is known to be dead (134). In most cases, open-chest cardiac compression should only be considered after delivery of the fetus because delivery may result in rapid resuscitation and because the complications associated with emergency cesarean delivery will likely be less severe than those associated with emergency open-chest CPR.

Even a successful resuscitation may result in significant maternal and fetal problems. Potential maternal complications include brain injury, a variety of cardiopulmonary complications, laceration of the liver, uterine rupture, and preterm labor. Fetal complications can include CNS depression from antiarrhythmic drugs, intrauterine fetal demise due to inadequate uteroplacental perfusion or cardiac arrest from maternal defibrillation attempts. If the fetus is delivered during resuscitation attempts, problems associated with prematurity, hypoxia, and acidosis are likely to necessitate intensive neonatal resuscitation. In such circumstances, a neonatologist is an invaluable member of the resuscitation team.

## Neurologic Complications

### *Unduly High Segmental Blockade*

#### *Etiology*

Higher-than-anticipated block can be a complication of spinal or epidural anesthesia. Following spinal anesthesia, it may be due either to abnormal spread of the therapeutic dose or to injection of an excessive dose. With epidural anesthesia, the cause is excessive dose or unintentional subdural or subarachnoid injection of the local anesthetic. The most common complication associated with high block is hypotension. In the case of "total spinal anesthesia" loss of consciousness, respiratory insufficiency, and cardiovascular collapse can occur.

There is controversy regarding local anesthetic requirement of pregnant patients having epidural or spinal anesthesia (136). It is generally believed that the epidural and subarachnoid dose requirements of the parturient are approximately one-third those of nonpregnant women (137–139). In the case of epidural blocks, this may be due to wider spread of anesthetic solution because of epidural venous engorgement. Similarly, spinal cerebrospinal fluid (CSF) volume may be reduced, resulting in greater spread of anesthetic solution administered into the lumbar subarachnoid space. Recently, a number of studies have indicated that peripheral neuronal tissue in gravid animals (140) and humans (141) may be more sensitive to the effects of local anesthetics. Although there exists some controversy about the local anesthetic requirements for pregnant patients, it is evident from clinical experience that there can be great variability in the extent of blockade achieved with usual doses of a local anesthetic in parturients. Numerous factors influence the distribution of local anesthetics within the subarachnoid and epidural spaces (142,143). Even appropriate doses of local anesthetic can result in abnormally high blocks if hyperbaric anesthetic solutions are injected with the patient in Trendelenberg position.

### Unintentional Subdural Block

The subdural space is a potential space between the dura and the arachnoid membranes. A number of reports have confirmed the unintentional catheterization of this potential space, as well as delayed subdural migration of an epidural catheter (144–147). Subdural injection as a complication of epidural block had been estimated to occur with a frequency of 0.82% (148). Typically, the onset of block is more similar to epidural anesthesia than to spinal anesthesia, and for this reason typical test doses to rule out subarachnoid block may not detect a subdural injection (145). The extent of block produced from a given volume of local anesthetic is, however, usually much greater with subdural injection. It is not uncommon to have spread of block to the cervical level with 6 to 10 ml of local anesthetic solution (145,146). When small volumes of water-soluble contrast media are injected into the subdural space, they rapidly spread over a large number of segments, usually in a cephalad direction. Subdural blocks may be patchy or asymmetric (146). The subdural administration of morphine was reported in the management of a patient with cancer pain (149). The authors noted a significantly reduced dose requirement compared to that required by the epidural route, suggesting the potential for respiratory depression with unintentional subdural morphine administration. In a recent in vivo study, investigators found that the arachnoid is the primary diffusion barrier for opioids traversing the meninges (150). This would suggest that optimum subdural opioid doses may be similar to epidural dose requirements. However, because of the potential for serious respiratory depression, we recommend extreme caution when faced with uncertainty regarding catheter location (150A).

## Unintentional Subarachnoid Block

Unintentional dural puncture during epidural placement is a relatively common complication with a reported frequency of 1.6 to 2.9%; (144) however, the frequency can vary widely depending on the skill and experience of the practitioner. It is usually recognized at the time of occurrence and has a high likelihood of resulting in subsequent postdural-puncture headache (PDPH). Unrecognized injection of local anesthetic into the subarachnoid space either through an epidural needle or catheter is a much less common, although a potentially fatal complication if improperly managed. If large volumes of local anesthetic are injected, the result is sudden and massive spinal blockade (total spinal) characterized by severe hypotension, loss of consciousness and apnea.

### *Pathophysiology*

The most common complication associated with high block is hypotension. The hypotension can be sudden in the case of extensive subarachnoid block or can occur more slowly as in the case of subdural or extensive epidural block. If hypotension is severe, loss of consciousness will occur due to CNS ischemia. Accompanying the loss of consciousness is the loss of protective airway reflexes. Nausea and vomiting are commonly associated with hypotension and in the presence of depressed airway reflexes may lead to pulmonary aspiration of gastric contents. If subarachnoid block extends into the cervical segments, respiratory insufficiency can occur from intercostal and diaphragmatic paralysis. However, it is unlikely that the concentration of local anesthetic in the cervical region is sufficient to block completely the large motor fibers of the phrenic nerve. In such cases, it is more likely that apnea results from hypotension and consequent medullary ischemia (3).

### Prevention

It deserves reemphasis that before initiating any regional procedure, all necessary equipment for proper airway management and resuscitation be available for immediate use. This means that an intravenous infusion and appropriate monitors (e.g., ECG and blood pressure measuring devices) should be in place and shown to be working before starting the procedure. Supplemental oxygen administration is encouraged. Proper patient positioning is important for any regional anesthetic procedure. For subarachnoid anesthesia using hypo- or hyperbaric solutions, proper positioning is critical. It behooves the practitioner to be aware of potentially decreased anesthetic requirements in the pregnant patient and to take a conservative approach with dosing. Identify and double check the drug and amount to be injected. Maintain continuous verbal contact with the patient. This will aid in prompt diagnosis of ascending paralysis and in detecting signs of cerebral circulatory insufficiency. Frequently check vital signs and progression of block, especially during the first 20 minutes.

For epidural anesthesia, it is important to use an appropriate test dose (e.g., 30 to 60 mg lidocaine or 5 to 10 mg bupivacaine) to rule out subarachnoid needle or catheter placement. At least 3 to 5 min should elapse for a subarachnoid injection to manifest itself. We discourage the use of single-shot techniques and advocate incremental injection of local anesthetic through an appropriately placed catheter. The epidural block should be initiated slowly with incremental doses (e.g., 5 ml) of local anesthetic solution. It is advisable to stop and wait approximately 10 minutes after the first 5 to 10 ml of local anesthetic has been injected. In the event of a subdural injection, a much greater spread of local anesthetic will become apparent and the potential complications of additional anesthetic injection will be avoided (150A).

### *Treatment*

The treatment for high segmental block will depend on the extent to which problems associated with this complication manifest themselves. The priorities are to ensure adequate ventilation, protect the airway, and to maintain adequate perfusion pressure. In the event of a high epidural or subdural block, the onset may be relatively slow and extent of the block may be such that careful observation, fluid administration, and reassurance are all that is required. Motor strength in the upper extremities must be checked frequently to assess progression of the block.

The sudden onset of a "total spinal" constitutes an anesthetic emergency. To avoid catastrophic consequences, the airway must be immediately secured and effective ventilation established. Blood return to the heart must be facilitated by lateral uterine displacement, placing the patient in the 5° head down position and raising the lower limbs, and rapid intravenous fluid administration. Under no circumstances should the patient be placed in a head up position in an effort to stop further upward spread of the block (1,3). Vasopressors should be used as required to restore adequate perfusion pressure. In the event of cardiovascular collapse, cardiopulmonary resuscitation must be immediately initiated as outlined above. If the "total spinal" was due to the injection of a large volume of local anesthetic into the subarachnoid space, one should consider draining cerebrospinal fluid to decrease elevated subarachnoid pressure with the associated risk of spinal cord ischemia and to minimize potential neurotoxic effects from high concentration of local anesthetic (1,151).

## ***Headaches***

Headache is a common complaint in parturients. Although headaches are often attributed to anesthesia, especially if a regional anesthetic was employed, there are many causes of headaches in the peripartum period (152). Well recognized headache syndromes (e.g., migraine, cluster headaches, and tension headaches) are often modified by pregnancy and may be exacerbated in the early

**Table 16–5.** Differential Diagnosis for Headache in the Parturient

| | |
|---|---|
| Acute migraine | Cortical vein thrombosis |
| Cluster headache | Pseudotumor cerebri |
| Tension (psychogenic headache) | Tumor |
| Chronic paroxysmal hemicrania | Preeclampsia/eclampsia |
| Meningitis | Subarachnoid hemorrhage |

(Taken from: Chadwick HS, Ross BK: Causes and consequences of maternal-fetal perianesthetic complications. In Anesthesia and Perioperative Complications. Edited by JL Benumof, LJ Saidman. St. Louis, Mosby Yearbook, p. 533, 1992)

postpartum period. The syndrome of postpartum headache occurs in 30 to 40% of women by the end of the first postpartum week (153,154). The etiology of these headaches is not known although they are most common in women with a prior history or family history of migraine (83%) (153). Table 16–5 lists some potential causes of headaches in pregnancy (155). The most common cause of an anesthetic-induced headache is postdural-puncture headache (PDPH). Other potential causes may include meningeal irritation or infection.

### *Postdural-puncture Headache*

In the first report on spinal anesthesia published by Bier in 1899, prominent reference was made to the occurrence of headache following the procedure (156). Although nearly a century has passed, headache remains one of the most common complications of spinal anesthesia, especially in obstetric patients. The incidence of PDPH varies greatly depending on the criteria used for diagnosis, the patient population studied, and the technique used for dural puncture. Table 16–6 summarizes data from a variety of older studies (152). More recent studies, however, report higher frequencies even when small gauge needles were used (157,158). Our own data indicate an incidence of about 10% using 25- or 26-gauge Quincke tip needles in obstetric patients (159). When a headache occurs after spinal or epidural anesthesia, it must be considered a potentially serious complication and must be differentiated from other causes of headache in the perinatal period. A study of malpractice claims filed against anesthesiologists providing obstetric anesthesia care found that 12% of the claims were due to headache. This was the third most common injury for which a claim was brought. The only injuries for which more claims were filed were maternal death and newborn brain injury (Table 16–7) (76).

**Table 16–6.** Influence of Size and Bevel of Needle on Incidence of Postpuncture Headache

| Author | Needle | Incidence (%) |
|---|---|---|
| Arner | 24 gauge | 3.2 |
| | 22 gauge | 5.4 |
| Greene | 20 gauge | 41 |
| | 22 gauge | 26 |
| | 24 gauge | 8 |
| | 26 gauge | 0.4 |
| Harris and Harmel | 18 gauge and larger | 24 |
| | 20 gauge | 8 |
| | 24 gauge | 3.5 |
| Krueger | 20-gauge regular bevel | 22 |
| | 20-gauge "pencil" point | 7 |
| Hart and Whitacre | 20-gauge regular bevel | 5 |
| | 20-gauge "pencil" point | 2 |
| Ebner | 25 gauge | 1.0 |
| Phillips et al | 25 gauge | 0.9 |
| Myers and Rosenberg | 20 gauge | 0.33 |
| Tarrow | 25 or 26 gauge | 0.2 |

(From Bonica JJ: Principles and Practice of Obstetric Analgesia and Anesthesia. 1st Ed. Philadelphia, F. A. Davis, 1967.)

### *Etiology and Pathophysiology*

Bier (156) in 1899 first suggested that the headache may be caused by leakage of cerebrospinal fluid through the hole created in the dura. This is still considered to be the primary cause of PDPH. The most convincing evidence is that provided by the experimental studies of Kunkle, Ray, Wolff and their associates (160). In these studies, the acute removal of CSF in upright patients resulted in headache, and when the fluid was reinjected the headache was promptly relieved. Two mechanisms have been proposed to explain the origin of the painful stimulus. If the fluid leak rate is greater than the CSF formation rate, CSF volume will be less than normal. When the patient assumes an erect position, the brain will tend to shift in a caudad direction thereby placing traction on blood vessels and other innervated structures that anchor the brain to the cranium. Pain pathways for the headache include the trigeminal nerve for stimuli originating above the tentorium and the glossopharyngeal, vagus, and upper cervical nerves for stimuli originating below the tentorum. Another theory of mechanism proposes that as CSF volume is decreased, the cerebral blood volume increases proportionately. This results in abnormally dilated cerebral blood vessels, which may be the source of the painful stimulus.

PDPH is characterized as a mild, moderate, or severe discomfort that is dull, aching, or throbbing in nature. It is typically described as being frontal, occipital, or diffuse in location. Frequently, the headache is associated with moderate pain and stiffness of the neck that may radiate inferiorly along the trapezius ridge to the shoulders and down between the scapulae. Other symptoms that may be elicited are photophobia, nausea and vomiting, and visual disturbances. On rare occasions, the headache is associated with cranial nerve dysfunction, resulting in diplopia. PDPH usually occurs 1 to 5 days after dural puncture and characteristically persists for 3 to 5 days. On rare occasion, the headache lasts for months (161,162). The most important characteristic of the headache is that it occurs or is aggravated by sitting or standing and resolves or is improved when the patient lies down. Table 16–8 lists those clinical features found to be most useful in differentiating PDPH from typical postpartum headache syndrome (153,163).

Persistent or atypical headaches following lumbar

**Table 16–7.** Most Common Injuries in the Obstetric Anesthesia Claims

| | Non-OB Claims (n = 1351) | OB Claims (n = 190) | OB Regional (n = 124) | OB General (n = 62) |
|---|---|---|---|---|
| Patient/maternal death | 39% (524)* | 22% (41) | 12% (15)* | 42% (26) |
| Newborn brain damage | NA | 20% (38) | 19% (23) | 24% (15) |
| Headache | 1% (10)* | 12% (23) | 19% (23)* | 0% (0) |
| Newborn death | <0.5% (1)* | 9% (17) | 7% (8) | 10% (6) |
| Pain during anesthesia | <0.5% (5)* | 8% (16) | 13% (16)* | 0% (0) |
| Patient/maternal nerve damage | 16% (209)* | 8% (16) | 10% (12) | 7% (4) |
| Patient/maternal brain damage | 13% (174)* | 7% (14) | 7% (9) | 8% (5) |
| Emotional distress | 2% (30) | 6% (12) | 7% (9) | 5% (3) |
| Back pain | 1% (8) | 5% (9) | 7% (9)* | 0% (0) |

*$p \leq 0.01$

The most common injuries for which claims were made in obstetric anesthesia are shown in order of decreasing frequency. Percentages are based on the total claims in each group. Some claims had more than one injury and are represented more than once. Cases involving brain damage only include patients who were alive when the claim was closed. Statistical comparisons are made between OB and non-OB claims and between OB regional and OB general anesthetics. (Table from: Chadwick HS, et al.: A comparison of obstetric- and non-obstetric anesthesia malpractice claims. Anesthesiology 74:242–249, 1991.)

punctures should be carefully evaluated. Low cerebrospinal fluid pressure associated with PDPH may be responsible for some intracranial pathologic events or may lead to the diagnosis of unrelated conditions. The incidence of spontaneous subarachnoid hemorrhage is five times higher during pregnancy than it is in nonpregnant women (164). Most of these hemorrhages are due to rupture of cerebrovascular aneurysms or arteriovenous malformations. However, dural punctures for diagnostic or anesthetic purposes have been implicated in causing intracranial subdural and subarachnoid hematoma. Three cases of intracranial bleeding have been reported in parturients following accidental dural puncture during attempted epidural anesthesia (165). Sometimes, the evaluation of a headache following spinal anesthesia leads to the diagnosis of a condition unrelated to the anesthetic. In our own practice, we have seen two women with persistent headache following obstetric regional anesthesia who were eventually diagnosed as having pseudotumor cerebri. Others have reported diagnoses of a true intracranial tumor in the course of evaluating a parturient with postspinal headache and abducens nerve palsy (166).

**Table 16–8.** Clinical Features of Postdural Puncture and Postpartum Headache

| Postdural-Puncture Headache: | Postpartum Headache: |
|---|---|
| Onset: within first 5 days following dural puncture (90% within 3 days) | Onset: between 3 to 6 days postpartum |
| Duration: usually 3 to 5 days, seldom longer than 1 week | Duration: may last 12 hours |
| Characteristics: | Characteristics: |
| 50% frontal | primary bi-frontal |
| 25% occipital | |
| 25% diffuse | |
| severity dependent upon patient position | patient position unimportant |
| throbbing in nature | continuous in nature |
| Associated Symptoms: | Associated Symptoms: |
| blurred and/or double vision | vision rarely affected |
| photophobia | mild photophobia |
| dizziness, tinnitus, decreased hearing | no auditory component |
| nausea and vomiting | mild nausea and vomiting |
| unresponsive to minor analgesics | responds to minor analgesics |
| | previous family history common |

(Modified from: Chadwick HS, Ross, BK: Causes and consequences of maternal-fetal perianesthetic complications. *In* Anesthesia and Perioperative Complications. Edited by Benumof JL, Saidman LJ. St. Louis, Mosby Year Book, p 533, 1992.)

### *Prevention*

The problem of PDPH is better avoided than treated. Anesthesiologists should be familiar with the factors that have been associated with the development of PDPH. The size of the needle used for dural puncture determines the size of the dural rent and consequently the CSF leak rate. Although the incidence of PDPH varies widely in various studies, the greater incidence of headache with larger gauge needles is a consistent observation (Table 16–6). The orientation of the needle bevel to the dural fibers has also been shown to be important in determining the incidence of headache. Greene (167) in 1926 postulated that inserting the bevel parallel to the dural fibers would separate rather than cut the fibers. Laboratory and clinical studies have confirmed a lower leak rate (168) and lower incidence of headache (169) when the needle bevel is inserted parallel to the long axis of the body. The angle at which a needle punctures the dura has been shown to be an important factor in determining incidence of headache. Hatfalvi (170), in a series of over 600 spinal anesthetics using a lateral approach, reported no cases of PDPH. He attributed this to reduced CSF leakage as a result of tangential puncture of the dura. The lower CSF leakage rate was confirmed by Ready, et al using an in vitro model (168).

Needle tip design has long been thought to influence the incidence of PDPH. Greene (167) and Hart and Whita-

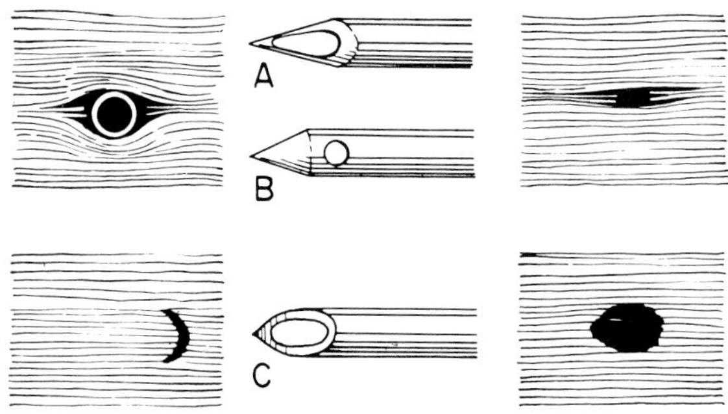


**Fig. 16–9.** The type of postpuncture hole in the dura produced by different types of spinal needles. Greene **(A)** and Whitacre **(B)** needles separate rather than cut longitudinal fibers of the dura mater. When the needle is removed, fibers tend to approximate and only a small hole remains. When the Pitkin, or regular spinal needle **(C)**, is inserted with the bevel of the needle at right angles to the longitudinal fibers of the dura, it produces a crescent-shaped cut involving many longitudinal fibers. When the needle is removed, a large hole remains through which cerebrospinal fluid leaks out of the subarachnoid space. The size of the hole can be decreased by inserting the needle with its bevel parallel to the longitudinal fibers of the dura mater. (From Moore DC: Complications of Regional Anesthesia. Charles C. Thomas Publisher, Springfield IL., 1955.)

cre (171) each developed noncutting tipped needles to separate instead of cut dural fibers (Figure 16–9). Such needles have been shown to reduce the incidence of PDPH (Table 16–6). Recently, disposable small gauge conical tipped needles have become available. We have found a significantly reduced incidence of PDPH in obstetric patients using 24-gauge Sprotte (modified Whitacre) needles compared to conventional 25- or 26-gauge Quincke tip needles (159). Other factors associated with PDPH include: gender, higher incidence in females; age, higher incidence in younger patients; number of dural punctures, higher incidence with increased number of punctures; and history of prior PDPH, higher incidence in patients with a previous history of PDPH (172). The obstetric patient is at particular risk of developing PDPH because these patients are young, female, and many will experience a period of bearing down that may increase the headache incidence (173). This latter finding, however, has not been observed by others (174).

### *Treatment*

Because PDPH usually resolves spontaneously within 1 week, initial treatment can be conservative, consisting of patient education, reassurance, and oral analgesics (e.g., acetaminophen, codeine). However, one must remember that the headache can be incapacitating and significantly impair mother-infant bonding and the parturient's ability to care for her newborn. Bed rest is advisable because of the postural nature of the symptoms, but does not reduce the incidence of headache (175,176). Prolonged bed rest may actually be contraindicated in the postpartum period because of the risk of deep venous thrombosis. In an effort to foster CSF production, fluid intake should be encouraged. This is important because many parturients may be dehydrated in the postpartum period. Tight abdominal binders have been recommended (177) but are often uncomfortable and impractical. Epidural saline, either by bolus injection or preferably by continuous infusion (e.g., 20 ml/hr for 24 hrs) has been shown, in some studies, to be effective in controlling the symptoms of PDPH (173,178,179).

Recently, the use of caffeine has regained popularity in managing PDPH. The cerebral vasoconstrictor activity of caffeine is thought to be responsible for the relief of symptoms, which are seen in about 80% of patients (180). Caffeine therapy has been shown to be an effective and inexpensive treatment both in intravenous and oral forms (181–183). A typical treatment regimen consists of 500 mg of caffeine sodium benzoate given over 4 hours by intravenous infusion or 300 mg caffeine given orally. One disadvantage of caffeine treatment is that it may result in only temporary relief of symptoms.

The most effective treatment of PDPH is to stop the leakage of CSF with the injection of autologous blood into the epidural space, "the epidural blood patch." The description of the epidural blood patch technique for the treatment of PDPH by DiGiovanni and Dunbar in 1970 (184) was a boon to both patients and anesthesiologists. Epidural blood patch has been shown to be efficacious in 95 to 100% of patients (185,186). Much has been written regarding the optimum volume of blood to use (186–188), the spinal level at which the blood should be injected (189), and the optimal timing of the procedure following dural puncture. In one study, epidural blood patch within 24 hours had a failure rate of 71% compared to 4% if performed after 24 hours (188). However, in another study, prophylactic epidural blood patch was effective at preventing a significant number of PDPH (190). Epidural blood patch has been shown to be effective months after dural puncture (191). Current practice at many institutions is to perform an epidural blood patch 24 to 48 hours after the onset of moderate or severe headache symptoms. Typically, 10 to 15 ml of fresh, aseptically drawn, autologous blood is slowly injected into the epidural space near the level of the original dural puncture. If the patient complains of paresthesia or of pain between the scapulae, the injection is stopped.

Because epidural blood patches are simple, effective, and relatively free of serious complications, there is little reason to delay treatment, particularly when headache is severe. However, the injection of blood into the epidural space is commonly associated with backache and mild signs of meningeal irritation. Potential complications, although very rare, include epidural infection, and nerve root compression. The unintentional injection of blood into the subarachnoid space may result in adhesive arachnoiditis.

## *Neurologic Sequelae of Pregnancy and Regional Anesthesia*

Some of these are causally related to the anesthetic while others are coincident with, but unrelated to, the anesthetic. These complications may involve the cranial nerves, the spinal cord and spinal nerves, as well as surrounding structures. Because the mechanisms of injury vary considerably, each is considered separately.

### Cranial Nerve Palsies

A variety of cranial nerve palsies have been associated with pregnancy but by far the most common is idiopathic facial paralysis or Bell's palsy. The incidence of this condition is 17 per 100,000 per year in women of all ages. The incidence during pregnancy and the first 2 postpartum weeks is 57 per 100,000 per exposure year (192). Bell's palsy is caused by an inflammation or compression of the facial (VII) nerve along its course, usually in the temporal bone. It is typically unilateral and results in facial weakness or complete paralysis; if the lesion is proximal to the branching of the chorda tympani, taste is lost in the anterior two-thirds of the tongue. Prognosis for recovery is good if paralysis is partial. The prognosis is less favorable if taste is lost or if the paralysis is complete. Neuropathies of other cranial nerves such as the trigeminal, trochlear, oculomotor, abducens, and optic nerve have been reported in pregnancy but are very rare and usually mild (192).

Cranial nerve dysfunction is a recognized but uncommon complication following spinal anesthesia. The incidence of this complication cited in the literature varies considerably. Thorsen (193) collected from the literature a total of 173 cases in a series of 68,179 spinal anesthetics reported between 1906 and 1947, and included seven cases communicated by colleagues from different Swedish hospitals. Virtually all of these data were obtained from questionnaires without follow-up examinations. Subsequently, Arner (194), using close follow-up in the immediate and long term postoperative period, noted no cases of cranial nerve palsies among 21,230 spinal anesthetics carried out during the period 1940–1950 in the Department of Anesthesiology at the Karolinska Sjukhuset in Stockholm. In the United States, Nicholson and Eversole (195) and Greene (196) also reported no cranial nerve palsies in a combined total of nearly 30,000 spinal anesthetics. Vandam and Dripps (197) reported six cases of abducens nerve palsy in a series of 9277 spinal anesthetics, all of which occurred following the use of 16-gauge needles for continuous spinal anesthesia. Paresis of the abducens (VI) nerve has been reported most frequently. Involvement of the oculomotor (III), trochlear (IV), facial (VII), auditory (VIII), and trigeminal (V) nerves has been less frequently linked to spinal anesthesia (198). The relatively high incidence of cranial nerve palsies that were reported in some studies published before 1950 probably relates to the large gauge spinal needles that were often used at that time. Cranial nerve dysfunction is very rarely seen as a complication of obstetric regional anesthesia today.

### Etiology and Pathophysiology

Almost all cases of cranial nerve dysfunction following spinal anesthesia have been associated with postdural-puncture headache (PDPH). The cause of the neuropathy is thought to be due to the same mechanism that is responsible for the headache, i.e., low CSF volume. The brain is normally suspended in CSF with the only fixed connections to the cranium being bridging vessels and cranial nerves. The falx and tentorum further help to stabilize the brain. When CSF is lost at a faster rate than it is produced, e.g., through a puncture in the dura, then the brain is thought to sag, especially when the patient is upright, thereby placing tension on the bridging vessels and cranial nerves. The abducens nerve is particularly vulnerable because of its relatively long extracerebral course and anatomic position. It emerges near the ventral midline at the junction of the pons and medulla oblongata, then passes superior to the anterior inferior cerebellar artery traveling upward, where it makes a sharp turn over the petrus temporal bone. When the brain is displaced downward, the abducens nerve becomes stretched over the petrus temporal ridge.

The trochlear nerve is vulnerable because it is the most slender cranial nerve with the longest intracranial course. Nerve palsy is usually unilateral and is preceded by headache. It may last from days to months. Symptomatology varies depending on which nerve is effected. When any of the nerves involving extraocular muscle function are involved, the most common symptom is diplopia. Numbness of the face can result from involvement of the trigeminal nerve (198). Hearing disturbances such as tinnitus, dizziness, and perhaps nausea and vomiting may indicate auditory nerve involvement or perhaps effects on the cochlea, which has a direct connection with the CSF. Cranial nerve symptoms are often orthostatic in nature and are improved when the patient is recumbent.

### Prevention

The risk of cranial nerve dysfunction can be minimized by taking those steps outlined below to prevent PDPH. This involves using small gauge spinal needles. If a needle with a cutting bevel tip is used, it should be oriented so that the bevel will be parallel to the longitudinal axis of the spine. As mentioned above, using a shallow angle of needle insertion may further reduce the risk of PDPH and associated complications. Perhaps the single most effective preventative measure is to use the newly available small gauge disposable spinal needles with atraumatic tips, such as Whitacre- and Sprotte-type needles. Because PDPH may be the forerunner of a cranial nerve problem, parturients who develop severe and persistent postural headaches should be encouraged to remain in the recumbent position and the headache actively treated.

### Treatment

If a parturient develops cranial nerve dysfunction as a complication of regional anesthesia, she should be encouraged to remain at bed rest. If the patient neglects the symptoms and remains upright, permanent neurologic injury can result (199). Consultation and diagnostic work-up should be considered to rule out other potential causes of the problem. If the cause is thought to be due to CSF leak and low CSF volume, then an epidural blood patch procedure should be performed as outlined previously.

## Spinal Cord and Peripheral Nerve Injuries

Among complications of childbirth, neurologic injury can result from both obstetric and anesthetic causes. Regional anesthesia always carries some risk of neurologic injury. Because of this, a postpartum neurologic deficit in a patient having a regional anesthetic will often focus suspicion on the anesthetic. The obstetric anesthesiologist should, therefore, be able to distinguish among symptoms of pre-existing disease, symptoms attributable to pregnancy or delivery, and complications related to the anesthetic. Postpartum neurologic complications are much more likely to arise from obstetric or natural causes than from peripartum regional anesthesia. The incidence of neurologic complications after regional anesthesia is estimated at 1 in 11,000 (200) to 1 in 20,000 (201), well below the 1 in 3000 that may be expected in parturients not having an anesthetic (202).

## Neuropathies in the Peripartum Period

Any form of neuropathy may occur in pregnancy. The reader is referred to a number of excellent articles reviewing both the common neuropathies of pregnancy and those associated with the administration of anesthesia in the parturient (192,202–205). Although many neuropathies have unknown etiologies, some are due to unsuspected trauma, excessive weight gain, fluid retention during pregnancy, the hormonal changes of pregnancy, and underlying medical conditions often aggravated by pregnancy. Peripartum polyneuropathies are usually the result of one of these factors and are unlikely to be related to anesthetic administration. The differential diagnosis in parturients with diffuse peripheral polyneuropathy is similar to that of nonpregnant women and includes postinfectious polyneuritis, metabolic disease, collagen vascular disease, and drug induced conditions.

*Mononeuropathies* in the peripartum period can present diagnostic challenges to the anesthesiologist, as these can mimic complications of general or regional anesthesia. Any of the cranial nerves can be affected. *Brachial plexus neuropathy* may be due to nerve compression between the clavical and first rib due to the increased weight of the breasts and abdomen combined with sagging of the shoulder. Sensory loss, and pain and shoulder wasting may ensue. Ulnar neuropathy, sometimes in association with median nerve involvement, has been described in the peripartum period. Full recovery usually follows delivery. Median neuropathy at the wrist (carpal tunnel syndrome), the most common mononeuropathy in the upper extremity, occurs in 7% or more of parturients (206). Conservative therapy, such as nocturnal wrist splinting, is effective in about 80% of pregnant patients. Surgery is rarely necessary for carpal tunnel syndrome associated with pregnancy but may be necessary if motor weakness develops.

*Lateral femoral cutaneous nerve neuropathy*, also known as meralgia parasthetica, can occur during the course of pregnancy (207,208). Symptoms of hypalgesia or dysesthesia are seen over the lateral aspect of the thigh. As this nerve is purely sensory, there is no associated motor impairment. Symptoms usually begin in the last trimester of pregnancy (207). The lateral femoral cutaneous nerve has a very long course and thus may be stretched by the increased weight and exaggerated lordosis of pregnancy (208). The exact cause of damage to the nerve is unknown but injury may occur within the pelvis, as it passes beneath the inguinal ligament, or at the fascia lata. Symptoms may persist permanently, but most often resolve within 3 months after delivery.

*Femoral neuropathy* occurs due to injury during vaginal delivery, cesarean section, hysterectomy, or other lower abdominal surgical procedures (209–211). This nerve is vulnerable to compression from retractors positioned against the greater psoas muscle, hemorrhage into the iliopsoas muscle causing nerve compression, and from trauma as it exits the abdomen next to the femoral artery. The prognosis is good in most cases; however, on occasion there may be pain and persistent weakness for several months. *Obturator neuropathy* is rare but may be caused by a difficult labor, hematoma, or by compression from the fetal head or high forceps.

*Sciatic neuropathy* may occur during pregnancy particularly during the last trimester as the sacral plexus is compressed by the fetus (211). Pain is sometimes severe enough to warrant bed rest. Permanent injury is rare and symptoms usually resolve quickly after delivery.

*Lateral peroneal neuropathy* is due to compression as it crosses the fibular head by poorly positioned leg supports, resulting in foot drop (192). Another cause of foot drop is compression of the lumbosacral trunk as it crosses the sacral ala, which form the posterior brim of the true pelvis (Figure 16–10). This injury is likely in short primigravida with a platypelloid pelvis, particularly following prolonged labor and midforceps delivery. Foot drop, in these circumstances, is usually unilateral and on the same side as the infant's brow. Prognosis is good for complete resolution of this injury.

## Bladder Dysfunction

Bladder dysfunction is frequently seen in the obstetric patient. Although bladder symptoms are common during pregnancy, neurologic lesions causing these symptoms are infrequent. Prolonged pressure on the pelvic nerves by the fetal head in the second stage of labor or during a difficult delivery can lead to partial denervation of the bladder, resulting in a hypotonic, distended bladder with frequency, and postvoid residual volume. In one study, the incidence of bladder dysfunction following delivery was 2 to 4 times greater following forceps delivery compared to spontaneous delivery (212). There was no difference in the incidence when regional anesthesia was used.

## Backache

Backache is frequently attributed to spinal or epidural anesthesia. Grove (213) investigated the incidence of backache following nonepidural vaginal deliveries and found it to be 40% in patients with spontaneous deliveries and 25% in patients with instrumented deliveries. Crawford (212) found the incidence of backache to be 45% in parturients having epidural anesthesia, which is similar to the incidence reported in Grove's study. A more recent study in one British hospital wherein nearly 12,000 deliv-

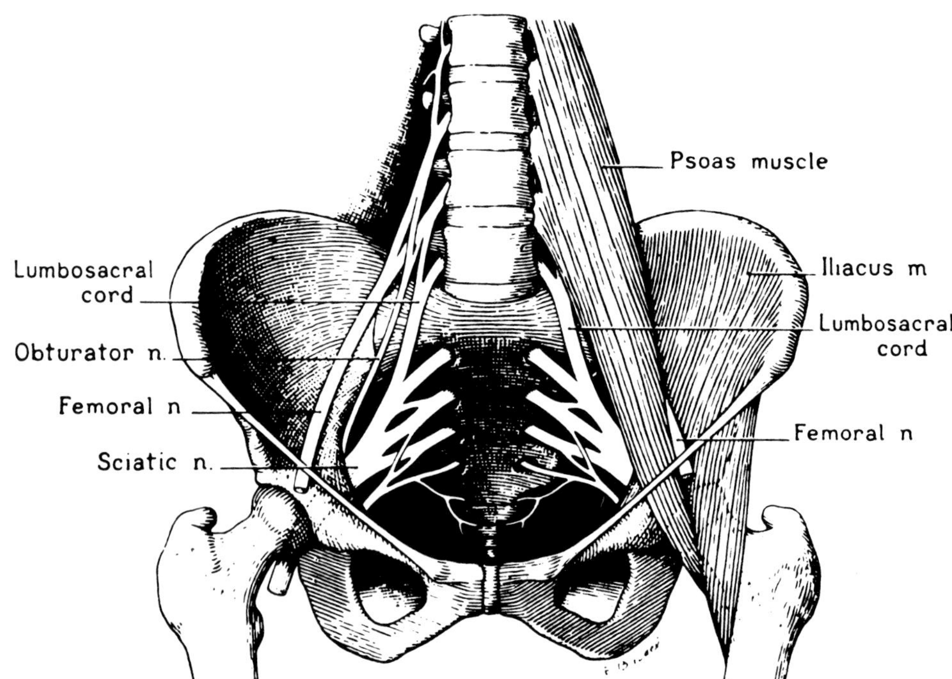


**Fig. 16–10.** Relationship of the lumbar-sacral plexus to the plexus and psoas major muscle. The position of the plexus makes it vulnerable to traumatic pressure produced by the presenting part. (From Cole JT: Maternal obstetric paralysis. Am. J. Obstet. Gynecol. 52: 374, 1946.)

eries were performed, revealed that backache lasting for more than 6 weeks occurred in 10.5% of women delivered by natural childbirth (214). A similar incidence occurred after delivery by elective cesarean section, whether general or regional anesthesia was used. However, in gravidae who had had epidural analgesia for labor and vaginal delivery or for cesarean section following a failed trial of labor, the incidence of prolonged backache rose to near 19%. Bromage (215) attributed this highly significant difference to ligamentous damage arising from tolerance of potentially damaging posture and straining movements in the presence of analgesia produced by relatively high (0.375 to 0.5) concentration of bupivacaine, which was used by British anesthetists at the time.

Although the incidence of lumbar disc disease during pregnancy is unknown, radicular pain is relatively common. Radicular symptoms have been noted to appear during pregnancy or early puerperium in 39% of parous females with surgically proven, lumbar disc protrusions, most often involving L5-S1 discs (216). Symptoms may occur at any time during pregnancy, labor, delivery, or early postpartum period. Treatment should consist of strict bed rest, local heat and massage, and analgesics. If sphincter function is impaired or if pain and motor weakness persist for more than 2 weeks, then neuroradiologic study and surgery may be indicated.

## Anesthetic Related Neuropathies

### Etiology and Pathophysiology

Neurologic injury due to regional anesthesia can be the result of a variety of causes. A review of cases that have been reported in the literature reveals that the complications may have been due to one or more of the following factors: 1) direct needle trauma during the procedure; 2) neurotoxicity from drugs or contaminants; 3) infection; 4) spinal hematoma; 5) spinal cord ischemia due to vasoconstrictors; and 6) exacerbation of pre-existing disease. Spinal hematoma, infection, and chemical neurotoxicity will be addressed separately in the following sections.

Failure of anesthetic block to resolve as expected may sometimes be related to local anesthetic effects. Prolonged neural blockade due to local anesthetic action must be considered with any of the local anesthetic agents used for spinal or epidural anesthesia. However, prolonged neural blockade (greater than 48 hours), to our knowledge, has only been reported following repeated epidural injections of bupivacaine for labor (215,217,218). The extended duration of blockade has been attributed to accumulation of highly lipid-soluble agents. The block usually resolves without long-lasting untoward effects.

Trauma to neural tissue from spinal or epidural needles and catheters is extremely rare (200,219). If nerve roots are injured, signs and symptoms are found at the spinal segment(s) involved. Sensory roots are more likely to be affected than motor roots. Nerve root injury is more common after spinal than after epidural anesthesia. Direct trauma to the spinal cord can be avoided if dural puncture or epidural placement is below the conus medullaris. The conus medullaris is usually located above the L1-L2 interspace but in some instances may extend to the L2-L3 interspace. Nerve root trauma is usually indicated by severe lancing radicular pain with needle placement.

Epidural and intrathecal catheters are also suspected of causing trauma to spinal roots, although there is little objective evidence in the literature of trauma caused by epidural catheters. In recent years, 26- to 32-gauge spinal microcatheters that can be passed through 25- or 26-gauge spinal needles became available. These catheters showed promise for increasing the popularity of continuous subarachnoid anesthesia in obstetrics. However, in May of 1992, the FDA issued a safety alert and removed these catheters from the market. A report by Rigler, et al described four cases of cauda equina syndrome following continuous spinal anesthesia (220). Microcatheters were used in three of these cases. The authors speculated that maldistribution and relatively high doses of local anesthetic exposed neural tissue to toxic concentrations of anesthetic. Laboratory studies using spinal cord models lend support to this theory (221–223). In addition, the breakage of microcatheters during removal has been reported. The future of small subarachnoid catheters in anesthesia is uncertain at this time.

Ischemic injury to the spinal cord can occur from direct action of excessive high concentration of epinephrine in the local anesthetic solution, especially if the anesthetic is associated with significant hypotension. The blood supply to the lower part of the spinal cord may be quite tenuous in some individuals. In patients in whom the blood supply is already compromised by disease or anatomic factors, vasoconstrictor effect, together with hypotension, may cause sufficient ischemia in the spinal cord to produce an anterior spinal artery syndrome or transverse myelitis (199).

Many complications associated with regional anesthesia in obstetrics have been attributed to exacerbation of pre-existing neurologic disease (224). In some cases, the relationship seems quite obvious, e.g., a patient with a bleeding dyscrasia who develops a spinal hematoma following an epidural anesthetic. In other cases, the relationship is purely speculative, e.g., worsening of neurologic symptoms in a patient with multiple sclerosis. In a study of 10,098 patients, Vandam and Dripps found 11 cases in which the anesthetic may have exacerbated pre-existing disease (224). The cases included meningioma, viral diseases affecting the nervous system, patients with metastatic tumors, and two elderly diabetic patients. Several neurologic diseases (e.g., multiple sclerosis) may be exacerbated in the postpartum period, which may implicate any anesthetic that was given for labor and delivery. Although a cause and effect relationship between regional anesthesia and exacerbation of pre-existing disease may be only speculative, it may be prudent to avoid regional anesthesia in such patients. However, this should not be considered an absolute contraindication, especially in cases in which the advantages of regional anesthesia are clear and the patient is informed and has given consent.

### *Prevention*

The most important means of avoiding spinal nerve injury are to rigidly adhere to the basic principles of good regional anesthesia. Patients should be carefully evaluated before regional anesthetics. Those who refuse or who are reluctant to have spinal or extradural anesthesia should not be forced to undergo the procedure. The risks and benefits of regional anesthesia should be carefully weighed in patients who have systemic disease that may involve the nervous system.

To avoid contamination, it is best to use disposable needles, syringes, and catheters. The packaging should be carefully checked to ensure sterility and up-to-dateness. Regional anesthetic techniques must be carried out under strict aseptic conditions. Care must be exercised to avoid contamination of the local anesthetic by the antiseptic solution. The local anesthetic and any other drugs must be accurately identified and the lowest therapeutic amount and concentration used. Solutions that have become turbid or that contain undissolved crystals should be discarded. Vasoconstrictor drugs should be avoided in patients with vascular disease. The anesthesiologist should not persist beyond reasonable attempts to place a regional block. If the patient experiences paresthesia during puncture or injection of the drug, the needle should be withdrawn and repositioned. If paresthesia persists, it is best to discontinue the procedure.

### *Diagnosis and Treatment*

The anesthesiologist should have an organized and thorough approach to the patient presenting with neurological symptoms. Appropriate questions to ask include: what is the nature of the symptom (sensory, motor, both; unilateral, bilateral)?; what is the location of the suspected lesion? can it be explained on an anatomic and physiologic basis?; does it follow a peripheral nerve distribution or a spinal segmental distribution?; are there related medical conditions that might explain the symptoms?; are there circumstances surrounding the pregnancy, labor, and delivery that might be the cause of the suspected lesion (i.e., protracted labor, difficult or instrument delivery, cesarean section and use of retractors)?; and were there any difficulties during the anesthetic that might explain the lesion?

A careful physical examination should document any sensory and motor deficits as either segmental or peripheral. The results of the history and physical exam will dictate the need for additional consultation and diagnostic tests. Electromyography, nerve conduction studies, and somatosensory evoked potentials may be helpful in localizing the lesion and determining a prognosis. Electromyography should be conducted immediately after the injury becomes apparent and again 2 to 3 weeks following the injury. This can help differentiate new injury from pre-existing lesions because it takes about 2 weeks for electromyographic denervation potentials to appear.

Treatment for acute neurologic injury is primarily supportive, including good nursing care and rehabilitation therapy. Prognosis depends on the type and extent of injury. Neuropractic injuries involve damage to the myelin sheaths surrounding axons. Prognosis for recovery with such injuries is excellent, as the myelin sheaths are repaired over a period of weeks. In the case of neurotmesis, axons have been damaged and Wallerian degeneration occurs. The prognosis is poor because the axons must regenerate along the length of the nerve, a very slow process that is rarely complete (225).

## ***Spinal Hematoma***

### *Etiology and Pathophysiology*

Spinal hematoma formation whether epidural, subdural, or subarachnoid can result in devastating neurologic injury. Such hematoma may occur spontaneously without any apparent precipitating event or condition. They can occur at any age and at any spinal cord level (226,227). Sudden spinal cord compression caused by spontaneous epidural hematoma without evidence of a pre-existing vascular anomaly has been reported during pregnancy (228,229). Risk factors for spinal hematoma formation include coagulopathy, trauma, spinal tumors, and vascular malformations.

The potential risks of epidural, subdural, or subarachnoid hematoma caused by neuraxial blocks or diagnostic lumbar punctures seem obvious, although it is difficult to quantify such risk. Neuraxial hematoma formation has been reported following epidural anesthetics and lumbar punctures, usually in association with anticoagulation therapy (226,230). The incidence of this complication is unknown but is very low. Spinal hematoma are more likely to be spontaneous than to be associated with epidural anesthesia (225).

Spinal hematoma of any type can result in cord compression and cord ischemia. The presenting symptom is usually severe localized back pain, sometimes with a radicular component. This is usually followed by rapidly progressing sensory loss, paraplegia, and bladder and bowel dysfunction. Sometimes signs and symptoms may progress more slowly, making diagnosis more difficult. Except for subarachnoid hemorrhage, CSF analysis is not diagnostic and, consequently, of little help. Computed tomography, magnetic resonance imaging, and myelography are the most useful studies to confirm the diagnosis.

### Prevention

Coagulopathy has been considered an absolute contraindication to regional anesthesia in the obstetric patient (231). This is especially true for labor analgesia in which there may be no clear medical indication for the procedure other than the relief of pain associated with a normal physiologic process (i.e., labor and delivery). A significant number of parturients without any known risk factors may present with thrombocytopenia (232). Furthermore, a number of conditions such as preeclampsia, infection, autoimmune disease, etc., are associated with low platelet counts. For these reasons, the obstetric patient may be at increased risk of spinal hematoma formation. However, we are not aware of any case reports in which a regional anesthetic procedure in an obstetric patient with thrombocytopenia resulted in neurologic injury as a result of spinal hematoma (233). However, this may be because regional anesthetics are avoided in such patients, or because such cases have not been reported in the literature.

Anesthetic interventions in obstetric patients are frequently required on an urgent or emergent basis, often before laboratory results and coagulation studies are available. Retrospective studies have indicated that many parturients have received neuraxial anesthetics with platelet counts that are considerably below normal (233,234). This can be a particular problem in preeclamptic women who, in addition to thrombocytopenia, often have a defect in platelet function, which can prolong bleeding time (235). None of the above studies have found neurologic injury as a result of spinal hematoma even in the obstetric patient at risk. A review of the ASA closed-claims data base containing over 250 malpractice claims involving obstetric anesthesia for the years 1976 to 1989 found no claims related to spinal hematoma formation. Although spinal hematoma is a devastating complication, the incidence appears to be exceedingly low. Prudence dictates avoiding regional anesthetic procedures in parturients with abnormal coagulation parameters; however, in cases where conduction anesthesia offers particular advantages, the benefits may outweigh the potential risks (233).

### Treatment

Evolving spinal cord compression constitutes a surgical emergency necessitating immediate decompressive laminectomy. Osmotic diuretics and steroids have been used as adjuncts. The severity of preoperative symptoms and time from first symptoms to surgery influence the prognosis. For this reason, neurosurgical consultation should be immediately obtained if spinal hematoma is suspected.

## Spinal Infection

### Etiology and Pathophysiology

Spinal infection can be the result of poor aseptic technique while performing the regional anesthetic block. Skin infections near the site of needle insertion may allow spread of infection to the epidural space or to the subarachnoid space. Vascular trauma during regional procedures may allow blood-borne organisms to seed infection in the epidural or subarachnoid space, resulting in epidural abscess or meningitis. The potential for spreading infection to the neuraxis has been the main contraindication to regional anesthetic techniques in patients with active infections.

Epidural abscess is usually the result of osteomyelitis or spontaneous hematogenous spread (236). The spontaneous occurrence of a Staphylococcus aureus epidural abscess has been reported in the postpartum period (237). The risks of epidural abscess due to neuraxial anesthesia are very low. One estimate places the incidence at less than 0.0015% (238). Most cases related to regional anesthesia were reported in the early days of caudal anesthesia for labor (239). Epidural abscess may be more common when catheters are left in place for prolonged periods such as for chronic pain management or when epidural steroids are also injected (240).

Meningitis following regional anesthesia is also rare, although three cases were recently reported in association with epidural anesthesia. One case may have involved the introduction of blood-borne bacteria into the CSF during unintentional subarachnoid puncture or during a subsequent blood patch procedure (241). The second case involved an uncomplicated epidural for labor and delivery with subsequent meningitis caused by a bacteria common in dental carries (242). In the third case, introduction of bacteria from the skin surface may have been the likely cause of meningitis (242). In another recent case report, meningitis was described following obstetric spinal anesthesia for removal of a retained placenta (243). In that case, it was not clear whether the etiology was due to chemical irritation or a partially treated bacterial infection. Although such cases are very rare, the potential for neuraxial infection, either introduced from the skin or from organisms in the blood, must be considered.

Signs and symptoms of acute bacterial meningitis include fever, headache, nuchal rigidity, Kernig's and Brudzinski's sign, altered mental status, and convulsions. Diagnostic lumbar puncture reveals elevated cerebrospinal fluid pressure, CSF pleocytosis, elevated CSF protein, and depressed CSF glucose. CSF cultures will usually be positive for the offending organism. Epidural abscess presents with fever and localized pain and tenderness, sometimes with a radicular component. If not promptly diagnosed and treated, lower extremity weakness and sphincteric dysfunction develop over a period of days to weeks. CSF examination may reveal elevated protein and moderate pleocytosis but may be otherwise unremarkable.

#### Prevention

Prevention of spinal infections involves using strict aseptic technique, avoiding inserting needles near areas of superficial infection, and avoiding neuraxial anesthetic procedures in septic patients. The cerebrospinal fluid is an excellent culture medium and the subarachnoid space has limited defenses against infection. The person performing the block should wear cap and face mask as well as sterile gloves. Breaks in sterile technique should not be ignored or treated lightly. The back should be prepared with antiseptic solution in the proper manner. Because chemical arachnoiditis has been caused by antiseptic solutions, it is important to wipe the skin before the needle is introduced. When performing a spinal anesthetic, it is advisable to use an introducer through which the spinal needle can be directed. This prevents the spinal needle from coming into direct contact with the skin. The introducer also acts as a guide and prevents the needle from deflecting. The operator should avoid holding or touching the part of the needle that will enter the subarachnoid space, thereby diminishing the risks of contaminating the needle.

The use of regional anesthesia in patients with chorioamnionitis is controversial (244). Because these patients frequently have positive blood cultures, the risk of seeding infection is a possibility (245). Many anesthesiologists will, however, initiate regional anesthetics if parturients are not grossly septic and are receiving antibiotic therapy when the procedure is initiated (246). This practice has not resulted in reports of epidural abscess or meningitis.

Similar concerns about spreading infection by needle trauma have been raised in pregnant patients with herpes infections. Herpes simplex virus type 2 (HSV-2) is an increasingly common infection in women of childbearing age. In the greater-Seattle area, approximately 30% of women of childbearing age are seropositive for HSV-2 and 8 to 10% have symptoms consistent with recurrent outbreaks (Brown ZA, personal communication, 1990). Approximately 30 to 50% of women with a history of recurrent HSV-2 infections are delivered by cesarean section. (247) Regional anesthesia seems to be safe in patients with recurrent HSV-2 infections (248,249) perhaps because recrudescence is not associated with viremia. However, because primary infections are associated with viremia and often severe generalized symptoms such as fever, lymphadenopathy, and headache, we advise avoiding regional anesthesia in patients with primary infections.

#### Treatment

Treatment for spinal infections consists of rapid initiation of intravenous antibiotic therapy. This should be based on the type of organism responsible for the infection and sensitivity studies, although initiation of antibiotic therapy should not be delayed. Analgesics, antipyretics, and sedatives are used as necessary. Anticonvulsants may be required in some cases of meningitis. Epidural abscess usually requires prompt surgical intervention to decompress the spinal cord and remove infected and necrotic tissue.

### Chemical Meningitis and Neurotoxicity

#### Etiology and Pathophysiology

Meningeal irritation and neurotoxicity from clinically used concentrations of local anesthetics are extremely rare. Drug manufacturers go to great lengths to ensure that their products cause a minimal amount of local tissue reaction. Nonetheless, it is clear that virtually all local anesthetics in sufficiently high concentration will cause injury to nerve tissue (250,251). Case reports have linked neurologic injury from spinal anesthesia with a wide variety of local anesthetics (252), although it has not always been clear if the local anesthetic or a contaminant was the cause of the injury. In the past, detergents and other solutions used for cleaning reusable needles and syringes have been implicated in causing aseptic meningitis and neurologic injury (253). One of the most serious potential sequelae is adhesive arachnoiditis. This condition involves a gradual proliferation of the arachnoid, resulting in scarring and obliteration of the subarachnoid space. The signs and symptoms of the resulting caudal equina syndrome may be progressive over months or years and usually involve numbness and weakness in the perineum and lower extremities with bowel, bladder, and sexual dysfunction.

In recent years, the local anesthetic most often linked with neurotoxicity has been 2-chloroprocaine. This agent has been very popular in obstetrics because of its rapid onset, short duration of action, and very low systemic toxicity. In some of the reported cases of neurologic injury, it appears that the local anesthetic was unintentionally injected into the subarachnoid space (254), although this may not have occurred in all cases (255). A considerable amount of research has been directed at determining if the cause of neurotoxicity was the drug itself or the antioxidant, sodium bisulfite, with which the local anesthetic was formulated to minimize oxidation. Some laboratory (256) as well as animal studies (257) have indicated that the sodium bisulfite was the most likely cause of neurotoxicity. Other studies, however, indicate that the drug itself may be more neurotoxic than other commonly used local anesthetics (258). Presumably because of the concern regarding sodium bisulfite, the manufacturers now use EDTA as the antioxidant in commercially available 2-chloroprocaine. The drug continues to be available to the practitioner but due care should be exercised in its use. Recent reports have indicated that the epidural use of the new formulation 2-chloroprocaine may be associated with severe spasmodic back pain (259,260).

### Prevention

All local anesthetics should be used in the appropriate fashion using the minimum dose necessary for the procedure. Before injecting significant volumes of local anesthetic with epidural techniques, a test dose should be given to rule out subarachnoid as well as intravascular placement. Care should be taken to avoid contaminating needles, catheters, and syringes with antiseptic solutions used for cleaning the skin. In addition, it is advisable to use disposable equipment whenever possible, to minimize the risk of introducing contaminants, such as detergents or cleaning solutions, during regional anesthetic procedures.

### Treatment

The management of chemical meningitis is based on supportive care and treatment of symptoms. Antibiotics are not indicated although they are often started because of diagnostic uncertainty. In cases where an inappropriate drug or a large dose of local anesthetic is known to have been injected into the subarachnoid space, it may be advisable to drain as much CSF as possible to remove as much of the substance as possible and to lower subarachnoid pressure (if large volumes were injected).

## Shivering

Shivering is a minor but annoying accompaniment of labor and delivery in 23% of normal parturients without extradural analgesia (261) and 20 to 75% of women who have extradural analgesia for labor and delivery (215,262). Although it is not a true complication of obstetric anesthesia, shivering can have adverse effects. Metabolic rate and oxygen consumption can increase 200%, thereby substantially increasing the demands on an already stressed pulmonary and cardiovascular system (263). Parturients with cardiopulmonary disease or those with stressed infants may be adversely affected by shivering. In addition to these concerns, shivering can complicate monitoring, heighten anxiety, and add to fear and stress during labor and delivery.

### Etiology

The etiology of shivering during normal labor and delivery is not known, although a number of mechanisms have been proposed. There is a correlation between the occurrence of postpartum chills and fetal-maternal transfusions, although there does not seem to be a correlation with blood-incompatibility (264). A possible immunologic reaction to emboli of fetal or trophoblastic cells has been suggested but not confirmed. Other suggestions include: amniotic fluid embolism, bacteremia or the release of other toxins, maternal thermogenic response to sudden thermal imbalance from the rapid removal of the fetus and placenta, vasomotor reactions, and nervous excitement.

Epidural-related shivering typically begins 5 to 15 minutes after the injection of the local anesthetic into the epidural space. A variety of mechanisms have been suggested to explain shivering in association with epidural anesthesia: Vasodilation from sympathetic blockade can result in a drop in core temperature leading to thermoregulatory shivering. The absorption of local anesthetic may cause a nonthermoregulatory tremor or may cause central disinhibition of spinal cord reflexes producing tremors similar to those seen during recovery from general anesthesia. Absorption of local anesthetics may raise the hypothalamic thermoregulatory set point. Differential blockade of warm and cold afferent thermoreceptor fibers at the dorsal roots of the spinal cord may cause shivering. Cold receptors in the epidural space may be stimulated by cold anesthetic solution. A number of recent studies have addressed the likely mechanics involved (263,265–267). At this time, the most attractive hypothesis is that the sympathectomy caused by epidural anesthesia results in peripheral vasodilation leading to central hypothermia and normal thermoregulatory shivering.

A number of methods have been used in an attempt to minimize shivering during epidural anesthesia in obstetrics. The use of warmed intravenous fluids, warm ambient temperature, and warmed local anesthetic injectate have all been used with variable success (262,265,268,269). Intravenous meperidine 50 mg given at the time of cesarean delivery has been found to be effective in treating this problem (270). Epidurally administered opioids have also been found to be effective in treating and preventing shivering in this setting (262,271–273). In one study, epidural fentanyl 25 mg given prophylactically to patients undergoing cesarean delivery resulted in a 50% reduction in shivering (274). In our experience, the use of epidural lidocaine without epinephrine (except for the test dose), prophylactic epidural fentanyl 50 μg, and warm intravenous fluids has virtually eliminated shivering associated with the onset of epidural anesthesia for cesarean section.

## REFERENCES


1. Bonica JJ: Principles and Practice of Obstetric Analgesia and Anesthesia. Philadelphia, F.A. Davis Co., 1967, pp. 689–712.
2. Chadwick HS, Ross BK: Causes and consequences of maternal-fetal perianesthetic complications. *In* Anesthesia and Perioperative Complications. Edited by JL Benumof, LJ Saidman. St. Louis, Mosby Year Book, 1992.
3. Greene NM: Physiology of Spinal Anesthesia. Baltimore, Williams and Wilkins Co., 1981.
4. Mason DT: The autonomic nervous system and regulation of cardiovascular performance. Anesthesiology 29:670, 1968.
5. Braunwald E: The control of ventricular function in man. Br. Heart J. 27:1, 1965.
6. Bromage PR: Physiology and pharmacology of epidural anesthesia. Anesthesiology 28:592, 1967.
7. Bromage PR: Physiology of Epidural Anesthesia. *In* Epidural Analgesia. Philadelphia, W.B. Saunders Co., 1978, pp. 347–442, 664–709.
8. Defalque RJ: Compared effects of spinal and extradural an-

esthesia upon blood pressure. Anesthesiology 23:627, 1962.
9. Shimosato S, Etsten BE: The role of the venous system in cardiocirculatory dynamics during spinal and epidural anesthesia in man. Anesthesiology 30:619, 1969.
10. Otton PE, Wilson EJ: The cardiocirculatory effects of upper thoracic epidural analgesia. Can. Anaesth. Soc. J. 13:341, 1966.
11. McLean APH, Mulligan GW, Otton P, MacLean LD: Hemodynamic alterations associated with epidural anesthesia. Surgery 62:79, 1967.
12. Ward RJ, Bonica JJ, Freund FG, Akamatsu et al: Epidural and subarachnoid anesthesia: cardiovascular and respiratory effects. JAMA 191:275, 1965.
13. Bonica JJ, Kennedy WF Jr, Ward RJ, Tolas AG: A comparison of the effects of high subarachnoid and epidural anesthesia. Acta. Anaesth. Scand. Suppl. 23:429, 1966.
14. Kennedy WF Jr, Bonica JJ, Akamatsu TJ, Ward RJ, et al: Cardiovascular and respiratory effects of subarachnoid block in the presence of acute blood loss. Anesthesiology 29:29–35, 1968.
15. Berges PU, Morikawa K, Bonica JJ: Effects of various levels of subarachnoid block on hemodynamics and ventilation. Abstracts of Annual ASA Meeting, p. 58, 1970.
16. Bonica JJ, Berges PU, Morikawa K: Mechanism of hemodynamic response to intravenous lidocaine. Abstracts of ASA Annual Meeting, p. 53, 1970.
17. Bonica JJ, Akamatsu TJ, Berges PU, Morikawa K, et al: Circulatory effects of peridural block: I. Effects of level of analgesia and dose of lidocaine. Anesthesiology 33:619–626, 1970.
18. Bonica JJ, Akamatsu TJ, Berges PU, Morikawa K, et al: Circulatory effects of peridural block: II. Effects of epinephrine. Anesthesiology 34:514–522, 1971.
19. Bonica JJ, Kennedy WF Jr, Akamatsu TJ, Gerbershagen HU: Circulatory effects of peridural block. III. Effects of acute blood loss. Anesthesiology 36:219–227, 1972.
20. Ueland K, Gills RE, Hansen JM: Maternal cardiovascular dynamics: I. Cesarean section under subarachnoid block anesthesia. Am. J. Obstet. Gynecol. 100:42, 1968.
21. Ueland K, Akamatsu TJ, Eng M, Bonica JJ, et al: Maternal cardiovascular dynamics: VI. Cesarean section under epidural anesthesia without epinephrine. Am. J. Obstet. Gynecol. 114:775–780, 1972.
22. Akamatsu TJ, DerYuen D, Ueland K, Bonica JJ: Cardiovascular effects of epidural anesthesia with epinephrine for cesarean section. Obstet. Gynec. News. 9:3, 1974.
23. Bonica JJ: Cardiovascular side effects and complications of local and regional anesthesia. Journèes D'Enseignement Post-Universitaire D'Anesthesie Et Reanimation: Anesthesiques Locaux En Anesthesie Et Reanimation, Paris Librairie Arnette, p 373, 1974.
24. Bonica JJ: Cardiovascular effects of peridural block. *In* Regional Anesthesia: Recent Advances and Current Status. Edited by JJ Bonica. Philadelphia, F.A. Davis Co., pp. 64–81, 1971.
25. Akamatsu TJ: Cardiovascular response of spinal anesthesia. *In* Regional Anesthesia: Recent Advances and Current Status. Edited by JJ Bonica. Philadelphia, F.A. Davis Co., pp. 84–96, 1971.
26. Akamatsu TJ, Bonica JJ: Spinal and extradural analgesia-anesthesia for parturition. Clin. Obstet. Gynecol. 17 (2): 183–198, 1974.
27. Tucker GT, Mather LE: Clinical pharmacokinetics of local anesthetics. Clin. Pharmacokinet. 4:241, 1979.
28. Kao FF, Jalar UH: The central action of lignocaine and its effect on cardiac output. Br. J. Pharmacol. 14:522, 1959.
29. Jorfeldt L, Lofstrom B, Pernow B, Persson B, et al: The effect of local anaesthetics on the central circulation and respiration in man and dog. Acta. Anaesth. Scand. 12:153, 1968.
30. Becket AH, Boyes RN, Appleton PJ: The metabolism and excretion of lidocaine. J. Pharm. Pharmacol. 18:76S, 1966.
31. Moore FD, Dagher FJ, Boyden CM, et al: Hemorrhage in normal man: I. Distribution and dispersal of saline infusions following acute blood loss: clinical kinetics of blood volume support. Ann. Surg. 163:485–504, 1966.
32. Assali NS, Prystowsky H: Studies on autonomic blockade. II. Observations on the nature of blood pressure fall with high selective spinal anesthesia in pregnant women. J. Clin. Invest. 29:1367–1375, 1950.
33. Howard BK, Goodson JH, Mengert WF: Supine hypotensive syndrome in late pregnancy. Obstet. Gynecol. 1:371–377, 1953.
34. Kerr MG: Cardiovascular dynamics in pregnancy and labour. Br. Med. Bull. 24:19–24, 1968.
35. Kerr MG, Scott DB, Samuel E: Studies of the inferior vena cava in late pregnancy. Br. Med. J. 1:532–533, 1964.
36. Bieniarz J, Crottogini JJ, Curuchet E, Romero-Salinias G, et al: Aortocaval compression by the uterus in late human pregnancy. Am. J. Obstet. Gynecol. 100:203–217, 1968.
37. Zilianti M, Salazar JR, Aller J, Aguero O: Fetal heart rate and pH of fetal capillary blood during epidural analgesia in labor. Obstet. Gynecol. 36:881–886, 1970.
38. Amussen E, Christensen EH, Neilsen M: Regulation of circulation in different postures. Surgery 8:604, 1940.
39. Bletka M, Hlavat Y, Trnkova M, Bendl J, et al: Volume of whole blood and absolute amount of serum proteins in the early stage of late toxemia of pregnancy. Am. J. Obstet. Gynecol. 106:10–13, 1970.
40. Lechner RB, Chadwick HS: Anesthetic care of the patient with preeclampsia. Anesth. Clin. North. Am. 8:95–114, 1990.
41. Wetstone DL, Wong KC: Sinus bradycardia and asystole during anesthesia. Anesthesiology 41:87–89, 1974.
42. Caplan RA, Ward RJ, Posner K, Cheney FW: Unexpected cardiac arrest during spinal anesthesia: a closed claims analysis of predisposing factors. Anesthesiology 68:5–11, 1988.
43. Chester WL: Spinal anesthesia, complete heart block, and the precordial chest thump: an unusual complication and a unique resuscitation. Anesthesiology 69:600–602, 1988.
44. Mackey DC, Carpenter RL, Thompson GE, Brown DL, et al: Bradycardia and asystole during spinal anesthesia: a report of three cases without morbidity. Anesthesiology 70: 866–868, 1989.
45. Eckenhoff JE, Hafkenschiel JH, Folz EL, Driver RL: Influence of hypotension on coronary blood flow, cardiac work, and cardiac efficiency. Am. J. Physiol. 152:545–553, 1948.
46. Hackel DB, Sancetta SM, Kleinerman J: Effect of hypotension due to spinal anesthesia on coronary blood flow and myocardial metabolism in man. Circulation 13:92–97, 1956.
47. Sivarajan M, Amory DW, Lindbloom LE, Schwettman RS: Systemic and regional blood-flow changes during spinal anesthesia in the Rhesus monkey. Anesthesiology 43: 78–88, 1975.
48. Palmer CM, Norris MC, Giudici MC, Leighton BL, et al: Incidence of electrocardiographic changes during cesarean delivery under regional anesthesia. Anesth. Analg. 70: 36–43, 1990.
49. Greene NM, Bucker JP, Kerr WS, von Felsinger JM, et al: Hypotensive spinal anesthesia: respiratory, metabolic, he-

patic, renal, and cerebral effects. Ann. Intern. Med. 140: 641, 1954.

50. Papper EM, Habif DV, Bradley SE: Studies of renal and hepatic function in normal man during thiopental, cyclopropane, and high spinal anesthesia. J. Clin. Invest. 29:838, 1950.

51. Lynn RB, Sancetta SM, Simeone FA, Scott RW: Observations on the circulation in high spinal anesthesia. Surgery 32: 195–213, 1952.

52. Stenger V, Anderson T, De Padna C, Eitzman D, et al: Spinal anesthesia for cesarean section. Physiological and biochemical observations. Am. J. Obstet. Gynecol. 90:51, 1964.

53. Vasicka A, Hutchinson HT, Eng M, Allen CR: Spinal and epidural anesthesia, fetal and uterine response to acute hypo- and hypertension. Am. J. Obstet. Gynecol. 90: 800–810, 1964.

54. Schellenberg JC: Uterine activity during lumbar epidural analgesia with bupivacaine. Am. J. Obstet. Gynecol. 127: 26–31, 1977.

55. Griess FC Jr: Pressure-flow relationship in the gravid uterine vascular bed. Am. J. Obstet. Gynecol. 96:41–47, 1966.

56. Ebner H, Barcohana J, Bartoshuk AK: Influence of postspinal hypotension on the fetal electrocardiogram. Am. J. Obstet. Gynecol. 80:569–576, 1960.

57. Hon EH, Reid BL, Hehre FW: The electronic evaluation of fetal heart rate. II. Changes with maternal hypotension. Am. J. Obstet. Gynecol. 79:209–215, 1960.

58. Moya F, Smith B: Spinal anesthesia for cesarean section: clinical and biochemical studies of effects on maternal physiology. JAMA 179:609–614, 1962.

59. Abboud TK, Blikian A, Noueihid R, Nagappala S, et al: Neonatal effects of maternal hypotension during spinal anesthesia as evaluated by a new test. Anesthesiology 59:A421, 1983.

60. Lewis M, Thomas P, Wilkes RG: Hypotension during epidural analgesia for caesarean section. Anaesthesia 38: 250–253, 1983.

61. Wollman SB, Marx GF: Acute hydration for prevention of hypotension of spinal anesthesia in parturients. Anesthesiology 29:374–380, 1968.

62. Menendiola J, Grylack OJ, Scanlon JW: Effects of intrapartum maternal glucose infusion on the normal fetus and newborn. Anesth. Analg. 61:32–35, 1982.

63. Lanier WL, Stangland KJ, Scheithauer BW, Milde JH, et al: The effects of dextrose infusion and head position on neurologic outcome after complete cerebral ischemia in primates. Examination of a model. Anesthesiology 66: 39-47, 1987.

64. Crawford JS, Burton M, Davies P: Time and lateral tilt at caesarean section. Br. J. Anaesth. 44:477–484, 1972.

65. Gutsche BB: Prophylactic ephedrine preceding spinal anesthesia for cesarean section. Anesthesiology 45:462–465, 1976.

66. Wright RG, Shnider SM: Hypotension and regional anesthesia in Obstetrics. 3rd Ed. *In* Anesthesia for obstetrics. Edited by SM Shnider, G Levinson. Baltimore, Williams & Wilkins, 1993, pp. 397–408.

67. Shnider SM, Levinson G: Anesthesia for cesarean section. *In* Anesthesia for Obstetrics, 3rd edition. Edited by SM Shnider, G Levinson. Baltimore, Williams & Wilkins, 1993, pp. 211–246.

68. Marx GF, Cosmi RV, Wollman SB: Biochemical status and clinical condition of mother and infant at cesarean section. Anesth. Analg. 48:986–994, 1969.

69. Datta S, Alper MH, Ostheimer GW, Weiss JB: Method of ephedrine administration and nausea and hypotension during spinal anesthesia for cesarean section. Anesthesiology 56:68–70, 1982.

70. Berges PU, Bonica JJ, Morikawa K: Hemodynamic effects of the Trendelenburg and leg-up position during low and high spinal anesthesia. Abstracts of ASA Annual Meeting, 1971, p 149.

71. Ralston DH, Shnider SM, deLorimier AA: Effects of equipotent ephedrine, metaraminol, mephentermine and methoxamine on uterine blood flow in the pregnant ewe. Anesthesiology 40:354–370, 1974.

72. Lechner RB, Droste S, Chadwick HS: Lumbar epidural analgesia and changes in the fetal heart rate pattern: a blinded study of 139 patients. Anesthesiology 71:A853, 1989.

73. Smith BE, Hare FW, Hess OW: Convulsions associated with anesthetic agents during labor and delivery. Anesth. Analg. 43:476, 1964.

74. Albright GA: Cardiac arrest following regional anesthesia with etidocaine or bupivacaine. Anesthesiology 51: 285–287, 1979.

75. Albright GA: Local anesthetics. *In* Anesthesia in obstetrics. Edited by G Albright, IJ Ferguson, IT Joyce. Boston, Butterworth, 1986, pp. 115–150.

76. Chadwick HS, Posner K, Caplan RA, Ward RJ, et al: A comparison of obstetric and nonobstetric anesthesia malpractice claims. Anesthesiology 74:242–249, 1991.

77. Bromage PR: Epidural analgesia. Philadelphia, W.B. Saunders Co., 1978, pp. 55–58.

78. deJong RH, Ronfeld RA, deRosa RA: Cardiovascular effects of convulsant and supraconvulsant doses of amide local anesthetics. Anesth. Analg. 61:3–9, 1982.

79. Liu PL, Feldman HS, Giasi RG, Patterson MK, et al: Comparative CNS toxicity of lidocaine, etidocaine, bupivacaine, and tetracaine in awake dogs following rapid intravenous administration. Anesth. Analg. 62:375–379, 1983.

80. Liu P, Feldman HS, Covino BM, Giasi R, et al: Acute cardiovascular toxicity of intravenous amide local anesthetics in anesthetized ventilated dogs. Anesth. Analg. 61:317–322, 1982.

81. Rosen MA, Thigpen JW, Shnider SM, Foutz SE, et al: Bupivacaine-induced cardiotoxicity in hypoxic and acidotic sheep. Anesth. Analg. 64:1089–1096, 1985.

82. Chadwick HS: Toxicity and resuscitation in lidocaine- or bupivacaine-infused cats. Anesthesiology 63:385–390, 1985.

83. Kotelko DM, Shnider SM, Dailey PA, Brizgys RV, et al: Bupivacaine-induced cardiac arrhythmias in sheep. Anesthesiology 60:10–18, 1984.

84. Morishima HO, Pedersen H, Finster M, Hiraoka H, et al: Bupivacaine toxicity in pregnant and nonpregnant ewes. Anesthesiology 63:134–139, 1985.

85. Sage DJ, Feldman HS, Arthur GR, Doucette AM, et al: The cardiovascular effects of convulsant doses of lidocaine and bupivacaine in the conscious dog. Reg. Anesth. 10: 175–183, 1985.

86. Clarkson CW, Hondegham LM: Mechanism for bupivacaine depression of cardiac conduction: fast block of sodium channels during the action potential with slow recovery from block during diastole. Anesthesiology 62:396–405, 1985.

87. Heavner JE: Cardiac dysrhythmias induced by infusion of local anesthetics into the lateral cerebral ventricle of cats. Anesth. Analg. 65:133–138, 1986.

88. Thomas RD, Behbehani MM, Coyle DE, Denson DD: Cardiovascular toxicity of local anesthetics: An alternative hypothesis. Anesth. Analg. 65:444–450, 1986.

89. Bromage PR: Choice of local anesthetics in obstetrics. *In* Anesthesia for Obstetrics. 3rd edition. Edited by SM

Shnider, GL Levinson, GL. Baltimore, Williams & Wilkins, 1993, pp. 83–102.
90. Avery T, Redon D, Schaenzer G, Rusy BF: The influence of serum potassium on cerebral and cardiac toxicity of bupivacaine and lidocaine. Anesthesiology 61:133–138, 1984.
91. Sage DJ, Feldman HS, Arthor GR, Datta S, et al: Influence of lidocaine and bupivacaine on isolated guinea pig atria in the presence of acidosis and hypoxia. Anesth. Analg. 63: 1–7, 1984.
92. Santos AC, Pedersen H, Harmon TW, Morishima HO, et al: Does pregnancy alter the systemic toxicity of local anesthetics? Anesthesiology 70:991–995, 1989.
93. Kasten GW, Martin ST: Resuscitation from bupivacaine-induced cardiovascular toxicity during partial inferior vena cava occlusion. Anesth. Analg. 65:341–344, 1986.
94. Moore DC, Crawford RD, Scurlock JE: Severe hypoxia and acidosis following local anesthetic-induced convulsions. Anesthesiology 53:259–260, 1980.
95. Moore DC, Thompson GE, Crawford RD: Long-acting local anesthetic drugs and convulsions with hypoxia and acidosis. Anesthesiology 56:230–232, 1982.
96. Morishima HO: Toxicity and distribution of lidocaine in nonasphyxiated and asphyxiated baboon fetuses. Anesthesiology 54:182–186, 1981.
97. Epstein BS, Banerjee S, Chamberlain G, Coakley CS: The effect of the concentration of local anesthetic during epidural anesthesia on the forces of labor. Anesthesiology 29: 187, 1968.
98. Greiss FC, Still JG, Anderson SG: Effects of local anesthetic agents on the uterine vasculatures and myometrium. Am. J. Obstet. Gynecol. 124:889–899, 1976.
99. Moore BC, Batra MS: The compounds of an effective test dose prior to epidural block. Anesthesiology 55:693–696, 1981.
100. Chadwick HS: Obstetric anesthesia closed claims update. Am. Soc. Anesthesiol. Newslett. 57:12–18, 1993.
101. Hood DD, James III DM: Maternal and fetal effects of epinephrine in gravid ewes. Anesthesiology 64:610–613, 1986.
102. Chestnut DH, Weiner CP, Martin JG, Herrig JE, et al: Effect of intravenous epinephrine on uterine artery blood flow velocity in the pregnant guinea pig. Anesthesiology 65: 633–636, 1986.
103. Cartwright PO, McCarroll SM, Antzaka C: Maternal heart rate changes with a plain epidural test dose. Anesthesiology 65:226–228, 1986.
104. Leighton BL, Norris MC, Sosis M, Epstein R, et al: Limitations of epinephrine as a marker of intravascular injection in laboring women. Anesthesiology 66:688–691, 1987.
105. Moore DC, Batra MS, Bridenbaugh LD, Brown DL, et al: Maternal heart rate changes with a plain epidural test dose: validity of results open to question. Anesthesiology 66: 854, 1987.
106. Talledo OE, Chesley LC, Zuspan FP: Renin-angiotensin system in normal and toxemic pregnancies. III. Differential sensitivity to angiotensin II and norepinephrine in toxemia of pregnancy. Am. J. Obstet. Gynecol. 100:218–221, 1968.
107. Hom M, Johnson P, Mulroy M: Blood pressure response to an epinephrine test dose in beta-blocked subjects. Anesthesiology 67:A268, 1987.
108. Popitz-Bergez F, Datta S, Ostheimer GW: Intravascular epinephrine may not increase heart rate in patients receiving metoprolol. Anesthesiology 68:815–816, 1988.
109. Grice SC, Eisenach JC, Dewan DM, Mandell G: Evaluation of 2-chloroprocaine as an effective intravenous test dose for epidural anesthesia. Anesthesiology 67:A627, 1987.
110. Roetman KJ, Eisenach JC: Evaluation of lidocaine as an intravenous test dose for epidural anesthesia. Anesthesiology 69:A669, 1988.
111. Leighton BL, Gross JB: Isoproterenol is an effective marker of intravenous injection in laboring women. Anesthesiology 71:206–209, 1989.
112. Leighton BL, Gross JB: Air: an effective indicator of intravenously located epidural catheters. Anesthesiology 71: 848–851, 1989.
113. Kasten GW, Martin ST: Successful cardiovascular resuscitation after massive intravenous bupivacaine overdosage in anesthetized dogs. Anesth. Analg. 64:491–497, 1985.
114. DePace NC, Betesh JS, Koller MN: 'Postmortem' caesarean section with recovery of both mother and offspring. JAMA 248:971–973, 1982.
115. Marx GF: Cardiopulmonary resuscitation of late-pregnant women. Anesthesiology 56:156, 1982.
116. de Jong RH, Davis NL: Treating bupivacaine arrhythmias: preliminary report. Reg. Anesth. 6:99–103, 1981.
117. Kasten GW, Martin ST: Bupivacaine cardiovascular toxicity: comparison of treatment with bretylium and lidocaine. Anesth. Analg. 64:911–916, 1985.
118. Long WB, Rosenblum S, Grady IP: Successful resuscitation of bupivacaine-induced cardiac arrest using cardiopulmonary bypass. Anesth. Analg. 69:403–406, 1989.
119. Aldrete JA, Johnson DA: Allergy to local anesthetics. JAMA 207:354–357, 1969.
120. Brown DT, Beamish D, Wildsmith JAW: Allergic reactions to an amide local anesthetic. Br. J. Anaesth. 53:435–437, 1981.
121. Aldrete JA, Johnson DA: Evaluation of intracutaneous testing for investigation of allergy to local anesthetics. Anesth. Analg. 49:173–181, 1970.
122. Cavanagh D, DeCenzo JA, Ferguson JH: Cardiac arrest and the obstetrician-gynecologist. Obstet. Gynecol. 22:56–67, 1963.
123. Gold EM: Cardiac arrest in obstetrics. Clin. Obstet. Gynecol. 3:114–130, 1960.
124. Tomkinson J, Turnbull A, Robson G, Dawson I, et al: Report on confidential enquiries into maternal deaths in England and Wales 1976–1978. London, Her Majesty's Stationary Office, 1982.
125. Turnbull AC, Tindall VR, Robson G, Dawson IMO, et al: Report on confidential enquiries into maternal deaths in England and Wales 1979–1981. London, Her Majesty's Stationary Office, 1986.
126. Lee RV, Rodgers BD, White LM, Harvey RC: Cardiopulmonary recuscitation of pregnant women. Am. J. Med. 81: 311–318, 1986.
127. Rees GAD, Willis BA: Resuscitation in late pregnancy. Anaesthesia 43:347–349, 1988.
128. Emergency Cardiac Care Committee and Subcommittees, American Heart Association: Guidelines for Cardiopulmonary Resuscitation and Emergency Cardiac Care. JAMA 268:2171–2302, 1992.
129. Albarran-Sotelo R, Atkins JM, Bloom RS, Campbell F, et al: Textbook of advanced cardiac life support. Dallas, Texas, American Heart Association, 1987.
130. Selden BS, Burke TJ: Complete maternal and fetal recovery after prolonged cardiac arrest. Ann. Emerg. Med. 17: 346–349, 1988.
131. Curry JJ, Quintana FJ: Myocardial infarction with ventricular fibrillation during pregnancy treated by direct current defibrillation with fetal survival. Chest 58:82–84, 1970.
132. Sullivan JM, Ramanathan KB: Management of medical problems in preganacy-severe cardiac disease. N. Engl. J. Med. 313:304–309, 1985.

133. Rotmensch HH, Elkayam U, Frishman W: Antiarrhythmic drug therapy during pregnancy. Ann. Intern. Med. 98: 487–497, 1983.
134. Lindsay SL, Hanson GC: Cardiac arrest in near-term pregnancy. Anaesthesia 42:1074–1077, 1987.
135. Oates S, Williams GL, Rees GAD: Cardiopulmonary resuscitation in late pregnancy. Br. Med. J. 297:404–405, 1988.
136. Grundy EM, Zamora AM, Winnie AP: Comparison of spread of epidural anesthesia in pregnant and nonpregnant women. Anesth. Analg. 57:544–546, 1978.
137. Shnider SM, Levinson G: Obstetric anesthesia. *In* Anesthesia. Edited by RD Miller. New York, Churchill Livingstone, 1986, p 1688.
138. Bromage PR: Epidural analgesia. Philadelphia, W.B. Saunders Co., 1978, pp. 522–525.
139. Cheek TG, Gutsche BB: Maternal physiologic alterations during pregnancy. *In* Anesthesia for Obstetrics. Edited by SM Shnider, G Levinson. Baltimore, Williams & Wilkins, 1987, p. 9.
140. Flanagan HL, Datta S, Lambert DH, Gissen AJ, et al: Effect of pregnancy on bupivacaine-induced conduction blockade in the isolated rabbit vagus nerve. Anesth. Analg. 66: 123–126, 1987.
141. Butterworth JF, Walker OF, Lysak SZ: Pregnancy increases median nerve susceptibility to lidocaine. Anesthesiology 72:962–965, 1990.
142. Greene NM: Distribution of local anesthetic solutions within the subarachnoid space. Anesth. Analg. 64: 715–730, 1985.
143. Park WY: Factors influencing distribution of local anesthetics in the epidural space. Reg. Anesth. 13:49–57, 1988.
144. Boys JE, Norman PF: Accidental subdural analgesia: A case report, possible clinical implications and relevance to "massive extradurals." Br. J. Anaesth. 47:1111–1113, 1975.
145. Lee A, Dodd KW: Accidental subdural catheterization. Anaesthesia 41:847–849, 1986.
146. Manchanda VN, Murad SHN, Shilyansky G, Mehringer M: Unusual clinical course of accidental subdural local anesthetic injection. Anesth. Analg. 62:1124–1126, 1983.
147. Hartrick CT, Pither CE, Pai U, Raj PP, et al: Subdural migration of an epidural catheter. Anesth. Analg. 64:175–178 1985.
148. Lubenow T, Keh-Wong E, Kristof K, Ivankovich O, et al: Inadvertent Subdural Injection: a complication of an epidural block. Anesth. Analg. 67:175–179, 1988.
149. Brown G, Atkinson GL, Standiford SB: Subdural administration of opioids. Anesthesiology 71:611–613, 1989.
150. Bernards CM, Hill HF: Morphine and alfentanil permeability through the spinal dura, arachnoid, and pia mater of dogs and monkeys. Anesthesiology 73:1214–1219, 1990.
150A. Chadwick HS, Bernards CM, Kovarik DW, Tomlin JJ: Subdural injection of morphine for postcesarean analgesia: a report of three cases. Anesthesiology 77:590–594, 1992.
151. Shnider SM, Levinson G, Ralston DH: Regional anesthesia for labor and delivery. *In* Anesthesia for obstetrics. Edited by SM Shnider, G Levinson. Baltimore, Williams & Wilkins, 1987, p. 115.
152. Bonica JJ: Principles and Practice of Obstetric Analgesia and Anesthesia. Philadelphia, F.A. Davis, 1967, pp. 721–725.
153. Stein G, Morton J, Marsh A, Collins W, et al: Headaches after childbirth. Acta. Neurol. Scand. 69:74–79, 1984.
154. Pitt B: Maternity blues. Br. J. Psychiatry. 122:431–433, 1973.
155. Reik L: Headaches in pregnancy. Semin. Neurol. 8: 187–192, 1988.
156. Bier A: Versuche uber Cocainisirung des Ruckenmakes. Deutsch Ztschr Chir 51:361, 1899.
157. Snyder G, Person D, Flor C, Wilden R: Headache in obstetrical patients; comparison of Whitacre needle versus Quincke needle. Anesthesiology 71:A860, 1989.
158. Cesarini M, Torrielli R, Lahaye F, Mene J, et al: Sprotte needle for intrathecal anaesthesia for caesarean section: incidence of postdural puncture headache. Anaesthesia 45: 656–658, 1990.
159. Ross BK, Chadwick HS, Mancuso JJ, Benedetti C: Sprotte needle for obstetric anesthesia: decreased incidence of post dural puncture headache. Reg. Anesth. 17:29–33, 1992.
160. Kunkle E, Ray B, Wolff H: Experimental studies on headache: analysis of the headache associated with changes in intracranial pressure. Neurol. Psychiatr. 49:323–358, 1943.
161. Abouleish E: Epidural blood patch for the treatment of chronic post-lumbar puncture cephalgia. Anesthesiology 49:291–292, 1978.
162. Abouleish E, deLaBega S, Blendinger I, T10, T: Long-term follow-up of epidural blood patch. Anesth. Analg. 54: 459–463, 1975.
163. Gielen M: Postdural puncture headache (PDPH): A review. Reg. Anesth. 14:101–106, 1989.
164. Fox MW, Harms RW, Davis DH: Selected neurologic complications of pregnancy. Mayo Clin. Proc. 65:1595–1618, 1990.
165. Newrick P, Read D: Subdural haematoma as a complication of spinal anaesthetic. Br. Med. J. 285:341–342, 1982.
166. Alfery DD, Marsh ML, Shapiro HM: Post-spinal headache or intracranial tumor after obstetric anesthesia. Anesthesiology 51:92–94, 1979.
167. Greene HM: Lumbar puncture and the prevention of postpuncture headache. JAMA 86:391–392, 1926.
168. Ready LB, Cuplin S, Haschke RH, Nessly M: Spinal needle determinants of rate of transdural fluid leak. Anesth. Analg. 69:457–460, 1989.
169. Mihic D: Postspinal headache and relationship of needle to longitudinal dural fibers. Reg. Anesth. 10:76–81, 1985.
170. Hatfalvi BI: The dynamics of post-spinal headache. Headache 17:64–67, 1977.
171. Hart JR, Whitacre RG: Pencil-point needle in prevention of postspinal headache. JAMA 147:657–658, 1951.
172. Lybecker H, Moller JT, May O, Nielsen HK: Incidence and prediction of postdural puncture headache. Anesth. Analg. 70:389–394, 1990.
173. Okell RW, Sprigge JS: Unintentional dural puncture. A survey of recognition and management. Anaesthesia 42: 1110–1113, 1987.
174. Ravindran RS, Viegas OJ, Tach MD, Cline PJ, et al: Bearing down at the time of delivery and the incidence of spinal headache in parturients. Anesth. Analg. 60:524–525, 1981.
175. Jones RJ: The role of recumbency in the prevention and treatment of postspinal headache. Anesth. Analg. 53: 788–796, 1974.
176. Carbaat PAT, vanCrevel H: Lumbar puncture headache: controlled study on the preventive effect of 24 hours' bed rest. Lancet 2:1133–1135, 1981.
177. Moore DC: Anesthetic Techniques for Obstetrical Anesthesia and Analgesia. Springfield, IL, Charles C. Thomas, 1964, p. 155.
178. Baysinger CL, Menk EJ, Harte E, Middaugh R: The successful treatment of dural puncture headache after failed epidural blood patch. Anesth. Analg. 65:1242–1244, 1986.
179. Usubiaga JE, Usubiaga LE, Brea LM, Goyena R: Effect of saline injections on epidural and subarachnoid space pres-

sures and relation to postspinal anesthesia headache. Anesth. Analg. 46:293–296, 1967.

180. Jarvis AP, Greenawalt JW, Fagraeus L: Intravenous caffeine for postdural puncture headache. Anesth. Analg. 65: 316–317, 1986.
181. Sechzer PH, Abel L: Post-spinal anesthesia headache treated with caffeine. Evaluation with demand method. Curr. Ther. Res. 24:307–312, 1978.
182. Baumgarten RK: Should caffeine become the first-line treatment for postdural puncture headache? Anesth. Analg. 66:913–914, 1987.
183. Camann WR, Murray RS, Mushlin PS, Lambert DH: Effects of oral caffeine on postdural puncture headache; a double-blind, placebo-controlled trial. Anesth. Analg. 70:181–184, 1990.
184. DiGiovanni AJ, Dunbar BS: Epidural injections of autologous blood for postlumbar-puncture headache. Anesth. Analg. 49:268–271, 1970.
185. Brownridge P: The management of headache following accidental dural puncture in obstetric patients. Anaesth. Intensive Care 11:4–15, 1983.
186. Ostheimer GW, Palahniuk RJ, Shnider SM: Epidural blood patch for post-lumbar-puncture headache. Anesthesiology 41:307–308, 1974.
187. Crawford JS: Experiences with epidural blood patch. Anaesthesia 35:513–515, 1980.
188. Loeser EA, Hill GE, Bennet GM, Sederberg JH: Time vs. success rate for epidural blood patch. Anesthesiology 49: 147–148, 1978.
189. Szeinfeld M, Ihmeidan IH, Moser MM, Machado R, et al: Epidural blood patch: evaluation of the volume and spread of blood injected into the epidural space. Anesthesiology 64:820–822, 1986.
190. Cheek TG, Banner R, Sauter J, Gutsche BB: Prophylactic extradural blood patch is effective; a preliminary communication. Br. J. Anaesth. 61:340–42, 1988.
191. Wilton NCT, Globerson JH, DeRosayro AM: Epidural blood patch for postdural puncture headache: it's never too late. Anesth. Analg. 65:895–896, 1986.
192. Massey EW: Mononeuropathies in pregnancy. Semin. Neurol. 8:193–196, 1988.
193. Thorsen G: Neurological sequelae after spinal anesthesia. Acta. Chir. Scand. Suppl. 121:1–272, 1947.
194. Arner O: Complications following spinal anesthesia: their significance and a technic to reduce their incidence. Acta. Chir. Scand. Suppl. 167:1–145, 1952.
195. Nicholson MJ, Eversole UH: Neurologic complications of spinal anesthesia. JAMA 132:679–685, 1946.
196. Greene NM: Neurological sequelae of spinal anesthesia. Anesthesiology 22:682–698, 1961.
197. Vandam LD, Dripps RD: Long-term follow-up of patients who received 10,098 spinal anesthetics. Syndrome of decreased intracranial pressure (headache and ocular and auditory difficulties). JAMA 161:586–591, 1956.
198. Lee JJ, Roberts RB: Paresis of the fifth cranial nerve following spinal anesthesia. Anesthesiology 49:217–218, 1978.
199. Moore DC: Complications of regional anesthesia. Springfield, IL, Charles C. Thomas, 1955.
200. Usubiaga JE: Neurological complications following epidural anesthesia. Int. Anesthesiol. Clin. 13:1–153, 1975.
201. Hellmann K: Epidural anaesthesia in obstetrics: a second look at 26,127 cases. Can. Anaesth. Soc. J. 12:398–404, 1965.
202. Hill EC: Maternal obstetric paralysis. Am. J. Obstet. Gynecol. 83:1452–1460, 1962.
203. Massey EW, Cefalo RC: Neuropathies of pregnancy. Obstet. Gynecol. Surv. 34:489–492, 1979.
204. Brown JT, McDougall A: Traumatic maternal birth palsy. J. Obstet. Gynaecol. Br. Emp. 164:431–435, 1957.
205. Philip BK: Complications of regional anesthesia for obstetrics. Reg. Anesth. 8:17–30, 1983.
206. Massey EW, Cefalo RC: Managing the carpal tunnel syndrome in pregnancy. Contemp. Ob. Gyn. 9:39–42, 1977.
207. Rhodes P: Meralgia paraesthetica in pregnancy. Lancet 2: 831, 1957.
208. Pearson MG: Meralgia paraesthetica with reference to its occurrence in pregnancy. Obstet. Gynaecol. Br. Emp. 64: 427–430, 1957.
209. Donaldson JO: Neuropathy. *In* Neurology of Pregnancy. Edited by JO Donaldson. London, W.B. Saunders Co., 1989, pp. 23–59.
210. Adelman U, Goldberg GS, Puckett JD: Postpartum bilateral femoral neuropathy. Obstet. Gynecol. 42:845–850, 1973.
211. Whittaker WG: Injuries to the sacral plexus in obstetrics. Can. Med. Assoc. J. 79:622–627, 1958.
212. Crawford JS: Lumbar epidural block in labour: a clinical analysis. Br. J. Anaesth. 44:66–74, 1972.
213. Grove LH: Backache, headache, and bladder dysfunction after delivery. Br. J. Anaesth. 45:1147–1149, 1973.
214. MacArthur C, Lewis M, Knox EG, Crawford JS: Epidural anaesthesia and long term backache after childbirth. Br. Med. J. 301:9–12, 1990.
215. Bromage PR: Neurologic complications of regional anesthesia for obstetrics. *In* Anesthesia for Obstetrics. 3rd edition. Edited by SM Shnider, G Levinson. Baltimore, Williams & Wilkins, 1993, pp. 433–453.
216. O'Connell JEA: Lumbar disc protrusions in pregnancy. J. Neurol. Neurosurg. Psychiatry. 23:138–141, 1960.
217. Cuerden C, Buley R, Downing JW: Delayed recovery after epidural analgesia for labour. Anaesthesia 32:773–776, 1977.
218. Pathy GV, Rosen M: Prolonged block with recovery after extradural analgesia for labour. Br. J. Anaesth. 47:520–522, 1975.
219. Vandam LD, Dripps RD: A Long-term follow-up of 10,098 spinal anesthetics. II. Incidence and analysis of minor sensory neurological defects. Surgery 38:463–469, 1955.
220. Rigler ML, Drasner K, Krejcie TC, Yelich SJ, et al: Caudal equina syndrome after continuous spinal anesthesia. Anesth. Analg. 72:275–281, 1991.
221. Lambert DH, Hurley RJ: Caudal equina syndrome and continuous spinal anesthesia. Anesth. Analg. 72:817–819, 1991.
222. Ross BK, Coda B, Heath CH: Local anesthetic distribution in a spinal model: a possible mechanism of neurologic injury after continuous spinal anesthesia. Reg. Anesth. 17: 69–77, 1992.
223. Rigler MR, Drasner K: Distribution of catheter-injected local anesthetic in a model of the subarachnoid space. Anesthesiology 75:684–692, 1991.
224. Vandam LD, Dripps RD: Exacerbation of pre-existing neurologic disease after spinal anesthesia. N. Engl. J. Med. 255: 843–849, 1956.
225. Donaldson JO: Neuropathy. *In* Neurology of Pregnancy. Edited by JO Donaldson. London, W.B. Saunders Co., 1989, pp. 23–59.
226. Costabile G, Husag L, Probst C: Spinal epidural hematoma. Surg. Neurol. 21:489–492, 1984.
227. Dawson BH: Paraplegia due to spinal epidural haematoma. J. Neurol. Neurosurg. Psychiatry 26:171–173, 1963.
228. Bidzinski J: Spontaneous spinal epidural hematoma during pregnancy: case report. J. Neurosurg. 24:1017, 1966.
229. Yonekawa Y, Medhorn HM, Nishikawa M: Spontaneous

spinal epidural hematoma during pregnancy. Surg. Neurol. 3:327–328, 1975.
230. Owens EL, Kasten GW, Hessel EA, II: Spinal subarachnoid hematoma after lumbar puncture and heparinization: a case report, review of the literature, and discussion of anesthetic implications. Anesth. Analg. 65:1201–1207, 1986.
231. Shnider SM, Levinson G, Ralston DH: Regional anesthesia for labor and delivery. *In* Anesthesia for Obstetrics. 3rd edition. Edited by SM Shnider, G Levinson. Baltimore, Williams & Wilkins, 1983, pp. 150.
232. Burrows RF, Kelton JG: Thrombocytopenia at delivery: a prospective survey of 6715 deliveries. Am. J. Obstet. Gynecol. 162:731–734, 1990.
233. Rasmus KT, Rottman RL, Kotelko DM, Wright WC, et al: Unrecognized thrombocytopenia and regional anesthesia in parturients: A retrospective review. Obstet. Gynecol. 73:943–946, 1989.
234. Rolbin SH, Abbott D, Musclow E, Papsin F, et al: Epidural anesthesia in pregnant patients with low platelet counts. Obstet. Gynecol. 71:918–920, 1988.
235. Kelton JG, Hunter DJS, Neame PB: A platelet function defect in preeclampsia. Obstet. Gynecol. 65:107–109, 1985.
236. Baker AS, Ojeman RG, Swartz MN, Richardson EP: Spinal epidural abscess. N. Engl. J. Med. 293:463–468, 1975.
237. Male CG, Martin R: Puerperal spinal epidural abscess. Lancet, March 17, 1973:608–609, 1973.
238. Loarie DJ, Fairley HB: Epidural abscess following spinal anesthesia. Anesth. Analg. 57:351–353, 1978.
239. Bromage PR: Epidural Analgesia. Philadelphia, W.B. Saunders Co., 1978, pp. 682–690.
240. Strong WE: Epidural abscess associated with epidural catheterization: a rare event? Report of two cases with markedly delayed presentation. Anesthesiology 74:943–946, 1991.
241. Berga S, Trierweiler MW: Bacterial meningitis following epidural anesthesia for vaginal delivery: A case report. Obstet. Gynecol. 74:437–439, 1989.
242. Ready LB, Helfer D: Bacterial meningitis in parturients after epidural anesthesia. Anesthesiology 71:988–990, 1989.
243. Roberts SP, Petts HV: Meningitis after obstetric spinal anaesthesia. Anaesthesia 45:376–377, 1990.
244. Behl S: Epidural analgesia in the presence of fever. Anaesthesia 40:1240–1241, 1985.
245. Carp H, Bailey S: The association between meningitis and dural puncture in bacteremic rats. Anesthesiology 76: 739–742, 1992.
246. Chestnut DH: Spinal anesthesia in the febrile patient. Anesthesiology 76:667–669, 1992.
247. Brown ZA, Berry S, Vontver LA: Genital herpes simplex virus infections complicating pregnancy; natural history and peripartum management. J. Reprod. Med. 31:420–425, 1986.
248. Ramanathan S, Sheth R, Turndorf H: Anesthesia for cesarean section in patients with genital herpes infections: A retrospective study. Anesthesiology 64:807–809, 1986.
249. Crosby ET, Halpern SH, Rolbin SH: Epidural anaesthesia for caesarean section in patients with active recurrent genital herpes simplex infections: a retrospective review. Can. J. Anaesth. 36:701–704, 1989.
250. Meyers RR, Kalichman MW, Reisner LS, Powell HC: Neurotoxicity of local anesthetics. Anesthesiology 65:119–120, 1986.
251. Ready LB, Plumer MH, Haschke RH, Austin E, et al: Neurotoxicity of intrathecal local anesthetics in rabbits. Anesthesiology 63:364–370, 1985.
252. Marx GF: Maternal complications of regional anesthesia. Reg. Anesth. 6: 104–107, 1981.
253. Goldman WW, Sanford JP: An "epidemic" of chemical meningitis. Am. J. Med. 29:94–101, 1960.
254. Reisner LS, Hochman BN, Plumer MH: Persistent neurologic deficit and adhesive arachnoiditis following intrathecal 2-chloroprocaine injection. Anesth. Analg. 59: 452–454, 1985.
255. Ravindran RS, Bond VK, Tasch MD, Gupta CD, et al: Prolonged neuronal blockade following regional analgesia with 2-chloroprocaine. Anesth. Analg. 59:447–451, 1980.
256. Gissen AJ, Datta S, Lambert D: The chloroprocaine controversy. II. Is chloroprocaine neurotoxic? Reg. Anesth. 9: 135–145, 1984.
257. Wang BC, Hillman DE, Spielholz NI, Turndorf H: Chronic neurological deficits and Nesacaien-CE: an effect of the anesthetic, 2-chloroprocaine, or the antioxidant, sodium bisulfite? Anesth. Analg. 63:445–447, 1984.
258. Meyers RR, Kalichman MW, Reisner LS, Powell HC: Neurotoxicity of local anesthetics: Altered perineural permeability, edema, and nerve fiber injury. Anesthesiology 64: 29–35, 1986.
259. Fibuch EE, Opper SE: Back pain following epidurally administered Nesacaine-MPF. Anesth. Analg. 69:113–115, 1989.
260. Ackerman WE III: Back pain after epidural Nesacaine-MPF. Anesth. Analg. 70:224–226, 1990.
261. Jaameri K, Jahkola A, Perttu J: On shivering in association with normal delivery. Acta. Obstet. Gynecol. Scan. 45: 383–388, 1966.
262. Shehabi Y, Gatt S, Buckman T, Isert P: Effect of adrenaline, fentanyl and warming of injectate on shivering following extradural analgesia in labour. Anaesth. Intens. Care 18: 31–37, 1990.
263. Sessler DI, Ponte J: Shivering during epidural anesthesia. Anesthesiology 72:816–821, 1990.
264. Goodlin R, O'Connell L, Gunther R: Childbirth chills are they an immunological reaction? Lancet ii (7506):79–80, 1967.
265. Ponte J, Collett BJ, Walmsley A: Anaesthetic temperature and shivering in epidural anaesthesia. Acta. Anaesthesiol. Scand. 30:584–587, 1986.
266. Ponte J, Sessler DI: Extradurals and shivering: Effects of cold and warm extradural saline injections in volunteers. Br. J. Anaesth. 64:731–733, 1990.
267. Glosten B, Sessler DI, Ostman LG, Faure EAM, et al: Intravenous lidocaine does not cause shivering-like tremor or alter thermoregulation. Reg. Anesth. 16:218–222, 1991.
268. Workhoven MN: Intravenous fluid temperature, shivering, and the parturient. Anesth. Analg. 65:496–498, 1986.
269. Aglio LS, Johnson MD, Datta S, Ostheimer GW: Warm intravenous fluids reduce shivering in parturients receiving epidural analgesia. Anesthesiology 69:A701, 1988.
270. Casey WF, Smith CE, Katz JM, O'Loughlin K, et al: Intravenous meperidine for control of shivering during emergency cesarean section under epidural anesthesia. Anesth. Analg. 67:S27, 1988.
271. Brownridge T: Shivering related to epidural blockade with bupivacaine in labor, and the influence of epidural pethidine. Anaesth. Intensive Care 14:412–417, 1986.
272. Matthews NC, Corser G: Epidural fentanyl for shaking in obstetrics. Anaesthesia 43:783–785, 1988.
273. Sevorino FB, Johnson MD, Lema MJ, Datta S, et al: The effect of epidural sufentanil on shivering and body temperature in the parturient. Anesth. Analg. 68:530–533, 1989.
274. Liu WHD, Luxton MC: The effect of prophylactic fentanyl on shivering in elective Caesarean section under epidural analgesia. Anaesthesia 46:344–348, 1991.

Section D

# PHARMACOLOGY AND TECHNIQUES OF GENERAL ANALGESIA AND ANESTHESIA

# Chapter 17

# OPIOIDS, SEDATIVES, HYPNOTICS, ATARACTICS

COSTANTINO BENEDETTI

This chapter discusses the pharmacology and clinical application of the medications, except local anesthetics and inhalation agents, used in obstetrics to provide the mother with comfort during the predelivery period. Because all these drugs cross the placenta, the fetus and the newborn also experience the drug's pharmacologic effects, which often are even more pronounced in them than in the mother. Because of the depressant effects caused by these drugs on the newborn, they are not used as frequently as in the past, especially before delivery. The main exception is the use of low doses of intraspinal opioids given in combination with intraspinal local anesthetic agents to induce a synergistic analgesic effect.

It is essential that all members of the obstetric team be knowledgeable of medications and their effects because successful obstetric analgesia and anesthesia rests on the fine balance between relief of pain for the mother without risk to her, the fetus, and the infant. In the first edition of this book Bonica stated:

> "The primary mission of the physician is to select indicated drugs and techniques and to use them in a way that causes the least alteration of the maternal and fetal physiology. How effectively such a great responsibility is discharged depends primarily on application of the knowledge of how each drug affects every function of the mother and infant, and on the physician's skill, experience and judgment (1)."

This still holds true today and, in medical centers where expert anesthesiologists are available 24 hours a day, the use of regional analgesia, obtainable with different techniques and drug combinations, is preferable to the systemic administration of a number of medications.

The intensity of parturition's pain varies greatly in relation to the various stages of labor and delivery of the infant. In the latent phase of the first stage, most women report a mild to moderate pain, which gradually increases to become severe and at times excruciating during the active phase of delivery. As for any painful experience, there is a great variation among patients. Recent statistics from the United States, Canada, and Sweden report that 20% of patients experience mild to moderate pain throughout delivery, 30% of patients experience moderate to severe pain, and 15% of patients experience severe to excruciating pain during the active phase of the first stage (2).

(From J Jones, F Smith, G Rabbit: Acute pain: A review of its effects and therapy with systemic opioids. *In* Advances In Pain Research and Therapy: Opioid Analgesia. Vol. 2. Edited by C Benedetti, CR Chapman, G. Geron. New York, Raven Press, 1990)

Surgical interventions are employed more frequently for the delivery of neonates. In some centers, cesarean sections are used in 40% of all deliveries. In these situations, anesthesia has to be provided to the mother for the delivery and analgesia provided after the surgical intervention. It is clear, therefore, that during the predelivery period, a continuum of different intensity of analgesia, up to surgical anesthesia, may have to be provided. For this reason, it is of paramount importance that the physician be familiar with the pharmacology and application of opioids and sedatives to employ them properly and to be aware of the differences these medications have on the mother and the neonate in both effect and intensity.

This chapter comprises several topics. After brief historical notes and terminology, opioids will be described, including their general principle of pharmacology, clinical effects, and general indications of the most frequently used opioids with a particular focus on the effects on the mother, labor, and fetus/newborn. The clinical application of these substances will then be illustrated. Sedatives, hypnotics, and ataractics will be discussed succinctly, as they are no longer used extensively due to the depressive effects on the neonate, though still employed when general anesthesia for the mother is indicated (see Chapter 19). Ketamine, a dissociative analgesic/anesthetic agent, which has different applications in obstetrics both as an analgesic and an anesthetic agent, will be described.

## HISTORICAL NOTES

### *Opioids and Their Derivatives*

In the history of humanity very few substances have enjoyed such a prolonged and widespread use as the extract of Papaver somniferum and the substances related to it. Its pharmacologic effects were well known over 5000 years ago when, at the dawn of recorded history, the Sumerians mentioned the poppy in their pharmacopeia (3) and called it "HU GIL," the plant of joy. The word "opium," first used by Plinius the Elder in the first century A.D., derives its meaning from the Greek "opus," which means vegetable juice (4). Greek and Roman physicians used preparations containing opium to alleviate arthritic pain, chest pain, uncontrollable cough, to induce sedation, and for its styptic effect (5). Opium was used extensively to treat dysentery, which ravaged Europe and the Middle

East during the first millenium A.D. In ancient Hebrew medicine, opium is included as the main substance of at least two different potions. One was used to induce analgesia and sleep during surgical operation, and another, containing also wine or vinegar, was given to condemned people to alleviate the pain of death (3,4).

The use of opium for inducing analgesia during surgical operations is described in the records of the medical school of Salerno which flourished in the 9th Century A.D. Nicolaus Salernitanus gives a precise description of how to prepare the "Spongia somnifera," sleeping draught (6,7). In the 13th Century, Boccaccio mentions such a preparation in one of the novels of the "Decameron (8)," and in the 15th Century, Hugo from Lucca and other physicians of the medical school of Bologna are reported to have used such potions (9–11). While sporadic attempts were made in this period to alleviate the pain of surgery, the concept of relieving pain suffered from parturition were highly unpopular, as its use was thought to contradict the revelation of the Old Testament. In 1591, Eufame MacAlyane, of Edinburgh, was buried alive for seeking relief of pain during the delivery of her two children (12). Great advances have been made in our searches since then. We have only recently appreciated the life-threatening effects that intense pain can have on a mother with severe cardiovascular disease or on a fetus with a borderline functioning placenta (see Chapters 31 and 41).

In the 16th Century, Paracelsius introduced Laudanum, a mixture of 10% opium in a hydroalcoholic extract, which is still used today in several countries for the treatment of pain. In 1803, a young German pharmacist, F.A.W. Sertürner, isolated an alkaloid of opium and called it "morphium" from the Greek god of sleep and dreams, Morpheus (13,14). Later, it was renamed "morphia" and then "morphine." We now know that about 25 alkaloids can be extracted from the juice of the Papaver somnifurum. The content of the most important alkaloids will vary depending from the area of the world where the plant was grown: morphine content can vary from 4 to 21%, codeine 0.8 to 2.5%, papaverine 0.5 to 2.5%, and thebaine 0.5 to 2% (15). Introductions of the hypodermal needle by Wood and the hypodermic syringe by Pravaz in 1853 opened the way to the widespread clinical application of morphine (16). During both the Franco-Prussian and the American Civil wars dependency to morphine became known as the "soldiers' disease" (15).

In 1901, Dr. Katawata (17) of Japan reported the injection of 10 mg of morphine combined with 20 mg eucaine, a local anesthetic, into the subarachnoid space of two patients with uncontrollable back pain. The patients obtained excellent pain relief, which lasted in one of them for 2 days and for several days in the other. Katawata reported no side-effects from the procedure; however, this technique was not used again until 75 years later.

Pohl, in 1915, discovered an antagonist of morphine, but it was not until 1951 that Wikler and Eckenhoff independently used an antagonist for the first time to reverse the effect of morphine overdose in man, opening an era of greater safety in the use of opiates (18–20). In the 1950s, several opioid antagonists and agonist/antagonists were developed; however, it was not until the late 1960s and early 1970s that careful investigations were begun to elucidate the effects of opioids on the central nervous system (21). The discovery of endogenous opioids in the mid-1970s further stimulated basic and clinical research on these substances. At the same time, opioid receptors were identified in the spinal cord of animals. These discoveries prompted, in 1974, the study of injection of morphine in the subarachnoid space of animals. Yaksh and Rudy (22) reported in 1976 that opioids, applied to the subarachnoid space of rats, induced significant analgesia with distribution that paralleled the segment of the spinal cord exposed to the opioid. The next step was the application of this technique in humans. Wang and associates, in 1979 (23), reported the intrathecal injection of 0.5 to 1 mg of morphine in eight patients suffering from severe, intractable cancer pain. The results were very encouraging, as morphine was able to produce fast, profound, and long-lasting pain relief. The average duration of relief was reported to be of 20 hours (12 to 24 hours), and the onset of maximum analgesia was within 15 to 45 minutes from injection. Of greater importance, other somatosensory, motor, and sympathetic functions were not affected by the intrathecal opioids. This made its use preferable to the use of local anesthetic because this technique afforded cardiovascular stability and the ability of the patient to ambulate. This first report was soon followed by many others from various parts of the world. Also in 1979, Behar, et al (24) and Cousins, et al (25) reported that injection of morphine in the epidural space afforded similar pain relief in cancer patients. In 1980, Bromage, et al (26) reported the use of epidural opiates for postoperative pain; Pasqualucci, et al (27) used intrathecal morphine for myocardial infarction pain and Scott, et al (28) for labor pain. Since then, most opioids have been used with success: morphine (29–31), fentanyl (32), meperidine (33), Beta-endorphin (34), buprenorphine (35), methadone (26), and diamorphine (36).

## Psychotropic Agents

Mind- and consciousness-altering drugs have been a part of human life since earliest times, as evidenced by the use of such drugs as alcohol in the form of beer from cereal, wine from fruits and berries, and mead from honey (37).

For over a 1000 years the dried rhizome and roots of Valeriana officinalis have been used for their calmative effects to allay nervousness and hysteria. Some active constituents, called valepotriates, have mild but definite tranquilizing activity. Most important, this effect is not synergistic with other sedatives like alcohol and barbiturate (38).

Another class of psychotropic agents known for centuries both in America and Europe is the tropane alkaloids, which are mostly derived from plants of the potato family, the Solanaceae, to which the genus Datura belongs. Many species of this genus contain pharmacologic active compounds such as scopolamine (hyoscine) and atropine [(+) hyoscyamine] that have been used for centuries for cosmetic and ritual purposes (15). These compounds act as blocking agents of the postganglionic cholinergic neurons. They first stimulate then depress the medulla and higher cerebral centers; inhibit gastric secretion and motility, increase heart rate, decrease glandular secretion of the nasal-oral mucosa and of the respiratory tract; and relax the muscles of the bronchi and cause vasodilatation. In the Middle Ages, women of southern Europe learned that the instillation in the eyes of the juice of the berry would produce a striking appearance by causing mydriasis, while the ingestion of the entire plant could cause severe symptoms and even death. They called the plant Atropa belladonna (38) (Atropos was the Greek Fate that cut the thread of life, and underscores the deadly effects of the plant, while bella donna, from Italian meaning "beautiful lady" refers to its effects if used properly (38)). The active substance of Atropa belladonna was later called atropine. While atropine does not cross the blood-brain barrier and therefore no effect on the CNS, scopolamine does and its effects on the CNS can be intense. At high doses it induces unconsciousness preceded and followed by vivid, colorful hallucinations. Native American medicine men have used the extracts of either Datura stramonium or meteloides to initiate young men to magic and religious rites for centuries. In Europe, it was learned that by boiling plants of this type and mixing the extract with fats and oils, powerful mixtures could be obtained. By rubbing these ointments on the skin or inserting into body orifices, people could escape from the often difficult reality to the most vivid of dream states. The dreams most frequently described were of flying freely in the air. The familiar pictures of witches flying on a broomstick are derived from the description of these hallucinations and the use of an anointed broom staff to apply the mixture to the perivaginal area, from where it was readily absorbed. Equally, the derivative of tropane could lead users to believe that they were lycanthropes (werewolves) (15). We read from a 1602 report by Boguet: "... Thus, for some the solanaceous ointment was a means of metamorphosing to werewolves while others for experiencing the witches flight (39)." The use of these substances was strongly opposed by the Christian religion and their use never became widespread for medical use. Atropine and scopolamine are now used at low doses mostly for their anticholinergic action. Scopolamine, together with an opioid, was used extensively in obstetrics in the 1950s and early 1960s to induce analgesia, sedation, and amnesia during labor and delivery, and scopolamine and an opioid were the main components of the so called Twilight Sleep (40). Because of its predictable, violent delirium, this technique is no longer used in most parts of the world. Presently, the only recommended use of scopolamine is the transdermal preparation used to treat nausea induced by motion sickness and opioids.

In 1869, Oskar Liebriech introduced chloral hydrate as an hypnotic agent, which is still widely used. Paraldehyde was another notable sedative that followed. In 1864, Adolf von Baeyer synthesized malonyl urea, later known as barbituric acid. Barbiturates, of which several hundred analogues were synthesized, have been used extensively since the beginning of this century as sedative-hypnotics. Rauwolfia serpentina extracts were reported in Indian medical literature describing sedating and hypotensive properties with a long history of use (37). Although phenothiazines (active derivatives of Rauwolfia) were independently synthesized as part of the development of aniline dyes in the 1800s, their medicinal use was not explored until the 1940s (41). In 1960, Chlordiazepoxide (Librium) was the first benzodiazepine introduced into clinical use as an anxiolitic, for preoperative sedation and to treat alcohol withdrawal. The following year, Diazepam (Valium) was marketed and, due to its rapid onset, oral availability, and very low acute toxicity, became one of the most frequently prescribed drugs. In 1978, Midazolam was introduced for clinical use and has gained significant popularity due to its relatively short duration and lack of venous irritability. The discovery in 1977 of specific benzodiazepine receptors in both the animal and human brain has greatly increased our knowledge of the pharmacology of these compounds.

## TERMINOLOGY

### *Opioids (Narcotics)*

The term narcotic is now outdated and a new terminology is preferred for these substances. Exogenous and endogenous ligands with morphine-like effects have varyingly been termed opiates or opioids. A ligand is a substance that binds to a receptor (Latin "legare" = to bind). The current consensus is that the term opiate should be used only for morphine and other substances with the morphinan or related chemical structures (direct derivatives of morphine), and that the term opioid should apply to all substances with morphine-like properties, including the endogenous peptides. Hence, opioid receptor is used instead of opiate receptor. In the same manner, the use of endogenous opioids or opioid peptides as a generic term should be preferred to endorphins (42).

To induce their pharmacologic effects, most drugs must bind with specific macromolecules located on the cell membrane, called receptors with which a ligand interacts. The binding site is the part of this macromolecule at which the binding interaction takes place. Coupled to the binding site is an effector mechanism and, usually, an amplifier system. The drug-receptor interaction is characterized by at least two parameters, the affinity of the drug toward the binding site and the efficacy (or intrinsic activity) of the drug (i.e., the ability of the drug to activate the effector mechanism when bound to the receptor). Thus, by definition, a pure antagonist has receptor affinity but zero efficacy. The multiple forms of receptor for a specific class of drug (i.e. opioids) are called types (42).

### *Sedative/hypnotic—Tranquilizer—Ataractics*

Sedative-hypnotic refers to the same class of drugs that when given at a certain dose provides sedation (Latin "sedare" = to allay, to calm) and, at higher doses, sleep (Greek "hypnos" = to sleep). A tranquilizer (Latin "tranquillitas" = stillness, calmness) is a more recent word used to designate the newer psychotropic drugs, mostly the benzodiazepines (43). Benzodiazepines are also referred to as anxiolytic (Latin "anxietas" = a troubled state" + Greek "lysis" = a loosening) (43). The older term ataraxics, which is seldom used today, comes from ataraxia (Greek "a" = without + "taraktos" = disturb; meaning, therefore, calmness of mind). Ataraxics was employed by Stoics and Skeptics to denote a freedom from the emotions which proceed from vanity and self conceit (43).

## Opioid Analgesics

This section describes the general pharmacology of opioids, including the mechanism of analgesia, other therapeutic effects, and the undesirable effects and complications induced by this group of drugs. This description is followed by a more detailed discussion of the most important opioid analgesics.

### *General Principles of Pharmacology*

Opioids have pharmacologic effects on almost every organ and function in the human body (44). Some of these effects are beneficial and some are not. One specific action can be beneficial in one circumstance but not in another. For instance, the constipating effect is useful to treat diarrhea, but bothersome during analgesic therapy. The most important targets of this group of drugs are the central nervous system and the gastrointestinal system. The effects on the central nervous system are remarkably diverse and include analgesia, euphoria or dysphoria, sedation, drowsiness, emesis, dizziness, hypoventilation, myosis, and pruritus. All opioids cause the above stated effects but the intensity of these effects may vary even when individual opioids are given in equianalgesic doses.

Opioid effects are mediated by specific receptors located on cell membranes. In the central nervous system, these receptors have been identified both pre- and postsynaptically. While we do not know all the details, several physical-biochemical steps are involved from the first interaction of the agonist opioid with the receptor to the observable biological changes. What follows is a simplistic description of some of the known events (42).

As previously mentioned, opioid receptors are macromolecules composed of at least two parts: a binding site, which interacts with the opioid molecule, and a triggering mechanism, which activates a number of sequential biochemical reactions that lead to the final neuronal effect of the opioid. The basic effect of opioids is that of neuronal inhibition, accomplished either by blocking the release of neurotransmitters or by hyperpolarization of the cell. Inhibition of neurotransmitter release is caused by changes in the CA + + channels, and this effect occurs in neurons with presynaptic receptors.

Conversely, hyperpolarization of the neuron is due to alterations of the K+ channel induced by activation of postsynaptic receptors. If, after the application of an opioid, a stimulating effect is observed in vivo, this is due to the inhibition of inhibitory neurons in a polyneuronal system. The union of the opioid agonist with the receptor and the sequential reactions may be described as follows (42).

Once the molecules of an opioid have reached the proximity of the neural cell in the central nervous system, they come in repeated contact with the neuronal cell membrane as they float in the extracellular fluid. If, during these contacts an opioid binding site (part of the receptor macromolecule) is encountered, a brief union occurs causing a conformational change in the other part of the receptor macromolecule. This change triggers the first of a sequential series of auto-activating biochemical reactions that leads to the final neuronal effect of inhibition.

Many opioid receptors are located on each cell membrane and a fixed, albeit partial, number of them must be activated by a specific opioid to obtain the pharmacologic effect. Different agonists, acting on the same type of receptors, have to activate a particular number of them to elicit the same neuronal effect. To illustrate this concept more clearly, let us compare two opioids: morphine and fentanyl. Morphine has to activate a larger number of mu receptors than fentanyl to cause the final inhibitory effect. Morphine has therefore been defined as having low efficacy compared to fentanyl for the mu receptor. This concept of efficacy is important in explaining some of the clinical observations related to opioid tolerance. As a receptor is exposed to many unions with opioid molecules, the part of macromolecule involved with the triggering of the sequential biochemical intracellular reactions becomes inactive so that the union between the binding site and the opioid is not followed by any reaction. These receptors have been called silent, as they are unable to activate the transduction and effector mechanisms. As an increasing number of normally functioning receptors exhaust their ability to induce the biological reactions (and therefore become silent receptors), the chances that the required fixed number of active receptors interact with opioid molecules gradually decrease unless an increased number of opioid molecules (increased dose) are exposed to them. However, as more receptors become silent even the highest dose of opioids will be ineffective. Because opioids with low efficacy need to activate a larger number of receptors, they will become ineffective sooner than high-efficacy opioids. This concept can be used clinically to treat patients who have become tolerant to low-efficacy opioids (morphine) by switching to one with high efficacy (fentanyl) (Figure 17–1).

#### *Opioid Receptor Types*

For many years it has been hypothesized that several opioid receptors exist and up to five receptors have been implicated in opioid induced analgesia: mu, kappa, delta, epsilon, and sigma (44–48). Recently, however, just the mu, kappa, and delta are considered true opioid receptors.

In brief, the mu receptors, believed by Pasternak to be two subtypes, $mu_1$ and $mu_2$ (49), mediate supraspinal analgesia, euphoria, respiratory depression, constipation, pruritus, urinary retention, nausea and vomiting, and physical dependence; the delta receptors mediate analgesia, show little or no cross tolerance with mu agonists and, when partially activated by a subanalgesic dose of delta agonists, greatly potentiate morphine analgesia; the kappa receptors mediate spinal analgesia, myosis, sedation and have cross tolerance with mu receptors. The identity and existence of the epsilon receptor are presently in question (47). The sigma receptors mediate dysphoria,

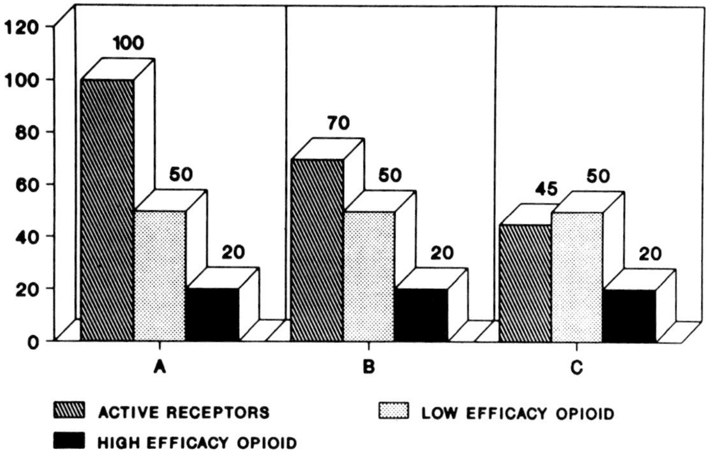


**Fig. 17–1.** Conceptual model of opioid ligands and receptors interaction in naive **(A)**; moderately **(B)**; and highly **(C)** tolerant patients. A discreet number of receptors are present on the cell membrane; they change from active to silent as they are exposed to prolonged opioid interaction (see text). Different opioids must activate a definite number of receptors to produce the biochemical effect. A low efficacy opioid will have to activate more receptors than a high efficacy one. In **(A)** (naive patient) 100 hypothetical active receptors are present and both high and low efficacy drugs will cause a biological response. In **(B)**, as tolerance develops, the number of active receptors will decrease so that the number of receptors to be activated by a low efficacy drug will be close to the number of active receptors present, therefore an increased dose of the drugs will be needed to obtain the same response. In **(C)**, with high tolerance, the number of active receptors is less than the number of receptors needed for a low efficacy drug to produce the effect; therefore, at any dose, this drug will be ineffective. However, a high efficacy drug will still be able to provide an effect because the number of active receptors is higher than the number of receptors needed to be occupied. (Redrawn from Benedetti C: Acute pain: A review of its effects and therapy with systemic opioids. *In* Advances in Pain Research and Therapy: Opioid Analgesia. Vol. 14. Edited by C Benedetti, CR Chapman, G Giron. New York, Raven Press, 1990.)

hallucination, and stimulation of respiratory and vasomotor centers (Table 17–1). Recent findings suggest that sigma receptor agonists, which include ketamine and phencyclidine (PCP, "angel dust"), are potent agonists of excitatory transmitters at the spinal cord level and are not reversed by naloxone. These characteristics suggest that the sigma receptor does not belong to the family of opioid receptors (48). Specific opioids have different affinities for each of these receptors (Table 17–2), which in turn have a heterogeneous distribution in the organism and different functions.

Recent clinical observations indicate that agonists for different opioid receptors might relieve different types of pain syndromes. Pancreatic pain, for example, is poorly relieved by average doses of morphine but is well controlled by standard doses of buprenorphine. (Arner, personal communication, 1987)

## *Pharmacokinetics and Pharmacodynamics*

When studying the action of a drug on a living organism, several factors must be considered. Absorption, distribu-

**Table 17–1.** Opiate Receptor Effects

| $Mu_1$ | $Mu_2$ | Kappa | Sigma | Delta |
|---|---|---|---|---|
| Morphine | | bremazocine | *N*-allylcyclazocine | morphine |
| β-Endorphin | | dynorphin | | leu-enkephalin |
| Analgesia | no analgesia | analgesia; excessive heat | no analgesia | no analgesia |
| Apnea?? | apnea | apnea ± | tachypnea | apnea$^{++}$ |
| Indifference | sedation | sedation | delirium | ? |
| Miosis | | miosis | mydriasis | |
| Nausea and vomiting | | | | nausea and vomiting |
| Constipation | | | | |
| Urine retention | | diuresis | | |
| Pruritus | | no change | no change | pruritus |
| Change in temperature | | | | |
| δ cross | | no cross | | μ cross |
| Tolerance | | tolerance | | cross-tolerance |

(From Benedetti C: Acute pain: a review of its effects and therapy with systemic opioids. *In* Advances In Pain Research and Therapy, Vol. 14. Edited by C Benedetti. New York, Raven Press, 1990.)

**Table 17–2.** Opiate Receptor Interactions

| Drug | Receptor | | | | |
|---|---|---|---|---|---|
| | Mu | Kappa | Sigma | Delta | Epsilon |
| Exogenous | | | | | |
| morphine | + + + | + | | + + | |
| fentanyl | + + + + | | | + | |
| alfentanil | + + + | | | ? | |
| sulfentanil | + + + + | | | + | |
| lofentanil | + + + | | | ? | |
| meperidine | + + | | | + + | |
| hyromorphone | + + + | | | + + | |
| methadone | + + + | | | + + | |
| naloxone | − | − | − | − | |
| naloxazone | − − − − | | | | |
| naloxonazine | − − − − | | | | |
| nalbuphine | | + + + | + | | |
| pentazocine | − | + + + | + + | ? | − − |
| nalorphine | | + + | + + + | + + | |
| bremazocine | | + + + | | | |
| ketocyclazocine | | + + + | | | |
| butorphanol | | + + | + + | | |
| phencycladine | | | + + + | | |
| Endogenous | | | | | |
| β-endorphin | + + + | | | + + | + + + |
| D-Ala-D-Leu-enkephalin | | | | + + + | |
| leu-enkephalin | + | | | + + + | + + |
| met-enkephalin | + + + | | | + + + | |
| dynorphin (small) | | + + + + | | | |
| dynorphin (large) | | + + + | | | |
| α-neoendorphin | | + + + | | | |

(From Benedetti C: Acute pain: a review of its effects and therapy with systemic opioids. In Advances In Pain Research and Therapy, Vol. 14. Edited by C Benedetti. New York, Raven Press, 1990.)

tion, and elimination comprise the study of pharmacokinetics, a dynamic parameter relating to the concentration of a drug in the blood, cerebrospinal fluids (CSF), or tissues. Pharmacodynamics relates to the mechanism of action and to the strength of the pharmacologic effects of a drug (50). Even though this is a general term, in 1981 Holford succinctly said: "Pharmacokinetic is what the body does to the drug, while pharmacodynamics is what the drug does to the body (51)." It is easy to visualize the complexity of the interrelation between these two branches of pharmacology.(52). Depending on the dose, on the amount of absorption, amount and type of proteins in the plasma (53), and variations in metabolism and excretions, different concentrations of a drug reach the site of action that influence but do not determine the intensity and duration of the effects (54).

After IV injection or absorption into the vascular system from other routes of administration, an opioid is immediately affected by plasma pH and by its propensity to bind to various circulating elements (e.g., red blood cells, plasma proteins). To induce its pharmacologic effects, the substance must leave the plasma, diffuse into the tissues, reach the receptors, and activate them. Several factors favor movement of the drug to its sites of action: lower protein binding; lower ionization; and higher lipid solubility.

In plasma, only the unbound and nonionized portion of the drug, called the diffusible fraction, is free to leave the vasculature. The diffusible fraction determines the initial concentration gradient and therefore the rate of diffusion. The other factor in determining the rate of movement of the drug from plasma and extravascular fluid to tissues is lipid solubility. For rapid access to the CNS, an opioid must have both a high diffusible fraction and a high lipid solubility.

The product of the diffusible fraction and the lipid solubility of an opioid is known as the diffusion potential into the CNS. The ratio of the diffusion potential of an opioid compared to that of morphine is called the lipid diffusion index or LDI. Thus, the lipid diffusion index of morphine is 1, meperidine, 14, and of fentanyl, 160.

After an IV bolus of fentanyl, the opioid enters the brain rapidly because of its high diffusion potential. As the plasma concentration falls, the result of removal of the drug by tissues and biotransformation, the gradient reverses and fentanyl leaves the brain equally rapidly. Meperidine follows the same process of forward and then reverse transfer, to and from the brain, but more slowly because of its lower diffusion potential. Morphine has the lowest diffusion potential of all the common opioids that results in some delay between IV morphine injection and development of maximal brain concentration (and onset of maximal effect). Morphine leaves plasma so slowly that biotransformation or elimination lowers plasma concentration and further decreases the "driving concentration" during the onset period, causing a further reduction of its rate of diffusion into the CNS. However, due to its low lipid solubility, less drug will be nonspecifically bound by

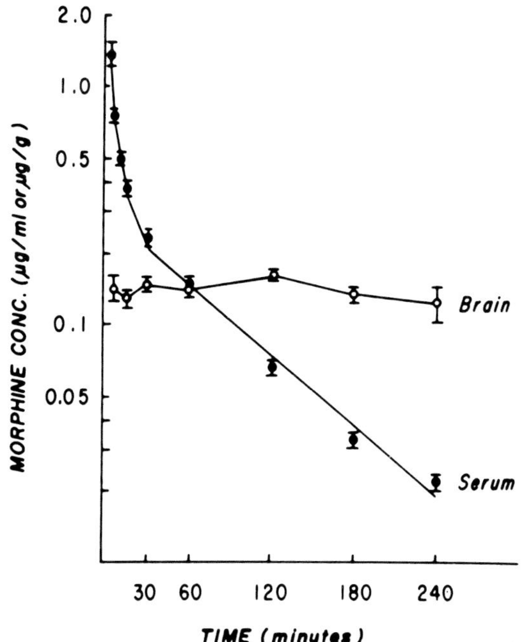


**Fig. 17–2.** Lack of relationship between serum and brain concentration of morphine in normocarbic dogs. After 4 hours the brain concentration remains almost constant while the serum is dramatically decreased. (From Nishitateno K, Ngai SH, Finck AD, Berkowitz BA: Pharmacokinetics of morphine: Concentrations in the serum and brain of the dog during hyperventilation. Anesthesiology. 50:520–523, 1979.)

brain lipids and less will be needed in the CNS to exert the same effects. This low lipid solubility is responsible for a slow dynamic interaction between the plasma and the CNS. Once morphine has penetrated the CNS tissue, the diffusion back to the plasma is slow. In 1979, Nishitateno (55) elegantly demonstrated that the plasma concentration of morphine does not parallel the brain concentration of the drug. The brain concentration remains at higher levels compared to the decreasing plasma concentration over time (Figure 17–2).

## Pharmacokinetics

Opioids are often inactivated by biotransformation and elimination. Biotransformation, which facilitates elimination, refers to the structural change of a substance through enzymatic transformation. It occurs in various organs of the body (56) but primarily in the liver and to a lesser extent in the kidneys.

The process involves mostly synthetic reactions (conjugation) caused primarily by activity of microsomal enzyme systems. These microsomal enzyme systems have various rates of activity depending on genetic factors and on the influence of other compounds or chemicals, which can cause enzyme systems to produce faster rates of metabolism.

The main conjugation reaction in the detoxification process is glucuronide synthesis. The glucuronide compounds are excreted primarily in the urine but also in the feces through the biliary system. Some of these compounds have pharmacologic actions of their own. Morphine 6 glucoronide, for instance, has a powerful antalgic effect.

Elimination is primarily through renal excretion by glomerular filtration and active tubular secretion. Many drug metabolites formed in the liver are also added to bile and excreted by the gastrointestinal tract.

Once a specific concentration of opioid has been reached in the plasma, cerebral spinal fluid or CNS, the final effect is not equal for every individual. This varied response is best illustrated by considering the wide range that exists among patients in regard to the minimal effective analgesic concentration (MEAC) for each specific opioid. The minimal effective analgesic concentration is the minimal plasma level of an opioid that can control severe pain in a particular patient. For example, while a patient with a plasma concentration of meperidine of 410 ng/ml may still experience severe pain, the pain is relieved significantly when a concentration of 460 ng/ml has been reached. This concentration of 460 ng/ml will be the minimal effective analgesic concentration for meperidine for that patient (Figure 17–3) (57). While minimal effective analgesic concentration is fairly consistent for each individual patient (Mather found, at most, a twofold intrasubject variation), there is a great intersubject variation. Austin and colleagues (57) found that, in six patients, the intersubject minimal effective analgesic concentration varied from 270 to 700 ng/ml for meperidine (Figure 17–4), while Tamsen (58,59) found a similar variation ranging from 94 to 754 ng/ml. In practical terms, this represents an eightfold difference in intersubject requirement for meperidine confirming the empirical clinical observations of a seven- to eightfold difference in opioid requirements between patients. Morphine has a mean minimal effective analgesic concentration of 16 ng/ml with a range of 6 to 33 ng/ml (60). Table 17–3 reports the minimal effective analgesic concentration of several opioids.

If opioids were to have analgesic properties only, it would be easy to provide analgesia for all patients just by maintaining the plasma concentration 2 to 3 standard deviations above the mean minimal effective analgesic concentration. Unfortunately, these medications induce

**Table 17–3.** Minimum Effective Analgesic Plasma Concentration

| Analgesic | Minimum Effective Analgesic Concentration (MEAC) Mean ± SD (ng/ml) | Range |
|---|---|---|
| Hydrocodone | 6 | |
| Ketobemidone ($n = 15$) | 25 ± 11 | 10–51 |
| Morphine ($n = 10$) | 16 ± 9 | 6–33 |
| Meperidine (Pethidine) ($n = 20$) | 455 ± 174 | 94–754 |
| Fentanyl | 1 | |
| Alfentanil | 10 | |

(From Benedetti C: Acute pain: a review of its effects and therapy with systemic opioids. *In* Advances In Pain Research and Therapy, Vol. 14. Edited by C Benedetti. New York, Raven Press, 1990.)

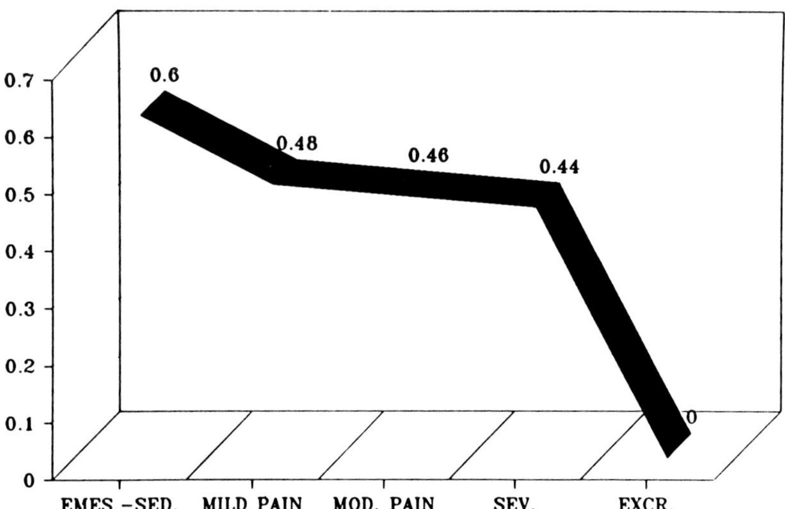


**Fig. 17–3.** There is no linear relationship between plasma concentration of an opioid and the relief of severe pain that it produces. Instead, until a certain plasma concentration is reached the change in pain intensity is minimal. After this critical value is reached, small changes in plasma concentrations will achieve significant reduction in pain intensity. This may be considered a therapeutic window for the opioid and it has been called Minimal Effective Analgesic Concentrations (MEAC). Side effects, such as emesis and sedation, occur in many patients at concentrations within the therapeutic window. (From Benedetti C: Acute pain: A review of its effects and therapy with systemic opioids. *In* Advances in Pain Research and Therapy: Opioid Analgesia. Vol. 14. Edited by C Benedetti, CR Chapman, G Giron. New York, Raven Press, 1990.)

multiple effects on the organism. Emesis, sedation, and dizziness, for instance, occur at plasma concentrations equal or slightly above the minimal effective analgesic concentration of each individual patient and, at somewhat higher concentration, respiratory depression ensues. Therefore, the therapeutic window for the analgesic effect is very narrow. From the above discussion it is clear that the optimal control of severe pain is achieved only by maintaining the plasma concentration of the opioid at a constant value just above the minimal effective analgesic concentration for specific patients. All this underscores the necessity of individualizing the dosage of opioids to the response and need of each individual patient. The concept of minimal effective analgesic concentration refers to pain of a specific intensity; most data refers to severe pain. Lower plasma concentration of opioids is needed to relieve pain of lower intensity. It should be noted, however, that the concept of an all or none effect applies for different pain intensities. Excruciating pain will have a minimal effective analgesic concentration higher than that for severe pain, while for moderate pain relief the minimal effective analgesic concentration will be lower.

## *Sites and Mechanism of Analgesia*

Although great advances have been made in elucidating the functioning of the opioid system, especially with regard to analgesia, our knowledge is far from complete. A detailed and clear understanding of the intrinsic mechanism of action of opioids is still lacking. Several factors prevent the elucidation of this mechanism: (1) the multiplicity of opioid substances, each of which interacts with more than one site of the macromolecules that form the opioid receptors (46,47); (2) the ability of one substance to act as an agonist in one animal tissue and as an antagonist in another, adding further confusion; (3) the difficulty

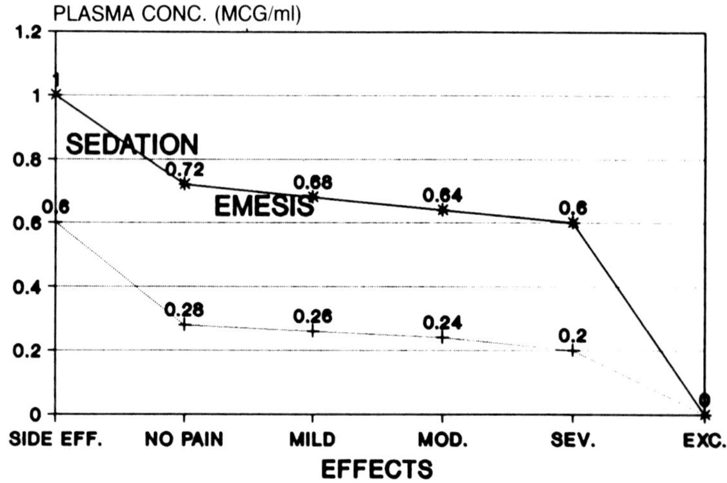


**Fig. 17–4.** One standard deviation above and below the mean of the minimal effective analgesic concentration shows the great variation among patient population. (From Benedetti C: Acute pain: A review of its effects and therapy with systemic opioids. *In* Advances in Pain Research and Therapy: Opioid Analgesia. Vol. 14. Edited by C Benedetti, CR Chapman, G Giron. New York, Raven Press, 1990.)

of finding not only agonists that bind to one opioid receptor but also finding antagonists that are receptor-specific. Naloxone, for instance, is a mu antagonist at low doses (up to 15 nmol) but at higher doses antagonizes also sigma and kappa agonists (46); and (4) the recent discovery (but lack of physiologic significance), that animal tissues can transform the nonpeptide, nonmorphinan reticuline to morphine and codeine, and that these substances are present in low doses in animals (61–64). Despite these difficulties, we now have considerable information regarding this complex system.

Unlike the nonsteroidal anti-inflammatory drugs (NSAIDs), which have a ceiling effect for analgesia, opioids act in a dose-dependent manner and can usually control all types of pain (up to the induction of surgical analgesia). The limiting factor is the severity of the side-effects such as sedation and respiratory depression, which increase proportionately with the dose.

One of the major topics of contention has been the site of action of opioids with regard to analgesia. Some authors argued that they act on the brain, others that they act on the spinal cord. Still others asserted that opioids alter only the appreciation of pain at the conscious level, while opponents contended that they decreased the intensity of the noxious impulses that reach consciousness. Herz and Teschemacher (65) suggested that morphine-induced analgesia in the intact animal by activating a descending inhibitory system (originating in the brain stem) inhibited the transmission of noxious stimuli at the level of the spinal cord. However Calvillo, et al (66) reported that in decerebrated spinalized cats, opioids given IV in high doses depressed the firing of activated nociceptive spinal neurons, and that this effect was reversed by naloxone. Calvillo also observed that even at very high doses, opioids had no effect on transmission of noxious impulses on peripheral nerves and nociceptive receptors.

We now know that systemic opioids induce analgesia by acting at different levels of the central nervous system (67). At the spinal cord level they impair or inhibit the transmission of nociceptive input from the periphery to the central nervous system, probably by inhibiting release of substance P. This occurs when an opioid activates the receptors located presynaptically on the primary nociceptive neurons. Nociceptive transmission is further impaired when an opioid activates postsynaptic receptors causing hyperpolarization of the neuron. At the level of the basal ganglia, opioids, probably by removing inhibition, activate a serotoninergic descending system that impairs, at the spinal cord level, peripheral nociceptive input. By acting on the limbic system, opioids alter the emotional response to pain, thus making it much more bearable (68). Therapeutic analgesic doses of opioids control dull, prolonged, aching pain better than sharp, colicky pain (69). At very high doses (e.g., 2 to 4 mg morphine/kg body weight, in human), however, they induce a state of analgesia, with obliteration of autonomic responses to the most intense nociceptive stimuli (70). This intense analgesia can be explained by the activations of more than one antinociceptive system by the high doses of opioids.

One recent report indicated that the descending antinociceptive system, activated mainly by the interaction of opioids with receptors in the anterior part of the periaqueductal gray of the brain stem, requires a much lower concentration of these drugs to produce analgesia than the analgesia elicited strictly by the activation of the receptors in the spinal cord (71). Therefore, opioids at low cerebral spinal fluid concentrations, such as those obtainable after therapeutic doses of oral, intramuscular, or intravenous administration, act mostly through the descending antinociceptive system. Whenever high cerebral spinal fluid concentrations are obtained, for instance, after intraspinal administration, the activation of opioid receptors in the spinal cord constitute the major mechanism of analgesia (71). This was illustrated clearly by Satoh and Takagi who in 1971 reported that in intact animals 2 to 4 mg/kg of morphine induced analgesia, but that in the C1, spinalized animal analgesia could be induced only if the dosages were increased to 10 mg/kg, indicating that a spinal antinociceptive mechanism is activated only by high dosages of opioids (72). The use of very high doses of IV opioids or the use of epidural opioids will activate both the spinal and supraspinal antinociceptive systems providing intense analgesia.

## Clinical Effects of Opioids

Clinical trials have shown that potent opioids, administered in equianalgesic doses to the general population, produce a statistically similar incidence and degree of effects. The response, however, is highly heterogeneous, with some patients developing more intense side-effects from one particular opioid than from another. Thus, patients receiving opioid therapy should be monitored closely for adverse side-effects and complications; if effects are particularly intense with one opioid, others should be tried at equianalgesic doses.

### *Euphoria and Sedation*

Euphoria, which at times may be desirable, occurs in some patients receiving opioid therapy; however, other patients may experience unpleasant dysphoria. Excessive sedation, drowsiness, confusion, dizziness, and unsteadiness can develop during the first few days of opioid therapy but usually clears in 3 to 5 days. Persistent sedation and drowsiness can be ameliorated by reducing the dose and increasing the frequency of the opioid administration to ensure sustained analgesia, by the concomitant use of CNS stimulants like amphetamines (73–74) or caffeine, or both. This is appropriate for relatively short-term therapy and for patients with terminal cancer.

### *Seizures*

Multifocal myoclonic seizures can occur in patients who erroneously receive chronic meperidine therapy. Seizures result from the accumulation of its active metabolite normeperidine, which produces central nervous system hyperexcitability and lowers the seizure threshold (75). This hyperirritability is not reversed by naloxone but may be suppressed by the administration of intravenous anticonvulsants and by switching to another opioid.

### Constipation

This is the most frequent and most uncomfortable side-effect of opioids, and tolerance does not develop. Therefore, with the onset of opioid therapy, measures should be instituted to ensure a regular bowel regimen by administering cathartics, stool softeners, and fluids to avoid constipation, which can lead to frank bowel obstruction.

Opioids also produce biliary spasm and urinary retention. These side-effects should be considered when prescribing opioids to patients with pathologic changes involving these specific organs. Fentanyl, meperidine, morphine, and pentazocine have been studied with regard to effects on the sphincter of Oddi and it was found that they increase the intrabiliary pressure of common duct of 99%, 61%, 53%, and 15%, respectively (76).

### Nausea and Vomiting

Nausea and vomiting are common and highly disliked side-effects of opioid therapy. Patients can refuse these analgesics if the emesis is not treated. This effect is potentiated by vestibular stimulation; ambulatory patients suffer more emesis than supine patients. Nausea and vomiting can be prevented or must be effectively treated. Nausea can be prevented by the concomitant use of hydroxyzine (77), by giving a reduced dose of opioids, or by the concomitant use of perchlorperazine or haloperidol. Transdermal scopolamine (Transderm-SCOP-CIBA), commonly used to prevent emesis associated with motion sickness, is also an effective treatment of opioid-induced nausea and vomiting. However, this preparation should be used cautiously in the elderly because it produces disorientation and confusion (personal observation). If the patient is vomiting, the antiemetic drug should be given intravenously, intramuscularly, or rectally.

### Pruritus

Pruritus is mostly limited to the face, alae of the nose, palate, and torso. This side-effect is much more evident with intraspinal opioids (78). Its mechanism of action is not known but it appears to be centrally mediated. It is controlled by small, carefully titrated doses of naloxone. Recent reports that nalbuphine, a mu antagonist-kappa agonist, reverses the pruritus caused by intraspinal morphine imply that this side-effect is mu-mediated (79,80). Also, we have used Hydroxizine with success in treating this bothersome side-effect.

### Tolerance

Tolerance is a normal response to chronic opioid therapy. It is characterized by the development of decreasing analgesic effects and other actions of a drug (42). Tolerance develops at different rates for various effects. Tolerance to the sedative effects of morphine, for example, develops much more rapidly than tolerance to its constipating effects. Tolerance develops faster when opioids are administered intravenously by continuous infusion than does it by patient controlled analgesia (PCA) (81).

The earliest sign of tolerance is the patient's complaint that the duration or degree of analgesia, or both, has decreased, although no increase is seen in the nociceptive input. This is treated by increasing the frequency or dose of the drug, or both. Cross tolerance among opioids occurs but it is not complete; therefore, switching to an alternative opioid often results in adequate pain relief. This effect is explained by the relative efficacy that different opioids have, as explained earlier. When changing opioid, the switch should be made from one of low-efficacy to a high-efficacy one and titrated to a dose that produces analgesia, as the conversion table for equianalgesic doses for naive patients does not apply to tolerant patients.

### Physical Dependence

Physical dependence represents a neuroadaptive response to the pharmacologic effects of chronic opioid use. The biochemical mechanism is mediated by cyclic AMP. Adenylate cyclase is inhibited by opioids. With chronic treatment, adaptation occurs that consists of increased cyclase activity to return cAMP to pretreatment level. Sudden removal of the opioid effect, caused either by abrupt discontinuation of an opioid or administration of an antagonist, leads to a state of over production of cAMP until the cyclase activity slowly returns to normal. Clinically, physical dependence is characterized by the development of the abstinence syndrome on abrupt withdrawal of the drug. The syndrome consists of yawning, lacrimation, frequent sneezing, agitation, tremors, insomnia, fever, tachycardia, and other signs of hyperexcitability of the sympathetic nervous system. The time of onset and the characteristics of the abstinence syndrome vary. Often it develops gradually with only signs of restlessness and irritability, which then lead to the full picture of abstinence syndrome. Some patients, though, may not experience the early signs and suddenly develop all the symptoms of sympathetic hyperactivity. Longer-acting opioids, methadone and buprenorphine, tend to cause less intense withdrawals than shorter-acting drugs. The abstinence syndrome can be prevented by slowly tapering the dose of the opioid at a rate of 15 to 20% daily, and it can be effectively treated by reinstituting the drug in doses of about 25 to 40% of the previous daily dose (82). Because the syndrome is mediated by the adrenergic system, $\alpha$-2 agonists, such as clonidine, also prevent its development.

### Psychologic Dependence

Psychologic dependence, a better term than addiction, is characterized by an abnormal behavior pattern of drug use, by craving of a drug for effects other than pain relief, by becoming overwhelmingly involved in the procurement and use of the drug, and by the tendency to relapse after withdrawal (83). Fear of addiction has been an important factor in the underdosing of opioids in patients with severe pain, but opioid addiction rarely occurs in patients receiving opioids for medical purposes. Porter and Jick (84) monitored 40,000 hospitalized medical patients for psychologic dependence. They found that, among the nearly 12,000 patients who received one or more doses of opioids and who had no previous history of this syndrome, only four developed psychologic dependence. In another study of cancer patients receiving chronic opioid therapy, Kanner and Foley (85) found that drug abuse and psychologic dependence did not occur in this population. These and other data suggest that the medical use of opioids is rarely associated with development of psychological dependence.

### *Respiratory Depression*

Opioids, in particular the mu receptor agonist, depress respiration. This is noticeable even at therapeutic doses of morphine and increases progressively with higher doses. The effect of opioids on respiration is multifaceted: opioids depress both respiratory rate and tidal volume and, as a consequence, decrease minute ventilation. The major effect is a decrease in responsiveness of the medullary respiratory centers to carbon dioxide tension. Pain counteracts some of this depression.

Provided that the opioid is titrated to achieve adequate pain relief, clinically significant respiratory depression usually does not occur. On the other hand, this complication occurs whenever the minimal effective analgesic concentration for the particular patient and drug is significantly exceeded. Also, sudden deterioration of hepatic and renal functions decreases the elimination of an opioid and causes it to accumulate. Respiratory depression is preceded by significant sedation. Therefore, an increase in patient sedation is a premonitory sign of hypoventilation and impending apnea.

Maternal ventilation is usually maintained within normal limits during the period of painful contraction when judicious therapeutic doses of opioids are given; however, between contractions the effect of the drugs may become evident. If an excessive dose has been administered and the interval between contractions is long, the depressant effect may result in significant hypoxia and hypercarbia, which may be deleterious to both the mother and the fetus.

Respiratory depression or even arrest can occur in patients given high doses of opioids to relieve the pain and in patients who subsequently receive an epidural or spinal block that abruptly eliminates all of the pain and, therefore, its respiratory stimulating effects. It is therefore especially important to watch such patients closely after these procedures (82). Because the residual volume is decreased in the gravida, there is less respiratory reserve, so that opioid-induced respiratory depression produces more prompt and greater alteration of ventilatory function.

Mild respiratory depression can be terminated by reducing the drug dosage, whereas moderate or severe depression should be treated with naloxone given in doses of 0.1 to 0.4 mg IV. Because naloxone is a fast but short-acting agent, repeated administration or an IV drip might be necessary to prevent severe respiratory depression or arrest from recurring in patients on long-acting opioids. For patients who have been on chronic opioid therapy, it is important to administer the naloxone slowly, or it could precipitate severe withdrawal symptoms. Physicians should also be aware that naloxone has, on rare occasions, produced pulmonary edema (86).

### *Circulation*

Even a therapeutic dose of opioids may cause a vasodilation that may lead to orthostatic hypotension. The vasodilation is probably produced by release of histamine, especially by morphine, and a depression of the homeostatic reflex mechanism. If patients are given therapeutic dosages and they are normovolemic, hypotension usually is not significant, especially if the woman is supine. Parturients who have received significant doses of opioids should not be made to walk or sit up because hypotension may cause nausea, vertigo, vomiting and, at times, loss of consciousness with consequent injury to the patient.

The hypotensive effect of opioids is exaggerated in parturients with hypovolemia, either acute or chronic, caused by blood loss, traumatic shock, malnutrition, eclampsia or pregnancy-induced hypertension (PIH). These patients usually have a compensatory vasoconstriction that is altered even by therapeutic dosages of opioids therefore causing significant decrease in blood pressure, even when patients are in a supine position. In such patients, opioids should be used in very small dosages, possibly IV, and titrated to effect with frequent monitoring of blood pressure. The effect of the compression of the inferior vena cava caused by the pregnant uterus may also decrease venous return and therefore significantly reduce the blood pressure. It is highly recommended that the patient be placed in the lateral position or the uterus displaced away from the vena cava.

Phenothiazine drugs are potent with vasodilators, and the combination of opioids with phenothiazine, which is often used in obstetrics, is more likely to be followed by hypotension than when each of these drugs is used alone.

Cardiac output does not change significantly after the administration of therapeutic doses of opioids, even in patients with heart disease. However, the rapid administration of intravenous opioids, even at therapeutic dosages, may result in cardiovascular depression with bradycardia, decreased cardiac output, and marked hypotension even in supine parturients. This can be obviated by slow intravenous administration of 3 to 5 mg of morphine or an infusion of diluted solutions. If hypercarbia develops due to respiratory depression, cerebral blood flow and coronary blood flow are indirectly increased when opioids are given to patients. This may cause an increase of 25 to 50% of the cerebral spinal fluid, an increase which is usually not significant unless there is already increased intracranial pressure.

### *Effects on Labor*

Systemic therapeutic doses of opioids decrease uterine contractions and can prolong labor (87). Uterine hyperactivity is decreased by this class of drug, which tends to return contractility to normal. In this particular situation, the duration of labor and delivery can be shortened by opioids. If the opioid is given during the latent phase of the first stage of labor, there is a tendency for it to slow cervical dilatation and it may even result in uterine inertia. An optimum dose given after 4 to 5 cm of dilatation does not produce such effects and may even enhance labor by eliminating the inhibiting effect of fear and pain. The depressant effect of opioids on labor is less evident in multigravidae than primigravidae and less evident also when dosage is given after the membrane has been ruptured. The effects of intraspinal opioids on labor have not yet been carefully studied.

An optimum dose has no significant depressant effect, while an excessive dose delays labor. The overdose may be absolute (for instance, morphine 15 or 25 mg) or relative (rapid intravenous injection of 5 mg of morphine). This is also related to the time of administration: the same dose of a drug that inhibited uterine contraction early in labor when the pain was mild to moderate may not depress contractions when the labor is more advanced and uterine contraction and pain are stronger.

Obviously, all of these factors are interrelated and the effects dependent upon the influence that the drug has under the circumstances existing at the time of administration. This strongly emphasizes the importance of individualizing the administration of opioids and to avoid standard use.

### Effects on the Infant

All opioids pass to the fetus after they are administered to the mother and all of them exert a direct depressant effect on the respiratory center of the infant. When given in excessive dosages, they may also have an indirect effect on the fetus by depressing the respiration and circulation of the mother with subsequent decrease of oxygen and carbon dioxide. Moreover, perfusion experiments conducted on human placenta indicate that morphine, meperidine, codeine (and probably other opioids) have a direct vasoconstriction action on the placental vessels. This action may impair transfer of oxygen and carbon dioxide. The degree of neonatal depression caused by all opioids during their peak action is about the same, when given to the mother in equianalgesic dosages. Several studies have indicated that opioids have an increased depressive effect on the newborn, more so than on the adult (88–90). Depending on how the medication is given to the mother, the effect on the newborn may be almost concomitant or delayed. If the opioid is injected subcutaneously or intramuscularly to the mother, usually the peak effect of respiratory depression to the newborn occurs 2 to 4 hours after the injection. This is because of the slow intravascular absorption from the injection site. On the other hand, if the opioid is given intravenously, the opioid reaches the fetus faster and, therefore, if the delivery of the baby occurs shortly after the peak depressive effect, it will be noted in the neonate. However, a small dose of morphine given epidurally (3 mg) before delivery of the neonate does not have a depressant effect on either the mother or infant (91).

The degree of respiratory depression produced by opioids also depends on the gestational age and the condition of the infant. The greater the degree of prematurity,

**Table 17–4.** Different Classification Systems for Opioids

| Weak or Strong Opioids | Opium and its Derivatives | Agonists and Antagonists |
|---|---|---|
| Weak | Natural opium alkaloids | Agonists |
| Codeine | Phenanthrene derivatives | Alfentanil |
| Propoxyphene (Darvon) | Morphine | Alphaprodine |
| Strong | Codeine | Codeine |
| Alfentanil (Alfenta) | Thebaine (nonanalgesic) | Diacetylmorphine |
| Alphaprodine (Nisentil) | Benylisoquinoline derivatives | Dihydromorphinone |
| Buprenorphine (Bupronex; Temgesic) | (nonanalgesic) | Dihydrohydroxymorphinone |
| Butorphanol (Stadol; Dorphanol) | Papaverine | Etorphine |
| Cholecystokinin | Noscapine | Fentanyl |
| Diacetylmorphine (heroin) | Semisynthetic derivatives of opium alkaloids | Levorphanol |
| Dihydromorphinone, hydromorphone (Dilaudid) | Morphine derivatives | Meperidine |
| Dihydrohydroxymorphinone, oxymorphone (Numorphan) | Diacetylmorphine | Methadone |
| Fentanyl (Sublimaze) | Dihydromorphinone | Morphine |
| Etorphine | Dihydrohydroxymorphinone | Oxycodone |
| Levorphanol (Levo-Dromoran) | Thebaine derivatives | Propoxyphene |
| Meperidine (Demerol) | Buprenorphine | Sufentanil |
| Methadone (Dolophine) | Oxyocodone | Partial agonists, agonist-antagonists |
| Morphine | Synthetic compounds | Buprenorphine |
| Nalbuphine (Nubain) | Morphinans | Butorphanol |
| Naloxone (Narcan) | Levorphanol | Nalbuphine |
| Naltrexone (Trexan) | Nalbuphine | Pentazocine |
| Oxycodone (Percocet; Tylox) | Naloxone | Antagonists |
| Pentazocine (Talwin) | Naltrexone | Cholecystokinin |
| Sufentanil (Sufenta) | Phenylheptylamines | Naloxone |
| | Methadone | Naltrexone |
| | Propoxyphene | |
| | Phenylpiperidine | |
| | Alfentanil | |
| | Alphaprodine | |
| | Fentanyl | |
| | Meperidine | |
| | Sufentanil | |

(From Benedetti C: Acute pain: a review of its effects and therapy with systemic opioids. *In* Advances In Pain Research and Therapy, Vol. 14. Edited by C Benedetti. New York, Raven Press, 1990.)

**Table 17–5.** Opioid Analgesics Used for Moderate to Severe Pain. Pharmacokinetic and Pharmacodynamic Data[a]

| Class Generic Name; Proprietary Names | Routes[b] | Equianalgesic Dose[c] (mg) | Peak[d] (hr) | Duration[d] (hr) | Half-life (hr) | Comments | Precautions |
|---|---|---|---|---|---|---|---|
| Agonists | | | | | | | |
| Naturally occurring opium derivatives | | | | | | | |
| Morphine | IM[e] | 10–15 | 0.5–1 | 3–5[f] | 2–3.5 | Standard of comparison for opioid-type analgesics | Impaired ventilation; bronchial asthma; increased intracranial pressure; liver failure; renal failure |
| | PO[e] | 30–60[c] | 1.5–2 | 4 | | | |
| Codeine | IM | 120 | 0.5–1 | 4–6 | 3 | Less potent than morphine; excellent oral potency | Like morphine |
| | PO | 30–200 | | 3–4 | | | |
| Partially synthetic derivatives of morphine | | | | | | | |
| Hydromorphone (Dilaudid) | IM | 1–2 | 0.5–1 | 3–4 | 2–3 | Slightly shorter acting than morphine, possibly less sedation, N/V | Like morphine |
| | PO | 2–4 | 1.5–2 | 4–6 | | | |
| Oxymorphone (Numorphan) | IM | 1–1.5 | 0.5–1 | 3–5 | NA | Like morphine | Like morphine |
| Heroin | IM | 4 | 0.5–1 | 3–4 | 2–3 | Slightly shorter acting | Like morphine |
| | PO | 4–8 | 1.5–2 | 3–4 | | | |
| Oxycodone | PO | 30 | 1 | 4–6 | NA[b] | Available only (5-mg doses) in combination with acetaminophen (Percocet) or aspirin (Percodan), which limits dose escalation | Like morphine |
| Synthetic compounds | | | | | | | |
| Morphonans | | | | | | | |
| Levorphanol (Levo-Dromoran) | IM | 2 | 0.5–1 | 5–8 | 12–16 | Like methadone | Like methadone |
| | PO | 4 | 1.5–2 | | | | |
| Phenylheptylamines | | | | | | | |
| Methadone (Dolophine) | IM | 8–10 | 0.5–1 | 4–8 | 15–30 | Good oral potency; long plasma half-life | Like morphine, accumulative with repeated doses |
| | PO | 10 | 1.5–2 | 4–12 | | | |
| Propoxyphene HCl (Darvon) | PO | 32–65 | | 4–6 | 3.5 | "Weak" opioid, often used in combination with nonopioid analgesics | Accumultive with repeated doses, convulsions with overdose |
| Phenylpiperidines | | | | | | | |
| Meperidine (Demerol) | IM | 75–100 | 0.5–1 | 2–3 | | Shorter acting and about 10% as potent as morphine; has mild atrophine-like anti-spasmatic effects | Normeperidine accumulates with repetitive dosing, causing CNS excitation; not for patients with impaired renal function or for those receiving monoamine oxidase inhibitors |
| | PO | 200–300 | 1–2 | 2–3 | | | |
| Alphaprodine (Nisentil) | IM | 40 | | 1.5–2 | | Similar to meperidine but shorter acting, low placental transfer—not available in USA | Like meperidine |
| Fentanyl | IV | 50–100 μg | | 0.75–1 | | Short-acting potent opioid, mostly used in anesthesia or continuous infusion | More severe side effects than morphine |
| Sufentanil | IV | 5–10 μg | | | | | |
| Diffentanil | IV | 500–1000 μg | | 0.25–0.4 | | | |
| Agonist-Antagonists | | | | | | | |
| Buprenorphine (Temgesic) | IM | 0.3–0.6 | 0.5–1 | 6–8 | NA | Partial agonist of the morphine-type, less abuse liability than morphine | Can precipitate withdrawal in narcotic-dependent patients |
| | SL | 0.4–0.8 | 2–3 | 6–8 | | | |
| Butorphanol (Stadol) | IM | 2 | 0.5–1 | 4 | 2.3–3.5 | Like nalbuphine | Like pentazocine |
| Pentazocine (Talwin) | IM | 40–60 | 0.5–1 | 3–4 | 2–3 | Mixed agonist-antagonist; less abuse liability than morphine; included in Schedule IV of Controlled Substances Act | Can cause psychotomimetic effects; might precipitate withdrawal in narcotic-dependent patients, not for those with myocardial infarction |
| | PO | 50–200 | 1.5–2 | 3–4 | | | |
| Nalbuphine (Nubain) | IM | 10–20 | 0.5–1 | 4–6 | 5 | Like pentazocine but not scheduled | Incidence of psychotomimetic effects lower than with pentazocine |

[a] Adapted from ref. 69a.
[b] IM, intramuscular; PO, oral; SL, sublingual; NA, not available; IV, intravenous.
[c] These doses are recommended starting doses from which the optimal dose for each patient is determined by titration and the maximal dose is limited by adverse effects.
[d] Peak time and duration of analgesia are based on mean values and refer to the stated equianalgesic doses.
[e] For a single oral dose the ratio of IM/oral is 1:6; for repeated doses the ratio is closer to 1:3.
[f] Plasma half-life at least for morphine is age-dependent; it increases with age.
(From Benedetti C: Acute pain: a review of its effects and therapy with systemic opioids. *In* Advances In Pain Research and Therapy, Vol. 14. Edited by C Benedetti. New York, Raven Press, 1990.)

**Table 17–6.** Opioid Analgesics Used for Moderate to Severe Pain. Systemic Pharmacologic and Toxicologic Eff

| | Central Nervous System | | | | | | Cardiova |
|---|---|---|---|---|---|---|---|
| **Class; Generic Name; Proprietary Names** | **Analgesia** | **Mood** | **Sedation** | **Emetic Center** | **Cough Center** | **Respiratory Center** | **Cardiac Rate** |
| Agonists | | | | | | | |
| Naturally occurring opium derivatives | | | | | | | |
| Morphine | ↑ ↑ ↑ ↑ | ↑ = ↓ | ↑ ↑ ↑ | ↑ ↑ ↑ | ↓ ↓ ↓ | ↓ ↓ ↓ | = ↓ |
| Codeine | ↑ ↑ | = ↑ | ↑ | ↑ | ↓ ↓ ↓ | ↓ | NA |
| Partially synthetic derivatives of morphine | | | | | | | |
| Hydromorphone (Dilaudid) | LM[b] | LM | ↓ ↓ | LM | LM | LM | LM |
| Oxymorphone (Numorphan) | LM | LM | LM | LM | LM | LM | LM |
| Heroin | LM | = ↓ | LM | LM | LM | LM | LM |
| Oxycodone | ↑ ↑ ↑ | = ↑ | LM | LM | LM | LM | LM |
| Synthetic compounds | | | | | | | |
| Morphonanes | | | | | | | |
| Levorphanol (Levo-Dromoran) | ↑ ↑ ↑ | = | ↑ | ↑ | ↓ ↓ ↓ | ↓ ↓ ↓ | LM |
| Phenylheptylamines | | | | | | | |
| Methadone (Dolophine) | ↑ | NA | ↑ ↑ | ↑ ↑ | | ↓ ↓ | ↑ ↑ ↑ |
| Propoxyphene HCl (Darvon) | | | | | | | |
| Phenylpiperidines | | | | | | | |
| Meperidine (Demerol) | ↑ ↑ ↑ | ↑ ↑ | ↑ ↑ | ↑ ↑ | ↓ ↓ | ↓ ↓ ↓ ↓ | = ↑ |
| Alphaprodine (Nisentil) | LM | LM | LM | LM | LM | LM | LM |
| Fentanyl | ↑ ↑ ↑ ↑ ↑ | | ↑ ↑ ↑ | ↑ ↑ ↑ ↑ | ↓ ↓ ↓ | ↓ ↓ ↓ ↓ | ↓ ↓ ↓ |
| Agonist-Antagonists | | | | | | | |
| Buprenorphine (Temgesic) | ↑ ↑ ↑ | ↑ ↓ | ↑ ↑ ↑ | ↑ ↑ ↑ | | ↓ ↓ ↓ | LM |
| Butorphanol (Stadol) | ↑ ↑ | = | ↑ ↑ ↑ ↑ | ↑ ↑ ↑ | NA | ↓ ↓ ↓ | ↑ ↑ ↑ |
| Pentazocine (Talwin) | ↑ | ↓ ↓ ↓ | ↑ ↑ ↑ ↑ | ↑ ↑ | | ↓ ↓ ↓ | ↑ ↑ ↑ |
| Nalbuphine (Nubain) | ↑ ↑ | ↓ ↓ | ↑ ↑ ↑ ↑ | ↑ ↑ | NA | ↓ ↓ | = ↓ |

[a] some toxic effects are quite different among opioids, e.g., fentanyl increases common bile duct pressure 99% above predrug level whereas effect of an opioid may be statistically identical to morphine but on an individual basis there may be considerable difference to warrant chan

[b] LM like morphine.

(From Benedetti C: Acute pain: a review of its effects and therapy with systemic opioids. *In* Advances In Pain Research and Therapy, Vol. 14.

the greater is the effect. These drugs should be avoided in the delivery of premature babies.

Fetal and neonatal depressant effects of opioids are potentiated by hypoxemia. Hypoxia and hypercarbia are a normal occurrence at time of birth though these conditions are readily corrected in the normal newborn; in the presence of opioids or other CNS depressants, however, the recovery is slow. It has also been shown that in human newborns the depressant effects of opioids on the brain persist for 2 to 4 days after birth, a period considerably longer than expected based on adult responses to these drugs. The depressant effect of opioids on the fetus and newborn is also potentiated by other analgesics, hypnotics and anesthetic agents, hypotension, prolonged labor, cesarean section, and trauma during delivery. In this respect, it is important to remember that opioids are eliminated slowly and the infant may have subclinical amounts, which in themselves produce no effect, but which may have a synergistic effect with one or more of the above factors to produce residual neonatal depression.

## Description of Single Opioids

Opioids have been classified in different ways. One method subdivides them into weak opioids (with low dependency potential) versus stronger opioids (with higher dependency potential). Another system is to consider opioids for their agonist, partial agonist, and agonist/antagonist activities. Opioids can also be divided into naturally occurring, semisynthetic, and synthetic groups (Table 17–4). The naturally occurring opioids are the alkaloids of opium and they are divided into two chemical classes. One class contains the three rings of the phenanthrene nucleus. Members of this class are morphine, codeine, and thebaine. The other class consists of the benzylisoquinoline alkaloids, which lack any analgesic activity. Representatives of this class are papaverine and noscapine. The semisynthetic opioids are obtained by simple modification of a naturally occurring alkaloid. Heroin, for example, is derived from morphine, while etorphine and buprenorphine are derived from thebaine. Synthetic opioids contain the phenanthrene nucleus of morphine, but they are completely synthesized. The synthetic opioids have further been subdivided into several groups based on their chemical structure (i.e., morphinans, phenylheptylamines, and phenylpiperidines).

The opioids used most frequently for labor analgesia are described in some detail in this section, while the others will be described briefly because though they may not be used for labor, they may find an application in ects of Opioid Analgesics Used for Moderate to Severe Pain[a]

| scular System | | | | Genitourinary System | | |
|---|---|---|---|---|---|---|
| Blood Pressure | Gastrointestinal Peristalsis | Biliary Common Duct Pressure | Bronchial Constriction | Ureter Tone | Bladder Tone | Histamine Release |
| = ↓ | ↓ ↓ ↓ | ↑ ↑ | ↑ ↑ ↑ | ↑ ↑ | ↑ ↑ ↑ | ↑ ↑ ↑ ↑ |
| ↓ ↓ ↓ ↓ (if given IV) | ↓ | ↑ | NA | NA | NA | ↑ ↑ ↑ ↑ ↑ |
| LM | LM | LM | LM | LM | LM | NA |
| LM | LM | LM | LM | LM | LM | NA |
| LM | LM | LM | LM | LM | LM | LM |
| LM | LM | LM | LM | LM | LM | LM |
| LM | LM | LM | LM | LM | LM | ↑ |
| | ↓ ↓ | NA | NA | NA | NA | |
| ↓ ↓ ↓ | ↓ ↓ | ↑ ↑ ↑ | NA | ↑ | ↑ | |
| LM | LM | LM | LM | LM | LM | NA |
| ↓ ↓ ↓ | ↓ ↓ ↓ | ↑ ↑ ↑ ↑ ↑ | NA | | = | |
| LM | ↓ ↓ ↓ | ↑ ↑ ↑ ↑ | NA | NA | NA | NA |
| ↑ ↑ ↑ | ↓ ↓ | ↑ | NA | NA | NA | NA |
| ↑ ↑ ↑ | ↓ ↓ | ↑ | NA | NA | NA | NA |
| ↑ = ↓ | ↓ | NA | NA | NA | NA | NA |

pentazocine only 15%; IV morphine causes a wide variation in histamine release whereas fentanyl does not. In other cases, the toxic
ıge of opioid if some side effects are particularly intense with one specific drug.

Edited by C Benedetti. New York, Raven Press, 1990.)

obstetric patients. (Significant amounts of data in this section are derived from Chapter 11 on narcotics, found in the first edition of this book.) Tables 17–5 and 17–6 report data for comparison of opioids. Table 17–7 reports equianalgesic doses for some opioids in nontolerant patients. As mentioned several times, because of great intersubject variability, the dosages indicated after each drug are only for orientation and represent an average dose to control moderate to severe pain in adult patients. In the clinical setting, the dose for each individual must be titrated with regard to amount, to frequency, and to the specific need for adequate pain control.

**Table 17–7.** Equivalent Analgesic Doses of Narcotics

| Drug | Oral Dose (mg) | Intramuscular Dose (mg) |
|---|---|---|
| Alphaprodine (Nisentil) | | 45.0 |
| Anileridine (Leritine) | | 35.0 |
| Codeine | 200.0 | 130.0 |
| Diacetylmorphine (heroin) | | 3.0 |
| Fentanyl (Sublimaze) | | 0.1 |
| Hydromorphone (Dilaudid) | 7.5 | 1.5 |
| Meperidine (Demerol) | 400.0 | 100.0 |
| Methadone | 10.0 | 8.0 |
| Morphine | 30.0 | 10.0 |
| Oxycodone (Percodan) | 30.0 | 15.0 |
| Oxymorphone (Numorphan) | | 1.5 |
| Pentazocine (Talwin) | 180.0 | 6.0 |

(From Benedetti C: Acute pain: a review of its effects and therapy with systemic opioids. *In* Advances In Pain Research and Therapy, Vol. 14. Edited by C Benedetti. New York, Raven Press, 1990.)

## Agonist Opioids

The binding of an agonist to the stereospecific receptors causes the pharmacologic effects detailed above. Agonist opioids include morphine, codeine, meperidine, dihydromorphone, methadone, among others.

## Morphine

Morphine is the standard of comparison for all the potent opioid analgesics. It is used mostly by the IM or IV route for the treatment of acute severe pain in which a definite end to the episode is anticipated.

Since 1979, morphine has been used extensively by the intraspinal route to induce a more intensive and prolonged analgesia than that capable of being induced when given by the systemic route.

In obstetrics, when morphine is used judiciously, it does not have any significant or worse side-effects than other opioids (92,93) (Keats, AS: Personal communication.) When given either intramuscularly or intravenously, dosages of 5 mg to a maximum 10 mg will provide good analgesia especially in the early phase of labor. It is not recommended that the medication be given close to the time of delivery as this may produce significant hypoventilation in the newborn. During the last several years, intraspinal morphine has been used to effect labor analgesia. When given at the beginning of labor, at doses of 3 to 5 mg epidurally or at 0.3 to 0.5 mg subarachnoid, intraspinal morphine provides significant analgesia that is often sufficient until the later phases of the first stage. At these dosages, there is no significant depressive effects on the newborn. For a rough approximation, intrathecal morphine should be given at a dose 1/10 of the epidural dose and thus 1/10 of the IM or IV dose.

When given intramuscularly or intravenously, morphine may produce orthostatic hypotension due to vasodilatation and histamine release (93,94). The other side effects on other organs in the central nervous system are similar to those described for the entire group. It must be reemphasized that, on the average, at equianalgesic dosages the degrees of side effect of morphine are no greater than that of meperidine and other potent opioids.

### Effect on Labor

There is no general consensus on the effect on labor by morphine because several studies performed during the last 65 years have failed to provide a reliable answer (95). One study (96) indicated that morphine depresses uterine forces, another (97) that it enhances them, and still others that it has no effect on uterine contractions (Figure 17–5) (95–100). In patients with uterine inertia caused by apprehensions, anxiety and pain, morphine or any other opioids may enhance contractions and thus shorten labor (1).

### Effect on the Infant

Morphine, like other opioids, crosses the placenta membrane readily (101–103). It may also produce constriction of placental vessels, a constriction that is antagonized by naloxone or nalorphine (104). There is no indication that morphine has a greater depressant effect on the respiration of the newborn than other opioids, and, therefore, this should not be a consideration in avoiding its use as long as proper dosages are employed (101–106).

### Partially Synthetic Derivatives of Morphine

#### Dihydromorphone (Dilaudid)

Hydromorphone (Dilaudid) is a semisynthetic derivative of morphine, approximately 6 to 8 times as potent but with slightly shorter activity (3 hours); its equianalgesic dose, therefore, compared to 10 mg of morphine, is 1.5 mg. It is absorbed easily by the gastrointestinal tract and, therefore, effective after oral and rectal administration. The analgesic effect appears approximately 15 minutes after parenteral administration and 30 minutes after

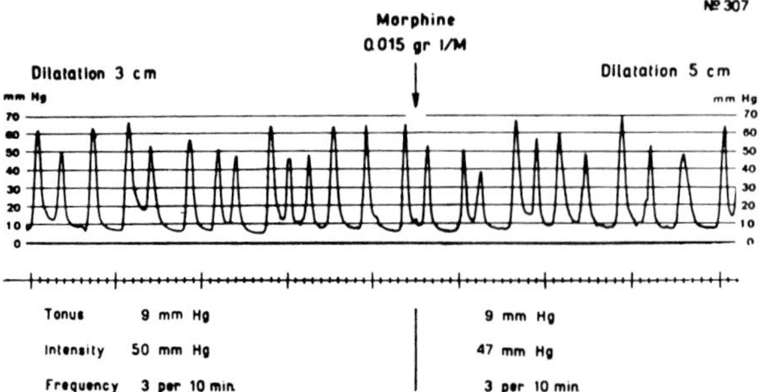


**Fig. 17–5.** Action of morphine on uterine contractility. Tone, intensity, and frequency of contractions are normal, and morphine does not significantly modify them. (From Caldeyro-Barcia R, Alvarez H, Poseiro JJ: Action of morphine on the contractility of the human uterus. Arch. Int. Pharmacodyn. 101:171, 1955.)

oral administration. Because this drug induces less bothersome side effects than morphine, particularly nausea and vomiting, it is often preferred by patients.

#### Meperidine

Meperidine (Pethidine; Demerol) is a synthetic phenylpiperidine opioid analgesic often used interchangeably with morphine. It produces less smooth muscle contraction than morphine (107). In equianalgesic doses, it appears to have the same central side-effects and the mechanisms of action appear to be the same. Meperidine is absorbed by the gastrointestinal tract but the oral dose is about 50% less effective than when given intramuscularly. The major disadvantage of the drug is that its duration of action is almost 50% shorter than morphine, a factor very often overlooked by physicians. The drug is usually given every 4 to 6 hours; the analgesia produced is unacceptable, especially 2.5 to 3 hours after administration. As mentioned earlier, chronic administration of meperidine has been associated with seizures due to accumulation of its metabolite normeperidine, which lowers the seizure threshold and causes CNS hyperirritability. Meperidine given at the dose of 15 to 25 mg IV prevents or controls the shivering associated with volatile anesthetics, subarachnoid/epidural block, and chemotherapy, an effect not reproducible with other opioids.

In obstetrics, meperidine has been used in the last 4 decades more frequently to relieve labor pain than any other opioids. Control studies indicate that 50 mg, 75 mg, and 100 mg of meperidine are approximately equivalent to 6 mg, 8 mg, and 10 mg of morphine (108), respectively, and in equianalgesic doses meperidine provides relief that is in every way comparable to that of morphine (109). A single dose of 50 mg given intramuscularly provides satisfactory analgesia to more than 80% of parturients during the early stages of labor (110–113). More prompt and intense analgesia can be produced in a single intravenous dose given during the early stages of labor (114). Epidural meperidine has been used for the relief of labor pain. The intraspinal use of meperidine seems well indicated because the substance does not only act as an opioid agonist but possesses also inherent local anesthetic properties. It has been reported that when combined with 0.125% or 0.25% of bupivacaine, it provides excellent analgesia and also prevents shivering often associated with intraspinal local anesthetics (115–118).

## Effects on the Mother

In the past it was believed that meperidine caused less respiratory depression than morphine, though the available data indicate that such is not the case (Figure 17–6) (93,94,119). In contrast with morphine, meperidine causes a pulse rate increase that may be excessive for cardiac patients, though it causes orthostatic hypotension similar to morphine. The rapid intravenous administration of 50 to 100 mg of meperidine produces significant vasodilations, possibly through histamine release and such administration may also depress the myocardium and the vasomotor center (120). Some of these effects are offset by the central nervous system stimulation and consequent activation of the sympathoadrenal response evoked by meperidine (120). This response may be partially blocked if the sympathetic system has been interrupted, as happens with high intraspinal block. Meperidine should be avoided or used with great caution in patients being treated chronically with monoamino oxidase inhibitor (Isocarboxazid-Marplan, Pargyline-Eutonyl, Phenelzine-Nardil, Tranylcypromine-Parnate). These medications, used to treat psychotic depression, act by blocking the oxidative deaminations of endogenous catecholamine, which, therefore, are not inactivated and accumulate. Meperidine, given to these patients, may cause a variety of symptoms that include either severe, prolonged hypotension, respiratory depression, and coma or signs of excitation of the CNS with hypertension, delirium, and convulsions (121). Meperidine has similar effects as morphine on smooth muscle. (94,121). Other undesirable side effects include profuse sweating, dryness of mouth, and

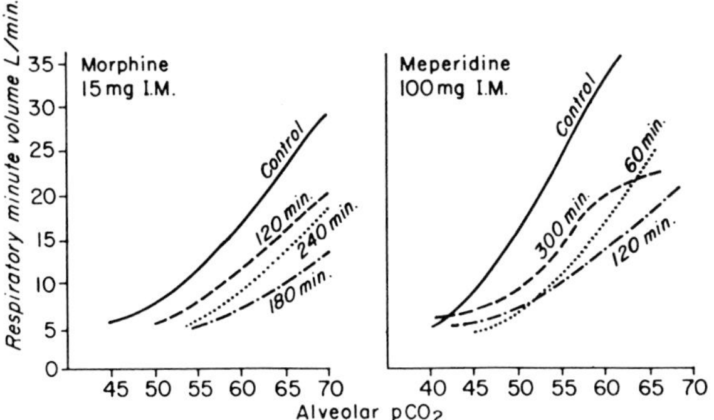


**Fig. 17–6.** Respiratory depressant effects of morphine and meperidine determined by the respiratory response to carbon dioxide. Graphs show relation between end expiratory carbon dioxide tension (horizontal) and respiratory minute volume (vertical). Carbon dioxide tension was increased by permitting the endogenous $CO_2$ to accumulate by removing the soda lime canister from the system. Both drugs diminished significantly the response to carbon dioxide, indicating depression of the respiratory center. (Redrawn from Eckenhoff JE, Helrich M, Rolpf WD Jr: Anesthesiology. 18:703, 1957.)

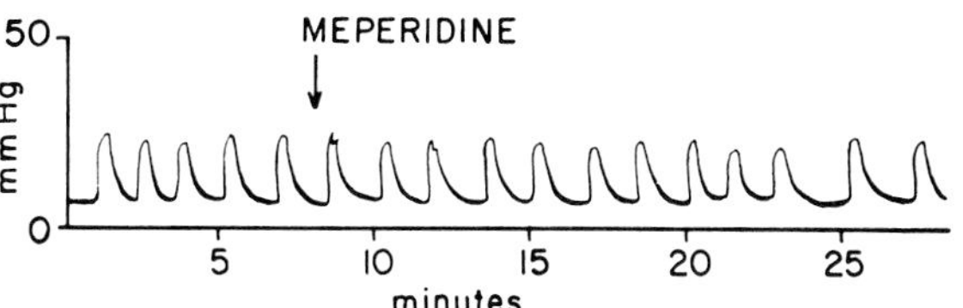


**Fig. 17–7.** Lack of effect of meperidine on uterine contractions. At time of injection the cervix was 3 to 4 cm dilated. No alteration of the intensity, frequency, or pattern of contraction is noted. (Redrawn from Alfonsi PL, Massi GB: Obstet. Gynecol. 18:37, 1963.)

flushing on the face. The incidence of nausea and vomiting and vertigo is similar to that of morphine (92).

## Effect on Labor

The effect of meperidine on the effect on labor is similar to that of morphine. One tokodynamometric study indicated no effect on uterine contractions (Figure 17–7) (99), while others show a uterine depressant action (122–124). This difference in results may be due to the time of application of the medication. It appears that the injection of meperidine during the very early stage of labor may indeed slow down uterine contractions (1), but if given at the proper time, it has no hampering effect and may actually enhance the progress of labor.

## Effect on the Newborn

The plasma level of meperidine in the newborn is approximately 60 to 70% of that in the maternal blood. However, there is little correlation between the blood level and the clinical condition of the infant. Well-conducted studies show that 15% of the infants delivered of mothers given meperidine failed to breathe adequately within 2 minutes, while others showed that the minute ventilation was decreased 10 to 15% (125). Continuous measurement of oxygen saturation demonstrates a residual depressant effect that persists for several hours (126). Many studies show that meperidine is no better and sometimes worse than other opioids (105,127,128).

### *Alphaprodine (Nisentil)*

This opioid is no longer available in the United States but may still be available in other countries in the world. Alphaprodine is a synthetic compound that is structurally similar to meperidine and has been used extensively in obstetrics. When given subcutaneously, it produces faster analgesia than other opioids (129). At doses ranging from 30 to 60 mg, alphaprodine produces very satisfactory analgesia in 80 to 90% of the parturients, especially in the early stages of labor (111,129–131). Well-controlled clinical trials in patients with postoperative pain suggested that 30, 40, or 50 mg of this medication have the approximate analgesia potency of 6, 8, or 10 mg of morphine or 50, 75, or 100 mg of meperidine, respectively (Keats, AS: Personal communication). Using a double-blinded technique, Gillam and associates (111) found no difference in the degree, time of onset, and duration of analgesia produced by 50 to 100 mg of meperidine or by 20 to 40 mg of alphaprodine in obstetric patients. These results suggest that the advantage of a more rapid absorption and, therefore, more prompt analgesia following subcutaneous administration of this medication is not reproducible when the medication is given either intramuscularly or intravenously.

#### Side Effects on Mother

There is no significant difference in the side effects afforded by this medication versus other opioids on the mother. The only significant difference is the shorter duration of the side effects, and possibly less vomiting than other opioids.

#### Effect on Labor

Most clinical reports indicate that alphaprodine does not interfere with labor. Gillam and co-workers found no significant difference of the effect of alphaprodine and meperidine on the length of labor (111). Using intrauterine tokodynamometric measurements, Ekelman and Reynolds (132) noted a decrease in the intensity of uterine contractions in 50% of patients who received various amounts of alphaprodine intravenously. This effect was greater in primiparous than multiparous patients and in patients whose membranes were intact. As pointed out, the effects of alphaprodine on uterine contraction may or may not be of sufficient duration or magnitude to delay the progress of labor.

#### Effect on the Infant

Contrary to the enthusiastic claims found in most clinical reports, well-conducted studies indicate that alphaprodine is not the void of neonatal respiratory depression, but is similar in that respect to other opioids (111,131,132). Gillam and associates (111) found that neonatal depression was not encountered among those parturients who delivered over 1 hour of the time of the last dose of alphaprodine.

### *Fentanyl*

Fentanyl is a synthetic opioid related to phenylpiperidine and is approximately 80 to 100 times as potent as morphine. It is used mostly for general anesthesia in combination with other anesthetic agents. Fentanyl in doses of 100 to 300 μg is often given to mothers under general anesthesia for cesarean section after the neonate is born. Since 1980, fentanyl has been used epidurally (133). Being highly lipophilic, fentanyl, or other lipophilic opioids, does not accumulate when given at the appropriate doses in the cerebral spinal fluid (134,135). When applied intraspinally, these opioids should be injected as close as possible to the spinal segments where the primary nociceptive afferents, carrying the nociceptive impulses from the involved dermatomes, enter the spinal cord. When this is accomplished, small doses of the drug will produce significant analgesia. The injection of relatively large doses of epidural fentanyl (50 to 100 ug) below the termination of the spinal cord produces analgesia but, very likely, the effect in this particular instance is mostly systemic due to absorption via the epidural venous plexi. In fact, the intravenous injection of 100 μg of fentanyl is also very effective in relieving intense acute pain (136).

Sufentanil, which is 8 to 10 times more potent then fentanyl, and alfentanil, which is about 10 times less potent than fentanyl, have not been studied yet as systemic analgesic for acute pain but they may offer some advantages over fentanyl due to their short duration of action and therefore easier titrability by continuous IV infusion. Over the last several years, small doses of sufentanil have often been mixed with low concentrations of bupivacaine (0.125% to 0.0625%) to be infused epidurally for labor pain control.

## Less Commonly Used Opioids

The following opioids are not used often in labor and delivery by the systemic route but they are listed because of their possible use in obstetric patients.

### *Codeine*

Except for aspirin, codeine is probably the most widely used analgesic and is the most commonly used prescription opioid in the world. This is due to its high oral efficacy and low incidence and degree of physical dependence in most individuals who are given the drug for prolonged periods. Tolerance can develop necessitating an increase in dosage and/or frequency of administration. Its mode of action is similar to all opioids and the side effects are similar but less intense than those of other opiates. These include nausea, vomiting, sedation, dizziness, and constipation. The major drawback to codeine is that it is not as effective in treating severe pain and therefore stronger opioids must be used in those cases.

### *Partially Synthetic Derivatives of Morphine*

#### *Dihydrohydroxymorphone (Numorphan)*

Oxymorphone (Numorphan) is a parenteral opioid with a potency 7 to 10 times that of morphine and with pharmacologic effects quite similar to those of morphine. A rectal suppository preparation containing 5 mg of oxymorphone is available.

#### *Diacetyl-morphine (heroin)*

Heroin is not available for clinical use in the United States. However, it is used in many parts of the world, especially for the treatment of terminal cancer pain. Intramuscular heroin is approximately two times as potent as morphine. It has a slightly faster onset of action but shorter duration than morphine (137). Heroin is readily absorbed by the oral, nasal, and gastrointestinal routes. However, heroin is rapidly metabolized to morphine in the liver during its first pass, before it enters the CNS where its pharmacologic effects are mediated (138). As a consequence, equal milligram doses of morphine provide slightly more blood morphine than heroin (139). Several studies have failed to show the advantage of this drug over morphine when used at equipotent dosages, either by oral or other routes (140).

## Partially Synthetic Derivatives of Codeine

### Oxycodone

Oxycodone is a semisynthetic codeine analogue derived from thebaine. Its potency is similar to morphine; 10 mg of oxycodone are equivalent to 10 mg of oral morphine. The effects are qualitatively similar to morphine, with a duration of action from 4 to 6 hours. Oxycodone, 5 mg, is available in the United States in combinations with either 325 mg of aspirin (Percodan) or 325 mg of acetaminophen (Percocet). These combinations are quite effective in relieving moderate pain as experienced several days after an operation.

## Synthetic Compounds

***Levorphanol.*** Levorphanol (Levo-Dromoran) is a synthetic opioid (a morphinan) with a potency approximately four times that of morphine. Side effects and mode of action are very similar to morphine with the possible exception of less nausea and vomiting. It is quite ineffective when given orally and therefore is usually not used by this route.

***Methadone.*** Methadone (Dolophine) is a synthetic opioid slightly more potent but less dependence producing than morphine. Methadone produces less euphoria and less sedation than many other opioids. The central mechanism of action is very similar to morphine. It is well absorbed when taken orally so there is little advantage to parenteral administration. Methadone has a long half-life and consequently a longer duration of action than any of the other aforementioned opioids (141). This property makes it an ideal drug for long-term administration. For these reasons, methadone is commonly used in maintenance programs and is a very useful drug in managing pain problems necessitating prolonged treatment with opioids. Its longer duration of action is primarily because the majority of the drug is first protein bound and then slowly released back to the plasma as diffusible fraction. To reach a steady state, several days of administration are needed. During the first 2 to 3 days, therefore, methadone should be given every 4 to 6 hours and thereafter every 6, 12, and even 24 hours. The range of dosage and frequency varies according to the severity of the pain and the patient's tolerance. Oral doses of 5 to 10 mg every 6 to 8 hours are quite common. However, dosages in the order of 20 to 30 mg every 4 hrs have been given without ill effects in terminal cancer patients.

Its efficacy has been proven in the management of terminal cancer patients with pain, administration lasting up to 2 years without any significant abuse manifestation. There are less clear indications for its long-term use in chronic nonmalignant pain problems, and, in general, long-term opioid administration should be avoided in these cases. However, patients with chronic pain such as low back pain, with cyclic variations of intensity and severity, time-limited bouts of pain can certainly be treated with methadone (or any other long-acting opioids) on a recurrent basis.

***Propoxyphene.*** Propoxyphene (Darvon) was first introduced under the premise that it had the same analgesic potential as codeine but without the dependence liability or side effects. Several clinical trials have shown, however, that 90 to 120 mg orally are equipotent to 60 mg of codeine and doses of 60 mg are no more effective than 600 mg of aspirin. Doses of 32 mg or lower are no more efficacious than placebo. From clinical experience propoxyphene appears to have an abuse potential but it is not clear if this is physiological or psychologic. The drug is often compounded with other medications such as acetylsalicylic acid or acetaminophen. Unless the drug has been used at high dosages, such as 800 to 1200 mg per day, there is no clear evidence that withdrawal reactions will ensue after acute cessation of the drug. Thus, propoxyphene appears to be less effective as an analgesic than codeine and has enjoyed some popularity because of its alleged lower dependence potential, a property not observed in practice. In addition to being less potent, its higher cost should discourage clinicians from prescribing it as a substitute for codeine.

## Agonist-antagonist Derivatives

Agonist-antagonist opioids are less efficacious than the pure agonists but they can produce analgesia with less respiratory depression and have a lower abuse potential. With this class of opioids, there tends to be a ceiling effect on respiratory depression as well as on analgesia.

In recent years, in an attempt to isolate a drug with high analgesic activity and a low incidence of side effects, several drugs with agonist/antagonist activity, or partial agonistic activity, have been introduced to clinical practice.

***Buprenorphine.*** Buprenorphine (Buprenex; Temgesic) is a semisynthetic derivative of thebaine; it is highly lipophilic and binds strongly to the mu class opiate receptor. Buprenorphine is about 20 to 30 times more potent than morphine when given intramuscularly and therefore its equianalgesic dose, for 10 mg of morphine, is 0.3 mg. It is also easily absorbed from the oral mucosa. A sublingual preparation has been developed and used in most parts of the world for several years. The drug produces its analgesic effect 45 to 60 minutes after parenteral administration. The duration of action varies from 3 to 14 hours after a single dose. Data from over 9000 patients indicate that the mean duration of action is a little more than 8 hours (142). The drug has proven effective in postoperative (143) and myocardial infarction pain, pain of neoplastic and orthopedic origin, labor pain, and as an adjunct to anesthesia. The side effects are very similar to those of morphine, though euphoria seems to be less frequent while a "responsive" sedation is more evident (142).

In countries where sublingual buprenorphine is available, chronic-pain patients have received it for several months without the need to increase the dosage, indicating that the development of tolerance to its analgesic effect may be slower than with other opioids (144). Some patients chose to discontinue the drug because of side effects, especially sedation and nausea, rather than discontinue due to failure to obtain analgesia. Abrupt withdrawal of buprenorphine in dependent patients causes a mild to moderate abstinence syndrome much less severe than that after morphine withdrawal. The abstinence syndrome peaks approximately 2 weeks after discontinuation of buprenorphine and lasts for over a week.

Patients using other mu agonist opioids should not be abruptly switched to buprenorphine as this may precipitate an abstinence syndrome (see Table 17–2).

A clinical observation indicates that in about 20% of patients treated, buprenorphine does not induce significant analgesia even if doses are increased. In these patients, switching to another opioid is advised, though patients in which buprenorphine affords good pain relief and administered by Patient-Controlled Analgesia pumps, it is the drug with higher indices of preference by patients (145).

***Butorphanol.*** Butorphanol (Stadol; Dorphanol) is a morphinan with characteristics similar to pentazocine, but with a greater analgesic efficacy and fewer side effects. The parenteral use is associated with significant sedation even though patients remain responsive (146). It produces approximately 50% less nausea and vomiting than morphine and such side effects as constipation and urinary retention are less frequent after chronic administration than with morphine if used at therapeutic doses. This drug has been available for over 10 years and few cases of drug abuse have been reported. A transnasal preparation of the drug is available for the treatment of acute pain (147). Each nasal spray delivers 1 mg of butorphanol. Its pharmacokinetic profile is very similar to IV administration of the drug. After transnasal application, 70% of the drug is available if compared to IV injection (Figure 17–8). This preparation has been tested for postcesarean pain with good results (147).

***Nalbuphine.*** Nalbuphine (Nubain) is an analgesic derivative of the agonist oxymorphone and the antagonist naloxone. It is a kappa and sigma agonist and a moderately potent mu antagonist. While nalbuphine is well-absorbed after oral, intramuscular, or subcutaneous administration, the oral form is not presently marketed. The analgesic effect after intramuscular administration appears after 45 to 60 minutes and has a duration slightly longer than morphine. When used in equipotent dosage, the respiratory depression is of similar degree to that produced by morphine. However, there seems to be no further increase in respiratory depression with doses above 30 mg of nalbuphine (146).

The drug has been used successfully in the management of cancer patients and in this situation seems to act like morphine (148). Euphoria is observed after 8 mg of nalbuphine IM, and dysphoria and psychotomimetic reactions are usually not problematic until a dose of 70 mg is reached. A primary side effect is sedation similar to that induced by butorphanol. The plasma half-life of nalbuphine is approximately 5 hours, and it is mostly metabolized in the liver. Tolerance and physical dependence have been described. High doses of the drug tend to produce irritability, inability to concentrate, depression, and headaches after approximately 1 week. Because nalbuphine is a mu antagonist, it may precipitate an abstinence syndrome in patients taking large doses of morphine over

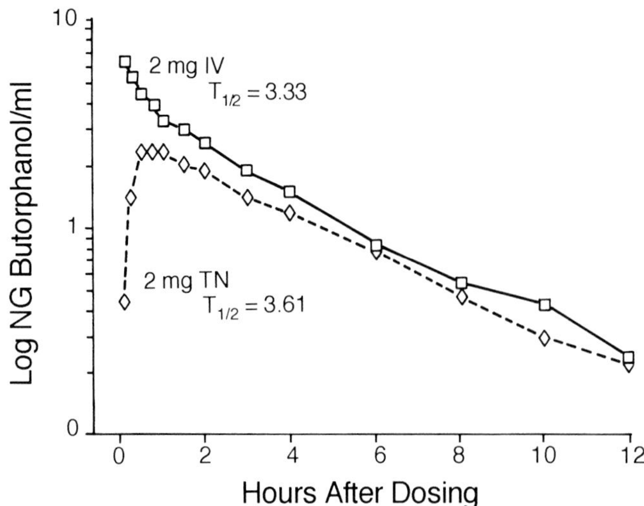


**Fig. 17–8.** Transnasal butorphanol pharmacokinetics. Fourteen normal volunteers received transnasal (TN) and intravenous (IV) butorphanol in a study sponsored by the Department of Metabolism and Pharmacokinetics, Bristol-Myers Company. Plasma samples were taken from peripheral vein. $T_{1/2}$, half-life. (Redrawn from Cool WM, Kurtz NM, Chu G: Transnasal delivery of systemic drugs. *In* Advances in Pain Research and Therapy: Opioid Analgesia. Vol. 14. Edited by C Benedetti, CR Chapman, G Giron. New York, Raven Press, 1990.)

time, and therefore these patients should not be abruptly switched to nalbuphine. Nalbuphine, at doses of 2 to 5 mg IV, is effective in reversing the pruritus caused by intraspinal morphine.

***Pentazocine (Talwin).*** This drug is a benzomorphine derivative with both opioid agonist and antagonist properties. It was first introduced with the claim that it was a good opioid with no dependence potential. Its mechanism of action is similar to that of other opioids, and it has the advantage that it can be administered both parenterally and orally. It displays the same side effects as other opioids, including respiratory depression, somnolence, decreased cough reflex, nausea, and in many patients, unpleasant hallucinations. After prolonged use, abrupt discontinuation of the drug causes a severe abstinence syndrome that is often worse than that caused by morphine or other opioids (149). Another problem with this drug is that some physicians administer opioids on a rotating, weekly basis using three or four different opioids alternately with the mistaken assumption that this decreases the possibility and incidence of dependence and tolerance. The alternate use of an agonist with an agonist/antagonist may cause severe problems both in the management of pain and in the appearance of abstinence symptoms. The use of pentazocine after a pure agonist may induce reversal of the analgesic effect by its antagonistic action.

## *Opioid Antagonists*

In 1915, Pohl produced the first opioid antagonist by providing minor change of the codeine molecule (150). Minor changes done to other opioid agonists have produced chemical substances that bind to one or more opioid receptors and produce no pharmacologic effect. These substances have the ability to displace competitively an opioid agonist from the receptor and, therefore, reducing or abolishing, in a dose dependent basis, the pharmacologic effect caused by the opioid agonist. Naloxone, the (N-Allyl) derivative of oxymorphone, and naltrexone are two opioid antagonists. They both have high affinity for the mu receptors but they also interact lightly with the delta and kappa receptor. To antagonize the effect of delta and kappa ligands, high doses of naloxone must be used.

***Naloxone.*** Naloxone is often used to reverse the respiratory depression induced by an overdose of opioids. It is administered IV at the dose of 1 to 5 μg/kg. The effect is rapid and the respiratory depression promptly corrected. Intraveneous naloxone, carefully titrated, is often used after administration of intraspinal opioids to abolish unwanted side effects such as pruritus, urinary retention, nausea, and vomiting without significantly affecting the analgesics. If used judiciously, it will not cause significant reversal of the analgesia. Naloxone is a short-acting medication (30 to 45 minutes) and therefore supplemental doses may be needed in patients with respiratory depression caused by long-acting opioids. Intramuscular injections of twice the initial intravenous dose may provide longer therapeutic plasma levels (151). Alternatively, a continuous infusion of 5 μg/kg/hr of naloxone may be used for long-term treatment of respiratory depression such as that induced by a high dose of intraspinal opioid.

A rapid injection of IV naloxone may cause nausea and vomiting. This may be reduced by giving the therapeutic dose over 2 to 3 minutes. Cardiovascular stimulation has occurred following administration of opioid antagonists. Tachycardia, hypertension, pulmonary edema (152–156), and cardiac dysrhythmia up to ventricular fibrillation have occurred following the administration of naloxone. This has been attributed to a sudden increase in sympathetic nervous system activity (157).

***Naltrexone.*** Naltrexone also acts predominantly as a mu antagonist, though in contrast to naloxone, it is quite active after oral administration and its effect is sustained up to 24 hours.

***Cholecystokinin.*** The duodenal mucosa secretes an octapeptide, cholecystokinin, which increases the contractility of the gallbladder and relaxes the sphincter of Oddi. When administered in the central nervous system, this substance antagonizes the analgesic effect of opioids. It has been suggested that this may be an endogenous opioid antagonist. This hypothesis is further substantiated by the fact that proglumide, a cholecystokinin antagonist, potentiates opioid analgesia in animals (158).

## General Principles of Application of Analgesics

The preceding section is a very concise summary of the enormous amount of data available on the pharmacology of opioids. However, even with this knowledge, providing a patient with the most effective analgesia and precise dosing schedule for a specific acute pain problem is a difficult and time-consuming task. The major reasons for these difficulties are the subjectiveness of pain and the difficulties in measuring it (159,160), the paucity of pharmacodynamic knowledge about both the analgesic and side effects elicited by these drugs, and the great individual variation in drug requirement which, at present, does not seem to follow any specific pattern. To reach a therapeutic plan for an individual patient, great care should be taken in obtaining a detailed history that focuses on the effects of the opioids previously used, on the effects experienced, on the possibility of previous long-term use of them and therefore the presence of tolerance as well as the present use of drugs that may interact with opioids (for example, MAO inhibitor and meperidine).

In treating the pain of an obstetric patient, several factors must be taken into consideration, though the most important is the relationship between the administration of the opioid and the time of delivery of the newborn. If the pharmacologic effects are still present in the mother at the time of delivery, then the newborn will also be affected. Respiratory depression is, in reality, the only significant negative side effect that the opioid may induce on the newborn. If this should occur, it is easily treatable by assisting the ventilation and injecting 0.01 mg/kg of naloxone intramuscularly. Naloxone should not be given to neonates born of mothers who have a physical dependency to opioids as it can trigger withdrawal symptoms.

The use of systemic opioids during a normal delivery should be quite limited. Morphine at a dose of 5 to 15 mg of IM or IV or the equianalgesic dose of meperidine or hydromorphone can be given during the very early phase of labor, up to 3 to 4 cm of cervical dilatation. Afterward its use should be curtailed to prevent significant neonatal depression. As the labor progresses and the intensity of pain increases, intraspinal administration of analgesic should be instituted.

In the early 1980s, some authors described the use of intraspinal opioids for labor and delivery and reported unsatisfactory analgesia (161–164). This should not be surprising because the intensity of labor pain, especially during the accelerating phase of cervical dilatation, is such that the intraspinal opioids cannot provide complete pain relief. It should be remembered that during the second stage, sacral anesthesia, not analgesia, is needed! It was soon discovered that, by adding local anesthetic, one could achieve satisfactory labor and delivery analgesia/anesthesia (165–168). The advantage of combining the two types of drugs is due to the synergistic effect that these two classes of medications have on each other. As a consequence, the concentration of the local anesthetic can be decreased to the point that it prevents the development of a significant motor blockade, and the miniscule doses of opioids needed do not cause significant depression of the mother and the neonate (167,169–179).

To understand why such small doses of intraspinal opioids provide such an intense analgesia, one must consider the pharmacokinetics of opioids, not in the plasma where it is usually measured, but instead, in the cerebral spinal fluid. The concentration of an opioid in the cerebral spinal fluid reflects much more closely the concentration in the CNS, the actual site of action of opioids for the purpose of analgesia. In particular, we must remember that intraspinal opioids cause analgesia or hypoalgesia by binding to the spinal opioid receptors, which are distributed throughout the length of the spinal cord. They are located both pre- and postsynaptically (between the first and second order neurons) and in the substantia geletinesa. The interaction between the opioid and its receptors interferes with or blocks the transmission of nociceptive impulses carried by the peripheral neurons. The action is segmental in nature, that is, the opioid receptors located around the synapses of the activated nociceptors must be exposed to the opioid to induce analgesia. It is important, therefore, that an effective concentration of opioid be present in the cerebral spinal fluid, bathing that segment of the spinal cord where the activated peripheral nerve enters.

Soon after the publication of the first articles describing the use of intraspinal opioids in humans (23–26), it was reported that the plasma concentration of epidurally administered morphine was very similar to the plasma concentration of a similar IM dose (Figure 17–9). In 1984, Nordberg (71) published a monogram as a supplement

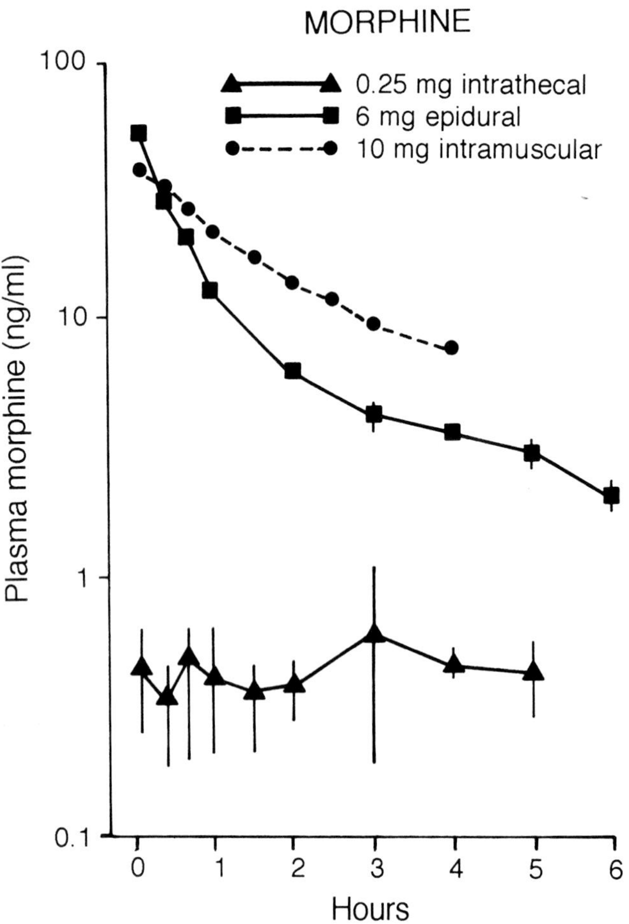


**Fig. 17–9.** Plasma concentrations of morphine after administration of 0.25 mg intrathecally, 6 mg epidurally, and 10 mg intramuscularly. Means ± SEM are shown. (Redrawn from Nordberg G: Pharmacokinetic aspects of spinal morphine analgesia. Acta. Anaesthesiol. Scand. 28(Suppl 79):1–38, 1984.)

of *Acta Anaesthesiologica Scandinavica*, in which he reported the results of several studies and provided a simple and clear pharmacologic explanation for the clinical observations that 0.2 to 0.5 mg morphine given intrathecally or 4 to 6 mg of morphine given epidurally provide intense analgesia for 12 to 36 hours (Figure 17–10).

Other studies showed the relationship between some physical characteristics of the opioids and the type of analgesia they could provide: either generalized or segmental pain relief. In particular, several studies (180–182) indicated that morphine, a hydrophilic medication, is not easily absorbed by the nervous tissue and therefore remains in the cerebral spinal fluid, which, as we know, is subjected to a slow, passive circulation. This permits any hydrophilic drug to be carried to different areas of the spinal cord and even the brain (Figure 17–11 and Figure 17–12) (71,183), and, in so doing, it provides generalized analgesia. Fentanyl and sufentanil, on the other hand, are lyophillic medications and provide a segmental analgesia, as their prompt absorption in the nervous tissues prevents their accumulation in the cerebral spinal fluid, and, therefore, do not reach dermatomes distant from the epidural site of injection of the drug. This is particularly true if the appropriate dose of the lipophilic drug is given. When high doses of lipophilic drugs are given epidurally, a significant amount will be absorbed by the epidural venous plexi to produce a generalized effect similar to parenteral injection.

What follows is the description of several protocols used to deliver the two opioids intraspinally.

## Continuous Epidural

Continuous epidural blockade is the technique of choice for the relief of labor and delivery pain (see Chapter 13 for a detailed discussion). The addition of an opioid to the analgesic solution has become fashionable in the last 7 years because it has allowed the anesthesiologist to decrease the concentration of the local anesthetic significantly and provide equally effective analgesia.

Fentanyl was used extensively in combination with low concentration of the local anesthetic bupivacaine (Marcaine) to provide good analgesia for parturition (163,165–167,172,184–186). The combination of the two medications is only warranted if it is associated with a significant decrease in the total amount of each drug used to achieve equal analgesia, so that the side effects induced by higher doses of either drug are diminished. The usual dosage consists of 2 μg/ml of fentanyl with either 0.625 mg or 1.25 mg/ml (0.0625% or 0.125% ) of bupivacaine. This combination is given at an infusion rate ranging from 8 to 15 mL per hour. Although there is no consensus among the experts, it is advisable to stop the fentanyl-containing solution 1 to 2 hours before the delivery of the baby so that the concentration of the opioid in the newborn will be significantly lower than if the infusion is continued up to the delivery of the neonate. When the fentanyl-containing solution is stopped, bupivacaine, at a concentration of 0.125% or 0.25%, is infused at 8 to 15 mL per hour to provide analgesia to the mother for the delivery.

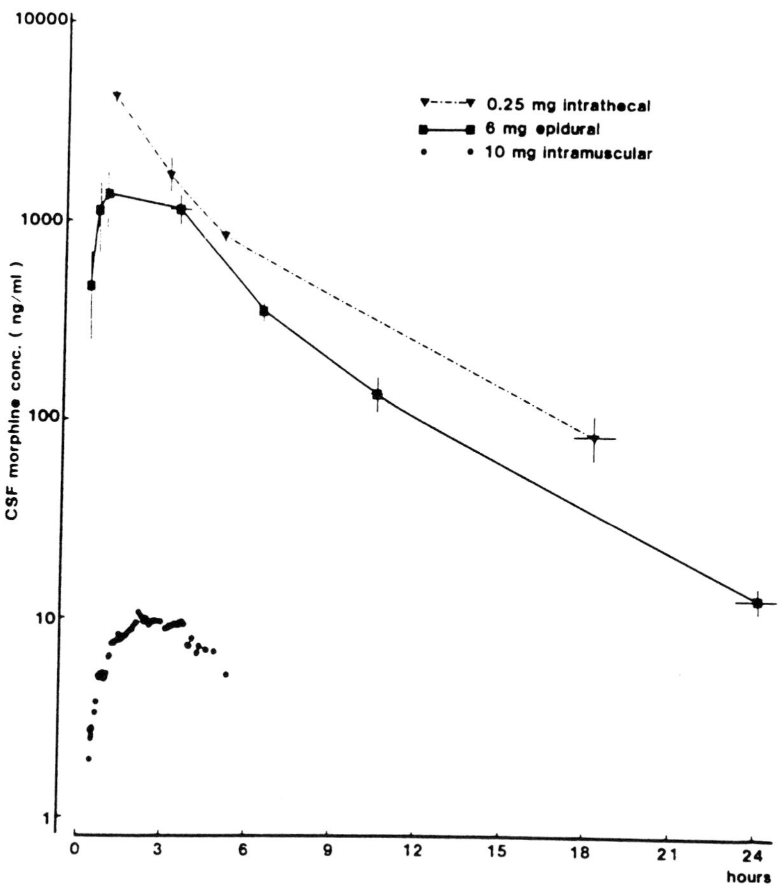


**Fig. 17–10.** Cerebral spinal fluid concentrations of morphine after administration of 0.25 mg intrathecally, 6 mg epidurally, and 10 mg intramuscularly. Means ± SEM are shown. (From Nordberg G: Pharmacokinetic aspects of spinal morphine analgesia. Acta. Anaesthesiol. Scand. 28(Suppl 79):1–38, 1984.)

In the last several years, numerous reports in the literature have described the use of sufentanil instead of fentanyl as an adjunct of local anesthetic for labor pain control (169,170,187–189). A recent article reported that the addition of up to 30 μg of sufentanil with 0.125% bupivacaine reduced the total amount of local anesthetic used for labor while producing equal analgesia, and provided less motor block and less instrumental deliveries (190). In our institution (The Ohio State University Hospitals), we use a bolus of 8 to 10 ml of 0.125% bupivacaine plus 0.5 μg/ml sufentanil before starting a continuous infusion of 8 to 15 ml of 0.625% bupivacaine plus 0.5 μg/ml sufentanil with very good results.

## *Continuous Intrathecal*

Continuous subarachnoid block was first proposed by Lemmon (191) in 1940 as a new anesthetic technique that would allow prolonged surgery to be performed under spinal anesthesia. The difficulty with the technique was the unavailability of proper equipment. Dr. Tuohy (192) suggested, a few years later, the introduction of a Number 4 urethral catheter in the subarachnoid space via a large needle. In 1951, Carpenter and associates (193) described the continuous subarachnoid infusion of diluted procaine solution for labor and delivery analgesia using a Vinylite catheter that could pass through an 18-gauge Quincke spinal needle. These authors reported a 10% incidence of postspinal headache. In 1962, Bizzarri and associates (194) reported on 27 patients treated with a thinner subarachnoid catheter inserted via a special 21-gauge spinal needle. One of the major reasons that continuous subarachnoid block did not achieve widespread application was the side effect of spinal headache, which many patients developed. A recent study, which compared the incidence of headache using two different-sized needles, found that in young people, a smaller-gauge needle, such as 25 to 26 gauge, significantly decreased the chance of postspinal headache (195).

The development of very small catheters (28 and 32 gauge) reactivated the interest in continuous intrathecal anesthesia and analgesia for obstetrics.

There are several advantages of a continuous subarachnoid block versus a continuous lumbar epidural:

1. First and foremost is that the amount of medication needed to obtain the desired analgesia is approximately one order of magnitude less with subarachnoid block than with epidural block. This translates in less medication not only to the mother but also to the fetus;
2. One of the risks of performing lumbar epidural blocks is the inadvertent injection of large quantities of local anesthetic either intravascularly or subarachnoid. In the event of these occurrences, the patient may develop a toxic effect from high dosages of intravenous local anesthetic (convulsions) or develop a very high or total subarachnoid block that

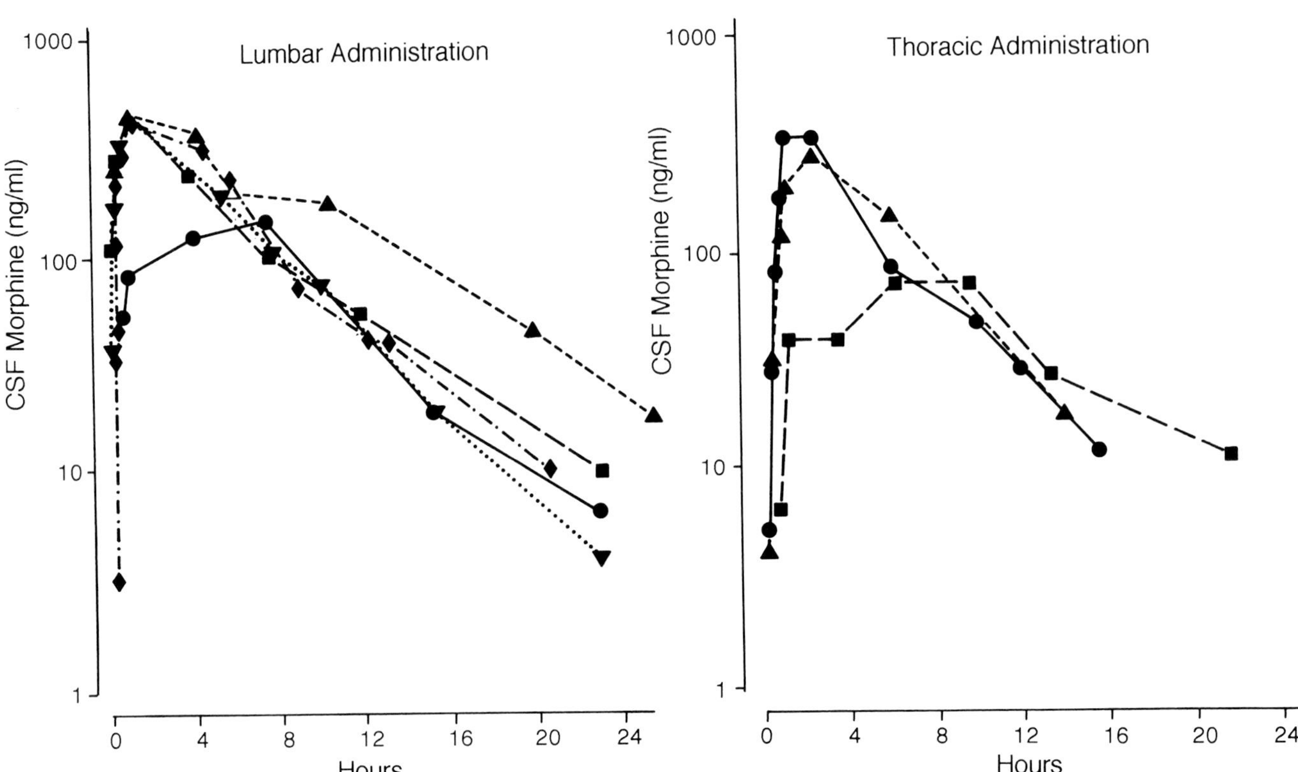


**Fig. 17–11.** Morphine concentrations in lumbar cerebral spinal fluid (L3–L4) after epidural injection of 2 mg in 10 ml saline in the lumbar (L2–L4) and thoracic region (T7–T8), respectively. Individual values are shown. (Redrawn from Nordberg G: Pharmacokinetic aspects of spinal morphine analgesia. Acta. Anaesthesiol. Scand. 28(Suppl 79):1–38, 1984.)

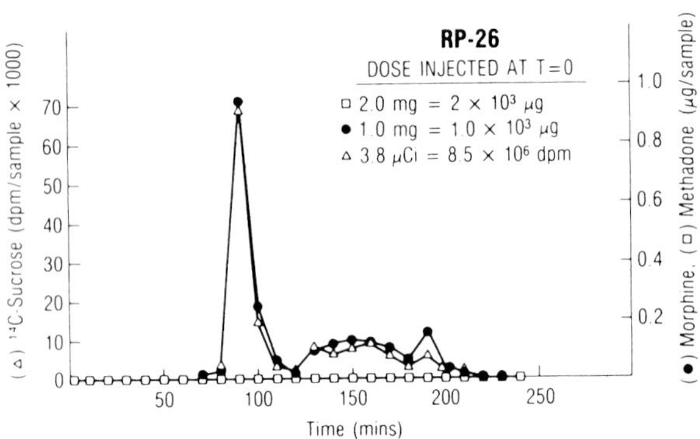


**Fig. 17–12.** Cisternal cerebral spinal fluid concentration of C-14 sucrose, morphine, and methadone after lumbar subarachnoid administration. Cisternal cerebral spinal fluid is collected by ventriculo-cisternal perfusion. C-14 sucrose and morphine appear and peak simultaneously in cisternal cerebral spinal fluid at 90 minutes after lumbar administration. Methadone is cleared completely from cerebral spinal fluid before reaching the cisterna magna. (From Payne R: Cerebral spinal fluid distribution of opioids in animals and man. Acta. Anaesthesiol. Scand. 31(Suppl 85):38–46, 1987.)

requires assisted ventilation and support of the blood pressure with vasoactive drugs;

3. Lumbar epidural blocks have a higher failure rate than subarachnoid blocks, and subarachnoid block has a faster onset of action than that associated with epidural block. For this reason, it is particularly useful if an urgent cesarean section is to be performed. Especially in the pregnant woman, unilateral or "spotty blocks" develop with an annoying frequency. The reason is not presently very clear, and;
4. Continuous subarachnoid blocks can be more carefully titrated to the desired duration and location of analgesia by using varying concentrations of local anesthetics and baricity of the solution.

We studied 26 parturients using the continuous spinal technique, delivered via a 32-gauge microcatheter (196). All had excellent pain control during parturition, and the incidence of instrumental delivery was not different from the use of epidural analgesia. Three patients developed a mild postspinal headache, which was treated conservatively. Seven other patients received a combination of 0.3 mg (0.3 ml) of preservative-free (PF) morphine together with 7 mg of isobaric lidocaine (0.7 ml of 1% lidocaine) injected through the spinal needle before the insertion of the microcatheter. Analgesia developed within 2 contractions from the injection of the mixture. If the continuous spinal had been started early during the labor (3 to 4 cm of cervical dilatation), the patients did not require any other analgesic until onset of the rapid phase of the first stage. At that point, 5 to 10 mg of isobaric lidocaine (1%) provided excellent analgesia. This dose was repeated several times until the end of the second stage (unpublished data).

The important advantages of continuous subarachnoid block have been somewhat overshadowed by several factors. At times, the insertion of the microcatheter is somewhat laborious, particularly with the 32-gauge catheter that had to be introduced using a paramedian approach, a technique which is not as popular as the midline approach. The report (197) that several elderly patients developed caudal equina syndrome after the use of 5% hyperbaric lidocaine given at dosages above 100 mg has induced the Food and Drug Administration of the United States to withdraw these catheters from the U.S. market. Presently, studies are being conducted to establish the limitations and dangers of this technique. A recent study (198) showed that due to the extremely small size of the microcatheters, the injections of local anesthetics into the cerebrospinal fluid is not associated with turbulence and mixing of the two liquids, resulting in that the local anesthetic tends to accumulate undiluted in the sacral conus of the subarachnoid space. It is quite likely that the undiluted solution of high concentration lidocaine has a neurolytic effect on the small sacral nerves traveling in the subarachnoid space.

Intraspinal opioids, in particular intrathecal opioids, are drugs of choice in patients with severe cardiovascular diseases such as severe aortic stenosis, pulmonary hypertensions, coarctation of the aorta, intraventricular defects, and Eisenmenger's syndrome. In these patients, the increased release of catecholamines induced by the intense pain of parturition as well as the decrease in peripheral vascular resistance caused by the sympatholytic effect of the local anesthetic can have deleterious effects on the well-being of the mother. In these cases, the intense analgesia provided by intrathecal morphine has great advantages in the management of these patients. If needed, the addition of a small dose of local anesthetic injected via a caudal epidural catheter will greatly increase the analgesic effect needed for the delivery without causing significant sympathetic blockade.

### *Needle through Needle*

The observations that subarachnoid morphine can provide excellent analgesia for early labor but that supplemental analgesia provided by a local anesthetic is often required as labor progresses, have prompted the development of the needle-through-needle technique. This technique consists of localizing the epidural space in the usual manner. Once the epidural space has been identified, a thin, 25-to 27-gauge, 12-cm spinal needle is passed through the epidural needle and inserted in the subarachnoid space and 0.25 to 0.5 mg of preservative-free morphine is injected. The spinal needle is then removed, and the epidural catheter passed through the epidural needle, which is then removed. With this technique, a very small dosage of intrathecal morphine provides very good analgesia, especially for the early phase of the first stage, and if needed, supplemental analgesia can be provided by activating the epidural catheter with local anesthetics. Using this technique, a study by Rawal, et al (199) has demonstrated much less local anesthetic can be used to provide equal pain relief when compared to the technique of continuous epidural without an opioid and only with local anesthetic. Another study (200) found that this was the only real advantage, as all the other parameters were similar between the two groups. This author has obtained very similar analgesia by injecting 4 to 5 mg of preservative-free morphine epidurally immediately after the test dose. With this technique, there is no need of a subarachnoid puncture and the plasma concentration of morphine at time of delivery is low in both the mother and neonate.

Intraspinal opioids cause several side effects. Table 17–8 summarizes the incidence of the side effect of using either 0.5 mg or 1 mg of morphine.

**Table 17–8.** Percentages of Patients Having Adverse Side Effects after Intrathecal Injection of 0.5 mg or 1 mg Morphine[a]

| Side Effects | Morphine 0.5 mg ($n$ = 12) (%) | Morphine 1 mg ($n$ = 18) (%) | Combined Data ($n$ = 30) (%) |
|---|---|---|---|
| Pruritus[b] | 58 | 94 | 80 |
| Nausea/vomiting | 50 | 56 | 53 |
| Urinary retention | 42 | 44 | 43 |
| Drowsiness/dizziness | 33 | 50 | 43 |
| Respiratory depression | 0 | 6 | 3 |
| Headache | 0 | 5 | 3 |

[a] This table demonstrates the incidence of side effects demonstrated by one study, but is representative of what might be expected. Pruritus is the most common side effect, Incidence of urinary retention is very high and probably related to labor and delivery. (Adapted from Abboud TK, Shnider SM, Dailey PA, Raya JA, Sarkis F, Grobler NM, Sadri S, Khoo SS, DeSousa B, Baysinger CL, Miller F: Intrathecal administration of hyperbaric morphine for the relief of pain in labor. Br J Anaesth 56: 1351–1360, 1984.)

[b] $P$ = 0.02: 0.5 mg vs. 1 mg.

## *Treatment of Nonparturition Acute Pain Syndromes in the Obstetric Patient*

After the delivery of the neonate or if the obstetric patient needs opioids during the pregnancy as in post-traumatic pain or surgical procedures during pregnancy, she can be treated like a typical patient. The one concern, in the postdelivery period, is that opioids are excreted in the milk; therefore, if the neonate is to be breast-fed, opioids should be used sparingly.

Moderate to severe pain in the obstetric patient, as after cesarean section, is best treated, if the professional expertise is available, with intraspinal opioids, which offer intense, excellent analgesia with a low degree of sedation and mental clouding, and allow not only early ambulation and activity of the parturient but also normal interaction of the mother with the neonate after the surgical delivery. If a single injection subarachnoid block is used for the cesarean section, the addition of 0.2 to 0.4 mg of preservative-free morphine to the solution will provide analgesia for 18 to 36 hours. If an epidural block is used instead as the anesthesia for the procedure, 3 to 5 mg of epidural preservative-free morphine will provide very good postoperative analgesia for 8 to 20 hours. Also, due to the low doses of opioids used to provide good analgesia, the concern of opioids in the breast milk is greatly decreased. When opioids cannot be used intraspinally, systemic administration still provides good pain control. For the majority of patients, the most appropriate method of providing systemic opioids is through Patient-Controlled Analgesia.

## *Patient-Controlled Analgesia*

In the early 1970s, the first reports appeared in the medical literature describing a new modality for the administration of analgesics to patients with acute and cancer pain (142,201–212). Patient-controlled analgesia consists of the self-administration of analgesics, mostly intravenously, via an infusion pump that can deliver a predetermined bolus dose whenever activated by the patient. Obviously, the parameters and limits are set by the physician. Patient-controlled analgesia was developed to help solve the problem of inadequate analgesia for hospitalized patients. During the past several years, the use of this technique has become popular in many medical centers around the world and more patients and medical personnel are accepting it as a satisfactory method of pain control (205,206,209,210–212). It is becoming apparent that 85% of the patients treated with this modality obtain good to excellent analgesia, 10% fail to understand how to use the patient-controlled analgesia pump, and 5% state that they prefer the attention of the nurse versus the self-administration of analgesics.

When properly used, patient-controlled analgesia is a good analgesic technique because it bypasses the complexities of individual pharmacokinetics and pharmacodynamics, which are responsible for the enormous interpatient variation in drug requirement, and provides a clear profile of doses needed for comfort (Figure 17–13) (213). Because the ideal opioid does not exist, as all have more or less severe and annoying side effects, we are seeing that patients tend to reach a level of comfort that usually is a balance between acceptable pain and minimal side effects. With patient-controlled analgesia, patients are able to maintain plasma concentration of opioids close to their minimal effective analgesic concentration (Figure 17–14).

For the application of this technique, special patient-controlled analgesia pumps are required. Several patient-controlled analgesia pumps are now available with different features. Intelligently designed patient-controlled analgesia pumps have the capability of providing both boluses on demand and a baseline continuous infusion that can be used either singularly or in combination; have a way of recording the patient's activation of the pump and

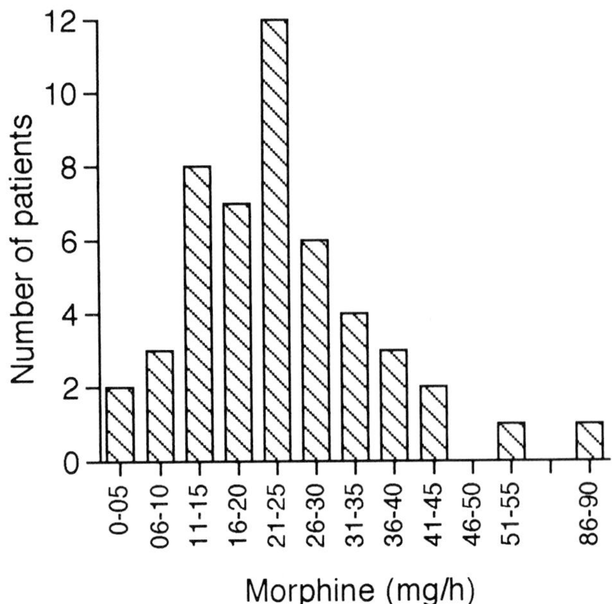


**Fig. 17–13.** Doses of morphine self-administered for postoperative pain by 49 patients using the Cardiff Palliator. (Redrawn from Dodson ME: Aspects of anaesthesia. A review of methods for relief of postoperative pain. Annals of the Royal College of Surgeons of England 64:324–327, 1982.)

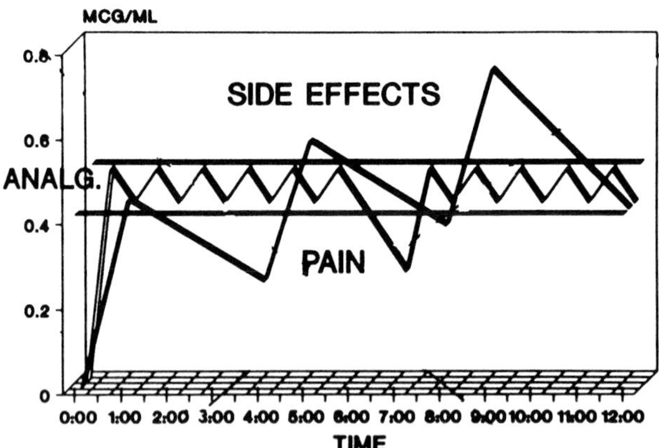


**Fig. 17–14.** Conceptual graph of plasma concentration achievable with patient controlled analgesia versus intramuscular injection of 100 mg of meperidine every 4 hours. The plasma concentration of intramuscular meperidine varies more than that obtainable with patient controlled analgesia. If the patient fails to activate the patient-controlled-analgesia device for a period of time (because of sleep, for instance) the plasma concentration will decrease below the therapeutic window. Because of this inconvenience, a continuous infusion proportional to the previous patient controlled analgesia use of the opioid will prevent this occurrence. (From Benedetti C: Acute pain: A review of its effects and therapy with systemic opioids. *In* Advances in Pain Research and Therapy: Opioid Analgesia. Vol. 14. Edited by C Benedetti, CR Chapman, G Giron. New York, Raven Press, 1990.)

the total amount of drug used; and all this information can and should be easily printed for proper recording. The availability of these pumps implies an initial capital investment on the part of the hospital. This cost is offset by the time saved by nursing personnel, who do not have to administer drugs on a routine basis, and by better analgesia, an important factor in preventing postoperative or post-traumatic complications (214–218), and therefore decreasing time of hospitalization and cost (216,217). A recent study has shown that patients being treated postoperatively with patient-controlled analgesia decreased the hospital cost by about 10% over similar patients treated with IM opioids, due to a shorter hospital stay (Table 17–9) (216). Morphine is commonly used for patient-controlled analgesia, although other opioids have been used. Table 17–10 summarizes the quality of analgesia provided by the most frequently used opioids versus side effects and patient acceptance.

The most effective protocol for the use of patient-controlled analgesia is to begin with an IV bolus of morphine, starting with 2 to 4 mg for a 70 kg adult, and then to slowly titrate within the next 20 to 30 minutes sufficient IV morphine to have the patient comfortable. At this point, the parameters of the patient-controlled analgesia pump are set to deliver a 1 or 2 mg bolus of morphine with each request and a lock-out period of 6 to 15 minutes. The lock-out period prevents redosing before the drug has time to take effect.

After an 8-hour period, the total use of morphine is calculated and the comfort of the patient is assessed. A comfortable, not overly sedated patient indicates proper use of the patient-controlled analgesia. At this point, the pump is set to deliver a continuous infusion of morphine with an hourly rate of one-eighth of the total dose used during the preceding 8 hours, and the patient still allowed to use the patient-controlled analgesia feature of the pump if pain reoccurs.

Reevaluation every 24 hours of the patient's comfort, sedation, and usage of the drug will permit adjustments of the continuous infusion to the patient's requirements. This technique provides good analgesia and has an advantage over single patient-controlled analgesia boluses in that the patient's plasma level of opiate does not fall much below the minimal effective analgesic concentration especially during sleep.

Although most studies using patient-controlled analgesia employed the intravenous route, if no intravenous access is available, the patient-controlled analgesia concept may be used with good effects via the intramuscular and even the subcutaneous route. Allowing the patient who can take oral analgesia to keep a small number of analgesic pills at the bedside and instructing her to take a pill when the pain becomes bothersome, the patient-controlled analgesia concept can be applied even for oral therapy (a quite accepted form of therapy when the patient is prescribed analgesic for home use!).

Although intraspinal opioids and patient-controlled analgesia are the techniques that provide the best and most satisfactory analgesia for the control of acute pain, they are not available in all medical centers. Good pain relief can still be provided with the use of a continuous infusion of opioids or even, more simply, with intramuscular opioids, provided that these are carefully titrated to the individual's need and a "cookbook" approach to pain management is avoided.

**Table 17–9.** Comparison of Cost of Hospitalization for Selected Surgical Procedures Using Patient-Controlled Analgesia (PCA) or Intramuscular As-Needed Injections of Opioids[a,b]

| Procedure | Average Cost | | | | |
|---|---|---|---|---|---|
| | Non-PCA | ($n^1$) | PCA | ($n^2$) | D |
| Lumbar laminectomy | $ 9,257 | 17 | $ 8,225 | 9 | $1,032 |
| Cholecystectomy | 8,876 | 25 | 7,892 | 15 | 984 |
| Thoracotomy | 20,626 | 20 | 18,891 | 5 | 1,735 |

[a] Adapted from ref. 117.
[b] $n$, number of patients ; $n^2$, number of patients; D, difference in cost.
(From Benedetti C: Acute pain: a review of its effects and therapy with systemic opioids. *In* Advances In Pain Research and Therapy, Vol. 14. Edited by C Benedetti. New York, Raven Press, 1990.)

**Table 17–10.** Postoperative Intravenous On-Demand Analgesia[a,b]

| Analgesic | Pain Score | Emesis (%) | Patient's View (%) + | = | − | Preferred Nurse (%) |
|---|---|---|---|---|---|---|
| Fentanyl | 1.07 | 32.5 | 81.0 | 19.1 | 0.0 | 17.5 |
| Alfentanil | 1.37 | 10.0 | 80.0 | 13.3 | 6.7 | 15.0 |
| Piritramide | 1.42 | 17.5 | 73.3 | 15.4 | 15.4 | 17.5 |
| Buprenorphine | 1.57 | 10.0 | 92.9 | 7.1 | 0.0 | 5.0 |
| Pentazocine | 1.60 | 15.0 | 68.4 | 15.8 | 15.8 | 5.0 |
| Morphine ($n$ = 21) | 1.95 | 4.8 | 81.8 | 9.1 | 9.1 | 9.5 |
| Pethidine | 2.22 | 7.5 | 47.1 | 35.3 | 17.7 | 5.0 |
| Tramadol | 2.27 | 7.5 | 36.0 | 24.0 | 40.0 | 20.0 |
| Nefopam | 2.90 | 2.5 | 46.2 | 7.7 | 46.2 | 15.0 |
| Metamizole | 3.02 | 22.5 | 11.1 | 37.0 | 51.9 | 22.5 |

[a] From ref. 85, with permission.
[b] Forty patients per group.
(From Benedetti C: Acute pain: a review of its effects and therapy with systemic opioids. In Advances In Pain Research and Therapy, Vol. 14. Edited by C Benedetti. New York, Raven Press, 1990.)

## *Continuous Infusion*

Acute pain can be treated effectively with continuous infusions of opioids, but the patient must be carefully monitored because of the possibility of overdosing. The infusion rate should be constantly modified in response to the patient's comfort and presence of side effects. The most effective way of using this technique is to initially give a loading dose of the chosen opioid so that the minimal effective analgesic concentration is rapidly achieved. One way of accomplishing this in a 70-kg adult patient is to give IV 2 to 4 mg of morphine, 20 to 30 mg of meperidine or 0.5 to 1 mg of dihydromorphone slowly (1 to 2 minutes). Another equal bolus may have to be given 10 to 15 minutes later should the desired analgesia not be obtained. This is followed by a continuous infusion at a rate per hour equal to one-fourth the total dose of morphine used to achieve analgesia with the loading dose, one-third that of meperidine or dihydromorphone. It deserves reemphasis that patients must be carefully monitored to observe any signs of drug accumulation and toxicity.

### *Intramuscular Administration*

The most frequent route of administration of opioids for treatment of pain is still IM injection because of its relative ease of administration. Several studies and clinical observations indicate that it provides variable results from the point of view of time of onset, intensity, and duration of analgesia (219–221). Austin, et al (222) have shown that the IM administration of 100 mg meperidine produces a peak meperidine concentration (PMC) which varies fivefold in different patients (Figure 17–15) and that any one patient given meperidine at different times of the day may show a twofold difference in peak meperidine concentration. If we combine these data on absorption with the concepts of minimal effective analgesic concentration and its large intrapatient variation, we can easily appreciate how unpredictable it is to obtain not only a reproducible pharmacokinetic picture among patients but a predictable pharmacodynamic response (Figure 17–16).

It is difficult to explain all the factors that can influence the plasma level and onset of analgesia, but certainly an important one is the site of the IM injection. Injection into a well-perfused muscle such as the deltoid will provide a faster and higher plasma level than an injection into a less well-perfused muscle or even into adipose tissue. This may occur when the injection is done in the gluteal region, and it will certainly influence the uptake of the drugs into the vascular system (223). Similarly, in hypovolemic or hypothermic patients, peripheral blood flow is reduced significantly and absorption impaired or abolished until reversal of the pathogenic state. Cases of delayed overdosage due to this mechanism have been reported (224). The basic fact still remains that the patient has to be carefully followed, the analgesia evaluated, and the dosages regimen revised so that the proper amount is given at regular intervals 20 to 30 minutes shorter than the duration of analgesia provided by that particular drug to that particular patient.

### *Other Routes of Administration*

Besides parenteral routes, other routes of administration are presently available and new ones are being developed. For painful syndromes in which oral intake is not curtailed, most opioids are available as oral preparations either as pills or tablets or as elixir.

***Transnasal.*** Butorphanol has had several clinical trials involving dental and episiotomy (225–227). They show that it has a long linear dose response analgesia with the same side effects of the injectable drug. In a comparison study between IV and transnasal butorphanol for post-cesarean section pain (228), 2 mg transnasal and 1 + 1 mg 60 minutes later gave more prolonged analgesia than 2 mg IV (Figure 17–17).

Sublingual buprenorphine is used extensively in the countries in which it is available, providing effective, long-lasting analgesia in at least 80% of the patients who use it properly (143,144). The tablets must be allowed to dissolve sublingually and be absorbed by the oral mucosa to provide the desired effect.

Rectal opioids can be used with success (229) and with good patient compliance should patients be unable to take oral medications.

## Sedatives

Parturition is often associated with fear and apprehension. Fear may be caused by the expected pain of labor and apprehension by the unknown outcome both with relation to the neonate and to the patient health. It is

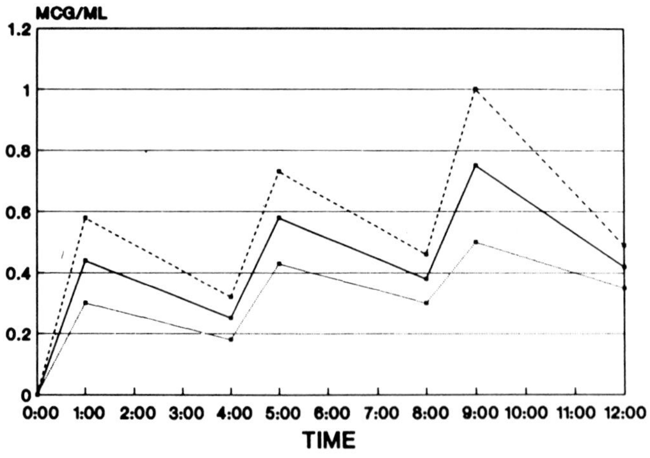


**Fig. 17–15.** Intramuscular injections of 100 mg of meperidine every 4 hours produce greatly fluctuating plasma concentrations, as shown in this chart. Of interest is the large individual variations of absorption and disposition of the drug from different patients. ——, mean; ------, +1 SD; and ·····, −1 SD. (Adapted from Austin KL, Stapleton JV, and Mather LE: Multiple intramuscular injections: A major source of variability in analgesic response to meperidine. Pain. 8:47–62, 1980.)

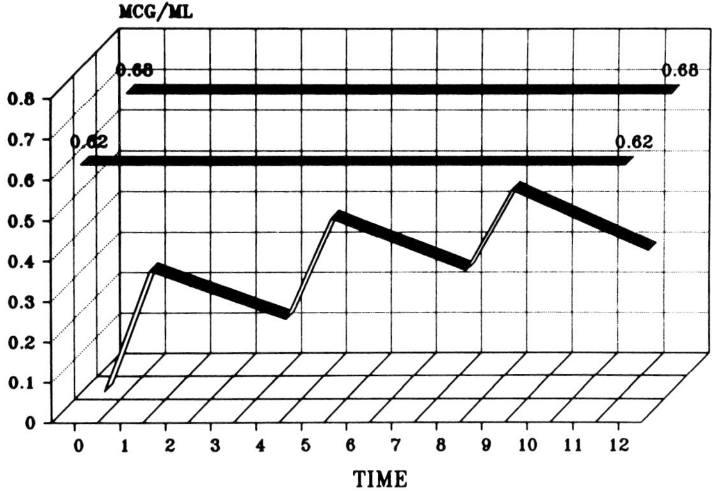


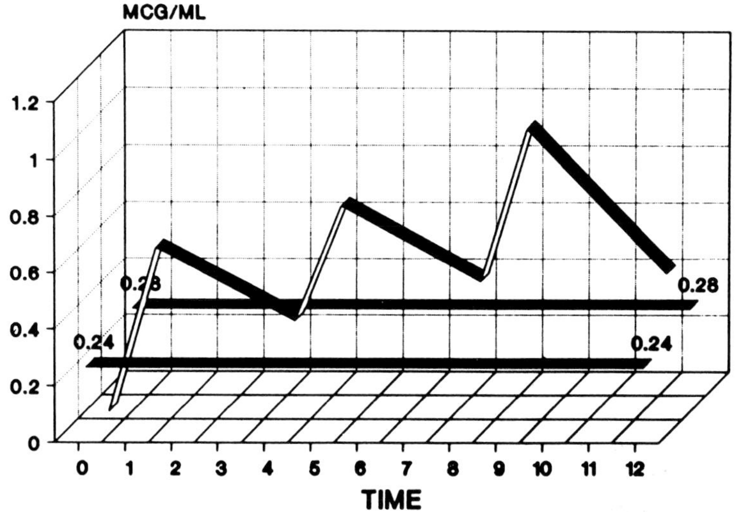


**Fig. 17–16.** The combination of the data relative to the meperidine plasma concentration after intramuscular injection and the minimal effective analgesia concentration of meperidine provides us with an extremely wide range of interaction between the two variables. **A:** Shows that a patient with a minimal effective analgesic concentrations 1 standard deviation from the mean who also obtained plasma concentrations (after 100 mg of meperidine IM every 4 hours) 1 standard deviation below the mean. In this patient the therapeutic window will not be reached even after 12 hours of drug administration, and there will be no pain relief. **B:** On the opposite side of the spectrum, a patient with a minimal effective analgesic concentrations 1 standard deviation below the mean and the absorption 1 standard deviation above the mean will reach toxic level of meperidine immediately after the first injection. Between these two extremes, the majority of the patient population will fall. From these illustrations it is clear that opioid therapy should be tailored to the patient's desired effect. (From Bendetti C: Acute pain: A review of its effects and therapy with systemic opioids. *In* Advances in Pain Research and Therapy: Opioid Analgesia. Vol. 14. Edited by C Benedetti, CR Chapman, G Giron. Raven Press, New York, 1990.)

therefore of great importance to alleviate these emotions. The most basic and effective anxiolytic therapy is the one provided by proper psychological preparation of the patient: this includes a detailed explanation of the physiology of labor and the expectations of the mother. In some parturients, however, anxiolytic medications may be needed. As briefly mentioned in the section on physiopathology, anxiety plays a major role in intensifying the pain perceived by patients and antianxiety medications are, at times, very useful. The addiction of anxiolytics to opioids has been shown to increase their analgesic effects while decreasing some of their side effects. Because all of the sedatives cross the placenta, they produce undesired pharmacologic effects on the fetus/neonate and therefore must be prescribed, just as we have mentioned with opioids, judiciously and during the early phase of labor. Short-acting drugs are preferred to long-acting ones. The drugs that have mostly been used for anxiolytic medication during labor are the barbiturates, the benzodiazepines and, in some parts of the world, scopolamine. Table 17–11 summarizes the optimal doses and therapeutic effects of this class of medications (230). It must be noted, however, that, at least in the United States, these medications are used much less frequently now than in the past. For this reason, these drugs will not be described in great depth. Some of these medications, when used at higher doses, induce general anesthesia and are further described in Chapter 18.

## Barbiturates

Since the introduction of the benzodiazepines, barbiturates have been used less frequently. Short-acting barbiturates can still be useful as obstetric sedatives in place of the more expensive, nonbarbiturate hypnotics. These medications should not be used in excessive dosages as done 30 or 40 years ago in an attempt to produce complete amnesia of the event, as these medications have significant pharmacologic effects on the neonate. At the doses of 50 to 200 mg, both secobarbital (Seconal) and pentobarbital (Nembutal) are effective during the early phase of the first stage to relieve anxiety (230).

***Therapeutic effects:*** When used at the above stated equipotent doses, barbiturates produce a sense of relaxation and tranquility but are not analgesic (231,232). At higher dosages they may even cause disorientation and

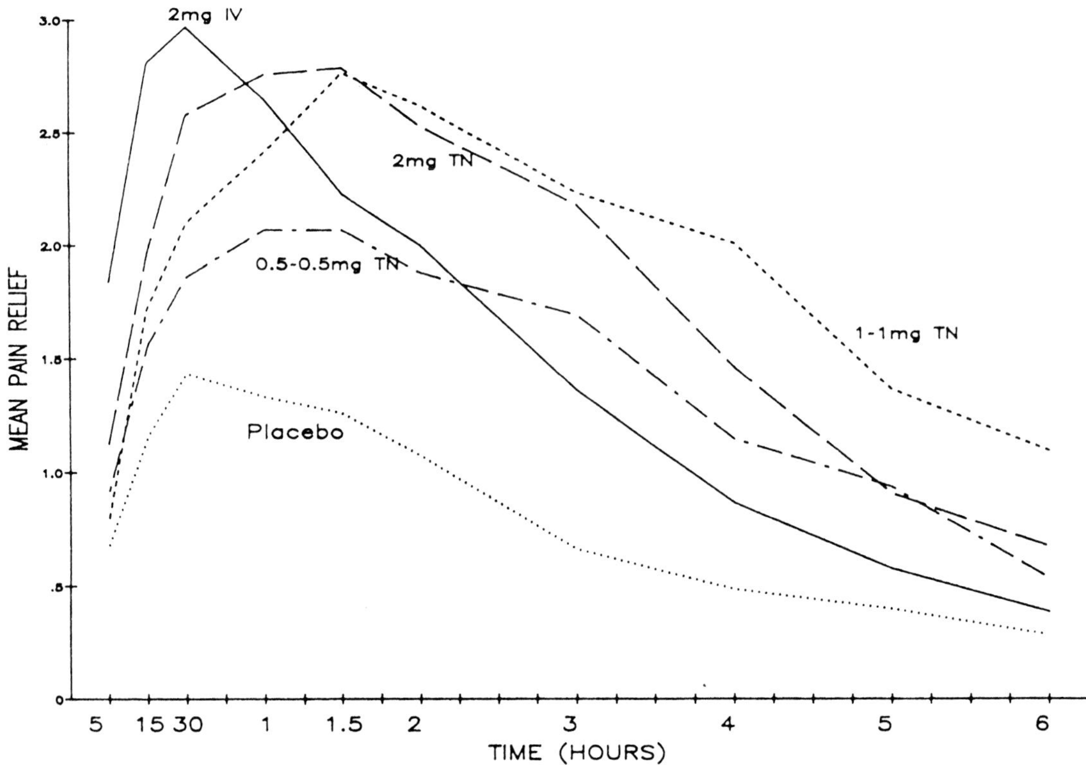


**Fig. 17–17.** Transnasal butorphanol in moderate to severe postoperative cesarean section pain. Time-effect curve for transnasal butorphanol: placebo (n = 37); 2 mg intravenous (IV) butorphanol (n = 37); 2 mg transnasal (TN) butorphanol (n = 38); 1 mg transnasal butorphanol followed by 1 mg at 60 minutes (n = 37); 0.5 mg transnasal butorphanol followed by 0.5 mg at 60 minutes (n = 38). Mean pain relief scores on the ordinate are plotted against time in hours on the abscissa. All treatments were double-dummy. (From Cool WM, Kurtz NM, Chu G: Transnasal delivery of systemic drugs. *In* Advances in Pain Research and Therapy: Opioid Analgesia. Vol. 14. Edited by C Benedetti, CR Chapman, G Giron. New York, Raven Press, 1990.)

an apparent hyperalgesic response to the pain of strong contractions (233). Therefore, barbiturates should be used, if at all, during the early phase of the first stage to relieve anxiety and promote sleep between the mildly painful contractions that are present during this phase of labor. When the pain becomes more intense and severe, regional anesthesia with local anesthetic or a mixture of local anesthetic and opioids, is indicated. If these techniques are not available then opioids, either orally, intramuscularly or intravenously, may be given, following the guidelines described in the earlier section, to diminish the pain.

Barbiturates are readily absorbed from the gastrointestinal tract (234). After oral administration, the peak effect is reached within 1 to 1½ hours and lasts approximately 4 hours; after intramuscular injections, the effect is present after 30 minutes and lasts approximately 2 hours. For faster effect, between 2 to 4 minutes, the intravenous route is needed. While the oral administration is more practical to use, especially if the woman is attended by a midwife, the intravenous route is safer because the medication can be carefully titrated to the need. In so doing, overdosages are easily prevented.

### *Side Effects on the Mother*

While small to moderate dosages of barbiturates (50 to 200 mg of pentothal or secobarbital) have no significant effect on the physiological parameters of the mother, (Figure 17–18) higher dosages, such as 300 mg and over, may cause instead a decrease in ventilation (235–237), cardiovascular depression, and a decrease in most maternal functions. Large doses of barbiturates administered to the mother also have a deleterious effect on the newborn.

### *Effect on Labor*

Proper doses of barbiturates given to anxious patients can have a beneficial effect on labor by counteracting the inhibitory role that anxiety plays on uterine contraction (237). At higher dosages, though, barbiturates may influence uterine contractions in a negative way (237) (see Figures 17–19 and 17–20).

### *Effect on Infant*

Within a few minutes of intravenous injection of a barbiturate to the mother, it appears in the fetal circulation. The metabolic process of barbiturate in the neonate is similar to that of the process in the mother (238). Barbiturates have a synergistic depressant effect not only when associated with opioids but even with asphyxia or other depressive states in the infant. This is much more evident in premature infants in which extreme care should be used in providing these drugs to the mother. When given

**Table 17–11.** Sedatives, Hypnotics, and Ataractics

| Drug | Synonym | Dose (mg.) | Therapeutic Effect* | | | | | |
|---|---|---|---|---|---|---|---|---|
| | | | Sedation | Sleep | Tranquilizer | Antiemetic | Antihistaminic | Analgesia |
| A. Barbiturates | | | | | | | | |
| 1. Secobarbital | Seconal | 50–200 | 4 | 4 | 2 | 2 | 0 | — |
| 2. Pentobarbital | Nembutal | 50–200 | | | | | | |
| 3. Cyclobarbital | Phanodorn | 100–300 | | | | | | |
| 4. Vinbarbital | Delvinal | 50–200 | | | | | | |
| B. Ataractics | | | | | | | | |
| 1. Phenothiazines | | | | | | | | |
| a. Chlorpromazine | Thorazine<br>Largactil | 25 | 3 | 1 | 4 | 3 | 1 | 1 |
| b. Promethazine | Phenergan | 25–50 | 3 | 1 | 4 | 3 | 4 | — |
| c. Promazine | Sparine | 25–50 | 3 | 1 | 3 | 1 | 1 | 1 |
| d. Perphenazine | Trilafon<br>Fentazin | 10 | 2 | 1 | 3 | 4 | 1 | — |
| e. Prochlorperazine | Compazine<br>Stemetil | 15 | 3 | 1 | 4 | 4 | 1 | — |
| f. Triflupromazine | Vesprin<br>Vespral | 50 | 3 | 1 | 4 | 3 | 1 | — |
| g. Mepazine | Pacatal<br>Pecazine | 50 | 2 | 1 | 3 | 0 | 0 | — |
| 2. Propanediols | | | | | | | | |
| a. Meprobamate | Equanil<br>Miltown | 500 | 3 | 3 | 2 | 0 | 0 | 0 |
| 3. Diphenylmethanes | | | | | | | | |
| a. Hydroxyzine | Atarax<br>Vistaril | 100 | 3 | 1 | 4 | 0 | 0 | 1 |
| C. Nonbarbiturate sedative-hypnotics | | | | | | | | |
| 1. Ethinamate | Valmid | 500–1000 | 3 | 3 | 1 | 0 | 0 | 0 |
| 2. Glutethimide | Doriden | 250–500 | 3 | 3 | 1 | 0 | 0 | 0 |
| 3. Ethchlorvynol | Placidyl | 250–500 | 3 | 3 | 1 | 0 | 0 | 0 |
| 4. Methyprylon | Noludar | 200–400 | 3 | 3 | 1 | 0 | 0 | 0 |
| 5. Chloral Hydrate | | 1–2 gm. | 4 | 3 | 1 | 0 | 0 | 0 |
| 6. Scopolamine | Hyoscine | 0.3 mg (gr.1/200) | 2 | 1 | 2 | 0 | 0 | 0 |

* 0, no effect; 1, minimum effect; 2, moderate effect; 3, good effect; 4, maximum effect; —, analgesic effect.

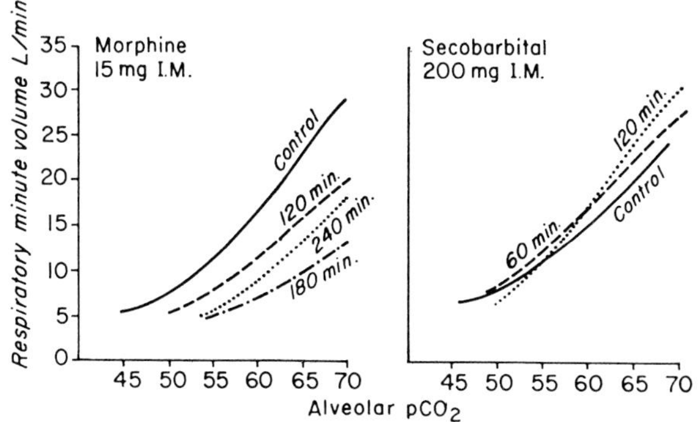


**Fig. 17–18.** The effects of secobarbital on respiration compared with those of morphine. Graph shows the relation between the end-expiratory carbon dioxide tension (horizontal) and respiratory-minute volume (vertical). The carbon dioxide tension was increased by permitting the endogenous $CO_2$ to accumulate by removing the soda lime cannister from the system. Note that though morphine depressed respiration (the $CO_2$ response curve is shifted to the right), secobarbital had no significant effect. (Modified from Echenhoff JE, et al: Anesthesiology. 18:703, 1957.)

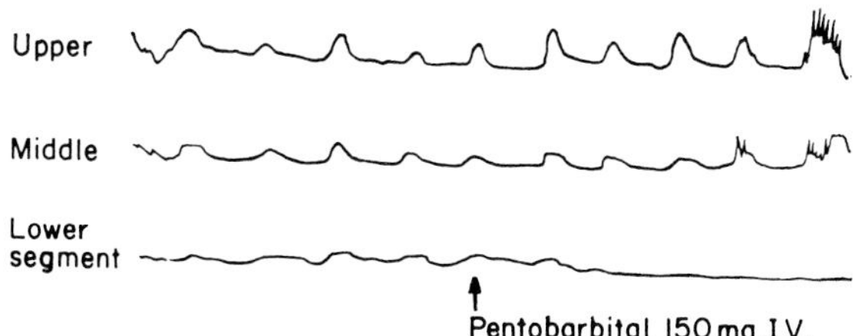


**Fig. 17–19.** Enhancement of labor following intravenous administration of 150 mg of pentobarbital. Note that before the injection there was good synchronism and good profile of contractions, but some irregularity in strength, slight fundal dominance, and active lower uterus. Following injection, the patient became sleepy and her contractions became stronger, more frequent, more regular in rhythm and intensity, and of much better gradient. Note also that during the last contraction registered on the record, the parturient bore down. She continued to do so with subsequent contractions, and had a precipitate delivery 4 contractions later. (Redrawn from Reynolds SRM, Harris JS, Kaiser IH: Clinical Measurement of Uterine Forces in Pregnancy and Labor. Charles C. Thomas, Springfield, IL. 1954.)

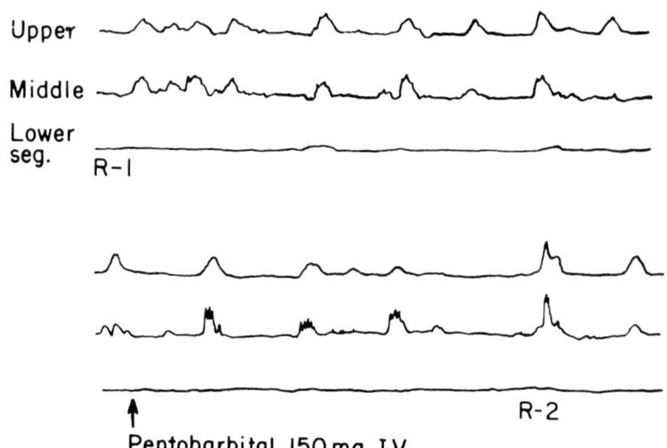


**Fig. 17–20.** Adverse effect of intravenous pentobarbital administered in early labor. At $R_1$ the cervix was 3 cm dilated. Note that contractions are of moderate intensity, regular, and occurring every 4 minutes with a fair gradient. The patient was given 150 mg of pentobarbital. Within 5 minutes there was a decrease in amplitude, rate, and regularity of uterine contractions that lasted 22 minutes. At $R_2$ the cervix was still 3 to 4 cm dilated. (Redrawn from Reynolds SRM, Harris JS, and Kaiser IH: Clinical Measurement of Uterine Forces in Pregnancy and Labor. Springfield, IL. Charles C. Thomas, 1954.)

at the recommended low dosages to the mother, (see Table 17–11) barbiturates do not have significant long-term neurobehavioral effects on the mature infant or on the onset of respiration or the Apgar scores (238–242). However, these medications may delay slightly the rate of recovery from birth asphyxia (243) and the newborn attention may be depressed for as long as 2 to 4 days (244). Signs of overdosages in the infant include somnolence, sluggish reflexes, flaccidity, bradycardia, hypothermia, and indifference to nursing that may persist for up to 2 days (233). Irving and associates reported (245,246) severe depressions in over 40% of newborns delivered to mothers who had received 600 to 750 mg of pentobarbital. These dosages are not recommended and are not used any more in most centers of the world because they induce sleep in the mother who often likes to actively participate in the delivery of the baby.

### *Benzodiazepines*

Benzodiazepines [Diazepam (Valium), Lorazepam (Ativan), Midazolam (Versed)] have several pharmacologic effects, including sedation, anxiolytic and anticonvulsant effect, muscular relaxation, amnesia and, possibly, an antiemetic action. Most benzodiazepines have a prolonged plasma half-life and therefore are not well-suited for use in obstetrics. These medications should not be used in early pregnancy because of an increased risk of congenital malformation, such as cleft palate and harelip, has been reported after the use of diazepam and chlordiazepoxide.

Benzodiazepines' proposed mode of action and detailed suggestion for their clinical use is explained in Chapter 18.

### *Scopolamine*

Scopolamine (hyoscine) is abundant, particularly in the plants Datura fastuosa var. alba and in Datura meteloides (15). Because of its sedative and amnestic effects, scopolamine has been used widely in the past (247) alone or together with an analgesic to produce a twilight sleep. This technique is highly discouraged now because it prevents the participation of the mother to the delivery and may precipitate delirium in the mother who then becomes difficult to control. Possibly, the only useful application of scopolamine is in the transdermal preparation that helps in the control of emesis caused by motion sickness or by therapeutic doses of opioids. When used in this form, the patch is usually applied over the mastoid process. Scopolamine is absorbed throughout the skin and reaches a therapeutic level after 4 to 6 hours and lasts for 72 hours.

### *Phenothiazine*

Phenothiazines are synthetic major tranquilizers first used clinically in the 1950s. Promethazine (phenergan) and propiomazine (Largon) are both useful to relieve anxiety during labor. They should be preferred to the other phenothiazides such as chlorpromazine (Thorazine), promazine (Sparine) and prochlorperazine (Compazine), as these later drugs tend to induce hypotension due to their alpha adrenergic blocking effects. Promethazine can be given IV at a dose of 25 to 50 mg for an anxiolytic effect (248), though many controlled studies have shown that it has an antianalgesic effect (249–252) and should therefore be used only in the early labor in which the pain is of mild intensity. This medication should not be injected intra-arterially because it can cause severe arterial constriction with tissue necrosis and gangrene.

### *Hydroxyzine*

Hydroxyzine (Vistaril, Marax, Atarax) at a dose of 25 to 50 mg is an effective medication to treat anxiety and, at a dose of 75 to 100 mg, it has hypnotic properties. It is not related chemically to the other known anti-anxiety medications, and its mechanism of action is not known. Beaver (253) has reported that Hydroxyzine, 25 to 100 mg per OS or IM, increases the analgesic effect of morphine by at least 50% and decreases the anxiety associated with acute pain. The antiemetic action decreases the incidence and may even abolish the nausea and vomiting induced by opioids (254). It has also been used effectively against pruritus caused by opioids. At high dosages, this drug can induce sedation and dryness of the mouth. It has a minimal effect on the circulatory system, though if taken for an extended period of time, it can cause electrocardiographic alteration similar to that induced by tricyclic antidepressant drugs.

As very high doses given to pregnant rats cause fetal malformation, it is not recommended for pregnant women during the early pregnancy. Because it still is not known if it is secreted in milk, it should be taken with caution by breast-feeding mothers.

## Dissociative Drug

### *Ketamine*

Ketamine is an interesting injectable anesthetic agent belonging to the class of the arylcyclohexylamines. When injected intravenously, ketamine produces smooth, rapid onset of surgical anesthesia with no cardiovascular or respiratory depression. At subanesthetic dosages, it provides intense analgesia. Its widespread use is hampered by two bothersome side effects: (1) significant stimulation of the cardiovascular system; and (2) a high incidence of emergency reaction which, at times, is frightening to the patient. A comprehensive review article was written by White, et al in 1982 (255).

Ketamine induces a condition known as dissociative anesthesia (255). It is apparently produced by a functional electrical physiologic dissociation between the limbic system and the thalamocortical pathways (256). The anesthetic state appears to be characterized by catalepsy with slow nystagmus, intact corneal and light reflexes, and associated at times with movement that may not be related to painful stimuli (255). At subanesthetic levels, the patient may respond to surgical stimuli but will not remember any painful experience.

The mechanism of action of ketamine appears to be complex and is not completely understood. In part, it is mediated by its interactions with the phencyclidine receptors, which are found predominantly in the corticothalamic and limbic areas. At high concentrations, ketamine may bind to opioids receptors (257).

Recent studies indicate that ketamine acts also as a channel blocker of N-methyl-D-aspartate (NMDA) receptor located on the postsynaptic membrane between the I and II order sensory neurons in the dorsal horn of the spinal cord. This receptor, so named because N-methyl-D-aspartate is the most effective agonist, is acted upon by the endogenous excitatory amino acids (EAA) L-glutamate and L-aspartate (258,259). These amino acids are widely distributed in the CNS and are believed to be neurotransmitters. Willcockson, et al showed in 1984 that nociceptive neurons in the spinal cord increased firing after iontophoretic application of glutamate (260). Cahusac, et al, also in 1984 (261), reported that the intrathecal administration of an N-methyl-D-aspartate antagonist in conscious rats repressed the behavioural responses to adverse electrical stimuli. In 1987, Aanonsen and Wilcox (262) reported that intrathecal administration of excitatory amino acids in conscious mice caused adverse behaviors and hyperalgesia to noxious stimuli. In 1990, Sher and Mitchell (263) showed that ketamine in small doses significantly decreased the ischemia-induced hyperanalgesic response to noxious pinching. In the field of clinical research, Maurset, et al in 1989 (264), reported that 0.3 mg/kg of ketamine provided good, nonopioid-type of analgesia after impacted molar teeth removal. Oshima, et al in 1990 (265) reported prolonged use of 2.5 to 15 mg per hr of ketamine in patients with pain associated with advanced cancer who were no longer responding to opioids analgesia.

The pharmacologic preparation of ketamine is in its racemic form. This form, however, is a combination of two optical isomers or enantiomers. They are the (+) ketamine hydrochloride and the (−) ketamine hydrochloride (255). The (+) ketamine produces more intense analgesia with fewer emergence reactions than the (−) isomer (266,267). This finding is of particular interest, and it is hoped that further research is done in isolating the most effective enantiomer with the least side effects. The ability of ketamine to induce intense analgesia even at subanesthetic dosages has provided a useful drug for obstetric use. Early studies, however, indicated a number of maternal complications and infants with low Apgar scores (268–270). This was later understood to be caused by excessive dosages of the medication and, at lower dosages (0.2 to 0.5 ml/kg IV), ketamine produced nondepressed neonates and little side effects to the mother (271,272). The use of ketamine as subanesthetic dosages often causes dream states in the patient; however, in the great majority of patients, these dreams are quite pleasant and acceptable. Ketamine, at a dose of 15 to 25 mg IV, can be used to supplement a neural block for labor and delivery that is not providing satisfactory analgesia (273). The use of larger doses of ketamine (1 to 2 mg/kg IV) for induction of surgical anesthesia for cesarean sections or instrumental delivery of the baby provides rapid, good surgical anesthesia, and amnesia. Because at this high dose a significant number of patients may have unpleasant emergent reactions, it is advisable, unless contraindicated by other reasons, to inject, after the delivery of the baby, midazolam at the dosage of 2 to 4 mg IV (273). This drastically decreases the emergence reaction caused by the medication.

When compared with thiopental, ketamine provides better analgesia and amnesia with comparable incidence of unpleasant emergence reactions. Bunodiere, et al (274) used only ketamine as the anesthetic for cesarean section. This author reported that fetal mortality was less than half than the one seen with other anesthesia techniques. Due to anticonvulsant properties, ketamine could be useful in the preeclamptic patient (275). However, it should be used carefully due to its cardiac stimulating effect. A comparison with ketamine and thiopental for rapid IV induction of surgical anesthesia for cesarean section showed less of a fall over arterial neonatal blood pressure (276). Neonatal neurobehavioral testing after vaginal delivery was better after ketamine/nitrous oxide than thiopental/nitrous oxide (277).

## Conclusions

Intense pain can now be effectively controlled with the medications at our disposal. Fears that have been associated with the use of opioids continue to interfere with their proper use. Only with the proper education of physicians and healthcare personnel will we be able to overcome this problem. For this reason, I will reiterate the following points:

1. Psychological dependence should be clearly differentiated from physical dependence. The former is very uncommon in patients with pain. Physical dependence to opioids develops in patients treated for over 2 weeks on high doses of opioids and, therefore, they must be tapered gradually to prevent opioid withdrawal.
2. Significant respiratory depression does not occur until there is significant relief of pain or the patient becomes sedated significantly.

3. There is a wide variation of dose requirement among patients (up to tenfold). Therefore, the dose should be individualized.
4. The analgesic window overlaps that of side effects such as sedation, dizziness, and nausea. Therefore, complete analgesia, without side effects, is difficult to achieve with only systemic opioids.
5. Different opioids, even those that are believed to bind to the same receptor, may induce side effects of different intensities in particular patients. Often a change to another opioid reduces the side effects while providing analgesia.
6. Efforts should be made to maintain a steady-state plasma level and prevent peaks and valleys in the plasma concentration, as this predisposes to side effects during the period of high plasma levels in pain during periods of low levels.

Another obstacle to proper opioid therapy is patient compliance to the prescribed therapeutic regimen. If the side effects are too intense, patients will not follow medical instructions. Severe emesis, marked sedation and constipation, and side effects inherent to opioid therapy, should be properly prevented and treated. Constipation is very common and should be treated aggressively with regular bowel regimen by administering cathartics, stool softeners, and proper hydration. Anti-emetics should be given preventively. Transdermal scopolamine patch has been effective in abating emesis associated with opioid therapy. Sedation should be treated by decreasing the dose of single doses and increasing the frequency or by giving mild stimulants.

In summary, severe acute pain experience by women in the predelivery period can be effectively treated with the medications and techniques at our disposal, but this requires dedication and profound knowledge on the action and side effects of analgesics. It is therefore the duty of each physician called to treat a parturient suffering unrelenting severe pain to have the knowledge and expertise to alleviate that patient's suffering. Intense pain experience during parturition is not only humiliating for the mother but can indeed cause increased morbidity and mortality to both the mother and neonate if a severe pathological state preexists.

## REFERENCES


1. Bonica JJ: Principles and Practice of Obstetric Analgesia and Anesthesia, 1st Edition. Philadelphia, F.A. Davis Co., 1967, p. 234.
2. Bonica JJ: Management of pain of childbirth: the nature of childbirth and its relief by continuous epidural analgesia. (Monograph) St. Paul, Pharmacia Deltec Inc., 1992.
3. Kritikos PG, Papadaki SP: The history of the poppy and of opium and their expansion in antiquity in the eastern Mediterranean area. Bull. Narc. XIX:July-September: 17–38, 1967.
4. Plinio C: Della storia naturale. Vol. secondo, Venezia, L. XX, 76–80, 1844.
5. Benedetti C, Premuda L: The history of opium and its derivatives. *In* Opioid Analgesia—Recent Advances in Systemic Administration. Advances in Pain Research and Therapy, Vol. 14. Edited by C Benedetti, CR Chapman, G Giron. New York, Raven Press, 1990.
6. Castiglioni A: A History of Medicine. New York, Alfred A. Knopf, 1947.
7. Keys TE: The History of Surgical Anesthesia. New York, Schuman's, 1945.
8. Boccaccio: Il Decamerone (Firenze, Adriano Salani), v. I. Giornata Quarta, Novella Decima, 1928, pp. 436–437.
9. De Renzi S: Storia della medicina in Italia. Tomo quinto, Napoli, 1848.
10. Gualino L: Saggi di medicina storica. Torino, 1930.
11. Premuda L: Storia della Medicina. Padova, 1975.
12. Heaton CE: The history of anesthesia and analgesia in obstetrics. J. Hist. Med. 1:567, 1946.
13. Sertürner FW: Uber das Morphium, eine neue salzfähige Grundlage, und die Mekonsäure, als Hauptbestandteile des Opiums. Gilbert's Annalen der Physik, 55:56, 1817.
14. Sertürner FW: Ueber eins der fürchterlichsten Gifte der Pflanzenwelt, als ein Nachtrag zu meiner Abhandlung über die Mekonsäure und das Morphium. Gilbert's Annalen ser Physik 57:183, 1817.
15. Lewis WH, Elvin-Lewis MPF (Eds): Medical Botany: Plants Affecting Man's Health. New York, John Wiley & Sons, 1977.
16. Fülöp-Miller R: Triumph over Pain. New York, Literary Guild of America, 1938.
17. Matsuki A: Nothing new under the sun—A Japanese pioneer in the clinical use of intrathecal morphine (Editorial). Anesthesiology 58:289–290, 1983.
18. Eckenhoff JE, Elder JD, King BD: N-Allyl-normorphine in the treatment of morphine or demerol narcosis. Am. J. Med. Sci. 223:191–197, 1952.
19. Eckenhoff JE, Hoffman GL, Driipps RK: N-Allyl-normorphine: An antagonist to the opiates. Anesthesiology 13: 242–251, 1952.
20. Wikler A: Effect of large doses of N-Allyl-normorphine on man. Fed. Proc. (abstr.) 10:345, 1951.
21. Way EL: Review and overview of four decades of opiate research. *In* Neurochemical Mechanisms of Opiates and Endorphins (Adv Biochem Psychopharmacol, vol. 20). Edited by HH Loh, DH Ross. New York, Raven Press, 1979.
22. Yaksh TL, Rudy TA: Analgesia mediated by a direct spinal action of narcotics. Science 192:1357–1358, 1976.
23. Wang JK, Nauss LA, Thomas JE: Pain relief by intrathecally applied morphine in man. Anesthesiology 50:149–151, 1979.
24. Behar M, Olshwang D, Magora F, Davidson JT: Epidural morphine in treatment of pain. Lancet 1:527–528, 1979.
25. Cousins MJ, Mather LE, Blynn CJ, Wilson PR, et al: Selective spinal analgesia. Lancet 1:1141–1142, 1979.
26. Bromage PR, Camporesi E, Chestnut D: Epidural narcotics for postoperative analgesia. Anesth. Analg. 59:473–480, 1980.
27. Pasqualucci V, Moricca G, Solinas P: Intrathecal morphine for the control of pain of myocardial infarction. Anesthesia 36:68–69, 1981.
28. Scott PV, Bowen FE, Cartwright P, Mohan RAO, et al: Intrathecal morphine as sole analgesic during labour. Br. Med. J. 2:351–353, 1980.
29. Howard RP, Milne LA, Williams NE: Epidural morphine in terminal care. Anaesthesia 36:51–53, 1981.
30. Zenz M, Schappler-Scheele B, Nehaus R, Piepenbrock S, et al: Long-term peridural morphine analgesia in cancer pain. Lancet 1:91, 1981.
31. Mandaus L, Blomberg R, Hammar E: Long-term epidural morphine analgesia. Acta. Anaesthesiol. Scand. (Suppl.) 74: 149–150, 1982.

32. Wolfe MJ, Davies GK: Analgesic action of extradural fentanyl. Br. J. Anaesth. 52:357–358, 1980.
33. Glynn CJ, Mather LE, Cousins MJ, Wilson PR, et al: Peridural meperidine in humans: analgesic response, pharmacokinetics and transmission into CSF. Anesthesiology 55: 520–526, 1981.
34. Oyama T, Fukushi S, Jin T: Epidural Beta-endorphin in treatment of pain. Can. Anaesth. Soc. J. 29:24–26, 1982.
35. Cahill J, Murphy D, O'Brien D, Mulhall J, et al: Epidural buprenorphine for pain relief after major abdominal surgery. A controlled comparison with epidural morphine. Anaesthesia 38:760–764, 1983.
36. Jacobson L, Phillips PD, Hull CJ, Conacher ID: Extradural versus intramuscular diamorphine: a controlled study of analgesic and adverse effects in the postoperative period. Anaesthesia 38:10–18, 1983
37. Lewis WH, Elvin-Lewis MPF: Depressants. *In* Medical Botany: Plants Affecting Man's Health. New York, Wiley & Sons, 1977, pp. 432–448.
38. Tyler VE, Brady LR, Robbers JE: Pharmacognosy. Philadelphia, Lea & Febiger, 1988.
39. Harner MJ: The role of hallucinogenic plants in European witchcraft, 125–150. *In* Hallucinogens and Shamanism. Edited by MJ Harner. New York, Oxford University Press, 1974, pp. 130–1, 133–4, 138–9.
40. Weil A, Rosen W: Chocolate to Morphine: Understanding Mind-Active Drugs. Boston, Houghton Mifflin Company, 1983.
41. Siddiqui S, Siddiqui RH: Chemical examination of the roots of Rauwolfia serpentina Benth. J. Ind. Chem. Soc. 8:667, 1932.
42. Neil A: Tolerance and dependence. *In* Advances in Pain Research and Therapy, Vol. 14: Opioid Analgesia. Edited by C Benedetti, CR Chapman, G Giron. New York, Raven Press, 1990, pp. 121–142.
43. Haubrich WS: Medical Meanings: A Glossary of Word Origins. New York, Harcourt Brace Jovanovich, Publishers, 1984.
44. Akil H, Watson SJ, Young E, Lewis ME, et al: Endogenous opioids: biology and function. Ann. Rev. Neurosci. 7: 223–55, 1984.
45. Bonica JJ, Benedetti C: Lesson 15: postoperative pain. Anesthesiology News, 10(Feb):9–16. Lesson 15, conclusion: postoperative pain. Anesthesiology News, 10(Mar):8–17, 1984.
46. Kosterlitz HW, Paterson SJ: Types of opioid receptors: relation to antinociception. Philos. Trans. R. Soc. Lond. (Biol.), 308:291–297, 1985.
47. Kosterlitz HW: Opioid peptides and their receptors. The Wellcome Foundation Lecture, 1982. Proc. R. Soc. Lond. (Biol.), 225:27–40, 1985.
48. Neil A, Terenius L: Receptor mechanisms for nociception. *In* Regional Opioids in Anesthesiology and Pain Management. Edited by Sjostrand, N Rawal. Boston, Little, Brown and Co, 1986, pp. 1–15.
49. Pasternak GW, Childers SR, Snyder SH: Opiate analgesia: Evidence for mediation by a subpopulation of opiate receptors. Science 208:514–516, 1980.
50. Ross EM, Gilman AG: Pharmacodynamics: mechanisms of drug action and the relationship between drug concentration and effect. *In* The Pharmacological Basis of Therapeutics. Edited by LS Goodman, AG Gilman, TW Rall, F Murad. New York, MacMillan Publishing Company, 1985, pp. 35–48.
51. Holford NHG, Sheiner LB: Understanding the dose-effect relationship: clinical application of pharmacokinetic-pharmacodynamic models. Clin. Pharmacokinet. 6:429–453, 1981.
52. Dahlström BE, Paalzow LK, Segre G, Agren AJ: Relation between morphine pharmacokinetics and analgesia. J. Pharmacokinet. Biopharm. 6:41–53, 1978.
53. Kinniburgh DW, Boyd NO: Isolation of peptides from uremic plasma that inhibit phenytoin binding to normal plasma proteins. Clin. Pharmacol. Ther. 30:276–280, 1981.
54. Hull CJ: Pharmacokinetics and pharmacodynamics. Br. J. Anaesth. 51:579–618, 1979.
55. Nishitateno K, Ngai SH, Finck AD, Berkowitz BA: Pharmacokinetics of morphine: concentrations in the serum and brain of the dog during hyperventilation. Anesthesiology 50:520–523, 1979.
56. Benet LZ, Sheiner LB: Pharmacokinetics: the dynamics of drug absorption, distribution, and elimination. *In* The Pharmacological Basis of Therapeutics. Edited by LS Goodman, AG Gilman, TW Rall, F Murad. New York, MacMillan Publishing Company, 1985.
57. Austin KL, Stapleton JV, Mather LE: Relationship of meperidine concentration and analgesic response. A preliminary report. Anesthesiology 53:460–466, 1980.
58. Tamsen A, Hartvig P, Fagerlund C, Dahlström B: Patient-controlled analgesic therapy, part one: pharmacokinetics of pethidine in the perioperative and postoperative periods. Clin. Pharmacokinet. 7:149–163, 1982.
59. Tamsen A, Hartvig P, Fagerlund C, Dahlström B: Patient-controlled analgesic therapy, part two: individual analgesic demand and analgesic plasma concentrations of pethidine in postoperative pain. Clin. Pharmacokinet. 7:252–265, 1982.
60. Dahlström B, Tamsen A, Paalzow L, Hartvig P: Patient-controlled analgesic therapy, part IV: pharmacokinetics and analgesic plasma concentrations of morphine. Clin. Pharmacokinet. 7:266–279, 1982.
61. Donnerer J, Cardinale G, Coffey J, Lisak CA, et al: Chemical characterization and regulation of endogenous morphine and codeine in the rat. J. Pharmacol. Exp. Ther. 242: 583–587, 1987.
62. Donnerer J, Oka K, Brossi A, Rice KC, et al: Presence and formation of codeine and morphine in the rat. Proc. Natl. Acad. Sci. U.S.A. 83:4566–4567, 1986.
63. Weitz CJ, Faull KF, Goldstein A: Synthesis of the skeleton of the morphine molecule by mammalian liver. Nature 330: 674–677, 1987.
64. Weitz CJ, Lowney LI, Faull KF, Feistner G, et al: Morphine and codeine from mammalian brain. Proc. Natl. Acad. Sci. U.S.A. 83:9784–9788, 1986.
65. Herz A, Teschemacher H: Activities and sites of antinociceptive action of morphine-like analgesics and kinetics of distribution following intravenous, intracerebral and intraventricular application. Adv. Drug. Res. 6:79–119, 1971.
66. Calvillo O, Henry JL, Neuman RS: Effects of morphine and naloxone on dorsal horn neurones in the cat. Can. J. Physiol. Pharmacol. 52:1207–1211, 1974.
67. Duggan AW, North RA: Electrophysiology of opioids. Pharmacol. Rev. 35:219–282, 1983.
68. Benedetti C: Neuroanatomy and biochemistry of antinociception. *In* Advances in Pain Research and Therapy, Vol 2. Edited by JJ Bonica, V Ventafridda. New York, Raven Press, 1979.
69. Arnér S, Bolund C, Rane A, Ronnback L: Narcotic analgesics in the treatment of cancer and postoperative pain. Acta. Anaesthesiol. Scand. 26(Suppl. 74):1–178, 1982.
70. Lowenstein E: Morphine "anesthesia"—a perspective. Anesthesiology 35:563–564, 1971.

71. Nordberg G: Pharmacokinetic aspects of spinal morphine analgesia. Acta. Anaesthesiol. Scand. 28(Suppl. 79):1–38, 1984.
72. Satoh M, Takagi J: Enhancement by morphine of the central descending inhibitory influence on spinal sensory transmission. Eur. J. Pharmacol. 14:60–65, 1971.
73. Bonica JJ: The Management of Pain. Philadelphia, Lea & Febiger, 1953.
74. Forrest WH, Brown BW Jr, Brown CR, Defalque R, et al: Dextroamphetamine with morphine for the treatment of postoperative pain. N. Engl. J. Med. 296:712–715, 1977.
75. Halpern LM, Bonica JJ: Analgesics. *In* Drugs of Choice. Edited by W Modell. St. Louis, C.V. Mosby, 1984.
76. Radnay PA, Brodman E, Mankikar D, Duncalf D: The effect of equianalgesic doses of fentanyl, morphine, meperidine, and pentazocine on common bile duct pressure. Anaesthetist 29:26–29, 1980.
77. Beaver WT: Comparison of analgesic effects of morphine sulfate, hydroxyzine and other combinations in patients with postoperative pain. *In* Advances in Pain Research and Therapy. Edited by JJ Bonica, V Ventrafridda. New York, Raven Press, 1976, pp. 553–557.
78. Benedetti C: Intraspinal analgesia: an historical overview. Acta. Anaesth. Scand. 31(Suppl. 85):17–24, 1987.
79. Henderson SK, Cohen H: Nalbuphine augmentation of analgesia and reversal of side effects following epidural hydromorphone. Anesthesiology 65:216–218, 1986.
80. Wakefield RD, Mesaros M: Reversal of pruritus, secondary to epidural morphine, with the narcotic agonist/antagonist nalbuphine (NubainR) (abstract). Anesthesiology 63: A255, 1985.
81. Hill HF, Chapman CR, Kornell JA, Sullivan KM, et al: Self-administration of morphine in bone marrow transplant patients reduces drug requirement. Pain 40:121–129, 1990.
82. Bonica JJ, Benedetti C: Management of cancer pain. *In* Comprehensive Textbook of Oncology. Edited by AR Moossa, MC Robson, SC Schimpff. Baltimore, Williams & Wilkins, 1985, pp. 443–477.
83. Cancer Pain. Geneva, Switzerland. World Health Organization, 1986.
84. Porter J, Jick H: Addiction rare in patients treated with narcotics. N. Engl. J. Med. 302:123, 1980.
85. Kanner RF, Foley KM: Patterns of narcotic drug use in a cancer pain clinic. Ann. N.Y. Acad. Sci. 362:161, 1980.
86. Flacke JW, Flacke WE, Williams GD: Acute pulmonary edema following naloxone reversal of high-dose morphine anesthesia. Anesthesiology 47:376–378, 1977.
87. Campbell C, Phillips OC, Frazier TM: Analgesia during labor: a comparison of pentobarbital, meperidine, and morphine. Obstet. Gynecol. 17:714–718, 1961.
88. James LS: The effect of pain relief for labor and delivery on the fetus and newborn. Anesthesiology 21:405, 1960.
89. Bonica JJ: Effects of analgesia and anesthesia on the fetus and newborn. *In* Effects of Labor and Delivery on the Fetus and Newborn. Edited by R Caldyro-Barcia. New York, Pergamon Press, 1967.
90. Moya F, Thorndike D: The effects of drugs used in labor on the fetus and newborn. Clin. Pharmacol. Ther. 4:628, 1962.
91. Capogna G, Celleno D, Costantino P, Sebastiani M, et al: Epidural morphine and buprenorphine for analgesia during and after cesarean section: maternal effects and neonatal outcome. Reg. Anesth. 15(S):26, 1990.
92. Beecher HK: Measurement of Subjective Responses. New York, Oxford University Press, 1959.
93. Eddy NB, Halbach H, Braenden OJ: Synthetic substances with morphine-like effect: Clinical experience: potency, side effects, addiction liability. Bull. W.H.O., 17:569, 1957.
94. Eckenhoff JE, Oech SR: The effects of narcotics and antagonists upon respiration and circulation in man. Clin. Pharmacol. Ther. 1:483, 1960.
95. Caldeyro-Barcia R, Alvarez H, Poseiro JJ: Action of morphine on the contractility of the human uterus. Arch. Int. Pharmacodyn. 101:171, 1955.
96. Bourne AW, Burn JH: Action on the human uterus of anaesthetics and other drugs commonly used in labour. Brit. Med. J. 2:87, 1930.
97. Bickers W: Uterine contractions in labor: effects of analgesic drugs. Virginia Med. Monthly 69:15, 1942.
98. Dodek SM: External hysterographic studies of the effect of certain analgesics and anesthetics upon the parturient human uterus. Anesth. Analg. 13:8, 1934.
99. Eskes TKAB: Effect of morphine upon uterine contractility in late pregnancy. Am. J. Obstet. Gynecol. 84:281, 1962.
100. Hensen H: Uber den Einfluss Morphiums und des Aethers auf die Wehenthatigkeit des Uterus. Arch. F. Gynaek. 55: 129, 1898.
101. Bonica JJ: Effects of analgesia and anesthesia on the fetus and newborn. *In* Effects of Labor and Delivery on the Fetus and Newborn. Edited by R Caldeyro-Barcia. New York, Pergamon Press, 1967.
102. Moya F, Thorndike D: The effects of drugs used in labor on the fetus and newborn. Clin. Pharmacol. Ther. 4:628, 1962.
103. Shute E, Davis M: The effect on the infant of morphine administered in labor. Surg. Gynecol. Obstet. 57:727, 1933.
104. Gautieri RG, Ciuchta HP: Effect of certain drugs on perfused human placenta. J. Pharm. Sci. 51:55, 1962.
105. Campbell C, Phillips OC, Frazier TM: Analgesia during labor: a comparison of pentobarbital, meperidine, and morphine. Obstet. Gynecol. 17:714, 1961.
106. Myers JD: A preliminary clinical evaluation of dihydrocodeine bitartrate in normal parturition. Am. J. Obstet. Gynecol. 75:1096, 1958.
107. Radnay PA, Brodman E, Mankikar D, Duncalf D: The effect of equianalgesic doses of fentanyl, morphine, meperidine, and pentazocine on common bile duct pressure. Anaesthetist 29:26–29, 1980.
108. Wallenstein SL, Houde RW: Clinical evaluation of relative analgesic potencies of anileridine, meperidine and morphine. J. Pharmacol. Exp. Ther. 122:81, 1958.
109. Foldes FF, Swerdlow M, Siker ES: Narcotics and Narcotic Antagonists. Springfield, IL, Charles C. Thomas Publisher, 1964.
110. Crawford JS: Principles and Practice of Obstetric Anaesthesia. Springfield, IL, Charles C. Thomas Publisher, 1959.
111. Gillam JS, Hunter GW, Darner CB, Thompson GR, et al: Meperidine hydrochloride and alphaprodine hydrochloride as obstetric analgesic agents. Am. J. Obstet. Gynecol. 75:1105, 1958.
112. Hingson RA, Hellman LM: Eight thousand parturients evaluate drugs, techniques, and doctors during labor and delivery. Am. J. Obstet. Gynecol. 68:1, 262, 1954.
113. Holmes JM: Forceps delivery under pethidine narcosis and pudendal block. J. Obstet. Gynaec. Brit. Emp. 67:115, 1960.
114. Harris H, Tafeen CH, Freedman HL, Fogarty E: The intravenous use of demerol, scopolamine and nalline in labor. Am. J. Obstet. Gynecol. 75:39, 1958.
115. Brownridge P: Shivering related to epidural blockade with bupivacaine in labour, and the influence of epidural pethidine. Anaesth. Intensive Care 14:412–417, 1986.

116. Matthews NC, Corser G: Epidural fentanyl for shaking in obstetrics. Anaesthesia 43:783–785, 1988.
117. Johnson MD, Sevarino FB, Lema MJ: Cessation of shivering and hypothermia associated with epidural sufentanil. Anesth. Analg. 68:70–71, 1989.
118. Sevarino FB, Johnson MD, Lema MJ, Datta S, et al: The effect of epidural sufentanil on shivering and body temperature in the parturient. Anesth. Analg. 68:530–533, 1989.
119. Wikler A: Sites and mechanism of actin of morphine and related drugs in the central nervous system. Pharmacol. Rev. 2:435, 1950.
120. Sugioka K, Boniface KW, Davis DA: The influence of meperidine on myocardial contractility in the intact dog. Anesthesiology 18:623, 1957.
121. Goodman LS, Gilman A: The Pharmacological Basis of Therapeutics. 3rd Ed. New York, The Macmillan Co., 1965.
122. Friedman EA: Primigravid labor. Obstet. Gynecol. 6:6, 567, 1955.
123. Lindgren L: The influence of anaesthetics and analgesics on different types of labour. Acta. Anaesth. Scand. Suppl. II:49, 1959.
124. Reynolds SRM, Harris JS, Kaiser IH: Clinical Measurement of Uterine Forces in Pregnancy and Labor. Springfield, IL. Charles C. Thomas Publisher 1954.
125. Roberts H, Kane KM, Percival N, Snow P, et al: Effects of some analgesic drugs used in childbirth. Lancet 1:128, 1957.
126. Taylor ES, von Fumetti HH, Essig LL, Goodman SN, et al: The effects of demerol and trichlorethylene on arterial oxygen saturation in the newborn. Am. J. Obstet. Gynecol. 69:348 1955.
127. Cappe BE, Himel SZ, Grossman F: Use of a mixture of morphine and N-allylnormorphine as an analgesic. Am. J. Obstet. Gynecol. 66:1231, 1953.
128. Shnider SM, Moya F: Effect of meperidine on newborn infant. Am. J. Obstet. Gynecol. 89:1009, 1965.
129. Emich Jr JP: Nisentil—an obstetric analgesic. Am. J. Obstet. Gynecol. 69:124, 1955.
130. Kane WM: The results of nisentil in 1000 obstetrical cases. Am. J. Obstet. Gynecol. 65:1020, 1953.
131. Powell PO Jr, Savage JE: Nisentil in obstetrics. Obstet. Gynecol. 2:658, 1953.
132. Ekelman SB, Reynolds SRM: Effect of the analgesic nisentil on uterine contractions: considered by parity, stage of labor and status of membranes. Obstet. Gynecol. 6:644, 1955.
133. Wolfe MJ, Davies GK: Analgesic action of extradural fentanyl. Br. J. Anaesth. 52:357–358, 1980.
134. Payne R: CSF distribution of opioids in animals and man. Acta. Anaesthiol. Scand. 31(Suppl.85):38–46, 1987.
135. Payne R, Foley KM: Advances in the management of cancer pain. Cancer Treat. Rep. 68:173–183, 1984.
136. Loper KA, Ready LB, Downey M, Sandler AN, et al: Epidural and intravenous fentanyl infusions are clinically equivalent after knee surgery. Anesth. Analg. 70:72–5 1990.
137. Kaiko RF, Wallenstein SL, Rogers AG, Grabinski PY, et al: Clinical analgesic studies of intramuscular heroin and morphine in postoperative and chronic pain. *In* Advances in Pain Research and Therapy, Vol 8. Edited by KM Foley, CE Inturrisi. New York, Raven Press, 1986, pp. 107–116.
138. Umans JG, Chiu TSK, Lipman RA, Schultz MF, et al: Determination of heroin and its metabolites by high-performance liquid chromatography. J. Chromatogr. 233: 213–225, 1986.
139. Inturrisi CE: Pharmacokinetics of oral, intravenous, and continuous infusions of heroin. *In* Advances in Pain Research and Therapy, Vol 8. Edited by KM Foley, CE Inturrisi. New York, Raven Press, 1986, pp. 117–127.
140. Inturrisi CE, Max M, Umans J, Schultz M, et al: Heroin: disposition in cancer patients. Clin. Pharmacol. Ther. 31: 235–241, 1982.
141. Gourlay GK, Wilson RR, Glynn CJ: Methadone produces prolonged post-operative analgesia. Br. Med. J. 284: 630–631, 1982.
142. Lewis JW, Rance MJ, Sanger DJ: The pharmacology and abuse potential of buprenorphine: a new antagonist analgesic. Adv. Substance Abuse 3:103–154, 1983.
143. Bullingham RES, McQuay HJ, Porter EJB, Allen MC, et al: Sublingual buprenorphine used postoperatively: ten hour plasma drug concentration analysis. Br. J. Clin. Pharmacol. 13:665–673, 1982.
144. Ventafridda V, De Conno F, Guarise G, Tamburini M, et al: Chronic analgesic study on buprenorphine action in cancer pain. Comparison with pentazocine. Arzneimittelforsch 33:587–90, 1983.
145. Lehmann KA: Patient-controlled analgesia for postoperative pain. *In* Advances in Pain Research and Therapy: Opioid Analgesia. Vol. 14. Edited by C Benedetti, CR Chapman, G Giron. New York, Raven Press, 1990, pp. 297–324.
146. Jaffe JH, Martin WR: Opioid analgesics and antagonists. *In* The Pharmacological Basis of Therapeutics. Edited by LS Goodman, AG Gilman, TW Rall, F Murad. New York, MacMillan Publishing Company, 1985, pp. 491–531.
147. Cool WM, Kurtz NM, Chu G: Transnasal delivery of systemic drugs. *In* Advances in Pain Research and Therapy: Opioid Analgesia. Vol. 14. Edited by C Benedetti, CR Chapman, G Giron. New York, Raven Press, 1990, pp. 241–258.
148. Wallenstein SL, Rogers AG, Kaiko RF, Houde RW: Nalbuphine: clinical analgesic studies. *In* Advances in Pain Research and Therapy Vol 8. Edited by KM Foley, CE Inturrisi. New York, Raven Press, 1986, pp. 247–252.
149. Jasinski DR, Martin WR, Hoeldtke RD: Effects of short- and long-term administration of pentazocine in man. Clin. Pharmacol. Ther. 11:385–403, 1970.
150. Benedetti C: Intraspinal analgesia: an historical overview. Acta. Anaesth. Scand. 31(Suppl.85):17–24, 1987.
151. Heisterkamp DV, Cohen PJ: The use of naloxone to antagonize large doses of opiates administered during nitrous oxide anesthesia. Anesth. Analg. 53:12–18, 1974.
152. Vitalone V, Lopresti C: Acute pulmonary edema after intravenous naloxone. Minerva Anestesiol. 58(4):225–7, 1992.
153. Bromacombe J, Archdeacon J, Newell S, Martin J: Two cases of naloxone-induced pulmonary edema—the possible use of phentolamine in management. Anaesth. Intensive Care 19:578–80, 1991.
154. Silverstein JH, Gintautas J, Tadoori P, Abadir AR: Effects of naloxone on pulmonary capillary permeability. Prog. Clin. Biol. Res. 328:389–92, 1990.
155. Wride SR, Smith RE, Courtney PG: A fatal case of pulmonary edema in a healthy young male following naloxone administration. Anaesth. Intensive Care 17:374–7, 1989.
156. Bigo P, Manno E, Matani A, Franci I: Important side-effects of naloxone as an antagonist of neuroleptoanalgesia. Minerva Anesthesiol. 49:389–91, 1983.
157. Delle M, Ricksten SE, Haggendal J, Olsson K, et al: Regional changes in sympathetic nerve activity and baroreceptor reflex function and arterial plasma levels of catecholamines, renin and vasopressin during naloxone-precipitated morphine withdrawal in rats. J. Pharmacol. Exp. Ther. 253: 646–54, 1990.
158. Price DD, von der Gruen A, Miller J., Rafii A, et al: Potentiation of systemic morphine analgesia in humans by pro-

glumide a cholecystokinin antagonist. Anesth. Analg. 64: 801–806, 1985
159. Beecher HK: Measurement of Subjective Responses. New York, Oxford University Press, 1959.
160. Houde RW: Methods for measuring clinical pain in humans. Acta. Anaesthesiol. Scand. 74(Suppl.):25–29, 1982.
161. Husenmeyer RP, O'Connor MC, Davenport HT: Failure of epidural morphine to relive pain in labour. Anaesthesia 35: 161–163, 1980.
162. Crawford JS: Experiences with epidural morphine in obstetrics. Anaesthesia 36:207–209, 1981.
163. Carrie LES, O'Sullivan GM, Seegobin R: Epidural fentanyl in labour. Anaesthesia 36:965–969, 1981.
164. Writer WDR, James FM, Wheeler AS: Double-blind comparison of morphine and bupivacaine for continuous analgesia in labor. Anesthesiology 54:215–219, 1981.
165. Youngstrom P, Eastwood D, Patel H, Bhatia R, et al: Epidural fentanyl and bupivacaine in labor: double-blind study (abstract). Anesthesiology 61:A414, 1984.
166. Skerman JH, Thompson BA, Goldstein MT, Jacobs MA, et al: Combined continuous epidural fentanyl and bupivacaine in labor: a randomized study (abstract). Anesthesiology 63:A450, 1985.
167. Cohen SE, Tan S, Albright GA, Halpern J: Epidural fentanyl/bupivacaine mixtures for obstetric analgesia. Anesthesiology 67:403–407, 1987.
168. Naulty JS, Malinow A, Hunt CO, Hausheer J, et al: Epidural butorphanol-bupivacaine for analgesia during labor and delivery (abstract). Anesthesiology 65:A369, 1986.
169. Van Steenberge A, Debroux HC, Noorduin H: Extradural bupivacaine with sufentanil for vaginal delivery: a double-blind study. Br. J. Anaesth. 59:1518–1522, 1987.
170. Phillips GH: Combined epidural sufentanil and bupivacaine for labor analgesia. Reg. Anesth. 12:165–168, 1987.
171. Cellano D, Capogna G: Epidural fentanyl plus bupivacaine 0.125 per cent for labour: analgesic effects. Can. J. Anaesth. 35:375–378, 1988.
172. Chestnut DH, Owen CL, Bates JN, Ostman LG, et al: Continuous infusion epidural analgesia during labor: a randomized, double-blind comparison of 0.0625% bupivacaine/0.0002% fentanyl versus 0.125% bupivacaine. Anesthesiology 68:754–759, 1988.
173. Phillips G: Continuous infusion epidural analgesia in labor: the effect of adding sufentanil to 0.125% bupivacaine. Anesth. Analg. 67:462–465, 1988.
174. Reynolds F, O'Sullivan G: Epidural fentanyl and perineal pain in labour. Anaesthesia 44:341–344, 1989.
175. Hunt CO, Naulty JS, Malinow AM, Datta S, et al: Epidural butorphanol-bupivacaine for analgesia during labor and delivery. Anesth. Analg. 68:323–327, 1989.
176. Jones G, Paul DL, Elton RA, McClure JH: Comparison of bupivacaine and bupivacaine with fentanyl in continuous extradural analgesia during labour. Br. J. Anaesth. 63: 254–259, 1989.
177. Rodriquez J, Payne M, Afrasiabi A, Abboud TK, et al: Continuous infusion epidural anesthesia during labor: a randomized, double-blind comparison of 0.0625% bupivacaine/0.002% butorphanol and 0.125% bupivacaine. Reg. Anesth. 15:300–303, 1990.
178. Lysak SZ, Eisenach JC, Dobson CE: Patient-controlled epidural analgesia during labor: a comparison of three solutions with a continuous infusion control. Anesthesiology 72:44–49, 1990.
179. Naulty JS, Smith R, Ross R: Effect of changes in labor analgesic practice on labor outcome (abstract). Anesthesiology 69:A660, 1988.
180. Payne R, Inturrisi CE: CSF distribution of morphine, methadone and sucrose after intrathecal injection. Life Sci. 37: 1137–1144, 1985.
181. Bullingham RES, McQuay HJ, Moore RA: Extradural and intrathecal narcotics. *In* Recent Advances in Anaesthesia and Analgesia. Edited by RS Atkinson, CL Longton Hewer. Edinburgh, Churchill Livingstone, 1982, 141–156.
182. Tung AS, Yaksh TL: The antinociceptive effects of epidural opiates in the cat: studies on the pharmacology and the effects of lipophilicity in spinal analgesia. Pain 12: 343–356, 1982.
183. Payne R: CSF distribution of opioids in animals and man. Acta. Anaesthesiol. Scand. 31(Suppl.85):38–46, 1987.
184. Justins DM, Francis D, Houlton PG, Reynolds F: A controlled trial of extradural fentanyl in labour. Br. J. Anaesth. 54:409–414, 1982.
185. Justins DM, Knott C, Luthman J, Reynolds F: Epidural versus intramuscular fentanyl: analgesia and pharmacokinetics in labour. Anaesthesia 38:937–942, 1983.
186. Vella LM, Willatts DG, Knott C, Lintin DJ, et al: Epidural fentanyl in labour: an evaluation of the systemic contribution to analgesia. Anaesthesia 40:741–747, 1985.
187. Phillips GH: Epidural sufentanil/bupivacaine combinations for analgesia during labor. Effect of varying sufentanil doses. Anesthesiology 67:835–838, 1987.
188. Leysen JE, Gommeren W, Nienegeers CJE: (3H) Sufentanil, a superior ligand for $\mu$-opiate receptors: binding properties and regional distribution in rat brain and spinal cord. Eur. J. Pharmacol. 87:209–225 1983.
189. de Sousa H, de la Vega S: Spinal sufentanil. Reg. Anesth. 13:23, 1988.
190. Vertommen JD, Vandermeulen E, Van Aken H, Vaes L, et al: The effects of the addition of sufentanil to 0.125% bupivacaine on the quality of analgesia during labor and on the incidence of instrumental deliveries. Anesthesiology 74: 809–814, 1991.
191. Lemmon WG: A method for continuous spinal anesthesia. Ann. Surg. 111:141–144, 1940.
192. Tuohy EB: The use of continuous spinal anesthesia utilizing the ureteral catheter technic. JAMA 128:262–264, 1945.
193. Carpenter SL, Ceravolo AJ, Foldes FF: Continuous-drop subarachnoid block with dilute procaine solution for labor and delivery. Am. J. Obstet Gynecol. 61:1277–1284, 1951.
194. Bizzarri D, Giuffrida JG, Bandoc L, Fierro FE: Continuous spinal anesthesia using a special needle and catheter. Anesth. Analg. 43:393–399, 1964.
195. Rasmussen BS, Hansen LBP, Mikkelsen SS: Postspinal headache in young and elderly patients. Anaesthesia 44: 571–573, 1989.
196. Benedetti C, Chadwick HS, Mancuso JJ, Ross BK, et al: Incidence of postspinal headache after continuous subarachnoid analgesia for labor using a 32-gauge microcatheter. Anesthesiology 73(3A):A922, 1990.
197. Rigler ML, Drasner K, Krejcie TC, Yelich SJ, et al: Cauda equina syndrome after continuous spinal anesthesia. Anesth. Analg. 72:275–281 1991.
198. Ross BK, Coda B, Heath CH: Local anesthetic distribution in a spinal model: a possible mechanism of neurologic injury after continuous spinal anesthesia. Reg. Anaesth. 17: 69–77, 1992.
199. Rawal N, Schollin J, Wesstrom G: Epidural versus combined spinal epidural block for cesarean section. Acta. Anaesthesiol. Scand. 32:61–66, 1988.
200. Abouleish E, Rawal N, Shaw J, Lorenz T: Intrathecal morphine 0.2 mg versus epidural bupivacaine 0.125% or their combination: effects on parturients. Anesthesiology 74: 712–716, 1991.
201. Forrest WH, Smethurst PWR, Kienetz ME: Self-administra-

tion of intravenous analgesics. Anesthesiology 33: 363–365, 1970.
202. Graves DA, Foster TS, Batenhorst RL, Bennett RL, et al: Patient-controlled analgesia. Ann. Intern. Med. 99: 360–366, 1983.
203. Keeri-Szanto M: Apparatus for demand analgesia. Can. Anaesth. Soc. J. 18:581–582, 1971.
204. Keeri-Szanto M: Demand analgesia. J. Med. 13:3, 241–246, 1982.
205. Lehmann KA: Autoregulation de l'analgesie postoperatoire. Cahiers d'Anesthesiologie 33:119–123, 1985.
206. Lehmann KA: Practical experience with demand analgesia for postoperative pain. *In* Patient-Controlled Analgesia. Edited by M Harmer, M Rosen, MD Vickers. Oxford, Blackwell Scientific Publications, 1985 pp. 134–139.
207. Rosen M, Slattery P, Vickers MD: Cardiff Palliator. Br. J. Anaesth. 55:9, 922, 1983.
208. Tamsen A: Patient Control Analgesic Therapy. Doctoral Thesis, University of Uppsala, Uppsala, Sweden, 1981.
209. Tamsen A: Patient characteristics influencing pain relief. *In* Patient-Controlled Analgesia. Edited by M Harmer, M Rosen, MD Vickers. Oxford, Blackwell Scientific Publications, 1985 pp. 30–37.
210. Tamsen A, Hartvig P, Fagerlund C, Dahlström B: Patient-controlled analgesic therapy, part one: Pharmacokinetics of pethidine in the perioperative and postoperative periods. Clin. Pharmacokinet. 7:149–163, 1982.
211. Tamsen A, Hartvig P, Fagerlund C, Dahlström B: Patient-controlled analgesic therapy, part two: Individual analgesic demand and analgesic plasma concentrations of pethidine in postoperative pain. Clin. Pharmacokinet. 7:252–265, 1982.
212. Tamsen A, Sjoestroem S, Hartvig P: The Uppsala experience of Patient-Controlled Analgesia. *In* Advances in Pain Research and Therapy, Vol 8. Edited by KM Foley, CE Inturrisi. New York, Raven Press, 1986, pp. 325–332.
213. Dodson ME: Aspects of anaesthesia. A review of methods for relief of postoperative pain. Ann. R. Coll. Surg. Engl. 64:324–327, 1982.
214. Anand KJS, Phil D, Hickey PR: Pain and its effects in the human neonate and fetus. N. Engl. J. Med. 317:1321–1329, 1987.
215. Anand KJS, Sippell WG, Aynsley-Green A: Randomized trial of fentanyl anesthesia in preterm babies undergoing surgery: effects on the stress response. Lancet, 1:243–248, 1987.
216. Anand KJS, Sippell WG, Schofield NM, Aynsley-Green A: Does halothane anaesthesia decrease the metabolic and endocrine stress responses of newborn infants undergoing operation? Br. Med. J. 296:668–672, 1988.
217. Ross EL, Perumbeti P: PCA: Is it cost effective when used for postoperative pain management? Anesthesiology 69: A710, 1988.
218. Yeager MP, Glass DD, Neff RK, Brinck-Johnsen T: Epidural anesthesia and analgesia in high-risk surgical patients. Anesthesiology 66:729–736, 1987.
219. Kaiko RF, Wallenstein SL, Rogers AG, Grabinski PY, et al: Clinical analgesic studies and sources of variation in analgesic responses to morphine. *In* Advances in Pain Research and Therapy. Opioid Analgesics in the Management of Clinical Pain, Vol 8. Edited by KM Foley, CE Inturrisi. New York, Raven Press, 1986, pp. 13–23.
220. Mather LE, Denson DD: Pharmacokinetic considerations for drug dosing. *In* Practical Management of Pain. Edited by P Raj. Chicago, Mosby Year Book Medical Publishers, 1986, pp. 489–502.
221. Mather LE, Lindop MJ, Tucker GT, Pflug AE: Pethidine revisited: plasma concentration and effects after intramuscular injection. Br. J. Anaesth. 47:1269–1275, 1975.
222. Austin KL, Stapleton JV, Mather LE: Multiple intramuscular injections: a major source of variability in analgesic response to meperidine. Pain 8:47–62, 1980.
223. Grabinski PY, Kaiko RJ, Rogers AG, Houde RW: Plasma levels and analgesia following deltoid and gluteal injections of methadone and morphine. J. Clin. Pharmacol. 23: 48–55, 1983.
224. Beecher HK: Resuscitation and Anesthesia for Wounded Men; The Management of Traumatic Shock. Springfield, IL, Charles C. Thomas, 1949.
225. Chu G, Cool WM, Kurtz NM: Analgesic efficacy and safety of butorphanol in dental pain: a metered dose nasal spray. Pain S4:S154, 1987.
226. Cool WM, Chu G, Kurtz NM, Abboud T, et al: Intranasal butorphanol: comparison of analgesic efficacy measures in different pain models. Clin. Pharmacol. Ther. 41:8, 1987.
227. Kurtz N, Chu G, Cool M, Abboud T, et al: Analgesic efficacy and safety of intranasally administered butorphanol in post-partum episiotomy pain. Pain S4:S153, 1987.
228. Cool WM, Kurtz NM, Chu G, Abboud T: Intranasal butorphanol in postoperative pain. Pain S4:S153, 1987.
229. Hanning CD: Non-parenteral techniques. *In* Acute Pain. Edited by G Smith, BG Covino. London, Buttersworth, 1985, pp. 180–204.
230. Bonica JJ: Principles and Practice of Obstetric Analgesia and Anesthesia, 1st Edition. Philadelphia, FA Davis Co., 1967, p. 260–276.
231. Clutton-Brock JC: Some pain threshold studies with particular reference to thiopentone. Anesthesia 15:71, 1960.
232. Dundee JW: Alterations in response to somatic pain associated with anesthesia. II. The effect of thiopentone and pentobarbitone. Brit. J. Anaesth. 32:407, 1960.
233. Snyder FF: Obstetric Analgesia and Anesthesia. Philadelphia, W.B. Saunders Co., 1949.
234. Goodman L, Gilman A: The Pharmacological Basis of Therapeutics. 3rd Ed. New York, Macmillan Co., 1965.
235. Rucker E: Intravenous anesthesia for obstetrical delivery. J. Med. Assoc. Alabama 23:59, 1953.
236. Korn RJ, Rock W, Zimmerman HJ: Studies of hepatic function in patients receiving promazine. Amer. J. Med. Sci. 235:431, 1958.
237. Reynolds STM, Harris JS, Kaiser IH: Clinical Measurement of Uterine Forces in Pregnancy and Labor. Springfield, IL, Charles C. Thomas Publisher, 1954.
238. Root B, Eichner E, Sunshine I: Blood secobarbital levels and their clinical correlation in mothers and newborn infants. Amer. J. Obstet. Gynecol. 81:948, 1961
239. Cambell T, Phillips OC, Frazier TM: Analgesia during labor: a comparison of pentobarbital, meperdine, and morphine. Obstet. Gynecol. 17:714, 1961.
240. Fealy J: Placental transmission of pentobarbital sodium. Obstet. Gynecol. 11:342, 1958.
241. Fitzpatrick MJ, deBlois JA, Kushner DH: Reduction of fetal depression intravenous use of promazine for sedation during labor. Obstet. Gynecol. 16:78, 1960.
242. Moya F, Thorndike V: Effects of drugs used in labor on the fetus and newborn. Clin. Pharmacol. Ther. 4:628, 1963.
243. James SL: Biochemical alterations observed in the neonate. *In* Perinatal Pharmacology. Report of the Forty-first Conference on Pediatric Research. Edited by CD May. Columbus, OH, Ross Laboratories, 1962, p. 35.
244. Stechler G: Newborn attention as affected by medication during labor. Science 144:315, 1964.
245. Clifford SH, Irving FC: Analgesia, anesthesia and the newborn infant. Surg. Gynecol. Obstet. 65:23, 1937.

246. Irving FC: Advantages and disadvantages of barbiturates in obstetrics. Rhode Island Med. J. 28:493, 1945.
247. vonSteinbuchel H: Vorlaufige Mittheilung uber die Anwendug von Skopolamin-Morphium-Injectionen in der Gebursshilfe. Z. Geburtsh. Gynaek 26:1304, 1902.
248. Carroll JJ, Moir RS: The use of promethazine (Phenergan) hydrochloride in obstetrics. JAMA 168:2218, 1958.
249. Powe CE, et al: Propiomazine hydrochloride in obstetrical analgesia. JAMA 181:290, 1962.
250. Keats AS, Telford J, Kurosu Y: "Potentiation" of meperidine by promethazine. Anesthesiology 22:34, 1961.
251. Moore J, Dundee JW: Alterations in response to somatic pain associated with anesthesia. V. The effect of promethazine. Brit. J. Anesth. 33:3, 1961
252. Moore J, Dundee JW: Alterations in response to somatic pain associated with anesthesia. VII. The effect of nine phenothiazine derivatives. Brit. J. Anesth. 33:422, 1961.
253. Beaver WT: Comparison of analgesic effects of morphine sulfate, hydroxyzine and other combinations in patients with postoperative pain. *In* Advances in Pain Research and Therapy. Edited by JJ Bonica, V Ventafridda. New York, Raven Press, 1976, pp. 260–275.
254. Bare WW: Double-blind evaluation of hydrozyzine hydrochloride for labor and delivery. Amer. J. Obstet. Gynecol. 83:18, 1962.
255. White PF, Way WL, Trevor AJ: Ketamine—Its Pharmacology and Therapeutic Uses. Anesthesiology 56:119–136, 1982
256. Corssen G, Miyasaka M, Domino EF: Changing concepts in pain control during surgery: dissociative anesthesia with CI-581. Anesth. Analg. 47:746–759, 1968.
257. Reich DL, Silvay G: Ketamine: an update on the first twenty-five years of clinical experience, Can. J. Anaesth. 36(2): 186–97, 1989.
258. Anis NA, Berry SC, Burton NR, Lodge D: The dissociative anaesthetics, ketamine and phencyclidine, selectively reduce excitation of central mammalian neurones by N-methyl-aspartate. Br. J. Pharmacol. 79:565–75, 1983.
259. Thomson AM, West DC, Lodge D: An N-methylaspartate receptor-mediated synapse in rat cerebral cortex: a site of action of ketamine? Nature 313:479–81, 1985.
260. Willcockson WS, Chung JM, Hori Y, Lee KH et al: Effects of iontophoretically released amino acids and amines on primate spinothalamic tract neurons. J. Neuro. Sci. 4: 732–740, 1984.
261. Cahusac PMB, Evans RH, Hill RG, Rodriquez RE et al: The behavioral effects of an N-Methyl-aspartate. Br. J. Pharmacol. 79:565–75, 1984.
262. Anonsen LM, Wilcox GL: Nociceptive action of excitatory amino acids in the mouse: effects of spinally administered opioids, phencyclidine and sigma agonists. J. Pharmacol. Exp. Ther. 243:9–19, 1987.
263. Sher GD, Mitchell D: N-Methyl-D-aspartate receptors mediate reponses of rat dorsal horn neurones to hindlimb ischemia. Brain Res. 522:55–62, 1990.
264. Maurset AM, Skoglund LA, Hustveit O, Oye I: Comparison of ketamine and pethidine in experimental and postoperative pain. Pain 36:37–41, 1989.
265. Oshima E, Tei K, Kayazawa H, Urabe N: Continuous subcutaneous injection of ketamine for cancer pain. Can. J. Anaesth. 37:385–6, 1990.
266. Marietta MP, Way WL, Castagnoli N, et al: On the pharmacology of the ketamine enantiomorphs in the rat. J. Pharmacol. Exp. Ther. 202:157–65, 1977.
267. White PF, Ham J, Way WL, et al: Pharmacology of ketamine isomers in surgical patients. Anesthesiology 52:231–39, 1980.
268. Jackson APF, Dhadphale RP, Callaghan ML: Haemodynamic studies during induction of anesthesia for open-heart surgery using diazepam and ketamine. Br. J. Anaesth. 50: 375–77, 1978.
269. Carrel R: Ketamine: A general anesthetic for unmanageable ambulatory patients. ASDC J. Dent. Child. 40:288–292, 1973.
270. Cohenour K, Gamble JW, Metzgar MT, et al: A composite general anesthesia for pediatric outpatients. J. Oral Surgery 36:594–598, 1978.
271. Chodoff P, Stella JC: Use of CI-581, a phencyclidine derivative for obstetric anesthesia. Anesth. Anal. 45:527–530, 1966.
272. Akamatsu TJ, Bonica JJ, Rehmet R: Experiences with the use of ketamine for parturition. 1. Primary anesthetic for vaginal delivery. Anesth. Analg. 53:284–7, 1974.
273. Hodgkinson R, Robinson, DA: The role of ketamine in obstetric anesthesia. Presented at the Ketalar Roundtable, New Orleans, 1984.
274. Bunodiere M, Green M, Bunodieve N, et al: Le chlorhydrate de ketamine pour l'anesthesie en obstetrique. Anesth. Analg.(Paris) 32:197, 1975.
275. Rucci FS, Caroli G: Ketamine and eclampsia. Br. J. Anaesth. 46:546, 1974.
276. Marx GF, Cabe CM, Kim YI, et al: Neonatal blood pressures. Anaesthetist 25:318–322, 1976.
277. Hodgkinson K, Marx GF, Kim SS, et al: Neonatal neurobehavioral tests following vaginal delivery under ketamine, thiopental, and extradural anesthesia. Anesth. Analg. 56: 548–53, 1977.

Chapter 18

# PHARMACOLOGY OF INHALATIONAL AND INTRAVENOUS ANESTHETICS

K.C. WONG
JON R. SUNDIN

---

Clinical pharmacology is the essence of anesthetic practice. In the words of John J. Bonica, "An anesthesiologist is a clinical pharmacologist who practices medicine in its most intense and dynamic form." The administration of drugs and anesthetics to the parturient represents an even greater challenge to the anesthesiologist because, regardless of the route of administration, a drug is always carried by the blood to the receptor site to exert its pharmacologic action, and the fetus is also dependent upon maternal blood supply for its homeostasis. Therefore, the fetus will invariably receive drugs carried by maternal circulation. It is imperative, then, that the obstetric anesthesiologist have a thorough understanding of the drug administered to the mother as well as the drug unintentionally received by the fetus. Although a great deal is known with regard to the maternal pharmacologic effects of inhalational and intravenous anesthetics, far less direct data are available about their effects on the human fetus. This chapter will review some basic principles about pharmacokinetics of inhalational and intravenous anesthetics, and pharmacodynamics of drug concentration and drug receptor interaction. The discussion on the pharmacology of the drugs will be focused on information of clinical interest regarding the mother and the fetus.

Because all inhalational anesthetics and intravenous anesthetics are carried by the blood to the receptors at which they are active, they are also carried to organ systems and receptor sites for which they are not intended. Structural specificity of a drug results in more discreet responses; unfortunately, there are no 100%-receptor-specific drugs. Therefore, other drug receptor interactions may be elicited concurrently with the primary desired response. Side effects are thus inherent in all drugs administered to a patient. For example, analgesia from opiates is commonly accompanied by sedation and respiratory depression; hypnosis from halothane or thiopental is commonly associated with myocardial depression. Optimal anesthetic management is achieved when there is maximal desired drug effect with minimal side effects. The effects of drugs on the fetus may be thought of as a side effect of drugs administered to the mother. Figure 18–1 demonstrates the uptake distribution of drugs, with IV and inhalation drugs compared and contrasted in parts A and B.

The amount of the drug that finally reaches the receptor site following access into the blood is influenced by how the drug is distributed, biotransformed, and eliminated from the body. Pharmacokinetics deal with all of the processes that affect the drug during its journey through the body. Pharmacodynamics deal with the mechanism of drug action and the relationship between drug concentration and receptor interaction. These principles are applied to the mother as well as to the fetus.

## Pharmacokinetics of Intravenous and Inhalational Anesthetics

Pharmacokinetics is the quantitative study of drug disposition in the body or "what the body does to the drug." To produce a desired pharmacologic response, an appropriate concentration of the drug must be delivered to the receptor site. Onset and duration of drug effects will be related to the rise and fall of the drug concentration at its site of action. The concentration of drug in plasma plays an essential role in the disposition of the drug throughout the body (1). Factors that influence the concentration of the drug in the body are absorption, distribution, biotransformation, and excretion. The interrelationship of these factors determines the concentration of a drug at its locus of action. Figure 18–2 demonstrates these influential factors.

The absorption, distribution, biotransformation, and excretion of a drug are all involved with passage of the drug across cell membranes (Figure 18–3). Routes of penetration include bulk flow through intercellular pores, passive diffusion through the membrane lipid bilayer, and carrier-mediated membrane transport, and pinocytosis. Most drugs penetrate membranes by passive dissolution and diffusion across membranes down a concentration gradient. Such transfer is directly proportional to the magnitude of the concentration gradient across the membrane, the lipid:water partition coefficient, and the molecular size of the drug (1,2).

Lipid solubility is the most important property. The greater the lipid solubility, the more rapidly the drug penetrates the lipoprotein membrane.

Ionization of a drug limits its rate of penetration because ionization decreases lipid solubility and creates an ionic force that may be repelled or bound by similarly

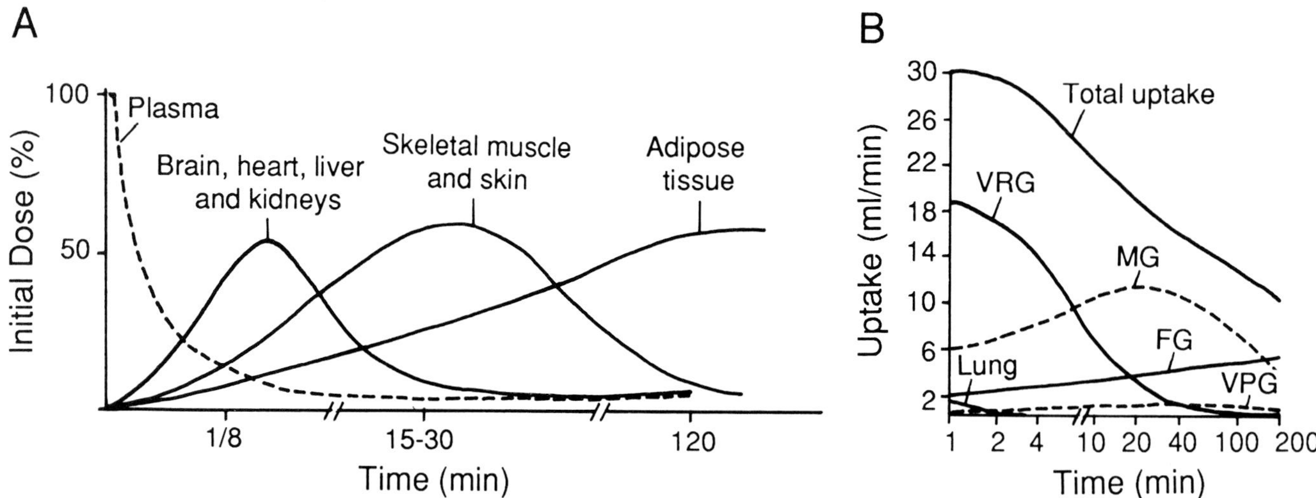


**Fig. 18–1.** Uptake distribution of drugs. **(A)** The distribution of thiopental following IV injection. Note the redistribution of the drug with time to tissues with lower rates of blood flow. (Redrawn from Price HL, et al: Clin. Pharmacol. Ther. 1:16, 1960.) **(B)** The distribution of halothane when 1% halothane is inspired. (Redrawn from Eger EI II: Brit. J. Anaesth. 36:155, 1964.)

charged membrane components (1,2). Most drugs are weak acids or bases existing in both ionic and nonionic forms. The nonionic forms are usually lipid soluble and able to penetrate the membrane while the ionic form has decreased lipid solubility and is unable to penetrate. The degree of ionization is determined by the pKa of the drug, which is defined as the pH at which the number of ionized and nonionized molecules in the solution are equal. This relationship is defined by the Henderson-Hasselback equation, as shown in Figure 18–4. Ionization is complete for certain drugs (e.g., muscle relaxants) with little resultant penetration across any lipid membrane. Weakly acidic or weakly basic drugs with pKas close to physiologic pH will have un-ionized forms that readily penetrate and cross lipid membranes. The driving force results from the concentration gradient of the un-ionized form. As the un-ionized form moves across the membrane, it dissociates into ionized form based on the ratio determined by the Henderson-Hasselback equation. If the pH on both sides of the membrane is the same, the total amount of drug, ionized and un-ionized, will be equal on both sides.

However, if the pH differs as may happen in a laboring patient with fetal distress, the concentration of the non-ionized drug will be equal, but total concentration may be widely different. This is due to a higher concentration of ionized form, as described by the Henderson-Hasselback equation, being present on the fetal side of the membrane. For example, bupivacaine with a pKa of 8.1 will be 15% nonionized at the maternal pH of 7.4, but only 11% nonionized in a distressed fetus with a pH of 7.2. In this situation, the fetus will act as an ion trap for bupivacaine, and the total amount at equilibrium will be higher in the fetus than in the mother.

Molecular size determines drug movement via intercellular pores of capillary endothelial membranes (except within the central nervous system, which has tight junctions) (Figure 18–5). Most drugs used by anesthesiologists are too large to penetrate parenchymal membranes (4 A°), but are small enough to penetrate capillary membranes (1). Ionization limits drug passage across parenchymal membranes, but not across the intercellular pores of the capillary endothelium. These intercellular pores are sufficiently large (40 A°) so that diffusion is limited by blood flow and concentration and not by lipid solubility or pH gradients (1,2). Proteins are large enough that they are limited by the size of capillary intercellular pores. Most drugs are bound by plasma proteins to some extent, and the protein bound drugs are unable to cross membranes, and are not capable of further distribution (Figure 18–6).

Finally, while passive diffusion through lipoprotein membranes is dominant in the absorption and distribution of most drugs, active transport of many drugs occurs across neuronal membranes, the choroid plexus, renal tubular cells, and hepatocytes. The characteristics of active transport (selectivity, competitive inhibition, energy requirements, saturability, and movement against an electrochemical gradient) may be important in the mechanism of action of drugs (1,2). For example, cocaine and imipramine inhibit the reuptake of norepinephrine at adrenergic nerve terminals; furosemide inhibits chloride and sodium transport in the ascending limb of the loop of Henle; and digitalis inhibits NaK ATPase, thus the transport of Na and K across cell membranes.

### Absorption

Absorption deals with the process of delivery of drug from its site of administration to the circulation. Clinically, it is useful to think in terms of bioavailability, which indicates the extent to which a drug reaches its receptor site of action. Bioavailability can change drastically for the same drug if different routes of administration are used.

Factors that greatly affect absorption are solubility, drug concentration, circulation, and absorptive surface.

Drugs given in an aqueous solution are absorbed more

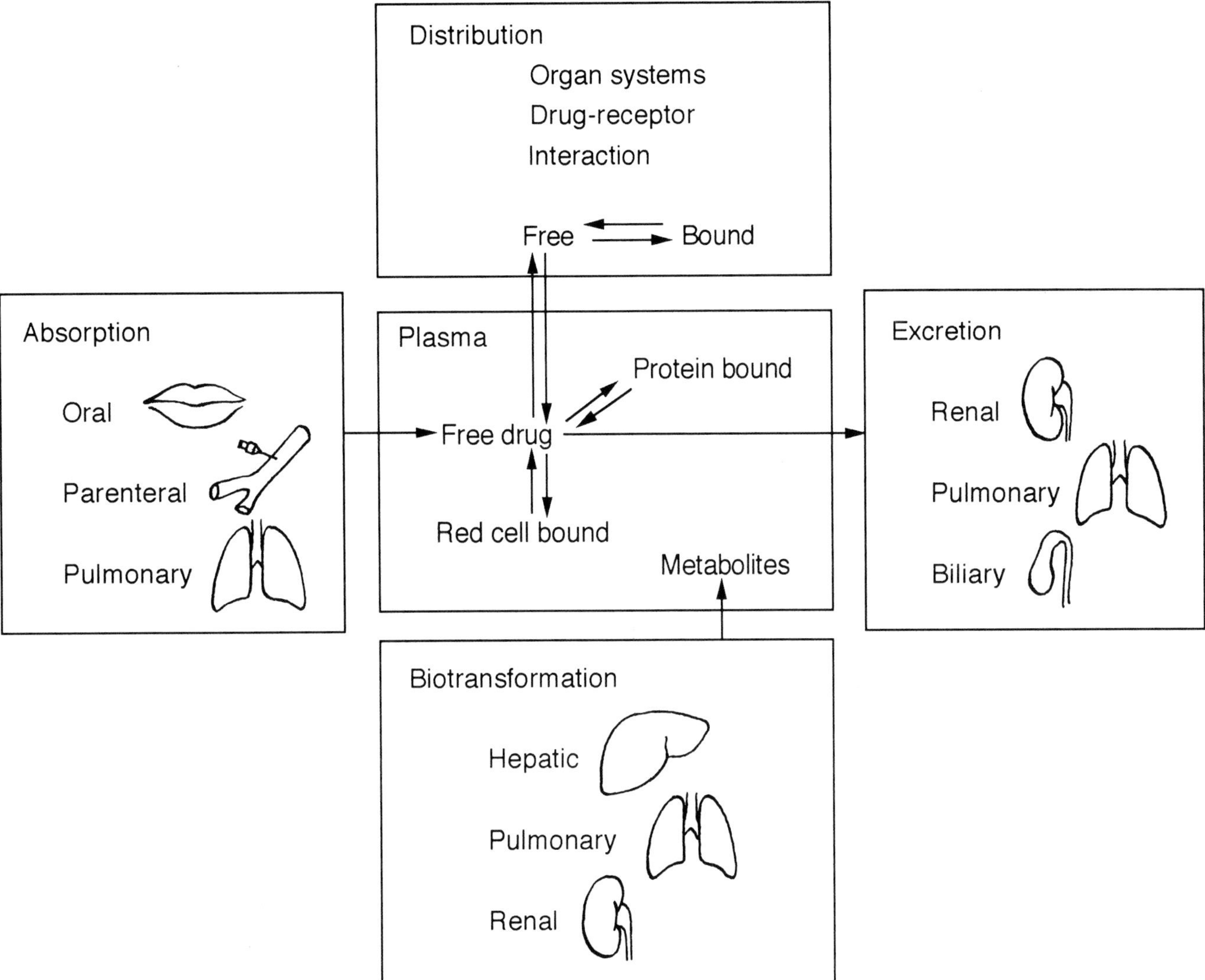


**Fig. 18–2.** The pharmacokinetics of absorption, distribution, biotransformation, and excretion of a drug. Important considerations are: (1) bound drugs are inactive and unable to cross biologic membranes; (2) distribution to unintended organ systems account for side effects of drugs; (3) biotransformation generally results in deactivation of drugs and increased water solubility for renal excretion. (Redrawn from Wong KC: Pharmacology. *In* Marshall BE, Longnecker DE, Fairly HB: Anesthesia for Thoracic Procedures. Boston, Blackwell Scientific Publishers, 1988.)

readily than drugs in oily solution because they mix more readily with the aqueous phase at the absorptive site (2). Higher concentrations are absorbed more rapidly due to increased availability and diffusion driving force. Massage, local application of heat and vasodilators increase absorption, whereas decreased blood flow due to shock, hypothermia, and vasoconstrictors will decrease absorption. Drugs are absorbed rapidly from large absorptive surfaces such as the pulmonary alveoli and intestinal mucosa.

### *Oral Ingestion*

Absorption from the gastrointestinal tract is more variable, less predictable, and slower than with parenteral administration. Therefore, the only medicines routinely given orally by anesthesiologists are preoperative medications.

Other important factors affecting absorption after oral ingestion are drug form, resistance to gastric acid degradation, gastrointestinal motility, and degree of ionization.

Most oral drugs are given in tablet form. Both the carrier substance and the drug itself must first dissolve to be available for absorption. Enteral coatings are often added to decrease gastric irritation. If complete dissolution does not occur, much of the administered dose will pass through the gastrointestinal tract without absorption. Many drugs are sensitive to and broken down by gastric acid into inactive forms, again limiting absorption of the active drug (1). Many surgical patients are in pain and as a result have decreased gastrointestinal motility with decreased delivery of the drug to the absorptive surface (1). Because most drug absorption from the gastrointestinal surface is by passive processes, the un-ionized form

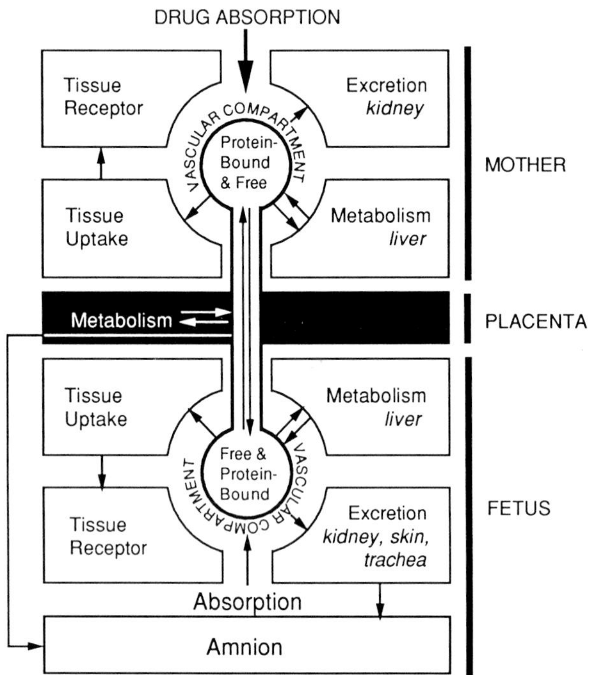


**Fig. 18–3.** Absorption distribution of biotransformation and difference between maternal and fetal penetration. (Redrawn from Rajchgot P, MacLeod SM: Perinatal pharmacology. *In* Principles of Medical Pharmacology. Edited by H Kalant, WHE Roschlau, EM Sellers. 4th Ed. New York, Oxford University Press, 1985.)

will diffuse more readily. Weak acids such as barbiturates and salicylates are less ionized in the stomach and therefore are thought to be more readily absorbed here than in the intestine due to the availability of greater nonionized molecules in the acidic stomach. However, the stomach has a thick mucous covered wall with high electrical resistance and a small surface in contrast to the intestine, which has a thin epithelium with low electrical resistance and an extremely large surface (1). As such, the rate of absorption from the intestine will be greater than from the stomach even when the degree of ionization in the intestine is greater than in the stomach (2).

After absorption from the stomach and intestine, the drug must first pass through the liver before it gains access into the systemic circulation. The extent by which the drug is metabolized into an inactive form or excreted by the bile from this process will determine the bioavailability of the drug. This is called the first pass effect (1).

**Henderson-Hasselbalch equation:**

$$pH = pK_a + \log \frac{[nonionized]}{[ionized]}$$

**$pk_a$ is the degree of ionization.**
**Nonionized is also described as undissociated drug.**
**Ionized is also described as dissociated drug.**
**The $pk_a$ for weak acids is high, and for weak bases is low.**

**Fig. 18–4.** Drug ionization, defined as the Henderson-Hasselbalch equation. (From Baden JM, Rice SA: Metabolism and toxicity. *In* Anesthesia. 3rd Ed. Edited by RD Miller. New York, Churchill Livingstone, 1990.)

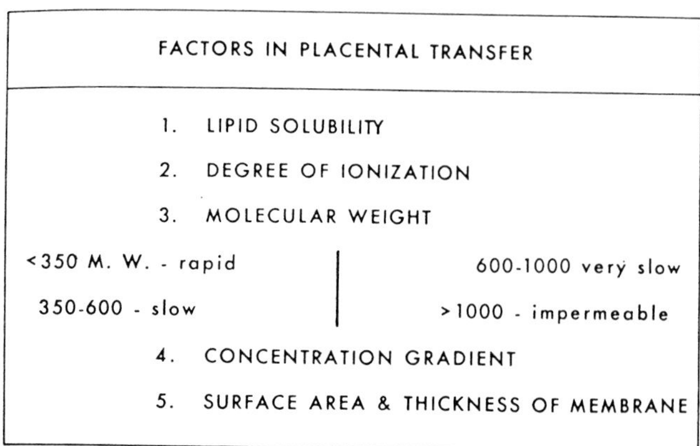
FACTORS IN PLACENTAL TRANSFER

1. LIPID SOLUBILITY
2. DEGREE OF IONIZATION
3. MOLECULAR WEIGHT

| | |
|---|---|
| <350 M. W. - rapid | 600-1000 very slow |
| 350-600 - slow | >1000 - impermeable |

4. CONCENTRATION GRADIENT
5. SURFACE AREA & THICKNESS OF MEMBRANE

**Fig. 18–5.** Molecular size. (From Shnider SM. Obstetrical anesthesia current concepts and practice. Baltimore, Williams & Wilkins, 1970.)

## *Mucosal Administration*

Sublingual, nasal, and rectal routes of administration of drugs are common. Absorption of drugs via the sublingual and nasal mucosal routes could be rapid and also avoids first pass hepatic metabolism as the blood supply in these areas flows into the superior vena cava. Rectal absorption is not as reliable, but is still useful especially for sedating or inducing anesthesia in young children.

## *Parenteral Injection*

Parenteral injection is the most reliable and fastest route for delivery of drugs to the receptor site of action.

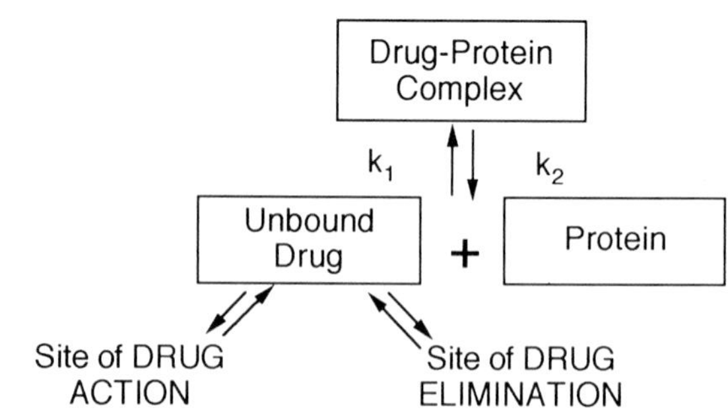


**Fig. 18–6.** Effect of protein binding on drug disposition. (Redrawn from Endrenyi L: Drug distribution. *In* Principles of Medical Pharmacology. 5th Ed. Edited by H Kalant, WHE Roschlau. Philadelphia, BC Decker Inc, 1989.)

Drugs are already in solution and diffuse readily from the circulation through the intercellular pores of the capillary endothelium. Speed of diffusion depends on the concentration gradient between the interstitial space where the drug is deposited and the area of blood flow through the capillary network exposed to the drug.

### *Intramuscular Injection*

Intramuscular injection has reliable absorption due to the relatively vascular nature of muscle (Figure 18–7). This route is often used to deliver preoperative medications such as antisialagogues, sedatives, and narcotic analgesics. Intramuscular injection of ketamine and succinylcholine is commonly used in routine pediatric cases to induce anesthesia and facilitate endotracheal intubation.

The factors that limit the absorption of drugs delivered by the routes outlined above are avoided by intravenous administration. Reliable concentrations can rapidly and reliably be delivered by the intravenous route. This immediacy and reliability of delivery is crucial to the anesthesiologist because administration of intravenous anesthetics requires moment-to-moment titration in response to the patient's reaction.

Many irritating drugs can only be given parenterally by the intravenous route because the blood both dilutes and buffers the irritating drug. For example, thiopental, with a pH of 10.5, is harmful to subcutaneous tissue and small arterioles; norepinephrine, with its potent vasoconstrictor property, can produce tissue ischemia if given intramuscularly or subcutaneously; and diazepam causes pain and is absorbed poorly when given intramuscularly.

### *Inhalation*

Pulmonary absorption of inhaled anesthetics and drugs is rapid and reliable due to the tremendous surface area, immediate proximity to capillary endothelium, and high blood flow (Figure 18–8). Absorption of inhaled anesthetics is rapid, easily regulated with modern equipment, and also has the advantage of rapid clearance by the same route with minimal metabolism or accumulation of metabolites. Factors directly affecting uptake and distribution of inhalational anesthetics will be discussed later.

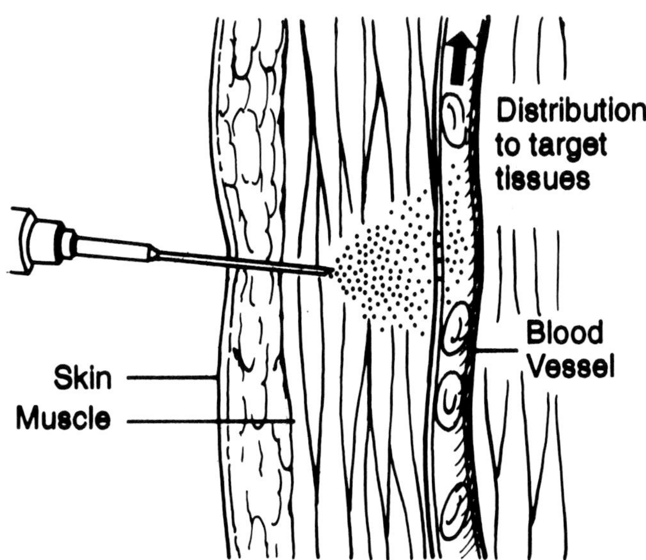


**Fig. 18–7.** Intramuscular injection. (Redrawn from Seeman P, Kalant H: Drug solubility, absorption, and movement across body membranes. *In* Principles of Medical Pharmacology. 5th Ed. Edited by H Kalant, WHE Roschlau. Philadelphia, BC Decker Inc, 1989.)

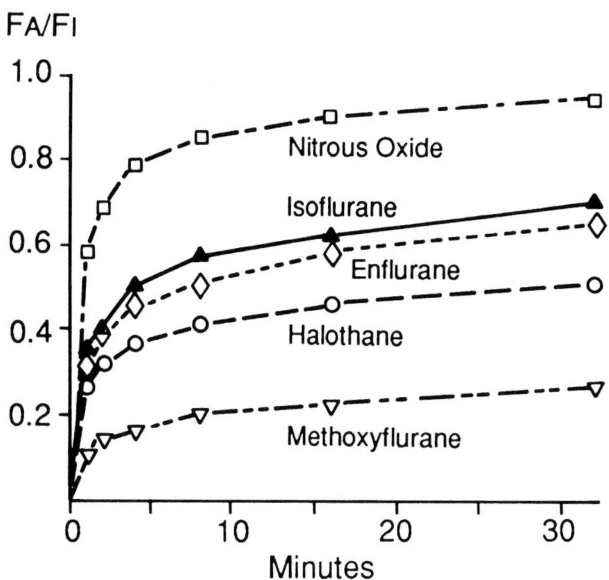


**Fig. 18–8.** Alveolar uptake of inhalation anesthetics. (Redrawn from Eger II EI: Uptake and distribution. *In* Anesthesia. 3rd Ed. Edited by RD Miller. New York, Churchill Livingstone, 1990.)

## *Distribution*

The distribution of drugs to tissues can be characterized in terms of rate and capacity. After a drug is absorbed or is injected into the blood stream, it will first be distributed to organ systems with the greatest blood flow. Because blood flow to the brain, heart, and viscera is large, these organs receive also a larger portion of the drug administered. Therefore, it is reasonable to expect myocardial depression as a common side effect during rapid induction by inhalational or intravenous anesthetics.

Distribution of a highly lipid soluble drug is most dependent on concentration in the blood and blood flow itself. Effects of ionization, molecular size, and protein binding are influential factors. As will be discussed in the section on kinetics, uptake by nontarget tissue, redistribution, and elimination all delay the onset of desired target tissue concentration. Conversely, when administration of a drug is stopped and elimination is desired, tissue depots such as muscle and especially fat will delay elimination and recovery, due to reversal of concentration gradients within the different tissue groups with resultant redistribution of drug. An example of this is thiopental. Thiopental is a short-acting drug due to initial redistribution from the vessel-rich group to muscle and fat, but with repeated injections and accumulation within fat it can become a long-lasting agent.

There are two special barriers that are germane for this

discussion. The blood-brain barrier has tight junctions and lacks pinocytotic vesicles, restricting the entry of drugs into the central nervous system extracellular space and cerebrospinal fluid (Figure 18–9). Ionized drugs are severely limited in their ability to cross the blood-brain barrier where only lipophilic drugs may gain access. Similarly, drugs are able to cross the placenta by simple diffusion. The basic concepts of placental transfer of drugs and fetal disposition of anesthetic drugs will be discussed in more detail in Chapter 8. However, it is important to point out the complexity of the maternal hemodynamic factors that alters the delivery of a drug to the placenta. During the peak of a uterine contraction, uterine arterial blood flow ceases, preventing further delivery of drug to the placenta. On the other hand, drug concentrations in the intervillous space of the placenta could increase by inhibiting uterine venous outflow, thus promoting placental transfer of the drug to the fetus. Factors such as maternal hypotension or hypertension, which influence the uterine blood flow, would also influence drug concentration in the placenta. Placental drug transfer is facilitated by a high concentration of nonionized, lipid soluble, and nonprotein bound drug. High molecular weight, poor lipid solubility, and increased ionization of a drug will retard the transfer of a drug across the placenta (Table 18–1). Molecular weights of greater than 1000 have difficulty crossing the placenta. Most of the drugs used by the anesthesiologist are less than 1000 and may gain easy access through the placenta. Therefore, to a large extent, the fetus is exposed to the same drugs given to the mother.

**Table 18–1.** Factors Determining Placental Drug Transfer

| Factor | Effect on Transfer |
|---|---|
| Placental blood flow | Increased drug delivery to placental membranes as blood flow increases. |
| Molecular size of drug | Decreased transfer of drug across placental membrane as molecular size increases. |
| Lipid solubility of drug | Increased transfer of drug across placental membrane as lipid solubility increases. |
| $pK_a$ of drug—basic drugs: | Increased ion trapping on fetal side. |
| —acidic drugs: | Decreased ion trapping on fetal side. |
| Fetal pH (which is slightly less than maternal pH) | Increased ion trapping of basic drugs on fetal side. |

(From Rajchgot P, MacLeod SM: Perinatal pharmacology. *In* Principles of Medical Pharmacology. 4th Ed. Edited by H Kalant, WHE Roschlau, EM Sellers. New York, Oxford University Press, Inc. 1985.)

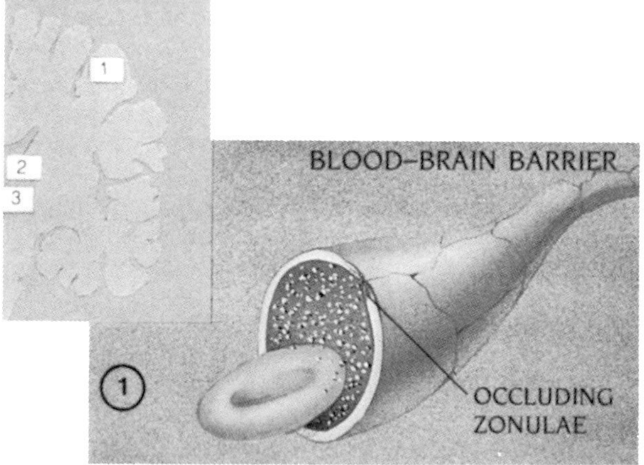


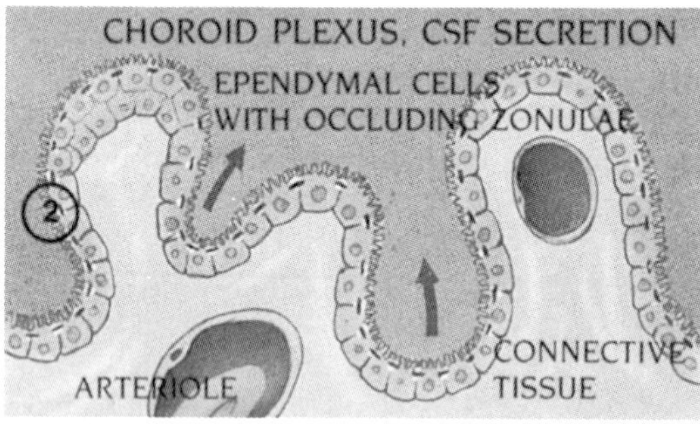


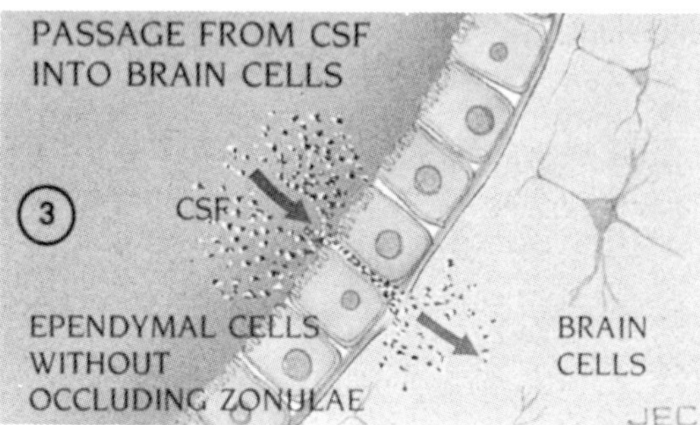


**Fig. 18–9.** Blood brain barrier. (From Seeman P, Kalant H: Drug solubility, absorption, and movement across body membranes. *In* Principles of Medical Pharmacology. 5th Ed. Edited by H Kalant, WHE Roschlau. Philadelphia, BC Decker Inc, 1989.)

Concentration within the fetus varies depending on timing of injection, number of injections, infusions, cardiac output, dilution within the fetal circulation, amount of fetal circulation, and amount of fetal metabolism (3). Theoretically, the percentage of the intravenous dose that is transferred to the fetus should approach the percentage of maternal cardiac output (10% to 15%) to the placenta. Injections should be timed to uterine contractions, which decrease drug delivery to the uteroplacental unit, and injections should be given in a slow, incremental fashion to avoid a bolus effect to the fetus by allowing the initial high concentration to dilute out into maternal circulation and tissues.

### *Biotransformation*

It is beyond the scope of this discussion to include many of the biochemical mechanisms by which drugs or substances are metabolized in the body. There are books and reviews devoted specifically to this topic (2–4). A practical conception for the metabolism of drugs by the body is that drugs in their active form are generally lipid soluble and un-ionized, which are relatively insoluble in water. Metabolism renders these substances more polar, therefore more water soluble than its original drug form, thus promoting renal excretion via urine. Inhalational anesthetics are generally more inert than intravenous anesthetics and resist metabolism. Furthermore, the lungs are efficient organs for the uptake as well as the elimination of inhalational anesthetics.

Metabolism usually produces inactive metabolites of the parent substance or drug; however, some intermediate metabolites are pharmacologically active. For example, morphine is converted to codeine, and thiopental to pentobarbital. The types of biochemical reaction that result in biotransformation of drugs may include conjugation, oxidation, reduction, and hydrolysis. Hepatic conjugation with glucuronic acid is a common pathway by which many drugs used in anesthesia are rendered water soluble and less active (opiates, for example). Other examples involving these biochemical reactions are oxidation of meperidine to meperidinic acid; reduction of chloralhydrate to trichloroethanol; and hydrolysis of succinylcholine to succinic acid and choline. The hepatic smooth endoplasmic reticulum represents the major site of enzyme systems for biotransformation of drugs and substances; however, the lungs and the kidney are also important sites of extrahepatic metabolism. Glucuronides are generally inactive and are rapidly excreted by the urine and the bile. However, glucuronides eliminated in the bile may he subsequently hydrolyzed by intestinal or bacterial glucuronides and the liberated, free drug may be reabsorbed by the intestine. This enterohepatic recycling may prolong the drug action of certain drugs, thus being an additional factor for the prolonged pharmacologic effects of morphine and other opiates.

The barbiturates and many hydrocarbons, including some inhalational anesthetics, are known to stimulate the hepatic smooth endoplasmic reticulum. This increase in hepatic enzyme activity is attributable to the induced synthesis of cytochrome $P_{450}$ reductase and other enzymes involved in drug metabolism. Of clinical interest is that several fluorinated inhalational anesthetics are defluorinated by cytochrome $P_{450}$ to produce nephrotoxic concentrations of fluoride ion (5). The role of enzyme induction in the biotransformation of intravenous anesthetics is still unclear, but could be important because microsomal enzyme systems are involved in oxidative reactions and glucuronide synthesis (4).

It is common to find elevated serum glutamic oxaloacidic transaminase, lactic dehydrogenase, alkaline phosphatase, and cholesterol levels in normal parturients. Although these abnormal liver function test results do not necessarily indicate hepatic disease, both total protein and the albumin:globulin ratio are decreased during pregnancy. The reduction in minimal alveolar concentration (MAC) and increased sensitivity to central nervous system (CNS) depressant drugs may be in part related to a reduced hepatic metabolism of drugs during pregnancy (6). An elevation in progesterone and beta-endorphin levels during pregnancy is an important factor for an increased tolerance to pain and decreased need for anesthetic and analgesic drugs.

Hepatic microsomal enzyme systems are poorly developed in newborns, particularly in premature infants (3). The combination of poorly developed drug metabolizing enzyme systems, as well as ineffective blood-brain barrier and immature mechanisms for excretion via the hepatobiliary and renal systems, makes the infant vulnerable to the toxic effects of drugs (Figure 18–10). Although not well-studied, it would be reasonable to suggest that the fetus would even be more vulnerable to the toxic effects of drugs than the mother.

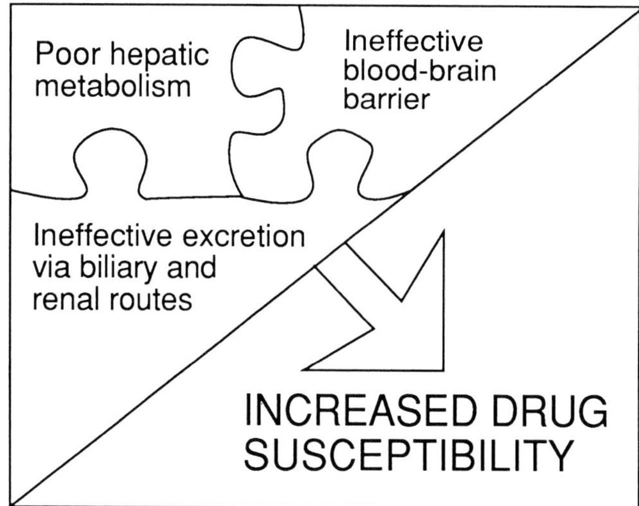


**Fig. 18–10.** Premature neonate's sensitivity to drugs.

### *Excretion*

Whereas inhalational anesthetics are generally eliminated by the lungs with minimal metabolism of the inhalational anesthetic, intravenous drugs are eliminated from the body either unchanged or following a metabolic transformation. Metabolism usually renders the drug more polar and water soluble, which allows the metabolic product to be more readily eliminated by the kidneys or the hepatobiliary system. Lipid soluble drugs are thus not easily eliminated from the body until they have been made more water soluble. Excretion of drugs and metabolites by the kidneys involves three processes of the nephron:

1. glomerular filtration
2. active tubular secretion
3. passive tubular reabsorption

These processes are usually intact in the normal parturient but compromised during certain disease processes, most commonly diabetes and preeclampsia. Other routes of excretion of drugs are in sweat, saliva, tears, and milk.

### *Clinical Pharmacokinetics*

The pharmacokinetics of absorption, distribution, biotransformation, and excretion contribute to the variation of drug concentration in the plasma. Typical curves illustrating the rate of disappearance of a drug in the plasma are shown in Figure 18–11. These curves are usually constructed from measurements of the rate of disappearance of the drug from the plasma following a bolus intravenous injection of the drug. The present discussion is aimed at providing useful clinical information to the reader. For a detailed discussion of the theoretical and mathematical

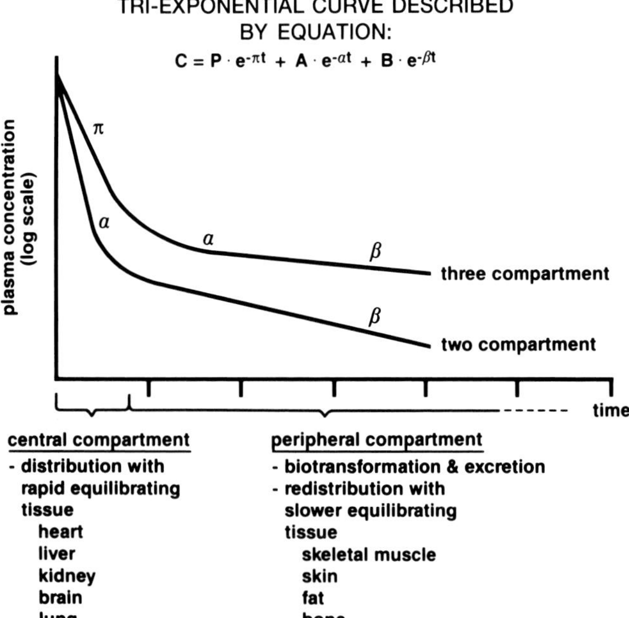


**Fig. 18–11.** Typical curves of disappearance of a drug in plasma. The initial rapid fall is from distribution with rapid equilibrating tissues. The slow pulse of disappearance represents a combining effect from biotransformation and excretion as well as redistribution with slow equilibrating tissues. The plasma-concentration curves illustrate when two and three compartment models are used. (From Wong KC: Pharmacology. *In* Anesthesia for Thoracic Procedures. Edited by BE Marshall, DE Longnecker, HB Fairly. Boston, Blackwell Scientific Publishers, 1988.)

consideration of pharmacokinetics, the reader is referred to excellent reviews and textbooks (2,3,7,8).

## *Distribution and Elimination Half-Life ($T_{1/2}$)*

The initial decrease in drug concentration in the plasma is from distribution with rapid equilibrating tissues, such as heart, liver, brain, kidney, and lungs (Figure 18–11). The slow phase of drug concentration reduction of plasma represents biotransformation and excretion, as well as redistribution with slower equilibrating tissues such as skeletal muscle, skin, fat, and bone. For many of the drugs administered intravenously during anesthesia, the plasma concentration time curve can be described by two lines and therefore a "two compartment" model will mathematically describe the process. For some drugs, a one-compartment model may be sufficient; for others, a three-compartment model is necessary (Figure 18–11). Most drugs used in clinical anesthesia have plasma concentration curves that can be described by a two- or three-compartment model. The plasma concentration curves for most opiates and intravenous (IV) induction drugs have been described by three-compartment models characterized by the algebraic sum of three single exponential curves designated by π (pi), α (alpha), and β (beta) components (Figure 18–11). The tri-exponential curve is described by the equation:

$$c = p * e^{-\pi t} + A * e^{-\alpha t} + B * e^{-\beta t} \quad (1)$$

From each rate constant a corresponding distribution half-life or elimination half-life can be calculated, so that:

$$T_{1/2\pi} = \frac{0.693}{\pi}$$
$$T_{1/2\alpha} = \frac{0.693}{\alpha} \quad (2)$$
$$\text{and } T_{1/2\beta} = \frac{0.693}{\beta}$$

Although the slower decline phase of the concentration time curve has been commonly described as the beta-equilibration half-life ($T_{1/2\beta}$, biotransformation and redistribution with slower equilibrating tissues contribute to the slope of this portion of the curve (Figure 18–11).

## *The Volume of Distribution ($V_d$)*

The volume of distribution of a drug is the apparent volume in which the drug is distributed during the steady state when the concentration of the drug in the plasma is the same throughout the body. Clearly, a vast amount of detailed information with regard to tissue equilibration will be required to characterize the distribution pattern. A gross simplification, but clinically useful approach, is to assume that the body is a single compartment. Thus,

$$V_d = \frac{\text{total amount of drug in the body}}{\text{concentration of drug in plasma}} = \frac{\text{dose/weight}}{\text{dose/volume}} = \frac{\text{volume}}{\text{weight}} \quad (3)$$

If a drug is highly lipid soluble in tissues, for example, its volume of distribution may be greater than that estimated for the total body water. Obviously, appropriate interpretation must be made of such a seemingly abnormal physiologic calculation.

## *Plasma Drug Clearance*

Another useful calculation for the removal of the drug from the body is drug clearance (Cl). Drug clearance is the volume of blood or plasma from which the drug is completely removed per unit of time. Plasma clearance may be estimated by measuring plasma concentrations repeatedly after a single dose of the drug until it is completely eliminated. Thus:

$$Cl = \frac{\text{mean rate of removal}}{\text{mean plasma concentration}} = \frac{\text{dose/time}}{\text{dose/volume}} = \frac{\text{volume}}{\text{time}} \quad (4)$$

### *Summary*

In sum, the concepts of compartmental analysis, drug distribution, elimination half-life, volume of distribution, and drug clearance are useful pharmacokinetic principles to assist anesthesiologists in the selection and adjustment of intravenous drug dosage schedule and to facilitate interpretation of measured plasma concentration of a drug.

A listing of these common pharmacokinetic parameters is summarized below:

1. Distribution half-life in minutes: $T_{1/2\pi}$, $T_{1/2\alpha}$; this parameter represents the fast declining phase of drug in plasma representing distribution with rapid equilibrating tissues.
2. Elimination half-life in minutes: $T_{1/2\beta}$; this parameter represents the slow phase of the drug disappearing from the plasma from biotransformation, excretion, and redistribution with slow equilibrating tissues.
3. Drug clearance in ml/kg/min: Cl; representing the rate of elimination of a drug from the plasma.
4. Volume of distribution in liters/kg: $V_d$; representing the apparent volume in which a drug is distributed during the steady state.

It would be instructive to compare the pharmacologic and pharmacokinetic parameters of several intravenous hypnotics (Table 18–2) to illustrate the utility of these numbers for estimating the onset and duration of drug effect. Thiopental, methohexital, and propofol all have a short distribution phase ($T_{1/2\pi}$, on the order of 2 to 4 minutes following intravenous injection. This short distribution phase is representative of the rapid uptake of these drugs by the brain and other well-perfused organs (Figure 18–11). The rapid onset of action of these hypnotics is apparently related to their lipid solubility and therefore to their ability to penetrate the blood-brain barrier. By comparison, thiopental has a longer beta elimination half-life ($T_{1/2\beta}$ and a slower clearance rate in comparison with methohexital and propofol. Therefore, following repeated injections of these drugs, thiopental will be expected to accumulate in the body, thus exerting a prolonged hypnotic effect. In contrast, methohexital, with a high clearance rate and a low volume of distribution, does not tend to accumulate in the body even with a repeated injection (Table 18–2). A large volume of distribution should contribute to prolonged duration of drug action. In the case of propofol, in spite of adequate clearance rate, the large volume of distribution results in accumulation of the following prolonged infusion (Table 18–2) drug. It should be remembered that such other influential factors as protein binding, lipid solubility, ionization, biotransformation, etc, also contribute to the duration and intensity of the drug action (Figure 18–2). Thus, pharmacokinetic data should be used in conjunction with physiologic data for optimal patient care.

**Table 18–2.** Pharmacokinetics of Intravenous Anesthetics

| Drug | $T_{1/2\pi}$ (min) | $T_{1/2\alpha}$ (min) | $T_{1/2\beta}$ (h) | Vd (l/kg) | Cl (ml/kg/min) |
|---|---|---|---|---|---|
| Thiopental | 2.4 | 47.0 | 5.1 | 1.6 | 1.6 |
| Methohexital | 4.8 | 60.0 | 1.5 | 1.1 | 9.9 |
| Propofol | 2.3 | 50.0 | 4.7 | 2.3 | 2.0 |
| Diazepam | — | 30.0 | 24.0 | 1.0 | 0.24 |
| Midazolam | — | 6.0 | 1.7 | 1.8 | 6.4 |
| Ketamine | — | 13.0 | 2.5 | 3.2 | 20.0 |
| Etomidate | 2.6 | 28.1 | 5.6 | 4.5 | 25.8 |

(From data in Prys-Roberts C, Hug CC Jr: Pharmacokinetics of Anesthesia. Cambridge, MA, Blackwell Scientific Publications, 1984; White PF: Propofol: pharmacokinetics and pharmacodynamics. Seminars in Anesthesia 7:4, 1988; and Shafer A, Doze VA, Shafer SL, White PF: Pharmacokinetics and pharmacodynamics of propofol infusions during general anesthesia. Anesthesiology 69:348, 1988.)

## Pharmacodynamics

Pharmacodynamics deals with mechanisms of drug action and the relationship between drug concentration and receptor interaction (what the drug does to the body) (9). In general, drugs interact with functional macromolecular components of the organism and inhibit or facilitate an existing biochemical or physiologic process. It should be emphasized that drugs do not produce a "new pharmacologic response in the body." Drugs only enhance or inhibit existing physiologic responses. Drugs that produce effects from direct alteration of the functional properties of the receptor with which they interact are called agonists; while drugs are called antagonists when they are devoid of intrinsic pharmacologic action, but cause inhibition of the action of a specific agonist (for example, antagonism of opiate receptors by naloxone).

### *Dose Response Relationship*

A certain number of drug receptor interactions must take place before a response is observed. The intensity of this response should be directly related to the number of drug receptor interactions. It is necessary to describe a drug with respect to its dose response curve because communications with regard to drug potency as well as effectiveness are most accurately compared at the concentration in which 50% of the subjects will exhibit the sought-after response ($ED_{50}$) (Figure 18–12). Minimal alveolar concentration (MAC) is the $ED_{50}$ of an inhalational anesthetic agent. This is a value extrapolated from the dose response curve that provides a meaningful and precise expression of the effective dose of the drug. Because 50% of the subjects are expected not to produce a desired response at this dose, clinical anesthesia is concerned with finding the correct dose so that the patient receives just enough and is never overdosed. Another index of drug potency is the Median Lethal Dose ($LD_{50}$), which is usually determined in laboratory rodents and defined as the dose of a drug at which 50% of the animals will succumb. Therapeutic index is defined by the ratio of $LD_{50}/ED_{50}$ (Figure 18–12). A large therapeutic index suggests relative safety of the drug ( narcotics generally have therapeutic indices in the range of 100 to 5000, for example, while inhalational anesthetics generally are in the range of 5 to 10).

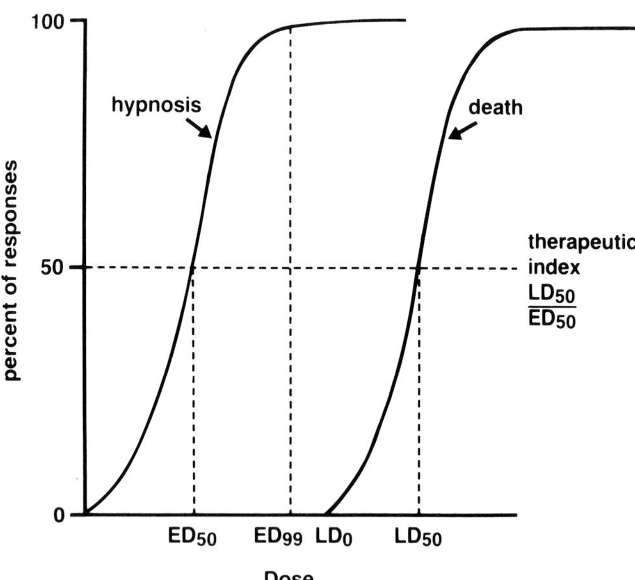


**Fig. 18–12.** Relationship between effective dose and lethal dose. The ideal range for clinical anesthesia is between $ED_{50}$ and $ED_{99}$. (From Wong KC: Pharmacology. *In* Anesthesia for Thoracic Procedures. Edited by BE Marshall, DE Longnecker, HB Fairly. Boston, Blackwell Scientific Publishers. 1988.)

### *Influence of Age, Sex, and Pathophysiology*

Many factors can influence the response of a patient to a drug. Even among a group of patients homogeneous with respect to age, sex, weight, physical status, among other factors, variability in response is expected to occur. $ED_{50}$ thus represents a mean about which the frequency of different responses is normally distributed. Clinical anesthesia, however, is rarely practiced in a homogeneous group. Therefore, it is important to understand physiologic differences among patient groups so that optimal anesthesia can be practiced.

In general, very young and elderly patients are sensitive to neurodepressants. Metabolism and excretion are poorly developed in the fetus and newborn and may be compromised in the elderly. The female body habitus and hormonal variations can influence physiologic and pharmacologic responses. Disease processes that influence the pharmacokinetics and pharmacodynamics of drugs will produce profound dose response effects. The American Society of Anesthesiology physical status classification system describes the severity of pathophysiology, which may reflect the potential degree of anesthetic risk.

### *Influence of Pregnancy*

Pregnancy produces significant physiologic and anatomic changes, which influence the pharmacodynamics of drugs. These factors are discussed in detail elsewhere in Chapter 2. It is important to emphasize that the parturient is more sensitive to neurodepressants and more tolerant of pain, in comparison to her nonpregnant status (6). Biochemical bases for this phenomenon may be related to an elevated level of β-endorphin and progesterone during pregnancy. Both endogenous substances have been well-demonstrated to have analgesic properties (10,11).

**Table 18–3.** MAC Presented as Per Cent End-Tidal Anesthetic Concentration

| | Nonpregnant Ewes (n = 6) | Pregnant Ewes (n = 6) | Change (Per Cent) |
|---|---|---|---|
| Halothane | 0.97 ± 0.04 | 0.73 ± 0.07 | −25 |
| Isoflurane | 1.58 ± 0.07 | 1.01 ± 0.06 | −40 |
| Methoxyflurane | 0.26 ± 0.02 | 0.18 ± 0.01 | −32 |

All values between nonpregnant and pregnant group are significantly different ($P < 0.025$).
(From Palahniuk RJ, Shnider SM, Eger EI II: Pregnancy decreases the requirement for inhaled anesthetic agents. Anesthesiology 41:82, 1974.)

No data are available for the effect of pregnancy on minimal alveolar concentration in humans. Palahniuk reported a 25 to 40% decrease in minimal alveolar concentration for near-term pregnant ewes (Table 18–3) (6). It is generally assumed that a similar reduction for minimal alveolar concentration occurs in humans.

### *Receptor Specificity and Side Effects*

Specificity of drug receptor interaction may be directly related to potency and the lack of side effects. However, there are no known 100%-receptor-specific drugs. On the other hand, there may be multiple similar receptor sites exerting different physiologic effects. For example, acetylcholine through its ubiquitous distribution in the autonomic nervous system can stimulate both sympathetic and parasympathetic ganglia, as well as postganglionic parasympathetic receptors. Acetylcholine is also the neurotransmitter for the neuromuscular junction. It is not surprising then, that succinylcholine, structurally similar to acetylcholine, can produce tachycardia and bradycardia, as well as neuromuscular blockade. The opiate Mu receptor is perhaps the most important receptor for analgesia. Mu receptors also exist in the medullary areas for the modulation of respiratory drive. The administration of a Mu receptor opiate will invariably produce respiratory depression.

Many factors in the operating room can enhance side effects exerted by general or regional anesthesia. Some of these factors include: surgical manipulation, cardiopulmonary bypass, hypothermia, acid-base balance, mechanical ventilation, and position of the patient. Inferior vena caval compression by the uterus in a supine parturient is a well-known factor that inhibits cardiac filling and produces supine hypotension.

## INHALATIONAL AGENTS

### *Historical Perspectives*

Inhalational analgesia and anesthesia constitute a major part of modern anesthetic practice. Surgery was uncommon before 1846. Not only was there concern for the surgical trespass of anatomy and physiology, but the lack of effective anesthesia was a major deterrent. The discovery of the anesthetic properties of nitrous oxide, diethylether (ether) and chloroform constituted the beginning of surgical anesthesia. On January 19, 1847, Sir James Young Simpson first used ether in his obstetric practice and on November 8, 1847, he used chloroform to alleviate the pain of labor. The anesthetic qualities of these three inhalational anesthetics were apparently so well-accepted that no significant additional inhalational anesthetics were introduced in the ensuing 80 years. Chloroform fell out of clinical practice because of its hepatotoxic effects similar to carbon tetrachloride, and ether lost popularity in the 1950s because of the introduction of halothane, which has better patient acceptance, faster onset of anesthetic action, and lack of flammability. In spite of these undesirable effects of ether, it remains the safest, most potent inhalational anesthetic for the patient because of its protective effects on the cardiovascular and respiratory system. Nitrous oxide remains the most widely used inhalational anesthetic for obstetric analgesia as well as an adjunct to other potent inhalational anesthetics, or to intravenous anesthetics. Ether is discussed in this book because of its important application to impoverished countries worldwide, still today.

### Diethyl Ether

Diethyl Ether (ether) was the first anesthetic used clinically. Ether's use is now limited to countries without access to the newer, more expensive agent. The advantages of ether are:

1. low cost
2. can be given by open drop method obviating the need for expensive delivery systems
3. wide margin of safety
4. stability

The disadvantages of ether are:

1. slow and unpleasant induction and emergence
2. increased airway secretions due to irritation of mucosal linings
3. high incidence of emesis
4. explosive in usual anesthetic concentrations

Ether produces analgesia with concentrations of 0.6 to 1.7 vol%. Induction of anesthesia requires concentrations of 5 to 10 vol% with maintenance levels of 2 to 4 vol% for light anesthesia (12,13).

Light anesthesia with ether is associated with an increase in alveolar ventilation (14). Bronchodilation is produced through its sympathomimetic effects. Increased salivation is caused by its irritating effects on mucosal linings and can lead to laryngospasm and bronchospasm with high concentrations at induction. Pretreatment with atropine or scopolamine is standard practice to help decrease secretions.

The myocardium is directly depressed by ether with no change or a slight increase in heart rate and cardiac output (15,16). There is a decrease in peripheral resistance; therefore, blood pressure decreases or remains unchanged. Ether does not sensitize the myocardium to epinephrine.

Ether anesthesia can cause a slight increase in lactic acid production due to increased sympathetic activity. However, in patients with thyrotoxicosis, Cushing's disease, and liver disease, lactate metabolism is impaired and severe metabolic acidosis can develop.

Ether produces a direct myometrial depression (17). Even light planes of anesthesia with ether can abolish uterine contractions. This may be beneficial in treating patients with abnormally increased uterine tone or for internal version or extractions, but potential problems are created when ether is used because its effects on the uterus can last up to 20 minutes after cessation of administration. This could lead to decreased uterine activity at time of delivery with resultant postpartum hemorrhage.

### Fluroxene and Halothane

The desirable qualities of ether to maintain homeostasis of the surgical patient have led the search for new agents with an ether molecule. Fluroxene is a fluronated diethylether discovered in 1951 that possesses most of the cardiopulmonary desirable effects of ether and has higher potency. However, fluroxene frequently caused nausea and vomiting, and is flammable at higher anesthetic concentrations (18,19). So, it also has rapidly fallen out of clinical use.

Halothane was developed in the mid 1950s as a result of careful structural design with predictions about the molecular structure that would provide nonflammability, molecular stability, and anesthetic potency. Halothane was found to produce excellent patient acceptance with rapid onset of anesthetic action and minimal nausea and vomiting, which was common among patients anesthetized with ether and fluroxene (19,20). Nevertheless, these desirable qualities of halothane were counterbalanced by its potent respiratory and cardiovascular depression, arrhythmogenic effects with the use of epinephrine, and its association on occasions with hepatonecrosis. Thus, the search for ether anesthetic molecules continues.

### Methoxyflurane

It was found that the reduction of one methyl group from the diethylether molecule vastly increased potency in comparison with the diethylether and its derivative, but also eliminated flammability. Methoxyflurane is a fluronated methylethylether, which was an improvement over the myocardial irritability and cardiopulmonary instability effects of halothane. However, methoxyflurane was more susceptible to biodegradation and produced renal and hepatic injury (5,21). It retained its high blood and tissue solubility as diethylether, and thus has also fallen out of general operating room use. Because of its pleasant odor and high potency, it is still widely accepted in some parts of the world as an inhaler for obstetric analgesia during the first stage of labor.

### Enflurane

Enflurane was synthesized by R.C. Terrell in 1962 of Ohio Medical Products and was the next methylethylether available for clinical anesthesia (18,19). Similar to methoxyflurane, it also provided stable cardiovascular system and good muscle relaxation in the surgical patient. In contrast to halothane and methoxyflurane, enflurane resists biodegradation and thus reduces the possibility of producing harmful metabolites (22,23). However, enflurane, unlike all of the previously known inhalational anesthetics, can produce seizure-like electrocardiograms at anesthetic concentrations. Furthermore, enflurane is prone to reduce blood pressure by virtue of vasodilation. Enflurane was the most widely used potent inhalational anesthetic in North America until the introduction of isoflurane in 1965 by R.C. Terrell (18).

### *Isoflurane*

Isoflurane is an isomer of enflurane and represents a further improvement over enflurane in several respects. Isoflurane is more potent, even less biodegradable than enflurane, and does not produce seizure-like activity of electroencephalogram in the anesthetized patient. However, its introduction to clinical anesthesia was temporarily halted by the preliminary study of Corbett who suggested that isoflurane might be a hepatocarcinogen in mice (24). As a consequence, approval of isoflurane was denied by the Food and Drug Administration pending confirmation of Corbett's initial findings. The subsequent studies of Eger, et al failed to confirm that isoflurane was a hepatocarcinogen (25). Isoflurane was finally released for clinical use in 1980 and is probably the most widely used potent inhalational anesthetic in North America today.

Although the above inhalational anesthetics available to the clinician allow a choice and the appropriate management of anesthetized patients in a variety of clinical settings, there is not an anesthetic that would satisfy the following criteria of what might be considered the ideal anesthetic: the agent is physically stable, nonflammable, potent (able to induce surgical anesthesia in adequate oxygen concentration), rapid in onset, stable to the cardiovascular and pulmonary system, an excellent muscle relaxant, resists biodegradation, no acute or chronic toxicity to organ systems, no teratogenic effect to the fetus, patient acceptance for induction, and economical to use. Obviously, such an ideal anesthetic does not exist today. So the search for the ideal inhalational anesthetic continues.

### *Sevoflurane and Desflurane (I-653)*

Two potentially useful new inhalational anesthetics are being intensely studied at present. Sevoflurane is a fluronated methylisopropyl ether whose solubility in blood approaches that of nitrous oxide. Therefore, the speed of induction of sevoflurane is rapid, and because it is a potent anesthetic, unlike nitrous oxide, sevoflurane can produce surgical anesthesia in adequate oxygen concentrations (26,27). The minimal alveolar concentration of sevoflurane in humans is 1.71%. Its rapid induction is also facilitated by the absence of pungency that exists with isoflurane as an induction agent. Unlike all of the other halogenated inhalational agents, sevoflurane does not increase heart rate and, apparently, does not increase cerebral blood flow (28). Its primary disadvantage appears to be its chemical instability and the potential toxic effects of the degradation products in humans.

Desflurane is a fluorinated methylethylether identical to isoflurane except for the substitution of a fluorine for the chlorine on the alpha methylcarbon. It is even less soluble than nitrous oxide and sevoflurane (partition coefficient of 0.42), and therefore has demonstrated rapid induction and emergence from anesthesia with desflurane in rats. Desflurane is about one-half to one-third as potent as sevoflurane, and in rats the minimal alveolar concentration of sevoflurane is 5.7%. Unlike sevoflurane, desflurane is chemically stable in soda lime and produces minimal degradation products (29). Desflurane is similar to isoflurane in every respect on both the cardiopulmonary system and electrocardiogram effects, and does not seem to present any major disadvantage clinically over isoflurane.

A summary of the physical and physiologic properties of these inhalational anesthetics is presented in Table 18–4. The pharmacology of the inhalational anesthetics on the organ systems of the parturient will be presented by a comparative pharmacology format. Fetal effects and teratogenicity will be presented where published data are available.

## ***Uptake***

The large pulmonary alveolar area not only provides an efficient surface for gaseous exchange, but also poses essentially no barrier to the transfer of anesthetic gases in either direction. However, any pathological condition that increases the distance between alveoli and the plasma capillary membrane is expected to interfere with the uptake of gases from the alveoli into the blood. Severe preeclampsia can lead to pulmonary edema and inadequate pulmonary gaseous exchange. In the absence of abnormal pulmonary conditions, three factors determine how rapidly gaseous anesthetics pass from the inspired gases into the blood:

1. solubility of the anesthetic in the blood
2. rate of blood flow through the lungs
3. partial pressure of the anesthetic in the arterial and mixed venous blood (30)

### *Solubility of the Anesthetic in the Blood*

The more soluble an inhalational anesthetic is in the blood, the slower is the rate of achieving an equilibrium between the alveolar and blood concentrations of the anesthetic. The blood volume then acts as the first reservoir that must be filled before an effective partial pressure of the anesthetic can be exerted on the central nervous system (Figure 18–2). Therefore, the speed of induction is slow, as such inhalational anesthetics as methoxyflurane with a gas partition coefficient of 13 in contrast to that of nitrous oxide with a blood gas partition coefficient of 0.47 demonstrates. (Table 18–4 and Figure 18–13) (31). However, it should be emphasized that the speed of induction of an inhalational anesthetic is not only dependent upon its solubility in the blood, but also its potency, which

**Table 18–4.** Properties of Inhalational Anesthetics

| Properties | Isoflurane<br>F H F<br>F—C—C—O—C—H<br>F Cl F | Desflurane<br>F H F<br>F—C—C—O—C—H<br>F F F | Enflurane<br>Cl F F<br>H—C—C—O—C—H<br>F F F | Sevoflurane<br>H $CF_3$<br>H—C—O—C—H<br>H $CF_3$ | Halothane<br>Br F<br>H—C—C—F<br>Cl F | Methoxyflurane<br>Cl F H<br>H—C—C—O—C—H<br>Cl F H | Nitrous Oxide<br>N≡N═O |
|---|---|---|---|---|---|---|---|
| Molecular weight (g) | 184.5 | 168.0 | 184.5 | 182.0 | 197.4 | 165.0 | 44.0 |
| Boiling point (760 torr) | 48.5 C | 23.5 C | 56.5 C | 58.5 C | 50.2 C | 104.7 C | — |
| Specific gravity | 1.50 | 1.45 (25 C) | 1.52 (25 C) | 1.50 | 1.86 | 1.41 (25 C) | — |
| Vapor pressure (torr) | 250.0 | 663 (20 C) | 175.0 (20 C) | 160 (20 C) | 243.0 (20 C) | 25.0 (20 C) | — |
| | | — | 356.0 (37 C) | 200 (25 C) | 480.0 (37 C) | 56.0 (37 C) | — |
| Odor | Pleasant, pungent | Pleasant, pungent | Pleasant, ethereal | Pleasant, ethereal | Pleasant, sweet | Pleasant, fruity | Pleasant, sweet |
| Preservative | No | No | No | Yes | Yes | Yes | No |
| React to: | | | | | | | |
| Metal | No | No | No | Yes | Yes | Yes | No |
| Alkali | No | No | No | Yes | Yes | Yes | No |
| Ultraviolet light | No | No | No | Yes | Yes | Yes | No |
| Explosiveness | No | No | No | No | No | No | No |
| Partition coeff. | | | | | | | |
| Blood/gas | 1.4 | 0.42 | 1.9 | 0.68 | 2.3 | 13.0 | 0.47 |
| Brain/gas | 2.09 | 0.54 | 2.6 | 1.15 | 4.79 | 22.1 | 0.50 |
| Fat/gas | 64.2 | 12.0 | 105.0 | 34.0 | 136.0 | 890.0 | 1.22 |
| Liver/gas | 2.34 | 0.55 | 3.8 | 1.25 | 5.13 | 24.8 | 0.38 |
| Muscle/gas | 4.40 | 0.94 | 3.0 | 2.38 | 9.49 | 20.8 | 0.54 |
| Oil/gas | 97.8 | 18.7 | 98.5 | 53.4 | 224.0 | 930.0 | 1.4 |
| Water/gas | 0.61 | 0.22 | 0.8 | 0.36 | 0.7 | 4.5 | 0.47 |
| Rubber/gas (23 C) | 0.62 | — | 74.0 | — | 120.0 | 630.0 | 1.2 |
| Minimum alveolar concentration (MAC) for man (age 19–55) as atm % in: | | | | | | | |
| Oxygen | 1.15 | 5.7 | 1.68 | 1.71 | 0.75 | 0.16 | 110 |
| 70% $N_2O$ | 0.50 | — | 0.57 | 0.65 | 0.29 | 0.07 | — |
| Approx % recovered as metabolites | 0.2 | 0.2 | 2.4 | 2.3 | 15–20 | 50 | — |

(Data adapted from references 18, 30, 38)
(From Terrell RC: Physical and chemical properties of anesthetic agents. Br. J. Anaesth. 56:3S, 1984.)
(From Yasuda N, Targ AG, Eger EI II: Solubility of I-653, sevoflurane, isoflurane, and halothane in human tissues. Anesth. Analg. 69:370–373, 1989.)
(From Eger IE II: Isoflurane (Forane): A Compendium and Reference. Madison, Wisconsin, Ohio Medical Products, 1981.)

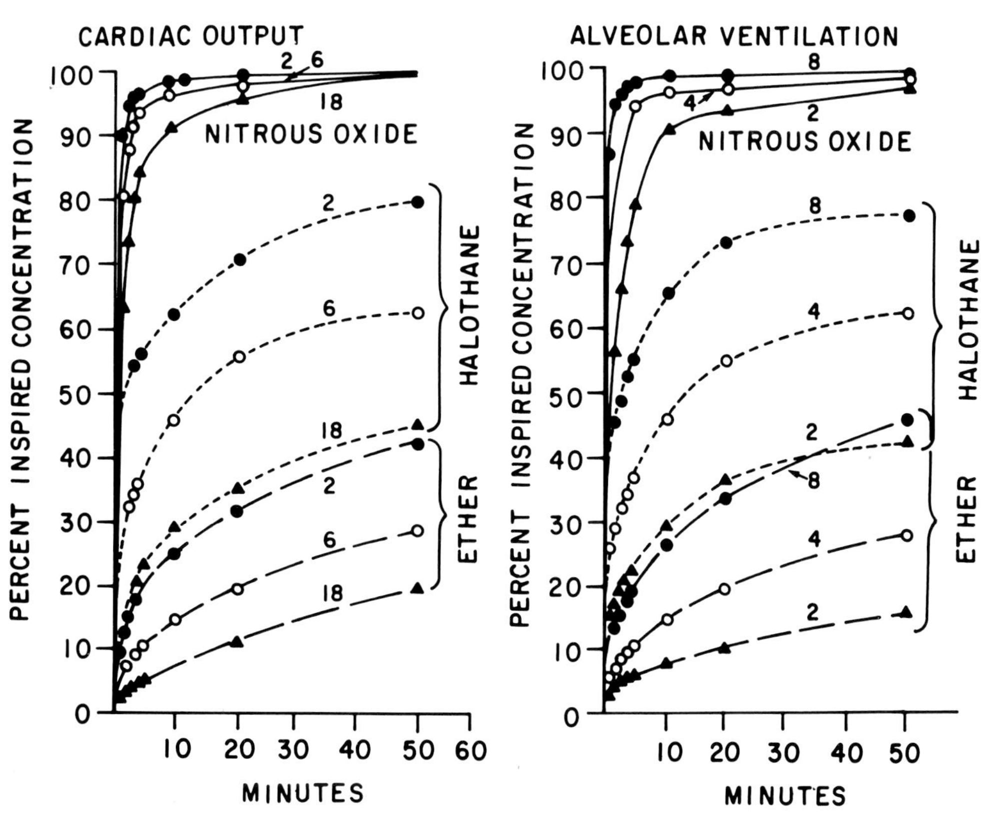


**Fig. 18–13.** The left side shows the effect on alveolar concentration of varying cardiac output from 2 to 16 to 18 liters/min as indicated on each graph. Relative distribution of output is unchanged. The top three graphs are those of nitrous oxide, the middle three halothane, and the lower three ether. The right side similarly illustrates the effect of alteration of alveolar ventilation from 2 to 4 to 8 liters/min. (Redrawn from Eger EI II: Applications of a mathematical model of gas uptake. Papper EM, Kitz RJ. *In* Uptake and Distribution of Anesthetic Agents. McGraw-Hill Book Co., New York, 1963.)

is best correlated by its oil/gas partition coefficient (Table 18–4).

### Rate of Blood Flow Through the Lungs

Cardiac output is the principal determinant for the amount of pulmonary blood flow and thus the rate at which anesthetics pass from the alveoli to the arterial blood. An increase in cardiac output augments the uptake of anesthetics and, likewise, the converse. A highly soluble anesthetic will be more influenced than a poorly soluble anesthetic because the blood gas equilibration of the latter is more rapidly attained at any cardiac output. This concept is illustrated in Figure 18–13, which compares $N_2O$, halothane, and ether.

### Partial Pressure of Anesthetic in Arterial and Mixed Venous Blood

Following the uptake of the anesthetic into the blood, the anesthetic is distributed to all organ systems that receive blood. The mixed venous blood returned to the lungs carries the balance of what has been distributed to tissues, accumulating more anesthetic gas with each passage through the body. As the concentration gradient between the mixed venous blood and the alveolar blood reduces, so too does the transfer of anesthetic from the alveoli into the blood.

## Distribution

Distribution of inhalational anesthetics is determined initially by the blood flow to the tissue. Tissues with larger proportions of blood flow will receive initially larger doses of the anesthetic. Tissue/blood partition coefficients are nearly uniform when measured in lean tissues; however, the tissue/blood coefficient for all anesthetics is generally larger for fatty tissues. Therefore, obese patients will always be a better depot for the highly lipid soluble agents. The oil/gas partition coefficient not only reflects lipid solubility, but also potency (Table 18–4). The larger its value, the more slowly the anesthetic equilibrates in the fatty tissue, and, conversely, the rate of elimination from the fatty tissue is slower.

## Metabolism and Excretion

Most inhalational anesthetics are eliminated largely unchanged via pulmonary exhalation, but a variable amount of the absorbed anesthetic is metabolized primarily by liver microsomal enzymes and other tissues of the body such as blood, intestinal tract, kidneys, and lungs (1,4). Both nitrous oxide and isoflurane are exhaled virtually unchanged by the lungs. About 82% of absorbed enflurane is eliminated by the lungs unchanged, and less than 3% undergoes metabolism to difluoro methoxy, difluoro acetic acid, and fluoride ion (23,32). About 20% of absorbed halothane is metabolized to trifluoroacetic acid and chloride, bromide, and fluoride ions (32). Sevoflurane is metabolized to about the same extent as enflurane (27,32), and, like other potent volatile anesthetics, isoflurane and sevoflurane metabolism is increased by drugs that induce hepatic enzymes, such as phenobarbital or ethanol (4,32).

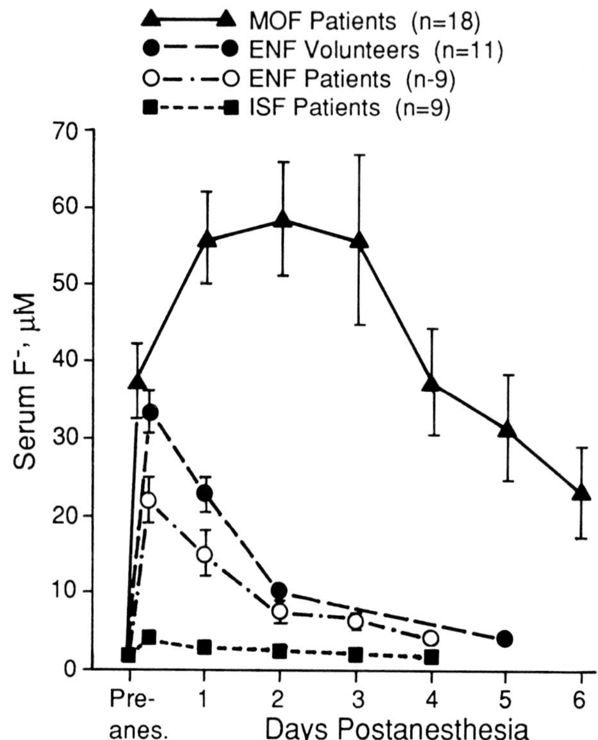


**Fig. 18–14.** Fluoride ion nephrotoxicity. (Redrawn from Baden JM, Rice SA: Metabolism and toxicity. *In* Anesthesia. 3rd Ed. Edited by RD Miller. New York, Churchill Livingstone, 1990.)

### Nephrotoxicity of Fluoride Ion

Although the addition of fluoride to the anesthetic molecule tends to decrease flammability and to improve anesthetic qualities, the fluoride-carbon bond is susceptible to metabolic breakdown (Figure 18–14). In 1966, vasopressin resistant, high output renal failure was reported by Crandall, et al in patients receiving methoxyflurane anesthesia (21). The fluoride ion, a metabolite of methoxyflurane, has been well-defined as the causative agent. The serum fluoride ion threshold level for renal dysfunction in humans is about 50 µm/L. The fluoride ion is also a metabolite of enflurane and halothane; however, the amount is small, especially for halothane. Because of the risk of fluoride renal toxicity, Methoxyflurane is rarely used in the operating room today. However, the use of a methoxyflurane inhaler for pain relief during labor does not produce toxic levels of fluoride ion concentration when a total dose of not more than 10 ml is used.

## Pharmacodynamics

### Cardiovascular System

There is an enormous number of publications concerning the cardiovascular system and inhalational anesthetics. It is not the intent here to provide an exhaustive review of the literature, but rather to point out pertinent comparative pharmacology of several useful inhalational agents of clinical interest. The ultimate goal of the anesthesiologist is to ensure adequate organ perfusion of the patient during general anesthesia. However, in clinical situations direct assessment of organ perfusion is impossible. The measurement of urinary output from an indwelling catheter is helpful in assessing renal function and intravascular volume in the anesthetized patient, and the production of urine itself may suggest adequate perfusion of other organs as the body tends to sacrifice renal perfusion for perfusion of more vital organs, such as the brain and the heart. But there is no certainty of the correlation between adequate urinary output and adequate perfusion of other organ systems.

The more common intraoperative measurement of the blood pressure assumes that adequate blood pressure is indicative of adequate organ perfusion. But this is also not always true because mean blood pressure is a product of cardiac output and systemic vascular resistance. A decreased cardiac output compensated by an increased peripheral resistance will maintain mean arterial pressure. Furthermore, cardiac output is a function of stroke volume and heart rate. Therefore, although useful and convenient, the indirect measurement of blood pressure is not a reliable means of assessing the cardiovascular system, especially in a high-risk patient whose hemodynamic status may be changing rapidly. Interpretation of cardiovascular data must take into consideration the interrelationship of these variables. Comparison of data from published reports is complicated by differences in experimental design and animal models. Comparison of studies in humans is even more difficult because of variables and limitations in clinical settings. These limitations pose a problem in attempting to summarize the cardiovascular effects of inhalational anesthetics that are clinically relevant.

In general, all inhalational anesthetics are dose-related direct myocardial depressants (Figure 18–15). Myocardial contractility and conduction velocity of excitable cells are depressed. Although hard data are limited, published reports suggest a direct vasodilatory effect of halogenated inhalational anesthetics on the blood vessel (33,34). In other words, direct effects of inhalational anesthetics on the heart and on the blood vessels are qualitatively similar. Any difference observed on the heart rate and blood pressure in vivo is the result of extra cardiac effects from reflex compensatory mechanisms, central nervous system effects, and humoral effects. A summary of some cardiovascular effects of halothane, enflurane, isoflurane, sevoflurane, and nitrous oxide is presented in Table 18–5.

In vitro studies suggest that halothane is more depressant than isoflurane or enflurane in the isolated cat papillary muscle preparation (35,36). Papillary muscle from cats with congestive heart failure, however, are more sensitive to the depressant effects of isoflurane and other anesthetics (36). In contrast to these in vitro results, in vivo animal studies and studies in human volunteers suggest that isoflurane produced substantially less depression of myocardial contractility and left ventricular ejection performance than did either halothane or enflurane (37). In

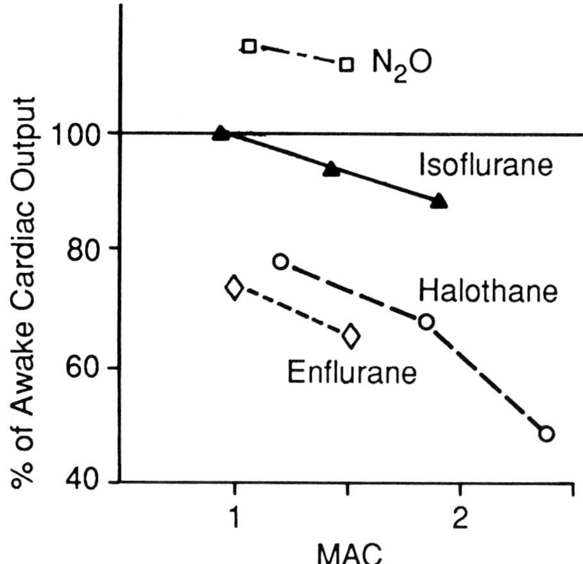


**Fig. 18–15.** Myocardial depressant effects of anesthetics. (Redrawn from Eger EI II: Isoflurane [Forane]. A Compendium and Reference. Madison, WI, Ohio Medical Products, 1985.)

unmedicated human volunteers, during normocapnea, 1 to 2 minimal alveolar concentration isoflurane did not depress the pre-ejection period, the mean rate of ventricular ejection, or ejection time. These concentrations also did not decrease the IJ (internal jugular) wave of the ballistocardiogram. In contrast, halothane and enflurane depressed the ballistocardiogram IJ wave in a dose-related fashion (38).

Whereas halothane tends to decrease heart rate and cardiac output, isoflurane tends to increase heart rate and maintains cardiac output (38). The bradycardic effect of halothane may be related to a depression of the baroreflex mechanism while the tachycardic effect of isoflurane may be the result of central sympathetic stimulation to the heart. Enflurane also produces dose-dependent arterial blood pressure decreases in a fashion similar to halothane, from direct myocardial depression and vasodilation. Cardiac electrophysiologic studies in dogs suggest that enflurane prolongs AV nodal conduction time both in spontaneously beating and during incremental increases in atrial paced rate similar to halothane (39). In contrast to halothane, enflurane did not prolong His-Purkinje or ventricular conduction time. The higher incidence of ventricular arrhythmias during halothane anesthesia may be related to its prolongation of ventricular conduction time.

The cardiovascular effects of sevoflurane have advantages over other inhalational anesthetics (Table 18–5). Sevoflurane appears to decrease blood pressure less than isoflurane, and the heart rate appears to decrease rather than increase (26,38). More epinephrine is required to produce ventricular arrhythmias during sevoflurane in comparison with isoflurane or halothane (40). Myocardial ischemia is exacerbated by an elevation in heart rate. Although there is still concern with regard to the use of isoflurane in patients with myocardial ischemia, two recent prospective randomized studies of 2106 patients re-

**Table 18–5.** Some Cardiovascular Effects of Inhalational Anesthetics

| Drug | Cardiac Output | Heart Rate | Mean Arterial Pressure | Peripheral Vascular Resistance | Arrythmogenicity to Epinephrine |
|---|---|---|---|---|---|
| Isoflurane | +1, 0, −1 | +2 | −1 | −3 | −1 |
| Enflurane | −1 | +2 | −3 | −2 | −1 |
| Sevoflurane | +1, 0, −1 | 0, −1 | 0, −1 | 0, −1 | 0 |
| Halothane | −2 | −1, 0 | −2 | −1 | −3 |
| Methoxyflurane | −1, 0 | 0 | 0, −1 | −1 | 0 |
| Nitrous oxide | +1 | +1 | +1 | +1 | 0 |

+ = increased, 0 = no effect, − = decreased.

ceiving coronary artery surgery suggested no difference among outcomes of a variety of general anesthetic techniques, including primary opiate or halogenated inhalational anesthetics (41,42). Minimizing significant tachycardia and hypotension is essential in the management of patients with ischemic heart disease, regardless of the choice of inhalational anesthetic.

Nitrous oxide administered with oxygen in humans produces a dose-related increase in sympathetic activity, reflected by an increase in cardiac output and peripheral vascular resistance (43). Nitrous oxide remains as the most common adjunct used with a potent inhalational anesthetic. The addition of nitrous oxide to a primary inhalational or opiate anesthetic tends to decrease cardiac output, increase peripheral vascular resistance, and maintain mean arterial pressure.

Drugs, which tend to depress myocardial tissue in general, are antiarrhythmic in nature. In contrast to the other inhalational anesthetics, halothane is known to sensitize the myocardium toward the arrhythmogenic effects of epinephrine, in the experimental lab, and the anesthetized patient (40,44). A comparison of the pharmacological effects of these inhalational anesthetics on the cardiovascular system is summarized in Table 18–5.

## Respiratory System

All of the inhalational anesthetics produce profound dose-related respiratory depression. Nitrous oxide is the least depressant of the inhalational anesthetics under discussion (45,46). In laboratory animals halothane, enflurane, and isoflurane produce significant depression of hypoxic ventilatory response at 1 minimal alveolar concentration, and enflurane is more depressing than isoflurane (47,48). On the other hand, hypercapnic drive is reduced significantly by 1 minimal alveolar concentration halothane ≥ enflurane ≥ isoflurane (48).

The clinical significance of these findings is as follows: hypoxia and hypercapnia during anesthesia with these inhalational agents reduced optimal stimulation of respiratory functions. Furthermore, reductions of pulmonary compliance and functional residual capacity as well as inhibition of hypoxic pulmonary vasoconstriction also contribute to inefficient gas exchange that occurs with all of the halogenated inhalational anesthetics. The respiratory effects of sevoflurane were recently studied in patients for minor surgery (49). At 1.1 minimal alveolar concentration, sevoflurane produced almost the same degree of respiratory depression as halothane, but at 1.4 minimal alveolar concentration, sevoflurane produced more profound respiratory depression than halothane (49).

It is important to emphasize here that all obstetric patients who are rendered unconscious by general anesthetics should receive an endotracheal tube for protection of the airway and an effective means to support their pulmonary functions. It is prudent to assume that all parturients in active labor have a full stomach, and furthermore, that all patients must receive cricoid pressure before and during induction procedures, as in Figure 18–16.

## Central Nervous System

Cerebral blood flow is generally increased during halothane, enflurane, and isoflurane anesthesia, while cerebral metabolism is reduced in a dose-related fashion (50). The cerebral circulation is most sensitive to changes in $CO_2$ tensions in the blood and remains responsive to vasodilation and vasoconstriction of hypercapnia and hypocapnia, respectively, during surgical anesthesia. In contrast to the above inhalational anesthetics, sevoflurane does not appear to increase cerebral blood flow in isocapneic swine

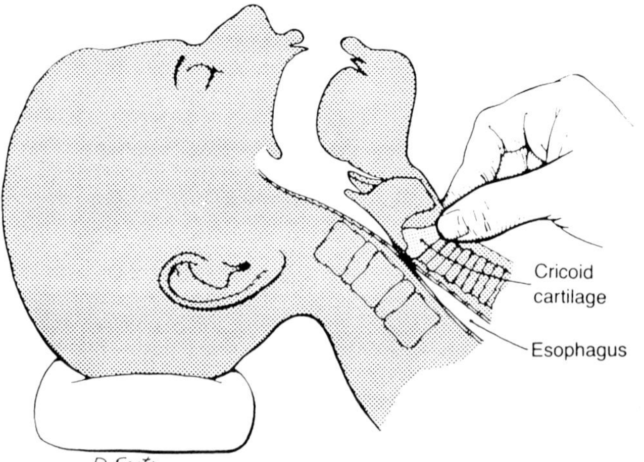


**Fig. 18–16.** Sellick's maneuver (cricoid pressure). (Redrawn from Stehling LC: Management of the airway. *In* Clinical anesthesia. Edited by PG Barash, BF Cullen, RK Stoelting. New York, JB Lippincott Company, 1989.)

(29). Cerebral vasodilation and increased cerebral blood flow are associated with increased intracranial pressure, but this can be controlled by reduced concentration of the inhalational anesthetic administered, and by controlled hyperventilation. All of the inhalational agents produce progressive electroencephalogram changes with an increase in the voltage and decrease in frequency. Unique to enflurane is its ability to induce high voltage, fast frequency (14 to 18 Hz) pattern progressing to spike dome complex with periods of electrical silence or frank seizure activity with motor movements (50). The seizure activity is generally of short duration, self-limited, and may be prevented by avoiding deep anesthesia and/or hypocapnia. Enflurane, therefore, should be avoided in patients with history of seizures.

### Kidney

Anesthesia with inhalational anesthetics produces dose-dependent reductions of renal blood flow, glomerular filtration, and urinary output. These effects can be attenuated by optimal hydration and the maintenance of mean arterial blood pressure. Inhalational anesthetics probably do not interfere with autoregulation of renal blood flow per se, but it is the hypotension below which autoregulation cannot occur that is primarily responsible for reduced renal function and reduced production of urine.

In contrast to other inhalational anesthetics, methoxyflurane can produce a vasopressin-resistant high-output renal failure, resulting in polyuria, dehydration, hypernatremia, and azotemia (5,21). This renal toxic syndrome is associated with plasma fluoride concentration of 50 μM/L or more, which can be expected in patients receiving 1 minimal alveolar concentration methoxyflurane for more than 2 hours. The use of a methoxyflurane inhaler for pain relief of the first stage of labor is not expected to produce toxic levels of fluoride concentration in the plasma. Justification of its use for analgesia in labor is also based upon its intermittent administration of subcutaneous concentrations immediately preceding a painful uterine contraction.

### Liver and Gastrointestinal Tract

The incidence and duration of postoperative nausea and vomiting are far less with the fluorinated inhalational anesthetics in comparison with older inhalational agents such as ether and cyclopropane (51). The obstetric population is more prone to postoperative nausea and vomiting following general anesthesia (52). Splanchnic and therefore hepatic blood flow are reduced by all inhalational anesthetics as a passive consequence of reduced perfusion pressure. Hepatocellular functions are, however, depressed, and the ability of microsomal enzymes to metabolize drugs is reduced following halothane administration. The extent of this hepatocellular depression is similar among all of the inhalational anesthetics and is generally reversible following complete elimination of the inhalational anesthetic from the body.

Halothane continues to attract attention as a potential hepatotoxic agent. However, hepatitis that occurs in the postoperative period is most often due to the transmission of a hepatitis virus in transfused blood (53,54). There are no hard data to support the clinical notion that patients with known liver disease or exposure to hepatotoxic drugs are more prone to hepatitis following an inhalational anesthetic than the healthy patient (55). A typical course consists of fever some 3 to 5 days following anesthesia and surgery, with anorexia, nausea, and vomiting. Occasionally, a rash and eosinophilia may be present. Progressive hepatic failure and death occur in about 50% of these patients, but the overall incidence is approximately 1:10,000 general anesthetics (55). Because this hepatic failure is most often seen after repeated administrations of halothane over a short period of time, halothane hepatitis has been used to describe this illness. Hepatic necrosis associated with repeated administrations of enflurane has also been reported. Bromsulphalein (BSP) retention is increased significantly 1 day after administration of 11.7 minimal alveolar concentration/hours of halothane, but not 1 day after administration of 8.8 minimal alveolar concentration/hours of isoflurane or 9.6 minimal alveolar concentration/hours of enflurane in volunteers not undergoing surgery (56).

In contrast to the change in bromsulphalein function test, no change in serum LDH or SGOT followed halothane anesthesia. Isoflurane also did not alter either of these indices of hepatic function. However, both indices increased 1 day after anesthesia with enflurane. None of these volunteers displayed clinically significant hepatic dysfunction. These studies suggest that prolonged duration of anesthesia with these inhalational agents do not significantly impair liver function or cause hepatic damage, and also suggest that intraoperative events may play a significant role in iatrogenically induced hepatic failure (56). Isoflurane has been extensively used over the past 8 years in surgical patients, and the incidence of postsurgical hepatic failure has been small in comparison with enflurane and halothane. This finding lends support to the hypothesis that metabolites of halothane and enflurane may contribute to hepatic dysfunction and failure. Sevoflurane has not been approved for clinical use; therefore, comments with regard to sevoflurane-induced hepatic dysfunction are tenuous. However, because of its chemical instability and metabolism, the potential for hepatotoxicity exists.

### Obstetric Anesthesia Considerations

At clinical concentrations, $N_2O$ does not affect uterine contractility; however, isoflurane, enflurane, and halothane all produce significant dose-related depression of contractility of human uterine muscle in vitro (57). Significant uterine depression, however, is seen only when the concentration of the inhalational anesthetics exceed 1 minimal alveolar concentration in oxygen.

The use of halothane 0.5%, enflurane 1.0%, and isoflurane 0.75% in combination with nitrous oxide has not been shown to increase intraoperative bleeding from the uterus during cesarean section (58). At these concentrations, the myometrium will respond to exogenously administered oxytocin (59). At higher concentrations of these inhalational anesthetics, uterine contractile response to oxytocin is diminished. Likewise, halothane 0.5% with $N_2O$ 75% in oxygen, has been shown to decrease blood loss by 40% in comparison with halothane 1% in oxygen, during therapeutic abortion (60). The number of patients in this study and another study done in 1972 (61) is small, and there is little doubt that halogenated, inhalational anesthetics produce dose-related uterine muscle relaxation. It is prudent to minimize the anesthetic concentration above minimal alveolar concentrations of inhalational anesthetics for elective therapeutic abortion to prevent excessive bleeding. Nitrous oxide supplemented with intravenous thiopental or opiates, or regional anesthesia, remain the best choices for therapeutic suction abortion. In contrast, the uterine muscle relaxant effect of halogenated inhalational anesthetics is used to advantage during breech delivery or internal version of the second twin after the first has been delivered.

Because all of the halogenated, inhalational anesthetics are highly lipid soluble, they all easily cross the placental barrier (62). In the pregnant ewe, isoflurane and halothane are indistinguishable in their effects on maternal and fetal cardiovascular and acid-base effects (63). When both maternal blood pressure and cardiac output decreased by more than 35% from 2 minimal alveolar concentrations of isoflurane and halothane, uterine vasodilation and uterine blood flow decreased and the fetus became hypoxic and acidotic (63). Enflurane crosses the placental barrier and produces results similar to isoflurane and halothane in the fetus and the newborn (64). Because of its lower blood solubility, isoflurane is expected to leave the neonate faster than halothane and enflurane when neonatal pulmonary ventilation has been established. The low solubility and low cardiovascular depressant effects of sevoflurane would be desirable for use in obstetric anesthesia (Table 18–5).

### Carcinogenicity

As noted earlier, the preliminary data of Corbett suggested that isoflurane might be a carcinogen in mice, resulting in subsequent studies of several modern inhalational anesthetics and the delayed release of isoflurane for clinical use (24). Using the same strain of Swiss mice as Corbett, Eger, et al tested the carcinogenicity of enflurane, isoflurane, halothane, methoxyflurane, and nitrous oxide with a wide range of minimal alveolar concentration levels during the last half of pregnancy and after delivery. Pulmonary adenomas, lymphomas, hepatocyte lesions, and liver vascular lesions were found in both treatment and controlled animals. There was no indication that any specific anesthetic or anesthetic dose was carcinogenic (25). These data not only vindicated isoflurane, but also suggested that the modern inhalational anesthetics are not carcinogens in mice.

### Mutagenicity

The Ames test, devised by Dr. Bruce Ames, measures the conversion of bacteria, salmonella typhomurium, from a histadine-dependent to histadine-independent organism when the bacteria are exposed to a suspected mutagen (65). The sensitivity of the test is increased by the inclusion in the test mixture of microsomes from livers of animals pretreated to induce liver enzymes. The Ames test measures not only the effect of parent compound but also that of its metabolites, and has been widely accepted as a reliable in vitro test of mutagenicity and carcinogenicity. The Ames test indicates that isoflurane, enflurane, methoxyflurane, and nitrous oxide are not mutagens (66,67). Although halothane gave a negative result, its supposed metabolites gave a positive result (68).

### Teratogenicity

Sprague Dawley rats were exposed to isoflurane, enflurane, halothane, nitrous oxide or xenon at a wide range of clinical concentrations from 2 to 24 hours per day during the middle trimester of pregnancy. Halothane and nitrous oxide were found to produce skeletal abnormalities, while the other anesthetics including xenon did not (38). The earlier studies of Fink and coworkers had already demonstrated skeletal abnormalities induced by halothane or nitrous oxide in pregnant rats (69,70). Obviously, no prospective study can be ethically designed to define the risk to the fetus associated with anesthesia and surgery during pregnancy. A retrospective study of 2565 women undergoing surgery during pregnancy were compared with pregnant females not undergoing surgery (71). No significant difference in the rate of congenital anomalies was found between the two groups suggesting no teratogenic effect. However, there was an increased risk of spontaneous abortion in those undergoing surgery with general anesthesia in the first or second trimester of pregnancy. The epidimiological studies on reproductive disease are inconclusive. They have not shown a cause and effect relationship between trace concentrations of anesthetics and reproductive disease (72). Although there are no prospective studies in pregnant human beings, the general clinical belief is that all inhalational anesthetics should be avoided in the parturient during the first two trimesters of pregnancy.

## Intravenous Agents

### *Barbiturates*

Thiopental has been the gold standard for induction agents since its introduction into clinical practice by Lundy in 1935 (73). When compared with other general anesthetics, barbiturates are well-suited for induction due to pleasant induction and emergence, less nausea and vomiting , no effect on uterine contraction, and, when used in concentrations of less than 4 mg/kg, they have little effect on the fetus.

#### Mechanism of Action

The barbiturates exert a dose-response sedative and hypnotic effect by depression of the reticular activating system. Barbiturates exert presynaptic depression by decreasing release of neurotransmitters such as acetylcholine (74) and postsynaptic inhibition via gamma aminobutyric acid (GABA) enhanced actions (75). Barbiturates enhance GABA receptor binding causing an increase in chloride conductance resulting in neuronal hyperpolar-

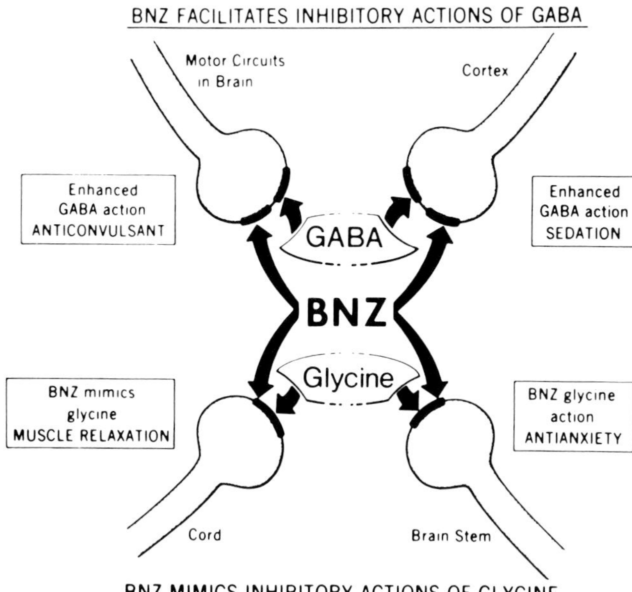


**Fig. 18–17.** Pharmacologic sites of benzodiazepines and receptor interaction. Sedation, anticonvulsant, antianxiety, and muscle relaxation are elicited at different central nervous system sites sharing similar physiological effects of endogenous gamma amino butyric acid (GABA) and glycine. (From Richter JJ: Current theories about the mechanisms of benzodiazepines and neuroleptic drugs. Anesthesiology. 54:66–72, 1981.)

ization and, hence, inhibition of the postsynaptic neuron. This facilitation of GABA-ergic inhibition is similar to benzodiazepine facilitation. However, barbiturates do not displace benzodiazepines from their receptors sites, but do increase benzodiazepine affinity for benzodiazepine receptors (Figure 18–17).

### *Pharmacokinetics*

Table 18–2 reviews the pharmacokinetics of thiopental and methohexital. Methohexital elimination half-life is one-third that of thiopental, due mainly to its increased clearance. Early awakening from a single dose of either agent is similar. However, return of psychomotor function from repeated doses will be quicker with methohexital due to its 4 to 5 times greater metabolism and clearance (Table 18–2).

Thiopental and methohexital undergo maximum brain uptake within 30 seconds due to 20 to 25% of the total cardiac output going to 10% of body mass, of which the brain comprises. Early awakening is from the rapid redistribution to other tissues (76).

Barbiturates are almost entirely metabolized. Less than 1% is removed unchanged in the urine. The increased clearance of methohexital is partly due to its lower lipid solubility in comparison with thiopental and, therefore, its greater availability in the plasma for delivery to the liver for metabolism (76).

### *Pharmacodynamics*

#### Cardiovascular System

Barbiturates produce dose-dependent decreases in cardiac output, cerebral blood flow, mean arterial pressure, and increases in system vascular resistance and heart rate. In the healthy, well-hydrated patient, these changes are minimal at the usual induction dose. Direct cardiac depression occurs only when doses several times that normally used to induce anesthesia are administered. When congestive heart failure or hypovolemia is present with the sympathetic system already at maximal output, barbiturate administration can cause an exaggerated fall in blood pressure. In general, the cardiovascular depressant effects of barbiturates are much less than the cardiovascular depressant effects of the volatile inhalation agents (77–79).

The reduction in blood pressure and increase in heart rate seen with induction doses of barbiturates are the result of venous pooling from dilation of the peripheral capacitance vessels with a resultant increase in heart rate due to baroreceptor-mediated increase of sympathetic nervous system activity (80). Patients taking beta-antagonists or central-acting alpha antihypertensive agents may have accentuated responses to the blood pressure lowering effects of intravenous barbiturates.

#### Respiratory System

Anesthetic doses of barbiturates produce dose-dependent depression of the medullary and pontine respiratory centers. With lighter planes of anesthesia, laryngeal and cough reflexes are not well-depressed. Coughing, sneezing, hiccoughing, and laryngospasm occur when inadequate amounts are used without adequate paralysis.

#### Liver

Barbiturates are well-known for their ability to alter the microsomal drug metabolizing system. They combine with cytochrome p-450, competitively interfering with the metabolism of several drugs and steroid substances. Barbiturates cause a significant increase in enzyme, protein, and lipid content of the hepatic smooth endoplasmic reticulum. The rate of metabolism of several drugs, steroid hormones, cholesterol, bile salts, and vitamin K is increased. This microsomal enzyme induction also increases the metabolism of barbiturates themselves resulting in increased tolerance. Cross-tolerance also occurs with many sedatives, ethanol, and anesthetic drugs, which may result in increased dosage requirements.

#### Kidney

Induction doses of barbiturates result in decreased renal blood flow and glomular filtration rate. This occurs most likely secondary to the reduction of cardiac output, and reduced mean arterial pressure caused by barbiturate along with the resultant stimulation of antidiuretic hormone secretion.

### *Obstetric Anesthesia Considerations*

The main differences between thiopental and methohexital are methohexital's more rapid clearance, greater potency, and excitatory phenomenon resulting in skeletal muscle movement and hiccoughing.

Barbiturates readily cross the placenta with peak umbilical vein concentrations 1 minute after administration. Fetal exposure is, therefore, rapid, but neonatal effects are remarkably benign. Fetal concentrations are substantially less than maternal concentrations (81). Lower concentrations in the fetal brain are attributed to dilution by blood returning from the viscera and extremities and clearance by the fetal liver (82). Woods, et al calculated fetal hepatic extraction ratio in fetuses of pregnant ewes and could not demonstrate a significant role for the fetal liver in protecting the fetal brain from thiopental (83). Regardless of the mechanism, doses of less than or equal to 4 mg/kg of thiopental do not result in excessive concentrations in the fetal brain (84).

## Propofol

Propofol is one of a group of alkylphenols with anesthetic properties from the research laboratories of ICI Pharmaceuticals in Maxfield, England. Because phenol compounds are virtually insoluble in aqueous solutions, propofol is prepared in an aqueous emulsion (intralipid) containing 10% soybean oil, 2.25% glycerol, and 1.1% purified egg phosphotide, which provides a "milky appearance" (Figure 18–18). This intravenous agent has been used in Europe for several years and is gaining popularity as a complete intravenous anesthetic for ambulatory surgery.

### Mechanism of Action

Similar to the barbiturates and benzodiazepines, propofol produces a dose-dependent sedative hypnotic effect on central nervous system functions. The mechanism of central nervous system depression has not been characterized but with an induction dose of 2 to 2.5 mg/kg intravenously, there is loss of consciousness within one circulation time (less than 60 seconds) and recovery is also rapid, even following multiple doses or continuous infusion for short surgical procedures of less than 1 hour duration (84).

### Pharmacokinetics

Pharmacokinetic-modeling studies of propofol suggest a rapid blood-brain equilibration half-life of around 2 to 3 minutes and a distribution half-life of 2 to 4 minutes (85). A comparison of propofol with other induction intravenous agents is shown in Table 18–2. The volume of distribution for propofol, as well as the clearance rate, is large suggesting a highly lipophilic compound that is extensively distributed to well-perfused tissue during the early rapid phase of distribution with subsequent redistribution to other body tissues and accumulation in fat similar to the thiobarbiturates (Table 18–2).

Propofol is metabolized in the liver to produce water soluble glucuronide and sulphate conjugates, which are primarily excreted in the urine. Metabolism of propofol is rapid with less than 20% of an induction bolus dose of propofol recovered as unchanged drug after only 30 minutes. The total body clearance rate of propofol has been reported to exceed liver blood flow, suggesting that there are extra hepatic biotransformation and/or extra renal elimination processes that may occur (84). These properties are desirable especially for short ambulatory surgical procedures.

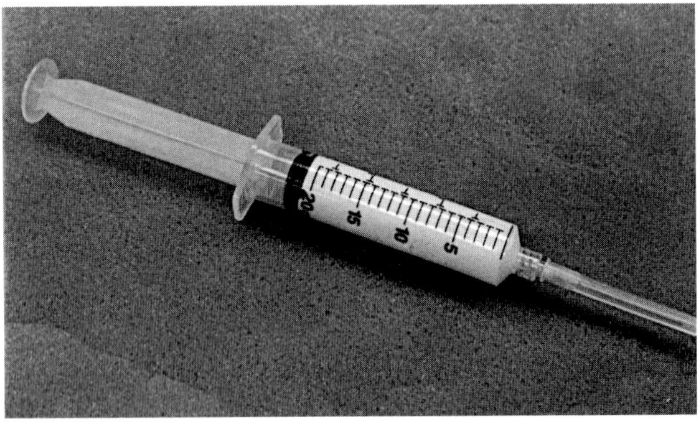

**Fig. 18–18.** Propofol injection.

### Pharmacodynamics

#### Central Nervous System

The quality and duration of an induction dose of intravenous propofol are also dependent upon the physical status of the patient, similar to other intravenous agents. The elderly and debilitated patient are more sensitive to the central nervous system, as well as cardiopulmonary effects of propofol. With a usual induction dose of 1.5 to 2.5 mg/kg IV, the duration of hypnosis is from 5 to 10 minutes (84,85). A maintenance infusion of or in combination with inhalational anesthetic agents is necessary to maintain surgical anesthesia (86).

When propofol was compared to thiopental or methohexital for induction followed by a volatile anesthetic agent and nitrous oxide for maintenance of anesthesia, the recovery profile of propofol compared favorably in comparison with the thiobarbiturates. Recovery was generally faster from propofol than was it from methohexital or thiopental (84,85).

#### Cardiovascular System

Hemodynamic effects of propofol 2.5 mg/kg intravenously have been compared to thiopental 4 mg/kg IV. The cardiovascular depressant properties of propofol are similar to or greater than those of thiopental (Table 18–6) (84,85). Propofol produced a 15 to 30% decrease in systolic, diastolic, and mean arterial blood pressure, and this hypotensive effect was accentuated when propofol was administered with an opiate analgesic. In elderly and hypovolemic patients, as well as patients with impaired left ventricular function, propofol can produce profound depression of the cardiovascular system (84,86). The decrease in blood pressure was associated with a decreased stroke volume, cardiac index, and systemic vascular resistance. Heart rate that was decreased insignificantly in this study was depressed significantly during maintenance infusion of propofol in comparison with methohexital and thiopental/enflurane in another study (86).

**Table 18–6.** Some Cardiovascular Effects of Intravenous Anesthetics

| Drugs | Cardiac Output | Heart Rate | Mean Arterial Pressure | Peripheral Vascular Resistance | Left Ventricular End Diastolic Pressure |
|---|---|---|---|---|---|
| Thiopental | −2, −1, 0 | 0, +1, +2 | −1, 0, +1 | 0, +1 | 0 |
| Methohexital | −1, 0 | 0, +1 | −1, 0, +1 | 0, +1 | 0 |
| Propofol | −2, −1, 0 | −2, −1, 0 | −2, −1, 0 | −2, −1, 0 | 0, +1 |
| Diazepam | 0 | −1, 0, +1 | −1, 0 | 0 | 0 |
| Midazolam | 0 | −1, 0, +1 | −1 | 0 | 0, +1 |
| Etomidate | 0, +1 | 0, +1, +2 | −1, 0 | −1, 0 | 0, +1 |
| Ketamine | 0, +1, +2 | 0 to +3 | 0, +1, +2 | +2 | 0 |

+ = increased, 0 = no effect, − = decreased.
(From White PF: Propofol: pharmacokinetics and pharmacodynamics. Seminars in Anesthesia 7:4, 1988; and Shafer A, Doze VA, Shafer SL, White PF: Pharmacokinetics and pharmacodynamics of propofol infusions during general anesthesia. Anesthesiology 69:348, 1988.)

## Respiratory System

Propofol produces a dose-related depression of the respiratory system (87). When a bolus dose of propofol of 2 to 2.5 mg is administered rapidly for induction, transient apnea of 30 to 90 seconds occurs in about 50% of unpremedicated patients. If an opiate analgesic is administered for premedication or as an adjuvant during the induction period, apnea is produced in all patients unless the propofol induction dose is slowly titrated. Typically, there is a rapid reduction in tidal volume with tachypnea preceding the apneic period. Carbon dioxide response curve is depressed by 40 to 60% during maintenance infusion of propofol (87). Similar to the barbiturates, surgical stimulation counteracts the respiratory depressant effects of propofol during anesthetic induction.

### *Obstetric Anesthesia Considerations*

The use of propofol for obstetric anesthesia has been limited. The fast recovery of propofol for short surgical procedures should also be advantageous for cesarean section.

A preliminary study compared propofol (2.5 mg/kg) with thiopentone (5.0 mg/kg) as induction agent for elective cesarean section in 50 ASA physical status I or II patients (88). The quality of awakening of the mothers given propofol was far superior to those given thiopentone, but the neonates were slower to start spontaneous respiration and had lower Apgar scores at 1 and 5 minutes in comparison with the thiopentone group. However, neonates had Apgar scores of 10 by 20 minutes (88). Celleno, et al, using propofol 2.8 mg/kg also reported lower Apgar scores at 1 and 5 minutes. They also carried out neurobehavioral exams at 1, 4, and 24 hours after delivery. Twenty-five percent of the infants had muscular hypotonus at 5 minutes (89). In contrast, using propofol 2.15 ± 0.26 mg/kg as the induction dose, Moore, et al reported no difference in infant well-being as assessed by Apgar score and cord blood analysis of thiopentone or propofol. Factors associated with uterine relaxation and bleeding were also similar in the two groups (90). Using propofol 2 mg/kg followed by 6 mg/kg/hr infusion with nitrous oxide 50% in oxygen or 9 mg/kg/hr with 100% $O_2$, Gregory, et al reported Apgar scores and umbilical blood gas analysis being similar in both groups, but the neurologic and adaptive capacity scores (91) at 2 hours were poor in the higher infusion propofol group (92).

The total body clearance of propofol following a 2 mg/kg induction dose is increased in women undergoing cesarean section in comparison with women undergoing laparoscopic sterilization as control (93). This is caused partly by removal of drug following delivery of the neonate and placenta, although increased extrahepatic metabolism is an additional possibility. Apparent volumes of distribution and half-lives are similar to those found in nonpregnant patients (93).

Dailland, et al studied the placental transfer and neonatal effects of propofol in women undergoing elective cesarean section (94). Following propofol 2.5 mg/kg with either 50% nitrous oxide in oxygen and halothane (group 1) or propofol infusion 5 mg/kg/hr (group 2), the umbilical venous blood concentration of propofol was 0.13 to 0.75 μg/ml and 0.78 to 1.37 μg/ml, respectively. At delivery, the ratio of the drug concentration in umbilical venous blood to that in maternal blood was 0.70 ± 0.06 for group 1 and 0.76 ± 0.10 for group 2. A trace amount of propofol was also found in the mother's milk. Propofol is cleared rapidly from the neonatal circulation and exposure of the neonate through breast milk would be negligible compared to the placental transfer of the drug (94).

Although the use of propofol for cesarean section has apparent advantages for the mother, published data suggest that higher doses of propofol may cause neonatal depression. The use of propofol for cesarean section needs further classification.

## *Benzodiazepines*

Benzodiazepines have a broad range of clinical application. They are used for their sedative, amnestic, and anesthetic properties by the anesthesiologist. Other favorable properties include minimal effects on the cardiovascular and respiratory systems, anticonvulsant activity, and a wide margin of safety.

Diazepam is limited by a slow onset, prolonged recovery compared to thiopental, high incidence of thrombophlebitis, and possibility of recurrent sedation.

Midazolam more closely approaches the speed of thiopental, but still requires 30 to 60 seconds longer for full effect. Onset of anesthesia with thiopental is 50 to 100% faster (95) and recovery 1 to 2 1/2 times slower with midazolam (96).

### Mechanism of Action

Receptors for benzodiazepines and GABA are not identical because they do not show competition at respective receptor sites (97). The distribution of benzodiazepine receptors is highest in the cerebrocortex, hypothalamus, cerebellum, corpus triatum, and medulla (97). This distribution parallels the distribution of GABA receptors. The parallel anatomic distribution of benzodiazepine and GABA receptors suggests that benzodiazepines might influence the activity of GABA-containing neurons (Figure 18–17).

GABA is an important inhibitory neurotransmitter. High concentrations of GABA are found in both the central and peripheral nervous system. Inhibitors of GABA synthesis (e.g., allylglycine) and GABA antagonist (e.g., picrotoxins and viculline) prevent the normal inhibitory activity of GABA and upper motor neurons. Seizures induced by these substances can be prevented by benzodiazepines. The anticonvulsant activity of benzodiazepines results from facilitation of GABA postsynaptically. This facilitation takes place when benzodiazepine binds its receptor postsynaptically causing an allosteric change in the GABA receptor. This results in increased binding and increased effect of GABA (98). Benzodiazepines have no direct GABA-mimetic action.

The sedative properties of benzodiazepines are probably due to the same mechanism responsible for the anticonvulsive activity via GABA facilitation in the cortex (98).

The antianxiety effect of benzodiazepines seems to be mediated by glycine-mimetic effects at the brain stem level (Figure 18–17) (99). Muscle relaxation is also probably mediated by glycine-mimetic effects at the spinal cord level (Figure 18–17) (98). Benzodiazepine mechanisms for amnesia have not been elucidated (97,99).

### Pharmacokinetics

Pharmacokinetic data of both midazolam and diazepam are found in Table 18–2.

The elimination half-life of both increase with increasing age. Plasma clearance of midazolam is much more rapid than that of diazepam, leading to a much more rapid normalization of mental function (100). The prolonged effect of diazepam is due to slower clearance (Table 18–2), possible enterohepatic circulation, and the active metabolite desmethyldiazepam (100). Neither potency nor duration of action of midazolam's metabolites have been elucidated.

Liver dysfunction increases the elimination half-life of both diazepam and midazolam by decreasing metabolism and also by increasing the volume of distribution due to decreased protein binding associated with cirrhosis or severe hepatic disease. Decreased hepatic blood flow would also contribute to decreased clearance (100).

### Pharmacodynamics

#### Central Nervous System

Benzodiazepines cause anterograde amnesia, but not retrograde amnesia. Midazolam (5 mg) and diazepam (10 mg) intravenously give similar onset (2 to 8 minutes) and duration (50 to 60 minutes) of anterograde amnesia (101,102).

Both midazolam and diazepam reduced cerebral metabolic oxygen requirements and cerebral blood flow in dog and human studies (103,104). Midazolam in the dog study gave a greater degree of protection compared to diazepam, suggesting that it may protect against ischemic damage to a greater extent.

#### Cardiovascular System

Benzodiazepines have been widely used for induction of anesthesia in critically ill patients because of their minimal cardiovascular effects when used alone (Table 18–5). When other agents such as narcotics are added, hypotension often ensues due to a transient depression of baroreflex function and a sustained decrease in sympathetic tone. This effect of diazepam and midazolam on the sympathetic nervous system may limit the ability to compensate for hemodynamic changes due to hypovolemia (105).

Unlike narcotics, addition of nitrous oxide following induction of anesthesia with diazepam does not result in cardiac depression (106).

#### Respiratory System

Diazepam causes a decreased expired minute volume due mainly to a decreased tidal volume with an associated increased $PaCO_2$ (107). Midazolam also causes a decreased tidal volume, but is compensated for by an increased respiratory rate so that the minute volume does not change in conscious patients (108). With loss of consciousness, $CO_2$ sensitivity is lost in most subjects, resulting in a depression of the ventilatory drive. Benzodiazepines do not shift the $CO_2$ response curve to the right, as with opioids, but flatten the slopes of response.

Addition of other central nervous system depressants to benzodiazepines results in exaggerated or prolonged depression of respiration. Patients who have chronic obstruction pulmonary disease (COPD) may also exhibit exaggerated respiratory depression when given diazepam or midazolam.

### Obstetric Anesthesia Considerations

Benzodiazepines have been used as sedatives, anxiolytics, anticonvulsants, and induction agents in the obstetric suite. In small doses, benzodiazepines have minimal fetal and neonatal effects (109). Small doses of diazepam (5 to 10 mg) do significantly decrease beat-to-beat variability of the fetal heart rate; however, there are no adverse effects on fetal acid-base or clinical status (110).

Neonates did not have altered Apgar scores, nor altered umbilical vein, nor artery acid-base status when diazepam doses of 2.5 to 10 mg were used as an anxiolytic in women undergoing cesarean section with regional anesthesia.

The neonates did have decreased motor tone after delivery, but the altered motor tone returned to normal by 24 hours of age.

When diazepam is used in large doses, there may be persistence of neonatal hypotonia, hypoactivity, decreased eating, and hypothermia.

Midazolam has a more rapid onset of action than diazepam when used intravenously, and a much shorter duration of action. As with diazepam, minimum cardiovascular or respiratory effects are seen in the mother. Midazolam rapidly crosses the placenta in the ewe, but not to the same extent as with diazepam, probably due to its water solubility and higher protein binding.

When comparing midazolam 0.3 mg/kg with thiopental 4 mg/kg, there were no significant maternal differences found in neurological status, systolic blood pressure, or heart rate (111).

In comparing fetal outcome between midazolam and thiopental, there were significant differences. Body tone, arm recoil, and body temperature were inferior in the midazolam group, only within the first 2 hours however (112).

Placental transfer of midazolam is slower than that of valium or thiopental (113,114).

## Ketamine

Ketamine has a broad range of clinical application due to its ability to produce profound analgesia, amnesia, and dissociative anesthesia. Other attributes that make ketamine an attractive agent are its ability to give central sympathetic stimulation, which leads to support of the cardiovascular system as well as maintaining respiratory drive.

Because of these properties, ketamine has been used as an adjunct to other agents for supplemental analgesia, as an adjunct to induction of anesthesia, or as the sole induction agent, especially in situations in which hemodynamic stability is in question.

### Mechanisms of Action

Ketamine produces a cataleptic-like state by dissociating the thalamus and limbic system.

The intense analgesia induced by ketamine could be due to a variety of interactions: (1) depression of specific thalamic nuclei; (2) depression of specific spinal afferent pathways associated with pain perception; (3) highly selective depression of nuclei within the medullary reticular formation; (4) lamina-specific depression of spinal cord activity; (5) ketamine binding to opiate receptors; and (6) interaction with cholinergic and muscarinic receptors (115).

### Pharmacokinetics

The pharmacokinetic profiles of nonbarbiturate induction agents are outlined in Table 18–2. Ketamine's pharmacokinetic profile resembles that of thiopental with high lipid solubility, rapid onset of action, and short duration of action.

Ketamine is 5 to 10 times more lipid soluble than thiopental. This, along with the increased cerebral blood flow induced by ketamine and low protein binding, ensures a rapid onset of action.

Like thiopental, redistribution from the brain to peripheral tissue sites is responsible for termination of unconsciousness. Tissue accumulation with repeated doses can turn a short-acting agent into a long-acting agent.

Liver metabolism within the microsomal enzyme system is primarily responsible for clearance of ketamine.

### Pharmacodynamics

#### Central Nervous System

Ketamine produces a dissociative anesthesia manifested by a cataleptic-like state if no other anesthetics or neuromuscular blockers are used.

Ketamine is a potent cerebral vasodilator. Cerebral blood flow increases up to 60%, which along with increased blood flow to the spinal cord, can cause an increase in CSF pressure (115,116). As such, ketamine should be used with caution, if at all, in patients with intracranial pathology, e.g., space occupying lesions, severe preeclampsia or eclampsia.

Ketamine causes increased activity of both the thalamic and limbic systems but does not alter the seizure threshold in epileptic patients, (117) and it may in fact have anticonvulsant activity (118).

#### Cardiovascular System

When ketamine is injected directly into the cerebral circulation, an immediate increase in blood pressure, heart rate, and cardiac output is produced (Table 18–6). This central mechanism is supported by the fact that pentobarbital, inhaled anesthetics, ganglionic blockade, cervical epidural blockade, and spinal cord transection prevent ketamine-induced changes of heart rate and blood pressure.

Ketamine, when used in conjunction with other anesthetic agents, has less cardiac stimulating effects. Enflurane and halothane block the cardiovascular-stimulating properties of ketamine and can result in significant cardiovascular depression when ketamine is administered. In the absence of autonomic control, spinal cord lesions, or in critically ill patients, the direct cardiovascular depressant effects of ketamine can be unmasked and can result in further cardiac instability.

Ketamine causes an increase in coronary blood flow from its direct dilation of vascular smooth muscle (119). Despite the increased supply caused by ketamine, the net $O_2$ extraction remains unchanged due to the increased myocardial oxygen consumption caused by the increased cardiac work (120). Pulmonary artery pressure and right ventricular stroke work are increased as the result of increased pulmonary vascular resistance induced by ketamine. Ketamine produces up to a 40% increase in pulmonary vascular resistance (121).

#### Respiratory System

Ketamine does not produce significant respiratory depression except when rapid intravenous boluses are given, or when used in conjunction with narcotics. Transient increases in intrapulmonary shunting are caused by ketamine administration but usually last less than 10 minutes (121).

Ketamine has bronchodilating properties that appear to be separate from $beta_2$ receptor mechanisms. Propranolol blocks the relaxant effect of epinephrine but not of ketamine (122). In dog studies, ketamine was shown to be as effective as halothane or enflurane in preventing induced bronchospasm. The respiratory response to $CO_2$ is maintained during ketamine anesthesia (123).

Upper airway secretions are increased by intravenous or intramuscular ketamine and can be offset by the use of anticholinergics. Despite reactivity of the airway during ketamine anesthesia, the usual airway precautions taken for other full stomach cases should be employed during ketamine anesthesia, e.g., cricoid pressure and rapid sequence intubation with a cuffed endotracheal tube.

### Obstetric Anesthesia Considerations

Ketamine can be used in many obstetric anesthesia settings. These range from analgesia and sedation to supplementation of regional block to full induction and maintenance of anesthesia.

Doses of 0.2 to 0.4 mg/kg IV work well for analgesia with good patient acceptance and no neonatal depression (124). Ketamine doses of less than 1 mg/kg IV have not been shown to cause neonatal depression. Unlike thiopental, ketamine does not cause depression of blood pressure in acidotic neonates and is associated with better neurobehavioral scores (125). Infants with known intrauterine asphyxia had excellent Apgar scores after cesarean section in mothers induced with 1.2 mg/kg of ketamine (126).

### Emergence Delirium

The incidence of emergence delirium ranges from 5 to 30%. Age less than 16 years, female sex, doses of ketamine greater than 2 mg/kg, and a history of personality disorders or frequent dreaming seem to be associated with an increased frequency of emergence delirium. The delirium itself is associated with visual, auditory, proprioceptive, and confusing illusions. Dreams and hallucinations may occur and last up to 24 hours. Central effects of ketamine result in misinterpretation of auditory and visual stimuli and loss of skin and musculoskeletal sensations resulting in decreased sensations of gravity and proprioception with a resultant sensation of detachment and floating (115,127).

Prevention of delirium is aided by discussing the possible side effects of ketamine before and after the use of this anesthetic with the patient. The administration of a benzodiazepine premedication and of intraoperative use of thiopental or inhalation agents seem to decrease the incidence of this side effect. There is no evidence that allowing quiet emergence in a darkened room alters the incidence of emergence reactions (128).

## Etomidate

Etomidate is a water soluble hypnotic agent that produces a rapid induction of anesthesia with minimal cardiovascular or respiratory changes (129).

### Mechanism of Action

The mechanism of action of etomidate is similar to that of barbiturates. Etomidate exerts depressive effects in the reticular activating system and has a facilitatory action on spinal nerves (130). Etomidate has also been shown to have a GABA-mimetic action that can be reversed by GABA antagonists (131).

### Pharmacokinetics

Etomidate penetrates the brain rapidly, reaching peak levels within 1 minute after intravenous injection. Awakening occurs within 2 to 3 minutes after a single intravenous dose and is probably due to rapid redistribution of the drug from the brain to other tissues. Plasma clearance of etomidate is rapid, thus reducing potential for accumulation (see Table 18–2). Seventy-six percent of etomidate is bound to albumin, therefore, hypoalbuminaria can greatly potentiate its clinical effects (132).

Hepatic microsomal enzymes and plasma esterases are responsible for the metabolism of etomidate. The overall clearance of etomidate is far greater than that for the barbiturates.

### Pharmacodynamics

#### Central Nervous System

Etomidate is a potent hypnotic with rapid onset and resolution of action. This effect is mediated primarily via a GABA-mimetic action. Recovery is rapid, usually within 3 to 5 minutes of intravenous dosing. There is a higher incidence of postoperative nausea and vomiting when compared to thiopental, but this can be decreased by prophylactic administration of intravenous droperidol (133).

Etomidate has no analgesic action, therefore, as with barbiturates, it has little effect toward oblating the hemodynamic response stimulated by laryngoscopy and intubation.

#### Cardiovascular System

Etomidate is usually described as a drug that changes hemodynamic variables the least when compared to other induction agents (Table 18–6).

In normal patients and patients with compensated ischemic heart disease, heart rate, pulmonary artery pressure, pulmonary capillary wedge pressure, right atrial pressure, pulmonary vascular resistance, systemic vascular resistance, and systolic time intervals are not significantly altered after doses of 0.15 to 0.3 mg/kg (134). In addition, compared to other agents, etomidate produces the least change in the balance of myocardial oxygen supply and demand.

In comparing etomidate and thiopental in animal models of hypovolemia, there is significantly more hemodynamic depression in the thiopental group, and increased survival in the etomidate group (135).

#### Respiratory System

As with ketamine, if given slowly, etomidate does not cause apnea. A 25% reduction of tidal volume is seen,

(136) but this is offset somewhat by an increase in respiratory rate. When used in conjunction with other intravenous or inhalation anesthetics, the respiratory depression observed may be exaggerated.

## Adrenocortical Suppression

Etomidate inhibits 11-beta hydroxilase activity (137) for up to 8 hours after an induction dose of etomidate. This suppression may lead to decreased cortisol and aldosterone production in the early postoperative period (138). Whether this is clinically significant at this time is not clear. However, it would be theoretically undesirable to pharmacologically suppress these protective responses to perioperative stress.

## Myoclonic Movements

Involuntary myoclonic movements occur in up to 40% of patients administered etomidate. There was no epileptoform activity on electrocardiogram associated with these movements (139). The incidence of these movements can be reduced with prophylactic administration of fentanyl or benzodiazepines. It was also noted that the incidence of these movements decreased with the change of the carrier solvent to propylene glycol.

### *Obstetric Anesthesia Considerations*

There are several potential situations in obstetric anesthesia when etomidate could be of benefit. These would include potential hypovolemic states as found with placenta previa or abruptio, uterine ruption, postpartum bleeding or with preeclamptic or eclamptic patients when minimal cardiovascular insult or upset is desirable.

In one study, it was found the maternal-to-fetal base excess differences and the degree of biochemical correlation between the mother and infant were more favorable following etomidate than were they following thiopental inductions (140). An abstract reported at the 1986 Society of Obstetric Anesthesiologists and Perinatology did not confirm this finding (141).

Also of concern is the possible adrenal suppression of the neonate by placental transfer of etomidate.

## ***Opiates***

Opiates are widely used in clinical anesthesia as a primary and supplemental agent.

Stereospecific opiate receptors were proven to exist in the early 1970s. There is a complex system and distribution of opiate receptors throughout the brain, spinal cord, peripheral nerves and ganglia, adrenal medulla, and intestinal tract with multiple afferent and efferent interconnections, which result in a wide array of target-organ effects (Figure 18–19). Table 18–7 lists five major subclasses of opiate receptors felt to be responsible for a wide array of effects and side effects.

### *Endogenous Opiates*

A close correlation exists between locations of high densities of opiate receptors and locations of the endogenous opiate substances.

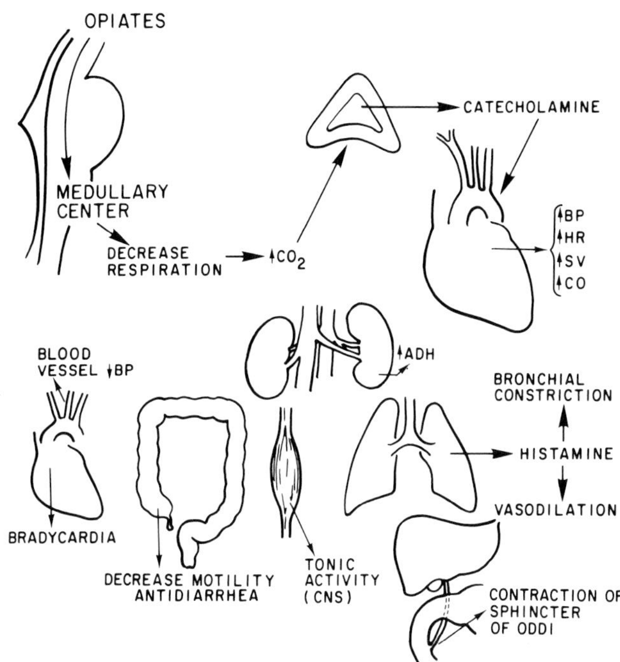


**Fig. 18–19.** Some common sites of nonanalgesic opiate and receptor interaction. Subclasses of opiate receptors have been described by the array of opiate effects. See Table 18–7.

Endorphin cells are limited to the medial basal and uncinate region of the hypothalamus, the pituitary intermediate lobe, and the adenohypophysis. Their pattern of distribution and mode of synthesis and release is suggestive of a hormonal function.

Enkephalinergic cells are found in many nuclei of the brain and spinal cord, in peripheral ganglia and nerves, and the adrenal medulla and gut. The fact that enkephalins are found in areas of the central nervous system in close association with opiate receptors suggests that they may play a role as transmitters at these sites and may function

**Table 18–7.** Association of Opiate Subclass Receptors with Physiological Functions

| | | |
|---|---|---|
| Mood: | Euphoria | mu |
| | Dysphoria | sigma |
| | Hallucinations/Excitement | sigma |
| | Sedation | kappa |
| Analgesia: | | mu, delta, kappa, epsilon |
| Respiratory: | Depression | mu, delta |
| | Tachypnea | sigma |
| Cardiac: | Tachycardia | sigma |
| | Bradycardia | mu |
| Endocrine: | Decreased ADH | kappa |
| | Increased Prolactin | mu |
| | Increased GH | delta |
| Body Temperature: | Hyperthermia | delta |
| | Hypothermia | mu |
| Miscellaneous: | Addiction | mu |
| | Miosis | mu |
| | Hypertonia | sigma |

as modulators of physiologic parameters that are influenced by the administration of exogenous opiates.

## *Pharmacodynamics*

### Analgesia

Opiates affect primary afferent sensory input, influence dorsal horn cells, and produce a modulation of dorsal horn activity by activating descending pathways from the brainstem.

The ability of opiates to modulate the sensation of pain appears to rely upon a complex system of opiate receptors involved with both afferent and efferent neural pathways with each level of the neuroaxis.

### Central Nervous System

Changes in mood or emotional reactions after opiate administration are thought to be mediated by the limbic system and also on the multiple afferent pathways synapsing in the limbic system. Euphoria and sedation are the common effects of opiates; however, dysphoria has been described occasionally in the female patient. The mechanism of action for the dysphoria is unknown, although opiates are known to produce varied central nervous system responses in laboratory animals (e.g., sedation in dogs, catatonia in rats, and unusual behavior in cats, including catatonia, irritability, and fear).

### Respiratory System

Respiratory depression is due to suppression of spontaneous activity of medullary inspiratory and expiratory neurons. Depression of these cells seems to be the main cause of respiratory depression, but other sites may also be involved.

Opiates also have a potent antitussive effect mediated through suppression of neurons in the rostral pons and/or medulla (142).

### Cardiovascular System

Opiates are well-known for their lack of direct cardiac depression when used alone. Their major effects on the circulation are exerted peripherally and via central nervous system effects.

Opiates decrease heart rate via vagal mediation (143). After vagotomy, heart rate remained at control values after fentanyl administration. Opiates also have a direct effect upon the SA node, causing a decrease in heart rate (144). Vagotomy, atropine or propranolol did not block this negative chronotropic activity.

Opiates cause arterial and venous vasodilation with limitations in the ability of the cardiovascular system to respond to postural changes. Vasodilation caused by opiates is hypothesized to be due to direct vasodilatory properties (145), neurally mediated vasodilation (146), and/or histamine release (147).

Fentanyl and sufentanil are known to cause vagally mediated bradycardia via a central effect. This mechanism appears to be mediated by opiate receptors in the medulla, which excite cardioinhibitory vagal fibers and depress sympathetic efferents (148).

Rapid narcotic administration can result in tachycardia and hypertension from stimulation of adrenal medulla (149). Hypotension can also be caused by narcotics secondary to vasodilation (150).

Morphine causes transient decreases of vascular resistance in arterioles and a prolonged dilatory effect on capacitance vessels (151). High-dose morphine anesthesia also dramatically increased fluid requirements to maintain perfusion and urine output.

Opiates exert changes in cerebral blood flow by both direct and indirect effects. Small preanesthetic doses have no significant effect on the cerebral circulation. As the dose of narcotic is increased, respiratory depression increases with the associated $CO_2$ retention and increased cerebral blood flow. When ventilation is controlled, this effect is prevented.

Higher doses of narcotics can also cause decreased arterial blood pressure, especially when used in conjunction with other anesthetics. This decrease in blood pressure results in decreased cerebral perfusion pressure.

### Gastrointestinal Tract

The major effects of narcotics on the gastrointestinal tract are on motility, secretion, and vasodilation.

Morphine has been studied the most. Food passing through the duodenum may be delayed up to 12 hours (152). This delay is thought to be due to contraction of the proximal portion of the duodenum. Gastric emptying may be delayed up to 12 hours in patients treated with narcotics. This increases the risk of aspiration at the time of induction and emergence.

### Liver

Opiates that cause spasm of the sphincter of Oddi resulting in symptoms of biliary colic are of concern (Figure 18–19). Intraoperative measurements of common bile duct pressures revealed increases in pressure of 99.5% with fentanyl, 52.7% with morphine, 61.3% with meperidine, and 15% with pentazocine (153).

### Kidney

Effects of narcotics on the kidneys are not easy to elucidate. A few facts do appear clear:

1. Narcotic administration that is subsequently followed by decreased glomerular filtration rate (GFR), which may or may not result in decreased urine output. This appears to be independent of antidiuretic hormone (ADH) release in man.
2. When $N_2O$ is used in conjunction with narcotics, a further decrease in glomerular filtration rate is seen with an associated decrease in urine output. This effect is due primarily to decreased cardiac output and increased vasoconstriction from sympathetic stimulation.
3. High levels of ADH can be associated with $N_2O$/narcotic anesthesia in the setting of surgical stress.

The above changes in urine output and glomerular filtration rate still maintain adequate urine production in healthy volunteers (154). These changes may be of clinical significance in patients with compromised renal function, hypovolemia, infection, or in association with nephrotoxic drugs.

### Obstetric Analgesia and Anesthesia Considerations

***Morphine.*** Babies delivered less than 1 hour or more than 6 hours after maternal morphine administration seldom showed signs of narcosis, while the peak incidence of neonatal depression occurred approximately 3.5 hours after administration (155).

Morphine has been shown to have a greater effect on fetal respiratory depression (156), fetal heart rate (157), and fetal heart rate variability, effects that lasted longer than that produced by other narcotics (158).

***Meperidine.*** Despite meperidine's inferior sedative properties and its increased incidence of nausea and vomiting when compared with morphine, there has been a sustained clinical impression that meperidine is less likely to cause neonatal narcosis.

Maternally administered meperidine is not benign in its effect on the fetus. Meperidine can cause changes in fetal heart rate variability, in fetal electroencephalogram, $O_2$ saturation, minute ventilation, alveolar ventilation, Apgar scores, and neurobehavioral scores.

Not all neonates were depressed after maternal meperidine administration. The degree of depression correlates with the total dose given and the time interval between maternal administration and delivery. Delivery within 1 to 5 hours after maternal meperidine administration showed no significant depression when compared to controls (159). If delivered 2 to 3 hours after a dose, there was significant depression, with greater depression occurring in those mothers who received higher doses.

The proposed mechanisms for this delay in depression is the role of the active metabolite normeperidine that is formed in the mother then transferred to the fetus (160,161). The delay is due to the time required for the mother to produce these metabolites and transfer them to the fetus.

Meperidine is metabolized to normeperidine, which has a long half-life, has more convulsive and respiratory depressant effects than meperidine, and is less effectively antagonized by naloxone. Note also that meperidine metabolism in the infant is defective. The half-life in the neonate is 22 hours, versus 3 hours in the parturient.

***Alphaprodine.*** Alphaprodine has good analgesic and sedative properties with a lower incidence of nausea and vomiting than meperidine.

Alphaprodine has a greater respiratory depressant effect than morphine in adults (162), causes decreased fetal heart rate variability (158), and causes a high incidence of sinusoidal-type fetal heart rate (163).

***Fentanyl.*** Fentanyl has become popular for analgesia in obstetric practice because it is potent, short acting, and highly protein bound. Neonatal blood levels were determined at 2 and 7 minutes after delivery in infants delivered of mothers who had received 1 μg/kg of fentanyl intravenously within 10 minutes of delivery by cesarean section (164). Fentanyl concentrations in the newborn were 2 ng/ml at 2 minutes and 1 ng/ml at 7 minutes after delivery. Apgar scores were greater than 8 at 1 minute (except for one at 1 minute due to obstetric difficulties) and neurobehavioral scores were normal at 4 and 24 hours.

When anesthesia is required during pregnancy for surgery that cannot be done with local or regional techniques, narcotic-based anesthesia is a safe alternative.

Narcotics can be used as an adjunct to inhalational techniques or as the primary agent with 100% $O_2$, as might be needed in cardiac anesthesia for maximal cardiovascular stability.

Balanced anesthesia today consists of combining several agents to produce anesthesia, analgesia, amnesia, muscle relaxation, and maintenance of cardiovascular homeostasis. The inclusion of narcotics in a balanced anesthesia technique includes less fluctuation of cardiovascular dynamics, lower requirements for inhaled anesthetics, gives the advantage of rapid supplementation for unexpected stimuli or preventing response to expected stimuli by acute intravenous bolus of the narcotic being used.

The main disadvantage of using narcotics to supplement anesthesia is respiratory depression postoperatively. If not carefully titrated, narcotics can cause nausea, vomiting, bradycardia, and hypotension.

### Pharmacokinetics and Clinical Anesthesia

The use of narcotics as the primary anesthetic was described by Scheidevlein in 1900 (165). He used 2 mg/kg of morphine with 1 to 3 mg of scopolamine. This method was soon abandoned because 70% of the patients had to be restrained during surgery, and several deaths occurred, probably due to respiratory depression (165).

Lowenstein reported that 0.5 to 1 mg/kg of morphine with 100% $O_2$ produced minimal hemodynamic changes in surgical patients without cardiac disease and frequently increased the cardiac index in patients with aortic valvular disease (166). Because of this, morphine anesthesia became very popular in the early 1970s. As this technique was more widely used, deficiencies became apparent: (1) hypotension; (2) vasodilation with increased fluid and blood requirements; (3) generalized edema; (4) hypertension and tachycardia during times of maximal surgical stimulation; (5) intraoperative awareness; and (6) prolonged somnolence and respiratory depression.

Newer narcotics are now in use that have overcome many of these unacceptable side effects. Alfentanil, fentanyl, and sufentanil, discussed below, among them. The application of these drugs in the obstetric suite will usually be in the pregnant patient with cardiac disease. Their pharmacokinetic profiles are outlined in Table 18–8.

## Alfentanil

Alfentanil is a synthetic opioid one-fourth as potent as fentanyl with a high therapeutic index of 1080 (167). Alfentanil also has a smaller volume of distribution, lower clearance, and shorter elimination half-life than fentanyl or sufentanil (Table 18–8) (168).

**Table 18–8.** Pharmacokinetics of Opiates

| Drug | IV Dose | $T_{1/2\pi}$ (min) | $T_{1/2\alpha}$ (min) | $T_{1/2\beta}$ (h) | Vd (l/kg) | Cl (ml/kg/min) |
|---|---|---|---|---|---|---|
| Morphine | 1 mg/kg | 1.3 | 20.0 | 4.5 | 4.7 | 12.0 |
| Meperidine | 50 mg | — | 3.3 | 3.1 | 2.6 | 12.0 |
| | 100 to 200 mg | — | 3.0 | 4.7 | 4.3 | 8.8 |
| Fentanyl | 3 μg/kg | 0.7 | 55.1 | 1.7 | 0.7 | 3.6 |
| | 30 μg/kg | 1.6 | 21.0 | 5.8 | 2.0 | 5.2 |
| Alfentanil | 50 μg/kg | 1.4 | 9.5 | 1.5 | 1.0 | 7.7 |
| | 125 μg/kg | 1.0 | 13.0 | 1.4 | 0.59 | 5.1 |
| Sufentanil | 5 μg/kg | 1.4 | 17.7 | 2.7 | 1.7 | 12.7 |

(From Prys-Roberts C, Hug CC Jr: Pharmacokinetics of Anesthesia. Cambridge, MA, Blackwell Scientific Publications, 1984; and Stanley TH: Opiate anaesthesia. Anaesthesia Intensive Care 15:38, 1987.)

These characteristics suggest that it is a more desirable agent for short, outpatient procedures. Its main side effects are nausea and vomiting, chest wall rigidity, and postoperative respiratory depression if not properly titrated (169).

Maintenance infusion rates of alfentanil must be titrated carefully to the patient's response because of interpatient variability in pharmacodynamic responses.

## Fentanyl

Fentanyl is well-known for maintenance of hemodynamic stability at induction when used as a supplemental analgesic (2 to 15 μg/kg), even in patients with poor cardiovascular function. Hypotension occurs occasionally, due usually to bradycardia, but can be prevented by administering prophylactically an anticholinergic or antagonized by use of ephedrine or pancuronium.

When used in balanced anesthesia for cases of 2 to 3 hours duration, loading doses of 7 to 7.5 μg/kg have been used followed by maintenance doses of 3.5 to 4.5 μg/kg every 30 to 40 minutes, giving a total dose of approximately 15 μg/kg in conjunction with 60 to 67% $N_2O$. Approximately 30% of the patients require supplemental halogenated inhalational agent to overcome tachycardia and hypertension not prevented by fentanyl. Eighteen percent of these patients required naloxone reversal to maintain adequate respiration at the end of anesthesia (170).

Fentanyl has been studied extensively and used for open heart surgery because of its lack of myocardial depression. Doses of 50 to 120 μg/kg are used and supplemented with vasodilator therapy and/or inhalation anesthesia for control of breakthrough hypertension, which is often seen at time of sternotomy and aortic root manipulation (167).

## Sufentanil

Sufentanil is 4 to 7 times more potent than fentanyl and has greater efficacy in attenuating the hypertensive response to surgical stress in both balanced techniques and when used in anesthetic concentrations for open heart surgery.

Loading doses of approximately 1.5 μg/kg with thiopental give smooth inductions with little hemodynamic response. Maintenance doses of 0.3 to 0.4 μg/kg every 25 to 30 minutes with nitrous oxide 60 to 67% maintained stable hemodynamic status without additional inhalational agents being required (170). The average dose for a 2 to 3 hour case is 2 to 2.8 μg/kg. Naloxone reversal was required in 41% of these patients to maintain adequate ventilation after the end of surgery.

Sufentanil doses of 10 to 20 μg/kg used with $O_2$ for cardiac anesthesia have a much lower incidence of hypertension when compared to fentanyl (171). The cardiovascular actions of sufentanil are similar to those of fentanyl.

## Stiff Man Syndrome

When used for induction, narcotics cause an apparent increase in chest wall muscle tone resulting in rigidity that impedes spontaneous and controlled ventilation. The mechanism of muscle rigidity is probably of central nervous system origin, as thiopental has been shown to reduce motor neuronal discharge (H reflex) induced by morphine 2 mg/kg in human volunteers (172).

Slow titration of muscle relaxant along with slow titration of the induction dose of narcotic will reduce the incidence of this side effect. If it does occur, succinylcholine administration causes rapid relaxation.

### *Reversal of Narcotic Anesthesia*

Naloxone is the most widely used narcotic antagonist at this time. It is used to treat deliberate opiate overdoses, opiate-induced respiratory depression in the postoperative period, newborn opiate-induced respiratory depression, and the untoward side effects of subarachnoid and epidural opiates.

Side effects include severe hypertension (164), arrhythmias (173,174), pulmonary edema (175,176), and cardiac arrest (174,176). The cause of these serious side effects is unknown. A suggested etiology is abrupt withdrawal of analgesia with a resultant increase in sympathetic activity due to the sudden perception of pain. Most reports of complications with naloxone have occurred after cardiac surgery, but some have also occurred in young healthy women (176), with doses as small as 100 μg IV (174). Other more minor side effects of naloxone include emesis, restlessness, and shivering.

## REFERENCES

1. Benet LZ, Sheiner LB: Pharmacokinetics: The dynamics of drug absorption, distribution and elimination. *In* The Pharmacological Basis of Therapeutics. 7th Ed. Edited by AG Gilman, LS Goodman, TW Rall, F Murad. New York, MacMillan Publishing Co., 1985, pp. 3–34.
2. Levine RR: Pharmacology: Drug Actions and Reactions. 3rd Ed. Little, Brown and Co., Boston, 1983.
3. Green TP, O'Dea RF, Mirkin, BL: Determinants of drug disposition and effect in the fetus. Ann. Rev. Pharmacol. Toxicol. 19:285, 1979.
4. La Du BN, Mandel HG, Way EL: Fundamentals of Drug Metabolism and Drug Disposition. Baltimore, Williams and Wilkins, 1971.
5. Mazze RI, Caverly RK, Smith NT: Inorganic fluoride neph-

rotoxicity: prolonged enflurane and halothane anesthesia in volunteers. Anesthesiology 46:265, 1977.
6. Palahniuk RJ, Shnider SM, Eger EI II: Pregnancy decreases the requirement for inhaled anesthetic agents. Anesthesiology 41:82, 1974.
7. Hull CJ: Pharmacokinetics and pharmacodynamics. Br. J. Anaesth. 51:579, 1979.
8. Prys-Roberts C, Hug CC Jr: Pharmacokinetics of Anesthesia. Cambridge, MA, Blackwell Scientific Publications, 1984.
9. Ross EM, Gilman AG: Pharmacodynamics: Mechanisms of drug action and the relationship between drug concentration and effect. *In* The Pharmacological Basis of Therapeutics. 7th Ed. Edited by AG Gilman, LS Goodman, TW Rall, F Murad. New York, MacMillan Publishing Co., 1985, pp. 35–48.
10. Merryman W: Progesterone "anesthesia" in human subjects. J. Clin. Endocrinol. Metab. 14:1567, 1954.
11. Stoelting RK: Opiate receptors and endorphins: their role in anesthesiology. Anesth. Analg. 59:874, 1980.
12. Ebersole CM, Artagio JF Jr: Ether analgesia: inspired concentrations, flammability and levels in arterial blood. Anesthesiology 19:607–610, 1958.
13. Faulconer A Jr: Correlation of concentrations of ether in arterial blood with electroencephalograms patterns occurring during ether oxygen and during nitrous oxide oxygen and ether anesthesia of human surgical patients. Anesthesiology 13:361–369, 1952.
14. Dripps RD, Severinghaus JW: General anesthesia and respiration. Physiol. Rev. 35:741–777, 1955.
15. Jones RE, Linde HW, Deutsch S, Dripps RD, et al: Hemodynamic actions of diethyl ether in normal man. Anesthesiology 23:299–305, 1962.
16. Kubota Y, Scheizer HJ, Vndam LD: Hemodynamic effects of diethyl ether in man. Anesthesiology 23:306–314, 1962.
17. Vasicka A, Kretchmer H: The effect of conduction and inhalation anesthesia on uterine contractions. Am. J. Obstet. Gynecol. 82:600–611, 1961.
18. Terrell RC: Physical and chemical properties of anesthetic agents. Br. J. Anaesth. 56:3S, 1984.
19. Vitcha JF: A history of Forane. Anesthesiology 35:4, 1971.
20. Haumman JL, Foster PA: The antiemetic effect of halothane. Br. J. Anaesth. 35:114, 1963.
21. Crandell WB, Pappas SG, Macdonald A: Nephrotoxicity associated with methoxyflurane anesthesia. Anesthesiology 27:591, 1966.
22. Dooley JR, Mazze RI, Rice SA, Borel JD: Is enflurane defluorination inducible in man? Anesthesiology 50:213, 1979.
23. Chase RE, Holady DA, Fiserova-Bergerova V: The biotransformation of ethrane in man. Anesthesiology 35:262, 1971.
24. Corbett TH: Cancer and congenital anomalies associated with anesthetics. Ann. N. Y. Acad. Sci. 271:58, 1976.
25. Eger EI II, White AE, Brown CL, Brava CG, et al: A test of the carcinogenicity of enflurane, isoflurane, halothane, methoxyflurane and nitrous oxide in mice. Anesth. Analg. 57:678–694, 1978.
26. Holaday DA, Smith FR: Clinical characteristics and biotransformation of sevoflurane in healthy human volunteers. Anesthesiology 54:100, 1981.
27. Katoh T, Ikeda K: The minimum alveolar concentration (MAC) of sevoflurane in humans. Anesthesiology 66:301, 1987.
28. Manohar M: Regional brain blood flow and cerebral cortical $O_2$ consumption during sevoflurane anesthesia in healthy, isocapneic pigs. J. Cardiovasc. Pharmacol. 8:1268, 1986.
29. Eger EI II: Stability of I-653 in soda lime. Anesth. Analg. 66:983, 1987.
30. Yasuda N, Targ AG, Eger EI II: Solubility of I-653, sevoflurane, isoflurane, and halothane in human tissues. Anesth. Analg. 69:370–373, 1989.
31. Eger EI II: Applications of a mathematical model of gas uptake. *In* Uptake and Distribution of Anesthetic Agents. Edited by EM Papper, RJ Kitz. New York, McGraw-Hill Book Co., 1963, p. 96.
32. Van Dyke R: Biotransformation of volatile anesthetics with special emphasis on the role of metabolism in the toxicity of anesthetics. Can. Anaesth. Soc. J. 20:21, 1973.
33. Price HL, Price ML: Effects of general anesthetics on contractile response of rabbit aortic strips. Anesthesiology 23: 16, 1962.
34. Longnecker DE, Harris PD: Dilation of small arteries and veins in the rat during halothane anesthesia. Anesthesiology 37:423, 1972.
35. Sugai N, Shimosato S, Etsten BE: Effect of halothane on force velocity relationship and dynamic stiffness of isolated heart muscle. Anesthesiology 29:267, 1968.
36. Kemmotsu 0, Hashimoto Y, Shimosato S: Inotropic effects of isoflurane on mechanics of contraction in isolated cat papillar muscles from normal and failing hearts. Anesthesiology 39:470, 1973.
37. Stevens WC, Cromwell TH, Halsey MJ, Eger EI II, et al: The cardiovascular effects of a new inhalation anesthetic, Forane, in human volunteers at constant arterial carbon dioxide tension. Anesthesiology 35:8, 1971.
38. Eger EI II: Isoflurane (Forane): A Compendium and Reference. Madison, Wisconsin, Ohio Medical Products, 1981.
39. Atlee JL, Rusy BF: Atrioventricular conduction times and atrioventricular conductivity during enflurane anesthesia in dogs. Anesthesiology 47:498, 1977.
40. Imamura S, Ikeda K: Comparison of the epinephrine-induced arrhythmogenic effect of sevoflurane with isoflurane and halothane. J. Anesth. Japan 1:62, 1987.
41. Slogoff S, Keats AS: Randomized trial of primary anesthetic agents on outcome of coronary artery bypass operations. Anesthesiology 70:179, 1989.
42. Tuman KJ, McCarthy RJ, Spiess BD, DaValle M, et al: Does choice of anesthetic agent affect outcome after coronary artery surgery? Anesthesiology 70:189, 1989.
43. Kawamura R, Stanley TH, English JB, Hill GE, et al: Cardiovascular response to nitrous oxide exposure for two hours in man. Anesth. Analg. 59:93, 1980.
44. Johnston RR, Eger EI II, Wilson CA: A comparative interaction of epinephrine with enflurane, isoflurane and halothane in man. Anesth. Analg. 55:709, 1976.
45. Saidman LJ, Hamilton WK: We should continue to use nitrous oxide. *In* Nitrous Oxide/$N_2O$. Edited by Eger EI II. New york, Elsevier Publishers, 1985, p. 345.
46. Eger EI II: Should we not use nitrous oxide? *In* Nitrous Oxide/$N_2O$. Edited by Eger EI II. New york, Elsevier Publishers, 1985, p. 339.
47. Hirshman CA, Edelstein G, Peetz S, Wayne R, et al: Mechanism of action of inhalational anesthesia on airways. Anesthesiology 56:107, 1982.
48. Hirshman CA: Depression of hypoxic ventilatory response by halothane, enflurane and isoflurane in dogs. Br. J. Anaesth. 49:957, 1977.
49. Matsuyuki DM, Kazuyuki I: Respiratory effects of sevoflurane. Anesth. Anal. 66:241, 1987.
50. Wade JG, Stevens WC: Isoflurane: an anesthetic for the eighties? Anesth. Analg. 60:666, 1981.
51. Collins VJ: Antiemetic drugs, vomiting and aspiration. *In*

Principles of Anesthesiology. 2nd Ed. Philadelphia, Lea & Febiger, 1976, p. 1598.

52. Bellville JW: Postanesthetic nausea and vomiting. Anesthesiology 22:773, 1961.
53. Grady GF, Bennett AJ: Risk of post transfusion hepatitis in the United States. JAMA 220:692, 1973.
54. Aach RD, Kuhn RA: Post-transfusion hepatitis: current perspectives. Ann. Intern. Med. 92:539, 1982.
55. Dykes MHM: Anesthetic Hepatotoxicity. ASA refresher course in Anesthesiology 10:75, 1982.
56. Stevens WC, Eger EI II, Joas TA, et al: Comparative toxicity of isoflurane, halothane, fluroxene and diethyl ether in human volunteers. Can. Anaesth. Soc. J. 20:357, 1973.
57. Munson ES, Embro WJ: Enflurane, isoflurane and halothane and isolated human uterine muscle. Anesthesiology 46:11, 1977.
58. Warren TM, Datta S, Ostheimer GW, Naulty JS, et al: Comparison of the maternal and neonatal effects of halothane, enflurane and isoflurane for cesarean delivery. Anesth. Analg. 62:516, 1983.
59. Max GF, Kim YL, Lin CC, et al: Postpartum uterine pressure under halothane or enflurane anesthesia. Obstet. Gynecol. 51:695, 1978.
60. Cullen BF, Margolis AJ, Eger EI II: The effects of anesthesia and pulmonary ventilation on blood loss during elective therapeutic abortion. Anesthesiology 32:108, 1970.
61. Dolan WM, Eger EI II, Margolis AJ: Forane increases bleeding in therapeutic suction abortion. Anesthesiology 36:96, 1972.
62. Gibb CP, Munson ES, Min KT: Anesthetic solubility coefficients for maternal and fetal blood. Anesthesiology 43:100, 1975.
63. Palahniuk RJ, Shnider SM: Maternal and fetal cardiovascular and acid-base changes during halothane and isoflurane anesthesia in the pregnant ewe. Anesthesiology 41:462, 1974.
64. Dick W, Knocke E, Trant E: Clinical studies on the use of Ethrane in obstetrical anesthesia. Anaesthetist 26:381, 1977.
65. Ames BN, McCann J, Yamasaki E: Methods for detecting carcinogens and nitrogens with the salmonella/mammalian microsome mutagenicity test. Mutat. Res. 31:347, 1975.
66. Baden JM, Kelley M, Wharton RS, Hitt BA, et al: Mutagenicity of halogenated ether anesthetics. Anesthesiology 46: 346, 1977.
67. Waskell L: A study of the mutagenicity of anesthetics and their metabolites. Mutat. Res. 57:141, 1978.
68. Sachder K, Cohen EN, Simmons VF: Genotoxic and mutagenic assays of halothane metabolites in Bacillus subtilis and Salmonella typhimurium. Anesthesiology 53:31, 1980.
69. Fink BR, Shepard TH, Blandau RJ: Teratogenic activity of nitrous oxide. Nature 214:146, 1967.
70. Basford AB, Fink BR: The teratogenicity of halothane in the rat. Anesthesiology 29:1167, 1968.
71. Duncan PG, Pope WDB, Cohen MM, Greer N: Fetal risk of anesthesia and surgery during pregnancy. Anesthesiology 64:790, 1986.
72. Ferstanding LL: Trace concentrations of anesthetic gases. A critical review of their disease potential. Anesth. Analg. 57:328, 1978.
73. Lundy JS: Intravenous anesthesia: preliminary report of the use of two new thiobarbiturates. Proc. Staff Meet. Mayo Clin. 10:536, 1935.
74. Richter J, Waller MB: Effects of pentobarbitol on the regulation of acetylcholine content and release in different regions of rat brain. Biochem. Pharmacol. 26:609, 1977.
75. Ransom BR, Barker J: Pentobarbitol selectively enhances GABA mediated postsynaptic inhibition in tissue cultured mouse spinal neurons. Brain Res. 114:530, 1976.
76. Breimer DD: Pharmacokinetics of methohexitone following intravenous infusion in humans. Br. J. Anaesth. 48:643, 1976.
77. Eger EI II, Smith NT, Stoeling RK, Cullen DJ, et al: Cardiovascular effects of halothane in man. Anesthesiology 32: 396, 1970.
78. Calverly RK, Smith NT, Prys-Roberts C, et al: Cardiovascular effects of enflurane anesthesia during controlled ventilation in man. Anesth. Analg. 47:619, 1978.
79. Becker KE, Tonneson AS: Cardiovascular effect of plasma levels of thiopental necessary for anesthesia. Anesthesiology 49:197, 1978.
80. Yamamura T, Kimura T, Furukawa K: Effects of halothane, thiamylal and ketamine on central sympathetic and vagal tone. Anesth. Analg. 62:129, 1983.
81. Kosaka Y, Takahashi T, Mark LC: Intravenous thiobarbiturate anesthesia for cesarean section. Anesthesiology 31:489, 1969.
82. Finster M, Morishima HO, Mark LC, Perel JM, et al: Tissue thiopental concentrations in the fetus and newborn. Anesthesiology 36:155, 1972.
83. Woods W, Stanski DR, Curtis J, Rosen M, et al: The role of the fetal liver in the distribution of thiopental from mother to fetus. Anesthesiology 57:A390, 1982.
84. White PF: Propofol: Pharmacokinetics and pharmacodynamics. Seminars in Anesthesia 7:4, 1988.
85. Shafer A, Doze VA, Shafer SL, White PF: Pharmacokinetics and pharmacodynamics of propofol infusions during general anesthesia. Anesthesiology 69:348, 1988.
86. Coates DP, Monk CR, Prys-Roberts C, Turtle M: Hemodynamic effects of infusions of the emulsion formulation of propofol during nitrous oxide anesthesia in humans. Anesth. Analg. 66:64, 1987.
87. Goodman NW, Black AMS, Carter JA: Some ventilatory effects of propofol as a sole anaesthetic agent. Br. J. Anaesth. 59:1497, 1987.
88. Couper JL, Lombard TP: Comparison of propofol (Diprivan) with thiopental as induction agent for elective caesarean section. Can. J. Anaesth. 35:S132, 1988.
89. Celleno D, Capogna G, Tomassetti M, Costantino P, et al: Neurobehavioral effects of propofol on the neonate following elective cesarean section. Br. J. Anaesth. 62:649–654, 1989.
90. Moore J, Bill KM, Flynn RJ: A comparison between propofol and thiopentone as induction agents in obstetrical anaesthesia. Anaesthesia 44:753–757, 1989.
91. Gregory MA, Gin T, Yau G, Raymond KW, et al: Propofol infusion anaesthesia for cesarean section. Can. J. Anaesth. 37 (5):514–20, 1990.
92. Amiel-Tison C, Barrier G, Shnider SM, Levinson G, et al: A new neurologic and adaptive capacity scoring for evaluating obstetric medications in full term newborn. Anesthesiology 56:340, 1982.
93. Gin T, Gregory MA, Chan K, Buckley T, et al: Pharmacokinetics of propofol in women undergoing elective caesarean section. Br. J. Anaesth. 64:148, 1990.
94. Dailland P, Cockshott ID, Lirzin JD, Jacquinot P, et al: Intravenous propofol during cesarean section: placental transfer, concentration in breast milk, and neonatal effect. A preliminary study. Anesthesiology 71:827, 1989.
95. Sarnquist FH, Mathers WD, Brock-Utne J, Carr B, et al: A bioassay of water soluble benzodiazepines against sodium thiopental. Anesthesiology 52:149, 1980.
96. Jensen S, Schon-Olesen A, Hattel MS: Use of midazolam as

an induction agent: comparison with thiopentone. Br. J. Anaesth. 54:605, 1982.

97. Mohler H, Okada T: Benzodiazepine receptor: demonstration in the central nervous system. Science 198:849, 1977.
98. Richter JJ: Current theories about the mechanism of benzodiazepines and neuroleptic drugs. Anesthesiology 45:66, 1981.
99. Barchas JD, Akil H, Elliot GR: Behavioral neurochemistry: neuroregulators and behavioral states. Science 200:964, 1978.
100. Reves JG, Fragen RJ, Greenblatt DJ: Midazolam: pharmacology and uses. Anesthesiology 62:310–324, 1985.
101. Dundee JW, Pandit SK: Anterograde amnesic effects of pethidine, hyoscine and diazepam in adults. Br. J. Pharmacol. 44:140, 1972.
102. Dundee JW, Wilson DB: Amnesic action of midazolam. Anaesthesia 35:459, 1980.
103. Forster A, Juge O, Morel D: Effects of midazolam on cerebral blood flow in human volunteers. Anesthesiology 56: 453, 1982.
104. Nugent M, Artru AA, Michenfelder JD: Cerebral metabolic, vascular and protective effects of midazolam maleate. Anesthesiology 56:172, 1982.
105. Adams P, Gelman S, Reves JG, Greenblatt DJ, et al: Midazolam pharmacodynamics and pharmacokinetics during acute hypovolemia. Anesthesiology 63:140, 1985.
106. Ebert TJ, Kotrly KJ, Madsen KE, Bernstein JS, et al: Fentanyl-diazepam anesthesia with or without $N_2O$ does not attenuate cardiopulmonary baroreflex-mediated vasoconstrictor response to controlled hypovolemia in humans. Anesth. Analg. 67:548, 1988.
107. Catchlove RFH, Kafer ER: The effects of diazepam on the ventilatory response to carbon dioxide and on steady-state gas exchange. Anesthesiology 34:9, 1971.
108. Morel D, Forster A, Bachman M, Suter PM: Changes in breathing patterns induced by midazolam in normal subjects. Anesthesiology 57:A481, 1982
109. Scher J, Hailey DM, Beard RW: The effects of diazepam on the fetus. J. Obstet. Gynaecol. Br. Commonwealth 79:635, 1972.
110. Conklin KA, Graham CW, Murad S, Randal FM, et al: Midazolam and diazepam: maternal and fetal effects in the pregnant ewe. Obstet. Gynecol. 56:471, 1980.
111. Crawford ME, Carl P, Bach V, Ravlo O, et al: A randomized comparison between midazolam and thiopental for elective cesarean section anesthesia. I. Mother. Anesth. Analg. 68:229, 1989.
112. Ravlo O, Carl P, Crawford ME, Bach V, et al: A randomized comparison between midazolam and thiopental for elective cesarean section anesthesia. II. Neonates. Anesth. Analg. 68:234, 1989.
113. Kanto J: Use of benzodiazepines during pregnancy, labour and lactation, with particular references to pharmacokinetics considerations. Drugs 23:354, 1982.
114. Bach V, Carl P, Ravlo O, Crawford ME, et al: A randomized comparison between midazolam and thiopental for elective cesarean section anesthesia. III. Placental transfer and elimination in neonates. Anesth. Analg. 68:238, 1989.
115. White PF, Way WL, Trevor AJ: Ketamine—its pharmacology and therapeutic uses. Anesthesiology 56:119, 1982.
116. Takeshita H, Okuda Y, Sori A: The effects of ketamine on cerebral circulation and metabolism in man. Anesthesiology 36:69, 1972.
117. Celesia GG, Chen RC, Bamforth BJ: Effects of ketamine in epilepsy. Neurology 25:196, 1975.
118. Reder BS, Trapp LD, Troutman KC: Ketamine suppression of chemically induced convulsions in the two-day-old white leghorn cockerel. Anesth. Analg. 59: 406, 1980.
119. Diaz FA, Bianco A, Bello N, et al: Effects of ketamine on canine cardiovascular function. Br. J. Anaesth. 48:941, 1976.
120. Smith G, Thorburn J, Vance JP, et al: The effects of ketamine on the canine coronary circulation. Anesthesiology 34:555 1979.
121. Gooding JM, Dimick AR, Tavakoli M: A physiologic analysis of cardiopulmonary responses to ketamine anesthesia in noncardiac patients. Anesth. Analg. 56:813, 1977.
122. Hirshman CA, Downes H, Farbood A, Bergman NA: Ketamine block of bronchospasm in experimental canine asthma. Br. J. Anaesth. 51:713, 1979.
123. Soliman MG, Brinale GF, Kuster G: Response to hypercapnia under ketamine anesthesia. Can. Anaesth. Soc. J. 22: 486, 1975.
124. Akamatsu TJ, Boreca JJ, Rehmet R: Experiences with the use of ketamine for parturition. I. Primary anesthetic for vaginal delivery. Anesth. Analg. 53:284, 1974.
125. Marx GF, Cabe CM, Kim YI, et al: Neonatal blood pressures. Anaesthetist 25:318, 1976.
126. Dich-Nielsen J, Holasek J: Ketamine as induction agent for cesarean section. Acta. Anesthesiol. Scand. 26:139, 1982.
127. Collier BB: Ketamine and the conscious mind. Anaesthesia 27:120, 1972.
128. Hejja P, Galloon S: A consideration of ketamine dreams. Can. Anaesth. Soc. J. 22:100, 1975.
129. Patschke D, Brückner JB, Eberlein HJ, Hess W, et al: Effects of anaesthesia, etomidate and fentanyl on haemodynamics and myocardial consumption in man. Can. Anaesth. Soc. J. 24:57, 1977.
130. Baiker-Heberlein M, Kenius P, Kikillus H, et al: Investigations on the site of the central nervous system action of the short acting hypnotic agent "etomidate" in cats. Anaesthetist 28:78, 1979.
131. Evans RH, Hill RG: GABA-mimetic action of etomidate. Experientia 34:1325, 1978.
132. Meuldermans W, Heykants J: The plasma protein binding and distribution of etomidate in dog, rat, and human blood. Arch. Int. Pharmacodyn. Ther. 221:150, 1976.
133. Holdcroft A, Morgan M, Whitman JG, Lumley J: Effect of dose and premedication on induction complications with etomidate. Br. J. Anaesth. 48:199, 1976.
134. Kaplan JA: Cardiac Anaesthesia, Vol 2: Cardiovascular Pharmacology. New York, Grune and Stratton, 1983, p. 13.
135. Tarabadkar S, Kopriva CJ, Sreenivasan N, Lescovich F, et al: Hemodynamic impact of induction in patients with decreased cardiac reserve. Anesthesiology 53:(S)543, 1980.
136. Choi SD, Spaulding BC, Gross JB, Apfelbaum JL: Comparison of the ventilatory effects of etomidate and methohexital. Anesthesiology 62:442, 1985.
137. Owen H, Spence AA: Etomidate. Br. J. Anaesth. 56:555, 1984.
138. Wagner RL, White PF, Kan PB, Rosenthal MH, et al: Inhibition of adrenal steroidogenesis by the anesthetic etomidate. N. Engl. J. Med. 310:1415, 1984.
139. Ghoneim MM, Yamada T: Etomidate: a clinical and electroencephalograms comparison with thiopental. Anesth. Analg. 56:479, 1977.
140. Downing JW, Buley RJB, Brock-Utne JG, et al: Etomidate for induction of anaesthesia at cesarean section: comparison with thiopental. Br. J. Anaesth. 51:135, 1979.
141. Suresh MS, Solanski DR, Andrew JJ, et al: Comparison of etomidate with thiopental for induction of anesthesia at cesarean section. Society of Obstetric Anesthesia and Perinatology, 18th annual meeting, 1986, p. 23.

142. Chou DT, Wong SC: Studies on the localization of central cough mechanisms. Sites of action of antitussive drugs. J. Pharmacol. Exp. Ther. 194:499, 1975.
143. Reiton JA, Stengert KB, Wymore ML, Martucci RW: Central vagal control of fentanyl induced bradycardia during halothane anesthesia. Anesth. Analg. 57:31, 1978.
144. Urthaler F, Isobe JH, James TN: Direct and vagally mediated chronotropic effects of morphine studied by selective perfusion of the sinus node of awake dogs. Chest 68:222, 1975.
145. Lowenstein E, Whiting RB, Bittar D, Sanders CA, et al: Local and neurally mediated effect of morphine on skeletal muscle vascular resistance. J. Pharmacol. Exp. Ther. 180:359, 1972.
146. Lowenstein E, Hallowell P, Levine FH, et al: Cardiovascular response to large doses of intravenous morphine in man. N. Engl. J. Med. 281:1389, 1969.
147. Thompson WL, Walton RP: Elevation of plasma histamine levels in the dog following administration of muscle relaxants, opiates, and macromolecular polymers. J. Pharmacol. Exp. Ther. 143:131, 1966.
148. Kitahata LM, Collins JG: Narcotic Analgesics in Anesthesiology. Baltimore, Williams and Wilkins, 1982.
149. Monk J: Sufentanil: a review. Drugs 36:249–381, 1988.
150. Sethna DH, Moffitt EA, Gray RJ, Bussell J, et al: Cardiovascular effects on morphine in patients with coronary arterial disease. Anesth. Analg. 61:109, 1982.
151. Henney RP, Vasko JS, Brawley RK, et al: The effects of morphine on the resistance and capacitance vessels of the peripheral circulation. Am. Heart J. 72:242, 1966.
152. Gilman AG, Goodman LS, Rall TW, Murad F: The Pharmacological Basis of Therapeutics. 7th Ed. New York, MacMillan Publishing Company, 1985, pp. 502–503.
153. Radnay PA, Brodman E, Mankikar D, et al: The effect of equianalgesic doses of fentanyl, morphine, meperidine and pentazocine on common bile duct pressure. Anaesthetist 29:26, 1980.
154. Papper S, Papper EM: The effects of preanesthetic, anesthetic and postoperative drugs on renal function. Clin. Pharmacol. Ther. 5:205, 1963.
155. Shute E, Davis ME: The effect on the infant of morphine administered in labor. Surg. Gynecol. Obstet. 57:727, 1933.
156. Way WL, Castle EC, Way EL: Respiratory sensitivity of the newborn infant to meperidine and morphine. Clin. Pharmacol. Ther. 6:454, 1965.
157. Grimwade J, Walker D, Wood C: Morphine and the fetal heart rate. Br. Med. J. 3:373, 1971.
158. Petrie RH, Yeh SY, Murata Y, et al: The effect of drugs on fetal heart rate variability. Am. J. Obstet. Gynecol. 130:294, 1978.
159. Shnider SM, Moya F: Effects of meperidine on the newborn infant. Am. J. Obstet. Gynecol. 89:1009, 1964.
160. Morrison JC, Whybrew WD, Rosser SI, et al: Metabolites of meperidine in the fetal and maternal serum. Am. J. Obstet. Gynecol. 126:997, 1976.
161. Morrison JC, Wiser WL, Rosser SI, et al: Metabolites of meperidine related to fetal depression. Am. J. Obstet. Gynecol. 115:1132, 1973.
162. Forrest WH, Bellville JW: Respiratory effects of alphaprodine in man. Obstet. Gynecol. 31:61, 1968.
163. Gray JH, Codmore DW, Luther ER, et al: Sinusoidal fetal heart rate pattern associated with alphaprodine administration. Obstet. Gynecol. 52:678, 1978.
164. Eisele JH, Wright R, Rogge P: Newborn and maternal fentanyl levels at cesarean section. Anesth. Analg. 61:179, 1982.
165. Kaplan JA: Cardiac Anesthesia, Volume 2. Cardiovascular Pharmacology. New York, Grune and Stratton, 1983, p. 38.
166. Lowenstein E: Morphine "anesthesia"—a perspective. Anesthesiology 35:563, 1971.
167. Stanley TH: Opiate anesthesia. Anaesthesia Intensive Care 15:38, 1987.
168. Bovill JG, Sebel PS, Blackburn CL, Oei-Lim V, et al: The pharmacokinetics of sufentanil in surgical patients. Anesthesiology 61:502, 1984.
169. Shafer A, Sung M-L, White PF: Pharmacokinetics and pharmacodynamics of alfentanil infusions during general anesthesia. Anesth. Analg. 65:1021, 1986.
170. Flacke JW, Bloor BC, Kripke BJ, Flacke WE, et al: Comparison of morphine, meperidine, fentanyl, and sufentanil in balanced anesthesia. Anesth. Analg. 64:897, 1985.
171. de Lange S, Boscoe MJ, Stanley TH, Pace N: Comparison of sufentanil $O_2$, and fentanyl $O_2$ for coronary artery surgery. Anesthesiology 56:112, 1982.
172. Freund FG, Martin WE, Wong KC, Hornbein TF: Abdominal muscle rigidity induced by morphine and nitrous oxide. Anesthesiology 38:358, 1973.
173. Azar I, Turndorf H: Severe hypotension and multiple atrial premature contractions following naloxone administration. Anesth. Analg. 58:524–525, 1979.
174. Michaelis LL, Hickey PR, Clark TA, et al: Ventricular irritability associated with the use of naloxone hydrochloride. Ann. Thorac. Surg. 18:608–614, 1974.
175. Flacke JW, Flacke WE, Williams GD: Acute pulmonary edema following naloxone reversal of higher dose morphine anesthesia. Anesthesiology 47:376, 1977.
176. Andrea RA: Sudden death following naloxone administration. Anesth. Analg. 59:782, 1980.

# Chapter 19

# BASIC PRINCIPLES OF GENERAL ANALGESIA AND ANESTHESIA FOR OBSTETRICS

MARK A. MORGAN
JOHN I. FISHBURNE, JR

This chapter contains a comprehensive discussion of the general principles and techniques of providing analgesia and anesthesia to gravidae and parturients with inhalation, intravenous, and other parenteral agents.

Systemic drugs such as opioids and inhalation agents, in subanesthetic concentrations, are used primarily to provide partial relief of pain for the first stage of labor, and frequently also for the second stage and the postpartum period. The advantages of analgesia are that the mother remains awake through the process of parturition, can cooperate and maintain protective pharyngeal and laryngeal reflexes, while accruing the advantage of partial pain relief. General anesthesia is the administration of intravenous, inhalation, and other agents with intent to produce unconsciousness for the purpose of performing cesarean section or operative vaginal delivery.

These methods of producing analgesia and anesthesia have been used in obstetric practice since Sir James Simpson first administered diethyl ether to a parturient in January 1847, and for the first century thereafter these techniques were preeminent in obstetric practice. Although the use of regional analgesia has increased progressively during the past 50 years, analgesia achieved with systemic opioids and other drugs and/or subanesthetic doses of inhalation agents is still being used widely in the United Kingdom, Scandinavia, and a number of developing countries. Even in the United States it is still used during the first stage of labor, as illustrated by the Gibbs, et al survey, which showed that in 1986 inhalation and/or systemic analgesia was used in approximately 50% of parturients, the largest portion with systemic analgesia (1). Certainly, the use of analgesic inhalation agents is rare today for normal vaginal delivery in both the United States and the United Kingdom; nevertheless, inhalation analgesia and general anesthesia may remain important methods of providing pain relief during labor and vaginal delivery in other countries throughout the world, as well as for cesarean section and surgical procedures in pregnancy. Tables 19–1, 19–2, 19–3, and 19–4 indicate obstetric anesthesia procedures and personnel performing them.

The object of this chapter is to present a discussion of general basic principles and technique of administration of various agents to achieve analgesia and anesthesia for parturients. The information is presented in two major sections: (1) analgesia achieved primarily with inhalation agents, but often complemented with opioids and other systemic drugs; and (2) balanced general anesthesia. Each section will consider the "Pharmacology in Parturients," including efficacy and side effects on the mother, fetus, and newborn, with descriptions of the technical aspects of their administration. A detailed description of the pharmacology, including pharmacokinetics and pharmacodynamics of inhalation and intravenous agents and muscle relaxants, is found in Chapter 18, while a detailed discussion of placental transfer of these agents and their

**Table 19–1.** Anesthetic Procedures Used for Labor and Personnel Performing Them

| | Hospitals (%) | | | |
|---|---|---|---|---|
| **Procedure** | **Stratum I (>1500 births)** | **Stratum II (500–1,499 births)** | **Stratum III (<500 births)** | **All Strata** |
| No anesthesia | 27 | 33 | 45 | 32 |
| Intermittent inhalation | 0 | 0 | 0 | 0 |
| Narcotics/barbiturates/tranquilizers | 52 | 53 | 37 | 49 |
| Paracervical | 5 | 5 | 6 | 5 |
| Epidural | 22 | 13 | 9 | 16 |
| Anesthesiologist or CRNA directed by one | 70 | 61 | 35 | 62 |
| CRNA directed by an obstetrician | 4 | 8 | 10 | 6 |
| Obstetric specialist or resident | 26 | 31 | 46 | 30 |
| Other personnel | 0 | 0 | 10 | 1.3 |
| Total | 106* | 104* | 97† | 102* |

* Values add to greater than 100% because in some cases more than one procedure was used.
† Values add to less than 100% because some respondents failed to answer all questions.
(From Gibbs CP, Krischer J, Peckham BM, Shart H, et al: Obstetric anesthesia: a national survey. Anesthesiology 65:298–306, 1986.)

**Table 19–2.** Anesthetic Procedures Used for Cesarean Section and Personnel Performing Them

| Procedure | Hospitals (%) | | | |
|---|---|---|---|---|
| | Stratum I (>1500 births) | Stratum II (500–1,499 births) | Stratum III (<500 births) | All Strata |
| Epidural block | 29 | 16 | 12 | 21 |
| Anesthesiologist or CRNA directed by one | 89 | 83 | 61 | 84 |
| CRNA directed by an obstetrician | 4 | 11 | 15 | 7 |
| Obstetric specialist or resident | 8 | 6 | 20 | 9 |
| Other personnel | 0 | 0 | 3 | 0.4 |
| Spinal Block | 33 | 35 | 37 | 34 |
| Anesthesiologist or CRNA directed by one | 94 | 86 | 49 | 83 |
| CRNA directed by an obstetrician | 4 | 8 | 39 | 12 |
| Obstetric specialist or resident | 2 | 5 | 7 | 4 |
| Other personnel | 0 | 0 | 6 | 1 |
| General anesthesia | 35 | 45 | 46 | 41 |
| Anesthesiologist or CRNA directed by one | 86 | 74 | 44 | 74 |
| CNRA directed by an obstetrician | 14 | 27 | 55 | 25 |
| Other personnel | 0.1 | 0.1 | 2 | 0.4 |
| Total | 97* | 96* | 95* | 96* |

* Values add to less than 100% because some respondents failed to answer all questions.
(From Gibbs CP, Krischer J, Peckham BM, Shart H, et al: Obstetric anesthesia: a national survey. Anesthesiology 65:298–306, 1986.)

**Table 19–3.** Personnel Performing Newborn Resuscitation

| Personnel | Hospitals | | | |
|---|---|---|---|---|
| | Stratum I (>1500 births) | Stratum II (500–1,499 births) | Stratum III (<500 births) | All Strata |
| Vaginal delivery (n)* | 112 | 56 | 56 | 224 |
| Anesthesiologist or CRNA directed by one (%) | 18 | 9 | 1 | 12 |
| CRNA directed by an obstetrician (%) | 5 | 12 | 12 | 9 |
| Obstetrician (%) | 37 | 47 | 32 | 37 |
| Pediatrician (%) | 36 | 26 | 13 | 28 |
| Other personnel (%) | 4 | 6 | 43 | 14 |
| Cesarean section (n)* | 125 | 70 | 58 | 253 |
| Anesthesiologist or CRNA directed by one (%) | 22 | 20 | 12 | 19 |
| CRNA directed by an obstetrician (%) | 2 | 3 | 11 | 4 |
| Obstetrician (%) | 4 | 5 | 6 | 5 |
| Pediatrician (%) | 70 | 70 | 46 | 64 |
| Other personnel (%) | 2 | 2 | 24 | 7 |

Questionnaire responses adding to more than 100% excluded.
* (n) refers to number of valid responses.
(From Gibbs CP, Krischer J, Peckham BM, Shart H, et al: Obstetric anesthesia: a national survey. Anesthesiology 65:298–306, 1986.)

effects on the fetus and newborn is contained in Chapter 8.

## Inhalation Analgesia

### *Introduction*

Analgesia during labor attained sovereign and ecclesiastical approval when Queen Victoria announced she would have chloroform, administered on a silk handkerchief by John Snow, during her labor and for the delivery of Prince Leopold (2). Since then, many different inhalation analgesics have been used during the labor process. Historically, chloroform, diethyl ether, and nitrous oxide were most commonly utilized as described in Chapter 1. More recently, three other agents have been used for inhalation analgesia; trichloroethylene, nitrous oxide, and methoxyflurane. Other volatile inhalation agents such as halothane and isoflurane can also be used as analgesics during labor.

Inhalation analgesia is popular in the United Kingdom and in other countries where regional analgesia is infrequently administered. Many of these agents are used as the sole analgesic in labor. However, they can be used, under careful supervision, with intravenous narcotics and occasionally as a supplement to regional analgesia. Patients for whom inhalation analgesia may be used include those who have refused regional analgesia, and those for whom its use may be contraindicated.

### *Clinical Pharmacology*

Characteristics of the commonly used inhalation analgesia agents, those agents most used in the past, and other potential agents, are given in Table 19–5. Although it had been initially reported that methoxyflurane was more effective at producing analgesia than nitrous oxide or trichloroethylene (3–5), more extensive investigations have shown that each of these agents produces complete analgesia in only 10% of patients, while 30% experience little or no analgesia (6–8).

As illustrated in Table 19–5, nitrous oxide is a relatively insoluble gas, thus limiting its accumulation in maternal blood. As a result, analgesia will only be acquired after breathing nitrous oxide for approximately 45 seconds (Figure 19–1). This is in sharp contrast to trichloroethylene (Figure 19–2) and methoxyflurane, which are relatively soluble agents. Because of their delayed clearances, a more prolonged time of inhalation is required to achieve analgesia. Maternal and fetal accumulations of trichloroethylene and methoxyflurane make them unsuitable for more than 2 hours of use (9,10). None of the inhalation analgesic agents adversely affect the progress of labor

**Table 19–4.** Availability of In-house Anesthesia Personnel for Labor and Delivery

| | Stratum I (>1500 births) | | | Stratum II (500–1,499 births) | | | Stratum III (<500 births) | | | Total | | |
|---|---|---|---|---|---|---|---|---|---|---|---|---|
| | % | N* | Total† | % | N* | Total† | % | N* | Total† | % | N* | Total† |
| Full time‡ | | | | | | | | | | | | |
| Anesthesiologist | | | | | | | | | | | | |
| Weekdays | 38 | 86 | 226 | 8 | 13 | 168 | 3 | 2 | 83 | 21 | 101 | 481 |
| Nights/weekends | 27 | 58 | 215 | 7 | 12 | 168 | 2 | 2 | 82 | 15 | 69 | 463 |
| CRNA | | | | | | | | | | | | |
| Weekdays | 19 | 40 | 209 | 8 | 13 | 160 | 6 | 5 | 86 | 13 | 59 | 457 |
| Nights/weekends | 21 | 45 | 212 | 10 | 16 | 158 | 8 | 7 | 88 | 15 | 69 | 463 |
| Others | | | | | | | | | | | | |
| Weekdays | 5 | 9 | 174 | 2 | 3 | 134 | 6 | 4 | 71 | 5 | 19 | 383 |
| Nights/weekends | 4 | 7 | 174 | 3 | 4 | 134 | 6 | 4 | 71 | 4 | 15 | 376 |
| Shared time§ | | | | | | | | | | | | |
| Anesthesiologist | | | | | | | | | | | | |
| Weekdays | 51 | 114 | 223 | 54 | 96 | 177 | 20 | 16 | 81 | 45 | 216 | 481 |
| Nights/weekends | 49 | 109 | 223 | 44 | 75 | 170 | 16 | 13 | 82 | 40 | 190 | 175 |
| CRNA | | | | | | | | | | | | |
| Weekdays | 17 | 31 | 185 | 27 | 41 | 151 | 29 | 25 | 86 | 23 | 97 | 420 |
| Nights/weekends | 19 | 36 | 190 | 25 | 37 | 149 | 27 | 23 | 86 | 23 | 98 | 426 |
| Others | | | | | | | | | | | | |
| Weekdays | 6 | 10 | 163 | 4 | 5 | 124 | 11 | 8 | 69 | 6 | 21 | 352 |
| Nights/weekends | 5 | 8 | 163 | 4 | 5 | 124 | 11 | 8 | 69 | 6 | 21 | 358 |

* Number of positive responses.
† Total number of responses.
‡ Assigned only to labor and delivery without other duties.
§ Assigned to labor and delivery and other duties.
(From Gibbs CP, Krischer J, Peckham BM, Shart H, et al: Obstetric anesthesia: a national survey. Anesthesiology 65:298–306, 1986.)

(10–12). Similarly, when nitrous oxide, trichloroethylene, and methoxyflurane have been used in analgesic concentrations, no adverse fetal/neonatal effects have been observed (10). More detail on the pharmacologic effects of these agents can be found in Chapter 18.

### *Technical Considerations*

Nitrous oxide can be delivered in an intermittent flow, self-administered manner, using the Lucy Baldwin apparatus. This apparatus employs gas cylinders of oxygen and nitrous oxide, with mixing occurring in a separate chamber. A variable amount of oxygen, 30 to 50%, can be delivered to the patient along with nitrous oxide. This apparatus has been useful in managing painful labor (13,14). More recently, nitrous oxide has been delivered to the laboring patient with the Entonox apparatus developed by Tunstall (15). Nitrous oxide and oxygen in a 50:50 mixture are contained in one cylinder, which is equipped with a pressure gauge, demand valve, and pressure-reducing valve. The pressure-reducing valve is connected by corrugated tubing to the face mask or mouth piece. An exhalation valve is also in the circuit (Figure 19–3) (16). The Entonox cylinder should be kept at a temperature that does not fall below −7° C to prevent separation of the gases (17). If cooling below this temperature is a pos-

**Table 19–5.** Inhalation Analgesia Agents in Obstetrics

| Agent | MW | Solubility Coefficient Blood/Gas | % Inhaled |
|---|---|---|---|
| Nitrous oxide | 44 | 0.47 | 50.00 |
| Trichloroethylene | 131 | 9.20 | 0.35 to 0.50 |
| Methoxyflurane | 165 | 13.00 | 0.35 |
| Halothane | 197 | 2.54 | 0.75 |
| Isoflurane | 185 | 1.38 | 0.50 |
| Enflurane | 185 | 1.90 | 0.50 |
| Cyclopropane | 42 | 0.42 | 5.00 |
| Diethyl ether | 74 | 12.10 | 1.00 |
| Desflurane | 168 | 0.42 | 3.00 |
| Sevoflurane | 200 | 0.68 | 0.75 |

MW = molecular weight

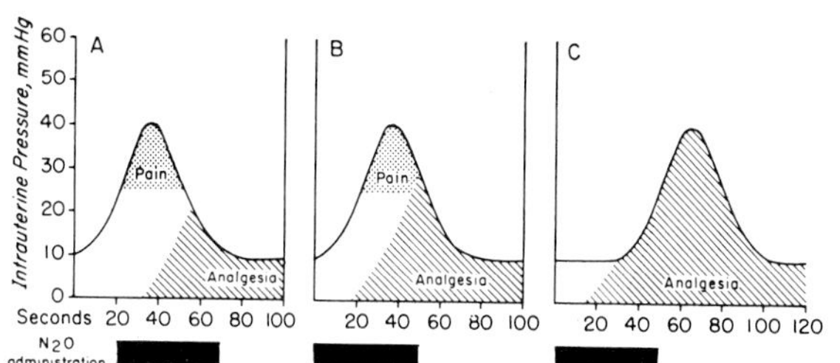


**Fig. 19–1.** Relation between time of onset of uterine contraction, of pain due to the contraction, and of analgesia produced with intermittent administration (six big breaths) of nitrous oxide during mid-first stage of labor. **A,** The nitrous oxide is started at the time the patient feels the pain. **B,** The nitrous oxide is started at the time the contraction starts. **C,** The nitrous oxide is started 30 seconds before the predicted time of onset of contraction, so that the patient experiences analgesia for the entire contraction.

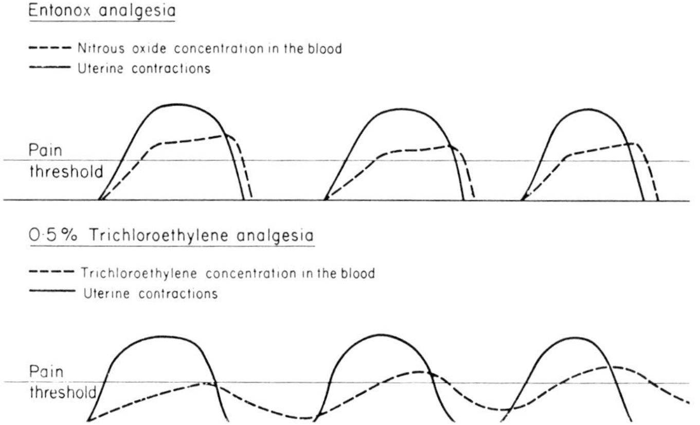


**Fig. 19–2.** A diagrammatic representation of the analgesic action of Entonox and trichloroethylene. (Modified from Moir DD, Carty MJ: Pain relief in labour—systemic and inhalation analgesia. In Obstetric Anaesthesia and Analgesia. Edited by DD Moir, MJ Carty. London, Bailliere Tindall, 1980.)

sibility, then the cylinders should be stored in a horizontal position, which allows for less differential gas delivery.

Trichloroethylene, due to its low volatility, is best administered with a vaporizer. Many devices are available, including the Duke inhaler, the Airlene vaporizer, the Tecota Mark VI vaporizer, and the Emotril automatic trilene inhaler. These devices all permit self-administration of the agent. The Duke inhaler, when filled, contains 15 ml of trichloroethylene and is lightweight, allowing it to be hand-held (Figure 19–4). This inhaler is not temperature compensated and should only be used in a controlled environment. In contrast, the Airlene vaporizer is temperature compensated and has three settings, delivering concentrations of 0.35, 0.5 or 1.1%. The only two approved inhalers in the United Kingdom are the Tecota Mark VI and the Emotril automatic trilene inhaler (10). These inhalers are similar and are temperature compensated (Figure 19–5 and 19–6).

Methoxyflurane, with its similarity in physical properties to trichloroethylene, can also be delivered by hand-held vaporizer. The Cardiff inhaler (Figure 19–7) has been the only delivery device approved in the United

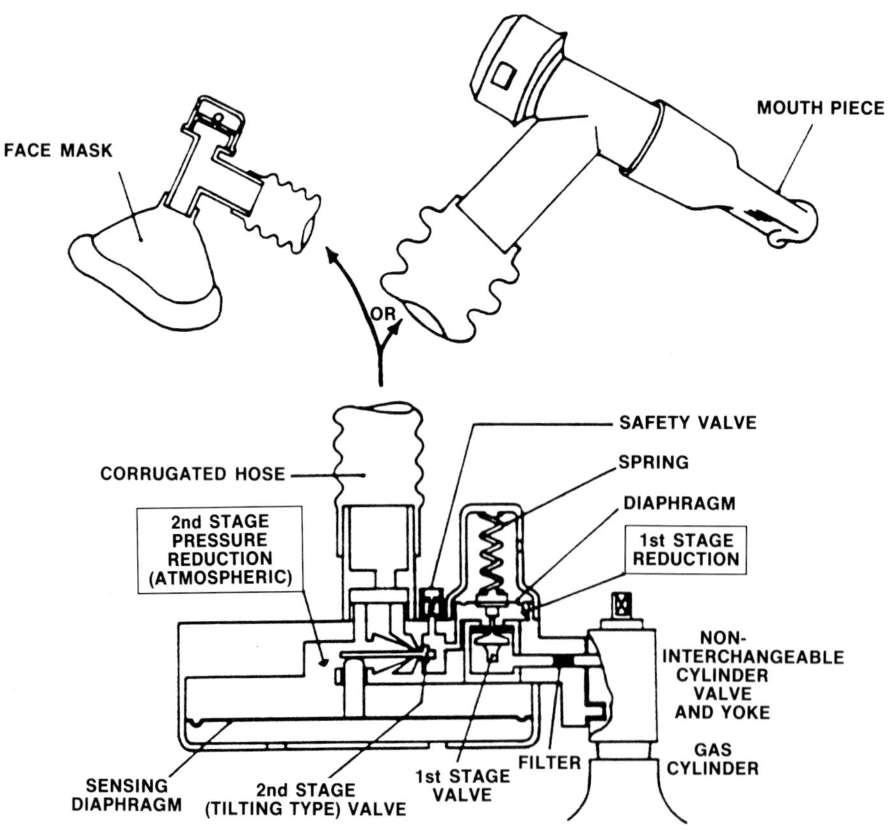


**Fig. 19–3.** Entonox apparatus for $N_2O$ inhalation analgesia during. labor. (From Crawford JS: Principles and Practice of Obstetric Anesthesia. 5th Edition. Cambridge, MA, Blackwell Scientific, 1984.)

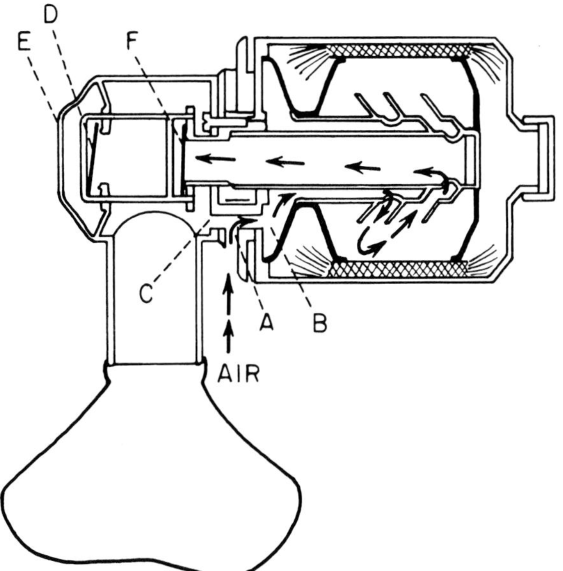


**Fig. 19–4.** Cross section of a Cyprane Inhaler, a semi-open, non-rebreathing vaporizer used for trichloroethylene and other volatile anesthetics. As the patient inspires, air is drawn through the hose located in the mixture-adjusting collar **(A)**. It is then directed down into the mixing chamber through slots in **(B)** as shown by arrows, or directed upward toward the face piece through slots in **(C)** or through both, depending on the setting of the mixture-adjusting collar. Rotating the mixture-adjusting collar alters the relative areas of opening for the parts in (B) and (C) so that more or less air bypasses the vaporizing chamber. On expiration, the gases are directed to the atmosphere through the valve **(D)** and holes in the side of the cover **(E)**. Non-return valve **(F)** prevents the expired gases from passing through the vaporizing chamber.

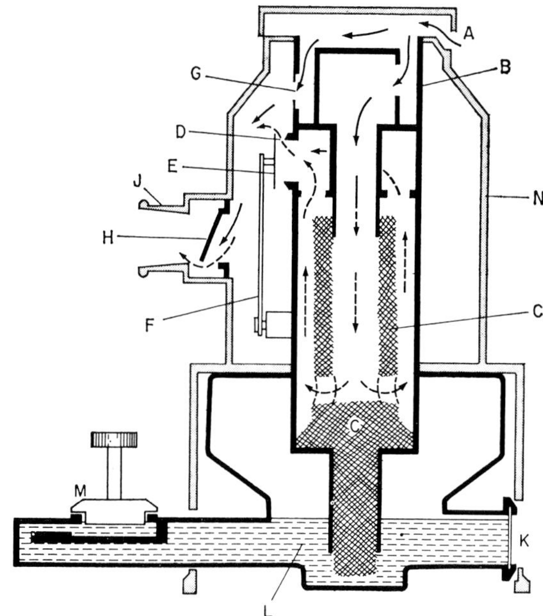


**Fig. 19–5.** Cross sectional diagram of the Tecota Mark 6 Inhaler. Air enters at **(A)** and forms two streams. One stream passes directly to the one-way valve **(H)** and onwards to the patient. The other stream enters the vaporizing chamber **(B)** and picks up trichloroethylene vapor from the wicks **(C)**. The trichloroethylene and air mixture now leaves the vaporizing chamber through orifice **(D)**. The size of orifice **(D)** is controlled by a valve **(E)** which is operated by the expansion or contraction of the bimetal strip **(F)** in response to temperature changes. The patient thus receives a mixture of trichloroethylene and air whose composition is unaffected by temperature. The two air streams merge and are inhaled by the patient. **(J)** is the breathing tube mount. **(M)** is the filler orifice and **(K)** is a window for observation of the liquid level. (Moir DD, Carty MJ: Pain relief in labour—systemic and inhalation analgesia. In: Obstetric Anaesthesia and Analgesia. Edited by DD Moir, MJ Carty. London, Bailliere Tindall, 1980.)

Kingdom for inhalation analgesia with methoxyflurane (18), and is temperature controlled. If it were not, an excessively high concentration of methoxyflurane could be delivered. Methoxyflurane in analgesic concentrations has not been known to cause fluoride nephrotoxicity (19).

### *Technique of Administration*

Many techniques have been used for administration of inhalation analgesia. These have included intermittent use by the patient herself, by an anesthesiologist, and/or by continuous administration. The timing of administration is dependent on several factors. These include the patient's progress in labor, the intensity of her pain, the specific obstetric requirements, the other agents that have been, or will be administered for analgesia or anesthesia, and whether the inhalation analgesia is administered by the patient herself or by an anesthesiologist. Each of the three previously discussed inhalation analgesics will be addressed as to their mode of administration.

Nitrous oxide can be administered either continuously or intermittently. Continuous administration has the advantage of maintaining an even concentration (20). Analgesia should be initiated with 35% nitrous oxide and 65% oxygen by face mask and increased as required. Usually, 40% to 45% nitrous oxide with oxygen is sufficient to provide analgesia if psychologic support is also given. The intermittent administration of nitrous oxide is more complicated. When the pattern of 4 or 5 contractions is observed, nitrous oxide in oxygen is begun 20 to 30 seconds before the predicted time of the onset of each subsequent contraction. This method is best used toward the end of the first stage and in the early second stage of labor.

Trichloroethylene and methoxyflurane are commonly administered in a similar manner. Analgesia is initiated with 10 to 12 breaths of the agent and continued on an intermittent basis beginning 15 to 20 seconds before each contraction. Because these agents can build up over time and have potentially adverse effects, their administration should be limited to 2 hours (9,10).

## General (Balanced) Anesthesia

### *Introduction*

Anesthesia for the obstetric patient has long been a subject of controversy. Gibbs, et al surveyed anesthesiologists

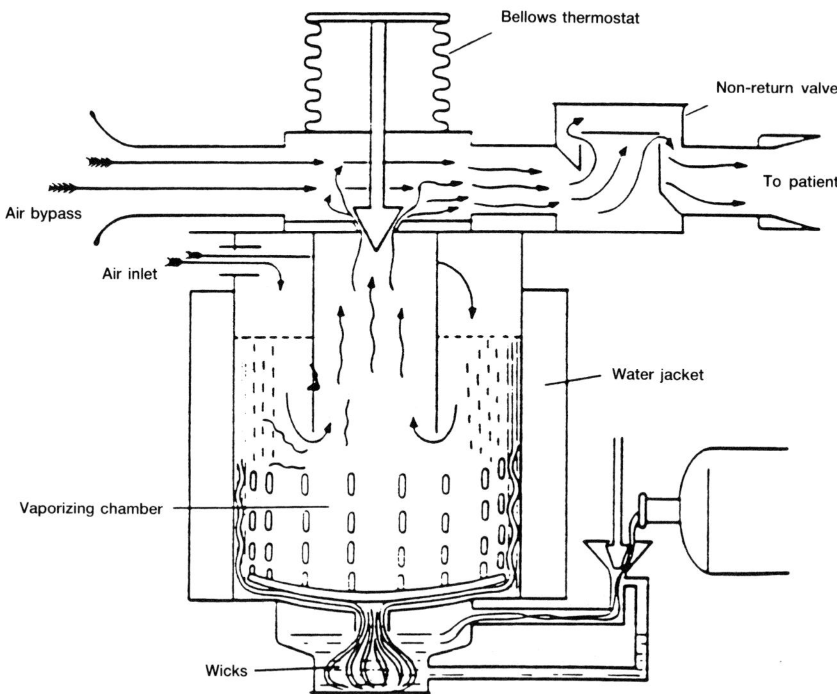


**Fig. 19–6.** The vaporizing chamber of the Emotril Inhaler. (Moir DD, Carty MJ: Pain relief in labour—systemic and inhalation analgesia. In: Obstetric Anaesthesia and Analgesia. Edited by DD Moir, MJ Carty. London, Bailliere Tindall, 1980.)

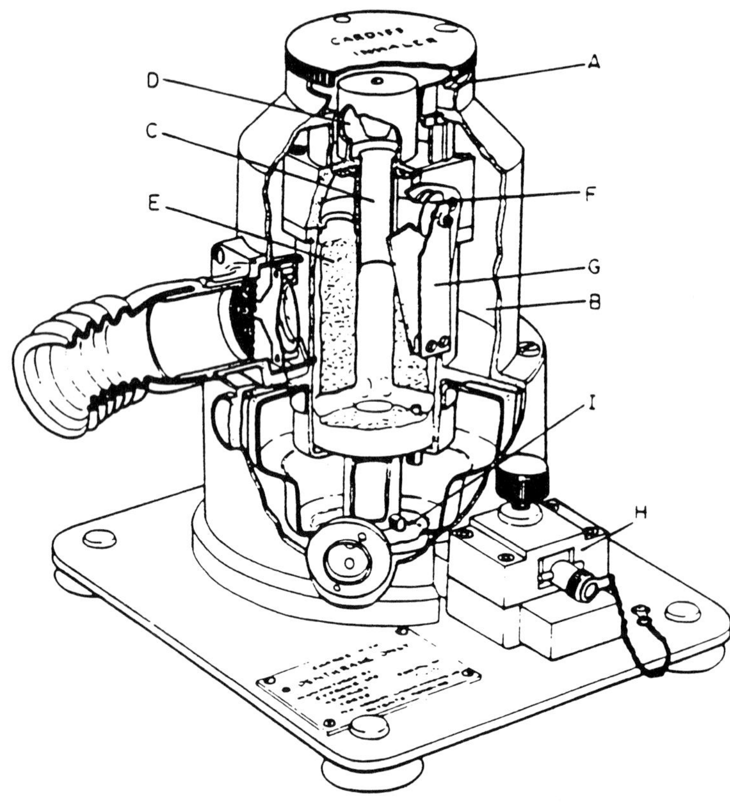


**Fig. 19–7.** A circuit diagram of the Cardiff Inhaler. Air enters at ports **(A).** Some of this air enters the mixing chamber **(B)** directly. The remainder of the air enters the vaporizing chamber **(C)** through port **(D)** and is saturated with methoxyflurane vapor as it passes over the surface of the wick **(E).** This saturated air now emerges through port **(F)** into the mixing chamber **(B)** where it is diluted with air. The final concentration of methoxyflurane vapor is maintained at 0.35% in air, despite fluctuations in environmental temperature, by variations in the size of the port **(F)** effected by a bimetal strip device strip device **(G).** The inhaler is filled from a Penthrane bottle with filler attachment. The liquid is poured in at **(H)** where there is a Frazer-Sweatman pin index fitting, enters the sump **(I)** and is soaked up in the wick **(E).** (Moir DD, Carty MJ: Pain relief in labour—systemic and inhalation analgesia. In: Obstetric Anaesthesia and Analgesia. Edited by DD Moir, MJ Carty. London, Bailliere Tindall, 1980.)

and obstetricians in an attempt to identify why they no longer practiced obstetric anesthesia. Unpredictability of working hours and isolation of labor and delivery from general operating suites, along with family members' presence in labor and delivery rooms were identified as the major factors. The view that obstetric anesthesia is not as challenging professionally as general operating room anesthesia, the poor remuneration for anesthesia services, and the increasing malpractice risk were also identified by these two groups. Gibbs concluded that these factors should be addressed by hospitals that provided obstetric services, and that obstetricians and anesthesiologists should each become more aware of the practices of the other (1).

Life threatening events for which general anesthesia may be required, such as severe "fetal distress," cord prolapse, and shoulder dystocia occur unpredictably. The major difference between obstetric anesthesia and nonobstetric anesthesia is that with the former the anesthesiologist is responsible for two lives, namely, the mother and her baby. Thus, of fundamental importance is the maintenance of uteroplacental perfusion, incorporating both acute maternal intravascular volume expansion and avoidance of aortocaval compression, treatment with antacids to alter the pH of her gastric contents to reduce the hazards of aspiration, and appropriate monitoring of the parturient and her fetus (21).

Modern general obstetric anesthesia is a combined technique utilizing an intravenous induction agent, muscle relaxant, various mixtures of nitrous oxide and oxygen, endotracheal intubation, and prolonged maintenance with either narcotics or inhalation agents. Variations of this technique can be used to provide general anesthesia for cesarean section, difficult vaginal delivery, or to produce uterine relaxation for various obstetric maneuvers. This technique is reserved for situations where local, regional or low-dose ketamine analgesia are not appropriate for vaginal delivery. These include "fetal distress," where rapid vaginal delivery is necessary; a severely mentally retarded or extremely uncooperative patient, who might injure herself or her fetus during delivery; and during situations requiring uterine relaxation (intrauterine exploration, manual removal of a retained placenta, vaginal delivery of a second twin, delivery of an after-coming breech, and replacement of the inverted uterus) (22).

The Gibbs study of 1986 revealed that at that time 30 to 50% of obstetrical anesthesia services were provided by physicians, or other personnel, not trained or certified as anesthesia specialists (1). Moreover, Gibbs found that the preanesthetic assessment of the obstetric patient was viewed differently from that of the surgical patient going to the operating room. Pregnant women and their neonates deserve to receive the highest current standards of anesthesia and analgesia care. Early consultation with the anesthesiologist by the obstetrician and completion of a preanesthetic assessment are essential for provision of optimal care within the labor and delivery suite. Finally, it is desirable that obstetricians understand the important contributions that anesthesiologists can make to the care of their patients. As Shnider stated, "the ultimate success of an obstetric anesthesia service will depend in large part on the rapport between anesthesiologist and obstetrician. Both must enter the partnership wholeheartedly and with mutual understanding and respect for each other's problems" (23). Only through understanding of both the needs of the obstetrician and the problems presented by a high-risk situation can optimum peripartum anesthetic care of mother and fetus be provided.

## Clinical Pharmacology

Although the pharmacology of agents used during general anesthesia is extensively discussed in Chapter 18, a brief review of the effects of these agents on mother, labor, fetus, and neonate is provided here. Sodium thiopental (Pentothal) and methohexital (Brevital) are the intravenous induction agents most frequently used in the United States (24). The elimination half-life of sodium thiopental is significantly increased in pregnant women at term because there is a larger than normal volume of distribution (25). Anesthetic doses have been reported to cause disappearance of uterine activity (26). Sodium thiopental rapidly crosses the placenta, and fetal concentrations reach their peak between 2 and 4 minutes after maternal intravenous injection (27).

Jouppila, et al observed a 22 to 50% reduction in intervillous blood flow during induction of general anesthesia, with 4 mg/kg of thiopental, in 10 healthy gravid women, using the intravenous 133 Xenon method (28). Despite this significant reduction in intervillous blood flow, it has been observed that normal fetuses are not significantly affected (29).

Because it decreases uterine contractility, it has been surmised that uterine blood flow may be improved and placental intervillous perfusion increased by thiopental, as long as the maternal blood pressure is maintained (26). Thus, if used in appropriate doses, barbiturates are unlikely to compromise the fetus when the patient is otherwise healthy (24).

Ketamine, a phencyclidine derivative, produces excellent analgesia, amnesia, and anesthesia by dissociation of the afferent pathways from cortical perception. Ketamine causes a release of catecholamines, which stimulate the cardiovascular system to increase heart rate, systemic and pulmonary vascular pressure, and cardiac output, and may, therefore, be useful in situations of maternal hypotension or hemorrhage (27). However, because of the catecholamine release, this agent should not be used in the hypertensive patient (30).

When administered during the first trimester, ketamine causes a significant increase in uterine pressure, equal to that of ergotrate (24,31). Likewise, during the second trimester of pregnancy, ketamine causes an increase in uterine tone, which is dose-related. Therefore, induction of anesthesia with ketamine during the first or second trimester would be expected to increase the intrinsic vascular resistance in the myometrium, decreasing placental blood flow. However, unlike thiopental, no human placental blood flow studies have been performed. The effect of ketamine on the term uterus is somewhat different. The baseline uterine pressures do not increase. Although the intensity and frequency of contractions usually increase slightly, there appears to be little overall effect (24,31). However, doses greater than 1 mg/kg have been reported to increase uterine tone and the incidence of neonatal respiratory depression. Therefore, this drug should not be used in any situation in which "fetal distress" is a factor (27–29). In the absence of further evidence, ketamine, as an induction agent, should be avoided throughout pregnancy, except when its advantages, such as blood pressure support, the rare case of porphyria, or barbiturate allergy, outweigh the potential disadvantages (24,30).

Nitrous oxide rapidly crosses the placenta. The fetal/maternal concentration ratio is 0.8 after just 3 minutes, and the umbilical artery/vein concentration ratio is almost 0.9 after 15 minutes of inhalation (32). Although nitrous oxide has little effect on uterine contractility (33), Shnider, et al have observed that as the length of fetal exposure increases in the term infant, the percent of Apgar scores less than 7 increases (34). Premature neonates are more sensitive to the effects of transplacental nitrous oxide than are term neonates (35).

The use of 70% nitrous oxide in thiopental-nitrous oxide anesthesia in animals has been associated with progressive fetal acidosis by decreasing uterine blood flow. This has led some investigators to recommend avoiding nitrous oxide concentrations of greater than 50% (29).

Halothane, enflurane, and isoflurane are considered to be complete anesthetics because they provide hypnosis, amnesia, analgesia, and muscle relaxation. These agents can produce hypotension by lowering cardiac output via direct depression of the myocardium, or by vasodilation (24), and thus can lead to reduced placental blood flow. However, Palahniuk and Shnider have demonstrated, in the gravid ewe, that systemic hypotension, with its resultant decrease in uterine blood flow, is only achieved at greater than 1.5 MAC of halothane or isoflurane (Figure 19–8). Decreased uterine blood flow was associated with fetal hypoxia and acidosis (36). It appears, however, that low to moderate concentrations of these halogenated anesthetics have few fetal sequlae and can even increase placental blood flow by their ability to reduce systemic

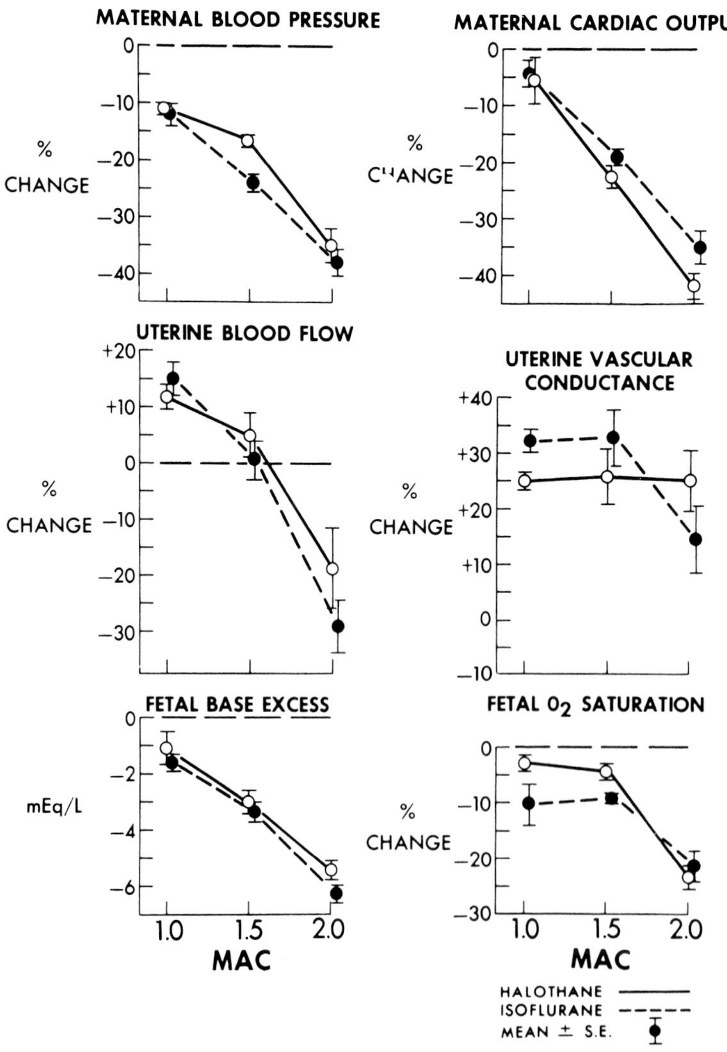


**Fig. 19–8.** Changes from control values in mean maternal arterial blood pressure, cardiac output, uterine blood flow, uterine vascular conductance, fetal arterial base excess, and fetal arterial $O_2$ saturation at 1.0, 1.5, and 2.0 MAC halothane and isoflurane. (From Palahnuik RJ, Shnider SM: Anesthesiology. 41:462–72, 1974.)

catecholamine levels and uterine tone (24,29). The uterine relaxation effect has been observed at MAC levels of only 0.5% of halothane and can be induced within 2 minutes, lasting for 5 minutes after discontinuation. This effect has been shown with the other halogenated agents as well.

Other new, and/or yet, not fully studied inhalational agents are desflurane and sevoflurane. The latter agent, sevoflurane, is another fluronated ether with blood solubility so low as to rival nitrous oxide. Its immediate appeal, then, as an induction agent is further enhanced by the fact that it does not have an offensive odor. Desflurane is also a fluronated ether and is very similar to isoflurane, currently very popular. Its blood solubility is even less than sevoflurane. The problem with desoflurane is its potency, because its MAC is estimated to be 5.7%, compared to sevoflurane, which is only 1.7%. The reception and application of these new drugs await the full gamut of animal and human trials over the next few years to determine their safety.

Although increased blood loss due to anesthetic-induced uterine atony may occur at delivery (37), the use of oxytocin and rapid ventilation to blow off the anesthetic agent will allow normal uterine contractions and hemostasis to be achieved (26). The immediate uterine relaxation produced by these agents is an advantage in various intrapartum crises, such as shoulder dystocia, intrauterine manipulation, vaginal delivery of breech or second twin, and in pelvic surgery during early pregnancy (24,27,38).

Since its first use in clinical anesthesia, the muscle relaxant succinylcholine has been the drug of choice in situations in which it is crucial to rapidly secure the airway, such as in patients with "full stomach" who are at high risk of regurgitation during induction of anesthesia (30,39). Whenever succinylcholine is used for tracheal intubation in the pregnant patient, cricoid pressure should be applied to obstruct the esophagus to prevent regurgitation (Figure 19–9) (24).

Succinylcholine has not been found in fetal umbilical cord blood unless the mother has received a bolus of 300 mg or more. Therefore, with the use of usual clinical doses, succinylcholine will not cross the placental barrier in sufficient amounts to affect the Apgar score (40). Because of their high degree of ionization at a physiologic pH, all of the currently used muscle relaxants have insufficient placental transfer to cause any clinical effects in the neonate (41).

Edrophonium, neostigmine, and pyridostigmine are all quarternary ammonium compounds and therefore are unlikely to cross the placenta. Rapid intravenous administration of these anticholinesterase agents to reverse nondepolarizing muscle relaxants may cause direct release of acetylcholine and could, theoretically, stimulate uterine contractions. Increased salivation, bradycardia, and possibly bronchospasm are associated with their administration and therefore either atropine or glycopyrrolate should be given prophylactically with these drugs (24). There is no evidence that single clinical doses of common muscle relaxants are teratogenic in the human (29).

Severe neonatal depression is usually related to obstetric factors rather than to the anesthetic drugs when general obstetric anesthesia, for either vaginal or cesarean delivery, is properly administered (22). Anesthesia-related factors, such as aspiration of gastric contents, failed tracheal intubation, and intravascular injection of local anesthetic agents during attempted epidural anesthesia, contribute to 8 to 10% of obstetric anesthetic mortality (42). In the instance of obstetric anesthesia, when it is understood at the outset that the patient has a greater risk, the anesthesiologist is placed in a difficult situation in management of the airway: errors can lead to severe hypoxemia, whereas in the positioning of the patient, errors can lead to peripheral nerve injury (43). The previously cited national survey by Gibbs and colleagues indicated that the availability of obstetric anesthesia services has only minimally increased compared to previous survey findings spanning 25 years (1). The complications related to the administration of analgesia and anesthesia that result in maternal death are often considered preventable when reviewed by maternal-mortality committees. Because obstetric anesthesia is potentially hazardous, it is necessary that well-trained, experienced anesthesia personnel be available to avoid serious complications.

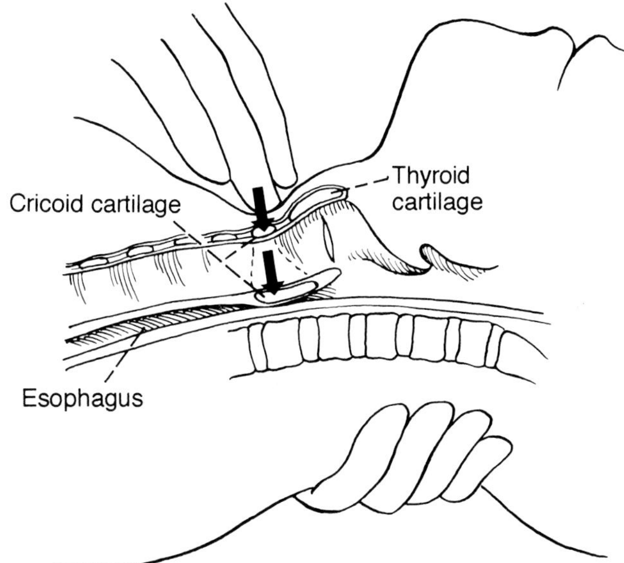


**Fig. 19–9.** Proper application of hands to apply cricoid pressure. (Modified from Fezer SJ: Cricoid pressure. How, when, and why. AORN Journal. 45:1374–7, 1987.)

## *Technical Considerations*

### *Preanesthetic Preparation*

The preoperative evaluation of the obstetric patient is the same as that of the nonobstetric patient requiring general anesthesia. However, as previously stated, anesthesia personnel must always be aware that they are caring for two patients; a mother and her fetus. The initial evaluation of the mother includes a complete medical, surgical, and obstetric history. If the presence of medical complications of pregnancy is ascertained, further maternal evaluation is needed.

**Table 19–6.** The Three Levels of the Final Five Risk Factors. (* 5 cm is approximately three fingers' breadth)

| Risk Factor | Level | |
|---|---|---|
| Weight | 0 | < 90 kg |
| | 1 | 90–110 kg |
| | 2 | > 110 kg |
| Head and neck movement | 0 | Above 90° |
| | 1 | About 90° (ie. ± 10°) |
| | 2 | Below 90° |
| Jaw movement | 0 | IG ≥ 5 cm* or SLux > 0 |
| | 1 | IG < 5 cm and SLux = 0 |
| | 2 | IG < 5 cm and SLux < 0 |
| Receding mandible | 0 | Normal |
| | 1 | Moderate |
| | 2 | Severe |
| Buck teeth | 0 | Normal |
| | 1 | Moderate |
| | 2 | Severe |

(From Wilson ME, Spiegelhalter D, Robertson JA, Lesser P: Predicting difficult intubation. Br. J. Anaesth. 1988;61:211–6.)

During a preanesthetic examination of the obstetrical patient, the oral cavity is checked for loose teeth and any anatomical abnormality that may likewise be associated with a difficult endotracheal intubation (Table 19–6). Two simple observations can predict those patients who may be difficult to intubate. First, the patient should be asked to open her mouth widely and to protrude her tongue as far as possible. Inability to visualize the faucial pillars and uvula, because they are hidden by the base of the tongue, identifies a patient who is potentially difficult to intubate (44). Second, one should measure the distance between the lower incisors and the temporomandibular joint (TMJ) and likewise measure the distance between the alveolus (immediately behind the last molar) and the lower border of the mandible. If the distance between the lower incisors and temporomandibular joint, divided by the distance between the alveolus and lower border of the mandible, is 3.6 or greater, difficulty in intubation can be anticipated. At the Ohio State University Hospital, a preoperative evaluation scoring system has been devised. This is used to determine those who may require an awake intubation (Figure 19–10).

Aspiration associated with general anesthesia is an ever present danger with all techniques. Every pregnant woman beyond the first trimester should be considered to have a full stomach. Therefore, when possible, these patients should have had no oral intake for at least 8 hours before general anesthesia (45).

In preparation for induction of general anesthesia, prophylactic hydration with at least 800 ml of Ringer's lactate or normal saline is recommended.

The most common cause of maternal death related to general anesthesia is aspiration pneumonia (46,47). Since Mendelson first described this complication of obstetric general anesthesia (48), many animal studies have been performed to discover the etiology of this process and to develop preventive measures. It has been observed that raising the pH of the gastric contents reduces complications of aspiration (23,42,48,49). It has also been hypothesized that a volume of gastric contents of 25 ml or greater is a second etiology of aspiration pneumonia (42,50). These two etiologies constitute reasons for the commonplace usage of antacids, $H_2$-receptor blockers, and/or gastrointestinal tract stimulants as premedication for general obstetric anesthesia.

Although antacids have been demonstrated to raise the pH of the gastric contents (30,47,51–53), aspiration of a particulate antacid alone has been observed to cause severe pneumonia (54). Taylor and Pryse-Davies observed that 43% of patients who did not receive antacid therapy had a gastric pH less than 2.5 (55). However, the use of oral antacids reduces gastric pH level by some 5 to 20%, depending on the choice of agent, its volume, concentration, and timing of administration.

O'Sullivan and Bullingham, using radiotelemetric continuous measurement of intragastric pH, observed that 15 ml of sodium citrate solution elevated the pH of the gastric contents above 3.0 for 26 minutes. Doubling the dose did not prolong its effectiveness (56). Sodium citrate causes 95% of patients to have a gastric contents pH greater than 2.5. Based on these studies, routine prophylactic administration of 15 ml of 0.3 M sodium citrate solution is recommended. Because the duration of action of this antacid is limited, it must be administered within 30 minutes of the expected time of anesthesia.

$H_2$-receptor antagonists effectively reduce gastric contents volume and acidity (57), but they require a period of time to first achieve a pharmacologically active blood concentration, and then to exert an inhibiting effect. Thorburn, et al observed cimetidine, combined with sodium citrate, to rapidly and safely raise the gastric contents pH and recommended that they be used to treat only those patients at risk of acid aspiration, thus avoiding routine administration to laboring patients not requiring cesarean section (Table 19–7) (58).

Cimetidine, administered parenterally, has been associated with severe cardiac arrythmias, hypotension, reduction in hepatic blood flow, and impaired hepatic metabolism of drugs (42). Ranitidine, however, does not appreciably alter liver function. Mykleby, et al found that cimetidine given intramuscularly 30 minutes before induction resulted in a significantly higher gastric pH and reduced gastric volume, when compared to those receiving 15 ml of sodium citrate and controls (59). Johnston, et al found that oral cimetidine did not increase the gastric acidity to 2.5 or greater in those cases in which anesthesia was required within 60 minutes of the loading dose (60). Both cimetidine and metoclopramide directly inhibit vascular smooth muscle and may therefore cause systemic hypotension, especially when used together. If there is time to attempt gastric emptying, the combination of $H_2$-receptor antagonists and gastric motility stimulants, such as metoclopramide and nonparticulate antacid, all may be justified, when solid food has been recently ingested.

Despite such widespread usage of these prophylactic regimens, it remains to be proven whether aspiration pneumonia is actually prevented. It has been observed that despite the routine use of antacids for premedication in England and Wales, maternal deaths due to aspiration still occur (47). Although the routine use of drugs to re-

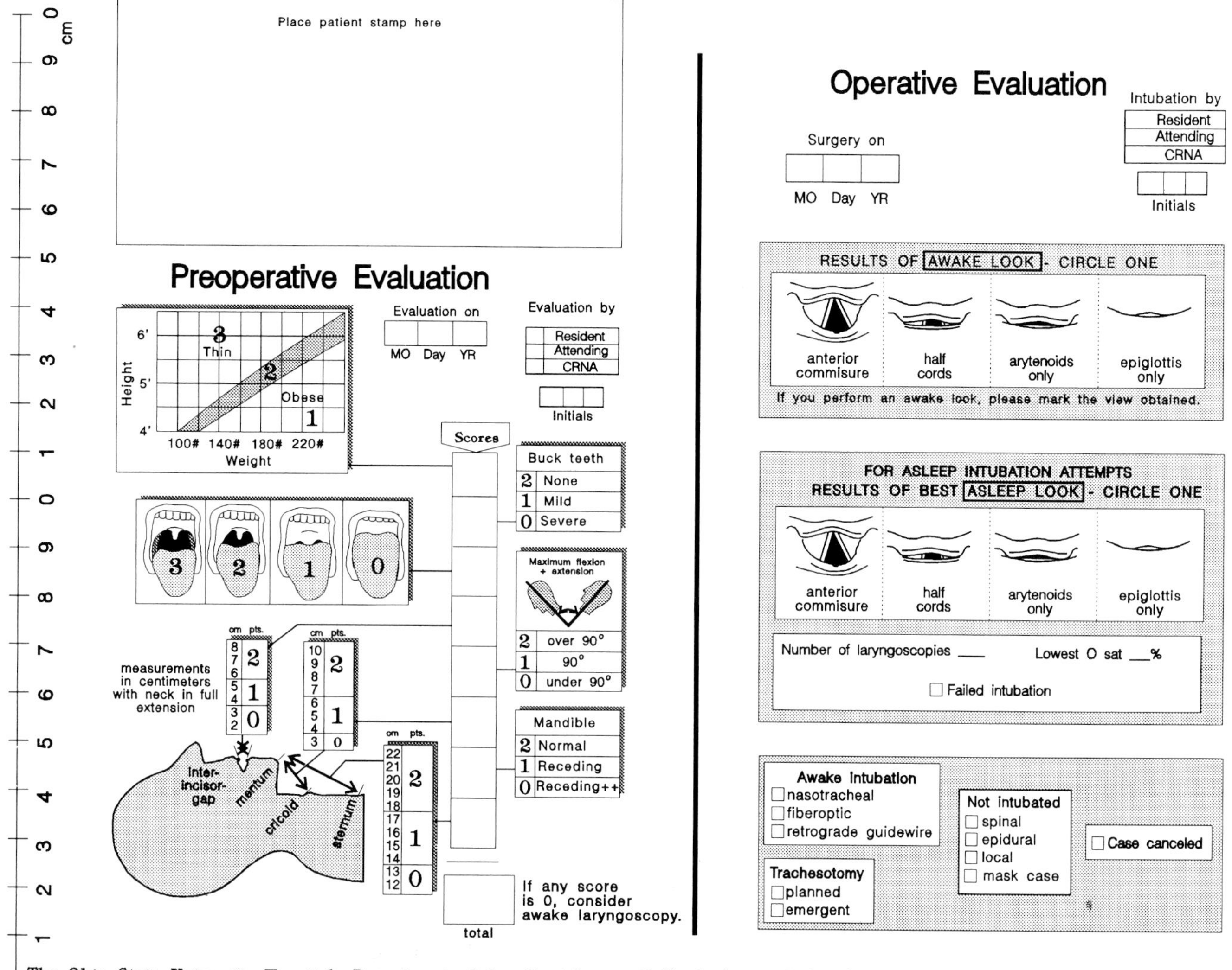

Place patient stamp here

**Preoperative Evaluation**

Height 6' 5' 4'
3 Thin
2
Obese 1
100# 140# 180# 220#
Weight

3 2 1 0

Evaluation on
MO Day YR

Evaluation by
Resident
Attending
CRNA
Initials

Scores

Buck teeth
2 None
1 Mild
0 Severe

Maximum flexion + extension
2 over 90°
1 90°
0 under 90°

Mandible
2 Normal
1 Receding
0 Receding++

measurements in centimeters with neck in full extension

cm pts.
8 7 6 — 2
5 4 — 1
3 2 — 0

cm pts.
10 9 8 — 2
7 6 5 4 — 1
3 — 0

cm pts.
22 21 20 19 18 — 2
17 16 15 14 — 1
13 12 — 0

Inter-incisor-gap
mentum
cricoid
sternum

If any score is 0, consider awake laryngoscopy.
total

**Operative Evaluation**

Surgery on
MO Day YR

Intubation by
Resident
Attending
CRNA
Initials

RESULTS OF AWAKE LOOK - CIRCLE ONE
anterior commisure | half cords | arytenoids only | epiglottis only
If you perform an awake look, please mark the view obtained.

FOR ASLEEP INTUBATION ATTEMPTS
RESULTS OF BEST ASLEEP LOOK - CIRCLE ONE
anterior commisure | half cords | arytenoids only | epiglottis only

Number of laryngoscopies ___ Lowest O sat ___%
☐ Failed intubation

Awake Intubation
☐ nasotracheal
☐ fiberoptic
☐ retrograde guidewire

Not Intubated
☐ spinal
☐ epidural
☐ local
☐ mask case

☐ Case canceled

Tracheotomy
☐ planned
☐ emergent

The Ohio State University Hospitals Department of Anesthesiology -- Difficult Airway Index Evaluation Form --

**Fig. 19–10.** Preoperative evaluation scoring sheet.

**Table 19–7.** Antacid Therapy for Emergency Cesarean Section

| | No Sedation ($n$ = 39) | Not in Labor ($n$ = 22) | Sedation Only ($n$ = 17) | Sedation and Epidural ($n$ = 6) | Epidural ($n$ = 16) |
|---|---|---|---|---|---|
| Gastric volumes | | | | | |
| Mean natural logarithm (volume in ml) | 3.24 (26) | 2.58 (13) | 3.11 (22) | 3.48 (32) | 2.59 (13) |
| SD | 0.93 | 1.1 | 1.01 | 1.35 | 1.2 |
| pH of first gastric sample | | | | | |
| Mean | 6.26 | 6.81 | 6.81 | 6.78 | 6.98 |
| SD | 1.11 | 0.92 | 0.68 | 0.78 | 0.53 |

Mean and standard deviation of pH of the first gastric samples and of the natural logarithms of the gastric volumes, characterized by the method of sedation. Figures in parentheses are the mean gastric volumes. The differences among the gastric volumes were significant ($F$ value 2.522, $p < 0.05$), but not among their pH values (analysis of variance).
(From Thorburn J, Moir DD: Antacid therapy for emergency cesarean section. Anesthesia 1987;42:352–5.)

duce gastric contents pH and volume has not been proven effective, it still remains the standard of care.

Atropine and glycopyrrolate are postganglionic blocking agents that are used before induction of general anesthesia because of their anticholinergic activity. They protect against reflex bradycardia during intubation, drying of secretions, and counter the muscarinic effects that occur when nondepolarizing muscle relaxants are reversed. Atropine, a tertiary amine, easily crosses the placental and blood-brain barriers of the fetus. Potential side-effects include fetal bradycardia via a central effect and fetal tachycardia via a vagolytic effect. In addition, atropine has been shown to cause relaxation of the lower uterine segment (26).

Glycopyrrolate, a quaternary ammonium compound, does not cross the placenta or the blood-brain barrier (31). In contrast to atropine, it does not produce as much maternal tachycardia, has a longer duration of action, and if administered 30 to 40 minutes before induction, elevates the pH of the maternal gastric contents (27). Glycopyrrolate is not associated with the high incidence of bradyarrhythmias, AV block, or ventricular extrasystole experience with atropine (24).

When short-term memory was tested postoperatively in patients who had received either atropine or glycopyrrolate, only those who had received atropine were observed to have a significant deficit (61). Therefore, glycopyrrolate appears to be the preferred drug for administration to the pregnant patient (24).

All instruments and equipment to be utilized during general anesthesia should be checked for proper functioning before placing the patient in the operating room. Adequacy of oxygen, nitrous oxide, and quantity of halogenated agent should be determined. The ventilator should be checked for proper functioning, and proper flow of gases through the ventilation bag and tubing should be confirmed. Confirmation that adequate devices to assist with a difficult intubation are readily available is also important.

Once the gravid patient has been placed on the operating table, all monitoring devices should be applied. Similarly, the patient should have left lateral tilt or uterine displacement. Aortocaval compression has been observed to decrease uteroplacental perfusion through direct compression of the aorta, which reduces blood flow to the uterine arteries, and by decreased cardiac output secondary to impedance of venous return (21). Studies have confirmed that neonatal Apgar scores were improved when women were placed in left lateral tilt position during cesarean section rather than maintained in the supine position (62,63). Therefore, displacement of the uterus from the inferior vena cava and aorta is of prime importance in the conduct of both general and regional obstetric anesthesia (64).

### *Induction of Anesthesia*

Preoxygenation of the pregnant patient before induction of general anesthesia is very important. Oxygen consumption is increased and functional residual capacity is decreased during pregnancy, resulting in the susceptibility of the gravid patient to hypoxia during periods of induced apnea (22). Archer and Marx determined the arterial blood gas changes during 60 seconds of apnea in gravid and nongravid women undergoing surgery (65). They observed a significantly greater decrease in arterial oxygen tension in the gravid women. Although use of the four-breath preoxygenation technique has been shown to effectively denitrogenate the lungs (34), it will not eliminate the extensive tissue stores of nitrogen in pregnant women (42). Recently, Byrne, et al demonstrated that complete pulmonary nitrogen washout during pregnancy requires at least 3 minutes of breathing 100% oxygen (66). Due to the fetal oxygen content lag, abbreviated maternal preoxygenation may result in reduced fetal oxygenation. Consequently, if time permits, a full 3-minute preoxygenation should be performed.

Sellick is credited with first describing the use of cricoid pressure in preventing regurgitation of stomach contents into the lungs during induction of general anesthesia (67). With the patient in slight reverse Trendelenberg position during preoxygenation, the assistant identifies the thyroid cartilage prominence and gently places his/her thumb and second finger on either side of the cricoid cartilage, which is the first tracheal cartilage located one finger's width below this anatomical landmark. It is important to avoid premature application of cricoid pressure (prior to anesthetic induction) as this may induce vomiting and cause patient discomfort. Therefore, cricoid pressure should be applied during anesthesia induction, as soon as the patient loses consciousness. Lateral movement of the trachea is prevented while downward pressure is applied compressing the esophagus between the cricoid cartilage and the sixth cervical vertebra. Pressure should not be exerted over the thyroid or the tracheal cartilages because they are incomplete rings and will not occlude the esophagus (Figure 19–9). Wraight, et al determined that 44 Newtons of externally applied force were sufficient to protect the majority of patients from the hazards of aspiration (68).

Cricoid pressure is continued until intubation is accomplished, the endotracheal tube cuff has been inflated, and tube placement has been verified by auscultation. Premature release could be followed by aspiration before the airway has been secured. If the patient should vomit, cricoid pressure must be released and the patient turned to her side with her head down so that the mouth and larynx can be suctioned. Cricoid pressure held during active vomiting may lead to esophageal rupture (69).

Petito and Russell studied the ability of cricoid pressure to prevent the patient's stomach from inflating during mask ventilation (70). In their study, 50 patients were randomly divided between either the presence or absence of cricoid pressure during a 3-minute period of standardized mask ventilation. They observed that in those patients in whom cricoid pressure was applied, there was less gastric inflation. However, cricoid pressure was less successful in a subgroup of patients who were considered difficult to ventilate. It is important that a skilled assistant perform this maneuver because incorrect application can make intubation of the trachea difficult or impossible, while perhaps failing to prevent regurgitation.

## General Anesthesia

Thiopental (3 to 4 mg/kg) and ketamine (1 mg/kg) are the most commonly used agents for induction of general anesthesia. Thiopental crosses the placenta rapidly (71) making it impossible for the fetus not to be exposed to the drug before delivery. The peak concentration of thiopental is achieved in umbilical venous blood within 1 minute and in umbilical arterial blood in 2 to 3 minutes (34). Kosaka, et al observed that 60% of neonatal Apgar scores were 7 or greater when a thiopental dose of 8 mg/kg was used for induction. However, by decreasing the dose to 7 mg/kg, 75 to 90% of neonatal Apgar scores were 7 or greater (71). Other investigators have demonstrated that thiopental in 4 mg/kg doses has no contribution to low Apgar scores (64,72). Similarly, Petrikovsky demonstrated that intravenous barbiturates and muscle relaxants administered during anesthesia induction were not associated with fetal heart rate changes (73). However, Jouppila demonstrated that thiopental, in conjunction with succinylcholine, lowered uterine blood flow by 35% during induction (28).

Ketamine centrally mediates an increase in sympathetic tone, increasing both heart rate and blood pressure. Although ketamine has been associated with hallucinations and postoperative excitement, less maternal recall and neonatal neurobehavioral depression have been observed than with thiopental (74,75). Ketamine is particularly useful in hemorrhagic shock but should be avoided in patients with pregnancy-induced hypertension. A minor advantage of ketamine is that when mixed with succinylcholine, a precipitate does not form, as it does with thiopental (51). The cardiovascular effects of ketamine and thiopental are compared in Table 19–8.

A new induction agent, propofol, is now becoming very popular as an intravenous anesthetic in many ambulatory settings because of its rapid central nervous system (CNS) depression/recovery cycle. Unconsciousness now can occur as rapidly as 30 to 60 seconds, yet return to consciousness can be as rapid as 5 to 15 minutes (76). The latter is due largely to an extremely fast blood-brain half-life of less than 3 minutes, a quick vascular distribution half-life of less than 4 minutes, and quick biotransformation and clearance rates. Its metabolism is hepatic and other extra hepatic sites (76).

When propofol, which is prepared in a milky lipid medium because penol-based compounds are relatively water insoluble, is contrasted with thiopental, the recovery times are faster (76). A composite of studies in obstetrics reveal advantages of propofol versus thiopental, but some questions were raised about neonatal recovery, though one study showed no differences in neonatal well-being (77). Future studies will most likely determine its applicability to obstetrics. It is difficult to imagine any induction agent superseding thiopental, which has been the classic standard for some 50 years now. New agents, propofol and ketamine (before it continued to challenge the supremacy of thiopental) have yet to succeed thiopental. If any agent can, it is possible propofol may be the one, based upon its beneficial pharmacodynamics. For a more detailed discussion of propofol, please see Chapter 18.

Etomidate, another induction agent with excellent characteristics suited for obstetrics, is a water soluble agent that has minimal cardiovascular depression associated with its use. Its pharmacodynamic profile is such that it effects almost immediate (1 minute) unconsciousness followed by rapid clearance and awakening within 3 to 5 minutes. Its other advantage is its great hemodynamic stability in comparison to other hypnotic agents. Therefore, its greatest potential contribution could be in those emerging hypovolemic situations that threaten the lives of both the mother and fetus, such as placenta previa, abruptio placenta, and uterine rupture. However, from the negative standpoint, the use in obstetrics most likely will come only after the concern about its potential suppression of the adrenals is ruled out (78). Further reference to etomidate can be found in Chapter 18.

The preadministration of a small dose of a nondepolariz-

**Table 19–8.** Cardiovascular Effects of Anesthetic Induction

| | Systolic Blood Pressure (mm Hg) | | | Diastolic Blood Pressure (mm Hg) | | | Heart Rate (beats/min) | | |
|---|---|---|---|---|---|---|---|---|---|
| | Ketamine | Thiopental | Combination | Ketamine | Thiopental | Combination | Ketamine | Thiopental | Combination |
| Before hospitalization | 110 ± 10.6 | 116 ± 10.5 | 110 ± 5.7 | 66 ± 8.2 | 70 ± 7.9 | 63 ± 9.6 | — | — | — |
| During hospitalization but before cesarean section | 109 ± 8.5 | 121 ± 11.8 | 118 ± 10.5 | 69 ± 6.6 | 75 ± 9.0 | 72 ± 4.8 | 87 ± 9.1 | 84 ± 11.4 | 84 ± 6.2 |
| Before anesthetic induction | 125 ± 13.4 | 143 ± 12.3[d] | 133 ± 9.8 | 71 ± 12.5 | 84 ± 8.5 | 82 ± 10.2 | 90 ± 11.6 | 91 ± 11.9 | 88 ± 16.5 |
| Endotracheal intubation | 158 ± 24.7[b] | 167 ± 39.8[b] | 161 ± 33.1[b] | 101 ± 17.3[b] | 116 ± 19.0[b] | 98 ± 20.9 | 101 ± 12.0 | 121 ± 17.8[b] | 108 ± 25.9[b] |
| Incision | 147 ± 14.1[b] | 163 ± 30.6[b] | 156 ± 23.0[b] | 95 ± 13.9[b] | 100 ± 18.4[b] | 96 ± 15.4 | 103 ± 13.6[b] | 112 ± 16.9[b] | 105 ± 13.3[b] |

Values are means ± SD.
[a] $p < 0.05$ compared with values during hospitalization but before cesarean section within groups.
[b] $p < 0.05$ compared with values before anesthetic induction within groups.
(From Schultetus RR, Hill CR, Dharamraj CM, Banner TE, et al: Wakefulness during cesarean section after anesthetic induction with ketamine, thiopental, or ketamine and thiopental combined. Anesth. Analg. 1986;65:723–8.)

ing muscle relaxant has been recommended to avoid succinylcholine-induced fasciculations and possibly the concomitant increases in intragastric pressure produced by these fasciculations (42). Anticholinergic drugs should be avoided for premedication and at induction because they rapidly lower esophageal sphincter tone, increasing the risk of reflux and aspiration (79). With regard to physically reducing the volume of gastric contents, suction intubation of the stomach has not been observed to be reliable (30,80,81).

Prior to intubation, intravenous administration of muscle relaxants, such as succinylcholine (80 to 100 mg), offers optimal conditions to allow rapid endotracheal intubation. Although pregnancy reduces plasma cholinesterase activity (82), metabolizing of a moderate succinylcholine dose is not usually prolonged (83). Because serum cholinesterase activity of a specific obstetric patient is generally unknown, return of neuromuscular function should be monitored before the administration of another muscle relaxant (84). Maintenance of muscle relaxation throughout a cesarean section operation is generally assured by administration of nondepolarizing muscle relaxants that are easily reversible and/or have a short duration of action (39,84–86). These are preferred by some over continuous succinylcholine infusion (34). No neonatal adverse effects, as determined by Apgar scores, umbilical cord blood gases or neonatal neurobehavioral scores, have been observed with moderate doses of these drugs (34,42).

### *Tracheal Intubation*

The technique of tracheal intubation of the obstetric patient is no different than that for any other patient requiring general anesthesia. The use of a laryngoscope with either a Miller or MacIntosh blade is mandatory. These blades allow the direct observation of the endotracheal tube while it passes through the vocal cords. An endotracheal tube with internal diameter of 7.0 to 7.5 mm is usually adequate in size; however, a 6.5-mm tube should be kept close at hand. Pregnancy may present some unique problems for the anesthetist performing endotracheal intubation. Large and pendulous breasts can press against the laryngoscope handle, and mucosal edema of the larynx, in the preeclamptic patient, can make this a challenge (87).

Traditionally, confirmation of tracheal intubation and equal ventilation of both lungs has been ascertained by auscultation over the lung fields and stomach. This confirmation should occur before proceeding with the surgical procedure, because repositioning or reinsertion of the endotracheal tube can be difficult, once surgery has begun. However, utilizing auscultation alone to confirm proper endotracheal tube placement is not 100% reliable. The introduction of carbon dioxide gas analyzers that continuously sample the content of expired carbon dioxide have allowed rapid detection of the presence of $CO_2$ in the trachea or its absence in the esophagus (85,86). This allows immediate verification of proper endotracheal tube position in the patient for whom intubation may have been difficult.

Similarly, pulse oximetry has permitted continuous noninvasive analysis of arterial hemoglobin oxygen saturation, providing instantaneous warning of hypoxemia. This technology alerts the anesthesiologist when desaturation is occurring during repeated attempts at intubation. Likewise, Campbell and Paulette have reported that the pulse oximeter recording of hypoxemia has enabled early identification of aspiration (89).

Wilson, et al estimated that in obstetric anesthesia 2.7% of intubations are reported to be difficult and that failed intubation occurs in approximately 0.05 to 0.3% of intubations (44). If a Grade 3 laryngoscopic view is encountered (Figure 19–11c), no more than a few attempts at endotracheal intubation should be performed before beginning a failed intubation drill.

The initial maneuver in the failed intubation drill is dependent on the obstetric indication for cesarean section. If the operation is elective, the patient can be awakened and a regional anesthetic performed. If a regional anesthetic is not possible, an awake blind oral or nasal intubation can be considered. Another alternative is bronchofiberscope-directed tracheal intubation (34,42,89,90). However, if the obstetrical indication for cesarean section is serious fetal distress, the next maneuver is dependent on the skill and experience of the anesthesiologist and his or her ability to easily ventilate the patient with bag and mask. If the patient is easily ventilated with a mask, anesthesia may be maintained with nitrous oxide, oxygen, and halothane throughout the cesarean section. Although mask anesthesia can often be administered successfully, the continuation of cricoid pressure along with adequate patient paralysis is extremely important in reducing the maternal risk of aspiration.

The anesthesiologist's skill is further challenged if the patient is either difficult or impossible to ventilate with bag and mask. Not only is the fetus seriously jeopardized, but the apneic pregnant patient rapidly becomes cyanotic, and hypoxic injury or death may supervene (91). Therefore, oxygenation is the first priority. Although in this situation several maneuvers are available to achieve maternal oxygenation, the maneuver chosen is dependent on the anesthesiologist's skill and the availability of equipment and assisting personnel. Possibly the simplest maneuver, and one requiring the least amount of equipment and no need for experienced assisting personnel, is the cricothyroidotomy (34,42). Other maneuvers include the use of transglottic jet ventilation (92), placement of a 14- to 16-gauge cannula through the crico-thyroid membrane coupled with jet ventilation (42), placement of an esophageal gastric tube airway (90), and laryngeal mask (Figures 19–12 and 19–13) (93). None of these maneuvers is clearly optimal; therefore, it is essential that every anesthesiologist have many maneuvers he or she can comfortably perform when this life threatening situation arises.

Failure to perform endotracheal intubation after multiple attempts was considered responsible for 16 maternal deaths, reported from the United Kingdom, in 1982 (94) and 11 maternal deaths reported over a 2-year period in New York City (95). Wallace and Cunningham have suggested that whenever a difficult intubation is anticipated, use of preanesthetic direct laryngoscopy could greatly re-

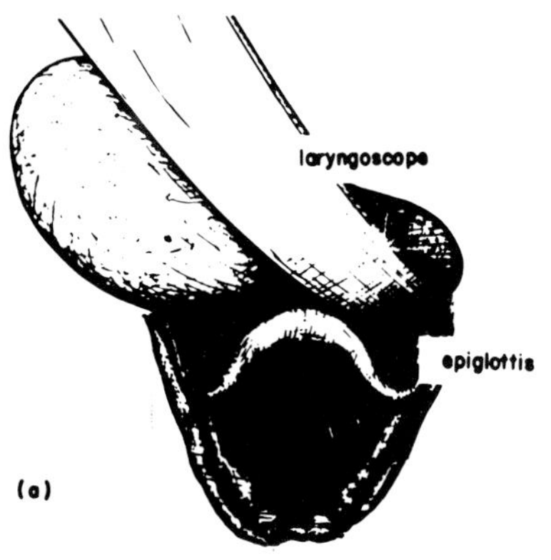


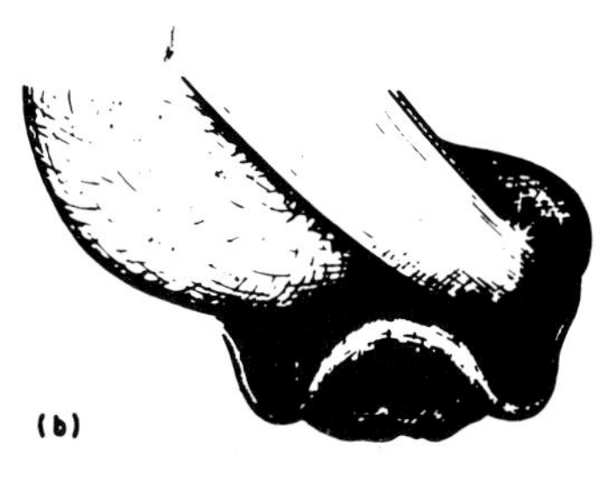


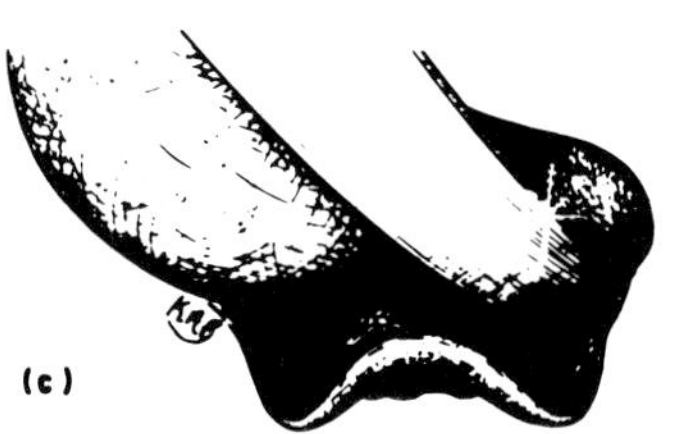


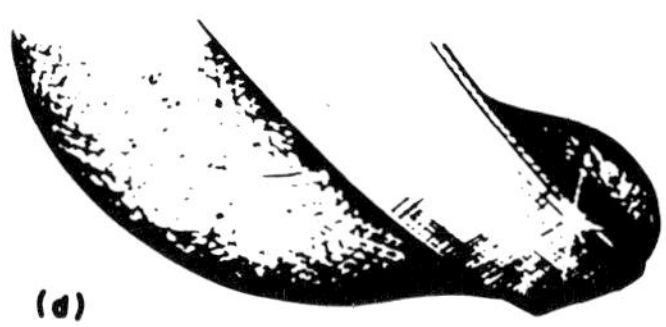


**Fig. 19–11.** The best views obtainable at laryngoscopy, assuming correct technique. Grade 1(a), grade 2(b), grade 3(c), grade 4(d). (From Cormack RS, Lehane J: Difficult tracheal intubation in obstetrics. Anaesthesia. 39:1105–11, 1984.)

duce the number of occasions when a failed intubation drill would be needed (79).

Cormack and Lehane graded the appearance of the posterior pharynx at laryngoscopy and related this to the likelihood of difficult intubation (96). In Grade 1, most of the glottis is visible and no difficulty during intubation should be anticipated. In Grade 2, only the posterior extremity of the glottis is visible and slight difficulty during intubation may be encountered. Usually, light pressure on the larynx brings at least the arytenoids, if not the vocal cords themselves, into view. In Grade 3, no part of the glottis is visible and only the epiglottis can be seen. In this situation, severe difficulty may be encountered during intubation. In Grade 4, not even the epiglottis can be seen and intubation is impossible, except through the use of the previously described special methods (Figure 19–11).

Cormack and Lehane believe Grade 3 visualization to be the most likely cause of maternal death due to failed intubation, because these cases are often not obvious in advance. Because the inability to visualize the cords can lead to an inappropriate reaction, these authors have urged anesthesiologists to deliberately simulate the Grade 3 condition. This can be accomplished by lowering the laryngoscope blade to where the epiglottis descends, hiding the vocal cords, and thus allowing the anesthetist to practice controlled blind intubation (96).

Although many techniques have been advocated for blind intubation, Cormack has endorsed the use of an Oxford tube placed over a flexible introducer. The introducer is inserted anteriorly, keeping it against the epiglottis to ensure that it will not enter the esophagus. If the introducer is kept in the midline, it will usually enter the tra-

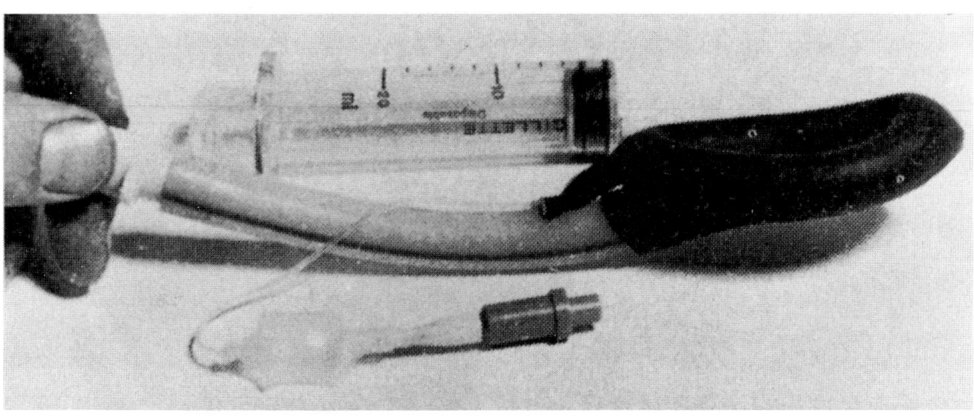

**Fig. 19–12.** Laryngeal mask prototype. (From Brain AIJ, McGhee TD, McAteer EJ, Thomas A, et al: The laryngeal mask airway. Development and preliminary trials of a new type of airway. Anaesthesia. 40:356–61, 1985.)

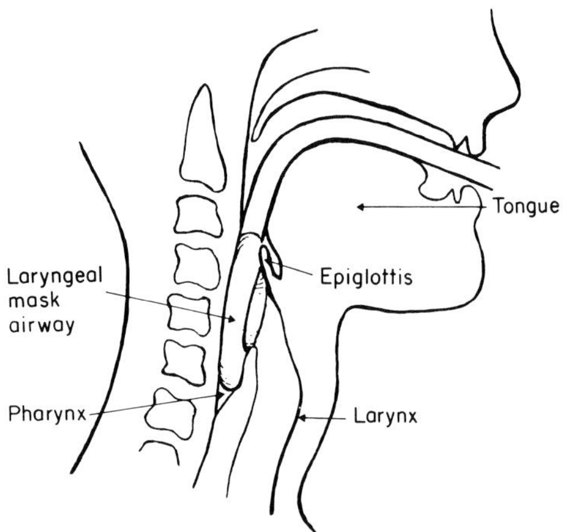


**Fig. 19–13.** The laryngeal mask in position. (From Brain AIJ, McGhee TD, McAteer EJ, Thomas A, et al: The laryngeal mask airway. Development and preliminary trials of a new type of airway. Anaesthesia. 40:356–61, 1985.)

chea. Enough of the introducer should protrude from the patient's mouth to allow the Oxford tube's passage over it, through the larynx and into the trachea, without any movement of the introducer.

In 1951, King, et al reported a hypertensive response to laryngoscopy and endotracheal intubation during general anesthesia (97). This response to stimulation of the epipharynx and laryngopharynx is a sympathetic reflex that produces hypertension and tachycardia. Although this hypertensive response may be of a transient nature, usually lasting less than 10 minutes, the response is variable and often unpredictable. These episodes of hypertension and tachycardia, following endotracheal intubation, may be responsible for complications that occur throughout the subsequent course of anesthesia. Hypertensive patients are particularly susceptible to significant increases in blood pressure during endotracheal intubation. In the patient with preeclampsia, this response may lead to pulmonary edema, compromised left ventricular function, and loss of cerebral blood flow autoregulation with associated intracerebral edema, hemorrhage and/or seizure (98–101).

Several methods have been described to reduce the pressor response of intubation. These methods can be divided into three categories, according to their site of action. Regional and/or topical analgesia can be used to block afferent pathways. Intravenous or "deep" inhalation anesthesia can be used to modify the central nervous system response. Rapidly acting antihypertensives can be used to blunt the peripheral effects (101).

The use of lidocaine spray, applied topically to the larynx to block the afferent pathways, has been popular in the past (99). Intravenous lidocaine at doses of 1 mg/kg given 120 seconds before intubation has been observed not only to blunt the hypertensive response to laryngoscopy and intubation but also to prevent intracranial hypertension (21,102–104).

Recently, intravenous narcotics have been found to effectively obtund the hypertensive responses to intubation (105), but concern over neonatal depression has limited their use for cesarean section. Alfentanil, with a short duration of action, high protein binding, and low lipid solubility, offers some advantages over other narcotics for potential reduction of neonatal depression (100). However, use of higher doses of alfentanil, while blunting the hypertensive maternal response to endotracheal intubation, has been shown to result in neonatal depression (106). Dann, et al have observed that 10 ≤ g/kg of intravenous alfentanil, administered before induction, significantly reduced the hypertensive response to endotracheal intubation without producing any neonatal depression (100). Connell, et al believe that the safest way to obtund the hypertensive response to endotracheal intubation in patients with preeclampsia is to use either fentanyl or alfentanil before induction of general anesthesia (107). The alternative of deep inhalation anesthesia is not an option for the obstetrical patient due to the significant risk of aspiration before endotracheal intubation, and the increased likelihood of anesthesia-related depression of the newborn.

For the hypertensive obstetrical patient, blood pressure must be well controlled before induction and laryngoscopy. The goal before intubation, in such a patient, is to decrease the diastolic blood pressure to 90 to 100 mm Hg. Various antihypertensive drugs have been used, such as hydralazine by intravenous bolus, or continuous infusions of trimethaphan, nitroprusside, nitroglycerin, or labetalol, to acutely decrease blood pressure and also to ablate the hypertensive response to endotracheal intubation (21).

Of these, the most commonly used is hydralazine. Its major advantage is that it reduces substantially systemic blood pressure through direct vasodilation. It has been demonstrated in the gravid ewe that this occurs without compromise of uterine blood flow (108). The major disadvantage of this drug is that hypotension may be excessive, reducing uteroplacental circulation and producing fetal distress. The onset of the hypotensive effect is slow to occur, gradually developing over 15 to 20 minutes following intravenous administration. In addition, its low molecular weight (160 daltons) promotes placental passage, so hypotension of the newborn is likely (109).

Trimethaphan has likewise been employed for this purpose. This drug has a high molecular weight (597 daltons), which somewhat limits its placental transmission. It also releases histamine and decreases cardiac output (110). Furthermore, prolonged respiratory paralysis may occur synergistically with succinylcholine administration (111). Trimethaphan acts more rapidly than hydralazine and reduces systemic arterial blood pressure without significantly affecting maternal cerebral blood flow (112).

Sodium nitroprusside has also been employed to manage this condition. This agent has a very rapid onset of action and does not increase cerebral blood flow. On occasion, however, preeclamptic patients may become significantly hypotensive, resulting in reduction of uteroplacental blood flow with consequent fetal distress (113). The chief objection to the use of nitroprusside relates to its potential for fetal cyanide toxicity. Although demonstrated in fetal lambs, short term usage in humans has failed to produce neonatal toxicity (114).

**Table 19–9.** Maternal Arterial and Umbilical Cord Blood Gas Values at the Time of Delivery in the Control and NTG Treatment Groups

| | Control (n = 10) | NTG (n = 9) |
|---|---|---|
| Maternal pH | 7.40 ± 0.02 | 7.40 ± 0.01 |
| Maternal $Pa_{O_2}$ (mm Hg) | 119 ± 15 | 118 ± 19 |
| Maternal $Pa_{CO_2}$ (mm Hg) | 34.0 ± 2.8 | 34.1 ± 1.2 |
| Maternal $H_{CO_3}$ (meq/l) | 22.6 ± 1.4 | 20.3 ± 0.7 |
| Umbilical artery pH | 7.29 ± 0.02 | 7.26 ± 0.02 |
| Umbilical artery $Pa_{O_2}$ (mm Hg) | 12.8 ± 2.2 | 8.0 ± 1.8 |
| Umbilical artery $Pa_{CO_2}$ (mm Hg) | 52.2 ± 2.1 | 55.1 ± 1.1 |
| Umbilical artery $H_{CO_3}$ (mEq/l) | 24.7 ± 0.4 | 24.7 ± 0.4 |
| Umbilical vein pH | 7.33 ± 0.02 | 7.30 ± 0.02 |
| Umbilical vein $Pa_{O_2}$ (mm Hg) | 24.0 ± 2.3 | 18.1 ± 3.0 |
| Umbilical vein $Pa_{CO_2}$ (mm Hg) | 46.4 ± 1.7 | 48.7 ± 1.7 |
| Umbilical vein $H_{CO_3}$ (mEq/l) | 23.4 ± 0.6 | 23.6 ± 0.4 |

Data are mean ± SEM.
No statistical differences between groups.
(From Hood DD, Dewan DM, James FM III, Floyd HM, et al: The use of nitroglycerine in preventing the hypertensive response to tracheal intubation in severe preeclampsia. Anesthesiology 63:329–32, 1985.)

Nitroglycerin has a rapid onset of action leading to a smooth decrease in systemic blood pressure. Comparison of data for nitroglycerin treatment and control groups is listed in Table 19–9. Nitroglycerine's molecular weight is low (227 daltons) but neonatal depression and hypotension have not been observed (115). Studies of uterine blood flow are contradictory, but for the most part suggest sparing of the uteroplacental circulation, with preservation of blood flow (116). Autoregulation of cerebral blood flow is diminished by nitroglycerin such that subsequent increase in blood pressure may dramatically and detrimentally increase intracranial pressure (117).

Labetalol is a nonselective beta adrenergic and selective alpha 1 adrenergic blocking agent with intrinsic beta-2 agonist activity. Administered intravenously, it is seven times more potent as a beta blocker than it is as an alpha blocker (118). It crosses the placenta with a fetal-maternal ratio of 0.5, but has only minimal hypotensive effects on the newborn (119). In preeclampsia, labetalol lowers the blood pressure rapidly, without causing tachycardia, or increasing cerebrospinal fluid (CSF) pressure, but has only a moderate antihypertensive effect that is, nonetheless, sufficient to protect the maternal CNS from dangerously high blood pressure during intubation (119).

## *Maintenance of Balanced Anesthesia*

Maternal awareness under general anesthesia during cesarean section is a regrettable but sometimes necessary or unavoidable complication. In situations in which there is fetal compromise and urgency for delivery, it may be necessary to communicate frankly with the mother and make her aware that to save the baby's life she may have to undergo uncomfortable situations for a hastily performed emergency abdominal delivery. For example, it may be necessary to *not* use nitrous oxide so as to provide 100% oxygen concentration. All efforts should be undertaken to reduce the incidence of this phenomenon of maternal awareness. Anesthesia maintained with equal proportions of nitrous oxide and oxygen results in a 10 to 20% incidence of intraoperative awareness (121). By increasing the concentration of nitrous oxide to 75%, the frequency of maternal awareness is reduced to 5% (122). This occurs however, at the expense of neonatal oxygenation (123). When halothane 0.1 to 0.65%, enflurane 0.5 to 1.5%, methoxyflurane 0.1%, or isoflurane 0.75% is com-

**Table 19–10.** Acid Base and Blood Gas Data*

| Sample site | $N_2O$ n = 16 | Halothane 0.25% n = 16 | Halothane 0.5% n = 18 | Enflurane 0.5% n = 18 | Enflurane 1% n = 13 |
|---|---|---|---|---|---|
| Maternal artery | | | | | |
| pH | 7.39 ± 0.01* | 7.41 ± 0.01 | 7.37 ± 0.02 | 7.40 ± 0.01 | 7.40 ± 0.02 |
| $Po_2$ (mm Hg) | 142 ± 14 | 147 ± 11 | 141 ± 9 | 137 ± 9 | 135.8 ± 13 |
| $Pco_2$ (mm Hg) | 32.5 ± 1 | 28 ± 1 | 30.6 ± 1 | 30.9 ± 1 | 29.1 ± 2 |
| BE (mEq/l) | −4.9 ± 0.6 | −6.5 ± 0.5 | −6.1 ± 0.6 | −5.3 ± 0.3 | −6.3 ± 0.6 |
| Umbilical vein | | | | | |
| pH | 7.31 ± 0.01 | 7.33 ± 0.01 | 7.32 ± 0.01 | 7.31 ± 0.01 | 7.34 ± 0.01 |
| $Po_2$ (mm Hg) | 29.3 ± 2 | 30.5 ± 2 | 31.1 ± 2 | 31.7 ± 2 | 33.1 ± 2 |
| $Pco_2$ (mm Hg) | 39.3 ± 2 | 37.5 ± 1 | 39.9 ± 1 | 39.8 ± 2 | 36.2 ± 1 |
| BE (mEq/l) | −4.7 ± 0.5 | −5.1 ± 0.5 | −5.1 ± 0.5 | −5.3 ± 0.5 | −5.8 ± 0.9 |
| Umbilical artery | | | | | |
| pH | 7.26 ± 0.01 | 7.25 ± 0.01 | 7.24 ± 0.01 | 7.27 ± 0.01 | 7.24 ± 0.01 |
| $Po_2$ (mm Hg) | 16.9 ± 1 | 17.7 ± 1 | 16.4 ± 1 | 18.8 ± 2 | 16.1 ± 2 |
| $Pco_2$ (mm Hg) | 48.6 ± 2 | 50.5 ± 2 | 50.5 ± 2 | 49.9 ± 2 | 49.7 ± 3 |
| BE (mEq/l) | −3.9 ± 0.5 | −4.4 ± 0.5 | −3.9 ± 0.6 | −3.3 ± 0.5 | −5.5 ± 0.6 |

* Values are mean ± s.e.mean. No significant differences between groups by Student's *t*-test.
(From Abboud TK, Kim SH, Henriksen EH, Chen T, et al: Comparative maternal and neonatal effects of halothane and enflurane for cesarean section. Acta. Anaesth. Scand. 29:663–668, 1985.)

**Table 19–11.** Assessment of Blood Loss*

| | $N_2O$ n = 16 | Halothane 0.25% n = 16 | Halothane 0.5% n = 18 | Enflurane 0.5% n = 18 | Enflurane 1% n = 13 |
|---|---|---|---|---|---|
| Estimated blood loss (ml) | 803 ± 16* | 673 ± 73 | 709 ± 57 | 677 ± 57 | 785 ± 62 |
| Hematocrit (%) ante-partum | 35.5 ± 0.6 | 35.2 ± 0.8 | 38.7 ± 0.7 | 37.0 ± 0.6 | 37.4 ± 0.8 |
| Hematocrit (%) 3rd postoperative day | 30.5 ± 0.8 | 31.3 ± 0.8 | 32 ± 1 | 33.6 ± 0.9 | 31 ± 1 |
| EBL > 1000 ml (no. of patients) | 2 | 3 | 0 | 2 | 0 |

* Values are mean + s.e.mean. No significant difference between groups by Student's *t*-test.
(From Abboud TK, Kim SH, Henriksen EH, Chen T, et al: Comparative maternal and neonatal effects of halothane and enflurane for cesarean section. Acta. Anaesth. Scand. 29:663–668, 1985.)

bined with an equal mixture of nitrous oxide and oxygen, antepartum maternal awareness is eliminated (121,122,124–129). Tables 19–10 and 19–11) compare data on nitrous oxide, halothane (0.25% and 0.5%), and enflurane (0.5% and 1%).

Because pregnancy causes a reduction of pulmonary functional residual capacity, reduced amounts of anesthetic are required. Palahniuk, et al observed the minimal alveolar concentration of halothane and isoflurane to be 25 to 40% less in gravid, as compared to nongravid, ewes (36). Halothane in higher concentrations, 0.8% or more, has been associated with reduced Apgar scores (40).

Occasionally, maternal awareness occurs despite appropriate anesthetic management. Maduska advises the anesthetist to discuss this complication honestly and matter-of-factly with the patient because few initiate litigation when they understand the important relationship between anesthetic management and neonatal outcome (22).

The use of halogenated anesthetic agents to supplement nitrous oxide during cesarean section gives rise to the possibility of increased postpartum blood loss because of the potent uterine relaxant properties of these agents (131,132). See Table 19–12 for data on isoflurane and halothane. However, several studies have failed to support this hypothesis when analgesic amounts of halothane, enflurane or isoflurane were utilized during cesarean section (34,64,124,128,133,134). It is suggested that caution be used in patients at high risk for bleeding and in those with a low preoperative hematocrit. In these patients, judicious use of inhalation agents combined with prompt postpartum administration of oxytocin and meticulous surgical technique reduces the risk of postpartum blood loss and eliminates maternal awareness. Once delivery has occurred, intravenous narcotic analgesics may be added and the level of anesthesia can be deepened with increased nitrous oxide concentrations.

### *Termination of General Anesthesia*

Anesthesia reversal and extubation are crucial events during which the avoidance of both aspiration of gastric contents and maternal hypertension is required. An awake extubation avoids maternal aspiration; however, blood pressure must be closely monitored and prompt treatment initiated for those patients who experience a hypertensive response.

During the postpartum period major fluid shifts occur as the extravascular volume that has accumulated during pregnancy begins to be mobilized and excreted. A postanesthetic visit is recommended to ascertain the patient's experience with the anesthetic.

## General Anesthesia for Special Indications

### *Operative Vaginal Delivery*

There is virtually no place in modern obstetrics for inhalation anesthesia during abnormal vaginal delivery. Inhalation anesthesia today is usually part of the general anesthetic regimen that includes intravenous anesthetic induction agents, muscle relaxants, and endotracheal intubation. General anesthesia of this nature is reserved for cesarean section, occasional very difficult vaginal deliveries or situations in which uterine relaxation is required (22). Induction of general anesthesia for uterine relaxation is becoming less frequent, with increased use of ce-

**Table 19–12.** Mean Apgar Scores (Range) at 1 and 5 Minutes Together With Mean (SD) Maternal Arterial and Umbilical Venous and Arterial pH, $Po_2$ and $Pco_2$ at delivery

| | Apgar Scores | | Maternal Arterial | | | Umbilical Arterial | | | Umbilical Venous | | |
|---|---|---|---|---|---|---|---|---|---|---|---|
| Treatment | 1 minute | 5 minutes | pH | $Po_2$, kPa | $Pco_2$, kPa | pH | $Po_2$, kPa | $Pco_2$, kPa | pH | $Po_2$, kPa | $Pco_2$, kPa |
| Isoflurane (*n* = 25) | 7.4 (5–8) | 8.9 (7–9) | 7.36 (0.05) | 19.1 (8.9) | 4.2 (1.0) | 7.26 (0.05) | 3.5 (1.0) | 6.1 (1.0) | 7.30 (0.05) | 4.6 (1.4) | 5.6 (1.2) |
| Halothane (*n* = 25) | 6.7 (4–8) | 8.8 (8–10) | 7.37 (0.05) | 21.9 (5.7) | 4.4 (0.8) | 7.27 (0.04) | 3.2 (0.7) | 6.6 (1.1) | 7.30 (0.03) | 4.9 (0.8) | 5.9 (0.8) |

(From Ghaly RG, Flynn RJ, Moore J: Isoflurane as an alternative to halothane for cesarean section. Anesthesia 1988;43:5–7.)

sarean delivery for most breech presentations and multifetal gestations. Indications for this technique include delivery of a second twin, delivery of the after-coming head of a breech presentation, transvaginal uterine exploration for uterine rupture, retained placenta, and replacement of an inverted uterus (22).

### *Preterm Gestation*

Operative vaginal deliveries are occasionally needed for preterm gestations, i.e. before completion of the thirty-seventh week of pregnancy. These deliveries comprise between 5 and 8% of all births and account for up to 80% of all neonatal mortality (135). General anesthesia can be administered safely for these preterm deliveries if the caveats applicable to all pregnant patients are followed. The primary anesthetic goal in the management of the premature gestation is maternal safety and, secondarily, protection of the preterm fetus. General anesthesia techniques and drugs are similar for delivery of both the premature and term infant and, therefore, the time between induction and delivery should be minimized to decrease possible anesthetic exposure of the neonate.

Patients with preterm labor are often delivered abdominally because of the higher incidence of breech presentations and multiple gestations. When not otherwise contraindicated, some obstetricians prefer vaginal delivery with forceps to protect the immature cranium of the preterm neonate from birth trauma. Both of these delivery routes require anesthetic intervention. The preterm gestation will most likely have received tocolysis with a beta adrenergic agent such as ritodrine hydrochloride. This produces uterine relaxation by increasing intracellular cyclic 3 to 5 AMP which can cause increased cardiac irritability. The perinatal team (pediatrician, obstetrician, anesthesiologist) should be prepared to treat any neonatal anesthetic or drug exposure that might occur with maternal general anesthesia.

### *Breech Presentations*

The breech fetus presents three potential problems for obstetricians and anesthesiologists: (1) prematurity, (2) possible traumatic delivery, and (3) coexistent maternal illness or fetal anomaly. A major concern is the manner in which anesthesia may impact the delivery process. Umbilical cord prolapse occurs in 5 to 7% of all breech presentations (136). For this reason, the anesthesia team must be informed when a patient with a breech presentation is in labor, so that they may be prepared to administer general anesthesia should an emergency operation be required. Preparation should include a preanesthetic interview, assessment of the patient's risk status for anesthesia, and a discussion with the patient of the types of anesthesia and their complications. Communication is essential. "Fetal distress" of the breech presentation mandates rapid delivery, but not at the expense of maternal safety. Often, general anesthesia is most expedient; however, no single anesthetic technique is suitable for every patient. Both teams must be flexible and willing to alter the obstetric and anesthetic plans at a moment's notice.

General anesthesia has the advantage of using high concentrations of potent inhalation agents, which provide profound uterine relaxation for intrauterine manipulations, such as breech extraction. However, significant maternal risks, as well as the potential for associated fetal drug depression, accompany its administration. Bodmer, et al observed that neonates delivered as breech presentations, under general anesthesia, experienced a two to threefold higher rate of depression, when compared with those delivered under lumbar epidural anesthesia. Even with lumbar epidural anesthesia, however, cesarean sections for breech presentation had similar depression rates as breech vaginal deliveries (137).

### *Vaginal Delivery of Multiple Fetuses*

Multi-fetal gestations, compared to singleton gestations, are associated with increased fetal morbidity and a three to sixfold increase in fetal mortality. This increased morbidity/mortality is most often due to prematurity and malpresentation. The gravida with a multi-fetal gestation demonstrates altered physiology as compared to her counterpart with a singleton gestation. These alterations include more profound aortocaval compression and upward displacement of the diaphragm by the enlarged uterus, resulting in further decrease in functional residual capacity and dyspnea. Thus, ventilation-perfusion mismatch and arterial hypoxemia more readily occur.

Today, as the number of fetuses increases beyond two, primary cesarean section becomes a certainty. Also, the need for version or extraction increases in twin gestations when the second twin is in a nonvertex presentation. Therefore, general anesthesia with endotracheal intubation may be needed to relax the uterus for internal podalic version and breech extraction. Any of the potent halogenated inhalation agents will achieve adequate relaxation of the uterus. A regional block, such as spinal or lumbar epidural anesthesia, may provide adequate analgesia, but it does not provide uterine relaxation. When such relaxation is a primary need, a regional block should not be used alone (51).

## Cesarean Section

There is no single "ideal" anesthetic method for cesarean section. The choice depends upon the indications for delivery, the degree of urgency, maternal preference, and the experience and skill of the anesthesiologist. A successful anesthetic requires expert technical skills and a thorough understanding of maternal and fetal physiology and pharmacology. Because general anesthesia can be induced quickly, and support of the maternal cardiovascular system can be readily accomplished, this technique may be the method of choice for emergent situations such as "fetal distress" and maternal hemorrhage. However, the choice is less obvious for more common and less urgent indications, such as dystocia, repeat cesarean section, and breech presentation. Although a brief discourse on the use of general anesthesia for cesarean section follows, a more detailed discussion is provided in Chapter 30.

### *Elective Cesarean Section*

Lumbar epidural anesthesia is considered by many to be the anesthetic technique of choice for elective repeat

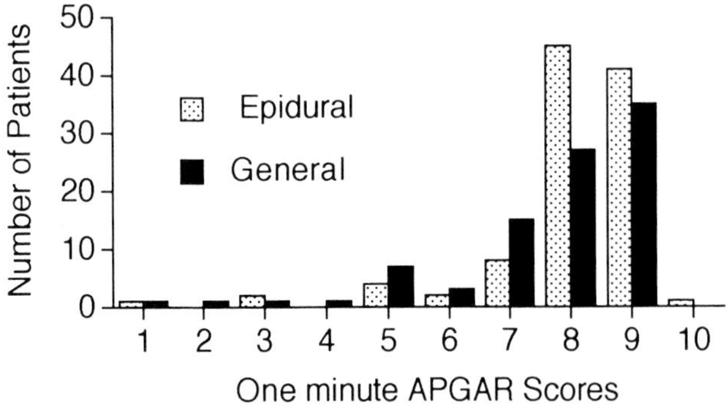


**Fig. 19–14.** One minute Apgar scores with patients under epidural and general anesthesia. (Modified from Zagorzycki MT, Brinkman CR: The effect of general and epidural anesthesia upon neonatal Apgar scores in repeat cesarean section. Surg. Gynecol. Obstet. 155:641–5, 1982.)

cesarean delivery. Zagorzycki and Brinkman reviewed 195 uncomplicated repeat cesarean section deliveries performed with either lumbar epidural anesthesia or general anesthesia. They observed similar numbers of neonates in each group with Apgar scores of less than 7. This occurred despite the fact that the mean incision to delivery time for the patients having epidural anesthesia was significantly longer when compared with those given a general anesthetic (Figure 19–14 and Figure 19–15). Zagorzycki and Brinkman concluded that general anesthesia for elective repeat cesarean section does not produce a higher incidence of newborn depression, as reflected by the 1- and 5-minute Apgar scores (64). Similarly, Gale, et al reported no differences in neonatal outcome related to the mode of anesthesia in 205 elective cesarean sections (138). James, et al could not strongly recommend one method over another and felt that for the routine

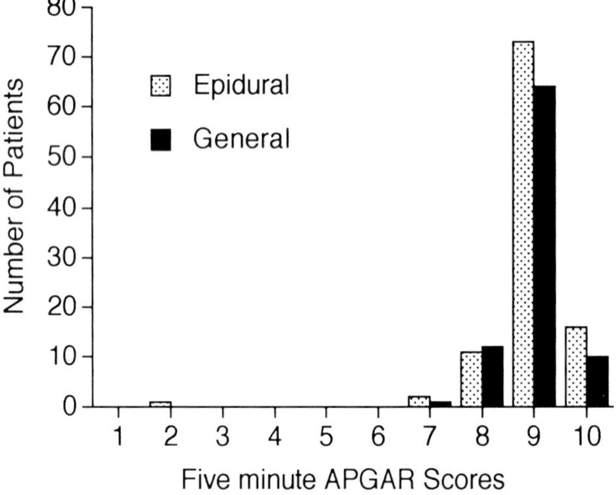


**Fig. 19–15.** Five minute Apgar scores with patients under epidural and general anesthesia. (Modified from Zagorzycki MT, Brinkman CR: The effect of general and epidural anesthesia upon neonatal Apgar scores in repeat cesarean section. Surg. Gynecol. Obstet. 155:641–5, 1982.)

elective cesarean section the mother's desires should be respected (63).

Chestnut observed that general anesthesia for repeat cesarean section did not increase postpartum febrile morbidity (including fever index), diagnosis of infection, or use of therapeutic antibiotics; nor did it lengthen the postoperative hospital stay (139). In contrast, Neilson and Hokegard reported a higher incidence of acute respiratory disorders in neonates delivered by cesarean section with general anesthesia as compared to those whose mothers received lumbar epidural anesthesia (140).

Maternal plasma norepinephrine and beta-endorphin levels, in patients undergoing induction of general anesthesia for cesarean section, are increased compared to those in patients receiving lumbar epidural anesthesia. These elevations are believed to be a response to maternal stress (141). It has been observed that elevated catecholamine levels reduce uterine blood flow (Figure 19–16) (142). This has led to the conclusion, by some investigators, that infant well-being will be least compromised by using a regional technique for repeat cesarean section (143).

Fetal acidosis has been observed in diabetic patients undergoing cesarean section with regional anesthesia, as compared to general anesthesia. Rapid hydration with intravenous solutions containing glucose has been implicated. Although under these circumstances acidosis also occurs in neonates of normal mothers, it is not as severe

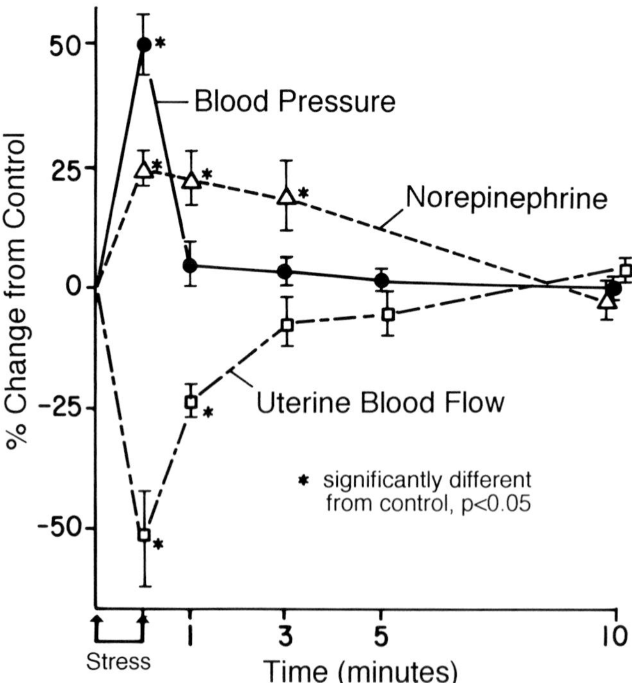


**Fig. 19–16.** Effects of electrically induced stress (30 to 60 seconds) on maternal mean arterial pressure, plasma norepinephrine levels, and uterine blood flow. All values subsequent to control are given as mean percentage changes ± SE. (Modified Shnider SM, Wright RG, Levinson G, Roizen MF, et al: Uterine blood flow and plasma norepinephrine changes during maternal stress in the pregnant ewe. Anesthesiology. 50:524–7, 1979.)

as in the neonates of diabetics. It has been recommended that because any glucose load may be detrimental to the fetus, solutions containing glucose should be avoided during prehydration for regional anesthesia and for volume resuscitation following hemorrhage (51).

## *Emergent Cesarean Section*

Emergent cesarean sections are more likely to result in maternal mortality. Anesthesia-related mortality in the United Kingdom most commonly occurs with emergent procedures (anesthesia for forceps deliveries, emergency cesarean section, and postpartum dilatation and curettage) and when inexperienced anesthetists perform general anesthesia without adequate supervision (51). Therefore, it would seem prudent for anesthetists to evaluate all patients admitted to the labor unit, regardless of the anticipated future need for anesthesia services. As previously stated, for elective cesarean section, the choice of anesthesia for emergent cesarean section depends on the reason for the operation, the degree of urgency, the desires of the patient, and the judgment of the anesthesiologist. Because there is no single "ideal method" of anesthesia for cesarean section, the anesthesiologist must choose the method deemed safest and most comfortable for the mother, least depressant of the neonate, and conducive to optimal working conditions for the obstetrician (33). General anesthesia has the theoretical advantages of a more rapid induction, less hypotension and cardiovascular instability, and better control of the airway and ventilation. Properly conducted general anesthesia for cesarean section provides protection for both fetus and mother. Fetal protective benefits include maintenance of normal uterine blood flow, increased fetal oxygenation, and limited anesthetic depression. Adequacy of oxygenation-ventilation, hemodynamic stability, muscle relaxation, and amnesia offer maternal protection (144). Although general anesthesia possesses these theoretical advantages, expeditious delivery is necessary to minimize neonatal depression. Unnecessary delay in delivery creates a dilemma for the anesthesiologist. To maintain adequate anesthesia, administration of depressant drugs or increasing concentrations of volatile agents is necessary, accelerating the time-dependent transfer of these agents to the fetus. To restrict their use enhances awareness.

Crawford, et al believe that the clinical and biochemical status of the neonate is directly related to the uterine incision-to-delivery time interval, when cesarean section is performed under general anesthesia (145). Datta, et al studied 60 patients receiving general anesthesia for cesarean section. They observed that when the induction-to-delivery interval was 8 minutes or greater and the uterine incision-to-delivery interval was more than 180 seconds, Apgar scores and the pH of the umbilical artery and vein were significantly reduced (Table 19–13). Irrespective of the induction-to-delivery time, uterine incision-to-delivery intervals of longer than 3 minutes, in those whose cesarean section was performed with regional anesthesia, were also associated with umbilical vein and artery acidosis, and low Apgar scores (146). Therefore, prolonged uterine incision-to-delivery intervals must be avoided because intrauterine manipulation appears to cause constriction of the umbilical and placental blood vessels and may also stimulate fetal respiration, leading to fetal meconium and/or amniotic fluid aspiration (42).

It is important for obstetricians, before they find themselves in emergency situations, to understand the capabilities and limitations of the available anesthesia personnel and, whenever possible, endeavor to use those most experienced and knowledgeable in obstetric anesthesia (51).

## Nonobstetric Surgical Diseases

It is estimated that between 0.5% and 2.0% of pregnant women will undergo anesthesia at some time during pregnancy for a surgical procedure for an incidental illness. Although a brief review of general anesthesia for nonobstetrical disorders is given here, a more detailed discussion of anesthesia for surgical diseases complicating pregnancy may be found in Chapter 39.

No single anesthetic agent or technique has been found to be superior with regard to fetal outcome. However,

**Table 19–13.** Neonatal Acid-Base Values and Apgar Scores After Undergoing General Anesthesia*

| Parameter | I-D < 8 min<br>U-D < 90 sec<br>(n = 23) | I-D < 8 min<br>U-D 91–180 sec<br>(n = 16) | I-D < 8 min<br>U-D 91–180 sec<br>(n = 10) | I-D < 8 min<br>U-D > 180 sec<br>(n = 11) |
|---|---|---|---|---|
| Umbilical vein | | | | |
| pH | 7.36 ± 0.01 | 7.37 ± 0.01 | 7.35 ± 0.01 | 7.30 ± 0.01[†] |
| $pO_2$ | 40 ± 2 | 35 ± 2 | 26 ± 2[†] | 33 ± 4 |
| Umbilical artery | | | | |
| pH | 7.31 ± 0.01 | 7.30 ± 0.01 | 7.29 ± 0.01 | 7.22 ± 0.01[†] |
| $pO_2$ | 25 ± 1 | 20 ± 2 | 19 ± 2 | 15 ± 2[†] |
| $pCO_2$ | 54 ± 2 | 57 ± 2 | 57 ± 2 | 64 ± 2 |
| Base deficit | 2 ± 0.5 | 2 ± 1 | 2 ± 1 | 5 ± 1[†] |
| Percent apgar score < 7 | | | | |
| 1 minute | 4 | 38 | 60 | 73 |
| 5 minute | 0 | 6 | 10 | 27 |

I-D = induction-to-delivery interval; U-D = uterine incision-to-delivery interval
* mean ± standard error
[†] $p < 0.05$
(Modified from Datta S et al: Obstet. Gynecol. 1981;58:331–5.)

the basic objectives are first, maternal safety and second, the avoidance of drugs that may threaten fetal well-being. The "ideal" anesthetic would be one that produces a desired maternal effect, yet would have minimal undesirable fetal effects. To date no direct proof of a clear link between maternal exposure to anesthesia and undesirable reproductive outcome is available. Efforts to detect the effects of exposure to volatile anesthetics on human reproduction are currently limited to epidemiologic surveys.

Brodsky, et al reported on 287 gravid patients who had general anesthesia for surgical procedures. The incidence of fetal loss in women who had anesthesia and surgery during the first trimester was observed to be greater than the rate of first trimester spontaneous abortion in a nonoperated control group (8% versus 5.1%). Similarly, the incidence of fetal death following anesthesia and surgery during the second trimester was higher than that of the control group (6.9% versus 1.4%). Although these data were controlled for smoking, maternal medical illness, and parity, all of which may have a bearing on pregnancy outcome, no information was given as to the indication for, or the type of, operation performed (147).

Duncan and colleagues surveyed the entire population of Manitoba and found the incidence of anomalies among 2565 children of women who had undergone surgical procedures during the first or second trimester to be 1.68%, and that among a similarly sized group of controls to be 1.52% (148). Crawford and Lewis reported the incidence of abnormalities to be 3.6% among the offspring of pregnancies in which general anesthesia had been administered during the first 16 weeks (excluding cases of abortion). On the other hand, it was 8.0% among cases that had been conducted under lumbar epidural anesthesia during the same gestational period (149). For an anesthetic agent to double the incidence of a congenital defect that occurs spontaneously at the rate of 1 per 1000 pregnancies, it would have to be given to over 23,000 pregnant women before the increase could be detected at a 5% level with 95% confidence (150).

Although regional techniques have been recommended for the pregnant patient, there is no definitive evidence to support the use of one anesthetic technique over another with regard to spontaneous abortion or congenital anomalies, as long as maternal blood pressure and oxygenation are adequately maintained. Similarly, for surgery that cannot be postponed, there is no conclusive evidence that any anesthetic drug (premedicant, intravenous agent, local anesthetic or inhalational agent) or technique (regional versus general) is safer than another (150).

## REFERENCES


1. Gibbs CP, Krischer J, Peckham BM, Shart H, et al: Obstetric anesthesia: a national survey. Anesthesiology 65:298–306, 1986.
2. Roberts RB: General analgesia and anesthesia. *In* Pain control in obstetrics. Edited by E. Abouleish. Philadelphia, J.B. Lippincott Co., 1977, 357.
3. Major V, Rosen M, Mushin WW: Methoxyflurane as an obstetric analgesic: a comparison with trichloroethylene. Br. Med. J. 2:1554, 1966.
4. Jones PL, Rosen M, Mushin WW, Jones EV: Methoxyflurane and nitrous oxide as obstetric analgesics. I. A comparison with continuous administration. Br. Med. J. 3:255, 1969.
5. Jones PL, Rosen M, Mushin WW, Jones EV: Methoxyflurane and nitrous oxide as obstetric analgesics. II. A comparison with self-administered intermittent inhalation. Br. Med. J. 3:259, 1969.
6. Rosen M, Mushin WW, Jones P, Jones EV: Field trial of methoxyflurane, nitrous oxide and trichloroethylene in obstetric analgesia. Br. Med. J. 3:263, 1969.
7. Cole PV, Crawford JS, Doughty AG, Epstein HG, et al.: Specifications and recommendations for nitrous oxide/oxygen apparatus to be used in obstetric analgesia. Anaesthesia 25: 317, 1970.
8. Holdcroft A, Morgan M: An assessment of the analgesic effect in labour of pethidine and 50% nitrous oxide in oxygen (Entonox). J. Obstet. Gynaecol. Br. Commonw. 81: 603, 1974.
9. Latto IP, Rosen M, Molloy MJ: Absence of accumulation of methoxyflurane during intermittent self-administration for pain relief in labour. Br. J. Anaesth. 44:391, 1972.
10. Moir DD, Carty MJ: Pain relief in labour—systemic and inhalation analgesia. *In* Obstetric Anaesthesia and Analgesia. Edited by DD Moir, MJ Carty. Bailliere Tindall, London, 1980, p. 116.
11. Dodek SM: New methods for graphically recording contractions of parturient human uterus, study of effects of sedatives, anesthetics and stimulants upon uterus in labor. Surg. Gynecol. Obstet. 55:45, 1932.
12. Lindgren L: The influence of anaesthetics and analgesics on different types of labor. Acta. Anaesthesiol. Scand. (Suppl. II);3:49, 1959.
13. McAneny TM, Doughty AG: Self-administered nitrous oxide/oxygen analgesia in obstetrics. Anaesthesia 18:488, 1963.
14. Moir DD, Bissett WIK: An assessment of nitrous oxide apparatus used for obstetric analgesia. J. Obstet. Gynaecol. Br. Commonw. 72:265, 1965.
15. Tunstall ME: Use of a fixed nitrous oxide and oxygen mixture from one cylinder. Lancet 2:964, 1961.
16. Crawford JS: Principles and Practice of Obstetric Anaesthesia. 5th Ed. Cambridge, MA, Blackwell Scientific, 1984.
17. Gale CW, Tunstall ME, Wilton-Davies CC: Pre-mixed gas and oxygen for midwives. Br. Med. J. 1:732, 1964.
18. Jones PL, Molloy MJ, Rosen M: The Cardiff penthrane inhaler. A vaporizer for the administration of methoxyflurane as an obstetric analgesic. Br. J. Anaesth. 43:190, 1971.
19. Ramanathan S: Labor analgesia. *In*: Obstetric Anesthesia. Edited by S Ramanathan. Philadelphia, Lea & Febiger, 1988.
20. Wilson RD, Priano LL, Allen CR, Phillips MT, et al: Demand analgesia and anesthesia in obstetrics. South. Med. J. 65: 556–562, 1972.
21. Malinow AM, Ostheimer GW: Anesthesia for the high-risk parturient. Obstet. Gynecol. 69:951–64, 1987.
22. Maduska AL: Inhalation analgesia and general anesthesia. Clin. Obstet. Gynecol. 24:619–33, 1981.
23. Shnider SM: Obstetric anesthesia coverage: problems and solutions. Obstet. Gynecol. 34:615–20, 1969.
24. Gaba DM, Baden JM: Physiological effects of drugs used in anesthesia. *In* The Pregnant Surgical Patient. Edited by JM Baden, JB Broadsky. Mt. Kisco, New York, Futura Publishing Company, Inc., 1985, pp. 105–32.
25. Morgan DJ, Blackman GL, Paull JD, Wolf LJ: Pharmacokinetics and plasma binding of thiopental: II. Anesthesiology 54:474–80, 1981.
26. Hutson JM, Petrie RH: Drug effects on uterine activity and labor. Clin. Obstet. Gynecol. 1982; 25:189–201.

27. McDonald JS: Anesthesia and the high-risk fetus. *In* Gynecology and Obstetrics. Edited by R Deep, DA Eschenbach, JJ Sciarra. Philadelphia, J.B. Lippincott Co., 1988, Vol. 3, (Chapter 91), pp. 1–16.
28. Jouppila P, Kuikka J, Jouppila R, Hollmen AI: Effect of induction of general anesthesia for cesarean section on intervillous blood flow. Acta. Obstet. Gynecol. Scand. 1979; 58: 249.
29. Delaney AG: Anesthesia in the pregnant woman. Clin. Obstet. Gynecol. 1983; 26:795–800.
30. Stirrat GM, Thomas TA: Prescribing for labour. Clin. Obstet. Gynecol. 1986; 13:215–29.
31. James FM: Anesthesia for nonobstetric surgery during pregnancy. Clin. Obstet. Gynecol. 1987; 30:621–8.
32. Marx GF, Joshi CW, Orkin LR: Placental transmission of nitrous oxide. Anesthesiology 1970; 2:429–32.
33. Heyman JH, Barton JJ: Safety of local versus general anesthesia for second-trimester dilatation and evacuation abortion. Obstet. Gynecol. 1986; 68:877–8.
34. Shnider SM, Levinson G: Anesthesia for Cesarean Section. 2nd Ed. Baltimore, Williams and Wilkins, 1987, pp. 159–78.
35. Vatashsky E, Hochner-Celnikier D, Beller U, Ron M, Aronson HB: Neonatal outcome in cesarean section under general anesthesia, related to gestational age, induction-delivery and uterus-delivery intervals. Isr. J. Med. Sci. 1983; 19: 1059–63.
36. Palahniuk RJ, Shnider SM, Eger EI: Pregnancy decreases the requirements for inhaled anesthetic agents. Anesthesiology 1974; 41:82–83.
37. Soyannwo OA, Elegbe EO, Odugbesan CO: Effect of flunitrazepam (Rohypol) on awareness during anesthesia for cesarean section. Afr. J. Med Sci. 1988; 17:23–6.
38. Robie GF, Payne GG Jr, Morgan MA: Selective delivery of an acardiac acephalic twin. N. Engl. J. Med. 1989; 320: 512–3.
39. Famewo CE: Conditions for endotracheal intubation after atracurium and suxamethonium. MEJ Anesth. 1986; 8: 371–7.
40. Zagorzycki MT: General anesthesia in cesarean section: effect on mother and neonate. Obstet. Gynecol. Surv. 1984; 39:134–7.
41. Biehl D, Palahniuk RJ: Update on obstetrical anesthesia. Can. Anaesth. Soc. J. 1986; 33:238–45.
42. Ramanathan S: Anesthesia for cesarean section. *In* Obstetric Anesthesia. Philadelphia, Lea & Febiger, 1988, pp. 132–148.
43. Cheney FW, Posner K, Caplan RA, Ward RJ: Standard of care and anesthesia liability. JAMA 1989; 261:1599–1603.
44. Wilson ME, Spiegelhalter D, Robertson JA, Lesser P: Predicting difficult intubation. Br. J. Anaesth. 1988; 61:211–6.
45. Blouw R, Scantliff J, Craig PB, Palahniuk RJ: Gastric volume and pH in postpartum patients. Anesthesiology 1976; 45: 456–7.
46. Moir DD: Maternal mortality and anaesthesia. Br. J. Anaesth. 1980; 52:1–3.
47. Spielman FJ, Corke BC: Anesthesiologists' practice of obstetric anesthesiology. J. Reprod. Med. 1984; 29:683–5.
48. Mendelson CL: Aspiration of stomach contents into the lungs during obstetric anesthesia. Am. J. Obstet. Gynecol. 1946; 52:191–205.
49. Burgess GE: Antacids for obstetric patients. Am. J. Obstet. Gynecol. 1975; 123:577–9.
50. James CF, Gibbs CP, Banner T: Postpartum perioperative risk of aspiration pneumonia. Anesthesiology 1984; 61: 756–9.
51. Shaw DB, Wheeler AS: Anesthesia for obstetric emergencies. Clin. Obstet. Gynecol. 1984; 27:112–24.
52. Abboud TK, Earl CS, Henriksen EH, Hughes SC, et al: Efficacy of clear antacid prophylaxis in obstetrics. Acta. Anaesthesiol. Scand. 1984; 28:301–4.
53. Finn WF: Maternal welfare—Nassau County, New York, 1957–81. Obstet. Gynecol. Surv. 1984; 39:127–33.
54. Gibbs CP, Schwartz DJ, Wynne JW, Hood CI, et al: Antacid pulmonary aspiration in the dog. Anesthesiology 1979; 51: 380–5.
55. Taylor G, Pryse-Davies J: The prophylactic use of antacids in the prevention of the acid-pulmonary-aspiration syndrome (Mendelson's syndrome). Lancet 1966; 1:288–91.
56. O'Sullivan GM, Bullingham RE: The assessment of gastric acidity and antacid effect in pregnant women by a noninvasive radiotelemetry technique. Br. J. Obstet. Gynaecol. 1984; 91:973–8.
57. Coombs DW, Hooper D, Colton T: Preanesthesia cimetidine alteration of gastric fluid volume and pH. Anesth. Analg. 1979; 58:183–8.
58. Thorburn J, Moir DD: Antacid therapy for emergency cesarean section. Anesthesia 1987; 42:352–5.
59. Mykleby CCM, Kallar SK, Ciresi SA: The effect of oral bicitra compared with intramuscular cimetidine on gastric volume and pH in outpatient surgery. J. Am. Assoc. Nurse Anesth. 1988; 56:515–9.
60. Johnston JR, Moore J, McCaughey W, Dundee JW, et al: Use of cimetidine as an oral antacid in obstetric anesthesia. Anesth. Analg. 1983; 62:720–6.
61. Simpson KH, Smith RJ, Davies LF: Comparison of the effects of atropine and glycopyrrolate on cognitive function following general anesthesia. Br. J. Anaesth. 1987; 59:966–9.
62. Crawford JS, Burton M, Davies P: Time and lateral tilt at caesarean section. Br. J. Anaesth. 1972; 44:477–84.
63. James FM, Crawford JS, Hopkinson R, Davies P, Naiem H: A comparison of general anesthesia and lumbar epidural analgesia for elective cesarean section. Anesth. Analg. 1977; 56:228–35.
64. Zagorzycki MT, Brinkman CR: The effect of general and epidural anesthesia upon neonatal apgar scores in repeat cesarean section. Surg. Gynecol. Obstet. 1982; 155:641–5.
65. Archer GW Jr, Marx GF: Arterial oxygen tension during apnea in parturient women. Br. J. Anaesth. 1974; 46: 358–60.
66. Byrne F, Oduro-Dominah A, Kipling R: The effect of pregnancy on pulmonary nitrogen washout: a study of preoxygenation. Anaesthesia 1987; 42:148–50.
67. Sellick BA: Cricoid pressure to control regurgitation of stomach contents during induction of anaesthesia. Lancet 1961; 2:404–6.
68. Wraight WJ, Chamney AR, Howells TH: The determination of an effective cricoid pressure. Anaesthesia 1983; 38: 461–6.
69. Fezer SJ: Cricoid pressure. How, when, and why. AORN Journal 1987; 45:1374–7.
70. Petito SP, Russell WJ: The prevention of gastric inflation. A neglected benefit of cricoid pressure. Anaesth. Intens. Care. 1988; 16:139–43.
71. Kosaka Y, Takahashi T, Mark LL: Intravenous thiobarbiturate anesthesia for cesarean section. Anesthesiology 1969; 31:489–506.
72. Finster M, Poppers PJ: Safety of thiopental used for induction of general anesthesia in elective cesarean section. Anesthesiology 1968; 29:190–1.
73. Petrikovsky B, Cohen M, Fastman D, Tancer ML: Electronic fetal heart rate monitoring during cesarean section. Int. J. Gynecol. Obstet. 1988; 26:203–7.

74. Schultetus RR, Hill CR, Dharamraj CM, Banner TE, et al: Wakefulness during cesarean section after anesthetic induction with ketamine, thiopental, or ketamine and thiopental combined. Anesth. Analg. 1986; 65:723–8.
75. Hodgkinson R, Bhatt M, Kim SS, Grewal G, et al: Neonatal neurobehavioral tests following cesarean section under general and spinal anesthesia. Am. J. Obstet. Gynecol. 1978; 132:670–4.
76. Shafer A, Doze VA, Shafer SL, White PF: Pharmacokinetics and pharmacodynamics of propofol infusions during general anesthesia. Anesthesiology 69:348–356, 1988.
77. Joyce TH III, Loon M: Pre-eclampsia: effect of albumin 25% infusion. Anesthesiology SS:A313, 1981.
78. Reddy BK, Pizer B, Bull PT: Neonatal serum cortisol suppression by etomidate compared with thiopentone for elective caesarean section. Eur. J. Anaesth. 5:171–176, 1988.
79. Wallace D, Cunningham FG: Obstetrical anesthesia. *In* Williams Obstetric Supplement, No. 20. Edited by NF Gant, J Pritchard, P MacDonald. Baltimore, Williams and Wilkins, 1988.
80. Adeljoj B, Petring OU, Hagelsten JD: Inaccuracy of preanesthetic gastric intubation for emptying liquid stomach contents. Acta. Anaesthesiol. Scan. 1986; 30:41–3.
81. Kempen PM: Cricoid pressure, awake intubation, or both? Anesthesiology 1986; 64:831–2.
82. Shnider SM: Serum cholinesterase activity during pregnancy, labor and puerperium. Anesthesiology 1965; 26: 335–9.
83. Blitt CD, Petty WC, Alberternst EE, Wright BJ: Correlations of plasma cholinesterase activity and duration of action of succinylcholine during pregnancy. Anesth. Analg. 1977; 56:78–83.
84. Baraka A: Neuromuscular blockade of atracurium versus succinylcholine in a patient with complete absence of plasma holinesterase activity. Anesthesiology 1987; 66: 80–1.
85. Cook WP, Schultetus RR, Caton D: A comparison of d-tubocurarine pretreatment and no pretreatment in obstetric patients. Anesth. Analg. 1987; 66:756–60.
86. Astley BA, Hackett H, Hughes R, Payne JP: Recovery of respiration following neuromuscular blockade with atracurium and alcuronium. Br. J. Anaesth. 1986; 58(Supp. 1): 75S-79S.
87. Heller PJ, Scheider EP, Marx GF: Pharyngolaryngeal edema as a presenting symptom in preeclampsia. Obstet. Gynecol. 1983; 62:523–4.
88. Campbell RL, Paulette SW: Pulmonary aspiration during general anesthesia. Anesthesia Progress (March/April): 98–101, 1986.
89. American College of Obstetricians and Gynecologists. Technical Bulletin 112, Anesthesia for cesarean section, 1982.
90. Tunstall ME, Geddes C: Failed intubation in obstetric anesthesia. An indication for the use of the "Esophageal Gastric Tube Airway." Br. J. Anaesth. 1984; 56:659–61.
91. Archer GW Jr, Marx GF: Arterial oxygen tension during apnoea in parturient women. Br. J. Anesth. 1974; 46: 358–60.
92. Satyanarayana T, Capan L, Ramanathan S, Chalon J, Turndorf H: Bronchofiberscopic jet ventilation. Anesth. Analg. 1980; 59:350–4.
93. Brain AIJ, McGhee TD, McAteer EJ, Thomas A, et al: The laryngeal mask airway. Development and preliminary trials of a new type of airway. Anaesthesia 40:356–61, 1985.
94. Paull J: International overview of obstetric anaesthesia. Clin. Anaesthesiology 4:429, 1986.
95. Marx GF, Finster M: Difficulty in endotracheal intubation associated with obstetric anesthesia. Anesthesiology 1979; 51:364–5.
96. Cormack RS, Lehane J: Difficult tracheal intubation in obstetrics. Anaesthesia 1984; 39:1105–11.
97. King BD, Harris LC, Greifenstein FE, Elder JD, et al: Reflex circulatory responses to direct laryngoscopy and tracheal intubation performed during general anesthesia. Anesthesiology 1951; 12:556–66.
98. Hodgkinson R, Husain FJ, Hayashi RH: Systemic and pulmonary blood pressure cesarean section in parturients with gestational hypertension. Can. Anaesth. Soc. J. 1980; 27: 389–94.
99. Burns AM, Dorje P, Lawes EG, Neilsen MS: Anaesthetic management of cesarean section for a mother with preeclampsia, the Klippel-Feil syndrome and congenital hydrocephalus. Br. J. Anaesth. 61:350–4, 1988.
100. Dann WL, Hutchinson A, Cartwright DP: Maternal and neonatal responses to alfentanil administered before induction of general anesthesia for cesarean section. Br. J. Anaesth. 59:1392–6, 1987.
101. Fox EJ, Sklar GS, Hill CH, Villanneva R, et al: Complications related to the pressor response to endotracheal intubation. Anesthesiology 1977; 44:524–5.
102. Denlinger JK, Ellison N, Ominsky AJ: Effects of intratracheal lidocaine on circulatory responses to tracheal intubation. Anesthesiology 1974; 41:409–12.
103. Jones MM, Joyce TH: Anesthesia for the parturient with pregnancy-induced hypertension. Clin. Obstet. Gynecol. 30:591–600, 1987.
104. Donegan MF, Bedford RF: Intravenously administered lidocaine prevents intracranial hypertension during endotracheal suctioning. Anesthesiology 1980; 52:516–8.
105. Dahlgren N, Messeter K: Treatment of stress response to laryngoscopy and intubation with fentanyl. Anaesthesia 1981; 36:1022–6.
106. Redfern N, Bower S, Bullock E, Hull CJ: Alfentanil for cesarean section complicated by severe aortic stenosis. Br. J. Anaesth. 59:1309–12, 1987.
107. Connell H, Dalgleish JG, Downing JW: General anaesthesia in mothers with severe pre-eclampsia/eclampsia. Br. J. Anaesth. 59:1375–80, 1987.
108. Ring G, Krames E, Shnider SM, Wallis KL, Levinson G: Comparison of nitroprusside and hydralazine in hypertensive pregnant ewes. Obstet. Gynecol. 1977; 50(5):598–602.
109. Marx GF, Cabe CM, Kim YI, Eifelman AI: Neonatal blood pressures. Anaesthetist 1976; 25:318–22.
110. Goodman LS, Gillman AG: Goodman and Gilman's The Pharmacological Basis of Therapeutics. 8th Ed. New York, Pergamon Press, 1990.
111. Poulton TJ, James FM III, Lockridge O: Prolonged apnea following trimethaphan and succinylcholine. Anesthesiology 1979; 50:54–6.
112. Fahmy NR, Soter NA: Effects of trimethaphan on arterial blood histamine and systemic hemodynamics in humans. Anesthesiology 62:562–6, 1985.
113. Stempel JE, O'Grady JP, Morton MJ, Johnson KA: Use of sodium nitroprusside in complications of gestational hypertension. Obstet. Gynecol. 1982; 60(4):533–8.
114. Naulty J, Cefalo RC, Lewis PE: Fetal toxicity of nitroprusside in the pregnant ewe. Am. J. Obstet. Gynecol. 1981; 139(6):708–11.
115. Hood DD, Dewan DM, James FM III, Floyd HM, et al: The use of nitroglycerine in preventing the hypertensive response to tracheal intubation in severe preeclampsia. Anesthesiology 63:329–32, 1985.
116. Wheeler AS, James FM III, Meis PJ, Rose JC, et al: Effects

of nitroglycerin and nitroprusside on the uterine vasculature of gravid ewes. Anesthesiology 1980; 52:390–4.
117. Writer WDR, James FM III, Stullken EH Jr, Koontz FA: Intracranial effects of nitroglycerin—an obstetrical hazard? Anesthesiology 1980; 33(3):S309.
118. MacCarthy PE, Bloomfield SS: Labetalol, a review of its pharmacology, pharmacokinetics, clinical uses and adverse effects. Pharmacotherapy 1983; 3:193–219.
119. Macpherson M, Broughton PF, Rutter N: The effect of maternal labetalol on the newborn infant. Br. J. Obstet. Gynaecol. 93:539–42, 1986.
120. Ramanathan J, Sibai BM, Mabie WC, Chauhan D, et al: The use of labetalol for attenuation of the hypertensive response to endotracheal intubation in preeclampsia. Am. J. Obstet. Gynecol. 159:650–4, 1988.
121. Abboud TK, Kim SH, Henriksen EH, Chen T, et al: Comparative maternal and neonatal effects of halothane and enflurane for cesarean section. Acta. Anaesthesiol. Scand. 29: 663–668, 1985.
122. Palahniuk RJ, Scatliff J, Biehl D, Wieve H, et al: Maternal and neonatal effects of methoxyflurane, nitrous oxide and lumbar epidural anesthesia for cesarean section. Can. Anaesth. Soc. J. 1977; 24:586–96.
123. Marx GF, Mateo CV: Effects of different oxygen concentrations during general anesthesia for cesarean section. Can. Anaesth. Soc. J. 1971; 18:587–93.
124. Moir DD: Anaesthesia for caesarean section: an evaluation of a method using low concentrations of halothane and 50% of oxygen. Br. J. Anaesth. 1970; 42:136–42.
125. Warren TM, Datta S, Ostheimer GW, Naulty JJ, et al: Comparison of the maternal and neonatal effects of halothane, enflurane and isoflurane for cesarean delivery. Anesth. Analg. 1983; 62:516–20.
126. Crawford JS, Burton OM, Davies P: An anaesthesia for section: further refinements of a technique. Br. J. Anaesth. 1973; 45:726–31.
127. Galbert MW, Gardner AE: Use of halothane in a balanced technique for cesarean section. Anesth. Analg. 1972; 51: 701–4.
128. Coleman AJ, Downing JW: Enflurane anesthesia for cesarean section. Anesthesiology 1975; 43:354–57.
129. Wilson J: Methoxyflurane in caesarean section. Br. J. Anaesth. 1973; 45:233.
130. Latto IP, Waldron BA: Anaesthesia for caesarean section. Br. J. Anaesth. 1977; 49:371–78.
131. Munson ES, Embro WJ: Enflurane, isoflurane, and halothane and isolated human uterine muscle. Anesthesiology 1977; 46:11–14.
132. Gilstrap LC, Hauth JC, Hankins GDV, Patterson AR: Effect of type of anesthesia on blood loss at cesarean section. Obstet. Gynecol. 69:328–32, 1987.
133. Hood DD, Holubec DM: Elective repeat cesarean section: effect of type of anesthesia on blood loss. J. Reprod. Med. 1990; 35:368–72.
134. Ghaly RG, Flynn RJ, Moore J: Isoflurane as an alternative to halothane for cesarean section. Anesthesia 1988; 43: 5–7.
135. Dewan DM: Anesthesia for preterm delivery, breech presentation, and multiple gestation. Clin. Obstet. Gynecol. 1987; 30:566–78.
136. Collea JV: Current management of breech presentation. Clin. Obstet. Gynecol. 23:525, 1980.
137. Bodmer B, Benjamin A, McLean FH, Usher RH: Has use of cesarean section reduced the risks of delivery in the preterm breech presentation? Am. J. Obstet. Gynecol. 1986; 154:244–50.
138. Gale R, Zalkinder-Luboshitz I, Slater PE: Increased neonatal risk from the use of general anesthesia in emergency cesarean section. A retrospective analysis of 374 cases. J. Reprod. Med. 1982; 27:715–9.
139. Chestnut DH: Effect of anesthesia for repeat cesarean section on postoperative infectious morbidity. Obstet. Gynecol. 1985; 66:199–202.
140. Neilson TF, Hokegard KH: The incidence of acute neonatal respiratory disorders in relation to mode of delivery. Acta. Obstet. Gynecol. Scand. 1984; 63:109–14.
141. Abboud TK, Noueihed R, Khoo S, Hoffman DI, et al: Effects of induction of general and regional anesthesia for cesarean section on maternal plasma beta-endorphin levels. Am. J. Obstet. Gynecol. 1983; 146:927–30.
142. Shnider SM, Wright RG, Levinson G, Roizen MF, et al: Uterine blood flow and plasma norepinephrine changes during maternal stress in the pregnant ewe. Anesthesiology 1979; 50:524–7.
143. Loughran PG, Moore J, Dundee JW: Maternal stress response associated with cesarean delivery under general and epidural anaesthesia. Br. J. Obstet. Gynecol. 1986; 93: 974–9.
144. McDonald JS, Mateo CV, Reed EC: Modified nitrous oxide or ketamine hydrochloride for cesarean section. Anesth. Analg. 1972; 51:975–85.
145. Crawford JS, James FM, Davies P, Crawley M: A further study of general anaesthesia for cesarean section. Br. J. Anaesth. 1976; 48:661–7.
146. Datta S, Ostheimer GW, Weiss JB, Brown WU, et al: Neonatal effect of prolonged anesthetic induction for cesarean section. Obstet. Gynecol. 1981; 58:331–5.
147. Brodsky JB, Cohen EN, Brown BW, Wu ML, et al: Surgery during pregnancy and fetal outcome. Am. J. Obstet. Gynecol. 1980; 138:1165–7.
148. Duncan PG, Pope WDB, Cohen MM, Greer N: Fetal risk of anesthesia and surgery during pregnancy. Anesthesiology 1986; 64:790–4.
149. Crawford JSA, Lewis M: Nitrous oxide in early human pregnancy. Anaesthesia 1986; 41:900–5.
150. Brodsky JB: Anesthesia and surgery for the pregnant patient and fetal outcome. *In* The Pregnant Surgical Patient. Edited by JM Baden, JB Brodsky. Mt. Kisco, New York, Future Publishing Co., Inc., 1985, pp. 247–57.

# Chapter 20

# COMPLICATIONS OF GENERAL ANESTHESIA

JOHN S. McDONALD
JAY JACOBY

This chapter reviews the various complications associated with general anesthesia for obstetrics. An attempt has been made to include as many complications as reasonable, so that the reader will be familiar with them, be able to recognize them, and most importantly, be able to avoid them as much as possible. Included are complications of induction, aspiration, difficult airways, failed intubation, problems of alternative airway methods, human error, maternal disease, pulmonary embolism, emergencies, safety in anesthesia today, and the anesthetic contribution to maternal mortality. Emphasis is upon those complications of anesthesia that are related specifically to obstetrics.

## History

General anesthesia was rarely used in obstetrics until Dr. John Snow gave chloroform to Queen Victoria for the birth of Prince Leopold in 1853 and Princess Beatrice in 1857. Though these were vaginal births, they paved the way for a remarkable early history of appreciation for the value of the method. Today, over 100 years later, general anesthesia is not used often for vaginal birth, and it is infrequently used for cesarean section; by far the most popular method is regional anesthesia.

The prevailing attitude was that anesthesia was not needed for obstetric patients for two reasons: (1) childbirth is a natural process, occurring since creation; and (2) anesthesia had never been needed before. The scriptures state that painful childbirth was humanity's punishment for Eve's disobedience with the forbidden fruit. Most deliveries were done without anesthesia. When it was administered, it was usually done by an untrained person who gave a few breaths of chloroform.

Dr. Robert Hingson was the ground-breaking pioneer in obstetric anesthesia. After service on a destroyer in WW II, he was stationed at a Marine Hospital that had a large obstetric service, caring for the wives of sailors. He promoted continuous caudal anesthesia and popularized all forms of regional anesthesia, showing that it was better for both mothers and babies. As an academician and as a charismatic public speaker for decades, he did much to change the practice of obstetric anesthesia (1,2).

In the early to mid 1960s, Columbia University was the seat of interest in obstetric anesthesiology because of individuals such as Dr. Virginia Apgar, Dr. Stanley James, Dr. Frank Moya, Dr. Sol Shnider, and others at this institution who developed a dedication to improvement of care in that area. About the same time in metropolitan New York, Dr. Gertie Marx at Mt. Sinai Hospital developed a fellowship in obstetric anesthesia. Meanwhile, on the west coast in Seattle, in the mid 1960s, Dr. John J. Bonica was beginning to write the first edition of what would become known as the 'Bible of Obstetric Anesthesia,' "Principle and Practice of Obstetric Analgesia and Anesthesia." Shortly after that, Dr. Sol Shnider accepted a position at the University of California as chief of obstetric anesthesia.

By 1968, Dr. John S. McDonald was already in residency in anesthesiology at the University of Washington, having just completed a residency in Obstetrics and Gynecology at the University of Iowa. At the same time another obstetrician was taking an anesthesia residency at Emory University. This individual was Dr. George Jackson, who soon left academia to go into private practice. This brief chronology places into perspective the resurgence of interest in this specialty that really only began in the mid to late 1960s after the initial interest was developed in this country by pioneers such as Dr. Robert Hingson and Dr. John Cleland in the early 1940s.

Before the 1970s, there was little interest in the subspecialty area of obstetric anesthesia. It was recognized as an area to itself, but that was mainly because of deselection, not selection, by anesthesiologists in the private community and even in most of the academic centers around the country. It was shunned.

Interest in obstetric anesthesia was promoted by the formation of the Society of Obstetric Anesthesiology and Perinatology, spearheaded by Dr. Sol Shnider and colleagues. It also became generally accepted that this area of care for the mother and her unborn baby was of vital concern to all of us. A recurrent problem, which is diminishing, has been to find qualified anesthesiologists with a dedicated interest in this subspecialty.

## Philosophy

It is important to identify the special problems, and solutions for management, of obstetric patients. It is vital that any individual who administers anesthesia for obstetrics not only is a facile person with regional analgesia, but that he/she is also capable and experienced with general anesthesia, and an expert in maintaining the airway in difficult situations. Many adverse outcomes and malpractice cases involve three areas: (1) difficult airway; (2) difficult intubation; and (3) ventilation problems.

### *Preference for Mother or Baby*

Some have suggested that if the life of the baby is at stake, and intubation is impossible, the anesthesiologist can have someone administer cricoid pressure, and continue the case with general anesthesia via mask. We are opposed to this for the reason that no one can guess which patients may regurgitate, aspirate, and perhaps eventually die because of complications. In such a scenario, the life of the mother is being traded for the "life saving emergency of delivery of the baby." We seriously doubt that any mother or father would agree to a gamble with the woman's life for the possibility that an unborn baby may be saved. We believe that, if all aspects of all possibilities were really explained to them, they would opt first and foremost, for the safety of the mother. But such a choice is flawed from the beginning, because we never know whether in fact the baby's life is threatened and will only be saved with an immediate cesarean section; nor, for that matter, do we know if the baby has already been seriously damaged. Last, though there have been individual reports of general anesthesia being administered in this fashion, we cannot confirm its complete safety. Until proven otherwise, it is a method that sets the mother up for regurgitation and aspiration, and we would prefer not to be a party to it.

### *Loss of Enjoyment*

One of the chief disadvantages of general anesthesia is loss of maternal enjoyment of the moment of birth of her baby. This is a major highlight in any woman's life, and it makes little sense to miss the entire birth scene. This is an excellent time for bonding with the newborn. Absence of this bonding period is also said to be a possible cause of postpartum mental disturbance. A woman experiences all sorts of problems, joys, and travails during the 9 months of gestation, and to be unconscious when the big moment arrives is not a fitting climax to the long process.

A memorable example of the importance that the mother gives to the moment of birth is illustrated by the history of a diabetic patient who had suffered two fetal losses before her current pregnancy of 33 weeks. It was decided to deliver the patient by cesarean section, and the technique of anesthesia was discussed with the patient. The mother decided upon regional anesthesia so that she would be able to interact with the baby immediately after birth, be able to touch it, be able to see it breathe, and be able at last to see a live baby. Regional anesthesia was used successfully and a live baby was delivered, and handed to the tearful and appreciative mother. She confided later that she was so thankful to be able to see and touch her newborn baby just after delivery. She mentioned that if she had had general anesthesia, if she had not been able to see her baby, and if something happened to the baby without her being able to bond with it, she would have been devastated. Thus, this interaction between the mother and newborn must not be undervalued or taken lightly by any of the health care team.

### *Summary*

We must emphasize the importance of detailed knowledge of pregnancy-associated physiologic changes before working in and administering obstetric anesthesia. Please see Chapter 2 for detailed descriptions of the physiologic changes. To summarize briefly, pregnant patients are: (1) more sensitive to inhalation drugs due to the ventilation changes (functional residual capacity, residual volume, and total lung volumes all diminished) and to the diminished requirements of alveolar concentration of anesthetics during pregnancy; (2) more predisposed to oxygen desaturation due to increased oxygen consumption, increased cardiac output, and reduced functional residual capacity, which acts as the body's oxygen reservoir; and (3) more liable to suffer from pulmonary aspiration due to decreased tone of the gastroesophageal sphincter, because of hormonal changes and mechanical factors. Finally, the administration of a general anesthetic must be accomplished by an individual who is an expert in laryngoscopy and intubation, and capable of exercising alternative methods of obtaining airway patency, as well as knowledgeable about the advantages of regional anesthesia, and adept in its administration.

## Special Problems in Obstetrics

The unique problems of obstetric anesthesia are related to lack of trained anesthesia personnel, the frequency of emergencies, multiple patients, physiologic changes of pregnancy, diseases of pregnancy, and obesity.

Because of manpower problems, there have been many instances of inadequately trained individuals administering anesthesia for obstetric patients, with occasional catastrophic results, due to improper application of drugs and techniques, and inadequate detection, diagnosis, and definitive therapeutic measures.

### *Emergencies*

There are situations in obstetric anesthesia unlike any others, which may be precipitated in the middle of the night, when the anesthetist has no skilled help. There is a tremendous difference between an elective operation and a declared emergency cesarean section. The mental disadvantages in regard to the emergency case include lack of flexibility, lack of preparedness, lack of control, and, finally, the stress of the ticking clock in regard to salvation of the fetus at risk. This is an extremely important matter, and one in which the cooperation and understanding between the two disciplines of obstetrics and anesthesiology must be closely coordinated.

Certainly, the anesthesiologist does not want to be in the position of questioning the decision-making basis of obstetricians. To them, an emergency is an emergency, and in the case of the obstetric one, the scenario is stat. The anesthesiologist is well aware of the fact that the fetus is at risk due to one or a combination of many maternal, fetal, or placental complications. The response time must be swift and the decision making in haste, due to the fact that the physician must quickly obtain analgesia so that surgery can begin and the fetus can be delivered and removed from the threat of severe damage or even demise. This is one of the factors that tends to turn many anesthesiologists away from the practice of obstetric anesthesiology.

To compound the problems, anesthesiologists often work alone and are thrust into a confusing clinical picture in which they have to assure an adequate intravenous route, monitor blood pressure, place EKG pads and begin cardiac monitoring, attach other monitors, establish an airway, anesthetize the patient, and then stabilize her as surgery begins. If extra complications occur that distract the anesthesiologist, or if problems occur during any phase of the induction and preparation for delivery, then some aspect of the protective steps for the patient's benefit may be omitted. The mother, baby, or both may pay for distraction at such a crucial time.

The stat cesarean is also traumatic from the nursing and surgical viewpoints. The care and consideration needed for every patient is often disrupted by such emergency procedures. For surgeons, nurses, and other personnel, these may be minor nuisances, but in the case of the speciality of anesthesiology, it can mean the patient's life and even the baby's life. Thus, it behooves the obstetrician to call for assistance as early as possible when a problem is developing, to alert people, so that the anesthesiologist and nurses can all begin to work together and plan strategically for a successful outcome for everyone concerned.

There has been a standing philosophy for some time in many centers that the only method of analgesia possible in such emergencies is general anesthesia. The reasoning behind this is simple and is linked to the timing problem. It is often stated that subarachnoid analgesia takes too long and is not suitable for some emergencies. Yet there have been many situations in which administration of a spinal took no longer than it would have taken to induce general anesthesia. In circumstances in which the airway may be questionable and the intubation suspect, a subarachnoid block should be attempted after quick discussion with the obstetrician and the patient. Such a step could go far to save a mother's life and protect the life of the unborn baby at the same time.

## *Local Anesthesia for Emergencies*

This is a situation in which local anesthesia must also be mentioned. It is a clear possibility and should be made a clear probability in centers where there are many patients with morbid obesity who are pregnant. Local analgesia may be the one thing that will work best in a difficult situation, in which anesthesiologists believe they are faced with an impossible airway-management problem, the obstetrician demands delivery as quickly as possible, and the fetus continues to deteriorate. There may not be time to attempt an awake intubation. The anesthesiologist may determine that it would be a lethal threat to the patient's life if he or she followed the usual rapid sequence induction technique.

This is the time when optimal communication, coordination, cooperation, and compromise must be operative. A time when the anesthesiologist and obstetrician must put aside any of their biases and work together to effect a safe outcome for both the mother and baby. The point here is that in this situation the obstetrician must not become frantic and threatening and demand "anesthesia immediately or the life of this baby will be lost, and it will be your fault." This type of unprofessional conduct does nothing to solve a difficult situation and only ignites the tempers of all who are involved, and distracts them from performing at their best level.

In this scenario of one of the most difficult situations possible, in which the fetus is in distress and the mother is morbidly obese and presents as a possible difficult intubation, the obstetrician can inject the local anesthetic before the formal prepping and draping, before gowning and gloving. The obstetrician can proceed swiftly with a cutaneous block of the dermatome distribution of T-10, T-11, and T-12, the dermatome distribution of the ilioinguinal nerves bilaterally, and infiltrate the line of incision (Figure 20–1). Another possibility would be as depicted in Figure 20–2. In this case, a 22-gauge spinal needle is used, with two lines of infiltration, one on either side of the vertical incision beneath the umbilicus to the pubis. In case of a Pfannenstiel incision, a different type of injection technique is necessary, as depicted in Figure 20–3 and 20–4, and that is basically the blockade of the ilioinguinal and iliohypogastric nerves bilaterally. The nurse should prep the patient while the obstetrician gowns and gloves and prepares for the incision. In this way, the local anesthetics will have some time to become effective. The anesthesiologist should prepare a dilute solution of ketamine, and administer small intermittent doses of ketamine if necessary to help with the patient's pain control, but more im-

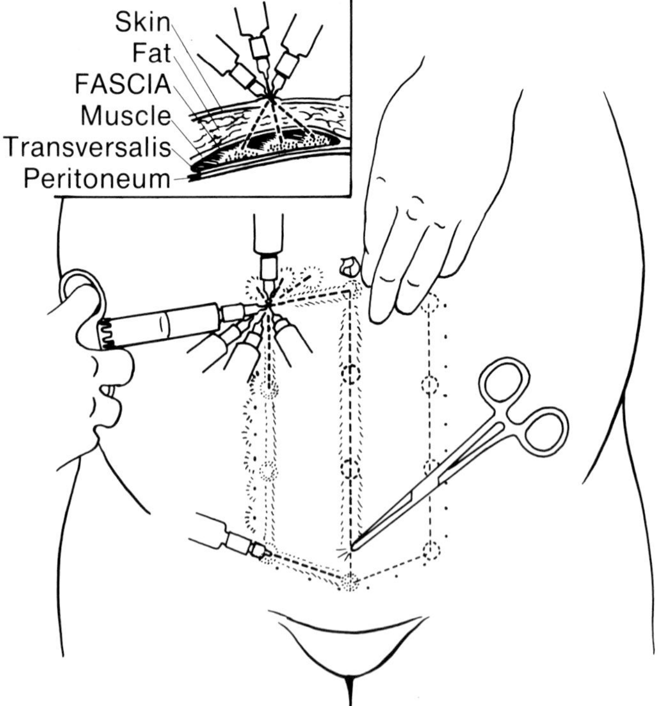


**Fig. 20–1.** Abdominal field block. Infiltration of the abdominal wall for cesarean section. This blocks the T10, T11, and T12 dermatomes, the ilioinguinal nerve distribution, and the line of incision. (Redrawn from Ranney B, Stonage WF: Advantages of local anesthesia for cesarean section. Obstet Gynecol 45:162, 1975.)

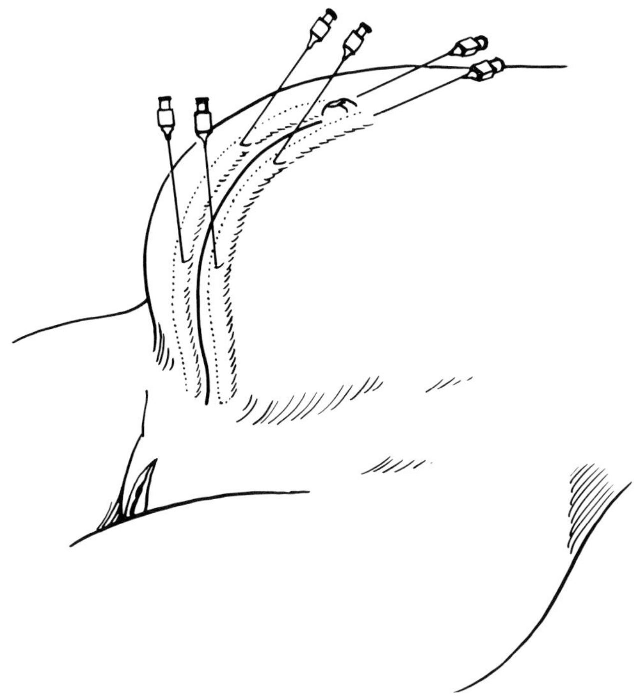

**Fig. 20–2.** Local infiltration of the lower abdominal wall. A long 22-gauge needle is used to infiltrate in parallel lines from the umbilicus to the pubis. The incision is made between them. (Redrawn from Gordh T: Infiltration anaesthesia for cesarean section. *In* Illustrated Handbook in Local Anaesthesia. Edited by E Eriksson. Philadelphia, WB Saunders, 1980.)

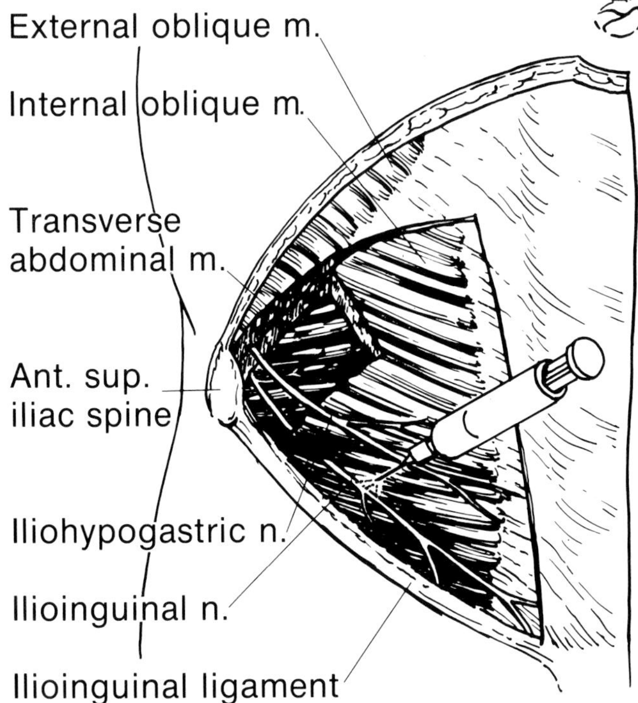


**Fig. 20–3.** Ilioinguinal nerve blockade. This is useful for a Pfannenstiel incision, along with infiltration of the site of incision. (Redrawn from Gordh T: Infiltration anaesthesia for cesarean section. *In* Illustrated Handbook in Local Anaesthesia. Edited by E Eriksson. Philadelphia, WB Saunders, 1980.)

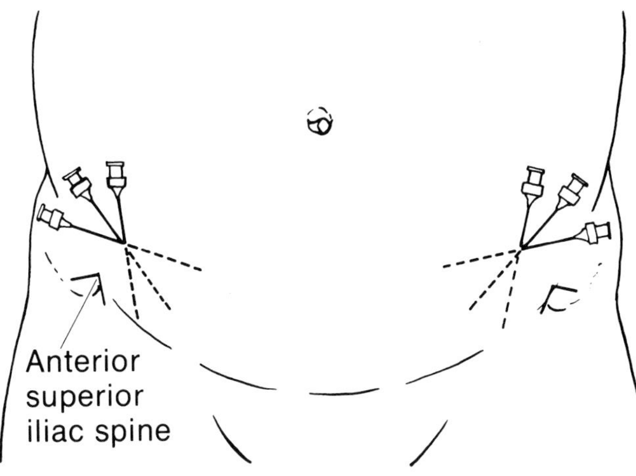


**Fig. 20–4.** Iliohypogastric nerve block. This is also used before a Pfannenstiel incision. (Redrawn from Gordh T: Infiltration anaesthesia for cesarean section. *In* Illustrated Handbook in Local Anaesthesia. Edited by E Eriksson. Philadelphia, WB Saunders, 1980.)

portantly, the anesthesiologist serves as a facilitator to calm the patient and to assuage her fears of the procedure.

Fifty years ago, cesarean operations were routinely performed under local anesthesia. The performance of a cesarean section under local is not very difficult, as it necessitates only the incision of the skin, entry of the peritoneum, followed by entry of the uterus, which is quite superficial, and delivery of the baby. Of course, such a procedure is not simple and cannot be performed without planning and practice. Therefore, it is wise to plan early for such a possibility, and teach the obstetric residents to use regional block techniques, the anatomic courses of the superficial abdominal nerves, local infiltration, maximum doses and safe levels of local anesthetic drugs. This is an area in which the anesthesiologist can assume a leadership role, solve a big problem in regard to the health and welfare of a mother and her baby, and receive appreciation from obstetricians because of their help in teaching the technique of local anesthesia. This could be a very valuable contribution and could serve as an important adjunct for the obstetrician at some time in the future.

### *The Principal Physiologic Changes of Pregnancy*

Some of the more important physiologic changes associated with pregnancy are summarized below:

Respiratory System (3)
- *Increased* tidal volume and minute ventilation
- *Decreased* lung capacity, residual volume, functional residual capacity

Cardiovascular System (4)
- *Increased* blood volume, cardiac output and cardiac size
- *Decreased* peripheral resistance, blood pressure
- Dilutional anemia
- Hemodynamic instability due to the uterus compressing the aorta and vena cava (5,6)

**Table 20–1.** Administration of Intravenous Fluid

| Route of Delivery (Anesthesia) | During Birth (ml/hr) | Delivery (ml/hr) | After Birth (ml/hr) |
|---|---|---|---|
| Vaginal delivery (local) | 361 ± 264 | 757 ± 422 | 70 ± 50 |
| Vaginal delivery (conduction) | 330 ± 119 | 1046 ± 860 | 82 ± 48 |
| Cesarean section (conduction) | 430 ± 463 | 838 ± 543 | 142 ± 41 |
| Cesarean section (general) | 595 ± 858 | 1088 ± 394 | 157 ± 36 |

Values reported as mean ± SD.
(From Cotton DB, Gonik B, Spillman T, Dorman KF: Intrapartum to postpartum changes in colloid oncotic pressure. Am. J. Obstet. Gynecol. 149:174–176, 1984.)

- Gastrointestinal System
  - Displacement
  - Delayed emptying (7–10)
  - Increased incidence of hiatal hernia (11,12)
  - Relaxation of gastroesophageal sphincter (13,14)
- Renal Function
  - Ureters and renal pelvis dilate
  - Renal blood flow and glomerular filtration increase
  - Lower renal threshold for sugar causes glycosuria
- Anesthetic Sensitivity
  - Increased endorphin activity (15)
  - MAC for inhaled anesthetics is reduced (16,17)
  - Speed of induction is increased
  - Muscle relaxant drug duration is often increased
- Water Balance
  - Plasma protein and colloid oncotic pressure decrease (18)
  - There is an increase of extracellular fluid, and peripheral edema develops (19,20)

Pulmonary water balance is in a tenuous state. Fluid loading may be deliberate before regional anesthesia, or inadvertent during labor, particularly with inductions. Pulmonary edema is a hazard. Sudden fluxes in pulmonary water balance can cause lung water to accumulate rapidly, if more fluid is formed than can be swept away by normal channels. Intravenous fluids at the time of vaginal delivery and cesarean section must be used judiciously so that the patient is not overloaded. Intravenous boluses before the use of regional anesthesia have been extremely important in offsetting the hypotension that may occur due to the sympathectomy that is associated with the regional block techniques. However, administration of intravenous fluid for vaginal delivery today follows a more conservative route, which is illustrated in Table 20–1. Comparisons of intrapartum and postpartum colloid oncotic pressures according to the vaginal delivery or the cesarean section route are shown in Table 20–2. Note that the changes of colloid oncotic pressure are not significantly different, regardless of whether the patient is delivered vaginally or abdominally, or whether the anesthetic was a regional or a general.

Fluid overload is a serious threat to the mother's health and well-being. The pertinent physiologic changes that are associated include those we have already discussed in this chapter, primarily the increase in cardiac output by more than 40%, the greatly expanded blood volume, and the associated increased plasma volume. In addition, there is a significant increase in extracellular fluid in the connective tissue spaces. This may be as much as 2 liters. This results in a reduction in oncotic pressure of 7 cm of water. These related physiologic changes can be important because pulmonary water can accumulate rapidly. This phenomenon may be better understood if a formula is used to demonstrate the aforementioned variables, as in Table 20–3 (21). The initial colloid oncotic pressure is seemingly the *crucial parameter* that promotes fluid absorption, thus preventing alveolar flooding in spite of an occasional overload of the interstitial spaces in pregnancy.

These physiologic changes result in a more rapid induction of anesthesia, and more importantly, a more rapid development of a hypoxic state. If one adds to this the fact that the anesthesiologist cannot predict which patients may have difficult airways and be difficult to intubate, it is clear that avoidance of general anesthesia should be a factor in providing safe anesthesia for the mother. Unfortunately, problems relating to the fetus may make the situation more difficult and require general anesthesia for the mother.

## Morbid Obesity

The patient with morbid obesity is viewed as the most difficult and threatening patient to manage and care for in

**Table 20–2.** Comparison of Intrapartum and Postpartum Colloid Osmotic Pressure Changes by Route of Delivery

| Colloid Osmotic Pressure (mm Hg) | Vaginal Delivery | | Cesarean Section | |
|---|---|---|---|---|
| | Anesthesia | | Anesthesia | |
| | Local (n = 18) | Conduction (n = 18) | Conduction (n = 18) | General (n = 18) |
| Intrapartum | 21.8 ± 1.8 | 20.7 ± 2.4 | 21.1 ± 2.1 | 20.5 ± 2.0 |
| Postpartum | 16.5 ± 2.1 | 15.1 ± 1.4 | 15.5 ± 2.0 | 14.4 ± 1.5 |
| Δ Change | −5.2 ± 2.0 | −5.6 ± 2.1 | −5.6 ± 1.8 | −6.1 ± 2.4 |

The postpartum values were all significantly ($p < 0.01$) decreased from the intrapartum values in each group. The degree of reduction was not significantly different in any of the groups when compared by route of delivery or type of anesthesia. Values are expressed as mean ± standard deviation.
(From Cotton DB, Gonik B, Spillman T, Dorman KF: Intrapartum to postpartum changes in colloid oncotic pressure. Am. J. Obstet. Gynecol. 149: 174–176, 1984.)

**Table 20–3.** The Starling Formula

$$\dot{Q}f = Lp \cdot A[(Pmv - Pis) - \sigma(\pi mv - \pi is)]$$

| | |
|---|---|
| $\dot{Q}f$ | = transvascular water flow |
| Lp | = hydraulic conductivity of the membrane (increased in the hydrated states of pregnancy) |
| A | = surface area of exchange (thought not to rise with pregnancy) |
| Pmv | = microvascular hydrostatic pressure (great capacity for expansion) |
| Pis | = interstitial hydrostatic pressure (opposes filtration of fluid) |
| $\sigma$ | = Staverman reflection coefficient (membrane permeability) |
| $\pi$mv | = plasma oncotic pressure (falls in pregnancy so flow out of vessels is promoted) |
| $\pi$is | = interstitial oncotic pressure (unknown, but less than plasma) |

(Modified by Robert Kirby, M.D., From MacLennan FM. Maternal mortality from Mendelson's Syndrome: an explanation. *Lancet.* March 15, 1986:587.)

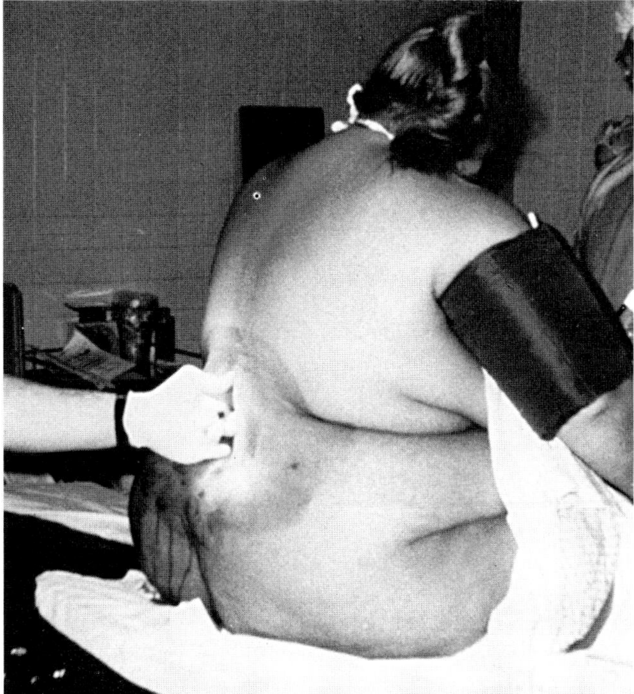

**Fig. 20–5.** Morbid obesity. This patient is in sitting position for continuous epidural. Block was accomplished successfully using a 5-inch needle. (From The Ohio State University, Department of Anesthesiology, 1992.)

obstetric anesthesia. Not only is regional anesthesia more difficult, but so is general anesthesia more difficult and menacing, from the viewpoint of airway management, intubation problems, and safety. It must be stated at the outset that the authors of this chapter and the editors of this book believe firmly in the concept of regional anesthesia for most applications of anesthesia for obstetrics. Not only does this allow the mother awareness during her delivery, be it either vaginal or abdominal, but it also affords assurance of patient control over her airway, and avoids the need to be dependent upon another individual for oxygenation and ventilation. The importance of this cannot be overstated. It is wise to make sure that this one subtle point is clear to all obstetric patients and other lay people.

Being able to maintain constant control over one's own breathing may represent the difference between life and death. Also, it must be appreciated that many patients, because of extreme obesity, cannot breathe unless they are in a 30 to 45° sitting position. This is illustrated in Figure 20–5. Both the surgery and anesthesia plans must take this into account; the standard supine position may be untenable.

Epidural and spinal anesthesia are more difficult to accomplish because the anatomic landmarks are obscured. Longer needles and the paramedian approach are often required. Sonographic guidance may help to place the epidural needle (22).

If any consideration is given to general anesthesia, awake intubation with local anesthesia should be used. A surgeon skilled in performing a tracheostomy should stand by to assist if needed.

## *Not So Morbidly Obese Patient*

Not so morbid obesity refers to the person whose body weight is 30 to 100 pounds greater than normal. This individual, when not pregnant, is unlikely to cause insuperable difficulties with anesthesia. When she becomes pregnant, the difficulties increase, probably due to the edema that so often develops. For regional anesthesia, it is more difficult to palpate and locate the bony landmarks. If there is a problem, the paramedian approach provides a better chance of success. For general anesthesia, maintaining the airway before intubation is more difficult, and intubation is much more difficult due to edema of the airway tissues and enlargement of the breasts. If there is any doubt about success of intubation, it should be done with the patient under local anesthesia, conscious but sedated, and breathing spontaneously. A surgeon skilled in performing tracheostomy should be on hand, ready to intervene if necessary.

## *Effects on the Fetus*

Among the complications of general anesthesia in obstetrics, we must consider possible adverse effects on the fetus. Anything harmful to the mother affects also the fetus. Any drug given to the mother is transmitted to the fetus through the placenta (Figure 20–6 and Table 20–4) (16,23–27). Even conditions that do not have an adverse effect on the mother may inflict injury upon the neonate (Table 20–5) (28,29). This is most likely to occur in situations that result in diminished uterine blood flow, or transmission of depressant drugs to the fetus that later affect the neonate. The depressant effect on the mother may be insignificant, but the neonate, subjected to the trauma of delivery, severed from its umbilical life-line, changing its pattern of blood circulation, must also initiate breathing, clear its lungs and adjust to the cold world. The neonate often needs help to get started, and even a little depressant drug may be too much for it. This is where the neonatologist shines.

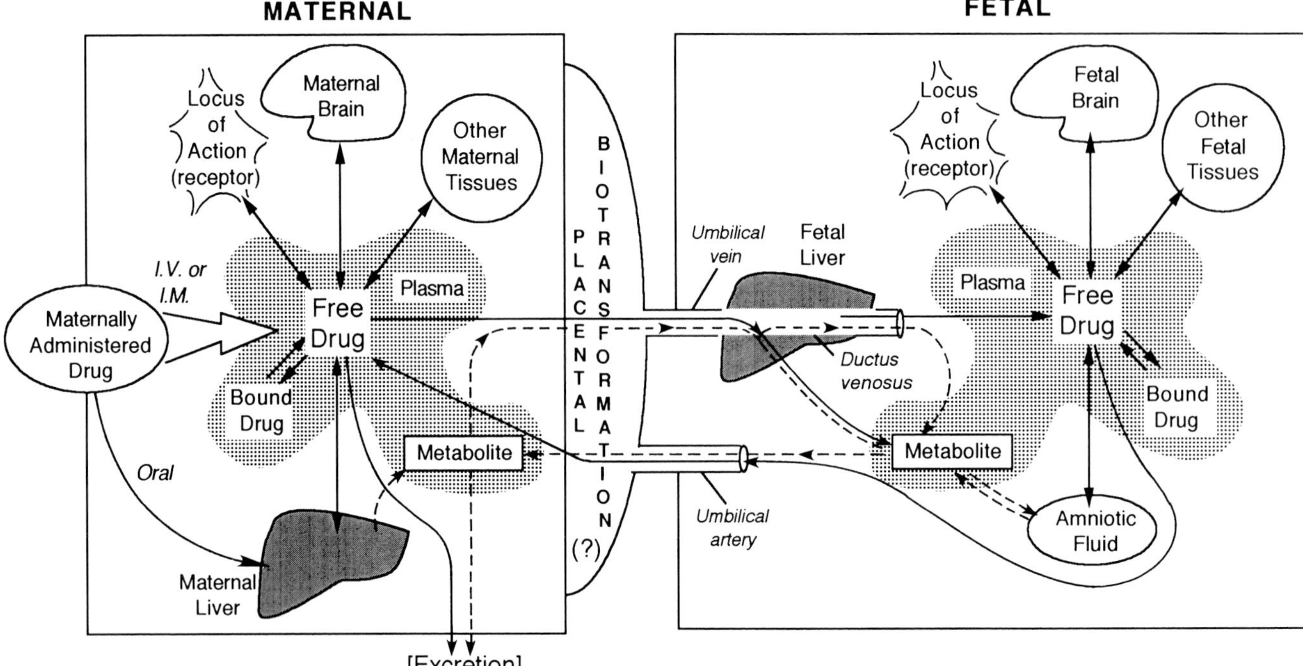


**Fig. 20–6.** Placental transmission of drugs. Any drug given to the mother is transmitted to the fetus through the placenta. A complex equilibrium is established. (Redrawn from Mirkin BL: Perinatal pharmacology: placental transfer, fetal localization, and neonatal disposition of drugs. Anesthesiology. 43:156–170, 1975.)

## Other Potential Problems

Induction is almost always accomplished with intravenous medication. If the intravenous line infiltrates, the patient does not lose consciousness as expected; the site of infiltration is painful and becomes inflamed. There may be tissue damage.

When the patient does lose consciousness, she may develop obstruction of the air passages, and be unable to breathe. It may be impossible to give artificial respiration. It may also be impossible to insert an endotracheal tube. Progressive asphyxia may develop (30). At any time, the patient may have active or passive regurgitation, followed by aspiration. The regurgitated material may add mechanical blockage of the airway, or cause laryngeal spasm.

The endotracheal intubation may be traumatic, the tube may be misplaced, or it may be impossible to insert the tube.

The patient's vital signs may change dramatically, because of the effect of the drugs, because of inability to ventilate or intubate, because of aspiration or of reflex stimulation. The doses of drugs may be inadequate or excessive. If there are any medical problems present before the induction, they may become worse because of it.

**Table 20–4.** Protein Binding of Drugs

$$[P] + [D] \underset{k_2}{\overset{k1}{\rightleftharpoons}} [PD]$$

[P] = free protein concentration
[D] = free drug concentration
[PD] = drug-protein complex concentration

At equilibrium:

$$k_1[P][D] = k_2\,[PD]$$

$$\frac{[PD]}{[P]\,[D]} = \frac{k_1}{k_2} = K = \text{association or affinity constant}$$

(From Mirkin BL: Perinatal pharmacology: placental transfer, fetal localization and neonatal disposition of drugs. Anesthesiology 43:156–170, 1975.)

## Venous Access

Any patient having general anesthesia should have a good intravenous infusion that runs freely without signs of infiltration. If there is any possibility that significant bleeding may occur, the size of the catheter should be adequate for rapid blood transfusion, ordinarily a 16 gauge.

The intravenous should be tested before beginning, by momentarily opening the control clamp and observing a rapid, free flow of fluid, without swelling at the intravenous site. If the patient complains of pain at the site when medication is injected, the administration of medication should be stopped, and a new intravenous should be started.

If there are not any good peripheral veins, it is tempting to consider insertion of a catheter into the subclavian or internal jugular vein. Either of these approaches may cause problems, especially a pneumothorax. During an emergency procedure, this may be undiagnosed, with se-

**Table 20–5.** Modifications of Anesthetic Technique Resulting in Improved Neonatal Outcome

| Study | No. Patients | Type of General Anesthesia | Lateral Tilt | Results |
|---|---|---|---|---|
| Marx and Mateo (16) | | 33–67% Nitrous oxide | | |
| | | $6\frac{1}{2}$% Cyclopropane or $1\frac{1}{4}$–$2\frac{1}{2}$% fluroxene | | |
| | 25 | 28–33% Oxygen | —* | Apgar $\leq 7$ in 48% of patients |
| | 25 | 65% Oxygen | — | Apgar $\leq 7$ in 16% of patients |
| | 25 | 93–97% Oxygen | — | Apgar $\leq 7$ in 8% of patients |
| Crawford et al. (5) | 87 | 67% Nitrous oxide-33% oxygen | No | 1 min A-C† $<8$ in 51% of patients<br>5 min A-C $<8$ in 15% of patients |
| | 63 | 67% Nitrous oxide-33% oxygen | Yes | 1 min A-C $<8$ in 33% of patients<br>5 min A-C $<8$ in 8% of patients |
| Moir (17) | 75 | 70% Nitrous oxide-30% oxygen | — | 2 min Apgar $<8$ in 45% of patients |
| | | 50% Nitrous oxide-50% oxygen, 0.5% halothane | — | 2 min Apgar $<8$ in 11% of patients |
| Robertson et al. (23) | | 67% Nitrous oxide-33% oxygen | | |
| | 9 | I-D‡ $<16$ min | — | 1 min A-C $<8$ in 33% of patients<br>5 min A-C $<8$ in 22% of patients |
| | 9 | I-D 16–42 min | — | 1 min A-C $<8$ in 88% of patients<br>5 min A-C $<8$ in 67% of patients |
| Zagorzycki and Brinkman (26) | 90 | 50% Nitrous oxide, 50% oxygen, 0.5% halothane | | |
| | | I-D $<15$ min | Yes | 1 min Apgar $<7$ in 15% of patients<br>5 min Apgar $<7$ in 0% of patients |
| | | I-D $\geq 15$ min | Yes | 1 min Apgar $<7$ in 20% of patients<br>5 min Apgar $<7$ in 0% of patients |

* —, no specific effort to tilt the patient was noted.
† A-C, Apgar minus color score (thus, the maximum value is 8).
‡ I-D, induction to delivery interval.
(From Zagorzycki MT: General anesthesia in cesarean section: effect on mother and neonate. Obstet. Gynecol. Survey. 39:134–137, 1984.)

rious consequences. It is safer to rely upon a peripheral vein cutdown.

## Airway Obstruction

All patients having general anesthesia should be preoxygenated, by breathing oxygen from a mask for several minutes, or by several deep breaths from a mask while oxygen is flowing at a high rate. This fills the lungs with oxygen and provides a small reservoir for safety.

Loss of consciousness causes loss of control of the airway, which is normally maintained by the tone of voluntary striated muscle. Airway obstruction may be caused by normal tissue when the muscles become either flaccid or tense. It may be caused by abnormal tissue that encroaches on the air passages because of enlargement by edema, infection, hematoma, or tumor. It may be caused by bony abnormalities, scarring, trauma, or foreign bodies. Airway obstruction is always worse in obese pregnant patients.

Opening the obstructed airway may be accomplished or aided by extension of the head, support of the mandible, pushing the mandible forward (jaw thrust), or pulling the tongue out. Airway obstruction can be one of the greatest threats to the mother's life. The maneuvers just described, such as thrusting the mandible forward, in some emergent situations, i.e., in a patient who does not have an airway and with the patient becoming hypoxic, may be facilitated by someone assisting the anesthesiologist. While the anesthesiologist is attempting with a mask to get positive oxygen pressure into the patient, a second person may assist by placing their fingers behind the mandible, raising it, and pulling forward as forcibly as they can, to help get the tongue forward enough so that an adequate airway is obtained. The assistance of a second person, to lift the mandible forward, is often very valuable. A curved oral airway or a soft rubber nasal airway often helps.

When none of these is effective, unplanned endotracheal intubation is performed as an emergency. Endotracheal intubation is almost always planned for the obstetric patient, so the obstructed airway at the induction is only a transient and unimportant matter, should the intubation be successful. If it is not, other steps must be taken swiftly.

## Mendelson's Aspiration Syndrome

Dr. Curtis L. Mendelson read a now famous paper at the New York Obstetrical Society in December of 1945 (31). In that historic presentation he related that the incidence of gastric aspiration in 44,016 deliveries over the previous 13 years at his hospital was 0.15%, and that aspiration causes pneumonitis. What is remarkable is that there were only 2 deaths in the 66 cases of aspiration, which accounted for a 3% fatality rate. The mortality rate due to aspiration was 1 in 22,000. It should be recalled that in those days the typical anesthetic was chloroform or gas-oxygen-ether, administered without use of an endotracheal tube. It is likely that many cases of aspiration were not counted due to inability to identify them. In fact, the incidence of nonfatal Mendelson's syndrome is essentially unknown even today. A recent study in Sweden (32) in the specialty of anesthesia generally revealed 87 aspirations in 185,000 cases, an incidence of only 0.05%,

**Table 20–6.** Concomitant Anaesthetic Complications

| Complication | Cases |
|---|---|
| Laryngospasm | 19 |
| Intubation difficulties | 8 |
| Vomiting | 41 |
| Ventilatory problems | 7 |
| Bronchospasm | 12 |
| Cardiac arrest | 3 |
| Hypotension | 2 |
| Serious arrhythmia | 2 |
| Insufficient anaesthesia | 3 |
| Technical difficulties | 2 |
| Unspecified | 2 |
| No other complication | 22 |

(From Olsson GL, Hallen B, Hambraeus-Jonzon: Aspiration during anaesthesia: a computer-aided study of 185,358 anaesthetics. Acta. Anaesthesiol. Scand. 30: 84–92, 1986.)

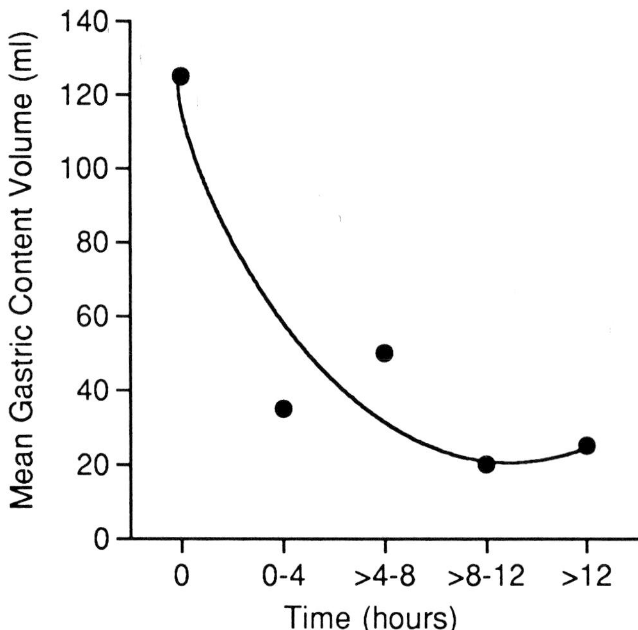


**Fig. 20–7.** Volume of material removed from stomach by suction during cesarean section. Means from 51 patients in labor, related to time interval between last meal and onset of labor. * Nine patients ate after labor began. (Redrawn from Roberts RB, Shirley MA: Reducing the risk of acid aspiration during cesarean section. Anesth. Analg. 53:859–868, 1974.)

or 1 in 2131 cases. Among the 87 who aspirated, 65 had concomitant anesthetic complications. There were 4 deaths in the 87 who aspirated, a 4.7% fatality rate. This translates to a mortality rate due to aspiration of only 1 in 46,000 anesthetics. This study substantiates that deaths from aspiration are rare, and when they do occur, they are often associated with poor physical condition of the patient or other complicating medical problems that may be patient related or care related (Table 20–6) (32).

Although the frequency of deaths from aspiration is low, each occurrence is a catastrophe. The end result of aspiration is pneumonitis, which was first reported by Hall in 1940 (33). He stated then that it may well be the prime cause of maternal mortality. The predominant physical findings in Mendelson's report were cyanosis, tachycardia, and dyspnea; in addition, there was a high frequency of asthma-like reactions. Mendelson's aspiration pneumonitis is one cause of Adult Respiratory Distress Syndrome (ARDS).

A number of preventions have been instituted to lessen the incidence of this disease process, including reduction of gastric volume, elevation of gastric pH, induction of patients in the head up position, use of cricoid pressure during induction, use of a rapid sequence induction regimen, prevention of gastric dilatation by avoiding or limiting mask positive pressure, and the use of potent, rapidly acting muscle relaxants just prior to laryngoscopy and intubation (Figure 20–7 and Table 20–7) (34–39).

Despite these preventative regimens, it appears that there has not been a substantial reduction in maternal morbidity and mortality due to this syndrome. Three significant elements of the aspiration equation are pH, volume of aspirate, and quality of aspirate. Despite widespread use of antacids and other gastric acid neutralizers, aspiration syndrome still looms as one of the most significant anesthetic causes of maternal morbidity and mortality.

This portion of the chapter looks at several aspects of the aspiration syndrome, including pathophysiology and preventative suggestions directed specifically at improvement of maternal outcome. In addition, it discusses the current consensus for detection, diagnosis, and definitive therapy for the aspiration syndrome.

## *Pathophysiology*

The foundation for aspiration syndrome is laid in the first trimester, when the gastroesophageal sphincter loses some of its tone, presumably due to early hormonal changes. In the second and third trimesters, this foundation is added upon by notable anatomic changes that eventually result in significant upward displacement of the stomach. This compounds the problem of incompetence of the gastroesophageal sphincter. Delayed gastric emptying associated with pregnancy, and the higher than normal residual gastric volume, both become added concerns. Active or passive regurgitation, and aspiration of gastric material, trigger the onset of the disease process. The material may be clear liquid with a low pH value or contain solid particulate matter, as well as large pieces of inadequately chewed food. The onset and course of the syndrome, and eventual survival of the patient, are dependent upon the nature and amount of the aspirated material, in addition to any other complicating factors such as a preexisting infection or conditions of medical significance .

Mendelson reported his initial investigative work with instillation of various materials into the lungs of adult rabbits. It was that study that spotlighted the importance of

**Table 20–7.** Steps That Have Been Recommended to Minimize Risks of Aspiration in Parturients, and Disadvantages Thereof (From Various Sources)

| Recommended Step | Disadvantages |
|---|---|
| 1. NPO during labor | Patient may eat before admission. Gastric contents increased during long labor. |
| 2. Preanesthetic emptying of stomach by | |
| a. N-G tube | Theoretically ideal; unpleasant; effectiveness doubtful; time-consuming. False sense of security. |
| b. Apomorphine | Circulatory collapse reported. Undiagnosed esophageal pouch or hiatus hernia possible. |
| 3. Awake intubation | Barbaric without local anesthesia. Vomiting and aspiration possible if laryngeal reflexes obtunded by local anesthetic. |
| 4. Head-up or anti-Trendelenburg | Intubation difficult. If regurgitation or vomiting occurs, aspiration inevitable. Intragastric pressure high after succinylcholine. |
| 5. Cricoid pressure | Skilled assistant needed. Rupture of esophagus with vomiting. |
| 6. Head-down and/or inhalational induction | Flammable agents often used. Fetal depression. Unprotected trachea. |
| 7. Lateral position | Obstructed airway enhances vomiting. |
| 8. Mandatory endotracheal intubation | Inexperienced intubators not always successful. Aspiration still possible before, during, and after intubation. |
| 9. Oral antacids | May not be effective with large gastric volumes. |
| 10. Regional anesthesia | Aspiration still possible, especially if patient is also sedated. Other complications may be higher than with general anesthesia. |

(From Roberts RB, Shirley MA: Reducing the risk of acid aspiration during cesarean section. Anesth. Analg. 53:859–868, 1974.)

the pH of the aspirated gastric material, because it revealed that hydrochloric acid was responsible for bronchiolar spasm, peribronchiolar congestion, and an exudative reaction that interfered with normal pulmonary circulation and led to cardiac failure. Interestingly enough, Mendelson referred to early work by Winternitz in 1920, who described similar pulmonary changes that occurred following war gas-poisonings with chlorine and phosgene (40). It may well have been this very piece of work that stimulated Dr. Mendelson to do his study.

The above all serve as pathophysiologic elements related to patient causes of the disease process. In addition, there are also important physician-related causes. One of these is the lack of appreciation of the need for rapid establishment of the orotracheal airway followed by airway security obtained by use of an endotracheal tube with an inflated cuff. The rapid sequence induction is just what it means: rapid. This is defined as intubation immediately after the succinylcholine fasciculations subside. Thus, the single salient aspect of airway security is identified with rapid, sure intubation and endotracheal tube cuff inflation while cricoid pressure is maintained. If this does not happen on the first pass, then aspiration has a significantly greater chance of occurring. Often, the importance of the first-pass success is not appreciated, and the case is treated as just another routine cesarean section. It would be wise to emphasize to all those responsible anesthesiologists working in this area to keep these two important facts in mind: (1) the importance of rapidity of action; and (2) the importance of success on the first attempt at intubation. It is now timely to encourage all obstetricians to be aware of this aspect of patient care, which is not normally understood or even known by those who are not directly responsible for anesthesia care.

The problem, of course, is that it just is not possible to obtain 100% successful laryngoscopy and intubation on the first pass. To date there have not been established foolproof criteria for preoperative identification of those patients who are difficult to intubate, despite many attempts by many to do so. Therefore, this is the single most uncontrolled factor in the pathophysiology of the aspiration syndrome today, and, it is unlikely that it will be eradicated as the most important factor in the near future, unless a sure method of intubation is discovered that simultaneously maintains patient control of the airway and breathing.

### Prevention

One of the most important measures in preventing regurgitation was reported by Dr. Sellick in a rather modest fashion, in the Preliminary Communications section of the Lancet in 1961. This was his now famous paper on "Cricoid Pressure to Control Regurgitation of Stomach Contents During Induction of Anaesthesia" (41). It was here that he first described pressing the cricoid cartilage against the fifth cervical vertebra, effectively shutting off the esophagus (Figures 20–8 through 20–10). He reported the initial study of 26 high-risk cases, most with intestinal obstruction, in which he used the technique successfully and without incident. Only two of the 26 were obstetric patients, and both had forceps deliveries. This maneuver, conceived, developed, and studied at the Middlesex Hospital in London, is no doubt one of the great advances in the prevention of gastric aspiration generally, and in obstetric anesthesia particularly.

A recent study of the effect of Ranitidine and sodium citrate on the status of the gastric volume and pH concluded that the best combination was the use of intramuscular doses of Ranitidine (50 mg) every 6 hours during the labor period, and sodium citrate (30 ml) before induction, for those who went on to have general anesthesia. Patients with the lowest volumes of gastric juice and the highest pH values were found in the group that had this combination treatment (35). Even a single oral dose of Ranitidine administered the night before surgery elevated

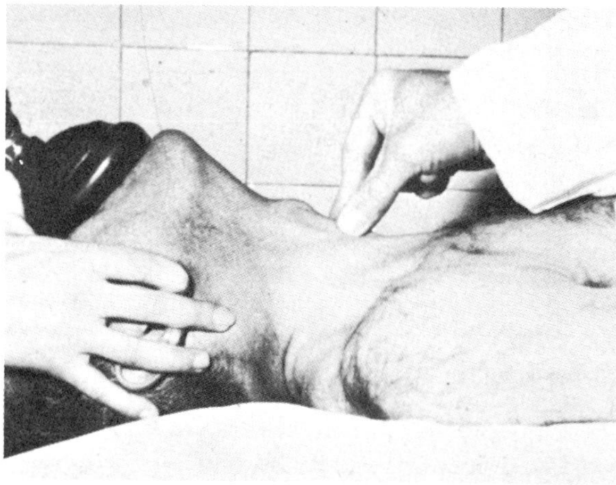

**Fig. 20–8.** The Sellick maneuver: Extension of the head and neck, and application of pressure over the cricoid cartilage. (From Sellick BA: Cricoid pressure to control regurgitation of stomach contents during induction of anaesthesia. Lancet. August 19, 404–406, 1961.)

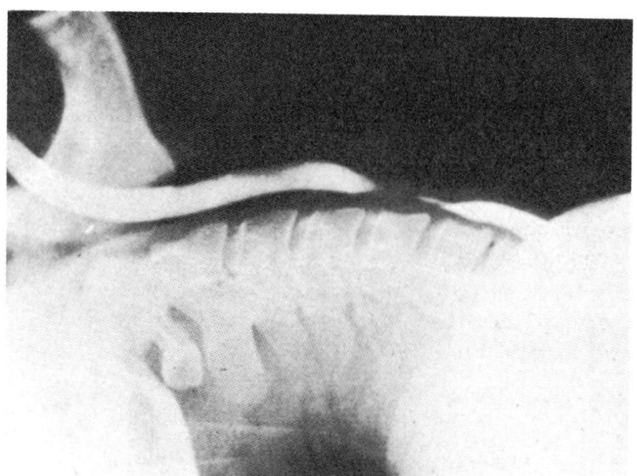

**Fig. 20–10.** Obliteration of esophageal lumen by pressure over the cricoid cartilage. Technique as in figure 20–11. (From Sellick BA: Cricoid pressure to control regurgitation of stomach contents during induction of anaesthesia. Lancet. August 19, 404–406, 1961.)

the pH to 6.74 and reduced the volume to a mean of 8 ml (Table 20–8) (36,42–44).

Measures to prevent aspiration have been in use for over a decade, with very little reduction in the incidence or severity of the aspiration syndrome of pregnancy. A few preventative measures have been adopted as routine in most centers, and include:

1. Reduction of gastric volume by the use of Ranitidine given as prophylaxis early in labor;
2. Elevation of gastric pH by the use of repeated doses of sodium citrate;
3. Increasing the tone of the gastroesophageal sphincter by the use of Metoclopromide, especially in diabetic patients;
4. Prevention of gastric reflux by the use of cricoid pressure;
5. Reduction of the volume and pressure of gas in the stomach by avoiding positive pressure breathing during induction;
6. Rapid sequence induction with thiopental/succinylcholine;
7. Immediate laryngoscopy within seconds after fasciculations cease;
8. Endotracheal tube placement quickly;
9. Immediate cuff inflation; and
10. Immediate confirmation of proper tube placement by observation of $CO_2$ wave form.

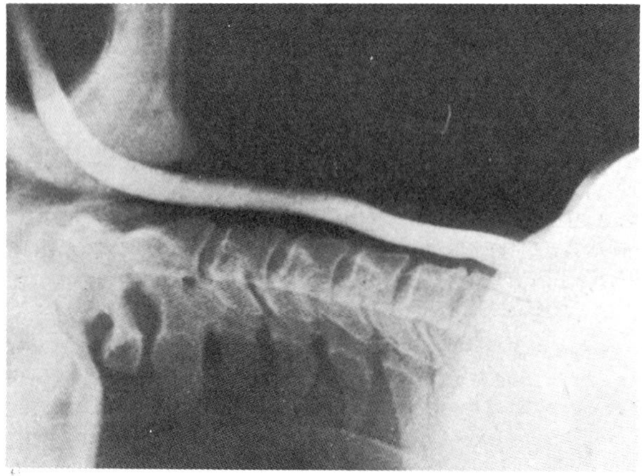

**Fig. 20–9.** Lateral x ray showing the lumen of the esophagus containing a rubber tube filled with contrast material. (From Sellick BA: Cricoid pressure to control regurgitation of stomach contents during induction of anaesthesia. Lancet. August 19, 404–406, 1961.)

One of the more distasteful methods of prevention of aspiration during induction is first to insert a gastric tube and suction out the gastric contents. This has been popular in England, but a recent study (34) concluded that the merits of performing orogastric suction of gastric contents

**Table 20–8.** pH and Volume of Gastric Aspirates After Induction of Anaesthesia in Patients Who Received Famotidine 40 mg, Ranitidine 300 mg or Placebo on the Evening Before Surgery

| | Famotidine | Ranitidine | Placebo |
|---|---|---|---|
| pH, median (range) | 6.17* (1.48–8.18) | 6.74* (1.31–8.20) | 2.45* (1.29–8.14) |
| Volume, ml; median (range) | 8† (0–50) | 8† (0–65) | 10† (0–210) |
| Bile contamination, *n* (%) | 31 (27) | 27 (23) | 13 (23) |

* Active as compared with placebo, $p < 0.01$; famotidine as compared with ranitidine, NS.
† Active as compared with placebo, NS.
(From Gallagher EG, White M, Ward S, Cottrell IJ, et al: Prophylaxis against acid aspiration syndrome. Single oral dose of $H_2$-antagonist on the evening before elective surgery. Anaesthesia 43:1011–1014, 1988)

were outweighed by the unpleasantness of the procedure. The bottom line of the study was that the procedure did not decrease the risk of aspiration. The one exception to this, i.e., when the use of the orogastric suction might be indicated, is for the patient who is known to have had solid food shortly before labor began. Suction must not be relied upon, however, because it cannot empty the stomach completely, because food chunks are swallowed that are larger than the diameter of the suction tube.

The inability to determine which patients may be difficult to intubate means that any obstetric patient may be exposed to the hazard of the acid aspiration syndrome or to asphyxia, due to the fact that endotracheal tube placement may not occur on the first pass, and may not occur on the second or even third pass, necessitating positive pressure ventilation between episodes of laryngoscopy and attempted intubation. Administration of more thiopental and succinylcholine in itself presents a certain hazard, even a lethal one, and this issue will be discussed later, in the section on failed intubation.

### Oral Intake

It is becoming more common to allow laboring patients to have some oral intake, particularly ice chips, water, and perhaps a small amount of a carbonated soft drink. In recent literature, there have been discourses on both sides of the issue of allowing oral intake during labor. For the most part, anesthesiologists are adamant about not allowing such a trend to advance any further. This is based upon their fear of what can happen during any intubation in obstetrics, especially with the pathophysiologic changes being foremost in their minds. On the other hand, obstetricians hear the complaints of the patients who wish to have some limited intake, and they seem to favor a more liberal stand that would allow clear liquids only (45,46). In a random poll during the summer of 1991, it was discovered that three tertiary centers had a policy of allowing clear liquids and ice chips during early labor.

### Diagnosis

Most often, the diagnosis of aspiration is made before symptoms develop by the anesthetist who is attempting to intubate. The anesthetist sees fluid or food particulate matter in the vicinity of the cords. The patient may or may not exhibit immediate signs of respiratory distress. These may develop over the next several hours, and be accompanied by a decrease in the $AaDO_2$ and pulmonary shunt. Changes in oxygenation and pulmonary function will be diagnosed with pulse oximetry and frequent determinations of arterial blood gases. It is important to follow the patient with chest x rays to watch for typical changes of pulmonary edema or pneumonia. These changes begin to appear in the first 24 hours and may progress to a full lung "white out." The patient's color may be clinically less than optimal, with signs of desaturation peripherally and blue discoloration of the fingers, toes, lips, conjunctiva, and ears. In addition, the patient may complain of shortness of breath, chest pain, and inability to take a deep breath. There may be a feeling of lassitude or even confusion and total disorientation, depending upon the severity of the illness.

### Treatment

Immediate treatment for aspiration consists of rapid endotracheal intubation despite the presence of fluid in the pharynx. The cuff must be inflated immediately. The trachea and bronchi should be suctioned. One-hundred percent oxygen should be administered with some inhalational agent for amnesia, but no nitrous oxide. In addition, positive pressure ventilation should be used. This will aid in keeping the highest possible level of pulmonary function in effect for the mother during the operation, which should be abbreviated as much as possible. Positive end-expiratory pressure (PEEP) and continuous positive airway pressure (CPAP) may minimize further damage and deterioration at the pulmonary capillary interface.

Immediately after surgery, the patient should be moved to an intensive care area in which the physician is expert in the management of such patients. Often this is a surgical intensive care unit that is attuned to postsurgical pulmonary and cardiovascular management. During this time, the patient may need to have bronchoscopy and therapeutic suctioning of the airways to dislodge and remove particulate matter. If only clear fluid aspiration has been noted, this is not necessary. Other recommended treatments have been shown to be of no value: immediate washing of the bronchi with saline or bicarbonate, and administration of steroids and antibiotics. The patient should be treated as a classical case of adult respiratory distress syndrome.

## Difficult Airway and Failed Intubation

The incidence of difficult intubations generally is very low (0.5% to 2%). These data are from the general surgical population and are not very reliable for obstetrics. In the obstetric population, it may be much higher; especially in morbidly obese patients who are pregnant, the incidence may be exceeding high (47,48). However, there are no definite studies to confirm this. What is certain in the obstetric population is that there is really a need for rapid and sure intubation on the very first pass, so as to prevent the possibility of regurgitation and aspiration. For all the many reasons already mentioned in this chapter, the pregnant patient is at greater risk of such a complication. One retrospective obstetric study in the recent literature quoted the incidence of difficult intubation as 7 cases out of 1980 cases, for a 0.35% incidence rate (49). This study also emphasized that patients who were found to have difficult intubations presented without any skeletal abnormalities. Simple examination, however, revealed that six of the seven primiparae scheduled for cesarean section were graded with preclinical assessment of class IV using the Mallampati criteria, and with laryngoscopy only one of seven was graded better than III.

Not publicized but of great concern are the consequences of failed intubation in the obstetric patient. These consequences are dependent upon whether a patent airway is readily provided or not. In many cases, especially in the morbidly obese patient, this may be most difficult or even impossible. In short, previously unsuspected obstructed airways may simply overwhelm the anesthesiologist who is often without skilled help in the middle of the night. When laryngoscopy is difficult and the cords cannot be visualized, the patient is much more likely to vomit and aspirate, and has a very short tolerance for apnea due to the rapid desaturation that is accelerated in pregnancy.

Failed intubation is one of the important causes of the acid aspiration syndrome as well as cerebral hypoxia. It is also one of the most important problems of lethal consequence. The inability to insert an endotracheal tube is always distressing, but it is not always an emergency issue, unless it is associated with inability to establish a mask airway. In such an emergency, the anesthesiologist must maintain as tight a mask fit as possible, using both hands and a high flow of oxygen. Someone must be recruited to give intermittent strong positive pressure on the breathing bag, even if it does not seem to expand the patient's chest. The patient becomes progressively more desaturated until she can ventilate on her own again. For the obstetric patient, this usually means somewhere between 4 to 5 minutes of apnea before the succinylcholine wears off, and then the patient can begin to generate some small muscular activity on her own. This should enable her to take in fresh oxygen and gradually reoxygenate her blood.

The real problem arises when the anesthesiologist decides to use additional doses of short-acting muscle relaxant to provide "more optimal conditions" for laryngoscopy, prolonging the apnea time to 8 to 10 minutes. This scenario can become a lethal one, should no pulmonary ventilation be established. This condition should not arise, however, because a second dose of muscle relaxant should not be administered if the mask airway is not deemed adequate or satisfactory, especially if the patient has obvious morbid obesity. What can happen in reality, moreover, is that the anesthesiologist in charge becomes stressed and excited; this may lead to reflex reinjection of succinylcholine in the empty hope that it will provide better conditions for laryngoscopy and intubation.

### Pathophysiology

The primary anatomic causes of difficult intubation are:

1. receding jaw;
2. small mouth;
3. high arched palate;
4. prominent frontal incisors;
5. short and thick neck;
6. large tongue;
7. large tonsils or other mass in the throat;
8. reduced mobility of the mandible; or
9. reduced mobility of the cervical spine.

Other causes of a miscellaneous nature can include acromegaly, myxedema, goiter, and morbid obesity associated with pregnancy (50). In addition, there are many congenital causes such as Pierre Robin Syndrome, Treacher Collins Syndrome, congenital tracheal stenosis, and laryngeal webs.

**Table 20–9A** Complications of Difficult Airway

| |
|---|
| Soft-tissue lacerations with subsequent swelling and air way problems |
| Dislodged and broken teeth, with possibility of aspiration and subsequent bronchial complications like atelectasis and abscess |
| Gastric content aspiration and aspiration pneumonitis and abscess |
| Temporomandibular joint dislocation |
| C-spine injury and subluxation |
| Hypoxia, with resultant brain damage and cardiac arrest |
| Hypercarbia—causing varying degrees of cardiac arrhythmias, hypertension, and intracranial pressure changes |

**Table 20–9B** Management of Difficult Intubation

| |
|---|
| Awake intubation |
| Blind—nasal |
| Direct laryngoscopy |
| nasal intubation |
| oral intubation |
| Fiberoptic endoscopy |
| Rigid optical stylet |
| Rigid bronchoscopy |
| Anterior commissure laryngoscopy |
| Retrograde translaryngeal intubation |
| Translaryngeal jet ventilation |
| Cricothyroidotomy |
| Tracheostomy |
| Mask ventilation |

(From Gupta B, McDonald JS: The difficult airway. Hospital Physician 65: 69–71, 74, January 1986.)

The problem of difficult mask airway is similar in some respects to and is associated with mandibular configuration, prognathism, micrognathism, macroglossia, hypertrophied tonsils and other pharyngeal tissues, size and width of the mouth, and palate configuration. The problem is exacerbated with the obese patient because, not only is maintenance of the airway difficult, but also the ability to ventilate the lungs is impaired due to passive resistance factors. Thus, the unexpected inability to ventilate a patient may take the practitioner by surprise at a time when other compounding circumstances may well put the patient's very life at hazard (Table 20–9).

### Prediction

The presence of the anatomic characteristics associated with difficult airways and intubations may arouse concerns. Reliable gradation of anticipated difficulty would be very helpful (Figures 20–11, 20–12 and Table 20–10).

One source suggests cataloging the difficult intubations into four grades. These grades are based upon an awake look before anesthesia and consist of those outlined in Table 20–11. It was concluded that the chief problems came with Grade 4 and Grade 3, in which the epiglottis could be visualized but the cords could not be seen (49–55). Because these comprise only 0.05% or 1 in 2000 cases, it is possible that the anesthesiologist may

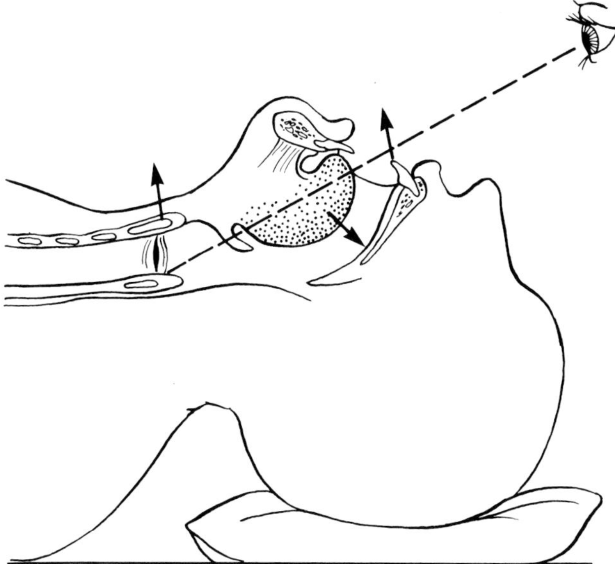

Fig. 20–11. Anatomy of difficult intubation. Difficult intubation may occur if the vocal cords, the upper teeth, or the tongue are displaced in the direction of the arrows. Such displacement may be due to variations in normal anatomy. The laryngoscope must provide a clear line of vision to the vocal cords. It does so by compressing the entire tongue so that the line of sight is cleared. (Redrawn from Cormack RS, Lehane J: Difficult tracheal intubation in obstetrics. Anesthesia. 39:1105–1111, 1984.)

practice sometime before he/she encounters such a case. If this happens during the night, with no warning and in a stressful situation, it is easy to see that mistakes could be made. On the other hand, this should popularize the

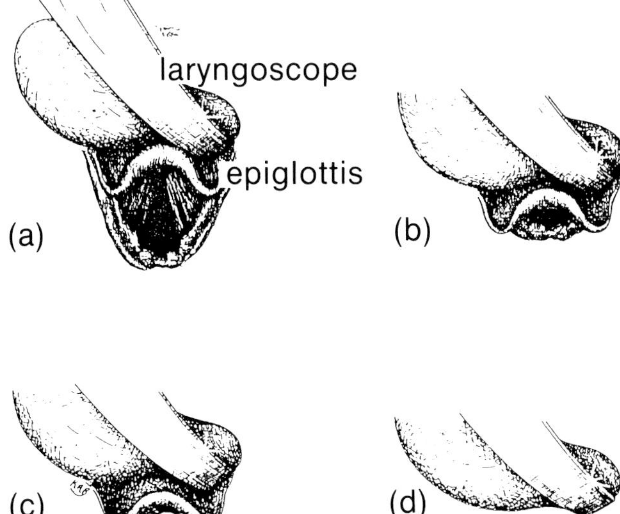


Fig. 20–12. The best obtainable views at laryngoscopy, with correct technique and with no pathologic changes. The incidence of each grade: **(a)** Grade 1: 99%; **(b)** Grade 2: 1%; **(c)** Grade 3: 1:2,000; **(d)** Grade 4: 1:100,000. (From Cormack RS, Lehane J: Difficult tracheal intubation in obstetrics. Anesthesia. 39:1105–1111, 1984.)

**Table 20–10.** The Three Levels of the Final Five Risk Factors

| Risk Factor | Level | |
|---|---|---|
| Weight | 0 | <90 kg |
| | 1 | 90–110 kg |
| | 2 | >110 kg |
| Head and neck movement | 0 | Above 90° |
| | 1 | About 90° (i.e. ± 10°) |
| | 2 | Below 90° |
| Jaw movement | 0 | IG ≥5 cm* or SLux >0 |
| | 1 | IG <5 cm and SLux = 0 |
| | 2 | IG <5 cm and SLux <0 |
| Receding mandible | 0 | Normal |
| | 1 | Moderate |
| | 2 | Severe |
| Buck teeth | 0 | Normal |
| | 1 | Moderate |
| | 2 | Severe |

IG = inter-incisor gap
SLux =sublaxation or maximal forward protrusion of lower incisors beyond upper incisors.
Important risk factors. Level 2 is the most serious risk. (Modified by Jay Jacoby, M.D. From Wilson ME, Spiegelhalter D, Robertson JA, Lesser P: Predicting difficult intubation. Br. J. Anaesth. 61:211–216, 1988)

practice of preinduction awake looks in questionable patients (Figures 20–13 through 20–16 and Table 20–12).

Preparation for failed intubation has been in the past, and remains today, unsatisfactory. The reason for this seems to be the lack of any dependable guidelines for anticipation and detection of the problem. Many different methods have been explored. There are two good prospective studies on prediction of difficult intubation: (1) by Mallampati (52), who subsequently developed the four grades of visualization of the uvula and tonsilar pillars as a predictive instrument; and (2) by Wilson (55), who developed a 5-division scale related to range of motion of the neck, jaw movement, recessive mandible, prominent teeth, and obesity.

The most recent attempt to develop some type of anthropometric index was at The Ohio State University (56). This was a 2-year prospective study of over 1500 cases, encompassing all of the suggested parameters mentioned in the past, which appeared useful for a predictive index. The final conclusion of their study was that there just was no one factor and not even a constellation of factors, which would serve as reliable predictors for patients who would be difficult to intubate. Too many times, patients with no definite hint of problems on preoperative examination turn out to be difficult to intubate. Furthermore, there was no factor discovered to predict patients whose airways would be difficult to maintain during the induction. Despite the development of the "awake look" policy part way through the study, they still did not find good, solid criteria to aid in prediction. However, this may be the most comprehensive and most reliable index available (Figure 20–17).

What makes the anticipation and preparation more difficult is the fact that most intubations are really easily performed. The problem is encountered so seldom that there is a relaxed attitude toward the subject among anesthesi-

**Table 20–11.** Correlation Between Visibility Without Instruments of Facial Pillars, Soft Palate and Uvula, and Exposure of Glottis by Direct Laryngoscopy

| Visibility of Structures Without Instruments no. pts (%) | Laryngoscopy Grade | | | |
|---|---|---|---|---|
| | Grade 1 no. pts (%) | Grade 2 no. pts (%) | Grade 3 no. pts (%) | Grade 4 no. pts (%) |
| Class 1 | | | | |
| 155 (73.8%) | 125 (59.9%) | 30 (14.3%) | — | — |
| Class 2 | | | | |
| 40 (19%) | 12 (5.7%) | 14 (6.7%) | 10 (4.7%) | 4 (1.9%) |
| Class 3 | | | | |
| 15 (7.14%) | — | 1 (0.5%) | 9 (4.3%) | 5 (2.4%) |

Visibility without instruments noted as Class 1, 2 or 3
Visibility with a laryngoscope noted as Grade 1, 2, 3 or 4
Class 1: Faucial pillars, soft palate and uvula could be visualized. Class 2: Faucial pillars and soft palate could be visualized, but uvula was masked by the base of the tongue. Class 3: Only soft palate could be visualized.
Grade 1: Glottis (including anterior and posterior commissures) could be fully exposed. Grade 2: Glottis could be partly exposed (anterior commissure not visualized). Grade 3: Glottis could not be exposed (corniculate cartilages only could be visualized). Grade 4: Glottis including corniculate cartilages could not be exposed.
(Modified by Jay Jacoby, M.D. From Mallampati SR, Gatt SP, Gugino LD, Desai SP, et al: A clinical sign to predict difficult tracheal intubation: a prospective study. Can. Anaesth. Soc. J. 32:429–434, 1985).

ologists. Certainly, the moment of difficulty generates considerable stress and mental trauma, but even the individual involved becomes lulled into a sense of security and inaction during the next several weeks of more routine, easily performed laryngoscopy and intubation.

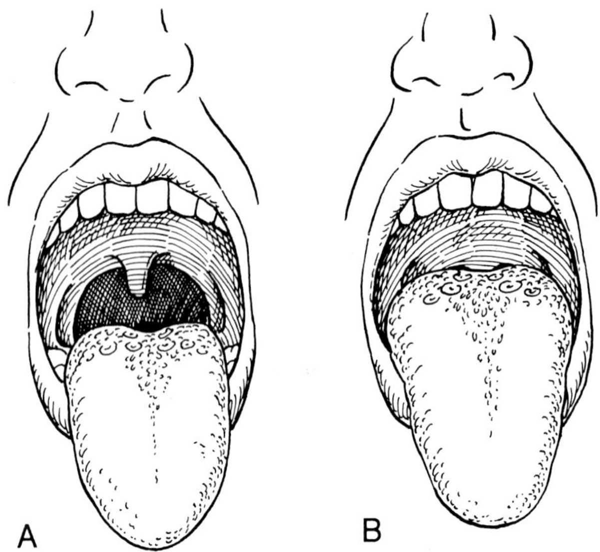


**Fig. 20–13.** Prediction of intubation ease or difficulty. **(A)** Uvula, soft palate, and facial pillars are visible: easy intubation. **(B)** Uvula, soft palate, and facial pillars are *not* visible: difficult intubation. (Redrawn from Mallampati SR, Gatt SP, Gugino LD, Desai SP, et al: A clinical sign to predict difficult tracheal intubation: A prospective study. Can. Anaesth. Soc. J. 32:429–434, 1985.)

## *Management*

Obstetric patients in the greater New York metropolitan area who had difficult intubations and bad results were reviewed by Marx, who recommended strict adherence to several principles to aid in the management of this problem (57). First, careful assessment of the airway, including the possibility of a difficult intubation. Second, when such a possibility exists, alternative anesthetic techniques should be used, such as awake placement of an endotracheal tube or regional anesthesia. Third, operative intervention should not begin until there is confirmation of bilateral aeration of the lungs. Fourth, if difficulty with intubation occurs without warning, the anesthetic should be discontinued, the patient awakened, and an alternative technique used for delivery. Fifth, obstetric anesthesia units should have a means of emergency transtracheal ventilation available to them, including a tube device and a tracheostomy kit (57–59).

**Table 20–12.** Correlation of Mallampati Classes and Laryngoscopy Grades. Mallampati Class (1–3) and Laryngoscopy Grades (1–5) in 675 Patients

| Mallampati Class | Laryngeal View | | | | |
|---|---|---|---|---|---|
| | 1 | 2 | 3 | 4 | 5 |
| 1 | 398 | 84 | 17 | 5 | 1 |
| 2 | 49 | 4 | 2 | 1 | 0 |
| 3 | 76 | 33 | 0 | 3 | 2 |

(From Oates JDL, Macleod AD, Oates PD, Pearsall FJ, et at: Comparison of two methods for predicting difficult intubation. Br. J. Anaesth. 66: 305–309, 1991).

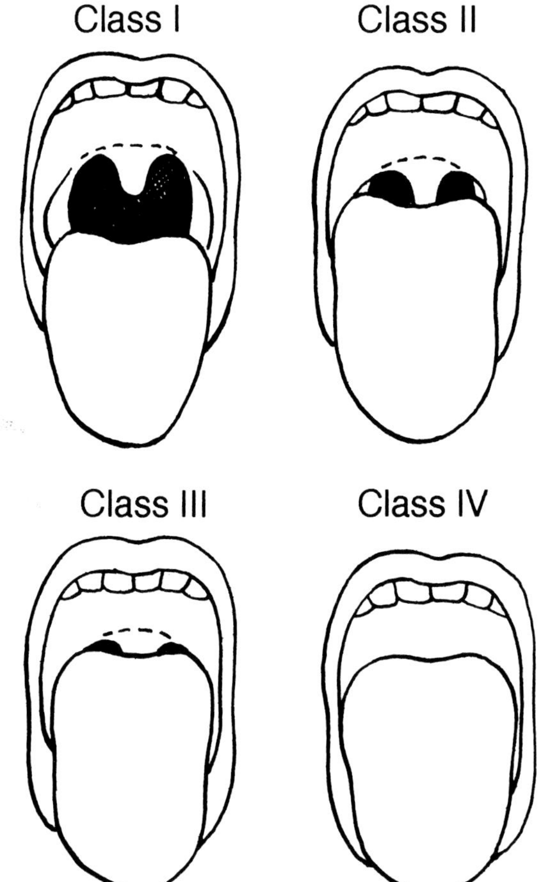


Fig. 20–14. Prediction of intubation ease or difficulty. Pictorial designation (modified) of Mallampati scores. Class I: facial pillars, soft palate, and uvula visible. Class II: soft palate and uvula visible. Class III: soft palate visible. Class IV: none of the landmarks visible. (Redrawn from Samsoon GLT, Young JRB: Difficult tracheal intubation: A retrospective study. Anaesthesia. 42: 487–490, 1987.)

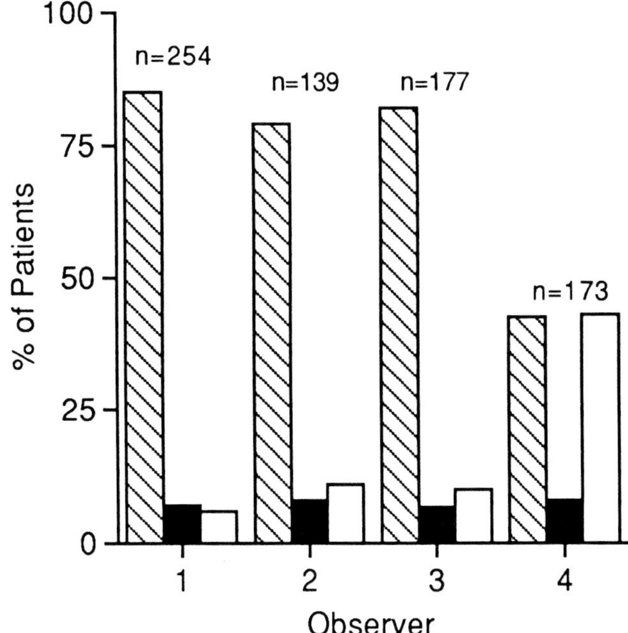


Fig. 20–15. Prediction of intubation ease or difficulty. Mallampati class scores assigned by four observers: n = number of patients observed; striped bars: easy; solid bars: moderately difficult; clear bars: difficult. (Redrawn from Oates JDL, Macleod AD, Oates PD, Pearsall FJ, et al: Comparison of two methods for predicting difficult intubation. Br. J. Anaesth. 66:305–309, 1991.)

### Prevention of Failure

The elements of prevention include careful planning, anticipation of the problem, and a management program to handle the problem when it does arise. There are no reliable means of identification of patients who are difficult to intubate. Even more serious is the fact that sometimes after administration of a muscle relaxant it may be difficult or even impossible to establish an airway and ventilate the patient. This may well be the case, despite the fact that the airway was adjudged adequate after administration of thiopental. One thing, however, is certain: the patient who is morbidly obese should be classified as probable trouble with regard to difficult or impossible airway and difficult or impossible intubation. In addition to this reflection on body habitus, there are concerns about certain anatomic features such as retrognathia, narrowing of the posterior oropharyngeal area, enlargement of the tongue, a low or narrow soft palate, and redundant pharyngeal tissue in and around the tonsilar area. Morbidly obese pregnant women may have such large breasts that they interfere with insertion of the laryngoscope.

When it is anticipated that airway or intubation difficulties may occur, do not administer general anesthesia. Instead, apply local anesthesia to the airway (60). Use a laryngoscope and look in the throat to determine ease of exposure of the vocal cords. If you can, insert the endotracheal tube. When there is assurance that the tube is in the trachea (exhaled $CO_2$ curve, good breath sounds), general anesthesia may be started.

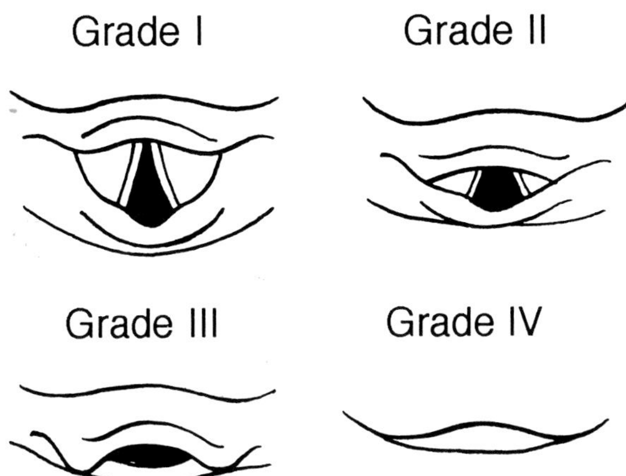


Fig. 20–16. The classification of laryngoscopic views. Grades used by Cormack and Lehane. Modified. (From Samsoon GLT, Young JRB: Difficult tracheal intubation: A retrospective study. Anaesthesia. 42:487–490, 1987.)

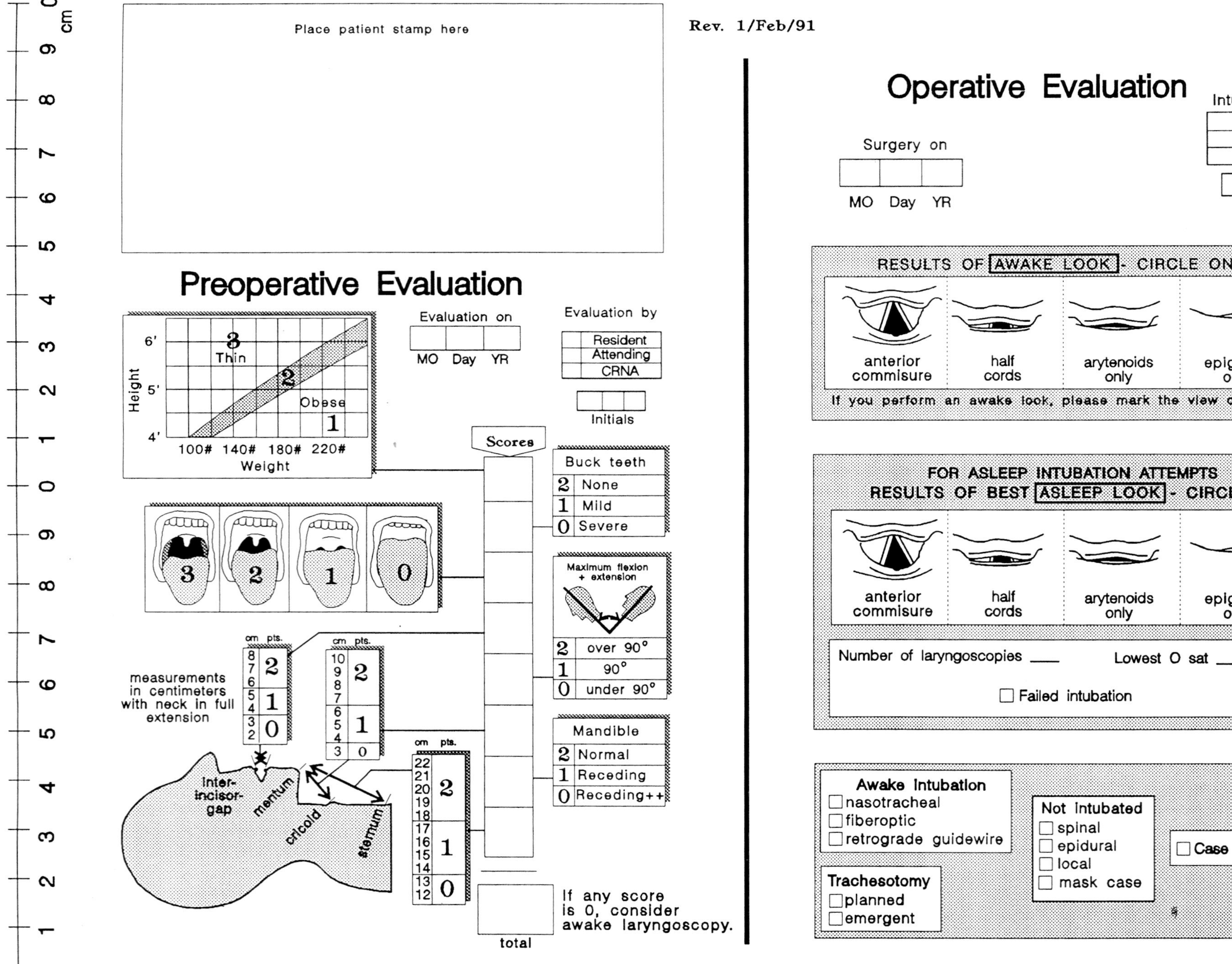

Place patient stamp here

Rev. 1/Feb/91

# Preoperative Evaluation

Evaluation on: MO | Day | YR

Evaluation by: Resident / Attending / CRNA — Initials

Height (4', 5', 6') vs. Weight (100#, 140#, 180#, 220#): 3 Thin — 2 — Obese 1

Mallampati views: 3, 2, 1, 0

Scores — total

| Buck teeth | |
|---|---|
| 2 | None |
| 1 | Mild |
| 0 | Severe |

| Maximum flexion + extension | |
|---|---|
| 2 | over 90° |
| 1 | 90° |
| 0 | under 90° |

| Mandible | |
|---|---|
| 2 | Normal |
| 1 | Receding |
| 0 | Receding++ |

measurements in centimeters with neck in full extension

| cm | pts. |
|---|---|
| 8 7 6 | 2 |
| 5 4 | 1 |
| 3 2 | 0 |

| cm | pts. |
|---|---|
| 10 9 8 7 | 2 |
| 6 5 4 | 1 |
| 3 | 0 |

| cm | pts. |
|---|---|
| 22 21 20 19 18 | 2 |
| 17 16 15 14 | 1 |
| 13 12 | 0 |



If any score is 0, consider awake laryngoscopy.

# Operative Evaluation

Surgery on: MO | Day | YR

Intubation by: Resident / Attending / CRNA — Initials

RESULTS OF AWAKE LOOK - CIRCLE ONE

anterior commisure | half cords | arytenoids only | epiglottis only

If you perform an awake look, please mark the view obtained.

FOR ASLEEP INTUBATION ATTEMPTS
RESULTS OF BEST ASLEEP LOOK - CIRCLE ONE

anterior commisure | half cords | arytenoids only | epiglottis only

Number of laryngoscopies ___ Lowest O sat ___%

☐ Failed intubation

**Awake Intubation**
☐ nasotracheal
☐ fiberoptic
☐ retrograde guidewire

**Trachesotomy**
☐ planned
☐ emergent

Not Intubated
☐ spinal
☐ epidural
☐ local
☐ mask case

☐ Case canceled

A valuable technique for prevention of failed intubation is the use of the fiberoptic laryngoscopy method of intubation. The prudent approach would be via the oral cavity. This may necessitate use of a special oral airway to facilitate passage of the fiberoptic instrument through the mouth. The nasal route should not be used in the pregnant patient due to the very vascular tissues in the nasopharynx during gestation and the danger of causing bleeding.

The retrograde wire or catheter method of intubation may also be used. The retrograde catheter should be passed into the trachea two rings down from the cricothyroid membrane. The method of retrograde fiberoptic guidance is described in more detail in the treatment section of this chapter.

Regardless of the efforts to identify patients and the experience of the anesthesiologist involved, there will still be failures in intubation. Such failures demand a prearranged agreement between the anesthesiologist and obstetrician on a plan for immediate treatment. The reason for close communication, coordination, and cooperation between these two primary care givers is that the life of both the mother and baby may hang in the balance. In an attempt to get as good an outcome as possible, careful forethought of every aspect of the problem is warranted. It has become popular to advocate the use of cricothyrotomy as a life saving maneuver for the mother in such situations. This method may have merit and may result in some oxygenation of the mother that may be lifesaving. However, there may still be inability to get adequate flows of oxygen into the lungs of the mother, due to very high and unexpected resistance factors. Therefore, we advocate that all Labor and Delivery Units establish what we refer to as "Labor and Delivery Failed Intubation Exercises." In these exercises, the Failed Intubation Alert is practiced (Table 20–13).

We have developed plans of management of patients who are to be intubated. These have been developed with simplicity in mind. In elective cases, the decision-making process may follow that outlined in Figure 20–18, "Anticipated Easy Intubation." In emergency cases, the decision-making process is more abbreviated, and follows the logical flow of maintaining safety for the mother at all times, as in Figures 20–19 and 20–20. There are other possibilities that also should be reviewed, such as those in Table 20–14. Outlines like these may serve as a beginning point for discussion with obstetric and anesthesia groups. Modifications may be made based upon local rules and regulations. This is entirely reasonable and logical, because they reflect what is right for individual doctors and hospitals, and patients' best interests.

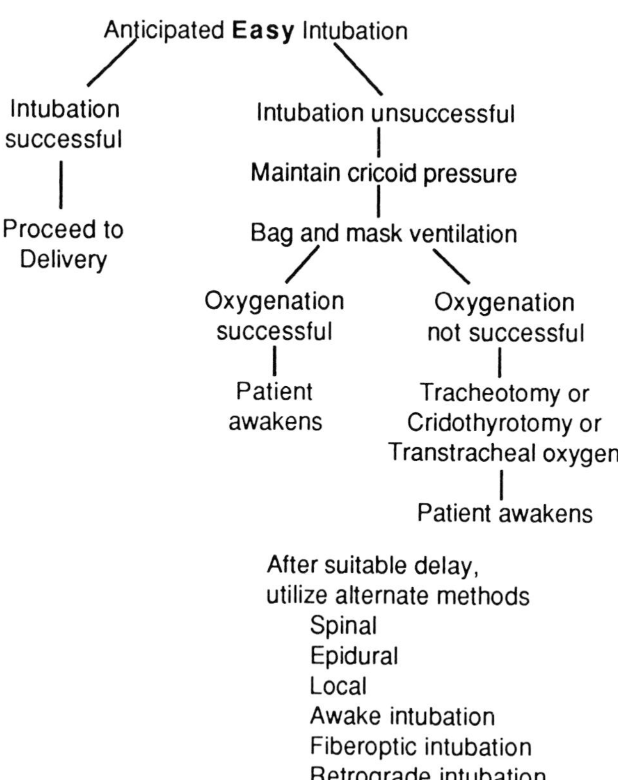


**Fig. 20–18.** Algorithm for intubation. Elective cesarean section. Anticipated easy intubation. (Redrawn from The Ohio State University Hospitals, Department of Anesthesiology.)

**Table 20–13.** Failed Intubation Drill

1. Ventilate by face mask with 100-percent $O_2$ maintaining cricoid pressure.
2. If no element of fetal distress is present, allow patient to awaken:
   a. If not contraindicated, use a regional technique.
   b. May attempt intubation using fiberoptic bronchoscope.
3. If surgery continues:
   a. Maintain mask ventilation with $O_2$ and 0.5 MAC halothane or isoflurane, continuing to apply cricoid pressure. Intravenous ketamine may also be administered.
   b. Decide whether to use further relaxants or to allow spontaneous ventilation to return.
   c. Following delivery of neonate, decide whether to make further attempts to intubate.
4. If mask ventilation fails:
   a. Perform cricothyrotomy using a cricothyrotomy cannula.
   b. A 12-gauge intravenous cannula with a 4.5-mm endotracheal tube adaptor suffices if specific cricothyrotomy cannulas are not available.

(From Messeter KH: Endotracheal intubation with the fiberoptic bronchoscope. Anaesthesia 35:294–298, 1980.)

This cannot be practiced effectively without a serious, open, discussion among the anesthesiologists, obstetricians, and nurses. The procedure must be initiated by the anesthesiologist who diagnoses a problem with intubation. Alternative methods of anesthesia should be used, such as continuous spinal or lumbar epidural, so that the plan need not be put into use. If there is an attempt to induce general anesthesia and the intubation cannot be accomplished, then the exercise should be immediately activated.

It cannot be overemphasized how important it is that the management of this problem requires a team effort. The team consists of anesthesiologists, nurse anesthetists,

**Table 20–14.** Causes of Anticipated Difficult Intubation

- Anatomic Variations
  - Receding jaw
  - Small mouth
  - High arched palate
  - Protruding prominent incisor teeth
  - Short neck
- Congenital Causes
  - Pierre Robin syndrome
  - Trisomy 18 syndrome
  - Mandibulo facial dysostosis
  - Treacher Collins' syndrome
  - Unilateral malar, maxillary, and mandibular hypoplasia
  - Temporomandibular joint malformation
  - Hemifacial microsomia
  - Goldenhar's syndrome
  - Marqui's syndrome
  - Cockayne's syndrome
  - Congenital tracheal stenosis
  - Laryngeal webs
  - Pseudoxanthoma elasticum—rigid epiglottis
- Infections
  - Epiglottis
  - Croup
  - Intraoral abscess
  - Retropharyngeal abscesses
  - Ludwig's angina
  - Trismus—any etiology
  - Airway distortions
  - Cellulitis of tongue
- Tumors
  - Cystic hygroma
  - Oropharyngeal tumors
  - Laryngeal tumors
- Postsurgical
  - Hemilaryngectomy
  - Radical neck surgery
- Postradiation
  - Postradiation fibrosis and airway distortion
  - Temporomandibular joint movement restriction due to fibrosis of masseter and other muscles
- Trauma
  - Facial injuries and lacerations—mid-face and lower face
  - Facial features—mid-face and mandible
  - C-spine injury
  - Laryngeal injury
- Arthritis
  - Ankylosing spondylitis of C-spine and temporomandibular joint
  - Rheumatoid arthritis
  - Atlanto occipital instability
  - Subluxation of cervical vertebrae
  - Cricoarytenoid cartilage stenosis
  - Cervical spondylosis
- Endocrine
  - Acromegaly
  - Myxedema
  - Big goiter
  - Obesity
- Technical Difficulties
  - Poor technique
  - Improper equipment
  - Inadequate experience
- Miscellaneous
  - Recent burns of face and oral cavity
  - Postburn fibrosis
  - Halo traction after C-spine injury
  - Masseter spasm-malignant hyperthermia after succinylcholine

(From Gupta B, McDonald JS: The difficult airway. Hospital Physician 65:69–71, 74, January 1986).

obstetricians, pediatricians, nurses, nurse specialists, and all the other support people in the labor and delivery area who work together harmoniously every day. There is no question that a competent team can handle even the most difficult of problems when everyone is working and pulling in the same direction, with the goals clearly outlined. On the other hand, a problem can cause chaos and confusion and result in a bad outcome in cases in which the team is not prepared, and in which no leadership exists during a crisis. This is not to say that a bad outcome cannot occur with a prepared team. On the contrary, in medicine, we all know that a bad outcome can occur, regardless of the excellence of care and with logical medicine practiced at every step of the way (61).

### *Fiberoptic Intubation*

Oral fiberoptic intubation is best done by using one of the three oral airways constructed to allow passage of the fiberoptic bundle. These are the Berman, Patel-Syracuse, and Williams airways (Figure 20–21). In preparation, a fiberoptic scope is inserted through an endotracheal tube, which then rides over it, near the eyepiece. If necessary, a small amount of sedative may be used to help provide a calm and more relaxed patient (62–64).

First, adequate transtracheal analgesia is obtained. Second, anesthesia of the mouth, pharynx, and supraglottic area is effected by having the patient gargle small amounts of lidocaine two or three times. Next the airway is placed in the patient's mouth. The fiberoptic scope is passed through the airway, toward the back of the tongue. The scope is then reflected acutely forward to visualize the cords and larynx. At that time, supplemental analgesia can be obtained by spraying small aliquots of local anesthetic through the injection or suction port of the fiberoptic scope. As the fiberoptic bundle approaches the cords, the patient is asked to take a deep breath, and the scope can then be passed smoothly through the cords and into the trachea. At that moment, one should be able to visualize the tracheal rings. Farther down, there is an unmistakable view of the carina. The oral airway is then carefully removed. The endotracheal tube, which is riding over the fiberoptic bundle near the eyepiece, is gently slid down the bundle into the mouth, through the cords and into position in the trachea. This maneuver requires the cooperation of the patient, who must be encouraged to remain calm throughout the procedure. The fiberoptic scope is then withdrawn. The tube is checked for proper position. The cuff is inflated, bilateral breath sounds and $CO_2$ waveforms verified, and thiopental injected to induce uncon-

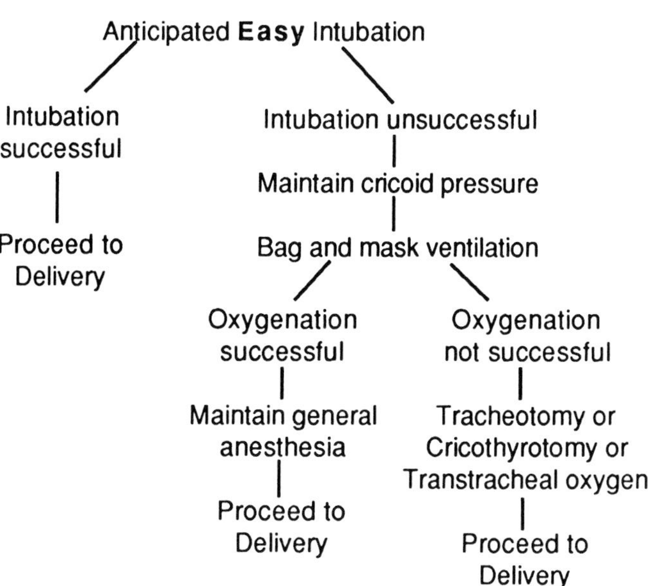


**Fig. 20–19.** Algorithm for intubation. Emergency cesarean section. Anticipated easy intubation. (Redrawn from The Ohio State University Hospitals, Department of Anesthesiology.)

sciousness. General anesthesia is then continued as planned, and the operation is begun.

### *Nasal Intubation*

If there is an overriding reason to use the nasal route for intubation, the Gupta-McDonald technique will minimize bleeding and facilitate passage. Have the patient sniff through each nostril to determine which is most patent. Prepare the nose using a spray or droplets of lidocaine and neosynephrine to shrink the mucous membranes and

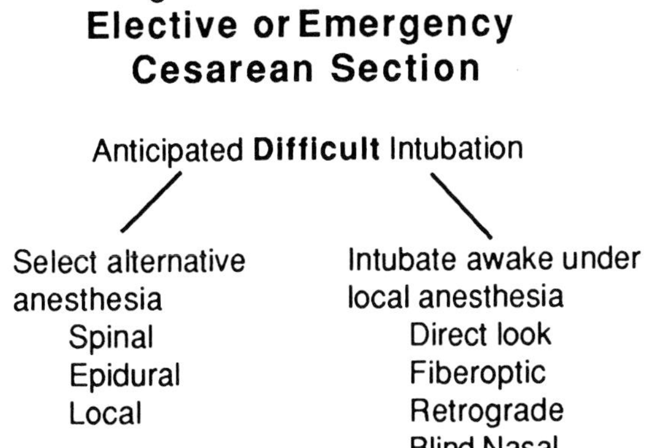


**Fig. 20–20.** Algorithm for intubation. Elective or emergency cesarean section. Anticipated difficult intubation. (Redrawn from The Ohio State University Hospitals, Department of Anesthesiology.)

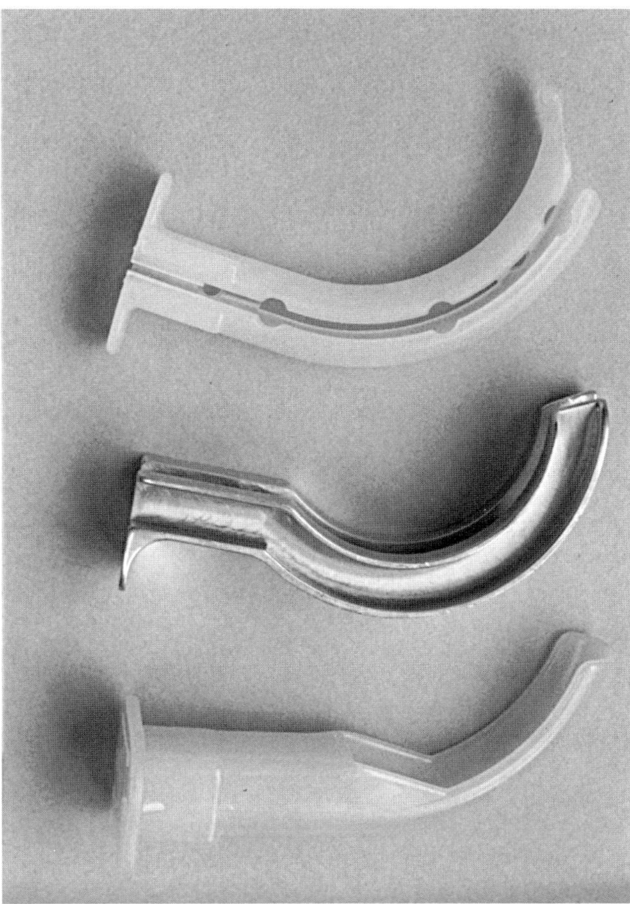

**Fig. 20–21.** Oral airways designed to facilitate passage of a fiberoptic scope. These are from top to bottom: Berman, Patel-Syracuse, and Williams. (From The Ohio State University, Department of Anesthesiology, 1993.)

provide local anesthesia. This substitute for cocaine is made by mixing 3 ml of 4% lidocaine and 1 ml of 1% neosynephrine, yielding 3% lidocaine and 0.25% neosynephrine (65,66). Place lidocaine jelly or the viscous solution in the patient's mouth and throat and have her hold it there. Select a soft rubber nasal trumpet airway, and cut it lengthwise, along its concave aspect, from end to end. Coat it with lidocaine jelly, and insert it gently into the nostril along the floor of the nose, not upward into the apex. Use slight back and forth rotating motion as it advances. When it is fully in place, the fiberscope and then the endotracheal tube can be inserted through it. The split rubber opens to accommodate the larger diameter endotracheal tube, and yet protects the adjacent vascular mucus membrane (Figure 20–22). The nasal airway is then withdrawn.

### *Retrograde Intubation*

Other important management possibilities include the use of the retrograde intubation method (59,67–71). The idea is to do a percutaneous puncture of the trachea, and insert a wire or catheter in a retrograde fashion up through the cords, pharynx, and finally out of the mouth.

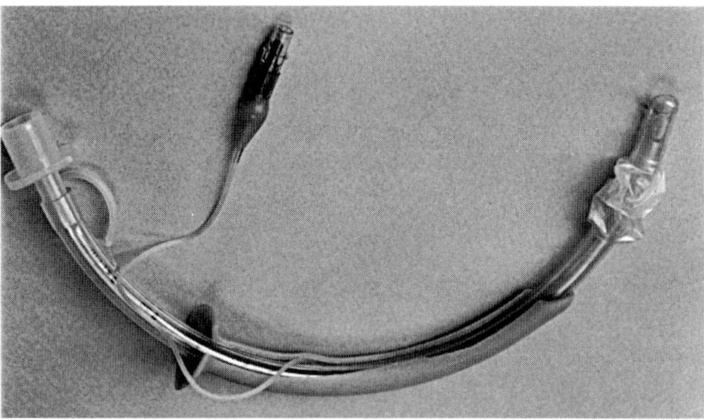

**Fig. 20–22.** A rubber nasal airway is cut along its convex curve. After it is in the patient's nose, a lubricated endotracheal tube is passed through it. The airway opens to allow the endotracheal tube to slide through. (From McDonald JS, Gupta B: From The Ohio State University, Department of Anesthesiology, 1992.)

The tube is advanced over the wire into the trachea. With this technique, there have been failures due to hang-up of the tube at the entrance to the larynx. The Weaver technique, which is a modification of the Rosenberg technique (72), is a possible solution to that problem. Instead of inserting the guidewire through the end opening of the endotracheal tube, it is inserted through the Murphy eye, the lateral opening. This effectively allows the tube to be guided into the larynx without striking an obstacle at the orifice. Figure 20–23 demonstrates this point.

Lechman described the use of the combination of the fiberoptic bronchoscope with a percutaneous transtracheal retrograde wire for visual and mechanical aid during intubation. He cleverly used the suction port, through which the guidewire was run, for help in guiding the end of the bronchoscope into the trachea (71). The bronchoscope could be advanced down the pharynx and literally passed through the center of the cords, over the guidewire. All of this could be accomplished despite poor visualization due to blood, mucus, and particulate debris. Sometime after the description of the bronchoscopic technique, a fiberoptic laryngoscope became available with a suction port. It was used successfully instead of the bronchoscope in both general surgical cases and obstetric cases (71). The method of fiberoptic laryngoscopic intubation over a guidewire is described in detail in Figure 20–24. The guidewire method avoids some of the disadvantages of the standard nasopharyngeal fiberoptic and the standard blind nasotracheal tube placement. The operator can be more successful at an earlier stage of learning the fiberoptic technique, due to the "guidance of the wire," and there is less hemorrhage and trauma than associated with the tube through the nose.

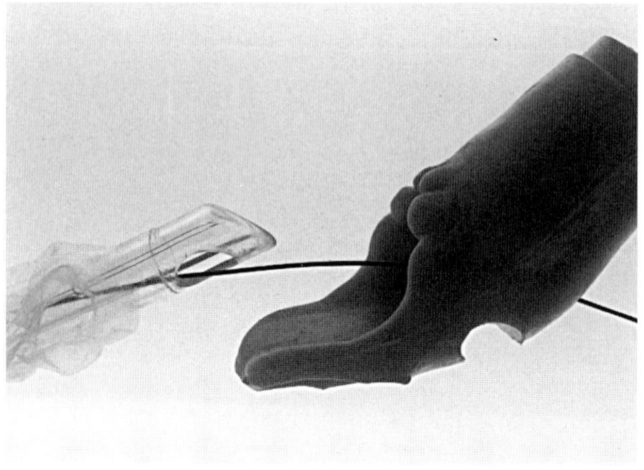

**Fig. 20–23.** Retrograde wire passed through the Murphy eye to increase depth of passage of the tube into the trachea before removing the wire. (From Weaver J, The Ohio State University, Department of Anesthesiology, 1992.)

Intubation procedures for pregnant women should be performed through the oral cavity instead of the nose. The use of the nose for tube insertion may cause serious bleeding, due to the very rich vascular plexuses in the nasopharynx during pregnancy. However, a soft rubber nasopharyngeal trumpet airway can usually be inserted without trauma or bleeding. An aid in the management of the difficult airway and intubation is to very gently place a soft lubricated nasopharyngeal airway in the nose after applying a vasoconstrictor and local anesthetic. Insert a connector taken from an appropriately sized endotracheal tube into the outer end of the nasopharyngeal

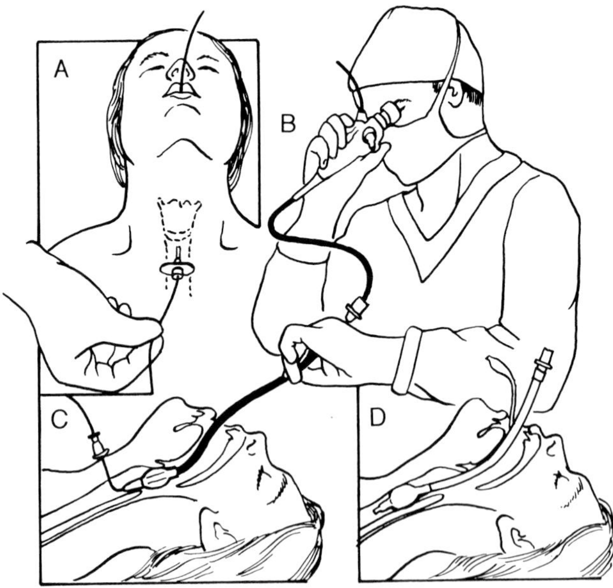


**Fig. 20–24.** Guided fiberoptic endotracheal intubation. **(A)** A guidewire is inserted percutaneously through the neck and retrieved from the mouth. The end at the neck is secured with a clamp. **(B)** The endotracheal tube is mounted on the fiberscope and the guidewire is inserted retrograde through the biopsy part. **(C)** The fiberscope is advanced over the guidewire into the trachea. The endotracheal tube is then advanced over the fiberscope. **(D)** The tube is in the trachea; fiberscope and guidewire are then removed. (Redrawn from Goldman E, McDonald JS: Continuous oxygenation during nasotracheal intubation. Anesthesiology. 61:352, 1984.)

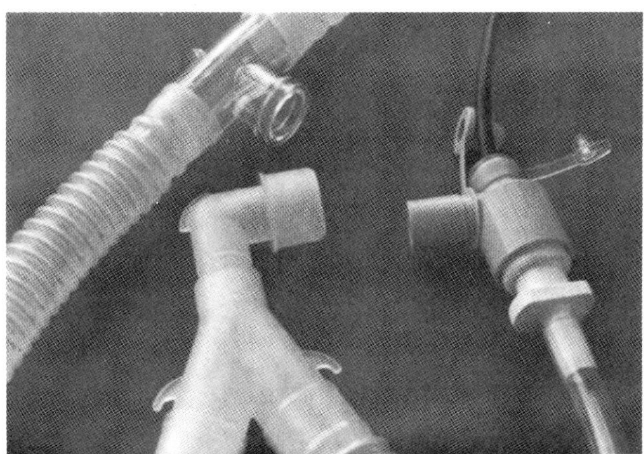

**Fig. 20–25.** Oxygen is administered during the intubation procedure. A swivel adapter allows free movement between the tube and the oxygen source—a T–piece or the anesthetic circuit. (From Goldman E, McDonald JS: Continuous oxygenation during nasotracheal intubation. Anesthesiology. 61:352, 1984.)

airway. This allows one to hook up the anesthesia circuit to it, and administer 100% oxygen via the circle system to the patient through one nostril, while passing the retrograde wire and tracheal tube through the mouth. Because it has been found that increasing maternal $FiO_2$ increases fetal $PaO_2$, it would seem to be prudent to use this modification when contemplating fiberoptic management techniques (Figure 20–25) (26,73,74).

### *When All Else Fails*

Airway obstruction, with inadequate oxygenation and ventilation, is one of the most urgent of all life-threatening emergencies. The most effective treatment is immediate establishment of the airway by mechanical means, either intubation or tracheostomy. The problem is that such emergencies arise without warning, and a skilled surgeon may not be available to perform the tracheostomy. That is why alternatives should also be considered. Establishment of a needle orifice through the cricothyroid membrane or through a tracheal ring and a flow of oxygen through it, may serve as a lifesaving, temporizing measure (75–78). Intermittent jets of high pressure oxygen through a large bore needle entrain increased flows of air down into the lungs (79–81). The jet may be effective when there is incomplete airway obstruction. However, when airway obstruction is complete, the jet does not effect entrainment of air into the lungs. In such a condition, it may be necessary to use a much larger 2.3- to 3.5-mm cannula and an Ambu bag assist for oxygen delivery (78). In one study (79), it was possible to use a smaller transtracheal catheter (2.4 mm or 10 gauge) with a portable pressure device for ventilation control and to maintain adequate blood gases for a limited time period (Table 20–15). The findings from this study reinforce the admonition that a critical transtracheal orifice of about 2.5 mm diameter is mandated to assist or control ventilation during complete airway obstruction. Several devices have been described for jet ventilation (Figures 20–26 through 20–28).

Oxygen should be administered under pressure through the largest catheter or device available. Even an 18-g needle will admit enough oxygen to sustain life, although pulmonary ventilation is minimal and carbon dioxide retention occurs. In desperate circumstances, oxygen delivery is important, $CO_2$ removal is not. In both animals and humans, it has been possible to maintain adequate ventilation through a 16-gauge cannula. When 50 psi pres-

**Table 20–15.** Arterial Blood Gases and Cardiovascular Parameters With and Without Oscillatory Pressure Ventilation Through a 10-g Catheter in Complete Upper Airway Obstruction (mean ± SD)

| | | Time (Sec) after Tracheal Occlusion | | | | | | | | | |
|---|---|---|---|---|---|---|---|---|---|---|---|
| | | **Baseline** | **90** | **120** | **180** | **240** | **300** | **360** | **600** | **960** | **1,800** |
| pH | Group 1 | 7.39 ± .03 | 7.42 ± .06 | 7.39 ± .04 | 7.37 ± .04 | 7.36 ± .03 | 7.33 ± .05 | 7.31 ± .05 | 7.25 ± .07 | — | — |
| | Group 2 | 7.37 ± .05 | 7.36 ± .06 | 7.37 ± .06 | 7.39 ± .06 | 7.38 ± .08 | 7.37 ± .07 | 7.39 ± .06 | 7.40 ± .08 | 7.41 ± .07 | — |
| | Ambu | 7.45 ± .02 | 7.40 ± .06 | 7.40 ± .05 | 7.41 ± .05 | 7.40 ± .05 | 7.40 ± .04 | 7.40 ± .06 | 7.39 ± .08 | 7.38 ± .1 | 7.41 ± 0 |
| $PaCO_2$ (mm Hg) | Group 1 | 36 ± 14 | 36 ± 4 | 44 ± 4 | 47 ± 4 | 49 ± 4 | 52 ± 3* | 52 ± 5 | 62 ± 10 | — | — |
| | Group 2 | 38 ± 3 | 43 ± 5 | 42 ± 4 | 41 ± 4 | 41 ± 4 | 41 ± 5 | 41 ± 5 | 41 ± 6 | 39 ± 6 | — |
| | Ambu | 33 ± 3 | 41 ± 5 | 41 ± 5 | 40 ± 6 | 41 ± 6 | 41 ± 7 | 42 ± 6 | 42 ± 9 | 45 ± 11 | 40 ± 8 |
| $PaO_2$ (mm Hg) | Group 1 | 72.8 ± 9 | 192 ± 27 | 110 ± 33 | 51 ± 11 | 27 ± 10 | 13 ± 5† | 6.7 ± 2 | 5 ± 4 | — | — |
| | Group 2 | 89 ± 10 | 333 ± 54 | 425 ± 31 | 473 ± 33 | 475 ± 44 | 461 ± 41 | 477 ± 35 | 474 ± 32 | 500 ± 59 | — |
| | Ambu | 90 ± 6 | 233 ± 21 | 250 ± 22 | 277 ± 10 | 289 ± 11 | 293 ± 13† | 287 ± 30 | 291 ± 20 | 289 ± 28 | 272 ± 4 |
| HR (beats/min) | Group 1 | 98 ± 16 | 96 ± 16 | 96 ± 16 | 105 ± 19 | 124 ± 18 | 124 ± 4 | 102 ± 17 | 76 ± 9 | — | — |
| | Group 2 | 116 ± 23 | 115 ± 28 | 108 ± 27 | 114 ± 25 | 113 ± 25 | 113 ± 24 | 113 ± 23 | 110 ± 21 | 107 ± 19 | — |
| | Ambu | 152 ± 22 | 152 ± 22 | 154 ± 30 | 151 ± 30 | 150 ± 29 | 148 ± 27 | 146 ± 26 | 150 ± 20 | 138 ± 31 | 148 ± 2 |
| MAP (mm Hg) | Group 1 | 89 ± 18 | 94 ± 18 | 95 ± 18 | 106 ± 18 | 104 ± 24 | 62 ± 19 | 43 ± 15 | 22 ± 12 | — | — |
| | Group 2 | 101 ± 12 | 94 ± 8 | 91 ± 7 | 87 ± 10 | 88 ± 10 | 86 ± 11 | 85 ± 12 | 86 ± 12 | 85 ± 12 | — |
| | Ambu | 100 ± 9 | 92 ± 10 | 94 ± 5 | 93 ± 8 | 91 ± 6 | 90 ± 11 | 87 ± 11 | 82 ± 8 | 79 ± 21 | 80 ± 1 |
| MPAP (mm Hg) | Group I | 16 ± 2 | 12 ± 3 | 13 ± 4 | 16 ± 8 | 22 ± 8 | 25 ± 4* | 21 ± 5 | 17 ± 6 | — | — |
| | Group 2 | 20 ± 3 | 24 ± 4 | 22 ± 4 | 22 ± 4 | 21 ± 4 | 21 ± 3 | 20 ± 3 | 20 ± 2 | 19 ± 3 | — |
| | Ambu | 14 ± 2 | 16 ± 3 | 16 ± 3 | 15 ± 3 | 15 ± 2 | 14 ± 3† | 14 ± 2 | 15 ± 3 | 18 ± 8 | 16 ± 5 |

HR = heart rate, MAP = mean arterial pressure, MPAP = mean pulmonary arterial pressure.
Comparison of data at 1,800 sec and 300 sec vs. 90 sec after occlusion: * = $p < 0.05$ and † $p < 0.001$.
(From Goldman E, McDonald JS, Peterson SS, Stock MC, et al: Transtracheal ventilation with oscillatory pressure for complete upper airway obstruction. J. Trauma. 28: 611–614, 1988).

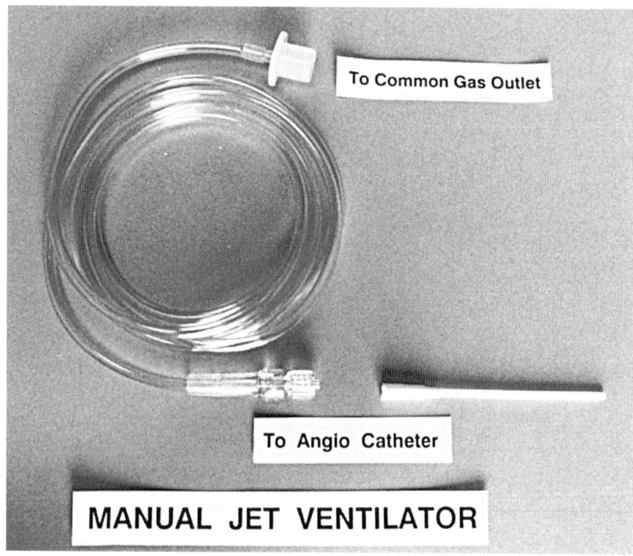


**Fig. 20–26.** Sample equipment for transtracheal oxygen delivery. (From The Ohio State University, Department of Anesthesiology, 1992.)

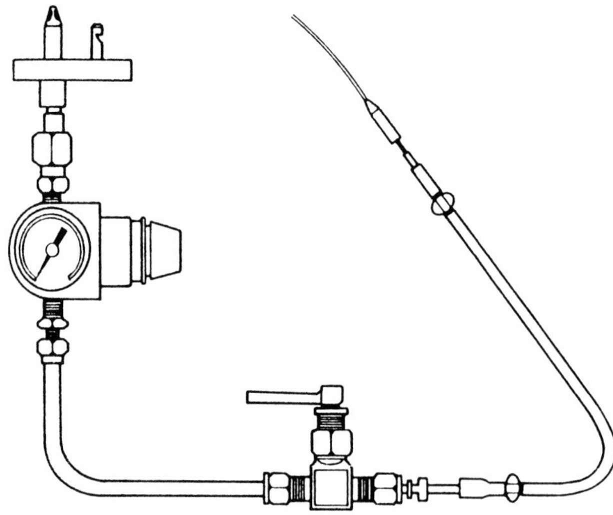

**Fig. 20–28.** A simple jet ventilator. (From Swartzman S, et al.: Percutaneous transtracheal jet ventilation for cardiopulmonary resuscitation: Evaluation of a new jet ventilator. Crit. Care Med., 12(1):8, 1984.)

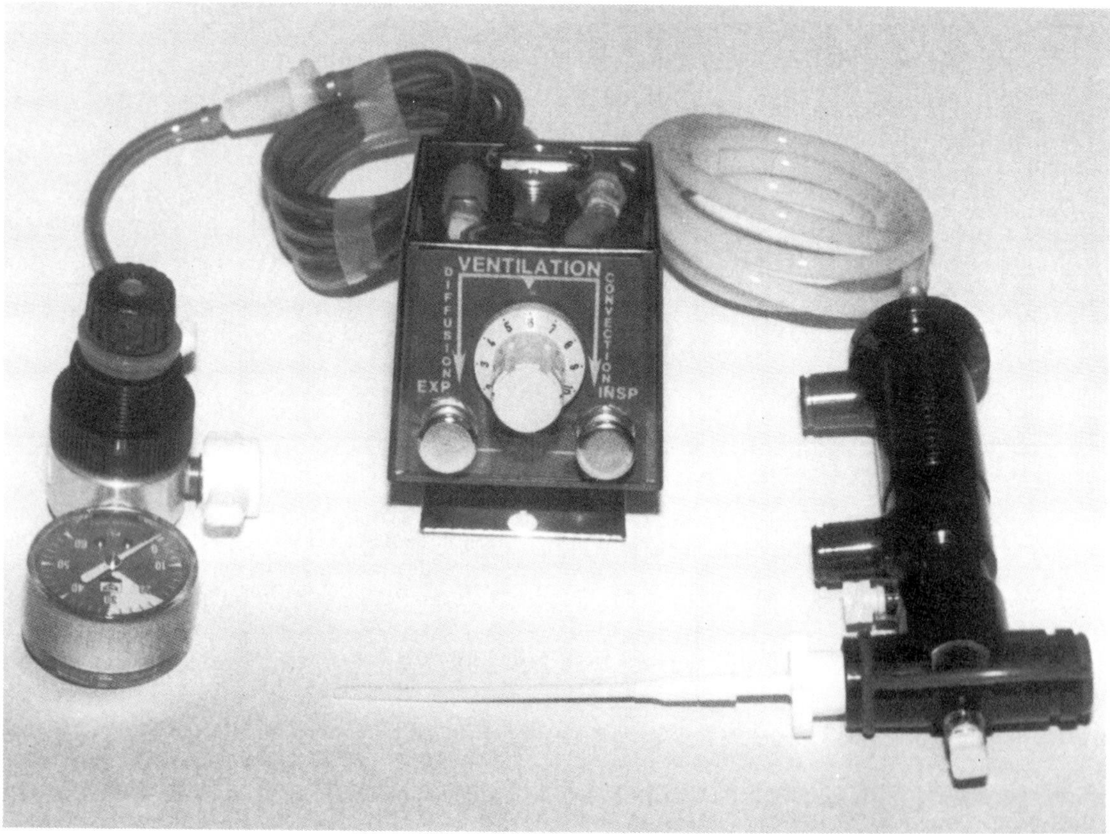


**Fig. 20–27.** Oscillatory pressure assembly for transtracheal ventilation. **Left:** Inflow high-pressure line. **Center:** The logic center and controls. **Right:** Inspiratory/expiratory valve attached to a 10 g plastic catheter and a 3 mm endotracheal tube connector. (From Goldman E, McDonald JS, Peterson SS, Stock MC, et al: Transtracheal ventilation with oscillatory pressure for complete upper airway obstruction. J. Trauma. 28:611–614, 1988.)

sure is applied to a 16-gauge cannula, oxygen flow of 500 ml/second is obtained.

Providing anesthesia for operative delivery must be viewed, from the anesthesiologist's standpoint, as a threat to the very life of the patient predicted to have a difficult airway and difficult intubation problem. In such instances, the logical alternatives must be explored, including use of regional analgesia by spinal or epidural methods, or by use of local infiltration analgesia.

## *Alternative Routes to Airway Management*

The complementary goals of airway management are to keep the passageway to the trachea open and the passageway to the stomach closed. Besides the commonly used techniques of the anesthetist, several other options have been developed, some for use primarily by paramedics during emergencies.

Another option that may be considered, though not highly recommended, is the Esophageal Gastric Tube Airway (Figure 20–29). A tube is passed into the esophagus and a cuff is inflated. The cuff prevents regurgitation into the pharynx. Gastric contents may come up through the tube to the exterior. The outer end of the tube goes through a hole in the mask, and a gastric tube may be passed through it for suction. The mask over mouth and nose permits spontaneous or controlled ventilation, the oxygen entering through the patient's mouth and nose (82).

The Esophageal Obturator blocks the esophagus, preventing stomach contents from entering the pharynx and preventing air from entering the stomach. A face mask is used with this to provide pulmonary ventilation. The drawback is that if the obturator enters the trachea, the airway is completely blocked.

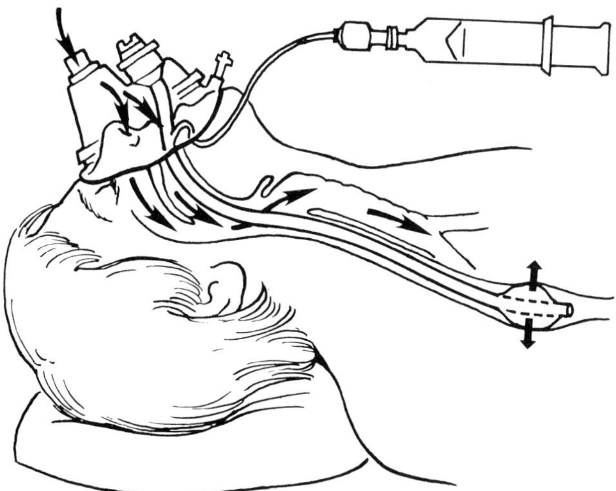

**Fig. 20–29.** The Esophageal Gastric Tube Airway (EGTA). The tube is threaded down the esophagus and the cuff is inflated, preventing regurgitation of gastric contents. A smaller nasogastric tube may be passed into the stomach for suction. The esophageal gastric tube is connected to an orifice in the mask. A second orifice in the mask attaches to a breathing circuit, and positive-pressure oxygen may be given, with the oxygen flowing through the nose, mouth, and pharynx into the larynx. (Redrawn from Tunstall ME, Geddes C: Failed intubation in obstetric anesthesia. Br. J. Anaesth. 56:659–661, 1984.)

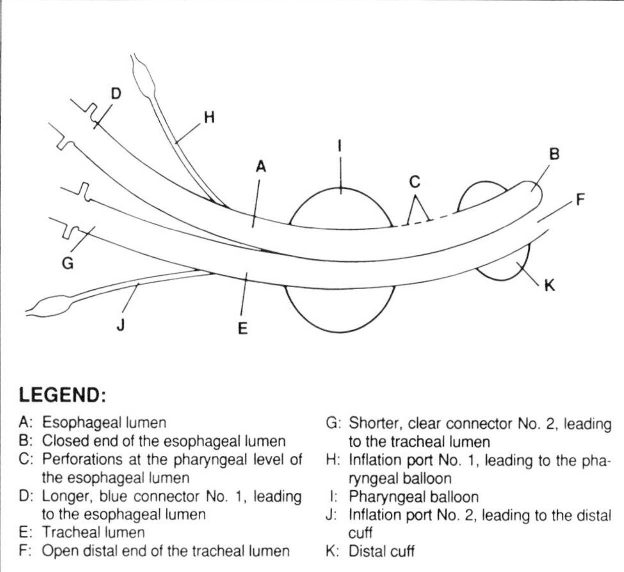


**Fig. 20–30.** The Esophageal Tracheal Combitude (ETC). The diagram shows that ETC consists of two concentric tubes with cuffs. The outer tube has multiple perforations. (From Johnson JC and Atherton GL: The esophageal tracheal combitube. An alternative route to airway management. J.E.M.S. May:29–34, 1991.)

Several ingenious methods have been devised to overcome this problem. The best seems to be the Esophageal Tracheal Combitube (Figures 20–30 through 20–32). This is essentially a double lumen tube with two cuffs, one at the tip of the tube and one at the midpoint. When the tube is inserted, the midpoint cuff inflates in the pharynx. The tube itself may enter either the trachea or esophagus. If it enters the trachea, it is used like a regular endotracheal tube. If it enters the esophagus, it is used for gastric drainage, while pulmonary ventilation is accomplished through an accessory pathway.

The Laryngeal Mask airway was developed by Dr. A.I.J. Brain (Figures 20–33 through 20–35). It is a wide-bore tube that is inserted through the mouth into the pharynx. A large elliptical cuff at its tip is inflated, sealing the orifice of the esophagus, and allowing the air to pass freely between the tube and the larynx. The tube is inserted without use of a laryngoscope, and is effective in providing a clear airway in 95% of patients. It is not as reliable as an endotracheal tube, but can be used when tracheal intubation is impossible.

## Unusual Causes of Airway Obstruction

This is an interesting example of a complication not related to anesthesiology at all but causing airway obstruction nevertheless. The patient was in labor, with a diagnosis of toxemia. She had low platelets and elevated bleeding times. A cesarean section was decided upon for fetal indi-

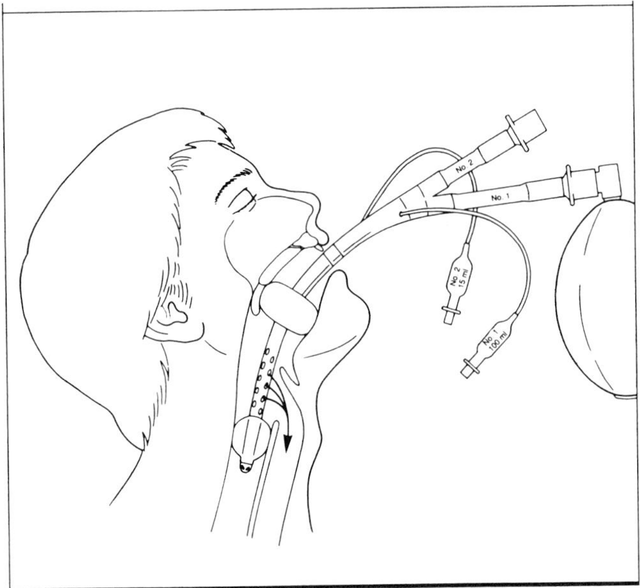


**Fig. 20–31.** The Esophageal Tracheal Combitube in the esophageal position. The esophagus is sealed off from the pharynx. Air or oxygen travels in the outer of the concentric tubes, exits through the perforations, and enters the trachea. A suction tube may be passed through the inner of the concentric tubes. (From Johnson JC, Atherton GL: The esophageal tracheal combitube. An alternative route to airway management. J.E.M.S. May: 29–34, 1991.)

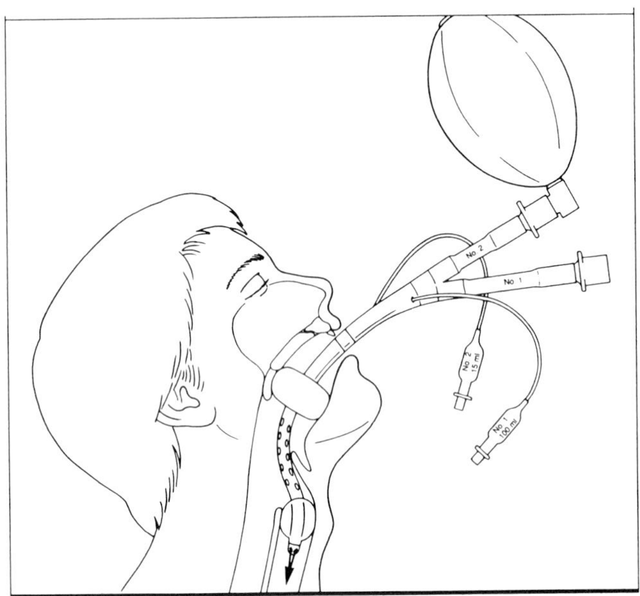


**Fig. 20–32.** The Esophageal Tracheal Combitube in the tracheal position. The inner lumen is used like a regular endotracheal tube. Suction may be applied to the outer lumen to remove secretions of the pharynx. (From Johnson JC, Atherton GL: The esophageal tracheal combitube. An alternative route to airway management. J.E.M.S. May:29–34, 1991.)

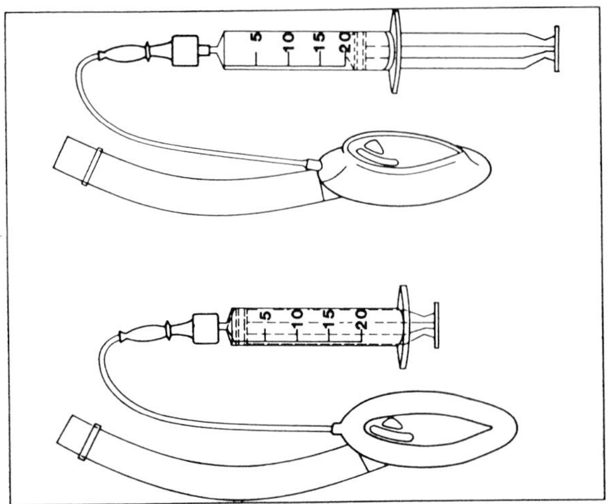


**Fig. 20–33.** The Laryngeal Mask Airway (LMA). **(A)** Large cuff deflated before insertion. **(B)** Cuff inflated with 20 ml of air after placement in the pharynx. The outer end has a standard circuit adapter. (From Maltby JR: The laryngeal mask airway. Anesthesiology Review XVIII:55–57, 1991.)

cations. At the time of standard induction and attempt at intubation, cannulation of the trachea was not successful due to poor visualization. The patient had some difficulty breathing after being awakened. A fiberoptic laryngoscope was then used. As is often the case, there was too much blood to visualize the cords and pass the scope into the trachea, but the operator could see that there was deviation of the trachea due to a mass in the retropharyn-

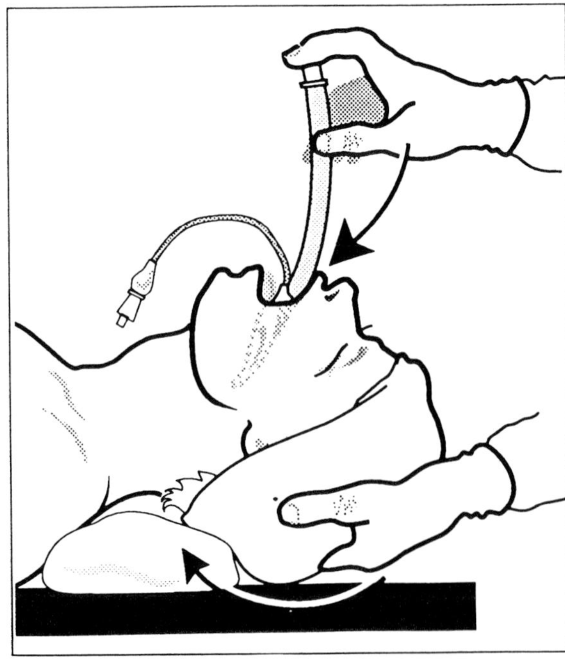

**Fig. 20–34.** Technique for insertion of the LMA. The cuff is deflated and the lubricated tube gently advanced until its tip is behind the thyroid cartilage. (From Maltby JR: The laryngeal mask airway. Anesthesiology Review XVIII:55–57, 1991.)

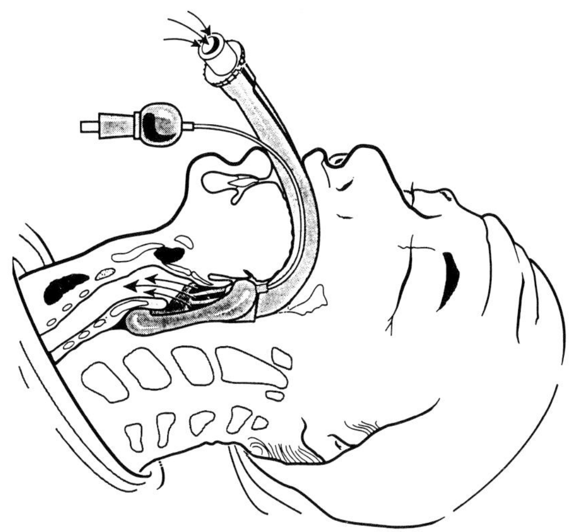

**Fig. 20–35.** The LMA in position, with the cuff inflated. (Visualization is not required.) The anesthetic circuit is attached to the outer end, and the patient is managed as though she had an endotracheal tube in place. (From Maltby JR: The laryngeal mask airway. Anesthesiology Review XVIII:55–57, 1991.)

geal area on the right side. A consult was obtained from the ENT physician, and a tracheostomy was performed with some difficulty; thereafter, the cesarean section proceeded without incident. The surgeon did mention at the time of the tracheostomy that there was significant deviation of the trachea to the left side, and he graded the procedure as difficult. In the postpartum period, after satisfactory return of normal clotting and bleeding times, the patient was again seen by the ENT physician, and they diagnosed and removed a large retropharyngeal hematoma (83).

A second illustration involves a woman who suffered a bee sting at a picnic while drinking from a soda can. She dropped the can with a shriek; a bee had crawled into the can and was not visible to her; it stung her tongue, which rapidly became swollen. She was rushed to the hospital, suffering significant airway obstruction. While a tracheotomy set was being opened, the anesthesiologist rapidly did a blind nasal intubation, which made tracheotomy unnecessary. Small doses of epinephrine and Benadryl were administered. Uterine contractions began, and labor progressed rapidly. Because she was already intubated, an anesthetic machine was attached, inhalation analgesia was administered, and an uneventful delivery took place.

Various foreign objects may be in a patient's mouth when she presents for general anesthesia, such as: loose teeth, hard candy, chewing gum, chewing tobacco. It is wise to verify that no foreign objects are present before starting.

Massive scar tissue under the chin and over the neck may make the tissues rigid and immovable. Thermal burn scars are easily identified. A patient who has had radiation therapy to her neck will have changes not noticeable to casual observation: the tissues are rock-hard, making it impossible to use an oral airway or a laryngoscope.

Pharyngeal and laryngeal edema causing airway obstruction may also occur as a complication of preeclamptic toxemia or pregnancy induced hypertension (84,85).

## Complications of Alternative Airway Methods

Each alternative airway method, i.e., methods other than use of the oral tracheal tube placed during normal induction, may cause problems, that include nasal bleeding, tissue emphysema, cricothyrotomy, and tracheotomy complications. If they fail, asphyxia and cardiac arrest follow.

### *Nasal Bleeding*

Even without the passage of a nasotracheal tube, there has been a report in the literature of a serious threat to the life of a woman due to severe epistaxis in pregnancy. There is well-recognized hyperemia of the nasal mucosa during pregnancy. In addition, there also is a specific mass that may grow in the nasal area, referred to as nasal granuloma gravidarum (Figure 20–36), which is also a potential serious bleeding problem. It is not prudent to pass a nasotracheal tube or a nasogastric tube in a pregnant patient because of the nasal hyperemia. Furthermore, with the adjuncts available today for oral intubation, there is no need to place the patient at risk for major nasal bleeding (86).

### *Retropharyngeal Perforation*

This is a rare but potentially lethal complication of an attempt to pass a nasotracheal tube. In the one incident reported personally to the author, a standard induction was followed by poor visualization of the cords, and the endotracheal tube could not be inserted. The patient was awakened and her nose was prepared for nasal intubation. After adequate local anesthetic and lubrication, the tube was passed with ease through the nose back into the nasopharynx. A slight obstruction was noted, but with a small amount of pressure there was a sudden loss of resistance to its movement. Because the patient complained vociferously and became combative, it was thought that she was suffering from shortness of breath. A mask was placed over the nose and mouth, and several breaths of positive pressure oxygen were administered to try to help the patient. She became even more combative, and a small dose of ketamine was given to calm her. A few more breaths were administered before a laryngoscope was inserted to visualize the tube. The tube was not seen at all. In fact, there was a gross amount of bleeding and so much "tissue bulging out into the pharynx" that it was not possible to visualize the larynx. The tube was removed, and after the patient awakened, she related that a tremendous pain had developed as the tube was passed through her nose. This pain was accentuated even more after she was given mask oxygen. She still complained of pain while describing the incident.

Because this was an elective cesarean section, it was cancelled and rescheduled for another day. It was noted that the patient had subcutaneous crepitus in the left suprascapular area. An x ray subsequently showed a substantial amount of air in the mediastinum. In this case, there

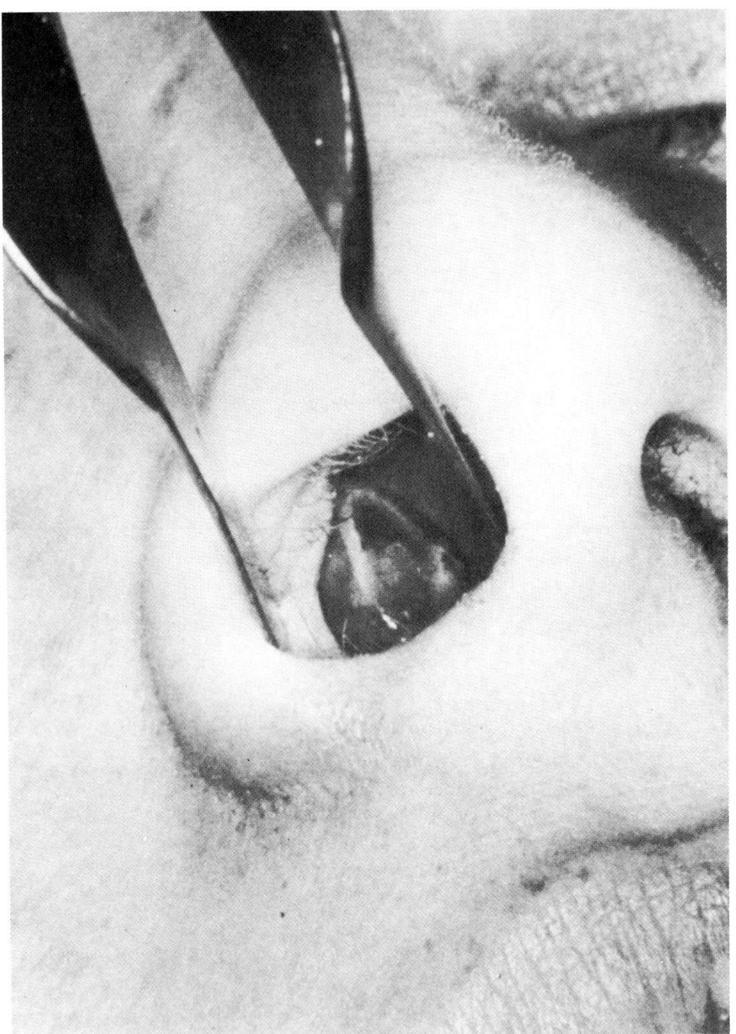

**Fig. 20–36.** Enlarged photo of nasal granuloma gravidarum. The illustration shows a large granuloma of the nasal mucous membrane, which causes obstructive symptoms and bleeds easily. (From Skau NK, Pilgaard P, Neilsen G. Granuloma gravidarum of the nasal mucous membrane. J. Laryngol. Otol. 101:1286–1288, 1987.)

was no significant detrimental effect upon cardiac output because efforts to ventilate were discontinued, and the tube was removed. The tip of the tube had pierced the mucosa of the nasopharynx, and dissected down between the mucosa and the prevertebral fascia.

### *Cricothyrotomy Complications*

It is to be expected that complications will occur when a surgical approach is made to the airway. In two reports of cricothyrotomy, the complication rates were 40% in one and 31% in the other (87,88). Complications were bleeding, obstruction, and incorrect placement. However, all those who have evaluated the procedure concur that if conventional airway methods fail, this surgical approach is justified and can be lifesaving. Furthermore, it can be performed by the physician/nurse team with little training or instruction (89). It is well-established that this technique is effective, causes only few serious complications, can be learned swiftly, and may be the only method available to save a patient's life.

## Rapid Induction Sequelae

These problems are mentioned because they are common sequelae of induction of general anesthesia. The rapid sequence induction process is one of the most poorly understood aspects of general anesthesia. It is the swift, total, overwhelming physiologic robbery of a patient's basic defense mechanisms, so that a quiet and relaxed field is obtained for placement of a laryngoscope followed by insertion of an endotracheal tube.

Many years ago it was common to induce anesthesia by slowly administering ether to a patient until she would gradually reach the level of surgical anesthesia. Shortly after the introduction of intravenous barbiturates and muscle relaxants in the late 1940s, it became popular to use endotracheal tubes for airway protection. This often necessitated the placement of the endotracheal tube as part of the rapid sequence induction of anesthesia. There have been problems associated with such an induction, namely, hypertension, hypotension, cerebrovascular accident, esophageal intubation, and cardiac arrest. These problems will be discussed in this section.

### *Hypertension*

The majority of patients who suffer from hypertension in pregnancy have essential hypertension. It is blamed for many aspects of both maternal and fetal problems. For example, maternal hypertension is found to be frequently associated with intrauterine growth retardation (IUGR). In a recent study, it was found that 86% of the perinatal deaths were in the intrauterine growth retardation group. In addition to maternal hypertension, smoking, low weight gain during pregnancy, low prepregnancy weight, and premature delivery were found (90). Pregnancy-induced hypertension may be associated also with hypovolemia and even organ failure. New findings are just evolving about a specific gene linkage to hypertension (91–96).

Induction of general anesthesia and intubation have been associated with a hypertensive response even in the normotensive patient. In the patient who suffers from hypertension, the response is greater. Of course, it is of concern to the anesthesiologist, who does not want to place his patient at risk of a cerebral accident from such an acute cardiovascular reaction. It is possible to protect against a hypertensive spike during induction and intubation by the use of alpha blockers, beta blockers, deeper anesthesia, or opioids, which blunt the patient's stress response (97–100).

The hypertensive response to induction and intubation is exaggerated in women with severe pregnancy-induced hypertension. The ideal anesthetic for such a patient may be regional, should minimal fetal risk be present. For patients who cannot withstand even small fluctuations in cerebral pressures and who have some fetal compromise in addition, making haste necessary, general anesthesia with an opioid plus an effective beta blocker may be best. Thus, the cardiovascular response to tracheal intubation, i.e., the usual hypertension after laryngoscopy and intubation, can now be reduced to minor fluctuations, with application of the proper pharmacologic agent. It is still a concern, however, because such changes have been responsible for decreasing uterine blood flow, elevating pulmonary artery pressure, elevating systemic arterial pressure, and even precipitating pulmonary edema.

In developing a plan to reduce the hypertensive response to induction and intubation, it should be determined what category the patient is in. There are four important questions: Was there a prepregnancy diagnosis of hypertension? Was she on regular medication with good control? Is there any evidence of superimposed toxemia with this pregnancy? Is there any evidence of fetal compromise? If answers to all of these questions are negative, then the patient is in a low-risk category. It is expected that the rise in blood pressure after a normal rapid sequence induction will be mild and transient. This category of patient need not be managed in any fashion out of the ordinary.

If two or more of the above questions are answered in the affirmative, then the patient should be considered for a carefully planned induction that affords protection against a severe hypertensive response. It is no longer important today to be concerned about the administration of respiratory depressant drugs, which will provide substantial protection to the mother, but which will also affect the newborn. This is the case with fentanyl, which is very effective in blocking the pressor response to laryngoscopy and intubation, but is also a respiratory depressant for the newborn. Of course, it is necessary to consult and inform the pediatrician, and have him/her stand by for immediate resuscitation and long term treatment of the newborn.

The choice of anesthetic technique for mothers with hypertension must be decided upon after careful consideration of several factors. These include the mother's preference to be awake or asleep for her delivery, the extent of her disease, the severity of her hypertension with current treatment, the health of the fetus, and the sophistication of the neonatal unit in the hospital. One notable study (91) of 106 patients with severe hypertension, who were delivered at 26 to 35 weeks' gestation because of either fetal distress or unstable maternal blood pressure, showed 80% well-baby survival at 1 year followup. Antepartum management was with hydralazine and methyldopa, with delivery by cesarean section when indicated. All mothers survived and left the hospital well, in spite of three severely affected mothers who had postpartum eclampsia, pulmonary edema, and transient renal failure. The primary survival factors for the baby were gestational age and birth weight. A secondary factor was intraventricular hemorrhage, which was correlated with prolonged maternal hypertension and low gestational age. The primary anesthetic technique for these patients was general anesthesia.

Recent investigative work shows that pregnancy-induced hypertension is associated with a vasodestructive process at the placental level, leading to a new diagnosis of hemorrhagic endovasculitis (HEV). Clinicopathologic studies reveal relationship to still-births, intrauterine growth retardation babies, and live-born infants with a high incidence of neurologic abnormalities. It should be obvious from this that whatever method of anesthesia is decided upon, the maternal blood pressure should be maintained at near "normal" levels, so that further placental insufficiency is not precipitated by an episode of hypotension. It should also be noted that whatever anesthetic is chosen, it cannot compensate for the damage that has already been done to the fetus in utero (101).

For the past 40 years, the induction agent of choice has been thiopental. There are two important problems with thiopental: (1) a tendency to cause cardiac depression and hypotension; this in turn reduces cardiac output and delivery of blood to the placenta; and (2) just the opposite problem of a significant hypertensive response to induction and intubation. This may be due to an inadequate dose. A favorite induction agent in Europe, Propofol, resulted in a lessened hypertensive response after intubation, in one series of 40 cesarean patients (102). Other induction agents useful for blunting the pressor response to intubation may be the newer synthetic opioids, fentanyl and alfentanil.

### Hypotension

It is well-recognized that during regional anesthesia, hypotension is worsened by the pressure of the uterus on the vena cava and aorta. The lateral tilt is used to help prevent it. This tends to be ignored during general anesthesia, to the detriment of the patient.

Maternal hypotension associated with the induction of

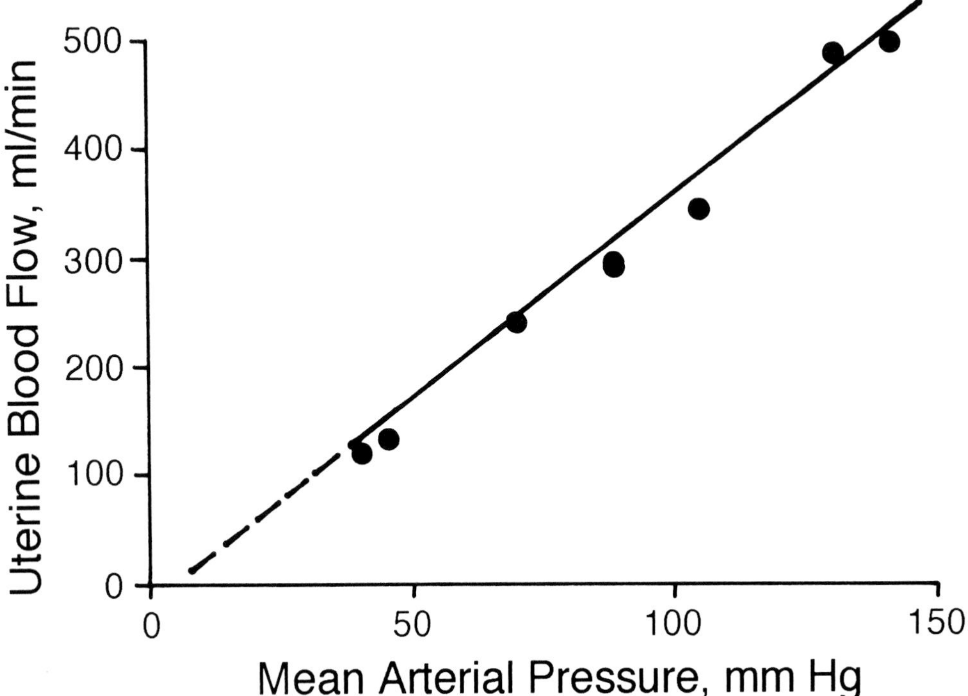


**Fig. 20–37.** Uterine blood flow/Mean arterial pressure.

general anesthesia is due to vasodilation and the cardiac depressant effect of the anesthetic drug. This lowers cardiac contractility, which in turn decreases cardiac output. These cause a reduction in systemic blood pressure, which is dependent upon both cardiac output and peripheral vascular resistance. This relatively transient effect of induction agents is often not appreciated or well-recognized, except by obstetric anesthesiologists. It is especially important when there is evidence of fetal compromise. In such situations, even small reductions in placental blood flow due to maternal hypotension may be detrimental to the well-being of the fetus. A review of Figure 20–37 also shows the interesting relationship between maternal blood pressure and uterine blood flow. Note that a 50% fall in maternal blood pressure may result in a significantly greater percentage fall in uterine blood flow. This supports the concept that maintenance of maternal pressure at or near baseline levels is important. Although hypotension may occur from time to time regardless of what the anesthesiologist may do to prevent it, the important point is that detection and diagnosis must occur promptly and that timely and effective treatment be instituted. Thus, the fact that hypotension occurred is not so important as is early recognition and institution of effective therapy.

In the early 1970s, Dr. John S. McDonald did a prospective study of over 1000 cesarean sections, comparing regional anesthesia and general anesthesia. Parameters included maternal blood pressure and various fetal and neonatal factors, including umbilical blood gases and Apgar scores. The final conclusion was that there was no significant difference in outcome of neonates based solely on anesthetic technique. An important aspect of this study was that induction doses of thiopental were small (2.5 mg/kg), and that immediate detection and treatment of hypotension was instituted. In a recent similar study on comparison of regional and general anesthesia, the same conclusion was reached. They emphasized attention to preoperative infusion, and a table tilt plus left uterine displacement to prevent vena caval compression (28,102,103).

Maternal hypotension is associated ordinarily with regional anesthesia because of loss of peripheral vascular resistance. However, hypotension can and does occur also with general anesthesia. This must be appreciated, and attention must be given to its prompt detection and treatment. Comparison of general versus regional anesthesia showed that the disadvantages of general include a nonresponsive mother who does not interact with her newborn baby, a higher maternal mortality, and use of more drugs; while the disadvantages of regional include hypotension and postspinal puncture headache. The choice of anesthetic must depend upon the interaction of the knowledge of these factors plus the preference of the mother, the capability of the anesthesiologist, and the obstetric indications for the cesarean delivery.

## Complications Due to Human Error

General anesthesia for obstetrics has many valuable attributes, including swiftness, cardiac and pulmonary stability, and low frequency of hypotension. Yet, there are certain inherent problems associated with this technique, the most serious of which is the hazard of hypoxia after induction. If intubation is difficult or impossible, panic may develop. Additional succinylcholine may be administered, prolonging the inability of the patient to resume spontaneous breathing. This causes further desaturation and hypoxia, cardiac arrhythmias, and even cardiac arrest.

In this section, we discuss hypoxia, hypercarbia its counterpart, and problems caused by drugs.

### *Inadvertent Esophageal Intubation*

Correct placement of the endotracheal tube should be a simple matter to confirm, and in most instances, it is. In the past, this has been done by careful observation of chest movement and careful auscultation of the chest on both sides. Now confirmation is technologically oriented toward determining $CO_2$ exhalation (104,105). This may be done by seeing a color change on an indicator or by viewing the $CO_2$ wave form on a screen. A characteristic wave form is absolutely confirmatory of tracheal intubation. The former clinical methods were sometimes in error, and failures to detect improper location of the endotracheal tube placed patients in lethal jeopardy. The problem with the older clinical method is that it may be very difficult to detect changes in chest movement and breath sounds due to obesity and other disease processes. Unrecognized esophageal intubation is one of the most common causes of death in general anesthesia. Now, the verification of correct intubation by immediate observation of the $CO_2$ output is a requisite to safe general anesthesia (Figure 20–38).

The effects of unrecognized esophageal intubation are more rapidly devastating in pregnant women because of more rapid desaturation, due to reduced functional residual capacity and elevated metabolic rate (30). There also are complications of gastric distention, regurgitation, and aspiration.

In a recent report of closed-claims studies of insurance cases, it was noted that esophageal intubation, difficult intubation, and inadequate ventilation were responsible for 75% of the problems. It is significant that listeners thought they heard breath sounds in 48% of cases in which the tube actually was in the esophagus. Monitoring of $CO_2$ output would have prevented the errors (106). Intubations under urgent or arrest conditions might be considered analogous to emergency obstetric conditions. In a recent study of such conditions, the incidence of difficult intubations was nearly 6%. Correct placement of the endotracheal tube occurred in 96% of the cases, but esophageal intubation occurred in 4% (104). This problem will continue to frustrate clinicians as long as the current methods of intubation are in vogue.

### *Hypoxia*

For many years, there has been little progress made in regard to general anesthesia and its associated difficulties causing life-threatening problems. In 1978, Moir stated that most deaths in obstetrics that occur in association with anesthesia are preventable, and that hypoxic cardiac arrest accounts for most maternal anesthetic deaths (107). Hypoxia associated with general anesthesia is most often due to placement of the endotracheal tube in the esophagus of a patient who is paralyzed (30). Failure to recognize the misplacement is the principle error. Other causes include obstruction of the airway, disconnection of the breathing system, failure of the oxygen supply, and

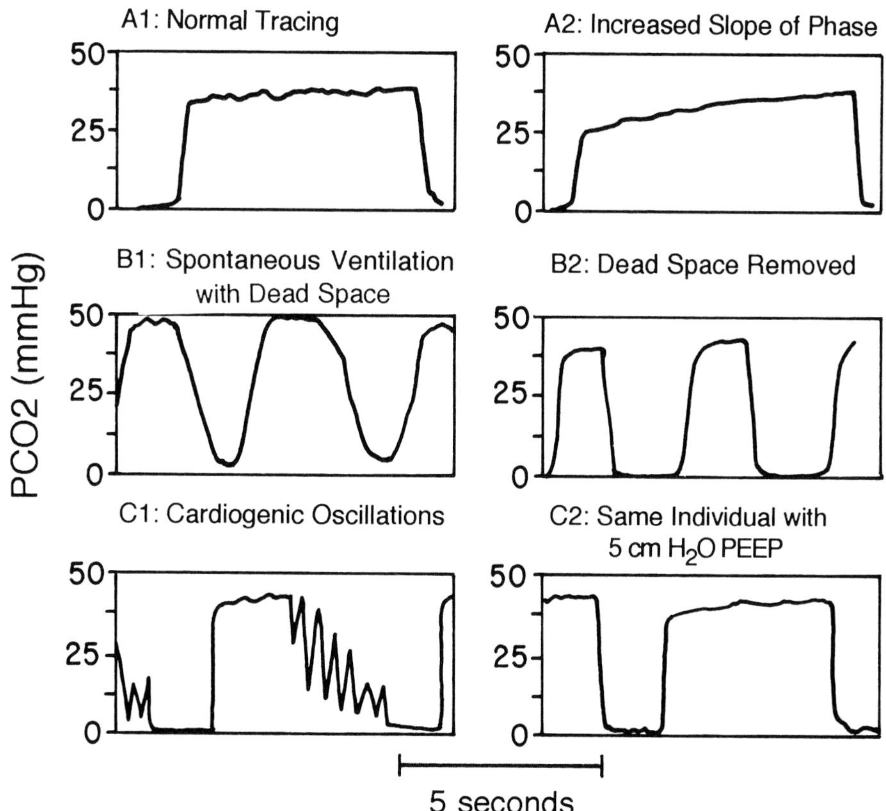


**Fig. 20–38.** Capnograph tracings. **(A1)** normal; **(A2)** increased slope usually caused by uneven gas mixing in the lungs; **(B1)** added dead space; **(B2)** removal of dead space gives sharper waveforms and return to normal concentrations; **(C1)** The rapid rise and fall of the curve is caused by the impact of the heart on the lung. **(C2)** The addition of PEEP increases the lung expansion, making the lung resistant to change of volume. (From Moon RE, Camporsei EM: Respiratory monitoring. *In* Anesthesia. 3rd Ed. Edited by RD Miller. New York, Churchill Livingstone, 1990.)

pulmonary edema resulting from either aspiration or fluid overload.

### Hypercarbia

The most common causes for hypercarbia are the same as those mentioned for hypoxia, with the addition of inadequate ventilation. Hypocarbia is the more common occurrence during general anesthesia, due to overzealous alveolar ventilation, but it is not usually a basis for problems. On the other hand, improper tube placement, tube disconnects, and other errors of airway management can be life threatening to the patient. Inadequate reversal of narcotics and muscle relaxants may cause hypoxia and hypercarbia in the recovery period. They must be avoided by making sure that all postanesthetic patients are managed by the same standards of recovery care and use of the same monitoring equipment, as is found in the main operating room suite of the general hospital.

Hypercarbia alone causes respiratory acidosis, which is usually well-tolerated, and is rarely a cause of serious difficulty.

### Unintentional Awareness During Surgery

An interesting case report describes a mother who wished to remain awake and aware after induction and intubation, until after the delivery of her baby. This request was entirely unexpected. Because the patient was awake and cooperative, the anesthesiologist granted her request. Subsequently, the patient recalled the procedure and the delivery of her baby with no unpleasant or painful memory (108). Similar awake analgesia with ether was used for heart surgery by Artusio at Cornell in the 1950s.

Unintentional awareness as a phenomenon of concern to the anesthesiologist resulted from the liberal use of muscle relaxants and the move away from potent inhalational agents to $N_2O$ with opioids, barbiturates, and other injectables. Parkhouse described and coined the term "awareness during surgery" in 1960 (109–113). It was nearly 19 years later that Tunstall described the Isolated Forearm Technique, or IFT, as a means of assessing wakefulness during the intraoperative period. A tourniquet isolates the forearm from the muscle relaxant. The muscles are able to function. The hand moves if anesthesia is inadequate.

Maternal awareness during surgery was identified in the mid1970s as a problem relating to the tendency to minimize the thiopental dosage during induction for a cesarean birth. In most of these cases, the $N_2O$ concentration was also reduced from 70% to 50%. The incidence of awareness was significant, perhaps in the 20 to 25% range, and this was believed to be excessively high. The suggestion then was to add a small percentage of inhalation agent, such as halothane 0.4%, enflurane 0.8%, or isoflurane 0.6% (113,114). Since then, there have been few articles on the subject, so one can surmise that there is no longer a real problem with maternal awareness due to deliberately low doses of anesthetics (115–118).

The problem of maternal awareness today focuses on "human error" associated with a paralyzed patient who, by mistake, does not receive any analgesic or amnestic agent. Thus, the patient may have significant recall, not only for the incision, but also the delivery, announcement of the sex of the baby, and the entire closure process. These incidents frequently trigger malpractice suits against the anesthetist, who really has little defense under such circumstances. Many of the patients report later distorted sleep patterns, interruption of family relationships, disharmonious sexual relationships, and depression. These incidents are very unusual and are nearly always due either to faulty devices for administration of inhalation agents or intravenous injection of the wrong agents for induction and analgesia, and inability to judge the adequacy of anesthesia during the procedure.

It is wise to check the patient's pupils after delivery of the baby, to note if they are widely dilated due to strong sympathetic stimulation because of poor analgesia. Dilated pupils are less likely to be noted now that the use of opioids and potent inhalation agents has become common.

Signs of inadequate anesthesia in a paralyzed patient may include: increases in pulse rate and blood pressure, cardiac arrhythmias, sweating, tearing, and bronchospasm. In addition to recording pupil size, the anesthetist should record peak inspiratory pressure.

### Adverse Effects of Drugs

There was a time when the statement was made that deliveries presented conflicting requirements for two separate patients, i.e. the mother and the baby. The conflict arose out of the necessity to provide anesthesia for the mother while not unduly depressing the central nervous system of the fetus. This is really not a major problem today, since the development of sophisticated neonatal care. Neonates can obtain adequate and extended oxygenation and ventilation, based upon solid principles used successfully for many years in adult respiratory management. Such sophistication and the years of experience with outstanding survival statistics have been the most exciting, forward reaching developments in perinatology over the past 2 decades. Today, if the mother needs general anesthesia with significant CNS depression to protect her, similar depression of the baby should not be a contraindication.

Injudicious use of oxytocics just after delivery may cause detrimental effects on the mother. One example is the use of a large bolus dose of oxytocin to effect placental expulsion after delivery. There are examples in the literature of maternal hypotension and even cardiac arrest after such treatment. In addition to its immediate vasodepressive effect, it must also be recalled that oxytocin has an impressive antidiuretic effect, and produces a decrease in urine flow. This may cause water overload and hyponatremia. Pitocin in dextrose solution without balanced salt content, used for prolonged inductions, may also cause dilutional hyponatremia.

The basis of the adverse effect of oxytocin upon the mother's cardiovascular system is vasodilation, but it is just the opposite for ergotamine. With the latter, the primary physiologic effect is vasoconstriction, due to stimulation of both the alpha and beta receptors. This is the cause of the elevated blood pressures seen after its use to counteract uterine atony. The overlap effects of ergotamine and ephedrine have been known to cause such severe hypertension as to result in cerebrovascular accidents.

Prolonged apnea may occur following administration of either depolarizing or nondepolarizing relaxants. Pregnant women have reduced levels of pseudocholinesterase, causing increased sensitivity to succinylcholine and delay in recovery. Obstetric patients who have pregnancy-induced hypertension are often treated with magnesium, a time-honored therapy for toxemia of pregnancy. Patients who receive magnesium and general anesthesia often show altered reactions to muscle relaxant drugs. They are more sensitive to succinylcholine, becoming relaxed with smaller doses, and the effect may be prolonged. They are also more sensitive to nondepolarizing relaxant drugs, and again, the effect may be prolonged. This is probably caused by decreased amount of acetylcholine liberated at the neuromuscular junction.

## Maternal Disease

Whether due to pregnancy or not, maternal disease may be confused with anesthetic accident or adverse effect. Maternal disease may make adverse reactions to anesthesia become more severe. Maternal disease may cause fetal death, which might then be attributed to an anesthetic complication.

### *Embolism*

Pregnant women, as all other patients, may suffer embolism of blood clots, fat droplets, and air. Also, they may develop amniotic fluid embolism.

Thrombotic pulmonary embolism occurs more frequently in pregnant women. However, it is not particularly associated with general anesthesia, nor is fat embolism.

Air embolism does occur as a complication at the time of delivery (119). The torn uterine veins readily allow air to enter, should a negative pressure develop in the veins. This occurs when the torn veins are at a level higher than the heart, as in Trendelenburg position, or if the fundus of the uterus is lifted out of the abdominal cavity during a cesarean. It can be detected with a stethoscope over the heart, an esophageal stethoscope, or a Doppler. Specific treatment is to change the posture, occlude the open veins with a wet towel, and to aspirate the air from the heart by means of a CVP catheter.

Amniotic fluid embolism may occur as a sudden, rapidly catastrophic event, manifested by cyanosis, dyspnea, hypotension, and other evidences of the adult respiratory distress syndrome. It is treated as adult respiratory distress syndrome, and has a high mortality rate. It may occur after a tumultuous labor or during or shortly after a cesarean operation. Frequently, there is confusion as to whether there was an anesthetic accident or an obstetric catastrophe. Definitive proof is the demonstration of lanugo hairs or fetal squames in the maternal pulmonary vessels (120).

### *Neurologic Disorders*

Because obstetric and other direct causes of maternal mortality have decreased over the past 2 decades, there has been an increased interest in nonobstetric causes for maternal mortality. Cerebrovascular accident is an example of such a cause, with hemorrhagic and ischemic strokes responsible for much of the mortality. At one busy obstetric unit during the latter part of the 1980s, the incidence of stroke was about 1 in 6000 pregnancies. It is important to realize how serious this malady is: there was a 20% mortality during that time period, and another 40% of the survivors had residual neurologic deficits. This experience demonstrated that specific management and success in reduction of the morbidity and mortality could only be achieved with aggressive workup and understanding of the problem that precipitated the crisis (121).

In addition to the common neurologic disorders, hemorrhagic and ischemic cerebrovascular problems, subarachnoid hemorrhage, and eclampsia, unusual disorders occur, such as pseudotumor cerebri, obstetric nerve palsies, and pituitary tumors (122).

The incidence of subarachnoid hemorrhage during pregnancy is 1 in every 10,000 patients, a rate five times higher than in nonpregnant women. Maternal mortality from this can vary considerably (from 0 to 14%), and the fetal mortality is also considerable (from 10 to 28%). It is thought to be related primarily to less-than-adequate placental perfusion.

An example of the ischemic cerebrovascular problem is a report of multiple cerebral infarcts in a young pregnant woman who had neurofibromatosis with thrombotic tendencies. This particular patient also had laboratory evidence of a positive lupus anticoagulant with anticardiolipin antibody (123).

One sobering statistic is that the risk of stroke in pregnant women is thirteen times greater than in nonpregnant women of the same age. The major causes of stroke in pregnant women are arterial occlusion and cerebral venous thrombosis.

In addition to the disorders just described, the pregnant state can precipitate many other neurologic conditions that may have predated the pregnancy, including epilepsy, headaches, multiple sclerosis, myasthenia gravis, spinal cord injury, and even dormant brain tumors. It is thought that the activation of these problems is caused by the edema and hyperdynamic vascular state that is common to pregnancy (122).

Nerve palsies may be due to pressure on the nerves of the lumbosacral plexus. They may also be caused by faulty positioning on the delivery table for a prolonged period, in an unfeeling patient. The anesthetist must assure that there is adequate padding and no pressure upon or stretching of the nerves.

### *Cardiac Arrest*

Cardiac arrest as a sequel of general anesthesia is caused almost exclusively by the problems discussed in this chapter, namely, failed intubation and inability to establish an adequate airway. These result in rapid desaturation of the patient's blood due to her pregnant state. Asphyxia causes first tachycardia then bradycardia, then arrhythmia, due to insufficient oxygenation of the myocardium. This is followed by complete cardiovascular collapse and arrest within a very few minutes. No greater calamity or emergency exists. The anesthesiologist must take direct and forceful control of the situation, and begin aggressive therapy, which is somewhat different from the management of cardiac arrest for a nonpregnant person.

A woman at term has a distorted cardiac axis due to diaphragm elevation. This places the left ventricle outside the line between the sternum and the vertebral bodies. The effectiveness of closed cardiac resuscitation in nonpregnant patients is based upon the ability to compress the ventricle between these two bony structures, and produce a cardiac output. Because closed chest compression is ineffective for a woman at term, the anesthesiologist may also need to call for open cardiac resuscitation, which is done by opening the chest and directly compressing the ventricles with the hand. During resuscitation, epinephrine 0.5 mg to 1.0 mg should be administered every 5 minutes, in accordance with the Advanced Cardiac Life Support (ACLS) guidelines.

During the first year of his academic medicine career, Dr. John S. McDonald found a patient who had a cardiac arrest after a spinal anesthetic for cesarean section. It was obvious that it was a very high spinal, and had resulted in respiratory arrest followed by cardiac arrest. This was undetected by the resident, who was distracted in the operating room. The patient was intubated, and external cardiac massage was begun. However, carotid pulsations were not adequate, despite heroic external massage. The chest of the patient was immediately opened, and a hand was inserted to administer internal cardiac massage. At the same time, the obstetrician was instructed to deliver the baby. The baby was delivered within 2 to 3 minutes, and the patient responded favorably and recovered uneventfully. The life of the patient was most likely preserved due to detection of the inadequacy of external cardiac massage, and the combined application of internal cardiac massage and immediate delivery of the baby.

The point to emphasize here is to ask the obstetrician to deliver the baby immediately, so that its resuscitation can be started independently, and so that the vena caval obstruction is alleviated. Furthermore, the mother's resuscitation can be more effective when the fetus is delivered.

Aggressive efforts must be made to reestablish pulmonary ventilation and oxygenation, including intubation or use of a large bore needle in the trachea, a cricothyrotomy, a jet ventilator, or a tracheostomy.

Nurses should be recruited to help with supplies, and to call for assistance from surgeons, ENT specialists, and obstetricians.

## Malignant Hyperthermia

This disease process is a potentially lethal complication of general anesthesia (mortality from less than 5% to 30%), regardless of whether or not a patient is pregnant. The disease process was described originally in the 1950s. Since then, there have been innumerable incidents of malignant hyperthermia reported, many of them culminating in death (124–128). The underlying mechanism is an alteration of calcium metabolism in muscle cells that causes phenomenal release of energy and heat. The patient suffers from both hyperthermia and muscle rigidity. The classical clinical features include hyperthermia, muscle rigidity, perspiration, cardiac arrhythmias, tachycardia, increased $O_2$ utilization, increased $CO_2$ production, hyperventilation, cyanosis, and acidosis. Triggering agents can include anesthetic agents, muscle relaxants, and stress reactions. The absolute diagnosis depends upon a skeletal muscle biopsy and a positive contracture test.

### *History*

The preanesthetic history is important. Some individuals recount having had hyperthermic episodes. The condition is familial, so inquiry should be made as to whether anyone in the family is known to have had it, or whether anyone in the family died during operation of unknown cause. If a suspicious history is elicited, a blood CPK level may help to establish whether the patient is likely to be susceptible. When in doubt, it is advisable to avoid the most common triggering agents, halothane and succinylcholine.

### *Prophylaxis*

For a person who is known to have malignant hypothermia, or thought to be susceptible, a preemptive, preoperative management strategy has been developed. Regimens have been developed for administration of Dantrolene orally several days before the expected delivery or need for anesthesia, with a loading dose immediately before anesthesia. The oral dose of Dantrolene is 100 mg twice daily. If the patient has been untreated until hospital admission, administer a 150 mg loading dose, followed by 100 mg every few hours until a satisfactory level is obtained (128).

As in all threatening disease processes that complicate the application of anesthesia to the patient, there must be strict adherence to the three basic tenets of sound practice that have been the central theme in this book. To reiterate, these are: (1) detection; (2) diagnosis; and (3) definitive therapy.

### *Detection*

In the case of malignant hyperthermia, the detection must be early and swift, and requires continuous monitoring of: (1) body temperature; (2) $CO_2$ output; (3) $O_2$ saturation; and (4) EKG. The clinical observer looks for muscle hyperactivity or rigidity on induction or during the procedure, perspiration, cyanosis, spontaneous hyperventilation, and excessively warm soda lime container.

### *Diagnosis*

In making the diagnosis, one must rule out other problems that may mimic malignant hypothermia, such as an ongoing infection, an unrecognized underlying neurologic disease process, or a variant of a seizure disorder. The detection of increased $CO_2$ production may be the earliest warning of malignant hyperthermia, a substantial increase occurring several minutes and even an hour before other signs (129). When in doubt, the diagnosis must always be in favor of the obvious, and the most life-threatening possibility, in this case, malignant hyperthermia

## *Definitive Therapy*

In the early management of this disease, there were two primary strategies. From the obstetric viewpoint, there was emphasis on cesarean section delivery rather than vaginal delivery. From the anesthesia viewpoint, there was emphasis on regional analgesia with use of an ester instead of an amide local anesthetic agent. Amides may be triggering agents, whereas esters are not (130–132). If general anesthesia is indicated for a susceptible patient, a "clean" anesthesia machine should be used to avoid any potential contamination by anesthetic vapors that might act as triggering agents for malignant hyperthermia. Succinylcholine should be avoided; rapid onset of intense paralysis for intubation can be obtained by administration of atracurium or vecuronium (133). These careful considerations, and the early use of Dantrolene, have provided a margin of safety (134).

Definitive therapy must be instituted immediately to offer the patient as much protection as possible (135). Dantrolene is rapidly effective and life saving, and acts by preventing calcium release from the sarcoplasmic reticulum in the skeletal muscle (136). It should be used as soon as the diagnosis is made. Administered intravenously at 1 mg/kg/min, the mean effective dose is around 2.5 mg/kg. Larger amounts are often needed. Response to treatment includes slowing of the heart rate to near normal and some notable decrease in muscle tone.

Additional therapy includes the administration of 100% oxygen and cooling of the body with ice, ice water externally or used intraperitoneally if this is an option at the time, or by gastric lavage. In addition, hyperventilation is necessary to keep ahead of the tremendous production of $CO_2$. If cardiac arrhythmia develops, do not use lidocaine; instead, procaine or Dilantin are acceptable. Treatment of the metabolic phase of the acidosis with sodium bicarbonate and institution of adequate diuresis to make sure the kidneys are functioning normally rounds out the immediate treatment regimens. Active cooling should be stopped when the temperature is down to 101°, as there is some overshoot. The patient should be observed in an intensive care unit for 48 hours. All the family members should be warned of susceptibility.

As in the case of many life-threatening emergencies, it would be prudent to organize a drill or procedure to follow, so that all involved parties would know their responsibilities. One of the chief advantages of such a plan is to demonstrate before a disaster how much cold sterile water is needed, and how many assistants are needed to perform the reconstitution of Dantrolene. The anesthesiology department should have available a "clean" machine with new tubing and support materials that are kept in reserve for such an occasion, and this is demonstrated at the drill. For treatment of a patient suspected to have malignant hyperthermia, refer to Tables 20–16 and 20–17. The survival of the patient with malignant hyperthermia is dependent upon early detection and institution of aggressive therapy.

There are reports that relate excellent results in man-

**Table 20–16.** Treatment of Malignant Hyperthermia During General Anesthesia

1. Administer Dantrolene. Repeat as needed.
2. Discontinue all anesthetic agents.
3. Change to a clean machine.
4. Hyperventilate with 100% oxygen.
5. Begin vigorous cooling.
6. Place arterial and CVP lines.
7. Check ABG's repeatedly.
8. Monitor ECG, $ETCO_2$, $O_2$ saturation, CPK, Ca, temperature.
9. Adjust fluid administration to maintain CVP and urine output.
10. Administer bicarbonate if necessary.
12. Transfer to intensive care unit.

(From Jacoby, JJ. Procedure used at The Ohio State University Hospitals.)

**Table 20–17.** Treatment of Malignant Hyperthermia During Regional Anesthesia

1. Administer Dantrolene. Repeat as needed.
2. Discontinue all amide type drugs.
3. Discontinue epinephrin.
4. Begin vigorous cooling.
6. Administer 100% oxygen.
7. Place arterial and CVP lines.
8. Check ABG's repeatedly.
9. Monitor ECG, $ETCO_2$, $O_2$ saturation, CPK, Ca, temperature.
10. Adjust fluid administration to maintain CVP and urine output.
11. Administer bicarbonate if necessary.
12. Transfer to intensive care unit.

(From Jacoby, JJ. Procedure used at The Ohio State University Hospitals.)

**Table 20–18.** Maternal Mortality Figures Obtained From the Confidential Enquiries into Maternal Deaths In England and Wales

| Years | Maternal Mortality per 1000 Total Births | Number of Deaths from Anaesthesia | Percentage True Maternal Deaths from Anaesthesia | Percentage with Avoidable Factors* |
|---|---|---|---|---|
| 1952–54 | 0.53 | 49 | 4.5 | — |
| 1955–57 | 0.43 | 31 | 3.6 | 77 |
| 1958–60 | 0.33 | 30 | 4.0 | 80 |
| 1961–63 | 0.26 | 28 | 4.0 | 50 |
| 1964–66 | 0.20 | 50 | 8.7 | 48 |
| 1967–69 | 0.16 | 50 | 10.9 | 68 |
| 1970–72 | 0.13 | 37 | 10.4 | 76 |
| 1973–75 | 0.11 | 31 | 13.2 | 90 |
| 1976–78 | 0.11 | 30 | 13.2 | 93 |
| 1979–81 | 0.11 | 22 | 12.2 | 100 |

* This term has been replaced by "substandard care", first used in 1979–81

(From Morgan M: Anaesthetic contribution to maternal mortality. Br. J. Anaesth. 59:842–855, 1987.)

agement of these patients, with no episodes of temperature elevation, changes in myoglobin or CPK values, and with no untoward effects upon the fetus. Dantrolene does pass through the placenta with the same efficiency as many other drugs, in the range of 0.4 F/M ratio (137,138).

Although the mother is the focus of attention in regard to malignant hyperthermia, neonatal muscle rigidity triggered by succinylcholine administration to the mother has been described (139). It is prudent to offer only regional anesthesia to the mother, using an ester-type local anesthetic, except in instances in which general anesthesia is strongly indicated. If general anesthesia is the technique of choice, induction can be performed with thiopental and a nondepolarizing relaxant, and maintenance of balanced anesthesia with $N_2O$ and opioids. The pediatrician must be alerted to the change of anesthetic agents and the reasons for it.

## Maternal Mortality

Death of pregnant women, or serious jeopardy, has been mentioned several times in this chapter. The prevention of death is an even more important goal than the provision of complete anesthesia (Figure 20–39 and Tables 20–18 through 20–22) (45,46,106,107,111, 140–153).

When vaginal delivery is imminent and there is no time to administer regional anesthesia, and general anesthesia is too dangerous, the following is an effective technique: Tell the patient you are going to relieve the pain, but she must follow instructions. Encourage her repeatedly to take deep breaths from the mask, which you place over her face while there is a high flow of oxygen, with or without a little nitrous oxide. Hyperventilation and suggestion are effective in producing some analgesia. If nothing else, the mask muffles the screams; the technique makes everyone feel better. The patient's recall is that she did obtain pain relief.

In considering maternal mortality, it appears that complications of general anesthesia were the most susceptible to prevention. In a series of individual state reports, general anesthesia for morbidly obese patients was implicated as a prime causative factor for obstetric mortality (147).

**Table 20–19.** Causes of Maternal Death and Associated Conditions by Outcome of Pregnancy, United States, 1979–1986

| Cause of Death/Associated Condition | Outcome of Pregnancy | | | | | | | |
|---|---|---|---|---|---|---|---|---|
| | Live Birth | Stillbirth | Ectopic | Abortion* | Molar | Undelivered | Unknown | Total |
| Hemorrhage | 249 (18.3%) | 89 (33.8%) | 305 (88.9%) | 43 (34.7%) | 2 (14.3%) | 30 (20.5%) | 81 (20.7%) | 799 (30.2%) |
| Ruptured ectopic | 0 | 0 | 295 | 0 | 0 | 0 | 0 | 297 |
| Uterine rupture/laceration | 14 | 20 | 0 | 6 | 0 | 9 | 19 | 68 |
| Abruptio placentae | 52 | 42 | 0 | 0 | 0 | 7 | 25 | 126 |
| Placenta previa | 28 | 4 | 0 | 0 | 0 | 5 | 8 | 45 |
| Retained placenta and products of conception | 16 | 1 | 0 | 13 | 0 | 0 | 6 | 36 |
| Disseminated intravascular coagulation | 32 | 8 | 0 | 6 | 1 | 5 | 5 | 57 |
| Uterine bleeding | 54 | 4 | 0 | 14 | 1 | 0 | 10 | 83 |
| Other/unspecified | 53 | 10 | 8 | 4 | 0 | 4 | 8 | 87 |
| Pulmonary embolism | 370 (27.1%) | 47 (17.9%) | 10 (2.9%) | 24 (19.4%) | 2 (14.3%) | 60 (41.1%) | 106 (27.1%) | 619 (23.4%) |
| Thrombotic | 207 | 13 | 8 | 13 | 1 | 31 | 46 | 319 |
| Amniotic fluid | 151 | 32 | 1 | 7 | 1 | 18 | 54 | 264 |
| Air | 6 | 2 | 1 | 4 | 0 | 9 | 4 | 26 |
| Other/unspecified | 6 | 0 | 0 | 0 | 0 | 2 | 2 | 10 |
| Pregnancy-induced hypertension complications | 307 (22.5%) | 59 (22.4%) | 1 (0.3%) | 1 (0.8%) | 2 (14.3%) | 17 (11.6%) | 92 (23.5%) | 479 (18.1%) |
| Preeclampsia | 159 | 25 | 1 | 0 | 0 | 6 | 34 | 225 |
| Cerebrovascular/CNS complications† | 57 | 7 | 0 | 0 | 0 | 4 | 16 | |
| Other/unspecified | 102 | 18 | 1 | 0 | 0 | 2 | 18 | |
| Eclampsia | 131 | 30 | 0 | 0 | 2 | 10 | 53 | 226 |
| Cerebrovascular/CNS complications† | 87 | 16 | 0 | 0 | 0 | 7 | 31 | |
| Other/unspecified | 44 | 14 | 0 | 0 | 2 | 3 | 22 | |
| Other/unspecified | 17 | 4 | 0 | 1 | 0 | 1 | 5 | 28 |
| Infection | 101 (7.4%) | 22 (8.4%) | 6 (1.7%) | 35 (28.2%) | 2 (14.3%) | 8 (5.5%) | 28 (7.2%) | 202 (7.6%) |
| Genital tract | 20 | 4 | 0 | 11 | 0 | 0 | 2 | 37 |
| Chorioamnionitis | 10 | 7 | 0 | 0 | 0 | 4 | 10 | 31 |
| General septicemia | 34 | 9 | 2 | 11 | 2 | 1 | 6 | 65 |
| Other/unspecified | 37 | 2 | 4 | 13 | 0 | 3 | 10 | 69 |
| Cardiomyopathy | 53 (3.9%) | 4 (1.5%) | 0 | 1 (0.8%) | 0 | 2 (1.4%) | 30 (7.7%) | 90 (3.4%) |
| Anesthesia complications | 65 (4.8%) | 3 (1.1%) | 4 (1.2%) | 11 (8.9%) | 0 | 0 | 3 (0.8%) | 86 (3.3%) |
| Aspiration | 19 | 0 | 0 | 0 | 0 | 0 | 2 | 21 |
| Other/unspecified | 46 | 3 | 4 | 11 | 0 | 0 | 1 | 65 |
| Other/unspecified | 218 (16.0%) | 39 (14.8%) | 17 (5.0%) | 9 (7.3%) | 6 (42.9%) | 29 (19.9%) | 51 (13.0%) | 369 (14.0%) |
| Total maternal deaths | 1363 (100.0%) | 263 (100%) | 343 (100.0%) | 124 (100.0%) | 14 (100.0%) | 146 (100.0%) | 391 (100.0%) | 2644 (100.0%) |

CNS = central nervous system.
* Includes induced (legal and illegal) and spontaneous abortions.
† Includes cerebrovascular accidents (hemorrhage, embolism) and other central nervous system conditions.
(From Morgan M. Anaesthetic contribution to maternal mortality. Br. J. Anaesth. 59:842–855, 1987.)

**Table 20–20.** Number and Percent of Selected Causes of Maternal and Nonmaternal Deaths and of Deaths Occurring More Than 42 Days After Pregnancy Ended, United States, 19 Reporting Areas, 1980–1985

| Cause of Death | All Deaths | No. Died After Pregnancy Ended* | Died More Than 42 Days After Pregnancy Ended | |
|---|---|---|---|---|
| | | | *N* | % |
| Maternal—direct | | | | |
| Embolism | 102 | 80 | 7 | 9 |
| Hypertensive disease | 74 | 63 | 1 | 2 |
| Ectopic pregnancy | 60 | 53 | 2 | 4 |
| Hemorrhage | 55 | 47 | 2 | 4 |
| Cerebrovascular accident | 51 | 35 | 2 | 6 |
| Anesthesia complications | 42 | 40 | 4 | 10 |
| Abortions (all types) | 31 | 24 | 3 | 13 |
| Cardiomyopathy | 25 | 19 | 11 | 58 |
| Obstetric infection | 21 | 19 | 1 | 5 |
| Hydatidiform mole | 3 | 3 | 2 | 67 |
| Other direct causes | 41 | 31 | 3 | 10 |
| Total direct | 507 | 414 | 38 | 9 |
| Maternal—indirect | | | | |
| Infectious conditions | 31 | 22 | 3 | 14 |
| Cardiovascular | 31 | 22 | 6 | 27 |
| Other | 29 | 14 | 3 | 21 |
| Total indirect | 94 | 58 | 12 | 21 |
| Total maternal | 601 | 472 | 50 | 11 |
| Nonmaternal | | | | |
| Injury | 90 | 16 | 5 | 31 |
| Other | 21 | 13 | 2 | 15 |
| Total nonmaternal | 111 | 29 | 7 | 24 |
| All Deaths† | 712 | 501 | 57 | 11 |

* Excludes women who died with an undelivered infant or whose outcome of pregnancy was unknown.
† Excludes two deaths of unknown cause.
(From Rochat RW, Koonin LM, Atrash HK, Jewett JF: The Maternal Mortality Collaborative. Obstet. Gynecol. 72:91–97, 1988.)

**Table 20–21.** Maternal Mortality Ratios* and Relative Risks for Age and Race by Cause of Death, United States, 19 Reporting Areas, 1980–1985

| Cause of Death | Age Group | | | Race Group | | |
|---|---|---|---|---|---|---|
| | <30 Ratio | ≥30 Ratio | RR | White Ratio | Black and Others Ratio | RR |
| Embolism | 2.0 | 5.5 | 2.7 | 1.7 | 4.4 | 2.6 |
| Indirect† | 2.0 | 4.8 | 2.3 | 1.6 | 4.1 | 2.5 |
| Hypertensive disease | 1.5 | 3.7 | 2.5 | 1.1 | 3.4 | 3.0 |
| Ectopic pregnancy | 1.1 | 3.3 | 3.0 | 0.7 | 3.5 | 5.3 |
| Hemorrhage | 0.8 | 3.2 | 3.8 | 1.1 | 1.5 | 1.3 |
| Cerebrovascular accident | 1.1 | 2.7 | 2.4 | 1.3 | 1.8 | 1.4 |
| Anesthesia | 0.9 | 2.1 | 2.4 | 0.6 | 2.3 | 4.2 |
| Abortion (all types) | 0.7 | 1.5 | 2.1 | 0.4 | 1.8 | 4.1 |
| Cardiomyopathy | 0.3 | 2.0 | 7.1 | 0.4 | 1.2 | 3.2 |
| Infection | 0.7 | 0.4 | 0.6 | 0.4 | 0.8 | 1.8 |
| Other | 1.2 | 2.1 | 1.8 | 0.7 | 1.9 | 2.7 |
| All causes | 12.3 | 31.3 | 2.5 | 10.0 | 26.7 | 2.7 |

RR = relative risk.
* Crude cause-specific ratio per 100,000 live births for each age group or race group.
† Indirect maternal deaths, coded as ICD-9 647–648.
(From Rochat RW, Koonin LM, Atrash HK, Jewett JF: The Maternal Mortality Collaborative. Obstet. Gynecol. 72:91–97, 1988.)

The obese individual has several reasons for a higher morbidity and mortality from general anesthesia, including: (1) greater difficulty with airway management after muscle relaxation, due to pharyngeal closure; (2) greater difficulty with intubations; (3) greater incidence of gastric aspiration, due to reduction of the esophageal/gastric bar-

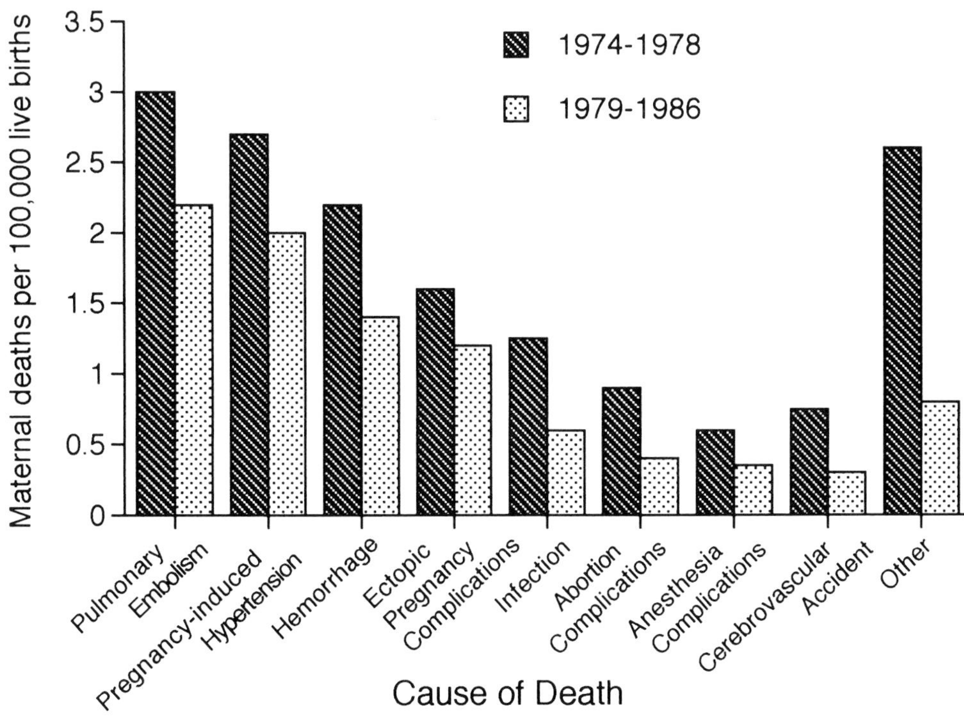


**Fig. 20–39.** Maternal mortality, 1974–78 and 1979–1986. Maternal deaths per 100,000 live births is given for each major cause of death during the designated time periods. All deaths decreased in frequency. Anesthetic deaths decreased from 0.5 to 0.3 per 100,000, a 40% decrease. These figures include abortions, whether spontaneous or induced, legal or illegal. (Redrawn from Atrash HK, Koonin LM, Lawson HW, Franks AL, et al: Maternal mortality in the United States, 1979–1986. Obstet. Gynecol. 76:1055–1060, 1990.) For 1992 data, see Table 20–22.

**Table 20–22.** Maternal Deaths and Maternal Mortality Rates for Selected Causes by Race: United States, 1989 (Maternal deaths are those assigned to Complications of pregnancy, childbirth, and the puerperium, category numbers 630–676 of the *Ninth Revision International Classification of Diseases, 1975*. Rates per 100,000 live births in specified group. Beginning in 1989, race for live births is tabulated according to race of mother; see Technical notes]

| Cause of Death (Ninth Revision International Classification of Diseases, 1975) | | Number | | | | Rate | | | |
|---|---|---|---|---|---|---|---|---|---|
| | | All Races | White | All Other: Total | All Other: Black | All Races | White | All Other: Total | All Other: Black |
| Complications of pregnancy, childbirth, and the puerperium | 630–676 | 320 | 180 | 140 | 124 | 7.9 | 5.6 | 16.5 | 18.4 |
| Pregnancy with abortive outcome | 630–638 | 50 | 21 | 29 | 26 | 1.2 | 0.7 | 3.4 | 3.9 |
| Ectopic pregnancy | 633 | 34 | 14 | 20 | 19 | 0.8 | * | 2.4 | * |
| Spontaneous abortion | 634 | 3 | 1 | 2 | — | * | * | * | * |
| Legally induced abortion | 635 | 3 | 1 | 2 | 2 | * | * | * | * |
| Illegally induced abortion | 636 | — | — | — | — | * | * | * | * |
| Other pregnancy with abortive outcome | 630–632, 637–638 | 10 | 5 | 5 | 5 | * | * | * | * |
| Direct obstetric causes | 640–646, 651–676 | 241 | 144 | 97 | 85 | 6.0 | 4.5 | 11.4 | 12.6 |
| Hemorrhage of pregnancy and childbirth | 640–641, 666 | 43 | 30 | 13 | 10 | 1.1 | 0.9 | * | * |
| Toxemia of pregnancy | 642.4–642.9, 643 | 58 | 29 | 29 | 27 | 1.4 | 0.9 | 3.4 | 4.0 |
| Obstructed labor | 660 | — | — | — | — | * | * | * | * |
| Complications of puerperium | 670–676 | 89 | 60 | 29 | 26 | 2.2 | 1.9 | 3.4 | 3.9 |
| Other direct obstectric causes | 642.0–642.3, 644–646, 651–659, 661–665, 667–669 | 51 | 25 | 26 | 22 | 1.3 | 0.8 | 3.1 | 3.3 |
| Indirect obstetric causes | 647–648 | 29 | 15 | 14 | 13 | 0.7 | * | * | * |
| Delivery in a completely normal case | 650 | — | — | — | — | * | * | * | * |

(Modified by Jay Jacoby, M.D. From U.S. Department of Health and Human Services, Centers for Disease Control Public Health Service. Monthly Vital Statistics Report 40(8):S2, 1992.)

rier; and (4) greater difficulty in establishing positive pressure oxygenation and ventilation, due to enormous resistance factors of abdominal pressure and chest wall pressure secondary to the obese status. The best preventive measure would be to restrict the anesthesia techniques for morbidly obese patients to either regional anesthesia or local anesthesia with systemic supplementation by the anesthesiologist. The anesthesiologist can teach the use of local anesthetics to obstetric colleagues, including their toxic doses, the proper placement for maximal effect, and the use of the peritoneal "spray" technique for sensitive intraperitoneal structures.

The authors of this book again state their strong opinion in favor of the use of regional anesthesia for such cases when possible. The use of the epidural catheter method of administration of drugs allows slow development of the level of block, and thus causes less of a problem with hypotension due to sympathetic blockade. Another choice might be use of the continuous spinal, again with the catheter method. The catheter may be placed during the early phase of labor, and used for pain relief during labor. Supplemental doses of local anesthetics may be given to provide satisfactory analgesia for cesarean section. The patient and the surgeon should be informed that the lower T-8 to T-10 level of block is used to protect the mother from problems with oxygenation and ventilation, and thus the usual profound analgesia associated with higher T-6 to T-4 levels may be absent.

We must not rest until the incidence of death due to anesthesia is reduced.

## REFERENCES


1. Hingson RA, Edwards WB: Continuous caudal anesthesia during labor and delivery. Anesth. Analg. 21:301–311, 1942.
2. Hingson RA, Southworth JL: Continuous caudal anesthesia. Am. J. Surg. 48:93–96, 1942.
3. Cugell DW: Pulmonary function in pregnancy. Am. Rev. Tuberc. 67:568, 1953.
4. Bader RA: Hemodynamics in normal pregnancy. J. Clin. Invest. 34:1524, 1955.
5. Bieniarz J, Crottogini JJ, Curuchet E, Romero-Salinas G, et al: Aortocaval compensation by the uterus in late human pregnancy. Am. J. Obstet. Gynecol. 100:203–217, 1968.
6. Marx GF: Aortocaval compression: incidence and prevention. Bull. N.Y. Acad. Med. 50:443–446, 1974.
7. Davison JS, Davison MC, Hay DM: Gastric emptying time in late pregnancy and labour. J. Obstet. Gynaecol. Br. Commonw. 77:37–41, 1970.
8. Nimmo WS, Wilson J, Prescott LF: Narcotic analgesics and delayed gastric emptying during labour. Lancet 1(7912): 890–893, 1975.
9. Simpson KH, Stakes AF, Miller M: Pregnancy delays paracetamol absorption and gastric emptying in patients undergoing surgery. Br. J. Anaesth. 69:24–27, 1988.
10. Wilson J: Gastric emptying in labour: some recent findings and their clinical significance. J. Int. Med. Res. 6(Suppl1): 54–62, 1978.
11. Lind JF, Smith AM, McIver DK, Coopland AT, et al: Heartburn in pregnancy—A manometric study. Can. Med. Assoc. J. 98:571–574, 1968.
12. Spence AA, Moir DD, Finlay WEI: Observations on intragastric pressure. Anaesthesia 22:249–256, 1967.
13. Brock-Utne JG, Rubin J, Downing JW, Dimopoulos GE, et

al: The administration of metoclopramide with atropine. Anaesthesia 31:1186–1190, 1976.
14. Brock-Utne JG, Rubin J, Welman S, Dimopoulos GE, et al: The action of commonly used antiemetics on the lower oesophageal sphincter. Br. J. Anaesth. 50:295–298, 1978.
15. Gintzler AR: Endorphin-mediated increases in pain threshold during pregnancy. Science 210:193–195, 1980.
16. Maduska AL: Inhalation analgesia and general anesthesia. Clin. Obstet. Gynecol. 24:619–633, 1981.
17. Palajhniuk RJ, Shinder, SM, Eger EI II: Pregnancy decreases the requirements for inhaled anesthetic agents. Anesthesiology 41:82, 1974.
18. Cotton DB, Gonik B, Spillman T, Dorman KF: Intrapartum to postpartum changes in colloid oncotic pressure. Am. J. Obstet. Gynecol. 149:174–176, 1984.
19. Caton WL: Plasma volume and extravascular fluid volume during pregnancy. Am. J. Obstet. Gynecol. 5:471, 1949.
20. Haley HB, Woodbury JW: Observations on body composition and body water metabolism in normal pregnancy. J. Clin. Invest. 31:635, 1952.
21. MacLennan FM: Maternal mortality from Mendelson's Syndrome: an explanation. Lancet 1(8481):587–589, 1986.
22. Wallace DH, Currie JM, Gilstrap LC, Santos R: Indirect sonographic guidance for epidural anesthesia in obese pregnant patients. Reg. Anesth. 17:233–236, 1992.
23. Castro MI, Eisenach JC: Maternally administered esmolol produces fetal β-blockade and hypoxemia. Anesthesiology 69:A708, 1988.
24. Kuhnert BR: Effects of maternal epidural anesthesia on neonatal behavior. Anesth. Analg. 63:301–308, 1984.
25. Mirkin BL: Perinatal pharmacology: Placental transfer, fetal localization and neonatal disposition of drugs. Anesthesiology 43:156–170, 1975.
26. Nicholas JF: Increasing maternal $FIO_2$ increases fetal $PaO_2$. Can. J. Anaesth. 34:S55, 1987.
27. Ostman LGP, Chestnut DH, Robillard JE, Weiner CP, et al: Assessment of transplacental passage and hemodynamic effects of esmolol in the gravid ewe. Anesthesiology 97: A63, 1987.
28. Hollman AI, Jouppila R, Koivisto M, Maatta L, et al: Neurologic activity of infants following anesthesia for cesarean section. Anesthesiology 48:350–356, 1978.
29. Zagorzycki MT: General anesthesia in cesarean section: effect on mother and neonate. Obstet. Gynecol. Survey. 39: 134–137, 1984.
30. Archer GW Jr, Marx GF: Arterial oxygen tension during apnoea in parturient women. Br. J. Anaesth. 46:358–360, 1974.
31. Mendelson CL: The aspiration of stomach contents into the lungs during obstetric anesthesia. Am. J. Obstet. Gynecol. 52:191–205, 1946.
32. Olsson GL, Hallen B, Hambraeus-Jonzon: Aspiration during anaesthesia: a computer-aided study of 185,358 anaesthetics. Acta. Anaesthesiol. Scand. 30:84–92, 1986.
33. Hall GC: Aspiration pneumonitis as an obstetric hazard. JAMA 114:728, 1940.
34. Brock-Utne JG, Rout C, Moodley J, Mayat N: Influence of Preoperative Gastric Aspiration on the volume and pH of gastric contents in obstetric patients undergoing caesarean section. Br. J. Anaesth. 62:397–401, 1989.
35. Colman RD, Frank M, Loughnan BA, Cohen DB, et al: Use of I.M. ranitidine for the prophylaxis of aspiration pneumonitis in obstetrics. Br. J. Anaesth. 61:720–729, 1988.
36. Gallagher EG, White M, Ward S, Cottrell IJ, et al: Prophylaxis against acid aspiration syndrome. Single oral dose of $H_2$—antagonist on the evening before elective surgery. Anaesthesia 43:1011–1014, 1988.
37. Wynne JW, Modell JH: Respiratory aspiration of stomach contents. Ann. Int. Med. 87:466–474, 1977.
38. Nimmo WS: Aspiration of gastric contents. Br. J. Hosp. Med. 34(3):176–179, 1985.
39. Roberts RB, Shirley MA: Reducing the risk of acid aspiration during cesarean section. Anesth. Analg. 53:859–868, 1974.
40. Winternitz, MC: Collected Studies On The Pathology Of War Gas Poisoning. New Haven, Yale University Press, 1920.
41. Sellick BA: Cricoid pressure to control regurgitation of stomach contents during induction of anaesthesia. Lancet 2:404–406, 1961.
42. Attia RR, Ebert AM, Fischer JE: Gastrin: Placental, maternal, and plasma cord levels, its possible role in maternal residual gastric acidity. Abstracts of Scientific Papers, Annual Meeting, American Society of Anesthesiologists, San Francisco, 1976, p. 547.
43. Brock-Utne JG, Rubin J, Welman S, Dimopoulos GE, et al: The effect of gylcopyrrolate (Robinul) on the lower oesophageal sphincter. Can. Anaesth. Soc. J. 25:144–146, 1978.
44. Roberts RB, Shirley MA: The obstetrician's role in reducing the risk of aspiration pneumonitis. Am. J. Obstet. Gynecol. 124:611–728, 1976.
45. Elkington KW: At the water's edge: where obstetrics and anesthesia meet. Obstet. Gynecol. 77:304–308, 1991.
46. Chestnut DH, Cohen SE: At the water's edge: where obstetrics and anesthesia meet. Obstet. Gynecol. 77:965–967, 1991.
47. Crawford JS: Difficulty in endotracheal intubation associated with obstetric anesthesia. Anesthesiology 51:475, 1979.
48. Lyons G: Failed intubation: six years' experience in a teaching maternity unit. Anaesthesia 40:759–672, 1985.
49. Samsoon GLT, Young JRB: Difficult tracheal intubation: a retrospective study. Anaesthesia 42:487–490, 1987.
50. Cormack RS, Lehane J: Difficult tracheal intubation in obstetrics. Anesthesia 39:1105–1111, 1984.
51. Gupta B, McDonald JS: The difficult airway. Hospital Physician 65: 69–71, 74, January 1986.
52. Mallampati SR, Gatt SP, Gugino LD, Desai SP, et al: A clinical sign to predict difficult tracheal intubation: a prospective study. Can. Anaesth. Soc. J. 32:429–434, 1985.
53. Oates JDL, Macleod AD, Oates PD, Pearsall FJ, et al: Comparison of two methods for predicting difficult intubation. Br. J. Anaesth. 66:305–309, 1991.
54. Shorten GD, Roberts JT: The prediction of difficult intubation. Anesthesiology Clinics of North America 9:63–67, 1991.
55. Wilson ME, Spiegelhalter D, Robertson JA, Lesser P: Predicting difficult intubation. Br. J. Anaesth. 61:211–216, 1988.
56. McDonald JS, Gupta B, Cook R: Rationale and methodology for development of difficult airway index. Unpublished data, 1993.
57. Marx GF, Finster M: Difficulty in endotracheal intubation associated with obstetric anesthesia. Anesthesiology 51: 364–365, 1979.
58. Tunstall ME, Geddes C: "Failed intubation" in obstetric anesthesia. Br. J. Anaesth. 56:659–661, 1984.
59. Waters DJ: Guided blind endotracheal intubation for patients with deformities of the upper airway. Anaesthesia 18:158–162, 1963.
60. Gold MI, Buechel DR: Translaryngeal anesthesia: a review. Anesthesiology 20:181–185, 1959.
61. James FM, Wheeler AS, Dewan DM: Obstetric Anesthesia:

The Complicated Patient. Philadelphia, F.H. Davis Co., 1988, p.113.

62. Messeter KH: Endotracheal intubation with the fiberoptic bronchoscope. Anaesthesia 35:294–298, 1980.
63. Ovassapian A, Doka JC, Romsa DE: Acromegaly—Use of fiberoptic laryngoscopy to avoid tracheostomy. Anesthesiology 54:429–430, 1981.
64. Ovassapian A, Yelich SJ, Dykes MHM: Fiberoptic nasotracheal intubation: incidence and causes of failure. Anesth. Analag. 62:692–695, 1983.
65. Goldberg HE, Jacoby J: A substitute for cocaine. Anesth. Analg. 64:457–458, 1988.
66. Mokriski BLK, Malinow AM, Gray WC, McGuinn WJ: Topical nasopharyngeal anaesthesia with vasoconstriction in preeclampsia-eclampsia. Can. J. Anaesth. 35:641–643, 1988.
67. Akinyemi OO, John A: A complication of guided blind intubation. Anaesthesia 29:733–735, 1974.
68. Akinyemi OO: Complications of guided blind endotracheal intubation. Anaesthesia 34:590–592, 1979.
69. Butler FS, Cirillo AA: Retrograde tracheal intubation. Anesth. Analg. 39:333–338, 1960.
70. Gupta B, McDonald JS, Brooks JHJ, Mendenhall J: Oral fiberoptic intubation over a retrograde guidewire. Anesth. Analg. 68:1–3, 1989.
71. Lechman MJ, Donahoo JS, MacVaugh H III: Endotracheal intubation using percutaneous retrograde guidewire insertion followed by antegrade fiberoptic bronchoscopy. Crit. Care. Med. 14:589–590, 1986.
72. Rosenberg MB, Levesque PR, Bourke DL: Use of the LTA kit as a guide for endotracheal intubation. Anesth. Analg. 56(2):287–8, 1977.
73. Goldman, E, McDonald, JS: Continuous oxygenation during nasotracheal intubation. Anesthesiology 61:352, 1984.
74. Humphrey D, Brock-Utne JG: Suggested solutions to the problem of T-piece anaesthesia breathing system. Can. J. Anaesth. 34:S130, 1987.
75. Reed JP, Kermph JP, Hamelberg HA, Jacoby JJ: Studies with transtracheal artificial respiration. Anesthesiology 15: 28–41, 1954.
76. Jacoby J, Hamelberg W, Ziegler CH, Flory FA, et al: Transtracheal resuscitation. JAMA 162:625–628, 1956.
77. Hughes RK: Needle tracheostomy. Arch. Surg. 93:83–86, 1966.
78. Neff CC, Pfister RC, VanSonnenberg E: Percutaneous transtracheal ventilation: experimental and practical aspects. J. Trauma 23:84–90, 1983.
79. Benumof JL, Scheller MS: The importance of transtracheal jet ventilation in the management of the difficult airway. Anesthesiology 71:769–778, 1989.
80. Goldman E, McDonald JS, Peterson SS, Stock MC, et al: Transtracheal ventilation with oscillatory pressure for complete upper airway obstruction. J. Trauma 28: 611–614, 1988.
81. Swartzman S, Wilson MA, Hoff BH, Bunegin L, et al: Percutaneous transtracheal jet ventilation for cardiopulmonary resuscitation: evaluation of a new jet ventilator. Crit. Care. Med. 12:8–13, 1984.
82. Tunstall ME, Geddes C: Failed intubation in obstetric anesthesia. Br. J. Anaesth. 56:659–661, 1984.
83. Buonafede D: Expanding neck hematoma: an uncommon cause of failed intubation. Anesth. News February 1991, 8, 15.
84. Heller PJ, Scheider EP, Marx GF: Pharyngeal edema as a presenting symptom in preeclampsia. Obstet. Gynecol. 62: 623–629, 1983.
85. Mackenzie AI: Laryngeal edema complicating obstetric anesthesia. Anaesthesia 33:271–277, 1978.
86. Skau NK, Pilgaard P, Neilsen G: Granuloma gravidarum of the nasal mucous membrane. J. Laryngol. Otol. 101: 1286–1288, 1987.
87. Erlandson MJ, Clinton JE, Ruiz E, Cohen J: Cricothyrotomy in the emergency department revisited. J. Emerg. Med. 7: 115–118, 1989.
88. Spaite DW: Pre-hospital cricothyrotomy: an investigation of indications, technique, complications, and patient outcome. Ann. Emerg. Med. 19:279–285, 1990.
89. Miklus RM, Elliott C, Snow N: Surgical cricothyrotomy in the field: experience of a helicopter transport team. J. Trauma 29:506–508, 1989.
90. Callan NA, Witter FR: Intrauterine growth retardation: characteristics, risk factors and gestational age. Int. J. Gynaecol. Obstet. (Ireland) 33:215–220, 1990.
91. Derham RJ, Hawkins DF, DeVries LS, Aber VR, et al: Outcome of pregnancies complicated by severe hypertension and delivered by 34 weeks; stepwise logistic regression analysis of prognostic factors. J. Obstet. Gynaecol. Br. Commonw. 96:1173–1181, 1989.
92. Joyce TH III, Debnath KS, Baker EA: Preeclampsia—Relationship of CVP & epidural analgesia. Anesthesiology 51: S297, 1979.
93. Joyce TH III, Loon M: Pre-eclampsia: effect of albumin 25% infusion. Anesthesiology 55:A313, 1981.
94. Soder G, Grenroth C, Noree LO, Willund PE: Treatment of preeclampsia and eclampsia as a hypoperfusion syndrome. Acta. Anaesth. Scand. Suppl. 57:71–78, 1975.
95. Benedetti TJ, Kates R, Williams V: Hemodynamic observations in severe preeclampsia complicated by pulmonary edema. Am. J. Obstet. Gynecol. 152:330–334, 1985.
96. Berkowitz RI, Rafferty TD: Invasive hemodynamic monitoring in critically ill pregnant patients: role of Swan-Ganz catheterization. Am. J. Obstet. Gynecol. 137:127, 1980.
97. Fenakel K, Fenakel G, Appelman Z, Lurie S, et al: Nifedipine in the treatment of severe preeclampsia. Obstet. Gynecol. 77:331–337, 1991.
98. Ludlow SW, Davies N, Davey DA, Smith JA: The effect of sublingual nifedipine on uteroplacental blood flow in hypertensive pregnancy. Br. J. Obstet. Gynaecol. 95: 1276–1281, 1988.
99. Lurie S, Fenakel K, Friedman A: Effect of nifedipine on fetal heart rate in the treatment of severe pregnancy-induced hypertension. Am. J. Perinatol. 7:285–286, 1990.
100. Vink GJ, Moodley J, Philpott RH: Effects of dihydralazine on the fetus in the treatment of maternal hypertension. Obstet. Gynecol. 55:519–522, 1980.
101. Sibai BM, Spinato JA, Watson DL, Hill GA, et al: Pregnancy outcome of 303 cases with severe preeclampsia. Obstet. Gynecol. 64:319–325, 1984.
102. Yau G, Gin T, Ewart MC, Kotur CF, et al: Propofol for induction and maintenance of anaesthesia at caesarean section. A comparison with thiopentone/enflurane. Anaesthesia 46:20–23, 1991.
103. Lees MM, Taylor SH, Scott DB: A study of cardiac output at rest throughout pregnancy. J. Obstet. Gynaecol. Br. Commonw. 74:319–328, 1967.
104. Vukmir RB, Heller MB, Stein KL: Confirmation of endotracheal tube placement: a miniaturized infrared qualitative CO2 detector. Ann. Emerg. Med. 20:726–729, 1991.
105. Birmingham PK, Cheney FW, Ward RW: Esophageal intubation: a review of detection techniques. Anesth. Analg. 65: 886, 1986.
106. Caplan RA, Posner KL, Ward RJ, Cheney FW: Adverse respi-

ratory events in anesthesia: a closed claims analysis. Anesthesiology 72:828–833, 1990.
107. Moir DD: The contribution of anaesthesia to maternal mortality. J. Int. Med. Res. 6(Suppl. 1):40–44, 1978.
108. Tunstall ME: On being aware by request. Br. J. Anaesth. 52:1049–1051, 1980.
109. Parkhouse, J: Awareness during surgery. Postgrad. Med. J. 36:674–677, 1960.
110. Brahams D: Cesarean section: pain and awareness without negligence. Anaesthesia 45:161–162, 1990.
111. Green RA: Changes in obstetric anaesthesia in the last twenty-five years. J. Int. Med. Res. 6(Suppl. 1):33–39, 1978.
112. Matthews P, Dann WL, Cartwright DP: Awareness during cesarean section. Anaesthesia 46:157–158, 1991.
113. Warren TM, Datta S, Ostheimer GW, Naulty JS, et al: Comparison of the maternal and neonatal effects of halothane, enflurane and isoflurane for cesarean delivery. Anesth. Analg. 62:516–520, 1963.
114. Wilson J, Turner DJ: Awareness during cesarean section under general anesthesia. Br. Med. J. 1:280–283, 1969.
115. Baraka A, Louis F, Dalleh R: Maternal awareness and neonatal outcome after ketamine induction of anaesthesia for cesarean section. Can. J. Anaesth. 37:641–644, 1990.
116. Crawford JS: Fetal well-being and maternal awareness. Br. J. Anaesth. 61:247–249, 1988.
117. Leicht CH: Anesthesia for the pregnant patient undergoing nonobstetric surgery. Anes. Clin. of North America 8: 131–142, 1990.
118. Abboud TK, Kim SH, Henriksen EH, Chen T, et al: Comparative maternal and neonatal effects of halothane and enflurane for cesarean section. Acta. Anaesth. Scand. 29: 663–668, 1985.
119. Handler JS, Bromage PR: Venous air embolism during cesarean delivery. Regional Anesthesia 15:170–173, 1990.
120. Clark SL, Montz FJ, Phelan JP: Hemodynamic alterations associated with amniotic fluid embolism: a reappraisal. Am. J. Obstet. Gynecol. 151:617–621, 1985.
121. Simolke GA, Cox SM, Cunningham FG: Cerebrovascular accidents complicating pregnancy and the puerperium. Obstet. Gynecol. 78:37–42, 1991.
122. Fox MW, Harms RW, Davis DH: Selected neurologic complications of pregnancy. Mayo Clin. Proc. 65:1595–1618, 1990.
123. Carr ME Jr, Howe CW: Lupus anticoagulant and cerebrovascular accident in a patient with neurofibromatosis. South. Med. J. 82:921–923, 1989.
124. Britt BA: Recent advances in malignant hyperthermia. Anesth. Analg. 51:841–850, 1972.
125. Brown RC: Hyperpyrexia and anaesthesia. Br. Med. J. 1526–1527, 1954.
126. Editorial. Cause of death: malignant hyperpyrexia. Br. Med. J. 3:5772:441–442, 1971.
127. Saidman LJ, Harvard ES, Eger EJ II: Hyperthermia during anesthesia. JAMA 90:1029–1032, 1964.
128. Morison, DH: Placental transfer of dantrolene. Anesthesiology 59:265, 1983.
129. Meier-Hellmann A, Römer M, Hannemann L, Kersting T, et al: Early recognition of malignant hyperthermia using capnometry [in German]. Anaesthetist 39:41–43, 1990.
130. Adragna MG: Medical protocol by habit—the avoidance of amide local anesthetics in malignant hyperthermia susceptible patients. Anesthesiology 62:99–100, 1985.
131. Moore DC: Ester or amide local anesthetics in malignant hyperthermia—who knows? Anesthesiology 64:294–296, 1986.
132. Wingard DW: Malignant hyperthermia: a human stress syndrome? Lancet 2:1450–1451, 1974.
133. Bevan DR: Atracurium and vecuronium. Can. Anaesth. Soc. J. 32:317–319, 1985.
134. Douglass MJ, McMorland GH: The anaesthetic management of the malignant hyperthermia susceptible parturient. Can. Anaesth. Soc. J. 33:371–378, 1986.
135. Harrison GG: Anaesthetic-induced malignant hyperpyrexia: a suggested method of treatment. Br. Med. J. 3: 454–456, 1971.
136. Britt BA: Dantrolene. Can. Anaesth. Soc. J. 31:61–75, 1984.
137. Houvenaeghel M, Achilli-Cornesse E, Jullian-Papouin H, Martin-Meyssonier A, et al: Oral dantrolene in a parturient with myotonic dystrophy and susceptibility to malignant hyperthermia. Ann. Fr. Anesth. Reanim. (France) 7: 408–11, 1988.
138. Shime J, Gare D, Andrews J, Britt B: Dantrolene in pregnancy: lack of adverse effects on the fetus and newborn infant. Am. J. Obstet. Gynecol. 159:831–834, 1988.
139. Sewall K, Flowerdew RMM, Bromberger P: Severe muscular rigidity at birth: malignant hyperthermia syndrome? Can. Anaesth. Soc. J. 27:279–282, 1980.
140. Atrash HK, Koonin LM, Lawson HW, Franks AL, et al: Maternal mortality in the United States, 1979–1986. Obstet. Gynecol. 76:1055–1060, 1990.
141. Beecher HK, Todd DP: A study of the deaths associated with anesthesia and surgery based on a study of 599,548 anesthesias in ten institutions 1948–1952, inclusive. Ann. Surg. 140:2–35, 1954.
142. Benedetti TJ, Starzyk P, Frost F: Maternal deaths in Washington state. Obstet. Gynecol. 66:99–101, 1985.
143. Cheney FW, Posner K, Caplan RA, Ward RJ: Standard of care and anesthesia liability. JAMA 261:1599–1603, 1989.
144. Conklin KA: Can anesthetic-related maternal mortality be reduced? Am. J. Obstet. Gynecol. 163:253–254, 1990.
145. Endler GC, Mariona FG, Sokol RJ, Stevenson LB: Anesthesia-related maternal mortality in Michigan 1972 to 1984. Am. J. Obstet. Gynecol. 159:187–193, 1988.
146. Hunter AR: The contribution of anaesthesia to maternal mortality. Proc. Royal Soc. Med. 67:905–910, 1974.
147. May WJ, Greiss FC Jr: Maternal mortality in North Carolina: a forty-year experience. Am. J. Obstet. Gynecol. 161: 555–561, 1989.
148. Moir DD: Anaesthesia and maternal deaths. Scot. Med. J. 24:187–189, 1979.
149. Morgan M: Anaesthetic contribution to maternal mortality. Br. J. Anaesth. 59:842–855, 1987.
150. Petitti DB: Maternal mortality and morbidity in cesarean section. Clin. Obstet. Gynecol. 28:763–769, 1985.
151. Rochat RW, Koonin LM, Atrash HK, Jewett JF: The Maternal Mortality Collaborative. Obstet. Gynecol. 72:91–97, 1988.
152. Rubin GL, Peterson HB, Rochat RW, McCarthy BJ, et al: Maternal death after cesarean section in Georgia. Am. J. Obstet. Gynecol. 139:681–685, 1981.
153. Sachs BP, Yeh J, Acker D, Driscoll S, et al: Cesarean section-related maternal mortality in Massachusetts, 1954–1985. Obstet. Gynecol. 71:385–388, 1988.

Section E

# NONPHARMACOLOGIC METHODS OF OBSTETRIC ANALGESIA AND ANESTHESIA

Chapter 21

# PSYCHOLOGIC AND OTHER NONPHARMACOLOGIC TECHNIQUES

PENNY SIMKIN

This chapter describes and evaluates psychologic and physical approaches to the management of childbirth pain. Childbirth education classes offer information and rehearsal of numerous self-help methods for pain management. In addition, various pain-relieving modalities from the field of physical therapy and psychologic approaches to modify the effects of mental state on bodily processes are gaining widespread acceptance. Finally, greater attention to the emotional needs of the laboring woman indirectly reduces childbirth pain by motivating and assisting the woman in the use of self-help measures, while increasing her sense of mastery and general satisfaction with her birth experience. Childbirth education, physical therapy, and emotional support are used as a substitute for or an adjunct to pharmacologic methods to reduce or eliminate labor pain. The anesthesiologist, anesthetist, obstetrician, family physician, and midwife should be aware of their place in obstetrics.

This chapter describes and discusses in three sections the pain-relieving effects and other effects of: Childbirth Education, Emotional Support in Labor, and Physical Therapy Modalities and Psychologic Techniques. Birth never changes; that is, the physiological functioning of the human body in reproduction remains essentially the same from one culture to another and from one era to the next. Our understanding of this process does change, however, as our scientific knowledge increases; our perceptions of reproduction also change with the attitudes of the society and the culture.

In the twentieth century, western society has undergone massive shifts in attitudes toward reproduction associated with such major historical events as several major wars, the Industrial Revolution, and the increasing mobility of the family. The large close-knit extended family (consisting of parents, grandparents, aunts, uncles, in-laws, and children) of the past was replaced by the smaller nuclear family (parents and children), and more recently by single parent families, blended families, foster families, and other alternative family configurations. Traditionally, knowledge and customs of childbearing and childrearing were transferred informally from mother to daughter, and woman to woman through role modeling, day-to-day interactions, and social conversations.

These strong women's networks of support and education broke down as family members moved away from each other and changed location many times in a lifetime. Furthermore, the expertise of experienced females became less applicable to the rapidly changing perceptions of birth from primarily women's social work at home to men's medical work in the hospital. Women who had given birth in their own homes, surrounded by experienced, familiar, and caring females were baffled as their daughters entered the hospital and were delivered of their babies among strangers of both sexes. Older women's experience and knowledge were of little benefit to their daughters as birth was transformed into a complex medical event. The new experts, physicians and nurses, shaped and controlled a new attitude and approach to reproductive care, and became the new disseminators of information.

Significant improvements in maternal and infant mortality, as well as improvements in techniques and agents of pharmacologic pain relief have occurred over the past 2 decades because of the commitment of so many dedicated health care individuals, including physicians in obstetrics, anesthesiology and neonatology, and nurses in related fields. No advances such as the many that have occurred over this time period come without some who believe problems exist with patient fulfillment and autonomy.

## CHILDBIRTH EDUCATION

The natural childbirth and childbirth education movement in Europe and North America originated from within the medical profession and was quickly adopted by a vocal lay public. Grantly Dick-Read, Fernand Lamaze, Robert Bradley, Pierre Vellay, all medical doctors, are the most prominent names associated with the origins of natural childbirth as we know it today. These men shared a common belief that labor and birth do not have to be painful, if women are informed, relaxed, well-supported in labor, and if they know self-help measures to deal with labor pain. These men and their followers practiced, wrote, and taught their methods in the 1930s and 1940s in Europe, and in the 1950s and 1960s in the United States. Controversial figures within their own professions, each developed a substantial following among the public as a result of their popular books and speaking engagements.

During the 1950s, the public began to express dissatisfaction with the obstetric care of the day. This era was described in Chapter 1 as the end of the "Period of Neglect (1860–1940): Dark Ages of Obstetric Analgesia and Anesthesia," and the beginning of the "Renaissance of Obstetric Anesthesia (1945-present)." Ironically, an anonymous letter from a registered nurse to the *Ladies' Home Journal*, in November, 1957, may have catalyzed the consumer movement in childbirth. In this letter, titled, "Sadism in the Delivery Rooms?" the author described some horrors she had witnessed and asked the magazine "to investigate the tortures that go on in the modern delivery rooms." In 1958, the *Journal* published two articles and numerous letters to the editor. "Few full-length articles have elicited such a flood of letters from *Journal* readers." This popular magazine revealed a degree of "cruelty in the maternity wards" that had until then been unsuspected by both the medical profession and the public. Thus, the stage was set for childbirth education classes and greater participation by patients in their own maternity care. While most classes at the time were focused on either the Read or Lamaze method, a variety of other programs also appeared at about the same time, all with the primary aim to prevent or self-manage childbirth pain through the use of psychologic or physical nonpharmacologic modalities. Grantly Dick-Read, a British physician, described the vicious fear-tension-pain cycle: culturally induced fear of labor leading to tension during contractions, which then led to pain and in turn to greater fear. To combat this cycle, he proposed education to dispel fear of the unknown and muscular relaxation to relieve tension. In addition, he prescribed specific, progressive breathing patterns for the woman to learn and practice during pregnancy, and to use during labor, as well as physical exercises to improve her general health, muscle tone, and sense of well-being. He also advocated "understanding attention" directed toward the laboring woman as essential for minimizing the discomforts of labor. The term, "natural childbirth" was coined by Read. Robert Bradley, began using the Read method in the United States in the late 1940s and later introduced modifications to adapt the method to the needs of Americans. Bradley introduced the concept of the father as a "coach" for the laboring woman, a role designed to help her carry out the prescribed breathing and relaxation routines.

"Psychoprophylaxis" (literally "mind prevention"), based on Pavlov's concepts of conditioned reflexes, originated in the Soviet Union in the mid-1940s and introduced to the west by Fernand Lamaze and Pierre Vellay. Psychoprophylaxis has become so closely associated with the name of Fernand Lamaze that in some quarters "Lamaze" has become an eponym for all forms of childbirth education. "The Lamaze Method" was popularized in North America by Marjorie Karmel, Elisabeth Bing and colleagues. Psychoprophylaxis was "aimed very definitely at abolishing the so-called unavoidable pain associated with uterine contractions during labor." Conceptually, it recognized the potentially painful stimulus of the uterine contraction, but suggested that by the development of new conditioned reflexes, pain transmission or perception could be inhibited or blocked. In practice, like "natural childbirth," psychoprophylaxis includes lectures or discussions for imparting knowledge and attitudes, training in voluntary muscle relaxation, body building exercises, and a progression of specific breathing techniques. The emphasis is on the importance of a strong focus of attention and prescribed activities during contractions to blot out unwanted sensations. Lamaze, like Read, recognized the importance of human support during labor, writing: "in the labor ward each parturient should be helped, right through labor, by a qualified person, doctor, midwife or specially trained nurse."

Sheila Kitzinger, a British anthropologist, criticized the Lamaze method and emphasized greater awareness of the psychologic, sexual, and sociological significance of childbearing, incorporating them into her psychosexual approach. She also promoted a model of acceptance of labor pain as opposed to the avoidance model, which characterized the other major methods in the sixties and seventies. Kitzinger helped women to perceive labor pain as a "side-effect of a task willingly undertaken of pain with a purpose."

Over the years, as childbirth education matured, there was much cross-fertilization among educators and influential practitioners, resulting in constant innovation and modification of the various approaches. Disagreement among leaders in the field has always existed, as educational methods and pain relief measures are proposed, debated, tested, and either adopted or discarded. Childbirth education, at first a subspecialty of physical therapy and nursing, evolved into an independent profession, represented by several professional organizations, all founded in the 1960s: the American Society for Prophylaxis in Obstetrics (Lamaze method), the American Academy of Husband-Coached Childbirth (Bradley method), and the International Childbirth Education Association (no method orientation, but has as its motto, "Freedom of Choice Based on Knowledge of Alternatives").

Despite the conceptual differences that differentiate these approaches, there is a remarkable similarity in their practical applications. All share the approach of group sessions to establish a community of experience and include the provision of accurate and reliable information about pregnancy, birth and the experiences that women will undergo or encounter, techniques for voluntary muscular relaxation, and specific breathing patterns to serve as a vehicle for distraction and relaxation, as well as physical comfort measures. Over the years, childbirth education has become more complex and has expanded its focus beyond its primary goal of the reduction of labor pain. The development of safer regional anesthetics, the rise of feminism and patients' rights, the holistic health movement, the greatly increased popularity of antenatal classes among all social classes, the changing economics of health care, emphasis on reduction of maternal and neonatal morbidity, and the increasingly technologic approach to perinatal care have exerted profound influences on expectant parents and their educators.

Whereas in the 1950s and 1960s the goal of pain reduction was universal in childbirth education, this is no longer the case. Childbirth education no longer attracts only highly motivated people who wish to avoid pain medication, although this small and vocal minority of expectant parents still exists. These latter "influential consumers" carefully investigate and select the childbirth classes that encourage natural childbirth, read extensively, exercise their right to choose their caregivers and places for birth (changing in midpregnancy if they feel unsatisfied), and expect full participation in the decision-making concerning their own and their baby's care. They feel capable of understanding the issues and want to take responsibility for becoming informed and making choices. But today, vast numbers of people attend classes for other reasons as well: simply to learn what to expect in labor and afterward; to learn about procedures, interventions, and hospital routines; to obtain advice and answers to questions; to reduce anxiety; to meet other expectant parents; and to learn baby care and feeding. Many parents know little or nothing about classes before they attend; they come because they are told to, by their doctor, midwife, friend or spouse. Therefore, childbirth classes today are not unified in the goal of pain reduction; they vary in ideology, objectives, quality, structure, methods, content, and qualifications of the instructors, reflecting the diversity of the clientele who attend.

Childbirth education is sometimes perceived as a vehicle for those outside the mainstream of medical thinking (both lay and professional) to influence or change the course and philosophy of maternity care. Indeed, this was the original purpose of childbirth education. Independent childbirth educators, parents, and unconventional medical care providers have banded together for decades to ensure the availability of the maternity care options they desire. On the other hand, childbirth education is also utilized as a way to maintain control of maternity care by the providers of that care. Katona traces the history of childbirth education, showing how obstetricians and midwives dealt with the threat of "natural childbirth" by offering their own classes in offering reassurance, relieving anxiety and encouraging compliance and acceptance of the existing models of care. Depending on the ideology, preferences, and biases of the teacher, childbirth education may either promote or discourage parent decision-making, use of medications, acceptance of routine interventions, formula or breast feeding, and anxiety or confidence in the caregiver and place of birth.

Regardless of orientation, most childbirth classes today attempt to accomplish these other goals: good health habits, stress management, anxiety reduction, enhancement of family relationships, feelings of "mastery," enhanced self-esteem and satisfaction, successful infant feeding, smooth postpartum adjustment, and family planning. With the broadened emphasis of today's childbirth classes, educators look outside the obstetric literature to the biological and social sciences, to psychotherapy, to physical therapy, to alternative healing disciplines, to Eastern philosophies and meditation techniques, to athletics, to the disciplines of law, ethics and history, to poetry, music, theatre, dance, and art for guidance and new applications, in hopes of better preparing women to give birth with fulfillment and satisfaction.

## Content of Childbirth Classes

Although it is the mainstay of prenatal education, preparation for childbirth is only one of many types of courses offered for expectant parents. Prenatal classes are available on pregnancy self-care, breastfeeding, newborn care, cesarean birth preparation, postpartum recovery and adjustment, prenatal exercise, fathering, infant safety, grandparenting, sibling preparation, preparation for vaginal birth after a previous cesarean, and more. After the birth, classes are available on infant care and development, mother-infant exercise, infant massage, and more.

Childbirth education, the subject of this chapter, usually consists of 10 to 20 hours of classes spanning 4 to 10 weeks, or one intensive weekend. Classes vary in size from a few to 20 women and their husbands or loved ones. The International Childbirth Education Association (ICEA) has set the following minimum standards for content of classes for those who never have attended classes before.

Classes should provide a minimum of 12 class hours divided among a minimum of six class sessions.

Class content should include:

The natural physiologic and psychologic patterns of pregnancy, labor, birth, and post partum;
Common abnormal or unexpected variations on the usual patterns of the childbearing year;
Maternal and infant nutrition, including breastfeeding;

Common medical interventions and procedures during the labor and birth process, as well as: obstetric procedures and technologies; vaginal and cesarean birth and vaginal birth after previous cesarean; analgesia and anesthesia; indications, contraindications, benefits and risks for the above; alternatives to the above, whether or not available in the community.

Adequate class time must be allotted for demonstration, return demonstration, practice and review of: coping methods for labor, including: relaxation skills; breathing, either in a pattern or as a natural response to the forces of labor; comfort measures; body awareness and conditioning exercises for pregnancy, birth, and postpartum.

Content varies, however, according to the goals and underlying philosophy of teachers and sponsors. Classes sponsored by hospitals with high epidural rates place less emphasis on self-help pain management techniques than those sponsored by most independent educators or non-profit childbirth education organizations, or by hospitals or birth centers in which there are no round-the-clock anesthesia services. Most midwives and physicians encourage their clients to take classes that match their own philosophy regarding clinical management, participation by clients in decision-making, and pain management. Public agencies serving socially deprived clients who may lack knowledge of hygiene, healthy living, and parenting may devote a larger proportion of their time to these topics and on motivation toward positive change than the other classes described here.

Figure 21–1 is a sample of a topic outline used by this author for an 8-week series that offers complete preparation for unmedicated childbirth. It also covers pain medications for those who desire them or who will have to use them in cases of difficulty or complicated labor. Approximately 6 of the total of 20 hours are spent actively

## 8-WEEK (PLUS REUNION) CHILDBIRTH CLASS OUTLINE

**Penny Simkin, P.T.**

**Class 1:**

Introductions: Teacher, assistant, and class members
Philosophy & Purposes of Classes
Decisions: Health care for baby, birth plan, feeding the baby, return to employment, child care
Preparation for Breastfeeding: Anatomy of breast; identifying and treating flat or inverted nipples
*Refreshment break*
Childbirth film
Conditioning Exercises; passive relaxation with slow breathing

**Class 2:**

Review of Anatomy (slides)
Events of Late Pregnancy for Placenta, Mother, Fetus
Prematurity
*Refreshment break*
Conditioning exercises (cont.); Relaxation: The Roving Body Check; slow breathing in labor positions; light breathing

**Class 3:**

Normal Labor: Onset & Signs, Physiological Events, Stages & Phases (slides)
*Refreshment break*
Perineal Massage; Touch Relaxation and Roving Body Check (cont); Attention Focusing; Adaptation exercise for light breathing; Acupressure and hand massage

**Class 4:**

Normal Labor: Emotional needs of the laboring woman, stress points, partner's role in labor support
*Refreshment break*
Relaxation countdown; review slow breathing; light breathing in contraction pattern variable breathing

**Class 5:**

Childbirth film
Labor variations, complications; very rapid & very long labors; self-help strategies; emergency delivery; labor interventions—indications, risks, and benefits
*Refreshment break*
Review relaxation & breathing in variety of maternal positions; practice with pain stimulus; back labor techniques (positions, counterpressure, cold, movement, hydrotherapy)
Pain medications preference scale

**Class 6:**

Medications for pain: Names, when used, how given, desired and undesired effects on mother, labor, fetus, and newborn.
*Refreshment break*
Review of previously learned techniques; scramble breathing, handling the "urge to push"

**Class 7:**

Discussion of Birth Plans
Cesarean Birth (slides): Indications, procedure, anesthesia, recovery, options
The Newborn (slides): Appearance, routine procedures and their rationale, abilities
*Refreshment break*
Second stage techniques; role play of labor and practice in labor support

**Fig. 21–1.** 8-Week (plus reunion) Childbirth Class Outline.

**8-WEEK (PLUS REUNION) CHILDBIRTH CLASS OUTLINE**

**Penny Simkin, P.T.**

**Class 8:**

Guest speakers: New parents from earlier class who discuss their birth and postpartum experiences
Postpartum—what to expect
Video on initiating breastfeeding
*Refreshment break*
Review of all labor techniques

**Reunion Class**

Reunion, after all babies have been born
Potluck Meal
Sharing of labor stories, questions, and answers
Trouble shooting present problems
Group photo of all babies

**Fig. 21–1.** *(Continued).*

rehearsing the comfort measures and labor enhancement measures. Reading assignments supplement the class material.

By providing information on the anatomy, physiology, and the emotional experience of labor, appropriate medical terminology, exposure to realism of birth through films, role play, and discussion with new parents, childbirth class members learn what to expect. Through discussion and social contact with other expectant parents, they form a support network. From discussions and descriptions of complications and the common interventions ranging from self-help measures to cesarean section, parents gain a realistic understanding of the unpredictable nature of labor and the role of medical personnel. Thorough discussions of various types of pharmacologic pain relief and their risks and benefits enable parents to make informed decisions that can be especially beneficial in helping to develop a healthy attitude toward the supplemental effect that regional analgesia can have in conjunction with childbirth preparation. Thorough preparation of the husband or companion enhances his personal experience of the birth as well as his ability to comfort and assist the laboring woman. Lastly, discussion of what to expect of a newborn baby and of the postpartum recovery, along with an introduction to breastfeeding, helps with adjustment during the early days and weeks of parenthood. A reunion class is held after all the babies are born to renew the social network and review the childbirth and postpartum experiences of the class members.

## Labor Support as an Adjunct to Childbirth Education

Other influences, such as the quality of labor support from her partner or others and staff attitudes, may determine whether or not a woman uses the techniques she learns. If not encouraged by her partner and the experts around her to use her coping techniques, even a well-prepared and highly motivated woman may experience doubts and be unable to continue using the techniques. On the other hand, if she is encouraged and reassured, and is complimented on how well she is coping, she is more likely to continue. Therefore, a combination of effective teaching and consistent followup in labor, encouraging use of the learned strategies, help ensure that women do indeed use what they learn.

Read, Lamaze, and Vellay believed in the value of following up their teaching with effective labor support. Read himself, or one of his trained educators, accompanied his patients in labor. Lamaze insisted on bedside assistance for all trained women. Vellay instituted the use of monitrices, professional nurses providing continuous labor support. Though monitrices never were widely used in North America or the United Kingdom, husbands and loved ones have been encouraged to attend classes and provide continuous labor support. Five research teams investigated the effects of labor support as an adjunct to childbirth classes. Brant stated, "Previous experience had shown that, during labor, patients frequently forgot what they have been taught antenatally." In his study, all women received childbirth education. The treatment group of 123 primigravidae was randomly selected from among women booked for care at the hospital clinic. The control group consisted of 66 primigravidae who delivered within a prescribed period of time. The treatment group received four additional individual half-hour sessions with a trained assistant who then accompanied each throughout labor. Preparation emphasized the sensations and emotional reactions to be expected at the various phases of labor. Relaxation and patterned breathing were also emphasized. The control group received lectures and exercise classes and the usual support during labor. Length of labor was similar in the two groups, although the second stages were shorter in the treatment group, as were incidences of low and mid forceps operations. The dosage of pethidine during first stage and the percentage and length of time trilene analgesia was used during second stage were all markedly lower in the treatment group. Apgar scores were higher in the treatment group. The author concluded that realistic expectations of pain and emotional stress during labor combined with expert labor support brought superior results.

Henneborn and Cogan studied two groups of husband-wife Lamaze-prepared couples: in one group, the husbands attended only the first stage of labor; in the other, they attended both labor and birth. When husbands were present throughout, the women received less medication and reported more positive feelings about the birth. The study was limited by a low return of completed questionnaires (49 of 317 couples contacted completed all three of the questionnaires that comprised the study) and the self-selection factor that separated the two groups. The possibility exists, however, that the greater participation and satisfaction was related to the continuous labor support.

Campbell and Worthington compared two types of training for husbands to assist their wives with labor and delivery. One group engaged in unstructured discussion. The other received behaviorally explicit structured training, reviewing techniques from class and other techniques for handling discouragement, panic, and conflict. Results indicated that the men preferred the structured training, the women had more confidence in the men who had the structured training, and those men managed the women's panic in labor better than the men in the discussion group.

Copstick, Taylor, Hayes, and Morris found similar results in their study of the relationship between the type of labor support provided to women receiving an epidural block and those not receiving an epidural block. The women who received an epidural block had been less likely to use the pain-control measures learned in class than those who did not receive an epidural. They also had received a different type of labor support. Those who had an epidural received more "general support" hand holding, verbal encouragement, and reassurance. The partners of those who did not use an epidural gave more specific and directive support timing of contractions, massage, and active encouragement to use breathing, distraction, relaxation, and other pain-relieving techniques.

Bennett, Hewson, Booker, and Holliday studied 398 primiparae 3 weeks after birth and found that women's perceptions of good support from doctor, midwives, and partner were related to decreased use of epidural anesthesia and higher satisfaction ratings.

In these five studies, the quality of labor support appears to have been an important variable in the women's abilities to utilize what they learned in childbirth classes. By the same token, as Shearer points out, "Bedside practices can make prenatal education appear to be effective, or to have made no difference, or to have actually caused harm to patients. Regardless of how comparable or randomly chosen the class and no-class groups are in a study, obstetric management will completely dominate any effects of teaching."

## EFFECTIVENESS IN REDUCING USE OF PAIN MEDICATIONS

### *Comparison of Different Methods of Childbirth Preparation*

There are few studies comparing pain-relieving effects of different methods of childbirth preparation. The two major methods, Read's natural childbirth and Lamaze's psychoprophylaxis, have never been compared with each other systematically, using random assignment and a control group. Other comparisons have been made, however, between psychoprophylaxis and some less-popular methods of preparation, either combined with psychoprophylaxis or not, such as respiratory autogenic training, biofeedback systematic desensitization, generic "hospital classes," and self-hypnosis.

These studies comparing different types of preparation have failed to show significant differences in use of pain medications, with the exception of possible advantages from Respiratory Autogenic Training over Traditional Psychoprophylaxis, and of Psychoprophylaxis over hospital classes.

### *Comparisons of Prepared Versus Unprepared Women*

Numerous studies comparing outcomes in prepared and unprepared women have appeared since the early 1950s. Early reports, as well as some more recent ones of childbirth preparation classes, are descriptive, anecdotal, and uncontrolled. Those reporting benefits from classes may have testified more to the enthusiasm of their proponents than to the effectiveness of the approaches. It is important, however, to bear in mind that at the time these studies were reported, massive narcosis and virtually universal general anesthesia for delivery had become accepted as standard obstetric practice, in North America and elsewhere. In this setting, Thoms and Karlovsky's report of 2000 consecutive deliveries among women who participated in childbirth education classes, of which 34 percent of these consecutive deliveries were conducted without analgesia and 29 percent without anesthesia, was most impressive, despite the self-selection of the women who chose to attend their clinic and the possibly distorting effect of the enthusiasm of the investigators. Other investigators of that period reported similar findings.

Quite contrary findings were published a few years later from the same clinic as Thoms and Karlovsky's by Davis and Morrone. They compared 355 self-selected prepared women with 108 women who had not attended classes, and found no differences between the two groups in the use of analgesia or anesthesia. In contrast to the findings of Thoms and Karlovsky in the same clinic 8 years previously, only 8% of their patients did not receive analgesia, and only 0.2% avoided anesthesia for the second stage of labor. These authors suggested that "with the passage of time, the original evangelical zeal is gone." As stated earlier, differences in class content and in followup support in labor may also have contributed to the vastly different outcomes. The recent studies of Patton and colleagues and Storrock and Johnson described earlier in this chapter had similar findings.

A major problem with the early and many recent studies is the lack of comparability between those women who chose to attend classes and those who did not. Davis and Morrone found that those who elected to attend classes were older, better educated, and of a higher socioeconomic group. Similar studies have addressed the specific question of the differences between those who chose to attend classes and those who did not. As motivation to take classes may, in itself, be a significant determining factor in the results obtained, several studies attempted to control for that variable.

The groups in Patton, English, and Hambleton's study groups were comparable in age, childbirth risk score, ethnic group, and socioeconomic group, but the retrospective nature of their study precluded them from learning how many classes were attended, the content of the class, (which may very well have included a bias toward the use of anesthesia) or other important factors. In other words, class attendance or nonattendance, as indicated by a "Yes" or "No" in the chart, may not have represented a real difference between the groups.

Huttel, Mitchell, Fischer, and Meyer took the opportunity of working in a cultural setting in which psychoprophylaxis was completely unknown. This precluded any preconditioning of either hospital staff or women. One hundred thirty-two primiparae due to give birth within an 8-week span were randomly allocated to an experimental or control group. All were invited to the hospital via letter; 95 women appeared. The 49 women who had been allocated to the control group were given the opportunity to meet the obstetrician and to visit the delivery room; the 46 women allocated to the experimental group were offered a five-session course of psychoprophylactic training. Women who did not complete the training, or who had a cesarean section, were excluded from the study.

The final sample contained 31 women in the experimental group and 41 in the control group. Medication was used significantly less often, and in smaller quantities, in the trained (experimental) group than in the control group. Unfortunately, the validity of this study was marred by failure to report on the women who were excluded: inevitably, this failure introduced a serious selection bias into the samples.

Enkin, Smith, Dermer, and Emmett compared women who took psychoprophylactic preparation classes with two control groups: those who requested classes, but could not be accommodated because the classes were full; and a group of women drawn from the general hospital population. For analysis, the three groups were matched into triads according to age, parity, and date of delivery. Having requested and applied for classes, it was presumed that the women in both the trained group and the first control group would have been similarly motivated, thus correcting for self-selection. Possible bias on the part of the physician was reduced by excluding the author's patients from the study. The trained group used significantly less analgesia and anesthesia than either of the control groups. There was no statistically significant difference between the two control groups. This would indicate that the effects of the training outweighed those of motivation. Other studies have confirmed the findings of reduced need for pharmacologic analgesia in women who have had some formal training in childbirth preparation.

Doering and Entwisle chose their subjects by "acquaintance networks" to provide a sample from a wide variety of doctors and hospitals, and thus a diversity of childbirth experiences. One hundred sixteen doctors and 38 hospitals were represented in the final sample. Most of their trained women were contacted through childbirth preparation classes. They chose the subjects randomly from the lists of women who registered for classes and then contacted them after delivery. In this way, they avoided the risk of contacting only "success stories." At the close of the interview, the interviewee was asked if she knew any other pregnant women. These women were contacted in turn. All of the untrained women, and a few trained ones, were located by referral from other women.

Of a total of 290 women invited, 269 (93%) participated; 132 had Lamaze training, 137 did not. The two groups did not differ significantly in age, parity, socioeconomic status or education. The outcome measures related to analgesia were based on the woman's report of the medication she had received. The women were classified into three groups: fully conscious (including no medication, pudendal block or local infiltration); semiconscious (including first stage sedatives or analgesics and major regional blocks, such as epidural or spinal); and unconscious (general anesthesia). There was a strong association "both in statistical and practical terms" between Lamaze training and reduced use of analgesia and anesthesia. Other cohort studies have also suggested a reduced need for pharmacologic analgesia in women who have had some formal training in childbirth preparation, thus adding additional support to the conclusions of the few small randomized trials. In a case-controlled study Hetherington matched 52 class-attending couples with 208 matched "nonattending" control couples. Classes were 6 weeks long, and all 52 couples attended all of the classes. Significant differences were found: the attendees used one-third less pain medication and two-thirds less conduction anesthesia, and had twice as many spontaneous deliveries than the nonattendees.

Nichols conducted a randomized trial of prenatal classes on 49 single adolescents, but reported on only 16 in the class group and 10 in the control group who completed the study. No differences between the groups were found in the psychologic tests of self-esteem or evaluation of labor and delivery, conducted at 7 and 9 months of pregnancy and 1 month after childbirth.

According to Beck and Hall, the minimum essentials for an adequate trial of childbirth preparation for childbirth should be: random assignment of subjects, the raters' unawareness of the subject's group membership; and a three-group design to include no-treatment controls and attention-placebo controls, as well as the experimental subjects. Both the necessity for trials of this nature and the difficulties involved in mounting them are acknowledged. Only one such trial has been reported to date.

Timm studied a group of very low income women attending two urban hospital clinics in Pittsburgh. Medical records of all women attending the clinics were reviewed. The study excluded those who attended for pregnancy termination, had major complications, were scheduled for elective cesarean, or who planned to attend a prenatal class. Of those eligible, all who agreed to be in the study were stratified according to age, race, and parity, and randomly assigned to one of three treatment groups: prenatal classes of a standard format; knitting classes, as an attention-placebo in which each woman was guided in knitting a shirt for the expected infant; and a group that did not attend classes but were encouraged to consult the physicians and nurses if they had any questions regarding any aspect of childbearing. To encourage continued participation, women were paid for their attendance at a series of six prenatal classes or knitting classes, or for serving as controls.

Of the 146 women who agreed to participate, 28 delivered before completing the study, leaving 40 who were assigned to the prenatal class, 31 to the knitting class, and 47 to the no-class program. At the time of entry into the hospital, study participants were not identified as such but were treated as all other women using the hospital facility. The women who had attended the prenatal class used significantly smaller amounts of medication than did those in the two control groups. This is an important finding because this low-income population group is recognized to be at high perinatal risk. In reducing the medications used in labor, added risk to the infant may be minimized.

### *Relationship Between Medication Use and Experience of Pain*

A reduction in the use of pain medications was found in the best-designed trials, including those that were partially or fully controlled for possible inherent differences between women who took classes and those who did not. These findings were reported in different countries, different cultures, and with different study designs. It cannot be assumed, however, that a reduction in use of pain medication is necessarily associated with reduced pain. The use of pain medications is related only in part to the pain experienced by the woman. Factors such as availability (many hospitals do not have 24-hour anesthesia services), quality of labor support, wish of the mother, or hospital customs, partially determine whether she will receive medication, what kind, and how much.

For these reasons, many investigators have attempted to evaluate the pain of labor using outcome variables other than medication use. Questionnaires such as the McGill Pain Questionnaire and other verbal descriptive scales, visual scales, such as pain thermometers, and observed behavior are all examples of methods used to assess labor pain, and each method has its avid supporters. Labor pain has been assessed both during labor, by observing or questioning women, and afterward by asking them to recall their pain. Two consistent findings have been reported: there is a wide variation in the pain experienced by women, with some reporting little or no pain, while others report very severe pain; also, the mean level of pain in labor is very high. No recent systematic trials have reported consistently low levels of pain among prepared women. For many women, childbirth pain is willingly accepted, even if medications are freely available, for various reasons: fear of side effects on mother or baby; a high motivation and adequate support to have a "natural" childbirth; or perception of the pain as manageable, normal, and nonthreatening.

While confirming the expected negative correlation between class attendance and the use of anesthesia, Davenport-Slack and Boylan found no correlation between class attendance and the woman's subjective report of pain during childbirth, concluding that these unexpected and seemingly inconsistent findings may have reflected the way in which the pain was measured. The wording of the questions designed to evaluate pain is important. When women in the Davenport-Slack and Boylan study were asked how painful childbirth was in comparison to other painful experiences, 97% said it was the most painful experience they had ever had. Yet, when asked to describe childbirth in terms of a range from "extremely painful" to "not painful at all," only 27 percent placed childbirth in the former category.

The problem of pain in labor was addressed directly in a study by Melzack and his colleagues. Using the McGill Pain Questionnaire (MPQ), which discriminates between the sensory, affective, and evaluative aspects of pain as well as giving a total pain rating index, they studied 141 successive women in active labor. The group was a representative sample of the women who gave birth in that hospital. It consisted of 87 primiparae, 61 of whom had attended prenatal classes, and 54 multiparae, of whom 30 had attended the classes.

They found the average intensity of labor pain to be extremely high, higher than that for other clinical pain syndromes studied, including cancer, phantom limb pain, postherpetic neuralgia, and toothache. However, there was a wide range of scores, with the pain varying from "mild" to "excruciating." In all dimensions of pain, as well as in the total index, labor was significantly more painful for first births than for later births.

Among the primiparae, prepared childbirth training and practice were associated with lower pain scores for the sensory, affective, miscellaneous, and total pain rating measures. Similar but less significant differences were found for the multiparae. Other factors associated with lowered mean pain scores were complications during pregnancy, age, and socioeconomic status. Using multiple regression analysis to determine statistically reliable predictors of pain, they found that in the primiparae, prepared childbirth practice accounted for 8% of the variance in the sensory component, 13% in the affective component, and 10% in the total pain index. The prepared women experienced significantly but not dramatically lessened pain even though they had elected to have the training, and therefore represented a self-selected sample with positive attitudes. In this study, use of epidural analgesia was extremely high, both among the prepared women (82%) and the unprepared (81%).

Niven and Gijsbers also studied labor pain, administering the McGill Pain Questionnaire once during the first stage of labor to describe present pain, and again 24 to 48 hours postpartum to recall the pain experienced during the first and second stages. As others have found, labor pain varied greatly among the 29 subjects, but the average level was severe. The postpartum assessments tended to be higher, suggesting that the pain of late labor was more severe than the pain experienced during first stage when the first assessment was made. The authors found no correlation between childbirth education and lowered pain scores, but did find the pain scores of those using various pain medications to be similar to those using psychoprophylaxis alone.

Lower pain scores were reported by women who had previously experienced significant levels of pain unrelated to childbirth (for example, dysmenorrhea, headache, and migraine). The authors suggest that the repetitious and long-lasting nature of such pain may result in hormonal adaptations or cause the woman to establish coping strategies that she draws opon during labor. The authors believe that women with little experience with repeating or long-lasting pain are particularly vulnerable to childbirth pain and need careful preparation and emotional support during labor.

In the study mentioned earlier, Copstick asked 80 prepared primiparae 1 to 4 days after birth to assess their labor pain on a scale of 0 to 100. Their mean pain rating was 99, and was no different between those who received an epidural block, i.e., in the pain experienced before the epidural, and those who did not.

## Analogues of Labor Pain

The search to establish the true value of childbirth classes has taken the form of testing each component of Lamaze instruction in the laboratory, in simulated pain situations. Subjects are taught various pain coping techniques and compared with a control group for their ability to tolerate pain as created by various measurable analogues for pain: for example, plunging the forearm in ice water (the cold pressor) for a measured length of time; increasing pressure on the distal index finger (the Forgione-Barber pain stimulator), and others. Research on the analgesic effectiveness of many of the component strategies of prepared childbirth has been reviewed by Stevens and Heide. Geden, Brouder, Glaister, and Pohlman reviewed previous labor analogue research and the problems inherent in generalizing the findings to clinical childbirth settings. The pain induced in labor analogue research is of short duration and cannot compare with that experienced in a labor of average length. Furthermore, labor analogue research lacks the reward at the end (the baby) that is inherent with childbirth pain. The ethical requirement that subjects in analogue research be allowed to drop out at any time precludes generalization of findings to labor. Finally, the social context of pain influences perception, "and there are obvious differences between the environment of an experimental pain laboratory and that of a labor room in a hospital."

The motivation for finding a reliable analogue for labor pain stems from the desire to develop new labor coping strategies and to improve their effectiveness in reducing pain. Worthington tested the validity of the cold pressor as an analogue for the pain of early labor by comparing the effectiveness of Lamaze techniques (relaxation, patterned breathing, and attention-focusing) and other techniques with groups of women, first with the cold pressor and later with labor pain. There was a significant correlation between the women's performances in the cold pressor test and in early labor. Lamaze classes improved performance when compared to Red Cross classes and a control group. The influence of self-selection of those in the Lamaze group was not controlled, but the matter of self-selection was addressed by testing two other groups of nonpregnant students who were randomly assigned to receive either brief Lamaze training or none. The former performed better on the cold pressor test.

In a later report using the cold pressor as the labor pain analogue with nulliparous women, Worthington, Martin, and Shumate tested coping strategies taught in childbirth classes. They found that the combination of structured breathing, attention focal points, and coaching provided the strongest treatment. Practice under stress was also found to be more effective than imaginal practice or no practice. They found effleurage to be ineffective with the cold pressor. The external validity of this finding on effleurage may be questioned, because one's sense of touch is profoundly altered by cold in a way not at all similar to the labor situation. Relaxation as a coping strategy was not examined. Although the authors simulated childbirth preparation as closely as they could, they acknowledge differences in anxiety levels between the experimental groups and laboring women. Length of training, strength of contractions, amount of practice, and the fact that women in the experimental group could stop the pain by removing their hand from the ice water when they wished, while laboring women cannot stop contractions when they wish, all raise questions on the application of these findings to childbirth education.

Geden and colleagues tested components of Lamaze preparation (relaxation training, breathing exercises, and information) in all possible combinations, using repeated exposure over a 1-hour period to a pain stimulus (pressure on the distal index finger). They found the relaxation component to be the most efficacious of the three components tested. They suggest that if the less effective components of Lamaze preparation are deleted, more emphasis can then be placed on the more effective components, and on different new pain coping strategies. A clinical trial comparing those strategies found to be most effective in the laboratory setting with the standard Lamaze preparation may provide clinically relevant findings.

### Other Effects

Childbirth education has received credit for a number of other obstetric advantages, such as decreased blood loss, decreased operative intervention, and improved condition of the baby. However, these findings are not confirmed by other studies, and, when present, are probably secondary to decreased use of medication. Some studies have reported a shortening of labor; others have found no differences. Scott and Rose and Storrock and Johnson found labor to be slightly longer in the mothers who had received the training. The best controlled mothers found no difference in length of labor or in birth weight, the only outcome variables measured in addition to use of medication.

While they are important, psychologic variables such as an enhanced feeling of self esteem, a sense of achievement or a positive feeling about the birth experience, are extremely difficult to measure. Roberts, Wooten, Kane and Harnett stated that "It would be a grave mistake to be guided by figures alone, because there does not appear to be any satisfactory yardstick by which we can measure the peace of mind and sense of security that mothers derive from the childbirth classes." Morris asked, "How can we produce statistics to show how many women emerge from labor exalted rather than demoralized, confident rather than afraid?" Daunted by the difficulty, many researchers have simply ignored the issue and restricted their study to obstetric outcome.

Kondas and Scetnicka studied two groups of 20 anxious pregnant women, as determined on Taylor's "manifest anxiety scale." The groups were matched for age, parity, education, and level of anxiety. One group received standard psychoprophylactic preparation, in which information about labor and delivery was given in full; the other group was subject to systematic desensitization, and only spontaneous questions were answered. Both groups showed a decrease in anxiety related to childbirth, but those having systematic desensitization showed it more strongly. Slight or no pain was recorded for 68% of the systematic desensitization group, compared with 21% of the psychoprophylactic group. The level of anxiety and the amount of pain were assessed by the therapist, and the possibility of observer bias must be acknowledged.

Despite the difficulties involved in devising satisfactory methods of measurement, several studies have attempted to assess the impact of childbirth training on the experience of childbirth. Davenport-Slack and Boylan found childbirth training to be highly correlated with an unstructured account of childbirth by the mother as a "positive rewarding experience." Tanzer found that attendees at a natural childbirth class experienced a significantly higher ratio of positive to negative emotions than nonattendees. Enkin and colleagues used a rating scale applied to a series of positive and negative adjectives describing labor, delivery, and the overall experience. Compared with a control group that had requested but not received training, the women who attended the classes had a significantly more positive experience of labor and delivery; the difference between the class group and the group who had not requested classes was even greater. There was no significant difference between the two control groups.

Huttel and others evaluated mothers' ratings of their delivery experience by means of a series of questions administered immediately postpartum. The answers given were recorded, transcribed verbatim, and ranked by observers who were unaware of the group to which the mothers had been allocated. Significant differences were found in favor of the instructed group, specifically in their impression of birth as having been "mastered actively" rather than "experienced passively," and in the fact that their wish for further children tended to be enhanced rather than weakened by the delivery experience.

Mother's attitudes to childbirth and to their babies were scored by independent raters in the study by Doering and Entwisle. These authors found that childbirth preparation leads to increased awareness during childbirth, and that such awareness had a larger impact on the mothers' experience and reactions than did the direct effect of the preparation itself.

Two papers relating to a study of psychologic outcomes of childbirth education point out that enjoyment in childbirth is not totally dependent upon decreased pain. The authors used independent scales to evaluate separately the subjective pain a woman felt and her enjoyment of the childbirth experience. They found that women who had taken classes experienced both less pain and more enjoyment during the birth than those who had not, but that the difference in the enjoyment index was greater than the difference in the pain index. In other words, reduction in pain was not the only factor determining the woman's enjoyment. Prepared women also had continuous bedside support from their husbands, which contributed to their enjoyment. Unfortunately, despite the use of two-way analysis of variance to allow for the effects of parity, socioeconomic status, self-confidence, and some other variables, the lack of comparability between the experimental and the control groups impaired the validity of what otherwise would have been a most illuminating approach.

Humenick proposed that if pain management is the key to satisfaction in childbirth, then it logically follows that "epidural or other analgesia is the best answer" to coping with childbirth, as it is more effective in reducing pain than relaxation, patterned breathing, and other coping techniques. She hypothesized that mastery, mobilizing inner resources, being self-reliant, independent, and self-controlled during childbirth is the key to childbirth satisfaction.

In a study designed to test this hypothesis, Humenick and Bugen found that among 37 Lamaze-prepared women, more active participation in labor and women's ratings of their birth experience were significantly correlated with increases in instrumentality scores. Instrumentality included "independence, activity (versus passivity), competitiveness, decisiveness, confidence, and ability to stand up well under pressure." The study suffered from selection bias and lack of a control group, but may demonstrate areas worthy of further research.

Lowe reviewed studies of the importance of maternal confidence in coping with labor and described the role of childbirth education in aiding the development of such confidence. She pleaded for more research to develop a sensitive instrument for measuring maternal confidence and to evaluate educational and other interventions.

Felton and Segelman studied beliefs about personal control in new mothers and fathers who had Lamaze training as compared to Red Cross training or no training. Pretests using Rotter's Internal-External scale were administered approximately 6 to 8 weeks before due dates and before the trained couples took their classes. Posttests (the same test) were administered to some participants after their classes were finished but before they gave birth; others took the posttest after the births of their children. Results indicated that the Lamaze-trained women who completed the posttest after the birth and the Lamaze-trained men who completed the posttest after the classes but before the birth, showed significant shifts in beliefs about personal control in the direction of greater belief in themselves as the origin of control. There were no significant differences in any of the other groups.

In discussing the differences in the Lamaze-trained men's and women's feelings about personal control before and after the birth, the authors stated that before the birth, the women were concerned about unexpected complications in labor over which they would have no control. After the birth, when those complications had not arisen, they then began to feel greater personal control. The men, before birth, perceived themselves as responsible for their partners' welfare, and thus perceived themselves as having greater personal control. But after birth, with the full impact of total responsibility for the baby's welfare, and the great unpredictable demands, they felt less in control.

In studying the effects of childbirth education on young, low-income, minority women, Masterpasqua compared an experimental group of 30 women who selected childbirth education with two control groups of 30 women each: one group chose not to take the available classes; the other had attended the clinic during the year before classes became available and thus could not take classes. There were no differences between the groups in perinatal complications, maternal behaviors, or mothers' perceptions of their infants. However, when the groups were further categorized into "at risk" (for subsequent psychiatric problems for the child) and "no risk" groups, Masterpasqua reported significantly reduced risk among male infants and infants of multiparae in the group who received childbirth education. The psychologic benefit of childbirth education in an at-risk group deserves further exploration.

Unfortunately, this author failed to find studies published since the early 1980s on satisfaction with the childbirth experience as a function of attendance or nonattendance at childbirth classes. The many papers on satisfaction with childbirth did not consider class attendance as a variable to assess.

## *Adverse Effects*

If the benefits of childbirth education are difficult to document in a systematic manner, the adverse effects and potential hazards are even more elusive. Rumors abound, like those of women who suffered untold agony unnecessarily because they had been brainwashed by their childbirth educators into believing that all medication was harmful, or others of the babies who died because their mothers insisted of "natural childbirth" and refused necessary operative intervention. While such events may indeed have occurred in isolated instances, there has been little documentation of them in the literature. Such sensational rumors rarely are followed up, and the stories often become more outrageous in the telling.

The dearth of documented cases of obstetric ill-effects caused by childbirth education has not deterred criticism. From the earliest beginnings of consumer interest in prepared childbirth, highly placed opponents have been numerous and vocal.

Reid and Cohen, in 1950, were scathing in their criticism of what they called "present day trends in obstetrics," pointing out that "the very basis of modern obstetrics, with its fiveold decrease of maternal mortality in the past 2 decades "was being challenged by the concept that "what was natural must be good." They described the fallacies in the beliefs that childbirth among primitive peoples is always easy, and that uterine contractions are not actually painful. They went on to point out the (then) lack of evidence that any maternal medication adversely affects the newborn, or that separation of mother and newborn does any harm.

The discussion following the paper by Davis and Morrone, which found neither beneficial nor adverse effects from childbirth education, was an opportunity for the acknowledged leaders of American obstetrics to voice their opinions. The concerns that they expressed indicate the degree of resistance to childbirth education at the time, which remains to some degree today: "The elaborate program of preparation tends to create rather than allay apprehension;" "If there is nothing to be afraid of, why raise such a fuss about it?" "If truly natural childbirth is to be fostered, the key figure must be a wise, kindly understanding obstetrician who generates such an atmosphere of happiness and assurance that apprehension is inevitably dispelled." Or again, "Some patients who give the most vocal support to childbirth without aid end up by requiring large amounts of medication." "In any preparation program some patients might yield to psychologic pressures to carry on their labors the way the group intended." "The unmedicated patient limits or introduces compromise in the selection of the type of anesthesia when it is truly indicated." Fielding and Benjamin claimed that "the truth can be stated simply, 'Natural childbirth's basic principle carries with it definite dangers to mother and child. It is a positive decision to let the destructive side of nature take its course.'" However, nowhere in their book did they give any specific examples of these hazards. They agreed, however, that there are "no charts or statistics on 'natural childbirth' failures beyond those relating to women who drop out of prenatal training programs before completion of their courses."

More recently, MacDonald contemptuously cited anecdotes of a woman who wished to eat her placenta; a duty registrar (physician) who asked that the senior registrar relieve him so that he could accompany his wife in labor; a father who refused medication at first on behalf of his wife. The author says, "My professional and personal experiences of childbirth have led me to believe that far too much is made of the emotional aspects, bonding, etc., and not enough of safety."

Such opinions would have been more authoritative had they been cited with evidence, either case reports or studies. The answers to the following questions are completely unknown: the extent to which fear is created rather than alleviated by childbirth classes; the proportion of prepared women who end up taking increased medication; whether women succumb to peer or educator pressures to conform, or refuse needed medication or intervention.

Stewart described psychiatric symptoms following attempted natural childbirth. Stewart's earlier report describes five women and four men whose expectations for natural childbirth were not met and who sought psychiatric treatment within 6 months of the birth. Generally, the women expressed feelings of depression, inadequacy, and guilt at receiving interventions (or, in one case, refusing them), which they believed were unnecessary or harmful. Two of the women worried that their babies were brain damaged, one after refusing nonstress testing and later delivering a postmature baby with breathing difficulties and neurologic sequelae; the other, after accepting epidural anesthesia and requiring forceps for delivery.

The men had accompanied their wives into the delivery room, but felt faint and anxious when there. Depression, anger at their wives, and feelings of inadequacy led them to seek psychiatric treatment. In all cases, the patients responded to psychotherapy lasting between 3 and 12 months.

Stewart cites childbirth classes that are inflexible and intolerant of medications and interventions as the underlying causes for these cases of depression. All the referred patients had received their childbirth training from community-based organizations whose teachers' backgrounds were nonmedical and whose classes emphasized natural childbirth and expected participation of the partner.

In a letter responding to Stewart's 1982 article, Campbell questions the assumption that childbirth education causes such psychiatric symptoms. Because Stewart had no comparison group, it is impossible to predict whether some parents attending natural childbirth classes are more likely than others to suffer postnatal psychiatric symptoms. Second, the author failed to consider other psychosocial factors that may influence one's reactions to childbirth or one's interest in attending natural childbirth classes.

Last, Campbell states that nurses and doctors need to be more flexible in their care of parents, anticipating that they may have disappointment or depression should the birth be unsuccessful in their eyes. Not only childbirth educators, but staff, as well, may play an important role in shaping postpartum feelings about the birth.

As if to answer Campbell's objections to her 1982 conclusions, Stewart reported that the percentage of patients seeking psychiatric treatment for symptoms related to their childbirth experience dropped precipitously after the hospital instituted its own childbirth classes in 1983. From 1972 to 1980, of 504 patients with postpartum neurosis or psychosis, only 3 attributed their symptoms to the birthing experience. By 1981, the number of community-based prenatal programs had doubled, and in 1981 and 1982, 18 of 125 patients attributed their postpartum symptoms to their birthing experience. All had taken the community based classes. In 1983, the hospital began offering and encouraging attendance at their own classes. Only 6 of 130 referrals were women attributing their postpartum symptoms to their birthing experiences. The author did not state which classes the six patients had taken.

Stewart offers convincing evidence that the community-based classes, at least those being offered during 1981 and 1982, may have prepared people unrealistically for the experience they would have in her hospital. The classes offered by her hospital appear to have performed that role better, because they prepared women to fit into their system. Those women who questioned the status quo may have set up a confrontational situation or hostility with the staff which could lead to poor staff-patient relationships and later depression in the new mother. Some hospital staffs are more receptive than others to individual preferences. Stewart's findings may be a reflection of hostile or intolerant staff attitudes and the effect they may have on a woman who asks for a different type of care than the caregiving staff usually administers.

Sandelowski also discussed feelings of failure engendered in women whose high expectations are not met: "The women who appear to be most susceptible to feelings of failure . . . are those who belong to what can loosely be described as the 'natural childbirth culture' . . . . In an important sense, the proponents of alternative childbirth have expectations that are too high or unrealistic when viewed against prevailing obstetric practice." She pointed out that when expectations are high, changes in maternity practices frequently result, but many women suffer disappointment. When expectations are lowered, women are less likely to be disappointed, but change cannot occur.

The dilemma so well described by Sandelowski illustrates the differing views toward childbirth education and their purposes. Yet there has been little systematic evaluation of the extent to which negative feelings of anger, guilt or inadequacy are engendered when a woman's or her partner's expectations are not met. Nor has the role of childbirth classes been systematically evaluated in creating these high expectations. Nelson found positive effects of childbirth education in her study of approximately 300 women: "Visions of childbirth that are most distinct from the prevailing medical model can be found among the women who remain unprepared . . . . Middle class women might well find that childbirth preparation has the unanticipated consequence of bringing their ideology into line with the established protocol of the hospital in which they are preparing to give birth."

Hott investigated pre- and postpartum attitudes toward self, spouse, and the ideal self or spouse among 47 couples who chose the Lamaze method of childbirth. Thirty-four of the couples shared the delivery as planned; the other 13 were prevented from doing so by complications resulting in cesarean section. Hott found that both men and women who did not achieve their goal of a shared experience held both themselves and their various ideal concepts in lower esteem than did those whose experience went as planned. No studies comparing these concepts among trained and untrained couples have been carried out.

Hott's findings disagree with those of Christensen-Szalansky, who followed 18 prepared women's preferences regarding the use of anesthesia in labor longitudinally, surveying them at 1 month before labor, during early and late labor, and again 1 month post partum. His sample, taken from independent childbirth classes, expressed a rather strong desire to avoid anesthesia 1 month before labor. This desire remained during early labor, but diminished from this period until complete dilatation. In other words, their desire to avoid anesthesia was strongest when they had no pain and, not surprisingly, diminished when they had severe pain. Eleven of the 18 women received anesthesia (8 primiparae, 3 multiparae). However, when interviewed 1 month later, the women who used anesthesia were shifting back dramatically toward avoiding anesthesia in the future. Among those who did not receive anesthesia, the desire to avoid it in the future was as strong as it had been 1 month before their due date. These findings indicate that the women's expectations and desires for future births were changed little by their actual experiences with present births.

The differences in the findings of Hott and Christiansen-Szalansky are difficult to explain, but may reflect differences in study design, in the content of classes or the quality of emotional support available to each group.

For the individual expectant mother, the benefits and risks of the prenatal class depend to a large extent on the same factors that determine the benefits and hazards of any other obstetric intervention: the individual's or couple's needs; how appropriate the class is for the those involved; and the skill and sensitivity with which the class is conducted.

## Conclusions on Childbirth Education

This discussion of childbirth education has reviewed studies of its effectiveness. By itself, the single variable of childbirth preparation cannot guarantee the reduction in pain medication use that is often claimed for it.

As this chapter indicates, there are at least four factors that must be present if a laboring woman is to avoid pain medications in a setting in which they are freely available:

1. A desire to avoid pain medications. Obviously if a woman wants or plans to use them, it would be unkind and unfair to withhold them. Among women who prefer to avoid pain medications, there are varying degrees of commitment. Some are motivated and able to use self-help measures and labor support throughout a long and challenging labor; others will rely on self-help measures only if labor is short and straightforward. The latter group is more likely to use pain medications for a more demanding labor.
2. Childbirth preparation. She needs to know some alternatives to pain medications, and those are taught and rehearsed in good childbirth classes and include relaxation techniques, physical and emotional support measures (for partners), comfort measures, and psychologic techniques.
3. Support in her efforts to use self-help comfort techniques not only from her partner, but more importantly from the professional caregiving staff. A woman in labor is highly vulnerable to either positive or negative suggestion, especially from those whom she perceives as experts, nurses, midwives, and physicians. If her caregivers are neutral or unsupportive of her efforts, she is less likely to avoid pain medications.
4. A reasonably normal labor. If labor is prolonged or complicated, the chances increase that she will require pain medications. Even the most highly motivated woman must recognize that a change in plans may be necessary in particular circumstances.

Besides reducing use of pain medication, childbirth education has a variety of other goals, as well: knowledge of reproductive anatomy and physiology; reduction of fear; reduction of cesarean sections and other potentially risky interventions; informed consent and enhancement of patient-caregiver communication; promotion of a healthy lifestyle for mother and family; breastfeeding; social support; and responsible participation in decision-making. Thus, even when reduction in use of pain medications is not a goal for a woman, she may attend childbirth classes for other reasons.

The widespread popularity of childbirth education would suggest that participants in classes must feel it has some benefit. The number of women attending prenatal classes is now substantial: while few nationally collected data are available, figures from a number of communities indicate that between 30 and 70% of all expectant mothers in the English speaking world attend some form of childbirth class.

The full impact of childbirth education cannot be assessed solely by its effect on the individual parturient, for there may be indirect effects that engender significant changes in the ambience in which women give birth. Among such indirect effects are the proliferation of newspapers and magazine articles and books on subjects relating to pregnancy, birth, infant feeding, and childcare. A recent mail-order catalog of books specializing in childbearing and early parenting lists approximately 300 titles on the subject of pregnancy and birth and another 500 on related subjects (newborn care, breastfeeding, parenting, women's health, and more.) Such literature reflects both public interests and influences public thinking.

### *Summary*

In sum, we have seen that the perceived need for childbirth education classes rises with changes in society, as some changes weakened the extended family's role in education and support, while also increasing the complexity of maternity care. Childbirth education began as a way to restore simplicity and satisfaction to the birth experience by increasing the participation of the mother and reducing her use of pain medications. Validation of the effectiveness of childbirth training has been difficult, due to the difficulty in designing and conducting well-controlled trials. The attitudes conveyed in classes, the quality of instruction, and the specific techniques being taught all vary, making it impossible to generalize about the effects of childbirth classes.

The existing evidence suggests that women who attend childbirth education classes use somewhat less analgesic medication and feel somewhat less pain in labor, although pain levels can still be very high. The wide variation in results from different studies may depend not only on differences in the classes, but also on the support provided by the caregivers in labor. Adverse effects of childbirth education classes have not been evaluated systematically . The very existence of classes and their growing popularity appear to have contributed to significant changes in maternity care.

## EMOTIONAL SUPPORT IN LABOR

Customarily, when birth took place in the home laboring women were surrounded by other experienced women who advised, reassured and encouraged them, massaged them and provided them with hot packs, poultices and nourishment, and generally looked after their needs for comfort and emotional support. All that was removed when birth moved to the hospital. Busy nurses and heavily medicated women left little opportunity for such care. No one, until recently, has investigated the benefits of the type of support described above; few had ever suspected that it could make a difference in outcomes. In fact, the acceptance of husbands in the maternity area for the purpose of coaching the mothers and witnessing the births of their own children was a hard-won consumer victory in the 1960s. Professionals at first could see no good reason for the fathers' presence, though many reasons to oppose it. But by the late 1970s, most resistance had subsided and fathers were a mainstay in the birthing environment.

The husband or father was originally designated by the childbirth educators as the "coach" and was trained for a dominant role in labor in which he was responsible for the woman's reactions to her contractions. He was supposed to fill the role played by the experienced woman years before, keeping his wife relaxed and quiet and dictating her breathing patterns during contractions. In natural childbirth, the father was seen as essential to the mother's ability to avoid pain medications.

But, as Keirse, Enkin, and Lumley demonstrate in their review of this subject, only a few men could comfortably and competently meet their mates' needs. Some women resented being coached; some men did not want to coach. Many childbirth classes failed to motivate and prepare the average father to be a coach. In fact, the coaching role ceased even to be a major topic in many childbirth classes.

Perhaps it is too much to expect of most men to witness their loved one's pain and lead her in coping with it, to act as her advocate, and to maintain perspective and confidence in a strange environment filled with busy authoritative professional people. For most men, keeping out of the way, cooperating with the staff, and letting the staff do what they feel is best, has seemed to be the most suitable role. In fact, recent descriptive studies of men at birth confirmed that many men play a relatively minor support role in labor, providing companionship but not exerting leadership as a "coach."

Thus, a dilemma has arisen. As described in the first part of this chapter, actively involved partners or labor coaches can positively influence the woman's ability to continue using the coping techniques learned in childbirth classes though few men can actually fulfill that role. The mothers' needs for emotional support and physical comfort are great and surpass the capabilities of most fathers and busy nurses. Today, increasingly, expectant mothers and couples are recruiting the services of a "doula" or labor support person whose responsibility is emotional support and physical comfort of the mother and her partner.

## Labor Support

"Doulas," experienced labor support providers who may or may not have professional training, have demonstrated their value in improving outcomes in six different studies in five different countries. For the purposes of this chapter, two of these studies are particularly relevant, as they were the only studies that took place in hospitals in which epidural anesthesia was freely available. Lay labor support providers usually provide only emotional support and, depending on their experience or guidance from the caregiver, some physical support.

Hodnett and Osborn conducted a stratified, randomized trial to determine effects of continuous professional support in labor in 103 married (or "partnered") middle-class primigravidae who had attended childbirth education classes (either Lamaze [n = 47] or General [n = 56]) and who had vaginal births. Of the 145 women originally entered in the study, 42 were excluded, mostly because of cesarean sections (n = 25), withdrawal (n = 8), late developing pregnancy complications (n = 5), and other reasons (n = 4). Hodnett describes professional labor support as involving the following four dimensions:

- emotional support (encouragement, reassurance, continuous physical presence);
- informational support (instructions, explanations, and advice);
- physical support (comfort measures, such as massage, cool compresses, ice chips);
- advocacy (interpreting the woman's or couple's wishes to hospital staff, acting on their behalf).

Several personal and social variables were included in the analysis of outcomes: prenatal anxiety (measured by the Spielberger State-Trait Anxiety Inventory before and after childbirth classes); expected and experienced control during labor (measured by Hodnett and Simmons-Tropea Labor Agency Scale prenatally before and after childbirth classes, and postnatally 2 to 4 weeks after birth); and Commitment to Unmedicated Birth (measured with Christensen-Szalansky's instrument at 38 to 39 weeks gestation and compared postnatally with actual medication usage). The 103 women were randomly allocated to a control group (accompanied by husband or partner, but no professional labor support person, n = 54) or an experimental group (accompanied by husband or partner and a professional labor support person, n = 49).

Findings included less use of epidural anesthesia (61% versus 81%) and fewer episiotomies (61% versus 85%) in the experimental group. In addition, perceptions of control during childbirth were increased in the women who had greater expectations of control (as measured by the Labor Agentry Scale), who had a support person, and who did not receive pain relief medication.

The type of prenatal class, the state/trait anxiety scores, and the level of commitment to unmedicated birth had little impact on outcomes, when considered independently of the presence of a labor support person. Outcomes such as length of labor and oxytocin usage were not different in the supported and unsupported groups. Of the 25 women who were excluded because of cesarean sections, the rate was the same for those allocated to the experimental group (17%) as for the control group (18%).

This is the only study published to date of the effect of a labor support person accompanying middle class women who took childbirth classes and whose husbands or partners also accompanied them in labor. The group with a professional labor support person clearly benefited, although not as dramatically as those women in the studies of low-income women who did not take classes or have their partners present.

The first randomized controlled trial of labor support in a United States hospital was conducted in Houston, Texas, in a busy, modern, teaching hospital that did not permit the presence of a companion for the women during labor. The hospital was fully equipped with all the obstetric equipment and personnel to perform all obstetric procedures. Of the 412 healthy normal nulliparae who agreed after admission to the hospital in early labor to participate in the study, 212 (the experimental group) received continuous emotional support from a trained doula from 3- or 4-cm dilation through the delivery of the baby. A group of 200 women were randomly assigned to an "observer" group. They were accompanied throughout labor by an inconspicuous research person who was there only to observe and record staff procedures and interactions. This person provided no emotional support or verbal or other interaction. In addition, 204 women comprised a control group that had neither a doula nor an observer; this group received only routine care from the staff. Hospital staff interacted with patients during an average of 21% of the time. Results are summarized in Table 21–1.

In their discussion, the authors speculate that the reasons for the improved outcomes and decreased use of interventions and epidurals in the supported group may be found in the causal relationship between maternal anxiety or stress and levels of stress hormones. The soothing and calming effects of the doula reduce maternal anxiety and its harmful side effects.

The same may be said, to a lesser degree, of the observed group. Although the observers said and did nothing to the laboring women, their mere presence may have exerted a calming effect. In addition, the observers may have had an effect on the behavior of the hospital staff, who may "have followed hospital protocol more closely for the use of obstetric interventions, such as anesthesia and oxytocin, which could explain the decreased use of these agents in the supported and observed groups . . . "

**Table 21–1.** Comparisons of Outcomes in Supported, Observed, and Control Groups

| Outcome | Supported | Observed | Control | p Value* |
|---|---|---|---|---|
| Narcotic Analgesia | 21.7% | 28% | 25.5% | no difference |
| Epidural Anesthesia | 7.8% | 22.6% | 55.3% | <0.0001 |
| Oxytocin Augmentation | 17% | 23% | 43.6% | <0.0001 |
| Mean Duration of Labor | 7.4 hrs | 8.4 hrs | 9.4 hrs | =0.0001 |
| Cesarean Delivery | 8% | 13% | 18% | =0.009 |
| Forceps Delivery | 8.2% | 21.3% | 26.3% | <0.0001 |
| Prolonged Newborn Hospital Stay | 10.4% | 17% | 24% | <0.001 |
| Sepsis Evaluation | 4.2% | 9.5% | 14.7% | <0.001 |
| Maternal Fever | 1.4% | 7% | 10.3% | =0.0007 |

* p Values for Supported vs. Control Groups
(From Kennell J, Klaus MH, McGrath S, Robertson S, Hinkley C: Continuous emotional support during labor in a U.S. hospital. JAMA 265(17): 2197–2201, 1991.)

The lower incidence of maternal fever in the supported group was associated with lower epidural use; this finding was consistent with that reported by Fusi, that epidural anesthesia is associated with maternal fever. In this study, almost twice as many women who received epidural anesthesia developed a fever as those without an epidural. The chief reason for neonatal sepsis evaluations and the resulting prolonged hospitalizations was maternal fever.

Cesareans for "failure to progress" were most common in the control group (25 of 37 versus 5 of 17 in the supported group, and 10 of 26 in the observed group).

The authors conclude that medical costs will be reduced when supportive companions (doulas) are continuously available for all laboring women. The doula reduces use of anesthesia, cesarean deliveries, and newborn septic workups, all of which add substantially to maternity care costs.

Doulas work for hire with couples who can afford their services, or voluntarily with single or poor women. They arrive in early labor and remain with the women until a few hours after the birth. If the woman's partner is comfortable in an active coaching role, the doula assists him. If not, she relieves him of that responsibility. The modern doula is typically a woman, young to middle-aged, who has given birth (though there are many childless doulas), and who has had intensive training in labor support. Many are also childbirth educators.

Though a young profession, labor support is attracting substantial interest from the public and the medical profession, especially caregivers of socioeconomically deprived women. Two professional organizations, the National Association of Childbirth Assistants and Doulas of North America, offer certification, continuing education, and promotion of the acceptance of the doula as a contributing member of the maternity care team.

## PHYSICAL THERAPY MODALITIES AND PSYCHOLOGIC TECHNIQUES

From the beginnings of recorded history, the avoidance or mastery of childbirth pain has predominated the minds of childbearing women and their caregivers. The pharmacologic management of childbirth pain and the purview of a major medical subspecialty constitutes the major portion of this text. The nonpharmacologic management of childbirth pain also has a long history: palliative care, empirical remedies, and physical comfort measures have been passed on through the generations without much scientific scrutiny. Generally harmless, many of these measures provide some measure of relief from pain even though the mechanism through which they operate is not completely understood. In more recent times, the study of pain transmission and its modulation have provided theoretical explanations of the mechanisms at work with the older techniques and produced many exciting findings that are today being applied to new techniques for relieving pain.

The following contains a description of the many physical and psychologic tools for childbirth pain management, with theoretical explanations of how they might work and a review of the scientific evidence (where available) about their effectiveness.

## Labor Pain and Its Modification

The origins of labor pain and its transmission have been described elsewhere in this volume. The complex nature of pain is summarized by Gilman and Winans: "Pain is composed of a distinctive sensation and the individual's reaction to this sensation with accompanying emotional overtones, activity in both somatic and autonomic systems, and volitional efforts of avoidance or escape."

Efforts to modulate pain may be directed toward any one or a combination of the components that contribute to the perception of pain: for example, removing or diminishing the stimulus causing the sensation; providing innocuous sensory stimulation to compete with and inhibit pain awareness; modifying the individual's reaction to it; diminishing or replacing the accompanying negative emotional overtones; controlling somatic and autonomic activity. Because of the numerous variables influencing pain sensations and the numerous approaches to pain relief, evaluation of pain-relieving measures is extremely complex and dependent on psychologic as well as physical variables. The Gate Control Theory for modulation of pain sensation provides a helpful conceptual framework for classifying and for understanding the numerous nonpharmacologic methods for reducing pain awareness.

### Modification of Pain: The Gate Control Theory

The pain message received by the brain is modified in numerous ways between the site of the stimulus (for example, the contracting uterus or dilating cervix) and the cortex. The Gate Control Theory of Wall and Melzack postulates that the dorsal horn in the spinal cord is the site where impulses converge, some excitatory to noxious (painful) impulse transmission and others inhibitory. Depending on the balance of impulses, the conscious perception will be of greater or lesser pain.

While small thinly myelinated and unmyelinated afferent fibers transmit pain impulses relatively slowly, the opposite is true for the large myelinated A fibers that run adjacent to them, transmitting innocuous stimuli, such as touch and pressure. These "fast" fibers activate cells, located in the substantia gelatinosa in the dorsal horn, inhibit transmission of noxious impulses and decrease pain perception at the level of the spinal cord. The faster transmission over these fibers helps to "close" the gate to pain sensations. In addition, descending fibers from centers in the brain stem and cortex to the dorsal horn can modulate (increase or decrease) the excitability of the cells that transmit pain information. Therefore, the brain receives messages about injury by way of a gate-controlled system, which is influenced by (1) injury signals, (2) other types of afferent impulses and (3) descending control.

Findings indicate that synthesis and release of endorphins in the dorsal horn and in higher centers of the brain stem are part of the pain modulation system. Endorphins bind to receptor sites at the synapse and are thought to inhibit the release of neurotransmitters of noxious impulses.

Thus, according to the Gate Control Theory, one's perception represents the net effect of influences that diminish pain awareness and that augment pain awareness.

Pain can be modified or reduced in numerous nonpharmacologic ways. Familiar examples abound: the athlete or soldier who is injured, but does not even notice the pain when involved in the heat of competition or battle; the headache of which one is unaware when engrossed in a movie or play, but which "comes back" when it is over; and the massage or bath that soothes the aching back or feet. These well-known observations do not lend themselves to easy interpretation and explanation. People respond to pain stimuli in different ways; they even respond differently at different times and under different circumstances.

An understanding of the reasons for such varying responses to painful stimuli is the basis for many of the nonpharmacologic methods of pain relief utilized in childbirth. These methods vary widely in how they affect the nervous system and in how effective they are. They may be classified by the way they alter the transmission of pain impulses or how they modify the pain sensation. The general classifications are as follows:

1. Those techniques that reduce the painful stimuli.
2. Those techniques that excite sensory receptors in the skin, bombarding the "gate" in the dorsal column with competing stimuli.
3. Those techniques that enhance activity in the descending inhibitory pathways from the brain to the synapses in the dorsal horn.

The techniques to be described herein include: physical therapy techniques of movement and maternal positioning, counterpressure, application of heat and cold, hydrotherapy, various kinds of massage, intracutaneous injections of sterile water, acupuncture and acupressure, transcutaneous electrical nerve stimulation; and psychologic techniques of patterned breathing, relaxation, distraction, visualization, attention-focusing, audio-analgesia, and hypnosis. Each of these techniques is claimed to benefit the laboring woman by reducing pain. How might they alter transmission of pain stimuli? What is the evidence of their effectiveness? How good is the evidence?

### Techniques That Reduce Painful Stimuli

The most obvious solution to the problem of pain is to remove or avoid it. If one cannot avoid it (and few pregnant women can avoid the contractions that cause labor pain), one can use techniques that reduce the painful stimuli elicited by uterine contractions or a particular position of the presenting part. This is the designated purpose of various maternal body positions, movement, counterpressure, and hydrotherapy.

### *Maternal Movement and Position Changes*

Laboring women find that they experience less pain in some positions than others, and, if left to their own devices, will select those body positions that are least painful.

In 1882, Engelmann published Labor Among Primitive Peoples, a book describing birth customs in a variety of cultures. He gathered his information by direct observation, library research, and by collecting observations from physicians and travelers in foreign countries. He found that women "whose parturition is governed by instinct and not by modern obstetric custom" tend to labor in more upright or "inclined" postures, as opposed to recumbent or horizontal postures. Atwood's review confirmed Engelmann's earlier findings.

Today, laboring women in western society are usually restricted to bed because of cultural expectations and obstetric customs, such as electronic fetal monitoring, intravenous hydration, and medications, which make movement out of bed difficult or unsafe. Despite these restraints, modern women seem to prefer freedom of movement when it is allowed. In their observational study, Carlson, Diehl, Sachtleben-Murray, McRae, and colleagues found that when given freedom to assume any position in or out of bed during the course of their labor without interference or instruction by attendant personnel, the laboring women assumed an average of 7.5 positions during labor. These women changed positions more frequently in late first stage and second stage than they did earlier in labor. Caldeyro-Barcia has reported that women's spontaneous behavior during labor includes changing among various upright postures: sitting, standing, and walking. Although women's reasons for changing positions were not sought, it can be assumed that they were far more likely to seek greater comfort than greater discomfort.

Through trial and error and observations of the instinctive tendency of laboring women to seek comfort, caregivers have learned that some positions (sitting, walking, standing, or kneeling and leaning forward) are usually more comfortable than others, and women naturally prefer those. There is, however, no universal acceptance of a particular position or positions by all laboring women. When the mother changes positions, she alters the relationships between gravity, the uterine contractions, the fetus, and her pelvis, which may be advantageous in reducing pain and enhancing labor progress. For example, back pain caused by pressure of the fetal head against the sacroiliac joint may be relieved if the mother moves from a supine or semirecumbent to a hands and knees posture. Pain from an occiput posterior position of the fetus may be relieved by rotation of the fetal head, which is sometimes accomplished by the same posture, combined with pelvic rocking and abdominal stroking.

Various devices are used to assist women in positioning. The "birthing bed" is a highly versatile bed that can be configured in numerous positions through either electronic or hydraulic controls. Numerous maternal positions are possible on this bed: lying flat; semi reclining, Trendelenberg, kneeling and leaning forward, lithotomy, and modified lithotomy. A squatting bar comes with these beds. It allows the unanesthetized mother to squat with stable support. Rocking chairs are standard equipment in many birthing rooms. Beanbag chairs and large therapy balls (sometimes referred to as Birth Balls in this context) are also used sometimes. All these devices allow comfortable movement or positioning.

The perceived pain-relieving effects of maternal body positions and movement are influenced by numerous factors, including fetal size, position, fetal head size and shape, size and shape of the maternal pelvis, and the quality of uterine contractions. Experienced caregivers, therefore, trust the mother's ability to find pain-reducing positions. They try not to restrict her movement, and encourage her to seek comfort, suggesting possible positions and trusting her judgment.

Beyond the potential mechanical advantages of alleviating the source of pain, position changes and ambulation also offer distraction and activation of joint receptors as stimuli to compete with pain stimuli for recognition at the level of the cortex.

### *Counterpressure and Bilateral Hip Pressure*

Counterpressure and bilateral hip pressure alleviate low back pain in the laboring woman. Counterpressure consists of steady strong force applied to a spot (designated by the woman) on the low back during contractions, using one's fist, heel of hand or a firm object. Bilateral hip pressure involves steady pressure with both hands applied to the lateral surfaces of the hips and directed toward the center. While there are no controlled trials of the effectiveness of these types of pressure, the techniques are widely taught in childbirth classes and testimonials from users as to their benefits abound. These pressure techniques are most effective when a woman suffers back pain, which is thought to be related to an occiput posterior position of the fetus. The steady pressure probably relieves strain against the sacroiliac ligaments caused by the fetal occiput.

Reasonable speculation suggests that counterpressure probably moves the sacrum slightly, helping to restore a more normal and less painful alignment of the sacrum and ilium. The bilateral hip pressure may alter the relationship of the ilia to the sacrum, lessening joint pain.

## Techniques that Activate Peripheral Sensory Receptors

### *Superficial Heat and Cold*

The use of hot compresses applied to the low abdomen, groin or perineum, a warm blanket over the entire body, or ice packs on the low back, anus or perineum provide pain relief in labor. The therapeutic use of heat and cold, because of their widespread empirical acceptance and low incidence of harmful side effects when used reasonably (that is, at safe temperatures that cause neither burns nor frost damage), have not been subjected to randomized controlled trials to their efficacy.

Superficial heat is generated from hot or warm objects, such as hot water bottles, hot moist towels, electric heating pads, heated silica gel packs, warm blankets, baths, and showers. Superficial cold is generated from ice bags, blocks of ice, frozen silica gel packs, and towels soaked in cool or ice water, and other cold objects.

### *Mechanism of Pain Relief Achieved with Heat or Cold*

Transmission of temperature sensations takes place over the same small nerve fibers that transmit pain stimuli (the A delta fibers). As hypothesized by Melzack, the higher brain centers discriminate between peripheral heat or cold stimuli and visceral pain stimuli, perceiving heat as a pleasant "counter-stimulant" or cold at "counter-irritant." These counter-stimuli then compete for recognition at the conscious level.

In addition to possible direct effects on pain perception, several well-known physiologic responses elicited by heat and cold indirectly result in pain relief. These indirect effects may be achieved through reduction of painful muscle spasms or cramps, changes in circulation to an area, a decreased inflammatory response, relaxation of tiny muscles in the capillaries and hair follicles in the skin. In other words, the application of heat or cold may reverse some conditions that create pain or are associated with it.

Table 21–2 summarizes the physiological effects of heat and cold. As can be seen, heat and cold have the capacity for altering autonomic responses that may be associated with pain or injury, or with anxiety.

Cold packs are particularly useful for musculoskeletal and joint pain; thus, low back pain in labor responds especially well to cold therapy. Perineal pain in the postpartum period is also greatly relieved by the application of cold packs.

Some caution should be exercised when using heat and cold with laboring women. The temperature of the hot or cold object should never exceed levels of tolerance of the person applying it. The laboring woman's pain threshold is sometimes altered to the point that tissue damage from extreme heat or cold could occur without her awareness. A protective layer or two of cloth should be placed between the source of cold and her skin, to allow for a gradual increase in cold sensation from a pleasant cool sensation to cold. Lastly, a laboring woman will find application of cold intolerable if she is already chilled. If she is shivering or if her hands or feet are cold, she should become comfortably warm before a cold pack is applied. As comfort measures, heat and cold are widely accepted if not fully understood. Because they provide only partial relief from labor pain, they might at best be considered only as adjunct therapy.

**Table 21–2.** Physiologic Effects of Heat and Cold

| Heat | Cold |
|---|---|
| 1. Increased local blood flow | 1. Decreased local blood flow |
| 2. Increased local skin and muscle temperature | 2. Decreased local skin and muscle temperature |
| 3. Increased tissue metabolism | 3. Decreased tissue metabolism |
| 4. Decreased muscle spasm | 4. Decreased muscle spasm (longer lasting than with heat) |
| 5. Relaxation of tiny muscles in skin (capillaries, hair follicles) | 5. Slows transmission of impulses over afferent neuron, leading to decreased sensation |
| 6. Raises pain threshold | |

### *Hydrotherapy: Baths and Showers*

The healing and pain-relieving properties of water hot or cold, whirling or still, sprayed or poured have been hailed over the centuries. A common household remedy for numerous ailments aches and pains, sores and burns, fatigue and tension baths, showers or whirlpools are not available to most women laboring in hospitals. Most obstetric units have few such facilities because they were designed and built when women were routinely confined to bed and sufficiently drugged to make bathing impossible. While that remains the case to a large extent today, some new and remodeled birthing facilities provide bath tubs and showers (even whirlpool baths) for laboring women.

### *Potential Benefits of Hydrotherapy in Labor*

Odent, writing about extensive use of the bath by laboring women in his obstetric unit, said, ". . . Immersion during the second half of the first stage of labor is helpful, particularly for parturients having painful and inefficient contractions . . . . We hope that other experiences would confirm that immersion in warm water is an efficient, easy, and economical way to reduce the use of drugs and the rate of intervention in parturition."

Brucker, Brown, and Balaskas and Gordon, and Milner advocate hydrotherapy to relieve pain, promote relaxation, reduce psychologic tension, lower blood pressure, and to improve efficiency of contractions.

Smith described the effects of warm tub baths on 31 low-risk women in labor. The women used standard residential tubs with inflatable pillows. Their abdomens were not immersed. They had cold cloths for their foreheads, and water was poured over their abdomens. They left the tub in time for the second stage. Smith measured nine variables at these three times: before the women entered the tub, and 15 and 60 minutes after entering the tub. The time spent in the tub ranged from 12 to 202 minutes (mean 60 minutes). Women left the tub usually either to change position or to deliver.

Mean arterial blood pressure and anxiety level were statistically, significantly decreased after 15 minutes in the tub, and remained at the lower level. Maternal pulse and estimated uterine activity decreased after 1 hour in the tub. Maternal temperature and fetal heart rate did not change with bathing. Pain and distress decreased significantly after 15 minutes, but returned close to the pretub level by 1 hour. Nine primigravidae in active labor dilated at an average rate of 2.7 cm per hour. Smith concluded that warm tub baths in labor are a "useful and safe practice for low-risk women."

A comparative study from Scandinavia of the use of baths during labor indicated more rapid dilation in 88 women who entered the tub for 1/2 to 2 hours after 5-cm dilation when compared with a self-selected control group who did not use the bath during labor (2.5 cm/hourversus 1.26 cm/hour, $p<0.05$). Descent of the vertex was also more rapid in the bath group, averaging 1.39 units of station/hour in the bath group versus .45 units of station/hour. Pain scores as measured on a visual analogue scale decreased markedly in the bath group while the women were in the water and increased markedly once they left the tub.

The same group of researchers compared 13 infants of mothers who had taken a tub bath with 9 infants of mothers who did not. Plasma catecholamines, pH, $PCO_2$, base excess, and beta-endorphin-like immunoreactivity in the two groups did not differ significantly.

Church describes their birth center's experience with 831 women who used warm water immersion during active labor, 483 of whom gave birth in the water. The bath is used primarily for pain relief and relaxation, but sometimes also to lower elevated blood pressure. Writes Church: "... we have noticed numerous times that an elevated blood pressure can be reduced dramatically within minutes of immersion in a heated pool of water ...." They have had one case of maternal infection among the 483 underwater births. The multiparous woman's membranes ruptured spontaneously during the birth of the head. She developed fever 48 hours after the birth and responded well to oral amoxicillin therapy.

It is beyond the scope of this chapter to discuss birth in the water, suffice it to say that this innovation has become a rather popular option in out-of-hospital birth settings. Most hospitals require the woman to leave the tub in the second stage of labor.

The dramatic pain relieving and relaxing effects of hydrotherapy can be explained as follows: A warm bath, shower or whirlpool bath exerts a soothing action on cutaneous nerve endings, causing vasodilation in the skin, relaxation of tiny muscles at the base of the hair follicles, and a reversal, generally, of the sympathetic nervous system response (stress of "fight or flight response"), which frequently arises in labor. By reducing stress in labor, the bath enhances the woman's sense of well-being and reduces her pain perception. The higher brain centers (thalamus and cortex) send inhibitory impulses to the dorsal column to inhibit transmission of pain signals. In addition, the physical effects of immersion buoyancy and hydrostatic pressure result in a feeling of weightlessness and a relief of pressure on the abdomen. These effects often produce relaxation and dramatic reduction of pain.

Last, thermal receptors and tactile receptors are activated by immersion in water, and more so by the spray of a shower or the swirling water of the whirlpool bath. Thus, the dorsal column receives stimuli from throughout the periphery, and the gate to pain is closed, inhibiting transmission of pain impulses to the cortex.

### Potential Adverse Effects of Hydrotherapy in Labor

Resistance to immersion in water centers on concerns for safety. The question of maternal and newborn infection troubles many caregivers, especially if the laboring woman remains in the bath with ruptured membranes. Waldenstrom and Nilsson carried out a comparative retrospective study of 89 women who took a warm bath after spontaneous rupture of the membranes and 89 others who had the same interval between spontaneous rupture of the membranes and delivery, but who did not take a bath. They found no significant differences between the groups with respect to infections, asphyxia or respiratory problems in the infant, or maternal signs of amnionitis.

Reinke, Johnston, Hile, Cunnington, and Carr carried out a chart review of 1337 patients who actively labored in their hospital during 1989, 732 of whom used the tubs during labor. Of these, 376 used the tubs after rupture of membranes. The investigators found no difference in incidence of chorioamniotis, endometritis, or neonatal infection between those who bathed only before and those who bathed after rupture of membranes. Furthermore, there were no differences between those who did not bathe at all and those who did. They describe their rigorous cleansing protocols and the type of tub they used, which was originally designed for hospital or home use by geriatric and invalid patients, and is therefore equipped with a backwash mechanism that effectively cleans the internal plumbing that cannot be reached with ordinary cleaning methods.

This important matter requires further research on incidence of infection with and without bathing in labor, and also rigid infection control protocols in cleaning the tubs. Another concern arises over monitoring of the fetal heart if the mother is immersed in water. This task is carried out with a doppler. The mother merely lifts her abdomen out of the water. Elevated maternal body temperature due to the warm water can be prevented by checking the mother's vital signs and taking appropriate action.

Last, the concern arises for the baby's safety should the mother give birth in the water. This most unconventional practice shocks most medical professionals who worry that the baby will breathe in water as it is being born. Odent describes 100 water births in his hospital, with no untoward effects on the baby or mother. Church describes their delivery practices in the water. The woman pushes instinctively with her urge to push. Once the head is out, in the absence of meconium, they do not pull to assist the shoulders until the next contraction. Then, the infant is immediately lifted up to the mother. If the baby cannot be delivered, the mother stands so that the infant's head is out of the water to allow further manipulation. "We have not observed gasping efforts of the infant while it is left alone waiting for the next contraction; it seems to gasp only once it has reached air."

### Touch and Massage

Use of touch in various forms conveys pain reducing messages, depending on the quality and circumstances of the touch. A hand placed on a painful spot, a pat of reassurance, stroking one's hair or cheek in an affectionate gesture, a tight embrace, holding a hand, or more formal purposeful massage techniques all communicate to the receiver a message of caring, of wanting to be with her, and to help her. While massage is used for numerous purposes other than pain relief, the object of most massage is to make people feel better, or to relieve pain and facilitate relaxation.

Hedstorm and Newton reported that touch and physical contact during labor are widely practiced in numerous cultures today as they have been in the past. Whereas much of the physical contact in the past and in non-Western cultures is for purposes of positioning, support, massage, and compression of the abdomen to promote descent, in the West today, the major purpose is to convey caring and reassurance. Childbirth educators today also teach various forms of touch and massage as pain-relieving measures.

A recent study investigating the work activities of the nurses in a Toronto teaching hospital found that nurses do not touch laboring patients for the purpose of expressing caring and reassurance. In fact, this work-sampling study detected only two instances of reassuring touch in a total of 616 observations of work activities! Furthermore, less than 10% of their activities were categorized in any way as "supportive." Most of these supportive activities were in the form of instruction or information to the patient. Approximately ½ of their work activities did not involve the patient. If these findings are typical of the nursing care in other institutions, the tasks of comforting, reassuring touch, and other palliative measures must be performed by people the mother brings into labor with her.

Massage in labor takes numerous forms. Hilbers and Gennaro describe how various types of massage stimulate different mechanoreceptors in the skin, increasing neural activity in the larger myelinated fibers. Stimuli are transmitted more rapidly over these pathways than are they over the pain pathways. The effect of "bombarding" the central nervous system with innocuous or pleasing stimuli is to bias cortical perceptions away from the awareness of pain. Such competitive large-fiber stimulation probably provides relief for only as long as it is being administered. When discontinued, the woman's awareness of her pain increases. In addition, the phenomenon of adaptation may diminish the pain-relieving effects of massage over a period of time. Therefore, use of intermittent massage, or variation in the type of stroke and location of the touch probably prolong the pain-reducing effects of massage.

Massage takes the form of: light or firm stroking; vibration; kneading; deep circular pressure; continual steady pressure; joint manipulation; use of fingertips, entire hands, or various devices that roll, vibrate, or apply pressure. In theory, the various forms of massage stimulate different sensory receptors, thus occupying numerous pathways to inhibit pain stimuli at the level of the dorsal horn.

The sense of well-being afforded by soothing touch also reduces pain perception by enhancing the descending inhibitory pathways from the limbic system in the midbrain, where the motivational-affective component of response to pain originates. The autonomic nervous system is controlled by the limbic system; thus, if a woman interprets her sensations as dangerous, painful or fearful, the limbic system activates a sympathetic "fight or flight" response, which facilitates transmission of pain impulses and increases pain perception. In labor, it is easier to prevent than to relieve the effects of a stress response.

How effective are touch and massage in controlling or relieving pain? Are women less likely to require pain medications if they receive touch and massage during labor than if they do not? These questions have not been pursued in a systematic scientific way, although experience strongly suggests that touch and massage relieve many types of pain. Penny interviewed 150 women and Birch interviewed 30 nurse-midwifery clients within 2 days after they gave birth, asking them about their perceptions of touch received during labor. The results of the two surveys were very similar. All subjects felt the touch they had received was positive (except for abdominal palpation and vaginal exams); most stated that touch helped them cope with labor. Rubbing, holding, pressure, and patting were the types of touch most often described as helpful. Most said they felt less or somewhat less pain when they were touched. Nearly half stated their husbands or relatives were the people providing the comforting touch; the midwife and nurse were also identified by a significant minority. In Penny's survey, the doctor who did vaginal exams was identified most often as one providing "negative touch." When asked to describe the meaning of touch, more than 80% reported the following: being supported, comforted, cared for, reassured, safe, accepted, encouraged, understood, closer to the person touching them, and able to rely on that person.

As for negative effects of touch, besides those mentioned above, many women in Birch's study reported that their perception of the therapeutic value of touch changed as labor progressed. Most reported that touch was perceived as less therapeutic with the passage of time. Rubbing and massaging were the types of touch most likely to diminish in therapeutic value, whereas pressure was more likely to continue its effectiveness.

Both those authors emphasized that touch is a powerful means of nonverbal communication, and they encourage caregivers to use touch as a means of providing reassurance and caring, and not only as a method for accomplishing procedures.

In an attempt to quantify benefits of touch during labor, Saltenis studied 21 primigravid mothers in active labor. For alternating blocks of three contractions, each patient received a low degree of physical contact with the nurse, then a high degree of physical contact. A low degree of physical contact was described as clinical touch (e.g., palpation, procedural touch, assistance in changing position). A high degree of physical contact included hand holding, stroking the patient's brow or shoulder, patting her back, in addition to clinical touch. Patients' behavioral reactions to the contractions (vocal, nonverbal activity, physical activity, extent of control of breathing, and verbal expressions of attitude toward the contractions) and their vital signs (blood pressure and pulse) were compared.

Findings included improvements in patients' coping ability and comfort along with drops in systolic blood pressure and pulse rate when the patients had a high degrees of physical contact with the nurse. The apparently harmless intervention is well-received by laboring women and easily discontinued if she wishes; therefore, it seems unlikely to occupy a high priority in anyone's list of research questions.

Another form of touch, referred to somewhat deceptively as "therapeutic touch," does not necessarily include physical contact between healer and patient. As described by Krieger, it is the "simple placing of the hands for about 10 to 15 minutes on or close to the body of an ill person by someone who intends to help or heal that person."

The technique is based on the premise that each person is surrounded by an energy field that can be assessed and altered by the hands of the healer. The field of a person in pain can theoretically be "unruffled" and pain reduced if healers move their hands in stroking motions a few inches away from the body. This approach, as strange as it seems to those who embrace the Western approach to pain and illness, is gaining interest, not only among alternative health care providers, but in university medical settings as well. One application of therapeutic touch in labor is for the woman who is tense, agitated and in pain, but who does not want to be touched.

## Acupuncture

Acupuncture, as practiced in China for over 2500 years, consisted of the insertion of strategically placed needles in any of more than 365 points along the twelve meridians of the body. Acupuncture treats disease and pain by correcting "blockages, excesses, or imbalances in the flow of the vital life force." Acupuncture therapy is a product of ancient Chinese philosophy, in which man is perceived as a microcosmic image of the universe, subject to the same tensions and disruptions of Yin and Yang as nature itself. Beginning in 1958, under Mao Tse Tung's direction, the application of acupuncture was broadened to include analgesia for surgery and childbirth. Today, it is sometimes combined with electrical current, which augments the pain-relieving effect. It is only since the Cultural Revolution that Western physicians have taken acupuncture seriously as a therapy. Renewed contact between Westerners and the Chinese has resulted in efforts to understand and evaluate Chinese medical customs in the context of the Western scientific approach.

The precise technique of obstetric acupuncture varies among practitioners in selection of points, size of needle, and method of insertion. Some operators stimulate traditional acupuncture points and others use points in the dermatomes supplied by the same spinal cord segments that supply the cervix and pelvis. Abouleish and Depp utilized electroacupuncture at eight points for first stage: four on the abdomen, one on the hand, and three on the leg below the knee. For second stage, points were located in the perineal body and behind the anus, with two "accessory" points beside the vagina. The authors complained that the needles placed in these points were in the way, restricted movement, and tended to become dislodged. They called for further studies to find fewer and more effective points further away from the uterus and perineum.

Umeh studied acupuncture for labor, using only two points on the sacrum along the bladder meridians in 30 pregnant Nigerian women. She reported adequate pain relief in 19 subjects. Despite the fact that the procedure was time-consuming, and the results somewhat inconsistent, she felt the simplicity, safety, and low cost make it worthwhile, especially in the developing world.

### Mechanism for Pain Relief with Acupuncture

Acupuncture blocks both sensory and emotional components of pain. Chapman described acupuncture as having a strong psychologic component, which he feels is largely responsible for the analgesic effects. The technique is not used routinely for all patients, and after patients are carefully selected, they are thoroughly prepared physically, mentally, and emotionally for the procedure. In fact, he draws a parallel between preparation for acupuncture and preparation for childbirth. He cites the following features shared by the two: provision of information about the upcoming procedures and expected sensations; social support and moment-by-moment coaching; successful pain control and testimonials from others who have utilized the procedures; relaxation techniques.

Those receiving acupuncture analgesia, then, have complete faith in the effectiveness of the technique. Expressed in the terms of the Gate Control Theory, the higher brain centers transmit strong inhibitory impulses to the dorsal horn, serving to close the gate to pain. This hypothesis is consistent with another, which proposes that endogenous opioid (endorphin) production is enhanced with acupuncture and blocked by a narcotic antagonist (naloxone).

In an attempt to further clarify the mechanism by which acupuncture reduces pain, Yang Cai and Wu compared the inhibitory effects of acupuncture on separate sensory and emotional components of pain. Using nine volunteers, they established the intensity of electrical stimulation of the sural nerve required to achieve seven sensory levels for each person: touch, the sensory threshold; slight numbness; severe numbness; slight pain (pain threshold); medium pain; intense pain (threshold of unbearable pain); extreme unbearable pain. Emotional components were evaluated as well through subjects' reports of what they felt and observation of their overt behavior (language, actions, and facial expression). In addition, the character and extent of sweating were noted.

Then electroacupuncture was applied to the sural nerve proximal to the pain source for 30 minutes while repeating the electrical stimulation. The pain stimulus was then continued for another 30 minutes after electroacupuncture was discontinued.

Both the sensory and emotional components of pain were inhibited markedly during acupuncture, and although sensory components reverted to the original when acupuncture was stopped, the emotional component (or degree of emotional upset with the pain) remained as low as it had been with acupuncture. "The subjects could bear the stimulus of intense pain primarily because electroacupuncture had improved the emotional experience of pain and had reduced the reactions associated with negative emotion; nervousness, dread, ill-ease, anxiety. Accordingly, the endurance of pain rose. We contend, therefore, that the primary effect of acupuncture is to assuage the emotional component of pain, especially under the conditions of intensely painful stimuli."

Obstetric and gynecologic applications of acupuncture include induction of labor, prevention of preterm labor, treatment of dysmenorrhea, cesarean section, instrumental deliveries, and management of labor pain.

### *Effectiveness of Acupuncture for Relief of Labor Pain*

Acupuncture during labor has not been well or frequently studied, and no controlled trials have been published, despite indications that it might provide good analgesia. Descriptive studies of acupuncture for relief of pain in labor have given little useful information. Of 15 women to whom he administered electroacupuncture during labor, Ledergerber reported that six had total relief of pain in labor and birth, and three had total relief in labor but required a small amount of Novocaine around the rectum during delivery. In the six remaining women, acupuncture was unsuccessful.

Abouleish and Depp utilized electroacupuncture during childbirth with 12 parturients and produced an "average of 60% analgesia" in active labor in seven patients. They neglect to mention how they measured pain. In the other five, four received no pain relief, and one discontinued very early because of her dislike of the needles. Ten of the 11 received regional anesthesia. Nine were "delighted" with the experiment and wanted acupuncture for future deliveries, because they received no drugs and were alert and free from aftereffects. This degree of satisfaction seems surprising because each woman had eight needles inserted in her abdomen, hand, and leg. Although the authors of the study found acupuncture impractical, time-consuming, restrictive of the patient, and interfering with electronic fetal monitoring, 9 of 12 patients were pleased with it. In light of patient satisfaction, it seems ironic that the authors had such a negative reaction.

Skelton and Flowerdew compared electroacupuncture for 85 women in labor with conventional analgesia, including epidural block, in a matched sample of 85. Of the 10 women in the acupuncture group who dropped out because of inadequate analgesia, eight were already extremely distressed on admission. Satisfaction with analgesia and with the "birth experience" was higher in the acupuncture group than with the analgesia (control) group, although those who reported the greatest pain relief were those who received an epidural block. This uncontrolled study may have been biased by the fact that one of the authors, who has an acupuncture service, was both the care provider and the postnatal evaluator.

A recent well-designed trial of acupuncture for management of primary dysmenorrhea indicated considerable improvement in a group of 11 women receiving Real Acupuncture for 3 months when compared with a Placebo Acupuncture group (in which needles were placed on points other than acupuncture points), a standard control group, and a visitation control group (who saw their doctor frequently, but had no acupuncture treatment). The Real Acupuncture group reduced their medication use by an average of 41% at the end of the study period. No other group changed their medication use. Acupuncture has also been studied for its potential in inducing labor and inhibiting premature labor, and was found promising for both indications. The use of acupuncture in obstetrics has not garnered a great deal of interest, especially in acute conditions like labor. The techniques involved are complex and time-consuming, and also less consistent and less effective than epidural analgesia; therefore, it is doubtful that its use will grow significantly.

## ***Acupressure***

Acupressure has been called "acupuncture without needles." The technique, also called shiatsu, involves the application of pressure or deep massage to the traditional acupuncture points, with thumb, fingertip, fingernail or palm of hand. Practitioners who use acupressure assume that it works in the same way as acupuncture by raising local endorphin levels in the treated area or possibly by activating the central biasing mechanism in the brain to inhibit painful stimuli. This has never been substantiated. In fact, the only references to acupressure for obstetric application seem to exist in the lay literature and childbirth education literature. Only barest mention can be found in medical and nursing literature.

The new Lamaze method, an adaptation of the Lamaze method, now includes the teaching of acupressure for discomforts of pregnancy and for control of anxiety, back labor, and ineffective contractions. Specific pain-relieving shiatsu techniques for labor described by Ohashi include thumb pressure at strategic points of the sacrum, occiput, and medial surface of the tibia. Sometimes combined with vibratory massage, shiatsu is applied for 5 to 10 seconds at a time and repeated several times.

Of the new Lamaze method's effectiveness, either anecdotal or scientific, such evidence is lacking in the literature at this time. Acupressure is easy to learn and can be applied by a nonprofessional companion of the laboring woman. Formal evaluation of its effectiveness would be worthwhile to establish its place as a comfort measure for labor.

### *Intradermal Sterile Water Blocks*

Odent described "lumbar reflex therapy" for low back pain and arrest of labor. It involves injecting small amounts of water intradermally in the lumbar area. "After an intense momentary local pain, this type of therapy usually brings immediate relief for this specific back pain and also allows dilation to progress." Two recent randomized placebo controlled trials of this technique demonstrated significant reduction of pain in the experimental groups in both trials. Ader, Hansson, and Wallin randomized 45 laboring women with low back pain into 2 groups: One group received four intracutaneous injections of 0.1 ml sterile water in the lumbosacral region. The other group, the placebo group, received subcutaneous injections of isotonic saline in the same region. Both the patient and her midwife were blinded to the type of injection.

Both groups experienced pain relief, as measured on a visual analogue scale, but the sterile water group experienced significantly greater relief of pain at 10 ($p<0.001$), 45 ($p<0.02$), and 90 ($p<0.05$) minutes following the treatment. The midwives' assessments based on observations of the women concurred with the women's assessments.

Trolle, Moller, Kronborg, and Thomsen carried out a similarly designed trial of 272 randomly assigned women. Twice as many women in the sterile water group noticed an analgesic effect ($p<0.0005$), and the effect was significantly greater. The median time before the effect was apparent was 2 minutes. When the injection of either type of water is given, there is some immediate pain, which is far greater in the group receiving sterile water; it lasts for about 20 to 30 seconds. The authors of both papers suggested that stimulation of fast conducting nerve fibers may inhibit the visceral pain of the contractions either at the level of the dorsal column of the spinal cord or the midbrain, as described in the gate control theory. Second, they postulated a rise in Beta-endorphin levels produced by the painful injections. This promising method for relief of back pain in labor is efficient and simple to administer, is inexpensive, and has no observed side effects other than a momentary burning pain.

## *Transcutaneous Electrical Nerve Stimulation (TENS)*

Transcutaneous electrical nerve stimulation (TENS) is a method of pain management that is noninvasive, portable, easy to use, and quickly discontinued if necessary. Used originally for the relief of chronic pain, trauma, and postsurgical pain, transcutaneous electrical nerve stimulation has recently been introduced on a small scale for pain relief in labor.

The transcutaneous electrical nerve stimulation unit consists of a hand-held box containing a 9-volt battery-powered generator of electrical impulses, some characteristics of which (pulse width, frequency, and amplitude or intensity) may be varied. A low-voltage electric current is transmitted to the skin via surface electrodes, which results in a "buzzing," tingling or prickling sensation. The therapist may preset certain characteristics; the laboring woman may vary some, such as the intensity, pulse frequency, and patterns of stimulation, so that she can increase, decrease, or pulse the sensations as she wishes.

Most transcutaneous electrical nerve stimulation units used in obstetrics contain two channels, each of which is connected to an independently controlled pair of electrodes. Thus, the woman may experience different sensations from the two pairs of electrodes. Quality of sensation is also varied by the placement and the size of the electrodes. When the intensity of electrical stimulation increases, the sensation of buzzing or tingling intensifies and the muscles beneath the electrodes may contract involuntarily. Intensity can reach painful levels, especially if the electrodes are small in area.

Usually, the transcutaneous electrical nerve stimulation unit is set just below the pain threshold intensity of the woman. This level may remain continuous or may be lowered between contractions. During contractions, the woman or her partner may increase the intensity to a level that competes successfully with the pain of her contractions.

In all reported investigations of transcutaneous electrical nerve stimulation for labor, one pair of electrodes was placed paravertebrally at the level of T10 to L1, to correspond to the spinal segments where the afferents, carrying painful stimuli from the uterus, enter the spinal cord. The second pair of electrodes was placed either paravertebrally at S2 to S4 or at either the sacral or suprapubic sites.

Safety concerns have focused on theoretically possible effects of high intensity transcutaneous electrical nerve stimulation on the fetus' heart function, especially when electrodes are placed on the low abdomen close to the fetus. Further concerns arose when interference with electronic fetal monitor tracings were reported.

Though no untoward effects on the fetus have been reported, there has been only one investigation of the safety aspects of transcutaneous electrical nerve stimulation, especially as applied to the fetus. Bundsen and Ericson proposed and studied a preliminary safety norm for transcutaneous electrical nerve stimulation. In 15 supervised births, they established a limit on maximum current density level at 0.5 microamperes per square millimeter when transcutaneous electrical nerve stimulation is used in the suprapubic region, and there were no adverse fetal effects. In addition, they tested a filter to suppress the electrical disturbances of the electronic fetal monitor, which had previously occurred. Less concern has been raised when electrodes are placed only on the back, which is where they have been placed in most studies.

### Pain-relieving Mechanisms of TENS

Transcutaneous electrical nerve stimulation is thought to work by bombarding the large-diameter afferent fibers with innocuous stimuli, thus closing the gate to pain. Furthermore, evidence suggests that levels of endorphins are increased in cerebrospinal fluid after low-frequency and high-intensity transcutaneous electrical nerve stimulation.

### Effectiveness of TENS

Transcutaneous electrical nerve stimulation for childbirth pain, although hardly ever used clinically, has been subjected to more controlled trials than any of the other modalities discussed in this chapter. This somewhat surprising situation can perhaps be explained by the fact that transcutaneous electrical nerve stimulation was conceptualized in the laboratory by scientists whose vocations center on understanding pain mechanisms. Most other nonpharmacologic methods of pain relief are based on age-old beliefs, discovered through trial and error and handed down through the generations. Scientific validation of their effectiveness has yet to be established. Transcutaneous electrical nerve stimulation, however, is one modality that has been extensively tested before being widely adopted. Ironically, the results of the trials remain inconclusive as to the value of transcutaneous electrical nerve stimulation for labor pain.

To date there have been at least four randomized controlled trials of transcutaneous electrical nerve stimulation in labor. In summary, the pooled overviews suggest paradoxical conclusions: that the effect of transcutaneous nerve stimulation is to increase the incidence of reported intense pain, yet to decrease the likelihood of use of epidural anesthesia, and to be favorably assessed by the women who use it. It has no obvious effect on the use of other forms of analgesia.

Harrison and colleagues carried out the only randomized double-blind, placebo-controlled trial of transcutaneous electrical nerve stimulation reported to date. They studied 100 primigravidae (49 in transcutaneous electrical nerve stimulation group; 51 in transcutaneous electrical nerve stimulation placebo group) and 50 para 2, gravida 3 women (27 in transcutaneous electrical nerve stimulation group; 23 in transcutaneous electrical nerve stimulation placebo group). The results of this, the methodologically best trial, coincided with those of the pooled overviews.

Although the difference in frequency of the most intense pain scores between the groups was not statistically significant, there was a strong trend toward increased pain in the women who had the transcutaneous electrical nerve stimulation, and this also agreed with independent assessment made by the midwives. They found no statistically significant differences in the proportion of women who used no other analgesia besides transcutaneous electrical nerve stimulation or placebo. Among the primigravidae, 6 of 49 (12%) of the women in the transcutaneous electrical nerve stimulation group and 7 of 51 (14%) of the placebo group used no other analgesia. In the multigravidae, 13 of 27 (48%) of the transcutaneous electrical nerve stimulation and 9 of 23 (39%) of the placebo group took no other analgesia. The authors explained that at their hospital, self-administered nitrous oxide (Entonox) was readily available and routinely accepted by many women. If use of Entonox is disregarded, the proportion of primigravidae not using other analgesia rises to 20 of 49 (41%) and 12 of 51 (24%) in the transcutaneous electrical nerve stimulation and placebo groups, respectively. For multigravidae the proportions were 22 of 27 (81%) and 15 of 23 (65%), respectively.

Use of epidural analgesia was lower in the transcutaneous electrical nerve stimulation group than the control; all but three epidurals were used by primigravidae. The women's postpartum assessments of transcutaneous electrical nerve stimulation were more favorable in the transcutaneous electrical nerve stimulation groups compared to the placebo groups. Thirty-eight of 49 (78%) of the transcutaneous electrical nerve stimulation primigravidae and 25 of 35 (81%) of the transcutaneous electrical nerve stimulation multigravidae had favorable assessments of transcutaneous electrical nerve stimulation, compared with 15 of 51 (29%) and 7 of 23 (30%) of the women in the placebo groups. In Nesheim's placebo-controlled, but unblinded study, a wide variety of analgesics was available and extensively used by all the women in both groups, but the women's assessments of pain relief and of transcutaneous electrical nerve stimulation's value were more positive in the transcutaneous electrical nerve stimulation group than in the placebo group. Although paracervical block was used for more (20/35) women in the placebo group than in the active treatment group (10/35), the author believed that this was primarily due to observer bias, "the midwives tending to pity the patients receiving mock stimulation," and concluded that "... no clinically significant beneficial effects of transcutaneous nerve stimulation during labor could be demonstrated in this study."

A smaller randomized trial by Bundsen and colleagues compared the effects of transcutaneous electrical nerve stimulation on 15 induced labors with 9 induced controls, finding a trend toward lesser analgesia use in the former. Erkkola and colleagues studied 100 laboring women with transcutaneous electrical nerve stimulation, comparing them to a randomly selected group of 100 patients without transcutaneous electrical nerve stimulation. At all phases of labor, the transcutaneous electrical nerve stimulation group rated their pain higher than the control group, and they used more analgesia. Despite this, 96 of the transcutaneous electrical nerve stimulation group judged transcutaneous electrical nerve stimulation to have provided good or moderate pain relief!

In addition to the randomized trials, a number of uncontrolled studies and nonrandomized cohort studies have also yielded conflicting results, no doubt reflecting the characteristics of the women who chose the modality as much as its effectiveness per se.

These trials suggest that some women tend to find transcutaneous electrical nerve stimulation helpful in labor, but that it does not stand alone as an adequate method of pain relief. The question remains as to whether transcutaneous electrical nerve stimulation's effectiveness might be improved if it were used differently, with different physical parameters, electrode size and placement, or if it were used more in conjunction with childbirth preparation. In addition, time of administration in labor may influence its effectiveness. Early initiation (that is, during latent or early active labor) brings better results than late initiation.

## Techniques that Enhance Descending Inhibitory Pathways

These techniques include education about the birth process and what to expect, along with re-education or indoctrination to a perception of birth as a normal healthy process, the pain of which is "different from ordinary pain," "positive" of "functional" pain, "pain with a purpose" of "creative pain." Goals of childbirth education include helping women achieve a sense of confidence and optimism in their abilities to give birth, along with competence in the use of comfort measures. They and their partners also learn specific pain-relieving measures. Thus, the cognitive and evaluative abilities of the woman are enlisted in the effort to reduce pain perceptions.

If one is fearful or anxious, the descending afferents facilitate transmission of pain impulses to the cortex, thus opening the gate to pain. Measures to inhibit autonomic arousal that which takes place at the midbrain level—the relaxation response to pain—are incorporated to combat pain perception. Emotional support, discussed earlier in this chapter, a comfortable environment, presence of loved ones, relaxation techniques, hypnosis, and visualization all contribute to a woman's sense of well-being, and help close the gate to pain.

It is known that the subcortical levels of the brain, where autonomic arousal and primitive responses to pain originate, contain heavy concentrations of endogenous opioid receptors, which suggests that the mechanism of pain inhibition at this level involves release of endorphins or similar substances. The effectiveness of the cognitive techniques taught in conventional childbirth classes are discussed earlier in this chapter. Here, other specific techniques which enhance the descending inhibitory pathways and thus reduce pain—attention-focusing, hypnosis, audio-analgesia and music—will be discussed.

### Attention Focusing and Distraction

Numerous methods exist for coping with pain by involving the conscious participation of the individual in attention-focusing or mind-diverting activities designed to "take one's mind off the pain." Using the principles of the Gate Control Theory, such strategies close the gate to pain by bombarding the synapses at the dorsal horn with impulses that inhibit transmission of pain stimuli.

Attention-focusing may be accomplished by deliberate intentional activities on the part of the laboring woman. Examples include patterned breathing, attention to verbal coaching, visualization and self-hypnosis, performing familiar tasks, such as grooming and eating, and concentration on a visual, auditory, tactile or other stimulus. Attention-focusing may be more passive, with stimuli from the environment or from other people distracting the woman from her pain. Television, a walk out-of-doors, a massage or shower stimulate receptors in the brain, which also send inhibitory messages to the dorsal horn. Passive distraction does not require as much mental concentration as deliberate attention-focusing measures and is probably ineffective when pain is severe. Attention-focusing and distraction are usually used in combination with other strategies. Discussion of the effectiveness of attention-focusing is included in the section on childbirth education, earlier in this chapter.

### Hypnosis

Hypnosis was first used in obstetrics in the early nineteenth century and has been used on a limited scale and in various ways ever since. While the popularity and acceptability of hypnosis in childbirth have fluctuated, it seems to have been most widely accepted by the medical profession in the 1950s and 1960s, as indicated by the number of papers appearing in the medical literature during that period.

Hypnosis is defined as "a temporarily altered state of consciousness in which the individual has increased suggestibility." Under hypnosis, a person demonstrates the following characteristics: physical and mental relaxation (deeper than can be achieved without hypnosis); increased focus of concentration; ability to modify perception; ability to modify memory (increase or decrease memory); ability to control normally uncontrollable physiologic responses (such as blood pressure, blood flow, heart rate, and the healing process); and trance logic (tolerance of logical inconsistencies).

Hypnosis is used in two ways to control pain perception in childbirth. Most hypnotherapists teach self-hypnosis so that women may enter a trance during labor to reduce awareness of painful sensations. Among the techniques they use are: relaxation; visualization (helping the client to imagine a pleasant safe scene and placing herself there, or symbolizing her pain as an object that can be disposed of, or picturing herself as in control or free of pain); distraction (focusing on something other than the pain); glove anesthesia (through suggestion, creating a feeling of numbness in one of the client's hands, and then spreading that numbness wherever she wishes by placing her numb hand on the desired places of her body). The client is taught to induce these techniques herself. Rarely do hypnotherapists accompany their clients in labor.

Other therapists rely on posthypnotic suggestion almost completely. They use "hypnoreflexogenous techniques," which combine hypnosis and Lamaze training, giving posthypnotic suggestions that will allay their fears about the pain and difficulty of labor and modify their interpretation of and reaction to contractions. The laboring woman will be "relaxed, fearless, happily expectant." These hypnotherapists do not teach their clients to routinely enter a hypnotic state during labor, because they will not need to. Most, they claim, will be comfortable as a result of the effectiveness of the posthypnotic suggestions. Exceptions to this are extraordinary circumstances such as forceps delivery or episiotomy and repair, when going into a trance would be necessary.

The mechanism by which hypnosis alters the laboring woman's perceptions of pain during contractions and descent continues to puzzle both its advocates and its critics. A theoretical explanation, using the Gate Control Theory, might be that hypnosis works in at least three ways. First, by not recognizing painful stimuli or by reinterpreting them as benign sensations, the brain centers are prevented from sending impulses that further open the gate. In other words, the cortex and brain stem are prevented from augmenting the perception of pain. Second, hypnosis actually dampens the perception of pain by enhancing the descending inhibitory pathways from the brain to the dorsal horn, where the "gate" is theoretically located. Hypnosis influences the cortex and lower brain centers to replace the usual pain messages (which can increase pain perception by opening the gate to pain impulses) with messages of calm and well-being (which close the gate). Third, the autonomic nervous system response is also dampened, and stress hormones (epinephrine, norepinephrine, dopamine, and cortisol), which increase pain perception, are not produced as they usually are in labor.

Therefore, through hypnosis, deep relaxation can be achieved along with inhibition of the stress response and alteration of the perception of contractions from being painful or frightening to being a "pleasant hardening" of the uterine muscle. The "gate" to pain is thus closed by the bombardment from above by innocuous impulses.

Peterson used "body-centered hypnosis" in which she strives to "create a subjective experience of already having mastered the birth process." Rather than focusing on dissociation from the bodily experience of labor, "body-centered hypnosis deepens a woman's bodily sensation, and mediates a woman's fears through bodily sensation and physical memory." Her unusual approach has only been studied anecdotally.

### Effectiveness of Hypnosis

Just how effective is hypnosis in reducing pain in childbirth? In their 1982 review article on hypnosis in obstetrics, Werner, Schauble, and Knudsen cited eight studies that found reductions in the amount of chemical analgesia used in labor by women who used hypnosis when compared with various norms; ten reported lower perceived pain in women using hypnosis; and five reporting reduced anxiety before and during labor in women using hypnosis. Although the findings are impressive, because the methods of selection, observation, and analysis of subjects in all the cited trials were retrospective and subject to bias, the reports of benefit from hypnosis have to be considered, not as authoritative, but simply as indications of the desirability of further study.

There is one prospective randomized trial of hypnosis in labor. This trial evaluated the effect of self hypnosis on pain relief, satisfaction, and analgesic requirements for women in their first labor. Eighty-two primigravidae were randomly allocated to either a hypnosis group or a control group. Both groups received routine childbirth classes. Those in the hypnosis group were also seen individually each week for hypnosis training in relaxation and pain relief.

Thirteen women were ultimately excluded, leaving 29 women in the hypnosis group and 36 in the control group. Hypnotic depth was assessed in the experimental group. Five patients were good hypnotic subjects; 19 moderate; and five poor. There was no difference in analgesia use between the two groups, although within the hypnosis group, significantly fewer epidurals were used by the good or moderate hypnotic subjects than by the poor subjects ($p<0.01$). As for satisfaction, 52% of the hypnosis group were "very satisfied" with labor, compared to 23% of the control group ($p=0.08$).

Mean duration of pregnancy and mean duration of labor were found to be significantly longer in the hypnosis group ($p<0.05$), although in neither case did the longer times reach levels of clinical concern. Similar findings have been reported elsewhere; in fact, hypnosis has been used to stop premature labor in the belief that one cause of premature labor is psychosocial stress, which can be reduced through hypnosis. Werner, Schauble, and Knudson also reported longer labors among Werner's patients, and asked, "Why should labor be hurried and intense?" Because the time factor alone is not of clinical concern, as long as mother and fetus are in good condition, it is possible that a longer labor may be better paced for the mother, providing more rest between contractions without raising her levels of anxiety or pain.

One might conclude from this trial that hypnosis may increase women's satisfaction with labor, that it may lengthen both pregnancy and labor, and that, among good or moderate hypnotic subjects, it may reduce analgesic use.

The fact that hypnosis lost its popularity among obstetricians by the early 1970's was probably due to a combination of factors that had little to do with demonstrated safety or effectiveness. The development of better methods of anesthesia, combined with the fact that adequate hypnosis preparation is time-consuming and expensive, probably persuaded obstetricians toward greater use of anesthesia and away from hypnosis. Coupled with these factors were warnings from the American Medical Association and the American Psychiatric Association that hypnosis is a powerful and potentially harmful technique that should be used only by physicians with extensive post-graduate psychiatric training. Even though there were few cited examples of harm done by hypnosis, (for example, damage to patients' mental health, alleged sexual improprieties) these statements acted as a deterrent. Because few obstetricians had psychiatric training, many withdrew their use of hypnosis in favor of other less controversial or "dangerous" methods.

## Music and Audio-Analgesia

Music and audio-analgesia are used to control pain in numerous situations, including dental work, postoperative pain, treatment of burns, physiotherapy exercises, and occasionally in childbirth. Many childbirth educators use music in childbirth classes to create a peaceful and relaxing environment, and also advocate it for use during labor as an aid to relaxation. They suggest that expectant parents select music that the mother finds soothing and rehearse relaxation to those tapes, and then play them in labor as one way to reinforce their ability to relax under the duress of labor. Music therapists have advocated that music in labor be used for more than achieving a calm environment. They suggest that properly chosen music (pleasing to the mother and containing appropriate rhythms) reinforces the mother's efforts at patterned breathing, assists her with relaxation, and provides distraction from discomfort and disturbing hospital sounds.

Other pain specialists advocate the use of audio-analgesia in various pain situations, including childbirth. This involves the use of white noise (sound consisting of all frequencies, suggesting the noise of a waterfall or the ocean) the volume of which can be controlled by the person in pain. Theoretically, the white noise dampens other incoming stimuli from the environment and from other parts of the body, thus decreasing pain perception.

## Music, Audio-Analgesia, and the Gate Control Mechanism

The Gate Control theory, when applied in the case of auditory stimulation, would explain the pain relieving mechanism in terms of enhancement of descending inhibitory pathways. Probably a variety of factors are at play:

distraction, if the music or sound is loud enough or compelling enough for the subject to be consciously aware of it; endorphin production, if the music is well-liked, pleasing or familiar to the subject; relaxing, if the sound or music is soothing and is associated with pleasant memories; and reinforcing of other behaviors, such as rhythmic breathing.

Both music and white noise, alone or in combination, have been studied for their effectiveness in reducing childbirth pain. Obstetric applications were inspired by the success in controlling dental pain reported during the 1950's, before the use of local anesthesia or nitrous oxide for dental procedures became routine.

### *Audio analgesia*

Audio analgesia for pain relief in obstetrics consists of the use of soothing music between contractions combined with white noise, the volume of which is controlled by the laboring woman, during contractions. The volume of the white noise supersedes the music during contractions. After learning of the success of audio analgesia in reducing pain associated with dental procedures, investigators from several different institutions became interested in testing its effectiveness in reducing labor pain. The purpose of two of these studies was to discover whether the quantity of pain-relieving drugs used in labor could be reduced through the use of audio analgesia. McDowell reported no reduction in drug use, although he quoted the physician supervising the study, who said that might be because "we tend to prescribe analgesia at a predetermined rate." Satisfaction expressed by the women was high, with 76% stating that they would use audio analgesia again.

Burt and Korn, reported decreased use of analgesic drugs in 100 women who used audio analgesia in labor when compared to another group of 100 women who did not. In fact, 47% of the women using audio analgesia used no analgesic drugs, as compared with 32% of the control group. They found that approximately two-thirds of the women had either an excellent or a good result. Reports from the women were consistent with those from the nurses and doctors. Glass reported similar findings.

None of the reports described above made an effort to randomize the subjects or to blind the groups from the observers. Therefore, biases in the investigators were not controlled for and the results may have been skewed.

Moore attempted to control for potential bias by providing each of the 25 women participating in the study with earphones and audio analgesia: the control group (12 women) received background music between contractions and self-controlled "sea noise" up to 90 decibels during contractions. Ninety decibels is considered to be louder than heavy traffic and almost as loud as subway noise. At that level the music could no longer be heard. The experimental group (13 women) had a similar arrangement, except that their "sea noise" could be turned up to 120 decibels, the point of "auditory discomfort." In other words, the only difference between the two groups was that the experimental group could attain a higher level of white noise. Thus, the authors believed they could account for the placebo effect; they assumed that the music and relatively low noise level would have no beneficial effects in themselves; any benefits would stem from a placebo effect. Pain-relieving medications were available "if the midwife considered the pain-relief was inadequate."

Results were obtained from two questionnaires, one answered by the midwife in attendance, the other administered by another midwife who had not been present during labor to each woman on the third day postpartum. The primiparae seemed to derive better pain relief from the audio analgesia than from the multiparae. The midwives reported complete or good pain relief (as opposed to fair or poor) in 3 of the 5 primiparae in the experimental group, and in 0 of 6 primiparae in the control group ($p = 0.06$). There was no difference in the midwives' assessments of pain relief among the multiparae.

All five primiparous women in the experimental group reported that the "sea noise" helped them considerably or completely, as compared with only two of the six in the control group ($p = 0.04$). Four of the primiparae in the experimental group were satisfied with the amount of pain relief they had with sea noise (compared with two of the six in the control group, $p = 0.07$) and would like to use it in their next labor (compared with three in the control group, $p = 0.17$). The fifth in the experimental group said she "didn't know" to both the last two questions. There was no difference among the multiparae in both groups in their assessment of how much help the sea noise afforded them, or if they were satisfied with the amount of pain relief they received.

Interestingly, both the experimental and the control groups of multiparae were overwhelmingly in favor of having sea noise again in future labors. In fact, 11 of the 13 multiparae in both groups and 7 of 11 of the primiparae wanted to have sea noise again. This finding shows that even the audio analgesia as used in the control group was found to be pleasant. One wonders if the investigators' control criteria were too similar to the experimental criteria, thus preventing a true test of the value of audio analgesia. Almost as many multiparae in the control group (three of six) as in the experimental group (four of seven) found relief from the audio analgesia they used. This might be either a comment on the ineffectiveness of audio analgesia or an indication that there was too little difference between the two protocols, with both of them affording some pain relief, with a trend in the direction of the experimental group.

The investigators assumed that music alternating with sea noise reaching no more than 90 decibels has no effect on pain. Yet they did not adequately explain or defend this assumption. It is possible that the "placebo" dose of audio analgesia had beneficial effects similar to those of the experimental dose, thus explaining the high rate of satisfaction among multiparae.

Moore, Brown, and Hill discontinued their study of audio analgesia partly because it was time-consuming for the physicians (the equipment was complicated and technical problems arose frequently), the earphones were cumbersome and uncomfortable for the women, who would need to rest from them periodically, and because they felt their results did not warrant continuing. With today's improvements in tape recorders, earphones, and sound reproduction, the technical difficulties would be eliminated. Their findings, though somewhat equivocal, merit further trials with study designs modified to provide a clearer difference between the experimental and control groups.

### Music

Judging from the absence of recently published papers on the subject, the interest in audio analgesia or white noise for labor pain has faded, while the use of music has elicited a modest degree of interest, especially among the childbearing public, childbirth educators, and a few care providers. The pleasing qualities of music may offer an added dimension beyond the distraction brought by white noise. Music from a tape recorder or phonograph creates a pleasant and relaxing ambience; or if the mother uses earphones, music blocks out disturbing, distracting or unpleasant sounds. Many birthing rooms today are furnished with compact disks and compact disk players for use by laboring women. When carefully chosen, music may be used to reinforce rhythmic breathing patterns and massage strokes, or to facilitate visualizations and induction of hypnosis. Thus, music may have the potential to reduce stress and to enhance other pain-relieving measures. Music may also elicit more relaxed and positive behavior from the staff and support people.

Music also increases endorphin production in a sizable minority of people. Goldstein found that music, primarily that with "special emotional meaning for a person," elicited "thrills" in the majority of people responding to his questionnaire. A "thrill" was described as an unusually pleasurable chill, shudder, tingling or tickling, invariably associated with sudden changes in mood or emotion. In a controlled trial comparing the effects of injectable saline and naloxone (a narcotic antagonist) on music-induced thrills, Goldstein found that naloxone significantly attenuated thrills repeatedly in 3 of 10 subjects. Because naloxone is known to block the effects of endorphins, Goldstein's findings imply that in some people, music causes increased production of endorphins, endogenous pain-relieving substances. The few trials of pain-relieving effects of music in labor found positive effects.

Having selected seven women who would act as their own controls, Hanser, Larson, and O'Connell provided them with two individual music therapy training sessions in addition to their Lamaze training. The women were taught the purposes of background music during labor: to cue rhythmic breathing; to assist relaxation; and to use the music as an auditory focal point, diverting attention from discomfort and anxiety-raising hospital sounds. The music therapist selected music that would fulfill those purposes and match the individual tastes of each woman. She also instructed each woman and her labor partner to use the music to help them carry out the Lamaze breathing and relaxation techniques.

The music therapist was present in labor for at least 35 contractions. She played music appropriate to the circumstances for 10 contractions, alternating with silence for five contractions. She recorded negative and positive pain-related behaviors (for example, tension or relaxation in specific body parts; irregular, broken breathing patterns or rhythmic Lamaze breathing; negative or positive verbalizations, or vocalizations expressing doubt, pain, or tension) on an observation form during each contraction and the interval following. An independent observer was present for at least five contractions of each labor to determine observer reliability. The resulting interobserver reliability was 97%. Within 1 week following delivery, each mother completed an open-ended questionnaire inquiring about her perceptions and preferences for music or no music.

All seven women demonstrated fewer negative pain responses during the music periods ($p<0.05$). Six of the seven women stated on the questionnaire that they believed the music fulfilled the purposes of helping them relax, cueing breathing, or distracted them from the pain. The other respondent stated she was not always aware of the music, but when she "thought about it," the music helped her relax.

Clark, McCorkle, and Williams compared a group of women who had received prepared childbirth training with a group who had received the training plus music relaxation techniques and who were also assisted during labor by a music therapist. The latter were more positive in their responses to a questionnaire about their labors than the former.

Sammons investigated the likelihood that women from Lamaze classes would use music in labor if they had a single labor rehearsal with musical accompaniment than if they did not. Fifty-four women attending Lamaze classes were randomly assigned to either a music-rehearsal or nonmusical-rehearsal group. Both groups received Lamaze training, were told that music during labor was an option, and answered a postpartum questionnaire asking about their feelings on the use of music in labor. In addition, the experimental group had musical accompaniment during one labor rehearsal in class. There was "scant elaboration on the potential benefits of music in labor," even in the experimental group. In fact, most of those from both groups who did not use music (79% of the total sample, and 42% of the experimental group) stated that they had not thought about it as option for labor, which suggests that the instructor was ineffective in her discussion of music. Although the 24 women in the experimental group were more likely to intend to or use music in labor (40% versus 20%), the difference was not statistically significant.

The questionnaire responses indicated that all eight women who used music in labor would do so again, and 61% of the total sample would consider it. If the instructor were to "make a more definitive statement about the efficacy of music for analgesia and relaxation, greater use might be seen."

These small studies of childbirth pain, when combined with findings of the effects of music or auditory stimulation on other types of pain (for example, postoperative pain, dental pain, pain associated with burn therapy indicate that music has the capacity to reduce pain, at least in selected patients. Its efficacy, however, seems to depend on the degree of prior education, preparation, and accommodation to the personal musical tastes of each patient.

## Impact of Nonpharmacologic Methods of Relief of Labor Pain

In today's climate, all methods of labor pain relief need to be measured against the current "gold standard" of pain relief, the epidural block, which boasts a high rate of success (from 67% to 90%). Disadvantages of the procedure exist, however, in the form of financial cost, requirements for complex adjunct care, subtle but definite effects on the neonate, and a myriad of possible undesirable side effects on the woman or alterations of her labor pattern. The side effects, the unavailability of anesthesia services in many less densely populated areas, as well as a desire among many women to experience their labors, mandate continuing development of labor pain relief measures.

Satisfaction in childbirth is not necessarily equated with absence of pain. Many women are willing to experience pain in childbirth, but do not want the pain to overwhelm them. Techniques such as the ones described in this chapter cannot match epidural analgesia for effectiveness, but they are simple, inexpensive, have fewer potentially harmful side effects, and some are well-liked by the women. For those women whose goals for childbirth include the use of self-help measures to manage pain with minimal drug use, and for those who have little or no access to pharmacologic methods of pain relief, the methods described here are the available alternatives. All that needs to be said about them is that they seem to help some women. Many of them require time and effort to learn and master, and their effectiveness is unpredictable, partly because of the vast complexities of the pain system and the even more vast complexities of the human personality. Others are simple and can be used by the staff without prior preparation of the woman. For all these reasons, the need remains to continue to explore and adequately study nonpharmacologic methods of pain relief for safety, satisfaction, and effectiveness in producing desired results.

## SELECTED READINGS


Abouleish E, Depp R: Acupuncture in obstetrics. Anesth. Analg. 54:83, 1975.

Ader L, Hansson B, Wallin G: Parturition pain treated by intracutaneous injections of sterile water. Pain 41:133, 1990.

American Psychiatric Association: Training in medical hypnosis: a statement of position by the APA. Document available from the Central Office, Washington, D.C.:3, 1961.

Andrews C: Nursing intervention to change a malpositioned fetus. Adv. Nurs. Sci. 3:53, 1981.

Anonymous: Sadism in delivery rooms? Ladies' Home Journal: 74:6, 1957.

Atwood R: Parturitional posture and related birth behaviour. Acta. Obstet. Gynecol. Scand. 57:5, 1976.

Augustinsson L, Bohlin P, Bundsen P, Carlsson C, et al: Pain relief during delivery by transcutaneous electrical nerve stimulation. Pain 4:59, 1977.

Balaskas J, Gordon Y: Water Birth: The Concise Guide to Using Water During Pregnancy, Birth, and Infancy. London, Unwin Hyman Ltd., 1990.

Bean C: Methods of Childbirth. 3rd Ed. Garden City, NY, Doubleday, 1990.

Beck N, Hall D: Natural childbirth—a review and analysis. Obstet. Gynecol. 52:371, 1978.

Beck N, Siegel L: Preparation for childbirth and contemporary research on pain, anxiety, and stress reduction: a review and critique. Psychosom. Med. 42:429, 1980.

Bennett A, Hewson D, Booker E, Holliday S: Antenatal preparation and labor support in relation to birth outcomes. Birth 12:9, 1985.

Bernat S, Woolridge P, Marecki M, Snell L: Biofeedback-assisted relaxation to reduce stress in labor. J. Obstet. Gynecol. Neonat. Nurs. 21:295, 1992.

Bertsch T, Nagashima-Whalen L, Dykeman S, et al: Labor support by first-time fathers: direct observations with a comparison to experienced doulas. J. Psychosom. Obstet. Gynecol. 11: 251, 1990.

Bing E, Karmel M, Tanz A: A Practical Course for the Psychoprophylactic Method of Childbirth. New York, ASPO, 1962.

Bing E: Six Practical Lessons for an Easier Childbirth. New York, Bantam, 1967.

Birch ER: The experience of touch received during labor. Postpartum perceptions of therapeutic value. J. Nurse Midwifery 6:270, 1986.

Birth and Life Bookstore: Imprints, 36. Seattle, Birth and Life Bookstore, 1992.

Bonica J: Acupuncture anesthesia in the People's Republic of China: implications for British medicine. Acupuncture Anesth. 229:1317, 1974.

Bonica J: Obstetric Anesthesia and Analgesia. Amsterdam, World Federation of Societies of Anesthesiologists, 1980.

Bonnel A, Boureau F: Labor pain assessment: validity of a behavioral index. Pain 22:81, 1985.

Bradley R: Husband-Coached Childbirth. New York, Harper and Row, 1965.

Brant H: Childbirth with preparation and support in labor: an assessment. N. Z. Med. J. 61:211, 1962.

Brown C: Therapeutic effects of bathing during labor. J. Nurse Midwifery 27:13, 1982.

Brucker M: Nonpharmaceutical methods for relieving pain and discomfort during pregnancy. Matern. Child. Nurs. J. 9:390, 1984.

Bundsen P, Ericson K: Pain relief in labor by transcutaneous electrical nerve stimulation: safety aspects. Acta. Obstet. Gynecol. Scand. 61:1, 1982.

Bundsen P, Peterson L, Selstam U: Pain relief during delivery: an evaluation of conventional methods. Acta. Obstet. Gynecol. Scand. 61:289, 1982b.

Bundsen P, Peterson LE, Selstam U: Pain relief in labor by transcutaneous electrical nerve stimulation: a prospective matched study. Acta. Obstet. Gynecol. Scand. 60:459, 1981.

Burt R, Korn G: Audio analgesia in obstetrics: "White sound" analgesia during labor. Am. J. Obstet. Gynecol. 88:361, 1964.

Buxton CL: A Study of Psychophysical Methods for Relief of Childbirth Pain. Philadelphia, W.B. Saunders, 1962.

Caldeyro-Barcia R: Physiological and psychological bases for the modern and humanized management or normal labor. *In* Recent Progess in Perinatal Medicine and Prevention of Congenital Anomaly. Tokyo Ministry of Health and Welfare Government of Japan, 77, 1979.

Campbell A, Worthington E Jr: A comparison of two methods of training husbands to assist their wives with labor and delivery. J. Psychosom. Res. 25:557, 1981.

Campbell D: Psychiatric symptoms following attempted natural childbirth (Letter). Can. Med. Assoc. J. 128:517, 1983.

Carlson J, Diehl J, Sachtleben-Murray M, McRae M, et al: Maternal position during parturition in normal labor. Obstet. Gynecol. 68:443, 1986.

Castallo M: Preparing parents for parenthood. JAMA 166:1970, 1958.

Cave C: Social characteristics of natural childbirth users and nonusers. Am. J. Public Health 68:898, 1978.

Chamberlain G, Chave S: Antenatal education. Community Health 9:11, 1977.

Chapman C: New directions in the understanding and management of pain. Soc. Sci. Med. 19:1261, 1984.

Chapman L: Expectant fathers' roles during labor and birth. J. Obstet. Gynecol. Neonat. Nurs. 21:114, 1991.

Charles A, Norr K, Block C, Meyering S, et al: Obstetric and psychological effects of psychological effects of psychoprophylactic preparation for childbirth. Am. J. Obstet. Gynnecol. 131:44, 1978.

Charles A, Norr K, Block C, Meyering S, et al: Obstetric outcomes and psychoprophylactic preparation for childbirth. Am. J. Obstet. Gynecol. 131:44, 1978.

Christensen-Szalanski J: Discount functions and the measurement of patients' values: women's decisions during childbirth. Med. Decis. Making. 4:47, 1984.

Church L: Waterbirth: one birthing center's observations. J. Nurse Midwifery 34:165, 1989.

Clark M, McCorkle R, Williams S: Music therapy assisted labor and delivery. J. Music Ther. 18:88, 1981.

Cogan R, Henneborn W, Klopfer F: Predictors of pain during prepared childbirth. J. Psychosom. Res. 20:523, 1976.

Cogan R: Variations in the effectiveness of childbirth preparation. Perinatal Press 7:4, 1983.

Copstick S, Hayes R, Taylor K, Morris N: A test of a common assumption regarding the use of antenatal training during labor. J. Psychosom. Res. 29:2, 1985.

Copstick S, Hayes R, Taylor K, Morris N: Partner support and the use of coping techniques in labor. J. Psychosom. Res. 30: 4, 1986.

Council on Mental Health: Medical use of hypnosis. JAMA 168: 2, 1958.

Davenport-Slack B, Boylan C: Psychological correlates of childbirth pain. Psychosom. Med. 36:215, 1974.

Davis C, Morrone F: An objective evaluation of a prepared childbirth programme. Am. J. Obstet. Gynecol. 84:1196, 1962.

Doering S, Entwisle D: Preparation during pregnancy and ability to cope with labor and delivery. Am. J. Orthopsychiatry 45: 825, 1975.

Eastman N: Discussing Davis and Morrone, 1962. Am. J. Obstet. Gynecol. 84:1201, 1962.

Engelmann G: Labor Among Primitive Peoples. St. Louis, J.H. Chambers and Co., 1882.

Enkin M, Smith S, Dermer S, Emmett J: An adequately controlled study of the effectiveness of PPM training. *In* Psychosomatic Medicine in Obstetrics and Gynecology. Edited by N Morris. Basel, Karger, 1972.

Erkkola R, Pikkola P, Kanto J: Transcutaneous nerve stimulation for pain relief during labour: a controlled study. Ann. Chir. Gynaecol. 69:273, 1980.

Evans T: Discussing Davis and Morrone, 1962. Am. J. Obstet. Gynecol. 84:1202, 1962.

Felton G, Segelman F: Lamaze childbirth training and changes in belief about personal control. Birth Family J. 5:141, 1978.

Fenwick L, Simkin P: Maternal positioning to prevent or alleviate dystocia in labor. Clin. Obstet. Gynecol. 30:83, 1987.

Fielding W, Benjamin L: The Childbirth Challenge, Commonsense Versus 'Natural' Methods. New York, Viking Press, 1962.

Fields H, Levine J: Pain-mechanisms and management. West. J. Med. 141:347, 1984.

Freeman R, Macaulay A, Eve L, Chamberlain G: Randomised trial of self hypnosis for labour. Br. Med. J. 292:657, 1986.

Fusi L, Maresh M, Steer P, Reard R: Maternal pyrexia associated with the use of epidural analgesia in labor. Lancet I:1250, 1989.

Gardner W, Licklider J, Weisz A: Suppression of pain by sound. Science 132:32, 1960.

Geden E, Beck N, Brouder G, Glaister J, et al: Self-report and psychophysiological effects of Lamaze preparation: an analogue of labor pain. Res. Nurs. Health 8:155, 1985.

Gilman S, Winans S: Essentials of Clinical Neuroanatomy and Neurophysiology. 6th Ed. Philadelphia, F.A. Davis, 1982, p. 36.

Glass L: Discussion following Burt and Korn's paper. Am. J. Obstet. Gynecol. 88:366, 1964.

Goldstein A: Thrills in response to music and other stimuli. Physiol. Psychol. 8:126, 1980.

Gradert Y, Hertel J, Lenstrup C, Bach F, et al: Warm tub bath during labor: effects on plasma catecholamine and beta endorphin-like immunoreactivity concentrations in the infants at birth. Acta. Obstet. Gynecol. Scand. 66:681, 1987.

Gregg R: Biofeedback relaxation training effects in childbirth. Behav. Eng. 4:57, 1978.

Grim L, Morey S: Transcutaneous electrical nerve stimulation for relief of parturition pain: a clinical report. Phys. Ther. 65: 337, 1985.

Hanser S, Larson S, O'Connell A: The effect of music on relaxation of expectant mothers during labor. J. Music Ther. 20: 50, 1983.

Hanvey L: A national review of prenatal education programs. *In* Pre-pregnancy and Pregnancy Care and Education: Proceedings of the 6th Symposium on the Prevention of Handicapping Conditions, Alberta: Edmonton, 1984, p. 188–196.

Harrison R, Woods T, Shore M, Mathews B, et al: Pain relief in labour using TENS. A TENS placebo controlled study in two parity groups. Br. J. Obstet. Gynaecol. 93:739, 1986.

He L: Involvement of endogenous opiod peptides in acupuncture analgesia. Pain 31:99, 1987.

Heardman H: A Way to Natural Childbirth. Edinburgh, Livingstone, 1948.

Hedstorm L, Newton N: Touch in labor: a comparison of cultures and eras. Birth 13:181, 1986.

Helms J: Acupuncture for the management of primary dysmenorrhea. Obstet. Gynecol. 69:51, 1987.

Hemminki E, Virta A, Koponen P, Malin M, et al: Atrial on continuous human support during labor: feasibility, interventions and mothers' satisfaction. J. Psychosom. Obstet. Gynaecol. 11:239, 1990.

Henneborn W, Cogan R: The effect of husband participation on reported pain and probability of medication during labor and birth. J. Psychosom. Res. 19:215, 1975.

Hetherington A: A controlled study of the effect of prepared childbirth classes on obstetric outcome. Birth 17:86, 1990.

Highsmith A, Kaylor B, Calhoun M: Microbiology of Therapeutic Water. Clin. Management 11:34, 1991.

Hilbers S, Gennaro S: Nonpharmaceutical pain relief. NAACOG Update Series 5:2, 1986.

Hodnett E, Osborn R: Effects of continuous intrapartum professional support on childbirth outcomes. Res. Nurs. Health 12:289, 1989.

Hofmeyr B, Nikodem V, Wolman W, Chalmers B, et al: Companionship to modify the clinical birth environment: effects on progress and perceptions of labour and breastfeeding. Br. J. Obstet. Gynaecol. 98:756, 1991.

Hott J: Best laid plans. Pre- and post-partum comparison of self and spouse in primiparous Lamaze couples who share delivery and those who do not. Nurs. Res. 29:20, 1980.

Hughey M, McElin T, Young T: Maternal and fetal outcome of Lamaze-prepared patients. Am. J. Obstet. Gynecol. 51:643, 1978.

Humenick S, Bugen L: Mastery: the key to childbirth satisfaction? A study. Birth Family J. 8:84, 1981.

Humenick S: Mastery: the key to childbirth satisfaction? A review. Birth Family J. 8:79, 1981.
Humenick S: Mastery: the key to childbirth satisfaction? A review. Birth Family J. 8:84, 1981.
Huttel F, Mitchell I, Fischer W, Meyer A: A quantitative evaluation of psychoprophylaxis in childbirth. J. Psychosom. Res. 16:81, 1972.
ICEA: The Role of the Childbirth Educator and the Scope of Childbirth Education. Minneapolis, International Childbirth Education Association, Inc., 1986, p. 4.
Jensen D: The Human Nervous System. New York, Appleton-Century-Crofts, 1980, p. 320.
Jiminez S: The Pregnant Woman's Comfort Guide. Englewood Cliffs, Prentice Hall, 1983.
Jungman R: Acupressure. *In* Childbirth Education: Practice, Research, and Theory. Edited by F Nichols, S Humenick. Philadelphia, W.B. Saunders, 1988.
Jungman R: Education for Childbirth. A New Lamaze Handbook. San Antonio, Education of Childbirth, Inc., 1982.
Karmel M: Thank You, Dr. Lamaze. Dolphin, Garden City, NY, 1959.
Katona C: Approaches to antenatal education. Soc. Sci. Med. 15A: 225, 1981.
Keirse M, Enkin M, Lumley J: Social and professional support during childbirth. *In* Effective Care in Pregnancy and Childbirth. Edited by I Chalmers, M Enkin, M Keirse. New York, Oxford University Press, 1989.
Kennell J, Klaus M, McGrath S, Robertson S, et al: Continuous emotional support during labor in a U.S. hospital. J. Am. Med. Assoc. 265:2197, 1991.
Kitzinger S. Pain in childbirth. J. Med. Ethics 4:119, 1978.
Kitzinger S: The Complete Book of Pregnancy and Birth. 2nd Ed. New York, Alfred A. Knopf, 1989.
Kitzinger S: The Experience of Childbirth. New York, Taplinger, 1962.
Klaus M, Kennell J, Robertson S, Sosa R. Effects of social support during parturition on maternal and infant morbidity. Br. Med. J. 293:585, 1986.
Kondas O, Scetnicka B: Systematic desensitization as a method of preparation for childbirth. J. Behav. Ther. Exp. Psychiatry 3:51,1972.
Krieger D: Therapeutic touch: the imprimateur of nursing. Am. J. Nurs. 75(5):784–787, 1975.
Lamaze F, Vellay P: L'accouchement sans douleur par la méthod psychophysique. Quoted in Buxton (1962).
Lamaze F: Painless Childbirth: The Lamaze Method. 2nd Ed. Chicago, Contemporary Books, 1984.
Ledergerber C: Electroacupuncture in obstetrics. Acupunct. Electrother. Res. Int. J. 2:105, 1976.
Lederman R, Lederman E, Work E, MacCann D: The relationship of maternal anxiety plasm catecholamines and plasma cortisol to progress in labor. Am. J. Obstet. Gynecol., 132:495, 1978.
Lenstrup C, Schantz A, Berget A, Feder E, et al: Warm tub bath during delivery. Acta. Obstet. Gynecol. Scand. 66:709, 1987.
Leonard R: Evaluation of selection tendencies of patients preferring prepared childbirth. Obstet. Gynecol. 42:371, 1973.
Letters: Should we have published "Cruelty in maternity wards"? Ladies' Home Journal 75:4, 1958.
Lieberman A: Easing Labor Pain. Boston, Harvard Common Press, 1992
Love N. Explaining the pain of active labor: the importance of maternal confidence. Res. Nurs. Health 12:237,1989.
Lowe N. Maternal confidence in coping with labor: A self-efficacy concept. J. Obstet. Gynecol. Neonat. Nurs. 20:457, 1991.
Lumley J, Astbury J: Birth Rites Birth Rights: Childbirth Alternatives for Australian Parents. Melbourne, Sphere, 1980.
Macdonald R: Personal view. Br. Med. J. 287:1544, 1983.
Maslar P: The effect of music on the reduction of pain: a review of the literature. The Arts in Psychotherapy 13:215, 1986.
Masterpasqua F: The effectiveness of childbirth education as an early intervention program. Hosp. Community Psychiat. 33: 56, 1982.
McCaffery M: Nursing Management of the Patient with Pain. Philadelphia, Lippincott, p. 119.
McDowell C: Obstetrical applications of audio analgesia. Hosp. Topics 44:102, 1966.
McNiven P, Hodnett E, O'Brien-Pallas L: Supporting women in labor: a work sampling study of the activities of labor and delivery nurses. Birth 19:3, 1992.
Melzack R, Kinch R, Dobkin P, Lllebrun M, et al: Severity of labour pain: influence of physical as well as psychological variables. Can. Med. Assoc. J. 130:372, 1984.
Melzack R, Taenzer P, Feldman P, Kinch R: Labour is still painful after prepared childbirth training. Can. Med. Assoc. J. 125: 357, 1981.
Melzack R: How acupuncture can block pain. *In* Pain: Clinical and Experimental Perspectives. Edited by M Weisenberg. St. Louis, C.V. Mosby Co., 1975.
Melzack R: The Puzzle of Pain. New York, Basic Books, Inc., 1973.
Miller H: Education for childbirth. Obstet. Gynecol. 17:120, 1961.
Miller Jones C: Forum: transcutaneous nerve stimulation in labour. Anaesthesia 35:372, 1980.
Milner I: Waterbaths for pain relief in labor. Nurs. Times 84:38, 1988.
Moore D: Prepared childbirth and marital satisfaction during the antepartum and postpartum period. Nurs. Res. 32:73, 1983.
Moore W, Browne J, Hill I: Clinical trial of audio analgesia in childbirth. J. Obstet. Gynaecol. Br. Common. 72:626, 1965.
Morgan B, Bulpitt C, Clifton P, Lewis P: The consumer's attitude toward obstetric care. Br. J. Obstet. Gynaecol. 91:624, 1982.
Morgan B: The consumer's attitude toward obstetric care. Br. J. Obstet. Gynaecol. 91:624, 1984.
Morris N: Human relations in obstetric practice. Lancet 1:913, 1960.
Nelson M: The effect of childbirth preparation on women of different social classes. J. Health Soc. Behav. 23:339, 1982.
Nesheim B: The use of TENS for pain relief during labour: a controlled clinical study. Acta. Obstet. Gynecol. Scand. 60: 13, 1981.
Nettelbladt P, Fagerstrom C, Uddenberg N: The significance of reported childbirth pain. J. Psychosom. Res. 20:215, 1976.
Nichols FH: The psychological effects of prepared childbirth on self esteem, active participation during childbirth, and childbirth satisfaction of single adolescent mothers. J. Obstet. Gynecol. Neonat. Nurs. 16:207, 1987.
Niven C, Gijsbers K: A study of labor pain using the McGill Pain Questionnaire. Soc. Sci. Med. 19:1347, 1984.
Norr K, Block C, Charles A, Meyering S, et al: Explaining pain and enjoyment in childbirth. J. Health Soc. Behav. 18:260, 1977.
Odent M: Birth Reborn. New York, Pantheon, 1984.
Odent M: Birth under water. Lancet, ii:1476, 1983.
Ohashi W, Hoover M: Natural Childbirth the Eastern Way. New York, Ballantine Books, 1983.
Olson H: Hypnosis in the treatment of pain. Individual Psychol. 40:412, 1984.
Omer H, Friedlander D, Palti Z: Hypnotic relaxation in the treatment of premature labor. Psychosom. Med. 48:351, 1986.
Patton L, English E, Hambleton J: Childbirth preparation and outcomes of labor and delivery in primiparous women. J. Family Practice 20:375, 1985.
Penny K: Postpartum perceptions of touch received during labour. Res. Nurs. Health 2:9, 1979.

Perkins E: The pattern of women's attendance at antenatal classes: Is this good enough? Health Educ. J. 39:3, 1980.

Peterson G: Body-centered hypnosis for pregnancy and childbirth. Mothering 1:81–85, Spring 1992.

Pomeranz B, Chiu D: Naloxone blockade of acupuncture analgesia: endorphin implicated. Life Sci. 19:1757, 1976.

Read GD: Natural Childbirth Primer. New York, Harper and Row, 1956.

Read GD: Natural Childbirth. London, W. Heinemann, 1933.

Reading A, Cox D: Psychosocial predictions of labor pain. Pain 22:309, 1985.

Reid D, Cohen M: Evaluation of present day trends in obstetrics. J. Am. Med. Assoc. 142:615, 1950.

Reinke C, Johnston M, Hile C, Cunnington K, et al: Endometritis, chorioamniotis, neonatal sepsis as complications of bathing after rupture of membranes. Unpublished manuscript, 1992.

Ringrose C: Lamaze preparation for childbirth. N. Engl. J. Med. 295:1966, 453:1976.

Roberts H, Wooton I, Kane K, Harnett W: The value of antenatal preparation. J. Obstet. Gynecol. Br Empire 60:404, 1953.

Robson J: Forum: transcutaneous nerve stimulation for pain relief in labour. Anaesthesia 34:357, 1979.

Saltenis I: Physical touch and nursing support in labor. Unpublished Masters Thesis, Yale University, 1962.

Sammons L: The use of music by women during childbirth. J. Nurse Midwifery 29:266, 1984.

Sandelowski M: Expectations for childbirth versus actual experiences: the gap widens. Matern. Child. Nurs. J. 9:237, 1984.

Scott J, Rose N: Effects of psychoprophylaxis (Lamaze Preparation) on labor and delivery in primiparas. N. Engl. J. Med. 294:1205, 1976.

Shealy C, Maurer D: Transcutaneous nerve stimulation for control of pain. Surg. Neurol. 2:45, 1974.

Shearer M, Editor: Effects of prenatal education depend on the attitudes and practices of caregivers. Birth 17:73, 1990.

Shultz G: Cruelty in maternity wards. Ladies' Home Journal 75: 44, 1958.

Shultz G: Journal mothers testify to cruelty in maternity wards. Ladies' Home Journal 75:58, 1958.

Simkin P, Enkin M: Antenatal classes. *In* Effective Care in Pregnancy and Childbirth. Edited by I Chalmers, M Enkin, M Keirse. New York, Oxford University Press, 1989 Sjolund B, Eriksson M: The influence of naloxone on analgesia produced by peripheral conditioning stimulation. Brain Res. 173:295, 1979.

Sjolund B, Terenius L, Eriksson M: Increased cerebrospinal fluid levels of endorphins after electro-acupuncture. Acta. Physiol. Scand. 100:382, 1977.

Skelton I, Flowerdew M: Acupuncture and labour—A summary of results. Midwives Chronicle & Nursing Notes: 134, 1988.

Smith L: The effect of warm tub bathing during labour. Presentation to the 3rd International Congress on Pre- and Perinatal Psychology. San Francisco, July 9–12, 1987.

Sosa R, Kennell J, Klaus M, Robertson S, et al: The effect of a supportive companion on perinatal problems, length of labor, and mother-infant interaction. N. Engl. J. Med. 303:597, 1980.

St. James-Roberts I, Chamberlain G, Haran F, Hutchinson C: Use of electomyographic and skin-conductance biofeedback relaxation training to facilitate childbirth in primiparae. J. Psychosom. Res. 26:455, 1982.

Stevens R, Heide F: Analgesic characteristics of prepared childbirth techniques: attention focusing and systematic relaxation. J. Psychosom. Res. 21:429, 1977.

Stevens R: Psychological strategies for management of pain in prepared childbirth. I: A review of the research. Birth Family J. 3:157, 1976.

Stevens R: Psychological strategies for management of pain in prepared childbirth. II: A study of psychoanalgesia in prepared childbirth. Birth Family J. 4:4, 1977.

Stewart D: Possible relationship of post-partum psychiatric symptoms to childbirth education programmes. J. Psychosom. Obstet. Gynecol. 4:295, 1985.

Stewart D: Psychiatric symptoms following attempted natural childbirth. Can. Med. Assoc. J. 127:713, 1982.

Stewart P: Transcutaneous nerve stimulation as a method of analgesia in labour. Anaesthesia 34:361, 1979.

Sturrock W, Johnson J: The relationship between childbirth education classes and obstetric outcome. Birth 17:82, 1990.

Thoms H, Karlovsky E: Two thousand deliveries under a training for childbirth program. Am. J. Obstet. Gynecol. 68:279, 1954.

Timm M: Prenatal education evaluation. Nurs. Res. 28:338, 1979.

Toronto Task Force on High Risk Pregnancy: Report: City of Toronto, Department of Public Health, 1980. p. 93.

Trolle B, Moller M, Kronborg H, Thomsen S. The effect of sterile water blocks on low back labor pain. Am. J. Obstet. Gynecol. 164 (5, part 1):1277–81, 1991.

Tsuei J, Lai Y, Sharma S: The influence of acupuncture stimulation during pregnancy. Obstet. Gynecol. 50:479, 1977.

Umeh B: Sacral acupuncture for pain relief in labour: initial clinical experience in Nigerian women. Acupunct. Electrother. Res. Int. H. 11:147, 1986.

Van Auken W, Tomlinson D: An appraisal of patient training for childbirth. Am. J. Obstet. Gynecol. 66:100, 1953.

Vardurro J, Butts P: Reducing the anxiety and pain of childbirth through hypnosis. Am. J. Nurs. 82:620, 1982.

Velvovsky I, Platonov K, Ploticher V, Shugom E: Painless Childbirth Through Psychoprophylaxis. Moscow, Foreign Languages Publishing House, 1960.

Waldenstrom U, Nilsson C: Warm tub bath after a spontaneous rupture of the membranes. Birth 19:57, 1992.

Wall P: The gate control theory of pain mechanisms: a re-examination and re-statement. Brain 101:1, 1978.

Werner W, Schauble P, Knudson M: An argument for the revival of hypnosis in obstetrics. Am. J. Clin. Hypnosis 24:149, 1982.

Worthington E, Martin G, Shumate M: Which prepared-childbirth coping strategies are effective? J. Obstet. Gynecol. Neonatal Nurs 11:45, 1982.

Worthington E: Labor room and laboratory: clinical validation of the cold pressor as a means of testing preparation for childbirth strategies. J. Psychosom. Med. 26:223, 1982.

Yahia C, Ulin P: Preliminary experience with a psychophysical program for childbirth. Am. J. Obstet. Gynecol. 93:942, 1965.

Yang M, Kok S: Further study of the neurohumoral factor endorphin in the mechanism of acupuncture analgesia. Am. J. Clin. Med. 7:143, 1979.

Yang Z, Cai T, Wu J: Psychological aspects of components of pain. J. Psychol. 118:135, 1984.

Zax M, Sameroff A, Farnum J: Childbirth education, maternal attitudes, and delivery. Am. J. Obstet. Gynecol. 123:185, 1975.

Zimmermann-Tansella C, Dolcetta G, Azzini V, Zacche G, et al: Preparation course for childbirth in primiparae: a comparison. J. Psychosom. Res. 23:227, 1979.

PART III

# CLINICAL CONSIDERATIONS

Section F

# ANALGESIA AND ANESTHESIA FOR NORMAL LABOR AND VAGINAL DELIVERY

Chapter 22

# ANTEPARTUM MANAGEMENT AND ANALGESIA FOR NORMAL LABOR AND VAGINAL DELIVERY

L. WAYNE HESS
JOHN C. MORRISON

This chapter discusses aspects of obstetric antepartum management and sedation and analgesia for both the first stage of labor and delivery in a normal gravida with a full-term pregnancy in whom there are no obvious obstetric or medical complications. The discussion on antepartum management is to acquaint nonobstetrician physicians with current-day obstetric concepts. The discussion of anesthetic management is for all who are involved in the delivery care of the mother and newborn. The chapter is divided into three major sections:

1. obstetric antepartum care;
2. obstetric intrapartum care; and
3. anesthetic antepartum, intrapartum, and postpartum care.

## OBSTETRIC ANTEPARTUM CARE

### *General Principles*

The expectations of the pregnant patient have changed tremendously in the past 25 years. The poorly educated or poorly informed gravida has the expectation that pregnancy and childbirth are associated with little or no maternal or fetal risk. The risks for poor pregnancy outcome, an inherent possibility in all gestations, are not discussed or considered when pregnancy is contemplated. Yet, statistics fail to validate these expectations, as approximately 25% of all clinically apparent, low-risk pregnancies will end with suboptimal fetal or maternal outcomes, even when prenatal care has been excellent. Risks include a 15% risk of spontaneous abortion (1), 1% risk of stillbirth (2), 3 to 4% risk of congenital anomaly (3), and a 5 to 10% risk of preterm delivery (4). In addition, approximately 5% of low-risk gravidae (5) will have significant morbidity during pregnancy or the puerperium, including eclampsia, postpartum hemorrhage, and endometritis.

The highly motivated, well-informed, and well-educated parturient, on the other hand, has different expectations of her pregnancy and obstetric health care providers. She places major emphasis on an informed, organized antepartum care continuum, on an informative and organized educational course for pregnancy, on an emotionally positive birth experience, and on adequate informed consent (6). Additionally, these women expect a personal commitment and accountability on the part of the health care team; to both provide quality prenatal care and to alter this care periodically in keeping abreast of changing social customs and advances in medical science (7). They also expect that pregnancy or anesthetic complications will be prevented if possible and that such complications will be recognized early if they do occur and treated appropriately to minimize or eliminate sequelae for mother or infant. The mother will not opt for anesthesia if she believes there will be a risk to her unborn baby. She will withstand whatever pain is necessary during labor to make sure her fetus is not placed at risk just for the purpose of her having less pain or a pain-free labor. Thus, it is imperative that during the early discussions of childbirth and alternative analgesic methods, both the positive and negative be mentioned to the mother.

Prenatal care was first introduced into clinical practice in Europe in the early 1900s, and it rapidly became common practice throughout the world (8). Reduction in health care complications by application of preventive medicine, enhanced patient education, and improved communication between patients and health care providers have become established goals of prenatal care. The studies in both Britain and the United States (9) have demonstrated that prenatal care is both efficacious and cost-effective. However, which health care provider renders the most cost-effective prenatal care is still unresolved (10). Also, whether the patient should travel to the health care provider or the health care provider travel to the patient through the provision of neighborhood clinics has become of prime financial importance, with increasing governmental regulations to regionalize prenatal care, minimize the number of unplanned, single, or teenage pregnancies, and decrease the number of gravidae who fail to obtain pregnancy care.

#### *Definitions*

The following general definitions will acquaint those less familiar with the terminology of some specific word usage:

A **nulligravida** is a woman who is not now and never has been pregnant.

A **gravida** is a woman who is or has been pregnant irrespective of the pregnancy outcome.

A **nullipara** is a woman who has never completed a pregnancy beyond an abortion.

A **primipara** is a woman who has been delivered once of a fetus or fetuses that have reached viability beyond the stage of abortion.

A **multipara** is a woman who has completed two or more pregnancies beyond the stage of abortion. The number of pregnancies, not the number of fetuses, determines parity.

A **parturient** is a woman in labor.

A **puerpera** is a woman who has just given birth.

The **first trimester** begins at conception and ends 13 weeks from the last menstrual period.

The **second trimester** is the period from 13 to 26 weeks from the last menstrual period in a gravida.

The **third trimester** begins 27 weeks following the last menstrual period and ends with delivery in the gravida. The mean duration of pregnancy is 280 days or 40 weeks from the first day of the last normal menstrual period.

A **preterm** delivery occurs when an infant delivers prior to 37 weeks gestation.

A **postterm** delivery occurs when an infant delivers after 42 weeks gestation. A **term** delivery occurs between 37 and 41 weeks gestation.

**Obstetrical history.** It is common to summarize a woman's past obstetric history by a series of four numbers as follows: 6, 1, 1, 1. The first number refers to the number of **full term** deliveries, the second to the number of **preterm** deliveries, the third to the number of **abortions**, and the fourth to the number of children presently **living**.

**Maternal death** is the death of a woman during pregnancy or within 42 days of pregnancy termination regardless of the site of pregnancy implantation. The **maternal mortality** (death rate) refers to the number of maternal deaths that occur as a result of the pregnancy state, labor, or the puerperium or medical intervention thereof. An **indirect maternal death** is an obstetric death occurring as the result of a previously existing disease state. A **nonmaternal death** is an obstetric death from accidental or incidental causes in no way related to the pregnancy.

An **abortion** is the delivery of a fetus that weighs less than 350 grams or has completed less than 20 weeks gestation from the last menstrual period.

The **stillbirth** (fetal death rate) expresses the number of stillborn infants per 1000 infants born.

**Neonatal death** occurs when the live-born infant dies before 29 days of life. The **neonatal mortality (death rate)** is the number of neonatal deaths per 1000 live-born infants.

The **perinatal mortality rate** is the number of fetal deaths (stillbirths) plus neonatal deaths per 1000 total births.

## Psychologic Preparation

Normally, women go through numerous psychologic changes during pregnancy. In the first trimester of pregnancy, most women experience either excitement and fulfillment or disappointment and regret (11). Their impressions of their family relationships change from that of the nuclear to the extended family (11). In the second trimester, the gravida's intrapsychic equilibrium changes with identity reformulation and an increased need for love and affection (11). Most women in the third trimester experience heightened anxiety, introversion, narrowing of interests, depression, and impatience (11).

Through careful observation of the psychologic changes that gravidae undergo during pregnancy, their anesthesia and analgesia needs during labor can be predicted. Various motivational factors, coping style, personality traits, and attention-distraction patterns will determine the amount and types of anesthesia that will be requested by these women.

Numerous psychologic methods to minimize the pain and anxiety occurring with labor have been popularized recently . Most of these methods begin during prenatal care and involve observational modeling, feedback and relaxation training, operant conditioning, cognitive coping strategies, stress inoculation, among other things (12). Anxiety and misconception diminution and patient education are also extremely important in most of these methods. The most popular of these methods are the Dick-Read, Lamaze, Harris, Bradley, and Leboyer methods (12). Scott, et al (13) demonstrated convincingly the effectiveness of these methods in selected gravidae. These methods are reviewed extensively in Chapter 21 on psychoprophylaxis.

As mentioned in the first edition, optimal results for the parturient can best be achieved by the establishment of a warm, supportive, committed doctor-patient relationship. The modern mother-to-be wants to participate in her gestation in an active, concrete manner, and, furthermore, she wants to have an adult, responsible relationship with her doctor who she considers her health care manager, guide, friend, and counselor combined. Such an interaction with a sound foundation based upon confidence, faith, and respect empowers the patient, eliminates her fears of the unknown and untested travails of pregnancy and labor. Anesthesiologists become the third leg on the stool, so to speak, as they lay the final solidarity of support when they meet with the patient to discuss intrapartum pain. It is often the fear of this that preys on the mind of the parturient, so the earlier this discussion can be held the better. At the time the anesthesiologist gains the complete confidence of the patient by being attentive, by displaying a sense of understanding and compassion, and by offering unconditional positive reinforcement to the patient, the parturient leaves the meeting with a great weight lifted from her shoulders. She leaves feeling that she and her baby are the most important agenda facing the anesthesiologist. Herein lay the importance of the great psychological impact anesthesiologists have upon their patients in obstetrics.

### Education and Counseling

In recent years, there has been increasing emphasis in establishing prenatal care before the onset of pregnancy in reproductive-age women. This emphasis has occurred in an attempt to further lower maternal and fetal risks of pregnancy. For example, fetal organogenesis begins approximately day 15 following conception and is essentially complete by day 57 following conception (14). Therefore, before missing a menstrual period and before a woman realizes she is pregnant, fetal organogenesis has begun. To minimize the risk of malformation to the fetus all teratogenic agents must, therefore, be eliminated before conception. It is therefore optimal to explain potential maternal and fetal risks to the reproductive-age woman before conception.

Women with diabetes mellitus should have excellent regulation of their blood glucose before conception to minimize the risks of fetal anomalies (15). Breast masses and abnormal pap smears should be thoroughly evaluated and corrected before conception, as should sexually-transmitted diseases. Women susceptible to rubella should be immunized and appropriate genetic counseling completed. Vitamin supplementation to minimize the risks of fetal neural tube or other defects may be begun before gestation (16).

Preconception education should also be a vital portion of prenatal care. Known hazardous exposures to the fetus should be discussed. Explaining the importance of landmarks to date the pregnancy should be emphasized. Indications, limitations, and time constraints for prenatal diagnosis, chorionic villus sampling, and abortion can also be discussed with these women. The known medical risks associated with pregnancy (i.e., spontaneous abortion, stillbirth, fetal anomaly, cesarean birth, preeclampsia, etc.) should be outlined. Signs and symptoms of ectopic pregnancy may also be discussed. Limitations of present technologies to diagnose and treat fetal anomalies or maternal disease should be outlined in preparation for future pregnancy.

## Preparation for Analgesia and Anesthesia

The many visits the patient makes to her obstetrician allow the development of a strong and trusting relationship. Some patients are even loath to have their deliveries performed by their doctor's colleagues because of the strong bond that develops between the patient and doctor. Obstetricians, thus, are in a powerful position with regard to the level of respect and admiration that develops. They, therefore, should tell the parturient about the anesthesiology team at the hospital that is dedicated to the management of the obstetrician's patients. The obstetrician's office should arrange an early meeting between the patient and the anesthesia spokesperson who guides the introductory obstetric/anesthesia lectures. The first meeting might be by group (including the spouse), limited to 20 or 30 people, and be held in the evening during the week or on the weekend. A subsequent private appointment for an antepartum history and physical might be scheduled for the patient to be completed on the labor floor by an anesthesiologist on duty or by his/her assistant. As previously mentioned, this visit may serve as the most important interactive session the patient will have regarding her fears and, thus, must be taken very seriously by the anesthesiologist.

### The First Prenatal Visit

The first prenatal visit should include a thorough history which includes a problem-oriented prenatal risk assessment. Obstetric, medical and surgical, social, genetic, occupational, and psychologic risks should all be adequately assessed. The American College of Obstetricians and Gynecologists (ACOG) Antepartum Record system (Figures 22–1 through 22–5) provides an excellent method of assessing and detailing these problems. In addition, a financial risk assessment should be performed to determine the patient's ability to pay for health care; instruction for the patient to stop working if complications occur during the pregnancy; and discussion about the financial provisions for a newborn baby. The first prenatal visit should also include a thorough physical examination to include a pelvic examination and clinical pelvimetry. Thirty milligrams of elemental oral iron supplementation should be provided to all gravidae at the first prenatal visit (17).

Laboratory analyses are performed on all pregnant patients (18). Such analyses typically includes: (1) cervical cytology; (2) complete blood count; (3) urinalysis and culture; (4) blood type, Rh, and indirect Coombs; (5) serologic test for syphilis; (6) rubella antibody titer; (7) sickle cell prep (for all black patients); (8) blood glucose screen; (9) Neisseria gonorrhea and chlamydia culture; (10) serum alpha-fetoprotein (either performed or patient advised of availability of the test); and (11) hepatitis B surface antigen (19) for women at risk (see Table 22–1). Other laboratory studies that are possibly indicated depending on maternal risks include: (1) hemoglobin electrophoresis if mean corpuscular volume (MCV) is less than 80, to screen for hemoglobinopathies; (20) (2) tuberculin skin testing; (3) cervical cultures for group B beta streptococci or herpes virus; (4) toxoplasmosis titer (for cat owners); (5) urine drug screen; (6) HIV (AIDS) titer in at-risk individuals; (7) estriol, alpha-fetoprotein, and beta hCG to screen for Down's syndrome; (21) and (8) fetal ultrasonic examination.

Risk factors for the occurrence of gestational diabetes (22) are included in Table 22–2. Only 50% of gestational diabetics have risk factors. Therefore, most obstetricians recommend screening all gravidae during pregnancy for glucose intolerance with a 1-hour post 50 g glucose challenge blood sugar or a 2-hour assessment following a meal containing 100 g of carbohydrate. A plasma glucose greater than 140 mg/dL on these tests would require a 3-hour 100 g oral glucose tolerance test for these gravidae. The National Institutes of Health established normal values for the 100 g oral glucose tolerance test in pregnancy (Table 22–3) (23). Two abnormal test values on this glucose tolerance test establishes the diagnosis of gestational diabetes.

### Anticipatory Counseling

All gravidae should receive anticipatory counseling during early prenatal care. Precautions concerning exercise,

# ACOG ANTEPARTUM RECORD

DATE ______________________

NAME ________________________________________________
LAST FIRST MIDDLE

ID # _______________ HOSPITAL OF DELIVERY ____________________

NEWBORN'S PHYSICIAN ______________ REFERRED BY ______________

FINAL EDD ______________________

| BIRTH DATE<br>MO DAY YR | AGE | RACE | MARITAL STATUS<br>S M W D SEP | ADDRESS: |
|---|---|---|---|---|
| OCCUPATION<br>☐ HOMEMAKER<br>☐ OUTSIDE WORK ____________<br>☐ STUDENT Type of Work | | | EDUCATION<br>(LAST GRADE COMPLETED) | ZIP: PHONE: (H) (O)<br>INSURANCE CARRIER/MEDICAID # |
| EMERGENCY CONTACT: | | | RELATIONSHIP: | PHONE: |

| TOTAL PREG | FULL TERM | PREMATURE | ABORTIONS INDUCED | ABORTIONS SPONTANEOUS | ECTOPICS | MULTIPLE BIRTHS | LIVING |
|---|---|---|---|---|---|---|---|
| | | | | | | | |

## MENSTRUAL HISTORY

LMP ☐ DEFINITE ☐ APPROXIMATE (MONTH KNOWN) MENSES MONTHLY ☐ YES ☐ NO FREQUENCY: Q ______ DAYS MENARCHE ____________(AGE ONSET)

☐ UNKNOWN ☐ NORMAL AMOUNT/DURATION PRIOR MENSES ______ DATE ON BCP'S AT CONCEPT. ☐ YES ☐ NO hCG + _____ / _____ / _____

## PAST PREGNANCIES (LAST SIX)

| DATE MO / YR | GA WEEKS | LENGTH OF LABOR | BIRTH WEIGHT | TYPE DELIVERY | ANES. | PLACE OF DELIVERY | PERINATAL MORTALITY YES / NO | TREATMENT PRETERM LABOR YES / NO | COMMENTS / COMPLICATIONS |
|---|---|---|---|---|---|---|---|---|---|
| | | | | | | | | | |
| | | | | | | | | | |
| | | | | | | | | | |
| | | | | | | | | | |
| | | | | | | | | | |
| | | | | | | | | | |

## PAST MEDICAL HISTORY

| | O Neg + Pos. | DETAIL POSITIVE REMARKS INCLUDE DATE & TREATMENT |
|---|---|---|
| 1. DIABETES | | |
| 2. HYPERTENSION | | |
| 3. HEART DISEASE | | |
| 4. RHEUMATIC FEVER | | |
| 5. MITRAL VALVE PROLAPSE | | |
| 6. KIDNEY DISEASE / UTI | | |
| 7. NEUROLOGIC/EPILEPSY | | |
| 8. PSYCHIATRIC | | |
| 9. HEPATITIS / LIVER DISEASE | | |
| 10. VARICOSITIES / PHLEBITIS | | |
| 11. THYROID DYSFUNCTION | | |
| 12. MAJOR ACCIDENTS | | |
| 13. HISTORY OF BLOOD TRANSFUS. | | |

| | AMT/DAY PREPREG | AMT/DAY PREG | #YRS USE |
|---|---|---|---|
| 14. TOBACCO | | | |
| 15. ALCOHOL | | | |

| | O Neg + Pos. | DETAIL POSITIVE REMARKS INCLUDE DATE & TREATMENT |
|---|---|---|
| 16. Rh SENSITIZED | | |
| 17. TUBERCULOSIS | | |
| 18. ASTHMA | | |
| 19. ALLERGIES (DRUGS) | | |
| 20. GYN SURGERY | | |
| 21. OPERATIONS / HOSPITALIZATIONS (YEAR & REASON) | | |
| 22. ANESTHETIC COMPLICATIONS | | |
| 23. HISTORY OF ABNORMAL PAP | | |
| 24. UTERINE ANOMALY | | |
| 25. INFERTILITY | | |
| 26. IN UTERO DES EXPOSURE | | |
| 27. STREET DRUGS | | |
| 28. OTHER | | |

**COMMENTS:** ________________________________________________

**Fig. 22–1.** ACOG prenatal records. (From The American College of Obstetricians and Gynecologists, Washington, DC 20024, 1989.)

Patient Addressograph

**GENETICS SCREENING**
INCLUDES PATIENT, BABY'S FATHER, OR ANYONE IN EITHER FAMILY WITH:

| | YES | NO | | YES | NO |
|---|---|---|---|---|---|
| 1. PATIENT'S AGE ≥ 35 YEARS | | | 10. HUNTINGTON CHOREA | | |
| 2. THALASSEMIA (ITALIAN, GREEK, MEDITERRANEAN, OR ORIENTAL BACKGROUND): MCV < 80 | | | 11. MENTAL RETARDATION | | |
| | | | IF YES, WAS PERSON TESTED FOR FRAGILE X? | | |
| 3. NEURAL TUBE DEFECT (MENINGOMYELOCELE, OPEN SPINE, OR ANENCEPHALY) | | | 12. OTHER INHERITED GENETIC OR CHROMOSOMAL DISORDER | | |
| 4. DOWN SYNDROME | | | 13. PATIENT OR BABY'S FATHER HAD A CHILD WITH BIRTH DEFECTS NOT LISTED ABOVE | | |
| 5. TAY-SACHS (EG, JEWISH BACKGROUND) | | | | | |
| 6. SICKLE CELL DISEASE OR TRAIT | | | 14. ≥3 FIRST-TRIMESTER SPONTANEOUS ABORTIONS, OR A STILLBIRTH | | |
| 7. HEMOPHILIA | | | 15. MEDICATIONS OR STREET DRUGS SINCE LAST MENSTRUAL PERIOD | | |
| 8. MUSCULAR DYSTROPHY | | | IF YES, AGENT(S): | | |
| 9. CYSTIC FIBROSIS | | | 16. OTHER SIGNIFICANT FAMILY HISTORY (SEE COMMENTS) | | |

**COMMENTS:** ______________________________

______________________________

______________________________

______________________________

| INFECTION HISTORY | YES | NO | | YES | NO |
|---|---|---|---|---|---|
| 1. HIGH RISK AIDS | | | 4. PATIENT OR PARTNER HAVE HISTORY OF GENITAL HERPES | | |
| 2. HIGH RISK HEPATITIS B | | | 5. RASH OR VIRAL ILLNESS SINCE LAST MENSTRUAL PERIOD | | |
| 3. LIVE WITH SOMEONE WITH TB OR EXPOSED TO TB | | | 6. HISTORY OF STD, GC, CHLAMYDIA, HPV, SYPHILIS | | |
| | | | 7. OTHER (SEE COMMENTS) | | |

**COMMENTS:** ______________________________

______________________________

______________________________ **INTERVIEWER'S SIGNATURE** ______________

**INITIAL PHYSICAL EXAMINATION**

DATE ____ / ____ / ____ PREPREGNANCY WEIGHT ______ HEIGHT ______ BP______

| | | | | | | |
|---|---|---|---|---|---|---|
| 1. HEENT | ☐ NORMAL | ☐ ABNORMAL | 12. VULVA | ☐ NORMAL | ☐ CONDYLOMA | ☐ LESIONS |
| 2. FUNDI | ☐ NORMAL | ☐ ABNORMAL | 13. VAGINA | ☐ NORMAL | ☐ INFLAMMATION | ☐ DISCHARGE |
| 3. TEETH | ☐ NORMAL | ☐ ABNORMAL | 14. CERVIX | ☐ NORMAL | ☐ INFLAMMATION | ☐ LESIONS |
| 4. THYROID | ☐ NORMAL | ☐ ABNORMAL | 15. UTERUS | ☐ NORMAL | ☐ ABNORMAL | ☐ FIBROIDS |
| 5. BREASTS | ☐ NORMAL | ☐ ABNORMAL | 16. ADNEXA | ☐ NORMAL | ☐ MASS | |
| 6. LUNGS | ☐ NORMAL | ☐ ABNORMAL | 17. RECTUM | ☐ NORMAL | ☐ ABNORMAL | |
| 7. HEART | ☐ NORMAL | ☐ ABNORMAL | 18. DIAGONAL CONJUGATE | ☐ REACHED | ☐ NO | ______ CM |
| 8. ABDOMEN | ☐ NORMAL | ☐ ABNORMAL | 19. SPINES | ☐ AVERAGE | ☐ PROMINENT | ☐ BLUNT |
| 9. EXTREMITIES | ☐ NORMAL | ☐ ABNORMAL | 20. SACRUM | ☐ CONCAVE | ☐ STRAIGHT | ☐ ANTERIOR |
| 10. SKIN | ☐ NORMAL | ☐ ABNORMAL | 21. ARCH | ☐ NORMAL | ☐ WIDE | ☐ NARROW |
| 11. LYMPH NODES | ☐ NORMAL | ☐ ABNORMAL | 22. GYNECOID PELVIC TYPE | ☐ YES | ☐ NO | |

**COMMENTS** (Number and explain abnormals): ______________________________

______________________________

______________________________

______________________________ **EXAM BY** ______________

**Fig. 22–2.** ACOG prenatal records. (From The American College of Obstetricians and Gynecologists, Washington, DC 20024, 1989.)

## ACOG ANTEPARTUM RECORD

NAME ______________________________________________
LAST FIRST MIDDLE

DRUG ALLERGY:

ANESTHESIA CONSULT PLANNED ☐ YES ☐ NO

| PROBLEMS/PLANS | MEDICATION LIST: | Start date | Stop date |
|---|---|---|---|
| 1. | 1. | | |
| 2. | 2. | | |
| 3. | 3. | | |
| 4. | 4. | | |

**EDD CONFIRMATION**

INITIAL EDD:

LMP ____/____/____ = EDD ____/____/____

INITIAL EXAM ____/____/____ = ____ WKS = EDD ____/____/____

ULTRASOUND ____/____/____ = ____ WKS = EDD ____/____/____

INITIAL EDD ____/____/____ INITIALED BY ____________

**18–20-WEEK EDD UPDATE:**

QUICKENING ____/____/____ + 22 WKS = ____/____/____

FUNDAL HT. AT UMBIL. ____/____/____ + 20 WKS = ____/____/____

FHT W/FETOSCOPE ____/____/____ + 20 WKS = ____/____/____

ULTRASOUND ____/____/____ = ____ WKS = ____/____/____

FINAL EDD ____/____/____ INITIALED BY ____________

**32–34-WEEK EDD–UTERINE SIZE CONCORDANCE** (± 4 OR MORE CM SUGGESTS THE NEED FOR ULTRASOUND EVALUATION)

| VISIT DATE (YEAR ____) | | | | | | | | | | | | | | | |
|---|---|---|---|---|---|---|---|---|---|---|---|---|---|---|---|
| WEEKS GEST. (BEST EST.) | | | | | | | | | | | | | | | |
| FUNDAL HEIGHT (CM) | | | | | | | | | | | | | | | |
| PRESENTATION | | | | | | | | | | | | | | | |
| FHR PRESENT: F=FETOSCOPE D=DOPTONE | | | | | | | | | | | | | | | |
| FETAL MOVEMENT: +=PRESENT O=ABSENT | | | | | | | | | | | | | | | |
| PREMATURITY: SIGNS/SYMPTOMS:* +=PRESENT O=ABSENT | | | | | | | | | | | | | | | |
| CERVIX EXAM (DIL./EFF./STA.) | | | | | | | | | | | | | | | |
| BLOOD PRESSURE: INITIAL | | | | | | | | | | | | | | | |
| BLOOD PRESSURE: REPEAT | | | | | | | | | | | | | | | |
| EDEMA +=PRESENT O=ABSENT | | | | | | | | | | | | | | | |
| WEIGHT (PREPREG: ________) | | | | | | | | | | | | | | | |
| CUMULATIVE WEIGHT GAIN | | | | | | | | | | | | | | | |
| URINE (GLUCOSE/ ALBUMIN/KETONES) | | | | | | | | | | | | | | | |
| NEXT APPOINTMENT | | | | | | | | | | | | | | | |
| PROVIDER (INITIALS) | | | | | | | | | | | | | | | |
| TEST REMINDERS | 8–18 WEEKS CVS/AMNIO/MSAFP | | | | | 24–28 WEEKS GLUCOSE SCREEN/RhIG | | | | | | | | | |

**COMMENTS:** ______________________________________________

*For example: vaginal bleeding, discharge, cramps, contractions, pelvic pressure.

**Fig. 22–3.** ACOG prenatal records. (From The American College of Obstetricians and Gynecologists, Washington, DC 20024, 1989.)

## LABORATORY AND EDUCATION

| INITIAL LABS | DATE | RESULT | REVIEWED |
|---|---|---|---|
| BLOOD TYPE | / / | A B AB O | |
| Rh TYPE | / / | | |
| ANTIBODY SCREEN | / / | | |
| HCT/HGB | / / | ______ % ______ g/dl | |
| PAP SMEAR | / / | NORMAL / ABNORMAL / ____ | |
| RUBELLA | / / | | |
| VDRL | / / | | |
| GC | / / | | |
| URINE CULTURE/SCREEN | / / | | |
| HBsAg | / / | | |
| **8–18-WEEK LABS (WHEN INDICATED)** | **DATE** | **RESULT** | |
| ULTRASOUND | / / | | |
| MSAFP | / / | ____________ MOM | |
| AMNIO/CVS | / / | | |
| KARYOTYPE | / / | 46, XX OR 46, XY / OTHER____ | |
| ALPHA-FETOPROTEIN | / / | NORMAL____ ABNORMAL____ | |
| **24–28-WEEK LABS (WHEN INDICATED)** | **DATE** | **RESULT** | |
| HCT/HGB | / / | ______ % ______ g/dl | |
| DIABETES SCREEN | / / | 1 HR______________ | |
| GTT (IF SCREEN ABNORMAL) | / / | ____FBS ____1 HR<br>____2 HR ____3 HR | |
| Rh ANTIBODY SCREEN | / / | | |
| RhIG GIVEN (28 WKS) | / / | SIGNATURE ____________ | |
| **32–36-WEEK LABS (WHEN INDICATED)** | **DATE** | **RESULT** | |
| ULTRASOUND | / / | | |
| VDRL | / / | | |
| GC | / / | | |
| HCT/HGB | / / | ______ % ______ g/dl | |
| **OPTIONAL LAB (HIGH-RISK GROUPS)** | **DATE** | **RESULT** | |
| HIV | / / | | |
| HGB ELECTROPHORESIS | / / | AA AS SS AC SC AF ↑$A_2$ | |
| CHLAMYDIA | / / | | |
| OTHER | / / | | |

**COMMENTS/ADDITIONAL LAB**

**PLANS/EDUCATION** (COUNSELED ☐)

- ☐ ANESTHESIA PLANS ____________
- ☐ TOXOPLASMOSIS PRECAUTIONS (CATS/RAW MEAT) ____________
- ☐ CHILDBIRTH CLASSES ____________
- ☐ PHYSICAL ACTIVITY ____________
- ☐ PREMATURE LABOR SIGNS ____________
- ☐ NUTRITION COUNSELING ____________
- ☐ BREAST OR BOTTLE FEEDING ____________
- ☐ NEWBORN CAR SEAT ____________
- ☐ POSTPARTUM BIRTH CONTROL ____________
- ☐ ENVIRONMENTAL/WORK HAZARDS ____________
- ☐ TUBAL STERILIZATION ____________
- ☐ VBAC COUNSELING ____________
- ☐ CIRCUMCISION ____________
- ☐ TRAVEL ____________

**REQUESTS** ____________

**TUBAL STERILIZATION** DATE INITIALS

CONSENT SIGNED ___/___/___ ________

AA128 2 / 2

**Fig. 22–4.** ACOG prenatal records. (From The American College of Obstetricians and Gynecologists, Washington, DC 20024, 1989.)

Patient Addressograph

## ACOG ANTEPARTUM RECORD

NAME ______________________________________
LAST FIRST MIDDLE

ID # ______________________________________

### Progress Notes

Fig. 22–5. ACOG prenatal records. (From The American College of Obstetricians and Gynecologists, Washington, DC 20024, 1989.)

**Table 22–1.** Risk Factors for Hepatitis B Infection

1. Asian ancestry
2. Health care provider
3. Prior history of hepatitis
4. Intravenous drug abuse
5. Prostitution
6. Tattoo
7. Prior blood transfusion
8. Employment in a dialysis unit or institute for the mentally retarded
9. Sexual contact with person presently or previously infected with hepatitis B virus

(From Baker DA, Polk BF: Hepatitis B: a controllable disease. Obstet. Gynecol. 62:105, 1983.)

work, travel, sexual intercourse, drug, alcohol or cigarette use, seat belt use, etc., should be explained. Danger signals that should be brought to the immediate attention of the health care provider, such as vaginal bleeding, persistent headache, blurred vision, abdominal pain, dysuria, frequent uterine contractions before 36 weeks gestation, and change of fetal movement patterns, are emphasized. Routine practice and habits in prenatal care of the particular health care provider, i.e., use of episiotomy, enema, vulvar preparation, ambulation during labor, electronic fetal monitoring, etc., should be conveyed to the gravida. Methods of contacting the health care provider at any time, cesarean delivery or vaginal birth after prior cesarean delivery (VBAC) practices, and methods of fetal health assessment (oxytocin challenge test) (24), nonstress test (25), fetal acoustic stimulation (26), biophysical profile (27), and fetal movement counting (28) should be appropriately discussed.

**Table 22–2.** Risk Factors for Gestational Diabetes

1. Maternal age greater than 25 years
2. Obesity
3. Family history of diabetes mellitus
4. Previous infant weighing more than 4000 g
5. Previous stillborn infant
6. Previous infant with congenital anomaly
7. Present or previous hydramnios
8. History of recurrent abortions

(Modified from O'Sullivan JB, Mahan CM, Charles D, Dandrow RV: Screening criteria for high-risk gestational diabetic patients. Am. J. Obstet. Gynecol. 116:895, 1973.)

**Table 22–3.** Normal Glucose Levels for the 100 Gram Oral Glucose Tolerance Test

| | |
|---|---|
| Fasting plasma glucose | 105 mg/dl |
| 1-hour plasma glucose | 190 mg/dl |
| 2-hour plasma glucose | 165 mg/dl |
| 3-hour plasma glucose | 145 mg/dl |

(From Carpenter MW, Couston DR: Criteria for screening tests for gestational diabetes. Am. J. Obstet. Gynecol. 144:768, 1982.)

Equally important in anticipatory counseling is the discussion of the possible need for forceps or abdominal delivery and the availability of various methods of analgesia or anesthesia. Optimally, the gravida should be introduced to the anesthesiologist during the prenatal period before the onset of labor or pregnancy complications. This is even more critical in high-risk patients. It is important that both the obstetrician and anesthesiologist communicate similar philosophies concerning pain management during labor. For the most part, this is simple in cases in which care is provided by obstetric anesthesiologists in a highly developed center, because the information can be given by the anesthesiologist, and the obstetricians can, for the most part, be spared having to spend considerable time and effort on it. In these cases, they are supportive of the plan put forth by their obstetric anesthesiologists. In cases in which first stage analgesia is managed exclusively by obstetricians, they should be responsible for informing the patient of alternatives for analgesia and for outlining a plan.

Many medical and obstetric conditions can be anticipated to complicate dramatically the patient's anesthetic management. Early (rather than third trimester) consultation with the health care provider who will administer the patient's anesthesia will frequently minimize the gravida's risks during the pregnancy. For example, when a gravida presents to her obstetric health care provider with serious medical or obstetric illness, she should be referred for consultation with the anesthetist as soon as is feasible. This will allow the anesthetist to plan an approach to the patient's anesthetic care before obstetric complications occur. Nothing frustrates the anesthetist more than to be called to evaluate a new patient (such as one with uncorrected tetralogy of Fallot) with severe hemorrhage secondary to an incomplete first or second trimester spontaneous abortion who requires immediate operative intervention. In this situation, no plan has been formulated previously for her anesthetic management, and the patient's morbidity and mortality could be expected to increase. This is probably one of the most frustrating and more important areas of conflict in good patient management, i.e., the lack of communication and referral at an early time for the parturient at risk. A clear message must be given to the obstetric colleague and that is: the anesthesiologist wants to be informed of high-risk patients and have them referred at an early time so that a complete history, physical, and evaluation of the primary problem can be identified and a plan for anesthesia contemplated.

In today's medicolegal climate, the discussion of drug use in pregnancy has assumed increasing importance. There is substantial misunderstanding among the public concerning the risks of drug exposure. Approximately 3 to 4% of infants are born with major congenital anomalies. Most of these anomalies are secondary to random mutations and are not preventable. However, drugs, chemical, and x ray exposure are incorrectly implicated by the lay public as the major causes of birth defects. Yet most data show that drugs, chemical or x ray exposure account for only a small percentage of the 3 to 4% of infants with birth defects (29). The Food and Drug Administration, in an effort to establish risks of drugs to the pregnant patient,

**Table 22–4.** Risk Categories of Drugs Utilized During Pregnancy

| | |
|---|---|
| Category A: | Controlled studies in women fail to demonstrate a risk to the fetus in the first trimester (and there is no evidence of a fetal risk in later trimesters), and the possibility of fetal harm appears remote. |
| Category B: | Either animal reproduction studies have not demonstrated at fetal risk (but there are no controlled studies in pregnant women) or animal reproduction studies have shown an adverse effect (other than a decrease in fertility) that was not confirmed in controlled studies in women in the first trimester (and there is no evidence of a risk in later trimesters). |
| Category C: | Either studies in animals have revealed adverse effects on the fetus (teratogenic or embryocidal or other) and there are no controlled studies in women or studies in women and animals are not available. Drug should be given only if the potential benefit justifies the potential risk to the fetus. |
| Category D: | There is positive evidence of human fetal risk, but the benefits from use in pregnant women may be acceptable despite the risk (e.g., if the drug is needed in a life-threatening situation or for a serious disease for which safer drugs cannot be used or are ineffective). |
| Category X: | Studies in animals or human beings have demonstrated fetal abnormalities or there is evidence of fetal risk based on human experience or both, and the risk of the use of the drug in pregnant women clearly outweighs any possible benefit. The drug is contraindicated in women who are or may become pregnant. |

(From Federal Register 44:37434, 1980.)

has classified drugs into five categories (30). Table 22–4 lists these drug categories.

## *Quality Assurance and Risk Management*

The Joint Commission for the Accreditation of Hospitals and various other health regulatory boards have imposed increasing requirements to document the quality of inpatient medical care. This trend is moving rapidly to the outpatient setting. Policy and procedure manuals for ambulatory, medical, nursing, and administrative services have become increasingly important and are recommended by the American College of Obstetricians and Gynecologists (31).

More recently, cocaine (or other drug) addiction and HIV infection occurring during pregnancy have become important epidemiologic issues. The pregnancy and health-related risks of these problems should ideally be discussed before achieving a pregnancy. Both of these issues are discussed in depth in Chapter 35.

Table 22–5 lists parameters that are used to establish the estimated date of confinement for a gravida. The 95% confidence limits for these parameters, as established by Jimenez (32), Anderson (33,34), and others (35,36), are also included. The use and agreement of a multiple of these parameters increases further the accuracy of the estimated date of confinement. Table 22–6 lists criteria established by the American College of Obstetricians and Gynecologists (37) for performing a cesarean delivery without amniotic fluid analysis to determine fetal pulmonary maturity. Two of these clinical criteria and one of the laboratory criteria must be met. Use of these parameters and guidelines will reduce dramatically the risk of iatrogenic prematurity.

Since the late 1970s, medicolegal and ethical considerations in prenatal care have assumed increasing importance. Fetal therapy and elective or therapeutic abortion have polarized segments of the population into vocal political action groups that attempt to legislate moral and ethical issues in prenatal care. It follows, therefore, that medicolegal issues concerning the administration of various forms of intrapartum analgesia have also assumed increasing importance in recent years. It seems that many times the easiest aspect of care to blame is that which affects both the mother and fetus, which is shrouded by misunderstanding and mystery, and which most nonanesthesia personnel and lay persons both find unnecessary and unanticipated, i.e., the anesthetic management. Potential litigation could be minimized by a sincere, honest, empathetic discussion of the patient's diagnosis, prognosis with or without analgesia, indications, risks, limitations, alternatives, and expected outcome of analgesia administration with the gravida during pregnancy and before administration during labor.

Quality assurance and risk management concerns mandate that resuscitation equipment and a health care provider skilled in resuscitation be immediately available whenever intrapartum analgesia is administered. Ideally, policies and procedures should be well-documented concerning obtaining, storing, administering, and disposing of narcotics and other drugs in the labor and delivery suite. Each hospital should have written guidelines detailing which health care providers may administer intrapartum analgesia. Continuing medical education and current certification in basic cardiopulmonary life support (CPR) and advanced cardiac life support (ACLS) should be encouraged for all health care providers who employ intrapartum analgesia.

## *Women's Concerns About Prenatal Care*

A small number of women express dissatisfaction with pregnant care as it is delivered in the United States. Most of these concerns involve a lack of a personal approach to the patient, the doctor's time portrayed as more important than the patient's, and specific goals being ill-defined for each clinic visit (38). Gravidae may feel that health care providers are more interested in analysis of health problems than are they in getting to know them as people (38). Women dissatisfied with pregnant care also complain that the actual experience of prenatal care is below their expectations.

Many of these concerns over prenatal care could be eliminated by common sense analysis of the medical system and appropriate interventions and changes to the medical system. The provision of consistent information by prenatal and anesthesia health care providers in an environment that is sensitive to the patient's needs improves tremendously the patient's satisfaction. This improved satisfaction would translate into improved medical care for the patient and diminished medicolegal risks to obstetric and anesthesia health care providers. The au-

**Table 22–5.** Parameters to Establish the Estimated Date of Confinement

| Parameter | Median Time for First Detection (Weeks From LMP) | Confidence Limits (Weeks) |
|---|---|---|
| 1. LMP | — | ±2 |
| 2. Basal body temperature rise | 2 | ±3 days |
| 3. Home ovulation (LH surge) test | 2 | ±3 days |
| 4. Beta hCG (radioimmunoassay) | 3 | ±1 |
| 5. Urine hCG (hemagglutination inhibition) | 5 | ±10 days |
| 6. Uterine size on pelvic examination between 8 to 16 weeks gestation | — | ±2 |
| 7. Fetal heart tones | | |
| Doppler stethoscope | 11 | ±2 |
| DeLee-Hillis stethoscope | 20 | ±2 |
| 8. Quickening | | |
| Primigravida | 19.5 | ±17 days |
| Multigravida | 17 | ±18 days |
| 9. MacDonald measurements of uterine height (20 to 30 weeks gestation) | — | ±4 |
| 10. Abdominal ultrasound measurements | | |
| Gestational sac | 5 | ±10 days |
| Crown-rump length | 7 | ±5 days |
| BPD 12 to 24 weeks | 12 | ±10 days |
| 24 to 30 weeks | — | ±2 |
| 30+ weeks | — | ±3 |
| Femur length 12 to 26 weeks | 12 | ±10 days |
| 26+ weeks | — | ±3 |

(Modified from American Academy of Pediatrics/American College of Obstetricians and Gynecologists: Guidelines for Perinatal Care, Washington, DC, 1983; Jiminez JM, Tyson JE, Reisch JS: Clinical measures of gestational age in normal pregnancies. Obstet. Gynecol. 61:438, 1983; Andersen HF, Johnson TRB, Barclay ML, Flora JD: Gestational age assessment I: analysis of individual clinical observations. Am. J. Obstet. Gynecol. 139: 173, 1981; Andersen HF, Johnson TRB, Flora JD, Barclay ML: Gestational age assessment II: analysis of individual clinical observations. Am. J. Obstet. Gynecol. 139:173, 1981; Johnson TRB Jr, Work BA Jr: A dynamic graph for documentation of gestational age. Obstet. Gynecol. 54:115, 1979; O'Brien GD, Queenan JT: Growth of the ultrasound fetal femur length during normal pregnancy I. Am. J. Obstet. Gynecol. 141:833, 1981.)

thors also believe firmly that the pregnant patient can have many of her fears and concerns alleviated by adequate emphasis on pain relief methods during labor. After delivery, many parturients express that much of their fear and anxiety had centered on the fact that they were not sure they would be able to endure the pain or that they would make a fool of themselves or embarrass their mate during labor because of their reaction to pain and the threat of labor. With adequate exposure to anesthesiologists who are skilled informants and good communicators, these patients and their husbands can look forward with much of this anxiety and apprehension removed. This is another reason a carefully considered and presented antepartum-pain lecture needs to be woven into the standard antepartum lecture and tour that most centers now have for patients.

**Table 22–6.** Criteria to Perform Elective Cesarean Delivery Without Verification of Fetal Pulmonary Maturity

**Clinical criteria:**
- LMP—normal, regular, well established
- Twenty weeks have elapsed since first detection of fetal heart tones by DeLee-Hillis stethoscope
- Uterine size determined by pelvic examination by an experienced examiner prior to 16 weeks gestation

**Laboratory criteria:**
- Thirty-six weeks have elapsed since the occurrence of a positive beta hCG
- Crown-rump measurement between 6 to 14 weeks' gestation consistent with clinical criteria
- BPD measurement prior to 20 weeks' gestation consistent with clinical criteria

(From the American Academy of Pediatrics/American College of Obstetricians and Gynecologists: Guidelines for Perinatal Care. Washington, DC, 1983, p. 66.)

## OBSTETRIC INTRAPARTUM CARE

Knowledge of the pertinent anatomy and of the many different postures in which the fetus may be found in utero is essential for accurate diagnosis and for an understanding of the mechanisms of labor and the proper conduct of parturition. Figures 22–6 and 22–7 are included

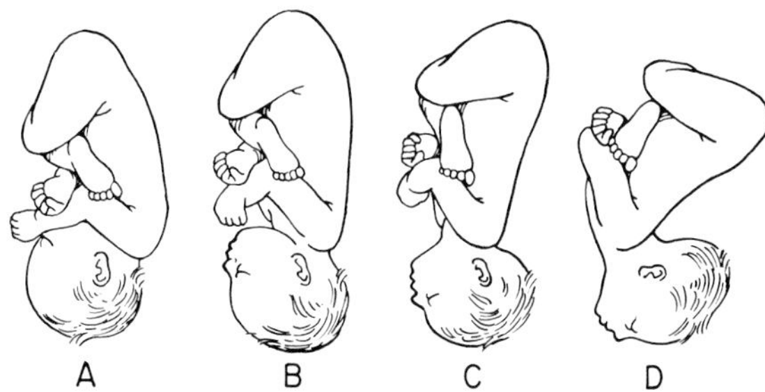


**Fig. 22–6.** Attitudes of the fetus in **A,** vertex, **B,** sinciput, **C,** brow, and **D,** face presentations. (Modified from Eastman NJ, Hellman LM: Williams Obstetrics. 12th Ed. New York, Appleton-Century-Crofts, 1961.)

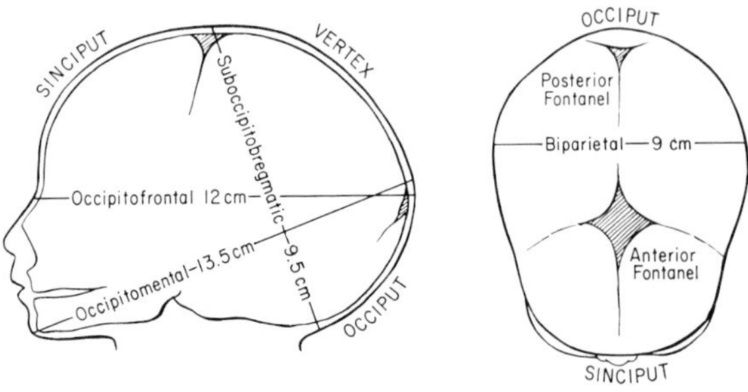


**Fig. 22–7.** Diameters of the fetal head.

for a quick review. The postures are depicted and described in terms of attitude, presentation, presenting part, position, and lie. Because there are differences in usage of these terms, they are defined here.

## *Fetal Postures*

### *Attitude*

Attitude is the posture of the fetus in relation to itself and with no regard to its relation to the mother. In the normal attitude, the fetus's back is arched, the head flexed, the chin touching the chest, the arms folded across the chest, thighs flexed on the abdomen, knees flexed with the legs crossed, and the feet flexed on the legs.

### *Presentation*

Presentation refers to the relationship between the long axis of the fetus to the long axis of the mother. In a longitudinal presentation, the fetal and maternal spines are parallel; in a transverse presentation, the fetal and maternal spines are at right angles; in an oblique presentation, the fetal spine crosses the mother's at an acute angle.

### *The Presenting Part*

This is the part of the fetus that descends first through the birth canal and, therefore, that part which the examining finger first contacts. In cephalic presentation, the presenting part varies with the posture of the child: in a normal posture, there is a vertex presentation, termed occiput; in partial extension, there is sinciput presentation; in greater extension, there is a brow presentation, designated frontum; and in complete extension, there is a face presentation, designated mentum (Figure 22–6).

### *Position*

Position is the relationship of the presenting part to the maternal pelvis. The presenting part is usually in relation to the obliquely anterior, transverse, or obliquely posterior aspect of either side of the pelvis. Accordingly, six positions are generally considered: left anterior, left transverse, left posterior, right anterior, right transverse, and right posterior. Table 22–7 summarizes the classification and incidence of types of presentations. At the onset of labor, the fetal head is in the transverse position in over 60% of the cases. Diagnosis of presentation or position is made by inspection and palpation of the abdomen, vaginal or rectal examination, auscultation, and, in unusual or doubtful cases, by fetal ultrasonographic examination. Figure 22–7 presents the diameters of the fetal head with their average diameters. The cardinal movements of labor generally present the smallest diameters of the fetal head to the smallest maternal pelvic measurements.

**Table 22–7.** Types and Incidence of Presentation

| Presentation | Percentage |
|---|---|
| Longitudinal Presentation (lie) | 99 |
| Cephalic (head) | 96 |
| Vertex (occiput), the head completely flexed | 95 |
| Occipito-anterior (OA) | 2 |
| Left occipito-anterior (LOA) | 12 |
| Left occipitotransverse (LOT) | 35 |
| Left occipitoposterior (LOP) | 3 |
| Occipitoposterior (OP) | 1 |
| Right occipitoposterior (ROP) | 9 |
| Right occipitotransverse (ROT) | 25 |
| Right occipito-anterior (ROA) | 8 |
| Face (chin), the head is completely extended | 0.5 |
| Mento-anterior (MA) | |
| Left mento-anterior (LMA) | |
| Left mentotransverse (LMT) | |
| Left mentoposterior (LMP) | |
| Mentoposterior (MP) | |
| Right mento-anterior (RMA) | |
| Right mentotransverse (RMT) | |
| Right menotoposterior (RMP) | |
| Brow (frontal), the head is partially extended | 0.5 |
| Fronto-anterior (FA) | |
| Left front-anterior (LFA) | |
| Left frontotransverse (LFT) | |
| Left frontoposterior (LFP) | |
| Frontoposterior (FP) | |
| Right front-anterior (RFA) | |
| Right frontotransverse (RFT) | |
| Right frontoposterior (RFP) | |
| Breech or Pelvic | 3 |
| Sacro-anterior (SA) | |
| Left sacro-anterior (LSA) | |
| Left sacrotransverse (LST) | |
| Left sacroposterior (LSP) | |
| Sacroposterior (SP) | |
| Right sacro-anterior (RSA) | |
| Right sacrotransverse (RST) | |
| Right sacroposterior (RSP) | |
| Transverse Presentation | 1 |
| Left scapulo-anterior (LScA) | |
| Left scapuloposterior (LScP) | |
| Right scapulo-anterior (RScA) | |
| Right scapuloposterior (RScP) | |

(From Bonica JJ: Principles and Practice of Obstetric Analgesia and Anesthesia. F.A. Davis, Philadelphia, 1967.)

### *Lie*

The lie refers to the relationship of the long axis of the fetus to the mother and is either longitudinal, which is the ordinary lie in 99% of the cases, or transverse which is unacceptable for vaginal delivery, or oblique which is also incompatible with delivery from the vaginal route.

## Pelvimetry

Figures 22–8 and 22–9 depict the planes and diameters of the maternal bony pelvis. Figure 22–10 shows the major internal and external muscles of the pelvic sling. The configuration and natural tone of these muscles influence the cardinal movements of labor, allowing the larger and smaller diameters of the fetal head to be matched to the larger and smaller diameters of the maternal pelvis, respectively. Table 22–8 demonstrates the types and characteristics of the maternal pelvis. The prognosis for vaginal delivery is generally good for a gynecoid or anthropoid pelvis; however, it is less optimistic for a gravida with either an android or platypelloid pelvis.

Clinical pelvimetry is generally performed on all gravidae at their first prenatal visit and at the onset of labor. While this assessment is a qualitative evaluation and gives a subjective impression of the adequacy of the pelvis, it is the best clinical assessor of the ability of the patient to undergo successful vaginal delivery. The parameters thought to imply an increased success rate for vaginal delivery are a diagonal conjugate greater than 11.5 cm, a bi-ischial diameter greater than 8.5 cm, a pubic arch greater than 90°, blunt ischial spines, a sacrospinous notch greater than 2 cm, a mobile coccyx, and a hollow (round) sacrum. Other forms of pelvimetry (ultrasound, x ray, CT scan) are rarely used, but may be indicated for breech presentations when considering a trial of labor, when prior pelvic trauma and fractures have occurred, for example. Routine x ray pelvimetry is no longer used because of the fetal risks of x ray exposure and its poor prediction of delivery route.



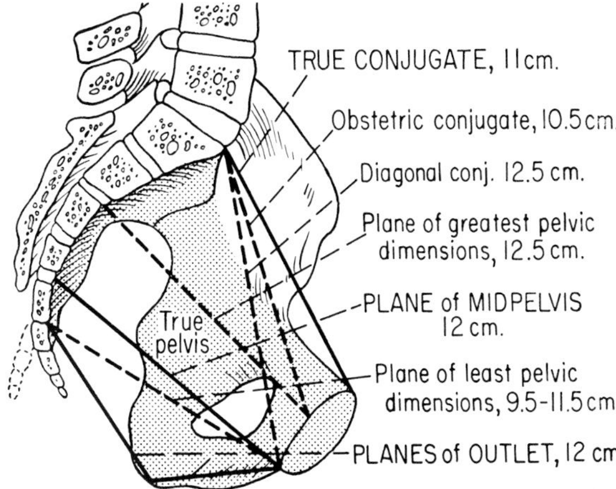


**Fig. 22–8.** Sagittal view of the pelvis showing important anteroposterior diameters (solid lines and large letters) and subordinate diameters.

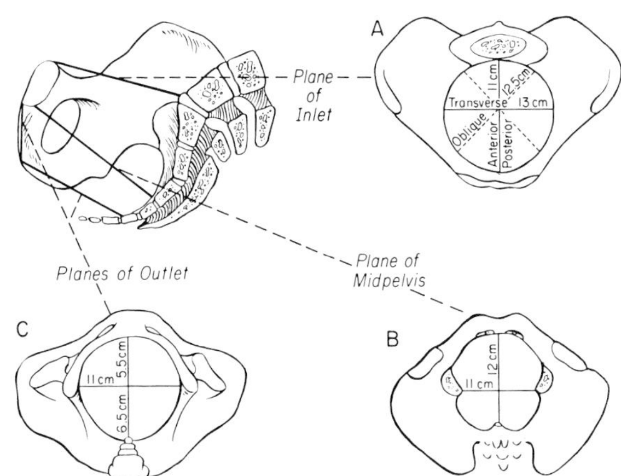


**Fig. 22–9.** Planes and diameters of the pelvis. **A,** Superior plane or obstetric inlet, bound posteriorly by the promontory of the sacrum, laterally by the iliopectineal line, and anteriorly by the rami of pubic bones and the upper margin of the symphysis pubis. **B,** Midpelvic plane bound posteriorly by the sacrum near the junction of the 3rd and 4th sacral vertebrae, laterally by the ischial spines, and anteriorly by the inferior aspect of the symphysis. **C,** Inferior plane or obstetric outlet composed of two triangular components: the posterior is bound behind by the sacrococcygeal joint, laterally by the sacrotuberous ligament, and bound by the bi-ischial diameter; the anterior component is bound by the bi-ischial diameter behind, the inner margin of the pubic arch laterally, and anteriorly by the inferior margin of the symphysis. The floor or the pelvic outlet is composed of the soft tissues of the perineum and the structures making up the urogenital diaphragm.

## Mechanisms of Labor in Occipito-Anterior Presentation

Mechanisms of labor (cardinal movements of labor) is the term applied to a series of changes in the attitude and position of the fetus that permit it to progress through the irregularly-shaped pelvic cavity. A thorough understanding of how this is accomplished is essential not only to good obstetric care but also to optimal anesthetic management. This progress is the result of the activity of the uterus and the auxiliary forces, and the resistance of the soft tissue and the bony pelvis to the descent of the fetus. The steps in the mechanism are descent, flexion, internal rotation, extension, restitution, and external rotation. These do not occur separately but rather are a combined process. Figure 22–11 with its accompanying legend contains a summary of the mechanisms of labor in left occipito-anterior presentation. The right occipito-anterior presentation is, of course, similar.

### Engagement

The phenomenon by which the presenting part enters the superior strait occurs during the last weeks of pregnancy in primigravidae, whereas in many multiparae it does not take place until after the onset of labor. During prelabor and the first stage of labor, uterine contractions efface and dilate the cervix. In occiput positions, the longest diameter of the infant's head, the anteroposterior, en-

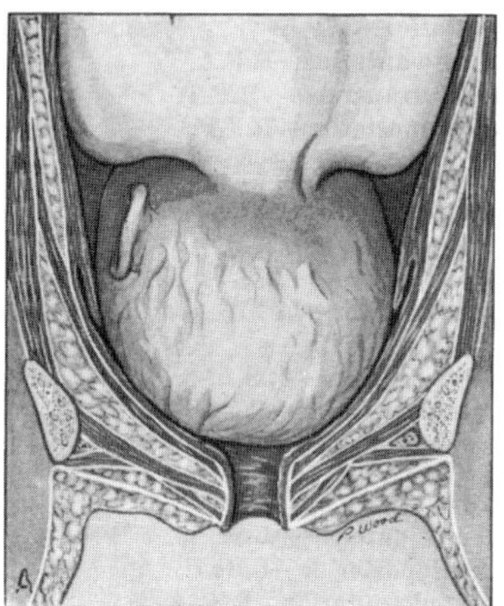

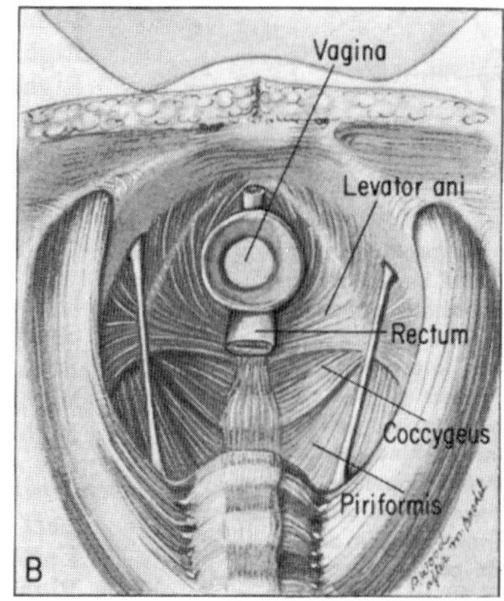

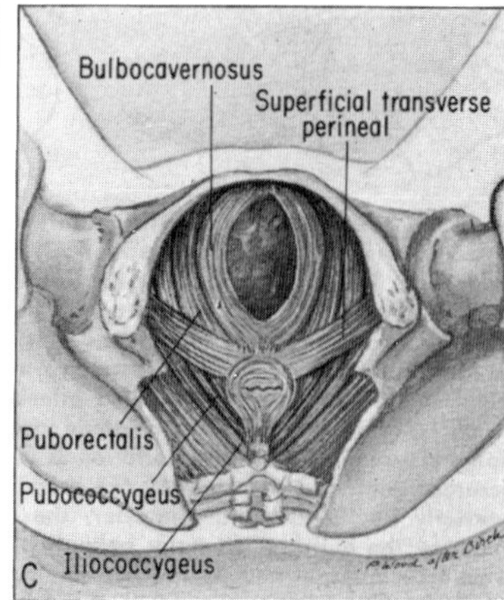


**Fig. 22–10.** The pelvic floor. **A,** Coronal section showing the fetal head on the pelvic floor during early labor. **B,** Superior view showing the musculature of the pelvic floor, which makes up the V-shaped trough that is so important in rotation of the head. **C,** Inferior view of the muscular pelvic floor just before birth.

ters the pelvis in the longest diameter of the inlet, the transverse, in most parturients. If the sagittal suture is equidistant from the symphysis and the sacral promontory, the head is said to be entering the inlet in a synclitic manner. Some degree of asynclitism is present in most parturients (Figure 22–12).

### Descent

Descent, the first movement for the birth of the child, is constant throughout the mechanisms of flexion, internal rotation, extension, restitution, and external rotation. Descent can be delayed by an incompletely dilated cervix, resistant soft tissue, disproportion between the size of the pelvic cavity and the fetus, and weak ineffective uterine contractions. Descent usually occurs more gradually in primigravidae than in multiparae, because the cervix dilates more slowly, and the soft tissue resistance is greater. The degree of descent is gauged by the station of the presenting part, which is its relationship to the plane of the ischial spines (Figure 22–13).

### Flexion

As soon as the descending head meets with resistance, it becomes more and more flexed and brings the chin into more intimate contact with the thorax, thereby substituting the suboccipitobregmatic diameter of 9.5 cm for the occipitofrontal diameter, which usually measures 11.5 cm. Flexion is said to occur because the force applied by the resistance of the soft tissues to the anterior portion of the head is greater than the force applied by the resistance of the soft tissues to the posterior portion. During descent the fetal trunk is gradually straightened out, while the head, generally, preserves its spatial orientation. Flexion is an essential prerequisite to descent, because it greatly reduces the diameters of the fetal head that present themselves to the birth canal.

**Table 22–8.** Pelvic Types

| Type | Pelvic Inlet Shape | Midpelvic Posterior Sagittal Diameter* |
|---|---|---|
| Gynecoid | round | average |
| Anthropoid | long, oval | long |
| Android | heart-shaped | short |
| Platypelloid | flat, oval | short |

* The posterior sagittal diameter is this distance of the anteroposterior diameter of the midpelvis between the sacrum and its intercept with the interspinous diameter.
(From Friedman EA: Labor: clinical evaluation and management. 2nd Ed. New York, Appleton-Century-Crofts, 1978.)

### Internal Rotation

Internal rotation refers to the first part of the passage of the head through the lower parturient canal, in which there is a progressive rotational movement of the head simultaneous with its progression through the birth canal. This is an absolutely essential movement in the completion of labor, except when the fetus is abnormally small. It usually begins when the preceding part of the head is in the pelvic outlet and continues while the rest of the head passes through the lower part of the bony pelvis. Although the movement is conditioned by both the pelvis and the soft parts inside and outside the pelvis, the soft parts play the primary role. The musculature of the pelvic floor constitutes a V-shaped trough, the inclined sides of which diverge anteriorly and superiorly (see Figure 22–10). This favors spiraling in accordance with the lines of least resistance. As the head descends to the pelvic floor in transverse position, both the muscular trough of the pelvic floor and the bony configuration of the pelvis direct the head into an anteroposterior position. Because the occiput is first to meet the inclined side of the levator ani muscles, and because the normal forepelvis at the lower level is more spacious than the posterior segment, the larger occipital and parietal portions of the vertex necessarily rotate anteriorly. With each uterine contraction, the head descends slightly and the occiput is pushed

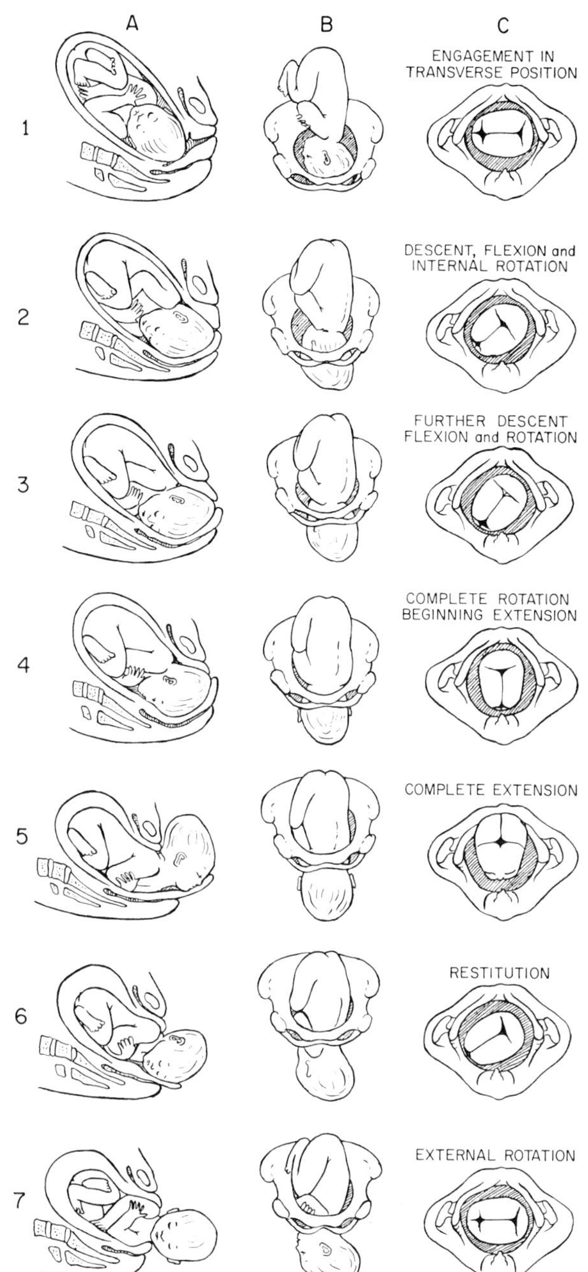


**Fig. 22–11.** Mechanism of labor and delivery for left occipito-anterior position. **A,** sagittal view; **B,** anterior view; C, as seen from below.

anteriorly a bit more by the pressure of the ischial spines and the sacrococcygeal platform. With the rotation, there is further descent until the vertex rests firmly against the perineum. In parturients in whom the pelvic muscles are paralyzed by subarachnoid, caudal or epidural block, the incidence of persistent posterior position is increased.

## *Extension*

Extension is another movement absolutely essential to the birth of the fetal head. After the occiput has rotated to an anterior position, the suboccipital area impinges be-

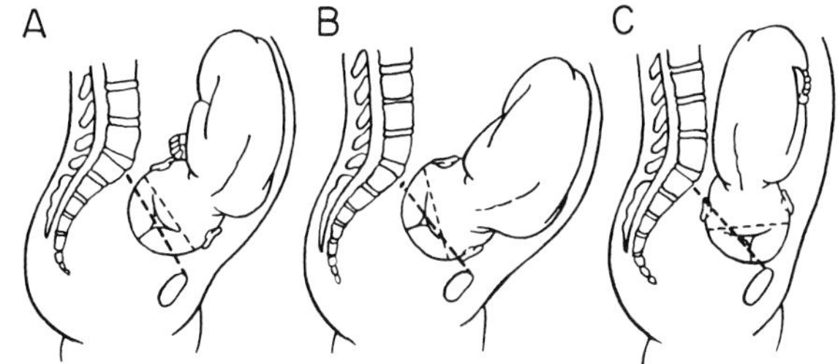


**Fig. 22–12.** Synclitism (A) and asynclitism (B) and (C). **A,** Sagittal suture of the fetus lies exactly midway between the symphysis and sacral promontory. **B,** Sagittal suture is close to the sacrum and the anterior parietal bone is felt by the examining finger—anterior asynclitism or Ngele's obliquity. **C,** Posterior parietal presentation or posterior asynclitism or Litzmann's obliquity. (From Eastman NJ, Hellman LM: Williams Obstetrics. 12th Ed. New York, Appleton-Century-Crofts, Inc., 1961.)

neath the pubis and the parietal bossae on the levator ani muscles and the descending pubic rami. With the increasing distension of the perineum and vaginal opening, a larger and larger portion of the occiput gradually appears. With further extension, the bregma, forehead, nose, mouth and finally the chin, emerge from the introitus by extension. Immediately after its birth, the head falls posteriorly, freeing the occiput.

## *Restitution*

As soon as the head is released from the grasp of the vulvovaginal ring, the neck untwists and restitution of the head occurs. The occiput, accordingly, turns 45° to the left to its original position and the sagittal suture comes to lie obliquely.

## *External Rotation*

When the anterior shoulder meets the resistance of the pelvic floor on the right side, it is shunted downward, forward, and inward to the symphysis. This causes the occiput to rotate 45° more to the left. The anterior shoulder remains impinged beneath the pubic arch while the fetal spine bends laterally to permit the posterior shoulder

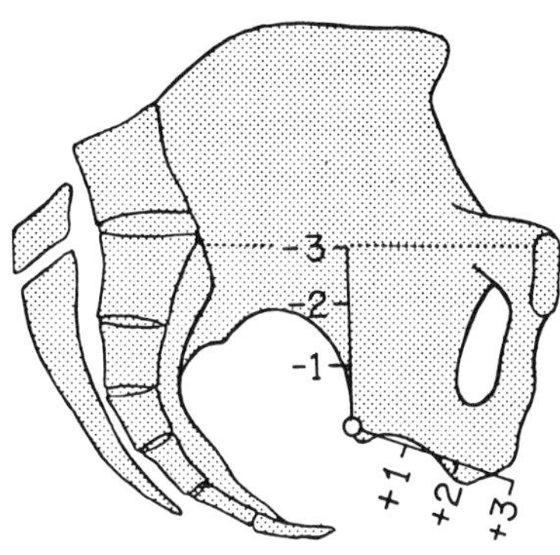


**Fig. 22–13.** Station of the presenting part gauged by its relationship to the ischial spine. Numbers indicate the distance (cm) above (−) or below (+) the spine.

to be forced over the perineum. When the posterior shoulder is free, it falls backward and the opposite one is pushed out from beneath the pubic arch. The body of the infant is then delivered without any particular mechanism.

## Labor

### Stages of Labor

Labor is a continuous process; however, for purposes of study it has been divided into three stages. The first stage is the period from the onset of labor until complete cervical dilation. The first stage of labor has been subdivided into various phases by Friedman (39). The second stage begins with complete cervical dilation and ends with expulsion of the fetus. The third stage begins with expulsion of the fetus and ends with expulsion of the placenta. Table 22–9 lists the mean duration and confidence limits for these stages and phases of labor.

### Disorders of Labor

Labor progression becomes abnormal when it falls outside the 95% confidence limits for normal women who undergo successful vaginal delivery. Friedman has labelled these disorders of labor progression as a prolonged latent phase, protracted active phase, secondary arrest of cervical dilation, among others. Table 22–10 includes these definitions of labor disorders.

### Induction and Augmentation of Labor

Oxytocin induction or augmentation of labor is indicated for a number of standard obstetric indications. Seitchik (40) has outlined standard dosage regimens for oxytocin utilization. The physiology and progression of labor with oxytocin utilization is similar to that of normal, spontaneous labor. Analgesia and anesthesia requirements of the gravida receiving oxytocin infusion are similar to those undergoing spontaneous labor (41).

### Food and Fluids

The only safe oral fluid that can be offered the parturient is water, because it is the only liquid that is rapidly absorbed in the stomach. Fortunately, withholding of food is rarely a problem, because most parturients in active labor do not desire food, and many of them are not able to keep it down. Many parturients do request to eat ice or hard candy while in labor and these should not interfere with the patient's management nor increase her anesthetic risks.

Following admission to the labor suite and after determining that the patient is in labor, an intravenous infusion of lactated Ringer's solution should be started. This not only replenishes the fluids and restores the energy that has been lost but also provides a ready avenue for medication. The fluid intake and output should be carefully recorded with particular attention to the amount of vomitus, urine, and degree of diaphoresis. Fluid recording is especially important in patients in prolonged labor. Patients who are to receive subarachnoid or epidural block should have received 500 ml of fluid in excess of that which was lost. This will do much to prevent or minimize arterial hypotension.

**Table 22–10.** Patterns of Abnormal Labor

| Pattern | Diagnostic Criteria |
|---|---|
| Prolonged latent phase | |
| nulliparae | latent phase duration ≥ 20 hr |
| multiparae | latent phase duration ≥ 14 hr |
| Protracted active phase | |
| nulliparae | rate of dilation ≤ 1.2 cm/hr |
| multiparae | rate of dilation ≤ 1.5 cm/hr |
| Protracted descent | |
| nulliparae | rate of descent ≤ 1.0 cm/hr |
| multiparae | rate of descent ≤ 2.0 cm/hr |
| Secondary arrest of dilation | cessation of active phase progression ≥ 2 hr |
| Arrest of descent | cessation of descent progression ≥ 1 hr |
| Failure of descent | lack of expected descent during second stage |
| Precipitate dilation | |
| nulliparae | dilation ≥ 5 cm/hr |
| multiparae | dilation ≥ 10 cm/hr |
| Precipitate descent | |
| nulliparae | descent ≥ 5 cm/hr |
| multiparae | descent ≥ 10 cm/hr |

(From Friedman EA: Labor: clinical evaluation and management. 2nd Ed. New York, Appleton-Century-Crofts, 1978.)

**Table 22–9.** Progression of Spontaneous Labor

| | Mean | | 95% Confidence Limit | |
|---|---|---|---|---|
| | Nulliparae | Multiparae | Nulliparae | Multiparae |
| Total duration of labor | 10.1 hr | 6.2 hr | 25.8 hr | 19.5 hr |
| Stages of labor | | | | |
| First | 9.7 | 8.0 hr | 24.7 hr | 18.8 hr |
| Second | 33.0 min | 8.5 min | 117.5 min | 46.5 min |
| Third | 5.0 min | 5.0 min | 30.0 min | 30.0 min |
| Latent phase | 6.4 hr | 4.8 hr | 20.6 hr | 13.6 hr |
| Maximum cervical dilation | 3.0 cm/hr | 5.7 cm/hr | 1.2 cm/hr | 1.5 cm/hr |
| Fetal descent | 3.3 cm/hr | 6.6 cm/hr | 1.0 cm/hr | 2.1 cm/hr |

(From Friedman EA: Labor: clinical evaluation and management. 2nd Ed. New York, Appleton-Century-Crofts, 1978.)

### Monitoring

The mother, fetus, and progress of labor are monitored frequently. Although the monitorings may be carried out by different individuals, it is important that all of the information be integrated and available to the obstetric team. To achieve this, the data must be promptly and accurately recorded on appropriate charts that are readily available to each member of the obstetric team. Maternal vital signs should be carefully measured every hour with the patient in the lateral position between contractions (42). These parameters should also be measured just before administration of drugs and at frequent intervals for 30 minutes after the drug is given. The maternal temperature should also be taken and recorded every 4 hours (42). The fluid intake and output must be carefully measured and recorded. Monitoring of the fetus consists of either continuous electronic fetal monitoring or listening to the fetal heart rate with a DeLee-Hillis stethoscope every 30 minutes during the latent phase, every 15 minutes during the active phase (first stage of labor), and every 5 minutes during the second stage of labor, with a manual recording of this rate (42). Uterine contractions are monitored by either continuous electronic recording or by abdominal palpation every 15 to 30 minutes (42). The duration and interval between contractions should be noted and recorded accurately. Periodic vaginal examinations are made to determine the amount of cervical dilation, effacement, descent, position of the presenting part, and station (Figure 22–13). The progress of labor is best assessed by a cervicographic method as suggested by Friedman and others (43,44). If the patient's labor falls outside the 95% confidence limits for normal (Table 22–9) and is abnormal (Table 22–10), the patient may require further evaluation for oxytocin augmentation of labor or cesarean delivery. Analgesia/anesthesia requirements for the parturient may also require reevaluation when the labor becomes abnormal.

Records are an essential part of good medical practice. In obstetrics, a careful record of the course of pregnancy and of the events of labor are necessary for the proper evaluation of obstetric management and the correlation of circumstances surrounding delivery, anesthesia, and their consequences to the newborn. In anesthetic practice, accurate records are necessary to: (1) provide information on the reaction of the parturient, the fetus, and the forces of labor to analgesia and anesthesia and to other drugs which may be used; (2) establish a time relationship so that undesirable responses and complications can be looked for; (3) provide data for teaching that can be studied for the benefit of subsequent patients; and (4) provide a medicolegal record. To be of maximum use, all data must be promptly recorded after they are obtained. One should not rely on memory. Each member of the obstetric team should be well-acquainted with all of the records. Please refer to Figures 22–1 through 22–5.

## ANESTHETIC MANAGEMENT

### *Preanesthetic Care*

It is now generally accepted that the best anesthetic management begins with preanesthetic care. Every individual who is to receive an anesthetic should be seen by the anesthetist. During the preanesthetic phase, the anesthesiologist: (1) establishes rapport with and instills confidence in the health care team; (2) familiarizes himself/herself with the patient's medical and anesthesia history, physical findings, and obstetric conditions; (3) evaluates the physiologic and emotional status of the parturient; (4) discusses with both the obstetrician and the parturient the anesthesia and obstetric plans and makes arrangements for analgesia and anesthesia; and (5) participates actively in the psychologic preparation of the gravida and, if necessary, helps the obstetrician with transfusions and other prepartum therapy. Ideally, the anesthesiology team will have an organized approach to the educational and "first exposure of the patient to them." This can best be done by having regular scheduled meetings with gravidae as they progress through gestation. It may be a good idea to first meet them in the late second trimester, for example. After this first meeting, which could be accomplished in a group fashion, the patients should be scheduled individually for a brief history and physical examination in the labor and delivery suite. This can often be done conveniently while the anesthesiologist is covering the labor and delivery suite in the late afternoon.

One visit by the anesthesiology team should be made soon after the parturient enters the hospital. Postponing this visit until the parturient needs analgesia precludes achieving the aforementioned objectives. Before seeing the patient, anesthesiologists should review the parturient's record and talk to the obstetrician and obstetric nurse to learn about the obstetric conditions and any additional information pertinent to the anesthetic management. Such information permits the anesthesiologist and staff to talk to the parturient with confidence, giving the parturient the impression that the anesthesiologist knows her condition well. This has a most reassuring effect and enhances development of rapport.

If both convenient and possible, it is especially nice to have the obstetrician introduce the anesthesiologist in charge, unless, of course, this person happens to be the anesthesiologist who gave the introductory anesthesia lectures earlier in pregnancy. If the patient and the anesthesiologist have not yet met each other and it is not possible to have the obstetrician introduce them, then the anesthesiologist should make his or her own introduction, welcome the patient, and begin to alleviate many of the parturient's fears concerning analgesia, anesthesia, pain, and how it is controlled. The visit should be unhurried and tactful, and the parturient encouraged to provide the necessary information. There is no substitute for talking to the parturient, listening to her patiently, and observing her. The visit should be a subtle educational process for both the anesthesiologist and the patient.

The medical history, including the function of the cardiovascular, respiratory, gastrointestinal, and nervous systems, should be reviewed. The patient should be asked specifically about recent colds or cough, dyspnea, orthopnea, palpitation, ankle edema, response to routine activities, and the occurrence of dizziness, lightheadedness, and weakness when supine. It is important to ascertain whether or not the patient has received corticosteroids, insulin, anticoagulants, tocolytic agents, antihypertensive agents, or other drugs that influence the action of anesthesia. She should be asked if she has had any drug reactions, allergy, or other abnormal response to previous therapy, and when and what she last ate and how close this was to the onset of labor.

The anesthesia history should include details about her previous experience with obstetric and surgical anesthetics, and how she feels about them. She should also be asked about the experiences her husband and relatives have had with anesthesia and encouraged to divulge her impressions about anesthesia. Because most patients have a subconscious fear of death, the anesthesiologist should make a point of emphasizing the safety of modern anesthesia. Citing impressive statistics is effective most of the time.

Physical examinations should be performed by anesthesiologists not only to obtain additional information but, equally important, to enhance rapport, for it manifests their interest and concern for the patient's welfare. The survey of the head and neck, including inspection of the mouth for loose dentures, bridges, carious teeth, and palpation of the neck provides information about possible problems during a general anesthesia. Inspection of the chest and auscultation of the heart and lungs should be done on every patient. The blood pressure and pulse must be measured with the patient supine and again with her in the lateral position to ascertain the degree of compression of the inferior vena cava and aorta by the uterus (supine hypotensive syndrome). Inspection and palpation of the lumbar spine, if epidural or subarachnoid block is planned, are carried out.

Selection of analgesia-anesthesia can only be done after evaluation of the history, physical findings, obstetric conditions, and the practices and philosophy of the obstetrician. The patient should be reassured repeatedly that because there are many agents and techniques available she will be provided with maximal relief consistent with complete safety to her and her baby. If possible, the patient should be given what she prefers. However, if her preference or what has been promised her is not the best form of analgesia-anesthesia, it is best to defer the decision until the matter has been thoroughly discussed with the obstetrician. Once this is done, the anesthesiologist should talk to the patient, giving her the reasons why another method has been chosen. If the reasons are properly presented, there is usually no problem convincing the patient about the selected analgesia-anesthesia. If after thorough discussion the patient still refuses or shows great concern or fear about the proposed method, it is best to choose another technique compatible with all concerned.

## Intrapartum Care

Like all other aspects of obstetric care, optimal sedation-analgesia requires a well-coordinated plan that should be initiated or completed by the obstetric anesthesiologist when one is available at a given center or, failing this, by the attending obstetrician who has responsibility for the first stage analgesia requirements. Morgan, et al's survey of 1000 patients undergoing vaginal delivery found that only 8% of parturients received no analgesia (45). Today, at most well-developed centers the overwhelming preference of many patients and physicians is for regional anesthesia; yet at other centers, where obstetric anesthesiologists are not available and even access to anesthesiologists is limited to operative cases, systemic analgesics are still the primary form of pain relief used in obstetrics in the United States and most of this is provided by obstetricians (46).

Most investigators have described the pain of labor and attempted to quantify that pain by measuring plasma concentrations of adrenocorticotropic hormone (ACTH), cortisol, catecholamines, and β-endorphins. These studies have demonstrated increased ACTH, cortisol, epinephrine, norepinephrine, and β-endorphins throughout labor (47,48). These responses are similar to those reported for surgical stress or hypoxia. In baboons, monkeys, and sheep, these stress and pain responses have been shown to detrimentally influence uteroplacental blood flow and fetal environment (49). There is convincing data in both man and monkeys that anesthesia, sedation, or both, can reduce the harmful effects of the stress and pain of labor for the fetus (50,51). As was mentioned earlier, the overwhelming preference at developed centers for delivery is for regional analgesia in the form of the lumbar epidural method. This practice necessitates the placement of a catheter in the epidural space of the patient early in labor when the patient is still comfortable. Management thereafter is by continuous, low-concentration administration by a pump device such as shown in Figure 22–14.

### Psychologic Analgesia

Everyone should consider the emotional and psychologic aspects of obstetric management to be very important. Because labor is emotionally the most critical phase of the entire pregnancy, everything must be done by the patient's attendants to help her maintain emotional homeostasis. The obstetrician should exploit every opportunity to reinforce the antepartal preparation throughout labor and during the delivery. One of the most effective psychotherapeutic tools in this initial phase of labor is careful explanation of the sensations that she is experiencing and of the status of her labor is. Vaginal examinations, vaginal "preps," and other, new procedures for the primigravida can frequently provide embarrassment and apprehension, which may be minimized by explaining the procedure before it is done. Reassuring the patient that what she is experiencing is normal and telling her of her condition is important for emotional well-being. These methods of psychologic analgesia are covered extensively in Chapter 21, in which psychoprophylaxis is discussed.

### Systemic Analgesia

Ideally, through encouragement and participation in childbirth classes, gravidae will be able to minimize their need for intrapartum analgesia. When analgesia is required, the method employed will have to be individualized depending on the particular hospital, training and skills of the available health care provider, and desires of the parturient. The ACOG Committee on Obstetrics (52)

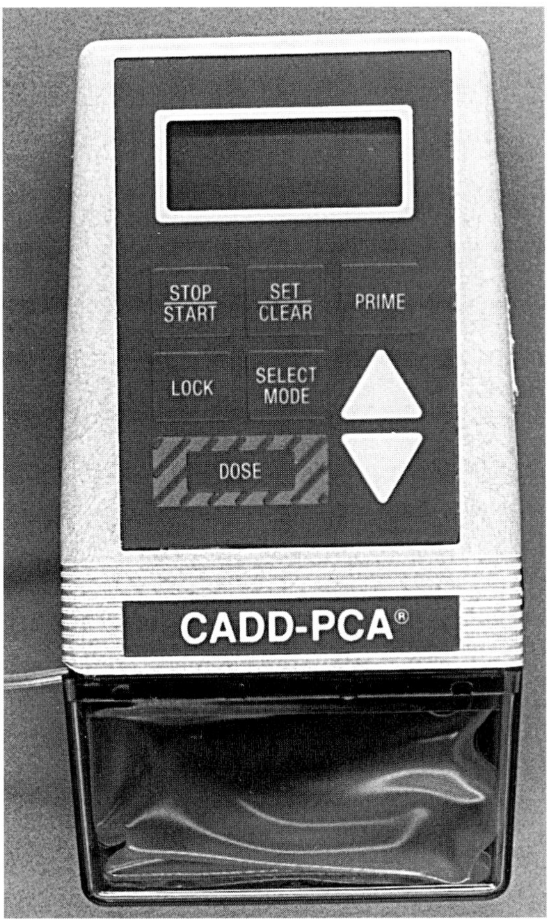


**Fig. 22–14.** Pharmacia pump. (From the Ohio State University Hospitals, Department of Anesthesiology, 1992.)

has recommended that the minimum effective form or dose of analgesia/anesthesia be employed for the laboring patient. This minimum effective analgesia/anesthesia may be either a regional or parenteral method. When parenteral analgesia is chosen, the intramuscular route of administration should be generally avoided because high maternal blood levels are not obtained, absorption is variable and erratic, and larger doses are required. In general, incremental intravenous doses of meperidine (25 mg) or butorphanol (1 mg) with or without promethazine (25 mg), promazine (20 mg), or hydroxyzine (50 mg—intramuscular only) should suffice it in providing adequate systemic analgesia for most parturients. As a general rule, drugs that are not FDA approved or manufacturer-recommended for intrapartum analgesia should be avoided unless they are a part of an ongoing study.

Petrie, et al (53) have studied the effects of various analgesics on the fetal heart rate recorded via electronic fetal monitoring. All narcotics and sedatives have been shown to decrease beat-to-beat variability of the fetal heart rate (53). This decrease in beat-to-beat variability occurs 10 minutes following intravenous administration of meperidine and begins to recover approximately 30 minutes following injection (53). Teramo noted that this decrement of fetal beat-to-beat heart variability was not associated with changes in acid-base status of the fetus (54). Additionally, all narcotics (particularly alphaprodine) have produced a sinusoidal fetal heart rate pattern following intravenous administration (55). This sinusoid pattern has not been shown to be of pathologic consequence to the fetus (56). Kliger and Nelson administered meperidine with and without promazine and found no significant change in Apgar score until greater than 200 mg of meperidine was administered intrapartum (57).

In 1970, Brazelton drew attention to the possibility that drug administration to the mother intrapartum might interfere with imprinting responses in both mothers and infants (58). Since 1970, many studies using the Brazelton neonatal behavioral assessment scale (59), the Scanlon early neonatal neurobehavioral scale (60), the Brackbill habituation rate of the orienting reflex (61), and the Bayley mental and motor infant scales (62) have failed to demonstrate significant neonatal effects when usual clinical doses of parenteral analgesic drugs are administered to the laboring patient.

### *Drugs Used Frequently*

The following drugs are used frequently in management of the parturient. They are mentioned here in conjunction with management of the first stage of labor in centers that are not highly developed and have full-time anesthesia personnel. In these centers, the obstetrician still has to be responsible for the first stage of labor analgesia and often for the second stage as well. There has been quite a definite tendency over the past few years to administer these drugs to patients via the intravenous route in small dosages rather than the intramuscular route in large dosages as was the custom in the past.

***Meperidine hydrochloride (Demerol).*** Meperidine was isolated in Germany in 1939. It rapidly supplanted morphine for intrapartum analgesia because it causes less nausea and does not penetrate the blood-brain barrier of the fetus as completely as does morphine (63). It has remained the most commonly-employed narcotic and the reference standard for obstetric analgesia since the 1940s. It is approved by the Food and Drug Administration (FDA) and recommended by all manufacturers for obstetric analgesia. The drug is a FDA class B drug for use during labor and a class D drug for use in early pregnancy. The parenteral forms available are 2.5, 5.0, 7.5, and 10% solutions containing 25, 50, 75, and 100 mg/ml, respectively. The drug is also available in 50 mg tablets. The drug is FDA approved for oral (PO), intramuscular (IM), subcutaneous (SC), intermittent IV, and continuous IV use. Following an intramuscular injection, the onset of action occurs in 15 minutes, the peak action in 40 to 60 minutes, and the duration of action for 2 to 4 hours. The distribution half-life of meperidine occurs 7.6 minutes following intravenous administration. The clearance rate of the drug is unrelated to pregnancy. Sixty percent of meperidine is plasma protein bound in the mother and 28% in the fetus and neonate (64). The drug exerts little if any effect on uterine activity (65). The principal metabolites of meperidine include normeperidine, meperidinic acid,

**Table 22–11.** Drugs Utilized for Intrapartum Analgesia

| Drug and Year of Introduction | Protein Binding (%) | Half-Life (hr) | Opioid Receptors Affected* | Average IV Dose (mg) | Dosage Interval (hr) | Onset (min) | Duration (hr) |
|---|---|---|---|---|---|---|---|
| Meperidine (Demerol), 1939 | 60 | 2.4–4.0 | mu(+), kappa(+) | 25–50 | 2–4 | 3–5 | 2–3 |
| Morphine (Duramorph), 1806 | 10–34 | 2.0–3.0 | mu(+), kappa(+) | 2–4 | 3–4 | 10 | 4–5 |
| Butorphanol (Stadol), 1978 | 65–90 | 2.5–4.0 | kappa(+), sigma(+) | 1–2 | 3–4 | 2–3 | 3–4 |
| Nalbuphine (Nubain), 1979 | 60–70 | 3.0–6.0 | mu(−), kappa(p), sigma(?) | 2–4 | 3–4 | 2–3 | 3–6 |
| Pentazocaine (Talwin), 1967 | 35–64 | 2.0–3.0 | mu(−), kappa(p), sigma(?) | 20–30 | 3–4 | 2–3 | 2–3 |

(+) = stimulation
(−) = inhibition
(p) = partial stimulation
(?) = effect not well established
(Modified from Dilts PV Jr: Selection of analgesia and anesthesia. Clin. Obstet. Gynecol. 24:521, 1981; Abboud TK, Artal R, Henriksen EH, Earl S, et al: Effects of spinal anesthesia on maternal circulating catecholamines. Am. J. Obstet. Gynecol. 142:252, 1982; Kliger B, Nelson HB: Analgesia and fetal depression with intravenous meperidine and propriomazine. Am. J. Obstet. Gynecol. 92:850, 1965; Hogg MIJ, Wiener PC, Rosen M, Mapleson WW: Urinary excretion and metabolism of pethidine and norpethidine in the newborn. Br. J. Anaesth. 49:891, 1977; Morrison JC, Whybrew WD, Rosser SI, Bucovaz ET, et al: Metabolites of meperidine in the fetal and maternal serum. Am. J. Obstet. Gynecol. 126:997, 1976; Powe CE, Kiem IM, Hagen C, Cavanagh D: Propiomazine hydrochloride in obstetrical analgesia. JAMA 181:290, 1962.

normeperidinic acid, and meperidine N-oxide. In general, only intravenous meperidine should be utilized during labor. Standard dosages and other information for utilization of meperidine is included in Table 22–11. The umbilical cord to maternal blood ratio of meperidine following IV injection and equilibration is 0.75 to 1 (66). Fetal equilibrium is reached 6 minutes following intravenous administration to the mother (67). There are three metabolic patterns for maternal elimination of meperidine with neonatal depression occurring more frequently with the type III pattern (68). Chronic maternal phenobarbital administration can induce hepatic microsomal enzyme production, increasing metabolism of meperidine to normeperidine, thereby increasing neonatal depression (normeperidine is probably responsible for most neonatal depression) (69). Maximum neonatal depression occurs 2 to 4 hours following intravenous administration to the mother. The degree of neonatal depression is dependent upon neonatal gestational age and the presence or absence of asphyxia (70). The earlier the gestational age, the greater the neonatal depression for a given degree of asphyxia. The elimination half-life of meperidine in the neonate is 18.1 hours (2.4 hours in the mother) while the half-life of normeperidine is 62 hours (71). Ninety-five percent of meperidine is eliminated from the neonate in 2 to 3 days, with the greatest excretion occurring in the first day (72). Neurobehavioral changes last up to 60 to 72 hours following delivery in neonates whose mothers received demerol analgesia; however, these changes do not appear if less than 2 mg/kg meperidine is given to the mother (73). When more than 200 mg meperidine is given to the mother, hypercarbia appears in the neonate but this does not significantly alter pH (74). This hypercarbia appears related predominantly to the presence of normeperidine. Feeding, rooting, and sucking reflexes do not appear to be altered with meperidine administration to the gravida (75).

***Butorphanol (Stadol).*** Butorphanol (Stadol) is a synthetic parenteral analgesic with agonist-antagonist properties. This drug was first introduced in 1978. It is approved by the FDA and the manufacturer for use as an obstetric analgesic. The drug is an FDA class B drug for labor and class D for use in early pregnancy. The drug is FDA approved for intramuscular and intermittent intravenous use. It is available in solutions containing either 1 or 2 mg/ml. Butorphanol has a potency that is 5 times that of morphine, 20 times that of pentazocine, and 40 times that of meperidine. Butorphanol is 80% protein bound in the mother. The onset of action of the drug occurs 10 minutes following intravenous injection and its action persists for 3 to 4 hours with a half-life of elimination of 2.7 hours. Butorphanol is metabolized predominantly in the liver by dealkylation and hydroxylation followed by conjugation to inactive metabolites. Excretion of the drug occurs mainly via the kidney by glomerular filtration with a small contribution by the biliary system. The respiratory-depression effects of 2 mg of butorphanol are similar to 10 mg of morphine. However, there appears to be a plateau effect with further administration of butorphanol. Four milligrams of butorphanol produce substantially less respiratory depression than 20 mg of morphine. Both the respiratory and narcotic effects of butorphanol are reversed with naloxone. Butorphanol rapidly crosses the placenta. The umbilical venous to maternal venous ratio is 0.84 following equilibration 1 1/2 hours after administration to the mother (76). Quilligan, et al (77) compared meperidine and butorphanol for relief of pain occurring during labor and found that butorphanol provided superior analgesia. Hodgkinson, et al (78) noted that butorphanol provided excellent analgesia for labor with no neurobehavioral effects on the neonate. Many consider butorphanol to be the analgesic of choice for the parturient, and this drug is rapidly gaining in popularity for this indication. Its advantages include: (1) the drug is an excellent, potent analgesic; (2) its metabolites are inactive; (3) there is minimal risk of maternal respiratory depression; and (4) no demonstrable neonatal neurobehavioral effects have been observed. The recommended dosage and other information are included in Table 22–11.

***Nalbuphine (Nubain).*** Nalbuphine (Nubain) was first introduced in 1979. The drug is approved by the FDA and the manufacturer for intrapartum analgesia. There have been very few studies evaluating this drug as an obstetric analgesic and it has failed to gain popularity for this indication (79). The drug is available in either 10 or 20 mg/ml solutions. It is FDA approved for intramuscular, subcutaneous, or intermittent intravenous use. Nalbuphine is a synthetic agonist-antagonist with pharmacologic properties similar to pentazocine and butorphanol. Its potency is equivalent to morphine on a milligram basis. The onset of action of the drug following intravenous injection is 2 to 3 minutes, its duration of action 5 to 6 hours, and its half-life of elimination 5 hours. Similar to butorphanol, nalbuphine has a plateau effect for respiratory depression reached when 30 mg of the drug has been administered. It is metabolized predominantly by the liver and excreted by the kidney. Dosages for administration and other data is contained in Table 22–11. Naloxone reverses the respiratory depression that can occur secondary to nalbuphine.

***Pentazocine (Talwin).*** Pentazocine is a synthetic analgesic with both opioid agonist and weak antagonist properties. The drug is approved by both the FDA and the manufacturer for intrapartum analgesia. Analgesia occurs 2 to 3 minutes following intravenous injection. The elimination half-life of the drug is 2 hours. There is extensive variation in metabolism of the drug by various individuals. Sixty percent of the drug is excreted predominantly as metabolites in the urine within 24 hours of administration. Doses in excess of 60 mg may be associated with psychomimetic effects such as hallucinations and nightmares. Advantages claimed for pentazocine include less nausea, emesis, and postural hypotension than meperidine (80). Less placental transfer of pentazocine than meperidine occurs; however, the incidence of neonatal depression appears equal with equipotent dosages of the two drugs (81). The respiratory-depressant effects of Talwin also appear to plateau compared to morphine. Pentazocine has failed to gain popularity as an obstetric analgesic secondary to its lack of clear advantages and its psychomimetic effects. Table 22–11 lists drug dosages for use intrapartum and other information. Naloxone reverses the respiratory depression that can occur secondary to this drug.

***Meperidine—promethazine (Mepergan).*** Meperidine in combination with promethazine has been utilized extensively for intrapartum analgesia. The use of promethazine appears to decrease the amount of meperidine required to achieve adequate obstetric analgesia without increasing the risk of neonatal depression (82). In general, the total dose of promethazine should be limited to 50 mg during labor. Mepergan supplies 25 mg meperidine and 25 mg promethazine per milliliter. Mepergan is approved by both the manufacturer and the FDA for intrapartum analgesia.

***Fentanyl—droperidol (Innovar).*** The manufacturer recommends against the use of Innovar in laboring patients. Ovadia and Halbrecht (83) administered Innovar to 100 laboring patients and found the drug more effective than meperidine-promethazine combinations, and none of the neonates required resuscitation. However, data are insufficient to make routine use of Innovar in the laboring patient advisable. Fentanyl has been used by itself successfully in labor as an analgesic and has been well-received to-date with no adverse maternal or fetal effects noted, although it is not approved by the FDA or the manufacturer for this indication.

***Naloxone (Narcan).*** Naloxone has been employed in three ways for laboring patients: (1) to the mother with each dose of narcotic; (2) to the mother 10 to 15 minutes before delivery; and (3) routinely to the neonate immediately after delivery. All of these methods for naloxone utilization are now considered inadvisable. Narcan should be administered only when narcotic overdosage is considered likely. The usual dosage of Narcan for the gravida is 0.4 mg intravenously and 0.01 mg/kg for the neonate.

***Phenothiazines.*** These drugs are major tranquilizers believed to act by blocking receptors to dopamine and norepinephrine in the brain. The exact mechanism of action remains poorly defined, but is probably centered in the basal ganglia and limbic portions of the forebrain (84). Most phenothiazines are potentially associated with extrapyramidal side effects as evidence of interference with the normal actions of dopamine. Phenothiazines are metabolized principally by oxidation and conjugation in the liver. Most metabolites are pharmacologically inactive. Metabolites appear predominantly in urine for elimination. The predominant immediate side effects of phenothiazines that are of consequence to the laboring patient are cardiovascular responses, extrapyramidal reactions, lowered seizure threshold, and allergic reactions. Intravenous administration of phenothiazines can cause a significant reduction in blood pressure due to: (1) hypothalamic or brain stem-mediated depression of vasomotor reflexes; (2) peripheral-adrenergic blockade; (3) direct relaxant effects on vascular smooth muscle; and (4) direct myocardial depression. EKG changes, which can occur secondary to phenothiazines, include prolongation of the PR and QT intervals and S-T segment depression. Acute dystonic reactions characterized by facial grimacing, torticollis, lateral jaw movements, smacking of the lips, and sudden forward thrusts of the tongue may occur with the administration of phenothiazines. Phenothiazines lower the seizure threshold and may prompt seizures in some patients. EEG changes that occur following administration of phenothiazines include an increase in burst and spike activity and decreased amplitude of sensory-evoked potentials. Finally, approximately 1% of patients given an intravenous phenothiazine will experience an allergic reaction. These reactions most commonly are mild and self- limited. Long-term consequences of phenothiazine therapy that may be of concern to the obstetrician/anesthesiologist include the neuroleptic malignant syndrome and obstructive jaundice (85,86). Neuroleptic malignant syndrome develops typically over 24 to 72 hours and is characterized by hyperthermia, hypertonicity of skeletal muscles, instability of the autonomic nervous system manifest by alterations in blood pressure, tachycardia or cardiac dysrhythmia, and fluctuating levels of consciousness; this occurs in 0.1% of patients treated with phenothiazines. Obstructive jaundice is considered to be an allergic reaction. It occurs in 1% of patients treated with phenothiazines 2 to 4 weeks following the administration of phenothiazines and is self-limiting if no additional phenothiazines are administered.

## Drugs Used Infrequently for Analgesia

The following drugs are used infrequently or no longer used today in management of the parturient. They are mentioned here not only for historical footnote and background but also to emphasize the point that they are better not used in current day management of laboring patients.

***Barbiturates.*** Because barbiturates are not analgesics, these agents may interfere with normal coping mechanisms, and when used alone may worsen the laboring gravida's perception of pain (87). The combination of a narcotic and barbiturate increases the degree of neonatal depression (88) and may alter the neonate's attention span for 2 to 4 days (89). Additionally, barbiturates may produce excitement, restlessness, and disorientation in some gravidae (90). For these reasons, barbiturates are no longer popular, nor advisable during labor for most women.

***Benzodiazepines.*** The most common benzodiazepines in use in clinical medicine are diazepam, lorazepam, midazolam, flurazepam, and chlordiazepoxide. Similar to barbiturates, these drugs are not analgesics and have the potential for altering normal pain-coping mechanisms in gravidae. Diazepam is the best studied of this class of drugs in the laboring patient (91). Diazepam, given to parturients, alters normal temperature regulation in newborns rendering them less capable of maintaining their body temperature (92). This effect in the newborn may persist for as long as 1 week (93). Additionally, diazepam competes with bilirubin for binding to albumin, increasing the likelihood of hyperbilirubinemia or kernicterus in the newborn (94). For these reasons, this class of drugs is considered inadvisable in the laboring gravida.

***Scopolamine.*** Scopolamine is an anticholinergic sedative with amnesic effects. It has no analgesic properties and frequently prompts bizarre behavior. It generally has no place in the modern practice of obstetrics.

***Promethazine.*** Promethazine (Phenergan), propiomazine (Largon), and hydroxyzine (Vistaril) are approved by the FDA and manufacturer for use in the laboring patient and are frequently employed and popular agents in combination with narcotics. These drugs, by relieving anxiety, reduce the narcotic requirements of parturients. Additionally, their antiemetic properties are valuable to reduce the nausea and vomiting that may occur in laboring patients. They are most commonly employed in combination with narcotics. Neither promethazine nor hydroxyzine in combination with narcotics has been found to produce additional neonatal depression (95,96) Table 22–12 summarizes dosages, dosage intervals, etc., of commonly employed phenothiazines.

***Others.*** Once popular narcotic analgesics such as alphaprodine (Nisentil) and anileridine (Leritine) are no longer marketed in the United States. Other marketed narcotics such as fentanyl (Sublimaze), sufentanil (Sufenta), codeine, buprenorphine (Buprenex), oxymorphone (Numorphan), hydromorphone (Dilaudid) are not approved by the FDA nor recommended by the manufacturer for use as intrapartum analgesics.

***Morphine (Duramorph).*** Morphine is approved by the FDA and the manufacturer for use as an obstetric analgesic. In equianalgesic doses, morphine produces more neonatal depression than meperidine (63). Because of its increased neonatal depression, delayed onset of action, and prolonged duration of action, it is infrequently employed for obstetric analgesia presently and generally considered inadvisable for this indication.

## Basic Pharmacology of Narcotic Analgesics

Narcotic analgesics act as agonists to specific stereoreceptors and saturable receptors present in the brain and other tissues. The L-isomer of the opioid appears to be the main isomer that produces analgesia. For the opioid to exert its effect, a tertiary positively-charged nitrogen, a quaternary carbon that is separated from this nitrogen by an ethane chain, and an aromatic ring must be present in the body of the opioid.

Opioid receptors were first described in 1973 (97). The highest concentrations of the receptors appear to be present in the limbic system, thalamus, hypothalamus, and the substantia gelatinosa of the spinal cord (98). These receptors have been divided into five classes: Mu ($\mu$), Delta ($\delta$), Kappa ($\kappa$), Sigma ($\sigma$), and Epsilon ($\epsilon$) (99). Mu receptors are further subdivided into $\mu 1$ and $\mu 2$ receptors. $\mu 1$ receptor-mediated responses include supraspinal analgesia (periaqueductal gray, nucleus raphe, magnus, and locus coeruleus), prolactin release, free and depriva-

**Table 22–12.** Adjunctive Drugs for Intrapartum Analgesia

| Drug and Year of Introduction | Average IV Dosage (mg) | Dosage Interval (hr) | Onset (min) | Duration (hr) |
|---|---|---|---|---|
| Promethazine (Phenergan), 1955 | 25–50 | 4–6 | 5 | 4–6 |
| Propiomazine (Largon), 1961 | 20–40 | 4–6 | 5 | 4–6 |
| Hydroxyzine (Vistaril), 1960 | (50–100)* | 4–6 | 15–30 | 4–6 |

* Intramuscular only.

(Modified from Scher J, Hailey DM, Beard RW: The effects of diazepam on the fetus. J. Obstet. Gynecol. Br. Commonw. 79:635, 1972; McAllister CB: Placenta transfer and neonatal effects of diazepam when administered to women just before delivery. Br. J. Anesthesia 52:423, 1980; Cree IE, Meyer J, Hailey DM: Diazepam in labor: Its metabolism and effect on the clinical condition and thermogenesis of the newborn. Br. Med. J. 4:251, 1973.)

tion-induced feeding, acetycholine turnover in the brain, and catalepsy. μ2 receptors mediate respiratory depression, growth hormone release, dopamine turnover in the brain, gastrointestinal tract motility, euphoria, and most cardiovascular effects of narcotics, including decreased heart rate. Delta (δ) receptors appear to function mainly as modulators of μ receptors but they also appear vital for spinal analgesia. Stimulation of Sigma (σ) receptors appears to produce mainly pyschotomimetic effects in patients. Epsilon (ε) receptors are responsible for most of the hormonal actions of opioids. It would appear that various receptor-specific opioids could produce maximal analgesia while minimizing undesirable side effects of opioids. Numerous research investigations are presently underway to identify receptor-specific agents.

In 1975, enkephalin, an endogenous opioid-like ligand that is produced by the body, was first reported (100). Since that time, numerous other endorphins have been reported: (1) leu-enkephalin, (2) met-enkephalin, (3) β-endorphin, (4) Dynorphin A, (5) Dynorphin B, (6) α-neo-endorphine, and (7) β-neo-endorphine (101). All of these ligands appear to modulate a person's pain response by binding to the five classes of opioid receptors previously described.

Painful sensations are transmitted to the spinal cord through nerve fibers that synapse in the dorsal horns in laminae I, II, and V where they ascend to the brain through the spinothalamic tract. The spinothalamic tract is composed of two divisions, the neospinothalamic tract and the paleospinothalamic tract. The neospinothalamic tract terminates in the ventral posterolateral nucleus of the thalamus which projects to the somatosensory cortex allowing determination of quality, intensity, and location of pain. The paleospinothalamic tract, conversely, is polysynaptic with connections to the reticular and limbic systems and subcortical areas of the brain. This system carries the "hurt" associated with painful stimuli. These two systems mediate so-called "first" and "second" pain. Stimulation of opioid receptors modulate both of these traits; however, the paleospinothalamic tract is influenced to a greater degree. This accounts for why patients who receive narcotics still perceive their pain but do not "care" as much about the pain.

Direct effects experienced by patients who receive narcotics include drowsiness, mental clouding, sleepiness, difficulty in mentation, euphoria, and apathy. Continuous dull pain appears to be relieved more effectively than is sharp intermittent pain. Patients continue to recognize that they are experiencing pain but their physical and emotional response to that pain is significantly blunted.

The side effects of most narcotics can be divided into cardiovascular, respiratory, neural, renal, gastrointestinal, and hormonal. Most narcotics can produce significant hypotension with intravenous injection. This hypotensive response may be worsened by the concomitant administration of phenothiazines. This hypotension appears mediated predominantly by direct arterial and venous dilation and by the release of endogenous histamine. Other cardiovascular side effects of narcotics include bradycardia, supraventricular tachycardia, decreased A-V conduction, and cardiac arrest (102–104). Respiratory actions of narcotics include decreased hypoxic ventilatory drive, altered respiratory rhythmicity, decreased bronchial ciliary activity, and decreased cough reflex (102–104). These respiratory effects are rarely of clinical significance in the young, healthy parturient. Renal effects of narcotics, again of minimal clinical significance, include increased release of ADH, decreased renal blood flow, reduced urine output with increased urinary osmolality, and increased ureteral and detrusor tone (102–104). Gastrointestinal (GI) actions of narcotics include nausea and emesis secondary to stimulation of the chemoreceptor trigger zone, decreased hydrochloric acid secretion by the stomach, decreased overall secretions by the gastrointestinal tract, decreased gastrointestinal motility, and increased sphincter tone and biliary tract pressure (102–104). Well-established hormonal effects of narcotics include blunting of the "surgical stress response," decreased plasma cortisol, lactate, luteinizing hormone and thyrotropin, and increased plasma catecholamines and prolactin.

Most narcotics are metabolized in the liver by hydrolysis and/or N-demethylation followed by conjugation with gluconic acid. Small amounts of free narcotic and the conjugated metabolites are excreted predominantly through the kidney by glomerular filtration. Approximately 10% of an administered dose of a narcotic is also eliminated in feces. Enterohepatic circulation of narcotics does occur.

Narcotics are contraindicated in patients receiving monoamine oxidase inhibitors (104). These drugs should be used with caution in patients with myxedema, multiple sclerosis, emphysema, kyphoscoliosis, obesity, cor pulmonale, asthma, seizure disorders, Addison's disease, liver disease, renal disease, chronic lung disease, hypercapnia, and supraventricular tachycardia. Narcotic antagonists and resuscitation equipment should be immediately available whenever narcotics are employed. When phenothiazines or other central nervous system depressants are concomitantly used, the narcotic dosage should be reduced by 25 to 50%. Adverse reactions to narcotics are generally responsive to control of the respiration via a patent airway; IV naloxone, oxygen therapy, intravenous fluids, and vasopressors are indicated.

### *Regional Analgesia*

The use of epidural analgesia utilizing either local anesthetic agents or opioids is covered extensively in Chapters 13 and 17. Pharmacology of the local anesthetics is covered in Chapter 11. However, because this method is really the most popular analgesic method in demand today in highly developed centers that have anesthesia coverage, and because it is such a superb method of analgesia for the normal laboring patient who is anticipating a vaginal delivery, it will be mentioned here also. In addition, caudal epidural, spinal, paracervical block, and pudendal block will be discussed here as other analgesic methods for pain relief for combined labor and delivery.

### *Lumbar Epidural Block*

This method of analgesia for both labor and delivery when available at highly developed regional centers is today by far the most popular method of pain relief from both the viewpoints of the patient and the obstetrician (105). Over 2 decades ago, around the time of the first edition of this book, this method was still struggling for respectability. It was even then the most powerfully effective method of pain relief and it was demonstrative in its effect, but it was also labor intensive and demanded skilled administrators who just were not available at that time. Now, many more anesthesiologists have dedicated themselves to providing obstetric care and so many training programs have emphasized the use of the method that there now exists new practitioners all over the country who are skilled in use of lumbar epidural for obstetrics.

The catheter is usually placed soon after the patient is admitted to labor and delivery and in progressive labor. Before this, of course, the patient has had the opportunity to discuss the method with her anesthesiologist or a member of his team. Obstetricians who are practicing at centers where the method is used frequently are very enthusiastic and supportive. Activation of the catheter is done only after consultation with the obstetrician and a discussion of the labor progress, any intercurrent problems, and the need as demonstrated by the patient's reaction to the stress of labor. Activation is by use of a small dose of 8 to 10 ml of 0.25 % bupivacaine after a test dose. The patient is then evaluated for effective analgesia, level of blockade, and any reactions. If all is well, the patient is then given a continuous dosage of a combination of bupivacaine, sufentanil, and epinephrine. This mixture is pumped continuously throughout labor. The patient is reevaluated every 1, 2, or 3 hours depending on need, and the mixture is continued if all goes well. Often for delivery, the patient will have an effective sacral block so that supplemental perineal analgesia will not be necessary. If this is not the case, then either a pudendal block, a subarachnoid block, or $N_2O$ can be used for the perineal supplement.

As mentioned, this is the most popular method of anesthesiologists for first and second stage obstetric analgesia. The reason for this popularity is straightforward from both the physician and patient viewpoints. The physician views it as an effective and a proven, safe technique for pain relief. The patient views it as being compatible with the desire to be awake and alert during the birth process. Like the caudal block, it entails local anesthetic injection into the epidural space; in contrast with the caudal technique, puncture is made in the lumbar or lower thoracic spinal region. Spinal epidural block was first achieved unintentionally by Corning in 1884 (106) but the technique was not used clinically until 1921, when Pages used it for surgery (107). A decade later, Dogliotti reported on his extensive studies, which placed the technique on a sound anatomic and pharmacodynamic basis, and made it popular in some surgical centers (108). In 1938, Graffagnino and Seyler reported the results of its use in obstetrics (109). Despite these and other sporadic reports, its use in obstetrics remained limited for another 2 decades. During this interval, two important developments took place that later contributed to the popularity of epidural block. One of these was the introduction of lidocaine, chloroprocaine, and other more penetrant local anesthetics; the other was the introduction of the continuous catheter technique. Soon after Lemmon's description of continuous spinal anesthesia, Hingson and Southworth considered use of the same equipment for epidural block, but technical difficulties in keeping the needle in place convinced them to abandon the idea in favor of continuous caudal block. The needle placement problem was solved by Curbelo, who threaded a ureteral catheter through a Tuohy needle. In 1949, he reported use of the continuous epidural block for surgery (110). Also in 1949, Flowers, Hellman, and Hingson (111) described the use of vinyl plastic tubing for continuous epidural block in obstetric patients, and Cleland (112) described a refinement of the technique—use of the double catheter technique. In 1954, Bromage published his excellent monograph on epidural block and subsequently studied and clarified many of the physicochemical bases of the method (113). During the past decade, the method has become increasingly popular among anesthesiologists. It is currently the most widely used technique in obstetrics. Hellmann (114) and Eisen and associates (115) published results on its use in over 26,000 vaginal and cesarean section deliveries. Reports on its use in large obstetric series have also been published by Bodell and associates (116), Chaplin and Renwick (117), Lund and associates (118), MacMillan (119), Moore and his associates (120), Schaudig (121), and Volpi (122) among others. During the past decades, the editors and many of the authors of chapters in this book have used this method for thousands of vaginal and abdominal deliveries.

## Caudal Block

This method of epidural offers a very special advantage for patients who abhor the idea of having a needle placed "into their back or spine." These patients can be told that this method is similar to the epidural technique but different from the placement or administration of the needle into the epidural space.

***Low Caudal Block.*** This block of segments S1 through S5 relieves the pain of perineal distention and provides excellent second stage analgesia for vaginal manipulations, but it is not effective for relief of the pain of uterine contractions. Separate analgesia for uterine pain can be obtained with the segmental epidural method of analgesia. Low caudal block can begin as soon as the parturient has moderate to severe perineal distension and discomfort.

***Mid-Caudal Block.*** When a caudal block is properly carried out and includes all the sensory fibers of spinal nerves T10 through S5, it relieves labor pain completely in 90 to 95% of parturients. However, 5 to 10% will have some discomfort in the back, and flanks if the fetal occiput is posterior in the pelvis. In such patients, pain impulses of labor from specified areas may either reach the spinal cord through segments higher than the tenth thoracic neurotome, or the intensity of analgesia may not be sufficient to block the strong second stage noxious impulses.

In past years, caudal block was often administered only at the last moment, i.e., sometime at the end of the first stage of labor. If little or ineffective analgesia was present at that time, the administrator was incumbered by movement of the patient and distress of the situation in general. Today, preplanning and consideration of catheter insertion at an early time in the first stage of labor, before the patient is uncomfortable, is recommended. This offers many advantages, including:

1. early catheter insertion is initiated when labor discomfort is minimal;
2. early catheter placement minimizes inadequate analgesia if labor progresses rapidly;
3. early catheter insertion minimizes the risk of the most serious complication caudal block puncture of the fetal head.

Consideration number two is especially important in multiparae, who are often deprived of the benefit of caudal analgesia because the procedure is postponed until there is not enough time to perform the technique and obtain analgesia. It is prudent to consider the catheter technique to be used exclusively for obstetrics, and that the single-dose technique be rarely used. Activation of the block with injection of local anesthetic depends on:

1. whether labor is spontaneous or induced;
2. severity of the pain;
3. obstetric conditions such as use of oxytocins, manual rotation, and use of outlet forceps; and,
4. special indications such as maternal cardiac disease.

For induced labor, caudal block may be started at the beginning of the induction or sometime during the latent phase (123–125). However, caudal in conjunction with lumbar epidural block is the ideal method during induction of labor, because both provide differential continuous pain relief without altering the response of the uterus to oxytocin (126). By administering the oxytocic physiologically, one ensures that labor progresses at a near normal rate, even though the caudal block may interfere with Ferguson's reflex and result in delayed second stage completion. When properly applied and rigidly supervised, the combination of elective induction of labor and early continuous caudal analgesia combined with lumbar epidural is especially useful when maternal or obstetric conditions dictate induction of labor such as toxemia or diabetes.

For spontaneous labor uncomplicated by maternal disease or obstetric difficulty, the conditions outlined in Table 22–13 should exist before caudal block is started.

**Table 22–13.** Mandatory Conditions Before Establishment of Caudal Block

1. parturient should be in active labor and experiencing moderate to severe pain during uterine contractions;
2. contractions should be regular, of good intensity, and occurring at intervals of 3 minutes or less and lasting 35 to 40 seconds or longer;
3. presenting part should be engaged in the pelvis; and
4. cervix should be dilated to 4 to 5 cm in multiparae and 5 to 6 cm in primiparae.

(Developed from data in Bonica JJ: Principles and Practice of Obstetric Analgesia and Anesthesia. Philadelphia, F.A. Davis Co., 1967, p. 575.)

Characteristically, it is not necessary to start the caudal block earlier, because most parturients can be sustained with psychologic support and small doses of sedatives and narcotics. However, analgesia can be started earlier if the parturient has heart disease or other disorders that require reduction of the hemodynamic and metabolic effects of labor. Caudal block can also be started early if the infant is premature or if other obstetric complications preclude the use of narcotics during early labor. It may also be prudent to postpone caudal block until the beginning of the second stage of labor if the obstetrician prefers not to use oxytocics to augment uterine contractions or manual/forceps rotation of the fetus, as caudal block may interfere with both mechanisms.

## *Spinal Block*

This technique is used now for the second stage of labor and in a continuous manner for the first and second stage. It offers great flexibility and is the only method of administration of local anesthetics in which the drug is screened from the fetus by being compartmentalized by the subarachnoid space. The spinal block is again another example of a method given originally by the obstetrician for the delivery stage when there was not adequate coverage in obstetrics by anesthesiologists. The method may have been designed initially for the primiparous patient who after laboring for hours could look forward to an assisted, comfortable delivery by the obstetrician giving a saddle block in the sitting position. The primary goal is to effect second stage pain relief and to do it in a safe manner; thus, it is necessary to monitor blood pressure carefully so that trends toward any hypotension can be detected early. Management of this type of hypotension is quite simple and effective by just position alone usually and sometime by injection of a mild vasopressor such as 10 mg of ephedrine intravenously.

In some centers still not staffed by anesthesiologists, the obstetrician does perform saddle block for delivery with close monitoring done by CRNAs; or monitoring in some instances by RNs who are specially trained by CRNAs or the anesthesiologists to attend to and diagnose and report important changes immediately. Here, again, is another example of an area in which the nurse has a very much appreciated and important role in the framework of the team effort. It must be emphasized that the obstetrician *must not* perform this method of analgesia if adequately trained assistance is not available. There were many examples of serious complications in the 1940s and 1950s because of just such a scenario.

There was a time when spinal block was administered for either multiparous or primiparous patients near complete dilation so that they could benefit from analgesia for the last few centimeters of dilatation and also benefit from an effective perineal block for delivery. Today this is not recommended. However, a modification does now exist that is extremely attractive and that is placement of a small catheter during labor and periodic injection for pain relief and injection for perineal block used exclusively for development of a perineal block. This method was described in detail in Chapter 13 on spinal anesthesia, but suffice it to say, it has definite appeal and offers a degree of flexibility heretofore never achieved. Small aliquots of tetracaine may be used for the second stage after use of small doses of morphine or fentanyl for labor pain relief. In addition, if cesarean section becomes necessary, the method can be used for administration of local anesthetic for a spinal effect for satisfactory analgesia for abdominal delivery.

### *Paracervical Block*

The paracervical block is now exceedingly unpopular because there have been so many undisputed reports of adverse fetal-neonatal effects that have caused a full spectrum of problems from minor newborn depression to full-blown severe cerebral incapacitation and even fetal death (127). This is extremely unfortunate because this technique was the primary one available and used by obstetricians for first stage pain relief and because it was used with only a small percent of severe complications. Furthermore, it is believed that those reported adverse effects were due to inappropriate administration with either too rapid administration or too deep administration of drug. It is still a technique that may be performed by the obstetrician in certain parts of the country, but it is rapidly falling into disrepute as an effective alternative nerve block method. Certainly, it can still be an effective maternal analgesic, but unless medications other than local anesthetics, which have been implicated in the aforementioned cerebral damage cases, are developed, paracervical block is unlikely to remain a viable choice for first stage pain relief.

### *Pudendal Block*

The pudendal block is another technique the obstetrician mastered because it is similar to the local infiltration block of the perineum. Again, it is a method that can be used by the obstetrician this time for second stage analgesia. There must be an appreciation of the fact that the pudendal nerve block necessitates careful deposition of local anesthetic in a narrowly circumscribed area of the pudendal nerve where it closely approaches the ischial spines in its course through the pelvis and on out to the perineum. In skilled hands, it produces a very impressive perineal block for complete pain relief for the second stage of labor. Most often, 10 ml of 2% lidocaine or 10 ml of 0.25% bupivacaine is injected on each side to obtain an adequate block. Though this technique is usually very safe, there have been reports of maternal toxic responses and even maternal infection and abscess formation. Because the pudendal nerve is the major peripheral nerve supplying the lower vagina and perineum, it is sufficient to produce perineal anesthesia for spontaneous delivery, low forceps delivery, episiotomy and repair. It is simply not necessary to block other adjacent located nerves such as the ilioinguinal, genital branch of the genitofemoral, and perineal branch of the posterior femoral cutaneous nerve. This, of course, simplifies the technique and adds to its popularity. Because it is a peripheral nerve, one can obtain satisfactory analgesia with use of dilute solutions of local anesthetics, such as 0.5% lidocaine or 0.125% bupivacaine; this adds an advantage of little muscle relaxation occurring.

Maternal alterations of any of the major physiologic systems, such as respiratory and cardiovascular, are not of consequence unless a mistake in injection occurs in which the anesthetic is deposited intravenously. Therefore, maternal complications that have been reported include: (1) the aforementioned systemic toxic reaction; (2) local nerve trauma; (3) vaginal hematoma; (4) infection through the greater sciatic foramen into the joint capsule of the ipsilateral femur; and (5) inadvertent injection of an epinephrine solution that resulted in maternal/fetal death.

Because the pudendal block is administered late or at the very end of the first stage of labor, its effect upon labor is of little or no consequence. In brief summary, though it does not alter the intensity, frequency, or duration of uterine activity, it has been blamed for interruption of the afferent limb of the perineal reflex, and thus it may eliminate the urge to utilize the Valsalva's maneuver effectively.

To a large degree, the prime advantage of the pudendal block is its negligible effect upon the fetus/neonate. This assumes, of course, that the technique is properly applied and that the dosages are reasonable. Nevertheless, rapid absorption by the previously mentioned accidental intravascular injection can result in severe problems for both the mother and fetus/neonate.

The pudendal block is effective as a perineal analgesic technique because both the labia majora and minora are supplied primarily by the posterior labial branch of the perineal nerve which is a branch of the pudendal. Only the most inferior aspect of the labia is supplied by the posterior femoral cutaneous nerve and the mons pubis by branches of the ilioinguinal and genitofemoral nerve. These three nerves, of course, are not at all related to the pudendal nerve and subserve as the only nonpudendal nerve structures that innervate the perineum. It is thus apparent that the pudendal nerve is the largest and most important branch of the pudendal plexus that innervates the female perineum and that its structure is complex, composed of somatic sensory, somatic motor, and autonomic vasomotor fibers.

The technique of pudendal nerve block is not simple because of the partial obstruction of the descending fetal head and the anatomic differences in the configuration of the ischial spinous process, which is the landmark for deposition of the local anesthetic, which effectively blocks the pudendal nerve. The most popular of the local anesthetic agents is 1% lidocaine for this deposition. More recently, 1% chloroprocaine has also been used because it offers the advantage of low toxicity. Bupivacaine may also be used and is of longer duration, which may be advantageous in multiparae in which the block is many times performed before complete dilatation. Most often, 10 ml of drug is injected on each side for a total of 20 ml. Performance of the block by the transvaginal approach is certainly the most common and preferred method of pudendal block. In this method, the operator uses the second and third finger of the opposite hand from the side he or she is blocking to position the needle guide into place at

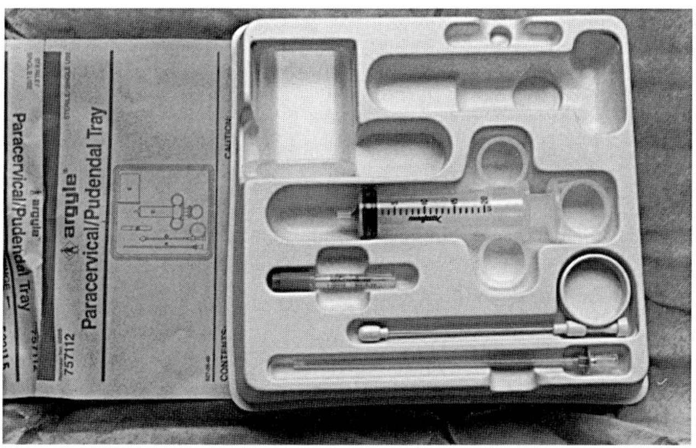


**Fig. 22–15.** Currently available disposable pudendal block set. (From the Ohio State University Hospitals, Department of Anesthesiology, 1992.)

the ischial spine. The needle guide is referred to as the "Iowa trumpet" and is vital to the success of the block, as otherwise, the needle catches repeatedly in the vaginal folds. Note Figure 22–15 which depicts a typical, currently available disposable pudendal block set. After the guide is in place, the operator inserts the needle until the mucosa is contacted. Note Figure 22–16. Then the needle is inserted just a few millimeters and the entire 10 ml slowly injected over 20 to 30 seconds. It is important not to drive the needle as deeply as possible, which may create one of the aforementioned errors in administration; this is due to the fact that the local anesthetic may then

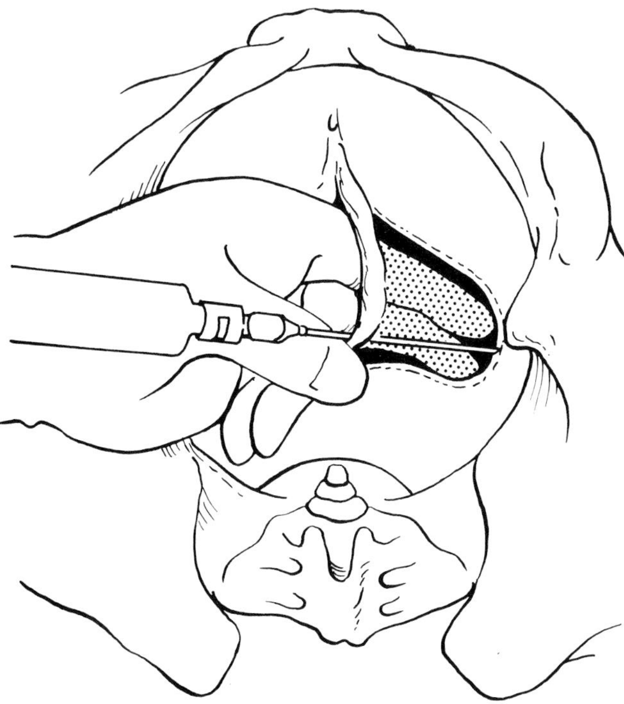

**Fig. 22–16.** Insertion of needle from Figure 22–15, just until the mucosa is contacted.

be deposited behind the course of the pudendal nerve as it sweeps behind the ischial spine on its course down the vagina to the perineum.

## *Local Infiltration Block*

The local infiltration block is accomplished by subcutaneous injection of a local anesthetic. Its primary use is for episiotomy pain. It is typically administered just before maximum perineal distension by injection of 5 to 10 ml of 1% lidocaine without epinephrine. The primary advantage is that small amounts of local anesthetic can be rather indiscriminately injected into the subcutaneous compartment where small nerve endings innervate peripheral tissues. The action is swift because the nerves are small and extremely sensitive to even dilute concentrations of local anesthetic.

One of the first uses of local infiltration or field block was by an obstetrician, Greenhill (128). Although it is a most simple technique to master, its practical application is not always satisfactory because of the difficulty in production of complete second stage pain relief. The primary explanation for this is that although local relief may be adequate for the actual episiotomy, it is not intense enough to obliterate perineal distension pain. It, of course, has no effect on labor, no detrimental maternal effects when properly applied in accepted drug amounts, and no untoward fetal/neonatal effects.

The best method of infiltrating the subcutaneous tissues is to use a small bore (22 gauge), long needle (2 inch), which can be in the form of a spinal needle. This allows point penetration with skin wheal analgesia and subcutaneous infiltration along a path which the needle follows with concomitant local analgesic injection. In this fashion a solid line or block of analgesia can be created subcutaneously for subsequent incision. A few minutes only are required to assure adequate analgesia is obtained by the action of the local anesthetic.

## *Inhalation Analgesia*

When inhalation analgesia is discussed, attention is immediately focused on the Duke Inhaler, a relic of the past, but an instrument so interesting that fascination with it never ends. This device allowed intermittent administration of anesthetic gases such as methoxyflurane or nitrous oxide to be administered by the patient during the first stage, and the so called "safety device" was the inclusion of a wrist strap which would allow the patient to drop the mask from her face upon achieving a satisfactorily deep enough level to lose consciousness (129).

Much more important than the Duke Inhaler is the administration of $N_2O$ as a second stage supplement even today. Actually, even today the use of inhalation analgesia is very effective when administered by an anesthesiologist and when the patient is kept in the first stage or analgesic level. It can be extremely effective as an adjunct to second stage analgesia, which is spotty or incomplete for various reasons. This is today still one of the most underused and underpopularized methods of analgesia, in spite of the fact that it is immediate in onset and quite effective in nearly 100% of cases. It also has minimal deleterious effect on the mother and fetus. For the most part, $N_2O$ is still the agent of choice and is usually administered in 25 to 40% concentration with oxygen either continuously or intermittently as the case necessitates. There is some skill needed in its administration, but this can be learned in a short time with good instruction and a skilled student who is motivated to learn. The method is quite versatile because it can be administered on its own as a sole analgesic for second stage or it can be administered as an adjunct to other methods such as pudendal block, epidural block or subarachnoid block. In the latter two instances, of course, the method would be used to "smooth over" an incomplete block with perhaps an area of skipped analgesia.

Inhalation analgesia refers to the pain relief for a brief period of time during the expulsion phase of the second stage of labor. This method of second stage pain relief is quite old and was used primarily in the 1940s, 1950s, and 1960s for brief periods of pain relief for the mother when no regional technique was available. For the most part, the administration was either by nurse anesthetists, or even by nurses who were simply schooled in the technique of applying a mask to a patient and administration of nitrous oxide/oxygen for a brief period of time during expulsion of the child. Nitrous oxide and oxygen were the favorite combination of inhalation drugs utilized. However, for a period of time, methoxyflurane was available for use and it became quite popular as an agent to combine with pure oxygen. It is no longer used. Earlier, cyclopropane and oxygen were used almost exclusively for this type of second stage analgesia. It should be pointed out that there is a major difference between anesthesia with loss of consciousness and analgesia only with full awareness. The latter technique provides for patient cooperation and alertness, yet because of the small concentrations of the drug being administered offers benefits of pain relief. The technique of inhalation has been and still is quite popular in dental anesthesia in which nitrous oxide and oxygen in 20 to 40% concentrations are still used to ameliorate dental pain. Of course, primary concerns in use of this technique include careful maintenance of the airway and maintenance of a light plane of analgesia. It can also be used today to supplement inadequate blocks for perineal discomfort during second stage expulsion. One of the greatest concerns relevant to use of this technique is making sure the patient does not enter the second stage in which unwanted reflexes such as vomiting occur. Naturally, all obstetric patients are asked to maintain an NPO (nothing by mouth) status when they go into labor, but anyone working in the area of obstetric anesthesia knows their first concern always is to prevent vomiting and this can only be done when it is constantly anticipated. This technique when used in skilled hands can provide an important adjunct for pain relief for the mother while presenting little or no threat to the fetus.

Any of the above-mentioned methods for analgesia for both labor and delivery can be used for successful control of pain, and they can be individualized for the patient so that she feels she is getting the best for herself and her unborn baby. No mother wants to risk the health and welfare of her fetus for pain relief for herself, but if pain relief can be obtained in an environment safe for the fetus, then she will feel comfortable with the concept of pain relief and be appreciative of it and the ability to enjoy the birthing process at the same time.

## POSTPARTUM CARE

### *Patient-Controlled Analgesia*

This modern method of postoperative pain relief is quite dissimilar to the old method of intramuscular injection of opioids, and it is much better due to the fact that only a small portion of the drug is injected into the intravascular compartment at any one time, affording immediate relief to the patient and doing so at smaller dosages than was needed when the intramuscular method was used. The latter method was classically a deposition method whereby a large dose (more than was required at the time) was given in the muscle so that it could be slowly leaked out into the body over time in the intervening 30 to 90 minutes to 120 minutes. The added improvement of the patient-controlled analgesia method (PCA) is that the patient herself remains in control and is able to decide when to administer another dosage based upon pain intensity. Naturally, there are lockout times to protect the patient from overdosing, but for the greatest majority of patients there is a tendency to underdose—not overdose—when it comes to self-medication.

A typical regimen might be:

1. morphine sulphate—1.2 to 2.0 mg per 10 minutes, with maximum of 30 mg in 4 hours;
2. demerol (meperidine)—15 to 20 mg per 10 minutes, with maximum of 200 to 300 mg in 4 hours;
3. dilaudid—0.2 to 0.5 mg per 10 minutes, with maximum of 5 mg in 4 hours.

The patient is able to control injection of analgesia based on her interpretation of her own pain intensity. Lock out times, with maximums being protected by the electronic mechanism of the pump, are for the patient's protection in regard to prevention of respiratory depression. The beauty of pain controlled analgesia method is it places control in the hands of the patient who is experiencing the pain.

### *Continuous Lumbar Epidural Analgesia*

Administration of analgesic concentrations of dilute drugs into the epidural space has become a favorite method of postoperative pain relief. This method offers the ideal situation of blockade of the nociceptive signal before it can reach the central nervous system for recognition. Thus, the signal is blocked at the spinal level and the patient can literally go about her daily routine with little interruption. The patient can ambulate normally, can deep breathe and cough, and can sponge bathe without difficulty. This latter method is said to be the one method that can set the stage for an earlier recovery of the patient and perhaps result in earlier discharge home with less complications. If an epidural was used successfully for labor and delivery, it can be left in place for a small continuous delivery of opioid to achieve just enough pain relief that the patient is happy and comfortable.

Only preservative-free opioids are used for epidural analgesia. This is based on evidence showing preservatives cause neurotoxicity. The epidural opioids are administered to the patient using a combination technique. Initially, the patient is given a bolus followed by a continuous infusion. This method has proven to be the safest and most effective approach.

A typical regimen for this method might be:

1. morphine sulphate—preservative free (PF)—2 to 5 mg diluted to 5 to 10 ml in saline;
2. dilaudid (Hydromorphone HCL)—preservative free (PF)—0.5 to 1.2 mg diluted to 5 to 10 ml in saline;
3. fentanyl citrate—50 to 100 mg diluted to 5 to 10 ml in saline.

A typical regimen for continuous infusion doses might be:

1. morphine sulphate PF—200 to 500 μg/hour;
2. dilaudid (Hydromorphine HCL) PF—80 to 200 μg/hour;
3. fentanyl—50 to 100 μg/hour.

### Patient-Controlled Lumbar Epidural

This is a new approach to postoperative pain relief and is a modification of the lumbar epidural method but by control of the patient similar to the control exercised by the patient controlled analgesia method. Again, the lumbar epidural catheter is left in place and the patient learns to activate the delivery button based upon pain signals. Soon the rhythm of administration is learned and the patient can anticipate the need for a larger or an earlier delivery of medication from time to time. Again, the patient is protected from over-administration by a lock-out device, which is similar to that used in the patient-controlled analgesia method. This latter method may turn out to be the best because it is often discovered that the patients have a great deal of variation in regard to their postoperative pain needs, and there is usually only a very short time for pain to be a major bother in the early recovery period. This method is the newest addition to the pain relief methods and will be evaluated with interest.

## REFERENCES

1. Christiaens GCML, Stoutenbeek PH: Spontaneous abortion in proven intact pregnancies. Lancet 2:572, 1984.
2. Stubblefield P, Berek J: Perinatal mortality in term and postterm births. Obstet. Gynecol. 56:676, 1980.
3. Hook EB: Incidence and prevalence as measures of the frequency of birth defects. Am. J. Epidemol. 116:743, 1982.
4. Kessel SS, Villar J, Berendes HW, Nugent RP: The changing pattern of low birth weight in the United States: 1970 to 1980. JAMA 251:1978, 1984.
5. Sibai BM, Taslimi M, Abdella TN, Brooks TF, et al: Maternal and perinatal outcome of conservative management of severe preeclampsia in midtrimester. Am. J. Obstet. Gynecol. 152:32, 1985.
6. Garcia R, Garcia J: Women's views of care during pregnancy and childbirth. *In* Effective Care in Pregnancy and Childbirth. Vol 1. Edited by I Chalmers, M Enkin, MJNC Keirse. New York, Oxford University Press, 1989, p. 131.
7. Keirse MJNC: Interaction between primary and secondary care during pregnancy and childbirth. *In* Effective Care in Pregnancy and Childbirth. Vol 1. Edited by I Chalmers, M Enkin, MJNC Keirse. New York, Oxford University Press, 1989, p. 197.
8. Chalmers I: Evaluating the effects of care during pregnancy and childbirth. *In* Effective Care in Pregnancy and Childbirth. Vol 1. Edited by I Chalmers, M Enkin, MJNC Keirse. New York, Oxford University Press, 1989, p. 3.
9. Chalmers I, Hetherington J, Elbourne D, Keirse MJNC, etal: Materials and methods used in synthesizing evidence to evaluate the effects of care during pregnancy and childbirth. *In* Effective Care in Pregnancy and Childbirth. Vol 1. Edited by I Chalmers, M Enkin, MJNC Keirse. New York, Oxford University Press, 1989, p. 39.
10. Robinson S: The role of the midwife: opportunities and constraints. *In* Effective Care in Pregnancy and Childbirth. Vol 1. Edited by I Chalmers, M Enkin, MJNC Keirse. New York, Oxford University Press, 1989, p. 162.
11. Ramito P: Unhappiness after childbirth. *In* Effective Care in Pregnancy and Childbirth. Vol 1. Edited by I Chalmers, M Enkin, MJNC Keirse. New York, Oxford University Press, 1989, p. 1433.
12. Shearer MH: Maternal patients' movements in the United States, 1820–1985. *In* Effective Care in Pregnancy and Childbirth. Vol 1. Edited by I Chalmers, M Enkin, MJNC Keirse. New York, Oxford University Press, 1989, p. 110.
13. Scott JR, Rose NR: Effect of psychoprophylaxis (Lamaze preparation) on labor and delivery in primiparas. N. Engl. J. Med. 294:1205, 1976.
14. Shepard TH: Teratogens: An update. Hosp. Pract. 19:191, 1984.
15. Miller E: Elevated maternal hemoglobin A1c in early pregnancy and major congenital anomalies in infants of diabetic mothers. N. Engl. J. Med. 304:1331, 1981.
16. Smithells RW, Sheppard S, Schorah CJ, Seller MJ, et al: Possible prevention of neural-tube defects by periconceptional vitamin supplementation. Lancet 1:339, 1980.
17. Recommended Dietary Allowances, ed 10. National Academy of Sciences, Washington, DC, 1989.
18. Standards of Obstetrics/Gynecology Services, ed 7. The American College of Obstetricians and Gynecologists, Washington, DC, 1989.
19. Baker DA, Polk BF: Hepatitis B: a controllable disease. Obstet. Gynecol. 62:105, 1983.
20. Kan YW, Golbus MS, Trecartin R: Prenatal diagnosis of sickle cell anemia. N. Engl. J. Med. 294:1035, 1976.
21. Nebiolo L, Ozturk M, Brambati B, Miller S, et al: First-trimester maternal serum alpha-fetoprotein and human chorionic gonadotropin screening for chromosome defects. Prenatal Diagnosis 10:575, 1990.
22. O'Sullivan JB, Mahan CM, Charles D, Dandrow RV: Screening criteria for high-risk gestational diabetic patients. Am. J. Obstet. Gynecol. 116:895, 1973.
23. Carpenter MW, Couston DR: Criteria for screening tests for gestational diabetes. Am. J. Obstet. Gynecol. 144:768, 1982.
24. Collea J, Hollis W: The contraction stress test. Clin. Obstet. Gynecol. 25:707, 1982.
25. Lavery J: Nonstress fetal heart rate testing. Clin. Obstet. Gynecol. 25:689, 1982.
26. Smith CV, Phelan JP, Broussard P, Paul RH: Fetal acoustic stimulation resting III: predictive value of a reactive test. J. Reprod. Med. 33:217, 1988.

27. Platt LD, Eglinton GS, Sipos L, Broussard PM, et al: Further experience with the fetal biophysical profile. Obstet. Gynecol. 61:480, 1983.
28. Sadovsky E, Ohel G, Havazeleth H, Steinwell A, et al: The definition and the significance of decreased fetal movements. Acta. Obstet. Gynecol. Scand. 62:409, 1983.
29. Leck I: Correlations of malformation frequency with environmental and genetic attributes in man. *In* Handbook of Teratology. Edited by JG Wilson, FC Fraser. New York, Plenum Press, 1977, p. 243.
30. Federal Register 44:37434, 1980.
31. American Academy of Pediatrics/American College of Obstetricians and Gynecologists: Guidelines for Perinatal Care, Washington, DC, 1983.
32. Jimenez JM, Tyson JE, Reisch JS: Clinical measures of gestational age in normal pregnancies. Obstet. Gynecol. 61:438, 1983.
33. Andersen HF, Johnson TRB, Barclay ML, Flora JD: Gestational age assessment I: analysis of individual clinical observations. Am. J. Obstet. Gynecol. 139:173, 1981.
34. Andersen HF, Johnson TRB, Flora JD Jr, Barclay ML: Gestational age assessment II: prediction from combined clinical observations. Am. J. Obstet. Gynecol. 140:770, 1981.
35. Johnson TRB Jr, Work BA Jr: A dynamic graph for documentation of gestational age. Obstet. Gynecol. 54:115, 1979.
36. O'Brien GD, Queenan JT: Growth of the ultrasound fetal femur length during normal pregnancy I. Am. J. Obstet. Gynecol. 141:833, 1981.
37. American Academy of Pediatrics/American College of Obstetricians and Gynecologists: Guidelines for Perinatal Care. Washington, DC, 1983, p. 66.
38. Robinson J: The role of the social sciences in perinatal care. *In* Effective Care in Pregnancy and Childbirth. Vol 1. Edited by I Chalmers, M Enkin, MJNC Keirse. New York, Oxford University Press, 1989, p. 81.
39. Friedman EA: Labor: Clinical Evaluation and Management. 2nd Ed. New York, Appleton-Century-Crofts, 1978.
40. Seitchik J, Amico J, Robinson AG, Castillo M: Oxytocin augmentation of dysfunctional labor. IV. Oxytocin pharmacokinetics. Am. J. Obstet. Gynecol. 150:225, 1984.
41. Dilts PV Jr: Selection of analgesia and anesthesia. Clin. Obstet. Gynecol. 24:521, 1981.
42. American Academy of Pediatrics/American College of Obstetricians and Gynecologists: Guidelines for Perinatal Care. Washington, DC, 1992, p. 76–8.
43. Friedman EA: The therapeutic dilemma of arrested labor. Contemp. Ob/Gyn. 11:34, 1978.
44. O'Driscoll K, Meagher P: Active Management of Labor. London, W.B. Saunders, 1980.
45. Morgan B, Bulpitt CJ, Clifton P, Lewis PJ: Effectiveness of pain relief in labour: survey of 1000 mothers. Br. Med. J. 285:689, 1982.
46. Gibbs CP, Krischer J, Peckham BM, Sharp H, et al: Obstetric anesthesia: a national survey. Anesthesiology 65:298, 1986.
47. Tuimala RJ, Kauppila AJI, Haapalahti J: Response of pituitary-adrenal axis on partal stress. Obstet. Gynecol. 46:275, 1975.
48. Goland RS, Wardlaw SL, Stark RI, Frantz AG: Human plasma β-endorphin during pregnancy, labor, and delivery. J. Clin. Endocrinol Metab 52:74, 1981.
49. Roman-Ponce H, Thatcher WW, Caton D, Barron DH, et al: Effects of thermal stress and epinephrine on uterine blood flow in ewes. J. Anim. Sci. 46:167, 1978.
50. Abboud TK, Artal R, Henriksen EH, Earl S, et al: Effects of spinal anesthesia on maternal circulating catecholamines. Am. J. Obstet. Gynecol. 142:252, 1982.
51. Myers RE, Myers S: Use of sedative, analgesic, and anesthetic drugs during labor and delivery: Bane or boon? Am. J. Obstet. Gynecol. 133:83, 1979.
52. American College of Obstetricians and Gynecologists: Obstetric Anesthesia and Analgesia. Tech. Bull. 112, Washington, DC, 1988.
53. Petrie RH, Yeh S-Y, Murata Y, Paul RH, et al: The effect of drugs on fetal heart rate variability. Am. J. Obstet. Gynecol. 130:294, 1978.
54. Teramo K: Fetal monitoring during maternal analgesia. *In* Gynecology and Obstetrics. Edited by L Castelazo-Ayala, C MacGregor. Amsterdam, Excerpta Medica, 1977, p. 398.
55. Gray JH, Cudmore DW, Luther ER, Martin TR, et al: Sinusoidal fetal heart rate pattern associated with alpha prodine administration. Obstet. Gynecol. 52:678, 1978.
56. Busacca M, Gementi P, Ciralli I, Vignali M: Sinusoidal fetal heart rate associated with maternal administration of meperidine and promethazine in labor. J. Perinatol. Med. 10: 215, 1982.
57. Kliger B, Nelson HB: Analgesia and fetal depression with intravenous meperidine and propriomazine. Am. J. Obstet. Gynecol. 92:850, 1965.
58. Brazelton TB: Effect of prenatal drugs on the behavior of the neonate. Am. J. Psychiatry 126:1261, 1970.
59. Caldwell J: The placental transfer of drugs during childbirth: a possible influence on the newborn. J. Psychosom. Res. 20:267, 1976.
60. Scanlon JW, Brown WU Jr, Weiss JB, Alper MH: Neurobehavioral responses of newborn infants after maternal epidural anesthesia. Anesthesiology 40:121, 1974.
61. Brackbill Y, Kane J, Manniello RL, Abramson D: obstetric premedication and infant outcome. Am. J. Obstet. Gynecol. 118:377, 1974.
62. Bayley N: Manual for the Bayley Scales of Infant Development. New York, Psychological Corp, 1969.
63. Way WL, Costley EC, Way EL: Respiratory sensitivity of the newborn infant to meperidine and morphine. Clin. Pharmacol. Ther. 6:454, 1965.
64. Kuhnert BR, Kuhnert PM, Tu A-SL, Lin DCK, et al: Meperidine and normeperidine levels following meperidine administration during labor. I. Mother. Am. J. Obstet. Gynecol. 133:904, 1979.
65. Kuhnert BR, Kuhnert PM, Tu A-SL, Lin DCK: Meperidine and normeperidine levels following meperidine administration during labor. II. Fetus and neonate. Am. J. Obstet. Gynecol. 133:909, 1979.
66. Rothberg RM, Rieger CH, Hill JH, Danielson J, et al: Cord and maternal serum meperidine concentrations and clinical status of the infant. Biol. Neonate. 33:80, 1978.
67. Shnider SM, Way EL, Lord MJ: Rate of appearance and disappearance of meperidine in fetal blood after administration of narcotic to the mother. Anesthesiology 27:227, 1966.
68. Morrison JC, Wiser WL, Rosser SI, Gayden JO, et al: Metabolites of meperidine related to fetal depression. Obstet. Gynecol. 115:1132, 1973.
69. Stambaugh JE, Hemphill DM, Wainer IW, Schwartz I: A potentially toxic drug interaction between pethidine (meperidine) and phenobarbitone. Lancet 1:398, 1977.
70. Kliger B, Nelson HB: Analgesia and fetal depression with intravenous meperidine and propriomazine. Am. J. Obstet. Gynecol. 92:850, 1965.
71. Hogg MIJ, Wiener PC Rosen M, Mapleson WW: Urinary excretion and metabolism of pethidine and norpethidine in the newborn. Br. J. Anaesth. 49:891, 1977.
72. Morrison JC, Whybrew WD, Rosser SI, Bucovaz ET, et al: Metabolites of meperidine in the fetal and maternal serum. Am. J. Obstet. Gynecol. 126:997, 1976.

73. Kuhnert BR, Kuhnert PM, Philipson EH, Syracuse CD: Disposition of meperidine and normeperidine following multiple doses during labor. II. Fetus and neonate. Am. J. Obstet. Gynecol. 151:410, 1985.
74. Kuhnert BR, Philipson EH, Kuhnert PM, Syracuse CD: Disposition of meperidine and normeperidine following multiple doses during labor. I. Mother. Am. J. Obstet. Gynecol. 151:406, 1985.
75. Kuhnert BR, Linn PL, Kennard MJ, Kuhnert PM: Effects of low doses of meperidine on neonatal behavior. Anesthesia Analgesia 64:335, 1985.
76. Maduska AL, Hajghassemali M: A double-blind comparison of butorphanol and meperidine in labor: maternal pain relief and effect on the newborn. Can. Anesth. Soc. J. 25:398, 1978.
77. Quilligan EJ, Keegan KA, Donohue MJ: Double-blind comparison of intravenously injected butorphanol and meperidine in parturients. Int. J. Obstet. Gynaecol. 18:363, 1980.
78. Hodgkinson R, Huff RW, Hayashi RH, Husain FJ: Double-blind comparison of maternal analgesia and neonatal neurobehavior following intravenous butorphanol and meperidine. J. Int. Med. Res. 7:224, 1979.
79. Gal TJ: Analgesic and respiratory depressant activity of nalbuphine: a comparison with morphine. Anesthesiology 55: 367, 1982.
80. Moore J, Ball HG: A sequential study of intravenous analgesic treatment during labor. Br. J. Anesth. 46:365, 1974.
81. Refstad SO, Lindbaek E: Ventilatory depression of the newborn of women receiving pethidine or pentazocine. Br. J. Anaesth. 52:265, 1980.
82. Potts CR, Ullery JC: Maternal and fetal effects on obstetric analgesia. Intravenous use of promethazine and meperidine. Am. J. Obstet. Gynecol. 81:1253, 1961.
83. Ovadia L, Halbrecht I: Neuroleptanalgesia: a new method of anesthesia for normal childbirth. Harefuah 72:143, 1967.
84. Attia RR, Grogono AW, Domer FR: Practical Anesthetic Pharmacology. 2nd Ed. Norwalk, CT, Appleton-Century-Crofts, 1987, p. 156.
85. Clayton BD: Mosby's Handbook of Pharmacology. 4th Ed. Washington, C.V. Mosby, 1987, pp. 460.
86. Rayburn WF, Zuspan FP: Drug Therapy in Obstetrics and Gynecology. 2nd Ed. Norwalk, CT, Appleton-Century-Crofts, 1986, pp. 211.
87. Dundee JW: Alterations in response to somatic pain associated with anesthesia. II. The effect of thiopentone and pentobarbitone. Br. J. Anaesthesia 32:407, 1960.
88. Shnider SM, Moya F: Effects of meperidine on the newborn infant. Am. J. Obstet. Gynecol. 89:1009, 1964.
89. Root B, Eichner E, Sunshine I: Blood secobarbital levels and their clinical correlation in mothers and newborn infants. Am. J. Obstet. Gynecol. 81:948, 1961.
90. Clutton-Brock JC: Some pain threshold studies with particular reference to thiopentone. Anaesthesia 15:71, 1960.
91. Scher J, Hailey DM, Beard RW: The effects of diazepam on the fetus. J. Obstet. Gynecol. Br. Commonw. 79:635, 1972.
92. McAllister CB: Placenta transfer and neonatal effects of diazepam when administered to women just before delivery. Br. J. Anaesthesia 52:423, 1980.
93. Cree IE, Meyer J, Hailey DM: Diazepam in labor: its metabolism and effect on the clinical condition and thermogenesis of the newborn. Br. Med. J. 4:251, 1973.
94. Schiff D, Chan G, Stern L: Fixed drug combinations and the displacement of bilirubin from albumin. Pediatr. 48: 139, 1971.
95. Powe CE, Kiem IM, Hagen C, Cavanagh D: Propiomazine hydrochloride in obstetrical analgesia. JAMA 181:290, 1962.
96. Zsigmond ER, Patterson RL: Double-blind evaluation of hydroxyzine hydrochloride in obstetric anesthesia. Anesthesia Analgesia 46:275, 1967.
97. Pert CB, Snyder SH: Opiate receptor: demonstration in nervous tissue. Science 179:1011, 1973.
98. Pasternak GW: Multiple morphine and enkephalin receptors and the relief of pain. JAMA 259:1362, 1988.
99. Goodman RR, Pasternak GW: Multiple opiate receptors. *In* Analgesics: Pharmacological and Clinical Perspectives. Edited by MJ Kuhar, GW Pasternak. New York, Raven Press, 1984, p. 69.
100. Hughes JT: Isolation of an endogenous compound from the brain with pharmacological properties similar to morphine. Brain Res. 88:295, 1975.
101. Chretien M, Benjannet S, Dragon N, Seidah NG, et al: Isolation of peptides with opiate activity from sheep and human pituitaries: Relation to α-lipotropin. Biochem. Biophys. Res. Commun. 72:472, 1976.
102. Wood M: Opioid agonists and antagonists. *In* Drugs and Anesthesia: Pharmacology for Anesthesiologists. 2nd Ed. Edited by M Wood, AJJ Wood. Baltimore, Williams & Wilkins, 1990.
103. Kalant H: Opioid analgesics and antagonists. *In* Principles of Medical Pharmacology. 5th Ed. Edited by H Kalant, WHE Roschlau. Philadelphia, B.C. Decker Inc., 1989.
104. Jaffe JH, Martin WR: Opioid analgesics and antagonists. *In* Goodman and Gilman's The Pharmacological Basis of Therapeutics. 8th Ed. Edited by AG Gilman, TW Rall, AS Nies, P Taylor. Pergamon Press, Tarrytown, NY, 1990.
105. Shnider SM, Levinson G, Ralston DH: Regional anesthesia for labor and delivery. *In* Anesthesia for Obstetrics. 3rd Ed. Edited by SM Shnider, G Levinson. Baltimore, Williams & Wilkins, 1993.
106. Corning JL: Spinal anesthesia and local medication of the cord. N.Y. J. Med. 42:483, 1885.
107. Pages F: Metameric anesthesia. Rev. Sanid. Milit. 11:351, 1921.
108. Dogliotti AM: A new method of block anesthesia: segmental peridural spinal anesthesia. Am. J. Surg. 20:107, 1933.
109. Graffagnino P, Seyler LW: Epidural anesthesia in obstetrics. Am. J. Obstet. Gynecol. 35:597, 1938.
110. Curbelo MM: Continuous peridural segmental anesthesia by means of ureteral catheter. Curr. Res. Anesth. Analg. 28:1, 1949.
111. Flowers CE Jr, Hellman LM, Hingson RA: Continuous peridural anesthesia/analgesia for labor, delivery and cesarean section. Curr. Res. Analg. 28:181, 1949.
112. Cleland JGP: Continuous peridural and caudal analgesia in obstetrics. Curr. Res. Analg. 28:61, 1949.
113. Bromage PR: Spinal Epidural Analgesia. Baltimore, Williams & Wilkins Co., 1954.
114. Hellmann K: Epidural anaesthesia in obstetrics: a second look at 26,127 cases. Canad. Anaesth. Soc. J. 12:398, 1965.
115. Eisen SM, Rosen N, Winesanker H, Hellman K, et al: The routine use of lumbar epidural anaesthesia in obstetrics: a clinical review of 9532 cases. Can. Anaesth. Soc. J. 7:280-289, 1960.
116. Bodell B, Tisdall LH, Ansbro FP: Epidural anesthesia for cesarean section: a report on 800 cases. Anesth. Analg. 41: 453, 1962.
117. Chaplin RA, Renwick WA: Lumbar epidural anaesthesia for vaginal delivery. Can. Anaesth. Soc. J. 5:414, 1958.
118. Lund PC, Cwik JC, Quinn JR: Experiences with epidural anesthesia, 7730 cases. Analg. Anesth. 40:153, 1961.
119. MacMillan A: Peridural anaesthesia for obstetrics. Can. Anaesth. Soc. J. 1:75, 1954.
120. Moore DC, Bridenbaugh LD, Owen CK, MacDougall MP,

et al: Lumbar epidural block: anesthetic of choice for cesarean section. Report of 100 cases. Western J. Surg. 61:459, 1953.

121. Schaudig H: On problems and current technic of peridural anaesthesia in obstetrics and gynecology. Anaesthetist 10: 152, 1961.
122. Volpi I: Sulle indicazioni dell'anestesia peridurale nel taglio cesareo. Minerva Anest 24:227, 1958.
123. Cantarow JH: Planned, rapid labor-elective induction of labor by intravenous pitocin following caudal anesthesia. Obstet. Gynecol. 4:213, 1954.
124. Friedman A, Schantz S, Page HR: Continuous caudal analgesia and anesthesia in obstetrics. A critical evaluation of 510 consecutive cases. Am. J. Obstet. Gynecol. 80:1181, 1960.
125. Nohill WK, Howland RS: Pitocin-caudal anesthesia method or artificial induction of labor. N.Y. J. Med. 58:198, 1958.
126. Hallet RL: The conduct of labor and results with continuous caudal anesthesia. Int. J. Anesth. 1:91, 1953.
127. Ralston DH, Shnider SM: The fetal and neonatal effects of regional anesthesia in obstetrics. Anesthesiology 48: 34–64, 1978.
128. Greenhill PJ: Shall spinal anesthesia be used in obstetrics? 11:283, 1950.
129. Artusio JF Jr, Van Poznak A, Kass A, McGoldrick KEA, et al: A triple crossover, partly blind comparison of the performance and effect on CNS function of three hand-held methoxyflurane inhalers. Anesth. Analg. 50:776–784, 1971.

# Chapter 23

# MANAGEMENT OF THE MOTHER AND NEWBORN

JOHN S. McDONALD
H. MODANLOU

## MANAGEMENT OF THE MOTHER

This portion of the chapter deals with maternal care during the puerperium and the immediate postpartum period. Included are physiologic changes due to application of anesthesia during the delivery period. The application of adequate care for the mother necessitates the full understanding of the normal physiologic changes associated with the birth process so that the pathologic changes can be anticipated and treatment programs developed. This discussion, as in the first edition, will be divided into three periods: (1) the immediate puerperium just after delivery during which complications from anesthesia and delivery can occur; (2) the intermediate puerperium extending until discharge during which complications from anesthesia and delivery can occur; and (3) the remote puerperium extending from discharge until 6 weeks postpartum during which complications associated with involution and normalization of the genital tract can occur. Also during this latter period, many significant changes occur in circulation, respiration, and in renal, hepatic, and other bodily functions that are of particular interest to the anesthesiologist.

### Basic Considerations

The term puerperium strictly defined refers to the period of time from the delivery through 6 weeks postpartum. This is usually the time the patient comes back to her obstetrician for the 6-week followup exam. During this period of time, many of the complications which can occur as a direct result of parturition are predominant, yet there are some complications that are directly linked to the delivery of anesthesia itself. For purposes of discussion in this portion of the chapter on maternal management, the puerperium will be handled as divided entities as mentioned above. The first portion of the puerperium is the immediate puerperium, which involves the period of time within 3 to 6 hours just after delivery. This is the period of time in which the mother is usually observed more closely, under more direct view of the nursing staff who are alert to look for: (1) bleeding problems, many of which may be due to episiotomy incisions and repair; (2) hypotensive problems; and (3) problems related to respiration. The second portion of the puerperium is the intermediate puerperium, which involves the period of time after the first 6 hours until discharge occurs. In the writing of this edition, this period of time has become abbreviated significantly due to the policy of early discharge now used throughout this country. Often, now the patients are discharged on the second or third day after delivery, whereas in the past, discharge was typically the fifth or six day postdelivery. This intermediate puerperium is a period of time when some of the later bleeding problems can occur due to faulty involution of the uterus. The third portion of the puerperium is the late puerperium, which involves the period from discharge until the 6-week examination referred to earlier. Once again, bleeding problems can surface here due to involution of the placental site (1), which may even necessitate hospitalization, or postpartum depression problems may surface that may also be severe enough to place a patient on medication after careful examination. Of course, it must be kept in mind that just as changes are occurring rapidly in the genital tract, they are also occurring in the other organ systems such as in the cardiovascular, respiratory, and metabolic systems. Such changes are of importance to the obstetrician and the anesthesiologist who may be confronted with a diagnostic problem.

### Anatomic and Physiologic Changes

#### *Reproductive Changes*

##### *The Uterus*

The immediate postpartum uterus can be described as a hard, globoid structure 15 cm long, 12 cm wide, and 10 cm thick, weighing about 1 kg (2). The anterior and posterior uterine walls, each of which is 4 to 5 cm thick, are closely opposed, and this effects compression of the rich uterine vascular plexuses of pregnancy, and through this mechanism blood loss is controlled until subsequent thrombosis of the vessels occurs. The cervix, during this time, is soft, bruised, and edematous with evidence of small lacerations. The uterus decreases rapidly in size so that it weighs approximately 500 grams at 1 week, 350 grams at 2 weeks, and 50 to 70 grams when complete involution has taken place by the end of the puerperium. The height of the fundus at different stages of the puerperium is shown in Figure 23–1. The process of involution of the uterus is remarkable in that the tremendous cellular expansion of pregnancy must now involute and attempt to regain near the status quo before inception. This involution is due to resorption of all the cellular building blocks

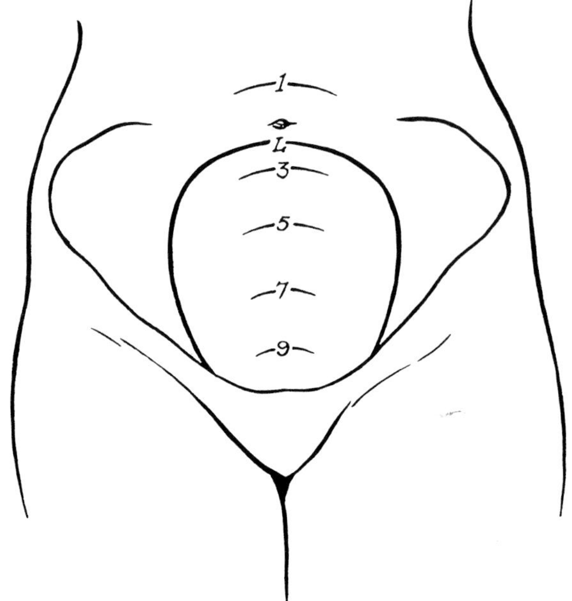


**Fig. 23–1.** The height of the fundus of the uterus at the end of labor (L) and at 1, 3, 5, 7, and 9 days postpartum. (Modified from Greenhill JP: Obstetrics 13th Ed. Philadelphia, WB Saunders Co., 1965.)

laid down during the remarkable stage of pregnancy and also involves some breaking down or autolysis of these units. During the puerperium, there is a tenfold decrease in the size of the hypertrophied myometrial cells characteristic of pregnancy, which is detailed in Chapter 5 on uterine physiology. Immediately after delivery of the baby, the height of the uterus begins to shorten considerably due to the fact that the uterine muscle is contracting around what is left in the uterine cavity—namely the placenta. The umbilical cord extends noticeably out of the vagina and often a "mound" is visible in the maternal abdomen due to the intense contraction of the uterus. These are all positive signs that mark the beginning of the expulsion of the placenta so that the uterus can contract upon itself, stop the bleeding at the placental attachment site, and begin the long process of involution over the next 6 weeks. The uterine contractions are quite intense during this time and may well exceed the intrauterine pressures such as found in labor in the 70 to 80 mm Hg range. This is also a time when uterine contraction efforts often are augmented by administration of either oxytocin, which cause rhythmic contractile patterns, or methergine, which cause tetanic contractile patterns. The administration of exogenous oxytocin can be the prime source of discomfort to the mother in the immediate puerperium due to the intensity of these uterine contractions, as described above.

## The Placenta

The site of former attachment of the placenta must undergo remarkable changes early after detachment of the placenta. This is necessary to gain control of the free loss of blood from this rich site of vascular attachment. The area, which at first is elevated and composed of a combination of necrotic decidual tissues and thrombosed vessels, soon becomes overtaken by phagocytic cellular units, which are responsible for the involution process over the next several days and even weeks. During this time, the necrotic debris is cast off in the form of discharge, referred to as lochia. The conversion of lochia types and their duration is illustrated in Figure 23–2 (3). During this time, gradual undermining of the placental site occurs by growth of the endometrial cells that, through the process of necrotic slough and replacement by new growth of cells, soon nearly cover the entire placental site. Over the next several weeks, the placental site continues to involute until the thrombosed vessels noted above become converted to fibroblasts and, later, the entire site becomes merely a fibrous scar. This involution is extremely important and its failure to fully involute may be responsible for late hemorrhage problems in the puerperium. The classic work done by Williams so many years ago (4) was challenged by Anderson (1) only to the point that placental site slough is comparable to any damaged tissue site in the body. Lochia, mentioned above, is the result of the uterine expulsion of the necrotic decidual outer layer that occurs throughout the immediate, intermediate, and late puerperium, i.e., between delivery and 7 days (5). For approximately the first 7 days, it is described as lochia rubra due to its being composed of decidua, blood, and membrane remnants. During this period, sometime around the seventh day, it is described as lochia alba due to its composition, primarily, of cast-off leucocytes and sera.

## The Cervix and Vagina

The cervix, which is impacted by parturition to a major degree, recovers slowly over the first several weeks of the puerperium, with the various associated changes, including hyperplasia, hypertrophy, ulceration, laceration, and ecchymotic injuries that improve day-to-day (6,7). The vagina also pays a price for the birth process: massive stretching, hyperplasia, hypertrophy, and laceration. It too slowly recovers near its normal size and shape during the late puerperium period.

## The Perineum

The perineum, impacted by stretching, laceration, and surgical episiotomy incision, accomplishes a good repair within a few weeks after delivery. The old admonition to refrain from intercourse until after the 6-week visit is now replaced by a more practical admonition: engage in it when so inclined after the cessation of the lochia rubra period (8). In addition, it may be prudent to use a condom barrier for both infection and fertility protection in these early periods during which many of the women's reproductive organs return to normal. Certainly, the supporting tissues of the muscles of the perineum, pelvis, and abdomen must not be left out, as they are also undergoing dramatic recovery and a return to normal as each play such an important supportive role in the pregnancy process.

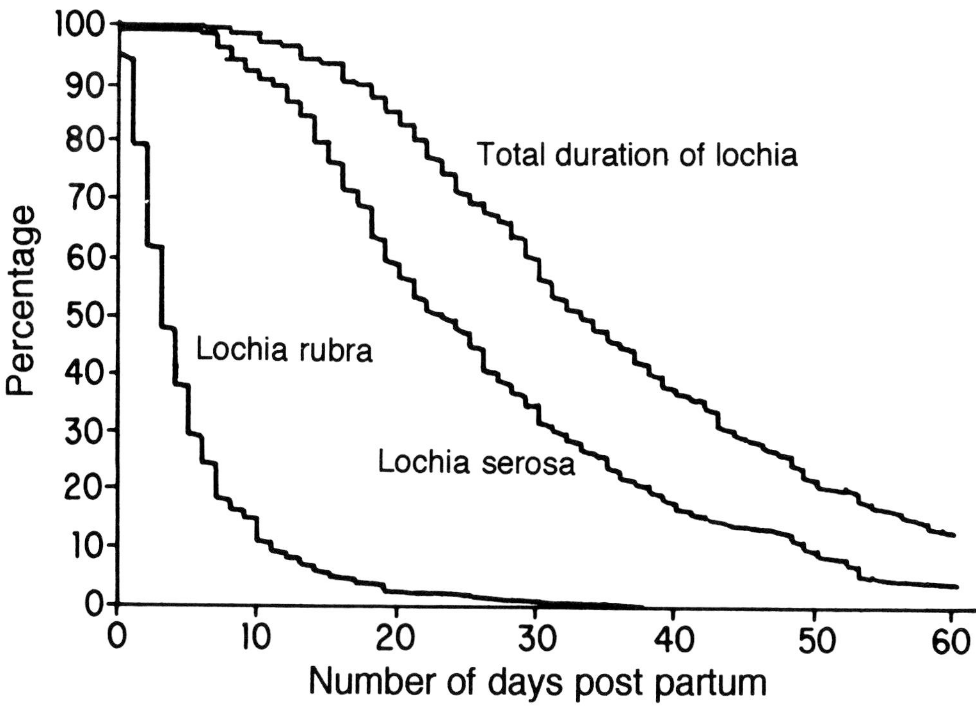


**Fig. 23–2.** Lochia types in the postpartum period described as percentage over time. (Redrawn from Oppenheimer LW, Sherriff EA, Goodman JDS, Shah D, et al: The duration of lochia. Br. J. Obstet. Gynaecol. 93:754, 1986.)

*The Breasts*

The breasts are each made up of multiple lobes, which, in turn, are made up of lobules that contain very large numbers of acini glands (9). It is these acini glands that form the actual milk product. They undergo major enlargement during pregnancy by means of strong endocrine stimulation by estrogen and progesterone. During the immediate puerperium (10), they become increasingly stimulated by means of the baby's sucking, which promotes milk letdown by prolactin secretion from the anterior pituitary, stimulating uterine contractions at the

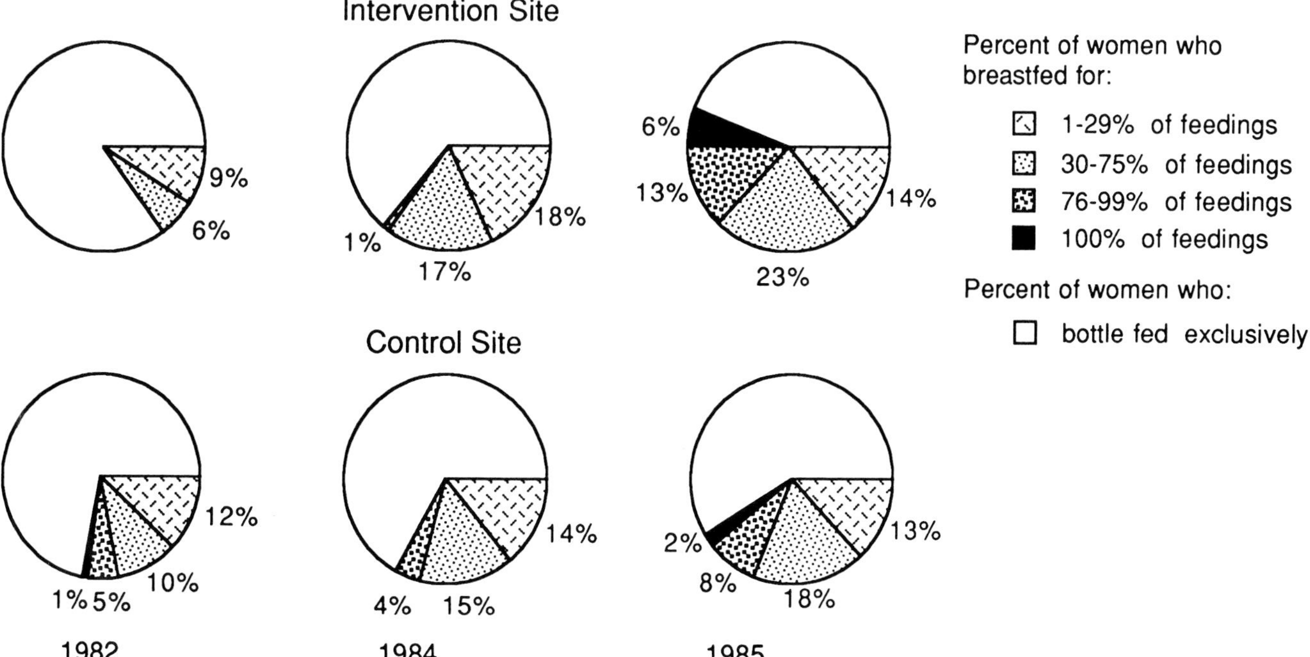


**Fig. 23–3.** Breast-feeding patterns shown as percentage over the various years (Redrawn from Winikoff B, Myers D, Laukaran VH, Stone R: Overcoming obstacles to breast-feeding in a large municipal hospital: applications of lessons learned. Pediatrics 80:423, 1987.)

same time (11). One of the most exciting changes in this immediate puerperium has been, in fact, the tremendous increase in the numbers of mothers now opting to breast feed their babies as compared to a decade or two ago (12–14). It is estimated that over these last 10 to 20 years, the incidence of breast feeding has doubled. The chief reason for this increase in breast feeding is the use of international programs in promoting its acceptance by patients and hospitals alike (Figure 23–3) (14). Released first from the breast is colostrum, a high protein, high salt milk, but which gives rise to the onset of normal milk secretion by the third day postpartum, which by then contains proteins, fats, and sugar in addition to small amounts of salt. Very important to a successful breast feeding program is the atmosphere developed in the postpartum rooms and the attitude and support received from the nursing staff.

## Respiratory Changes

The entire respiratory tract, including the nasopharynx, the larynx, the trachea, the bronchi, and the alveoli all undergo significant reduction in capillary engorgement and vascularity, so prominent in pregnancy, during the puerperium. In fact, one of the most serious consequences and even a lethal one can be the well-meaning anesthesiologist who may attempt to establish an airway via the nasopharynx. Such an attempt may be met with copious bleeding due to the changes of pregnancy just alluded to, the capillary engorgement and swelling. The intrusion of the tube may cause unexpected heavy bleeding , which may be difficult to control. There is also reduction in pulmonary blood volume and reflective decreases in the expanded lung markings, the latter of which sometimes is interpreted as pulmonary edema during pregnancy (15–17). In the early chapter on respiratory changes in pregnancy (Chapter 2), it became immediately apparent that many respiratory changes occur in concert with the developing gestation (Figure 23–4). Just as these physiologic changes increase due to the demands of pregnancy, so also do they return to normal, nonpregnant values during the intermediate and late puerperium. Data detailing the rapidity of change right at the moment delivery is still not available; thus, it still is not clear when each parameter returns to its nonpregnant level. Note in Table 23–1 that at 1 month postpartum, the values are still abnormal, while by 6 months all values are within limits of normal. Significant alterations also occur in the acid-base balance of the mother just after delivery. In the early puerperium, the respiratory alkalosis and metabolic acidosis are normalized with the greatest changes occurring during the first 5 to 7 days after delivery, during the first portion of the late puerperium. These changes in ventilation reflect the changes in the ovarian hormones, and progesterone and estrogen, which are believed to be responsible for the hyperventilation of pregnancy (18–21). The alveolar and arterial blood carbon dioxide tensions rise rapidly at first and then return gradually to normal values (Figures 23–5 and 23–6). Table 23–2 shows the results obtained by Sjøstedt 3 to 7 days after parturition when $PCO_2$ and pH levels were between those noted during pregnancy and the normal nonpregnant level. The mild metabolic acidosis, however, had disappeared because the base excess values were normal and the buffer base value increased even above normal owing to the disappearance of hydremia. Similar changes were reported by others (22,23).

## Circulatory Changes

### Cardiac Output

The cardiac output increase associated with pregnancy is one of the best known changes that occurs during gestation. Its increase of some 40% helps to generate the essential increase in blood flow necessary to sustain the continued growth phase during pregnancy. This change in cardiac output remains in effect during the second and

**Table 23–1.** Effect of Pregnancy on Lung Volumes and Other Ventilatory Variables in Man (Ranges in Parentheses are Estimate "B" of the 95% Range)

| Variable | Pregnancy, Lunar Month | | | | | | | Postpartum, Month | |
|---|---|---|---|---|---|---|---|---|---|
| | 4 | 5 | 6 | 7 | 8 | 9 | 10 | 1 | 6 |
| Respiratory rate (breaths/min) | 16 | 15 | 16 | 16 | 16 | 16 | 16 (12–20) | 17 | 15 (11–19) |
| Tidal volume, L | 0.56 | 0.59 | 0.61 | 0.61 | 0.65 | 0.70 | 0.7 (0.4–1.0) | 0.55 | 0.5 (0.2–0.8) |
| Minute volume, L/min | 8.7 | 9.1 | 10.0 | 9.7 | 10.3 | 11.0 | 10.3 (7.3–13.6) | 9.5 | 7.3 (4.3–10.3) |
| Ventilatory equivalent, (ml air/ml $O_2$) | 3.3 | 3.5 | 3.6 | 3.5 | 3.6 | 3.7 | 3.3 (1.3–5.3) | 3.4 | 3.0 (1.0–5.0) |
| Maximum breathing capacity, L/min | 97 | 99 | 97 | 96 | 97 | 97 | 96 (74–118) | 92 | 102 (80–124) |
| Total lung capacity, L | 4.2 | 4.2 | 4.2 | 4.1 | 4.3 | 4.1 | 4.1 (3.5–4.7) | 4.1 | 4.2 (3.6–4.8) |
| Vital capacity, L | 3.2 | 3.2 | 3.2 | 3.2 | 3.3 | 3.3 | 3.3 (2.9–3.7) | 3.1 | 3.3 (2.8–3.8) |
| Inspiratory capacity, L | 2.6 | 2.7 | 2.7 | 2.7 | 2.7 | 2.7 | 2.7 (2.3–3.1) | 2.5 | 2.6 (2.2–3.0) |
| Expiratory reserve volume, L | 0.65 | 0.65 | 0.65 | 0.61 | 0.63 | 0.56 | 0.55 (0.3–0.8) | 0.56 | 0.65 (0.4–0.9) |
| Functional reserve capacity, L | 1.6 | 1.6 | 1.6 | 1.5 | 1.5 | 1.4 | 1.3 (1.0–1.6) | 1.5 | 1.6 (1.3–1.9) |
| Residual volume, L | 1.0 | 1.0 | 1.0 | 0.9 | 0.9 | 0.8 | 0.8 (0.6–1.0) | 1.0 | 1.0 (0.8–1.2) |

(From Handbook of Respiration, 1958, National Research Council. Adapted from Cugell DW, Frank NR, Gaensler EA, Badger TL: Pulmonary functions in pregnancy; serial observations in normal women. Amer. Rev. Tuberc. 67:568, 1953.)

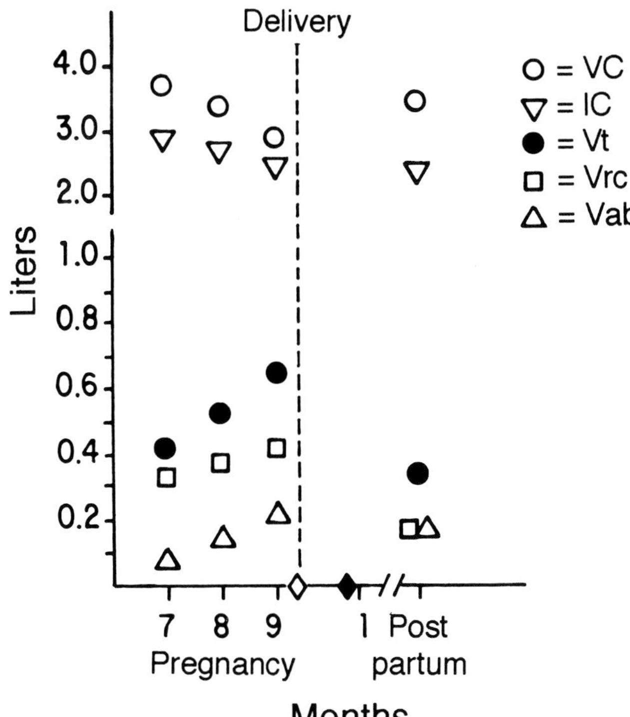


**Fig. 23–4.** The decline in vital capacity and inspiratory capacity in the last few months of pregnancy. This chart shows the relationship between breathing by displacement of the rib cage versus displacement of the abdomen. That is, late in pregnancy there is a tendency to use the rib cage for expansion. VC = vital capacity; IC = inspiratory capacity; $V_T$ = tidal volume; Vrc = volume displaced by rib cage during tidal breathing; Vab = volume displaced by abdomen during tidal breathing; open triangle = date of delivery; closed triangle = estimated date of confinement; vertical lines trisecting the abscissa = dates of study; F = statistics; subscripts to F = appropriate degrees of freedom for that subject. (Redrawn from Gilroy, RJ, Mangura, BT, Lavietes, MH: Rib cage and abdominal volume displacement during breathing in pregnancy. Am. Rev. Respir. Dis. 137: 668, 1988.)

third trimesters and even into the early puerperium. In fact, just after separation and delivery of the placenta, there is a surge in cardiac output that exceeds that of the third trimester. The studies of Ueland, which correlated

**Table 23–2.** Acid-Base Changes in Pregnancy

| Patient | pH | $PCO_2$ (mm Hg) | Buffer Base (mEq/L) | Standard Bicarbonate (mEq/L) | Base Excess (mEq/L) |
|---|---|---|---|---|---|
| Control | 7.423 | 37.1 | 46.2 | 23.9 | +1.1 |
| During pregnancy | 7.443 | 32.1 | 43.8 | 21.4 | 0 |
| Labor | 7.462 | 26.7 | 44.2 | 21.2 | −1.7 |
| Puerperium | 7.441 | 34.3 | 47.1 | 23.1 | +0.8 |

(From Sjøstedt S: Acid-base balance of arterial blood during pregnancy, at delivery, and in the puerperium. Am. J. Obstet. Gynecol. 84:775, 1962.)

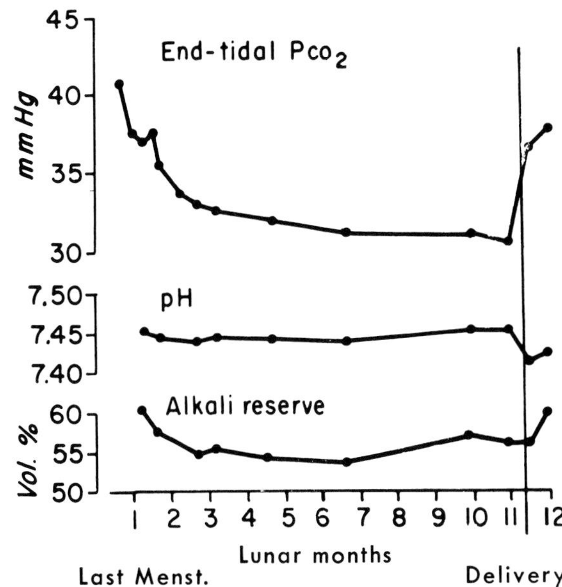


**Fig. 23–5.** Progressive changes of alveolar carbon dioxide tensions, pH, and alkali reserve of one individual studied repeatedly before conception, throughout pregnancy, and in the postpartum period. (Modified from Prowse CM, Graensler EA: Respiratory and acid-base changes during pregnancy. Anesthesiology 26:381, 1965.)

the magnitude of this change, revealed that following vaginal delivery, there were increases in cardiac output of some 80% without regional anesthesia and some 60% with regional anesthesia (Figure 23–7) (24). This change in cardiac output was found to be due to an increase in stroke volume not rate. Due to simultaneous reduction in peripheral resistance, there was no significant change

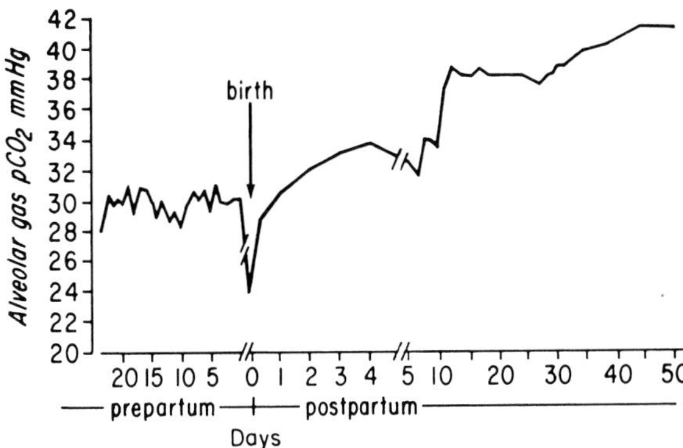


**Fig. 23–6.** Typical changes in maternal alveolar carbon dioxide levels before, during, and after labor. Note the marked decrease during labor (from hyperventilation) and the rapid increase immediately thereafter. (Adapted from Boutourline-Young H, Boutourline-Young E: Alveolar carbon dioxide levels in pregnant, parturient and lactating subjects. Obstet. Gynaec. Brit. Emp. 63:509, 1956.)

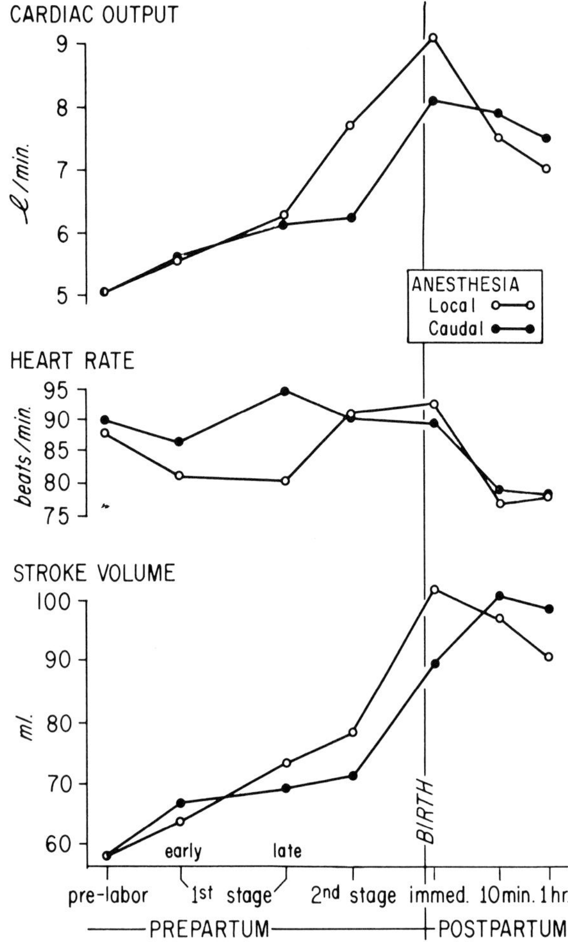


**Fig. 23–7.** Effect of local and continuous caudal analgesia on maternal hemodynamics. Extradural analgesia modifies the cumulative effects of parturition on cardiac output during labor, but not during the immediate puerperium. (Modified from Ueland K, Hansen JM: Maternal cardiovascular dynamics. 3. Labor and delivery under local and caudal analgesis. Am. J. Obstet. Gynecol. 103:8, 1969.)

in blood pressure (25,26). This increase is transient, of course, but nevertheless must be recognized due to its threat to maternal stability at that time, especially in parturients who may suffer from other problems such as cardiac or respiratory in nature. During labor some of the most amazing changes occur due to the superimposed increase in cardiac output secondary to uterine contractions. Without the benefit of regional anesthesia, there are notable increases in heart rate due to the pain of the uterine contraction. The other factors important in determining just how much of an increase in cardiac output occurs include the intensity and duration of the contraction and the position of the patient, i.e., is she on her back or on her side. The latter is the preferred position for all laboring patients due to the obviation of the problems associated with vena caval obstruction and even aortic compression. By one-half hour after delivery, the cardiac output is reduced to near 50% at which it remains over the next week or so. After that the decline is gradual, with normal cardiac output regained by the second week postpartum. The maternal blood pressure normally returns to near nonpregnant values in the early puerperium. The frequency distribution for maximal systolic and diastolic pressures is shown in Figure 23–8.

## Hematologic Changes

There are also significant changes occurring in regard to blood volume in the pregnant patient. Other than those changes associated with cardiac output, the changes in blood volume are perhaps the most dramatic. By the end of the puerperium, there has been a gradual fall in blood volume from the normal pregnant level of nearly 6 liters to 3 or 4 liters. Of the near 35% increase in blood volume associated with pregnancy, the largest component is plasma volume. Naturally, with delivery the greatest reduction in blood volume occurs with approximately 1000 ml lost over time (27). However, within 72 hours there is another increase in plasma volume of nearly 1000 ml due to the shift in fluid from the extracellular to the intravascular space (28). Nevertheless, there is still a net decline in blood volume of close to 15% by the third day postpartum, which means some slight, but insignificant rise in measurable hematocrit. Actually, the relative loss of plasma volume and red cell volume varies among different patients and at different times of the puerperium depending on the rate of return of this excess extracellular fluid into the circulation (27,28).

Among other cellular changes, there is the white blood cell count, which acutely rises to as high as 15,000 and remains there until after the second day postpartum (29). From this point on there is a gradual return to nonpregnant levels within 1 month. However, it must be appreciated that during stresses of labor a leukocyte count can rise to as high as 25,000 with no clinical evidence of infection. The physiologic leukocytosis is accompanied by an increase in polymorphonuclear leukocytes that may number up to 87% (30). There are other interesting changes associated with labor, delivery, and the puerperium; the eosinophil count, for example, falls abruptly during delivery, but then rises during the early puerperium, reaching a peak at about the fifth or sixth day, then gradually returning to normal, nonpregnant levels by the end of the second to the fourth week (Figure 23–9).

With regard to coagulation factors, there is some increased fibrinolytic action in the first 3 to 4 days, with a rapid return to normal by the end of the first week. The fibrinogen, which increases significantly during pregnancy, gradually returns to normal within the 2 weeks just after delivery. Also, by 2 weeks postpartum there is an increase in platelet count (30). See Chapter 26 for details.

## Excretory Tract Changes

Both the urinary tracts and digestive tracts will be discussed in this section. During the 12 to 18 hours after delivery, many urinary tract changes are seen. The bladder mucosa is edematous and hyperemic, but the edema rarely causes obstruction of the urethra. Shortly after completion of delivery, the bladder may suffer from sluggish

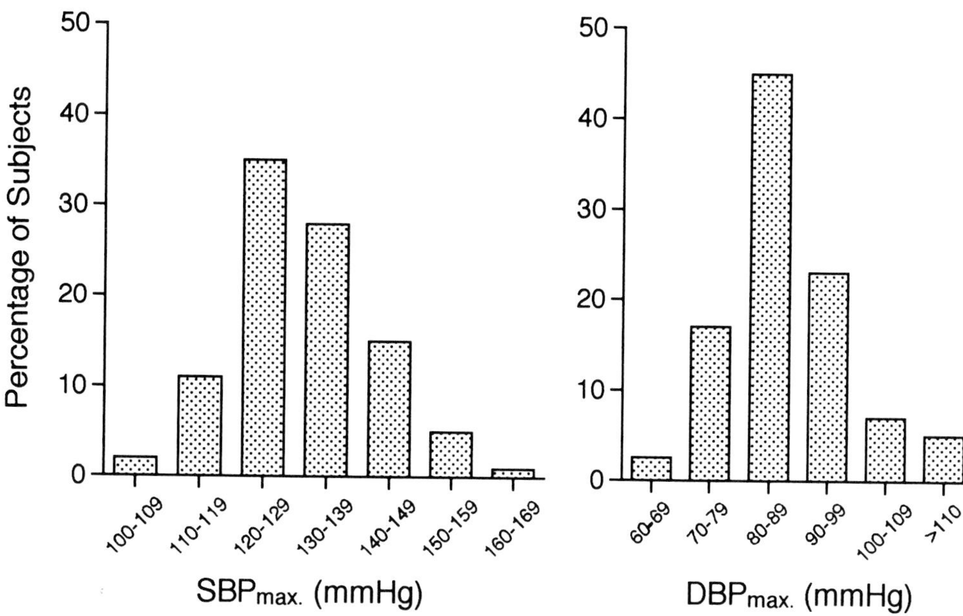


**Fig. 23–8.** Distribution of systolic and diastolic blood pressures in 136 women after vaginal delivery. (Redrawn from Walters BNH, Thompson ME, Lea E, DeSwiet M: Blood pressure in the puerperium. Clin. Sci. 71:589, 1986.)

action due to its being distended with less-than-normal sensation and, thus, overdistension due to incomplete emptying may occur. This leads to urinary retention and even the necessity for catheterization in some instances. Dilation of the upper excretory tracts, including ureters and even the renal pelvis, is thought to be due to a combination of hormonal and mechanical factors. Qualitative changes in the right and left kidneys are reported in Table 23–3 (31). Actual urographic studies during this period demonstrate urethral and upper calycyx dilatation thought to be due to iliac artery pressure. For the most part, the aforementioned changes subside within 1 to 2 weeks after delivery. The 25% increase in renal plasma flow begins to fall in the late third trimester and continues after delivery to values below normal. The continued fall for some 4 to 6 months after delivery is the most prolonged change of all (32). The 50% increase in glomerular filtration rate returns to nonpregnant levels soon after delivery, and the filtration fraction, which also rises about 50%, remains inconsistently increased during the immediate puerperium and gradually decreases to nonpregnant levels by 6 weeks postpartum. It may be that this mechanism is very important in helping to get rid of the large flux in extracellular fluid in those 48 to 72 hours postpartum as mentioned above. The blood urea nitrogen (BUN) and creatinine that are reduced by nearly one-half in pregnancy, also revert to normal soon after delivery.

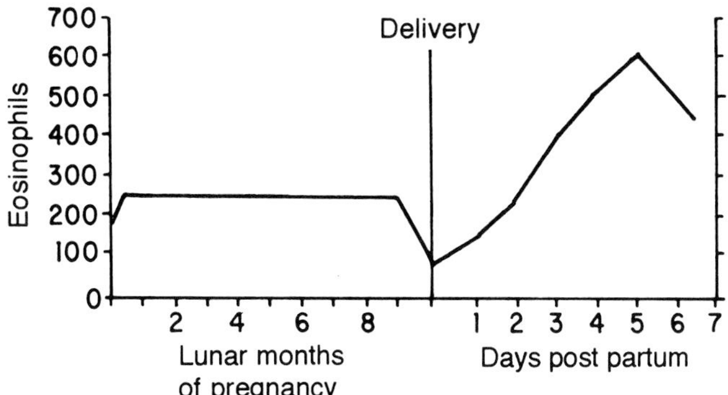


**Fig. 23–9.** Effect of pregnancy, labor, and the puerperium on the eosinophil count. Note particularly the abrupt fall caused by delivery and the rise during the early puerperium. In prolonged or traumatic delivery the fall is much greater and the postpartum rise is slower. (The eosinophil count is shown in $mm^3$.)

As mentioned above, there is a large flux of extracellular fluid that shifts into the intravascular space soon after deliver. Fortunately, diuresis begins promptly and continues for the first 4 to 5 days. The postpartum urine output may be phenomenal, reaching volumes as high as 3000 ml per day. This diuresis aids in a rapid return of the increased interstitial fluid to normal nonpregnant levels. Some proteinuria may be noted in patients, i.e., as high as 40% of women, but this, too, soon disappears by somewhere around 24 hours. Sugar is often spilled in the urine during the first weeks of the puerperium. Most mothers will also have a significant increase in the amount of acetone in the urine just after delivery, but this too disappears over the next 3 days. The reason for such urinary metabolic byproducts may be due to excessive but necessary carbohydrate consumption from the increased muscular activity during labor and at the same time the lack of normal dietary supplement.

The gastrointestinal tract sustains significant decreases in both tone and motility in the early portion of the puerperium. This may be a reflex due to the stress of labor and its various noxious stimuli evoked by uterine contractions and unrelieved by regional analgesia methods. In such instances, gastric emptying can be delayed similar to that found during pregnancy. Also in the first few days constipation is common. In these days with fewer and fewer extensive operative vaginal deliveries and thus fewer and fewer large perineal incisions for delivery, there is less

**Table 23–3.** Pregnancy Kidney Changes Throughout Gestation

| | % Incidence | | | |
|---|---|---|---|---|
| **Right Kidney** | **No Change** | **Stasis** | **Hydronephrosis** | **Hydronephrosis With Clubbing** |
| Gestation weeks | | | | |
| 12 | 75.0 | 25.0 | 0.0 | 0.0 |
| 16 | 51.4 | 45.7 | 2.9 | 0.0 |
| 20 | 11.4 | 74.3 | 14.3 | 0.0 |
| 24 | 5.9 | 47.0 | 41.2 | 5.9 |
| 28 | 3.0 | 30.4 | 33.3 | 33.3 |
| 32 | 3.3 | 40.0 | 16.7 | 40.0 |
| 36 | 3.0 | 33.3 | 15.2 | 48.5 |
| Post-partum | | | | |
| 2 days | 12.1 | 51.5 | 15.2 | 21.2 |
| 6 weeks | 31.2 | 68.8 | 0.0 | 0.0 |
| 12 weeks | 25.0 | 75.0 | 0.0 | 0.0 |

| | % Incidence | | | |
|---|---|---|---|---|
| **Left Kidney** | **No Change** | **Stasis** | **Hydronephrosis** | **Hydronephrosis With Clubbing** |
| Gestation weeks | | | | |
| 12 | 85.7 | 14.3 | 0.0 | 0.0 |
| 16 | 77.1 | 22.9 | 0.0 | 0.0 |
| 20 | 42.9 | 57.1 | 0.0 | 0.0 |
| 24 | 44.1 | 44.1 | 8.8 | 3.0 |
| 28 | 24.2 | 60.6 | 12.2 | 3.0 |
| 32 | 16.7 | 63.3 | 13.3 | 6.7 |
| 36 | 18.2 | 63.6 | 12.1 | 6.1 |
| Post-partum | | | | |
| 2 days | 24.2 | 72.7 | 0.0 | 3.1 |
| 6 weeks | 53.1 | 46.9 | 0.0 | 0.0 |
| 12 weeks | 45.8 | 54.2 | 0.0 | 0.0 |

Note the incidence of the four grades of renal change during and after pregnancy and also the difference between the two sides.
(From Cietak, KA, Newton, JR: Serial qualitative maternal nephrosonography in pregnancy. Br. J. Radiol. 58:399, 1985.)

pain after delivery and less immobility. This fact and the fact that better methods of pain relief for the immediate puerperium are now in vogue, all help to reduce the associated problems with the gastrointestinal tract. The modern mother should be up and around, have a hearty appetite, and be relatively pain-free throughout her short hospital stay.

## *Physiologic Changes*

The thyroid increases in size by about one-third during pregnancy and returns to normal size very slowly over a period of time well beyond the puerperium (Table 23–4) (33). The thyroxine and triiodothyronine are both elevated during gestation and return to baseline sometime in the first 4 weeks after delivery. The basal metabolic rate and the most reliable measurement of metabolic function, oxygen consumption, return to normal within some 14 days of delivery. The actual metabolism of proteins, carbohydrates, fats, and minerals return to nonpregnant levels more gradually. Water balance also returns to normal nonpregnant levels over the first 14 days. When all fluid losses are added, such as blood, amniotic fluid, and insensible loss, there is a phenomenal fluid loss of nearly 6 liters at delivery Further, another 6 liters are lost during the puerperium. During the immediate puerperium, water loss through the kidneys and from the skin is accentuated. An average loss of about 13 pounds follows delivery of the infant and placenta and loss of the amniotic fluid. A further loss of about 5 to 7 pounds occurs during the puerperium.

Unless there is a superimposed infection, the body temperature remains within the normal range during the postpartum period. In some patients who experienced long labors, there may be transient elevation of body temperature, but persistent fever must be taken seriously. Puerperal morbidity is said to be present if the oral temperature exceeds 100.4° F on any 2 days between the second and eleventh postpartum days. The common problems of the postpartum chills, which appear shortly after completion of the third stage of labor, occur in many patients. Their cause is unknown but thought to be related to either losses of large amounts of heat at delivery with all the fluid shifts or, possibly, due to breakdown of maternal-fetal barriers and mild sensitization of the mother by fetal foreign proteins.

## *Psychologic Changes*

One of the best-known phenomena of pregnancy is that associated with the postpartum blues or mild emotional changes just after delivery (Figure 23–10) (34). These changes are not believed related to any anesthetic agent or technique used for delivery because they are also found in mothers who receive no analgesia for delivery. The mother may become teary eyed upon the slightest provocation; she may become irritable and apprehensive with-

**Table 23–4.** Ultrasonic Volume Changes in the Thyroid at Delivery and 6 Months Postpartum

| Subject | Initial Postpartum Thyroid Volume ($cm^3$)* | Thyroid Volume Six Months Postpartum ($cm^3$) |
|---|---|---|
| 1 | 4.9 | 4.1 |
| 2 | 6.2 | 4.6 |
| 3 | 9.4 | 9.1 |
| 4 | 5.7 | 4.6 |
| 5 | 6.6 | 8.0 |
| 6 | 7.2 | 6.3 |
| 7 | 9.4 | 9.5 |
| 8 | 5.0 | 4.5 |
| 9 | 7.6 | 7.4 |
| 10 | 6.3 | 5.4 |
| Mean | 6.83 | 6.35 |

* Thyroid volume was measured within four days after delivery.
(Modified from Nelson M, Wickus GC, Caplan RH, Beguin EA: Thyroid gland size in pregnancy: an ultrasound and clinical study. J. Reprod. Med. 32:888, 1987.)

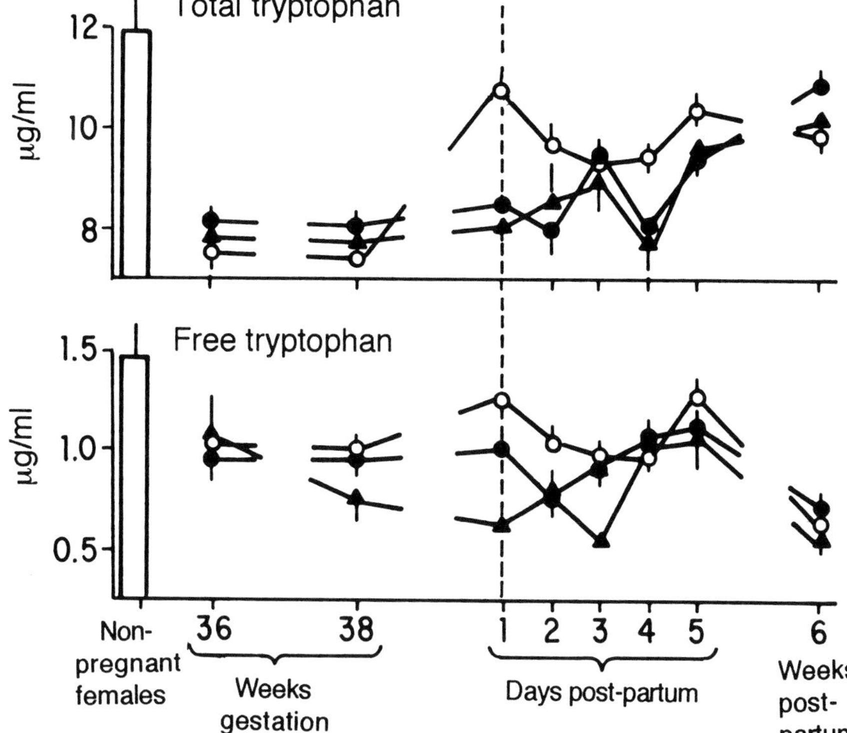


**Fig. 23–10.** Note the antepartum total tryptophan was low and experienced a rapid rise on postpartum days 1 and 2. This rise was absent in 37% of the patients. This absence was related to the occurrence of postpartum blues. (Redrawn from Handley SL, Dunn TL, Waldron G, Baker JM: Tryptophan, cortisol and puerperal mood. Br. J. Psychiat. 136: 498, 1980.)

out a suggestion of its cause (35). Symptoms most frequently associated with postpartum depression are shown in Table 23–5. This would appear to be a truly happy and even euphoric time: delivery of her newborn baby and determination that the baby was normal and healthy; but somehow, these blues and emotional changes are quite common, occurring in as high as 40 to 60% of parturients. The period is fortunately very short in duration, lasting as short as 1 day to 3 days. In some mothers such a feeling of being blue and slightly depressed may be replaced by a development of apprehension and tension due to the realization that they have an onerous responsibility for the care of their newborn. Some of the apprehension may also be attributable to re-living tumultuous childhood relationships with their own mother and father and the fear that they too could become a failure in raising their own baby. It is interesting to note that the psychologic impact of delivery is quite different in the male, who usually floats on air for several days after the delivery. He is the proud father of a newborn baby; he feels elated, relaxed, successful, even euphoric at times. There must, therefore, be something to the fact that the many changes in the hormonal relationships at delivery play a certain, major role in this very common postpartum problem for women.

If this period of time is not short lived as noted, there may be other deeper problems of a more serious psychologic nature. There are some women who have been given a general anesthetic for a delivery at a time when there were some emergency problems. Obviously, some of these emergencies were situations in which the baby's life was at risk and the obstetricians had to make a judgment decision to effect an emergency delivery. Many times this emergency delivery is an unexpected cesarean section with a rapid sequence induction, minimal anesthetic, and rapid delivery. In the postpartum, some mothers may complain of not having an adequate level of anesthesia or that they were either not asleep or not pain free. Other mothers, who lost the life of their baby despite the emergency cesarean, may have problems for some time in their attempt to come to grips with the lack of completion or closure they had had in regard to their baby. One moment

**Table 23–5.** Symptoms of Depression

| Symptom | % of Patients Experiencing Symptom* |
|---|---|
| Feeling sad | 93 |
| Poor concentration | 93 |
| Loss of interest | 89 |
| Appetite loss | 87 |
| Weight loss | 85 |
| Feeling worthless | 74 |
| Somatic complaints | 74 |
| Irritability | 67 |
| Waking early | 61 |
| Trouble falling asleep | 59 |
| Trouble staying asleep | 46 |
| Feelings of hopelessness | 61 |
| Feelings of self-reproach | 59 |
| Indecision | 59 |
| Restless | 59 |
| Tired all the time | 57 |

* N = 54

(Modified from Garvey MJ, Tollefson GD: Postpartum depression. J. Reprod. Med. 29:113, 1984.)

they could feel their baby moving vigorously within their abdomen, the next, they are awakening and someone is telling them their baby did not live. This has to be a tremendous psychologic burden. It behooves us to be sensitive to this issue and to be alerted to it so that some professional and effective means of helping to handle this burden can be arranged for her before the mother awakens. This type of approach should also be considered in instances of prematurity, congenital defects, or other serious medical disorders of the newborn. The new mother should receive all the emotional support possible from a caring, committed staff of doctors, nurses, and other health care professionals, all of whom are vital links in the management of the psychologically destitute puerpera who does not have the mental skills or the physical stamina to handle such stressful situations.

The rare postpartum psychotic reaction occurs in women who have had evidence of preexisting psychopathology. In the modern healthy and open psychiatric approach to a patient's problem, it is now generally agreed that the isolated neurotic or psychotic reaction that surfaces during the puerperium is not separate and distinct from those occurring among nonpregnant patients. A psychotic reaction, rare as it may be, is very disturbing to all of those concerned on the health care team, and immediate attention, support, and a concerned, understanding attitude is necessary. The emotional upheaval of the delivery can bring on a psychosis just as any marginally compensated patient with psychopathology can experience a problem due to other types of stress.

## Management of the Postpartum Mother in the Immediate Puerperium

It is most important that the recovery room in obstetrics be staffed by nurses who are responsive to and have been trained by anesthesiologists to be alert for the various key issues involved in patient recovery from normal spontaneous delivery, forceps delivery, and cesarean delivery. The early puerperium can be a confusing time due to the fact that mothers are exposed to complications from the delivery experience and also the anesthetic experience. It is therefore necessary that these nurses be especially trained to understand the complex, interactive environment during this special period of time. The patient must be signed out of the recovery room in the operating room area. This rule should also apply to the obstetric area when there has been an anesthetic involvement. In anesthetic involvement, the reference is to either general or major regional block, including epidural or spinal types of blocks. The most serious complications that manifest in this immediate puerperium period include problems of the airway, problems related to cardiovascular function such as hypo-or hypertension, problems associated with nausea and emesis, hemorrhagic problems (36), and problems related to inadequate pain relief. One of the most serious, life-threatening challenges can be postpartum hemorrhage. Ten of the most frequent factors associated with this condition are noted in Table 23–6. There is certainly not a place in today's practice of medicine in this country for a double standard of recovery between the operating room environs and the delivery room environs. In the past, however, many obstetric recovery areas have acted on such a differential standard. As noted by Dr. Bonica in the first edition, the archaic concept of obstetrics receiving depreciated, outmoded equipment and handed-down monitoring units must be vigorously opposed by the obstetric team. Such a policy used to be the rule rather than the exception. Each year new equipment acquisitions were made for operating rooms and the old equipment dutifully moved to the obstetric suite. In recent years, there have been many new advances in equipment and monitoring that make management of the trauma patients much easier. Some of these include the recent advances in fluid infusers, which are capable of large volume/small time constant infusion of blood and blood byproducts. This equipment is usually kept in the main operating suite due to high usage in trauma cases. The equipment is very expensive and demands high level technical upkeep and operation; therefore, to duplicate such equipment and personnel for the rare usage in the obstetric suites is questionable from a hospital-budget viewpoint. Of course, the risk is relegation of certain operative obstetric cases to the operating suite for optimum management of high volume infusion and optimum monitoring by the most sophisticated, highly technical equipment available. Some would admonish that the personnel in the operating room are also better geared toward management of the high-end and high-risk cases due to their training and constant use of such equipment.

**Table 23–6.** Predisposing Factors for Postpartum Hemorrhage

| |
|---|
| Dystocia |
| Macrosomia (>4000 g) |
| Preeclampsia |
| Chorioamnionitis |
| Precipitous labor |
| Prolonged labor |
| Over distended uterus |
| Eclampsia |
| General anesthesia |
| Grand multiparity/twinning |

(Modified from Hayashi R, Castillo M, Noah M: Management of severe postpartum hemorrhage due to uterine atony using an analog of prostaglandin F2$\alpha$. Obstet. Gynecol. 58:426, 1981.)

### *Airway Problems*

Most of the airway problems encountered in the immediate puerperium period are related to residual effects of the anesthetic, especially in reference to the general technique. These problems may include inadequate muscle relaxant reversal, inadequate handling of secretions with reflex laryngospasm and bronchospasm, or inadequate sedation recovery following general anesthesia or even regional anesthesia with supplemental sedation. Most all of these can be handled with ease after detection of the problem. It is important to emphasize at this point how imperative it is to see a patient when a nurse summons with a concern regarding the airway. There is just no substitute for coming directly to the bedside and fully evaluating a patient. This defines good medical practice, allays the nurses' alarm, and solidifies the fact that they have backup and support from their medical staff who are supervising the recovery room area. Some of the problems are so simple as to only require anatomic positioning to prevent airway obstruction by the tongue, while others may need reversal of medication as mentioned above to effect improved ventilation and oxygenation. Today, adequate monitoring of both oxygenation and ventilation are requisites to good care and both will be detailed further later on in this discussion. Hypoventilation, atelectasis, and secretion buildup can all be due to excessive depression of the respiratory center and the airway reflexes in general. The latter can be responsible ultimately for hypoxemia due to intrapulmonary shunting. Again, the key is to make sure the detection of the problem is made, the call to the appropriate medical staff is made, and a visit by that staff person or their directives given to the staff nurse in charge for active intervention that will correct the problem. Finally, it must be emphasized that whenever delirium, excitement, or restlessness occur in this early period during anesthetic recovery, problems in oxygenation must be ruled out before the assumption is made that the patient is merely suffering from pain or anesthetic emergence confusion.

## Cardiovascular Problems

Of the two major problems in this area, hypertension and hypotension, hypotension is far and away the most frequently encountered and serious problem. Hypotension demands immediate detection and institution of corrective measures to restore normative function. There are many basic aspects of patient recovery that are important to teach, but perhaps the most important are the simple ones related to detection of hypotension and immediate elevation of the patients legs to effect improved vascular volume within seconds; the second is the detection of the obstructed airway and immediate forward displacement of the mandible so as to alleviate the obstruction of the tongue, which is the major causative factor. Many times the hypotension in the recovery room can be traced to excessive unrecognized blood loss in the delivery room that was partially masked due to the patients legs being elevated in the Sims' position. When the patient's legs are placed flat and she is transported to recovery, there is time for the hypovolemic problem to fully manifest itself. The venous pooling results in a decrease in cardiac output and, as a result, a reduction in blood pressure. In addition to the immediate corrective step of legs elevation, the patient should receive generous fluid boluses until the pressure normalizes. In some instances, it may even be necessary to use a vasopressor such as 5 to 10 mg of ephedrine in the very early stages of diagnosis and treatment, but for the most part, this is rarely indicated due to the very effective maneuver of elevation of the legs. Elevation of the legs is thought to result in an immediate transfusion of from 400 to 500 ml of blood volume into the circulatory pool for immediate distribution. The maneuver can be best carried out by grasping the patients feet just behind the lower legs and gently elevating them to a 60° or even a 90° position if necessary. This author has utilized this technique for over 2 decades now, and it has never failed to restore within seconds of its institution the maternal blood pressure. This refers to the use in a patient without blood volume who has a hypotensive threat from regional anesthesia.

Hypertension can also be a problem for management in this early period, but it is, as mentioned, certainly less often encountered. When it does occur though it necessitates immediate detection and action on the part of the health care team. It may be a serious warning of an impending hypertensive crisis associated with pregnancy-induced hypertension or it may be the forerunner of a hypertensive crisis associated with a full blown eclamptic situation. The latter is catastrophic and often can be fatal due to massive intracranial hemorrhage. In either case, as mentioned, it demands immediate treatment with antihypertensive medication to protect the patient from irreversible sequalea as mentioned above. A small amount of hydralazine up to 10 mg in a patient without baseline tachycardia can be repeated every 10 minutes; in a patient with tachycardia, 10 mg of labetelol can also be used and can be doubled every 10 minutes until a satisfactory reduction can be induced. For longer term management, these patients may well be best managed with a central venous pressure (CVP) and a nitroprusside drip for their potent afterload and preload reduction effect. It is important to keep the central venous pressure maintained due to its preload reducing effects.

## Nausea and Emesis Problems

Nausea may be low grade in many patients just after delivery due to the intense vaginal stimulation associated with delivery. The nausea is often short lived, but in some patients lingers, and the need for administration of an antiemetic may be obvious. The use of droperidol in small intravenous aliquots of 2 to 3 mg has been the mainstay in the past to reverse the uncomfortable sensation of nausea and to prevent the sequela of emesis. The addition of a new effective drug, ondansetron, has greatly improved our ability to control this problem (37). The great concern is unobserved emesis of a patient who may be not fully awake and incapable of secretion handling. This may lead to silent aspiration and possibly severe consequences including hypoxia, hypercarbia, pulmonary edema, sustained irreversible hypoxia, cardiac arrest, and even death. To prevent such a serious problem, all patients must be monitored carefully by well trained and schooled nurses and staff. There must be immediate access to and consultation with the anesthesiologist and/or his/her direct delegates. In addition, there should be state of the art monitoring equipment available in the obstetric labor and delivery suite to equal that used in the operating room environs.

## Hemorrhagic Problems

Hemorrhage is always a concern in this immediate puerperium period both from the uterus, which can become flaccid due to atonic contractions, and from the incision, whether from the abdomen or perineum. Perhaps this problem and the problem of the airway are the two most urgent ones that can cause significant patient harm and injury if detection, diagnosis, and definitive therapy are not immediately instituted. Most obstetric recovery rooms have considerable experience and expertise in detection and management of hemorrhage because it is the primary concern and most frequently encountered problem in the immediate puerperium. The reason for this experience and expertise is that over the years obstetricians have repeatedly emphasized hemorrhage as the most important problem they should be on the lookout for. It would seem to be a simple process to record the amount of bleeding on the postpartum pads in the recovery room and use this as the primary indicator for uterine atony and hemorrhage, but the problem is that sometimes an occult hemorrhage may occur. Bleeding may be concealed within the uterus without external evidence. Prompt diagnosis of this concealed bleeding can be made by frequent palpation of the fundus at regular intervals by an experienced person during the first few hours postpartum. This atonic condition must be treated without delay by administration of oxytocic drugs, either oxytocin by continuous drip or methergine by intramuscular injection. In some instances, the obstetrician may opt for the latter, which can provide the added benefit of sustained tetanic-like contractions, which are effective in hemorrhage control. During such times, the patient's airway must also be evaluated and her adequacy of respiration checked frequently because one serious complication must not be overlooked due to the distraction caused by another serious one. Sudden obstetric shock can and does occur during the immediate puerperium due to uterine inversion, amniotic fluid embolism, and air or thrombotic embolism. Such a condition is life threatening, especially in a situation in which preparation for immediate aggressive intravenous therapy has not been considered. Nevertheless, all concerned must answer the call to save the life of the mother by establishing adequate intravenous access ports by cutdowns if necessary, administration of blood or blood byproducts, or crystalloid solutions. At times, arterial lines, a central venous pressure line, a Swan-Ganz line, administration of vasopressors, cardiotonics, bicarbonate solutions, and other all-out regimens must be exhausted in an attempt to save the life of the mother (38,39). Patients who necessitate such intensive monitoring are best managed in units familiar with all aspects of such care. The main indications for admission of patients to intensive care units are denoted in Table 23–7 (40). Once again, please refer to Chapter 26 for details.

**Table 23–7.** Main Indications for Intensive Care Unit Admissions

| |
|---|
| Hypertensive disorders (eclampsia, pulmonary edema) |
| Massive hemorrhage (abruptio placentae, placenta accreta) |
| Medical problems of pregnancy |
| Cardiac |
| Pulmonary |
| Renal |
| Sepsis |
| Gastrointestinal |
| Endocrine |
| Central nervous system |
| Other |

(Modified from Mabie WC, Sibai BM: Treatment in an obstetric intensive care unit. Am. J. Obstet. Gynecol. 162:1, 1990.)

## *Pain Problems*

The mother must be given the respect and consideration necessary in the immediate puerperium for the benefit of the mother and baby and the bonding and intimacy needed in this sensitive time period. In addition, it must be appreciated that the mother acts as a hostess to all of her and her husband's family and friends who visit daily to see the newborn baby. She must be at her peak; she is already exhausted and somewhat weakened by the blood loss, labor episode, and the interruption of her normal sleep pattern, and to add pain to these problems is just not acceptable. The old method of medicating patients who suffered from postoperative pain was time and labor intensive, and often resulted in delays in relief of pain. This scenario is described in Figure 23–11. Fortunately, today we have more effective and efficient alternatives for postoperative pain management. In counseling before delivery, it should be pointed out that there are various options that the patient may choose from so that she may "control" the pain perceived after delivery. This is a tremendous step forward for anesthesia and a truly humanitarian contribution. The methods offered can also help to prevent oversedation and somnolence, which only add to the problems noted above. The primary methods recommended for postoperative analgesia consist of: (1) lumbar epidural method for administration of analgesic agents;

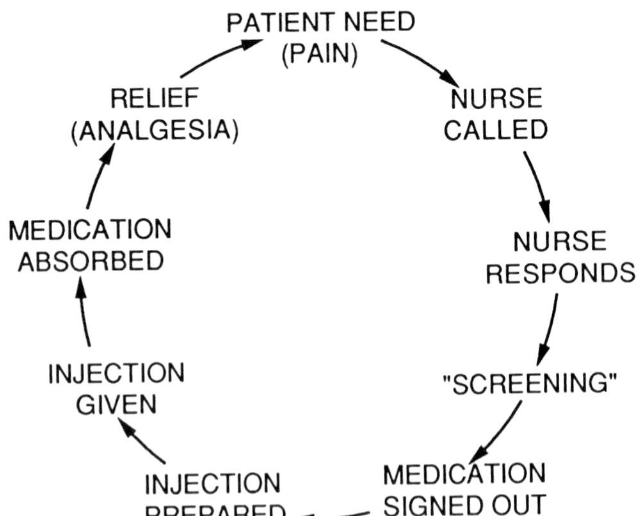


**Fig. 23–11.** Circular sequence to combat pain in antepartum period. Note that it may take from minutes up to an hour for pain relief to be realized because of delays built into the various components of the cycle. (Redrawn from Graves DA, Foster TS, Batenhorsts RL, Bennett RL, et al: Patient-controlled analgesia. Ann. Intern. Med. 99:360, 1983.)

(2) spinal method of administration of analgesic agents; and (3) patient controlled administration of analgesic agents via the systemic route. Of course, such treatment modalities should not be offered without setting up careful patient protective guidelines and an official service to administer to the needs of patients. The primary side effects presently include pruritus, urinary retention, nausea, and delayed respiratory problems. It is the latter that is of serious enough concern to be viewed as the primary determinant driving the development of the patient protective guidelines and necessity for keeping such a service under the administration of those who are skilled and familiar with usage and treatment of all such complications.

## Management of the Postpartum Mother in the Intermediate Puerperium

The type of complications that occur after the first 6 hours of delivery until the time of discharge include early onset of infections, postpartum hemorrhage, thromboembolism, postpuncture headache, backache, atelectasis, edema of the larynx and pain of the retropharyngeal area, and psychological depression, which is known more commonly as the postpartum blues. The early infections are centered chiefly in the uterus with endometritis being the most frequent offender by far. Second in line are infections of the bladder and urethra. Third are pulmonary infections, and last are thrombophlebitis and thromboembolism. Other associated anesthetic complications include postpuncture headaches, which often become clinically apparent by the second to the fourth postpartum day, backaches, and atelectasis. Edema of the larynx may be due to placement of the orotracheal tube during a general anesthetic . The psychologic depression, which is so prevalent, is associated with malaise, anorexia, feelings of helplessness, and a melancholic attitude. Finally, to round out the problems one may see in this intermediate period—after 6 hours and before discharge home, there must be a mention of wound infections and wound dehiscence. This section will focus on the problems of psychologic depression, wound infections, and wound dehiscence because the other problems have already been discussed in an earlier section or will be covered in the later part of this chapter.

### *Psychologic Depression*

The normal "blues" or "postpartum blues," as it is often referred to, is really quite common, usually short in duration, and mild in intensity. Its incidence has been recorded as high as 50%. The more severe and prolonged depressions labeled usually as postpartum depression, occur in less than 10% of patients. The early onset of irritability, anxiousness, and crying herald usually the onset of the normal postpartum blues. Apprehension, tension, or full realization that a new life must be now committed to may be predisposing reasons for this reaction. Some have said that there are generous hormonal shifts during this time also and that may be partly responsible. Whatever the etiology, which is still not well-defined, the time course is usually only a few days in length. The patient may have more general body complaints during this period, with complaints centering upon problems related to back pain, low abdominal pain, headache, and fatigue. The more serious emotional illnesses are rare fortunately, occurring less than 1% of the time. Serious emotional illness includes the psychoneuroses, such as anxiety reaction, conversion reaction, phobic reaction, dissociative reaction, obsessive-compulsive reaction, and the depressive reaction. Serious emotional illness also includes the more serious psychoses such as schizophrenia, paranoid reactions, and affective reactions.

### *Wound Infections*

Wound complications are an important part of the concern for speedy recovery in the postpartum mother. Some factors that contribute to such complications occur prior to surgery, some during the surgery itself, and some afterward. Prior to surgery, there are, of course, some medical factors that can increase the risk of wound infections and poor wound healing; two of the most notable are metabolic and include diabetes mellitus and faulty nutrition during gestation. In addition, the use of extended steroid therapy can impede substantially the patient's ability to counter an insidious infectious process. More important, and certainly more frequent from the causative standpoint, are intraoperative factors that concern surgical technique, including: (1) the surgical technique itself; (2) the attention to detail in regard to hemostasis; (3) the length of surgery; (4) the type of closure and type of suture material used in closure; and (5) the use of prophylactic antibiotics after surgery in patients of high infection potential. Postoperative factors include a variety of pulmonary complications and associated stimuli, which evoke a vigorous cough/Valsalva maneuver and include active upper respiratory infections, asthma, and flu syndromes that result in emesis. Actual infection percentages postoperatively after cesarean section are as small as 2 to 3% to as large as 14 to 15% depending on a host of interactive complex factors, including the ones mentioned above and others such as the patient's resistance, length of time in labor, and length of time of membrane rupture (41). With full recognition of the many interactive factors that can cause wound infection, the severity of same can be reduced with careful attention to detail and full realization of the risk and early detection and treatment. The various methods to be considered include identification of all patients at risk, careful surgical technique and swiftness, and early recognition of the signs and symptoms of wound infection followed by aggressive immediate intervention.

### *Wound Dehiscence*

The word dehiscence comes from the Latin word dehiscere, which means "to gape." It refers to the problem of wound disruption caused most often by infection and suture tearing through anchoring tissues. The anchoring tissues are most often restricted to the fascia which causes a major problem because it is the fascia that serves as the barrier for the abdominal region and all of its contents. Smaller wound dehiscences can also occur, and these are above the fascia in the investing muscular layers or even more superficial in the subcutaneous layers. The most superficial fascia is made up of Camper's fascia, a subcutaneous fatty layer, and Scarpa's fascia, the next membraneous, deeper layer. If a wound infection causes disruption of the sutures in this layer, it is a simple matter of cleaning up the wound daily until it heals from the deeper layers on up. The next deeper fascial plane is made up of the anterior layer of the rectus sheath and the posterior layer of the rectus sheath. A wound infection in this layer causes the involvement of the rectus muscle layers, which adds another dimension to the healing and cleaning process that must occur before healing can occur from the deeper layers on up. The last fascial plane is the transversalis fascia itself, which is just above the peritoneum. A disruption in this deepest layer is a major problem and life threatening because abdominal contents may be exposed and actually spill out extraperitoneally. Such a problem is detected by a large discharge that is actually peritoneal fluid. The detection of such a complication must signal immediate action consisting of covering of the wound by sterile dressings and taking the patient to the operating room for adequate anesthesia, prepping and draping of the wound, and exposure and inspection of the wound margins so that retention-type sutures can be placed for re-approximation of the wound margins, closure of the fascial defect, and a thorough cleansing of all the tissues superficial to that plane (42).

### *Pulmonary Infections*

The more common pulmonary infections include the pneumonias due to a preexistent bacterial or viral etiology, or a superimposed pneumonia in an area of pulmonary infarct (43). There are, of course, the aspiration syndromes with obvious contamination of the lungs with aspirated debris and with it secondary infections due to the local damage and cellular destruction. The most frequent cause of the bacterial pneumonias is Streptococcus pneumoniae but others include pneumococcal pneumonia and mycoplasma pneumonia. Detection is usually by clinical symptomatology including cough, chest pain, purulent sputum, and temperature elevation. Diagnosis should be by chest x ray and gram staining and culture of the sputum. In one recent study of the problem, the author concluded that in spite of early diagnosis and treatment, there was a relatively high rate of complications including respiratory failure and even intubation management. Some of these complications were respiratory support in nearly 20% and a bacteremia in 16% (42). The improvement in maternal survival from pneumonia is shown in Table 23–8. In addition to pulmonary infections, other widespread puerperal infections can occur as a result of hematogeneous spread, and these include some of the areas highlighted in Figure 23–12.

**Table 23–8.** Maternal Death Rates Reported by Different Studies

| Author | Incidence | Maternal Deaths No. | % |
|---|---|---|---|
| [1] Finland and Dublin, 1939 | 164/25,891 | 18/74 | 24 |
| [2] Oxorn, 1955 (before antibiotics) | 35/ND | 7/35 | 20 |
| Oxorn, 1955 (after antibiotics) | 29/ND | 1/29 | 3.5 |
| [3] Hopwood, 1965 | 23/2,720 | 2/23 | 8.7 |
| [4] Collaborative Perinatal Study, 1972 | 119/39,215 | ND | |
| [5] Benedetti et al, 1982 | 39/89,219 | 0/39 | 0 |
| Current Series | 25/32,179 | 1/25 | 4 |
| Subtotals | | | |
| Preantibiotic era | NC | 25/109 | 23 |
| Antibiotic era | 206/163,333 | 4/116 | 3.4 |

NC, not calculable
ND, no data reported
[1] Finland M, Dublin TD: Pneumococcic pneumonias complicating pregnancy and the puerperium. JAMA 112:1027–32, 1939.
[2] Oxorn H: The changing aspects of pneumonia complicating pregnancy. Am. J. Obstet. Gynecol. 70:1057–63, 1955.
[3] Hopwood HG: Pneumonia in pregnancy. Obstet. Gynecol. 25:875–9, 1965.
[4] Niswander KR, Gordon M: The women and their pregnancies. *In* The Collaborative Perinatal Studies of the National Institute of Neurological Diseases and Stroke. Philadelphia, W.B. Saunders, 1972, pp. 230–3.
[5] Benedetti TJ, Valle R, Ledger WJ: Antepartum pneumonia in pregnancy. Am J. Obstet. Gynecol. 144:413–7, 1982.
(Modified from Madinger NE, Greenspoon JS, Ellrodt AG: Pneumonia during pregnancy: has modern technology improved maternal and fetal outcome? Am. J. Obstet. Gynecol. 161:657, 1989.)

## Management of the Postpartum Mother in the Remote Puerperium

The remote puerperium extends from time of discharge from the hospital until the 6-week examination by the obstetrician. This is the period of time when delayed problems such as postpartum infections referable to the parturition can occur; additionally, some delayed hemorrhagic problems can occur also during this time period. Finally, problems associated with thromboembolic disease and delayed postpuncture headaches can also manifest themselves even during this late period. The following discussion will view these in more detail.

### *Postpartum Infection Problems*

Genital tract infections are still the most frequently encountered of the postpartum infectious processes. The causative agent, in descending order of frequency, is: streptococcus, E. coli, staphylococcus, clostridium, fragilis, and the prevotella bivia (bacteroides) or prevotella disiens. Most infection sites are limited to the cervix and vaginal area, and uterine cavity. When the latter is involved an endometritis is diagnosed with associated signs of temperature elevation, tachycardia, uterine tenderness, and foul-smelling lochia. Endometritis is often caused by a combination of microbes, including the aerobic and anaerobic gram-negative bacilli, the anaerobic gram-positive cocci, and the aerobic streptococci (44). The immediate concern is local spread via the fallopian tubes with seeding and involvement of the parametria. Treatment, therefore, must be immediate and definitive. A culture is taken during examination and the patient is placed on wide spectrum antibiotic coverage until return of the culture. Most often ampicillin or amoxocillin can be used as a first line coverage. The patient is also asked to observe pelvic rest and reduced activity status for a few days. Most pa-

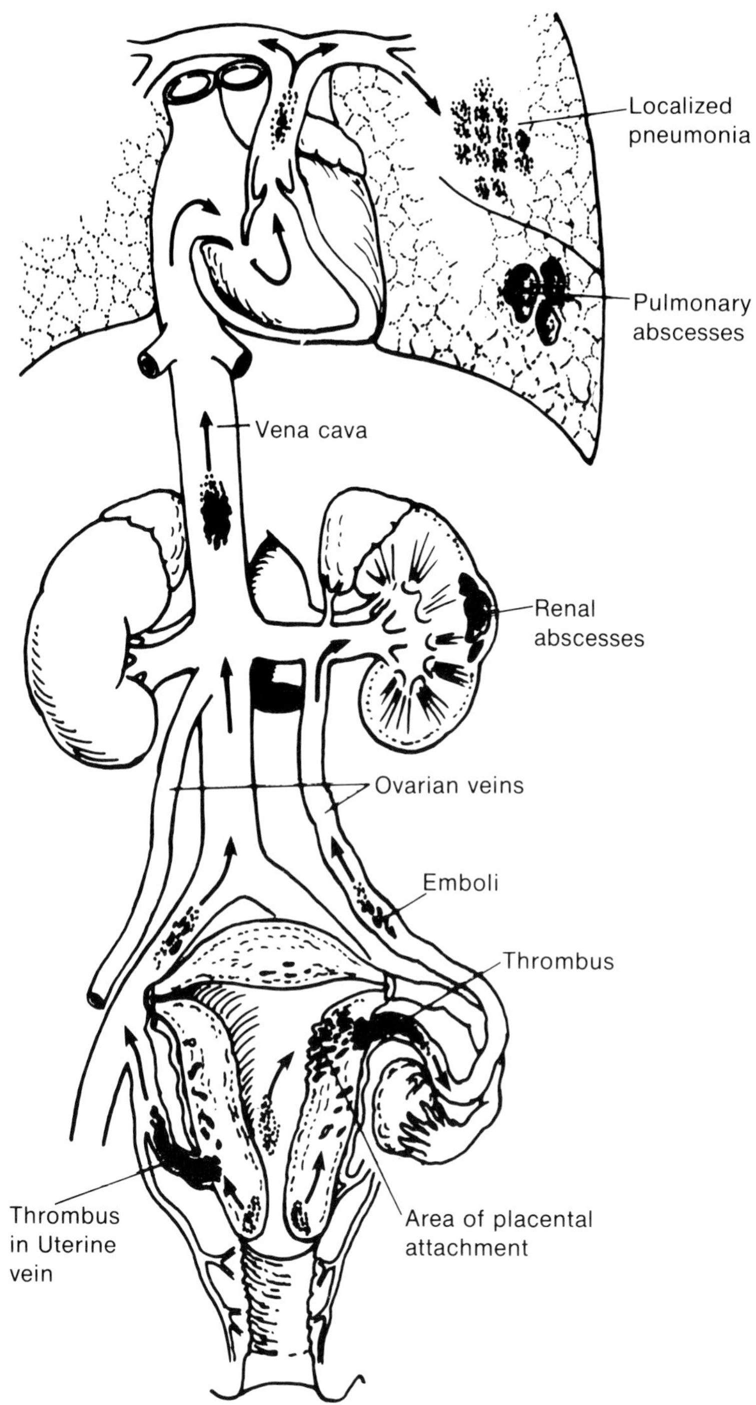


**Fig. 23–12.** An illustration of the wide-spread effect of puerperal infections on the body.

tients can be treated on an outpatient basis, but, clinically, if the response of the patient is not immediate, then hospitalization and treatment with intravenous antibiotics should be considered. For cesarean section coverage, first line agents would most likely consist of clindamycin and gentamycin (45). Some of the variables associated with wound infections are revealed in Table 23–9. For vaginal complications, cefoxitin or amoxicillin would be the first line agents, unless the patient is allergic to penicillin, in which case clindamycin and gentamycin would be substituted. Urinary tract infections are the next most frequent problem causing postpartum infections with most of these being confined to a cystitis caused by E. coli or other coliform bacteria. Typical signs and symptoms noted early in the disease process include pain over the suprapubic area, frequency, and dysuria. A diagnosis is easily confirmed with urine analysis and microscopic analysis revealing white cells and bacteria. Treatment consists of a reduced activity status and a broad spectrum antibiotic until the urine culture is returned with the predominant organism identified and sensitivities outlined. Mastitis is the third common problem noted as far as postpartum

**Table 23–9.** Wound Abscess After Cesarean Delivery

| Variable | Wound Abscess (N = 64) | P | Control (N = 64) |
|---|---|---|---|
| Labor duration (h)* | 7.1 ± 5.6 | <.001 | 3.7 ± 4.7 |
| Rupture of membrane interval (h)* | 9.9 ± 13.1 | <.005 | 4.4 ± 5.5 |
| No. of vaginal examinations* | 5.9 ± 3.7 | <.005 | 3.7 ± 4.0 |
| Internal fetal monitoring duration (h)* | 6.8 ± 5.9 | <.001 | 2.5 ± 3.7 |
| Operating time (min)* | 61.2 ± 26.4 | <.02 | 53.2 ± 15.0 |
| Estimated blood loss (ml)* | 821.8 ± 386.2 | <.01 | 674.2 ± 235.7 |
| Indication—dystocia | 37 (59%) | <.001 | 16 (25%) |
| Endometritis—chorioamnionitis | 44 (70%) | <.001 | 18 (28%) |
| Fever in labor | 7 (11%) | <.02 | 0 |
| Abdominal incision, percent transverse | 20 (31%) | .08† | 11 (17%) |

* Data expressed as mean ± SD.
† See text.
(From Gibbs RS, Blanco JD, St Clair PJ: A case-control study of wound abscess after cesarean delivery. Obstet. Gynecol. 62:498, 1983.)

infections are concerned. The causative agent is most often Staphylococcus aureus. The diagnosis is relatively simple due to the fact that exquisite breast tenderness, actual pain on milk expression, and redness of the area focus the attention to the breast. Mastitis today is best treated by administration of oral antibiotic therapy awaiting culture results. Dicloxacillin, an example of a penicillinase-resistant antibiotic, should be used if penicilin-resistant Staph. aureus is suspected (46). Breast-feeding may accelerate resolution of nonepidemic mastitis through decompression of the breasts, and is not harmful to the infant (46–48).

## Delayed Hemorrhagic Problems

The problems of postpartum hemorrhage are major and life threatening as noted in the earlier discussion of the immediate puerperium. In the delayed variation of the postpartum hemorrhage, most of the problems are caused by retained placental fragments or even an accessory cotyledon with inability of the uterus to contract around that area and continued bleeding from the exposed uterine lining. Another possibility is subinvolution of the placental site, or submucosal fibroid tumors which also result in continued bleeding from the uterine lining. The bleeding can vary between minimal to severe according to the size of the area involved and number of active vessels included. The treatment is diagnosis that rules out other causes of genital tract bleeding such as perineal, vaginal, or cervical, followed by therapy that consists of a D&C or other method to remove the offending barrier to effective contraction, administration of oxytocin, and replacement of fluid in appropriate quantities and quality as indicated.

## Thrombolembolic Disease Problems

Pregnancy produces a relative state of hypercoagulation and complications of a thromboembolic nature are not unexpected. Yet, because of the activity of most postpartum mothers, this complication is rare, occurring in less than 1 to 2% of postpartum mothers. When it does occur, the site of the disease process can be in the leg veins of the saphenous, popliteal and femoral area via the so called DVT or deep venous thrombosis route, or in the pelvis via the ovarian, the uterine, and the hypogastric veins. When the disease process is restricted to the lower extremity only and thrombophlebitis is predominant, there may be signs and symptoms of fever, tachycardia, and local area pain. Propagation of the thrombosis from the lumen of the vessel of origin toward the heart means embolism that can be sudden and life threatening; fortunately, this happens rarely. Certainly, the incidence of thromboembolism has an incidence lower than that found after general surgical procedures, perhaps due to the motivation for motion and activity stimulated by the birth of the newborn baby.

## Delayed Postpuncture Headache Problems

Most of the problems associated with postpuncture injuries are manifest very early in the puerperium, such as the immediate or, more commonly, the intermediate puerperium. However, the practitioner should be cognizant of the potentially threatening problems that may surface late. One of these is the delayed postpuncture complication of subdural hematoma. This manifests itself as a chronic headache due to tentorial pressure and pain associated with excessive subarachnoid fluid loss over many days and even weeks. The reservoir system of cerebral spinal fluid (CSF) and the support pad for the cranial structures become significantly reduced with resultant sagging of the brain and its covering including the meninges. It is believed that it is this phenomena that elicits the symptom of pain of the postpuncture headache. To take this pathophysiologic process a bit further, a vascular rupture may occur due to this intracranial displacement with resultant formation of subdural blood. Diagnosis must be made by obtaining either a magnetic resonance image (MRI) or a CT scan of the head that clearly show the subdural hematoma. Magnetic resonance imaging is preferred for definition of small subdural hematomas, but of course it is twice the price of the cat scan. The CT scan would be acceptable in suspected large subdurals only.

Intracranial bleeding after lumbar puncture with subdural hematoma is unusual, but the following 23-year-old G1 P1 patient is an illustration of such a problem. The patient received lumbar epidural analgesia for labor pain relief, but an inadvertent dural puncture occurred with an 18-gauge needle. The patient complained of headache with assumption of the vertical position on the first postpartum day. She was treated symptomatically and had some improvement over 4 days. She was discharged home only to return 4 days later with a history of severe headache of bursting proportions and transient dysarthria and loss of vision in her right eye. CT scan and carotid angiograms revealed a right-sided subdural hematoma that was confirmed at the time of operation with evacuation of a bilateral frontoparietal subdural hematoma. The magnetic resonance imaging technology was not available for use at the time of this case in 1975. The patient recovered uneventfully. It is possible that the loss of cerebrospinal fluid cushion resulted in some considerable shift of the brain tissue that may have ruptured local vessels and resulted in subdural accumulation large enough to cause pressure in the right hemispheric area.

There are also instances in which postpuncture headaches do not show up until after the patient is discharged. Thus, by definition, they would be classified in the remote puerperium. These are the slow leak problems that only manifest themselves as significant headaches after the patient is discharged home. They can follow a typical course, however, with postural headache beleaguering the patient hourly until she calls her obstetrician to complain because she cannot function adequately. When these headaches are of the severe nature, they are really incapacitating to the point where the patient must maintain a horizontal position or even maintain the head below the heart position to obtain relief. The headaches due to postlumbar puncture leakage of the spinal fluid and spontaneous hypoliquorrheia are secondary to reduced spinal fluid pressure. As mentioned above, the mechanism behind the headache is most likely tension on sensitive intracranial structure. The syndrome of low spinal fluid headache was first described by Bier in 1899 (49). His original descriptive was a headache augmented by vertical position due to leakage of cerebral spinal fluid. There is some question as to whether there is a place for conservative therapy this late in the diagnosis cycle of such a problem, but some may still opt for the conservative route and use bed rest, fluids, and caffeine sodium benzoate regimens as opposed to the more aggressive route of bringing the patient in for an epidural blood patch. The latter seems more humanitarian as most of these patients have already suffered enough and are deserving of the more aggressive regimen by this late time period. It must be mentioned at this time that all patients with problems such as the ones enumerated in this section must be seen personally by a physician for a physical exam and evaluation. There is just no place for management of these problems over the phone. This reassures the patient, the husband and other relatives, assures you that you are not missing something not evident by verbal description, and makes sure you are fulfilling your medical responsibility to the patient.

## MANAGEMENT OF THE NEWBORN

This section will describe comprehensively the clinical management of the newborn infant from the instant of birth through the period of stable clinical condition at which time the newborn infant can maintain physiologic homeostasis and/or at which further care is provided in an observation nursery or the newborn intensive care unit. Provision of appropriate care should be based on the understanding of normal as well as pathologic fetal and neonatal conditions as the result of transition from fetal to neonatal life. A brief description of fetal and neonatal circulatory and respiratory changes occurring with the birth process is given. Our present understanding of pathologic conditions affecting physiologic homeostasis is briefly discussed.

Preparation for the care of the newborn infant at birth is preceded by a description of the personnel, facilities, and equipment necessary for successful management of distressed newborn infants at birth. For a continuum of care from fetus to neonate, the role of individual members of the perinatal team, comprised of an obstetrician, anesthesiologist, nurse, and pediatrician, is briefly described. Clinical appraisal of the newborn infant at birth and medical management based on physiopathologic considerations will also be discussed. The reader is encouraged to review other chapters of this book for related information pertinent to successful management of the newborn at birth.

### Basic Considerations

The importance of proper care and effective resuscitation of the newborn needs no elaboration. Approximately 50% of neonatal deaths occur during the first day of life. A significant number are the result of cardiorespiratory problems, particularly in preterm newborn infants (50). Morbidity and even mortality of a certain number of newborn infants may be due to inadequate and/or ineffective resuscitation at birth. Despite major advances in perinatal care over the past 2 decades, a significant number of newborn infants are depressed at birth and require skilled resuscitative measures. The detection of fetal distress by means of electronic fetal monitoring, fetal acid-base and blood gas measurements, and proper use of anesthesia and analgesia may have contributed to a decline in the incidence of neonatal depression, but a considerable number of infants still require resuscitation (51–54). Recently, we have examined this point in a regional perinatal center based on the method of delivery. Table 23–10 shows the incidence of low Apgar scores, and the number and percent of newborn infants requiring resuscitation by means of positive pressure ventilation by bag and mask and/or via the endotracheal tube separated by the delivery methods. From this table, one notes that 30% of the newborn infants were delivered by cesarean section. This fact, to a greater extent, is due to a more aggressive approach by obstetricians to prevent perinatal asphyxia by operative intervention.

When considering pathologic conditions at birth due to a variety of causes, one should examine specific factors that may interfere with fetal/neonatal adaptation during the intrapartum period. Several publications have emphasized the importance of maternal, fetal, and intrapartum elements that may adversely influence the fetal/neonatal condition (55–60). Knowledge of these specific maternal and fetal high-risk factors will enhance one's ability to anticipate problems and to provide effective preparation for successful resuscitation.

The neonatal team's understanding of these factors and their influence on the condition of the neonate, as well as consideration for neonatal pathophysiology, is essential for an effective and successful resuscitation in the delivery room.

**Table 23–10.** Method of Delivery and the Distribution of Apgar Scores

| | Type of birth | | | | | | | | | |
|---|---|---|---|---|---|---|---|---|---|---|
| | Vertex Vaginal | | Breech Vaginal | | Cesarean Repeat | | Cesarean Primary | | Total Births | |
| **Infant Characteristics** | # | % | # | % | # | % | # | % | # | % |
| Male infant* | 3613 | 50.2 | 37 | 46.3 | 533 | 49.8 | 1092 | 54.2 | 5275 | 50.9 |
| Female infant | 3589 | 49.8 | 43 | 53.8 | 538 | 50.2 | 923 | 45.8 | 5093 | 49.1 |
| Infant born alive | 7155 | 99.3 | 51 | 63.8 | 1067 | 99.6 | 2011 | 99.8 | 10284 | 99.2 |
| Fetal death | 48 | 0.7 | 29 | 36.3 | 4 | 0.4 | 4 | 0.2 | 85 | 0.8 |
| Apgar at 1 min: 1–3** | 115 | 1.6 | 33 | 41.3 | 37 | 3.5 | 153 | 7.6 | 338 | 3.3 |
| Apgar at 1 min: 4–6** | 429 | 6.0 | 9 | 11.3 | 76 | 7.1 | 271 | 13.4 | 785 | 7.6 |
| Apgar at 1 min: 7–10 | 6607 | 91.7 | 9 | 11.3 | 954 | 89.1 | 1585 | 78.7 | 9155 | 88.3 |
| Apgar at 5 min: 1–3** | 40 | 0.6 | 17 | 21.3 | 4 | 0.4 | 11 | 0.5 | 72 | 0.7 |
| Apgar at 5 min: 4–6** | 34 | 0.5 | 8 | 10.0 | 19 | 1.8 | 59 | 2.9 | 120 | 1.2 |
| Apgar at 5 min: 7–10 | 7077 | 98.2 | 22 | 27.5 | 1044 | 97.5 | 1940 | 96.3 | 10079 | 97.2 |
| Resus (PPV)*** mask or ETT | 518 | 7.2 | 27 | 33.8 | 134 | 12.5 | 496 | 24.6 | 1175 | 11.3 |
| Admitted to NICU**** | 481 | 6.7 | 27 | 33.8 | 112 | 10.5 | 461 | 22.9 | 1081 | 10.4 |

Long Beach Memorial Medical Center, California, 1984 to 1985.
* Significantly more frequent ($P < 0.05$) in primary section vs. vaginal vertex.
** Significantly more frequent ($P < 0.01$) in primary and repeat cesarean section vs. vaginal vertex.
*** Significantly more frequent ($P < 0.001$) in primary and repeat cesarean section vs. vaginal vertex.
**** Significantly more frequent in primary cesarean section vs. vaginal vertex.

## *Fetal and Neonatal Circulation*

### Physiologic Changes at Birth

Understanding of the fetal circulatory pathways and the function of fetal lungs is very important to our understanding of normal cardiorespiratory adaptation at birth. Both fetal circulation and fetal lungs undergo a maturation process during the course of gestation. This maturation process involves morphological and functional changes in preparation for extrauterine life. During the growth and maturation process, the placenta maintains gaseous exchanges between fetus and maternal compartments. At birth the respiratory functions of the placenta are assumed by the neonatal lungs.

Gaseous exchanges occur at the microvillous space of the placenta. Oxygenated blood returns to the fetus through the umbilical vein via the portal system. At the level of placenta to portal vein, fetal blood oxygen tension is about 32 to 35 mm Hg in normal physiologic condition. Oxygen saturation at this point is 80% (61). The umbilical vein joins the portal sinus at the liver. After preferential perfusion of the left lobe of the liver, umbilical vein blood mixes with portal vein blood and enters the inferior vena cava via the ductus venosus. The latter seems to decrease the umbilical venous pressure by producing a low-resistance shunt, and is not sensitive to changes in $PO_2$, $PCO_2$, or fetal pH. After mixing with blood from the inferior vena cava coming from the lower fetal body, the flow enters the right atrium. The crista dividens directs part of the inferior vena cava return through the foramen ovale into the left atrium. This blood, with that returning from the pulmonary veins, constitutes the total blood volume entering the left ventricle. The remainder from the inferior vena cava and blood from the superior vena cava enters the right ventricle. Because of intracardiac and extracardiac shunts, the right and left ventricle work in parallel rather than in series, which normally occurs during postnatal life. Cardiac output from the right ventricle constitutes about two-thirds of combined fetal cardiac output, of which about 90% is shunted through the ductus arteriosus to the descending aorta. Based on studies in mammals, particularly in fetal lambs, during the second half of gestation, fetal lungs receive approximately 10% of right ventricular output for their metabolic needs and growth. As the oxygenated blood of the umbilical vein mixes with other less oxygenated fetal blood via extracardiac and intracardiac shunts, its oxygen content decreases gradually. The blood in the descending aorta has a $PO_2$ of 20 to 22 mm Hg and an $O_2$ saturation of 55 to 60%. The myocardium, forelimbs, head, and brain receive blood from the left ventricle with $PO_2$ ranging from 26 to 28 mm Hg with $O_2$ saturation of about 65%, while the abdominal organs, lower body, and placenta are supplied with the lowest oxygenated blood (62–64). However, the proportions of blood distributed to the various organs change as gestation progresses. The distribution of combined cardiac output to different organs and physiologic shunts is due to the high pulmonary vascular resistance. The systemic circulation with significant cardiac output to the placenta (about 40% of combined cardiac output) constitutes a low-resistance circulation. At birth, with separation from the placenta and the initiation of breathing, the neonatal circulation gradually becomes the adult circulatory pattern. With the establishment of breathing and the clearing of fetal lung fluid, pulmonary vascular resistance gradually decreases while the pulmonary blood flow increases simultaneously. The systemic vascular resistance increases with the elimination of the placenta, and the right and left ventricle work in series. The output of the two ventricles becomes similar. Transitional neonatal circulation from fetal to adult circulatory pathways is influenced by the autonomic nervous system, as well as humoral factors such as catecholamines and prostaglandins, although the exact role of the individual humoral substance has yet to be fully understood. Initially, functional closure of intracardiac and extracardiac fetal shunts occurs, followed by the anatomic closures. Functional closure of the ductus arteriosus may occur a few hours after birth unless pathologic conditions, such as hypoxemia and persistence of high pulmonary vascular resistance, interfere with its closure. In such cases, persistence of fetal circulatory pathways or left-to-right shunting occur, as in preterm infants with respiratory distress syndrome.

The onset and maintenance of respiration after birth is dependent upon: (1) integrity of the respiratory center; (2) responsiveness to biochemical respiratory stimuli; (3) clearance of lung fluid; (4) normal respiratory systems and their supporting structures, from the thoracic cage to the cardiovascular system; and (5) an adequate supply of oxygen.

### Pathologic Conditions

Normal adaptation from fetal to neonatal life may be adversely affected by interference with fetal gaseous exchange. As noted above, the fetus is completely dependent opon placental respiratory function, i.e., uptake of $O_2$ and elimination of $CO_2$. Decreased placental respiratory function due to maternal and/or uteroplacental factors adversely affect the condition of the fetus. The effects of asphyxia/hypoxia have been studied in chronic preparation of lambs, close-to-term gestation by allowing the ewe to breathe low oxygen-gas mixture and/or interfering with umbilical blood flow. A fetus stressed in this manner has the ability to compensate for hypoxia by redistribution of cardiac output to different organs (65). The fetal circulatory adaptation to hypoxia is accomplished by increased perfusion to essential organs such as the myocardium, brain, and adrenal glands, with a concomitant decrease in perfusion of the lungs, skin, muscle, gastrointestinal tract, kidneys, and limbs. Apparently, the percentage of combined cardiac output to placenta is maintained. The redistribution of cardiac output in response to hypoxia appears to be associated with, or perhaps mediated by, increased plasma catecholamines, arginine vasopressin concentration, and a rise in endorphins. The role of the autonomic nervous system and other neurohumoral factors in modulating redistribution of fetal cardiac output in response to hypoxia has yet to be clarified. The integrity of the cellular function of individual organ systems depends on the degree and duration of hypoxia. In humans, particularly during the intrapartum period, the interference with fetoplacental gas exchange more frequently occurs as intermittent episodes related to uterine contractions rather than as a total or persistent asphyxial insult (66). Therefore, results of animal experiments dealing with persistent and/or total asphyxia may not duplicate the pathologic findings in the human fetus and newborn. Despite the ability to redistribute cardiac output to essential organs during hypoxia insult, a significant degree of hypoxia will reduce organ perfusion, affecting cellular integrity and function. Occurrence of cellular damage may relate to the duration and magnitude of the insult. Hypoxia, hypercarbia resulting in metabolic, and, to a lesser degree, respiratory acidosis, will interfere with cellular function and eventually lead to cellular death (66,67). Although organs such as the myocardium and brain may be partially spared, prolonged asphyxial insult will adversely affect these organs. Prolonged fetal asphyxia will result in systemic hypertension and hypervolemia. Altered functions of myocardial, pulmonary, renal, and other organ systems, as a consequence of asphyxia, should be kept in mind when therapeutic measures are being considered. Specific discussion on the pathology of these organ systems is beyond the scope of this chapter.

## Neonatal Heart Rate and Blood Pressure

### Heart Rate

During the course of gestation, heart rate gradually decreases. This decrease in baseline fetal heart rate is due to maturation of the parasympathetic nervous system, which becomes dominant by term gestation. The baseline heart rate at term gestation ranges between 120 and 150 beats per minute. Fetal heart rate response to asphyxia/hypoxia is initially mediated by the baroreflex mechanism, resulting in bradycardia. With persistence of asphyxia/hypoxia, fetal bradycardia may be related to aortic chemoreceptor responses to hypoxemia. Persistent hypoxemia will not only influence the baseline heart rate but will depress vagal influence on modulating baseline heart rate variability (53). Fetal bradycardia as the result of hypoxemia will reduce cardiac output, thus interfering with fetoplacental gas exchange and further aggravate the already reduced fetal oxygen supply, resulting in progressive metabolic acidosis.

Postnatally, in the normal newborn infant heart rate increases soon after birth, resultant from a surge in catecholamines. After the first few minutes, there is a gradual decline in neonatal heart rate. By 30 to 60 minutes of life, neonatal heart rate ranges about 130 to 140 beats per minute (BPM) (68). Moderately depressed and acidotic newborn infants have a more drastic tachycardic response soon after birth. The baseline remains somewhat higher during the first 30 minutes of life compared to normal newborn infants. Conversely, severely acidotic and asphyxiated newborns' heart rate response after birth is more attenuated than moderately depressed and acidotic newborn infants (Figure 23–13). The lack of somewhat lower cardiac response in severely acidotic newborn infants is most likely due to myocardial dysfunction as a result of prolonged fetal hypoxia and acidosis. Because neonates increases their cardiac output mostly by an increase in heart rate and to a lesser degree by increasing stroke volume, severely asphyxiated newborn infants have less cardiac reserve and may not withstand intravascular volume expansion, particularly with colloids. A rapid postnatal volume expansion may aggravate already increased afterload (systemic hypertension) and preload (increase in placental blood flow), which have existed just before the birth of a severely hypoxic/acidotic fetus. Treatment for infants with this condition should consist of

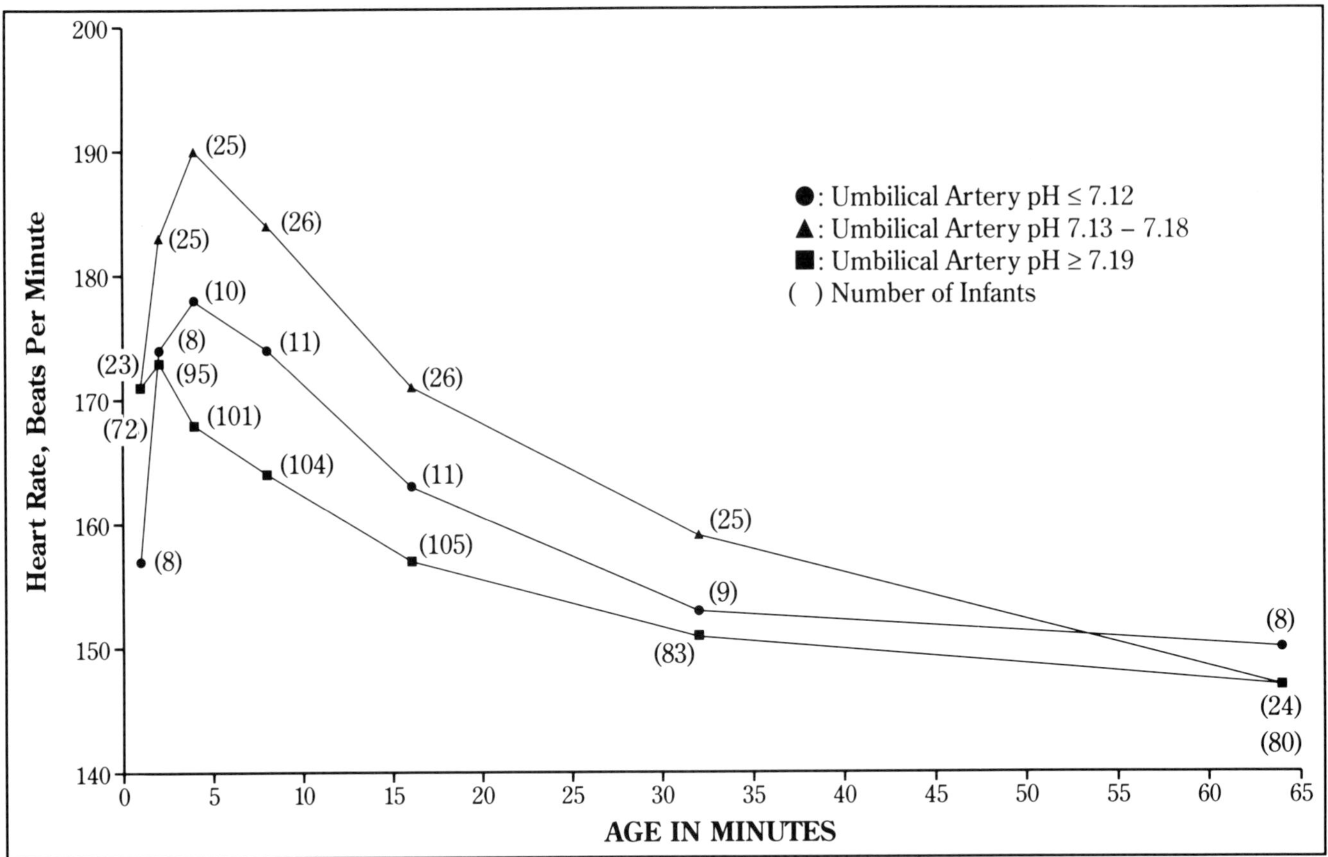


**Fig. 23–13.** Mean neonatal pH during the first 64 minutes of life in normal (umbilical artery pH ≥ 7.19), moderately acidotic (umbilical artery pH 7.13 to 7.18), and severely acidotic (umbilical artery pH ≤ 7.12) infants at birth.

establishment of appropriate ventilation and oxygenation with 100% $O_2$ and possible correction of metabolic acidosis with alkali rather than volume expansion with colloids. The latter may further aggravate decreased lung fluid clearance and lead to cardiac failure (69). Cardiopulmonary distress as the result of perinatal asphyxia/hypoxia should be distinguished (although it is not always possible to do so) from shock as the result of septicemia and hypovolemia (70). Figure 23–14 depicts correction of acidosis, during the first hour after delivery, with appropriate ventilation and oxygenation at birth.

### Blood Pressure

Dramatic circulatory changes at birth will induce hemodynamic changes such as increased peripheral vascular resistance and rise in systemic vascular pressure. The latter will gradually become higher than pulmonary vascular pressure, usually within minutes to hours after birth (62,65). Little information regarding systemic blood pressure exists in newborn infants during the first few minutes of life. Many years ago, we studied direct arterial blood pressure during the first hour of life in well and depressed newborn infants (Figure 23–15). Similar to the heart rate changes after birth, blood pressure in depressed newborns, particularly systolic blood pressure, is somewhat higher than in normal newborns. This is probably secondary to catecholamine surge, increased peripheral vascular resistance, and hypervolemia as the result of asphyxia/hypoxia. Only newborn infants with severe hypovolemia or cardiogenic shock are found to be hypotensive at birth. Neonatal heart rate and blood pressure findings in depressed and acidotic infants suggest that sudden volume expansion soon after birth may be harmful rather than beneficial. Exceptions are newborn infants with true hypovolemia due to feto-fetal, feto-maternal or vaso previa hemorrhage. Severe hypoxemia may also lead to myocardial dysfunction. When the practitioner uses therapeutic modalities in the treatment of asphyxiated infants, the possibility of myocardial dysfunction must be considered.

## Fetal and Neonatal Acid-Base Balance and Blood Gases

Because of structural and functional characteristics of the human placenta, fetal umbilical venous $PO_2$ is considerably less than that of the adult or the neonate after birth. Despite its low $PO_2$, fetal blood is capable of transporting large quantities of oxygen from the placenta to the fetal organs (63,64). This is aided by a high level of fetal hemoglobin in fetal red blood cells, which have a high affinity to oxygen (at a $PO_2$ of 32 to 35 mm Hg, fetal blood has a saturation of 80% at the pH of 7.40) and results in a higher rate of perfusion to the fetal organs. Apparently,

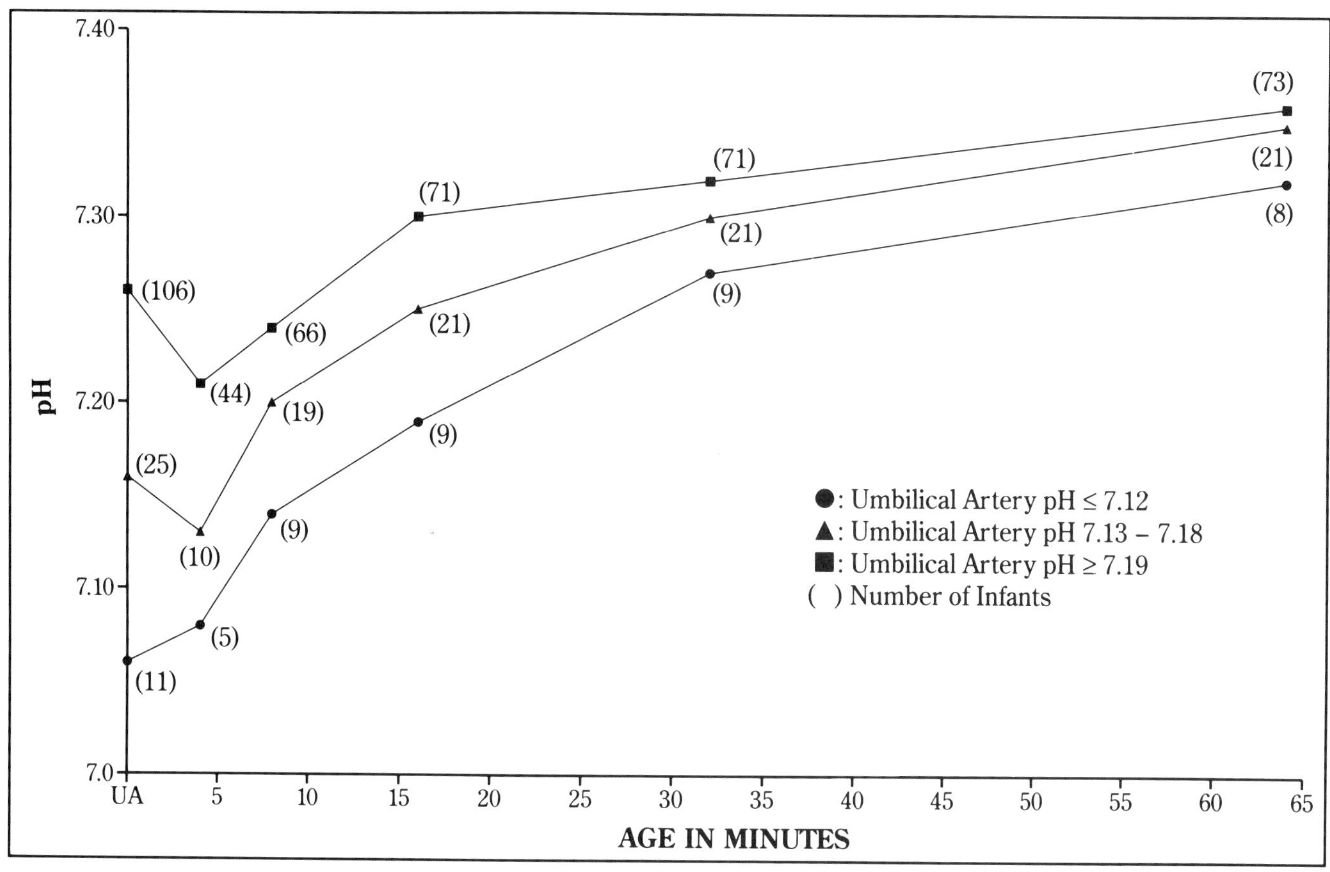


**Fig. 23–14.** Mean heart rate during the first 64 minutes of life in normal (umbilical artery pH ≥ 7.19), moderately acidotic (umbilical artery pH 7.13 to 7.18), and severely acidotic (umbilical artery pH ≤ 7.12) infants at birth.

the low fetal $PO_2$ is physiologically useful in keeping the ductus arteriosus open and the pulmonary vascular system constricted. Within a few minutes after birth, descending aortic blood $PO_2$ rises to about 60 mm Hg while the quantity of fetal hemoglobin remains the same. Again the rise of neonatal $PO_2$ and hemoglobin saturation is part of the complexity of factors responsible for the functional and later anatomical closure of the ductus arteriosus and decreasing pulmonary vascular resistance. Table 23–11 depicts values of fetal scalp, umbilical vein, umbilical artery, and neonatal descending aorta blood pH, $PO_2$, $PCO_2$, and base deficit during the intrapartum period, delivery, and the first 64 minutes of life in neonates with 1-minute and 5-minute Apgar scores of 7 or more. Note the value of the umbilical artery $PO_2$ and its rapid rise by 4 minutes from birth. Considering no significant changes in oxygen carrying capacity of the neonatal hemoglobin soon after birth, this rapid rise of $PO_2$, soon after birth, will increase the neonatal blood $O_2$ content and $O_2$ delivery to its organ systems.

Fetal $PCO_2$ is similar to that of an adult but there is a gradient of $CO_2$ tension between the fetus and the mother with the former being slightly higher. With the initiation of normal breathing, descending aortic blood $PCO_2$ falls to about 40 mm Hg within the first few minutes. Subsequently, a further decrease in $PaCO_2$ occurs until a mean of approximately 35 mm Hg occurs during the first hour (see Table 23–11).

Fetal pH ranges between 7.30 and 7.40 during the intrapartum period. There is a gradual decline in fetal pH during labor that accentuates during the second stage. This is due predominantly to lactic acid accumulation. The metabolic acidosis that develops with the progression of labor is due to a decrease in oxygen supply to the fetus. With the increased intensity and duration of intermittent uterine contractions, placental intervillous blood flow will be decreased resulting in proportional decrease in oxygen exchange. The decreased $O_2$ supply to fetal organs, although physiologic during labor, will reach a critical point at which it will not maintain aerobic metabolism. The resultant anaerobic metabolism leads to the production of lactic acid and metabolic acidosis. At birth, the mean umbilical arterial pH has been reported to range between 7.259 (71) and 7.28 (72). Umbilical arterial pH tends to be higher (7.32) in those infants delivered by elective cesarean section without labor (64). Neonatal descending aorta blood pH drops further, from the value of the umbilical artery, during the first few minutes after birth. As it was discussed earlier, this drop is the result of increased organ perfusion associated with the rise in systemic blood pressure. Increased tissue perfusion results in an influx of lactic acid in the circulation. Because

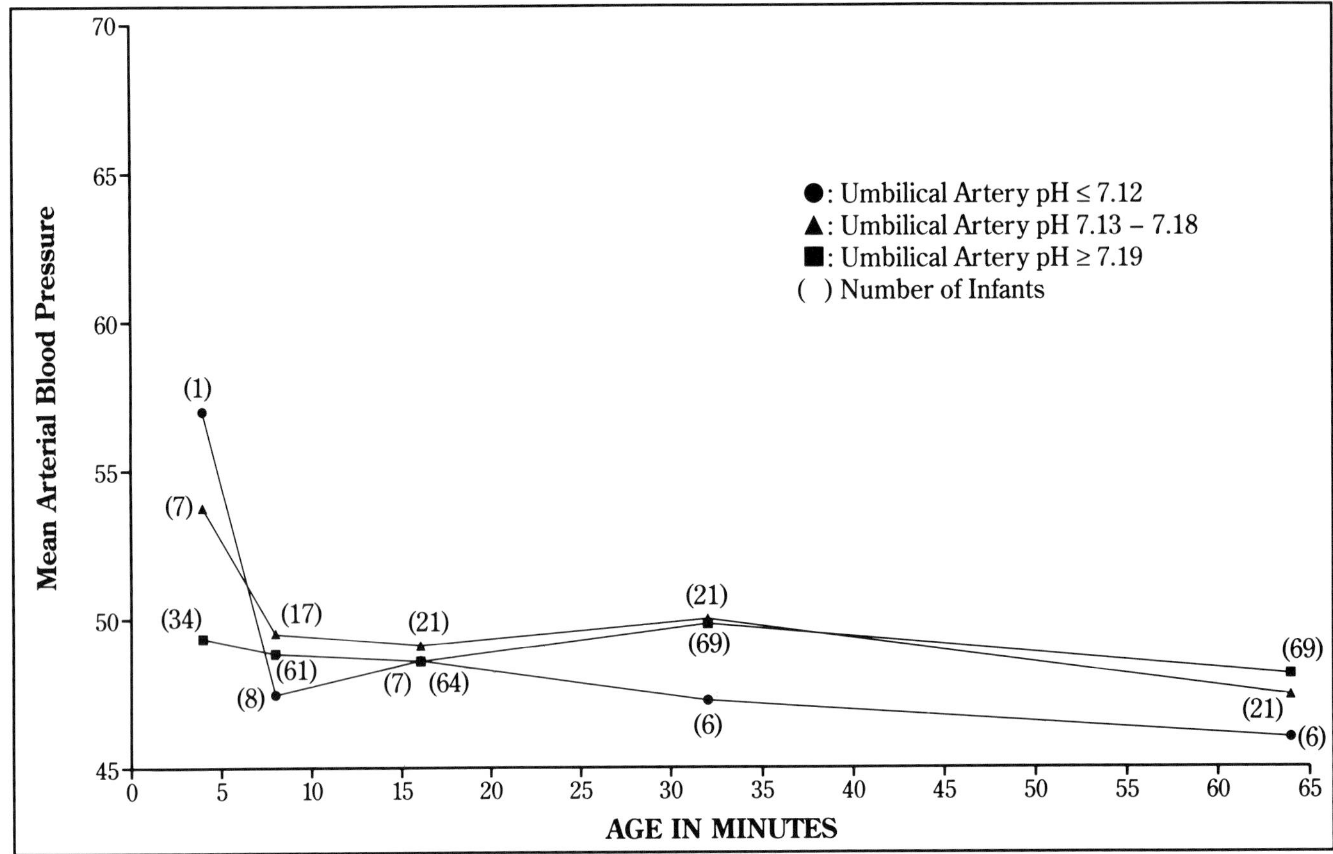


**Fig. 23–15.** Mean arterial blood pressure during the first 64 minutes of life in normal (umbilical artery pH ≥ 7.19), moderately acidotic (umbilical artery pH 7.13 to 7.18), and severely acidotic (umbilical artery pH ≤ 7.12) infants at birth.

**Table 23–11.** Changes in Fetal Scalp Blood, Umbilical Artery, Umbilical Vein and Neonatal Descending Aorta pH, $PO_2$, $PCO_2$ and Base Deficit During the First 64 Minutes of Life. All Figures Are Given ± 1 SD

| Time | pH | $PO_2$ | $PCO_2$ | Base Deficit |
|---|---|---|---|---|
| Early labor* | 7.30 ± 0.05 | 19.7 ± 2.9 | 45.5 ± 6.8 | 6.4 ± 2.1 |
| Midlabor** | 7.30 ± 0.04 | 21.1 ± 3.0 | 45.1 ± 5.5 | 5.4 ± 2.6 |
| Full cervical dilation | 7.28 ± 0.05 | 19.1 ± 3.8 | 47.8 ± 7.8 | 6.1 ± 2.5 |
| Umbilical artery at birth | 7.24 ± 0.06 | 17.6 ± 4.6 | 48.7 ± 7.3 | 8.8 ± 2.6 |
| Umbilical vein at birth | 7.32 ± 0.05 | 27.8 ± 5.5 | 38.9 ± 5.8 | 6.6 ± 2.5 |
| 4 min*** | 7.20 ± 0.06 | 53.3 ± 15.8 | 46.1 ± 7.2 | 10.5 ± 2.9 |
| 8 min*** | 7.24 ± 0.06 | 62.4 ± 16.7 | 39.7 ± 7.8 | 9.3 ± 2.9 |
| 16 min *** | 7.30 ± 0.06 | 62.4 ± 16.7 | 39.7 ± 7.8 | 9.3 ± 2.9 |
| 32 min*** | 7.32 ± 0.05 | 68.0 ± 15.4 | 35.4 ± 6.0 | 7.9 ± 2.9 |
| 64 min*** | 7.36 ± 0.04 | 70.3 ± 13.9 | 34.4 ± 6.7 | 4.2 ± 2.3 |

* Cervical dilation ≤ 4 cm.
** Cervical dilation 5 cm.
*** Arterial blood.

of increased tissue perfusion with higher $O_2$ content of the blood and aerobic metabolism, tissue pH will rise gradually, although such a physiologic change has not been studied. In a normal newborn infant, arterial pH will rise above 7.30 within the first 15 minutes (see Table 23–11) and will steadily increase to a mean value of 7.35 to 7.40 by 1 hour of age. Table 23–11 also shows the values of base deficit during the intrapartum period and during the first hour after birth.

This brief review emphasizes the fact that physiologic acidosis, mostly metabolic, occurs during the process of labor and delivery in the normal fetus and newborn. Analysis of umbilical cord blood (in particular umbilical artery blood), acid-base and blood gases, along with the infant's Apgar scores, will provide guidelines to assist the physician in assessing the infant soon after birth. Those involved in the delivery room care of neonates should be very familiar with perinatal physiologic changes, particularly at birth, to plan appropriate treatment modalities.

### *Temperature Control*

Biologic adjustment from fetal to neonatal life involves adaptation to the extrauterine environment. Human newborn infants must adapt to a cooler extrauterine environment by shivering and nonshivering (chemical) thermogenesis (73–75). The latter mechanism of thermogenesis is the predominant method of heat production by the newborn infant. The process of heat production translates to substrate utilization and an increase in oxygen consumption (76). Before birth, fetal temperature exceeds maternal temperature. The body temperature of the fetus is about 0.5° C higher than the mother's core temperature, i.e., about 37.8° C (77). The temperature gradient between the fetus and the mother permits heat transfer from fetus to mother via placenta (74). Although the heat transfer is from fetus to mother, maternal body temperature determines fetal temperature, i.e., with maternal fever, the fetal temperature increases proportionally to maintain the temperature gradient. One of the manifestations of this phenomenon is fetal tachycardia and decrease in fetal heart rate variability. Theoretically, this phenomenon is associated with increased fetal oxygen consumption.

Transfer to the extrauterine life of the delivery room, where the environmental temperature is set mostly for the comfort of the attending personnel, imposes a significant challenge to the newborn infant's ability to maintain body temperature. Understanding of the mechanisms of heat loss by the neonate in the delivery room is essential to provide a thermal environment that will make biologic adaptation less stressful. The mechanisms of heat loss are four in number: (1) convection, a function of surrounding air temperature; (2) radiation, a function of temperature of objects near neonates; (3) evaporation, via lungs and body surface; and (4) conduction, a function of temperature of objects in contact with the neonate's body.

To achieve minimal heat loss in the delivery room, the neonate should be placed in a positive thermal environment. This is achieved by maintaining delivery room temperature at a high comfort zone for the attending personnel, maintaining a radiant warmer on at all times, quickly drying the neonate, and, finally, using warmed blankets to care for the infant.

The consequence of thermal imbalance has deleterious effects because the human infant has a limited source of energy at birth, particularly in the form of carbohydrates, and at the same time must meet the higher metabolic requirements of the cold stress (77). Oxygen consumption increases significantly over the basal metabolic rate during cold exposure. Experimental studies in animals have shown that cerebral metabolic rate increases significantly during cold exposure (77). A similar phenomenon appears to occur in human neonates exposed to cold stress (78). Excessive cooling will result in an obligatory increase in substrate use, higher oxygen consumption, and $CO_2$ productivity.

Even under desired environmental temperature, the body temperature of the newborn infant falls. The fall is most rapid in the initial minutes after birth (74). Healthy, full-term newborn infants will maintain body temperature by increasing metabolic rate. Perinatal asphyxia/hypoxia, hypotension, and depression of the central nervous system by sedatives, analgesics, and anesthetics impair the newborn's thermal regulatory responses and further reduce thermal stability. Resulting hypothermia affects changes in acid-base homeostasis that favor the development of metabolic acidosis (79). Metabolic effects of severe acidosis are the occurrence of hypoglycemia, systemic and pulmonary vasoconstriction, lower arterial oxygen tensions, and anaerobic metabolism. For decades it has been known that prolonged exposure to cold in premature infants is associated with increased mortality. The concept of deep hypothermia, as used in surgical situations, has been considered to reduce metabolic demands. As the body temperature falls 10° C, metabolism will decrease by a factor of 2½ times. This kind of deep hypothermia can be achieved only through the use of strictly regulated and adequately controlled methods and should not be confused with ill-advised and contraindicated efforts to just "cool the baby a little" (75).

## General Considerations for Neonatal Resuscitation

### *Personnel: Obstetrics and Neonatal Team*

Provision of appropriate care of the infant in the delivery room requires collaborative efforts among obstetric and pediatric physicians, anesthesiologists, nurses, and respiratory therapists. Specialization in perinatal care has separated individual care takers into specific aspects of maternal and neonatal care; therefore, commitment to collaborative efforts with open communication is necessary if a perinatal center expects to provide appropriate neonatal care in the delivery room. Based on perinatal center philosophy, team members assigned to neonatal care in the delivery room may differ. In the perinatal center with a Neonatal Intensive Care Unit (NICU), the NICU team should be responsible for care of the neonate in the delivery room. This team should consist of a physician experienced in neonatal resuscitation (pediatrician, senior pediatric resident, neonatal fellow, and neonatologist), a nurse, and a respiratory therapist. The team can be supported by the obstetric anesthesiologist present in the delivery room. In hospitals with maternity services but without NICU or without 24-hour coverage of the delivery room by the NICU team, a team of physicians, nurses, and respiratory therapists should be identified to provide skilled 24-hour basis delivery room coverage. Although the presence of a physician may not be possible, a maternity unit should have at least two skilled individuals (neonatal nurse practitioner, respiratory therapist) trained in neonatal resuscitation and available within the hospital. The resuscitation team has to be aware of impending high-risk delivery as well as be prepared at a moment's notice to assemble in the delivery room ready for unforeseen emergencies.

### *Delivery Room Facilities*

Traditional labor, delivery and recovery (LDR) rooms should be constructed mainly for the comfort and safety of the mother and the infant. The initial care and any resuscitation measures should be done in the delivery room. Each delivery room should have a place for the care of the newborn that is close to the sources of oxygen and suction and is well lighted.

The presence of the father and other significant family members in the delivery room should not be a deterrent to the initial care or resuscitation of the infant. The table on which the infant is placed for the immediate care and

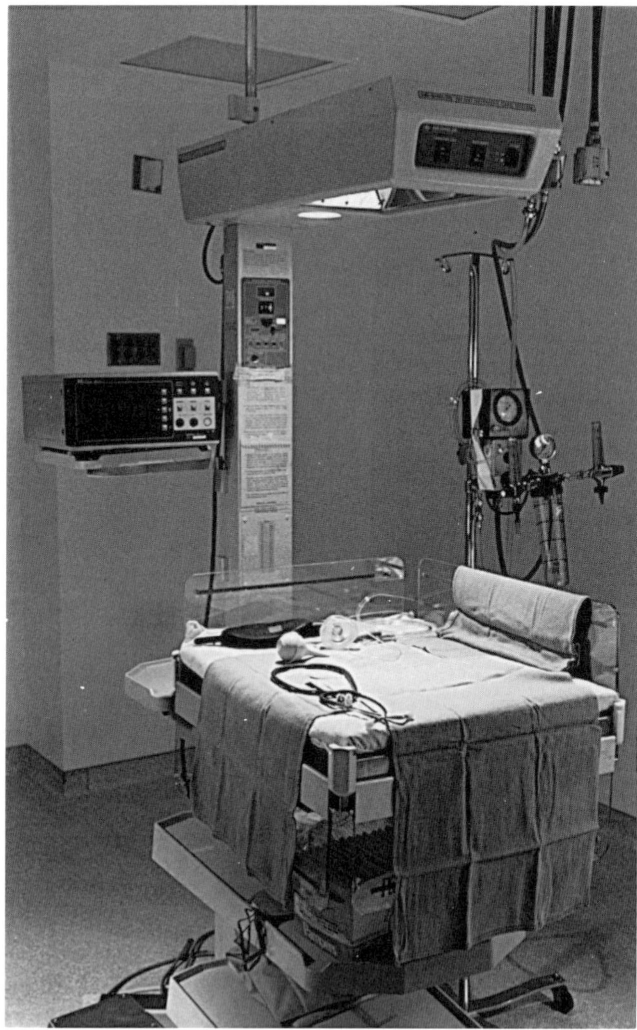

**Fig. 23–16.** Radiant warmer and other needed equipment in the delivery room. Emergency medicine cart is not shown.

any resuscitation measures should be heated to prevent temperature loss in the infant. An open radiant warmer (Figure 23–16) provides heat and easy access to the infant. The radiant warmer should have an attachment for the delivery of oxygen and suction. Sterile equipment for possible use should be immediately available in each delivery room (Figures 23–17 and 23–18). Such equipment includes suction catheters of different sizes, DeLee suction (DeLee suction trap should be used by the obstetrician in case of meconium-stained amniotic fluid with the delivery of the head before delivery of the shoulders), masks and endotracheal tubes of different sizes, a laryngoscope with numbers zero and 1 blades, bags, preferably with a pop-off valve, and an oxygen source, preferably from the wall. Also, an umbilical vessel catheterization and an emergency drug tray should be available (the tray should contain medications for eye and umbilical cord prophylaxis). After each delivery, the used equipment should promptly be replaced with sterile equipment, which is kept in the resuscitation area ready for immediate use.

After the initial stabilization and/or resuscitation of the infant in the delivery room, the physician member of the team is responsible for deciding whether to leave the infant with the mother or to transfer the infant to either the transition or term nursery or to the NICU. Transfer of the infant to the nursery or NICU should be done in a transport incubator. If the decision is made to transfer the infant to the NICU, NICU personnel should be notified and be prepared to receive the infant for further care. If, after resuscitation, the decision is made to transfer the infant to the term nursery, the physician should reevaluate the infant within a reasonable period of time to assure proper care of the infant based on labor, delivery, and the initial assessment.

### *Responsibility*

Communication between the obstetric team and the neonatal team responsible for resuscitation is the first step in planning effective neonatal resuscitation. Other important factors in resuscitation are preparation of the personnel, appropriate equipment in the delivery room, and the experience and effectiveness of the neonatal team attending the delivery. Individual team members should be familiar with their roles in the delivery room. The physician member of the team assumes overall responsibility for the conduct of neonatal resuscitation. During the resuscitation, the physician is responsible for airway management and intubation, while the respiratory therapist, if present, assists in suctioning, oxygen delivery and bagging, and stabilization of the endotracheal tube. The attending nurse is responsible for drying the infant, taking vital signs, and assessing the effectiveness of the ventilation.

Upon arrival in the delivery room, the physician member of the team should introduce himself to the mother, the father, if he is present, and to the other personnel in the delivery room. After stabilization and/or resuscitation, the physician should communicate his/her assessment of the infant to the obstetrician and to the parents. If medication is used, the nurse is responsible for its preparation and administration under the direction of the physician.

## General Management of the Newborn

Management of all newborn infants should include: (1) immediate care; (2) clinical appraisal of the infant's condition; and, if need be, (3) resuscitation. Efforts should be made to maintain normal body temperature during resuscitative efforts. A general physical examination is needed prior to transfer of the infant from the delivery room. The general examination is done after respiration is well established and maintained. The initial care, appraisal of the infant's condition, and any resuscitation measures should be done in the delivery room.

### *Immediate Care*

The first step in the care of the newborn is to establish and maintain a clear airway. As soon as the head is delivered, the upper airway, mouth, and nose should be suctioned. If there is thick meconium or blood in the mouth or nose, they are removed before the infant's first gasp

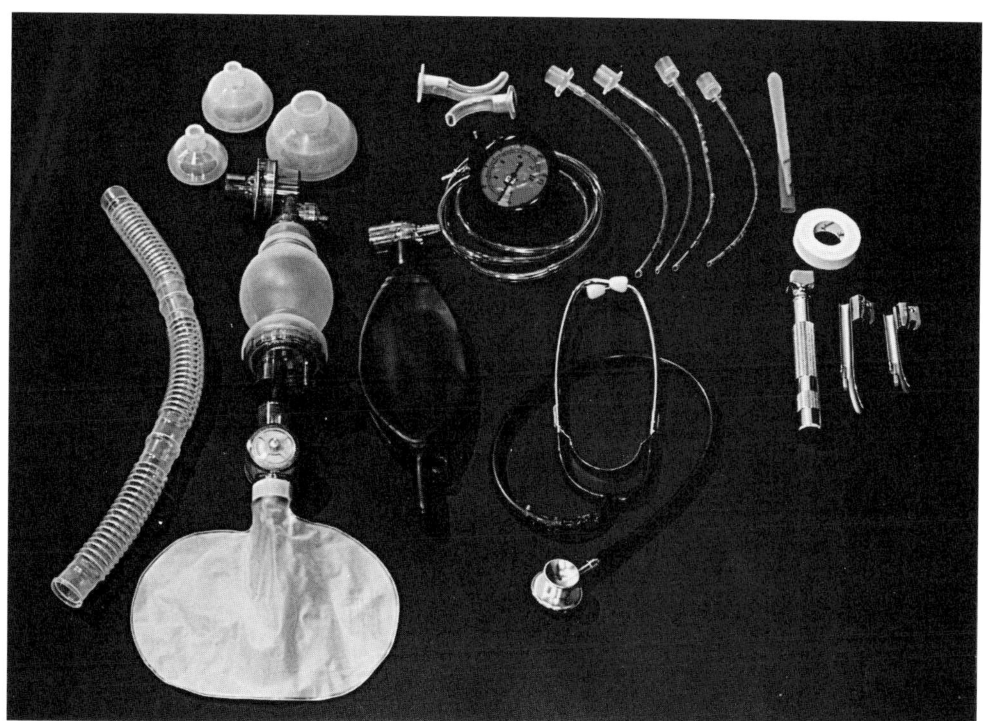

**Fig. 23–17.** Equipment needed in the delivery room for assisted ventilation during neonatal resuscitation. Note the two different ventilation bags, different sized masks, endotracheal tubes, and pencil-handle laryngoscope with number 0 and 1 straight blades.

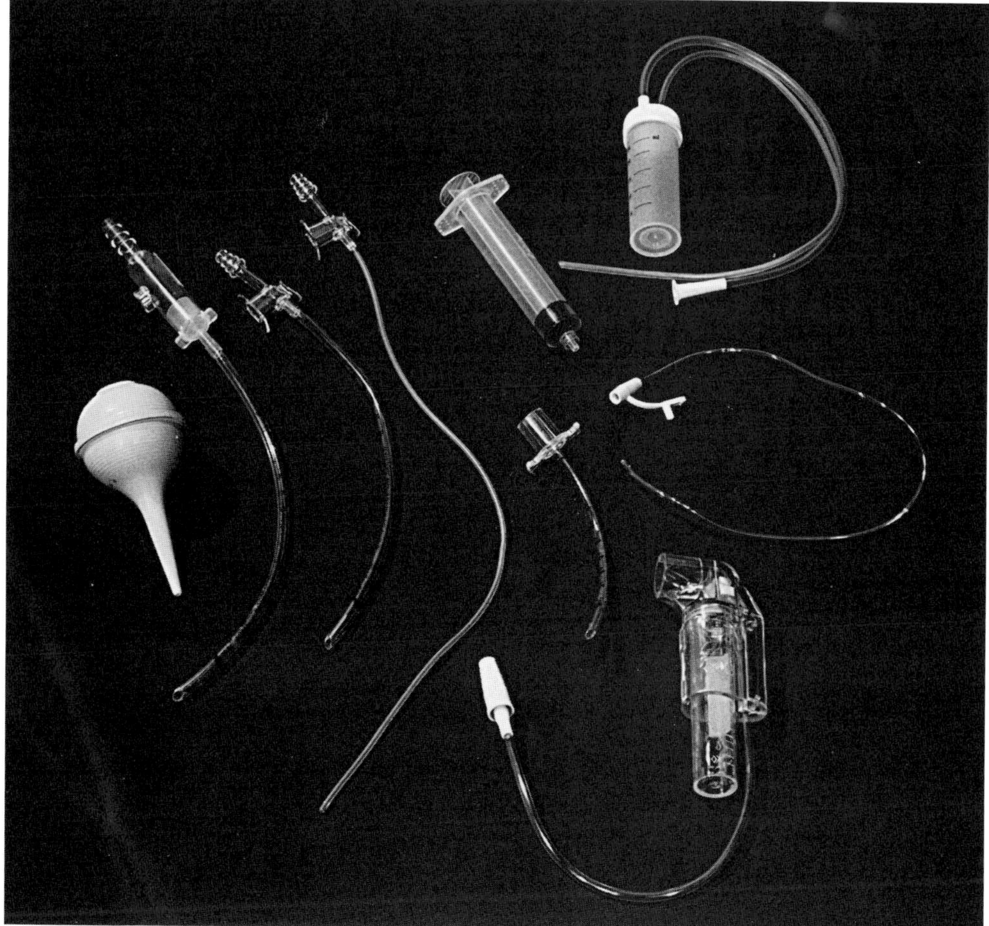

**Fig. 23–18.** Equipment needed in the delivery room for appropriate suctioning of meconium-stained amniotic fluid. Note DeLee suction for the obstetrician and three different apparatus for neonatal tracheal suctioning.

to prevent aspiration of the material into the lower air passages. The mouth must be suctioned before the nose, because in vigorous infants, suction of the anterior nares usually evokes an inspiratory gasp that may result in aspiration if the mouth is full of amniotic fluid. The practice of "milking" the trachea (by stroking the upper trachea and larynx toward the head with the operator's second finger) is traumatic, ineffective, and may lead to fracture of the larynx and, therefore, should be avoided (51).

The position of the newborn's head is extremely important in establishing and maintaining a patent airway. The optimal position on the table is with a slight tilt of the head to the side for proper suctioning of the oropharynx. To keep the airway patent, it is important that the head is in slight extension maintained by placing a towel under the upper back. Excessive extension of the head and keeping the infant in a steep head-down position for gravity drainage should be avoided, as the weight of the intra-abdominal organs, particularly the liver, will impede motion of the diaphragm during inspiration and decrease lung expansion. This is particularly important in the depressed infant. In addition, in very depressed neonates, venous return to the heart may be further compromised.

Further suctioning of the mouth, pharynx, and nose with a catheter is carried out to be sure that all secretions and blood have been removed. Suctioning should be brief and gentle, but effective. As newborn infants exhibit strong vagal response, prolonged suctioning of the pharynx and nose is avoided because it may produce either laryngospasm and/or profound bradycardia, as described by Cordero and Hon (80). As, too, infants are obligatory nose breathers, special care should be taken to ensure that the nares are clear and provide the infant with a patent airway. The cardiac rate can be monitored by palpation or stethoscope. This is done by the attending nurse and indicated to the physician in attendance by motion of his/her index finger. From birth to completion of suctioning should take about 1 minute. Most infants have already had the initial gasp and cry. If a fairly regular breathing pattern has not been established, some mild tactile stimulation may be needed. Any vigorous stimulation or slapping of the soles of the feet should be avoided.

## Clinical Appraisal of the Newborn

Clinical appraisal of the newborn begins with birth. The time of the first gasp, first cry, and the onset of sustained respiration are noted and recorded. The time for sustained respiration denotes the time period following delivery that elapses before the infant begins to maintain a regular and adequate ventilatory activity. Normal newborns generally achieve sustained respiration with adequate ventilation by 1 minute of age, when the initial Apgar score is assigned (81).

### Apgar Scores

Sixty seconds after the complete birth of the infant (disregarding the cord and placenta) the infant is evaluated using the Apgar scoring system (Table 23–12). A score of 10 indicates an infant in the best possible condition; a score of 0 to 2 indicates an infant in very poor condition. Based on 1-minute Apgar scores, infants can be divided into 3 general categories: vigorous, score of 7 to 10; moderately depressed, score of 4 to 6; and severely depressed, score of 0 to 3. As the infant's condition deteriorates, the usual order of disappearance of the component of the Apgar score's signs is as follows: color, respiration, tone, reflex activity, heart rate (51). Although minor variations occur in this order, in general, it does permit for more ready evaluation of the infant. For example, if an infant is crying or breathing regularly and moving all limbs (i.e., scores of 2 each for respiration and muscle tone), one can be reasonably certain that reflex activity and heart rate will have maximal scores. However, the most accurate way of using the Apgar score is to monitor and record each parameter carefully.

**Table 23–12.** Apgar Scoring System

| Sign | Score 0 | Score 1 | Score 2 |
|---|---|---|---|
| Heart rate | Absent | Slow (below 100) | Over 100 |
| Respiratory effort | Absent | Weak cry; hypoventilation | Good; strong cry |
| Muscle tone flexed | Limp | Some flexion of limbs | Active motion; limbs well |
| Reflex irritability* | No Response | Grimace | Cry |
| Color | Blue; pale | Body pink; limbs blue | Completely pink |

* Response to stimulation of sole of foot.

The heart rate is the most important of the five parameters in the Apgar scoring system. A rate below 100 indicates severe asphyxia requiring prompt resuscitation. Weak heart sounds or absent pulsation of the umbilical artery at the junction of the umbilical cord and skin indicates low arterial blood pressure and poor cardiac output and also suggests the need for immediate resuscitation.

Respiratory effort is the second most important sign. If respiration is vigorous and regular, a score of 2 is given; if it is present but irregular and ineffective, 1 is given; if apnea is present, a score of 0 is recorded. Infrequent gasps, even though they might be deep and accompanied by a cry, do not qualify for the maximal score. Moreover, a score of 2 cannot be given for respiratory effort if the infant has failed to achieve its sustained respiration at the time the Apgar score is taken. Apnea is not serious if artificial ventilation is being carried out effectively. However, as noted, untreated apnea is serious and can be fatal if allowed to persist.

Muscle tone is the third most important sign. Active flexion of the arms and legs as they resist extension, with good motion in all limbs, is scored 2; moderately good or fair is scored 1; and if the infant is limp the score is 0.

Often, tone evaluation is visual because the tonus of a vigorous infant moving all limbs is readily obvious, as is the absence of tonus in a flaccid infant. Anything in-between is given a score of 1. In the absence of neuromuscular disease, persistence of hypotonia beyond the first few hours of life may be an important sign of perinatal asphyxia.

Reflex irritability can be tested in two ways. One method is the response of the infant to a brisk and gentle slap on the sole of the foot. A prompt cry is scored 2; a grimace, 1; and no response, 0. Another method is to place the tip of the suction catheter just inside the nares after the pharynx has been cleared. If the infant coughs or sneezes, the score is 2; if it merely grimaces, the score is 1, and if no reaction occurs, the score is 0. This technique is no longer used, however, because the sneeze-cough is often preceded by a significant inspiratory effort with the consequent increased risk of aspiration.

Color is the least important sign. If, within 60 seconds, the infant is completely pink, a score of 2 is assigned, but this occurs in only about 15% of newborns. Usually, all of the infant is pink except for the hands and feet, which remain blue, thus giving a score of 1 for this parameter. If the entire body is blue or pale, the score is 0.

The Apgar score is repeated at 5 minutes and, if a score of 8 has not been achieved by this time, scoring is continued at 10, 15 and 20 minutes. Clinical studies reported in the 1960s (51) have shown that at 1 minute, about 5% of newborn infants have a score of 0 to 3; 15% have a score of 4 to 6; and 80% have a score of 7 to 10. The same studies noted that by 5 minutes, fewer infants have lower scores: 2%, 3%, and 95%, respectively. A more recent study in our institution (see Table 23–10) showed Apgar score distribution as follows: score of 1 to 3, 3.3%; 4 to 6, 7.6%; and 7 to 10, 88.3% at 1 minute. By 5 minutes, only 0.7% had scores of 1 to 3, 1.2% had scores of 4 to 6, and 97.25 had scores of 7 to 10. To be useful, the assessment must be made accurately and at the correct time. It is worthwhile to train nurses and house officers in the proper technique of assessing the newborn. Although a wall clock with a second hand is usually adequate to time the score, it is best to have a watch with a buzzer that is set to ring at 1 and 5 minutes.

Although it has limitations, the Apgar scoring system, first introduced by Virginia Apgar in 1952, is considered the simplest and most practical method to quantitate the clinical condition of the newborn (82). The 1-minute score is especially useful in judging the need for resuscitation. The value of each parameter in indicating the mechanisms of neonatal depression varies considerably. There is general agreement that the color can be influenced by many factors extraneous to neonatal depression and provides little significant information. Because the respiratory effort is influenced by narcotics, general anesthetics, and other respiratory depressant analgesics, this measurement may not be useful to indicate the degree and duration of intrauterine asphyxia. Thus, it may be possible for the infant delivered of a mother given these drugs to have a weak or absent respiratory effort and still have normal acid-base values characteristic of the vigorous infant. Impairment of muscle tone, when not resolving, probably reflects a degree of metabolic acidosis from perinatal asphyxia. Finally, because reflex response to noxious stimulation is usually more difficult to depress than either respiratory effort or muscle tone, a score of less than two for reflex irritability reflects moderate to severe perinatal asphyxia.

## *Resuscitation of the Depressed Newborn*

### *Mildly to Moderately Depressed Infant*

The mildly depressed newborn at 1 minute shows cyanosis, has not established regular respiration, and may have only fair muscle tone, so that the total Apgar score is about 6 or 7. Such an infant usually requires little more than stimulation, provided upper airway suctioning has been performed. Drying the infant, handling, and environmental temperature will generally provide adequate stimulation. Nothing more than slapping of the soles of the feet should be necessary for additional stimulation. If this does not produce sustained respiration, oxygen should be administered. Unheated oxygen blown to the face will provide strong stimulation. Prolonged unheated oxygen administration by blowing oxygen to the face should be avoided. Mestyan, et al (79) have shown that the newborn's face is particularly sensitive to thermal stimulation, as the local application of a cold stimulus to the face results in a distinct metabolic rise and an increased oxygen consumption. Oxygen can be used with the appropriate size mask and bag system with an oxygen flow of 6 to 8 liters/min. This system also permits the use of intermittent positive pressure ventilation. Usually, 10 to 20 cm $H_2O$ pressure applied for 1 second is adequate to assist ventilation. In an apneic infant, higher pressures are required initially to expand the alveoli. After initial expansion has been produced with 3 to 4 short puffs, pressures of 5 to 10 cm $H_2O$ for 0.5 seconds are sufficient to assist ventilation in mildly depressed infants. This technique is especially useful in newborn infants delivered of mothers given general anesthesia, because the assisted ventilation increases the rate of elimination of the anesthetic by the infant.

The face mask must be appropriate to the size of the infant and should cover the mouth and the nose. If it is the proper size, it will fit snugly to the face and be nearly leakproof without the need to have it pressing tightly against the skin. Each delivery room should be equipped with masks of different sizes. Figures 23–16 and 23–17 show basic resuscitation equipment of masks, endotracheal tubes, bags and laryngoscope with blades of two sizes. During bagging, care should be exercised not to occlude the trachea with the finger that supports the mandible. The use of an oropharyngeal airway during bagging is discouraged unless there is suspicion of airway obstruction. The abdomen should be carefully observed for evidence of the inflation of the stomach with the inspired oxygen mixture. A small gavage-type catheter should be placed in the stomach if assisted ventilation via bag and mask is continued.

Moderately depressed newborns have Apgar scores of 4 to 6 by 1 minute of age. Individuals in charge of resuscitation should not wait for 1-minute Apgar scores before initiating resuscitation. A team of two individuals, preferably a nurse and a physician, are needed for effective resuscitative efforts. The nurse will quickly dry the infant with a warm blanket while the physician clears the oropharynx and nasopharynx by suction. Based on the respiratory efforts of the infant, the physician will initiate bag and mask ventilation with 100% $O_2$. The initial pressure applied should be about 40 cm $H_2O$ applied for approximately 1 second. Subsequent pressure should be of 15 to 20 cm $H_2O$ for a term infant with normal lungs. Term, postterm, and preterm infants with lung diseases such as meconium aspiration, respiratory distress syndrome, or congenital pneumonia will require higher pressures for adequate ventilation. A tidal volume of 6 to 8 ml/kg and a rate of 40 breaths per minute is appropriate. Proper positioning of the infant under a radiant warmer is important in ventilating infants with bag and mask. Improvement in color with a rapid rise in heart rate are the evidence of adequate ventilation. Moderately depressed infants will respond to properly applied bag and mask ventilation by establishing a regular breathing pattern. The adequacy of ventilation is associated with the rising of the chest, rather than the abdomen. The attending nurse should check for adequate air exchange by listening to the lateral aspect of the chest at the midaxillary area. After 20 to 30 seconds of ventilation, the heart rate should be auscultated. If the heart rate does not improve and is accompanied by a lack of improvement in the infant's color and respiratory effort, the infant should be checked for proper positioning and/or airway obstruction. In the absence of the latter problem, endotracheal intubation will be necessary to provide proper ventilation and oxygenation. In cases of persistent neonatal depression and the history of maternal narcotic use during labor, a narcotic antagonist such as naloxone at a dose of 0.1 mg/kg should be administered. Generally, one dose of naloxone is sufficient to reverse the effect of narcotics given during labor but the drug may be repeated if the history of narcotic use is convincing.

### *Management of Severely Depressed Infant*

The severely depressed neonate at birth will have an Apgar score of 3 or less by 1 minute of age. As was mentioned above, resuscitation efforts should start at birth rather than by 1 minute of life. After the clearing of the airway, endotracheal intubation followed by intermittent positive pressure ventilation with 100% $O_2$ is the most appropriate method of resuscitation. This requires skill and expertise by the individual attending the delivery. The process of endotracheal intubation should not require more than 20 to 30 seconds. If the operator is not successful in intubation, bag and mask ventilation should be used as described above. Endotracheal intubation may be attempted again if prolonged assisted ventilation is anticipated. In severely depressed newborn infants not responding with improved muscle tone to endotracheal intubation and positive pressure ventilation, and with a heart rate continuing less than 60 beats per minute, external cardiac massage should be performed at a rate of 120 times per minute while ventilation is maintained and coordinated with external cardiac massage.

Periodic evaluation of the heart rate should be done to assess the infant's response. An increase in heart rate above 80 beats per minute and rising should be an indication for discontinuation of external cardiac massage. Very depressed neonates needing external cardiac massage and prolonged positive pressure ventilation will benefit from the endotracheal administration of epinephrine at a dosage of 0.1 to 0.2 ml/kg of 1:10,000 solution (82). Epinephrine is readily absorbed by the epithelial layer of the bronchial tree. Correction of metabolic acidosis with the use of neonatal solution of sodium bicarbonate may be considered while appropriate ventilation is maintained. There are significant controversies over the use of sodium bicarbonate, particularly in preterm infants, because administration may be associated with an increased incidence of central nervous system hemorrhage (83).

Small preterm infants who are moderately to severely depressed at birth should be ventilated and oxygenated after endotracheal intubation. The application of positive pressure ventilation via bag and mask is more cumbersome and less effective in tiny infants. This group of infants more frequently requires assisted ventilation after the initial resuscitation in the delivery room.

Infants suspected to have diaphragmatic hernia or esophageal atresia with possible tracheoesophageal fistula should be intubated for resuscitation rather than ventilated with bag and mask because the distension of the stomach and bowel will further compromise expansion of the lungs in diaphragmatic hernia (as the bowel in the chest will fill up with air) or result in overdistension of the stomach and interference with the motion of the diaphragm during inspiration.

During prolonged use of bag and mask ventilation, an orogastric tube should be placed to decompress the stomach of air.

A recent textbook published jointly by the American Academy of Pediatrics and the American Heart Association described in detail the recommended equipment in the delivery room for neonatal resuscitation, including the types and sizes of masks and bags and endotracheal tubes, as well as the technique of bag and mask ventilation and endotracheal intubation (84).

After the initial delivery room resuscitation of severely depressed infants and admission to NICU, those infants thought to be in cardiogenic shock as the result of severe metabolic acidosis will benefit from drugs with the properties to improve myocardial contractility and improve renal perfusion (85,86). Dopamine at a dosage of 2.5 to 5.0 μg/kg/min will be an effective agent. The use of atropine and calcium gluconate have not shown to be effective and their use should be discouraged.

Severely depressed infants with prolonged metabolic acidosis are subject to severe hypoglycemia because of anaerobic metabolism. Correction of hypoglycemia should be included in the resuscitative plan. Infants with persistent hypoglycemia do not respond well to resuscitative efforts. However, excessive administration of glucose may result in further production of lactic acid if these infants continue with persistent metabolic acidosis and poor tissue perfusion. Myers (65) has suggested that excessive lactic acid accumulation as the result of anaerobic metabolism may be deleterious to the central nervous system.

### Volume Expanders

Infants who are volume depleted as a result of bleeding to mother (feto-maternal hemorrhage), twin to twin transfusion, vasa previa, and bleeding or third spacing as a result of severe perinatal asphyxia, require judicious volume expansion. In infants with severe perinatal asphyxia with persistent metabolic acidosis associated with myocardial dysfunction and hypotension, sudden expansion of blood volume without pharmacologic support of the myocardium may result in further deterioration of the myocardial function and result in pulmonary edema.

The choice of volume expander should be based on the attending physician's assessment of the infant's condition. If anemia occurs, O Rh-negative blood should be given. In known cases of Rh-sensitization and fetal anemia with hydrops, O Rh-negative sedimented red cells matched with mother's plasma should be available before the delivery of the infant. A small aliquot of blood transfusion followed by partial exchange transfusion should be carried out. The Rh-sensitized infant with hydrops should not have a double volume exchange transfusion initially, as these infants tend to have persistent metabolic acidosis. The extra load of phosphated and citrated blood may cause further deterioration of the metabolic acidosis and worsen the infant's condition.

Crystalloid solutions, i.e., normal saline and lactated Ringer's solutions, should be readily available. These isotonic solutions are distributed to the extracellular space. A volume of 10 to 20 ml/kg should be used to achieve the desired vascular volume expansion. The choice of these solutions should be weighed against the possibility of hypernatremia and overexpansion of the blood volume when renal function is severely compromised.

Blood products, such as plasma, albumin, and plasma protein fraction, are available but relatively expensive and should be judiciously used because of colloid-osmotic effects and expansion of the intravascular volume, which may result in pulmonary edema, particularly when myocardial dysfunction exists.

To improve vascular volume and improve blood pressure resulting in better organ perfusion and oxygen carrying capacity, sedimented or packed red cells appear to be the best choice, particularly when anemia is documented. The attending caretaker should be aware that the fundamental aspects of resuscitation of a depressed and asphyxiated infant are appropriate ventilation and oxygenation while maintaining body temperature and glucose homeostasis. Adjuvant therapies, i.e., correction of the metabolic acidosis, improving myocardial contractility, and volume expansion, should be considered complementary to the basic fundamentals of neonatal resuscitation rather than as a primary therapeutic approach.

### Documentation

Appraisal of the infant's condition at birth and the resuscitation efforts should be well documented in the chart. The most experienced caretaker in the delivery room should assign the Apgar scores by noting each component separately. If by 5 minutes after birth the Apgar score is less than 7, one should determine Apgar scores at 10, 15, and 20 minutes, if necessary. This approach will give the caretakers the opportunity for continuous evaluation of the infant until the infant is clinically stable.

To document the degree and type of acidosis and hypoxia, determination of umbilical arterial and venous pH, base deficit, and blood gases should be done (87). The techniques of umbilical arterial and venous blood gases are simple and require only double clamping of the umbilical cord at the time of delivery. Two heparinized 1-ml syringes can be used to aspirate umbilical arterial and venous blood for pH and blood gas determinations. Determination of umbilical arterial pH and blood gases provides information about the degree of metabolic acidosis that may require therapeutic intervention.

## Prevention of Meconium Aspiration Syndrome

Prevention of meconium aspiration requires combined obstetric and pediatric intervention. Although antenatal aspiration of meconium is possible, it is generally agreed that the syndrome of meconium aspiration usually occurs during the process of delivery and immediately after birth (88–95). The prevention procedure is carried out as follows: while the infant's head is on the perineum, before the onset of respiration, the obstetrician will suction the oropharynx and nasopharynx with DeLee suction. When particulate matter is present in the amniotic fluid, even during cesarean section, the above procedure should be performed with the delivery of the infant's head. During cesarean section, mechanical suction may be used if excessive negative suction is not applied. The pediatric team, in turn, should perform routine suctioning of the trachea with direct vision after delivery. Carson, et al (95), describing this combined approach, suggested that routine suctioning of the trachea is necessary only when meconium is visualized at the vocal cords. We recommend direct tracheal suctioning when particulate meconium is present in the upper airway. Direct mechanical suction attached to the endotracheal tube, along with the use of a meconium suction adapter, is preferred rather than the use of a separate suction catheter. It should be emphasized that the procedure of endotracheal intubation, particularly in the vigorous infant, requires a skilled pediatric team in attendance. A recent clinical study suggested that vigorous infants at birth whose 1-minute Apgar scores may be 8 or greater will not benefit from direct endotracheal suctioning (96). The use of tracheobronchial lavage with saline has not been shown to be beneficial and may cause respiratory deterioration.

## Examination in the Delivery Room

Although a thorough physical examination should be carried out in the nursery, a brief physical examination of the infant in the delivery room should be performed. This brief physical, as well as neurological assessment, particularly the appraisal of the muscle tone, will provide the pediatrician with further evaluation of the physical condition, detection of congenital anomalies, evolving morbidity, and disposition of the infant. The depressed newborn requiring resuscitation, if sent to a regular or transition nursery, should be reevaluated within a reasonable time period by the pediatric team involved in the care in the delivery room to assure the infant's well-being. When in doubt, severely depressed infants should be taken to the NICU for further evaluation and care. Specific therapies should be based on obstetrical, intrapartum, resuscitation efforts, and clinical findings at birth.

Communication with both parents and the obstetrician together with the proper documentation of care and therapies provided constitute appropriate neonatal care. Successful outcome will depend on anticipation, preparation, and provision of skilled care in the delivery room.

## REFERENCES


1. Anderson WR, Davis J: Placental site involution. Am. J. Obstet. Gynecol. 102:23, 1968.
2. Hytten FE, Cheyne GA: The size and composition of the human pregnant uterus. J. Obstet. Gynaecol. Br. Commonw. 76:400, 1969.
3. Oppenheimer LW, Sherriff EA, Goodman JDS, Shah D, et al: The duration of lochia. Br. J. Obstet. Gynaecol. 93:754, 1986.
4. Williams JS: Regeneration of the uterine mucosa after delivery, with especial reference to the placental site. Am. J. Obstet. Gynecol. 22:664, 1931.
5. Chang YL, Madrozo B, Drukker BH: Ultrasonic evaluation of the postpartum uterus in management of postpartum bleeding. Obstet. Gynecol. 58:227, 1981.
6. Glass M, Rosenthal AH: Cervical changes in pregnancy, labor, and puerperium. Am. J. Obstet. Gynecol. 60:353, 1950.
7. Coppleson M, Reid BL: A colposcopic study of the cervix during pregnancy and the puerperium. J. Obstet. Gynaecol. Br. Commonw. 73:575, 1966.
8. Reamy K, White SE: Sexuality in pregnancy and the puerperium: a review. Obstet. Gynecol. Surv. 40:1, 1985.
9. Ferguson DJP, Anderson TJ: A morphological study of the changes which occur during pregnancy in the human breast. Virchows. Arch. Pathol. Anat. 401:163, 1983.
10. Helminen HJ, Ericsson JLE: Studies on mammary gland involution. I-III. J. Ultrastruct. Res. 25:193–214, 1968.
11. Brown MS, Hurloch JT: Preparation of the breast for breast feeding. Nurs. Res. 24:449, 1975.
12. Martinez GA, Dodd DA: Milk feeding patterns in the United States: first 12 months of life. Pediatrics 71:166, 1983.
13. Jelliffe DB, Jelliffe EFP: "Breast is best:" modern meanings. N. Engl. J. Med. 297:912, 1977.
14. Winikoff B, Myers D, Laukaran VH, Stone R: Over-coming obstacles to breast-feeding in a large municipal hospital: applications of lessons learned. Pediatrics 80:423, 1987.
15. Gilroy RJ, Mangura BT, Lavietes MH: Rib cage and abdominal volume displacement during breathing in pregnancy. Am. Rev. Respir. Dis. 137:668, 1988.
16. Weinberger SE, Weiss ST, Cohen WR, Woodrow W, et al: Pregnancy and the lung. Am. Rev. Respir. Dis. 121:559, 1980.
17. Baldwin GR, Moorthi DS, Whelton JA, MacDonnell KF: New lung functions and pregnancy. Am. J. Obstet. Gynecol. 127: 235, 1977.
18. Goodland RL, Reynolds JG, Pommerenke WT: Alveolar $CO_2$ tension levels during pregnancy and early puerperium. J. Clin. Endocr. 14:522, 1954.
19. James LS, Weisbrot IM, Prince CE, Holaday DA, et al: The acid-base status of human infants in relation to birth asphyxia and the onset of respiration. J. Pediat. 52:379, 1958.
20. Prytowsky H, Hellegers A, Bruns P: Fetal Blood Studies. XIV. A comparative study of the oxygen dissociation curve of non-pregnant, pregnant, and fetal human blood. Am. J. Obstet. Gynecol. 78:489, 1959.
21. Sjøgfstedt S: Acid-base balance of arterial blood during pregnancy, at delivery, and in the puerperium. Am. J. Obstet. Gynecol. 84:775, 1962.
22. Alward HC: Observations on the vital capacity during the last month of pregnancy. Am. J. Obstet. Gynecol. 20:373, 1930.
23. Biesenski JJ: Antifibrinolytic activity in normal pregnancy. J. Clin. Path. 13:220, 1960.
24. Ueland K: Maternal cardiovascular dynamics. VIII. Intrapartum blood volume changes. Am. J. Obstet. Gynecol. 126: 671, 1976.
25. Walters WAW, MacGregor WG, Hills M: Cardiac output at rest during pregnancy and the puerperium. Clin. Sci. 30:1, 1966.
26. Walters BNH, Thompson ME, Lea E, DeSwiet M: Blood pressure in the puerperium. Clin. Sci. 71:589, 1986.
27. Walters WAW, Limm VL: Blood volume and haemodynamics in pregnancy. Clin. Obstet. Gynaecol. 2:301, 1975.
28. Landesman R, Miller MM: Blood volume changes during the immediate Postpartum period. Obstet. Gynecol. 21:40, 1963.
29. Monheit AG, Cousins L, Resnick R: The puerperium: anatomic and physiologic readjustments. Clin. Obstet. Gynecol. 23:973, 1980.
30. Ygge J: Changes in blood coagulation and fibrinolysis during the puerperium. Am. J. Obstet. Gynecol. 104:2, 1969.
31. Cietak KA, Newton JR: Serial qualitative maternal nephrosonography in pregnancy. Br. J. Radiol. 58:399, 1985.
32. Sims EAH, Kratz KE: Serial studies of renal function during pregnancy and the puerperium in normal women. J. Clin. Invest. 37:1764, 1958.
33. Nelson M, Wickus GC, Caplan RH, Beguin EA: Thyroid gland size in pregnancy: an ultrasound and clinical study. J. Rerpod. Med. 32:888, 1987.
34. Handley SL, Dunn TL, Waldron G, Baker JM: Tryptophan, cortisol and puerperal mood. Br. J. Psychiat. 136:498, 1980.
35. Garvey MJ, Tollefson GD: Postpartum depression. J. Rerpod. Med. 29:113, 1984.
36. Hayashi R, Castillo M, Noah M: Management of severe postpartum hemorrhage due to uterine atony using an analog of prostaglandin F2$\alpha$. Obstet. Gynecol. 58:426, 1981.
37. Kenny GN, Oates JD, Leeser J, Rowbotham DJ, et al: Efficacy of orally administered ondansetron in the prevention of postoperative nausea and vomiting: a dose ranging study. Br. J. Anaesth. 68:466–70, 1992.
38. Cotton DB, Gonik B, Dorman KF, Harrist R: Cardiovascular alterations in severe pregnancy-induced hypertension: relationship of central venous pressure to pulmonary capillary wedge pressure. Am. J. Obstet. Gynecol. 151:962, 1985.
39. Robin ED: The cult of the Swan-Ganz catheter. Ann. Intern. Med. 103:445, 1985.
40. Mabie WC, Sibai BM: Treatment in an obstetric intensive care unit. Am. J. Obstet. Gynecol. 162:1, 1990.
41. Mead PB: Managing infected abdominal wounds. Contemp. Ob/Gyn. 14:69, 1979.
42. Madinger NE, Greenspoon JS, Ellrodt AG: Pneumonia during pregnancy: has modern technology improved maternal and fetal outcome? Am. J. Obstet. Gynecol. 161:657, 1989.
43. Hopwood HG: Pneumonia in pregnancy. Obstet. Gynecol. 25:875, 1965.
44. Hoyme UB, Kiviat N, Eschenbach DA: Microbiology and

treatment of late postpartum endometritis. Obstet. Gynecol. 68:226, 1986.
45. Gibbs RS, Blanco JD, St Clair PJ: A case-control study of wound abscess after cesarean delivery. Obstet. Gynecol. 62: 498, 1983.
46. Isada NB, Grossman JH III: Perinatal infections. [In] Obstetrics: Normal and Problem Pregnancies. 2nd Ed. Edited by SG Gabbe, JR Niebyl, JL Simpson. New York, Churchill Livingstone, 1991.
47. Marshall B, Hepper J, Zirbel C: Sporadic puerperal mastitis: an infection that need not interrupt lactation. JAMA 233: 1377, 1975.
48. Thomsen A, Espersen T, Maigaard S: Course and treatment of milk stasis, noninfectious inflammations of the breast, and infectious mastitis in nursing women. Am. J. Obstet. Gynecol. 149:492, 1984.
49. Bier A: Versuche uber Cocainisirung des Ruckenmakes. Deutsch Ztschr Chir 51:361, 1899.
50. Bonica JJ, Oliver TK Jr: Management of newborn. *In* Principles and Practice of Obstetric Analgesia and Anesthesia. Edited by JJ Bonica, Philadelphia, F.A. Davis, 1969, p. 895.
51. Beard RW, Filshie GM, Knight CA, Roberts GM: The significance of the changes in the continuous fetal heart rate in the first stage of labor. J Obstet. Gynecol. Br. Commonw. 78:865, 1971.
52. Kubli FW, Hon EH, Khazin AF, Takemura H: Observations in heart rate and pH in the human fetus during labor. Am. J. Obstet. Gynecol. 104:1190, 1969.
53. Yurth DA: Placental transfer of local anesthetics. Clin. Perinatol. 9:13, 1982.
54. Fishburne JI: Systemic analgesia during labor. Clin. Perinatol. 9:29, 1988.
55. Parer JT: The current role of intrapartum fetal blood sampling. Clin. Obstet. Gynecol. 23:565, 1980.
56. Miller FC: Prediction of acid-base values from intrapartum fetal heart rate data and their correlation with scalp and funic values. Clin. Perinatol. 9:353, 1982.
57. James LS, Weisbrot IM, Prince CE, Holaday DA, et al: The acid-base status of human infants in relation to birth asphyxia and the onset of respiration. J. Pediatr. 52:379, 1958.
58. Modanlou H, Yeh S-Y, Hon EH, Forsythe A: Fetal and neonatal biochemistry and Apgar score. Am. J. Obstet. Gynecol. 117:942, 1973.
59. Tejani N, Mann L, Bhakthavathsalan A: Correlation of fetal heart rate patterns and fetal pH with neonatal outcome. Obstet. Gynecol. 48:460, 1976.
60. Bowe ET, Beard RW, Finster M, Poppers PJ, et al: Reliability of fetal blood sampling. Am. J. Obstet. Gynecol. 107:279, 1970.
61. Rudolph AM: The fetal circulation. In: Congenital Disease of the Heart. Chicago, Yearbook Medical Publishers, Inc., 1974, p. 1.
62. Meschia G: Placental respiratory gas exchange and fetal oxygenation. *In* Maternal-Fetal Medicine: Principles and Practice. Edited by RK Creasy, R Resnik. Philadelphia, W.B. Saunders Company, 1984, p. 274.
63. Rurak D, Selke P, Fisher M, Taylor S, et al: Fetal oxygen extraction: comparison of the human and sheep. Am. J. Obstet. Gynecol. 156:360, 1987.
64. Phibbs RH: Delivery room management of the newborn. *In* Neonatology. 3rd Ed. Edited by GB Avery. Philadelphia, J.B. Lippincott Company, 1987, p. 212.
65. Myers RE: Experimental models of perinatal brain damage: relevance to human pathology. *In* Intrauterine Asphyxia and the Developing Fetal Brain. Edited by L Gluck. Chicago, Year Book Medical Publishers, Inc., 1977, p. 37.
66. Rosen MG: Factors during labor and delivery that influence brain disorders.*In* Prenatal and Perinatal Factors Associated with Brain Disorders. Edited by JM Freeman. Bethesda, MD, U.S. Department of Health and Human Services, NIH Publication No. 85–1149, April, 1985, p. 237.
67. Brann AW Jr: Factors during labor and delivery that influence brain disorders.*In* Prenatal and Perinatal Factors Associated with Brain Disorders. Edited by JM Freeman. Bethesda, MD, U.S. Department of Health and Human Services, NIH Publication No. 85–1149, April, 1985, p. 237.
68. Modanlou H, Yeh S-Y, Siassi B, Hon EH: Direct monitoring of arterial blood pressure in depressed and normal newborns during the first hour of life. J. Pediatr. 85:533, 1974.
69. Benitz WE, Frankel LR, Stevenson DK: The pharmacology of neonatal resuscitation and cardiopulmonary intensive care. Part I: Immediate resuscitation. West. J. Med. 144:704, 1986.
70. Thibeault DW, Hall FK, Sheehan MB, Hall RT: Postasphyxial lung disease in newborn infants with severe perinatal acidosis. Am. J. Obstet. Gynecol. 150:393, 1984.
71. Wible JL, Petrie RH, Koons A, Perez A: The clinical use of umbilical cord acid-base determinations in perinatal surveillance and management. Clin. Perinatol. 9(2):387, 1982.
72. Yeomans ER, Hauth JC, Gilstrap LC III, Strickland DM: Umbilical cord pH, $PCO_2$, and bicarbonate following uncomplicated term vaginal deliveries. Am. J. Obstet. Gynecol. 151: 798, 1985.
73. Adamsons K Jr: The role of thermal factors in foetal and neonatal life. Pediatr. Clin. North. Am. 13:599, 1966.
74. Stern L, Lees MH, Leduc J: Environmental temperature, oxygen consumption, and catecholamine excretion in newborn infants. Pediatrics 36:367, 1965.
75. Sinclair JC: Mechanisms of neonatal thermoregulation. *In* Physiological and Biochemical Basis for Perinatal Medicine. Edited by M Monset-Couchard, A Minkowski. Paris, S. Karger, 1979, p. 180.
76. Hein T: Energy requirements of thermoregulatory heat production in the newly born. *In* Physiological and Biochemical Basis for Perinatal Medicine. Edited by M Monset-Couchard, A Minkowski. Paris, S. Karger, 1979, p. 180.
77. Mann TP: Observations on temperatures of mothers and babies in the perinatal period. J. Obstet. Gynecol. Br. Commonw. 75:316, 1968.
78. Stratton D: Aural temperature of the newborn infant. Arch. Dis. Child. 52:865, 1977.
79. Mestyán J, Járai I, Bata G, Fekete M: The significance of facial skin temperature in the chemical heat regulation of premature infants. Biol. Neonate 7:243, 1964.
80. Cordero L Jr, Hon E: Neonatal bradycardia following nasopharyngeal stimulation. J. Pediatr. 78:441, 1971.
81. James LS: Emergencies in the delivery room. *In* Neonatal-Perinatal Medicine. 4th Ed. Edited by AA Fanaroff, RJ Martin. St. Louis, The C.V. Mosby Company, 1977, p. 360.
82. Linderman R: Resuscitation of the newborn. Endotracheal administration of epinephrine. Acta. Paediatr. Scand. 73: 210–212, 1984.
83. Howell JH: Sodium bicarbonate in the perinatal setting: revisited. Clin. Perinatol. 14:807, 1987.
84. Bloom RS, Cropley C: Textbook of neonatal resuscitation. American Heart Association and the American Academy of Pediatrics, Dallas, 1987.
85. DiSessa TG, Leitner M, Ti CC, Gluck L, et al: The cardiovascular effects of dopamine in the severely asphyxiated neonate. J. Pediatr. 99:772, 1981.
86. Fiddler GI, Chatrath R, Williams GJ, Walker DR, et al: Dopamine infusion for the treatment of myocardial dysfunction associated with a persistent transitional circulation. Arch. Dis. Child 55:194, 1980.

87. Tejani N, Verma U: Neonatal depression and birth asphyxia in the low birthweight neonate. Am. J. Perinatol. 5:85, 1988.
88. Brown BL, Gleicher N: Intrauterine meconium aspiration. Obstet. Gynecol. 57:26, 1981.
89. Hageman JR, Conley M, Francis K, Stenske J, et al: Delivery room management of meconium staining in the amniotic fluid and the development of meconium aspiration syndrome. J. Perinatol. 8:127, 1988.
90. Milner AD: ABC of resuscitation: resuscitation at birth. Br. Med. J. 292:1657, 1986.
91. Leake RD, Gunther R, Sunshine P: Perinatal aspiration syndrome: its association with intrapartum events and anesthesia. Am. J. Obstet. Gynecol. 118:271, 1974.
92. Gage JE, Taeusch Jr HW, Treves S, Caldicott W: Suctioning of upper airway meconium in newborn infants. JAMA 246: 2590, 1981.
93. Ting P, Brady JP: Tracheal suction in meconium aspiration. Am. J. Obstet. Gynecol. 122:767, 1975.
94. Gregory GA, Gooding CA, Phibbs RH, Tooley WH: Meconium aspiration in infants: a prospective study. J. Pediatr. 85:848, 1974.
95. Carson BS, Losey RW, Bowes WA Jr, Simmons MA: Combined obstetric and pediatric approach to prevent meconium aspiration syndrome. Am. J. Obstet. Gynecol. 126:712, 1976.
96. Linder N, Aranda JV, Tsur M, Matoth I, et al: Need for endotracheal intubation and suction in meconium-stained neonates. J. Pediatr. 112:613, 1988.

Section G

# ANALGESIA AND ANESTHESIA FOR MAJOR OBSTETRIC PROBLEMS

# Chapter 24

# INDUCTION OF LABOR AND MANAGEMENT OF NORMAL AND ABNORMAL LABOR

KENT UELAND

This chapter discusses cervical priming, the physiology of labor, the management of induction of labor, and normal and abnormal labor patterns. Although these are primarily obstetric problems, optimal anesthesiologic care is an integral and essential part of the care of parturients and their infants. It deserves reemphasis that the obstetric anesthesiologist must know the indications, contraindications, and techniques for the induction of labor and the etiology, pathophysiology, and obstetric management of parturients with various abnormal labor patterns. The information is presented with the first half of the chapter devoted to cervical priming and induction of labor, and the second part to the physiology of labor and management of abnormal labor patterns. More detailed information of these subjects can be found elsewhere (1–6).

## INDUCTION OF LABOR

Induction of labor has long been an important part of the methodology of obstetricians. Artificial rupture of the membranes, the oldest technique for the induction of labor, was reportedly performed by Soranus of Greece in 100 A.D., but it was not until 1906 that the effect of posterior pituitary extract was documented by Dale (7). In the early 1900s, numerous mechanical and medical means of dealing with uterine dystocia existed, but all produced variable and inconsistent effects. Consequently, Hofbauer's published account in 1911 of six successful inductions with pituitary extract aroused tremendous interest (8). A few successful case histories were recorded but abuse soon produced reports of serious maternal and fetal morbidity and mortality. Watson's criteria, illustrating the misuse of pituitary extract, included administration in instances of pelvic contracture to obviate the need for forceps and in cases of placental previa to minimize hemorrhage (9). Physicians then claimed that use of pituitary extract obviated forceps delivery in hundreds of instances (10–12). In 1918, DeLee introduced an era of moderation and advised extreme caution when using the drug (13). He developed guidelines, such as careful administration, close monitoring of the contractions, and avoidance of the technique in patients with pelvic contractures and abnormal fetal presentations. This conservative attitude was endorsed by many other obstetricians who believed that the use of pituitary extract before delivery of the fetus was extremely dangerous. In 1928 a major contribution was made by Kamm and his associates, who separated the pressor fraction from the oxytocic fraction, which was given the proprietary name Pitressin (14). Despite the admonition, pituitrin continued to be used widely until the late 1940s, when a series of publications reporting various serious cardiovascular reactions and even deaths following administration, resulted in the increased use of purified oxytocin extract Pitocin. In 1953, du Vigneaud and his associates elucidated the structure of oxytocin and its chemical synthesis, which was the first synthesis of a peptide hormone (15). Two years later, Boissonnas and his associates developed an entirely new method for the synthesis of oxytocin (16). During the ensuing 3 decades, the use of intravenous oxytocin for the induction of labor had become common practice.

In 1980, the U.S. Food and Drug Administration recommended against the use of oxytocin for elective induction of labor, reasoning that available data and information were inadequate to define the benefit-to-risks consideration. The FDA defined elective induction as the initiation of labor in a term pregnancy in a patient who is free of medical indication for the initiation of labor. They further required the package insert for all oxytocics to contain this warning. The initiating factor for this recommendation was probably iatrogenic prematurity from elective induction of labor. This has led to a substantial increase in inductions for quasi-medical-obstetric reasons, i.e., augmentation of labor, geographic, psychosocial indications, and overdiagnoses of medical-obstetric complications. As a result, we will now be unable to collect adequate data on the efficacy of elective induction of labor.

As with spontaneous labor, when labor is induced artificially, optimal anesthetic management is an integral part of total obstetric care. Although the obstetrician decides on the induction, the anesthesiologist needs to be informed and fully understand the induction, potential underlying problems, and possible complications. The first part of our discussion will center upon preinduction cervical priming along with indications and contraindications. Prerequisites, technical considerations, and various induction techniques will also be addressed. A discussion of anesthetic management will follow.

### *Preinduction Cervical Priming*

The success rate of electively induced labor with oxytocin directly relates to the condition of the cervix as ex-

**Table 24–1.** Bishop Score

| Factor | Score 0 | 1 | 2 | 3 |
|---|---|---|---|---|
| Dilation (cm) | Closed | 1–2 | 3–4 | 5 |
| Effacement (%) | 0–30 | 40–50 | 60–70 | 80 |
| Station | −3 | −2 | −1, 0 | +1, +2 |
| Consistency | Firm | Medium | Soft | — |
| Position | Posterior | Midposition | Anterior | — |

(From Bishop EH: Pelvic scoring for elective induction. Obstet. Gynecol. 24:266, 1964.)

pressed by the Bishop Score (Table 24–1) (17). This investigator found that if the score was unfavorable (i.e., 1 to 4), the failure rate of induction in multiparous patients was approximately 20%, as opposed to 5% when the score was intermediate (i.e., 5 to 8), and 0% when 9 or greater. The author prefers to use the Wingerup modification of the Bishop Score because it is more definitive and reduces the chance of examiner differences (Table 24–2) (18). With the Wingerup Score, 0 to 5 is considered unfavorable and 6 to 10 favorable. With the advent of the prostaglandins, an unfavorable cervix that has not undergone the natural priming process during the last few weeks of pregnancy can be primed. Much of the work with prostaglandin $E_2$ ($PGE_2$) cervical priming has been done by Ulmsten and coworkers in Sweden (1,19–21). These workers, using mostly intracervical $PGE_2$ in viscous gel in 0.5 mg doses, have demonstrated a very high success rate in achieving priming. Most encouraging is the fact that this priming appears to mimic the natural process that takes place in the last 3 weeks of normal pregnancy morphologically, physically, and biochemically (21–24). The success rate from a subsequent oxytocin induction improves substantially. It has been shown that intracervical $PGE_2$ priming shortens labor as well, most likely because of the significant softening of the cervix that changes its compliance and resistance to dilatation (25). $PGE_2$ has been tested in varying dosages intracervically (0.25 to 1.0 mg) and intravaginally (2 to 4 mg), but the ideal preparation appears to be the intracervical viscous gel in a dose of 0.5 mg (20,26).

**Table 24–2.** Wingerup Score (Modified Bishop Score)

| Factor | Score 0 | 1 | 2 |
|---|---|---|---|
| Cervical dilatation | < 0.5 cm | 0.5–1.5 cm | > 1.5 cm |
| Cervical effacement | None | < 50% | > 50% |
| Station of fetal head | Above or in pelvic inlet | Above spines | At or below spines |
| Cervical consistency | Firm | Medium | Soft |
| Cervical position | Posterior | Mid | Anterior |

(From Wingerup L: Ripening of Cervic Uteri Induced by Single Intracervical Application of Prostaglandin $E_2$ in Viscous Gel. Malmo, Litos Reprotryk, 1979, p. 20.)

**Table 24–3.** Methods Used to Attempt Cervical Priming

- Mechanical
  - Bougie
  - Foley catheter
  - Laminaria
- Hormones locally
  - Purified porcine relaxin
  - Estradiol vaginal gel
- Hormones systemically
  - Oxytocin
  - Estradiol 17-Beta
- Prostaglandin $E_2$ locally
  - Vaginal tablets, gel
  - Intracervical gel
  - Extra-amniotic gel
- Prostaglandin $F_2$ alpha locally
  - Intravaginal gel
  - Extra-amniotic gel
- Prostaglandin $E_2$, $F_2$ alpha systemically
  - Oral $PGE_2$
  - Intravenous $PGE_2$, $PGF_2$ alpha

(Modified from Steiner AL, Creasy RK: Methods of cervical priming. Clin. Obstet. Gynecol. 26:37, 1983.)

Intravaginal application, because of systemic absorption and the required higher dosage, induces uterine contractions not desirable under many clinical circumstances. Intracervical deposition, on the other hand, if confined within the endocervical canal, has essentially no effect on uterine activity (25,26). Because the highest concentration of $PGE_2$ is naturally found in the endocervix, the direct application to the target organ appears to physiologically mimic the natural priming process (2). Table 24–3 shows a partial list of the various prostaglandins, hormones (including routes of administration), and mechanical methods that have been used in the past to attempt to prime the cervix. Only intracervical $PGE_2$ viscous gel has withstood the test of time and appears to have all of the characteristics of an ideal priming agent listed in Table 24–4. The clinical benefits of cervical priming are numerous and include shortening of the duration of labor, decrease in the incidence of maternal pyrexia, decrease in the incidence of asphyxia, fewer instrumental deliveries, and a lower cesarean section rate (25,27,28).

**Table 24–4.** Characteristics of the Ideal Cervical Priming Agent

| |
|---|
| Cervical change same as natural priming |
| No uterine contractions |
| No systemic side effects |
| No fetal/neonatal effects |
| No effect on future pregnancies |
| Effective |
| Safe |
| Practical |
| Inexpensive |
| Patient/staff acceptance |

## BASIC CONSIDERATIONS

### *Indications*

Table 24–5 lists the more common maternal-fetal indications for induction of labor. Another indication that deserves consideration is induction of labor based on geographic reasons, i.e., history of rapid labor, or a patient living a long distance from the hospital. In the ACOG Technical Bulletin, elective induction is included and defined as the initiation of labor for convenience, and is not recommended (6).

### *Prerequisites*

#### Fetal Maturity

In many instances of indicated induction of labor, fetal maturity should be established. Ultrasound is a well-established noninvasive technique that is frequently used to determine gestational age. In a regularly menstruating woman with a known last menstrual period (LMP), one ultrasound scan at 20 to 22 weeks for biparietal diameter (BPD), femur length, and abdominal circumference that agrees with menstrual age is sufficient. If a discrepancy exists and/or the last menstrual period is unknown or periods are irregular, an early (first trimester) scan is preferred with a follow up at 20 to 24 weeks. If an early scan is not available, a scan should be done near the initial visit and repeated at least 4 to 6 weeks later. If both concur, no further evaluation is deemed necessary. However, if any doubt exists, an amniocentesis can be performed to establish fetal lung maturity with a lecithin/sphingomyelin (L/S) ratio greater than 2 and/or a positive phosphatidyl glycerol (PG). If the gestational age is below 34 weeks and the lecithin/sphingomyelin ratio is below 2, the use of steroids in the mother should be considered prior to attempted induction if the maternal or fetal clinical condition will permit.

When using the lecithin/sphingomyelin ratio, a value of 2 or more indicates a low risk of respiratory distress syndrome even below 35 weeks gestation. However, it does not preclude the development of respiratory distress syndrome. Unfortunately, the basic test has been modified by many laboratories and, if standards have not been reestablished based on the changes in procedure and the predictability of respiratory distress syndrome based on the modified test has not been reevaluated, inaccuracies in predicting respiratory distress syndrome could result from the use of improper numbers. It is imperative that managing obstetricians acquaint themselves with the numeric criteria used by the laboratory performing the test.

**Table 24–5.** More Common Indications For Induction of Labor

| |
|---|
| Medical |
| Diabetes |
| Hypertension |
| Renal disease |
| Deteriorating maternal illness (i.e., malignancy, SLE) |
| Obstetrical |
| Pregnancy-induced hypertension (PIH) |
| Prolonged pregnancy |
| Abruptio placentae |
| Premature rupture of membranes (PROM) |
| Chorioamnionitis |
| Fetal |
| Erythroblastosis |
| Intrauterine fetal demise (IUFD) |
| Intrauterine growth retardation (IUGR) |
| Fetal anomalies |
| Other fetal disorders (i.e., discordant twins) |

#### Fetal Presentation

Most physicians currently feel that a vertex presentation should exist prior to entertaining an induction of labor. However, a frank breech presentation with the buttocks dipping into the pelvis along with an adequate pelvis and an average sized fetus, should not totally preclude an attempted indicated induction and vaginal delivery in a fully informed patient, as long as trained personnel are available along with adequate anesthesia. In patients with an unstable lie or breech presentation, external version under ultrasound guidance might be considered. Many institutions now have set protocols for these procedures with a success rate that approaches 75% (29–31). In experienced hands and with the use of tocolysis, major maternal and fetal complications are rare.

#### Maternal Pelvis

Another prerequisite for induction of labor should be an adequate pelvis, with no evidence of cephalopelvic disproportion (CPD). The presenting part should be dipping into the pelvis or engaged. Careful clinical evaluation of the maternal pelvis is imperative before any attempted induction. On rare occasions CT pelvimetry should be considered if contemplating induction with a frank breech presentation.

#### Maternal Cervix

In a patient requiring a therapeutic induction of labor for one of the indications listed in Table 24–5, and with an unfavorable cervix, priming should be entertained as discussed previously. If the Wingerup Score is 6 or greater, an intravenous oxytocin induction is recommended.

### Contraindications

Table 24–6 lists some of the more frequently encountered absolute and relative contraindications to induction of labor. Because oxytocin is likely to aggravate fetal distress, it is absolutely contraindicated if there is evidence of fetal compromise. Total placental previa is an indication for cesarean section. Proven cephalopelvic disproportion (CPD) and a scar in the myometrium are also contraindications to induction of labor.

Depending on individual clinical circumstances, an attempt at induction can be undertaken with judicious use of oxytocin in patients with grand multiparity, an overdistended uterus, and in those with a previously known low transverse cesarean section scar. If one is a proponent of vaginal birth after cesarean (VBAC), then one should not

**Table 24–6.** Contraindications to the Use of Oxytocics

Absolute
1. Fetal distress
2. Central placental previa
3. Proven cephalopelvic disproportion
4. Scar in myometrium

Relative
1. Overdistended uterus (i.e., twins, hydramnios)
2. Grand multiparity
3. Breech presentation
4. Previous low transverse cesarean section (VBAC)
5. Prematurity
6. Unengaged presenting part
7. Malposition
8. Fetal anomalies (i.e., hydrocephalus)

hesitate to use oxytocin judiciously to effect vaginal delivery when indicated. Similarly, with careful monitoring, some patients with an unengaged vertex can be induced. In others, a malpresentation could be reduced by manipulation under ultrasound guidance and fetal heart rate monitoring to a position that is relatively favorable for attempted induction.

## Technical Considerations

Currently accepted techniques for induction of labor include drugs, such as oxytocin and prostaglandins, and mechanical means, such as stripping of membranes and artificial rupture of membranes (AROM).

### Medical (Pharmacologic) Induction

The only approved drug for use in induction of labor in the United States is oxytocin, the only accepted route of administration is intravenously and with the use of an electronically controlled infusion device. Although not approved for use for the pharmacologic induction of labor in this country, prostaglandins are commonly used worldwide and will be discussed here for completeness.

### Oxytocin

Oxytocin is best administered by using a tandem or piggyback arrangement in which the oxytocin containing device is inserted into the proximal end of an already established intravenous infusion of a glucose or electrolyte containing solution. This allows for a safe and exact rate of infusion of oxytocin. The recommended starting dose of oxytocin is between 0.5 and 2 mU/minute (32,33). When there is evidence of uterine irritability, the lowest dose should be utilized. However, one must keep in mind that uterine sensitivity to oxytocin is increased at term and that there is great individual variation in myometrial sensitivity to oxytocin. In addition, uterine tachyphylaxis may occur at any time during oxytocin infusion; therefore, it must always be used cautiously and titrated in relation to clinical response. The object is to administer the drug in physiologic doses sufficient to produce uterine activity similar to that found in spontaneous labor. At term, this is ordinarily accomplished with infusion rates of 4 to 6 mU/minute (33). It is not surprising that the condition of the cervix not only determines the success rate of induction, but also the number of contractions and total uterine work necessary to achieve complete dilatation (33,34).

If the desired contraction pattern is not reached with the initial dose of oxytocin, it can safely be increased in 1 to 2 mU/minute increments every 30 to 60 minutes (35–37). Approximately 90% of patients will achieve normal progress in labor with the administration of 16 mU or less.

Several reports in the literature indicate that patients undergoing oxytocin-induced labor have contractions of higher mean amplitude (52 to 55 mm Hg) when compared to patients in spontaneous labor or oral $PGE_2$ induced labor (37 to 45 mm Hg) (38–40). However, significant differences do not appear in the frequency of contractions or uterine tonus between contractions. The increase in intensity of contractions is supported clinically by the fact that oxytocin-induced contractions appear to be more painful and patients require more analgesia when compared to patients undergoing oral $PGE_2$ inductions (40,41).

All patients undergoing induction of labor with oxytocin should have close intrapartum monitoring, i.e., auscultation by stethoscope or Doppler ultrasound or continuous electronic fetal monitoring as recommended by the American College of Obstetricians and Gynecologists (42). In addition, resting uterine tone and frequency and duration of contractions should be checked and recorded frequently. Experienced labor personnel need to be in constant attendance. If there is any suspected deviation from normal, internal contraction monitoring and electronic fetal heart rate monitoring are recommended.

Although continuous intravenous infusion of oxytocin for induction of labor is currently the standard, a few investigators have recently suggested that pulsed administration of oxytocin intravenously may have more merit, as it seems to mimic physiologic production by the mother in labor (6). It also substantially reduces the amount of drug necessary. This clinical approach was first studied in England over a decade ago by Pavlou and coworkers (43). They randomized a small group of patients at term, inducing one group with amniotomy and pulsed oxytocin infusion (1 minute in every 10) and another group with amniotomy and continuous oxytocin infusion. Induction to full dilatation and induction to delivery intervals were similar for both groups. However, the former required a significantly lower dose of oxytocin and the maximum effective dose rate was much higher, reaching 64 mU/minute, in over half of the latter group. This remains somewhat experimental and needs further study before considering it a legitimate clinical alternative to continuous intravenous administration of oxytocin.

### Prostaglandin $E_2$

The literature is replete with studies showing successful induction of term labor using prostaglandin $E_2$ by varying routes of administration (19,20,26,28,38,41). Karim and

Sharma (44) were the first to report the results of a clinical trial with the use of oral $PGE_2$. Successful induction has also been achieved with intravenous, intracervical, intravaginal, and extra-amniotic $PGE_2$. The intracervical application has been used extensively in Sweden and other European countries. To date, $PGE_2$ has not been approved by the U.S. Food and Drug Administration, but it is, nonetheless, being extensively used in this country for both cervical priming and induction of labor. Unfortunately, the varying preparations, different dosage schedules, and routes of administration preclude gathering standardized meaningful data about efficacy, appropriate dosage schedules, factors affecting outcome, side effects, and the like.

In the author's experience of over 300 cases of induction of labor with oral $PGE_2$, both elective and indicated, efficacy similar to or better than, oxytocin was established (38,45). Several important advantages became evident from these studies: (1) delivery was achieved with less total uterine work; (2) the rate of cervical dilatation in the active phase of labor was faster than that reported for ideal spontaneous labor, 2.73 cm/hr compared to 2.12 cm/hr (46) (both of these factors are directly attributed to the marked softening of the cervix that occurs which in turn decreases resistance to dilatation); (3) the contractions mimicked in intensity those of women in spontaneous labor, and the mean amplitude was substantially below those reported in the literature during oxytocin induction of labor; (4) less analgesia was required during labor; (5) induction was safe; (6) no serious side effects occurred; and (7) patient acceptance was high. It is no wonder that this alternate approach to inducing labor is so popular in Europe, Canada, and many other developed countries. Success rate with oral $PGE_2$ induction can be substantially improved by early amniotomy (47–50) escalating dosage schedules (43,46,48,49,51), shorter intervals between successive doses (48,50), and continued intermittent administration until delivery (43,48). The standard dose of oral $PGE_2$ tablets for induction of labor is 0.5 to 2.0 mg/hour. The initial and continued dosage schedule should be dictated by individual clinical circumstances and responses.

Ulmsten and coworkers have provided us with the most valuable information regarding the use of intracervical $PGE_2$. They used a special viscous gel for cervical priming and induction of labor (1,19,20,24,26). Their extensive experience in over 1000 patients has shown both efficacy and safety with the intracervical application of 0.5 mg $PGE_2$ gel. In term patients with a favorable cervix, 97% will deliver within 7 hours following only a single application. The major advantages of the technique are its simplicity and patient acceptability, as patients are able to ambulate during early labor (26). In patients with an unfavorable cervical state, labor is induced successfully in approximately 25%. If extreme care is employed and the gel confined entirely to the endocervical canal, few patients exhibit any increase in uterine activity (25,26). Within 5 hours the cervix has been primed in the majority of patients and induction of labor can be safely and successfully undertaken using conventional intravenous oxytocin. The author and coworkers have achieved similar results with improved oxytocin induction success rates and a significantly shortened labor with normal uterine activity (25).

The primary goal of intracervical application of $PGE_2$ gel is cervical priming in patients requiring induction of labor and who have an unfavorable cervical state. This topic was discussed in more detail earlier in the chapter in the section on preinduction cervical priming.

### *Surgical Induction*

#### Stripping of Membranes

Stripping of membranes to induce labor consists of digitally separating the chorioamniotic membrane from the lower uterine segment. It is the least successful approach to the induction of labor. It can only be used in patients with a favorable cervical state, when success rates are highest regardless of technique used to initiate labor. This mechanical stimulation results in the release of prostaglandins locally (52). There are some potential risks to the procedure, such as bleeding from an unsuspected low lying placenta and inadvertent rupture of membranes with a high presenting part that could result in a prolapsed cord. As efficacy has not been clearly established, there is an unpredictable latent period before labor ensues, and there are some risks to the procedure. The author does not recommend this approach.

#### *Amniotomy*

Artificial rupture of the membranes (AROM) has been the most popular and dependable mechanical technique for inducing labor. It is particularly successful when the cervix is favorable. Artificial rupture of the membranes has been shown to substantially increase plasma prostaglandin levels, which may account for the high success rate in initiating labor (51,53). Certain prerequisites should pertain before artificial rupture of the membranes: (1) the presenting part should be tightly applied to the cervix or dipping well into the pelvis and (2) the procedure must be performed in the labor and delivery area and with close fetal heart rate monitoring. With a favorable cervix, the majority of patients will be in established labor within 6 to 12 hours. If not, an oxytocin induction should be started.

There are some advantages to amniotomy. It is relatively easy to perform and less confining for patients in early labor. It allows for the direct evaluation of amniotic fluid and for the placement of internal monitors. Last, it allows for a more physiologic onset of labor and tends to shorten the total duration of labor (54,55).

## *Anesthesiologic Management*

When the induction of labor is done for medical or obstetric reasons, particular problems arise, which are related to the problem for which the induction was done. Anesthesia in these conditions becomes a major concern in the conduct of labor. The importance of a meeting with all patients in the antepartum period with the anesthesiologist needs to be stressed at this point. As was emphasized in Chapter 22 (Antepartum Management and Analgesia for Normal Labor and Vaginal Delivery), this type of meeting between the anesthesiologist and the patient is very important. It can be held anytime in the antepartum period, but there is a preference for the late second or third trimester. Then the anesthesiologist has the opportunity to present the various methods of pain relief as well as agents available for producing such relief. In addition, the anesthesiologist assuages many fears of the patient regarding unknown physiologic changes and poor understanding of analgesic methods. This meeting helps to educate the patient and also helps her understand that another physician colleague has a primary and focused interest in her and her baby.

This session emphasizes some simplistic points about physiologic changes in pregnancy and effectiveness of labor pain relief and its low complication rate. It provides the patient with a time to discuss the many questions and considerations that concern her, which she could not discuss before because she felt they were either silly or unimportant to others in regard to her management.

Early consultation with the anesthesiologist is important in all labor cases, but becomes essential when induction is performed for medical/obstetric reasons. The obstetrician should inform the anesthesiologist thoroughly about the course of labor and the condition of the mother and fetus. The anesthesiologist should have an adequate opportunity to visit the patient before the induction and to carry out a thorough preanesthetic evaluation and preparation. Obviously, this requires that an anesthesiologist be readily available for this purpose, for the institution of emergency anesthesia if this should become necessary and to begin the anesthetic at the optimal time.

To provide maximum benefit to the mother and the fetus, the basic principles of anesthetic management must be adhered to. In addition to providing maximum relief of pain, the analgesic-anesthetic must fulfill the following criteria: (1) it should not impede the progress of labor; (2) it should not relax the perineum until flexion and internal rotation of the presenting part have taken place; (3) it should not impair the auxiliary forces of labor so that during the second stage the mother can effectively bear down and deliver either spontaneously or with the aid of forceps; (4) it should produce minimal or no side effects on the mother and infant. Obviously, whenever a medical or obstetric indication exists, anesthetic management should be tailored according to the principles identified in regard to those problems as outlined in many of the chapters in this book.

Before and during induction of labor the patient is reassured and prepared psychologically for the delivery. This preparation should also have been carried out in the physician's office during pregnancy. This may be supplemented with sedatives/analgesics administered in small doses, intravenously. When the patient begins to have moderate discomfort, relief may be provided by: (1) regional analgesia; (2) systemic analgesics; or (3) a combination of these. It is important to avoid premature administration or overdosage of sedative-narcotics or too-early administration of conduction analgesia, because initial labor patterns may be impaired or the onset of active labor prolonged or even stopped. Proper anesthetic management not only allows for maximal patient comfort but in many instances also effects a shorter labor.

### *Regional Analgesia-Anesthesia*

Regional analgesia, as modified by today's continuous pump technique, is almost the ideal method because it provides complete relief of pain without disturbing maternal functions and without depressing the fetus provided no complications develop. Techniques that may be used include: (1) continuous extradural block by either the lumbar or caudal route; or (2) continuous subarachnoid block.

### *Continuous Extradural Analgesia*

Used by an obstetric team skilled in its execution and application, continuous caudal or continuous lumbar epidural or the combined double catheter extradural technique provides the best method of producing analgesia during labor and anesthesia for delivery (56–58). Of the three, the double catheter method is the most refined. The low-dose continuous epidural block does not interfere with the Ferguson reflex and, therefore, does not impair uterine contractility. The caudal block, if used, is withheld until full cervical dilation has taken place and perineal distention with consequent pain develops.

The "continuous" feature of extradural analgesia provides maximum flexibility as far as the time when analgesia can be started, as well as control of duration, extent, and intensity of the block. A catheter can and should be inserted during the latent phase of labor, before the patient becomes uncomfortable and at a time when she can best cooperate. Some clinicians prefer to insert a catheter even before labor is induced in patients committed to delivery at the time. This does not cause a problem; however, if induction of labor is unsuccessful and the patient is sent home, the catheter should be removed. The fact that the catheter is in place provides a ready means of anesthesia should cesarean section become necessary.

With these techniques, one is able to provide both complete relief of pain and optimal conditions for uterine response to oxytocin. For optimal results, injection of the first therapeutic dose is withheld until the cervix becomes 4 to 5 cm dilated and the patient has entered the active phase of labor. One may encounter a rare exception to this rule; for example, the patient who is experiencing moderate to sever pain that is not relieved with small doses of sedative. In these patients a segmental epidural block can be started. Use of the continuous dilute solutions of local anesthetics overcame the former problem of reduction in effective uterine contractions due to the mass anesthetic effect of previously administered large bolus doses. At the same time, the oxytocin infusion can be increased to achieve optimum uterine activity during the pain control period with the continuous infusion method (59).

In any case, it is advisable to use dilute solutions of local anesthetics so as not to produce perineal relaxation which, as mentioned, may interfere with internal rotation. Moreover, the patient will be able to move her legs. After internal rotation has taken place, a higher concentration of the local anesthetic is used to produce perineal relaxation, which will facilitate delivery. Even though the block interrupts the reflex urge to bear down, the patient can be coached as to when and how long to do so to effect a spontaneous delivery.

There are some who believe that it is dangerous to use a technique that produces complete relief of pain. It is alleged that a tetanic contraction or rupture of the uterus might go unrecognized; however, such serious complications would go unrecognized only if the attending physician were not present or alert. Obviously, untrained personnel should not be responsible for the conduct of these labors. Moreover, it is unlikely that continuous extradural analgesia will mask the pain of a ruptured uterus because some of this pain is caused by irritation of the peritoneum, which is supplied by segments above the tenth thoracic dermatome.

Accurate figures on the safety and incidence of complications from extradural block anesthesia in obstetrics are difficult, at best, to come by. However, a recent study out of England involving over half a million procedures suggests a complication rate of 1 per 4000 to 5000 blocks (60). The complications ranged from severe to minor. Among the most frequent complications listed were three cases of cardiac arrest, 38 cases of damage to single spinal nerve or nerve root causing temporary neuropathy, 21 cases of acute toxicity with convulsions, eight high or total spinals, 16 cases of severe headache after accidental dural puncture, and two cases of spinal cord compression (one abscess, one hematoma). With the large number of procedures performed, this study certainly points to the safety of extradural anesthesia in obstetrics. Few patients with the above listed complications suffered permanent damage.

### *Paracervical or Lumbar Sympathetic Block Combined with Pudendal Block*

The pain pathways from the uterus may be interrupted in their course through the lumbar sympathetic chain or in the paracervical region. Either procedure can be repeated as necessary.

Paracervical block (PCB) was used extensively in the 1970s but has now fallen into disfavor because of several fetal deaths that were attributed to its use along with a high incidence of fetal bradycardia following its use (61). This form of regional anesthesia has not been used at Stanford Medical Center for the past 15 years. This is in part due to the fact that 24 hour anesthesia coverage is available and epidural anesthesia can be administered at any time by fully trained anesthesiologists. In low-risk patients, paracervical block anesthesia is sometimes used at institutions where epidural anesthesia is not available. This book is for the benefit of many different health care personnel. Therefore, PCB is mentioned because some obstetricians or family physicians may still use this analgesic method in low-risk cases. Any PCB must be performed with caution and skill only after the mother is fully informed of the risk-benefit ratio and concerns. Certain careful guidelines should be adhered to as mentioned in Chapter 15. If used, the smallest amount of local anesthetic possible should be used and meticulous attention must be paid to details of administration. Close fetal heart monitoring should always accompany its use.

As soon as perineal distention causes pain, bilateral transvaginal pudendal block may be carried out. This combination provides complete relief of pain. The advantages of these techniques are that they are simple, effective, and can be carried out by the obstetrician. As with extradural analgesia, care must be used not to begin analgesia prematurely, and not to use excessive doses of local anesthetics, because they depress uterine contractility and also may affect the fetus adversely.

### *Subarachnoid Block*

Subarachnoid block may be used to provide relief of pain during the latter stages of the first stage and during the second and third stages of labor. Although some physicians believe that spinal anesthesia should be reserved for the actual delivery, there is no good reason why it cannot be started much earlier in selected patients, e.g., those with 7 to 8 cm cervical dilation, depending, of course, on the progress of labor. The effects on uterine contractility are similar to those of standard extradural anesthesia except that spinal anesthesia causes paralysis of the perineal muscles and the lower limbs. However, like other techniques of regional anesthesia, it does not depress uterine contractility or seem to alter uterine response to oxytocin. It does interfere with the Ferguson reflex. With dibucaine (Nupercaine) one is able to produce analgesia for as long as 3 to 4 hours — sufficiently long in most patients to last until the delivery. If shorter-acting anesthetics are used, the procedure can be repeated. If necessary, or more convenient, a continuous subarachnoid block may be instituted. This is achieved by use of a subarachnoid catheter. There is no good reason why a second or third lumbar puncture cannot be done, provided fine (25 gauge or 26 gauge) needles are used.

### *Special Circumstances*

There may be special circumstances that exist in some centers where full time regional analgesia/anesthesia is not available. In those circumstances, we may consider use of various combinations of sedative/opiate combinations as described in Chapters 15 and 17; or for later second stage analgesia, we may consider $N_2O/O_2$ in 0.3/0.7 to 0.5/0.5 ratios so that some maternal analgesia is obtained with severe contractions and bearing-down efforts. The latter may elicit considerable perineal dilatation and distension with severe pain. Other methods no longer relied upon to any significant degree include lumbar sympathetic block and general anesthesia per se for vaginal delivery. Paracervical block combined with pudendal block is still utilized today in some centers to provide later first stage and second stage analgesia, respectively.

## Normal Labor

Labor can be defined as regular painful uterine contractions that lead to the expulsion of the fetus. The uterine contractions of labor have the following major character-

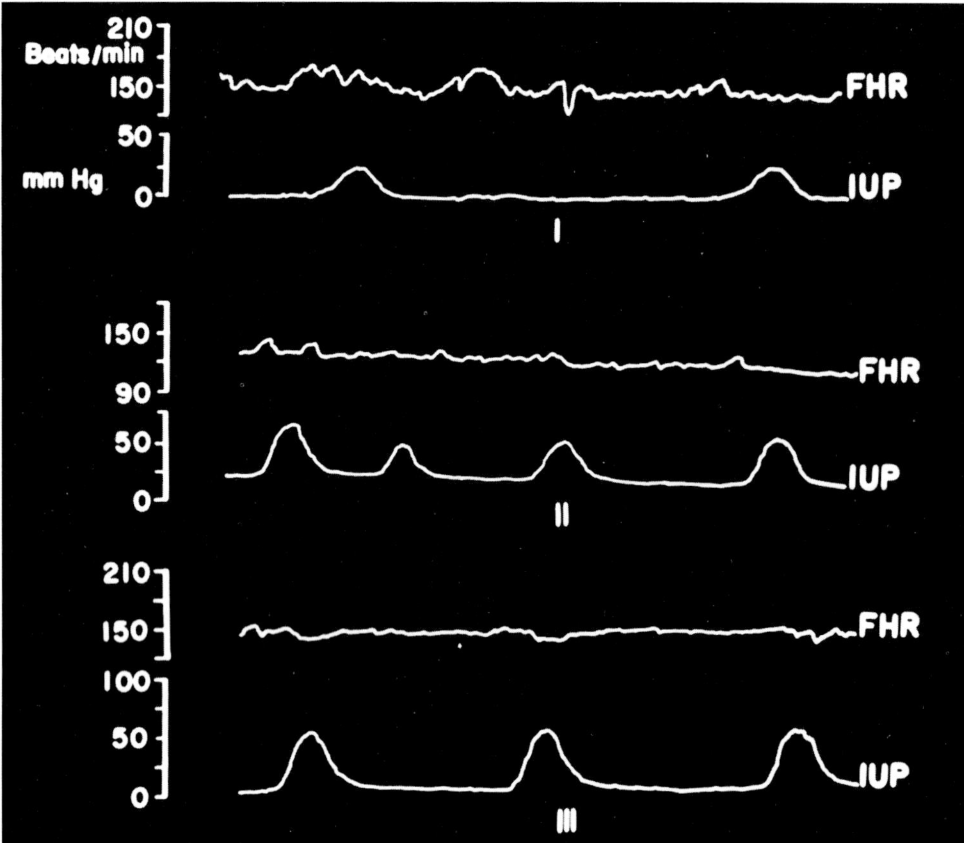


**Fig. 24–1.** Uterine contractility at the spontaneous onset of normal term labor. Note the infrequent and somewhat irregular contractions at the beginning (I) followed by increased frequency, intensity, and regularity (II) with the ensuing first stage of labor (III). FHR—fetal heart rate, IUP—intrauterine pressure.

istics: (1) frequency, (2) intensity, and (3) duration. In normal active labor, contractions should occur with a frequency of 2 to 5 times every 10 minutes. As labor progresses, they tend to become more frequent. Figure 24–1 depicts uterine activity at the onset of spontaneous labor and the early first stage of labor. During the early first stage of labor, the intrauterine pressure generated by a contraction reaches an average of 40 to 60 mm Hg. This intensity normally increases as labor advances, and it is not unusual to see contractions as strong as 70 to 90 mm Hg or more late in the first stage and in the second stage of labor. The duration of normal contractions ordinarily vary between 45 to 90 seconds. Generally, the more intense the contraction, the longer it lasts. Hence, as labor progresses the duration tends to increase. Uterine muscle also has another characteristic called tonus. This is defined as the pressure that remains in the uterus between contractions during labor. The average tonus in early labor approximates 5 to 7 mm Hg, whereas in late labor it reaches 10 to 12 mm Hg. Although contractions are rhythmical, they do not normally occur at regular set intervals. Similarly, the intensity and duration may vary, but a contraction following the longest pause is usually the strongest and longest (Figure 24–2).

## Spontaneous Labor

There is no simple explanation for the initiation of spontaneous labor in the human. It has become increasingly apparent that it is a complex integration of numerous factors that effect coordinated uterine activity that ultimately results in the evacuation of the uterus. Although we have made great strides in understanding the physiology of labor in many animals, including initiating factors, we have not been able to elucidate this in the human. There are many reasons for this including the complexity of the process itself, as well as ethical considerations, limiting investigative techniques in the human (2,3).

### *Uterine Physiology*

The concept of considering labor in terms of only smooth muscle function is no longer tenable. There are clearly two distinct forces of labor. These include uterine contractions and the resistance of the cervix. It is the coordinated interplay between these two forces that produces the ultimate successful outcome—delivery. During the last decade, the nonmuscular cervical factor or lower uterine segment has received much attention, and rightly so, because without a compliant cervix successful vaginal delivery cannot be accomplished (19). During the last few weeks of normal pregnancy, significant anatomical, biochemical, and physical changes transform the lower uterine segment and cervix from a collagenous sphincter that safely retains the conceptus into a compliant structure that allows for nearly resistance-free dilatation during labor.

The physiology of human labor in general remains far from being fully understood. However, we do have some knowledge of basic uterine muscle physiology. Uterine

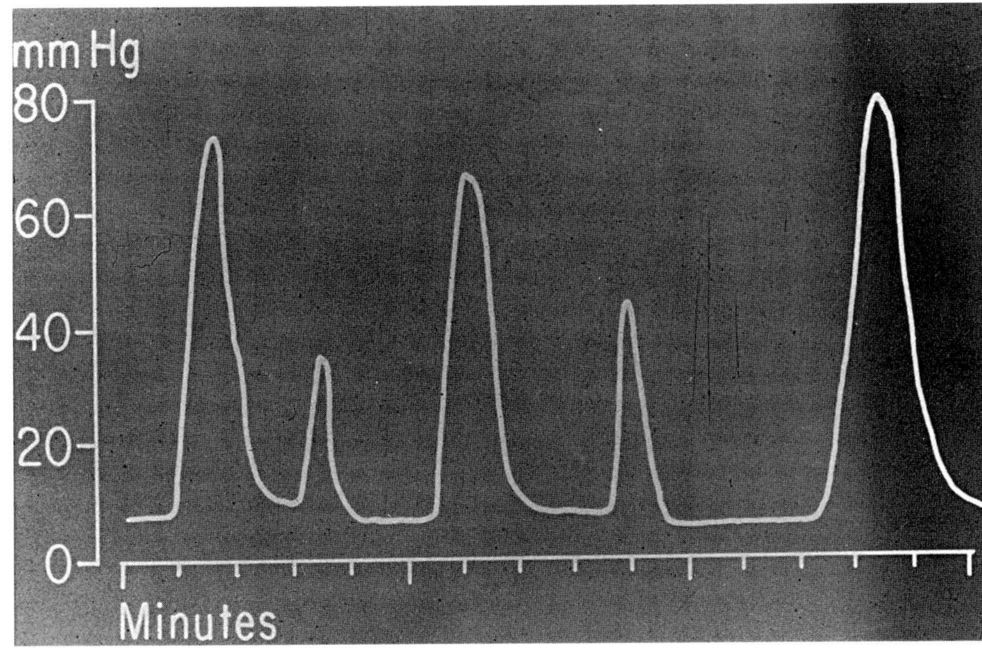


**Fig. 24–2.** This schematic represents uterine activity during normal labor. Contractions may vary as to intensity, frequency, and duration, and, unlike other contractible organs, uterine contractions do not occur at set intervals. The longer the interval between contractions, the more likely a more intense contraction of longer duration.

muscle, or smooth muscle in general, has several unique general characteristics which allow it to accommodate to its specific roles of pregnancy and parturition. It has the properties of being able to change in length without changing tension. It contracts and relaxes. Finally, at the onset of normal labor, incoordinate activity (Braxton Hicks contractions), which originate in various parts of the myometrium, gradually are transformed into coordinate contractions with fundal dominance. As labor progresses, the contractions increase in frequency, intensity, and duration and ultimately result in the successful evacuation of the fetus. This is the same structure that for 9 months adjusted its volume to a rapidly growing conceptus without changing its tension and with little effect on contractility.

During labor, contractions of uterine muscle (myometrium) result in progressive shortening of that muscle (i.e., it never returns to its original precontractile length). Although the uterus does not have an identifiable pacemaker like the heart, it does have spontaneous rhythmic contractile activity of varying frequency, duration, and intensity in both the pregnant and nonpregnant state. Normal uterine contractions at term pregnancy exhibit fundal dominance. The contractions originate in the fundus (at either cornua) and propagate down the uterus to the lower uterine segment and cervix (Figure 24–3)(4). The contractions are longest and most intense in the fundus and, as a result, the muscle retracts toward it thickening the fundus while thinning the collagenous laden lower uterine segment and cervix. For a detailed discussion of the physiologic aspects of uterine muscle activity, please refer to Chapter 4.

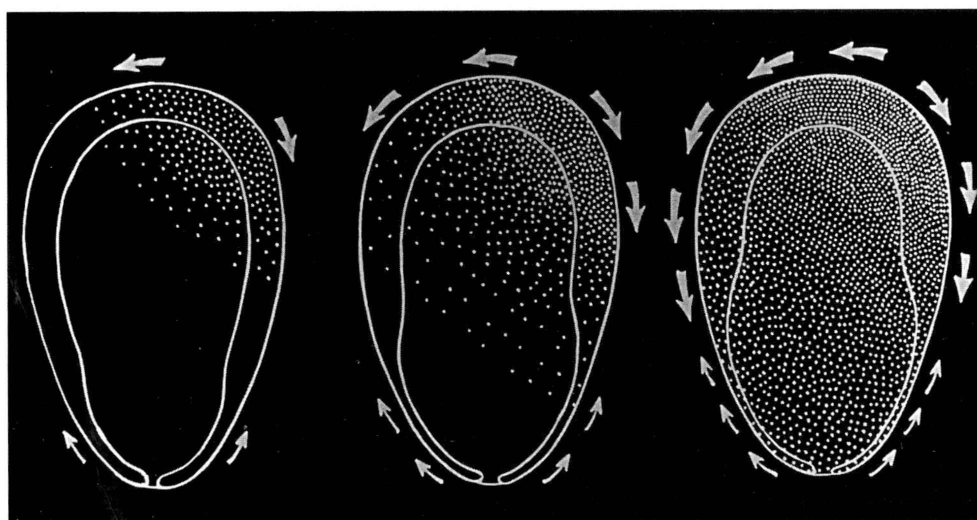

**Fig. 24–3.** A schematic representation of the propagation of fundally dominant contractions in normal spontaneous labor. Most frequently these contractions originate at either cornua. The arrows represent propagation of the contraction while the dots depict intensity.

## *Types of Uterine Contractions*

There are three types of uterine contractions: normal, subnormal, and abnormal. The characteristics of normal contractions have already been described.

Subnormal contractions tend to occur less frequently than normal contractions, have an amplitude of less than 40 mm Hg, and a duration of less than 30 to 40 seconds. However, as with normal contractions, they have fundal dominance. Subnormal contractions respond well to oxytocin augmentation, which converts them to normal contractions. Abnormal contractions, on the other hand, lack fundal dominance and the foci initiating the contractions may be located anywhere in the uterus. Ordinarily, they are less intense and occur less frequently than normal contractions. Rarely do they constitute the only type of contraction occurring for any length of time. Typically, they are mixed with either normal and/or subnormal contractions. Understandably, the higher the percentage of abnormal contractions, the more protracted the labor. Abnormal contractions are ineffective in dilating and effacing the cervix because of their reversed gradient of propagation. Figure 24–4 presents schematically the characteristics of the three major types of uterine contractions. Note the frequency of contractions as well as the amplitude in both the fundus and lower uterine segment for each.

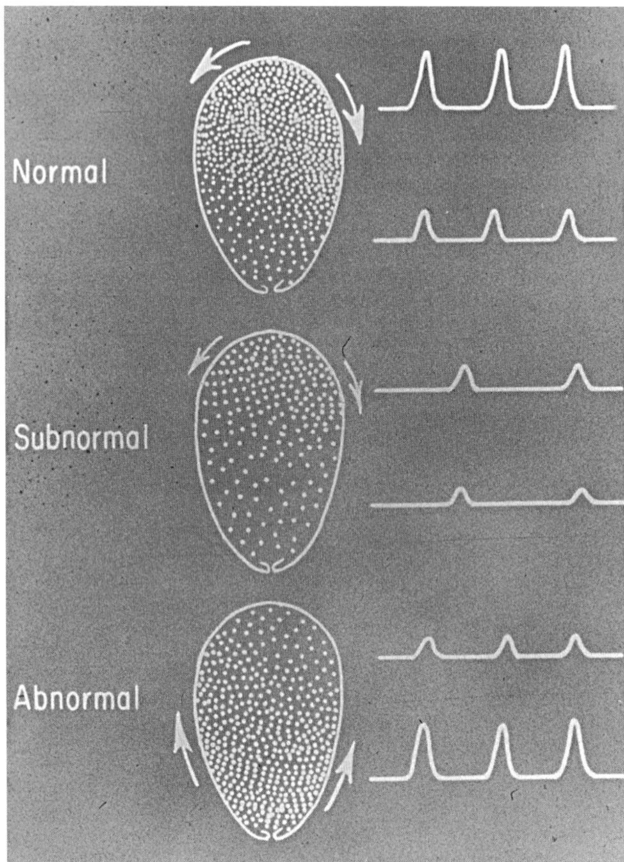


**Fig. 24–4.** A schematic representation of the three types of contractions that may be encountered during labor. Fundal dominance is the most important component in leading to a successful outcome.

The three types of uterine contractions can be identified clinically. During the peak of a normal contraction, the uterus cannot be readily indented upon abdominal palpation. Vaginal examination at the height of a normal contraction shows the cervix to be tightly applied to the presenting part. This indicates fundal dominance, as the cervix and lower uterine segment are being retracted cephalad. During subnormal contractions, on the other hand, the uterus is readily indentible abdominally, and on vaginal examination the cervix is not as firmly applied to the presenting part as in a normal contraction. Abnormal contractions may or may not be indentible abdominally; frequently they are. However, on vaginal examination during the peak of the contraction, the cervix hangs loose and the examining fingers can readily be inserted between the cervix and the presenting part.

## *The Phases and Stages of Labor*

Labor is divided into three stages. The first stage begins with the onset of regular painful uterine contractions and ends when the cervix is completely dilated and retracted. The first stage of labor can be subdivided into two major phases, the latent phase and the active phase (Figure 24–5) (62). The latent phase begins with the onset of labor and ends when the cervix begins to dilate progressively at approximately 4-cm dilatation. This phase is characterized mostly by effacement and softening of the cervix. In primigravida, the duration of the latent phase should not exceed 10 hours, while in multigravida it should not exceed 6 hours. The active phase of the first stage of labor begins when the cervix starts dilating at a steady state, normally at approximately 4 cm of dilatation, and ends with complete dilatation and retraction of the cervix. In the active phase, cervical dilatation should proceed at a rate of at least 1.5 cm/hour in both primigravida and multigravida (63). In ideal labor, it occurs at a rate in excess of 2 cm/hour (61).

If one can accurately time the onset of labor, the total duration of the first stage of term labor is approximately 12 hours in primigravidae and 7 hours in multigravidae (4). However, it is frequently difficult to pinpoint exactly when labor began, making it impossible to accurately establish the duration. In general, the main determinant of the total duration of labor is the length of the frequently elusive latent phase.

The second stage of labor may also be subdivided into two major phases: a descent phase and a pelvic floor phase (4). The descent phase begins with complete cervical dilatation and retraction, and ends when the presenting part reaches the pelvic floor or + 4 station (approximately 4 cm below the plane of the ischial spines). In both primigravidae and multigravidae, this should be achieved normally with no more than 10 uterine contractions. Frequently, the presenting part is already on the pelvic floor at the time of complete cervical dilatation and retraction. At other times only 3 or 4 contractions are required to achieve it. A low presenting part at the onset of labor or rapid descent early in labor are both favorable signs and

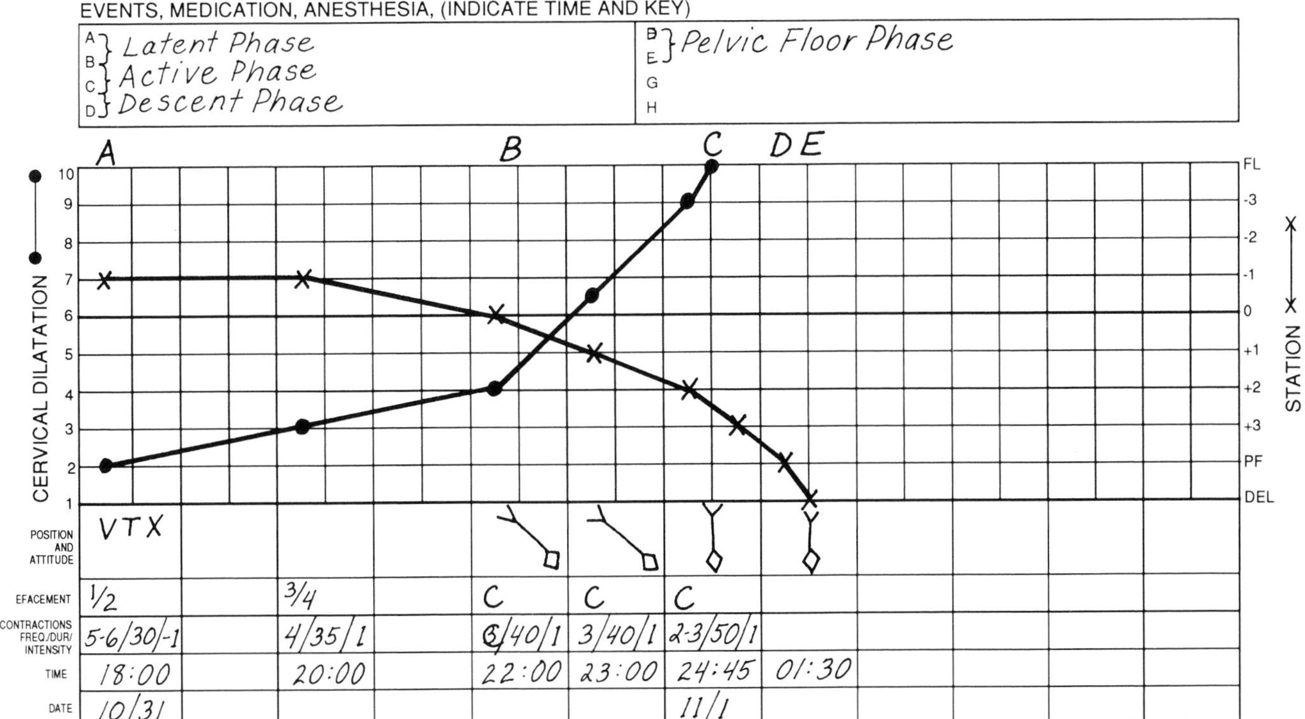


**Fig. 24–5.** Labor flow-sheet showing a normal "ideal" labor curve. Note cervical dilatation in the active phase of the first stage of labor occurs at a rate of 2.5 cm/hour.

frequently signify a short labor. A persistent high station, on the other hand, may indicate impending cephalopelvic disproportion. The pelvic floor phase starts when the presenting part reaches the pelvic floor (between contractions) and ends with the delivery of the fetus. In primigravidae, this phase should be completed in no more than 20 contractions, while in multigravidae no more than 10 contractions should be required. This phase is frequently achieved in 10 contractions or less in primigravidae and in 3 to 4 contractions in the multigravidae with the assistance of normal bearing-down efforts. Figure 24–6 shows the labor chart of cervical dilatation and descent of the presenting part in a normal primigravida labor.

The third stage of labor begins with the delivery of the fetus and ends with the delivery of the placenta. Placental separation invariably occurs with the first 1 or 2 uterine contractions following delivery. This stage of labor should usually be completed within 4 to 6 minutes, rarely longer than 10 minutes. Active management of this stage minimizes postpartum blood loss.

## *The Forces of Labor*

In the first stage of normal labor as mentioned earlier, two major forces are involved: uterine contractions; and resistance of the cervix (Figure 24–7) (1,19,26). In the second stage of labor, three major forces are normally evident: uterine contractions, maternal bearing down, and resistance of the bony pelvis. Maternal bearing-down efforts are vital and constitute approximately 50% of the expulsive forces.

Normally, primigravidae will have an engaged presenting part at the onset of labor. In vertex presentation, the presenting part is at the level of the plane of the ischial spines (0 station), and the biparietal diameter has negotiated the inlet of the pelvis (Figure 24–8). In multigravidae, this occurs less commonly and the vertex may remain unengaged (at a − station) during early labor. As labor progresses, the presenting part normally descends into the pelvis. The type of pelvis frequently determines the position of the vertex during descent. The position of the vertex of the fetus refers to the relationship of the fetal occiput to the mother's side. If the sagittal suture is directly transverse, and the fetal occiput on the maternal right side, the position is occiput right transverse (OLT). If, on the other hand, the occiput is to the right and anterior, and the sagittal suture oblique, the position of the vertex is occiput right anterior (ORA) (Figure 24–9).

With a normal gynecoid pelvis, descent occurs in the transverse position or the largest diameter of the pelvis. However, in women with an anthropoid pelvis, (a long anterior-posterior diameter) descent of the vertex occurs either in the occiput anterior (OA) or occiput posterior (OP) position, again oriented to the largest pelvic diameter (Figure 24–10). As the head descends, it normally flexes and rotates when it encounters the resistance of the soft tissues of the pelvis, and normally the vertex appears on the pelvic floor in the occiput anterior position. In patients receiving conduction anesthesia, the soft tissues of the pelvic diaphragm are relaxed so that normal rotation may either be delayed or does not take place, resulting in a higher incidence of abnormal positions, i.e.,

EVENTS, MEDICATION, ANESTHESIA (INDICATE TIME & KEY)

| | | |
|---|---|---|
| A External monitor, IV started | E Internal monitor | I |
| B PGE2 0.5 mg. p.o. | F Caudal injected | J |
| C PGE2 1.0 mg. p.o. | G | K |
| D AROM – clear fluid | H | L |

A B C C DE B F B

CERVICAL DILATATION 10 9 8 7 6 5 4 3 2 1

STATION FL −3 −2 −1 0 +1 +2 +3 PF DEL

POSITION & ATTITUDE Vtx

*INITIALS OF EXAMINER

EFFACEMENT 3/4 C

CONTRACTIONS FREQ./DUR./INTENSITY ō irreg. 3-4/40/-1 2-3/50/1 2-4/45/1

BP

PULSE

DTR'S

TEMP

FHR

OUTPUT

OXYTOCIN MU/MIN

*NURSE'S INITIALS

TIME (HRS.)

DATE

HR ½ HR ½ HR ½ HR ½ HR ½ HR ½ HR ½ HR ½ HR ½ HR ½ HR ½ HR ½

*RECORD SIGNATURE ON BACK

UNIVERSITY OF WASHINGTON HOSPITALS
HARBORVIEW MEDICAL CENTER
UNIVERSITY HOSPITAL
SEATTLE, WASHINGTON

LABOR FLOW SHEET
UH 0458 REV APR 77

ELECTIVE $PGE_2$ INDUCTION

NORMAL LABOR CURVE

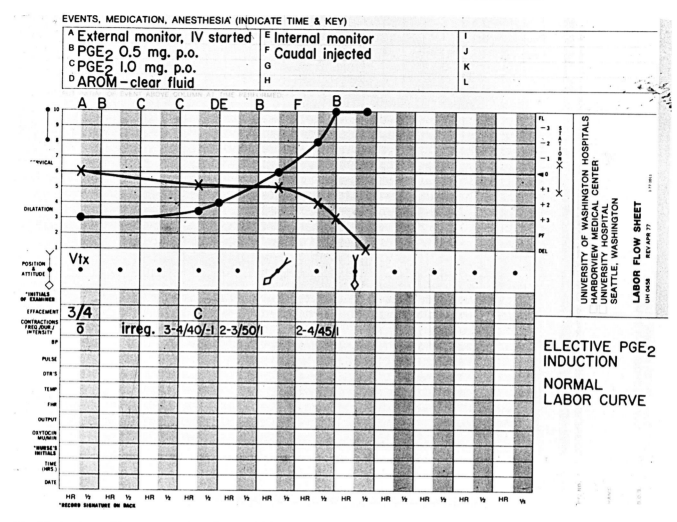

**Fig. 24–6.** A graphic representation of normal labor. Note that the curve of cervical dilatation and descent normally intersect between 5 to 7 cm dilatation.

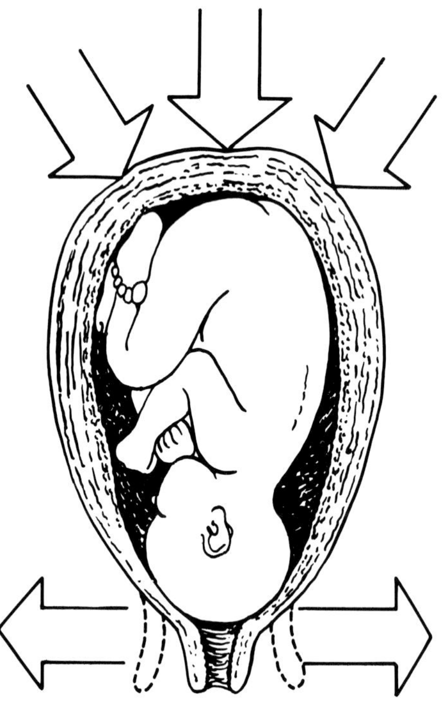

**Fig. 24–7.** The two major forces of the first stage of labor are depicted schematically: uterine contractions and cervix resistance.

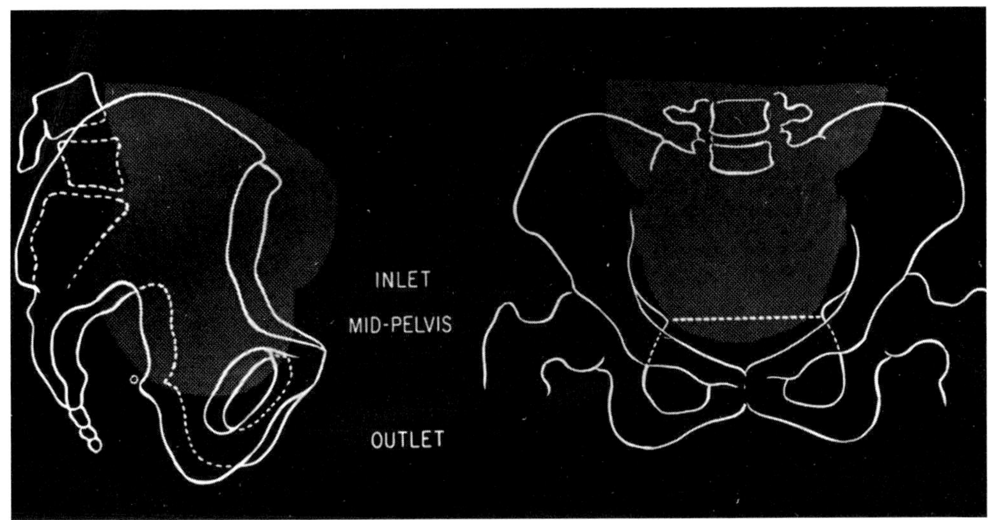


**Fig. 24–8.** Zero station signifies engagement of the fetal vertex, indicating that the biparietal diameter (the largest diameter of the fetal head) has negotiated the pelvic inlet.

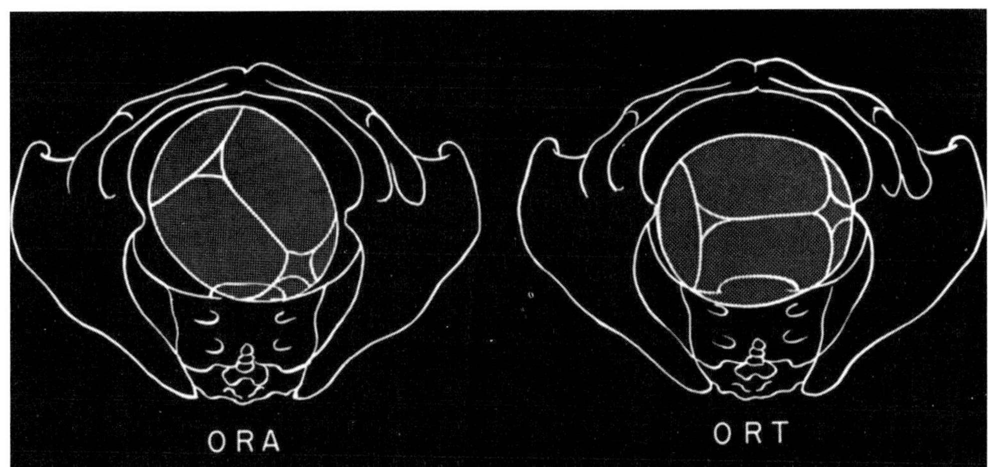


**Fig. 24–9.** A schematic representation of the position of the fetal vertex. ORA is occiput right anterior, ORT is occiput right transverse. Both signify the relationship of the fetal occiput to the maternal pelvis.

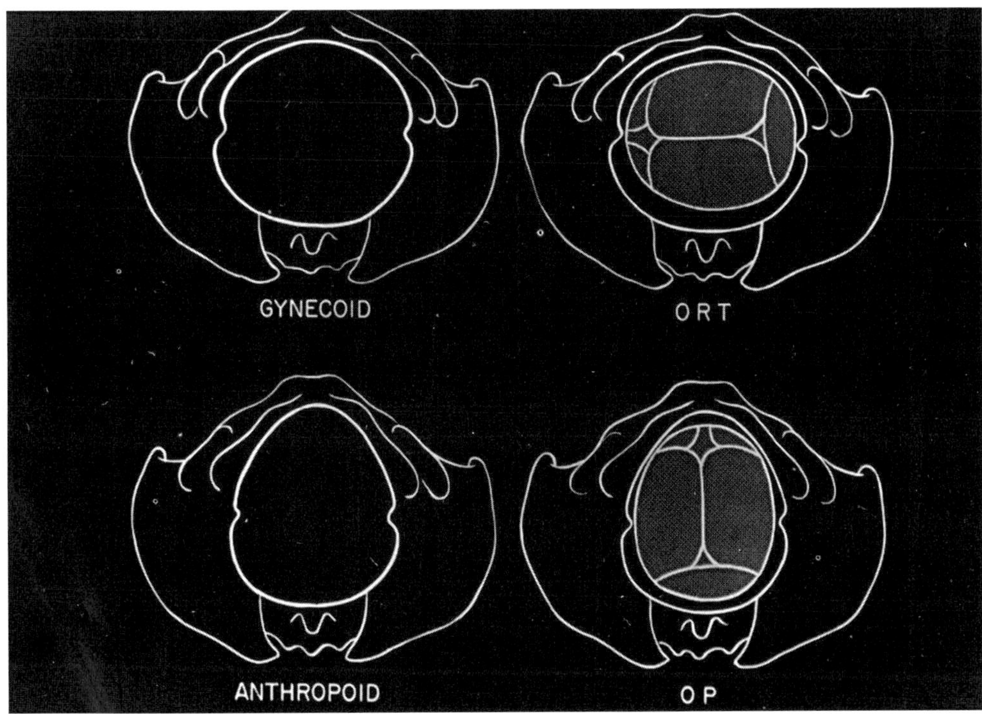


**Fig. 24–10.** As the occiput descends in the maternal pelvis, it accommodates to the largest diameter. In a normal gynecoid pelvis, the occiput descends in a transverse position, while in an anthropoid pelvis, it will be directly occiput posterior (OP) or occiput anterior (OA).

**Table 24–7.** Useful Concepts Regarding Labor

1. The mean duration of normal labor is 14 hours for nulliparae and 8 hours for multiparae.
2. The latent phase of the first stage of labor is the main determinant of the length of labor.
3. The mean rate of cervical dilatation in the active phase of the first stage of ideal labor is 2.5 cm/hour regardless of parity.
4. The forces of labor in the first stage are uterine contractions and the resistance of the cervix.
5. The forces of labor in the second stage are uterine contractions, maternal bearing-down efforts, and the resistance of the pelvis.
6. There are three types of uterine contractions: normal, subnormal, and abnormal.
7. Normal contractions during labor vary as to intensity, duration, and frequency.
8. Every patient has her own unique labor pattern.
9. Always equate uterine activity with progress in labor.
10. The most clinically useful information is obtained by a vaginal examination performed at the peak of a contraction.

occiput posterior or occiput transverse. If there are concomitant subnormal contractions, this can be corrected readily by the judicious use of intravenous oxytocin to augment the contractions.

The mean duration of labor for primigravidae is 14 hours, eight for multigravidae. Alterations or abnormalities in any of the following, power, i.e., uterine contractions, maternal bearing down; passage, i.e., cervix, bony pelvis; or (3) passenger, i.e., fetus (size or position), may prolong labor at any stage and produce major deviations from the expected normal. Understanding the normal physiology of labor enables one to identify the underlying cause, or causes, of significant abnormalities and direct appropriate therapy to correct the problem. This subject will be covered below.

Table 24–7 lists 10 basic concepts pertaining to labor for use as a guide toward a better understanding of the entire process.

## ABNORMAL LABOR PATTERNS

### *Precipitate Labor*

This is the term used for any spontaneous labor that results in delivery in less than 3 hours duration. Frequently, these short labors result in the spontaneous delivery of a healthy newborn from a thankful mother. However, if accompanied by significant increased uterine activity, including sustained hypertonus, fetal hypoxia can occur as can fetal and maternal injury from a rapid and unattended delivery. Hypertonic uterine activity may be controlled to some extent with systemically administered tocolytics. However, events occur so rapidly that there is frequently no time for any form of therapy. This is a relatively rare aberration of labor.

### *First Stage of Labor*

#### *Prolonged Latent Phase (Primary uterine inertia, primary uterine dysfunction).*

The great majority of aberrations of labor are due to prolonged or dysfunctional labor (5). Prolongation of the latent phase of the first stage of labor is considered if it lasts beyond 10 to 12 hours in primigravidae and 6 to 8 hours in multigravidae (Figure 24–11). Possible primary causes include false labor (recognized in retrospect), inability to accurately discern the onset of labor, uterine dysfunction (abnormal uterine contractions), and an unfavorable (unprimed), cervix at the onset of labor.

Secondary causes such as repeated sedation, fatigue, and prematurely administered anesthesia should all be infrequent events in today's obstetric practice.

Therapy, of course, should be directed at the underlying cause. Methods of cervical priming have been discussed previously in detail. This provides us with a therapeutic means to reduce the resistance of a firm, unprimed cervix. The one-time administration of intravenous analgesia (i.e., 10 mg morphine sulfate) may be useful. In some cases, this will allow a patient to rest, while in others provide comfort during early labor with an unfavorable cervix or possibly convert abnormal uterine contractions to subnormal which can, in turn, be successfully augmented with intravenous oxytocin. If contractions cease with this approach, a retrospective diagnosis of false labor can certainly be entertained. Expectant management is frequently indicated. In the vast majority of patients with prolonged latent phase, a normal active phase is achieved and the overall incidence of cesarean section is not significantly increased.

#### *Protracted Active Phase (Primary dysfunctional labor)*

In the active phase of the first stage of labor, if cervical dilatation does not progress at greater than 1.5 cm/hour in both primigravida and multiparous patients, protraction is diagnosed. Figure 24–12 depicts a protracted active phase in a patient with a malposition (OP) relative cephalopelvic disproportion (CPD). This is subsequently overcome by spontaneous rotation of the vertex due to amniotomy and improved uterine contractions. Relative cephalopelvic disproportion is the most common primary cause of this labor abnormality, be it positional, as in the case depicted, or due to a large fetus or borderline pelvis. Abnormal uterine activity such as subnormal contractions or abnormal contractions can also be etiologic factors. The most common secondary cause is conduction anesthesia or excessive sedation, which can be overcome readily with discreet intravenous oxytocin administration to augment subnormal contractions. With this aberration of labor, careful clinical evaluation of the configuration and size of the maternal pelvis is imperative. In addition, a careful determination of fetal position is important, along with a gross estimation of fetal size. Clinical evaluation of uterine contractions should also be undertaken to detect abnormal or subnormal uterine activity. Under rare circumstances, CT pelvimetry might be considered in questionable cases.

Management again depends on identifying the etiology of the problem. If amniotomy can be performed safely (i.e., vertex engaged or tightly applied to the cervix and lower uterine segment), one might improve uterine contractions. Additionally, it would allow for the insertion

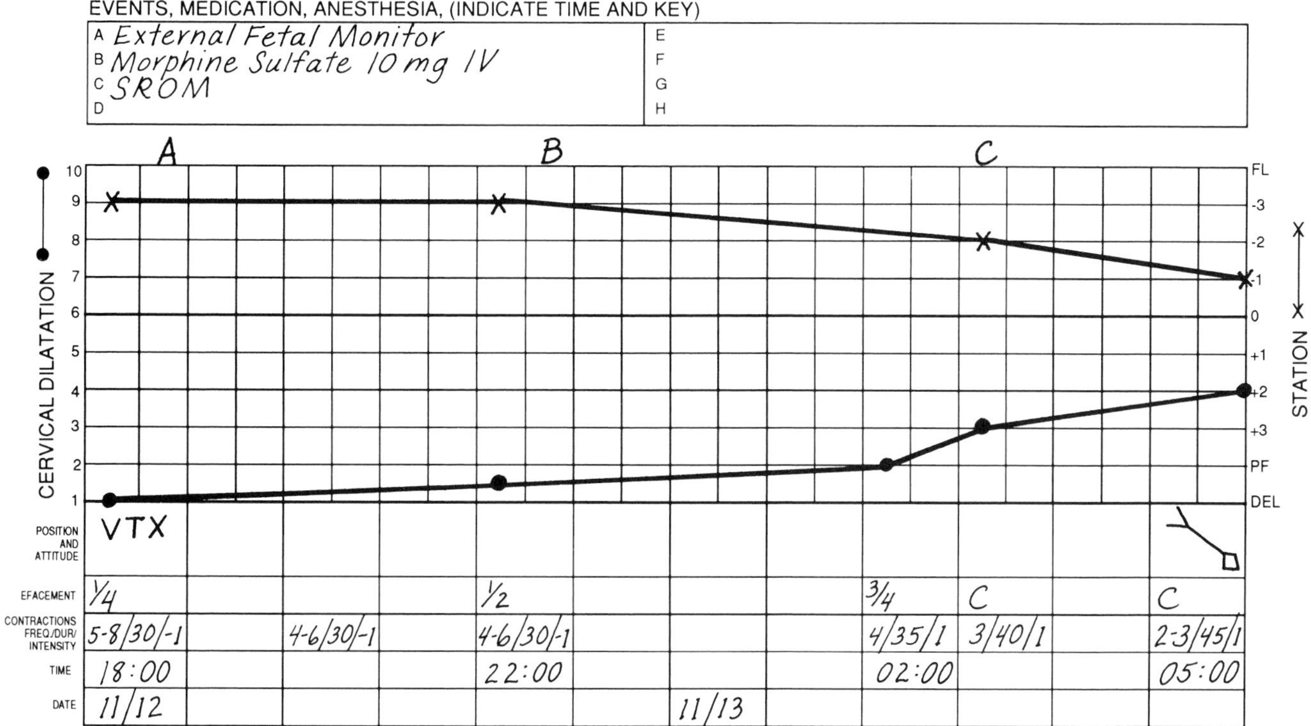


**Fig. 24–11.** Labor flow-sheet depicting a prolonged latent phase in a patient who enters labor with a high presenting part, unfavorable cervix, and mild irregular contractions.

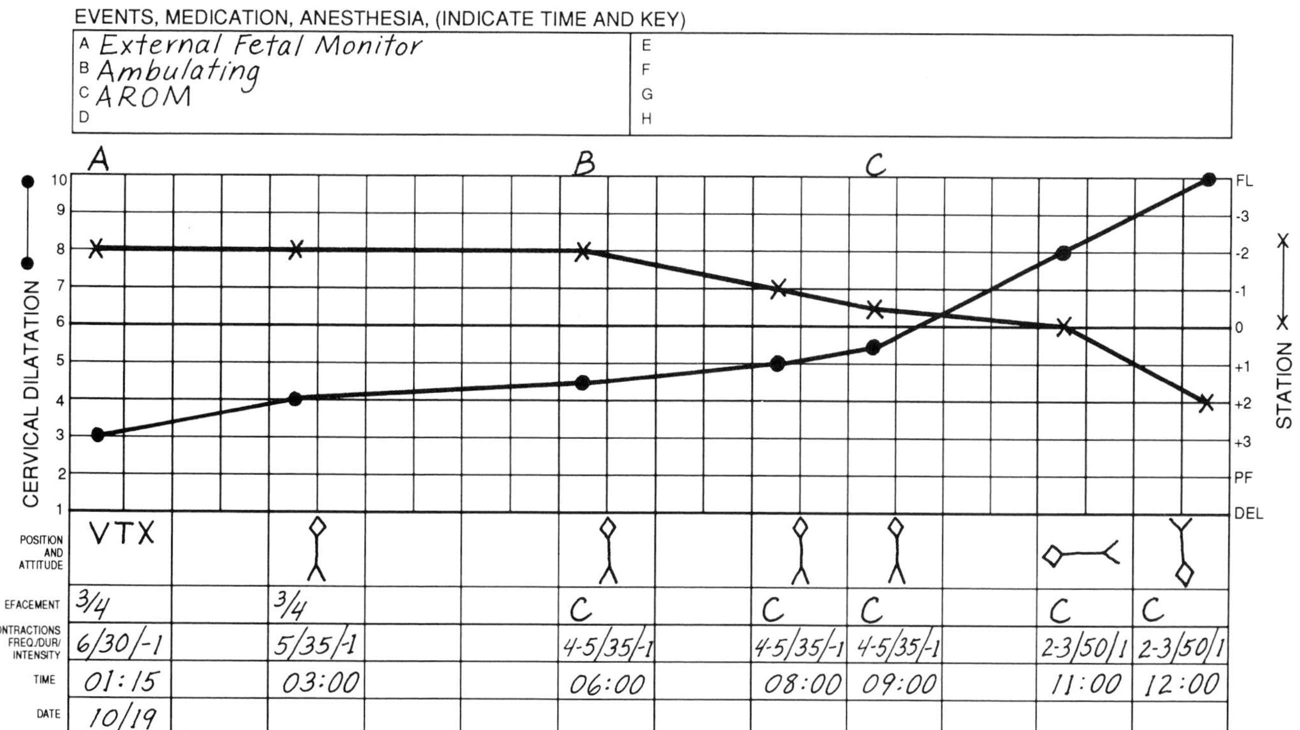


**Fig. 24–12.** Labor flow-sheet depicting protracted active phase of the first stage of labor. Note the deflexed occiput posterior (OP) position of the fetus with subsequent spontaneous rotation resulting from amniotomy and improved uterine function.

of an intrauterine catheter to better evaluate objectively uterine activity. If there is no concrete evidence of cephalopelvic disproportion and subnormal uterine contractions are present, intravenous oxytocin augmentation is appropriate. Similarly, if there is malposition cephalopelvic disproportion, improved uterine activity with cautious use of oxytocin can frequently overcome this relative problem. If we are dealing with abnormal uterine contractions, the use of segmental epidural anesthesia can at times convert these to subnormal contractions which will, in turn, respond to oxytocin augmentation. Figure 24–13 depicts a patient having abnormal uterine contractions who was incorrectly augmented with intravenous oxytocin causing hypertonic abnormal uterine activity (Figure 24–14). The oxytocin was discontinued and the patient was given an epidural anesthetic that converted the abnormal contractions to subnormal (Figure 24–15), which were in turn successfully augmented with oxytocin to effect normal labor and vaginal delivery (Figure 24–16). If this approach is utilized, one must carefully rule out evidence of any significant fetal-maternal disproportion that would obviously preclude a successful outcome.

When protracted active phase is superimposed on a prolonged latent phase of labor, one should suspect the presence of cervical dystocia. A stiff, noncompliant cervix can be detected clinically, and if associated with abnormal uterine activity, can lead to cervical edema and the potential for laceration later in labor. This is especially true if one attempts oxytocin augmentation. Under these circumstances, surgical delivery seems indicated.

If there is firm clinical evidence of cephalopelvic disproportion, cesarean section should be performed. However, most causes of isolated protraction are identifiable and clinically treatable, and the overall cesarean section rate is not significantly increased in these group of patients.

### Secondary Arrest of Dilatation

This abnormality is confined to the active phase of the first stage of labor. It is defined as no detectable cervical dilatation for 2 hours or more. It is most commonly encountered in patients between 6 to 8 cm of cervical dilatation. The overwhelming primary cause is cephalopelvic disproportion. As an isolated pattern, it results in the highest cesarean section rate. Figure 24–17 depicts the cervical dilatation and descent patterns characteristic of cephalopelvic disproportion. Of importance is failure of descent combined with arrest of dilatation in spite of normal uterine activity.

Clinical evaluation is similar to that for protraction disorders. Cephalopelvic disproportion must be ruled out clinically and, on occasion, CT pelvimetry may be useful. If present, cesarean section is indicated. If, on the other hand, the secondary arrest of dilatation appears to be related to conduction anesthesia or possibly to sedation, and subnormal contractions are present, oxytocin augmentation is indicated. Amniotomy with or without oxytocin augmentation could be an alternative approach, as this will also allow for the insertion of an intrauterine catheter to better monitor uterine activity. Figure 24–18 represents secondary arrest of dilatation related to subnormal contractions. Oxytocin augmentation promptly corrects the arrest abnormality.

If cephalopelvic disproportion is suspected but clinically not clearly evident, amniotomy, insertion of an intrauterine catheter, and careful oxytocin augmentation seems appropriate. Minor degrees of cephalopelvic dis-

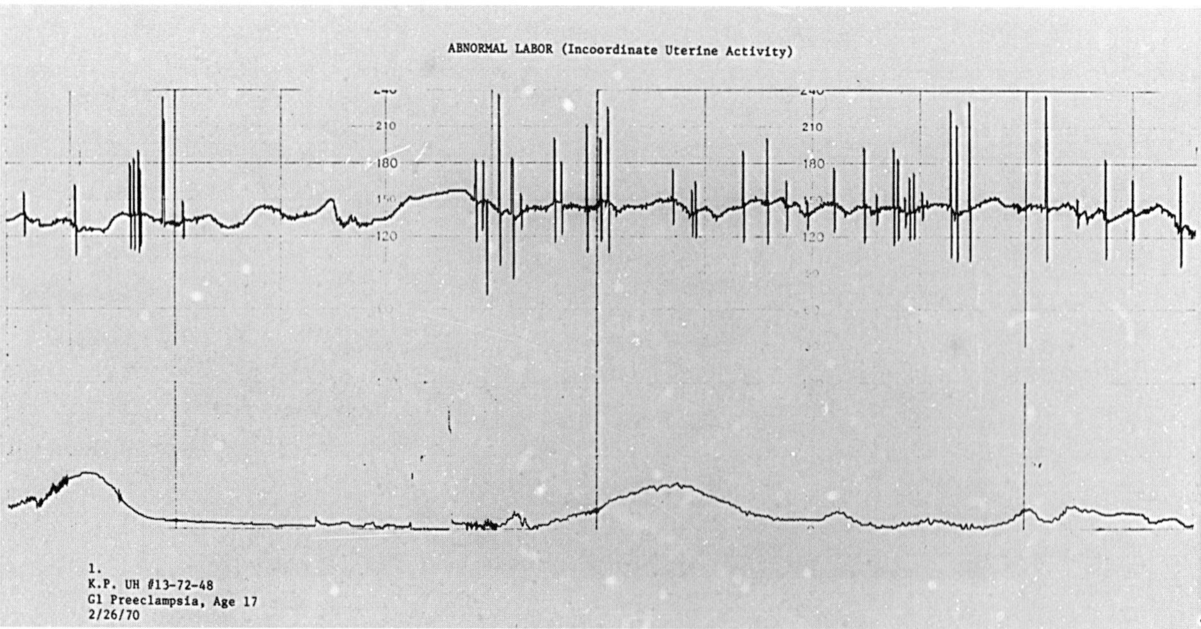


**Fig. 24–13.** Labor flow-sheet showing secondary arrest of dilatation. This pattern of cervical dilatation and descent is characteristic of cephalopelvic disproportion (CPD). [From author]

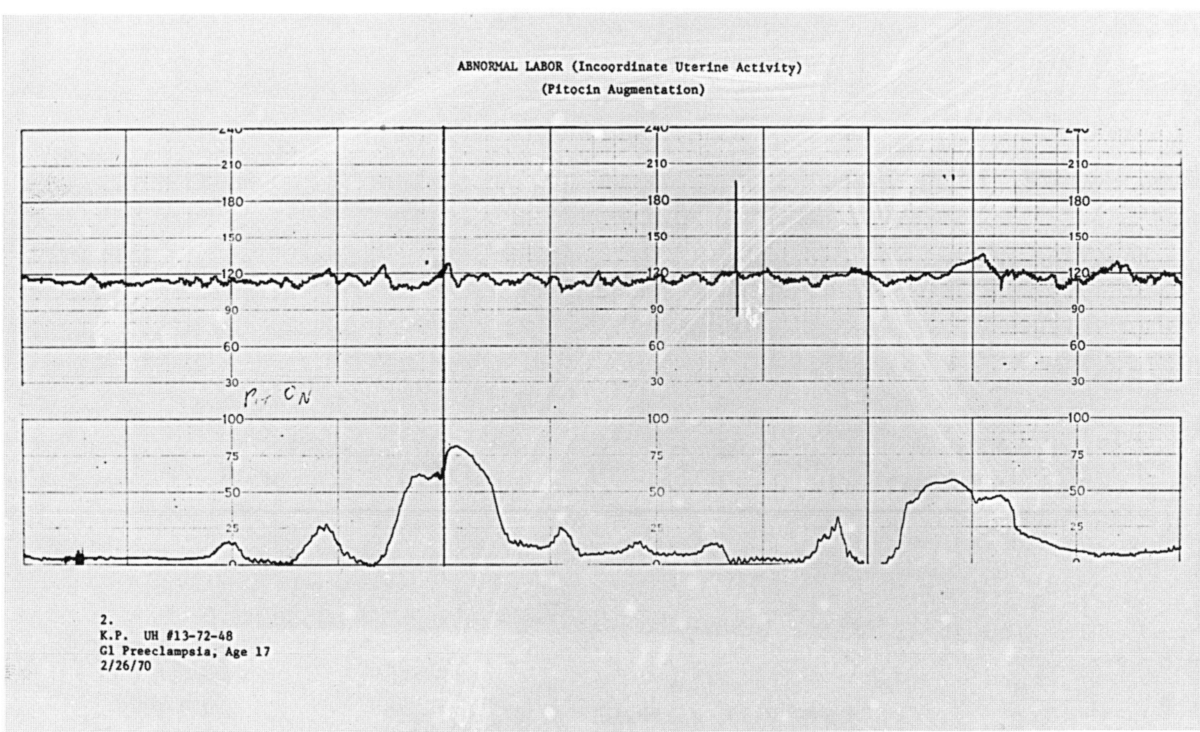


**Fig. 24–14.** Labor flow-sheet showing secondary arrest of dilatation because of subnormal contractions resulting from administration of an epidural. Prompt response to oxytocin augmentation is evident. [From author]

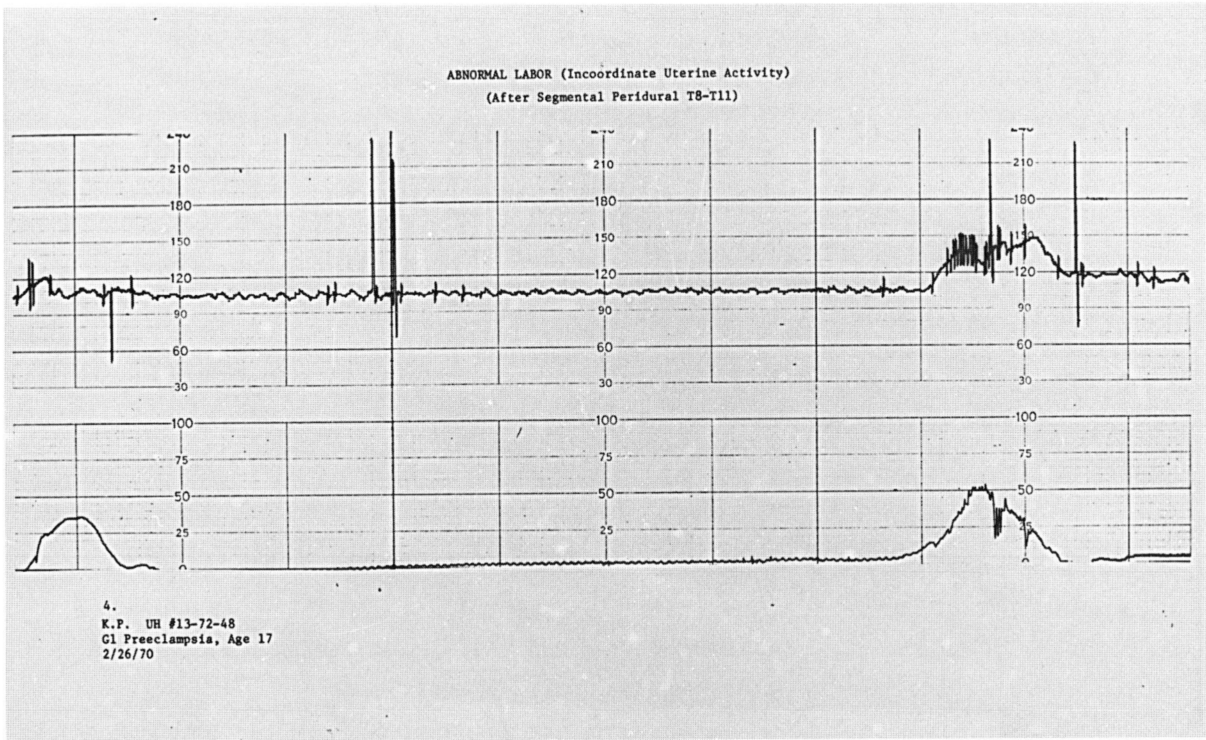


**Fig. 24–15.** Spontaneous abnormal uterine contractions (top) followed by hypertonic abnormal uterine activity due to intravenous oxytocin augmentation (next to top). The oxytocin was discontinued and a segmental epidural administered converting abnormal contractions to subnormal (next to bottom). These contractions subsequently responded to oxytocin augmentation (bottom) resulting in normal labor and vaginal delivery. [From author]

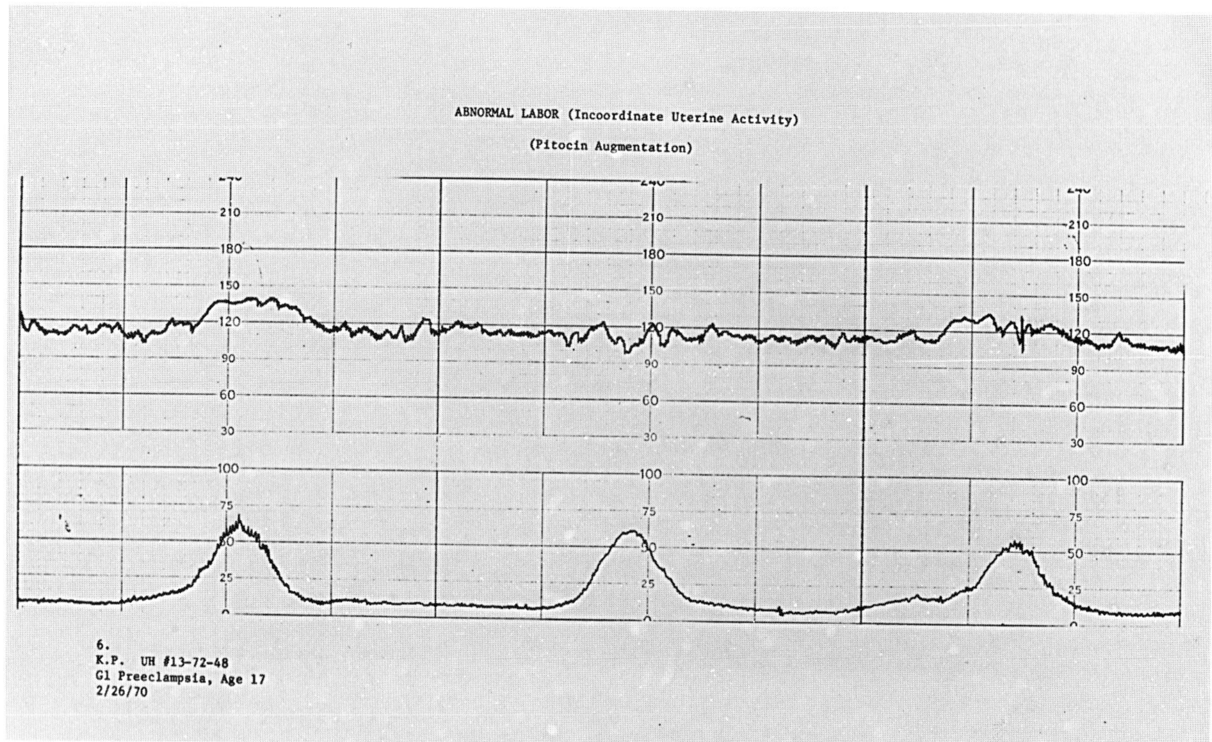


**Fig. 24–16.** Labor flow-sheet showing protracted descent in the second stage of labor due to malposition (OP) of the fetal vertex. Oxytocin augmentation resulted in spontaneous rotation to occiput anterior and spontaneous delivery. [From author]

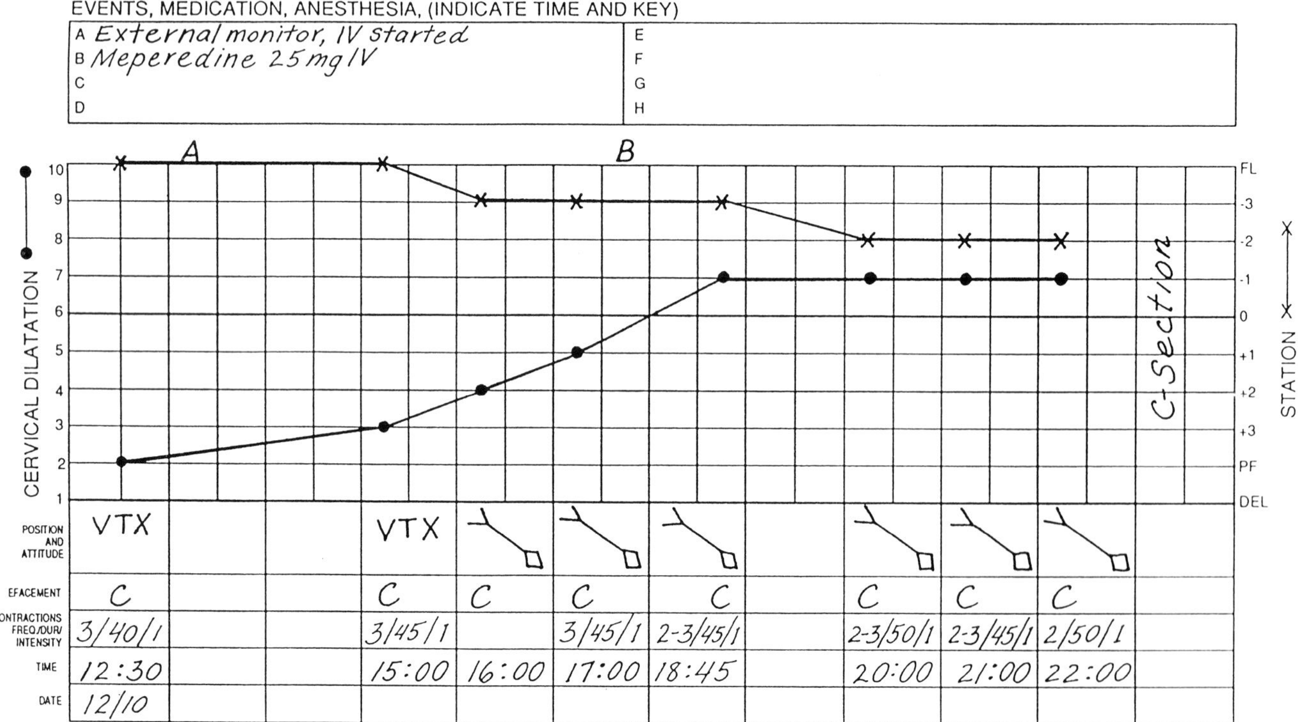


**Fig. 24–17.** Labor curve with cervical dilatation (y-axis) versus time (x-axis). This is a case in which labor analgesia was meperdine 25 mg IV very early in labor. Note the onset of dilatation at 6 cm.

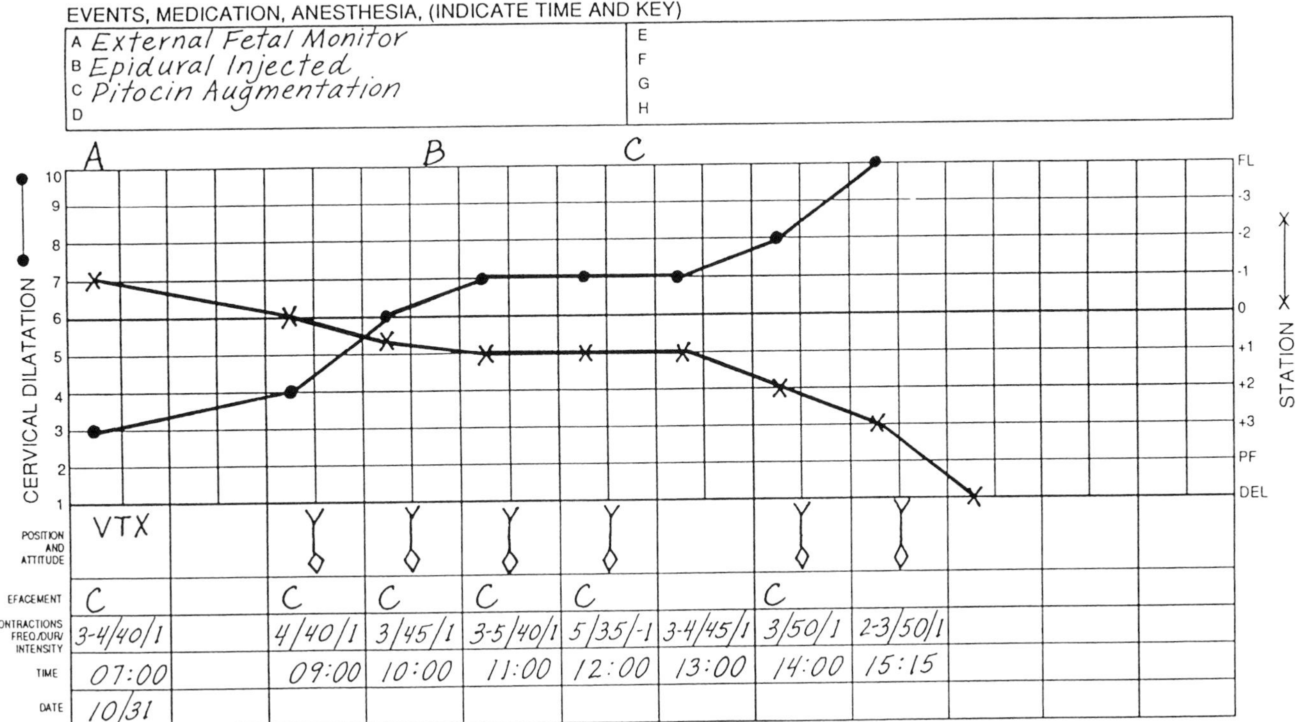


**Fig. 24–18.** Labor curve with cervical dilatation (y-axis) versus time (x-axis). This is a case of secondary onset of dilatation due to inadequate contractions. Note the continued dilatation after 13:00 hours.

proportion can be overcome with improved uterine function, especially if it relates to fetal malposition.

If secondary arrest of dilatation is superimposed on a protracted active phase and the etiology is not readily apparent (i.e., subnormal contractions due to conduction anesthesia or analgesia) serious cephalopelvic disproportion must be entertained and immediately ruled out. The vast majority of these labors result in a cesarean section delivery.

## *Second Stage of Labor*

There are two major phase abnormalities of the second stage of labor, and the following discussion is aimed at early delineation of problems and more prompt therapy to correct them. The important forces to consider now are the expulsive forces of uterine contractions and maternal bearing down and the resistance of the pelvis and, terminally, the maternal soft tissues.

### *Protracted Descent Phase (or Arrest of Descent).*

The failure of descent to the pelvic floor within 10 contractions after entering the second stage of labor in all patients (nulliparous and multiparous) is defined as protracted descent. Frequently, abnormalities in the second stage are preceded by abnormal dilatation patterns in the active phase of the first stage of labor. Figure 24–19 depicts protracted descent in the second stage of labor, likely due to malposition (OP).

Clinical evaluation not only includes clinical pelvimetry, determining fetal position and the presence or absence of molding, and the quality of uterine contractions, but also the effectiveness of maternal bearing-down efforts. Because 50% of expulsive forces in the second stage of labor are attributed to maternal pushing, it deserves careful evaluation. When the vertex is engaged, a contraction with maternal bearing down should normally cause the vertex to descend one station. This is a good clinical indicator of an adequate maternal pelvis. If this does not occur and careful clinical pelvimetry has been carried out, one must then evaluate uterine contractions and the efficacy of the maternal bearing-down efforts. Because abnormal contractions are relatively infrequent in the second stage of labor, the patient could be experiencing subnormal uterine activity. This can be detected clinically and corrected with oxytocin augmentation. If maternal bearing-down efforts are not appropriately directed, this could be the main problem. Generating high intra-abdominal (intrauterine) pressure and protruding the abdomen are not necessarily related to effective well-oriented pushing. On occasion, heavy sedation and anesthesia can interfere with adequate pushing. At other times, pain with the descent of the presenting part deeper into the pelvis will cause poor bearing-down efforts.

The most common cause of delay in descent is ineffectiveness in one or both of the expulsive forces. Another cause may be minor cephalopelvic disproportion, frequently positional. The most serious is cephalopelvic disproportion, which is invariably heralded by abnormal cervical dilatation patterns in the active phase of the first stage of labor. Cesarean section is the treatment of choice if it exists.

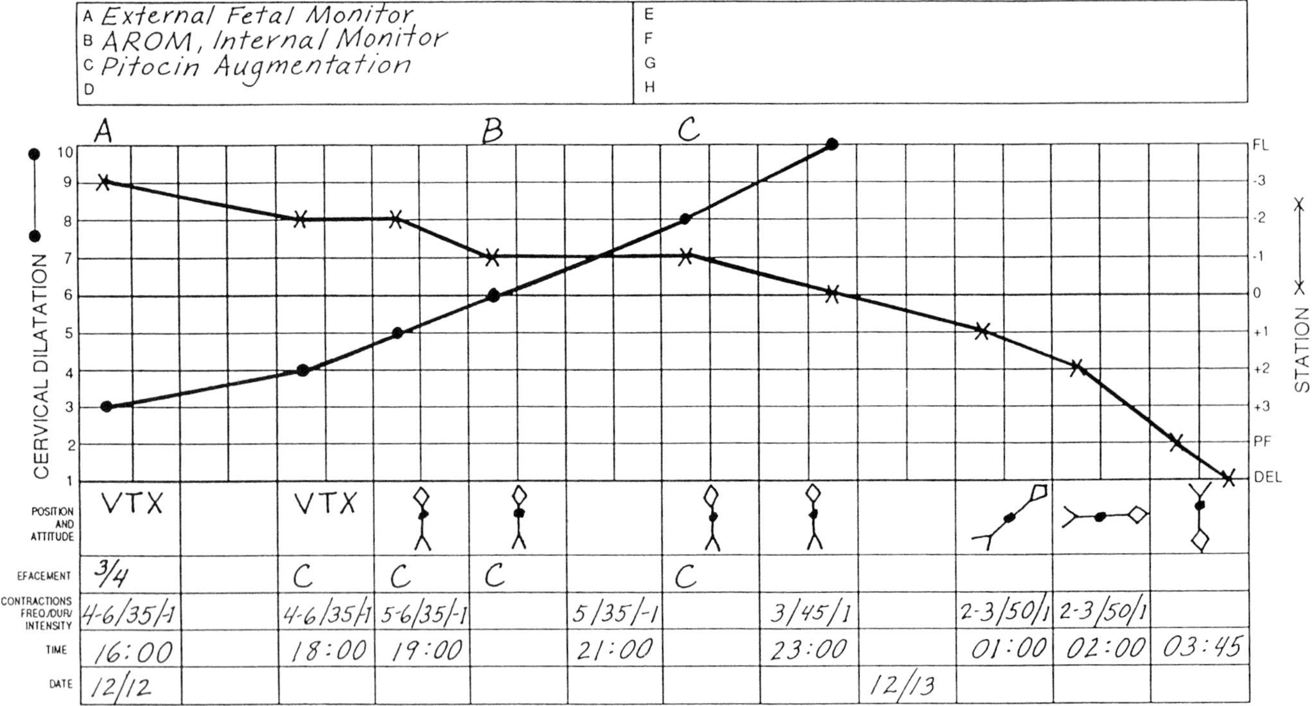


**Fig. 24–19.** Labor curve with cervical dilatation (y-axis) versus time (x-axis). This case illustrates a protraction of descent of fetus even though cervical dilatation is within normal range. This particular case was found to be a persistent OP.

### *Prolonged Pelvic Floor Phase*

Delay in this phase of late labor is invariably related to the ineffectiveness of expulsive forces. Subnormal contractions late in labor must be corrected to prepare the uterus for the third stage of labor and the prompt separation and expulsion of the placenta. Normal uterine activity in late labor will minimize blood loss during placental separation and the immediate puerperium by effectively clamping down the uterus and the major blood vessels traversing the myometrium. Ineffective bearing-down efforts may be overcome by proper coaching or with the use of low or outlet forceps. On occasion, a well-timed episiotomy may help shorten the pelvic floor phase at a time when the only resistance is the maternal soft tissues of the vulva and perineum.

Table 24–8 lists the causes, both primary and secondary, of the various abnormal labor patterns most commonly encountered, discussed in detail in the preceding pages.

## *Anesthetic Management*

Here in the anesthetic management of abnormal labor patterns, it is most important for the anesthesiologist to maintain close communication with the obstetrician. It is clear from this section that different cases and issues are involved that result in the use of varied applications of anesthetic agents and techniques.

Often, a clinically abnormal labor pattern can be rectified with the use of a local anesthetic administered via lumbar epidural or caudal epidural technique. Whether

**Table 24–8.** Etiology of Abnormal Labor Patterns

| | | |
|---|---|---|
| **First Stage** | | |
| Prolonged latent phase | | |
| | Primary: | False labor |
| | | Question of onset |
| | | Unfavorable cervix |
| | | Uterine contractions—abnormal, subnormal |
| | Secondary:* | Anesthesia |
| | | Fatigue—dehydration |
| | | Oversedation |
| Protracted active phase | | |
| | Primary: | CPD—relative |
| | | Abnormal pelvis |
| | | Large infant |
| | | Malposition |
| | | Uterine contractions—abnormal, subnormal |
| Secondary arrest of dilatation | | |
| | | Same as protraction disorders above |
| **Second Stage** | | |
| Protracted descent phase | | |
| | Primary: | CPD—usually combined with abnormal active phase |
| | | Malposition |
| | | Poor bearing down |
| | | Uterine contractions—subnormal |
| | Secondary: | Full bladder |
| Prolonged pelvic floor phase | | |
| | Primary: | Same as protracted descent excluding cephalopelvic disproportion |
| | | No episiotomy |

* Secondary causes pertain to all three aberrations of the first stage of labor and protracted descent phase of the second stage.

the reason is sympathetic blockade, which allows diminished sympathetic uterine effects and then development of more coordinated uterine contractions, or altered blood flow to the uterine muscle results in modified, more effective contractions is not completely understood. What is important is that this anesthetic technique be considered in such a circumstance.

During ineffective expulsive efforts by the mother, satisfactory sensory perineal block should be considered because many primaparae experience such intense pain with perineal distension and dilatation that they cannot "bear down" effectively. Initiation of a low caudal or a saddle block as noted in Chapter 13 will provide excellent pain relief and allow the patient to catch her breath and become an active participant in successful completion of the second stage. Many patients have voiced that they could not even consider pushing until they had sensory perineal blockade, and some of these patients were female anesthesiologist colleagues who were quite amazed by the difference in their ability to cooperate before and after regional block.

For the most part, the other abnormal labor pattern should not really be influenced by the present day continuous epidural infusion method as detailed in Chapter 13. This dilute anesthetic solution is very effective at offering pain relief while not suppressing uterine activity or having any fetal effect because of its dilution and low-dose delivery mode.

Naturally, there are other agents and techniques that can be considered for management of these abnormal labor patterns; and these include continuous spinal method, one-shot low epidural, or saddle block type of subarachnoid block, or single shot or continuous low caudal method.

## Vaginal Birth After Cesarean Delivery

Vaginal birth after cesarean delivery has become very popular recently because of its success in the past decade in regard to vaginal birth without associated fetal or maternal morbidity or mortality. Although serious consideration must be given to possible injuries, careful maternal and fetal monitoring will prevent such predicaments. For a more detailed discussion of vaginal birth after cesarean delivery (VBAC), refer to Chapter 4 and current obstetric textbooks, e.g., OBSTETRICS: NORMAL AND PROBLEM DELIVERIES, edited by Gabbe, Niebyl, and Simpson; WILLIAMS OBSTETRICS, edited by Cunningham, MacDonald, and Gant; and Zuspan's and Quilligan's MANUAL OF OBSTETRICS AND GYNECOLOGY.

### *Anesthetic Management*

For some period of time, there has been concern regarding epidurals for vaginal birth after cesarean delivery, as epidurals would inhibit maternal pain associated with uterine rupture. Extensive studies, which corroborate careful attention to maternal and fetal monitoring, prove safety can be possible to both the mother and baby (64).

## REFERENCES


1. Ulmsten U, Ueland K: The forces of labor: uterine contractions and the resistance of the cervix. Clin. Obstet. Gynecol. 26:1, 1983.
2. Liggins GC: Initiation of spontaneous labor. Clin. Obstet. Gynecol. 26:47, 1983.
3. Danforth DN, Ueland K: Physiology of uterine action. *In* Obstetrics and Gynecology. Edited by DN Danforth, JR Scott. Philadelphia, J.B. Lippincott Co, A1989, p. 582.
4. Calkins LA: Normal Labor. Springfield, IL, Charles C. Thomas, 1955.
5. Ueland K, Ueland FR: Dystocia due to abnormal uterine action. *In* Obstetrics and Gynecology. Edited by DN Danforth, JR Scott. Philadelphia, J.B. Lippincott Co., 1989, p. 711.
6. ACOG Technical Bulletin, No. 157, July 1991.
7. Dale HH: On some physiological actions of ergot. J. Physiol. 34:163, 1906.
8. Hofbauer J: Hypophysenextract als Wehenmittel. Abl. Gynaek. 35:137, 1911.
9. Watson BP: Pituitary extract in obstetric practice. Canad. Med. Assn. J. 3:739, 1913.
10. Hamm A: Ueber ein Neues Wehenmittel. Deutsch Med Wsschr 38:487, 1912.
11. Madill DG, Allan RM: The use of pituitary extract in labor. Surg. Gynecol. Obstet. 19:241, 1914.
12. Voigts J: Erfahrunges ueber Pituitrinwirkung in der Klinik und Poliklinik. Deutsch Med Wschr 37:2286, 1911.
13. DeLee JB: Discussion of paper by Kosmak, GW: the use and abuse of pituitary extract. JAMA 71:1119, 1918.
14. Kamm O, Aldrich TB, Grote IW, Row W, Bugbee EP: The active principles of the posterior lobe of the pituitary gland. J. Amer. Chem. Soc. 50:573, 1928.
15. du Vigneaud V, Ressler C, Swan JM, Roberts CW, et al:. Synthesis of octopeptide amide with hormonal activity of oxytocin. J. Amer. Chem. Soc. 75:4878, 1953.
16. Boissonnas RA, et al: Une nouvelle synthase de l'oxytocine. Helv. Chir. Acta. 38:1491, 1955.
17. Bishop EH: Pelvic scoring for elective induction. Obstet. Gynecol. 24:266, 1964.
18. Wingerup L: Ripening of Cervix Uteri Induced by Single Intracervical Application of Prostaglandin $E_2$ in Viscous Gel. Litos Reprotryk, Malmo, 1979, p 20.
19. Ulmsten U, Wingerup L, Beifraye P, Ekman G, Wiquist N: Intracervical application of prostaglandin gel for induction of term labor. Obstet. Gynecol. 59:336, 1982.
20. Ekman G, Forman A, Marsal K, Ulmstein UIF: Intravaginal versus intracervical application of prostaglandin $E_2$ in viscous gel for cervical priming and induction of labor at term in patients with an unfavorable cervical state. Am. J. Obstet. Gynecol. 147:657, 1983.
21. Forman A, Ulmsten U, Banyai J, Wingerup L, Uldbjerg N: Evidence for a local effect of intracervical prostaglandin $E_2$ gel. Am. J. Obstet. Gynecol. 143:756, 1982.
22. Conrad JT, Ueland K: The stretch modulus of human cervical tissue in spontaneous, oxytocin induced, and prostaglandin $E_2$ induced labor. Am. J. Obstet. Gynecol. 133:11, 1979.
23. Conrad JT, Ueland K: Reduction of the stretch modulus of human cervical tissue by the prostaglandin $PGE_2$. Am. J. Obstet. Gynecol. 126:218, 1976.
24. Uldbjerg N, Ekman G, Malmstrom A, et al: A quantitative study of the action of synthetic oxytocin on the pregnant human uterus. J. Pharmacol. Exp. Ther. 121:18, 1957.
25. Ferguson JE II, Ueland FR, Stevenson DK, Ueland K: Oxytocin-induced labor characteristics and uterine activity after preinduction cervical priming with prostaglandin $E_2$ intracervical gel. Obstet. Gynecol. 72:739, 1988.
26. Ulmsten U, Wingerup L, Ekman G: Local application of prostaglandin $E_2$ for cervical ripening or induction of term labor. Clin. Obstet. Gynecol. 26:95, 1983.
27. Calder AA: The management of the unripe cervix. *In* Human Parturition. Edited by MJNC Keirse, ABM Anderson, J Benne-

broek Gravenhorst. Leiden, Leiden University Press, 1979, p. 201.
28. Shepherd JH, Knuppel RA: The role of prostaglandins in ripening the cervix and inducing labor. Clin. Perinatol. 8: 49, 1981.
29. Edwards RL, Nicholson HO: The management of the unstable lie in late pregnancy. J. Obstet. Gynaecol. Br. Commonw. 76:713, 1969.
30. Dyson DC, Ferguson JE, Hensleigh P: Anterpartum external cephalic version under tocolysis. Obstet. Gynecol. 67:63, 1986.
31. Morrison JC, Myatt RE, Martin JN Jr: External cephalic version of the breech presentation under tocolysis. Am. J. Obstet. Gynecol. 154:900, 1986.
32. Turnbull AC: Influencing uterine contractility with oxytocin. *In* Human Parturition. Edited by MJNC Keirse, Martinus Nijhoff Publishers, 1979, p.143.
33. Caldeyro-Barcia R, Sica-Blanco Y, Poseiro JJ, Gonzalez Panizza V, et al: A quantitative study of the action of synthetic oxytocin on the pregnant human uterus. J. Pharmacol. Exp. Ther. 121:18, 1957.
34. Caldeyro-Barcia R, Sereno JA: The response of the human uterus to oxytocin throughout pregnancy. *In* Oxytocin. Edited by R Caldeyro-Barcia, H Heller. New York, Pergamon Press, 1961.
35. Seitchik J: The management of functional dystocia in the first stage of labor. Clin. Obstet. Gynecol. 30:42, 1987.
36. Seitchik J, Amico J, Robinson AG, Castillo M: Oxytocin augmentation of dysfunctional labor. IV. Oxytocin pharmacokinetics. Am. J. Obstet. Gynecol. 150:225, 1984.
37. Thomford PJ, Dziuk PJ: Low dose oxytocin infusion at term alters endogenous oxytocin pulses. Scientific Program and Abstracts, 34th Meeting Soc. Gynec. Invest., Abstract No. 151, p. 102, March 18–21, 1987.
38. Ueland K, Conrad JT: Characteristics of oral prostaglandin $E_2$-induced labor. Clin. Obstet. Gynecol. 26:87, 1983.
39. Roux JF, Mofid M, Moss PL, Dmytrus KC: Effect of elective induction of labor with prostaglandins $F_2$ Alpha and $E_2$ and oxytocin on uterine contractions and relaxation. Am. J. Obstet. Gynecol. 127:718, 1977.
40. Murray CP, Clinch J: Comparative study of labor induced by oral prostaglandin $E_2$ and intravenous oxytocin. J. Irish Med. Assoc. 68:135, 1975.
41. Kelly J, Flynn AM, Bertrand PV: A comparison of oral prostaglandin $E_2$ and intravenous oxytocin in the induction of labour. J. Obstet. Gynaecol. Br. Commonw. 80:923, 1973.
42. ACOG Technical Bulletin, No. 132, September, 1989.
43. Pavlou C, Barker GH, Roberts A, Chamberlain GV: Pulsed oxytocin infusion in the induction of labour. Brit. J. Obstet. Gynaecol. 85:96, 1978.
44. Karim SMM, Sharma SD: Oral administration of prostaglandins for the induction of labour. Br. Med. J. 1:260, 1971.
45. Ueland K: Unpublished material, 1989.
46. Hendricks CH, Brenner WE, Kraus G: Normal cervical dilatation pattern in late pregnancy and labor. Am. J. Obstet. Gynecol. 106:1065, 1970.
47. Murnaghan GA, Lamki H, Rashid S, Pinkerton JHM: Induction of labour with oral prostaglandin $E_2$. J. Obstet. Gynaecol. Br. Commonw. 81:141, 1974.
48. Thiery M, Yo Le Sian A, de Hemptinne D, Derom R, Martens G, Van Kets H, Amy JJ: ). Induction of labour with prostaglandin $E_2$ tablets. J. Obstet. Gynaecol. Br. Commonw. 81:303, 1974.
49. Lauersen NH, Wilson KH: Induction of labor with oral prostaglandin $E_2$. Obstet. Gynecol. 44:793, 1974.
50. Craft I: Oral prostaglandin $E_2$ and amniotomy for induction of labor. Adv. Bio. Sci. 9:593, 1973.
51. Miller JF, Welply GA, Elstein M: Prostaglandin $E_2$ tablets compared with intravenous oxytocin in induction of labour. Br. Med. J. 1:14, 1975.
52. Sellers SM, Hodgson HT, Mitchell MD, Anderson AB, Turnbull AC: Release of prostaglandins after amniotomy is not mediated by oxytocin. Br. J. Obstet. Gynaecol. 87:43, 1980.
53. Mitchell MD, Flint APF, Bibby J, Brunt J, et al: Rapid increases in plasma prostaglandin concentrations after the vaginal examination and amniotomy. Br. Med. J. 2:1183, 1977.
54. Keetel WC: Inducing labor by rupturing membranes. Postgrad. Med. 44:199, 1968.
55. Stewart P, Kennedy JH, Calder AA: Spontaneous labour: when should the membranes be ruptured? Br. J. Obstet. Gynaecol. 89:39, 1982.
56. Cantarow JH: Planned rapid labor: elective induction of labor by intravenous Pitocin following caudal anesthesia. Obstet. Genecol. 4:213, 1954.
57. Nowill WK, Howland RS: Pitocin-caudal anesthesia method of artificial induction of labor. New York J. Med. 58:198, 1958.
58. Stubblefield CT, Harer WB Jr: Elective induction of labor and long-acting caudal analgesia. Obstet. Gynecol. 20:468, 1962.
59. Friedman EA, Sachtleben MR: Caudal anesthesia. The factors that influence its effect on labor. Obstet. Gynecol. 13:442, 1959.
60. Scott DB, Hibbard BM: Serious nonfatal complications associated with extradural block in obstetric practice. Br. J. Anaesth. 64:537, 1990.
61. Ralston DH, Shnider SM: The fetal and neonatal effects of regional anesthesia in obstetrics. Anesthesiology 48:34, 1978.
62. Friedman EA: Primigravida labor: a graphic statistical analysis. Obstet. Gynecol. 6:567, 1955.
63. Hendricks CH, Brenner WE, Kraus G: Normal cervical dilatation pattern in late pregnancy and labor. Am. J. Obstet. Gynecol. 106:1065, 1970.
64. Cunningham FG, MacDonald PC, Gant NF. Cesarean section and cesarean hysterectomy. *In*: Williams Obstetrics. East Norwalk, Appleton & Lange, 1989A p. 446.

# Chapter 25

# PREECLAMPSIA

THOMAS J. BENEDETTI
HEATHCLIFF S. CHADWICK
THOMAS EASTERLING

---

Preeclampsia is a common complication of pregnancy. Six percent of nulliparous women will become preeclamptic; an additional 20% will manifest some degree of hypertension (1). Women with medical complications such as diabetes, chronic hypertension, and renal insufficiency may also become hypertensive. Frequently, these women will become hypertensive earlier in pregnancy and manifest more severe disease. Hypertensive disease is a leading cause of maternal mortality (2), frequently due to intracerebral hemorrhage or cerebral edema (3,4). When hypertension becomes severe prior to term, premature delivery results in significant neonatal morbidity and mortality. Premature infants born to hypertensive women experience more complications than those delivered by normotensive women (5).

Anesthesia services are often required in the management of women with hypertensive disease in pregnancy. Women with severe preeclampsia, in particular, can present the anesthesiologist with a wide range of challenges and potential risks. Among the potential problems are a variable and uncertain degree on intravascular volume depletion increasing the risks of hypotension, coagulopathy with the possibility for neuraxial hematoma formation, and airway edema complicating tracheal intubation. Anesthetic interventions can increase the risks of maternal pulmonary, cardiac, and neurologic complications. To optimize patient care and minimize complications, anesthesiologists must understand the pathophysiology of the disease and actively collaborate in patient care.

This chapter consists of comprehensive discussion of the most important, basic aspects of preeclampsia and its obstetric and anesthesiologic management. The material is presented in three parts: (1) Basic Considerations, including classification, epidemiology or incidence, etiology and pathophysiology, effects on uterine contractility and placenta, and effects on the fetus; (2) Obstetric Management; and (3) Anesthesiologic Management. More detailed information on these various aspects of the subject can be found elsewhere (6–8).

## BASIC CONSIDERATIONS

### Classification of Hypertension

#### *Classification/Definition*

Young women entering their first pregnancy often have surprisingly low blood pressures. The average value of arterial blood pressure in the sitting position at first trimester is about 105 to 110/50 to 55. Blood pressure varies somewhat depending on the gestational age; diastolic blood pressure tends to fall in the second trimester. This observation has resulted in some confusion when attempting to define hypertension in previously normotensive young women. The definitions accepted by the Committee on Terminology of the American College of Obstetricians and Gynecologists in 1952 serve as a framework from which to build one's thinking regarding diagnosis and management in a particular patient.

#### *Hypertension*

Hypertension is defined as either a systolic rise of at least 30 mm Hg or absolute value of 140 mm Hg, or alternatively, a diastolic rise of at least 15 mm Hg or absolute value of 90 mm Hg. The pressure rise must be from a previously established baseline or usual value. The pressures must also be sustained and observed on at least 2 occasions 6 or more hours apart. Korotkoff phase 5 sound should be used for the diagnosis of diastolic hypertension.

#### Gestational Hypertension

Gestational hypertension is a category developed to include women who meet the blood pressure criteria for hypertension but who fail to develop any of the other signs and symptoms of preeclampsia (pathologic edema or proteinuria greater than 300 mg/24 hours). The blood pressure must return to normal within 10 days of delivery. Women within this category have a high rate of recurrence in later pregnancies and are at increased risk to develop chronic hypertension later in life.

#### *Preeclampsia*

Preeclampsia is a disorder peculiar to human pregnancy. The diagnosis is made by the appearance of hypertension after the twentieth week of gestation combined with edema of the hands or face or the occurrence of proteinuria (greater than 300 mg/24 hours). Preeclampsia is further divided into categories of mild and severe.

#### Mild Preeclampsia

Mild preeclampsia is defined by the absence of all of the preceding factors that indicate severe disease.

**Table 25–1.** Signs/Symptoms of Severe Preeclampsia

- Systolic blood pressure of at least 160 mm Hg or diastolic of at least 110 mm Hg on two occasions at least 6 hours apart
- Proteinuria levels of at least 5 grams in a 24-hour urine collection
- Oliguria, less than 400 to 500 ml in a 24-hour urine collection
- Cerebral or visual disturbances
- Pulmonary edema or cyanosis
- Right upper quadrant or epigastric pain
- Impaired liver function
- Thrombocytopenia or coagulopathy

(From the American College of Obstetricians and Gynecologists, Management Of Preeclampsia. ACOG Technical Bulletin No. 91, February, 1986.)

### Severe Preeclampsia

Severe preeclampsia is diagnosed by the presence of one or more of the signs or symptoms indicated in Table 25–1.

### *Eclampsia*

Eclampsia is defined by the presence of convulsions in a woman with preeclampsia when convulsions cannot be definitely ascribed to another cause.

### *Pregnancy-Induced Hypertension (PIH)*

In the late 1970s, the term "pregnancy-induced hypertension" (PIH) became popularized (9,10). Although this term, which includes preeclampsia, eclampsia, and gestational hypertension, may help to simplify the approach to clinical management of these disorders, it may also serve to lump separate disease processes together.

Often the impression is given that only nulliparous patients should be included in the study of pregnancy-induced hypertension (11). However, much of the available data on cardiovascular function does not differentiate between multiparous and nulliparous patients. As a consequence, there is no alternative but to generalize from data that are known to include some patients whose hypertensive pathophysiology may be different from that associated with preeclampsia.

### *Chronic Hypertension*

Chronic hypertension is diagnosed when there is persistence of blood pressures in excess of 140/90 before and after pregnancy. The finding of pressures exceeding this level during the first 20 weeks of pregnancy is also diagnosed as chronic hypertension.

### *Epidemiology*

Preeclampsia is the major category of hypertensive diseases of pregnancy in terms of maternal and fetal morbidity and mortality. Toxemic diseases are the second leading cause of maternal mortality in the United States, accounting for 5 to 12% of all maternal deaths (12). As pointed out in the first edition, the incidence of toxemia or preeclampsia varies with the race, age, parity, and socioeconomic status of the patient. In private obstetric practice in the 1970s, it occurred in approximately 1 to 1.5% of gravidae, while in charity clinics the incidence was approximately 5 to 10% (13,14). Over 75% occurred in primigravidae, 80 to 90% occurred in patients under 30 years of age, and 90 to 95% occurred after 30 weeks of pregnancy (13–17). The incidence was several times higher in multiple pregnancy, 3 to 4 times higher should there have been hydatidiform mole, and considerably increased in gravidae with hydramnios or diabetes (13,14).

In 1989, the maternal mortality ratio (number of maternal deaths/number of live births) for toxemic pregnancy was 1.4/100,000. The majority of deaths from hypertension are the result of intracranial hemorrhage. This cause is underreported in the vital statistics (Figure 25–1) (18), and it is likely that some of the maternal mortalities reported under the category "stroke" are misclassified hypertensive disorders of pregnancy. In addition, the numbers of patients in the categories "anesthesia" and "hemorrhage" are probably augmented by the inclusion of critically ill patients with hypertensive diseases of pregnancy. In a recent critical review of maternal mortalities, 48% of deaths had multiple causes of death (18). It is hoped that an understanding of this complex clinical condition will lead to further reductions in maternal and fetal mortality.

## Etiology and Pathophysiology

### *Etiology*

The etiology and pathophysiology of preeclampsia are poorly understood. Early in pregnancy, before the onset of hypertension, women destined to become preeclamptic have been demonstrated to have higher blood pressures (19,20), increased sensitivity to angiotension II (21), increased metabolic clearance of dehydroisoepiandrosterone (22), and increased levels of plasma fibronectin (23). Although the clinical presentation of preeclampsia is often abrupt, these studies indicate that the underlying disease process is chronic with observable pathophysiologic changes in the first and second trimesters.

Endothelial injury has been hypothesized to mediate the observed multi-system dysfunction (24). A reduction in plasma prostacyclin/thromboxane ratio is present in the acute phase of preeclampsia and has also been postulated to mediate the disease process (25). However, reduced prostacyclin production has been reported to occur only as the clinical manifestations of the disease become evident (26).

Early treatment of hypertension with a B-blocker (27) and prophylaxis with aspirin (28,29) have each been demonstrated to decrease the incidence of proteinuric preeclampsia in selected patients at high risk of developing preeclampsia. Neither has been demonstrated to improve the perinatal mortality. The possible causes of preeclampsia are summarized in (Figure 25–2).

### *Maternal Effects*

Preeclampsia is a multi-system disease. Although its hallmarks are hypertension and proteinuria, patients may

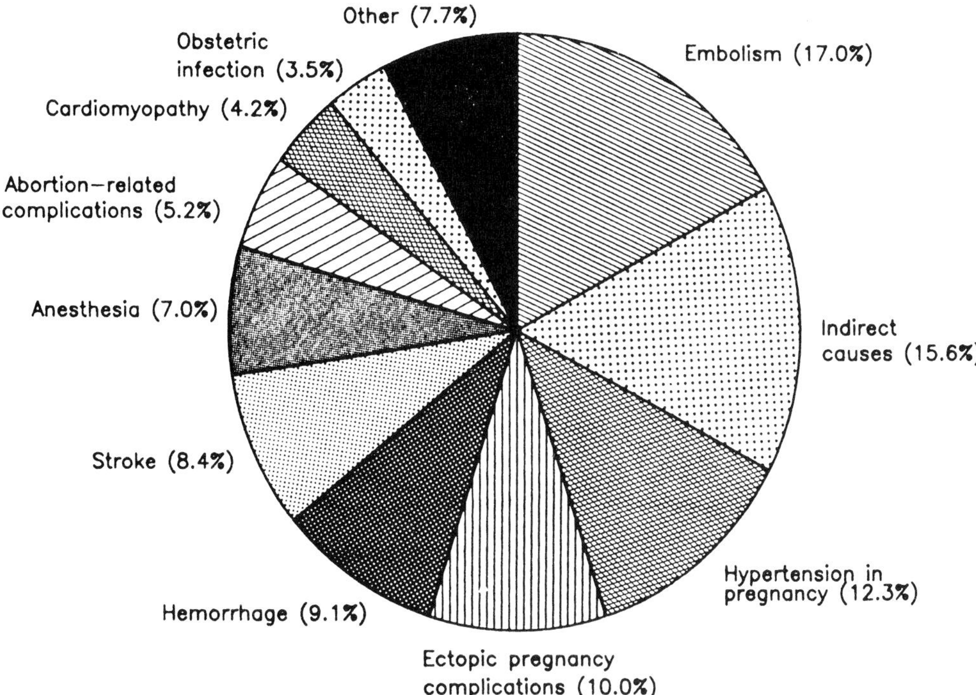


**Fig. 25–1.** Causes of maternal mortality in the United States, 1980–1985. (From Koonin LM, et al: Maternal mortality surveillance U.S. 1980–85. MMWR CDC Surveill Sum 37:19, 1988.)

actually develop renal insufficiency, thrombocytopenia, hemolysis, hepatic dysfunction, and central nervous system involvement.

## *Cardiovascular Changes*

Pregnancy-induced hypertension may present a wide spectrum of disease severity. Assessment of cardiovascular function is made more difficult by the fact that patients with severe hypertension may show different hemodynamic status than patients with mild hypertension. Despite these reservations, new information regarding the cardiovascular pathophysiology has increased our understanding of this disease and has provided new insights, even as it has raised many unanswered questions. Figure 25–3 is a graphic representation of the overlap among these categories.

In the last 8 years, many authors have published data regarding cardiac output in patients with varying severities of preeclampsia (30). One problem with the data regarding cardiac output in preeclampsia is the indexing of values. While cardiac output is frequently adjusted for body surface area in nonpregnant studies, it has been shown that there is no relationship between cardiac output and body surface area in pregnant patients using the standard Dubois formula (Figure 25–4) (31). Further, most authors have included at least a few multiparous patients in their studies; these patients are known to be more likely to have chronic renal diseases and other causes of their hypertension than have been unmasked by pregnancy. Whether the pathophysiology in this circumstance is the same as the nulliparous patient without previous renal disease has never been determined.

## *Cardiac Output*

Patients with early-onset preeclampsia/eclampsia are at highest risk of having placental dysfunction, intrauterine growth retardation, and perinatal death. Two-thirds of primigravid patients with early onset preeclampsia have renal abnormalities other than changes characteristic of preeclampsia on renal biopsy, excretory urography, or intravenous pyelogram (IVP) (32). They may have a hemodynamic picture different from that of the patient who has mild preeclampsia at term. Our own hemodynamic studies have shown that more of these patients have increased systemic vascular resistance rather than elevated cardiac output, as opposed to the usual finding in patients with late-onset preeclampsia (Figure 25–5) (31). Even when one limits the studies to those using thermodilution-measured cardiac output or the recently developed Doppler techniques, considerable variation exists in the reported values. Cardiac outputs as low as 4 liters/minute and as high as 13 liters/minute have been reported. Up to the present time, no clear picture of the hemodynamic status has emerged. Two studies revealed no increase in the cardiac output in comparison with normal pregnant patients (33,34). In both reports, however, many of the patients had severe, advanced disease.

The hemodynamic picture of severe hypertension may not be the same as that of milder forms of hypertension. Other studies have reported large numbers of patients who had cardiac outputs higher than in normal pregnancy. This is true even in patients who have not been previously treated with antihypertensives or intravenous fluids (32,35–37). The cardiac output is apparently elevated above normal nonpregnant levels at some point in the pathogenesis of preeclampsia depending on the stage of gestation and the duration of the disease process. Our own studies and those of others have shown an increase in the cardiac output in some patients with severe preeclampsia (Figure 25–6) (38).

An increase in cardiac output in the early stages of pre-

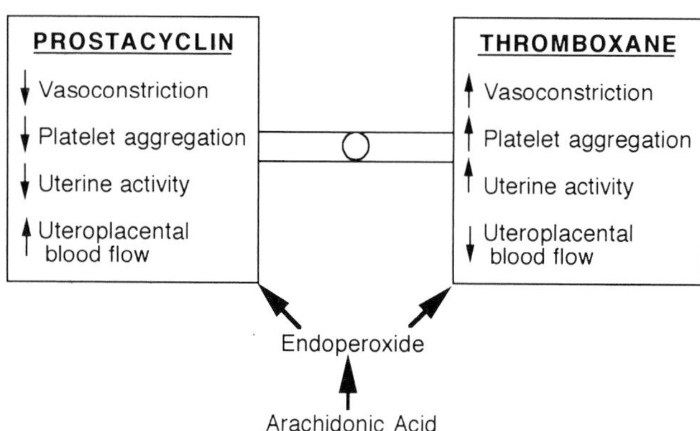


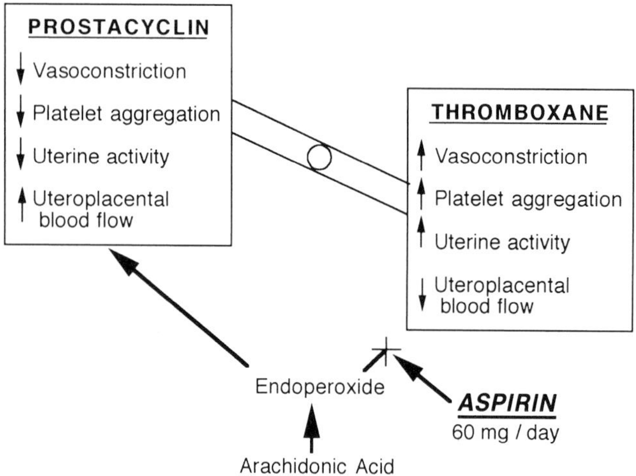


**Fig. 25–2.** Comparison of the balance in the biologic actions of prostacyclin and thromboxane in normal pregnancy with the imbalance of increased thromboxane and decreased prostacyclin in the preeclamptic patient. If the patient at risk for the development of preeclampsia is given aspirin, 60 mg a day, from the end of the first trimester throughout the remaining gestation, it may block the production of thromboxane without significant effect on the formation of prostacyclin. This may attenuate the effects of preeclampsia. (Redrawn from Walsh SW: Preeclampsia: An imbalance in placental prostacyclin and thromboxane production. Am. J. Obstet. Gynecol. 152:335–240, 1985. *In:* Schnider, SM, Levinson, G (eds): Anesthesia for Obstetrics, ed 3. Williams & Wilkins, Baltimore, 1993, p. 307.)

eclampsia has been previously hypothesized (39,40). This could produce an elevation in blood pressure as it does in a nonpregnant woman with renal hypertension. Increased cardiac output would help explain the findings of increased dehydroepiandrosterone sulfate (DHEA-S) clearance in patients with altered vascular sensitivity to angiotensin II. When the arterial pressure finally becomes elevated, cardiac output could have a variable response, depending on the extent of endothelial injury. This injury could be influenced by a number of factors including, antihypertensive administration, volume infusion or prolonged treatment with bed rest. In a recently concluded longitudinal study of 200 primigravid patients, we have

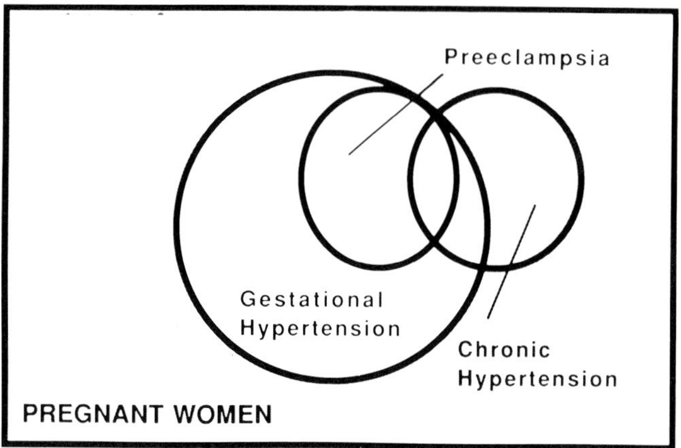


**Fig. 25–3.** Schematic representation of hypertensive disorder of pregnancy.

shown a significant elevation in cardiac output in patients destined to develop preeclampsia (Figures 25–7 and 25–8) (41). This elevated cardiac output persists throughout gestation and is present as early as 10 weeks from the last menstrual period. We believe that elevations in cardiac output may represent a primary factor in the development of preeclampsia (41).

The hemodynamic picture of preeclampsia probably changes over the course of the pregnancy and with the severity of the disease. We have longitudinally studied a patient during the early course of pregnancy who eventually developed severe preeclampsia. While she was normotensive, she had a cardiac output of over 11 liters/minute. By the time severe preeclampsia was apparent,

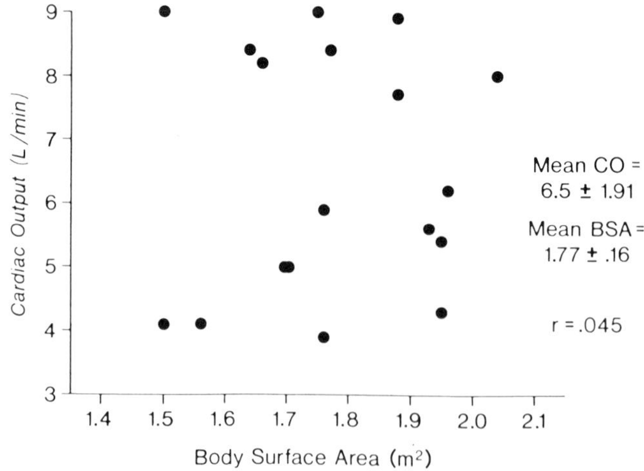


**Fig. 25–4.** Body surface area versus cardiac output in normotensive third trimester patients. No correlation between these two variables is observed. (From Easterling TR, Watts DH, Schmucker BC, Benedetti TJ: Measurement of cardiac output during pregnancy. Validation of Doppler technique and clinical observations in preeclampsia. Obstet. Gynecol. 69:845, 1987.)

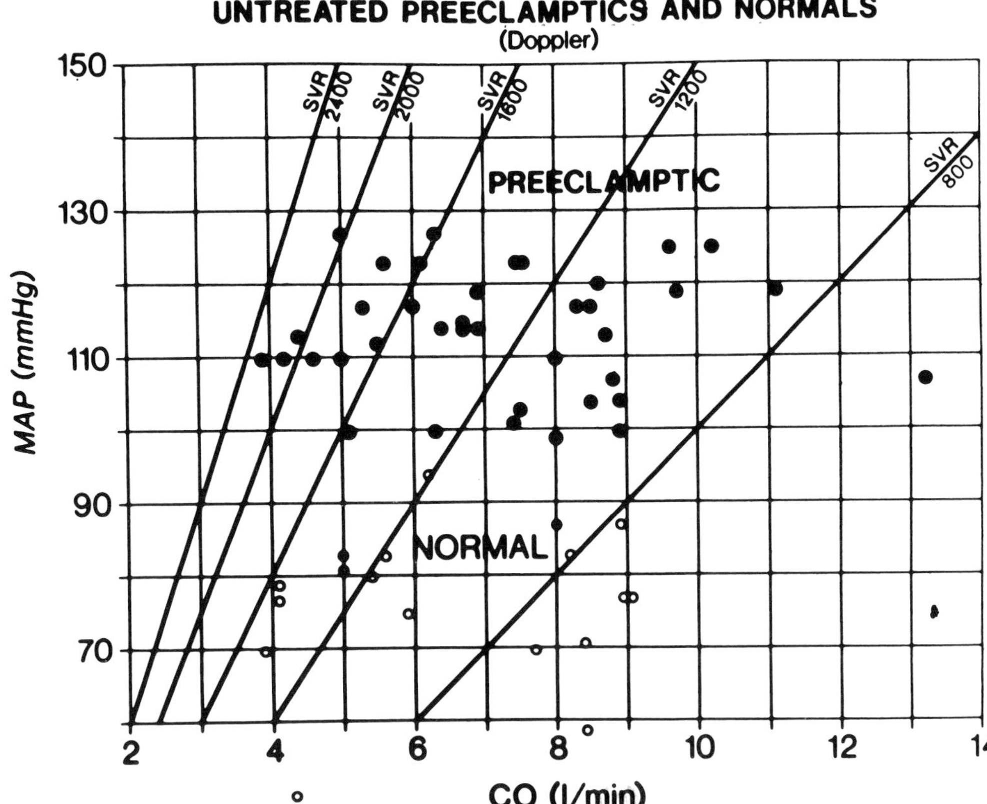


**Fig. 25–5.** Cardiac output, (CO) mean arterial pressure (MAP), and systemic vascular resistance in normal and preeclamptic pregnant patients. Cardiac output is measured noninvasively with Doppler technique. (From Easterling TR, Watts DH, Schmucker BC, Benedetti TJ: Measurement of cardiac output during pregnancy. Validation of Doppler technique and clinical observations in preeclampsia. Obstet. Gynecol. 69:845, 1987.)

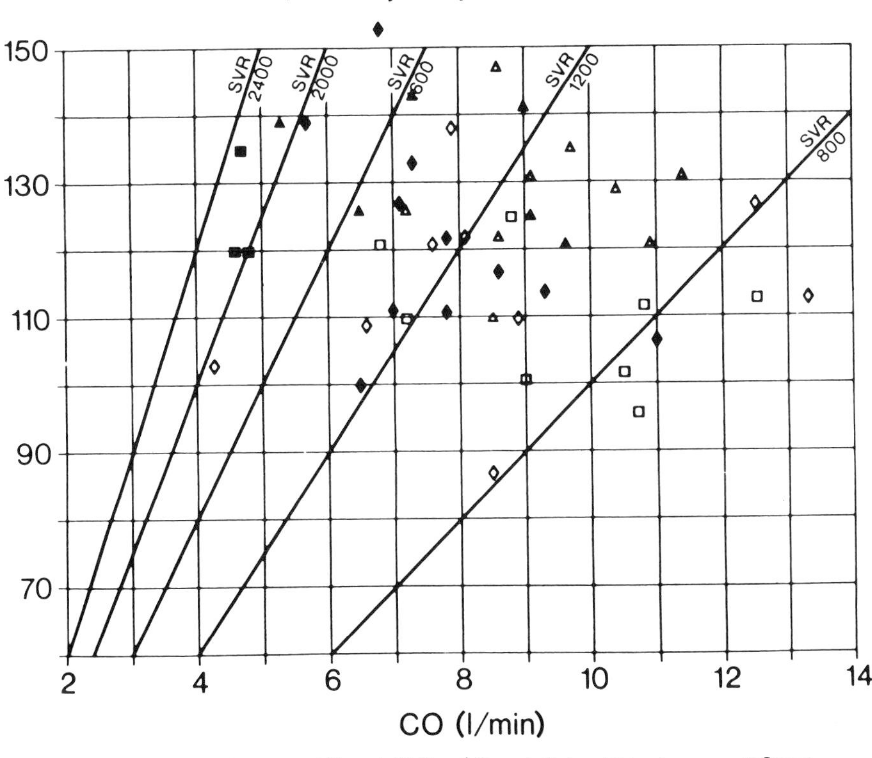


**Fig. 25–6.** Cardiac output mean arterial pressure and systemic vascular resistance in preeclamptic patients. Summary of published patients studied with invasive catheterization. (From Easterling TR, Watts DH, Schmucker BC, Benedetti TJ: Measurement of cardiac output during pregnancy. Validation of Doppler technique and clinical observations in preeclampsia. Obstet. Gynecol. 69:845, 1987.)

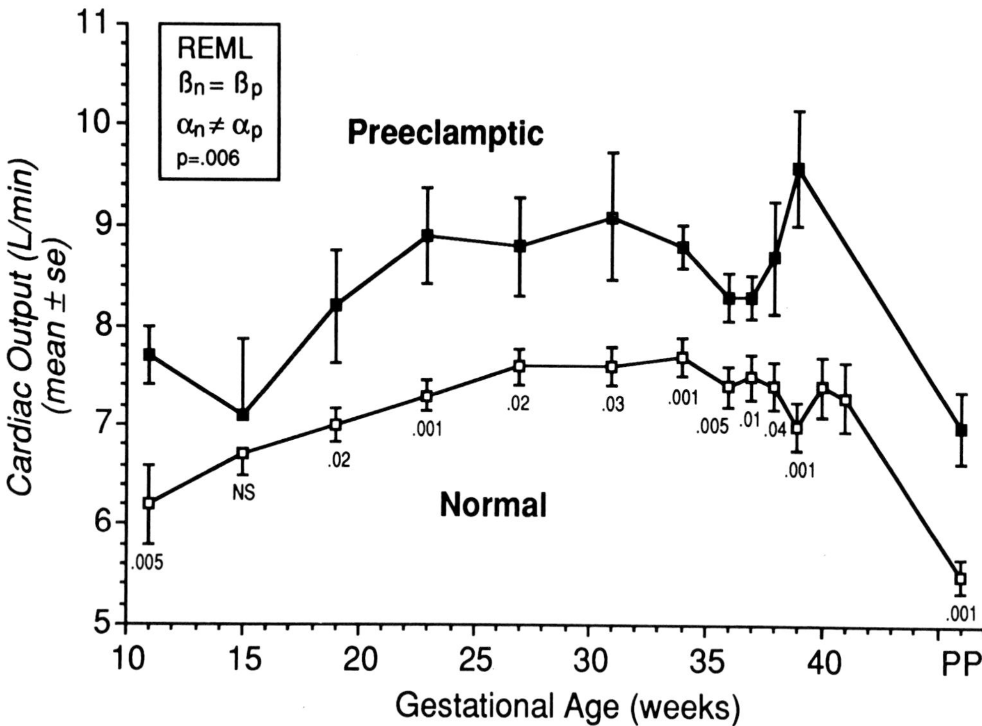


**Fig. 25–7.** Longitudinal measurement of cardiac output in pregnancy. All patients were normotensive in the first trimester. The bottom line shows the cardiac output of patients who remained normotensive. The top line shows the cardiac output of patients who eventually developed preeclampsia. (From Easterling TR, Benedetti TJ: Maternal hemodynamics in normal and preeclamptic pregnancies. A longitudinal study. Obstet. Gynecol. 76:1061–1069, 1990.)

her cardiac output had fallen to below 6 liters/minute (Figure 25–9). If the disease process had been further observed, it is possible that the cardiac output may have fallen to lower levels. Thus, in a given patient, cardiac output could range from high to low values.

### *Pulmonary Artery Pressure*

Pulmonary artery pressures in preeclampsia are not increased and the pulmonary vascular resistance is low to low-normal for pregnancy (38). When measured, pulmonary artery wedge pressure (PAWP) in patients with preeclampsia has been found to vary with the severity of change in systemic vascular resistance. If the resistance is high, then the pulmonary artery wedge pressure is usually low (34,38). If cardiac output is high, there is a tendency for the pulmonary artery wedge pressure to be in the low-normal to normal range for pregnancy. Pulmonary artery wedge pressure increases with uterine contractions

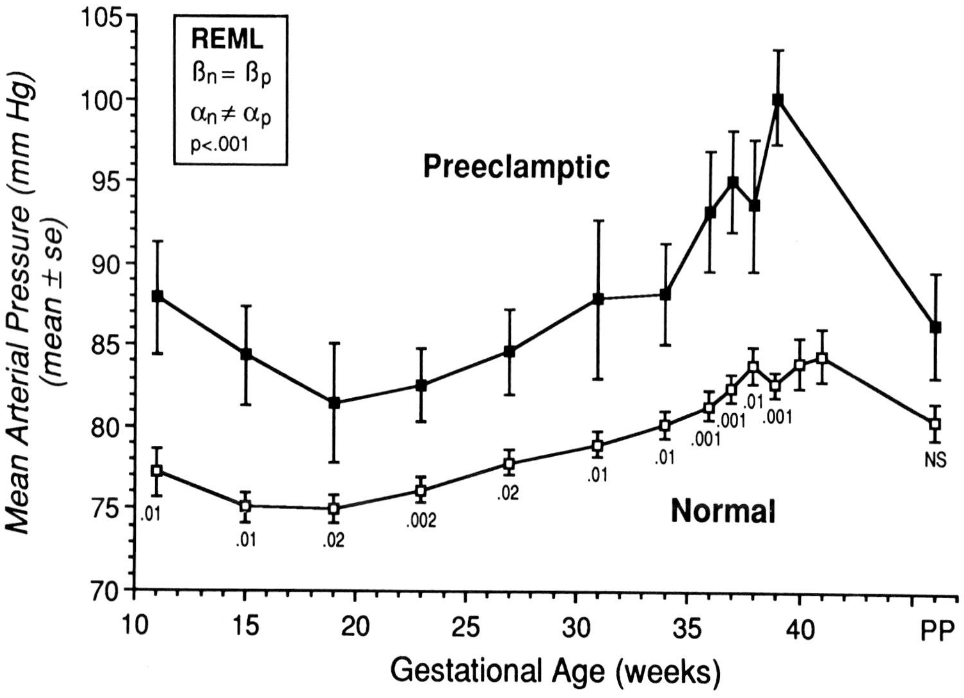


**Fig. 25–8.** Mean arterial pressure in the same patients as studied in Figure 25–7. Blood pressure is statistically higher in patients who eventually developed preeclampsia, confirming studies of others. However, all blood pressures were, at levels in the first trimester, generally accepted as normal. (From Easterling TR, Benedetti TJ: Maternal hemodynamics in normal and preeclamptic pregnancies. A longitudinal study. Obstet. Gynecol. 76: 1061–1069, 1990.)

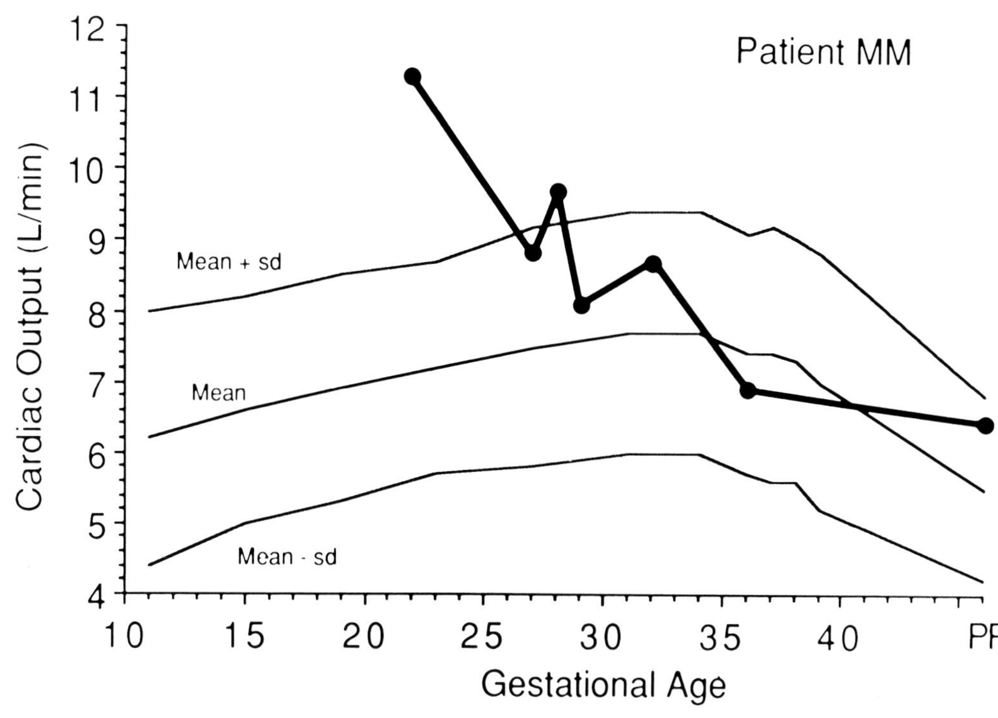


**Fig. 25–9.** Longitudinal graph of cardiac output in one patient who showed progressive falls in cardiac output during pregnancy from very high levels. She was lost to follow-up at 31 weeks while still normotensive. She returned at 35 weeks with severe preeclampsia. (From Easterline TR, Benedetti TJ: Maternal hemodynamics in normal and preeclamptic pregnancies. A longitudinal study. Obstet. Gynecol. (in press).)

and increases transiently after delivery (42). Left ventricular function is usually not impaired in patients with severe preeclampsia. The initial PAWP will often depend on the fluid balance status before initial hemodynamic measurements. In the case of severe volume depletion, whether iatrogenic or self-induced, the PAWP will usually be low. If aggressive volume therapy precedes measurements, PAWP will be elevated to more normal levels, but ventricular function is usually maintained. Figure 25–10 illustrates these two subsets of patients.

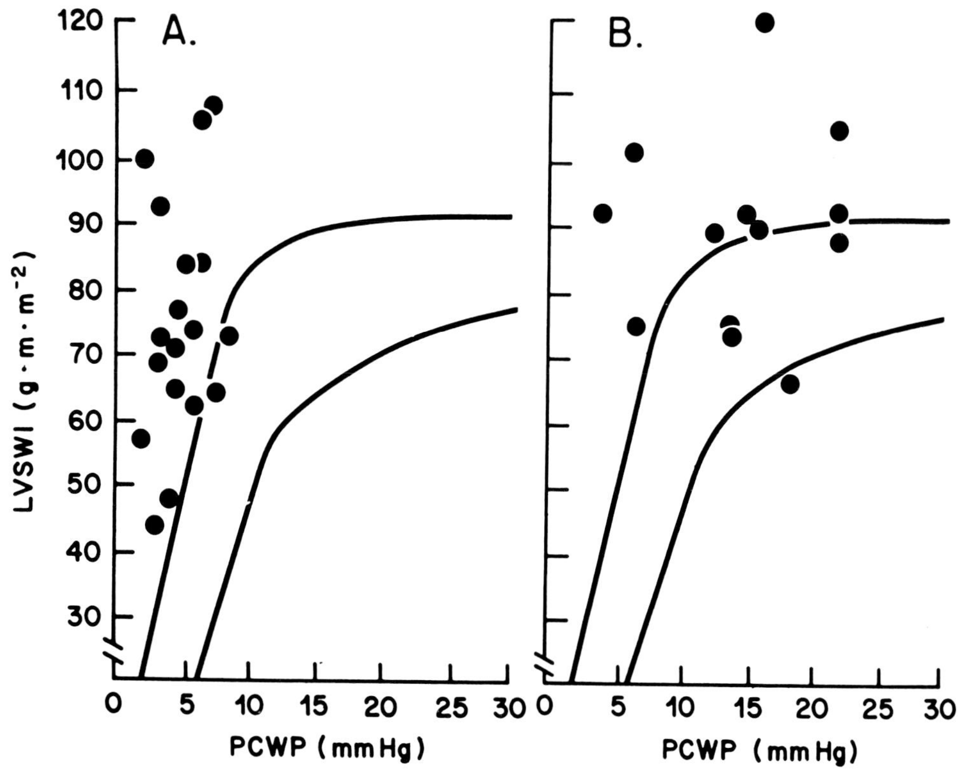


**Fig. 25–10. A,** left-ventricular-function curves in women managed with fluid restriction to 125 cc/hr contrasted to **B,** a woman managed with more aggressive fluid management. (PCWP—pulmonary capillary wedge pressure.) (From Hankins GD, Wendel GD, Cunningham FG, Leveno KJ: Longitudinal evaluation of hemodynamic changes in eclampsia. Am. J. Obstet. Gynecol. 150:506, 1984.)

### Blood Volume

Total blood volume is reduced in preeclampsia (43). This reduction appears to be proportional to the severity of the hypertensive disorder. Colloid osmotic pressure (COP) is reduced in pregnancy and is further reduced in preeclampsia (44,45), proportional to the severity of this disease. Oian, et al investigated the mechanism of plasma volume reduction with direct measurement of plasma colloid osmotic pressure, interstitial colloid osmotic pressure, and interstitial pressure in normal patients and in patients with preeclampsia (46,47). They found an increase in the interstitial colloid osmotic pressure in patients with severe preeclampsia compared to those with mild forms of preeclampsia and normotensive patients. They concluded that this could be secondary to reduced capillary hydrostatic pressure, increased microvascular permeability to protein, or reduced lymph flow. In a follow-up study, Bhatia, et al demonstrated a strong correlation between reduced capillary colloid osmotic pressure and plasma fibronectin level (45). This suggests that altered capillary permeability is the cause of reduced plasma colloid osmotic pressure in preeclampsia. Further studies of patients with mild preeclampsia without proteinuria, using a quantitative method for determination of proteinuria, would help clarify this issue. Figures 25–11 and 25–12 show a schematic representation of how these findings could lead to the commonly recognized clinical findings.

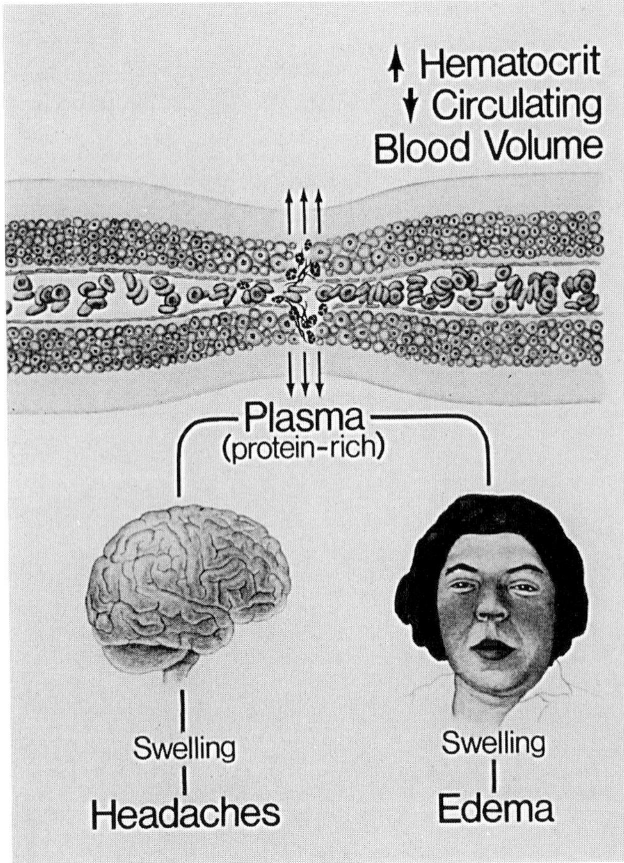


**Fig. 25–11.** Schematic representation of pathophysiologic changes at capillary level and their relationship to commonly observed clinical findings in preeclampsia.

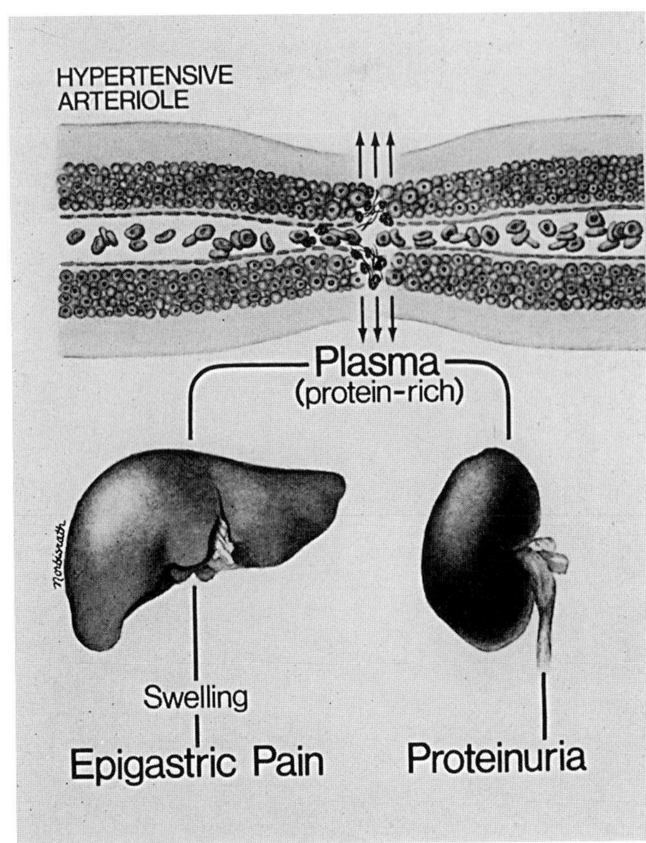


**Fig. 25–12.** Schematic representation of pathophysiologic changes at capillary level and their relationship to commonly observed clinical findings in preeclampsia.

No static theory can encompass all the hemodynamic observations made in patients with preeclampsia. Preeclampsia develops over a period of weeks or months with hypertension and proteinuria being relatively late occurrences. Gant, et al have shown an altered response to the pressor effect of angiotensin II infusion long before the mean arterial pressure becomes elevated (Figure 25–13) (9). In addition, Worley has shown that concomitant with the altered pressure response, there is an increase in DHEA-S clearance (Figure 25–14) (48). This is consistent with an increased placental flow at an early stage in the disease. Increased placental flow could be the result of increased cardiac output, or it could be secondary to some alteration of autoregulation of flow to the uterus and placenta. In nonpregnant patients, the hemodynamic alterations associated with hypertension encompass a spectrum. The picture depends on when in the course of the disease the study is performed. It may be that the same will eventually be found to be true in preeclampsia.

### Pulmonary Edema

Pulmonary edema in the pregnant hypertensive patient has been reported to occur by three different mecha-

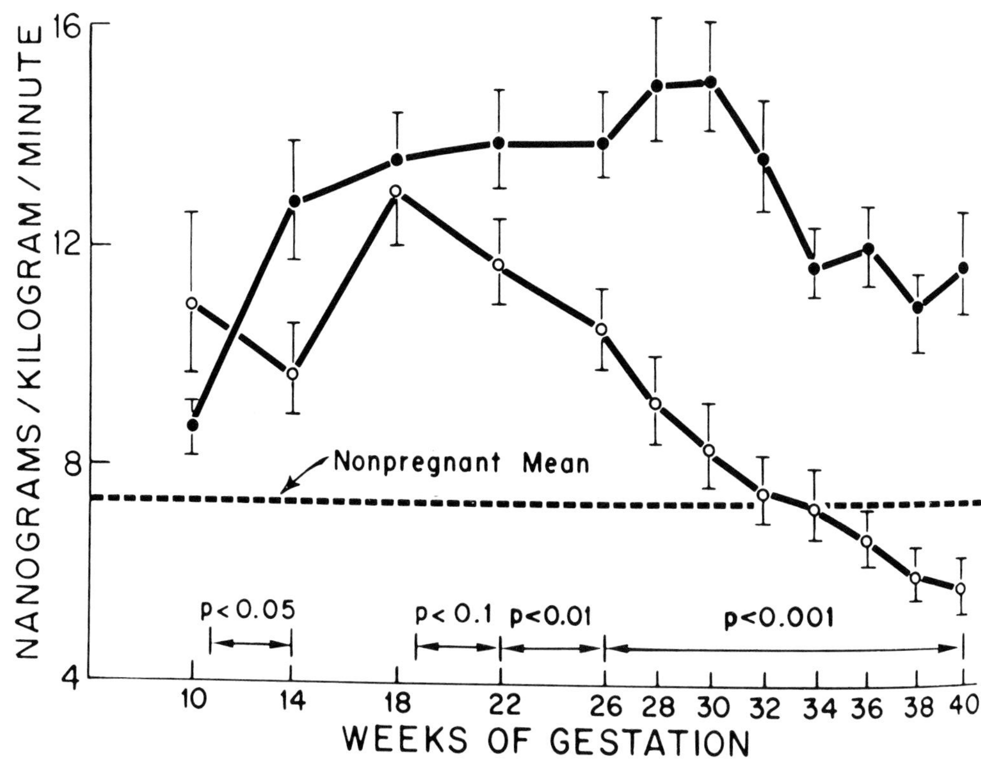


**Fig. 25–13.** Longitudinal study showing loss of resistance to infused effects of angiotensin II in patients who eventually developed pregnancy-induced hypertension (bottom curve). (From Gant NF, et al: A study of angiotensin II pressure response throughout primigravid pregnancy. J. Clin. Invest. 52: 2682, 1973.)

nisms: (1) altered capillary permeability; (2) left ventricular dysfunction; and (3) altered hydrostatic oncotic forces. Clinical differentiation between cardiogenic and noncardiogenic pulmonary edema is difficult, if not impossible, in pregnant patients. Permeability pulmonary edema has been reported in hypertensive pregnant patients (49–51). This diagnosis can usually be made with the use of a pulmonary artery catheter by documentation

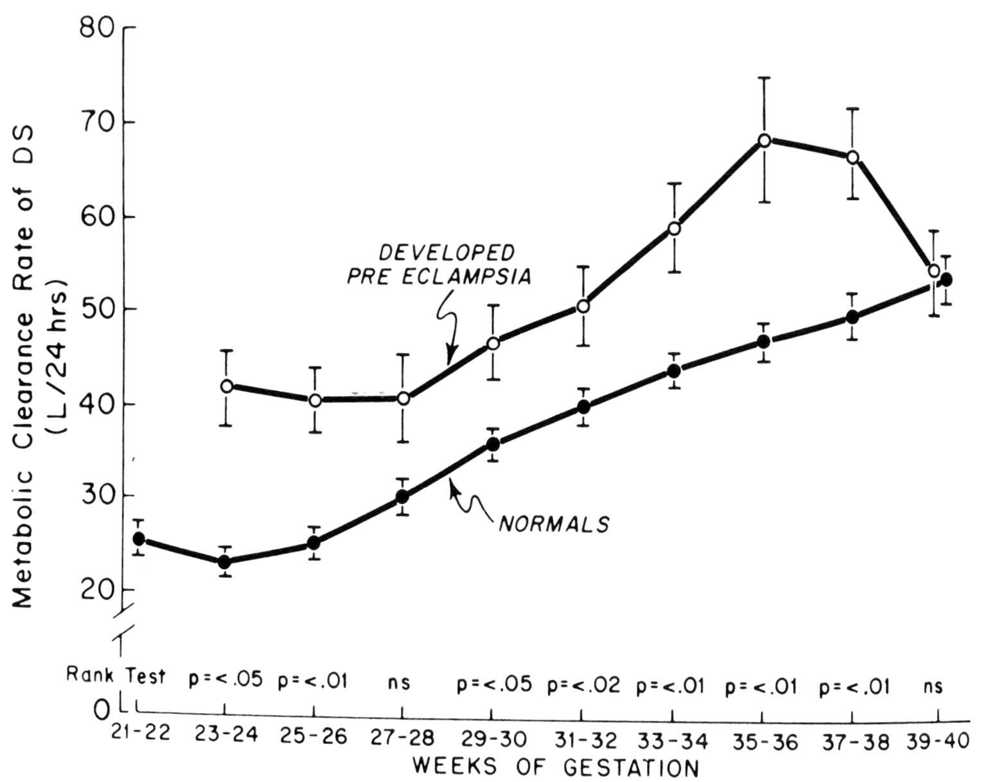


**Fig. 25–14.** Longitudinal study showing elevated metabolic clearance of DS in patients who eventually developed preeclampsia. (From Worley RJ, et al: Fetal considerations. Metabolic clearance rate of maternal plasma dehydroisoandrosterone sulfate. Semin. Perinatol. 12:15, 1978.)

of normal cardiac filling pressures with normal left ventricular performance and/or evidence of abnormal protein content in the pulmonary secretions. Treatment in this instance should center on supporting cardiac and respiratory function. Supplemental oxygen, positive end-expiratory pressure, and mechanical ventilation are usual essential therapeutic modalities. Volume status in these patients must be monitored very carefully. Over-expansion of the intravascular volume in this instance may contribute to increased pulmonary shunting. In contrast, vigorous diuresis may aggravate hypovolemia and have an adverse effect on cardiac output and subsequently vital organ perfusion. Clinically, the former (hypervolemia) is a much more common occurrence than the latter (hypovolemia).

In most preeclamptic patients, intubation and ventilation will not be required. If a hypertensive patient develops pulmonary edema, a reasonable first step in therapy is to administer a diuretic. If oxygenation and ventilation improve, the precise measurement of filling pressures and cardiac output may not be necessary. However, if the pulmonary edema is severe or if the clinical picture does not improve with diuretic therapy, invasive monitoring should be instituted.

Left ventricular dysfunction is the least common mechanism in which pulmonary edema in the pregnant hypertensive patient is reported to occur. Increased afterload appears to be the usual cause of left ventricular dysfunction. In this situation, afterload reduction will correct impaired myocardial performance and reduce pulmonary artery wedge pressure (Figure 25–15) (52). Intravenous hydralazine has been the traditional drug used in hypertensive episodes in obstetrics. It is probably the drug of choice because of its lack of adverse fetal effects. Nitroprusside may be used in the postpartum period if tachycardia limits the effectiveness of hydralazine therapy. Nitroprusside has been reported to cross the placenta in animals with lethal fetal effects (53). Nitroprusside is best given for short periods of time, if at all, to parturients with a fetus in utero.

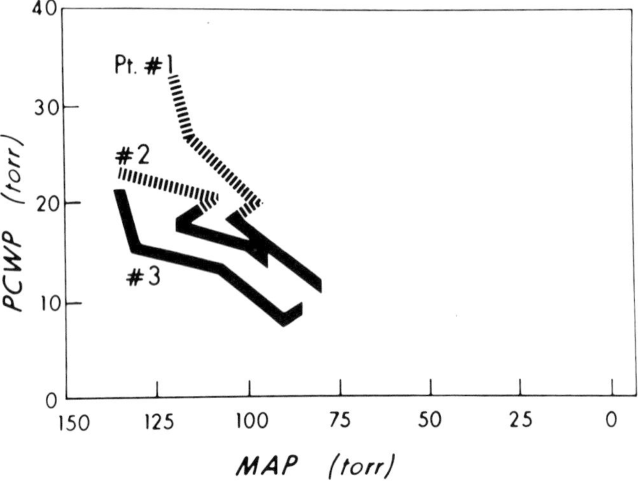


**Fig. 25–15.** Graph of mean arterial pressure MAP versus pulmonary capillary wedge pressure (PCWP) in three patients with pulmonary edema and severe hypertension. Reduction in MAP results in falls in pulmonary capillary wedge pressure in each case. (From Strauss RG, Keefer JR, Burke T, Civetta JM: Hemodynamic monitoring of cardiogenic pulmonary edema complicating toxemia of pregnancy. Obstet. Gynecol. 55:170, 1980.)

Pulmonary edema has also been reported in hypertensive pregnant patients and is associated with a reduction in the intervascular colloid osmotic pressure (44). When the colloid osmotic pressure is reduced to less than 16 mm Hg, a small rise in the pulmonary artery wedge pressure can result in a reversal of the normal Starling forces and result in the accumulation of extravascular lung water.

Several recent studies have clarified the factors related to the development of pulmonary edema in preeclampsia. As many as 3% of patients with severe preeclampsia may develop pulmonary edema (54). Older patients with prior chronic hypertension appear to have an increased risk compared to patients who were previously normotensive. About 70 to 80% of pulmonary edema cases first become clinically apparent in the postpartum period (51,54). It usually accompanies other end-organ damage associated with the severest forms of the preeclampsia. Ventricular function is usually, but not always, preserved.

Figure 25–16 shows the hemodynamic performance of 10 patients with pulmonary edema (51). Only 2 patients had myocardial failure while myocardial performance was normal in 8 patients. Three patients were found to have pulmonary capillary endothelial injury leading to pulmonary edema. However, the most common causes of pulmonary edema were an alteration in hydrostatic oncotic forces. In these patients, simultaneous elevation of the pulmonary capillary wedge pressures and reduction in plasma colloid oncotic pressure was found to be the only alteration in hemodynamics.

Elevated filling pressures were usually secondary to volume therapy. In addition, Hankins has shown that in some patients filling pressures may become elevated postpartum in the face of conservative (less than 100 cc/hr) fluid therapy (35). This observation is best explained by a discrepancy between the timing of extravascular fluid mobilization and the return of normal renal function. When fluid mobilization occurs before the kidney is able to filter and excrete the excess volume, filling pressures will rise. Figure 25–17 illustrates this phenomenon in a severely preeclamptic patient and shows the hemodynamic responses to diuretic therapy.

## Other Maternal Effects

### Renal Effects

Renal function is normal during the early weeks of a preeclamptic pregnancy, but changes can be detected with appropriate tests by the time the first clinical signs become apparent.

The urine contains an abnormal amount of protein, and occasionally blood. As the severity of preeclampsia-eclampsia increases and renal function deteriorates, the daily urine output diminishes and may even progress to anuria.

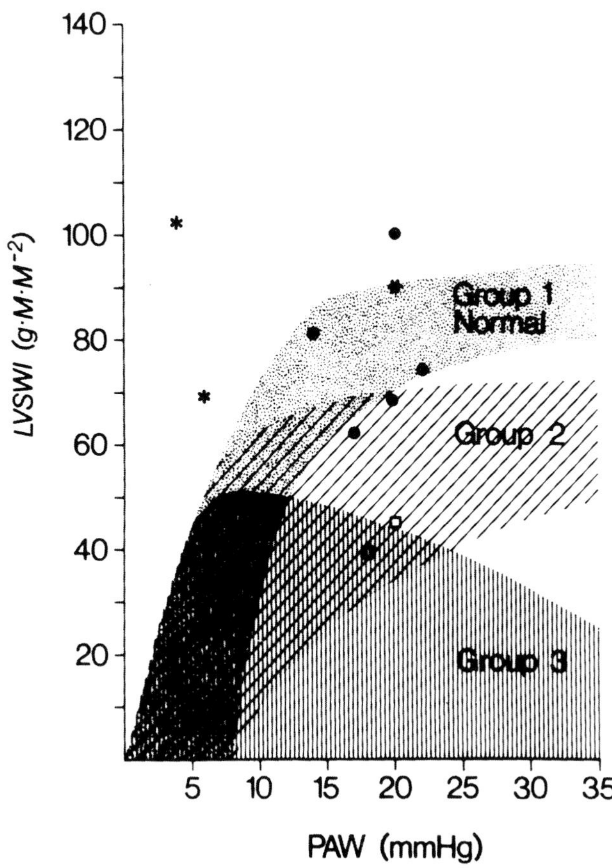


**Fig. 25–16.** Ventricular-function curve showing three groups of patients with pulmonary edema. The (*) represents the patients with capillary permeability injury. Circles represent patients with altered hydrostatic oncotic forces. Open square represents patients with left ventricular dysfunction. (From Benedetti TJ, Kates R, Williams V: Hemodynamic observations in severe preeclampsia complicated by pulmonary edema. Am. J. Obstet. Gynecol. 152:330, 1985.)

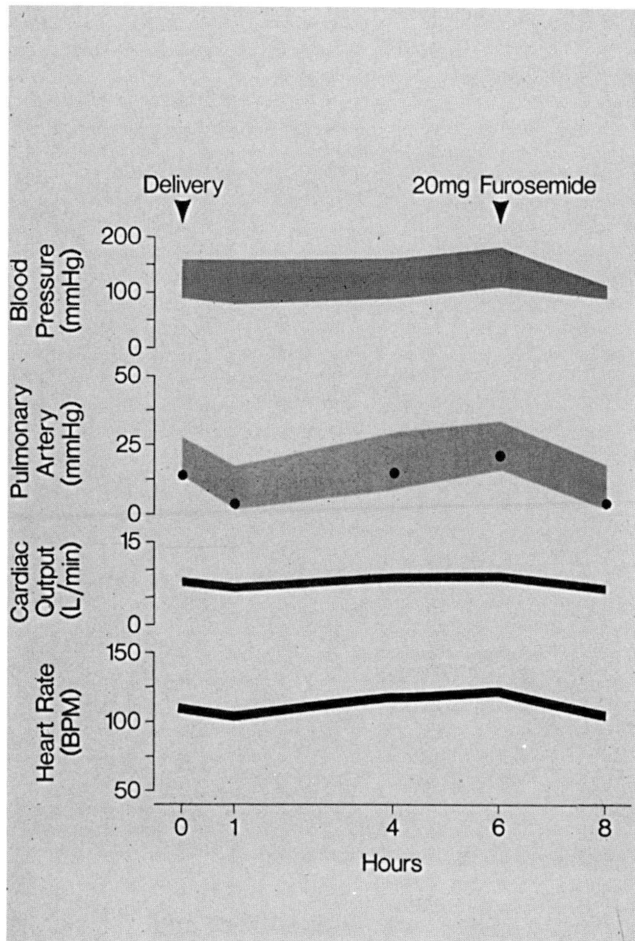


**Fig. 25–17.** Longitudinal hemodynamic data on one patient following delivery. Gradual rise in pulmonary capillary wedge pressure and pulmonary artery wedge pressure (circle) are paralleled by gradual rise in blood pressure. When the pulmonary artery wedge pressure reached 15, furosemide was administered and both pulmonary artery wedge pressure and blood pressure returned to more acceptable levels over the next 2 hours.

## *Oliguria*

Oliguria is classically defined in preeclampsia as urine output of less than 500 cc/24 hours. This output is one of the markers of severe disease and is often used as an absolute indication for delivery. Oliguria has been thought to be secondary to either severe volume depletion or decreased renal perfusion secondary to renal arteriospasm. Until recently, little hemodynamic data were available on which to base treatment.

Lee described urinary diagnostic tests commonly used to identify renal hemodynamics in patients with preeclampsia and oliguria (less than 30 cc/hr × 2 hours) (55). He found that the urine sodium values were high and pointed to an intrarenal cause. However, nearly all the other tests (urine osmolality, urine/plasma creatinine, fractional excretion of sodium) suggested a prerenal etiology. However, when he examined intracardiac filling pressures, he found the pulmonary artery wedge pressure to be normal to slightly elevated in five of the seven patients studied. Urinary diagnostic studies appear to have little clinical value in the assessment and treatment of preeclamptic patients.

Clark studied nine preeclamptic patients with oliguria (less than 30 cc/hr × 3 hours) (56). Using invasive hemodynamic monitoring, he found a variety of hemodynamic abnormalities. The majority of patients showed low pulmonary artery wedge pressures, hyperdynamic cardiac function, and moderately elevated systemic resistance. These patients all responded to volume infusion. A second group of patients had higher PAWPs and lower systemic vascular resistance. These patients had previous volume infusion but had failed to increase urine output. They were thought to have renal arteriospasm as the etiology of their oliguria and were treated with hydralazine to relieve the oliguria. Two patients had high wedge pressures but dissimilar systemic vascular resistance (SVR). One had normal systemic vascular resistance (920), while the other had a high systemic vascular resistance (2790). In the first patient, oliguria resolved with nitroglycerine therapy, used to reduce both preload and afterload. In the other patient, hydralazine was used to reduce afterload and improve myocardial function.

When evaluating an oliguric patient, one must first be sure that the diagnosis is correct. If the patient has been in the supine position, it is important to change her to the lateral position and be sure that she moves from side to side on an hourly basis. Mild to moderate degrees of caval compression and ureteral compression associated with position can falsely lead to the diagnosis of oliguria.

If the oliguria persists despite optimal positioning, then the two described studies form the basis of a clinical approach to the oliguric patient. At present, renal diagnostic studies seem to provide no clear information on which to base clinical management. If there is no hemodynamic information on which to base clinical management, then a fluid challenge of 500 cc of crystalloid solution should be performed. At least 1 to 2 hours should be allowed to determine a response after the fluid administration. If oliguria persists, then invasive hemodynamic monitoring can be performed to guide therapy. The choice of whether to use a central venous pressure (CVP) or a Swan-Ganz catheter is often necessary. In hospitals where central venous pressure is used as the first line of evaluation, it should be remembered that a low central venous pressure usually means a low PAWP. However, if the central venous pressure is greater than 6 cm $H_2O$, then there is no consistent relationship between the central venous pressure and the PAWP (Figure 25–18). In cases in which the central venous pressure is low, fluid administration can proceed using relative change in the central venous pressure as an indicator of volume response. If the patient is still oliguric when the central venous pressure reaches or exceeds 6 cm of $H_2O$, further fluid therapy should be administered on the basis of the PAWP and the cardiac output values obtained from the Swan-Ganz catheter. If the PAWP is less than 6 to 7 mm Hg, then continued fluid administration should be done to raise the PAWP to that level. Once that level is reached, at least 1 to 2 hours should be allowed to assess the response. If oliguria continues, therapy with hydralazine could be undertaken. If the PAWP is high normal or high (more than 12 mm Hg), an alternative therapy would be diuretic therapy with furosemide. In the case of the patient with high systemic vascular resistance, hydralazine therapy should be the treatment of choice.

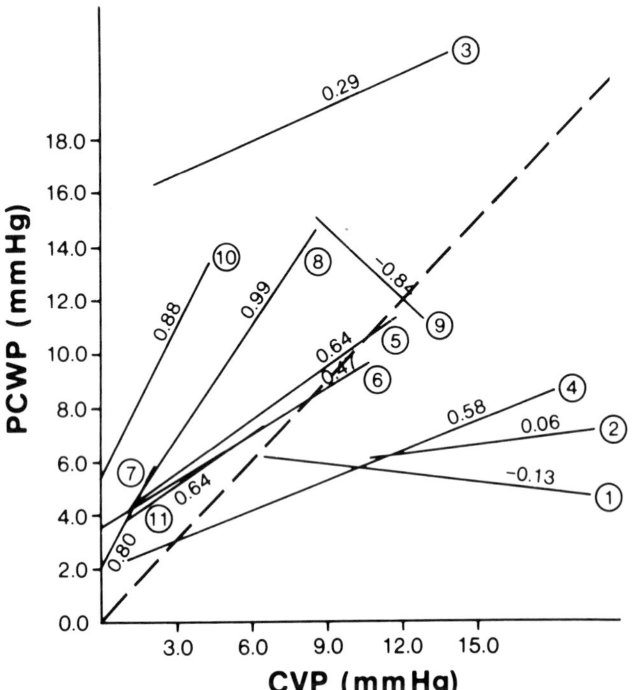


**Fig. 25–18.** Regression lines and correlation coefficients for 11 patients with severe preeclampsia. Poor correlation is seen in several patients, usually when the central venous pressure (CVP) exceeds 6 cm $H_2O$. (From Newsome LR, Bramwell RS, Curling PE: Severe preeclampsia. Hemodynamic effects of lumbar epidural anesthesia. Anesth. Analg. 65:31, 1986.)

## *Convulsions*

The presence of grand mal convulsions distinguishes eclampsia from preeclampsia. In the United States, the incidence has fallen from approximately 1% of births in 1940 to 0.1% in 1960 and to 0.03% in 1980 (57,58). These numbers can be strongly influenced by the population of a given hospital, with the figures being higher at institutions serving large numbers of patients without adequate prenatal care. The incidence is sevenfold higher in patients with pathologic proteinuria than in those without proteinuria. However, present data show that as many as 20% of patients with eclampsia have little or no proteinuria at the time of the first seizure. This finding is usually related to the health care provider's under-appreciation of the risk of eclampsia in a patient with mild elevations of blood pressure. Eclampsia almost always occurs after 20 weeks gestation but has been reported as early as 16 weeks. Half of the cases occur before the onset of labor, 33% during labor, and 17% occur after delivery. When eclampsia occurs postpartum, it is usually within the first 24 to 48 hours after delivery (59). However, in one study (60), the number of patients seizing 48 hours after delivery was nearly equal to the number seizing between delivery and 48 hours (17 versus 19). In this study, most of the patients suffering late postpartum eclampsia had had magnesium sulfate discontinued prior to the convulsion.

The cause of eclamptic convulsions is unknown. There are no clear data that the level of blood pressure elevation has any relationship to the development of eclamptic seizures. One reason for this may be that severe elevations of blood pressure are usually recognized as representing a risk for eclampsia and seizure prophylaxis instituted. Another could be the well-accepted principle of treating diastolic blood pressures above 110 mm Hg. Systolic blood pressures above 200 mm Hg should also be treated even if the diastolic is under 110 mm Hg, as the mean arterial pressure is usually above 130 mm Hg.

Factors that enhance the chances of death from eclampsia include advanced maternal age (more than 35 years), multiparity, systolic hypertension greater than 200 mm Hg, coagulopathy, and delivery delay in the presence of severe maternal illness. Eclampsia is often said to be the most severe form of hypertensive disease in pregnancy.

At the present time, this needs to be reexamined. In one study, more women died from hypertensive disease of pregnancy without having suffered eclampsia then died after having suffered an eclamptic seizure (61). In addition, it has been shown that patients who have eclampsia, but have only mild hypertension, can occasionally be safely treated in a conservative manner without resorting to immediate delivery (62). In the present era, prolonging pregnancy after eclamptic seizure is not usually justified. The special circumstances that have to exist to adopt this approach are mild blood pressure elevation after seizure control, absence of significant maternal end-organ dysfunction (normal hematologic, renal, and hepatic function studies), and normal results on fetal evaluation (adequate growth, normal antepartum testing). The majority of patients suffering eclamptic seizures will not meet these criteria. However, in the unusual circumstance in which gestation is less than 28 weeks and the criteria are satisfied, careful observation can be considered. However, this strategy should only be considered when the patient is very remote from term and the expected perinatal mortality and morbidity are high.

### *Effects on the Fetus and Newborn*

#### *Respiratory Distress Syndrome (RDS)*

In patients with severe preeclampsia/eclampsia, severe perinatal morbidity and mortality are related, in large part, to the forced delivery of the fetus at high risk for the development of respiratory distress syndrome (RDS) (63). Although some authors have reported accelerated pulmonary maturity in patients with preeclampsia (64), this does not appear to be a consistent observation, especially in patients between 28 and 32 weeks of gestation (63,65,66). A previous report indicated that glucocorticoid therapy to accelerate fetal pulmonary maturity may have an adverse effect on the fetus and result in an increased incidence of fetal demise (67). This was subsequently found to be related to inordinate delivery delay rather than a specific effect of antenatal glucocorticoid administration. Subsequent reports suggested that glucocorticoids can be safely administered with intensive and continuous fetal monitoring (68,69). Maintenance of maternal homeostasis during 48 hours to allow acceleration of fetal pulmonary maturity has involved the use of magnesium sulfate and hydralazine therapy.

The national collaborative study on antenatal steroid therapy found a higher rate of RDS in pregnancies of hypertensive mothers than controls (27% versus 14%), but failed to detect a significant reduction in RDS associated with steroid therapy (27% versus 21%) in hypertensive patients (70). From the currently available data, it would appear that delaying delivery for 48 hours to accelerate fetal pulmonary maturity in severe preeclampsia may not be effective. The same study demonstrated a much greater beneficial affect for vaginal delivery as opposed to cesarean section in reduction of RDS, 24% versus 12%. It would appear that the fetus of a mother with severe hypertensive disease, especially when complicated by multiple end-organ failure, might benefit more from vaginal delivery than from antenatal steroid therapy.

If the mother is not critically ill and the fetus shows no signs of compromise, antenatal steroid therapy should still be considered at gestational ages between 26 and 32 weeks. However, severe maternal hypertension requiring repetitive administration of intravenous antihypertensive medications or the presence of significant renal, hematologic or liver abnormalities indicating advanced maternal disease should be considered indications for delivery. The recent studies of neonatal surfactant therapy for the premature fetus offer much promise in reducing the pulmonary complications of the premature infant of the hypertensive mother.

## OBSTETRIC MANAGEMENT

The ultimate objective of obstetric and anesthesiologic management is to deliver as normal a fetus as possible. Until this can be accomplished, the obstetric objective is to control the disease process and continue this control as long as the intrauterine environment is adequate to support growth and maturation of the fetus without endangering the mother. This requires control of hypertension, improvement in circulation particularly in the uterus, placenta, and kidneys to improve intravascular volume, to correct acid base and nitrogen imbalances, and to decrease or eliminate hyperactivity of the central nervous system and reflexes.

### Prevention of Preeclampsia

Prevention of clinically recognizable preeclampsia has not been achieved until recent years. Efforts at prevention have been focused on affecting the thromboxane-prostacyclin rating, with low-dose aspirin or other platelet altering agents. Beaufils, et al (71) randomized 102 women at risk for preeclampsia and/or intrauterine growth retardation (IUGR) based on past obstetric history to either aspirin 150 gm and dipyridamole 300 or no treatment starting at 12 weeks gestation. The treated group had a decreased incidence of preeclampsia, fetal loss, and intrauterine growth retardation. Wallenberg (72) randomized a group of 46 nulliparous patients with abnormal angiotensin infusion tests to either ASA (60 mg/day) or placebo from 28 weeks gestation. The treated group had a reduced incidence of preeclampsia but not intrauterine growth retardation. Schiff (73) studied 65 women with positive rollover tests and either nulliparity, twins, or previous preeclampsia. These women were randomized to either ASA (100 mg/day) or placebo. The treated group had a reduced incidence of preeclampsia. Benigni (74) studied women with either chronic hypertension or previous poor obstetric history. He randomized patients to either ASA (60 mg/day) or placebo from 12 weeks of gestation. The treated patients had an increase in fetal birthweight. McFarland (75) studied nulliparous women with abnormal uterine artery Doppler wave forms at 24 weeks gestation. One-hundred women were randomized to ASA (75 mg/day) or placebo. The ASA group had a decreased incidence of preeclampsia. Finally, a meta-analysis of six controlled treatment trials concluded that ASA decreased the incidence of low birthweight (less than 10 percentile) and reduce the incidence of preeclampsia. However,

McFarland found no reduction in either fetal or neonatal death in the ASA treated groups. Unfortunately, the predictive value of current methods in identifying preeclampsia is poor. Current, large scale trials in nulliparous women in the USA and Europe are nearing completion. These studies will provide answers regarding the role of ASA in prevention of preeclampsia and whether there are significant maternal costs associated with this form of therapy. Until the results of these trials are known, its therapy should be considered experimental.

## Management of Mild Preeclampsia

The definitive treatment of preeclampsia is delivery. The goal of therapy is to prevent severe maternal complications and to deliver the fetus in the best possible condition. Preeclampsia will abate shortly after delivery in nearly all patients. When a patient presents with preeclampsia after 38 weeks, there is little justification for treatment other than delivery. On occasion, patients will show improvement in blood pressure or resolution of mild degrees of proteinuria after a variable period of hospitalization. If the patient has an unfavorable cervix for induction of labor, there is a tendency to delay delivery until the cervix is more favorable. This is probably not justified, as accelerated hypertension of acute fetal deterioration can occur at any phase of gestation.

## Management of Severe Preeclampsia

Severe preeclampsia is defined by severe hypertension (greater than 160/110) and proteinuria or by the presence of mild-to-moderate hypertension (greater than 140/90) and the presence of significant end-organ dysfunction. These end organs include the kidneys (proteinuria 5 grams/24 hours), blood (platelet counts less than 100,000 red cell hemolysis), liver (abnormal serum glutamic-oxaloacetic transaminase (SGOT), Bilirubin, lactate dehydrogenase (LDH), CNS (severe headache, visual disturbances), or pulmonary (pulmonary edema). Traditional teachings have called for delivery whenever the diagnosis of severe preeclampsia was made, regardless of gestational age of the fetus. In the past 5 years, more evidence has accumulated suggesting that selected patients with severe preeclampsia can benefit from delivery delay if appropriate maternal and fetal monitoring is undertaken (76).

In patients greater than 32 weeks gestation or in lower gestational ages in the presence of fetal pulmonary maturity, delivery of the fetus is usually the optimal therapy. In patients with pulmonary immaturity or gestational ages less than 32 weeks, conservative therapy can be undertaken. Requirements for this form of therapy include the absence of fetal compromise on antenatal testing and stable or improving hematologic, liver, and CNS parameters. Increasing amounts of proteinuria in the absence of other deteriorating maternal or fetal parameters are not an indication for delivery in very early gestational ages. Periodic assessment of maternal and fetal well-being are the cornerstones of conservative therapy. This is usually best accomplished in a tertiary care perinatal center in a maternal fetal intensive care environment. Unless these principles are followed, disastrous maternal and fetal outcomes may result.

In the unusual case of onset of severe preeclampsia at gestational ages less than 24 weeks, maternal risks for continuation of pregnancy usually outweigh the potential for fetal benefit. At these low gestational ages, sufficient time gain in utero to allow enhanced fetal survival is unusual. Termination of pregnancy is chosen by many women faced with this choice. Termination can be accomplished with prostaglandin $E_2$ suppositories. We have encouraged the induction of labor be preceded by lethal potassium chloride (KCL) injection of the fetal umbilical cord to prevent the delivery of a liveborn but asphyxiated fetus, which presents a no-win ethical dilemma for obstetric and pediatric management.

### *Expansion of Plasma Volume*

The observation that the plasma volume is reduced has caused much debate in the obstetric literature. The controversy revolves around the possible treatment implications of this observation. The major debate centers on whether volume infusion has a beneficial or potentially adverse effect in preeclampsia. Some observers maintain that slightly reduced blood volume has no hemodynamic significance (77). They feel that reduced volume is "merely fitting a contracted vascular bed. Volume infusion in this instance will result in vascular overload with resultant cardiac failure and pulmonary edema."

A number of recent studies have questioned this traditional concept. One study showed that volume infusion with colloidal fluids was associated with a movement of fluid from the extravascular extracellular space to the intravascular space. Associated with this finding was a reduction in measured mean arterial pressure (78). These acute volume loads resulted in a mild pressure reduction for only short periods (2 to 3 days).

Expansion of the plasma volume is an important factor for fetal growth (79). Intravenous volume infusion could not be expected to have an influence on fetal growth unless given repeatedly over a number of weeks. There would appear to be logistic and cost factors that would weigh against this approach. Nonselective B-blockade with oxyprenolol has been shown to be associated with an increased plasma volume (80,81). Treatment with $\alpha$-methyldopa was not associated with a similar expansion in plasma volume. However, many of the patients in this study were multiparous and probably had chronic hypertension, not preeclampsia.

### *Control of Blood Pressure*

These studies suggest that pharmacologic control of blood pressure with B-blockade can allow plasma volume expansion and result in improved fetal growth. Previous case reports have suggested impaired fetal growth with B-receptor blockade with propranolol (82,83). Most investigators now feel that these initial case reports were examples of the disease process (hypertension) affecting fetal growth rather than a separate drug effect. Therapy with selective B-1 blockade with a drug such as metoprolol or atenolol has not been hazardous to fetal growth.

These new observations are consistent with what is known regarding cardiovascular physiology and the control of arterial blood pressure during pregnancy.

A major unanswered question in this regard involves attempted long-term conservative treatment. Traditional teaching regarding pregnancy-induced hypertension maintains that while antihypertensive medications may control the blood pressure, major end-organ damage will still progress. Thus, fetal and maternal metabolic aberrations may still occur despite a well-controlled blood pressure. This was challenged by Rubin in 1983 (84). He did a randomized controlled study of pregnancy-induced hypertension remote from term in previously normotensive patients. He found a significant reduction in the development of new proteinuria and fewer patients with accelerated hypertension requiring delivery. Probably because of these observations, the only infants developing respiratory distress syndrome were in the placebo control group. The most significant finding was the 80% incidence of hospital readmission among the control group (33/39) compared to only 40% of the treated group (16/40).

In another study, Sibai used labetolol, a combination α-blocker and ß-blocker, in a study design similar to Rubin's (85). However, unlike atenolol, which lowers blood pressure by reducing cardiac output, the main cardiovascular effect of labetolol is reduction in systemic vascular resistance. He was unable to show any significant improvement in perinatal outcome with the use of labetolol to control mild hypertension remote from term. The actual place of long-term antihypertensive therapy in patients with preeclampsia is yet to be clearly defined.

The arteries, arterioles, and capillaries exert a major influence on the total peripheral resistance. They are a low-compliance system. The veins are a high-compliance system and contain 60 to 70% of the total blood volume at low pressures. Vasomotor tone in the two systems can vary independently, and there can be vasoconstriction in the resistance vessel without affecting the capacitance vessels (86). It is possible for the venous system to be underfilled at the time the arterial system is vasoconstricted. The traditional concept that the blood volume reduction in preeclampsia reflects a reduced vascular capacity may not be correct.

## Management of Eclampsia

The pregnant patient who suffers one or more seizures in the preeclamptic phase is considered to be an eclamptic patient as of that time. A seizure may be short-lived and minor, but is often a major episode and of a severe, life-threatening nature. The occurrence of seizures in this clinical setting increases the maternal and fetal mortality by tenfold (87). Outcome in this instance closely parallels the place in which the seizure occurs. Out-of-hospital seizures are more likely to be recurrent due to lack of medical attention, and the fetal and maternal outcome is usually poorer than in an in-hospital seizure. The patient, after such an episode, obviously must have CNS monitoring and baseline evaluation by a team of physicians including, at a minimum, neurologist, obstetrician who is taking care of the patient, and the anesthesiologist who will be involved in pain relief and/or anesthesia for the imminent delivery by cesarean section, if so chosen. After the seizure has ended, the patient needs to be monitored in an intensive care setting. She needs to have careful monitoring of intravenous fluids, monitoring of blood pressure, heart rate, and ventilation status by some type of saturation monitor.

Antepartum cardiovascular studies should be completed according to their indication. At times, there can be electrolyte disturbances, and at times there can be respiratory acidosis and/or superimposed metabolic acidosis, which may need to be detected, diagnosed, and treated within a short period of time to maintain the health and well-being of the patient. In addition, other organs such as the liver need to be evaluated and the hematologic system needs to be carefully evaluated. Because the description of the HELLP (Haemolysis, Elevated Liver and Low Platelets) syndrome is associated with eclampsia, it has been recognized that serious problems occur in regard to platelets, fibrinogen, and electrolytes, in addition to those problems that occur because of ventilatory insufficiency, which affects arterial blood gas values.

### *Role of Magnesium Sulfate*

Magnesium sulfate has been used for decades to prevent eclamptic seizures in preeclamptic patients. Standard therapy included a 4-gram intravenous loading dose and a 2-gram per hour maintenance dose as long as patients had adequate renal function to produce 150 ml every 4 hours. It is common for magnesium levels to be monitored periodically, but this is probably not necessary, as an absent patellar reflex provides a good bioassay of toxicity (7 to 10 mEq/L). Naturally, careful monitoring of the patient's reflexes and respiratory status is important when administration of intravenous magnesium is considered. The use of magnesium sulfate to prevent seizures has caused significant controversy among internists and other nonobstetrical physicians because it is not regarded as a central-acting anticonvulsant and because of its slow passage across the blood-brain barrier. There is widespread enthusiasm in the USA for its use based on substantial empirical observation. Recently, controlled trials of magnesium versus other agents in patients experiencing a prior eclamptic seizure have been conducted. One study showed a clear advantage of magnesium as opposed to hydontoin (88). The other showed equivalent results of both magnesium and diazepam (89). Table 25–2 shows

**Table 25–2.** Seizure Prevention: Comparison of Seizure Rates with Specific Agents

| Agent Used | Researcher | Seizure Frequency | # Treated/ # Seized |
|---|---|---|---|
| MgSO4 | Sibai | 16% (11/67) | |
| MgSO4 | Crowther | 21% (5/24) | 16% (16/102) |
| MgSO4 | Dommisse | 0% (0/11) | |
| Diazepam | Crowther | 26% (7/27) | |
| Phenytoin | Dommisse | 36% (4/11) | |
| Phenytoin | Coyaji | 36% (12/33) | |

**Table 25–3.** Seizure Prevention: Incidence of Seizures Over Time

| Institution | Year | Seizure Frequency | # Treated/ # Seized |
|---|---|---|---|
| 7 East Coast Hosp | 1937–40 | 3.6% | (3417/124) |
| 7 East Coast Hosp | 1947–50 | 1.9% | (4748/90) |
| Univ. Tennessee | 1977–80 | 0.4% | (1870/8) |
| Univ. Washington | 1980–90 | 0.2% | (1050/2) |

(Modified from Dieckmann WJ: Incidence of eclampsia and other toxemias. *In* Toxemias of Pregnancy. St. Louis, C.V. Mosby, 1952, pp. 32–57. Sibai BM, McCubbin JH, Anderson GD, et al: Eclampsia. I: Observation from 67 recent cases. Obstet. Gynecol. 58:608, 1981; Benedetti T, unpublished data, 1992.)

a comparison of the recurrent seizure rates in recent clinical publications. It would appear that the newer agents offer no significant advantage over magnesium in preventing recurrent seizures.

It is now nearly impossible to study the prevention of primary seizures because of the low frequency of eclamptic seizures in modern day obstetrics. Table 25–3 shows the incidence of eclampsia over time, as reported in the literature. The early reports were of untreated patients or patients treated with sedation and quiet observation. Recent studies from Sibai (90) and Benedetti (Benedetti TJ: Unpublished data) show the risk of eclampsia in patients treated with standard doses of magnesium to be on the order of 0.2 to 0.4%. Clinical trials showing an improvement in outcome would require thousands of patients and are not likely to be conducted because of the high cost and the general good outcome for both mother and fetus associated with magnesium use.

### *Clinical Management*

Over the decades, certain principles have become apparent as instrumental in reducing maternal and fetal compromise from eclamptic seizures. These principles are:

1. Do not attempt delivery for the usual fetal bradycardia that accompanies a maternal seizure. Allow the fetus to self-resuscitate after the cessation of the seizure. In the absence of placental abruption, the fetal heart rate will return to normal within 10 minutes.
2. Protect the maternal airway and protect against the patient from biting or swallowing her tongue, while instituting immediately some type of oxygenation and ventilation. This is best done with an oral airway. Use of tongue blades can lead to dental damage and stimulate gag reflex, resulting in vomiting and aspiration.
3. Administer an anticonvulsant. If the patient has not received magnesium sulfate previously, a 4- to 6-gram loading dose should be given over 15 to 20 minutes. If the patient has previously received magnesium sulfate, a level should be drawn and another 2 grams given intravenously. No other form of anticonvulsant has been shown to be superior to magnesium sulfate in abolishing recurrent eclamptic seizures. If the patient suffers a third seizure despite magnesium bolus therapy, then a short-acting barbiturate such as amobarbital can be used.
4. In general, acute anticonvulsant therapy during a maternal seizure is unnecessary and potentially harmful. By the time the drug is at the bedside, the usual eclamptic seizure has ended. In the unusual event of prolonged seizures or status, a short-acting barbiturate may be titrated to control the seizure. To minimize aspiration, preparation should then be made for endotracheal intubation and ventilatory support.
5. Prevent maternal injury as a result of excessive muscular contractions or prevention of anoxia. If the patient is in bed, the side rails should be raised to prevent a fall.
6. Monitor the magnesium sulfate levels and/or effects on the patient so that the patient may receive optimal levels for relief of convulsions while at the same time not having excessive amounts of magnesium sulfate administered; and
7. Identify and correct any maternal acidosis, either respiratory or metabolic, by use of blood gas determination, institution of oxygenation, ventilation, and use of intravenous buffering solutions to counteract immediate metabolic acidosis.

After an eclamptic episode, a decision needs to be made aggressively as soon as possible for management of the patient. Generally speaking, after control of maternal convulsions, the sooner the delivery, the better the patient's chance of recovery. Although many attempts at setting time limits for delivery of the fetus have been entertained, each patient should be evaluated individually. However, delivery should be imminent, either by a shortened labor by induction of oxytocin or by abdominal delivery by cesarean section. Fetal heart rate and uterine contraction monitoring are obvious necessities. Often during this period of time, the fetus shows abnormal heart rate tracings, including bradycardia and periodic changes such as late deceleration, which are indicative of some placental deficiency. This may at times precipitate the use of the abdominal delivery, chosen over continued induction, especially if the latter is not going well from the standpoint of progressive cervical dilatation. Fetal outcome can be quite good; however, the mother's condition is always guarded. With convulsions often come massive injuries in regard to the CNS, including intracranial bleeding, hypertensive signs such as cerebral edema, and even, in some, anoxia.

As mentioned before, the convulsions associated with the eclamptic patient are certainly life-threatening to the patient. Convulsions are to be avoided at all cost. Certainly, superimposed complications such as pulmonary edema can also occur with severe hypoxia, followed by generalized anoxia and even asphyxia. In the case of persistent maternal coma (greater than 6 hours) after seizures, the most intensive, world-experienced advocates deliver by cesarean section unless vaginal delivery is imminent (91). This policy has resulted in an improved outcome when compared to past experience by the same authors. Whether improved outcome is due to other improvements in care of early delivery is unclear, its causes will probably never be subjected to a controlled trial. Other important elements of such rare patients with persistent coma are radiologic brain imaging (CT or MRI) and close attention to fluid status to limit the cerebral edema that is often present. On occasion, intracranial pressure monitoring to optimize cerebral perfusion may be necessary.

## ANESTHETIC MANAGEMENT

### General Remarks

Anesthetic management of the patient with preeclampsia remains controversial in the early 1990s. However, most of the controversy lies with anesthetic management of cesarean section, not with anesthetic management of labor and delivery as it was in the 1970s and early 1980s. By the late 1980s, the more conservative attitudes in obstetrics and anesthesia were counter-balanced by the minimal effect upon blood pressure of the mother due to significant improvements in labor epidural management. Most of these improvements had to do with the reduced maternal hazard directly related to the use of continuous analgesia delivery methods with minimal local anesthetic and opioid combinations.

The reason for the continuous controversy in anesthetic management for cesarean section has to do with the continued hypotensive hazard associated with the T-4 level needed for incision and delivery during cesarean section. Some authors adamantly believe conduction anesthesia is contraindicated due to fetal compromise (92). In fact, this one criticism of regional anesthesia for cesarean section, namely hypotension, the lack of it with general anesthesia, and the touted safety of the latter may have given a false sense of security in regard to general anesthesia (93). On the other hand, the safety of regional anesthesia is also attested to by literature documentation of both maternal and fetal safety (63,94).

### Management for Labor and Vaginal Delivery

#### *Maternal Status Abnormal/Fetal Status Normal*

In this scenario, the mother carries a diagnosis of preeclampsia but has no significant associated problems such as reduced extracellular volume in which her blood pressure is elevated slightly, however consistent with a diagnosis of mild eclampsia, but she has no hyper-reflexia. In this case, with no evidence of any fetal compromise whatsoever, one may consider use of regional anesthetic technique such as lumbar epidural for the first stage and use of the same catheter to obtain a sacral block for delivery anesthesia. Another alternative might be lumbar epidural for the first stage followed by caudal epidural for the second stage, or even a saddle block for the second stage. Use of small doses in the beginning with current applications have reduced greatly the sympathetic blockade formerly associated with maternal hypotension and fetal jeopardy.

#### *Maternal Status Abnormal/Fetal Status Abnormal*

In this scenario, there is evidence of some fetal jeopardy, probably associated with some reduction in maternal/fetal perfusion. Again, regional analgesia may be used if careful attention to detail is maintained. This refers specifically to maintenance of maternal intracellular volume, and again, use of minimal doses of local anesthetic such as 8 ml of local anesthetic initially, followed by a continuous dosage of local anesthetic and sufentanil and dilute vasoconstrictive combination. The latter has been used for the past several years and offers several advantages in which there is concern about the fetal status. The chief advantage of this combination is the reduced volume of local anesthetic needed to obtain maternal relief, which reduces also the chances of maternal hypotension during the labor process. If good labor progress is made with gradual cervical dilatation, effacement, and descent, then plans can be considered for analgesia for delivery or the second stage. There are several options possible with pudendal block with or without supplemented $N_2O$, local analgesia with $N_2O$ supplemented caudal analgesia, or again, a saddle block for delivery analgesia.

It must be recalled at all times that maternal analgesia in these scenarios *must* afford fetal protection from the most damaging iatrogenic challenge—hypotension—at all costs. Therefore, if the obstetrician/anesthesiologist is not suitably skilled or feels uncomfortable with management of the preeclamptic patient with regional anesthesia, then he/she should opt for the other nonregional-based techniques, which do not carry as great a threat of hypotension.

Finally, in the case of the mother with the fetus in jeopardy, it must be recalled that close attention be paid to monitoring of the fetus throughout the first and second stages, and if at any time a serious fetal threat would become superimposed, then an orderly but facilitated delivery by cesarean section should be considered. The delivery by cesarean section of the distressed fetus will be discussed later in "Management for Cesarean Section—Emergency Status," which follows "Elective Status," below.

### Management for Cesarean Section—Elective Status

As with other aspects of preeclampsia, there is controversy regarding appropriate anesthetic management of affected patients. Pritchard feels that conduction anesthesia is contraindicated because of the risk of maternal hypotension and subsequent fetal compromise (92). He reports using general anesthesia for cesarean section and narcotic analgesic for labor in 154 patients with preeclampsia/eclampsia; no maternal mortality among these patients would appear to speak for the safety of this method of anesthesia (93). There are many studies demonstrating the maternal and fetal safety of carefully conducted epidural anesthesia of preeclampsia (63,94).

The hemodynamic consequences of epidural and general anesthesia have been reported. During tracheal intubation and extubation, there is a significant rise in the mean arterial pressure (45 mm Hg), pulmonary artery pressure (20 mm Hg), and pulmonary artery wedge pressure (20 mm Hg), as shown in Figure 25–19 (94). These elevations may persist for as long as 10 minutes before the

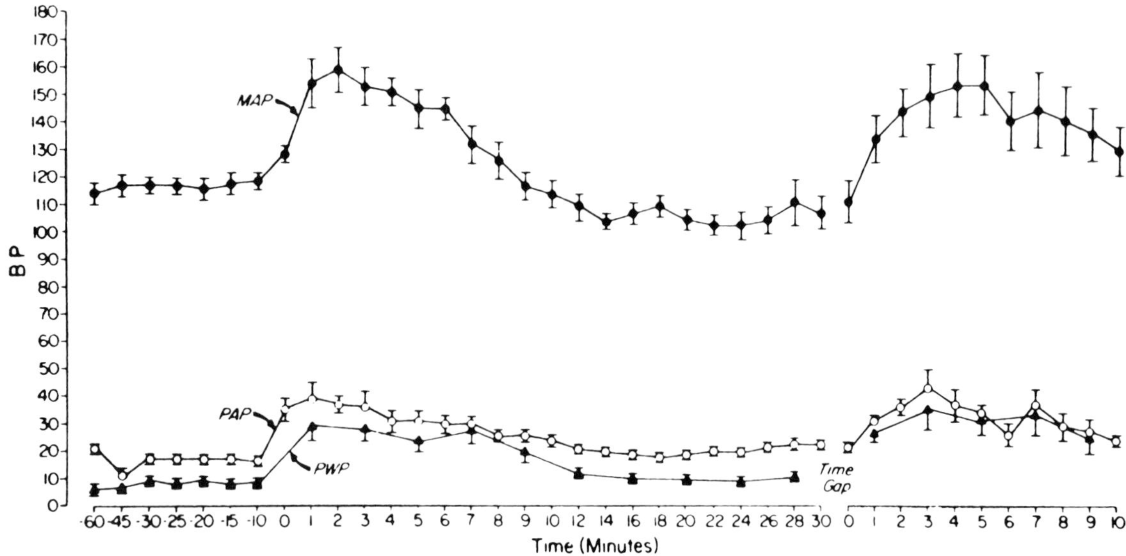


**Fig. 25–19.** Mean arterial pressure (MAP), pulmonary artery pressure (PAP), and pulmonary artery wedge pressure (PAWP) in a patient receiving general anesthesia for cesarean section. Note marked rises during intubation and extubation. (From Hodgkinson R, Husain J, Hayashi R: Systemic and pulmonary blood pressure during cesarean section in parturients with gestational hypertension. Can. Anaesth. Soc. J. 27:389, 1975.)

return to baseline. Such large increases in mean arterial pressure and pulmonary artery pressure may precipitate cerebral hemorrhage, cerebral edema, and pulmonary edema. We have observed acute decreases in pulmonary compliance associated with general anesthesia and tracheal intubation that may be secondary to these rapid increases in pulmonary artery wedge pressure (63). These effects could be altered by the use of deeper general anesthesia, but this could have adverse fetal effects. Another approach would be to use continuous infusion of a long-acting or short-acting antihypertensive prior to the induction of anesthesia. Hydralazine can be used in this instance, and it has been used successfully to limit the hypertensive response in nonpregnant patients during induction before tracheal intubation (95). Hydralazine has the advantage of improving uteroplacental blood flow but is relatively slow in onset compared with the newer antihypertensive agents. Nitroglycerin has been shown to be useful in this instance. Blood pressure is initially reduced with nitroglycerin infusion, and the resultant increase during tracheal intubation simply returns to preintubation baseline. Another agent that has been used to acutely lower blood pressure is trimethaphan (Arfonad). Some have hypothesized that because this drug has a higher molecular weight than nitroglycerine (597 versus 227), it would be less likely to cross the placental barrier (96). However, this theoretical consideration has never been investigated, and most drugs of molecular weight less than 1000 have adequate placental transmission. Nitroprusside also has been used to control episodes of maternal hypertension, but there is a stated theoretical concern regarding fetal cyanide accumulation with longer maternal administration. However, this is not substantiated in the literature. In sheep studies, maternal tachyphylaxis developed at a mean dose of 254 μg/kg/min and 50% of the fetal lambs died. On the basis of these studies, the authors cautioned that nitroprusside should be discontinued if more than 0.5 μg/kg/minute was required for blood pressure control or if maternal tachyphylaxis developed. Intravenous propranolol for blood pressure control just prior to the delivery of the fetus should be avoided because it has been shown to adversely effect fetal transition to extrauterine life (97).

Epidural anesthesia preceded by adequate volume expansion is not associated with a significant negative impact upon hemodynamic parameters (Figure 25–20) (94,98). However, just what constitutes an adequate intravascular volume and how to monitor this is the subject of some debate. Hodgkinson studied severe preeclamptic patients who had previously been treated with magnesium sulfate, hydralazine, and an undescribed amount of intravenous fluid. The patients had an average wedge pressure of 8 mm Hg prior to the induction of epidural anesthesia for cesarean section with either 12 or 20 cc of 0.75% bupivacaine. He observed no significant hemodynamic effects on mean maternal pulmonary artery pressure or on pulmonary artery wedge pressure despite a mean fall in maternal mean arterial pressure of 20 mm Hg (16%) (99). Graham studied 10 preeclamptic patients, most of whom had severe preeclampsia. They administered only 700 cc of crystalloid solution prior to epidural block with either 12 ml of 3% chloroprocaine (vaginal delivery) or chloroprocaine plus 12 ml of 0.5% bupivacaine for cesarean section. They found no change in cardiac output after induction of anesthesia to T-6 level. They did not report maternal blood pressure, nor did they report pulmonary artery pressures. They reported good Apgar scores and no signs of fetal distress (36). Newsome reported on 11 patients with severe preeclampsia in whom epidural anesthesia was used. Patients received up

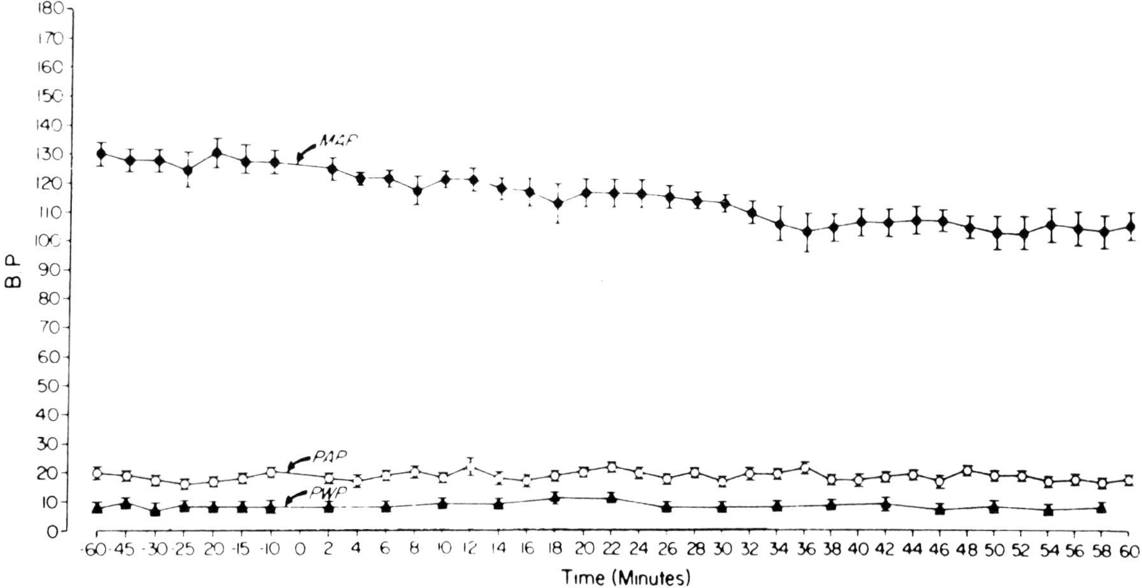


**Fig. 25–20.** Mean arterial pressure (MAP), pulmonary artery pressure (PAP), and pulmonary artery wedge pressure (PAWP) in a patient undergoing cesarean section under epidural anesthesia. (From Hodgkinson R, Husain J, Hayashi R: Systemic and pulmonary blood pressure during cesarean section in parturients with gestational hypertension. Can. Anaesth. Soc. J. 27:389, 1975.)

to 1000 cc of Ringers lactate to achieve a pulmonary artery wedge pressure of 8 to 12 mm Hg. In the vaginally delivered patients, 5 to 10 ml of 0.125% bupivacaine was used and in the cesarean section patients, 18 to 25 ml of 0.5% bupivacaine was used. There was no significant change in cardiac index, pulmonary artery wedge pressure, or mean pulmonary artery (PA) pressure after anesthesia, but there was a significant drop in maternal mean arterial pressure from 120 mm Hg to 97 mm Hg. No mention was made of fetal heart rate changes, but all Apgar scores were reported to be greater than 8 at 5 minutes (98).

These relatively small amounts of preanesthetic fluids are in sharp contrast to the report of Joyce, et al (100). Unfortunately, this work, although widely quoted, has never withstood peer review and is published only in abstract form. It advocates large amounts of fluid before epidural anesthesia, the volumes of which are proportional to the maternal blood pressure. These volumes ranged from 1000 cc of crystalloid to 2 liters of crystalloid plus 750 cc of plasminate. We are reluctant to give large saline loads to patients with preeclampsia because of the reported propensity for the saline to quickly exit from the intravascular space. We have reported previously three patients in whom massive cerebral edema was associated with large volume infusions of crystalloid fluids (101). In a similar vein, we view the use of large volumes of colloid solution as equally hazardous in the development of postpartum pulmonary edema (51). The optimal solution to this problem seems to be a slow onset regional anesthetic that can be conducted with a modest preload with crystalloid solution. This is usually able to be accomplished in severe preeclamptics without resorting to more than 2000 cc of crystalloid and usually without the use of colloidal solutions.

Caution must be used with conduction anesthesia, however, in patients with severe preeclampsia/eclampsia. Thrombocytopenia is a frequent occurrence in the severe forms of the disease, and clinically significant bleeding is uncommon in patients with preeclampsia, despite altered coagulation studies, unless there is evidence of placental abruption. However, when the platelet count is reduced, some anesthesiologists are reluctant to perform lumbar epidural anesthesia. Recent data regarding modest thrombocytopenia in normal patients have shown that epidural anesthesia is probably administered to patients every day with platelet counts of 90,000 to 150,000 (102). No adverse effects were seen in either hypertensive or normotensive patients receiving epidural anesthesia when the platelet count was within this range. The exact lower limit of platelet counts that allow safe conduction anesthesia is unknown. There is only one case report in the literature alluding to bleeding in the epidural space in a preeclamptic who had conduction anesthesia. In this case, the mother had multiple end-organ dysfunction and the outcome was not described (103).

Bleeding times have been used to identify patients who could safely tolerate epidural anesthesia. However, it has been shown that bleeding time can be abnormal in preeclamptic patients regardless of the absolute platelet count (104). Lumbar epidural anesthesia has been performed in patients with abnormal bleeding times but normal platelet counts without complication (105). The bleeding time may be too sensitive to provide clinically useful information regarding patients at risk from bleeding into the epidural space. To date, there have been no reported cases of bleeding complications after lumbar epidural anesthesia in patients with severe preeclampsia. The appropriate place for the bleeding time in selecting patients for lumbar epidural anesthesia is still unclear.

**Table 25–4.** Serum Magnesium Levels and Clinical Side Effects

| | Serum Magnesium Levels | |
|---|---|---|
| | mEq/liter | mg/100 cc |
| Term pregnancy | 1.24 to 1.65 | 1.5 to 2.0 |
| Therapeutic | 4 to 7 | 5.0 to 8.5 |
| Loss of tendon reflex | 7 to 10 | 8.5 to 12.0 |
| Respiratory depression | 15 | 18 |
| Cardiac arrest | 30 | 36 |

Intravenous or intramuscular magnesium sulfate is usually used for seizure control in patients with preeclampsia. Although the exact mechanism is still not understood, enormous clinical experience with this medication supports its use for prophylaxis and treatment of eclamptic convulsions. Intravenous therapy is usually accomplished with a loading dose of 4 grams over 20 minutes followed by a continuous infusion of 1 to 3 g/hour, depending on renal function and urine output. Table 25–4 lists the therapeutic and toxic ranges of this medication. Magnesium sulfate therapy results initially in a transient afterload reduction but compensatory tachycardia soon restores blood pressure to preinfusion levels. It is not an effective antihypertensive medication.

Magnesium inhibits the presynaptic calcium-facilitated transmitter release at the neuromuscular junction. Patients receiving magnesium sulfate are more sensitive to neuromuscular blocking drugs (106). When general anesthesia is required, reduced dosages of neuromuscular blocking drugs should be used. Careful attention to the degree of motor blockade is necessary to avoid overdosage. Because many anesthetic agents have antihypertensive and anticonvulsant properties, some anesthesiologists have chosen to discontinue magnesium therapy intraoperatively and to resume therapy just prior to recovery. If this strategy is used, care should be taken to remember to resume magnesium therapy after delivery as a significant number of eclamptic seizures take place in the postpartum period. Magnesium sulfate therapy is usually continued for 24 hours after delivery. However, in mild cases, therapy may be discontinued after 12 hours should blood pressure return to normal and a good diuresis apparent. In a similar manner, unusually severe cases of preeclampsia may require 36 to 48 hours of therapy in the puerperium.

In summary, anesthesia for elective cesarean section presents an opportunity for development of unique interactions between the anesthesiologist and the mother. The opportunity offers a unique chance for the anesthesiologist to educate the patient. This education can begin with the discussion about the inherent risks of general anesthesia, which most all patients are uninformed about. Such discussion can also serve to point out and identify the benefits of regional anesthesia to both the mother and baby. It is regrettable that the early days of regional analgesia for cesarean section began with a negative rather than a positive history. Most of this early negative history was due to the poor or inadequate sterilization of needles and the resultant infections; some of these infections were due to chemical meningitis caused by poor cleansing of the needles during processing for reuse over and over again. This negative history focuses primarily on the 1950s and 1960s. In the latter 1960s and 1970s, the focus was again negative, but this time centered around the residual effect of the regional anesthetic upon the newborn in the first 24 to 48 hours. There was great emphasis placed upon the development of sensitive enough indicators so that repeatable evaluations could be made to compare various anesthetic agents one against the other. Such work helped to emphasize the point that the only acceptable regional anesthetic was the one that did not have significant depressive or residual depressive effects upon the neonate. This argument was especially active in the area of anesthesia for cesarean section for patients with preeclampsia. In preeclampsia, the major point made was that the fetus in utero was a captive of his/her environment and that regional anesthesia meant decreased uteroplacental blood flow with possible serious side effects for the fetus. Naturally, more focus was centered upon cesarean section anesthesia because a large sympathetic block meant more harm to the fetus due to large falls in maternal blood pressure. There were several reports of bad fetal effects due to such consequences, and these were held as examples of how bad the selection of regional anesthesia could be for preeclampsia. Of course there is no argument with the fact that hypotension of a severe or prolonged nature can have significant deleterious effects upon the fetus and neonate. On the other hand, there must also be recognition that some instances of faulty administration of general anesthesia also has caused serious maternal and fetal effects. This section will discuss the options available to the practitioner in cases of preeclampsia when cesarean section is indicated.

### *Regional Anesthesia*

This form of anesthesia provides the safest form of anesthesia for the mother because it involves only the administration of a local anesthetic to the area of the spinal cord, thereby blocking sensory input from the abdominal area. As mentioned above, there can be instances of untoward reactions to regional anesthesia, including the three most common ones: hypotension, convulsions due to CNS toxic effect, and respiratory arrest. These complications are typical of lumbar epidural block, while total spinal with shock and respiratory arrest are more typical of spinal block. In a search of the literature for the incidence of complications of epidural and spinal block for the general population, there appears to be a consensus that epidural has considerably lower complication rates than spinal (107). For those with preeclampsia, Newsome, et al found that lumbar epidural anesthesia did not significantly alter the incidence of complications (98). While the authors realize it is important to have general knowledge of the percentage of errors associated with various techniques, they also appreciate that decisions on given techniques for given situations must be highly individualized and that the rule always must be safety of the mother and baby before all else.

In this regard, the application of regional anesthesia to patients with preeclampsia for cesarean section can be considered a reasonable option due to the fact that these specific instances are of an elective nature and that means for that the most part the fetus is not adjudged to be in jeopardy. Therefore, if the mother has mild or moderate preeclampsia with no evidence of fetal compromise, lumbar epidural can and should be considered an option. In such cases, two regional techniques could be considered, namely, lumbar epidural or continuous spinal anesthesia. In lumbar epidural, the advantage is placement of the catheter early at a convenient time with test doses and therapeutic doses injected only when surgery is eminent. The safety in regard to epidural lies in the intermittent spaced injections, which means that there is a greatly reduced incidence of CNS toxic convulsions and inadvertent subarachnoid block. Hence, there is also a reduced opportunity for fetal complications, including subjection to insufficient uteroplacental blood flow, and, thus, hypoxemia. In situations of preeclampsia, there has always been great concern that the baseline condition consist of a reduced uteroplacental reserve, thus less of a fall in maternal blood pressure could be tolerated and for a shorter period of time. The use of continuous spinal technique, which was really introduced in 1898 by Dr. Bier, is undergoing a new surge in popularity, and may actually offer the ideal method of control and safety for the mother and fetus/neonate because of: (1) compartmentalization effect with minimal or no drug effect on the fetus due to the fact that the local anesthetic does not enter the venous system; and (2) use of fractionated, spaced injections of local anesthetic with all the advantages enumerated in regard to epidural spaced injections mentioned above. It would appear that studies in the near future will address the issue of advantages and disadvantages of continuous spinal anesthesia in regard to its application in preeclampsia. Suffice it to say that the methods mentioned are valid, reasonable considerations that should be mentioned and considered in regard to anesthesia for elective cesarean section in the mother with preeclampsia.

## *General Anesthesia*

General anesthesia has always been considered a strong contender as the choice for anesthesia for cesarean section patients with preeclampsia. This has been due primarily to the fact that hypotension was not as much of a threat with this method compared to that with regional anesthesia. Of course, this is not true; in fact, general anesthesia is associated with an increase in maternal blood pressure instead of a decrease, and this is in response to an increased vascular resistance in the face of minimal analgesic conditions. What has not been considered an issue is the serious danger of general anesthesia in regard to failure of the airway, aspiration, and hypoxia and cardiac arrest. For example, even though there are references to situations in which regional analgesia may have been implicated in instances of fetal morbidity, there are no references regarding instances in which airway problems may have been encountered during induction of general anesthesia for cesarean section. This is one of the major problems with general anesthesia today; in spite of many years and studies to predict which patients may have airway difficulties on induction, we are left today without a reliable predictive instrument. This means that any given patient may present with a difficult-to-intubate scenario that may turn into a difficult or even an impossible airway management situation. Coupled with the various changes in respiratory physiology as pointed out in Chapter 2, such a challenge may result in disaster, especially when performed in the even more stressful backdrop of an emergent obstetric problem.

In a situation in which stress, obesity, pregnancy, and a normal airway and easy intubation are put together, the technique of general anesthesia is certainly reliable and effective. The current method of rapid sequence induction with cricoid pressure, quick inflation of an endotracheal tube, and avoidance of positive pressure makes the technique safe for the mother. At the same time, the use of minimal anesthetic drugs for both induction and maintenance of anesthesia also makes the technique safe for the fetus. Since the early 1970s, there have been several articles that attest to the use of general anesthesia in cesarean section. Before this time of general standardization, different anesthesiologists would often use general anesthesia much the same way they did in their surgical patients, and this often meant the use of major inhalation anesthetics, such as cyclopropane, halothane, and fluroxene, which were popular at that time. Naturally, all of these gases passed quickly from the mother to the fetal compartment, and thus resulted in fetal depression in relation to the degree of usage of the general anesthetic. It was only by restriction of the use of potent anesthetics and use of minimal dosages of all drugs in relation to both induction and maintenance that comparable neonatal conditions were shown between regional anesthesia and general anesthesia (108,109). The problem now has become that the technique is perfected from the viewpoint of minimization of fetal depression, from where it was considered that general anesthesia be used in many situations for its rapidity and seemingly easy application. What was not factored into the situation of cesarean section choice were those problems of difficult-to-predict and manage airway crises. As mentioned earlier, most of these isolated incidents were considered to be just that, i.e., isolated instances, and thus were not reported in those days before better communication of problems in the area of obstetric anesthesiology. It would appear, then, that even in situations of mild to moderate preeclampsia that the anesthetic technique of choice is regional anesthesia should no evidence of fetal compromise be evident. In an elective cesarean section situation with some evidence of fetal compromise, one should consider use of general anesthesia to avoid any fear of hypotension. Of course, one of the very important inputs in regard to the final decision must be the mother's choice. If she is adamant about being awake and being able to experience the interaction and bonding between mother and baby, then every possibility of regional anesthesia should be given.

## Management for Cesarean Section—Emergency Status

In this scenario, the stage is clearly set for expeditious delivery. It is the condition that often precipitates both maternal and fetal morbidity and even mortality. Often the mother's status is unchanged except for situations of abruptio placenta or placenta previa, in which even maternal health and welfare is threatened. One must remember that the latter is superimposed upon the preeclamptic state, so even a greater hazard exists. Even though there is general distaste for the use of general anesthesia in obstetrics for cesarean section, this may be one of those instances in which general anesthesia could provide: (1) an expeditious delivery; and (2) anesthetic state without risked hypotension.

However, in an absolute emergency in which the obstetrician announces that a cesarean section must be performed on an emergency basis to save the life of the baby, the anesthesiologist, when forced with a precarious situation such as (1) a morbid obese patient or (2) an unstable maternal cardiovascular status, may declare that a general anesthetic may itself cause maternal mortality and may insist on a delivery under local anesthesia. The latter, of course, is not ideal, takes a longer time for delivery, results in less than ideal maternal analgesia, and results in less than ideal surgical conditions; yet it is preferred over a situation in which the mother's life may be at a significant hazard.

To prevent such a situation, the preeclamptic obese patient may be managed in early labor with placement of a subarachnoid catheter. In the declared emergency situation, the anesthesiologist could then consider use of that catheter with small injections of local anesthetic until adequate analgesia exists for surgical incision. This method would offer a viable alternative for anesthesia in a compromised condition in which the anesthesiologist could feel reasonable maternal protection was afforded. It must be appreciated that the foregoing scenario is one of the most difficult of all clinical challenges. It touches on the very important aspect of the importance of decision making in crisis conditions. And it involves the crucial judgment of protection of the life of the mother versus the life of the unborn fetus.

One of the better methods of assuring improved management of difficult problems in obstetrics such as the one just outlined is to have regular communication sessions established between obstetricians and anesthesiologists with the prime purpose to identify all high-risk patients such as the ones mentioned. In this way, the patients could be tracked and their appearance in the obstetric wards or antepartum areas identified. As patients are identified, their management could be discussed and planned in some logical fashion. This will serve to reduce some of the unplanned and unexpected high-risk patients early in the morning.

Of course, the final decision in regard to the anesthetic lies in the hands of the anesthesiologist who must make the decision on the basis of the problem presented, the stress of the moment, and his/her own comfortability and ability. What must be emphasized is the close communication and understanding that must exist between the obstetrician and anesthesiologist. Both are interested in the welfare of their patient. Sometimes, however, the obstetrician may become focused upon the urgency for operative delivery and not recognize the risk to the mother, which the anesthesiologist must point out and protect. It is hoped that more obstetric programs will teach their residents to operate under local anesthesia so that they will develop confidence and competence in the method. In the final analysis, successful management of the preeclamptic mother who is in need of emergency cesarean section is really the combined effort of both key medical team members at this time—the anesthesiologist and the obstetrician. Naturally, soon the pediatrician also joins the team to make it a triple team effort on behalf of the mother and baby. No where in medicine is there more satisfaction when an emergency has been successfully managed and the result is good for both mother and baby. There is a great sense of relief and good feelings of satisfaction that a difficult situation and challenge has been met and handled to the best of everyone's capabilities. On the other hand, there is no more depressing situation than that in which the life of the mother or baby is lost due to such an emergency. A bad effect may occur despite all best efforts of everyone involved. In both situations, it is best to have a review of the problems encountered, the management instituted, and the outcomes monitored so that difficult cases such as these can build on better management philosophies each time.

## Postpartum Anesthetic Considerations

The revolution in thinking about and providing for better care in the postsurgical period came about in the 1980s and early 1990s. The same consideration was naturally transferred to pain relief for the parturient after cesarean section. In many centers, the birth and development of acute pain services really began in the postpartum wards. It became a natural extension of care to leave an epidural catheter in place to administer narcotics for pain relief. The problems that soon developed, however, caused concern about the validity of providing such pain relief due to the complications which developed, such as pruritis and bladder atony. Bladder atony presented the biggest problem, as postpartum stays were reduced to only 3 to 4 days at most and because inability to void meant more diagnostic problems for the obstetrician and labor-intensive care for the nurses. Thankfully, several centers began to use different combinations of narcotics that would minimize those complications. This was fortunate because not only did the patient get pain relief to an excellent degree, but she also did not suffer anywhere near the problems with bladder atony and pruritus.

At the same time that the epidural catheter was used for pain relief, the PCA or patient controlled analgesia method was also popular. It provided the patient with pain relief less effective than that with epidural, but the patients were not unhappy because they did not have a comparative scale against which they could judge their degree of relief. Typical examples of pain relief regimens for both the PCA method and the epidural method are

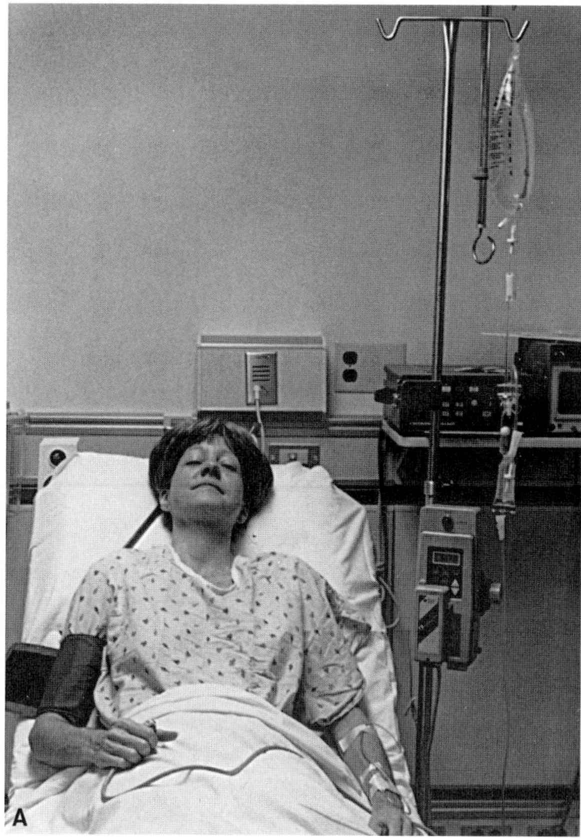


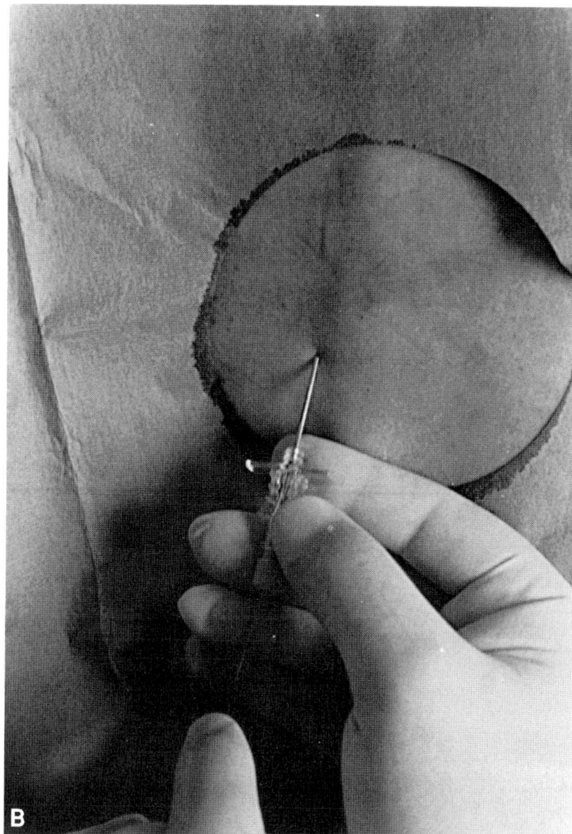


**Fig. 25–21.** Examples of pain relief regimens for **(A)** the PCA method and **(B)** the epidural method. (From The Ohio State University, Department of Anesthesiology, 1992.)

shown in Figure 25–21. The parturient has many stresses on her just after delivery: she must assume the role of mother to her newly born child; she must hold court for everyone who comes to visit and pay regards to her relatives, her friends, and her newborn. In addition, she must recover from an operative procedure and recoup a tremendous amount of lost energy. Therefore, it is very beneficial to have a pain relief method that can help to make this aspect of the mother's recovery easier and more expedient.

## REFERENCES


1. MacGillivray I: Some observations on the incidence of preeclampsia. J. Obstet. Gynaecol. Br. Emp. 65:536–539, 1958.
2. Kaunitz AM, Hughes JM, Grimes DA, Smith JC, et al: Causes of maternal mortality in the United States. Obstet. Gynecol. 65:605–612, 1985.
3. Hibbard LT: Maternal mortality due to acute toxemia. Obstet. Gynecol. 42:263–270, 1973.
4. Benedetti TJ, Starzyk P, Frost F: Maternal deaths in Washington State. Obstet. Gynecol. 66:99–101, 1985.
5. Brazy JF, Grimm JK, Little VA: Neonatal manifestations of severe maternal hypertension occurring before the thirty-sixth week of pregnancy. J. Ped. 100:265–271, 1982.
6. Cunningham FG, MacDonald PC, Gant NF: Williams Obstetrics. 18th Ed., East Norwalk, Appleton & Lange, 1989.
7. Shnider SM, Levinson G: Anesthesia for Obstetrics. 3rd Ed., Baltimore, Williams & Wilkins, 1993.
8. Gabbe SG, Niebyl JR, Simpson JL: Obstetrics: Normal & Problem Pregnancies. 2nd Ed., New York, Churchill Livingstone, 1991.
9. Gant NF, Daley GL, Chand S, Whalley PJ, et al: A study of angiotensin II pressor response throughout primigravid pregnancy. J. Clin. Invest. 52:2682, 1973.
10. Gant NF, Worley RJ, Whalley PJ, Crosby UD, et al: A clinical test useful for predicting the development of acute hypertension of pregnancy. Am. J. Obstet. Gynecol. 120:1, 1974.
11. Chesley L: History and epidemiology of preeclampsia-eclampsia. Clin. Ob. Gyn. 27:801–820, 1984.
12. Rochat RW, Koonin LM, Atrash HK, Jewett JF: The maternal mortality collaborative: maternal mortality in the United States. Report from the maternal mortality collaborative 72:91, 1988.
13. Eastman NJ, Hellman LM: Williams Obstetrics. 13th Ed., New York, Appleton-Century-Crofts, 1966.
14. Levitt MF, Altchek A: Hypertension and toxemia of pregnancy. *In* Medical, Surgical, and Gynecological Complications of Pregnancy. Edited by JJ Rovinsky, EF Guttmacher. Baltimore, The Williams & Wilkins Co., 1960.
15. Greenhill JP: Obstetrics. 13th Ed. Philadelphia, W.B. Saunders Co., 1965.
16. Clough WS: The young primipara. Obstet. Gynecol. 12: 373, 1958.
17. Gemmell AA, Logan WPD, Benjamin B: The incidence of toxaemia. J. Obstet. Gynaecol. Brit. Emp. 61:458, 1954.
18. Koonin LM, Atrash HK, Rochat RW, Smith JC: Maternal mortality surveillance U.S. 1980–85. MMWR CDC Surveill. Sum. 37:19, 1988.

19. Reiss RE, O'Shaughnessy RW, Quilligan TJ, Zuspan FP: Retrospective comparison of blood pressure course during preeclamptic and matched control pregnancies. Am. J.Obstet. Gynecol. 156:894–898, 1987.
20. Moutquin JM, Rainville C, Giroux L, Raynauld P, et al: A prospective study of blood pressure in pregnancy. Prediction of preeclampsia. Am. J.Obstet. Gynecol. 151:191–6, 1985.
21. Gant NF, Daley GL, Chand S, Whalley PJ, et al: A study of angiotension II pressor response throughout primigravid pregnancy. J. Clin. Invest. 52:2682–2689, 1973.
22. Gant NF, Madden JD, Siiteri PK, MacDonald PC: Fetal-placental maternal interrelationships: a sequential study of the metabolism of dehydroisoandrosterone sulfate in primigravid pregnancy. Excerpta Medica 273:1026–1031, 1972.
23. Lockwood CJ, Peters JH: Increased plasma levels of EDT cellular fibronectin precede the clinical signs of preeclampsia. Am. J.Obstet. Gynecol. 162:358–362, 1990.
24. Roberts JM, Taylor RN, Nusci TJ, Rodgers GM, et al: Preeclampsia: an endothelial cell disorder. Am. J. Obstet. Gynecol. 161:1200–1204, 1989.
25. Friedman SA: Preeclampsia: a review of the role of prostaglandins. Obstet. Gynecol. 71:122–137, 1988.
26. Ylikorkala O, Pekonen F, Viinkka L: Renal Prostacyclin and thromboxane in normotensive and preeclamptic pregnant women and their infants. J. Clin. Endocrinol. Metab. 63: 1307–1312, 1986.
27. Rubin PC, Butters L, Clark DM, Reynolds B, et al: Placebo-controlled trial of atenolol in treatment of pregnancy-associated hypertension. Lancet 1:431–434, 1983.
28. Wallenberg HCS, Dekker GA, Makovitz JW, Rotmans P, et al: Low-dose aspirin prevents pregnancy-induced hypertension and pre-eclampsia in angiotension-sensitive primigravidae. Lancet 1:1–3, 1986.
29. Schiff E, Peleg E, Goldenberg M, Rosenthal T, et al: The use of aspirin to prevent pregnancy-induced hypertension and lower the ratio of thromboxane $A_2$ to prostacyclin in relatively high risk pregnancies. N. Engl. J. Med. 321: 351–356, 1989.
30. Dildy GT, Phelan J, Cotton DB: Complications of pregnancy induced hypertension. *In* Critical Care Medicine. 2nd Ed. Edited by S Clark. Boston, Blackwell Scientific Publications, 1991, pp. 251–279.
31. Easterling TR, Watts DH, Schmucker BC, Benedetti TJ: Measurement of cardiac output during pregnancy: validation of Doppler technique and clinical observations in preeclampsia. Obstet. Gynecol. 69:845, 1987.
32. Lhle BM, Long D, Oats, J: Early onset preeclampsia: recognition of underlying renal disease. Br. Med. J. 294:79, 1987.
33. Groenendijk R, Trimbos MJ, Wallenberg HC: Hemodynamic measurements in preeclampsia: preliminary observations. Am. J.Obstet. Gynecol. 150:232, 1984.
34. Assali NS, Holm L, Parker H: Systemic and regional hemodynamic alterations in toxemia. Circulation 29,30 (Suppl II):53, 1956.
35. Hankins GD, Wendel GD, Cunningham FG, Leveno KJ: Longitudinal evaluation of hemodynamic changes in eclampsia. Am. J.Obstet. Gynecol. 150:506, 1984.
36. Graham C, Goldstein A: Epidural anesthesia and cardiac output in severe preeclamptics. Anaesthesia 53:709, 1980.
37. Cotton DB, Lee W, Huhta JC, Dorman KF: Hemodynamic profile of severe pregnancy induced hypertension. Am. J. Obstet. Gynecol. 158:523, 1988.
38. Benedetti TJ, Cotton DB, Read JC, Miller FC: Hemodynamic observations in severe preeclampsia using a flow directed pulmonary artery catheter. Am. J. Obstet. Gynecol. 136:465, 1980.
39. Benedetti TJ: Pregnancy-induced hypertension. *In* Cardiac Problems in Pregnancy. Edited by H Elkayam, N Gleicher. New York, Alan R. Liss, 1990, pp. 323–340.
40. Easterling TR, Benedetti TJ: Preeclampsia: a hyperdynamic disease model. Am. J. Obstet. Gynecol. 160: 1447, 1989.
41. Easterling TR, Benedetti TJ: Maternal hemodynamics in normal and preeclamptic pregnancies: a longitudinal study. Obstet. Gynecol. 76:1061–9, 1990.
42. Rafferty TD, Berkowitz RL: Hemodynamics in patients with severe toxemia during labor and delivery. Am. J. Obstet. Gynecol. 138:263–270, 1980.
43. Soffronoff EC, Kauffman DM, Connaughton JF: Intravascular volume determination and fetal outcome in hypertensive disease of pregnancy. Am. J. Obstet. Gynecol. 127:4, 1978.
44. Benedetti TJ, Carlson RW: Studies of colloid osmotic pressure in pregnancy-induced hypertension. Am. J. Obstet. Gynecol. 135:308, 1979.
45. Bhatia RK, Bottoms SF, Saleh A, Norman GS, et al: Mechanism for reduced colloid osmotic pressure in preeclampsia. Am. J. Obstet. Gynecol. 157:106, 1987.
46. Oian P, Maltau JM, Noddeland H, Fadnes HO: Oedema-preventing mechanisms in subcutaneous tissue of normal pregnant women. Br. J. Obstet. Gynecol. 92:1113, 1985.
47. Oian P, Maltau JM, Noddeland H, Fadnes HO: Transcapillary fluid balance in preeclampsia. Br. J. Obstet. Gynaecol. 93:235, 1986.
48. Worley RJ, Everett RB, Madden JD, MacDonald PC, et al: Fetal considerations: metabolic clearance rate of maternal plasma dehydroisoandrosterone sulfate. Semin. Perinatol. 2(1):15–28, 1978.
49. Berkowitz R, Rafferty D: The use of the Swan-Ganz catheter in obstetrics and gynecology. Am. J. Obstet. Gynecol. 137: 127, 1980.
50. Andersen FH, Lynch JP, Johnson TRB: Adult respiratory distress syndrome in obstetrics and gynecology. Obstet. Gynecol. 55:291, 1980.
51. Benedetti TJ, Kates R, Williams V: Hemodynamic observations in severe preeclampsia complicated by pulmonary edema. Am. J. Obstet. Gynecol. 152:330, 1985.
52. Strauss RG, Keefer JR, Burke T, Civetta JM: Hemodynamic monitoring of cardiogenic pulmonary edema complicating toxemia of pregnancy. Obstet. Gynecol. 55:170, 1980.
53. Stempel JE, O'Grady JP, Morton MJ, Johnson KA: Use of sodium nitroprusside in gestational hypertensive emergencies. Obstet. Gynecol. 60:533, 1982.
54. Sibai BM, Mabie BC, Harvey CJ, Gonzalez AR: Pulmonary edema in severe preeclampsia-eclampsia: analysis of thirty-seven consecutive cases. Am. J. Obstet. Gynecol. 156:1174, 1987.
55. Lee W, Gonik B, Cotton DB: Urinary diagnostic indices in preeclampsia-associated oliguria: correlation with invasive hemodynamic monitoring. Am. J. Obstet. Gynecol. 156: 100, 1987.
56. Clark SL, Greenspoon JS, Aldahl D, Phelan JP: Severe preeclampsia with persistent oliguria: management of hemodynamic subsets. Am. J. Obstet. Gynecol. 154:490, 1986.
57. Pritchard JA, Stone SR: Clinical and laboratory observations on eclampsia. Am. J. Obstet. Gynecol. 99:754, 1967.
58. Gedekoh RH, Hayashi TT, MacDonald HM: Eclampsia at Magee Women's Hospital, 1970–1980. Am. J. Obstet. Gynecol. 40:860, 1981.

59. Redman CWG: Eclampsia still kills. Br. Med. J. 296:1209, 1988.
60. Watson DL, Baha SM, Shaver DC, Dacus JV, et al: Late postpartum eclampsia: an update. South. Med. J. 76:1487, 1983.
61. Benedetti TJ, Starzyk P, Frost F: Maternal deaths in Washington State. Obstet. Gynecol. 66:23, 1985.
62. Harbert GM, Claiborne HA, McGaughey JR: Convulsive toxemia: a report of 168 cases managed conservatively. Am. J. Obstet. Gynecol. 100:336, 1968.
63. Benedetti TJ, Benedetti JK, Stenchever MA: Severe preeclampsia: maternal and fetal outcome. Clin. Exp. Hypertens. B1(2&3):401, 1982.
64. Gluck L, Kulovich MV: Lecithin/sphingomyelin ratios in amniotic fluid in normal and abnormal pregnancy. Am. J. Obstet. Gynecol. 115:539, 1973.
65. Yoon J, Kohl S, Harper RG: The relationship between maternal hypertensive disease of pregnancy and the incidence of idiopathic respiratory distress syndrome. Pediatrics 65:735, 1980.
66. Skjaerassen J: Amniotic fluid phospholipid concentrations in pregnancies with preeclampsia and/or intrauterine growth retardation. Acta. Obstet. Gynecol. Scand. 58:191, 1979.
67. Liggins GC, Howie RN: A controlled trial of antepartum glucocorticoid treatment for prevention of respiratory distress syndrome in premature infants. Pediatrics 50:515, 1972.
68. Nochimson DJ, Petrie RH: Glucocorticoid therapy for the induction of pulmonary maturity in severely hypertensive gravid women. Am. J. Obstet. Gynecol. 133:449, 1979.
69. Ricke PS, Elliott JP, Freeman RK: Use of corticosteroids in pregnancy-induced hypertension. Obstet. Gynecol. 55: 206, 1980.
70. Collaborative group on antenatal steroid therapy: effect of antenatal dexamethasone administration on the prevention of respiratory distress syndrome. Am. J. Obstet. Gynecol. 141:276, 1981.
71. Beaufils M, Donsimoni R, Uzan S, Colau JC: Prevention of preeclampsia by early antiplatelet therapy. Lancet 2:840, 1985.
72. Wallenberg H, Dekker G, Makowitz J: Lowdose aspirin prevents pregnancy induced hypertension and preeclampsia in angiotensin sensitive primigravidae. Lancet 1:1, 1986.
73. Schiff E, Peleg E, Goldenberg M, Rosenthal T, et al: The use of aspirin to prevent pregnancy-induced hypertension and lower the ratio of thromboxane $A_2$ to prostacyclin in relatively high risk pregnancies. N. Engl. J. Med. 321: 351–356, 1989.
74. Benigni A, Gregorini G, Frusca T, Chrabrando C, et al: Effect of lowdose aspirin on fetal and maternal generation of thromboxane in women at risk for pregnancy induced hypertension. N. Engl. J. Med. 321:357, 1989.
75. McFarland P, Pearce JM, Chamberlin GVP: Doppler ultrasound and aspirin in recognition of pregnancy induced hypertension. Lancet 335:1552–1555, 1990.
76. Sibai BM, Taslimi M, Abdella TN, Brooks TF, et al: Maternal and perinatal outcome of conservative management of severe preeclampsia in midtrimester. Am. J. Obstet. Gynecol. 152:32–37, 1988.
77. Assali N, Vaughn R: Blood volume in preeclampsia: fantasy and reality. Am. J. Obstet. Gynecol. 129:355, 1977.
78. Gallery ED, Boyce ES, Saunders DM, Gyry AZ: The effect of volume expansion on blood pressure, plasma and extracellular fluid volumes in hypertensive pregnancy. Aust. N. Z. J. Obstet. Gynaecol. 20:189, 1980.
79. Arias F: Expansion of intravascular volume and fetal outcome in patients with chronic hypertension and pregnancy. Am. J. Obstet. Gynecol. 123:610, 1975.
80. Gallery ED, Saunders DM, Hunyor SN, Gyry AZ: Randomized comparison of methyldopa and oxyprenolol for treatment of hypertension in pregnancy. Br. Med. J. 1:1591, 1979.
81. Gallery ED, Saunders DM, Hunyor SN, Gyry AZ: Improvement in fetal growth with treatment of maternal hypertension in pregnancy. Clin. Sci. Mol. Med. 55:359S, 1978.
82. Habib A, McCarthy JS: Effects on the neonate of propranolol administered during pregnancy. J. Pediatr. 91:808, 1971.
83. Sabom M, Curry C, Wise D: Propranolol therapy during pregnancy in a patient with idiopathic hypertrophic subaortic stenosis: is it safe? South. Med. J. 71:328, 1978.
84. Rubin PC, Clark DM, Sumner DJ, Low RA, et al: Placebo-controlled trial of atenolol in treatment of pregnancy associated hypertension. Lancet 1:431, 1983.
85. Sibai BM, Gonzalez AR, Mabie WC, Moretti M: A comparison of labetalol plus hospitalization versus hospitalization alone in the management of preeclampsia remote from term. Obstet. Gynecol. 70:323, 1987.
86. Shepherd RT: Role of the veins in circulation. Circulation 33:484, 1966.
87. Dieckmann WJ: Incidence of eclampsia and other toxemias. *In* Toxemias of Pregnancy. St. Louis, C.V. Mosby, 1952, pp. 32–57.
88. Dommisse J: Phenytoin sodium and magnesium sulfate in the management of eclampsia. Br. J. Obstet. Gynaecol. 97: 104–109, 1990.
89. Crowther C: Magnesium sulfate versus diazepam in the management of eclampsia: a randomized controlled trial. Br. J. Obstet. Gynaecol. 97:110–117, 1990.
90. Sibai SM: Magnesium sulfate is the ideal anticonvulsant in preeclampsia. Am. J. Obstet. Gynecol. 162:1141–1145, 1990.
91. Moodley AM, Graham DI, Bullock MR: Active management of the unconscious eclamptic patient. Br. J. Obstet. Gynaecol. 93:554–562, 1986.
92. Pritchard J: Management of severe preeclampsia and eclampsia. Semin. Perinatol. 2:83, 1978.
93. Pritchard JA: Standardized treatment of 154 consecutive cases of eclampsia. Am. J. Obstet. Gynecol. 123:543, 1975.
94. Hodgkinson R, Husain J, Hayashi R: Systemic and pulmonary blood pressure during cesarean section in parturients with gestational hypertension. Can. Anaesth. Soc. J. 27:389, 1980.
95. Davies M, Cronin K, Cowie R: The prevention of hypertension at intubation. Anaesthesia 36:147, 1981.
96. Diaz SF, Marx GF: Placental transfer of nitroglycerin. Anesthesiology 51:475, 1979.
97. Tunstall ME: The effect of propranolol on the onset of breathing at birth. Br. J. Anaesth. 51:792 1969.
98. Newsome LR, Bramwell RS, Curling PE: Severe preeclampsia: hemodynamic effects of lumbar epidural anesthesia. Anesth. Analg. 65:31, 1986.
99. Hodgkinson R, Husain FJ, Hayashi RH: Systemic and pulmonary blood pressure during caesarean section in parturients with gestational hypertension. Can. Anaesth. Soc. J. 27:389, 1980.
100. Joyce TH, Debnath KS, Baker EA: Preeclampsia: the relationship of CVP and epidural anesthesia. Anesthesiology S51:297, 1979.
101. Benedetti TJ, Quilligan EJ: Cerebral edema in severe PIH. Am. J. Obstet. Gynecol. 137:860, 1980.
102. Burrows RF, Kelton JG: Incidentally detected thrombocy-

topenia in healthy mothers and their infants. N. Engl. J. Med. 319:142, 1988.

103. Sibai BM, Taslimi MM, El-Nazer A, Mabie BC, et al: Maternal-perinatal outcome associated with the syndrome of hemolysis, elevated liver enzymes and low platelets in severe preeclampsia-eclampsia. Am. J. Obstet. Gynecol. 155:501, 1986.

104. Kelton J, Hunter DJ, Neame PB: A platelet function defect in preeclampsia. Obstet. Gynecol. 65:107, 1985.

105. Rolbin SH, Abbott D, Musclow E, Papsin F, et al: Epidural anesthesia in pregnant patients with low platelet counts. Obstet. Gynecol. 71:918, 1988.

106. Skaredoff MN, Roaf ER, Data S: Hypermagnesemia and anesthetic management. Can. Anaesth. Soc. J. 29:35, 1982.

107. Douglas MJ: Potential complications of spinal and epidural anesthesia for obstetrics. Semin. Perinatol. 15:368–374, 1991.

108. Abboud TK, Zhu J, Afrasiabi A, Reyes G, et al: Epidural butorphanol augments lidocaine sensory anesthesia during labor. Reg. Anesth. 16:265–7, 1991.

109. Olson CL, Chaska BW, Grambsch PM, Wiltgen CM, et al: Intrapartum intervention and delivery outcome in low-risk pregnancy. J. Am. Board. Fam. Pract. 4:83–8, 1991.

# Chapter 26

# HEMORRHAGE: RELATED OBSTETRIC AND MEDICAL DISORDERS

JACK M. SCHNEIDER

Hemorrhage is the leading cause of death in pregnant women (1). Perinatal death, as well as maternal and perinatal morbidity, are even more common with maternal hemorrhage, especially if hypovolemic shock ensues (2). A vital statistics approach under-reports maternal deaths and fails to define contributory factors (1–4). For example, review of maternal deaths with a live birth outcome ranks hemorrhage third after pulmonary embolism and pregnancy-induced hypertension complications even though hemorrhage often antedated the demise attributed to these two conditions (1).

A definition for antepartum hemorrhage is lacking. Clinically measured blood loss of 500 ml or more and/or bleeding requiring two or more units of blood replacement to maintain a desired hematocrit level may be used. With vaginal birth-related hemorrhage defined as blood loss of 500 ml or greater in the first 24 hours postpartum and cesarean birth-related hemorrhage defined as a loss of 1000 ml or greater, the threshold blood-loss levels for the definition of hemorrhage in pregnancy are the same as the average blood loss in vaginal and cesarean births (5–8). The true incidence of postdelivery hemorrhage is unknown. Subjective assessment lacks rigor and underestimates particularly the higher volumes of blood loss (Figure 26–1) (9–12). Combs and co-workers chose a hematocrit decrease of 10 points or more from admission to the first day postpartum as an objective, clinically relevant definition of postpartum hemorrhage (13,14). This definition is in accord with the American College of Obstetricians and Gynecologist's clinical indicators for quality assurance (15).

The persistence of hemorrhage as a major risk factor for the pregnant woman is in part reflective of a clinical lack of awareness of the potential threat, late diagnosis of the causative abnormality, and, thereby, delay in instituting appropriate management. Further, the expertise of most obstetricians and many anesthesiologists is lacking with regard to nonobstetric conditions coincident with pregnancy that may be associated with excessive blood loss. Table 26–1 lists the factors that can be reasonably known before onset of labor in predicting hemorrhage.

This chapter classifies bleeding complicating pregnancy as obstetric or medical disorder-related (Table 26–2 and Table 26–3). In presenting the diagnosis and management of conditions associated with unfavorable impacts of excessive bleeding on the mother-baby dyad, emphasis is placed on prevention of hemorrhage through an understanding of hemostasis and the timely initiation of appropriate interventions.

## Normal Hemostasis

The four major subdivisions of the hemostatic system interact in a remarkably precise manner to effect thromboregulation. These subdivisions are: (1) the vascular wall and endothelium; (2) platelets; (3) plasma and tissue hemostasis factors, inhibitors, modulators; and (4) the fibrinolytic process.

### *Vascular Component*

Normal endothelial cells lining the blood vessels present a smooth, dynamic surface to blood components that protects against platelet adherence and factor activation. Endothelial cells synthesize heparin-like molecules and thrombin binding sites, which impart anticoagulant and local fibrinolysis activities to the vascular surface (16,17). Endothelial cells are also a major source of tissue-type plasminogen activator (t-PA) and prostacyclin ($PGI_2$), a potent inhibitor of platelet aggregation (18,19). With vascular injury, spasm and retraction of the vessel wall ensues, in part secondary to serotonin and thromboxane $A_2$ ($TXA_2$) release from the platelets, exposing subendothelial tissue.

### *Platelet Component*

The platelet is responsible typically for initiating clot formation. Adherence of platelets to exposed subendothelial tissue is facilitated by von Willebrand factor (vWf), which forms an adhesive bond between platelet surface glycoprotein (GPIb) and extracellular matrix macromolecule in the high flow/high shear conditions operative in the arterial circulation.

Platelet aggregation follows platelet adherence and requires: (1) activation of the platelet with release of platelet agonists such as adenosine diphosphate (ADP), calcium, and serotonin from thrombocyte granules; (2) exposure of platelet surface binding sites (GPIIb/IIIa complex) for adhesive proteins; and (3) the presence of an adequate quantity of a soluble adhesive protein (e.g., fibrinogen, vWf, fibronectin) (20). Thrombin, factor XII,

**Table 26–1.** Postpartum Hemorrhage Predictor

| Factor | Adjusted OR | 95% CI | *P* |
|---|---|---|---|
| Preeclampsia | | | |
| Present vs absent | 4.57 | 2.89–7.22 | <.0001 |
| Parity | | | |
| Nulliparous vs parous | 3.20 | 2.43–4.21 | <.0001 |
| Multiple gestation | | | |
| Twins vs singleton | 3.02 | 1.07–8.47 | <.05 |
| Previous postpartum hemorrhage | | | |
| Present vs absent | 2.85 | 1.07–7.60 | <.05 |
| Previous cesarean* | | | |
| Present vs absent | 2.67 | 1.44–4.95 | <.01 |
| Ethnic group | | | |
| Asian vs not Asian | 1.87 | 1.37–2.55 | <.01 |
| Hispanic vs not Hispanic | 1.67 | 1.10–2.53 | <.05 |

OR = odds ratio; CI = confidence interval.
Factors considered but removed by stepwise elimination: accoucheur, induced labor.
* Probably a surrogate variable related to hemorrhage because of association with augmented labor. See text.
(From Combs CA, Murphy EL, Laros RK: Factors associated with postpartum hemorrhage with vaginal birth. Obstet. Gynecol. 77(1):69–76, 1991.)

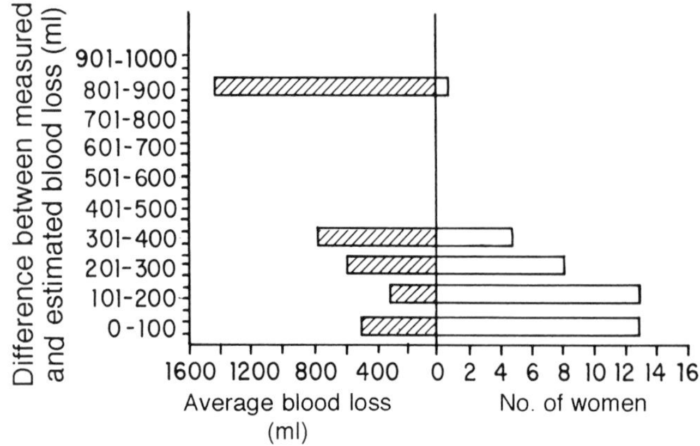


**Fig. 26–1.** Difference between measured and estimated blood losses during elective cesarean sections. (Modified from Duthie SJ, Ghosh A, Ng A, Ho PC: Intra-operative blood loss during elective lower segment cesarean section. Br. J. Obstet. Gynaecol. 99:364–7, 1992.)

**Table 26–2.** Etiology of Obstetric Bleeding

- Antepartum
  - Placental Abruption
  - Placenta Previa
  - Hypotensive Disorders
  - Molar Pregnancy
  - Dead Fetus Syndrome
- Postpartum
  - Uterine Atony
  - Uterine/Vaginal Lacerations
  - Uterine Rupture/Inversion
  - Placental Abruption
  - Placenta Previa/Accreta
  - Preeclampsia (HELLP syndrome)
  - Dead Fetus Syndrome
  - Amniotic Fluid Embolism
  - Dilutional Coagulopathy

**Table 26–3.** Etiology of Medical Disorder-Related Hemorrhage

- Thrombocytopenia
  - Isoimmune
  - Alloimmune
  - Thrombotic Thrombocytopenic Purpura
  - Drug-associated
- Sepsis/Septic Shock
- Systemic Lupus Erythematosus
- Coagulopathies
- Factor Deficiency States
- Clotting Component Inhibitors
- Acquired inhibitors

and epinephrine are also important platelet agonists for the reorientation of the binding sites for fibrinogen, a major adhesive protein involved in platelet aggregation (21,22). The platelet plug formed by fibrinogen's platelet to platelet cross-linkage constitutes what is termed primary hemostasis.

Platelets provide binding sites for factors V, VII, and activated X (FXa). Factor XI is activated by platelets. The Va/Xa complex on the platelets' surface accelerates the activation of prothrombin (23). Clot retraction is also a predominate role of platelets (24).

### *Hemostatic Factors/Modulators/Inhibitors*

There are two initiating pathways—intrinsic and extrinsic—to the waterfall or cascade sequencing of blood clotting (Figure 26–2). Either path converges upon a common track with the end result development of a fibrin clot (25,26). The cascade of proteolytic enzyme activity exhibits biochemical amplification in that more protein is activated at each step than at the previous (26).

The intrinsic pathway (contact-activated) is so named because all of the components are in the vasculature. Factor XII (FXII) converts prekallikrein to kallikrein which in turn activates factor XII (FXIIa). High molecular weight kininogen (HMWK) appears to enhance the activation of prekallikrein, the effect of kallikrein on FXII, and the activation of factor XI (FXIa) (27). Factor VIIa activates factor XI (FXIa) which in turn activates factor IX (FIXa). Factor IXa in the presence of platelet factor 3 ($PF_3$), calcium, factor VIII, and platelet phospholipid activates factor X (FXa), the entry to the common pathway of coagulation.

The extrinsic pathway (tissue factor-dependent) does not require intrinsic components although factor VII activation (FVIIa) appears to be enhanced by kallikrein, FXIIa, and FIXa (28,29). Activation of factor VII (FVIIa) occurs after binding to tissue thromboplastin (TF). The resultant VIIa/TF then activates factors IX and X. Activation of factor X (Xa), the entry to the common pathway, is both direct (VIIa/TF) and indirect (IXa/VIIIa/platelet phospholipid)

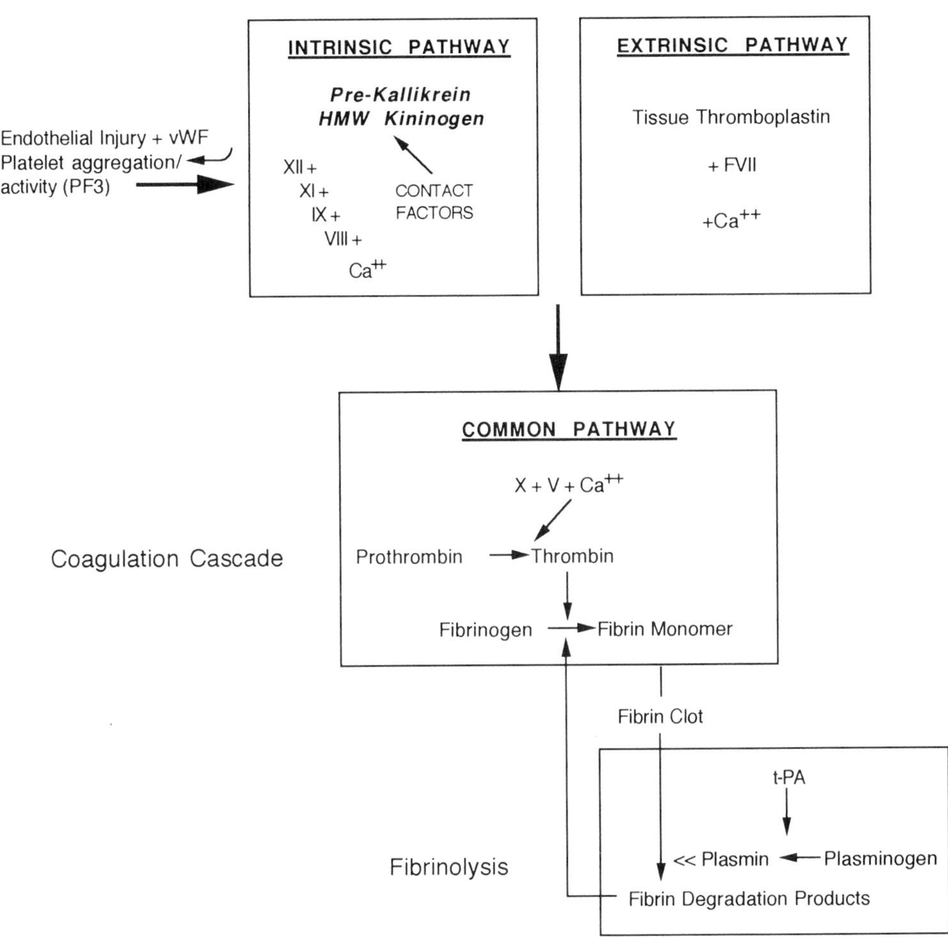


**Fig. 26–2.** Outlines coagulation and fibrinolytic pathways.

(30). The latter activation mechanism addresses the inhibition of factor X activation by VIIa/TF complex as clot formation progresses (31).

The common pathway in the cascade effects the conversion of prothrombin to thrombin by FXa, factor V (FV), and calcium on a matrix of $PF_3$ phospholipid. Thrombin cleaves two peptides (A and B) from fibrinogen to form fibrin monomers. Thrombin also directly impacts on platelet aggregation. Factor XIII (fibrin stabilizing factor) imparts covalent cross-linkage to the fibrin strands in the clot. This stabilized fibrin clot constitutes secondary hemostasis.

Most of the procoagulant factors in the cascade are synthesized by the liver. The reduced-form of Vitamin K functions as a cofactor in the hepatocyte conversion of the N-terminus glutamic acid residues of prothrombin and factors VII, IX, and X into gamma-carboxyglutamic acid (32,33). This amino acid configuration imparts metal binding properties. In the presence of calcium ions, these proteins undergo conformational change that results in the expression of negatively-charged phospholipid membrane binding properties (34).

Coagulation is controlled or modulated by other proteins. Antithrombin III, a circulating active anticoagulant, inhibits thrombin as well as factors XIIa, XIa, IXa, and Xa by forming 1:1 complexes with these enzymes (35). This inhibition is catalyzed by heparin sulfate proteoglycans on the endothelial surface (36,37). Thrombomodulin, an endothelial cell membrane protein receptor-cofactor for thrombin, inhibits the ability of thrombin to clot fibrinogen, activate factor V, or activate platelets (17,38–40). Furthermore, the thrombin/thrombomodulin complex operative in the microcirculation activates factor C at a rate 20,000-fold faster than free thrombin (17).

Factor C and its cofactor protein S are vitamin K-dependent proteins (41–43). In contrast to antithrombin III, protein C is inactive in plasma and requires activation on the endothelial surface (phospholipid) in a calcium ion environment. Activated protein C (Ca) exhibits its anticoagulant effect by degrading both platelet-bound and free factors Va and VIIIa, thereby preventing further thrombin generation (44–46). The rate of factor Va degradation by Ca is enhanced by the formation of Ca/protein S complex on the surface of phospholipid vesicles (47). To further fine tune thromboregulation, plasma contains an inhibitor of protein Ca that inactivates this anticoagulant by forming 1:1 complexes (48,49).

Fibrin acts as a local control factor by capping or sealing the platelet plug and subendothelial tissues, thus limiting continued platelet adhesion and aggregation. It also neutralizes thrombin by adsorption (50).

### *Fibrinolysis Component*

Plasminogen is activated to plasmin by tissue-type plasminogen activator (t-PA) released from endothelial cells or other tissue (19,51,52). Plasmin degrades fibrinogen and fibrin, thus lysing the fibrin clot. Interestingly, plasminogen is closely bound to fibrinogen in the clot so that thrombolysis begins hand in hand with thrombosis. The endothelial cells appear to control the assembly of fibrinolytic components on the cell membrane (53). Activated protein C apparently enhances fibrinolysis by neutralizing a circulating t-PA inhibitor, thus accelerating the conversion of plasminogen to plasmin (54).

## Pregnancy-Related Anatomy/Physiology

### *Anatomy*

The structural and physiologic changes the uterus undergoes in pregnancy are well designed to minimize postpartum bleeding. Uterine muscle hypertrophies, and there is also concomitant increase in elastic tissue (55). There is a zonal preponderance of muscle in the upper segment of the uterus, the usual implantation site of the placenta. Further, the muscle fibers are generally S-shaped with varying polarity to one another, which during the contractile state postpartum produces a tourniquet-like effect on the vasculature of the uterine fundus, thus minimizing blood loss (56). In contrast, the preponderance of connective tissue in the lower uterine segment is associated with less control of blood loss with injury in this area due to lacerations or placental invasion.

A spiral rather than straight design to the arteries of the uterus, although somewhat attenuated in pregnancy, favors retraction with injury and further facilitates effective hemostasis with contraction of the uterine musculature. Further, intrauterine release of endothelin-1, a vasoconstrictor peptide, at delivery may play a key role in causing constriction of the placental bed blood vessels (57).

### *Physiology*

#### *Hematologic*

Blood volume expands an average 45% (1000 to 2000 ml) with the predominant change occurring in the second trimester of pregnancy (58,59). Multiple gestation generally expands both the plasma volume and the red blood cell volume greater than does a singleton gestation. The plasma volume component increases to a greater extent than the increase in red blood cell volume so that there is a decrease in hematocrit, which is most significant in the second trimester (60). Blood leukocyte counts increase up to approximately 12,000/μL by the third trimester. The increase is due predominantly to an increase in segmented neutrophils. Labor, delivery, and the early postpartum period impart a further increase to as high as 20,000 to 30,000/μL (61). The platelet count does not change appreciably from the nonpregnant range during pregnancy, although there is evidence of an increased rate of destruction (aggregation) and slightly shortened lifespan near the end of the pregnancy (Figure 26–3) (62–64).

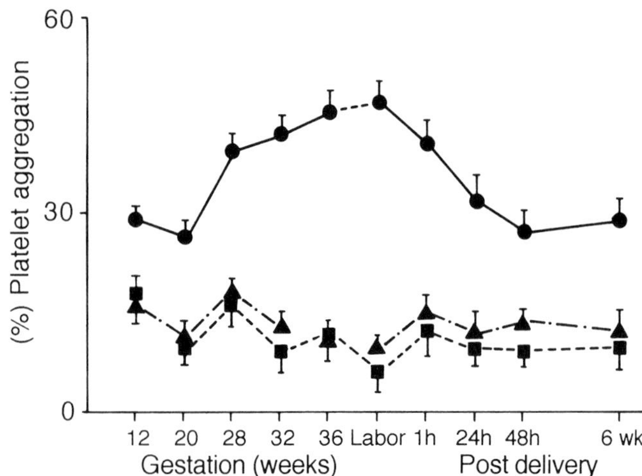


**Fig. 26–3.** Demonstrates percentage of platelet coagulation at various times of gestation and post delivery period. (Modified from Norris LA, Sheppard BL, Bonnar J: Increased whole blood platelet aggregation in normal pregnancy can be prevented in vitro by aspirin and dazmegrel (UK38485). Br. J. Obstet. Gynaecol. 99:253–7, 1992.)

#### *Cardiovascular*

##### Peripheral Resistance

There is an overall decrease in peripheral resistance that is maximal in the second trimester of pregnancy. The decrease is predominantly expressed in a lowering of diastolic blood pressure. It probably reflects the impact of the low-resistance arterial-venous "shunt" of the placenta, pregnancy hormones, and increased heat production by the fetus (65,66). An increase in vascular capacitance, particularly on the venous side, is secondary to hormonal impacts on the vascular musculature, which lowers peripheral resistance. Vasodilation is likely also influenced by the increase in prostacyclin in pregnancy. Central venous pressure is unchanged at approximately 10 cm $H_2O$, and this continues through the third trimester (67). Pulmonary capillary wedge pressure (PCWP) is not altered significantly in pregnancy (6 to 12 mm Hg). The physiologic decrease in plasma albumin concentration imparts a decrease in the colloid oncotic pressure (COP), which falls from a mean in the nongravid state of 21 to 25 mm Hg to around 18 to 22 mm Hg at term (68,69). In normal pregnancy, thereby, the colloid oncotic pressure-pulmonary capillary wedge pressure (COP-PCWP) gradient remains at 10 mm Hg or greater, which is adequate to prevent pulmonary edema.

##### Blood Pressure

Blood pressure is lowered with the maximal decrease seen in the second trimester associated with the timing of maximal decrease in the peripheral resistance. The decrease in diastolic blood pressure is of the order of 10 to 15 mm Hg. During labor, diastolic blood pressure may rise into the 90s mm Hg range secondary at times to pain as well as to the increased venous return to the heart with uterine contractions (70,71).

Clinical assessment of blood pressure in pregnancy is recommended to be done with the patient in the left lateral position to minimize impact of the gravid uterus on venous return and thus cardiac output. The point of muffling of Korotkoff sounds, the fourth phase, is recommended as the diastolic end point in pregnancy (72,73). With the patient on the left side, the arterial blood pressure, if measured in the superior arm, will be found to be approximately 10 mm Hg lower than that found at the level of the heart (74). Further, the size of the sphygmomanometer cuff relative to arm circumference is important, with inadequately sized cuffs associated with the false impression of increased blood pressure when arm circumference is great (75).

## Heart

Heart size increases by about 10% due to hypertrophy (76). Systolic ejection-type murmurs are definable in 90% or more of pregnant women by the second trimester (77). Assessments of cardiac output show overall increases of the order of approximately 30 to 50% with some women showing a decrease at or near term (78). Echocardiographic assessment of the heart reveals a shift to the hyperdynamic range with normal ejection fractions (79). There is an increase in heart rate of 10 to 15 beats per minute and an increase in stroke volume due to the increased blood volume and likely the inotropic effect of estrogen on myocardial contractibility (80,81). Aortocaval compression by the gravid uterus decreases cardiac output because of decreased return of blood to the heart.

## Regional Blood Flow

While there is no significant change in uterine perfusion/gm total tissue weight, uterine blood flow increases to about 500 to 800 ml/min as a function of uteroplacental perfusion, which is directly reflective of maternal cardiac output (82). Renal plasma flow increases about 50%, imparting increased clearance of plasma creatinine (83). There is increased blood flow to the skin with little or no change in blood flow to the liver, spleen, or gut.

## Labor/Delivery Impact

Labor is associated with a further increase in cardiac output especially with pushing efforts during the second stage of labor. Heart rate decreases and stroke volume increases or changes little (59,78,84). These changes are influenced by the mother's position, hydration, and anesthesia/analgesia status.

Following vaginal delivery, there is a short-lived increase in cardiac output by up to 60% over prelabor levels. Stroke volume also increases 60 to 70%, which is approximately two to three times the increase associated with pregnancy. Heart rate may fall up to 15 to 20 beats per minute with any decrease persisting for several days (84). Within hours after delivery, blood volume falls from the previously noted pregnancy increase by approximately 5 to 15%, dependent on blood loss at delivery and intravenous fluid administration (78,85).

## Coagulation

From a coagulation standpoint, pregnancy is characterized as a state of chronic, compensated, disseminated intravascular coagulation (DIC).

## Vasculature

The reactivity of blood vessels to injury does not appear to be altered in normal pregnancy. The spiral arteries of the uterus, however, appear to have increased sensitivity to vasopressors in the antepartum period. The protective function of the endothelial cells as an interface between the blood and subendothelial tissues is not altered.

## Platelets

Significant quantitative or qualitative changes in platelets are not evidenced by the platelet count or the Ivy bleeding time in pregnancy although platelet survival decreases (62,86,87). The increase in thrombin generation in pregnancy may in part reflect alterations in platelet function (62,63).

## Factors/Modulators/Fibrinolysis

There is an overall increase in the activity of several of the coagulation factors, especially factor VII, fibrinogen, and factor VIII (88–91). There is a lesser increase in factors II, X, and XII and a possible increase in factors V and IX (Table 26–4) (89,92–96). The increase in factor VII reflects the presence of a phospholipase C sensitive form of factor VII present in pregnant women, but not demonstrable in the nonpregnant woman (89). Not only does

**Table 26–4.** Antepartum Clotting Factor Changes in Pregnancy

| Factor Number | Synonym | Vitamin K-Dependent | Pregnancy Change |
|---|---|---|---|
| I | Fibrinogen | | ↑ ↑ ↑ |
| II | Prothrombin | X | ↑ |
| III | Tissue thromboplastin | | ↓ |
| IV | Calcium ions | | →, ↓ |
| V | Proaccelerin | | →, (↑)* |
| VII | Factor VII | X | ↑ ↑ ↑ ↑ |
| VIII | Antihemophilic factor | | ↑ ↑ ↑ |
| IX | Christmas factor | X | →, (↑)* |
| X | Stuart factor, Prower factor | X | ↑ |
| XI | Plasma thromboplastin antecedent | | ↓ |
| XII | Hageman factor | | ↑ |
| XIII | Fibrin-stabilizing factor | | ↓ |

* (↑) Factor *may* be increased in pregnancy.

factor VIII coagulant (VIII:C) increase in pregnancy, but the von Willebrand factor component of the factor VIII complex increases progressively in pregnancy as well (90–92,97–99). Other factors, including factors III, calcium ions (FIV), XI; and XIII are either unchanged or lowered in pregnancy (88,91,92,96,100,101). The major circulating anticoagulant proteins in pregnancy appear to remain at normal levels with the exception of free protein-S, which is significantly reduced (102–106). Although antithrombin III activity is not functionally changed, a significant decrease in activity is seen in the pregnant woman with systemic infection in contrast to the nonpregnant patient (104).

Most studies have shown fibrinolytic activity during early pregnancy to increase with decline in the third trimester (107,108). Assessment of whole blood rather than plasma fibrinolysis, however, suggests that fibrinolytic activity is still very robust at term (109,110). Any decrease in fibrinolytic activity is thought to be mediated through the placenta (88,111–114). Plasminogen activator inhibitors are increased in pregnancy (107,108,110,115). Fibrinolytic activity in pregnancy, however, does not appear to correlate with the increase in inhibitors (110).

### *Impacts—Labor/Delivery*

In labor there is a further increase in fibrinogen, factor VII complex, factor VIII, factor VIII complex, and fibrin degradation products from the increases already expressed during pregnancy. Platelet aggregation is increased (64). As expected, fibrinolysis increases (109). Protein C and protein S do not change appreciably from levels in the third trimester (105).

Delivery of the placenta imparts tissue and vascular injury, with attendant transient decreases in the platelet count and fibrinogen followed by a further increase in fibrin and fibrinogen degradation products, particularly fibrinopeptide-A (64,116–120). The FVIII:C and the von Willebrand factor components of factor VIII complex also decrease rapidly after delivery (97,121–124). There is a gradual fall in FII and FX postpartum, but factor VII decreases significantly during the first 30 minutes after placental delivery (89). The platelet count and platelet activity are increased gradually in the postpartum recovery period (64,125). Fibrinolytic activity rapidly normalizes (i.e., rises) postpartum (107,109,110). Free protein S does not return to normal for several weeks after delivery (105).

## Laboratory Assessors of Coagulation in Pregnancy

The history and, to a lesser degree, the physical assessment are the most sensitive methods of screening for a bleeding disorder. Laboratory assessments of coagulation play only a supplemental role. Further, in these times of monetary constraint on health care costs, a case can be made for a true "need-to-know" approach to the ordering of laboratory tests. Normal pregnancy values for any test should be known to the practitioner, as should there be an understanding that there are only three possibilities to the forthcoming test result report—no change, an increase, or a decrease. Laboratory testing should not follow a routinized approach. Coagulation testing should be ordered only when the history and physical assessments fail to provide a diagnosis or to assess the course of the disease process and the impact of interventions.

With the advent of automated cell counters, the platelet count as a part of the complete blood count became the most available coagulation assessment to the obstetrician. The most frequently obtained assessments of coagulation have been the prothrombin time (PT) and the activated partial thromboplastin time (APTT). In fact, most often both of these tests have been obtained at the same time as screening assessments for coagulation. Yet neither of these tests has a significant positive predictive value in asymptomatic patients (126,127). Even application of expanded American College of Physicians guidelines for ordering these tests found less than 30% of the tests to have been appropriately ordered (128,129). Routinization of laboratory assessments often leads to repetition of an abnormal test result without further action. Inappropriate interventions such as the administration of fresh frozen plasma for a prolonged activated partial thromboplastin secondary to the presence of lupus anticoagulant may also result (129).

In pregnancy, fibrinogen depletion is far and away the predominant determinant of hemorrhage associated with abnormal coagulation. With severe hyprofibrinogenemia from any cause, abnormal bleeding ensues because fibrinogen is not available for binding platelet to platelet via the IIb/IIIa complex. The prothrombin time does not assess fibrinogen, and the activated partial thromboplastin is not sensitive to hypofibrinogenemia until levels associated with significant hemorrhage—namely, a fibrinogen level of less than 100 mg/dl. Even in massive hemorrhage (i.e., loss of greater than or equal to total prehemorrhage blood volume over 24 hours), it is rare to have significant factor deficiency other than fibrinogen. Far more often, there is an inadequacy of normal functioning platelets (130). Unless there is a specific clinical indication for other studies, the CBC (platelet count) and serum fibrinogen levels are the most important laboratory assessments of coagulation in the obstetric patient.

The routine type and cross match of units of blood prior to vaginal or cesarean birth is not appropriate (131,132). A type and screen has been recommended for preoperative assessment (132). A type and hold approach imparts about 30 minutes longer for cross-matching but at one-half the cost. Lacking a positive historical or physical notation that poses a high risk for excessive blood loss, coagulation studies and/or whole blood or blood components should not be obtained.

## *Specific Tests*

### *Complete Blood Count/Platelet Count*

The blood count determines the hemoglobin and hematocrit, which assess baseline red blood cell reserve. A decreased mean red blood cell volume ($\leq$ 79 fl) may be indicative of risk for one of the thalassemia syndromes. An elevated leukocyte count may suggest a hematopoietic disorder as an underlying cause of bleeding, while a decreased leukocyte count in the face of the expected increase seen in normal pregnancy suggests an immune disorder. Although the platelet count from venipuncture-obtained blood is reported out as a part of the CBC result, normal platelet function can not be implied with counts of less than 100,000/μL. Accurate platelet counts are not determinable from blood obtained by finger stick. When a complete blood count is obtained, a smear should also be prepared to assess the morphology of each cell line. Macrothrombocytes suggest increased consumption of platelets, fragmented erythrocytes are typically representative of microangiopathic anemia, and abnormal leukocyte distribution and/or morphology suggests a leukemic process.

### *Prothrombin Time (PT)*

The prothrombin time, in assessing the Vitamin K-dependent clotting factors, is a test of the extrinsic pathway (FVII) and the common pathway (FV, FX and prothrombin). Hypofibrinogenemia is not assessed by the prothrombin time. Prothrombin time is not changed in pregnancy with a normal range of no greater than 3 seconds over control. This author restricts this assessment to the clinical situations of evident or implied liver dysfunction, Vitamin-K deficiency, or oral anticoagulant therapy.

### *Activated Partial Thromboplastin Time (APTT)*

The activated partial thromboplastin time tests the intrinsic (contact-activated) pathway and is sensitive to factor VIII and IX deficiency, but usually not until the concentration of these factors is below 30% of normal. The activated partial thromboplastin time does not assess factor VII. Neither the prothrombin nor the activated partial thromboplastin times assess for factor XIII. The activated partial thromboplastin time, as does the prothrombin time, assesses for factors X, V, and prothrombin (FII).

Hypofibrinogenemia is not reflected in prolongation of the activated partial thromboplastin time until values are less than 100 mg/dl. This author generally restricts the activated partial thromboplastin time to the clinical situation of assessing heparin anticoagulant therapy or liver dysfunction and as a screening assessment for lupus anticoagulant.

### *Fibrinogen*

As noted above, fibrinogen deficient states are not defined by either the prothrombin time or the activated partial thromboplastin time at clinically significant low levels.

The fibrinogen concentration increases two- to threefold in pregnancy to be typically at 450 mg/dl or greater. Because most laboratories use normative male values for laboratory test results, the practitioner must be very suspicious from a clinical viewpoint of a "normal" value of 350 mg/dl or less. Similarly, high values ($\geq$ 600 mg/dl) are suspect because they are most often seen early in fibrinogen consumptive processes such as severe preeclampsia and sepsis.

Fibrinogen concentration is the test to obtain in obstetric-related hemorrhage in contrast to the prothrombin time and/or activated partial thromboplastin time.

### *Bleeding Time (BT)*

The bleeding time assesses vascular integrity and, in particular, platelet function. Dysfunctional platelets leading to prolongation of the bleeding time are usually not seen until the platelet count falls below 50,000/μL. Nonsteroidal anti-inflammatory agents, such as full-dose aspirin and von Willebrand factor deficiency may prolong the bleeding time.

Pregnancy does not significantly alter the bleeding time. Normal values range from 3 to 10 minutes (133). The bleeding time should be performed using the Ivy method on the forearm, employing a standardized template (134). This test is recommended before regional anesthesia with thrombocytopenia (less than 100,000/μL), a history of certain drug(s) usage, von Willebrand disease, and active vasculitis syndromes.

### *Thrombin Clotting Time (TCT)*

This test assesses the conversion of fibrinogen to fibrin by the addition of thrombin to the blood sample. This assessor of hypofibrinogenemia can be done at the bedside by the addition of 2 ml of the patient's whole blood to 0.1 ml of freshly prepared topical thrombin, which can be prepared in advance and frozen. With normal fibrinogen levels, a firm clot forms in seconds. With moderately depressed fibrinogen in the 100 to 150 mg/dl range, there is a discernible clot initially, but it retracts to a volume of no more than 50% of the total of the liquid and clot. The liquid phase appears hemolyzed as the clot does not entrap many of the red blood cells. Severely depressed fibrinogen (less than 50 to 100 mg/dl) is expressed by lack of formation of a clot or by formation of a soft coagulum, which retracts to be barely visible within 30 minutes.

The normal thrombin time is less than 2 seconds longer than the control with a normal range of 10 to 15 seconds. The bedside assessment is particularly useful in clinical states in which frequent serial assessments of fibrinogen is required.

### *Whole Blood Clot Time*

This test, the placement of 5 ml of blood into a "red top" silicone coated tube, should be done by the staff instituting an intravenous route in cases of excessive bleeding or frank hemorrhage. A firm clot should form within a 10-minute time period. Either the thrombin clotting time or this test should be performed at the bedside to activate the timely request of blood and blood components rather than to await the subsequent laboratory coagulation reports, which typically are not available for 45 minutes or longer. A prolonged thrombin or whole blood clot time with lysis of the coagulum over the next 15 to 30 minutes usually is reflecting an excess of fibrin degradation products.

### *Fibrin Degradation Products (FDP)/D-Dimer*

These products result from the plasmin degradation of both fibrinogen and fibrin. As noted earlier, normal pregnancy physiology increases fibrin degradation products, and their production is accentuated in labor and delivery, particularly with delivery of the placenta. This author rarely obtains this commonly requested test in pregnancy-related hemorrhagic conditions, because the characteristic rapid consumption of fibrinogen in these conditions is uniformly reflected in an increase in these potent coagulation inhibitors.

It is not atypical for fibrin degradation products evaluated postpartum to be mildly elevated (20 to 40 μg/ml range). No import to an elevated level should be made until values of 5 mg or more per deciliter are evident. D-dimer assessment is required if one wishes to define that the fibrin degradation products are secondary to fibrinolysis rather than from primary fibrinogenolysis.

### *Fibrinopeptide A (FPA)*

Fibrinopeptide A is the first peptide cleaved from fibrinogen during fibrin generation. As already noted, fibrinopeptide A is increased during normal pregnancy, reflecting thrombin activity and fibrin generation (120). It is a particularly useful test to evaluate fibrin generation in sepsis (119).

### *Antithrombin III (AT III)*

Antithrombin III, the natural anticoagulant for many of the activated clotting components, is the best test for the diagnosis of disseminated intravascular coagulation and the monitoring of its therapy (135).

### *Factor Assay*

Factor XIII is not assessed by the prothrombin or activated partial thromboplastin times, and requires a specific fibrin stabilization assay. While all of the factors can be specifically assayed for, fibrinogen and factor VIII are the ones most commonly measured. von Willebrand factor is assessed in the circumstance of a prolonged bleeding time and a normal platelet count. Factor assays are reported as a percentage of the activity of plasma pooled from normal donors. The normal range for any factor is 60 to 160%.

### *Type and Screen*

While an indirect assessor of risk, the type and screen or cross match may identify agglutinins, inhibitors, or antibodies, which may play an undesirable role in abnormal bleeding and/or its management.

### *Euglobulin Lysis Time (ELT)*

This test measures the presence of plasminogen activators. Under 90 minutes' time reflects fibrinolytic activity.

### *Acquired Anticoagulants*

Lupus anticoagulant (LAC), an antiphospholipid autoantibody, binds to the phospholipid portion of the preformed prothrombin-activator complex, resulting in a prolongation of the activated partial thromboplastin time (136). It also appears to inhibit production of prostacyclin by vascular tissues (137). While lupus anticoagulant is not associated with abnormal bleeding except when hypoprothrombinemia, thrombocytopenia, or qualitative platelet defect is present, it is important to distinguish the prolongation of laboratory assessors of coagulation due to the presence of this "anticoagulant" from antibodies reacting with coagulation factors and causing bleeding (138–140).

The details of the coagulation assays for lupus anticoagulant and other antiphospholipid antibodies are reported (141).

## Coagulopathies

History is the most sensitive assessor of risk for abnormal coagulation.

### ***Differentiation of Disorders***

#### *Coagulation Factors*

Inherited coagulation factor deficiencies, more common in males than in females, are associated with deep (hematoma), large, and solitary bleeds typically occurring late (intraprocedure/postprocedure) in the course of the abnormal bleeding.

#### *Platelet/Vessel*

In contrast, platelet/vessel disorders are more common in females and are associated with superficial and multiple bleeds (petechiae/ecchymoses) typically occurring early in the course of abnormal bleeding.

### ***Disseminated Intravascular Coagulation (DIC)***

#### *Laboratory Tests for Disseminated Intravascular Coagulation*

Disseminated intravascular coagulation denotes systemic thrombin activation with consumption of predominantly fibrinogen and to a lesser degree factors VIII, V, and platelets. There is widely disseminated microvascular fibrin deposition. Remembering the close association of fibrinogen and plasminogen, it should be appreciated that the rapid consumption of fibrinogen is associated with rapid activation of the fibrinolytic system with both fibrinogenolysis and fibrinolysis.

Disseminated intravascular coagulation is not an independent entity, but rather an associated feature of certain conditions. Building on the already hypercoagulable state of pregnancy as the starting point for this consumption, conditions that activate coagulation by either altering endothelial cell function or damaging endothelium (preeclampsia, endotoxin) include; releasing tissue thromboplastin (abruptio placenta, accreta placenta, dead fetus syndrome, amniotic fluid embolism); or imparting quantitative or qualitative alteration to platelets (preeclampsia, endotoxin). All these conditions make pregnancy the greatest risk time in the women's life cycle for both disseminated intravascular coagulation and thromboembolic disease.

Laboratory diagnosis of disseminated intravascular coagulation requires demonstration of hypofibrinogenemia and fibrinogen and fibrin degradation products. While the clinical diagnosis of acute disseminated intravascular coagulation and frank hemorrhage is often obvious, the diagnosis of the subclinical state is the key to prevention of massive hemorrhage. The prothrombin and activated partial thromboplastin times are insensitive assessors of hypofibrinogenemia and, indeed, in compensated disseminated intravascular coagulation conditions, such as preeclampsia, the activated partial thromboplastin time may actually be shortened reflective of the hypercoagulable state characterized by significant elevation in fibrinogen and platelet number. This phenomenon may also be expressed in the postrecovery phase of disseminated intravascular coagulation.

Antithrombin III is the most sensitive laboratory indicator of disseminated intravascular coagulation; normal AT III level is not consistent with a diagnosis of disseminated intravascular coagulation (135). The presence of fibrin degradation products per se does not provide insight as to the severity of the hypofibrinogenemia. This information is obtained by serial assessment of fibrinogen levels, either directly or indirectly by the thrombin clot time. These assessments should be done every 2 to 4 hours when disruption of vascular integrity is a potential, such as during the labor and delivery process. Platelet counts are required to assess the severity of the thrombocytopenia. Again, the AT III level is a critical indicator of the effectiveness of therapy.

### *Treatment*

While it is accepted that the key to management of acute disseminated intravascular coagulation is successful treatment of the primary initiating cause, anticipation of risk and prevention of the disseminated intravascular coagulation syndrome is the prima facie element. Fibrinogen replacement is usually what is required in obstetric-related disseminated intravascular coagulation. Much less common is the need for factor VIII administration. The need for other factor replacement is unusual except in the instance of massive hemorrhage or secondary to sepsis-associated disseminated intravascular coagulation. Platelets should not be given prophylactically regardless of the platelet count or anticipated cesarean birth. Prophylactic platelets are consumed with further fibrin generation and increase in fibrin degradation products with further negative impact on coagulation by their anticoagulant activity.

Specific treatment approaches for the disseminated intravascular coagulation are covered under the individual condition.

## *Specific Factor-Deficient States*

A congenital factor-deficient state has been described for all of the coagulation factors, although clinically significant deficiencies in pregnancies predominantly reside with factors VIII and IX. The von Willebrand factor, while not a procoagulant protein, also poses pregnancy-related hemorrhage risk. Pertinent facts regarding these conditions are presented in the general order of sequencing of factor action in the intrinsic and common pathways.

### *Factor XII*

Hemorrhage is not a risk with factor XII deficiency, although the activated partial thromboplastin time is prolonged (142). Indeed, thromboembolic disease may be an increased risk for these patients (143).

The von Willebrand factor plays an essential role in clotting as the key adhesive protein in platelet aggregation with vascular injury (144). It also binds and stabilizes factor VIII from proteolysis and plasma and imparts properties to the platelets to enable them to withstand high shear forces (145–147). vWf plays a role in the adhesion of endothelial cells to basement membrane (148). That this role is critical to formation of a platelet plug is evidenced by the prolongation of the bleeding time in deficient states.

von Willebrand's disease is the most common congenital coagulopathy affecting women (97,149). Major types of the disease are clinically manifest: Type I—a quantitative deficiency of vWf; Type II—a qualitative abnormality of vWf activity; and Type III—a severe disorder with vWf antigen or activity absent (150,151).

Most cases of clinically significant von Willebrand disease are known before pregnancy because of a history of menorrhagia. Some, however, are not defined until bleeding complicates pregnancy because of the acceptance by the woman that her menses are normative by family standards. Although the factor VIII/vWf complex increases in pregnancy, ristocetin co-factor concentration and bleeding time changes are more variable (97,152). However, individual response over several pregnancies appears to be consistent (97).

The major risks in pregnancy are birth-related hematoma and postpartum hemorrhage as noted by von Willebrand (153). Unfortunately, there is poor correlation between the rise in factor VIII:C and vWf in pregnancy and bleeding complications (154). A normal bleeding time done immediately before delivery is predictive of adequate hemostasis during labor and delivery. A normal antepartum bleed time, however, does not assure a risk-free condition for postpartum hemorrhage because of the rapid fall in vWf after placental delivery (97,122,154).

Even though factor VIII continues to increase during pregnancy to about 38 weeks gestation, abortion and ectopic implantation may still pose a significant hemorrhage risk in the first half of pregnancy (121,123,124). An abnormal bleeding time in the first trimester of pregnancy then must prompt measurement of vWf-ristocetin co-factor. After approximately 26 weeks gestation, monthly repetition of this assessment should be done should the bleeding time not be corrected ($\leq$ 12 min) by the physiologic increases in co-factor as the pregnancy progresses.

Type I disease patients should be given prophylactic cryoprecipitate prior to vaginal delivery if the ristocetin cofactor concentration is less than 50%. A single dose of 10 units will often suffice it. All patients who are to undergo cesarean section with vWf-related prolongation of bleeding time, regardless of level of co-factor, as well as those patients with a past history of postpartum hemorrhage, should receive prophylaxis (97,152). Fifteen to twenty packs of cryoprecipitate may be required. To address the known risk for delayed postpartum hemorrhage in these patients, cryoprecipitate therapy should be continued every 12 to 24 hours for about 4 days postpartum (152,155). Patients with Type IIB disease may also manifest thrombocytopenia, requiring platelet transfusion in addition to cryoprecipitate (156).

DDAVP (1-deamino-8-D-arginine vasopressin), a synthetic antidiuretic hormone, has been used in stable nonpregnant patients with mild or moderate Type I disease, but its associated risk of thrombosis probably precludes its use in pregnancy except in the postpartum patient who refuses cryoprecipitate therapy.

## Factor XI

Deficiency of the contact components including factor XI may prolong the activated partial thromboplastin time, but it does not appear to have evident impact on clinical coagulation.

## Factor IX; Factor VIII

Factor IX (Hemophilia B) and the more common factor VIII (Hemophilia A) deficiencies are X-linked recessive disorders predominantly restricted to males. The physiologic increase in factor VIII in pregnancy in the carrier state has associated mean values of ~50% (97,98). Factor IX activity levels do not increase to near this degree in pregnancies complicated by the carrier state (95).

The "deficiency" in these conditions is more in decreased activity of the factor than in the quantity of factor produced. Clinical severity correlates with the level of activity: a severe course is experienced with 1% or less normal activity, a moderate course with 2 to 5% activity, and a mild course with 6 to 50% activity (157). The predominant risk in pregnancy is postpartum hemorrhage followed by postsurgical bleeding (95,97,158).

A carrier with factor VIII activity of less than 30% should receive cryoprecipitate or factor VIII concentrate to increase the factor VIII level to 50% of nonpregnant normal values prior to birth (159). Lower threshold levels for factor IX activity therapy are operative. Cryoprecipitate does not contain a significant amount of factor IX activity. Fresh frozen plasma or factor IX concentrate should be used as required in patients with hemophilia B (97). Severe factor IX activity deficient states may be treated with prothrombin-complex concentrates, but heparin must be used with the concentrate to minimize thrombosis risk.

DNA technology has enhanced the assessment for the maternal carrier state and the prenatal diagnosis of fetal disease, but coagulation activity measurement to assess the carrier state is still required in some cases (160).

The risk of hepatitis and AIDS viral transmission attendant to nonpasteurized cryoprecipitate has been addressed by monoclonal antibody-derived factor VIII and IX products (161,162). This more purified factor VIII product has not addressed, however, the issue of the formation of inhibitors (162). Treatment of patients with von Willebrand's disease or hemophilia A with pasteurized factor VIII is shown in Table 26–5.

## Factor XI

Factor XI deficiency has been reported mainly in Ashkenazi Jews with the predominant risks being blood loss

**Table 26–5.** Hemophilia Treatment with Postfactor 8 Concentrate in 155 Total Patients

| | Age at First Infusion yr | Observation Period mo | Total Dose of Factor VIII IU |
|---|---|---|---|
| Median | 3.00 | 45.00 | 17,100 |
| Maximum | 82.00 | 110.00 | 2,155,375 |
| Minimum | 0.20 | 4.00† | 500 |
| Mean | 9.40 | 49.23 | ND |
| Sample covariance | 11.98 | 4.91 | ND |

* Patients were treated with pasteurized factor VIII concentrate exclusively. ND denotes not done.
† Only four patients had observation periods of less than 15 months.
(From Schimpf K, Brackmann HH, Breuz W, Kraus B, et al: Absence of antihuman immunodeficiency virus types 1 and 2 seroconversion after the treatment of hemophilia A or von Willebrand's disease with pasteurized factor VII concentrate. N. Engl. J. Med. 321(17):1148–52, 1989.)

with birthing lacerations or postpartum hemorrhage (100,163). Plasma provides an adequate resource when needed.

## Factor V

Deficiency of factor V appears to pose little risk in pregnancy. A low incidence of postpartum hemorrhage has been reported but it may be severe (164,165). Fresh frozen plasma provides sufficient factor V in cases of hemorrhage.

## Factor VII

Factor VII deficiency has been reported. It does not appear to pose a risk for hemorrhage in pregnancy, probably because of the production of a phospholipid-factor VII complex with increased specific activity when compared to the nonpregnant form of factor VII (87).

## Factor X

Factor X deficiency rarely complicates pregnancy, although postpartum hemorrhage has been reported (100,166). Fresh frozen plasma is used in cases of hemorrhage.

## Factor XIII

Postpartum hemorrhage and bleeding from the umbilical stump have been reported with factor XIII deficiency (100). Repeated miscarriages are also reported (101). Fresh frozen plasma provides factor XIII in cases of hemorrhage.

## Inherited Hypofibrinogenemia

This disorder is almost never a problem because fibrinogen levels increase as a physiologic response in pregnancy. There is a lowered reserve, however, that may contribute to earlier expression of hemorrhage secondary to disseminated intravascular coagulation.

## Vitamin-K Deficiency

Vitamin-K is a necessary cofactor for carboxylation of prothrombin, factors VII, IX, X, protein C, and protein S. Severe liver disease, vitamin-K malabsorption, nutritional inadequacy, and antibiotic effects (either by direct action in the liver, as seen with N-methyl-thiotetrazole conformed cephalosporins or indirectly by suppression of intestinal flora) may be associated with factor deficiencies of a degree leading to severe hemorrhage.

Fresh frozen plasma is a source for factor abnormality secondary to vitamin-K deficiency.

## Liver Disease

Almost all of the factors involved in normal hemostasis are produced in the liver. Severe functional impairment of the liver can lead to severe hemorrhage secondary to deficiency of one or more of these critical clotting factors. This is most commonly seen in obstetrics with fulminant viral hepatitis, cirrhosis, or acute fatty liver.

## Thrombin Inhibitors

Antithrombin III and protein C are the major inhibitors of thrombin activity. Deficiencies of either of these or protein C's cofactor, protein S, pose high risk for thrombosis (167,168,169). Most cases of thromboembolic disease in pregnancy that are secondary to one of these deficiencies are associated with antithrombin III activity. Thrombosis risk usually presents at an early age prompting the advise that young patients with venous thrombosis, those with recurrence of deep vein thrombosis without other obvious causes, and those with a family history of thrombotic disease should be screened for deficiency of AT III and, if normal, for protein C and protein S deficiencies (Figure 26–4). The risk of thrombosis with a deficiency is enhanced in the thrombogenic state of pregnancy (170,171). A clue to the presence of antithrombin III or protein C-S deficiency may be provided by the requirement of very high doses of heparin to effect the desired prolongation of the activated partial thromboplastin time in patients being managed for thrombosis.

While AT III and protein C are unchanged in uncomplicated pregnancy, both free and bound protein S are decreased (172). Deficiency of any of these three proteins in a pregnant woman with prior thromboembolic disease must be treated with prophylactic heparin (173,174). High doses of heparin, particularly in the aggravated hypercoagulable state associated with thrombogenesis, are required (175). Heparin dosage is adjusted to prolong the activated partial thromboplastin time patient to control ratio to 1.3 to 1.5. High-dose heparin ($\geq$ 20,000 units/day) administration for several months in pregnancy carries some risk for osteopenia (176,177). In severe AT III deficiency, fresh frozen plasma (a relatively poor source of AT III) or AT III concentrate in combination with heparin may be required, reflective of heparin's anticoagulant action being mediated through antithrombin III by changing its molecular configuration (96,175,178–180). Fresh frozen plasma is the source for protein C replacement. Purified protein C from human plasma or recombinant protein C is available (181). Aspirin should not be used in protein S deficiency because it inhibits protein S release from platelets (169).

Postthrombosis management of patients with protein C or S deficiency requires long-term warfarin therapy after completion of the pregnancy (182). Coumarin derivative use is contraindicated during pregnancy, particularly in the first trimester because of the potential for severe injury to the embryo. Vitamin-K administration has been recommended to prevent warfarin-induced skin necrosis when used for protein C deficiency (183).

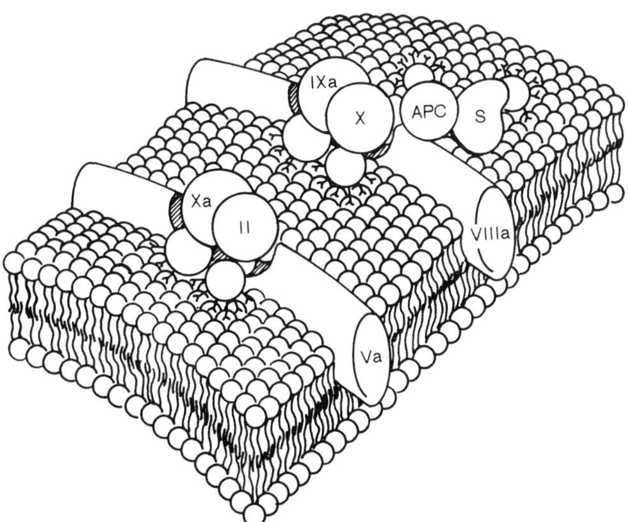


**Fig. 26–4.** Demonstrates various complexes of coagulation factors on the surface of a membrane. Note that factors V and VIII are substrates for activated protein C. (Modified from Rick ME: Protein C and Protein S: Vitamin K-dependent inhibitors of blood coagulation. J.A.M.A. 263(5):701–3, 1990.)

## Factor Inhibitors

Factor VIII inhibitors may develop as autoantibodies in postpartum women or as alloantibodies following factor VIII transfusion (184). Inhibitors to factors V, IX, XI, and XIII have also been described (185–187).

Inhibitors are usually IgG and therefore may cross the placenta. Spontaneous remission may occur in almost 40% of patients with factor VIII autoantibodies (188). Clinical distinction from factor VIII or IX deficits typically follows a severe delayed postpartum hemorrhage. Diagnosis is made by adding various dilutions of the patient's plasma to a constant amount of factor VIII either from concentrate or pooled normal plasma.

Treatment with factor VIII concentrates in patients with low levels of inhibitor usually suffices. In those with high levels of inhibitor, however, factor VIII concentrate infusion response is unsatisfactory. Plasmapheresis can temporarily reduce inhibitor levels by up to 50% (189). Pooled gamma globulin may also neutralize the autoantibodies (184).

## Acquired Inhibitors

Lupus anticoagulant and its kindred anticardiolipin (ACA) are antibodies to negatively charged phospholipid,

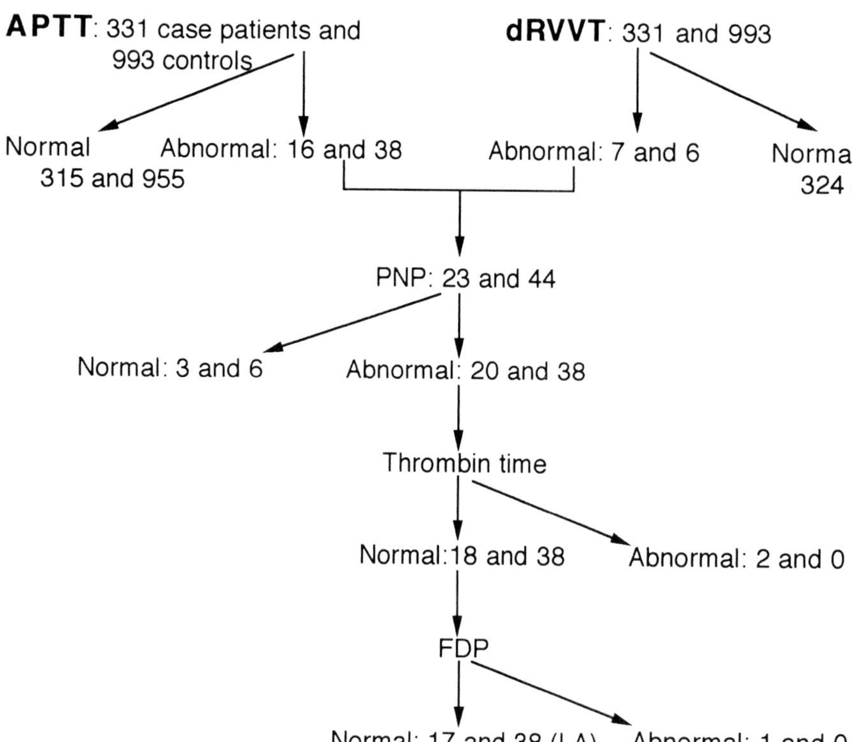


**Fig. 26–5.** Shows the screening steps for lupus anticoagulant in women with and without fetal loss. APTT = activated partial thromboplastin time. dRVVT = dilute Russels viper venom time. PNP = platelet neutralizing procedure. FDP = fibrinogen degradation products. (Modified from Infante-Rivard C, David M, Gauthier R, Rivard GE: Lupus anticoagulants, anticardiolipin antibodies, and fetal loss. N. Engl. J. Med. 325(5):1063–6, 1991.)

which are associated with fetal loss and such adverse pregnancy outcomes as early onset severe preeclampsia and intrauterine growth retardation (141,190–194). The fetal loss issue in asymptomatic women is somewhat controversial (195). The anticardiolipin antibody does not appear to have as firm a relationship to thrombotic disease as has been ascribed to lupus anticoagulant. Lupus anticoagulant—a name applied before its function was defined—is a misnomer in that lupus anticoagulant does not contribute to bleeding except when hypoprothrombi-

**Table 26–6.** Clinical and Serological Data

| Age | Clinical Data | RBNP* Qualitative | Positive Anticardiolipin Isotypes (SD) | Serum ANA |
|---|---|---|---|---|
| 23 | SLE, DVT | Pos | IgG 31.0; IgM 3.6; IgA 5.0 | 1:160 |
| 30 | | | IgM 2.9 | <1:20 |
| 36 | | Pos | IgG 6.6; IgM 3.0 | 1:640 |
| 34 | | Pos | IgM 4.6 | <1:20 |
| 35 | | Neg | IgM 7.0 | <1:20 |
| 36 | | Neg | IgM 3.5 | 1:40 |
| 32 | DVT | Pos | All isotypes negative | <1:20 |
| 32 | SLE, T | Pos | IgG 22.5; IgM 19.8; IgA 20.0 | 1:80 |
| 32 | SLE, TIA | Pos | IgG 7.0 | 1:320 |
| 29 | SLE, DVT | Pos | IgG 23.0; IgA 3.6 | 1:160 |
| 29 | | Neg | IgM 7.0 | 1:80 |
| 39 | | Neg | IgM 5.0 | 1:160 |
| 28 | | Neg | IgG 13.0; IgM 5.0 | <1:20 |
| 27 | SLE | | IgG 4.4; IgM 8.0; IgA 4.0 | 1:5120 |

RBNP = rabbit brain neutralization procedure; STS = nontreponemal serologic test for syphilis; ANA = antinuclear antibodies; SLE = systemic lupus erythematosus; DVT = deep vein thrombosis (lower extremity); pos = positive; Ig = immunoglobulin; ND = not done; neg = negative; T = thrombocytopenia; TIA = transient (cerebral) ischemic attack.
* Values exceeding the mean +2 SD of normal subjects (≥0.17) are reported as qualitatively positive.
† False positive, based on a negative fluorescent treponemal antibody test.
(Modified from Rosove MH, Tabsh K, Wasserstrum N, Howard P, et al: Heparin therapy for pregnant women with lupus anticoagulant or anticardiolipin antibodies. Obstet. Gynecol. 75(4), 630–4, 1990.)

nemia or quantitative/qualitative platelet abnormality are present (138,139). About 4% of pregnant women test positive for one of these antiphospholipid antibodies (196).

Antepartum therapy has been advocated in patients with high antibody levels and/or prior pregnancy-related loss (Figure 26–5 and Table 26–6) (139,190–195,197). I have observed resolution of elevated levels of lupus anticoagulant and anticardiolipin between pregnancies as well as with first testing in a subsequent pregnancy. I therefore recommend obtaining levels of these "antibodies" prior to conception, if possible, and if low or negative, then repeat testing at about monthly intervals from 12 to 24 weeks gestation. Interlaboratory reproducibility of "titers" to lupus anticoagulant remain a problem clinically, requiring that the clinician assure the reliability of the test results. Careful monitoring of fetal status appears to be of at least equal import in improving pregnancy outcome (198).

Heparin was first recommended as a therapeutic intervention referable to recurrent pregnancy loss but it does not appear to have advantage over prednisone in this regard (191–193). Low-dose aspirin, which may also have an ameliorating effect on the development of severe preeclampsia, has also been advocated (Table 26–7) (192,194,199–203). Aspirin in a dosage of 40 to 80 mg/day is effective in normalizing the prostacyclin-thromboxane ratio (Figure 26–6) (203–206). Further, this impact on these prostanoids qualitatively and favorably affects the pressor response to angiotensin II in women with preeclampsia (Figure 26–7) (207).

Thromboembolic disease may also be reduced in mothers receiving heparin. This effect is not so with low-dose aspirin. Further, heparin use may lead to thrombocytopenia and, in high dosage use, to osteopenia (176,177,208). Because the activated partial thromboplastin time is already prolonged in patients with lupus anticoagulant, heparin dosage is monitored by thrombin time ($\geq$ 100 seconds) and prothrombin time (less than 2 seconds prolongation over control) (191).

Prednisone lowers the activated partial thromboplastin time (190,209). Complications with prednisone include increase in glucose intolerance, requiring insulin therapy in about 15% of patients, as well as an increase in pregnancy-induced hypertension and preterm birth secondary to premature rupture of membranes (137,193,210).

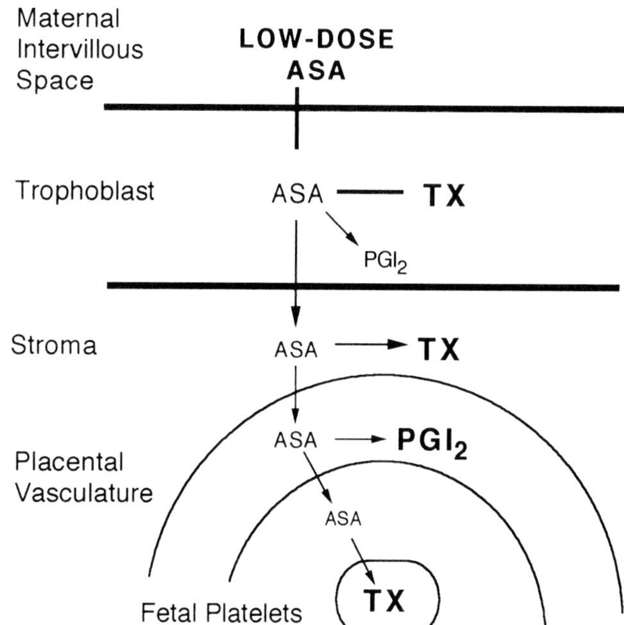


**Fig. 26–6.** Demonstrates comparison of thromboxane (TX) and prostacyclin ($PGI_2$) in human placenta. It also demonstrates the effect of low-dose aspirin (ASA) during pregnancy to inhibit placental thromboxane production. (Modified from Walsh SW: Physiology of low-dose aspirin therapy for the prevention of preeclampsia. Semin. Perinatol. 14(2):152–70, 1990.)

## *Fetal/neonatal Risk*

The predominate risk for the fetus in pregnancies complicated by coagulopathy is injury secondary to inadequate oxygenation when hypovolemic shock ensues in the mother. Fetal injury can also follow inadequate placental perfusion such as may occur in abruption of the placenta. Neonatal bleeding with factor deficiencies is usually secondary to trauma or surgical procedures such as circumcision. The acquired inhibitors are associated with fetal loss secondary predominantly to thrombosis in

**Table 26–7.** Pregnancy Treated with Corticosteroids and Low Dose Aspirin

| | | | Outcome* | | | |
|---|---|---|---|---|---|---|
| Author and Year | No. of Patients | No. of Pregnancies | Live Births | Fetal Deaths | Spontaneous Abortions | |
| Lubbe, 1988 | 19 | 19 | 15 (78%) | NA | NA | |
| Gatenby, 1989 | 27 | 27 | 17 (63%) | NA | NA | Includes some pregnancies treated without LDA |
| Ordi, 1989 | 7 | 9 | 7 (78%) | 2 (22%) | 0 | |
| Lockshin, 1990 | 10 | 11 | 2 (18%) | 6 (55%) | 3 (27%) | Includes three patients not treated with LDA |
| Cowchock, 1991 | 19 | 19 | 13 (68%) | NA | NA | |
| Reece, 1991 | 18 | 18 | 14 (78%) | 1 (5%) | 3 (17%) | |
| Branch, 1991 | 31 | 38 | 25 (66%) | 7 (18%) | 6 (16%) | |

* Fetal deaths defined as intrauterine death of a fetus proven to be alive after 10 weeks of gestation.
(From Branch DW: Antiphospholipid Syndrome: laboratory concerns, fetal loss, and pregnancy management. Semin. Perinatol. 15(3):230–7, 1991.)

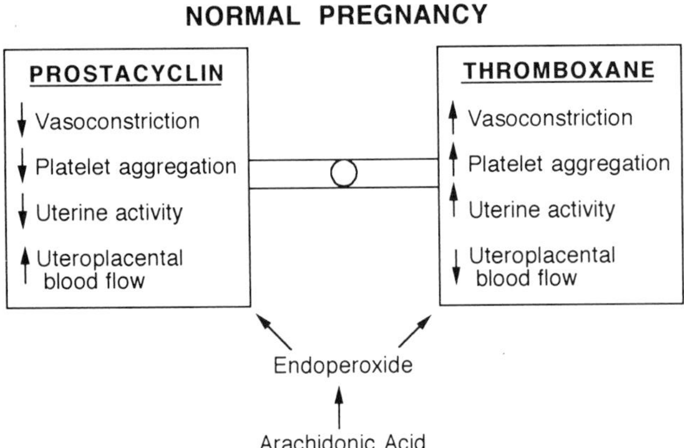


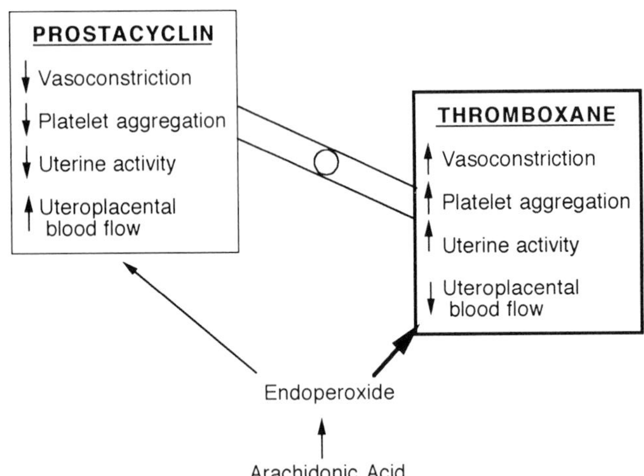


**Fig. 26–7.** Compares the prostacyclin and thromboxane components in normal pregnancy (Top) to the imbalance of the increased thromboxane and decreased prostacyclin in preeclampsic pregnancy. (Modified from Walsh SW: Physiology of low-dose aspirin therapy for the prevention of preeclampsia. Semin. Perinatol. 14(2):152–70, 1990.)

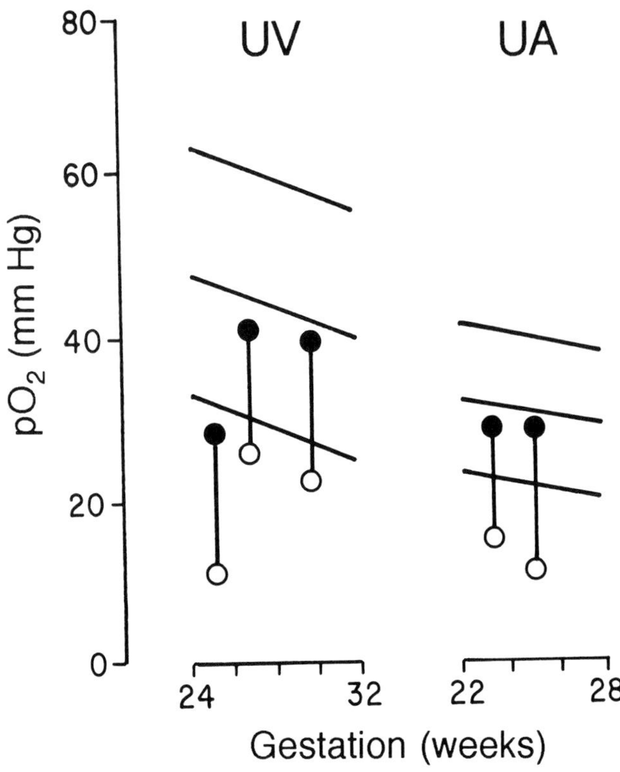


**Fig. 26–8.** Demonstrates the effect of 10 minutes of maternal hyperoxygenation on changes elicited in $PO_2$ of hypoxic fetuses. Open circles = values before hyperoxygenation. Closed circles = values after hyperoxygenation. (Modified from Nicolaides KH: Cordocentesis. Clin. Obstet. Gynecol. 32(1):123–35, 1988.)

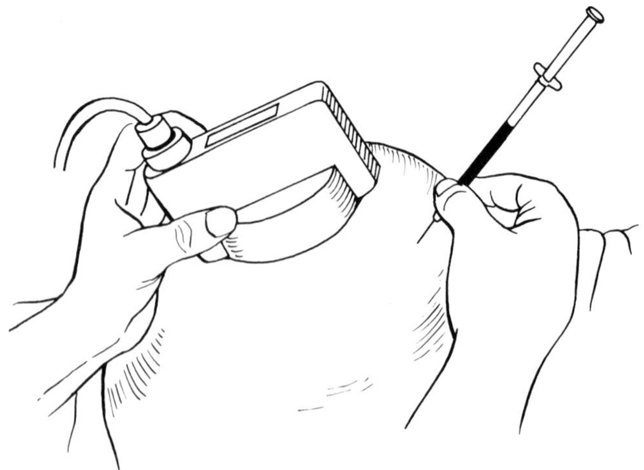

**Fig. 26–9.** Demonstrates the method of cordocentesis fetal-blood sampling by use of ultrasonography. (From Nicolaides KH: Cordocentesis. Clin. Obstet. Gynecol. 32(1):123–35, 1988.)

the placental bed (211–213). Antithrombin III and protein C have caused thrombosis in the fetus and the newborn (96,214–217). Lupus anticoagulant and anticardiolipin antibody have been so implicated in the newborn as well (215,218,219).

The hemophilia and the severe form (type-III) of von Willebrand syndrome in the fetus may have associated intracranial hemorrhage particularly with traumatic birth (220–223). DNA analysis is available for carrier detection of hemophilia (224). Similarly, analysis from cells obtained at chorionic villus sampling (CVS) can define type-III vWf disease with high confidence. While percutaneous umbilical blood sampling (PUBS) may be used to define the fetal/neonatal risk, and even to provide therapeutic intervention (Figure 26–8), this procedure is not without risk in these cases (Figure 26–9) (225,226). Fetal scalp trauma that occurs with scalp electrode placement or blood sampling must be avoided. Although vWf factor levels tend to be elevated in the newborn from those levels that will be operative at a later date, the vWf level should be obtained before any surgery. Definition of a hemophilia in the newborn dictates diligent attempts to avoid trauma as well as satisfactory correction of the factor deficiency before any operative interventions.

## Obstetric Hemorrhage

Dysfunction of the musculature of the uterus contributes more to pregnancy-related hemorrhage than do specific disease states. Even in instances of hemorrhage secondary to nonobstetric conditions, the predominant volume of blood loss is from the uterus. The predominant factor loss in obstetric hemorrhage is fibrinogen, followed to a much lesser degree by factor VIII. While platelets may be decreased, they rarely play a role in significant failure of hemostasis except during or after massive hemorrhage.

Perfusion inadequacy and/or hypoxemia are the predominant risks for the fetus/newborn with maternal hemorrhage.

### *Antepartum Conditions*

Antepartum hemorrhage is less common than abnormal bleeding in the intrapartum or postpartum periods. Most cases of antepartum bleeding are secondary to disruption of the placenta-uterine interface.

#### *Abruptio Placentae*

Some degree of abruption or premature separation of the placenta occurs in approximately 1% of pregnancies (227). The clinical presentation is most often one of vaginal bleeding often associated with pain, but more often with uterine contraction activity. Uterine tenderness to palpation is present in approximately 50% of cases. The quantification of external bleeding often significantly underestimates the total blood loss, because much of the blood remains retroplacental.

Abruption of the placenta is more common in patients with a history of prior abruption, particularly with associated hypertension. Abruption risk, as well as related perinatal mortality, is increased significantly in smokers of cigarettes (228). High parity and lower uterine segment implantation sites also increase the risk for placental abruption. Trauma to the abdomen and uterus, particularly secondary to motor vehicle accident with seat-belt in place, may produce a separation of the placenta. In most instances of trauma with abruption, there is no external blood loss from the uterus requiring a high index of suspicion and a protocol approach to the diagnosis of the abruption. Such an approach includes at initial patient contact the monitoring of the fetal heart rate, obtaining of a fetal red blood cell assessment in maternal blood (i.e., a Kleihauer-Betke), fibrin split products and, finally, the obtaining of a fibrinogen. If the fibrinogen level is greater than 350 mg/dl, the test level should be repeated to assure stability in 8 to 12 hours. Fibrin split products should be positive in virtually all cases of abruption with clinical import.

Preterm labor may be associated with or heralded by placental abruption. All patients with preterm labor, as well as those with clinical suspicion of abruption of the placenta, should have uterine ultrasonography to assess placental status. Unfortunately, ultrasound assessment will fail to confirm placental abruption in about one-half of the cases in which it is subsequently demonstrated at delivery. A normal ultrasound study does not rule out abruption of the placenta.

As previously noted, fibrinogen concentration rises significantly during the course of normal pregnancy. Abruption of the placenta may be suggested in pregnancy by relative hypofibrinogenemia, i.e., a level of less than 350 mg/dl. The fibrinogen level can fall very rapidly (229,230). If the patient is having continued heavy bleeding at the time of admission, a whole blood clot or a thrombin clot tube should be obtained at the bedside. With less severe bleeding, fibrinogen levels should be obtained serially every 2 hours should the patient be having uterine contraction activity.

The consumption of fibrinogen is secondary to placental-uterine tissue injury with release of tissue thromboplastin and activation of factor VII, i.e., initiation of the extrinsic pathway of the clotting cascade. Activation of the fibrinolytic system causes release of fibrinogen-fibrin degradation products. While absence of fibrin degradation products in the circulation makes the diagnosis of clinically significant abruption unlikely, the level of fibrin degradation products does not proffer any indication as to the degree of hypofibrinogenemia.

Thrombocytopenia (platelet count less than 100,000/μL) occurs in about one-quarter of patients with abruption. It is extremely rare for the platelet count to fall to less than 10,000 and therefore the thrombocytopenia rarely contributes to the hemorrhage except with massive blood loss (231). Platelet transfusion is not indicated regardless of the platelet count or anticipated cesarean birth unless active bleeding, not responsive to blood and volume replacement, is ongoing. Prophylactic platelets are simply consumed with further fibrin generation, increase in fibrinogen-fibrin degradation products, and further enhancement of their fibrin degradation products anticoagulant activity. Following delivery of the placenta, fibrinogen levels rise at an average rate of about 9 mg/dl/hour (232). A depressed platelet count is slower to recover, often taking 4 or more days to obtain a level $\geq$ 100,000 μL.

Time is of the essence as regards the diagnosis and initial management in severe cases of placental abruption as evidenced by the fact that almost three-quarters of the fetal deaths occur more than 90 minutes after admission to the hospital (227). Patients admitted with preterm labor secondary to placental abruption who are stable and with fibrinogen levels of greater than 150 mg/dl may be treated with magnesium sulfate tocolytic therapy if there is fetal immaturity. The milder clinical presentations can be managed with volume replacement and serial assessment of maternal fibrinogen level as well as fetal status during labor and planned vaginal birth.

More seriously affected patients characterized by blood that is not clotting at the time of admission or unstable cardiovascular status with hypofibrinogenemia ($\leq$ 150 mg/dl) should be given volume replacement as crystalloid-colloid, 10 to 15 cryoprecipitate packs, and packed red blood cells, as needed. The cryoprecipitate is preferred over fresh frozen plasma as the source of large amounts of fibrinogen because of its lower volume. Furthermore, obtaining fresh frozen plasma commonly takes 45 minutes or longer rather than the 10 to 15 minute time to obtain cryoprecipitate and initiate infusion. Patients with hemorrhage and associated severe hypofibrinogenemia should be stabilized and have the cryoprecipitate infusing before operative intervention to effect cesarean birth. Heparin should not be employed in these patients. The key to prevention of acute tubular or bilateral cortical renal necrosis is rapid and aggressive restoration of blood volume (233).

### Placenta Previa and Accreta

Placenta previa complicates approximately 0.5% of pregnancies (234). Vaginal bleeding in these patients is generally painless, although suprapubic tenderness to palpation and uterine contraction activity from partial separation of the low-lying placenta often complicate the bleeding. The bleeding is rarely complicated by disseminated intravascular coagulation as may be the case with abruption of the placenta. Rather, the blood loss is from maternal veins. Marginal abruption of a low-lying placenta previa is an associated risk.

Diagnosis of placenta previa has been greatly facilitated by the availability of ultrasonography. This diagnosis is more common in earlier pregnancy with retreat of some of the noncentrally placed placentas from the cervical opening with progression of the gestation. With documented placenta previa and no bleeding by 34 weeks gestation, the clinician should suspect concomitant placenta accreta, which increases in occurrence significantly in patients with previous cesarean section (235).

Conservative management with delivery of the baby by cesarean section after attainment of fetal lung maturity is recommended (236,237). Selection of delivery time with placenta previa and/or placenta accreta typically follows the obtaining of fetal lung maturity tests beginning at about 34 weeks gestation (238).

The subject of not removing the placenta at the time of cesarean section is discussed later in the section on Retention of the Placenta. The reader is referred to Chapter 38 and the section on Placenta Accreta.

### Dead Fetus Syndrome

The hypofibrinogenemia associated with retained dead fetus is typically not manifest until 3 to 4 weeks following intrauterine death (239). The exception to this is in the case of fetal death with associated hydropic changes, presumably because of the increased thromboplastin release from the hydropic fetal tissue. This complication is predominantly one of singleton fetal demise, although coagulopathy following the death of one fetus in a multiple gestation has been reported (240).

A fibrinogen level should be obtained on all patients with intrauterine fetal death before initiation of labor. Again, the activated partial thromboplastin time and the prothrombin time will not delineate clinically significant hypofibrinogenemia until the issue becomes obvious by the hemorrhage of nonclottable blood. Serial fibrinogen assessments should be done every 2 hours during labor in the patients who have low values (150 to 350 mg/dl). For values greater than 350 mg/dl, assessments can be done every 4 hours.

Prelabor administration of heparin will correct significant hypofibrinogenemia over a 1 to 2 day period of time (241). In multiple gestation, awaiting adequate fetal maturity for the living fetus(es) to ensue, subcutaneous heparin on a twice a day basis is employed. When fetal maturity is not an issue and maternal fibrinogen level is less than 150 mg/dl, continuous heparin infusion in an amount (800 to 1200 units/hour, with higher amounts in the more obese patient) to prolong the activated partial thromboplastin time 1.2 to 1.4 times the control is employed. Weiner suggests individualizing the heparin dose to reflect normalization of the level of fibrinopeptide A (242). Ultrasonography should address not only the issue of fetal demise, but whether or not there is associated placental abruption and/or hydropic change in the fetus that can additionally impact on the coagulopathy.

### Molar Pregnancy

Hemorrhage secondary to molar pregnancy is mainly caused by rapid blood loss from the noncontractile distended uterus at the time of evacuation of the mole by a combination of suction and sharp curettage. Disseminated intravascular coagulation has been reported, however (104,243). Blood fibrinogen concentration and platelet count should be known before elective intervention for molar pregnancy. Cryoprecipitate is used in those instances in which the preoperative fibrinogen level is less than 150 mg/dl.

### Preeclampsia/Eclampsia

Preeclampsia—classically a triad of pregnancy-associated hypertension and variably severe edema and proteinuria—is restricted to pregnancy (244,245). The etiology of the disorder remains unknown, although an immune-type process is supported by much circumstantial evidence (246–249). Although characterized as a hypertensive disorder, the clinical presentations wherein thrombocytopenia or rarely disseminated intravascular coagulation lead to abnormal maternal bleeding do not typically manifest severe hypertension ($\geq$ 110 mm Hg) (250,251).

The disease process of preeclampsia is established well before its clinical presentation. Current understanding of the sequence of events in this disorder include a failure of the decidual vessels to undergo their normal pregnancy changes so that vascular resistance is not significantly lowered (252,253). Vascular resistance is further increased by athetosis in the vessels, suggestive of an immune-type response (245,254,255). The resultant decrease in perfusion of trophoblast causes generation or activation of placentally-derived "toxin(s)," which in turn induces vasospasm and endothelial cell injury (256–258). Lipid peroxides and thromboxane are generated by the placenta in abnormal amounts in women with preeclampsia

(259–263). The peroxides activate cyclo-oxygenase and inhibit prostacyclin synthetase contributing to the decrease in $PGI_2/TxA_2$ ratio characteristic of severe preeclampsia (260,262,264). With damage of the vascular endothelium, platelets are activated with resultant diffuse fibrin thrombus formation and propagation. The vasospastic and fibrin deposition components of this disease add additional impact to tissue hypoperfusion with hypoxemic accentuation of the endothelial injury and initiation of coagulation. Elevated plasma vasoactive peptide levels have been reported in pregnancies complicated by preeclampsia (Figure 26–10) (265–267). This regulatory peptide not only possesses potent vasodilator properties, but it has been shown to inhibit platelet aggregation and increase production of prostacyclin.

Before attaining the threshold blood pressure level (i.e., 140/90 mm Hg) to be defined as hypertensive, women with preeclampsia demonstrate increased sensitivity to pressor substances (Figure 26–11), decreased plasma volume, increased cardiac output, and statistically significant elevation in blood pressure as early as 18 weeks gestation (268–273). Once disease is clinically evident, total peripheral resistance and blood pressure are increased and cardiac output is normal or decreased (258,274). Venous tone is increased (275). Epigastric, right upper quadrant pain or both is the presenting complaint in about 90% of cases of severe preeclampsia with progressive thrombocytopenia (falling levels to ≤ 100,000/μL) (244,276–279). Other common symptoms include malaise and nausea, sometimes with vomiting. This collection of symptoms, coupled with the often present sign of right upper quadrant tenderness to palpation, commonly leads to initial mis-diagnosis as a gastrointestinal disorder (279–281). Conversely, incorrect diagnosis of medical-surgical cases as an obstetric disorder may cause delay of appropriate therapy and iatrogenic premature birth (282). Again, hypertension is not essential to the diagnosis of severe preeclampsia (250,251,277).

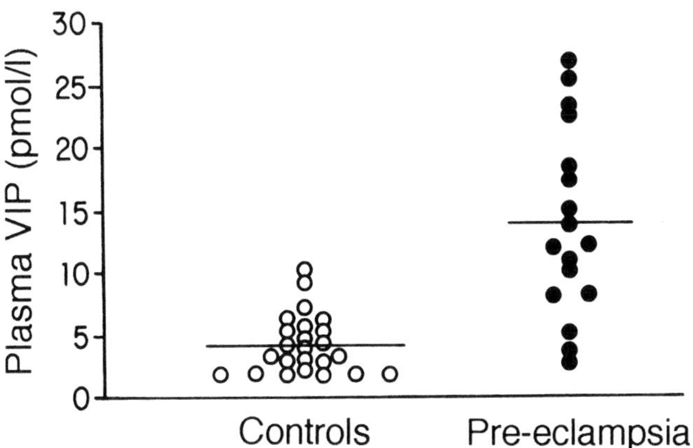


**Fig. 26–10.** Demonstrates the plasma vasoactive intestinal polypeptide in both control and preeclamptic patients. Mean values are denoted by horizontal lines. (Modified from Holst N, Oian P, Aune B, Jenssen TG, Burhol PG: Increased plasma levels of vasoactive intestinal polypeptide in pre-eclampsia. Br. J. Obstet. Gynaecol. 98:803–6, 1991.)

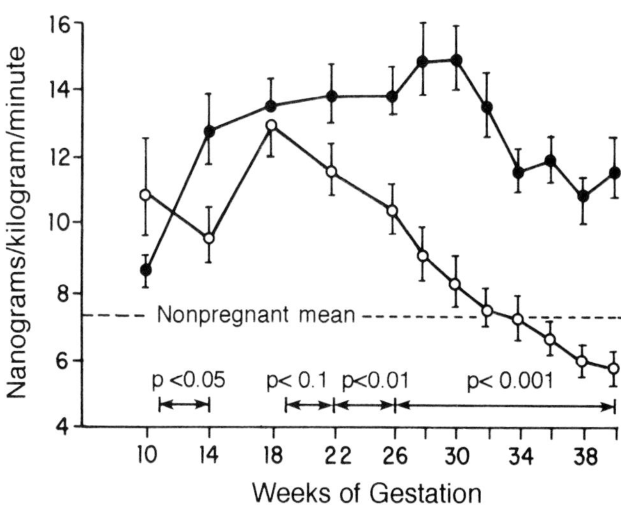


**Fig. 26–11.** Comparison of angiotensin necessary to elicit pressor response in primigravidas who had normal blood pressure (BP) (black circles) compared to those with pregnancy-induced hypertension (HIP) (open circles). (Modified from Gilstrap LC, Gant NF: Pathophysiology of preeclampsia. Semin. Perinatol. 14(2):147–51, 1990.)

That the compensated hypercoagulability of pregnancy is aggravated by preeclampsia is evidenced by further reduced levels of AT III and a decrease in the factor VIII activity to antigen ratio (244,250,283–286). Further, the platelet count decreases, and turnover as well as content and activity are altered (287–292). Preeclampsia reflects a platelet rather than a thrombin-driven consumption. Accordingly, the plasma fibrinogen concentration, the prothrombin time, and the activated partial thromboplastin time are almost always normal unless there is severe liver dysfunction. The bleeding time is often prolonged in severe preeclampsia in association with the thrombocytopenia, but rarely to threatening levels of ≥ 15 minutes (133,277). Eclampsia may further aggravate the bleeding tendency and its complications but, unless the increased risk for placental abruption eventuates, disseminated intravascular coagulation is still a rare complication (293).

Prolongation of the prothrombin time usually reflects the association of acute fatty liver with decreased synthesis of factor VII. Factors XI and XII may also reach critically low levels as can others of the procoagulants produced by the liver causing a prolongation of the activated partial thromboplastin time. Liver failure is also reflected in reduced synthesis of inhibitors to coagulation, in particular AT III, further aggravating the coagulation process. Prolongation of the prothrombin time or partial thromboplastin time (PTT) must prompt investigation as to causation, as 1% or less of severe preeclamptic patients are thus represented.

Thrombocytopenia (less than 100,000/μL) occurs secondary to platelet consumption in 15 to 20% of patients with preeclampsia (250,276,293,294). Classic disseminated intravascular coagulation with consumption of fibrinogen and coagulation factors is rare, and when disseminated intravascular coagulation is present, it usually represents a complication of placental abruption, which is more common in the hypertensive conditions of pregnancy, and/or as a terminal event following adult respiratory distress syndrome (ARDS) (250,295). Maternal mortality is very high if disseminated intravascular coagulation develops.

The most severe presentation—characterized by more or less significant microangiopathic hemolysis (H), elevated liver enzymes (EL), and low platelets (LP)—complicates approximately 10% of preeclampsia cases (277,278,293). The ascribed acronym HELLP is a superb one for this presentation of the disease process, as both the patient and the practitioner may benefit from any help they get (278).

Timely delivery is the standard of care for preeclampsia. The deportment of the women with HELLP syndrome often belies the severity of their illness. It is mandatory that the caretakers understand that women with severe preeclampsia (Table 26–8) have a life-threatening illness. There is no place for procrastination as regards instituting aggressive, supportive care, or in effecting delivery. Once liver enzymes are elevated (SGOT ≥ 100 units) and/or severe thrombocytopenia (≤ 50,000/μL) is manifest, there is very high perinatal/maternal morbidity and mortality. Hemolysis, when severe or continuing, portends an even worse prognosis for the mother. Conservative management, as advocated by some for this progressive disease process, is warranted only in cases of significant fetal immaturity and then only when the hospital-based platelet count remains ≥ 75,000, the SGOT remains at ≤ 100, and there are no other maternal-fetal complications (293,296). Because these laboratory-based parameters may quickly change, they should be checked in the stable patient at least twice a day once they are found to be abnormal.

Hospital-based treatment in the main consists of $MgS0_4$ infusion and antihypertensive therapy for severe hypertension. $MgS0_4$ is preferred over phenytoin by obstetricians for prophylaxis against convulsions and for its other salutary effects (244,258,297). While this in part likely reflects the comfort of experience with the clinical use of $MgS0_4$, phenytoin metabolism is dependent on normal hepatic function and exhibits saturation kinetics, thereby, in severe preeclampsia, posing an inordinate risk for toxicity (298,299).

**Table 26–8.** Expanded List of Severe Preeclampsia Features

| Features | Parameters |
|---|---|
| Blood pressure | ≥160/110 mmHg (at bed rest) |
| Proteinuria | ≥5G/24 hr |
| Cerebral/visual abnormalities | Present |
| Upper abdominal pain | Present |
| Oliguria | <500 ml/24 hr |
| Pulmonary edema/cyanosis | Present |
| *(H): Hemolysis | Present |
| *(EL): ↑ Liver Enzymes | SGOT ≥100 Iu/L |
| *(LP): Thrombocytopenia | <100,000/μL |

* Presence of all three features constitutes HELLP syndrome.

Women with severe preeclampsia, especially when severe hypertension (≥ 110 mm Hg diastolic blood pressure at bedrest) and or hemoconcentration (hematocrit ≥ 40%) are manifest, are at particular risk for development of pulmonary edema (245,300,301). The well-intended attempt to enhance tissue perfusion/oxygenation by the expansion of plasma volume with crystalloid solutions poses a high order of risk for iatrogenic pulmonary edema with an opposite to desired effect on oxygenation. More severe clinical presentations of the preeclampsia are more likely to be associated with this untoward response to even small volume preloading (i.e., 500 ml). Increased capillary permeability secondary to hypoxic injury and the reduction in colloid oncotic pressure secondary to hypoalbuminemia, crystalloid, and occasionally $MgS0_4$. Large-volume ascites combined with cesarean birth may portend a greater intolerance for intravenous fluid challenges in patients with HELLP syndrome (304).

A central, indwelling arterial catheter is required to differentiate those patients who may benefit from low volume (i.e., ≤ 500 ml), high molecular weight fluid preloading prior to vasodilative, antihypertensive therapy (305). Further, therapeutic interventions in patients with established cardiac or renal failure and/or pulmonary edema not responsive to diuresis may be more appropriately guided by information garnered from centrally-obtained data. The decision for the use of this intervention requires (in prioritized order): (1) normal coagulation values; (2) initiation of appropriate blood products in instances of associated hemorrhage; (3) a practitioner experienced in interpretation of the data obtained; and, (4) a practitioner skilled in catheter placement. Catheterization of large centrally-placed vessels must NOT be done until coagulation homeostasis is assured.

Severe hypertension (≥ 110 mm Hg diastolic after initiation of bedrest and $MgS0_4$ infusion is treated with intravenous hydralazine·HCl (244,297,306). Nitroglycerin has also been recommended especially when there is associated pulmonary edema (307). Sublingual nifedipine (10 to 20 mg), a calcium channel blocker, appears to be effective without adverse impact on fetal or maternal blood flow (Figure 26–12 and 26–13) (308–312). Captopril, an angiotensin converting enzyme (ACE) inhibitor, should not be used because of potential for life-threatening injury to fetal kidneys (313). Sodium nitroprusside, used in the past when the elevated blood pressure was not responsive to hydralazine, is cumbersome to use and poses potential risk for the fetus by the formation of cyanohemoglobin, although the clinical import of this is controversial (244,314–317). Intravenous labetalol or verapamil have been employed for management of severe hypertension refractory to hydralazine therapy (305,306,317–319).

The blood pressure lowering effect and the dosage relationship of the specific antihypertensive medicine is very individual. Titrated infusion rates and lower dosages than are used in other antihypertensive emergencies are employed to avoid relative maternal hypotension (≤ 95 mm Hg, diastolic). Acute and/or significant decreases in mean

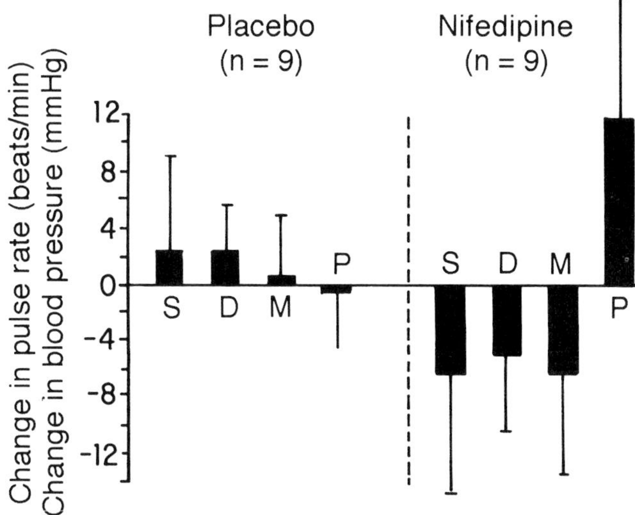


**Fig. 26–12.** Changes in systolic and diastolic mean arterial pressure and pulse rate after placebo or nifedipine treatment. (Modified from Lindow SW, Davies N, Davey DA, Smith JA: The effect of sublingual nifedipine on uteroplacental blood flow in hypertensive pregnancy. Br. J. Obstet. Gynaecol. 93: 1276–1281, 1988.)

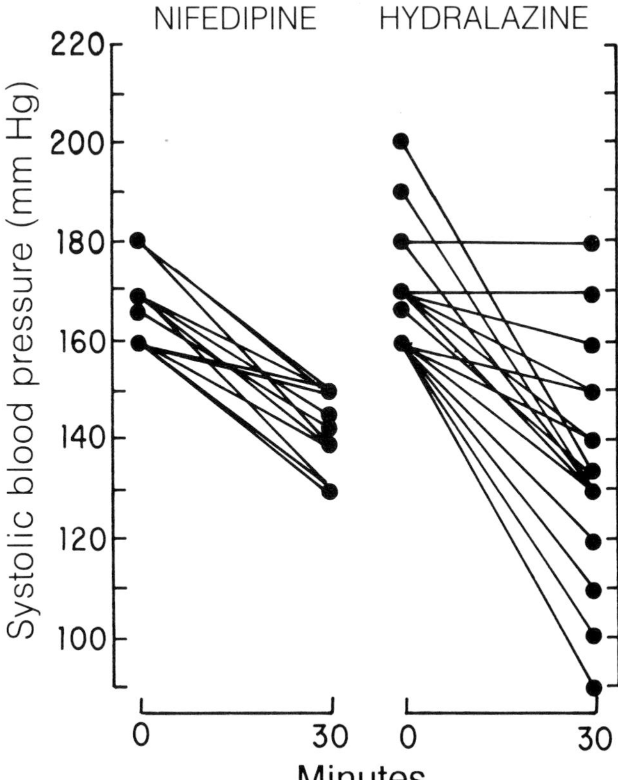


**Fig. 26–13.** Systolic pressure changes with nifedipine versus hydralazine. (Modified from Fenakel K, Fenakel G, Appelman Z, Lurie S, et al: Nifedipine in the treatment of severe preeclampsia. Obstet. Gynecol. 77(3):331–7, 1991.)

arterial pressure (MAP) have the potential for associated maternal or fetal morbidity due to a further decrease in organ perfusion. While hydralazine infusion, for example, may enhance the cardiac output while lowering blood pressure, it may be at the expense of uteroplacental perfusion (320,321).

Drug-induced reduction of maternal blood pressure without prior volume expansion with low volume (~ 400 ml), high molecular weight fluid may reduce oxygen delivery and consumption even with hyperdynamic cardiac function (305,322). Extreme caution is required in giving these hypertensive women any fluid challenge, even when faced with further hypovolemia secondary to hemorrhage. Attention to detail as to the type and the quantity of a fluid to be infused is essential.

Maternal prognosis with HELLP syndrome is associated less with the severity of thrombocytopenia, more with the plasma level of liver enzymes and most critically with the severity of the microangiopathy. The most critical element for restoration of maternal health is the expertise of the caretakers. All interventions for these severely ill patients must be timely and thoughtful. The opportunities for iatrogenic maternal demise run rampant in this presentation of the disease.

The consumptive process in these women is predominantly one impacting on the quantity of platelets. Regardless of the platelet count or the planned route of delivery, the thrombocytopenia should not be treated with prophylactic platelets. Any additional platelets are rapidly consumed with aggravation of the microvascular thromboses and tissue perfusion and oxygenation are further compromised. When progressive hemolytic anemia (falling HCT, less than 28%) is evident, packed red blood cells may be required. In the vary rare instance of confirmed disseminated intravascular coagulation and hemorrhage, cryoprecipitate should be used. When the coagulopathy is associated with severe liver disease, such as acute fatty liver, wherein factor levels of less than 30% may be operative, fresh frozen plasma may be required. Packed red blood cells and cryoprecipitate are used rather than whole blood, crystalloid or plasma when possible to minimize the intravascular volume load to the patient. Platelet transfusion is restricted to cases of hemorrhage refractory to the above therapy. Plasmapheresis has a role in factor deficiency states when the volume load attendant to deficiency correction with fresh frozen plasma is excessive for the patient. This therapy in severe cases of hemolysis or significantly elevated liver enzymes [SGOT (AST) $\geq$ 2000 IU/L; SGPT (ALT) $\geq$ 3000 IU/L] may be life-saving (323). It has also been recommended in cases of progressive disease not responding to intensive, interventive therapy (324,325). Intravenous immunoglobulin may offer another alternative (326).

Eclampsia, perhaps because of the aggravation of hypoxia/acidosis, trends to a more severe coagulopathy. Cesarean sections should not be done in response to fetal distress documented during and/or immediately after maternal seizure activity. Likewise, central catheter placement should not be undertaken. To perform either of these two interventions prior to maternal stabilization and therapy (typically 4 to 8 hours time postseizure) as well

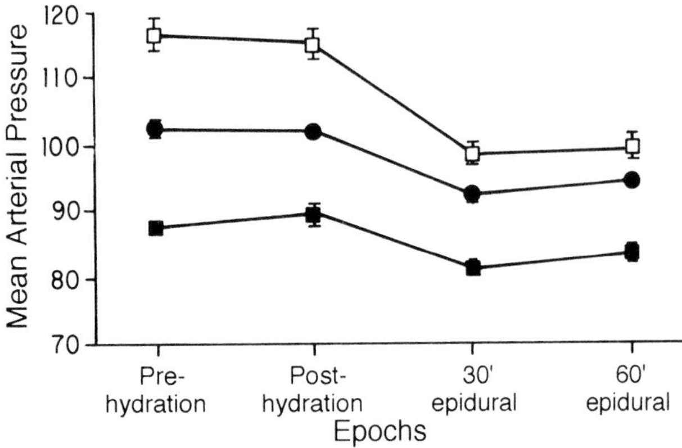


Fig. 26–14. MAP during time periods (pre, post, 30 minutes after, and 60 minutes after epidural block). (Modified from Ramos-Santos E, Devoe LD, Wakefield ML, Sherline DM, et al: The effects of epidural anesthesia on the Doppler velocimetry of umbilical and uterine arteries in normal and hypertensive patients during active term labor. Obstet. Gynecol. 77(1):20–6, 1991.)

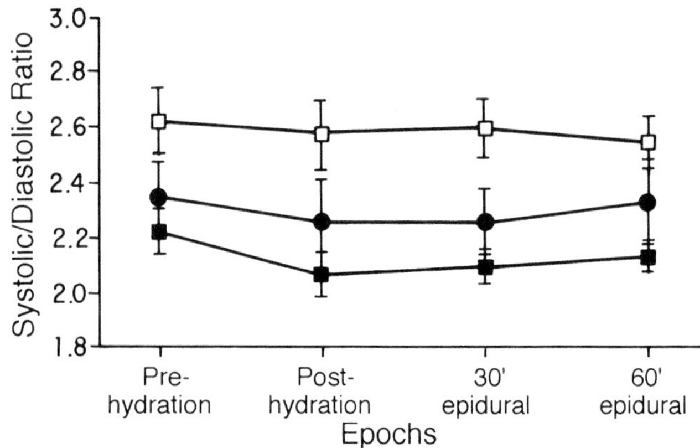


Fig. 26–16. Systolic and diastolic ratios during pre, post, 30 minutes and 60 minutes after epidural block. (Modified from Ramos-Santos E, Devoe LD, Wakefield ML, Sherline DM, et al: The effects of epidural anesthesia on the Doppler velocimetry of umbilical and uterine arteries in normal and hypertensive patients during active term labor. Obstet. Gynecol. 77(1):20–6, 1991.)

as prior to obtaining assurance of normal coagulation parameters, carries an inordinate risk for maternal death.

Epidural anesthesia is often advocated for its maternal blood pressure lowering effects (Figure 26–14). It may also have a salutary effect on uterine artery vasospasm, thus benefitting fetal well-being (327). The complications of maternal hypotension with attendant decrease in cardiac output and underperfusion of maternal and fetal tissues may be prevented by volume preloading (Figure 26–15 and 26–16). As this is fraught with the previously cited risk for pulmonary edema in the severely ill patient, slow, deliberate development of the desired anesthesia and avoidance of the typical rapid 1 to 2 liter, lactated Ringer's infusion is highly recommended. Because the platelets are commonly dysfunctional in this condition, platelet counts less than 100,000/μL demand an Ivy bleeding time determination (Figure 26–17) (328,329). Epidural anesthesia should not be done if the bleeding time is in excess of 11 minutes. "Significant" epidural space bleeding may occur when the platelet count is greater than 90,000/μL, but the bleeding time is greater than 15 minutes (293).

Perinatal morbidity includes intrauterine growth retardation (IUGR), thrombocytopenia, and neutropenia (330–333). Changes in red blood cell morphology have

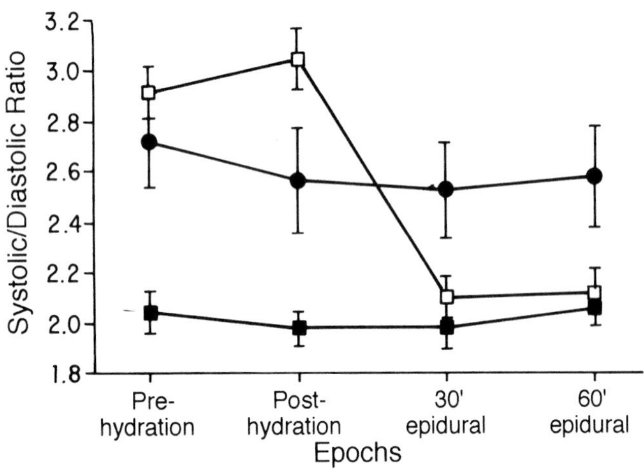


Fig. 26–15. Systolic and diastolic ratios during pre, post, 30 minutes and 60 minutes after epidural block. (Modified from Ramos-Santos E, Devoe LD, Wakefield ML, Sherline DM, et al: The effects of epidural anesthesia on the Doppler velocimetry of umbilical and uterine arteries in normal and hypertensive patients during active term labor. Obstet. Gynecol. 77(1):20–6, 1991.)

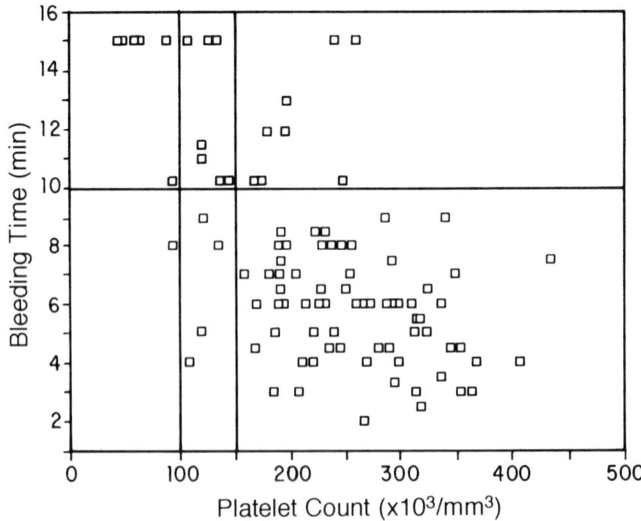


Fig. 26–17. Bleeding time as platelet count in preeclamptic women. (Modified from Ramanathan J, Sibai BM, Vu T, Chauhan D: Correlation between bleeding times and platelet counts in women with preeclampsia undergoing caesarean section. Anesthesiology 71:188–91, 1989.)

also been noted (334). Respiratory distress syndrome, adjusted to gestationally-dated risk, seems to be less likely in babies from mothers with severe maternal hypertension (335).

## Intrapartum Conditions

### Abruptio Placentae

Bleeding from abruption of the placenta often precipitates uterine contraction activity, which cannot or should not be altered by tocolytic therapy should there be probable adequacy of fetal lung maturity. Further, many marginal or partial abruptions of the placenta occur during labor. Most of these are associated with increased uterine bleeding but rarely with the development of disseminated intravascular coagulation, a risk predominantly restricted to placental abruption occurring in the antepartum period. Preterm labor and/or labor associated initially with uterovaginal bleeding or fetal distress should prompt investigation for abruption of the placenta including obstetric ultrasonography, CBC, and fibrinogen assessment. Similarly, the "irritable uterine contraction pattern" (low amplitude contractions with ~ one (1) minute interval between) on electronic monitoring suggests the diagnosis of placental abruption.

The management of the mother and baby during labor and delivery as regards coagulation assessments and treatment of excessive bleeding is the same as that covered in the antepartum section.

### Rupture of Uterus

Rupture of the uterus most often follows abdominal trauma. As an isolated obstetric-related event, it may occur before the onset of labor in patients with previous cesarean section, particularly when the uterine scar extends into the upper segment of the uterus (336).

More commonly, uterine rupture not associated with trauma occurs after labor ensues. As a complication of vaginal birth after cesarean section (VBAC), it occurs at a rate of 1 to 2/1000 births (337). Uterine rupture during labor is more common in multiparous women experiencing an abnormal labor pattern. Risk appears to be further increased by oxytocin augmentation of dysfunctional labor particularly in women of parity ≥ seven (338,339).

Rupture of the unscarred uterus often takes place laterally where the arterial vasculature enters the uterine wall. Bleeding into the broad ligament and retroperitoneally may be extensive with shock out of proportion to any externally evident blood loss. While sudden, acute abdominal pain usually heralds rupture of the uterus during labor, conduction anesthesia may completely mask this pain. Electronic fetal heart rate and contraction monitoring should be used in all labors with previous cesarean section, with dysfunctional labor, and with pitocin augmentation of labor, particularly should conduction anesthesia be employed. With rupture of the uterus during electronic monitoring, there is an initial onset of severe variable decelerations followed by a fall in the fetal heart rate. An associated topping off of the uterine contraction pressure documentation, which may be followed by an apparent uterine contraction pressure of zero also occurs. Amniotic fluid embolism may occur at the time of uterine rupture with the rapid evolution of the profound cardiorespiratory and coagulation complications described below.

Emergency cesarean birth may be life-saving for the baby if carried out within 10 minutes of uterine rupture. Prompt operative response also minimizes the risk of shock in the mother. Therapy of hypovolemic shock with or without disseminated intravascular coagulation should be initiated and ongoing before hysterectomy or other operative interventions except primary repair of the uterine musculature if deemed appropriate.

### Amniotic Fluid Embolism

While amniotic fluid embolism (AFE) is associated with placental abruption, placenta previa/accreta, rupture of the membranes, and tumultuous labor/delivery, none of these associated risk factors is useful in either predicting or preventing this complication. There is often no prodrome. Many patients will say they are not feeling well, will sit up in the bed and vomit followed shortly by dyspnea, tachypnea, and cyanosis. The cardiopulmonary collapse presents as a shock state, typically without significant blood loss initially.

The pathophysiology of the cardiopulmonary changes, no less the subsequent, rapidly progressive disseminated intravascular coagulation is not well defined. While obstruction of the pulmonary vasculature by fetal debris and subsequent cor pulmonale was thought in the past to be the initiating characteristics of the cardiopulmonary failure, in fact, it appears that left ventricular rather than right ventricular failure is present (340).

Clinically significant hemorrhage is preceded by laboratory evidence of coagulopathy by 30 to 60 minutes providing a brief opportunity for obtaining the blood components required for therapy (341). Amniotic fluid contains thromboplastin, which activates the coagulation cascade by the activation of factor X (342). The addition of amniotic fluid void of particulate matter to plasma still effects the activation of factor X (343). Thrombin consumption follows the pulmonary endothelial damage secondary to particulate matter from the amniotic fluid, but this consumptive process appears to be transient and not the predominant contributor to the coagulopathy. Amniotic fluid also contains plasmin proactivator, which may contribute to the thrombin generation (344). The very high concentration of fibrin degradation products has lead to the suggestion that primary fibrinogenolysis may contribute significantly to the disseminated intravascular coagulation (345). The hypoxia-acidosis that follows the significant resistance to pulmonary distention as well as the profound arteriolar vasoconstriction in the pulmonary bed, further aggravates the disseminated intravascular coagulation. Amniotic fluid's procoagulant effect also correlates with it's phospholipid content (343).

The management of suspected amniotic fluid embolism must be prompt. With suspected diagnosis at the time of the cardiopulmonary manifestations, blood components, in particular cryoprecipitate, and platelet concentrates,

**Table 26–9.** Blood Components' Volumes and Content

| Component | Approximate Volume in ml | Approximate in vivo Increase/Unit of Component | Other Factors |
|---|---|---|---|
| Packet Red Blood Cells (PRBC) | 300 | 3% Hct ↑ | some stable factors |
| Fresh Frozen Plasma (FFP) | 200 | ↑ factors ≈ equal to one unit whole blood | stable and labile factors (VIII, V) |
| Cryoprecipitate (C:AHF) | 15 | 10–15 mg/dl ↑ fibrinogen | FVIII, FXIII, vWf |
| Platelet Concentrate | 30 | 5–10,000/μL | platelet-bound FVIII and FV and stable factors* |

* Eight to 10 platelet concentrates may contain the equivalent of stable clotting factors in two units of plasma.
(From Circular of information for the use of human blood and blood components. American Red Cross. American Association of Blood Banks, and the Council of Community Blood Centers, March 1989.)

should be ordered rather than awaiting the results of laboratory testing or remarkable hemorrhage. Oxygen delivery to the mother is often times difficult because of the significant smooth muscle constriction of airway. In the past, positive end expiratory pressure was recommended, but this may further impair left ventricular dysfunction (340). Because of the salutary effect of heparin on thrombin generation as well as its antiserotonin impact on the smooth muscle of the respiratory tree, give a bolus of 10,000 units of heparin in that grace period from the onset of cardiopulmonary symptoms and hemorrhage (88,346). Heparin should not be used in the face of hemorrhage secondary to the coagulopathy (347). Of the obstetric-related disseminated intravascular coagulation states, amniotic fluid embolism imparts the most significant fibrinogenolysis. Use of an antifibrinolytic agent has been suggested (348).

Pulmonary edema is a common associated complication in surviving patients as is adult respiratory distress syndrome. Pulmonary edema further aggravates the associated hypoxemia attendant to efforts at pulmonary resuscitation. Cryoprecipitate, 15 to 20 units, initially is preferred to fresh frozen plasma because its infusion can be initiated more rapidly and also because there are significant differences in the volume of blood product delivered to the patient (Table 26–9). Once hemorrhage is manifest secondary to disseminated intravascular coagulation, the use of platelet concentrates is inevitable and therefore they should be ordered at the same time as the initial laboratory work, cryoprecipitate, packed red blood cells, and fresh frozen plasma are ordered.

## *Postpartum Conditions*

History repeats itself in obstetrics as elsewhere. Any patient with a history of postpartum hemorrhage should be delivered in a setting in which blood will be immediately available when postpartum hemorrhaging occurs following birth.

### *Atony of Uterus*

Uterine atony is the leading cause of obstetric hemorrhage (1). Even in coagulation factor deficient states, excessive, life-threatening blood loss usually follows completion of the third stage of labor. Combs and associates confirmed others' experiences in showing that nulliparity, prolongation of the third stage of labor, augmentation of labor, instrumental delivery, twin gestation, and previous postpartum hemorrhage with vaginal birth and abnormal labor, general anesthesia, and amnionitis with cesarean birth to be associated with postpartum hemorrhage (7,13,14,349–353). Preeclampsia also increases postpartum hemorrhage risk (13,14). This is likely in part due to the uterine musculature-relaxing effect of magnesium sulfate, and, in part, it reflects platelet dysfunction as well as the increased mean arterial pressure complicating severe cases of preeclampsia.

The active management of the third stage of labor, characterized by administration of an oxytocic agent after early cord clamping followed by controlled cord traction, has been shown to decrease the incidence of postpartum hemorrhage, transfusion, and hemorrhage-related anemia (354–356). This accords with the experience at the time of cesarean section wherein manual removal of the placenta immediately after cord clamping and administration of an intravenous oxytocic agent typically is followed by prompt, firm contraction of the uterine musculature.

When uterine atony occurs, the uterine cavity should be explored for retained placental tissue and the uterus gently massaged. Initially, 10 units of oxytocin are given intravenously over 2 to 3 minutes' time and continuous intravenous infusion of oxytocin-containing fluid is continued for 6 or more hours as required. Rapid intravenous administration of oxytocin done in this fashion does not appear to be associated with hypotension or cardiac arrhythmias, although bolus-push oxytocin in the face of massive hemorrhage may induce hypertension (357). Prostaglandin-$F_2\alpha$ (0.25 mg), injected intramuscularly or intra-myometrially, should be used if uterine atony does not respond to these interventions (358–360). Continued bleeding after uterine tone normalizes must immediately prompt an investigation as to the origin of the blood loss and maternal coagulation status. Procrastination approaches, such as ordering additional oxytocin administration and/or intravenous fluid therapy until forced to respond to hypovolemic shock, are inappropriate. Uterine packing can play a significant role in those women who either desire to maintain reproductive capability and/or when there is massive hemorrhage in the face of unavailability or refusal to receive blood and blood components (361,362).

## Retention of Placenta

Retention of a portion of the placenta may produce postpartum blood loss directly or indirectly by contributing to uterine atony. Incomplete separation of the placenta from the uterine wall may denote placenta accreta. Postpartum hemorrhage secondary to uterine atony that is unresponsive to therapy, or recurs after an initially good response to therapy, requires cervical and intrauterine evaluation, including uterine cavity curettage. With persistent bleeding, uterine packing may be effective following manual removal of the placenta and curettage for the management of low-lying placental implant or placenta accreta.

Continuing bleeding in the face of normal coagulation requires surgical intervention. In women desirous of retaining reproductive capability, hysterotomy and placement of parallel rows of continuous, locking, vertical mattress sutures through the uterine wall from endometrium to serosa may arrest bleeding or, at least, decrease it to an extent to facilitate a positive impact from a thrombogenic material such as topical thrombin (Parke-Davis, Morris Plains, NJ) placed on packing gauze against the lower uterine segment tissues. Surgical interventions including curettage of the uterus and selective arterial embolization increase the risk for postpartum uterine and pelvic infection. Antibiotics should be selected to address the typical, multiple organisms involved in postpartum uterine infection. Packing should be removed in 12 to 24 hours after hemostasis is obtained. Prophylactic heparin (5 to 6000 units subcutaneous every 12 hours for 48 hours or until fully ambulatory) may decrease the risk for thromboembolic disease, particularly when pelvic infection complicates postpartum hemorrhage.

Finally, the finding of an accretal placenta that does not come free of the uterine attachment with ease on intrauterine exploration and attempted removal does not necessarily require removal and/or hysterectomy. In women who desire maintenance of reproductive capability, the placenta sans cord may be left in situ should hemorrhage secondary to uterine atony not be a continuing feature. Patients with the placenta left in place should receive a complete course of appropriate antibiotic coverage. Methotrexate therapy may also play a role in placenta resorption (363). Delayed bleeding from a retained placenta may be able to be addressed by targeted arterial embolization.

## Uterine Inversion

Inversion of the uterus is almost uniformly associated with cord traction on a fundally implanted placenta (364). Hemorrhage may be significant if the placenta has separated. With early recognition of this complication of placental delivery and before there is significant tissue edema, intravenous tocolytic therapy may facilitate uterine muscle relaxation and vaginal reinversion of the uterus (365,366). Once hypovolemic shock is manifest, however, $MgSO_4$ tends to lower blood pressure and β-mimetics may be associated with cardiac complications and/or pulmonary edema.

If celiotomy is required, the sequential traction on the round ligaments with ring forceps and/or the reduction of the inversion through a posterior midlevel lower uterine segment incision usually is successful (367,368). Intramyometrial injection of 15-methyl $F_2\alpha$ (0.25 to 0.50 mg) should be given after abdominal reinversion. The uterus should be observed before surgical closure until uterine tonus recurs and hemorrhage and/or recurrent inversion are no longer issues. Occasionally, intrauterine packing will be required because the uterus will require several hours before there is a return of adequate function of the muscle.

## Lacerations: Birth Canal/Uterine

Lacerations during birthing with associated hemorrhage occur most commonly in the perineal area followed by vaginal, cervical, and uterine tissues. Extensive blood loss may occur even without laceration as a complication of local anesthesia, pudendal nerve block, operative delivery or simply, spontaneous vaginal delivery when the woman has abnormal coagulation function such as occurs with von Willebrand disease or thrombocytopenic conditions.

The perineum, vagina, and cervix should be routinely inspected visually after each and every birth for lacerations and/or bleeding. Further, the vagina should be palpated for hematoma formation. Vaginal packing should be employed in those instances of coagulation dysfunction with diffuse, continued vaginal wall bleeding not amenable to primary repair. Selective arterial embolization has also been used (369–371).

Hypovolemic shock out of proportion to blood loss in association with appropriate uterine tonus requires initiation of resuscitative therapy and prompt identification of the source of the blood loss. Hidden bleeding with subsequent shock may result from cervical or uterine lacerations that extend into the broad ligament. Diagnosis of this condition often requires exam under anesthesia and/or exploratory celiotomy. Ultrasonography, CT, or MRI study of the parauterine tissues may be required for definition of a hematoma.

## Dead Fetus Syndrome

The bleeding associated with delivery of a dead fetus almost always occurs after delivery. While uterine atony, birth canal, or uterine trauma, particularly secondary to associated shoulder dystocia management, may occur as with any vaginal birth, the hypofibrinogenemia secondary to the dead fetus should be defined before the delivery of the placenta to avoid inordinate blood loss. As noted in the antepartum section, serial fibrinogen assessment and appropriate interventions with low levels of plasma fibrinogen are required to prevent extraordinary maternal blood loss. This approach is further mandated when the fetal demise is secondary to abruption of the placenta and especially if fetal hydrops is present.

## Coagulopathies

As noted earlier, while various factor deficiencies may contribute to obstetric hemorrhage, clinically significant hemorrhage usually is in association with uterine atony or loss of vascular integrity in the birth canal.

Dilutional coagulopathy implies complete exhaustion of coagulation factors with major hemorrhage and replacement therapy. In the past, this concept mandated the prophylactic infusion of fresh frozen plasma, even with arrested hemorrhage, when five units or more of whole blood or packed red blood cells were transfused. Platelet concentrates infusion were also advocated when ten or more units of blood were transfused. In fact, especially in pregnancy, platelet consumption or dysfunction to a degree to require platelet transfusion is very rare. Further, the procoagulants are not uniformly consumed or lost if liver function is not seriously impaired. Component therapy is the desired approach to the replacement of coagulation factor deficiency. Again, fibrinogen and factor VIII replacement (as cryoprecipitate) are the typical need in obstetric hemorrhage. Prophylactic platelet transfusion often poses more risks than benefit.

## *Maternal Trauma*

Motor vehicle accidents (MVA) are the most common cause of nonobstetrical maternal mortality (1). Three-point constraints and lap belts, in that order, significantly decrease the risk of maternal-fetal demise over that associated with motor vehicle accidents when the mother is unrestrained (372–375). Acute head injury with subdural hematoma may lead to disseminated intravascular coagulation with high mortality risk when serum fibrinogen level is low (376).

Although placental abruption is increased with seat-belt use, the far greater contributor to fetal demise is maternal death that occurs predominantly in women who are unrestrained at the time of injury (372,373). Because of its lack of elastic tissue compared to the uterus, placental abruption may occur following acute maternal deceleration without other evidence of maternal trauma (377). The frequency of abruption of the placenta as a complication of motor vehicle accidents is directly related, however, to the severity and multiplicity of the maternal injuries (372).

Ultrasonography, CBC, and plasma fibrinogen concentration, as assessors of abruption of the placenta, should be obtained on all abdominal trauma cases. It is important to remember that sonography often times will not diagnose a clinically significant abruption (378,379). Pelvic ultrasonography may give guidance, however, to appropriate interventions by defining fetal demise, gestational age, and amniotic fluid volume. Further, a clinically significant quantity of intraperitoneal blood will typically collect in the pelvis and may be detected by the ultrasonogram.

Uterine contraction monitoring appears to be more sensitive than ultrasonography for the presumptive diagnosis of placental abruption (378). Most abruption-associated fetal deaths occur in the first 48 hours posttrauma, suggesting the critical period for continuous electronic fetal heart rate monitoring in viable (~ 25 weeks gestation) pregnancies (372). Electronic uterine contraction and fetal heart rate monitoring in minor maternal injury without evidence of uterine tenderness, uterine contractions, uterine-vaginal bleeding, rupture of amniotic membranes, or a nonreassuring fetal heart rate pattern (including tachycardia) may be discontinued within 6 hours and the patient discharged (380).

Almost one-third of pregnant women with blunt abdominal trauma have a positive Kleihauer-Betke (377). All Rh-negative women sustaining abdominal trauma should receive anti-D immune globulin. While evidence of a high volume fetal-maternal bleed must prompt additional anti-D immune globulin therapy for the mother and serial ultrasonographic evaluation for hydropic changes, a negative Kleihauer-Betke does not preclude a sensitizing fetal-maternal bleed.

Splenic rupture, even with apparently trivial trauma, and extensive retroperitoneal hemorrhage secondary to uterine or other pelvic tissue injury are increased in the pregnant woman, particularly after 20 weeks gestation (381–383). Other diagnostic studies, including those imparting irradiation exposure to the fetus and drug therapy mandated by the extent of the maternal injuries, must be carried out without regard to the pregnancy (383,384). Peritoneal lavage has been performed in pregnancy, but exploratory celiotomy should not be delayed by the performance of this procedure should the index of suspicion for significant intraperitoneal bleeding be high (385,386).

Hypovolemic shock in the mother may be relatively delayed in presentation reflecting the expanded blood volume in pregnancy. But when it occurs, its appearance is sudden and portends a potential for a catastrophic outcome for mother and baby. Blood volume replacement requirements for trauma-related hemorrhage is typically much greater than nonobstetric caretakers are accustomed to, thus setting the stage for inadequate fluid resuscitation. In instances in which the woman must be kept in a fixed supine position, movement of the uterus off of the vena cava by lateral displacement facilitates venous return to the heart and thereby increased cardiac output to optimize oxygenation for mother and fetus.

Antithrombin III falls significantly after severe trauma (387). Heparin prophylaxis, once maternal coagulation is normal, should be employed in the immobilized, bed-restrained woman with pelvic injury to address the significantly increased risk in pregnancy of thromboembolic disease.

Preterm labor is a common complication of uterine trauma and should be managed with magnesium sulfate infusion as required. Significant uterine contractions may be initiated by placental abruption. In addition, preterm labor often follows abdominal exploratory interventive procedures after about the twenty-fourth week of gestation. In such cases, prophylactic magnesium sulfate infusion is recommended for its tocolytic effect.

Most penetrating abdominal trauma in obstetrics follows gunshots or stabbings (382,388). Perinatal mortality is significantly higher than maternal death in penetrating tissue injuries (388,389). Exploration of the abdomen is recommended in patients sustaining gunshot wounds to the abdomen and in those women regardless of trauma type who do not become or remain stable with appropriate resuscitative intervention. A conservative (i.e., nonsurgical) approach has been recommended by Franger and associates for the stable maternal-fetal dyad in cases of gunshot entry wound below the level of the uterine fundus. Subsequent celiotomy is dependent on radiographic evaluation of the projectile's resting place with continued observation advised if the bullet resides within the uterus (389).

In the maternal code situation, with uterine enlargement to the umbilicus or above (approximately 24 weeks gestation), emptying of the uterus may be lifesaving for the woman as it optimizes cardiac venous return and pulmonary gases exchange. In the instance in which hysterotomy is being performed after failed initial resuscitative interventions in the mother, it is inappropriate to waste time on antiseptic procedures or operative hemostasis until resuscitation becomes successful. Postmortem cesarean birth for fetal survival is best effected within 5 minutes of maternal demise (390).

### *Fetal/Neonatal Risks*

Antepartum maternal hemorrhage leading to shock places the fetus and a surviving newborn at significant risk for hypoxemia-related injury secondary to decreased uterine perfusion. Uterine blood flow near term approximates 10% of total maternal cardiac output. A decrease in maternal intravascular volume not only decreases cardiac output and thus uterine blood flow, but the compensatory vasoconstriction in the mother decreases uterine flow to a further degree.

With adequate uterine perfusion, fetal $PO_2$ remains in the normal range until maternal $PO_2$ falls to 60 mm Hg or less (391). Because of the oxygen-dissociation curve characteristics for fetal blood, administering oxygen to the mother does increase fetal $PO_2$ to a small degree (392). Even small changes may be beneficial to the fetus. Maternal hyperventilation, as may be seen in hypovolemic shock, may produce a further decrease in uterine blood flow (393).

## Blood Loss in Medical Disorders Complicating Pregnancy

Most cases of inherited coagulopathy, which may contribute blood loss in pregnancy, are discernible by obtaining appropriate intake history before conception. Further, a prior obstetric history of recurrent pregnancy losses and/or second trimester presentation of severe preeclampsia should ideally prompt preconceptional investigation for an immune-type disorder. Counseling before pregnancy will not define all risks, however, because many of the immune-disorder syndromes are more common in women during the child-bearing years and may first present coincident with the index pregnancy.

### *Immune Disorders*

Thrombocytopenia is probably the leading coagulation abnormality associated with excessive bleeding in pregnancy. Frank hemorrhage, however, is rare as a complication of thrombocytopenia alone. Specifically, medical disorders typically impact on blood loss in pregnancy because of associated thrombocytopenia. When the medical disease-based thrombocytopenia is added to other hemorrhagic states in pregnancy, it may make a significant contribution to total blood loss. Postpartum blood loss is the major hazard.

#### *Antiphospholipid Antibodies*

Lupus anticoagulant and anticardiolipin antibodies are associated with an increased risk for recurrent pregnancy loss, fetal death, and remote-from-term, severe preeclampsia (190–193). As is the case for the false-positive serologic test for syphilis, these antiphospholipid antibodies are more commonly present in women with other positive autoantibody tests such as the antinuclear antibody associated with lupus erythematosus and platelet-specific antibody associated with thrombocytopenia.

Lupus anticoagulant and anticardiolipin antibodies although typically associated with a high incidence of thrombosis may contribute to significant bleeding when hypoprothrombinemia or quantitative/qualitative platelet abnormalities are present (138,139). In general, the thrombocytopenia induced by these antiphospholipids is not severe and per se does not cause hemorrhage in pregnancy.

#### *Autoimmune Thrombocytopenia*

Autoimmune thrombocytopenia (ATP) is the most common autoimmune disorder in pregnancy (394). Because of the frequent association of thrombocytopenia with other conditions, (e.g., drug-induced thrombocytopenia, bacteriemia, preeclampsia, lupus erythematosus, and leukemia), autoimmune thrombocytopenia is primarily a diagnosis of exclusion. A thorough history regarding drug use of a kind associated with thrombocytopenia and laboratory assessments for lupus erythematosus, preeclampsia or other possible abnormality is warranted. Pregnancy does not alter the occurrence rate nor does it exacerbate chronic autoimmune thrombocytopenia (395). Although the platelet count in normal pregnancy is thought to show little if any change, mild (100 to 150,000/μL), so called gestational or periparturient, thrombocytopenia is seen in up to 8% of pregnancies (396–398). These patients do not, however, have significant maternal or perinatal morbidity.

Diagnosis of autoimmune thrombocytopenia in pregnancy is often suggested by the platelet count done as part of a routine prenatal CBC. Automated blood cell counters have undoubtedly increased the discovery of thrombocytopenia in pregnancy. They may also falsely suggest autoimmune thrombocytopenia because of a low platelet count secondary to clumping of platelets caused by the anticoagulant EDTA (399). All cases of suspected thrombocytopenia require the performance of a peripheral blood smear to confirm the platelet count as well as to look for large platelets (megathrombocytes). The absence of large platelets in the peripheral smear makes the diagnosis of autoimmune thrombocytopenia tenuous and should prompt other studies including bone marrow aspiration, particularly with a platelet count of under

50,000/μL. Platelet-associated IgG antibodies (PA-IgG) are thought to confirm the diagnosis, but about 60% of nonthrombocytopenic pregnant women have a positive PA-IgG assay (396,400).

The increased platelet destruction in autoimmune thrombocytopenia is effected by the cells of the reticuloendothelial system following binding of IgG antiplatelet autoantibodies to platelet membrane. Antibody production and platelet destruction are predominantly functions of the spleen. Maternal splenomegaly, however, is not associated with autoimmune thrombocytopenia, and, in fact, if discovered during physical examination or at ultrasonography, a lymphoproliferative disorder must be considered. Aspirin and alcohol may aggravate the bleeding tendency in autoimmune thrombocytopenia. Therefore, they should be avoided. There are placental receptors for IgG antiplatelet antibody, thus facilitating the passage of antibody to fetal platelets.

Once a diagnosis of autoimmune thrombocytopenia is made, laboratory studies include serial assessments of the platelet count. Thyroid function and antinuclear antibody (ANA) titer screening is necessary because some patients with autoimmune thrombocytopenia also have thyroid dysfunction or lupus (401). Although the bleeding time is usually normal in autoimmune thrombocytopenia, a preprocedure bleeding time is recommended in women with a bleeding history in the pregnancy and/or in cases of a platelet count less than 50,000/μL. All cases of frank hemorrhage with autoimmune thrombocytopenia require appropriate clotting studies to rule in the culpable coagulation abnormality. It is extremely rare for even moderately severe thrombocytopenia (15,000 to 50,000/μL) to be the sole cause of hemorrhagic diathesis in autoimmune thrombocytopenia, perhaps reflecting the increased hemostatic competence of the young, large platelets typical of this disorder (402).

Maternal risks are predominantly those of birth canal hematoma and wound bleeding (e.g., episiotomy and suprafascial abdominal incision sites), particularly with platelet counts less than 20,000. Severe thrombocytopenia (≤ 20,000/μL) may significantly contribute to other causes of postpartum hemorrhage (403).

Fetal and neonatal risk is predominantly related to intracranial hemorrhage. Autoimmune thrombocytopenia does not increase the spontaneous abortion rate, intrauterine growth retardation, or preeclampsia (394,404). The apparent increase in fetal mortality secondary in part to intracranial hemorrhage has led some investigators to the conclusion that the fetus with thrombocytopenia (less than 50,000/μL) should be delivered by cesarean section (395,405). Others suggest that cesarean birth does not protect against intracranial hemorrhage (406–408). Laros, in fact, suggests the risk for intracranial hemorrhage to be higher with cesarean birth (406).

The severity of fetal/neonatal thrombocytopenia is not predicted by the maternal platelet count or the antiplatelet antibody levels (400,409–412). Further, post-splenectomy status women typically have a platelet count exceeding 100,000/μL but may be at higher risk of delivering a thrombocytopenic baby than the women with autoimmune thrombocytopenia who possess a spleen (413,414).

Fetal scalp sampling has been recommended for direct assessment of fetal platelet count but may underestimate the count particularly if the operator errs in using a heparinized collecting system (415–417). Clotting of the fetal scalp wound does not assure a platelet count greater than 50,000/μL (418). Further, when there is severe thrombocytopenia, the scalp wound may continue to bleed. Cordocentesis at about 38 weeks gestation has also been advocated for accurate assessment of fetal platelet count and to select those babies for whom cesarean birth is deemed appropriate, but its clinical utility is questionable in autoimmune thrombocytopenia (395,407,419,420).

Initial therapy for the asymptomatic pregnant woman with a platelet count consistently under 30,000/μL is oral prednisone in a dose of 60 to 80 mg per day with gradual tapering to a dosage that maintains the maternal platelet count above or near 50,000/μL. About 70% of patients with acute disease in pregnancy respond favorably within 3 weeks' time to allow gradual tapering of the steroid medication (421). The prednisone's impact on the platelet count appears to be due to increased platelet production (422). Pregnancy-associated hypertension and glucose intolerance sufficient to require insulin therapy are complications of corticosteroid use. Because only a small percentage of the prednisone crosses the placenta, a dosage of 60 milligrams or more per day for a few weeks prior to delivery or use of another steroid such as dexamethasone, which crosses the placenta to a higher degree, have been employed but without absolute assurance of a positive effect on the perinatal platelet count (423–426). Such high doses of prednisone, moreover, further enhance the risk for hypertensive disease of pregnancy and/or further deterioration in glucose tolerance.

High-dose hyperimmune globulin intravenous infusions are employed in patients in whom steroids are not effective (395,407,427–429). Even with a predictable, rapid, and positive response in the mother, perinatal thrombocytopenia may persist (430–432). Recent experience with the less costly Rh-immune globulin suggests that it be tried before the gamma-globulin (433,434). Splenectomy in the mother is reserved for the rare patient with intracranial hemorrhage and more commonly for those failing steroid and immune globulin therapies in the first two trimesters of pregnancy (395,404,407,435). After this time (~ 26 weeks gestation), plasmapheresis is employed (404,407). As with the failed therapies, splenectomy only corrects the mother's thrombocytopenia. It does not reduce any risk for the fetus and newborn. Polyvalent pneumococcal vaccine should be administered about 2 weeks before and repeated every 10 years after splenectomy (436,437).

Platelet infusions are restricted to the management of excessive blood loss explained solely by thrombocytopenia. Ten platelet packs should be available for patients with a platelet count less than 20,000/μL. But I do not advocate prophylactic platelet infusion against some arbitrary selected platelet count unless some other coagulation defect is also evident. Suprafascial, negative-pressure abdominal wound drainage, and pressure dressings may minimize bleeding into the incised tissues after cesarean section.

Route of delivery remains the enigma in patients with autoimmune thrombocytopenia. Cesarean birthing has associated maternal morbidity following perioperative bleeding. Vaginal birth supposedly carries a high risk for fetal intracranial hemorrhage, although any such risk is unpredictable, unpreventable, and perhaps unreal (438). The breech presenting and/or the preterm fetus (≤ 34 weeks gestation) should probably be delivered by cesarean section to minimize the risk of intracranial damage, but data to support this view are lacking.

### *Isoimmune Thrombocytopenia*

Isoimmune thrombocytopenia is a disease process wherein the mother produces antibodies against the PLA1 (PLSI) antigen on fetal platelets following sensitization by paternal antigen. The impact of this disease is fetal/neonatal—not maternal—unless the autoimmune and isoimmune thrombocytopenia are coexistent (439). The isoimmune type of thrombocytopenia poses a significantly greater risk than the autoimmune type for intracranial hemorrhage in the newborn. Evidence suggests a platelet membrane abnormality in the isoimmune variant that increases the risk for perinatal hemorrhage over that experienced with autoimmune thrombocytopenia at the same platelet count. Thus, the antenatal diagnosis of intracranial hemorrhage in the fetus is far more common in this condition than in autoimmune thrombocytopenia (440,441). Ultrasonogram is advocated to assess for intracranial hemorrhage before any prophylactic or therapeutic procedures to preclude unwarranted and unrewarding interventions (406). In contrast to autoimmune thrombocytopenia, cordocentesis for diagnosis and fetal therapy, as well as selection of the fetus for delivery by cesarean section, although not uniformly protective against intracranial hemorrhage, is consistently advocated (395,407,442–444). Maternal and fetal IgG infusion has been used in selected cases in an attempt to ameliorate the severity of the fetal thrombocytopenia (407,445,446).

### *Thrombotic Thrombocytopenic Purpura (TTP)*

Thrombotic thrombocytopenic purpura (TTP) is a syndrome of thrombocytopenia, microangiopathic hemolytic anemia, and neurologic abnormalities with varying occurrence of fever and renal dysfunction that occurs most commonly in young women (447,448). Hemolytic uremic syndrome (HUS) is most likely a variant of the same disorder. In contrast to disseminated intravascular coagulation which is thrombin-driven, thrombotic thrombocytopenic purpura is a platelet-vessel wall interactive dysfunctional syndrome. Its etiology and pathogenesis are at this time unclear (449). Thrombotic thrombocytopenic purpura, hemolytic uremic syndrome, and HELLP may represent a spectrum of clinical presentations from a common process (450). All three conditions exhibit platelet activation, aggregation, and consumption. Platelet aggregates produce ischemia and infarction of tissues leading to expressivity of the specific disorder.

It is important to differentiate thrombotic thrombocytopenic purpura and hemolytic uremic syndrome from toxemia of pregnancy early in the clinical course to initiate appropriate therapy in a timely fashion. While initial clinical presentation and subsequent course may be helpful, the prenatal course of the women before the onset of symptoms offers the best clues. Severe preeclampsia more commonly follows the progressive appearance of edema and some increase in blood pressure followed by proteinuria. In contrast, thrombotic thrombocytopenic purpura typically presents in a fulminant manner in a woman who was previously completely healthy. Findings that may aid the presumptive diagnosis of thrombotic thrombocytopenic purpura and HELLP are presented in Table 26–10 with the caveat that at any given moment in the clinical course, either presentation may mimic the other. In distinction to thrombotic thrombocytopenic purpura, the large von Willebrand multimers are not common in HELLP syndrome (451–454).

Plasma exchange by plasmapheresis with fresh frozen plasma is the therapy of choice for thrombotic thrombocytopenic purpura (450,455–457). This therapeutic approach has reversed the associated mortality from over 90% to less than 10% (456). Such therapy should be considered as well in patients thought to have severe toxemia and who are either worsening postpartum or do not show evidence of initial resolution of platelet consumption within 48 hours (323,324,450). Fresh frozen plasma infusion used alone for thrombotic thrombocytopenic purpura is not as efficacious as plasma exchange. It does play a role, however, as initial therapy when plasmapheresis is not available as well as for prophylaxis against relapse (455,457–461). Plasma exchange is discontinued with persistent platelet counts ≥ 150,000/μL and cessation of hemolysis reflected in a stable hematocrit and progressive

**Table 26–10.** Comparison of TTP and HELLP

| Finding | TTP | HELLP |
|---|---|---|
| Atypical CNS behavior | Yes | No |
| Neurologic signs | Common | Uncommon, except brisk DTR's |
| Headache | Uncommon | More common |
| Seizures associated | Uncommon | More common |
| Coma | More common | Rare |
| Purpura, bleeding | Very common | Rare |
| Abdominal pain | Uncommon | More common |
| Fever | Common | No |
| Anemia, (Hct ↑, ↓): ANTEPARTUM | Yes, (↓) | Uncommon, (↑) |
| RBC: abnormal forms | Severe | Common, but less marked |
| Leukocytosis | Common | Uncommon |
| SGOT/SGPT ↑ | ↑ | ↑ ↑ ↑ |
| Creatinine ↑ >1.5 mg/dl | More common | Less common |
| Placental Abruption | Risk not increased | Risk increased |
| Large vWb multimers | Common | Rare, if at all |
| **Clinical Course** | | |
| Relapse | Fairly common | Rare |
| Spontaneous resolution postdelivery | Rare | Almost always by 96 hours |

clearing of the abnormal red blood cells in the peripheral smear.

While some traditionally employ corticosteroids in the initial treatment of thrombotic thrombocytopenic purpura even with plasma exchange, we and others do not (448,450,455,462). While early favorable results often occur, relapse after this initial response to corticosteroid therapy alone may be associated with rapid deterioration and death (462).

As with other disorders impacting unfavorably on platelets, high-dose immune globulin and vincristine therapy have been used in persistent disease (463–466). Heparin therapy was advocated in the past for the early therapy of postpartum hemolytic uremic syndrome but a higher mortality in the heparin-receiving group of a controlled study among children leaves this advocacy suspect (467).

Even though the thrombocytopenia may be severe (less than 20,000/μL) in thrombotic thrombocytopenic purpura and bleeding is increased as in other thrombocytopenia-vascular syndromes, frank hemorrhage is rare. It is critical to appreciate that thrombotic thrombocytopenic purpura may be significantly aggravated by platelet transfusions including lethal consequence because of the rapid sequestration of the platelets in the microvasculature with subsequent severe hypoxic-anoxic tissue injury (448,461,462,468,469). Plasmapheresis in all cases is the favored alternative to platelet transfusion. Platelet transfusion in thrombotic thrombocytopenic purpura cases MUST be restricted to the rare instance of hemorrhage unresponsive to other therapies.

## *Systemic Lupus Erythematosus (SLE)*

Systemic lupus erythematosus is the most common collagen vascular disorder complicating pregnancy, reflecting its increased frequency in childbearing age women (470,471). The diagnosis of this disorder requires the serial or simultaneous presence of four or more symptoms, signs or laboratory abnormalities. However, recurrent pregnancy wastage (not on the criteria list), a false-positive test for syphilis, or a history of severe preeclampsia presenting in the second trimester of pregnancy (not on the list), may be the sole clue that leads to a clinical impression of lupus erythematosus (472,473). Less obvious presentations of systemic lupus erythematosus in pregnancy are much more common than fully expressive disease (474). Antinuclear antibody testing is almost always positive in patients with systemic lupus erythematosus (470,474).

Pregnancy in the absence of active multisystem disease or lupus nephritis does not aggravate systemic lupus erythematosus; in contrast, systemic lupus erythematosus, particularly in the 10%, or more, of cases with antiphospholipid antibodies, poses significant risk for the pregnancy (470,475–481). Preeclampsia is more common with positive antinuclear antibody and/or lupus anticoagulant/anticardiolipin (LAC/ACA) tests and even more so when chronic hypertensive renal disease is present at the outset of pregnancy. The differential diagnosis of acute lupus erythematosus versus preeclampsia is usually not difficult. The proteinuria of systemic lupus erythematosus typically antedates hypertension and urine cellular casts are usually present at initial presentation of any proteinuria. Although hematuria may complicate severe preeclampsia, particularly with an indwelling bladder catheter, erythrocyte casts are not present as they almost always are with initial hematuria complicating systemic lupus erythematosus.

Thrombocytopenia complicating systemic lupus erythematosus usually has associated leukopenia and may have hemolytic immune-type anemia as well—unusual findings in preeclampsia. Further, the thrombocytopenia of systemic lupus erythematosus typically responds to corticosteroid therapy, while this is not usually the case in preeclampsia (475). Clinically significant elevation of serum creatinine levels (≥ 1.5 mg/dl) are much less likely in preeclampsia. If doubt persists, management approaches should reflect a working diagnosis of preeclampsia superimposed on systemic lupus erythematosus (470).

Lupus-associated thrombocytopenia is present in about 15% of cases (394). It is typically not severe and does not cause maternal hemorrhage. Any blood loss is greater when the thrombocytopenia is associated with hemolytic anemia and particularly so if acute vasculitis is also present.

As in autoimmune thrombocytopenia, platelet counts less than 50,000/μL on serial testing are treated with prednisone. In severe thrombocytopenia (≤ 20,000/μL) not responsive to corticosteroid therapy, high-dose gamma globulin infusions, splenectomy or plasmapheresis may be effective (482–486). Depressed platelet counts but greater than 50,000/μL in association with high-titer anticardiolipin antibody are said to be responsive to low-dose aspirin (80 mg every day) (487,488).

Perinatal complications constitute the bulk of the risk during pregnancy. Early pregnancy loss is increased with active nephritis and with the presence of antiphospholipid antibodies (489–498). Similar to autoimmune thrombocytopenia, neither the maternal platelet count nor the PA-IgG antibody level are predictive of perinatal thrombocytopenia. Although neonatal thrombocytopenia may occur, the low risk for intracranial hemorrhage in the fetus precludes cordocentesis or cesarean birth as a mandate of contemporary perinatal care. However, preeclampsia, intrauterine growth retardation, complications of fetal heart block, or other obstetric issues may dictate delivery by cesarean section. When thrombocytopenia is present, perioperative bleeding is greater. Interventions to minimize surgical wound bleeding are the same as suggested for autoimmune thrombocytopenia.

Corticosteroid therapy is the mainstay of management in systemic lupus erythematosus with its attendant risk of hypertension and increased glucose intolerance. The administration of low-dose aspirin in those patients with antiphospholipid antibodies is probably warranted whether or not steroid therapy is required (478). Subcutaneous heparin bid, intravenous gamma globulin, and plasmapheresis have been used with high antiphospholipid antibody titers but adequate data to match up a specific therapy with the specific patient is lacking. Women on chronic steroid therapy for systemic lupus erythematosus should receive increased dosage over the 72 hours of labor, delivery, and postpartum periods with tapering of the dosage over about 1 week's time back to prelabor levels should there be no evidence of active nephritis.

### *Drug-Associated Thrombocytopenia*

In addition to the ubiquitous aspirin, a host of other drugs and agents are implicated in the causation of thrombocytopenia (394,487). In contrast to the nonpregnant state wherein epistaxis, petechiae, or other bleeding is the presenting feature, the thrombocytopenia in pregnancy most often is an incidental finding at the time of routine CBC determination. Maternal hemorrhage is rare although aspirin use within 10 days before delivery and carbenicillin may be associated with excessive blood loss (488).

With most drugs, resolution of the thrombocytopenia occurs within days after stopping the offending substance. Corticosteroid may be required. Prophylactic platelet transfusion is not indicated. In those instances wherein platelet-associated IgG antibody is produced, there is theoretical bleeding risk to the fetus, but such risk has not been defined.

### *Sepsis/Septic Shock*

In obstetrics, sepsis—the clinical evidence of infection plus evidence of a systemic response to infection—occurs predominantly secondary to postpartum endometritis (489,490). While topical cultures taken from the uterus usually reveal more than one organism, positive blood cultures typically show a single organism. Pyelonephritis is the most common antenatal cause of bacterial sepsis, with E. Coli, a gram-negative aerobic coliform, the predominant organism (490). Septic shock and adult respiratory distress syndrome may complicate the pyelonephritis (491).

Septic shock in under age-forty adults is almost exclusively restricted to pregnant women (492). Mortality in the obstetric population is 25% or higher (493). Survival requires that the caretaker recognize the condition early and promptly institute resuscitative and drug intervention. Accurate early identification of the offending organism(s) and selection of appropriate antibiotics with effective removal of the infection source as necessary are of equal import. The clinical presentation before the heralding shaking chill and temperature spike seen with septic shock includes a decrease in blood pressure, increase in respiratory rate, decrease in urine output, and a decreased (for pregnancy) WBC, with neutropenia. Setting absolute blood pressure values for the diagnosis of shock rather than a fall of the mean arterial pressure from the patient's baseline level may lead to missing the early diagnosis of septic shock, particularly in pregnancy (494,495). Subtle, mental status changes may be the sole clue of impending life-threatening shock (496). At times, the patient's responses are almost clairvoyant regarding life and death.

Shock secondary to sepsis is of the distributive type. There is initially lowered systemic vascular resistance with pooling of blood secondary to increased venous capacitance in the face of normal or even increased cardiac output (494,497). This maldistribution and pooling of blood, in addition to decreasing preload, lead to increasing acidosis that further adversely affects cardiac function (498). A specific myocardial depressant factor in the patient's blood adds to the myocardial dysfunction (499).

Only those therapeutic approaches that may impact on the prevention of disseminated intravascular coagulation and hemorrhage are noted here. Prompt administration of $O_2$, by nonrebreathing mask if necessary, to maintain $O_2$ saturation at $\geq$ 94% ($pO_2$ greater than 75 mm Hg), and intravenous fluids are imperative to maintain tissue oxygenation and to avoid progressive acidosis that may initiate or aggravate coagulopathy and adult respiratory distress syndrome. Because of the increased clearance of serum albumin, if initial intravenous fluid loading (2 L of normal saline or lactated Ringer's) does not maintain adequate blood pressure and tissue perfusion, a colloid fluid (albumin) is used in addition to the crystalloid for continuing fluid therapy (500). Because of increased capillary permeability, this approach carries some risk of pulmonary edema and further aggravation of hypoxemia. My experience, however, is in accord with others in that the use of large volumes of crystalloid poses a greater risk for pulmonary edema/adult respiratory distress syndrome (501,502). Others disagree with the use of colloid solutions (494,503). A diuretic is sometimes required in the fluid management phase in these patients regardless of the type of intravenous fluid chosen.

I also administer intravenous corticosteroid (12 mg dexamethasone) and heparin (8 to 10,000 units) at the outset of the septic shock should hemorrhage not be established because of the impact these drugs have on preventing activation of intravascular coagulopathy. Antithrombin III may be useful along with the heparin. Study results assessing a significant impact of corticosteroid on the survivability of the patient with septic shock are varied and in humans may be flawed by the failure to administer the steroid until shock status is advanced (504–506). The rationale for heparin therapy early in the management of septic shock includes: (1) septic shock in this age group of patients is almost exclusively seen in pregnancy; (2) thrombin generation is increased in uncomplicated pregnancy; (3) AT III appears to decrease more dramatically with infection in pregnancy then with disseminated intravascular coagulation in the nonpregnant patient; (4) disseminated intravascular coagulation in pregnancy-related infection is a higher order risk than in the nonpregnant condition; (5) because amplification occurs in the coagulation process, less inhibitor (AT III and thus, heparin dosage) is needed early to block the continuing cascade; and (6) the thrombogenic changes of pregnancy require a higher initial dose of heparin for the desired impact—i.e., there is, again, an underlying thrombogenic process.

A central arterial pressure catheter can be invaluable in monitoring fluid resuscitation and cardiac function by assessment of pulmonary artery wedge pressure. Initiation of $O_2$, intravenous fluids, and intravenous drug therapies must not await, however, the availability of the expert to place the central arterial catheter. Hypotension and hypoxemia not responsive to intravenous fluids may require intravenous pressor agents and inotropic agents, e.g., digoxin (507–509). Dopamine is the drug of choice should a pressor be required but it may decrease uteroplacental perfusion (2,510,511).

While blood cultures are recommended, they neither require sampling at the time of fever and/or chills nor should they be obtained without the obtaining of samples for Gram stain and microscopic assessment for potential identification of the offending organism(s) (492). A Gram stain of the buffey-coat (WBC layer of a centrifuged blood sample obtained at the time of blood culture) will define the characteristics of the causative organism in over 50% of cases in which a blood culture is subsequently reported as positive—a report that may come days later. Early knowledge of the offending organism can prompt highly selective antibiotic therapy rather than the usual two- or three-drug approach to cover all expected possibilities.

Surgical debridement and/or drainage of infected tissues should be done early to constitute a favorable outcome. Either curettage of the infected uterus or much less frequently removal of the uterus or other infected organs/tissues must be done to stop continuing sepsis. Curettage of an infected uterus may lead to Asherman's syndrome, but this intervention should not be withheld in the face of continuing sepsis (512). Specific antibodies against the bacterial endotoxins and/or other shock-related agents to prevent the sequence of events leading to irreversible shock may improve survival in the future (513).

Adult respiratory distress syndrome complicates sepsis in almost 40% of cases and has been reported with pyelonephritis even without demonstrable bacteremia (514,515). The adult respiratory distress syndrome doubles the mortality rate associated with the primary disorder without respiratory distress syndrome. When adult respiratory distress syndrome is a result of gram-negative sepsis, mortality exceeds 70% (516,517).

Thrombocytopenia, generally of a mild degree, is a common associate of bacteremia. In contrast, the coagulation abnormality in septic shock is a classic disseminated intravascular coagulation following the direct and indirect effects of toxin on the compliment cascade and the coagulation cascade in activating factor XII and stimulating platelet activating factor (518). Thrombomodulin activity is decreased promoting coagulation (519).

The treatment of the disseminated intravascular coagulation is not different than outlined earlier except that fibrinogen depletion in contrast to depletion of other coagulation factors is not as profound as that seen with placental abruption or dead fetus syndrome. Thereby, the use of fresh frozen plasma over cryoprecipitate is favored in continuing hemorrhage status with septic-driven disseminated intravascular coagulation. Platelet transfusion is also more likely to be required should hemorrhage complicate septic shock, more than is the case in obstetric-related hemorrhage. Vitamin K should be given if liver function is compromised.

### *Leukemia*

Acute leukemia may lead to bleeding by inadequate production of platelet by the bone marrow, by disseminated intravascular coagulation (more common in the promyelocytic variety), or by disseminated intravascular coagulation secondary to associated sepsis. Platelet transfusions may be life-saving but their positive impact on coagulation is short-lived. The maternal and perinatal outcomes with acute leukemia have been reviewed (520). As a general rule, aggressive medical therapy, as in the nonpregnant state, is warranted, with delivery at or beyond 24 weeks gestation and when the mother is in a state of remission. Although long-term survivors among young women with leukemia are rare, survival through the pregnancy is common and the outlook for the fetus, if carried to viability, is good.

## Prevention of Hemorrhage and its Complications

Prevention of hemorrhage is preferable to cure. The woman's caretakers must possess a high order of suspicion to anticipate the risk of hemorrhage, and, when it occurs, they must formulate a logical, rapid, and prioritized response. Approaches to prevent hemorrhage and minimize the risk for its associated complications are summarized in Table 26–11. The risk for development of adult respiratory distress syndrome is minimized by rapid correction of the hypovolemic shock and by careful attention to resuscitative fluid type and quantity, particularly in such conditions as severe preeclampsia and septic shock wherein there is microvascular endothelial injury.

Pulmonary embolism is the leading cause of maternal death in pregnancies ending in a live birth (1). Many of these cases of thrombotic disease follow either the recovery phase of severe hemorrhage or the surgery and, often times, coincident, pelvic infection associated with the interventions taken to resolve the bleeding. Table 26–12 lists the risk factors for venous thrombosis and pulmonary embolism (521). It is notable that the immobilized, older pregnant woman in the peripartal period with pelvic surgery and infection following hemorrhage constitutes a phenomenal risk for thromboembolic disease. Should the patient have severe preeclampsia with its decreased AT III levels and/or lupus anticoagulant, the risk is increased still further (104,521). The listed inherited factors (Table 26–12), of course, enhance the risk for thromboembolism in pregnancy over that experienced in the nonpregnant state.

Virchow defined the triad of factors initiating intravascular coagulation: vessel wall injury, venous stasis of blood, and local clotting alterations (522). The antepartum changes in the clotting factors, inhibitors, modulators, and fibrinolytic activity have been elucidated above. Postpartum changes in the platelets and fibrinogen, as well as the rapid decrease in fibrinolytic activity back to prepregnancy levels, impart further risks to make the postpartum period the predominant time for thromboembolism (107,109,126,523).

As there is no convincing evidence that imposed immobilization in the form of complete bed rest significantly lowers maternal/fetal morbidity or mortality, avoidance of ambulation for women with a complicated pregnancy should not be absolute (524,525). When maternal condition precludes modest ambulation, however, graduated compression elastic stockings should be used to address

**Table 26–11.** Approaches to Prevent or Minimize the Risk of Massive Hemorrhage and its Complications

| Complication | Intervention |
|---|---|
| Postpartum Hemorrhage Secondary To: | |
| Uterine atony | Active management third stage of labor; massage of uterine fundus; early use 15-methyl $F_{2\alpha}$; gravity suit |
| Placental retention | Routine inspection of placenta; bimanual exploration of uterine cavity ± curettage with continued bleeding post vaginal delivery |
| Placenta previa/accreta | Antepartum diagnosis; suture; packing; fibrin glue; hysterectomy; gravity suit |
| Vaginal/cervical laceration(s) | Routine assessment for lacerations with vaginal birth; appropriate repair before excessive blood loss |
| Uterine inversion | Early recognition and reduction of inversion |
| Post cesarean uterine artery bleeding | Incorporation of uterine artery branches into angle stitches |
| Coagulopathies, inherited | Prelabor/delivery diagnosis and specific prophylactic intervention when indicated |
| Intrapartum Hemorrhage Secondary To: | |
| Placental abruption | Avoidance of smoking; treatment of hypertension; serial fibrinogen; cryoprecipitate with bleeding and fibrinogen ≤100 mg/dl |
| Uterine Rupture | Definition of previous uterine scar direction early in pregnancy; appropriate use of pitocin for labor induction/augmentation; repeat cesarean birth before the onset of labor with prior classical (vertical) uterine incision; delivery rather than aggressive tocolytic therapy when preterm labor and previous vertical uterine incision |
| Antepartum Hemorrhage Secondary To: | |
| Dead fetus syndrome | Serial assessment fibrinogen; heparin infusion pre-labor if fibrinogen ≤150 mg/ml; cryoprecipitate with hemorrhage |
| Maternal trauma—motor vehicle accident | Belt restraints; air-bag; thorough evaluation for abruption of placenta and other causes of hypovolemia; early diagnosis and therapy of DIC in head trauma |
| ARDS | Rapid restoration of intravascular volume and $O_2$ transport to tissues |
| Pulmonary Embolism | Ambulation/elastic stockings; pneumatic compression lower extremity veins; prophylactic heparin |

the stasis in the leg veins occurring during pregnancy (521,526,527). In cases of the strict immobilization required in multisystem trauma, or the moribund or paralyzed respirator-dependent patient, external pneumatic compression to the lower extremities is recommended.

The use of prophylactic heparin in patients who lack an inherited risk factor but have a prior history of deep vein thrombosis or pulmonary embolism is advocated by most obstetric-based authors (96,528,529). Studies in the laboratory and in vivo have demonstrated that pregnancy requires higher doses of heparin to impart the equivalent anticoagulation effect that occurs in the nonpregnant state at lower dosage (120,530,531).

**Table 26–12.** Risk Factors for Venous Thrombosis and Pulmonary Embolism

| |
|---|
| Acquired Factors |
| Reproductive-age women > men |
| Pregnancy > nonpregnant state |
| Postpartum > antepartum |
| Obesity |
| Prolonged bed rest |
| Advancing age |
| Varicosities |
| Dehydration; shock (hypovolemic and cardiac) |
| Infection, sepsis |
| Cesarean birth > vaginal birth |
| Prior deep vein thrombosis, thromboembolism |
| Estrogen therapy |
| Microvascular disease as in diabetes, lupus erythematosus |
| Lupus anticoagulant |
| Inherited Factors |
| Antithrombin III deficiency |
| Protein C and/or S deficiency |
| Dysfibrinogenemia |
| Disorders of plasminogen and plasminogen activation |

Surgery, particularly in the pelvis, for a duration of over 30 minutes increases the risk of thromboembolism (521). Cesarean birth increases the risk ninefold over vaginal birth (528). Given the increased risk for thromboembolism in the postpartum patient who has restricted ambulation and/or is obese (≥ 200 lbs.), had pelvic surgery (i.e., cesarean section), has pelvic infection, has preeclampsia, has chronic microvascular disease, or has lupus anticoagulant, prophylactic heparin should be given. Again, in preeclampsia, AT III decreases, thus predisposing to the risk of thrombosis (120,283,286). I also administer heparin to all postpartum patients who have had a significant hemorrhage (clinical shock and ≥ two units transfusion required). While it may seem paradoxical to order drug therapy that may cause bleeding for a patient just recovering from severe hemorrhage, the postpartum woman who has been in hypovolemic shock (immobilization, stasis, hypercoagulable state) and given birth (increased hypercoagulable state), particularly if by cesarean section (vascular injury, increased hypercoagulable state), it is at extremely high risk for thromboembolic disease. A dosage of 6000 to 8000 units of heparin is used subcutaneously every 8 hours for the first 24 hours and then every 12 hours until the woman is fully ambulatory. The higher dosage is employed for the obese (≥ 200 lbs) patient and/or for the woman who is restricted to strict bed rest. The first dose is given about 2 hours after any surgery and after removal of an epidural catheter. In the posthemorrhage patient, only a normal activated partial thromboplastin time before initiation of the heparin is required. Continuous intravenous heparin (typically 400 to 600 units/hour) to keep the twice per day assessed activated partial thromboplastin time at 1.2 to 1.3 times the control can be used if deemed necessary. If there is renal disease with decreased heparin clearance implied, continuous intravenous heparin (200 to 300 units/hour) with every 4 hour activated partial thromboplastin time assessments is initially employed. Subcutaneous, low-molecular-weight heparin may afford as effective antithrombotic efficacy with a requirement for less frequent dosing and less risk for major bleeding complications (181,532,533).

Although the diagnosis and therapy of pulmonary embolism are outside the scope of this chapter, it must be noted that over half of the approximately 15% of patients that ultimately die from pulmonary embolism do so within 30 minutes of the onset of acute symptoms, which makes prevention paramount (534,535). Should the diagnosis of pulmonary embolism be suspected, 15,000 units of heparin should be given by intravenous push and then the patient evaluated for a diagnosis—a workup that may take hours to complete.

## *Management of Hemorrhage*

When prevention approaches for excessive bleeding either cannot be applied or are unsuccessful, appropriate and rapid responses must be directed to preventing progression to secondary or irreversible shock. While hemorrhage remains a major contributor to maternal mortality, it is much more often associated with significant morbidity (2). As noted earlier, even primary (reversible) shock may portend grave risk for the fetus and/or newborn.

Otherwise uncomplicated obstetric patients demonstrate the classic signs associated with blood loss, but it is important to appreciate that these signs present after a greater absolute blood loss because of the expanded intravascular blood volume of pregnancy. Further, tachycardia ($\geq$ 110 BPM) and systolic hypotension ($\leq$ 90 mm Hg) tend to be relatively late signs, occurring typically only after a loss of approximately 40% (i.e., 2.5 to 3 L) of the normal pregnancy blood volume. This contrasts to the nonpregnant patient for whom a loss of 15 to 25% of blood volume is associated with the presentation of primary shock signs (536). When the systolic blood pressure exceeds 90 mm Hg, orthostatic testing is a more reliable indicator of significant hypovolemia. A 10 mm Hg decrease in the systolic pressure roughly equates to a circulating volume loss of 20%—in pregnancy, a one liter or greater deficit.

Estimation of blood loss associated with uncomplicated parturition is notoriously inaccurate (9,11). When hemorrhage is manifest, the difference between estimated blood loss and actual blood loss is often sizable. The higher the blood loss, the greater the underestimate (10,12). Blood loss should be quantified by volume (i.e., ml in the bedpan or suction bottle) or weight (1 mg equates to 1 ml of blood). Fruit-sizing of clots or other volumes is clinically useless and should not be employed.

All obstetric services should have a succinct, clearly stated Code Red protocol. Similar to the cardiac resuscitation code blue, the code red document should define the accountable staff and the diagnostic/therapeutic steps in a prioritized manner (Table 26–13). It is critically important to define the responsibilities of each member of the code-red team before the emergency situation to maintain interprofessional exchanges that are directed to maximizing timely, efficient responses for the patient(s) rather than working through, during the precious early minutes of the response, who is in charge and who is responsible, as well as accountable, for what (537). An experienced anesthesiologist's involvement may be life-saving.

ORDER—a mnemonic for Oxygenate, Restore circulatory volume, Drug therapy, Evaluate and Remedy the underlying problem—has been suggested for the priorities in the management of shock in obstetric patients (538). The "laws" and "rules" outlined in Table 26–14, while seemingly mundane, if applied consistently, will minimize many of the risks attendant to the resuscitation of the pregnant woman with hypovolemic shock.

Oxygenation of maternal blood should be accomplished by whatever means is required—mask; nonrebreathing mask; endotracheal intubation or tracheostomy for assisted and/or positive pressure ventilation. In the antepartum situation, $O_2$ administration to the mother

**Table 26–13.** Construct of Code-Red Protocol for Massive Maternal Hemorrhage

| Action | Responsible Professional |
|---|---|
| $O_2$ Administration to mother | Nurse #1; (anesthesiologist, obstetrician, other) |
| 2-IV ports, 16-Ga catheter | Nurse #1, #2; (anesthesiologist, obstetrician, other) |
| * "Bedside" whole blood or thrombin clot time | Nurse #1, #2; (anesthesiologist, obstetrician, other) |
| * Stat labs order entry: CBC, fibrinogen, other | Unit secretary; Nurse #2, #3 |
| Initiate Infusion therapy | Nurse #1, #2, (anesthesiologist, obstetrician, other) |
| Obtain blood; components | Technician; aide; nurse #4 |
| Set-up operating room | Nurse #2, #3 |
| Set-up blood warmer | Nurse #4, (anesthesiologist #2) |
| Set-up cell-saver unit | Nurse #4; technician; (anesthesiologist) |

* Drawn when IV infusion(s) started.

**Table 26–14.** Laws and Rules Regarding Hemorrhage and its Therapy

Laws
- Blood loss is often underestimated
- If the patient is white, not pink, she needs red (blood cells)
- Crystalloid does not bind $O_2$
- Lactated Ringer's does not clot

Rules
- Blood for blood
- Blood component for blood component
- Warm all infusates ASAP
- Minimize crystalloid; use colloid
- Assure normal coagulation before central placement of venous catheter
- Cryoprecipitate use early in abruption; dead fetus syndrome
- Selective use fresh frozen plasma
- 5/2/10 replacement relationships
- No prophylactic platelet transfusions
- Rh-immune globulin if Rh-positive platelet source to Rh-negative patient
- Focus on mother most appropriate for baby as well

may enhance available oxygen for the fetus (392,494). Definitive surgery (e.g., hysterectomy) for hemorrhage should not be initiated until adequate oxygenation of the mother is effected.

Restoration of circulatory volume is critical for tissue perfusion and oxygenation. A normal human can survive only a 30% loss of intravascular volume without fluid replacement, while should normovolemia be maintained, up to an 80% red blood cell mass loss is tolerated (539). While the choice of restorative intravenous fluids remains controversial, this author supports the general dictum that the fluids used should match the fluids lost as closely as possible.

### *Laboratory Assessments*

In obstetric hemorrhage cases, laboratory assessments ordered by the physician almost routinely include the prothrombin time, partial thromboplastin time, and fibrin split products (FSP). Again, the presence of fibrin split products particularly in the postpartum patient is normal. The prothrombin time and partial thromboplastin time are poor indicators of factor deficiency until clinically critical levels are met (≤ 80 mg/dl fibrinogen; ≤ 20% factor activity). These tests are only useful in massive hemorrhage or liver disease. When the plasma fibrinogen is adequate (i.e., ≥ 100 mg/dl), in massive hemorrhage, a prothrombin time (factor VII, factor V) or partial thromboplastin time (factor VIII, factor IX) ratio to control of greater than 1.8 does correlate with factor activity less than 20%. Hemorrhage secondary to nonheredity factor deficiency occurs rarely, if at all, with normal fibrinogen levels (130).

A bedside whole blood or thrombin clot time, complete blood count for the platelet estimate, plasma fibrinogen, and glucose level should be obtained. Hyperglycemia, secondary to increased insulin resistance, may follow hypovolemic shock. A baseline glucose assessment is even more germane to pregnancy with its inherent tendency to glucose intolerance. Four to six units of whole blood or packed red blood cells should be ordered at the onset of the management of obstetric hemorrhage. If the bedside clot is abnormal, 10 units of cryoprecipitate should also be made ready.

### *Volume/Perfusion/Blood Products*

#### Crystalloid and Colloid Infusates

In hemorrhagic shock, there is increased albumin turnover and increased capillary permeability leading to a shift of fluid from the intravascular to extravascular spaces. Coupled with this indirect loss of albumin is the direct loss in the hemorrhaged blood resulting in a fall in the plasma colloid osmotic pressure further increasing the loss of intravascular fluid to extravascular compartments (540).

Following the dictum to replace what intravascular fluids are lost and because albumin has been lost along with water and electrolytes, I believe the restorative fluids should reflect this loss. I therefore administer colloid in the form of 5% albumin when more than 2 liters of crystalloid are required for fluid resuscitation (541). Dextran is not used because of its potential negative impact on coagulation.

There is no advantage of lactated Ringer's (LR) solution over 0.9% NaCl as regards re-expansion of plasma volume. Indeed, with the large volumes of crystalloid employed in obstetric hemorrhage cases, the lactated Ringer's may be less favorable than NaCl because the lactate may add unnecessary burden to acid-base metabolism in the patient who already has severe lactic acidosis, as occurs in cases of severe preeclampsia and eclampsia.

The quantity of crystalloid required to restore intravascular volume and effect adequate tissue perfusion is 3 to 5 times the calculated blood loss (540–542). Sodium chloride infusion decreases colloid osmotic pressure by over 30%, and it decreases oxygen transport when contrasted to colloid (501,541,543–547). It must be noted that pregnancy is already characterized by a decrease in colloid oncotic pressure (COP), which is lowered further in conditions with proteinuria. Postpartum colloid osmotic pressure is most notably decreased, posing increased risk for pulmonary interstitial fluid leakage in this period (548–550). Furthermore, the severely hypertensive patient may have a significant increase in the pulmonary capillary wedge pressure further enhancing the potential for pulmonary edema.

Patients with prehemorrhage, contracted plasma volumes for pregnancy (as may occur in preeclampsia and cyanotic cardiopulmonary disease) are at particular risk for death following volume overload and pulmonary edema. Such patients should not receive multi-liter infusions of crystalloid alone for the management of hemorrhage requiring replacement of blood or blood components. In pregnancy, with little margin between an appropriate pulmonary capillary wedge pressure-colloid osmotic pressure gradient and an abnormal one leading to the formation of pulmonary edema, a balanced crystalloid/colloid volume restoration approach should be used (540,547,550). Dextran is not used because of its undesirable effect on platelet and factor VIII function.

Albumin and hetastarch do not pose infectious disease risk. Albumin may decrease the levels of ionized calcium in the blood, however (551). Even though the routine addition of intravenous calcium is not advised in massive transfusion management, when albumin is used for the resuscitation, calcium should be administered (1.0 g IV as 10% Ca gluconate for every 5 units of red blood cells) (552). The risks/benefits for crystalloid versus colloid use in the nonpregnant patient have been summarized (501,502,547,553).

Hypertonic saline solutions have been employed in the attempt to decrease infusion volumes and minimize pulmonary edema risk, but experience in pregnancy is lacking and potential for life-threatening complications contraindicates this approach at present (501,554). None of these nonblood fluids provide a substitute for the red blood cells' oxygen-transport function; perfluorocarbons remain experimental (555).

### *Blood and Blood Component Infusates*

Present day guidelines regarding blood transfusion include: (1) limiting use to symptomatic and/or defined clinical circumstances; (2) not using whole blood or its components solely for volume expansion; (3) using components rather than whole blood; (4) reserving fresh frozen plasma use for clotting factor deficiencies for which no concentrate is available (556,557). In fact, fresh whole blood is the ideal infusate for hemorrhage wherein both hypovolemia and symptomatic oxygen-carrying capacity deficit are features of the shock (130). Whole blood, however, is not available in many clinical settings. Factors V and VIII are unstable and platelets are short-lived making stored whole blood a poor choice for the management of disseminated intravascular coagulation.

Packed red blood cells (P:RBC's) are the blood component of choice for patients with a symptomatic deficit in oxygen transport. Every labor and delivery unit should have at least two dedicated units of type O, Rh-negative packed red blood cells for use without delay in hemorrhagic shock patients.

With adequate intravascular volume, 7 gm of hemoglobin is considered necessary for adequate tissue oxygenation. This value, however, relates to red blood cells with normal levels of 2, 3 diphosphoglycerate (DPG). Although the stored packed red blood cells undergo less of the negative impacts of storage observed with whole blood, decreased 2, 3 diphosphoglycerate is still evident (556,558). The oxygen available to the tissues is lowered to less than is expected from the associated hemoglobin level. This is a particularly significant change in the antepartum patient when one appreciates that 2, 3 diphosphoglycerate is increased by 30% to facilitate $O_2$ delivery to the fetus (559).

Intraoperative salvage of autologous red blood cells employing a cell-saver unit has been employed in pregnancy (Cell Saver: Haemonetics, Braintree, MA). The fact that the red blood cells are washed before infusion should make this approach a safe consideration in massive blood loss, as may occur in abdominal trauma, abdominal pregnancy, ectopic pregnancy, placenta percreta, and placental abruption with disseminated intravascular coagulation.

## *Complications of Blood Transfusions*

Massive hemorrhage may be defined as the loss of 10 or more units of blood or as the loss of one blood volume or more in 24 hours. Massive transfusion is then defined as the replacement of 10 or more units of blood (or ≥ one blood volume) in 24 hours (558,560). Obstetric hemorrhage of this magnitude typically occurs over a short time span of 1 to 2 hours.

Throughout this chapter, the author has pervasively advocated early, appropriate intervention, including the administration of blood and blood components. This is not to say that transfusions do not themselves pose a life-threatening risk for the recipient (Table 26–15). A conservative bent is clinically appropriate as regards initiation of transfusion therapy, but procrastination in assessing the cause of the hemorrhage and/or in initiating an appropriate response, including transfusion, is untenable.

Any and all of the complications of homologous blood transfusion can occur from packed red blood cells. However, febrile reactions and fluid overload are less of a problem with the red blood cells than with whole blood. Microaggregates—although of unclear import as regards pulmonary complications—are also less of a problem than with stored whole blood, and thus a special microfilter is not required when administering packed red blood cells for obstetric hemorrhage.

**Table 26–15.** Risks of Rapid, Multiple-Unit Homologous Transfusions

- Minor reactions (allergic; febrile)
- Hemolytic reaction (mismatched blood)
- Alloimmunization
- Infections
  - Viral
    - Hepatitis, B, C, D, F
    - Cytomegalovirus
    - Epstein-Barr virus
    - HTLV-1
    - HIV
    - Bacterial
    - Parasitic
  - Pulmonary edema
  - Microaggregates
  - Metabolic complications (hypothermia; citrate toxicity; acidoses; ↑, ↓$K^+$; ↓$Ca^{++}$; ↑$Mg^{++}$)

(Modified by author. From Circular of information for the use of human blood and blood components. American Red Cross. American Association of Blood Banks, and the Council of Community Blood Centers. March 1989.)

Hypothermia secondary to infusion of large quantities of cold blood components has many adverse effects on the mother, including the risk for cardiac arrhythmias and increasing acidosis (556). Further, tissue delivery of oxygen is impaired by shifting the oxygen-dissociation curve to the left, increasing blood viscosity, and decreasing red blood cell deformity (561). Coagulation is impaired with factor activity depressed, bleeding time increased, and thrombaxane $B_2$ production decreased (562,563). In transfusions that exceed 3 units of crystalloid and/or 2 units of packed red blood cells over a short time, all infusates should be warmed to no more than 37° C.

Routine administration of calcium is not required unless albumin is employed as noted above or liver dysfunction is significant with impaired citrate clearance (552). Hypokalemia is more common than hyperkalemia, although the latter may occur early in massive transfusion (560,564,565). Serial serum potassium monitoring and with renal compromise, continuous EKG monitoring are recommended in massive transfusion.

Viral infection disease transfer may complicate transfusion of packed red blood cells, cryoprecipitate, fresh frozen plasma, and platelets. While most cases of post-transfusion, chronic hepatitis are due to the hepatitis C virus, there is now an implicated hepatitis F virus with a new viral infection perhaps as threatening as HIV awaiting presentation in the future (566,567). For this reason, if no other, purely prophylactic blood component infusions should not be done.

Fresh frozen plasma should not be used solely for intravascular volume expansion. To do so poses a doubled risk for infectious disease transfer when used with packed red blood cells. I do continue, however, to use the five units (packed red blood cells) x two (fresh frozen plasma) units = ten (platelet) packs rule in the management of hemorrhage when there is continued bleeding of nonclotting blood over a rapid time frame and ≥ five units of packed red blood cells replacement is already accomplished. This approach is in accord with others who support the use of fresh frozen plasma when one blood volume is expended within 2 to 3 hours; when with a normal plasma fibrinogen level, the prothrombin time or partial thromboplastin time are greater than 1.8 times the control or when a nonstable factor deficiency exists for which a specific concentrate is not available (130,556–558). Further, with the more rapid blood loss and replacement requirement typical of massive obstetric hemorrhage, it is much more likely that less than 30% factor activity is manifest.

Fresh frozen plasma contains the labile and stable components of the coagulation, fibrinolytic, and complement systems with the exception of platelets. It also has the proteins that maintain intravascular oncotic pressure as well as AT III, which is decreased with preeclampsia, infection, and surgery—frequent associates of obstetric hemorrhage. When the hemorrhage is associated with severe HELLP syndrome, thrombotic thrombocytopenic purpura, or some of the other thrombocytopenic conditions, plasma infusion or pharesis may be life-saving.

Cryoprecipitate is the preferred source for fibrinogen replacement. Each unit contains at least 150 mg of fibrinogen and 80 units factor VIII. The infused volume is appreciably less than that of fresh frozen plasma (Table 26–9), and the thaw time is much shorter allowing for faster response without fluid overload in hypofibrinogenemic states.

It is important to remember that most obstetric-related hemorrhage is associated with depletion of fibrinogen first, followed by factor VIII, and lastly platelets. Further, even in nonobstetric massive transfusion, critical levels of factor deficiency are not seen without hypofibrinogenemia (130).

Platelet concentrates are more likely to be required in massive transfusion than is specific factor replacement to address continuing microvascular bleeding (130,556–568). Undoubtedly, however, the positive impact seen with platelet concentrates is in part reflective of the fibrinogen, platelet-bound factor V, factor VIII and factors IX, X, and XI present in the packs (556,558,569). A microaggregate filter can not be used with platelet transfusion because it traps the platelets. A single platelet pack can be expected to raise the patient's count 5000 to 10,000/μL (Table 26–9). Infection transfer risk is the same as for blood. The Rh-negative woman must be given Rh-immune globulin to avoid sensitization when Rh-positive donor platelet concentrates are used.

In sum, fibrinogen inadequacy is usually the single coagulation deficiency in obstetric-related hemorrhage and should be corrected by early use of cryoprecipitate. If hemorrhage of nonclotting blood continues after packed red blood cells and fibrinogen infusion, then fresh frozen plasma and platelet concentrates should be employed, particularly if rapid, massive transfusion is required. Waiting for hematology results to give defined direction to component selection is often times not possible with the rapid blood loss attendant to obstetric hemorrhage.

**Table 26–16.** Alternatives to Banked Homologous Transfusion

| |
|---|
| Prevention of excessive blood loss. |
| Restoration of intravascular volume without blood or blood components. |
| Directed-donor specific (*not* from husband's family) packed red blood cells. |
| Autologous red blood cells. |
| Intraoperative salvage (cell-saver unit). |
| Others: research re: hypertonic saline, $O_2$-transporter fluids. |

Alternatives to homologous transfusion are noted in Table 26–16. Use of directed-donor specific blood components should minimize the risk of infection transfer. The husband's family members are not used as donors to minimize the risk of subsequent pregnancy isoimmune disease.

Predeposition of blood by obstetric patients to an autologous donor program to afford maternal/fetal safety from infectious diseases remains impractical. In most situations, no more than two units of maternal blood can be withdrawn from the mother before the need (570–572). This is predominantly due to the fact that blood banks use a hematocrit of ≥ 34% rather than the notation of the physiologically increased red blood cell mass of pregnancy as the threshold for donor status (573). Few obstetric patients require blood transfusion with parturition regardless of delivery route. Those who do typically need far more blood than two units (574,575).

## *Drug Therapy*

Drug therapy for protracted hypotension is generally restricted to the use of vasopressors. Such agents including dopamine are avoided antenatally unless clearly required for vital organ function because they decrease uterine blood flow (2,510,511,538). Furosemide (20 to 40 mg IV bolus) with high volume (greater than 3 L) crystalloid use and/or persistent oliguria may decrease the risk of pulmonary edema experienced in massive transfusion. Hypokalemia should be ruled out before induced diuresis in the patient who has received a massive transfusion. In the postpartum patient, dopamine at low dosage (2 to 5 μg/kg/min) may improve persistent oliguria after adequate fluid resuscitation (576).

After coagulation is normalized and to minimize the risk of thromboembolism, heparin should be administered as described in the section on prevention of hemorrhage complications.

## *Evaluation of Maternal/Fetal Status*

In massive hemorrhage, ongoing blood pressure; pulse; respiratory rate; $O_2$ saturation and $pO_2$; CBC (for hematocrit and platelet count); fibrinogen; prothrombin time, partial thromboplastin time (for factor deficiency); and serum potassium should be obtained. Serial measurement of serum glucose to detect the need for insulin therapy should also be done. A finger-stick source sample should not be used because of erroneous results in the peripheral hypoperfusion stage of the shock.

A foley catheter should be placed and urinary output assessed every 2 hours with expected output of at least 40 ml every 2 hours. Little, if any, useful information is obtained by the often recommended hourly measurement of urine output. Rather, it wastes several minutes of precious nursing care time. Except in the patient with severe renal disease or cardiac failure, urinary output is a more critical indicator of the adequacy of tissue perfusion than is the pulmonary capillary wedge pressure. Daily weights should be used to assess delta intake-output.

Evaluation of the woman for the cause of blood loss must be done promptly, but after blood clot status assessment(s) and $O_2$/volume resuscitation are initiated. More often than not, appropriate anesthesia is required to allow for adequate vaginal, intrauterine, and/or intra-abdominal definition of the source of the bleeding.

As in the management of distributive shock, a centrally-placed intravascular catheter to monitor pressure is considered by many to be helpful. Unfortunately, the central venous pressure does not fall discriminately with even large intravascular volume losses. Although the pulmonary arterial wedge pressure does fall with severe hypovolemia, it does not correlate well with circulating blood volume. Many patients considered to have had appropriate intravascular volume resuscitation according to the wedge pressure value remain significantly hypovolemic (577).

Central venous catheter placement in the hemorrhaging patient then should not be a cause celebre unless no other vessel for rapid infusion of resuscitative fluids is available. A central arterial catheter is not required unless the woman has underlying pulmonary or cardiac dysfunction. In the initial resuscitation of massive blood loss, it is irrational to waste time in attempts at preload, afterload differentiation when there is no load. No central arterial catheter should be placed via the subclavian or internal jugular vein—no matter the operator's experience—until coagulation is determined to be adequate. Other complications than traumatic hemorrhage can occur with these catheters, including thrombosis, arrhythmias, and right-sided endocardial lesions (578–591). The advantages of their use must clearly outweigh the attendant risks before catheter placement is initiated.

In the prebirth circumstance, the only available indication—and a poor one at that—of adequacy of fetal oxygenation is electronic fetal heart rhythm monitoring. Because the fetus is dependent on the mother for oxygenation, the earlier the appropriate interventions for maternal tissues perfusion and oxygenation, the better for the baby. Cesarean section for fetal well-being should not be undertaken in an unstable mother. To do so may result in cardiac arrhythmia and arrest.

### *Remedial Interventions*

The management of postpartum hemorrhage secondary to uterine atony dictates that all obstetric units must have immediate access to oxytocin (20 units in 100 ml, 0.9% NaCl IV), methylergonovine (0.2 mg IM), and 15-methyl prostaglandin $F_2\alpha$ (0.25 mg IM or 0.25 to 0.50 mg intramyometrial) (359,360). Care must be taken to be certain only Hemabate (The Upjohn Co., Kalamazoo, MI) is stocked on labor/delivery to avoid inadvertent administration of the $E_1$ rather than the $F_2\alpha$ prostaglandin. Prostaglandin $E_1$ may produce life-threatening responses, including disseminated intravascular coagulation (580). Each and every unit should have in-house resuscitative supplies and crystalloid fluids as well as cryoprecipitate (10 units), 5% albumin (4 units), type O, Rh-negative packed red blood cells (2 to 4 units), platelet concentrates (10 packs), and fresh frozen plasma (2 units), for instances of hemorrhage secondary to abnormal coagulation.

Mechanical interventions include direct massage of the uterine fundus should uterine atony be evident. When the uterus remains hypotonic, transvaginal elevation of the uterus with compression of it between the vaginally and abdominally placed hands may significantly decrease blood loss. Direct transabdominal compression of the aorta against the vertebrae in massive hemorrhage until operative intervention is possible and may be life-saving.

Autotransfusion may be effected by direct elevation of the lower extremities or placement of the patient in the Trendelenburg position. Antishock trousers have been used to enhance autotransfusion in the hemorrhage patient refusing blood components (581). The gravity-suit, which imparts transabdominal pneumatic compression to lower vessel wall tension and reduce blood flow, has been successfully employed in abdominal and in ectopic pregnancies as well as to decrease blood loss in placenta previa, uterine atony, and postcesarean/hysterectomy bleeding (582–585).

Surgical interventions may be required to address continued bleeding. Any evident lacerations of the birth canal that have associated bleeding must be repaired. Vaginal packing is required in some cases of continued bleeding from multiple lacerations of the vagina, especially in patients with a coagulopathy. Following vaginal birth, should uterine bleeding persist in the face of adequate bimanual intrauterine examination, curettage should be done. Previous cesarean birth patients with normal uterine tonus but continued, excessive uterine bleeding require transabdominal reopening of the uterine incision for direct exploration of the uterus. Most often, the bleeding is from a branch of the uterine artery that was not incorporated in one of the angle-stitch sutures.

Hemorrhage from a lower uterine segment placental site can often times be controlled by placing parallel rows of through-and-through (serosa to endometrium), locking, # 1 absorbable suture. An interrupted suture technique has been described but obviously will take more operative time (586). Gelfoam pads (The Upjohn Co.) or microfibrillar collagen (Avitene: Alcon, Inc., Humacao, Puerto Rico) applied to continued oozing sites may be effective. The use of packing to which fibrin sealant "glue"—a combination of fibrinogen (as cryoprecipitate) and thrombin—has been applied as a viable alternative to hysterectomy with continued bleeding from a placental site or atonic uterus for the woman desirous of maintaining reproduction capability (361,581,588). This approach has been used in several patients to control bleeding from the lower uterine segment after placental delivery or an atonic uterus. The patient is given antibiotic coverage and the packing removed in 12 to 24 hours.

Hypogastric artery ligation is unsuccessful in adequately controlling uterine source hemorrhage in the majority of cases (589,590). Further, there are more serious complications in those patients subsequently requiring hysterectomy after hypogastric artery ligation (591). This vascular ligation should be employed only in the stable patient strongly desirous of further pregnancies. In the unstable patient, especially with coagulopathy, a 3/4" to 1" penrose drain can be tied around each of the common iliac arteries to prevent maternal death from hemorrhage until the coagulopathy can be corrected and cardiovascular stability attained. Absent blood flow to the lower extremities is tolerated for long periods of time in this generally young female population.

Hysterectomy may be deemed necessary even in the woman desiring future procreation. The mean, hysterectomy-associated blood loss exceeds 2000 ml (591). This procedure should not be undertaken in the face of coagulopathy or an unstable patient because of the high association of maternal death. Temporizing measures that can be done until the woman's blood does clot and stability is sufficient for hysterectomy are listed in Table 26–17. Ligation of the uterine arteries, and the ovarian arteries as well, if bleeding continues, employs a # 0-absorbable suture that is passed around the vessel and through the myometrium from front to back of the uterus at approximately 1 to 2 cm from the lateral serosal border (592). A large needle (e.g., CTX) is required to facilitate the placement of the suture through the uterus.

Hemorrhage from placenta previa or placenta accreta implantation sites in the lower uterine segment is typically not amenable to subtotal hysterectomy because the blood source is the anastomosis of branches of the vaginal and pudendal arteries with cervical branches of the uterine artery. Otherwise, a subtotal procedure is an appropriate consideration for massive hemorrhage patients.

Pelvic artery embolization—employing particulate matter such as Gelfoam or a stainless steel minicoil—has been used in pregnancy for postoperative and postvaginal delivery bleeding (369–371,593). It is not helpful in the acute, unplanned, hypovolemic shock phase because of the long period of time required for the procedure. Predelivery vascular embolization may become a consideration in the future for placenta accreta with extension into the bladder and contiguous vasculature in an attempt to moderate the hemorrhage attendant in such cases.

**Table 26–17.** Temporizing Measures to Minimize Further Uterine Blood Loss from Placental Implantation Site

| |
|---|
| Direct compression of the uterus between the operator's hands |
| Through and through suture of lower uterine segment |
| Pressure packing of venous bleeding sites (± fibrin glue) |
| Penrose drain constriction of the common iliac arteries |
| Ligation of the uterine arteries without vessel transection |
| Ligation of ovarian uterine arteries without vessel transection |

## Anesthetic Considerations

Antepartum consultation should be obtained from an anesthesiologist trained and experienced in regional and general anesthesia techniques in pregnancy whenever the clinical setting suggests increased risk for anesthetic complications and/or obstetric hemorrhage.

Emergency general anesthesia complications, including failed intubation and pulmonary aspiration, are greatly increased when the woman's neck is shortened or immobile as well as with abnormalities of the mouth and/or teeth (594). The obstetrician has the responsibility to examine the patient for such risks during the antenatal period. Maternal medical conditions as well as obstetric complications, ranging from cardiac disease to twin gestation, may have important implications for anesthetic technique as well. Known conditions in which the risk for massive hemorrhage is significantly increased include placenta previa, suspected placenta accreta, severe preeclampsia, and prior history of excessive blood loss secondary to uterine atony.

Too often, anesthesiologists are not afforded care-team membership before an emergency. Neither they nor the patient should be thrust into a life-threatening circumstance when prior, appropriate preparation would have avoided such a situation. Rather, the anesthesiologist should be asked by the obstetrician to jointly develop a plan of management that addresses possible risk prevention interventions, the place of delivery (which hospital and what operating room), the optimal anesthesia approach, and the timing of the initiation of anesthesia relative to labor and delivery (537,594,595).

Following placement of an intravenous catheter and attainment of normal coagulation assessment(s), women known to be at significant risk for maternal/fetal complications during labor and delivery should have a functional catheter placed for subsequent epidural or spinal anesthesia. When the risk consideration is one of a potential complication of emergency general anesthesia, "strong consideration should be given to antepartum referral of the patient" should 24-hours/day, immediately available, competent, emergency anesthesia capability not be in place at the hospital where delivery is initially planned (594).

In cases of hemorrhage, the anesthesiologist should insist on the accurate measurement of blood loss and not be confused with gross subjective estimates. As presented above, crystalloid should not be the sole resuscitative fluid used in massive hemorrhage. Time should not be wasted packing red blood cells should whole blood be immediately available in the symptomatic, hypovolemic patient. In the life-threatening situation, O, Rh-negative packed red blood cells should be used until type-specific blood or blood components are available. Cryoprecipitate should be obtained and given promptly in instances of hemorrhage in which the blood is not clotting.

Fetal distress based upon a nonreassuring fetal heart rhythm tracing is an often stated indication for emergency cesarean birth. The term is not precise, and it rarely provides insight into fetal oxygenation and acid-base status over and above that clinically surmised in such conditions as maternal hypovolemic shock or transient fetal bradycardia secondary to maternal seizure. Maternal mortality or life-threatening morbidity should not be assumed by the anesthesiologist because of the issue of fetal distress.

Posteclamptic-seizure patients should be stabilized for an extended period before induction of anesthesia without regard to fetal status. Oxygen, intravenous fluid resuscitation, and critical drug therapies should precede anesthesia for surgery directed to the management of hemorrhage. It is inappropriate to add an anesthesia-related risk to the mother, for example, in a situation of an extremely morbidly obese patient who is believed to have difficulty with obtaining an airway during rapid induction. There may be alternatives to general anesthesia, such as local anesthetic techniques with stand-by anesthesia support with mask oxygenation. If appropriate, even small doses of an amnesia drug may be used, such as ketamine hydrochloride. Such a maneuver may be helpful in saving the mother's life. The anesthesiologist's responses should be appropriate as well as deliberate in keeping with the tenet: primum non nocere—first of all, do no harm.

Anesthesia site bleeding may occur with general anesthesia (endotracheal tube trauma) or regional anesthesia (needle introducer or catheter trauma). With soft cuff endotracheal tubes, oral intubation rarely poses hemorrhagic complications. In contrast, nasotracheal intubation is more frequently associated with significant bleeding and is best avoided in the patient with a coagulopathy.

Bleeding at the site of spinal or epidural anesthesia may lead to hematoma formation and spinal cord injury. While a platelet count of greater than 50,000/μL portends little or no risk for epidural hematoma formation at the time of lumbar catheter placement in the pregnant woman, this is only true if responses to vascular injury, including platelet function, are intact (596). Epidural and subdural hematomas have occurred with platelet counts over 50,000/μL, including the occurrence in patients who have undergone preprocedure restoration of platelet counts to normal (293,597). An Ivy bleeding time must be done on all patients with a platelet count under 100,000/μL as well as those who have received platelet transfusion, even if the most recent platelet count exceeds 100,000/μL immediately before catheter placement.

Again, it is important to accept the facts that in preeclampsia/eclampsia, the platelets are often dysfunctional and, further, that quantitative (platelet count) as well as qualitative (bleeding time) platelet assessments can change from normal to abnormal within a couple of hours. In the rare circumstance in which there is no choice regarding epidural catheter placement, its use in the face of abnormal coagulation requires that postprocedure the catheter be removed and no epidural or intrathecal analgesic agents be employed to allow for accurate neurologic assessments during at least the first 24 hours. If there is any question regarding spinal neurologic status, magnetic residence imaging is the diagnostic technique of choice to access for spinal hematoma (598).

Preoperative antiplatelet therapy has been reported to be associated with spontaneous or traumatic epidural hematomas but this risk is extremely low in the reproductive-age woman (599–603). The low-dose aspirin used alone increasingly in complicated pregnancy does not pose such a risk. Alcohol and various drugs such as nafcillin, however, may lead to epidural space hematoma secondary to platelet dysfunction. Again, a thorough history for the use of any drug impacting on platelet function and an Ivy bleeding time before catheter placement is recommended (394,487,604).

Oral, vitamin-K antagonist anticoagulants are rarely used in pregnancy. Their use in pregnancy for AT III deficiency is considered avoidable (96). When required, as in highly selected cases of severe factor C or factor S deficiency, the oral agent should be switched to intravenous heparin therapy and regional anesthesia avoided (602).

An activated partial thromboplastin time should be obtained before epidural catheter placement in patients on heparin therapy. Although the risk of hematoma with subcutaneous heparin prophylaxis alone in doses of 5000 to 6000 units twice per day in pregnancy does not appear to be a significant issue, some authors advise against epidural anesthesia in these patients because there is no test sensitive enough to detect the risk for abnormal bleeding (602,605–607). When used with aspirin, however, a bleeding time should also be obtained to detect any cases of heparin potentiation (608). In contrast to subcutaneous heparin, even low-dose intravenous bolus heparin use may lead to hematoma formation regardless of whether the heparin administration proceeds or follows the catheter placement (602).

Coagulation status, as noted previously, impacts significantly on the potential mortality/morbidity associated with central venous catheter placement, especially by the internal jugular or subclavian routes. In addition to assuring that coagulation is adequate before placing a central venous catheter, the anesthesiologist must be certain that the postoperative caretakers are knowledgeable about and experienced with such lines. If this is not the case, the anesthesiologist—or, whoever placed the catheter—must either continue to monitor and manage the woman's hemocardiovascular status or remove the catheter. Finally, neither the central venous nor the pulmonary artery capillary wedge pressures should be expected to provide definitive data regarding blood volume adequacy (577), only the pulmonary capillary wedge.

Perivascular local anesthesia, such as pudendal block, may result in sizable hematoma formation when thrombocytopenia is present.

Epidural anesthesia is considered safe as regards extradural hematoma formation should the platelet count be ≥ 50,000/μL and the bleeding time normal (407). General anesthesia is not without complication because airway bleeding from mucosal trauma attendant to endotracheal tube placement may occur. Again, the bleeding time is usually not deranged with auto-immune thrombocytopenia as it may be, for example, in severe preeclampsia.

## REFERENCES

1. Koonin LM, Atrash HK, Lawson HW, Smith JC: Maternal Mortality Surveillance-United States, 1979–1986. *In* CDC

Surveillance Summaries, July 1991. MMWR 40 (No.SS-2): 1, 1991.
2. Paull J: Resuscitation in obstetrics and gynaecology. RACS Foundation Symposium on Fluid Replacement. Excerpta Medica: 1985, p. 95.
3. Allen MH, Chavkin W, Marinoff J: Ascertainment of maternal deaths in New York City. Am. J. Public Health 81:380, 1991.
4. CDC, Enhanced maternal mortality surveillance-North Carolina, 1988 and 1989. MMWR 40:469, 1991.
5. Pritchard JA, Baldwin RM, Dickey JC, Wiggins KM: Blood volume changes in pregnancy and the puerperium. II. Red blood cell loss and changes in apparent blood volume during and following vaginal delivery, cesarean section, and cesarean section plus total hysterectomy. Am. J. Obstet. Gynecol. 84:1271, 1962.
6. Gahres EE, Albert SN, Dodek SM: Intrapartum blood loss measured with $Cr^{51}$-tagged erythrocytes. Obstet. Gynecol. 19:455, 1962.
7. Newton M, Mosey LM, Egli GE, Gifford WB, et al: Blood loss during and immediately after delivery. Obstet. Gynecol. 17:9, 1961.
8. Wilcox CF, Hunt AB, Owen CA Jr: The measurement of blood lost during cesarean section. Am. J. Obstet. Gynecol. 77:772, 1959.
9. Newton M: Postpartum hemorrhage. Am. J. Obstet. Gynecol. 94:711, 1966.
10. Brant HA: Precise estimation of post partum haemorrhage: difficulties and importance. Brit. Med. J. 1:398, 1967.
11. Wallace G: Blood loss in obstetrics using a haemoglobin dilution technique. J. Obstet. Gynecol. Brit. Comm. 74:64, 1967.
12. Duthie SJ, Ghosh A, Ng A, Ho PC: Intra-operative blood loss during elective lower segment caesarean section. Br. J. Obstet. Gynaecol. 99:364, 1992.
13. Combs CA, Murphy EL, Laros RK: Factors associated with postpartum hemorrhage with vaginal birth. Obstet. Gynecol. 77:69, 1991.
14. Combs CA, Murphy EL, Laros RK: Factors associated with hemorrhage in cesarean deliveries. Obstet. Gynecol. 77: 77, 1991.
15. American College of Obstetricians and Gynecologists. Quality Assurance In Obstetrics and Gynecology. Washington, DC, 1989.
16. Rosenberg RD, Damus PS: The purification and mechanism of action of human antithrombin-heparin cofactor. J. Biol. Chem. 248:6490, 1973.
17. Esmon NL, Owen WG, Esmon CT: Isolation of a membrane bound cofactor for thrombin-catalyzed activation of protein C. J. Biol. Chem. 257:859, 1982.
18. Marcus AJ, Weksler BB, Jaffe EA: Enzymatic conversion of prostaglandin endoperoxide H2 and arachidonic acid to prostacyclin by cultured human endothelial cells. J. Biol. Chem. 253:7138, 1978.
19. Bachman F, Kruithof KO: Tissue plasminogen activator: chemical and physiological effects. Semin. Thromb. Hemost. 10:6, 1984.
20. Shattil SJ, Bennett JS: Platelets and their membranes in hemostasis: physiology and pathophysiology. Ann. Intern. Med. 94:108, 1981.
21. Hawiger J: Hemostasis and Thrombosis. *In* Basic Principles and Clinical Practice. 2nd Ed. Edited by RW Colman, J Hirsch, VJ Marder, EW Salzman. Philadelphia, J.B. Lippincott 1987, p. 182.
22. Weiss HJ, Rogers J: Fibrinogen and platelets in the primary arrest of bleeding. Studies in two patients with congenital afibrinogenemia. N. Engl. J. Med. 285:369, 1971.
23. Miletich JP, Jackson CM, Majerus PW: Properties of the factor $X_\alpha$ binding site on human platelets. J. Biol. Chem. 253:6908, 1977.
24. Bettex-Galland M, Trescher EF: Thrombosthenin, the contractile protein from blood platelets and its relation to other contractile proteins. Adv. Protein Chem. 20:1, 1965.
25. Davie EW, Ratnoff OD: Waterfall sequence for intrinsic blood clotting. Science 145:1310, 1964.
26. McFarlane RG: An enzyme cascade in the blood clotting mechanism and its function as a biochemical amplifier. Nature 202:498, 1964.
27. Griffin SH, Cochmane CG: Mechanisms for the involvement of high molecular weight kinogens in surface dependent reactions of Hageman factor. Proc. Natl. Acad. Sci. U.S.A. 73:2554, 1976.
28. Nemerson Y: Biological control of factor VII. Semin. Thromb. Hemost. 35:96, 1976.
29. Sauto H, Ratnoff OD: Alterations of factor VII activity by activated Fletcher factor (a plasma kallikrein); A potential link between intrinsic and extrinsic clotting systems. J Lab Clin Med 85:405, 1975.
30. Nemerson Y: Tissue factor and hemostasis. Blood 71:1, 1988.
31. Rapaport SI: Inhibition of factor VIIa/tissue factor-induced blood coagulation: With particular emphasis upon a factor $X_\alpha$ dependent-inhibitory mechanism. Blood 73:359, 1989.
32. Stenflo J, Fernlund P, Egan W, Roepstorff P: Vitamin K-dependent modifications of glutamic acid residues in prothrombin. Proc. Natl. Acad. Sci. U.S.A. 71:2730, 1974.
33. Nelsesteun GL, Zytkovicz TH, Howard JB: The mode of action of vitamin K. Identification of gamma-carboxyglutamic acid as a component of prothrombin. J. Biol. Chem. 249:6347, 1974.
34. Borowski M, Furie BC, Bauminger S, Furie B: Prothrombin requires two sequential metal-dependent conformational transitions to bind phospholipid. J. Biol. Chem. 261: 14969,1986.
35. Bick RL: Clinical relevance of antithrombin III. Semin Thromb Hemost. 4:276, 1982.
36. Marcum JA, McKenny JB, Rosenberg RD: Acceleration of thrombin-antithrombin complex formation in rat hindquarters via heparin-like molecules bound to the endothelium. J. Clin. Invest. 74:341, 1984.
37. Marcum JA, Atha DH, Fritze LMS, Nawroth P, et al: Cloned bovine aortic endothelial cells synthesize anticoagulantly active heparin sulfate proteoglycan. J. Biol. Chem. 261: 7507, 1986.
38. Esmon CT, Owen WG: Identification of an endothelial cell cofactor for thrombin-catalyzed activation of protein C. Proc. Natl. Acad. Sci. U.S.A. 78:2249, 1981.
39. Esmon CT, Esmon NL, Harris KW: Complex formation between thrombin and thrombomodulin inhibits both thrombin-catalyzed fibrin formation and factor V activation. J. Biol. Chem. 257:7944, 1982.
40. Esmon NL, Carroll RC, Esmon CT: Thrombomodulin blocks the ability of thrombin to activate platelets. J. Biol. Chem. 258:12238, 1983.
41. Stenflo J: A new vitamin K-dependent protein: purification from bovine plasma and preliminary characterization. J. Biol. Chem. 251:355, 1976.
42. Seegers WH, Novoa E, Henry RL, Hassouna HI: Relationship of "new" vitamin K-dependent protein C and "old" autoprothrombin II-A. Thromb. Res. 8:543, 1976.
43. Di Scipio RG, Hermodson MA, Yates SG, Davie EW: A comparison of human prothrombin, factor IX (Christmas factor), factor X (Stuart factor), and protein S. Biochemistry 16:698, 1977.

44. Marlar RA, Kleiss AJ, Griffin JH: Mechanism of action of human activated protein C, a thrombin-dependent anticoagulant enzyme. Blood 59:1067, 1982.
45. Comp PC, Esmon CT: Activated protein C inhibits platelet prothrombin-converting activity. Blood 54:1272, 1979.
46. Dahlbck B, Stenflo J: Inhibitory effect of activated protein C on activation of prothrombin by platelet-bound factor $X_{\alpha}$. Eur. J. Biochem. 107:331, 1980.
47. Walker FJ: Regulation of activated protein C by protein S: the role of phospholipid in fact Va inactivation. J. Biol. Chem. 256:11128, 1981.
48. Marlar RA, Griffin JH: Deficiency of protein C inhibitor in combined factor V/VIII deficiency disease. J. Clin. Invest. 66:1186, 1980.
49. Suzuki K, Nishioka J, Hashimoto S: Protein C inhibitor: purification from human plasma and characterization. J. Biol. Chem. 258:163, 1983.
50. Ogston D, Bennett B: Naturally occurring inhibitors of coagulation. *In* Haemostasis: Biochemistry, Physiology and Pathology. Edited by D Ogston, B Bennett. London, John Wiley & Sons, 1977, 230.
51. Castellino FJ: Biochemistry of human plasminogen. Semin. Thromb. Hemost. 10:18, 1984.
52. Loskutoff D: The fibrinolytic system of cultured endothelial cells: Insights into the role of endothelium in thrombolysis. *In* Vascular Endothelium in Hemostasis and Thrombosis. Edited by MA Gimbrone. Edinburgh, Churchill Livingstone, 1986, 120.
53. Nachman RL, Hajjar KA: Endothelial Cell Fibrinolytic Assembly. *In* Progress in Vascular Biology, Hemostasis, and Thrombosis. Edited by ZM Ruggeri, CA Fulcher, J Ware. New York, New York Academy of Sciences, 1991, p. 240.
54. van Hinsbergh VWM, Bertina RM, van Wijngaarden A, van Tilburg NH, et al: Activated protein C decreases plasminogen activator-inhibitor activity in endothelial cell-conditioned medium. Blood 65:444, 1985.
55. Cunningham FG, MacDonald PC, Gant NF: Maternal Adaptations to Pregnancy. *In* Williams Obstetrics. Edited by FG Cunningham, PC MacDonald, NF Gant. Norwalk, Appleton & Lange, 1989, p. 129.
56. Cunningham FG, MacDonald PC, Gant NF: Maternal Adaptations to Pregnancy. *In* Williams Obstetrics. Edited by FG Cunningham, PC MacDonald, NF Gant. Norwalk, Appleton & Lange, 1989, 130.
57. Hakkinen LM, Vuolteenaho OJ, Leppaluoto JP, Laatikainen TJ: Endothelium in maternal and umbilical cord blood in spontaneous labor and at elective cesarean delivery. Obstet. Gynecol. 80:72, 1992
58. Pritchard JA: Changes in the blood volume during pregnancy and delivery. Anesthesiology 26:393, 1965.
59. Ueland K: Maternal cardiovascular dynamics: VII. Intrapartum blood volume changes. Am. J. Obstet. Gynecol. 126: 671, 1976.
60. Lange RD, Dynesius R: Blood volume changes during normal pregnancy. N. Engl. J. Med. 266:877, 1962.
61. Cunningham FG, MacDonald PC, Gant NF: The Puerperium. *In* Williams Obstetrics. Edited by FG Cunningham, PC MacDonald, NF Gant. Norwalk, Appleton & Lange, 1989, 252.
62. Tygart SG, McRoyan DK, Spinnato JA, McRoyan CJ, et al: Longitudinal study of platelet indices during normal pregnancy. Am. J. Obstet. Gynecol. 154:883, 1986.
63. Fay RA, Hughes AD, Farron NT: Platelets in pregnancy: hyperdestruction in pregnancy. Obstet. Gynecol. 61:238, 1983.
64. Norris LA, Sheppard BL, Bonnar J: Increased whole blood platelet aggregation in normal pregnancy can be prevented in vitro by aspirin and dazmegrel (UK38485). Br. J. Obstet. Gynecol. 99:253, 1992.
65. Metcalfe J, Ueland K: Maternal cardiovascular adjustments to pregnancy. Prog. Cardiovasc. Dis. 16:363, 1974.
66. Cruikshank DP, Hays PM: Maternal Physiology in Pregnancy. *In* Obstetrics: Normal and Problem Pregnancies. 2nd Ed. Edited by SG Gabbe, JR Niebyl, JL Simpson. New York, Churchill Livingstone, 1991, p. 134.
67. O'Driscoll K, McCarthy JR: Abruptio placentae and central venous pressures. J. Obstet. Gynaecol. Br. Commonw. 73: 923, 1966.
68. Wu PYK, Udani V, Chan L, Miller FC, et al: Colloid osmotic pressure: variations in normal pregnancy. J. Perinatol. 11: 193, 1983.
69. Clark SL, Cotton DB, Lee W, Bishop C, et al: Central hemodynamic assessment of normal term pregnancy. Am. J. Obstet. Gynecol. 161:1439, 1989.
70. Ueland K, Hansen JM: Maternal cardiovascular dynamics. III. Labor and delivery under local and caudal analgesia. Am. J. Obstet. Gynecol. 103:8, 1969.
71. Lees MM, Scott DB, Kerr MG: Haemodynamic changes associated with labour. J. Obstet. Gynaecol. Br. Commonw. 77:29, 1970.
72. Petrie JC, O'Brien E, Littler WA, de Swiet M: Recommendations on blood pressure measurement. Br. Med. J. 293:611, 1986.
73. Davey DA, MacGillivray I: The classification and definition of the hypertensive disorders of pregnancy. Am. J. Obstet. Gynecol. 158:892, 1988.
74. Webster J, Newnham D, Petrie JC, Lovell HG: Influence of arm position in measurement of blood pressure. Br. Med. J. 288:1574, 1984.
75. Linfors EW, Feussner JR, Blessing CL, Starmer CF, et al: Spurious hypertension in the obese patient. Effect of sphygmomanometer cuff size on prevalence of hypertension. Arch. Intern. Med. 144:1482, 1984.
76. Ihrman K: A clinical and physiological study of pregnancy in material from northern Sweden: VII. The heart volume during and after pregnancy. Acta. Soc. Med. Upsal. 65:326, 1960.
77. Cutforth R, MacDonald CB: Heart sounds and murmurs in pregnancy. Am. Heart J. 71:741, 1966.
78. Metcalfe J, McAnulty JH, Ueland K: Cardiovascular physiology. Clin. Obstet. Gynecol. 24:693, 1981.
79. Mashini IS, Albazzaz SJ, Fadel HE, Abdulla AM, et al: Serial noninvasive evaluation of cardiovascular hemodynamics during pregnancy. Am. J. Obstet. Gynecol. 156:1208, 1987.
80. Rubler S, Damani PM, Pinto ER: Cardiac size and performance during pregnancy estimated with echocardiography. Am. J. Cardiol. 40:534, 1977.
81. Tanz RD: Inotropic effects of certain steroids upon heart muscle. Rev. Can. Biol. 22:147, 1963.
82. Wallenburg HCS: Maternal haemodynamics in pregnancy. Fetal Med. Rev. 2:45, 1990.
83. Dunlop W, Davison JM: Renal haemodynamics and tubular function in human pregnancy. Clin. Obstet. Gynaecol. 1: 769, 1987.
84. Lee W, Pivarnik J: Hemodynamic studies during pregnancy. J. Maternal-Fetal Med. 1:75, 1992.
85. Ueland K, Novy MJ, Peterson EN, Metcalfe J: Maternal cardiovascular dynamics. IV. The influence of gestational age on the maternal cardiovascular response to posture and exercise. Am. J. Obstet. Gynecol. 104:856, 1969.
86. Pekonen F, Rasi V, Ammala M, Viinikka L, et al: Platelet function and coagulation in normal and preeclamptic pregnancy. Thromb. Res. 43:553, 1986.
87. O'Brien WF, Saba HI, Knuppel RA, Scerbo JC, et al: Altera-

tions in platelet concentration and aggregation in normal pregnancy and preeclampsia. Am. J. Obstet. Gynecol. 155: 486, 1986.

88. Bonnar J: Blood coagulation and fibrinolysis in obstetrics. Clin. Haematol. 2:213, 1973.
89. Dalaker K: Clotting factor VII during pregnancy, delivery and puerperium. Br. J. Obstet. Gynaecol. 93:17, 1986.
90. Kasper CK, Hoag MS, Aggeler PM, Stone S: Blood clotting factors in pregnancy: Factor VIII concentrations in normal and AHF-deficient women. Obstet. Gynecol. 24:242, 1964.
91. Stirling Y, Woolf L, North WRS, Seghatchian MJ, et al: Haemostasis in normal pregnancy. Thromb. Haemost. 52:176, 1984.
92. Todd ME, Thompson JH, Bowie EJW, Owen CA: Changes in blood coagulation during pregnancy. Mayo. Clin. Proc. 40:370, 1965.
93. Beardsley DS: Hemostasis in the perinatal period: Approach to the diagnosis of coagulation disorders. Semin. Perinatol. 15:25, 1991.
94. Bonnar J, McNicol GP, Douglas AS: Coagulation and fibrinolytic mechanisms during and after normal childbirth. Br. Med. J. 2:200, 1970.
95. Briet E, Riesher HM, Blatt PM: Factor IX levels during pregnancy in a woman with haemophilia B. Hemostasis 11:87, 1982.
96. Sipes SL, Weiner CP: Venous thromboembolic disease in pregnancy. Semin. Perinatol. 14:103, 1990.
97. Greer IA, Lowe GDO, Walker JJ, Forbes CD: Haemorrhagic problems in obstetrics and gynaecology in patients with congenital coagulopathies. Brit. J. Obstet. Gynecol. 98:909, 1991.
98. Rizza CR, Rhymes JL, Austen DEG, Kernoff PBA, et al: Detection of carriers of haemophilia in a "blind study." Brit. J. Haematol. 30:447, 1975.
99. Thornton CA, Bonnar J: Factor VIII-related antigen and factor VIII coagulant activity in normal and pre-eclamptic pregnancy. Br. J. Obstet. Gynaecol. 84:919, 1977.
100. Czapek EE: Coagulation Problems. Int. Anesthesiol. Clin. 11:175, 1973.
101. Briet E, Tilberg NH, Veltkamp JS: Oral contraceptives and the detection of carriers of hemophilia B. Thromb. Res. 13:279, 1978.
102. Weiner CP, Sabbagha RE, Vaisrub N: Distinguishing preeclampsia from chronic hypertension using antithrombin III. Proceedings of the Society for Gynecologic Investigation, Washington, DC, 1983, abstr 29.
103. de Boer K, Cate JW, Sturk A, Borm JJJ, et al: Enhanced thrombin generation in normal and hypertensive pregnancy. Am. J. Obstet. Gynecol. 160:95, 1989.
104. Weiner CP, Brandt J: Plasma antithrombin III activity: an aid in the diagnosis of preeclampsia-eclampsia. Am. J. Obstet. Gynecol. 142:275, 1982.
105. Bremme K, Ostlund E, Almqvist I, Heinonen K, et al: Enhanced thrombin generation and fibrinolytic activity in normal pregnancy and the puerperium. Obstet. Gynecol. 80:132, 1992.
106. Gonzales R, Alberca J, Vicente V: Protein C levels in late pregnancy, postpartum and in women on oral contraceptives. Thromb. Res. 39:637, 1985.
107. Bonnar J, McNichol GP, Douglas AS: Fibrinolytic enzyme system and pregnancy. Br. Med. J. 3:387, 1969.
108. Fletcher AP, Alkjaersig NK, Burstein R: The influence of pregnancy upon blood coagulation and plasma fibrinolytic enzyme function. Am. J. Obstet. Gynecol. 134:743, 1979.
109. Arias F, Andrinopoulos G, Zamora J: Whole blood fibrinolytic activity in normal and hypertensive pregnancies and its relation to placental concentration of urokinase inhibitor. Am. J. Obstet. Gynecol. 133:624, 1979.
110. Kruithof EKO, Tran-Thang C, Gudinchet A, Hauert J, et al: Fibrinolysis in C pregnancy: a study of plasminogen activator inhibitors. Blood 69:460, 1987.
111. Walker JE, Gow L, Campbell DM, Ogston D: The inhibition by plasma of urokinase and tissue activator-induced fibrinolysis in pregnancy and the puerperium. Thromb. Haemost. 49:21, 1983.
112. Astedt B: Significance of placenta in depression of fibrinolytic activity during pregnancy. J. Obstet. Gynaecol. Br. Commonw. 79:205, 1972.
113. Astedt B: Fibrinolytic activity of veins in the puerperium. Acta. Obstet. Gynecol. Scand. 51:325, 1972.
114. Wright JG, Cooper P, Astedt B, Lecander I, et al: Fibrinolysis during normal human pregnancy: complex interrelationships between plasma levels of tissue plasminogen activator and inhibitors and the euglobulin clot lysis time. Br. J. Haematol. 69:253, 1988.
115. Uszynski M, Abildgaard U: Separation and characterization of two fibrinolytic inhibitors from placenta. Thromb. Haemost. 25:580, 1971.
116. Basu HK: Fibrinolysis and abruptio placenta. Br. J. Obstet 76:481, 1969.
117. Stiehm ER, Kenna AL, Schelble DT: Split products of fibrin in maternal serum in the perinatal period. Am. J. Obstet. Gynecol. 108:941, 1970.
118. Hathaway WE, Bonnar J: Perinatal Coagulation. New York, Grune & Stratton, 1978, p. 27.
119. Weiner CP, Kwaan H, Hauck WW, Duboe FJ, et al: Fibrin generation in normal pregnancy. Obstet. Gynecol. 64:46, 1984.
120. Weiner CP: The treatment of clotting disorders during pregnancy. *In* Gynecology and Obstetrics, Vol 3. Edited by JJ Sciarra. Philadelphia, J.B. Lippincott, 1988, p. 1.
121. Noller KL, Bowie EJW, Kempers RG, Owen CA: von Willebrand's disease in pregnancy. Obstet. Gynecol. 41:865, 1973.
122. Krishnamurthy M, Miotti AB: von Willebrand's disease and pregnancy. Obstet. Gynecol. 49:244, 1977.
123. Sorosky J, Klatsky A, Nobert GF, Burchill RC: von Willebrand's disease complicating second trimester abortion. Obstet. Gynecol. 55:253, 1980.
124. Punnonen R, Nyman D, Gronroos M, Wallen O: von Willebrand's disease and pregnancy. Acta. Obstet. Gynecol. Scand 60:507, 1981.
125. Sagi A, Creter D, Goldman J, Djaldetti M: Platelet functions before, during and after labor. Acta. Haematol. 65:67, 1981.
126. Eisenberg JM, Clarke JR, Sussman SA: Prothrombin and partial thromboplastin times as pre-operative screening tests. Arch. Surg. 117:48, 1982.
127. Rohrer MJ, Michelotti MC, Nahrwold DL: A prospective evaluation of the efficacy of preoperative coagulation testing. Ann. Surg. 208:554, 1988.
128. Sox HC: Common Diagnostic Tests: Use and Interpretation. American College of Physicians, Philadelphia, 1987, p. 350.
129. Erban SB, Kinman JL, Schwartz JS: Routine use of the prothrombin and partial thromboplastin times. JAMA 262: 2428, 1989.
130. Ciavarella D, Reed RL, Counts RB, Baron L, et al: Clotting factor levels and the risk of diffuse microvascular bleeding in the massively transfused patient. Br. J. Haematol. 67: 365, 1987.
131. American College of Obstetricians and Gynecologists: Blood Component Therapy. Technical Bulletin #78, Washington, DC, 1984.
132. Hill ST, Lavin JP: Blood ordering in obstetrics and gynecol-

ogy: recommendations for the type and screen. Obstet. Gynecol. 62:236, 1983.

133. Ivankovic M, Germain AM, Mezzano D, Pereira J, et al: Bleeding time in normal pregnancy and preeclampsia. 39th Annual Meeting of Society for Gynecologic Investigation, San Antonio, Texas, Abstract #126, p. 171, 1992.

134. Mielke CH Jr, Kaneshiro MM, Maher IA, Weiner JM, et al: The standardized normal Ivy bleeding time and it's prolongation by aspirin. Blood 34:204, 1969.

135. Bick RL: Disseminated intravascular coagulation: clinical laboratory characteristics in 48 patients. Ann. N.Y. Acad. Sci. 370:843, 1981.

136. Thiagarajah P, Shapiro SS, De Marco L: Monoclonal immunoglobulin M coagulation inhibitor with phospholipid specificity: mechanism of a lupus anticoagulant. J. Clin. Invest. 66:397, 1980.

137. Carreras LO, Defreyn G, Machin SJ, Vermylen J, et al: Arterial thrombosis, intrauterine death and "lupus" anticoagulant: detection of immunoglobulin interfering with prostacyclin formation. Lancet 1:244, 1981.

138. Feinstein DI: Lupus anticoagulant, thrombosis, and fetal loss. (editorial) N. Engl. J. Med. 313:1348, 1985.

139. Canoso RT, Hutton RA, Deykin D: A chloropromazine-induced inhibitor of blood coagulation. Am. J. Hematol. 2: 183, 1977.

140. Bajaj SP, Rapaport SI, Fierer DS, Herbst KD, et al: A mechanism for the hypoprothrombinemia of the acquired-lupus anticoagulant syndrome. Blood 61:684, 1983.

141. Branch DW: Antiphospholipid antibodies and pregnancy: maternal implications. Semin. Perinatol. 14:139, 1990.

142. Bennett B, Ratnoff OD, Holt JB, Roberts HR: Hageman trait (factor XII deficiency): a probable second genotype inherited as an autosomal dominant characteristic. Blood 40: 412, 1972.

143. McPherson RA: Thromboembolism in Hageman trait. Am. J. Clin. Pathol. 68:420, 1977.

144. Girma JP, Meyer D, Verweij CL, Pannekoek H, et al: Structure-function relationship of human von Willebrand factor. Blood 70:605, 1987.

145. Weiss HJ, Sussman II, Hoyer L: Stabilization of factor VIII in plasma by the von Willebrand factor: studies on post-transfusion and dissociated factor VIII and in patients with von Willebrand's disease. J. Clin. Invest. 60:390, 1977.

146. Turitto VT, Weiss HJ, Baumgartner HR: Platelet interaction with rabbit subendothelium in von Willebrand's disease: altered thrombus formation distinct from defective platelet adhesion. J. Clin. Invest. 74:1730, 1984.

147. Bolhuis PA, Sakariassen KS, Sander HJ, Bouma BN, et al: Binding of factor VIII-von Willebrand factor to human arterial subendothelium precedes increased platelet adhesion and enhances platelet spreading. J. Lab. Clin. Med. 97:568, 1981.

148. Dejana E, Lampugnani MG, Giorgi M, Gaboli M, et al: von Willebrand factor promotes endothelial cell adhesion via an Arg-Gly-Asp-dependent mechanism. J. Cell. Biol. 109: 367, 1989.

149. Silver J: von Willebrand's disease in Sweden. Acta. Paedriatr. Scand. (Suppl.) 238:5, 1973.

150. Berkowitz SD, Ruggeri ZM, Zimmerman TS: von Willebrand disease. *In* Coagulation and Bleeding Disorders. The Role of Factor VIII and von Willebrand Factor. Edited by TS Zimmerman, ZM Ruggeri. New York, Marcel Dekker, 1989, p. 215.

151. Sadler JE, Mancuso DJ, Randi AM, Tuley EA, et al: Molecular Biology of von Willebrand Factor. *In* Progress in Vascular Biology, Hemostasis, and Thrombosis. Edited by ZM Ruggeri, CA Fulcher, J Ware. New York, New York Academy of Sciences, 1991, p. 114.

152. Lipton RA, Ayromlooi J, Coller BS: Severe von Willebrand's disease during labor and delivery. JAMA 248:1355, 1982.

153. von Willebrand E, Jurgens R, Dahlberg U: Konstitionell trombopati en ny arftlig blodarsjukdom. Fin Lakaresalls Handl 75:193, 1934.

154. Takahashi N: Studies on the pathophysiology and treatment of von Willebrand's disease VI. Variant von Willebrand's disease complicating placenta previa. Thromb. Res. 31:285, 1983.

155. Weiner CP: Treatment of Coagulation and Fibrinolytic Disorders. *In* Hematologic Problems in Pregnancy. Edited by DZ Kitay. Oradell, NJ, Medical Economics Books, 1987, p. 331.

156. Rick ME, Williams SB, McKeown LP: Thrombocytopenia associated with pregnancy in a patient with type IIB von Willebrand's disease. Blood 11:786, 1987.

157. Gitschier J: The Molecular Basis of Hemophilia A. *In* Progress in Vascular Biology, Hemostasis, and Thrombosis. Edited by ZM Ruggeri, CA Fulcher, J Ware. New York, New York Academy of Sciences, 1991, p. 89.

158. Bunschoten EM, van Houwelingen JC, Visser EJMS, van Dijken PJ, et al: Bleeding symptoms in carriers of haemophilia A and B. Thromb. Haemost. 59:349, 1988.

159. Weiner CP: Treatment of Coagulation and Fibrinolytic Disorders. *In* Hematologic Problems in Pregnancy. Edited by DZ Kitay. Oradell, NJ, Medical Economics Books, 1987, p. 333.

160. Mibashan RS, Peak IR, Rodeck CH, Thumpston JK, et al: Dual diagnosis of prenatal haemophilia A by measurement of fetal factor VIIIC and VIIIC antigen (VIIICAg). Lancet 2:994, 1980.

161. Schimpf K, Brackmann HH, Kreuz W, Kraus B, et al: Absence of anti-human immunodeficiency virus types 1 and 2 seroconversion after the treatment of hemophilia A or von Willebrand's disease with pasteurized fact VIII concentrate. N. Engl. J. Med. 321:1148, 1989.

162. Roberts HR: Factor VIII replacement Therapy: Issues and Future Prospects. *In* Progress in Vascular Biology, Hemostasis, and Thrombosis. Edited by ZM Ruggeri, CA Fulcher, J Ware. New York, New York Academy of Sciences, 1991, p. 109.

163. Purcell G, Nossel HL: Factor XI (PTA) deficiency: surgical and obstetric aspects. Obstet. Gynecol. 35:69, 1970.

164. Phillips LL, Little WA: Factor V deficiency in obstetrics. Obstet. Gynecol. 19:507, 1962.

165. Langer R, Caspi E, Kaufman S, Freid K, et al: Management of labor in a patient with factor V deficiency. Isr. J. Med. Sci. 18:701, 1982.

166. Rizza CR: The clinical features of clotting factor deficiencies. The management of patients with coagulation factor deficiencies. *In* Human Blood Coagulation, Hemostasis and Thrombosis. Edited by R Biggs. London, Blackwell Scientific Publications, 1976.

167. Thaler E, Lechner K: Antithrombin III deficiency in thromboembolus. Clin. Haematol. 10:369, 1981.

168. Comp PC: Hereditary disorders predisposing to thrombosis. *In* Progress in Thrombosis and Hemostasis. Edited by BS Coller. Orlando, FL, Grune & Stratton, Orlando, 1986, p. 71.

169. Rick ME: Protein C and Protein S: vitamin K-dependent inhibitors of blood coagulation. JAMA 263:701, 1990.

170. Brandt P, Stembjerg S: Subcutaneous heparin for thrombosis in pregnant women with hereditary antithrombin deficiency. Br. Med. J. i:449, 1980.

171. Winter JH, Fenech JA, Ridley W, Bennett B, et al: Familial antithrombin III deficiency. Quart. J. Med. 51:373, 1982.
172. Comp PC, Thurnau GR, Welsh J, Esmon CT: Functional and immunologic protein S levels are decreased during pregnancy. Blood 68:881, 1986.
173. Greer IA: Thromboembolic problems in pregnancy. Fetal. Med. Rev. 1:79, 1989.
174. Carter CJ, Bellem PJ: Management of protein C deficiency in pregnancy. Fibrinolysis. Suppl. 1:161, 1988.
175. Hellgren M, Tengborn L, Abildgaard U: Pregnancy in women with congenital antithrombin III deficiency: experience of treatment with heparin an antithrombin. Gynecol. Obstet. Invest. 14:127, 1982.
176. Wise PH, Hall AJ: Heparin induced osteopenia in pregnancy. Br. Med. J. 281:110, 1980.
177. de Swiet M, Ward PD, Fidler J, Horsman A, et al: Prolonged heparin therapy in pregnancy causes bone demineralization (heparin-induced osteopenia). Br. J. Obstet. Gynaecol. 90:1129, 1983.
178. Brandt P: Observations during the treatment of antithrombin III deficient women with heparin and antithrombin concentrate during pregnancy, parturition, and abortion. Thromb. Res. 22:15, 1981.
179. Wessler S, Yen ET: Theory and practice of minidose heparin in surgical patients. Circulation 47:671, 1973.
180. Tengborn L, Bengtsson T: Case report: antithrombin III concentrate. Acta. Obstet. Gynecol. Scand. 65:375, 1986.
181. Salzman EW: Low-molecular-weight heparin and other new antithrombotic drugs. N. Engl. J. Med. 326:1017, 1992.
182. Broekmans AW, Veltkamp JJ, Bertina RM: Congenital protein C deficiency and venous thromboembolism: a study in three Dutch families. N. Engl. J. Med. 309:340, 1983.
183. McGehee WJ, Klotz TA, Epstein DJ, Rapaport SI: Coumarin necrosis associated with hereditary protein C deficiency. Ann. Intern. Med. 100:59, 1984.
184. Kasper CK: Complications of Hemophilia A Treatment: factor VIII Inhibitors. *In* Progress in Vascular Biology, Hemostasis, and Thrombosis. Edited by ZM Ruggeri, CA Fulcher, J Ware. New York, New York Academy of Sciences, 1991, p. 97.
185. Greenwood RJ, Rabin SC: Hemophilia-like postpartum bleeding. Obstet. Gynecol. 30:362, 1967.
186. Marengo-Rowe AJ, Murff G, Leveson JE, Cook J: Hemophilia-like disease associated with pregnancy. Obstet. Gynecol. 40:56, 1972.
187. Fisher DS, Clyne LP: Circulating factor XI antibody and disseminated intravascular coagulation. Arch. Intern. Med. 141:515, 1981.
188. Green D, Lechner K: A survey of 215 non-hemophilic patients with inhibitors to factor VIII. Thromb. Haemost. 45: 200, 1981.
189. Francesconi M, Korniger C, Thaler E, Niessner H, et al: Plasmapheresis: its value in the management of patients with antibodies to factor VIII. Haemostasis 11:79, 1982.
190. Lubbe WF, Palmer SJ, Butler WS, Liggins GC: Fetal survival after prednisone suppression of maternal lupus anticoagulant. Lancet 1:1361, 1983.
191. Rosove MH, Tabsh K, Wasserstrum N, Howard P, et al: Heparin therapy for pregnant women with lupus anticoagulant or anticardiolipin antibodies. Obstet. Gynecol. 75: 630, 1990.
192. Branch DW: Antiphospholipid syndrome: laboratory concerns, fetal loss and pregnancy management. Semin. Perinatol. 15:230, 1991.
193. Cowchock FS, Reece EA, Balaban D, Branch DW et al: Repeated fetal losses associated with antiphospholipid antibodies: a collaborative randomized trial comparing prednisone to low-dose heparin treatment. Am. J. Obstet. Gynecol. 166:1318, 1992.
194. Lubbe WF, Liggins GC: Role of lupus anticoagulant and autoimmunity in recurrent pregnancy loss. Semin. Reprod. Endocrinol. 6:181, 1988.
195. Infante-Rivard C, David M, Gauthier R, Rivard G-E: Lupus anticoagulants, anticardiolipin antibodies, and fetal loss: a case-control study. N. Engl. J. Med. 325:1063, 1991.
196. Robinson RD, Polzin WJ, Kozakowski MH, Kopelman JN, et al: The incidence of antiphospholipid antibodies in the obstetric population. Abstract, 40th Annual Meeting of the American College of Obstetricians and Gynecologists. April 1992, p. 1.
197. Frampton G, Cameron JS, Thom M, Jones S, et al: Successful removal of antiphospholipid antibody during pregnancy using plasma exchange and low-dose prednisolone. Lancet 2:1023, 1987.
198. Trudinger BH, Stewart GJ, Cook CM, Connelly A, et al: Monitoring lupus anticoagulant-positive pregnancies with umbilical artery flow velocity waveforms. Obstet. Gynecol. 72:215, 1988.
199. Beaufils M, Uzan S, Donsimoni R, Colan JC: Prevention of pre-eclampsia by early antiplatelet therapy. Lancet 1:840, 1985.
200. Wallenburg HCS, Dekker GA, Makovitz JW, Rotmans P: Low-dose aspirin prevents pregnancy-induced hypertension and pre-eclampsia in angiotensin-sensitive primigravidae. Lancet 1:1, 1986.
201. Hadi HA, Treadwell EL: Lupus anticoagulant and anticardiolipin antibodies in pregnancy: a review. II. Diagnosis and Management. Obstet. Gynecol. Surv. 45:786, 1990.
202. Schiff E, Peleg E, Goldenberg M, Rosenthal T, et al: The use of aspirin to prevent pregnancy-induced hypertension and lower the ratio of thromboxane $A_2$ to prostacyclin in relatively high risk pregnancies. N. Engl. J. Med. 321:351, 1989.
203. Walsh SW: Physiology of low-dose aspirin therapy for the prevention of preeclampsia. Semin. Perinatol. 14:152, 1990.
204. Weksler BB, Pett SB, Alonso D, Richter RC, et al: Differential inhibition by aspirin of vascular and platelet prostaglandin synthesis in atherosclerotic patients. N. Engl. J. Med. 308:800, 1983.
205. Spitz B, Magness RR, Cox SM, Brown CEL, et al: Low dose aspirin. I. Effect of angiotensin II pressor response and blood prostaglandin concentrations in pregnant women sensitive to angiotensin II. Am. J. Obstet. Gynecol. 59:1035, 1988.
206. Masotti G, Galanti G, Poggesi L, Abatte R, et al: Differential inhibition of prostacyclin production and platelet aggregation by aspirin. Lancet 2:1213, 1979.
207. Caruso A, Ferrazzani S, De Carolis S, Pomini F, et al: Low-dose aspirin qualitatively affects the vascular response to angiotensin II in hypersensitive pregnant women. Clin. and Exper. Hyper. in Pregnancy B11:81, 1992.
208. Cines DB, Tomaski A, Tannenbaum S: Immune endothelial-cell injury in heparin-associated thrombocytopenia. N. Engl. J. Med. 316:581, 1987.
209. Exner T, Rickard KA, Kronenberg H: A sensitive test demonstrating lupus anticoagulant and its behavioral patterns. Br. J. Haematol. 40:143, 1978.
210. Landy HJ, Kessler C, Kelly WK, Weingold AB: Obstetric performance in patients with the lupus anticoagulant and/or anticardiolipin antibodies. Am J. Perinatol. 9:146, 1992.
211. Dewolf F, Carreras LO, Moerman P, Vermylen J, et al: Decidual vasculopathy and extensive placental infarction in

a patient with repeated thromboembolic accidents, recurrent fetal loss, and lupus anticoagulant. Am. J. Obstet. Gynecol. 142:829, 1982.
212. Abramowski CR, Vegas MC, Swinehart G, Gyves MT: Decidual vasculopathy of the placenta in lupus erythematosus. N. Engl. J. Med. 303:668, 1980.
213. Hadi HA, Treadwell EL: Lupus anticoagulant and anticardiolipin antibodies in pregnancy: a review. I. Immunochemistry and clinical implications. Obstet. Gynecol. Surv. 45: 780, 1990.
214. Schneider JM, Haesslein HC: Fetal thrombosis with antithrombin III and protein C deficiencies. Unpublished cases.
215. Finazzi G, Cortelazzo S, Viero P, Galli M, et al: Maternal lupus anticoagulant and fatal neonatal thrombosis. Thromb. Haemost. 57:238, 1987.
216. Melissari E, Nicolaides KH, Scully MF, Kakkar VV: Protein S and C4b-binding protein in fetal and neonatal blood. Br. J. Haematol. 70:199, 1988.
217. Marlar RA, Montgomery RR, Broekmans AW: Diagnosis and treatment of homozygous protein C deficiency: report of the Working Party on Homozygous Protein C and Protein S, International Committee on Thrombosis and Haemostasis. J. Pediatr. 114:528, 1989.
218. Sheridan-Pereira M, Porreo RP, Hays T, Burke MS: Neonatal aortic thrombosis associated with the lupus anticoagulant. Obstet. Gynecol. 71:1016, 1988.
219. Silver RK, MacGregor SN, Pasternak JF, Neely SE: Fetal stroke associated with elevated maternal anticardiolipin antibodies. Obstet. Gynecol. 80:497–9, 1992.
220. Baehner RL, Strauss HS: Hemophilia in the first year of life. N. Engl. J. Med. 275:524, 1966.
221. Yoffe G, Buchanan GR: Intracranial hemorrhage in newborn and young infants with hemophilia. J. Pediatr. 113: 333, 1988.
222. Kletzel M, Miller CH, Becton DL, Chadduck WM, et al: Postdelivery head bleeding in hemophilic neonates: causes and management. Am. J. Dis. Child. 143:1107, 1989.
223. Bray GL, Luban NL: Hemophilia presenting with intracranial hemorrhage. Am. J. Dis. Child. 141:1215, 1989.
224. Peake IR, Furlong BL, Bloom AL: Carrier detection by direct gene analysis in a family with haemophilia B (factor IX deficiency). Lancet 1:242, 1984.
225. Nicolaides KH: Cordocentesis. Clin. Obstet. Gynecol. 31: 123, 1988.
226. Ash KM, Mibashan RS, Nicolaides KH: Diagnosis and treatment of feto-maternal hemorrhage in a fetus with homozygous von Willebrand's disease. Fetal. Ther. 3:189, 1988.
227. Knab DR: Abruptio placentae: an assessment of the time and method of delivery. Obstet. Gynecol. 52:625, 1978.
228. Raymond E, Mills JL: Placental abruption: effects of maternal behavior and associated fetal problems. Abstract, 40th Annual Meeting of the American College of Obstetricians and Gynecologists. April 1992, p. 23.
229. Kleiner GJ, Merskey C, Johnson AJ, Markus WB: Defibrination in normal and abnormal parturition. Br. J. Haematol. 19:159, 1970.
230. Pritchard JA: Haematological problems associated with delivery, placental abruption, retained dead fetus and amniotic fluid embolism. Clin. Haematol. 2:563, 1973.
231. Odendaal HJ, Brink S, Steytler JG: Clinical and haematological problems associated with severe abruptio placentae. S. Afr. Med. J. 54:476, 1978.
232. Pritchard JA, Brekken AL: Clinical and laboratory studies on severe abruption placenta. Am. J. Obstet. Gynecol. 97: 681, 1967.
233. Pritchard J, Mason R, Corley M, Pritchard S: Genesis of severe placental abruption. Am. J. Obstet. Gynecol. 108: 22, 1970.
234. American College of Obstetricians and Gynecologists: Hemorrhagic shock. Technical Bulletin #82, Washington, DC, 1984.
235. Clark SL, Koonings PP, Phelan JP: Placenta previa/accreta and prior cesarean section. Obstet. Gynecol. 66:89, 1985.
236. Crenshaw C, Jones DED, Parker RT: Placenta previa: a survey of twenty years experience with improved perinatal survival by expectant therapy and cesarean delivery. Obstet. Gynecol. Survey 28:461, 1973.
237. Cotton DB, Read JA, Paul RH, Quilligan EJ: The conservative aggressive management of placenta previa. Am. J. Obstet. Gynecol. 137:687, 1980.
238. Korwen Z, Zuckerman H, Brzezinski A: Placenta previa accreta with afibrinogenemia: report of three cases. Obstet. Gynecol. 18:138, 1961.
239. Pritchard JA: Fetal death in utero. Obstet. Gynecol. 14:573, 1959.
240. Skelly H, Marivate M, Norman R, Kenoyer G, et al: Consumptive coagulopathy following fetal death in a triplet pregnancy. Am. J. Obstet. Gynecol. 142:595, 1982.
241. Jimenez JM, Pritchard JA: Pathogenesis and treatment of coagulation defects resulting from fetal death. Obstet. Gynecol. 32:449, 1968.
242. Weiner CP: Treatment of Coagulation and Fibrinolytic Disorders. *In* Hematologic Problems in Pregnancy. Edited by DZ Kitay. Oradell, NJ, Medical Economics Books, 1987, p. 321.
243. Talbert LM, Easterling WE, Flowers CE, Graham JB: Acquired coagulation defects of pregnancy: including a case of a patient with hydatiform mole. Obstet. Gynecol. 18: 69, 1961.
244. Cunningham FG, MacDonald PC, Gant NF: Hypertensive disorders in pregnancy. *In* Williams Obstetrics. Edited by FG Cunningham, PC MacDonald, NF Gant. Norwalk, Appleton & Lange, 1989, p. 653.
245. Sibai BM: Preeclampsia-eclampsia. Current problems in obstetrics. Gynecol. Fertil. 13:1, 1990.
246. Sibai BM: Immunologic aspects of preeclampsia. Clin Obstet. Gynecol. 34:27, 1991.
247. Stirrat GM: The immunology of hypertension in pregnancy. *In* Hypertension in pregnancy. Edited by F Sharp, EM Symonds. Ithaca, Perinatology Press, 1987, p. 249.
248. El-Roeiy A, Gleicher N: The immunologic concept of preeclampsia. *In* Handbook of hypertension. Vol. 10. Edited by PC Rubin. Amsterdam, Elsevier Science, 1988, p. 257.
249. Redman CWG: Immunology of Preeclampsia. Semin. Perinatol. 15:257, 1991.
250. Pritchard JA, Cunningham PG, Mason RA: Coagulation changes in eclampsia: Their frequency and pathogenesis. Am. J. Obstet. Gynecol. 124:855, 1976.
251. Killam AP, Dillard SH, Patton RC, Pederson PR: Pregnancy-induced hypertension complicated by acute liver disease and disseminated intravascular coagulation. Am. J. Obstet. Gynecol. 123:823, 1975.
252. Ramsey EM, Harris HWS: Comparison of ureteroplacental vasculature and circulation in the rhesus monkey and man. Contrib. to Embryol. No. 261, 38:59, 1966.
253. Robertson WB, Khong TY, Brosens I, DeWolf F, et al: The placental bed biopsy: review from three European centers. Am. J. Obstet. Gynecol. 155:401, 1986.
254. Zeek PM, Assali NS: Vascular changes in the decidua associated with eclamptogenic toxemia. Am. J. Clin. Pathol. 20: 1099, 1950.
255. Kitzmiller JL, Benirschke K: Immunofluorescent study of

placental bed vessels in preeclampsia. Am. J. Obstet. Gynecol. 115:248, 1973.

256. Gilstrap LC, Gant NF: Pathophysiology of preeclampsia. Semin. Perinatol. 14:147, 1990.

257. Roberts JM, Taylor RN, Musci TJ, Rodgers GM, et al: Preeclampsia: an endothelial cell disorder. Am. J. Obstet. Gynecol. 161:1200, 1989.

258. Roberts JM, Taylor RN, Freidman SA, Goldfien A: New developments in preeclampsia. Fetal Medicine Review 2:125, 1990.

259. Ishihara M: Studies on lipoperoxide of normal pregnant women and of patients with toxemia of pregnancy. Clin. Chim. Acta. 84:1, 1978.

260. Moncada S, Vane R: Pharmacology and endogenous roles of prostacyclin endoperoxides, thromboxane $A_2$, and prostacyclin. Pharmacol. Rev. 30:293, 1979.

261. Hubel CA, Roberts JM, Taylor RN, Musci TJ, et al: Lipid peroxidation in pregnancy: new perspectives on preeclampsia. Am. J. Obstet. Gynecol. 161:1025, 1989.

262. Walsh SW, Wang Y, Maynard EL, Jesse RL: Low-dose aspirin (ASA) inhibits abnormally increased levels of both thromboxan (TX) and lipid peroxides (LPO) in preeclamptic placentas. 39th Annual Meeting of the Society for Gynecologic Investigation, Abstract #128, San Antonio, 1992, p. 172.

263. Johnson RD, Raz A, Walsh SW, Nelson M: Cyclooxygenase regulation and thromboxane production by cultured human trophoblast from term placental villi. 39th Annual Meeting of the Society for Gynecologic Investigation, Abstract #130, San Antonio, 1992, p. 173.

264. Walsh SW: Preeclampsia: An imbalance in placental prostacyclin and thromboxane production. Am. J. Obstet. Gynecol. 152:335, 1985.

265. Holst H, Oian P, Aune B, Jenssen TG, et al: Increased plasma levels of vasoactive intestinal polypeptide in preeclampsia. Br. J. Obstet. Gynecol. 98:803, 1991.

266. Ercal N, O'Dorisio M, Vinik A, O'Dorisio TM, et al: Vasoactive intestinal peptide receptors in human platelet membrane. Characterization of binding and functional activity. Ann. N.Y. Acad. Sci. 527:663, 1988.

267. Haugen G, Stray-Pedersen S, Bjoro K: Vasoactive intestinal peptide and prostanoid production in normal and single umbilical artery cords in normotensive and hypertensive pregnancies. Clin. Exper. Hypertens. B9:69, 1990.

268. Zuspan FP, Nelson GH, Ahlquist RP: Epinephrine infusions in normal and toxemic pregnancy. I. Nonesterified fatty acids and cardiovascular alterations. Am. J. Obstet. Gynecol. 90:88, 1964.

269. Talledo OE, Chesley LC, Zuspan FP: Renin-angiotensin system in normal and toxemic pregnancies III. Differential sensitivity to angiotensin II and norepinephrine in toxemia of pregnancy. Am. J. Obstet. Gynecol. 100:218, 1968.

270. Gant NF, Daley GL, Chand S, Walley PJ, et al: A study of angiotensin II pressor response throughout primigravid pregnancy. J. Clin. Invest. 52:2682, 1973.

271. Gallery EDM, Saunders DH, Boyce ES, Gyory AZ: Relation between plasma volume and uric acid in the development of hypertension in pregnancy. *In* Pregnancy Hypertension. Edited by J Bonnar, I MacGillivary, EM Symonds. Baltimore, University Park Press, 1980.

272. Easterling TR, Benedetti J: Increased cardiac output prior to the development of the disorder, preeclampsia: a hyperdynamic disease model. Am. J. Obstet. Gynecol. 160:1447, 1989.

273. Gallery EDM, Hunyor SN, Ross M, Gyory AZ: Predicting the development of pregnancy-associated hypertension: the place of standardized blood-pressure measurement. Lancet i:1273, 1977.

274. Groenendijk R, Trimbos JB, Wallenburg HC: Hemodynamic measurements in preeclampsia: preliminary observations. Am. J. Obstet. Gynecol. 150:232, 1984.

275. Goodlin RC: Venous reactivity and pregnancy abnormalities. Acta. Obstet. Gynecol. Scand 65:345, 1986.

276. Giles C, Ingles TCM: Thrombocytopenia and macrothrombocytopenia in gestational hypertension. Br. J. Obstet. Gynaecol. 88:115, 1981.

277. Weinstein L: Hematology of Toxemia. *In* Hematologic Problems in Pregnancy. Edited by DZ Kitay. Oradell, NJ, Medical Economics Books, 1987, p. 360.

278. Weinstein L: Syndrome of hemolysis, elevated liver enzymes and low platelet count: a severe consequence of hypertension in pregnancy. Am. J. Obstet. Gynecol. 142: 159, 1982.

279. Goodlin RC: Severe preeclampsia: another great imitator. Am. J. Obstet. Gynecol. 125:747, 1976.

280. Goodlin RC: Beware the great imitator-severe preeclampsia. Contrib. Obstet. Gynecol. 20:215, 1982.

281. Goodlin RC: Hemolysis, elevated liver enzymes and low platelet syndrome. Obstet. Gynecol. 64:449, 1984.

282. Goodlin RC: Preeclampsia as the great impostor. Am. J. Obstet. Gynecol. 164:1577, 1991.

283. Weiner CP, Kwaan HC, Xu C, Paul M, et al: Antithrombin III activity in women with hypertension during pregnancy. Obstet. Gynecol. 65:301, 1985.

284. Saleh AA, Bottoms SF, Welch RA, Ali AM, et al: Preeclampsia, delivery and the hemostatic system. Am. J. Obstet. Gynecol. 157:331, 1987.

285. Redman CWG, Denson KWE, Beilin LJ, Bolton FG: Factor VIII consumption in preeclampsia. Lancet ii:1249, 1977.

286. Weenink GH, Borm JJJ, ten Cate JW, Treffers PE: Antithrombin III levels in normotensive and hypertensive pregnancy. Gynecol. Obstet. Invest. 1983:230.

287. Bonnar J, McNichol GP, Douglas AS: Coagulation and fibrinolytic systems in preeclampsia and eclampsia. Brit. Med. J. 2:12, 1971.

288. Redman CW, Bonnar J, Beilin L: Early platelet consumption in preeclampsia. Br. Med. J. 1:467, 1978.

289. Ahmed Y, Sullivan MHF, Elder MG: Increased platelet turnover in a patient with previous recurrent preeclampsia and failure of aspirin therapy. Br. J. Obstet. Gynecol. 98:218, 1991.

290. Inglis TCM, Stuart J, George AJ, Davies AJ: Haemostatic and rheological changes in normal pregnancy and preeclampsia. Br. J. Haematol. 50:461, 1982.

291. Douglas JT, Shah M, Lowe GDO, Belch JJF, et al: Plasma fibrinopeptide A and beta-thromboglobulin in preeclampsia and pregnancy hypertension. Thromb. Haemost. 7:54, 1982.

292. Louden KA, Broughton-Pipkin F, Heptinstall S, Fox SC, et al: Platelet reactivity and serum thromboxane $B_2$ production in whole blood in gestational hypertension and preeclampsia. Br. J. Obstet. Gynecol. 98:1239, 1991.

293. Sibai BM, Taslimi MM, El-Nazer A, Amon E, et al: Maternal-perinatal outcome associated with the syndrome of hemolysis, elevated liver enzymes and low platelets in severe preeclampsia-eclampsia. Am. J. Obstet. Gynecol. 155:501, 1986.

294. Gibson B, Hunter D, Neame PB, Kelton JG: Thrombocytopenia in preeclampsia and eclampsia. Semin. Thromb. Hemost. 8:234, 1982.

295. Weinstein L: Hematology of Toxemia. *In* Hematologic Problems in Pregnancy. Edited by DZ Kitay. Oradell, NJ, Medical Economics Books, 1987, p. 370.

296. Thiagarajah S, Bourgeois FJ, Harbert GN, Caudle MR: Thrombocytopenia in preeclampsia: associated abnormalities and management principles. Am. J. Obstet. Gynecol. 150:1, 1984.
297. Pritchard JA, Cunningham FG, Pritchard SA: The Parkland Memorial Hospital protocol for treatment of eclampsia: evaluation of 245 cases. Am. J. Obstet. Gynecol. 148:951, 1984.
298. Ryan G, Lange IR, Naugler MA: Clinical experience with phenytoin prophylaxis in severe preeclampsia. Am. J. Obstet. Gynecol. 161:1297, 1989.
299. Winter ME, Tozer TN: Phenytoin. *In* Applied Pharmacokinetics—Principles of Therapeutic Drug Monitoring. 2nd Ed. Edited by WE Evans, JJ Schentag, WJ Jusko. San Francisco, Applied Therapeutics, 1986, p. 493.
300. Benedetti TJ, Kates R, Williams V: Hemodynamic observations in severe preeclampsia complicated by pulmonary edema. Am. J. Obstet. Gynecol. 152:330, 1985.
301. Sibai BM, Mabie BC, Harvey CJ, Gonzales AR: Pulmonary edema in severe preeclampsia: Analysis of 37 consecutive cases. Am. J. Obstet. Gynecol. 156:1174, 1987.
302. Oian P, Maltau JM, Noddeland H, Fadnes HO: Transcapillary fluid balance in preeclampsia. Br. J. Obstet. Gynaecol. 93:235, 1986.
303. Zinaman M, Rubin J, Lindheimer MD: Serial plasma oncotic pressure levels and echoencephalography during and after delivery in severe pre-eclampsia. Lancet i:1245, 1985.
304. Woods JB, Blake PG, Perry KG Jr, Magann EF, et al: Ascites: a portent of cardiopulmonary complications in the preeclamptic patient with the syndrome of hemolysis, elevated liver enzymes, and low platelets. Obstet. Gynecol. 80:87, 1992.
305. Belfort M, Anthony J, Kirshon B: Respiratory function in severe gestational proteinuric hypertension: the effects of rapid volume expansion and subsequent vasodilatation with verapamil. Br. J. Obstet. Gynecol. 98:964, 1991.
306. Mabie WC, Gonzalez AR, Sibai BM, Amon E: A comparative trial of labetalol and hydralazine in the acute management of severe hypertension complicating pregnancy. Obstet. Gynecol. 70:328, 1987.
307. Cotton DB, Jones MM, Longmire S, Dorman KF, et al: Role of intravenous nitroglycerin in the treatment of severe pregnancy-induced hypertension complicated by pulmonary edema. Am. J. Obstet. Gynecol. 154:91, 1986.
308. Hanretty KP, Whittle MJ, Howie CA, Rubin PC: Effect of nifedipine on doppler flow velocity waveforms in severe pre-eclampsia. Br. Med. J. 299:1205, 1989.
309. Lindow SW, Davies N, Davey DA, Smith JA: The effect of sublingual nifedipine on uteroplacental blood flow in hypertensive pregnancy. Br. J. Obstet. Gynecol. 95:1276, 1988.
310. Martins-Costa S, Ramos JG, Barros E, Bruno RM, et al: Randomized, controlled trial of hydralazine versus nifedipine in preeclamptic women with acute hypertension. Clin. and Exper. Hyper. In Pregnancy B11:25, 1992.
311. Fenakel K, Fenakel G, Appelman Z, Lurie S, et al: Nifedipine in the treatment of severe preeclampsia. Obstet. Gynecol. 77:331, 1991.
312. Barton JR, Prevost RR, Wilson DA, Whybrew WD, et al: Nifedipine pharmacokinetics and pharmacodynamics during the immediate postpartum period in patients with preeclampsia. Am. J. Obstet. Gynecol. 165:951, 1991.
313. Boutroy MJ: Fetal effects of maternally administered clonidine and angiotensin-converting enzyme inhibitors. Dev. Pharmacol. Ther. 13:199, 1989.
314. Stempel JE, O'Grady JP, Morton MJ, Johnson KA: Use of sodium nitroprusside in complications of gestational hypertension. Obstet. Gynecol. 60: 533, 1982.
315. Goodlin RC: Fetal and maternal effects of sodium nitroprusside. Am. J. Obstet. Gynecol. 146:350, 1983.
316. Shoemaker CT, Meyers M: Sodium nitroprusside for control of severe hypertensive disease of pregnancy: a case report and discussion of potential toxicity. Am. J. Obstet. Gynecol. 149:171, 1984.
317. Riley A, Symonds EM: The investigation of labetalol in the management of hypertension in pregnancy. Exerpta Medica, Amsterdam, 1982.
318. Pirhonen JP, Erkkola RU, Makinen JI, Ekblad UU: Single dose of labetalol in hypertensive pregnancy: effects on maternal hemodynamics and uterine and fetal flow velocity waveforms. J. Perinat. Med. 19:167, 1991.
319. Garden A, Davey DA, Dommisse J: Intravenous labetalol and intravenous dihydralazine in severe hypertension in pregnancy. Clin. Exp. Hypertens. B 1:371, 1982.
320. Gant NF, Madden JD, Siiteri PK, MacDonald PC: The metabolic clearance rate of dehydroisoandrosterone sulfate: IV. Acute effect of induced hypertension, hypotension, and natruresis in normal and hypertensive pregnancies. Am. J. Obstet. Gynecol. 124:143, 1976.
321. Lipshitz J, Ahokas RA, Reynolds SL: The effect of hydralazine on placental perfusion in the spontaneously hypertensive rat. Am. J. Obstet. Gynecol. 156:356, 1987.
322. Cotton D, Longmire S, Jones M, Dorman K, et al: Cardiovascular alterations in severe pregnancy-induced hypertension: Effects of intravenous nitroglycerin coupled with blood volume expansion. Am. J. Obstet. Gynecol. 154: 1053, 1986.
323. Catanzarite VA: HELLP syndrome and its complications. Contemp. Obstet. Gynecol. 36:13, 1991.
324. Martin JN Jr, Files JC, Blake PG, Norman PH, et al: Plasma exchange for preeclampsia. 1. Postpartum use for persistently severe preeclampsia-eclampsia with HELLP syndrome. Am. J. Obstet. Gynecol. 162:126, 1990.
325. Watson WJ, Katz VL, Bowes WA Jr: Plasmapheresis during pregnancy. Obstet. Gynecol. 476:451, 1990.
326. Pourrat O, Ducroz B, Magnin G: Intravenous immunoglobulins in postpartum, persistently severe HELLP syndrome: a safe alternative to plasma exchange? Am. J. Obstet. Gynecol. 166:766, 1992.
327. Ramos-Santos E, Devoe LD, Wakefield ML, Sherline DM, et al: The effects of epidural anesthesia on the doppler velocimetry of umbilical and uterine arteries in normal and hypertensive patients during active term labor. Obstet. Gynecol. 77:20, 1991.
328. Kelton JG, Hunter DJ, Neame PB: A platelet function defect in preeclampsia. Obstet. Gynecol. 65:107, 1985.
329. Ramanathan J, Sibai BM, Vu T, Chauhan D: Correlation between bleeding times and platelet counts in women with preeclampsia undergoing cesarean section. Anesthesiol 71: 188, 1989.
330. Long PA, Abell DA, Beischer NA: Fetal growth retardation and pre-eclampsia. Br. J. Obstet. Gynaecol. 87:13, 1980.
331. Kleckner HB, Giles HR, Corrigan JJ: The association of maternal and neonatal thrombocytopenia in high-risk pregnancies. Am. J. Obstet. Gynecol. 128:235, 1977.
332. Brazy JE, Gumm JK, Little VA: Neonatal manifestations of severe maternal hypertension occurring before the thirty-sixth week of pregnancy. J. Pediatr. 100:265, 1982.
333. Easterling TR, Benedetti TJ, Carlson KC, Brateng DA, et al: The effect of maternal hemodynamics on fetal growth in hypertensive pregnancies. Transactions of the 11th Annual Meeting of the Society of Perinatal Obstetricians. Am. J. Obstet. Gynecol. 165:902, 1991.

334. Weinstein L: Hematology of Toxemia. *In* Hematologic Problems in Pregnancy. Edited by DZ Kitay. Oradell, NJ, Medical Economics Books, 1987, p. 371.
335. Yoon JJ, Kohl S, Harper RG: The relationship between maternal hypertensive disease of pregnancy and the incidence of idiopathic respiratory distress syndrome. Pediatr. 65:735, 1980.
336. Eden RD, Parker RT, Gall SA: Rupture of the pregnant uterus: a 53 year review. Obstet. Gynecol. 68:671, 1986.
337. Finley B, Gibbs C: Emergent cesarean delivery in patients undergoing a trial of labor with a transverse lower-segment scar. Am. J. Obstet. Gynecol. 155:936, 1986.
338. Phelan JP: Uterine Rupture. Clin. Obstet. Gynecol. 33:433, 1990.
339. Fuchs K, Peretz BA, Marcovici R, Paldi E, et al: The "grand multipara"—is it a problem? A review of 5785 cases. Int. J. Gynaecol. Obstet 23:321, 1985.
340. Clark SL, Montz FJ, Phelan JP: Hemodynamic alterations associated with amniotic fluid embolism: a reappraisal. Am. J. Obstet. Gynecol. 151:617, 1985.
341. Graeff H, Kuhn W: Coagulation Disorders in Obstetrics-Pathobiochemistry, Pathophysiology, Diagnosis, Treatment. Philadelphia, W.B. Saunders Co., 1980.
342. Phillips LL, Davidson EC: Procoagulant properties of amniotic fluid. Am. J. Obstet. Gynecol. 113:911, 1972. 343. Weiner CP, Brandt J: A modified activated partial thromboplastin time with the use of amniotic fluid. Am. J. Obstet. Gynecol. 144:234, 1982.
344. Albrechtsen OK, Trolle D: A fibrinolytic system in human amniotic fluid. Acta. Haematol. 14:376, 1955.
345. Beller FK, Douglas GW, Debrovner CH, Robinson R: The fibrinolytic system in amniotic fluid embolism. Am. J. Obstet. Gynecol. 87:48, 1963.
346. Maki M, Tachita K, Kawasaki Y, Nagasawa K: Heparin treatment of amniotic fluid embolism. Tohoku. J. Exp. Med. 97155, 1969.
347. Resnik R, Swartz WH, Plumer MH, Benirschke K, et al: Amniotic fluid embolism with survival. Obstet. Gynecol. 47:295, 1976.
348. Weiner CP: Treatment of Coagulation and Fibrinolytic Disorders. *In* Hematologic Problems in Pregnancy. Edited by DZ Kitay. Oradell, NJ, Medical Economics Books, 1987, p. 325.
349. Gilbert L, Porter W, Brown VA: Postpartum haemorrhage: a continuing problem. Br. J. Obstet. Gynaecol. 94:67, 1987.
350. Prendiville W, Elbourne D, Chalmers I: The effects of routine oxytocic administration in the management of the third stage of labour: an overview of the evidence from controlled trials. Br. J. Obstet. Gynaecol. 95:3, 1988.
351. Hall MH, Halliwell R, Carr-Hill R: Concomitant and repeated happenings of complications of the third stage of labour. Br. J. Obstet. Gynaecol. 92:732, 1985.
352. Dewhurst CJ, Dutton WAW: Recurrent abnormalities of the third stage of labour. Lancet ii:764, 1957.
353. Gilstrap LC, Hauth JC, Hankins GDV, Patterson AR: Effect of type of anesthesia on blood loss at cesarean section. Obstet. Gynecol. 69:328, 1987.
354. Prendiville WJ, Harding JE, Elbourne DR, Stirrat GM: The Bristol Third Stage Trial: active versus physiological management of third stage of labour. Br. Med. J. 297:1295, 1988.
355. Poeschmann RP, Doesburg WH, Eskes TKAB: A randomized comparison of oxytocin, sulprostone and placebo in the management of the third stage of labor. Br. J. Obstet. Gynaecol. 98:528, 1991.
356. Rooney I, Hughes P, Calder AA: Is continued administration of syntometrine still justified in the management of the third stage of labour? Health Bulletin 43:99, 1985.
357. Hendricks CH, Brenner WE: Cardiovascular effects of oxytocic drugs used postpartum. Am. J. Obstet. Gynecol. 108: 751, 1970.
358. Thiery M, Parewijck W: Local administration of (15S)-15 methyl $PGF_2$ alpha for management of hypotonic postpartum hemorrhage. Zeitschrift Fur Geburtshilfe and Perinatologie 189:179, 1985.
359. Hayashi RH, Castillo MS, Noah ML: Management of severe postpartum hemorrhage with a prostaglandin F2 analogue. Obstet. Gynecol. 63:806, 1984.
360. Buttino L Jr, Garite TJ: The use of 15 methyl $F_2$ alpha prostaglandin (Prostin 15M) for the control of postpartum hemorrhage. Am J. Perinatol. 3:241, 1986.
361. Hester JD: Postpartum hemorrhage and re-evaluation of uterine packing. Obstet. Gynecol. 45:501, 1975.
362. Escamilla JO, Chez RA: When a patient requires postpartum uterine packing. Contemp. Obstet. Gynecol. 37:42, 1992.
363. Raziel A, Golan A, Ariely S, Herman A, et al: Repeated ultrasonography and intramuscular methotrexate in the conservative management of residual adherent placenta. J. Clin. Ultrasound 20:288, 1992.
364. Watson P, Besch N, Bowes WA Jr: Management of acute and subacute puerperal inversion of the uterus. Obstet. Gynecol. 55:12, 1980.
365. Grossman RA: Magnesium sulfate for uterine inversion. J. Reprod. Med. 26:261, 1981.
366. Catanzarite VA, Moffitt KD, Baker ML, Awadalla SG, et al: New approaches to the management of acute uterine inversion. Obstet. Gynecol. 68:78S, 1986.
367. Huntington JL: Acute inversion of the uterus. Boston Med. Surg. J. 15:376, 1921.
368. Haultain FWN: The treatment of chronic uterine inversion by abdominal hysterotomy with a successful case. Br. Med. J. 2:974, 1901.
369. Yamashita Y, Takahasi M, Ito M, Okamura H: Transcatheter arterial embolization in the management of postpartum hemorrhage due to genital tract injury. Obstet. Gynecol. 77:160, 1991.
370. Rosenthal DM, Colapinto R: Angiographic arterial embolization in the management of postoperative vaginal hemorrhage. Am. J. Obstet. Gynecol. 151:227, 1985.
371. Gilbert WM, Moore TR, Resnick R, Doemeny J, et al: Angiographic embolization in the management of hemorrhagic complications of pregnancy. Am. J. Obstet. Gynecol. 166: 493, 1992.
372. Crosby WM: Trauma during pregnancy: maternal and fetal injury. Obstet. Gynecol. Survey 29:683, 1974.
373. Pepperell RJ, Rubenstein E, Macisaac IA: Motor-car accidents during pregnancy. Med. J. Aust. 1:203, 1977.
374. Crosby WM, Costiloe JP: Safety of lap-belt restraint for pregnant victims of automobile collisions. N. Eng. J. Med. 284:632, 1971.
375. Crosby WM, King AI, Stout LC: Fetal survival following impact: improvement with shoulder harness restraint. Am. J. Obstet. Gynecol. 112:1101, 1972.
376. Kumura E, Sato M, Fukuda A, Takemoto Y, et al: Coagulation disorders following acute head injury. Acta. Neurochir. 85:23 1987.
377. Rose PG, Strohm PL, Zuspan FP: Fetomaternal hemorrhage following trauma. Am. J. Obstet. Gynecol. 153:844, 1985.
378. Pearlman MD, Tintinalli JE, Lorenz RP: A prospective controlled study of outcome after trauma during pregnancy. Am. J. Obstet. Gynecol. 162:1502, 1990.
379. Goodwin TM, Breen MT: Pregnancy outcome and fetomat-

ernal hemorr [illegible] atastrophic trauma. Am. J. Obstet. Gyneco [illegible]

380. Mostello DJ [illegible] ddiqi TA: Surveillance after noncatastro [illegible] ne pregnant patient: How much is en [illegible] 7. Society of Perinatal Obstetricians [illegible], January 1990.

381. Elliott M: [illegible] nd pregnancy. Aust. N. Z. J. Obstet. [illegible].

382. Lavin JP, [illegible] rauma during pregnancy. Clin. Peri [illegible]

383. America [illegible] ans and Gynecologists: Trauma [illegible] OG Technical Bulletin, #161, W [illegible] er, 1991.

384. National [illegible] rotection and Measurements. [illegible] re of pregnant women. NCRP R [illegible] DC: NCRPM, 1977.

385. Rothenb [illegible] W, Zabel J, Fischer RP: Diagno [illegible] unt trauma in pregnant women [illegible] 29:479, 1977.

386. Esposit [illegible] corpio R: Evaluation of blunt [illegible] g during pregnancy. J. Traum [illegible]

387. Seyfer [illegible], Urbaniak JR: Coagulation c [illegible] nd trauma. Ann. Surg. 193:21 [illegible]

388. Buchsb [illegible] of the abdomen. *In*: Traum [illegible] Buchscbaum. Philadelphia, [illegible] 9, p. 82.

389. Frange [illegible] n AM: Abdominal gunshot w [illegible] Obstet. Gynecol. 160: 1124, [illegible]

390. Buchs [illegible] tmortem cesarean section. [illegible] ed by HJ Buchsbaum. Philad [illegible] ny, 1979, p. 236.

391. Sobre [illegible] n A, Malaga JM: Human fetal a [illegible] nd acid-base status during de [illegible] Obstet. Gynecol. 111: 1111, [illegible]

392. Wulf [illegible] nical aspects of placental gas [illegible] as Exchange and Blood Flow i [illegible] ongo, H Bartels. DHEW public [illegible] C, 1972.

393. Motoy [illegible] F, Cook CD: The effect of char [illegible] $O_2$ and the $pO_2$ of fetal lambs. [illegible] 67.

394. Patriar [illegible] al thrombocytopenia in pregna [illegible] 41:661, 1986.

395. Moise [illegible] ocytopenic purpura in pregna [illegible] 34:51, 1991.

396. Hart D, [illegible] es RF, et al: An epidemic of mate [illegible] ssociated with elevated antiplate [illegible] unt and antiplatelet antibody in [illegible] ncies: relationship to neonatal plat [illegible]. Gynecol. 154:878, 1986.

397. Freedman [illegible] B, Abbott D: Unexplained peripartu [illegible] nia. Am. J. Hematol. 21:397, 1986.

398. Burrows RF, [illegible] entally detected thrombocytopenia in h [illegible] and their infants. N. Engl. J. Med. 319:142, [illegible]

399. Pegels JG, Bruy [illegible] ngelfriet CP, von dem Borne AE: Pseudothrombocytopenia: an immunologic study on platelet antibodies dependent on ethylene diamine tetra-acetate. Blood 59:157, 1982.

400. Burrows RF, Kelton JG: Platelets and pregnancy. Contemp. Rev. Obstet. Gynaecol. 1:26, 1988.

401. Kelton JG, Cruickshank M: Hematologic disorders of pregnancy. *In* Medical Complications During Pregnancy. Edited by GN Burrow, TF Ferris. Philadelphia, W.B. Saunders Company, 1988, p. 81.

402. Harker LA, Slichter SJ: The bleeding time as a screening test for evaluation of platelet function. N. Engl. J. Med. 287: 155, 1972.

403. Noriega-Guerra L, Aviles-Miranda A, Alvarez de la Cadena O, Espinosa LZ, et al: Pregnancy in patients with autoimmune thrombocytopenic purpura. Am. J. Obstet. Gynecol. 133:439, 1979.

404. Martin JN, Morrison JC, Files JC: Autoimmune thrombocytopenic purpura: current concepts and recommended practices. Am. J. Obstet. Gynecol. 150:86, 1984.

405. O'Reilly RA, Taber B: Immunologic thrombocytopenic purpura and pregnancy. Obstet. Gynecol. 51:590, 1978.

406. Laros RK, Kagan R: Route of delivery for patients with immune thrombocytopenic purpura. Am. J. Obstet. Gynecol. 148:901, 1984.

407. Browning J, James D: Immune thrombocytopenia in pregnancy. Fetal Med. Rev. 2:143, 1990.

408. Cook RL, Miller RC, Katz VL, Cefalo RC: Immune thrombocytopenic purpura in pregnancy: a reappraisal of management. Obstet. Gynecol. 78:578, 1991.

409. Kelton JG, Inwood MJ, Barr RM, Effer SB, et al: The prenatal prediction of thrombocytopenia in infants of mothers with clinically diagnosed immune thrombocytopenia. Am. J. Obstet. Gynecol. 144:449, 1982.

410. Scott JR, Rote NS, Cruikshank DP: Antiplatelet antibodies and platelet counts in pregnancies complicated by autoimmune thrombocytopenic purpura. Am. J. Obstet. Gynecol. 145:932, 1983.

411. Kelton JG: Management of the pregnant patient with idiopathic thrombocytopenic purpura. Ann. Intern. Med. 99: 796, 1983.

412. Cines DB, Dusak B, Tomaski A, Mennuti M, et al: Immune thrombocytopenic purpura and pregnancy. N. Engl. J. Med. 306:826, 1982.

413. Jones RW, Asher MI, Rutherford CJ, Monro HM: Autoimmune (idiopathic) thrombocytopenic purpura in pregnancy and the newborn. Br. J. Obstet. Gynecol. 84:679, 1977.

414. Samuels P, Tomaski A, Bussel J, Druzin M, et al: The natural history of immune thrombocytopenic purpura in pregnancy. *In*: Proceedings of the ninth annual meeting of the Society of Perinatal Obstetricians. February 1989.

415. Ayromlooi J: A new approach to the management of immunologic thrombocytopenic purpura in pregnancy. Am. J. Obstet. Gynecol. 130:235, 1978.

416. Scott JR, Cruikshank DP, Kochenour NK, Pitkin RM, et al: Fetal platelet counts in the obstetric management of immunologic thrombocytopenic purpura. Am. J. Obstet. Gynecol. 136:495, 1980.

417. Christiaens GC, Helmerhorst FM: Validity of intrapartum diagnosis of fetal thrombocytopenia. Am. J. Obstet. Gynecol. 157:864, 1987.

418. Moise KJ, Patton DE, Cano LE: Misdiagnosis of a normal fetal platelet count after coagulation of intrapartum scalp samples in autoimmune thrombocytopenic purpura. Am J. Perinatol. 8:295, 1991.

419. Daffos F, Forestier F, Kaplan C, Cox W: Prenatal diagnosis and management of bleeding disorders with fetal blood sampling. Am. J. Obstet. Gynecol. 158:939, 1988.

420. Scioscia AL, Grannum PA, Copel JA Hobbins JC: The use of percutaneous umbilical blood sampling in immune thrombocytopenic purpura. Am. J. Obstet. Gynecol. 159: 1066, 1988.

421. Knuppel RA, McNancy H: Idiopathic thrombocytopenic

purpura and pregnancy. *In* Controversy in Obstetrics and Gynecology. Edited by D Reid. Philadelphia, W.B. Saunders, 1983, p. 3.

422. Gernsheimer T, Stratton J, Ballem PJ, Slichter SJ: Mechanisms of response to treatment in autoimmune thrombocytopenic purpura. N. Engl. J. Med. 320:974, 1989.
423. Karpatkin M, Porges RF, Karpatkin S: Platelet counts in infants of women with autoimmune thrombocytopenia: effect of steroid administration to the mother. N. Engl. J. Med. 305:936, 1981.
424. Strother SV, Wagner AM: Prednisone in pregnant women with idiopathic thrombocytopenic purpura. N. Eng. J. Med. 319:178, 1988.
425. Levitz M, Jansen V, Dancis J: The transfer and metabolism of corticosteroids in the perfused human placenta. Am. J. Obstet. Gynecol. 132:363, 1978.
426. Yin CS, Scott JR: Unsuccessful treatment of fetal immunologic thrombocytopenia with dexamethasone. Am. J. Obstet. Gynecol. 152:316, 1985.
427. Fabris P: Successful treatment of a steroid-resistant form of idiopathic thrombocytopenic purpura in pregnancy with high doses of intravenous immunoglobulins. Acta. Haematol. 77:107, 1987.
428. Lavery JP, Koontz WL, Liu YK, Howell R: Immunologic thrombocytopenia in pregnancy: use of antenatal immunoglobulin therapy: case report and review. Obstet. Gynecol. 66S:424, 1985.
429. NIH Concensus Conference: Intravenous Immunoglobulin: Prevention and treatment of disease. JAMA 264:3189, 1990.
430. Newland AC, Boots MA, Patterson KG: Intravenous IgG for autoimmune thrombocytopenia in pregnancy. N. Engl. J. Med. 310:261, 1984.
431. Mizunuma H, Takahashi Y, Taguch H, Arai A, et al: A new approach to idiopathic purpura during pregnancy by high-dose immunoglobulin G infusion. Am. J. Obstet. Gynecol. 148:218, 1984.
432. Pappas C: Placental transfer of immunoglobulins in immune thrombocytopenic purpura. Lancet 1:389, 1986.
433. Boughton BJ, Chakraverty R, Baglin TP, Simpson A, et al: The treatment of chronic idiopathic thrombocytopenia with anti-D (Rho) immunoglobulin: its effectiveness, safety and mechanism of action. Clin. Lab. Haematol. 10:275, 1988.
434. Moise KJ, Cano LE, Sala DJ: Resolution of severe thrombocytopenia in a pregnant patient with rhesus-negative blood with autoimmune thrombocytopenic purpura after intravenous rhesus immune globulin. Am. J. Obstet. Gynecol. 162:1237, 1990.
435. Woerner SJ, Abildgaard CF, Grench BN: Intracranial hemorrhage in children with idiopathic thrombocytopenic purpura. Pediatrics 67:453, 1981.
436. Leads from the MMWR. Recommendations of the immunization practices advisory committee pneumococcal polysaccharide vaccine. JAMA 261:1265, 1989.
437. Mufson MA, Krause HE, Schiffman G, Hughey DF: Pneumococcal antibody levels one decade after immunization of healthy adults. Am. J. Med. Sci. 293:279, 1987.
438. Laros RK, Sweet RL: Management of idiopathic thrombocytopenic purpura during pregnancy. Am. J. Obstet. Gynecol. 122:182, 1975.
439. Van Leeuwen EF, Von Dem Borne AE, Oudesluijs-Murphy AM, Ras-Zeijlmams GJ: Neonatal alloimmune thrombocytopenia complicated by maternal autoimmune thrombocytopenia. Br. Med. J. 281:27, 1980.
440. Herman G, Jumbelic M, Ancona R, Kickler TS: In utero cerebral hemorrhage in alloimmune thrombocytopenia. Am. J. Pediatr. Hematol. Oncol. 8:312, 1986.
441. Burrows RF, Caco CC, Kelton JG: Neonatal alloimmune thrombocytopenia: spontaneous in utero intracranial hemorrhage. Am. J. Hematol. 28:98, 1988.
442. Kaplan C, Daffos F, Forestier F, Cox WL, et al: Management of alloimmune thrombocytopenia: antenatal diagnosis and in utero transfusion of maternal platelets. Blood 72:340, 1988.
443. Daffos F, Forestier F, Muller JY, Habibi B, et al: Prenatal treatment of alloimmune thrombocytopenia. Lancet 2:632, 1984.
444. Sia CG, Amigo NC, Harper RG, Farahain G, et al: Failure of cesarean section to prevent intracranial hemorrhage in siblings with isoimmune neonatal thrombocytopenia. Am. J. Obstet. Gynecol. 153:79, 1985.
445. Bussel JB, Berkowitz RL, McFarland JG, Lynch L, et al: Antenatal treatment of neonatal alloimmune thrombocytopenia. N. Engl. J. Med. 319:1374, 1988.
446. Lynch L, Bussel JB, McFarland JG, Chitkara U, et al: Antenatal treatment of alloimmune thrombocytopenia. Obstet. Gynecol. 80:67, 1992.
447. Amorosi EL, Ultman JE: Thrombotic thrombocytopenic purpura: report of 16 cases and review of the literature. Medicine 45:139, 1966.
448. Ridolfi RL, Bell WR: Thrombotic thrombocytopenic purpura: report of 25 cases and review of the literature. Medicine 60:413, 1981.
449. Schmidt JL: Thrombotic thrombocytopenic purpura: successful treatment unlocks etiologic secrets. Mayo Clin. Proc. 64:956, 1989.
450. Caggiano V, Fernando LP, Schneider JM, Haesslein HC, et al: Thrombotic Thrombocytopenic Purpura: report of fourteen cases—Occurrence during pregnancy and response to plasma exchange. J. Clin. Apheresis 1:71, 1983.
451. Moake JL, Byrnes JJ, Troll JH, Rudy CK, et al: Effects of fresh-frozen plasma and its cryosupernatant fraction on von Willebrand factor multimeric forms in chronic relapsing thrombotic thrombocytopenic purpura. Blood 65: 1232, 1985.
452. Katz JA, Moake JL, McPherson PD, Weinstein MJ, et al: Relationship between human development and disappearance of unusually large von Willebrand fact multimers from plasma. Blood 73:1851, 1989.
453. Moore JC, Murphy WG, Kelton JG: Calpain proteolysis of von Willebrand factor enhances its binding to platelet membrane glycoprotein IIb/IIIa: an explanation for platelet aggregation in thrombotic thrombocytopenic purpura. Br. J. Haematol. 74:457, 1990.
454. Thorp JM, White GC, Moake JL, Bowles WA: von Willebrand factor multimeric levels and patterns in patients with severe preeclampsia. Obstet. Gynecol. 75:163, 1990.
455. Rock GA, Shumak KH, Buskard NA, Blanchette VS, et al: Comparison of plasma exchange with plasma infusion in the treatment of thrombotic thrombocytopenic purpura. N. Engl. J. Med. 325:393, 1991.
456. Shepard KV, Fishleder A, Lucas FV, Goormastic M, et al: Thrombotic thrombocytopenic purpura treated with plasma exchange or exchange transfusions. West. J. Med. 154:410, 1991.
457. Moake JL: TTP—Desperation, empiricism, progress. N. Engl. J. Med. 325:426, 1991.
458. Katz VL, Watson WJ, Thorp JM, Hansen W, et al: Treatment of persistent postpartum HELLP syndrome with plasmapheresis. Am J. Perinatol. 9:120, 1992.
459. Ansell J, Beaser RS, Pechet L: Thrombotic thrombocytope-

nic purpura fails to respond to fresh frozen plasma infusion. Ann. Intern. Med. 89:647, 1978.

460. Aster RH: Plasma therapy for thrombotic thrombocytopenic purpura: sometimes it works, but why? N. Engl. J. Med. 312:985, 1985.

461. Moake JL: Thrombotic thrombocytopenic purpura and the hemolytic-uremic syndrome. *In*: Hematology: Basic Principles and Practice. Edited by R Hoffman, E Benz, S Shattil, B Furie. New York, Churchill Livingstone, 1991, p. 1495.

462. Bell WR, Braine HG, Ness PM, Kickler TS: Improved survival in thrombotic thrombocytopenic purpura—hemolytic uremic syndrome. N. Engl. J. Med. 325:398, 1991.

463. Viero P, Cortelazzo S, Buelli M, Comotti B, et al: Thrombotic thrombocytopenic purpura and high-dose immunoglobulin treatment. Ann. Intern. Med. 104:282, 1986.

464. Finn NG, Wang JC, Hong KJ: High-dose intravenous gamma-immunoglobulin infusion in the treatment of thrombotic thrombocytopenic purpura. Arch. Intern. Med. 147: 2165, 1987.

465. Raniele DP, Opsahl JA, Jensen NJ, Crosson JC, et al: Treatment of thrombotic thrombocytopenic purpura (TTP) with intravenous immunoglobulin G (IgG): 88% response rate. *In*: Internal Society for Blood Transfusion and American Association of Blood Banks book of abstracts. Vol. 1 American Association of Blood Banks, Arlington, VA, 1990, p. 90.

466. Gutterman L: Treatment of thrombotic thrombocytopenic purpura (TTP) with exchange plasmapheresis (EP), vincristine (VCR), and methylprednisolone (MP): a standardized initial treatment in 11 patients. Blood 76: Suppl 1: 509a, 1990.

467. Beattie JJ, Murphy AV, Willoughby MLN, Belch JJF: Prostacyclin infusion in haemolytic-uraemic syndrome in children. Br. Med. J. 283:470, 1981.

468. Harkness DR, Byrnes JJ, Lian ECY, Williams WD, et al: Hazard of platelet transfusion in thrombotic thrombocytopenic purpura. JAMA 246:1931, 1981.

469. Gordon LI, Kwaan HC, Rossi EC: Deleterious effects of platelet transfusions and recovery thrombocytosis in patients with thrombotic microangiopathy. Semin. Hematol. 24:194, 1987.

470. Gimovsky ML, Montoro M: Systemic lupus erythematosus and other connective tissue diseases in pregnancy. Clin. Obstet. Gynecol. 34:35, 1991.

471. Gimovsky ML, Montoro M, Paul RH: Pregnancy outcome in women with SLE. Obstet. Gynecol. 63:686, 1984.

472. Cohen SS, Reynolds WE, Franklin EC, Kulka JP, et al: Preliminary criteria for the classification of lupus erythematosus. Bull. Rheum. Dis. 21:643, 1971.

473. Tan EM, Cohen AS, Fries JF, Masi AT, et al: The 1982 revised criteria for the classification of systemic lupus erythematosus. Arthritis Rheum. 25:1271, 1982.

474. Montoro M: Systemic lupus erythematosus during pregnancy. *In* Critical Care Obstetrics. Edited by S Clark, J Phelan. Oradell, NJ, Medical Economics Books, 1987, p. 332.

475. Lockshin MD: Pregnancy associated with systemic lupus erythematosus. Semin. Perinatol. 14:130, 1990.

476. Out JH, Derksen RHWM, Christiaens GCML: Systemic lupus erythematosus and pregnancy. Obstet. Gynecol. Surv. 44:585, 1989.

477. Fort JG, Cowchock FS, Abruzzo JL, Smith JB: Anticardiolipin antibodies in patients with rheumatic diseases. Arthritis Rheum. 30:752, 1987.

478. Scott JR, Rote NS, Branch DW: Immunologic aspects of recurrent abortion and fetal death. Obstet. Gynecol. 70: 645, 1987.

479. Varner MW: Autoimmune disorders and pregnancy. Semin. Perinatol. 15:238, 1991.

480. Mintz G, Niz J, Gutierrez G, Garcia-Alonso A, et al: Prospective study of pregnancy in systemic lupus erythematosus. Results of a multidisciplinary approach. J. Rheumatol. 13: 732, 1986.

481. Feinstein DI, Rapaport SI: Anticoagulants in systemic lupus erythematosus. *In* Lupus Erythematosus (suppl 2). Edited by EL Dubois. Los Angeles, University of Southern California Press 1974, p. 438.

482. Stafford-Brady FJ, Gladman DD, Urowitz M: Successful pregnancy in systemic lupus erythematosus with an untreated lupus anticoagulant. Arch. Intern. Med. 148:1647, 1988.

483. Carreras LO, Perez GN, Vega HR, Casavilla F: Lupus anticoagulant and recurrent fetal loss: successful treatment with gammaglobulin. Lancet 2:393, 1988.

484. Scott JR, Branch DW, Kochenour NK, Ward K: Intravenous immunoglobulin treatment of pregnant patients with recurrent pregnancy loss caused by antiphospholipid antibodies and Rh immunization. Am. J. Obstet. Gynecol. 159: 1055, 1988.

485. Burkett G: Lupus nephropathy and pregnancy. Clin. Obstet. Gynecol. 28:310, 1985.

486. Fine LG, Barnett EF, Danovitch GM, Nissenson AR, et al: Systemic lupus erythematosus in pregnancy. Ann. Intern. Med. 94:667, 1981.

487. Anderson H: Maternal hematologic disorders. *In* Maternal-Fetal Medicine: Principles and Practice. Edited by RK Creasy, R Resnik. Philadelphia, W.B. Saunders Company, 1989, p. 907.

488. Anderson H: Maternal hematologic disorders: the effect of maternal ITP on the fetus. *In* Maternal-Fetal Medicine: Principles and Practice. Edited by RK Creasy, R Resnik. Philadelphia, W.B. Saunders Company, 1989, p. 911.

489. Bone RC: Sepsis, the sepsis syndrome, multi-organ failure: a plea for comparable definitions. Ann. Intern. Med. 114: 332, 1991.

490. Lee W, Clark SL, Cotton DB, Gonick B, et al: Septic shock during pregnancy. Am. J. Obstet. Gynecol. 159:410, 1988.

491. Cunningham FG, Lucas MJ, Hankins GD: Pulmonary injury complicating antepartum pyelonephritis. Am. J. Obstet. Gynecol. 156:797, 1987.

492. Shubin H, Weil MN: Bacterial shock. JAMA 235:421, 1976.

493. Duff P: Pathophysiology and management of septic shock. J. Reprod. Med. 24:109, 1980.

494. Clark SL: Shock in the pregnant patient. Semin. Perinatol. 14:52, 1990.

495. Bone RC: A critical evaluation of new agents for the treatment of sepsis. JAMA 266:1686, 1991.

496. Young LS: Gram negative sepsis. *In* Principles and Practice of Infectious Diseases. Edited by GL Mandell, RG Douglas, JE Bennett. New York, John Wiley & Sons, 1985, p. 452.

497. Parker MM, Parillo JE: Septic shock, hemodynamics and pathogenesis. JAMA 250:3324, 1983.

498. Ognibene FB, Parker MM, Natanson C, Keenan A, et al: Depressed left ventricular performance in response to volume infusion in patients with sepsis. Clin. Res. 32:679A, 1984.

499. Parillo JE, Buuch C, Shelhamer JH, Parker MM, et al: A circulatory myocardial depressant substance in humans with septic shock. J. Clin. Invest. 76:1539, 1985.

500. Wilson RF: The diagnosis and management of severe sepsis and septic shock. Heart Lung 5:422, 1976.

501. Moss GS, Gould SA: Plasma expanders: an update. Am. J. Surg. 155:425, 1988.

502. Gammage G: Crystalloid versus colloid: is colloid worth the cost? Int. Anesth. Clin. 25:37, 1987.
503. Shire KI, Kuhn M, Young LS, Tillisch JH: Aspects of the management of shock. Ann. Intern. Med. 93:723, 1980.
504. Sprung CL, Caralis PV, Marcial EH, Pierce M, et al: The effects of high dose corticosteroids in patients with septic shock. N. Engl. J. Med. 311:1137, 1984.
505. Bore RC, Fisher CJ, Clemmer TP, Slotman GJ, et al: A controlled clinical trial of high-dose methylprednisolone in the treatment of severe sepsis and septic shock. N. Engl. J. Med. 317:653, 1987.
506. The Veterans Administration Systemic Sepsis Cooperative Study Group. Effect of high-dose glucocorticoid therapy on mortality in patients with clinical signs of systemic sepsis. N. Engl. J. Med. 317:659, 1987.
507. Dopamine for treatment of shock. Med. Lett. Drugs Ther. 17(4):13, 1975.
508. Innes IR, Nickerson M: Norepinephrine, epinephrine and the sympathomimetic amines. *In* The Pharmacological Basis of Therapeutics. 5th Ed. Edited by LS Goodman, A Gilman. New York, MacMillan, 1975, p. 494.
509. Thompson WL: Dopamine and other vasoactive agents in shock. Scot. Med. J. 24:89, 1979.
510. Callender K, Levinson G, Shnider SM, Feduska NJ, et al: Dopamine administration in the normotensive pregnant ewe. Obstet. Gynecol. 51:586, 1978.
511. Rolbin SH, Levinson G, Shinder SM, Biehl DR, et al: Dopamine treatment of spinal hypotension decreases uterine blood flow in pregnant ewes. Anesthesiology 51:36, 1979.
512. Asherman JG: Traumatic intrauterine adhesions. J. Obstet. Gynecol. Br Empire 57:892, 1950.
513. Wolff SM: Monoclonal antibodies and the treatment of gram-negative bacteremia and shock. N. Eng. J. Med. 324: 487, 1991.
514. Pepe PE, Potkin RJ, Reus DH, Hudson LD, et al: Clinical predictors of the adult respiratory distress syndrome. Am. J. Surg. 144:124, 1982.
515. Elkington KW, Greb LC: Adult respiratory distress syndrome as a complication of acute pyelonephritis during pregnancy: a case report and discussion. Obstet. Gynecol. 67:18, 1986.
516. Montgomery AB, Stager MA, Carrico CJ, Hudson LD: Causes of mortality in patients with the adult respiratory distress syndrome. Am. Rev. Respir. Dis. 132:485, 1985.
517. Kaplan RL, Sahn SA, Petty TL: Incidence and outcome of the respiratory distress syndrome in gram-negative sepsis. Arch. Intern. Med. 139:867, 1979.
518. Young LS: Gram-negative sepsis. *In* Edited by GL Mandell, RG Douglas, JE Bennett. Principles and Practice of Infectious Diseases. 3rd Ed. New York, Churchill Livingstone, 1990, p. 611.
519. Moore KL, Andreoli SP, Esmon NL, Esmon CT, et al: Endotoxin enhances tissue factor and suppresses thrombomodulin expression of human vascular endothelium in vitro. J. Clin. Invest. 79:124, 1987.
520. Catanzarite VA, Ferguson JE: Acute leukemia and pregnancy: a review of management and outcome, 1972–1982. Obstet. Gynecol. 39:663, 1984.
521. U.S. Dept of Health and Human Services: Prevention of venous thrombosis and pulmonary embolism. National Institutes of Health Concensus Development Conference Statement. Vol. 6 #2, Bethesda, 1986.
522. Virchow R: Die cellularpathologie in ihrer begrundung auf physiologiche und pathologiche gewebslehre. Berlin, A Hirschwald, 1858.
523. Bonnar J: Venous thromboembolism. *In*: Recent Advances in Obstetrics Gynecol. London, Churchill Livingstone, 1979.
524. Crowther CA, Bouwmeester AM, Ashurst HM: Does admission to hospital for bed rest prevent disease progression or improve fetal outcome in pregnancy complicated by non-proteinuric hypertension? Br. J. Obstet. Gynaecol. 99: 13, 1992.
525. Bedrest in obstetrics. (editorial) Lancet 1:1137, 1981.
526. McCausland AM, Hyman C, Winsor T, Trotter AD: Venous distensibility during pregnancy. Am. J. Obstet. Gynecol. 81:472, 1961.
527. Wright HP, Osborn SB, Edmonds DG: Changes in the rate of flow of venous blood in the leg during pregnancy, measured with radioactive sodium. Surg. Gynecol. Obstet. 90: 481, 1950.
528. Alger LS, Laros RK: Thromboembolic disease in pregnancy. JCE Obstet. Gynecol. 13, 1978.
529. Hellgren M, Nygards EB: Long term therapy with subcutaneous heparin during pregnancy. Gynecol. Obstet. Invest. 13:76, 1982.
530. Whitfield LR, Lele AS, Levy G: Effect of pregnancy on the relationship between concentration and anticoagulant action of heparin. Clin. Pharmacol. Therap. 34:23, 1983.
531. Tengborn L, Bergqvist D, Matzsch T, Bergvist A, et al: Recurrent thromboembolism in pregnancy and puerperium: is there a need for thromboprophylaxis? Am. J. Obstet. Gynecol. 160:90, 1989.
532. Hull RD, Raskob GE, Pineo GF, Green D, et al: Subcutaneous low-molecular-weight heparin compared with continuous intravenous heparin in the treatment of proximal-vein thrombosis. N. Engl. J. Med. 326:975, 1992.
533. Levine MN, Hirsh J, Gent M, Turpie AG, et al: Prevention of deep vein thrombosis after elective hip surgery: a randomized trial comparing low molecular weight heparin with standard unfractionated heparin. Ann. Intern. Med. 114:545, 1991.
534. Wessler S: Heparin as an antithrombotic agent—Low-dose prophylaxis. JAMA 236:389, 1976.
535. Donaldson GA, Williams C, Scanell J, Shaw RS: An appraisal of the application of the Trendelenberg operation to massive fatal pulmonary embolism. N. Engl. J. Med. 268:171, 1963.
536. Hardaway RM: Monitoring of the patient in a state of shock. Surg. Gynecol. Obstet. 148:339, 1979.
537. Gibbs CP, Krischer J, Peckham BM, Sharp H, et al: Obstetric anesthesia: a national survey. Anesthesiology 65:298, 1986.
538. Cavanaugh D, Knuppel RA, Marsden DE: Hemorrhagic shock in obstetrics. *In* Managing OB/GYN Emergencies. 2nd Ed. Edited by JT Queenan. Oradell, NJ, Medical Economics Books, 1985, p. 100.
539. Isbister JP: Blood Transfusion. *In* Intensive Care Manual. 3rd Ed. Edited by TE Oh. Boston, Butterworths, 1990, p. 532.
540. Traverso LW, Lee WP, Langford MJ: Fluid resuscitation after an otherwise fatal hemorrhage. I. Crystalloid solutions. J. Trauma. 26:168, 1986.
541. Rackow EC, Falk JL, Fein IA: Fluid resuscitation in circulatory shock: a comparison of the cardiorespiratory effects of albumin, hetastarch and saline solutions in patients with hypovolemic and septic shock. Crit. Care Med. 11:839, 1983.
542. American College of Surgeons Committee on Trauma. Advanced trauma life support student manual. Chicago: ACS, 1988, p. 72.
543. Tait AR, Larson LO: Resuscitation fluids for the treatment of hemorrhagic shock in dogs: effects on myocardial blood flow and oxygen transport. Crit. Care Med. 19:1561, 1991.

544. Pascual JM, Watson JC, Runyon AE, Wade CE, et al: Resuscitation of intraoperative hypovolemia: a comparison of normal saline and hyperosmotic/hyperoncotic solutions in swine. Crit. Care Med. 20:200, 1992.
545. Gisselsson L, Rosberg B, Ericsson M: Myocardial blood flow, oxygen uptake and carbon dioxide release of the human heart during hemodilution. Acta. Anaesthesiol. Scand. 26:589, 1982.
546. Rosburg B, Wulff K: Regional blood flow in normovolemic and hypovolemic hemodilution. Br. J. Anaesth. 51:423, 1979.
547. Hauser CJ, Shoemaker WC, Turpin I, Goldberg SJ: Oxygen transport responses to colloids and crystalloids in critically ill surgical patients. Surg. Gynecol. Obstet. 150:811, 1980.
548. Gonik B, Cotton DB: Peripartum colloid osmotic pressure changes: influence of intravenous hydration. Am. J. Obstet. Gynecol. 150:99, 1984.
549. Cotton DB, Gonik B, Spillman T, Dorman KF: Intrapartum to postpartum changes in colloid osmotic pressure. Am. J. Obstet. Gynecol. 149:174, 1984.
550. Hughson WG, Friedman PJ, Feigin DS, Resnik R: Postpartum pleural effusion: a common radiologic finding. Ann. Intern. Med. 97:856, 1982.
551. Nearman HS, Herman ML: Toxic effects of colloids in the intensive care unit. Crit. Care Med. 7:713, 1991.
552. Abbott TR: Changes in serum calcium fractions and citrate concentrations during massive blood transfusions and cardiopulmonary bypass. Br. J. Anaesthesiol. 55:753, 1983.
553. Tranbaugh RF, Lewis FR: Crystalloid versus colloid for resuscitation of hypovolemic patients. Adv. In Shock Res. 9: 203, 1983.
554. Shackford SR: Hypertonic saline and dextran for intraoperative fluid therapy: more for less. Crit. Care Med. 20:160, 1992.
555. Mitsuno T, Ohyanagi H, Nasio R: Clinical studies of a perfluorochemical whole blood substitute (Fluosol-DA). Ann. Surg. 195:60, 1982.
556. Circular of information for the use of human blood and blood components. American Red Cross. American Association of Blood Banks, and the Council of Community Blood Centers. March 1989.
557. Fresh frozen plasma: indications and risks. National Institutes of Health Consensus Development Conference Statement Vol. 5, #5. Bethesda, DHHS Publication (NIH), 1984.
558. Nolan TE, Gallup DG: Massive Transfusion: a current review. Obstet. Gynecol. Surv. 46:289, 1991.
559. Yeomans ER, Hankins GDV: Cardiovascular Physiology and Invasive Cardiac Monitoring. Clin. Obstet. Gynecol. 32:3, 1989.
560. Rutledge R, Shelton GF, Collins ML: Massive transfusion. Crit. Care Clin. 2:791, 1986.
561. Collins JA: Massive blood transfusion. Clin. Haematol. 5: 201, 1976.
562. Bunker IF, Goldstein R: Coagulation during hypothermia in man. Proc. Soc. Exp. Biol. Med. 97:199, 1958.
563. Valeri CR, Cassidy G, Khuri S, Feingold H, et al: Hypothermia-inducted reversible platelet dysfunction. Ann. Surg. 205:175, 1987.
564. Carmichael D, Hosty T, Kastl D, Beckman D, et al: Hypokalemia and massive transfusion. South. Med. J. 77:315, 1984.
565. Linko K, Tigerstedt I: Hyperpotassemia during massive blood transfusion. Acta. Anaesth. Scand. 28:220, 1984.
566. Lynch-Salamon DI, Combs CA: Hepatitis C in obstetrics and gynecology. Obstet. Gynecol. 79:621, 1992.
567. Hibbs JR, Frickhofen N, Rosenfeld SJ, Feinstone SM, et al: Aplastic anemia and viral hepatitis: Non-A, Non-B, Non-C? JAMA 267:2051, 1992.
568. Miller RD, Robbins TO, Tong MJ, Barton SL: Coagulation defects associated with massive blood transfusions. Ann. Surg. 174:794, 1971.
569. Ciavarella D, Lavallo E, Reiss RF: Coagulation factor activity in platelet concentrates stored up to seven days: an in vitro and in vivo study. Clin. Lab. Haematol. 8:233, 1986.
570. Herbert WN, Owen HG, Collins ML: Autologous blood storage in obstetrics. Obstet. Gynecol. 72:166, 1988.
571. McVay PA, Hoag RW, Hoag MS, Toy PTCY: Safety and use of autologous blood donation during the third trimester of pregnancy. Am. J. Obstet. Gynecol. 160:1479, 1989.
572. Druzin ML, Wolf CFW, Edersheim TG, Hutson JM, et al: Donation of blood by the pregnant patient for autologous transfusion. Am. J. Obstet. Gynecol. 159:1023, 1988.
573. American Association of Blood Banks. Standards for Blood Banks and Transfusion Services. 11th Ed. Arlington, VA, American Association of Blood Banks, 1984.
574. Simon TL: Postpartum blood requirements: should autologous donations be considered? JAMA 259:2021, 1988.
575. Andres RL, Piacquadio KM, Resnick R: A reappraisal of the need for autologous blood donation in the obstetric patient. Am. J. Obstet. Gynecol. 163:1551, 1990.
576. Henderson IA, Beattie TJ, Kennedy AC: Dopamine hydrochloride in oliguric states. Lancet 2:827, 1980.
577. Shippy CR, Appel PL, Shoemaker WC: Reliability of clinical monitoring to assess blood volume in critically ill patients. Crit. Care Med. 12:107, 1984.
578. Robin ED: The cult of the Swan-Ganz catheter. Ann. Intern. Med. 103:445, 1985.
579. Rowley KM, Clubb S, Smith GJW, Cabin HS: Right-sided infective endocarditis as a consequence of flow-directed pulmonary artery catheterization. N. Engl. J. Med. 311: 1152, 1984.
580. Reedy MB, McMillion JS, Engvall WR, Sulak PJ, et al: Inadvertent administration of prostaglandin $E_1$ instead of prostaglandin $F_{2\alpha}$ in a patient with uterine atony and hemorrhage. Obstet. Gynecol. 79:890, 1992.
581. Haesslein HC, Schneider JM: Antishock trousers: use in obstetrics for patients refusing blood transfusions. Unpublished experience.
582. Hall M, Marshall JR: The gravity suit: a major advance in management of gynecological blood loss. Obstet. Gynecol. 53:247, 1979.
583. Sandberg EC, Pelligra R: The medical antigravity suit for management of surgically uncontrollable bleeding associated with abdominal pregnancy. Am. J. Obstet. Gynecol. 146:519, 1983.
584. Gardner WJ, Taylor HP, Dohn DF: Acute blood loss requiring 59 transfusions: the use of the antigravity suit as an aid in postpartum intra-abdominal hemorrhage. JAMA 167: 985, 1958.
585. Gunning JE: For controlling intractable hemorrhage: the gravity suit. Contemp. Obstet. Gynecol. 22:23, 1983.
586. Cho JY, Kim SJ, Cha KY, Kay CW, et al: Interrupted circular suture: bleeding control during cesarean delivery in placenta previa accreta. Obstet. Gynecol. 78:876, 1991.
587. Rovsov J: Fibrin Glue: An effective hemostatic agent for nonsuturable intraoperative bleeding. Ann. Thorac. Surg. 38:409, 1984.
588. Lupinetti F, Stoney WS, Alford WC Jr, Burrus GR, et al: Cryoprecipitate-topical thrombin glue. J. Thorac. Cardiovasc. Surg. 90:502, 1985.
589. Clark SL, Phelan JP, Yeh SY, Bruce SR, et al: Hypogastric artery ligation for obstetric haemorrhage. Obstet. Gynecol. 66:353, 1985.
590. Evans S, McShane P: The efficacy of internal iliac artery

ligation in obstetric hemorrhage. Surg. Gynecol. Obstet. 160:250, 1985.

591. Clark SL, Yeh S-Y, Phelan JP, Bruce S, et al: Emergency hysterectomy for obstetric hemorrhage. Obstet. Gynecol. 64:376, 1984.
592. O'Leary JA: Pregnancy following uterine artery ligation. Obstet. Gynecol. 55:112, 1980.
593. Greenwood LH, Glickman MG, Schwartz PE, Morse SS, et al: Obstetric and nonmalignant gynecologic bleeding: treatment with angiographic embolization. Radiology 164: 155, 1987.
594. Committee on Obstetrics: Maternal and Fetal Medicine, American College of Obstetricians and Gynecologists: Anesthesia for emergency deliveries. ACOG No. 104, 1992.
595. American Society of Anesthesiologists: Joint statement on the optimal goals for anesthesia care in obstetrics. *In* Handbook for Delegates. Chicago, ASA, 1988, 618.
596. Crosby ET: Obstetrical anaesthesia for patients with the syndrome of haemolysis, elevated liver enzymes and low platelets. Can. J. Anaesth. 38:227, 1991
597. Mapstone TB, Rukate HL, Shurin SB: Quadriplegia secondary to hematoma after lateral C-1, C-2 puncture in a leukemic child. Neurosurgery 12:230, 1983.
598. Tekkok IH, Cataltepe O, Tahta K, Bertan V: Extradural haematoma after continuous extradural anaesthesia. Br. J. Anaesth. 67:112, 1991.
599. Mayumi T, Dohi S: Spinal subarachnoid hematoma after lumbar puncture in a patient receiving antiplatelet therapy. Anesth. Analg. 62:777, 1983.
600. Locke GE, Giorgio AJ, Biggers SL, Johnson AP, et al: Acute spinal epidural hematoma secondary to aspirin-induced prolonged bleeding. Surg. Neurol. 5:293, 1976.
601. Horlocker TT, Wedel DJ, Offord KP: Does preoperative antiplatelet therapy increase the risk of hemorrhagic complications associated with the regional anesthesia? Anesth. Analg. 70:631, 1990.
602. Wille-Jorgensen P, Jorgensen LN, and Rasmussen LS: Lumbar regional anaesthesia and prophylactic anticoagulant therapy. Is the combination safe? Anaesthesia 46:623, 1991.
603. Mishima K, Aritake K, Morita A, Miyagawa N, et al: A case of acute spinal epidural hematoma in a patient with antiplatelet therapy. No Shinkei Geks 17:849, 1989.
604. Jeter EK, Scott A, Kizer J, Lazarchick J: Impaired platelet function associated with parenteral nafcillin. Ann. Clin. Lab. Sci. 20:79, 1990.
605. Metzger G, Singbartl G: Spinal epidural hematoma following epidural anesthesia versus spontaneous spinal subdural hematoma. Two case reports. Acta. Anaesthesiol. Scand. 35:105, 1991.
606. Mattingly SB, Stanton-Hicks M: Low-dose heparin therapy and spinal anesthesia. JAMA 246:886, 1981.
607. Owens EL, Kasten GW, Hessel EA: Spinal subarachnoid hematoma after lumbar puncture and heparinization: a case report, review of the literature, and discussion of anesthetic implications. Anesth. Analg. 65:1201, 1986.
608. Gurewich V, Nunn T, Kuriakos TTX, Hume M: Hemostatic effects of uniform, low-dose subcutaneous heparin in surgical patients. Arch. Intern. Med. 138:41, 1978.

# Chapter 27

# ANALGESIA AND ANESTHESIA FOR FORCEPS DELIVERY

RICHARD DEPP

The introduction of obstetric forceps into the methodology of the obstetrician in the eighteenth century represented a major advance in the management of difficult labor. For the first time, a tool was available to resolve "obstructed" labors. Of great philosophical importance was the fact that the goal of this new instrument was to save both mother and infant. However, controversy has surrounded the use of these instruments since their inception.

This controversy has been fueled through the years by the subjective nature of clinical opinions; the inconsistent definitions of forceps operations, thereby limiting comparisons between procedures and between studies; the studies that suffer from small sample size, retrospective methodology, and lack of proper controls; and most recently, the consumer movement that has popularized noninterventional childbirth.

Analgesia and anesthesia play a critically important role in influencing maternal and perinatal outcome among parturients delivered with the aid of forceps. Properly administered analgesia and anesthesia enhance the results obtained by the obstetrician because they permit effective pain relief and provide the obstetrician with optimal conditions for the orderly application of forceps. Improperly applied, however, anesthesia may produce direct deleterious effects on the mother and the fetus and indirectly may significantly increase the need for forceps delivery or may provide inadequate conditions for the optimal application of forceps. In this chapter, we discuss various important aspects of forceps delivery. The first part consists of Basic Considerations, including history of the development of forceps and evolution of their indication, the purpose of forceps delivery, and the management of labor as prerequisites to considering the use of forceps delivery. This is followed by clinical considerations of forceps delivery, including classification, prerequisite and indications for forceps, clinical conditions of the mother and the infant that may indicate their use, and recently established indications. A third section pertains to technical aspects of forceps delivery, including classification, selection, technique of application and possible risks. The last section pertains to anesthesiologic management. More detailed information on the subject of forceps delivery is found elsewhere (1–3).

## BASIC CONSIDERATIONS

### *History of Obstetric Forceps*

The history of the development of forceps and the historical evolution of forceps indications are among the most interesting, albeit changing, aspects in the field of obstetrics. Here we will briefly discuss this history.

#### *Development of Obstetric Forceps*

The development of modern obstetric forceps heralded the onset of a new philosophical approach to difficult childbirth. Early innovations to overcome obstructed labor were designed simply to evacuate the uterus, hopefully saving the mother. The invention of the modern obstetric forceps represented an attempt to resolve difficult labors while saving both the mother and the child.

The modern obstetric forceps were invented by the Chamberlen family in England in the early seventeenth century (4). Before their invention, the only way of managing obstructed labor was by cesarean delivery, which was uniformly fatal, or by destructive embryotomy. The Chamberlens were an influential family of male obstetricians who dominated the world of European obstetrics for four generations due to the successful and secretive use of their invention. The original Chamberlen instrument possesses several of the characteristics of our modern forceps, most notably a cephalic curve and the ability to disarticulate the two shanks of the instrument (Figure 27–1). It was a very short instrument with no pelvic curve; these two features severely limited its utility and contributed to much of the morbidity and mortality associated with it.

The Chamberlen forceps underwent its first important modification in the mid-eighteenth century. Andre Levret and William Smellie independently lengthened the shank of the instrument and added a pelvic curve. This allowed a more anatomic application to the fetal head and also allowed the use of the instrument at high stations, reducing the likelihood of injury to maternal soft tissue. In addition, Smellie invented the articulation known as the English lock, which is still in use today. These modifications were extraordinarily successful, and the use of the Levret-Smellie type forceps became widespread (Figure 27–2).

Little advance was made over the Levret-Smellie modifications until 1845, when Sir James Simpson introduced

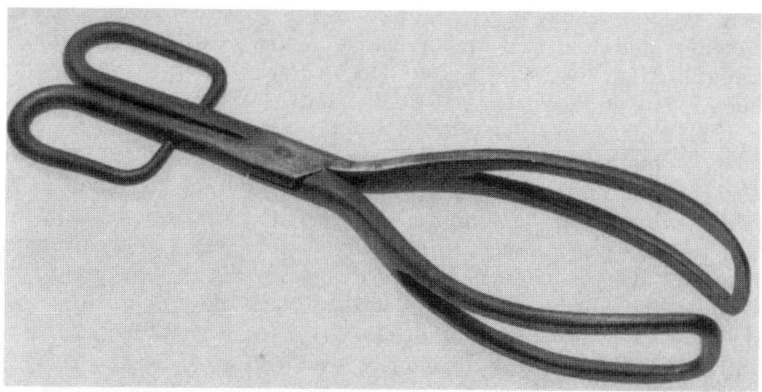

**Fig. 27–1.** Chamberlen delivery forceps. (From Grady JP: Modern Instrumental Delivery. Baltimore, Williams & Wilkins, 1988.)

the first obstetric forceps with scientifically calculated cephalic and pelvic curves, designed to minimize both maternal and fetal injury. He recognized that maternal and infant mortality increased with increasing duration of labor, and therefore encouraged the use of forceps to shorten labor.

The next major advance occurred in 1877, when Etienne Tarnier enunciated the principle of "axis traction." This principle states that force must be applied in a direction perpendicular to the plane of the pelvis at which the head is stationed. The Tarnier forceps (Figure 27–3), which were designed for use at very high stations, were the first forceps designed to adhere to the principle of axis traction, thereby imitating the natural mechanism of labor. The principle of axis traction is still very much in use today in modern obstetric forceps technique.

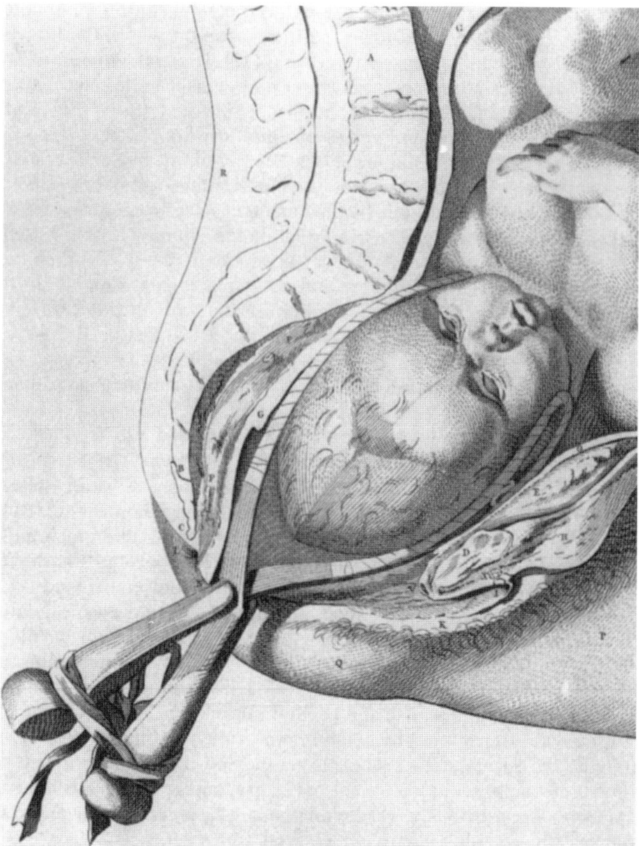

**Fig. 27–2.** Application of Leveret-Smellie forceps for assisted delivery with fetus' head in occiput transverse position. (From Grady, JP: Modern Instrumental Delivery. Baltimore, Williams & Wilkins, 1988.)

There has been little substantial change in the classical instrument since 1877; however, several special instruments have been developed to deal with highly individual situations. In 1915, Christian Kielland introduced a specialized instrument to facilitate forceps rotation in labors complicated by deep transverse arrest of the fetal head. In 1924, Lyman Barton introduced a second instrument to deal with deep transverse arrest (Figure 27–4). Both the Kielland and Barton forceps were revolutionary in their approach to the problem of transverse arrest in the midpelvis, and both are in use today. The Piper forceps were introduced in 1929 by Edward Piper, and are designed for delivery of the after-coming head in the breech presentation.

## *Historical Evolution of Forceps Indications*

Historically, forceps operations have sustained the ebb and flow of the historical pendulum in a pattern common to many medical procedures. Originally, forceps procedures were limited to maternal and obstetric indications for the termination of difficult labors. In the 1920s, routine prophylactic forceps became commonplace upon the recommendations of DeLee (5). More recently, the pendulum has swung more to use of forceps primarily for obstetric indications. This historical cycle limits the ability to compare the efficacy and complications of forceps deliveries in different time frames. Medical science has advanced considerably; in addition, routine use may result in a lower rate of complications and better outcome than use only for maternal or fetal indication. Forceps usage only in cases in which obstetric indications exist may preselect a population in which a higher rate of complications would be anticipated under any circumstances.

Indications for operative vaginal delivery have evolved substantially over the decades. DeLee (5) believed that the routine elective use of outlet forceps reduced the sustained compressive forces of the pelvic tissues against the fetal head that are known to cause molding of the head and increased intracranial pressure. DeLee (5) reasoned that the application of well-placed outlet forceps resulted in less cumulative localization of pressure to the presenting head than did continued labor (6). Due to his influence, "prophylactic" or "elective" forceps operations became very popular in the 1920s. Many institutions reported that over 50% of their deliveries were associated with the use of forceps. In addition, DeLee believed that interventional delivery to shorten the second stage of labor resulted in less perineal trauma, which would decrease the incidence of pelvic relaxation in multiparous women. He recommended routine use of an episiotomy to better preserve the functional integrity of the perineum

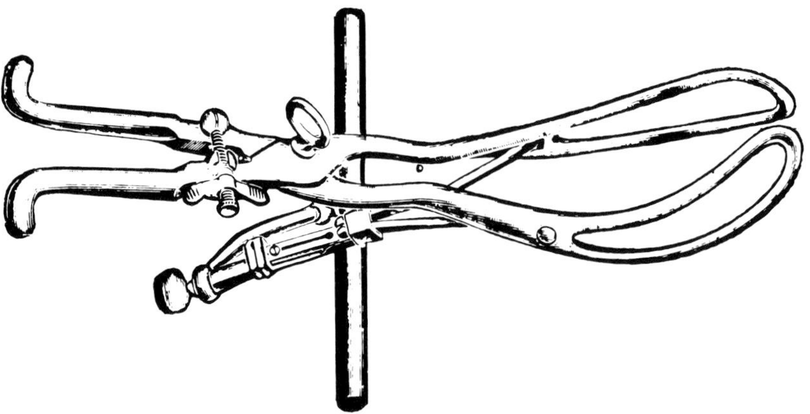

**Fig. 27–3.** Example of Tarnier forceps. (Laufe LE, Berkus MD: Assisted Vaginal Delivery: Obstetric Forceps and Vacuum Extraction Techniques. New York, McGraw-Hill, Inc., 1992.)

through surgical incision, as opposed to the occurrence of unpredictable tearing.

Use of prophylactic forceps remained popular throughout the late 1960s and probably increased short-term in the early 1970s with more common use of lumbar epidural block. At that time, use of either lumbar epidural or subarachnoid block commonly resulted in paralysis of pelvic floor and perineal muscles with resultant failure of internal rotation of the fetal vertex. Alterations in uterine blood flow and decreased uterine contractility were common, as well as decreased incentive for the patient to push with contractions as a result of anesthetic blockade of the afferent limb of the bearing-down reflex. As it was generally accepted that elective (outlet or low) forceps in experienced hands had little if any risk for mother or fetus, forceps were widely accepted as a safe and efficacious means of resolving many of these problems.

The first use of the vacuum extractor was popularized by Malmstroñ in the 1950s and soon became a favorite method of assisting vaginal delivery in Europe. Its acceptance in the U.S. has been sporadic, but by 1992 it seems generally accepted as a reasonable method of assisted delivery. The instrument itself has undergone significant modification since its first introduction, as noted in Figures 27–5 and 27–6. The principle is the same, however, with formation of a caput succedaneum inside the cup for purposes of downward traction force and stability. Over a period of years, comparisons of forcep delivery to vacuum delivery have not identified one technique superior over the other. There is, however, certainly a vocal preference

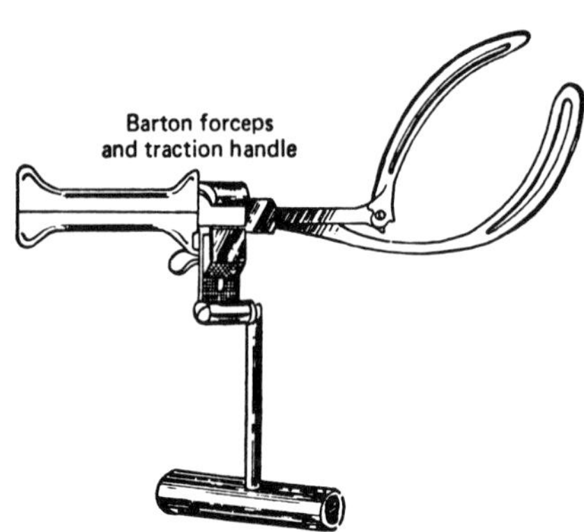


**Fig. 27–4.** The Barton forceps showing application of traction handle. (Modified from Benson RC: Handbook of Obstetrics & Gynecology. 8th Ed. Norwalk, CT, Appleton & Lange, 1983.)

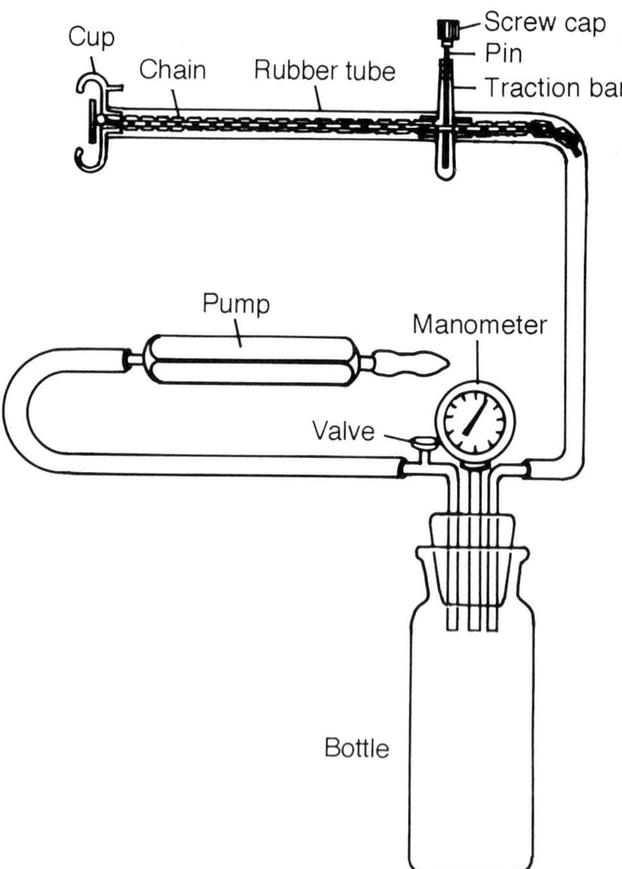


**Fig. 27–5.** Modified Malstroñ vacuum extractor. (Redrawn from Benson RC: Handbook of Obstetrics & Gynecology, 8th Ed. Norwalk, CT, Appleton & Lange, 1983.)

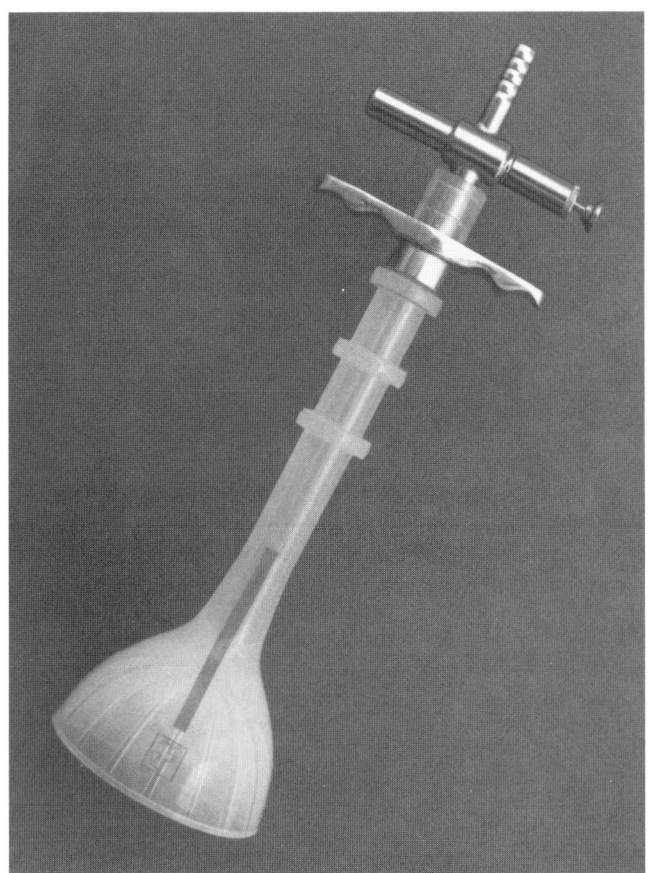

**Fig. 27–6.** Example of "Vac-u-nate Silicone Vacuum Cup" forceps. (From Gesco International Inc., San Antonio, Texas.)

given by the individual who is dedicated to one or the other. The comparisons are noted in Table 27–1.

For optimal application of forceps and the analgesia and anesthesia required, it is essential to know well and keep in mind the stages and phases of labor, the forces of labor, especially the expulsive forces during the second stage, and the impact on the mechanisms of descent that effect the station and engagement of the presenting part. Although these are discussed in detail in both Chapters 4 and 22, they are briefly recapitulated here for the convenience of the reader.

**Table 27–1.** Analgesia for Forceps versus Vacuum Delivery

| | Forceps | Vacuum |
|---|---|---|
| Analgesia | Moderate | Minimal |
| Application | Several steps | Single step |
| Difficulty | Moderate | Simple |
| Speed of use | Fast | Slow |
| Setup | Several steps | None |
| Delivery | Rapid | Slow |

(From author)

## *Definition of Stages and Forces of Labor*

### Stages of Labor

It is agreed generally that the first stage of labor consists of a latent phase, which begins with the onset of labor, characterized by regular, painful contractions, while the cervix is usually 2 cm dilated and ends when the cervix is 4 cm dilated. The mean duration of the latent phase is 10 hours in nulliparae and 6 hours in multiparae, although it may persist as long as 20 and 14 hours, respectively. The second phase of the first stage, the active phase, is characterized by a progressive cervical dilatation that begins at 4 cm and ends at complete (10 cm) cervical dilatation. Although Freidman (7) (Figure 27–7) subdivides the active phase into three components consisting of the acceleration phase, defined as the junction between the late and active phase of labor, the phase of maximum cervical dilatation and the deceleration phase, many obstetricians do not believe that the first and third of these occur in most parturients, but rather there is a progressive acceleration throughout the active phase. The statistical lower limits (mean − 2 SD) of the cervical dilatation for the active phase in nulliparous parturients is 1.2-cm per hour and in multiparae 1.0-cm per hour (7–9), although others insist that the rate is similar for both nulliparae and multiparae. If one can time the onset of labor, the total duration of the first stage of term labor is approximately 12 hours in nulliparae and 7 hours in multiparae.

The second stage, defined as the period of time from full cervical dilatation to delivery, can be subdivided into the descent phase and pelvic floor phase. The descent phase begins with complete cervical dilatation and traction and ends when the presenting part reaches the pelvic floor or plus 4 station. During the latter part of the first stage and during the second stage, the cardinal mechanisms of flexion, internal rotation, and extension take place. These mechanisms are impaired in parturients

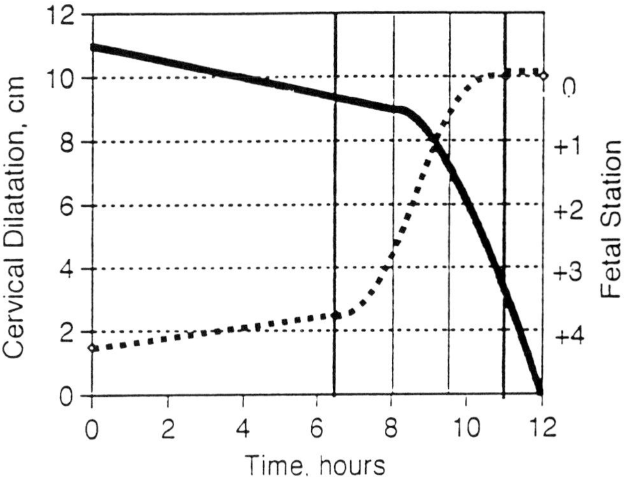


**Fig. 27–7.** The descent versus dilatation curve for labor. (From Cunningham FG, MacDonald PC, Gant NF: Williams Obstetrics. 18th Ed. Norwalk, CT, Appleton & Lange, 1989. Redrawn from Friedman: Labor: Clinical Evaluation and Management, 2nd Ed. New York, Appleton, 1978.)

whose pelvic musculature is relaxed by regional anesthesia, which may impair rotation and prolong the second stage. In the past, the upper limits of second stage duration were determined on the basis of statistical association with fetal outcome. Historically, it was noted that fetal outcomes were less favorable if the second stage was allowed to continue beyond 2 hours in a nulliparous patient, and 1 hour in a multiparous patient (2). However, these observations were made before the advent of continuous fetal monitoring and fetal scalp blood pH sampling during the second stage of labor. Currently, the limits of second stage labor are less rigidly defined and are more dependent upon fetal cardiovascular status than upon arbitrary limits.

## The Natural Expulsive Pressures of Labor

In Chapter 4, the important role of the auxiliary forces of labor during the latter part of the second stage to help the uterus expel the infant and the reflex mechanisms were discussed in detail. As mentioned there, these forces usually generate 25 to 60 mm Hg or higher pressure, which superimposed upon the pressure generated by uterine contraction, produced a total intramniotic pressure of 120 to 155 mm Hg or higher. The forces generated by "bearing down" play little or no role during the first stage of labor, but usually in the second stage, the additional force necessary to expel the infant is provided by the reflex contraction of the diaphragm, the abdominal and intercostal muscles, and the accessory muscles of expiration.

The magnitude of the total pressure generated to expel the fetus is individual-dependent, varying according to the intensity, duration, and frequency of uterine contractions, the power generated by the auxiliary muscles, and the type and amount of analgesia and anesthesia employed. To be effective, the forces of "bearing down" must be superimposed upon the force generated by the contracting uterus, so that together the two forces generate enough intrauterine pressure to expel the fetus through the completely dilated and retracted cervix, the vagina, pelvic floor, and perineum. Because the reflex that mobilizes the auxiliary forces is initiated by afferent input of nociceptive and pressoreceptive fibers contained in the sacral segments, analgesia/anesthesia of these segments eliminates the reflex. Moreover, in the event that regional anesthesia weakens the lower abdominal muscles, the force generated is decreased. Moreover, heavy sedation and confusion interfere with coordination of the process and impair the ability of the patient to cooperate. On the other hand, with proper coaching an enthusiastic and cooperative patient, the parturient can generate as much, if not more force, by contracting the auxiliary muscles.

## Station and Engagement

Before discussing the classification of forceps procedure, it is important to define station (engagement), which is one of the determinants of the classification of forceps. Station of the presenting part refers to the level of the leading bony edge of the fetal vertex (or presenting part in the case of a breech) in the maternal pelvis. When the leading edge is at the level of the ischial spines, the station is referred to as zero. Levels that are 1, 2, or 3 cm above or below the level of the spines are referred to as: station −1, −2, −3 or, alternatively, +1, +2, +3, respectively.

"Engagement of the vertex occurs when the biparietal diameter has passed through the pelvic inlet. It is generally assumed that the biparietal diameter lies approximately 2 to 3 centimeters above the leading edge of the fetal skull in flexed occiput anterior positions. In a practical sense, engagement is clinically diagnosed when the leading bony portion of the fetal head is at or below the level of the ischial spines (station 0 or more)" (10).

Under certain circumstances, descent of biparietal diameter may be overestimated by using the leading edge as an indicator because of the presence of one or more of the following: cephalic molding; caput succedaneum; or occiput posterior position. Consequently, the head may be engaged in some cases at a minus one station, but, alternatively, unengaged at a zero or in some cases at +1 station in an occiput posterior with considerable molding and protruding caput succedaneum.

## Labor Disorders

The term "failure to progress" is a nonspecific one that is often and primarily used clinically to describe active phase of labor disorders. In early labor, (latent phase of first stage) before 4 cm dilation, causation of failure to progress may be secondary to false labor, in the case of induction, an unripe or unresponsive cervix, or in some cases oversedation.

More specific terms to describe failure to progress have been defined by Friedman (11). Under this scheme, disorders of labor include: (1) prolonged latent phase; (2) prolonged active phase (slope less than threshold); (3) arrest of active phase; (4) arrest of descent; (5) prolonged descent; and (6) failure to descend. The obstetric anesthesiologist is most concerned with the latter five disorders of labor.

In the first stage of labor, prolongation of active dilatation is diagnosed if rate of dilatation is less than 1.2 cm/hour in a nullipara, or less than 1.5 cm/hour in a multipara once active phase labor has begun. In the active phase,many obstetricians take a more pragmatic approach in patient management, setting 1 cm/hour as a threshold for satisfactory progress in cervical dilation in the phase of maximum slope. An active phase arrest is diagnosed when there is no progress in cervical dilatation for 2 hours. Failure to progress in the active phase of the first stage of cervical dilatation may be attributed to either suboptimal uterine contractions or the "relative" versus "absolute" continuum of cephalopelvic disproportion (CPD).

There are several disorders primarily associated with the second stage of labor. Failure to descend is diagnosed when the head fails to descend into the true pelvis at all. Prolonged descent is diagnosed when the rate of descent (generally in the late portion of the active phase of labor or in second stage) is less than 1 cm/hour for nulliparous patients and less than 2 cm/hour in multiparous patients.

Arrest of descent is diagnosed when there is no descent for 1 hour. In the second stage, both relative cephalopelvic disproportion and impairment of pushing forces may be operative in causation of descent disorders. In the second stage, prolongation or arrest of descent may be the indication for forceps delivery.

## Assessment and Management of Labor

A brief discussion of the assessment and proper management of labor is considered desirable at this point to better understand current limitations of our understanding of the impact of analgesia and anesthesia on the progress of labor.

### *Assessment of Uterine Activity*

Continuous external tocodynamometry is the most common method to measure intrapartum uterine activity (contraction frequency and duration). This method is simple, noninvasive, and inexpensive. However, only a properly calibrated intrauterine pressure transducer can measure contraction intensity. For scientific purposes, the most complete evaluation of uterine activity is obtained by quantitatively measuring the area under the uterine activity curve produced by an internal pressure transducer. Using these uterine activity assessment techniques, Miller, et al (12) and Huey, et al (13) made several observations that must be addressed in any clinical research study involving determinants of labor progress. They noted that: normal uterine activity increases with progressive labor; uterine contractions become more efficient with progressive cervical dilatation; and the total uterine activity required for multiparous patients to progress is less than that required for nulliparous patients. As a consequence, any study of the pharmacologic effects of an agent on labor must control for cervical dilation, parity, prior contraction pattern, and prior labor curve. Medication effect may vary significantly depending solely upon the point in the curve of labor when the agent is given; furthermore, uterine activity is not the sole determinant of progress of labor. The issue is made even more complex by the observation that one may alter uterine activity without actually altering labor progress.

### *Diagnosis of Failure to Progress*

In the first stage, to individualize the management of failure to progress, the physician ordinarily will assess contraction, frequency and duration, and, when possible, intensity; assess the station and position of the presenting part; assess the flexion of the head as reflected by the position of the fontanelles in the cervical canal where possible; assess pelvic capacity through clinical pelvimetry; and assess descent of the presenting part in response to bearing-down efforts. Most fetuses will deliver in a flexed, occiput anterior position. This position allows the smallest diameter of the fetal head to traverse the maternal pelvis. However, it is not uncommon for the fetal head to persist in a malposition or malrotation due to factors such as configuration of the maternal pelvis or improperly administered anesthesia of the sacral segments that relax the perineal muscle sling. Such malpositions include occiput transverse and occiput posterior positions, as well as deflexed positions. When these occur, a larger diameter of the fetal head (e.g., occipitofrontal) must traverse the pelvis. These labors are often more prolonged and difficult, and may demonstrate prolongation or arrest disorders.

Suboptimal uterine contractions (inadequate contraction frequency and/or less frequently insufficient intensity) are the most common cause of the disorders of active phase labor. Varying degrees of relative cephalopelvic disproportion are also operative in many cases but cannot be assessed directly. Instead, if there is failure of cervical progress or descent of the presenting part once adequate uterine artery is achieved with or without oxytocin stimulation, relative CPD is inferred. Uterine activity may be evaluated by either manual palpation or evaluation of the uterine activity channel of the continuous fetal heart rate monitor. In most cases, continuous electronic external tocodynamometry is adequate to assess timing and frequency of contractions. In some cases, it may be necessary to insert an intrauterine pressure catheter.

### *Management*

A common objective in management, in which some optimal uterine contractions are suspected, is to have the parturient achieve about 4 contractions per moving 10-minute window, each contraction lasting approximately 60 seconds. If intrauterine pressure is available, progress is more likely with contraction intervention measuring approximately 50 to 75 mm Hg; however, some patients achieve progress with contractions of lesser intervention. In most cases, inadequate uterine activity can be managed by judicious oxytocin augmentation. Once adequate contractile activity is achieved, a reasonable approach is to observe the patient for an additional 1 to 2 hours to assess rate of cervical progress with adequate uterine activity.

Past approaches to second stage of labor management stressed the value of absolute time limits of the second stage. If the second stage extended beyond 2 hours in the nullipara or 1 hour in the multipara, delivery by forceps or cesarean was indicated. More recently, the American College of Obstetrics and Gynecology (ACOG) has provided guidelines that are more judgement dependent and in line with practice realities. "When these intervals (Primigravida: greater than 3 hours with regional anesthetic or greater than 2 hours without a regional anesthetic) (Multigravida: greater than 2 hours with regional anesthetic or greater than 1 hour without a regional anesthetic) are exceeded, the risks and benefits of allowing labor to continue should be assessed and documented."

## Clinical Considerations of Forceps Delivery

### *Classification of Forceps Procedures*

Classification of forceps procedures have not been consistent even in recent history. In large part, this is a reflection of the controversies surrounding their perceived risks and benefits. Inconsistencies in classifications also reflect the concern that classification should in some way communicate the degree of difficulty of the procedure, which is dependent, not only on the relation of fetal size to maternal pelvic capacity, but also to the station and position of the fetal vertex.

Before 1965, forceps classifications were divided into outlet forceps, low forceps, mid forceps, (low-mid and high-mid) and high forceps. High forceps are not considered acceptable therapy and have no place in modern obstetrics. In 1965, the ACOG simplified the classification into three broad categories: outlet forceps, mid forceps, and high forceps. The former "low forceps" designation was no longer to be used. The 1965 classification required that the suture be in the anterior/posterior diameter to be designated as "outlet forceps." There was also no allowance for the designation of "low-mid" and "high-mid" categories of mid forceps deliveries, as had been common practice before 1965. This classification, although recommended, did not reflect the degree of difficulty inherent in various procedures, and made comparisons of outcomes difficult, if not impossible. Consequently, it was not accepted by many practicing obstetricians.

### Current ACOG Classification

In 1988, the ACOG reorganized the classification system into one more similar to the pre-1965 status listed in Table 27–2. The major thrust has been to better define the categories of forceps procedures. The hope is that better classification will lead to more accurate statistics on frequency and outcome of forceps operations of comparable difficulty. The current classifications are quoted below:

1. Outlet forceps. The application of forceps when: (1) the scalp is visible at the introitus without separating the labia; (2) the fetal skull has reached the pelvic floor; (3) the sagittal suture is in the anterior-posterior diameter or in the right or left occiput anterior or posterior position; and (4) the fetal head is at or on the perineum. According to this definition, rotation cannot exceed 45°. Forceps delivery under these conditions may be desirable to shorten the second stage of labor.
2. Low forceps. The application of forceps when the leading point of the skull is at station +2 or more. Low forceps have two subdivisions: (1) rotation 45° or less (e.g., left occipitoanterior to occiput anterior, left occipitoposterior to occiput posterior); and (2) rotation more than 45°.
3. Mid forceps. The application of forceps when the head is engaged but the leading point of the skull is above station + 2.

**Table 27–2.** History of Procedure Classification

| Classification | ACOG, 1965–1988 | ACOG, 1988–present |
|---|---|---|
| Outlet forceps | Anterior-posterior diameter only | Anterior, posterior, or oblique |
| Scalp | Visible | Visible |
| Presenting part at | Pelvic floor on perineum | |
| Rotation | Not acceptable | <45° |
| Low forceps | Not acceptable | Reinstated |
| a. Station | ≥+2 | |
| b. Rotation | | |
| c. ≤45° | Not apply | Subdivision |
| d. ≤45° | Not apply | Subvidision |
| Mid forceps | | |
| Station | 0, +1 | |
| Forceps rotation | All No longer a determinant | |
| Comment | Unusual at +2 | Rare at 0, +1 |

(From ACOG Committee Opinion. Number 59, February, 1988.)

### "Trial" of Forceps vs. "Failed" Forceps

It is generally accepted that when judiciously used, outlet and low forceps operations have outcomes comparable to spontaneous vaginal deliveries. In addition, most operators have excellent outcomes with "easy" mid forceps deliveries. However, there is often considerable difficulty in determining prospectively if a given mid forceps procedure in a particular patient will be easy or difficult. It is under these circumstances that the cautious "trial of forceps" has a role. The term trial of forceps implies a cautious attempt at operative vaginal delivery, with alteration of the management plan should the attempt prove more difficult than anticipated. A trial of forceps is not appropriate in cases of known cephalopelvic disproportion, an unengaged presenting part, brow or mentum posterior presentations, or other clinical situations in which lack of success may be anticipated. However, if the clinician judges, after evaluation of all available clinical data, that there is a reasonable chance of success with an operative vaginal delivery, a trial of forceps is justified. Cesarean deliveries must be available in the event of an unsuccessful attempt. A careful attempt at application, rotation, and employing moderate traction will not injure the infant. The attempt should be abandoned if any unexpected resistance or difficulty in forceps application is encountered. Injuries occur when the operator attempts to overcome resistance with force or persists in attempts to achieve a favorable application.

The term "failed forceps" has been used to designate those trial procedures that were abandoned due to lack of success. Dennen (14) believes that this term should be retired, implying as it does a procedure abandoned after multiple attempts proved it to be impossible. To many practitioners, the term "failed forceps" may suggest bad judgement or poor medical practice.

## Prerequisites and Indications for Forceps Operations

### Prerequisites

Forceps delivery is referred to as an operative delivery. As such, it is of paramount importance to accord it the respect, deliberation, and care that would be accorded any surgical procedure.

There are few contraindications and/or prerequisites to the application of forceps. However, there is little disagreement as to their validity. Disregard for past experience increases the likelihood of adverse outcome. The six

**Table 27–3.** Forceps Application Prerequisites

1. The head must be engaged, (preferably, deeply engaged).
2. The fetus must present either by the vertex or by the face with the chin anterior (except in the use of Piper forceps for the after-coming head in a breech presentation).
3. The position of the head must be precisely known so that the forceps may be appropriately applied.
4. The cervix must be completely dilated.
5. The membranes must be ruptured.
6. There should be no (absolute) disproportion between the size of the head and that of the pelvic inlet, the midpelvis, or the outlet. (In practice, this is very difficult to ascertain prospectively).

(From Pritchard JA, MacDonald PC, Gant NF: Williams Obstetrics. 17th Ed. Norwalk, Appleton-Century-Crofts, 1985, pp. 840–841.)

prerequisites to forceps application are listed in (Table 27–3) (15).

### Clinical Considerations that Influence Forceps Indications

Much of the deliberation involved in the decision to perform forceps delivery entails balancing the risks to the fetus and to the mother from forceps delivery with those resulting from cesarean delivery and associated anesthesia requirements. Here we have discussed the evolution of present day indications for forceps. Next we will consider the risks incurred by the fetus in late labor and delivery, particularly in the presence of factors that prolong labor or produce a traumatic process.

In the preelectronic monitoring era, clinical studies suggested that there was a higher risk of fetal morbidity and mortality when the second stage of labor exceeded 2 hours. Forceps were often used at the conclusion of the 2-hour interval to reduce this potential morbidity. The origin of the morbidity associated with a prolonged second stage may have been the result of one or more complications, including the following: unsuspected intrapartum asphyxia, central nervous system (CNS) damage predating labor, or trauma arising from forceps intervention to effect delivery.

Today, the capability for continuous intrapartum fetal heart rate surveillance improves the ability to identify the fetus that may not tolerate labor or a prolonged second stage. As a result, the length of the second stage of labor is not in itself an absolute indication for operative termination of labor. However, it must be realized that, despite our ability to minimize the occurrence of severe fetal acidemia at birth, we currently do not have the means to identify the fetus with significant preexisting CNS damage prior to the onset of labor. Fetal CNS damage leading to cerebral palsy predating the onset of labor is estimated to represent approximately 80 to 90% of total cases. The remaining 10 to 20% originates during labor and in the neonatal period, largely correlated with preterm birth and intrauterine growth retardation. The fraction contributed by any trauma arising out of the intrapartum application of obstetric forceps is likely to be minimal should forceps be applied judiciously and used within the context of the definitions, indications, and conditions discussed below.

### Maternal Risks Attendant to Cesarean Delivery

The cesarean delivery rate in the United States has risen significantly in the past 2 decades; this has been paralleled by an increased number of anesthetic procedures. One of the benefits has been the demand for an increasing number of anesthesiologists with formal specialized training in obstetric anesthesia. Despite the increased availability of qualified individuals with special training in this area, maladministered anesthesia continues to account for 7% of maternal mortality (16).

One of the major advantages of forceps operations is the avoidance of cesarean delivery and its associated morbidity. Maternal postpartum morbidity, especially infectious, is clearly more prominent following cesarean birth than mid forceps, which is in turn more prominent than that following low and outlet forceps. Although few data exist relative to anesthetic complications resulting from forceps delivery, the risk can be inferred to be considerably less than that arising out of anesthesia for cesarean delivery, as anesthesia needs are less and general anesthesia is seldom required.

The anesthetic risks of cesarean delivery are significant, and it is likely that anesthetic-related deaths are underestimated (17,18). There is, however, some controversy in this area. Kaunitz noted that anesthesia accounted for 4% of all United States maternal deaths between 1974 and 1978 (18). Turnbull, et al subsequently reported that anesthetic deaths were responsible for 12.5% of maternal deaths in England and Wales from 1979 to 1981 (19). Moldin, in reporting on similar data collected in Sweden between 1973 and 1979, reported no anesthetic deaths in more than 65,000 cesarean sections (20).

It is likely that much of the anesthetic risk attendant to cesarean delivery relates to the availability of discretionary and planning time prior to cesarean delivery. Hood and Dewan reported that the risk of anesthesia related to cesarean delivery increases approximately fourfold if the cesarean section is emergent in nature (21). Although it is arguable that many of these deaths are preventable by "appropriate anesthetic management," there is value in avoiding cesarean delivery where possible by less invasive procedures so as to minimize the likelihood of a need for general anesthesia. Further reduction may be possible, for instance, by making contingency plans for cesarean delivery when mid forceps delivery is considered.

### Factors Responsible for Recent Changes in Indications and Use

In recent years, many factors have contributed to the decline of operative vaginal delivery, as well as some of anesthesia side effects that may impinge on the second stage of labor, increasing their usage. They include to a lessor degree, the "natural childbirth" movement; development of protocols for the safe and efficacious use of oxytocin to resolve many cases of uterine dysfunction; ability to carefully monitor fetal status, thereby eliminating the need for arbitrary end points in second stage labor; and to a greater degree, more expert use of epidural anesthesia to minimize the labor consequences of perineal and pelvic floor muscle paralysis. Furthermore, the advent of the antibiotic era, the availability of blood products, and the development of new anesthetic techniques have also contributed to the safety of cesarean section, often making it a preferable alternative to a difficult vaginal delivery. In the 1980s, with decreased educational exposure to forceps delivery, there has been a further decrease in forceps use in some centers.

### *Current Indications for Forceps*

It is indisputable that in the proper hands, carefully performed and selective use of operative vaginal delivery is associated with lower maternal morbidity and mortality than is associated with caesarean delivery. It is therefore incumbent upon the medical profession to continue to perform these procedures properly, and to train young practitioners in the art and "science" of obstetric forceps.

Current indications for forceps deliveries may be maternal, fetal, or elective. Elective, or prophylactic forceps, may be considered to be either maternal or fetal in indications. Although these have declined significantly in popularity, it is this author's opinion that the elective forceps delivery may be a necessary and desirable procedure for educating young practitioners in the art of operative vaginal delivery. It is in these patients that the ideal combination of fetal status and position, maternal cooperation, and anesthetic adequacy may be achieved thus providing a controlled and low-risk setting for the education of the young obstetrician.

### *Maternal Indications*

Maternal indications may include exhaustion, failure to progress, bleeding, or medical indications. Maternal exhaustion may ensue after long or difficult labors or a long second stage involving strenuous pushing efforts, or ineffectual pushing as a result of weak abdominal musculature, a pendulous abdomen, or respiratory difficulties that disrupt efficient generation of the adequate forces ordinarily provided by the diaphragm and abdominal muscles. In some instances, the pain and maternal discouragement generated by the pressure of the presenting part against the pelvic floor may be contributory. Under such circumstances, if the presenting part is well into the pelvis, and the prerequisites for forceps delivery are met, forceps delivery may be employed to overcome these difficulties; cesarean delivery is seldom necessary. In other instances, particularly in the absence of adequate anesthesia, the patient may be unwilling or unable to tolerate the pain generated as the head impinges upon the pelvic floor. Anesthesia, support, and forceps is a reasonable approach to this problem.

Should there be an arrest of descent in the second stage of labor, the pelvic dimensions judged to be adequate to accommodate the involved fetus, and the vertex is at +2 station, mid forceps is a reasonable option. Should the fetal vertex be malpositioned (e.g., occiput transverse or occiput posterior), or deflexed, the application of forceps will not only allow the operator to rotate the head to a more optimal position, but will also allow flexion of the fetal head, thereby decreasing the effective diameter of the presenting part. Two caveats are pertinent, particularly in nulliparae: (1) beware of macrosomia of 4500 g or more; and (2) be prepared for shoulder dystocia, particularly if estimated fetal weight is more than 4500 g. Unfortunately, it is only possible to estimate fetal weight plus or minus 400 to 500 g for that weight range.

More rarely, maternal complications may be an indication for forceps delivery. In several medical conditions, the stress of second stage labor with its increased intracranial, intrathoracic, and intraabdominal pressures pose an increased risk to the mother. Relatively common examples include significant functional maternal cardiac or pulmonary impairment, cerebral vascular anomalies, detached retina, or spontaneous pneumothorax. In such cases, there may be advantage in not allowing the patient to push any longer than is absolutely necessary. Another maternal indication may be the presence of profuse bleeding, in the second stage associated with placental abruption. If hemorrhage or shock are present, an expeditious delivery is desirable, as the source of the bleeding may then be more easily identified and corrected.

#### *Fetal Indications*

Fetal complications, indicating a need for more expeditious delivery, may be acute in origin such as placental abruption, cord prolapse, significant cord compression as indicated by persistent nonremediable moderate to severe variable decelerations, or even acute onset late decelerations following an identifiable and remediable precipitating event such as hypotension or excess uterine activity. Alternatively, fetal complications reflecting a chronic uteroplacental insufficiency may be present, indicated by repetitive (commonly associated with decreased baseline variability) nonremediable, uniform late decelerations.

Should the cervix be incompletely dilated, the condition not correctable, and the anticipated time of vaginal delivery in excess of 30 minutes, cesarean delivery may be indicated. However, in the event that the ordinary prerequisites for forceps delivery are present and delivery is indicated because of fetal jeopardy, a reasonable option is to apply forceps to expedite delivery. Under these circumstances, it may be useful to counsel the patient, partic-

**Table 27–4.** Current (1988) ACOG Committee Indications

1. Shortening the second stage of labor: Outlet forceps may be used to shorten the second stage of labor in the best interests of the mother or the fetus, as long as the criteria for outlet forceps are met. (No specific indications are provided.)
2. Prolonged second stage: The following durations are approximate; when these intervals are exceeded, the risks and benefits of allowing labor to continue should be assessed and documented:
   a. Primigravida: More than 3 hours with a regional anesthetic or more than 2 hours without a regional anesthetic.
   b. Multigravida: More than 2 hours with a regional anesthetic or more than 1 hour without a regional anesthetic.
3. "Fetal distress." (No objective criteria provided).
4. Maternal indications (e.g., cardiac, exhaustion).

(From ACOG Committee Opinion. Number 59, February, 1988.)

**Table 27–5.** Comparison of Common Forceps

| Characteristics | Simpson | Elliott | Kielland | Piper |
|---|---|---|---|---|
| Length | 35 cm | N/A | 40 cm | 44.5 cm |
| Shanks | Parallel | Overlapping | Overlapping | Parallel |
| Locks | English | N/A | Sliding | N/A |
| Blade length | 18 cm | 15 cm | 15 cm | N/A |
| Fenestration | Yes | Yes | Yes | Yes |
| Pelvic curve | N/A | N/A | N/A | N/A |
| Cephalic curve | Shallow | Accentuated | Shallow | Shallow |
| Modifications | DeLee-Short | Tucker-McLean<br>Tucker-Luikart<br>Long-Elliott | Luikart-Kielland | None |

N/A: Not applicable.

ularly in cases in which there are repetitive significant decelerations preceding the application of the forceps, that there may be fetal depression that will be independent of the forceps' use (see Table 27–4) for 1988 ACOG Committee Indications.

## Technical Considerations

### *Classification and Selection of Instruments*

#### *General Design*

Forceps may be divided into two broad instrument categories, conventional and special. Conventional forceps include the Simpson and Elliott types with their subsequent modifications, including the DeLee forceps, the Tucker-McLean forceps, and the Tucker-Luikart modifications. Conventional forceps are used primarily for outlet and low forceps, as well as occasional mid forceps delivery (Scanzoni rotation). Special forceps include the Kielland and Barton types for forceps rotations, instruments with axis traction handles, and Piper forceps for application to the after-coming head of the breech. Table 27–5 compares the most common forceps.

#### *Instrument Selection*

Table 27–6 summarizes clinical fetal characteristics that may modify forceps selection. Many obstetricians develop significant experience and comfort with a single classical instrument, and use that instrument for virtually all procedures. This approach has been criticized by some who feel that forceps selection should be determined by such factors as the shape of the fetal head; the presence or absence of molding and caput formation; the size of the fetal head; and the purpose for which the forceps are being used (traction and/or rotation, flexion of the head, correction of asynclitism, etc).

**Table 27–6.** Criteria for Forceps Selection

| Clinical Findings | Forceps | | | |
|---|---|---|---|---|
| | Elliott | Simpson | Kielland | Piper |
| Molding | Extensive | Little | Yes | Little |
| Head | Large | Round | N/A | Round |
| Purpose | Outlet forceps | Outlet forceps | Asynclitism | Breech |
| Outlet | Yes | Yes | Rare | No |
| Low | Yes | Yes | Rare | No |
| Mid | Yes | Yes | Yes | No |
| Asynclitism | Seldom | Seldom | Yes | No |
| Breech | N/A | N/A | No | Yes |

N/A: Not applicable.

The most commonly used forceps, particularly for low and outlet procedures, are the Elliott and Simpson forceps and their common derivatives. Kielland forceps are commonly used for forceps rotation, particularly of deep transverse arrest or occiput posterior; they are particularly useful in the treatment and resolution of asynclitism. Some obstetricians prefer the Barton forceps, particularly for an occiput transverse position in a platypelloid (wide and flat) pelvis. In most instances, Piper forceps are used for the delivery of the after-coming head of breech presentations. Some obstetricians in the United States use the Kielland or other forceps types for the after-coming head.

### *Techniques of Application*

Because this is not an obstetric text, the actual description of forceps application and techniques of delivery are not presented. Rather, the author presents an overview of techniques so that the anesthesiologist may be more familiar with the cues and progress of the procedure. One cannot discuss forceps technique without reiterating the importance of the experience, judgment, clinical examination, and skill of the operator. Forceps application, particularly mid forceps, is more than a simple surgical procedure.

Even in today's consumer-oriented world, most patients undergoing low or mid forceps delivery are prepared and draped using traditional techniques. The managing obstetrician should perform a pelvic exam to check for the presence of prerequisites and/or contraindications to delivery. Of great significance is the station and position of the presenting part, as well as the pelvic contour. Before applying the forceps, adequacy of anesthesia should be determined. This may be done by the obstetrician or the anesthesiologist. Inadequate anesthesia will often result in an uncooperative patient and make the procedure far more difficult than necessary. In addition, inadequate anesthesia is extremely upsetting to the patient. In applying the forceps, the obstetrician should avoid, where possible, displacing the head to a higher station. In some instances, it is quite difficult to determine the actual position of the fetal head by traditional techniques such as location of suture lines and fontanelles; it may be necessary to locate the fetal ears relative to their anatomical proximity to the fetal occiput.

All modern forceps applications are cephalic applications. In prior years it was acceptable to apply forceps in a pelvic application; in the past, forceps actually may have been placed intentionally across the face. This is no longer an acceptable practice. Subsequent to careful application of the forceps, the obstetrician will check to determine that the forceps are properly applied with regard to the sagittal and the lambdoidal sutures.

If rotation is necessary, this is accomplished following flexion of the fetal head to reduce the diameter of the presenting cephalic presentation. Once the fetal vertex is in the desired position, traction may be applied in a manner to mimic uterine contractions. This, however, does not imply that traction need be limited to the contracting phase. Rather, the obstetrician commonly applies traction for a number of cycles of traction and relaxation until delivery is effected. In the instance of mid forceps delivery, the actual traction process may extend over 5 minutes and occasionally as long as 15 minutes. It is better to be patient in this process as the objective of the entire process is to simply speed up the normal labor process.

In most instances, the episiotomy incision is delayed until the forceps are applied, the application is confirmed, and traction is performed providing descent of the vertex and some distention of the perineum. At this time, the perineum has thinned out, is less vascular, and can be surgically incised, minimizing blood loss.

Upon completion of the forceps procedure, the clinician should record an operative summary description in the patient's medical record, including: the indications for the forceps operation, the position and station of the vertex at the time of application of the forceps, the amount of traction required (mid forceps), maternal complications, and fetal outcome.

### *Possible Risks of Forceps Deliveries*

Fetal and maternal injury may arise as complications associated with forceps operations. Maternal injury is mainly limited to soft tissue trauma and includes: cervical, vaginal, and lower uterine segment lacerations; bladder and urethral trauma; hematomas; and perineal lacerations. Fetal injuries include facial marks from the forceps, which are usually transient; facial nerve paralysis; bruises and lacerations; cephalohematomas; and skull fractures. The role of forceps delivery in the development of newborn neurologic damage is highly questionable. This is particularly true in individual cases in the absence of a depressed skull fracture and/or subdural hematoma. As mentioned earlier, approximately 80% of cases of cerebral palsy are thought to result from fetal neurologic damage antedating the onset of labor. The remaining 20% are largely correlated with preterm birth and intrauterine growth retardation.

There is general agreement that uncomplicated outlet and low forceps deliveries have fetal and maternal outcomes and complication rates similar to those of spontaneous vaginal deliveries. However, there is still considerable controversy regarding the potential effects of mid forceps operations. Friedman, et al (22) compared long-term intelligence quotient scores in children born by spontaneous vaginal delivery with scores of children born by both low and mid forceps procedures. While he found no difference in long-term intelligence quotient scores between spontaneous vaginal deliveries and low forceps deliveries, he noted a statistically significant decrement of 6 points in the mid forceps group. However, the data of Friedman do not establish a cause and effect relationship.

The risks associated with mid forceps deliveries remain debatable. However, mid forceps deliveries are the repertoire in carefully selected cases managed by experienced personnel. In large part this conclusion is based upon absence of well-controlled prospective studies reflecting a clinically significant disadvantage to forceps delivery.

A sensible control group to evaluate the complications of mid forceps operations would include patients undergoing cesarean delivery as an alternative to mid forceps delivery. Using such a group, Dierker, et al (23) retrospectively evaluated outcomes in 176 mid forceps deliveries and compared them to spontaneous vaginal deliveries, low forceps deliveries, and cesarean delivery. He found that mid forceps deliveries were associated with a higher risk of cervical and third-degree perineal lacerations and excessive maternal bleeding when compared to the general population; he suggested, however, that this increased incidence must be balanced with the potentially more serious sequelae of cesarean delivery. He also found an increase in cephalohematomas and depressed 1-minute Apgar scores in the mid forceps group; however, the incidence of depressed 1-minute Apgar scores was the same as that in the cesarean birth group, and the incidence of depressed 5-minute Apgars was lower in the mid forceps group than in the cesarean group. He concluded that judicious use of mid forceps is not associated with increased short-term risk to mother or infant. Gilstrap, et al (24) compared outcomes of 177 elective, 293 indicated low, and 234 indicated mid forceps deliveries with 303 spontaneous deliveries and 111 cesarean sections. He found a lower incidence of depressed Apgar scores with low and mid forceps deliveries when compared with cesarean birth. The only significant difference found between low and mid forceps deliveries was an increased rate of maternal vaginal lacerations and post delivery maternal anemia in the mid forceps group. He concluded that the continued usage of judicious mid forceps deliveries is justifiable.

## ANESTHESIOLOGIC MANAGEMENT

### *Preliminary Considerations*

To provide optimal anesthesiologic care to parturients who may require forceps delivery, it is necessary for the obstetrician and anesthesiologist to consider the following issues: (1) the effects of the drugs and techniques used for pain relief on uterine contractility and other forces of parturition that are necessary to produce a normal progress of labor and spontaneous delivery; (2) how these effects interact with preexisting obstetric conditions to influence (increase or decrease) the need for forceps delivery; and (3) once the decision is made that forceps delivery is required, it is necessary to consider many factors in selection of the anesthesia and to adhere to certain basic principles essential for optimal results.

As the first two issues are discussed in great detail in Chapters 4 and 22 of this book, only a brief recapitulation will be presented here under the following headings: (1) Effects of Opioid Inhalation Analgesia; (2) Effects of Local Anesthetics and Regional Anesthesia on the Progress of Labor; and (3) The Effects of Continuous Epidural and Subarachnoid Block on the Forces of Labor During the Second Stage.

### Effects of Opioid Inhalation Analgesia

Administered in analgesic concentration, inhalation agents have no effect on uterine contractility or other forces of labor, and therefore have no influence on cervical dilatation and the duration of labor. The effects of meperidine, the most commonly employed analgesic during labor in the United States, and other opioids depend on the phase of labor and the dose and route of administration. Generally administered in the prodomal or latent phase of labor, opioids will decrease the rate of cervical dilatation and thus prolong labor, whereas administration of Opioids in the well established active phase of labor usually do not inhibit cervical change, but actually can increase progress, provided of course that the drug is given in optimal doses. Although some authors have reported a marked decrease in uterine activity following injection of meperidine (25), most studies document an increased amount of uterine activity following intravenous administration (26–29).

### Effects of Local Anesthetics and Regional Anesthesia on the Progress of Labor

Numerous articles containing information on the effects of local anesthetics and epidural anesthesia on uterine contractility (as measured by internal tokodynamometry) and the progress of labor are summarized in Chapter 22. Some of the well-controlled studies showed that the injection of single boluses of 8 to 10 ml of lidocaine or bupivacaine to initiate continuous epidural analgesia produced a transient (15 to 20 minutes) decrease in uterine contractility, but this effect was significantly less in the second injection and disappeared after the third or fourth injection. Moreover, most of these studies showed that notwithstanding the transient effects, the duration of the first stage of labor was not increased. Inclusion of 1:200,000 epinephrine in the local anesthetic solution enhanced the transient inhibitory effect of the local anesthetic but did not increase the duration of the first stage (30). In contrast, repeated injections of 18 to 22 ml of lidocaine or other local anesthetic containing 1:200,000 (90 to 100 ug) of epinephrine was used for continuous caudal anesthesia did prolong the duration of labor. Other factors that were found to enhance the inhibitory effect of local anesthetic and epinephrine were the supine position, maternal arterial hypotension, severe maternal metabolic acidosis consequent to prolonged labor, the use of excessive amounts of local anesthetics and consequent absorption that may have direct myometrial depressant effect, accidental intravenous injection of local anesthetics or use of a large amount for paracervical block with consequent delivery or high concentration of the local anesthetic to the uterine musculature that increases uterine tone while decreasing rate and strength of contractions (31–37). Obviously, in such situations, the myometrial depressant effect and the effect on the progress of labor is due to technical errors that can and must be avoided.

In conclusion, there seems to be a general concensus among obstetricians and anesthesiologists that a continuous epidural block that extends no higher than T-10 spinal segment (8,9,38) does not have a consistent or more than a transient effect upon uterine activity or the progress of the first stage of labor in the absence of confounding variables such as cephalopelvic disproportion or maternal hypotension.

### Local Anesthesia with Paracervical Block (PCB) Anesthesia

Local anesthetics generally have little or no effect on uterine contractility in the concentrations ordinarily used in clinical practice (31). In certain situations, such as inadvertent intravenous injection or PCB, delivery of high concentrations of local anesthetic to the uterine vasculature may increase uterine tone while decreasing rate and strength of contractions (32). Local anesthetics may have a direct effect on the uterus. Greiss (33) has demonstrated a dose-related increase in uterine tone following injection of local anesthetics into the uterine artery of pregnant ewes.

High concentrations of local anesthetic placed in direct proximity to the uterine artery may be absorbed intravascularly and may increase uterine tone (33). Both Baxi (35) and Miller (36) noted transient increases in uterine activity following PCB. Jenssen (37) observed a decrease in uterine activity following PCB, with a reduction in contraction frequency and a reduction in total uterine activity; however, he noted an enhanced rate of cervical dilatation in the group receiving PCB. See Chapter 22 for further discussion regarding paracervical block.

### The Effects of Continuous Epidural and Subarachnoid Block on the Forces of Labor During the Second Stage

Review of the data published before 1980 on the effects of continuous epidural, continuous caudal or subarachnoid block on second stage labor is much more controversial. Some clinicians reported that continuous lumbar epidural analgesia had no inhibitory effects on uterine contraction and, if properly managed, did not significantly influence the resistant forces and the auxiliary forces of labor so that it had little or no effect on the incidence of spontaneous delivery. Other reports suggest that epidural analgesia did not effect the progress of cervical dilatation, but increased significantly the incidence of lack of adequate (i.e., malrotation of the presenting part) and the need for instrumental delivery. The discrepant results can be attributed to: (1) different obstetric conditions existing at the time the block was initiated; (2) in many instances, continuous epidural block used in the United Kingdom and in Scandinavian countries was reserved for patients with dysfunctional labor that by its nature is longer and often requires oxytocin stimulation, uterine contraction, and forceps delivery; (3) the posture of the parturient during labor differed; (4) difference in the obstetrician's preference concerning the use of oxytocin and outlet forceps; and (5) the technique of epidural block used but particularly the extent of the block and the amount and concentration of the local anesthetic used.

It has long been recognized that continuous caudal anesthesia, standard epidural block with anesthesia extending from T-10 to S-5, and subarachnoid block (T-10 to S-5) initiated before mid-second stage produces premature sensory and motor blockade of the sacral spinal segments. This in turn produces: (1) block of the afferent limb of Ferguson's reflex with consequent decrease in the secretion of endogenous oxytocin that is said to play a particularly important role during the second stage; (2) premature weakness or paralysis of the perineal muscles that interferes with the resistant forces and thus impairs the cardinal mechanisms of internal rotation resulting in nonrotation; (3) block of the afferent limb of the reflex urge to bear down; and (4) if motor block extends much above L-1, decreases the force of the contraction of the lower abdominal muscles with consequent decrease in the bearing-down expulsive forces. These, in turn, have the potential of prolonging the second stage, increasing the incidence of persistent fetal malrotations, and thereby increasing the incidence of operative delivery for disorders of descent.

During the period 1945 to 1975, the incidence of forceps delivery was high, especially in the United States, ranging from 50 to 85% in nulliparae and between 47 and 65% in multiparae. This increase in forceps delivery was in part due to the fact that in the United States episiotomy and outlet forceps delivery were considered the hallmark of American obstetric practice. Many experienced American clinicians believed that these adverse effects of major regional anesthesia were offset by the fact that a relaxed perineum facilitated manual rotation and also delivery of the infant. This was in contrast to the obstetric practice in the United Kingdom, in Scandinavia, and in other continental European countries where the use of forceps delivery was equated with increased risk to the mother and infant. While most obstetricians in those countries appreciated the value of obstetric anesthesia for the mother and to the fetus, they repeatedly expressed concern that the use of lumbar epidural anesthesia and subarachnoid block increased the number of instrumental deliveries and malrotation. This prompted a large number of reports that expressed great concern about the relatively high incidence of malrotation and forceps delivery published by obstetricians and anesthesiologists in the United States, the United Kingdom, and Scandinavia.

These concerns prompted obstetric anesthesiologists and some obstetricians, who realized the value of epidural analgesia in providing effective pain relief and as a therapeutic measure for incoordinate uterine contractions, to modify the technique and also to modify the obstetric management to decrease the incidence of the undesirable side effects on the forces of the second stage of labor. These modifications included: (1) the use of "selective" lumbar epidural analgesia in the first and second stage of labor and the avoidance of perineal analgesia and anesthesia together; (2) time allowed for the blockade in the perineum to wear off during the second stage so that the parturient could bear down forcibly in patients who had developed perineal analgesia during the latter part of the first stage; (3) the progressive increase and refinement of continuous lumbar epidural infusion analgesia achieved with very low concentration of local anesthetics alone or combined with opioids; (4) the use of double-catheter technique; (5) the delay of the bearing-down efforts until the fetal head was in the introitus, discarding the concept that the second stage should be limited to less than 1 hour and allowing the parturient to continue the second stage until spontaneous delivery occurred; and (6) the emphasis on "active management of labor," an integrated program that includes augmentation of uterine contractions with oxytocin during the second stage of labor.

After some experience, the first two modifications were discounted because having the parturient experience severe pain during the second stage is not only cruel to the mother, but is actually counter-productive because it may be associated with higher incidence of forceps delivery, probably because of the imposed maternal distress—a fact demonstrated by the study of Phillips and Thomas (39). These investigators compared a group of patients who received intermittent epidural anesthesia right up to delivery with a group in whom anesthesia was halted at full dilatation. They found no difference in duration of first or second stage, and no significant difference in forceps use between the two groups. They found a significant increase in persistent malrotations in the group receiving no additional anesthesia for second stage, as well as an increased level of maternal dissatisfaction. They concluded that maintenance of selective analgesia throughout the second stage was beneficial to the patient.

The most important advances made during the past decade that were intended to reduce the incidence of malrotation and forceps delivery were a step in the refinement of lumbar epidural analgesia. The first of these was reducing the concentration of the local anesthetics: instead of using intermittent doses of 0.25 to 0.375% bupivacaine, a number of workers used 0.0625% bupivacaine with 0.0002% fentanyl for labor and vaginal delivery and noted excellent analgesia in virtually all parturients who developed minimal motor block and who had normal second stage labor with spontaneous delivery in a high percent of parturients (40). The next step was the use of continuous infusion of low concentration of local anesthetics entailing the use of precise infusion pumps for drug delivery. Next, with the advent of intraspinal opioid analgesia for the treatment of acute and cancer pain, obstetric anesthesiologists began to use subarachnoid and epidural injection of morphine and other opioids during the first stage of labor. While these techniques provided fairly effective analgesia during the first stage and permitted the retention of the bearing-down efforts, the perineal analgesia was often inadequate for spontaneous delivery and totally unsatisfactory for instrumental delivery.

The latest modification, initiated in 1985, was the use of continuous epidural infusion of low concentration of local anesthetic and opioids (40). The excellent series of studies of Chestnut and his associates are described in detail in Chapter 13. The current technique, again described in detail in Chapter 13, entails the use of continuous epidural infusion of 0.625% bupivacaine with 0.002% fetanyl administered throughout labor and delivery. This technique produces little or no motor blockade so that the incidence of spontaneous delivery and the duration of the second stage are within normal limits. The disadvantage of this technique is that during the second stage only about three-fourths of patients have good to excellent analgesia and have little relaxation. These disadvantages can be obviated by a terminal injection of 10 ml of 0.25% bupivacaine with the patient sitting or the use of double-catheter technique described in Chapter 13.

Another modification that has decreased the incidence of malrotation and forceps delivery was delaying the bearing-down efforts until the fetal head is seen as in the parted introitus. Thus, if progress in descent is being made and fetal well-being documented via continuous heart monitoring, the second stage of labor may be allowed to continue beyond the traditional 2-hour limit for nulliparae and 1-hour limit for multiparae. Maresch (41), for example, has proposed that second stage labor may be allowed to continue for up to 4 hours without major risk to either mother or fetus. In 1988, the ACOG issued a recommendation that it is reasonable to allow a second stage of approximately 3 hours in nulliparae receiving regional anesthetics.

### *Conclusion*

Although some studies (41) report increased rates of forceps deliveries, this may be partially due to individual obstetric practice patterns, the practical realities of a busy obstetric practice when confronted with a prolonged second stage, hesitancy by some to administer oxytocin, and nurse staffing problems for ideal coaching of patients relative to second stage pushing. Furthermore, increased use of forceps delivery is not necessarily bad for the patient; there is no evidence that differences in outcome exist between properly performed outlet or low forceps and spontaneous delivery. The same, however, may not be true for elective mid forceps deliveries, which may be associated with increased maternal and fetal risk.

## General Principles of Anesthetic Management

Before briefly discussing the objectives and selection of an anesthetic, some mention should be made of the importance of a team approach in the selection of the proper technique and agent. Together, the team, consisting of obstetrician, anesthesiologist with input from neonatology, may consider the effect of the technique chosen on both the fetus and mother, as well as the labor forces. Obstetric requirements and other obstetric determinants for agent selection are presented in tabular form in Table 27–7.

Bonica, in his 1969 edition of PRINCIPLES AND PRACTICES OF OBSTETRIC ANALGESIA AND ANESTHESIA alluded to six cardinal "Cs." They are: consultation, cooperation, coordination, communication, courtesy, and compromise (Table 27–8). All are important goals for both the anesthesiologist and obstetrician, and when accomplished are more likely to foster long-term positive relations between team members. In some instances, the anesthesiologist or obstetrician is frankly uncomfortable with certain anesthetic approaches. In such instances, physicians should communicate their discomfort in frank terms, and the obstetrician, as a courtesy, should compromise and respect the anesthesiologist's recommendation unless there is concern that the approach is likely to be detrimental.

The anesthesiologist, particularly those with special interest and experience in obstetric anesthesia, is commonly more knowledgeable regarding the selection of individual agents and subtleties of dilution and dose. While the obstetrician may be at a disadvantage in the former area, he/she has commonly accumulated significant practical experience with the advantages and complications of the variety of anesthetic techniques for each of the forceps delivery types (outlet, low, mid, and mid rotations). Although it is certainly possible to perform an outlet delivery and some low forceps delivery with relative satisfac-

**Table 27–7.** Analgesic and Anesthetic Requirements According to Obstetric Forcep Procedure

| Requirements | Outlet Forceps | Low Forceps | Mid Forceps | Mid Forceps with Rotation |
|---|---|---|---|---|
| Analgesia | Minimal | Moderate | Significant | Significant |
| Analgesia site | Perineum & vagina | Perineum & vagina | Perineum, vagina, cervix, uterus | Perineum, vagina, cervix, uterus |
| Relaxation | Not required | Perineum | Highly desirable for perineum & vagina | Highly desirable for perineum & vagina |
| Labor forces | Desirable | Desirable | Not required/desired | Not required/desired |
| Manipulation | Minimal | Minimal | Moderate to "significant" | Moderate to "significant" |
| Traction | Mild to moderate | Mild to moderate | Moderate | Moderate |
| Duration | Short | Longer | Longer | Longer |
| Possible cesarean | Unlikely | Unlikely | Significant | More significant |

**Table 27–8.** The Six Cardinal "Cs"

| |
|---|
| 1. Consultation |
| 2. Cooperation |
| 3. Coordination |
| 4. Communication |
| 5. Courtesy |
| 6. Compromise |

tion simply by using a local and pudendal block, the more complex the forceps delivery (higher stations and need for rotation), the more likely the need for a more sophisticated anesthetic technique approach.

What can the obstetric and anesthesiology members of the team do to minimize delay in the second stage and decrease the incidence of malrotation and forceps delivery? The anesthesiologist can use continuous infusion of dilute solutions of local anesthetics and opioids as discussed in Chapter 13. It is now commonplace to use the most dilute concentration possible for relief of labor pain. The perineal dose of epidural should be withheld until descent and internal rotation of the fetal head has occurred, or, alternatively, use lower doses and concentrations during the second stage to maintain skeletal muscle tone and preserve the bearing-down efforts (42,43).

The obstetrician and labor-floor support team, on the other hand, can demonstrate patience in the second stage, allowing the second stage to continue beyond traditional limits as long as maternal and fetal well-being are maintained. They may also provide teaching and coaching for the parturient during pushing to ensure that adequate and timely pushing effort is maintained, even if sensation is lost. There is no need to discontinue the anesthetic at full cervical dilatation; this may be extremely distressing to the patient.

## Anesthesia Risk Associated with Labor Terminated by Forceps Delivery

The patient who is a candidate for forceps delivery may be at increased risk of regional-anesthesia related hypotension as a function of prolonged pushing and hyperventilation. In the past, the likelihood and degree of hypotension was in large part due to either a rapid onset of a generous sympathetic block or the lack of adequate hydration prior to the sympathectomy challenge, or in some cases a combination of both. The etiology of hypotension associated with lumbar epidural analgesia is detailed in Chapter 13, but, to briefly summarize here, please note the following two formulas:

$$\text{C.O.} = \text{H.R.} \times \text{R.A.P.} \quad (1)$$

$$\text{B.P.} = \text{C.O.} \times \text{P.V.R.} \quad (2)$$

In the case of the lumbar epidural, the administered drug reduces peripheral vascular resistance beyond the point of cardiac compensation by either heart rate changes or right arterial pressure changes. Thus, blood pressure falls according to the degree of peripheral vascular resistance reduction with rapid intravenous hydration. There is a transient increase in right arterial pressure before the sympathectomy, i.e., the decrease in PVR that helps offset the fall in BP.

Rapid administration of ½, 1, or even 2 liters of fluid before or during activation of a lumbar epidural block has been found to decrease the incidence of hypotension with minimal associated increase in central venous pressure (44,45). Lewis reported that only 6.7% of patients demonstrate transient hypotension if they receive 2 liters of crystalloid (44) versus a dramatically higher incidence of 30% by authors utilizing less than 1 liter for dehydration (46,47). Caritis and Aboulesh, on the other hand, provide supportive evidence for spinal anesthesia in cases in which dehydration of less than 1 liter was adequate (48). Because forceps deliveries may be more likely in association with maternal pregnancy diabetes, it is particularly important to avoid a dextrose-containing solution for prehydration as the induced maternal hyperglycemia may result in a reactive neonatal hypoglycemia (49).

However, current day practices with continuously pumped low-concentration anesthetics just do not present the hypotensive threat noted above. This is primarily because of the absence of any significant sympathectomy. Thus, the patient is kept on an analgesic, but without the need of the excessive fluid challenges heretofore utilized because of the previously noted altered physiology. If more motor effect, i.e., relaxation, is needed, a small dose, i.e., 8 to 10 ml of 2% lidocaine can be used without the fear of maternal hypotension. As mentioned earlier, the usual scenario with use of the continuous analgesic combination is a slowly diffusible sacral block to the point that forceps delivery or spontaneous delivery can be performed with little added agent.

## Anesthesia Objectives and Requirements for Forceps Delivery

There are three primary anesthetic objectives for forceps delivery. They include: maximum pain relief; optimal operative conditions for the surgical procedure; and minimal adverse effect on the fetus. Continuous epidural anesthesia also provides the advantage of potential postoperative analgesia, which may be of particular significance for the patient who has undergone mid forceps delivery, particularly should a mediolateral episiotomy be required.

An individualized selection of the proper anesthetic for the patient under consideration is a major consideration, particularly should mid forceps be considered. When selecting the proper anesthetic agent, the team must consider the statistical chance that the patient will need to proceed to cesarean delivery. Further, it is important that the deliberation process recognize that there are two patients involved, the mother and unborn fetus. There is a balance in the selection process; for example, regional anesthesia generally has less depressive effect on the newborn while certain patients with coagulation defects may not be appropriate candidates for epidural anesthesia.

The individual case requirements (Table 27–9) depend upon the indication for and complexity of the intended procedure, ranging between the extremes of a simple out-

**Table 27–9.** Indications for Forceps Use

| Requirements | Forceps | | | Mid Forceps |
|---|---|---|---|---|
| | Outlet | Low | Mid | |
| Elective procedure | Most | Some | Rare | None |
| Maternal exhaustion | Few | Common | Common | Some |
| Failure to progress | N/A | Most | Most | Most |
| Maternal bleeding | N/A | Few | Few | Few |
| Fetal distress | Few | Few | Few | Few |

let forceps versus a significantly more complex mid forceps rotation. The obstetrician requires that the patient lie quietly on the table to minimize the likelihood of vaginal tears and extension into the rectum and sphincter. Obviously, the procedure and agent chosen must consider the physiologic status of the mother and, where possible, the psychological status of the mother. Finally, the training, experience, and skill of both the obstetrician and the anesthesiologist are significant determinants of agent and route of anesthesia chosen.

All forceps deliveries should be approached in an individualized manner. When selecting the agent and technique, the obstetrician/anesthesiologist team needs to consider, in addition to the previously mentioned considerations, the indications for the procedure, the complexity of the procedure, the obstetric requirements, the procedure time requirements, the skill and experience of the anesthesiologist with regard to these techniques, as well as the experience of the obstetrician with the variety of anesthetic techniques under the specific circumstance at hand.

The presence or absence of maternal complications can be the most important determinant of anesthetic selection. Common examples would be shock and hypovolemia, abruptio placenta with disseminated intravascular coagulation, placenta previa with hemorrhage, or even severe maternal anemia. Other maternal risk factors may include such complicating medical conditions as functional heart impairment and significant pulmonary dysfunction. In such circumstances, avoidance of sympathetic blockade, which may aggravate hypotension, is an important goal. At this point, we would remind the reader that a special situation occurs in the case of the morbidly obese patient. These patients may deliver from below, but may be in need of cesarean section conversion also. As mentioned in Chapter 14, this patient may be best served by use of a continuous 22-gauge spinal technique with opioid or even small doses of local anesthetic used for the first stage and more potent local anesthetic concentrations substituted if the need for cesarean section does materialize.

Fetal determinants must also be considered. Should forceps be indicated to hasten the delivery of a fetus with nonremediable late decelerations or significant variable decelerations, the obstetrician will desire an anesthetic technique with predictable rapid onset with minimal chance to impair uteroplacental blood gas exchange.

Finally, the urgency of the procedure is a common and important determinant. Ideally, urgency should be a minor, not major issue if good communication is adhered to. In many cases, the anesthetic team may opt for second stage control with predelivery placement of an epidural and caudal catheter. Should delivery be required within a short interval, a saddle block or general anesthesia may be desirous in the absence of a previously placed epidural catheter because of the rapidity of onset and certainty of effect. On the other hand, the obstetrician must be flexible enough to be able to perform local analgesia if necessary in situations in which time demands rapid fetal delivery, but in which the anesthesiologist determines general anesthesia may be a severe threat to the patient's life. See Chapter 13 for a detailed description of how the obstetrician and anesthesiologist can work together in such a situation. In some instances, the obstetrician may desire assistance via the pushing efforts of the mother, and thus will desire an agent that will not impair either uterine contractile activity and yet allow the patients to generate effective pushing activity. Some patients do not push effectively between contractions; should the administration of the anesthetic agent reduce uterine activity, it may be necessary for the obstetrician to administer oxytocin to augment uterine activity.

## *Special Considerations For Mid Forceps Operations and Trial of Forceps*

Many of the above considerations are appropriate in selection of a proper agent and technique for mid forceps delivery. However, mid forceps delivery, particularly when rotation is required, increases the complexity of the anesthetic requirements. Unlike low forceps delivery, there is little expectation that maternal pushing efforts will have beneficial effect. Rather, the obstetrician is more concerned that the pelvic muscles be totally relaxed and the patient completely immobile during the often complex procedure. As in the case of selection of an anesthetic for fetal distress, the obstetrician's main concern is the certainty of adequate anesthesia and promptness of its onset.

In selecting the anesthetic agent and procedure for mid forceps delivery, the anesthesiologist should also consider the increased likelihood of a cesarean delivery should the intended mid forceps procedure be unsuccessful. Inherent in the decision to proceed with mid forceps delivery is the need to move to cesarean section should forceps application be difficult or should traction produce minimal descent in the face of subjectively adequate traction. Further, because there is increased likelihood of cesarean delivery, it may be wise to perform the procedure in the operating room, particularly if the obstetrician anticipates that delivery may be difficult or unsuccessful. Here again, the use of a continuous subarachnoid technique provides analgesia requirements for both the second stage vaginal delivery and immediate conversion to cesarean section, if indicated.

Finally, maternal and fetal complications are more common in the case of mid forceps delivery due to either the indication for the procedure or as a complication of the procedure. In some instances, there may be trauma resulting in significant maternal hemorrhage while in others, there may be either trauma to or asphyxia of the fetus, which requires immediate support and resuscitation of the newborn. The number and training of individuals available in the delivery room and operating room are thus also important determinants in planning anesthesia agent and technique.

Regional anesthetic techniques that may be considered for forceps delivery include: pudendal block, saddle block, spinal block, continuous spinal block, intermittent lumbar epidural or continuous lumbar epidural. Should spinal (as opposed to saddle) block be employed, the frequency of hypotension due to sympathetic blockade aggravated by aortocaval compression may become a major clinical problem, particularly for a patient who must lie in the supine position for prolonged periods of time during the preparation for and application of the forceps. In such cases, it is essential to displace the uterus laterally to minimize the magnitude of aortocaval compression.

Epidural anesthesia has become a very popular method for managing the analgesic and anesthetic needs of laboring patients. Not only is it useful during the labor process, but it provides excellent anesthesia for virtually any type of forceps procedure. Continuous lumbar epidural anesthesia is particularly suited for the combination of events and procedures that one may potentially encounter during labor and delivery. Although there is a chance that the supine patient may develop postural hypotension, preinduction hydration, and uterine displacement, supplemented as needed with ephedrine, should minimize the effects of hypotension.

### *Fetal Surveillance*

Because administration of the epidural block and patient preparation and application of forceps may take a considerable amount of time, it is important to maintain continuous surveillance of the fetal heart rate. Under these circumstances, fetal heart rate abnormalities occur with enough frequency to be of concern. These abnormalities usually consist of either a prolonged deceleration of several minutes duration or, alternatively, of repetitive late decelerations with an onset 10 to 15 minutes after injection of the local agent. These late decelerations usually demonstrate variability within the deceleration and, upon recovery, baseline variability is generally maintained. This acute onset uteroplacental insufficiency is generally thought to be secondary to decreased uterine blood flow secondary to sympathetic blockade and alterations of blood flow distribution. In some cases, there is an observable increase in uterine contraction activity and tone immediately before the onset of the fetal heart rate deceleration.

Finally, it is well-established that local agents used for regional anesthesia readily cross the placenta attaining significant blood levels in the unborn fetus (50). Because there is concern regarding the potential effect of these agents on neonate, the anesthesiologist should maintain the lowest possible effective dose as possible.

## Overview and Summary

Obstetric application of forceps to effect vaginal delivery is one of the art forms that separates the specialist in obstetrics and gynecology from family practitioners and midwives, who also devote a portion of their medical activities to obstetrics. It is a procedure that has seen its popularity ebb and flow throughout the years. Nowhere in medicine is the complete evaluation of the patient (both psychologically and physically), judgment, experience, and skill more important. While some institutions discourage the use of forceps, the procedure is still taught. In a survey conducted in 1981 involving 144 directors of Canadian and United States residency programs, the incidence of mid forceps deliveries ranged between 1 to 4% in more than 50% of the programs (51). Under proper circumstances and in the right hands, a properly conducted forceps delivery can effect a safe vaginal delivery avoiding the requirement for cesarean section and the maternal complications that may result from that procedure. Conversely, forceps delivery may result in trauma to both mother and fetus. It is not possible to guarantee that forceps application will necessarily result in a completed vaginal delivery, nor that trauma to either mother or fetus will not occur. Certainly, no surgical procedure is without those hazards. Nonetheless, an orderly and logical approach to the indications, use, and anesthesia requirements of obstetric forceps offers the opportunity of great benefit to both mother and newborn, including the satisfaction of a vaginal delivery at reduced physical, psychological, and economic cost when compared to cesarean delivery.

## REFERENCES


1. Shnider SM, Levinson G: Anesthesia for Obstetrics. 3rd Ed. Baltimore, Williams & Wilkins, 1993.
2. Cunningham FG, MacDonald PC, Gant NF: Williams Obstetrics. 18th Ed. Norwalk, Appleton & Lange, 1989.
3. Gabbe SG, Niebyl JR, Simpson JL: Obstetrics: Normal and Problem Pregnancies. 2nd Ed. New York, Churchill Livingstone, 1991.
4. Aveling HJ: The Chamberlens and the Midwifery Forceps. London, Churchill, 1882.
5. DeLee JB: The prophylactic forceps operation. Am. J. Obstet. Gynecol. 1:34, 1920.
6. Bonica JJ: Obstetric Analgesia and Anesthesia. New York, Springer-Verlag, 1972.
7. Friedman EA: Primigravida labor: a graphicostatistical analysis. Obstet. Gynecol. 6:576, 1959.
8. Friedman EA: Labor on multiparous: a graphicostatistical analysis. Obstet. Gynecol. 8:691, 1959.
9. Friedman EA: Labor: Clinical Evaluation and Management, 2nd Ed. New York, Appleton-Century-Crofts, 1978.
10. ACOG Committee Opinion. Number 59, February 1988.
11. Friedman EA, Sachtelben-Murray MR, Daharoughe D: Long-term effects of labor and delivery on offspring: a matched-pair analysis. Am. J. Obstet. Gynecol. 250:941, 1984.
12. Miller FC, Yeh SY, Schifrin BS: Quantitation of uterine activity in 100 primiparous patients. Am. J. Obstet. Gynecol. 124: 398, 1976.
13. Huey JR, Al-Hadjiev A, Paul RH: Uterine activity in the multiparous patient. Am. J. Obstet. Gynecol. 126:682, 1976.
14. Dennen PC: Dennen's Forceps Deliveries. Philadelphia, F.A. Davis, 1989, pp. 7–8.
15. Pritchard JA, MacDonald PC, Gant NF: Williams Obstetrics. 17th Ed. Norwalk, Appleton-Century-Crofts, 1985, pp. 840–841.

16. Friede AM, Rochat RW: Maternal mortality and perinatal mortality: an epidemiologic perspective. And Sachs B, Acker D: Clinical Obstetrics: A Public Health Perspective. Littleton, MA, PSG Publishing Company, Inc., 1986. (MMWR: Maternal mortality: pilot surveillance in seven states. JAMA 255:184, 1986.)
17. Rubin G, McCarthy B, Shelton J, Rochat RW: The risk of childbearing re-evaluated. Am. J. Public Health 71:712–716, 1981.
18. Kaunitz AM, Hughes JM, Grimes DA, Smith JC: Causes of maternal mortality in the United States. Obstet. Gynecol. 65:605, 1985.
19. Turnbull AC, Tindall VR, Robson SG, Dawson IMP, et al: Report on confidential enquiries into maternal deaths in England and Wales, 1979–1981. Department of Health and Social Security, Report on Health and Social Subjects No. 29. Her Majesty's Stationery Office, London, 1986.
20. Moldin P, Hokegard KH, Neilson TF: Cesarean section and maternal mortality in Sweden 1973–1979. Acta. Obstet. Gynecol. Scand. 63:7, 1984.
21. Hood DD, Dewan DM: Obstetric anesthesia. *In* Risk and Outcome in Anesthesia. Edited by DL Brown. Philadelphia, J.B. Lippincott, 1988.
22. Friedman EA, Neff RK: Labor and Delivery: Impact on Offspring. Littleton, MA, PSG Publishing Company, Inc., 1987.
23. Dierker LJ, Debanne S: The mid forceps: maternal and neonatal outcomes. Am. J. Obstet. Gynecol. 152:176, 1985.
24. Gilstrap LC, et al: Neonatal acidosis and method of delivery. Obstet. Gynecol. 63:681, 1984.
25. Petrie RH, et al: The effect of drugs on uterine activity. Obstet. Gynecol. 48:431, 1976.
26. Ballas S, Taoff ME, Taoff R: Effects of intravenous meperidine and meperidine with promethazine on uterine activity and fetal heart rate during labor. Isr. J. Med. Sci. 12:1141, 1976.
27. DeVoe SJ, Rigsby WC, DeVoe SJ, et al: Effects of meperidine on uterine contractility. Am. J. Obstet. Gynecol. 105:1004, 1969.
28. Filler WW Jr, Hall WC, Filler NW: Analgesia in obstetrics: the effects of analgesia on uterine contractility and fetal heart rate. Am. J. Obstet. Gynecol. 98:832, 1967.
29. Riffel HD, Nochimson DJ, Paul RH, Hon EHG: Effects of meperidine and promethazine during labor. Obstet. Gynecol. 42:738, 1973.
30. Chestnut DH, Bates JN, Choi WW: Continuous infusion epidural analgesia with lidocaine: efficacy and influence during the second stage of labor. Obstet. Gynecol. 69:323–327, 1987.
31. Epstein BS, Banerjee S, Chamberlain G, Coakley CS: The effect of the concentration of local anesthetic during epidural anesthesia on the forces of labor. Anesthesiology 29: 187, 1968.
32. McGaughey HS Jr, Corey EL, Eastwood D, Thorton WM Jr: Effects of synthetic anesthetics on the spontaneous motility of human uterine muscles in vitro. Obstet. Gynecol. 19:233, 1962.
33. Greiss FC, Still GA, Anderson SG: Effects of local anesthetic agents on the uterine vasculatures and myometrium. Am. J. Obstet. Gynecol. 124:889, 1976.
34. Reference deleted.
35. Baxi LV, Petrie RH, James LS: Human fetal oxygenation following paracervical block. Am. J. Obstet. Gynecol. 135: 1109, 1979.
36. Miller FC, Quesnel G, Petrie RH, Paul RH, et al: The effects of paracervical block on uterine activity and beat-to-beat variability of the fetal heart rate. Am. J. Obstet. Gynecol. 130:284, 1978.
37. Jenssen H: The effect of paracervical block on cervical dilatation and uterine activity. Acta. Obstet. Gynecol. Scand. 52: 13, 1973.
38. Berges PU: Regional anesthesia for obstetrics. *In* Clinical Anesthesia. Edited by JJ Bonica. Philadelphia, F.A. Davis, 1971, p. 141.
39. Phillips KC, Thomas TA: Second stage of labour with or without extradural analgesia. Anaesthesia 38:972, 1983.
40. Chestnut DH, Owen Bates JN, Choi WW: Continuous infusion epidural analgesia during labor: a randomized, double-blind comparison of 0.0625% bupivacaine/0.0002% fentanyl versus 0.125% bupivacaine. Anesthesiology 68: 754–759, 1988.
41. Maresch M, Choong KH, Brard RW: Delayed pushing with lumbar epidural analgesia in labour. B. J. Obstet. Gynaecol. 90:623, 1983.
42. Berges PU: Regional anesthesia for obstetrics. *In* Clinical Anesthesia. Edited by JJ Bonica. Philadelphia, F.A. Davis, 1971, p. 141.
43. Akamatsu TJ: Advances in obstetric anesthesiology during the period 1960–1970. *In* Clinical Anesthesia: A Decade of Clinical Progress. Edited by LW Fabian. Philadelphia, F.A. Davis, 1971.
44. Lewis GF, Thomas P, Wilkes RG: Hypotension during epidural analgesia for cesarean section. Anesthesia 38:250, 1983.
45. Thomas P, Buckley P: Maternal and neonatal blood glucose after crystalloid loading for epidural cesarean section. Anesthesia 39:1240, 1984.
46. Brizgys RV, Dailey PA, Shnider SM, Kotelko DM, et al: The incidence and neonatal effects of maternal hypotension during epidural anesthesia for cesarean section. Anesthesiology 67:782–786, 1987.
47. Shnider SM, Levinson G: Anesthesia for cesarean section. *In* Anesthesia for Obstetrics. Edited by SM Shnider, G Levinson. Baltimore, Williams & Wilkins, 1987.
48. Caraitis SN, Abouleish E, Edelstone DI, Mueller-Heubach E: Fetal acid-base state following spinal or epidural anesthesia for cesarean section. Obstet. Gynecol. 56:610, 1980.
49. Kenepp NB, Shelley WC, Gabbe SG, Kumar S, et al: Fetal and neonatal hazards of maternal hydration with 5% dextrose before cesarean section. Lancet 1:1150, 1982.
50. Scanlon JW, et al: Neurobehavioral responses of newborn infants after maternal epidural anesthesia. Anesthesiology 40:121, 1974.
51. Healy LD, Laufe LE: Survey of obstetric forceps training in North America in 1981. Am. J. Obstet. Gynecol. 151:54, 1985.

# Chapter 28

# BREECH AND OTHER ABNORMAL PRESENTATIONS

EDWARD J. QUILLIGAN
KIRK A. KEEGAN, JR.
JOHN S. McDONALD

The dilemma of breech presentation and its subsequent management is not an uncommon event for the obstetrician as approximately 1 in 25 women entering labor will do so with a breech presentation. This fact was confirmed by Morgan and Kane (1), who analyzed 404,817 patients from 117 hospitals during the years 1961 to 1962. They noted 16,327 breech births for an incidence of roughly 4%. Subsequent authors noted a 2.6% incidence at term, and a 4.2% incidence overall, with the higher incidence reflecting the higher prevalence of breech presentation in preterm delivery (2,3). Hickok (4) reporting on 127,171 births in the state of Washington, confirmed the highest incidence of breech (20.6%) at 25 to 26 weeks, and the lowest incidence (1.7%) at greater than 40 weeks gestation (Table 28–1). Ultrasound data (5) in undelivered patients at varying gestational ages suggested similar percentages as that reported by Hickok (Table 28–1). The dilemma is deepened because of the severe complications associated with breech presentation, such as severe threats to maternal and fetal viability with placental previa and cord prolapse complications; such as an increased perinatal morbidity and mortality with prematurity and growth retardation complications; and such as delayed problems with developmental complications that only show up after many years. This chapter will discuss current aspects of breech presentation and aspects of anesthesia for breech delivery, and other abnormal presentations and their anesthesia requirements.

## ETIOLOGY OF BREECH PRESENTATION

Why babies present as breech remains, in part, enigmatic. By design and by nature, as term approaches, the fetus becomes aligned most often in a polar presentation with its long axis parallel to the long axis of the mother. Additionally, the vertex settles in the most dependent portion of the uterine cavity with the breech occupying the top portion. Tompkins (6) reported that previous suspected etiologies such as multiparity and contracted pelvis are noncontributory, and, that in 80% of cases, an etiology is unknown. He did show a correlation with uterine malformations, placenta previa, and fetal anomalies. Fetuses with skeletal and neuromuscular defects limiting fetal mobility have a higher frequency of breech presentation. In fact, fetuses with congenital anomalies, overall, have a higher incidence of breech presentation regardless of birth weight or gestational age (7) (Table 28–2). Brenner (8) reported a threefold increase in anomalies, 6% versus 2%, when comparing breech versus vertex deliveries (Table 28–3).

### Types of Breech Presentation

Breech presentation may be categorized in three ways: (1) frank breech, in which the thighs are flexed against the abdomen and the lower legs are extended; (2) complete breech, in which the thighs are flexed against the abdomen and the lower legs are flexed at the knee; and (3) footling breech, in which one or both legs are extended at the hip and knee. Frank breech is the most common presentation, with an approximate incidence of 38% in infants weighing less than 2500 grams. In those infants weighing greater than 2500 grams, the incidence varies from 51 to 73% (9–11). Complete breech is less common in both infants weighing less than 2500 grams, 12%, and in infants weighing over 2500 grams, ranging from 5 to 12%. Footling breech presentations represent 50% of all breech infants weighing less than 2500 grams, and 20 to 24% of infants weighing greater than 2500 grams. Type of breech presentation, as seen below, impacts greatly on subsequent obstetric management of delivery.

### Rationale for Delivery—Vaginal or Cesarean Section?

The management of breech presentation has undergone a significant change in the past 30 years. Prior to 1970, the majority of breech presentations were delivered vaginally. While many obstetricians viewed a breech vaginal delivery with trepidation, it was also felt to be a mark of skill if one could successfully conduct such a delivery. In 1939, Joseph B. D. Lee wrote: "Let me watch a man conduct a breech case and I will give you his obstetrical rating." A shift toward delivery of a breech by cesarean section began in the 1960s, and by the late 1970s, most breeches were being delivered by cesarean section. Three major factors influenced this change in management: (1) the improved safety of cesarean section for both mother and child; (2) a legal climate in which any damaged infant was cause for malpractice litigation; and (3) a number of articles pointing out a significant increase in morbidity and mortality in the infant presenting as a breech.

**Table 28–1.** Breech Presentation by Gestational Age at Delivery

| Weeks Gestation | % Breech (Scheer) n = 2276 | % Breech (Hill) n = 4024 | % Breech (WA State) n = 127,171 |
|---|---|---|---|
| 25–26 | 31.8+ | N.A. | 20.6 |
| 27–28 | 24.9 | 24.4 | 21.7 |
| 29–30 | 16.0 | 18.7+ | 11.5 |
| 31–32 | 12.7+ | 13.3+ | 7.4 |
| 33–34 | 10.8+ | 9.4 | 6.3 |
| 35–36 | 7.0 | 6.8 | 4.9 |
| 37–38 | 7.0+ | 3.7* | 3.6 |
| 39–40 | 6.1+ | N.A. | 2.6 |
| >40 | N.A. | N.A. | 1.7 |

* reported for 37–40 weeks
+ two-sided p value $< 0.05$ ($X^2$ test comparing each study with Washington state)
(From Hickok DE, Gordon DC, Milberg JA, Williams MA, et al: The frequency of breech presentation by gestational age at birth: a large population-based study. Am. J. Obstet. Gynecol. 1992;166:851–2.)

In Morgan and Kane's large study of over 16,000 breech births, the overall perinatal mortality rate (PMR) for breech birth was 151/1000 live births compared to a rate of 28/1000 live births for the entire study population. Much of this increase in perinatal mortality associated with breech delivery was attributed to a significantly higher percentage of babies weighing less than 2500 grams, 32% in the breech group, as compared to only 8.7% in the entire series. However, even when the low-birthweight infant was excluded, the perinatal mortality rate for breech term infants was 30/1000 live births while that for the entire study group was 8.4/1000 live births. This fourfold increase in perinatal mortality in term breech infants was also confirmed by Todd and Steer (2). Patterson, et al (11) correcting for antepartum stillbirth, lethal anomalies, and maternal and fetal complications unrelated to fetal position such as abruption and erythroblastosis, showed a fivefold increase in mortality rates for breech, 19.1/1000 versus 4.1/1000 live births in vertex presentations. They suggested that this increase in perinatal mortality in breech births was due to an increase in low-birthweight infants, congenital malformations, umbilical cord prolapse during labor, and, most importantly, birth trauma.

Ruben and Grimm (12) reported a thirteen-fold increase in the incidence of birth trauma in vaginal breech deliveries, 6.7% versus 0.05% when compared to cephalic deliveries. Gold, et al (13), in an analysis of 157,969 live births in New York City, reported 274 cases of severe birth injury for an overall incidence of 1.7/1000 live births. Breech deliveries in this series sustained severe birth injury at a rate of 14/1000 live births, significantly higher than cephalic presentations, but at a lower rate than that reported by Ruben and Grimm. Types of injuries most frequently described in the Gold, et al series were tentorial tears, cephalohematomas, disruptions of the spinal cord, brachial plexus palsys, fractures of the long bones, and rupture of the sternocleidomastoid muscles. Tentorial tears were more frequently associated with breech extraction. The more common injuries associated with assisted breech deliveries were nerve and spinal cord injuries. These injuries in general result from excessive traction on the infant during the delivery. The brachial plexus is particularly susceptible to injury during breech delivery. Tan (14), in an analysis of 90,436 births over a 3-year period, documented 57 cases of brachial plexus palsy for an overall incidence of 0.6/1000 live births. This incidence rose to 24.5/1000 live births for breech deliveries. Brans and Cassady (15) reported actual transections of the spinal cord and fractures of the cervical vertebra in two-thirds of the spinal cord lesions associated with breech delivery. Earlier, Wilcox (16) had made the association of spinal cord damage during the delivery process and hyperextension of the fetal head. This correlation was confirmed by Caterini, et al (17) who studied 73 breech infants delivered vaginally with hyperextended heads. Injuries to the central nervous system resulted in death in 10, (13.7%), compared to no deaths in a similar group of 35 infants delivered by cesarean section. They also noted a significant reduction in the incidence of medullar or vertebral injuries in those babies born by cesarean sec-

**Table 28–2.** Frequency of Breech Presentation in Disorders

| Disorder | No. of Cases | Percentage of Breech Presentation | Expected Percentage for Birthweight | Relative Difference |
|---|---|---|---|---|
| Prader-Willi syndrome | 22 | 50 | 3.9 | 12.8 |
| 18 trisomy syndrome | 14 | 43 | 7.1 | 6.1 |
| Smith-Lemil-Opitz syndrome | 20 | 40 | 3.2 | 12.5 |
| Fetal alcohol syndrome | 10 | 40 | 8.2 | 4.9 |
| Potter anomaly | 87 | 36 | 7.7 | 4.7 |
| Zellweger syndrome | 15 | 27 | 3.7 | 7.2 |
| Myotonic dystrophy | 14 | 21 | 3.7 | 5.7 |
| 13 trisomy syndrome | 8 | 12 | 6.0 | 2.0 |
| Werdnig-Hoffman syndrome | 10 | 10 | 2.6 | 3.8 |
| de Lange syndrome | 52 | 10 | 5.6 | 1.7 |
| 21 trisomy syndrome | 39 | 5 | 2.7 | 2.0 |

(From Braun FT, Jone KL, Smith DW: Breech presentation as an indicator of fetal abnormality. J. Pediatrics. 1975;86:419.)

**Table 28–3.** Rates of Congenital Abnormalities Among 1016 Breech and 29,343 Nonbreech Consecutive Deliveries

| | Over-all (%) | | 36 or More Weeks' Gestation (%) | |
|---|---|---|---|---|
| | Breech | Nonbreech | Breech | Nonbreech |
| Central nervous system | 0.8 | 0.2 | 0.8 | 0.2 |
| Hydrocephalus | 0.5 | 0.1 | 0.7 | 0.0 |
| Anencephalus | 0.2 | 0.0 | 0.1 | 0.0 |
| Urinary system | 0.8 | 0.6 | 0.7 | 0.5 |
| Cardiovascular system | 1.0 | 0.5 | 0.7 | 0.5 |
| Respiratory and gastrointestinal systems | 1.5 | 0.4 | 1.1 | 0.3 |
| Inguinal hernia | 0.9 | 0.1 | 0.4 | 0.0 |
| Down's syndrome | 0.2 | 0.1 | 0.3 | 0.1 |
| Skeletal system | 0.9 | 0.5 | 0.8 | 0.5 |
| Multiple abnormalities | 1.1 | 0.1 | 0.6 | 0.1 |
| Central nervous system predominant | 0.3 | 0.0 | 0.1 | 0.0 |
| Cardiovascular system predominant | 0.3 | 0.0 | 0.0 | 0.0 |
| Total congenital abnormalities | 6.3 | 2.4 | 5.0 | 2.1 |

(From Brenner WE, Bruce RD, Hendricks CH: The characteristics and perils of breech presentation. Am. J. Obstet. Gynecol. 1974;118:700–709.)

tion, (5.7%) as compared to a 20.6% incidence in the 73 babies born vaginally. Furthermore, the incidence of meningohemorrhages was 6.8% in the vaginal group and 0.0% in the cesarean section group.

It was, therefore, this increase in perinatal morbidity and mortality associated with breech presentation, plus the perception that both morbidity and mortality would be significantly decreased if the breech were delivered by cesarean section, that produced the significant shift in the mode of delivery during the 1970s. This shift in thinking has persisted to the present, with the vast majority of those babies in breech presentation when the mother enters labor being delivered by cesarean section.

Despite the apparent benefits of cesarean section delivery, it is clear that even under optimal circumstances, cesarean section is associated with a twofold increase in maternal death, increased maternal morbidity, and increased cost to the health care system. Are there alternative strategies that can be pursued? At least two such strategies need to be addressed: (1) reducing the incidence of breech presentation: and (2) vaginal delivery of selected breeches.

Reducing the incidence of breech presentation using external cephalic version has been in use by some obstetricians for many years. Initially, it was suggested that version be performed before the thirty-sixth week of gestation as the baby could then be more easily turned because of the increased ratio of amniotic fluid to baby. Ranney (18), utilizing this technique, reported a 1.1% incidence of breech presentation at term. He noted a higher success rate if the version was performed before 37 weeks, but unfortunately, one-third of babies verted to vertex at 36 weeks or less reverted to breech presentation by term. In 1974, Saling (19) suggested that external cephalic version might be more easily performed after 37 weeks if one utilized beta-sympathomimetic drugs for uterine relaxation. Using this technique, he found a success rate of 75% and a reduction from 3.8% to 1.6% in the incidence of breech presentation at term. Tocolytics are now invariably used for version attempts after 36 to 37 weeks gestation.

Van Dorsten, et al (20), in one of the first prospective randomized trials on external version, noted a 68% version success rate in the study group with all patients entering labor with a vertex presentation. In those patients in which version failed, all patients entered labor with breech presentation, and 75% were delivered by cesarean section. In the control, nonversion group, only 18% of babies spontaneously verted to a cephalic presentation after 37 weeks.

The management reported by Van Dorsten is the one most frequently followed today; that is, breech presentation is confirmed by ultrasound late at 36 to 37 weeks gestation, or early by examination at less than 20 weeks with normal interval growth. After this, a nonstress test is performed to confirm fetal reactivity, tocolysis is begun using ritodrine, terbutaline or magnesium sulfate, and following uterine relaxation, an external cephalic version is performed while monitoring the fetal heart rate with ultrasound. If there is fetal bradycardia, the version attempt is halted. If the fetal heart rate returns to normal, the version can be re-attempted. If the fetal heart rate remains slow, the baby is repositioned to a breech. Persistent fetal bradycardia is managed by immediate cesarean section. Following the version, either successful or unsuccessful, a repeat nonstress test is performed, and if reactive, the patient is discharged from the hospital. Rh-negative patients should receive Rh immune globulin.

Subsequent studies on external version have noted success rates varying from 48% to 77% (21,22). Several factors have been reported to impact upon the efficacy of external cephalic version and may explain the wide variation in success rates. Ferguson, et al (22) found that decreased amniotic fluid volume and fetal abdominal circumference less than the fifth percentile for gestational age in a nonfrank breech, were significant factors in decreasing the success rate in their series. Van Dorsten (20) found that the only factor decreasing success was maternal weight in excess of 175 lbs. Hellstrom (23) found the critical factors to be a reduction in the amniotic fluid volume, extended fetal legs, and the maternal primigravid state. Morrison, et al (24), on the other hand, found the only significant factor in his series to be a gestational age greater than 40 weeks.

The complications of external cephalic version are, fortunately, infrequent. Reversion, which occurs frequently before 36 weeks gestation, occurs in less than 5% of cases after 37 weeks gestation. Severe fetal maternal bleeding is rare; however, one massive hemorrhage resulting in fetal death has been reported (25). Small fetal-maternal transfusion occurs more commonly. Gjode (26) found that 28% of his 50 patients had significant increases in fetal red cells in the maternal circulation after attempted version. These bleeds were in the range of 0.1 to 1.5 ml. However, because as little as 0.1 ml of fetal blood can immunize an Rh-negative mother, it is important that consideration of Rh immune globulin be given in these cases. One can routinely give Rh immune globulin to all Rh-negative mothers following version attempts, or test maternal blood for fetal cells before and after the version and administer immune globulin if an increase in cells is noted.

Fetal bradycardia during version attempts occurs in up to 30% of cases, but it usually is transitory and does not constitute true fetal distress. However, in about 2% of cases, true fetal distress will occur. In these instances, prudent management demands immediate delivery, which will be perfectly safe for the fetus because it is beyond 37 weeks gestation. Fetal death from premature separation of the placenta and/or cord prolapse has been mentioned as a potential complication of version. However, Scaling reviewed eight studies (27) with 1144 version attempts after 37 weeks, and only one fetal death was noted (27,28). A failed version is not technically a complication, but its management requires discussion. Because the spontaneous version rate following a failed external version, in most series, is very low, 5%, the patient will usually enter labor with a breech presentation. If one follows the philosophy that all patients with breech presentations entering labor undergo cesarean section, immediate cesarean section following a failed version avoids the possibility of interval rupture of the membranes, with its attendant risk of significant fetal morbidity and/or mortality, particularly if it occurs in a nonhospital setting. It is therefore prudent to confirm fetal lung maturity using either accepted clinical or laboratory parameters, before attempting external version.

Despite the widespread philosophy of cesarean section for all breeches, there are a number of problems with proving this concept scientifically. The majority of studies demonstrating a significantly greater perinatal mortality in the vaginally born breech infant are retrospective, frequently group all gestational ages, and compare breech presentation to cephalic presentation. As an example, perinatal mortality as reported by Morgan and Kane was $5\frac{1}{2}$ times greater in the breech infant than in the nonbreech infant, and $3\frac{1}{2}$ times greater when the premature breech was excluded. Interestingly, however, when the mode of vaginal breech delivery (spontaneous) in infants weighing greater than 2500 grams was compared, the perinatal mortality was similar, 24/1000 in both vaginal and cesarean section groups. A significant reduction in perinatal mortality was noted only in the elective repeat cesarean section group. However, in the same study, if one looked at all weights, the perinatal mortality in breech spontaneous vaginal delivery was 242/1000 as compared to cesarean sections, which was 76/1000 live births. This huge difference can only be accounted for by an excess perinatal mortality in infants weighing less than 2500 grams. Brenner, et al (8) noted similar findings of a higher perinatal mortality rate in vaginally delivered breech infants at 39 weeks or less, and no difference in perinatal mortality when comparing vaginal delivery and cesarean section at 40 to 43 weeks. The first prospective randomized study of vaginal delivery versus cesarean section for the breech infant was performed by Collea, et al (9). They chose a group of "ideal" candidates in which the infants were term, with an estimated fetal weight (EFW) of less than 4000 grams, had frank breech presentations, adequate maternal pelvimetry by x ray, and then randomized them to either elective cesarean section or vaginal delivery. A total of 55 patients comprised the elective cesarean section group and 67 patients were randomized to vaginal delivery. In the latter group, 32 were sectioned for an inadequate pelvis and 5 for failed labor, leaving 30 patients who delivered vaginally. There was essentially no difference in the Apgar scores of the elective cesarean section versus the vaginal delivery group. However, there were two cases of mild Erbs' palsy in the vaginal delivery group. Gimovsky, et al (29), also in a prospective randomized fashion, expanded the series by including nonfrank breeches. Of the 70 patients randomized to a trial of labor, 31 subsequently delivered vaginally. There were essentially no differences in the outcomes of the two groups with the single exception of a perinatal mortality in the vaginal delivery group. This occurred in a patient who, without anesthesia, became hysterical on the delivery table; the fetal head was trapped for 5 minutes. An easily accomplished assisted breech delivery was accomplished after the administration of anesthesia.

Flanagan, et al (30) reviewed 716 cases of breech presentation that incorporated selected external version, trial of labor, and cesarean section without trial of labor. Those patients with trials of labor had to have an estimated fetal weight less than 3850 grams, a flexed fetal head, and normal pelvic capacity by x ray. External version was attempted in approximately 24% of the total group, with a success rate of 49%. Cesarean section was performed in 379 without a trial of labor, a failed trial of labor occurred in 69, and vaginal delivery was successful in 175 (28% of total). No differences were noted in perinatal outcome for any method of delivery. One infant in the vaginal delivery group had a facial nerve paralysis with a suspected prenatal etiology. Barlov and Larsson (31) prospectively analyzed 226 singleton term breech births at the Central Hospital in Karlskrona, Sweden. X-ray pelvimetry proved inadequate in 102 patients (45%), and these patients were delivered by cesarean section. A total of 124 patients underwent a trial of labor, of which 101 (82%) were successful. The remaining 23 patients underwent cesarean section for indications arising during labor. There were no neonatal mortalities in the vaginal delivery group. One infant in the cesarean section group expired from multiple malformations incompatible with life. There were in this study, however, more neurologic problems in the vaginally delivered group, including one baby with brachial plexus palsy, one with cerebral irritation, and two with intracranial hemorrhage. It would appear, therefore, that while there is essentially no difference in overall perinatal morbidity and mortality in the well-selected vaginally delivered infant compared to the abdominally delivered infant, there is a slightly higher incidence of transcient neurologic damage in the vaginal group.

Long-term assessment of morbidity in breech vaginal versus cesarean section delivery is more difficult to assess, as there are no prospective randomized studies available. Neligan, et al (32) reported on 185 children delivered as breech who attended normal schools in the district of Newcastle. There were two mild cases of cerebral palsy in this group, giving an incidence of 1.1%. This was compared with a 1.8/1000 incidence of cerebral palsy in the total Newcastle survey population. They found essentially no difference in the Goodonough IQ at 5 years and nonverbal IQ at 10 years between breech infants delivered vaginally and those by cesarean section. McBride, et al (33) compared 101 vertex presenting infants delivered by elective cesarean section with 100 breech presenting children (82 of which delivered vaginally) and found essentially no difference in IQ or coordination. Croughan-Minihane, et al (34) in a report from the Northern California Kaiser Hospital population, studied 1240 nonanomalous singleton breech infants delivered between 1976 and 1977. They found, using multiple logistic regression to control for confounding variables, essentially no difference in the relative risk for asphyxia, head trauma, neonatal seizures, cerebral palsy, or developmental delay in this predominantly term group of patients when they compared vaginally born with cesarean section delivered infants. Thus, based on the data which is neither prospective or controlled, it would appear that there is essentially no difference in long-term outcome in term vaginally delivered versus cesarean section delivered infants.

For the infant weighing less than 2500 grams, there is a rather general impression that the infant should be delivered by cesarean section. This is based on retrospective studies showing a significantly higher incidence of perinatal mortality in the vaginally delivered premature infant, as compared to that infant delivered by cesarean section (1,8). However, even in the premature infant, more recent studies are not uniform in demonstrating that cesarean section is the preferred method of delivery. Bodmer, et al (35) compared two time periods, 1961 to 1974, when the cesarean section rate for premature breeches was 8%, to 1978 to 1984, when 89% of premature breeches were delivered by cesarean section. They found, despite the increased cesarean section rate, no difference in the incidence of either severe depression at birth, or perinatal mortality between the two time periods when one compared breech and cephalic deliveries. They did note, however, a 13% incidence of trapped fetal heads in vaginal breech deliveries weighing less than 1000 grams. Kitchen, et al (36) examined 326 infants of which 117 were breech deliveries, born between 24 to 28 weeks gestation. They looked at 14 different obstetric variables and found no difference in those infants delivered vaginally as compared to those delivered by cesarean section. Gimovsky and Paul (37) reported a benefit of cesarean section in infants weighing less than 1500 grams. However, in an analysis of their article by Myers and Gleicher (38), it was pointed out that the majority of the deaths in the vaginally delivered group occurred in infants who weighed less than 750 grams. Oleajn, et al (39) also failed to document the benefit of more frequent cesarean section in the less than 1500-gram breech infant.

Conversely, Duenhoelter, et al (40) identified 44 breech pairs weighing between 1000 to 2499 grams delivered between 1972 to 1977 and matched them for mode of delivery. They noted seven deaths in the vaginally delivered group as compared to one death in the cesarean section group. Ingemarsson, et al (41) compared 42 preterm breech infants delivered by cesarean section between 1975 and 1977 with 48 preterm breech infants delivered vaginally between 1971 to 1974. These infants were followed for a minimum of 2 to 4 years. They found that cesarean section significantly reduced the frequency of prolonged asphyxia and neonatal mortality from 14.6% to 4.8%. At 12 months of age, 24% of those preterm infants delivered vaginally had developed mental or neurologic abnormalities, compared to 2.5% of those infants delivered by cesarean section. In a study such as this, however, it is almost impossible to control for changes in therapy during the two time periods, thereby diminishing the study's impact.

In sum, antepartum patients presenting with a breech at 37 weeks should be considered for external cephalic version. After appropriate informed consent, vaginal breech delivery of the selected term breech appears to be a viable alternative to universal cesarean section. In the premature infant (less than 1500 gms), there appears to be reasonable, but not absolute, evidence to recommend cesarean section as the optimal mode of delivery. In the 1500- to 2500-gram infant, there is no solid evidence that would preclude a trial of labor in selected breech presentations.

## Anesthetic Management of the Breech

The results obtained from a delivery of a breech may be in large part directly related to the anesthetic employed and the skill with which it was delivered. Many of the poor-outcome statistics noted in the earlier portion of this chapter may well have been due to forced delivery of a breech under conditions of little or no pelvic muscle relaxation and analgesia. Unfortunately, these statistics do not detail the type of anesthesia used, and the intensity of muscle relaxation will never be known. Under the most ideal conditions of breech delivery, good analgesia and good relaxation are vitally important to the maneuver.

Well administered analgesia and anesthesia facilitate the delivery and decrease the hazards to the mother and infant; however, improper administration may adversely affect the existing physiopathology, produce its own complications, and thus compromise the baby. For optimal results, it is necessary to adhere to certain logical principles. These principles are common sense and in line with those highlighted throughout this book and really distill down to careful, thorough, and thoughtful consideration of the condition of both the mother and fetus and all the other conditions that may impact on their safety before pain relief techniques are instituted. All of these considerations must be evaluated and discussed within the framework of the obstetric requirements so that once again it becomes apparent that both colleagues are closely involved in decision-making strategies in regard to the final welfare of the mother and her infant. In every breech delivery, it is desirable to provide: (1) adequate pain relief and a quiet operative field; (2) relaxation of the perineum and birth canal; and (3) effective maternal use of her own auxiliary forces of labor. In addition, there are times when uterine relaxation is required should manipulation or instrumentation be necessary. The importance of each of these requirements varies from patient to patient, so that each patient must be considered individually. This section of the chapter will discuss these issues for the breech for vaginal birth and for the breech for cesarean birth.

## Vaginal Breech Delivery

The obstetrician has the responsibility to communicate to the anesthesiologist his/her intention in regard to the plan for delivery. The delivery of a breech vaginally can basically be performed by three defined methods: (1) spontaneous breech delivery; (2) assisted breech delivery; and (3) complete breech extraction. Each method has its own requisites for analgesia and anesthesia, which will be discussed below.

### Spontaneous Breech Delivery

In the case of anticipated vaginal delivery with normal labor pattern, dilatation, and descent, the patient may be in need of pain relief for contractions. The strategy in spontaneous breech delivery is for the patient to spontaneously deliver the baby to the umbilicus, at which time the obstetrician can take over and assist the delivery of the head by positioning the baby correctly. But here, the mother pushes until birth of the head occurs, with positioning of utmost importance, of course. The particular requisites for pain relief and relaxation include the following: (1) pain relief for contractions; (2) no pain relief for vaginal and perineal distension; (3) no muscular relaxation of the vagina or pelvic musculature; and (4) a mother with an intact perineal reflex who can voluntarily push very hard to get the baby delivered spontaneously. A possible technique would be the epidural with the dilute combination of local anesthetic, opioid, and epinephrine with slow continuous infusion. This will allow adequate pain relief from contractions and full control of the mother's abdominal reflex musculature for pushing when deemed necessary. The one admonition is to do a perineal sensory check hourly to make sure that the sensory input from the perineum is still intact. Many times, after 3 to 4 hours of labor and by the time for delivery, the perineum has adequate sensory denervation so that distension of the lower birth canal and even perineal distension and episiotomy are painless due to the several hours of low-dose combination infusion mentioned above. In this case, we are in need of a completely intact perineum so that it can serve as an adequate stimulus for generation of a tremendous Valsalva to help descent and delivery spontaneously of the breech baby. If there is evidence of perineal sensory loss during the hourly exams, the continuous infusion can be turned off and the sensory input will return rapidly. Another technique that can be used is the continuous spinal, which allows small intermittent injections of isobaric or hyperbaric dilute local anesthetic so that just a few segments from T10 through T12 or L1 and L2 are denervated. This allows for pain relief for uterine contractions while again sparing the abdominal musculature that may be needed for maternal voluntary pushing during second stage descent of the breech. This method also allows for flexibility and control of the first stage requirements separate from those of the second stage. It is very plain by now that these requirements are quite different and thus demand the flexibility of timing and differential effect of analgesia versus muscular relaxation. When delivery is imminent, perineal analgesia can be achieved through pudendal block or inhalation analgesia using a $N_2O/O_2$ combination, an inhalation agent/$O_2$ combination, or by supplementation of the pudendal block with one of the latter inhalation techniques. It is important to keep in mind that these latter methods are truly analgesic concentrations with the patient being awake and conversant throughout the entire procedure. This is a method that is performed with the mask and demands experience and skill by the operator, but which is very safe when correctly administered. This is distinct from the rapid sequence induction and intubation, for use when uterine and pelvic and perineal relaxation is demanded short term during assisted breech delivery and complete breech extraction, of which will be described shortly.

### Assisted Breech Delivery

In earlier days, there were many who advocated local anesthetic perineal infiltration or pudendal block during spontaneous breech delivery; experience soon dictated that anesthesiologists were needed at that time for the performance of rapid institution of general anesthesia if it became necessary for assisted breech delivery. The latter is defined as assistance in delivery after the baby is spontaneously delivered to the umbilicus. In this method, the head is delivered by use of the Mauriceau-Smellie-Veit maneuver or by use of the Piper forceps applied to the aftercoming head. The particular requisites for pain relief and relaxation include the following: (1) pain relief for contractions; (2) pain relief for vaginal and perineal distension; (3) muscular relaxation of the vagina or pelvic musculature; and (4) a mother with an intact or ablated perineal reflex who does not need to voluntarily push after delivery to the umbilicus. A possible technique of anesthesia for this delivery method could be use of the epidural with the continuous infusion combination referred to above. In this case, in which assisted breech delivery is planned anyway, there is no need to be concerned about a sensory denervated perineum. Naturally, as in all of these breech deliveries, it is important that the anesthesiologist be present to work closely with the obstetrician in regard to progress of the delivery. When the obstetrician decides to assist the delivery, he/she wants there to be adequate perineal, vaginal, and uterine relaxation so that he/she can rotate the shoulders, sweep the arms down, and perform the Mauriceau-Smellie-Veit maneuver or apply the Piper forceps. There usually is this amount of relaxation, but if not, the anesthesiologist may be asked to quickly induce the patient and provide the same. This anesthetic task is performed by use of the rapid sequence induction and administration of a potent inhalation agent, such as isoflurane or enflurane. There may still be those who insist that halothane is the only effective uterine relaxant, but the literature now substantiates the fact that other agents are also effective as adequate uterine relaxants when given in adequate concentrations. For example, in Table 28–4, note the inclusion of "uterine relaxation" under the heading of disadvantages. Though this effect of isoflurane may be viewed as a disadvantage, in the case of desired relaxation, it may be adjudged an advantage. Also, it is important to realize that halothane is being used less and less today. With that recognition and the recognition that it still carries the stigmata of hepatic injury as a possibility, it probably will remain a poor choice for use in obstetrics in the future. One recent study confirmed the feasibility of use of either isoflurane 1.25% with 100% oxygen or enflurane 1.5% with 100% oxygen for obstetrics, and the requisites of no maternal awareness and no fetal depression were fulfilled.(42).

In the past, the regional techniques such as subarachnoid, caudal, and epidural blocks were considered contraindicated for use in breech delivery because they were alleged to: (1) decrease uterine contractions and thus prolong the first and second stages of labor; and (2) eliminate the auxiliary forces and thus make spontaneous delivery of the infant or the breech in partial extraction impossible.

There was also a paradoxical belief that these regional procedures increased uterine contractility and therefore were contraindicated in breech extractions. Serious consideration of the effects of these techniques makes it obvious that these are not valid arguments. If these procedures are not begun prematurely, uterine contractions are not diminished. Occasionally, there is diminished uterine contractility for a few minutes after the local anesthetic is started, but then very soon the uterus resumes contractions with the same intensity and duration. In some patients, contractions were found to be enhanced by the relief of pain and elimination of the effects of anxiety and fear. Moreover, the effective perineal relaxation provided by the block can aid rather than impede the progress of labor by eliminating the resisting forces of the perineum.

**Table 28–4.** Advantages and Disadvantages of Isoflurane

| Advantages | Disadvantages |
|---|---|
| No hepatic/renal toxicity | Pungent odor |
| Low blood gas solubility | Respiratory depression |
| Low arrhythmogenic potential | Uterine relaxation |
| Good muscle relaxation | Reduced blood pressure |

(From Wade JG, Stevens WC: Isoflurane: an anesthetic for the eighties. Anesth. Analg. Sept 1981, 60(9), pp. 666–682.)

The argument that extradural and subarachnoid blocks eliminate the auxiliary forces of labor is also not valid. It is true, of course, that these techniques eliminate the afferent limb of the reflex mechanism, which creates the patient's urge to bear down. It is also true that the auxiliary forces are necessary for spontaneous breech delivery and partial breech extraction. However, if the patient is not oversedated and is cooperative, she can be coached to bear down effectively. Certainly, she has the power to do so, for, if analgesia does not extend above the tenth thoracic dermatome, the diaphragm and intercostal and abdominal muscles are not affected if the concentration of the local anesthetic does not exceed analgesic doses. Even if maximum therapeutic concentrations such as 2% lidocaine are used, some of the muscles are not weakened because motor blockade usually extends only to two to three segments below the level of analgesia. For the patient to use these forces effectively, it is necessary that she be able to cooperate and that the obstetric nurse, anesthesiologist or obstetrician coach her so she will bring the forces into action at the optimal time, that is, when uterine contractions occur during the second stage. The fact that the urge to bear down is eliminated without significantly impairing the parturient's muscular ability to bear down permits better control of the rate of the delivery. The patient who is cooperative can be coached just when to push and when not to push, thus giving some individual control over the voluntary effort. This obviates the danger of hasty delivery, and thus reduces the incidence of intracranial hemorrhage, one of the primary causes of perinatal mortality and morbidity. There is no intent to try to equate the pushing force present when the breech reaches the sensory intact perineum, which is an overwhelming tremendous forceful effect, to the pushing force present when the breech reaches the sensory denervated perineum under coaching as just outlined. As admitted, the force of the former is certainly more impressive than the force of the latter. But the point is, that with good coaching, persistence, and a good attitude on the part of the patient, the latter method can also effectively result in adequate progress of descent and even delivery of the breech to a point at which an assisted breech delivery can be conducted.

There was also a camp of belief that regional anesthesia was contraindicated solely because there may be a need for general anesthesia in the middle of the delivery. At a national meeting attended by one of the authors (John S. McDonald), Crawford stated; "The superimposition of general anaesthesia upon regional block is neither aesthetically satisfying, nor conducive to ideal patient-doctor or anaesthetist-obstetrician relationship, especially when the change of course occurs in mid-operation." Although gen-

**Table 28–5.** Combined General and Regional Analgesia

1. The procedure is executed skillfully by one with sufficient experience with it;
2. The anesthetic management of the parturient, after the block is started and throughout labor and delivery, is in the hands of a physician who has no other duties;
3. Hypotension is minimized or prevented by an intravenous infusion of 300 to 500 ml of lactated Ringer's solution just before the block;
4. Oxygen is administered during the entire second stage of labor; and
5. Optimal obstetric care is given.

erally this statement is correct, there are instances in which it is absolutely necessary to protect the well-being of the mother and the baby, and that a general anesthetic may have to be superimposed on a regional anesthetic that is partially functional. In other words, this superimposition is of importance to the mother and the baby and also the obstetrician who needs to complete the operative maneuver or procedure. In another sense, the concommitant use of general and regional anesthesia is also interpreted as use of a balanced anesthesia technique, which, strictly defined, is the combined use of several agents for the purpose of exploiting their therapeutic actions while at the same time minimizing or eliminating their disadvantages. In this case, the spinal blocks fulfill more specifically the first three basic requirements for breech delivery rather than other methods without accompanying depression of the mother or fetus. That the blocks do not produce uterine relaxation does not detract from their value, because these blocks can be complemented with a potent inhalation anesthetic for the very short time that may be needed. By restricting use of the general anesthetic to the brief period in which uterine relaxation is needed, any of the depressant effects are significantly decreased.

That such benefits are derived by the fetus, newborn, and the mother from continuous caudal, continuous epidural, and subarachnoid blocks is attested by reports from all those medical centers where these techniques are used for breech delivery (43–47). In each of these centers, perinatal mortality in patients to whom regional anesthesia was given was consistently lower than that in those managed with general anesthesia, especially among premature births. Finally, neonatal depression and morbidity were significantly less because of lack of direct depressant action with this form of analgesia and because of better obstetric conditions (48–50). For those same reasons, maternal complications were less, and the length of labor often decreased (48,51).

These aforementioned benefits of the combination of the general technique superimposed upon a regional block accrue only if the conditions in Table 28–5 are met. Lack of skill and experience on the part of the physician who is to administer the anesthetic or the one who attempts delivery are contraindications to the use of this described method of anesthesia.

## *The Complete Breech Extraction*

Total extraction of the infant, defined as complete breech extraction, is simply not indicated today under any circumstances, with the lone possible exception of the delivery of a second twin. Wells, et al looked at twin deliverers over a 5-year period and concentrated specifically on those situations in which twin B was a nonvertex. They compared the three delivery routes: (1) primary abdominal delivery; (2) breech extraction of the second twin; and (3) external version of the second twin. There was no difference in neonatal outcome between the three delivery routes except for the fact that mothers in the external version group were more likely than those in the breech extraction group to undergo abdominal delivery (52). Gocke, et al looked at 682 consecutive twin deliveries. There were 136 sets of vertex, nonvertex twins whose birthweights were greater than 1500 gms. External version was attempted on 41 twins, 55 twins attempted breech extraction, and 40 had primary cesarean section. There was no difference in the neonatal morbidity or mortality among the modes of delivery. However, again external version was associated with a higher failure rate than was primary breech extraction, and there were more fetal complications than cesarean section or breech extraction (53).

Complete breech extraction is certainly not indicated during problems associated with labor, which are usually confined to the realm of descent, i.e., failure to descent. There may be some acute emergency occurring during breech delivery that may necessitate rapid breech extraction, e.g., prolapse of fetal part or umbilical cord with some evidence of fetal compromise.

Timing for interaction between the obstetrician and anesthesiologist is crucial in such maneuvers. Best results occur when both are completely informed and updated on the planned strategies of both obstetric and anesthetic viewpoints. To protect the fetus, a quiet, relaxed delivery field is needed, which includes uterine relaxation. The particular requisites for pain relief and relaxation include those listed in Table 28–6. In other words, the requisites for this delivery method are the same as those for the assisted breech delivery. From the obstetric viewpoint, the only difference is that in complete breech extraction, there is aggressive movement toward delivery from the breech onward, i.e., not waiting for the spontaneous delivery of the baby up to the umbilicus of the fetus. In essence, there is no difference from the viewpoint of the anesthesiologist.

When anesthesia of the perineum and birth canal and uterine relaxation have been achieved, a thorough vaginal examination is carried out to: (1) ascertain the degree of cervical dilation and the nature of the breech position; (2) rupture the membranes if they are still intact; and (3) carefully search for the umbilical cord. If the fetus is found

**Table 28–6.** Pain Relief Requisites

Requisites for pain relief and relaxation include:
1. pain relief for contractions;
2. pain relief for vaginal and perineal distension;
3. muscular relaxation of the vagina or pelvis musculature; and
4. a mother with an intact or ablated perineal reflex who does not need to voluntarily push after delivery to the umbilicus.

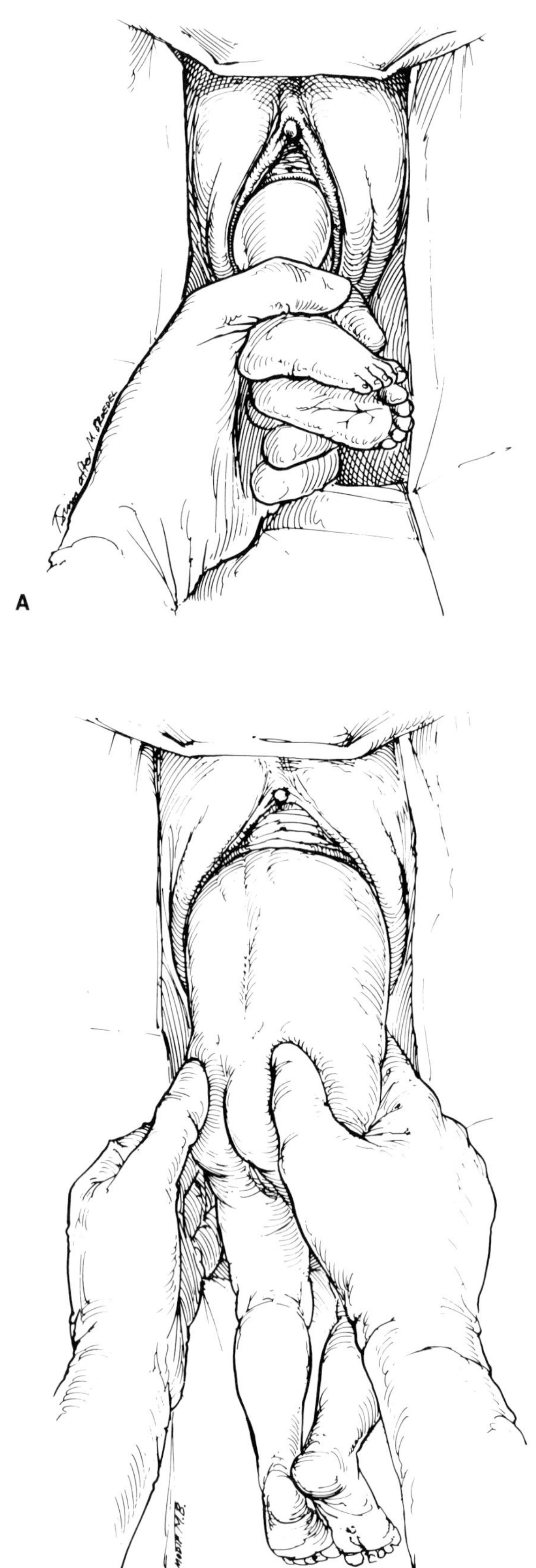

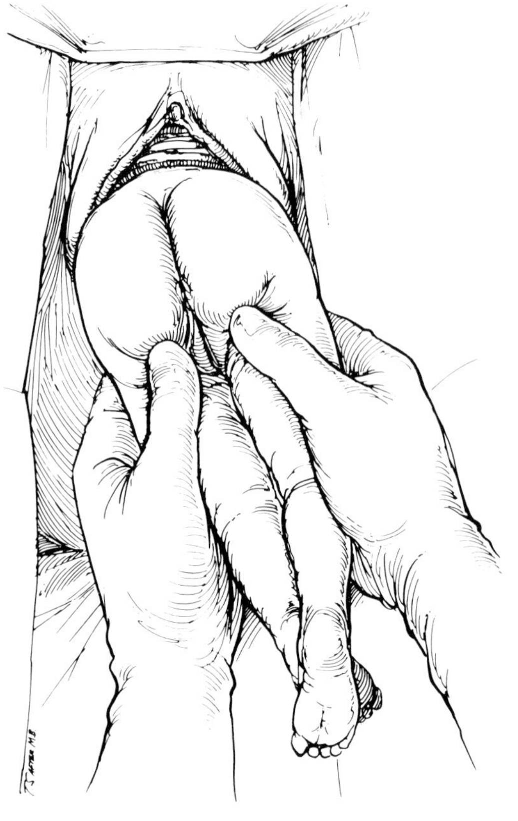

**Fig. 28–1.** Complete breech extraction. **(A)** The legs are locked securely between the operator's fingers and gentle downward pressure is exerted to aid in descent of the breech. **(B)** Both hands are adjusted to lock onto the upper femur so that continued downward pressure can be exerted to aid in delivery of the breech. **(C)** The breech is grasped by both hands with gentle downward pressure continued to effect delivery of the shoulder. (From Cunningham FG, MacDonald PC, Gant NF: Williams Obstetrics. 18th Ed. East Norwalk, Appleton & Lange, 1989, p. 394.)

to be astride the cord, the cord should be slipped over one of the buttocks before the legs are brought down. The breech delivery itself is divided into four maneuvers: (1) bringing out the breech and legs; (2) delivery to the shoulder; (3) engaging the shoulder girdle; and (4) delivery of the head. The first step (Figure 28–1 parts A, B, and C) is effected by introducing the entire hand into the vagina and grasping both ankles and drawing them through the vulva (Figure 28–1 part A). Downward traction is then applied, and as the legs emerge, they are grasped higher and higher (Figure 28–1 part B). When the breech appears at the vulva, first downward and then upward traction is made until it is delivered (Figure 28–1 part C). In frank breech, the Pinard maneuver is used for sweeping the legs down into the vagina and then out onto the perineum (Figure 28–2). The rest of the delivery is carried out as described for assisted breech delivery. With difficulty in delivery of the fetal head, one of the most important maneuvers is insertion of the hand of the operator into the uterine cavity and placement of the hand alongside the fetal head. This is done by coordinating anesthesia concommitant with lower uterine relaxant, i.e., inhalation anesthesia. Then the head and the rest of the baby's delivery is permitted through the lower uterine segment. Combining gentle downward traction from above and below may facilitate such a delivery.

## Balanced Regional Anesthesia

The preference is for balanced anesthesia consisting of continuous epidural or subarachnoid block, or for caudal block for analgesia and perineal relaxation, and inhalation anesthesia for uterine relaxation, should it be needed. For this purpose, isoflurane or enflurane effect surgical anes-

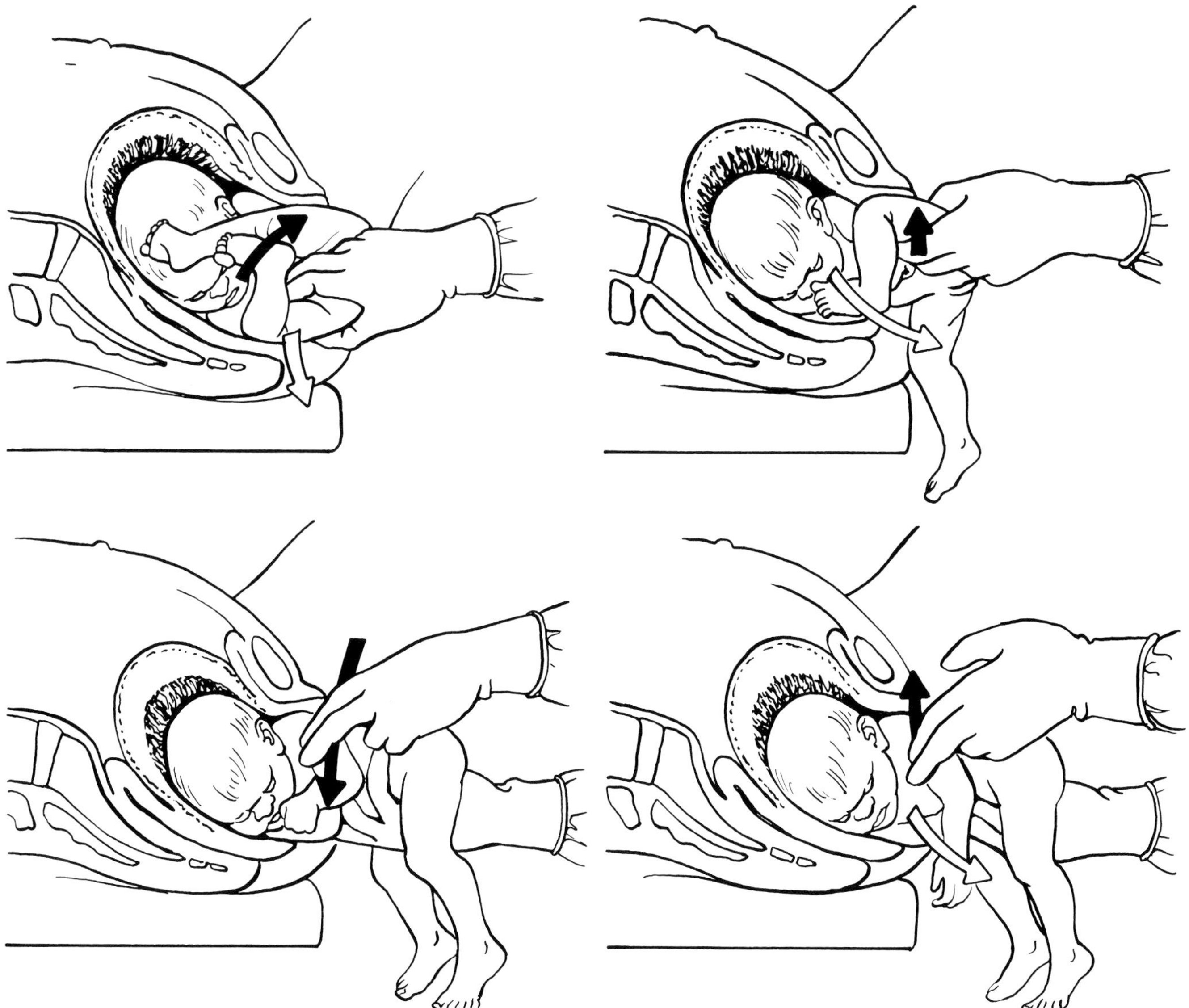

**Fig. 28–2.** Pinard's maneuver. (Redrawn from Seeds JW: Malpresentations. *In* Obstetrics: Normal and Problem Pregnancies. 2nd Ed. Edited by SG Gabbe, JR Niebyl, JL Simpson. New York, Churchill Livingstone, 1991, p. 554.)

thesia rapidly, and they both attain suitable uterine relaxation. These agents are beneficial also in that recovery is rapid after washout of the system.

If an epidural is in place for labor, it can be used for the purpose of obtaining a sacral block for adequate analgesia of the vagina and perineum. This is achieved by trying to concentrate the local anesthetic in the area of the sacrum by tilting the table into the reverse Trendelenburg position. The volume and concentration of the local anesthetic used should be sufficient to produce paralysis of the perineal muscles and perineal analgesia extending from S2 to S4. If the patient has not received regional analgesia during the first stage, a block can be begun for management of just the second stage; in this case, it is prudent to use the caudal block with 3% chloroprocaine or a subarachnoid block with 5% lidocaine. Both of these techniques will give rapid and dense analgesia.

In breech extraction, it is important for very close communication and coordination to exist between the anesthesiologist and the obstetrician. With adequate regional analgesia and effective analgesia and relaxation of the vaginal area and lower uterine segment, it may be possible for the obstetrician to perform breech extraction slowly, in cooperation with the patient and while speaking with her the entire time without any additional inhalation analgesia added. On the other hand, there may be situations in which the lower uterine segment is contracted tightly around the fetal parts and impossible for the obstetrician to perform the maneuver he/she needs to do. In the latter instance, an addition of a general anesthetic may be necessary for providing safety to the mother and baby. In such an instance, just before the obstetrician is ready for intrauterine maneuvers, the patient is given thiopental or propofol to effect a pleasant, smooth, and rapid sleep, and then either isoflurane or enflurane added for maintenance of anesthesia and for uterine relaxation (42). Sufficient inhalation drug is given over a short period of time to produce surgical anesthesia by the time the effect of the barbiturate disappears. If the parturient already has regional anesthesia of the birth canal, the obstetrician may introduce his/her hand into the canal to palpate the uterus and so advise the anesthesiologist about the degree of uterine relaxation needed. With this technique, uterine relaxation may be achieved in 4 to 8 minutes. If fetal distress requires that it be effected more rapidly, the technique of muscle relaxant-endotracheal intubation and hyperventilation with the chosen inhalation agent can be chosen.

It is important that during the induction of anesthesia the obstetrician not stimulate the patient by introducing his/her hand into the birth canal or any other maneuver that may excite the parturient, because this may provoke struggling, laryngospasm, and attendant cardiovascular responses. When deep surgical anesthesia is attained, the anesthesiologist asks the obstetrician to commence the procedure and the intrauterine maneuver is carried out. When this is completed, the obstetrician informs the anesthesiologist that the procedure is completed, and the inhalation agent is eliminated rapidly with the parturient maintained on nitrous oxide/oxygen until complete delivery and perineal repair is completed, or with the parturient awakened at that time.

### The Breech Delivery by Cesarean

The decision for a cesarean delivery removes much of the unknown from the scenario and is a signal for the anesthesiologist to proceed with the anesthetic technique of choice according to the wishes of the patient, just as in any other cesarean section. This, of course, assumes there is no urgency for delivery identified due to some unexpected fetal condition. If the latter is the case, then the anesthesiologist must be notified immediately so that plans can be made for an expedited but safe anesthetic. The anesthetic requirements for a nonemergent anesthetic for cesarean delivery of a breech are no different than any other elective cesarean section, but the delivery from the obstetrician's viewpoint may be modified in regard to the uterine incision depending upon how low the breech is lying and how difficult the delivery appears to be.

## OTHER ABNORMAL PRESENTATIONS

### Brow Presentation

When the area of the skull between the anterior fontanel and the bridge of the nose becomes the presenting part, it is referred to as a brow or frontal presentation (Figure 28–3). The incidence of brow presentation varies widely from as low as 1 in less than a 1000 to 1 in over 3000 (54,55). The etiologic factors are similar to those of face presentation. In fact, on a continuum, a bit less than normal flexion means brow presentation, while even less flexion means a face presentation. Once again, any condition that tends to prevent flexion and increase ex-

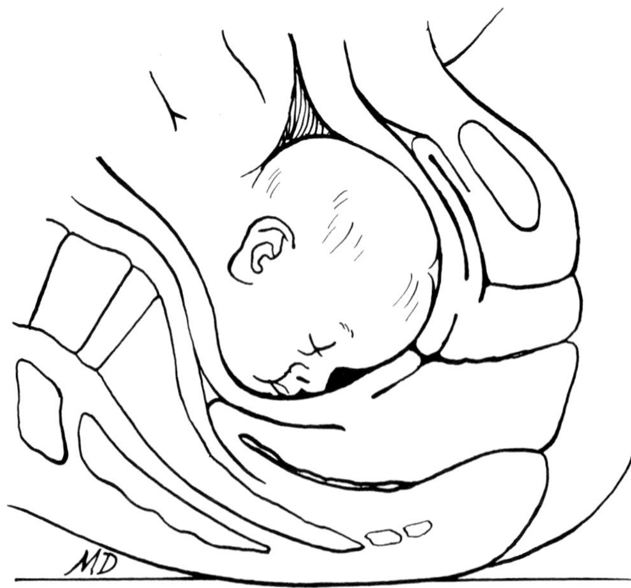


**Fig. 28–3.** Brow presentation. (Redrawn from Cunningham FG, MacDonald PC, Gant NF: Williams Obstetrics. 18th Ed. East Norwalk, Appleton & Lange, 1989, p. 359.)

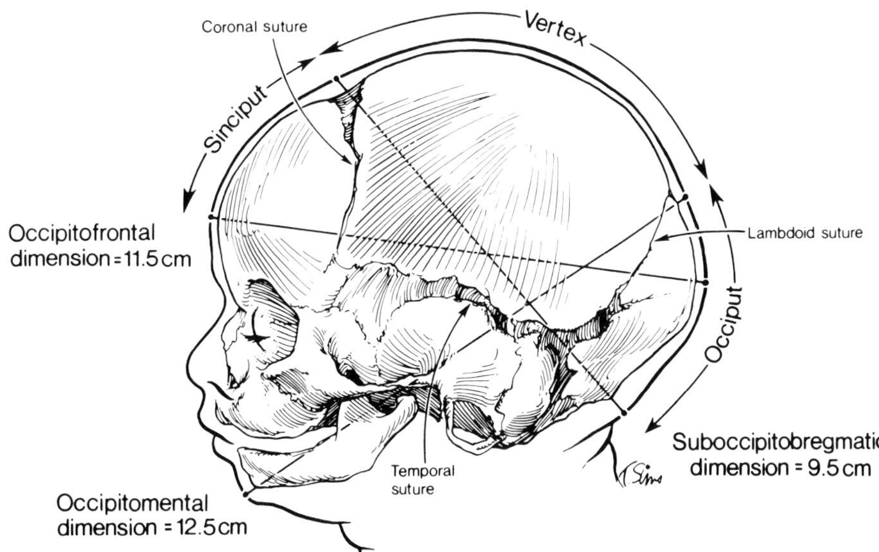


**Fig. 28–4.** Diameters of the fetal head. (From Cunningham FG, MacDonald PC, Gant NF: Williams Obstetrics. 18th Ed. East Norwalk, Appleton & Lange, 1989, p. 93.)

tension causes the brow to present. A condition might be a combination of large pelvis and a small fetus, but such conditions are rare, thus the rather rare incidence. The mechanism of brow presentation entails passage of the greatest anteroposterior diameter of the fetal head, the occipitomental diameter, which is 12.5 cm compared with the 9.5 cm of the suboccipitobregmatic diameter in normal occipital presentation, as noted in Figure 28–4. Consequently, engagement and descent are impossible until after significant molding has taken place, by which the occipitomental diameter has become diminished and the occipitofrontal diameter increased in length to allow pelvic passage. As the descent takes place, the mentum rotates so that this region of the face comes to lie behind the pubis. With continued descent and flexion of the neck, the occiput and vertex pass over the perineum, the head falls posteriorly, and the face slips from beneath the symphysis. As imagined, this is a complex mechanism that must transpire before spontaneous vaginal delivery can occur. That the completion of this maneuver does not frequently transpire is attested by the fact that vaginal delivery occurs in only about one-half of the brow presentations (56,57).

Maternal mortality is not affected, and there can be some slight increase in morbidity primarily due to manipulation and prolonged labor trial. Instrumentation and maneuvers necessary for delivery may produce complications unless they are done carefully. Because cesarean section is frequently performed, the morbidity associated with it is low, as it is in operative delivery today. Current thought is in regard to minimal manipulation, careful maternal and fetal monitoring in a trial of labor, and institution of cesarean section as indicated for the failures to progress.

The corrected perinatal mortality can range from as low as 1% to as high as 8% (57). Perinatal morbidity is also significantly increased. Cerebral hemorrhage can result from the significant overriding of the skull bones, excessive molding, and forceps manipulation. Prolonged labor adds to the normal birth asphyxia. Edema of the brow produces the characteristic deformed head.

### *Obstetric Management*

Brow presentation should be suspected when abdominal palpation reveals a straight fetal spine, but often it is not appreciated before labor and sometimes not until delivery is imminent. If the labor is progressing normally with no need for excessive oxytocin and no evidence of failure to progress in regard to dilatation and descent, the obstetric management is largely expectant in nature. In such a case, vaginal delivery may be possible with the conversion of the brow to a face or an occiput presentation. In the event of evidence of an abnormal labor pattern or in the event of fetal distress, a cesarean section should be performed without delay.

### *Anesthetic Management*

The anesthetic requirements and management of brow presentation are similar to those of face presentation. We prefer continuous epidural analgesia because it provides complete relief of pain, which is usually much needed by the parturient who is already fatigued by the prolonged labor. Again, we would emphasize the consideration for use of the continuous epidural low dose combination technique to help minimize complications for the fetus/newborn and mother. Even more important, these techniques do not depress the fetus nor newborn who have been exposed already to the effects of prolonged labor and, probably, several doses of narcotics. This method may also enhance uterine contractions if there is inertia. Continuous caudal analgesia may be used instead, provided it is applied as described under face presentation. An important advantage of continuous epidural block is that it can be extended cephalad to produce anesthesia for cesarean section. For the second stage of labor alone, the subarachnoid technique can also be used in the form of a saddle block for chiefly sacral effect, or in the form of a low spinal block to include the lumbar segments and the thoracic 10 to 12 segments. With relief of labor pains already blocked by use of the continuous epidural infusion, either of these two latter methods will work very effectively for delivery and enable the mother to use effective Valsalva maneuvers to push the baby out. If cesarean section is decided upon, then the epidural can be brought up to a T4 level by repeated injections of 3% chloroprocaine plain or 2% lidocaine with epinephrine, or 0.5% bupivacaine in 5 ml aliquots every 5 minutes until the desired level is reached.

## *Face Presentation*

Face presentations occur when complete head extension or deflexion occurs. In this situation, the chin becomes the lead portion, hence the descriptive of the position, left mento-anterior (L.M.A.), right mento-anterior (R.M.A.), and so forth (Figure 28–5). The occiput may nearly make physical contact with the fetal back as shown in Figure 28–6. This condition is pretty rare, with one occurrence in every 600 to 800 deliveries, an incidence of 0.17% (56). As mentioned above, face presentations may result from spontaneous brow conversions. Other factors that produce extension or prevent flexion of the head must also be considered possible causes. For example, contracted pelvis, large fetus, anencephaly, loops of cord around the neck, multiparity with lax abdominal walls, uterine dysfunction, hydramnios, and premature rupture of the membranes all can be considered important factors (58–61). Such a presentation is also seen whenever there is no need for flexion of the fetal head such as in premature infants and in patients with large pelves and small babies. By far the largest number of face presentations, about 70%, occur in multiparae (60,61).

Maternal mortality in face presentation is not increased above that of vertex presentation (60,61). However, maternal morbidity may be augmented because of prolonged labor and injury. Furthermore, deep tears in the perineum and birth canal occur more frequently and are probably due to the greater downward protrusion of the pelvic floor, because the presenting part must descend very deeply before flexion of the neck under the symphysis can occur (62).

There is a greater perinatal mortality and morbidity in face presentation than in occipito-anterior presentation (60,61). There may be cerebral hemorrhage due to excessive molding or forceps manipulation and asphyxia secondary to prolonged labor. Less frequent complications include facial paralysis, compression and fracture of the trachea and larynx, edema of the glottis, and vascular compression of the neck against the pelvis.

### Obstetric Management

The duration of labor in face presentation is usually prolonged (60,61). The biparietal diameter does not pass the pelvic inlet until the chin reaches the pelvic floor; consequently, engagement occurs late in labor. The descent is commonly slow and internal rotation does not occur until the pelvic floor is well distended by the advancing face. Uterine inertia occurs in about 15% of cases of face presentation. When the fetus descends into the pelvis in the mentoposterior or transverse positions during labor, it rotates to anterior positions spontaneously in most patients (61). In the past, many face presentations were not made until delivery because few vaginal exams were performed due to the tendency to use rectal exams for estimation of effacement and dilatation. Now, it is difficult to imagine that the diagnosis of face presentation is not made early; however, some of the first vaginal exams with little dilatation may not detect the condition due to the fact that the presence of the mentum has simply not appreciated. Obstetric management of face presentation

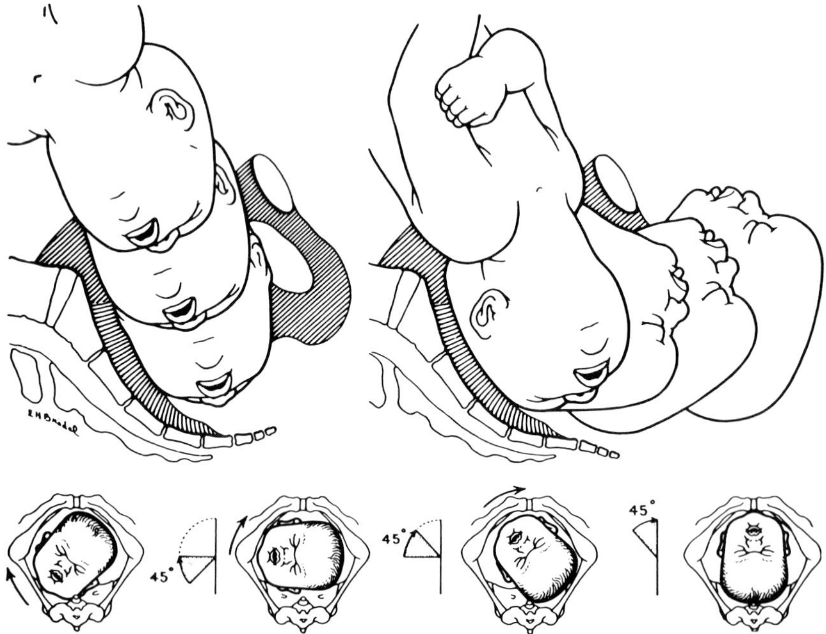


**Fig. 28–5.** Face presentations. (From Cunningham FG, MacDonald PC, Gant NF: Williams Obstetrics. 18th Ed. East Norwalk, Appleton & Lange, 1989, p. 358.)

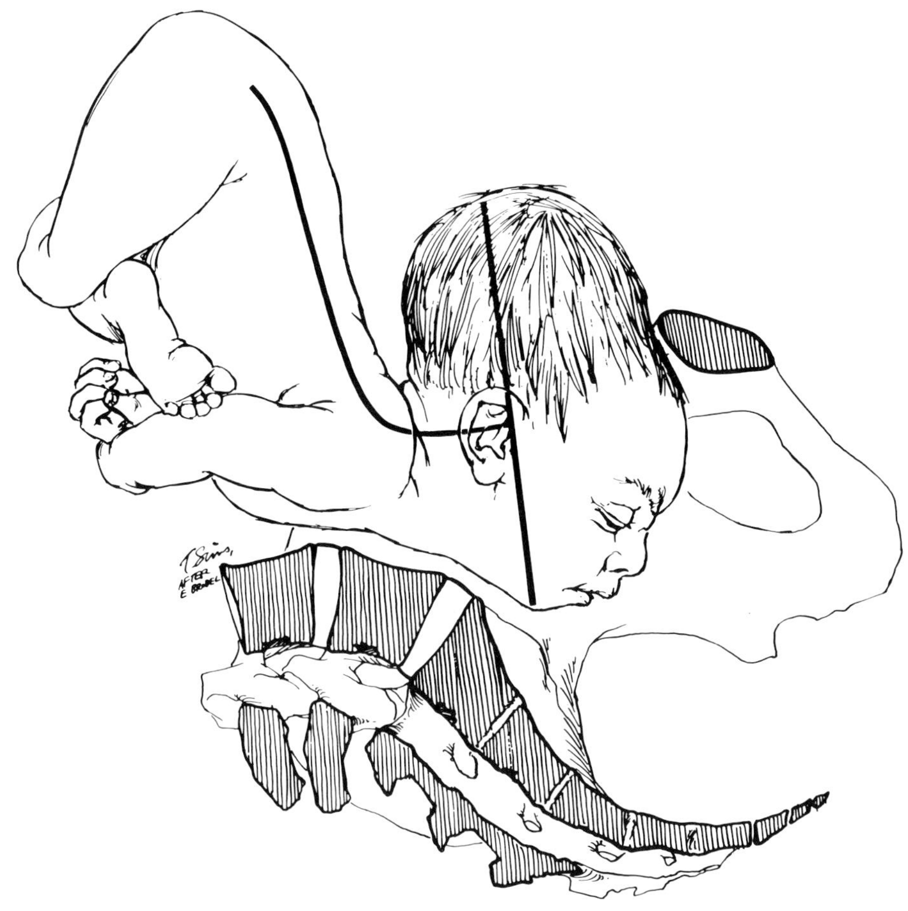

**Fig. 28–6.** Face presentation showing relationship between fetal back and occiput. (From Cunningham FG, MacDonald PC, Gant NF: Williams Obstetrics. 18th Ed. East Norwalk, Appleton & Lange, 1989, p. 358.)

varies (62–66). If the pelvis is normal, the infant not unusually large, and the position mento-anterior or transverse, no interference is needed; in most patients, the infant will deliver vaginally either spontaneously or by low forceps (60,61). If the fetal position is mentoposterior, one can expectantly wait for spontaneous anterior rotation and, occasionally, for spontaneous conversion to vertex. If this fails to occur within a short period of time, a cesarean section is done. Most believe that a mentoposterior position that persists after labor is well-established is best managed by cesarean section, regardless of parity or size of the baby.

### *Anesthetic Management*

Any anesthetic plan must take into consideration the needs of the obstetrician for delivery of the abnormal presentation either by vaginal delivery or by cesarean delivery. In addition, consideration must be given for the fetus perhaps already depressed by a prolonged labor. This is particularly important if the fetus is premature. For first stage, the single epidural catheter with the low dose continuous infusion technique affords excellent pain relief for the mother and safety for the fetus. Of course, the double-catheter technique, as described in Chapter 13, can also be used to advantage in these cases in which it is ideal to withhold perineal relaxation until just before delivery. Additionally, this latter regional method provides another level of safety for those mothers with organic disease processes such as pulmonary or cardiac problems. During second stage, in addition to analgesia for uterine contractions and perineal distention, it is essential to have perineal muscular relaxation. Parturients with face presentation and other obstetric complications require early involvement of their anesthesiologists in labor so that the analgesia-anesthesia is coordinated with the rest of the obstetric care. Finally, if cesarean section becomes necessary, the regional block can be extended to the upper thoracic dermatomes. Another cesarean anesthetic technique might be a spinal block or a general anesthetic. The coordinated management of cases such as these emphasize once again the beauty of the situation in which the skilled anesthesiologist and obstetrician work in concert for the benefit of the mother and baby.

## *Transverse Lie*

In transverse lie, the long axis of the fetus lies nearly perpendicular to the long axis of the mother. In variations of angles less than 90°, an oblique lie is diagnosed. Because the head and breech of the fetus are in the iliac fossae, the presenting part is the shoulder. Transverse lie occurs once in 300 to 600 deliveries—an incidence of 0.17 to 0.3% (67–69). The most frequent maternal factors associated with transverse presentations are multiparity with abnormal relaxation of the abdominal walls, uterine malformations, contracted pelvis, and pelvic masses (uterine or ovarian tumors or pelvic kidney). Fetoplacental factors include placenta praevia, implantation of the placenta directly over the fundus or in the lower segment decreasing the length of the uterine cavity, prematurity, multiple pregnancy, dead fetus, premature rupture of the membranes, and hydramnios. In about 10% of the patients, shoulder presentation is a recurrent phenomenon. In about 15 to 25% of the cases, the cause is unknown.

Maternal mortality is very low today due to the acceptance that transverse lie is a deliverable situation only with cesarean section. Most maternal deaths occurred in the past due to neglected cases from spontaneous rupture of the uterus or from traumatic rupture following belated and ill-advised version and extraction; many of these were also complicated by infection (62). However, maternal mortality is increased to a slight degree over normal due to the association of transverse lie with placenta praevia. Placenta previa, and all variations such as percreta and accreta, greatly increase the chance of serious bleeding, and the threat to life is significant. Maternal morbidity is also frequently increased by hemorrhage, and perineal and cervical lacerations.

Perinatal mortality in transverse lie has been quoted to be between 4 and 30% (70,71). In shoulder lie without interference, the fetal loss was close to 100% in 1952 (72). Because internal podalic version is now supplanted with cesarean section, the mortality and morbidity by manipulation is reduced. Neonatal morbidity is increased. Extreme flexion of the fetus and compression of the chest contribute to fetal asphyxia.

### Obstetric Management

Diagnosis before labor begins is now confirmed with ultrasound, which confirms the lie. Management of this condition is by attempt at external version, but if this fails, a cesarean section is performed (73). This is usually the scenario, as labor, ruptured membranes, or a tonic uterus all mitigate against external version. Furthermore, aggressive obstetric manipulations such as internal version and extraction or breech extraction are associated with an unacceptable maternal and fetal mortality and morbidity (70,74,75). The use of a longitudinal incision is recommended because a transverse one limits the uterine incision in length and direction.

### Anesthetic Management

Because the selection of the mode of delivery is already made, i.e., cesarean section, in all those transverse presentations that failed external version, the anesthetic management is relegated to a discussion of the anesthetic best for this operative procedure. Basically, this decision is usually given to the mother who is asked whether she wants to be awake or asleep for the operation. However, in this event, a very important admonition must be made regarding the selection of a regional technique in the case of transverse lie in which placenta previa, percreta, or accreta may co-exist. In the latter cases, it is recommended that general anesthesia be used to preserve the vasoconstrictive capabilities of the mother, who may suffer a tremendous blood loss after delivery of the baby and after manual removal of the placenta. The bleeding from the placental bed in this lower uterine segment can be incredibly brisk. This can pose a threat to the mother just after delivery, especially in instances in which regional analgesia has reduced the control of peripheral vascular resistance. The continued bleeding, the hypotension from blood loss, and reduction in vascular resistance all result in a fall in blood pressure, and the latter can result in arrhythmias and cardiac arrest. In this latter situation, the anesthesiologist can help to save the life of the patient by having at least two large bore venous lines, by being available to monitor and support the cardiovascular system, by administration of large quantities of blood and blood products during major hemorrhage, and by maintenance of ventilation.

## *Compound Presentations*

The most common compound presentation consists of a vertex with prolapse of an arm. Less common is a breech, accompanied by a prolapsed hand and a vertex with prolapse of one or both legs. When there is a small fetus, we have sometimes observed vertex presentation with prolapse of one hand and both feet, a situation that is not rare when the child is dead. Compound presentations occur between once in 377 and once in 1213 deliveries (56,76,77). Any condition that prevents complete filling and occlusion of the pelvic inlet by the presenting part is a predisposing cause of compound presentations (62). A multipara with a large pelvis, a small baby, and premature rupture of the membranes is an excellent candidate for a compound presentation. In 10 to 15% of the cases of compound presentation, no apparent cause is found.

Maternal mortality and morbidity are not increased significantly if the compound presentation is handled properly. The duration of labor is not affected, and the descent of the main presenting part, head or breech, proceeds while the prolapsed member remains behind. The fetus or newborn suffers little if the cord has not prolapsed. Occasionally, there may be trauma caused by attempts to replace the prolapsed limb, or because of fetopelvic disproportion. The most frequent (20%) and most serious complication of compound presentation is prolapse of the umbilical cord (78). When this occurs, birth asphyxia and perinatal morbidity are increased. Obviously, maternal and perinatal morbidity and mortality depend largely on the way this problem is managed.

Perinatal mortality is elevated, but the figures vary from as low as 9% to as high as 17% and 19% (56,79,80). The greatest percentage of the losses occur due to premature delivery, prolapse of the umbilical cord and its attendant mortality, and aggressive obstetric manipulations.

### Obstetric Management

If there is no prolapse of the cord, a compound presentation usually terminates in spontaneous vaginal delivery. When labor is progressing well and there is no fetal distress, one should wait for full dilation of the cervix and routine delivery. Normally, as the fetal presenting part descends, the hand ascends out of the way. When descent does not progress, the recommendation is for cesarean section. As mentioned above, a significant contribution to the morbidity and mortality of the fetus is due to the aggressive management methods by obstetricians in the past. Thus, internal version and extraction and delivery attempts by use of the forceps or vacuum extractor are not suggested.

### Anesthetic Management

For delivery in cases of compound presentation, the anesthetic requirements are essentially those needed in either vertex presentation or breech presentation. Similarly for cesarean section, the anesthetic used can be decided upon after consideration of all the possible problems, the mother's choice, and finally the decision must be made by the anesthesiologist who will administer the anesthetic and be responsible for it.

## Internal Podalic Version and Extraction

Internal podalic version and extraction has a strong historic heritage in obstetrics. Its value in instances of transverse lie, umbilical cord prolapse, abnormal presentation associated with uterine inertia, and the difficult delivery of the second twin in the years before antibiotics and oxytocics is not questioned. There was no alternative presented to the obstetrician then. However, version and extraction is clearly and consistently associated with both a high fetal morbidity and mortality and a high maternal morbidity in most reports in the literature. In addition, certain reports have recorded maternal mortality as high as 13% secondary to this procedure (79). Maternal morbidity and mortality are significantly increased after version and extraction (61). Uterine rupture, cervical and perineal laceration, hemorrhage, and attendant puerperal sepsis play the major role in complications. Rosensohn states that version and extraction is the most important factor responsible for traumatic uterine rupture (81). Keettel reported as high as 13% of all maternal deaths in 1 year were attributed to this technique. His review of 156 versions and extractions over a 25-year period revealed 28% of the parturients sustained lacerations, while 34% experienced puerperal morbidity (79). Maternal trauma is augmented by forceful obstetric manipulations in situations of poor uterine relaxation and incomplete cervical dilation. By its very nature, it is an emergency procedure and thus carries the disadvantages inherent in any technique hurriedly performed. There is little question as to who suffers most after version and extraction. The corrected fetal mortality statistics vary with figures of 4.6% (82), 6.7% (83), and 8.7% (84) recorded as the lowest, and 23% (85) and 38% (86) recorded as the highest. Perinatal mortality figures also vary, with 24% (83) recorded as the average low and 58% the maximum (81). This indictment of version and extraction as a potentially dangerous procedure derives from the combined morbidity and mortality of the mother and baby that is most likely due to a combination of obstetric trauma and deep level anesthesia, which was administered for adequate uterine relaxation. Because the ideal obstetric situation with a small or normal-sized infant, a large or normal pelvis, intact membranes with a normal amount of amniotic fluid, and a physician experienced with version and extraction, together with optimal anesthetic management provided by a skilled obstetric anesthesiologist rarely, if ever, exists, this technique is just not recommended today. Cesarean section has proved much safer and is currently preferred for management of all obstetric problems mentioned earlier.

### Anesthetic Management

As mentioned under the section on breech delivery by cesarean section, the anesthetic considerations and requirements become identical to situations of elective cesarean section with the anesthetic technique largely decided upon by preference expressed by the mother and input by the anesthesiologist. Optimal anesthetic care is, of course, a critical requirement as always if the mother and newborn are to be spared serious complications. If well administered, anesthesia facilitates the delivery and thus decreases the hazard to the mother and infant. On the other hand, improper administration may adversely affect the mother and the fetus, produce its own complications, and thus further compromise mother and fetus. Optimal anesthesia in this situation as in all difficult scenarios in obstetric anesthesiology requires not only a skilled and experienced anesthetic administrator but also good communication and close cooperation and coordination and understanding of the mutual problems by the obstetrician and anesthesiologist. In sum, either a regional technique using the epidural method or subarachnoid method, or a general technique is acceptable.

## External Version

In the past, the use of external version was popular for a period of time, then fell into disuse because of the recognized fetal hazard and the fact that many "conversions" to vertex occurred. Now, there is a renewed interest due to the use of ultrasound and the ability to use it as a guide during external version, and a willingness to cease efforts in lieu of evidence of fetal danger. When anesthesia was used for external version, the depth of anesthesia necessary to provide good uterine relaxation afforded an opportunity for placental separation, uterine rupture, and fetal trauma without recognition. Thus, there appears to be little indication for the use of anesthesia in external version as it is used today, certainly less than there was at the time of the first edition of this book. As always, however, it would be wise to have the anesthesiologists informed of the procedures to be performed and to have an anesthetic history and physical performed on the patients so that if some dire emergency should occur,the anesthesiologist in-house would at least have a working knowledge of the patient and be able to participate in a more rapid fashion to an emergency status.

## Interlocking and Twin Collision

This rare complication of multiple pregnancy has a quoted incidence of 1 in 1000 twin deliveries (87). Twin entanglement presents only one of the many hazards asso-

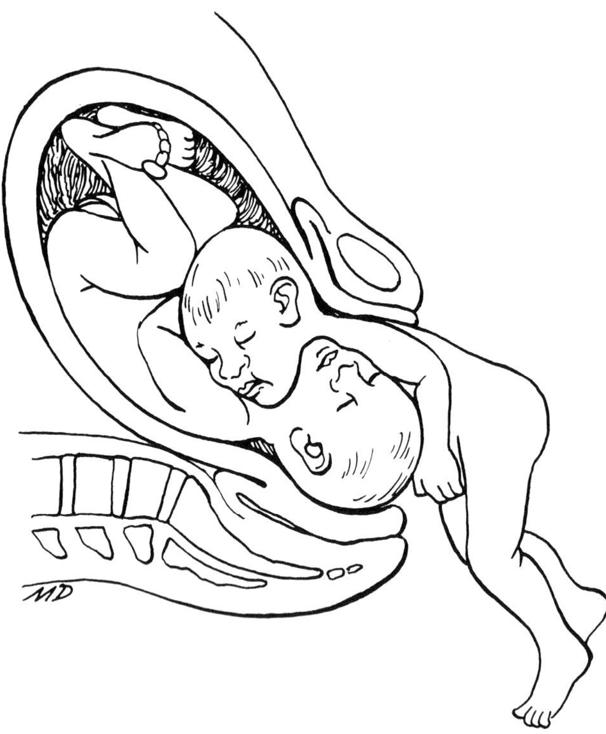

**Fig. 28–7.** Interlocking twins: chin-to-chin. (Redrawn from MacDonald JS: Other operative obstetric procedures. *In* Principles and Practice of Obstetric Analgesia and Anesthesia. 1st Ed., Vol. 2. Edited by JJ Bonica. Philadelphia, FA Davis Co., 1969, p. 1372.)

ciated with multiple gestation, yet its impact is sudden and distressing. An understanding of the various entanglements is necessary to provide the broad background necessary to cope with this unusual situation. Yet very few physicians will ever encounter a single case; therefore, a brief review follows. Chin-to-chin interlocking comprises a relatively small proportion of twin entanglements, yet has received relatively greater notice in the literature because of its rarity and particularly difficult management. It refers to the chin-to-chin apposition of the first fetus who is breech to the second who is vertex (Figure 28–7). This arrangement must occur above the true pelvis, and with subsequent descent, collision occurs—the simultaneous full engagement of two fetal poles—which usually precludes the delivery of two viable infants. The key to a successful management lies in the early detection of the problem, and with the universal use of ultrasound today, this should not present a problem. Thus, when detection of the potential setup for interlocking twins is made, the decision for cesarean section follows quickly behind.

Here again, anesthetic management is similar to that as mentioned previously, namely, the application of either regional or general techniques based upon the mutual agreement between the patient and the anesthesiologist.

### *Manual Removal of the Placenta*

Obstetric treatment of the third stage of labor presents a tremendous variation in management. It is often managed in a relaxed, unassuming manner because of a failure to appreciate that complications incurred from the third stage can be responsible for many maternal deaths. Hemorrhage, the one common denominator in third stage management, is also the major complication in the cause of maternal death (62). An appreciation of the factors involved in promoting third stage hemorrhage will enable the obstetric anesthesia team to anticipate and minimize their effect on the parturient. Labor and delivery complications that cause excessive uterine stretch and muscular fatigue promote third stage hemorrhage. These complications include hydramnios, excessive fetal size, multiple gestation, low placental implantation, maternal fatigue, and prolonged labor. Other factors, related to trauma and anesthesia, include mechanical trauma to any portion of the lower uterine segment, cervix and vagina, failure simply to control a major bleeder of an episiotomy, failure to administer oxytocics, and profound anesthesia usually associated with the more potent general anesthetics. Anticipation of such problems, combined with an adequate plan of active management, will circumvent many of these potential situations. Massive uterine hemorrhage is usually associated with incomplete placental separation, thus preventing spontaneous uterine compression of the local placental bed. Active management of third stage hemorrhage should include immediate manual removal of the placenta with uterine cavity exploration followed by vigorous, continuous bimanual uterine compression and rapid administration of appropriate concentrations of oxytocics, and at the same time adequate volume replacement. Today, the issue of blood transfusion is naturally of great concern, as many mothers now donate blood for their own use should blood be necessary, but most of these are patients who plan to have a cesarean delivery. Thus, most patients who have an unexpected third trimester hemorrhage will have had the foresight to have donated blood. Certainly, aggressive, active management of this situation at the very beginning will help prevent some use of blood bank blood, and active measures such as those mentioned can substantially reduce maternal hemorrhage and preserve many lives (88).

With persistent hemorrhage after uterine compression and oxytocic administration, one must assume lower uterine segment, cervical or vaginal canal laceration and perform an exploration of these areas. If there is one lesson to broadcast in this regard, it is not to waste valuable time trying to visualize and correct the problem vaginally. It is best to enter the abdomen and repair the laceration from above. This may seem to be aggressive but it may also be responsible for saving lives against persistent hemorrhage and complications that may arise due to the inability to stop the hemorrhage. Rarely will uterine packing, hypogastric artery occlusion by balloon tamponade (87) or ligation, or postpartum hysterectomy be necessary, but when indicated, they too are life-preserving techniques. In many obstetric centers, manual removal of the placenta is becoming an accepted procedure. In others, manual removal is usually resorted to if spontaneous separation has not occurred within 10 to 20 minutes.

Adequate anesthesia for removal of the placenta must offer analgesia for the uterus, vagina, and perineum. In addition, adequate uterine relaxation facilitates a manual separation and removal, but this is usually present provided oxytocics have not been administered or a delay has not occurred. It is recommended to use a rapid sequence induction and intubation and general anesthetic technique in these cases, because small amounts of inhalation anesthetic can provide uterine relaxation and access for the obstetrician to get his/her hand into the uterus for manual removal after adequate lower uterine relaxation. Generally, regional is not preferred unless it is already in place and the obstetrician announces that he/she can already enter the uterine cavity. In such case, the anesthesiologist can either use the epidural already in place and standby to see if that amount of analgesia is sufficient, or he/she can standby with inhalation anesthesia to be given to the patient should the obstetrician report a need for it due to a contracted lower uterine segment and inability to manually extract the placenta without the added help of relaxation. In the latter instance, general anesthesia is induced with the usual careful precautions to prevent aspiration by use of rapid sequence induction method. The inhalation agent used is again the call of the anesthesiologist, supplemented with nitrous oxide or entirely by itself with 100% oxygen. When the more potent inhalation agents are used in analgesic concentrations, the fear of excess bleeding is not serious, but it must be appreciated that this requires expert skill in administration by an anesthesiologist who has had experience in this area, because the deeper planes are easily attained and cause further uterine bleeding due to profound uterine relaxation.

## REFERENCES


1. Morgan HS, Kane SH: An analysis of 16,327 breech births. JAMA 1964; 187:262–265.
2. Todd WD, Steer CM: Term breech: review of 1,006 term breech deliveries. Obstet. Gynecol. 1963; 22:583.
3. Morley GW: Breech presentation, a 15-year review. Obstet. Gynecol. 1967; 30:745.
4. Hickok DE, Gordon DC, Milberg JA, Williams MA, et al: The frequency of breech presentation by gestational age at birth: a large population-based study. Am. J. Obstet. Gynecol. 1992; 166:851–2.
5. Hill LM: Prevalence of breech presentation by gestational age. Am. J. Perinatol 1990; 7:92–93.
6. Tompkins P: An inquiry into the causes of breech presentation. Am. J. Obstet. Gynecol. 1946; 51:595.
7. Braun FT, Jone KL, Smith DW: Breech presentation as an indicator of fetal abnormality. J. Pediatrics 1975; 86:419.
8. Brenner WE, Bruce RD, Hendricks CH: The characteristics and perils of breech presentation. Am. J. Obstet. Gynecol. 1974; 118:700–709.
9. Collea JV, Rabin SC, Weghorst GR, Quilligan EJ: The randomized management of term frank breech presentation: vaginal delivery versus cesarean section. Am. J. Obstet. Gynecol. 1978; 131:186–195.
10. Johnson CE: Breech presentation at term. Am. J. Obstet. Gynecol. 1970; 106:865.
11. Patterson SP, Mullinicks RC, Schreier PC: Breech presentation in the primigravida. Am. J. Obstet. Gynecol. 1967; 98: 404.
12. Ruben A, Grimm G: Results in breech presentation. Am. J. Obstet. Gynecol. 1963; 86:1048.
13. Gold EM, Clyman MJ, Wallace HM, Rich H: Obstetric factors in birth injury. With consideration of the value of birth certificate reporting. Obstet. Gynecol. 1953; 1:431–436.
14. Tan KL: Brachial palsy. J Obstet. Gynecol. British Commonwealth 1973; 80:60.
15. Brans YW, Cassady G: Neonatal spinal cord injuries. Am. J. Obstet. Gynecol. 1975; 123:918.
16. Wilcox HL: The attitude of the fetus in breech presentation. Am. J. Obstet. Gynecol. 1949; 58:478.
17. Caterini H, Langer A, Sama JC, Devanesan M, et al: Fetal risk in hyperextension of the fetal head in breech presentation. Am. J. Obstet. Gynecol. 1975; 123:631–636.
18. Ranney B: The gentle art of external cephalic version. Am. J. Obstet. Gynecol. 1973; 116:244.
19. Saling E, Muller-Holvew J: External cephalic version of a tocolysis. J. Perinatal Med. 1975; 3:115.
20. Van Dorsten JP, Schifrin BS, Wallace RL: Randomized control trial of external cephalic version with tocolysis in late pregnancy. Am. J. Obstet. Gynecol. 1981; 141:417–424.
21. Van Veelen AJ, Van Cappellen AW, Flu PK, Straub MJ, et al: Effect of external cephalic version in late pregnancy on presentation at delivery: a randomized controlled trial. Br. J. Obstet. Gynaecol. 1989; 96:916–921.
22. Ferguson JE II, Armstrong MA, Dyson DC: Maternal and fetal factors affecting success of antepartum external cephalic version. Obstet. Gynecol. 1987; 70:722–725.
23. Hellstrom AC, Nilsson B, Stange L, Nylund L: When does external cephalic version succeed? Acta. Obstet. Gynecol. Scand. 1990; 69:281–285.
24. Morrison JC, Myatt RE, Martin JN Jr, Meeks GR, et at: External cephalic version of the breech presentation under tocolysis. Am. J. Obstet. Gynecol. 1986; 154:900–903.
25. Luyet F, Schmid J, Maroni E, Duc G: Massive feto-maternal transfusion during external cephalic version, with fatal outcome. Arch. Gynk. 1976; 221:273.
26. Gjode P, Rasmussen TB, Jorgensen J: Fetomaternal bleeding during attempts at external version. British J. Obstet. Gynecol. 1980; 87:571–573.
27. Scaling ST: External cephalic version without tocolysis. Am. J. Obstet. Gynecol. 1988; 158:1424–1430.
28. Stine LE, Phelan JP, Wallace R, Eglinton GS, et at: Update on external cephalic version performed at term. Obstet. Gynecol. 1985; 65:642.
29. Gimovsky ML, Wallace RL, Schiffrin BS, Paul RH: Randomized management of the nonfrank breech presentation at term: a preliminary report. Am. J. Obstet. Gynecol. 146:34, 1983.
30. Flanagan TA, Mulchahey KM, Korenbrot CC, Green JR, et al: Management of term presentation. Am. J. Obstet. Gynecol. 1987; 156:1492–1502.
31. Barlov K, Larsson G: Results of a five-year prospective study using a feto-pelvic scoring system for term singleton breech delivery after uncomplicated pregnancy. Acta. Obstet. Gynecol. Scand 1986; 65:315–319.
32. Neligan GA, et al: Formative years. New York, Oxford University Press, 3:24, 1974.
33. McBride WG, Black BP, Brown CJ, Dolby RM, et al: Method of delivery and developmental outcome at five years of age. Med. J. Australia 1979; 1:301–304.
34. Croughan-Minihane MS, Petitti DB, Gordis L, Golditch I: Morbidity among breech infants according to method of delivery. Obstet. Gynecol. 1990; 75:821–825.
35. Bodmer B, Benjamin A, McLean FH, Usher RH: Has use of cesarean section reduced the risks of delivery in the preterm breech presentation. Am. J. Obstet. Gynecol. 1986; 154:244–250.
36. Kitchen W, Ford GW, Doyle LW, Rickards AL, et al: Cesarean section or vaginal delivery at 24 to 28 weeks gestation: com-

parison of survival of neonatal and two-year morbidity. Obstet. Gynecol. 1985; 66:149.
37. Gimovsky ML, Paul RH: Singleton breech presentation in labor experienced in 1980. Am. J. Obstet. Gynecol. 1982; 143:733.
38. Myers SA, Gleicher N: Breech delivery: why the dilemma? Am. J. Obstet. 1987; 6:156.
39. Oleajn AF, Shy KK, Luthy DA, Hickok D, et al: Cesarean birth and neonatal mortality in very low birthweight infants. Obstet. Gynecol. 1984; 64:267.
40. Duenhoelter JH, Wells CE, Reisch JS, Santos-Ramos R, et al: A paired control study of vaginal and abdominal delivery of the low birthweight breech fetus. Obstet. Gynecol. 1979; 54:310.
41. Ingemarsson I, Westgren M, Svenningsen NW: Long-term followup of preterm infants in breech presentation delivered by cesarean section: a prospective study. Lancet 1978; 2:172–175.
42. Tunstall ME, Sheikh A: Comparison of 1.5% enflurane with 1.25% isoflurane in oxygen for caesarean section: avoidance of awareness without nitrous oxide. Br. J. Anaesth. 1989; 62:138–143.
43. Levinson G, Shnider SM: Anesthesia for abnormal positions and presentations and multiple births. *In* Anesthesia for Obstetrics. 3rd Ed. Baltimore, Williams & Wilkins, 1993.
44. Confine E, Ismajovich B, Rudick V, David MP: Extradural analgesia in the management of singleton breech delivery. Br. J. Anaesth. 57:892–895, 1985.
45. Chada YC, Mahmood TA, Dick MJ, Smith NC, et al: Breech delivery and epidural analgesia. Br. J. Obstet. Gynaecol. 99: 96–100; 1992.
46. Songane FF, Thobani S, Malik H, Bingham P, et al: Balancing the risks of planned cesarean section and trial of vaginal delivery for the mature, selected, singleton breech presentation. J. Perinat. Med. 15:531–43, 1987.
47. Breeson AJ, Kovacs GT, Pickles BG, Hill JG: Extradural analgesia—the preferred method of analgesia for vaginal breech delivery. Br. J. Anaesth. 50:1227–30, 1978.
48. Boyson WA, Simpson JW: Breech management with caudal anesthesia. Amer. J. Obstet. Gynecol. 79:1121, 1960.
49. Malik SJ, Mir NA: Perinatal mortality in high risk pregnancy: a prospective study of preventable factors. Asia Oceania J. Obstet. Gynaecol. (Japan) 18:45–8, 1992.
50. Mahomed K, Seereas R, Coulson R: Outcome of term breech presentation. East Afr. Med. J. 66:819–23, 1989.
51. Klufio CA, Amoa AB: Breech presentation and delivery. PNG Med. J. 34:289–95, 1991.
52. Wells SR, Thorp JM Jr, Bowes WA Jr: Management of the nonvertex second twin. Surgery Gynecol. Obstet. 172: 383–385, May 1991.
53. Gocke SE, Nageotte MP, Garite T, Towers CV, et al: Management of the nonvertex second twin: primary cesarean section, external version, or primary breech extraction. Am. J. Obstet. Gynecol. 161:111–114, July 1989.
54. Meltzer RM, Sachtleban MR, Friedman EA: Brow presentation. Am. J. Obstet. Gynecol. 100:255, 1968.
55. Kovacs SG: Brow presentation. Med. J. Aust. 2:820, 1970.
56. Cruikshank DP, White CA: Obstetric Malpresentations: twenty years' experience. Am. J. Obstet. Gynecol. 116:1097, 1973.
57. Levy DL: Persistent brow presentation—a new approach to management. South Med. J. 69:191, 1976.
58. Quiel V: Face presentation in labor. Zentralbl. Gynakol. 113: 1380, 1385–7, 1991.
59. Schwartz Z, Dgani R, Lancet M, Kessler I: Face presentation. Aust. N.Z. J. Obstet. Gynaecol. 26:172–6, 1986.
60. Magid B, Gillespie CF: Face and brow presentations. Obstet. Gynecol. 9:450, 1957.
61. Schmitz HE, Cuccu U, Pavlic RS: Face presentation. Obstet. Gynecol. 13:641, 1959.
62. Eastman NJ, Hellman LM: Williams Obstetrics. 13th Ed. New York Appleton-Century-Crofts, Inc., 1966.
63. Willson JR: Management of Obstetric Difficulties. 6th Ed. St. Louis, The C.V. Mosby Co., 1961.
64. Greenhill JP: Obstetrics. 13th Ed. Philadelphia, W.B. Saunders Co., 1965.
65. Reid DE: Textbook of Obstetrics. Philadelphia, W.B. Saunders Co., 1962.
66. Taylor ES: Beck's Obstetrical Practice. 8th Ed. Baltimore, The Williams & Wilkins Co., 1966.
67. Johnson CM: Transverse presentation of the fetus. Amer. J. Obstet. Gynecol. 57:765, 1949.
66. Evaldson GR: The grand multipara in modern obstetrics. Gynecol. Obstet. Invest. 30:217–223, 1990.
67. Stein AL, March CM: Pregnancy outcome in women with mullerian duct anomalies. J. Reprod. Med. 35:411–414, 1990.
68. Yates JA, MacDonald PC: Williams Obstetrics. 16th Ed. New York, Appleton-Century-Crofts, 1980.
69. Hourihane MJ: Etiology and management of oblique lie. Obstet. Gynecol. 32:512, 1968.
70. Garies LC, Ritzenthaler JC: Transverse presentation. Am. J. Obstet. Gynecol. 63:583, 1952.
73. Hankins GDV, Hammond TL, Snyder RR, Gilstrap LC: Transverse lie. Am. J. Perinatol. 7(1):66–70, 1990.
74. Cockburn KG, Drake RF: Transverse and oblique lie of the foetus. Aust. N.Z. J. Obstet. Gynaecol. 8:211, 1968.
75. Pelosi MA, Apuzzio J, Fricchione D, Gowda VV: The intra-abdominal version technique for delivery of transverse lie by low segment cesarean section. Am. J. Obstet. Gynecol. 135:1009, 1979.
76. Weissberg SM, O'Leary JA: Compound presentation of the fetus. Obstet. Gynecol. 41:60, 1973.
77. Cunningham FG, MacDonald PC, Gant NF: Williams Obstetrics. 18th Ed. E. Norwalk, CT, Appleton & Lange, 1989.
78. Breen JL, Wiesmeien E: Compound presentation—a survey of 131 patients. Obstet. Gynecol. 41:60, 1973.
79. Keettel WC, Crealock FW: Place of version and extraction in present day obstetrics. J. Iowa State Med. Soc. 42:251, 1952.
80. Goplerud J, Eastman NJ: Compound presentation. Obstet. Gynecol. 1:59, 1953.
81. Rosensohn M: Internal podalic version at New York Lying-In Hospital (1932–1950). Am. J. Obstet. Gynecol. 68:916, 1954.
82. Assali NS, Zacharias LF: Fetal and maternal mortality. An eleven-year survey. Am. J. Obstet. Gynecol. 54:651, 1947.
83. Schmitz HE, Bremner JX, Towne JE, Baba GR: The management of prolonged labor. A four-year review from the Lewis Memorial Maternity Hospital. Am. J. Obstet. Gynecol. 54: 642, 1947.
84. Martin PL: Obstetrical complications. Major complications encountered in 10,708 obstetrical cases in the University of California Hospital. Calif. West Med. 53:74, 1940.
85. Nissen ED: Twins: collision, impaction, compaction, and interlocking. Obstet. Gynecol. 11:514, 1958.
86. Speiser MD, Speck G: An evaluation of the treatment of the persistently unengaged vertex in the multipara. Am. J. Obstet. Gynecol. 51:607, 1946.
87. Clark RJ: Personal communication with JS McDonald, 1985.
88. Randall JH: Bleeding during and after the third stage of labor. Lancet 75:237, 1955.

Chapter 29

# MULTIPLE GESTATION—PRETERM AND POST-TERM DELIVERY

JOHN S. McDONALD

Multiple births have always been viewed as special events, they occur infrequently, and are the focus of attention for everyone in the labor and delivery area during delivery. They also present some special challenges to each individual member of the perinatal team. In turn, multiple births increase the hazards to the fetuses and to the mother because of separate maternal and fetal implications.The extra weight gain by the mother, for example, can be a problem from the standpoint of administration of an anesthetic to the mother via either regional or general; the higher incidence of vena cava compression with multiple gestations can be a problem from the standpoint of a higher incidence of hypotension with effects on both the mother and fetus; and the positioning of twins can be a problem for the fetus from the standpoint of interlocking at the time of vaginal delivery.

As pointed out repeatedly in the first edition of this book, anesthesia can have profound effects upon the favorable outcome of both the mother and the baby; if carefully thought-out and given due consideration, the anesthetic plan can help to make the birth experience a most pleasant and memorable one and provide safety for the mother, fetus, and newborn. However, if poorly thought-out and poorly administered, the anesthetic can have significant unfavorable influences upon both the mother and baby and can, at times, result in devastating consequences. Therefore, in the instance of the multiple birth, anesthesiologists are behooved to carefully plan and coordinate their efforts well in advance with the obstetrician and pediatrician and to make sure that their efforts are well understood by nursing, the other important member of the perinatal team.

In the past decade, there has developed an interesting trend toward an increase in the number of multiple births due to the effectiveness of infertility methods. Infertility procedures increase the possibility for multiple births greatly. Infertility methods in the past decade have undergone major advances in effectiveness of treatment and in protection of the mother and fetus. Recent methodology has focused on highly selective treatment of infertility with clomid as the first drug of choice and pergonal as the second drug of choice in certain refractory pituitary problems. In cases of triplets, quadruplets, and quintuplets, the patient can be counseled in regard to selective embryo reduction with the final decision being made by the parents. The latter form of selective birth control offers a better margin of safety for the mother and surviving fetuses. This, of course, is another reason to stress the need for optimal anesthesia care for labor and delivery of multiple births. To emphasize this point, it is easy to understand why these births are of great concern to the mother and father who have had an infertility problem for some time, who finally have accomplished a pregnancy, and who now are faced with a multiple gestation situation. This naturally results in tremendous pressure upon the perinatal team to ensure that the highest level of anesthetic care is made available, which of course, in a practical sense, is the case for all patients in an equal, unbiased manner. In the early 1990s, several critical interactive management policies have helped to shape the optimum safety in management of the multiple gestation delivery. These policies and methods include: (1) heavy reliance on ultrasonic diagnosis of fetal problems; (2) use of Doppler flow methods for evaluation of the growth and development of the fetus; (3) use of fetal heart rate methodology for added information regarding fetal well-being; and (4) a policy of interactive cooperation among obstetrics, anesthesiology, and pediatrics in regard to decision making about high-risk management cases. As mentioned at the outset, this chapter will help to emphasize the treatment methods that we believe have the most beneficial effect upon the fetus and mother in the multiple gestation situation.

## BASIC CONSIDERATIONS

Multiple gestations create their own aura of excitement that culminates with delivery of twins, triplets, quadruplets, quintuplets, sextuplets, septuplets, or octuplets. Unfortunately, survival of multiple gestations are fraught with high morbidity and mortality in regard to the fetuses, and sometimes even the life of the mother is at risk. By far the largest proportion of twins are from dizygotic origin, i.e., from two eggs rather than from monozygotic origin, i.e., from one egg. Figure 29–1 depicts the placentation possibilities with respect to twins. The latter, monozygotic twins, are usually thought of as identical and are usually of the same sex with predominance in favor of females over males. Dizygotic twins are thought of as fraternal and have individual amounts of unique genetic coding so that they are truly like individual brothers and sisters. The incidence of multiple births as related to twins

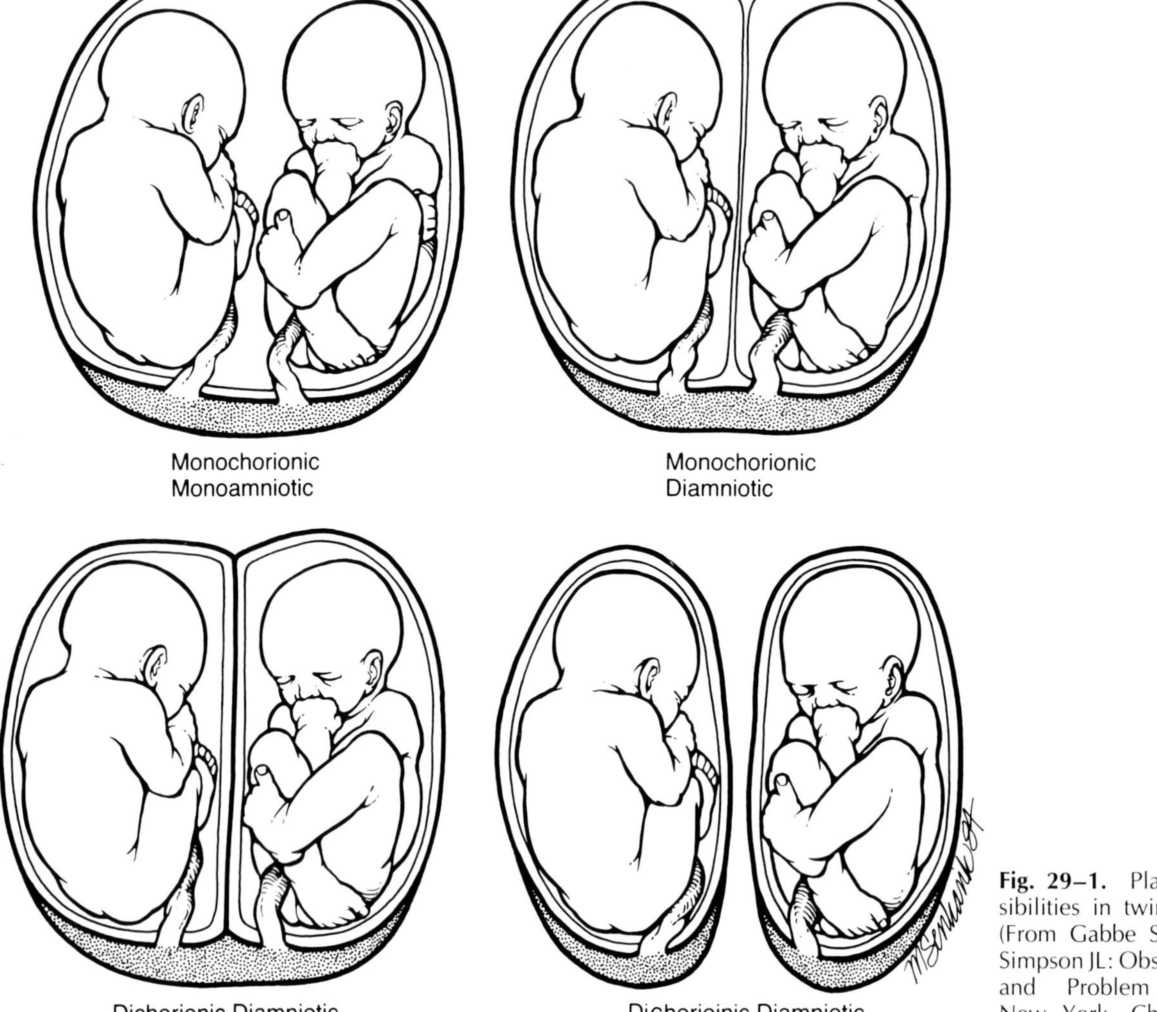


**Fig. 29–1.** Placentation possibilities in twin pregnancies. (From Gabbe SG, Niebyl JR, Simpson JL: Obstetrics: Normal and Problem Pregnancies. New York, Churchill Livingstone, 1991.)

is quoted as variable around the world and from 12 per 1000 in the United States, to only 1 per 155 in Japan, but to as high as 45 per 1000 in Africa (1,2). To approximate the frequency of occurrence of multiple pregnancies, the Hellin's hypothesis may be used: [frequency ($f$) of birth of $n$ infants is expressed as: $f = 80^{(n-1)}$], or see Table 29–1 (3,4). The cause of twinning is related more to the mother's genetic background than is it to the father's. Various factors have a positive effect upon dizygotic twinning, including age, parity, and use of ovulating induction drugs. Monozygotic twinning on the other hand is independent of age, parity, and racial background, and its incidence is remarkably consistent at a rate of nearly 1 per 250 throughout the world (5). See Table 29–2 for twinning rates by zygosity in five countries (6).

**Table 29–1.** Approximation of the Frequency of Occurrence of Multiple Pregnancies

| | |
|---|---|
| Twins | 1:80 |
| Triplets | $1:80^2$ = 1:6,400 |
| Quadruplets | $1:80^3$ = 1:512,000 |

(From Benson RC: Multiple pregnancy. *In* Current Obstetric and Gynecologic Diagnosis and Treatment 1987. Edited by ML Dernoll, RC Benson. Norwalk, CT, Appleton & Lange, 1987, p. 322.)

The most profound change over the last 20 years since the first edition of this book has been in the development and use of drugs to stimulate ovulation and the advances made in the area of infertility. The following paragraph from the first edition stated:

> "Some drugs used to stimulate ovulation in cases of infertility are known to increase the incidence of multiple gestations when pregnancy occurs, presumably by increasing the frequency of multiple simultaneous ovulation. These agents include human FSH, either as pituitary extract or menopausal serum, and clomiphene citrate, a synthetic estrogen homologue. Series

**Table 29–2.** Twinning Rates by Zygosity in Five Countries

| Country | Monozygotic | Dizygotic | Total |
|---|---|---|---|
| Niberia | 5.0 | 49 | 54 |
| United States | | | |
| Black | 4.7 | 11.1 | 15.8 |
| White | 4.2 | 7.1 | 11.3 |
| England and Wales | 3.5 | 8.8 | 12.3 |
| India (Calcutta) | 3.3 | 8.1 | 11.4 |
| Japan | 3.0 | 1.3 | 4.3 |

(From MacGillivray RT: Seminars In Perinatology. The Northwestern University Multihospital Twin Study.)

in the studies are still small, but one reports 33% twins with clomiphene and another 25% twins and 12% quadruplets with gonadotropin" (7–9).

Gonadotropins can have an incidence of multiple fetuses as high as 40% with the highest number of fetuses recorded as 11. The latter was a situation in which all were aborted (10).

It is interesting to note that ultrasound techniques performed early in the gestation have helped to identify that many twin conceptions never make it to term because a large number are largely resorbed prior to delivery of the viable fetus at or near term. There may be anatomic residual evidence of the nonviable twin at various stages of development described as fetus compressus or fetus papyraceous, or there may be such complete resorption that no evidence remains. Survival is remarkable, however, and there are examples of both sextuplets and octuplets surviving after gonadotropin therapy.

## Physiopathology

The maternal physiologic impact is significantly above that detailed in the changes of parturition in Chapter 2. Earlier work on physiologic changes associated with multiple gestation reports that the increase in plasma and blood volumes is as low as 10% greater to as high as 40% greater (11). The cardiac output is only slightly increased over that in singleton pregnancies, but the tendency toward anemia is more frequent and severe due to both the greater increase in blood volume and the increased iron and folate requirements as demanded by another fetus. In the third trimester, the baseline increase in heart rate and stroke volume both effect a further increase in cardiac output (Table 29–3) (12). Systemic vascular resistance increases about 10% above that in single pregnancies. Because of the larger-sized uterus, there are multiple maternal problems. One is the mechanical compression factor, with a greater incidence and degree of hypotension in the supine positions due to vena caval obstruction. Another is the encroachment upon the lung capacity with resultant respiratory embarrassment due to compression of the lung parenchyma, with shortness of breath in the mother except in the semi-sitting position. Uterine size can become enormous and reach double or even triple dimensions of that in single gestations. Another is the effect of the stretch of the uterine musculature upon labor. There may be hypotonic contractions during labor, which result in a failure to dilate the cervix effectively; and this same problem may result in one of the most serious complications of multiple gestations after delivery, namely, uterine hemorrhage. Finally, another problem is the reduced size of the epidural space due to increased uterine compression of the vena cava and resultant distension of all of its tributaries, including the azygos and hemiazygos system, which connects directly to the epidural venous complex.

The fetal physiological impact of multiple gestations is a measure greater than that just related for the mother. Past studies report significant elevations in neonatal deaths associated with multiple pregnancy. The perinatal mortality per 1000 births for single births, twins, triplets,

**Table 29–3.** Cardiovascular Parameters in Singleton and Twin Gestations

Note: $P \leq 0.005$

A. Second Trimester

| Gestation | HR | MAP | EDD (cm) | SV | CI |
|---|---|---|---|---|---|
| Singleton (n = 16) | 75 ± 10 | 77 ± 8 | 4.9 ± 0.3 | 76 ± 13 | 3.7 ± 0.7 |
| Twin (n = 6) | 86 ± 11 | 81 ± 10 | 4.9 ± 0.3 | 85 ± 15 | 4.6 ± 0.6 |

B. Third Trimester

| Gestation | HR | MAP | EDD (cm) | SV | CI |
|---|---|---|---|---|---|
| Singleton (n = 17)* | 74 ± 9 | 75 ± 6 | 4.9 ± 0.3 | 71 ± 12 | 3.3 ± 0.6 |
| Twin (n = 14)** | 83 ± 10 | 78 ± 4 | 5.0 ± 0.4 | 93 ± 16 | 4.9 ± 0.7 |

HR = Heart rate.
MAP = Mean arterial pressure (mm Hg).
EDD = Left ventricular end-diastolic dimension.
SV = Stroke volume (ml).
CI = Cardiac Index ($L \cdot min^{-1} \cdot m^{-2}$).
* = 16 of these subjects were also studied in the second trimester.
** = Four of these subjects were also studied in the second trimester.
(Modified from Veille JC, Morton MJ, Burry KJ: Maternal cardiovascular adaptations to twin pregnancy. Am. J. Obstet. Gynecol. 153:261, 1985.)

**Table 29–4.** Perinatal Mortality Rates in Multiple Pregnancy

| Singletons | Twins | Triplets | Quadruplets |
|---|---|---|---|
| 39 | 152 | 309 | 509 |

All rates are per 1000.
(From Benson RC: Multiple pregnancy. *In* Current Obstetric and Gynecologic Diagnosis and Treatment 1987. Edited by ML Pernoll, RC Benson. Norwalk, CT, Appleton & Lange, 1987.)

and quadruplets from the most recent U.S. statistics is shown in Table 29–4 (4). In addition to this, there is a greater risk of a fetus in a multiple gestation not making it to term because of the possibility of fetal death, and, as mentioned earlier, fetus compressus or papyraceous alongside the normal gestation that goes to term. The etiology of the higher perinatal mortality rate is partly due to the higher incidence of low-birthweight infants in multiple gestation. Modern advances in the area of diagnosis and antepartum monitoring due to ultrasound and Doppler methods and significant improvements in neonatal intensive care have had major impacts upon the poor perinatal mortality rate previously associated with multiple births. This improvement in the perinatal mortality has been due to a two-pronged attack. An example of improved antepartum care is the study of stillbirths from 1975 to 1979 compared to the period 1980 to 1983 in which the stillbirths were 23/1000 and 0/1000, respectively. An example of the impact of better neonatal care is the perinatal mortality in twins (1969 to 1979) of 95/1000, compared to the 1987 rate of 152/1000 (4,13). The dramatic improvement is due largely to the tremendous improvements in neonatal care, especially in management of those small babies whose weights are 1000 g to 1800 g. Similar improvements are also noted in the triplet series with a perinatal mortality of 93/1000 (1975 to 1988) falling to 51/1000 (1985 to 1988) (14,15). The study by Gonen, et al indicated that the probable, major determinants of improved outcome were: early diagnosis by ultrasonagraphy; meticulous antenatal care; early hospitalization; delivery by cesarean section; and on-site availability of a neonatologist for every baby at the time of delivery (14). Despite these improvements in the perinatal mortality due to advances in antenatal and neonatal care areas, the fact remains that the percentages of early births have not improved; in other words, the prematurity rate for twins, triplets, and more is the same now as it was 1 and 2 decades ago, as can be seen in the gestational age distribution graph of Figure 29–2.

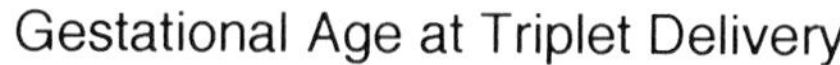


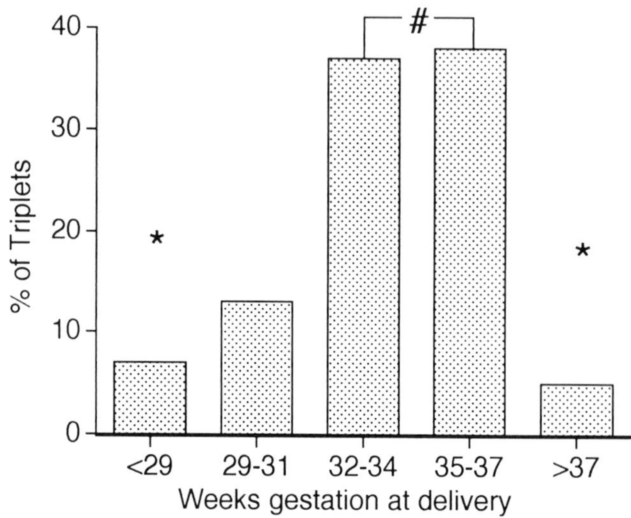


**Fig. 29–2.** Age distributions of 198 triplets reveals approximately 60% were between 32 and 37 weeks at the time of delivery. (Modified from Newman RB, Hamer C, Miller MC: Outpatient triplet management: A contemporary review. Am. J. Obstet. Gynecol. 161:547, 1989.)

## Obstetric Management

It is acknowledged that improvements in antepartum care have had tremendous beneficial effect upon survival of the multiple gestation pregnancy; however, because this is not an obstetric textbook, the reader is referred to those excellent texts of obstetrics and gynecology for the latest in the advances of antepartum care in a detailed fashion, to such works as: (1) Gabbe's "Obstetrics Normal and Problem Pregnancies, 2nd Ed."; (2) Pernoll's "Current Obstetric & Gynecologic Diagnosis & Treatment, 7th Ed."; and (3) "Cunningham's Williams Obstetrics, 18th Ed." Here the discussion will be limited to the intrapartum period.

One of the most apparent advances in intrapartum care has been the ability to monitor the status of the individual babies during the labor period (16). This, together with the ability to map out the relative positions of each baby and their relationship relative to each other, allows an unprecedented view of the potential problems that labor could precipitate. See Figure 29–3 for examples of both

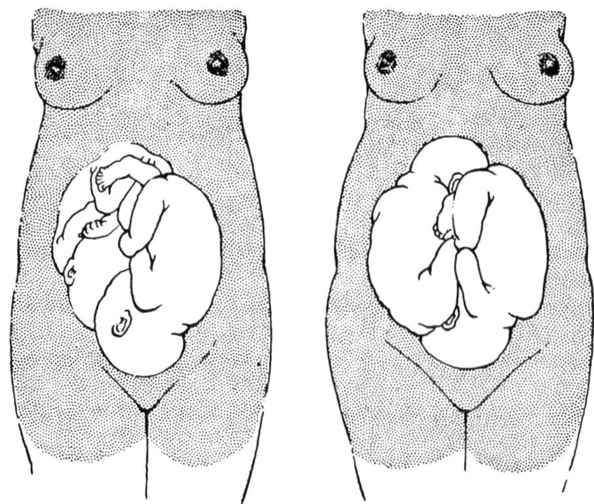

**Fig. 29–3.** Examples of both twins presenting by the vertex or one twin vertex and one breech. (From Benson RC: Handbook of Obstetrics & Gynecology. 8th ed. East Norwalk, Appleton & Lange, 1983.)

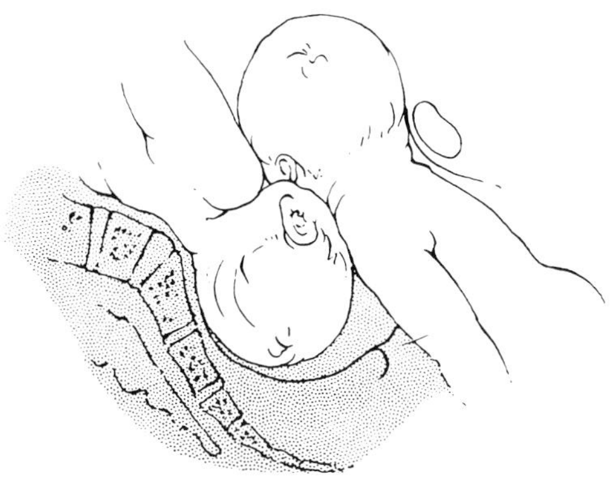

**Fig. 29–4.** Locked twins. (From Benson RC: Handbook of Obstetrics & Gynecology. 4th ed. East Norwalk, Appleton & Lange, 1971.)

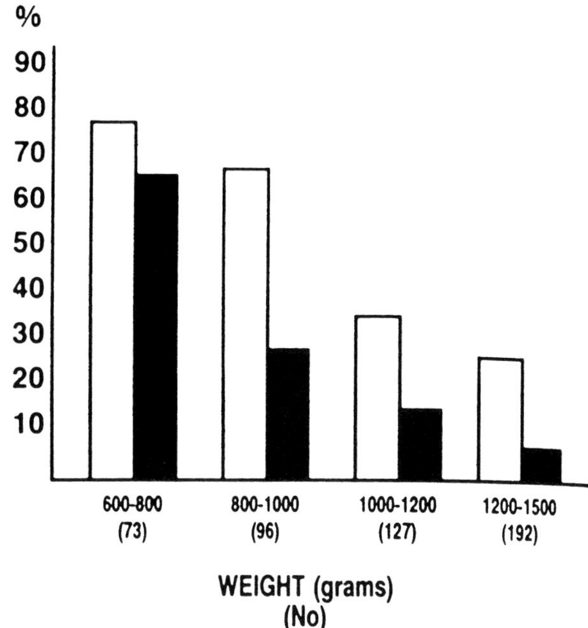


**Fig. 29–5.** Incidence of intraventricular hemorrhage (white bars) and mortality (black bars) according to birthweight groupings. (From Morales WJ, Koerten J: Obstet Gynecol 68:37, 1986.)

twins presenting by the vertex, or one twin vertex and one breech. Thus, vaginal delivery may well be planned for the first twin vertex and the second twin vertex alignment. On the other hand, cesarean section may be the choice in those situations in which the first twin is in a nonvertex position. The dreaded "locking twins position" is a potential situation should the nonvertex position combine with the second twin, a vertex and face-to-face apposition (Figure 29–4). This condition was responsible for a high fetal mortality in earlier years when it was more common to attempt vaginal delivery without the knowledge of the exact fetal reference positions. In one series of this problem, the mortality was greater than 25% because the problem was not diagnosed until too late, i.e., during delivery of the first breech whereafter delivery of the aftercoming head was impossible (17,18). Other combinations of fetal positions do occur, such as transverse and oblique, but the general philosophy today is toward cesarean section except in those instances in which both fetuses are vertex or in those instances in which close updating of the positioning and dependable monitoring is readily available and dependable (19,20). The problem of the low-birthweight baby must be addressed in reference to vaginal versus cesarean delivery also. Due to the poor results reported in singleton breech deliveries of less than 1500 g, current consensus appears to favor cesarean delivery in instances in which the birthweight is less than 1500 g (21,22). One of the primary concerns in regard to survival in these less-than-1500-g babies is the propensity for intraventricular hemorrhage with vaginal delivery, perhaps associated with the changes in the cephalic pressures during the actual mechanics of delivery (Figure 29–5).

External cephalic version is another strategy that must be considered in transverse and other malpositioning of the second twin (Table 29–5). Figure 29–6 shows the large majority (over 60%) of twins as being Cephalic-cephalic or Cephalic-breech in a series of 341 twin pregnancies (23). Studies reveal a high degree of failure rate, i.e., above 50%, and an associated higher rate of fetal distress. Thus, recommendations were for breech extraction in fetuses over 1500 g, or otherwise cesarean section delivery (Table 29–6) (24,25). It is possible to obtain a sonogram for estimated fetal weight on the second twin so that this latter decision can be supported by accurate data. Thus, after an attempt is made after delivery of the first twin to cephalic conversion of the second twin, and it is a failure, then vaginal delivery via breech extraction is reasonable in those fetuses proven to be over 2000 g. It is understood that some obstetricians will be loath to performing a vaginal delivery and then combining with a cesarean delivery. In other words, many practitioners will opt to deliver both by cesarean section from the beginning. This is a decision that must be individualized and is dependent upon the circumstances, the facilities, the

**Table 29–5.** Delivery Complications*

| | Complication | Outcome |
|---|---|---|
| External Version | | |
| Successful | Fetal distress | C/S |
| Successful | Fetal distress | C/S |
| Successful | Cord prolapse | C/S |
| Successful | Cord prolapse | C/S |
| Successful | Cord prolapse | C/S |
| Successful | Failure to descend | C/S |
| Successful | Compound presentation | C/S |
| Breech Extraction | | |
| Unsuccessful | Lower uterine segment contracted | C/S |
| Unsuccessful | Lower uterine segment contracted | C/S |

C/S: Cesarean section.
(From Gocke SE, Nageotte MP, Garite T, Towers CV, et al: Management of the nonvertex second twin: primary cesarean section, external version, or primary breech extraction. Am. J. Obstet. Gynecol. 161:111, 1989.)

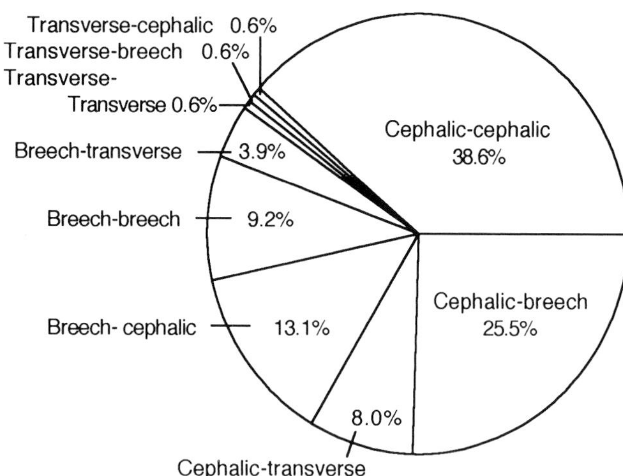


**Fig. 29–6.** Twin presentation at time of delivery. (Redrawn from Thompson SA, Lyons TL, Makowski EL: Outcomes of twin gestations at the University of Colorado Health Sciences Center, 1973–1983. J. Reprod. Med. 32:328, 1987.)

timing in regard to consultation and back up, and the preferences of the obstetrician based upon his/her past experience and comfort. For those mothers with three fetuses or more, the prevailing preference seems to be delivery by cesarean section, especially in an environment of learning in which less and less experience with complex maneuvers of intrauterine manipulation is gained. Such a preference seems a logical answer to the problem.

Another problem associated with twin deliveries is the time interval between deliveries. There are examples in the literature of remarkably long periods of time, even weeks between such deliveries, but these are truly unusual situations (Figure 29–7) (26–28). For the most part, current day recommendations are to deliver the second twin in an unhurried manner with no trauma to the mother or the fetus and with good analgesia for the mother (29). There are records of time periods that the second twin must be delivered within, but these are artifactual and made before the times of modern sophistication in monitoring with real-time ultrasound and Doppler (30,31). Patients are now benefiting from electronic monitoring of the first baby and Doppler monitoring of the second baby. There is no problem today with keeping track of the second baby with use of the real-time ultrasound when movement occurs and the Doppler signal is weak. In the following section, the coordination of the anesthesia and the obstetric management will be made and the application of the technique and the possible changes that must be made during labor will be discussed.

**Table 29–6.** Second Twin Delivery

| | Group A | Group B | *p* |
|---|---|---|---|
| Successful vaginal delivery | 19/41 (46%) | 53/55 (96%) | <0.001 |
| Cesarean section | 16/41* (39%) | 2/55 (4%) | <0.001 |
| Successful secondary breech extraction | 6/41 (15%) | — | — |
| Total | 41/41 (100%) | 55/55 (100%) | |

Group A = Attempted external version (n = 41).
Group B = Attempted breech extraction (n = 55).
* Seven successful and nine unsuccessful versions required cesarean section.
(Modified from Gocke SE, Nageotte MP, Garite T, Towers CV, et al: Management of the nonvertex second twin: primary cesarean section, external version, or primary breech extraction. Am. J. Obstet. Gynecol. 161:111, 1989.)

## Anesthetic Management

There is nothing magic about the management of the patient with a multiple gestation from the viewpoint of the anesthesia delivery. The same solid, basic or foundation aspects of management espoused for patients in other special categories such as breech presentation are used in the management of this special problem. First comes the decision of the choice of anesthetic technique, namely, use of general anesthesia, use of regional anesthesia such as lumbar epidural or spinal block, or use of local anesthesia. Next comes the decision of the choice of anesthetic agent. Then comes the planning stage, including explaining the preferences just mentioned to the mother and father. This stage also includes the communication link to the other members of the perinatal team, the obstetrician, the pediatrician, and the nurse. Finally, the coordination of the anesthesia team must be organized, i.e., which member will be responsible for what duty, who the induction assistant will be, who the resuscitator will be, and who will assist, etc. Provisions must also be made for exigencies such as sudden prolapse of the cord, hemorrhage, coordination with the blood bank, and a check on availability and time lags in blood and blood products. As is readily apparent, the planning stage for anesthetic management must be thought-out in advance and coordinated with the entire perinatal team and even other members of the medical team outside of obstetrics. It is a responsibility not to be taken lightly, and emphasizes the need for leadership in this area so that all of the complexities of interaction can be performed smoothly. Multiple gestation is a situation in which the close interaction of the involved specialties is vital to production of the desired result.

By far the largest number of multiple pregnancies are delivered via cesarean section. The reasons for this are the high number of complications associated with multiple gestations, including failures of labor, tendency toward premature labor, associated cord accidents, problems with second stage labor mechanics, and trends away from intrauterine manipulations in all obstetric practices all across the country today. Anesthetic Management for Vaginal Delivery, discussed later in this chapter, is really in regard to the management of twin deliveries. Triplets, quadruplets, and quintuplets are managed by cesarean delivery, for the most part, as mentioned above. Of course, the adverse litigious atmosphere does not help this situation, but even without this atmosphere, there exists a real appreciation of the fetal complications associated with the

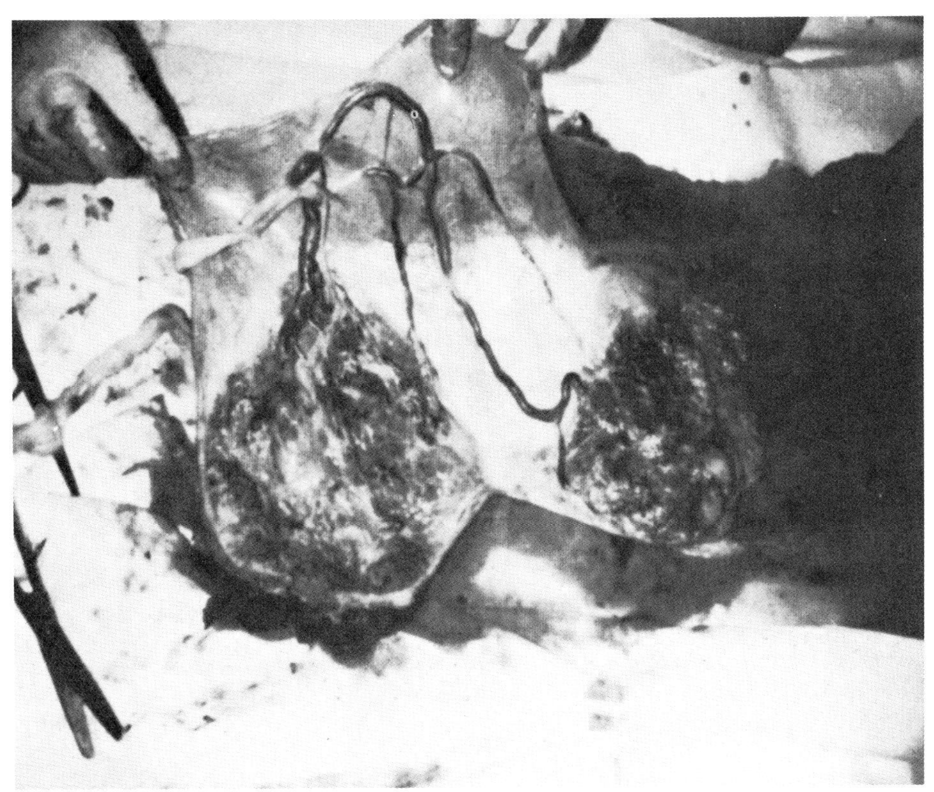

**Fig. 29–7.** The placenta of twin B (the surviving twin) is seen on the left; the placenta of twin A (the nonsurviving twin) is seen on the right. The latter placenta was left intact after delivery 12 weeks prior. Twin B survived because of tocolysis and cerclage and was released from the hospital in excellent condition. (From Feichtinger W, Breitenecker G, Fröhlich H: Prolongation of pregnancy and survival of twin B after loss of twin A at 21 weeks gestation. Am. J. Obstet. Gynecol. 161:891, 1989.)

more aggressive manipulations of the past and, as a result, obstetric decision making has steered away from this type of practice in recent years toward the more conservative approach. Naturally, the aforementioned use of the monitoring with early ultrasound estimation of fetal weight, with intrapartum localization of the fetuses with real-time ultrasound, with Doppler monitoring of the fetal heart beat, and with electronic monitoring as a supplemental method, all have contributed tremendously in providing a safer environment for the intrapartum course. All of these improvements over the years have helped to foster this attitude, and with it has come a much improved outcome for the products of the multiple gestation pregnancies.

Anesthesia selection and administration for the patient with a multiple gestation presents a challenge to the anesthesiologist for many reasons, some of which are due to exaggerated physiological changes such as in the respiratory and cardiovascular systems. One example is a problem with regional anesthesia. Because of the larger than normal uterine mass, there is often a threat of supine hypotension over and beyond that associated with singleton pregnancies. This threat is chiefly in regard to anesthesia for cesarean section, which necessitates a higher sensory block. Because hypotension is one of the important complications to avoid, the use of regional anesthesia in these patients may have to be modified or limited to deliberate, slow development of anesthetic block with small and divided doses of local anesthetic administered over 5-minute time periods. Otherwise, the systemic vascular resistance may plummet and result in significant hypotensive reactions due to the combined effect of the reduced vascular resistance, the reduction in return of venous volumes to the heart, and the fixed heart rate response associated with a T-4 block. Another example is a problem with general anesthesia. Falls in blood pressure in and around the time of the induction of the anesthetic can be secondary also to the larger than normal uterine mass, which may be difficult to elevate and deviate enough laterally to avoid vena cava and aortic compression regardless of the attempts at doing so. Thus, the patient may be refractory to lying on her back even for very brief periods of time and induction may have to be done with the patient in a slightly modified 45° lateral position.

## Anesthesia for Vaginal Delivery

In consideration of anesthesia for labor and delivery, the epidural is likely the most versatile method. One large series of 130 women with twins who received epidural analgesia was studied by Crawford, who found the second stage was increased threefold when compared to women without epidural analgesia. This study was completed before 1987, however, and there have been substantial changes in administration of the drug since then (Table 29–7)(32). The most successful change in administration has been the use of the continuous, low concentration local anesthetic with minute levels of opioid and epinephrine as described in Chapter 13. This provides excellent pain relief without the hazard of hypotension, and allows the mother to advance through the first stage of labor in comfort. The second stage is managed either with no additional anesthetic, as nearly 80% of patients receiving this continuous method had adequate perineal analgesia for delivery if the administration time was over 3 hours, or

**Table 29–7.** Distribution by Gestational Age, Mode of Delivery, and Type of Analgesia/Anesthesia of 196 Cases of Twin Pregnancy

| Gestational Age at Delivery | Vaginal Delivery | | Elective Cesarean Section | | Emergency Cesarean Section | | Vaginal 1/Cesarean Section 2 | |
|---|---|---|---|---|---|---|---|---|
| | Epidural | No Epidural | Epidural | General | Epidural | General | Epidural | No Epidural |
| ⩾38 | 33 | 8 | 8 | 1 | 6 | 11 | 2 | 2 |
| 37 | 25 | 4 | — | 1 | 1 | 2 | — | — |
| 36 | 15 | 1 | 1 | 1 | 2 | — | — | — |
| 35 | 8 | 4 | — | — | 1 | 3 | — | 1 |
| 34 | 9 | 2 | — | 3 | 2 | 4 | — | — |
| 33 | — | 1 | — | — | — | 3 | — | — |
| 32 | 5 | 1 | — | 1 | — | — | 1 | 1 |
| 31 | 5 | 1 | — | — | — | 3 | — | — |
| 30 | — | — | — | — | — | — | — | — |
| 29 | 1 | 1 | — | — | — | — | 1 | — |
| 28 | — | 1 | — | 1 | — | 2 | — | — |
| 27 | 1 | — | — | — | — | 1 | — | — |
| 26 | 2 | — | — | — | — | — | — | — |
| 25 | 1 | — | — | — | — | — | — | — |
| 24 | — | 1 | — | — | — | — | — | — |
| TOTALS | 105 | 25 | 9 | 8 | 12 | 29 | 4 | 4 |

(From Crawford JS: A prospective study of 200 consecutive twin deliveries. Anaesthesia 42:33, 1987.)

by administration of a sitting up, small, more concentrated dose of local anesthetic for the purpose of blocking the sacral fibers just before vaginal delivery. Another method that can also provide suitable analgesia is the use of small aliquots of opioid intravenously during labor for first stage analgesia and the addition of a pudendal block with $N_2O$ supplementation as needed for the actual delivery. The $N_2O$ can be given either intermittently or continuously with changes in concentration from 20% to 30% to 50% as indicated during painful periods.

### *Anesthesia for Cesarean Section*

Because of the increasing trend toward delivery of the fetuses of multiple gestations by the cesarean route rather than by vaginal delivery, the plan for the optimum anesthetic must be carefully considered. More recent reports have recorded nearly 50% of the multiple births were by cesarean section, not of vaginal delivery (23,33). Figure 29–8 depicts the mode of delivery for twin gestations, and Table 29–8 depicts the mode of delivery for triplets. It is important to discuss the issue of the type of anesthetic technique with the mother in detail so that she is aware of the advantages to her and to her babies. This may seem like a small consideration to the physician, but patients report repeatedly that they appreciate being informed of such detail, and by getting this information first hand from the anesthesiologist, such consideration greatly alleviates much of their anxiety and concern. It also gives them an opportunity to air some of their questions and eradicate any misconceptions they may have.

The types of anesthesia for consideration include regional anesthesia, general anesthesia, and local anesthesia. Regional anesthesia can be subdivided into spinal methods and epidural methods. The spinal methods include the usual single spinal injection of a local anesthetic into the subarachnoid space and the continuous spinal method by which separated, smaller aliquots of local anesthetic may be injected for desired effect. The former method has been by far the most common method used over the years because it is simple, fast to achieve the desired ef-

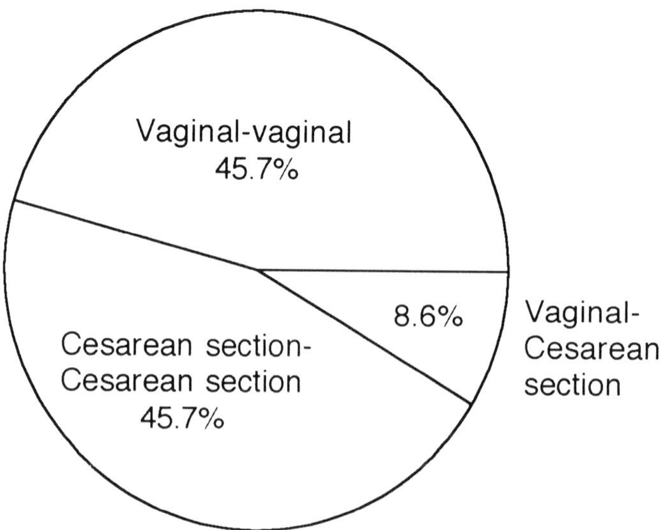


**Fig. 29–8.** Mode of delivery in twin gestation. (From Thompson SA, Lyons TL, Makowski EL: Outcomes of twin gestations at the University of Colorado Health Sciences Center, 1973–1983. J. Reprod. Med. 32:328, 1987.)

**Table 29–8.** Mode of Delivery in Triplets

| Patient | Mode of Delivery |
|---|---|
| 1 | Cesarean section |
| 2 | Cesarean section |
| 3 | Cesarean section |
| 4 | Cesarean section |
| 5 | Cesarean section |
| 6 | Cesarean section |
| 7 | Cesarean section |
| 8 | A. Midforceps<br>B. Breech extraction<br>C. Breech extraction |
| 9 | Cesarean section |
| 10 | Cesarean section |
| 11 | Cesarean section |
| 12 | A. Normal Spontaneous Vaginal Delivery<br>B. Midforceps<br>C. Cesarean section |
| 13 | Cesarean section |

(Modified from Keith LG, et al: The Northwestern University triplet study II: fourteen triplet pregnancies delivered between 1981 and 1986. Acta. Genet. Med. Gemellol. 37:65–75, 1988.)

fect, and was the first and most popularized method. The continuous spinal method, on the other hand, was introduced only in the 1900s and did not receive great reviews for the simple reason that we did not have adequate technology at that time to make the needles and catheters necessary to take full advantage of the method.

The continuous spinal has been repopularized now by recent literature reports including Benedetti, Kestin, et al, and Huckaby, et al. It is particularly suited to obstetrics and especially the areas that present difficult challenges, such as morbid obesity and the multiple gestation situation. The reason for its particular suitability is that it is the only method the anesthesiologist can use that will give full control of slow development of anesthesia and time for accommodation so that many of the complications common to regional anesthesia can be minimized or avoided altogether. For example, the most dramatic and life-threatening complication of regional anesthesia is the hypotension that accompanies the sympathetic block. This occurs because of the inability of the mother to accommodate and increase her vascular resistance above the level of the sympathetic block to offset the fall in vascular resistance below the level of the sympathetic block. With a catheter in the subarachnoid space, the local anesthetic can be injected at small amounts at a time and then a wait period inserted until the effect of that injection is fully manifest. During this wait period, the mother's physiological response to the sympathetic effect of the small amount of drug administered can be mobilized, offsetting any fall in blood pressure. The next injection can follow within minutes and so on until the desired dermatome level of block is attained for suitable analgesia for the cesarean section. The local anesthetic is enhanced by an opioid such as fentanyl, and this increases the effectiveness of the block and allows a lower level of block to be used for cesarean section analgesia. For example, with the opioid enhancement, the dermatome level may be only at the T-6 or even T-8 level, instead at the T-4 level. The effective analgesia is much improved with the opioid so that little or any perception of discomfort will be noted by the patient even when maximum stimulation of the visceral layer of the peritoneum occurs during dissection of the bladder flap and during exploration of the upper abdomen after delivery, and most notably during the time when the uterus may be exteriorized at closing procedures. In sum, the continuous spinal has been a welcome new addition to the scene of regional anesthesia because of the great control it brings to the anesthesiologist. The control comes in the ability to administer only the small amounts of drug necessary to get the desired effect and to give those dosages only when the timing is correct in accordance with safety for the mother and fetus. The continuous spinal has been discussed in detail in Chapter 14 in regard to its place in the management of high-risk obstetrics. This technique has been repopularized largely because of: (1) our tremendous advances in technology in regard to making of catheters and needles; (2) our recent favorable clinical experiences with long-term catheter usage; and (3) our better understanding of the use of opioid enhancement drugs in combination with local anesthetic drugs in the subarachnoid space to provide more intense analgesia.

The epidural method can also be considered for use in cesarean section for multiple gestations. It is also the sympathetic block and the resultant physiological changes associated with it that limit its usefulness here just as in the subarachnoid block. Of course, the advantage of the epidural being injected in increments with time adjustment periods interspersed has been in vogue only since the middle to latter years of the 1970s, well after the first edition of this book was published. The only other important modification invoked since then has been the addition of fentanyl to the local anesthetic. In the case of the epidural opioid enhancement, 50 μg are added to each 10 ml, or a total of 100 μg per 20 ml solution. This allows for substantial improvement in anesthetic potency and an intense sensory denervation even to the point that dissection of the bladder flap and stimulation of the peritoneum does not cause pain. The most common of complications, hypotension, can be reduced by careful attention to hydration of the patient before regional anesthetic challenge, use of the intermittent injection technique just mentioned above, and careful attention to positioning of the mother's uterus to avoid hypotension.

## Preterm and Post-term Delivery

Even in the 1990s, it is possible to have imprecise definition of the gestational age. The time-honored method of estimation of the expected date of confinement (EDC) is to use the "obstetric wheel," by placing the arrow on the last menstrual period. In essence, this is use of the Naegele formula for determining EDC, which was described as the addition of 7 days to the first day of the last menstrual period (LMP) and counting back 3 months.

The problem with both of these "mathematical" determinations is that many menstrual periods are not "normal," that many times small bleeding episodes may be interpreted as the last menstrual period or that many menstrual periods are the result of discontinuance of birth control pills with resultant anovulation for 1 or more months, or even more confusing periods of amenorrhea.

The most acceptable means for defining the EDC is by the following:

1. positive pregnancy test within 4 to 6 weeks of the last menstrual period (LMP);
2. detection of fetal heart tones (FHT);
3. identification of fetal movement;
4. biparietal diameter determination;
5. crown-rump measurement; and
6. ultrasound scan before the end of the second trimester.

These methods are not perfect by any means, but they are reported to be reliable within reasonable days of accuracy, and when combined so that agreement between two different methods exists, then the likelihood of prediction becomes much greater (34–37). For our purposes in this chapter, preterm will be used to describe those fetuses that deliver before 38 weeks, and postterm for those fetuses that deliver after 42 weeks. Because there have been remarkable improvements in neonatal care since the first edition of this book, and because the greatest risk group of preterm fetuses appears to be in the very low-birthweight neonates of less than 1500 g and in the extremely low-birthweight neonates of less than 1000 g, the discussion of the anesthetic management that follows will be restricted to this particularly high-risk group.

## Preterm Delivery

The successful arrest of preterm labor is a major part of the success rate in regard to survival of these special and very small babies. Arrest is usually only successful if it is instituted early in the diagnosis phase. The various discussions about differentiation of small growth retarded babies versus true premature babies is beyond the scope of this text, but the author would refer the reader to two other texts for an excellent coverage of the subject: "Williams Obstetrics" and "Obstetrics Normal and Problem Pregnancies."

The pharmacologic methods in use today include many different agents. The beta receptor agonist drugs have been in use since the early 1970s. Ritodrine was the first of these to be approved for use in arrest of premature labor. Its popularity has waxed and waned since then, and it seems that current opinion deems it though effective in delaying labor, it does so only for a brief period of time with little effect on the eventual perinatal survival statistics. In addition, there have been some significant side effects associated with its intravenous use. These include pulmonary edema, myocardial symptoms, and some metabolic effects, including some sodium and water retention. As a result of this brevity and side effects, its use is restricted to those few cases that seem reasonable and not complicated by a patient compromise at the outset. One of the older and well-established agents for depression of labor is magnesium sulphate. It is a well recognized and understood agent with widespread acceptance. Its problems are associated with central nervous system depression. Patients on such therapy must be carefully monitored for problems such as depressed respiration and depressed deep tendon reflexes. Terbutaline is another agent used before ritodrine, and even though it was popular, it also suffered from associated pulmonary problems such as pulmonary edema. The recent discovery that a reduction in calcium inhibits uterine contractility has encouraged interest in the calcium channel blocking drugs such as nifedipine, diltiazem hydrochloride, and verapamil hydrochloride. To date, these drugs have not been associated with some of the more serious cardiac and pulmonary side effects as noted with the other uterine motility inhibitory drugs as previously mentioned. A recent newcomer to this field has been the antiprostaglandins, which also appear to have a possible role in prevention of premature labor.

### Preterm Labor and Delivery Management

Current attitudes continued to favor conservative measures in regard to management of both labor itself and the actual delivery. It is now well appreciated that those fetuses under 1500 g are at risk from the ravages of prolonged labor, excessive uterine contractions, prolonged second stages, and difficult deliveries either by spontaneous vaginal delivery eventually or by forceps delivery. It would seem prudent to deliver these very small preterm babies by cesarean section whenever there is evidence of abnormal heart rate patterns, bleeding, infection, or failure to dilate and descend in a normal manner. A further recommendation is for fetal monitoring in such cases with special attention to changes not only in patterned responses to contractions but also to development of other ominous signs such as increases or decreases in the baseline heart rate or fixation of the baseline with little or no baseline variability. The mode of delivery has been an argumentative issue for some time with proponents on both sides of the issue discussing the dangers associated with fetal intracranial hemorrhage. Early interpretation of the excessively high rate of such hemorrhage hypothesized that it was: (1) secondary to the pressures experienced as a result of either maternal Valsalva maneuvers or delivery with forceps, which elicited undo pressure; or (2) secondary to the sudden changes in pressures inside and outside the sensitive fetal head upon actual delivery. Subsequent clinical reviews of vaginal delivery versus cesarean delivery have not verified that abdominal delivery reduces the incidence of this problem of intracranial hemorrhage (38–43).

### Preterm Anesthetic Management

The problem of preterm delivery presents an unusual challenge to the anesthesiologist. Preterm delivery is one of the examples of the absolute need for close communication and coordination of care methods used that must be understood and agreed upon by the obstetrician and the pediatrician. Many past suggestions for anesthetic management of the preterm were focused on the use of only regional anesthetic techniques because of the fear of "respiratory depression" secondary to the use of systemic medications or general anesthetic agents. These were days when superb methods of airway and ventilation and oxygenation were not possible. Furthermore, intensive care units either did not exist or were primitive. This is hardly a problem today with the sophistication that our colleagues have developed in management of such problems. Our preterm infants benefit from the finest neonatal care available in the world today. Thus, if regional anesthetic techniques would be contraindicated because of some unusual reason such as maternal bleeding, for example, the delivery could be managed nicely by use of perineal local and pudendal blocks in conjunction with $N_2O$ administration to lessen the pain associated with uterine contractions or to add to the analgesia of the incompletely blocked perineum. Of course, regional analgesia is still an excellent choice for both labor and vaginal delivery. Table 29–9 shows the intervals between twin deliveries with epidural and without epidural, and reveals little difference in the mean interval or range of intervals, regardless of the anesthetic. The modern modifications such as detailed in Chapter 13 can be used to major advantage here in which minimal exposure to hypotension is of paramount importance. The continuous analgesic block with the catheter offers a degree of freedom from this complication and at the same time excellent analgesia for the mother both in the first stage and the second stage. An excellent choice of anesthesia for cesarean section is the regional technique, i.e., lumbar epidural or continuous subarachnoid catheter for the preterm fetus; however, cesarean section can also be safely performed under the general technique, or by local technique. Regional anesthesia has

**Table 29–9.** Twin Delivery Intervals With and Without Epidural

| Birthweight (kg) | n | Mean Interval (minutes) | Range (minutes) |
|---|---|---|---|
| **Epidural** | | | |
| >3.0 | 15 | 13.7 | 4 to 33 |
| 2.5–3.0 | 27 | 13.0 | 5 to 27 |
| 2.0–2.5 | 35 | 11.6 | 3 to 52 |
| 1.5–2.0 | 22 | 11.3 | 4 to 56 |
| ≤1.5 | 6 | 7.3 | 2 to 13 |
| **No Epidural** | | | |
| >3.0 | 3 | 11.7 | 6 to 22 |
| 2.5–3.0 | 8 | 9.7 | 3 to 24 |
| 2.0–2.5 | 4 | 11.5 | 3 to 24 |
| 1.5–2.0 | 7 | 7.7 | 4 to 12 |
| ≤1.5 | 3 | 7.0 | 6 to 9 |

(Modified from Crawford JS: A prospective study of 200 consecutive twin deliveries. Anaesthesia 42:33, 1987.)

in the past and probably still does today, poses somewhat as a threat to the premature fetus if there is evidence of any other complications, such as fetal distress or placental insufficiency.

This threat is related to the hypotension that can occur in conjunction with the sympathetic block when a large volume of anesthetic is injected within a short period of time. This hypotension serves as another threat and, in the presence of complications such as mentioned above, may be additive enough to cause serious fetal jeopardy, morbidity, or even mortality. Nevertheless, this threat of hypotension associated with regional anesthesia can be significantly reduced by: (1) using small individual doses of local anesthetic injected over time with 5-minute wait periods between each injection; (2) making sure the patient's intravascular volume is adequate to withstand a sympathetic block; (3) making sure the patient does not have any supine hypotension due to faulty positioning; and (4) using adjuvant opioid enhancement so that a lower than usual sensory block can suffice it for the operative trespass. It is not recommended to use the standard subarachnoid block with single injection of a bolus of local anesthetic. The sympathetic block from such procedures may be excessive and result in the problem of hypotension alluded to above. It should be recalled that the most significant influence on hypotension is the rapidity with which the block comes on with little time to accommodate for the extensive sympathectomy by increasing the vascular resistance in the areas not affected by the sympathectomy.

## Post-term Delivery

### Post-term Labor and Delivery Management

Often this diagnosis is related more to an error in the estimated date of confinement than to a true postdate phenomena. In most patients, labor will begin sometime in the thirty-eighth week to the fortieth week if dating of conception is accurate. However, as expected, there is a considerable variation in the attempt to accurately date conception and, as a result, some patients may not begin spontaneous labor until 41 or even 42 weeks. The problem becomes one of accurate diagnosis, monitoring of the health of the intrauterine exposure, estimation of the fetal viability, and finally, making a decision on when to terminate the pregnancy. On the one hand, the postterm fetus may present a problem from the standpoint of excessive size, and, on the other hand, the postterm fetus may be in significant jeopardy due to exposure to insufficient oxygenation and other ingredients to maintain intrauterine growth and development. In either of the latter situations, it may be prudent to consider termination of pregnancy for the health and welfare of the fetus/newborn. In one series of patients with prolonged gestations, a policy of delivery by the forty-second week of gestation resulted in quite favorable outcomes for the neonates and no increased incidence of cesarean section for the mothers (44). Naturally, there may be some maternal indications that encourage delivery before even 42 weeks, and those of course include pregnancy with superimposed pregnancy-induced hypertension, diabetes, Addisons, certain

CNS disease processes, and many of the pulmonary- and cardiac-based problems. Today, there has been sufficient development of some of the antepartum test regimens so that at least there can be reasonable decisions made on the basis of definitive data that point to a healthier versus a less healthy intrauterine environment. Some of these tests include: (1) the contraction stress test; (2) the nonstress test; (3) the biophysical profile; (4) the aortic flow velocities; and (5) the volume changes of the amniotic fluid. The latter has recently been an intense area of interest in regard to amnio-infusion therapy. All of the postterm pregnancies should be carefully observed during labor for changes that indicate fetal distress. It is axiomatic that labor can be a serious threat to the postterm fetus, especially if any superimposed problems also exist. In such instances, it may be advantageous to insist upon the most conservative obstetric management, such as close monitoring of the fetal heart and close monitoring of maternal intrauterine cardiovascular and pulmonary parameters.

### *Post-term Anesthetic Management*

The problem of postterm delivery, likewise is distinct, just as it is in preterm labor. The anticipated anesthetic should be planned with due consideration for maternal/fetal safety and discussed in advance with the obstetrician and the pediatrician. Most of the concern in anesthetic management here lies in the hypotension that had been a given complication of regional analgesia from epidural blocks. The problem became simply one that while the postterm fetus may do well in labor if no other superimposed complications occurred, it would not do well in a situation in which marginal placental reserve would be further threatened by such hypotension. Thus, very often, most anesthetic techniques were viewed with concern that hypotension could not be adequately prevented. With the advent of minimal uses of the local anesthetics and thus minimal sympathetic blocks, the concern of hypotension has literally been eradicated in regard to relief of labor pain. Therefore, in the postterm fetus it is an obvious choice. Again, careful attention must be paid to reduce and even eliminate hypotension. In such cases in which that may be a consideration, then the general technique, or even the local technique can be considered viable options. With the continuous subarachnoid method, a slow onset of the sympathetic block allows for physiological compensation and maintenance of blood pressure and presumed maintenance of intervillous space blood flow. Naturally, the local method of analgesia can also be used for cesarean section with standby of the anesthesiologist who can help maintain patient comfort by verbal communication, physical contact, and periodic injection of ketamine for added analgesia and anesthesia during the uncomfortable periods. Supplemental inhalation of anesthetics with $N_2O$, enflurane, isoflurane, and desflurane can also be considered, but absolute attention to keeping the patient in the first stage is paramount. For further discussion on this subject, refer to Chapter 18.

## REFERENCES


1. Hrubec Z, Robinette CD: The study of human twins in medical research. N. Engl. J. Med. 310:435, 1984.
2. Marivate M, Norman RJ: Twins. Clin. Obstet. Gynaecol. 9: 723, 1982.
3. Kochenour NK: Obstetric management of multiple pregnancy and postmaturity. *In* Neonatal-Perinatal Medicine: Diseases of the Fetus and Infant. Edited by AA Fanaroff, RJ Martin. Toronto, The C.V. Mosby Company, 1987, p. 149.
4. Benson RC: Multiple pregnancy. *In* Current Obstetric & Gynecologic Diagnosis & Treatment 1987. Edited by ML Pernoll, RC Benson. Norwalk, CT, Appleton & Lange, 1987, pp. 321–331.
5. Vogel F, Motulsky AG: Human genetics: problems and approaches. New York, Springer-Verlag, 1979.
6. MacGillivray I: Epidemiology of twin pregnancy. Semin. Perinatal. 10:4, 1986.
7. Gemzell CA: *In* Control of ovulation. Edited by CA Villee. New York, Symposium Publications Division, Pergamon Press, 1961.
8. Naville AH, et al: Induction of ovulation with clomiphene citrate. Fertil. Steril. 15:290, 1964.
9. Neuwirth RS, et al: Successful quadruplet pregnancy in a patient treated with human menopausal gonadotropins. Am. J. Obstet. Gynecol. 91:982, 1965.
10. Jewelewicz R, Vande Wiele RL: Management of multifetal gestation. Contemp. Ob/Gyn. 6:59, 1975.
11. Rovinsky JJ, Jaffin H: Cardiovascular hemodynamics in pregnancy: III. Cardiac rate, stroke volume, total peripheral resistance, and central blood volume in multiple pregnancy: synthesis of results. Am. J. Obstet. Gynecol. 95:787, 1966.
12. Veille JC, Morton MJ, Burry KJ: Maternal cardiovascular adaptations to twin pregnancy. Am. J. Obstet. Gynecol. 153: 261, 1985.
13. Desgranges MF, DeMuylder X, Moutquin JM, et al: Perinatal profile of twin pregnancies: a retrospective review of 11 years (1969–1979) at Hospital Notre Dame, Montreal, Canada. Acta. Genet. Med. Gemollol. 31:157, 1982.
14. Gonen R, Heyman E, Asztalos EV, Ohlsson A, et al: The outcome of triplet, quadruplet, and quintuplet pregnancies managed in a perinatal unit: obstetric, neonatal, and follow-up data. Am. J. Obstet. Gynecol. 162:454, 1990.
15. Newman RB, Hamer C, Miller MC: Outpatient triplet management: a contemporary review. Am. J. Obstet. Gynecol. 161:547, 1989.
16. Laube DW: Multiple pregnancy, operative delivery, anesthesia, and analgesia. Current Opinion in Obstetrics and Gynecology 2:40–44, 1990.
17. Nissen ED: Twins: collision, impaction, compaction, and interlocking. Obstet. Gynecol. 11:514, 1958.
18. Khunda S: Locked twins. Obstet. Gynecol. 39:453, 1972.
19. Chervenak FA, Johnson RE, Berkowitz RL, et al: Is routine cesarean section necessary for vertex-breech and vertex-transverse twin gestation? Am. J. Obstet. Gynecol. 148:1, 1984.
20. Acker D, Lieberman M, Holbrook H, et al: Delivery of the second twin. Obstet. Gynecol. 59:710, 1982.
21. Duenhoelter JH, Wells CE, Reisch JS: A paired controlled study of vaginal and abdominal delivery of the low birth weight breech fetus. Obstet. Gynecol. 54:310, 1979.
22. Goldenberg RL, Nelson KG: The premature breech. Am. J. Obstet. Gynecol. 127:240, 1977.
23. Thompson SA, Lyons TL, Makowski EL: Outcomes of twin gestations at the University of Colorado Health Sciences Center, 1973–1983. J. Reprod. Med. 32:328, 1987.
24. Chervenak FA, Johnson RE, Berkowitz RL, Hobbins JC: Intrapartum external version of the second twin. Obstet. Gynecol. 62:160, 1983.
25. Gocke SE, Nageotte MP, Garite T, Towers CV, et al: Management of the nonvertex second twin: primary cesarean sec-

tion, external version, or primary breech extraction. Am. J. Obstet. Gynecol. 161:111, 1989.
26. Mashiach S, Ben-Rafael Z, Dor J, Serr DM: Triplet pregnancy in uterus didelphys with delivery interval of 72 days. Obstet. Gynecol. 58:519, 1981.
27. Woolfson J, Fay T, Bates A: Twins with 54 days between deliveries: case report. Br. J. Obstet. Gynaecol. 90:685, 1983.
28. Feichtinger W, Breitenecker G, Fröhlich H: Prolongation of pregnancy and survival of twin B after loss of twin A at 21 weeks' gestation. Am. J. Obstet. Gynecol. 161:891, 1989.
29. Rayburn WF, Lavin JP, Miodovnik M, Varner MW: Multiple gestation: time interval between delivery of the first and second twins. Obstet. Gynecol. 63:502, 1984.
30. Ferguson WF: Perinatal mortality in multiple gestations: a review of perinatal deaths from 1609 multiple gestations. Obstet. Gynecol. 23:861, 1964.
31. Spurway JH: The fate and management of the second twin. Am. J. Obstet. Gynecol. 83:1377, 1962.
32. Crawford JS: A prospective study of 200 consecutive twin deliveries. Anaesthesia 42:33, 1987.
33. Holcberg G, Baile Y, Lewenthal H, Insler V: Outcome of pregnancy in 31 triplet gestations. Obstet. Gynecol. 59:472, 1982.
34. Jimenez JM, Tyson JE, Reisch J: Clinical measurements of gestational age in normal pregnancies. Obstet. Gynecol. 61: 438, 1983.
35. Sholl JS, Sabbagha RE: Ultrasound detection. *In* Intrauterine Growth Retardation. Edited by C-C Lin, MI Evans. New York, McGraw-Hill, 1984.
36. Robinson HP, Fleming JEE: A critical evaluation of sonar crown-rump length measurements. Br. J. Obstet. Gynaecol. 82:702, 1975.
37. Crane JP, Kopta MM, Welt SI: Abnormal fetal growth patterns: ultrasonic diagnosis and management. Obstet. Gynecol. 50:205, 1977.
38. Hanigan WC, Kennedy G, Roemisch F, Anderson R, et al: Administration of indomethacin for the prevention of periventricular-intraventricular hemorrhage in high-risk neonates. J. Pediatr. 112:941, 1988.
39. Newton ER, Haering WA, Kennedy JL Jr, Herschel M, et al: Effect of mode of delivery on morbidity and mortality of infants at early gestational age. Obstet. Gynecol. 67:507 1986.
40. Pomerance JJ, Teal JG, Gogolok JF, Brown S, et al: Maternally administered antenatal vitamin K1: effect on neonatal prothrombin activity, partial thromboplastin time and intraventricular hemorrhage. Obstet. Gynecol. 70:235, 1987.
41. Morales WJ, Koerten J: Prevention of intraventricular hemorrhage in very low birth weight infants by maternally administered phenobarbital. Obstet. Gynecol. 68:295, 1986.
42. Sinha S, Davies J, Toner N, Bogle S, et al: Vitamin E supplementation reduces frequency of periventricular hemorrhage in very preterm babies. Lancet 1:466, 1987.
43. Tejani N, Verma U, Hameed C, Chayen B: Method and route of delivery in the low birth weight vertex presentation correlated with early periventricular/intraventricular hemorrhage. Obstet. Gynecol. 69:1, 1987.
44. Leveno KJ, Lowe TW, Cunningham FG, Wendel GD, et al: Management of prolonged pregnancy at Parkland Hospital. Proceedings of the Society for Gynecologic Investigation, [Abstract 290P], March, 1985b.

# Chapter 30

# CESAREAN SECTION

MARTIN L. PERNOLL
JEFF E. MANDELL

This chapter is devoted to cesarean section, defined as the delivery of the fetus, placenta, and membranes through abdominal and uterine incisions. The material is presented according to the following list of subjects and consists of three major sections: (1) Basic Considerations, including history, definitions, incidence, indications, and impact of the procedure on the mother, fetus, and newborn; (2) Surgical Considerations, including description of the types of operative procedures carried out; and (3) Anesthetic Management. The text retains the same format and some of the material found in the first edition, although most of the information in this chapter has been acquired during the past 3 decades.

The following discussion is based on the assumption that the reader is fully acquainted with the information in Part III that describes the various agents and techniques used for obstetric anesthesia with emphasis on cesarean section and also with the contents of Chapters 22 and 24. More detailed discussion of the obstetric aspects of the subject can be found elsewhere (1–3).

## BASIC CONSIDERATIONS

### History

Cesarean section is one of the oldest operations in recorded history. Over nineteen-hundred years ago, Pliny reported Scipio Africanus (273 to 183 BC), that the first of the Caesars was so named from having been removed by an incision in his mother's womb (4). Most early cesarean sections were accomplished after the death of the mother in an attempt to save the life of the child in accordance with the Roman code of law known as *lex sesarea*. Scattered reports relate to primitive, unsuccessful attempts to accomplish this operation on living subjects. The first successful operation of this kind was performed in 1500 by Jacob Nufer, a Swiss swinegelder, who delivered his wife abdominally after all efforts at vaginal delivery had failed (5). Rousset published the first treatise on cesarean section and included case reports on 15 successful sections. He was the first to use the expression cesarean section (6). During the ensuing 2 centuries, the operation was done with increasing frequency, and, because the uterine incision was not sutured, maternal mortality continued to remain extremely high—well over 50%. In 1882, Snger (7) and Kehrer (8) aggressively advanced the idea of suturing the uterus after delivery. This led to an improvement in surgical technique, and the reduction in maternal mortality associated with cesarean section has been truly phenomenal (9).

### *Definitions*

As stated in the introduction, cesarean section is the delivery of the fetus, placenta, and membranes through abdominal and uterine incisions. Cesarean section is distinguished from abdominal hysterotomy when the same procedure is employed, but the fetus is previable. Several adjectives may assist in the precise description of cesarean section: primary (first cesarean), repeat cesarean (any cesarean after the first), lower uterine segment or low segment (incision in the lower uterine segment), fundal or classical (incision in the uterine corpus), elective (versus mandatory), transverse (incision transverse to the long axis of the uterus), and vertical (incision parallel to the uterine long axis) (Figures 30–1 and 30–2).

### *Incidence*

This first edition reported the incidence of cesarean section to be somewhat variable, but averaging about 5% in most large studies (9). Prophetically, the beginning of this chapter indicated that today cesarean section is being done with increasing frequency (9). However, that the barely noticeable increase then would swell to the current level could scarcely have been anticipated. Indeed, the increased incidence of cesarean section deliveries in the United States is remarkable (Table 30–1 and Figure 30–3).

#### Causes of the Increase

Reasons for the rising incidence of cesarean since 1980 may be detailed as follows: approximately half (48%) of the increase is due to repeat cesareans; 29% is related to dystocia; 16% is due to fetal distress; 5% occurs with breech, and 2% occurs with other complications (10,11). Dystocia and breech presentation account for less of the recent rise than these diagnoses did before 1978 (12).

Unfortunately, such outcome-oriented data cannot measure the impact exerted by the medicolegal climate in the United States, which appears to be partially responsible for obstetricians who resort to cesarean section more quickly and for less defined reasons. The decline in perinatal mortality in the U.S. and the increase in incidence of cesarean can not be directly correlated because there has been a comparable decrease (during the same

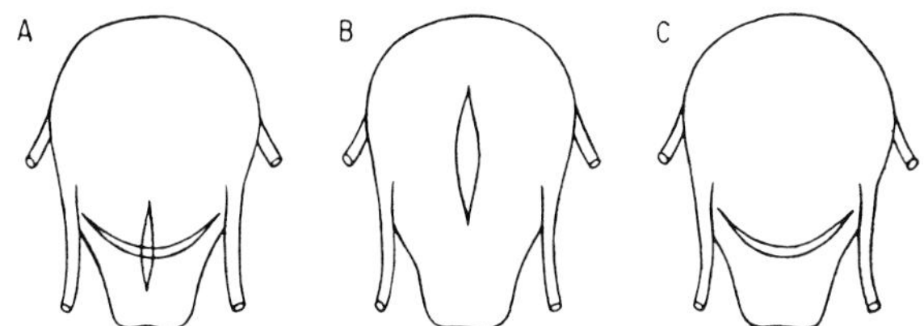


**Fig. 30–1.** Types of uterine incisions for cesarean section. **A,** Low vertical or transverse cervical. **B,** Classical. **C,** Water's extraperitoneal uterine incision.

time) in the perinatal mortality in other industrialized nations, which have not had the extraordinary increase in cesarean births (13).

However, where there was a wide range of cesarean rates between the industrialized countries of Europe, North America, and the Pacific, these countries had consistent increases in cesarean rates over the past decade. Now the annual rate of increase appears to be converging (12). Currently, there is no indication that cesarean delivery rates are leveling off or decreasing (12). Increasingly, successful reports of alterations in practice management to potentially decrease cesarean rates are occurring. This may be an early indication that the increases in cesarean rates may be nearing their end (13). Examples of the suggestions (with representative, not exhaustive, references) from several investigators that could limit the number of cesareans include: enhancing the rate of vaginal birth following a previous cesarean section (Table 30–2) (14), the use of active management of labor (as used in Ireland) (15), vaginal birth for selected breech presentations (16), antepartal external version to decrease the number of

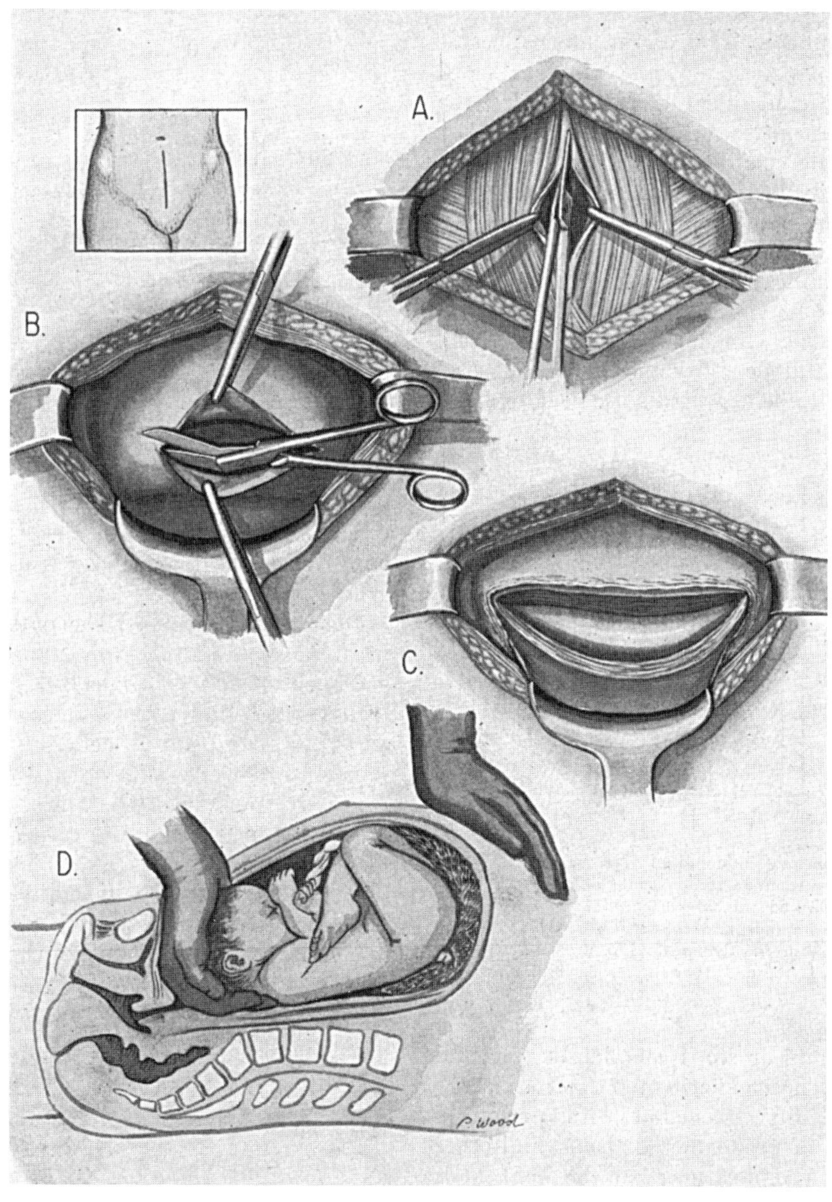


**Fig. 30–2.** Technique of low cervical cesarean section. Inset, Abdominal incision. **A,** Incision of the parietal peritoneum. **B,** Transverse incision through vesicouterine fold peritoneum. **C,** Transverse lower uterine incision. **D,** Delivery of the infant.

**Table 30–1.** Incidence of Cesarean Section in the United States (By Year for Mothers of All Ages)

| Year | Cesarean Rate (%) |
|---|---|
| 1965 | 4.5 |
| 1970 | 5.5 |
| 1975 | 10.4 |
| 1980 | 16.5 |
| 1985 | 22.7 |
| 1989 | 22.8 |

(1965 to 1985 data from Taffel SM, Placek PJ, Liss T: Trends in the United States cesarean section rate and reasons for the 1980–1985 rise. Am. J. Public. Health. 77:955, 1987.) (1989 data from National Center for Health Statistics. Advance report of new data from the 1989 birth certificate. Monthly Vital Statistics Report: 40(12S), Hyattsville, MD, Public Health Service, 1992.)

breech presentations (17), and the safe use of forceps in selected cases (18).

In 1981, the National Institutes of Health Consensus Development Task Force on Cesarean Birth studied the trend toward cesarean section delivery (19). They noted that vaginal delivery should be associated with fewer delivery risks, require less anesthesia, pose a lower potential for postpartum morbidity, involve a shorter hospital stay, save money, and encourage earlier and smoother interaction between mother and infant. As 30 to 40% of cesarean sections are performed solely because of previous cesarean section, a substantial and beneficial decrease in incidence will occur should vaginal delivery after previous cesarean section be more widely adopted in the absence of contraindications.

## *Vaginal Birth After Cesarean*

If the original indication for cesarean section is still present (i.e., true fetopelvic disproportion), obviously the cesarean must be repeated. However, several recent, large

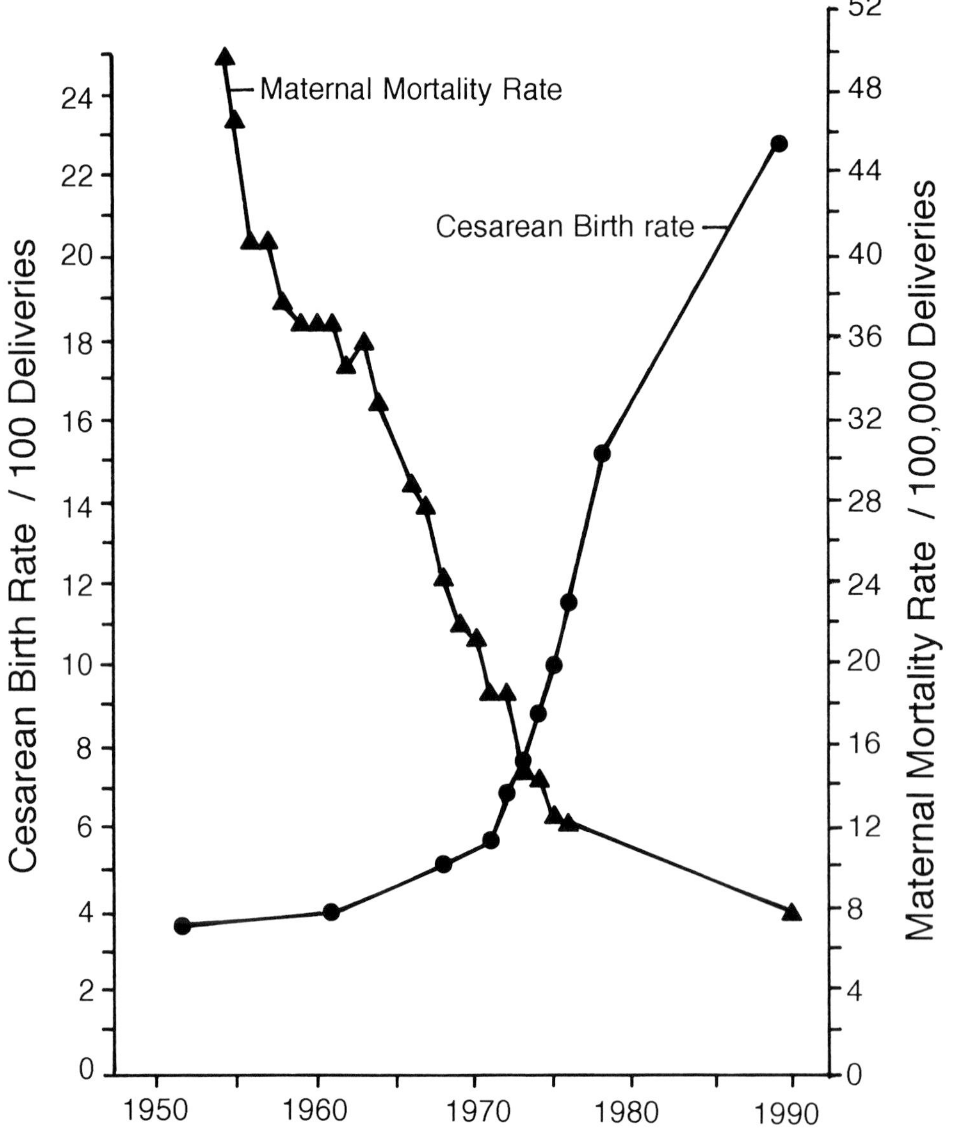


**Fig. 30–3.** Cesarean section rate and maternal mortality rate. (Redrawn from Bottoms SF, Rosen MG, Sokol RJ: Current concepts—The increase in the cesarean birth rate. N. Engl. J. Med. 302:559–563, 1980, and 1989 data from National Center for Health Statistics. Advance report of new data from the 1989 birth certificate. Monthly Vital Statistics Report: 40(12S), Hyattsville, MD, Public Health Service, 1992; Monthly Vital Statistics Report: 40(8S), Hyattsville, MD, Public Health Service, 1992.)

**Table 30–2.** Outcome of Trial of Labor Related to Number of Prior Cesarean Deliveries

**1982–1983**

| No. of Prior Cesarean Sections | No. | Trial of Labor | | Vaginal Delivery | |
|---|---|---|---|---|---|
| | | n | % | n | % |
| 1 | 923 | 726 | 76 | 595 | 82 |
| 2 | 226 | 23 | 10 | 16 | 70 |
| ≥3 | 60 | 2 | 3 | 2 | 100 |

(From Eglinton GS, Phelan JP, Yeh SY, Diaz FP, et al: Outcome after prior cesarean delivery. J. Reprod. Med. 29:3, 1984.)

**1983–1984**

| No. of Prior Cesarean Sections | No. | Trial of Labor | | Vaginal Delivery | |
|---|---|---|---|---|---|
| | | n | % | n | % |
| 1 | 1111 | 911 | 82 | 753 | 83 |
| 2 | 260 | 126 | 49 | 91 | 72 |
| ≥3 | 62 | 8 | 13 | 7 | 88 |

(From Phelan JP, Clark SL, Diaz F, Paul RH: Vaginal birth after cesarean. Am. J. Obstet. Gynecol. 157:1510, 1987.)

**Table 30–3.** Guidelines for Vaginal Delivery After a Previous Cesarean Birth

1. The concept of routine repeat cesarean birth should be replaced by a specific indication for a subsequent abdominal delivery, and in the absence of a contraindication, a woman with one previous cesarean delivery with a low transverse incision should be counseled and encouraged to attempt labor in her current pregnancy.
2. A woman with two or more previous cesarean deliveries with low transverse incisions who wishes to attempt vaginal birth should not be discouraged from doing so in the absence of contraindications.
3. In circumstances in which specific data on risks are lacking, the question of whether to allow a trial of labor must be assessed on an individual basis.
4. A previous classical uterine incision is a contraindication to labor.
5. Professional and institutional resources must have the capacity to respond to acute intrapartum obstetric emergencies, such as performing cesarean delivery within 30 minutes from the time the decision is made until the surgical procedure is begun, as is standard for any obstetric patient in labor.
6. Normal activity should be encouraged during the latent phase of labor; there is no need for restriction to a labor bed before actual labor has begun.
7. A physician who is capable of evaluating labor and performing a cesarean delivery should be readily available.

(From ACOG Committee Opinion: Guidelines for vaginal delivery after a previous cesarean birth. Number 64, October 1988. Reaffirmed 1991. The American College of Obstetricians and Gynecologists, 409 12th Street, SW, Washington, DC 20024-2188.)

studies of vaginal birth after cesarean (VBAC) indicate the same conclusions concerning the safety and efficacy of the method. Representative of these studies is a large recent report that disclosed that prior cesarean section was performed in 8.2% of their total population, and 66% of those with prior cesarean underwent trial of labor. Of these, 81% achieved a vaginal delivery. With vaginal birth, there was less maternal morbidity, a similar incidence of uterine dehiscence (1.9%), and an insignificantly different incidence of uterine rupture (0.3% with repeat cesarean and 0.5% with vaginal birth after cesarean) (20). The American College of Obstetricians and Gynecologists has issued guidelines for vaginal delivery following a cesarean birth, which are listed in Table 30–3.

As a result of this report and similar studies, the policy of "once a cesarean section, always a cesarean section" should be abandoned (20).

### *Indications and Contraindications*

There are, with notable exceptions, few contraindications to cesarean in the presence of a valid indication. The most common contraindications include: pyogenic infections of the abdominal wall, an abnormal fetus incompatible with life, a dead fetus (except to save the life of the mother), and lack of appropriate facilities, equipment and supplies, or personnel (21).

Generally, when vaginal delivery is not feasible or imposes risks exceeding those of cesarean to the mother or fetus, abdominal delivery is warranted. In some cases, the indications may be absolute, while in others, they are relative. Obviously, obstetric judgment plays a crucial role in distinguishing between these indications. It is not possible to discuss in detail all indications for cesarean section. The most important are listed in Table 30–4, and we will make brief comments on the first three major categories. Other of these major topics are discussed elsewhere in this book.

#### *Fetopelvic Disproportion*

#### Abnormalities of the "Passage"

Generally with fetopelvic disproportion (FPD), the vertex is presenting and is simply too large to come through the maternal pelvis. In the majority of cases, fetopelvic disproportion is only ascertainable after the onset of labor. If the baby is not oversized, this may indicate a maternal pelvis that is inadequate in one or more of the pelvic diameters. However, in industrialized countries it is more often caused by the fetus being large for its gestational age. Certain extreme cases of fetopelvic disproportion may be identified before labor. Fetopelvic disproportion may also apply when a careful evaluation for a vaginal breech delivery shows a fetus too large for the pelvis.

Inlet dystocia from either bony abnormalities or soft tissue problems may be suspected if a patient with empty bladder and rectum presents in labor with an unengaged vertex. With labor, the head can still be palpated above the symphysis, and it is not uncommonly asynclitic or occiput posterior. Soft tissue dystocia is much less common than other causes of fetopelvic disproportion, but it may be caused by congenital anomalies, scarring of the birth canal, genital tract masses, or a low-lying placenta.

Midpelvic disproportion is the most common abnormality of passage and is suspected if the ischial spines are closely spaced or very prominent, if the sidewalls are converging, or if the pelvic anteroposterior diameter is

**Table 30–4.** Usual Indications for Cesarean Section

I. Fetopelvic disproportion
- A. Pelvic (the Passage) insufficiency
  - 1. Bony pelvis
    - a. Pelvic inlet (usually anterior-posterior <10 cm)
    - b. Midpelvis (usually transverse, ie, ischial spines <9.5 cm)
    - c. Outlet (very unusual and then almost never seen in the absence of other pelvic contractures)
  - 2. Soft tissue obstruction
    - a. Low lying placenta (especially posteriorly implanted)
    - b. Uterine leiomyomata
    - c. Ovarian tumors
    - d. Other genital tract neoplasia (rare)
- B. Fetal complications (the Passenger)
  - 1. Normal fetus
    - a. Macrosomia (>4,000 g)
    - b. Malposition and malpresentation
      - i. Breech unfavorable for vaginal delivery
      - ii. Deflexed head
      - iii. Transverse or oblique lie
      - iv. Brow
      - v. Posterior mental position
      - vi. Shoulder presentations
      - vii. Compound presentations
  - 2. Anomalous fetus
    - a. Meningomyelocele
    - b. Hydrocephalus
    - c. Sacrococcygeal teratoma
    - d. Miscellaneous fetal anomalies
  - 3. Multiple gestation
    - a. Twins
      - i. Twin A any presentation except vertex
      - ii. Twin B not suitable for vaginal delivery
      - iii. Failure of intrapartum external version
      - iv. Fetal distress (even if Twin A has been delivered vaginally)
      - v. All monoamniotic twins
    - b. Triplets or greater number
- C. Abnormalities of the labor (the Powers)
  - 1. Primary uterine inertia
    - a. Prolonged latent phase (unusual, but >20 hr in a nullipara and >14 hr in a multipara)
    - b. Protraction disorders
      - i. Protracted active phase dilatation (nulligravida >1.2 cm/h, multigravida >1.5 cm/h)
      - ii. Protracted descent (nulligravida >1 cm/h, multigravida >2 cm/h)
    - c. Arrest disorders
      - i. Prolonged deceleration phase (nulliparas ≥3 h, multiparas ≥1 h)
      - ii. Secondary arrest of dilatation (no dilation for ≥2 h)
      - iii. Active phase arrest of descent (≥1 h)
      - iv. Failure of descent in the deceleration phase or second stage (≥1 h)
  - 2. Uterine inertia due to fetopelvic disproportion
  - 3. Failed induction

II. Fetal distress
- A. Uteroplacental insufficiency
- B. Cord accidents
- C. Metabolic acidosis

III. Obstetric hemorrhage (maternal and/or fetal)
- A. Abruptio placenta
- B. Placenta previa
- C. Ruptured uterus
- D. Vasa previa

IV. Infections
- A. Severe chorioamnionitis
- B. Active maternal genital herpes
- C. Active maternal condylomata acuminata

V. Maternal and/or fetal complications potentially adversely influenced by labor and/or vaginal delivery
- A. Antepartal testing indicative of labor intolerance
- B. Cervical dystocia
- C. Medical
  - 1. Fulminating preeclampsia-eclampsia
  - 2. Diabetes
  - 3. Erythroblastosis
  - 4. Severe maternal heart disease
  - 5. Other debilitating conditions
- D. Surgical
  - 1. Cervical or uterine scarring of extent that may rupture with labor (e.g., extensive myomectomy, trachelorrhaphy)
  - 2. Cervical cerclage
    - a. All abdominal cervical cerclages
    - b. Certain vaginal cerclages (e.g., cannot remove)
  - 3. Serious maternal problems (e.g., vesicovaginal or rectovaginal fistula)
  - 4. Prior extensive vaginal plastic operations
  - 5. Carcinoma of the cervix

VI. Repeat cesarean

short. Ultimately with midpelvic disproportion, the fetal vertex fails to advance beyond station + 2. Outlet disproportion is rare and is usually only associated with a pelvis that has other defects (22).

## Abnormalities of the "Passenger"

Fetal macrosomia (fetus larger than 4000 g) occurs in approximately 5% of deliveries and may merit cesarean section in the woman with an average or smaller-sized pelvis. Abnormalities of fetal position, presentation, attitude, or lie complicate approximately 5% of all labors. This category of abnormality includes, but is not limited to: occiput posterior position, occiput transverse position, face presentation, brow and sinciput presentation, breech and compound presentation, and transverse or oblique lies. Generally, these complications require detailed obstetric evaluation to ascertain proper delivery mode, but, taken as a group, there is an increasing tendency for cesarean delivery. In the case of the occiput posterior and occiput transverse positions, vaginal delivery may be attempted if the following criteria are met: (1) the operator has mid forceps skill and experience; (2) other criteria for use of mid forceps have been met; and (3) macrosomia and gross fetopelvic disproportion have been excluded.

The sinciput position usually converts to face, brow, or vertex position as labor progresses. However, fetopelvic disproportion, uterine inertia, and arrested progress of labor all occur with frequency and act to increase the incidence of cesarean section. In 60% of brow presentations, pelvic contracture, prematurity, and grand multiparity are associated. Thus, whereas this complication only occurs in 0.06% of deliveries, cesarean is often the result when it does occur. Face presentation occurs in 0.2% of cases and is associated with grand multiparity, advanced maternal age, pelvic masses, contracted pelvis, multiple gestation, polyhydramnios, macrosomia, congenital anomalies, prematurity, placenta previa, and premature rupture of the membranes. Mentum posterior is not deliverable vaginally. Moreover, the possibility for vaginal delivery is guarded in any face presentation, and it is only the occasional mentum anterior with a small baby in a multipara that will deliver vaginally.

Abnormalities of fetal lie (excluding breech) occur in 0.33% of deliveries, but are materially increased in premature labors. In patients with abnormal axial lies, a twentyfold increase in incidence of cord prolapse exists than of vertex delivery, and cesarean section is nearly always necessary for delivery. With breech presentations, the following may be safely delivered vaginally: near-term, frank breeches, weight between 2500 to 3500 g, flexed head, no concurrent congenital anomalies, maternal pelvis of adequate dimensions (by x-ray pelvimetry), and normal labor pattern without fetal distress. If all these criteria are not met, a cesarean section should be performed. Another group in this category are fetuses with malformations. Obviously in these categories, obstetric judgment plays a major role (23).

## Abnormalities of the "Powers"

In Chapter 4, the characteristics of uterine contraction and other forces of labor are discussed in detail. To recapitulate briefly here, during the active phase of the first stage and during the second stage, normal uterine contractions have the following characteristics: duration of 30 to 90 seconds (mean 60 seconds), a frequency of 3 to 5 per 10-minute period, and intensities of 25 to 60 mm Hg (mean 40 to 50 mm Hg). In addition, there must be a complete return to baseline tone, which is 5 to 7 mm Hg during the late first stage and second stage. This "resting phase" is very important for uterine blood flow. It is not uncommon for some parturients to have contractions that are more frequent or more forceful. In this circumstance, careful observation is warranted, but such contractions may not be deleterious unless fetal heart rate patterns indicate fetal compromise. Contraction patterns less than the above, associated with failure to progress, necessitate careful evaluation and, in the absence of fetopelvic disproportion, may warrant administration of oxytocics.

In the first stage of labor, aberrations are generally identified as "failure to progress." This diagnosis most commonly denotes either a secondary arrest of cervical dilatation or a prolonged active phase of labor (also called a primary dysfunctional labor). Both diagnoses refer only to the active phase of labor (after 3- to 4-cm dilatation in a nullipara and after 2- to 3-cm dilatation in a multipara). In an arrest of cervical dilatation, progress that has been occurring at the expected rate (nullipara at more than 1.2 cm/hour, multipara at more than 1.5 cm/hour) ceases. If there is no progress in dilatation for 2 hours in the face of adequate contractions, the diagnosis of failure to progress is made, and it may also be said that the patient has failed a trial of labor.

In these circumstances, the cause of failure to progress is most frequently fetopelvic disproportion, and cesarean delivery is usually necessary. A primary dysfunctional labor occurs when cervical dilatation is progressing at less than the rate noted above. If contractions are adequate, this pattern is generally observed closely with cesarean section performed for complications.

In the very late first stage (more than 8-cm dilatation) or second stage labor, failures to progress are much more commonly determined by either protracted or failed descent of the presenting part. During this time, descent should be occurring at 1 cm/hour in nulliparae and 2 cm/hour in multiparae. In the absence of abnormal contractions, failures of descent have a high rate of cephalopelvic disproportion, and cesarean delivery is common. It may be said that a patient has failed a test of labor when 2 hours pass in the second stage with ruptured membranes, normal uterine contractions, and good voluntary efforts without discernable progress in fetal descent (24).

Fetal monitoring is prudent in any case of suspected fetopelvic disproportion. In most tests of labor, signs of fetal distress appear usually before completion of the test; tests of labor are not commonly used today.

To control the increased rate of cesarean due to dystocia, work from Ireland, mentioned previously, suggests the success of a policy of active management of labor (15). This involves amniotomy once the diagnosis of labor is established, oxytocin augmentation if labor is progressing at less than 1 cm/hour, and continuous supportive nursing. The reports of this experience, subsequently confirmed in Canada, indicate a cesarean section rate of about 5%, without increased fetal morbidity or mortality. In one such study, the cesarean section rate was 4.3% versus 13% for controls ($p<0.005$) (25). Forceps delivery rate was 19.4% versus 29% ($p<0.005$), and labor more than 12 hours was 7% versus 20%.

Some differences in population may account for differences in cesarean rates and outcome. When 1 year of obstetric outcome at the National Maternity Hospital in Dublin, Ireland, and the Parkland Memorial Hospital in Dallas were compared using active management of labor, the cesarean rate was 18% in Dallas and 6% in Dublin. In addition, in Dallas there was a sevenfold decrease in intrapartum fetal death, and a twofold decrease in infant seizures for the first year when compared with previous experience (26).

### Fetal Distress

Fetal distress is a critical response to stress. It manifests through a complexity of signs and implies metabolic derangements, most notably hypoxia and acidosis, that may affect vital organ function to the point of temporary or permanent injury or death. Fetal distress may be chronic or acute, and potentially affects up to 20% of all pregnancies (27). Prompt recognition of the symptoms and signs, as well as correct and decisive intervention, are mandatory to reduce the perinatal morbidity (particularly central nervous system damage) and mortality associated with fetal distress.

### Chronic Fetal Distress

Chronic fetal distress implies sublethal fetal deprivation affecting growth and development. It may be caused by decreased placental perfusion (i.e., maternal vascular disease, maternal hypertension, inadequate maternal systemic circulation, inadequate oxygenation of maternal blood), increased fetal needs (i.e., multiple gestation), placental abnormalities (i.e., premature placental aging, diabetes mellitus), and a number of miscellaneous causes (congenital anomalies, congenital infections, erythroblastosis fetalis). Usually, these chronic conditions will be known antenatally or will be detected by serial fetal evaluations (i.e., biometric testing, fetal mensuration by ultrasound) (28). Chronic fetal distress usually warns that increased fetal monitoring and an aggressive program for determination of fetal well-being are necessary, and that labor may not be tolerated (thus necessitating cesarean section).

### Acute Fetal Distress

Unfortunately, the diagnostic criteria for acute fetal distress are often not precise and the proper diagnosis requires integration of several clinical parameters. The differential diagnosis also considers diverse possibilities (Table 30–5).

Acute fetal distress is usually suspected by fetal heart rate criteria, but as much as the adult heart rate is only one indicator of well-being, it must be interpreted in light of all information available. In some circumstances, it is desirable to use fetal scalp blood gas determinations to enhance precision in the diagnosis of acute fetal distress. More sophisticated methodology for accurately determining fetal distress may soon be forthcoming.

The fetal heart rate (FHR), which is normally 120 to 160 beats per minute (BPM), may remain within these limits even though severe fetal distress is occurring. However, in early or mild fetal distress the fetal heart rate may rise from the previous baseline. With severe fetal distress, the fetal heart rate may decline from previously noted levels or actually fall to bradycardic levels. By contrast, acceleration of 15 beats per minute lasting 15 seconds or more in response to fetal motion, acoustic stimulation, or tactile stimulation of the scalp are indicative of fetal well-being (29).

The beat-to-beat variability, both short and longer term, is a very useful guide to fetal distress and is usually the best guide to fetal oxygenation (30). Normally, it is present, but progressively decreases or is absent with increasing fetal compromise. Rarely, fetal heart rate variability will acutely increase with a sudden compromise (i.e., cord impingement) and then decrease after a few minutes unless the compromise is relieved.

With the membranes intact usually no response of fetal heart rate to uterine contractions is apparent. Fetal heart rate accelerations caused by fetal motion or stimulation are also indicators of well-being. If a membrane ruptures, the almost always benign fetal heart rate pattern of early deceleration is increased eightfold.

The fetal heart rate pattern of variable decelerations is a concern because this pattern represents umbilical cord compression. When the fetal heart rate with a variable deceleration pattern is depressed for more than 60 seconds or to severe levels (fewer than 90 beats per minute), fetal distress, as demonstrated by blood gas criteria, is usually present.

Inconsistent fetal heart rate late deceleration patterns merit close followup, and consistent late decelerations (occurring with three consecutive contractions) not responding to the usual therapeutic alterations are viewed as fetal distress. Combined patterns are particularly ominous, especially combined variable and late decelerations.

Fetal scalp blood pH determination is one of the most certain ways to ascertain fetal distress. Fetal scalp blood pH of 7.25 or more is considered normal. A pH between 7.20 and 7.24 is ominous and merits rapid delivery unless therapeutic modalities improve fetal status. Fetal scalp pH under 7.20 is indicative of fetal distress and merits rapid intervention.

***Therapy.*** The various therapies for acute fetal distress attempt to correct the unfavorable fetal gaseous exchange. The usual attempts to correct acute fetal distress include:

1. Maternal hyperoxygenation to raise maternal-fetal oxygen transfer by enhancement of the $PO_2$ gradient. Oxygen is usually administered by mask at a rate of 6 to 7 liters/min.

**Table 30–5.** The Differential Diagnosis of Acute Fetal Distress

| | Normal | Possible Fetal Distress | Probable Fetal Distress | Fetal Distress |
|---|---|---|---|---|
| FHR in beats/min | 120–160 | Tachycardia (probably normal) | Tachycardia (or normal) or | Tachycardia (or normal) or bradycardia |
| Beat-to-variability | Present | Present but may be decreased | Decreased or absent; rarely, increased | Absent |
| Response of FHR to uterine contraction | None, or if membranes ruptured mild to moderate early deceleration (acceleration with stimulation) | Mild variable decelerations | Prolonged or increasingly severe variable deceleration; (nonconsistent) late deceleration | Severe variable deceleration, late deceleration, or combined patterns |
| Fetal scalp blood pH anticipated | ≥7.25 | 7.20–7.24 | 7.20–7.24 | ≤7.20 |
| Meconium (term pregnancy) | Usually none | Perhaps | Often present | Often present |
| Probable fetal condition | Satisfactory | Mild compromised | Compromised | Often critical |

(From Catanzarite VA, Perkins RP, Pernoll ML: Assessment of fetal well being. *In* Current Obstetrics and Gynecologic Diagnosis and Treatment. 6th ed. Edited by ML Pernoll, RC Benson. Los Altos, Appleton & Lange, 1987, p. 292.)

2. Altering maternal position to the lateral recumbent or switching from side to side to relieve pressure on the umbilical cord, maternal aorta, and inferior vena cava to improve uterine blood flow.
3. Correction of hypotension involves several steps designed to restore the gravida's arterial pressure and increase the intervillous blood flow: altering position to the lateral recumbent; displacing the uterus off the abdominal great vessels by manually pushing it aside; elevating the legs; applying elastic leg bandages or other devices to decrease peripheral venous pooling; and rapid administration of intravenous fluids. If drugs are necessary, cardiotonic ones (i.e., ephedrine) are preferred.
4. Decreasing uterine activity permits better placental perfusion and is a laudable goal. However, this can currently only be accomplished by cessation of oxytocin when it is a contributing factor to uterine hyperactivity. However, as information and experience increase with various agents capable of creating uterine relaxation, it may be proven that their application has a role in treatment of fetal distress associated with uterine hyperactivity.
5. Other therapy that might be useful:
   a. Correcting maternal acidosis (using sodium bicarbonate) if that is the cause of fetal acidosis.
   b. Administering 50 g intravenously of hypertonic glucose, if there is maternal deprivation acidosis or hypoglycemia, although large prospective studies have not been performed (31).

Data concerning the reliability of meconium as an indicator of fetal distress indicate that it is neither specific nor sensitive. Thus, meconium is usually not a sound indicator of fetal distress, but is, nonetheless, a severe problem. Preventing the meconium aspiration syndrome requires a careful, combined obstetric and neonatal approach involving atraumatic delivery, suctioning the nasopharynx upon emergence of the head, and careful suctioning of the trachea below the vocal cords after delivery in selected cases (32). Saline lavage of the tracheobronchial tree will only be necessary occasionally.

### *Obstetric Hemorrhage*

Third trimester hemorrhage continues to be one of pregnancy's most ominous complications, and it is common, complicating approximately 5 to 10% of all pregnancies. However, it is only the 2 to 3% of these pregnancies that experience the serious hemorrhages that account for the three leading causes of maternal death and a major cause of perinatal morbidity and mortality in the United States. In such emergency circumstances, the use of cesarean is noncontroversial, affording both mother and fetus significantly greater safety than do attempts at vaginal delivery.

The major causes of serious hemorrhage are placenta previa and abruptio placenta. Only rarely (in about 1/2000 deliveries) does the catastrophic uterine rupture occur (33). In any hemorrhagic complication of pregnancy, it must be ascertained that a coagulopathy is not present and, if there is any sign of fetal compromise, that it is not from fetal blood loss (34).

## *Impact of Cesarean Section on the Mother, Fetus, and Newborn*

### *Effects on the Mother*

### Maternal Physiologic Changes

Cesarean section imposes on the mother greater stress from physiologic alterations and increased risks in morbidity and mortality than is associated with uncomplicated vaginal delivery. The magnitude of stress from physiologic alterations and increased risks depends on the indication for abdominal delivery. In women undergoing elective cesarean section, alterations and risks are limited to cardiovascular and respiratory changes, blood loss of about 1000 ml, and the slightly greater risk associated with intra-abdominal operation and the required anesthesia. Patients undergoing cesarean section for semi-emergency or emergency reasons are exposed to the added risk inherent in the complications that make cesarean section necessary. These complications that cause physiologic alterations are extensively discussed elsewhere (see Chapter 2) and are mentioned here only to reiterate their potential impact on anesthetic and surgical management.

### Cardiovascular Changes

Major hemodynamic changes occur during and immediately after abdominal delivery (35,36). The hemodynamic effects of low cervical cesarean section among 32 patients studied by Adams (36) are shown in Table 30–6

**Table 30–6.** Average Hemodynamic Values for 32 Patients Studied for the Effects of Low Cervical Cesarean Section

| | Before Cesarean Section | Promptly after Cesarean Section Change | | Seventh Day Postpartum Change | |
|---|---|---|---|---|---|
| | | Value | (%) | Value | (%) |
| Cardiac output (L/min) | 6.4 | 9.1 | 42 | 7.4 | 16 |
| Left ventricular work (kg-m/min) | 6.7 | 11.8 | 77 | 8.7 | 30 |
| Stroke volume (ml) | 74 | 118 | 60 | 106 | 43 |
| Blood pressure (mm Hg) | 107/68 | 125/78 | 17/14 | 112/72 | 5/6 |
| Mean blood pressure (mm Hg) | 85 | 98 | 15 | 89 | 5 |
| Heart rate (beats per min) | 92 | 81 | −12 | 75 | −18 |
| Circulation time (arm to leg in sec) | 16.6 | 13.3 | −20 | 14.5 | −13 |
| Pulmonary (central) blood volume (ml) | 1642 | 2058 | 25 | 1894 | 15 |
| Total peripheral resistance (dynes · sec/cm$^{-5}$) | 1095 | 955 | −13 | 981 | −10 |

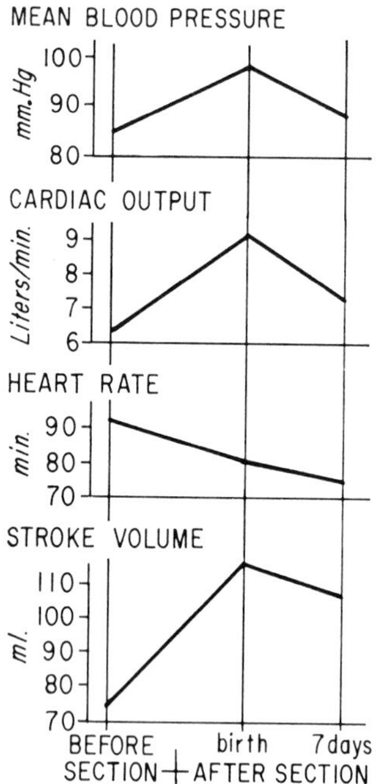


**Fig. 30–4.** Average values for mean arterial pressure, cardiac output, heart rate, and stroke volume before and immediately after elective cesarean section and on the seventh postoperative day. (Modified from Adams JQ: Hemodynamic effects of cesarean section. Am. J. Obstet. Gynecol. 82:673, 1961.)

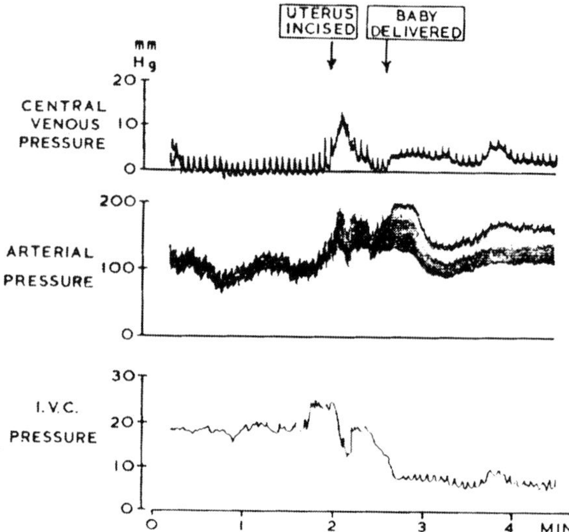


**Fig. 30–6.** Changes in central venous pressure, arterial pressure, and inferior vena cava pressure at delivery during cesarean section. The transient rise in venous pressure was associated with a marked rise in arterial pressure and an increase in pulse pressure. After delivery, the pressure in the inferior vena cava was promptly reduced to nonpregnant values. (Modified from Scott DB: Inferior vena caval occlusion in late pregnancy and its importance in anaesthesia. Br. J. Anaesth. 40:120, 1968.)

and Figure 30–4. Similar hemodynamic changes were reported by Ueland, Gills, and Hansen, (35) who have studied 20 parturients in great detail. On the basis of the available data, the "average" hemodynamic changes that occur during and after the abdominal delivery itself are as follows: cardiac output increases about 30 to 40%, (37), stroke volume increases about 60 to 70%, and cardiac rate usually decreases about 10 to 15%. Because of the decrease in peripheral resistance, the blood pressure increases only about 10 to 15% (Figure 30–5). In some patients, there is a transient, very significant rise in blood pressure, but it rapidly falls to normal postpartum levels

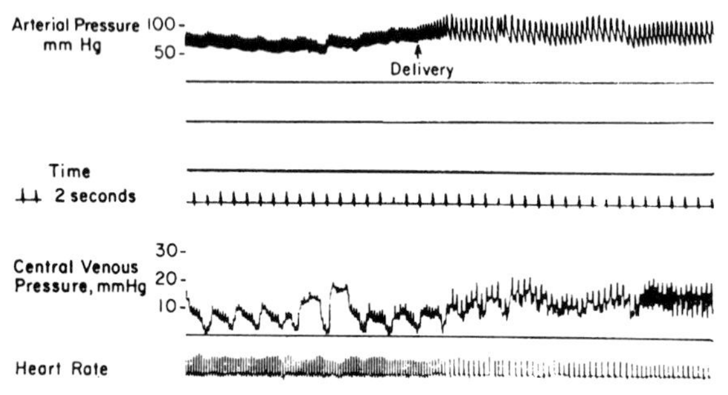


**Fig. 30–5.** Changes in arterial blood pressure, central venous pressure, and heart rate during elective cesarean section. Note the significant increase in pulse pressure and decrease in cardiac rate. (Modified from Ueland K, Gills RE, Hansen JM: Maternal cardiovascular dynamics, I: Cesarean section under subarachnoid block anesthesia. Am. J. Obstet. Gynecol. 100:42, 1968.)

(Figure 30–6). After delivery, the pressure in the inferior vena cava promptly decreases and the central venous pressure returns to nonpregnant levels. The increase in pulmonary blood volume may further decrease functional residual capacity of the lungs. This, in turn, results in more rapid changes in the concentration of gases in the alveoli—a consideration of great importance to the anesthesiologist.

The significant increase in cardiac output and in cardiac work is probably the result of sudden increase in venous return that occurs immediately on delivery of the infant. This is, in turn, the product of two factors: elimination of the pressure on the inferior vena cava by the large gravid uterus and extrusion of a sizable volume of blood (500 to 600 ml) into the systemic circulation as the uterus contracts during and following delivery of the infant. The degree of change or "swing" in maternal hemodynamics is greatly influenced by many factors, including position, apprehension, pain, oxytocics, coexisting problems such as dehydration hemorrhage, anemia and acidosis, and anesthesia.

Uterine involution is associated with an autotransfusion of 500 ml (38). While blood loss associated with cesarean section usually approximates 1200 ml, the potential for fluid overload may still occur because of pre-indication volume loading to offset the administration of sympatholytic anesthetics.

## Pulmonary Changes

Parturients have a diminished functional residual capacity, increased total lung capacity, and increased oxygen uptake (39,40). Thus, it requires comparatively little

**Table 30–7.** Physiological Dead Space in Pregnant and Nonpregnant Patients

| | Nonpregnant (NP) | Predelivery (Pre-d) | Pre-d vs NP (p) | Postdelivery (Post-d) | Post-d vs NP (p) | Pre-d vs Post-d (p) |
|---|---|---|---|---|---|---|
| $V_T$ (ml) | 674.41 ± 26.83 | 789.30 ± 30.70 | <0.01 | 778.29 ± 32.29 | <0.05 | NS |
| $V_D$ (ml) | 255.17 ± 20.41 | 201.36 ± 20.08 | 0.1–0.05 | 209.85 ± 22.91 | 0.1–0.05 | NS |
| $V_T$ ($ml \cdot kg^{-1}$) | 8.99 ± 0.33 | 9.48 ± 0.31 | NS | ** | ** | ** |
| $V_D$ ($ml \cdot kg^{-1}$) | 3.37 ± 0.23 | 2.46 ± 0.28 | <0.05 | ** | ** | ** |
| $V_D$ corrected (ml)* | 255.18 ± 18.82 | 201.36 ± 17.20 | <0.05 | ** | ** | ** |
| $V_D/V_T$ | 0.37 ± 0.02 | 0.25 ± 0.02 | <0.001 | 0.27 ± 0.02 | <0.01 | NS |
| $V_D$ anatomical | 166.89 ± 19.72 | 194.96 ± 17.13 | NS | 184.86 ± 14.03 | NS | NS |
| $V_D$ alveolar | 0.19 ± 0.01 | 0.01 ± 0.02 | <0.001 | 0.03 ± 0.03 | <0.001 | NS |
| $PaCO_2$ (kPa) | 3.41 ± 0.07 | 3.83 ± 0.09 | <0.001 | 3.34 ± 0.08 | NS | <0.001 |
| $P_ECO_2$ | 2.75 ± 0.09 | 3.76 ± 0.07 | <0.001 | 3.22 ± 0.09 | <0.001 | <0.001 |
| $CO_2$ output ($ml \cdot min^{-1}$) | 168.43 ± 6.72 | 271.18 ± 11.43 | <0.001 | 229.92 ± 10.11 | <0.001 | <0.001 |

n = 17 in pregnant and nonpregnant groups.
* $V_D$ corrected for $V_T$, age, and weight using multiple regression equations.
** Values could not be calculated due to variation in the weight following delivery of the baby.
(From Shankar KB, Moseley H, Vemula V, Kumar Y: Physiologic dead space during general anaesthesia for Caesarean section. Can. J. Anaesth. 34: 373, 1987.)

apnea to produce significant hypoxia in the parturient. Consequently, whether regional or general anesthesia is used, supplemental $O_2$ should be used liberally.

Shankar noted a significant decrease in physiological dead space in patients undergoing cesarean section under general anesthesia as compared to patients undergoing abdominal hysterectomy under general anesthesia (Table 30–7) (41). This may be due to increased cardiac output, which would diminish the amount of lung with high ventilation perfusion (V/Q) ratios. Shankar has also demonstrated a decreased gradient between arterial and end-tidal $CO_2$ tensions (42). With the increasing prevalence of end-tidal $CO_2$ monitoring, the anesthesiologist should be aware of this phenomenon and maintain end-tidal $CO_2$ levels several mm Hg higher than in the nonpregnant patient.

## Gastrointestinal Changes

Term parturients are known to have increased intragastric volumes, decreased gastric pH, increased intragastric pressure, and a delay in gastric emptying (43). These factors all act to enhance the risk of gastric aspiration. Indeed, the risk of aspiration of gastric contents cannot be overstated, as it remains one of the most common reasons for maternal demise.

## *Maternal Morbidity*

### Intraoperative

The intraoperative surgical complications with cesarean section are as high as 11.6% (9.5% minor complications, 2.1% major complications). Minor complications include blood transfusion, injury to the infant without sequelae, minor laceration of the isthmus, and difficulty in delivering the infant. Major complications include bladder injury, laceration into cervix and vagina, laceration through most of corpus uteri, laceration through the isthmus into the broad ligament, laceration of both uterine arteries, intestinal injury, and injury to the infant with sequelae. As might be anticipated, the complications are higher in emergency (18.9%) than in elective (4.2%) cases (44).

Shankar found six risk factors in the emergency (but not in elective) cases: (1) station of the fetal presenting part; (2) labor prior to surgery; (3) low gestational age; (4) rupture of fetal membranes (with labor) prior to surgery; (5) previous cesarean delivery; and (6) lack of skill of the operator. They concluded that the proportion of emergency operations needs to be reduced by converting to elective cesareans or allowing more vaginal births, and that emergency cesarean requires greater skill on the part of surgeons and should not be entrusted to young, inexperienced obstetricians (44).

### Postoperative

Complications following cesarean are not uncommon (14.5%) and over 90% of all complications are infectious (13.3%). The most common infections are endometritis, urinary tract infection, and wound infection. The complication rate in elective cases (4.7%) is much lower than in emergency operations (24.2%). The most significant factors predisposing to postoperative morbidity are duration of ruptured membranes prior to surgery, duration of labor prior to surgery, anemia, and obesity. A combination of risk factors increases the complication rate (45).

Many other factors may increase infectious risk, including socioeconomic factors (the lower socioeconomic groups are at greater risk), prenatal care (those with less prenatal care are at higher risk), age (the very young and possibly the very old are at increased risk), nutritional factors (the malnourished are at higher risk), gestational age (the lower the gestational age, the greater the risk), duration of the preoperative hospital stay (longer hospital stays predispose to risk), and systemic illnesses (e.g., diabetes, systemic lupus erythematosus, chronic renal disease all place the gravida at enhanced risk). Increasing numbers of vaginal examinations during labor increases the risk of infection, although the number that places the patient at risk has been variously reported from 3 to 7. These factors may exert their influence on, or be influenced by, the maternal immune system, vaginal flora, and antibacterial factors in the amniotic fluid (46). There are conflicting data about intrauterine catheter monitoring's effect on the risk of postcesarean infectious morbidity. Occasionally (in less than 2% of cases) postcesarean infections will become life-threatening through advanced complications such as septic shock, pelvic abscess, or septic pelvic thrombophlebitis (47).

In sum, the factors associated most significantly with postoperative infectious risk include rupture of the membranes for 8 or more hours, labor for 12 or more hours with cervical effacement and dilation to 4 or more cm, multiple vaginal examinations, low socioeconomic status, or complicating medical conditions (48). The use of prophylactic antibiotics materially decreases infectious morbidity and mortality (see below).

The most common noninfectious postoperative complications (less than 10% of the total) include paralytic ileus, intra-abdominal hemorrhage, bladder paresis, thrombosis, and pulmonary complications.

***Venous Air Embolus.*** Patients undergoing cesarean section are at risk of massive venous air embolus. Small amounts of air may be detected by precordial Doppler in at least 50% of cesarean sections, whether done with epidural or general anesthesia. Aside from the suggestion that small amounts of venous air may cause some of the complaints of dyspnea and chest pain experienced by parturients receiving epidural anesthesia, venous air embolus reaches the level of clinical significance in less than 1% of parturients (49,50).

Measures that will decrease the incidence of venous air embolus include adequate prehydration and avoidance of extreme Trendelenburg position. Precordial Doppler monitoring may aid in the early detection of air embolus, and end-tidal $CO_2$ monitoring may help assess the consequence of the embolus (51).

### *Maternal Mortality*

Cesarean section carries a maternal mortality rate from 40/100,000 to 80/100,000 (41). This mortality rate is more than 25 times that for vaginal delivery. Admittedly, those undergoing cesarean are usually at much higher risk, but infectious morbidity and mortality may be 80 times that of vaginal delivery.

Anesthetic complications' contribution to overall maternal mortality in the United States is 7% (52,53). However, both low-risk patients and high-risk patients may be affected. Thus, anesthesia consistently remains in the top seven causes of maternal mortality (54).

The issue of mortality with cesarean section is discussed in Chapter 20 under "Complications of General Anesthesia." In that chapter, it is mentioned that much of the mortality of general anesthesia is associated with airway patency and intubation problems in associated patients with morbid obesity. These are situations in which any difficulty can accentuate the problems associated with pregnancy and anesthesia, and these situations should be appreciated by the obstetric colleague. Often, the obstetrician may not be informed of the problems associated with such patients and only a good educational program and excellent communication and coordination between the anesthesiologist and his/her colleague obstetrician can overcome such difficulties.

It is hoped that this book will be one of the information bases from which such problems that are real and threatening to the life of the patient, but not well appreciated by one of the three interactive colleagues, i.e., obstetrician, anesthesiologist, or pediatrician, can be identified and discussed so that better management solutions can be worked out in advance of the problems anticipated. It is by such identification and intensive problem solving by all three disciplines that we can develop a healthier atmosphere for both the baby and the mother. If, for example, it is appreciated that the maternal and fetal mortality from an attempted intubation on a mother who is morbidly obese has an anticipated difficulty to visualize vocal cords, this patient may well be scheduled in advance for placement of continuous subarachnoid catheter so that some control over both analgesia for first stage discomfort and some control over immediate cesarean section due to fetal distress may be gained. This provides the patient with comfort and protection from having to undergo general anesthesia.

## Effects on the Fetus and Newborn

Properly done, cesarean section imposes less of a risk on the fetus and newborn than does complicated vaginal delivery. However, compared with normal vaginal birth, even uncomplicated cesarean section is associated with greater perinatal hazard. This risk is influenced by: (1) maturity of the fetus; (2) maternal and obstetric complications; (3) whether the operation is done electively or under emergency conditions; (4) type and duration of analgesia and anesthesia and the quality of anesthetic care; and (5) operative technique and duration of the procedure. In assessing statistics, it seems logical to consider these factors.

## Elective Cesarean Section

Elective cesarean section done at term is associated with a slight though definite increase in perinatal morbidity and mortality over uncomplicated vaginal birth. Using serial oxygen determinations of the newborn, Montgomery and associates (55) found oxygen saturation to be significantly lower following elective cesarean section than following vaginal delivery (Figure 30–7). A slightly greater perinatal asphyxia associated with elective cesarean section compared with normal vaginal birth has also been demonstrated by acid-base studies of newborn infants who generally manifest lower $PO_2$, oxygen saturation, pH, and buffer base, and higher $CO_2$ than neonates delivered vaginally (56,57). In an analysis of nearly 20,000 cases from the Collaborative Project, Benson and his associates (58) found that among 145 newborns near or at

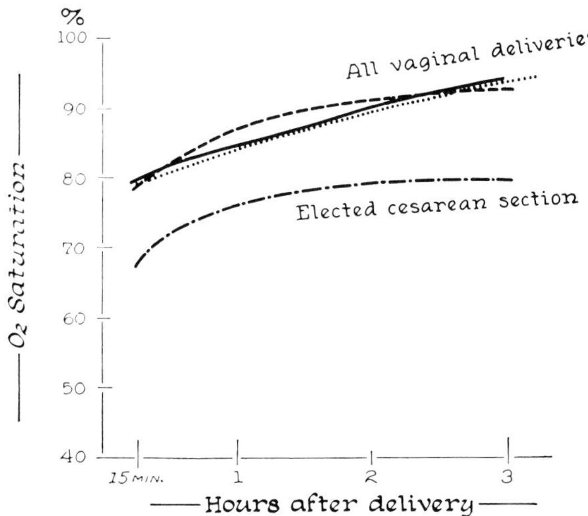


**Fig. 30–7.** Oxygen saturation during the first 3 hours of life among newborns delivered by elective cesarean section and normal vaginal delivery. The curves represent mean values of 8 infants in each of the two groups. (From Montgomery TL, Brandfass RT, First HE: Oxygen saturation determinations of the newborn in vaginal delivery and cesarean section. Am. J. Obstet. Gynecol. 71:1, 1956.)

term (37 to 40 weeks) delivered by elective cesarean section, the incidence of neonatal depression (Apgar score of 6 or less at 1 and 5 minutes) was higher than in a control group of 1883 infants delivered vaginally, regardless of the type of anesthesia used (Table 30–8).

**Table 30–8.** The Apgar Scores and Neurologic Status of Infants Delivered per Vaginam or by Elective Cesarean Section

| | Per cent of Total Infants Delivered | | | |
|---|---|---|---|---|
| | 1 Minute | | 5 Minutes | |
| Apgar Score | Cesarean Section | Vaginal Delivery | Cesarean Section | Vaginal Delivery |
| 0–3 | 7.0 | 4.6 | 2.3 | 0.5 |
| 4–6 | 15.4 | 12.7 | 6.2 | 1.8 |
| 7–10 | 78.6 | 82.7 | 91.5 | 97.7 |
| All scores | 100.0 | 100.0 | 100.0 | 100.0 |
| | 4 Months | | 1 Year | |
| Neurologic Examination | Cesarean Section | Vaginal Delivery | Cesarean Section | Vaginal Delivery |
| Abnormal or Suspect | 10.9 | 6.9 | 9.7 | 7.2 |
| Normal | 89.1 | 93.1 | 91.3 | 92.8 |
| All scores | 100.0 | 100.0 | 100.0 | 100.0 |

[Developed from data by Benson RC, Shubeck F, Clark WM, Berences H, et at: Fetal compromise during elective cesarean section. A report from the Collaborative Project. Am. J. Obstet. Gynec. 91:645, 1965. (Patients who were primigravidae, had complicated pregnancies, or had labor before cesarean section were excluded. Gestation was 37 to 40 weeks)]

They also found a slightly higher incidence of abnormal pediatric-neurologic examinations at 4 months and at 1 year.

### Perinatal Mortality and Morbidity

***General.*** There is little doubt that cesarean section carries less risk than a complicated vaginal delivery for the offspring; however, there is no conclusive proof that current liberal cesarean section has improved mental performance or reduced the overall incidence of neurologic problems.

***Iatrogenic Prematurity.*** Iatrogenic prematurity from elective repeat cesarean was a major concern before the currently available means of fetal assessment. Today, accurately determining gestational length (e.g., early pregnancy testing, early ultrasound examination) or determining fetal pulmonary maturity (e.g., lecithin/sphingomyelin ratio, phosphatidylglycerol) before any elective repeat cesarean should virtually eliminate iatrogenic prematurity from this cause.

## SURGICAL CONSIDERATIONS

### Operative Procedures

Currently, the two most commonly used methods of cesarean sections are the lower segment cesarean section and the classical cesarean section (Figure 30–1). Much less frequently employed, and then for very specific indications, is a variant of the lower segment cesarean, the extraperitoneal (in which the peritoneum is not entered) and cesarean hysterectomy (Figure 30–1). In all, save a few cases in which the classical cesarean is necessary (see below), the lower segment cesarean is the procedure of choice because there is less blood loss, the scar is less likely to rupture in a subsequent labor and delivery, and there is less chance of bowel adhesions to the incisional site.

As in all surgical procedures, the principles of hemostasis, accuracy of apposition, avoidance of tissue necrosis, minimization of suture material, reduced operating time and avoidance of infection will beneficially influence outcome. There is a temptation to attempt elective procedures coincident with cesarean section. Tubal ligation is probably the most frequent and is rarely contraindicated. However, the value of other procedures must be carefully considered relative to length operating time, prior transfusion, infection, etc. Incidental appendectomy is the second most common elective procedure with cesarean section, and may be safely accomplished should the appendix be readily accessible and the cesarean has no complicating factors. Myomectomy should be performed only for pedunculated tumors with a base that can be completely ligated. Attempting removal of other myomas nearly always leads to significant bleeding.

### Lower Segment Cesarean Section

The lower segment (low cervical) cesarean is performed in the lower uterine segment, an anatomical area influenced extraordinarily by late pregnancy and labor.

Thus, operative judgment is necessary to appropriately locate the incision.

In lower segment cesarean section, the abdomen is generally entered through a lower abdominal transverse or Pfannenstiel incision. After transversely incising the fascia, the midline raphe is grasped and by sharp dissection separated from the underlying tissues both superiorly and inferiorly. The rectus muscles are retracted laterally and the attenuated posterior fascia and parietal peritoneum entered by sharp dissection. The vesicouterine peritoneal fold is identified and the uterine peritoneum sharply incised transversely approximately 1 cm from its attachment to the bladder. The largely areolar connections between the bladder and the lower uterine segment are removed for 3 to 4 cm by blunt dissection and the bladder retracted toward the symphysis pubis to expose the lower uterine segment. The lower uterine segment is then carefully entered transversely by sharp dissection with a scalpel. Once the incision is started, it is generally extended laterally and cephalad by the use of bandage scissors. Direct visualization usually ensures that the uterine vessels are beyond the limits of the incision. Occasionally, a longitudinal midline lower uterine segment incision is substituted for the transverse incision should more access to the upper uterus be desirable. The major difficulty with this incision is frequent extension into the myometrium of the uterine corpus.

After delivery of the fetus and removal of the placenta and membranes, the uterine incision is commonly closed in two running or interrupted layers using 0 or 00 absorbable suture (e.g., polyglycolic). The bladder is replaced over the area of the incision and, although it is not necessary, the visceral peritoneum is generally closed using a running suture of 000 or 0000 absorbable suture. The abdomen is closed in the usual manner.

### Classical Cesarean Section

The usual indications for classical cesarean are placenta previa, transverse or oblique fetal lie, and cases in which extreme haste is necessary to deliver the fetus (59).

The classical cesarean section is the simplest to perform. Although a transverse abdominal incision may occasionally be used, the abdomen is usually entered through a low vertical midline incision extending from the umbilicus to the symphysis pubis. The midline raphe of the rectus abdominis is incised and the parietal peritoneum entered by sharp dissection. Using a scalpel, the uterus is entered to create a vertical incision through the visceral peritoneum into the myometrium of the uterine corpus. After the uterine cavity is entered,the incision is extended with bandage scissors to decrease the possibility of fetal injury. The delivery is effected and the placenta and membranes removed. The incision is usually repaired with three layers of absorbable suture (e.g., polyglycolic). Commonly, the two deeper layers are closed with a running or interrupted 0 or 00, while the most superficial layer is closed with a running (or "baseball") 00 or 000.

### Extraperitoneal Cesarean Section

A special lower uterine segment cesarean is designed to avoid entering the peritoneal cavity and is thus called extraperitoneal. This procedure may have had advantages before extensive use of antibacterial agents, but its use today is questionable.

### Cesarean Hysterectomy

The major indications for cesarean hysterectomy include: inability to control bleeding (e.g., from uncontrollable atony, from the placental implantation site of a previa, from the uterine incision), rupture of the uterus (with a repair being impractical), placenta accreta, massive infection of the uterus (usually involving tissue necrosis),and uterine or cervical tumors (e.g., uterine leiomyomata, cervical carcinoma in situ). Subtotal hysterectomy (i.e., leaving the cervix) is reserved for cases (usually hemorrhage) in which the patient's well-being is threatened by the operative time and risk of total hysterectomy.

Cesarean hysterectomy is technically the same as other hysterectomy except for the size of the uterus, the amount of edema, the friability of the tissues,and the extraordinary vascularity. Over two-hirds of cesarean hysterectomy patients must have transfusion (41).

## ANESTHETIC MANAGEMENT

The importance of optimal anesthetic care of parturients, emphasized throughout this book, is especially vital in patients with obstetric or medical complications and for operative delivery because of the additional physiologic and psychologic stress imposed by complications and the procedure. In the past, there have existed great differences of opinion regarding the "anesthetic of choice in cesarean section" due to the fact of the wide spectrum of training, competence, and philosophies of anesthesiologists and obstetricians. However, recent studies have provided much new data that have helped to clarify issues heretofore confusing and consequently there is some general agreement about the application of the major forms of obstetric analgesia and anesthesia. Here we will discuss three major methods in current use in general terms, so as to place them in proper perspective. We will first discuss their use for elective cesarean section. This will serve as a framework of reference for more complicated problems encountered in semi-emergency and emergency cesarean section.

### *Elective Cesarean Section*

For optimal anesthesiologic care in elective cesarean section, it is necessary to adhere to the basic principles of antepartal preanesthetic, intra-anesthetic, and postanesthetic care detailed in Chapter 22. Teamwork is critical. In many institutions, anesthesiologists have interaction with gravidae early in pregnancy to discuss obstetric anesthesia in general.

In most cases, patients are admitted to the hospital a day before the operation. Ideally, the obstetrician and anesthesiologist should discuss the course of pregnancy and the proposed plan for operation before the anesthesiologist sees the patients for preanesthetic evaluation and care.

## Preoperative and Preanesthetic Preparation

The importance of the preanesthetic visit by the anesthesiologist to develop rapport, obtain an adequate anesthetic history, evaluate the patient's physical and emotional status, provide psychologic support and prescribe preanesthetic medication has been stressed earlier in this book. The history should include an inquiry concerning the most comfortable position for the patient for when she is lying down. Gravidae with severe supine hypotension usually develop lightheadedness, dyspnea, and other symptoms of cerebral ischemia promptly after assuming the supine position, and by then most of them have already realized that they feel better on their side. In addition to examining the heart and lungs, the anesthesiologist should measure the blood pressure, pulse and respiration, and the fetal heart rate with the gravida in the supine and again in the lateral position to diagnose supine hypotension and to ascertain its severity. Following evaluation of the patient and discussion with the obstetrician, the decision is made about the anesthetic to be used.

Psychologic preparation for the anesthetic and the operation is extremely important in all patients scheduled for cesarean section, but especially in those who are to undergo abdominal delivery for the first time. Because these patients realize that abdominal delivery carries a slightly greater risk than does vaginal delivery, they are naturally more apprehensive about the operation and anesthetic. The anesthetic should be discussed in a reassuring manner and everything possible done to instill confidence.

Preoperative and preanesthetic orders are written by the obstetricians and include laboratory studies and prophylactic antibiotics, while the anesthesiologist leaves orders for fasting and for premedication, should these be essential.

## Laboratory Study

***Normal Gravida.*** A hematocrit or hemoglobin may be helpful in gauging the need for blood therapy in the event of large amounts of blood loss, but a differential count contributes little to the management of the normal patient. Blood should be typed and screened, i.e., ABO/Rh typed and screened for unexpected antibodies. The history and physical are generally sufficient predictors of derangements of electrolytes and coagulation profile. It is unlikely that a woman who has withstood the stress of pregnancy would have unsuspected abnormalities detectable by electrocardiogram; thus, in the majority of patients, a preoperative electrocardiogram is unnecessary. A chest x ray carries little fetal risk, but should nonetheless be obtained only if the history and physical suggest its necessity.

***High-Risk Gravida.*** The population of patients presenting for cesarean section includes a high proportion of high-risk pregnancies. For these patients, individualized studies will be required. For example, diabetics will need assessment of serum glucose. Preeclamptics may exhibit coagulation defects, both in the coagulation cascade and platelet function; therefore, assessment requires not only the usual platelet count, fibrinogen, prothrombin and partial thromboplastin times, but also an Ivy bleeding time (60).

The patients who have active bleeding, preeclampsia, overdistention of the uterus, coagulopathy, prolonged labor, or oxytocin stimulation are at risk for hemorrhage and should have at least two units of packed red cells available.

With concern about HIV, many obstetricians advise those gravidae who can do so to have one to two units of blood drawn during pregnancy, usually in the late second or early third trimester. This is stored for autotransfusion, should that become necessary.

## Prophylactic Antibiotics

There is some indication that prophylactic antibiotics used with all cesarean sections lower the infectious morbidity. The rationale for this broad usage is that current risk criteria fail to identify as many as 50% of cases that will subsequently become infected. This broad interpretation and extended use of prophylaxis is somewhat controversial. Moreover, even when all are given prophylactic antibiotics, approximately 20% of women will still require systemic antibiotic therapy for postoperative uterine infection and some serious postoperative pelvic infection will still occur (61). In addition, while prophylactic antibiotics do reduce significantly febrile morbidity and endomyometritis, the data are less conclusive for wound infections and urinary infections. However, the use of prophylactic antibiotics for risk groups (detailed above) is well accepted.

The time of administration of antibiotics must be coordinated with the obstetrician and pediatrician who provide neonatal care. Preoperative dosing of the mother yields therapeutic levels of antibiotics in the fetus, and this complicates the evaluation of the newborn at risk for sepsis. Thus, it has become more common to either administer intravenous antibiotics after the cord is clamped (intraoperatively) or to use intraoperative uterine wound and peritoneal cavity lavage with an antibiotic solution (59).

The most common groups of microorganisms involved in endometritis after cesarean section are group B streptococci, aerobic gram-negative bacilli, anaerobic gram-positive cocci, and anaerobic gram-negative bacilli (47).

There are several criteria used to choose prophylactic antibiotics. They should be effective against the contaminating organisms, inexpensive, nontoxic, and demonstrated to have clinical effectiveness. Prophylactic antibiotics should not be one of the antibiotics reserved for the treatment of specific severe infections nor a drug used against bacterial pathogens with acquired resistance (62). Although many antibiotics have been studied for their prophylactic efficacy, first- and second-generation cephalosporins are the most widely used. If more than one agent is used, they should be tailored to cover both anaerobic and aerobic organisms. To date, no single agent or combination of agents has emerged as the treatment of choice.

## Fasting

The practice in the United States is to maintain patients nothing by mouth (NPO) past midnight prior to elective cesarean section, while in the United Kingdom, the practice of a light breakfast of tea and toast has been advocated. Recent evidence suggests that fasts of less than 4 hours are associated with higher intragastric volumes and lower pH (63). Thus, the practice of the overnight fast appears sound.

## Premedications

With the exception of acid prophylaxis, there is little support for premedication of patients undergoing cesarean (57). Parturients have different expectations than do patients for elective surgery. It is now still justified to refer to withholding of maternal depressant drugs, which may have similar depressant effects upon the neonate. Of course, neonatal care has progressed to the point that ventilation and oxygenation can be administered and adjusted very well in the first days of life; nevertheless, it is unacceptable to suggest use of cerebral depressants that may have untoward effects upon a mother's newborn baby. In addition, there is just not the necessity for use of hypnotics, narcotics, or anilixotics before cesarean section. Furthermore, the modern mother is capable and expects to be awake and alert to be able to participate and enjoy the benefits of hearing and watching her newborn baby be born and enjoy the closeness of contact with her baby in those first few precious moments of life. In keeping with the general theme of this book, this chapter endorses the use of human interaction and reassurance by the anesthesiologist with the patient so that any anxiety can be identified and worked with just before and during the operative delivery period. Moreover, the use of drugs as premedication is certainly not in keeping with the special aspects of the management of the pregnant patient and her unborn baby. The following drugs are mentioned because of their use in the past as drugs that were given for tranquilization at a time when it was thought a necessary part of the practice of obstetric anesthesiology.

***Narcotics.*** Meperidine has been used in obstetrics since 1939, but has a potential for significant neonatal effects (64). Neonatal depression increases with longer drug-to-delivery interval. This has been attributed to the meperidine metabolite normeperidine, which is produced at a greater rate by mother than fetus (65,66). Thus, it is recommended that meperidine not be given as a premedicant for cesarean section.

Due to the greater respiratory depressant effects of morphine in the neonate, this drug is also not recommended as a premedicant. Butorphanol has been found to be relatively free of neonatal effects when used for labor analgesia, but its utility as a premedicant has not been examined (67).

Narcotics delay gastric emptying and produce nausea. Thus, there would seem to be little advantage in the use of narcotics as premedicants for cesarean section.

***Barbiturates.*** Barbiturates produce prolonged depression of neonates (68), and thus are not recommended for premedication of the parturient. Barbiturates are hypnotics and act by global cerebral depression of all central nervous system input. Such drugs have no place in the practice of obstetric anesthesiology as consideration as drugs to be used in the preoperative preparation of a patient.

***Benzodiazepines.*** Benzodiazepines are widely used in anesthetic practice to diminish anxiety associated with induction of general and regional anesthesia and to diminish the incidence of recall under general anesthesia. Crawford compared diazepam 5 mg, lorazepam 1 mg, ethanol (equivalent to a "'double gin,' British measure"), and placebo as premedicants for elective cesarean section. No significant neonatal depression was noted, and the incidence of recall under general anesthesia was reduced from 6.3% to 0.9% in the benzodiazepine groups. However, the proportion of patients reporting a greater sense of calmness was only marginally greater in the benzodiazepine groups. Other studies have confirmed the relative safety of diazepam in doses less than 10 mg (69). Diazepam is now no longer used because it produces neonatal hypotonia. Therefore, it is better to withhold these agents until they are needed during the procedure in the event that the mother exhibits undue anxiety and apprehension.

***Anticholinergics.*** Use of anticholinergics for premedication is a common practice, as these drugs are known to blunt bradycardic responses to tracheal intubation and to succinylcholine, diminish oral secretions, and possibly decrease gastric volume. Abboud compared the fetal and maternal responses to atropine 0.01 mg/kg and glycopyrrolate 0.005 mg/kg and found that in these doses, there were no significant effects on fetal heart rate. With administration of larger doses of atropine, tachycardia has been reported. Glycopyrrolate, which is less likely to cross the placenta due to its quaternary ammonium structure, produces antisialagogic effects with less maternal tachycardia and sedation, and thus may be preferable for those patients in which such therapy is desired (58,70). If antisialagogues are considered to be necessary because of their potent drying effect, and anesthesiologists believe this to be a necessity, they may be used preoperatively. In such a case, it might be preferred to use the intravenous medication just before induction so as to maximize its effect just after laryngoscopy intubation. In so doing, antisialagogues will also not cause the parturient to be uncomfortable due to the intense sensation of mucous membrane desiccation.

## Choice of the Optimal Anesthetic Technique for Cesarean Section

The choice of the anesthetic technique for cesarean section is dictated by many factors, including the reason for the operation, the degree of urgency, the impact of each anesthetic procedure on the mother and fetus including the presence of contraindications to each method, the desires and preference of the patient, and most importantly, the skill, experience, and judgment of the anesthesiologist. As previously mentioned, there is no ideal method of anesthesia for cesarean section and, indeed, studies of maternal and fetal outcome with general and regional anesthesia have not provided evidence of superiority of either method. Thus, it is difficult to conclude that a given anesthetic method will be optimal for a situation. In this chapter, we will discuss the advantages and disadvantages of epidural, subarachnoid (spinal), general anesthesia, and local infiltration. The anesthesiologist must choose the method that he/she believes is safest and most comfortable for the mother, is least depressing to the newborn, and provides the optimal working condition for the obstetrician. Before proceeding with the discussion of the specific techniques, we will consider the following issues that may help to assess the advantages and disadvantages of each of the techniques: (1) maternal mortality; (2) fetal effects; (3) maternal stress response; (4) operative bleeding; (5) postoperative infectious morbidity; (6) herpes infection; (7) preeclampsia; (8) intercurrent disease; (9) time considerations; and (10) the patient's desires and preferences.

## Maternal Mortality

The recent studies on maternal morbidity and mortality provide ample support for the contention that in patients for whom it is an option, continuous epidural anesthesia may be preferable. Maternal mortality, while relatively uncommon, provides a clear means of differentiating anesthetic techniques. In the United Kingdom, statistics demonstrate that general anesthesia is associated with a far greater incidence of maternal death than is regional anesthesia, and American surveys have supported this observation (71–74). These studies demonstrate that aspiration is the primary cause of maternal mortality, despite increased awareness of the risks of acid aspiration. It must be emphasized that without randomized, controlled studies, all studies are anecdotal. There is every reason to suspect that general anesthesia is more commonly employed in emergency situations, and such patients would be a higher risk group. Nonetheless, fewer maternal deaths attributable to hypoxia and acid aspiration occur in parturients undergoing regional anesthesia. While maternal demise does occur with regional anesthesia, this is often the result of errors in technique, vascular or subarachnoid injection, inadequate volume repletion, or unsuspected cardiac disease.

Despite the increased prevalence of prophylaxis for acid aspiration, maternal deaths due to aspiration have not diminished significantly, leading to the disturbing possibility that maternal mortality associated with general anesthesia may not be significantly reducible (59). Although rigid adherence to proper technique and honing of skills and vigilance may protect patients from iatrogenic death, a healthy respect for the risks associated with induction of general anesthesia in the parturient must be maintained.

Maternal mortality is further discussed in Chapter 20, and the importance of development of a plan to manage the problem patient early before admission to the labor and delivery suite for cesarean section is stressed. In most instances, the problems arise in situations in which an unsuspecting anesthesiologist is placed at a disadvantage by a request for a hurry-up anesthetic on a high-risk patient who has not been previously seen. To complete the scenario, this usually happens in the middle of the night when anesthesiologists are all by themselves. This places anesthesiologists at a tremendous disadvantage because they do not have someone else available to render a second opinion or to advise or even agree with a method of management. In many ways, the anesthesiologist feels uncomfortable, ill-prepared, and a little inadequate because of the circumstances. The aforementioned may cause him/her to make a decision to go ahead to facilitate delivery in spite of their concerns. In other words, in helping out in a situation, anesthesiologists take chances with a given technique on a given patient when in the back of their mind they have a worry about something going wrong. It must be emphasized here that the anesthesiologist must make decisions on safe, solid anesthetic techniques based upon the facts and, if the situation absolutely dictates that general anesthesia should not be performed, the anesthesiologist must maintain his/her stand and state the reasons for option for regional or local analgesia based upon safety of the mother.

## Fetal Effects

Anesthetics cannot be differentiated by fetal effects. Cord pH may be somewhat lower following regional anesthesia, possibly attributable to a period of enforced maternal hyperventilation under general anesthesia and also to maternal hypotension when hydration is inadequate and the patient is not optimally positioned. Crawford noted that infants delivered following epidural anesthesia exhibited higher Apgar scores and shorter times to sustained respiration, and opined that these infants were in "comparatively better condition" (75). Hollmen found that there was little difference in neurobehavioral outcome following epidural versus general anesthesia, except when maternal hypotension ensued (76). Datta demonstrated that while a prolonged interval from induction to delivery was associated with poorer fetal outcome under general anesthesia, this was not the case with subarachnoid anesthesia (77).

## Maternal Stress Response

Loughran and Moore (78,79) examined maternal stress responses to cesarean section, and found the increases in heart rate, blood pressure, and levels of plasma catecholamines, cortisol, and glucose seen when elective cesarean sections are performed under general anesthesia to be ablated by epidural anesthesia to the T-6 dermatome. Milsom (80) found similar effects on heart rate and blood pressure, and found that this was attributable to a lower systemic vascular resistance in patients undergoing epidural anesthesia, as there was no significant difference in cardiac output between the groups.

## Operative Bleeding

While in general it is believed that general anesthesia with nitrous oxide and low concentrations of inhalational agents does not cause increased uterine bleeding, Gilstrap, et al (81) found evidence of this phenomenon. There has been some suggestion of increased sensitivity of chorionic plate arteries to prostaglandin $E_2$ mediated vasoconstriction following epidural anesthesia, (82) but to ascribe the lower blood loss seen with epidural anesthesia to this phenomenon is speculative at best.

## Postoperative Infectious Morbidity

Anstey (83) demonstrated a significantly higher incidence of postoperative infectious morbidity in patients undergoing cesarean section with general anesthesia versus epidural anesthesia. However, Chestnut (84) found no evidence of an increase in postoperative infection as a result of choice of regional or general anesthesia.

## Herpes Infections

Ramanathan compared outcomes of a small group of patients with secondary herpes simplex virus 2 (HSV-2) infections undergoing cesarean section under general and epidural anesthesia and found no adverse outcomes attributable to either (85). It should be noted that the small number of patients limits the ability to conclude that either anesthetic is without complications. Ravindran obtained similar results with an equivalent number of patients (86). The Society for Obstetric Anesthesia and Perinatology (SOAP) has recently surveyed its membership regarding their practice for patients with herpes simplex virus 2 infections, and the results indicate a collective experience with 3000 such patients. One-third report they do not provide epidural anesthesia to patients with active primary lesions (87). Because the remaining two-thirds do provide epidural anesthesia to such patients, and case reports of significant complications attributable to herpes simplex virus 2 are lacking, it is a reasonable inference that herpes simplex virus 2 infection does not pose an excessive risk to the patient undergoing epidural anesthesia. Nonetheless, it would seem imprudent to administer an epidural through an area of active lesions or to a patient with active herpes simplex virus 2 viremia, due to the dire consequences of herpetic encephalitis.

## Preeclampsia

In patients with pregnancy-induced hypertension, some controversy exists on the preferred choice of anesthetic. Jouppila studied the effect of lumbar epidural anesthesia on intervillous blood flow, using (133) Xenon washout, and demonstrated a 77% improvement in blood flow, but only a 34% increase with segmental (T-10 to T-12) analgesia (88). From these studies, it can be concluded that epidural anesthesia has a beneficial effect on intervillous blood flow, which increases with the increasing extent of sympathectomy. It should be noted, however, that a wider sympathectomy may induce maternal hypotension, which this group has associated with decreased intervillous blood flow. Jouppila has also demonstrated a 20% reduction in intravillous blood flow with induction of general anesthesia in healthy parturients (89,90).

## Intercurrent Disease

Choice of anesthetic technique may be mandated by intercurrent disease. While no disease state provides an absolute contraindication to all forms of general anesthesia, contraindications to epidural and spinal anesthesia include coagulopathies and intercurrent infection. Several groups have studied the relationships of anesthesia, cesarean section, and diabetes (60,91,92).

## Patient's Desire

The desire of the patient to have or not have a given anesthetic clearly is an extremely important determinant. While some patients clearly are not interested in being awake during delivery, it is increasingly common for patients to perceive this experience in a positive light. Thus, increasingly, patients are choosing epidural anesthesia for cesarean section. In recent years, epidural anesthesia is used in approximately 40% of cesarean sections (93).

Although a recent quote of the percentage of regional anesthesia in cesarean section mentions a 40% figure, the figure is not representative of the incidence in university teaching centers today. In a survey of other Big Ten Schools, it was discovered that the average stated regional anesthesia rate for cesarean section was between 62.5 and 71.4%. (Survey conducted by John S. McDonald, July, 1992. Unpublished.) This rate reflects increased interest in mothers within the last few years who want to be awake and in control of their emotions, and the increased interest and capability of anesthesiologists in providing excellent pain relief by use of either epidural or subarachnoid block.

## Time Considerations

When emergency cesarean section is indicated, time considerations may prevent use of epidural anesthesia. In the previously cited studies, mean time from induction of anesthesia to delivery ranged from 7 to 16 minutes with general anesthesia, from 39 to 41 minutes with epidural anesthesia, and from 16 to 18 minutes with subarachnoid anesthesia. While it is clear that there is an irreducible time component with regional anesthesia due to the time required for effective neural blockade, there is good reason to believe that under regional anesthesia, the obstetrician might elect to proceed at a more deliberate pace. Knowledge that prolonged induction to delivery time has been associated with poorer outcome with general anesthesia and the lack of similar findings in epidural and subarachnoid anesthesia may be one explanation. Also, the obstetrician may be more gentle with the awake patient.

## *Immediate Preanesthetic Care*

### Acid Aspiration Prophylaxis

As noted previously, acid aspiration is one of the most common causes of maternal demise; thus, prophylaxis is mandatory. The two classes of prophylactics currently in use are nonparticulate antacids, such as sodium citrate, and type 2 histamine ($H_2$) antagonists, such as cimetidine and ranitidine (94). In addition, metoclopramide has been advocated in Britain as an agent to hasten gastric emptying (95). A recent survey of anesthetic practice in Britain indicates that nonparticulate antacids (sodium citrate and mist magnesium trisilicate) are the most prevalent form of prophylaxis in that country (96).

Sodium citrate, when given less than 1 hour preoperatively, has been demonstrated to be effective in raising gastric pH well above 2.5. Cimetidine and ranitidine, when given sufficiently before the procedure, are also capable of raising gastric pH. Due to the relative simplicity of use and its significantly lower cost, sodium citrate is currently the preferred antacid.

### Procedures on Arrival to Operating Room

Informed consent for the procedure is obtained before the patient receiving medication. On arrival at the operating suite, the patient is greeted warmly and reassured by the anesthesiologist. When she is transferred from the cart to the operating table, she should be made to lie on her side in which position she should remain until the induction of general anesthesia or after regional block is completed. The sphygmomanometer cuff and stethoscope are applied to the arm that is not to be used for the intravenous infusion. The maternal blood pressure, cardiac rate, respiration, and fetal heart rate are measured and recorded. Comparison with the blood pressure obtained the night before helps to evaluate the cardiovascular effects of preanesthetic medication and emotional stress. Preoperatively, a secure, large bore intravenous route (preferably 18 gauge or larger) must be established and an indwelling catheter placed in the bladder. No anesthetic should be started without having the infusion running. If subarachnoid or epidural block is contemplated, lactated Ringer's solution is started at a rapid rate so that a total of 500 to 700 ml has been administered by the time the block is established. If the patient appears apprehensive, small amounts (50 mg) of thiopental or pentobarbital may be given intravenously. The abdomen is usually surgically prepared after the administration of a regional anesthetic, but before the administration of a general anesthetic. To control blood loss immediately after delivery, sufficient oxytocin must be available to give both rapid infusions and to add to subsequent intravenous solutions.

All the equipment needed for the administration of anesthesia, including the apparatus for resuscitation, should be checked and made ready for prompt use before the induction of anesthesia. Moreover, no anesthetic should be started without having a well-instructed and experienced assistant who has no other responsibility but to provide psychologic support to the patient during induction and to help the anesthesiologist. Equally important, the anesthetic should not be started until the obstetrician has scrubbed and has the gown and gloves on. This is a precaution that should be taken in all instances even with elective cesarean section in the event unexpected complications require that the section be done immediately.

### Intravenous Hydration

***Crystalloids.*** Parturients often come to the operating room in a state of relative hypovolemia. Fasting and emesis may directly diminish intravascular volume, and aortocaval compression may create a state of inadequate venous return. In addition, complications such as toxemia and hemorrhage may be present. Therefore, volume repletion is an important part of anesthetic management of the parturient.

***The "Glucose Controversy."*** The use of glucose in volume expansion has been the subject of some controversy. Kenepp studied the effect of various amounts of glucose in a volume infusion of approximately 1 liter in patients undergoing epidural anesthesia for cesarean section. Addition of 25 or 57.5 g dextrose produced a significant rise in maternal and cord glucose concentrations, with a significant increase in fetal insulin levels and decrease in fetal glucagon levels. These changes were accompanied by a significant incidence of neonatal hypoglycemia at 2 hours age, and an increase in the incidence of neonatal jaundice. Use of 7.5 g dextrose was not associated with such effects (97).

Loong studied laboring patients, and found no significant difference in cord glucose levels in patients receiving 5% dextrose, Hartmann's solution, or no intravenous hydration (98). It should be noted that both the rate of glucose administration (1 g/hour) and the total glucose load were lower than that used in the previous study. Kenepp suggested that administration of glucose at rates less than 6 g/hour was not associated with adverse effects in the neonate (54).

In light of the work of Lu, which demonstrated a decrease in the dose of bupivacaine required to produce cardiovascular collapse in hypoglycemic rats (99), it seems prudent not to deprive the parturient of maintenance glucose infusion, but not to use solutions containing 5% dextrose for acute volume loading. In summary, dextrose administration of less than 6 g/hour or 7.5 g acutely should be considered safe. In other words, an infusion of 100 ml per hour will result in a maternal load of 5 g of glucose, which is under the standard 6 g per hour. In an acute situation, not more than 140 ml of D5LR or D5W should be administered, which would result in a 7-g load. To be sure, it would seem prudent to follow the accepted practice of keeping with use of lactated ringers for instances in which acute hydration is indicated in patients who are diabetic.

## CHOICE OF ANESTHETIC TECHNIQUES

### Introduction

Choice of anesthetic technique for cesarean section is dictated by many factors, including effect of anesthetic agents on the mother and fetus, the urgency for initiation of the cesarean section, the presence of contraindications to each technique, the skill and experience of the physician, and patient preference. In addition, studies of maternal and fetal outcome with general and regional anesthesia have not provided unequivocal evidence of superiority of either method. Thus, it is impossible to conclude that a given anesthetic technique will be optimal for all situations (100,101). Indications for employing epidural or general anesthesia for cesarean section are listed in Table 30–9.

Nevertheless, after more than a continuum of 4 decades of practice of obstetric anesthesiology and several thousand combined cesarean sections by both editors, it is again in keeping with the general theme of this book that in all instances, save those in which the mother really requests to be asleep, that the preferred choice of anesthetic technique is certainly regional. There is just no question that regional is safer for the mother, provides optimum conditions for the fetus, and provides one of the most exhilarating experiences of a mother's lifetime—the

**Table 30–9.** Cesarean Section Indications

| | Epidural | | General | |
|---|---|---|---|---|
| | n | % | n | % |
| Breech presentation | 16 | 46 | 16 | 28 |
| Transverse/oblique presentation | 1 | 3 | 2 | 3 |
| Dystocia | 6 | 17 | 14 | 25 |
| Fetal distress | 2 | 6 | 17 | 30 |
| Placental dysfunction | 1 | 3 | 0 | 0 |
| Placental praevia | 0 | 0 | 1 | 2 |
| Previous cesarean section | 3 | 8 | 2 | 3 |
| Previous dead child | 3 | 8 | 0 | 0 |
| Previous complicated labor | 1 | 3 | 1 | 2 |
| Protracted labor | 0 | 0 | 3 | 5 |
| Maternal disease | 2 | 6 | 1 | 2 |
| Total | 35 | | 57 | |

(From Juul J, Lie B, Nielsen F: Epidural analgesia versus general anesthesia for cesarean section. Acta. Obstet. Gynecol. Scand. 67:203–206, 1988.)

delivery of her own baby. It is just not the delivery of the baby, but the many moments of newborn-mother-father interaction that make it special. In certain high-risk cases, namely morbid obesity with a mother who is deemed to be a difficult laryngoscopy and intubation, the choice should be decisive in favor of regional or local analgesia. Local analgesia is often scoffed at by both obstetricians and anesthesiologists who have little if any experience with it, but have heard many "stories" recited about its inadequacies. The problem that has been in search of a solution for many years has finally been found at The Ohio State University where a course has been structured for the obstetricians by the anesthesiologists who teach three phases of local analgesia competency. Phase one is the lecture on various aspects of local anesthetic pharmacology; phase two is a demonstration in the cadaver dissection facility of the location and number of nerves that have to be denervated for adequate analgesia of the abdominal wall; and phase three is the actual performance of the local anesthetic blocks with the obstetricians on the patient chosen for the method.

## *Epidural Anesthesia*

### *Pathophysiologic Considerations*

One of the single most important complications of continuous epidural anesthesia for cesarean section is hypotension (102). A parturient is already at increased risk for hypotension due to aortocaval compression, and the sympathectomy that results from an appropriate level of epidural anesthesia may exacerbate the preexistent hypotension (103). Brizgys, et al found an 30% overall incidence of hypotension (systolic blood pressure less than 100 or more than 30% fall from baseline) in parturients undergoing epidural anesthesia for cesarean section. In patients not previously in labor, this incidence was 36%. Prophylactic use of intramuscular ephedrine 25 mg did not significantly diminish the incidence of hypotension (104). It is important to note that attention to hydration and left uterine displacement does not entirely eliminate this problem. Certain detailed information can be found in Chapters 13 and 15.

Attention must be directed to monitoring blood pressure following the induction of epidural anesthesia (Figures 30–8 and 30–9). While a patient may appear to be in no distress, significant hypotension can be developing (105). It is, of course, important to detect hypotension as soon as possible when it is associated with epidural anesthesia for cesarean section. Because the amount of anesthetic and, therefore, the level of blockade is higher for cesarean section than it is for labor, it is accepted that there may be some hypotension developed with epidural anesthesia for the operative procedure. However, with segmental injections or timed injections every 5 minutes over a period of 20 minutes, i.e., fractionation of the dosage, the tendency for hypotension is less because the parturient has an opportunity to adjust to the sympathetic blockade. Hollmen, et al noted that the assessment in their series of 30 patients was a sensitive indicator of the effects of stress factors that were associated with cesarean section, with one of those factors being hypotension. Their

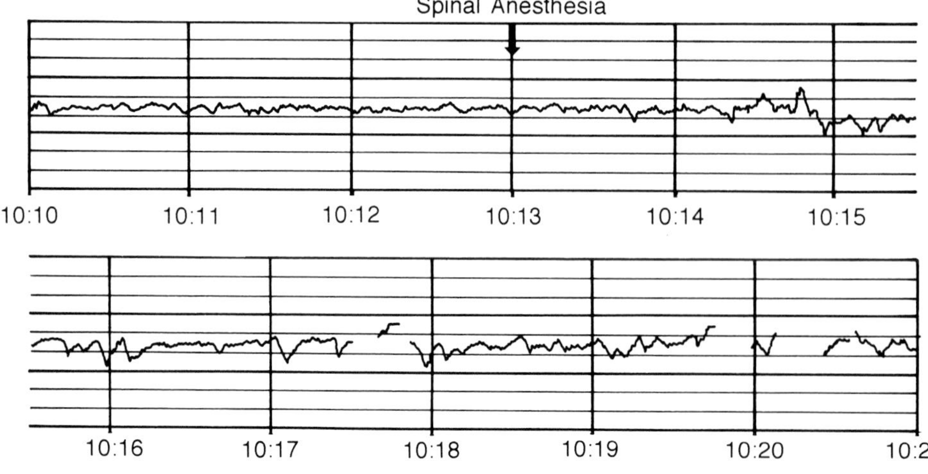


**Fig. 30–8.** Cesarean section case of hypotension for a few minutes. There was a normal heart rate prior to the spinal anesthetic being performed at 10:13 hours. At 10:15 hours through 10:20 hours, there are some fetal irregularities and loss of beat to beat variation. The fetal heart rate appears to be undulating.

| OB-OR-12 | 6-May-1992 | | | | | | | | |
|---|---|---|---|---|---|---|---|---|---|
| Vital Signs | 10:13 | 10:14 | 10:15 | 10:16 | 10:17 | 10:18 | 10:19 | 10:20 | 10:21 |
| Heart rate | | 76 | 80 | 58 | 54 | 68 | 70 | 70 | 74 |
| NBP-S | 110 | 102 | | 90 | | 116 | 115 | 112 | 113 |
| NBP-D | 52 | 59 | | 32 | | 59 | 51 | 50 | 48 |
| NBP-M | 81 | 80 | | 50 | | 77 | 73 | 75 | 77 |
| NBP-R | 75 | 84 | | 60 | | 60 | 74 | 73 | 75 |
| $SPO_2$-% | 100 | 100 | 100 | 99 | 97 | 100 | 100 | 100 | 100 |
| $SPO_2$-R | 72 | 76 | 80 | 58 | 56 | 68 | 68 | 72 | 74 |

**Fig. 30–9.** This figure shows intensive maternal monitoring every minute and details changes in the heart rate, systolic and diastolic pressure, and $O_2$ saturation. Notice mother's blood pressure is 110/52 at 10:13, 102/59 at 10:14, at 10:15 it could not be determined, 90/32 at 10:16, it could not be detected again at 10:17, and at 10:18 it came back to near normal at 116/59, and thereafter normalized. This is an example of an evanescent period of hypotension after spinal anesthetic for cesarean section, and proves the point that it is very important to monitor the patient minute by minute after challenging the patient with a spinal anesthetic.

study confirmed that periods of hypotension, which were even responsive to ephedrine, may be associated with varying periods of diminished intervillous blood flow in the neonate (106). Hypotension was thought to be of greatest importance in the presence of other factors that compromised placental blood flow, such as toxemia and diabetes.

As mentioned in the first edition of this book by Dr. Bonica, there is a reduced requirement for analgesic dosage in regard to the pregnant patient due to reduction in the size of the epidural space. Now it is widely accepted and understood within the field of obstetric anesthesiology that a diminished volume of local anesthetic is required to achieve a given level of anesthesia late in pregnancy.

As a result of the early studies by Bromage (107), Grundy (108), in a prospective, controlled study, failed to demonstrate such a phenomenon. He offered as an explanation that while in his study care was taken to avoid aortocaval compression, this entity was unknown at the time of Bromage's study, and occlusion of the inferior vena cava with consequent increased flow through the vertebral venous plexus has been demonstrated to increase the spread of previously injected contrast media in dogs (109).

## *Pharmacologic Considerations*

### Toxicity Factors of Local Anesthetics Peculiar to Pregnancy

The toxicity of local anesthetics may be influenced by numerous factors existing in the patient undergoing cesarean section. Pregnancy has been demonstrated to diminish the dose of bupivacaine necessary to produce cardiovascular collapse in sheep (110). Lu presented evidence that hypoglycemia diminished the dose of bupivacaine necessary for cardiovascular collapse in rats (57). Cimetidine, but not ranitidine, has been demonstrated to interfere with hepatic clearance of lidocaine (111,112). Bupivacaine clearance has been found to be unaltered by either cimetidine or ranitidine (113,114). Thus, it would seem that ranitidine, not cimetidine, be given as premedication for parturients who might be candidates for epidural lidocaine anesthesia.

Propranolol also interferes with lidocaine and bupivacaine metabolism, both by reduction in hepatic blood flow and diminution of hepatocyte drug metabolism (115). It is not recommended that patients receiving propranolol before delivery be discontinued from this medication, nor that epidural anesthesia be considered contraindicated; however, as Bowdle concluded, "caution should be exercised in administration of multiple doses of bupivacaine or lidocaine to patients receiving propranolol." (116). Preeclampsia has also been demonstrated to diminish lidocaine clearance, both by the two aforementioned mechanisms, and by diminution in plasma protein levels leading to higher unbound lidocaine concentrations (117). Caution should be exercised in such patients.

### Effect of Administration Method to Time of Block

Thompson noted that more rapid administration of 0.5% bupivacaine led to higher peak serum levels (118). Three groups, one receiving an initial bolus of 20 ml over 20 seconds and additional increments after 20 minutes (group A), the other two receiving an initial volume of 10 ml and further increments of 10 ml at 10 minute (group B) or 20 minute (group C) intervals, were titrated to an endpoint of a T-6 level (Table 30–10). The quality and incidence of nausea, vomiting, and hypotension were also studied by Thompson, and results are reported in Table 30–11.

Thus, greater safety may be obtained by a slow induction of epidural anesthesia, and a 20-minute interval between doses of bupivacaine does not limit subsequent spread. It is therefore recommended that after the test dose, 5 ml be administered every 5 minutes until a total of 20 ml is given. This technique has the added advantage of permitting assessment of the adequacy of the catheter placement, so that an improperly placed catheter will not be injected with a full dose of a given local anesthetic.

**Table 30–10.** Method of Bupivacaine Administration's Effect on Time to Block, Peak Level, and Hypotension

| Group | Dose (mg/kg) | Time to Block (min) | Peak Level (ng/ml) | Hypotension (%) |
|---|---|---|---|---|
| A | 1.7 | 40 | 1506 | 65 |
| B | 1.7 | 35 | 1273 | 24 |
| C | 1.3 | 45 | 1002 | 33 |

(Adapted from Thompson EM, Wilson CM, Moore J. McClean E: Plasma bupivacaine levels associated with extradural anaesthesia for caesarean section. Anaesthesia 40:427, 1985.)

## Fetal Effects of Local Anesthetics

Toxicity of local anesthetic agents in the fetus is affected by all factors that affect maternal toxicity. In addition, factors that cause fetal acidosis, i.e., maternal hypotension, hypoxia, uteroplacental insufficiency, etc., increase fetal local anesthetic levels by the mechanism of ion trapping. While it is not clear that local anesthetics in the concentrations seen in the newborn cause ill-effects, it would seem that the use of epidural anesthesia in obstetric emergencies, with rapid administration of local anesthetics to patients with fetuses at increased risk for acidosis, would entail increased risk of fetal local anesthetic toxicity (119,120). The message here is clear: do not be placed in a situation in which large volumes of local anesthetic must be given rapidly over short periods of time. This can increase both maternal and fetal toxicity.

## Choice of Agents

Various local anesthetic agents have been used safely for epidural anesthesia. Bupivacaine, lidocaine, 2-chloroprocaine, and mepivacaine have all been reported to be safe when used appropriately; however, questions have been raised about all of these drugs over the years (121–124).

Following reports of persistent neural blockade and adhesive arachnoiditis associated with epidural use of 2-chloroprocaine, this drug has experienced disfavor (125). Gissen presented data that demonstrated that sodium bisulfite at low pH, not 2-chloroprocaine, impaired function of isolated phrenic nerves (126). Kalichman, measuring morphologic alterations in intact nerves, found that 2-chloroprocaine and not bisulfite caused toxicity (127). He concluded that additional studies would be required to resolve the cause of the clinically observed toxicity. Regardless, a new solution of 2% chloroprocaine without bisulfate has been used for sometime now in obstetrics in surgical anesthesia with no reports of any sequelae. By now it is apparent that most of the problems associated with local anesthetics have been generated by their use dictated by clinical methodology. In other words, the problems associated with bupivacaine and the resultant cardiotoxicity were largely due to the large doses given over short periods of time. The problems associated with mepivacaine that had to do with fetal depression and toxic reactions were due to repeated doses given in short time periods inadequate for excretion of the previous dose. The problem with chloroprocaine was due to errors in subarachnoid spillage of epidurally injected agent. Nevertheless, all of the above named agents had basic problems related to their basic structure that precipitated the problems at the clinical level. For example, bupivacaine was shown to be relatively more cardiotoxic, mepivacaine shown to have a peculiarly difficult metabolic pathway, and chloroprocaine possibly will be shown to have been toxic due to the interaction between the preservative bilulfite and a low pH status as mentioned above. Although many who used 2% chloroprocaine switched over to other local anesthetic drugs after the initial scare of toxicity in the 1980s, the availability of a new solution for the most part has not been met with overwhelming popularity. Mepivacaine is rarely used in obstetrics in this country today, and most all of the recent literature documentation comes from abroad in relation to its clinical application (128–131). By far the most popular drugs currently used for the epidural route are lidocaine and bupivacaine.

In August 1983, responding to concerns regarding cardiac toxicity of bupivacaine, the United States Food and Drug Administration recommended that 0.75% concentration not be used in obstetrics. Marx notes that maternal deaths continue to be reported with epidural administration of bupivacaine in 0.5% and even 0.25% concentrations and concluded that the total dose in an acute administration may be more important than the concentration of the drug administered (132). It is therefore recommended that no more than 5 cc of any bupivacaine solution be injected in the period required to manifest premonitory signs of a toxic reaction (30 to 60 seconds). This practice is supported by the recommendations of authors from major centers, and, in light of the aforementioned results of Thompson, this restriction would not seem to increase the chances of inadequate blockade. Of course, the reasoning behind such a suggestion takes advantage of the uptake, distribution, biotransformation, and excretion pathways of all injected drugs. By 5 minutes, any injected drug that has a rapid fall in its peak concentration just after its maximum uptake and redistribution will experience a fall in its venous concentration levels, which are not a serious threat to either cardiotoxicity or central nervous system toxicity. This practice has been invoked by many teaching centers since the very early 1980s, and

**Table 30–11.** Quality of Extradural Anesthesia and Incidence of Nausea, Vomiting, and Hypotension

| | | Quality of Anesthesia | | Side Effects | | |
|---|---|---|---|---|---|---|
| Group | n | Excellent | Satisfactory | Nausea | Vomiting | Hypotension |
| A | 14 | 5 | 9 | 6 | 1 | 9 |
| B | 17 | 13 | 4 | 5 | 0 | 4 |
| C | 10 | 7 | 3 | 2 | 0 | 3 |

(From Thompson EM, Wilson CM, Moore J, McClean E: Plasma bupivacaine levels associated with extradural anaesthesia for caesarean section. Anaesthesia 40:427, 1985.)

it is an example of one of the very important modifications of clinical practice that can have substantial impact on clinical safety for the mother and fetus and newborn baby.

Scanlon reported that infants delivered following epidural analgesia with lidocaine, but not bupivacaine, had an increased incidence of neurobehavioral compromise characterized as "floppy but alert." (133). The effects were transient and were not associated with perceptible long-term sequelae (134). Abboud has subsequently been unable to demonstrate such an effect for lidocaine (135,136). Tronick followed infants for the first 10 days of life, and, while reporting the transient motor depression seen by Scanlon, found no persistent differences attributable to local anesthetics (137). Thus, there seems little reason to abandon lidocaine at this time.

## Use of Epinephrine

Use of epinephrine in obstetric epidural anesthesia is controversial. While some authors have reported that epinephrine will diminish the peak levels of lidocaine, etidocaine, and bupivacaine associated with induction of epidural anesthesia, (138) recent reports have questioned this finding with bupivacaine (Figures 30–10 and 30–11) (139). These authors do note a more profound blockade resulting from the addition of epinephrine. There is also evidence to indicate that epinephrine transiently depresses intravillous blood flow and uterine tone (140–142). Albright studied intervillous blood flow in humans using (133) Xe washout, and found no diminution of flow due to addition of 50 mg epinephrine to 2-chloroprocaine administered epidurally (143). Marx studied Doppler flow velocity in patients given epidural lidocaine and found no increase in uterine artery resistance in response to 40 mg epinephrine when resistance was not previously elevated (144). Veille, et al also found that pre- and postepidural umbilical artery waveforms were not significantly different (Figure 30–12) (145). Thus, it

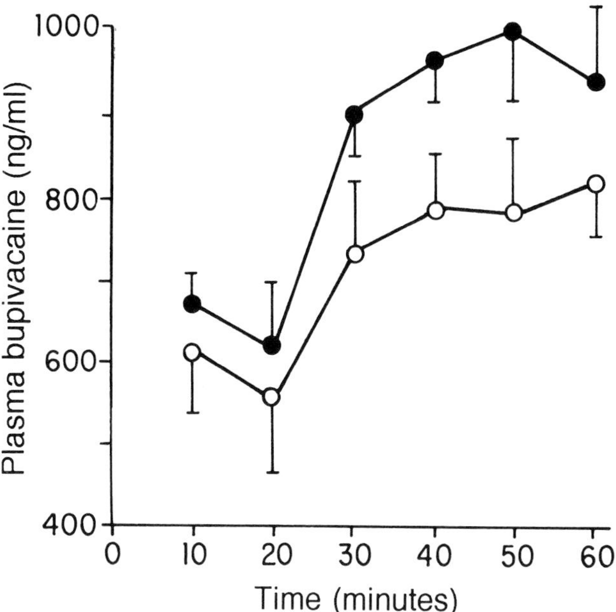


**Fig. 30–11.** Plasma bupivacaine levels (mean, SEM) during extradural analgesia for cesarean delivery after administration of plain bupivacaine. ●, Ranitidine pretreatment (n = 9); ○, no ranitidine pretreatment. (Redrawn from Wilson CM, Moore J, Ghaly RG, Flynn R, et al: Plasma concentrations of bupivacaine during extradural anaesthesia for caesarean section. The effect of adrenaline. Anaesthesia 43:12, 1988.)

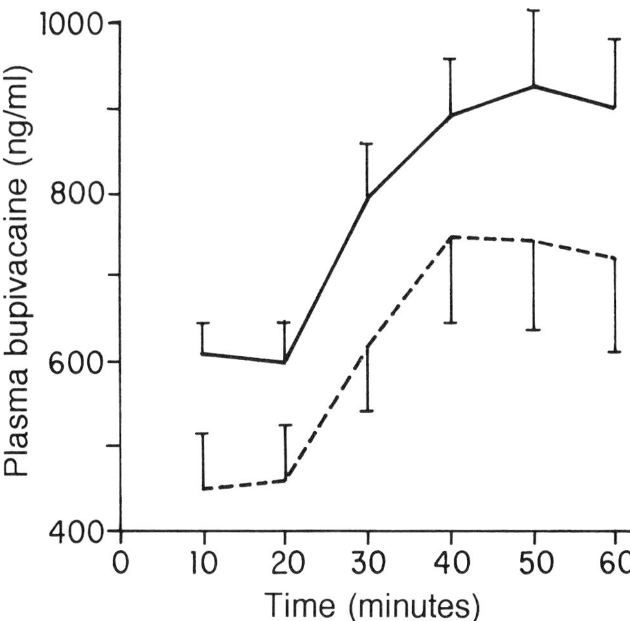


**Fig. 30–10.** Plasma bupivacaine levels (mean, SEM) during extradural analgesia for cesarean delivery in the two groups. ——, Plain bupivacaine: ––––, bupivacaine with adrenaline. (Redrawn from Wilson CM, Moore J, Ghaly RG, Flynn R, et al: Plasma concentrations of bupivacaine during extradural anaesthesia for caesarean section. The effect of adrenaline. Anaesthesia 43:12, 1988.)

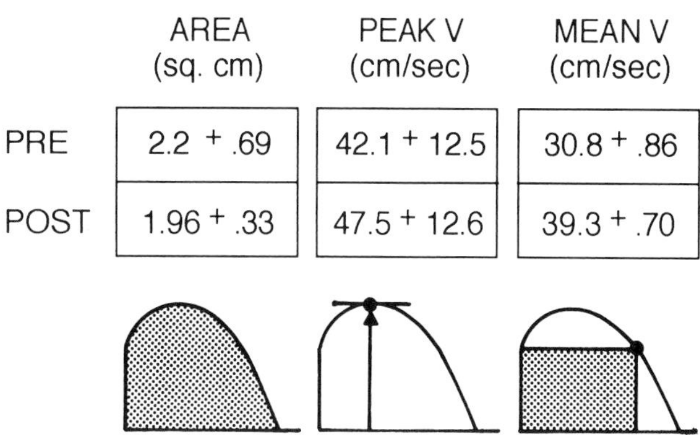

| | AREA (sq. cm) | PEAK V (cm/sec) | MEAN V (cm/sec) |
|---|---|---|---|
| PRE | 2.2 + .69 | 42.1 + 12.5 | 30.8 + .86 |
| POST | 1.96 + .33 | 47.5 + 12.6 | 39.3 + .70 |

**Fig. 30–12.** Digitalized value of the umbilical artery waveform obtained in the pre- and postepidural periods (N = 18 patients). Area = area of the curve; peak V = peak flow velocity; mean V = mean flow velocity; pre and post = pre-epidural and post-epidural. The values did not vary significantly, using the patient as her own control (mean ± SD). (Redrawn from Veille JC, Youngstrom P, Kanaan C, Wilson B: Human umbilical artery flow velocity waveforms before and after regional anesthesia for cesarean section. Obstet. Gynecol. 72:890, 1988.)

would seem that if one could be assured that the local anesthetic solution were being injected epidurally, extending the previously recommended maximum acute dose of 5 cc to any anesthetic solution containing 1: 200,000 epinephrine would be a safe practice.

In conclusion, no compelling evidence exists to suggest that epinephrine should be either excluded from or included in all local anesthetics used for cesarean section epidural anesthetics. If epinephrine decreases the risk of maternal local anesthetic toxicity while increasing the risk of diminution of placental blood flow, administration may be individualized to the patient's circumstances. In some cases, fetal distress will prove the overwhelming concern, while in others, the primary concern will be maternal well-being. However, in most normal parturients, it is unlikely that a difference in outcome could be demonstrated.

### Narcotics

Use of epidural narcotics for intraoperative management of patients undergoing cesarean section has been gaining increased interest in recent years. Addition of fentanyl 50 to 100 mg to the local anesthetic dose can be expected to improve the quality and duration of anesthesia, and has become routine practice in many institutions. With these small doses of narcotics, fetal depression has not been reported (146).

The use of the narcotic additive to the local anesthetic for cesarean section has resulted in one of the most dramatic beneficial effects noted in recent years. In past years, there would be many instances of maternal discomfort associated with dissection in and around the area of the bladder flap and at the time of delivery of the fetal head. This was always explained on the basis of the fact that innervation of the visceral peritoneum was vagal while innervation of the parietal peritoneum was segmental in nature. Thus, the latter would be adequately blocked by the level of the epidural or spinal, which was often at the T-2 through the T-4 level. Now, with merely the addition of this very small amount of fentanyl, i.e., 50 μg per 10 ml of injected local anesthetic or a total of 100 μg in a total epidural for cesarean section, the mother is remarkably comfortable throughout the entire procedure.

## TECHNICAL CONSIDERATIONS

### Preparation for Management of Complications

A disturbing tendency exists to perform obstetric anesthesia under "battlefield conditions." Despite the recognition of the potential for catastrophic outcomes in the obstetric suite, it is often the poorest-equipped anesthetizing location in the hospital. Thus, it is imperative that the ability to deliver oxygen under positive pressure, suction, and the equipment and drugs necessary for tracheal intubation be available at the location where any anesthetic is administered. Furthermore, it is clear that standards of monitoring adhered to in the operating room should apply to the patient undergoing epidural anesthesia for cesarean section. As of this time, this would include an electrocardiogram and blood pressure monitor, $SaO_2$, and $EtCO_2$ monitoring.

### The Effect of Positioning

Thorburn advocated the positioning of the patient undergoing epidural anesthesia in the sitting position, arguing that lack of sacral anesthesia was a significant cause of intraoperative pain (147). While this may be so, there are few data to support this conjecture. Merry found that maintaining patients sitting for 5 minutes following injection of 8 ml of bupivacaine produced little difference in the spread of analgesia compared to left lateral recumbency (148). Norris, using larger volumes of 2-chloroprocaine, demonstrated no significant difference in rate of onset of sacral blockade or extent of neural blockade on the basis of 30 to 40° head-up position (149). Hodgkinson noted that in lean patients, sitting position had no effect on anesthetic spread, but that in obese patients, the sitting position limited cephalad spread (150). While some authors have expressed concern that the left lateral position might compromise anesthetic spread to the right side, Datta compared patients in semi-sitting supine and semi-sitting left lateral position and found no difference in adequacy of anesthesia, but did find significantly better fetal acid-base and significantly lower fetal bupivacaine levels in the patients treated with lateral position (97). It is recommended that left uterine displacement be maintained during induction of epidural anesthesia, and that obese patients be placed somewhat head-up during this period, but it is not recommended to dose the patient in the sitting position.

A recent study of the lateral versus sitting positions used for placement of the epidural revealed that an initial prospective, randomized study of 144 patients suggested that the majority of anesthesiologists did better with patients placed in the sitting position with both needle entry into the epidural space and catheter threading into the epidural space. However, a prospective, nonrandomized, followup study of 152 patients, which minimized the subjective aspects involved, suggested that the real factor lies in the skill and experience of the person performing the procedure (151).

### Administration and Dosing Through the Needle

The question of whether or not to administer local anesthetics through the needle before placement of an epidural catheter should now be a question of the past. Extensive experience with single-shot epidurals have demonstrated the safety of injection through the needle, and one recent report demonstrates good results with a fractionated 20-cc dose of 0.5% bupivacaine given entirely through the needle (152). It is also widely held that injection through the needle results in a faster onset of blockade, and may distend the epidural space, allowing easier passage of the epidural catheter. Conversely, it is well established that the absence of adverse reactions following administration of local anesthetics through the needle does not preclude malposition of the epidural catheter. While it is unlikely that a study of outcome based on whether or not local anesthetics were injected through the needle before insertion of the epidural catheter will ever be performed, there exists some work upon which to base a choice.

Verniquet reported that by administration of 10 ml of 0.5% bupivacaine through the 16-gauge Tuohy needle, the incidence of intravascular catheter placement was reduced from 9% to 3% (153). These data can be interpreted to support the practice of administration of an initial dose of local anesthetic through the needle; Verniquet, however, found no evidence of venoconstriction being responsible for the lower incidence of venous catheterization.

This aspect of the technical matters of epidural placement can be found in more detail in Chapter 13. Suffice it to say at this point that there seems to be sufficient experience with the careful, slow placement of the catheter into the epidural space so that accidental dural entry does not occur. Furthermore, for the most part, it is always safer to place the epidural catheter, rather than the epidural needle, to check for the various errors during the first few minutes of the test dose, and then use that route for the graduated 5-ml injections of local anesthetic to prevent maternal complications as much as possible.

It could thus be argued that injection of an initial volume of normal saline through the epidural needle could produce equivalent results; however, no data are available to support this contention. Some practitioners employ a bolus of air through the needle to distend the epidural space. However, such a practice may be hazardous. Naulty studied healthy term parturients undergoing epidural placement for labor, and found a 43% incidence of Doppler-detectable venous air embolism following injection of 5 ml of air (154). Parturients are known to have increased pulmonary vascular pressure, and thus could be at increased risk for paradoxical embolism, although no reports of this are known. Thus, it would seem that some advantage could be expected from prior distension of the epidural space and that air not be the medium used for this procedure. Normal saline actually looms as an appealing medium for this purpose.

## Subarachnoid Injection

Injection of local anesthetics into the subarachnoid space in quantities intended for the epidural space has been associated with significant morbidity and mortality. While it would seem unlikely that the site of injection could be equivocal when dosing through the needle, the work of Mehta calls this into question (155). In 100 patients undergoing epidural placement in a pain clinic setting, the authors confirmed the loss of resistance by injection of radiocontrast dye. In these patients, 7% of the needles were placed such that contrast media was partially seen in the extra-arachnoid-subdural space. The significance of this finding was discussed by Hardy, who studied postmortem dura and arachnoid mater to discover whether epidural catheters could penetrate these tissues. Finding that the dura was too tough and resilient to be penetrated by epidural catheters, while the arachnoid could be penetrated with relative ease, he suggested that migration of epidural catheters into the subarachnoid space might actually be instances in which subdural catheters penetrated the arachnoid (156). There are several reports of radiologically confirmed subdural catheter placement in obstetric patients (157–159). Once it is known that catheters can be introduced into the subdural space, that epidural needles may be positioned partially in the subdural space with some frequency, and that it is easier to penetrate the arachnoid than it is the dura with an epidural catheter, it stands to reason that there are patients in whom the injection of an initial dose of local anesthetic through the needle will obscure the prompt recognition of a subdural or subarachnoid catheter. While such occurrences may be rare, unintended subarachnoid injection is a major cause of maternal morbidity attributable to epidural anesthesia, and the absence of cerebrospinal fluid flowing from the epidural needle does not preclude such an event.

Another issue regarding the injection of local anesthetics through the needle is what measures are to be taken when an adverse reaction is obtained. If an impending total spinal or convulsion were suspected, it would be injudicious to leave the needle in place while evaluating the patient. To quote Crawford, "It is of incomparably greater importance to be able to institute the appropriate resuscitation, should an injection be inadvertently made intravenously or intrathecally, than it is to employ any of the advocated techniques of test dosing" (160).

Finally, there exists the possibility of placing the initial dose of local anesthetic through the needle, with subsequent malposition of the epidural catheter. In such an instance, the detection of the malposition would be delayed by the prior injection of the initial dose. If the incision had been made on the basis of the belief that the catheter was functional and the initial dose inadequate for the entire procedure, general anesthesia might be required. Such occurrences, while uncommon, are known to the authors.

In sum, the general rule for safety regarding injection of local anesthetic into the epidural space is to place the needle safely and successfully in the epidural space with distension with use of a few milliliters of saline; the catheter is placed with the upmost of care with slow advancement by gentle but continuous pressure until it begins to slide into the epidural space. In instances in which some obstruction may be initially met, the operator may exert gentle, continuous pressure on the catheter and rotate the catheter in a clockwise fashion to expedite insertion. This maneuver will allow a catheter to come in contact with a venous structure and then allow it to roll over it often in an atraumatic manner, thus avoiding venous catheterization or tearing of the structure.

## The Epidural Test Dose

As noted above, in the absence of fluoroscopic confirmation, the exact location of an epidural catheter is not known. In reviewing the literature concerning obstetric epidural test doses, Prince noted that malposition of epidural catheters has been associated with two potentially lethal complications (total spinal blockade and intravascular injection) in 3 to 10/10,000 epidurals (161). Numerous techniques have been advanced for detecting malposition, and much highly spirited debate has occurred as to the proper technique. While there have been numerous recommendations (including the inclusion of succinylcholine 5 mg in a test dose), most adherents of the test dose use a combination of epinephrine and local anesthetics to detect intravascular and subarachnoid catheter placement, respectively (162).

Ordinarily, a 3-ml volume of 1.5% lidocaine with 1: 200,000 epinephrine is injected as the test dose with continuous monitoring of the pulse for some 5 minutes afterward. It is important today to be certain this test dose is also mixed in D10W to assure a hyperbaric medium. In case of subarachnoid spillage, this will result in restriction of the subarachnoid effect to the lower thoracic and lumbar areas. The lidocaine challenge consists of a total of 45 mg of lidocaine and 15 μg of epinephrine. This amount of lidocaine may not be adequate for definitive motor block; however, to detect a subarachnoid spill, the following maneuver may be used: the patient is asked to bend her knees. This maneuver is performed by use of the large posterior quadrant thigh muscles, which are innervated by the sacral fibers. Then resistance is exerted against the patient's tibias, and the patient is asked to straighten her legs. In case of subarachnoid spill, this is impossible for her to do because knee extension is accomplished by the anterior thigh muscles innervated by lumbar fibers. If the patient is able to perform both knee flexion and extension against resistance, then subarachnoid spill can be ruled out for the most part. In addition, the vascular spill can be attributed to a positive chronotropic effect upon the heart, because epinephrine is a potent chronotropic agent, and this effect will be noted within a 5 minute time span of injection.

The use of epinephrine is attributed to Moore, who recommended that epinephrine 15 mg be included with an initial dose of 3 ml of local anesthetic to detect intravascular injection as well as subarachnoid, noting an increase in heart rate of some 32 beats per minute with the intravenous administration of that dose (163). Cartwright noted heart rate increases of greater than 30 beats per minute in 12% of laboring women following administration of bupivacaine 3 ml without epinephrine, and concluded that this would lead to an unacceptable false positive rate (164). Leighton measured heart rate changes in laboring patients following intravenous administration of epinephrine 15 mg or normal saline in double-blind fashion, and found that while an experienced investigator correctly guessed the identity of the injectate in all cases, the criteria of baseline-to-peak rise in heart rate lacked sensitivity and specificity as a marker of intravascular injection. They recommended that if this was to be an effective test, "monitoring sophisticated enough to detect a transient 10 beats/min increase in the maximum maternal heart rate is required." (165). The risks of intravenous epinephrine administration were investigated by Hood, who administered epinephrine to gravid ewes and found a transient, dose-dependent diminution in uterine blood flow (166). It should be noted that in the study by Leighton, decelerations in the fetal heart rate were manifest in response to the epinephrine dose on two occasions. Given the inability of epinephrine-containing test doses to exclude all intravascular catheters and the possible risks of intravascular epinephrine administration can the epinephrine test dose be advised? (167). Intravascular placement may occur in 5.2% of obstetric epidural anesthetics, with nearly one-third unrecognized by aspiration. The complications of intravascular local anesthetic injection are real and life-threatening (168,169). Thus, the practice of epinephrine-containing test doses seems advisable in all patients. However, to obtain the maximum benefit from this technique, it is recommended that the following measures be observed: (1) careful aspiration of the catheter before injection (having first flushed the catheter with a minimal volume to clear any clot at the tip); and (2) limitation of the test dose to 15 mg of epinephrine and careful monitoring of heart rate for at least 5 minutes postinjection with an electrocardiographic monitor that has trending capability, if possible. If not, careful attention to heart rate changes must be noted throughout the first 5 minutes after injection.

If concern exists as to the ability of the fetus to withstand the diminution of blood flow associated with an intravascular injection of 15 mg of epinephrine, a reasonable alternative would be the use of lidocaine or 2-chloroprocaine in divided doses not to exceed 5 ml per injection, with careful attention to patient symptoms. It must also be noted that support can be found in the literature for reviling the use of epinephrine in the test dose. It is also essential that the lack of response to the initial test dose not diminish the vigilance of the anesthesiologist.

While epinephrine may help detect intravascular catheter placement, it has no known ability to detect subarachnoid placement. Thus, a local anesthetic is typically included in the test dose. Again, controversy exists as to the proper agent to use. Bupivacaine 0.5% has been advocated as an adequate solution for a subarachnoid test dose. However, the subarachnoid block produced with 3 cc of 0.5% bupivacaine and 15 mg of epinephrine may be slow in onset and difficult to distinguish at 5 minutes. Furthermore, Fine has reported an atypical high spinal with precisely this test dose (169). Bupivacaine 0.25% is probably not an adequate test dose for subarachnoid placement, due to the difficulty in assessing the blockade. Lidocaine has been advocated for the subarachnoid test dose, due to the typically rapid onset of the subarachnoid blockade it produces. Abraham has advocated the use of hyperbaric 1.5% lidocaine with epinephrine as an effective test dose to exclude subarachnoid placement, comparing the onset of 2 ml of this mixture deliberately injected into the subarachnoid to that instilled through an epidural catheter. All 15 patients dosed via the subarachnoid developed objective signs of blockade within 2 minutes, while only 1 of 250 patients dosed via the epidural route had such signs in less than 4 minutes (170). Again, the need for careful monitoring for sensory changes should be maintained for an appropriate period of time. A minimum of 5 minutes for detection of changes is recommended.

## Management of Complications

***Dural Puncture.*** Dural puncture is one of the most common forms of morbidity associated with epidural anesthesia for cesarean section. The incidence of unintended dural puncture in obstetric practice is reported to be 1 to 3%. Following epidural needle dural puncture, the incidence of postlumbar puncture headache is 30 to 78% (171). Controversy exists as to the preferred course of action following lumbar puncture. Prophylactic epidural blood patch has not proven to be effective (172); however, instillation of preservative-free saline has been advocated by several authors (60,173,174). The use of epidural saline injection presumes a subsequent successful epidural placement. While instillation of preservative-free saline in the recommended volumes (30 to 60 cc), limited by signs such as nuchal rigidity, seems a relatively benign way to significantly diminish the incidence of postlumbar puncture headache (175), it is unclear what effect the infusion of such a large fluid volume has on the safety and efficacy of epidural narcotics. Thus, it is recommended that saline boluses not be combined with epidural narcotics until there is evidence of the procedure's safety.

***Hypotension.*** Hypotension associated with epidural anesthesia is frequently due to aortocaval compression. Thus, the first preventive or therapeutic measure is left uterine displacement or left lateral recumbency. Adequate volume repletion with crystalloid should be assured (176). Failing this, pharmacologic intervention may be necessary. Ephedrine is the agent of choice because of both its cardiotonic and lack of uterine blood flow depression effects (177).

To maintain fetal well-being, prevention of maternal hypotension is preferable to correction. Conversely, overvigorous hydration may precipitate dyspnea and even pulmonary edema, and use of ephedrine may cause undesirable tachycardia and palpitations. Thus, it is recommended that patients be observed during volume loading and that reliance on routine standing orders to administer a fixed volume to all parturients be abandoned.

***Nausea.*** Droperidol has been found to be effective in ameliorating nausea and vomiting following spinal and epidural anesthesia for cesarean section (178,179). Metoclopramide 0.15 mg/kg, given immediately following clamping of the umbilical cord, also significantly reduced nausea without sedation (180). More recently, a quite effective agent to control nausea has been under study and now passed by the FDA. This drug is ondansetron. Ondansetron has been reported to be extremely effective in the relief of postoperative nausea and may well be the most efficacious drug yet today to combat this problem (181). In addition, the use of transdermal scopolamine has very recently been used in the control of perioperative nausea (182–185). Effectiveness in reducing postoperative nausea was 49% to 63% in recent studies.

***Inadequate Analgesia.*** Despite the best technique, up to 20% of patients will experience some pain while undergoing cesarean section under epidural anesthesia. In some cases, general anesthesia has been required; however, such cases can almost always be predicted by careful assessment of the quality of the block (186).

Many patients can be successfully managed without general anesthesia. Reassurance and emotional support are adequate in a surprisingly large number of patients. In addition, nitrous oxide in concentrations below 50%, ketamine (0.25 mg/kg), and fentanyl (1 mg/kg) have been demonstrated to be safe pharmacologic adjuncts (187).

***Shivering.*** Shivering is a frequent phenomenon in patients undergoing epidural anesthesia. Various forms of therapy have been tried with differing success: warming of intravenous fluids has been reported as both successful and unsuccessful (188,189); warming of local anesthetic solutions may or may not diminish the incidence of shivering (190,191); and meperidine may or may not be of benefit (192,193). Radiant heating of the face and chest has more rapidly terminated shivering associated with anesthesia than the application of warm blankets (194). Because all of the heating measures are benign and might work better in combination, it seems advisable to routinely warm intravenous and local anesthetic solutions and to apply radiant heat to the gravida's face and chest. If that fails, meperidine 25 to 50 mg may be given to those patients who have distressing shivering following delivery. Radiant warming should be employed in preference to warm blankets for those patients still uncomfortable postoperatively.

***Total Spinal.*** Unintentional introduction of doses of local anesthetics appropriate to the epidural space into the subarachnoid space is one of the complications of epidural anesthesia most commonly associated with maternal demise. Appropriate management depends on prompt recognition and rapid institution of supportive measures. The familiar ABCs of cardiopulmonary resuscitation are a useful guide. Assure the airway, preferably by endotracheal intubation. Ventilate with 100% $O_2$. Support circulation with positioning, fluids, and ephedrine as needed.

Following stabilization of the patient, consideration may be given to the consequences of the large volume of local anesthetic in the subarachnoid space, particularly if 2-chloroprocaine was the agent used. Exchange of the cerebrospinal fluid with preservative-free saline has been advocated to reduce the potential for long-term neurologic sequelae.

***Local Anesthetic Toxicity.*** Toxic levels of local anesthetics may be achieved either by cumulative absorption of local anesthetics injected into the epidural space or by unintended intravascular injection. Local anesthetic toxicity is typically manifested by generalized seizures, but cardiovascular collapse has been associated with bupivacaine and etidocaine. Often, the toxic reaction is accompanied by prodromal symptoms, such as tinnitus and perioral numbness.

If such symptoms are noted, immediate institution of oxygen therapy will provide a margin of safety against hypoxia should a seizure ensue. If the clinical suspicion of impending seizure is high, a small dose of thiopental (50 to 100 mg) may prevent the seizure. Consideration should be given to immediate induction of general anesthesia should prodromal symptoms continue to intensify.

If a generalized seizure or cardiovascular collapse ensues, CPR should be instituted promptly as outlined above.

Assessment of fetal status should be performed as soon as possible. If the fetus is delivered immediately, local anesthetic levels may be elevated due to ion trapping, and thus the anesthetist should be prepared for the need to provide cardiopulmonary resuscitation and supportive measures for both mother and baby.

## Subarachnoid Block

### Pathophysiology and Pharmacologic Considerations

Patients undergoing subarachnoid anesthesia are at greater risk for supine hypotension than those undergoing epidural anesthesia, perhaps due to the greater extent and speed of onset of the sympathectomy. Ueland found that patients undergoing subarachnoid anesthesia for cesarean section have a significant fall in cardiac output and blood pressure in the supine position, which was corrected by turning the patient in left lateral decubitus position (Figure 30–13)(35). Laboring patients undergoing subarachnoid anesthesia for cesarean section are at lower risk for hypotension than are nonlaboring patients, due to the transient autotransfusion of uterine contractions (195).

Volume preloading can be expected to reduce, but not eliminate, the risk of hypotension, and it is more effective when combined with uterine displacement. Prophylactic use of ephedrine has been advocated for prevention of hypotension; however, this will not eliminate the problem (196). Left uterine displacement should be considered essential in the safe conduct of subarachnoid anesthesia for cesarean section. With the exception of patients who are at risk for volume overload, preloading with approximately 1000 ml of crystalloid will also increase the safety of the technique. Despite these measures, as many as 50% of patients will still manifest significant hypotension, which should be promptly treated with ephedrine intravenously.

As mentioned in Chapter 14 concerning subarachnoid block, the most efficacious method of correction of hypotension is simultaneous left uterine displacement and elevation of the legs to the straight up position. The legs should remain in this position for a minute or two, but even during the first few seconds of such a maneuver, one should note a substantial improvement in blood pressure. Most of the time, this maneuver is all that is needed to quickly reverse the hypotensive effect. It satisfies all of the three important criteria for use in clinical troublesome situations, i.e., it is quick, simple, and effective. If in the rare instance this maneuver is not effective or effective only as long as the legs are left in an upright position, one can use supplemental small dosages of ephedrine, i.e., 5 to 10 mg intravenous.

Local anesthetic toxicity and placental transfer of local anesthetics are not problems associated with subarachnoid anesthesia, due to the doses given.

### Choice of Agents

The anesthetic agents for subarachnoid anesthesia in cesarean section are summarized in Table 30–12. Certainly, the most popular drugs used for anesthesia for cesarean section are bupivacaine and tetracaine (197). Table 30–13 depicts the level and duration of block achieved with varying volumes of 0.5% bupivacaine. It is common practice today to add a small amount of opioid for pain relief postoperatively. Intrathecal morphine sulfate in doses of 0.1 to 0.5 mg provides quality postcesarean analgesia with a duration of 18 to 36 hours (198,199). Pruritus, nausea, vomiting, and urinary retention are common with intrathecal opioids, but the severity is minimal at lower doses. Abboud, et al demonstrated that intrathecal morphine 0.1 to 0.25 mg provides 18 to 28 hours of analgesia with minimal side effects (198). This duration of action is optimal for postcesarean patients who usually can tolerate oral analgesics within 16 to 24 hours. While the potential for respiratory depression exists with any dose of intrathecal morphine, it is rare to absent at the

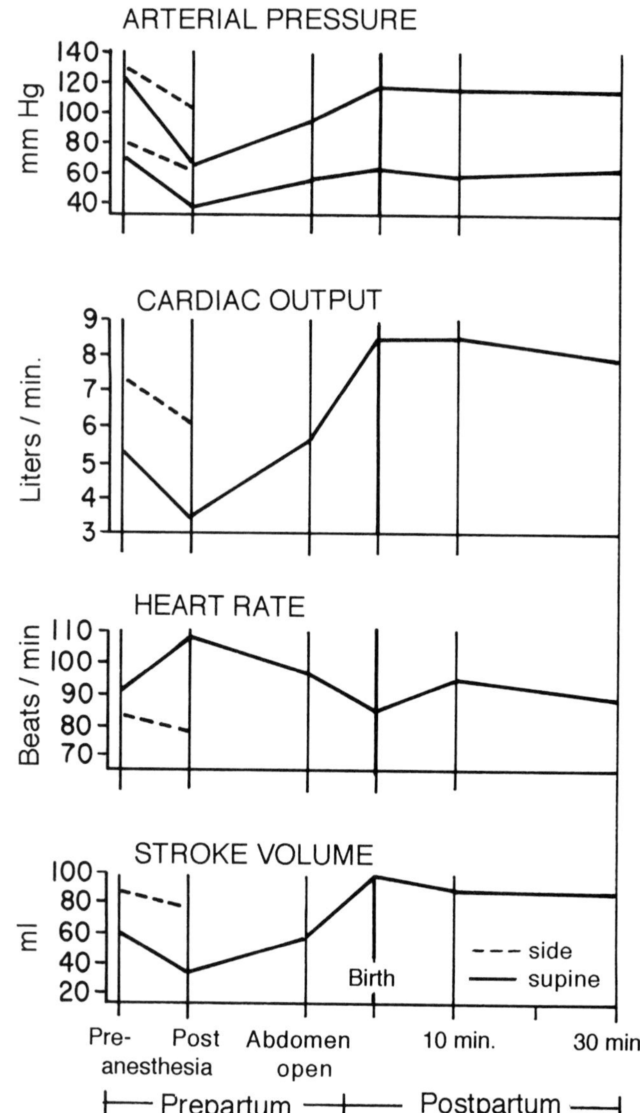


Fig. 30–13. Hemodynamic changes in patients undergoing cesarean section with subarachnoid block. Before the operation, measurements were made with the patient supine and on her side both before and after the induction of anesthesia. (Redrawn from Ueland K, Gills RE, Hansen JM: Maternal cardiovascular dynamics, I: Cesarean section under subarachnoid block anesthesia. Am. J. Obstet. Gynecol. 100:42, 1968.)

**Table 30–12.** Subarachnoid Local Anesthetic Agents for Cesarean Section

| Agent (mg & ml) | Height 5′ | 5′3″ | 5′6″ | 5′9″ | 6′ | Onset (min) | Duration (min) |
|---|---|---|---|---|---|---|---|
| Lidocaine 5% | 60 | 65 | 70 | 75 | 80 | 1–3 | 45–75 |
| (in 7.5% dextrose) | 1.2 | 1.3 | 1.4 | 1.5 | 1.6 | | |
| Tetracaine 0.5% | 7 | 8 | 9 | 10 | 11 | 3–5 | 120–180 |
| (in 5% dextrose) | 1.4 | 1.6 | 1.8 | 2.0 | 2.2 | | |
| Tetracaine 0.5% | 6/60 | 7/70 | 8/80 | 9/90 | 10/100 | 2–4 | 120–180 |
| (in 5% procaine) | 1.2 | 1.4 | 1.6 | 1.8 | 2.0 | | |
| Bupivacaine 0.75% | 7.5 | 10 | 12 | 14.25 | 15 | 2–4 | 75–120 |
| (in 5% dextrose) | 1.0 | 1.3 | 1.6 | 1.9 | 2.0 | | |

(Adapted from Hurley R: Anesthesia for Cesarean Delivery. *In* Common Problems in Obstetric Anesthesia. Edited by S Datta, GW Ostheimer. Chicago, 1987, p. 197. Year Book Medical Publishers, Inc.)

lower doses of 0.1 mg to 0.25 mg (198). This is described in greater detail in Chapter 14 concerning subarachnoid block.

## Tetracaine

Tetracaine has been a common agent for subarachnoid anesthesia; however, Chantigian noted this drug has a significant incidence of inadequate anesthesia. By combining tetracaine with 10% procaine (instead of 10% glucose) he produced a solution of greater baricity, which yielded greater patient comfort and reduced supplemental analgesia requirements (200).

## Bupivacaine

Bupivacaine has been used as 0.5% isobaric, 0.5% hyperbaric (201), and 0.75% hyperbaric solutions. With hyperbaric 0.5% bupivacaine given in doses of 7.5 mg, Santos noted incomplete analgesia in most patients (198), but with 12.5 mg, Michie found analgesia to be complete in all patients (199).

## Lidocaine

Hyperbaric lidocaine has been investigated for anesthesia when endotracheal intubation fails. While providing rapid onset, the duration of anesthesia is brief, and the incidence of dysphagia due to high blockade led the authors to discourage the use of subarachnoid lidocaine for cesarean section (200).

## Use of Epinephrine

Because duration of tetracaine and bupivacaine is adequate for virtually all cesarean sections, there would seem little motivation to add epinephrine to these agents. Prolongation of lidocaine anesthesia could be desirable. However, recent evidence suggests epinephrine does not prolong the duration of lidocaine analgesia in an obstetric population (201). Due to the potential for errors in dilution of epinephrine and the questionable benefits of its use, it is currently not widely used in subarachnoid anesthesia for cesarean section.

### *Technical Considerations*

Control of the level of subarachnoid anesthesia is crucial to its safe use. The various approaches advocated to achieve control of the level are summarized below.

## Single Dose Techniques

When using a single dose of subarachnoid local anesthetic, control of spread is achieved by baricity, volume

**Table 30–13.** Subarachnoid Bupivacaine 0.5% for Cesarean Section: Volume, Level of Block, and Duration of Block

| Volume of LA (ml) | Number of Patients* | Age (yr) | Weight (kg) | Height (m) | Level of Block (**) | Duration of Motor Block*** (min) |
|---|---|---|---|---|---|---|
| 2.25 | 9 | 27 | 68.4 ± 3.7 | 1.58 ± 0.01 | T5 (T2–T8) | 250.8 ± 18.6 |
| 2.5 | 21 | 28 | 72.4 ± 2.2 | 1.59 ± 0.01 | T4 (T2–T7) | 209.7 ± 8.7 |
| 2.75 | 13 | 29 | 70.4 ± 2.1 | 1.59 ± 0.02 | T4 (T1–T8) | 239 ± 15.7 |
| 3.0 | 3 | 26 | 76.1 ± 5.3 | 1.67 ± 0.03 | T2 (T2–T7) | 276.7 ± 41.5 |
| 3.25 | 1 | 23 | 71 | 1.73 | T6 | 311 |
| 3.5 | 1 | 24 | 90.4 | 1.61 | T1 | 360 |

LA Local Anesthetic
* Excludes the failures of the spinal through extradural needle technique (n = 4).
(**) Median and range of spread of sensory blockade.
*** Excludes patients who received extradural local anesthetic.
(From Carrie LES, O'Sullivan G: Subarachnoid bupivacaine 0.5% for Caesarean section. Euro. J. Anaesth. 1:275–283, 1984. Modified to exclude some standard deviations.)

of injection, and patient position. It should be noted that cerebrospinal fluid dynamics are altered at term, particularly during labor, due to engorgement of the epidural veins. Thus, conventional nonobstetric practices may result in high levels. Russell believed that the use of isobaric bupivacaine for cesarean section offered some advantage in that the patient could be maintained in left lateral position without developing a one-sided block (201). However, following further experience with the technique, he found that control of the level was not always possible (202). Thus, the use of isobaric solutions is not advised.

With hyperbaric solutions, maintaining the patient in the sitting position for 1 minute before assuming left lateral tilt slowed the onset of the block, but did not affect eventual level or duration of anesthesia (183). Using hyperbaric tetracaine, Sprague found that if patients were positioned in right lateral decubitus position during induction of subarachnoid anesthesia and promptly turned to left lateral tilt (12-cm wedge under right hip), adequate levels of anesthesia could be obtained for cesarean section (203). While if the patient was initially in left lateral decubitus, this was not always possible without placing the patient supine. Thus, it is recommended that subarachnoid anesthesia be induced with the patient in right lateral decubitus position. When technical considerations prevent this, the sitting position may be used, but onset will be delayed.

### Continuous Spinal Anesthesia

Interest in continuous spinal anesthesia with large-bore catheters declined, probably due to the incidence of postlumbar puncture headaches. Recent advances in catheter technology have led to micro-bore catheters, such as can be placed through a 25-gauge or 22-gauge needle. The experience to date with the 25-gauge technique and use of the very small catheter has been fraught with many problems, including: (1) inability to aspirate to check for placement; (2) difficulty in obtaining a good block due to streaming; (3) difficulty with injection; and (4) some concern about neural toxicity. However, experience with the 22-gauge needle with the 25-gauge catheter has been much more successful and seems to offer a practical solution to the past difficulties encountered with the larger bore needles and catheters, which were problems from the standpoint of postpartum headaches. Placement of the catheter using the paramedium approach allows a better angle for gliding the catheter into the subarachnoid space (Covino BG, personal communication).

## Subarachnoid/Epidural Combination

Rawal has described a technique for combined subarachnoid and epidural anesthesia (204). Following introduction of a 16-gauge Tuohy needle into the epidural space with the bevel-directed caudad, a long 26-gauge spinal needle is introduced through the Tuohy needle and hyperbaric local anesthetic is injected. The epidural needle is then rotated 180° and an epidural catheter passed. If the level of anesthesia obtained via the subarachnoid dose is inadequate, additional anesthetic can be given via the epidural catheter. In a study comparing this technique to conventional epidural anesthesia, patients receiving combined spinal-epidural anesthesia required significantly lower doses of local anesthetic to achieve a T-4 level, required supplemental analgesics significantly less frequently, had better subjective ratings of analgesia, and had lower maternal and cord local anesthetic concentrations (205). There were no postlumbar puncture headaches; however, with only 39 patients, the predictive power of this statement is limited. Despite the use of the sitting position, four patients exhibited initial anesthetic levels in excess of T-4. However, by decreasing the subarachnoid dose, this problem could possibly be reduced.

In sum, combined spinal-epidural anesthesia has the following advantages: control of anesthetic level, use of equipment currently available, rapid onset of anesthesia, and reasonable assurance of proper placement of the epidural needle. However, it has not gained wide acceptance.

### Management of Complications

With some exceptions, the complications of spinal anesthesia are similar to those of epidural anesthesia. The incidence of postlumbar puncture headache is understandably greater, even when using 25-gauge needles, and may be treated as noted above. The incidence of hypotension and high levels of blockade are also greater, but local anesthetic toxicity is rarely seen, due to the reduced dosage. Therapy for hypotension and high blockade levels is as noted previously.

## General Anesthesia

### Pathophysiology

Physiologic alterations of importance to induction and maintenance of general anesthesia for cesarean section revolve around maintenance of adequate maternal and fetal oxygenation. Intubation is rendered even more critical by the risks of aspiration detailed above. Indeed, general anesthesia during pregnancy should not be undertaken in the absence of endotracheal intubation.

### Pharmacologic Considerations

#### Induction Agents

***Thiopental.*** Thiopental has been used extensively for induction of anesthesia for cesarean section (206,207). Doses of 4 to 7 mg/kg are not associated with diminished Apgar scores; however, with larger doses, neonatal depression can be seen (208). Thiopental pharmacokinetics were studied by Christensen (209), who found a decreased requirement for loss of ciliary reflex in parturients (3.53 mg/kg) versus young women (5.43 mg/kg). Maternal terminal elimination half-life was found to be shorter than in the nonparturient. Neonatal elimination was significantly slower than in normal adults. Thus, it is recommended that somewhat smaller doses of thiopental be administered to the parturient.

Following a single dose of 5 mg/kg thiopental for anesthetic induction, levels in colostrum are less than 0.04 mg/100 ml (210). Thus, breast feeding should not preclude use of this agent.

**Table 30–14.** Umbilical Blood Gas Values and Apgar Scores

| | Ketamine (n = 12) | Thiopental (n = 13) | Combination (n = 11) |
|---|---|---|---|
| Apgar Score ≥7 (n) | | | |
| 1 min | 10 | 13 | 9 |
| 5 min | 12 | 13 | 10 |
| Umbilical blood gas values (means ± SD) | | | |
| Arterial | | | |
| pH | 7.31 ± 0.04 | 7.31 ± 0.04 | 7.32 ± 0.06 |
| $PCO_2$ (mm Hg) | 50.5 ± 6.9 | 50.8 ± 6.7 | 51.2 ± 10.1 |
| $PO_2$ (mm Hg) | 13.8 ± 3.3 | 15.2 ± 6.3 | 14.7 ± 4.8 |
| Venous | | | |
| pH | 7.36 ± 0.05 | 7.36 ± 0.05 | 7.38 ± 0.07 |
| $PCO_2$ (mm Hg) | 44.6 ± 6.2 | 44.8 ± 5.9 | 42.8 ± 7.8 |
| $PO_2$ (mm Hg) | 24.3 ± 5.2 | 25.3 ± 9.6 | 27.8 ± 5.2 |

(From Schultetus RR, Hill CR, Dharamraj CM, Banner TE, et al: Wakefulness during cesarean section after anesthetic induction with ketamine, thiopental, or ketamine and thiopental combined. Anesth. Analg. 65: 723–8, 1986.)

***Methohexital.*** Methohexital has been advocated as an induction agent for cesarean section, but Holdcroft found that there was a relatively narrow margin for error with this drug. While neonatal depression was not seen with induction doses of 1.0 mg/kg, doses of 1.4 mg/kg were associated with poorer neonatal status (211). Thus, this drug offers little advantage for cesarean anesthesia.

***Ketamine.*** Ketamine has increasingly become the induction agent of choice for cesarean section in situations of maternal hemorrhage, either alone or in combination with a small dose (1 mg/kg) of thiopental. Ketamine has been found to provide greater cardiovascular stability and lower incidence of intraoperative awareness (212,213). Neonatal status is no worse and is probably better than with thiopental (Table 30–14) (214,215). An induction dose of ketamine is typically 1 mg/kg. Ketamine has also been advocated as a complete anesthetic for cesarean section in developing nations.

***Etomidate.*** Etomidate (0.3 mg/kg) may offer some advantage over thiopental (3.5 mg/kg) in neonatal status when used for cesarean anesthesia. This agent has superior cardiovascular properties, but has not yet found wide acceptance in obstetrics (216).

***Midazolam.*** Midazolam (0.02 mg/kg) compared to thiopental (3.5 mg/kg) for induction of general anesthesia for cesarean section has a significantly greater incidence of neonatal respiratory depression (217). This agent is not recommended for use in cesarean section.

## Muscle Relaxants

Muscle relaxants are used for both induction and maintenance of anesthesia for cesarean section. Induction of general anesthesia implies rapid sequence induction, and maintenance often is as much to assist with light anesthesia as it is to allow surgical exposure. The commonly employed agents may all be given safely prior to cord clamping. Safe practice hinges on knowledge of the susceptibility of parturients to muscle relaxants, particularly when combined with magnesium sulfate (218).

***Succinylcholine.*** Plasma cholinesterase activity falls rapidly in the first 10 weeks of pregnancy and remains low, such that over 10% of patients are said to be at risk for prolonged duration of succinylcholine immediately postpartum (219). Conversely, while plasma cholinesterase levels are diminished in parturients, time to 90% twitch recovery following a single intubating dose is not prolonged (220). Thus, while prolonged paralysis should not be the norm with succinylcholine, it occasionally occurs. Thus, monitoring of the degree of neuromuscular blockade should be performed routinely, even when only a single intubating dose is contemplated.

Administration of succinylcholine has been associated with a number of unpleasant side effects, such as muscle fasciculations, myalgias, and increased intragastric pressure (221–223). Preadministration of a small dose of nondepolarizing muscle relaxation may prevent these effects (224). However, the necessity of such measures in patients undergoing cesarean section has been questioned (225). Myalgias are less common in pregnancy, whether succinylcholine is given by bolus or as a continuous infusion. Use of gallamine or d-tubocurarine pretreatment has not proven effective in reducing the incidence of myalgias in parturients (226). While fasciculations increase intragastric pressure, they may not increase the potential for regurgitation, as the esophagogastric pressure gradient is unchanged in normal patients. The intragastric pressure increases are well within the range that can be managed with cricoid pressure.

Thus, pretreatment provides only minimal advantage in management of the parturient and pretreatment has disadvantages. Pretreatment increases the time required to obtain optimal intubating conditions and results in less satisfactory intubating conditions. Parturients demonstrate increased susceptibility to nondepolarizing muscle relaxants, particularly preeclamptics undergoing magnesium sulfate therapy, and are at increased risk to develop hypoxemia with hypoventilation. Thus, parturients represent a population of patients who are less likely to obtain advantages from pretreatment, and are more prone to develop complications due to its use. It is not recommended that pretreatment be routinely applied, and when pretreatment is used, attention must be given to the potential for respiratory compromise.

Succinylcholine continuous infusions have been used widely for maintenance of muscle relaxation during cesarean section, but have been largely replaced by the short-acting nondepolarizing agents atracurium and vecuronium. Despite precautions such as blue dye markers and red labels, unintended connections of a muscle relaxant in place of the normal intravenous fluid line have occurred.

***Curare.*** Curare has been used successfully for maintenance of muscle relaxation in cesarean section. However, placental transfer of this drug may uncommonly cause demonstrable neonatal depression.

***Pancuronium.*** Pancuronium has also been used for maintenance of muscle relaxation in cesarean section. An umbilical venous to maternal venous ratio of 0.22 has been determined for this drug, but this value increases with prolongation of the incision to delivery interval. Neonatal depression associated with pancuronium is rare (227).

***Atracurium.*** Atracurium has been evaluated for maintenance of muscle relaxation in cesarean section, and has been found to provide good muscle relaxation with minimal neonatal effects when given in doses of "approximately 0.3 mg/kg." Due to the high ionization of this drug at physiologic pH and its high molecular weight, it does not significantly cross the placenta (228). While data concerning its utility as an induction agent are not yet available, it may well become acceptable as an induction agent when succinylcholine is contraindicated.

***Vecuronium.*** Vecuronium has also been evaluated for maintenance of muscle relaxation during cesarean section. The umbilical venous/maternal venous ratio for this drug is 0.11, and it has a half-life of 36 minutes in the neonate. Maternal clearance of vecuronium is increased in pregnancy; thus, there is rapid resolution of the blockade. In doses of 0.04 mg/kg, no adverse neonatal effects could be detected for vecuronium, or for pancuronium, by Apgar or neuroadaptive scores (229). Again, the data do not address the safety of vecuronium as an induction agent, but due to the short half-life and low maternal-fetal ratio, this drug may become acceptable when succinylcholine is to be avoided.

## Maintenance Agents—Narcotics

As discussed in the section on premedication, all narcotics cross the placenta. Thus, routine use of narcotics for obstetric anesthesia has been regarded as anathema. The advent of short-acting narcotics such as fentanyl and alfentanil has caused a reexamination of this philosophy. Fentanyl 1 mg/kg administered within 10 minutes of delivery has been found to produce no appreciable effect in neonates (230,231). Alfentanil 10 mg/kg administered 1 minute prior to induction of general anesthesia has been found to attenuate significantly the hypertensive response to intubation without respiratory depression in the neonate (232). In a single case involving cesarean section for a patient with severe aortic stenosis, 35 mg/kg of alfentanil was associated with apnea responsive to naloxone (Table 30–15) (233). Attenuation of the hypertensive response to intubation in pregnancy-induced hypertension by fentanyl 200 mg plus droperidol 5 mg has also been demonstrated (234).

**Table 30–15.** Alfentanil Concentrations and Percentage Binding to Plasma Proteins

| | Mother | Infant |
|---|---|---|
| Plasma alfentanil concentration at delivery (ng ml$^{-1}$) | 67 | 22.4 (cord blood) |
| Drug bound in plasma (%) | 88 | 67 |
| Free drug concentration in plasma (ng ml$^{-1}$) | 8.04 | 7.4 |
| Total alfentanil concentration in plasma 48 min after delivery (1 hr after alfentanil) (ng ml$^{-1}$) | | 12.5 |

(From Redfern N, Bower S, Bullock RE, Hull CJ: Alfentanil for caesarean section complicated by severe aortic stenosis. Br. J. Anaesth. 59:1309, 1987.)

**Table 30–16.** Important Components of Intraspinal Narcotic Orders

1. The patient has recieved the following:
   Morphine ________ mg
   Route: Epidural ________ Intrathecal ________
   Date ________
   Time ________
2. No PO, IM, IV, or SC narcotics are to be given for 20 hours, except by order of an anesthesiologist: telephone #________ beeper #________
3. Check and record respiratory rate every 30 minutes for 12 hours, then every hour until 24 hours following epidural or intrathecal narcotic administration.
4. Narcan (naloxone) ampule (1 ml, 0.4 mg) must be readily available at the nursing station for immediate administration.
5. Oxygen flow meter with nipple adapter and self-inflating bag with mask must be immediately accessible, either at nursing station or on emergency cart.
6. Call house officer or anesthesiologist (telephone #________ beeper #________) should the patient show evidence of airway obstruction, change in respiratory pattern, decreased respiratory effort, or respiratory rate below 11.
7. If respiratory depression is present, house officer or nurse may administer Narcan 0.1–0.2 mg IV, and repeat as necessary.
8. Call anesthesiologist (telephone #________ beeper #________) if patient complains of severe itching, urinary retention, excessive nausea, or vomiting or appears unexpectedly somnolent.

(From Hughes SC: Intraspinal opiates in obstetrics. *In* Shnider SM, Levinson G: Anesthesia for Obstetrics. 2nd Ed. Edited by S Shnider, G Levinson. Baltimore, 1987, p. 134. Williams & Wilkins.)

Despite the apparent lack of neonatal depression associated with administration of small doses of narcotics during induction of general anesthesia for cesarean section, this practice should be reserved for those patients in whom the benefits of diminution of cardiovascular response to intubation outweigh the risks of a depressed neonate. The availability of naloxone and a staff capable of managing the apneic newborn should be assured and the decision made in consultation with the obstetrician and pediatrician.

Following delivery, there is no contraindication to the administration of narcotics, and fentanyl in doses up to 5 mg/kg permits diminution of the inhalational anesthetic. All intraspinal narcotic orders should contain the important components listed in Table 30–16. Please see Chapter 20 for a more detailed description of local infiltration analgesia for cesarean section. However, following is a brief summary of field block for abdominal surgery that details equipment in the plan used for such a technique (235).

This is an advanced form of local anesthesia, which may be carried out by the surgeon in a few minutes. It is useful if there is no anesthetist available and an operation must be performed without delay. It is also most valuable when regional (spinal, epidural) or general anesthesia is too dangerous, too difficult, or not available. Almost any surgical procedure can be carried out in this way.

## Equipment

1. 10-ml syringe with finger-grip attachment.
2. 3-way stop cock.
3. 25 g, 1–1/2-inch needle.
4. 30-ml syringe with 18-gauge needle.
5. 250-ml pouch of 0.9% saline.
6. 30-ml vial of marcaine 0.75% with epinephrine 1:200,000.
7. IV administration set.

Using the large syringe and needle, withdraw and discard 55 ml of saline from the pouch. Then draw up the marcaine and inject it into the pouch. Shake to mix. Final content is 225 ml, containing Marcaine 1 mg per ml. Keeping the exterior of the IV tubing sterile, insert the dripper end of the IV administration set into the pouch.

Using sterile surgical precautions, insert other end of IV set into the 3-way stopcock. Turn stopcock to allow filling of the syringe from the pouch. Turn stopcock again to allow injection from syringe through needle.

## Plan

1. After the patient has been prepped for surgery, raise a skin wheal just below the umbilicus.
2. Insert needle through skin wheal and advance it laterally just under the skin, injecting about 2 ml of solution while the needle advances. It is not necessary to aspirate as long as the needle is in motion.
3. When the needle has advanced its full length, press the skin down over the tip and inject another 0.5 ml. This will produce a new wheal.
4. Use the same technique to produce lines of infiltrated skin and wheals on both sides (see diagram).
5. Infiltrate the skin of the midline in a similar manner, using 3 ml for each segment. About 40 ml of solution is required to produce this grid. By turning the stopcock, refill the syringe as necessary..
6. Through a lateral skin wheal, insert the needle perpendicularly and advance until it pierces the rectus fascia. Aspirate to be sure that the needle tip is not in a blood vessel. Inject 1 ml below the fascia. Retract the needle halfway and advance in a fanwise fashion through the fascia twice more, and inject 1 ml at each location, using a total of 3 ml at each site. Aspirate before each injection.
7. Repeat the subfascial injections at each lateral skin wheal site. This will consume about 30 ml of solution. Do not do subfascial injections through the midline wheals.
8. The subfascial injections may be done through each lateral skin wheal at the time it is made, before going on to complete the skin grid.
9. An extra 5 ml should be injected in the area of the mons pubis.
10. After testing the line of incision with an Allis clamp, the skin and fat are incised in the midline, exposing the fascia. Bleeders are coagulated.
11. Insert the needle tip just through the fascia and inject 1 or 2 ml. Repeat at every inch along the exposed areas. Use about 10 ml. Incise the fascia, exposing the peritoneum.
12. Infiltrate the peritoneum, and also inject, fanning laterally into the transversalis. Use about 15 ml. Incise the peritoneum, exposing the uterus.
13. Insert the needle through the visceral peritoneum on the uterus, and inject about 10 ml, forming a bleb of local anesthetic. Spread this with finger pressure over the lower uterine segment.
14. Spray 20 ml of the solution into the peritoneal cavity, coating the fundus of the uterus and the bowel to obtain topical anesthesia.

Only a little more than half the total amount of local anesthetic solution is required for this procedure. Because the 225 mg of marcaine (with epinephrine) represents the average maximum allowable dose (3 mg/kg) and only 125 mg has been used, there is an ample reserve that may be injected to reinforce the anesthetic wherever needed. Additional safety factors include that the drug is very dilute with a small diffusion gradient, that it is injected in increments, and that the rate of absorption is retarded by the epinephrine.

The sine qua non for success is gentle handling of the tissues.

Patients are always apprehensive before and during an operation. Modest sedation is desirable, making the procedure more tolerable and easier to accomplish, and it will not harm the fetus. Use an anticonvulsant sedative (valium, versed or a barbiturate) as an additional protection against local anesthetic toxic reaction. If the patient complains of pain, which is not relieved by additional local anesthetic, the anesthetist should administer ketamine in 10 mg doses until the patient is comfortable.

If no anesthetist is available, sedation can be given by a nurse, following the directions of the surgeon. Small appropriate doses of the drugs may be given, making sure that the patient does not lose consciousness. Examples of single doses are: valium 1 mg or versed 1 mg or pentobarbital (Nembutal) 25 mg or thiopental (Pentothal) 25 mg.

Any patient who needs an emergency operation also needs to breathe extra oxygen. If there is no anesthetist, the surgeon should see to it that oxygen is administered throughout the procedure, and that a nurse is assigned to monitor the patient continuously.

## Inhalational Agents

Inhalational agents uniformly pass from the mother to the fetus as a function of time and concentration administered. The use of inhalational agents permits adequate anesthesia at lower concentrations of nitrous oxide, permitting use of a higher $FIO_2$, providing greater safety (236).

***Halothane, Enflurane and Isoflurane.*** Halothane, enflurane, and isoflurane have all found acceptance in the United States for maintenance of cesarean section anesthesia. For example, anesthesia with 50% oxygen and nitrous oxide with an addition of only 0.5% halothane or the equivalent low concentration of enflurane or isoflurane from the time of induction through delivery is often effective in reducing some of the unacceptable side effects of the pure oxygen-nitrous oxide muscle relaxant anesthetic. Administration of these inhalational agents in doses less than one MAC is associated with a low, i.e., acceptable incidence of maternal recall, and is not associated with significant depression of uterine blood flow (237,238).

All three agents cause depression in uterine contractility in a dose-dependent fashion (239). Recently, there has been the suggestion that isoflurane may produce less uterine bleeding than halothane (240). Halothane and enflurane have been studied with regard to their potential for hepatic or renal toxicity in the preeclamptic, and have been found safe (241). Thus, the decision as to which of the three agents to use in the parturient would seem little different than the decision of which inhalational agent to use for an equivalent procedure in an equivalent nonpregnant patient. However, many prefer to use isoflurane; it has been shown that the use of 100% oxygen with isoflurane can lower the incidence of neonatal resuscitation and improves fetal oxygenation (Figure 30–14) (242).

***Nitrous Oxide.*** Nitrous oxide crosses the placenta rapidly, with a fetal-maternal ratio of 0.8 after 3 minutes. Prolonged administration of high concentrations of nitrous oxide have been associated with poor perinatal outcome, possibly due to diffusional hypoxia (243). It has been suggested that a ceiling effect exists, with no improvement in fetal oxygenation with an $FIO_2$ exceeding 0.5 (217,244,245). However, recent evidence suggests that if the decrease in concentration of nitrous oxide is compensated for by an increase in inhalational agent to assure ablation of sympathetic response, fetal oxygenation can be improved by high inspired oxygen tensions (246). Conversely, reduction of $FIO_2$ from 0.5 to 0.33 at a constant concentration of isoflurane (0.8%) has been demonstrated to produce no diminution in fetal oxygenation (Table 30–17). In assessing these studies, it should be noted that maternal hypocapnia, aortocaval compression, and maternal response to light anesthesia can adversely affect fetal oxygenation (247). Without optimization of these factors, manipulation of the $FIO_2$ is of limited value.

Despite concerns regarding inactivation of vitamin $B_{12}$ by nitrous oxide, placental methionine synthetase activity is unaffected by the administration of this drug for cesarean section (248). It is recommended that administration of nitrous oxide be limited to 50%, and that if delivery has not been effected within 15 minutes, discontinuation of nitrous oxide be considered. In the severely compromised fetus, elimination of nitrous oxide and use of increased concentrations of inhalational agent may be indicated. Normocarbia and uterine displacement should be assured.

## Agents for Control of Blood Pressure

As with epidural and subarachnoid anesthesia, the treatment of choice for hypotension is to relieve aortocaval compression, restore intravascular volume and use ephedrine when necessary.

Hypertension is most frequently a problem during intubation and is of short duration with little consequence to the normal parturient. When acute management of this response is required, either due to pregnancy-induced hypertension or coexisting cardiovascular disease, numerous options have been suggested. Short-acting narcotics have predictably attenuated the response to intubation, but may induce hypoventilation in the neonate. Nitroglycerine infusion has been successfully employed to obtund the hypertensive response without adverse neonatal effects (249); however, caution with this drug has been advised due to its ability to increase intracranial pressure (250).

Nitroprusside has been found to produce cyanide toxicity in ewes (251); however, it has been used in the management of intracranial aneurysm resection in 20-week pregnancies without adverse effects (252). If nitroprus-

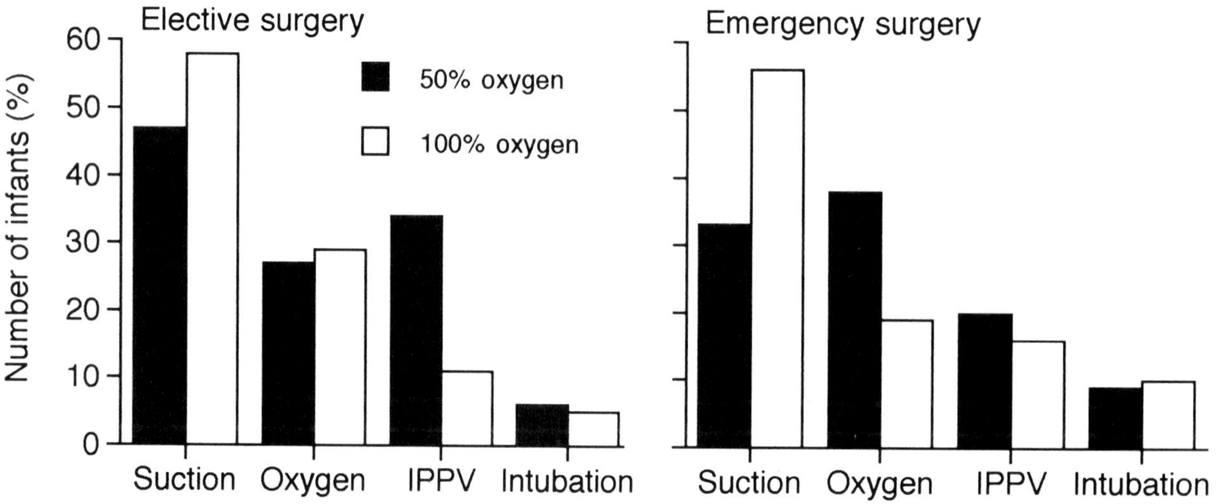


**Fig. 30–14.** Neonatal resuscitation of infants delivered by elective or emergency cesarean section performed under isoflurane anesthesia with 100% or 50% oxygen. The reduced requirement for oxygen in the emergency group is significant ($P < 0.05$). (Redrawn from Piggott SE, Bogod DG, Rosen M, Rees GAD, et al: Isoflurane with either 100% oxygen or 50% nitrous oxide in oxygen for caesarean section. Br. J. Anaesth. 65:325, 1990.)

**Table 30–17.** Comparison of Outcome Variables for 50% and 33% Oxygen Concentrations

| | Group A 50% Oxygen (n = 16) | Group B 33% Oxygen (n = 19) | Statistics | A-B | 95% CI for Diff |
|---|---|---|---|---|---|
| Umbilical vein | | | | | |
| Mean $PO_2$ (kPa) | 3.9 | 3.7 | t = 0.6, P = 0.5 | 1.5 | −3.3–6.1 |
| Mean $PCO_2$ (kPa) | 6.2 | 6.2 | t = −0.1, P = 0.9 | −0.2 | −5.3–4.8 |
| Mean pH | 7.30 | 7.31 | t = −0.9, P = 0.4 | −0.01 | −0.05–2.02 |
| Time to spontaneous ventilation(s) | | | | | |
| Median | 12.5 | 10.0 | w = 2.09, P = 0.5 | 2.5 | −5–90 |
| Range | 5–180 | 2–240 | | | |
| Apgar (minus) color: No. with scores 7 or 8 | | | | | |
| 1 min | 7 (43%) | 9 (47%) | $\chi^2$ = 0.002, P = 0.9 | −4% | −37–29% |
| 5 min | 16 (100%) | 17 (89%) | — | | — |
| Induction-Delivery interval (min) | | | | | |
| Median | 7.0 | 8.0 | w = 274, P = 0.7 | −1.0 | −3.0–1.7 |
| Range | 5–12 | 2–20 | | | |
| Uterine incision-delivery interval(s) | | | | | |
| Median | 80.0 | 87.0 | w = 270, P = 0.6 | −7 | −45–30 |
| Range | 15–240 | 30–480 | | | |

(From Lawes EG, Newman B, Campbell MJ, Irwin M, et al: Maternal inspired oxygen concentration and neonatal status for caesarean section under general anesthesia. Br. J. Anaesth. 61:250, 1988.)

side is being used for acute management of transient hypertension, cyanide toxicity is unlikely (253). However, if the patient proves resistant to the drug, or tachyphylaxis develops, the drug should be discontinued. Trimethaphan has also been advocated for this situation, but is not universally successful in ablating the response to intubation. Labetalol has been demonstrated to lower maternal blood pressure without compromising uterine blood flow when taken orally, but the applicability of this to acute management is unknown (254). Esmolol may offer some promise for such management, but has been demonstrated to produce fetal bradycardia and hypoxemia when infused in pregnant ewes (255).

## *Technical Considerations*

### Rapid Sequence Induction

Rapid sequence induction has become the induction of choice for general anesthesia for cesarean section. Because cricoid pressure is an accepted practice in such cases and preparation for the management of regurgitation is routine, the only real distinction between the rapid sequence and the deliberate sequence is the avoidance of positive-pressure mask ventilation. While positive-pressure ventilation by mask may produce gastric distension and regurgitation, application of cricoid pressure has been demonstrated to prevent gastric inflation in the absence of airway obstruction (256). In addition, mask ventilation with cricoid pressure is an accepted component of most failed intubations.

With the advent of pulse oximetry as a routinely applied component of monitoring in the operating room, it would seem prudent and acceptable therapy to use gentle (less than 35 cm $H_2O$) ventilation by mask with cricoid pressure to those parturients exhibiting desaturation during induction of general anesthesia.

### A Working Technique

There are many different approaches to the practice of general anesthesia for cesarean section. The following practice has met with success at our institution and we believe reflects a thorough consideration of current anesthetic knowledge. The reader should not interpret this as the only method, but simply one that works.

Patients are routinely administered sodium bicitrate (Bicitra) 30 cc before induction. Following preoxygenation, rapid sequence induction is performed using thiopental 1.0 mg/kg, ketamine 1.0 mg/kg, and succinylcholine 1.0 mg/kg. Intubation is accomplished with an appropriate-sized tracheal tube. Maintenance consists of oxygen 50%, nitrous oxide, and isoflurane 0.5 to 1.0%. Following return of twitch, muscle relaxation is maintained with atracurium or vecuronium. After clamping of the umbilical cord, isoflurane is decreased to 0.25% or discontinued, and fentanyl less than 5 mg/kg administered. At the completion of the procedure, neuromuscular blockade is reversed and patients are extubated following sustained head lift and responsiveness to command.

### Failed Endotracheal Intubation

Airway edema due to preeclampsia, bearing down during second-stage labor, or simply due to weight gain in pregnancy, may complicate airway management. A series of smaller endotracheal tubes should be available in the event of an inability to pass the selected size endotracheal tube. Attempting to intubate with a tube of greater size than 7.0 mm may meet with failure.

Failed endotracheal intubation is the bête noire of obstetric anesthesia, occurring in the majority of avoidable maternal deaths associated with anesthesia (257). Failed intubation has been reported to occur approximately 1:300 cesarean sections (258). Successful management of this problem requires a concerted plan of action. The reader is recommended to the section in this text (Chapter 20) or the excellent reviews by Tunstall (259) or Rosen (260).

### *Local Infiltration/Regional Block*

Local infiltration anesthesia has never been widely used and is so rare today that few obstetricians and surgeons have learned the technique. Thus, few have the technical skill or ability to properly select and prepare patients for this anesthetic method. Moreover, the patient must be carefully monitored by someone capable of administering anesthesia and there are few, if any, absolute contraindications to other anesthetics or absolute indications for local anesthesia. The procedure takes as much, or more, time as any other anesthetic technique. In addition, whereas this should be one of the safest techniques, it has two major risks: that the patient will experience severe pain or develop local anesthetic toxicity. Indeed, in an attempt to relieve pain, toxic levels are all too frequently administered.

To decrease the possibility of toxic levels, the local anesthetic is usually diluted with sterile saline for injection, and epinephrine is added (epinephrine raises the maximal safe limit). The limits (without epinephrine) that should not be exceeded are: bupivacaine 2.5 mg/kg, chloroprocaine 11 mg/kg, etidocaine 4 mg/kg, lidocaine 4 mg/kg, mepivacaine 5 mg/kg, and tetracaine 1.5 mg/kg. The limits that should not be exceeded with epinephrine (1:200,000) are: bupivacaine 3 mg/kg (261), chloroprocaine 14 mg/kg, etidocaine 5.5 mg/kg, and lidocaine 7 mg/kg (262).

The nerves supplying the area (T-6 to T-12 superiorly and the upper lumbar nerves inferiorly) may be anesthetized by field block, by rectus block, or paravertebral injections (9). The skin incision is usually anesthetized separately by intracutaneous injection using a 5-cm 25-gauge spinal needle. After injection of this, as well as subsequent layers of the abdominal wall, sufficient time should be allowed for anesthesia to develop before proceeding to the next step. Once the abdomen is opened, great care and gentleness are required to expose the uterus, to inject along the sites of incision, and to make the necessary incision and remove the baby (263).

### *Emergency Cesarean Section*

In selecting the anesthesia for emergency cesarean section, we must consider: (1) the degree of urgency; (2) the physiopathology associated with the indication for the operation; (3) the condition of the mother; (4) the condition of the fetus; (5) whether the patient has been in labor and, if so, the type of obstetric care and analgesia used; (6) the speed of the operator; and (7) the skill and experience of the persons available for administration of anesthesia. Although all of these are important, the first and last are the most critical.

## Conclusion

Cesarean section can be one of the most powerful tools in preventing maternal and perinatal morbidity and mortality. However, it is a double-edged sword and, applied without clear and unmistakable indications, can contribute to rather than subtract from morbidity and mortality of both mother and baby. Currently, it is one of women's most frequent operations, and whether current rates are too high will only be determined by time.

Because of the current trend of mothers wanting to be

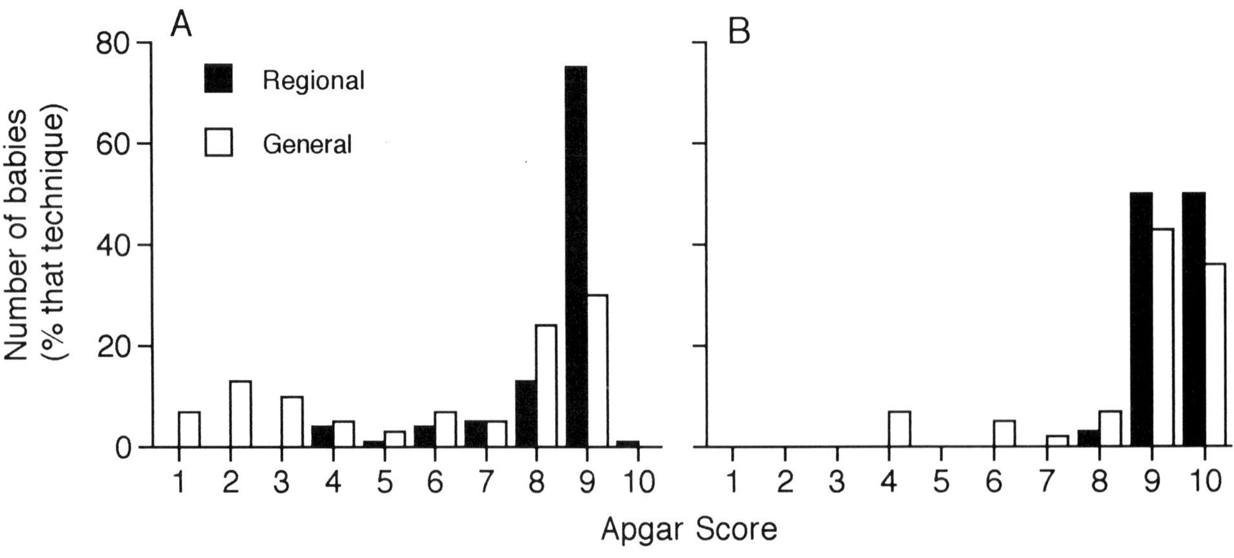


**Fig. 30–15.** Apgar scores at (A) 1 min and (B) 5 min for all deliveries: (□) general anesthetic; (■) regional anesthetic. Wilcoxon unpaired rank sum test results (mean ± SD): general anesthetic Apgar 1 min, 6.2 ± 2.7 (n = 91); regional anesthetic Apgar 1 min, 8.3 ± 1.4 (n = 123)(P < 0.001); general anesthetic 5 min, 8.7 ± 1.5 (n = 91); regional anesthetic Apgar 5 min, 9.4 ± 0.6 (n = 123)(P < 0.001). (Redrawn from Wauchob TD, Jessop JJ: A comparison of neonatal Apgar score following regional or general anaesthesia for Caesarean section. Eur. J. Anaesthesiol. 7:299, 1990.)

awake and participate in their baby's delivery at the time of cesarean section, and because recent studies confirm better newborn outcome with regional versus general anesthesia, and because of the general belief that regional is also safer for the mother, regional anesthesia is the choice for anesthetic technique (Figure 30–15) (264).

The safety of each cesarean, regardless of how many are performed, depends on teamwork between patients, nurses, obstetricians, anesthesiologists, and pediatricians or neonatologists. Each anesthetic technique has advantages, disadvantages, and limitations that must be clearly understood by all members of the team. Selection of the proper technique and precision and skill in its administration while caring for the patient's other needs materially enhances outcome.

Thus, this chapter is dedicated to furthering teamwork and enhancing maternal and perinatal outcome.

## REFERENCES


1. Depp R: Cesarean delivery and other surgical procedures. *In* Obstetrics Normal and Problem Pregnancies, 2nd Ed. Edited by SG Gabbe, JR Niebyl, JL, Simpson. New York, Churchill Livingstone, 1991, p. 635.
2. Shnider SM, Levinson G: Anesthesia for cesarean section. *In*: Anesthesia for Obstetrics. 3rd Ed. Edited by SM Shnider, G Levinson. Baltimore, Williams & Wilkins, 1993, p. 211.
3. Hales RW, Danforth DN: Operative Delivery. *In* Current Obstetric and Gynecologic Diagnosis and Treatment, 7th ed. Edited by ML Pernoll. East Norwalk, CT, Appleton & Lange, 1991, p. 536.
4. Plinius GS: Historiae Naturalis. Book 7, Chapter 9.
5. Cited by Bauhin C: Foetus vivi ex matre viva sine alterutrius vitae periculo caesura a Francisco Rousseto medico gallice conscripta. Basel, 1591.
6. Rousset F: Hysterotomotokias id est Caesarei partus assertio historiologica. Paris, 1590.
7. Snger M: Zur Rehabilitirung des classischen Kaiserschnittes. Arch F. Gynkol 19:370, 1882.
8. Kehrer FA: Ueber ein modificirtes Verfahren beim Kaiserschnitte. Arch. F. Gynkol. 19:177, 1882.
9. Finster M, Bonica JJ, Thompson IE: Cesarean Section. *In* Principles and Practice of Obstetric Analgesia and Anesthesia. Edited by JJ Bonica. F.A. Davis, Philadelphia, 1970, p. 1338.
10. Taffel SM, Placek PJ, Liss T: Trends in the United States cesarean section rate and reasons for the 1980–1985 rise. Am. J. Public Health 77:955, 1987.
11. Shiono PH, McNellis D, Rhoads GG: Reasons for the rising cesarean delivery rates: 1978–1984. Obstet. Gynecol. 69: 696, 1987.
12. Notzon FC, Placek PJ, Taffel SM: Comparisons of national cesarean section rates. N. Engl. J. Med. 316:386, 1987.
13. Shiono PH, Fielden JG, McNellis D, Rhoads GG, et al: Recent trends in cesarean birth and trial of labor rates in the United States. JAMA 257:494, 1987.
14. Phelan JP, Clark SL, Diaz F, Paul RH: Vaginal birth after cesarean. Am. J. Obstet. Gynecol. 157:1510, 1987.
15. O'Driscoll K, Foley M, MacDonald D: Active management of labor as an alternative to cesarean section for dystocia. Obstet. Gynecol. 53:485, 1984.
16. Collea JV, Chein C, Quilligan EJ: The randomized management of term frank breech presentation: a study of 208 cases. Am. J. Obstet. Gynecol. 137:235, 1980.
17. Brocks V, Philipsen T, Secher NJ: A randomized trial of external cephalic version with tocolysis in late pregnancy. Br. J. Obstet. Gynaecol. 91:653, 1984.
18. Dierker LJ, Rosen MG, Thompson K, Debanne S, et al: The midforceps: maternal and neonatal outcomes. Am. J. Obstet. Gynecol. 152:176, 1985.
19. NIH Consensus Development Task Force: Statement on cesarean childbirth. Am. J. Obstet. Gynecol. 139:903, 1981.
20. Paul RH, Phelan JP, Yeh SY: Trial of labor in the patient with a prior cesarean birth. Am. J. Obstet. Gynecol. 151: 297, 1985.
21. Danforth DN: Operative Delivery. *In* Current Obstetrics and Gynecologic Diagnosis and Treatment. 6th Ed. Edited by ML Pernoll, RC Benson. Los Altos, Appelton & Lange, 1987, p. 500.
22. Schlater S, Pernoll ML: Dystocia. *In* Current Obstetrics and Gynecologic Diagnosis and Treatment. 6th Ed. Edited by ML Pernoll, RC Benson. Los Altos, Appelton & Lange, 1987, p. 442.
23. Schlater S, Pernoll ML: Dystocia. *In* Current Obstetrics and Gynecologic Diagnosis and Treatment. 6th Ed. Edited by ML Pernoll, RC Benson. Los Altos, Appelton & Lange, 1987, p. 445.
24. Friedman EA: Labor: Clinical Evaluation and Management. 2nd Ed. New York, Appleton-Century-Crofts, 1978.
25. Akoury HA, Brodie G, Chaddick R, McLaughin VD, et al: Active management of labor and operative delivery in a nulliparous woman. Am. J. Obstet. Gynecol. 158:255, 1988.
26. O'Driscoll K, Foley M: Correlation of decrease in perinatal mortality and increase in cesarean section rates. Obstet. Gynecol. 61:1, 1983.
27. Pernoll ML, Benda GI, Babson SG: Indicators of Fetal Jeopardy. *In* Diagnosis and Management of the Fetus and Neonate at Risk. 5th Ed. C.V. Mosby Co., St. Louis, 1986, p. 45.
28. Herrera E, Pernoll ML: Complication of Labor and Delivery. *In* Current Obstetrics and Gynecologic Diagnosis and Treatment. 6th Ed. Edited by ML Pernoll, RC Benson. Los Altos, Appelton & Lange, 1987, p. 452.
29. Catanzarite VA, Rerkins RP, Pernoll ML: Assessment of Fetal Well Being. *In* Current Obstetrics and Gynecologic Diagnosis and Treatment. 6th Ed. Edited by ML Pernoll, RC Benson. Los Altos, Appelton & Lange, 1987, p. 285–301.
30. Paul RH, Suidan AK, Yeh S-Y, Schifrin BS, et al: Clinical fetal monitoring, VII: the evaluation and significance of intrapartum baseline fetal heart rate variability. Am. J. Obstet. Gynecol. 123:206, 1975.
31. Herrera E, Pernoll ML: Complication of Labor and Delivery. *In* Current Obstetrics and Gynecologic Diagnosis and Treatment. 6th Ed. Edited by ML Pernoll, RC Benson. Los Altos, Appelton & Lange, 1987, p. 452.
32. Kliegman RM, King KC: Intrauterine Growth Retardation: Determinants of Aberrant Fetal Growth. *In* Behrman's Neonatal Perinatal Medicine. 3rd Ed. C.V. Mosby, St. Louis, 1983, p. 70.
33. de Nully P, Tobiassen C: Rupture of the pregnant uterus. Ugeskr Laeger 152:170, 1990.
34. Pernoll ML: Third-trimester Hemorrhage. *In* Current Obstetrics and Gynecologic Diagnosis and Treatment. 6th Ed. Edited by ML Pernoll, RC Benson. Los Altos, Appelton & Lange, 1987, p. 413.
35. Ueland K, Gills RE, Hansen JM: Maternal cardiovascular dynamics, I: cesarean section under subarachnoid block anesthesia. Am. J. Obstet. Gynecol. 100:42, 1968.
36. Adams JQ: Hemodynamic effects of cesarean section. Am. J. Obstet. Gynecol. 82:673, 1961.
37. Ueland K, Novy MJ, Peterson EN: Maternal cardiovascular

dynamics, IV: the influence of gestational age on the maternal cardiovascular response to posture and exercise. Am. J. Obstet. Gynecol. 104:856, 1969.

38. Hendricks CH: Hemodynamics of a uterine contraction. Am. J. Obstet. Gynecol. 76:968, 1958.
39. Russell IF, Chambers IF: Closing volume in normal pregnancy. Br. J. Anaesth. 53:1043, 1981.
40. Pernoll ML, Metcalfe J, Schlenker TL, Welch JE, et al: Oxygen consumption at rest and during exercise in pregnancy. Resp. Physiol. 25:285, 1975.
41. Shankar KB, Moseley H, Vemula V, Kumar Y: Physiologic dead space during general anaesthesia for Caesarean section. Can. J. Anaesth. 34:373, 1987.
42. Shankar KB, Moseley H, Kumar Y, Vemula V: Arterial to end tidal carbon dioxide tension difference during caesarean section anaesthesia. Anaesthesia 41:698, 1986.
43. Moore PJ: Maternal Physiology During Pregnancy. *In* Current Obstetrics and Gynecologic Diagnosis and Treatment. 6th Ed. Edited by ML Pernoll, RC Benson. Los Altos, Appelton & Lange, 1987, p. 127.
44. Nielsen TF, Hokegard K-H: Cesarean section and intraoperative surgical complications. Acta. Obstet. Gynecol. Scand. 63:103, 1984.
45. Nielsen TF, Hokegard K-H: Postoperative cesarean section morbidity: a prospective study. Am. J. Obstet. Gynecol. 146:911, 1983.
46. Yonekura ML: Risk factors for postcesarean endomyometritis. Am. J. Med. 78(Suppl 6B):177, 1985.
47. Duff P: Pathophysiology and management of postcesarean endomyometritis. Obstet. Gynecol. 67:269, 1986.
48. Gibbs RS: Clinical risk factors for puerperal infection. Obstet. Gynecol. 55:178S, 1980.
49. Younker D, Rodriguez V, Kavanagh J: Massive air embolism during cesarean section. Anesthesiology 65:77, 1986.
50. Fong J, Gadalla F, Pierri MK, Koff H, et al: Incidence of venous air embolus during cesarean section. Anesthesiology 69:A655, 1988.
51. Malinow AM, Naulty JS, Hunt CO, Datta S, et al: Precordial ultrasonic monitoring during cesarean delivery. Anesthesiology 66:816, 1987.
52. Lehmann DK, Mabie WC, Miller JM, Pernoll ML: The epidemiology and pathology of maternal mortality: Charity Hospital of Louisiana in New Orleans, 1965–1984. Obstet. Gynecol. 69:833 1987.
53. Koonin LM, Atrash HK, Rochat RW, Smith JC: Maternal mortality surveillance U.S. 1980–85. MMWR CDC Surveill. Sum. 37:19, 1988.
54. Morgan M: Anaesthetic contribution to maternal mortality. Br. J. Anaesth. 59:842, 1987.
55. Montgomery TL, Brandfass RT, First HE: Oxygen saturation determinations of the newborn in vaginal delivery and cesarean section. Am. J. Obstet. Gynecol. 71:1, 1956.
56. James LS, Weisbrot IM, Prince CE, Holaday DA, et al: The acid-base status of human infants in relation to birth asphyxia and onset of respiration. J. Pediatr. 52:379, 1958.
57. Marx GF, Smith BE, Greene NM: Umbilical vein blood biochemical data and neonatal condition. J. Pediatr. 66:989, 1965.
58. Benson RC, Shubeck F, Clark WM, Berences H, et al: Fetal compromise during elective cesarean section. A report from the Collaborative Project. Am. J. Obstet. Gynecol. 91: 645, 1965.
59. Danforth DN: Operative Delivery. *In* Current Obstetrics and Gynecologic Diagnosis and Treatment. 6th Ed. Edited by ML Pernoll, RC Benson. Los Altos, Appelton & Lange, 1987, p. 506.
60. Kelton JG, Hunter DJS, Neame PB: A platelet function defect in preeclampsia. Obstet. Gynecol. 65:107, 1985.
61. Ledger WJ: Current problems in antibiotic treatment in obstetrics and gynecology. Rev. Infect. Dis. 4(S4):S679, 1985.
62. Cartwright PS, Pittaway DE, Jones III HW, Entman SS: The use of prophylactic antibiotics in obstetrics and gynecology. A review. Obstet. Gynecol. Survey 39:537, 1984.
63. Lewis M, Crawford JS: Can one risk fasting the obstetric patient for less than 4 hours? Br. J. Anaesth. 59:312, 1987.
64. Datta S, Alper MH: Anesthesia for cesarean section. Anesthesiology 53:142, 1980.
65. Kuhnert BR, Linn PL, Kennard MJ, Kuhnert PM: Effects of low doses of meperidine on neonatal behavior. Anesth. Analg. 64:335, 1985.
66. Way WL, Costley EC, Way EL: Respiratory sensitivity of the newborn infant to meperidine and morphine. Clin. Pharmacol. Ther. 6:454, 1965.
67. Hodgkinson R, Huff R, Hayashi R, Husain FJ: Double-blind comparison of maternal analgesia and neonatal neurobehaviour following intravenous butorphanol and meperidine. J. Int. Med. Res. 7:224–230, 1979.
68. Crawford JS: Premedication for elective caesarean section. Anaesthiology 34:892, 1979.
69. Rolbin SH, Wright RG, Shnider SM, Levinson G, et al: Diazepam during cesarean section P effects on neonatal Apgar scores, acid-base status, neurobehavioral assessment, and fetal plasma norepinephrine levels. ASA Abstracts, 1979.
70. Abboud T, Raya J, Sadri S, Grobler N, et al: Fetal and maternal cardiovascular effects of atropine and glycopyrrolate. Anesth. Analg. 62:426, 1983.
71. Moir DD: Anaesthesia and maternal deaths. Scott. Med. J. 24:187, 1979.
72. Hunter AR, Moir DD: Confidential enquiry into maternal deaths. Br. J. Anaesth. 55:367, 1983.
73. Moir DD: Maternal mortality and anaesthesia . Br. J. Anaesth. 52:1, 1980.
74. Eurard JR, Gold EM: Cesarean section and maternal mortality in Rhode Island: incidence and risk factors, 1965–1975. Obstet. Gynecol. 50:594, 1980.
75. Crawford JS, Davies P: Status of neonates delivered by elective caesarian section. Br. J. Anaesth. 54:1015, 1982.
76. Hollmen AI, Jouppila R, Koivisto M, Maatta L, et al: Neurologic activity of infants following anesthesia for cesarean section. Anesthesiology 48:350, 1978.
77. Datta S, Ostheimer GW, Weiss JB, Brown WU: Neonatal effect of prolonged anesthetic induction for cesarean section. Obstet. Gynecol. 58:331, 1981.
78. Loughran PG, Moore J, Dundee JW: Maternal stress response associated with caesarian delivery under general and epidural anesthesia. Br. J. Obstet. Gynaecol. 93:943, 1986.
79. Moore J, Dundee JW: A comparison of the maternal 'stress' response during caesarean delivery with general or epidural anesthesia. Anesth. Analg. 65:S104, 1986.
80. Milsom I, Forssman L, Biber B, Dottori O, et al: Maternal haemodynamic changes during caesarean section: a comparison of epidural and general anesthesia. Acta. Anaesthesiol. Scand. 29:161, 1985.
81. Gilstrap III, LC Hauth, JC Hankins, GDV Patterson AR: Effect of type of anesthesia on blood loss at cesarean section. Obstet. Gynecol. 69:328, 1987.
82. Parkin A, Pipkin FB: The effects of mode of delivery and type of anesthesia on the response of human chorionic plate arteries to prostaglandin $E_2$. Am. J. Obstet. Gynecol. 149:573, 1984.
83. Anstey JT, Sheldon GW, Blythe JG: Infectious morbidity

after primary cesarean sections in a private institution. Am. J. Obstet. Gynecol. 136:205, 1980.

84. Chestnut DH: Effect of anesthesia for repeat cesarean section on postoperative infectious morbidity. Obstet. Gynecol. 66:199, 1985.
85. Ramanathan S, Sheth R, Turndorf H: Anesthesia for cesarean section in patients with genital herpes infections: a retrospective study. Anesthesiology 64:807, 1986.
86. Ravindran RS, Gupta CD, Stoops CA: Epidural anesthesia in the presence of Herpes simplex virus (type 2) infection. Anesth. Analg. 61:714, 1982.
87. SOAP Newsletter 14(3):1–6, 1983.
88. Jouppila P, Jouppila R, Hollmen A, Koivula A: Lumbar epidural analgesia to improve intervillous blood flow during labor in severe preeclampsia. Obstet. Gynecol. 59:158, 1982.
89. Jouppila P, Jouppila R, Hollmen A: Epidural analgesia and placental blood flow during labor in pregnancies complicated by hypertension. Br. J. Obstet. Gynaecol. 86:969, 1979.
90. Jouppila P, Jouppila R, Kuikka J: Placental blood flow during caesarean section under lumbar extradural analgesia. Br. J. Anaesth. 50:275, 1978.
91. Datta S, Brown WU: Acid-base status in diabetic mothers and their infants following general or spinal anesthesia for cesarean section. Anesthesiology 47:272, 1977.
92. Datta S, Brown WU Jr, Ostheimer GW, Weiss JB, et al: Epidural anesthesia for cesarean section in diabetic parturients: maternal and neonatal acid-base status and bupivacaine concentration. Anesth. Analg. 60:574,1981.
93. Shnider SM, Levinson G: Anesthesia for Cesarean Section. *In* Anesthesia for Obstetrics. 2nd Ed. Edited by SM Schnider, G Levinson. Baltimore, William & Wilkins, 1987, p. 160.
94. Dewan DM, Floyd HM, Thistlewood JM, Bogard TD, et al: Sodium citrate pretreatment in elective cesarean section patients. Anesth. Analg. 64:34, 1985.
95. Howard FA, Sharp DS: Effect of metoclopromide on gastric emptying during labour. Br. Med. J. 1:446–8, 1973.
96. Sweeney B, Wright I: The use of antacids as a prophylaxis against Mendelson's syndrome in the United Kingdom. A survey. Anaesthesia 41:419, 1986.
97. Kenepp NB, Kumar S, Stanley CA, Gutsche GG, et al: Fetal and neonatal hazards of maternal hydration with 5% dextrose before caesarean section. Lancet 1:1150 1982.
98. Loong EPL, Lao TTH, Chin RKH: Effects of intrapartum intravenous infusion of 5% dextrose or Hartmann's solution on maternal and cord blood glucose. Acta. Obstet. Gynecol. Scand. 66:241, 1987.
99. Lu GP, Batiller GM, Marx GF: Hypoglycemia enhances bupivacaine cardiotoxicity in the rat. Anesthesiology 65(3A): A191, 1986.
100. James III FM, Crawford JS, Hopkinson R, Davies P, et al: A comparison of general anesthesia and lumbar epidural analgesia for elective cesarean section. Anesth. Analg. (Current Researches) 56(2):228,1977.
101. Downing JW, Houlton PC, Barclay A: Extradural analgesia for caesarean section: a comparison with general anaesthesia. Br. J. Anaesth. 51:367, 1979.
102. Rudick V, Galon A, Niv D, Leykin Y, et al: Anesthetic management of 646 consecutive cesarean section cases. Isr. J. Med. Sci. 21:18 1985.
103. Scott DB: Inferior vena caval occlusion in late pregnancy and its importance in anaesthesia. Br. J. Anaesth. 40:120, 1968.
104. Brizgys RV, Shnider SM, Kotelko DM, Dailey PA, et al: The incidence and neonatal effects of maternal hypotension during epidural anesthesia for cesarean section. Anesthesiology 57:A395, 1982.
105. Datta S, Alper MH, Ostheimer GW, Brown WU, et al: Effects of maternal position on epidural anesthesia for cesarean section, acid-base status, and bupivacaine concentrations at delivery. Anesthesiology 50:205, 1979.
106. Hollmen AI, Jouppila R, Koivisto M, Maatta L, et al: Neurologic activity of infants following anesthesia for cesarean section. Anesthesiology 48:350, 1978.
107. Bromage PR: Spread of analgesic solutions in the epidural space and their site of action. Br. J. Anaesth. 34:161, 1962.
108. Grundy EM, Zamora AM, Winnie AP: Comparison of spread of epidural anesthesia in pregnant and nonpregnant women. Anesth. Analg. 57:544, 1978.
109. Hehre FW, Yules RB, Hipona FA: Continuous lumbar peridural anesthesia in obstetrics, III: attempts to produce spread of contrast media by acute vena cava obstruction in dogs. Anesth. Analg. 45:551, 1966.
110. Morishima HO, Pedersen H, Finster M, Hiraoka H, et al: Bupivacaine toxicity in pregnant and nonpregnant ewes. Anesthesiology 63:134, 1985.
111. Feely J, Wilkinson GR, McAllister CB, Wood AJJ: Increased toxicity and reduced clearance of lidocaine by cimetidine. Ann. Intern. Med. 96:592, 1982.
112. Feely J, Guy E: Lack of effect of ranitidine on the disposition of lidocaine. Br. J. Clin. Pharmacol. 16:117, 1983.
113. Kim KC, Tasch MD: Effects of cimetidine and ranitidine on local anesthetic central nervous system toxicity in mice. Anesth. Analg. 65:840, 1986.
114. O'Sullivan GM, Smith M, Morgan B, Brighouse D, et al: $H_2$ antagonists and bupivacaine clearance. Anaesthesia 43:93, 1988.
115. Branch RA, Shand DG, Wilkinson GR, Nies AS: The reduction of lidocaine clearance by dl-propanolol: an example of hemodynamic drug interaction. J. Pharmacol. Exp. Ther. 184:515, 1973.
116. Bowdle TA, Freund PR, Slattery JT: Propranolol reduces bupivacaine clearance. Anesthesiology 66:36, 1987.
117. Ramanathan J, Bottorff M, Jeter JN, Khalil M, et al: The pharmacokinetics and maternal and neonatal effects of epidural lidocaine in preeclampsia. Anesth. Analg. 65:120, 1986.
118. Thompson EM, Wilson CM, Moore J, McClean E: Plasma bupivacaine levels associated with extradural anaesthesia for caesarean section. Anaesthesia 40:427, 1985.
119. Biehl D, Shnider SM, Levinson G, Callender K: Placental transfer of lidocaine: effects of fetal acidosis. Anesthesiology 48:409, 1978.
120. Abboud TK, Kim KC, Noueihed R, Kuhnert BR, et al: Epidural bupivacaine, chloroprocaine, or lidocaine for cesarean section—maternal and neonatal effects. Anesth. Analg. 62:914, 1983.
121. Abboud TK, Moore MJ, Jacobs J, Murakawa K, et al: Epidural mepivacaine for cesarean section: maternal and fetal effects. Reg. Anesth. 12:76, 1987.
122. Ravindran RS, Bond VK, Tasch MD, Gupta CD, et al: Prolonged neural blockade following regional anesthesia with 2-chloroprocaine. Anesth. Analg. 59:447, 1980.
123. Moore DC, Spierdijk J, vanKleef JD, Coleman RL, et al: Chloroprocaine neurotoxicity: four additional cases. Anesth. Analg. 61:155 1982.
124. Goins JR: Experience with mepivacaine paracervical block in an obstetric private practice. Am. J. Obstet. Gynecol. 167:342–4, 1992.
125. Reisner LS, Hochman BN, Plumer MH: Persistent neurologic deficit and adhesive arachnoiditis following intrathe-

cal 2-chloroprocaine injection. Anesth. Analg. 59:452, 1980.

126. Gissen AJ, Datta S, Lambert D: The chloroprocaine controversy, II: Is Chloroprocaine neurotoxic? Reg. Anesth. 9: 135, 1984.
127. Kalichman MW, Powell HC, Reisner LS, Myers RR: The role of 2-chloroprocaine and sodium bisulfite in rat sciatic nerve edema. J. Neuropath. Exp. Neurol. 45:566, 1986.
128. Raeder JC: Propofol anaesthesia versus paracervical blockade with alfentanil an midazolam sedation for outpatient abortion. Acta. Anaesthesiol. Scand. 36:31–7, 1992.
129. Kuhn S, Meier N, Godoy G, Aguilera R: Serum level determination of local anesthetics using high pressure liquid chromatography. Rev. Med. Chil. 118:662–6, 1991.
130. Klein CE, Gall H: Type IV allergy to amide-type local anesthetics. Contact Dermatitis 25:45–8, 1991.
131. Malmqvist LA, Tryggvason B, Bengtsson M: Sympathetic blockade during extradural analgesia with mepivacaine or bupivacaine. Acta. Anaesthesiol. Scand. 33:444–9, 1989.
132. Marx GF: Bupivacaine cardiotoxicity—concentration or dose? Anesthesiology 65:116, 1986.
133. Scanlon JW, Brown WU Jr, Weiss JB, Alper MH: Neurobehavioral responses of newborn infants after maternal epidural anesthesia. Anesthesiology 40:121, 1974.
134. Scanlon JW, Ostheimer GW, Lurie OA, Brown WU, et al: Neurobehavioral responses and drug concentrations in newborns after maternal epidural anesthesia with bupivacaine. Anesthesiol 45:400 1976.
135. Abboud, TK Khoo, SS Miller, F Doan, T, et al: Maternal, fetal, and neonatal responses after epidural anesthesia with bupivacaine, 2-chloroprocaine, or lidocaine. Anesth. Analg. 61:638, 1982.
136. Abboud TK, Sarkis F, Blikian A, Varakian L, et al: Lack of adverse neonatal neurobehavioral effects of lidocaine. Anesth. Analg. 62:473, 1983.
137. Tronick E, Wise S, Als H, Adamson L, et al: Regional obstetric anesthesia and newborn behavior: effects over the first ten days of life. Pediatrics 58:94, 1976.
138. Mather LE, Tucker GT, Murphy TM, Stanton-Hicks MD'A, et al: The effects of adding adrenaline to etidocaine and lignocaine in extradural anaesthesia, II: pharmacokinetics. Br. J. Anaesth. 48:989, 1976.
139. Reynolds FR, Taylor G: Plasma concentrations of bupivacaine during continuous epidural analgesia in labour: the effect of adrenaline. Br. J. Anaesth. 43:436, 1971.
140. Laishley RS, Morgan BM, Reynolds F: Effect of adrenaline on extradural anaesthesia and plasma bupivacaine concentrations during caesarean section. Br. J. Anaesth. 60:180, 1988.
141. Wilson CM, Moore J, Ghaly RG, Flynn R, et al: Plasma concentrations of bupivacaine during extradural anaesthesia for caesarean section. The effect of adrenaline. Anaesthesia 43:12, 1988.
142. Craft JB, Epstein BS, Coakley CS: Effect of lidocaine with epinephrine versus lidocaine (plain) on induced labor. Anesth. Analg. 51(2):243, 1972.
143. Albright GA, Jouppila R, Hollmen AI, Jouppila P, et al: Epinephrine does not alter human intervillous blood flow during epidural anesthesia. Anesthesiology 54:131, 1981.
144. Marx GF, Schuss M, Anyaegbunam A, Fleischer A: Effects of epidural block with lidocaine and lidocaine-epinephrine on umbilical blood flow velocity waveforms. Anesthesiology 65(3A):A377, 1986.
145. Veille JC, Youngstrom P, Kanaan C, Wilson B: Human umbilical artery flow velocity waveforms before and after regional anesthesia for cesarean section. Obstet. Gynecol. 72:890–3, 1988.
146. Eisele JH, Wright R, Rogge P: Newborn and maternal fentanyl levels at cesarean section. Anesth Analg 61:179, 1982.
147. Thorburn J, Moir DD: Epidural analgesia for elective caesarean section. Anaesthesia 35:3, 1980.
148. Merry AF, Cross JA, Mayadeo SV, Wild CJ: Posture and the spread of extradural analgesia in labour. Br. J. Anaesth. 55: 303, 1983.
149. Norris MC, Dewan DM: Effect of gravity on the spread of extradural anaesthesia for caesarean section. Br. J. Anaesth. 59:338, 1987.
150. Hodgkinson R, Husain FJ: Obesity, gravity, and spread of epidural anesthesia. Anesth. Analg. 60:421, 1981.
151. Stone PA, Kilpatrick AW, Thorburn J: Posture and epidural catheter insertion. Anaesthesia 45 (11):920–923, Nov. 1990.
152. Laishley RS, Morgan BM: A single dose epidural technique for caesarean section. Anaesthesia 43:100, 1988.
153. Verniquet AJW: Vessel puncture with epidural catheters. Anaesthesia 35:660, 1980.
154. Naulty JS, Ostheimer GW, Datta S, Knapp R, et al: Incidence of venous air embolism during epidural catheter placement. Anesthesiology 57:410, 1982.
155. Mehta M, Salmon N: Extradural block. Confirmation of the injection site by X-ray monitoring. Anaesthesia 40:1009, 1985.
156. Hardy PAJ: Can epidural catheters penetrate the dural mater? An anatomical study. Anaesthesia 41:1146, 1986.
157. Abouleish E, Goldstein M: Migration of an extradural catheter into the subdural space. A case report. Br. J. Anaesth. 58:1194, 1986.
158. Boys JE, Norman PG: A case report, possible clinical implications and relevance to 'massive extradurals.' Br. J. Anaesth. 47:111, 1975.
159. Bridle-Smith G, Barton FL, Watt, JH: Extensive spread of local anaesthetic solution following subdural insertion of an epidural catheter during labour. Anaesthesia 39:355, 1984.
160. Crawford JS: A reply. Anaesthesia 41:766, 1986.
161. Prince G, McGregor D: Obstetric epidural test doses. A reappraisal. Anaesthesia 41:1240, 1986.
162. Dawkins CJM: An analysis of the complications of extradural and caudal block. Anaesthesia 24:554, 1969.
163. Moore DC, Batra MS: The components of an effective test dose prior to epidural block. Anesthesiology 55:693, 1981.
164. Cartwright PD, McCarroll SM, Antzaka C: Maternal heart rate changes with a plain epidural test dose. Anesthesiology 65:226, 1986.
165. Leighton BL, Norris MC, Sosis M, Epstein R, et al: Limitations of epinephrine as a marker of intravascular injection in laboring women. Anesthesiology 66:688, 1987.
166. Hood DD, Dewan DM, Rose JC, James III FM: Maternal and fetal effects of intravenous epinephrine containing solutions in gravid ewes. Anesthesiology 59:A393, 1983.
167. Seidman SF, Marx GF: Epinephrine test dose is not warranted for confirmation of intravascular migration of epidural catheter in a parturient (letter). Can. J. Anaesth. 35: 104–5, 1988.
168. Kenepp NB, Gutsche BB: Inadvertent intravascular injections during lumbar epidural anesthesia (letter). Anesthesiology 54:172, 1981.
169. Fine PG, Wong KC: Cranial nerve block after test dose through an epidural catheter in a preeclamptic parturient. Can. Anaesth. Soc. J. 31:565, 1984.
170. Abraham RA, Harris AP, Maxwell LG, Kaplow S: The efficacy of 1.5% lidocaine with 7.5% dextrose and epinephrine as an epidural test dose for obstetrics. Anesthesiology 64:116, 1986.

171. Kalas DB, Hehre FW: Continuous lumbar peridural anesthesia in obstetrics, VIII: further observations on inadvertent lumbar puncture. Anesth. Analg. 51:192, 1972.
172. Palahnuik RJ, Cumming M: Prophylactic blood patch does not prevent postlumbar puncture headache. Can. Anaesth. Soc. J. 26:132, 1979.
173. Crawford JS: The prevention of headache consequent upon dural puncture. Br. J. Anaesth. 44:598, 1972.
174. Craft JB, Epstein BS, Coakley CS: Prophylaxis of dural-puncture headache with epidural saline. Anesth. Analg. 52:228, 1973.
175. Smith BE: Prophylaxis of epidural wet tap headache. Anesthesiology 51:S304, 1979.
176. Marx GF, Cosmi RV, Wollman SB: Biochemical status and clinical condition of mother and infant at cesarean section. Anesth. Analg. 48:986, 1969.
177. Ralston DH, Shnider SM, de Lorimer AA: Effects of equipotent ephedrine, metariminol, mephenteramine, and methoxamine on uterine blood flow in pregnant ewe. Anesthesiology 40:354, 1974.
178. Santos A, Datta S: Prophylactic use of droperidol for control of nausea and vomiting during spinal anesthesia for cesarean section. Anesth. Analg. 63:85, 1984.
179. Mandell G, Dewan D, Howard G, Floyd H: The effectiveness of low dose droperidol in controlling nausea and vomiting during epidural anesthesia for cesarean section. Anesthesiology 65(3A):A391, 1986.
180. Chestnut DH, Bates JN, Choi WW, Vandewalker GE: Administration of metaclopromide for prevention of nausea and vomiting during regional anesthesia for cesarean section: a randomized, double blind, placebo controlled study. Anesthesiology 65(3A):A390, 1986.
181. Kenny GN, Oates JD, Leeser J, Rowbotham DJ, et al: Efficacy of orally administered ondansetron in the prevention of postoperative nausea and vomiting: a dose ranging study. Br. J. Anaesth. 68:466–70, 1992.
182. Bailey PL, Streisand JB, Pace NL, Bubbers SJM, et al: Transdermal scopolamine reduces nausea and vomiting after outpatient laparoscopy. Anesthesiology 72:977–980, 1990.
183. Stromberg BV, Reines DH, Ackerly J: Transderm scopolamine for the control of perioperative nausea. Am. Surg. 57: 712–5, 1991.
184. Harris SN, Sevarino FB, Sinatra RS, Preble L, et al: Nausea prophylaxis using transdermal scopolamine in the setting of patient-controlled analgesia. Obstet. Gynecol. 78:673–7 1991.
185. Loper KA, Ready LB, Dorman BH: Prophylactic transdermal scopolamine patches reduce nausea in postoperative patients receiving epidural morphine. Anesth. Analg. 68: 144–6, 1989.
186. Spielman FJ, Corke BC: Advantages and disadvantages of regional anesthesia for cesarean section. J. Reprod. Med. 30:832, 1985.
187. Akamatsu TJ, Bonica JJ, Rehmet R, Eng M, et al: Experiences with the uses of ketamine for parturition: I. Primary anesthetic for vaginal delivery. Anesth. Analg. (Current Researches) 53:284, 1974.
188. Workhoven MN: Intravenous fluid temperature, shivering, and the parturient. Anesth. Analg. 65:496, 1986.
189. McCarroll SM, Cartwright P, Weeks SK, Donati F: Warming intravenous fluids and the incidence of shivering during caesarean section under epidural anaesthesia. Can. J. Anaesth. 33:S72, 1986.
190. Walmsley AJ, Giesecke AH, Lipton JM: Epidural temperature: a cause of shivering during epidural anesthesia. Anesth. Analg. 65:S164, 1986.
191. Webb PJ, James FM, Wheeler AS: Shivering during epidural analgesia in women in labor. Anesthesiology 55:706, 1981.
192. Casey WF, Smith CE, Katz JM, O'Laughlin K, et al: Intravenous meperidine for control of shivering during Caesarean section under epidural anaesthesia. Can. J. Anaesth. 35: 128, 1988.
193. Harris MM, Arnold WP, Lawson D, Ellis JE: Meperidine does not prevent shivering following epidural lidocaine. Reg. Anesth. 12:57, 1987.
194. Sharkey A, Lipton JM, Murphy MT, Giesecke AH: Inhibition of postanesthetic shivering with radiant heat. Anesthesiology 66:249, 1987.
195. Clark RB, Thompson DS, Thompson CH: Prevention of spinal hypotension associated with cesarean section. Anesthesiology 45:670, 1976.
196. Gutsche BB: Prophylactic ephedrine preceding spinal analgesia for cesarean section. Anesthesiology 45:462, 1876.
197. Van Gessel EF, Miege B, Forster A, Salvaj G, et al: Comparison of hyperbaric solutions of bupivacaine and tetracaine during continuous spinal anaesthesia. Can. J. Anaesth. 39: 323–9, 1992.
198. Abboud TK, Dror A, Zhu J, Mantilla M, et al: Minidose intrathecal morphine for the relief of post-cesarean section pain: safety, efficacy, and ventilatory responses to carbon dioxide. Anesth. Analg. 67:137–43, 1988.
199. Chadwick HS, Ready LB: Intrathecal and epidural morphine sulfate for postcesarean analgesia—a clinical comparison. Anesthesiology 68:925–9, 1988.
200. Chantigian RC, Datta S, Burger GA, Naulty JS, et al: Anesthesia for cesarean delivery utilizing spinal anesthesia. Tetracaine versus tetracaine and procaine. Reg. Anesth. 9:195, 1984.
201. Russell IF: Spinal anesthesia for caesarean section. The use of 0.5% bupivacaine. Br. J. Anaesth. 55:309, 1983.
202. Santos A, Pedersen H, Finster M, Edström H: Hyperbaric bupivacaine for spinal anesthesia in cesarean section. Anesth. Analg. 63:1009, 1984.
203. Michie AR, Freeman RM, Dutton DA, Howie HB: Subarachnoid anaesthesia for elective caesarean section. A comparison of two hyperbaric solutions. Anaesth 43:96, 1988.
204. Bembridge M, Macdonald R, Lyons G: Spinal anaesthesia with hyperbaric lignocaine for elective caesarean section. Anaesthesia 41:906, 1986.
205. Spivey DL: Epinephrine does not prolong spinal anesthesia in term parturients. Anesth. Analg. 64:468, 1985.
206. Russell IF: Inadvertent total spinal for caesarean section. Anaesthesia 40:199, 1985.
207. Sprague DH: Effects of position and uterine displacement on spinal anesthesia for cesarean section. Anesthesiology 44:164, 1976.
208. Rawal N: Single segment combined subarachnoid and epidural block for caesarean section. Can. Anaesth. Soc. J. 33: 254, 1986.
209. Rawal N, Schollin J, Wesström G: Epidural versus combined subarachnoid epidural block for cesarean section. Acta. Anaesthesiol. Scand. 32:61, 1988.
210. Finster M, Poppers PJ: Safety of thiopental used for induction of general anesthesia in elective cesarean section. Anesthesiology 29:190, 1968.
211. Shnider SM, Levinson G: Anesthesia for Cesarean Section. *In* Anesthesia for Obstetrics, 2nd Ed. Edited by SM Shnider, G Levinson. Baltimore, William & Wilkins, 1987, p. 175.
212. Kosaka Y, Takahashi T, Mark LC: Intravenous thiobarbiturate anesthesia for cesarean section. Anesthesiology 31:489, 1969.
213. Christensen JH, Andreasen F, Jansen JA: Pharmacokinetics

of thiopental in caesarean section. Acta. Anaesthesiol. Scand. 25:174, 1981.
214. Andersen LW, Qvist T, Hertz J, Mogensen F: Concentrations of thiopentone in mature breast milk and colostrum following an induction dose. Acta. Anaesthesiol. Scand. 31: 30, 1987.
215. Holdcroft A, Morgan M, Gordon HI: Comparison of effect of two induction doses of methohexitone on infants delivered by elective caesarean section. Br. Med. J. 2:472, 1974.
216. Peltz B, Sinclair DM: Induction agents for caesarean section. A comparison of thiopentone and ketamine. Anaesthesia 28:37, 1973.
217. Bernstein K, Gisselsson L, Jacobsson L, Ohrlander S: Influence of two different anaesthetic agents on the newborn and the correlation between foetal oxygenation and induction-delivery time in elective caesarean section. Acta. Anaesthesiol. Scand. 29:157, 1985.
218. Dich-Nielsen J, Holasek J: Ketamine as induction agent for caesarean section. Acta. Anaesthesiol. Scand. 26:139, 1982.
219. Zimmermann H: Ketamine drip anaesthesia for caesarean section. Trop. Doct. 18:60, 1988.
220. Downing JW, Buley RJR, Brock-Utne JG, Houlton PC: Etomidate for the induction of anaesthesia at caesarean section: comparison with thiopentone. Br. J. Anaesth. 51:135, 1979.
221. Bland BAR, Lawes EG, Duncan PW, Warnell I, et al: Comparison of midazolam and thiopental for rapid sequence anesthetic induction for elective cesarean section. Anesth. Analg. 66:1165, 1987.
222. Giesecke AH Jr, Morris RE, Dalton MD, Stephen CR: Of magnesium, muscle relaxants, toxemic parturients, and cats. Anesth. Analg. 47:689, 1968.
223. Evans RT, Wroe JM: Plasma cholinesterase changes during pregnancy. Anaesthesia 35:651, 1980.
224. Blitt CD, Petty WC, Alberternst EE, Wright BJ: Correlation of plasma cholinesterase activity and duration of action of succinylcholine during pregnancy. Anesth. Analg. (Current Researches) 56(2):78, 1977.
225. Churchill-Davidson HC: Suxamethonium and muscle pains. Br. Med. J. 1:74, 1954.
226. Thind GS, Bryson THL: Single dose suxamethonium and muscle pain in pregnancy. Br. J. Anaesth. 55:743, 1983.
227. Bryson THL, Ormston TOG: Muscle pains following the use of suxamethonium in caesarean section. Br. J. Anaesth. 34:476, 1962.
228. Cook WP, Schultetus RR, Caton D: A comparison of d-tubocurarine and no pretreatment in obstetric patients. Anesth. Analg. 66:756, 1987.
229. Cullen DJ: The effect of pretreatment with nondepolarizing muscle relaxants on the neuromuscular blocking action of succinylcholine. Anesthesiology 35:572, 1971.
230. Bennetts FE, Khalil KI: Reduction of post-suxamethonium pain by pretreatment with four nondepolarizing agents. Br. J. Anaesth. 53:531, 1981.
231. Duvaldestin P, Demetriou M, Henzel D, Desmonts JM: The placental transfer of pancuronium and its pharmacokinetics during caesarean section. Acta. Anaesthesiol. Scand. 22:327, 1978.
232. Flynn PJ, Frank M, Hughes R: Use of atracurium in caesarean section. Br. J. Anaesth. 56:599, 1984.
233. Dailey PA, Fisher DM, Shnider SM, Baysinger CL: Pharmacokinetics, placental transfer, and neonatal effects of vecuronium and pancuronium administered during cesarean section. Anesthesiology 60:569, 1984.
234. Eisele JH, Wright R, Rogge P: Newborn and maternal fentanyl levels at cesarean section. Anesth. Analg. 61:179, 1982.
235. Jacoby J: Field Block for Lower Abdominal Surgery. Columbus, Ohio, The Ohio State University.
236. Marx GF, Mateo CV: Effects of different oxygen concentrations during general anesthesia for elective cesarean section. Can. Anes. Soc. J. 18:587, 1971.
237. Crawford JS, Lewis M, Davies P: Maternal and neonatal responses related to the volatile agent used to maintain anaesthesia at cesarean section. Br. J. Anaesth. 57:482, 1985.
238. Palahnuik RJ, Shnider SM: Maternal and fetal cardiovascular and acid-base changes during halothane and isoflurane anesthesia in the pregnant ewe. Anesthesiology. 41:462, 1974.
239. Munson ES, Embro WJ: Enflurane, isoflurane, and halothane and isolated human uterine muscle. Anesthesiology 46:11, 1977.
240. Ghaly RG, Flynn RJ, Moore J: Isoflurane as an alternative to halothane for caesarean section. Anaesthesia. 43:5, 1988.
241. Crowhurst JA, Rosen M: General anaesthesia for caesarean section in severe preeclampsia. Br. J. Anaesth. 56:587, 1984.
242. Piggott SE, Bogod DG, Rosen M, Rees GAD, et al: Isoflurane with either 100% oxygen or 50% nitrous oxide in oxygen for caesarean section. Br. J. Anaesth. 65:325–329, 1990.
243. Marx GF, Cosmi EV, Woolman SB: Biochemical status and clinical condition of mother and infant at cesarean section. Anesth. Analg. 48:986, 1969.
244. Rorke NJ, Davey DA, Du Toit HJ: Foetal oxygenation during caesarean section. Anaesthesia. 23:585, 1968.
245. Baraka A: Correlation between maternal and foetal $PO_2$ and $PCO_2$ during caesarean section. Br. J. Anaesth. 42:434, 1970.
246. Bogod DG, Rosen M, Rees GA: Maximum $FIO_2$ during caesarean section. Br. J. Anaesth. 61:255, 1988.
247. Lawes EG, Newman B, Campbell MJ, Irwin M, et al: Maternal inspired oxygen concentration and neonatal status for caesarean section under general anaesthesia. Br. J. Anaesth. 61:250, 1988.
248. Landon MJ, Toothill VJ: Effect of nitrous oxide on placental methionine synthetase activity. Br. J. Anaesth. 58:524, 1986.
249. Hood DD, Dewan DM, James FM III, Bogard TD, et al: The use of nitroglycerin in preventing the hypertensive response to tracheal intubation in severe preeclamptics. Anesthesiology. 59:A423, 1983.
250. Writer WDR, James FM III, Stullken JR, EH, Koontz FA: Intracranial effects of nitroglycerin—an obstetrical hazard? Anesthesiology 53:S309, 1980.
251. Naulty J, Cefalo RC, Lewis PE: Fetal toxicity of nitroprusside in the pregnant ewe. Am. J. Obstet. Gynecol. 139:708, 1981.
252. Rigg D, McDonogh A: Use of sodium nitroprusside for deliberate hypotension during pregnancy. Br. J. Anaesth. 53: 985, 1981.
253. Connell H, Dalgleish JG, Downing JW: General anaesthesia in mothers with severe pre-eclampsia/eclampsia. Br. J. Anaesth. 59:13375, 1987.
254. Nylund L, Lunell N-O, Lewander R, Sarby B, et al: Labetalol for the treatment of hypertension in pregnancy. Acta Obstet. Gynecol. Scand. Suppl. 118:71, 1984.
255. Castro MI, Eisenach JC: Maternally administered esmolol produced fetal β-blockade and hypoxemia. Anesthesiology. 69:A708, 1988.
256. Lawes EG, Campbell I, Mercer D: Inflation pressure, gastric insufflation and rapid sequence induction. Br. J. Anaesth. 59:315, 1987.
257. Report on the confidential enquiries into maternal death

in England and Wales 1976–1978. Her Majesty's Stationery Office, 1983.

258. Lyons G: Failed intubation. Six years' experience in a teaching maternity unit. Anaesthesia. 40:759, 1985.
259. Tunstall ME, Sheikh A: Failed intubation protocol: oxygenation without aspiration. Clin. Anesth. 4:171, 1986.
260. Rosen M: Difficult and Failed Intubation in Obstetrics. *In* Difficulties in Tracheal Intubation. Edited by IP Latto, M. Rosen. London, Ballire Tindall, 1985.
261. Hurley R, Feldman H: Toxicity of local anaesthetics in obstetrics I: Bupivacaine—Research and clinical aspects. Clinics Anaesth. 4(1):93–9, 1986.
262. Gibbs CP: Obstetric Anaesthesia. *In* Obstetrics, Normal & Problem Pregnancies. Edited by SG Gabbe, JR Niebly, JL Simpson. New York, Churchill Livingstone, 1986, p. 424.
263. McDonald JS: Obstetric Analgesia and Anesthesia. *In* Current Obstetric and Gynecologic Diagnosis and Treatment. 6th Ed. Edited by ML Pernoll, RC Benson. Palo Alto, Appleton and Lange, 1987, p. 478.
264. Wauchob TD, Jessop JJ: A comparison of neonatal Apgar score following regional or general anaesthesia for Caesarean section. Eur. J. of Anaesthesiol. 7:299–308, 1990.

Section H

# NONOBSTETRIC MATERNAL COMPLICATIONS

# Chapter 31

# HEART AND OTHER CIRCULATORY DISEASES

JOHN H. McANULTY

This chapter addresses many of the problems associated with heart disease in pregnancy, including cardiovascular changes in normal pregnancy, symptoms and signs of heart disease, diagnostic cardiovascular drugs in pregnancy, the recognition and treatment of cardiovascular complications, and, finally, the complications of types of anesthetics in general and anesthesia for women with cardiovascular disease processes. The cardiovascular limitations and needs of the mother with heart disease will be reviewed, as will their effects on the fetus. Anesthesiologists and obstetricians should find this information useful as they manage this often fragile group of patients.

Heart disease in women of child-bearing age is becoming more common. This is not a measure of failure. Rather, young woman who once died before reaching the age of pregnancy now survive and are capable of conception. This population is unique—the treatment of one person so directly affects the health of two. Anesthesiologists are increasingly working with these patients in three situations and the concerns about anesthesia are somewhat different for each. These situations are nonobstetric surgery, labor and delivery, and cardiac surgery.

## BASIC PRINCIPLES

### Nonobstetric Surgery

During the course of a pregnancy, these patients with heart disease are similar to other women in that they will have anywhere between a 0.5 and 2% chance of requiring nonobstetrical surgery (1,2). With this, not only are maternal safety and fetal survival important considerations, but potential teratogenic effects of anesthetic drugs in the first trimester must also be considered.

### *Labor and Delivery*

While the teratogenicity of the anesthetic agents is no longer a major issue, maternal safety and the need for adequate fetal perfusion and newborn safety are essential.

### *Cardiac Surgery*

During their pregnancy, some women will have severe enough hemodynamic problems to require cardiac surgery. Additional attention is required to maintain adequate hemodynamics in protecting both the fetus and mother.

## IMPORTANT PRINCIPLES

### The Balance of Health Priorities

While the fetus and its development should be considered with all interventions, maternal safety should always take precedence. The mother's health is the highest priority.

### *Patient Fragility and the Need for Expert Care*

Pregnant women with heart disease have, or are at potential risk of, hemodynamic embarrassment. Because of this, whenever anesthesia is delivered, it should be done, if at all possible, by the anesthesiologist with the greatest experience in working with women and heart disease. A team comprised of the anesthesiologist, obstetrician, pediatrician, and cardiologist should be informed and available.

### *Identification of Women with Heart Disease at Particularly High Risk*

All pregnant women with heart disease are at high risk at the time of surgery. There is a subgroup in whom this is particularly true (3) (Table 31–1). In this subgroup, if there is a chance to avoid or interrupt pregnancy at any time, but particularly before surgery, that should be considered. When women with these problems require surgery, the administration of anesthesia is likely to be particularly dangerous.

### Cardiovascular Changes in A Normal Pregnancy

The remarkable changes that occur in the cardiovascular system during pregnancy are not fully understood. These changes result in adequate provision of oxygen and nutrients for normal fetal development and allow other maternal organs to adapt to the pregnancy. The mother's commitment to the fetus is exceptional. However, as much as she gives to the baby, when blood flow to essential maternal organs is threatened, blood is diverted from the uterus and the fetus. This may be the result of a relative increase in sensitivity of uterine arteries to elevated catecholamines (4,5). In a person with a normal cardiovascular system, blood flow to the fetus at times of stress remains adequate. In the woman with heart disease, when uterine flow may already be marginal, the chance of inadequate uterine and fetal perfusion increases. Surgery and

**Table 31–1.** Cardiovascular Abnormalities Placing a Mother and Infant at Extremely High Risk

| |
|---|
| **Advise Avoidance or Interruption of Pregnancy:** |
| Pulmonary hypertension |
| Dilated cardiomyopathy with congestive failure |
| Marfan Syndrome with dilated aortic root |
| Cyanotic congenital heart disease |
| Symptomatic obstructive lesions |
| **Pregnancy Counseling and Close Clinical Followup Required:** |
| Prosthetic valve |
| Coarctation of the aorta |
| Marfan Syndrome |
| Dilated cardiomyopathy in asymptomatic women |
| Obstructive lesions |

anesthesia are stresses likely to interfere with uterine blood flow.

## Cardiac Output

By the twentieth week of pregnancy, resting cardiac output increases to a level almost 50% above the nonpregnant level (6–12). From that point on, cardiac output is increasingly effected by maternal position and then by labor and delivery (Figures 31–1 and 31–2). Despite the increasing size of the uterus, the fetus, and the breasts, cardiac output gradually falls during the last half of pregnancy, to a level approximately 25% above baseline with the woman in a supine position. This fall in output is due, in part, to interference of venous return from compression of the enlarging uterus compressing the inferior vena cava. When cardiac output is measured with a woman on her left side, there is little or no fall in cardiac output during the last trimester (6,10,11).

A product of stroke volume and heart rate, cardiac output is influenced by both (Figure 31–1). The resting heart rate increases by approximately 20 beats per minute in a steady fashion throughout the pregnancy (6,10). Even at term, however, it rarely exceeds 100 beats per minute at rest in a woman with a normal heart. Stroke volume also gradually increases but is very dependent on venous return to the heart. With the patient at rest and on her left side, stroke volume increases steadily throughout the course of pregnancy to a level that is 20 to 25% above the nonpregnant value. Cardiac output is also directly related to oxygen consumption and inversely related to the arteriovenous oxygen concentration difference. Resting oxygen consumption increases during pregnancy and at term is approximately 30% above that in the nonpregnant woman (10,13). Because cardiac output increases more rapidly and peaks at the middle of pregnancy, maternal tissues extract less oxygen and the AV $O_2$ difference is decreased early in pregnancy. With the fall in cardiac output late in pregnancy in the supine position, maternal tissues must extract a higher percentage of oxygen and measured arteriovenous oxygen differences are increased at term.

With the beginning of labor, the cardiac output increases to a level that on average is 13% above the prelabor level by the time the cervix is dilated to 8 cm (14). Uterine contractions increase the cardiac output by another 34% due to heart rate changes and the extrusion of approximately 500 cc of blood into the circulation. Thus, a total of a 40 to 50% increase in cardiac output with each contraction results. Anesthesia affects these increases. With epidural anesthesia, the total increase in cardiac output with each contraction is reduced to 30 to 40% above the prelabor condition, and with general anesthesia, the increase in cardiac output with contraction totals only 25% above the prelabor values (14) (Figure 31–2).

In the few hours following a vaginal delivery, cardiac output can increase by as much as 80% of the prelabor level. This increase is approximately 50% following cesarean section (Figure 31–2). These values are similar whether epidural or general anesthesia is used (15). Cardiac output changes return to normal within a few weeks following delivery (13).

## Blood Pressure and Distribution of Blood Flow

The mean arterial pressure falls by about 10 mm Hg by the middle of pregnancy with diastolic pressure reduced more than systolic pressure. Thus, the pulse pressure increases. The pressures rise to nonpregnant levels by term. Because cardiac output rises to its maximum level by the twentieth week, and because blood pressure is a product of cardiac output and systemic vascular resistance, the resistance itself falls to two-thirds of its nonpregnant level by the twentieth week, rising toward normal during the last half of pregnancy. Regional vascular resistance changes result in a redistribution of the cardiac output during pregnancy (Figure 31–3). By the last trimester of pregnancy, the majority of the increase in cardiac output seen during pregnancy is distributed to the kidneys, the skin, the uterus, and to the breasts.

Like cardiac output, the blood pressure may also be affected by natural position. It may fall dramatically when a woman is in the supine position, particularly late in pregnancy, the result of a fall in return of venous return to the heart caused by compression of the inferior vena cava. This "supine hypotension in pregnancy" syndrome can be alleviated by left lateral recumbent positioning (Figure 31–4).

Attention to pulmonary vascular resistance is important when considering cardiovascular abnormalities. In woman without pulmonary vascular disease, the fall in pulmonary vascular resistance parallels that of systemic vascular resistance—an important concept in woman with intracardiac left to right shunts, which in general are not significantly altered by pregnancy.

## Uterine Blood Flow

While a discussion of blood flow to any region of the body could be expanded, uterine blood flow warrants particular discussion given the subject of this text. Uterine blood flow is approximately 100 cc per minute at rest (2% of the cardiac output) and increases to approximately 1200 cc per minute at term, approximately 17% of the cardiac output (Figure 31–2) (16–18). As noted earlier, if overall cardiac output falls, vascular resistance is altered to maintain cerebral and coronary blood flow with a compromise of uterine blood flow. Directly related

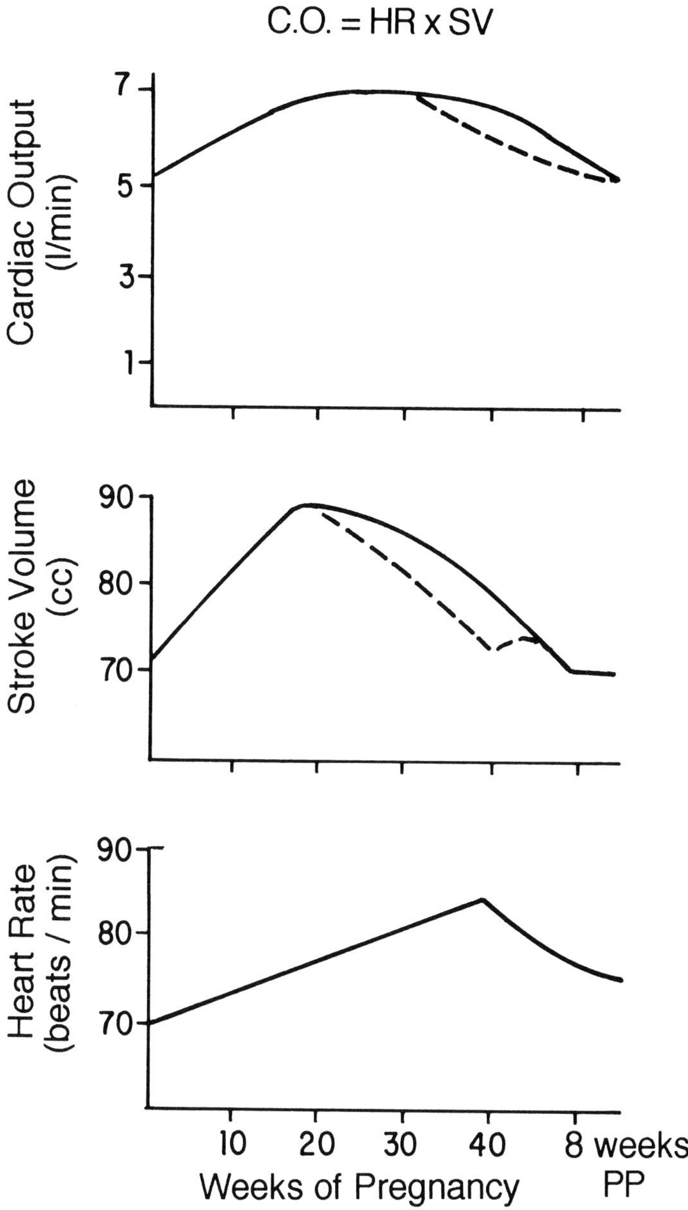


**Fig. 31–1.** These graphs depict the hemodynamic changes expected during a normal pregnancy (the specific changes in cardiac output seen with labor and delivery are depicted in Figure 31–2). The solid lines indicate resting values measured in the left lateral position and the dotted lines indicate resting values measured in the supine position. The information is the author's impression of what to expect based on information obtained by many investigators. (Redrawn from Ueland K, Novy MJ, Peterson EN, Metcalfe J: Maternal cardiovascular dynamics: IV. The influence of gestational age on the maternal cardiovascular response to posture and exercise. Am. J. Obstet. Gynecol. 104:856, 1969; Atkins AFJ, Watt JM, Milan P, Davies P, et al: A longitudinal study of cardiovascular dynamic changes throughout pregnancy. Eur. J. Obstet. Gynaecol. Reprod. Biol. 12: 215, 1981; Capeless EL, Clapp JF: Cardiovascular changes in early phase of pregnancy. Am. J. Obstet. Gynecol. 161:1449, 1989; Easterling TR, Benedetti TJ, Schumucker BC, Millard SP: Maternal hemodynamics in normal and pre-eclamptic pregnancies: A longitudinal study. Obstet. Gynecol. 76:1061, 1990; Robson SC, Hunter S, Boys RJ, Dunlop W: Serial study factors influencing changes in cardiac output during human pregnancy. Am. J. Physiol. 256:H1060, 1989; Clark SL, Cotton DB, Pivarnik JM, Lee W, et al: Position change and central hemodynamic profile during normal third-trimester pregnancy and post partum. Am. J. Obstet Gynecol. 164:883, 1991; Vered Z, Poler SM, Gibson P, Wlody D, et al: Noninvasive detection of the morphologic hemodynamic changes during normal pregnancy. Clin. Cardiol. 14:327, 1991; Sady MA, Haydon BB, Sady SP, Carpenter MW, et al: Cardiovascular response to maximal cycle exercise during pregnancy and at two and seven months post partum. Am. J. Obstet. Gynecol. 162: 1181, 1990.)

to perfusion pressure and uterine vascular resistance, uterine blood supply is affected by alterations in either one. For the most part, the uterine blood vessels are maximally dilated, and there is little additional favorable autoregulation that would improve uterine blood flow. An improvement in uterine blood flow for the most part has to be the result of increased maternal mean arterial perfusion pressure and flow. There are, however, ways in which uterine blood flow can be diminished (Table 31–2). A fall in maternal perfusion pressure or flow appears to be the most important. However, flow can also fall because of an increase in uterine vascular resistance. This can be due to a number of factors, including catecholamine excess (or an increased sensitivity to catecholamines), uterine contractions, maternal mechanical pulmonary ventilation, and drugs (see below). In the past, anesthesia has had a clear potential for adversely affecting fetal perfusion due to the hypotension secondary to the sympathetic effect associated with regional anesthesia. As mentioned in previous chapters, this complication, i.e., hypotension, has now been virtually eliminated by the use of continuous low dosage delivery of medication. Still, anesthesia has a clear potential for adversely affecting fetal perfusion.

## *Heart Changes During Pregnancy*

While many of the hemodynamic measurements are the results of alteration of the vascular beds, the heart itself also changes. The ejection fraction does not. Because the stroke volume increases by approximately 25%, the heart must enlarge to achieve the ejection fraction (ejection fraction being the stroke volume divided by the end dia-

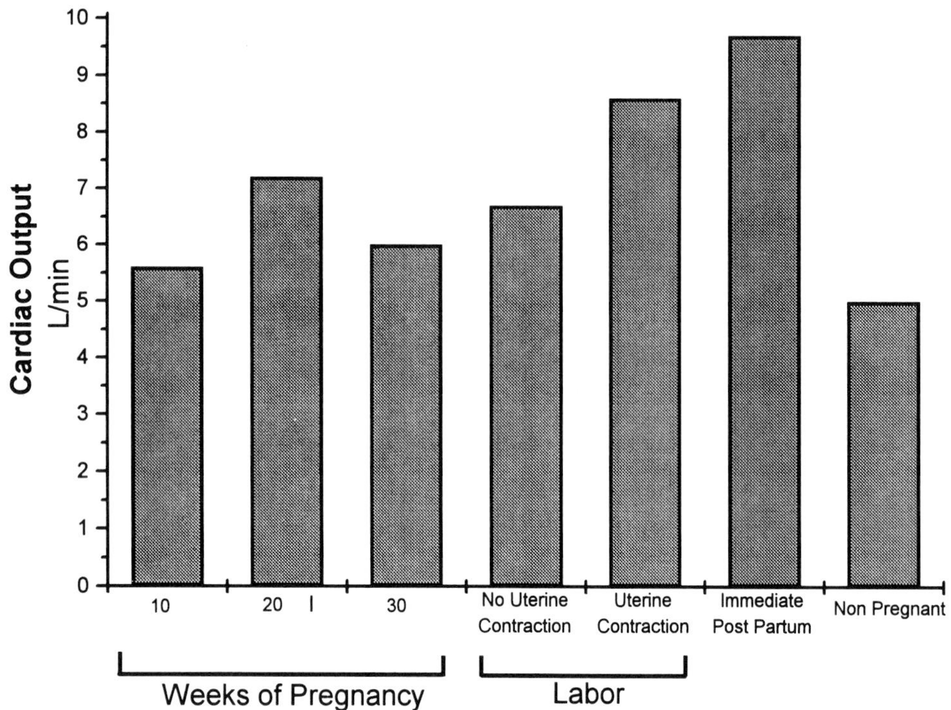


**Fig. 31–2.** This graft depicts the resting cardiac outputs measured in the left lateral position that are expected throughout pregnancy, with and without uterine contractions during labor, and after delivery. The information is the author's impression of what to expect based on information obtained by many investigators (From Ueland K, Novy MJ, Peterson EN, Metcalfe J: Maternal cardiovascular dynamics: IV. The influence of gestational age on the maternal cardiovascular response to posture and exercise. Am. J. Obstet. Gynecol. 104:856, 1969; Atkins AFJ, Watt JM, Milan P, Davies P, et al: A longitudinal study of cardiovascular dynamic changes throughout pregnancy. Eur. J. Obstet. Gynaecol. Reprod. Biol. 12:215, 1981; Capeless EL, Clapp JF: Cardiovascular changes in early phase of pregnancy. Am. J. Obstet. Gynecol. 161:1449, 1989; Easterling TR, Benedetti TJ, Schumucker BC, Millard SP: Maternal hemodynamics in normal and preeclamptic pregnancies: A longitudinal study. Obstet. Gynecol. 76:1061, 1990; Robson SC, Hunter S, Boys RJ, Dunlop W: Serial study of factors influencing changes in cardiac output during human pregnancy. Am. J. Physiol. 256:H1060, 1989; Clark SL, Cotton DB, Pivarnik JM, Lee W, et al: Position change and central hemodynamic profile during normal third-trimester pregnancy and post partum. Am. J. Obstet. Gynecol. 164:883, 1991; Vered Z, Poler SM, Gibson P, Wlody D, et al: Noninvasive detection of the morphologic hemodynamic changes during normal pregnancy. Clin. Cardiol. 14:327, 1991; Sady MA, Haydon BB, Sady SP, Carpenter MW, et al: Cardiovascular response to maximal cycle exercise during pregnancy and at two and seven months post partum. Am. J. Obstet. Gynecol. 162:1181, 1990).

stolic volume). Echocardiographic studies in humans show only mild increase in left ventricular end diastolic and systolic volumes. So, in addition to some enlargement, the heart must also become reconfigured (or remodeled). This occurs with only a 10 to 15% increase in myocardial mass during the pregnancy (19–21).

### Blood Volume Changes and Vascular Changes

Intravascular blood volume gradually increases by an average of 40% during pregnancy (22,23) (Figure 31–5). This increase is due mainly to a 50% increase in plasma volume. While red blood cell volume also increases, it does so by only 20%. One result of this is a fall in the normal maternal hematocrit to values of 32 to 36%. The other consequence of this increase in plasma volume could be a significant increase in intravascular pressures. However, this does not occur. Measured right atrial, pulmonary capillary wedge pressures, and intraventricular pressure measurements are normal. These measured pressures are the result of the changes in the vascular system with generalized increase in vascular capacitance, particularly in the venous bed (24). Increases in arterial compliance have been demonstrated as well (25). The advantage of this system is the maintenance of the hemodynamics as described. A disadvantage is that these changes increase vascular fragility; vascular accidents, when they occur in women, commonly do so during pregnancy.

### Mechanisms of the Cardiovascular Changes

While not completely understood, extensive animal studies and observations in humans suggest many of the changes are due to complex interactions of the reproductive hormones, particularly estrogen, as well as prostaglandins, the renin angiotensin-aldosterone system, and atrial natriuretic factor (26–28).

## Symptoms and Signs of Heart Disease in Pregnancy

It is often difficult to recognize heart disease in pregnancy. Many symptoms of a normal pregnancy—fatigue,

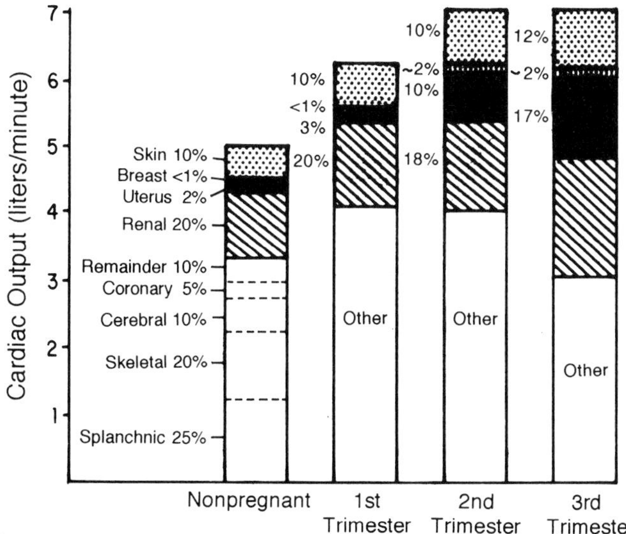


Fig. 31–3. Cardiac output and its distribution at rest. Resting cardiac output increases early in pregnancy from 5 liters in the nonpregnant state to 6 liters in the first trimester and 7 liters in the second and third trimesters. The data used for this diagram are incomplete, especially early in pregnancy. Values for each organ system are given as a percentage of total cardiac output. Changes in blood flow to "other" areas during pregnnacy have not been well defined. The graphs demonstrate that (1) resting cardiac output increases by 40% during pregnancy; (2) uterine blood flow increases progressively during pregnancy, reaching a value at term approximately tenfold greater than that of the nonpregnant uterus; (3) although the increase in uterine blood flow is dramatic, increased blood flow to other tissues accounts for most of the increase in cardiac output during pregnancy; and (4) renal blood flow increases early during pregnancy and the increase is maintained until delivery, when measurements are made with subjects in left lateral recumbency. The value given for uterine blood flow at term is substantially greater than that previously reported (110) and is based on radionuclide imaging (74b). (Redrawn from McAnulty JH, Ueland K. Heart disease and pregnancy. *In* The Heart. 6th ed. Edited by JW Hurst New York, McGraw-Hill, 1985, p. 1383.)

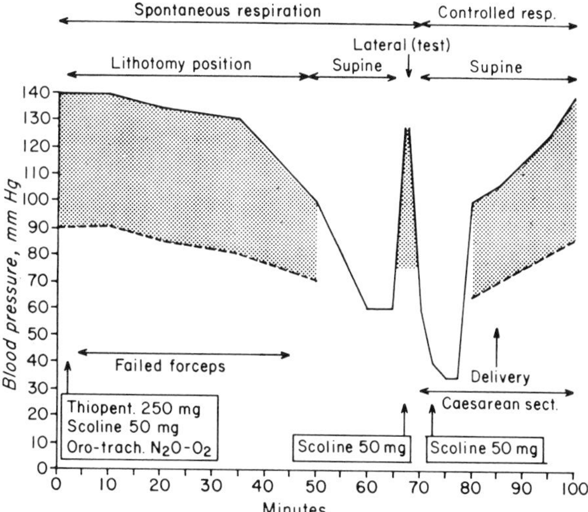


Fig. 31–4. An example of the supine hypotensive syndrome brought on by a patient placed in the supine position shows the dramatic fall in blood pressure that is reversed by left lateral displacement of the uterus.

dyspnea, orthopnea, pedal edema, and chest discomfort—are, of course, also those that suggest heart disease. Dyspnea severely limiting day-to-day activity, chest discomfort or syncopal spells occurring with exertion, and hemoptysis all exceed those symptoms accompanying a normal pregnancy and are worthy of evaluation. The cardiac examination is also difficult during pregnancy. A systolic murmur, an $S_3$ gallop, a dynamic precordium with a suggestion of cardiomegaly, and pedal edema can all be found in a normal pregnancy. A grade 3/6 systolic murmur or any diastolic murmur, a definitive CVP elevation (i.e., a mean pressure greater than 10 cm $H_2O$), rales, and/or organomegaly are all reasons to be concerned about heart disease.

## Diagnostic Cardiovascular Studies During Pregnancy

It is preferable to assess a woman's cardiac status using the history and physical examination alone. Occasionally, it will be necessary to resort to diagnostic testing. There are a number of reasons to avoid such studies during pregnancy. Some studies increase the risk to the fetus and subsequent live-born children, and they always carry the usual risk to the patient herself. Most are expensive. Many increase maternal apprehension. Misinterpretation is not unusual in that pregnancy can alter the findings of most cardiovascular studies. Any of the tests should be ordered and interpreted by an individual familiar with the changes that would be expected during a normal pregnancy.

### *Radiographic Procedures*

If essential for safety during surgery and anesthesia, these studies should be ordered to protect the mother. Because of the concern that they will alter the development of the fetus and because they may increase the chance of a subsequent malignancy in the child, there are a number of recommendations to consider when ordering a radiographic procedure (29). Every woman of childbearing age should be questioned about the possibility of pregnancy before any x-ray procedures are performed. If possible, the procedure should be delayed as long as possible during pregnancy or delayed, preferably, until termination of the pregnancy. The lowest amount of radiation as well as the optimal shielding of the fetus should always be used. Because the exposure to a child from a standard

**Table 31–2.** Causes of a Fall in Uterine Blood Flow

1. Maternal hypotension and low cardiac output syndrome
2. Uterine vasoconstriction:
   A. Due to increased endogenous catecholamines
   B. Due to exogenous vasoconstriction agents
   C. As part of hypertension syndrome: eclampsia or preeclampsia
   D. Uterine contractions and increased uterine tone

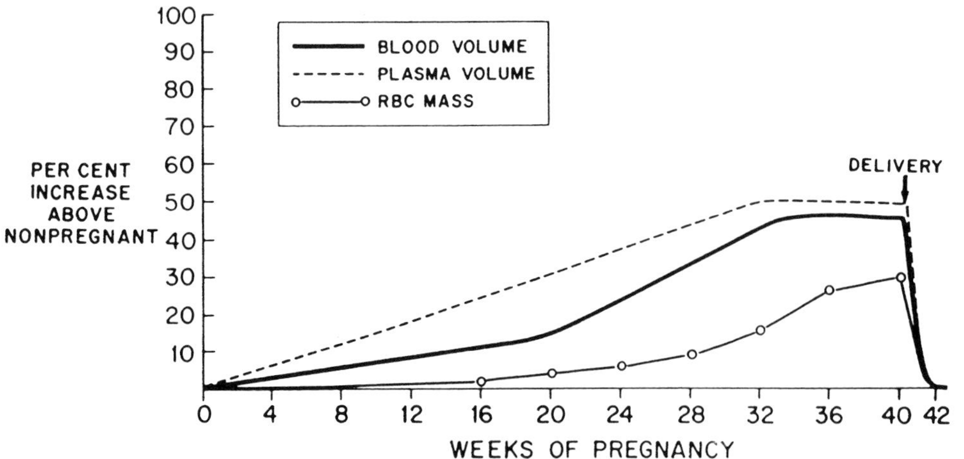


**Fig. 31–5.** Percentage increases (above nonpregnant values) in blood volume, plasma volume, and red blood cell mass during pregnancy. (With permission from Scott DE: Anemia in pregnancy. *In* Obstetrics and Gynecology Annual. Edited by RM Wynn. New York, Appleton-Century-Crofts, 1972, p. 219.)

x ray is so small (approximately 0.14 rads) and because this has not been associated with any recognizable increase of congenital deformations or malignancies, the risks are not prohibitive. If a chest x ray is ordered, interpretation should take into consideration the changes expected in a normal pregnancy—increased systolic and diastolic volumes and some increase in pulmonary vascular markings.

### *Radionuclide Studies*

Radionuclides cross the placenta and can be teratogenic. If possible, thallium cinematography as well as procedures using selenium, methionine, and strontium should be avoided. Even radionuclides that are thought to be bound to maternal albumen, can unbind and cross the placenta. Thus, radionuclide imaging should be limited to the situations in which such imaging is absolutely essential (29).

### *Electrocardiography*

The electrocardiogram and rhythm monitoring is safe for the mother and the fetus. The occasional difficulty of recognizing normal variations in young women can be made more difficult by the pregnancy. Mild inferior ST-T wave changes may have no clinical significance, but anterior changes should not exceed those expected in any normal young person. A horizontal QRS axis can result from the elevation of the diaphragm, but true left axis deviation should not be accepted—it is a clue for heart disease. Atrial and ventricular ectopy are as common during pregnancy as at other times and may be detected on the electrocardiogram.

### *Magnetic Resonance Imaging*

There is no information about the safety of this procedure during pregnancy in woman with heart disease. Evaluation of noncardiovascular disease has suggested reasonable safety (remembering that this procedure should not be performed, unless essential for maternal survival, in women with implanted pacemakers or defibrillators).

### *Echocardiography*

This procedure along with the Doppler evaluation of flow has proven optimal for cardiac evaluation of the pregnant woman. It permits evaluation of ventricular function, severity of valve disease, and the presence and degree of intracardiac shunts. This and its proven safety make echocardiography particularly helpful and particularly seductive. There are some disadvantages. It is expensive, approximately $500 in many centers. Additionally, misinterpretation is not uncommon. Changes associated with a normal pregnancy might otherwise be considered abnormalities (19,20). When performed, the procedure should be interpreted by an individual familiar with the expected changes of a normal pregnancy. There is little information available about the role or safety of transesophageal echo with pregnancy but when indicated, it would seem that the major risk would be from the anesthetic agent, and this is minor.

## Cardiovascular Drugs in Pregnancy

Cardiovascular drugs may be required to treat or prevent cardiovascular complications during the administration of anesthesia during pregnancy. Complete information about these drugs and their affect on pregnancy is unavailable, so it remains difficult to provide definitive recommendations about their use. Almost all of these drugs cross the placenta, with many causing physiologic changes in the fetus and, on occasion, some posing danger to the fetus. In Table 31–3 those cardiovascular drugs that are likely to be used during anesthesia are described with recommended dosage and administration. Some select comments about each drug group follow:

### *Inotropic Agents*

The digitalis preparation cross the placenta (in fact they have been used to treat fetal supraventricular tachyarrhythmias). Fetal intoxication can occur when maternal levels are in the toxic range. The digitalis preparations have not been shown, however, to cause congenital abnormalities, and pregnancy should not change the use of

**Table 31–3.** Cardiovascular Drugs and Their Effect on Uterine Blood Flow

| | Dose | Uterine Blood Flow | Comments |
|---|---|---|---|
| **Inotropic Agent** | | | |
| digoxin | Loading dose of 1.0 mg IV over 5 minutes | No change | Placental transfer; higher than usual maternal maintenance dose required |
| dopamine | Initiate with 1.0 μg/kg/min and titrate to effect (up to 10 μg/kg/min) | Direct effect ↓ UBF. Improved maternal hemodynamics may ↑ UBF | No adequate assessment of effects on fetus |
| dobutamine | Initiate with 1.0 μg/kg/min and titrate to effect (up to 15 μg/kg/min) | Direct effect ↓ UBF. Improved maternal hemodynamics may ↑ UBF | No adequate assessment of effects on fetus |
| epinephrine | Endotracheal—0.5 to 1.0 mg every 5 minutes IV—initiate with 0.5 mg bolus and follow with infusion of 2–10 μg/kg/min | Direct effect ↓ UBF. Improved maternal hemodynamics may ↑ UBF | No adequate assessment of effects on fetus |
| isoproterenol | Initiate at 1 μg/min and titrate up to 5 μg/min | | |
| amrinone | Initiate with .075 μg/kg over 2 minutes and follow with infusion of 2.5–10.0 μg/kg/min | Not evaluated | No adequate assessment of effects on fetus |
| **Vasodilator Agent** | | | |
| nitroprusside | Start at 0.5 μg/kg/min and titrate to effect (up to 10 μg/kg/min) | ↑ unless significant reduction maternal BP | Optimal drug because of ease in titration for optimal effects. Concern in animals about cyanide toxicity but not a concern in humans if infusion rate ≤ μg/kg/min |
| hydralazine | 5–10 mg IV dose given at 15–30 min intervals total dose | ↑ unless significant reduction maternal BP | Large experience without adverse fetal effects |
| nitroglycerin | 0.4–0.8 mg sublingual *or* 1–2 inches of dermal paste *or* IV infusion of 0.5 μg/min up to 40 μg/min | ↑ unless significant reduction maternal BP | With volume depletion, hypotension and a fall in uterine blood flow more likely |
| enalaprilat* | 1.25 to 5.0 mg IV given over 5 minutes with every 6 hour dosage | ↑ unless significant reduction maternal BP | Concerns about effects on development of fetal GU system |
| magnesium sulfate | 2.0 gm IV over 1 min. Repeat × 1 at 5 min | Not studied | Modest antihypertensive effect |
| **β Blockers** | **(Intravenous preparations)** | | |
| propranolol | 0.1 mg/kg IV over 5 min | May ↓ by ↑ uterine tone and/or lowering maternal BP | Premature labor and smaller than average birth weights. If taken at the time of delivery the newborn may have bradycardia and hypovolemia. Rapid metabolism of esmolol (11 min half life by the mother also occurs in the fetus) |
| labetalol | 20 mg IV followed by 20–80 mg IV every 10 min to total dose of 300 mg from IV infusion 1–2 mg/min | | |
| atenolol | 25 mg IV over 5 min | | |
| metoprolol | 15 mg IV over 1 min, repeat dose in 10 min | | |
| esmolol | 500 μg/kg IV dose with infusion rate of 50–300 μg/kg/min | | |
| **Calcium Channel Blockers** | | | |
| verapamil | 5–10 mg IV bolus, repeat PRN in 5 min then every 30 min PRN | Mild decrease | No evidence for teratogenicity or adverse fetal effects |
| nifedipine | 10 mg sublingual, repeat every 10 min PRN × 3 | Mild decrease | |
| diltiazem | 20 mg IV bolus | Little available data | |
| **Vasoconstrictor Agents** | | | |
| ephedrine sulfate | 5–15 mg IV bolus, repeat every 15 min p.r.n × 3 | No effect on UBF | Because it does not decrease UBF, from this group, ephedrine is the agent of choice. If improved ventricular function along with vasoconstriction is desired, then dopamine is preferable (see inotropic agents). Norepinephrine and phenylephrine should be used only when all other approaches to maintain BP have failed |
| metaraminol | Initiate with 0.1 mg/min and titrate to effect up to 2.0 mg/min | Mild decrease in UBF | |
| norepinephrine | Initiate with 2 μg/min and titrate up to effect (up to 4 μg/min) | Marked decrease in UBF | |
| phenylephrine | Initiate with 0.4 mg/min and titrate to effect (up to 0.8 mg/min) | Marked decrease in UBF | |

*(continued)*

**Table 31–3.** Cardiovascular Drugs and Their Effect on Uterine Blood Flow—*(continued)*

| | Dose | Uterine Blood Flow | Comments |
|---|---|---|---|
| **Antiarrhythmic Agents** | | | |
| lidocaine | Initial bolus of 1.0 mg/kg repeat ½ bolus at 10 min and drip at 0.05 mg/kg/min | None of these agents has a significant effect on uterine blood flow. | Each agent crosses the placenta. Greatest experience with lidocaine, procainamide and quinidine with no clear adverse fetal effects |
| procainamide | 15 mg/kg over 30 min and then drip at 0.08 mg/kg/min | | |
| quinidine | 15 mg/kg over 60 min and drip at 0.02 mg kg/kg/min | | |
| bretylium | IV bolus of 5 mg/kg then drip at 1–2 mg/min | | |
| phenytoin | 300 mg IV in central line then 100 mg every 5 min to total of 1000 mg | | |
| amiodarone | 5 mg/kg IV over 3 min then 10 mg/kg/day | | |
| **AV Node Blocking Agent** | | | |
| adenosine | 12 mg IV bolus | Transient decrease in UBF | |
| verapamil | 5–10 mg IV bolus | Mild decrease in UBF | |
| β blocking agent | (see above) | | |
| digoxin | (see above) | | |

* Available intravenous ACE inhibitor

these drugs (30). A higher than usual dose of digoxin may be necessary to achieve therapeutic levels in the mother.

When heart failure is severe, either dopamine or dobutamine can be used to improve myocardial performance. There is little experience with the effects of these drugs on a fetus because they are always used when the mother is at great risk and thus, the fetal loss and changes demonstrated may be due to the underlying syndrome rather than the drug itself. Dopamine is an inotropic agent and a vasodepressor agent with the advantage of having an increased chance of preserving renal blood flow. Dobutamine can achieve the same inotrope at a slightly lower left atrial filling pressure. Because both are alpha receptor stimulators, they can decrease uterine blood flow. The much hoped for improved cardiac output may counteract this decreased uterine blood flow with an overall beneficial effect on uterine perfusion. The direct effect of epinephrine is also to decrease uterine blood flow. If, however, this drug can achieve significant improvement in maternal hemodynamics, the overall effect may again be favorable in regards to uterine blood flow.

Newer inotropic agents, including those that act by inhibiting phosphodiesterase activity, have not been evaluated in pregnancy. They too should be reserved for extreme maternal needs.

Although recently shown to be of little benefit (31), ritodrine and terbutaline are occasionally used to quiet the uterus when premature labor occurs. Of interest, despite being beta agonists, (and thus inotropic agents) they can cause pulmonary edema. Should these drugs have been used in a patient who comes to anesthesia, diuretic therapy can be used to treat this complication.

## *Vasopressor Agents*

While dopamine, dobutamine, and epinephrine are often used for their vasoconstricting effects, occasionally a drug that preferentially increases blood pressure is required. Ephedrine sulphate is preferable. It has mixed alpha and beta stimulating effects and can increase maternal blood pressure without a definite decrease in uterine blood flow (32). Norepinephrine decreases perfusion of many maternal organs, including the uterus.

## *Vasodilator Drugs*

For hypertensive crises or for urgent afterload and preload reduction, nitroprusside is the vasodilator drug of choice. Despite a paucity of information about its use during pregnancy (33,34), this recommendation is made because nitroprusside is highly effective, works instantaneously, is easily titrated, and its effects dissipate immediately when the drug is stopped. The metabolite, cyanide, has been detected in the fetus, but this has not been demonstrated to be a significant problem in humans (33,34). The metabolite is a reason to limit the duration of use of this drug whenever possible. Intravenous nitroglycerin (35) and hydralazine (36,37) have also been used in pregnancy without clear adverse fetal effects. Intravenous angiotensin converting enzyme (ACE) inhibitors are now available. They should not be used when general surgery is required during pregnancy because they increase the risk of fetal renal development abnormalities and there is some concern about teratogenicity (38,39). However, if needed at the time of labor and delivery, these issues are not of concern and the angiotensin converting enzymes inhibitors can be used.

## *Calcium Channel Blocking Agents*

Nifedipine can be given sublingually as one way to lower blood pressure quickly (40,41). Detrimental fetal effects have not been described. Intravenous verapamil, the treatment of choice for some supraventricular tachyarrhythmias, can also be given for management of hypertension (42,43). There is no reported experience with intravenous diltiazem during pregnancy.

### *Beta Blocking Agents*

There are now five available intravenous beta-blocker agents that can be considered during pregnancy. If a beta (B)-blocker agent is used at the time of labor and delivery, the pediatrician should be advised of the potential need to treat the newborn infant for bradycardias and/or hypoglycemia. While there are some concerns about fetal adversity with the long-term use of oral agents, a large experience with their use to treat hypertension suggests the risk is very low (44–46).

### *Antiarrhythmia Drugs*

If antiarrhythmic drug therapy is required, the drugs can be used in the standard fashion. Lidocaine is as effective during pregnancy as at other times, and it has not been associated with fetal deformity (47,48). Because it has been shown to cause transient neonatal depression and possibly apnea when neonatal blood levels are greater than 2.5 μ/L (49), maternal blood levels should be kept below 4 μ/L (fetal levels are 60% of maternal levels). Intravenous procainamide and quinidine can cause hypotension but also have been free of recognizable adverse effects on the fetus (50,51). There is little experience with the remainder of the antiarrhythmic drugs during pregnancy. As a general rule, they should be avoided unless essential to protect the life of the mother (51–54). While there is little information about the use of adenosine during pregnancy, its short half-life and demonstrated efficacy with apparent safety make it a first-line therapy for supraventricular tachycardias (see below) (55,56).

### *Anticoagulants*

Warfarin therapy is contraindicated during pregnancy because it crosses the placenta and it has been associated with an increased risk of fetal developmental abnormalities as well as with bleeding (57,58). While heparin can cause maternal bleeding and uterine bleeding, it does not cross the placenta. It can be used in a standard manner when required during pregnancy.

## Cardiovascular Complications—Recognition and Treatment

Cardiovascular complications may occur at the time of anesthesia or because of the anesthesia. Some aspects of recognition and treatment apply no matter what the underlying cardiovascular etiology. The following information focuses on management of these syndromes during anesthesia and surgery, rather than on chronic management, which also may be difficult during pregnancy.

### *Pulmonary Hypertension*

Ideally, women with pulmonary hypertension should not become pregnant and thus should not require anesthesia during pregnancy. However, it happens. Some women are unaware of their pulmonary hypertension. Others elect to proceed despite the risks—up to a 50% maternal mortality and a still higher fetal loss (59,60). Pulmonary hypertension can occur without a recognizable cause. This "primary" pulmonary hypertension affects young adults with a 5 to 1 female-to-male preponderance. In others, pulmonary hypertension can be part of a congenital heart disease syndrome or secondary to chronic recurrent pulmonary emboli, to drugs (or their adulterants in the case of street drugs), or to an autoimmune syndrome.

Recognition of pulmonary hypertension is essential before the use of anesthesia. Some women will already have the diagnosis. In others, the clinical presentation will provide clues. Typical symptoms include weakness, fatigue, chest pain, syncope, dyspnea and Raynaud's phenomenon. On physical examination, a substernal lift caused by right ventricular hypertrophy and a loud pulmonic component of the second heart sound are common. Occasionally, there is a diastolic murmur due to pulmonary valve insufficiency. The electrocardiogram reveals right atrial and ventricular hypertrophy. On the chest x ray, the main, as well as the right and left, pulmonary arteries are enlarged and peripheral vascular markings are decreased. The echocardiogram can support the diagnosis, and, if there is associated tricuspid regurgitation, the jet velocity may help quantify the pulmonary artery pressure. When pulmonary hypertension occurs as a part, or result, of congenital heart disease, it can be severe enough to cause right to left shunting. This irreversible situation, the Eisenmenger complex, carries the same poor prognosis and presents as other pulmonary hypertension situations (60). Additional exam findings include clubbing and cyanosis.

Management during anesthesia should include insertion of a central venous line for administration of fluids and medications and for right atrial pressure monitoring. A pulmonary capillary wedge pressure recording line is a cautious second choice as it is difficult to record a wedge pressure tracing in these patients and arrhythmias are a common result of catheter manipulation. Meticulous attention to avoidance of air infusion through, or thrombus formation on, these lines is essential. Women with pulmonary hypertension and particularly those with right to left shunts, are at risk of cerebral embolization. A radial artery line is required for pressure monitoring as well as blood gas and chemistry analysis. Pressure monitoring as well as continuous rhythm monitoring should be initiated before anesthesia and maintained for 48 hours after surgery. Continuous oxygen delivery during that time is appropriate as well, not just to maintain optimal arterial saturation, but also to minimize pulmonary artery constriction.

Intravascular volume depletion puts these patients at greatest risk. Measurements to prevent this from occurring are essential (Table 31–4). The woman who is near term should undergo anesthesia while in the 45° left lateral position if at all possible. She should be given 1000 to 1500 cc of saline before surgery or labor and delivery, and fluid should be administered to maintain a high normal to elevated central venous pressure (5 to 20 mm Hg). If systemic hypotension occurs despite this, the patient should be put into the Trendelenburg position and ephed-

**Table 31–4.** Measures to Protect Against a Fall in Central Blood Volume

Position
- 45°–60° Left lateral
- 10° Trendelenburg

Volume Preloading
- 1500 cc of glucose free normal saline or Ringer's lactate solution just prior to anesthesia

Stockings
- Full leg stocking

Drugs
- Avoid vasodilator drugs
- Ephedrine for hypotension unresponsive to fluid replacement

Anesthesia
- Regional: serial small boluses
- General: emphasis on benzodiazepines and narcotics, supplementing with low dose inhalation agents

rine (1 mg/100 cc titrated to systolic BP greater than 90 minutes) or dopamine (1 to 10 μ/kg/min) should be administered. A persistent low cardiac output despite these measures can be treated with nitroprusside in the hope that it will decrease pulmonary vascular resistance favorably as compared to systemic vascular resistance. It can be titrated to a maternal systolic blood pressure of 90 mm Hg.

It is also essential to minimize any increase in pulmonary vascular resistance (Table 31–5). Measures should include prevention of acidosis, hypercarbia, hyperventilation, hypervolemia (this is difficult given the discussion above), as well as emboli.

For vaginal delivery or cesarean section, cautiously administered epidural anesthesia preceded by a benzodiazepine induction agent or low-dose narcotic results in optimal hemodynamics and oxygenation.

## *Congestive Heart Failure*

While it is difficult to find definitive studies suggesting that the control of congestive heart failure before going into a surgical procedure alters outcome, common sense suggests that this is appropriate when possible. Such control presumably increases the safety margin, will minimize the problems with maternal oxygenation, may minimize structural changes in the heart that predispose to arrhythmias, and makes the use of medications somewhat more predictable.

Treatment before anesthesia, particularly when congestive heart failure approaches the level of pulmonary edema, should not differ during pregnancy. Oxygen, morphine sulphate, diuretics, and vasodilating agents should be used to protect the mother. Confronted by labor and delivery, and/or the need for emergency surgery, management of congestive heart failure during anesthesia can be difficult. All of these women are at high enough risk to require constant rhythm monitoring during surgery or labor and delivery, and for at least 24 hours afterward. Hemodynamically significant rhythms should be treated aggressively (see below). An arterial pressure line allows pressure monitoring as well as rapid assessment of arterial blood gasses, and chemistries. This is one cardiac condition in which maintaining the woman in a supine position late in pregnancy may be beneficial (a form of preload reduction with obstruction of return of IVC blood through the inferior vena cava to the heart). Continuous $O_2$ administration to optimize arterial saturation is appropriate, and, in extreme cases of pulmonary edema if necessary, intubation with mechanical ventilation should be performed. Drug management generally should focus on three types:

1. Diuretics. Furosemide, in addition to being a diuretic, has an arterial vasodilator effect and is optimal. Initial 10 to 20 mg doses may be adequate.
2. Vasodilator Drugs. During surgery, nitroprusside, with its preload and afterload reducing properties, is the preferred agent. Beginning with 0.5 μ/kg/min it can be titrated up to 10 μ/kg/min with careful blood pressure monitoring. Morphine sulphate also has preload- and afterload-reducing effects; 4 to 12 mg doses may be particularly effective in the agitated patient and for treatment of pain.
3. Inotropic and Vasoconstrictor Drugs. If necessary to increase the cardiac output and to treat hypotension that does not respond to volume expansion, the inotropic agents dopamine (titrating from 0.5 to 10.0 μ/kg/min) or dobutamine (titrating from 0.5 to 10.0 μ/kg/min) should be used.

### Anesthesia

A number of issues concerning anesthesia are important. First, agents that decrease ventricular performance should be avoided—particularly the halogenated agents. Second, depending on the hemodynamics, anesthesia that causes a fall in systemic vascular resistance and in venous tone may have some advantages. Finally, it is worth remembering that in a patient with congestive heart failure, metabolism of a number of agents, particularly those metabolized in the liver, will differ from that which is expected.

### *Labor and Delivery*

A lumbar epidural is preferable for vaginal delivery as well as cesarean section.

**Table 31–5.** Measures to Minimize Pulmonary Vascular Resistance

1. Maintain optimal oxygenation
2. Avoid
   - Hyperinflation of lungs
   - Acidosis
   - Hypercarbia
   - Emboli from venous catheter
   - Vasoconstriction drugs

## *Low Cardiac Output Syndromes*

A low cardiac output is ominous. Recognized by signs of poor perfusion (obtundation, peripheral vascular constriction, low urine output) or by measurement, it is often due to intravascular volume depletion. This should be prevented when possible and corrected when present (Table 31–4). As emphasized earlier, this is particularly true in patients with pulmonary hypertension. It is also important in patients with other forms of obstructive disease—aortic stenosis, idiopathic hypertrophic subaortic stenosis (IHSS), mitral stenosis, or pulmonic valve stenosis. When any of these patients begin labor or require surgery, attention to volume status is essential. Arterial pressure lines and a central venous pressure or pulmonary capillary wedge pressure catheter should be used. Positioning is important in this group, particularly late in pregnancy, in which the left 45° lateral position is optimal. The patients should be monitored closely particularly for blood loss with adequate and quick replacement if necessary. Volume loss can also be replaced with normal saline or lactated Ringer's solution. If hypoperfusion persists despite volume replacement, dopamine or dobutamine may improve the cardiac output, especially if myocardial dysfunction is a contributing cause. If the systemic vascular resistance is elevated, nitroprusside may also improve perfusion.

## Hypertension

Hypertension can be present before and persist throughout pregnancy. When normotensive women become pregnant, 5 to 7% will develop hypertension for the first time. It has been called pregnancy induced hypertension (PIH) or "toxemia." In each case, management is somewhat controversial and there even continues to be disagreement on how best to name the syndromes (e.g., the Working Group on High Blood Pressure in Pregnancy suggests the term PIH not be used) (61). It is even unclear how best to measure the pressure, but use of phase V (disappearance) of the Korotkov sounds is recommended. During anesthesia, any uncertainty about the pressure should be resolved with an intra-arterial line.

If hypertension is associated with proteinuria, pedal edema, CNS irritability, elevation of liver enzymes, or coagulation disturbances, the syndrome has been labeled "preeclampsia." These associations, in combination with convulsions, have been called "eclampsia." Preeclampsia and eclampsia require recognition and treatment as both can result in fetal and maternal morbidity and mortality.

The rules for optimal hypertension management during anesthesia are not well defined. In the woman with hypertension before and during pregnancy, an argument could be made for keeping the systolic pressure below 160 mm Hg and the diastolic pressure less than 100 mm Hg. It may minimize complications and provide a margin of safety against severe hypertensive episodes due to anesthesia or surgery. Women with heart disease that are adversely effected by increased vascular resistance (mitral and aortic regurgitation, cardiomyopathies, left to right shunts, Marfan's syndrome, aortic dissection) should have the blood pressure kept in the range necessary to prevent low cardiac output syndromes, congestive heart failure, increased shunting, or vascular disruption. While patient status should dictate the degree of pressure control in this group, systolic pressure should be kept less than 120 mm Hg. Nitroprusside (titrated from 0.5 to 10.0 μ/kg/min) is the drug of choice. Alternative or additional agents include hydralazine (5 to 10 IV doses at 15 to 30 minute intervals), labetalol (20 mg IV as initial dose followed by 10 mg IV at 10 minute intervals to a total dose of 1.0 mg/kg), or nitroglycerin (0.4 to 0.8 mg sublingually, as a paste using 1 to 2 inches on the skin, or as an IV drip starting at 0.1 μ/kg/min and titrating to effect up to 40 μ/kg/min).

Hypertension associated with preeclampsia or eclampsia has at least two distinct features. First, it is associated with a unique and complex pathophysiology (61,62). An important feature of this pathophysiology is a diminished plasma volume, which is reason to avoid diuretic use. Volume replacement is not appropriate, however, since women with pregnancy-induced hypertension have an overall excess of extracellular volume, and they are prone to pulmonary edema. Treatment of the hypertension is the optimal way to expand the intravascular volume.

The second distinct feature of pregnancy-induced hypertension is the large clinical experience with magnesium sulfate as treatment for the hypertension as well as the symptoms of preeclampsia and eclampsia. Two to four grams intravenously is often used as first-line therapy for this syndrome. If a systolic pressure cannot be kept below 140 mm Hg in the perioperative period or during surgery, the treatment approach just outlined for patients with cardiovascular disease and hypertension is preferable. If convulsions occur and persist, intravenous diazepam should be used.

## Arrhythmias

Pregnancy, and the use of anesthesia during pregnancy, should not significantly alter the approach to arrhythmia therapy. While arrhythmias may be as frequent during pregnancy as at other times, suggestions that they may even be more common are not well substantiated. The rules for management during pregnancy are essentially the same. First, it is essential to document and define the rhythm. A 12 lead ECG is optimal. When an arrhythmia is recognized, a decision about the need for therapy is required. Occasionally, a tachycardia that looks very much like a supraventricular rhythm because of a presumed narrow QRS complex on one lead, can be clearly shown to be a wide QRS complex tachycardia on another. Second, when an arrhythmia is recognized, a decision about the need for therapy is required. If anything, the pregnancy should increase slightly the threshold for using therapy for rhythms sufficient to cause hemodynamic embarrassment because they will divert blood away from the fetus. Third, a search for a potentially reversible cause may reveal one that can be easily corrected without resorting to treating the rhythm itself (Table 31–6). Fourth, it is essential to balance the potential benefits of treatment against the potential risks.

### Tachyarrhythmias

While atrial premature beats and ventricular premature beats are a reason to look for a cause, treatment is not indicated unless they are clearly the cause of hemodynamic embarrassment. Treatment of the standard sus-

**Table 31–6.** Causes of Arrhythmias

Outside the Body
- Drugs, drugs, drugs
- Caffeine, alcohol

Inside the Body
- Metabolic abnormalities
- Oxygenation problems
- Endocrine abnormalities
  hyperthyroid, hypothyroid, and rarely pheochromocytoma, and Cushing's syndrome

Cardiac
- Any abnormality

tained tachycardias should be the same as in a nonpregnant woman:

1. Sinus tachycardia. This rhythm would not be treated. It is necessary to look for and correct the cause. Occasionally, it may be caused by the anesthetic agent or by hemodynamic effects of anesthesia.
2. Paroxysmal supraventricular tachycardia (PSVT). This old rhythm (paroxysmal atrial tachycardia or PAT) with a new name is common in young women of child-bearing age. It is not the result of acquired heart disease. It occurs because of a structural change, presumably present since birth. This change may be a "dual" atrioventricular node that allows AV nodal reentry rhythms or it may be an accessory atrioventricular pathway that can allow an atrial ventricular reentry rhythm. When this accessory pathway is used during sinus rhythm and causes a short PR interval with a wide QRS complex, the patient is said to have the Wolff-Parkinson-White syndrome. When not manifest on the electrocardiogram, it is considered a "concealed" accessory pathway.

Paroxysmal supraventricular tachycardia due to either mechanism results in an atrial rate generally between 150 and 250 beats per minute with one to one atrial to ventricular conduction. The QRS complex is most often narrow (less than 0.10 seconds) but may be wide if the patient has abnormal conduction through the normal pathway (e.g., bundle branch block) or if the ventricle is activated through an accessory pathway (so called antidromic conduction in patients with Wolff-Parkinson-White syndrome). In either event, because the atrioventricular node is involved in the rhythm mechanism, measures to block conduction at this site are most often effective. Carotid massage will stop the rhythm in some patients. If this does not work, adenosine is highly effective. It is essential to give a large enough dose and to give it rapidly by vein because the drug is metabolized rapidly (within 5 to 10 seconds). The initial dose is 12 mg unless the patient is very small (for example less than 90 pounds when 6 mg may be adequate). If 12 mg does not convert the rhythm, an attempt with 18 mg may succeed. Patients using theophylline may not respond to adenosine, and, in some, the drug may cause atrial fibrillation.

Intravenous verapamil is also very effective. The starting dose is 5 mg given intravenously, and, should there be no response in 5 minutes, another 10 to 15 mg dose should be given.

An intravenous B blocker is a third choice. If there is concern about the other effects of the B blockers, esmolol is the drug of choice (bolus of 0.5 mg/kg followed by a infusion of 1 to 2 mg/min, if necessary), not because it is a better B blocking agent, but rather because of its short half-life, approximately 11 minutes. If there are recurrent episodes of paroxysmal supraventricular tachycardia throughout the course of the anesthesia or postanesthesia, these drugs can be repeated. Recurrent chronic episodes require long-term oral drug treatment with digoxin, verapamil, or a B blocker. Should the drugs not work and the patient be hemodynamically compromised, direct current (DC) cardioversion can be performed.

### *Atrial Fibrillation and Atrial Flutter*

Management of these two rhythms should be the same. Unlike paroxysmal supraventricular tachycardia, they are more often an indication of heart or metabolic disease. Initial management should be aimed at slowing the ventricular response rate. The drug of choice is intravenous verapamil starting with 5 mg and then with a 10 or 15 mg bolus, if necessary. Verapamil can be administered every 1 to 3 hours. Hypotension with atrial fibrillation/flutter usually improves when the ventricular rate is slowed. If verapamil (a vasodilator with a negative inotropic effect) is suspected of exacerbating the hypotension, treatment with 10 cc of calcium chloride may reverse the effect. Intravenous diltiazem (0.2 mg/kg) is an alternative therapy should hypotension be of great concern, although it is untested in pregnancy. If the rate cannot be slowed or if hemodynamics remain suboptimal despite rate control, synchronized DC cardioversion is required. While adenosine is an effective AV node blocking agent, it does not convert atrial fibrillation and flutter, and the short half-life of the drug makes it an inappropriate choice because the ventricular response rate will return to a predrug level within a matter of 10 to 20 seconds. Recurrent episodes may require a trial of intravenous procainamide or quinidine. Long-term management of these rhythms should consider the use of an AV node blocking and/or an antiarrhythmic agent and should address the issue of thromboembolic concerns.

### *Multifocal Atrial Tachycardia*

Always a difficult rhythm to treat, it is essential to look for a potentially reversible cause. If the ventricular response rate is excessive, intravenous verapamil will have much the same effect that it does in atrial fibrillation.

### *Ventricular Tachycardia*

As with all other rhythms, the presence of ventricular tachycardia is a reason to look for a potentially correctable cause. If the patient is hemodynamically embarrassed, synchronized DC cardioversion is appropriate starting with 100 joules. If the rhythm is being tolerated and/or is recurrent, intravenous lidocaine is the therapy of choice. If this does not work, intravenous procainamide should be used.

A third choice is intravenous bretylium. A changing morphology ventricular tachycardia may be called *torsade de pointes*. A 12 lead ECG when the patient is not in tachycardia almost always reveals a prolonged QT interval, which is the reason patients with this tachycardia are labeled as having the Prolonged QT Interval Syndrome. Recognition is important because treatment is different than for other forms of ventricular tachycardia. If it is a congenital syndrome (often a family history of early sudden death or a history from the patient of previous unexplained syncope), optimal treatment is achieved with B blockade. If it is "acquired" (not suggested by history and caused by: 1) certain drugs—type 1A antiarrhythmic agents, calcium blockers, and tricyclic amines; and 2) metabolic abnormalities—hypokalemia or ischemia) isoproterenol (1–5 μ/min titrated to a rate of 100–200 beats per minute) or atrial pacing are optimal. Intravenous magnesium sulfate (2 grams over 1 minute followed by a second 2 gram dose in 5 minutes) will occasionally stop these often repetitive rhythms.

### *Ventricular Fibrillation*

Immediate nonsynchronized DC cardioversion with 360 joules and cardiopulmonary resuscitation (CPR) efforts are always the measures of choice. CPR during pregnancy should be similar to that used in a nonpregnant woman (63,64). If at all possible, the pelvis should be rolled toward the left to enhance blood return to the heart. The fetus is at risk from the maternal hemodynamics as well as the drugs used to treat the mother. If the mother can be treated, immediate assessment of fetal status (beginning with fetal heart rhythm monitoring) is essential. If the length of pregnancy has exceeded 24 weeks, emergency cesarean section should be considered, whether the mother survives or not. A neonatologist would hopefully be available to deal with the complications expected in the newborn as a result of the resuscitation.

### *Wide QRS Complex Tachycardias of Uncertain Type*

If a wide QRS complex tachycardia is consistently irregular, atrial fibrillation is the most likely cause with anomalous conduction through the normal pathway or, in a patient with WPW, with conduction through an accessory pathway. If the ventricular response rate is very rapid (for example, greater than 240 beats per minute), the latter is of particular concern. In this case, AV node blocking agents would not be expected to work and synchronized cardioversion should be performed. An irregular, wide QRS complex tachycardia should also raise the consideration of *torsade da pointes)* (see above under ventricular tachycardia).

If the wide QRS tachyrhythmia is regular, it may be difficult to know whether it is supraventricular versus ventricular in origin. Initial treatment should be a carotid massage maneuver—lack of a response would not be helpful, but if it is one of the supraventricular rhythms, this vagal maneuver may provide either the diagnosis or the treatment (Table 31–7). The second approach is a trial of intravenous adenosine. Again, a lack of a response would not help with the diagnosis, but if the rhythm is paroxysmal supraventricular tachycardia, it may terminate abruptly, or if it is atrial flutter with block, the diagnosis may become apparent. If adenosine does not help and the patient remains reasonably stable, a lidocaine or procainamide trial can be used. If the patient becomes unstable, synchronized DC cardioversion should be performed.

**Table 31–7.** Approach to a Regular Wide QRS Complex Tachycardia

Hemodynamic Instability
- Synchronized DC cardioversion

Hemodynamic Stability
Proceed in order
- Document with ECG
- Carotid massage
- Adenosine 12 mg IV
- Lidocaine 100 mg IV
- Synchronized DC cardioversion

### *Bradyarrhythmias*

These rhythms are also a reason to look for a reversible cause. Metabolic abnormalities, particularly hyperkalemia, acidosis, and hypoxemia, should be looked for and corrected. Drugs are common explanations, particularly the B blockers, calcium blockers, or digitalis. Anesthesia can also be a cause. Occasionally, an anesthetic agent can directly suppress sinus node function or atrioventricular conduction. More commonly, the bradyarrhythmic results from sympathetic withdrawal and a relative or absolute increase in parasympathetic effect. This is unpredictable and not a reason to avoid any particular agent or approach, but it is a reason to monitor for bradyarrhythmias. The bradyarrhythmias may be a warning of danger. In a large retrospective study, 26 of 27 episodes of "cardiac arrest" (presumably ventricular fibrillation) with anesthesia were preceded by a bradycardia. Two-thirds of these arrests occurred during induction, and anesthesia overdose or failure to ventilate were the implicated cause in each case (64).

A slow heart by itself is not a reason for treatment—it is only when the bradyarrhythmia is compromising the hemodynamics that treatment is necessary. Initial therapy of sinus bradycardia or atrioventricular block should include a trial of atropine (1.0 mg IV) and/or, if there are prolonged pauses, isoproterenol (1 to 5 μ/min). If the rhythm is persistent or recurrent, a temporary pacemaker may be necessary. An external pacemaker can be used, but it is worth remembering that it is often difficult to feel a pulse and to interpret the electrocardiogram when the device is in use. Thus, if the external device is used, attention to adequate perfusion is essential.

The chronic management of these rhythms depends on the cause and the potential reversible nature of the cause. Occasionally, a permanent pacemaker is required during pregnancy.

### *Arrhythmia Devices*

On occasion, a woman who has received a permanent pacemaker or implantable cardioverter defibrillator (ICD) will become pregnant. Management of the pregnancy does not have to be altered. If a cesarean section is performed (for obstetric reasons), cautery should be kept as far from the devices as possible. It is preferable to turn off the ICD during surgery. This can be done by taping a donut magnet over the device. Before removing the magnet, a person familiar with subsequent device status should be involved—some ICDs will remain off while others revert to the active mode.

## *Endocarditis*

If first recognized at the time that surgery and anesthesia are required, initial therapy should be as in any other patient with endocarditis. Long-term management will have to address the need for chronic medical therapy or surgery.

## Anesthesia

First, a reminder—uterine arteries are maximally dilated and local autoregulation can not improve flow. Thus, anything that lowers maternal perfusion pressure and flow, or causes uterine artery constriction, in this case anesthesia, is likely to decrease the availability of oxygen to the fetus. As mentioned earlier, when maternal needs present, it is uterine blood flow that will be compromised.

In general, for most cardiovascular lesions, the hemodynamics are so volume dependent that unless there is definite congestive heart failure, measures to avoid hypovolemia are always worth reemphasizing. This may seem paradoxical to the usual rule that always seems to emphasize the danger on volume overload. Increasingly, it is more apparent that the opposite may have more severe consequences. The general rules to consider in all cardiovascular patients undergoing general surgery and/or at the time of labor and delivery include the following:

1. When possible any procedure performed late in pregnancy should hopefully have the patient positioned in the left 30 to 45° lateral tilt position. This allows adequate venous return from the legs and minimizes aortic compression.
2. Unless there is congestive heart failure, a volume preload with 1000 to 1500 cc of normal saline or lactated Ringer's solution will minimize complications from anesthesia. If given at the time of labor and delivery, the fluid administration should not include glucose because it can cause subsequent hypoglycemia in the newborn. In women with known preeclampsia, this volume loading should be halved.
3. Hyperventilation decreases venous return and can reduce maternal cardiac output and blood pressure. It should be avoided in the ventilated woman with heart disease, in whom venous return, output, and pressure are already a concern.
4. Monitoring lines are helpful. In this population of fragile patients, monitoring lines allow instantaneous assessment of pressures, provide an avenue for rapid administration of fluids, and allow assessment of blood chemistries and gases. Monitoring lines also place some of these patients at risk. Of greatest concern are the lines that allow entry of air or thrombi into the venous system, which could potentially reach the arterial system. This is particularly true in people with intracardiac shunts and patients with pulmonary hypertension. It holds true in others as well because transient right to left shunting can occur with Valsalva maneuvers even in patients who have no recognizable shunts. Venous lines may also cause arrhythmias—the information to be obtained should be well worth the risks being taken.
5. Preoxygenation before induction and intubation is particularly important in these high-risk patients.
6. Women with structural cardiac abnormalities are at risk of endocarditis. Antibiotic prophylaxis before dental work, invasive procedures, or surgery is as appropriate during pregnancy as at other times. While the committee of the American Heart Association that has established the rules for this antibiotic prophylaxis has not recommended its use at the time of labor and delivery (65), many experts disagree. In the woman undergoing surgery (and having anesthesia), it seems appropriate to initiate antibiotic prophylaxis at the time of labor and continue it for 6 to 24 hours following delivery (Table 31–8) (65). A peripartum infection is reason to continue antibiotics for specific treatment.
7. Pain relief is particularly important in these patients. Increased pain results in increased catecholamine levels, which directly suppress uterine blood flow.
8. Fetal monitoring should be addressed in all pregnant women undergoing surgery and/or at the time of labor and delivery. This can be done usually, simply, with fetal heart rate monitoring. The fetal heart rate (generally variable with rates between 120 and 160 beats per minute) falls with fetal distress. While this fall can be due to a maternal drug (for example a beta blocker) or to maternal hypothermia, it can be due to fetal hypoxia caused by a fall in uterine blood flow.
9. Finally, because of the complexity of this patient population, the concept of a team of experts being involved in the surgery or at the time of labor and delivery is worth reemphasizing.

## *Type of Anesthesia*

The anesthesiologist well knows the advantages and disadvantages of various types of anesthesia. The following is only a brief discussion of the adverse hemodynamic effects on the mother with heart disease and her child.

### *General Anesthesia*

This approach to anesthesia obviously has two major advantages. First, maternal pain and apprehension, and the associated catecholamine response detrimental to women with heart disease, can be most effectively eliminated. Second, in an urgent situation in which protection of the

**Table 31–8.** Prevention of Bacterial Endocarditis: Recommendations by the American Heart Association

*FOR DENTAL/ORAL/UPPER RESPIRATORY TRACT PROCEDURES*

1. Standard Regimen in Patients at Risk (includes those with prosthetic heart valves and other high-risk patients):
   - Amoxicillin 3.0 g orally 1 hour before procedure, then 1.5 g 6 hours after initial dose.
   - For amoxicillin/penicillin-allergic patients:
     - Erythromycin ethylsuccinate 800 mg or erythromycin stearate 1.0 g orally 2 hours before a procedure, then one-half the dose 6 hours after the initial administration.
     - -OR-
     - Clindamycin 300 mg orally 1 hour before a procedure and 150 mg 6 hours after initial dose.
2. Alternate prophylactic regimens for dental/oral upper respiratory tract procedures in patients at risk:
   - A. For patients unable to take oral medications:
     - Ampicillin 2.0 g IV (or IM) 30 minutes before procedure, then ampicillin 1.0 g IV (or IM) *OR* amoxicillin 1.5 g orally 6 hours after initial dose.
     - -OR-
     - For ampicillin/amoxicillin/penicillin-allergic patients unable to take oral medications:
       - Clindamycin 300 mg IV 30 minutes before a procedure and 150 mg IV (or orally) 6 hours after initial dose.
   - B. For patients considered to be at high risk who are not candidates for the standard regimen:
     - Ampicillin 2.0 g IV (or IM) plus gentamicin 1.5 mg/kg IV (or IM) (not to exceed 80 mg) 30 minutes before procedure, followed by amoxicillin 1.5 g orally 6 hours after the initial dose. Alternatively, the parenteral regimen may be repeated 8 hours after the initial dose.
     - For amoxicillin/ampicillin/penicillin-allergic patients considered to be at high risk:
       - Vancomycin 1.0 g IV administered over 1 hour, starting 1 hour before the procedure. No repeat dose is necessary.

*FOR GENITOURINARY/GASTROINTESTINAL PROCEDURES*

1. Standard regimen:
   - Ampicillin 2.0 g IV (or IM) plus gentamicin 1.5 mg/kg IV (or IM) (not to exceed 80 mg) 30 minutes before procedure, followed by amoxicillin 1.5 g orally 6 hours after the initial dose. Alternatively, the parenteral regimen may be repeated once 8 hours after the initial dose.
   - For amoxicillin/ampicillin/penicillin-allergic patients:
     - Vancomycin 1.0 g IV administered over 1 hour plus gentamicin 1.5 mg/kg IV (or IM) (not to exceed 80 mg) 1 hour before the procedure. May be repeated once 8 hours after initial dose.
2. Alternate oral regimen for low-risk patients:
   - Amoxicillin 3.0 g orally 1 hour before the procedure, then 1.5 g 6 hours after the initial dose.

Prevention of Bacterial Endocarditis: Recommendations by the American Heart Association by the Committee on Rheumatic Fever, Endocarditis and Kawasaki Disease. JAMA 1990–264:2919–2922.

fetus or the mother requires emergency procedures or when a regional anesthetic is particularly dangerous (in the woman with a bleeding diathesis, anatomic variations making administration difficult, or localized infections), general anesthesia can result in greater control of hemodynamics. However, for most vaginal deliveries and cesarean sections in women with cardiovascular disease, general anesthesia is not the approach of choice. The hypertension that can accompany intubation and airway management can precipitate pulmonary edema in patients with myocardial dysfunction, regurgitant valve lesions, or intracardiac shunts, and the potential for hypotension can be determinant for women with obstructive lesions and pulmonary hypertension. Regional anesthesia is usually preferable. When cesarean section is performed, the balance between general anesthesia and regional anesthesia becomes closer, but unless an urgent procedure is required or the woman has particularly complex heart disease, again, regional anesthesia is favored.

### Regional Anesthesia

When nongynecologic surgery is required, local or regional anesthesia is preferable for all the reasons just mentioned. For routine labor and vaginal delivery, lumbar epidural anesthesia with pudendal nerve blocks to minimize pain is usually optimal. It, of course, is not perfect. Hypotension can occur in up to 25% of patients even with volume preloading (66). However, with attention to volume administration and positioning of the patient in the 45 to 60° left lateral position, this approach is least likely to cause significant peripheral vasodilation, can control pain, and has been shown to be effective and safe in large populations of women with heart disease. Concerns about prolongation of labor with epidural anesthesia are not appropriate should low concentration of local anesthetic without epinephrine be used in women protected against aortocaval compression (67). The potential for sudden rapid hypotension with spinal anesthesia makes it unsuitable for most women with heart disease. When regional epidural anesthesia is used, a mixture of a local narcotic agent with a local anesthetic has been proven to be effective and has minimized the side effects associated with each type of drug.

## Anesthetic Agents

### Induction Agents

With judicious administration, these agents are generally well tolerated in the woman with heart disease. One is not clearly preferable to the others although hemodynamic alterations are least likely with benzodiazepine derivatives (68–70) (See Table 31–9 for a full listing of anesthetic agents).

### Local Anesthetics

While each has been effectively and safely used in women with heart disease and pregnancy, most experience has been with lidocaine. It has proven to be safe and efficacious (68,71).

### Inhalation Agents

With light planes of anesthesia, there is little effect on maternal hemodynamics. With any agent, when deeper planes are achieved, falls in maternal cardiac output and blood pressure have a potential for limiting uterine blood flow. Because halothane has uterine-relaxant properties (and thus decreases the compression of uterine arteries), it has the potential for increasing uterine blood flow. In woman with myocardial dysfunction, the halogenated agents should be avoided as they have primary myocardial depressive effects (72–74).

**Table 31–9.** Anesthetic Agents

| | Maternal Hemodynamics | Uterine Blood Flow |
|---|---|---|
| Induction Agents<br>thiopental<br>diazepam<br>midazolam<br>ketamine<br>etomidate<br>propofol | Mild hypotension and decrease in CO *No* measurable effects with benzodiazepine. Tachycardia with ketamine. | Transient decrease or no change. |
| Local Anesthetics<br>lidocaine<br>etidocaine<br>mepivacaine<br>bupivacaine<br>chloroprocaine | No major direct drug effects. Hypotension with chloroprocaine. | No change at serum levels achieved with routine use. |
| Inhalation Agents<br>isoflurane<br>halothane<br>enflurane<br>methoxyflurane<br>nitrous oxide<br>desflurane | Light planes—little effect.<br>Deep planes—maternal hypotension and a fall in cardiac output, and a fall in HR.<br>Myocardial depression with halogenated agents (halothane, enflurane, methoxyflurane).<br>Peripheral vascular constriction with nitrous oxide. | Halothane increases uterine blood flow because of its uterine relaxant properties.<br>Deep planes lower flow due to maternal hypotension. |
| Narcotics<br>meperidine<br>fentanyl<br>morphine | May lower CO, hypotension. | Fall commensurate with fall in maternal BP |

In each case, variables such as stage of pregnancy or labor, other manipulations, including intubation and competing drug effects, can alter these affects. Most measurements of uterine blood flow were made in animal studies with little corroboration in humans.

### *Narcotics*

When given parentally, each narcotic may lower cardiac output and result in hypotension, and a fall in uterine blood flow can occur. With epidural infusion, analgesia can be achieved without significant maternal hemodynamic effects (68,75).

## Anesthesia For Women With Specific Cardiovascular Abnormalities

With the decline in incidence of rheumatic fever in the United States and the increasing size of the population of young adults surviving with congenital heart disease, the relative importance of mitral stenosis is decreasing in this country. When discussing specific lesions of the heart, it might, thus, seem better to discuss congenital abnormalities first. However, worldwide, it is still rheumatic heart disease that is most common, and mitral stenosis is the most common cardiac abnormality complicating pregnancy. Thus, this section of the chapter will start with valve disease.

### *Valve Disease*

A summary of the most important situations to avoid with each lesion (the "Avoid List") is given in Table 31–10.

### *Mitral Stenosis*

Whether or not there is a recognized history of rheumatic fever, mitral stenosis is due almost exclusively to this disease. The valve abnormality typically develops 5 to 20 years after the acute infection. Pregnancy has the potential for putting patients with mitral stenosis in danger because of three commonly associated situations: hypervolemia, tachycardia, and hypovolemia. Each of these situations present a potential risk of anesthesia. Danger increases with increasing severity of mitral stenosis and/or the associated pulmonary hypertension. Reported maternal mortality rates approach 1% with mitral stenosis, a number that is probably much higher in impoverished regions worldwide. Fetal loss also increases as the lesion becomes more severe. Thus, when considering anesthesia, it is important to recognize the presence of mitral stenosis. Common presenting symptoms include fatigue, dyspnea, chest pain, syncope, and occasionally hemoptysis. On physical examination, a loud $S_1$, an opening snap, an apical diastolic rumble, and often a parasternal lift can lead to the diagnosis. A chest x ray and electrocardiogram may reveal left atrial enlargement. The echocardiogram

**Table 31–10.** Valve Disease

| | *AVOID* |
|---|---|
| Mitral Stenosis | 1. Central volume depletion<br>2. Tachycardia<br>3. Major volume excess |
| Mitral Regurgitation | 1. Increases in systemic vascular resistance<br>2. Negative inotropic agents |
| Aortic Stenosis | 1. Central volume depletion<br>2. Significant fall in systemic vascular resistance<br>3. Bradycardia<br>4. Negative inotropic agents |
| Aortic Regurgitation | 1. Increases in systemic vascular resistance<br>2. Negative inotropic agents |

can confirm the diagnosis and help in the estimation of the severity of the disease.

Obstruction to blood flow from mitral stenosis can be severe enough that the increased cardiac output and intravascular volume of a normal pregnancy can result in pulmonary edema. This is most likely to occur after the twentieth week of pregnancy, during labor, or in the 24 hours after delivery (Figures 31–1 and 31–2). A tachycardia can exacerbate this because diastole is compromised more than systole; such compromise limits the time the blood has to flow from the left atrium to the left ventricle, increasing left atrial and pulmonary capillary wedge pressure. This can occur with a sinus tachycardia. If a woman develops atrial fibrillation, the problem can be particularly severe.

While volume overload is dangerous, the opposite extreme also places women at risk. Central volume depletion occurring intermittently with pregnancy (and with anesthesia) can decrease the left atrial filling pressure sufficiently to lower cardiac output to a level resulting in shock and possibly death. The pulmonary hypertension associated with mitral stenosis also suffers as a result of hypovolemia (see discussion on pulmonary hypertension above).

### Anesthesia

The need to avoid the volume extremes as well as to protect against tachycardia dictate the type of anesthesia. A central venous pressure line can help in the determination of the need for volume loading before delivery. The right atrial pressure should be maintained at a level above 6 mm Hg. If atrial fibrillation occurs, the ventricular rate response should be slowed immediately with verapamil or cardioversion, if necessary. A loading dose of digoxin before anesthesia (or labor) should be given, not because it prevents atrial fibrillation but because it will help control the ventricular response rate should the arrhythmia occur. If it is late in pregnancy, measures to avoid central volume depletion become more important (see Table 31–4).

***Labor and Delivery.*** To minimize the pain and the tachycardia associated with labor and to maintain venous tone, lumbar epidural anesthesia is optimal for most. Perineal analgesia with a pudendal nerve block can minimize the discomfort that results in the urge to push and thus decrease the hemodynamic swings occurring with labor.

Epidural anesthesia is also preferable for cesarean section. If general anesthesia is required, a benzodiazepine drug or propofol are the preferred induction agents: ketamine should be avoided because of its propensity for tachycardia. Pancuronium, epinephrine, and atropine are potentially detrimental for the same reasons. Light general anesthesia has been effective and well tolerated using halothane (unless there is ventricular dysfunction), with maintenance using fentanyl or nitrous oxide.

***Nonobstetric Surgery.*** For surgery, if local anesthesia can be used, it is optimal. If general anesthesia is required, the program outlined for labor and delivery is appropriate.

### Mitral Regurgitation

Women with mitral regurgitation classically present with the symptoms of fatigue and shortness of breath. Examination reveals an apical holosystolic murmur. If the regurgitation is due to mitral valve prolapse, a mid to late systolic click may precede a late systolic murmur.

No matter what the cause, mitral regurgitation is generally well tolerated during pregnancy. Should the patient develop congestive heart failure, arrhythmias, hypertension, or a low cardiac output syndrome, the measures outlined earlier are appropriate.

Mitral regurgitation is actually the most interesting of all valve lesions because it can result from alterations of any one of the parts of the mitral apparatus. This becomes somewhat important when considering anesthesia. If the mitral regurgitation is due to left ventricular dysfunction (with altering of the arrangement of the mitral apparatus resulting in regurgitation), the problem is not the mitral regurgitation itself, generally, but rather the left ventricular function. The halogenated anesthetics should be avoided. If a woman has been known to be fragile having had previous difficulty with congestive failure, a pulmonary capillary wedge monitoring line during surgery or during labor and delivery may help keep the hemodynamics even. If the regurgitation is due to rupture of a chordae tendineae (often of unknown cause, occasionally due to previous endocarditis or trauma) or is due to alteration of the valve itself (from rheumatic disease, from a prolapsing valve or from previous endocarditis), there are no specific management requirements.

Mitral valve prolapse was mentioned as one of the causes of mitral regurgitation. Because mitral valve prolapse exists in 5 to 10% of a young population, it is perhaps the most common cause. Associated with, or caused by, myxomatous degeneration and redundancy of the mitral valve, prolapse is diagnosed when a mid to late systolic click (or clicks) is heard on examination. If the click is followed by a late systolic murmur, regurgitation is present. Pregnancy can alter the exam finding, making them more or less prominent. An echocardiogram can confirm the diagnosis but adds little that is useful in regard to management and should not be ordered routinely. Interestingly, women with mitral prolapse may have an increased sensitivity to catecholamines, but anesthesia does not have to be altered in any specific way unless there is severe mitral regurgitation.

### Anesthesia

If congestive heart failure is present, it should be treated before surgery or to delivery. In addition to the use of inotropic agents and diuretics, afterload reduction makes particular sense. Lowering the pressure faced by the ventricle as it pumps blood from the ventricle to the aorta will decrease the amount of regurgitant blood flow through the mitral valve (see discussion of vasodilator agents).

***Labor and Delivery.*** Lumbar epidural is preferable for most vaginal deliveries. If general anesthesia is required, agents that depress ventricular function should be avoided. Agents exacerbating hypertension (e.g., nitrous oxide) can also be detrimental. If the mitral regurgitation is part of a syndrome of idiopathic hypotrophic subaortic stenosis (see discussion under cardiomyopathies), anesthesia considerations are important—not so much because of the regurgitation but because of the myocardial function.

***Nonobstetric Surgery.*** The recommendations described above for labor and delivery are applicable.

### Aortic Stenosis

More common in young men than women, this disease is almost exclusively congenital in etiology and could be included under "Congenital Heart Disease" for that reason. Still, it is valve disease. Women with aortic valve stenosis may present with chest pain, dyspnea, or syncope or they may be asymptomatic. Examination findings include a systolic murmur at the base that radiates to the carotid arteries. It is usually associated with a delayed upstroke of the carotid pulse contour. The electrocardiogram almost always reveals left ventricular hypertrophy. A chest x ray, particularly in a young woman, may be normal. The echocardiogram can confirm the diagnosis and can quantitate the severity of the stenosis.

Information about significance of aortic stenosis during pregnancy is sparse, although one review series suggested up to a 17% maternal mortality and a much higher fetal mortality (76). The mother's risk was highest at the time of interruption of pregnancy or at the time of labor and delivery—the times at which anesthesia may well have been used (this was not always clear). There are certain features about surgery and anesthesia that would seem to be particularly detrimental in the patient with aortic stenosis. Again, it is probably hypovolemia that creates the greatest risk. To maintain a cardiac output through a stenotic valve, the left ventricle thickens. To adequately fill the ventricle in diastole, increased diastolic ventricular volume and pressure are required. Redistribution or elimination of this volume can significantly decrease cardiac output, reduce coronary blood flow, and result in cascading problems of hypotension, arrhythmias, worsening perfusion, and death. Severe bradyarrhythmias can also be detrimental, they decrease the percentage of time the heart spends in systole—the time needed to eject blood through the stenotic valve.

### Anesthesia

Volume loading before anesthesia for surgery or for labor and delivery is important. If hypotension occurs, volume replacement is the treatment of choice. If volume replacement does not improve hypotension, intravascular monitoring lines may determine whether a high pulmonary capillary wedge pressure has been achieved (volume should not be discarded as the primary correctable cause of hypotension until the wedge pressure approaches 20 mm Hg). If hypotension persists despite volume replacement or if the patient continues to deteriorate as volume is being given, an inotropic agent or ephedrine should be given.

Occasionally, patients with aortic stenosis do get into difficulty with the opposite extreme, congestive heart failure. If they cannot maintain their oxygenation because of this problem, diuresis and inotropic support may be required.

While this section is about aortic valve stenosis, it is probably fair to say that surgical and anesthesiologic considerations also apply equally to women with supra-aortic valve stenosis and to those with a subaortic web. Both of these conditions are congenital abnormalities that may present in exactly the same manner and with the same physical exam findings as aortic stenosis. The echocardiogram can provide the clue that the problem is not in the valve itself. Another form of subaortic stenosis, idiopathic hypertrophic subaortic stenosis will be discussed under cardiomyopathies.

***Labor and Delivery.*** Lumbar epidural anesthesia is again preferable for labor and delivery. If general anesthesia is required, negative inotropic agents (halogenated compounds) should be avoided.

***Nonobstetric Surgery.*** The issues are the same as for labor and delivery.

### Aortic Insufficiency

Like the other major regurgitation valve lesion (mitral regurgitation), aortic insufficiency is well tolerated during pregnancy. While this may be a congenital abnormality, it also can be a part of the rheumatic heart syndrome, usually with associated mitral valve disease. A young woman with aortic insufficiency is often asymptomatic but she may present with dyspnea and fatigue. Physical examination will reveal a high pitched decrescendo diastolic murmur along the left sternal boarder. Often, there is a widened pulse pressure with brisk arterial pulses. The chest x ray may reveal cardiomegaly if compensatory ventricular dilation has occurred. The ECG may reveal left ventricular hypertrophy. Again, an echocardiogram can help confirm the diagnosis. It also may help determine the cause if it is not known with particular attention to the possibility that endocarditis or an aortic dissection can cause acute regurgitation.

### Anesthesia

Optimally, hypertension or congestive heart failure should be controlled before anesthesia. Acute exacerbation of either during anesthesia may be treated best with nitroprusside. Agents that increase blood pressure (e.g., nitrous oxide) can increase the degree of regurgitation and thus should be avoided. The halogenated compounds (negative inotropes) should also be avoided.

***Labor and Delivery.*** A vaginal delivery with lumbar epidural anesthesia is effective and safe. If cesarean section is required, lumbar epidural anesthesia is again preferable. If general anesthesia is required, hypertension created by endotracheal intubation should be treated with a vasodilator agent. The halogenated agents should be avoided because of their negative inotropic properties.

***Nonobstetric Surgery.*** The recommendations given for labor and delivery are applicable.

### Tricuspid Valve Disease

Isolated tricuspid valve stenosis is rare. Characterized by an elevated central venous pressure and evidence for right-sided heart failure, stenosis as part of other syndromes—rheumatic involvement of the mitral and aortic valves, Ebstein's anomaly (see below), or prosthetic valve disease (see below)—is occasionally encountered. The major theoretical and real concern is the need for adequate time and pressure to force enough blood through the valve to maintain the cardiac output. During anesthesia, it is essential to prevent a tachyarrhythmia or treat it emergently should it occur (as with mitral stenosis) and it is important to maintain high central venous pressure (greater than 10 cm of water).

While tricuspid regurgitation is a common echo Doppler finding during pregnancy. clinically significant disease is uncommon. Unfortunately, the incidence is increasing as intravenous drug abuse continues. The physical examination is diagnostic—an elevated central venous pressure with large V waves, an enlarged pulsatile liver, pedal edema, and, occasionally, ascites. Like the other regurgitation lesions, tricuspid regurgitation is generally well tolerated during pregnancy.

***Labor and Delivery.*** Elevation of pulmonary vascular resistance is potentially detrimental and again it is necessary to avoid hypovolemia, hypercarbia, acidosis, and hyperinflation of the lungs. Lumbar epidural anesthesia for vaginal delivery or cesarean section is the approach of choice. If general anesthesia is required, agents that potentially increase pulmonary vascular resistance (e.g., nitrous oxide) or that depress right ventricular function (e.g., the halogenated agents) would be less than optimal.

***Nonobstetric Surgery.*** The issues discussed for labor and delivery are applicable.

### *Pulmonary Valve Disease*

Pulmonary valve stenosis is almost exclusively congenital. It is most often recognized and "corrected" during childhood with surgery or, increasingly, with balloon valvuloplasty. There is always residual valve disease but persistent significant stenosis is uncommon. If stenosis is encountered (symptoms of fatigue, dyspnea, chest pain or syncope; a systolic murmur and possible ejections clicks, right ventricular lift, and possible elevated central venous pressure on exam; right ventricular hypertrophy on the ECG and chest x ray; usually quantifiable stenosis by an echo Doppler study), correction before surgery or labor and delivery is preferable. If this is not possible, this is still one more abnormality in which maintenance of a high and adequate central venous pressure is essential.

While isolated pulmonary valve insufficiency is rare, regurgitation is common, actually invariable, after surgery for pulmonary valve stenosis or for Tetralogy of Fallot, the cause of the decrescendo diastolic murmur along the left sternal border.

### *Anesthesia*

Measures to avoid central volume depletion are essential (Table 31–4).

***Labor and Delivery.*** Again lumbar epidural anesthesia is preferable for vaginal delivery and cesarean section. If general anesthesia is required, agents that depress right ventricular function (the halogenated agents) should be avoided.

### *Prosthetic Heart Valve Disease*

At the University of Oregon, this subject is of particular interest. The first insertion of a mitral prosthesis with relative, long-term success was performed at this center by Dr. Albert Starr on September 21, 1960. Excitement was followed by the sobering recognition of a new disease, prosthetic heart valve disease. Even today this disease, consisting of thromboembolic complications, anticoagulant complications, endocarditis, valve dysfunction, reoperation, and death affects patients at the rate of 5% per year. Still, the valves have saved lives and have improved functional capacity for many. Women with prosthetic valves can and do become pregnant (77).

Women with prosthetic valves may have residual stenosis or insufficiency, a condition that should be approached in the manner described for intrinsic valve disease. All patients with mechanical prostheses (and some with tissue valves) will be on antithrombotic agents. It is recommended that warfarin not be used at all during pregnancy, but some suggest that it can be used after the first trimester when organogenesis is closer to completion. Thus, some women approaching surgery or labor and delivery may be on this drug (57,58). If a woman is on warfarin, it is preferable not to reverse the warfarin effect because of the risk of subsequent thromboemboli, but rather to allow it to dissipate by stopping the drug for 3 to 4 days. If necessary for maternal safety, fresh frozen plasma or specific clotting factors can be used. Patients on aspirin will be at some increased risk of bleeding for up to 7 days after stopping the drug. Those treated with heparin (often as an outpatient using subcutaneous administration) will, of course, develop more rapidly a normal clotting status or can be treated with protamine.

Cardiac complications should be treated as previously described. In this group of patients in whom endocarditis is particularly likely and dangerous, it is worth reemphasizing attempts to prevent it by use of antibiotic prophylaxis.

### *Anesthesia*

It is the anticoagulant status along with the degree of ventricular dysfunction or pulmonary hypertension that influences optimal anesthesia. The risk of local bleeding with regional anesthesia has to be balanced against the risks of general anesthesia.

***Labor and Delivery.*** In most of the large series reporting on labor and delivery in women with prosthetic valves, the relationship between anticoagulation and type of anesthesia used is not given (58,78). Individual decisions will be required. When the degree of anticoagulation is significant and cannot safely be reversed, systemic analgesia for labor combined with inhalational analgesia for delivery is preferred because of the risk of bleeding with an epidural approach. In women with severe ventricular dysfunction or pulmonary hypertension, a lumbar epidural approach may be optimal.

***Nonobstetric Surgery.*** The same balance of issues required for labor and delivery is applicable when choosing anesthesia for nonobstetrical surgery.

## Congenital Heart Disease

Women who at one time would have never made it to childbearing age are not only surviving but are capable of conception. This population is increasing in size with each generation. In this country, congenital heart disease has already overtaken rheumatic heart disease as the most common type of heart disease seen with pregnancy. In the United States, congenital heart disease occurs in 0.8% of all live births. If either parent has a congenital heart abnormality, the chance of the child having a cardiac abnormality ranges from 2 to 50% depending on the lesion. When considering management, it is helpful to divide the traditional congenital abnormalities into intracardiac shunts, those abnormalities that obstruct blood flow through the heart, and into the complex cardiac abnormalities. Add to this the now large population of patients who have had a surgical correction of their congenital abnormality. They too often require special consideration when receiving anesthesia, either for surgery or for labor and delivery. The most basic important issues related to each type of abnormality are tabulated in Table 31–11).

### Intracardiac Shunts

Women with a left to right shunt tolerate surgery, pregnancy, and labor and delivery well. Any of these, in a woman with a right to left shunt, are associated with a high maternal and still higher fetal mortality.

### Left to Right Shunts

The degree of shunting of blood from left to right in women with intracardiac defects is influenced by the balance of resistances in the systemic and pulmonary vascular beds. During pregnancy, the resistance in both circuits declines proportionally during the various stages of pregnancy and, thus, the degree of intracardiac shunting does not change significantly. While not well studied, it appears that anesthetic agents for the most part also influence pulmonary and systemic arterial vascular resistances to a similar degree, and no particular approach to anesthesia has clearly exacerbated the degree of shunting during a surgical procedure. Theoretically, oxygen administration might be thought to exacerbate shunting because of its known ability to lower pulmonary vascular resistance, but this has not been shown to be detrimental during anesthesia. Potential complications of left to right shunting include arrhythmias, systemic emboli, right ventricular failure, and pulmonary hypertension. It is not clear that any are exacerbated by pregnancy or by the use of anesthesia during pregnancy.

**Table 31–11.** Congenital Heart Disease

| | AVOID |
|---|---|
| Left to Right Shunts | 1. Increases in systemic vascular resistance<br>2. Thromboemboli and air emboli from intravascular catheter |
| Right to Left Shunts | |
| Normal pulmonary vascular resistance—e.g. T.O.F. | a. Decreases in systemic vascular resistance<br>b. Severe hypoxemia<br>c. Emboli (thrombus or air) from intravascular catheter |
| Elevated pulmonary vascular resistance (Eisenmenger's) | —See pulmonary hypertension |
| Right or Left Ventricular Outflow Obstruction (including coarctation of the aorta) | 1. Volume depletion<br>2. Decreases in systemic vascular resistance<br>3. Bradycardia |
| Other Congenital Disease | |
| 1. Marfan's syndrome | a. Hypertension<br>b. High sympathetic tone |
| 2. Complex syndromes | a. Ebstein's—similar recommendations as for ASD, R to L shunts and outflow obstruction. |

***Atrial Septal Defects (ASD).*** Because women with an atrial septal defect can reach child-bearing age with few or no symptoms and because the classic examination findings (a systolic murmur at the base and a fixed split second heart sound) often go unrecognized, this lesion may first be identified at the time a woman is pregnant. Enlarged pulmonary arteries and increased pulmonary vascular markings on the chest x ray, a vertical QRS axis, and late right forces on the electrocardiogram and the usual criteria by echocardiography can confirm the diagnosis. The physiology and the exam findings are similar in the various types of the ostium secundum defects (the more common type of ASD), including those in which there is associated anomalous pulmonary venous return. An ASD caused by an endocardial cushion defect (an ostium primum defect) is more often associated with other cardiac abnormalities, increasing the risk of pregnancy, surgery, and anesthesia.

***Ventricular Septal Defects (VSD).*** Because the murmur associated with ventricular septal defects is generally more apparent, this abnormality is recognized more often in children and corrected before women reach child-bearing age. Up to 50% of VSDs close spontaneously before a child reaches age 5. The coarse systolic murmur, best heard along the left sternal boarder, often provides a clue for diagnosis. There may be evidence of increased pulmonary vascular flow on the chest x ray. An echocardiogram can confirm the diagnosis. The dangers of a VSD increase with associated cardiac lesions.

***Patent Ductus Arteriosus (PDA).*** The third common lesion causing a left to right shunt is the PDA. This abnormality often goes undetected if it is small. The classic physical examination finding for this lesion is a continuous murmur best heard in the upper left chest and along the left sternal boarder.

### Anesthesia for Left to Right Shunts

Management considerations during labor and delivery or for general surgery are essentially the same for each of these lesions. An exception is that bacterial endocarditis is so rare for an atrial septal defect that prophylaxis is not clearly indicated, particularly if the atrial septal defect is of the secundum type. Women with an ostium primum defect (usually with left axis deviation on the electrocardiogram and often with other associated cardiac abnormalities) do have an increased chance of endocarditis and they, like patients with a PDA or VSD, should receive antibiotic prophylaxis during surgery.

Anesthesia should be used with attempts to avoid shifts in vascular resistance and thus minimize changes of the intracardiac shunting.

***Labor and Delivery.*** Lumbar epidural anesthesia with its freedom from major changes in vascular resistance is most appropriate. If general anesthesia is required either for vaginal delivery or for cesarean section, cautious initiation with a benzodiazepine and oxygen followed by an inhalation agent can result in minimal vascular resistance changes. A significant increase in pulmonary vascular resistance can result in a secondary right to left shunt with an increased concern of inadequate systemic oxygen supply and paradoxical emboli, and measures to prevent this are important (Table 31–5). Note that for these left to right shunts, intracardiac pressure monitoring lines are not required. This recommendation should be reconsidered as lesions become more complex. If cyanosis is recognized either by examination or with an oximeter, 100% oxygen should be administered. When any of these abnormalities are complicated by pulmonary hypertension, the issues previously discussed in detail become increasingly important.

***Nonobstetric Surgery.*** The approach reviewed for labor and delivery is again optimal.

### Right to Left Shunts

These shunts are associated with high maternal and fetal morbidity and mortality and potential complications with anesthesia are great.

Shunting may be the result of an elevated pulmonary vascular resistance, a situation referred to as Eisenmenger's complex. Pregnancy results in up to a 50% maternal mortality and an 80% fetal loss. Pregnancy in these women is inadvisable but does occur. The syndrome is diagnosed when women have evidence of cyanosis and of pulmonary hypertension (see earlier discussion). Maternal deaths frequently occur in attempts to interrupt the pregnancy, with surgical procedures, at the time of delivery, and in the 48 hours following delivery. In each of these instances, anesthesia can contribute to and/or help prevent the mortality.

When right to left shunting occurs as a result of obstruction to pulmonary outflow (with normal pulmonary vascular resistance), the long-term consequences to the woman are better because it is a potentially correctable lesion. The most common syndrome with this physiology is Tetralogy of Fallot (the tetrad being obstruction to pulmonary outflow, a ventricular septal defect, an overriding aorta, and right ventricular hypertrophy). While correction of this lesion is preferable before any surgical procedure, occasionally, this is not possible. The hemodynamic consequences of this lesion are not related to pulmonary vascular resistance but rather to alterations in systemic vascular resistance. A fall can result in a significant increase in right to left shunting with severe hypoxemia. Prevention of sudden decreases in systemic vascular resistance is essential and, again, maintenance of central blood volume is important.

### Anesthesia for Right to Left Shunts

Continuous $O_2$ during anesthesia and for the next 24 to 48 hours is important. In women with elevated pulmonary vascular resistance, all of the issues discussed for pulmonary hypertension apply. Thus, prevention of a fall in central blood volume (Table 31–4), of an increase in PVR (Table 31–5), and of a fall in SVR is essential.

In women with pulmonary outflow obstruction and normal pulmonary vascular resistance, prevention of a fall in central blood volume (Table 31–4) should be combined with efforts to minimize a fall in systemic vascular resistance. Hypotension should be treated with volume and ephedrine.

***Labor and Delivery.*** For vaginal delivery, lumbar epidural anesthesia seems to be best tolerated, using a combination of both narcotics and local anesthetics as a way to minimize the degree of sympathetic blockade. For cesarean section, general anesthesia is preferable in this population, as it allows optimal airway management and titration of drugs to maintain vascular resistance and volume. Slow induction using fentanyl or sufentanil followed by inhalation agents has been used safely. Pudendal and pericervical block with local anesthetic agents should be used.

***Nonobstetric Surgery.*** The issues discussed for labor and delivery are applicable.

### Ventricular Outflow Tract Obstruction

The hemodynamic and volume changes of pregnancy are reasonably well tolerated by women with lesions causing obstruction to ventricular outflow. Many of the issues related to anesthesia have already been discussed.

### Right Ventricular Outflow Tract Obstructions

Pulmonary valve stenosis and pulmonary hypertension have two common causes of right ventricular outflow obstruction. The first has been discussed as a valve abnormality and the second (pulmonary hypertension) was discussed earlier because it is so dangerous, because it complicates so many disease processes, and because meticulous care during anesthesia is so critical for maternal safety. Other causes of obstruction to right ventricular outflow include peripheral pulmonary artery stenosis (one feature of the rubella syndrome) and obstruction due to subpulmonic valve muscular thickening.

***Anesthesia.*** The important issues for both labor and delivery, as well as for nonobstetrical surgery, are the same as those discussed for pulmonary valve stenosis.

### Left Ventricular Outflow Tract Obstruction

The surgical and anesthesiology considerations discussed for aortic valve stenosis apply equally to women with supra-aortic valve stenosis and to those with a subaortic web. Both of these may present with the symptoms and signs of valve stenosis. The echocardiogram can reveal that the valve is not the site of the obstruction. An important and common cause of left ventricular outflow obstruction is idiopathic hypertrophic subaortic stenosis, which is discussed later with the cardiomyopathies.

***Anesthesia.*** Management as reviewed for aortic stenosis is applicable for these lesions.

### Coarctation of the Aorta

This form of left ventricular outflow tract obstruction has some unique features. Patients may present with chest pain, but the diagnosis is often made when it is recognized that the woman has hypertension. This may be present in the right arm but not the left, or present in the arms and not the legs. Pulses distal to the coarctation may be reduced or absent. Affected women may have associated intracardiac disease, aortic valve disease, or intracranial aneurysms. Maternal mortality can approach 8% and is due to vascular rupture or to ventricular failure (79).

***Anesthesia.*** While severe hypertension must be treated to minimize the chance of vascular disruption, hypotension is also poorly tolerated. As with other ventricular outflow tract lesions, central blood volume must be maintained.

***Labor and Delivery.*** Vaginal delivery with lumbar epidural anesthesia is effective. If general anesthesia is required, the halogenated agents with their negative inotropic effects should be avoided.

***Nonobstetric Surgery.*** The recommendations outlined for labor and delivery are applicable.

### Complex Congenital Cardiac Abnormalities

There are many variants of congenital heart disease with mixtures of each of the abnormalities listed above. Additionally, patients who have endured surgery for congenital heart disease may have residual or new lesions. In the case of each of these abnormalities, it is often best to determine whether the patient has characteristics of a left to right shunt, a right to left shunt, pulmonary hypertension, obstruction within the heart, or myocardial dysfunction, and then determine the best anesthetic management based on which of these features seems most prominent.

### Ebstein's Anomaly

The hallmark of this abnormality is a malposition of the tricuspid valve within the right ventricular cavity rather than at the annulus. There are various spectrums of the disease. In some women, there is a mild displacement of the valve with no other abnormalities. The woman may be and remain asymptomatic. Associated abnormalities are common, however, and a woman may have symptoms as a result of an atrial septal defect, right ventricular hypoplasia, obstruction of the right ventricular outflow, or from arrhythmias resulting from accessory atrioventricular pathways (the Wolff-Parkinson-White syndrome). The obstruction to blood flow through the right ventricle can be sufficient to cause right to left shunting at the intra-atrial level. In the woman with cardiac symptoms, the echocardiogram can be diagnostic. Management considerations, including the use of anesthesia, should be based on assessment of which pathophysiology is predominant, e.g., if there is a right to left shunt, the approach to anesthesia previously discussed is applicable.

### Marfan's Syndrome

Women with this autosomal dominant disease are at increased risk of cardiovascular complications, especially during pregnancy. Maternal mortality rates between 4 and 50% have been reported with deaths due almost exclusively to vascular dissection or rupture (80). The risk is sufficient to recommend avoidance of pregnancy in women with this syndrome; some have felt that the risks are small enough to "allow" pregnancy, if there is no evidence of aortic dilation.

The patient with Marfan's syndrome has some combination of long extremities, sclerodactyly, hyperextensible joints, a high arched palate, mitral valve prolapse, a dilated ascending aorta on chest x ray, and ectopic lens. The diagnosis is often difficult. It has been suggested that the combination of vascular lesions with ectopic lens is required to diagnosis Marfan's syndrome (80). The echocardiogram can be used to estimate aortic root size (greater than 4.0 cm is classified as dilated).

***Anesthesia.*** Vascular disruption seems most likely to occur with hypertension or hyperdynamic states. Systolic blood pressure should be kept below 120 mm Hg. If a drug is necessary, nitroprusside is recommended. Beta blockers can help achieve this and will minimize the hyperdynamic effects of catecholamines.

***Labor and Delivery.*** Cesarean section is strongly recommended to avoid the hypertension associated with prolonged contractions during labor. Lumbar epidural anesthesia in combination with intravenous benzodiazepine is preferable. If general anesthesia is required, the potential hypertension associated with endotracheal intubation should be anticipated and hopefully prevented.

***Nonobstetric Surgery.*** The recommendations outlined for labor and delivery are applicable.

## Myocardial Disease

Most clinically encountered cardiomyopathies can be characterized as either "dilated" cardiomyopathies or "hypertrophic" cardiomyopathies.

### Dilated Cardiomyopathies

Women present most commonly with symptoms and signs of congestive heart failure. Less commonly, symptoms from an arrhythmia or a low cardiac output syndrome (fatigue and dizzy spells) or from a systemic embolus first suggest the diagnosis. Physical examination may reveal the heart failure, and there may be evidence for cardiomegaly by examination. A chest x ray will show cardiomegaly and an echocardiogram will reveal a dilated, thin-walled poorly contracting ventricle. When this diagnosis is made, a woman should be advised not to become pregnant because of the high chance of developing severe congestive heart failure in pregnancy; maternal mortality can exceed 10% (81). A cardiomyopathy may not be diagnosed until it becomes apparent in the tenth to twentieth week that the heart cannot tolerate the demands of the normal hemodynamic and volume changes of pregnancy.

The cause of most of the dilated cardiomyopathies is unknown. Many may begin as a myocarditis, an inflammatory disease presumed due to one of a variety of viruses, with subsequent myocardial cell damage and interstitial fibrosis. In South and Central America, myocarditis and the subsequent cardiomyopathy are more often due to the protozoa, Trypanosoma cruzi with the heart damage being part of Chagas' disease. Other common causes of a cardiomyopathy in this country are toxins, particularly alcohol and drugs.

A dilated cardiomyopathy may first be recognized in the third trimester of pregnancy or in the postpartum period, and when it first develops during this time it has been labeled a "peripartum cardiomyopathy" (82,83). While it is of interest that pregnancy indeed may be the cause when the cardiomyopathy develops during this time period, the management and the approach to the cardiomyopathy is no different than for that first recognized unrelated to a pregnancy.

Dilated cardiomyopathies put patients at risk of congestive heart failure, severe arrhythmias, thromboemboli, and early death. Recent studies have shown that the prophylactic use of the angiotensin converting enzyme inhibitor enalapril can decrease heart failure and improve survival (84). Because angiotensin converting enzymes inhibitors are relatively contraindicated in pregnancy (38), substitution with hydralazine may be preferable (although not of proven value). Arrhythmias do not require treatment unless they are the clear cause of hemodynamic distress or of symptoms. Warfarin has not been proven to prevent thromboemboli, still it is recommended unless a woman becomes pregnant (57). In that case, she should switch to aspirin (325 mg daily) or to heparin should she have had a previous embolus.

### Anesthesia

Congestive heart failure or arrhythmias should be treated as previously described. Volume preloading should be avoided if a woman has clinical evidence of congestive heart failure. Hypertension may cause pulmonary edema and should be treated aggressively.

***Labor and Delivery.*** Vaginal delivery or cesarean section with lumbar epidural anesthesia is effective. If general anesthesia is required, the halogenated agents should not be used.

***Nonobstetric Surgery.*** If congestive heart failure is present, it should be treated before the surgery, if possible. The anesthesia considerations discussed for labor and delivery are applicable.

### Hypertrophic Cardiomyopathies

These cardiomyopathies can be divided into two types: patients with concentric hypertrophy and those with asymmetric hypertrophy. There is little known about the former. A concentric hypertrophy can occur in a person with long-term hypertension or aortic stenosis. In these cases, treatment of the primary processes is appropriate. Occasionally, the hypertrophy is a familial characteristic and/or is of unrecognized etiology. In still others, an infiltrate process such as amyloidosis can be the cause. Patients with a concentric hypertrophy can present with chest pain (presumably the result of the thickened muscle outstripping even a normal blood supply), with heart failure due to poor muscle compliance, or with arrhythmias. It is difficult to make the diagnosis. Occasionally, the physical exam may be unremarkable except for evidence of heart failure. The electrocardiogram may show left hypertrophy, the echocardiogram can be diagnostic.

The most commonly encountered hypertrophic cardiomyopathy is "asymmetric." Affected women have disproportionate thickening of the intraventricular septum, called asymmetrical septum hypertrophy (ASH) (85,86). This can be an entity in itself and appears to be familial in etiology. When associated with an abnormal anterior motion of the mitral valve during systole [so called systolic anterior motion (SAM)], the patient has idiopathic hypertrophic subaortic stenosis (IHSS), also called hypertrophic obstructive cardiomyopathy (HOCM). This disease easily allows women to reach child-bearing age. Given its transmission as an autosomal dominant trait with variable penetration, it is already common and its prevalence is increasing. Women with idiopathic hypertrophic subaortic stenosis may be asymptomatic but can present with syncope, chest pain, or dyspnea. They have a 0.5 to 5.0% yearly risk of sudden death. Physical examination reveals a systolic murmur at the base with poor transmission to the carotid arteries. This murmur increases in intensity with a Valsalva maneuver. The carotid artery pulse contours are brisk and often bifid (rather than having the slow upstroke found with aortic valve stenosis). The chest x ray is usually normal. The electrocardiogram usually reveals left hypertrophy. The findings of asymmetrical system hypertrophy and systolic anterior motion on the echocardiogram are diagnostic.

The pathophysiology of idiopathic hypertrophic subaortic stenosis is complex. In some women, it is probably obstruction to the left ventricular outflow (due to opposition of the thickened septum with the mitral valve leaflet during systole), which causes both symptoms and perhaps death. In others, symptoms and the greatest risk may be due to the poor compliance of the thickened myocardium making them similar to others with hypertrophic cardiomyopathies.

### Anesthesia

Systolic function may be normal or even supernormal in many with a hypertrophic cardiomyopathy. Thus, inotropic support is not required. It is the diastolic function that is abnormal. To adequately fill the poorly "compliant" ventricle, increased left atrial pressure and volume are required. Therefore, during anesthesia, measures to maintain central blood volume are essential (Table 31–4). These women seem prone to develop atrial fibrillation and some do not tolerate it well. If it occurs and clearly affects cardiac output, urgent treatment with verapamil or cardioversion is required. Ventricular ectopy and even nonsustained ventricular tachycardia do not require treatment unless clearly deemed the cause of hemodynamic impairment.

In women with idiopathic hypertrophic subaortic stenosis, in addition to maintaining adequate central blood volume, avoidance of inotropic agents, vasodilator drugs, and diuretics is optimal unless heart failure is extreme, as each can increase the effects of outflow tract obstruction. Nitrous oxide, with its tendency to increase systemic vascular resistance, will also decrease the outflow gradient and has been safely used in women with this asymetric hypertrophy.

***Labor and Delivery.*** Vaginal delivery with lumbar epidural anesthesia has been effective and safe. This regional anesthesia is also preferable for cesarean section. If general anesthesia is required, halothane may be of benefit because its negative inotropic effect may be well tolerated and, in idiopathic hypertrophic subaortic stenosis, may actually decrease the outflow tract obstruction.

***Nonobstetric Surgery.*** The approach described for labor and delivery is applicable.

## Coronary Artery Disease

It is strange to consider coronary artery disease in young women, but, it can occur (87,88). This diagnosis should be entertained in patients with chest pain compatible with angina. On rare occasions, it is due to atherosclerosis (particularly if the person has a familial hyperlipidemia, diabetes, hypertension, a smoking history, or other risk factors). Other etiologies include spasm, vasculitis, dissection, or thromboemboli. The increasing prevalence of Kawasaki's disease as one cause of vasculitis raises the concern that the prevalence of coronary artery disease will be increasing (89).

### Anesthesia

The anesthesia considerations in the woman with known coronary artery disease should be the same as those in other patients with this problem. As with any patient with coronary artery disease, it is optimal to have ischemia under control before anesthesia is required. On occasion, coronary angioplasty or surgery is required during pregnancy. Hypertension or tachycardia should be avoided or, if present, treated aggressively.

***Labor and Delivery.*** The hemodynamic changes of labor (the increased cardiac output, and increase and then decrease of heart rate, and the occasional hypertensive response) along with the pain and anxiety can potentially cause ischemia symptoms. However, unless labor is clearly associated with angina, vaginal delivery with lumbar epidural anesthesia and pudendal nerve block is optimal. If general anesthesia is required, avoidance of hypertension (a slow intravenous induction is preferable) and of tachycardia (i.e., avoidance of agents like ketamine, pancuronium, epinephrine) will minimize ischemia.

***Nonobstetric Surgery.*** When possible, regional anesthesia is preferable with close attention to treatment of pain, anxiety, hypertension, and tachycardia.

## Anesthesia For Cardiovascular Surgery During Pregnancy

It is best to avoid major cardiovascular surgery during pregnancy. On occasion, this is not possible. When cardiac surgery is necessary, it is also preferable to avoid cardiopulmonary bypass because it has been associated with maternal mortality and with a 30 to 40% fetal loss. Again, on occasion, the bypass is required. In the woman requiring heart or vascular surgery, treatment of the complications of heart disease should be as discussed earlier. There has been much experience with cardiac surgery during pregnancy, but most information is anecdotal (66,90). During the course of cardiopulmonary surgery, fetal heart rate monitoring is essential, using inappropriate fetal bradycardia as an indication that there is inappropriate flow, acidosis or, metabolic abnormalities.

### Anesthesia

The anesthesia to be used should be taken into consideration on the type of heart disease with attention to the issues presented earlier.

### Cardiopulmonary Bypass

Clearly, the perfusionist and the anesthesiologist have to work closely with the cardiac surgery team. While information on which to base definitive recommendations is sparse, the following issues deserve attention.

1. Hypothermia. There has been some controversy about the use of hypothermia during pregnancy with some concerned that it will increase the incidence of premature labor and maternal arrhythmias. However, with close attention to arterial gases and perfusion pressures, hypothermia can be used with reasonable maternal and fetal safety (90). Maternal rectal temperature can be maintained between 26 and 32° C, while bearing in mind that fetal tissue will not cool as rapidly to the same level.
2. Perfusion Flow Rate. Ordinarily during extracorporeal circulation, flow is maintained at approximately 2.4 liters/minute/m$^2$ when surgery is performed at room temperature and at 1.6 liters/minute/m$^2$ during hypothermia. The distribution of blood flow during cardiopulmonary bypass surgery and particularly that to the uterus is not well defined. There is some suggestion that, to maintain uterine blood flow during pregnancy (as measured by fetal pulse rate monitoring), the flow rate should preferably be increased to 3 liters/minute/m$^2$ without hypothermia or 2.0 liters/minute/m$^2$ with hypothermia.
3. Pulsatile Flow. Pulsatile flow has resulted in successful surgery. It is unclear if the same results can be achieved with nonpulsatile flow. Thus, the pulsatile flow is recommended.
4. Cardioplegic Solutions. If a hyperkalemic solution is infused into the coronary circulation, efforts to collect the coronary vein drainage are important to avoid fetal exposure to the high potassium concentration.

These women are at sufficient risk to emphasize once again the concept of the team approach. An anesthesiologist with a large experience with both cardiac anesthesia and with pregnancy, a surgeon with expertise in managing the specific lesion requiring correction, an obstetrician familiar with fetal warnings, and a neonatologist can provide the care.

## REFERENCES


1. Brodsky JB, Cohen EN, Brown BW Jr, Wu ML, et al: Surgery during pregnancy and fetal outcome. Am. J. Obstet. Gynecol. 138:1165–1167, 1980.
2. Duncan PG, Pope WDB, Cohen MM, Greer N: Fetal risk of anesthesia and surgery during pregnancy. Anesthesiology 64:790–794, 1986.
3. McAnulty JH, Morton MJ, Ueland K: The Heart and Pregnancy. *In* Current Problems in Cardiology. Edited by RA O'Rourke. St. Louis, Mosby Year Book Medical Publishers, Inc., 9(13):596, 1988.
4. Rosenfeld CR, West J: Circulatory response to systemic infusion of norepinephrine in the pregnant ewe. Am. J. Obstet. Gynecol. 124:156, 1976.
5. Shnider SM: Serum cholinesterase activity during pregnancy, labor and the puerperium. Anesthesiology 26: 335–339, 1965.
6. Ueland K, Novy MJ, Peterson EN, Metcalfe J: Maternal cardiovascular dynamics: IV. The influence of gestational age on the maternal cardiovascular response to posture and exercise. Am. J. Obstet. Gynecol. 104:856, 1969.
7. Atkins AFJ, Watt JM, Milan P, Davies P, et al: A longitudinal study of cardiovascular dynamic changes throughout pregnancy. Eur. J. Obstet. Gynaecol. Reprod. Biol 12:215, 1981.
8. Capeless EL, Clapp JF: Cardiovascular changes in early phase of pregnancy. Am. J. Obstet. Gynecol. 161:1449–1453, 1989.
9. Easterling TR, Benedetti TJ, Schmucker BC, Millard SP: Maternal hemodynamics in normal and preeclamptic pregnancies: a longitudinal study. Obstet. Gynecol. 76:1061–1069, 1990.
10. Robson SC, Hunter S, Boys RJ, Dunlop W: Serial study of factors influencing changes in cardiac output during human pregnancy. Am. J. Physiol. 256:H1060–H1065, 1989.
11. Clark SL, Cotton DB, Pivarnik JM, Lee W, et al: Position change and central hemodynamic profile during normal third-trimester pregnancy and post partum. Am. J. Obstet. Gynecol. 164:883–887, 1991.
12. Vered Z, Poler SM, Gibson P, Wlody D, et al: Noninvasive detection of the morphologic hemodynamic changes during normal pregnancy. Clin. Cardiol. 14:327–334, 1991.
13. Sady MA, Haydon BB, Sady SP, Carpenter MW, et al: Cardiovascular response to maximal cycle exercise during pregnancy and at two and seven months post partum. Am. J. Obstet. Gynecol. 162:1181–1185, 1990.
14. Robson S, Dunop W, Boys R, Hunter S: Cardiac output during labour. Br. Med. J. 295:1169, 1987.
15. James C, Banner T, Caton D: Cardiac output in women undergoing cesarean section with epidural or general anesthesia. Am. J. Obstet. Gynecol. 160:1178, 1989.
16. Thoresen M, Wesche J: Doppler measurements of changes in human mammary and uterine blood flow during pregnancy and lactation. Acta. Obstet. Gynecol. 67:741–745, 1988.
17. Thaler I, Manor D, Itskovitz J, Rottem S, et al: Changes in uterine blood flow during human pregnancy. Am. J. Obstet. Gynecol. 162:121–125, 1990.
18. Lunell NO, Nylund LE, Lewlander R, Sarby B: Uteroplacental blood flow in preeclampsia, measurement with Indium-113m and a computer-linked gamma camera. Clin. Exp. Hypertension (B) 1:105, 1982.
19. Katz R, Karliner JS, Resnik R: Effects of a natural volume overload state (pregnancy) on left ventricular performance in normal human subjects. Circulation 58:434, 1978.
20. Rubler S, Damani PM, Pinto ER: Cardiac size and performance during pregnancy estimated with echocardiography. Am. J. Cardiol. 50:534, 1977.
21. Morton MJ, Tsang H, Hohimer AR, Ross D, et al: Left ventricular size, output and structure during guinea pig pregnancy. Am. J. Physiol. 246:R40, 1984.
22. Hytten FE, Paintin DB: Increase in plasma volume during normal pregnancy. J. Obstet. Gynaecol. Br. Commonw. 70: 402, 1963.
23. Letsky E: The haematological system. *In* Clinical Physiology In Obstetrics. Edited by F Hytten, G Chamberlain. Oxford, Blackwell, 1980.
24. Bader RA, Bader ME, Rose DJ, Braunwald E: Hemodynamics at rest and during exercise in normal pregnancy as studied by cardiac catheterization. J. Clin. Invest. 34:1524, 1955.
25. Hart MV, Morton MJ, Hosenpud JD, Metcalfe J: Aortic function during normal human pregnancy. Am. J. Obstet. Gynecol. 154:887, 1986.
26. Magness RR, Parker CR Jr, Rosenfeld CR: Does chronic administration of estradiol-17b (E2) reproduce the cardiovascular effects of pregnancy in nonpregnant ovariectomized sheep? Program and Abstracts, Endocrine Society 67th Annual Meeting, 1985, p 160.
27. Schrier RW: Pathogenesis of sodium and water retention in high-output and low-output cardiac failure, nephrotic syndrome, cirrhosis and pregnancy. N. Engl. J. Med. 319: 1065–1072, 1988.
28. Milsom I, Hedner J, Hedner T: Plasma atrial natriuretic peptide (ANP) and maternal hemodynamic changes during normal pregnancy. Acta. Obstet. Gynecol. Scand. 67:717–722, 1988.
29. Metcalfe JM, McAnulty JH, Ueland K: Heart Disease and Pregnancy. 2nd Ed. New York, Little, Brown and Company, 1986.
30. Rogers MC, Willerson JT, Goldblatt A, Smith TW: Serum digoxin concentrations in the human fetus, neonate, and infant. N. Engl. J. Med. 287:1010, 1972.
31. The Canadian Preterm Labor Investigators Group: Treatment of preterm labor with the beta-adrenergic agonist ritodrine. N. Engl. J. Med. 327:308–312, 1992.
32. Ralston DH, Shnider SM, deLorimier AA: Effects of equipotent ephedrine, metaraminol, mephentermine, and methoxamine on uterine blood flow in the pregnant ewe. Anesthesiology 40:354–370, 1974.
33. Shoemaker CT, Meyers M: Sodium nitroprusside for control of severe hypertensive disease of pregnancy: a case report and discussion of potential toxicity. Am. J. Obstet. Gynecol. 149:171, 1984.
34. Stempel JE, O'Grady JP, Morton MJ, Johnson KA: Use of sodium nitroprusside in complications of gestational hypertension. Obstet. Gynecol. 60:533, 1982.
35. Cotton DB, Longmire S, Jones MM, Dorman KF, et al: Cardiovascular alterations in severe pregnancy-induced hypertension: effects of intravenous nitroglycerin coupled with blood volume expansion. Am. J. Obstet. Gynecol. 154:1053, 1986.
36. Ferris TF: Toxemia and hypertension. *In* Medical Complications During Pregnancy. 3rd Ed. GN Burrow, TF Ferris. Philadelphia, W.B. Saunders, 1988.
37. Tamair I, Eldar M, Rabinowitz B, Neufeld HN: Medical treatment of cardiovascular disorders during pregnancy. Am. Heart J. 104:1357, 1982.
38. Hanssens M, Keirse MJ, Vankelecom F, Van Assche FA: Fetal and neonatal effects of treatment with angiotensin convert-

ing enzyme inhibitors in pregnancy. Obstet. Gynecol. 78: 128–135, 1991.
39. Fioccni R, Lijnen P, Fagard R, Staessen J, et al: Captopril during pregnancy. Lancet 2:1153 1984.
40. Constantine G, Beevers DG, Reynolds AL, Luesley DM: Nifedipine and a second line antihypertensive drug in pregnancy. Br. J. Obstet. Gynecol. 94:1136, 1987.
41. Lindow SW, Davies N, Davey DA, Smith JA: The effect of sublingual nifedipine on uteroplacental blood flow in hypertensive pregnancy. Br. J. Obstet. Gynecol. 95:1276, 1988.
42. Klein V, Repke JT: Supraventricular tachycardia in pregnancy: Cardioversion with verapamil. Obstet. Gynecol. 63: 16S, 1984.
43. Belfort MA, Moore PJ: Verapamil in the treatment of severe postpartum hypertension. S. Afr. Med. J. 74:265, 1988.
44. Ueland K, McAnulty JH, Ueland FR, Metcalfe J: Special considerations in the use of cardiovascular drugs. Clin. Obstet. Gynecol. 24:809, 1981.
45. Frishman WH, Chesner M: Beta-adrenergic blockers in pregnancy. Am. Heart J. 115:147–152, 1988.
46. Rubin PC, Buhters L, Clark DM, Reynolds B, et al: Placebo-controlled trial of atenolol in treatment of pregnancy-associated hypertension. Lancet 1:431, 1983.
47. Juneja MM, Ackerman WE, Kaczorowski DM, Sollo DG, et al: Continuous epidural lidocaine infusion in the parturient with paroxysmal ventricular tachycardia. Anesthesiology 71:305, 1989.
48. Biehl D, Shnider SM, Levinson G, Callender K: Placental transfer of lidocaine: effects of fetal acidosis. Anesthesiology 48:409, 1978.
49. Shnider SM, Way EL: Plasma levels of lidocaine in mother and newborn following obstetrical conduction anesthesia: clinical applications. Anesthesia 29:951, 1968.
50. Hill LM, Malkasian GD Jr: The use of quinidine sulfate throughout pregnancy. Obstet. Gynecol. 54:366, 1979.
51. Rotmensch HH, Elkayam U, Frishman W: Antiarrhythmic drug therapy during pregnancy. Ann. Intern. Med. 98:487, 1983.
52. Leonard RF, Braun TE, Levy AM: Initiation of uterine contractions by disopyramide during pregnancy. N. Engl. J. Med. 299:84, 1978.
53. Foster CJ, Love HG: Amiodarone in pregnancy. Case report and review of the literature. Int. J. Cardiol. 20:307–316, 1988.
54. Lownes HE, Ives TJ: Mexiletine use in pregnancy and lactation. Am. J. Obstet. Gynecol. 157:446–447, 1987.
55. Podolsky SM, Varon J: Adenosine use during pregnancy. Ann. Emerg. Med. 20:1027–1028, 1991.
56. Harrison JK, Greenfield RA, Wharton JM: Acute termination of supraventricular tachycardia during pregnancy. Am. Heart J. 123:1386–1388, 1992.
57. Hall JT, Pauli RM, Wilson KM: Maternal and fetal sequelae of anticoagulation during pregnancy. Am. J. Med. 68:122, 1980.
58. Iturbe-Alessio I, Fonseca MC, Mutchinik O, Santos MA, et al: Risks of anticoagulant therapy in pregnancy women with artificial heart valves. N. Engl. J. Med. 315:1390, 1986.
59. Spinnato JA, Kraynack BJ, Cooper MW: Eisenmenger's syndrome in pregnancy: epidural anesthesia for elective cesarean section. N. Engl. J. Med. 304:1215, 1981.
60. Gleicher N, Midwall JJ, Hochberger D, Jaffin H: Eisenmenger's syndrome and pregnancy. Obstet. Gynecol. Surv 34:721, 1979.
61. Cunningham FG, Lindheimer MD: Hypertension in pregnancy. Current Concepts 326:927–932, 1992.
62. Ferris TF: Toxemia and hypertension. *In* Medical Complications During Pregnancy. 3rd Ed. Edited by GN Burrow GN, TF Ferris. Philadelphia, W.B. Saunders, 1988.
63. Lee RV, Rodgers BD, White LM, Harvey RC: Cardiopulmonary resuscitation of pregnant women. Am. J. Med. 81: 311–318, 1986.
64. Keenan RL, Boyan CP: Cardiac arrest due to anesthesia. JAMA 253:2373–2377, 1985.
65. Prevention of Bacterial Endocarditis: Recommendations by the American Heart Association by the Committee on Rheumatic Fever, Endocarditis and Kawasaki Disease. JAMA 264: 2919–2922, 1990.
66. Brizgys RV, Dailey PA, Shinder SM, Kotelko DM, et al: The incidence and neonatal effects of maternal hypotension during epidural anesthesia for cesarean section. Anesthesiology 67:782–786, 1987.
67. Bates RG, Helm CW, Duncan A, Edmonds DK: Uterine activity in the second state of labour and the effect of epidural analgesia. Br. J. Obstet. Gynaecol. 92:1246, 1985.
68. Strickland RA, Oliver WC Jr, Chantigian RC, Ney JA, et al: Anesthesia, Cardiopulmonary Bypass, and the Pregnant Patient. Mayo Clin. Proc. 66:411–429, 1991.
69. Mofid M, Brinkman CR III, Assali NS: Effects of diazepam on uteroplacental and fetal hemodynamics and metabolism. Obstet. Gynecol. 41:364–368 1973.
70. Yau G, Gin T, Ewart MC, Kotur CF, et al: Propofol for induction and maintenance of anaesthesia at caesarean section. A comparison with thiopentone/enflurane. Anaesthesia 446: 20–23, 1991.
71. Biehl D, Shnider SM, Levinson G, Callender K: The direct effects of circulating lidocaine on uterine blood flow and foetal well-being in the pregnant ewe. Can. Anaesth. Soc. J 24:445–451, 1977.
72. Bonica JJ: Halothane in obstetrics. *In* The Anesthesiologist, Mother and Newborn. Edited by SM Shnider, F Moya. Baltimore, Williams & Wilkins, 1974.
73. Palahniuk FJ, Shnider SM: Maternal and fetal cardiovascular and acid-base changes during halothane and isoflurane anesthesia in the pregnant ewe. Anesthesiology 41:462–472, 1974.
74. Stevens WC, Kingston HGG: Inhalation anesthesia. *In* Clinical Anesthesia. Edited by PG Barash, BF Cullen, RK Stoelting. Philadelphia, J.B. Lippincott Company, 1989, pp 293–321.
75. Craft JB Jr, Robichaux AG, Kim HS, Thorpe DH, et al: The maternal and fetal cardiovascular effects of epidural fentanyl in the sheep model. Am. J. Obstet. Gynecol. 148: 1098–1104, 1984.
76. Arias F, Pineda J: Aortic stenosis and pregnancy. J. Reprod. Med. 20:229, 1978.
77. McAnulty JH, Morton MJ, Ueland K: The Heart and Pregnancy. *In* Current Problems in Cardiology. Edited by RA O'Rourke. St. Louis, Year Book Medical Publishers, Inc., 1988, (13)9:650–652.
78. Casanegra P, Aviles G, Maturana G, Dubernet J: Cardiovascular management of pregnant women with a heart valve prosthesis. Am. J. Cardiol. 36:802, 1975.
79. Deal K, Wooley CF: Coarctation of the aorta and pregnancy. Ann. Intern. Med. 78:706, 1973.
80. Pyeritz RE, McKusick VA: The Marfan syndrome: diagnosis and management. N. Engl. J. Med. 300:772, 1979.
81. Abelmann WH: Myocarditis. N. Engl. J. Med. 275:832–944, 1966.
82. Demakis JG, Rahimtoola SH: Peripartum cardiomyopathy. Circulation 44:1053, 1971.
83. Homans DC: Peripartum cardiomyopathy. N. Engl. J. Med. 312:1432, 1985.

84. The SOLVD Investigators: effect of enalapril on survival in patients with reduced left ventricular ejection fractions and congestive heart failure. N. Engl. J. Med. 325:293–302, 1991.
85. Kolibash AJ, Ruis DE, Lewis RP: Idiopathic hypertrophic subaortic stenosis in pregnancy. Ann. Intern. Med. 82:791, 1975.
86. McKenna WJ, Oakley CM, Krikler DM, Goodwin JF: Improved survival with amiodarone in patients with hypertrophic cardiomyopathy and ventricular tachycardia. Br. Heart J. 53:412, 1985.
87. Beary JF, Summer WR, Bulkley BH: Postpartum acute myocardial infarction: a rare occurrence of uncertain etiology. Am. J. Cardiol. 43:158, 1979.
88. Frenkel Y, Barkai G, Reisin L, Rath S, et al: Pregnancy after myocardial infarction: are we playing safe? Obstet. Gynecol. 77:822–825, 1991.
89. Taubert KA, Rowley AH, Shulman ST: Nationwide survey of Kawasaki disease and acute rheumatic fever. Pediatrics 119: 279–282, 1991.
90. McAnulty JH, Morton MJ, Ueland K: The Heart and Pregnancy. *In* Current Problems In Cardiology. Edited by RA O'Rourke. St. Louis, Year Book Medical Publishers Inc., 1988, (13)9.

# Chapter 32

# DIABETES AND OTHER ENDOCRINE DISORDERS

MICHAEL FOLEY
STEVEN G. GABBE

Endocrine disorders, including diabetes mellitus, are the most common medical complications of pregnancy. Each can produce significant alterations in the normal physiologic adaptation of the maternal-fetal unit. When unrecognized and untreated, disorders such as diabetic ketoacidosis, thyroid storm, and pheochromocytoma cause significant morbidity and mortality for both the mother and her infant. It is essential, therefore, that the obstetric anesthesiologist have a clear understanding of the pathophysiology and management of these endocrine disorders. This chapter discusses the etiology, pathophysiology, symptoms and signs, obstetric management and anesthetic management, diabetes mellitus, and other important endocrinologic disorders. A discussion of each condition will be presented in three parts: (1) Basic Considerations, which include basic information about the pathophysiology, incidence, and effects of each disorder; (2) Clinical Considerations, which include obstetric and medical management; and (3) Anesthetic Management. More detailed discussion of these subjects can be found elsewhere (1–4).

## The Pancreas: Diabetes Mellitis

Over the past 6 decades, significant advances have been made in the care of pregnancies complicated by diabetes mellitus. Improved understanding of the pathophysiology of diabetes in pregnancy as well as the development of techniques to prevent complications have reduced fetal and neonatal mortality to 2 to 5% at the present time. If one excludes deaths due to major congenital malformations, the perinatal mortality rate in diabetic women receiving optimal care is now equivalent to that observed in normal pregnancies.

### BASIC CONSIDERATIONS

#### *Pathophysiology of Diabetes in Pregnancy*

During pregnancy, maternal metabolism must adjust to provide adequate nutrition for both the mother and the developing fetoplacental unit. During the first trimester, glucose homeostasis is altered by increasing levels of estrogen and progesterone that cause beta-cell hyperplasia and an increased insulin response to a glucose load (5). The heightened peripheral use of glucose causes a fall in maternal fasting glucose levels and may contribute to more frequent episodes of hypoglycemia in the first trimester. This state of "accelerated starvation" is balanced by accelerated gluconeogenesis from amino acid precursors. The relative hyperinsulinemia observed early in pregnancy promotes lipogenesis and decreases lipolysis. Both maternal fat and protein stores are increased during the first half of pregnancy.

In the second half of pregnancy, rising levels of human placental lactogen (hPL) produced by the placenta stress maternal carbohydrate homeostasis. The actions of human placental lactogen are largely responsible for the "diabetogenic state" of pregnancy characterized by an exaggerated rate and amount of insulin release associated with insulin resistance. In addition, human placental lactogen stimulates lipolysis in maternal adipose tissue, sparing glucose for use by the fetus (6). Other hormones, including free cortisol, estrogen, and progesterone, contribute to the "diabetogenic state" of pregnancy (7). Should a pregnant patient have limited pancreatic reserve, her endogenous insulin production may be inadequate to meet the demands of pregnancy. Diabetes may then be revealed for the first time, a state known as gestational diabetes.

The placenta not only produces hormones that alter maternal metabolism, but the placenta also controls the transport of nutrients to the fetal compartment. Glucose transport across the placenta occurs by carrier-mediated facilitated diffusion. Therefore, glucose levels in the fetus are directly proportional to maternal plasma glucose concentrations. The placenta is essentially impermeable to protein hormones such as insulin, glucagon, growth hormone, and human placental lactogen. Ketoacids diffuse freely across the placenta and may serve as a fetal fuel during periods of maternal starvation (8).

Fetal glucose levels are normally maintained within narrow limits because maternal carbohydrate homeostasis is so well regulated. During pregnancy in the insulin-dependent diabetic woman, periods of hyperglycemia lead to fetal hyperglycemia. Persistent elevated levels of glucose may then stimulate the fetal pancreas, resulting in beta-cell hyperplasia and fetal hyperinsulinemia (9).

#### *Perinatal Morbidity and Mortality*

In the past, sudden and unexplained stillbirths occurred in up to 30% of pregnancies complicated by insulin-dependent diabetes (10). Stillbirths were most often observed during the final month of pregnancy, in patients with vascular disease, poor glycemic control, hydramnios, fetal macrosomia, or preeclampsia. In an effort to prevent intrauterine deaths, a strategy of scheduled preterm deliveries was established. Unfortunately, this approach led to many neonatal deaths from hyaline membrane disease (HMD).

Although uncommon today, the etiology of the excessive stillbirth rate in pregnancies complicated by diabetes mellitus remains unknown. Because extramedullary hematopoiesis is frequently observed in stillborn infants of diabetic mothers (IDMs), chronic intrauterine hypoxia has been suggested as a likely cause of these intrauterine fetal deaths. There is considerable evidence linking hyperinsulinemia and fetal hypoxia (11). Hyperinsulinemia can increase the metabolic rate of the fetus and heighten its oxygen requirements. In addition, several maternal factors, including hyperglycemia, ketoacidosis, preeclampsia, and vasculopathy can reduce placental blood flow and fetal oxygenation.

Excessive growth stimulated by hyperinsulinemia may predispose the fetus of the diabetic mother to shoulder dystocia, traumatic birth injury, and asphyxia. Macrosomia has been observed in as many as 50% of pregnancies complicated by gestational diabetes mellitus and 40% of insulin-dependent diabetic pregnancies (12). Fetal macrosomia in infants of diabetic mothers is reflected by increased adiposity, muscle mass, and organomegaly. The disproportionate increase in the size of the trunk and shoulders when compared to the head may contribute to the likelihood of a difficult vaginal delivery.

With the reduction in intrauterine deaths and a significant decrease in neonatal mortality related to hyaline membrane disease and traumatic delivery, congenital malformations have emerged as the most important cause of perinatal loss in pregnancies complicated by insulin-dependent diabetes mellitus (IDDM). At present, however, these malformations account for 30 to 50% of perinatal mortality (10). Most studies have documented a twofold to fourfold increase in major malformations in infants of insulin-dependent diabetic women. In general, the incidence of major malformations in worldwide studies of offspring of insulin-dependent diabetic mothers has ranged from 5 to 10%.

The insult that causes malformations in infants of diabetic mothers impacts on most organ systems and must act before the seventh week of gestation (13). The most characteristic congenital defects include sacral agenesis or caudal dysplasia, central nervous system malformations, particularly anencephaly, and open spina bifida and cardiac anomalies. It appears that a derangement in maternal metabolism, possibly in association with a greater genetic susceptibility, contributes to abnormal embryogenesis. Maternal hyperglycemia has been proposed by most investigators as the primary factor, but hyperketonemia and hypoglycemia have also been suggested (14).

After delivery, the neonate of the diabetic mother may suffer from a variety of metabolic abnormalities, including hypoglycemia, hypocalcemia, and hyperbilirubinemia.

## Maternal Classification

Over 40 years ago, Dr. Priscilla White pointed out that the age of onset of diabetes, its duration, and the severity of vascular disease influence perinatal outcome (15). Her classification scheme (Table 32–1) assumed tremendous importance because it allowed obstetricians to focus on those patients who are at greater risk during pregnancy.

Gestational diabetes, also labeled Class A diabetes, is a form of latent diabetes in which the stress of pregnancy reveals glucose intolerance characterized by postprandial hyperglycemia. These patients demonstrate carbohydrate intolerance during an oral 100-gram 3-hour glucose tolerance test (GTT) and are usually managed by dietary therapy alone.

Patients requiring insulin are designated by the letters B, C, D, R, and F (Table 32–1). Class B patients are those whose onset of disease is after age 20. Class B patients

**Table 32–1.** Modified White Classification of Pregnant Diabetic Women

| Class | Onset Age | Duration | Description | Management |
|---|---|---|---|---|
| A | any | any | Diabetes very mild<br>Diagnosis by glucose tolerance test which deviates only slightly from normal.<br>Highest chance for fetal survival. | Minimal dietary regulation. Delivery at term. No insulin. |
| B | >20 | <10 | Diabetes started at age of 20 years or above.<br>Duration of disease less than 10 years.<br>Free of vascular disease. | |
| C | 10–19 | 10–19 | Diabetes started between age 10–19.<br>Duration of disease 10–19 years.<br>Slight vascular disease. | Diet<br>Hospitalization during pregnancy as indicated<br>Termination at 36–37 weeks<br>Vaginal or cesarean section delivery<br>Insulin |
| D | <10 | >20 | Diabetes started before the age of 10 years.<br>Duration of disease 20 years or more.<br>Moderate vascular disease such as retinitis or transitory albuminuria or hypertension. | |
| F, R, H | any | any | All diabetic patients with nephritis, proliferative retinopathy, ischemic myocardial disease. | Chances for fetal survival guarded.<br>Interruption of pregnancy indicated on maternal and fetal criteria, i.e., insulin, or considered when there is evidence or progressive retinal or vitreous hemorrhage or aggravation of renal or cardiovascular impairment. |

have had diabetes less than 10 years and have no vascular complications.

Class C diabetes includes patients who have the onset of their disease between the ages of 10 and 19 years. Vascular disease is not present.

Class D includes women with disease of 20 years duration or greater, or whose onset occurred before age 10, or who have benign retinopathy. This includes microaneurysms, exudates, and venous dilatation.

Class F describes patients with renal disease. This includes those with reduced creatinine clearance and proteinuria of at least 400 mg in 24 hours measured during the first trimester. Several laboratory investigations suggest that diabetes nephropathy present prior to 20 weeks gestation is predictive of poor outcome (e.g., perinatal death or birth weight less than 1500 g) (16). These include proteinuria greater than 3.0 g/24 hr, serum creatinine above 1.5 mg/dL, anemia with hematocrit less than 25%, and hypertension. Several studies have failed to demonstrate a permanent worsening of diabetic renal disease as a result of pregnancy (17,18).

Class R diabetes designates patients with proliferative retinopathy. There is no difference in the prevalence of retinopathy in women who have or have not been pregnant. However, active proliferative retinopathy may worsen significantly during pregnancy.

Class H diabetes refers to the presence of diabetes of any duration associated with ischemic myocardial disease. There is evidence that the small number of women who have coronary artery disease are at an increased risk for mortality during gestation. While there are reports of successful pregnancies following myocardial infarction in diabetic women, cardiac status should be carefully assessed during early gestation or preferably prior to pregnancy.

## Obstetric Management

### Treatment of Maternal Diabetes Mellitus

Self glucose monitoring combined with aggressive insulin therapy has made the maintenance of maternal normoglycemia (levels of 60 to 120 mg/dL) a therapeutic reality in patients with insulin-dependent diabetes mellitus (19). Patients monitor their glucose control using glucose-oxidase impregnated reagent strips and a glucose meter. Glucose determinations are made in the fasting state and before lunch, dinner, and bedtime. During pregnancy, most insulin-dependent patients will require multiple insulin injections, usually a combination of intermediate-acting and regular insulin before breakfast and at dinnertime.

The efficacy of continuous insulin infusion therapy in pregnancy has been documented (20). A basal infusion rate of regular insulin is established, which is approximately 1 unit/hour. Bolus infusions are then given with meals and possibly snacks. Pump therapy requires close observation. Ketoacidosis has been observed in association with pump failure or maternal infection.

Most patients do well on a dietary program consisting of three meals and several snacks. Dietary composition should be 50 to 60% carbohydrate, 20% protein, and 25 to 30% fat with less than 10% saturated fats. Caloric intake is established based on prepregnancy weight and weight gain during gestation. Patients should consume approximately 35 kcal/kg body weight.

Most pregnant patients with insulin-dependent diabetes mellitus are followed with outpatient visits at 1 or 2 week intervals. At each visit, control is assessed and adjustments in insulin dosage are made to maintain a mean capillary glucose of less than 110 mg/dL (21). Fetal growth is evaluated by serial ultrasound examinations at 4 to 6 week intervals. Ophthalmologic examinations and 24-hour urine collections are performed during each trimester and are repeated more often if retinopathy or nephropathy is detected.

During the third trimester, when the risk of sudden intrauterine death increases, an outpatient program of fetal surveillance is initiated. Improved maternal control has played a major role in reducing perinatal mortality in diabetic pregnancies. Therefore, antepartum fetal monitoring tests have been used primarily to reassure the obstetrician and avoid unnecessary premature intervention. These techniques have few false-negative results. Therefore, in a patient who is well-controlled and exhibits no vasculopathy or hypertension, reassuring antepartum testing allows the fetus to benefit from further maturation in utero.

The nonstress test (NST) is the preferred screening method to assess antepartum fetal well being in the patient with diabetes mellitus (22). Maternal assessment of fetal activity may also be a helpful technique. The nonstress test evaluates the presence of accelerations of the baseline fetal heart rate. A reactive or reassuring nonstress test exhibits at least two accelerations of the fetal heart rate of 15 beats-per-minute amplitude and 15 seconds duration in a 20-minute period of monitoring. If these criteria are not met, further investigation with a contraction stress test (CST) or biophysical profile is undertaken.

### The Timing of Delivery

If the patient's diabetes is well-controlled and antepartum fetal surveillance remains normal, delivery should be delayed until fetal maturation has taken place. In general, elective induction of labor is usually planned at 38 to 40 weeks in well-controlled patients without vascular disease. Before elective delivery, an amniocentesis may be performed to document fetal pulmonary maturity with a mature lecithin-sphingomyelin ratio (L/S ratio or L/S) of greater than 2.0 and the presence of the acidic phospholipid phosphatidylglycerol (PG).

The route of delivery for the diabetic patient remains controversial. Delivery by cesarean section is usually favored when fetal distress is suggested by antepartum heart rate monitoring. The fetus estimated to weigh more than 4000 g is also best delivered by cesarean section to avoid shoulder dystocia and birth trauma.

During labor, continuous fetal heart rate monitoring is mandatory. Labor is allowed to progress as long as normal rates of cervical dilatation and descent are documented. Despite attempts to select patients with obvious fetal macrosomia for delivery by elective cesarean section, arrest of dilatation or descent should alert the physician of the possibility of cephalopelvic disproportion. About 25% of macrosomic infants (greater than 4000 g) delivered after a prolonged second stage will have shoulder dystocia (23).

Because neonatal hypoglycemia is directly related to maternal glucose levels during labor as well as to the degree of antepartum control, it is important to maintain maternal plasma glucose levels at approximately 100 mg/dL during labor (24). Continuous infusions of both insulin and glucose have proven most valuable during labor and delivery. Ten units of regular insulin may be added to 1000 ml of solution containing 5% dextrose. An infusion rate of 100 to 125 ml/hour will, in most cases, result in good glucose control. Insulin may also be infused from a syringe pump at a dose of 0.25 to 2.0 units/hour and adjusted to maintain normal glucose values (25). Another simplified regimen has been devised by Jovanovic and Peterson (26). In well-controlled patients, the usual dose of NPH insulin is given at bedtime, and the morning insulin dose is withheld. Once active labor begins or glucose falls below 70 mg/dL, the infusion is changed from saline to 5% dextrose at a rate of 2.5 mg/kg/minute. Glucose levels are recorded, and the infusion rate is adjusted accordingly. Regular insulin is administered should glucose values exceed 140 mg/dL. It is important to use a flow sheet that summarizes glucose values, insulin dosage, and other metabolic parameters during labor.

When cesarean section is to be performed, it should be scheduled for early morning. This simplifies intrapartum glucose control and allows the neonatal team to prepare for the care of the newborn. The patient is kept NPO and her usual morning insulin dose is withheld. Following surgery, glucose levels are monitored every 2 hours at the bedside using a glucose reflectance meter. An intravenous solution of 5% dextrose is administered at this time. It must be remembered that after delivery, insulin requirements are usually significantly lower than were pregnancy or prepregnancy needs.

## Anesthetic Management

### Basic Principles

Good anesthetic care is important to the diabetic mother and her infant because it permits better obstetric management. On the other hand, poor anesthesia may certainly be harmful to the mother and may be the critical factor in the infant's chances of survival. For optimal results, the anesthesiologist must be fully acquainted with the patient's disease, the present status of the diabetes, the condition of the fetus, the progress of labor, and the plan for medical and obstetric management. He/she needs to participate in the management of the patient from the beginning of hospitalization and, if possible, during the pregnancy. Certainly, he/she should see the patient even before labor is induced and discuss the possible anesthetic management.

One of the most important obligations of the anesthesiologist (as well as every other member of the obstetric team) is to provide the gravida psychologic support. This is essential in all patients, but it is especially useful in diabetics who are likely to be particularly concerned about the effects of anesthesia and labor. Therefore, educated childbirth and other suggestive techniques that have been carried out during pregnancy are reinforced during labor. In addition to the emotional benefit, psychologic support will decrease the amount of sedatives, narcotics, and other systemic agents required. If the parturient is a suitable candidate, hypnosis may be attempted for pain relief. When effective, this technique is associated with less biochemical and body-function deviation than with any other form of pain relief (27,28).

### General Principles

With regard to the fetus in selecting the method of analgesia, it is important to remember that: (1) placental blood flow is already compromised; (2) the infant is frequently premature and extremely delicate; (3) labor may be prolonged and the amount of birth asphyxia probably greater among fetuses delivered of diabetic, as compared with those delivered of nondiabetic, mothers; and (4) the fetus may have a serious anomaly. Every precaution should be taken to prevent maternal arterial hypotension, respiratory center depression, respiratory tract obstruction or hypoventilation, or extreme hyperventilation from any cause. It is best to avoid or minimize systemic depressants that pass the placental membrane and those that will prolong labor and thus increase the hazard of birth asphyxia. The anesthetic should permit atraumatic application of outlet forceps or facilitate breech delivery, should this be contemplated. Nylund, et al (29) compared the uteroplacental blood flow index in the last trimester of pregnancy for 26 women having diabetes mellitus with that of 41 healthy control parturients using indium—113 m intravenously—and a computer-linked gamma camera and found that uteroplacental blood flow decreased 35 to 45% in diabetic patients. Interestingly, the reduction in blood flow index in gestational diabetes did not suffer statistically from that in severe diabetes. Moreover, Bjork and Persson (30) showed that the villi in the placenta of diabetic patients were enlarged and, consequently, the placenta denser, thus reducing intervillous space and consequently uterine blood flow. In regard to impairment of oxygen transport, note that hemoglobin $A_{1C}$ is 2 to 3 times higher in insulin-treated diabetics than in normal controls. This has an effect on oxygen affinity, etc. Madsen and Ditzel (31) noted that red cell oxygen transport saturation and oxygen tension are impaired in insulin-dependent diabetic subjects. This, together with the decrease in concentration of 2,3 DPG tend to be lower so that oxygen release to tissue level may be impaired. In regard to the deranged buffered capacity, Brouillard, et al (32) reported that infants of diabetic mothers have a decreased buffering capacity and had different response to increased acid load. This multiplicity of problems makes the infant of diabetic mothers much more vulnerable to hypoxia and, hence, careful anesthetic management is mandatory.

Further impairment of uterine contractility must be avoided. Therefore, large doses of sedatives or narcotics and potent inhalation anesthetics should not be used and regional anesthesia should not be started too soon. It is also important not to interfere with the mechanism of internal rotation. This requires that relaxation of the perineal sling be avoided until after internal rotation has occurred and the patient is ready to deliver. For the actual delivery, relaxation of the perineum is desired to facilitate application of forceps. If the auxiliary forces will be required for spontaneous delivery, it is essential to avoid paralysis of the abdominal wall and to instruct the patient on how to bear down. These objectives can be achieved best with continuous epidural analgesia infusion containing dilute solution of local anesthetic and opioids as described in Chapter 13.

Whatever the method of analgesia used, it is important that the dose of each drug be individualized, an objective that requires careful evaluation of the parturient's needs in the expectation of delivery by the vaginal route, either by spontaneous, forceps, or vacuum methods.

## Analgesia and Anesthesia for Labor and Vaginal Delivery

Any pain in the latent phase should be managed by reassurance and psychologic support, and opioids should be avoided because of their depressant effect. If the patient in the latent phase has very severe pain, 1 mg of morphine intrathecally will provide very good pain relief without side effects on the mother or infant. As labor progresses to the active phase and the contractions become more painful, small doses of opioids may be used for analgesia. This pain-relief method can be very effective for some patients (33). Meperidine hydrochloride (Demerol), 40 to 75 mg IV over time (5 to 10 minute period) with careful maternal monitoring, or alphaprodine hydrochloride (Nisentil), 20 to 40 mg, may be used. In the past, the intramuscular route was typically used, but we now know the that intravenous route is better because smaller dosages can be used to titrate the optimum effect for the laboring mother. Unless the drugs are used in optimal doses, during the relaxation phase hypoventilation develops with consequent hypoxemia, hyperglycemia, acidosis, and fetal depression.

When labor pain is no longer adequately relieved with opioids, regional analgesia may be begun. Usually, this occurs when cervical dilation is 3 to 5 cm in the multigravida and 4 cm in the primigravida. Major regional analgesia is preferred in the form of continuous lumbar epidural because, when properly administered, it does not disturb the biochemical status of the mother, blunts or obviates the neuroendocrine stress response, has no direct effect on the fetus, and does not alter the course of labor. Hypotension and toxic reactions, the two complications of regional anesthesia, must be avoided, especially in diabetics, because these will cause disturbance of an already altered metabolism and acidosis. The exact type of regional anesthetic used depends on the skill of the administrator and the obstetric conditions. Other patients may need more intense analgesia and prefer little or no cerebral obtundation, and, for those patients, continuous lumbar epidural block is an excellent choice for pain relief during both labor and the subsequent delivery. This latter anesthetic technique may reduce the release of endogenous catecholamines, thereby limiting glycogenolysis and the resultant hyperglycemia (34).

When major regional anesthesia is used in a patient with diabetes mellitus, extreme care must be taken to avoid or to minimize the degree of maternal hypotension by promptly administering small doses (5 to 10 mg) of ephedrine intravenously or giving a continuous infusion that contains 100 mg of ephedrine per 500 mg of solution. Datta and coworkers have shown that the occurrence of untreated hypotension during epidural or spinal anesthesia in patients with diabetes mellitus is associated with significant neonatal acidosis, whereas when this is promptly treated, the effects on the fetus and newborn are minimal (35–37). The effects of untreated hypotension on the fetus are especially important in patients with diabetic vasculopathy.

## Prevention of Maternal Hypotension

To avoid or minimize the deleterious effects of the untreated maternal hypotension on the fetus, it is necessary to carry out routine left uterine displacement, prompt treatment with intravenous ephedrine, and ample hydration before the induction of anesthesia. Ample hydration with a 700 to 1000 ml dose to prevent hypotension is used before the induction of regional anesthesia. This hydration must be accomplished with nondextrose-containing solutions such as normal saline administered through a separate intravenous line.

One specific clinical investigation has demonstrated that the administration of large amounts of glucose-containing solutions to healthy women undergoing elective cesarean section may result in significant increases in umbilical vein glucose and insulin levels and a significant fall in umbilical arterial pH (38). The elevated insulin levels have been associated with neonatal hypoglycemia and a delayed release of glucagon at 2 hours of age (39). Most recently, Philipson (40) confirmed that normal women receiving 1 liter of 5% dextrose before the administration of epidural anesthesia delivered infants with reduced umbilical vein and arterial pH. The short-term administration of glucose to the mother results in fetal hyperglycemia that may increase fetal metabolic rate. With increased glucose consumption by the fetus, the production of lactic acid is increased. Fetal oxygen consumption is also raised, leading to a fall in fetal oxygen content and hypoxemia. Fetal hypoxemia may decrease fetal pH and lead to lactic acidosis. The fetus may then redistribute cardiac output in response to these metabolic changes, decreasing the blood flow to the placenta. In patients with diabetes mellitus whose fetuses may be hyperinsulinemic as well and in patients with vasculopathy in whom uteroplacental blood flow is reduced, a heightened fetal acidosis could develop. Certainly, all of these factors must be considered when choosing the optimal anesthetic for labor, and it is plain to see that such a decision cannot be made unless the obstetrician and the anesthesiologist communicate and coordinate their efforts. A very straightforward summation must be given about any jeopardy to the fetus so that the anesthesiologist and the obstetrician can decide if regional analgesia is safe in view of suspected or known preexisting fetal-placental compromise.

### Continuous Epidural and Continuous Caudal Block

Provided it is properly administered as described in Chapter 13, continuous epidural block achieved through an infusion pump undoubtedly is the best all-around technique in providing pain relief during labor, delivery, and the early puerperium for several reasons. For one, it produces analgesia that is more complete, more certain, and of longer duration than that of paracervical block, which should be avoided in these patients. By using continuous infusion of low concentration of local anesthetic and opioids, analgesia can be achieved without significant impairment of movement of the lower limbs and without relaxing the perineal sling before internal rotation takes place. Increasing the concentration of the local anesthetic just before delivery permits good relaxation, and thus facilitates the use of outlet forceps. In addition, this technique may increase placental blood flow (41), an effect that is especially beneficial to the infant of the diabetic mother. In patients with toxemia, this method also helps to control hypertension. Finally, the continuous method permits extension of anesthesia for cesarean section should this become necessary.

The disadvantages of continuous infusion include risk of toxic reaction and high block. These hazards can be minimized or even eliminated by skillful application, continuous observation of the patient, and prompt treatment of side effects. Serious hypotension can be avoided by having the parturient remain on her side during labor and by displacing the uterus to the left when the parturient is in position for the delivery. These techniques should not be used in the diabetic by the less experienced anesthetist.

***Subarachnoid Block.*** Continuous subarachnoid block with very small doses of local anesthetic and opioids can also be used for labor and vaginal delivery. Continuous subarachnoid block is best achieved by using a 32-gauge catheter inserted into the subarachnoid space, which permits repeated injections of very small amounts of local anesthetics and opioids, as necessary. In the event that an obstetric anesthesiologist is not available, true "saddle block" (see Chapter 14 for technique), which produces intense anesthesia and muscle relaxation of the lower lumbar and sacral segments, can be carried out by an obstetrician or general practitioner skilled in the application and initiated after internal rotation has occurred. Because this technique does not involve preganglionic or postganglionic sympathetic fibers, the risk of maternal hypotension is minimal. Hypotension must be prevented for optimal results, but it is also acceptable to be aware of this problem and to diagnose and treat it promptly; otherwise, it will disturb the diabetes, reduce placental blood flow, and compromise the fetus.

***Pudendal Block.*** This is an excellent method for the end of labor and preparation for delivery because it is relatively simple to carry out, causes less disturbance than do other techniques, permits full motion of the lower limbs, and can be executed by the same physician who is to carry out the obstetric management (provided, of course, he or she is skilled with the technique). Its disadvantages are that it requires vaginal examination for injection and that a small risk of toxic reaction exists after injecting the local anesthetic in these vascular regions. The latter can be obviated with correct technique.

### Management for Cesarean Section

Epidural anesthesia is preferred in the patient undergoing cesarean section (35). This technique allows the anesthesiologist to monitor the patient's mental status and detect the early signs of hypoglycemia (42). Datta and associates (36,37) have demonstrated that spinal anesthesia is associated with more acidosis than is associated with general anesthesia. Datta has shown that with spinal anesthesia, in which maternal hypotension is promptly treated with either frequent intravenous boluses of ephedrine or continuous ephedrine, the degree of maternal hypotension is minimal. In these cases, spinal anesthesia has the advantage in that it does not carry the risk of toxic reactions. In these cases, acidosis could be related to both maternal hypotension and the severity of maternal diabetes. While epidural anesthesia is favored, well-conducted general anesthesia may be used with good neonatal outcome.

The anesthesiologist must also be aware of the presence of severe maternal vasculopathy and/or gastropathy. While all patients with insulin-dependent diabetes mellitus would benefit from a predelivery anesthesia consult, in women with significant vasculopathy, a predelivery consultation is essential. The patient's cardiac status should be carefully evaluated and the risks of aspiration anticipated.

Cesarean section in a diabetic patient should be planned as a combined effort by the internist, obstetrician, and anesthesiologist. If the patient has been on long-acting insulin, this is withheld on the day of the operation. If the cesarean section is to be performed before noon, the patient is not allowed a breakfast. An intravenous glucose infusion is started and the patient is given a morning dose of soluble insulin equivalent to about two-thirds that of the quick-acting insulin given in her usual morning injection. If the cesarean section is to be performed in the afternoon, the gravida receives a full dose of quick-acting insulin with her normal breakfast, but is not allowed a lunch. No food or fluids by mouth are permitted during the 6 hours before the operation. It is particularly important to avoid drinks containing glucose, which apparently exaggerate delayed gastric emptying. All parturients should be given acid aspiration prophylaxis with one or more of the drugs currently available. Edwards and his coworkers (43) analyzed 100 reported maternal deaths associated with anesthesia and found that among this group were six diabetic patients whose deaths were caused by aspiration of gastric contents. All had received glucose drinks before the anesthetic was given.

### Anesthesia

***Regional Anesthesia.*** As mentioned at the beginning of this section, this technique of anesthesia for cesarean section is preferred today because it offers the mother the advantage of the awake state, it maximizes the bonding phenomenon, and it provides the anesthesiologist a continuous monitor of the awake cerebral state, which may become altered due to acidosis and other problems associated with the insulin-dependent diabetes mellitus state. Subarachnoid or lumbar epidural block is the method of choice. Prolonged hypotension must be avoided. The supine hypotensive syndrome should be diagnosed before starting the block. Arterial hypotension is minimized by procedures detailed in Chapters 13 and 31. Caudal anesthesia is not advisable unless the catheter is advanced so that its tip (the point of injection) is at the fifth lumbar vertebra. Otherwise, it will be necessary to inject large volumes (30 ml or more) of local anesthetic, thus increasing the risk of toxic reaction and hyperglycemia, especially if epinephrine is incorporated in the usual concentration. Infiltration or field block analgesia of the abdominal wall is excellent in elective cesarean section provided it is skillfully carried out. Unfortunately, this is not usually the case, and the patient experiences discomfort and sometimes sustains toxic reaction.

***General Anesthesia.*** General anesthesia is indicated in patients with severe hypovolemia or supine hypotensive syndrome and in those who have strong objections to regional techniques. In these patients, the following sequence produces good results: preliminary denitrogenation with 100% oxygen for 5 minutes; induction with intravenous injection of 125 to 200 mg of thiopental with concommitant application of cricoid pressure to prevent acid aspiration, promptly followed by 60 to 100 mg succinylcholine and tracheal intubation; maintenance of anesthesia with nitrous oxide-oxygen and muscle relaxant. General anesthesia is contraindicated in patients with food in their stomachs.

Emergency cesarean section for maternal bleeding or development of uncontrolled diabetes presents one of the greatest problems in obstetrics and anesthesia. Both maternal and fetal morbidity and mortality are high regardless of the technique used (44). The problems associated with hypotension secondary to blood loss or acidosis, in addition to the need for ventilatory assistance and supplementary oxygen, suggest that light general anesthesia with an endotracheal tube is the method of choice. Again, thiopental nitrous oxide muscle relaxant is the best method (45). Halothane and other potent inhalation agents are avoided because of greater risk of cardiovascular depression. Light general anesthesia suffices it, as control of ventilation and relaxation are obtained with the muscle relaxant. A cooperative obstetrician who will operate as rapidly as possible is essential for best results. Fetal mortality and morbidity increase with increasing duration or depth of anesthesia (46).

## The Adrenal Gland

Early advances in the medical and surgical management of disorders of the adrenal gland have led to an increased prevalence of these conditions in the obstetric population (47). A thorough understanding of normal adrenal physiology and alterations encountered during gestation is essential in the evaluation and treatment of the pregnant woman with suspected adrenal pathology.

## BASIC CONSIDERATIONS

### *Adrenal Physiology*

The adrenal gland consists of two distinct endocrine organs: the adrenal cortex and medulla. The adrenal cortex is divided into three functional zones: the outermost zona glomerulosa, which produces mineralcorticoids, of which aldosterone is of primary importance; and the zona

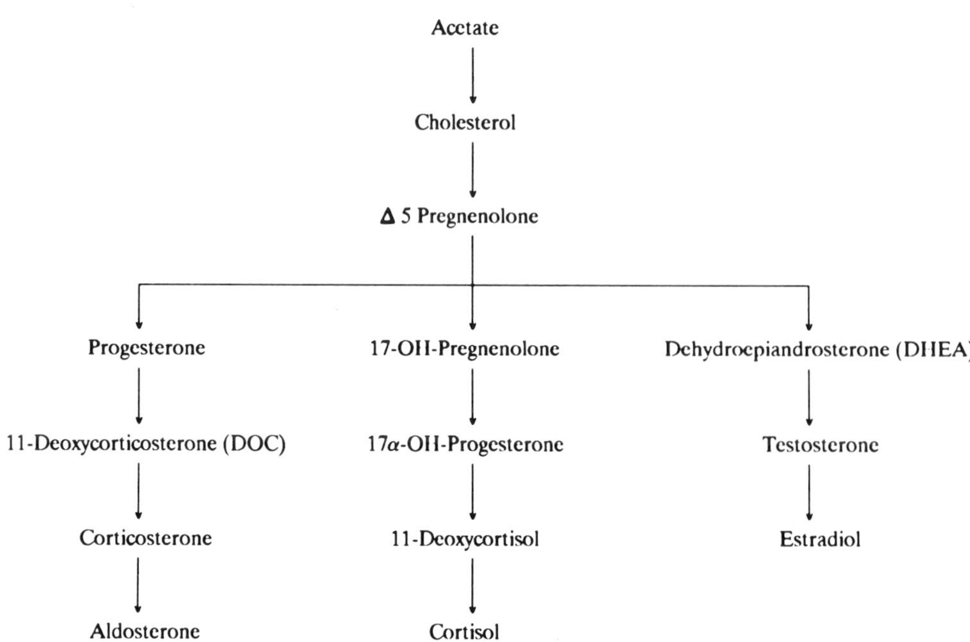


**Fig. 32–1.** Synthetic pathway of the adrenal cortex. Acetate molecules combine via coenzyme A to form the cholesterol nucleus. The side chain of cholesterol is cleared to form Δ5 pregnenolone, the primary precursor of all active adrenocortical hormones. A series of hydroxylations take place in the 17, 21, and 11 positions, resulting in the production of cortisol and aldosterone. Androgens are formed from 17 hydroxylated precursors and in turn serve as precursors for estrogens. (Adapted from Hollingsworth DR: Endocrine disorders of pregnancy. *In* Maternal Fetal Medicine: Principles and Practice. 1st ed. Edited by RK Creasy, R Resnik. Philadelphia, WB Saunders, 1984, p. 935.)

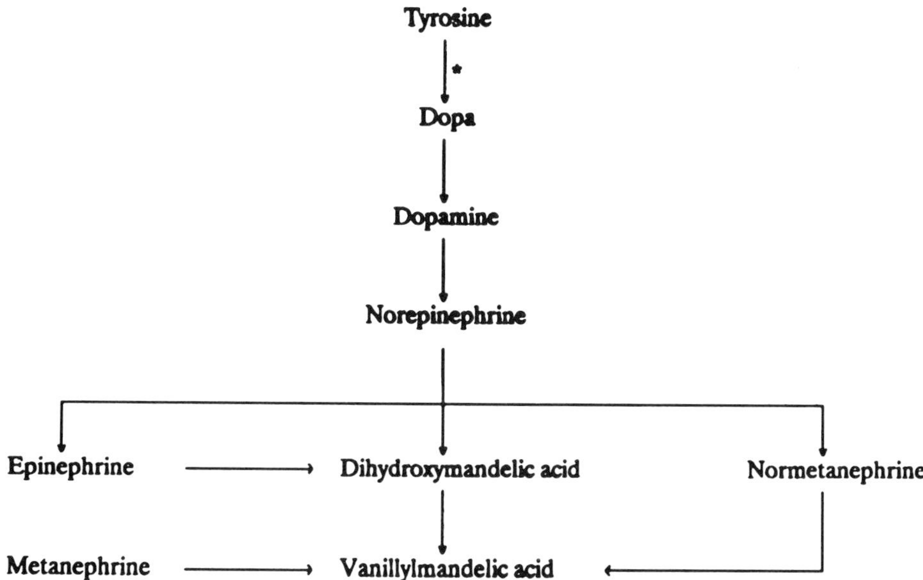


**Fig. 32–2.** The synthesis of endogenous catecholamines by the adrenal medulla; rate limiting step mediated by tyrosine hydroxylase. (Adapted from Tasch, MD: Endocrine diseases. *In* Anesthesia and Co-existing Disease. 1st ed. Edited by RK Stoelting, SF Dierdorf. New York, Churchill Livingstone, 1983, p. 465.)

fasciculata and zona reticularis, which produce glucocorticoids and androgens, respectively. Cholesterol serves as the precursor for steroid synthesis in the adrenal cortex (Figure 32–1) (48).

The adrenal medulla, a specialized organ of the sympathetic nervous system, synthesizes norepinephrine (49). The medulla is perfused by a portal venous system that drains the cortex exposing the medulla to a rich supply of glucocorticoids, primarily cortisol, which induce the various enzymes responsible for catecholamine synthesis (Figure 32–2). Therefore, cortisol secreted in the cortex ultimately regulates catecholamine output from the medulla.

### *Adrenocortical Function in Pregnancy and Labor*

#### Corticosteroid-Binding Globulin (CBG, Transcortin)

During pregnancy, increased estrogen production results in a significant elevation of plasma corticosteroid-binding globulin levels, which are reflected by increased plasma concentrations of total cortisol. Approximately 70% of plasma cortisol is bound by corticosteroid-binding globulin with the remaining 30% bound to albumin or in the free state. At term, the corticosteroid-binding globulin levels are three times the nonpregnant value. In data reported by De Moor, et al (50), the corticosteroid-binding globulin capacity increased from 24 μg cortisol/100 ml in normal nonpregnant females to a mean peak of 45 μg cortisol/100 ml at 28 to 31 weeks of gestation. Corticosteroid-binding globulin concentrations return to the normal nonpregnant level between 1 and 2 months after delivery.

#### Cortisol

Plasma cortisol concentrations rise progressively during pregnancy, surpassing the upper limits of normal nonpregnant values during the second trimester. Cortisol increases significantly during labor and vaginal delivery. This increase can be blocked if the anesthesia is raised to T8, which will reach the upper level of the nerve supply to the adrenal gland. Both bound and free cortisol are increased during labor and vaginal delivery (Figure 32–3). The elevated cortisol levels appear to be the result of both increased production and delayed plasma clearance by the maternal liver. While the increased levels of free cortisol in pregnancy approach those found in Cushing's syndrome, the diurnal variation of plasma cortisol is qualitatively similar to that in nonpregnant women (51).

#### Adrenocorticotropic Hormone (ACTH)

The secretion of hormones from the adrenal cortex is controlled by the pituitary adrenocorticotropic hormone (ACTH). The level of ACTH in plasma rises from early gestation until term (52). This rise has been postulated to occur as a result of placental ACTH that is not subject to negative feedback control by cortisol. Alternatively, increases in maternal clearance of free cortisol, as observed in pregnancy, may contribute to an increase in ACTH secretion.

#### Aldosterone/Deoxycorticosterone (DOC)

Aldosterone and deoxycorticosterone (DOC) rise early in pregnancy and increase approximately threefold during the last two trimesters (53). During gestation, deoxycorticosterone levels cannot be suppressed by dexamethasone and are unresponsive to ACTH. These findings suggest that the increased deoxycorticosterone secretion in pregnancy does not arise from the conventional ACTH-dependent pathways of the maternal adrenal (54).

## ***Cushing's Syndrome (Hypercortisolism)***

### *Basic Considerations*

In most instances, Cushing's syndrome develops as a result of excessive circulating corticosteroids stimulated

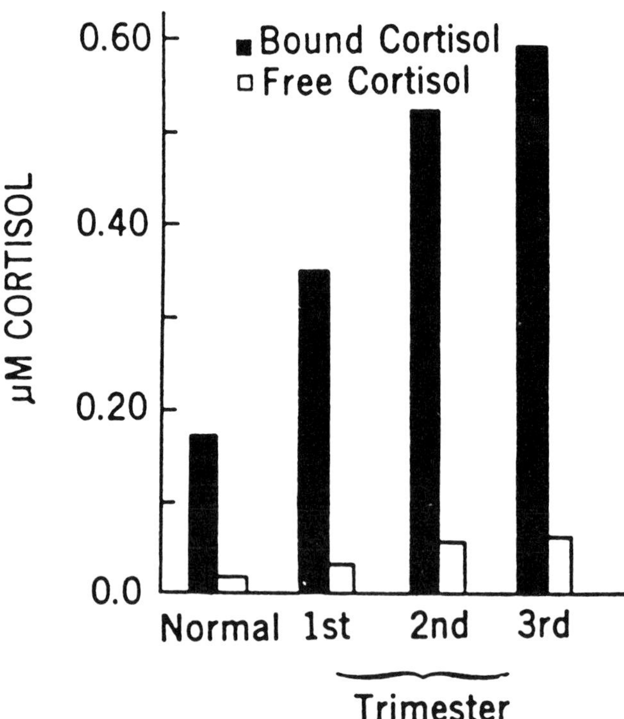


**Fig. 32–3.** Concentrations of free and bound cortisol with advancing gestation. (With permission from Rosenthal HE, Slaunwhite Jr WR, Sandberg AA: Transcortin: A corticosteroid-binding protein of plasma. X. Cortisol and progesterone interplay and unbound levels of these steroids in pregnancy. Clin. Endocrinol. Metab. 29:352, 1969.)

by specific adrenal tumors, bilateral adrenocortical hyperplasia, or exogenous corticosteroid therapy. The syndrome is observed predominantly among older women and is characterized by protein loss, central obesity, easy bruisability, emotional disturbances, hirsutism, acne, muscle weakness, osteoporosis, hypertension, and impaired glucose tolerance (55). This clinical presentation is identical to that of Cushing's disease, in which a basophilic adenoma of the pituitary gland causes excessive secretion of ACTH resulting in adrenocortical hyperfunction. The classical physical features of Cushing's syndrome include a round face with full cheeks (moon face) and an increased fat deposition over the upper dorsal vertebrae (buffalo hump).

Cushing's syndrome rarely complicates pregnancy, as these patients are commonly anovulatory and infertile. When pregnancy does occur, however, studies have reported a high rate of pregnancy loss due to preterm birth and intrauterine death (56). Kreines, et al (56) found that 4 of 16 pregnancies associated with Cushing's syndrome resulted in spontaneous abortions and another four in stillbirths. The other eight women all had preterm births. One premature infant, born at 30 weeks, required steroid therapy for adrenal insufficiency, while two prenatal deaths exhibited a significant reduction in adrenal size at autopsy. Clearly, Cushing's syndrome during pregnancy presents a significant perinatal risk.

### *Obstetric Management*

### Diagnosis in Pregnancy

It is often difficult to make an accurate diagnosis of Cushing's syndrome during pregnancy because central obesity, mild hypertension, fatigue, emotional lability, and glucose intolerance are common to both conditions. The abnormal striae in Cushing's syndrome, however, are often wider and more deeply purple. Progressive hirsutism and acne may also contribute to the clinical presentation of increased adrenal steroid production. The dexamethasone suppression test, which is frequently used to confirm the diagnosis of Cushing's syndrome in the nonpregnant population, has been shown to be both inaccurate and misleading during pregnancy (57). A 24-hour urine collection for free cortisol serves as a useful screening test. If the urinary free cortisol is elevated, a plasma ACTH determination should be obtained. Elevated or high normal levels suggest an abnormal increase in ACTH secretions during pregnancy. Undetectable or very low levels may indicate feedback suppression secondary to high cortisol production by an adrenal tumor. It is also helpful to document the presence or absence of the normal diurnal cortisol variation by obtaining a 24-hour profile of plasma cortisol (51). Ultrasonography and computed tomography (CT scan) of the adrenal glands and CT evaluation of the sella turcica may localize the adrenal or pituitary abnormality (55).

### *Treatment*

Because Cushing's syndrome represents a significant risk to the developing fetus, it should be treated if encountered during pregnancy (56). The traditional therapy for this disorder is surgical. If the etiology of the hyperadrenocorticism is excessive secretion of ACTH by a pituitary gland tumor, a transphenoidal microadenectomy may be indicated (58). Adrenalectomy is performed for patients with a benign adenoma of the adrenal cortex or carcinoma of the adrenal cortex. Irradiation of the pituitary gland or medical treatment with cyproheptadine has been used with varying degrees of success as alternatives to surgical management in patients with small pituitary adenomas (59). Gormley, et al (60) successfully managed a patient with an adrenal adenoma detected at 24 weeks gestation using metyrapone. These alternative treatment regimens represent isolated exceptions to the traditional rule of surgical management for this disorder.

### *Anesthetic Considerations*

An initial preoperative assessment of airway, cardiovascular function, blood pressure, electrolyte balance, acid-base status, and plasma glucose is imperative in the patient with Cushing's syndrome. Depending on the age of the patient, the extent of resultant osteoporosis must be considered for both proper intraoperative positioning and spinal access for regional anesthesia (61). The choice of drugs used for either preoperative medication or production of anesthesia is not influenced by the presence of hyperadrenocorticism (61). Attempts to reduce adrenal cortical activity with narcotics, barbiturates, or volatile anesthetics are generally not helpful because any drug-induced inhibition will be overridden by the stimulation associated with intense labor or surgery. In addition, regional anesthesia, although the preferred method of analgesia, may also be ineffective in preventing increased cortisol secretion during labor or surgery (62).

A significant intraoperative risk for aspiration exists in these patients due to obesity and the delayed gastric emptying time encountered in pregnancy. Preoperative $H_2$ blockers and antacids have been suggested as reasonable prophylactic measures. A continuous intravenous infusion of cortisol at a rate equivalent to 100 g/day should be initiated intraoperatively if a hypophysectomy or bilateral adrenalectomy has been performed (63). Mechanical ventilation during surgery is suggested, as skeletal muscle weakness, with or without coexisting hypokalemia, may diminish the strength of the respiratory muscles. Corticosteroid therapy is necessary in the postoperative period and should be instituted in consultation with an endocrinologist.

## Adrenocortical Insufficiency (Addison's Disease)

Addison's disease is probably the most common disorder of the adrenal gland encountered during pregnancy (64). It is, however, a relatively rare disease with an insidious onset that comes to a crisis following stress, e.g., surgery, acute infections, trauma, or termination of pregnancy. With adequate medical management, the prognosis for both mother and fetus is excellent.

### Chronic Adrenal Insufficiency

#### Etiology and Pathophysiology

Addison's disease may develop as a result of several processes (60). Autoimmune disease, hemorrhage, or granulomatous disease can destroy the adrenal cortex. Anterior pituitary dysfunction or panhypopituitarism can cause a deficiency of ACTH. Finally, administration of exogenous corticosteroids can result in adrenal-pituitary axis suppression.

#### Symptoms and Signs

Skeletal muscle weakness, weight loss, hypotension, and hyperpigmentation are common manifestations of primary adrenal insufficiency due to destruction of the adrenal cortex. Hyperpigmentation results from excessive production of melanocyte-stimulating hormone by the anterior pituitary. Any significant stress may result in Addisonian crisis, a true medical emergency manifested by fever, nausea and vomiting, diarrhea, abdominal pain, hypotension with circulatory collapse, hyperkalemia, hyponatremia, hypoglycemia, and intravascular hemoconcentration (65). The intravascular fluid compartment is contracted, and the clinical picture is characterized by hypovolemic shock. Hypoadrenocorticism secondary to anterior pituitary dysfunction is less likely to be associated with severe disturbances in electrolyte balance or volume status because aldosterone secretion is maintained. However, panhypopituitarism may be associated with signs and symptoms associated with absent growth hormone, thyroid-stimulating hormone, and gonadotropins, in addition to the numerous manifestations of ACTH deficiency.

#### Diagnosis

The clinical parameters for diagnosis during pregnancy are less reliable because weakness, fatigue, increased pigmentation, weight loss, anorexia, hypoglycemia, and nervousness occur both in normal pregnancy and in Addison's disease. In a review by Brent, et al, 4 of 39 cases (10%) were initially diagnosed in the puerperium when they developed adrenal crisis (66). Patients with untreated Addison's disease appear to tolerate pregnancy quite well. In a study by Drucker, et al, 55% of patients with adrenocortical insufficiency carried their pregnancies to term only to develop Addisonian crisis in the early postpartum period (67). Postpartum diuresis has been postulated to be an etiologic factor for the development of a crisis in the puerperium.

The laboratory diagnosis of Addison's disease, if not clinically apparent, rests primarily on the lack of rise in the plasma cortisol concentration after intravenous cortrosyn infusion (65). Two-hundred fifty milligrams of Cosyntropin, a synthetic subunit of ACTH (cortrosyn), is given as an intravenous bolus with serum cortisol levels being measured at baseline and 1 hour after the injection. Occasionally, it is necessary to prolong the test by giving 250 mg in 500 ml of 5% dextrose over 8 hours on 3 consecutive days. In normal women, the plasma cortisol level will increase to more than 20 μg/ml. ACTH levels are also helpful in differentiating Addison's disease from panhypopituitarism. Low-plasma cortisol and 24-hour urine free cortisol levels below normal pregnancy values provide additional laboratory evidence for the diagnosis of adrenocortical insufficiency during pregnancy.

#### Treatment

In the patient presenting with Addisonian crisis, one must confirm the diagnosis and immediately institute appropriate therapy. ACTH and cortisol levels should be determined and replacement therapy started immediately with an intravenous bolus of 100 to 200 mg of hydrocortisone sodium succinate (Solu-cortef) and a continuous infusion of normal saline and 5% dextrose (65). A central venous line or a pulmonary artery catheter may be helpful in guiding adequate hydration, which usually approaches 5 to 6 liters of fluid over the first 24 hours. The first liter is given over 30 minutes and should contain 50 g of glucose to prevent hypoglycemia. Each liter of fluid replacement should also contain 100 mg of Solu-cortef. The mineralocorticoid activity in this amount of cortisol makes administration of 9-alpha-fluorohydrocortisone (Florinef) or other mineralocorticoid unnecessary. Within 24 hours, one can usually change to once or twice daily intramuscular cortisone injections (25 to 50 mg) (68).

#### Maintenance During Pregnancy

During pregnancy, the usual dosage of adrenal steroid replacement is continued. Most patients' adrenal steroid requirements are adequately replaced with cortisone acetate, 25 mg in the morning and 12.5 mg at night, with 0.05 to 0.10 mg of 9-alpha-flurohydrocortisone daily. Alternatively, some patients may receive prednisone, 5.0 mg in the morning and 2.5 mg at night. The decreased mineralocorticoid activity of prednisone makes the 9-alpha-flurohydrocortisone even more important with this regimen. During labor, adequate hydration is a primary concern and cortisone acetate, 25 mg every 6 hours, should be given intravenously over several hours (55). In the early postpartum period, the patient should continue to receive parenteral steroids and fluids for several days to avoid a postpartum Addisonian crisis. The offspring of patients receiving steroids for Addison's disease have exhibited a tendency toward growth retardation attributed primarily to prolonged fetal hypoglycemia (69). On occasion, cortisol, 2 mg/kg every 8 hours, and 10% dextrose given intravenously are required to treat the rare infant who develops temporary iatrogenic adrenal insufficiency secondary to maternal steroid therapy (64).

### Anesthetic Considerations

The anesthetic management for the patient with known Addison's disease presents no unique problems, other than provision of exogenous corticosteroids as outlined above and a high index of suspicion for primary adrenal insufficiency should intraoperative hypotension occur. With the exception of etomidate, an imidazole sedative-hypnotic that exhibits a dose-related and time-related pattern of adrenal suppression, the selection of anesthetic drugs for preoperative and intraoperative administration is seldom influenced by the presence of treated hypoadrenocorticism (70). On occasion, skeletal muscle weakness may require the titration of muscle relaxants using monitored peripheral nerve stimulation. When using conduction anesthesia, careful attention should be directed to maintenance of volume status because these patients are especially susceptible to the hypotensive complications experienced with regional blockade.

## Primary Aldosteronism (Conn's Syndrome)

### Etiology and Pathophysiology

Primary hyperaldosteronism is due to excessive secretion of aldosterone from a functional adrenal tumor acting independently of a physiologic stimulus. This disease process occurs infrequently in pregnancy and is manifested by signs and symptoms reflecting the physiologic effects of aldosterone. Hypertension, paresthesia, headaches, periodic paralysis, polyuria, and polydipsia represent salient clinical features (71). As previously described under the section "Adrenocortical Function in Pregnancy," aldosterone excretion is increased in pregnancy, making the diagnosis of primary aldosteronism more difficult.

### Diagnosis

Confirmation of the diagnosis is demonstrated by an increased plasma aldosterone concentration above normal pregnant levels and elevated urinary potassium excretion. Measurement of plasma renin activity allows classification of the disease as primary (low renin activity) or secondary (elevated renin activity) (61). Selective adrenal gland venography and scanning studies may be helpful in differentiating hyperaldosteronism due to a functional tumor from that produced by adrenal cortical hyperplasia.

### Treatment

The definitive treatment for an aldosterone-secreting tumor is surgical excision. If there are multiple aldosterone-secreting tumors, bilateral adrenalectomy may be necessary. Spironolactone has been used successfully to manage hyperaldosteronism secondary to adrenal cortical hyperplasia (72). Caution should be exercised when using spironolactone in pregnancy, as animal studies have demonstrated an antiandrogenic effect in the fetus (73).

### Anesthetic Considerations

The primary anesthetic consideration is preoperative correction of hypokalemia and treatment of hypertension. Persistence of hypokalemia may modify the expected response to nondepolarizing neuromuscular blockers. With the exception of enflurane, which should be avoided in patients with hypokalemic nephropathy and polyuria, most inhaled or injected agents are acceptable for the maintenance of anesthesia (71). Meticulous attention to intravascular volume status is facilitated by a right atrial or pulmonary artery catheter. Acid-base status and serum electrolyte concentrations should be measured frequently in the perioperative period. Supplementation with exogenous cortisol is only necessary if surgery involves both adrenal glands. A continuous intravenous infusion of hydrocortisone sodium succinate (Solucortef) 100 mg every 24 hours may be initiated empirically if extensive surgery is anticipated. Although the data are limited, regional anesthesia appears to be a reasonable option for management of labor and delivery.

## Pheochromosytoma

### Etiology and Pathophysiology

Pheochromocytoma is a catecholamine-secreting tumor that originates in the adrenal medulla in over 90% of documented cases and has been described as arising from the sympathetic ganglia in the wall of the urinary bladder or among the paravertebral sympathetic chain (74). Approximately 10% of adrenal tumors are bilateral with less than 10% undergoing malignant change. Pheochromocytomas most commonly occur during the third or fourth decade of life which, in most instances, is outside the typical reproductive age group. If pheochromocytoma occurs during pregnancy, significant morbidity and mortality for both mother and fetus have been described. In a study by Schenker, et al, the maternal mortality was 55% when the diagnosis was made postpartum (75). In the same study, the overall fetal loss rate for patients with pheochromocytoma was 53% when diagnosed after delivery and 46% when the diagnosis was made during the antepartum period. Overall, only 50% of the diagnoses of pheochromocytoma are made prior to delivery. Durham reported a mortality rate of 48% and 58% for the mother and fetus, respectively, in 111 cases of pheochromocytoma (76). Most of the maternal deaths (58%) occurred before the diagnosis and resulted from severe pulmonary edema or cerebral vascular accidents.

#### Diagnosis

The signs and symptoms of pheochromocytoma during pregnancy include headache, epigastric pain, sustained or paroxysmal hypertension, chest pain, palpitations, perspiration, pallor, flushing, numbness, fainting, and dizziness. Postural hypotension is seen in approximately 50 to 60% of cases and cardiac hypertrophy, cardiomyopathy, sinus arrhythmias, and hypertensive encephalopathy have also been reported (77). The laboratory findings include hyperglycemia, hemoconcentration, and increased serum-free fatty acids secondary to alterations in catecholamine action. The definitive diagnosis depends on the demonstration of increased catecholamines, metanephrine, and vanillymandelic acid (VMA) in the urine or increased catecholamines in the blood. Urinary assays have been found to be more reliable because blood catecholamines may be elevated episodically or in other forms of hypertension. It is important to remember that methyldopa may interfere with catecholamine determination and should be discontinued before obtaining levels. Schenker described elevated urinary catecholamine levels in 43 of 48 (90%) of cases of pheochromocytoma (75).

#### Treatment

The high maternal and fetal mortality rates associated with pheochromocytoma in pregnancy mandate prompt treatment once the diagnosis has been established. All patients should be confined to strict bedrest and alpha-adrenergic blocking agents should be instituted. In the acute setting, phentolamine hydrochloride may be injected intravenously, 2 to 5 mg every 5 minutes, until the blood pressure stabilizes (68). Maintenance therapy with phenoxybenzamine in oral doses ranging from 4 to 100 mg/12 hr has been recommended to avoid the gastric side effects associated with phentolamine. Definitive treatment in most cases is surgical. If the diagnosis of pheochromocytoma is made before 24 weeks gestation, the tumor should be removed after medical stabilization (78). If the diagnosis is made after 24 weeks gestation, the mother should be treated with phenoxybenzamine until fetal lung maturity is established, and then delivery accomplished via cesarean section with concurrent excision of the adrenal tumors (79).

#### Anesthetic Considerations

The primary considerations in the pregnant patient with a pheochromocytoma is preoperative normalization of blood pressure and intravascular blood volume with alpha-adrenergic blockade (phenoxybenzamine) and control of tachyarrhythmias and ventricular ectopy with beta-adrenergic blockade (propranolol). With the exception of halothane, which should be avoided because it has been shown to sensitize the myocardium to catecholamines (80), enflurane, isoflurane, balanced nitrous oxide and narcotics, and regional anesthesia have all been successful anesthetic techniques. Using invasive hemodynamic monitoring has been suggested, as many of these patients display hemodynamic instability following excision of the tumor as a result of changing levels of plasma catecholamines and altered systemic vascular resistance. Postoperative surveillance in an intensive care unit also appears to be a prudent consideration.

## Pituitary Gland

### *Prolactin-Producing Adenomas*

#### Incidence and Symptomatology

The incidence of pituitary tumors presenting clinically in women of reproductive age has been reported to be 7.1/1000 (81). These women tend to have lower fertility rates secondary to disturbances in ovarian function caused by elevated prolactin levels. With the judicious use of bromocriptine, human menopausal gonadotropin, or clomiphene citrate, many patients now successfully achieve conception. Magyar and Marshal have reviewed the course of 91 pregnancies in 73 women with untreated pituitary tumors (82). The most common tumor-related symptoms were headache (23%) and visual disturbances (25%). The onset of visual disturbances tends to occur at approximately 14 weeks gestation, following the onset of headaches by 4 weeks. These problems arise secondary to the expanding pituitary adenoma, which impinges on the optic chiasma. In most cases, however, pregnancy will be uneventful, and few patients will experience symptoms or complications attributable to a pituitary adenoma. In studies by Gemzell, et al (83) Husami, et al (84), and Magyar, et al (82), 1 to 5% of patients with a pituitary adenoma experienced a complication that was directly related to the pituitary tumor. Most importantly, in those who were diagnosed as having a tumor less than 1 cm in size (a microadenoma), most were asymptomatic throughout pregnancy.

#### Diagnosis

In most cases, the diagnosis of a prolactin-secreting adenoma in pregnancy is a radiologic diagnosis. Computerized tomographic imaging of the sella turcica has replaced the conedown view as the diagnostic procedure of choice. Evaluation of serum prolactin levels during pregnancy is only marginally helpful because values greater than 200 ng/ml are frequently encountered with advancing gestation (85). A strong clinical suspicion aroused by a patient presenting with severe headaches, visual disturbances, or a history of oligo-ovulation or anovulation in which prolactin levels may have been elevated before conception, should prompt appropriate investigative measures.

#### Treatment

Most authorities agree that patients with a pituitary macroadenoma (larger than 1 cm) should receive adequate treatment consisting of surgery, bromocriptine, radiation, or a combination of modalities before pregnancy or induction of ovulation. Surgical or radiation therapy are now used less frequently due to the inherent complications of infection, diabetes insipidus, anosmia, visual field defects, and panhypopituitarism (86). At the present time, a more conservative medical approach using bromocriptine in doses ranging from 5 to 20 mg/day has become the therapy of choice for symptomatic pituitary adenomas. Recommendations for management of asymptomatic microadenomas include monthly serum prolactin determinations and visual field examinations. If visual field defects arise due to tumor enlargement in early pregnancy, bromocriptine or transsphenoidal hypophysectomy may be indicated. In the patient who is approaching term, however, the pregnancy may be terminated by elective induction of labor or cesarean section once fetal pulmonary maturity has been established (82).

### Anesthetic Considerations

The anesthetic considerations for this disease process entail concern for maintaining a quiet, pain-free state during the labor and delivery process. The possibility exists for systemic medication given in intravenous small quantities to relieve the maximum pain caused by the uterine contraction. This can be by small intravenous doses of demerol 25 mg, or fentanyl 1 mg, or nubaine 5 mg. The best method for excellent labor and delivery pain relief is the continuous epidural method with the pump and small doses of local anesthetic/opioid. For second stage pain relief, a perineal dose of nesacaine or 2% lidocaine or 0.5% bupivacaine for delivery through the indwelling epidural catheter can be used. If this is not possible or another method is preferred, then the saddle block for a selective perineal block or the pudendal block for the same reason can be substituted.

## Panhypopituitarism (Sheehan's Syndrome)

### Etiology and Pathophysiology

In 1939, Sheehan described a syndrome of panhypopituitarism occurring in 9/10,000 term pregnancies complicated by postpartum hemorrhage and shock (87). While the exact etiology is unknown, Sheehan postulated that anterior pituitary necrosis may result from an inadequate blood supply to the enlarged pituitary of a gravida during a hemorrhagic hypotensive episode. Sheehan reported that significant clinical manifestations of pituitary hypofunction became evident only after 75% of the entire gland was destroyed.

Classically, the clinical picture of pituitary deficiency follows a sequential loss of gonadotropins, growth hormone, thyroid stimulating hormone (TSH), and ACTH. Failure of lactation and rapid involution of the breasts are the earliest postpartum signs. These women with pituitary deficiency typically fail to regain strength and vigor in the postpartum period and are commonly misdiagnosed as having postpartum depression. Hypoglycemia secondary to growth hormone deficiency has been described in the postpartum period with blood glucose levels of 50 to 60 mg/dL (88). Secondary to a significant reduction in gonadotropin production, the uterus may be suprainvoluted, the menses scanty or absent, the ovaries and genitalia atrophic, and the patient's libido significantly reduced. In the later stages of severe disease, patients may experience adrenal insufficiency, hypothyroidism, hyperchromic anemia, and loss of axillary and pubic hair.

### Symptoms and Signs

Pituitary necrosis has been described in the antepartum period in patients with type I diabetes mellitus. Dorfman described eight patients with diabetes mellitus who suffered antepartum pituitary necrosis (89). Clinical suspicion should be aroused in the antepartum diabetic patient who has a persistent, deep, midline headache, nausea, vomiting, fatigue, lassitude, weakness, as well as an unexplained decrease in insulin requirement.

### Diagnosis

In the postpartum period, patients who fail to lactate, or in nonlactating patients, those who fail to menstruate 4 to 6 months after delivery, should have investigative measures initiated. Extensive diagnostic testing to evaluate all pituitary hormones is both unnecessary and impractical. Pregnancy alters the usual serum levels of various pituitary hormones as well as the responsiveness to TSH and ACTH. Evaluation of serum prolactin and thyroxine (T4) levels represents a good initial screening test. If these tests are abnormal, a more extensive protocol may be instituted. Serum T4 and TSH should be measured to distinguish between primary and pituitary or hypothalamic hypothyroidism. In the primary form, T4 levels are decreased (less than 6.0 μg/100 ml) and TSH levels elevated (more than 10 micronunits/ml). In pituitary or hypothalamic hypothyroidism, serum T4 levels are also decreased but the serum TSH is low or normal (less than 2 microunits/ml) (90). Serum cortisol levels may also be measured to evaluate the need for glucocorticoid replacement.

### Treatment

The treatment for Sheehan's syndrome consists of specific replacement of the deficient anterior pituitary hormones. Replacement hormones may include gonadotropins, cortisol, and thyroxine. Administration of a mineralocorticoid is usually unnecessary because the release of aldosterone is maintained in the absence of ACTH. While growth hormone is not needed in adults, those individuals experiencing urogenital atrophy may benefit from estrogen-replacement therapy (68).

### Anesthetic Considerations

Anesthetic management of patients with panhypopituitarism is simply the basic application of sound anesthetic principles. Because the primary loss of pituitary stimulation is in gonadotropins, growth hormone, thyroid-stimulating hormone, and ACTH, attention is directed toward the implicated physiological effects. These are noted in Table 32–2.

As evident from review of the anesthetic implications, the chief concerns in the treatment of Sheehan's syndrome are in the area of maintenance of normal heart

**Table 32–2.** Anesthetic Implications of Hormones

| Hormone | Effect | Anesthetic Implication |
|---|---|---|
| gonadotropins | sex organs | minimal or none |
| growth hormone | general growth | minimal or none |
| thyroid stimulating hormone | general energy | heart rate |
| ACTH | mineralocorticoid | electrolytes |

rate and balance of electrolytes. As mentioned, the clinical case may not be manifest until some 75% of the gland is destroyed. Replacement therapy may not include mineralocorticoid because aldosterone may be maintained in the absence of ACTH. Thus, chances are there will be little, if any, electrolyte problems. The chief problem is then reduced to the hypothyroid aspect, and this is not a strict contraindication to regional anesthesia in mild to moderate cases. Patients are normally able to accommodate to reductions in systemic vascular resistance with increasing resistance in nonaffected areas and by adjustments in heart rate. For labor, the continuous epidural method with the pump and small doses of local anesthetic/opioid can be very effective and free of complications. Otherwise for labor pain, small doses of systemic opioids can be given over a few minutes to note the analgesic effect and the effect upon the fetal heart rate. This may be 25 mg of demerol, 1 mg aliquots of fentanyl, or 5 mg of nubaine. For the actual delivery, local anesthetic injections in the form of pudendal blocks with small amounts of inhalation anesthetic can serve the need quite well. For cesarean section, the epidural can be used with small challenge doses given over several minutes with sensory level checks and accommodation to any blood pressure changes. The use of the subarachnoid block can precipitate the greatest fall in blood pressure in the shortest period of time and thus its use may best be limited to the continuous catheter method with small doses given and accommodation carefully evaluated over several minutes just as in the epidural scenario. Of course, cesarean section can also be done under the local anesthetic technique as described in Chapter 30.

## *Diabetes Insipidus*

### *Etiology and Pathophysiology*

Diabetes insipidus is a rare disease with an incidence in the general population of from 1 in 16,000 to 1 in 82,000 (91). This disorder is characterized by an absence of antidiuretic hormone (ADH) release secondary to destruction of the posterior pituitary, or failure of the renal tubules to respond to antidiuretic hormone, nephrogenic diabetes insipidus. Destruction of the posterior pituitary may result from Sheehan's syndrome, intracranial trauma, hypophysectomy, or pituitary neoplasia.

### *Signs and Symptoms*

The classic manifestations of diabetes insipidus are polydipsia and a high output of poorly concentrated urine (polyuria), despite normal or increased serum osmolality. Patients with diabetes insipidus usually exhibit normal fertility. However, this disorder may worsen during pregnancy, presumably secondary to an increased requirement for ADH, with the increased glomerular filtration seen as gestation advances.

### *Diagnosis*

The diagnosis is suspected when symptoms of polyuria and polydipsia are associated with urine-specific gravities below 1.010 and osmolalities less than that of plasma. The diagnosis may be confirmed by a water deprivation test during which the patient remains polyuric without having corresponding increases in urine osmolality. Treatment with exogenous vasopressin (ADH) results in a significant increase in urine osmolality, which substantiates the diagnosis. A CT scan is indicated to rule out a pituitary or hypothalamic lesion in the patient who presents with new onset disease during pregnancy.

### *Treatment*

The standard treatment for diabetes insipidus has changed from parenteral vasopressin to intranasal L-deamino-8-d-arginine vasopressin (DDAVP) (92). Dosage regimens of 0.1 ml intranasally up to 3 times daily have resulted in a reliable and immediate response. Although vasopressin has been postulated to cause uterine contractions, there have been no consistent reports of spontaneous abortion or premature labor associated with treatment during pregnancy (91). Several reports have documented good perinatal outcomes in pregnancies complicated by diabetes insipidus treated with appropriate therapy (93).

### *Anesthetic Considerations*

Aside from careful monitoring of urinary output and serum electrolytes during the perioperative period, there are no specific anesthetic considerations. Continuous epidural analgesia is the preferred technique for the management of labor and vaginal delivery. However, other regional techniques of inhalation analgesia anesthesia may also be used.

## Thyroid Gland

Thyroid disease is common among women of the reproductive age group and it occurs in approximately 0.2% of all pregnancies (94). The successful management of these patients is predicated on a thorough understanding of the disease processes and the potential effects that various treatment modalities may have on both the mother and fetus.

### *Thyroid Function In Pregnancy*

The metabolic demands encountered in pregnancy result in both an increase in the size and function of the thyroid gland. The enlargement of the gland is believed to represent a compensatory mechanism to maintain glandular activity despite decreases in plasma inorganic iodine

**Table 32–3.** Thyroid Function Tests in Pregnancy*

| Test | Normal Nonpregnant | Normal Pregnant | Hyperthyroidism | Comment |
|---|---|---|---|---|
| Total serum thyroxine | 4.5–12.5 μg/100 ml | Increased | Increased | Elevation is secondary to increased serum thyroxine binding globulin (TBG) |
| Resin triiodothyronine uptake (T3RU) | 25–35% | Decreased | Increased | Decrease is secondary to increase in TBG resulting in diminished resin uptake |
| Free thyroxine (FT4) | 1.0–2.1 ng/100 ml | Unchanged | Increased | Most sensitive indicator, diagnostic of hyperthyroidism if elevated |
| Total serum triiodothyronine (T3) | 90–120 ng/100 ml | Increased | Increased | Elevation is secondary to increased TBG |
| Thyroid stimulating hormone (TSH) | up to 7 μU/ml | Unchanged | Increased | Increase in primary hypothyroidism |
| Free thyroxine index (FT4I) | 3.5–11.0 μg/100 ml (Calculated value) | Not increased | Increased | $FT4I = Total\ T4 \cdot \frac{(T3RU\ of\ patient)}{Normal\ T3RU}$ (a calculated estimate of free thyroxine) |

* Normal values must be determined at the laboratory where performed.
(Modified from Cunningham FG, MacDonald PC, Gant NF: Williams Obstetrics. 18th Ed. Norwalk, Appleton & Lange, 1989, p. 154.)

(94). The increased metabolic demand coupled with significant hormonal changes in pregnancy result in dramatic alterations in the results of thyroid function tests (90,95). Secondary to a rise in estrogen, thyroxine binding globulin (TBG) reaches levels that are twice that of the nonpregnant woman by the twelfth week of gestation. While total thyroxine is elevated, free levels of T4 and triiodothyronine (T3) are generally not increased during pregnancy. Understanding these changes is important because many diagnostic and therapeutic decisions are based on the interpretation of these laboratory tests. Table 32–3 compares normal nonpregnant thyroid function test parameters with the changes expected during normal gestation (90).

## Hyperthyroidism

### Etiology and Pathophysiology

Hyperthyroidism results from excess secretion of T3 and/or T4 by the thyroid gland (96). While there is no clear evidence that pregnancy worsens the disease, control of hyperthyroidism is essential for maternal and fetal well-being. Uncontrolled hyperthyroidism has been reported to be associated with increased neonatal morbidity secondary to premature delivery and intrauterine growth retardation (94,96). Thyroid storm, a true endocrinologic emergency, may occur in the partially treated or undiagnosed patient. Grave's disease is by far the most common cause of hyperthyroidism in the pregnant patient. Other etiologies included in the differential diagnosis of hyperthyroidism are outlined in Table 32–4) (97).

### Symptoms and Signs

The clinical signs and symptoms of hyperthyroidism during pregnancy may be obscured by the normal hypermetabolic state of pregnancy. Heat intolerance, mild tachycardia, thyroid enlargement, and nervousness are common findings in many normal pregnancies. Thyrotoxicosis, however, should be suspected when a patient exhibits exophthalmos, lid lag (von Graefe's sign), tremor, obvious goiter, hyperreflexia, a resting tachycardia in excess of 100 beats per minute, or weight loss despite excellent dietary intake (68).

### Diagnosis

The laboratory diagnosis of hyperthyroidism in pregnancy is confirmed by an elevated free thyroxine index (FT4I) or free thyroxine. An assay for thyroid-stimulating immunoglobulin (TSIG, formerly LATS) is helpful in confirming the diagnosis of Grave's disease. Thyroid-stimulating immunoglobulins have resulted in fetal thyroid stimulation and resultant fetal/neonatal hyperthyroidism in approximately 1% of pregnant women with Grave's disease (98).

**Table 32–4.** Differential Diagnosis for Hyperthyroidism

1. Struma ovarii with hyperthyroidism
2. TSH-producing tumor
3. Pituitary resistance to thyroid hormone
4. Exogenous thyroid hormone
   a. Overzealous thyroid replacement
   b. Thyrotoxicosis factitia
   c. T3 suppression test
5. Plummer disease
6. Grave's disease
7. Jod-Basedow effect (hyperthyroidism due to exogenous iodide)
8. Toxic adenoma
9. Thyroiditis
   a. Subacute thyroiditis
   b. Silent thyroiditis
   c. Hashimoto's thyroiditis (early disease)
   d. Radiation thyroiditis
10. Albright syndrome (polyostotic fibrous dysplasia)
11. Metastatic thyroid carcinoma
12. Circulating thyroid stimulators (malignancies)
    a. Choriocarcinoma/hydatidiform mole
    b. Embryonal carcinoma

(Adapted from Lang R: New thyroid treatments, tests—even new diseases. Contemp. Obstet. Gynecol. 19:102, 1982, p. 104.)

### Treatment

The treatment of hyperthyroidism in pregnancy involves either antithyroid medication or surgery. Radioactive iodine therapy, a valuable treatment modality in the nonpregnant patient, is contraindicated during pregnancy. At 10 to 11 weeks gestation, the fetal thyroid undergoes colloid and follicle formation rendering it vulnerable to the destruction that may result from the uptake of radioactive iodine (99). The mainstay of medical treatment of hyperthyroidism in pregnancy is the thioamide, propylthiouracil (PTU) (100). This drug inhibits thyroid hormone synthesis by blocking the iodination of tyrosine molecules and by partially blocking the conversion of T4 to T3. Methimazole (tapazole) has been used interchangeably with propylthiouracil without significant therapeutic advantage; moreover, recent reports of aplasia cutis of the scalp in newborns of mothers taking tapazole have made propylthiouracil the drug of choice during pregnancy (101). The usual starting dose of propylthiouracil is 100 to 150 mg every 8 hours. Therapeutic effects are usually observed 2 to 4 weeks following the initiation of therapy. Once a therapeutic response has been achieved, as exemplified by a normalizing of free T4 or FT4I and a stabilizing clinical picture, the dose may be reduced to a level that results in a mildly hyperthyroid state (100). Overzealous treatment, resulting in hypothyroidism, must be avoided to allow appropriate fetal growth and development (102).

### Anesthetic Considerations

The first concern is for the status of the mother at the time of labor. By that time, hopefully, the patient's condition will be under control, specifically, the heart rate will be baseline or not greatly elevated. Pain relief for labor can be by systemic analgesics as noted in the previous section on Sheehan's syndrome. To reiterate, pain relief can be administered with small intravenous doses of demerol 25 mg, or fentanyl 1 mg, or nubaine 5 mg. Other alternatives are again the continuous epidural method with the pump and small doses of local anesthetic/opioid. Pain relief for delivery can be in the form of a perineal dose of nesacaine or 2% lidocaine or 0.5% bupivacaine for delivery through the indwelling epidural catheter. If this is not possible or another method is preferred, then the saddle block for a selective perineal block or the pudendal block for the same reason can be substituted. Because the epidural provides the most profound interruption of the nociceptive input of labor, it is the best choice for maintaining a relaxed, controlled, patient condition in this situation.

## Thyroid Storm

Thyroid storm is a severe exacerbation of hyperthyroidism due to an acute excessive release of thyroid hormone into the circulation. This uncommon condition may result from inadequate treatment of hyperthyroidism or may be the first clinical presentation of an undiagnosed hyperthyroid state. The clinical manifestations of thyroid storm include aberrations in the metabolic, hemodynamic, nervous, and gastrointestinal systems as outlined in Table 32–5. (103).

**Table 32–5.** Thyroid Storm: Clinical Presentation

| System | Manifestations |
|---|---|
| Cardiovascular | Tachycardia, arrhythmias, congestive heart failure |
| Metabolic | Fever, diaphoresis, warm skin, flushing |
| Gastrointestinal | Abdominal pain, vomiting, diarrhea, jaundice |
| Central nervous system | Agitation, disorientation, tremor, delirium, psychosis, coma, stupor |

(Adapted from Mestman JH: Severe hyperthyroidism in pregnancy. *In* Critical Care Obstetrics. Edited by SL Clark, JP Phelan, DB Cotton. Oradell, 1987. Medical Economics Co., Inc.)

### Management Of Thyroid Storm

The management of the patient in thyroid storm is both supportive and specific. The patient should be admitted to an intensive care unit where a search for a precipitating cause and proper treatment can be initiated. Intravenous fluids and electrolytes, cardiac monitoring, cooling measures, and oxygen therapy are the first steps taken along with routine laboratory tests, and blood and urine cultures (104). Drugs used to treat specific manifestations of excessive thyroid gland activity are outlined in Table 32–6 (105). If the patient fails to respond to conventional measures, removal of circulating hormones by plasmapheresis and peritoneal dialysis should be considered (106). When the patient shows clinical improvement, iodides and glucocorticoids may be discontinued. Treatment with antithyroid drugs should be maintained until the patient becomes euthyroid. Postpartum ablative therapy or antepartum subtotal thyroidectomy must be considered in all patients after an initial episode of thyroid storm.

### Anesthetic Considerations

Elective surgery should only be considered when the patient has been rendered euthyroid and the hyperkinetic circulation controlled with propranolol. Sedation in the preoperative period may be produced by administration of an oral barbiturate. Theoretically, narcotics should be avoided because they may stimulate the sympathetic nervous system. Anticholinergics interfere with normal heat-regulating mechanisms that may contribute to tachycardia (61). During the induction and maintenance of anesthesia, one should avoid drugs that result in excessive stimulation of the sympathetic nervous system, sensitize the myocardium to catecholamines, undergo biotransformation that may result in liver toxicity, or provide insufficient potency to offset surgical stimulation of the sympathetic nervous system. Monitoring during maintenance of anesthesia should be directed at early recognition of impending thyroid storm. It is prudent to be prepared by having the appropriate therapeutic measures available should a thyroid storm be encountered. In the patient with exophthalmos, care should be taken to avoid corneal ulceration

**Table 32–6.** Pharmacologic Management of Thyroid Storm

| Drug | Dose | Comments |
|---|---|---|
| Sodium iodide | 0.5–1.0 g IV q 8 hr | Acutely inhibits thyroid hormone secretion. Should be given one hour after initiation of PTU to avoid build-up of hormone stores within the gland. |
| Propylthiouracil | 600 mg p.o. then 300 mg q 6 hr | Reduces the synthesis of new thyroid gland hormones. |
| Propranolol | 1–2 mg/min *or* a dose sufficient to slow the heart rate to 90 bpm *or* 40–80 mg p.o. q 4 hr | Effective in controlling tachycardia and blocks peripheral conversion of T4 to T3. (If ineffective, consider using reserpine.*) |
| Hydrocortisone | 100–200 mg IV q 8 hr | Inhibits peripheral conversion of T4 to T3. |
| Acetaminophen | 10–20 gr rectally q 3–4 hr | Controls hyperpyrexia. Avoid salicylates; they increase free thyroid hormone by inhibiting binding to Thyroxine Binding Globulin (TBG). |

* (Anaissie E, Thome JF: Reserpine in propranolol-resistant thyroid storm. Arch. Intern. Med. 145:2248, 1985.)
(Adapted from Mestman JH: Severe hyperthyroidism in pregnancy. *In* Critical Care Obstetrics. Edited by SL Clark, JP Phelan, DBN Cotton. Oradell, 1987, p. 276. Medical Economics Co., Inc.)

and drying by providing adequate protection for the eyes during the perioperative period. Regional anesthesia, with its associated sympathetic blockade, may provide significant advantages over other methods of analgesia.

## *Hypothyroidism*

### *Etiology and Pathophysiology*

Hypothyroidism is seldom encountered during pregnancy because inadequate thyroid function is often associated with anovulation and infertility (107). Potential etiologies for hypothyroidism include Hashimoto's disease, dietary iodine deficiency (which is rare), and, more commonly, iatrogenic disease following surgical or medical treatment of hyperthyroidism. It is unclear whether maternal thyroid hormone is essential for normal fetal development. Potter has reported a series of severely hypothyroid patients giving birth to apparently normal offspring (107). In that study, however, extensive developmental testing of the offspring was not performed. In contrast, Man has demonstrated a higher incidence of mental retardation and congenital anomalies in children of mothers believed to be hypothyroid (108,109). The definitive diagnosis of hypothyroidism in this study, however, was questionable. Therefore, direct evidence supporting the concept that fetal development is directly altered by maternal hypothyroidism has yet to be reported.

### *Symptoms and Signs*

Clinical suspicion of hypothyroidism is based on nonspecific signs and symptoms, including lethargy, weakness, weight gain, cold sensitivity, hair loss, dry skin, and myxedematous changes. Confirmation of hypothyroidism is substantiated by the presence of low serum free T4 or FT4I and an elevated serum TSH level.

### *Treatment*

Once the diagnosis of hypothyroidism has been made in the pregnant patient, therapy consisting of sufficient replacement of thyroid hormone to achieve a euthyroid state should be initiated. L-thyroxine (Synthroid) is generally started at 0.05 to 0.1 mg/day increasing the dose over several weeks to a maximum of 0.2 mg/day. Optimal replacement may be accomplished by following TSH levels that may take as long as 4 to 8 weeks to normalize (100).

### *Anesthetic Considerations*

The infrequently-encountered hypothyroid pregnant patient presents the anesthesiologist with a daunting set of special considerations (61,110), as outlined in Table 32–7.

Monitoring the hypothyroid patient during operative intervention should be directed at early recognition of hypothermia and congestive heart failure. Regional anesthesia appears to be the ideal technique in the presence of hypothyroidism. Caution should be exercised when dosing local anesthetics due to decreased systemic biotransformation should systemic absorption occur. In addition, it would appear that the dose of local anesthetics necessary for peripheral nerve block is also reduced.

## Parathyroid Gland

### *Calcium Metabolism in Pregnancy*

Calcium homeostasis during pregnancy is a dynamic process. The daily requirement for calcium increases to 1200 mg (94). The net maternal accumulation of calcium by the end of gestation is estimated to be 25 to 30 g. The fetal skeleton represents the primary site of calcium uptake. Total calcium concentration, however, progressively falls reaching a nadir by the mid third trimester

**Table 32–7.** Anesthetic Considerations for Management of the Hypothyroid Parturient

1. Delayed gastric emptying time
2. Hypodynamic cardiovascular system
3. Slow biotransformation of narcotic agents
4. Extreme sensitivity to depressant drugs
5. Unresponsive baroreceptor reflexes
6. Contracted intravascular volume
7. Impaired free water clearance with resultant hyponatremia
8. Hypoglycemia
9. Anemia
10. Impaired ventilatory response to hypoxemia or hypercapnia
11. Hypothermia
12. Primary adrenal insufficiency

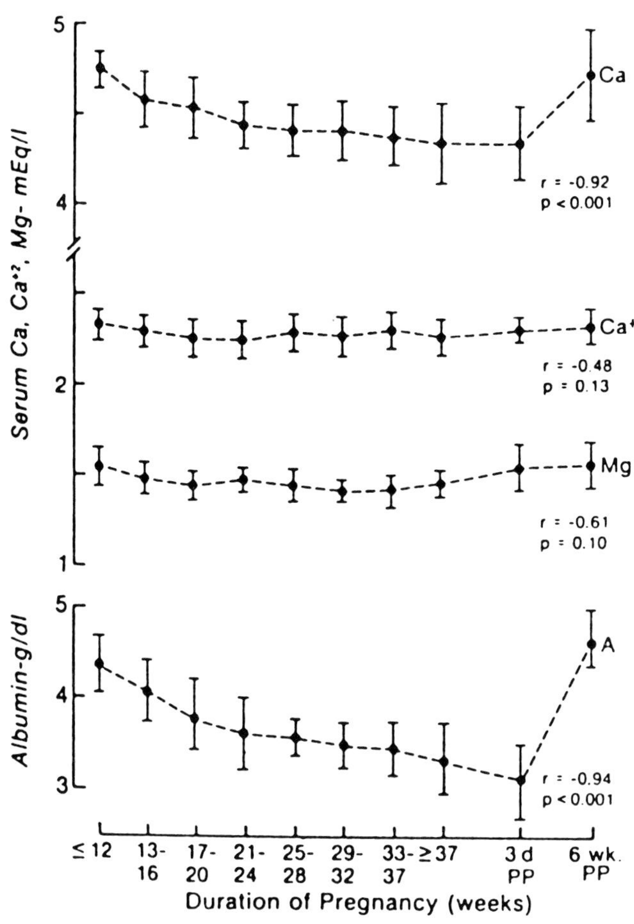


**Fig. 32–4.** Serum calcium, magnesium, and albumin in pregnancy. (With permission from Pitkin RM, Reynolds WA, Williams GA, Hargis GK: Calcium metabolism during pregnancy: A longitudinal study. Am. J. Obstet. Gynecol. 133:781, 1979.)

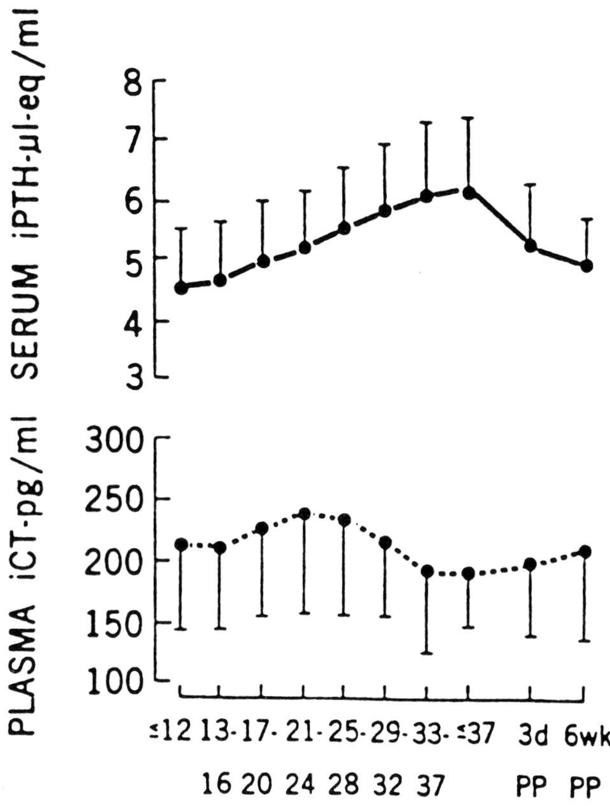


**Fig. 32–5.** Serum parathormone (iPTH) and calcitonin (iCT) levels during pregnancy. (Adapted with permission from Pitkin RM, Reynolds WA, Williams GA, Hargis GK: Calcium metabolism during pregnancy: A longitudinal study. Am. J. Obstet. Gynecol. 133:781, 1979.)

(Figure 32–4). The decrease in total serum calcium reflects a fall in the protein bound portion of the ion. Serum albumin, the most important carrier of plasma calcium, also falls progressively throughout pregnancy (Figure 32–4). The fall in serum albumin, coupled with increased glomerular filtration and excretion as well as an active placental transfer, all contribute to the fall in serum calcium levels with advancing gestation (111). Ionized serum calcium remains inappreciably changed during pregnancy. Pitkin has reported that levels of parathormone (PTH) increase progressively throughout pregnancy (Figure 32–5). Likely explanations for this observed increase include greater urinary calcium loss, facilitated placental transfer, and expanding intravascular volume. In contrast, calcitonin secretion would be expected to increase as a mechanism in response to the observed increases in PTH. Unfortunately, studies have been unable to substantiate consistent elevations in calcitonin with conflicting data, demonstrating no apparent change in serum levels of calcitonin (Figure 32–5) to a progressive increase during pregnancy (112). The placenta has also been implicated in playing a significant role in maternal-fetal calcium metabolism. Active transport of calcium to the fetal compartment serves as a protective measure ensuring adequate fetal calcium despite potentially inadequate maternal levels.

### *Hyperparathyroidism*

Primary hyperparathyroidism is an infrequent complication of pregnancy with only 90 to 100 cases reported in the literature (113). In the past, primary hyperparathyroidism was associated with a 45% incidence of stillbirths, neonatal deaths, or severe neonatal tetany. Over the last decade, as a result of early recognition and better management, this figure is now closer to 2%. Unfortunately, hypocalcemic tetany in the newborn often provides the only diagnostic clue to maternal hyperparathyroidism. The laboratory diagnosis rests primarily on demonstrating persistently elevated serum calcium levels with low serum and high urinary phosphorous values. In pregnancy, however, the diagnosis is suspected with lower serum calcium and phosphorous values and a higher PTH level than that found in the nonpregnant patient.

#### *Treatment*

Most authorities recommend prompt surgical excision of the abnormal parathyroid tissue at the time of diagnosis in any patient with progressive disease (113). The treatment of hyperparathyroidism during pregnancy should be individualized depending on the patient's gestational age, symptoms, and severity of disease. Medical treatment, including intravenous isotonic saline and furosemide to inhibit tubular reabsorption of calcium may be employed for short periods in anticipation of delivery. Importantly, thiazide diuretics should be avoided due to their calcium retentive properties. Mithramycin inhibits parathormone-induced osteoclastic activity and has been used effectively in hypercalcemic cancer patients. However, this drug should be avoided in pregnancy as its effects have not been well described. Oral phosphate may be used in patients with mild disease and normal renal function who, for whatever reason, are not surgical candidates (114).

### *Anesthetic Considerations*

Anesthetic management of the hyperparathyroid patient with hypercalcemia requires careful attention to intravascular volume, urine output, systemic manifestations such as osteoporosis, EKG changes, and drug interaction. There is no evidence that a specific anesthetic agent or technique offers a significant advantage. Aside from the effects that elevated serum concentrations of calcium may have on the efficacy of various nondepolarizing muscle relaxants, anesthetic management is otherwise routine (61). In the pregnant laboring patient, regional anesthesia appears to be ideal for both labor analgesia and cesarean delivery. Newborn hypocalcemic tetany may present at birth and should be anticipated by those responsible for resuscitative efforts.

## *Hypoparathyroidism*

Hypoparathyroidism is seldom encountered in pregnancy. Inadvertent parathyroidectomy at thyroid surgery has been reported to be the most common etiology of the disease. The diagnosis is suspected in a patient who presents with symptoms of lethargy, weakness, bone pain, irritability, carpopedal spasm (Trousseau's sign), and twitching of the upper lip elicited by tapping the facial nerve (Chvostek's sign). The diagnosis may be confirmed by observing low serum calcium levels and elevated serum phosphate. The principal concern in pregnancy is to prevent fetal bone demineralization, subperiosteal resorption, and osteitis fibrosa cystica described in infants born to hypoparathyroid mothers (115,116). Supplemental calcium in daily doses of 1 to 4 g as well as 100,000 to 150,000 IU of vitamin D is initiated after the diagnosis has been made. A short-acting oral form of vitamin D, calcitriol (1,25-dihydroxycholecalciferol), has recently been reported to provide a more predictable response in pregnancy. The usual recommended dose is 2 to 3 μg/day (117). During labor, careful attention to pain relief is paramount in preventing hyperventilation, which may result in exacerbation of hypocalcemia. Regional anesthesia is the ideal choice for management of the first and second stages of labor. Calcium may be given intravenously in the form of calcium gluconate should serum calcium levels fall dangerously low. Following delivery, the supplemental dosage of calcium and vitamin D can be reduced to prepregnancy levels in the nonlactating patient, which is due to normalization of the intravascular volume and absence of active placental transport. In patients who elect to breast feed, however, supplementation should continue at the antepartum level (95).

## Summary

With a clear understanding of the pathophysiology of the endocrine disorders that have been reviewed, the obstetric anesthesiologist can better contribute to the successful pregnancy outcomes now possible for most women with these problems. These favorable results also require a collaborative effort by all members of the perinatal team, including the obstetrician, pediatrician, obstetric anesthesiologist, and perinatal nurse.

## REFERENCES


1. Landon MB: Diabetes mellitus and other endocrine diseases. *In* Obstetrics Normal and Problem Pregnancies. 2nd Ed. Edited by SG Gabbe, JR Niebyl, JL, Simpson. New York, Churchill Livingstone, 1991, pp. 1097–1136.
2. Reese EA, Coustan DR (Eds): Diabetes Mellitus in Pregnancy: Principles and Practice. New York, Churchill Livingstone, 1988.
3. DeCherney AH, Dlugi AM, Caldwell BV: Endocrine emergencies during pregnancy. *In* Critical Care of the Obstetric Patient. Edited by RL Berkowitz. New York, Churchill Livingstone, 1983, pp. 385–410.
4. Cohen SE, Brose WG: Endocrine disease. *In* Obstetric Anesthesia: The Complicated Patient. 2nd Ed. Edited by FM James III, AS Wheeler, DM Dewan. Philadelphia, F.A. Davis Co., 1988, pp. 243–266.
5. Kalkhoff RK, Kissebah AH, Kim H-J: Carbohydrate and lipid metabolism during normal pregnancy: Relationship to gestational hormone action. *In* The Diabetic Pregnancy. Edited by IR Merkatz, PAF Adam. New York, Grune and Stratton, 1979, p. 3.
6. Spellacy WN: Human placental lactogen (HPL)—The review of a protein hormone important to obstetrics and gynecology. South. Med. J. 62:1954, 1969.
7. Yen SSC: Endocrine regulation of metabolic homeostasis during pregnancy. Clin. Obstet. Gynecol. 16:130, 1973.
8. Hay WW, Sparks JW: Placental, fetal, and neonatal carbohydrate metabolism. Clin. Obstet. Gynecol. 28:473, 1985.
9. Coustan DR: Hyperglycemia-hyperinsulinemia: Effect on the infant of the diabetic mother. *In* Diabetes and Pregnancy, Teratology, Toxicity, and Treatment. Edited by L Jovanovic, CM Peterson, K Fuhrmann. New York, Praeger, 1986, p. 131.
10. Gabbe SG: Management of diabetes in pregnancy: Six decades of experience. *In* The Yearbook of Obstetrics and Gynecology. Edited by RM Pitkin, F Zlatnik. Chicago, Yearbook Medical Publishers, 1980.
11. Carson BS, Philipps AF, Simmons MA, Battaglia FC, et al: Effects of sustained insulin infusion upon glucose uptake and oxygenation of the ovine fetus. Pediatr. Res. 14:147, 1980.
12. Modanlou HD, Komatsu G, Dorchester W, Freeman RK, et al: Large-for-gestational age neonates: anthropometric reasons for shoulder dystocia. Obstet. Gynecol. 60:417, 1982.
13. Mills JL, Baker L, Goldman AS: Malformations in infants of diabetic mothers occur before the seventh gestational week. Implications for treatment. Diabetes 28:292, 1979.
14. Sadler TW, Horton WE Jr: Mechanisms of diabetes-induced

congenital malformations as studied in mammalian embryo culture. *In* Diabetes and Pregnancy, Teratology, Toxicity, and Treatment. Edited by L Jovanovic, CM Peterson, K Fuhrmann. New York, Praeger, 1986, p. 51.

15. White P: Pregnancy complicating diabetes. Am. J. Med. 7: 609, 1949.
16. Main EK, Main DM, Landon MB, Gabbe SG: Factors predicting perinatal outcome in pregnancies complicated by diabetes nephropathy (Class F). Sixth Annual Meeting, Society of Perinatal Obstetricians, San Antonio, February, 1986.
17. Kitzmiller JL, Brown ER, Phillippe M, Stark AR, et al: Diabetic nephropathy and perinatal outcome. Am. J. Obstet. Gynecol. 141:741, 1981.
18. Reece EA, Coustan DR, Hayslett JP, Holford T, et al: Diabetic nephropathy: pregnancy performance and fetomaternal outcome. Am. J. Obstet. Gynecol. 159:56, 1988.
19. Landon MB, Gabbe SG: Glucose monitoring and insulin administration in the pregnant diabetic patient. Clin. Obstet. Gynecol. 28:496, 1985.
20. Coustan DR, Reece A, Sherwin RS, Rudolf MCJ, et al: A randomized clinical trial of the insulin pump vs intensive congenital therapy in diabetic pregnancies. JAMA 255:631, 1986.
21. Landon MB, Gabbe SG, Piana R, Mennuti MT, et al: Neonatal morbidity in pregnancy complicated by diabetes mellitus: predictive value of maternal glycemic profiles. Am. J. Obstet. Gynecol. 156:1089, 1987
22. Gabbe SG: Antepartum fetal surveillance in the pregnancy complicated by diabetes mellitus. *In*: Infant of the Diabetic Mother. Columbus, Ohio, Ross Laboratories, 1987, p. 86.
23. Benedetti TJ, Gabbe SG: Shoulder dystocia: a complication of fetal macrosomia and prolonged second stage of labor with midpelvic delivery. Obstet. Gynecol. 52:526, 1978.
24. Miodovnik M, Mimouni F, Tsang RC, Skillman C, et al: Management of the insulin-dependent diabetic during labor and delivery. Am. J. Perinatal. 4:106, 1987.
25. West TET, Lowy C: Control of blood glucose during labor in diabetic women with combined glucose and low dose insulin infusion. Br. Med. J. 1:1252, 1977.
26. Jovanovic L, Peterson CM: Management of the pregnant, insulin-dependent diabetic woman. Diabetes Care 3:63, 1980.
27. Werner WE, Schauble PG Knudson, MS: An argument for the revival of hypnosis in obstetrics. Am. J. Clin. Hypn. 24: 149 1982.
28. Fee AF, Reilley RR: Hypnosis in obstetrics: a review of techniques. J. Am. Soc. Psychosom. Dent. Med. 29:17, 1982.
29. Nylund L, Lunell N-O, Lewander R, Persson B, et al: Uteroplacental blood flow in diabetic pregnancy: measurements with indium 113m and a computer-linked gamma camera. Am. J. Obstet. Gynecol. 144:298–302, 1982.
30. Björk O, Persson B: Placental changes in relation to the degree of metabolic control in diabetes mellitus. Placenta 3:367–378, 1983.
31. Madsen H, Ditzel J: Changes in red blood cell oxygen transport in diabetic pregnancy. Am. J. Obstet. Gynecol. 143: 421–424, 1982.
32. Brouillard RG, Kitzmiller JL, Datta S: Buffering capacity and oxyhemoglobin affinity in infants of diabetic mothers. Anesthesiology 55:(3a)A319, 1981.
33. Gibbs CP, Gabbe SG: Diabetes. *In* Obstetric Anesthesia: The Complicated Patient. 2nd Ed. Edited by FM James III, AS Wheeler. Philadelphia, F.A. Davis Co., 1982, pp. 171.
34. Ho AM-H, Smedstad KG: Stress-free labor for the diabetic parturient. Diabetes Care 9:555, 1986.
35. Datta S, Kitzmiller JL: Anesthetic and obstetric management of diabetic pregnant women. Clin. Perinatol. 9:153, 1982.
36. Datta S, Brown WU Jr: Acid-base status in diabetic mothers and their infants following general or spinal anesthesia for cesarean section. Anesthesiology 47:272, 1977.
37. Datta S, Kitzmiller JL, Naulty JS, Ostheimer GW, et al: Acid-base status of diabetic mothers and their infants following spinal anesthesia for cesarean section. Anesth. Analg. 61: 662, 1982.
38. Jovanovic L, Peterson CM: Management of the pregnant, insulin-dependent diabetic woman. Diabetes Care 3:63, 1980.
39. Kenepp NB, Shelley WC, Gabbe SG, Kumar S, et al: Fetal and neonatal hazards of maternal hydration with 5% dextrose before cesarean section. Lancet 1:1150, 1982.
40. Philipson EH, Kalhan SC, Riha MM, Pimentel R: Effects of maternal glucose infusion on fetal acid-base status in human pregnancy. Am. J. Obstet. Gynecol. 157:866, 1987.
41. Jouppila P, Jouppila R, Hollmën A, Koivula A: Lumbar epidural analgesia to improve intervillous blood flow during labor in severe preeclampsia. Obstet. Gynecol. 59:158, 1982.
42. Cohen AW, Gabbe SG: Intrapartum management of the diabetic patient. Clin. Perinatol. 8:165, 1981.
43. Edwards G, Morton HJV, Pask EA, Wylie WD: Deaths associated with anesthesia. Anaesthesia 11:194, 1956.
44. Sachs BP, Oriol NE, Ostheimer GW, Weiss JB, et al: Anesthetic-related maternal mortality, 1954–1985. J. Clin. Anesth. 1:333, 1989.
45. McDonald JS, Mateo CV, Reed EC: Modified nitrous oxide or ketamine hydrochloride for cesarean section. Anesth. Analg. 51:975, 1972.
46. Albright GA (Ed): *In* Anesthesia in Obstetrics. Menlo Park, Addison-Wesley Publishing Co., 1978, pp. 155–156.
47. Bauknecht T, Krake B, Rechenbach U, Zahradnik HP, et al: Distribution of PGE and PGF2α receptors in human myometrium. Acta. Endocrinol. (Copenh). 98:446, 1981.
48. Bondy PK: The Adrenal Cortex. *In* Metabolic Control and Disease. 8th Ed. Edited by PK Bondy, LE Rosenberg. Philadelphia, W. B. Saunders, 1980.
49. Judzewitsh R: Thyroid and adrenal function. *In* Reproductive Physiology. Edited by RP Sherman. Oxford, Blackwell Scientific, 1979.
50. De Moor P, Steeno O, Brosens I, Hendrikx A: Data on transcortin activity in human plasma as studied by gel filtration. J. Clin. Endocrinol. Metab. 26:71, 1966.
51. Nolten WE, Lindheimer MD, Rueckert PA, Oparil S, et al: Diurnal patterns and regulation of cortisol secretions in pregnancy. J. Clin. Endocrinol. Metab. 51:466, 1980.
52. Carr BR, Parker Jr CR, Madden JD, MacDonald PC, et al: Maternal plasma adrenocorticotropin and cortisol relations throughout human pregnancy. Am. J. Obstet. Gynecol. 139:416, 1981.
53. Smeaton TC, Andersen GJ, Fulton IS: Study of aldosterone levels in plasma during pregnancy. J. Clin. Endocrinol. Metab. 44:1, 1977.
54. Nolten WE, Lindheimer MD, Oparil S, Ehrlich EN: Desoxycorticosterone in normal pregnancy. Am. J. Obstet. Gynecol. 132:414, 1978.
55. Burrow GN: Pituitary and adrenal disorders. *In* Medical Complications During Pregnancy. 3rd Ed. Edited by GN Burrow, TF Ferris. Philadelphia, W.B. Saunders, 1988.
56. Kreines K, DeVaux WD: Neonatal adrenal insufficiency associated with maternal Cushing's syndrome. Pediatrics 47: 516, 1971.
57. Grimes EM, Fayez JA, Miller GL: Cushing's syndrome and pregnancy. Obstet. Gynecol. 42:550, 1973.

58. Salassa RM, Laws Jr ER, Carpenter PC, Northcutt RC: Transphenoidal removal of pituitary microadenoma in Cushing's disease. Mayo Clin. Proc. 1978;53:24–8.
59. Hsu TH, Gann DS, Tsan KW, Russell RP: Cyproheptadine in the control of Cushing's disease. Johns Hopkins Med. J. 149:77, 1981.
60. Gormley MJJ, Hadden DR, Kennedy TL, Montgomery DAD, et al: Cushing's syndrome in pregnancy-treatment with metyrapone. Clin. Endocrinol. 16:283, 1982.
61. Tasch MD: Endocrine diseases. *In* Anesthesia and Co-existing Disease. 1st Ed. Edited by RK Stoelting, SF Dierdorf. New York, Churchill Livingstone, 1983.
62. Johnston IDA: Endocrine aspects of the metabolic response to surgical operation. Ann. R. Coll. Surg. Engl. 35: 270, 1964.
63. Symreng T, Karlberg BE, Kagedal B, Schildt B: Physiological cortisol substitution of long term steroid-treated patients undergoing major surgery. Br. J. Anaesth. 53:949, 1981.
64. Osler N: Addison's disease and pregnancy. Acta. Endocrinol. 41:57, 1962.
65. DeCherney AH, Dlugi AM, Caldwell BV: Endocrine emergencies during pregnancy. *In* Critical Care of the Obstetric Patient. Edited by R Berkowitz. New York, Churchill Livingstone, 1983, pp. 385–410.
66. Brent R: Addison's disease and pregnancy. Am J. Surg. 79: 645, 1950.
67. Drucker D, Shumak S, Angel A: Schmidt's syndrome presenting with intrauterine growth retardation and postpartum addisonian crises. Am. J. Obstet. Gynecol. 149:229, 1984.
68. Bacchus H: Metabolic and Endocrine Emergencies: Recognition and Management. Baltimore, University Park Press, 1977.
69. O'Shaughnessy RW, Hackett KJ: Maternal Addison's disease and fetal growth retardation. J. Reprod. Med. 29:752, 1984.
70. Duthie DJR, Fraser R, Nimmo WS: Effect of induction of anaesthesia with etomidate on corticosteroid synthesis in man. Br. J. Anaesth. 57:156, 1985.
71. Gangat Y, Triner L, Baer L, Puchner P: Primary aldosteronism with uncommon complications. Anesthesiology 45: 542, 1976.
72. McGuffin Jr WL, Gunnells Jr JC: Primary aldosteronism. Urol. Clin. North. Am. 4:227, 1977.
73. Messina M, Biffignandi P, Ghigo E, Jeantet MG, et al: Possible contraindication of spironolactone during pregnancy. J. Endocrinol. Invest. 2:222, 1979.
74. Sever PS, Roberts JC, Snell ME: Pheochromocytoma. J. Clin. Endocrinol. Metab. 9:543, 1980.
75. Schenker JG, Granat M: Pheochromocytoma and pregnancy: An updated appraisal. Aust. N.Z.J. Obstet. Gynecol. 22:1, 1982.
76. Durham JA: A noradrenaline pheochromocytoma complicating pregnancy. Aust. N.Z.J. Obstet. Gynecol. 17:53, 1977.
77. Cryer PE: Pheochromocytoma. J. Clin. Endocrinol. Metab. 14:203, 1985.
78. Venuto R, Burstein P, Schneider R: Pheochromocytoma: antepartum diagnosis and management with tumor resection in the puerperium. Am. J. Obstet. Gynecol. 150:431, 1984.
79. Fudge TL, McKinnon WMP, Geary WL: Current surgical management of pheochromocytoma during pregnancy. Arch. Surg. 115:1224, 1980.
80. Maddern PJ, Davis NJ, McGlew I, Oh T: Case report: pheochromocytoma. Aspects of management. Anesth. Intern. Care 4:156, 1976.
81. Coulam CB, Annegers JF, Abboud CF, Laws Jr ER, et al: Pituitary adenoma and oral contraceptives: a case-control study. Fertil. Steril. 31:25, 1979.
82. Magyar DM, Marshal JR: When your pregnant patient has a pituitary adenoma. Contemp. Obstet. Gynecol. 17:121, 1981.
83. Gemzell E, Wang CF: Outcome of pregnancy in women with pituitary tumors. Fertil. Steril. 31:363, 1979.
84. Husami N, Jewelewicz R, Vande Wiele RL: Pregnancy in patients with pituitary tumors. Fertil. Steril. 28:920, 1977.
85. Biswas S, Rodeck CH: Protein values in pregnancy. Br. J. Obstet. Gynaecol. 83:683, 1976.
86. McGregor AM, Scanlon MF, Hall K, Cook DB, et al: Reduction in size of a pituitary tumor by bromocryptine therapy. N. Engl. J. Med. 300:291, 1979.
87. Sheehan HL: Simmonds' disease due to Postpartum necrosis of the anterior pituitary. Q. J. Med. 8:277, 1939.
88. Smallridge RC, Corrigan DF, Thomason AM, Blue PW: Hypoglycemia in pregnancy. Arch. Intern. Med. 140:564, 1980.
89. Dorfman SG, Dillaplain RP, Gambrell Jr RD: Antepartum pituitary infarction. Obstet. Gynecol. 53(Suppl):215, 1979.
90. Hollingsworth DR: Endocrine Disorders of Pregnancy. *In* Maternal Fetal Medicine: Principles and Practice. 1st Ed. Edited by RK Creasy, R Resnik. Philadelphia, W.B. Saunders, 1984.
91. Hime MC, Richardson J: Diabetes insipidus and pregnancy: case report, incidence and review of literature. Obstet. Gynecol. Surv. 33:375, 1978.
92. Robinson AG: DDAVP in the treatment of central diabetes insipidus. N. Engl. J. Med. 294:507, 1976.
93. Burrow GN, Wassenaar W, Robertson GL, Sehl H: DDAVP treatment of diabetes insipidus during pregnancy and the postpartum period. Acta. Endocrinol. 97:23, 1981.
94. Mestman JH: Thyroid and parathyroid diseases in pregnancy. *In* Fetal and Maternal Medicine. Edited by EJ Quilligan, N Kretchmer. New York, Wiley, 1980.
95. Samuels P, Landon MB: Medical complications. *In* Obstetrics Normal and Problem Pregnancies. Edited by SG Gabbe, JR Niebyl, JL Simpson. New York, Churchill Livingstone, 1986.
96. Niswander KR, Gordon M: The Women and their Pregnancies. Philadelphia, W.B. Saunders, 1972.
97. Lang R: New thyroid treatments, tests—even new diseases. Contemp. Obstet. Gynecol. 19:102, 1982.
98. Munro DS, Dirmikis SM, Humphries H, Smith T, et al: The role of thyroid stimulating immunoglobulin of Grave's disease in neonatal thyrotoxicosis. Br. J. Obstet. Gynaecol. 85:837, 1978.
99. Chapman EM, Corner Jr GW, Robinson D, Evans RD: The collection of radioactive iodine by the human fetal thyroid. J. Clin. Endocrinol. Metab. 8:717, 1948.
100. Burrow GN: Thyroid diseases. *In* Medical Complications During Pregnancy. 3rd Ed. Edited by GN Burrow, TF Ferris. Philadelphia, W.B. Saunders, 1988.
101. Cheron RG, Kaplan MM, Larsen PR, Selenkow HA, et al: Neonatal thyroid function after propylthiouracil therapy for maternal Grave's disease. N. Engl. J. Med. 304:525, 1981.
102. Ramsey I, Kaur S, Krassas G: Thyrotoxicosis in pregnancy: results of treatment by antithyroid drugs combined with T4. Clin. Endocrinol. 18:73, 1983.
103. Nicoloff JT: Thyroid storm and myxedema coma. Med. Clin. North. Am. 69:1005, 1985.
104. Mestman JH: Severe hyperthyroidism in pregnancy. *In*

Critical Care Obstetrics. Edited by SL Clark, JP Phelan, JP, DB Cotton. Oradell, NJ, Medical Economics Co, Inc., 1987.

105. Anaissie E, Thome JF: Reserpine in propranolol-resistant thyroid storm. Arch. Intern. Med. 145:2248, 1985.
106. Singer PA, Mestman JH: Thyroid storm need not be lethal. Contemp. Obstet. Gynecol. 22:135, 1983.
107. Potter JD: Hypothyroidism and reproductive failure. Surg. Gynecol. Obstet. 150:251, 1980.
108. Man EB, Holden RH, Jones WS: Thyroid function in human pregnancy. VII. Developmemt and retardation of four year old progeny of euthyroid and hypothyroxinemic women. Am. J. Obstet. Gynecol. 109:12, 1971.
109. Man EB, Jones WS, Holden RH, Mellits ED: Thyroid functions in human pregnancy. VIII. Retardation of progeny aged 6 years; relationship to maternal age and maternal thyroid function. Am. J. Obstet. Gynecol. 111:905, 1971.
110. Myrkin JM: Anesthesia and hypothyroidism: a review of thyroxine physiology, pharmacology, and anesthetic implications. Anesth. Analg. 61:371–83, 1982.
111. Pitkin RM, Reynolds WA, Williams GA, Hargis GK: Calcium metabolism during pregnancy: a longitudinal study. Am. J. Obstet. Gynecol. 133:781, 1979.
112. Pitkin RM: Calcium and the parathyroid glands. *In* Medical Complications During Pregnancy. 3rd Ed. Edited by GN Burrow, TF Ferris. Philadelphia, W.B. Saunders, 1988.
113. Shangold MM, Dor N, Welt SI, Fleischmann AR, et al: Hyperparathyroidism and pregnancy: a review. Obstet. Gynecol. Surv. 37:217, 1982.
114. Montoro MN, Collea JV, Mestman JH: Management of hyperparathyroidism in pregnancy with oral phosphate therapy. Obstet. Gynecol. 55:431, 1980.
115. Stuart C, Aceto T Jr, Kuhn JP, Terplan K: Intrauterine hyperparathyroidism. Am. J. Dis. Child. 133:67, 1979.
116. Gradus (Ben-Ezer) D, Le Roith D, Karplus M, Zmora E, et al: Congenital hyperarathyroidism and rickets secondary to maternal hypoparathyroidism and vitamin D deficiency. Isr. J. Med. Sci. 17:705, 1981.
117. Salle BL, Berthezene F, Glorieux FH, Delvin EE, et al: Hypoparathyroidism during pregnancy: treatment with calcitrol. J. Clin. Endocrinol. Metab. 52:810, 1981.

# Chapter 33

# PULMONARY DISORDERS

ROBERT R. KIRBY

This chapter discusses the basics of pulmonary physiology as related to clinical considerations of pregnancy. In addition, clinical problems of a major impact that involve the pregnant patient will be discussed. These include various pulmonary embolus problems, such as amniotic fluid embolism, venous air embolization, fat embolization, and thromboembolism. Additional problems such as the major concerns always in regard to the pregnant patient, e.g., pulmonary aspiration, will be discussed. Finally, the more classic, long-studied pulmonary problems associated with respiration, e.g., acute respiratory failure, asthma, pulmonary edema, and pulmonary manifestations of cardiac disease, e.g., rheumatic and congenital problems, will be discussed. A more detailed treatise on pulmonary diseases in pregnancy can be found in current textbooks such as Kirby's "Critical Care" (1992), "Respiratory Failure" (1986), and Baum and Wolinsky's "Textbook of Pulmonary Diseases" (1986).

## BASIC CONSIDERATIONS

### Pulmonary Physiology in Pregnancy

Pregnant women undergo significant changes in cardiopulmonary function, the normal extremes of which must be appreciated by any anesthesiologist who cares for them (Table 33–1) (1). Minute ventilation increases significantly, and $PaCO_2$ values of 30 to 32 mm Hg are commonly reported. Functional residual capacity (FRC) is reduced by upward diaphragmatic and rib cage displacement. Bronchial smooth muscle is more reactive, and pharyngeal and airway mucosal edema are prominent features (1,2). Salivary gland activity is increased and secretions may be prominent during airway management and attempted trachea intubation.

These normal changes may be exacerbated by abnormal conditions such as preeclampsia (3). Pulmonary edema, in combination with the normally reduced functional residual capacity, predisposes to a rapid decrease in $PaO_2$. Mucosal edema and hyperemia contribute to airway bleeding and potentially rapid obstruction during intubation. Pulmonary vasoconstriction and the resulting increase of pulmonary microvascular pressure, coupled with a frequently noted decrease in colloid oncotic pressure, can trigger pulmonary edema. The pulmonary condition of the pregnant patient is worsened by a variety of other factors, including embolization syndromes, sepsis, shock, aspiration of gastric contents, and abruptio placentae.

#### *Ventilation/Perfusion*

##### *Lung Volume and Alveolar Ventilation*

When a normal adult lies supine, the functional residual capacity decreases by about 500 ml as a result of cephalad displacement of the diaphragm. This change is accentuated during pregnancy by the gravid uterus, causing still further reduction in functional residual capacity. As a result, anesthetic uptake is increased and hemoglobin desaturation more rapid when ventilation is impaired or interrupted.

Both tidal volume and respiratory rate increase at term (1,3). These changes are associated with a 50% increase of minute ventilation and a 70% increase of alveolar ventilation (see Table 33–1). The reduction of $PaCO_2$ is significant (about 25%), but not so great as would be predicted from the increase in ventilation. Hence, rather widespread ventilation/perfusion (V/Q) changes may be present. One would suppose that this apparent discrepancy is explained by an increase of dead space, yet the latter variable is reportedly unchanged. Hence, increased carbon dioxide production, in association with increased oxygen consumption, must be invoked to explain this phenomenon. Such variations result from increased metabolic activity (normal metabolic rate of the mother, products of conception, and work of carrying the fetus) and that of respiratory muscles, the work of which during labor may increase by as much as 300%.

##### *Pulmonary Blood Flow*

Maternal blood volume is approximately 40% above nonpregnant levels at term, and cardiac output increases by 30 to 40% above nonpregnant values between 20 and 30 weeks of gestation (3). Both heart rate and stroke volume are increased (see Table 33–1). A further increase in cardiac output of 15 to 45% above prelabor values occurs during labor (more so during uterine contractions). Finally, in the immediate postpartum period, it increases yet another 30 to 40% above values measured during labor and blood previously directed to the placenta is returned to the maternal systemic circulation.

Tachypnea in labor may be associated with significant alterations in pulmonary blood flow, although definitive studies in this regard are lacking. In nonpregnant individuals, the significant decrease in pleural pressure (Ppl) with tachypnea augments venous return and right ventricular filling, and is associated with displacement of the intraven-

**Table 33–1.** Cardiopulmonary Changes in Normal Pregnancy

| | |
|---|---|
| *Cardiovascular* | |
| Cardiac output | 30 to 40% at 20 to 30 weeks<br>additional 15 to 45% during labor<br>additional 10 to 40% during uterine contraction |
| RBC | 20 to 30% at term |
| Plasma volume | 45 to 55% at term |
| Hematocrit | Decreased |
| *Respiratory* | |
| Minute ventilation | 50% at term |
| Alveolar ventilation | 70% at term |
| $PaCO_2$ | 30 to 32 mm Hg |
| $PaO_2$ | Unchanged or slightly decreased |
| Oxygen consumption | Increased |
| Carbon dioxide production | Increased |
| Functional residual capacity (FRC) | Decreased |

tricular septum into the left ventricular cavity (4). Increased transmural pulmonary vascular pressure caused by pulmonary artery hypertension and decreased Ppl may result. In pregnancy, high peripheral venous pressure results from the gravid uterus, and venous return (in the absence of vena caval obstruction) is enhanced, further increasing transmural pulmonary vascular pressure. These changes are often reflected by an engorged pulmonary vascular bed noted on chest radiographs. The possibility of pulmonary edema, particularly in the presence of preexisting cardiopulmonary disease, is a real threat.

## Position Changes

In the supine position, spontaneous ventilation predominantly involves dependent lung areas because of greater shortening of the posterior diaphragm (5). Relatively little ventilation occurs in the nondependent lung fields. Pulmonary blood flow is distributed similarly, and a passive matching of ventilation and perfusion results.

If the patient is paralyzed and manually or mechanically ventilated during anesthesia, significant V/Q alterations occur. The flaccid diaphragm moves passively but is impeded in its posterior descent by the abdominal contents (5), an effect that is accentuated by the gravid uterus. Hence, most ventilation is nondependent. Pulmonary perfusion, however, remains largely dependent because of the relatively low-pressure characteristics of the pulmonary circulation. The high cardiac output of pregnancy may partially offset this V/Q imbalance. On the other hand, if vena caval compression significantly reduces venous return, as it does in 10% or more of supine pregnant patients, the V/Q imbalance may be increased (even less nondependent lung is perfused). Thus, the final V/Q relationship is unpredictable. In general, however, one would expect more dead space ventilation (nondependent lung) and greater shunt (dependent lung) than in nonpregnant individuals. When combined with the reduced functional residual capacity, increased oxygen consumption, and decreased hemoglobin, the potential for hypoxemia and tissue hypoxia—relative or absolute—is considerable.

## Airway Control

Many of the changes in airway morphology and function have been mentioned previously. Mucosal hypertrophy, alone or in conjunction with bronchospasm triggered by tracheal intubation, is problematic (1). It is perhaps trite to mention the fact that wheezing does not always represent bronchospasm. Endotracheal tube obstruction (kinking, secretions) or obstruction in any portion of the expiratory limb of the anesthesia/ventilator circuit can mimic small airway closure.

Obstetric patients are prone to aspiration of gastric contents (6), to amniotic fluid embolism, and to bronchospasm; wheezing is one of the earliest, yet nonspecific, signs in many cases. Pulmonary edema, associated with preeclampsia, drug reactions, congenital heart disease, and aspiration, also may provoke wheezing as a result of small airways partial obstruction. Remember, however, that wheezing may result from inadequate anesthetic depth. Increasing the delivered inhalational agent may be relatively contraindicated because of deleterious effects on uterine contractility and fetal depression. Conversely, the administration of beta agonists such as terbutaline or albuterol to offset wheezing caused by insufficient anesthetic depth may be unsatisfactory.

## Central Control of Respiration

Although much of the central nervous system's activity is depressed during pregnancy, respiratory-control mechanisms are activated. By the sixth week of gestation, reductions of alveolar and arterial $PaO_2$ occur and persist throughout pregnancy (1,2). This response is enhanced at high altitude, and $PaCO_2$ values in the low-to-mid 20 mm Hg range have been reported. Chronic hypocapnia is associated with renal excretion of bicarbonate, resulting in a return of arterial pH toward normal. Serum bicarbonate levels as low as 12 to 14 mEq/L may occur during hypoxia-induced hypocapnia in pregnancy, leading an inexperienced observer to believe that a significant nonrespiratory (metabolic) acidosis is present. In reality, such a change is a normal compensatory response to chronic hypoxia and hypocapnia. The decreased buffering capacity, however, may contribute to the dyspnea experienced by many women during pregnancy (1).

Hyperventilation in combination with a smaller than normal functional residual capacity leads to increased anesthetic uptake and a rapid equilibration of alveolar and inspired anesthetic partial pressures. This effect may not be appreciated with modern, rapid induction agents such as isoflurane, enflurane, and halothane. However, in years past, it was quite impressive with diethyl ether, which in nonpregnant individuals characteristically required a prolonged induction period.

In a related area, pregnancy decreased the requirement for potent inhalational agents, perhaps because of increased levels of progesterone (7) and endogenous opioids. Hence, the administrations of usual concentrations of anesthetic will have an unusually great effect on the rate of induction and depth of anesthesia.

## Anesthetic Considerations

It is apparent that the many significant changes in the physiology of respiration in pregnancy can alter responses of the mother to labor with and without analgesia. However, we want to emphasize that it is through the use of regional techniques that one can best approach the normative state. For example, $PaCO_2$ values in pregnancy of 30 to 32 are already below the usual nonpregnancy norm of 40, and without analgesia, they can be driven down into the 20s (Figure 33–1). This can cause other physiological changes, such as alteration in calcium ion availability and involuntary muscle spasms. Contrast this with patients who receive analgesia and who do not have associated respiratory changes due to hyperventilation

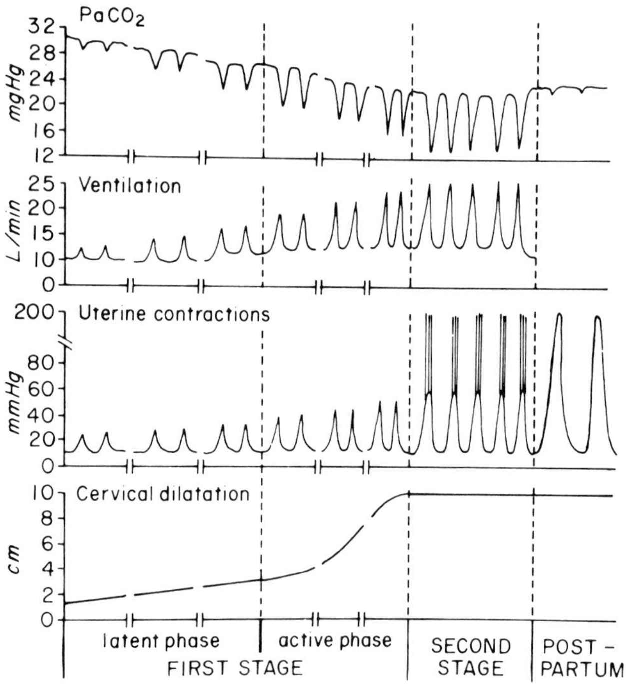


**Fig. 33–1.** Schematic representation of ventilatory changes during labor in an unpremedicated gravida. Note the correlation of the stages of labor as reflected by the Friedman's curve (bottom tracing), the frequency and intensity of uterine contractions, minute ventilation, and arterial carbon dioxide tension (top tracing). Early in labor, uterine contractions are slight and are associated with mild pain, causing only small increases in minute ventilation and decreases in $PaCO_2$. As labor progresses, however, the greater intensity of contractions causes greater changes in ventilation and $PaCO_2$. During the active phase, contractions with an increased intrauterine pressure of 40 to 60 mmHg causes severe pain, which acts as an intense stimulus to ventilation with a consequent reduction of the $PaCO_2$ to 18 to 20 mmHg. During the second stage, the reflex bearing-down efforts further increase intrauterine pressure and distend the perineum, producing consequent additional pain that prompts the parturient to ventilate at a rate almost twice that of early labor and causing a commensurate reduction in the $PaCO_2$ to levels as low as 12 to 16 mmHg. (Modified from Bonica JJ: Maternal respiratory changes during pregnancy and parturition. *In* Parturition and Perinatology. Clinical Anesthesia Series, Vol. 10, No. 2. Edited by GF Marx. Philadelphia, FA Davis, 1973.)

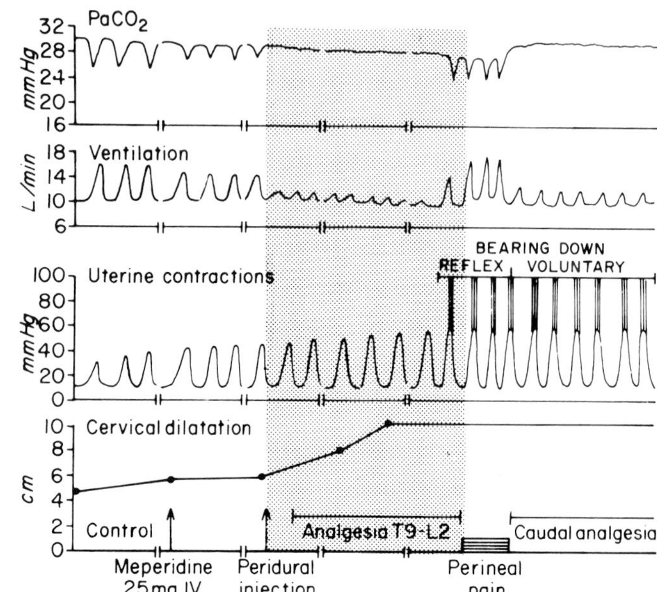


**Fig. 33–2.** Schematic representation of the effect of analgesia on ventilation based on measurements in a primipara. At 5 cm cervical dilatation, 25 mg of meperidine IV resulted in partial relief of pain and consequently produced smaller changes in ventilation and $PaCO_2$. Subsequent induction of segmental epidural analgesia produced complete pain relief, which eliminated maternal hyperventilation and $PaCO_2$ changes without affecting uterine contractions. During the second stage, the onset of perineal pain and initiation of reflex bearing-down efforts caused a concomitant increase in ventilation and a slight decrease in the $PaCO_2$, which were eliminated with the induction of low caudal (S1 to S5) analgesia. (Modified from Bonica JJ: Obstetric Analgesia and Anesthesia. 2nd ed. Seattle, University of Washington Press, 1980, p. 114.)

(Figure 33–2), and thus, no abnormal physiological changes of muscle spasm.

This is only one example, but there are other more demonstrative examples that have to do with the importance of maintaining the status quo in regard to normal physiology. Suffice it to say, the optimum management for patients to stay as near as possible to their physiologic norm is the use of regional analgesia technique, which abates the pain sensation of labor at the spinal cord level. Techniques that can accomplish this include lumbar epidural, caudal epidural, and spinal and paracervical blocks. Throughout this book, we have pointed out the advantages and disadvantages of regional analgesia/anesthesia for obstetrics. Naturally, the advantages far outweigh the disadvantages, and for the most part these techniques are ideally suited because they offer complete interruption of labor pain with minimal physiological embarrassment. At the time of the first edition of this book, the most serious concern about regional analgesia/anesthesia was the considerable physiological paybacks inherent, when one considers: (1) maternal hypotension due to sympathetic block; (2) maternal respiratory embarrassment due to a high block; (3) maternal convulsion due to the CNS toxic effect; and (4) maternal cardiovascular collapse due to the cardiac toxic effect. Almost 30 years later, the epidural

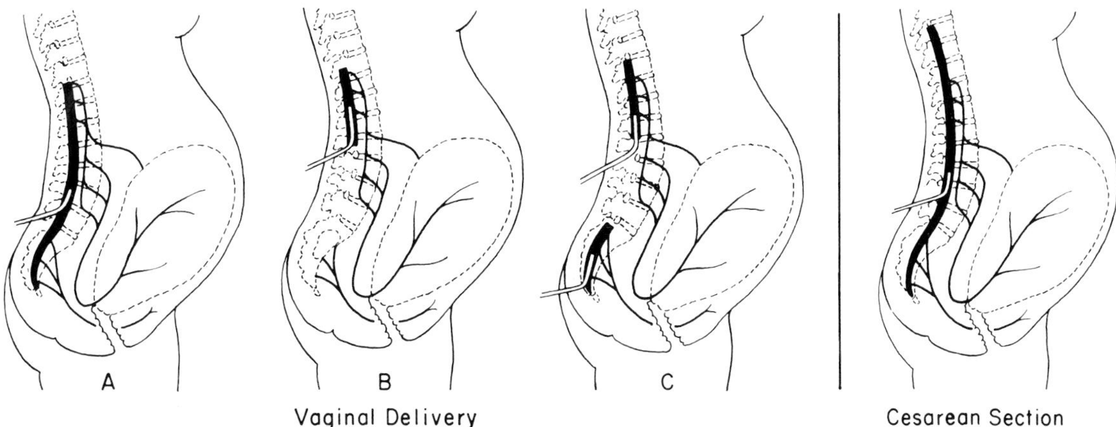


**Fig. 33–3.** Various techniques of spinal epidural block used in obstetrics. White tube indicates level of catheter. Black area in spinal canal indicates diffusion of local anesthetic. **A,** Standard technique for vaginal delivery (analgesia T10 to S5). **B,** Segmental epidural (T10, L1) block for analgesia during first stage of labor. **C,** Continuous epidural is same as **B,** but includes the pump.

has undergone multiple transformations from the standard widespread epidural to the segmental epidural, and now to the labor epidural with minimal doses given continuously via an external pump mechanism (Figure 33–3 and 33–4).

Therefore, today we can say that the current method of labor and delivery pain relief should be able to effect

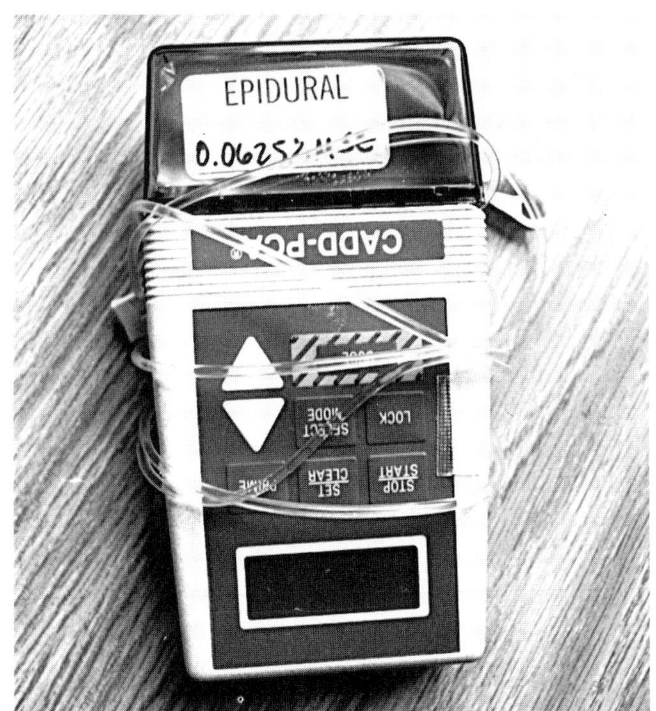


**Fig. 33–4.** One of the currently available pumps used for delivery of various medications. This pump has a specific subset of electronics that allows variable rates to be used according to need. In addition, bolus doses may be given with manual override. These pumps are available through Pharmacia Deltec Inc., St. Paul, MN.)

relief without significant maternal consequences. Certainly, labor epidural methods that are now available and in use that do consist of small, continuous dosages should not have deleterious effects upon pulmonary physiology as described in this section. Because there is not an elevated sensory level to worry about, there is no net decrease in lung volumes or alveolar ventilation. Pulmonary blood flow should also be unaffected, because there is no hypotension or reduced cardiac output. Finally, there is no concern about respiratory-control mechanisms being affected again because the levels are so low as to preclude high systemic central drug values.

There are still some anesthetic-induced complications to consider even today, when it comes to cesarean section pain relief, and this applies to both general and regional anesthetic techniques. For example, anesthetic-induced depression of cardiac output further limits pulmonary blood flow in nondependent lung regions, thereby increasing dead space. In addition, if cardiac output is severely reduced to the point that mixed venous oxygen content is decreased, any blood that passes through established right-to-left intrapulmonary shunts will further lower arterial oxyhemoglobin saturation (Table 33–2 and Figure 33–5) (8).

Although $PaCO_2$ is normally reduced in pregnancy, it can be further lowered by manual or mechanical ventilation. A low $PaCO_2$ may be associated with a decrease in cardiac output which, in combination with anesthetic cardiovascular depression and that associated with positive-pressure ventilation, is potentially significant. This effect is minimal with the low analgesic concentration of isoflurane, enflurane, or halothane commonly employed today. However, large falls in cardiac output sometimes follow spinal and peridural anesthesia, particularly in the absence of left uterine displacement and intravascular volume expansion. If the patient is severely preeclamptic with a reduced blood volume, the combination can be catastrophic. Blood volume repletion is essential if these techniques are used.

**Table 33–2.** Effects of Shunt (Qs/Qt) and Cardiac Output (CO) on $PaO_2$*

| | CO (L/min) | $PvO_2$ (mm Hg) | $CvO_2$ (ml/100 ml) | $CaO_2$ (ml/100 ml) | $C(a-v)O_2$ (ml/100 ml) | Qs/Qt | $PaO_2$ (mm Hg) |
|---|---|---|---|---|---|---|---|
| A (normal) | 5 | 47 | 14.8 | 19.8 | 5 | 0.02 | 600 |
| B (shunt) | 5 | 42 | 13.8 | 18.8 | 5 | 0.20 | 250 |
| C (cardiac output) | 2.5 | 18 | 7.5 | 17.5 | 10 | 0.20 | 90 |

* See Figure 33–5.

# CLINICAL CONSIDERATIONS

## *Pulmonary Embolization Syndromes*

### Thromboembolism

Pulmonary thromboembolization is the third leading cause of death in the United States, accounting for approximately 200,000 deaths annually (9). Pregnancy predisposes women to dependent venous stasis, and the majority of clots form in pelvic, iliofemoral, and popliteal vessels. Antepartum pulmonary embolization is rare, but the incidence increases dramatically in the postpartum period (10).

### Symptoms and Signs

Symptoms and signs are nonspecific and are dependent on the size of the embolus (Table 33–3) (9). Of major importance is fixed splitting of the second heart sound (right ventricular overload) and a flow murmur over the lung fields. A chest radiograph may show focal oligemia (Westermark's sign) and the EKG may reveal P pulmonale and a right axis deviation. Definitive diagnosis requires pulmonary angiographic studies. In severe cases, cardiovascular collapse can rapidly supervene.

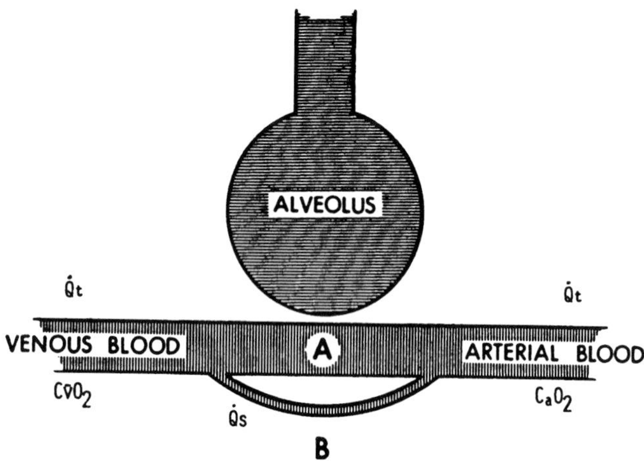


**Fig. 33–5.** Venous blood in the pulmonary circulation may pass through well ventilated areas **(A)** or areas of low or absent ventilation **(B).** If cardiac output is reduced and/or systemic oxygen extraction increases, the venous oxygen content ($CvO_2$) will be less than normal. Any blood passing through **B** will reduce arterial oxygen constant ($CaO_2$) below its normal value, and $PaO_2$ will decrease. (See Table 33–2). Qs = shunted blood; Qt = cardiac output. (With permission from Kirby RR: An overview of anesthesia and critical care medicine. *In* Anesthesia. 2nd ed. Edited by RD Miller. New York, Churchill Livingstone, 1986, p. 2161.)

### Therapy

Initial therapy is entirely supportive and includes oxygen, sometimes in conjunction with tracheal intubation and positive-pressure ventilation, fluid infusion, and cardiovascular support with inotropic agents. In severe cases, right ventricular failure (acute cor pulmonale) may be life-threatening. Thus, infusions must be carefully monitored. Although the classic V/Q abnormality is an increase in dead space, intrapulmonary shunting and hypoxemia also may be increased because of alterations in pulmonary capillary permeability, the development of interstitial pulmonary edema, and "pneumoconstriction." Improvement with PEEP/CPAP often is dramatic.

Heparin therapy for documented pulmonary thromboembolism is the preferred treatment, but can produce bleeding in obstetric patients. Initial doses are 5000 to 10,000 units followed by a continuous infusion of 500 to 1000 U/hour. A partial thromboplastin time of 1.5 to 2.0 times normal is the desired endpoint. Thrombolytic therapy with streptokinase or urokinase is associated with a high incidence of bleeding. Vena caval plication and insertion of caval filters have decreased in popularity (9). Pulmonary embolectomy is rarely, if ever, indicated.

### Amniotic Fluid Embolism

This symptomatic condition occurs once in 10,000 deliveries. It is most commonly seen with multiparity, pro-

**Table 33–3.** Signs and Symptoms of Pulmonary Thromboembolization

| | Percent* |
|---|---|
| *Signs* | |
| Tachypnea | 90 |
| Tachycardia | 45 |
| Increased $P_2$ | 53 |
| Localized crackles | 58 |
| Fever | 45 |
| Thrombophlebitis | 40 |
| Supraventricular dysrhythmias | 15 |
| *Symptoms* | |
| Dyspnea | 84 |
| Chest pain | 88 |
| Apprehension | 59 |
| Cough | 53 |
| Hemoptysis | 30 |

* Percentage of patients with pulmonary thromboembolization displaying sign or symptom.

longed and difficult labor, cephalopelvic disproportion, placenta previa, polyhydramnios, uterine tetany, precipitate delivery, following cesarean section, and with intrauterine fetal demise (11). Its onset may be heralded by cardiovascular collapse, and frequently entails dyspnea, cyanosis, shock, seizures, and coma (2). The maternal mortality rate is as high as 86%. Contrary to popular thinking, it does not appear to be related to induction of labor.

Differential diagnosis include other pulmonary embolic events, eclampsia, intracranial hemorrhage, and heart failure. Fetal squamous cells and other elements have been aspirated through central venous or pulmonary artery catheters (12). However, because the majority of such individuals do not have such catheters in place, diagnosis by this method is of limited value.

Therapy is generally supportive and includes oxygen, positive-pressure ventilation, fluids, vasopressors, and expeditious uterine evacuation. The latter is important to enhance venous return and also to allow closure of uteroplacental sinusoids and endocervical veins.

### Venous Air Embolization

Although commonly associated with sitting neurosurgical procedures (13), venous air embolization (VAE) has been reported in pregnant patients during orogenital sex (14,15) when the sexual partner blows air forcefully into the vagina, and during or following cesarean section (Figure 33–6). Placental separation followed by entry of air into the venous sinuses may be fatal in these circumstances. For obvious reasons, the former incident is unlikely to occur in the hospital setting. However, it should be considered as a possible etiology in pregnant patients brought to the emergency room in extremis for whom no other cause can be ascertained.

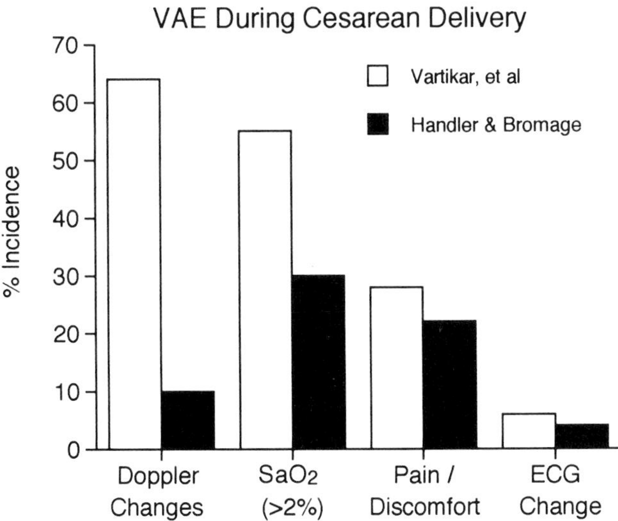


**Fig. 33–6.** This figure shows the percent incidence during cesarean section of venous air embolism from two different studies done in 1989 and 1990 (1989 data from Vartikar JV, Johnson MD, Datta S: Precordial Doppler monitoring and pulse oximetry during cesarean delivery: Detection of venous air embolism. Reg. Anesth. 14:145, 1989; 1990 data from Handler JS, Bromage PR: Venous air embolism during cesarean delivery. Reg. Anesth. 15:170, 1990.)

Following percutaneous vascular cannulation, significant venous air embolization can occur through large-bore needles/introducers in spontaneously breathing patients. Up to 100 ml air/second can be entrained through a 14-gauge needle in the subclavian or internal jugular vein during a deep and rapid inspiration. If such techniques are used, patients should be placed in a head-down position and instructed to hold their breath any time the needle/cannula hub is open to air.

Treatment includes aspiration of air if a central catheter is in situ and placement of the patient in a left lateral decubitus position. Vasopressors are desirable when hypotension is present. Oxygen should be administered, with positive-pressure ventilation if necessary. Paradoxical air embolism to the arterial circulation has been reported as a risk if pulmonary artery pressure is greatly increased. Hence, some investigators question the merits of manual or mechanical ventilation and PEEP during resuscitation because both modes of therapy can increase pulmonary vascular resistance (16).

### Fat Embolization

Fat embolization is likely only following trauma and fractures of the pelvis and long bones. It is mentioned here in an attempt to account for all possible differential diagnoses of embolization syndromes in general. Early stabilization and fixation of fractures is indicated in most cases. Treatment is largely supportive. No good evidence supports the prophylactic use of heparin or steroids. Prevention of hypoxia is essential to maternal and fetal well-being and is best achieved by oxygen administration and PEEP/CPAP, with or without mechanical ventilation.

## Pulmonary Aspiration of Gastric Contents

Of all of the pulmonary disorders in pregnancy, this entity is best known and perhaps most feared. Described by Curtis Mendelsohn in 1945 (7), it has been studied extensively since then. The reported mortality is high, although in the experience of this author, except when fecal aspiration occurs, the outcome is usually good. Parturients are at particular risk because of delayed gastric emptying, relaxed cardioesophageal sphincter tone, increased abdominal pressure, and what seems to be an inevitable fact that just before entering a phase of active labor, one discovers that the patient has eaten a full meal! Vomiting normally is increased during the first trimester of pregnancy, but sometimes persists as hyperemesis gravidarum.

Physical characteristics of aspiration syndromes depend upon what is aspirated and how much (Table 33–4) (17). With acid aspiration (classically stated to result from a volume of 25 ml or greater at a pH of 2.5 or less), wheezing, cyanosis, dyspnea, and tachypnea are noted. With particulate-matter aspiration (food chunks, etc.), airway obstruction with stridor, tachypnea, wheezing, and coughing predominate.

In severe cases, pulmonary edema may result from sudden increases of pulmonary capillary endothelial perme-

**Table 33–4.** Findings in Pulmonary Aspiration

| |
|---|
| Acid |
| Cyanosis |
| Tachypnea |
| Dyspnea |
| Wheezing |
| Bloody sputum (severe cases) |
| Suprasternal/intercostal retractions |
| Hypotension |
| Particulate |
| Stridor |
| Tachypnea |
| Wheezing |
| Coughing |

ability. Hypoxemia, hypercapnia, and nonrespiratory acidosis are prominent features and can be life-threatening. A chest radiograph is positive in approximately 90% of cases, although a delay in radiographic manifestation of up to 24 hours sometimes occurs (17). Most commonly involved is the right lower lobe, followed by the left lower and right middle lobes. Widespread and confluent infiltrates may be present and indistinguishable from other forms of the adult respiratory distress syndrome (ARDS).

Therapy is largely supportive and includes oxygen, establishment of an artificial airway in most cases, and positive airway pressure (PEEP/CPAP with or without mechanical ventilation). Except for the removal of food or other solid particles, do not waste time in an attempt to suction the aspirated material. Damage is immediate. Similarly, do not bother trying to neutralize a suspected acid aspiration with sodium bicarbonate or other alkali. The damage will only be made worse.

No valid evidence supports the use of corticosteroids in the amelioration of any aspiration syndrome (17). Antibiotics may be useful should the aspirated material be known to be infected. Otherwise, corticosteroids should be withheld until culture results document the source of infection. Aerosolized $B_2$ selective agents such as terbutaline, albuterol or fenoterol can be of value in alleviating bronchospasm. Mucosal and submucosal edema often are responsive to the nebulization of racemia epinephrine.

Prevention of aspiration is desirable but often difficult in pregnancy because patients usually are not "NPO." Remember that the time from which to consider that the stomach was full is not when the last meal was eaten, but when labor began (often several hours later). The safest rule-of-thumb is to assume every pregnant woman has a full stomach so as to prevent regurgitation during vaginal delivery by using forceful maneuvers such as shown in Figure 33–7.

Clear, nonparticulate antacids increase gastric pH, but must be administered within 1 hour of the projected anesthesia induction to be effective. Histamine antagonists decrease the volume and increase the pH of gastric secretions formed after they are administered, but do nothing for those already in situ.

If a rapid sequence induction is planned, a properly performed Sellick maneuver will prevent passive regurgitation and aspiration but will not stop active vomiting (17). Consideration should always be given to the possibility of using regional anesthesia for labor and delivery or for other operative procedures in pregnant patients. Keep in mind that even a properly placed cuffed endotracheal tube does not guarantee that aspiration will not occur (18).

## *Acute Respiratory Failure*

Differentiation between acute respiratory failure and embolization and aspiration syndromes is, in a sense, arbitrary, because the latter conditions obviously can produce life-threatening pulmonary insufficiency. However, mechanisms of damage and pathophysiologic changes vary somewhat, so the division into separate categories is reasonable.

A variety of lesions predispose to what has been termed the adult respiratory distress syndrome (19) (See Table 33–5). In many cases, the polymorphonuclear leukocyte seems to be a key factor (perhaps as a result of complement activation with production of C5a) (20). Leukoembolization and leukoagglutination within the pulmonary microvasculature, followed by neutrophil release of toxic-free radicals of oxygen, result in increased endothelial permeability, increased interstitial lung water, terminal airway closure, atelectasis, and right-to-left intrapulmonic shunting. The hallmark of this syndrome is hypoxemia, which is often severe and frequently refractory to the administration of oxygen and manual or mechanical ventilation (19,21).

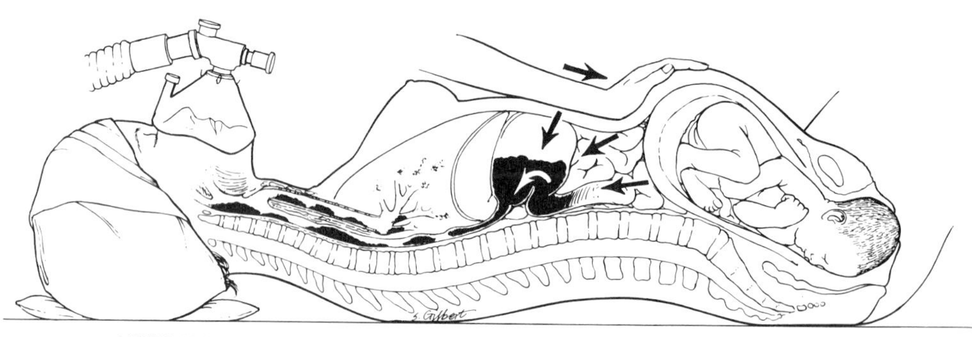


**Fig. 33–7.** Regurgitation of gastric contents caused by a marked increase in intra-abdominal and intragastric pressure from an attempt to place pressure on the uterus during delivery.

**Table 33–5.** Etiologic Factors in Adult Respiratory Distress Syndrome

| Type | Examples |
|---|---|
| Obstetrical | Eclampsia, amniotic fluid embolism |
| Sepsis | |
| Trauma | Burns, fat emboli, pulmonary contusion, nonthoracic trauma, near-drowning |
| Infection | Viral, bacterial, fungal, pneumonia, tuberculosis |
| Toxic gas inhalation | Oxygen, smoke, $NO_2$, $NH_3$, $Cl_2$, phosgene |
| Aspiration of gastric contents | |
| Drug injection | Heroin, methadone, barbiturates, thiazides, propoxyphene, salicylates, colchicine |
| Metabolic | Uremia, diabetic ketoacidosis |
| Miscellaneous | Pancreatitis, disseminated intravascular coagulation (DIC), bowel infarction, carcinomatosis, paraquat poisoning |

Because trauma tends to be a disease of young people (the leading cause of death in the under 40 age group), we see an increasing number of pregnant victims. Because the functional residual capacity is already reduced with pregnancy, one might suspect that the loss of functional residual capacity, characteristic of adult respiratory distress syndrome, is less well-tolerated in pregnancy compared to the nonpregnant state.

The $PaCO_2$ in adult respiratory distress syndrome is characteristically low in the early stages. Because the $PaCO_2$ is also low in pregnancy, a normal value (above 35 mm Hg) is cause for alarm and indicates the possibility of severe derangement of lung function. In view of the propensity for severe hypoxemia, all pregnant patients with adult respiratory distress syndrome (or any form of respiratory failure) should be continuously monitored with a pulse oximeter. Oxyhemoglobin saturations below 90% (a $PaCO_2$ of approximately 55 to 60 mm Hg during pregnancy) represent a serious threat to the fetus, and indicate major impairment of lung function.

Treatment is largely supportive. A few patients will respond to oxygen therapy, clearance of secretions, and chest physiotherapy. Many, however, should have their tracheas intubated and PEEP/CPAP applied, with or without mechanical ventilation (22). Because of the tendency in late pregnancy for compression of the inferior vena cava and a reduction of venous return, positive airway pressure may be poorly tolerated. Careful monitoring of cardiopulmonary function is mandatory.

Specific treatment is limited. All infectious processes (pneumonia, sepsis), if present, should be aggressively treated with appropriate antibiotics. Steroids are of no proven benefit and should not be used in any form of established adult respiratory distress syndrome. Some evidence suggests that they may be beneficial if administered prophylactically. However, because we usually do not have the luxury of knowing which patient will develop respiratory failure, prophylactic treatment is unlikely to be of much value.

## *Asthma*

The overall incidence and severity of asthma seems to be unaffected by pregnancy (2,10). Patients receiving long-term bronchodilator therapy should be continued on their established drug regimen. The importance of early medical intervention and aggressive treatment of severe asthmatic attacks cannot be overemphasized in view of the risk of fetal asphyxia. Commonly employed drugs are associated with a negligible risk of first trimester teratogenicity.

Pregnancy has a mixed effect on asthma. Forty-nine percent of patients are unchanged, 29% improve, and 22% become worse. Improvement may result from the increased release of progesterone and cortisol in pregnancy while upper airway edema, increased oxygen consumption, and decreased pulmonary reserve can produce exacerbations (23). Patients who are chronically symptomatic should continue effective drug therapy, if any (including theophylline, corticosteriods, beta-adrenergic agonists, and cromolyn). Intravenous aminophylline should be used during acute exacerbations, and oxygen therapy (nasal cannula, catheter, face mask) may be necessary during labor and delivery. Constant monitoring with a pulse oximeter is essential in this period, supplemented when necessary by arterial blood gas analysis.

## *Chronic Lung Disease*

In the previous edition of this book, bronchiectasis received major attention as a form of chronic lung disease (10). When it occurs, it can still present severe problems. However, its incidence since 1970 is definitely reduced, presumably as a result of better antibiotic therapy. This author has not seen a case in 13 years (and have never seen one in an obstetric patient). When a patient with bronchiectasis is encountered, aggressive antibiotic and chest physiotherapy are indicated. Tracheobronchial toiletry is of obvious importance, particularly should an endotracheal tube be inserted during general inhalational anesthesia.

Emphysema and chronic bronchitis in the child-bearing age group are rare (10). Because these are irreversible conditions, they can not be "cured." Nevertheless, any reversible component, i.e., airway edema and bronchospasm, should be treated aggressively with aerosolized topical vasoconstrictors and bronchodilators, respectively. Prevention or treatment of pulmonary infection is important. Any evidence of hypoxemia or hypercapnia (beyond baseline levels) necessitates hospitalization.

Chronic restrictive lung disease in pregnancy (pulmonary interstitial fibrosis, kyphoscoliosis) is rare (10). When severe, successful conclusion of the pregnancy represents a major threat to maternal survival. In the author's view, termination of pregnancy should be considered in advanced kyphoscoliotic lung disease. The best ventilator support therapy is largely ineffective in acute cor pulmonale, a very real risk with the superimposed cardiopulmonary stress of pregnancy.

Some years ago, cystic fibrosis in pregnancy was a rarely encountered problem, as few patients lived until their child-bearing years. Today, however, longer survival is

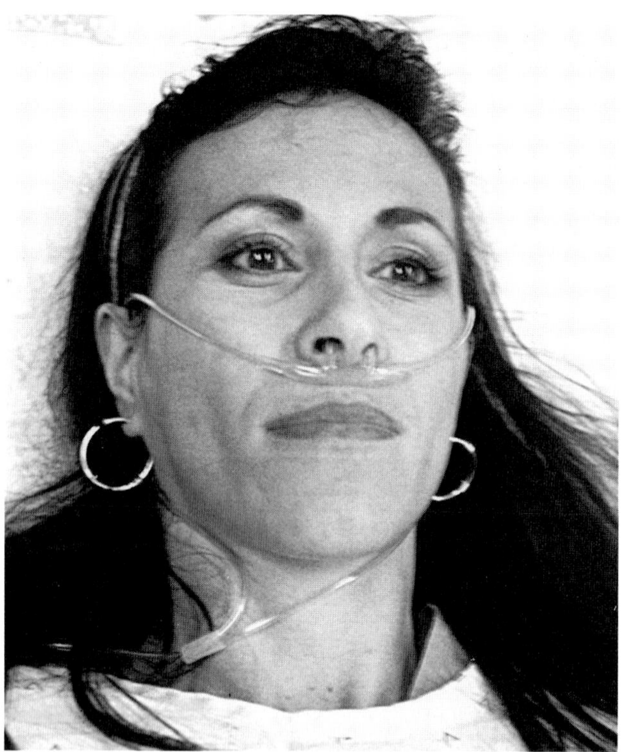

**Fig. 38–8.** Use of nasal prong for delivery of low rates of oxygen (ranges between 2 to 5 L/min). (From The Ohio State University Hospitals, Department of Anesthesiology, 1992.)

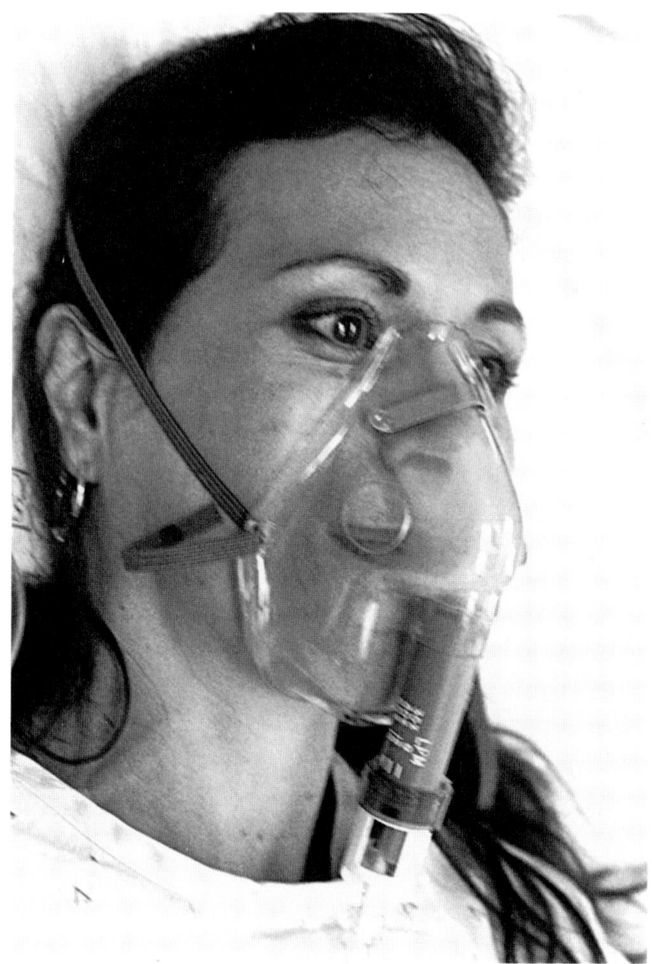

**Fig. 33–9.** Use of a Venturi mask, which is preferred for high oxygen rates (>5 L/min) to provide for a higher tracheal $PO_2$. This type of mask can be substituted for a reservoir system with a bag, which is used by many anesthesiologists. (From The Ohio State University Hospitals, Department of Anesthesiology, 1992.)

more common, and reports of successful completion of pregnancy in women with cystic fibrosis have been published (24). Interestingly, worsening of baseline pulmonary function often does not occur with pregnancy. Careful evaluation and close monitoring during gestation are essential, and hospitalization, vigorous pulmonary toilet, and aggressive antibiotic therapy are indicated at the first sign of pulmonary complications.

Acute respiratory failure, asthma, and chronic lung disease patients are all excellent candidates for regional anesthesia, and should be provided with such an option and be educated about the benefits to their well-being with such a technique. In each of these, supplemental $O_2$ can be administered by one of the several methods shown in Figures 33–8 through 33–11). It is important to use either lumbar epidural with slow advancement of the block or continuous subarachnoid block with fractionated small injections to prevent hypotension.

## *Anesthetic Considerations*

In the pulmonary embolization syndromes, there are a wide variety of considerations in regard to the choice of anesthetic technique. First, patients who are diagnosed as having thromboembolism and are in labor or are candidates for cesarean section delivery most likely will have some type of anticoagulant regimen already initiated. If these regimens are effective in prevention of continued thromboembolism episodes, they may also adversely affect the use of regional anesthetic techniques because of the fear of hematoma formation and bleeding into the lumbar epidural space. The first step, then, is to determine if a patient has been placed on an anticoagulant treatment regimen. The next step, if that indeed is the case, is to obtain a coagulation profile on the patient consisting of bleeding time, platelets, prothrombin time, thrombin time, and activated partial thromboplastin time. It is important to obtain these coagulation studies so that some reasonable decision can be made about the safety of use of regional anesthesia. Normal levels are shown in Table 33–6).

If the patient has been on subcutaneous heparin for some time, it is still possible to consider use of regional technique, especially if such as selection is preferred and also indicated. Many mothers may be on either daily injections or continuous subcutaneous pumps to keep their prothrombin time around 1.5 times normal with an endogenous heparin titer of 0.1 to 0.2 units/ml. It must be recalled that the pregnancy state is a state of relative

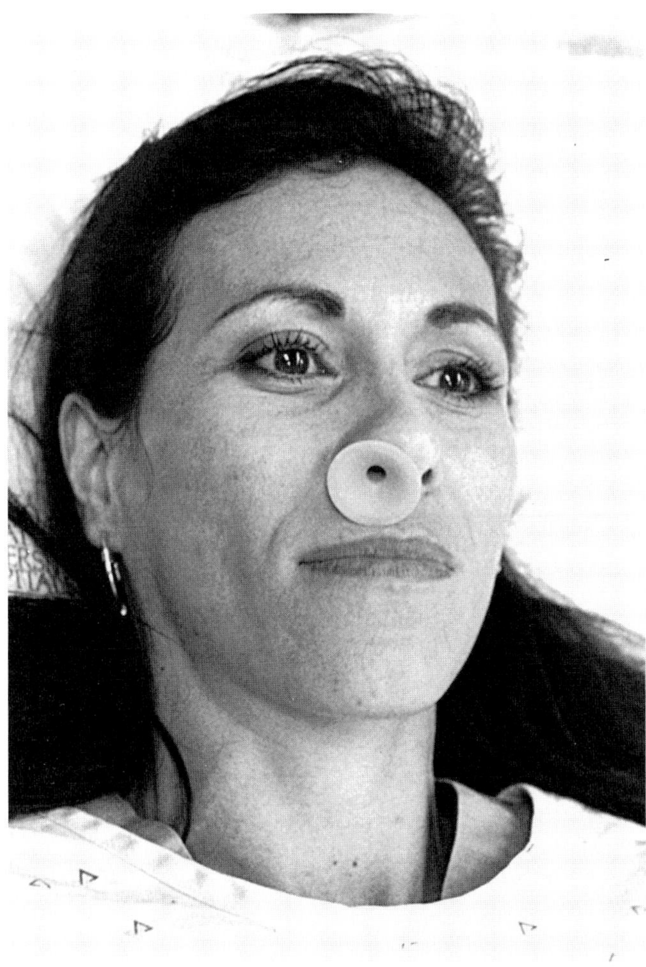

Fig. 33–10. Use of soft nasopharyngeal catheter, the end of which is located in the nasopharynx. (From The Ohio State University Hospitals, Department of Anesthesiology, 1992.)

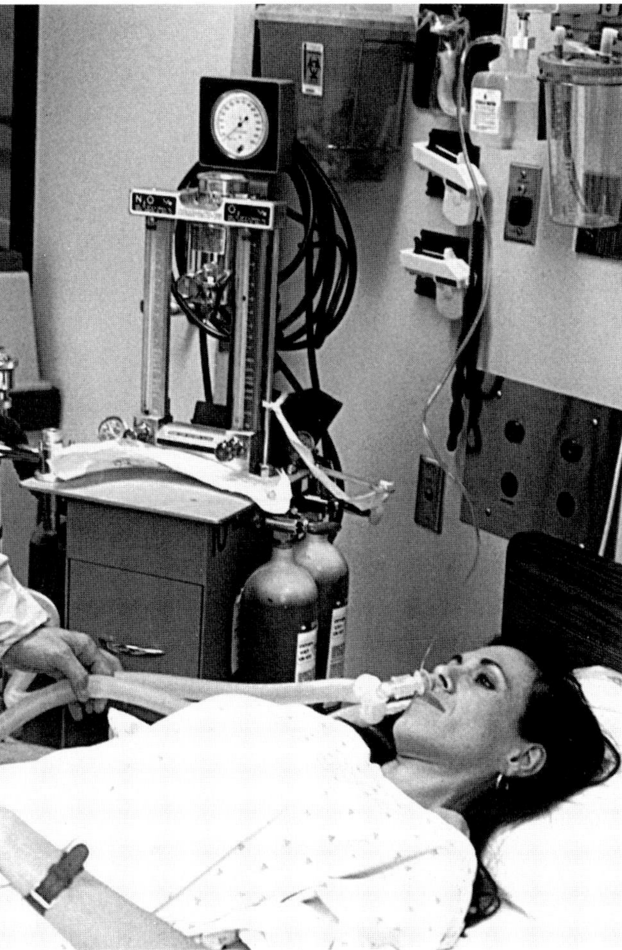

Fig. 33–11. This figure demonstrates the connection through the male fitting using an endotracheal tube connector that fits into the nasal opening of the nasopharyngeal catheter in Figure 33–10.

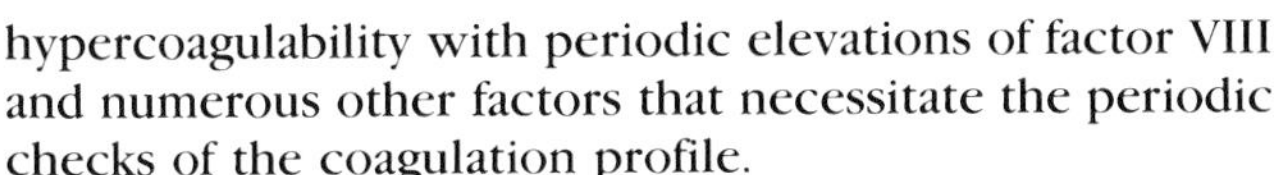

hypercoagulability with periodic elevations of factor VIII and numerous other factors that necessitate the periodic checks of the coagulation profile.

Moving on to the cesarean section candidates, for patients who have thromboembolism, the clinician is faced with a difficult decision. If the patient is adamant that she be awake to interact with her baby at delivery, and if the aforementioned coagulation profiles are not abnormal, then regional anesthesia can still be considered. A recent study of the influence of regional technique on the pathophysiology of deep venous thrombosis revealed the lumbar epidural and spinal had noticeable advantages over general anesthesia by increasing blood flow in the lower extremities, by decreasing the coagulation tendency, by improvement of the fibrinolytic action, and by reduction of operative blood loss (25). Of course, it is important to temper the enthusiasm for regional methods in the face of anticoagulant therapy should values be borderline-abnormal, as nontraumatic spinal/epidural hematomas are most always associated with needle trauma and subsequent closed-space blood formation and possible neurologic damage if not detected and treated early. If the decision is made in favor of regional anesthesia in the above noted scenario, it must be done only after full disclosure and information has been given to the patient and colleague obstetrician, and only when unanimous approval for same has been gotten.

The cesarean section experience can still be a quality

**Table 33–6.** Coagulation Profile

| Study | Normal | Abnormal |
|---|---|---|
| 1) Bleeding Time | 1 to 5 minutes* | >12 |
| 2) Platelets | 140,000 to 440,000 | <100,000 |
| 3) Prothrombin Time | 11 to 12 seconds* | >13 seconds |
| 4) Thrombin Time | 16 to 20 seconds* | >24 seconds |
| 5) Activated Partial Thromboplastin Time | 24 to 36 seconds* | >38 seconds |

* The normal levels stated here are for guidance only. The individual laboratories must be consulted for your normal ranges.
(From The Ohio State University Hospitals, Department of Anesthesiology, 1992.)

experience in cases in which the coagulation profiles are within normal limits and, in some instances, a local anesthetic can be proposed to the mother by the obstetrician who is skilled in the method and has support from the anesthesiologist who will administer small doses of ketamine and offer verbal support.

In the case of amniotic fluid embolism, venous air embolism, and fat embolism, there is usually little opportunity to consider alternate anesthetic techniques. For the most part, these problems occur suddenly, are cataclysmic in nature, and often are life threatening to the point that general anesthesia is the only method of consideration. All of these problems share similar pathophysiologic mechanisms, including: (1) immediate cardiac output reduction; (2) pulmonary hypertension and subsequent right heart failure; and (3) hypoxia due to drastic abnormalities in ventilation perfusion ratios. In all of these, maternal hypoxia and cardiovascular collapse may be a major threat to physiologic stability. General anesthesia affords a method of airway protection, a means of reversing pulmonary edema and hypoxia because of tracheal intubation, and positive pressure ventilation, and it offers a method of circulatory support because of fluid infusion and cardiovascular support with ionotropes. Finally, general anesthesia also offers a method of rapid fetal delivery, which may be life saving in such scenarios. These three entities, amniotic fluid embolism, venous air embolism, and fat embolism always stress the capabilities of the cardiovascular system to the maximum, and the outcome is often less than desirable for the mother or her fetus.

Pulmonary aspiration of gastric contents is also covered extensively in Chapter 43. This complication is most often associated with general anesthetic induction, but can occur spontaneously in labor in rare cases. Typically, this complication is diagnosed during attempts to intubate during the process of general anesthesia induction. Usually, the oral tracheal tube is in place and the anesthetic is continued for: (1) delivery of the fetus; (2) treatment of the aspiration with positive pressure ventilation; (3) and continued postoperative management of the patient with the oral tracheal tube left in place with added PEEP/CPAP, as previously mentioned.

Because there is always the possibility that airway instrumentation may precipitate acute bronchospasm, lumbar epidural is the preferred anesthetic choice for cesarean section. An inadequate level of sensory blocks, however, results in anxiety and pain, which can exacerbate the problem. Conversely, too high a sensory and motor blockade leads to increased dyspnea and can interfere with satisfactory ventilation. Properly administered and maintained epidural analgesia approaches the ideal for labor and vaginal delivery.

Should a general anesthetic be necessary for cesarean section, preoxygenation followed by cricoid pressure, and a rapid sequence induction with sodium thiopental or ketamine and succinylcholine is preferred. Although thiopental is worrisome to many anesthesiologists who fear its precipitation of an acute bronchospastic attack, this author feels the concern is vastly overrated. Ketamine is not associated with this problem, but it can lead to significant hypertension should the patient be already hypertensive. Following tracheal intubation, anesthesia can be maintained with isoflurane and a 50:50 nitrous oxide/oxygen mixture. Cardiac dysrhythmias in the face of theophylline, beta-adrenergic agents, and halothane preclude the latter. Short-acting nondepolarizing muscle relaxants (which, if used properly, should not require reversal) are preferable. A succinylcholine infusion is an accepted alternative.

Tuberculosis, which once was thought to have been largely eradicated, is now on the rise again. Hence, increasing numbers of cases are to be expected during pregnancy. Drug therapy with isoniazid and rifampin is effective and subjects the fetus to minimal risk. Appropriate isolation procedures during labor and delivery should be employed. Use of disposable ventilator and anesthesia circuits makes patient management and infection control much easier than was previously true. The risk of acquired immune deficiency syndrome (AIDS) has made anesthesiologists acutely aware of the importance of such measures. Similar precautions in cases of tuberculosis minimize the risk of patient/physician contact.

### Pulmonary Edema

Pulmonary edema has been mentioned repeatedly throughout this chapter. Certain facts should be kept in mind. First, it is not an entity unto itself. When it occurs, some predisposing factor is present (Table 33–7) (26). Second, two major concerns should be evident: (1) management of the effects (predominantly hypoxemia); and (2) establishment of the cause(s). The former problem is reasonably easy to address, because therapy is largely the same as for other forms of adult respiratory distress syndrome, the characteristic finding of which is pulmonary edema. However, in pregnant patients, particularly those with congenital heart disease, the problem may be cardiovascular in origin, and considerably more difficult to treat.

**Table 33–7.** Causes of Pulmonary Edema

| | |
|---|---|
| *Cardiogenic (High Pressures)* | |
| Cardiac dysfunction | Decreased left ventricular contractility, mitral stenoses, mitral regurgitation, intravascular volume overload, dysrhythmias |
| Pulmonary venous dysfunction | Venous occlusive disease, neurogenic pulmonary vasoconstriction |
| Pulmonary embolization | Amniotic fluid, thrombus, fat, air |
| Airway obstruction | Edema, asthma, foreign body |
| Preeclampsia | Pulmonary hypertension |
| Miscellaneous | Pneumothorax, tumor, one lung anesthesia (down lung syndrome) |
| *Noncardiogenic (Permeability)* | |
| Adult Respiratory Distress Syndrome (ARDS) | |
| Aspiration syndromes | |
| Pulmonary embolization | |
| Abruptio placentae | |
| Dead fetus syndrome | |
| Sepsis | |

Although this author's enthusiasm for pulmonary artery catheterization has waned in recent years (27) he feels that it is definitely indicated when the origin of pulmonary edema during pregnancy is not immediately clear (and sometimes even when it is) (28). A low pulmonary artery occlusion pressure (PAOP), for practical purposes, eliminates left ventricular failure as an etiologic factor. A high pulmonary artery pressure may reflect preeclampsia or other forms of noncardiogenic pulmonary edema. The distinction between these disease categories is clearly significant. Diuresis, which may be indicated for left ventricular failure, is an obvious threat to both maternal and fetal well-being in a mother who is hypovolemic and who has a noncardiogenic origin of her pulmonary edema. Sequential measurements of cardiac output, central venous pressure (CVP), pulmonary artery occlusion pressure, and mixed venous oxygen saturation, together with calculated values of systemic and pulmonary vascular resistance, can guide medical therapy based upon physiologic endpoints rather than a less rigidly informed guess (3).

When severe preeclampsia is present, inappropriate fluid therapy can precipitate significant elevation of pulmonary artery pressure and an increase of fluid deposition in the pulmonary interstitium. A lowering of plasma oncotic pressure postpartum will potentially exacerbate this problem, although the data in this regard are not altogether convincing. Should preeclampsia progress to eclamptic seizures, pulmonary aspiration of gastric contents can make the differential diagnosis problematic.

### Anesthetic Management

In the case of pulmonary edema, it must be appreciated that the management of anesthesia in such patients has been argued long, vociferously, and with much emotion. Whenever possible, blood pressure control should be achieved before the induction of anesthesia. Because this goal usually can be achieved very precisely with nitroglycerin or sodium nitroprusside, this author prefers these agents during acute hypertensive crises (Table 33–8).

Lumbar epidural offers many advantages. Blood pressure can be regulated. However, the anesthesiologist must bear in mind that severe preeclamptics are by definition hypovolemic. Too high a level of sensory and sympathetic blockage in combination with aortocaval compression by the gravid uterus can produce disastrous hypotension and cardiovascular collapse. In addition, 15% of even mild preeclamptic patients are thrombocytopenic; others may have abnormal platelet function.

**Table 33–8.** Sodium Nitroprusside Treatment of Hypertension in Pregnancy

| | CO | HR | MAP | CVP | PAM | PAW | SVR | PVR |
|---|---|---|---|---|---|---|---|---|
| 4 hours post-operatively | 4.2 | 82 | 90 | 5 | 53 | 9 | 1619 | 838 |
| SNP 0.25 μg/kg/min | 2.6 | 109 | 96 | 14 | 48 | 13 | 2521 | 1076 |
| SNP 0.75 μg/kg/min | 3.9 | 103 | 84 | 6 | 49 | 7 | 1598 | 861 |

SNP Sodium nitroprusside
(Modified from Roberts NV, Keast PJ: Pulmonary hypertension and pregnancy—a lethal combination. Anaesth Intens Care 18:366–374, 1990.)

Peripheral vasodilation, when properly controlled, decreases right ventricular preload and left ventricular afterload. In so doing, the tendency for further pulmonary edema formation is reduced. As blockage regresses in the postpartum period, however, centralization of the blood volume will follow, with a possible exacerbation of edema and lung dysfunction.

A general anesthesia will resolve some of these problems but presents others. Tracheal intubation is often difficult because of the edematous airway and the tendency toward bleeding. In addition, significant increases of mean arterial pressure, pulmonary artery pressure, and pulmonary artery occlusion pressure have led to further pulmonary edema and cerebral hemorrhage. If following a failed intubation, airway obstruction occurs, the patients inspiratory efforts may result in so-called negative pressure pulmonary edema. This condition sometimes results in severe hypoxemia and a radiographic picture similar to diffuse aspiration.

The origins of noncardiac (permeability) pulmonary edema, as has been mentioned, are multifactorial, and differentiation of one form from another is often difficult. For the reasons previously mentioned, flow-directed pulmonary artery catheterization can be useful both for diagnosis and therapeutic guide. Remember, however, that even if a permeability problem leads to the initial manifestations of pulmonary edema, pulmonary hypertension from any cause will make it worse. Careful fluid management during labor, anesthesia, and delivery is mandatory.

## Shock

Hemorrhage leading to cardiovascular insufficiency and shock is still a common problem in obstetrics (29). Causes include placenta previa, abruptio placentae, obstetric injuries (lacerations), retained products of conception, uterine atony, and major trauma. Historically, it has been thought that shock, per se, can lead to acute pulmonary insufficiency—an adult respiratory distress syndrome picture. This view formerly was so prevalent that the term *shock lung* frequently was applied. More recent studies, however, suggest that in the absence of sepsis or direct thoracic trauma, shock does not lead to lung dysfunction (30). Rather, conditions that can produce shock may also cause lung damage in a temporally related fashion, but not in a cause-and-effect one. It seems, then, that shock lung is a laboratory curiosity prevalent in lower vertebrates (i.e., dogs) but not in humans. Respiratory failure in sepsis, however, is a very real problem still associated with a high mortality.

### Anesthetic Management

All aspects of the management of shock are managed by the general anesthetic technique for reasons expressed in the management of amniotic fluid embolism, pulmonary embolism, fat embolism, and pulmonary edema, namely that this is an absolute emergency that must receive the fullest attention and dedication to detail regarding management of both pulmonary and cardiovascular systems. Immediate delivery of the fetus must also be accomplished and kept in the front of one's mind because it is only with delivery of the fetus that adequate resuscitative measures can be instituted. In such catastrophic emergencies superimposed upon pregnancy, the morbidity and mortality are understandably high. Shock conditions may be due to hemorrhagic problems such as placenta previa or abruptio placentae, but they may also be nonhemorrhagic—more often due to cardiogenic problems, such as congenital or acquired heart disorders as mentioned in the section on rheumatic heart disease or congenital heart disease. These latter cases are best handled in labor with a combined lumbar epidural/caudal epidural technique by which perfect separation of T10 to L1 and S2 to S4 inputs from first and second stage can be interrupted separately. The advantage, of course, is that no hypotension need occur because a small block in each instance avoids extensive sympathectomy and thus substantial reduction in peripheral vascular resistance. In past years, Dr. John S. McDonald has managed a series of a dozen patients with mixed mitral and aortic disease in this manner with excellent first and second stage analgesia and no changes in blood pressure or heart rate. In recent years, McDonald has managed to obtain labor pain relief and subsequent perineal relief for episiotomy and delivery with the continuous dilute solution of local anesthetic opioid combinations such as referred to in Chapter 13. If the administration time exceeds 2 hours, usually there is adequate perineal pain relief. This is likely due to the addition of sufentanil and epinephrine, both of which help to promote a more intense degree of analgesia, so much so that even the thick sacral fibers are penetrated.

## *Pulmonary Manifestations of Cardiac Disease*

### Rheumatic Heart Disease

Although decreased in incidence, rheumatic heart disease is still the most common heart disease in pregnancy (2). Mitral stenosis accounts for approximately 90% of the valvular lesions, and, in an advanced stage, is associated with pulmonary congestion, easy fatigability, and dyspnea. The condition is aggravated in pregnancy because of the increased blood volume and hyperdynamic state of the circulation. Pulmonary edema is a major complication. Control of the heart rate is essential, and avoidance of pain is a major consideration in this regard. Avoidance of conditions (including the administration of certain anesthetic agents such as ketamine and nitrous oxide) that induce pulmonary hypertension is also important.

Mitral insufficiency is the second most common valvular lesion in pregnancy (2). It is often manifested by left ventricular dysfunction and, in advanced conditions, pulmonary edema. Increases in systemic vascular resistance, which increase regurgitant flow, are poorly tolerated. Occasionally, mitral valve prolapse may lead to mitral insufficiency.

Aortic stenosis is rare but can be associated with left ventricular failure and pulmonary congestion. Depression of left ventricular function should be avoided by the use of minimally depressant anesthetic drugs. Aortic insufficiency is also rare and is accompanied by left ventricular volume overload and pulmonary congestion. As with mitral regurgitation, increased systemic vascular resistance, myocardial depression, and bradycardia are poorly tolerated.

### Congenital Heart Disease

Twenty-five percent of heart disease in pregnancy is congenital. Ventricular and atrial septal defects lead to left-to-right intracardiac shunts, which generally are well-tolerated in pregnancy. Nevertheless, left ventricular failure may occur with resultant pulmonary edema. Avoidance of tachycardia, increased systemic vascular resistance, and supraventricular dysrhythmias are important goals of management.

Right-to-left intracardiac shunts are serious problems during pregnancy. Profound hypoxemia may result and is exacerbated by pulmonary hypertension. Reduced blood volume, systemic vascular resistance, and venous return must be avoided. Pulmonary complications are not prominent unless the shunt is bidirectional.

## Diagnosis and Treatment

In general, both diagnostic and therapeutic modalities in pregnancy-associated respiratory failure are the same as in nonpregnant patients. Most have been considered earlier in this chapter. The availability of pulse oximetry should enhance monitoring capabilities and management (31). When combined with appropriately used fetal monitoring (32), maternal and fetal hypoxemia may be expected to be decreased in incidence and severity.

Mechanical or manual ventilation with PEEP/CPAP is effective in the treatment of many forms of acute respiratory failure. However, their potentially adverse effects on venous return, particularly when aortocaval compression is significant, can present major maternal and fetal problems. Conversely, noncardiogenic pulmonary edema can be acutely exacerbated by increased pulmonary arterial blood flow and pressure. Thus, sudden changes in the patient's condition, of an even greater magnitude than in the nonpregnant individual, are almost to be expected.

The clinical impression of this author is that obstetric patients are often managed as ward patients far too long before consultation is sought for respiratory (and other basically nonobstetric) conditions. If any patient should receive the benefits of critical care, it is the pregnant woman with serious or life-threatening disease. Unfortunately, many critical care practitioners have little or no experience in the management of sick obstetric patients. Improved communication and better interaction between specialists are essential to reduce maternal and fetal morbidity and mortality. Advances in this area should be no less than in perinatology.

## REFERENCES

1. Caton D: Pregnancy: essential physiologic concerns. *In* Critical Care. Edited by JM Civetta, RW Taylor, RR Kirby. Philadelphia, J.B. Lippincott, 1988, pp. 1341–1348.
2. James CF: Systemic disease in the obstetric patient: Anesthe-

sia and invasive monitoring. *In* Critical Care. Edited by JM Civetta, RW Taylor, RR Kirby. Philadelphia, J.B. Lippincott, 1988, pp. 1367–1376.
3. Hood DD: Hypertensive disorders of pregnancy: preeclampsia and eclampsia. *In* Critical Care. Edited by JM Civetta, RW Taylor, RR Kirby. Philadelphia, J.B. Lippincott, 1988, pp. 1349–1358.
4. Robotham JL, Scharf SM: Effects of positive and negative pressure ventilation on cardiac performance. Clin. Chest. Med. 4:161, 1983.
5. Froese AB, Bryan AC: Effects of Anesthesia and Paralysis on Diaphragmatic Mechanics in Man. Anesthesiology 41:242, 1974.
6. Mendelson CL: The aspiration of stomach contents into the lungs during anesthesia. Am. J. Obstet. Gynecol. 52:191, 1946.
7. Pfaff DW, McEwen BS: Actions of estrogens and progestins on nerve cells. Science 219:808, 1983.
8. Kirby, RR: Complications in anesthesia: respiratory system. *In* Handbook of Complications. Edited by N Gravenstein. Philadelphia, J.B. Lippincott, 1990.
9. Currie, RB: Pulmonary embolism. *In* Respiratory Failure. Edited by RR Kirby, RW Taylor. Chicago, Year Book Medical Publishers, 1986, pp. 335–348.
10. Prevention of venous thrombosis and pulmonary embolism. National Institutes of Health Consensus Development Conference Statement. Vol. 6, No. 2., 1986.
11. Morgan M: Amniotic fluid embolism. Anaesthesia 34:20, 1979.
12. Scharf RHM, de Campo T, Civetta JM: Hemodynamic alterations and rapid diagnosis in a case of amniotic-fluid embolus. Anesthesiology 46:155, 1977.
13. Pashayan AG: Monitoring the neurosurgical patient. *In* Problems In Anesthesia: Monitoring. Edited by N Gravenstein. Philadelphia, J.B. Lippincott, 1987, pp. 104–120.
14. Aronson ME, Nelson PK: Fatal air embolism in pregnancy resulting from an unusual sex act. Obstet. Gynecol. 30:127, 1967.
15. Kaufman BS, Kaminsky SJ, Rakow EC, Weil MH: Adult respiratory distress syndrome following orogenital sex during pregnancy. Crit. Care Med. 15:703, 1987.
16. Lucas WJ: How to manage air embolism. *In* Problems in Anesthesia: Perioperative Problems/Catastrophes. Edited by RW Vaughan. Philadelphia, J.B. Lippincott, 1987, pp. 288–303.
17. Goodwin SR: Aspiration syndromes. *In* Critical Care. Edited by JM Civetta, RW Taylor, RR Kirby. Philadelphia, J.B. Lippincott, 1988, pp. 1081–1090.
18. Stark DCC: Aspiration in the surgical patient. *In* International Anesthesiology Clinics: Pulmonary Aspiration. Edited by R Bryan-Roberts. Boston, Little, Brown and Co., 1977, pp. 13–48.
19. Maunder RJ: Clinical prediction of the adult respiratory distress syndrome. Clin. Chest Med. 6:413, 1985.
20. Tate RM, Pepine JE: Neutrophils and the adult respiratory distress syndrome. Am. Rev. Respir. Dis. 128:552, 1983.
21. Petty TL, Ashbaugh DG: The adult respiratory distress syndrome: clinical features, factors influencing prognosis and principles of management. Chest 60:233, 1971.
22. Taylor RW: The Adult Respiratory Distress Syndrome. *In* Respiratory Failure. Edited by RR Kirby, RW Taylor. Chicago, Year Book Medical Publishers, 1986, pp. 208–244.
23. Fitzsimmons R, Greenberger PA, Patterson R: Outcome of pregnancy in women requiring corticosteroids for severe asthma. J. Allergy Clin. Immunol. 78:349, 1986.
24. Brown MA, Taussig IM: Fertility, birth control and pregnancy in adult patients with cystic fibrosis. Pulmonary Perspectives 5:1, 1988.
25. Modig J: Influence of regional anesthesia, local anesthetics, and sympathicomimetics on the pathophysiology of deep vein thrombosis. Acta. Chir. Scand. Suppl. 550:119–127, 1988.
26. Mecca RS: Clinical aspects of pulmonary edema. *In* Respiratory Failure. Edited by RR Kirby, RW Taylor. Chicago, Year Book Medical Publishers, 1986, pp. 193–207.
27. Robin ED: Iatroepidemics: a probe to examine systematic preventable errors in (chest) medicine. Am. Rev. Respir. Dis. 135:1152, 1987.
28. Keefer JR, Strauss RG, Civetta JM, Burke T: Noncardiogenic pulmonary edema and invasive cardiovascular monitoring. Obstet. Gynecol. 58:46, 1981.
29. Gibbs CP: Hemorrhagic disorders in the obstetric patient. *In* Critical Care. Edited by JM Civetta, RW Taylor, RR Kirby. Philadelphia, J.B. Lippincott, 1988, pp. 1359–1366.
30. Horovitz JH, Carrico CJ, Shires GT: Pulmonary response to major injury. Arch. Surg. 108:349–355, 1974.
31. Cote CJ, Goldstein EA, Cote MA, Hoaglin DC, et al: A single-blind study of pulse oximetry in children. Anesthesiology 68:184, 1988.
32. Caton DD: Fetal Monitoring Concerns. *In* Critical Care. Edited by JM Civetta, RW Taylor, RR Kirby. Philadelphia, J.B. Lippincott, 1988, pp. 1377.

Chapter 34

# DISEASES OF THE GENITOURINARY SYSTEM AND GASTROINTESTINAL TRACT

JOHN P. ELLIOT
JOHN S. McDONALD

The anatomy and physiology of pregnant patients can be significantly different from nongravid women. Alterations in form and function of anatomy and physiology will occur in healthy individuals, but also in patients with various acute and chronic diseases. The medical approach to pregnant patients with diseases of the genitourinary and gastrointestinal tract must consider these changes. Specific considerations for anesthesia in these patients must also be adapted to the pregnant patient. In considering these problems, pregnancy may have an effect on the disease and likewise the disease may affect the pregnancy. Our discussion here will be presented from both perspectives.

To understand the patient with disorders of the excretory system (kidney and gastrointestinal), it is important to appreciate the normal physiological changes that occur in pregnancy.

## ANATOMY OF THE GENITOURINARY SYSTEM

Dilatation of the collecting system is the paramount change in pregnancy. The renal pelvis and the ureters are enlarged with progression from the first trimester until term. Ureteral dilatation starts at the pelvic brim distally and extends to the kidney. The etiology of these changes is not established, but both hormonal (estrogen and progesterone) and mechanical obstructive effects (uterine pressure at the level of the pelvic brim) are believed to play a role. Ureteral tone and function are unaffected by these changes. Renal size has been demonstrated to increase by 1 to 2 cm, which may be caused by the increased blood flow during pregnancy. There may also be an increase in vesicoureteral reflux during pregnancy which may explain the increase in infections. These anatomic changes often persist for several months following delivery and should be recalled when performing diagnostic ultrasound and intravenous pyelogram examinations.

## PHYSIOLOGY OF THE GENITOURINARY SYSTEM

There is a significant increase in the amount of blood delivered to the kidneys during pregnancy. Cardiac output is increased by 40 to 45% and the flow to the kidneys is increased by up to 30%. There is also a fall in renal vascular resistance.

The net effect of this increased blood flow to the kidneys, cardiac output, and decreased renal vascular resistance is an increase in renal plasma flow (RPF) and glomerular filtration rate (GFR) by as much as 50%. Laboratory tests of renal function are altered by these changes, with a lowering of BUN and creatinine values in the normal pregnant patient. The normal BUN in pregnancy is $8.7 \pm 1.5$ mg/100 ml (nonpregnant $13.0 \pm 3.0$ mg/100 ml), and creatinine in pregnancy is $0.46 \pm 0.06$ mg/100 ml (compared to nonpregnant $0.67 + 0.07$ mg/100 ml). Creatinine clearance is increased in pregnancy from nonpregnant values of 65 to 145 cc/min to 105 to 220 cc/minute; therefore, values below 100 cc/min are potentially pathological. Protein excretion is increased in pregnancy and proteinuria should not be considered abnormal until it exceeds 300 mg/24 hrs.

There are some important consequences of these physiologic changes in the pregnant female. The increase in the glomerular filtration rate causes a change in clearance for any substance that is eliminated by the kidney. Just as urea nitrogen and creatinine are more efficiently removed from the body during pregnancy, drugs and other medications will also be excreted more rapidly than in the nonpregnant patient. This has a profound effect on dosing medications in pregnancy. Epileptics on stable doses of phenytoin (Dilantin) may begin seizing when they become pregnant; likewise, doses of digitalis are considerably higher when the cardiac patient is pregnant. This more rapid excretion also affects antibiotics, narcotics, antiemetics, etc.

Renal disease is usually preexisting prior to the pregnancy; however, in an occasional patient, it may be first recognized during gestation. A patient history should be sought for hematuria, polyuria, and nocturia in addition to dysuria, urgency, and foul-smelling urine. A history of repeated urinary tract infections or kidney infection may be obtained. A complete blood count (CBC), urinalysis, and culture are generally performed at the first patient visit. This should screen the majority of patients for undiagnosed renal disease (Table 34–1) (1). Tests for specific renal problems are listed in Table 34–2, and confirmation tests for renal failure are listed in Table 34–3. Anemia may be caused by chronic renal disease and anemia and thrombocytopenia may indicate systemic lupus erythema-

**Table 34–1.** Tests for Determining Renal Problems

| Test | Diagnosis |
|---|---|
| Complete Blood Count | |
| Anemia | Chronic renal pathology |
| Anemia with leukocytosis | Polyarteritis nodosa |
| Anemia, leukocytosis thrombocytopenia | Systemic lupus |
| Urinalysis | |
| Increased pH | Adrenal pathology |
| Decreased specific gravity or osmolarity | Renal parenchymal disease |
| Proteinuria | Glomerular lesions (2 gm/day-interstitial nephritis)<br>Nephrosclerosis (0.5–2 gm/day) |
| Hematuria | Glomerulonephritis<br>Polycystic disease<br>Obstructive uropathy |
| Sediment greater than 5 RBC*/hpf | Glomerulonephritis<br>Collagen vascular disease<br>Polycystic disease |
| Excessive leukocytes | Chronic pyelonephritis<br>Polyarteritis nodosa |
| Casts (hyaline, granular, RBC) | Glomerulonephritis<br>Collagen vascular disease |
| Gram stain >5 bacteria (unspun urine one drop with bacteria equals $10^6$ organism per ml) | Chronic pyelonephritis |
| Blood chemistries elevated BUN and serum creatinine | Renal aprenchymal disease |
| Electrolytes | |
| [$Na^+$, $H_2CO_3^-$ increased, $K^+$ $Cl^-$ decreased] | Primary aldosteronism<br>Salt-losing nephritis |
| [$Na^+$, $H_2CO_3^-$, $K^+$ all decreased] | Renal failure |
| Increased uric acid, potassium, BUN, creatinine | |

* RBC, red blood cells
(From Gabert HA, Miller JM: Renal disease in pregnancy. Obstet. Gynecol. Surv. 40:449, 1985.)

tosis (SLE). The urinary sediment may reveal bacteriuria, proteinuria, hematuria or casts, which would necessitate further investigation. A positive culture would diagnose a urinary tract infection.

## INFECTIOUS DISEASE OF THE URINARY TRACT

### *Etiology*

The most common problem involving the urinary tract in pregnant patients is infection and it may affect 10% of all pregnancies (2). The majority of these are asymptomatic and consist of bacteriuria; however, acute cystitis may occur with symptoms of dysuria, urgency, and frequency. These lower tract infections should be treated vigorously with antibiotics to prevent upper tract infection (pyelonephritis). Because E. coli and Klebsiella-Enterobacter species account for 90% of all cases (3), treatment should be directed at these pathogens until culture results are available. Although pregnancy does not predispose to these lower tract infections, once present, the dilated ureters and increased reflux will predispose to upper tract infection.

**Table 34–2.** Specific Renal Problems and Appropriate Tests

| Diagnosis | Test |
|---|---|
| Infection, polynephritis | Urine culture |
| Impaired renal function | Intravenous pyelogram |
| GFR | 24-hour creatinine clearance<br>Inuline, radionucleotide clearance |
| Tubular | Urine concentration<br>PSP excretion |
| Renal plasma flow | PSP excretion |
| Renal artery occlusive disease | Plasma renin activity<br>Split renal function<br>Rapid sequence IVP<br>Transfemoral arteriography |
| Collagen vascular disease | 24-hour urine protein<br>Total serum proteins and electrophoresis<br>LE Prep and ANA test |
| Heavy proteinuria | Total protein<br>Cholesterol<br>Protein electrophoresis |
| Renal calculi | Intravenous pyelogram<br>Ultrasonography<br>Parathormone levels<br>Serum calcium |

| Urinary Electrolysis Problem | Urinary Value | Diagnosis |
|---|---|---|
| Volume depletion | Sodium 0 to 10 mEq/liter | Extra renal loss |
| | > mEq/liter | Renal salt-wasting adrenal deficiency |
| Acute oliguria | Sodium 0 to 10 mEq/liter | Prerenal azotemia |
| | > 30 mEq/liter | Acute tubular necrosis |
| Hyponatremia | Sodium 0 to 10 mEq/liter | Volume depletion<br>Edema |
| | Sodium loss > diet | Inappropriate ADH or adrenal deficit |
| Hypokalemia | Potassium 0 to 10 mEq/liter | Extrarenal loss |
| | >10 mEq/liter | Renal loss |
| Metabolic alkalosis | Chloride 0 to 10 mEq/liter | Responsive alkalosis |
| | Chloride-dietary imbalance | Resistant alkalosis |

(From Gabert, HA, Miller, JM: Renal disease in pregnancy. Obstet. Gynecol. Surv. 40:449, 1985.)

### *Clinical Course*

Acute pyelonephritis occurs in up to 2% of pregnancies and usually presents with fever, chills, and flank pain (usually right-sided). Nausea, vomiting, and dehydration are often present. Hospital admission for fluid replacement and antibiotic therapy is essential. Fever and potential endotoxin production may initiate labor (4) and have been associated with prematurity, so close observation and tocolytic treatment may be necessary. Treatment of acute pyelonephritis during pregnancy is shown in Table 34–4. Approximately one-third of the women with urinary tract infection will experience a recurrence, so frequent cultures should be a part of the followup. Culture-positive women should receive suppressive antibiotic therapy in the form of nitrofurantoin, 100 mg at bedtime, for the

**Table 34–3.** Confirmation Tests for Renal Failure

| Prerenal or Glomerulonephritis | Test | ATN or Obstruction |
|---|---|---|
| Less than 20 mEq/liter | Urinary sodium | Greater than 40 mEq/liter |
| Greater than 30 | Urine/plasma creatinine* | Less than 20 |
| Less than 1 | Renal failure index** | Greater than 1 |
| Less than 1 | Fractional excretion of sodium | Greater than 1 |
| Greater than 500 | Urinary osmolality | Less than 400 |

* U, urine; P, plasma; CR, creatinine
**[(Urine/Plasma) $Na^+$]/[(Urine/Plasma) Cr × 100]
(From Gabert HA, Miller JM: Renal disease in pregnancy. Obstet. Gynecol. Surv. 40:449, 1985.)

remainder of the pregnancy. The pathogenesis of acute pyelonephritis and the incidence of anemia and renal dysfunction in pregnant women with acute pyelonephritis is shown in Figure 34–1 and Table 34–5.

## Pregnancy-Induced Hypertension

### *Pathophysiology*

If there is no history of preexisting renal disease, the most common presentation of renal signs and symptoms in pregnancy is proteinuria and hypertension, and these signs must be distinguished between chronic renal disease and acute pregnancy-induced hypertension (PIH), also called preeclampsia. The renal lesion of pregnancy-induced hypertension is glomerular capillary endotheliosis. It was described by Farquhar (5) as a significant swelling of the endothelial cells of the glomerular capillaries with deposition of fibrinoid material within and under the endothelial cells.

Severe pregnancy-induced hypertension is associated with a decreased circulating volume, decreased renal blood flow, and decreased glomerular filtration rate. Proteinuria results from glomerular leakage of normal plasma proteins (6). Edema is the end result of increased blood pressure and decreased colloid oncotic pressure (COP) due to loss of protein in the urine. Most cases of proteinuria and hypertension in pregnancy will be caused by pregnancy-induced hypertension and not involve underlying renal pathology, but in atypical cases of pregnancy-induced hypertension, other factors should be sought that may influence treatment. Greater than 5 g of protein/24 hour indicates severe pregnancy-induced hypertension and may shift management to a more aggressive approach to delivery. Distinguishing between chronic renal disease with hypertension and proteinuria and pregnancy-induced hypertension is crucial, because the chronic disease may respond to aggressive antihypertensive therapy while pregnancy-induced hypertension generally does not. Delay in delivery may worsen the prognosis for mother and infant.

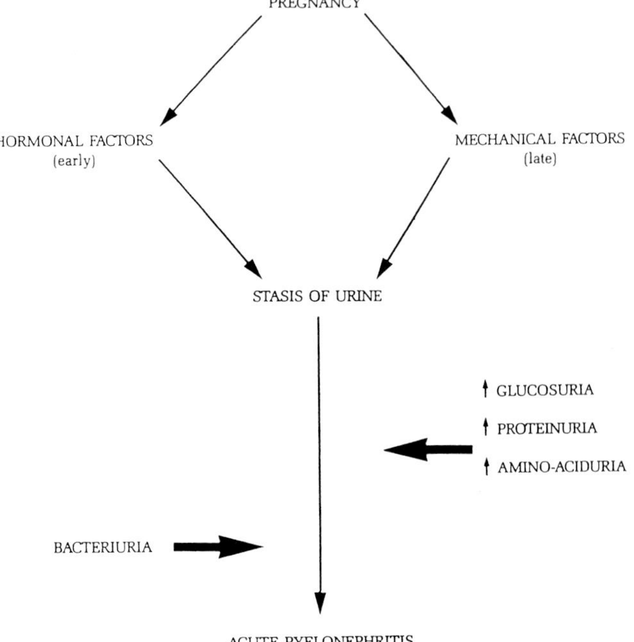


**Fig. 34–1.** Pathogenesis of acute pyelonephritis during pregnancy. Note: bacteriuria is present in two-thirds of cases on initial urine screen (From Gilstrap LC, Hankins GDV, Snyder RR, Breenberg RT: Acute pyelonephritis in pregnancy. Comp. Therapy 12:38, 1986.)

**Table 34–4.** Treatment of Acute Pyelonephritis During Pregnancy

Hospitalization
Parenteral Hydration
Parenteral Antibiotics
Ampicillin
Cephalosporin
Aminoglycoside
Frequent monitoring of vital signs
Urine and blood cultures
Complete blood cell count, serum creatinine levels
Clinic followup with frequent surveillance cultures
Suppressive antibiotic therapy

(From Gilstrap LC, Hankins GDV, Snyder RR, Breenberg RT: Acute pyelonephritis in pregnancy. Comp. Therapy. 12:38, 1986.)

**Table 34–5.** Incidence of Anemia and Renal Dysfunction in 36 Pregnant Women with Acute Pyelonephritis

| | No. | % |
|---|---|---|
| Anemia (Hematocrit < 30 volume %) | 24 of 36 | 66 |
| Decrease in hematocrit (≥ 6 volume %) | 13 of 36 | 36 |
| Renal dysfunction (Creatinine clearance < 80 mL/min) | 5 of 31 | 16 |

(From Gilstrap, LC, Hankins, GDV, Snyder, RR, Breenberg, RT: Acute pyelonephritis in pregnancy. Comp. Therapy. 12:38, 1986)

## Stones

Renal and ureteral calculi occur in about 0.3% of pregnancies. One-third are renal and two-thirds are ureteral in location. Most of these stones are calcium (90%) and their etiology is unclear. The diagnosis is difficult because pyelonephritis is present in most cases (7). Persistence of pain after the infection has cleared or left-sided costovertebral angle tenderness should suggest a possible calculus. Hematuria occurs in less than half of cases. Treatment is usually observational and supportive until the stone passes. Ultrasound is the most useful diagnostic tool.

## Acute Renal Failure

Acute renal failure (ARF) is defined as an accumulation of nitrogenous wastes that cannot be eliminated by extrarenal mechanisms. The causes of acute renal failure are divided into prerenal and postrenal, depending on the site of injury. Prerenal causes are usually due to inadequate perfusion of the kidney by a combination of volume depletion, hypotension, and decreased renal perfusion. Inadequate perfusion is usually reversible if the cause is corrected quickly. Categorically, problems that can cause acute renal failure in pregnancy include: volume depletion, disseminated intravascular coagulopathy, sepsis, obstruction, and renal parenchymal disease (Table 34–6) (8). Postrenal azotemia is due to obstruction distal to the kidneys and is treated by removal of the obstruction. In general, the treatment of acute renal failure involves identifying the etiology and treating that with constant attention to fluid and electrolyte changes and the potential need for dialysis.

## Chronic Renal Disease in Pregnancy

Significant renal disease is associated with an underlying problem with infertility, as many patients have irregular menstrual cycles, anovulation, or oligoovulation. However, good medical care has often improved fertility in these patients and they do become pregnant. In considering renal disease in pregnancy here, as the specific disease process that caused the renal impairment is usually not relevant, only the extent of the impairment will be discussed. Mild impairment is defined as a serum creatinine of less than 1.5 mg/100 ml. Moderate impairment is a serum creatinine between 1.5 mg/100 ml and 4.0 mg/100 ml. Severe renal failure is defined as the need for dialysis or a renal transplant.

**Table 34–6.** Causes of Obstetric Acute Renal Failure

| | |
|---|---|
| (a) Volume depletion | Hemorrhage:<br>Antepartum<br>Postpartum<br>Ectopic pregnancy<br>Abortion<br>Dehydration:<br>Hyperemesis gravidarum<br>Severe diarrhea |
| (b) Disseminated coagulopathy | Eclampsia<br>Abruptio placentae<br>Amniotic fluid embolus<br>Acute fatty liver of pregnancy<br>Postpartum hemolytic uremic syndrome<br>Drug/transfusion reactions |
| (c) Sepsis | Septic abortion<br>Acute pyelonephritis<br>Puerperal sepsis<br>Septicemia |
| (d) Obstruction | Uretereric damage<br>Bilateral pelvi-ureteral obstruction<br>Retroperitoneal hematoma |
| (e) Renal parenchymal disease | Acute glomerulonephritis<br>Renal involvement in multisystem disease |

(From Michael J: The management of renal disease in pregnancy. Clin. Obstet. Gynecol. 13:319, 1986.)

### *Mild Renal Impairment*

Women with mildly decreased renal function before pregnancy usually have a successful pregnancy outcome and their pregnancy does not adversely affect their renal function. Most patients will demonstrate an increase in glomerular filtration rate, although not as dramatic as a healthy pregnant female. Proteinuria is common (50%), especially with underlying glomerular disease.

#### *Pathophysiology*

Katz, et al (9) documented hypertension in 20% of their mildly impaired group. Hypertension influenced the obstetric complication rate, but pregnancy did not modify the natural course of glomerular disease. Fetal mortality is higher in patients having renal disease with hypertension than it is in renal disease without hypertension (10). Prognosis may be worse in patients who have membranoproliferative glomerulonephritis, who have a greater tendency to experience deterioration of renal function following pregnancy, and patients with IgA nephropathy who tend to develop persistent hypertension during and after pregnancy.

### *Moderate Renal Impairment*

There is much less data on patients with moderate renal impairment. Older studies were very pessimistic about outcome, but in the 1980s, perinatal mortality was about 10%; however, half of the pregnancies were delivered preterm (10). Hou, et al (11) reported on 23 pregnancies in women with moderate renal impairment. In 14 patients, renal function did not deteriorate or was consistent with expected decline, and seven women had a greater than expected decline (Table 34–7). Their conclusions were that pregnancy did not consistently cause a worsening of renal function, and that outcome was better than previously reported.

#### *Treatment*

Management of pregnancy in patients with mild to moderate renal insufficiency is generally targeted at control of blood pressure should the patient be hypertensive. Bed rest is important, and antihypertensive therapy should be used should diastolic blood pressure exceed 100 mm Hg. Superimposed pregnancy-induced hypertension occurs in about 25% of patients, and it may necessitate early delivery to protect the health of the mother and fetus. Intrauterine growth retardation can occur and should be fol-

**Table 34–7.** Changes in Serum Creatinine Concentration (mg/dl) During Pregnancy and After Delivery: Pregnancy-Related Decline in Renal Function

| Patient/Diagnosis | Before Conception 6 Months | Intrapartum | | | Postpartum | | Latest Follow-up |
|---|---|---|---|---|---|---|---|
| | | 1st | 2nd | 3rd | 0–3 Months | 4–6 Months | |
| 5/Focal sclerosis | | 1.8 | 2.1 | 3.5 | | 8.4 (5 months) | |
| 6/IgA nephropathy | 1.7 | 2.1 | 3.2 | Dialysis | | | Functioning transplant |
| 7/IgA nephropathy | 1.6 | 1.6 (early)<br>3.3 (12 weeks) | | | | 3.4 (6 months) | |
| 8/IgA nephropathy | 1.4<br>1.7 (at conception) | 1.6 | 1.7 | 1.6 | 2.6 (3 weeks)<br>2.9 (11 weeks) | 3.0 (4 months) | 3.4 (6 months) |
| 10/Chronic glomerulonephritis | 1.7 | 2.4 | 2.7 | 4.3 | | 5.0 (22 weeks) | |
| 12/Focal proliferative glomerulonephritis | | 2.7 | 3.0 | 2.5 | 3.9 (3 months) | | |
| 18/Medullary cystic disease | 2.5 (3 months)<br>2.5 (at conception) | 2.9 | 2.3 | 2.7–3.4 | 4.7 (1 month) | | 5.3 (8 months)<br>dialysis (19 months) |

(From Hou SH, Grossman SD, Madias NE: Pregnancy in women with renal disease and moderate renal insufficiency. Am. J. Med. 78:185, 1985.)

lowed closely with ultrasound examinations every 3 to 4 weeks. Fetal heart rate testing by contraction stress testing (CST) each week or nonstress testing (NST) twice a week should be initiated at the point of fetal viability (25 to 26 weeks). Delivery is often preterm, and should be at a tertiary-level hospital with excellent neonatal intensive care available. The timing of delivery is determined by either fetal or maternal deterioration or fetal lung maturity at 37 to 38 weeks.

## *Severe Renal Impairment*

Advances in medical care, including dialysis and renal transplantation programs, improved immunosuppressive therapy, and more powerful antihypertensive medications have led to an extended life span for patients with end stage renal disease (ESRD). Conception is difficult in these patients. The rate of spontaneous abortion approaches 50%. Surviving pregnancies are at risk for placental abruption, stillbirth, fetal distress, intrauterine growth retardation (IUGR), polyhydramnios, anemia, and hypertension.

### *Treatment*

Hemodialysis has been used since 1960 in end stage renal disease. Successful pregnancies on hemodialysis are limited to case reports. There are approximately 57 patients reported in the literature in which hemodialysis was used before pregnancy or to treat acute renal failure during pregnancy. Chronic ambulatory peritoneal dialysis (CAPD) (12) has been used successfully in patients with end stage renal disease and may represent a better alternative to hemodialysis. Chronic ambulatory peritoneal dialysis is associated with a live birth rate of 63% (12) compared to hemodialysis, which has a 20 to 25% survival rate (13). Fetal outcome for pregnant dialysis patients is shown in Table 34–8.

Both hemodialysis and peritoneal dialysis work on the principle of diffusion of solutes from an area of high concentration—the blood—through a semipermeable membrane to an area of low concentration. Hemodialysis is accomplished by inserting an arteriovenous shunt for vascular access. Blood is taken from this access through a dialysis membrane and then returned to the body. The dialysate solution contains physiologic levels of glucose, sodium, calcium, bicarbonate, and chloride. Urea and other toxic metabolites can be removed while maintaining normal electrolyte balance. The amount of fluid removed during hemodialysis can be controlled by changing the hydrostatic pressure across the semipermeable dialysis membrane.

Peritoneal dialysis allows passage of the toxic products from peritoneal capillaries across the peritoneum into the dialysate fluid instilled in the abdominal cavity. This is

**Table 34–8.** Fetal Outcome

| Patient No. | Gestation Age (wks) | Reason for Delivery | Weight (g) | Apgar Scores 1 & 5 Minutes |
|---|---|---|---|---|
| 1 | 34 | Fetal nonreactivity | 1340 | 9/10 |
| 2 | 33 | Spontaneous labor | 1410 | 7/9 |
| 3 | 36 | Elective cesarean section | 2780 | 8/10 |
| 4 | 20 | Spontaneous abortion | — | — |
| 4a | 32 | Fetal nonreactivity | 1065 | 9/9 |
| 5 | 19 | Spontaneous abortion | — | — |
| 6 | 34 | Fetal nonreactivity | 1720 | 1/3 |
| 7 | 29 | Thrombocytopenia | 780 | 5/9 |
| 8 | 18 | Spontaneous abortion | — | — |
| 9 | 38 | Elective cesarean section | 3120 | 9/9 |
| 10 | 36 | Spontaneous labor | 2044 | 9/9 |
| 11 | 36 | Spontaneous labor | 1750 | 5/9 |
| 12 | 35 | Spontaneous labor | 2218 | N/A |
| 13 | 16 | Spontaneous abortion | — | — |

(From Redrow M, Cherem L, Elliott J, Mangalat J, et al: Dialysis in the management of pregnant patients with renal insufficiency. Medicine 67: 199, 1988.)

accomplished by surgical placement of a permanent catheter into the abdominal cavity. One to three liters of dialysis fluid is then instilled into the abdomen and allowed to dwell, bathing the peritoneum for periods of 1 to 8 hours, and then removed. Excess fluid is removed with peritoneal dialysis by creating a dialysate hypertonic to the patient's plasma through the use of high glucose concentration in the dialysate solution.

Hemodialysis relies on high blood flow and a membrane that is highly permeable to small molecular weight substances such as urea and creatinine. In contrast, the peritoneal membrane has greater permeability to larger molecules, including proteins. The higher flow rates of hemodialysis allow for faster clearance and shorter treatment times. Some drawbacks to hemodialysis include the fact that the hemodialysis membrane is thrombogenic and requires anticoagulation. This membrane also can induce complement activation, hypoxemia, and leucopenia. There may be a difference in risks and outcome between patients conceiving with end stage renal disease and patients whose renal failure worsens during a pregnancy to the point of requiring dialysis support. Thirty-eight of the reported pregnancies were conceived while on hemodialysis, while 19 were dialyzed during a pregnancy.

Complications that have been reported with hemodialysis patients include prematurity, intrauterine growth retardation, fetal distress, anemia, hypertension, abruptio placentae, and spontaneous abortion (14). (Table 34–9) compares various complications between patients conceiving while on hemodialysis with patients started on dialysis in pregnancy. Different denominators are given because not all case reports detail the desired information. Intrauterine growth retardation is very common in patients who conceive while on hemodialysis, and when the pregnancy progressed to term, 5/5 (100%) had birth weight below the tenth percentile. Of interest, in the reported patients conceiving while on hemodialysis, hypertension did not lead to a worse outcome. Six of seven patients (86%) with hypertension delivered babies that lived compared to four survivors in seven pregnancies (57%) without hypertension.

**Table 34–9.** Complications of Dialysis in Pregnancy

| | Hemodialysis Prior to Conception (17) | Hemodialysis During Pregnancy (15) | CAPD(9)* |
|---|---|---|---|
| Polyhydramnios | 7/12 (58%) | 2/8 (25%) | 1/9 (11%) |
| Premature labor | 7/14 (50%) | 5/14 (36%) | 8/9 (89%) |
| Anemia | 11/11 (100%) | 8/8 (100%) | 8/9 (89%) |
| IUGR | 7/11 (64%) | 5/13 (38%) | 5/8 (63%) |
| Fetal distress | 1/7 (14%) | 3/14 (21%) | 4/7 (57%) |
| Hypertension | 7/14 (50%) | 7/12 (58%) | 9/9 (100%) |
| Fetal survival** | 12/17 (74%) | 14/15 (93%) | 6/9 (67%) |

* CAPD: Chronic Ambulatory Peritoneal Dialysis

** Hemodialysis data are collected case reports and are not representative of true survival rates, which indicate approximately 20% survival. (From Elliott JP, O'Keeffe DF, Schon DA, Cherem LB: Dialysis in pregnancy: a critical review. Obstet. Gynecol. Survey. 46:319, 1991.)

Chronic ambulatory peritoneal dialysis has been reported in eight pregnancies. Cattran, et al (15) reported the first pregnancy in 1983 that resulted in an intrauterine fetal demise at 32 weeks, and Kioko, et al (16) reported a successful delivery at 34 weeks in a diabetic pregnancy. Redrow, et al (12) reported six pregnancies in five patients on chronic ambulatory peritoneal dialysis, with four surviving babies. A summary of pregnancies with chronic ambulatory peritoneal dialysis is given in Table 34–9.

Obviously, statistical comparison is not scientific for these case reports, but of note is the high incidence of polyhydramnios in patients on hemodialysis, 9/20 (45%) compared to 1/9 (11%) with chronic ambulatory peritoneal dialysis. Published data reflect that fetal survival is also much higher with chronic ambulatory peritoneal dialysis (67%) when compared with hemodialysis (20%).

There does not appear to be any significant effect of pregnancy on end stage renal disease. If dialysis in a pregnant patient is needed, chronic ambulatory peritoneal dialysis appears to be a better alternative then does hemodialysis. If the patient is already on hemodialysis, she should be switched to chronic ambulatory peritoneal dialysis. The volume and frequency of exchange should provide a total creatinine clearance (considering dialysis and endogenous residual creatinine clearance) of greater than 15 cc/minute. The BUN should be kept under 60 mg/dl.

## Renal Transplants

End stage renal disease is often treated by renal transplantation. The donor may be related to the recipient, or may come from a deceased donor. Host rejection of the kidney is suppressed with drugs to maximize graft function and longevity. Prednisone, cyclosporine, and recently azathioprine are used in this sistuation. The successful transplant with a functioning kidney allows for a return of ovulation and increased libido. Pregnancy is a common occurrence in these patients who have not already completed their family.

Ideally, pregnancy in a transplant patient should be carefully planned. Two years should elapse from the time of the transplant to allow renal function to stabilize and to reduce immunosuppressive medications to moderate to low levels. There should be no proteinuria, no significant hypertension, and no evidence of rejection. The serum creatinine should be 2 mg/dL or less. Patients who could become pregnant should avoid warfarin oral anticoagulation, as this drug has caused documented teratogenicity (17).

### *Treatment*

It appears that the drugs used for immunosuppression are not teratogenic in humans. Prednisone has been well studied. It is metabolized to prednisolone in the placenta before passage to the fetus, and this weak steroid is poorly converted by the fetal liver into an active form (18). Azathioprine crosses the placenta poorly, and the fetal liver cannot convert it to its active form. There have been no reports of congenital anomalies associated with cyclosporine (19).

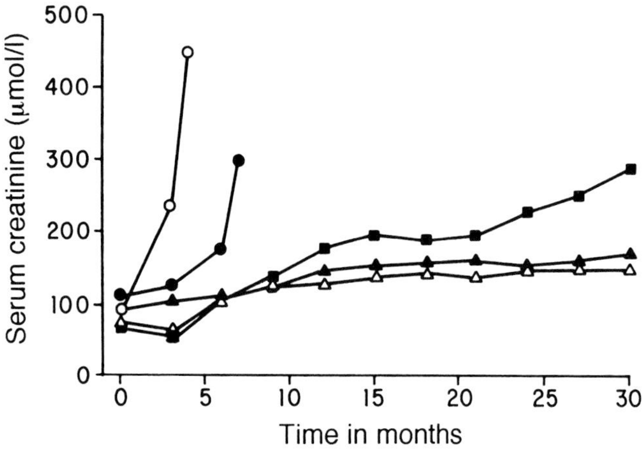


**Fig. 34–2.** Serum creatinine in five patients who suffered deterioration in renal function in pregnancy. (Redrawn from O'Donnell D, Meyers AM, Sevitz H, Botha JR, et al: Pregnancy after renal transplantation. Aust. N.Z. J. Med. 15:320, 1985.)

## *Clinical Course*

Outcome of pregnancy in renal transplant patients who fit the guidelines has been good. Accumulated data show outcome that is generally comparable to a normal population (18,20,21). Serum creatinine in patients with and without deterioration in renal function is shown in Figures 34–2 and 34–3, respectively. However, there may be increased risk of intrauterine growth retardation, preeclampsia, and prematurity. Ultrasound examinations to document fetal growth pattern should be performed every 4 weeks after 24 weeks gestation. Fetal heart rate testing by contraction stress test or nonstress test should be started at 25 to 26 weeks. Renal function should be followed frequently. Delivery usually can be accomplished vaginally, with cesarean section reserved for usual obstetric indications.

The outcome of pregnancy in patients with renal disease is certainly better today than in the past. Improved antihypertensive medications, better understanding of dialysis and its effects on the placenta and fetus, and improved transplant techniques have allowed the health care team to manage healthier patients with severe renal disease. Neonatal outcome has improved dramatically. Hou, et al (11) reported 23/27 (85%) long-term survival in patients with moderate renal insufficiency. In small numbers, chronic ambulatory peritoneal dialysis has resulted in a 63% fetal-survival rate (12). The effect of pregnancy on renal function is variable. Hou postulates that renal function will deteriorate in about one-third of women with moderate renal insufficiency (20). In transplant patients, about 8 to 15% will experience worsening of renal function associated with pregnancy (8). The motivated patient with severe renal impairment or a renal transplant should receive counselling concerning risks and complications of a pregnancy, but should not be coerced into an abortion against her desires.

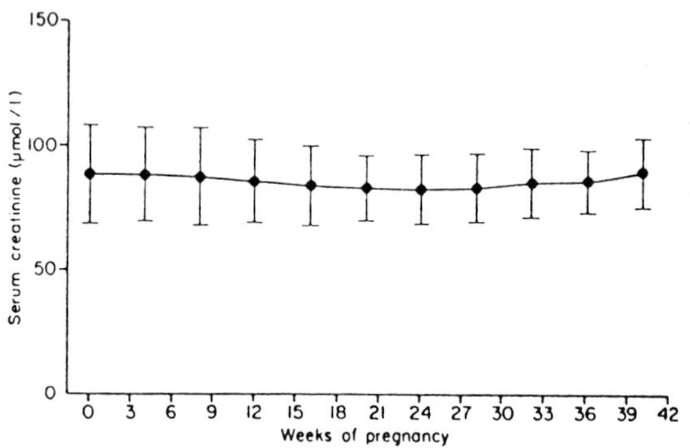


**Fig. 34–3.** Serum creatinine in those pregnancies completed without deterioration in renal function. (From O'Donnell D, Meyers AM, Sevitz H, Botha JR, et al: Pregnancy after renal transplantation. Aust. N.Z. J. Med. 15:320, 1985.)

# ANESTHETIC MANAGEMENT OF PATIENTS WITH GENITOURINARY SYSTEM DISORDERS

This section will include anesthetic considerations in regard to urinary infectious diseases, pregnancy-induced hypertension, stones, acute renal failure, chronic renal failure, and renal transplants. Because both general and regional anesthetic techniques alter renal function due to changes in circulation, electrolyte and acid-base balance, it is appropriate to consider patient management for obstetrics as very important to the health and welfare of both the mother and her unborn baby. As is apparent throughout this text, regional anesthesia is emphasized for its safety for the mother and the baby as long as hypotension is not a factor. Severe hypotension can reduce placental blood flow, but in today's practice the likelihood of this is minimized due to continuous low-dose regimens for labor and fractional dosing regimens for cesarean section.

## *General Anesthesia*

In earlier days when potent concentrations of inhalation anesthetics were used for cesarean section delivery, it was common to experience reductions in glomerular filtration rates with concomitant electrolyte and water excretion. This effect was due to the depression in renal blood flow, which was, in turn, secondary to depression in blood pressure and blood flow. The latter was typical of many volatile anesthetic agents, but today with uniform use of low concentrations of $N_2O$, oxygen, minimal thiopental, and only small concentrations of the volatile agents exclusive of methoxyflurane to offset any maternal recall, there tends to be, if anything, an increase in blood pressure and blood flow due to catecholamine release secondary to minimal anesthetic depth at the time of surgical stimulation. Of course, the level of such changes is also affected by the degree of maternal hydration, which, for the most part, is usually adequate. The aforementioned changes were short-lived and restricted to the time period of the anesthetic with compensatory diuresis occurring in the immediate postoperative period.

Inhalation anesthetics used today are not biochemically altered by liver metabolism and renal excretion as they were in past years. Thus, today's agents are "inert" and more or less excreted in the same form as they are administered. For the most part, significant changes in acid-base balance are due to retention of $CO_2$, which is due to inadequate ventilation during the anesthetic period. The latter is unusual and today unlikely because of the intense reliance upon monitoring of the $EtCO_2$ wave form, which gives indications of $CO_2$ on a breath-by-breath measure. Similarly, metabolic acidosis due to lack of oxygenation is unlikely today because of a similar reliance on intense monitoring of the $SaO_2$ wave form on a breath-by-breath measure.

Barbiturates are still used as induction agents with thiopental, by far, still the most popular agent. This agent causes a transient fall in blood pressure due to its negative ionotropic effect, but the episode is indeed short-lived with a reflex increase in blood pressure due to the release of catecholamines after surgical stimulation. Today, very small dosages of induction barbiturates are used so that the negative ionotropic effect is minimized as much as possible.

Narcotics are not used in cesarean section delivery today until after the delivery of the infant. They are then often used to provide adequate analgesia for the mother during the reparative process of uterine closure, and closure of the abdomen. Agents typically no longer used, or used infrequently, include tranquilizers and belladonna drugs, the latter because of their drying effect.

Muscle relaxants are still used today for help in maintaining a quiet surgical field without having to resort to deep levels of anesthesia. The earlier, more popular succinylcholine bolus and drip agents are now replaced by the newer, intermediate-acting muscle relaxants such as tracrium and norcuron. Tracrium and norcuron are also important in patients with severe renal disease with associated increases of potassium which, in the face of sudden and severe fasciculations, can release even more potassium and pose a significant cardiac threat.

Today's system of management most beneficial with regard to general anesthesia for the patient with renal disease would consist of the following: First, careful attention must be given to detail in regard to all monitoring means made available. These include at least those listed in Table 34–10.

Second, careful attention to maintaining the patient's blood pressure, which is not only beneficial to the patient from the standpoint of maintaining renal blood flow, but which is also beneficial to the fetus from the standpoint of maintaining uteroplacental blood flow. Third, control of ventilation and oxygenation to assure optimal maternal $paO_2$ and $paCO_2$; the latter, of course, also assures good fetal oxygen and carbon-dioxide levels. There may be instances in which preeclamptic patients have received magnesium for stabilization of blood pressure and protection from central nervous system (CNS) seizures. Such patients must be monitored carefully for return of muscular function after muscle relaxation. Generally speaking, a moderate dose of induction barbiturate is used with 50% nitrous-oxide/oxygen and adequate muscular relaxation until delivery of the baby. In some instances with evidence of inadequate maternal anesthetic depth as evidenced by tachycardia and sympathetic activity, small concentrations of isoflurane or enflurane may be added. The latter are particularly important to treat the hypertensive response that sometimes accompanies such light planes of anesthesia for cesarean section. In some patients with end stage renal disease, it may be wise to premedicate with an opioid, though ensure that communication with the neonatologist and obstetrician is made before doing so (22). Such a premedication may be adequate to offset some of the aforementioned hypertensive responses to induction. Naturally, it is imperative to monitor the urine output in the perioperative period, and, in the face of oliguria, aggressively manage with fluids or a diuretic such as furosemide, dopamine, or the more popular mannitol.

**Table 34–10.** Monitoring the Renal Disease Patient

(1) automated blood pressure (with a manual system backup);
(2) electrocardiogram (ECG);
(3) $EtCO_2$;
(4) $SaO_2$;
(5) temperature; and
(6) others preferred due to local circumstances.

In very ill patients, such as patients with pericarditis in end stage renal disease, careful planning and interaction with the management team are essential for optimization of the health and welfare of the mother and fetus. This interaction should include the nephrologist, the obstetrician, the anesthesiologist, and the neonatologist (23). Dialysis, close monitoring of the fluid and electrolyte status with quick response therapy, and echocardiography are all essential components in management. If pericardial effusion occurs despite such intensive therapy, a subxiphoid pericardiotomy may be necessary and should be performed under optimal conditions in the operating room with the anesthesiologist standing by ready for induction of anesthesia if necessary in anticipation of cesarean section delivery (24). A recent study of blood pressure responses to anesthetics revealed one excellent regimen to be fentanyl (12 μg/kg) and diazepam 0.25 mg/kg) with $N_2O$ 70% (Figures 34–4 and 34–5) (25). It seems reflex vasoconstrictor responses remained intact despite serious reductions in cardiac filling pressures.

Sevoflurane has recently been studied as a new replacement inhalational anesthetic because of its rapid onset, minimal disagreeable features, and its potent analgesia (Figures 34–6 and 34–7) (26). It has not yet been used in obstetric trials; however, one concern, as reflected in one study (26) that may contradict its use in patients with renal disease, is that 5 of 10 patients exceeded the 50 μmol/L nephrotoxic dose of inorganic fluoride (26). This lone study may not be a fair appraisal of the drug's use in patients with renal disease, however, because this study was performed in patients without renal disease and in cases that were of excessive duration. In contrast, enflurane resulted in inorganic fluoride levels of 22 μmol while maintaining renal blood flow, glomerular filtration rate, and urinary flow rates at 77%, 79%, and 67% of control

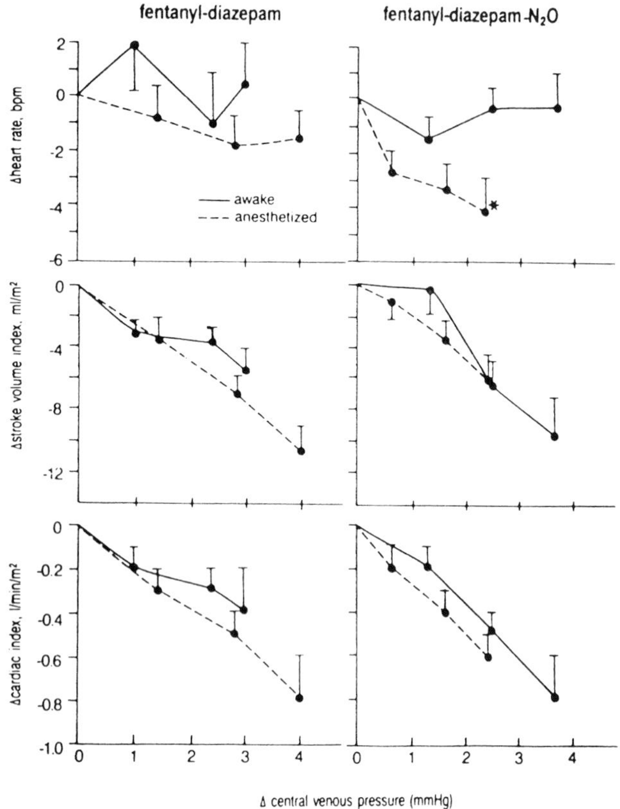


**Fig. 34–4.** Hemodynamic responses to controlled reductions in CVP were similar (except for heart rate) in awake and anesthetized patients. A slight but significant bradycardia was observed during lower-body negative pressure in patients anesthetized with fentanyl-diazepam-$N_2O$ ($p < 0.05$). (From Ebert TJ, Kotrly KJ, Madsen KE, Bernstein JS, et al: Fentanyl-diazepam anesthesia with or without $N_2O$ does not attenuate cardiopulmonary baroreflex-mediated vasoconstrictor responses to controlled hypovolemia in humans. Anesth. Analg. 67(6):548, 1988.)

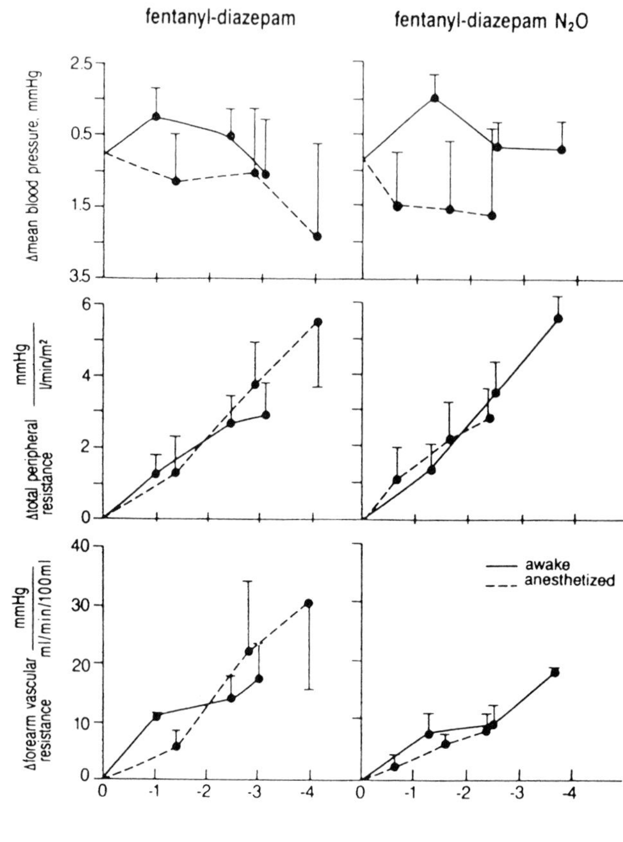


**Fig. 34–5.** Reflex vasoconstrictor responses to reduced CVP were maintained during anesthesia. Therefore, blood pressure did not decline (From Ebert TJ, Kotrly KJ, Madsen KE, Bernstein JS, et al: Fentanyl-diazepam anesthesia with or without $N_2O$ does not attenuate cardiopulmonary baroreflex-mediated vasoconstrictor responses to controlled hypovolemia in humans. Anesth. Analg. 67(6):548, 1988.)

values, respectively (27). Please see Chapter 19 for details on all aspects of general anesthesia.

## Regional Anesthesia

Regional anesthesia is the preferred anesthetic technique for patients with afflictions in the genitourinary system. The reasons for this preference are twofold, both of which stem from the standpoint of the woman, who, with the use of regional anesthesia, is able to enjoy: (1) the experience of the childbirth while at the same time enjoy the experience of being pain free during the operative intervention; and (2) the side benefit of increased renal blood flow during regional anesthesia.

The cause for this increased renal blood flow is the effect upon the sympathetic nerves in the abdomen, which help to control renal blood flow. With an increase in peripheral vascular resistance, which is more often the case with general anesthesia, there would be a decrease in renal blood flow. Conversely, with a decrease in peripheral vascular resistance, which is common with regional anesthesia, there is an increase in the renal blood flow. One of the most important aspects of administration of regional anesthesia to the pregnant patient with or without renal disease is to make certain that compression of the aorta by the uterus does not occur. Such a compression will lead to a decrease in uterine blood flow, perhaps at a level below that found in the nonpregnant state. The patient with renal disease realizes some advantage with the pregnant state, resulting in increased renal plasma flow and increased glomerular filtration rate; the latter effect reduces both blood urea nitrogen and serum creatinine levels during pregnancy. Yet, often the severity of the disease state negates any such advantage. Thus, when administration of regional anesthesia is performed, it must be done so with proper attention to details of prevention of reduction in maternal blood pressure, as the gain just mentioned in regard to increased renal plasma flow associated with regional anesthesia can be quickly offset with hypotension of a severe and prolonged degree.

In the patient with significant hypertension due to renal disease, its impact on end organs, including the brain, heart, lungs, liver, and kidney must also be considered. Of particular interest to the anesthesiologist is the effect

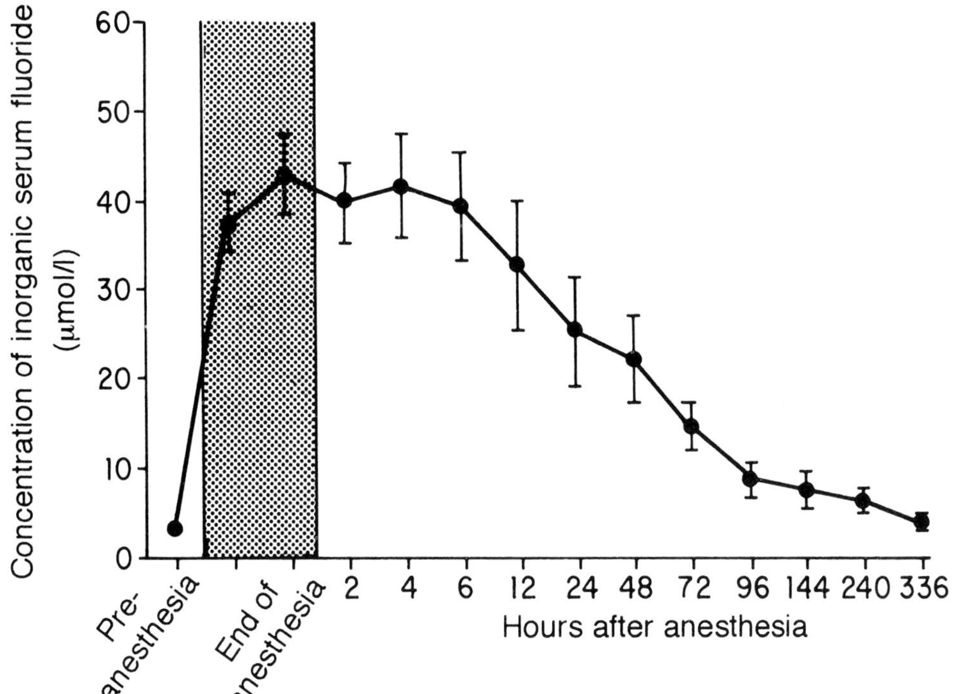


Fig. 34–6. Serum concentration of inorganic fluoride after inhalation of sevoflurane. Shadowed area represents the inhalation period. Data are presented as mean ± SE. (Redrawn from Kobayashi Y, Ochiai R, Takeda J, Sekiguchi H, et al: Serum and urinary inorganic fluoride concentrations after prolonged inhalation of sevoflurane in humans. Anesth. Analg. 74(5):753, 1992.)

upon the myocardium, i.e., as to whether left ventricular hypertrophy exists or if pulmonary hypertension is an issue. If myocardial compromise is prominent and associated pulmonary hypertension a significant concern, the anesthetic of choice may well be a carefully controlled general anesthetic with intubation under strict control of sympathetic reactivity, and consideration for obtundation of reflex cardiovascular changes that might ordinarily result in hypertension, hypotension, and pulmonary edema. This anesthetic technique may well be preferred over regional anesthesia due to the one concern that remains with with cesarean section, namely, that adequate sensory levels for analgesia do not result in serious loss of sympathetic control and thus hypotension. Imperative to the success of such a special general anesthetic regimen is the use of an agent effective in afterload reduction. Sodium nitroprusside may be the drug of choice; nitroglycerin might be considered also.

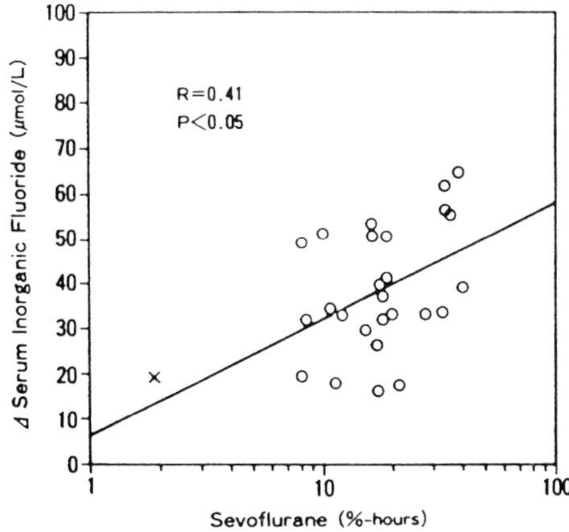


Fig. 34–7. Relationship between Δ serum inorganic fluoride and %-hours during anesthesia. Δ serum inorganic fluoride is the difference between preoperative and intraoperative values. For comparison, data (X) from a previous clinical study (Shiraishi Y, Ikeda K: Uptake and biotransformation of sevoflurane in humans: A comparative study of sevoflurane with halothane, enflurane, and isoflurane. J. Clin. Anesth. 2:377, 1990) in which patients received a 1-h inhalation of 1.88% sevoflurane are presented. (From Kobayashi Y, Ochiai R, Takeda J, Sekiguchi H, et al: Serum and urinary inorganic fluoride concentrations after prolonged inhalation of sevoflurane in humans. Anesth. Analg. 74(5):753, 1992.)

In the patient whose condition is not that serious, regional anesthesia may be used to benefit both the mother and the baby. In the past, lumbar epidural was preferred over the two regional methods, i.e., spinal or epidural, because there was less rapid and profound changes in blood pressure with the epidural. Now with renewed popularization of the use of the continuous spinal method and slow injection with separated boluses of local anesthetic, there is time for accommodation of the sympathetic denervation by balanced increases in vascular resistance above the level of the block. This should prevent any serious problem with regional anesthesia hypotension of a threatening nature. Thus, either technique, i.e., lumbar epidural or continuous subarachnoid block, can be used. The slower, more deliberate activation of the continuous subarachnoid block mentioned above is also prudent in patients with renal disease, as there has been some speculation in the literature that a more rapid spread of local anesthetic occurs in this disease process (28). If lumbar epidural is chosen, the level is also developed slowly, as indicated in Chapter 13, for safety of both the mother

**Table 34–11.** Lidocaine Pharmacokinetics in Various Disease States

| | Volume of Distribution at Steady State (liters/kg) | Clearance (ml/min/kg$^{-1}$) | Termination Elimination Half-Life |
|---|---|---|---|
| Normal | 1.32 | 10.01 | 1.8 |
| Cardiac failure | 0.88 | 6.3 | 1.9 |
| Hepatic disease* | 2.31 | 6.0 | 4.9 |
| Renal disease* | 1.20 | 13.7 | 1.3 |

* Note the difference between hepatic and renal disease.
(From Thomson PD, et al: Lidocaine pharmacokinetics in advanced heart failure, liver disease and renal failure in humans. Ann. Intern. Med. 78: 499, 1973.)

and the fetus. As noted in Table 34–11, the volume of distribution and clearance rate of lumbar epidural analgesia is not altered in renal disease (29). These unaltered volumes in renal disease will also protect the mother from high levels of local anesthetic due to what has been referred to in the literature as a "hyperdynamic circulation."

Our discussion thus far has been consideration of the mother's condition only. Of course, an important part of the equation is the condition of the fetus also. If there is evidence of serious fetal compromise, then serious consideration must be given to the anesthetic technique and agent so that the fetal reserve is protected. In situations in which maternal hypotension occurs, there is significant risk of fetal morbidity or mortality. Thus, again, in a case in which cesarean section is planned, there may be an advantage to use of the aforementioned general anesthetic technique for protection of the minimal fetal reserve remaining. On the other hand, one of these cases may be a situation in which the mother's safety is of concern. Specifically, maternal morbid obesity and concern in lieu of a possible difficult intubation may be of concern. In these cases in which the life of the mother is also at risk, agreement among the physicians to protect the life of the mother, first and foremost, must exist. This may mean selection of a regional anesthetic or, if this is not possible due to maternal obesity or other mitigating circumstances, then local anesthesia may be recommended by the anesthesiologist to the surgeon. In the latter case, the anesthesiologist should be available immediately for assistance with systemic medication such as ketamine and for assistance in verbal reassurance, which remains an area of support, often overlooked, throughout the entire case.

## Anatomy of the Gastrointestinal Tract

The anatomy of the gastrointestinal tract is altered by the enlarging uterus. Pressure is exerted on the colon, rectum, stomach, and esophagus, which can cause constipation, heartburn, and digestive difficulty. The intestines are gradually pressed into the upper abdomen, altering the location of organs such as the appendix. The anatomy of the liver is similar to the nonpregnant patient in both gross and microscopic detail. The normal liver is not palpable during pregnancy.

The enlarging uterus compresses the vena cava creating increased venous pressure below the level of the renal veins. Some of the blood dilates collateral circulation, such as the hemorrhoidal veins, sometimes causing symptomatic dilatation and thrombus formation due to stasis.

## Physiology of the Gastrointestinal Tract

The physiology of the gastrointestinal tract is significantly altered in pregnancy and is important in diagnosing and treating disease. Gastric emptying is prolonged in late pregnancy and during labor. The prolonged emptying time allows more water to be removed before excretion, which aggravates constipation. Gastric acid secretion may be slightly decreased or unchanged. Gall bladder function may be inhibited by hormonal effects of progesterone, which leads to an increased capacity, decreased contractility, and larger residual volume. The resulting biliary stasis may contribute to stone formation and pancreatic enzyme backup.

The liver demonstrates several physiologic changes in pregnancy. Mild cholestasis occurs, which is associated with a decrease in the excretion of sulfobromophthalein sodium (Bromsulphalein or BSP) and an increase in serum bile salts. The increased estrogen in pregnancy causes palmar erythema and spider angiomata in 50% of normal women, and this may be confused with liver disease.

## Laboratory Evaluation

Laboratory evaluation of hepatic function is altered by pregnancy. Total serum protein is decreased as are the albumin and globulin fractions. This is a dilutional effect of the increased plasma volume. Serum cholesterol is increased, and bilirubin is slightly increased. Alkaline phosphatase may double due to placental contribution. Aspartate aminotransferase (AST), also known as serum glutamic oxaloacetic transaminase (SGOT), and alanine aminotransferase (ALT), also known as serum glutamic pyruvic transaminase (SGPT), are normal. Clotting factors are elevated, specifically fibrinogen, and factors VII, X, and IX.

## Effect of Pregnancy on Drug Administration

The effects of pregnancy on the gastrointestinal tract are extended to changes in metabolic outcome for drugs and other substances entering the body. There are effects on absorption as well as excretion. Drugs or medications that are administered orally and are absorbed in the intestines will have a delay in absorption due to the prolonged emptying time for the stomach. In nonpregnant women, the hepatic blood flow averages 1548 ml/min/1.73m (30), which is 35% of cardiac output. In pregnancy, the hepatic blood flow is the same, 1544 ml/min/1.73m (22), but this is only 28% of cardiac output. Drugs that are cleared from the blood have a reduced clearance in the pregnant patient due to a larger volume of distribution.

## The Liver in Pregnancy

### *Cholestasis*

#### *Etiology*

Reduction in bile flow caused by elevated estrogen and progesterone results in reduced bile and bile-salt excretion. Extreme stasis in certain individuals leads to excessive cholestasis and results in jaundice or pruritus. There will be an increase in alkaline phosphatase, and total and unconjugated serum bilirubin, and bilirubin will appear in the urine. Serum bile salt assay will be elevated. The striking symptom is pruritus that is generalized and often worse at night. Fifty percent will demonstrate clinical jaundice.

### *Clinical Course*

Cholestasis tends to be recurrent and occurs in families with an autosomal dominant inheritance pattern. It usually occurs in the third trimester and disappears following delivery. The lack of other signs or symptoms of liver dysfunction generally excludes significant disease from the differential diagnosis. The incidence of cholestatic jaundice is less than 1/1000 pregnancies. The effects of extreme cholestasis on the pregnant woman are related to the severe pruritus, which is unresponsive to antipruritic medications. The psychological burden of this pruritus is impressive and may force the obstetrician to deliver the patient early, after determining fetal lung maturation.

### *Treatment*

Cholestyramine (Questran) may be helpful in reducing the pruritus, as it acts as an exchange resin in the intestines for bile acids. It should be given in doses of 4 g with meals, three times a day, and the total dose should not exceed 30 g per day. Phenobarbital may be useful for sedation and hepatic enzyme activation. Check patients for a prolonged prothrombin time (PT), as it may lead to postpartum hemorrhage and can he corrected by administration of vitamin K to the mother.

Cholestasis of pregnancy is associated with adverse fetal outcomes. There is an increased incidence of preterm deliveries (30 to 60%) (22,31), stillbirth (6 to 11%) (23,32), meconium in the amniotic fluid (66%) (22), and fetal distress in labor (11 to 33%) (23,24). The pathophysiology of these effects on the fetus is unknown. Maternal bilirubin does not cross the placenta but bile salts have been shown to be elevated in the fetal circulation (up to 3 times their normal level) (33). Bile salts also have an effect on colonic motility, which may explain the meconium passage in utero.

It is clear that these pregnancies should be monitored closely for preterm labor and uteroplacental insufficiency. Weekly contraction stress testing or twice weekly nonstress tests should be performed. Induction of labor following documentation of fetal lung maturation by amniocentesis should be attempted at 36 to 37 weeks in severe cases.

## Hyperemesis Gravidarum

### *Etiology*

Another common-symptom complex in pregnancy is nausea and vomiting. Nausea was reported to occur in 89% of pregnant women and vomiting is present in 55% of middle to upper class patients (34). Figure 34–8 demonstrates that there is a difference in the patterns of weight gain between patients who vomited and those who did not. The etiology of these symptoms is not clear but may be hormonal, perhaps involving sensitivity to estrogen (35). Treatment is not terribly effective, as standard antiemetics have little benefit in this condition. Because the nausea and vomiting occur in the first trimester, the potential teratogenesis of antiemetics must be considered. Bendectin was withdrawn from the U.S. market because of lawsuits concerning teratogenicity despite a lack of scientific evidence of problems. Phenothiazines are not as well studied but appear safe. Meclizine appears to be the drug of first choice, with dimenhydrinate as backup (36).

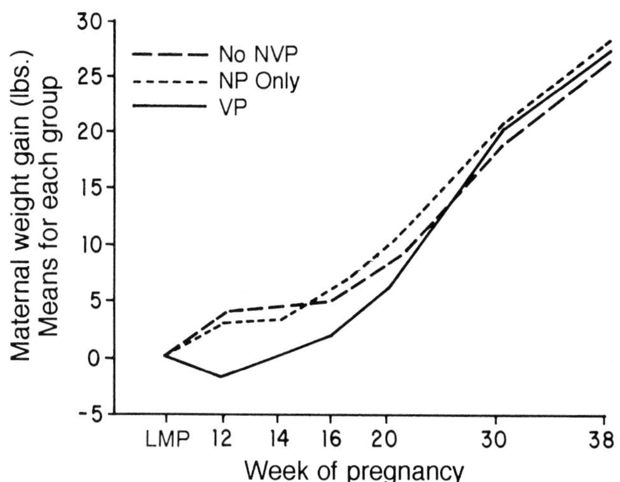


**Fig. 34–8.** Maternal weight gain during the course of pregnancy among three different nausea and/or vomiting of pregnancy exposure categories. No NVP = No nausea and/or vomiting of pregnancy; NP Only = Nausea only; VP = Vomiting of pregnancy. (Redrawn from Tierson FD, Olsen CL, Ernest BH: Nausea and vomiting of pregnancy and association with pregnancy outcome. Am. J. Obstet. Gynecol. 155:1017, 1986.)

Severe cases of nausea and vomiting are referred to as hyperemesis gravidarum. This occurs in about 3/1000 pregnancies. The etiology is unknown but there may be an underlying emotional disturbance, although elevated estrogen levels may be responsible (37). Of interest, in review of their patients in the Collaborative Perinatal Study, Depue, et al (37) found that patients with hyperemesis had a significantly reduced incidence of fetal loss. Clinically, the patient is dehydrated and suffers from malnutrition. Mild elevation in the SGOT and SGPT is sometimes seen.

### *Treatment*

Parenteral therapy is appropriate with intravenous hydration and correction of electrolyte abnormalities. Nutrition must be re-established to correct the ketosis and may have to be provided by parenteral hyperalimentation (total parenteral nutrition or TPN) (38). Total parenteral nutrition is generally supplied through a central vein with a surgically implanted indwelling catheter. Between 2000

**Table 34–12.** A Review of Published Cases of Acute Fatty Liver of Pregnancy*

| Number of Cases: | 140 | |
|---|---|---|
| Setting | | |
| Weeks of gestation at onset | 36, mean; range, 28 to 40 | |
| Nulliparity | 60/125 known | 48% |
| Twin gestation | 19 | 14% |
| Preeclampsia or eclampsia | 64 | 46% |
| Outcome | | |
| Fetal death | 66 | 47% |
| Maternal death | 62 | 44% |
| Normal subsequent pregnancy | 15 known | |

* Data are taken from cases reported in the literature. Patients known to be taking tetracycline were excluded. These data must be interpreted with the knowledge that cases that were unclear or doubtful were not included in the analysis. Also, there may be duplication of reports on single cases other than those acknowledged by the authors. Although this review encompasses a large number of reports, it may not be complete and all-inclusive.

(From Riely CA: Acute fatty liver of pregnancy. Semin. Liver. Dis. 7:47, 1987.)

**Table 34–13.** Acute Fatty Liver of Pregnancy: Proposed Diagnostic Criteria

| |
|---|
| Usual: possibly invariable |
| Third trimester |
| Abnormal transaminases: AST > 100, > 1000 |
| Delivery → → → decrease in AST, followed by clinical improvement |
| Suggestive |
| Preeclampsia or eclampsia |
| Nulliparity |
| Twin gestation |
| Decreased platelets |
| Elevated uric acid, relative to normally low values in pregnancy |
| CT positive for fat |
| Unlikely: suggests other diagnoses |
| Positive serologies for hepatitis A or B |
| Gallstones on ultrasound |
| Pruritus |
| History of drug use |
| Absolute |
| Liver biopsy positive for fat on special stains |

(From Riely CA: Acute fatty liver of pregnancy. Semin. Liver. Dis. 7:47, 1987.)

and 2400 calories per day are administered, along with dextrose and amino acid solutions. Insulin may be required to maintain normal blood sugars. Calcium and multivitamins are added. The addition of lipids to the hyperalimentation regimen is controversial but may not be necessary in the short course of hyperemesis gravidarum. With the advent of safe parenteral nutrition, recommendation for therapeutic termination of pregnancy because of hyperemesis is unwarranted.

## Acute Fatty Liver of Pregnancy

### *Pathophysiology*

Acute fatty liver of pregnancy in its worst form occurs in approximately 1/13,000 deliveries (Table 34–12) (39,40). It probably represents a spectrum of disease and occurs more frequently than is appreciated. The signs and symptoms are erroneously attributed to preeclampsia or other diseases. Acute fatty liver is a disorder presenting in the third trimester (mean gestational age 36 weeks). It is more common in primiparous women and has a higher incidence in twin gestations. The incidence of preeclampsia or eclampsia is significantly increased (46%) compared to the general population (7%). In severe cases, presenting complaints are those of acute hepatic failure. Nausea and vomiting and abdominal pain (right upper quadrant or epigastric) are frequent. Alternatively, the presenting symptoms may be those of preeclampsia, headache, or visual disturbances. Diagnostic criteria are listed in Table 34–13. The pathophysiology of fatal acute fatty liver of pregnancy is shown in Figure 34–9.

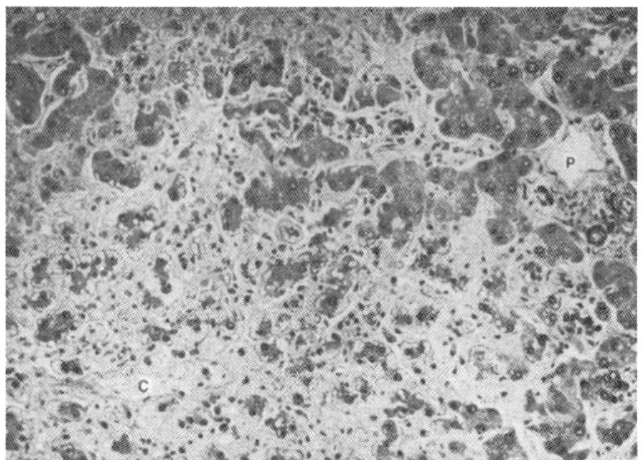


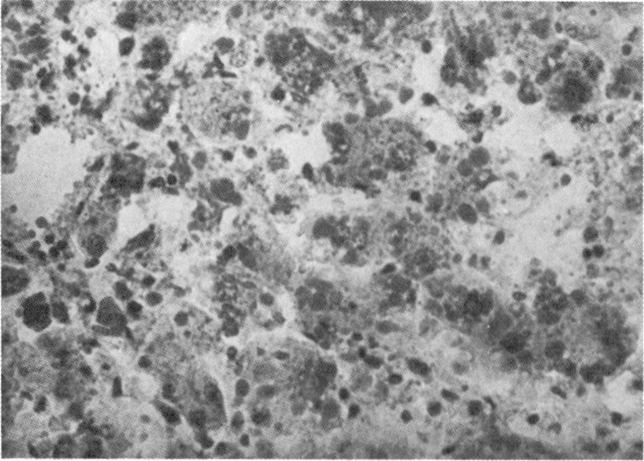

**Fig. 34–9.** Fatal acute liver of pregnancy. Autopsy specimen from 26-year-old woman (G2, P1) who presented at 36 weeks gestation with nausea and vomiting. Precipitous labor and delivery were followed by vaginal hemorrhage, ascites, coma, and death 6 days after admission. No history of preeclampsia. Peak AST, 136. **A:** there is centrizonal pallor with cell drop out and vacuolization of the remaining hepatocytes. The periportal hepatocytes are relatively spared; **C:** central vein; **P:** portal vein (Masson's trichrome; × 10); **B:** oil red stain of frozen section material demonstrates brightly stained, homogeneous dense fat droplets (Oil red O; × 25). (From Riely CA: Acute fatty liver of pregnancy. Semin. Liver Dis. 7:47, 1987.)

### *Clinical Course*

Jaundice is the most common physical finding. Hyperreflexia and edema with hypertension are often found. Transaminase values are elevated as are bilirubin and alkaline phosphatase levels. Coagulopathy is common and may range from a prolongation of prothrombin time due to loss of coagulation factors produced in the liver to disseminated intravascular coagulopathy (DIC). This picture may also be confused by the presence of HELLP syndrome (discussed under Pregnancy-Induced Hypertension, below) that involves thrombocytopenia. Blood loss after delivery may be severe due to disseminated intravascular coagulopathy, requiring transfusion and surgical ligation of the hypogastric arteries or hysterectomy. Other manifestations can include gastrointestinal hemorrhage, hypoglycemia, renal failure, pancreatitis, and coma.

### *Treatment*

Delivery of the pregnancy is the key to maternal survival. Although survival is expected, there is still mortality (8% maternal, 14% fetal) (41). In severe cases, delay of delivery worsens outcome. Treatment is generally supportive and should be in an intensive care unit. Signs of recovery usually occur in 2 to 3 days after delivery. Survivors have no permanent sequellae of their liver failure. There appears to be no evidence of recurrence in subsequent pregnancies, so patients who want another child need not fear this problem.

Fetal distress and fetal death are common. This appears to be due to fibrosis and infarction of the placenta. Expeditious delivery is recommended for fetal as well as maternal well-being.

## Pregnancy-Induced Hypertension (Preeclampsia)

### *Pathophysiology*

Pregnancy-induced hypertension (PIH) is a disease of pregnant women that occurs in approximately 5% of all gestations. In its classic form, the disease consists of hypertension, proteinuria, and edema. The liver may be affected by the generalized disease and arterial vasospasm. Edema of the liver capsule is thought to cause the symptoms of nausea and epigastric pain. In rare cases, subcapsular hepatocellular necrosis leads to subcapsular hematomas. Rupture of the liver can occur with catastrophic hemorrhage and death. Rupture has been associated with vomiting, contractions, or eclamptic seizures. This usually occurs very late in the course of the disease and can be prevented by good prenatal care and expeditious delivery. With rupture, maternal mortality is 70% and fetal mortality is 75% (42). Laparotomy is necessary, often with partial liver resection, to control the hemorrhage and prevent death.

A separate complication associated with some cases of severe pregnancy-induced hypertension is the HELLP syndrome. The name was given to describe the three major pathophysiological aspects of this syndrome—namely **H**emolysis, **E**levated **L**iver enzymes, and **L**ow **P**latelets (43). Often these are the only presenting signs. The patients may lack hypertension, proteinuria, and edema.

**Table 34–14.** Laboratory Findings

| Test | Mean ± 1 SD | Range |
|---|---|---|
| Platelet count × $10^3/mm^3$ | 55 ± 23 | 9–98 |
| Initial hematocrit (%) | 35.8 ± 5.5 | 12–48 |
| Postpartum hematocrit (%) | 25.3 ± 3.9 | 15–35 |
| Creatinine (mg/dl) | 1.7 ± 2.0 | 0.7–10.9 |
| Uric acid (mg/dl) | 8.3 ± 3.1 | 4.8–15.2 |
| Serum glutamic oxaloacetic transaminase (U/L) | 434 ± 556 | 72–4000 |
| Bilirubin (mg/dl) | 2.7 ± 2.5 | 1.2–16.7 |
| Albumin (gm/dl) | 2.8 ± 0.4 | 1.9–3.6 |

(From Sibai BM, Taslimi MM, El-Nazer A, Amon E, et al: Maternal-perinatal outcome associated with the syndrome of hemolysis, elevated liver enzymes, and low platelets in severe preeclampsia-eclampsia. Am. J. Obstet. Gynecol. 155:501, 1986.)

HELLP syndrome occurs more commonly in white patients than in blacks, which is the opposite of classic pregnancy-induced hypertension. Multiparae are also more commonly affected, which is also different than pregnancy-induced hypertension. Sibai, et al (44) reported on incidence of HELLP syndrome in 10% of patients with severe pregnancy-induced hypertension. Table 34–14 lists laboratory findings of all patients in this study before delivery, and Table 34–15 summarizes the related maternal complications. The perinatal outcome for these patients is listed in Table 34–16.

### *Clinical Course*

The pathophysiology of pregnancy-induced hypertension is unknown, but probably is related to release of vasoactive substances. The vascular changes result in damage to circulatory platelets and red blood cells. Arterial vasospasm may affect different organ systems more severely in different patients. Pregnancy-induced hypertension causes fibrin deposition in liver sinusoids that eventually causes the necrosis and hemorrhage that can lead to hematoma formation and capsule swelling (Figure 34–10) (45).

Most patients present with epigastric or right upper quadrant pain, nausea and/or vomiting, and headache. Lab-

**Table 34–15.** Maternal Complications (N = 110)

| Complication | No. | % |
|---|---|---|
| Abruptio placentae | 22 | 20 |
| Intravascular coagulopathy | 42 | 38 |
| Acute renal failure | 9 | 8 |
| Pleural effusions | 8 | 7.1 |
| Pulmonary edema | 5 | 4.5 |
| Ruptured liver hematoma | 2 | 1.8 |
| Maternal deaths | 2 | 1.8 |

(From Sibai BM, Taslimi MM, El-Nazer A, Amon E, et al: Maternal-perinatal outcome associated with the syndrome of hemolysis, elevated liver enzymes, and low platelets in severe preeclampsia-eclampsia. Am. J. Obstet. Gynecol. 155:501, 1986.)

**Table 34–16.** Perinatal Outcome (N = 114 Births)

| Outcome | No. | % |
|---|---|---|
| Perinatal deaths | 38 | 33.3 |
| Stillbirths | 22 | 19.3 |
| Neonatal deaths | 16 | 14.0 |
| Gestational age (wk) | | |
| ≥ 30 | 47 | 41.2 |
| 31–36 | 46 | 40.4 |
| > 36 | 21 | 18.4 |
| Small for gestational age | 36 | 31.6 |
| Apgar score | | |
| 1 min ≥ 4 | 39 | 34.0 |
| 5 min < 7 | 26 | 23.0 |

(From Sibai BM, Taslimi MM, El-Nazer A, Amon E, et al: Maternal-perinatal outcome associated with the syndrome of hemolysis, elevated liver enzymes, and low platelets in severe preeclampsia-eclampsia. Am. J. Obstet. Gynecol. 155:501, 1986.)

oratory findings include elevated LDH (above 600 IU/liter), SGOT, and bilirubin. The platelet count is below 100,000/mm$^3$ and the peripheral blood smear shows hemolysis. Renal abnormalities are frequent with elevated BUN and creatinine, and decreased creatinine clearance. Disseminated intravascular coagulopathy can complicate severe pregnancy-induced hypertension.

### Treatment

Obstetric management needs to be directed toward both the mother and the fetus because pregnancy-induced hypertension is potentially life-threatening to both. Mild pregnancy-induced hypertension may respond to bed rest for a period of time, but inevitably will get worse. A delay in delivery may be appropriate should fetal gestational age be immature and additional time helpful. Most cases of pregnancy-induced hypertension occur at term (more than 35 weeks) and delivery is the treatment of choice. Severe pregnancy-induced hypertension is treated by stabilization and delivery at any gestational age (See Table 34–17).

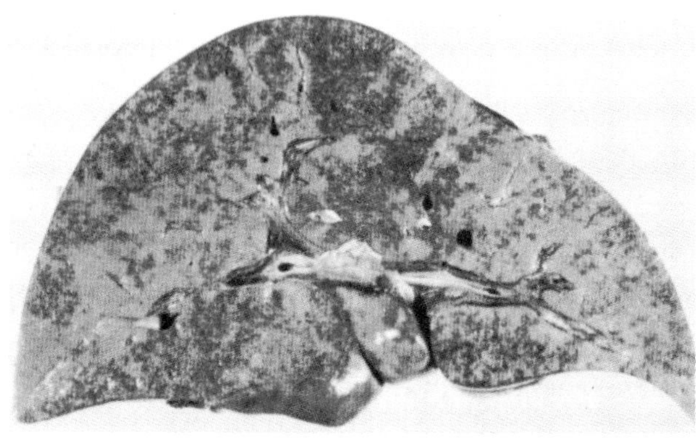

**Fig. 34–10.** Hepatic involvement in toxemia gives the liver a grossly mottled appearance due to areas of hemorrhage and necrosis in both lobes. (Rolfes DB, Ishak KG: Liver disease in toxemia of pregnancy. Am. J. Gastro. 81:1138, 1986.)

**Table 34–17.** Definition of Severe Pregnancy-Induced Hypertension

(1) blood pressure of more than 160 mm Hg systolic, or more than 110 mm Hg diastolic;
(2) proteinuria of more than 5 g in 24 hours;
(3) oliguria (500 ml or less per 24 hours;
(4) cerebral or visual disturbances;
(5) epigastric pain; or
(6) pulmonary edema or cyanosis

Magnesium sulfate is the drug of choice to suppress hyperactive neurological symptoms. Blood pressure can be controlled with hydralazine, and disseminated intravascular coagulopathy corrected with blood components (platelets, fresh frozen plasma, cryoprecipitate). The fetus must be monitored closely because the arterial vasospasm can affect the uterine blood supply leading to uteroplacental insufficiency.

*Gastrointestinal disease can occur before pregnancy or acutely during an ongoing pregnancy.*

## Hepatitis

### Etiology

Infectious disease involving the liver results in an inflammatory response termed hepatitis. These infections appear to be viral in origin and can be caused by: hepatitis A virus (HAV); hepatitis B virus (HBV); non-A, non-B virus; cytomegalovirus (CMV); Epstein-Barr virus (EBV); and rarely, herpes virus.

### Pathophysiology

Many cases may be asymptomatic, but others present with anorexia, nausea and vomiting, fatigue, myalgias, and low-grade fever. Symptoms and signs include jaundice, dark urine, light stools, and right upper quadrant pain. The disease affects pregnant women the same as nonpregnant and does not appear to affect the fetus in utero. One study (46) found that hepatitis had no effect on congenital malformations, stillbirth, abortion, or intrauterine growth retardation, but there was an increased risk of premature delivery, especially should infection occur in the third trimester.

Laboratory analysis typically shows large elevation of alanine aminotransferase and aspartate aminotransferase (often 10 times normal levels). Bilirubin is significantly elevated. The agent causing the inflammatory response can be identified by identifying antigens and antibodies in the mother's blood. This is important for the determination of the risk to the fetus at delivery.

### Clinical Course

Hepatitis A is transmitted by the fecal-oral route. The incubation period is 2 to 7 weeks and active disease lasts 2 to 3 weeks. Antibodies to hepatitis A virus confirm the diagnosis. IgM antibodies would indicate recent infection and IgG antibodies would reflect past exposure and immunity. Hepatitis A probably poses no risk for the infant, but treatment of the infant after delivery with immunoglobulin has been recommended.

Hepatitis B causes a more serious disease. Transmission is percutaneous or permucosal. The incubation period ranges from 1 to 6 months. Laboratory evaluation is more extensive. Both antigens and antibodies need to be determined to the hepatitis B surface antigen, core antigen, and e antigen. The presence or absence of antibodies and antigens in various combinations determines whether disease is active, in a chronic carrier state, or previous disease resolved. The presence of HbSAg indicates infection (either acute or chronic carrier state). Other antigens and antibodies refine the diagnosis. The presence of the HbeAg indicates a higher degree of infectivity. Acute hepatitis B or patients with a chronic carrier state can infect their child at delivery. Due to an approximate 0.1% incidence of asymptomatic carrier state in the U.S. and the devastating neonatal effects, the American College of Obstetrics and Gynecology has recommended that all pregnant patients be screened for hepatitis B carrier state. Long-term potential sequellae of chronic hepatitis B carrier state include cirrhosis and liver carcinoma.

If the mother is HbSAg-positive, the rate of transmission to her infant is about 40 to 69%, and 10% of the babies who develop hepatitis will be chronic carriers; however, if the mother also is HbeAg positive, transmission is about 90 to 95%, with a neonatal carrier rate of 85 to 90%. Neonatal therapy is recommended with hepatitis B immunoglobulin (HBIG) (0.5 ml intramuscularly) within 12 hours of birth and hepatitis B vaccine (Heptavax) 0.5 ml within 12 hours of birth and repeat 1 and 6 months later. The use of these two agents has been shown to reduce the chronic carrier state in the infant to 2 to 5% (47).

Non-A, non-B hepatitis is caused by an unknown virus. It is transmitted percutaneously and permucosally, and is the primary cause of post-transfusion hepatitis. There is a high carrier rate (10 to 50%). It is diagnosed after all other viruses and hepatotoxic drugs and chemicals have been eliminated. Vertical transmission to the neonate probably occurs and gammaglobulin prophylaxis should be given to the neonate.

The management of acute viral hepatitis in pregnancy is similar to that of nonpregnant patients. Supportive care should be given. Avoid all nonvital medications or drugs that may aggravate the liver damage. Unnecessary procedures and operations should be avoided. There is no benefit to the baby to unnecessarily deliver the patient by cesarean section (48). Unnecessary amniocentesis should be avoided because of the potential for introduction of the virus into the fetal compartment. Breast feeding, although a mode for spread of the disease, is permissible should the mother wish to breast feed. Prevention of spread should be achieved by immunoprophylaxis, not by isolation or restriction of activities.

## Cholecystitis and Cholelithiasis

### *Etiology*

Cholelithiasis (gallstones) is associated with elevations of estrogen and progesterone and pregnancy (49). The formation of stones is enhanced by elevated cholesterol levels, which exist in excess compared to bile salts in the gall bladder. The cholesterol precipitates into microcrystals, which grow into microscopic stones facilitated by the stasis that occurs in pregnancy. These stones then cause symptoms when they lodge in either the cystic duct or the common bile duct.

### *Pathophysiology*

Presenting symptoms include right upper quadrant pain, nausea and vomiting. Diagnosis is made by ultrasound demonstration of calculi or duct dilatation. Treatment is unaltered by pregnancy. Surgery is only recommended in cases of common duct obstruction; otherwise, definitive therapy is reserved for after delivery.

### *Clinical Course*

Cholecystitis is one of the most common nonobstetric problems seen in pregnancy. Symptoms include right upper quadrant pain (pain may be epigastric, right scapular, or left upper quadrant) that is episodic in nature, often triggered by meals. The pain may last a few minutes or several hours. There may be nausea and vomiting as well as fever. Palpable right upper quadrant tenderness is often present. White blood count is usually elevated. Serum aminotransferases are normal, and bilirubin is elevated along with alkaline phosphatase. Diagnosis is usually made by ultrasound. Management should be medical with surgery reserved for stone impaction and associated pancreatitis.

## Pancreatitis

Pregnant patients are similar to nonpregnant women with regard to pancreatitis. It is, apparently, a rare disease in pregnancy. At tertiary institutions the rate is approximately 1/1500 deliveries (50). The maternal mortality rate from single-institution series is about 3.4%. Cholelithiasis is the most commonly identified cause of pancreatitis; however, drugs, hyperlipidemia, and alcohol abuse may also elicit pancreatitis.

### *Pathophysiology*

Whatever the inciting event, pancreatitis represents release of activated digestive enzymes in the pancreas, leading to autodigestion. This may progress to necrosis and hemorrhage. Pancreatitis usually presents with abdominal pain, often epigastric in location, with radiation straight through to the back. It is exacerbated by food intake. Nausea and vomiting are common.

### *Clinical Course*

Ultrasound is very helpful in detecting such complications of pancreatitis as peritoneal fluid or pseudocyst. Diagnosis is usually based on an elevated serum amylase level; however, a 2-hour urine amylase may be necessary in mild cases because the increased clearance of amylase in pregnancy may lead to a normal serum amylase. Serum lipase is also elevated in acute pancreatitis.

### *Treatment*

Treatment is generally supportive. Intravenous fluids must be vigorously replaced and attention paid to calcium replacement. Nasogastric suction may provide some symptomatic relief. The surgical approach to gallstone pancreatitis should be reserved for resistant cases, with definitive surgical therapy reserved for after delivery.

## Acid Peptic Disease

Peptic ulcer disease seems to be more common in males and postmenopausal females. A protective effect of increased estrogen and progesterone is postulated, but the mechanism is unclear. The major symptom is dyspepsia. The pain is epigastric and is relieved by meals or antacids. Diagnosis is usually established in pregnancy by endoscopic examination and visualization. Treatment is generally with antacids (a magnesium-aluminum combination), cimetidine, and other acid blockers.

## Inflammatory Bowel Disease

### *Pathophysiology*

The effect of ulcerative colitis and Crohn's disease on pregnancy appears to be minimal. As is usually the case, inactive disease seems to not affect pregnancy, while active disease may be associated with higher rates of spontaneous abortion and preterm delivery (51,52).

### *Therapy*

Therapy of active inflammatory bowel disease is generally with sulfasalazine, either alone or in combination with steroids. Both drugs appear to be safe in pregnancy, and outcome in treated patients appears similar to outcomes in control groups that either had no inflammatory bowel disease or had untreated inflammatory bowel disease (53). Sulfasalazine interferes with folic acid absorption in the small bowel, and patients requiring therapy with this drug should receive supplemental folic acid therapy. Total parenteral nutrition may be useful in patients with severe exacerbations.

Surgical intervention is indicated for complications of inflammatory bowel disease—intestinal obstruction, gastrointestinal bleeding, colonic dilatation, and failure of medical therapy. Prior colonic resection does not prohibit pregnancy (54).

## Cirrhosis

Cirrhosis is a very uncommon complication in the pregnant female because chronic liver disease most often occurs after the childbearing age. Pregnancy does not appear to adversely affect the course of cirrhosis, as prognosis generally is related to the underlying disease. Ascites and edema, which complicate cirrhosis, are often troublesome because of the decreased albumin in normal pregnancy. Bleeding esophageal varices may be life-threatening and may rupture during the second stage of labor. Vaginal delivery under epidural analgesia without pushing (Valsalva) may lower the risk of life-threatening bleeding.

## Surgical Disease in Pregnancy

Diseases of the gastrointestinal tract that are treated primarily by surgical intervention include appendicitis and intestinal obstruction.

### *Appendicitis*

#### Pathophysiology

Acute appendicitis occurs in about 7/10,000 deliveries (55). Diagnosis in pregnancy is difficult and often leads to delay in surgical therapy, leading to increased mortality and morbidity for mother and baby. As the uterine size increases, the location of the appendix is changed; the more advanced the pregnancy, the higher and more lateral the location of the appendix. The uterus also tends to keep the appendix from contact with the abdominal wall, leading to milder and less well-localized symptoms.

#### Clinical Course

Diagnosis is not clear-cut in pregnancy (56). Nausea and right lower quadrant pain are not consistent. Temperatures are not usually elevated, and white blood cell counts are in the normal range for pregnancy, although a left shift is often noted.

#### Treatment

Management of appendicitis in pregnancy needs to be aggressive. Delay leads to perforation, which will affect morbidity and mortality. Perinatal loss will vary from 0.5% without perforation to 27% in the presence of pelvic peritonitis (57).

Controversy exists about the role of cesarean section at term in patients with appendicitis (58). Most authors agree that routine cesarean section is unwarranted in uncomplicated appendicitis. In the presence of generalized peritonitis, cesarean section is probably indicated as fetal death rate is high, possibly due to bacterial toxins; the incidence of labor within 24 hours is also high.

### *Intestinal Obstruction*

#### Pathophysiology

Intestinal obstruction in pregnancy is infrequent and results most commonly from the pressure of the growing uterus on adhesions from previous surgery. It is most common in the third trimester and presentation is with pain, vomiting, and constipation. A flat plate x ray of the abdomen is often helpful in making the diagnosis.

#### Treatment

Therapy consists of aggressive fluid replacement and surgical exploration. Cesarean section may be necessary should the large uterus prevent adequate evaluation of the bowel. As with appendicitis, early diagnosis and surgical intervention reduces the morbidity and mortality for mother and infant.

## ANESTHETIC MANAGEMENT OF PATIENTS WITH GASTROINTESTINAL TRACT DISEASES

Anesthesia for patients with disease of the gastrointestinal tract cannot be categorized for specificity in regard to the particular process or disease state. For the most part, the tenets of good anesthesia in such patients take foundation in the practical, sound principles espoused throughout this textbook. There are some special considerations that will be discussed in the following section that are of practical help when confronted with patients with certain afflictions. Some of these special considerations include anesthetic considerations of patients with liver and or biliary disease and in patients with acute intestinal tract disease.

In patients with liver and/or biliary disease, the changes in liver function must be detailed and the functional status of the patient considered. For example, there may be serious restrictions in regard to coagulation times, and, thus, unexpected problems regarding clot formation may increase the formation of an epidural hematoma. This situation may make regional anesthesia an undesirable choice under such circumstances. On the other hand, due to liver damage, there may be serious problems with drug metabolism, which effects drug disposition and dosage significantly, and this will be important knowledge for the anesthesiologist as he/she is planning the agent and amounts for induction of anesthesia. As one example, the level of pseudocholinesterase may be decreased and thus prolong the muscle paralysis after succinylcholine use. As another example, due to metabolism, the tolerance for inhalational agents may be increased due to facilitated biotransformation of the drugs, and thus the amount of drug may be increased for the same cerebral effect. This may be fine for the desired effect from the maternal viewpoint, but the uterine motility may also be effected with the increased dosage of inhalation drug and significant bleeding could result. The liver itself really does not affect extensively the initial response of the body to anesthetic agents such as the inhalation anesthetics, the muscle relaxants, and the vasopressor drugs. Yet, as mentioned, it can affect the metabolism and thus the length of time the drug acts. The drugs that are slightly potentiated include thiopental, which can still be used but should be used with caution and only in reduced dosages in patients with substantial liver disease. It is more of an academic point that the amide local anesthetics are detoxified by the liver and thus their effect may be intensified also in severe liver problems. Practically speaking, there are no reports of significant clinical effect of these local anesthetic agents in such disease processes, so it is doubtful that this is a point to be concerned about. Other local anesthetics such as the ester-type drugs are metabolized by estrases in the blood and are not so effected by changes in liver metabolism, even though plasma cholinesterase activity is low in patients with liver disease.

Generally speaking, regional analgesia is preferred in these patients if the aforementioned problems with coagulation are not a problem. Either lumbar epidural or spinal can effect good analgesia and not be effected by the problems of metabolism of the systemically used drugs alluded to above. Of course, one consideration to keep in mind is that some of these patients may be somewhat dehydrated and thus may need preload fluids administered before the sympathectomy associated with regional analgesia. Regional analgesia also gets around the problems associated with having to use higher levels of induction agents because of the tolerance factor just mentioned. Use of the higher dosages of drugs to prevent maternal recall and to increase comfort may have deleterious effects due to hypotension in the mother and uterine atony in the mother. Becasue prothrombin production is reduced in patients with liver disease, there needs to be documentation of normal clotting before the use of either epidural or spinal anesthesia in these patients. For a more in-depth discussion of indications and contraindication in cases of clotting abnormality, please see the discussion of this point in Chapter 13. In some very ill patients, there may be the complication of ascites intra-abdominal or even intraplueral. Consideration should be given toward aspiration on the effusion should there be evidence that it may affect the patient clinically, such as cause a substantial ventilation-perfusion gradient and impede oxygenation. One final, anatomically related point is that associated with esophageal varices. In such patients, it may be better to consider regional anesthesia should the clotting times be normal so as to prevent the increased pressure sometimes associated with the general anesthesia technique during times of intubation in a light plane of anesthesia or during the emergence period when nausea and even emesis may occur. If regional anesthesia is contraindicated for other purposes, then one should use general anesthesia with care being given to prevent increased tension or Valsalva maneuvers during induction. This can be done with administration of a generous preoperative narcotic with due warning to the neonatologist, of course, to be alert for neonatal respiratory depression. It can also be done with use of adequate topical sprays to the pharynx and translaryngeal analgesia. These two keystone methods of obtaining analgesia for awake intubation can be supplemented with superior laryngeal nerve block and lingual nerve block.

For labor then, one can consider use of systemic medications in moderation to obtain a suitable analgesic state for relief from labor contractions. In addition, a paracervical block can be considered for pain relief later in labor. Finally, pudendal block may be used for the actual delivery process. For cesarean section, one can consider either epidural or spinal or continuous spinal anesthesia should clotting mechanisms not be impeded. If general anesthesia is chosen, then one should use caution during induction to avoid the responses to intubation during the normal induction procedure with little, if any, protection against laryngeal reflex activity and little, if any, protection against cardiovascular reflexes such as hypertension.

## REFERENCES

1. Gabert HA, Miller JM: Renal disease in pregnancy. Obstet. Gynecol. Surv. 40:449, 1985.
2. Whalley PJ: Bacteriuria of pregnancy. Am. J. Obstet. Gynecol. 97:723, 1967.

3. Gilstrap LC, Cunningham FG, Whalley PJ: Acute pyelonephritis in pregnancy: an anterospective study of 565 women. Obstet. Gynecol. 57:409, 1981.
4. Gilstrap LC, Hankins GDV, Snyder RR, Breenberg RT: Acute pyelonephritis in pregnancy. Comp. Therapy 12:38, 1986.
5. Farquhar M: Ultrastructure of the nephron disclosed by electron microscopy. Section A—review of normal and pathologic glomerular ultrastructure. *In* Proceedings of the 10th Annual Conferences on the Nephrotic Syndrome. Edited by J Metcoff. New York, National Kidney Foundation, 1959, p. 2.
6. Robertson EG: Assessment and treatment of renal disease in pregnancy. Clin. Obstet. Gynecol. 28;279, 1985.
7. Harris RE, Duninlou DR: The incidence and significance of urinary calculi in pregnancy. Am. J. Obstet. Gynecol. 99: 237 1967.
8. Michael J: The management of renal disease in pregnancy. Clin. Obstet. Gynecol. 13:319, 1986.
9. Katz AI, Davison JM, Hayslett JP, Singson E, et al: Pregnancy in women with kidney disease. Kid. Int. 18:192, 1980.
10. Davison JM, Katz AI, Lindheimer MD: Kidney disease and pregnancy: obstetric outcome and long-term renal prognosis. Clin. Perinatol. 12:497, 1985.
11. Hou SH, Grossman SD, Madias NE: Pregnancy in women with renal disease and moderate renal insufficiency. Am. J. Med. 78:185, 1985.
12. Redrow M, Cherem L, Elliott J, Mangalat J, et al: Dialysis in the management of pregnant patients with renal insufficiency. Medicine 67:199, 1988.
13. Hou S: Pregnancy in women requiring dialysis for renal failure. Am. J. Kid. Dis. 9:368, 1987.
14. Elliott JP, O'Keeffe DF, Schon DA, Cherem LB: Dialysis in pregnancy: a critical review. Ob. Gyn. Survey 46:319, 1991.
15. Cattran DC, Benzie RJ: Pregnancy in a continuous ambulatory peritoneal dialysis patient. Peritoneal Dialysis Bulletin 3:13, 1983.
16. Kioko EM, Shaw KM, Clarke AD, Warren DJ: Successful pregnancy in a diabetic patient treated with continuous ambulatory peritoneal dialysis. Diabetes Care 6:298, 1983.
17. Barr M, Burdi AR: Warfarin—associated embryopathy in a 17 week abortus. Teratology 14:129, 1976.
18. Penn I, Makowski EL, Harris P: Parenthood following renal transplantation. Kid. Int. 18:221, 1980.
19. Davison JM, Lindheimer MD: Pregnancy in women with renal allografts. Semin. Nephrol. 4:240, 1984.
20. Hou S: Pregnancy in women with renal disease. N. Engl. J. Med. 312:836, 1985.
21. O'Donnell D, Meyers AM, Sevitz H, Botha JR, et al: Pregnancy after renal transplantation. Aust. N.Z. J. Med. 15:320, 1985.
22. Dyson D: Anesthesia for patients with stable end-stage renal disease. Vet. Clin. North. Am. Small. Anim. Pract. 22(2):469, 1992.
23. Weir PH, Chung FF: Anaesthesia for patients with chronic renal disease. Can. Anaesth. Soc. J. 31(4):468, 1984.
24. Rostand SG, Rutsky EA: Pericarditis in end-stage renal disease. Cardiol. Clin. 8(4):701, 1990.
25. Ebert TJ, Kotrly KJ, Madsen KE, Bernstein JS, et al: Fentanyl-diazepam anesthesia with or without $N_2O$ does not attenuate cardiopulmonary baroreflex-mediated vasoconstrictor responses to controlled hypovolemia in humans. Anesth. Analg. 67(6):548, 1988.
26. Kobayashi Y, Ochiai R, Takeda J, Sekiguchi H, et al: Serum and urinary inorganic fluoride concentrations after prolonged inhalation of sevoflurane in humans. Anesth. Analg. 74(5):753, 1992.
27. Cousins MJ, Greenstein LR, Hitt BA, Mazze RI: Metabolism and renal effects of enflurane in man. Anesthesiology 44(1): 44, 1976.
28. Orko R, Pitkänen M, Rosenberg PH: Subarachnoid anesthesia with 0.75% bupivacaine in patients with chronic renal failure. Br. J. Anaesth. 58:605, 1986.
29. Strasser K, Abel J, Breulmann M, Schumacher I, et al: Plasma level of etidocaine within the first two hours after axillary plexus block in healthy adults and patients with renal insufficiency. Anaesthetist 30:14, 1981.
30. Johnston WG, Baskett TF: Obstetric cholestasis: a 14 year review. Am. J. Obstet. Gynecol. 133:299 1979.
31. Wilson BR, Haverkamp AD: Cholestatic jaundice of pregnancy: new perspectives. Obstet. Gynecol. 54:648, 1979.
32. Reid R, Ivey KJ, Rencoret RH, Storey B: Fetal complications of obstetric cholestasis. Br. Med. Journal 1:870, 1976.
33. Laatikainen T: Fetal bile acid levels in pregnancies complicated by maternal intrahepatic cholestasis. Am. J. Obstet. Gynecol. 122(7):852–6, 1975.
34. Tierson FD, Olsen CL, Ernest BH: Nausea and vomiting of pregnancy and association with pregnancy outcome. Am. J. Obstet. Gynecol. 155:1017, 1986.
35. Järnfelt-Samsioe A, Samisoe G, Velinder GM: Nausea and vomiting in pregnancy: a review. Obstet. Gynecol. Surv. 4: 422, 1987.
36. Leathem A: Safety and efficacy of antiemetics used to treat nausea and vomiting in pregnancy. Clin. Pharm. 5:660, 1986.
37. Depue RH, Bernstein L, Ross RK, Judd HL, et al: Hyperemesis gravidarum in relation to estradiol levels, pregnancy outcome, and other maternal factors: a seroepidemiologic study. Am. J. Obstet. Gynecol. 156:1137, 1987.
38. Lee RV, Hatjis CG, Meis PJ: Total parenteral nutrition during pregnancy. Obstet. Gynecol. 66:585, 1985.
39. Riely CA: Acute fatty liver of pregnancy. Semin. Liver Dis. 7:47, 1987.
40. Moise KJ, Shah DM: Acute fatty liver of pregnancy: etiology of fetal distress and fetal wastage. Obstet. Gynecol. 69:482, 1987.
41. Snyder RF, Hankins GD: Etiology and management of acute fatty liver of pregnancy. Clin. Perinatol. 13:813, 1986.
42. Douvas SG, Meeks GR, Phillips O, Morrison JC, et al: Liver disease in pregnancy. Obstet. Gynecol. Surv. 38:531, 1983.
43. Weinstein L: Syndrome of hemolysis, elevated liver enzymes and low platelet count: a severe consequence of hypertension in pregnancy. Am. J. Obstet. Gynecol. 142:159, 1982.
44. Sibai BM, Taslimi MM, El-Nazer A, Amon E, et al: Maternal-perinatal outcome associated with the syndrome of hemolysis, elevated liver enzymes, and low platelets in severe preeclampsia-eclampsia. Am. J. Obstet. Gynecol. 155:501, 1986.
45. Rolfes DB, Ishak KG: Liver disease in toxemia of pregnancy. Am. J. Gastro. 81:1138, 1986.
46. Hieber JP, Dalton D, Shorey J, Combes B: Hepatitis and pregnancy. J. Pediatr. 91:545, 1977.
47. Wong VC, Ip HMH, Reesink HW, Lelie PN, et al: Prevention of the HbSAg carrier state in newborn infants of mothers who are chronic carriers of HbSAg and HbeAg by administration of hepatitis B vaccine and hepatitis B immunoglobulin. Lancet 1:921, 1984.
48. Rustgi VK, Hoofnagle JH: Viral hepatitis during pregnancy. Semin. Liver Dis. 7:40, 1987.
49. Shaffer EA: Current problems in obstetrics, gynecology, and fertility; The liver and pregnancy. Update, Vol. X, 1987.
50. Klein KB: Pancreatitis in Pregnancy in Gastrointestinal and Hepatic Complications in Pregnancy. *In* Gastrointestinal and Hepatic Complications in Pregnancy. Edited by VA Rustgi, JN Cooper. New York, Wiley and Sons, 1986.
51. Nielson OH, Andreasson B, Bondesen S, Jarnum S: Pregnancy in ulcerative colitis. Scand. J. Gastroenterol 18:735, 1983.

52. Khosla R, Willoughby CP, Jewell DP: Crohn's disease and pregnancy. Gut 25:52 1984.
53. Mogadam M, Dobbins WO, III Korelitz BI, Ahmed SW: Pregnancy in inflammatory bowel disease: effect of sulfasalazine and corticosteroids on fetal outcome. Gastroenterol. 80:72, 1981.
54. Hanan IM, Kirsner JB: Inflammatory bowel disease in the pregnant woman. Clin. Perinatol. 12:669, 1985.
55. Babaknia A, Parsa H, Woodruff JD: Appendicitis during pregnancy. Obstet. Gynecol. 50:40, 1977.
56. Bailey LE, Finley RK Jr, Miller SF, Jones LM: Acute appendicitis during pregnancy. Amer. Surg. 52:218, 1986.
57. Weingold AB: Appendicitis in pregnancy. Clin. Obstet. Gynaecol. 26:801, 1983.
58. Goldberg DN: Acute appendicitis in pregnancy. Can. J. Surg. 23:92, 1980.

# Chapter 35

# THE HEMATOLOGY OF PREGNANCY

MERLIN H. SAYERS
JAMES McARTHUR
JOHN S. McDONALD

During the last 20 years, remarkable advances have been made in virtually every area of hematology and oncology. These areas include: stem cell proliferation and maturation; a whole new field dealing with growth factors, their functions, and synthesis; the molecular-genetic basis for a large number of hematologic illnesses; hemostasis, including a modern appreciation of how platelets work, how thrombosis is prevented and facilitated; and a detailed appreciation of thrombolysis and use of thrombolytic agents. In addition, gains have been made in the understanding of the pathogenesis of many hematologic and nonhematologic malignancies and in developing countless new approaches to managing these diseases. Finally, there is the impact on all medical practice by newly defined and understood infectious diseases, of which acquired immune deficiency syndrome (AIDS) is certainly the prime example.

A complete grounding in basic hematology will help health care team members in all fields do the best they possibly can for their patients with illnesses represented by the areas of advancements mentioned. There are several excellent reviews of hematology and pregnancy, and the reader is referred to these for the kind of depth and practical information required for a detailed understanding. (1–3). In this section, we have chosen to give a general overview of normal hematology and then follow with a brief discussion and approach to common or prototype hematologic diseases. The second part of the chapter will review the effects of pregnancy on hematology and hematologic illnesses. This review will again be somewhat general but will target the major areas in hematology in which pregnancy either has a specific effect or in which it must be a special consideration. The final section of the chapter before General Anesthetic Considerations will concentrate on specific problems with which the obstetric anesthesiologist must be prepared to deal with.

Anesthesiologists are certainly specialists in their own field. However, in the case of associated hematologic difficulties, they are often the first to identify a clue to some hematologic impairment and must take action accordingly.

## REVIEW OF HEMATOPOIESIS

Decades of research work have gone into understanding the proliferation and maturation of the various hematopoietic cell lines, as is depicted in Figure 35–1. Similarly, significant research has produced an understanding of the variety of growth factors in existence and their relationship to the various steps in hematopoiesis. We can now identify with certainty what the various stages represent from uncommitted stem cells to mature hematologic cells. We can also describe quite clearly what changes are occurring before and after the cells and their progenitors can be distinguished on light microscopy. Equally, our understanding of each cell line's major functions has been broadened and enhanced. Coexistent with this research have been the developments in biochemistry, molecular biology, and genetics, which have resulted in an even more exact pinpointing of the various genetic factors involved in hematopoiesis. As each of these areas has been delineated, more information has been gleaned about the specific pathogenesis of a variety of hematologic problems. In many instances, this research has led to new and valuable treatments. It has also led to a wider understanding of how drugs, viruses, and other potentially harmful agents can exert their individual or collective effects.

### *The Erythroid System*

#### *Normal Erythropoiesis and Function*

The major functions of the red blood cells is to transport oxygen from the pulmonary circulation to the periphery, where oxygen is released to the tissues. Red blood cells also function, in part, to maintain a normal intravascular volume. Achieving these tasks requires a great deal of diversification in functionings from these non-nucleated cells. To illustrate, red blood cells must: have enzymatic systems allowing for both aerobic and anaerobic breakdown of glucose; have an internal system that keeps the oxygen molecules attached appropriately to its hemoglobin until the appropriate time for release; be deformable; and live for approximately 100 days before being destroyed in the spleen and other portions of the reticuloendothelial system. Erythropoiesis occurs, as is outlined in Figure 35–1, and a normal bone marrow response to loss of red cells—whether through anemia or bleeding—is essential for the patient to make up for such a loss. A handy indicator for the bone marrow's ability to respond to anemia is the doubly corrected reticulocyte count (or reticulocyte index). The reticulocyte is a

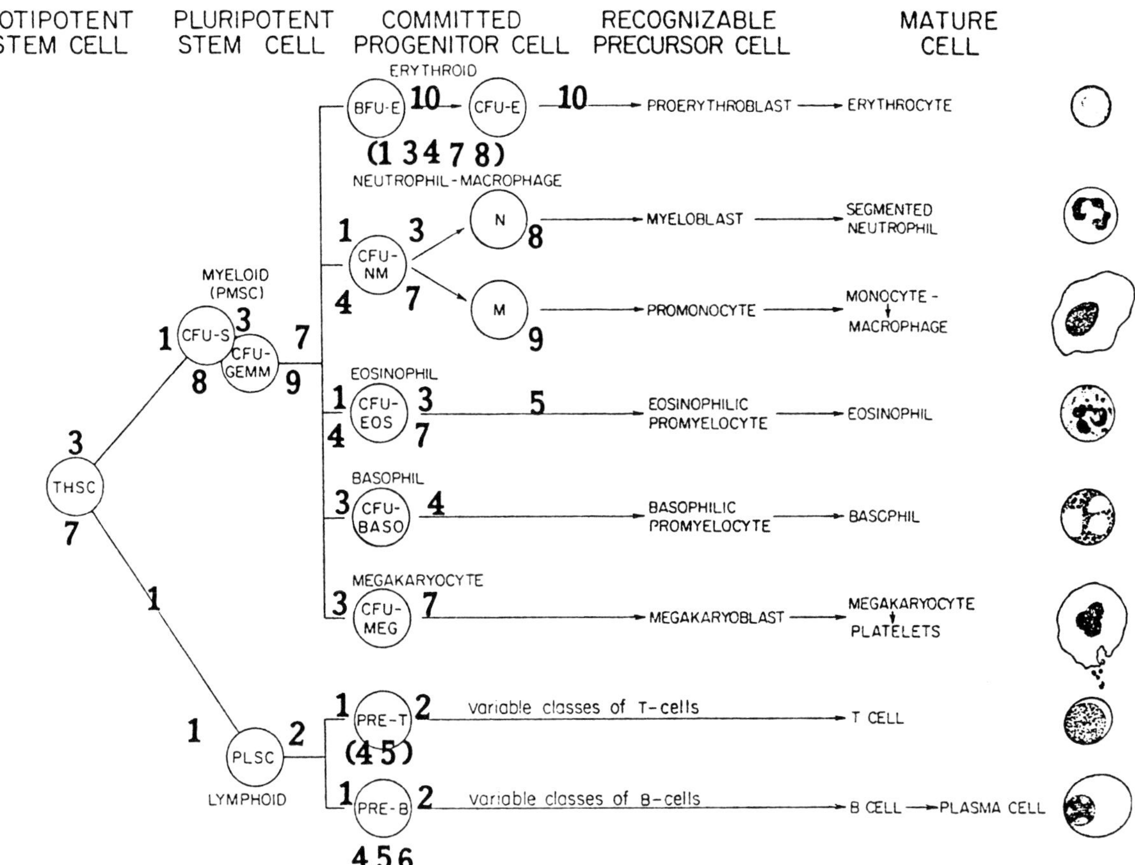


**Fig. 35–1.** A diagram of hematopoiesis showing steps in stem cell proliferation and maturation. THSC = totipotent hematopoietic stem cell; CFU = colony forming unit; PLSC = pluripotent lymphoid stem cell; S = spleen; GEMM = granulocyte, eosinophil, monocyte, megakaryocyte; BFUE = burst forming unit erythroid; E = erythroid; N = myeloid; M = monocyte; EOS = eosinophil; BASO = basophil; MEG = megakaryocyte; PRE-T = pre-T lymphoid progenitor; PRE-B = pre-B lymphoid progenitor. Numbers refer to growth factors, lymphokines, and monokines, which are involved in the regulation of hematopoiesis. 1 = lymphocyte activating factor or IL-1; 2 = T cell growth factor or IL-2; 3 = multi-CSF or IL-3; 4 = B cell stimulating factor or IL-4; 5 = eosinophil differentiation factor or IL 5; 6 = B cell differentiation factor or IL-6; 7 = granulocyte-macrophage colony stimulating factor or GMCSF; 8 = granulocyte CSF or G-CSF; 9 = macrophage CSF or M-CSF; 10 = erythropoietin. (Adapted from Hoffbrand AV, Pettit E: Sandoz Atlas—Clinical Hematology. New York, Gower Medical Publishing, 1988, pp. 2–5; Zuker-Franklin D, Greaves MF, Grossi CE, Marmont AM: Atlas of Blood Cells Function and Pathology. 2nd ed. Philadelphia, Lea and Febiger, 1988, pp. 6, 7, 11.)

slightly large grayish red cell that contains no nucleus but still has some residual reticular material in its cytoplasm. The existence of this material can be demonstrated by a special stain. It usually disappears during the red blood cell's first day in the peripheral blood. These cells normally spend 75% of their time in the bone marrow and are released for their final day into the peripheral blood. When the bone marrow production is Normal, any decrease in the red cell count will lead to a compensatory increase in the bone marrow's production rate. There is normally an inverse relationship of these two parameters. Thus, if a patient develops a severe anemia with a drop in hematocrit to 15, the bone marrow production rate increases to within 3 to 5 times normal; and this is indicated by a reticulocyte index of approximately 3 to 5. If, on the other hand, there is a specific bone marrow defect (such as iron deficiency, folic acid deficiency, $B_{12}$ deficiency, or the anemia of chronic disorders), the reticulocyte index will not increase appropriately in response to anemia. This proportional relationship forms a major and very important basis for the classification of anemias, which is depicted in Figure 35–2 and Table 35–1.

## *Erythrocytosis*

Erythrocytosis means an increased number of red cells above normal. This can occur either as a manifestation of polycythemia vera or as a physiologic response to increased erythropoietin.

Usually, patients with polycythemia vera have an associated thrombocytosis and leukocytosis, as well as splenomegaly. Should patients not present with the classical signs and symptoms of polycythemia vera, other tests can be done to confirm its presence.

Erythrocytosis secondary to increased erythropoietin can occur from a variety of causes. There is also an apparent erythrocytosis, which, in fact, is due to a decrease in plasma volume. This can be related to hypertension,

## Comments/Group

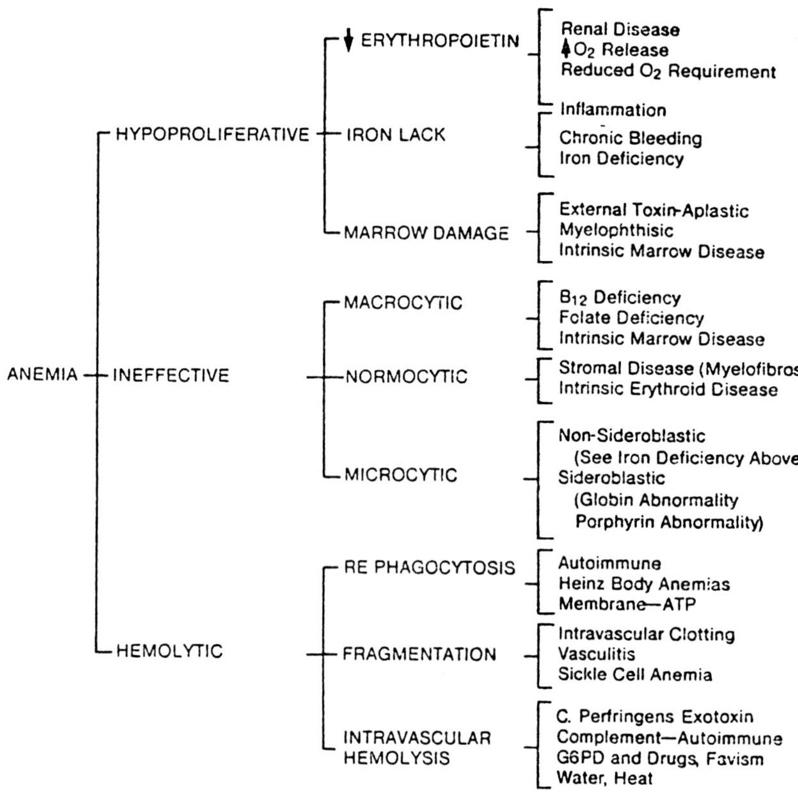


**Fig. 35–2.** A pathophysiologic approach to anemia. (With permission from Hillman, RS and Finch, CA: Red Cell Manual. 6th ed. Philadelphia, FA Davis Company, 1992, pp. 6–7.)

**Table 35–1.** Key Laboratory Tests in Some Common Anemias

| Anemia Type | Class^ | RI | MCV | MCH | Fe/TIBC | % Fe Saturation | Other |
|---|---|---|---|---|---|---|---|
| Aplastic/Hypoplastic | Hypoproliferative | ↓ | N or ↑ | N | N | N | Hypoplastic or aplastic marrow |
| Myelophthisic | Hypoproliferative | ↓ | N | N | Variable | Variable | BM invasion with tumor fibrosis<br>Teardrops, NRBC in smear |
| Chronic inflammation | Hypoproliferative | ↓ | N | N or Sl ↓ | ↓/↓ | N or Sl ↓ | ↑ RE iron stores<br>↓ Sideroblasts |
| Iron deficiency | Hypoproliferative +<br>Cytoplasmic maturation defect | ↓<br>↓ | ↓ | ↓ | ↓/↑ | <10% | ↓ RE iron stores<br>↓ Sideroblasts |
| Megaloblastic anemias | Nuclear maturation defect | ↓ | ↑ | N | ↑/↑ | ↑ ↑ | Megaloblasts in BM |
| Hemolytic anemias (uncomplicated) | Hemolysis | ↑ | N or ↑ * | N | Variable | Variable | May be normocytic or show characteristic abnormalities on blood smear<br>Unconjugated hyperbilirubinemia |
| Uncomplicated acute blood loss | Blood loss | ↑ | N or ↑ * | N | N | N | |
| Combined anemias | Variable | | | | | | |

^: Pathophysiologic
BM: Bone marrow
RE: Reticulo-endothelial
NRBC: Nucleated red blood cells
Sl: Slight
MCH: Mean cell hemoglobin
N: Normal
*: With marked reticulocytosis.
RI: Retic Index
MCV: Mean cell volume
Fe/TIBC: Iron/total iron binding capacity

stress, and certain medications. Performing a red cell mass will help delineate true erythrocytosis whether it is due to increased erythropoietin or polycythemia vera. It is essential for any patient with this problem to be evaluated before any obstetric procedures, if at all possible.

### Anemias

As outlined above, anemias can be classified on the basis of whether or not the bone marrow is responding normally to the degree of anemia. Patients who have blood loss or increased loss by hemolysis will have a reticulocyte index that is greater than 3. Patients who have some form of production problem—either hypoproliferation or ineffective erythropoiesis—will have a reticulocyte index that is usually 1 or less. The significant factor in this latter case is that the reticulocyte index is lower than would be expected from a normal marrow response to the degree of anemia.

The second major clue to evaluating a patient with anemia is the red cell size. Patients who have true hypoproliferative anemias such as aplastic anemia or the anemia of chronic renal disease will have normal-sized red cells that have the normal amount of hemoglobin in them. Patients who have disorders of iron metabolism—usually iron deficiency anemia, the anemia of chronic disease, or possibly thalassemia—will show small cells that have less than the normal amount of hemoglobin in them. The other major class of ineffective erythropoiesis is megaloblastic anemia, in which nuclear DNA synthesis is impaired, typically, by folate or $B_{12}$ deficiency. These patients with megaloblastic anemia again have a low reticulocyte index and large, oval to round red blood cells.

In some instances of hemolytic anemia, characteristic red cell shapes such as spherocytes, targets, schistocytes, helmet cells, or echinocytes will be seen. In each instance, characteristic cell shapes give a clue to the type of hemolytic process that is going on in the patient.

Other patients with hemolysis have no blood cell abnormalities on the peripheral blood smear, and the reason for suspecting their hemolysis is anemia in the face of an increased reticulocyte index. Usually, very special tests are required to identify this form of hemolysis.

Special mention must be made of glucose-6-phosphate dehydrogenase (G6PD) deficiency. It is an inherited biochemical defect that interferes with the patient's normal metabolism of glucose. The result is a condition in which hemolysis can occur de novo or as a result of exposure to certain oxidant drugs such as sulfa, phenacetin, and the like. In some cases, this hemolysis can be brisk, massive, and intravascular and can result in a life-threatening event. Its existence should be clearly established and worked up before any obstetric procedures.

Finally, there is a large number of refractory anemias which, while rare, require characterization and diagnosis as soon as they are detected. Aplastic anemias certainly fall within this category, as do the variety of refractory anemias that are characterized by myelodysplasia and some myeloproliferative syndromes. It is essential that such anemias be identified so that no unwarranted treatment is given to the patient.

## The Granulocyte-Macrophage System

### Normal Function, Proliferation, and Maturation

Granulocytes and macrophages phagocytose a variety of infectious and noninfectious material and either destroy, degrade, or store them. Granulocytes are produced in the marrow, as is noted in Figure 35–1, and require several growth factors for their maturation. They circulate in the blood for a relatively short time (less than 24 hours) before they migrate into the tissue to perform the phagocytic function. While in the blood, half of the granulocytes circulate while the other half stick to the inner margins of the capillaries. The former is referred to as the circulating pool and is equivalent to the resting granulocyte count. The latter is referred to as the marginal pool and is not part of the white count unless some specific stimulus causes this pool to demarginate. The main function of the marginal pool is to provide quick egress to tissue in response to specific inflammatory or other stimuli. When in the tissue, granulocytes' prime function is the ingestion of specific infectious, inflammatory, or degraded material, which they further destroy.

The monocyte-macrophage system is a bit more complex. These cells are related to the granulocytic or myeloid system and are produced in bone marrow. However, the monocytes seen in the peripheral blood are still immature cells. These must migrate from the blood where they then mature to become adult macrophages. They can now perform their functions as components of specific organs such as the lungs and liver. The circulating form in the blood does egress to tissue where it can phagocytose a wide range of materials and perform a wide variety of other functions (Figure 35–3). The monocyte-macrophage system is also responsible for antigen processing, and the system is also responsible for producing a wide variety of biologically active substances, including growth factors, hemostatic factors, and many other substances as shown in Figure 35–3.

### Disorders

There is no really good general schematic approach for dealing with granulocyte and macrophage problems. This is due, in part, to the absence of any parameter with the same value as the reticulocyte index. Therefore, disorders will be covered in terms of either too many or too few cells or cells that have lost their functional abilities.

Neutrophilia is the term given when one has too many granulocytes circulating in the peripheral blood. The causes of neutrophilia can generally be attributed to neoplastic and non-neoplastic or functional causes. In terms of the latter, infections, inflammations, anoxia, and severe stress to the body can all cause neutrophilia. When such is seen, there is usually an outpouring of somewhat younger neutrophils into the peripheral blood. This outpouring is a "shift to the left," and the cells are referred to as bands because the nuclei have no segments. Basophilic granulation can also be associated with this outpouring of younger neutrophils, and when one finds this clinically, it is imperative to look very hard for infection.

There are two major causes of neoplastic proliferation

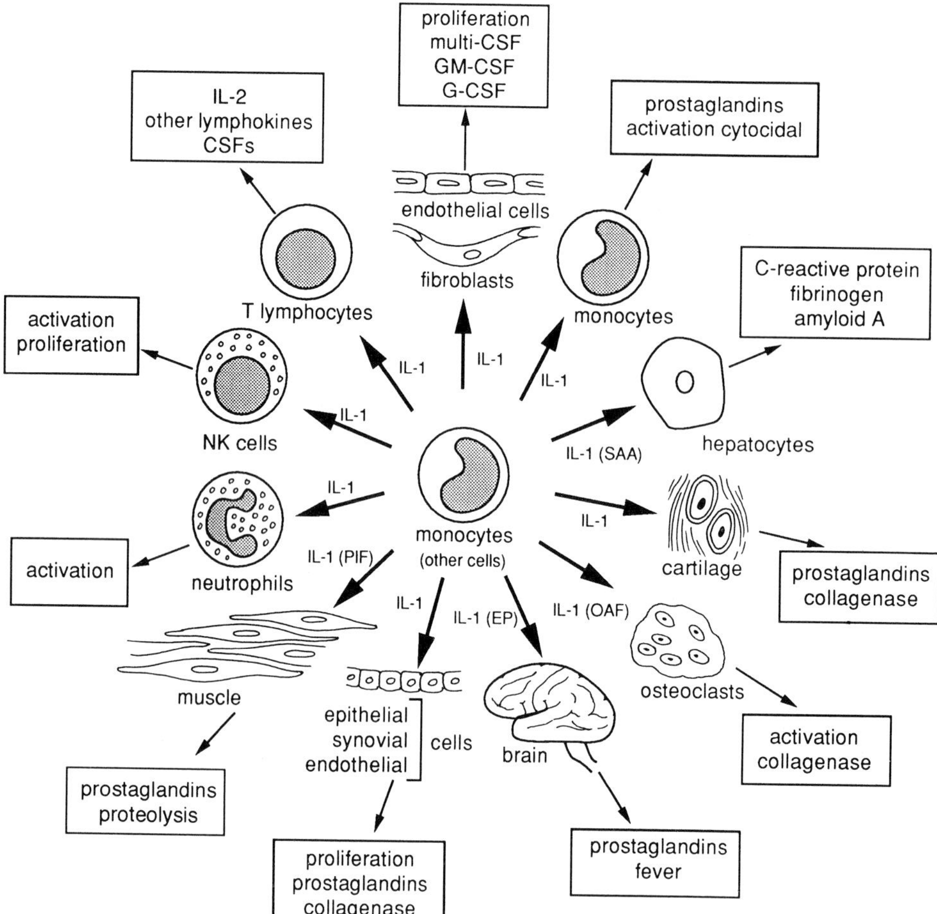


**Fig. 35–3.** One of the functions of the monocyte macrophage system is the production of interleukin-1. This, in turn, has a variety of important physiological effects. (With permission from Hoffbrand AV, Pettit E: Sandoz Atlas—Clinical Hematology. New York, Gower Medical Publishing, 1988, p. 6.)

of myeloid cells. Chronic granulocytic leukemia and acute nonlymphoblastic leukemia are often associated with increases in either mature or immature cells of the myeloid series. Chronic granulocytic leukemia has a more mature distribution of cells though a few very immature myeloblasts may be seen. Basophils and eosinophils are also commonly found. Acute myeloblastic leukemia is characterized by a monotonous collection of very young myeloid cells (usually myeloblasts, promyelocytes, or monoblasts) and is also associated with severe anemia and decreased platelet count.

The management of these diseases has undergone tremendous change in the last decade and cure is now being reported in over 50 to 70% of some selected series. Therefore, it is important to realize that patients with these problems must no longer be regarded as being in a hopeless situation.

Neutropenia refers to a decrease in the number of circulating granulocytes. This can again be the response to an overwhelming infection in which all of the granulocyte reserves are used up, to hematologic or nonhematologic malignancies involving the marrow, to sequestration in an enlarged spleen, to immunologic destruction, and to drug and viral causes. In this situation in which reserves are depleted, it is very important to determine whether or not other cell lines are involved. If they are, this could mitigate somewhat against either an infectious or a drug cause. Obviously, neutropenia can often be seen when patients are on chemotherapy for some form of malignancy, and in this situation, both their granulocytic function and lymphoid function are compromised. Chemotherapy patients require special care because of their increased susceptibility to a wide range of infections.

Monocytosis is the term used to designate too many monocytes in the peripheral blood, and this can be seen in a variety of infections, including tuberculosis. Monocytosis can also be seen in an unusual form of chronic leukemia as well as lymphomas and other neoplasms. There is also a variety of proliferative disorders caused by specific enzyme defects that lead to an increased number of macrophages—full of specific degradation products that cannot proceed through normal enzymatic processes—being deposited in various body organs. Finally, when one is evaluating a patient with monocytosis, it is always a good idea to make sure they have not had a splenectomy.

In terms of other neoplastic disorders, the acute nonlymphocytic leukemias have several subtypes whose blasts have the appearance of monoblasts or promonocytes. That which is observed for the myeloid abnormalities is observed for these diseases.

### The Lymphoid System

#### Normal Lymphopoiesis and Function

The two major lymphocyte families (T cells and B cells) are collectively responsible for the body's normal and abnormal immunologic responses. T cells, whose proliferation and maturation are shown in Figure 35–1, are responsible for cellular immunity and are also involved in many regulatory steps, which are important for the humoral immune function. There are several major families of T cells. Some actually kill specific organisms or cells. Others help immunologic reactions of the B cells to proceed. Still others suppress such reactions, and a final, large group of T cells are in a more generalized state in which they replicate a variety of their successors or predecessors. T cells also are important for the production of a variety of biologically active lymphokines.

Both B cells and T cells have primary and secondary lymphopoiesis. Primary lymphopoiesis refers to the first stages of proliferation and division of the cells; it precedes and is independent of any specific antigenic stimulation. Secondary lymphopoiesis begins when the cell is exposed to an antigen, becomes an active lymphocyte, and then differentiates into a specific cell with a specific series of functions or function.

B cells are responsible for antigen-antibody immunity, and the terminal cell of differentiation here is the plasma cell. Active B cells and plasma cells are capable of making immunoglobulin and have been preprogrammed during primary lymphopoiesis to respond to only one or a very few antigens of the millions to which they are exposed.

#### Disorders

Lymphocytosis can be either reactive or neoplastic and can reflect either a normal distribution of T and B cells and their subtypes or a monoclonal proliferation. Distribution or proliferation is easily distinguishable with currently available laboratory tests. Monoclonal lymphocytosis include such disorders as chronic B cell leukemia, lymphomas and acute lymphoblastic leukemias (B cell line), as well as chronic T cell leukemias, acute T cell leukemias, hairy cell leukemias, and Sezary syndrome. Reactive lymphocytoses can be seen in conditions such as whooping cough and infectious mononucleosis. Lymphocytopenia can again be a reflection of some infiltrative process that obliterates normal lymphocyte proliferation and maturation. It can also be seen on an immunologic basis, as well as being the result of certain specific lymphoid infections such as AIDS. With such lymphopenias, corresponding defects in immune functions occur and the patient again is unduly susceptible to a wide variety of infections from agents that are not usually pathogenic. In terms of functional disorders, when the finely tuned inter-reactions between T and B cells are disrupted, it is possible for autoantibodies or other antibodies to be produced against the patient's cells. In this situation, immune thrombocytopenia, immune hemolytic anemias, and immune neutropenias can be seen as a result of defective lymphoid function. Also, patients who receive chemotherapeutic agents have varying suppressions of their lymphoid function—largely depending upon the aggressiveness of the chemotherapy regimen used. In this situation, opportunistic infections are very common and again require specialized consultation and management.

## HEMOSTASIS

### Normal Hemostasis

The normal hemostatic process is a combination of vascular and platelet factors, which form a primary plug, and coagulation factors, which are involved in the formation of the final fibrin plug. At the same time, there is an active series of fibrinolytic and other anticoagulant activities going on, so that thrombus formation and dissolution are a finely tuned and balanced homeostatic series of mechanisms. The blood vessels supply an intact endothelial surface that—as long as it is not damaged—facilitates the smooth passage of blood in its fluid form. When vascular damage occurs, a variety of subendothelial tissues and released substances is responsible for the accumulation of platelets in the area of injury. The platelets, which have developed from megakaryocytes as shown in Figure 35–1, have a variety of functions, most of which are directed toward the formation of the primary plug:

1. Platelet shape change.
2. Platelet cohesion or aggregation.
3. Generation of lipid products both amplifying and dampening activations
4. Secretion of platelet granular contents.
5. Reorganization of the platelet membrane making phosphatidylserine available to interact with clotting factors and allowing clotting factors to bind to and generate thrombin on the platelet surface.
6. An oriented centripetal contraction of actomyosin that compacts the aggregated platelets and so consolidates the platelet hemostatic plug.

At this point, the formation of a thrombus begins and becomes facilitated by the intrinsic and extrinsic pathways of the coagulation cascade. These various reactions are shown in Figures 35–4, 35–5, and 35–6. Also shown are some details about the coagulation factors, including the extrinsic, intrinsic, and final common pathways. The relationship to the fibrinolytic system is also depicted. The initial laboratory evaluation for hemostasis is shown in Table 35–2.

### Abnormalities

Abnormal hemostasis can be divided into abnormal bleeding and abnormal thrombosis. Abnormal bleeding can occur when any of the three major factors outlined above is inoperative. Vascular abnormalities—either hereditary or acquired—can cause vascular purpura (Table 35–3). Classical examples of this are hereditary hemorrhagic telangiectasia, scurvy, senile purpura, or poor support of ground substance surrounding vessels. A variety of problems can involve the platelets (Table 35–4). Patients can have thrombocytopenia, which can be caused by impaired thrombopoiesis, sequestration of platelets in

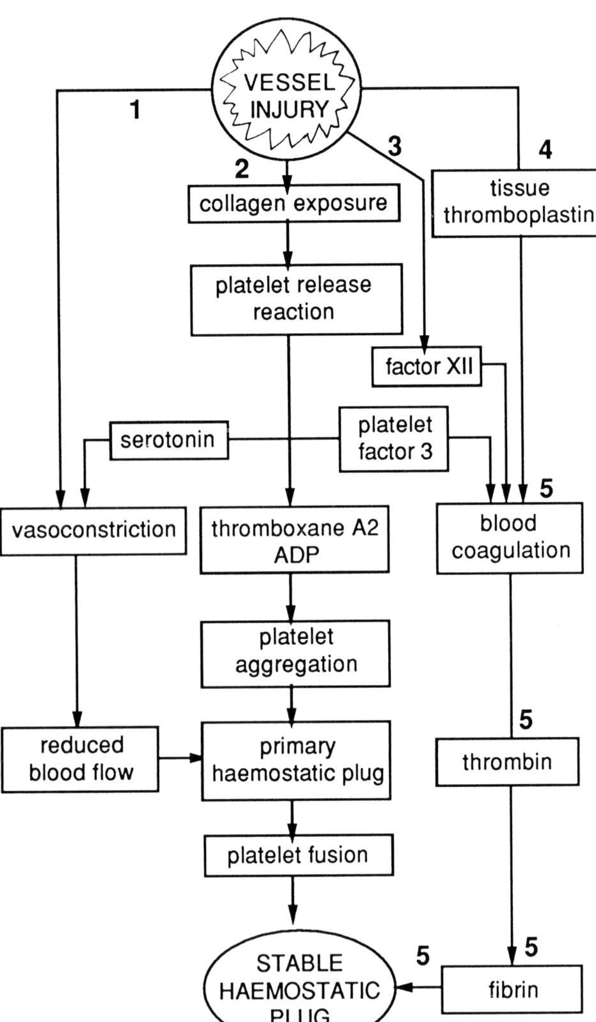


**Fig. 35–4.** A simplified diagram of normal haemostasis. Vascular factors (1) and platelet factors (2) contribute to primary haemostasis plug formation. Platelets and vascular and coagulation factors (3, 4, 5) contribute to the formation of a stable fibrin haemostatic plug. 3 = intrinsic pathway; 4 = extrinsic pathway, 5 = final common pathway. (Adapted from Hoffbrand AV, Pettit E: Sandoz Atlas—Clinical Hematology. New York, Gower Medical Publishing, 1988, p. 228.)

an enlarged spleen, or increased destruction of platelets. A large variety of drugs and infections can be responsible for impaired thrombopoiesis, as can the myelodysplastic and myeloproliferative syndromes referred to above. Certain infections and toxins can cause this problem as well.

Increased platelet destruction can be caused by a variety of infections, intravascular coagulation, or immune destruction of platelets. Immune destruction of platelets (ITP) itself can have a variety of causes, including autoimmune diseases and as an autoimmune response to the AIDS virus. One of the most frequently encountered hemolytic disorders in pregnancy is ITP; its association with primary separation of the placenta and complications

**Table 35–2.** Initial Laboratory Tests for Evaluation of Hemostatis

| Test | Evaluates |
|---|---|
| Platelet count and bleeding time | Vascular and platelet factors |
| Partial thromboplastin time and thrombin time | Intrinsic system |
| Prothrombin time and thrombin time | Extrinsic system |
| Thrombin time and fibrinogen | Final common path |

thereafter associated with the second and third trimesters, is often a major threat to mother and fetus (4).

Platelet functional impairments (Table 35–5) can be seen in a variety of hereditary conditions, of which von Willebrand's disease is the most common example. Patients can also have impairments of platelet function secondary to a variety of drugs, of which the classic example is aspirin. However, aspirin is not by any means the only drug that can impair platelet function (Table 35–4).

Coagulation factor deficiencies or inactivations can also lead to purpura and these are often times hereditary. The test result profiles of various hereditary syndromes are summarized in Table 35–6; those for acquired syndromes are summarized in Table 35–7. And, finally, a variety of conditions can be manifest by combined defects. von Willebrand's is a defect of factor VIII as well as platelet function; disseminated intravascular clotting again involves a wide variety of vascular, platelet, and clotting factor abnormalities, and can involve a vitamin K deficiency as well. The management of these disorders can be a very frustrating experience to even the most expert hematologist. The key to management is obviously clearly delineating the problem before trying to find the solution.

**Table 35–3.** Vascular Bleeding Disorders

Hereditary
- Hereditary hemorrhagic telangiectasia
- Ehlers-Danlos syndrome
- Marfan's syndrome
- Osteogenesis imperfecta
- Fabry's syndrome

Acquired
- Infections
  - Bacteial
  - Viral
  - Rickettsial
- Allergic
  - Henoch-Schönlein syndrome
  - Drugs
  - Food
- Atrophic
  - Senile purpura
  - Cushing's syndrome and steroid therapy
  - Scurvy purpura
  - Dysproteinemia
  - Amyloid
- Miscellaneous
  - Simple easy bruising
  - Factitious
  - Autoerythrocyte sensitization
  - Fat embolism

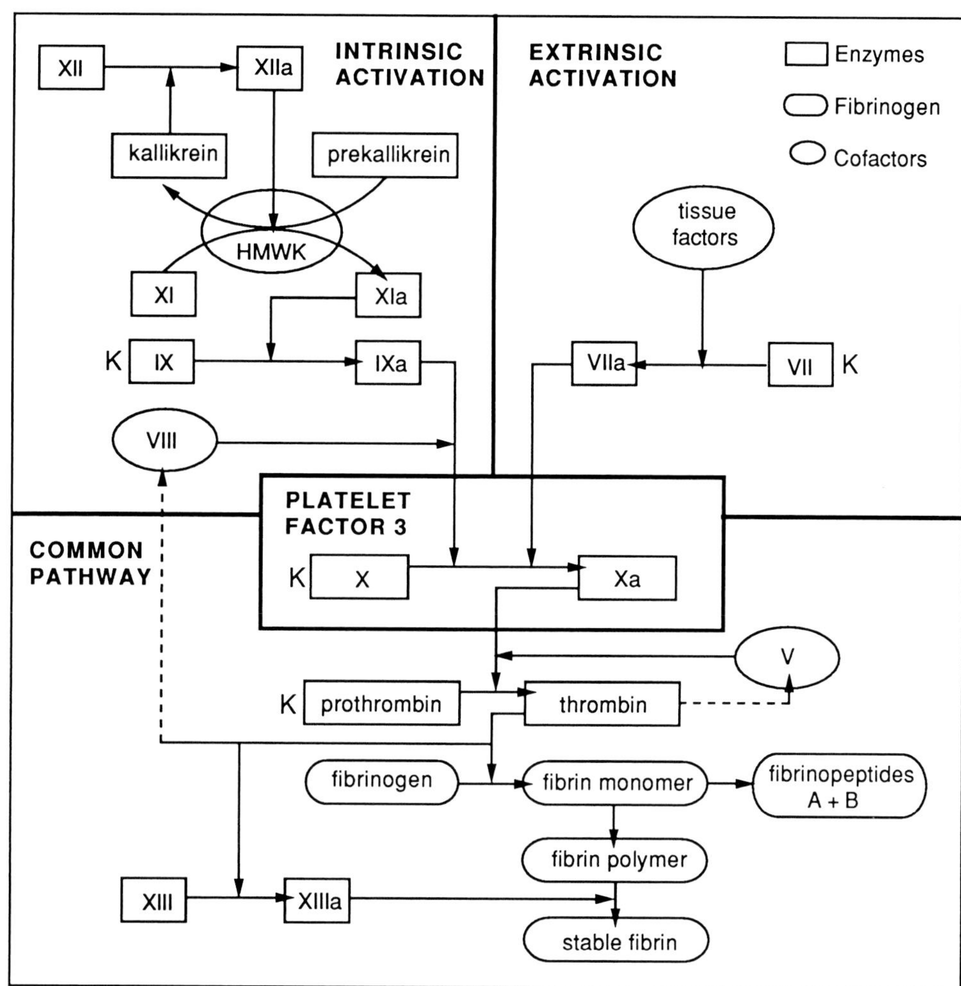


Fig. 35–5. A simplified diagram of blood coagulation. HWMK = high molecular weight kininogens; A = activated factor; K = vitamin K dependent factor. (With permission from Hoffbrand AV, Pettit E: Sandoz Atlas—Clinical Hematology. New York, Gower Medical Publishing, 1988, pp. 240, 247.)

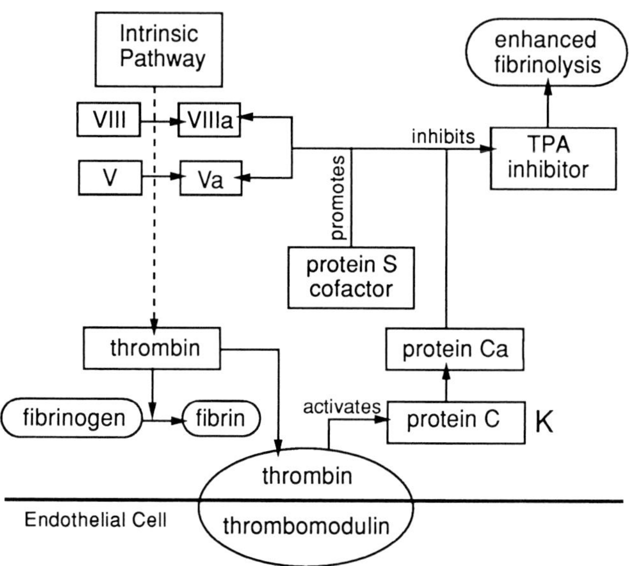


**Fig. 35–6.** A simplified diagram of fibinolysis. K = vitamin K dependent factor. (With permission from Hoffbrand AV, Pettit E: Sandoz Atlas—Clinical Hematology. New York, Gower Medical Publishing, 1988, pp. 240, 247.)

### *Thrombosis*

A variety of causes can be responsible deep venous thrombosis. Some of these include specific deficiencies that lead to hypercoagulable states such as Antithrombin 3 deficiency, Protein C and Protein S deficiency, and some lupus anticogulants. However, many patients with normal parameters in the above areas also have hypercoagulability, which is as yet unexplainable.

The basic management of thrombotic problems in pregnancy is outlined in the following section.

## PHYSIOLOGICAL CHANGES DURING PREGNANCY

### *Plasma and Red Cells*

Profound hematological changes occur during pregnancy that are both qualitative and quantitative. There is a progressive increase in blood volume that reflects changes not only in plasma volume, but also in the total volume of red cells, or red cell mass (4). The increase in plasma volume begins halfway through the first trimester and reaches a maximum at the end of the second trimester. By comparison, the increase in the red cell mass begins at the end of the first trimester and continues until term. The average increase is about 20% above the non-

**Table 35–4.** Causes of Thrombocytopenia

Failure of platelet production
- Generalized bone marrow failure
  - Leukemia
  - Myelodysplasia
  - Aplastic anemia
  - Myelofibrosis
  - Megaloblastic anemia
  - Uremia
  - Multiple myeloma
  - Marrow infiltration, eg carcinoma, lymphoma
- Selective megakaryocyte depression
  - Drugs
  - Alcohol
  - Chemicals
  - Viral infections
- Hereditary thrombocytopenias
  - May-Hegglin syndrome
  - Wiskott-Aldrich syndrome
  - Bernard-Soulier syndrome
  - Others

Abnormal distribution of platelets
- Splenomegaly

Increased destruction of platelets
- Immune
  - Alloantibodies
    - Neonatal
    - Post-transfusion
  - Autoantibodies
    - Primary
    - Secondary, e.g., systemic lupus erythematosus, chronic lymphocytic leukemia, post-infection, AIDS, post-bone marrow transplantation
- Drug-induced
  - Immune
  - Due to platelet aggregation
- Disseminated intravascular coagulation
  - Microangiopathic processes
    - Hemolytic-uremic syndrome
    - Thrombotic thrombocytopenic purpura
    - Extracorporeal circulation
  - Giant hemoangioma (Kasabach-Merritt syndrome)

Dilutional loss
- Massive transfusion of stored blood

**Table 35–5.** Disorders of Platelet Function

Inherited
- Plasma membrane defects
  - Thromboasthenia
  - Bernard-Soulier syndrome
  - PF3 deficiency
- Storage organelle deficiency
  - Dense body deficiency
    - Idiopathic storage pool disease
    - Hermansky-Pudlak, Wiskott-Aldrich, and Chdiak-Higashi syndromes
  - α-granule deficiency
    - Gray platelet syndrome
- Cyclooxygenase & thromboxane synthetase deficiencies
- von Willebrand's disease

Acquired
- Myeloproliferative disorders
- Myelodysplastic syndromes
- Acute myeloblastic leukemia
- Dysproteinemias
- Uremia
- Acquired storage pool deficiency
  - Disseminated intravascular coagulation
  - Hemolytic-uremic syndrome
  - Thrombotic thrombocytopenic purpura
  - Disseminated autoimmune disease
- Acquired von Willebrand's disease

Drugs, e.g., aspirin, dipyridamole, sulphinpyrazone, prostacylin, carbenicillin, imipramine, nonsteroidal anti-inflammatory.

pregnant state, but may reach 40% if iron supplements are taken. Proportionally, the increase in red cell mass is less than the increase in plasma volume, which averages 50%. This change in volume is proportional to the weight of the fetus and is larger with multiple pregnancies. As a result, there is a progressive decrease in the hemoglobin concentration during pregnancy until the increase in the plasma volume reaches a plateau. The influence that this phenomenon has on the hemoglobin cutoff values for the diagnosis of anemia during pregnancy can be seen in Table 35–8. A detailed discussion of this phenomenon can be found in Chapter 2.

Along with changes in red cell mass, there are more subtle changes that influence the erythrocytes of pregnant women. For example, osmotic fragility is increased and the cells tend to adopt a more spherocytic shape.

## White Cell Count

The total white cell count begins to rise early in pregnancy (5). The upper values for normal pregnant women have been reported as 9.9, 11.4, and 12.2 leukocytes/μl for each trimester. Most of the increase is accounted for by a doubling of the number of mature neutrophils. Increased concentrations of circulating cortisol and estrogen have been invoked to account for the leukocytosis.

## Platelets

While there is a progressive fall in the platelet count during pregnancy, frankly, thrombocytopenic levels are not reached (5). Mean values (± 1 standard deviation) for the first, second, and third trimester are, respectively,

**Table 35–6.** Hemostasis Tests in Hereditary Coagulation Disorders

| Test | Disease | | |
|---|---|---|---|
| | Hemophilia A | Hemophilia B | von Willebrand's Disease |
| Bleeding time | normal | normal | prolonged |
| Prothrombin time | normal | normal | normal |
| Activated partial thromboplastin time | prolonged | prolonged | prolonged |
| Thrombin clotting time | normal | normal | normal |
| Factor VIII | low | normal | low or normal |
| vWF | normal | normal | low |
| vwf:RiCof* | nomal | normal | low |
| Factor IX | normal | low | normal |

RiCof = Ristocetin cofactor activity

**Table 35–7.** Hemostasis Tests in Acquired Bleeding Disorders

| | Platelet Count | Prothrombin Time | Activated Partial Thromboplastin Time | Thrombin Time |
|---|---|---|---|---|
| Liver disease | low | prolonged | prolonged | normal* |
| Disseminated intravascular coagulation | low | prolonged | prolonged | grossly prolonged |
| Massive transfusion | low | prolonged | prolonged | prolonged |
| Heparin | normal** | mildly prolonged | prolonged | prolonged |
| Circulating anticoagulant | normal | normal or prolonged | prolonged | normal |

* rarely prolonged
** rarely low

$322 \pm 75$, $298 \pm 55$, and $278 \pm 75/\mu l$. This phenomenon occurs as a result of a number of contributing events, which include the dilutional effect of the increased plasma volume, shortened platelet survival, and increased platelet use in the expanded maternal intravascular compartment. These quantitative changes may be accompanied by qualitative changes, which include increased aggregation both in vivo and in response to known agonists.

### *Coagulation Factors*

During pregnancy, a number of the homeostatic mechanisms that determine the steady state between coagulation and fibrinolysis are reset in favor of modest hypercoagulability (6). This effect is, in part, a result of an increase in the concentration of clotting factors. While the increase may be 50% above the nonpregnant level for factors V, VII, VIII, and X, fibrinogen concentrations may increase dramatically. Mean values for the protein are 5.8 g/l at term compared to 3.6 for the nonpregnant female. Except for a short-lived decrease in the concentration of coagulation factors at delivery, the increase persists for at least 2 weeks during the postpartum period, returning to normal at about 1 month. Factors XI and XIII decrease in pregnancy.

Hypercoagulability in pregnancy is also a reflection of changes in protein S, Plasminogen, and antithrombin III. Protein S, a naturally occurring anticoagulant that is a cofactor for an inhibitor of activated factors V and VIII, is decreased in concentration during pregnancy and the postpartum period (7). Plasminogen, a proenzyme that binds to fibrin as an early step in the fibrinolytic process, is decreased in concentration at the same time an inhibitor, tissue plasminogen activator, is increased (8). Both of these events contribute to hypercoagulability. While antithrombin III concentration is unchanged or only slightly decreased in pregnancy, the level of this coagulation inhibitor declines much more precipitously in the pregnant woman, by comparison with her nonpregnant counterpart, after mild infection (9).

**Table 35–8.** Hemoglobin Concentrations for the Diagnosis of Anemia in Pregnancy*

| | Gestation (weeks) | | | | | | | |
|---|---|---|---|---|---|---|---|---|
| | 12 | 16 | 20 | 24 | 28 | 32 | 36 | 40 |
| Mean Hg (g/dL) | 12.2 | 11.8 | 11.6 | 11.6 | 11.8 | 12.1 | 12.5 | 12.9 |
| 5th percentile Hg values (g/dL) | 11.0 | 10.6 | 10.5 | 10.5 | 10.7 | 11.0 | 11.4 | 11.9 |

* (Data from Morbidity and Mortality Weekly Report June 9, 1989)

## Nutritional Considerations

### *Iron Balance*

The additional iron requirements that face the adult female are further increased during pregnancy, despite the reduction in iron loss that accompanies amenorrhea (10). Table 35–9 shows how the total iron requirements of about 1 g for an entire pregnancy are accumulated. For the woman who starts her pregnancy without any iron stores, a not uncommon event in the multiparous patient, daily iron requirements increase from 1.5 mg/day to 4 mg/day. This increased demand for iron is not spread evenly during gestation. The additional needs begin during the second trimester and reach a peak at the end of the third trimester. Iron requirements during the first trimester may actually be less than requirements in the nonpregnant woman because of the amenorrhea.

There is no doubt that iron supplements in pregnancy are effective in treating patients with iron deficiency anemia and in bolstering iron stores in women who start their pregnancies with storage-iron depletion. However, despite the substantial iron demand of pregnancy, routine supplementation of the diet with iron is difficult to justify (11,12). While women who are iron deficient at their first prenatal visit are obviously candidates for iron supplementation, it has proven very difficult to show that nutri-

**Table 35–9.** Iron Requirements of Pregnancy

| Source of Iron Loss | Mg Lost |
|---|---|
| "Obligatory" iron loss | $180 \pm 20$ |
| Increased red cell mass | $400 \pm 200$ |
| Fetal iron | $270 \pm 70$ |
| Placenta and cord | $100 \pm 70$ |
| Blood loss at delivery | $150 \pm 100$ |
| Total requirements | $1100 \pm 460$ |

tional supplements have any benefits for the well-nourished mother or her fetus.

Some physicians compromise and provide iron supplementation only during the second and third trimester, when iron requirements increase (13). Other physicians select only women with multiple pregnancies or those from a poor socioeconomic background. A conventional dose of iron is 30 to 60 mg/day. Providing iron tablets for the second or third trimesters only may encourage patient compliance, as gastrointestinal distress, the most common side-effect of iron tablets, is likely to be particularly intolerable during the first trimester.

In the fetus, the accumulation of hemoglobin and storage iron is rapid (14). Studies that show an inverse relationship between cord serum ferritin and hemoglobin concentration suggest that the amount of iron in fetal stores is influenced by the amount required for hemoglobin production. In mothers who have mild iron deficiency anemia, there is little or no effect on the concentration of hemoglobin in the fetus of newborns (15). However, when the mother has severe iron deficiency anemia during her pregnancy, the hemoglobin concentration in the newborn can be substantially decreased, though to a lesser degree than in the mother (16).

### *Folate and Vitamin $B_{12}$*

The daily requirements of folate during pregnancy are between 150 and 300 μg. This is a threefold increase over the daily requirement for the nonpregnant woman (17). Frequent childbirth and multiple pregnancy place additional demands on folate nutrition. These demands cannot be met by drawing on folate stores. Storage is limited and the liver reserve of folate, in the well-nourished woman, lasts only for about 4 weeks. Folate metabolism may be particularly precarious in pregnant women with a history of alcohol abuse. In addition, there is some evidence, albeit controversial, that suggests that women who have relied on oral contraceptive agents in the past are at risk of folate deficiency because of impaired absorption of the nutrient.

Even with a normal dietary folate intake, about 25% of pregnant women will have evidence of folate deficient erythropoiesis. Against this background, folate supplementation is routinely recommended at doses varying between 500 μg/day and 1 mg/day (18).

When folate deficiency leads to anemia, the disorder is often diagnosed in the third trimester or early in the postpartum period. At this time, there are increased folate requirements for lactation and for the enhanced erythropoiesis stimulated by maternal blood loss at birth.

Vitamin $B_{12}$ deficiency is a rare cause of anemia in the nonpregnant woman and rarer still during pregnancy because of the association between lack of the vitamin and infertility. An index of suspicion is aroused, however, when anemia occurs in pregnant women with a history of malabsorption (19). Strict vegetarians also run the risk of vitamin $B_{12}$ deficiency, but anemia may take many years of dietary restriction to develop. By comparison with folate, liver stores are normally robust and can provide for the daily $B_{12}$ requirement of 3 μg during pregnancy for 6 months to 1 year. Vitamin $B_{12}$ supplementation of the diet is indicated only for strict vegetarians who refuse any animal-derived food products.

With regard to implications for the fetus, adequate erythropoiesis is usually sustained despite maternal folate deficiency and anemia. This is not true for vitamin $B_{12}$. Fetal stores of the vitamin are decreased in step with maternal vitamin $B_{12}$ deficiency. Infants that are breast fed by vitamin $B_{12}$-deficient mothers run the risk of a $B_{12}$-deficiency syndrome between the ages of 4 months and 1 year. This syndrome is marked by anemia, changes in skin pigmentation, and developmental abnormalities.

## The Diagnosis of Anemia in Pregnancy

Anemia in pregnancy is so frequently due to iron deficiency that the attending physician is inclined to forget that the pregnant patient is heir to all the anemias that can be found in the nonpregnant state. For this reason, it is worth recalling the logical sequence of events that can be called upon to establish any cause for anemia (20).

Once it has been established that the patient's hemoglobin level is below the concentration shown in Table 35–8, the key investigation is the reticulocyte count. Depending on whether the count is appropriate or inappropriate to the anemia, there is a broad classification into two groups, namely, proliferative and hypoproliferative. While no classification of anemias is entirely satisfactory, Figure 35–7 attempts to combine two of the most common approaches, namely, morphological and pathophysiological. Difficulties arise when anemias have more than one component or when different mechanisms come into play as the anemia evolves. For example, red cell morphology may be unremarkable in the pregnant woman who has both folic acid deficiency and iron deficiency.

With regard to hypoproliferative anemias, the red cell indices are used to subdivide the anemias according to the mean cell volume as microcytic (mean cell volume under 76 fl), normocytic (mean cell volume 76 to 96 fl), or macrocytic (mean cell volume over 96 fl).

The most common microcytic anemia is due to iron deficiency. Table 35–10 lists the laboratory findings that confirm the diagnosis. While abnormalities of the values shown usually reflect a disparity between the amount of available dietary iron and the iron demands of the pregnancy, a relative iron deficiency can occur as a result of chronic infection. Under these circumstances, iron is not released from the reticuloendothelial system and, as a result, is unavailable for erythropoiesis. Patients whose anemia is on this basis tend to have a less significantly depressed saturation of their circulating transferrin and a serum ferritin level higher than it is in storage-iron depletion. In addition, the red cells tend to be normocytic and, quite often, the clinical features of the disorder that ac-

**Table 35–10.** Diagnosis of Iron Deficiency

(1) Plasma iron < 30 μg/dl.
(2) Transferrin saturation < 15%.
(3) Ferritin < 12 ng/ml.
(4) Red blood cell protroporphyrin elevated.

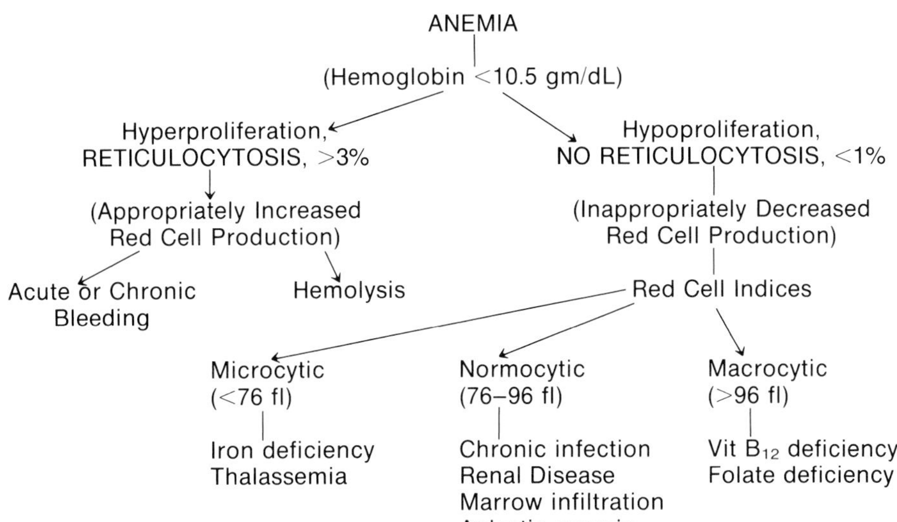


**Fig. 35–7.** Evaluation and classification of anemia in pregnancy.

count for the chronic inflammation are prominent, such as rheumatoid arthritis or lupus erythematosus. Other conditions that are associated with normocytic anemias include malignancies with or without infiltration of the marrow, chronic renal disease, and endocrinopathies such as hypothyroidism and hypogonadism. While a number of these diseases are obviously inconsistent with conception or sustained pregnancy, some primarily hematological malignancies that include features of normocytic anemia can, rarely, present in the obstetric patient, including leukemia, aplastic anemia, and myelofibrosis.

Macrocytic anemia is most often encountered in vitamin $B_{12}$ and folic acid deficiency but may be seen also in chronic liver disease and hemolytic states. Hemolysis is associated with macrocytosis because the reticulocyte, whose increased presence points to hyperproliferation in the marrow, is a larger cell than the mature erythrocyte.

## *Diagnosis of Inherited Blood Disorders*

Considerable experience has been accumulated with the antenatal diagnosis of such inherited disorders as thalassemia and hemoglobinopathies (21). Diagnosis can be made from a number of tissues. Fetal blood has been sampled early in the second trimester by one of two methods. Blood can be withdrawn from the umbilical vein under fetoscopy or, alternatively, a mixed sample of fetal and maternal blood can be aspirated from the placenta under ultrasound. Amniocentesis has also been employed to obtain a sample of fetal cells that can be examined biochemically. This approach has been used to diagnose red cell enzyme deficiencies. Amniocentesis is also useful in the analysis of DNA from fetal cells. DNA harvested in this way can be subjected to genome mapping. An alternative source of DNA is chorion biopsy.

## Specific Disease

### *Hemoglobinopathies and Thalassemia Syndromes*

Hemoglobulin consists of a globin, a polypeptide made up of two pairs of amino acid chains, and heme, an iron and protoporphyrin complex. Normally in the adult, there are four types of chains: alpha, beta, gamma, and delta. Most adult hemoglobin, which is designated HbA, is made up of two alpha and two beta chains. There are also small amounts of hemoglobin $A_2$, made up of two alpha and two delta chains, and fetal hemoglobin (HbF) made up of two alpha chains and two gamma chains. The differing amino acid structures of the chains confer different oxygen affinity on the hemoglobin molecule. In the term fetus, 75 to 90% of the hemoglobin is HbF, whose structure favors oxygen release at lower oxygen tension. By 1 year of age, however, most gamma chain production has been curtailed.

In terms of the inheritance of hemoglobin disorders, there may be structural abnormalities in hemoglobin or impaired production of the polypeptide chain, or both. The thalassemia syndromes comprise those disorders that are marked by impaired or suppressed chain synthesis. The structural abnormalities, which are due to amino acid substitution in the polypeptide chains, are referred to as hemoglobinopathies.

### *Hemoglobinopathies Sickle Hemoglobin*

The most common hemoglobinopathy in America is sickle hemoglobin (HbS). Sickle cell trait, the presence of the gene for HbS, is found in about 8% of American blacks. There are no clinical sequelae and the outcomes of pregnancies in patients with sickle cell trait are not adversely influenced (22). There is some evidence, though, that there is an increased risk for asymptomatic bacteriuria during pregnancy.

Patients who are homozygous for the sickle cell gene experience lifelong disease, the signs and symptoms of which are a reflection of intravascular sickling, decreased flow in the microcirculation, and tissue anoxia. Sickle cell crises are marked by pain and fever and occur as a result of tissue infarcts. In addition, the life span of sickle cells is shortened and these patients are anemic. While sickle cell disease is not compatible with long life, some women do achieve pregnancies, in which cases maternal and fetal morbidity and mortality are significantly increased (23). About 20% of the pregnancies end in spontaneous abortion, and in those pregnancies going to term, intrauterine growth retardation is a feature of another 25%.

### Hemoglobin C and SC Disease

About 2% of American blacks have the gene for hemoglobin C (HbC). Individuals heterozygous for the disease are asymptomatic, but homozygotes have a mild, chronic hemolytic anemia. While specific complications are rare, particular attention must be paid to the nutritional requirements of pregnancy in these patients, as chronic hemolysis itself superimposes additional demands for folate, $B_{12}$, and iron.

Hemoglobin SC disease occurs almost as frequently as sickle cell anemia, despite the lower frequency of the HbC gene. This is because life expectancy in SC disease is only slightly reduced. The patient who is a double heterozygote for hemoglobin S and C does, however, often suffer from thrombotic crisis. Such patients are also prone to aseptic necrosis of their femoral heads and may develop proliferative retinitis and renal medullary infarcts.

Although it might seem anomalous that patients who have one gene for hemoglobin C and one for adult hemoglobin, as well as those with one gene for hemoglobin S and one for adult hemoglobin, are asymptomatic, for reasons that are unclear, the simultaneous presence of hemoglobins S and C in an erythrocyte promotes polymerization of hemoglobin S.

### Thalassemia Syndromes

As was pointed out earlier, these syndromes are a consequence of inherited disorders in the production of the globin chains of hemoglobin (24). In alpha-thalassemia and beta-thalassemia, synthesis of the alpha and beta chains, respectively, is absent or reduced. The syndromes are especially common in Mediterranean populations and Asians and occur sporadically in American blacks.

Impaired polypeptide chain synthesis results in erythrocytes that are poorly hemoglobinized and, especially in the case of alpha-thalassemia, prone to hemolysis. This hemolysis occurs in the reticulo-endothelial system after the chains, which are present in relative excess, precipitate inside red cells, and damage the erythrocyte membrane.

The clinical severity of the thalassemia syndromes depends on whether the individual is homozygous or heterozygous for the disease. In heterozygous alpha-thalassemia or alpha-thalassemia trait, the disease is very mild and the major consideration is to ensure that the microcytic anemia is not confused with iron deficiency. By comparison, homozygous alpha-thalassemia is associated with fetal hydrops fetalis and an increased risk for preeclampsia in the mother.

Beta-thalassemia, which was previously referred to as Mediterranean anemia or Cooley's anemia, also presents in homozygous and heterozygous varieties. Homozygous beta-thalassemia is not inevitably associated with fetal death; however, the infant with this disorder inevitably becomes transfusion-dependent and life expectancy is significantly reduced. In the few beta-thalassemia major patients who do achieve pregnancy, there is an increased risk for spontaneous abortion.

Patients with beta-thalassemia minor are comparable to women with normal erythropoiesis in terms of pregnancy complications and outcome for the fetus. The disorder is asymptomatic, and the diagnosis is often made for the first time in a woman presenting with a mild anemia that fails to respond to iron therapy.

About 1 in 3000 American blacks are heterozygous for both beta-thalassemia and sickle hemoglobin. Perinatal mortality in these women is modestly increased as is the risk for maternal complications, including papillary necrosis and pyelonephritis.

## Nutritional Anemias

Some discussion of the most common causes of these anemias, namely iron and folate deficiencies, has been given in the preceding section on the nutritional requirements of pregnancy. More rarely, other deficiencies can either account for or contribute to anemia. In this regard, vitamins C and E, pyridoxine, and the metals copper and zinc play a role in hematopoiesis.

There are a number of conditions that should alert the physician to an increased risk for nutritional anemia. Women at either end of their reproductive careers are at a disadvantage. Teen-age pregnancies are often complicated by iron deficiency anemia when fetal requirements for the metal are superimposed on the requirements of adolescent growth. Women whose pregnancies occur in their late 30s or early 40s are also at risk of iron deficiency, especially if repeated pregnancies, menorrhagia, or dietary faddism have left them iron-depleted.

A history of alcohol abuse should also alert the physician to a likelihood that the patient will either present with a nutritional anemia during pregnancy or experience dramatic aggravation of preexisting anemia. The megaloblastic anemia of alcohol abuse is due to folate deficiency, both by virtue of a reduced dietary intake and because alcohol interferes directly with a number of folate derivatives. Folic acid deficiency is also more likely in women with multiple pregnancies, in those with a history of long-term oral contraceptive use, and in patients with epilepsy, since some anticonvulsants interfere with folate metabolism. In general, nutritional anemias are also more likely when pregnancy occurs against a background of such medical disorders as diabetes, renal disease, cardiovascular, and gastrointestinal disease.

Although vitamin $B_{12}$ is an important nutrient in hematopoiesis, it is an unlikely cause of nutritional anemia in pregnancy. This is because deficiency of the vitamin is associated with infertility. The common causes of deficiency include pernicious anemia, a failure of gastric parietal cells to secrete the intrinsic factor needed for absorption of the vitamin, chronic malabsorption in the ileum, the site of absorption for vitamin $B_{12}$ and intrinsic factor complexes, and strictly vegetarian diets that exclude all animal products.

With regard to symptoms, iron deficiency and folic acid deficiency are no different by comparison with other causes of anemia in giving rise to pallor, easy fatigability, weakness, palpitations, and shortness of breath. Although some of these symptoms could be attributed to the pregnant state, per se, a painful glossitis is sometimes a clue to an underlying folic acid depletion. This inflammation reflects impaired DNA synthesis in the oral epithelium. Laboratory features include a macrocytic anemia, that is, the erythrocytes have an increased mean cell volume, and neutrophils may have an increased number of lobes. Normally, neutrophils have three or four segments, but in folate deficiency the average may be five or six, and individual neutrophils may have 10 or 12 segments. Because folate deficiency is seldom a difficult diagnosis to make during pregnancy, sophisticated tests are unnecessary. Occasionally, in patients with anemia that may be contributed to by a number of factors, a serum folate assay is indicated, and a value less than 3 ng/ml indicates deficiency of the nutrient.

With regard to iron deficiency anemia, this disease shares the general symptoms of anemia referred to above. However, it may also be possible to elicit from these patients a history of pica. The abnormal substances that people with this disorder ingest include dirt, starch, ice, and ash. This dietary perversion is quite frequently abandoned once iron balance has been restored.

The laboratory diagnosis of iron deficiency anemia has to be made against the background of the physiological changes in the hemoglobin concentration that are seen during pregnancy (see Table 35–8). In particular, a fall in hemoglobin during the second trimester should not be automatically interpreted as developing anemia. When iron deficiency accounts for a pathological reduction in the hemoglobin concentration, the anemia is microcytic, that is, the mean cell volume is reduced. In addition, the serum iron is reduced, the unsaturated iron binding capacity is more than 500 μg/dl, and the transferrin saturation is less than 15%. Early in iron deficiency, before frank anemia is present, a clue to impending anemia can be obtained from the serum ferritin. A value less than 12 ng/ml implies a reduction in the amount of storage iron that would normally be available to contribute to the increased requirements for iron imposed by the pregnancy.

## Aplastic Anemia

The hallmark of aplastic anemia is pancytopenia, that is, a reduction in the number of circulating erythrocytes, granulocytes, and platelets. This reduction is a result of decreased output by the bone marrow, which is itself hypocellular. This hypocellularity is usually a consequence of either irreversible damage to hematopoietic stem cells by cytotoxic agents or immune suppression of their proliferative capabilities.

Some drugs predictably produce marrow aplasia, provided they are administered in sufficient dose. These drugs include many of the preparations used in the management of leukemia and lymphomas. Other drugs that are not cancer chemotherapeutic agents can produce the same effect in therapeutic doses in sensitive individuals. Included here are many drugs used in the management of epilepsy, such as phenytoin, trimethadione, and carbamazepine, and others such as chloramphenicol, sulfa drugs, phenylbutazone, and gold salts. Aplasia has also been associated with ionizing irradiation and exposure to benzene, and rarely the disorder has been seen as a complication of viral disorders such as hepatitis C and infectious mononucleosis.

When aplastic anemia occurs during pregnancy, maternal and fetal morbidity and mortality depend on the successful management of the infectious and hemorrhagic complications that are consequent on the neutropenia and thrombocytopenia respectively (25).

## Leukemia and Lymphoma

While diseases such as aplastic anemia are a result of damage to the hematopoietic stem cell, other diseases are a result of discrete pathology within the stem cell itself. These diseases, which include leukemia and lymphoma, are clonal in nature in that the entire tumor cell burden is derived from a single cell.

Leukemia is either lymphocytic or myeloid depending on the predominant cell type, and acute if the cells are immature, or chronic when the cells that accumulate are more mature. Accumulation of the malignant cells is at the expense of normal marrow elements, such as red blood cell and platelet precursors, so that patients presenting with leukemia are often anemic and have evidence of thrombocytopenia. With progression of the disease, there is infiltration of lymph nodes, liver and spleen, and increasing risk of infection due to impaired function of granulocytes. Untreated patients with acute leukemia survive, on average, less than 3 months. The goal of treatment is induction of remission by combination chemotherapy. Depending on when the leukemia presents, this treatment may have teratogenic implications for the fetus, especially if given during the first trimester (26). However, fetuses exposed during the second and third trimester do not appear to be vulnerable to the teratogenic effect of drugs.

By comparison with acute leukemia, the chronic form of the disease poses less risk for mother and fetus. Chronic myelocytic leukemia, which is more common than the lymphocytic variety in women of childbearing age, is marked by a more gradual loss of normal marrow function and resultant predisposition to infection and hemorrhage. During the chronic phase of myelocytic leukemia, which lasts 3 to 4 years, the aim of treatment is to reduce the number of circulating white cells, rather than to induce a remission. Because of the slowly progressive nature of the disease, this treatment can be delayed, in the interest of protecting the fetus from teratogenic side-effects, until the second trimester. While it does not appear that pregnancy, per se, accelerates the course of the disease, chronic myeloid leukemia eventually enters a second or blast phase when it behaves similarly to the acute type of disease. Sustained remissions, at this point, are rare despite aggressive chemotherapy and vigorous transfusion support.

Lymphomas are malignancies of B or T-lymphocytes that usually begin in lymph nodes. Occasionally, however, these neoplasms start in extranodal sites such as the skin, gastrointestinal tract, or ovaries. They are broadly divided into two types, Hodgkin's disease and non-Hodgkin's lymphoma. These diseases have in common the fact that prognosis depends on how widespread the disorder is at presentation and what histological subtype is identified.

Hodgkin's disease primarily affects lymph nodes, and a painless cervical lymphadenopathy is the common presenting finding. The diagnostic cell is the Reed-Sternberg cell, and the disease can be divided into four histological types: (1) nodular sclerosis, occurring in nearly three-fourths of patients; (2) mixed cellularity, which occurs in about one-fourth; and (3) and (4) lymphocyte-predominant and lymphocyte-depleted varieties, which occur rarely. Hodgkin's disease, in which lymphocyte-predominance or nodular sclerosis is featured on histology, carries the best prognosis. It is important to "stage" Hodgkin's disease at presentation. Staging aims to establish the extent to which the disease has spread, both within the lymphoreticular system and to extranodal sites. By comparison with non-Hodgkin's lymphoma, spread is to anatomically contiguous areas and it is only late in the disease that organs such as liver, spleen, and marrow are involved. More widespread disease is associated with a poorer prognosis, and this prognosis is even worse should constitutional symptoms, such as fever, weight loss and night sweats, be present. Staging for Hodgkin's disease includes a number of procedures, lymphangiography, intravenous pyelography, and whole body scanning, for example, that could have consequences for the fetus. Furthermore, under some circumstances, laparotomy and splenectomy are indicated when management choices depend on the presence or absence of abdominal disease. For these reasons, it is essential to find out if the female patient presenting with Hodgkin's disease is pregnant. For localized disease, radiation is the treatment of choice. When disease is present in lymph nodes on both sides of the diaphragm, or if there is diffuse involvement of the extralymphatic organs, chemotherapy is indicated. Because single-agent chemotherapy does not produce sustained remissions, combination chemotherapy with nitrogen mustard, vincristine sulfate (Oncovin), prednisone and procarbazine, is used routinely. Although pregnancy does not influence the prognosis in Hodgkin's disease, chemotherapy and radiation are hazardous to the fetus. No generalizations can be made, however, either about modifying the clinical workup and treatment regimens, or delaying management until after parturition. For some pregnant women, such approaches are justified (27,28).

Non-Hodgkin's lymphoma is less likely to be encountered during pregnancy because the disease typically affects people in their 50s and 60s (29). This disease also differs from Hodgkin's in that spread is less predictable and involvement of extralymphatic organs is more common. Histologically, these lymphomas are first categorized according to whether they are made up predominantly of small or large lymphocytes, and whether the cells are arranged diffusely or in nodules. The cells are further categorized according to whether they are well-differentiated, in which case they resemble typical small lymphocytes, or poorly differentiated lymphocytes. Some examples of non-Hodgkin's lymphomas have cells with prominently indented nuclei. These are referred to as cleaved cells.

Staging in non-Hodgkin's lymphoma frequently reveals widespread disease, and it is seldom necessary to subject patients to laparotomy to confirm this. Radiation therapy is occasionally indicated for the few patients in whom disease is localized. Chemotherapy choices vary widely. Patients with low-grade disease may require little or no treatment for many years. Those with high-grade disease are candidates for combination chemotherapy at presentation. By comparison with Hodgkin's disease, the goal here is to induce remission, as treatment is seldom curative.

### *Hemolytic Anemias*

Hemolytic anemias (Table 35–11) occur when red cell destruction is, for one reason or another, accelerated and there is a concomitant increase in erythropoietic activity in the marrow (30). Normally, erythrocytes survive for about 120 days in circulation before being taken up in the reticulo-endothelial system. The daily turnover of red cells is about 1%, which is reflected in the reticulocyte count. When red cells are destroyed prematurely, increased marrow activity results in an increase in the degree of reticulocytosis, which may be the first clue to the presence of hemolytic anemia.

Hereditary spherocytosis, which is characterized by autosomal dominant inheritance, is the most common form of inherited hemolytic anemia. Patients with this disease often have a history of intermittent jaundice, gallstones, and an enlarged spleen, which is the site of uptake of the red cells. Although the diagnosis can be confirmed by demonstrating that the spherocytes are particularly sensitive to osmotic stress, a family history and the appearance of spherocytes on the blood smear may be all that are necessary.

Pregnancy in a woman with hereditary spherocytosis may precipitate a crisis characterized by an increased rate of red cell destruction. While most women can be managed during crisis by blood transfusion, those with sustained periods of accelerated hemolysis are candidates for splenectomy. In general, however, most women with hereditary spherocytosis sustain pregnancies uneventfully. This assessment is particularly true for pregnant

**Table 35–11.** Classification of Hemolytic Anemia

- Hereditary
  - Structural abnormalities
    - Hereditary spherocytosis
    - Elliptocytosis
  - Thalassemia and hemoglobinopathies
  - Erythrocyte enzyme deficiencies
- Acquired
  - Autoimmune hemolytic anemia
  - Drug induced hemolytic anemia
  - Paroxysmal nocturnal hemoglobinuria
  - Infections (malaria and clostridia)
  - Microangiopathic hemolytic anemia

women with hereditary elliptocytosis, which usually runs an even milder course than hereditary spherocytosis.

With regard to the thalassemias and hemoglobinopathies, these diseases have already been discussed.

As far as red cell enzyme deficiencies are concerned, glucose is metabolized via two pathways, 90% in the glycolytic, or Embden-Meyerhof pathway and 10% in the hexose monophosphate shunt. The former pathway is responsible for adenosine triphosphate (ATP) synthesis, while the latter generates reduced nicotinamide adenine dinucleotide phosphate (NADP). NADP compound is essential for maintaining adequate levels of glutathione reductase, which buffers erythrocytes against oxidant injury.

Glucose-6-phosphate dehydrogenase is the most common inherited red cell enzyme deficiency and is found in about 3% of black American women. Because this enzyme is important for the hexose-monophosphate shunt, deficiency places red cells at particular risk of hemolysis when exposed to oxidants. A number of drugs, including acetylsalicylic acid, phenacetin, sulfonamides, and nitrofurantoin can act as oxidants and should be avoided by patients with glucose-6-phosphate dehydrogenase deficiency. Other patients with glucose-6-phosphate dehydrogenase deficiency experience hemolytic episodes after eating fava beans, or concomitantly with viral or bacterial infections.

Special attention should be paid to pregnant women with glucose-6-phosphate dehydrogenase deficiency during their last trimester. The activity of the enzyme may decrease at this time, with a resulting decrease in red cell survival and aggravation of anemia.

Pyruvate kinase (PK) deficiency is the most common erythrocyte enzyme deficiency in the Embden-Meyerhof pathway. As with other rarer enzyme deficiencies in this pathway, such as phosphoglycerate kinase and phosphofructokinase, the hemolysis tends to be more severe than that associated with glucose-6-phosphate dehydrogenase deficiency. The disease may present with anemia in childhood, and gallstones, jaundice, and x-ray abnormalities may also occur. Pregnancy may provoke a hemolytic crisis.

While specific tests are available to diagnose enzyme deficiencies, all share features of hemolytic anemia, namely, elevations in reticulocyte count, lactate dehydrogenase, and indirect bilirubin.

In some patients with hemolysis, autoimmunity accounts for the shortened red cell survival. Autoimmunity is confirmed when the Coombs' test, which detects IgG or complement on the red cell membrane, is positive.

There are two broad categories into which autoimmune hemolytic anemia can be subdivided, depending on whether the antibodies are warm-reacting or cold-reacting. The former are usually IgG antibodies and the latter IgM. IgM antibodies are not detected in the Coombs' test, but they do give rise to complement fixation on the erythrocyte membrane and, hence, a positive test.

Warm autoantibodies are sometimes found against a background of lupus erythematosus, viral infections, chronic lymphocytic leukemia, or lymphoma. Although the disorder may also be provoked by drugs such as penicillin and alpha methyl dopa, it is often not possible to pinpoint a cause. For patients in whom there is no underlying disease to treat, steroids and splenectomy are considered. This can be particularly problematical should presentation be during pregnancy. Transfusion is discouraged for two reasons. First, transfused cells will survive no longer than the patient's own short-lived population, and second, crossmatching is difficult because the broadly-specific autoantibody may mask an underlying alloantibody that the patient acquired during the current or an earlier pregnancy.

As with warm autoimmune hemolytic anemia, cold-reacting autoantibodies causing hemolysis may also be idiopathic or secondary. In the latter, the associated diseases are viral infections, including infectious mononucleosis, mycoplasma infections, or lymphoid malignancies. Patients who are symptomatic from cold-reactive antibodies may experience vaso-occlusive phenomena in their fingers and toes, such as acrocyanosis and ulcers. They may be chronically anemic, and bouts of hemolysis may be provoked by cold weather. In general, the course of the disease is relatively benign, especially in the postinfectious varieties, which are self-limited. In contrast to warm autoimmune hemolytic anemia, cold-reacting autoantibody disease is usually seen in older-aged groups and is a very rare complication of pregnancy. In those exceptional circumstances in which transfusion is contemplated, some authorities advise washed cells, the purpose being to reduce the likelihood of providing complement to a complement-depleted patient and thereby exacerbating the hemolysis.

In paroxysmal nocturnal hemoglobinuria (PNH), hemolysis occurs because of an acquired defect in the erythrocyte membrane that renders the cells particularly sensitive to complement lysis. Patients often present in their 30s or 40s with anemia and a history of episodes of dark urine (due to hemoglobinuria), fever, and chills. There is an increased risk of marrow aplasia, infection, and thrombosis in these patients, and the limited experience with pregnancy in individuals with paroxysmal nocturnal hemoglobinuria suggests that thrombotic complications are increased.

Fragmented red cells are the characteristic feature of microangiopathic hemolytic anemia. On the peripheral smear, these cells are seen either as deformed, irregularly-shaped schistocytes, or as crenated cells that resemble burrs. These abnormalities in red cell appearance are believed to result from damage to erythrocytes that occurs when their passage is partially obstructed by fibrin strands in the lumina of small vessels.

A number of conditions are associated with microangiopathic hemolytic anemia, including eclampsia, renal disease, thrombotic thrombocytopenic purpura, and the HELLP syndrome. HELLP, an acronym for hemolysis, elevated liver enzymes and a low platelet count, occurs in about 10% of patients with eclampsia. Most authorities agree that the management of the HELLP syndrome is by urgent delivery, as the disease is progressive and associated with a high risk for maternal and fetal complications (31).

### *Anesthetic Considerations*

This group of disorders is of concern to the anesthesiologist because of the basic underlying pathology, which may be the direct cause of some considerable maternal/fetal discomfort and even a threat to well-being; but this group is also of concern because of the impact they may have upon selection and administration of analgesia and anesthesia during the labor, at vaginal delivery, and at the time of cesarean section.

Certain basic anesthetic principles are important in the management of the patient who suffers from anemia due to the hemoglobinopathies, the Thalassemia syndromes, the nutritional anemias, the aplastic anemias, the leukemias and lymphomas, and the hemolytic anemias. As mentioned later in this chapter under "General Anesthetic Principles," these include attention to the three Ds of detection, diagnosis, and definitive therapy in regard to airway management, oxygenation, ventilation, hypotension, and blood loss. Naturally, all of these are important in regard to maintenance of healthy oxygen saturation in peripheral blood and support of adequate oxygenated blood to the peripheral tissues.

The hemoglobinopathies will have been screened previously by hemoglobin electrophoresis to identify specific problems such as sickle cell hemoglobin and hemoglobin C and SC disease. Hemoglobinopathies can be the cause of local anoxic phenomena due to the aforementioned sickling and interruption of flow in the microcirculation. Consistent with careful consideration and management of the patient is also the concern about the health of associated organ systems such as hepatic and renal systems. Further concerns may be brought up should these organ systems be also involved in the general disease process. Their presence can, of course, modify the decision making in regard to selection of the specific anesthetic technique and agents. It is, therefore, prudent to select an analgesic regimen that provides alleviation of anxiety and freedom from pain associated with uterine contractions. In most anesthesiologist's minds, this would be selection of regional analgesia, i.e., lumbar epidural for first stage pain relief; yet, it is important to consider the admonition to not use an anesthetic technique that might tend to promote local sequestration of blood should hypotension be a possible complication and, therefore, locales where the $pO_2$) may fall and precipitate red cell sickling, sludging, and more sequestration, which restarts the cycle all over again.

Hypotension has been viewed as the villain in this regard, and, in earlier days, this may have been a reasonable concern and logical criticism; however, one of the ways to circumvent such a complication might be to use the double catheter as devised by Dr. Cleland. By now, in the mid 1990s, with the move toward constant infusion therapy with minimal drug concentrations, there is little or no concern about hypotension of any degree that may precipitate such a cyclical disorder as just mentioned. Thus, the lumbar epidural management of the 90s, with continuous low dose infusion providing side-stepping of the stress of labor which stimulates the sympathetic nervous system causing vasoconstriction and just those circumstances, may set the stage for red blood cell sickling such as stress and vasoconstriction with reduced blood flow and hypotension.

Finally, another alternative is to use small aliquots of intravenous analgesic in the first stage with a pudendal block and/or local perineal block for second stage. It goes without saying that before the final decisions are made, consultation with the rest of the team as previously mentioned, to include the obstetrician, anesthesiologist, neonatologist, and hematologist should be made. The earliest concern has to be identification of anemia and correction with either infusion of packed red blood cells or a formal exchange transfusion. Other initial physiological comforts that are important include detailed attention to fluid replacement, maintenance of normovolemia, maintenance of normothermia, maintenance of normotension, and maintenance of normal ventilation and acid-base balance.

So far we have been discussing the management of labor and vaginal delivery only; cesarean section poses another completely different set of circumstances, which may serve as further threats to the safety and well-being of the mother and fetus. Cesarean delivery poses as an added threat primarily due to the fact that regional anesthetic techniques adequate for cesarean delivery may in themselves be a cause of the dreaded complication of hypotension as mentioned before. However, today the epidural, when activated in fractional injections spaced over time, can give enough time for accommodation of vascular resistance and a much smaller incidence of hypotension. Even the subarachnoid technique can be modified with use of a catheter so that small divided doses may be given over a short period of time, again allowing enough time for accommodation and a substantial reduction in the incidence of hypotension. Of course, it is vital for the anesthesiologist to maintain absolute vigilance in regard to monitoring of the cardiovascular system for early signs of any reduction, which can be treated immediately and successfully. Monitoring for such problems at cesarean section should include electrocardiogram, blood pressure, heart rate, and $SaO_2$. General balanced anesthesia for cesarean can also be successfully used and can provide the mother with comfort and adequate conditions for the surgeon and safety for the fetus/neonate. It goes without saying that it is imperative to maintain cardiovascular and pulmonary stability during induction and delivery of the baby to again prevent any possible intravascular crises.

The thalassemia syndromes are rarer but constitute the most common cause of genetic disorders in this group of hematological problems. The primary pathophysiological defect lies in synthesis of the special alpha globin or beta globin chains, and, thus, the disease's reference to either Alpha or Beta Thalassemia Disease. The alpha thalassemias chiefly have hypochromic or hemolytic type anemias with the severity usually being mild, but it can be severe depending on the degree of abnormal hemoglobins overall. Patients with alpha thalassemias are usually managed well with constant followup during gestation, with the internist and obstetrician working well together. Delivery precautions may include consideration regarding the degree of anemia and even the possibility of transfusion. The considerations outlined previously for the hemoglobinopathies apply to the alpha-thalassemic patients also.

The beta-thalassemias are usually classed as either "minor" when heterozygotic or "major" when homozygotic. Patients with thalassemia minor usually have no severe anesthetic problems and can be managed with just the usual good sense of practical application of sound obstetric anesthetic principles. Patients with thalassemia major can present significant anesthetic challenges, including the most serious concern of cardiomyopathy. Thus, these patients should be identified and carefully worked up for associated target organ disease such as the heart, liver, and kidneys. These patients can be managed similar to principles outlined in the section on hemoglobinopathies, but one important additional comment to keep in mind is that these patients may demand more consideration for monitoring of the cardiovascular status due to the possibility of a superimposed cardiomyopathy. To summarize again, first and second stage analgesia for vaginal delivery may be managed by the continuous mini infusion method, by the double catheter regimen, or by intravenous analgesia with supplemental pudendal and/or local perineal block being added for delivery (32). The cesarean sections may be conservatively managed by use of the balanced general technique and also a regional method, in the absence of any thrombocytopenia, using one of the modifications previously mentioned.

Patients with the leukemias and lymphomas are special challenges because of the sensitivity of the issues involved and the very much needed and appreciated compassion that must be shown. Otherwise, in the absence of thrombocytopenia, once again, the regional methods may be used to provide the mother with the valuable awake and participatory feelings that she will forever appreciate. Here is a situation in which the anemia component must be carefully assessed before a decision is made and the regional method used for either vaginal or cesarean delivery. It should be mentioned at this point that should one consider the hematological problem so severe from the standpoint of lack of clotting due to deficient platelets, then the use of the pudendal block should also be seriously considered contraindicated along with epidural because of the literature references to hematoma formation with pudendal block (33).

The nutritional, aplastic, and hemolytic anemias are all characterized by red cells with abbreviated life spans due to their specific disorders. The chief concern again is the level of anemia and the consideration for transfusion. Otherwise, again the basic sound principles and sound advice outlined earlier in this chapter can also be applied successfully here. The anesthesiologist must be able to be flexible and creative in the difficult patient management challenges of this chapter. At the same time, such attention to the special problems of the patients with hematological disease also enables anesthesiologists the opportunity to express their compassion for care of their patients, their completeness of understanding, and their eagerness to be of service to their fellow colleagues.

## COAGULATION ABNORMALITIES IN PREGNANCY

### Inherited Bleeding Disorders

The most common inherited coagulation disorder that may complicate pregnancy is von Willebrand's disease. It is characterized by impaired platelet adhesion and a low level of factor VIII. These abnormalities predispose to a risk of posttraumatic and postoperative bleeding, as well as postpartum hemorrhage (34).

Patients with von Willebrand's disease often have a history of prolonged bleeding after surgical or dental procedures. Menorrhagia is occasionally a feature. Typically, both the bleeding time and the partial thromboplastin time are prolonged. When the patient's platelets are challenged with known agonists, such as ristocetin, aggregation is impaired.

There are two approaches to the treatment of von Willebrand's disease. A vasopressin analog, 1-desamino-8-D-arginine vasopressin (DDAVP), can be used in patients with mild cases as an alternative to the use of blood products. DDAVP restores, temporarily, both the factor VIII coagulant activity and platelet function in these patients. Although there are some subtypes of von Willebrand's disease in which DDAVP is ineffective, the majority of patients experience at least a doubling of their factor VIII coagulant activity when DDAVP is administered. The implication is that, provided the patient has a baseline level of at least 10%, DDAVP will provoke a level that is high enough for surgery to be considered. For patients with severe von Willebrand's disease, the treatment of choice is cryoprecipitate, a concentrate of factor VIII prepared from volunteer whole blood donors. Commercially available preparations of factor VIII concentrate are ineffective in the management of von Willebrand's disease because they do not contain the factor that is necessary to repair the platelet defect in the disease. For most surgery patients, daily cryoprecipitate by intravenous infusion is adequate, although individuals with more severe disease may require cryoprecipitate twice a day.

When an uncomplicated vaginal delivery is expected in a patient with von Willebrand's disease, it is reasonable to monitor the patient in the postpartum period before routinely giving DDAVP or cryoprecipitate. Although there may be a high index of suspicion in those individuals with low levels of factor VIII coagulant activity, many physicians would observe the patient for untoward blood loss rather than administer prophylactic treatment.

Hemophilia A, an X-linked disorder, is exceptionally unusual in women, but can occur in the female offspring of carrier mothers and hemophiliac fathers. It can also occur when there is severe lyonization, or inactivation, of an X-chromosome in a woman who is a carrier for the disease. Treatment for women with hemophilia A is similar to that for women with von Willebrand's disease. In symptomatic patients, cryoprecipitate is indicated to cover cesarean section and the postoperative period. Women with milder disease who deliver vaginally can be managed expectantly and only given DDAVP or cryoprecipitate should excessive blood loss justify treatment.

Hemophilia B, or factor IX deficiency, is also an X-linked disorder that is only rarely diagnosed in women. The presentation of the disease in symptomatic women is identical to that of hemophilia A. Depending on the level of factor IX, there is an increased risk for hemorrhagic complications during cesarean section or following vaginal delivery. The treatment of hemophilia A and hemophilia

B differs in that there is no equivalent to cryoprecipitate for the management of factor IX deficient women. There are only two sources of factor IX that can be used in replacement therapy: fresh frozen plasma and commercial factor IX concentrates. The disadvantage to using fresh frozen plasma is that it requires large volumes to achieve therapeutic levels. This approach is often impossible in the patient whose pregnancy already results in a degree of hypervolemia.

## *Acquired Bleeding Disorders*

### Idiopathic Thrombocytopenia Purpura (ITP)

In this disease, an autoantibody is directed against an antigen expressed on platelets. These platelets are then taken up, prematurely, by the reticuloendothelial system. The role of an antibody in mediating the thrombocytopenia was suspected many years ago when it was recognized that some women with idiopathic thrombocytopenia purpura delivered children who were themselves temporarily thrombocytopenic.

Idiopathic thrombocytopenia purpura occurs in acute and chronic varieties. The acute disease is seen most often in childhood when it follows a variety of viral infections, including infectious mononucleosis and rubella. The disease is seldom fatal and spontaneous recovery usually occurs within 6 months. In patients who have significant decreases in their platelet counts, there may be spontaneous bleeding, particularly involving mucosal surfaces. In about one-fifth of patients, idiopathic thrombocytopenia purpura persists and enters a chronic phase.

Chronic idiopathic thrombocytopenia purpura in women is most often diagnosed in the 20- to 40-year-old age group. A history of a preceding infection is unusual. Many patients describe easy bruising, either spontaneously or after mild trauma, and there may be episodes of epistaxis, menorrhagia, hematuria, and gastrointestinal bleeding. Occasionally, chronic idiopathic thrombocytopenia purpura is seen in conjunction with other diseases such as lupus erythematosus or lymphoma.

Laboratory investigation shows the platelet counts to be between 10,000 and 70,000/μl. Occasionally, giant platelets are seen on the peripheral smear. A definitive diagnosis rests on the demonstration of antibodies that are either bound to the patient's platelets or free in the circulation. Treatment in acute idiopathic thrombocytopenia purpura may not be indicated in patients with relatively normal bleeding times in whom the platelet count is not profoundly suppressed. It is, however, important to avoid medications, such as aspirin, that interfere with platelet function. In chronic idiopathic thrombocytopenia purpura, there are initially two choices in patients who are symptomatically thrombocytopenic (35). In some studies, up to 50% of patients go into a sustained remission after treatment with prednisone. Patients who respond to this treatment usually reveal their sensitivities to steroids by a gradual rise in the platelet count that begins within 2 weeks of starting treatment. Splenectomy is indicated in those patients who fail steroid treatment or for those in whom the dose of steroids required to maintain a platelet count above 30,000 is intolerably high. Splenectomy benefits some 50% of individuals who fail steroids. Immunosuppression, with drugs such as cyclophosphamide and vinca alkaloids, are indicated for patients in whom splenectomy is ineffective.

### *Thrombotic Thrombocytopenic Purpura (TTP)*

The cause of this disease is unknown. It is characterized by thrombocytopenia, anemia, renal impairment, neurologic abnormalities, and fever. The disease is more common in women and can affect them during their reproductive years. Occasionally, thrombotic thrombocytopenic purpura is associated with a prodromal viral illness, and it has also been described in conjunction with drug allergies, lupus erythematosus, and toxemia. Although chronic varieties of thrombotic thrombocytopenic purpura have been described, the acute disease is often fatal when untreated.

A characteristic finding on the peripheral smear is the presence of schistocytes, abnormally-shaped red cells that have been damaged by fibrin plugs in the microvasculature. The platelet count is low, but because there are adequate numbers of megakaryocytes in the marrow, this decrease in number can be attributed to increased consumption rather than to decreased production. Clotting times, prothrombin times, and partial thromboplastin times are usually normal and the fibrinogen concentration is normal or increased. These findings serve to distinguish thrombotic thrombocytopenic purpura from disseminated intravascular coagulation in which the times are prolonged and the fibrinogen concentration is decreased.

The usual treatment for thrombotic thrombocytopenic purpura is a plasma exchange. Although it is tempting to suggest that exchange results in the removal of a circulating toxin, this seems unlikely because some patients go into remission with transfusions of plasma rather than exchange. This observation suggests that the disease may be caused by deficiency of a factor that prevents platelet aggregation and fibrin deposition. Some regimens call for the use of antiplatelet agents in addition to plasma exchange. Exchange is conducted on alternate days, until there is clinical improvement. A rise in platelet count is an early sign that continued plasma exchange may be beneficial.

The management of thrombotic thrombocytopenic purpura in pregnancy is complicated by the fact that the syndrome may be difficult to distinguish from severe eclampsia. Whereas thrombotic thrombocytopenic purpura is not improved by delivery, the opposite can be said for eclampsia. For this reason, when hypertension and proteinuria are prominent features, it would be more reasonable to proceed with prompt delivery.

### Disseminated Intravascular Coagulation (DIC)

This syndrome occurs when an underlying disease gives rise to widespread activation of the clotting system. The disorder is of particular interest to obstetricians because a number of the diseases that promote disseminated intravascular coagulation occur as complications of pregnancy or delivery. In this context, disseminated intravascular coagulation may be seen acutely in conjunction with amniotic fluid embolism, placental abruption, and pulmonary embolism. It may be seen subacutely with a retained dead fetus, and a chronic form of disseminated intravascular coagulation can be associated with preeclampsia and eclampsia. One theory of the pathogenesis of disseminated intravascular coagulation suggests that all of these conditions have in common the release into the blood stream of thromboplastins that activate clotting. Coagulation factors are consumed in this process and laboratory tests can be used to show that plasma fibrinogen concentration falls, along with concentration of other factors, especially factors V, VIII, and XIII. The platelet count also falls and fibrin-split products appear. It is the consumption of clotting factors that gives rise to the risk for hemorrhage.

Bleeding in disseminated intravascular coagulation may occur suddenly and extensively. Bleeding from venipuncture sites may be an early sign, followed by epistaxis, gastrointestinal bleeding, and hematuria. Postpartum hemorrhage may be dramatic.

The treatment of disseminated intravascular coagulation depends on both the treatment of the underlying condition and transfusion to restore the levels of coagulation factors and platelets (36). A number of the obstetric complications that trigger disseminated intravascular coagulation are best managed by delivery and in some patients this is all that is necessary to reverse the clotting process. Replacement therapy includes the use of cryoprecipitate, to restore the level of fibrinogen; fresh frozen plasma, to provide clotting factors; and platelets, to repair the thrombocytopenia. Although it has been theorized that this form of treatment merely provides more substrate for the coagulation cascade, clinical experience argues otherwise. Where there is controversy, however, is in the use of heparin. Some coagulation experts argue that heparin should be used because it interferes with clotting and should therefore "turn off" the process. There is a tendency not to use this anticoagulant in acute disseminated intravascular coagulation. A compromise position holds that heparin is occasionally indicated in patients who are severely ill with disseminated intravascular coagulation, for whom a period of time may be necessary before treatment of the underlying cause takes effect.

### Thromboembolic Disease (TED)

Thromboembolic disease, particularly deep venous thrombosis and pulmonary embolism, is the most important cause of obstetric morbidity and mortality (37). A number of factors contribute to the increased risk for thromboembolic disease in the obstetric patient, including stasis due to the pregnant uterus obstructing venous return, hypercoagulability, damage to vascular endothelium during vaginal delivery or cesarean section, and decrease in fibrinolytic activity.

With regard to the diagnosis of deep venous thrombosis, there are limitations to relying on the physical examination in that pain and swelling are variably present in the presence of established disease. The clinical diagnosis cannot be made exclusively on the results of physical findings. There are also difficulties with the diagnosis of pulmonary embolus. The majority of emboli do not give rise to symptoms. When symptoms are a feature, the patient may complain of dyspnea, chest pain, cough, tachypnea, or hemoptysis. With massive pulmonary embolization, the patient may present in right-sided heart failure and the electrocardiogram may show right axis shift with a strain pattern. About half of patients with a pulmonary embolus have pleural effusion on x ray.

With regard to more sensitive and specific tests for thromboembolic disease, it has to be borne in mind that the invasive procedures are not without risk to both mother and fetus. A diagnosis of deep venous thrombosis in the lower extremity is best made by venography. Although this is the investigation of choice, it is not without drawbacks. Pelvic veins are not visualized, calf veins may be difficult to fill, and chemical phlebitis can occur.

Impedance plethysmography can also be used to help in the diagnosis of deep venous thrombosis. This is a noninvasive method, involving the application of a pressure cuff to a thigh. When pressure in the cuff is released, the rate of return of blood that has gathered in the calf can be used to give a clue to the presence of venous obstruction. The procedure has the disadvantage that large thrombi can be missed should there be a well-developed collateral venous system. In addition, obstruction to the inferior vena cava by the uterus can be mistaken for venous obstruction by thrombus.

Doppler ultrasound is another noninvasive technique to measure changes in venous flow. Ultrasound does not detect distal thrombi, but it is reasonably sensitive for identifying obstruction in large veins above the knee.

With regard to pulmonary emboli, perfusion lung scans and, in selected patients, pulmonary angiograms are necessary to establish the diagnosis. Lung scans rely on the use of microspheres that have been radiolabelled with technetium, which can be given at a dose not harmful to the fetus. The microspheres become lodged in the pulmonary capillary vasculature and are highly sensitive in detecting pulmonary emboli. Specificity of this procedure is improved if it is combined with a ventilation scan. This procedure relies on the inhalation of xenon in conjunction with the perfusion study. A comparison can then be made of areas of the lung that are ventilated but not perfused.

The treatment of deep venous thrombosis rests on anticoagulation. Ideally, heparin is given, either subcutaneously or intravenously, in a dose to prolong the partial thromboplastin time to 1.5 to 2 times the control value. This treatment is continued for 10 days. If there has been recurrent thrombosis, subcutaneous heparin therapy can be continued until into the postpartum period. Anticoagulation with coumarin derivatives is not indicated in pregnancy. These agents are associated with multiple congenital abnormalities when given during the first trimester and fetal and placental hemorrhage is a risk when this form of anticoagulation is administered during the second and third trimesters.

Heparin is also indicated in the management of acute pulmonary embolus, preferably by the intravenous route. In patients with recurrent pulmonary emboli despite adequate heparinization, ligation of the inferior vena cava is indicated. In the face of massive embolization to the main pulmonary artery, pulmonary embolectomy may be indicated.

## *Anesthetic Considerations for the Patients with Coagulation Abnormalities*

In this section there is both the alpha and omega of the hematological dilemma: on the one hand, the disseminated intravascular coagulation problems with their flagrant bleeding disorder and, on the other hand, the thromboembolic disease or thrombo embolic disorders with their flagrant tendency to coagulate. Obviously, there is little to offer these patients for labor and delivery analgesia aside from supportive management and compassion for the problem at hand other than suggest use of local analgesia target directed at the specific area. This technique of management can be very nicely supported by addition of small 10 to 15 mg intravenous aliquots of ketamine during major uncomfortable periods. In addition, the supportive voice and touch of someone who understands and cares is often most appreciated and meaningful at such moments of great travail. The latter supportive move should be applied to all the aforementioned difficult management cases as suggested in the earlier text.

The Inherited Bleeding Disorders such as von Willebrand's disease and hemophilia A or B have a significant risk of continued bleeding after damage to small vessels such as could conceivably occur during epidural or spinal procedures. This, of course, brings up the entire problem of potential cord-compression damage and opens up the possibility of serious neurological injury subsequently. The editors of this text believe that it is very important to realize that no physician should take it upon themselves to "decide" to use major conduction techniques such as these when such serious neurologic sequelae could be possible. In other words, regardless of what the bleeding time is, regardless of what the platelets are, and regardless of apparent absence of clinical skin bruising, regional anesthesia should not be used on such high-risk patients unless the full story is outlined to the patient with all the possible sequalae and serious neurologic problems fully understood. In such cases, it is difficult to imagine why a patient would not opt for conservative management with use of local nerve blockade supplemented with small doses of ketamine to add to the comfort zone during major periods of discomfort. As mentioned earlier, these are times when the human voice and touch are absolutely vital to helping get the patient through a difficult time of challenge and stress. Thus, although many textbooks may suggest that regional anesthesia may be tried in certain circumstances, it just does not appear to be prudent to push a patient toward such use when there can be and may well be a possibility for serious irreversible damage. It must be recalled that these disease processes separate themselves entirely from other processes due to the fact that even though during labor and even delivery a torn epidural vessel may not bleed abundantly, it can do so during the postpartum period when the factor deficiencies fall significantly.

Idiopathic thrombocytopenia purpura or ITP and thrombotic thrombocytopenic purpura or TTP are disease entities characterized by thrombocytopenia. They are examples of disease processes in which conduction anesthesia is again questionable from the viewpoint of availability of other "alternative means" by which considerable comfort can be provided by use of local analgesic methods supplemented again by small dosages of ketamine for control of difficult periods of stress. Again, there are some who believe regional anesthesia is not contraindicated should a patient have normal bleeding time and platelets. As mentioned earlier, however, there is a difference between saying such a condition does not "contraindicate" regional anesthesia but quite a different thing to say go ahead and do it without the patient having complete information about the possible serious and irreversible neurologic sequelae that may result from such use. Regional anesthesia in patients with preeclampsia is a case in point. The same cautions are indicated here as they are for patients with other diseases that cause qualitative and quantitative platelet abnormalities. A patient with a platelet count less than 100,000/μl, or with other evidence of consumptive coagulopathy, is at risk of a hemorrhagic complication. While some have suggested that a bleeding time test could predict the degree of risk for patients with counts between 50,000 and 100,000/μl, the limitations of the test and its poor predictive value are deterrents to its usefulness.

In certain instances, these patients may also need cesarean section, and general anesthesia is the obvious choice for a compromised situation, but even with this technique, one must be careful in regard to intubation and use of the laryngoscope to make sure not to injure and cause a hematoma during intubation.

## Transfusion Considerations in Pregnancy

A good deal of attention has been paid recently to the level of hemoglobin at which surgical patients, in general, should be transfused. Whereas previously a level of 10 g/dl was required before it was felt that anesthesia could be given safely, there has been a significant revision downward of this figure. The feeling is that younger individuals are able to safely tolerate general anesthesia at a level much lower than this. This newer practice of setting a lower "transfusion trigger" has particular relevance for the pregnant woman. It should be remembered that she is well-adapted to her dilutional anemia, and a relatively low hemoglobin after an uncomplicated cesarean section, for example, should not be used prematurely as an indication for transfusion.

As it is, blood transfusion during cesarean section is seldom indicated, and for this reason, careful consideration should be given before autologous donations of blood are made during the last trimester of pregnancy. Many women, understandably concerned about the safety of blood transfusion, are keen to donate autologous units on their own behalf, even when routine vaginal delivery, rather than cesarean section, is expected. Although some blood programs recommend 1 or 2 unit autologous donations during the latter part of pregnancy, as "insurance," there is no justification for this procedure unless the patient has a complication, such as placenta previa, in which hemorrhage is the expected outcome. Autologous donation during pregnancy should not be regarded as routine. While some experience suggests that the procedure can be carried out safely, no large studies have been reported to confirm that the autologous donation is safe for both mother and fetus (38). While complications of blood donation occur only rarely, they include vasovagal attacks and seizures. It is not possible to predict that rare events like these will have no sequelae for the fetus.

When transfusion is justified during pregnancy, it is important to ensure that the cytomegaloviral antibody status of the mother is known. Women who are negative for antibodies to cytomegalovirus should be given cytomegalovirus seronegative blood products to avoid a primary cytomegalovirus (CMV) infection with possible deleterious consequences for the fetus (39).

A recent alternative to homologous blood transfusions has emerged in the form of directed donations. In this strategy, a transfusion recipient selects, usually from family and friends, the blood donors. As far as the woman in her child-bearing years is concerned, it is absolutely imperative, if directed donations are provided for transfusion during an elective surgery procedure, that the woman's husband, or his relatives, not be invited as directed donors. Unless this precaution is taken, the woman could be exposed to a red cell antigen that will set the stage for hemolytic disease of the newborn in subsequent pregnancies.

A number of patients are confused about the relative safety of immune globulin preparations. In particular, they may express anxiety about the risk of hepatitis or acquired immune deficiency syndrome from Rh immune globulin. It must be stressed that these products are safe from viral contamination.

With regard to the management of postpartum hemorrhage, a number of points are worth emphasizing. It is not necessary to obtain fresh blood for the individual requiring resuscitation from a massive hemorrhage. The concentration of coagulation factors in stored modified whole blood is well above the concentration required for hemostasis. In addition, if the patient is transfused to the point that dilutional thrombocytopenia is documented, then this should be treated with platelet infusions. Under some circumstances, it may be necessary to resuscitate the patient with severe hemorrhage using group O cells if the indications for transfusion are so urgent that there is no time to proceed with a conventional crossmatch. Some blood programs provide group O Rh positive red cells for use in these emergencies. The 15% of women who are Rh negative are likely to be immunized by this experience. If it is necessary to transfuse an Rh negative woman with Rh positive blood, then she becomes a candidate for Rh immune globulin. The globulin has to be given at a dose significantly in excess of the dose that would be required for postpartum prevention of Rh immunization. In this context, one vial of Rh immune globulin suppresses the immune response to 15 ml of Rh positive red blood cells.

## General Anesthetic Principles

In general, the severe reduction in blood-formed elements leads to severe oxygen desaturation due to the reduced oxygen carrying capacity. This results in a stress to the fetus and the mother. In the fetus, there are serious complications such as intrauterine fetal death, premature labor, and even very early abortion. In the mother, the risks are also related to oxygen carrying capacity restrictions and can result in serious increases in workload on the maternal myocardium secondary to elevated heart rate, elevated cardiac output, and elevated level of work for the heart, which can even terminate in cardiac failure. Naturally, one of the added stress periods during gestation is at the second trimester near the thirty-fourth week; a second stress period is during labor, and a third just after delivery of the baby. The anesthesiologist should also be cognizant of the fact that the mother who suffers from severe anemia can also suffer from abnormal labor patterns such as prolonged labor, uterine inertia, and cervical dystocia, and finally postpartum hemorrhage. Because the above noted added stress of pregnancy superimposed upon anemia can precipitate serious consequences such as cardiac failure, these patients may be considered for treatment of their anemia prior to the beginning of pregnancy stresses. One recognized treatment regimen consists of transfusion to a reasonable level of red cell mass over a graduated period of time.

Certain basic anesthetic principles are important in the management of the patient who suffers from hematologic problems. These include attention to the three Ds of detection, diagnosis, and definitive therapy in regard to airway management, oxygenation, ventilation, hypotension, and blood loss. Naturally, all of these are important in regard to maintenance of healthy oxygen saturation in peripheral blood and support of adequate oxygenated blood to the peripheral tissues. At the writing of the first edition of this book, it was necessary to mention that an intravenous line should be started either before labor or soon after it begins. Of course, now it is accepted practice that all parturients get an intravenous line during labor for their fluid support and for their protection in case of untoward complications such as hypotension or blood loss. This class of patient is also significantly more susceptible to the effects of the anesthetic drugs in general and therefore should receive small, divided doses of drugs for induction of anesthesia or for any other drug administration during labor. One safe method of determining the appropriate dose is to give only 40 to 60% of the usual dose on the first pass, observe the results, and then administer a small additional dosage for the desired effect. A similar caution should be exercised in regard to administration of the inhalation drugs, whereby smaller percentages of inhalation agents can be titrated to achieve the desired effect in the patient. High doses of anesthetic agents, regardless of what they might be, may precipitate sudden and severe cardiac depression, hypotension, and, consequently, rapid severe desaturation due to the underlying state of anemia. As mentioned before, regional anesthesia may be used if used discreetly and with caution regarding reduction in vasomotor blockade so that regional hypotension and stagnated flow does not produce hypoxia and resultant sickling of red cells. Of course, in today's management of labor, analgesia as outlined in Chapter 13 on lumbar epidural and caudal epidural, the slow titration of the local anesthetic obviates the development of such problems so common just 2 decades ago at the time of the first edition. In fact, an ideal management plan for patients in spontaneous labor or induced labor might be use of the lumbar epidural with the slow continuous infusion as elaborated upon in Chapter 13.

Regional and neuraxial anesthesia are contraindicated in the presence of coagulopathy as diagnosed by any one or combination of a platelet count less than 100,000/μl, a prothrombin time and/or a partial thromboplastin time greater than 1.5 times control, and a fibrinogen concentration less than 100 mg/100 ml. Under these circumstances, the risk for bleeding is increased along with the risk for irreversible neurological damage. With regard to platelet function, the value of a bleeding-time test is debatable when it is used in patients without a history of bleeding disorder. While the test result can predict the adequacy of hemostasis in a patient with a quantitative or qualitative platelet problem, the test is not a good predictor in patients who have no clinical history of a bleeding problem. The bleeding-time test has the added disadvantage that even the newer disposable devices, which introduce some standardization, are not standardized when it comes to the pressure that the technician uses to apply the device to the skin site where the test incision will be made.

The practice of the basic, safe principles of anesthesia and analgesia as described throughout this textbook are, of course, recommended for the management of the patient who may be suffering from hematological disorders that have been discussed in this chapter. Suffice it to say at this point, the anesthesiologist must be aware of the problems that the patient has in regard to these disorders and the best way to be sure that the entire picture is appreciated is to make sure good communication pathways are open with the patient's primary physician. This means good communication and coordination is maintained between the anesthesiologist and the obstetrician and/or internist at all times because the picture can change rapidly in these disorders without much warning. If there is sufficient time available for planning, then a management strategy can be designed to best suit the mother and fetus and assure the former reasonable comfort and the latter safety. In general, those principles just alluded to in regard to sound anesthesia management include protection of the mother's cardiovascular status, maintenance of oxygenation and ventilation, attention to details of dosage of drugs and the response effects, careful monitoring, including continuous $SaO_2$ determinations, and last, but not least, strict vigilance at all times.

## REFERENCES


1. Letsky EA: Haematological Disorders in Pregnancy. Clinics in Haematology, Vol. 14, No. 3. London, W.B. Saunders Company, 1985.
2. Laros RK: Blood Disorders in Pregnancy. Philadelphia, Lea and Febiger, 1986.
3. Kitay DZ: Hematologic Problems in Pregnancy. Oradell, NJ, Medical Economics Books, 1987.
4. Neri A, Pardo Y, Schoenfeld A, Zaizov R: Permature separation of placenta in a patient with idiopathic thrombocytopenic purpura. Fetal. Ther. 4:185–187, 1989.
5. Peck TM, Arias F: Hematologic changes associated with pregnancy. Clin. Obstet. Gynecol. 22:785, 1979.
6. Pitkin RM, Witte DL: Platelet and leukocyte counts in pregnancy. JAMA 242:2696, 1979.
7. Bonnar J: Hemostasis and coagulation disorders in pregnancy. *In* Hemostasis and Thrombosis. Edited by AL Bloom, DP Thomas. Edinburgh, Churchill Livingstone, 1981.
8. Comp PC, Thurnau GR, Welsh J, Esmon CT: Functional and immunologic protein S levels are decreased during pregnancy. Blood 68:881, 1986.
9. Gore M, Eldon S, Trofatter KF, Soong S-J, et al: Pregnancy-induced changes in the fibrinolytic balance: evidence for defective release of tissue plasminogen activator and increased levels of the fast-acting tissue plasminogen activator inhibitor. Am. J. Obstet. Gynecol. 156:674 1987.
10. Weiner CP, Brandt J: Plasma antithrombin III activity: an aid in the diagnosis of preeclampsia-eclampsia. Am. J. Obstet. Gynecol. 142:275, 1982.
11. Bothwell TH, Charlton RW, Cook JD, Finch CA: Iron Metabolism In Man. Cambridge, MA, Blackwell Scientific Publications, 1979.
12. Hemminki E, Starfield B: Routine administration of iron and vitamins during pregnancy: review of controlled clinical trials. Br. J. Obstet. and Gynaecol. 85:404, 1978.
13. Hibbard BM: Iron and folate supplements during pregnancy: supplementation is valuable only in selected patients. Br. Med. J. 297:1324, 1988.
14. Taylor DJ, Mallen C, McDougall N, Lind T: Effect of iron supplementation on serum ferritin levels during and after pregnancy. Br. J. Obstet. and Gynaecol. 89:1011, 1982.
15. Bridges KR: Iron imbalance during pregnancy. *In* Hematologic Disorders in Maternal-Fetal Medicine. Edited by MM Bern, FD Frigoletto. New York, Wiley-Liss, 1990.
16. Dallman PR, Siimes MA, Stekel A: Iron deficiency in infancy and childhood. Am. J. Clin. Nutr. 33:86, 1980.
17. Singla PN, Chand S, Agarwal KN: Cord serum and placental tissue iron status in maternal hypoferremia. Am. J. Clin. Nutr. 32:1462, 1979.
18. Pitkin RM: Vitamins and minerals in pregnancy. Clin. Perinatol. 2:221, 1975.
19. Chanarin I: Folate and cobalamin. Clinics in Haematology 14:629, 1985.
20. Gookin KS, Morrison JC: Nutritional anemias complicating pregnancy. *In* Blood disorders in pregnancy. Edited by RK Laros. Philadelphia, Lea & Febiger, 1986.
21. Hillman RS, Finch CA: The detection of anemia. *In* Red Cell Manual. 6th Ed. Philadelphia, F.A. Davis Company, 1992.
22. Weatherall DJ: Prenatal diagnosis of hematologic disorders. *In* Fetal and Neonatal Haematology. Edited by IM Hann, BES Gibson, EA Lafsky. London, Balliere Tindal, 1991.
23. Blattner P, Dar H, Nitowsky HM: Pregnancy outcome in women with sickle cell trait. JAMA 238:1392, 1977.
24. Charache S, Niebyl JR: Pregnancy in sickle cell disease. Clinics in Haematology 14:729, 1985.
25. Laros RK Jr: The hemoglobinopathies. *In* Blood Disorders in Pregnancy. Philadelphia, Lea & Febiger, 1986.
26. Mankad VN, Patel A: Leukemia and other malignancies. *In* Hematologic Problems in Pregnancy. Edited by DZ Kitay. Oradell, NJ, Medical Economics Books, 1987.
27. Sweet DL, Kinzle J: Consequences of radiotherapy and antineoplastic therapy for the fetus. J. Reprod. Med. 17:241, 1976.
28. Jacobs C, Donaldson S, Rosenberg SA, Kaplan HS: Management of the pregnant patient with Hodgkin's disease. Ann. Int. Med. 95:669, 1981.
29. Caligiuri MA: Leukemia and pregnancy: treatment and outcome. Adv. Oncol. 8:10, 1992.

30. Ward FT, Weiss MD: Managing lymphoma during pregnancy. Adv. Oncol. 8:18, 1992.
31. Perkins RP: Enzyme deficiency disorders. *In* Hematologic Problems in Pregnancy. Edited by DZ Kitay. Oradell, NJ, Medical Economics Books, 1987.
32. Weinstein L: Hematology of toxemia. Hematologic Problems in Pregnancy. Edited by DZ Kitay. Oradell, NJ, Medical Economics Books, 1987.
33. Meadows K: A successful pregnancy outcome in transfusion dependent thalassemia major. Aust. N.Z. J. Obstet. Gynaecol. 24:43, 1984.
34. Gaylord TG, Pearson JW: Neuropathy following paracervical block in the obstetric patient. Obstet. Gynecol. 60(4): 521–4, 1982.
35. Linker CA: Congenital disorders of hemostasis. *In* Blood Disorders in Pregnancy. Edited by RK Laros. Philadelphia, Lea & Febiger, 1986.
36. Kelton JG: Management of the pregnant patient with idiopathic thrombocytopenic purpura. Ann. Int. Med. 99:796, 1983.
37. Colvin BT: Thrombocytopenia. Clinics in haematology 14: 661, 1985.
38. Hirsh J, Ginsberg J, Turner C, Levine M: Management of thromboembolism during pregnancy: risks to the fetus. *In* Hematologic Disorders in Maternal-Fetal Medicine. Edited by MM Bern, FD Frigoletto Jr. New York, Wiley-Liss, Inc., 1990.
39. Sayers MH, Anderson KC, Goodnough LT, Kurtz SR, et al: Reducing the risk for transfusion-transmitted cytomegalovirus infection. Ann. Int. Med. 116:55, 1992.

# Chapter 36

# NEUROLOGIC DISORDERS

ALAN J. APPLEY
JOHN S. McDONALD
STEVEN L. GIANNOTTA

For women, the childbearing years are also a time during which most neurologic diseases first manifest themselves. The parturient will often first experience symptoms of her neurologic illness during pregnancy, and for those women with preexisting neurologic disorders, some will have dramatic alterations in the course of their illness. In addition, the physiologic effects of the neurologic disorder and its treatment can have a serious impact on the course of pregnancy and the developing fetus. In this chapter, we will explore the interactions of neurologic diseases and pregnancy and discuss the specific problems in the anesthetic management of these patients.

## EPILEPSY

At least 2% of the American population (4 million people) have epilepsy and approximately one-third of those affected are women in their childbearing years (1). Epilepsy is the most common, significant neurologic disorder encountered during pregnancy, and 0.5% of all pregnancies occur in women with epilepsy (2–7).

In its strictest sense, the term "gestational epilepsy" refers to a seizure disorder unrelated to eclampsia, which manifests itself during pregnancy only. Approximately 13% of epileptic women experience their first seizure during pregnancy (1,8). Nearly 40% of these women will not have seizures at any other time and probably best fit the criteria for gestational epilepsy (8). The etiology of gestational epilepsy is not well understood, but probably stems from a combination of an altered physiologic milieu in the face of an underlying, previously silent seizure disorder. It is well recognized that pregnancy can dramatically influence seizure frequency. The most recent data demonstrate that anywhere from one-fourth to one-third of pregnant women will experience an increased frequency of seizures (Figure 36–1) (8–10). The antecedent seizure pattern will often be predictive of a change in frequency during pregnancy (8) (See Figure 36–2). Nearly all patients who experience greater than one seizure/month have more frequent seizures during pregnancy, while only one-fourth of those with less than one seizure every 9 months experience an increased rate (8).

### *Seizure Patterns*

Hormonal, metabolic, and psychologic factors have been implicated in the alteration in seizure pattern during pregnancy. Although definite supporting evidence from human clinical studies is lacking, animal models have suggested that, while estrogen and chorionic gonadotropin may lower seizure threshold, progesterone raises this threshold (Figure 36–3) (11–13). Thus, the net hormonal effect on seizure threshold may vary depending on the relative ratios of these (and possibly other) hormones. A history of catamenial (perimenstrual) epilepsy does not seem to influence the effect of pregnancy on seizure frequency (8). A reduced requirement for both local and inhalation anesthetics has been observed during pregnancy, perhaps related to neuropeptides or other hormonal alterations (14,15). This phenomenon may alter the seizure threshold influencing the observed change in seizure frequency.

Other factors associated with pregnancy that have been implicated in an altered seizure frequency include electrolyte changes (sodium, calcium, and magnesium), alkalosis secondary to a progesterone-dependent hyperventilation, and sleep deprivation.

Clinically, the most relevant cause for an increased frequency of seizures in the parturient is subtherapeutic anticonvulsant blood levels. Physiologic alterations most likely responsible for this include: (1) increased volume of distribution; (2) decreased bioavailabilty; (3) increased clearance and excretion; and (4) variations in dosage (Figure 36–4) (16–20). Expanded intravascular and extravascular volumes with increased body weight during pregnancy increase the volume of distribution for most anticonvulsants. Decreased gastric emptying and intestinal transit time may alter bioavailability. Increased maternal liver capacity, coupled with fetoplacental metabolism and increased glomerular filtration, lead to more rapid metabolism and clearance of certain anticonvulsants. Decreased protein binding during pregnancy can also lower serum anticonvulsant levels so that monitoring of unbound anticonvulsant levels may be useful in selected patients (21). Variable dosing plays an important, if not the greatest, role in altered anticonvulsant drug levels (9). This can be a result of poor compliance (often because of maternal fear of fetal teratogenesis) or inability to tolerate oral medications in early pregnancy because of nausea and vomiting. The most effective strategy in minimizing the number of seizures during pregnancy is to stress early on the importance of proper anticonvulsant

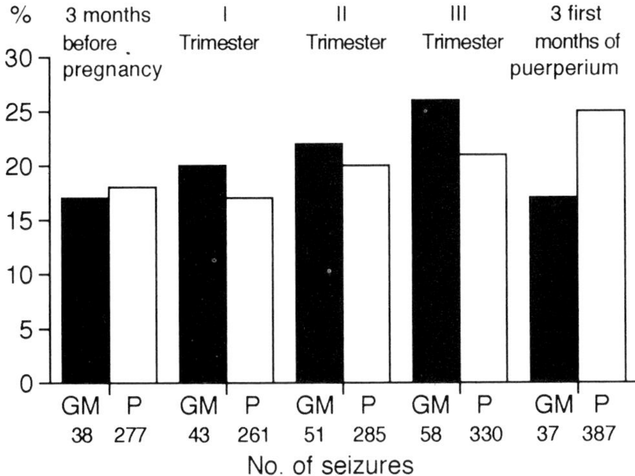


**Fig. 36–1.** The relative and absolute distribution of generalized convulsive (GM) and complex partial (P) seizures by 3-month periods. (Redrawn from Bardy AH: Incidence of seizures during pregnancy, labor and puerperium in epileptic women: A prospective study. Acta. Neurol. Scand. 75:356, 1987.)

dosing and close monitoring of serum anticonvulsant levels.

## Maternal Risks

Epilepsy and its treatment during pregnancy have been associated with an increased risk in complications of pregnancy (8,16,18,20–22). Some of the larger studies estimate that a pregnant epileptic is twice as likely to have an unfavorable outcome when compared to nonepileptic pregnant women (8,20–22). Need for induction of labor and intervention during delivery are probably more common in women with epilepsy. Bleeding at delivery is most likely increased in the pregnant epileptic because of an anticonvulsant-related vitamin K deficiency (20–22). Abruptio placentae, toxemia, and hyperemesis gravidarum probably occur equally in women with and without epilepsy (4).

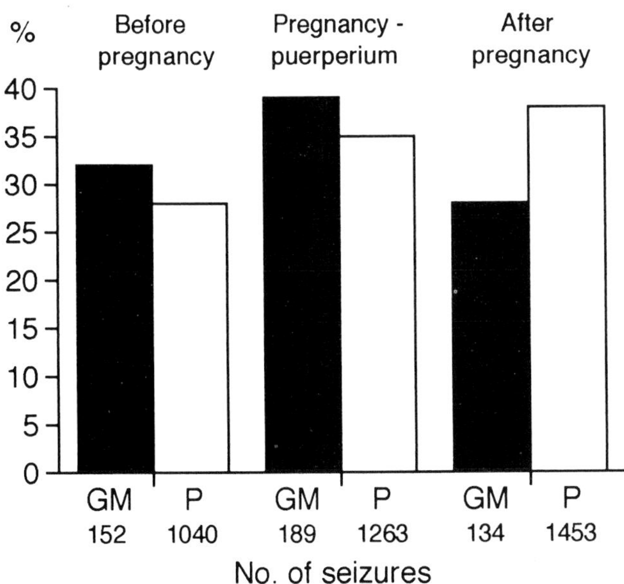


**Fig. 36–2.** The relative and absolute distribution of generalized convulsive (GM) and complex partial (P) seizures by 1-year periods. (Redrawn from Bardy AH: Incidence of seizures during pregnancy, labor and puerperium in epileptic women: A prospective study. Acta. Neurol. Scand. 75:356, 1987.)

## Fetal Risks

The effects of epilepsy and anticonvulsants on fetal outcome are not completely delineated. It is clear, however, that the incidence of preterm deliveries, low birth weight (below 2500 g), microcephaly, and developmental delay are higher in the offspring of epileptic mothers (1,18–21,23). Birth weight seems to be affected to a greater degree than can be accounted for by an increased incidence of premature births and may suggest a degree of intrauterine growth retardation (24).

The risk of congenital malformations is 1.25 to 3.00 times greater for children of epileptic mothers than it is for children of mothers without a seizure disorder (3–5,16,18,23). This phenomenon is statistically related to both seizure frequency and anticonvulsant use. Nakane, et al (23) found fetal anomalies were much less frequent in unmedicated mothers free from seizures (1.8%), and increasingly more common in unmedicated mothers with seizures (7.6%), followed by seizure-free medicated mothers (11.5%), followed by mothers receiving anticonvulsants but still having seizures (12.7%). The malformations most frequently reported in the children of treated epileptics include cardiac septal defects, cleft palate, and cleft lip (18). A constellation of anomalies characterized by limb defects, developmental delay, growth retardation, and craniofacial abnormalities has been reported as a fetal hydantoin syndrome (25). The specific relationship of this group of anomalies to hydantoins has not been confirmed in recent studies, (16,23) but it would seem that the offspring of epileptic mothers are at greater risk from the intrauterine exposure to anticonvulsants. A more clearly defined trimethadione syndrome exists (26), and valproic acid has been associated with neural tube defects, cleft palate, and urogenital anomalies (2,27). Although the adverse effects of single-drug anticonvulsant therapy are difficult to isolate, there is recent evidence that strongly suggests that multidrug therapy increases the incidence of an unfavorable outcome of pregnancy (23).

A well-recognized neonatal complication of maternal anticonvulsant use (almost exclusively due to phenytoin or phenobarbital) is a vitamin K-dependent coagulopathy (2–5,18,28). In contrast to hemorrhagic disease of the newborn, in which infants usually bleed from superficial sites 2 to 5 days postpartum, these infants often display evidence of hemorrhage intrapartum or within the first 24 hours after delivery (2,18,28). In addition, the bleeding sites are unusual, and fatal intracavitary (pleural, pericardial, peritoneal). Retroperitoneal or intracranial hemorrhages have been noted even after atraumatic normal delivery. The administration of oral vitamin K during the last several weeks of pregnancy or intravenously during

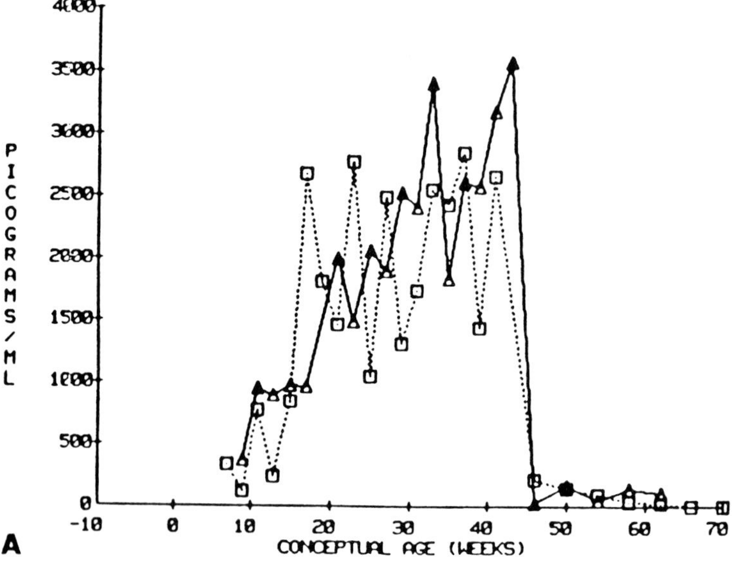


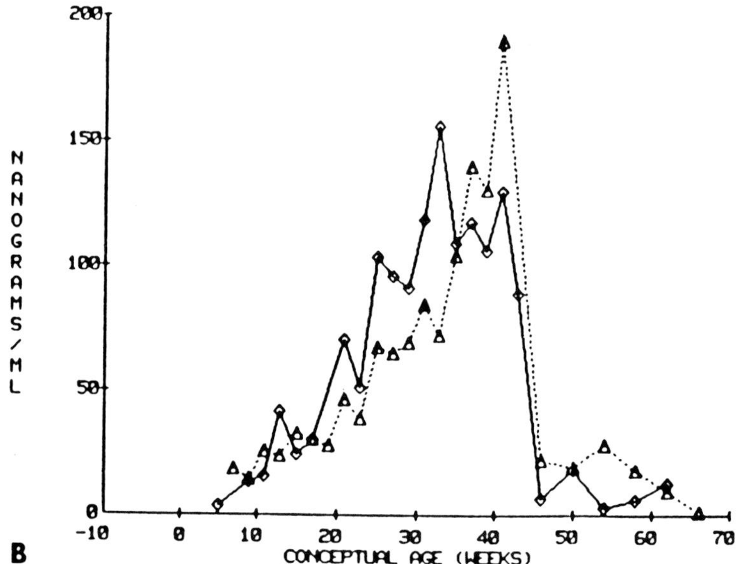


**Fig. 36–3.** Plot of mean total plasma estradiol **(A)** and progesterone **(B)** levels in epileptic women during and after pregnancy. Data are grouped by whether seizure frequency decreased (solid line) or increased (dotted line) during pregnancy. (From Ramsay RE: Effect of hormones on seizure activity during pregnancy. J. Clin. Neurophysiol. 4:23, 1987.)

labor should prevent this coagulopathy, but the infant should also routinely receive 1 mg of intramuscular vitamin K and clotting studies should be obtained from the cord blood with appropriate replacement of clotting factors if necessary (3,5).

Other neonatal complications of maternal anticonvulsant use include barbiturate withdrawal and sedation, and feeding difficulties due to antenatal phenytoin therapy (4,18).

Maternal seizures threaten not only the mother by major effects on the cardiovascular system in response to endogenous epinephrine and norepinephrine concentrations, but the fetus as well and are thought to cause hypoxia and decreased uteroplacental blood flow (2,29) (See Figure 36–5). Lactic acidosis and fetal hypoxia during a maternal seizure have also been documented (29,30). The most life-threatening example of generalized epilepsy is status epilepticus (31,32). This is infrequently encountered, but control of the airway and timely abatement of the seizures are imperative. Diazepam and lorazepam have been used to control status epilepticus with good success. Midazolam, a short-acting, water soluble imadobenzodiazepine, has recently been investigated for use in seizure control with good results from intramuscular, as well as intravenous, administration (33). The patient should also receive a loading dose of either phenytoin or phenobarbital immediately after administering diazepam or related agents. Refractory status epilepticus has been successfully and safely controlled with a continuous infusion of 7 to 12 mg/hr of midazolam after an initial 10 mg bolus injection (32).

## Eclampsia

Eclampsia, defined as the development of seizures or a neurologic deficit (including impairment of conscious-

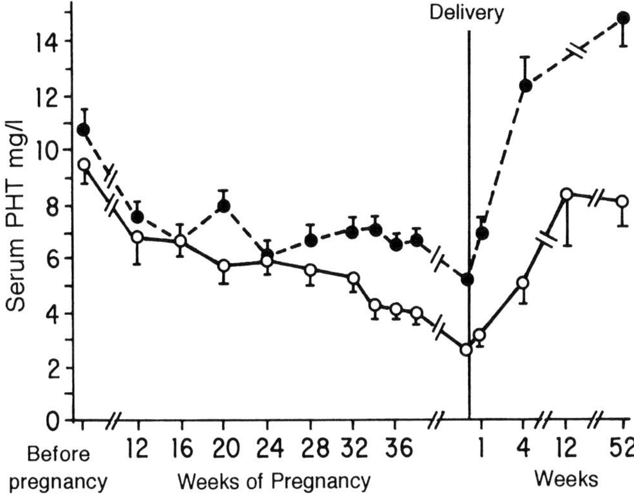


**Fig. 36–4.** Serum phenytoin (PHT) concentrations (mean ± standard error of mean) during pregnancy and puerperium in 58 cases on unchanged dosage (solid line) and 53 cases with increased drug dosage (broken line). Note the decrease in concentrations during pregnancy and at delivery and the rapid increase during first puerperal weeks. (Redrawn from Bardy AH, Hiilesmaa VK, Teramo KAW: Serum phenytoin during pregnancy, labor and puerperium. Acta. Neurol. Scand. 75:374, 1987.)

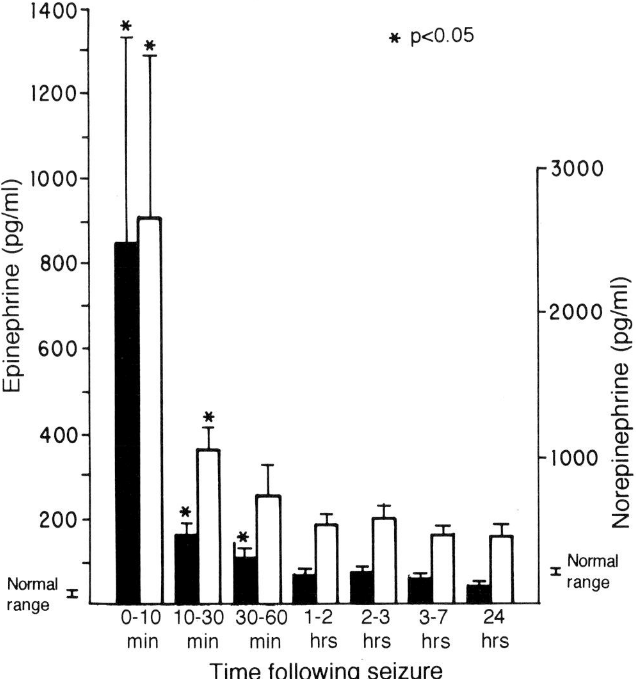


**Fig. 36–5.** Plasma epinephrine and norepinephrine concentrations following a single generalized tonic-clonic convulsion. Data are expressed as geometric means (± SE);* indicates $p < 0.05$. (Redrawn from Simon RP, Aminoff MJ, Benowitz NL: Changes in plasma catecholamines after tonic-clonic seizures. Neurology 34:255, 1984.)

ness) in parturients with preeclampsia, occurs in 0.05 to 0.2% of all deliveries (34). The seizures of eclampsia constitute a special class of epilepsy and are managed in a unique fashion. The pathogenetic mechanisms behind eclamptic seizures are not well understood. The degree of hypertension does not correlate well with the incidence of seizures (35,36). Hypertensive encephalopathy, disseminated intravascular coagulation (DIC) with resultant embolization of platelet-fibrin clots to the cerebral microcirculation, and severe cerebral vasospasm have also been implicated (36). The resultant cerebral ischemia with micro-hemorrhages, and even macro-hemorrhages, is one likely etiologic factor in eclamptic convulsions. Cerebral hemorrhage and edema account for 30 to 40% of maternal deaths due to eclampsia (36–38). Electroencephalography (EEG) is usually abnormal in the acute phase of eclampsia (39). However, the EEG pattern is nonspecific (diffuse slowing with or without focal slowing or paroxysmal spikes) and is similar to that observed in most metabolic encephalopathic states (33,39). CT scanning is usually not necessary in the evaluation of simple eclamptic convulsions, but persistent postpartum seizures, focal neurologic deficits, headache, nuchal rigidity, or a depressed level of consciousness warrant neuroradiologic investigation to rule out a space-occupying mass lesion.

The ideal treatment of eclamptic seizures relies on the prompt delivery of the fetus and placenta (33). Control of hypertension (primarily with hydralazine) and prevention or control of maternal seizures with parenteral magnesium sulfate are the cornerstones of the medical management of severe preeclampsia or eclampsia (33,36). The anticonvulsant effect of the magnesium is poorly understood, but probably relates to a central action partly because the therapeutic anticonvulsant serum levels of magnesium (6 to 8 mEq/l) are below the levels needed to produce skeletal muscle relaxation (12 to 17 mEq/l) (33,36). Dinsdale (40) and Kaplan, et al (41) recently reviewed the ongoing controversy regarding the role of magnesium in the treatment of eclamptic seizures.

## ANESTHETIC CONSIDERATIONS FOR EPILEPSY

Generally speaking, no specific anesthetic technique is contraindicated in epilepsy. This means local, regional, and general techniques can be considered for pain relief associated with either labor and delivery or cesarean section.

There are, however, certain important principles to be aware of in regard to use of agents in epilepsy. In a more general sense, the use of local anesthetic agents presents a certain threat to the mother in regard to the precipitation of seizures. We must recall that local anesthetics can have two quite opposite effects at the CNS level: one, of course, is at a lower level, where local anesthetics can have a potent anticonvulsant effect, but at a higher level, local anesthetics can produce convulsions on their own. This well-known paradoxical effect of local anesthetics at low blood concentrations as compared to high blood concentrations is a fact that is well-known to anyone working with local anesthetics. What is sometimes not appreciated is that there are other effects that influence the seizure threshold, i.e., the drug level at which an individual patient will experience a convulsion due to a certain milligram per milliliter blood level. Some of these other effects were previously mentioned, most notable of these include a patient who may be hypercapnic or have an elevated $pCO_2$. The question of whether a general anesthetic agent such as enflurane should be used for cesarean section in case of general anesthesia in a patient with a history of epilepsy is a question that is still in search of an answer. To this date, no published human data exist to confirm whether the administration of enflurane in such a circumstance would increase the risk of convulsions. However, recent evidence suggests that the effect of inhalational anesthetic agents on humans is more complex than initially viewed. Table 36–1 shows the various anesthetic agents in both epileptic and nonepileptic populations and the relationship to seizures in the two groups of patients; one group was a clinical group and the other group had an actual EEG study. In fact, Table 36–2 shows that even some of these agents can have an anticonvulsant effect, and this is documented by either the clinical or EEG study method, and as can be seen from the table, enflurane is designated as an anticonvulsant effect both by the clinical study and the EEG study. It would seem that, in spite of all the evidence that suggests that enflurane at higher dosages administered in the presence of a patient with a low $pCO_2$ may induce seizure activity, and, as this is counterbalanced against the effect that enflurane itself can act as an anticonvulsant drug in certain seizure disorders, the apparent conclusion is that enflurane, if used, should be used only in small concentrations and certainly those patients in which enflurane is used should not be hyperventilated as is sometimes the situation in the pregnant patient.

In regard to hyperventilation of the pregnant patient, there was a time when many of the patients who were in spontaneous labor, for example, would have evidence of $pCO_2$ in the low teens or upper teens because of hyperventilation due to pain. In addition, there was a period of time when anesthesiologists would hyperventilate the patient after an induction, and this might artificially cause a hypocapnic state and therefore subject the patient to a greater possibility of seizure from the use of enflurane. Even in patients without epilepsy, local anesthetic can precipitate a seizure by combination of central nervous system stimulation and reduced seizure threshold. A patient's condition is known to affect the pharmacodynamic and pharmacokinetic impact of a drug. We know, for example, that in the older age group, the half-life of a drug effect is increased due to the problems associated with biotransformation and excretion of drugs. Therefore, there may be a toxic effect of a drug due to a buildup of the drug as a result of its slow elimination over time. In addition, we know that the situation of acidosis or hypoxia also increases the toxic effects of drugs, such as local anesthetics. Certainly, recent clinical documentation has shown us that bupivacaine seems to have a greater cardiotoxicity in pregnancy than in the nonpregnant state. Patients who have the condition of epilepsy may or may not have a reduced incidence of reactions to local anesthetics, i.e., convulsions. It would appear that more important to management would be the drug interactions and the amount of local anesthetics used in patients and the avoidance of situations such as acidosis. Previous injection of local anesthetics for pain relief during either labor or at the time of cesarean section would certainly render such patients more prone to seizures or convulsions. Figure 36–6 shows the relationship between arterial $pCO_2$ and the dose of intravenous lidocaine in producing seizures. As is readily apparent from the figure, as the arterial $pCO_2$ increases, the dose of lidocaine needed to produce seizures decreases. Because most of the causes for acidosis are often respiratory acidosis, an increase in $pCO_2$, as just mentioned, would, therefore, make a patient more susceptible to central nervous system toxic effect or convulsion.

A review of factors that alter seizure frequency with pregnancy includes an alteration in electrolyte balance of sodium, calcium and magnesium, reduction in requirement of anesthetic agent, and subtherapeutic anticonvulsant blood levels. Of the three, subtherapeutic anticonvulsant blood level is the most relevant cause of seizures in the parturient, as mentioned at the outset of this the chapter. One of the series of questions during anesthetic workups of anticonvulsants should include: Was the patient underdosed because of nausea/vomiting, other causes? Did she get periodic serum anticonvulsant levels? With these questions in mind, the anesthesiologist should reduce his/her use of anesthetics to the minimal effective dosage warranted. This concept will provide adequate analgesia, enhance maternal comfort, and minimize exposure to seizures during the peripartum period.

Other physiologic factors effect the seizure threshold. One example of these other factors is shown in Figure 36–6, in which the relationship of $paCO_2$ with seizure levels in cats is demonstrated. Investigative work with local anesthetics, seizure thresholds, and cellular depressants has shown us that it is prudent to consider $paCO_2$ in cases of epilepsy for a membrane-stabilizing effect.

In a more specific sense, the volatile anesthetic agent enflurane should not be used as a cesarean section agent in cases of general anesthesia. This is the only volatile anesthetic agent that has been shown to have the potential of precipitating seizures.

## Labor Management

For the first stage, the lumbar epidural technique with continuous small dosages provides good pain relief while simultaneously exposing the mother to minimal drug levels. To complete the analgesia for second stage, one of three techniques may be considered. Because the pain and discomfort of second stage is due to lower vaginal and perineal distension, which is mediated via S-2 to 4 fibers, some type of blockade must be used to denervate this area. The three more classical techniques include: (1) injection of a more concentrated local anesthetic with greater volume to adequately penetrate those larger and more distant sacral fibers; (2) use of a caudal injection of local anesthetic to accomplish the same; and (3) use of a combined pudendal block with $N_2O/O_2$ inhalation analgesia administered just during the expulsive phase. The

**Table 36–1.** Proconvulsant Effects of Inhalation Anesthetics in Humans

| Agent | Population | Seizure Documentation: Clinical Report | Seizure Documentation: EEG Study | Type of EEG Electrodes Used in Study | Source |
|---|---|---|---|---|---|
| Nitrous oxide | Nonepileptic | + | – | Surface | A, B, C |
| | Epileptic | – | – | Depth | D |
| Halothane | Nonepileptic | – | – | Surface | E, F, G |
| | Epileptic | – | – | Surface | H |
| Enflurane | Nonepileptic | + | + | Surface | I, J, K, L, M, N, O |
| | Epileptic | + | + | Surface/depth | P, Q, R, S |
| Isoflurane | Nonepileptic | – | – | Surface | T, U, V, W |
| | Epileptic | N/A | N/A | | |
| Sevoflurane | Nonepileptic | – | – | Surface | X |
| | Epileptic | N/A | N/A | | |
| Desflurane (I-653) | Nonepileptic | N/A | N/A | | |
| | Epileptic | N/A | N/A | | |

+ Presence of seizures.
– Absence of seizures.
EEG Electroencephalographic.
N/A Information not available.
A (From Krenn J, Porges P, Steinbereithner K: Case of anesthesia convulsions under nitrous oxide-halothane anesthesia. Anaesthetists 16:83–5, 1967.)
B (From Steen PA, Michenfelder J: Neurotoxicity of anesthetics. Anesthesiology 50:437–53, 1979.)
C (From Yamamura T, Fukuda M, Takeya H, Goto T, et al: Fast oscillatory EEG activity induced by analgesic concentrations of nitrous oxide in man. Anesth. Analg. 60:283–8, 1981.)
D (From Ferrer-Allado T, Brechner VL, Dymond A, Cozen H, et al: Ketamine-induced electroconvulsive phenomena in the human limbic and thalamic regions. Anesthesiology 38:333–44, 1973.)
E (From Burchiel KJ, Stockard JJ, Calverley RK, Smith NT, et al: Electroencephalograms abnormalities following halothane anesthesia. Anesth. Analg. 57:244–51, 1978.)
F (From Backman LE, Lofstrom B, Widen V: Electroencephalography in halothane anesthesia. Acta. Anaesthesiol. Scand. 8:115–30, 1964.)
G (From Findeiss JC, Kien GA, Huse KOW, Linde HW: Power spectral density of electroencephalogram during halothane and cyclopropane anesthesia in man. Anesth. Analg. 48:1018–23, 1969.)
H (From Bennett DR, Madsen JA, Jordan WS, Wiser WC: Ketamine anesthesia in brain-damaged epileptics: electroencephalograms and clinical observations. Neurology 23:449–60, 1973.)
I (From Virtue RW, Lund LO, Phelps M Jr, Vogel JHK, et al: Difluoro-methyl 1,1,2-trifluoro-2-chloroethyl ether as an anesthetic agent: results with dogs, and a preliminary note on observations in man. Can. Anaesth Soc. J. 12:233–41, 1966.)
J (From Botty C, Brown B, Stanley V, Stephan CR: Clinical experiences with compound 347, a halogenated anesthetic agent. Anesth. Analg. 47:477–505, 1968.)
K (From Lebowitz MH, Blitt CD, Dillon JB: Clinical investigation of compound 347 (Ethrane) Anesth. Analg. 49:1–10, 1970.)
L (From Bart AJ, Homi J, Linde HW: Changes in power spectra of methoxyflurane and Ethrane. Anesth. Analg. 50:53–63, 1971.)
M (From Wollman H, Smith AL, Hoffman JC: Cerebral blood flow and oxygen consumption in man during electroencephalograms seizure patterns induced by anesthesia with Ethrane. Federation. Proc. 28:356, 1969.)
N (From Burchiel KJ, Stockard JJ, Myers RR, Smith NT, et al: Metabolic and electrophysiologic mechanisms in the initiation and termination of enflurane-induced seizures in man and cats. Electroencephalogr. Clin. Neurophysiol. 38:555, 1975.)
O (From Neigh JL, Garman JK, Harp JR: The electroencephalograms pattern during anesthesia with Enthrane: effects of depth of anesthesia, $Paco_2$, an nitrous oxide. Anesthesiology 35:482–7, 1971.)
P (From Niejadlik K, Galindo A: Electrocorticographic seizure activity during enflurane anesthesia. Anesth. Analg. 54:722–4, 1975.)
Q (From Fariello RG: Epileptogenic properties of enflurane and the clinical interpretation. Electroencephalogr. Clin. Neurophysiol. 48:595–8, 1980.)
R (From Flemming DC, Fitzpatrick J, Fariello RG, Duff T, et al: Diagnostic activation of epileptogenic foci by enflurane. Anesthesiology 52: 431–3, 1980.)
S (From Lebowitz MH, Blitt CD, Dillon JB: Enflurane-induced central nervous system excitation and its relation to carbon-dioxide tension. Anesth. Analg. 51:355–63, 1972.)
T (From Eger EI II, Stevens WC, Cromwell TH: The electroencephalogram in man anesthetized with Forane. Anesthesiology 35:504–8, 1971.)
U (From Homi J, Konchigeri HN, Eckenhoff JE, Linde HW: A new anesthetic agent—Forane: preliminary observations in man. Anesth. Analg. 51:439–47, 1972.)
V (From Clark DL, Hosick EC, Adam N, Castro AD, et al: Neural effects of isoflurane (Forane) in man. Anesthesiology 39:261–70, 1973.)
W (From Pauca AL, Dripps RD: Clinical experience with isoflurane (Forane). Br. J. Anaesth. 45:697–703, 1973.
X (From Avramov MN, Shimgu K, Omatsu Y, Osawa M, et al: Effects of different speeds of induction with sevoflurane on the EEG in man. J. Anesth. 1:1–7, 1987.)

latter technique is very useful and can be instituted in short order without extensive lead-time requirements. However, the use of the combined lumbar epidural and caudal epidural truly provides the ultimate in control of both the differential pain stimulus of first stage versus second stage, and the control of blood pressure. The latter looms as more and more important in instances of fetal compromise because maternal blood pressure reduction has such an impact on uterine placental blood flow.

A newcomer in management of current labor pain for both the patient and second stage has been very well accepted recently and consists of the continuous administra-

**Table 36–2.** Anticonvulsant Effects on Inhalation Anesthetics in Humans

| Agent | Anticonvulsant Documentation: Clinical Report | Anticonvulsant Documentation: EEG Study | Type of EEG Electrodes Used in Study | Source |
|---|---|---|---|---|
| Nitrous oxide | – | – | Surface | A |
| Halothane | + | + | Surface | B, C |
| Enflurane | + | + | Surface | B, D |
| Isoflurane | + | + | Surface | A, E, F, G |
| Sevoflurane | N/A | N/A | | |
| Desflurane (I-653) | N/A | N/A | | |

\+ Successful termination of status epilepticus reported.
– Failure to eliminate seizures reported.
EEG Electroencephalogram.
N/A Information not available.
A (From Ropper AH, Kofke WA, Bromfield EB, Kennedy SK: Comparison of isoflurane, halothane, and nitrous oxide in status epilepticus (letter). Ann. Neurol. 19:98–9, 1986.)
B (From Opitz A, Marschall M, Degan R, Kocj D: General anesthesia in patients with epilepsy and status epilepticus: *In* Edited by AV Delgado-Escueta, CG Wasterlain, DM Treiman, RJ Porter: Status Epilepticus: Mechanisms of Brain Damage and Treatment. New York, Raven Press, 1983, pp. 531–5.)
C (From Delgado-Escueta AV, Wasterlain CG, Treiman DM, Porter RJ: Management of status epilepticus. N. Engl. J. Med. 306: 1337–40, 1982.)
D (From Opitz A, Oberwetter WD: Enflurane or halothane anaesthesia for patients with cerebral convulsive disorders? Acta. Anaesthesiol. Scand. 71(Suppl):43–7, 1979.)
E (From Kofke WA, Snider MT, Young RSK, Ramer JC: Prolonged low flow isoflurane anesthesia for status epilepticus. Anesthesiology 62: 653–6, 1985.)
F (From Kofke WA, Snider MT, O'Connell BK, et al: Isoflurane stops refractory seizures. Anesthesiol. Rev. 15:58–9, 1987.)
G (From Kofke WA, Ropper A, Young RSK, Gray L, et al: Isoflurane for anesthesia status epilepticus. Neurology 37(Suppl 1):103, 1987.)

tion of a dilute local anesthetic (0.0625% bupivacaine) with a low-dose opioid (0.5% mcg/ml sufentanil) with epinephrine (1:200,000 concentration) via a mechanical pump. This sufentanil-bupivacaine-epinephrine solution, which was developed over a 2-year period by Dr. John S. McDonald and his colleagues at The Ohio State University, has been found to be the most efficacious clinically. It has been used for over 2000 lumbar epidural anesthetics recently without any notable maternal or fetal complications. Moreover, the obstetricians and labor nurses are avid proponents of the method and relate that satisfaction rates are higher for both first and second stage. The interesting aspect of this technique is that adequate second stage analgesia is the rule not the exception after first stage use for more than 2 hours.

## *Cesarean Section*

Anesthesia for cesarean section can be carried out under regional techniques, which the mother usually prefers because of the beauty of the neonatal bonding and ability to interact with the newborn baby and husband. In addition, the mother usually prefers to be awake and

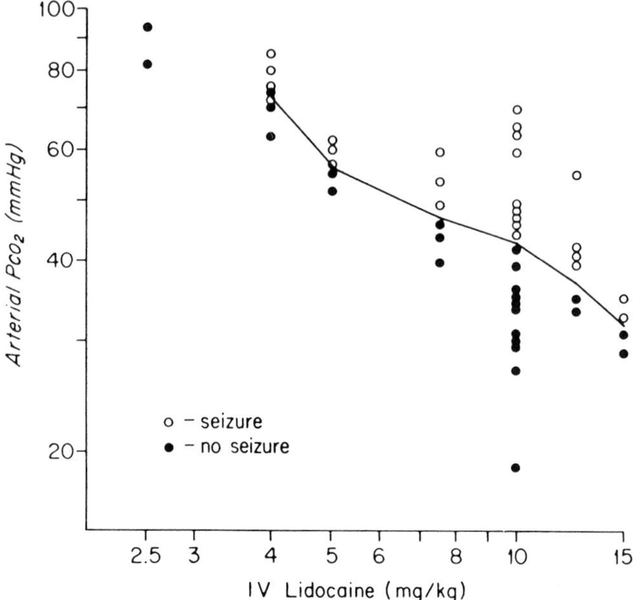


**Fig. 36–6.** The effect of $PCO_2$ on seizure threshold. (From de Jong RH, Wagman IH, Prince DA: Effect of carbon dioxide on the cortical seizure threshold to lidocaine. Exp. Neurol. 17:221, 1967.)

in control rather than to be asleep, as is the circumstance with general anesthesia.

The point has been made that the convulsive threshold may be lower in patients with seizure disorders, and, therefore, caution must be taken in injection of the local anesthetics for regional anesthesia. Today, however, there is much less a problem with maternal convulsion as a complication because local anesthetics are injected slowly and in a way that at any one time only 5 ml of drug is injected. Thus, initial therapy might consist of a 3 ml test dose followed by 5 ml of the chosen local anesthetic after a 4 to 5 minute wait. Another 4 to 5 minutes then must pass before an additional 5 ml of local anesthetic is again administered. This continues until the mother has received a full 20 ml dosage or until an adequate sensory level is detected with attention to skin testing for analgesic levels. In this fashion, a slow injection of the drug means the mother's central nervous system is not challenged with a single large dose as was the policy often in the past. Regional anesthesia for cesarean section can consist of either lumbar epidural, single-shot spinal, or continuous spinal. General anesthesia is also a choice for those mothers who do not prefer to be awake during their operative delivery. The usual rapid sequence induction with thiopental and a short-acting muscle relaxant is preferable, as documented in detail in Chapter 30. Please refer to that chapter for an in-depth discussion of the methods, concerns, and considerations of general anesthesia for cesarean section. Of course, this rapid sequence induction is somewhat modified for patients with cerebrovascular disease by use of adjunct drugs, e.g., esmolol or alfentanil, which are effective in blocking sympathetic induction effects. This admonition is repeated in "Anesthetic Considerations for Intracranial Hypertension and Neoplasms," which follows "Cerebrovascular Disease," below. One note of caution concerning enflurane: its use should be restricted in patients with seizure disorders because of the possibility of seizures with that drug (42).

## Cerebrovascular Disease

Cerebrovascular disease is relatively uncommon in young women, but it is well-recognized that pregnancy increases the risk of ischemic cerebrovascular events. In fact, pregnancy increases the risk of cerebral infarction approximately 13 times the expected rate for women of childbearing age (43). Certain selected physiologic changes that accompany pregnancy are probably responsible. There is a hypercoagulable state that reaches its peak during the third trimester, (44,45) but which may also be counteracted, at least in part, by an enhanced fibrinolytic state (44). Arterial occlusions and accompanying ischemic strokes occurring during the second and third trimesters of pregnancy and in the first postpartum week tend to coincide with these clotting alterations (46). In addition, an increase in fibrinogen and other plasma proteins (45) contributes to an increase in blood viscosity, while platelet aggregability increases in late pregnancy and the puerperium (47). The increase in plasma volume and cardiac output helps to counteract this hypercoagulable state (Figure 36–7) (48). However, the Valsalva maneuver accompanying labor can decrease cerebral blood flow (49) and, especially in the face of an underlying hematologic disorder such as sickle cell disease or thrombotic thrombocytopenic purpura, a thrombotic event may be more likely (50). In addition, extracranial cerebrovascular lesions may be more likely to present with symptomatic cerebral ischemia or infarction in the face of a hypercoagulable state and lowered cerebral blood flow.

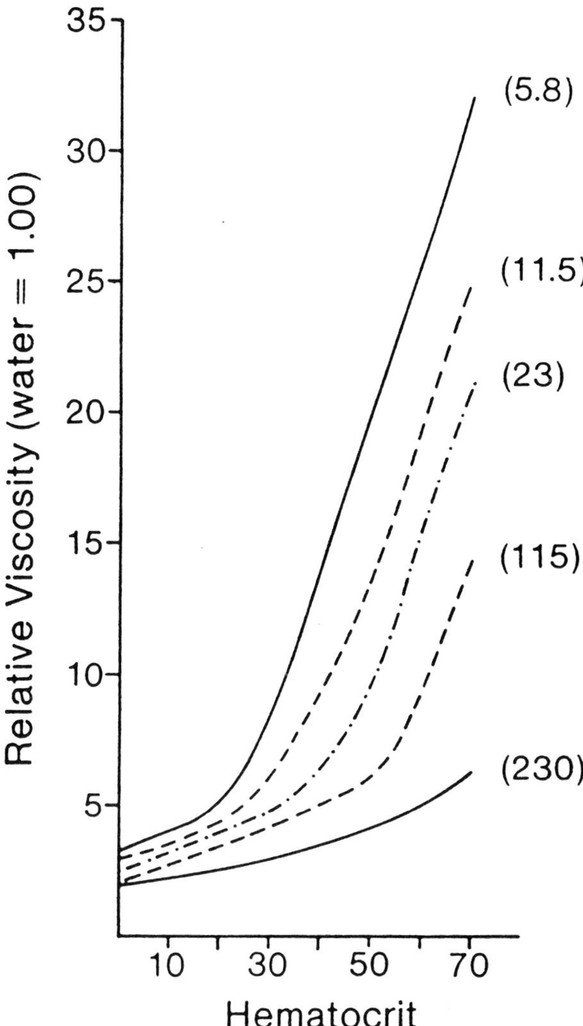


**Fig. 36–7.** Influence of hematocrit on viscosity at varying rates of shear (within parentheses by each curve). The steep portion of the curve representing a low shear rate is within the physiological range of hematocrit. (Modified from Stone HO, Thompson HK, Schmid-Nielson K: Influence of erythrocytes on blood viscosity. Am. J. Physiol. 214:913, 1968.)

## *Cardiac Disease*

Ischemic cerebrovascular events during pregnancy are often secondary to cardiac disease. Valve-related cerebral embolization can be due to endocarditis, rheumatic heart disease, or mitral valve prolapse (43). Rheumatic fever may be more likely to recur during pregnancy (51), and, as a result, all pregnant patients with a history of rheumatic fever or mitral valve prolapse should receive appropriate prophylactic antibiotic coverage during labor and delivery (52). Intracardiac thrombosis due to atrial fibrillation carries a 2 to 10% risk of cerebral embolization, and anticoagulation is recommended if sinus rhythm cannot be restored (43). Cardiomyopathy of pregnancy, if associated with embolic complications or if mural thrombi are noted on echocardiography, also necessitates the use of anticoagulants (43). Anticoagulation during pregnancy carries a heightened risk, both in terms of maternal hemorrhagic complications and fetal sequelae (53). Hall, et al (53) recently reviewed this subject. Coumarin derivatives and heparin seem to carry similar risks. The teratogenic effects of warfarin have been documented only in women who have received this drug in the first trimester of pregnancy (43).

## *Obstructive Intracranial and Extracranial Cerebrovascular Disease*

Approximately one-fourth of ischemic strokes in pregnancy are related to atherosclerosis and risk factors such as hypertension, hyperlipidemia, diabetes mellitus, and cigarette smoking, and the use of oral contraceptives are strongly implicated (43). Fibromuscular dysplasia can lead to ischemic stroke, although its management is controversial and has not been addressed in relation to pregnancy (43,53). Intracranial aneurysms, to be discussed later, are associated with fibromuscular dysplasia (54). Recently, an angiographically verified peripartum vasculopathy has been described and may be hormonally dependent (Figures 36–8, 36–9, and 36–10) (55–57).

Tuberculosis, syphilis, or other pyogenic leptomeningitides may lead to cerebral vasculitis, as can systemic

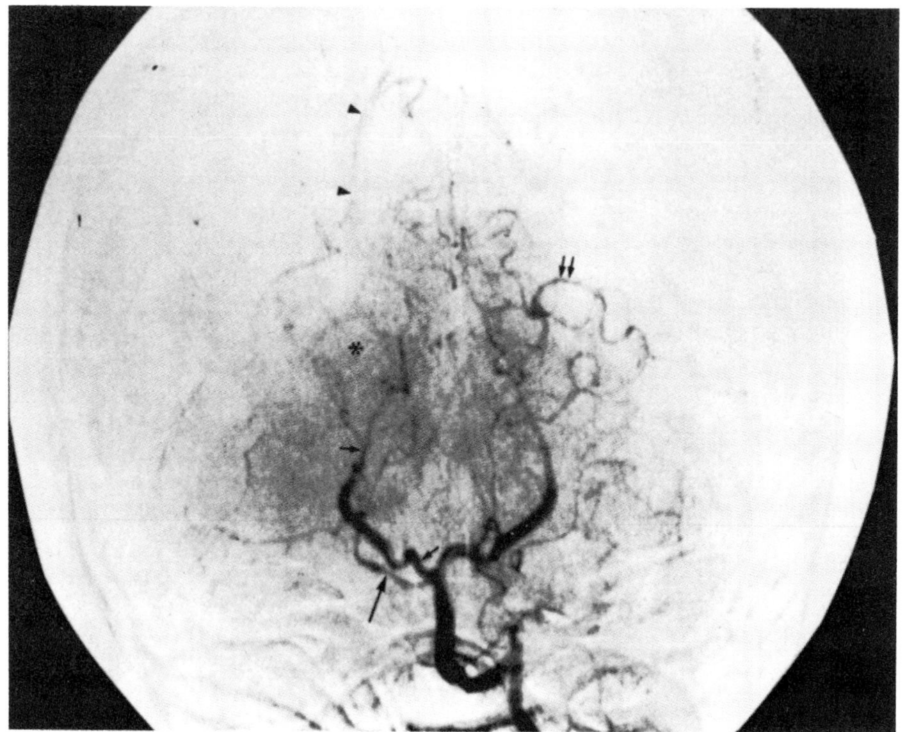

**Fig. 36–8.** Left vertebral injection demonstrates spasms of right posterior cerebral artery (arrows) with retrograde filling of peripheral branches (arrowheads) and paucity of right occipital vessels (*). Peripheral branches of left posterior cerebral artery are irregular (double arrows). Proximal right superior cerebellar artery shows marked spasm (long arrow) and the left side fails to fill. (From Trommer BL, Homer D, Mikhael MA: Cerebral vasospasm and eclampsia. Stroke 19: 326, 1988.)

lupus erythematosus (SLE) (43,58). The course of systemic lupus erythematosus may not be altered by pregnancy as was previously thought, (59) but there is a higher fetal-mortality rate among patients with systemic lupus erythematosus (58). The neuropsychiatric manifestations of systemic lupus erythematosus may be due to a generalized vasculitis or focal ischemic events, but cytotoxic antilymphocyte antibodies that cross-react with neurons and cause neurologic dysfunction in experimental animals have been identified (60).

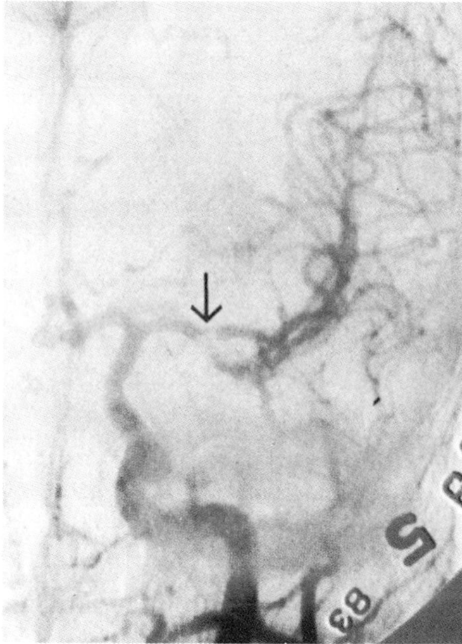

**Fig. 36–9.** Left internal carotid injection demonstrating stenotic lesion in the left middle cerebral artery (arrow). (From Brick JF: Vanishing cerebrovascular disease of pregnancy. Neurology 38:804, 1988.)

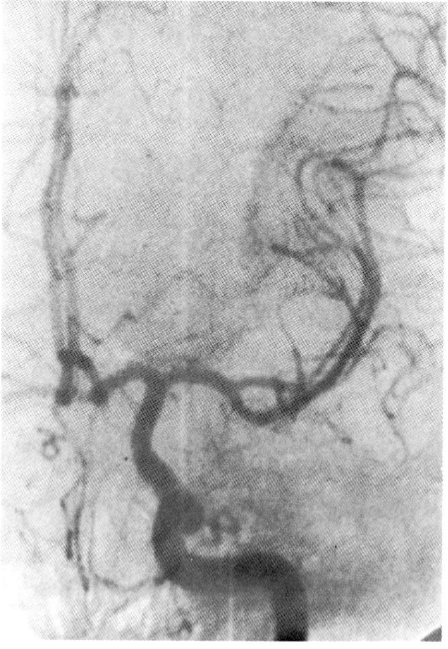

**Fig. 36–10.** Left internal carotid injection demonstrating resolution of the stenotic lesion 11 weeks after Figure 36–10. (From Brick JF: Vanishing cerebrovascular disease of pregnancy. Neurology 38:804, 1988.)

## *Intracranial Venous Thrombosis*

The incidence of cerebral venous thrombosis is approximately one case in 10,000 deliveries and occurs at least 10 times as frequently in India (61). With today's antibiotics, most cases of puerperal cerebral phlebothrombosis are aseptic (43). Prior oral contraceptive use, the hypercoagulable state of pregnancy, and other hyperviscosity syndromes such as polycythemia, leukemia, dehydration, malignancy, and sickle cell disease have been implicated as etiologic factors, but the precise cause in pregnancy is unknown (43,61,62).

The timing of the onset of cerebral phlebothrombosis is in contrast to that of arterial occlusions in pregnancy. Cerebral venous thrombosis most commonly occurs in the puerperium from 3 days to 4 weeks after childbirth, with over 80% of the cases occurring in the second and third weeks postpartum (43). With arterial lesions, 83% of cerebral venous thrombosis cases occur during pregnancy or within the first postpartum week (43,46). The clinical picture of intracranial venous thrombosis is characterized by a severe headache and a progression of variable motor and sensory disturbances. Seizures, impaired consciousness, and evidence of increased intracranial pressure are frequently encountered (43,61).

Treatment of cerebral phlebothrombosis includes hydration, anticonvulsants, and, in the absence of significant intracranial hemorrhage, anticoagulation (62,63) (See Table 36–3 for typical characteristics of three patients with cortical vein thrombosis). One of the mechanisms of stasis of intracerebral blood flow is demonstrated in

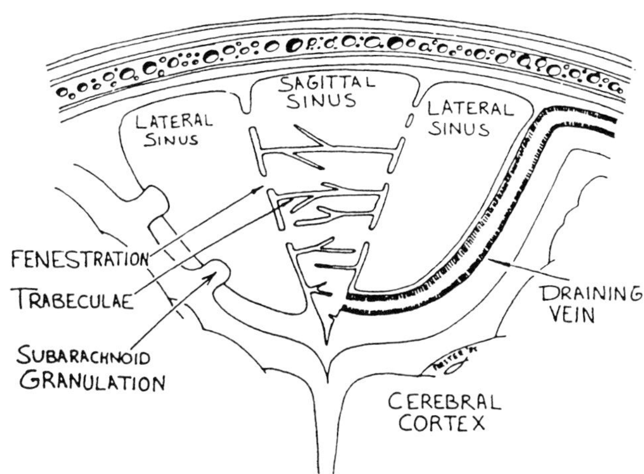


**Fig. 36–11.** Coronal view of the structures within the superior sagittal sinus with its draining cortical veins (artist's interpretation). (From Younker D, Jones MM, Adenwala J, Citrin A, et al: Maternal cortical vein thrombosis and the obstetric anesthesiologist. Anesth. Analg. 65:1007, 1986.)

Figure 36–11). In this instance, trabeculae cross longitudinally across the sagittal sinus. Anticoagulation in this setting is controversial, but Halpern, et al (64) reported an improved prognosis if the diagnosis can be established before hemorrhagic venous infarction has occurred. The mortality rate for this disease is approximately 25%, but those who survive tend to have less neurologic morbidity

**Table 36–3.** Characteristics of Patients with Cortical Vein Thrombosis

| | Patient | | |
|---|---|---|---|
| | 1 | 2 | 3 |
| Admission diagnosis | Intrauterine pregnancy | Eclampsia | Pregnancy-induced hypertension |
| Age | 20 | 15 | 18 |
| Parity | Gravida 1, para 0 | Gravida 1, para 0 | Gravida 1, para 0 |
| Weeks of gestation | 40 | 38 | 43+ |
| Medical history | Polio myelitic (poorly documented) mild right hemiparesis | Negative | Negative |
| Prior medication | None | None | None |
| Allergies | Penn G | None | None |
| Family history | None | None | None |
| Onset of symptoms | Fever, headache, weakness | Seizures, fever | Seizures, disseminated intravascular coagulation |
| Mode of delivery | Vaginal forceps | Cesarean section | Cesarean section |
| Anesthetic | Lumbar epidural; dural puncture ×2 | General endotracheal | General endotracheal |
| Apgar scores | 8/9 | 7/9 | 7/8 |
| Clinical | Seizures, hemiparesis, aphasia | Hypertension, seizures | Seizures, coagulopathy, hypertension |
| Radiologic findings | Cerebral arteriogram: positive | CAT scan: positive | CAT scan: positive |
| Urinalysis | 2+ bacteria | 1+ protein | 2+ protein |
| Outcome | Return to baseline neurologic status | Complete resolution | Complete resolution |
| Discharge diagnosis | Cerebral venous thrombosis | Cerebral venous thrombosis; eclampsia | Cerebral venous thrombosis |

(From Younker D, Jones MM, Adenwala J, Citrin A, et al: Maternal cortical vein thrombosis and the obstetric anesthesiologist. Anesth. Analg. 65:1007, 1986.)

than do those patients with infarcts due to arterial cerebrovascular disease (63).

## *Other Embolic Lesions*

Amniotic fluid, fat, air, and metastatic choriocarcinoma cells can occasionally embolize to the cerebral vasculature. Amniotic fluid emboli occur most commonly in older multiparous women with a uterine or birth canal tear. Metastatic choriocarcinoma can embolize to the cerebral vasculature and result in infarction or intracerebral hemorrhage due to erosion of the vessel wall (43,65). Systemic venous thromboembolism is more common in pregnancy because of the increased incidence of pelvic and lower extremity thrombophlebitis. This carries with it a 30% chance of paradoxical cerebral embolization due to a patent (or potentially patent) foramen ovale (43).

The laboratory evaluation of the patient with cerebral ischemia should include a complete blood count (including smear and platelet count), erythrocyte sedimentation rate, electrolyte determination, serum cholesterol and triglyceride levels, serologic studies, coagulopathy screening, β-HCG level, urinalysis, chest roentgenography, and electrocardiography (43). Neuroradiologic imaging should begin with magnetic resonance imaging (MRI) of the brain, if available and if the patient is stable; CT scanning otherwise is mandatory (66). The relative risks to the fetus of CT versus MRI have not been studied, but MRI poses less danger to the mother and fetus than does CT with intravenous contrast material. Echocardiography and Holter monitoring may be indicated should the clinical history, physical examination, and laboratory studies suggest cardiac pathology. Neurovascular imaging studies (noninvasive and invasive intravenous or intra-arterial angiography) may be undertaken and will help direct further medical or surgical management of the offending lesion.

## *Intracranial Hemorrhage*

Spontaneous intracranial hemorrhage during pregnancy can be associated with severe morbidity. The most common site of bleeding is into the subarachnoid space and its cause can usually be traced to an underlying aneurysm or arteriovenous malformation (AVM). Subarachnoid hemorrhage (SAH) accounts for approximately 12% of maternal mortality, occurs in 1 to 4 of every 10,000 deliveries, and is more common in preeclamptic than noneclamptic women (57,67). The clinical presentation is quite characteristic with the sudden onset of a severe headache, which is often accompanied by nausea, vomiting, photophobia, signs of meningeal irritation, depressed consciousness, seizure activity, and focal motor or sensory disturbances. Aneurysmal subarachnoid hemorrhage during pregnancy most commonly occurs in women between the ages of 25 and 35, and usually presents in the third trimester or up to 6 weeks postpartum (67,68). On the other hand, arteriovenous malformations are usually encountered in women under 25 years of age and are most likely to rupture in the second trimester and in the immediate peripartum period (68).

For the parturient suspected of an intracranial hemorrhage, timely neuroradiologic investigation is of the utmost importance. CT scanning without intravenous contrast accurately detects all but the smallest amount of subarachnoid blood. A lumbar puncture (LP) is indicated in the face of a normal CT scan (69). Cerebral angiography should be carried out as soon as possible once a subarachnoid hemorrhage has been documented, the patient is stabilized, and obstetric evaluation has been carried out to determine gestational age and fetal well-being (Figure 36–12) (70).

The initial medical management of a patient with a subarachnoid hemorrhage consists of bedrest, judicious use of analgesics, administration of anticonvulsants, and maintenance of at least a normovolemic state (71). Subarachnoid hemorrhage can have a number of serious sequelae, including hyponatremia, hydrocephalus, cardiac dysrhythmias, ischemia, and increased intracranial pressure. However, rebleeding and vasospasm with cerebral ischemia are two complications of subarachnoid hemorrhage that are responsible for most of the morbidity and

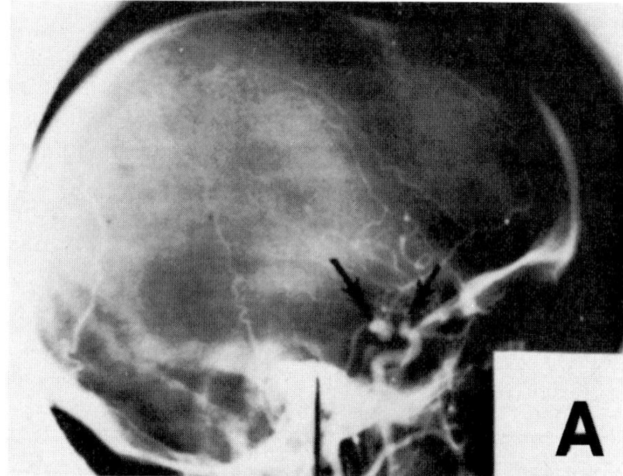


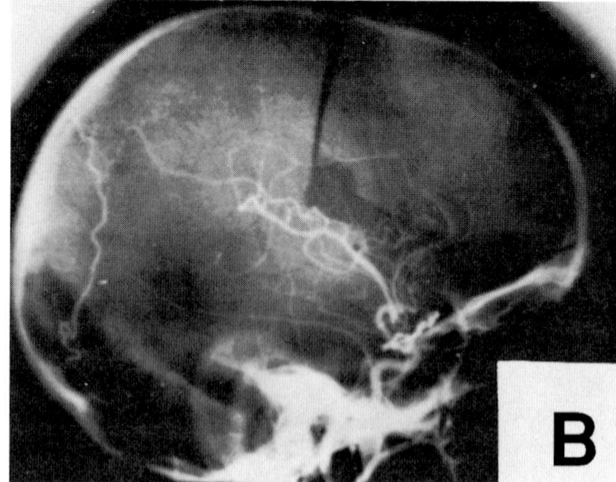


**Fig. 36–12.** **A,** Cerebral angiogram demonstrating two internal carotid artery aneurysms (straight arrows) and poor filling of cerebral vessels consistent with vasospasm. **B,** Postoperative cerebral angiogram in the same patient demonstrating successful clip ligation of both aneurysms. Vasospasm has resolved. (From Giannotta SL, Daniels J, Golde SH, Zelman V, et al: Ruptured intracranial aneurysms during pregnancy. A report of four cases. J. Reprod. Med. 31:139, 1986.)

mortality. Aneurysmal rebleeding is the most lethal consequence of subarachnoid hemorrhage and is responsible for as much as 70% of deaths (Figure 36–13) (70). The likelihood of rebleeding from a ruptured intracranial aneurysm is probably highest in the first 24 hours, but still poses a significant risk at any time until the aneurysmal sac is obliterated (Figure 36–14). Antifibrinolytic agents have been used to decrease the incidence of recurrent subarachnoid hemorrhage from ruptured aneurysms, but their use may be associated with an increased morbidity from ischemic complications of cerebral vasospasm (72). In addition, there is very little data on the use of antifibrinolytics in pregnancy and their effect on the fetus.

Cerebral vasospasm after subarachnoid hemorrhage is a complex subject that has been reviewed extensively recently (73–75). The signs of cerebral vasospasm are generally those of cerebral ischemia and infarction. Vasospasm generally does not occur before the fourth postbleed day and usually peaks between the seventh and tenth postbleed day. There is a trend today toward performing craniotomy for clip ligation of ruptured aneurysms as soon as possible after presentation to prevent early rebleeding and to allow optimal medical management of vasospasm, should it occur. This includes hypervolemia with intravenous colloid solutions and hypertensive/hyperdynamic therapy with phenylephrine, dopamine, or dobutamine. The morbidity and mortality of cerebral vasospasm remain unacceptably high and multicenter trials of various agents to prevent this phenomenon such as calcium channel blockers are currently underway. With today's fetal monitoring capabilities and neuroanesthetic techniques, surgical management of ruptured intracranial aneurysms during pregnancy should not differ significantly from that in a nonpregnant patient.

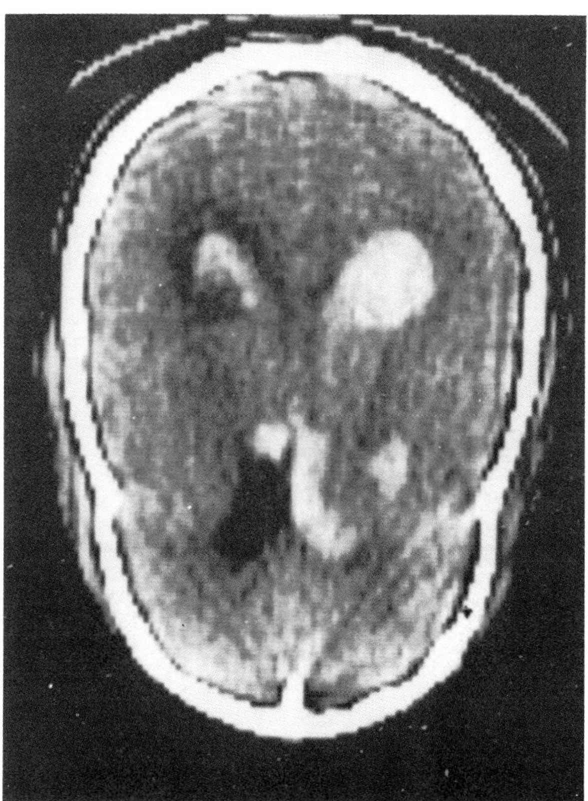

**Fig. 36–14.** CT scan showing massive intraventricular hemorrhage from aneurysmal rebleed. (From Giannotta SL, Daniels J, Golde SH, Zelman V, et al: Ruptured intracranial aneurysms during pregnancy. A report of four cases. J. Reprod. Med. 31: 139, 1986.)

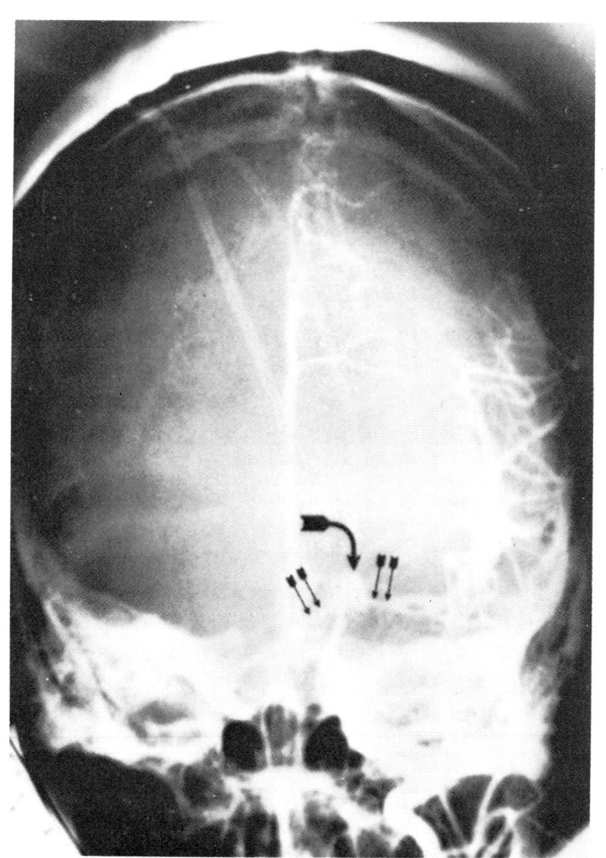

**Fig. 36–13.** Cerebral angiogram. Curved arrow points to aneurysm, straight arrows identify focal areas of vasoconstriction. (From Giannotta SL, Daniels J, Golde SH, Zelman V, et al: Ruptured intracranial aneurysms during pregnancy. A report of four cases. J. Reprod. Med. 31:139, 1986.)

## ANESTHETIC CONSIDERATIONS FOR CEREBROVASCULAR DISEASE

The anesthetic considerations in cerebrovascular disease states are of a specific nature that are geared to offer minimal fluxes in systemic blood pressure and reflex by minimal changes in central nervous system (CNS) pressure. For the most part, cardiac disease, obstructive intracranial disease processes, intracranial venous thrombosis, intracranial, and hemorrhage all are best managed with regional anesthesia with minimal effective doses and careful attention to avoid hypertensive changes for maternal protection while also concomitantly avoiding hypotension for fetal protection.

Often these patients have had surgical intervention at

some prior time, either in a previous pregnancy or the current one. All general management decisions must be made in consultation with the anesthesiologist, the obstetrician, and the neurosurgeon or neurologist whomever is the current physician relevant to the parturient's central nervous system problem. Patients with cerebrovascular disease personify the ultimate in close communication and coordination of care in a difficult medical disease state complicated by pregnancy and delivery. Many of the more seriously ill patients will undoubtedly be managed by cesarean section with general anesthesia, an obligatory choice due to concern about differential pressure changes between the intracranial/intraspinal spaces. Naturally, at all costs, the disorder of brain stem herniation must be avoided. If general anesthesia is used, it often must also be modified due to the previously mentioned requirement for avoidance of systemic pressure changes. Avoidance of systemic pressure changes is no problem and can be accomplished with larger than usual doses of thiopental, use of alpha blocking agents, or use of preinduction opioids. Again, close cooperation and communication and consultation among the neurosurgeon, the obstetrician, the anesthesiologist, and the pediatrician will allow satisfactory anticipation and management of the "sleepy newborn" in such a case. Management of the "sleepy newborn" is of no consequence in regard to management of the depressed neonate who does not spontaneously breathe well immediately postdelivery due to respiratory depression from drugs administered to the mother for the purpose of avoiding fluxes in maternal central nervous system pressure. Management of immediate neonatal respiratory depression is of little consequence if the delivery takes place in a level 4 center where there is an adequate neonatal intensive care unit management available. All of these complicated management cases in which close communication and coordination must take place among three or more levels of staff should be carried out in centers that are fully staffed and experienced with these complexities.

### *Labor Management*

For the care of those patients who are able to labor and deliver vaginally, two paramount rules must be kept in mind in regard to the parturient and her health and well-being: (1) the avoidance of either hypo-hypertensive changes associated with first or second stage analgesia; and (2) the avoidance of Valsalva maneuver in second stage.

The first problem can be solved by use of regional anesthesia, using, preferably, the lumbar epidural with small minimum effective doses that will provide adequate analgesia, while at the same time keeping the maternal blood pressure stable.

The second problem can be addressed by use of a sacral anesthetic dose given at the appropriate time in the second stage while discontinuing the lumbar epidural injections. The best methods of accomplishing this are: (1) use of the lumbar epidural catheter with the patient in the sitting position during injection of a small but more concentrated dose of local anesthesia, i.e., 8 to 10 ml of 0.5% bupivacaine or 2% lidocaine; (2) use of a caudal catheter with injections of 5 ml of 0.5% bupivacaine or 2% lidocaine; (3) use of a saddle block for perineal analgesia only; and (4) use of a pudendal block, again for selective perineal analgesia only.

A confounding problem that may arise is concern over a patient's coagulation status when she has been on autocoagulant therapy. Here again, careful, detailed consultation among the anesthesiologist, the obstetrician, and the neurosurgeon must be carried out with evaluation of the risks and benefits fully explored. In some cases, it may be acceptable to lower the autocoagulant exposure to a point at which regional anesthesia could be safely performed.

### *Cesarean Section*

Anesthesia for cesarean section can be carried out under regional techniques, which the mother usually prefers because of the beauty of the neonatal bonding and ability to interact with the newborn baby and husband. In addition, the mother usually prefers to be awake and in control rather than to be asleep as in the circumstance with general anesthesia.

Regional anesthesia for cesarean section can consist of either lumbar epidural, single shot spinal, or continuous spinal. General anesthesia is also a choice for those mothers who do not prefer to be awake during their operative delivery. The usual rapid sequence induction with thiopental and a short-acting muscle relaxant is preferable, as documented in detail in Chapter 30. Please see that chapter for an in depth discussion of the methods and concerns and considerations of general anesthesia for cesarean section. Of course, this rapid sequence induction is somewhat modified for patients with cerebrovascular disease by use of adjunct drugs, e.g., esmolol or alfentanil, which are effective in blocking sympathetic induction effects. This admonition is repeated later under "Anesthetic Considerations for Intracranial Hypertension and Neoplasms."

## Intracranial Hypertension and Neoplasms

Intracranial tumors are relatively uncommon, with an expected incidence for all ages of 4 to 5/100,000 population (76). During the early reproductive years, this incidence is much lower, but approaches the average incidence by age 40. Nonetheless, brain tumors do occur during the reproductive years and, in fact, may present or undergo accelerated growth during pregnancy. In addition, with the average age of parturients on the rise, there should be a concomitant rise in the incidence of intracranial neoplasms during pregnancy.

Brain tumors are not specifically related to pregnancy (Table 36–4), but the pregnant state can influence dramatically the growth and symptomatology of certain tumors. The sodium and water retention during pregnancy may hasten the symptomatic presentation of gliomas or meningiomas, and the altered hormonal milieu can affect the growth of meningiomas, pituitary tumors, and vascular neoplasms (77–80). See Table 36–5 for pregnancy-associated CNS tumors.

**Table 36–4.** Distribution of Brain Tumors in Nonpregnant and Pregnant Women Aged 20 to 40 Years

| | % of Brain Tumors | |
|---|---|---|
| **Tumor Type** | **Nonpregnant Women*** | **Pregnant Women**** |
| Meningioma | 29 | 29 |
| Plexus papilloma | 1 | 2 |
| Ependymoma | 5 | 2 |
| Cerebellar astrocytoma | 5 | 7 |
| Glioma | 36 | 38 |
| Vascular | 4 | 5 |
| Acoustic neurinoma | 15 | 14 |
| Medulloblastoma | 3 | 3 |

* (From Zulch KJ: Pathologische Anatomie der raumbeengenden intrakraniellen Prozesse. *In* Hanbuch der Neurochirurgie. Edited by Olivacrona H, Tönnis W. Berlin, Springer-Verlag, 1956, pp. 3, 45–69, 103, 104, 143–176.)
** (125,138,139–180,181–198,199–207)

### *Pituitary Tumors*

Until recently, pregnancy has been uncommon in patients with clinically symptomatic pituitary tumors. This is because most women with these tumors are infertile, usually because of hyperprolactinemia or hypopituitarism. However, since the advent of dopamine agonists (such as bromocriptine) and agents capable of inducing ovulation (such as clomiphene and gonadotrophins), there has been a dramatic rise in the number of pregnant women harboring a pituitary tumor.

The normal pituitary gland enlarges progressively during pregnancy, and by term its weight has nearly doubled (81). The hypertrophy and hyperplasia of prolactin-secreting cells (previously known as pregnancy cells) are responsible for this enlargement. Thus, it is not unexpected that tumors of the pituitary also enlarge during pregnancy.

Prolactinoma is the most common pituitary neoplasm encountered during pregnancy. The effects of pregnancy on both untreated and previously treated tumors have been recently reviewed by Molitch (78) who found that the risk of clinically important microadenoma enlargement during pregnancy was 1.6%. For macroadenomas (tumors greater than 1 cm in diameter), the risk of symptomatic tumor enlargement was 15.5%. Headaches and visual field deficits are the most common clinical findings in these patients. Should bromocriptine be unsuccessful in significantly reducing tumor size and in improving visual field loss, then a transsphenoidal adenomectomy is advocated. The effects of bromocriptine on the developing fetus are unknown, but adverse effects have not been reported.

Neither the previous treatment of a tumor, nor the presence of a tumor during pregnancy, seem to affect the spontaneous abortion rate or the perinatal mortality rate (79). A reported increased prematurity rate may be due to both the greater number of multiple pregnancies from ovulation induction and third trimester terminations in symptomatic patients. With today's neuroanesthetic tech-

**Table 36–5.** Pregnancy-Associated Central Nervous System Tumors

| | Tumor Site (References) | | |
|---|---|---|---|
| **Tumor Type** | **Supratentorial** | **Infratentorial** | **Spinal** |
| Meningioma | 55 | 2[125,151] | 5[139,152–155] |
| Convexity | 16[125,127–137] | | |
| Hypophyseal region | 15[125,137–146] | | |
| Sphenoid olfactorial | 20[125,138,139] | | |
| Not specified | 4[135] | | |
| Plexus papilloma | 3[125] | 2[135,165] | |
| Ependymoma | 0 | 3[133,135–137] | 3[153,176] |
| Cerebellar astrocytoma | 0 | 12* | 2 |
| Glioma | 55** | 7[125,138,170–175,177] | 1[177] |
| Vascular | 1[178] | 14[125,134,175–181] | 17[184–198] |
| Neurinoma | 0 | 30[125,138,199–201] | 0 |
| Medulloblastoma | | 6[125,135,137,202,204] | |
| Gangliocytoma | 1[205] | 0 | 0 |
| Pinealoma | 1[135] | | |
| Cholesteatoma | 3[126,206,207] | 0 | 0 |
| Total | 174 | 76 | 28 |

* (125,132,133,135,137,150,166–169)
** (125,132,134–138,146–149,127–207)

(Rest of data from Roelvink NCA, Kamphorst W, van Alphen HAM, Rao RB: Pregnancy-related primary brain and spinal tumors. Arch. Neurol. 44:209, 1987.)

niques, safe transsphenoidal adenomectomy should prevent early termination of pregnancy for symptomatic prolactinomas.

### Other Intracranial Neoplasms

Gliomas, which arise from the supportive glial cells and grow by infiltration of normal brain parenchyma, are the most common group of intra-axial neoplasms during the reproductive years. These tumors present with signs and symptoms of increased intracranial pressure (ICP), seizures, behavioral changes, or other focal neurologic deficits. Cerebral edema can be prominent and high-potency glucocorticosteroids (e.g., dexamethasone and methylprednisolone) are the mainstay in its treatment. Diuretics may also be necessary with significantly increased intracranial pressure or mass effect. Surgical decompression is then usually indicated and can be safely accomplished with appropriate neuroanesthetic management. Radiotherapy is usually administered in patients with high-grade tumors and can be delivered with proper shielding. The potential adverse effects of chemotherapy on the mother and the fetus outweigh the mostly theoretical benefits in malignant gliomas.

Usually slow-growing and highly vascular, meningiomas are extra-axial and become symptomatic by compression and distortion of the brain substance. In addition, there is a highly variable degree of associated cerebral edema quite sensitive to glucocorticoids. The rapid progression of symptoms in some parturients harboring meningiomas is well-recognized (77). Receptors specific for sex steroid hormones, as well as glucocorticoids, have been identified in varying relations in most meningiomas (80). Accordingly, hormonal therapy is under investigation for the adjunctive treatment of these tumors, but its role during pregnancy remains theoretical.

Hemangioblastoma, schwannoma, neurofibroma, craniopharyngioma, chordoma, epidermoid, dermoid, teratoma, choroid plexus papilloma, pineal region tumors, and colloid cysts can all occur during the reproductive years, but there is no evidence that their growth is influenced by pregnancy. Metastatic tumors are very uncommon in women of childbearing age, but choriocarcinoma deserves special note. Approximately 1 in 40,000 pregnancies in the United States precede the development of choriocarcinoma (77). The incidence of metastasis to the brain is approximately 20% (82). These lesions often present with an intracranial hemorrhage, either intratumoral or by rupture of a cerebral vessel wall following digestion by trophoblastic enzymes. The amount of mass effect produced by the lesion dictates the urgency of surgical intervention. Radiotherapy and chemotherapy have improved dramatically the survival of these patients (77). Serum human chorionic gonadotrophin determination should be performed on all patients presently or recently pregnant with a spontaneous intracranial hemorrhage.

### Benign Intracranial Hypertension

This syndrome is characterized by symptoms of increased intracranial pressure and visual obscurations without other focal neurologic signs and is due to an imbalance in the mechanisms of CSF production and absorption (77). The disease is usually self-limited and, during pregnancy, is less common than expected from age-matched and sex-matched controls (83). Some reports indicate that pregnancy does not alter the course of the disease (77,83), but other investigators have documented a definite worsening during gestation (84,85). Lumbar puncture reveals normal CSF under high pressure, and treatment includes diuretics, glucocorticoids, serial lumbar punctures and, in some cases, lumboperitoneal shunting. Close monitoring of the patients' visual status is of utmost importance.

### Head Trauma

The management of the pregnant patient with a head injury differs little from that of the nonpregnant patient. Intensive monitoring and medical management, including seizure control, diuresis, sedation, skeletal muscle relaxation, and hyperventilation may be required in the severely head-injured patient without a surgical lesion. In the presence of an operable mass lesion or penetrating trauma, surgical treatment should be carried out without delay.

There have been reports of pregnancies carried to term or near-term in vegetative and severely brain-injured patients (86,87). Hill, et al (86) cite the maintenance of maternal homeostasis, in a vegetative patient, from early in the second trimester to delivery of a normal fetus at 34 weeks gestation. Field, et al (88) recently reviewed this subject with special attention to medical and ethical issues.

## ANESTHETIC CONSIDERATIONS FOR INTRACRANIAL HYPERTENSION AND NEOPLASMS

In a broad sense, the primary concern and admonition in regard to anesthesia for patients with intracranial hypertension is prevention of any exacerbation of that state. Thus, any technique that increases intracranial pressure during induction is generally to be avoided. Examples of this might be standard induction of general anesthesia, which often can invoke remarkable increases in systemic pressure and also intracranial pressure. The mechanism for this is understood to be minimal analgesia and sedation that results in reflex physiological changes. These can be avoided by use of either preinduction administration of opioids for analgesia or by use of sympathetic blocking drugs such as esmolol or alfentanil, which prevent the increase in vascular resistance (89). Thus, with careful planning for avoidance of the aforementioned induction increases in central nervous system pressure, the general anesthetic technique may be used for cesarean section delivery with good results. Naturally, there is a need to confer with the obstetrician and pediatrician so that they will understand that the modifications to the induction may cause neonatal depression in the early neonatal period.

### Labor and Delivery

First of all, there probably are few instances in which labor and delivery will be the option taken in delivery of a patient who has life-threatening intracranial hypertension.

Most of these patients will be delivered by cesarean section. However, for those patients who are suffering from small increases, labor may be an option, and if it is, the following can be considered for pain relief. Local and regional anesthetic techniques can be considered for pain relief in labor and for delivery in patients with increased intracranial pressures and neoplasms. The key element here is to provide excellent pain relief so that there is minimal apprehension and stress from the mother's standpoint and minimal pain during contractions so that the reflex physiological changes associated with labor, documented in Chapter 13, are avoided. These consist chiefly of increases in heart rate, blood pressure, systemic vascular resistance, and respiratory rate. The best technique available for providing such an atmosphere during labor is the continuous epidural. The use of the catheter and injection of the combination local anesthetic and opioid as detailed earlier under "Anesthetic Considerations for Cerebrovascular Disease" could be one of the better methods for obtaining pain relief in labor. Please refer to that section for labor management.

### *Cesarean Section*

For intracranial hypertension and neoplasms, again, anesthesia for cesarean section can be carried out under regional techniques, as mentioned earlier. The mother usually prefers these techniques because of the beauty of the neonatal bonding and ability to interact with the newborn baby and husband. In this situation, the primary concern is any further increase in intracranial pressure; thus, the mother must be kept quiet and reassured that all is going well and under control. Regional anesthesia for cesarean section can consist of either lumbar epidural, single shot spinal, or continuous spinal. If there is any substantial increase in intracranial pressure and concern for producing a gradient between the intracranial compartment and the spinal compartment, then general anesthesia is the choice so that brainstem herniation can be avoided. As mentioned, there must be an induction that avoids any maternal physiological fluxes in blood pressure, heart rate, and intracranial pressure, and this is, essentially, the same concern as that voiced in the section on "Anesthetic Considerations for Cerebrovascular Disease." Here, just as in mothers who suffer from disorders of cerebrovascular disease, the induction of anesthesia must be smooth.

## SPINAL CORD LESIONS

### Trauma

Spinal cord injury occurs in approximately 25/1,000,000 men and women annually between the ages of 15 and 30 years. Cervical and thoracic injuries each comprise just under half of the lesions, with lumbosacral levels making up the remainder. Motor vehicle accidents are responsible for nearly half of the injuries in females (90).

Pregnancy can be a preexisting condition in a woman who sustains a spinal cord injury, and pregnancy is becoming increasingly more common in women with varying levels of preexisting paralysis. In the case of a pregnant patient sustaining a spinal cord injury, stabilization of both the patient's cardiorespiratory status and her spinal column is preeminent. Although spinal cord injury per se does not appear to alter fetal development, associated hypoxia, hypotension, infections (urinary tract, respiratory tract, and decubiti), anemia, and deep vein thrombosis can affect the fetus adversely (89,91).

**Table 36–6.** Level of Spinal Cord Lesion

T6 and above: 21 women—27 deliveries (1 intrauterine death, 1 set of twins).
- 13 vaginal and forceps
- 7 vaginal (1 breech)
- 7 C-sections (A)

During 22 of these deliveries, hyperreflexia was experienced. (1 patient developed a cerebral intraventricular bleed with coma.) (A; B; C; D)

Below T6: 12 women—23 deliveries (1 set of twins).
- 3 vaginal and forceps
- 8 vaginal
- 12 C-sections (1 patient 4; 1 patient 2; 5 patients 1) (1 set of twins)

Indication:
- 1 fear of bladder damage
- 1 ruptured membranes
- 1 premature twins with presenting cord

A (From Nath M, Vivian, Cherney W: Autonomic hyperreflexia in pregnancy and labor: a case report. Am. J. Obstet. Gynecol. 134: 390–392, 1979.)
B (From Oppenheimer W: Pregnancy in paraplegic patient: two case reports. Am. J. Obstet. Gynecol. 110:784–786, 1971.)
C (From Tabsh KMA, Brinkman CR, Reff RA: Autonomic dysreflexia in pregnancy. Obstet. Gynecol. 60(1):119–121, 1982.)
D (Ravindran RS, Cummins DF, Smith IE: Experience with the use of nitroprusside and subsequent epidural analgesia in a pregnant quadriplegic patient. Anesth. Analg. 60(1):61–63, 1981.)
(Rest of data from Verduyn WH: Spinal cord injured women, pregnancy and delivery. Paraplegia 24:231, 1986.)

Autonomic hyperreflexia is an important problem unique to patients with complete spinal cord injuries at T-6 and above (89). This syndrome is characterized by the acute onset of systolic and diastolic hypertension, sweating, skin blotching, and headache. The effects of a sudden reflex sympathetic outflow cannot be adequately compensated for by the intact parasympathetic system above the level of injury. This often results in bradycardia, although tachycardia is not uncommon in high quadriplegics (89). Verduyn (90) reported a series of 27 deliveries in 21 paraplegic women, 22 of which were complicated by autonomic dysreflexia. Bladder distension, if present, must be relieved (Table 36–6). Vasodilators are used to control hypertension, but the blood pressure can be very labile during labor. The hypertensive phase occurs during contractions and this swing in blood pressure during labor can help differentiate autonomic dysreflexia from pregnancy-induced hypertension (preeclampsia). Such a distinction can be difficult to make due to the frequent finding of proteinuria in spinal cord injured patients (89).

### *Tumors and Vascular Malformations*

Intramedullary, tumors such as astrocytomas and ependymomas do not have a specific association with pregnancy, and comprise only 15% of all spinal cord tumors (90,92). However, the incidence of vascular tumors such as hemangioblastoma seems to be increased during pregnancy, and hemangioblastoma have a tendency to become symptomatic during the third trimester (81). Although spinal meningiomas occur most commonly in women past childbearing age, pregnancy can stimulate rapid growth of these tumors, causing them to present much earlier.

Vascular malformations of the spinal cord (especially arteriovenous malformation and associated aneurysms) can cause subarachnoid hemorrhage or ischemic and compressive symptoms (i.e., back pain, lower extremity weakness, sensory changes, and bowel and bladder disturbances), that can fluctuate during pregnancy (93). Surgical management of intraspinal masses during pregnancy should not differ significantly from that during the nonpregnant state. The presence of progressive signs and symptoms of spinal cord compression or ischemia should dictate the urgency of the situation.

## Anesthetic Considerations for Spinal Cord Lesions

Anesthesia for the pregnant patient with spinal cord lesions presents an unusual opportunity for the specialist in this area to demonstrate talent in anesthesiology, medical judgment, and willingness to cooperate with both the obstetrician and the patient's neurologist or neurosurgeon, or whoever is managing the neurologic complications during the patient's gestation and delivery. Because the chief problem associated with spinal cord lesions is one of motor paralysis and sensory denervation, there may or may not be a need for anesthesia for either labor or delivery, depending on the level of sensory loss due to cord damage. Each case must be individualized, but in general terms, if the lesions are located in and around the T-10 level, then there is normally adequate sensory denervation so that regional or local blockade is not necessary. If, on the other hand, the extent of damage is below this level, then there may be some considerable preservation of sensation, which may necessitate some analgesia either by systemic medication or regional anesthesia should the first stage of labor be the problem, or regional anesthesia, local anesthetic blockade, or inhalation analgesia should the second stage be the problem. One of the serious problems that must be anticipated is autonomic hyperreflexia, which, as mentioned under the section on spinal cord lesions, is quite commonly a problem in patients with spinal cord injuries at T-6 and higher (Table 36–7).

**Table 36–7.** Treatment of Hyperreflexia

| | | |
|---|---|---|
| Epidural (A; B) | 6 | |
| Anaesthesia | 1 | (Patient reported physician stated she had hypertension.) |
| 5 C-sections (3 in C506 Tetraplegics, 2 in C6 Tetraplegics) | 2 | |
| Amyl Nitrate | 1 | |
| Ditropan Triple Anaesthesia, Guanethidine | 1 | |
| Arfonad | 1 | |
| Sodium Nitroprusside | 1 | |
| Magnesium Sulphate and Demerol | 1 | (Physician diagnosed pre-eclampsia) |
| Apresoline | 1 | (Only one dose after patient went into coma) |
| Diazepam plus Diphenhydramine (C) | 2 | |
| Hydralazine plus Diphendramine (C) | 1 | |
| Hydralizine plus Diphenhydramine and Promethazine (C) | 1 | |

A (From Nath M, Vivian J, Cherney W: Autonomic hyperreflexia in pregnancy and labor: a case report. Am. J. Obstet. Gynecol. 134: 390–392, 1979.)
B (From Tabsh KMA, Brinkman CR, Reff RA: Autonomic dysreflexia in pregnancy. Obstet. Gynecol. 60(1):119–121, 1982.)
C (From Young RK, Katz M, Klein SA: Pregnancy after spinal cord injuries: altered maternal and fetal response to labor. Obstet. Gynecol. 62(1):59–63, 1983.)
(Rest of data from Verduyn, WH: Spinal cord injured women, pregnancy and delivery. Paraplegia 24:231, 1986.)

### Labor and Delivery

If analgesia is needed for relief of labor pain, it can be provided by use of regional anesthesia, by use of local block anesthesia such as paracervical block and pudendal block, and by use of continuous subarachnoid block with opioids for first stage and then conversion to local anesthesia for actual delivery of the fetus. Of course, systemic analgesia by the use of opioids injected intravenously can also be effective for first stage analgesia. If the use of the local techniques proves to be inadequate for the delivery phase, then supplemental $N_2O$ analgesia can be given for added analgesia and comfort of the patient at the moment of birth. Epidural may also be used in the form of the minimal concentration dose, such as given by continuous pump as described in Chapter 13. Continuous pump allows for small doses to be administered over long periods of time. The net effect is analgesia due to the blockade of neural transmission without secondary side effects such as hypotension or toxicity due to large-dose exposures given over short periods of time.

### Cesarean Section

For cesarean delivery, any one of the methods mentioned earlier for cerebrovascular disease can be used here also, including regional anesthesia, general anesthesia, and local anesthesia. The regional techniques available include the epidural, the spinal single shot method, or the spinal continuous method. The general anesthetic technique includes the usual plan for intubation and securing of the airway, but the modification used in this special group of patients includes use of larger doses of thiopental for induction, use of larger percentages of inhalation anesthetics, and use of opioids before induction to obviate the usual stormy inductions typical of the low-dosage method that was developed to protect the fetus from depression after delivery. The local anesthetic technique is the same as that elaborated upon in Chapter 20, save that supplemental medication is used to obviate any problems that may be associated with pain or discomfort on incision and dissection and delivery of the fetus. In other words, both the general anesthetic technique and the local anesthetic technique are counterbalanced by supplementation of analgesia so that no increases in the central nervous system occur during the labor and delivery phases. The latter modification is to protect the mother from any changes that may eventually precipitate a deleterious change in the disease process at hand. The well-being and welfare of the fetus are not ignored and not threatened by such modifications because communication to the pediatrician and obstetrician by the anesthesiologist alerts them to the fact that some respiratory depression is to be expected in the newborn period and this is planned for accordingly. It is possible that the most favored technique may be epidural because it can be administered with great care and over longer intervals to prevent the possibility of a severe episode of hypotension.

## MYOPATHIES AND MYONEURAL JUNCTION DISORDERS

### Myasthenia Gravis

Myasthenia gravis (MG) is a disease of voluntary musculature that is characterized by weakness and fatiguability. Females experience approximately double the male incidence, with the peak occurrence in the third decade. The overall prevalence of this disease is 40 cases/million population (94).

The pathophysiology of myasthenia gravis is centered at the neuromuscular junction and is related to a reduction in acetylcholine receptors. An autoimmune phenomenon probably accounts for the neuromuscular junction defect, and at least in part, explains the close association of a thymic disorder with myasthenia gravis (93).

The effect of pregnancy on myasthenia gravis is unpredictable, with approximately one-third of patients showing no change in the status of their myasthenia. During pregnancy, 40% of patients will experience exacerbations, about 30% will undergo a remission, and 30% will also experience postpartum exacerbations. These postpartum exacerbations can have an acute onset with respiratory failure a frequent sequelae. The maternal mortality is 3.4/100 live births to myasthenic mothers (95).

The course of myasthenia during pregnancy, like epilepsy, can be altered by a variety of factors. The early gestational nausea can alter anticholinergic drug dosing. Anxiety can also exacerbate the symptoms of myasthenia. The relative hypoventilation in patients whose respiratory system is compromised can adversely affect the fetus and can lead to atelectasis and respiratory tract infections. These infections can, in turn, further exacerbate the myasthenic condition. Labor and delivery, with their attendant stress (emotional and physical) can exacerbate the myasthenic weakness, and respiratory compromise can occur rapidly (94).

In a study of 314 pregnancies in 217 myasthenic mothers, there was a 5% spontaneous abortion rate, an 8% perinatal death rate, while 19% of newborns experienced neonatal myasthenia gravis (myasthenic symptoms due to passive transfer of maternal antibodies specific for the acetylcholine receptor) (94). Neonatal myasthenia usually begins 12 to 48 hours after delivery and lasts an average of 3 weeks. Interestingly, α-fetoprotein can inhibit the anti-acetylcholine receptor (anti-AChR) antibody. Normal intrauterine fetal movements and the delay in onset of neonatal myasthenic symptoms are probably related to the newborn's falling α-fetoprotein levels. In addition, there seems to be evidence that a high maternal anti-AChR titer can increase the child's risk of neonatal myasthenia gravis and that these titers may be useful in predicting this (94).

The treatment of maternal myasthenia gravis should not differ greatly from that during the nonpregnant period and usually involves only manipulation of anticholinesterase and steroid dosages. Myasthenic crisis (myasthenic symptoms requiring mechanical ventilation) is managed with plasmapheresis and immunosuppression and does not differ in the parturient.

### *Myotonic Dystrophy*

Myotonic dystrophy is familial, transmitted as an autosomal dominant disorder, and has a prevalence rate between 3 to 5/100,000. The disease is characterized by myopathic weakness of the face, neck and hand, and by myotonia (failure of muscles to relax after a forceful contraction) of the muscles and tongue. Cataracts, developmental delay, alopecia, and respiratory failure are also characteristic features. Smooth muscle involvement affects the gastrointestinal tract and the uterus (96).

The disease worsens in pregnancy (usually during the second trimester) and improves significantly immediately postpartum. There have also been reports of the first appearance of clinical features occurring during pregnancy (97).

In pregnant women with myotonic dystrophy, there is a high incidence of spontaneous abortions and premature delivery related to abnormal uterine activity and polyhydramnios. Labor is affected (either prolonged or exceedingly rapid first and second stages) and excessive postpartum hemorrhage may result from an atonic uterus (95). Genetic counseling is aided by genetic-linkage studies performed after amniocentesis (98).

### *Other Myopathic Syndromes*

Myotonia congenita (Thomsen's disease) is an autosomal-dominant disorder characterized by myotonia and diffusely increased muscle bulk. The disease can worsen during the second half of pregnancy. Calcium carbonate can significantly decrease the cramps that occur during the second half of pregnancy in over 25% of women with Thomsen's disease. Restless legs syndrome, which occurs in 10% of these pregnant women, is characterized by an uncomfortable aching and an "urge to allow the legs to fidget" and is less likely to develop in women who supplement their diet with folate (37).

Connective tissue disorders such as polymyositis, dermatomyositis, and scleroderma can occur during the reproductive years causing the infant mortality rate to reach 50% when the mother's disease is severe (97).

### *Multiple Sclerosis*

Although the etiology of multiple sclerosis (MS) is unknown, immunologic abnormalities are associated with this demyelinating disease. MS affects mostly young white females living in higher latitudes. The disease usually is characterized by exacerbations and remissions of neurologic deficits, including visual impairment, ataxia, sensory disturbances, and bladder dysfunction (99).

Diagnosis rests on a characteristic clinical picture and associated laboratory abnormalities, including CSF immunoglobulin and myelin basic protein levels, MRI findings of demyelination, and abnormal evoked responses (visual, auditory, and somatosensory). The course of pregnancy does not seem to be adversely affected by MS (100,101).

The effect of pregnancy on the course of MS has been studied extensively, and it seems that fewer relapses can be expected during pregnancy. However, the risk of MS-onset, exacerbation, or progression is two to three times above the baseline rate up to 6 months postpartum (100). These data reflect the tendency for most immunologically mediated diseases (i.e., myasthenia gravis, systemic lupus erythematosus, and autoimmune thyroid disease) to improve during pregnancy (93,94). Although there is an apparent trend toward better prognosis for women with pregnancies after MS-onset, this is most likely due to the younger age of onset for these patients (100).

Therapy of MS has been less than satisfactory. Corticosteroids and ACTH seem to shorten the course of acute relapses and immunosuppressive therapy may stabilize or even reverse progression in chronically progressive MS. Plasmapheresis also plays a role in severe acute relapses. Corticosteroids and immunosuppressive agents have been associated with congenital anomalies in humans, and the antispasticity agents baclofen and dantrolene produce fetal anomalies in animals. However, a short course of corticosteroids is generally recommended in severe acute relapses during pregnancy (98).

## ANESTHETIC CONSIDERATIONS FOR MYASTHENIA, OTHER MUSCLE DISORDERS, AND MULTIPLE SCLEROSIS

Anesthetic considerations for this class of disorder are another challenge due to the special circumstances of the disease process itself. These myoneural junction abnormalities usually manifest themselves by slowness of movement and generalized motor weakness; this is not, however, a contraindication to any specific type of anesthesia. In fact, this disease process can be managed by general anesthesia, regional anesthesia, and even local anesthesia. An important part of the impaired function in myasthenia and other muscle disease processes is the unusual response to medications. This response must be kept in mind whichever anesthetic technique would be used, but the keyword here is use of minimal doses of medication and observance of the effect upon the patient before progressing onward with more medication. It must also be recalled that many patients will be receiving anticholinesterase drugs that may possibly interfere with the level and activity of endogenous cholinesterases, which are important in degradation of amide derivative local anesthetics. Because of this, in the past anesthesiologists have preferred use of only ester-derivative local anesthetics or use of spinal anesthesia in which the effect of the local anesthetic is compartmentalized and thus separated from a generalized systemic effect.

Multiple sclerosis is a poorly understood disease process that is also shrouded in mystery in regard to its remission and exacerbation history. There has been in the past a reluctance to administer regional anesthesia from fear that the patient may not recover fully and be even more severely impeded after the anesthetic wears off completely. In the first edition of this book, it was mentioned that because of this fear, regional anesthesia was not recommended. Since then, there have not been any definitive studies that indict regional anesthesia as the culprit in causing a deterioration in the patient's neurologic condition. It is still appreciated that the process or course of the disease processes cannot be predicted. It would seem prudent to make sure that the patient is aware of the fact that remissions and exacerbations occur throughout their lifetime and that it is not controlled by the fact that the patient would get a given regional anesthetic. In other words, it is wise to fully inform the patient, give her the options in regard to anesthetic techniques, and let her decide for herself whether she would prefer one method over the other. For the most part, the patient can be offered one of four alternatives that are not unlike those offered patients without neurologic disease. These alternatives consist of systemic medication, regional anesthesia, local anesthesia, and general anesthesia.

### *Labor and Delivery*

Analgesia for relief of labor pain can be provided by use of regional anesthesia such as epidural (102), by use of local block anesthesia such as paracervical block, and by use of continuous subarachnoid block with opioids for first stage pain relief. The epidural referred to for use in these patients with myasthenia and other muscular disorders is in the form of the minimal concentration dose such as given by continuous pump as described in Chapter 13. This allows for small doses to be administered over long periods of time. The net effect is analgesia due to the blockade of neural transmission, without secondary side effects such as hypotension or toxicity due to large-dose exposures given over short periods of time. Second stage analgesia completion after epidural as just described is often adequate for delivery, as is episiotomy even due to the 2 to 3 hour exposure of the sacral nerve roots to the local anesthetic, opioid, and epinephrine combination as outlined in Chapter 13. In the case of the continuous spinal in which opioid was used for first stage analgesia, either lidocaine or bupivacaine can be used for the local anesthetic analgesic effect for intense sensory denervation and muscle relaxation. This method of analgesia for labor and delivery is nicely suited for myasthenia and the other muscle disorders because, as pointed out earlier, in this disease process it is best to inject small aliquots of drug and note their effect before continuing with larger dosages. With the continuous spinal, small dosages can be injected at distinct intervals so that just the right level and intensity of block can be obtained. Systemic analgesia by the use of opioids injected intravenously is not the ideal method to be used in these patients because of the additive effect they can have upon respiration, bearing-down maneuvers, and other muscular movements that are necessary during both labor and at delivery. If the use of the local technique such as paracervical block prove to be adequate for labor, then the delivery phase can be covered by use of the pudendal block, and, if necessary, supplemented by $N_2O$ analgesia for the added analgesia and comfort at the moment of birth.

### Cesarean Section

For cesarean delivery, any one of the methods mentioned earlier in this chapter can be used, which includes regional anesthesia, general anesthesia, and local anesthesia. The regional techniques available include the epidural, the spinal single shot method, or the spinal continuous method. These regional techniques appear to be preferred in these patients with muscular disease processes because there seems to be slightly more control over the end effect of the drug. The general anesthetic technique includes the usual plan for intubation and securing of the airway, but the modification necessary in this special group of patients includes use of much smaller doses of thiopental for induction and small and judicious use of inhalation anesthetics for supplementation, if used at all. It may be necessary to invoke the verbal informed consent disclaimer to the patient in these cases because you are preferentially planning a light induction to avoid some of the complications the mother might experience if the larger, more normal dosages would be used to induce amnesia and analgesia for cesarean delivery. The local anesthetic technique is the same as that elaborated upon in Chapter 20, save that small supplemental doses should be used in these patients, again to avoid untoward maternal complications. The epidural for cesarean section in this group of patients is really very similar to that used in other patients, but smaller doses are injected with slightly greater time intervals to ensure that the desired effect of analgesia without substantial sympathetic block is occurring. After the catheter is placed, the patient is positioned with left lateral displacement of the uterus. The test dose is administered and the usual time interval of 4 to 5 minutes is observed before checking for subarachnoid spillage or intravenous spillage. Then 4 ml dosages of local anesthetic are administered with a full 6- to 7-minute interval before repeating until a level of T-6 to T-8 is obtained. If hypotension begins to develop, the patient's legs can be placed in the lithotomy position and small boluses of IV fluid can be given or, alternatively, small doses of ephedrine can be administered. The epidural as described offers the advantage of minimal homeostatic change for the mother and at the same time offers an awake delivery for the mother so that she can participate in the beauty of her child's birth and the interaction with her baby in those few precious moments after delivery.

## Disorders of the Peripheral Nervous System

### *Anterior Horn Cell Lesions*

Poliomyelitis during pregnancy has all but disappeared from the Western world, but pregnancy following childhood poliomyelitis can occasionally be encountered. Obstetric complications are directly related to degree of disability encountered (e.g., pelvic asymmetry from scoliosis and pelvifemoral, and pelvispinal and lower extremity muscle paralysis) (103). The presence of significant pelvic asymmetry necessitates delivery by cesarean section and patients with respiratory compromise can require ventilatory assistance until the gravid uterus no longer restricts diaphragmatic excursion (97,101).

Amyotrophic lateral sclerosis (ALS) is a rare degenerative disorder involving the anterior horn and lateral columns of the spinal cord and lower cranial nerve nuclei. The course of the disease, which is characterized by progressive weakness of the bulbar and distal musculature, is not altered by pregnancy. The uterine musculature is not involved and laxity of the perineal floor promotes a normal, spontaneous vaginal delivery (97,104).

### *Root and Plexus Lesions*

Back pain during pregnancy is experienced by nearly half of all women, often radiating down one or both lower extremities. Musculoskeletal causes are usually responsible, owing to increased stress by the enlarging uterus on the lumbosacral spine (105). Pelvic girdle relaxation syndromes can lead to mechanical instability and similar back pain. Transient osteoporosis of the hip, which usually develops in late pregnancy and may be a variant of reflex sympathetic dystrophy, can mimic pelvic girdle relaxation syndrome (97). Abscesses of the retropsoas or subgluteal spaces can result from pudendal or paracervical blocks and will produce postpartum back or pelvic pain (106).

Lower extremity radicular signs and symptoms during pregnancy suggest a herniated lumbar intervertebral disc. O'Connell (107) reviewed a series of women with herniated discs and found that of the women who had a history of pregnancy, 76% were asymptomatic before the pregnancy. Symptomatology developed during pregnancy in over one-half the patients and during the puerperium in another one-third. Conservative therapy (bedrest and analgesics) will usually suffice it, and surgery during pregnancy should be limited to those patients with a caudal equina syndrome due to a large centrally herniated disc or severe intractable radicular pain. Cervical radiculopathy is managed in a similar fashion and rarely requires surgical intervention during pregnancy.

Attacks of acute familial brachial plexus neuritis, although rare, have a striking tendency to occur during pregnancy and immediately postpartum (108). Lumbosacral plexus lesions during pregnancy are most commonly due to compression by the fetal head or obstetric forceps (37). The portion of the plexus containing elements of the L-4 and L-5 roots is most commonly injured, usually producing a unilateral foot drop on the side opposite the vertex presentation. Upper sacral roots can also be affected. Pain during delivery is common, but not universal, and the neurologic deficit may go unnoticed until the patient ambulates postpartum (especially after regional anesthesia). Prognosis is usually good for incomplete lesions, and these patients usually require cesarean section for future pregnancies, especially should dystocia develop (37).

### Peripheral Nerve Lesions

Other maternal obstetric palsies include obturator nerve compression intrapelvically, femoral nerve injury in the lithotomy position, and peroneal nerve palsy from improperly positioned leg straps (97).

Entrapment or compression syndromes are quite common during pregnancy. Symptoms of carpal tunnel syndrome have been reported in 25% of pregnant women that usually begin during the last two trimesters (107). Fluid retention is probably responsible for these compression syndromes, and the median nerve compression resolves spontaneously in up to 85% of cases (109). Two percent of parturients experience paresthesias in the fourth and fifth fingers resulting from ulnar nerve compression at the elbow (107). Tarsal tunnel syndrome (posterior tibial nerve compression) is also more common during pregnancy and results in pain and dysesthesias in the foot (107). Pain and dysesthesias are usually self-limited and abnormal posterior tibial nerve conduction almost always reverts to normal by 6 weeks postpartum (107).

Meralgia paresthetica, due to compression of the lateral femoral cutaneous nerve, is characterized by sensory disturbances over the anterolateral aspect of the thigh and is relieved by sitting or lying down. Symptoms are often bilateral, occur during the last trimester, and almost always regress after delivery (107).

Bell's palsy (idiopathic facial paralysis) is over three times more common in pregnant than in nonpregnant women. The onset is sudden and, depending on the severity of the paralysis, recovery can take 3 to 12 weeks or more. Complete lesions almost universally leave some residual deficit. Corticosteroids have been used safely in pregnancy for partial lesions that progress. Surgical decompression is controversial and rarely indicated. Pregnancy does not seem to affect the prognosis for recovery of facial nerve function (97,110).

Charcot-Marie-Tooth disease is a rare neuropathy with autosomal dominant transmission. There have been a number of reports concerning affected women who experienced exacerbation of their disease during pregnancy, probably secondary to endoneurial edema. Symptoms usually resolve after delivery, and the fetus should not be adversely affected (97).

### Polyneuropathies

The most common cause of metabolic polyneuropathy in the pregnant woman is nutritional deficiency. Although now uncommon in developed countries, this entity can also be seen with hyperemesis gravidarum, and patients can present with a thiamine deficiency and Wernicke's encephalopathy. Vitamin $B_{12}$ deficiency can also lead to a polyneuropathy as well as degenerative changes in the spinal cord (111).

The acute porphyrias present with abdominal symptoms followed by a peripheral neuropathy (including autonomic nerves) and attacks seem to be precipitated by pregnancy (97,112). Hormonal changes have been implicated in these pregnancy-related exacerbations as well as drugs, especially barbiturates and many other hepatically metabolized agents (97). Most of these exacerbations occur in early pregnancy and are usually not associated with increased fetal or maternal morbidity. However, prematurity and high fetal and maternal mortality rates can result from attacks later in pregnancy. Postpartum attacks are not uncommon and may be related to barbiturate therapy during pregnancy and labor (113). Phenothiazines are helpful with the abdominal symptoms, and beta-blocking agents are useful in managing the tachycardia and hypertension (97).

Landry-Guillain-Barré syndrome (acute inflammatory polyradiculoneuritis) is a demyelinating disease affecting 0.4/100,000 women and probably is immunologically mediated. An illness, surgical procedure, or inoculation within 8 weeks prior to the onset of symptoms is reported by over two-thirds of the patients (97).

A variable degree of generalized weakness with less prominent sensory changes, cranial nerve dysfunction and dysautonomia characterize this syndrome (110). Pregnancy does not seem to influence the course of this disease, but labor and delivery can be affected somewhat by pelvic and abdominal muscle weakness (111). Vaginal delivery, though usually safe, may require forceps or vacuum assistance (111). The risk of premature labor is increased, but there does not seem to be a significant effect of this disease on fetal well-being (97). The main risk to the mother and child is respiratory failure in advanced disease; these patients may require ventilatory assistance that is usually transient. Treatment is mainly supportive, although immunosuppression and plasmapheresis may be helpful.

Prognosis is generally good for a significant, if not full, recovery of neurologic function. However, approximately 3% of patients will experience one or more relapses and these episodes have been associated with pregnancy (112).

Diabetic neuropathy can occur in the pregnant patient, although this condition is not necessarily associated with pregnancy (97). The neuropathy is primarily sensory, although dysautonomia can be a prominent feature in advanced cases.

### Anesthetic Considerations for Disorders of the Peripheral Nervous System

The anesthetic considerations for this class of disorders include the anterior horn cell lesions, the root and plexus lesions, peripheral nerve lesions, and the polyneuropathies. The considerations here are, like the others in this chapter on neurologic disorders, important, impact significantly on the comfort of the patients, aid the medical decision-making process by the obstetrician, and are comforting to the neurologist or internist or family physician who is primarily responsible for the patient with the neurologic disorder. Most if not all of the patients with anterior horn lesions such as poliomyelitis or amyotrophic lateral sclerosis are not in serious danger of respiratory distress or collapse. These patients who have gotten pregnant have some muscular reserve and many times suffer from mid to lower cord lesions. As mentioned in the earlier section, if the lesion is at or above the T-10 level, there may be automatic sensory loss from the uterus and upper birth canal, and anesthesia for labor and delivery may not be necessary. There are many patients, however, who do need analgesia, and these patients deserve and demand careful consideration and application of the best of obstetric anesthesiology principles. The point was made in the last section that the patient should be given full informed consent regarding the benefit and side effects of regional analgesia techniques such as epidural and spinal blocks. There have been no definitive papers over the last 20 years that identify these regional techniques as being injurious to the underlying disease process or that offer proof that the disease process is exacerbated or activated. Thus, this edition will make a definite stand on suggesting that the patient be given full information in regard to this point and that she also be given the description of the alternatives such as local injection, systemic medication, and, in the case of cesarean delivery, general anesthesia. The patient thus should be able to make an informed decision in regard to which technique she desires. There may be certain mitigating circumstances that make epidural an unlikely method to use, such as the presence of an active inflammatory process (polyradiculoneuritis) in and around the nerve roots of T-10 to L-4, or there may be the unusual but possible scenario of a patient being in the throes of an active caudal equina syndrome. These latter clinical problems would naturally mitigate against use of the regional techniques, epidural block, or subarachnoid block for pain relief for labor. The individual nerve entrapment neuropathies should not restrict the possibility of use of the regional techniques because these neuropathies are a reflection of peripheral nerve entrapment between fascial planes or coming out of foraminae, and not an indication of an active inflammatory process.

### *Labor and Delivery*

Anesthesia for labor and delivery for these patients can consist of systemic medication, epidural, or local vaginal block such as paracervical.

### *Cesarean Section*

Again, anesthetic management for cesarean delivery or abdominal delivery can use regional anesthesia, general anesthesia, and, if necessary, local anesthesia techniques. As mentioned in prior sections, the regional techniques include both epidural and spinal methods, or as is more popular today, even the continuous spinal method. As discussed in previous sections of this chapter, regional techniques appear to be preferred in many of these patients as it allows for adequate analgesia and it allows concomitantly, reasonable muscle relaxation. The general anesthetic technique is identical to that described in other sections in this chapter, and it does include all the necessary safety aspects and preparations necessary before intubation and airway secureness. It is absolutely imperative that all these patients have the different anesthetic techniques and agents explained to them, including positives and negatives in relation to the disease process. Such explanation places the patient in a position to be an active decision maker, not a passive one. Most of these parturients, like any other parturient, are interested in being awake if possible to experience the beauty of the moment of birth. Again, the regional techniques by far offer the best anesthetic method to achieve this. As pointed out in another section, it is imperative to ensure that prior to regional anesthesia or local anesthesia in these patients, the disease process be identified and the area of involvement carefully outlined from the standpoint of both motor and sensory deficits. From the informed-patient viewpoint, it is necessary to mention to the patient that the placement of a local anesthetic is not going to have a negative or positive effect upon the disease process itself. Again, it is important to emphasize, that it is necessary to ensure that the patient does have complete information so she can make an intelligent and informed consent taking into account her needs as a mother in relationship to her spouse and her newborn baby. Neuropathies and singular nerve involvements certainly should not retard one from the use of the regional techniques once the aforementioned is fully explained to the patient and the patient requests the regional technique on the basis of informed consent and desire.

## Movement Disorders and Organic Mental Dysfunction

Chorea gravidarum refers to the movement disorder encountered during pregnancy as a sequela of infection with group A hemolytic streptococci. However, since the introduction of antibiotics, there has been a dramatic decline in the postinfectious form and, in its place, a significant proportion of cases related to systemic lupus erythematosus or underlying basal ganglia disease has emerged. Interestingly, chorea can be provoked by oral contraceptive use and an estrogen-dependent alteration in central dopaminergic activity has been implicated (114,115). In violent chorea, haloperidol may be required to prevent hyperthermia and rhabdomyolysis (37).

Wilson's disease (hepatolenticular degeneration) is an autosomal recessive disorder in which an accumulation of copper in the brain (among other organs) results in abnormal movements and mental impairment. Adequate chelation therapy with D-penicillamine (and Vitamin $B_6$ to counteract its antipyridoxine effect) allows pregnancy to proceed normally. Reduction of the D-penicillamine dose 6 weeks prior to a planned cesarean section is recommended due to the drug's impairment of wound healing (110).

Psychotic behavior can develop for the first time during pregnancy in a small group of patients. Over one-half of the psychotic patients display schizophrenic behavior, while the remainder are evenly split between manic-depression and psychoneurotic reactions. Psychotropic medications (phenothiazines, other antipsychotics and tricyclic antidepressants) can be used safely during pregnancy, but lithium can cause cardiac malformations (116). Please refer to Chapter 3 for more information on the psychologic aspects of pregnancy.

### *Headache*

Headache is a very common complaint during pregnancy, and its etiology falls into three main categories: (1) muscle-contraction (tension); (2) vascular; and (3) traction/inflammatory (117). Muscle-contraction headache is the most common variety encountered during pregnancy (37). It is characterized by a dull to sharp aching sensation or tightness, often bilateral, and localized to the vertex or suboccipt. The headache can appear at any time during the pregnancy and, although often present upon arising in the morning, usually worsens in the evening. There may be local scalp soreness and the patient may complain about poor concentration and dizziness. Cervical osteoarthritis and spondylosis, chronic myositis and myofascial pain, and depression or anxiety can all give rise to muscle-contraction headache. In addition, the specific mechanisms responsible for the headache are multifactorial and include excessive muscle activity, vascular dysfunction, defective serotonergic mechanisms, and psychological factors (116). The occasional muscle-contraction headache usually responds to local massage, heat or ice packs, and simple analgesics. Although some recommend diazepam for the relief of anxiety in this situation, amitriptyline can often improve the headache, especially if associated with other symptoms of depression (37).

Migraine headache is the most common cause of vascular headache and 70% of migraine sufferers are women of childbearing age (118). Classical attacks are unilateral, have a visual or sensorimotor prodrome, and are often accompanied by photophobia, nausea, and vomiting. The "common" variety, however, usually has no premonitory symptoms. Although the cerebral vasculature clearly undergoes alterations during an attack, the etiology is still unknown. Classical migraine is associated with a spreading cerebral oligemia (119) and the painful phase of migraine is associated with cranial arterial dilatation (116). In addition, headache-free migraineurs can have asymmetries in regional cerebral blood flow that may be related to a more labile control of the cerebral circulation (120). The clear association of migraine with menses, oral contraceptive use, and pregnancy points to an as yet undetermined hormonal influence (116).

Migraine is often dramatically improved during pregnancy and this usually begins during the second trimester. However, 20 to 50% of patients will not experience an improvement in symptoms, and some may experience their first attack during pregnancy (usually in the first trimester) (110). Neither pregnancy nor fetal outcome are adversely affected in women with migraine headaches (117).

If a history of precipitating factors can be elicited, then avoidance can significantly decrease susceptibility to attacks. Simple analgesics may provide relief, but prophylaxis with propranolol may be necessary in frequent classic migraine. There has been concern raised over fetal growth retardation and impaired neonatal B-adrenergic responsiveness in rats (110). Some patients may respond to propranolol given during the prodrome, often preventing the headache phase and thereby avoiding daily usage (121). Ergot alkaloids should be avoided because of the potential, serious adverse effects on the fetus and the gravid uterus (110).

Traction/inflammatory headache is due to traction, displacement, or inflammation of intracranial and extracranial structures, which are sensitive to pain (114). The headache of intracranial hypertension is the most serious example and is usually a deep, constant ache aggravated by coughing or straining and most prominent in the morning. Accompanying nausea, vomiting, and altered level of consciousness give further evidence that the headache may not have a benign etiology. Intracranial hypertension is discussed in greater detail earlier in this chapter.

### *Anesthetic Considerations for Movement Disorders and Organic Mental Dysfunction*

Patients with movement disorders are very special and may require supplemental sedation for control during labor and delivery. This can be used in addition to a baseline analgesic technique for labor and delivery such as described in the Cerebrovascular Disease section earlier in the chapter. Please see this section for specifics.

For cesarean section, the anesthetic of choice is a judgment call involving the obstetrician, patient, and anesthesiologist. In some instances with a calm patient who prefers to be awake and enjoy immediate bonding with her baby, a regional technique can be used with a small amount of sedation. Naturally, the latter must be communicated with other important members of the team, i.e., the neonatologist, so he/she is aware of the depressant effect of the aforementioned sedative.

## CENTRAL NERVOUS SYSTEM INFECTIONS

### *Bacterial Infections*

Bacterial meningitis, subdural empyema, and brain abscess can be encountered during pregnancy, but their presentation, diagnosis, and management are not altered by pregnancy. Most antimicrobial agents that are required to treat these life-threatening infections can be given safely during pregnancy. The exceptions are: (1) sulfonamides, which can lead to neonatal kernicterus if given in the third trimester; (2) chloramphenicol, which can cause the "grey baby syndrome" if given close to term; and (3) tetracyclines, which have toxic effects on fetal bone and tooth development and can lead to maternal hepatic failure (122).

Tuberculosis, if untreated, can reactivate in up to 15% of pregnancies, but adequately treated tuberculosis should not reactivate during pregnancy (123). Involvement of the central nervous system most commonly presents with meningitis, although in India and other developing countries, tuberculosis is often the most common cause of an intracranial mass lesion. If untreated, tuberculous meningitis leads to death within a few months and 20% of children born to these women will demonstrate clinical tuberculosis within the first month of life (121,122). The treatment of central nervous system tuberculosis requires therapy with at least three agents (e.g. isoniazid, rifampin, and ethambutol or pyrizinamide), and all have been used safely in pregnancy (122).

Syphilis can present in its secondary stage as a meningitis (often indistinguishable from viral meningitis except for positive CSF serologic studies), but more commonly central nervous system syphilis is latent and asymptomatic. Therapy is unchanged for the pregnant patient, although in penicillin-allergic patients, erythromycin does not significantly cross the placenta and neonatal penicillin treatment is then indicated (121).

### *Viral Infections*

Poliomyelitis has been discussed previously. Herpes encephalitis can present during pregnancy and can be successfully and safely treated with acyclovir. Cytomegalovirus (CMV) infection, while usually not a clinically important entity to the mother, is the most common cause of intrauterine infection (121). Maternal rubella, especially during the first trimester, can cause a congenital rubella syndrome with often devastating multisystem abnormalities (110).

Human immunodeficiency virus (HIV) is responsible for the acquired immunodeficiency syndrome (AIDS), which is becoming a significant problem for women of childbearing age. Intravenous drug use and sexual contact with infected males are the most common modes of transmission to women. The opportunistic infections associated with AIDS have a predilection for the central nervous system with toxoplasmosis, cryptococcosis, and cytomegalovirus infections occurring quite commonly. Toxoplasmosis can also affect pregnant women without AIDS, and is usually asymptomatic in these patients. Congenital toxoplasmosis results in more birth defects than herpes, rubella, and syphilis combined, with 1/1000 affected babies born each year (121). In addition, central nervous system lymphoma can also occur and present as a mass lesion. HIV can also involve the central nervous system directly and produce a dementia (with brain involvement), myelopathy (with spinal cord involvement), neuropathy, or any combination of these entities. Treatment is directed at symptomatic infections or malignancies and should not be affected by the pregnancy.

### *Miscellaneous Infections*

Cysticercosis cerebri (infestation with the pork tapeworm Taenia solium), is becoming increasingly more common in areas with a high immigrant population. The disease most commonly results in seizures or hydrocephalus, but parenchymal and cisternal lesions can present with a mass effect (124). Anticonvulsants and ventricular shunting are often required, but investigational use of praziquantel for active parenchymal disease has not yet been evaluated in the pregnant state. Cryptococcal meningitis and other fungal central nervous system infections have been reported during pregnancy. Coccidioidomycosis, if encountered during the last half of pregnancy, seems predisposed to dissemination and can infect the placenta (121).

### *Anesthetic Considerations for Central Nervous System Infections*

Any patients with evidence of an acute infectious disease process that affects the central nervous system certainly should not be offered regional anesthesia as a possible technique for pain relief for labor or for cesarean section. In such a case, the patient would undoubtedly be delivered by cesarean section to obviate the difficulty of labor under such circumstances. The anesthetic of choice would be general anesthesia with care being taken on induction to avoid large fluctuations in blood pressure by administration of supplemental opioid or even beta blockers to prevent the sympathetic overshoot due to laryngoscopy and intubation in lightly anesthetized patients, such as is often the case in cesarean section. Local anesthesia is not a pleasant option in such cases due to the lack of understanding and often great difficulty encountered in keeping such patients relaxed and in a trusting frame of mind.

## Summary

Although uncommon, neurologic diseases during pregnancy will confront the obstetric anesthesiologist. Therefore, a thorough understanding of the pathophysiology, signs, and symptoms of increased intracranial pressure and cerebral ischemia is of utmost importance. Fortunately, modern neuroanesthetic technique and aggressive monitoring have decreased significantly the risk to mother and fetus should surgery be required.

## REFERENCES


1. Bjerkdal T, Eganaes J: Outcome of pregnancy in women with epilepsy, Norway 1967–1978: Description of material. *In* Epilepsy, Pregnancy and the Child. Edited by D Janz, M Dam, A Richens, L Bossi. New York, Raven Press, 1982, p. 75.
2. Krumholz A: Epilepsy and pregnancy. *In* Neurological Disorders of Pregnancy. Edited by PJ Goldstein. Mount Kisco, NY, Futura Publishing, 1986, p. 65.
3. Montouris GD, Fenichel GM, McLain W Jr: The pregnant epileptic. A review and recommendations. Arch. Neurol. 36:601, 1979.
4. Philbert A, Dam M: The epileptic mother and her child. Epilepsia 23:85, 1982.
5. Dalessio DJ: Seizure disorders and pregnancy. N. Engl. J. Med. 312:559, 1985.
6. Forster FM, Booker HE: The epilepsies and convulsive disorders. *In* Clinical Neurology. Volume 3. Edited by AB Baker, RJ Joynt. Philadelphia, Harper and Row, 1986, Chapter 31.
7. Adams RD, Victor M: Principles of Neurology. 3rd Ed. New York, McGraw Hill, 1985, pp. 233–254.
8. Knight AH, Rhind EG: Epilepsy and pregnancy: a study of 153 pregnancies in 59 patients. Epilepsia 16:99, 1975.
9. Schmidt D, Canger R, Avanzini G, Battino D, et al: Change of seizure frequency in pregnant epileptic women. J. Neurol. Neurosurg. Psychiatry 46:751, 1983.
10. Bardy AH: Incidence of seizures during pregnancy, labor and puerperium in epileptic women: a prospective study. Acta. Neurol. Scand. 75:356, 1987.
11. Mattson RH, Cramer JA: Epilepsy, sex hormones, and antiepileptic drugs. Epilepsia 26 (Suppl 1): S40, 1985.
12. Schachter SC: Hormonal considerations in women with seizures. Arch. Neurol. 45:1267, 1988.
13. Ramsay RE: Effect of hormones on seizure activity during pregnancy. J. Clin. Neurophysiol. 4:23, 1987.
14. Pfaff DW, McEwen BS: Actions of estrogens and progestins on nerve cells. Science 219:808, 1983.

15. Nausieda PA: Estrogen and central dopamine receptor activity. Neurology 29:1605, 1979.
16. Janz D: Antiepileptic drugs and pregnancy: altered utilization patterns and teratogenesis. Epilepsia 23 (Suppl 1): S54, 1982.
17. Levy RH, Yerby MS: Effects of pregnancy on antiepileptic drug utilization. Epilepsia 26 (Suppl 1): S52, 1985.
18. Stempel LE, Rayburn WF: Anticonvulsant use during pregnancy. *In* Drug Therapy in Obstetrics and Gynecology. 2nd Ed. Edited by WF Rayburn, FP Zuspan. Norwalk, CN, Appleton-Century-Crofts, 1986, p. 53.
19. Bardy AH, Hiilesmaa VK, Teramo KAW: Serum phenytoin during pregnancy, labor and puerperium. Acta. Neurol. Scand. 75:374, 1987.
20. Bjerkdal T, Bahna SL: The course and outcome of pregnancy in women with epilepsy. Acta. Obstet. Gynecol. Scand. 52:245, 1973.
21. Levy RH, Schmidt D: Utility of free drug level monitoring of antiepileptic drugs. Epilepsia 26:199, 1985.
22. Eganaes J: Outcome of pregnancy in women with epilepsy, Norway, 1967 to 1978: Complications during pregnancy and delivery. *In* Epilepsy, Pregnancy and the Child. Edited by D Janz, M Dam, A Richens, L Bossi. New York, Raven Press, 1982, p. 81.
23. Nakane Y, Okuma T, Takahashi R: Multi-institutional study on the teratogenicity and fetal toxicity of antiepileptic drugs: a report of collaborative study group in Japan. Epilepsia 21:663, 1980.
24. Nelson KB, Ellenberg JH: Maternal seizure disorder, outcome of pregnancy, and neurologic abnormalities in the children. Neurology (NY) 32:1247, 1982.
25. Hanson JW, Smith DW: The fetal hydantoin syndrome. J. Pediatrics 87:285, 1975.
26. Zackai EH, Mellman WJ, Neiderer B, Hanson JW: The fetal trimethadione syndrome. J. Pediatrics 87:280, 1975.
27. Robert E, Guilband P: Maternal valproic acid and congenital neural tube defects. Lancet 2:1096, 1982.
28. Srinivasan G, Seller RA, Tiruvury A, Pildes RS: Material anticonvulsant therapy and hemorrhagic disease of the newborn. Obstet. Gynecol. 59:250, 1982.
29. Orringer CE, Eustace JC, Wynsch CD: Natural history of lactic acidosis after grand mal seizures. N. Engl. J. Med. 297:796 1977.
30. Teramo K, Hiilesmaa V, Bardy A, Saarikoski S: Fetal heart rate during a maternal grand mal epileptic seizure. J. Perinat. Med. 7:3, 1979.
31. Delgado-Escueta AV, Bajorek JG: Status epilepticus: Mechanisms of brain damage and rational management. Epilepsia 23 (Suppl 1): S29, 1982.
32. Simon RP: Physiologic consequences of status epilepticus. Epilepsia 26 (Suppl 1): S58, 1985.
33. Anson JA, Sundberg S, Stone JL: Treatment of status epilepticus with continuous midazolam infusion. Presented at the Annual Meeting of the AANS, Toronto, Canada, April 24–28, 1988.
34. Sibai BM, Anderson GD: Eclampsia. *In* Neurological Disorders of Pregnancy. Edited by PJ Goldstein. Mount Kisco, NY, Futura Publishing, 1986, p. 1.
35. Sibai BM, McCubbin JH, Anderson GD, Lipshitz J, et al: Eclampsia I. Observations from 67 recent cases. Obstet. Gynecol. 58:609, 1981.
36. Wright JP: Anesthetic considerations in preeclampsia-eclampsia. Anesth Analg 63:590, 1983.
37. Donaldson JO: Neurologic complications. *In* Burrow, GN, Ferris, TF (eds): Medical Complications During Pregnancy, ed 3. WB Saunders Co, Philadelphia, 1988, p 485.
38. Benedetti TJ, Quilligan EJ: Cerebral edema in severe pregnancy-induced hypertension. Am J Obstet. Gynecol. 137: 850, 1980.
39. Sibai BM, Spinnato JA, Watson DL, Lewis JA, et al: Effect of magnesium sulfate on electroencephalograms findings in preeclampsia-eclampsia. Obstet. Gynecol. 64:261, 1984.
40. Dinsdale HB: Does magnesium sulfate treat eclamptic seizures? Yes. Arch. Neurol. 45:1360, 1988.
41. Kaplan PW, Lesser RP, Fisher RS, Repke JT, et al: No, Magnesium sulfate should not be used in treating eclamptic seizures. Arch. Neurol. 45:1361, 1988.
42. Modica PA, Tempelhoff R, White PF: Pro- and anticonvulsant effects of anesthetics (part I and part II). Anesth Analg 70:303–15, 433–44, 1990.
43. Wiebers DO: Ischemic complications of pregnancy. Arch. Neurol. 42:1106, 1985.
44. Fletcher AP, Alkjaersig NK, Burstein R: The influence of pregnancy upon blood coagulation and plasma fibrinolytic enzyme function. Am J Obstet. Gynecol. 134:743, 1979.
45. Nilsson IM, Kullander S: Coagulation and fibrinolytic studies during pregnancy. Acta. Obstet. Gynecol. Scand. 46: 273, 1967.
46. Cross JN, Castro PO, Jennett WB: Cerebral strokes associated with pregnancy and puerperium. Br Med J 3:214, 1968.
47. Lewis PJ, Boylan P, Friedman LA, Hensby CN, et al: Prostacyclin in pregnancy. Br Med J 280:1581, 1980.
48. Wood JH, Kee DB Jr: Hemorheology of the cerebral circulation in stroke. Stroke 16:765, 1985.
49. Greenfield JC Jr, Rembert JC, Tindall GT: Transient changes in cerebral vascular resistance during the valsalva maneuver in man. Stroke 15:76, 1984.
50. Barnett HJM: Platelet and coagulation function in relation to thromboembolic stroke. Adv Neurol 16:45, 1977.
51. Ueland K, Metcalfe J: Acute rheumatic fever in pregnancy. Am J Obstet. Gynecol. 95:586, 1966.
52. Kaplan EL: AHA Committee report: Prevention of bacterial endocarditis. Circulation 56:139, 1977.
53. Hall JG, Pauli RM, Wilson KM: Maternal and fetal sequelae of anticoagulation during pregnancy. Am J Med 68:122, 1980.
54. Mettinger KL: Fibromuscular dysplasia and the brain. II. Current concept of the disease. Stroke 13:53, 1982.
55. Trommer BL, Homer D, Mikhael MA: Cerebral vasospasm and eclampsia. Stroke 19:326, 1988.
56. Brick JF: Vanishing cerebrovascular disease of pregnancy. Neurology 38:804, 1988.
57. Manelfe C, Guiraud B, Rascol A, Clanet M, et al: Postpartum cerebral angiopathy: angiographic study. Report of 6 cases (abstr). Am J Neuroradiol 4:1149, 1983.
58. Meyerhoff JD: Neurologic manifestations of the rheumatic diseases in pregnancy. *In* Neurological Disorders of Pregnancy. Edited by PJ Goldstein. Mount Kisco, NY, Futura Publishing, 1986, p. 121.
59. Lockshin MD, Reinitz E, Druzin ML, Murrman M, et al: Lupus pregnancy: Case-control prospective study demonstrating absence of lupus exacerbation during or after pregnancy. Am J Med 77:893, 1984.
60. Bluesten HG, Williams GW, Steinberg AD: Cerebrospinal fluid antibodies to neuronal cells: Association with neuropsychiatric manifestations of systemic lupus erythematosis. Am J Med 70:240, 1981.
61. Srinavasan K: Cerebral venous thrombosis and arterial thrombosis in pregnancy and puerperium. A study of 135 patients. Angiology 34:731, 1983.
62. Younker D, Jones MM, Adenwala J, Citrin A, et al: Maternal cortical vein thrombosis and the obstetric anesthesiologist. Anesth Analg 65:1007, 1986.

63. Krayenbuhl MA: Cerebral venous and sinus thrombosis. Clin Neurosurg 14:1, 1967.
64. Halpern JP, Morris JGL, Driscoll GL: Anticoagulants and cerebral venous thrombosis. Aust NZ J Med 14:643, 1984.
65. Aguilar MJ, Rabinowitch R: Metastatic chorionepithelioma simulating multiple strokes. Neurology 14:933, 1964.
66. Brant-Zawadzki M, Norman D (eds): Magnetic Resonance Imaging of the Central Nervous System. Raven Press, New York 1987.
67. Barno H, Freeman DW: Maternal deaths due to spontaneous subarachnoid hemorrhage. Am J Obstet. Gynecol. 125:384, 1976.
68. Robinson JL, Hall CS, Sedzinir CB: Arteriovenous malformations, aneurysms and pregnancy. J Neurosurg 41:63, 1974.
69. Adams HP Jr, Kassell NF, Torner JC, Sahs AL: CT and clinical correlations in recent aneurysmal subarachnoid hemorrhage: a preliminary report of the Cooperative Aneurysm Study. Neurology 33:981, 1983.
70. Giannotta SL, Daniels J, Golde SH, Zelman V, et al: Ruptured intracranial aneurysms during pregnancy. A report of four cases. J Reprod Med 31:139, 1986.
71. Neal JH, Giannotta SL: Surgical management of intracerebral hemorrhage. *In* Fisher M (ed): Medical Therapy of Acute Stroke. Marcel Dekker, New York, 1989.
72. Kasell NF, Biner JG, Adams HP: Antifibrinolytic agents and aneurysmal subarachnoid hemorrhage. Presented at the Annual Meeting of the AANS, Washington, DC, September 26, 1983.
73. Giannotta SL, McGillicuddy JE, Kindt GW: Diagnosis and treatment of postoperative cerebral vasospasm. Surg Neurol 8:286, 1977.
74. Heros RC, Zervas NT, Vasos V: Cerebral vasospasm after subarachnoid hemorrhage: An update. Ann Neurol 14:599, 1983.
75. Kassell NF, Sasaki T, Colohan ART, Nazar G: Cerebral vasospasm following aneurysmal subarachnoid hemorrhage. Stroke 16:562, 1985.
76. Butler AS, Brooks WH, Netsky MG: Classification and biology of brain tumors. *In* Youmans, JR (ed): Neurological Surgery, ed 2. WB Saunders, Philadelphia, 1982, p 2659.
77. Aronson NI, Kangolow S, Goldstein PJ: Brain tumors during pregnancy. *In* Neurological Disorders of Pregnancy. Edited by PJ Goldstein. Mount Kisco, NY, Futura Publishing, 1986, p. 41.
78. Molitch ME: Pregnancy and the hyperprolactinemic woman. New Eng J Med 312:1364, 1985.
79. Marshall JR: Pregnancy in patients with prolactin-producing pituitary tumors. Cln Obstet. Gynecol. 23:453, 1980.
80. Roelvink NCA, Kamphorst W, van Alphen HAM, Rao BR: Pregnancy-related primary brain and spinal tumors. Arch. Neurol. 44:209, 1987.
81. Golaboff LG, Etzin C: Effect of pregnancy on the somatotroph and the prolactin cells of the human adenohypophysis. J Clin Endocrinol Metab 29:15, 1969.
82. Bagshaine KD, Harland S: Immunodiagnosis and monitoring of gonadotrophin-producing metastases in the central nervous system. Cancer 38:112, 1976.
83. Kassam SH, Hadi HA, Fadel HE, Sims W, et al: Benign intracranial hypertension in pregnancy: current diagnostic and therapeutic approach. Obstet. Gynecol. Survey 38:314, 1983.
84. Powell JL: Pseudotumor cerebri and pregnancy. Obstet. Gynecol. 40:713, 1972.
85. Digre KB, Varner MW, Corbett JJ: Pseudotumor cerebri and pregnancy. Neurology 34:721, 1984.
86. Hill LM, Parker D, O'Neill BP: Management of maternal vegetative state during pregnancy. Mayo Clin Proc 60:469, 1985.
87. Dillon WP, Lee RV, Tronolone MJ, Buckwald S, et al: Life support and maternal brain death during pregnancy. JAMA 248:1089, 1982.
88. Field DR, Gates EA, Creasy RK, Jonsen AR, et al: Maternal brain death during pregnancy. Medical and ethical issues. JAMA 260:816, 1988.
89. Howie MB, Black HA, Zvara D, McSweeney TD, et al: Esmolol reduces autonomic hypersensitivity and length of seizures induced by electroconvulsive therapy. Anesth Analg 71:384, 1990.
90. Cohen BS, Hilton EB: Spinal cord disorders and pregnancy. *In* Neurological Disorders of Pregnancy. Edited by PJ Goldstein. Mount Kisco, NY, Futura Publishing, 1986, p. 139.
91. Verduyn WH: Spinal cord injured women, pregnancy and delivery. Paraplegia 24:231, 1986.
92. Connolly ES: Spinal cord tumors in adults. *In* Youmans, JR (ed): Neurological Surgery, ed 2. WB Saunders, Philadelphia, 1982, p 3169.
93. Aminoff MJ, Logue V: Clinical features of spinal vascular malformations. Brain 39:197, 1974.
94. Repke JT, Klein VR: Myasthenia gravis in pregnancy. *In* Neurological Disorders of Pregnancy. Edited by PJ Goldstein. Mount Kisco, NY, Futura Publishing, 1986, p. 213.
95. Plauche WC: Myasthenia gravis. Clin Obstet. Gynecol. 26: 592, 1983.
96. Jaffe R, Mock M, Abramowicz J, Ben-Aderet N: Myotonic dystrophy and pregnancy: A review. Obstet. Gynecol. Survey 41:272, 1986.
97. Shore RN: Myotonic dystrophy: Hazards of pregnancy and infancy. Dev Med Child Neurol 17:356, 1975.
98. Cohen BS, Felsenthal G: Peripheral nervous system disorders and pregnancy. *In* Neurological Disorders of Pregnancy. Edited by PJ Goldstein. Mount Kisco, NY, Futura Publishing, 1986, p. 153.
99. McArthur JC, Young F: Multiple sclerosis and pregnancy. *In* Neurological Disorders of Pregnancy. Edited by PJ Goldstein. Mount Kisco, NY, Futura Publishing, 1986, p. 197.
100. Poser S, Raun NE, Wikström J, Poser W: Pregnancy, oral contraception and multiple sclerosis. Acta. Neurol. Scand. 59:108, 1979.
101. Poser S, Poser W: Multiple sclerosis and gestation. Neurology 33:1422, 1983
102. Warren TM, Datta S, Ostheimer GW: Lumbar epidural anesthesia in a patient with multiple sclerosis. Anesth Analg 61:1022, 1982.
103. Daw E, Chandler G: Pregnancy following poliomyelitis. Postgrad Med J 52:492, 1976.
104. Levine MC, Michels RM: Pregnancy and amyotrophic lateral sclerosis. Ann Neurol 1:408, 1977.
105. Hellman JD: Managing musculoskeletal problems in pregnant patients. Musculoskeletal J Med 1:14, 1984.
106. Svancarek W, Chirino O, Schaefer G Jr, Blythe JG: Retropsoas and subgluteal abscesses following paracervical and pudendal anesthesia. JAMA 237:892, 1977.
107. O'Connell JEA: Lumbar disc protrusions in pregnancy. J. Neurol. Neurosurg. Psychiatry 23:138, 1960.
108. Voitk AJ, Mueller JC, Farlinger DE, Johnston RU, et al: Carpal tunnel syndrome in pregnancy. Can Med Assoc J 128: 277, 1983.
109. Massey EW: Carpal tunnel syndrome in pregnancy. Obstet. Gynecol. Survey 33:145, 1978.
110. Hilsinger RL Jr, Adour KK, Doty HE: Idiopathic facial paralysis, pregnancy and the menstrual cycle. Ann Otol 84:433, 1975.
111. Aminoff MJ: Maternal neurologic disorders. *In*: Maternal-

Fetal Medicine. Principles and Practice. WB Saunders Company, Philadelphia, 1984, p 1005.
112. Ahlberg G, Ahlmark G: The Landry-Guillain-Barré Syndrome and pregnancy. Acta. Obstet. Gynecol. Scand. 57: 377, 1978.
113. Jones MW, Berry K: Chronic relapsing polyneuritis associated with pregnancy. Ann Neurol 9:413, 1981.
114. Barber PV, Arnold AG, Evans G: Recurrent hormone dependent chorea: Effects of estrogens and progestogens. Clin Endocrinol 5:291, 1976.
115. Nausieda PA, Koller WC, Weiner WJ, Klawans HL: Chorea induced by oral contraceptives. Neurology 29:1605, 1979.
116. Dalessio PJ: Neurologic diseases. *In* Burrow, GN, Ferris, TF (eds): Medical Complications During Pregnancy. WB Saunders Company, Philadelphia, 1982, p 435.
117. Khurana RK: Headache. *In* Neurological Disorders of Pregnancy. Edited by PJ Goldstein. Mount Kisco, NY, Futura Publishing, 1986, p. 247.
118. Wainscott G, Sullivan FM, Volans GN, Wilkinson M: The outcome of pregnancy in women suffering from migraine. Postgrad Med J 54:98, 1978.
119. Lauritzen M, Olesen J: Regional cerebral blood flow during migraine attacks by xenon-133 inhalation and emission tomography. Brain 107:447, 1984.
120. Levine SR, Welch KMA, Ewing JR, Joseph R, et al: Cerebral blood flow asymmetries in headache-free migraineurs. Stroke 18:1164, 1987.
121. Spooner J: Personal communication, 1984.
122. Levin MI: Central nervous system infections and their treatment in pregnancy. *In* Neurological Disorders of Pregnancy. Edited by PJ Goldstein. Mount Kisco, NY, Futura Publishing, 1986, p. 89.
123. deMarch P: Tuberculosis and pregnancy. Chest 6:800, 1975.
124. Couldwell W, Zee C-Z, Apuzzo MLJ: Definition of the role of surgery in cisternal and parenchymatous cysticercosis cerebri. Presented at the annual meeting of the AANS, Toronto, Canada, April 25, 1988.
125. Tarnow G: Hirntumor und Schwangerschaft. Zentralbl Neurochir 1960;20:134–158.
126. Bernard H: Sarcome cérébral'a évolution rapide au cours de la grossesse et pendant les suites de couches. Bull Soc Obstet 1898;1:296–298.
127. Bailey P, Bucy PC: The origin and nature of meningeal tumors. Am J Cancer 1931;15:15–54.
128. Boshes B, McBeath J: Cerebral complications of pregnancy. JAMA 1954;154:385–389.
129. Gregory JR, Watkins G: Eclamptic manifestations occurring in pregnancy complicated by brain tumor. Am J Obstet Gynecol 1950;60:1263–1271.
130. Unger RR, Siedschlag WD, Bayer H: Raumfördernde intrakranielle Prozesse und Schwangerschaft. Zentralbl Neurochir 1976;37:177–189.
131. Shuanshoti S, Hongsaprabhas C, Netsky MG: Metastasizing meningioma. Cancer 1970;26:832–841.
132. Divry P, Bobon J: Tumeurs encéphalique et gravidité. Acta Neurol Psychiatr Belg 1949;49:59–80.
133. Reeves DL: Tumors of the brain complicating pregnancy. West J Surg Obstet Gynecol 1952;60:211–219.
134. Lorenz R: Der Einfluss auf raumfördernde intrakranielle Prozesse. Dtsch Med Wochenschr 1968;93:1787–1791.
135. Barnes JE, Abbott KH: Cerebral complications during pregnancy and the puerperium. Am J Obstet Gynecol 1961;82: 192–207.
136. Toakley G: Brain tumors in pregnancy. Aust NZ J Surg 1965;35:148–154.
137. Smolik EA, Nash FP, Clawson JW: Neurological and neurosurgical complications associated with pregnancy and the puerperium. South Med J 1957;50:561–572.
138. Kempers MD: Management of pregnancy associated with brain tumors. Am J Obstet Gynecol 1963;87:858–864.
139. O'Connell JEA: Neurosurgical problems in pregnancy. Proc R Soc Med 1962;55:577–582.
140. Enoksson P, Lundberg N, Sjöstedt S, et al: Influence of pregnancy on visual fields in suprasellar tumours. Acta Psychiatr Neurol Scand 1961;36:524–538.
141. Holmes G, Sargent P: Suprasellar endothelioma. Brain 1927;50:518–537.
142. Puccioni L: Contributo chimico allo studio dei tumori cerebrali in gravidanza. Riv Ital Ginecol 1935;18(suppl): 670–710.
143. Walsh FB: Clinical Neuro-Ophthalmology. Baltimore, Williams & Wilkins, 1947, p 1161.
144. Hagedoorn A: The chiasmal syndrome and retrobulbar neuritis in pregnancy. Am J Ophthalmol 1937;29: 690–698.
145. Fischer F: Über die Ursachen bitemporaler Hemianopsie bei Schwangerschaft. Z Augenheilkd 1935;85:88–108.
146. Bickerstaff ER, Small JM, Guest JA: The relapsing course of certain meningiomas in relation to pregnancy and menstruation. J Neurol Neurosurg Psychiatry 1958;21:89–91.
147. Haranghy L, Zoltan L, Szinay G, et al: Beiträge zum Verhalten extragenitaler Geschwülste während der Schwangerschaft. Acta Med Acad Sci Hung 1954;6:291–303.
148. Cushing H, Eisenhardt L: Meningiomas arising from the tuberculum sellae. Arch Ophthalmol 1929;1:1–41, 168–205.
149. Kloss K: Hirntumor und Schwangerschaft. Wien Z Nervenheilkd 1952;5:175–187.
150. Rand CW, Andler M: Tumors of the brain complicating pregnancy. Arch Neurol Psychiatry 1950;63:1–41.
151. Goldstein PJ, Rosenberg S, Smith RW, et al: Maternal death and brain tumor. Am J Obstet Gynecol 1972;112:297–298.
152. Rath S, Mathai KV, Chandy J: Multiple meningiomas of the spinal canal. J Neurosurg 1967;26:639–640.
153. Mealey J: Spinal cord tumor during pregnancy. Obstet Gynecol 1968;32:204–209.
154. Bogdanowitsch M: Entbindung bei vollständiger Lähmung des Rumpfes. Zentralbl Gynakol 1913;37:809–814.
155. Bailey P, Bucy PC: Tumors of the spinal canal. Surg Clin North Am 1930;10:233–257.
156. Hanssen A, Philippides D, Isch F: Glioblastome pendant la grossesse. Bull Fed Soc Gynecol Obstet 1951;3:465–466.
157. Lang W, Haering M: Hirntumor und Schwangerschaft: Diagnostische und therapeutische Probleme. Zentralbl Gynakol 1962;37:1449–1455.
158. Michelson JJ, New PF: Brain tumor and pregnancy. J Neurol Neurosurg Psychiatry 1969;32:305–307.
159. Von Seuffert E: Drei Fälle von Kaiserschnitt an der Toten. Arch Gynecol 1907;83:725–734.
160. Whitcher BR: Brain tumor complicating pregnancy. J Med Soc NJ 1956;53:112–114.
161. Mac Rae KSE: Survival of foetus after maternal death due to intracranial tumor. Br Med J 1939;1:978.
162. Jacobi W: Hirntumor und Schwangerschaft. Psychiatr Neurol Wochenschr 1921;23:237–239.
163. Cathala V: Opération césarienne post mortem. Bull Obstet 1908;11:144–150.
164. Ospelt M: Glioma cerebri und Schwangerschaft. Zentralbl Gynakol 1939;63:1401–1405.
165. Siegmund, cited by Tarnow G: Hirntumor und Schwangerschaft. Zentralbl Neurochir 1960;20:148.
166. Davis L, Martin J, Padberg F, et al: A study of 182 patients

with verified astrocytomas, astroblastomas and oligodendrogliomas of the brain. J Neurosurg 1950;7:299–312.
167. Cunningham JAK: Cerebral complications of pregnancy. NZ Med J 1961;60:180–184.
168. Shanks JA: Intracranial tumor in pregnancy. Practitioner 1957;50:561–572.
169. Höhne O: Tod intrapartum infolge von Kleinhirntumor. Zentralbl Gynakol 1927;51:2369–2371.
170. Leisewitz: Berichte aus gynäkologischen Gesellschaften und Krankenhäusern. Zentralbl Gynakol 1909;33:699.
171. Lichtenstein: Zur Klinik, Therapie und Aetiologie der Eklampsie nach einer neuen Statistik bearbeitet auf Grund von 400 Fällen. Arch Gynakol 1912;95:217–219.
172. Decio C: Tumore cerebellare in gravidanza. Zentralbl Neurol 1928;41:637.
173. Charlin C: Sehstörungen und Schwangerschaft. Zentralbl Ophthalmol 1931;24:570.
174. Tietze K: Zwei plötzlichè Hirntodesfälle an der gynäkologische-geburtshilflichen Praxis (sectio caesarea mortua). Med Welt 1935;9:1077–1078.
175. Vogt E: Gehirntumor im Wochenbett. Zentralbl Gynakol 1918;42:776–777.
176. Rogers L: Tumors involving the spinal canal and its nerve roots. Ann R Coll Surg Engl 1955;16:1–29.
177. Slooff JL, Kernohan JW, McCarty CS: Primary Intramedullary Tumors of the Spinal Cord and Filum Terminale. Philadelphia, WB Saunders Co, 1964, pp 11, 165–166.
178. King AB: Neurologic conditions occurring as complications of pregnancy. Arch Neurol Psychiatry 1950;63: 611–644.
179. Cushing H, Bailey P: Tumors From the Blood-Vessels of the Brain. Springfield, Ill, Charles C Thomas Publishers, 1928, pp 204–209.
180. Scarcella G, Allen MB, Andy OJ: Vascular lesions of the posterior fossa during pregnancy. Am J Obstet Gynecol 1961;82:836–840.
181. Bodechtel G: Differentialdiagnose neurologischer Krankheitsbilder. Stuttgart, West Germany, Georg Thieme Verlag, 1974, p 225.
182. Duperrat B: Tumeur Cérébral et grossesse. Presse Med 1945;53:118–119.
183. Hornet T, Duperrat R, Grépinet: Tumeur cérébral et grossesse: Etude anatomo-clinique d'un cas d'angioréticulome du cervelet se manifestant par des troubles circulatoires graves à l'occasion d'un accouchement. Rev Neurol 1938; 69:494–498.
184. Michon P, Lafont J: A propos du diagnostic de compression médullaire par hémangiome vertébral. Rev Neurol 1935; 63:565–571.
185. Newman MJD: Spinal angioma with symptoms in pregnancy. J Neurol Neurosurg Psychiatry 1958;21:38–41.
186. Fields WS, Jones JR: Spinal epidural hemangioma in pregnancy. Neurology 1957;7:825–828.
187. Delmas-Marsalet P: Poussées évolutive gravidique et image lipiodolée caractéristique des hémangiomes médullaire. Presse Med 1941;49:964–965.
188. Brion S, Netsky MG, Zimmerman HM: Vascular malformations of the spinal cord. Arch Neurol Psychiatry 1952;68: 339–361.
189. Schott B, Cotte L, Trillet M, et al: Sémiologie 'encéphalique' des hémorragies meningées spinales: A propos de deux observations de malformations vasculaires de la moelle. Rev Neurol 1963:109:654–657.
190. Aminoff MJ, Logue V: The prognosis of patients with spinal vascular malformations. Brain 1974;97:211–218.
191. Askenasy H, Behmoaram A: Neurological manifestations in hemangiomas of the vertebrae. J Neurol Neurosurg Psychiatry 1957;20:276–284.
192. Uiberall E, Politoff A: Gefäszmiszbildungen des Rückenmarkes. Acta Neurochir 1962;10:432–455.
193. Balado M, Morea R: Hemangioma extramedular produciendo paraplejias durante el embararo. Arch Argent Neurol 1928;1:345–351.
194. Lam RL, Roulhac GE, Erwin HJ: Hemangioma of the spinal canal and pregnancy. J Neurosurg 1951;8:668–671.
195. Bergamaschi P: Paraplegia de compressione midollare in gravidanza. Riv Obstet Ginecol Prat 1956;38:163–176.
196. Guthkelch AN: Hemangiomas involving the spinal epidural space. J Neurol Neurosurg Psychiatry 1948;11:199–210.
197. Girard PF, Garde A: Les angiomes de la moelle. Gaz Med Fr 1955;62:1175.
198. Glaser G: Ein Fall von zentralem Angiosarkom des Rückenmarks. Arch Psychiatr Nervenkrankh 1885;16:87–100.
199. Sjöquist O, cited by Haranghy L, Zoltan L, Szinay G, et al: Beiträge zum Verhalten extragenitaler Geschwülste während der Schwangerschaft. Acta Med Acad Sci Hung 1954; 6:291–303.
200. Cushing H: Tumors of the Nervus Acusticus and the Syndrome of the Cerebellopontine Angle. Philadelphia, WB Saunders Co, 1917, p 148.
201. Chimenti P: A proposito de un error de diagnostico: Tumor cerebeloso y vomitos incoercibles. Anal Ateno Buenos Aires 1945, pp 213–217.
202. Perez ML, Dixon J, Aranovich J, et al: Tumor cerebelar y embarazo. An Bras Ginecol 1941;12:271–279.
203. Mann B: Brain tumor complicating pregnancy. Am J Obstet Gynecol 1939;37:1051–1052.
204. Zülch KJ: Pathologische Anatomie der raumbeengenden intrakraniellen Prozesse, in Olivacrona H, Tönnis W (eds): Handbuch der Neurochirurgie. Berlin, Springer-Verlag, 1956, pp 3, 45–69, 103, 104, 143–176.
205. Christophe L, Divry P: Ganglioneurome (gangliocytome) parasagittal. J Belge Neurol Psychiatry 1940:40:340–352.
206. Halliday C: Pseudo-eclampsia, with two illustrative cases: I. Cerebral tumour; II. Meningitis. J Obstet Gynaecol 1939; 23:213–226.
207. Bickenbach W: Hirntumor und Schwangerschaft. Zentralbl Gynakol 1929;7:422–428.

# Chapter 37

# HIV-1 INFECTION IN WOMEN

JAMES A. McGREGOR

---

Human immunodeficiency virus is an increasingly common retroviral infectious disease caused by either HIV-1 or HIV-2.

All health care providers who serve women have important roles in providing reproductive health care and counseling to HIV-infected women and to women at risk for HIV infection. This discussion will summarize current information regarding the diagnosis, treatment, and anesthesia-related aspects of HIV infected women. This knowledge will enable care providers, especially anesthesia clinicians, to discuss diagnosis, natural history, and provide appropriate counseling and anesthesia-related services to HIV-infected women. This chapter also summarizes current data regarding how HIV infection can alter the course and manifestation of both obstetric and gynecological processes. Because only HIV-1 is prevalent in North America, this discussion will be limited to this infection.

To offer appropriate counseling and care, all care providers must know the risks for acquisition of HIV infection (Table 37–1). Both clinicians and specialists providing care for women should be able to educate their patients regarding HIV infection (Tables 37–2 and 37–2a). All care providers should become knowledgeable about choices for contraception, reproductive options, and aspects for fertility-related behaviors in regard to HIV infection. This chapter will provide a platform of knowledge with which to 1) derive proactive guidelines for care of HIV-infected pregnant women, and 2) keep abreast of our rapidly advancing knowledge regarding HIV infection and women, especially around the time of birth.

## Epidemiology

In 1987, Human Immunodeficiency Virus-1 (HIV-1) infection and Acquired Immunodeficiency Syndrome (AIDS) became two of the ten leading causes of death for women of reproductive age in the United States; by 1991, AIDS advanced to one of the five leading causes of death in this group (1). Assuming AIDS cases represent approximately 10% of HIV-infected people in the U.S., by mid-1989 1 million people, 100,000 of whom were women, had become infected with this virus (2). Heterosexual women and their birth children are the most rapidly increasing populations infected with HIV (2). The portion of women with AIDS who have acquired HIV through coitus has steadily increased to 19% through 1985 and to 32% in 1990 (3). For women attending sexually transmitted disease clinics in Baltimore from 1979 to 1989, HIV seroprevalence rose from less than 1% to 5%; the male-to-female ratio of HIV infection declined from 16:1 in 1979 to 1982, to 1:1 in 1988 to 1989 (4). The acquisition of HIV in women is most frequently associated with intravenous drug use (51%) and heterosexual coitus with a partner at risk (32%) (4).

The age, race, geographic distribution, and clinical outcome of women with AIDS are similar to that of heterosexual men with this infection (3). Women with AIDS are usually of reproductive age (85%) and live in large metropolitan areas (73%) (3). Three-fourths of infected women are black or Hispanic (3). Also, similar is the median time of AIDS diagnosis to death; for heterosexual men, it is 9.3 months, for women the median survival is 9.8 months (3). Three-year survival after AIDS diagnosis is 20% for women and 19% for men.

Like other reproductive-age individuals, many HIV-infected women will become pregnant and have children. Blinded seroprevalence studies of reproductive-age women estimate 1.5 per 1000 women who delivered live infants in 1989 were HIV infected (5); HIV antibody prevalence rates ranged from 0.0 to 2.28% (median, 0.22%), with rates over 1% occurring in many clinics in East Coast cities and in Puerto Rico (6). In these same cities, prevalence of serum HIV antibody was highest in clinics offering prenatal services and abortion when compared with family planning or general medicine clinics. Overall, risks of mother-to-child transmission of HIV range from 13 to 60% (7).

**Table 37–1.** Risk Factors for HIV Infection in Women or Sexual Partners

| |
|---|
| Sexual Transmission |
| Current or previous multiple sexual partners or use of sex for money or drugs |
| Bisexual activity |
| History of or current sexually transmitted diseases |
| Living in or having lived in countries where the incidence of HIV infection is high |
| Artificial insemination of semen not screened for HIV infection |
| Coitus with partner at risk of HIV infection without use of barrier contraception or spermicide |
| Blood-Borne Transmission |
| Transmission of blood or blood products before adequate screening began in the United States (between 1978 and 1985) |
| Injection, illicit drug use (especially if needles are shared) |

**Table 37–2.** Counseling for Women Infected with Human Immunodeficiency Virus (HIV)

Health Care Issues
- Describe the early clinical manifestations of HIV infection
- Inform about the current understanding of the prognosis of HIV
- Provide or refer to medical services for appropriate care for the asymptomatic, HIV-infected women for:
  - Immunologic testing
  - Antiviral therapy
  - Pneumocystis carinii pneumonia prophylaxis
- For pregnant women, inform about the risk of transmission from mother to fetus
- Stress the importance of the woman notifying her other health care providers of her HIV status

## Case Definition and Predictors of HIV Disease Progression

HIV is a retrovirus (lentivirus) that preferentially infects cells expressing CD4+ antigen on their surfaces. These include helper T lymphocytes, macrophages, and many cells in the central nervous system and in the placenta (8). Within 2 or 3 weeks of initial infection, approximately one-half of infected individuals experience a "flu-like" syndrome that may be accompanied by aseptic meningitis, central rash, arthralgia, diarrhea, fever, lymphadenopathy, and other nonspecific findings. In the vast majority of infected individuals, HIV-antibodies develop within 6 to 12 weeks after infection. Rarely, the virus-positive, antibody-negative period may be of considerably longer duration (9).

With time, HIV infection causes cell death and depletion of CD4+ T helper lymphocytes. This and other changes result in increasing susceptibility to characteristic "AIDS-defining" opportunistic infections and a number of characteristic neoplasias (Table 37–3). The adult AIDS case definition has been recently redefined as a group of severe illnesses, including specific opportunistic infections and cancers. This redefinition now includes invasive cervical cancer, recurrent pneumonia, and pulmonary tuberculosis (Table 37–3).

Risk of development of AIDS has been shown to be high for those infected individuals with 1) CD4+ cell count below 200/mm$^3$ or 2) below 20% of total circulating lymphocytes or 3) who demonstrate a rapid decline of CD4+ cells (2). The CDC has modified the AIDS case definition to include individuals with CD4+ lymphocyte counts less

**Table 37–2A.** Risk Reduction Counseling for HIV-Infection Women

- Reinforce the need for responsible sexual behavior, such as decreasing the number of partners and consistently usings condoms
- Reinforce the importance of avoiding the sharing of intravenous needles
- Encourange patient to notify sexual and needle-sharing partners of her HIV status and to advise them to be counseled and tested
- Inform of the prohibition from donating blood products or body organs
- Advise patient not to share toothbrushes, razors, or other personal items that might be contaminated with blood
- Discuss the possibility of transmission from mother to fetus

**Table 37–3.** 1993 Revised Classification System for HIV Infection and Expanded AIDS Surveillance Case Definition for Adolescents and Adults

| | Clinical Categories | | |
|---|---|---|---|
| CD4+ T-lymphocyte categories | A* | B† | C‡ |
| ≥500/μL | A1 | B1 | C1 |
| 200–499/μL | A2 | B2 | C2 |
| <200/μL§ | A3§ | B3§ | C3 |

* Clinical Category A—acute (primary) HIV infection, persistent generalized lymphadenopathy (PGL) and asymptomatic HIV-infected patients.

† Clinical Category B—symptomatic conditions occurring in an HIV-infected adolescent or adult, but not (A) or (C) conditions. Examples include:

- Candidiasis, vulvovaginal; persistent, frequent, or poorly responsive to therapy
- Candidiasis, oropharyngeal (thrush)
- Cervical dysplasia, moderate or severe/carcinoma in situ
- Constitutional symptoms, e.g. fever (≥38.5°C) or diarrhea lasting >1 month
- Hairy leukoplakia, oral
- Herpes zoster (shingles), involving at least two distinct episodes or more than one dermatome
- Idiopathic thrombocytopenia purpura
- Listeriosis
- Pelvic inflammatory disease; particularly if complicated by tubo-ovarian abscesses
- Peripheral neuropathy

‡ Clinical Category C—AIDS-indicator conditions
- Candidiasis of bronchi, trachea, or lungs
- Candidiasis, esophageal
- § Cervical cancer, invasive
- Coccidioidomycoses, disseminated or extrapulmonary
- Cryptococcosis, extrapulmonary
- Cryptosporidiosis, chronic intestinal (>1 month's duration)
- Cytomegalovirus disease (other than liver, spleen, or nodes)
- Cytomegalovirus retinitis (with loss of vision)
- Encephalopathy, HIV-related
- Herpes simplex: chronic ulcer(s) (>1 month's duration) or bronchitis, pneumonitis, or esophagitis
- Histoplasmosis, disseminated or extrapulmonary
- Isosporiasis, chronic intestinal (>1 month's duration)
- Kaposi's sarcoma
- Lymphoma, Burkitt's (or equivalent term)
- Lymphoma, immunoblastic (or equivalent term)
- Lymphoma, primary, of brain
- Mycobacterium avium complex or M. kansasii, extrapulmonary
- M. tuberculosis, any site (pulmonary or extrapulmonary)
- Mycobacterium, other or unidentified species, extrapulmonary
- Pneumocystis carinii pneumonia
- § Pneumonia, recurrent
- Progressive multifocal leukoencephalopathy
- Salmonella septicemia, recurrent
- Toxoplasmosis of brain
- Wasting syndrome due to HIV

§ New AIDS-defining conditions added as of January 1, 1993

From Centers for Disease Control and Prevention, 1993 revised classification system for HIV infection and expanded surveillance case definition for AIDS among adolescents and adults. MMWR 1992;41 (No. RR-17).

than 200 cells $mm^3$ regardless of symptomatology, because these patients appear to have a high risk of progression to an AIDS-defining illness (10). In a retrospective survey of 2748 men and women whose CD4+ counts fell below 200 CD4+ lymphocytes/$mm^3$, 46% developed AIDS-indicator diseases, compared with 6.5% of those with CD4+ lymphocyte counts of greater than 200 cells/$mm^3$ over a 12-month period (11). There were no differences in CD4+ counts and subsequent risk for development of AIDS among women and men, but few women were evaluated.

Increasing duration of HIV infection is also associated with increased risk for development of AIDS and AIDS-defining illnesses. For homosexual men, it has been possible to estimate the rate of progression by inferring the time of seroconversion from testing stored blood specimens (12). In 3% of those specimens tested, AIDS developed within 2 years of seroconversion; in 20% within 5 years; and in 40% within 7 years. Because for many individuals the duration of infection is not known, it has not been possible to study the rate of progression on the basis of duration of HIV infection in all risk or socioeconomic groups. Nevertheless, there is increasing evidence that a small portion, approximately 10% of HIV-infected individuals, do not necessarily (or only very slowly) progress to AIDS. These individuals appear to have a stable nonprogressive infection and remain healthy for prolonged periods. How this occurs and whether it is due to less virulent virus or to distinctive host factors is of intense interest.

In addition to changes in CD4+ lymphocyte counts, studies have suggested clinical and laboratory factors that may be associated with increased risk for development for progression to AIDS (13). Development of fever, weight loss, wasting, oral candidiasis, and hairy leukoplakia is associated with increased likelihood of progression. Lymphadenopathy alone does not seem to relate to rates of disease progression. AIDS is more likely to develop in HIV-infected patients who have p24 antigenemia or increased levels of neoptrin and/or beta-2 microglobulin (13). The impact of other factors, including intravenous drug use, smoking, intercurrent pregnancy and coinfections with STDs, cytomegalovirus or hepatitis needs to be evaluated. Rates and clinical predictors of progression to AIDS that are specific for women must be better characterized in prospective studies, including large numbers of women. Causes of death in females with AIDS are generally similar to men: drug abuse (27%), Pneumocystis carinii pneumonia (20%), other pneumonias (14%), septicemia (10%), as well as cervical cancer (<1%) and pelvic inflammatory disease (<1%) (1).

## Clinical Manifestations of HIV Disease and AIDS

Whether the clinical course of AIDS-related illnesses in women differs significantly from that in men also remains unclear because studies have included relatively few women. A large cohort of 200 women from Rhode Island has been reported that shows a wide spectrum of HIV-associated diseases in women (14). More than half of the women suffered from one or more reproductive-tract infections, including vaginal candidiasis, chronic or refractory herpes simplex infection, and/or genital warts. Pneumonitis, including P. carinii pneumonia, was also common: 44 developed AIDS.

Genital neoplasias have also been increasingly reported in HIV-infected women. For women in the Rhode Island cohort in which Papanicolaou (Pap) smear reports were available, squamous intraepithelial cervical lesions occurred in fully 35% (23 of 65); there were three women with lymphoma and one with Kaposi's sarcoma. Four additional women had a history of cervical or endometrial cancer before acquiring HIV infection.

Nine neoplasias were reported in another cohort study of 626 women (11). There were two cases each of cervical cancer and Kaposi's sarcoma, and one each of Hodgkins Disease, nonspecific lymphoma, leukemia, bladder cancer, and nasal cavity cancer. Overall, these findings are similar to men with HIV-disease, except for the relative absence of Kaposi's sarcoma and the often high rates of cervical intraepithelial abnormalities noted in women. Intraepithelial abnormalities, including dysplasia and squamous neoplasia, are now also noted in anal areas of homosexual men with HIV infection.

In the United States, there has been a dramatic increase in tuberculosis that has paralleled increases in HIV infection (15). This may, in part, be due to common sociodemographic factors (intravenous drug abuse, inner city residence, minorities, and poverty) for both HIV and tuberculosis. However, the lack of cell-mediated immunity associated with progressive HIV-infection disease likely hastens reactivation of previously healed tuberculosis infection (15). In addition, severe immunosuppression is associated with atypical presentation of tuberculosis, often characterized by cutaneous anergy and extrapulmonary pulmonary disease. For these reasons, it is particularly important to screen HIV-infected women for tuberculosis infection (Mantoux skin testing), as well as disease (chest x ray, etc.) and to provide appropriate isoniazid (INH) prophylaxis for infection or multiple drug therapy for disease. Pregnant women receiving INH should receive supplemental pyridoxine (vitamin $B_6$, 50 mg/day).

## Interactions Between Pregnancy and HIV Infection

Interactions between HIV infection during pregnancy are dynamic and multifaceted. The physiologic processes of pregnancy and parturition may be directly effected by HIV infection, with or without the presence of HIV disease and/or AIDS. Both the infected mother and the perinate can suffer consequences of ongoing HIV infection, including possibly increased early and late fetal loss, preterm birth, puerperal infection, and vertical transmission. Conversely, the natural course of HIV infection (to AIDS and possible death) could theoretically be accelerated due to immune alterations occurring during pregnancy.

Both the mother and fetus demonstrate immune alterations as part of mutual adaptations to support the pregnancy. While pregnant women are not "immunosuppressed," much anecdotal information suggests that pregnant women are at increased risk of "opportunistic" infection regardless of HIV status and that these infections are not so easily cleared or treated as in nonpregnant hosts. The combined immune alterations of HIV infection and pregnancy may increase risks of common infections (chorioamnionitis, endometritis, pyelonephritis, etc.) and/or rare infections (listeriosis, tuberculosis, etc.) during pregnancy and the puerperal period. Studies of all these possibilities are made difficult because of methodologic problems including: 1) the relatively few pregnant women followed so far; 2) ascertainment bias in case reporting; 3) inability to control for confounding variables, i.e. other concurrent infections, such as syphilis, gonorrhea, and chlamydia; and 4) inability to easily measure maternal immunosuppression as HIV infection progresses. In all populations studied, there appears to be the greatest HIV-associated morbidity and mortality in populations that have had HIV for longer durations or that have AIDS. As more women have HIV infection for longer durations, both obstetric and infectious HIV-related morbidity will likely increase.

Fertility is not impaired in HIV-infected women who are otherwise healthy. If these women are sexually active, they should be offered contraceptive and "safer sex" counseling.

Multiple cohort and some prospective studies show increased rates of spontaneous abortion. In the largest study reported, Temmerman examined 195 women admitted to a hospital in Kenya with abortion (16). Attempts were made to eliminate from analysis those with induced abortion. Spontaneous abortion was independently associated with HIV-antibody positivity (odds ratio = 2.2) as well as maternal syphilis and group B streptococcal infection. This suggested that predisposition to early pregnancy loss should be confirmed in better controlled studies.

Plausible mechanisms for increased reproductive loss during pregnancy include:

1) direct HIV infection of trophoblast cells;
2) embryonic infection;
3) alteration in maternal-embryonic/fetal mutual immune tolerance;
4) effects of other infections, nutrition, etc.

Early observations of a dysmorphic congenital syndrome associated with HIV infection (17) have not been confirmed in large studies (18). Whether HIV-infected pregnant women are at increased risk for such infection as cytomegalovirus, toxoplasmosis, herpes, hepatitis B primary, or infectious reactivation during pregnancy remains unknown.

Pregnancy complications such as preterm birth, low birth weight, perinatal death, and cesarean section, tend to show differing results in industrialized countries in comparison to Africa. Relatively small studies in New York (19) and Milan (20) do not show increased morbidity, at least in healthy HIV-infected women. Conversely, large studies in Africa tend to show increased risk of preterm birth and perinatal death, and possibly chorioamnionitis (21,22). Several studies suggest that increased risk of ascending intrauterine infection with histologic and clinical chorioamnionitis may account for these findings (21,22). Such ascending infection may be caused by microorganisms present in normal cervicovaginal flora or associated with sexually transmitted diseases, such as gonorrhea and/or chlamydia infection. Such confounding conditions may account for differences in outcome studies in different geographic regions. In these and other studies, infant birth weight is not correlated with eventual infection HIV status. In one study, fully one-fourth of HIV-infected women demonstrated elevated anticardiolipin antibodies suggesting that unanticipated associated factors can also play roles in HIV-associated pregnancy morbidity (23).

## Vertical Transmission of HIV

Embryos, fetuses, and infants may be vertically infected with HIV transplacentally (intrauterine) or intrapartum and postpartum (through breast-feeding and blood or blood products). The relative risks of each of these modes of transmission have varied during the course of the AIDS epidemic: in the early 1980s, U.S. children became infected primarily through blood or blood-product use. Currently, infection occurs principally during pregnancy or at the time of birth. Overall, (because blood products may now be considered "nearly safe"), the 13 to 60% (average 30%) rates of vertical transmission constitute the single most efficient and potent form of HIV transmission. Attempts to prevent vertical transmission can be a powerful means to decrease the prevalence and tragedy of HIV infection. Exact proportions of forms of transmission remain unknown but can be estimated to be one-fourth antenatal, one-half peripartum, and one-third breast feeding.

Intrauterine, transplacental infection may occur early in pregnancy. Many trophoblast cells express CD4+ HIV receptor molecules (24). Studies of aborted fetal materials suggest that HIV infection can be well-established in the first trimester (25). Fully 28% of 24 second trimester fetuses of HIV-positive mothers were positive for HIV nucleic acid (26).

Placental lesions, such as villitis, chorioamnionitis, abruption, or transplacental amniocentesis may increase placental "leakiness" and possible maternal-fetal bleeding. Other than avoiding invasive procedures (amniocentesis, cordocentesis, and fetoscopy) and use of prolonged antiretroviral agents (zidovudine) during pregnancy, it may be difficult to mitigate risks of transplacental infection.

That intrapartum transmission is important in mother-to-child-spread of infection is supported by considerable circumstantial evidence. Hepatitis B virus (HBV) is commonly transmitted at birth. Infectious HIV-1 virus is present in cervical and vaginal secretions (27) and in the copious amounts of blood released during placental separation, vaginal lacerations, or episiotomy. Insightful evidence comes from the European International Reports of HIV-exposed twins (28). In this study of 66 sets of twins, first borns (born either vaginally or by cesarean section) were significantly more likely to be infected than second born twins delivered by section or vaginal birth. This ongoing study suggests that passage through the birth canal is associated with increased risk of perinatal HIV acquisition. If substantiated, these observations suggest that perinates may be spared infections should: 1) they be delivered at term by planned section prior to labor; 2) fetal membranes be kept intact as long as possible during vaginal birth; or 3) the vagina and cervix could be irrigated with antiviral antiseptics so as to decrease the inoculum of HIV in the birth canal.

Newborns can presumably become vertically infected postpartum by continued contact with infectious maternal secretions. Thus, babies should be washed promptly after birth. HIV is detectable in both whole and cell-free human milk (29). In the European Collaborative Study, approximately 14% of infected newborns became infected by breast-feeding. Overall, rates of breast milk-linked infection remains unknown but are likely to be much higher should seroconversion (initial infection) occur during lactation, or should there be heavy antigenemia/viremia associated in advanced infection or AIDS (30). Healthy women with low levels of antigenemia viremia are presumably less likely to transmit infection through breast milk. At this time, recommendations are to avoid breast-feeding when safe alternatives exist (31). In many developing parts of the world, risk of death from contaminated-water induced diarrhea and other illnesses may outweigh risks of HIV infection from breast-feeding (31).

Confirming evidence of distinctive means of vertical transmission comes from observations of bimodal distribution of pediatric HIV infection. In the European Collaborative Study (18), survival analysis showed two distinctive groups in terms of earlier onset of infection and progressive illness: 83% of 64 infected children showed signs of infection within 6 months of birth. Of these, fully 26% developed AIDS by 12 months. These and other experiences (32) correlate with the hypothesis that infection early in pregnancy is manifested earlier and that a substantial number of these infected children have rapidly progressive illness and death. On the other hand, newborns infected late in pregnancy or after birth, when the immune system is more completely developed, may demonstrate less progressive, "adult-like" courses of infection. Means to reduce risk of infection would be most effective if designed to prevent each mode of vertical transmission, i.e. maternal zidovudine prophylaxis during pregnancy, zidovudine and passive immune globulin at birth, and avoidance of breast feeding after birth.

As noted, overall rates of mother-to-child transmission vary between 13 to 60% (average about 30%) (7). Rates differ with duration of followup, test criteria for infection (culture, PCR, p24 antigen), and populations studied. The European Collaborative Study (1988) followed children for 18 months and initially noted a transmission rate of 24%. This included children who were culture positive but antibody negative. This study was revised in 1991 to a risk ratio of 12.9% (95% CI, RR 9.5 to 16.3) based on 372 children (18). Importantly, 25 of these children with positive blood cultures remain seronegative and healthy. This observation suggests that aspects of either the infecting virus (virulence) or host responses (immune responses, MHC genotype, etc.) can play important roles in understanding how some individuals may remain infected but healthy for prolonged periods. Factors suggested to be associated with altered risks of transmission are noted in Table 37–4. Each of these factors is the subject of ongoing research.

**Table 37–4.** Factors Postulated (Unproven) to Affect Mother–Child HIV Transmission

Maternal:
- Advanced disease as measured by:
  - Clinical staging
  - Low CD4+ counts
  - p24 antigenemia
  - Elevated serum $B_2$-microglobulin, neoptrin, IgA
  - Increased age
  - Presence of other STDs, i.e., syphilis
- "Protective" antibodies against HIV epitopes
  - gp120
  - Principal neutralizing domain
  - V3 loop

Viral:
- Virulent strain or subspecies

Host:
- Coinfection: cytomegalovirus, etc.
- HLA tissue types

Obstetrics:
- Preterm birth
- Invasive procedures
- Vaginal delivery
- Break in child's skin: scalp sample, scalp electrode, etc.
- Fetal aspiration of blood, abruption, gasping, etc.

## Handling of the Perinate Intrapartum and Postpartum

There continues to be limited information regarding means to reduce intrapartum and/or postpartum HIV transmission from mother to babies. Empiric guidelines are suggested (Table 37–5), but remain speculative and essentially unevaluated. Steps should be employed to reduce amounts of infectious maternal blood fetuses and

**Table 37–5.** Suggestions to Reduce Antenatal, Intrapartum and Postpartum Exposure of Perinates to HIV (Unproven)

Antepartum
- Avoid invasive procedures:
  - Amniocentesis
  - Cordocentesis
  - Placental or chorion biopsies

Intrapartum
- Avoid:
  - Scalp electrodes, scalp sampling
  - Early rupture of fetal membranes
  - Skin abrasions, i.e. midforceps, multiple application of vacuum extractor
  - Overly vigorous suction, DeLee suction from wall

Postpartum
- Breast-feeding, if safe alternatives exist
- Wash newborn promptly in warm water
- Delay injections (vitamin K) and surgery (circumcision) until after bathing

Speculative
- Cesarean section prior to or early in labor
- Zidovudine prophylaxis
- High anti-HIV titer immune globulin, when available

babies are exposed to during and immediately after birth. Reasonable, but unproven, procedures include: 1) avoidance of fetal scalp sampling and/or use of fetal scalp monitoring electrodes; 2) avoidance of possibly skin-abrading procedures such as midforceps or use of Maelstrom vacuum extractor use; 3) DeLee suction for oral pharyngeal clearing should only be done with carefully adjusted suction available from the wall in the birthing room or from a suction machine to avoid traumatizing mucosal membranes and to avoid exposing the resuscitating care provider; 4) newborns born of possibly infected mothers should be handled with gloves and should be promptly bathed in soapy warm water; 5) routine injections for vitamin K for hepatitis B vaccination should be delayed until bathing is completed and the baby dried; 7) circumcision should be similarly delayed.

More speculative questions relating to reducing risks of perinatal transmission include: 1) use of preventive cesarean section performed before the onset of labor or before passage of the fetal head into the vagina; 2) administration of zidovudine to the mother during labor and to the newborn after birth as chemoprophylaxis; 3) use of high titer anti-HIV immune globulin for the newborn to augment passage of transplacental immunity immediately after birth. Breast-feeding by HIV-infected mothers should be avoided in areas where safe alternative nutritional sources are available for newborns.

Studies are ongoing to evaluate whether these or other suggestions can be effective in reducing risks of perinatal HIV transmission. Performance of cesarean section to possibly reduce risks of perinatal HIV transmission is undergoing investigation. Possible disadvantages include increased maternal mortality and costs and increased health care worker exposure to needle sticks (cesarean section surgery versus repair of lacerations or episiotomies). These are all factors that must be considered. Each of these possible interventions is based on identification of HIV-infected women before or during pregnancy through increased selective and, more helpfully, universal screening for HIV infection in women who are considering pregnancy or who are already pregnant. Such intervention may allow for identification of infected women. These women may be counselled regarding continuation of pregnancy and care plans for the pregnancy itself. Interventions to presumably reduce risks of peripartum HIV transmission may be then intelligently employed, including avoidance of lactation.

## Immunologic Monitoring

The correlation between the occurrence of AIDS-defining events and CD4+ cell counts below 500 cells mm$^3$ has led to the use of CD4+ T cell levels as the primary laboratory determinant for beginning both antiviral therapy and chemoprophylaxis against Pneumocystis carinnii pneumonia (10). A baseline CD4+ cell count should be obtained when the diagnosis of HIV is made. For individuals with CD4+ counts greater than 600 cells/mm$^3$, testing should be repeated in 6 months. If the CD4+ count is less than 600 cells/mm$^3$, another count should be obtained in 3 months. For those individuals with CD4+ counts that have rapidly declined since the previous measurement or counts that have approached a level at which either antiviral therapy or antipneumocystis prophylaxis should be initiated, counts should be repeated within 1 week (33). Rarely, patients may demonstrate an HIV-like immunosuppression with CD4+ T-lymphocyte depression but do not demonstrate any evidence of HIV infections. These patients may have another immunotrophic virus or other factor which remains to be detected. Chemoprophylaxis for P. carinii is still indicated in this setting.

## Therapy and Prophylaxis

Clinical trials of zidovudine (retrovir, AZT) have shown a delay in the progression of AIDS in asymptomatic HIV-infected patients with CD4+ counts less than 500 cells/mm$^3$ (34). For individuals with AIDS or CD4+ less than 200 cells/mm$^3$, zidovudine therapy has significantly decreased mortality frequency and severity of opportunistic infections. Clinical trials of zidovudine in HIV-infected women to date have been too small to demonstrate therapeutic efficacy (35). Other antiretroviral agents, including dideoxyinosine (ddI), have recently been approved as therapy for patients who either do not tolerate zidovudine treatment or have progression of HIV disease while taking zidovudine (36).

Although short-term benefits of zidovudine and ddI have been demonstrated in clinical trials, long-term effects of antiviral therapy, including improvement of life and overall delay of death, are still being evaluated. One clear-cut adverse effect of antiviral therapy has been the development of zidovudine drug resistance, which is observed especially after zidovudine has been received for longer than a year. Thus, extensive use of zidovudine early in HIV infection may eliminate its effectiveness when patients are more seriously ill.

As HIV-infected patients live longer, the spectrum of HIV-related disease will also change. For example, opportunistic non-Hodgkins lymphomas have been increasingly reported among severely immunocompromised HIV-infected patients who survive for long periods while receiving antiviral therapy (37).

Specific recommendations for zidovudine treatment and P. carinii pneumonia prophylaxis in pregnant women are evolving rapidly. A survey of zidovudine use in 43 HIV-infected pregnant women has been performed in which 12 of these women received zidovudine in the first trimester (38). In this small series, zidovudine was well tolerated and was not associated with malformations in newborns, premature labor or fetal distress. At this time, indications for retroviral therapy using AZT or zidovudine and P. carinii prophylaxis continue to be the same as in nonpregnant women.

## Prophylaxis for P. carinii Pneumonia

P. carinii pneumonia is the most frequent AIDS-defining event for both women and men in the United States (39). This is a major cause of death in HIV-infected women and men (40). The Public Health Service Recommends that antibiotic prophylaxis be instituted when patients are at high risk for P. carinii pneumonia to reduce both the frequency of initial episodes (primary prophylaxis) as well as the risks of relapse or recurrence (secondary prophylaxis) (41). High risk is defined as CD4+ T cell counts below 200/cells mm$^3$ or below 20% of the total circulating lymphocytes, or a prior occurrence of P. carinii pneumonia. Rapidly declining CD4+ T cells counts, the presence of HIV-related thrush, or unexplained fevers may also be associated with an increased risk of P. carinii pneumonia. Both trimethoprim-sulfa methoxazole (TMP-SMX) and aerosolized pentamidine are effective for primary and secondary prophylaxis. Trimethoprim-sulfa-methoxazole is more effective and less expensive than aerosol pentamidine in the prevention of recurrent P. carinii pneumonia, but it has been associated with a high frequency of adverse reactions. Nevertheless, there is considerably more experience with trimethoprim-sulfa methoxazole use in pregnancy and it remains the preferred method of chemoprophylaxis during pregnancy.

While concerns regarding sulfa-mediated kernicterus remain unsubstantiated, most clinicians discontinue TMP-SMX at term. The clinical efficacy of aerosolized pentamidine may depend on the nebulization device, drug dose, and patient characteristics such as the presence of preexisting lung disease. Administration of aerosolized pentamidine may also induce bronchospasm and coughing, which has been implicated in the spread of tuberculosis to both health care workers and other immunosuppressed patients. Therefore, it is especially important to evaluate the patient for the possibility of tuberculosis before beginning pentamidine therapy. Pregnant women with asthma should receive TMP-SMX as prophylaxis for P. carinii pneumonia.

## Immunization and Tuberculosis Testing

HIV-infected pregnant and nonpregnant women should receive pneumococcal, influenza, tetanus, and hepatitis B vaccines recommended for susceptible adults (42). In addition, tuberculosis skin testing [Mantoux test of purified protein derivative (PPD)] must also be accompanied by assessment of anergy using candida, mumps, or tetanus antigens (43).

## Female Reproductive Tract HIV-Associated Infections or Conditions Affecting Pregnant and Nonpregnant Women

### *Fungal*

Candidiasis may be the earliest and commonest cause of opportunistic mucosal infection in HIV-infected women. In a cohort of 29 HIV-infected women, chronic refractory vaginal candidiasis was reported in 7 (24%) (44). Women with refractory vaginal candidiasis were otherwise asymptomatic but had low CD4+ lymphocyte counts. However, the converse is not true, and uncomplicated vaginal candidiasis is not a useful risk marker for HIV infection.

The site of mucosal candida infection may relate to the degree of immunodeficiency, with vaginal candidiasis appearing early in the course of infection and esophageal candidiasis occurring late (in highly immunocompromised individuals). Women with thrush, with or without candidiasis, should be evaluated for HIV infection. In one study, local therapy for vaginal or oral candidiasis was effective for over 90% of individuals (45). Of those women who failed topical treatment, all responded to oral ketoconazole. Some treatment failures or episodes of recurrent yeast may relate to concomitant antibiotic prophylaxis against pneumocystis pneumonia. Diagnosis in HIV-infected women is the same as in noninfected individuals, primarily by microscopy.

### *HIV Infection*

HIV has been readily isolated from cervical and vaginal secretions of HIV-infected women (27). One study suggested that the presence of HIV in the lower genital tract secretions even during menses is independent of blood infections, as determined by peripheral blood cultures (45). In another study, HIV culture specimens were obtained from genital ulcers more frequently and in greater inocula than from cervical or vaginal secretions (46). The HIV-infected cells in cervical tissue, cervical vaginal secretions, and genital ulcers may play important roles in the transmission of HIV by heterosexual contact and possibly to perinates during their passage through the birth canal of HIV-infected women.

Studies have suggested that HIV can directly infect genital lymphocytes and epithelial cells (47). The inflammatory response to cervical or vaginal HIV infection may appear as cervicitis. One report has suggested that genital ulcers, not caused by other known genital ulcer diseases, may be due directly to HIV infection, and that these ulcers respond to zidovudine treatment (48). Conversely, HIV, by causing systemic or local immunosuppression or both, may worsen symptoms of other STDs and make them more difficult to treat.

## Herpes Virus

Both Herpes Simplex Virus (HSV) types 1 and 2 infections are common in the U.S. general population. Chronic mucocutaneous herpes infection secondary to either herpes simplex-2 or varicella zoster virus are common in HIV-infected women (39). Both case reports and clinical evidence suggest that HSV infections may be more severe in HIV-infected patients (49). For these patients, HSV infections may appear in atypical locations and are often extensive or persistent. In addition, the frequency of recurrences may increase as immunosuppression secondary to HIV progresses. Also of importance is that risks of HIV transmission may be increased by the presence of active HSV disease and epithelial ulceration.

The incidence of acyclovir-resistant HSV infection may also be increased among HIV infected patients who are immunosuppressed and who may have had multiple exposures to acyclovir (49). For these patients with acyclovir-resistant HIV, most respond to treatment with foscarnet or other agents. Long-term prophylaxis should be reserved for patients with multiple recurrences. Cytomegalovirus has also been reported as a cause of cervical ulceration in a woman with AIDS (50).

## Bacterial Sexually Transmitted Diseases

Relationships between HIV infection and STD pathogens, such as Neisseria gonorrhoeae and Chlamydia trachomatis are characterized by epidemiologic synergy. Because gonorrhea and chlamydia both cause an inflammatory responses, some studies have implicated them in the enhancement of HIV transmission. As noted, the immunosuppression produced by HIV may worsen symptoms or disease course caused by STDs. In addition, intimate sexual contact is a common mode of transmission for each agent. Choices of antibiotic treatment of these infections in HIV-infected women should follow guidelines for the general population (51).

The HIV seroprevalence of women admitted to gynecologic services in large American cities with pelvic inflammatory disease (PID) has increased. In a study from San Francisco, the prevalence increased from 0 in 1985 to fully 7% in 1988 (52). In New York in early 1989, the rate of HIV in women admitted with pelvic inflammatory disease was estimated to be fully 17% (53). In another study, HIV-infected women who had PID were less likely to have leukocytosis than uninfected women (54). These patients were more likely to have pelvic abscesses and require more surgical intervention (54). Immunosuppression secondary to HIV infection is increasingly common justification for inpatient treatment of pelvic inflammatory disease in HIV-infected women (51).

Chancroid is widely implicated in increasing risks of HIV transmission in African men and women because it causes large genital ulcers. Decreased responsiveness to standard therapy is documented in HIV patients with chancroid. Case reports also suggest an atypical presentation of chancroid with larger, multicentric or extragenital lesions. Combined treatment with a quinolone and trimethoprim-sulfamethoxazole or longer treatment period may be necessary.

An epidemic of syphilis is occurring in the United States (54). In HIV-infected individuals, the clinical presentations may be atypical and progression to neurosyphilis may be more frequent. In addition, standard therapy for early infection may be inadequate because standard benzathine penicillin therapy does not consistently achieve treponemicidal levels in the central nervous system (55). Because of the higher prevalence of neurosyphilis, some authorities recommend that a lumbar puncture be done routinely to select those individuals who might benefit from longer treatment.

## Human Papilloma Virus (HPV) Infection and the Risk of Cervical Cancer with HIV Infection

Recent studies in women with HIV and other immunodeficiency diseases show that HPV infection of the lower genital tract is common (56). HPV infection has been implicated as an important cofactor in the development of cervical dysplasia in lower genital tract cancer. HPV has been detected in cervical cancer specimens, and has been associated with cancer of the cervix in many epidemiologic studies (57). In fact, papilloma viruses have been shown to transform cells in vitro. Although more than 20 human papilloma virus types have been found to infect the genital tract, several types (6, 11, 16, 18, 31, 33, and 35) are more common and are associated with variable risks of progression to cervical cancer (58). HPV type 6 and 11 are found in benign condylomata, types 31, 33, and 35 may have an intermediate risk of progression to cancer, and types 16 and 18 are most clearly linked with invasive cervical neoplasia. One study has suggested that significant differences may exist between HPV types detected in patients with CIN-I as compared with those with CIN-II and III (59).

HPV, recognized by koilocytosis, perinuclear clearing, and parakeratosis on pap smear, biopsy, or Southern blot analysis of specific HPV genotype, is detected more frequently in HIV-infected women than HIV-negative women (60). HPV nucleic acid detection has also been correlated with symptomatic HIV infection and is present in 70% of symptomatic women, compared with 22% of asymptomatic and HIV-negative women (61). Sociodemographic characteristics common to women with cervical dysplasia and cancer, such as first intercourse at a young age, multiple sexual partners, low socioeconomic status, and a history of STDs are also common for women with HIV infection. Cervical dysplasia has been reported to be 5 to 10 times more common in HIV-infected women than among uninfected women living in the same communities (62). CIN is characteristically of a higher grade, more extensive, and more frequently involves other sites in the lower genital tract infection of HIV-positive women compared with HIV-negative women (62). HIV-infected women with CIN also may have lower CD4+ cell counts and CD4+ to CD8+ ratios than HIV-infected women without CIN (63). Cervical dysplasia and cervical cancer may be more common, more difficult to diagnosis, and more difficult to treat in HIV-infected women.

Cytologic diagnosis of cervical neoplasia may be more difficult to detect in HIV-infected women. In one study, pap smears were read as normal for 39% of HIV-infected who had CIN on histology (64). Although this discordance between colposcopically directed biopsy and pap smear suggests that all HIV-positive patients might benefit from colposcopy, previous reports (63) show concordance between pap smear and colposcopic biopsy histology. The multifocal nature of genital dysplasia in HIV-infected women suggests that a pap smear should be considered a reliable screening tool at this time. For pregnant or nonpregnant HIV-infected women who have severe dysplasia on pap smear, a thorough colposcopic evaluation of cervix, vagina, and vulva is indicated. If the report of false-negative pap results is confirmed by other researchers, routine baseline colposcopy may then be warranted. Other preliminary data suggest that CIN in HIV-infected women is significantly more likely to persist or recur within the first year after standard cryosurgical, laser, or electrocautery treatment.

One report suggests that HIV-infected women with cervical carcinoma are more likely to present at more advanced stages of cancer than HIV-negative women (63). In addition, stage-for-stage HIV-infected women experience a shorter time for recurrence, and their recurrence and death rates are higher than HIV-negative women. This report needs to be followed up by the other centers.

Despite these observations and concerns, the current impact of cervical cancer and morbidity and mortality in HIV-infected women remains small. In reports of cohorts of HIV-infected women who were not observed at gynecologic oncology referral centers, prevalence of cervical cancer has remained low (39). It may be that improvement in longevity of HIV-infected women may come from increased awareness of cervical dysplasia, implementation of universal pap smear screening in HIV-infected women, and further advances in medical therapy for the HIV patient.

Because HIV-infected women are at increased risk for cervical disease, the CDC recommends that pap smears be obtained for HIV-infected women at least annually. In light of the prevalence of cervical dysplasia in this population and the potential fulminant course of cervical cancer, biannual pap smears may be indicated throughout the patient's life.

## Counselling and Testing

Information to be discussed when a physician offers HIV testing to women has been previously outlined in the context of pregnancy and in well-woman care (64). Offering testing only to those who acknowledge risk factors for HIV infection (Table 37–1) is an insensitive (approximately 50%) predictor of HIV infection in studies of child-bearing women. Following the CDC-recommended paradigm to offer testing when the prevalence rate is greater than 1 in 1000, HIV testing should be universally offered to U.S. women of reproductive ages in areas in which this threshold of seroprevalence has been reached. These areas include inner city populations in all large to moderately large U.S. cities (65). Many authorities feel that the benefits of HIV testing should be offered to all pregnant women and women at risk. Obviously, diagnosis allows for positive steps to be taken in preventing spread to other individuals, including children exposed to breastfeeding who should receive timely chemoprophylaxis.

The current HIV counselling and testing model often offers HIV testing with one pretest and posttest counselling session. One meta-analysis of behavioral studies concerning the effects of HIV antibody counselling and testing on risk behaviors is suggested. To achieve substantial behavioral risks reduction, several sessions are suggested. (66). To facilitate behavioral change in this epidemic, care providers to women must develop strategies to incorporate risk-reduction counselling into everyday practice.

## Contraception

Contraceptive use must balance concerns regarding prevention of HIV and STD transmission and those of preventing unwanted pregnancies. Barrier contraceptives, including latex condoms and contraceptive foam, have been shown to reduce rates of transmission of STDs and to protect against HIV infection (66). The addition of the spermicide to condoms improves the protective effects against both STDs and HIV (67).

Alterations in immune responses in women who use oral contraceptives, Norplant or injections of medroxyprogesterone acetate (Depo-Provera), is theoretically possible, but clinically unlikely. One report from Africa suggested that the transmission of HIV infection to prostitutes is more likely to occur in those who use oral contraceptives (68). On the other hand, all studies from industrialized countries, including Northern Europe, do not show increased risks of HIV transmission or seroprevalence among oral contraceptive users. Impact of long-term exogenous hormones on the progression of HIV infection remains unknown. In any case, hormonal contraception does not offer protection against transmission of HIV or other STDs and may be a disincentive to use barrier contraception. The increased risk of ascending reproductive-tract infection and pelvic-inflammatory disease is a relative contraindication to the use of an intrauterine contraceptive device in HIV-infected women.

## Case Reporting and Partner Notification

The care provider's role in partner notification is rapidly evolving and may differ greatly according to the jurisdiction in individual patients' circumstances. Although the patient-physician relationship is privileged and confidential, some states have legislated a requirement to notify partners in an attempt to prevent HIV infection.

In the United States, the authority to require notification to partners of cases of clinical diseases belongs to each state's legislature. Most states require clinicians to report cases of AIDS, and in fewer states, HIV infection. Many state health departments have specially trained disease intervention specialists who can assist physicians in partner notification. Because HIV is an increasingly common STD that will be seen more often in women's health care practice, it is advisable that each clinician learn the state requirements for reporting HIV and AIDS and state laws requiring notification. In any case, it should be universal good practice for index patients to personally notify all partners. State-assisted partner notification and testing programs should be fully utilized. HIV is a frequently lethal STD that requires a full commitment by public and private health care providers in providing confidential testing and treatment.

## Preventing Transfusion-Acquired Transmission of HIV

Transfusion-acquired transmission of HIV infection has led to increased awareness of the infectious complications of blood and blood components. Screening blood for HIV antibody began in 1985 and has reduced the risk of HIV virus transmission to approximately 1 in 156,000 transfusions (69). The Red Cross has tried to decrease the likelihood that individuals with HIV will donate blood by routinely assessing risk behaviors, conducting a brief physical examination, and excluding individuals at high risk for HIV infection from donating blood. Because screening identifies only the presence of HIV antibody, recently infected individuals who donate blood, but have not developed antibody, may not be detected. Development of virus-specific tests, such as polymerase chain reaction (PCR) can further reduce the potential risk of HIV transmission. In the U.S., it is estimated that 70 to 200 of the 4 million blood recipients each year develop transfusion-

**Table 37–6.** Alternatives to Homologous Red Cell Transfusion in Obstetric or Gynecologic Surgery

| |
|---|
| Autologous transfusion program |
| Intraoperative blood salvage |
| Intraoperative blood dilution |
| Intraoperative controlled hypotension |
| Pharmacologic approaches to reduce blood loss |
| Recombinant erythropoietin to increase preoperative red cell mass |
| Synthetic oxygen transport media |

associated HIV infection, a rate similar to the risk of dying from hemolytic transfusion reaction (70). Women care providers and anesthesiologists frequently care for women undergoing surgical procedures for which transfusion of blood products may be necessary. Both surgeon's and anesthesiologist's roles in preventing transfusion-associated infection include minimization of blood loss, adherence to hospital procedures for transfusion, delay of transfusions until clinically indicated, encouragement of autologous (self) blood transfusions, and awareness of new alternatives to blood products and their proper use (Table 37–6) (71). Facilitating autologous donations and delaying transfusions are new strategies to decrease risks of transfusion-acquired infections. Patients can donate autologous blood before elective surgery when perioperative transfusions might be anticipated. This is also true for women contemplating birth by cesarean section. In nonpregnant women, one unit of blood can be donated every 72 hours as long as the hematocrit value is at least 33%, until 72 hours before surgery (72). Because the blood is not frozen, storage of autologous units is limited to 42 days. A National Institute of Health (NIH) consensus conference (1988) on the perioperative red blood cell transfusion has recommended lowering of hemoglobin levels at which transfusion would be indicated after acute blood loss from 10 g/dL hemoglobin to 8 g/dL or less for most patients (73).

## Reducing Risks of HIV Transmission for Health Care Workers

Risk of occupational transmission of HIV to anesthesia or obstetric-gynecologic personnel appears to be very low: no case reports of transmission in either group in prospective studies are available. This probably relates to the effectiveness of universal blood-infectious secretions precautions and overall low rates of HIV infection in women (Table 37–7). As noted, rates of HIV infection in women are increasing and efforts to reduce risk of HIV must be continuously maintained. Risks of skin-puncture injuries with contaminated needles are associated with an approximate 1–10/1000 rate of transmission: approximately 1/300 for solid needles and possibly as high as 1/100 for hollow needles contaminated with infected blood (74).

Universal precautions are mandatory and must be meticulously followed during provision of anesthesia, as well as obstetric and gynecological surgical procedures (Table 37–7). These precautions include mandatory use of gloves when initiating all intravenous or intra-arterial lines and during any possible exposure to potentially infectious secretions (blood contaminated saliva, bronchial fluid). Use of face shields, goggles, or glasses and face masks must be used so as to reduce the small risks of exposure during intubation or neonatal resuscitation. Such precautions must be fully followed regardless of HIV serostatus of the particular patient because HIV infection may be undiagnosed. If needle or other percutaneous exposure occurs, personnel should be carefully counselled, and prophylactic treatment with zidovudine considered, using updated protocols (Table 37–8). Risk of occupational HIV transmission to obstetrics and to anesthesia personnel can be minimized with continued vigilance and thorough application of universal precautions against all blood and bloody secretions.

**Table 37–7.** Keys of Universal Blood/Secretion Precautions

| |
|---|
| Treat *all* patients with universal precautions |
| Consider all patients possibly infected |
| Use extreme care with needles. Never recap. Use stop cocks and "safe needles" whenever possible. Always use needle disposal systems. |
| Wear gloves if contact with blood or secretions possible |
| Use protective eyewear (glasses or goggles or face shields) if secretion may be spread. Wear appropriate respiratory isolation masks if tuberculosis a possibility. |
| Pregnant personnel are not at increased risk, but should also take precautions against concomitant cytomegalovirus coinfection. |

## Special Concerns for Anesthesia Personnel

While providing patient care in labor and delivery areas, as well as in operating rooms, anesthesia personnel will inevitably care for HIV-infected women. Exposures can occur to undiagnosed HIV-infected patients as well as those who are identified with HIV infection or AIDS. Because anesthesia personnel provide care to patients with possible HIV infection and and because routine preoperative HIV-1 screening may not be logistically or ethically feasible, all patients should be treated as if they were carrying blood-born, potentially transmissible agents. So-called universal precautions are outlined in Table 37–7.

**Table 37–8.** Suggested Procedures If Exposed to Possibly Infectious Blood or Secretions

| |
|---|
| If mucosal "splash" wash with soap and water promptly. If needle, note type, presence of blood? |
| Report to appropriate area (employee health, emergency room, etc.) to initiate assessment, counselling, possible chemoprophylaxis and followup. |
| If serostatus unknown, ask patient (source) for permission to do HIV-antibody testing and counselling |
| Counselling regarding risks and precautions |
| Strongly consider zidovudine (AZT) prophylaxis at least until return of patient (donor) serology. |
| If patient (donor) refuses testing or is seropositive, obtain acute serum anti-HIV antibody test and repeat 6, 12, 24 weeks. |

Emphasis should be placed on avoiding contact with blood and bodily fluids. In particular, needle-stick injuries present the most significant risk of exposure for anesthesia personnel. Precautions to prevent needle-stick injury must be strenuously enforced. All personnel should avoid direct handling and recapping of contaminated needles. Use of puncture-resistent needle disposal units near the site of needle use and meticulous attention to needle handling will eliminate most risks of needle-stick injury. New needle designs that shield the used needle and obviate the need for "recapping" should be used in addition to stop cocks to reduce use of needle aspirations to obtain blood or inject medications. The most infectious bodily secretions appear to be blood, semen, and vaginal secretions (2). These fluids contain white blood cells, including potentially infected lymphocytes and thus represent increased risk for transmission of HIV. Other bodily fluids that are theoretical sources of HIV include cerebral-spinal, synovial, pleural, peritoneal, pericardial, and amniotic fluid. Secretions to which anesthesia personnel are routinely exposed, including sputum, saliva, nasal secretions, tears, urine, vomitus, and feces are much less likely to contain HIV, unless they contain visible blood. Use of gloves should be mandatory should exposure to bodily fluids be expected.

Anesthesia care providers are often asked questions regarding risks of HIV transmission during procedures. Patients having routine delivery or elective cesarean section often inquire about the safety of potential blood transfusions. As discussed, concern over transfusion-transmitted infection has dramatically changed transfusion practices and brought about innovative blood conservation techniques (Table 37–6). However, autologous transfusions are generally impractical in caring for pregnant women. The safety of the blood supply in North America has been secured by multiple programmatic changes in blood banking and serial testing of banked blood prior to use.

As noted, risks of anesthesia personnel acquiring HIV during the course of patient care must be extremely low. Transmission of HIV to anesthesia health care providers in the course of patient care has not been reported in prospective studies. Nevertheless, because approximately 80% of all occupationally related HIV infections occur subsequent to needle-stick injuries, anesthesia personnel must be vigilant. As noted, risk of seroconversion to HIV antibody after an injury with a needle contaminated with blood from an HIV-infected patient is likely less than 1%.

Routine antenatal screening of all patients for HIV has been advocated. As suggested, the reasonable "rule of thumb" is that should the prevalence of HIV infection be greater than 1 in a 1000, then antenatal populations should be screened at this time. Women who have risk factors for HIV infections should also be screened. A powerful case is made for screening routinely, as discovery of HIV infection will allow for patient counselling regarding the pregnancy, possible treatment during the pregnancy and for the baby in the newborn period, allow for precautions to be placed against sexual or other transmission of HIV into other individuals, and, finally, allow for medical personnel to adjust patient care appropriately. No evidence suggests a decrease in risk or improvement in care in patients who receive anesthesia or in those during pregnancy who receive "extraordinary vigilance" in order to avoid bodily fluid or needle stick contamination. Despite this, there are positive benefits for the woman who knows her HIV status, beneficence in the care of herself and her child.

Spill of blood or gross contamination with possibly infected secretions may be decontaminated with a variety of disinfectants. These include 70% alcohol, as well as dilute povidone-iodine-containing products (betadine) or chlorhexidine gluconate solutions. Bleach preparations also work equally as well for surface decontamination of HIV and other infectious viruses.

## Anesthetic Considerations

There is no general guideline for application of a standard anesthetic regimen for this disease process. The primary decisions for specific anesthetic technique and agent should be driven by the usual careful consideration for the patient's physical and mental state at the time of need and the usual care invoked to protect the anesthesia administrator. In other words, the use of local anesthetic techniques, the use of regional anesthetic techniques, and the use of full general anesthesia and monitored anesthesia care can be used to provide the analgesic and or anesthetic requirements necessary for labor and delivery or cesarean section delivery.

### *Local Anesthetic Techniques*

The use of the local anesthetic technique is perfectly acceptable and can provide reasonable analgesia in many situations for both vaginal delivery and for cesarean section delivery. Of course, it is not applicable for the first stage of delivery, but this can be managed with good success with low-dose intravenous medication. For the actual delivery moment, the anesthesiologist may want to stand by for administration of nitrous oxide and oxygen in a 50% ratio for a few appreciated moments of relief in case the local is not fully effective for the pain associated with perineal distension just at delivery. This is not in conflict with the previous admonition about nitrous oxide. The short period of delivery of a few minutes is not a threat to the immune system.

### *Regional Anesthetic Techniques*

The one area in controversial light at the present is the concern over spillage of HIV viruses into the CNS during performance of the epidural. This might be a possibility when a needle traverses a vein just before penetration of the cerebrospinal fluid during performance of the lumbar puncture. Yet, this concern is tempered with published evidence that confirms that the virus is already present in the CNS even in early AIDS infections (31). At the present time, there is no data on the effect of injected materials into the cerebrospinal fluid on the course of the disease process; these injected materials include saline, dextrose, opioids, local anesthetic drugs, and vasopressor drugs. Because of the unknown effects of these injected materials and because there are so many other important determinants to the course of the disease process, the decision for the use of the epidural technique—the flagship of current pain relief for obstetric anesthesia— should be determined on the basis of solid indication for pain relief and on the solid basis that the patient is desirous of having the technique performed. Naturally, such a determination sould take place only after the usual considerations for potential risks, hazards, and benefits have been weighed.

### General Anesthesia

There is published evidence to support that general anesthesia produces a decrease in the immune function response, which is both active and passive (77–81). The most flagrant general anesthetic immune suppressor is nitrous oxide, after which come the inhalation anesthetics such as enflurane, isoflurane, and the newer agents, desflurane and sevoflurane. All of the various safety measures must be invoked here, as outlined in Chapter 19 on general anesthesia in this textbook. Because of the possible complication of aspiration and later pneumonia in HIV-infected patients who already have considerable concern for pneumonia and pulmonary complications, it would seem prudent to avoid general anesthesia if at all possible. Problems that may make the decision to use general anesthesia difficult are those related to abnormal clotting or the actual coexistence of pulmonary complications as just mentioned. If general anesthesia is used, it is possible to avoid the inhalational anesthetics altogether by use of opioids for analgesia, muscle relaxants for relaxation, and oxygen in a full 100% concentration.

### Monitored Anesthesia Care

The additional help of the anesthesiologist during the use of local analgesia for delivery by either the vaginal route or the abdominal route is very helpful and much appreciated by the mother and the obstetrician. This assistance can be in the form of mere verbal support and in maintaining comfort with both visual and tactile methods, or, still, in the form of small dosages of analgesics or analeptics to relax the patient just during the delivery phase. Again, at this time consideration can be given for nitrous oxide for vaginal delivery during the few moments during the actual expulsion phase or consideration can be given to the use of ketamine in very small dosages.

### Summary

HIV infection and AIDS are significantly affecting the health and survival of women of reproductive age in the United States. Recent advances may prolong survival in women and change the natural history of HIV and associated infections. Most women who are HIV-infected are of reproductive age, and many of these will require care by health care providers specializing in women's care and anesthesia. Most studies of gynecological disease in HIV-infected women suggest that gynecological infections are more common and difficult to treat in this population than in uninfected women. Studies in pregnancy to-date do not suggest an overall worsening of outcomes; however, this may reflect more recent infection of women with HIV virus. Further information about HIV-related disease and studies of HIV-related therapies in women who are undergoing procedures, including anesthesia, remain a high priority. Women care providers and anesthesiology specialists should be able to counsel regarding contraception, reproductive decisions, and reducing at risk behaviors. Specific anesthesia implications include mandatory application of universal precautions against blood or bodily secretions. Clinical interest in HIV infection during pregnancy and in reproductive-age women and the care of these women and their children during pregnancy and parturition will continue to grow as HIV continues to become a heterosexual disease, the burdens of which are shared equally by women, their partners, and their children.

## REFERENCES


1. Chu SY, Buehler JW, Berkelman RL: Impact of the human immunodeficiency virus epidemic on mortality in women of reproductive age, United States. JAMA 164:225, 1990.
2. Centers for Disease Control. Update: Public Health Surveillance for HIV infection—United States, 1989 and 1990. MMWR 39:853, 1990.
3. Ellerbrock TV, Bush TJ, Chamberland ME, Oxtoby MJ: Epidemiology of women with AIDS in the United States, 1981 through 1990. JAMA 265:2971, 1991.
4. Quinn TC, Groseclose SL, Spence M, Provost V, Hook EW: Evolution of the human immunodeficiency virus epidemic among patients attending sexually transmitted disease clinics: A decade of experience. J Infect Dis 165:541, 1992.
5. Gwinn M, Pappaioanou M, George JR, et al: Prevalence of HIV infection in childbearing women in the United States—Surveillance using newborn blood samples. JAMA 265:1704, 1991.
6. Sweeney PA, Onorato IM, Allen DM, Byers RH: The Field Services Branch. Sentinel surveillance of human immunodeficiency virus infection in women seeking reproductive health services in the United States, 1988–1989. Obstet Gynecol 79:503, 1992.
7. Oxtoby MJ: Perinatally acquired human immunodeficiency virus infection. Pediatr Infect Dis J 9:609, 1990.
8. Maury W, Potts BJ, Rabson AB: HIV-1 infection of first-trimester and term human placental tissue: A possible mode of maternal-fetal transmission. J Infect Dis 160;583, 1989.
9. Ranki A, Valle SL, Krohn M, et al: Long latency precedes overt seroconversion in sexually transmitted human immunodeficiency virus infection. Lancet 2:589, 1987.
10. 1993 Revised Classification System for HIV Infection. MMWR 41:1–19, 1992.
11. Farizo KM, Buehler JW, Chamberland ME, et al: Spectrum of disease in persons with human immunodeficiency virus infection in the United States. JAMA 267:1798, 1992.
12. Biggar RJ: International registry of seroconverters. AIDS incubation in 1891 seroconverters from different exposure groups. J AIDS 4:1059, 1990.
13. Lifson AR, Hessol NA, Rutherford GW: Progression and clinical outcome of infection due to human immunodeficiency virus. Clin Infect Dis 14:966, 1992.
14. Carpenter CC, Mayer KH, Stein MD, Leibman BD, Fischer A, Fiore TC: Human immunodeficiency virus infection in North American women: Experience with 200 cases and a review of the literature. Medicine 70:307, 1991.
15. Barnes PF, Bloch AB, Davidson PT, Snider DE: Current concepts: Tuberculosis in patients with human immunodeficiency virus infection. N Engl J Med 324:1644, 1991.

16. Temmerman M, Plummer FA, Mirza NB: Infection with HIV as a risk factor for adverse pregnancy outcome. AIDS 4: 1087–1093, 1990.
17. Marian RW, Wiznia WW, Hutcheon G: Human T-cell lymphotropic virus III embryopathy. Amer J Dis Child 140(7): 638–640, 1986.
18. European Collaborative Study. Children born to women with HIV-1 infection: natural history and risk of transmission. Lancet 337:253–260, 1991.
19. Minkoff HL, Henderson C, Mendez H: Pregnancy outcomes among mothers infected with HIV and uninfected control subjects. Am J Obstet Gynecol 163:1598–1604, 1990.
20. Semprini AE, Ravizza M, Bucceri A: Perinatal outcome of HIV-infected women. Gynecol Obstet Invest 30;15–18, 1990.
21. Temmerman M, Kodvo T, Plummer FA: Maternal HIV infection as a risk factor for adverse obstetric outcome. VIII International Conference on AIDS, July, 1993, Abstract 4232.
22. Nyongo A, Gichange P, Temmerman M: HIV infection as a risk factor for chorioamnionitis in preterm birth. VIII International Conference on AIDS, July, 1993, Abstract # POB3469.
23. Johnstone FD, Kilpatrick DC, Burns SM: Anticardiolipin antibodies and pregnancy outcome in women with HIV infection. Obstet Gynecol 80:92–96, 1992.
24. Maury W, Potts BJ, Rabson AB: HIV-1 infection of first trimester and term human placental tissue: A possible mode of maternal-fetal transmission. J Infect Dis 160:583–588, 1989.
25. Lewis SH, Reynolds-Kohler C, Fox HE, Nelson JA: HIV-1 in trophoblast villous Hofbaur cells. Lancet 335:565–568, 1990.
26. Soeiro R, Rashbaum WK, Rubinstein A: The incidence of human fetal HIV infections as determined by presence of HIV-1 DNA in aborted tissues. International Conference on AIDS, July 1993, Abstract #WC3250
27. Wofsy CB, Cohen JB, Haver LB: Isolation of AIDS-associated retrovirus from genital secretions of women with antibodies to virus. Lancet 1:527–529, 1986.
28. Goedert JJ, Duliege AM, Amos CI, Felton S, Biggar RJ: High risk of HIV-1 infection for first born twins. Lancet 338: 1471–1475, 1991.
29. Thiry L, Sprecher-Goldberger S, Jonckhear T: Isolation of AIDS virus from cell free breast milk. Lancet 2:891–892, 1985.
30. Weinbreak P, Loustaud V, Denis F: Postnatal transmission of HIV infection. Lancet 1:492, 1985.
31. World Health Organization Global Programme on Aids 1992. Consensus statement on HIV transmission and breast feeding. Geneva 30 April-1May, 1992.
32. Blonche S, Tardieu M, Duliega A: Longitudinal study of 94 symptomatic infants with perinatally acquired HIV infection. Am J Dis Child 144:1210–1215, 1990.
33. State-of-the-Art Conference on azidothymidine therapy for early HIV infection. Am J Med 89:335, 1990.
34. CDC. Unexplained CD4+ T-lymphocyte depletion in persons without evident HIV infection—United Stated. MMWR 41:541–3, 1992.
35. Lagakos S, Fischl MA, Stein DS, Lim L, Volberding P: Effects on zidovudine therapy in minority and other subpopulations with early HIV infection. JAMA 266:2709, 1991.
36. Stein DS, Korvick JA, Vermund SH: CD4+ lymphocyte cell enumeration for prediction of clinical course of human immunodeficiency virus disease: A review. J Infect Dis 165: 352, 1992.
37. CDC Opportunistic non-Hodgkins lymphomas among severely immunocompromized HIV-1 infected patients surviving for prolonged intervals. MMWR 40:591, 1991a.
38. Sperling RS, Friedman F, Joyner M, Brodman M, Dottino P: Seroprevalence of human immunodeficiency virus in women admitted to the hospital with pelvic inflammatory disease. J Reprod Med 36;122, 1991.
39. Carpenter CC, Mayer KH, Stein MD, Leibman BD, Fischer A, Fiore TC: Human immunodeficiency virus infection in North American women: Experience with 200 cases and a review of the literature. Medicine 70:307, 1991.
40. Keonin LM, Ellerbrock TV: Pregnancy associated deaths due to AIDS in the U.S. JAMA 261:1306, 1989.
41. Centers for Disease Control. Recommendations for prophylaxis against Pneumocystis carinii pneumonia for adults and adolescents infected with human immunodeficiency virus. MMWR 41:1, 1992.
42. Centers for Disease Control. General recommendations on immunization. MMWR 38:205, 1989b.
43. Centers for Disease Control. Purified protein derivative (PPD)-tuberculin anergy and HIV infection: Guidelines for anergy testing and management of anergic persons at risk of tuberculosis. MMWR 40:27, 1991b.
44. Rhoads JL, Wright DC, Redfield RR, Burke DS: Chronic vaginal candidiasis in women with HIV infection. JAMA 297: 3105, 1987.
45. Vogt MW, Witt DJ, Craven DE, et al: Isolation patterns of the human immunodeficiency virus from cervical secretions during the menstrual cycle of women at risk for the acquired immunodeficiency syndrome. Ann Intern Med 106:380 1987.
46. Kreiss JK, Coombs R, Plummer F: Isolation of HIV from genital ulcers in Nairobi prostitutes. J Infect Dis 160:380–2, 1989.
47. Pomerantz RJ, de la Monte S, Donegan SP, et al: Human immunodeficiency virus (HIV) infection of the uterine cervix. Ann Intern Med 108:321, 1988.
48. Covino JM, McCormack WM: Vulvar ulcer of unknown etiology in a human immunodeficiency virus-infected woman: Response to treatment with zidovudine. Am J Obstet Gynecol 163:116, 1990.
49. Wasserheit JN: Epidemiological synergy: Interrelationships between human immunodeficiency virus infection and other sexually transmitted diseases. Sex Trans Dis 19:61, 1992.
50. Brown S, Senekjian EK, Montag AG: Cytomegalovirus infection of the uterine cervix in a patient with acquired immunodeficiency syndrome. Obstet Gynecol 71:489, 1988.
51. Peterson HB, Galand E, Zenilman J: Pelvic inflammatory disease: Review of treatment options. Rev Infect Dis 3:1135, 1990.
52. Safrin S, Dattel BJ, Hauer L, Sweet RL: Seroprevalence and epidemiologic correlates of human immunodeficiency virus infection in women with acute pelvic inflammatory disease. Obstet Gynecol 75:666, 1990.
53. Sperling RS, Friedman F, Joyner M, Brodman M, Dottino P: Seroprevalence of human immunodeficiency virus in women admitted to the hospital with pelvic inflammatory disease. J Reprod Med 36;122, 1991.
54. Hoegsberg B, Abulafia O, Sedlis A, et al: Sexually transmitted diseases and human immunodeficiency virus infection among women with pelvic inflammatory diseases. Am J Obstet Gynecol 163:1135, 1990.
55. Musher DM, Hamill RJ, Baughn RE: Effect of human immunodeficiency virus (HIV) infection on the course of syphilis and on the response to treatment. Ann Intern Med 113:872, 1990.
56. Byrne MA, Taylor-Robinson D, Munday PE, Harris JRW: The

common occurrence of human papillomavirus infection and intraepithelial neoplasia in women infected by HIV. J AIDS 3:379, 1989.
57. Reeves WC, Rawis WE, Brinton LA: Epidemiology of genital papillomaviruses and cervical cancer. Rev Infect Dis 11:436, 1989.
58. Franco EL: Viral etiology of cervical cancer: A critique of the evidence. Rev Infect Dis 13:1195, 1991.
59. Lungu O, Sun XW, Felix J, et al: Relationship of human papillomavirus type to grade of cervical intraepithelial neoplasia. JAMA 267:2493, 1992.
60. Feingold AR, Vermund SH, Burk RD, et al: Cervical cytologic abnormalities and papillomavirus in women infected with human immunodeficiency virus. J AIDS 3:896, 1990.
61. Vermund SH, Kelley KF, Klein RS, et al: High risk of human papillomavirus infection and cervical squamous intraepithelial lesions among women with symptomatic human immunodeficiency virus infection. Am J Obstet Gynecol 165:392, 1991.
62. Schafer A, Friedmann W, Mielke M, Schwartlander B, Koch M: The increased frequency of cervical dysplasia-neoplasia in women infected with the human immunodeficiency virus is related to the degree of immunosuppression. Am J Obstet Gynecol 164:593, 1991.
63. Maiman M, Fruchter RG, Serur E, et al: Human immunodeficiency virus infection and cervical neoplasia. Gynecol Oncol 38:377, 1990.
64. Minkoff HL, DeHovitz JA: Care of women infected with the human immunodeficiency virus. JAMA 266:2253, 1991.
65. Gwinn M, Pappaioanou M, George JR, et al: Prevalence of HIV infection in childbearing women in the United States—Surveillance using newborn blood samples. JAMA 265:1704, 1991.
66. Perlman JA, Kelghan J, Wolf PH, Baldwin W, Coulson A, Novello A: HIV risk difference between condom users and nonusers among U.S. heterosexual women. J AIDS 3:155, 1990.
67. Kestelman P, Trussell J: Efficacy of the simultaneous use of condoms and spermicides. Fam Plann Perspect 23:226, 1991.
68. Plummer FA, Simonses JN, Cameron DW, et al: Cofactors in male-female sexual transmission of human immunodeficiency virus type 1. J Infect Dis 163:233, 1991.
69. Menitove JE: Current risk of transfusion-associated HIV infection. Arch Pathol Lab Med 114:330, 1990.
70. Cummings P, Wallace EL, Schorr JB, Dobb RY: Exposure of patients to HIV through transfusion of blood products that test antibody negative. N Engl J Med 321:941, 1989.
71. Goodnough LT, Shuck JM: Risks, options and informed consent for blood transfusions in elective surgery. Am J Surg 159:602, 1990.
72. Holland P, ed. Standards For Blood Banks and Transfusion Service, ed 13. American Association of Blood Banks, Arlington, 1989.
73. National Institutes of Health Consensus Conference. Perioperative red cell transfusion. JAMA 260;2700, 1988.
74. Tokars JI, Marcus R, Culver D, et al: Surveillance of HIV infection and zidovudine use among health care workers after occupational exposure to HIV-infected blood. The CDC Cooperative Needlestick Surveillance Group. Ann Intern Med 118:913–9, 1993.
75. De Medici M, Damiani C, Consoli P, Camilli-Giammei T: Chronic exposure to inhalation anesthetics and immunity. Minerva Anestesiol (Italy) 58(12):1279–84, 1992.
76. Ianiushina VV: Evaluation of the effect of different anesthesia techniques on the immune status of pregnant women. Anesteziol Reanimatol 6:57–9, 1991.
77. Gadalov VP, Salo M, Mansikka M, Pellineimi TT: Mechanisms of the effect of general anesthesia with barbiturates on immunity. Anesteziol Reanimatol 3:26–30, 1990.
78. Markovic SN, Murasko DM: Anesthesia inhibits poly I:C induced stimulation of natural killer cell cytotoxicity in mice. Clin Immunol Immunopathol 56(2):202–9, 1990.
79. Whealon P, Morris PJ: Immunological responsiveness after transurethral resection of the prostate: general versus spinal anaesthetic. Clin Exp Immunol 48(3):611–8, 1982.

# Chapter 38

# UNUSUAL CASE MANAGEMENT PROBLEMS IN OBSTETRIC ANESTHESIA

JAY JACOBY
JOHN S. McDONALD

---

Diseases and abnormal conditions of every variety can exist in women who are pregnant. Management of the problems that arise is in the hands of the obstetrician and any consultants he/she calls in.

The anesthesiologist usually is involved only for acute intervention: pain relief to terminate pregnancy, to make labor tolerable, and for delivery. For very sick patients, he/she may be asked to insert invasive monitors and to manage ICU care. Pain relief in moderation for labor and the postcesarean period may be by systemic medication or regional block; for delivery, it may be by regional block or by general anesthesia.

In this chapter, we concentrate on the management of patients with complications, supplementing other chapters or adding short topics. We will review the gamut of abnormalities that may be encountered, focusing on the problems that the anesthesiologist is called upon to deal with while achieving pain relief for the delivery. The format follows thus: 1) a brief statement of the special problem, 2) how it affects the anesthetic considerations, and 3) our recommendations for management.

Pregnancy terminates by interruption, by delivery from below, or by cesarean section. Anesthesia for obstetric patients is essentially limited to a few possibilities:

For labor and vaginal delivery:

1. The obstetrician may give narcotics and/or some form of local anesthetic by paracervical block, pudendal block, or local infiltration. To supplement this, the anesthesiologist may be asked to give inhalation analgesia, mainly with low concentrations of nitrous oxide. The patient remains conscious and is not intubated.
2. The anesthesiologist may give a spinal or epidural anesthetic by single dose or continuous, depending on the time factor. Rarely, a caudal or a lumbar sympathetic block may be used.
3. The anesthesiologist may give full general anesthesia with intubation if an obstetric emergency develops.

For cesarean section:

1. The obstetrician may use local infiltration or a field block of the abdomen. At one time, this was standard; today it is rarely done because other methods given by the anesthesiologist are more convenient. However, local infiltration or field block has the virtue that it can be done in the absence of an anesthesiologist,when the common methods of anesthesia are inappropriate, or too dangerous, or too time-consuming. The anesthesiologist may be asked to supplement the local. Inhalation analgesia with low-dose nitrous oxide or very low-dose ketamine may be used, without intubation, while the patient remains conscious.
2. The anesthesiologist can administer a single-dose spinal or epidural, or continuous of either.
3. The anesthesiologist can administer full general anesthesia with rapid sequence induction and intubation, avoiding or minimizing the use of halogenated agents because of their effect on uterine contractility.

In summary, our choices are local or regional anesthesia such as spinal/epidural, or in some special cases, general anesthesia. The anesthetic must be tailored to meet the situation. Factors to be considered are maternal and fetal condition, mother's preference, obstetric problems, time constraints, and the anesthesiologist's preference.

The anesthesiologist's attitude must be sincere and sympathetic. Flexibility is essential. Rigidity in thinking makes for failure in performance. Swift adaptation to circumstances that change unexpectedly, is the sine qua non of obstetric anesthesia.

## PRINCIPLES OF ANESTHESIA FOR OBSTETRIC PATIENTS

1. Regional anesthesia is better than general.
2. Spinal anesthesia is more reliable than epidural for difficult cases.
3. Spinal anesthesia can be induced much more rapidly than can epidural.
4. Previous spinal (postdural puncture) headache is not so important as to preclude elective spinal anesthesia.
5. The paramedian approach may succeed when a midline approach fails.

6. For procedures of uncertain duration, the continuous catheter technique is better than a single dose.
7. The drug used for spinal or epidural anesthesia can be diluted to provide sensory analgesia without motor paralysis.
8. The dose of continuous spinal or epidural anesthetic should be titrated until the desired effect is achieved.
9. The most important aspect of general anesthesia is getting the endotracheal tube in place. All other features pale in comparison. If there is any doubt at all, about ability to get it in, use local anesthesia, and place it before the general anesthetic is started.

## SUBSTANCE ABUSE

People abuse themselves by deliberate and excessive intake of drugs, alcohol, tobacco, and food. The childbearing age is a most susceptible period, as the self-abuse may begin before puberty and continue through adulthood (1–3).

The substances used may have a variety of effects, depending upon the amount taken and the degree of tolerance. The amount required to achieve the desired effect tends to increase. The likelihood of damage increases with the amount taken and the duration of the abusive activity. Many individuals use a variety of substances, depending on availability. Abstinence produces distress and drug-seeking behavior. Denial is common, and the physician must be on the alert to detect signs of drug effects. A complete and honest history is often difficult to obtain.

Pregnant women who take drugs often fail to obtain proper prenatal care. The drugs may adversely affect the fetus by crossing the placenta (4). The fetus also is adversely affected by deleterious influences on the health of the mother, by poor nutrition, and the maternal complications of drug use, some of which are outlined below:

Infection: cellulitis, phlebitis, hepatitis, tetanus, osteomyelitis, endocarditis, infarction or abscess in brain or lung, AIDS.
Pulmonary: pneumonia, edema, hypertension.
Emboli: septic clots or foreign material.
Embryogenesis may be abnormal, and the fetus may be underweight, suffering from addiction and/or withdrawal, and unable to develop normally.
Infections may be transmitted across the placenta. A pediatrician should be alerted to the problems, and be present at the delivery to provide immediate care to the newborn.

Drug withdrawal is not advisable during the peripartum period. Withdrawal is stressful. Uterine blood flow may be reduced; fetal distress increased. Addicts require more analgesia and anesthesia than other patients. Enzyme induction by self-administered drugs may cause abnormal metabolic interactions.

The various drugs used by drug abusers include CNS depressants, antidepressants, and stimulants, as well as drugs that act on opiate receptors. Some stimulate and some depress the autonomic nervous system. Because many people take more than one substance, mixed effects are often seen. The physician must be prepared for unusual and bizarre combinations of effects. Treatment of acute problems must be symptomatic and supportive.

Acute problems that may require rapid response by the anesthesiologist include:

Pulmonary: Respiratory failure, aspiration, pneumonia, ventilation-perfusion mismatch, and chronic infection.
Cardiovascular: Cardiomyopathy, arrhythmia, ischemia, bradycardia or tachycardia, hypertension or hypotension.
Electrolytes: Changes of sodium, potassium, calcium and magnesium.
Gastrointestinal: Esophagitis, gastritis, pancreatitis, hepatitis, GI bleeding.
CNS: Agitation, confusion, convulsions, coma.
Hematologic: Dysfunction of all blood elements, coagulopathy.

Treatment must be tailored to the symptom presentation:

Respiratory: oxygen administration, airway protection, intubation, ventilation, specific antagonist administration, blood gas monitoring, and oximeter.
Circulatory: invasive monitors, fluids and vasoactive drugs, pacemaker, EKG monitoring.
CNS: control seizures with barbiturates, diazepam, or muscle relaxants; control agitation with sedatives; intubate and ventilate if necessary.

If the patient is not in acute drug-induced distress, but enters the hospital in labor or for elective cesarean, the following considerations should influence the choice of pain relief: Are there any physical abnormalities caused by the chronic drug intake? These may render the patient more susceptible to adverse effects of anesthetics, and the method chosen should bypass these problems if possible. Example: If there is a coagulopathy, do not perform an epidural block. If there is liver disease, do not use drugs that depend on liver function for detoxification, such as chloroprocaine or succinylcholine. If there is severe pulmonary dysfunction, do not use nitrous oxide.

An acutely intoxicated patient, with alcohol, narcotic, or sedative, requires less anesthetic than usual, because the intoxicant is synergistic with the anesthetic. All such patients must be treated as full-stomach cases.

Some degree of cross-tolerance may exist, so that patients habituated to one drug may require more of the anesthetic than expected to provide pain relief and/or unconsciousness. At the same time, the relaxing effect of inhalation anesthetics on uterine muscle is similar to that for normal people. The increased concentration required for anesthesia may cause uterine atony and bleeding. Therefore, do not use inhalation agents as principal anesthetic drugs. Enzyme induction and increased destruction of halogenated drugs are another reason to minimize their use.

Parenteral drug users may be infected with the AIDS or hepatitis virus, and should be isolated accordingly.

Venous access may be very difficult because the superficial veins have been thrombosed by drug injections. In such cases, the external jugular veins may still be available. The invasive techniques of venous access into the subclavian or internal jugular veins may cause serious complications such as pneumothorax or arterial bleeding with massive hematomas. A safer choice is a surgical cutdown.

When immediate control of an agitated patient must be obtained without venous access, the method of choice is intramuscular injection of ketamine, 10 mg/kg. The patient becomes quiet in 2 to 3 minutes; surgical anesthesia develops in 3 to 5 minutes. Intubation, then surgery can begin within 5 to 6 minutes. After anesthesia has begun, superficial veins tend to dilate and may become available for starting an infusion.

## Alcohol

### *Acute Intoxication*

Regional anesthesia may be difficult to perform, or is inadvisable, because the patient is uncooperative and combative. For general anesthesia, the alcohol already in the body acts like a basal anesthetic. The alcohol is synergistic with the anesthetic, and the dose of anesthetic drug required to reach surgical levels is reduced.

#### *Chronic Alcoholism*

Enzyme induction occurs and the individual develops tolerance and resistance to the effects of some anesthetics, particularly the inhalation agents. Tolerance or resistance to the injectable anesthetics is less noticeable; normal doses may be adequate.

If the patient is cooperative, pain relief may proceed in the normal manner, with regional anesthesia preferred unless there is coagulopathy. Before administering regional anesthesia, the patient should be told and a note should be made on the chart that signs of alcoholic polyneuropathy may appear later and that its appearance should not be attributed to the block but to the pathologic condition (5).

Myopathy makes the patient more susceptible to the neuromuscular blocking drugs and to the motor effect of regional anesthesia. Cardiomyopathy makes patients susceptible to cardiac depressant drugs (6). Pulmonary damage makes the patient more likely to develop hypoxia.

#### *Alcohol Withdrawal*

Autonomic hyperactivity develops in chronic alcoholics deprived of the drug. Agitation, hallucinations, tremor, tachycardia, and hypertension develop, called delirium tremens (DTs). Paraldehyde was the drug of choice for this condition; now benzodiazepines or barbiturates titrated intravenously, and clonidine, are preferred. The pediatrician should be informed prior to delivery, as these drugs may affect the fetus.

## Narcotics

Commonly used drugs include heroin, morphine, demerol, methadone, and fentanyl. Similar drugs having both agonist and antagonist effects are pentazocine, nalbuphine, butorphanol, and buprenorphine. The effects observed by physicians include euphoria, sedation, respiratory depression, unconsciousness, hypotension. The blood content of oxygen decreases and that of carbon dioxide rises. Overdose may cause death. Deprivation of the drug may cause severe withdrawal symptoms, increased sympathetic tone, and increased incidence of abruptio placenta. Hormone secretion is diminished, affecting ACTH, luteinizing hormone and testosterone, but prolactin increases.

Treatment depends upon the severity of symptoms. Naloxone is the most commonly used narcotic antagonist and may be satisfactory for moderately depressed patients, but its use may precipitate withdrawal symptoms. More aggressive treatment is needed for severe cases, namely intubation, ventilation, and circulatory-support measures.

Agonist-antagonist drugs produce mild effects, reversible by naloxone administration and act as agonists at Kappa receptors and antagonists at Mu receptors. Pain-relief measures may be similar to those for nonusers; if narcotic analgesia is used, larger doses probably will be needed.

Withdrawal symptoms of the mother include: anxiety, tremor, lacrimation and rhinorrhea, yawning, sweating, tachycardia, weakness, and vomiting. Withdrawal symptoms of the infant after birth include: excessive irritability, crying, tremor, seizures, fever, vomiting, poor sucking, and dehydration.

Anesthesia care for the mother includes administration of methadone or narcotic in sufficient amount to prevent withdrawal symptoms. Avoid or limit the dose of naloxone to prevent precipitating withdrawal symptoms. Coexisting pathology requires appropriate treatment. If the patient is cooperative, regional anesthesia is the best choice. If she is uncooperative, additional narcotic may be needed, and the delivery is accomplished with general anesthesia using the rapid sequence technique.

### *Intravenous Drug Use (Main Line Shooters)*

Intravenous injection often results in systemic infections and phlebitis, with sclerosis of veins. Hypoxia may follow an injection, and sympathetic tone rises between doses, perhaps causing an increase of placental abruption. The infants are often premature; meconium aspiration and fetal withdrawal symptoms are common. When possible, the opiate addict should be switched to methadone, with gradual reduction of dose. IV drug users should have isolation precautions for AIDS and hepatitis. During labor and delivery, narcotics should not be withheld to avoid precipitating withdrawal symptoms. However, intraspinal narcotics should not be used, as respiratory depression may be enhanced by the combination of methods of administration.

### *Analgesia for Labor and Delivery*

Coagulation problems and impaired immunity are contraindications to the use of large bore needles and catheters, and prolonged blocks. Single-dose epidural or spinal, using a small gauge needle, is acceptable for terminal labor and vaginal or cesarean delivery. The modern day use of dilute combination analgesia administered slowly by an external pump is also acceptable. This method obtains maximal analgesia with administration of minimal anesthetic concentration and dosages. Alternative: titrated narcotics for analgesia, 50% nitrous oxide and oxygen, and local or pudendal block for vaginal delivery.

## Sedatives

### *Barbiturates*

Acute intoxication requires resuscitative treatment as for a nonpregnant individual. If labor occurs or abdominal delivery is required, the unconscious patient requires no additional anesthetic. Ventilation through an endotracheal tube and a muscle relaxant is adequate for a cesarean.

Chronic intake of barbiturates causes an abstinence syndrome, so intake should not be stopped as term approaches. Residual effects of the drug make the patient more susceptible to any narcotics or general anesthetic drugs.

Regional anesthesia is preferred for labor and delivery of all patients who are chronic users of sedative drugs.

#### Meprobamate (Carbamates)

Sedation occurs. Narcotic effect is potentiated. Withdrawal symptoms develop.

#### Methaqualone (Ludes)

Sedative and anticonvulsant. Enzyme induction occurs. Overdose requires standard resuscitation. Convulsions may occur and should be controlled with muscle relaxants rather than barbiturates or benzodiazepines.

#### Antihistamines

As sedatives, they potentiate narcotics; large doses cause excitement, ataxia, hallucinations, flushing, convulsions, and dilated pupils. Barbiturates and benzodiazepines are satisfactory for treatment of convulsions. Major resuscitation is not normally required.

## Adjunct Abuse Drugs

### *Benzodiazepines, Phenothiazines, and Buterophenones*

These drugs are used to enhance the effects of narcotics or to relieve withdrawal symptoms. Their effects may be partially antagonized by physostigmine and flumazenil. If serious overdose occurs, the patient requires symptomatic support of respiration and circulation.

Benzodiazepines stimulate opiate receptors and produce drowsiness and ataxia. Physostigmine is a partial antagonist. Pain relief measures may be similar to those for nonusers.

Phenothiazines and buterophenones (droperidol, haldol) produce anticholinergic, antipsychotic, and neuroleptic effects. They have alpha-adrenergic blocking action. They enhance the effects of narcotics and sedatives.

These drugs reduce the doses of narcotics needed for labor. Epidural anesthesia is preferred over spinal because the patient may rapidly develop refractory hypotension. Blood pressure support with ephedrine or mephentermine should be started immediately. Bupivacaine should not be used because there may be synergistic myocardial depression.

To antagonize drug effects, physostigmine is best for the phenothiazenes and buterophenones, given intravenously in doses of 0.5 mg, up to 2 mg total. Flumazenil is best for benzodiazepines, given intravenously in doses of 0.2 mg, up to 1 mg total to reverse sedation, and up to 3 mg to reverse overdosage. An excess of flumazenil may cause convulsions. It has a shorter duration of action than do benzodiazepines, so recurrence of sedation may take place.

## Antidepressant Drugs

### *Tricyclic Antidepressants*

These drugs block uptake of norepinephrine in the CNS, decrease blood pressure, and have anticholinergic effects. Overdose causes fever, seizures, coma, and hypotension or hypertension. Useful for treatment are physostigmine, diazepam, and alpha-blocking drugs. Arrhythmias may be reversed with lidocaine, propranolol, or bretylium. Arrhythmia caused by amitriptyline can be reversed with bicarbonate. The patient is sensitive to sympathomimetic drugs as well as to anesthetic agents.

Pain relief measures for labor and delivery may be similar to those for nonusers. The patients are very susceptible to vasopressor drugs, and reduced doses should be titrated when needed.

### *MAO Inhibitors*

These are mood elevators (7). Overdose produces fever, agitation, convulsions, and fluctuations of blood pressure. Depressant drugs are potentiated, and their action is prolonged. Indirect-acting catecholamines are potentiated. If needed, direct-acting alpha agonists are recommended. Pain relief measures for labor and delivery may be similar to those for nonusers except for meperidine, which is contraindicated, as it may trigger severe hypertension.

### *Lithium*

This drug causes sodium retention, increased intravascular volume, and hypothyroidism. Low-salt diets reduce renal excretion of lithium and may trigger toxicity, manifested by coma, seizures, bradycardia, and circulatory collapse. General support measures should be supplemented by administration of osmotic diuretics and sodium bicarbonate. Fluid loss by vomiting or diarrhea should be replaced by intravenous salt solution and bicarbonate. Hypotension is relatively refractory to treatment; large doses of ephedrine are required. Lithium enhances the effects of sedatives, narcotics, and anesthetics.

The physiologic alterations of body water and electrolytes in pregnancy make lithium toxicity likely. Its use should be discontinued; treatment with tricyclic antidepressants is safer.

Pain relief for labor and delivery: reduced doses of narcotics are required, as the patient is more sensitive to general anesthetic drugs. Epidural anesthesia is preferable to spinal because the associated hypotension is refractory to treatment; large doses of ephedrine may be required.

## Hallucinogens

### *Marijuana*

This is a beta-adrenergic agonist, causing increased work of the heart, and tachycardia up to 140 beats per minute (8). Overdose produces hallucinations, delusions, and paranoia, which are best treated with diazepam. Postural hypotension occurs. It is synergistic with sedatives and general anesthetics, so reduced doses are needed. Fetal growth retardation and meconium staining occur.

Chronic bronchitis and bronchoconstriction make regional anesthesia preferable to general (9). Mephentermine is the preferred treatment for hypotension, because of the tendency for tachycardia. If general anesthesia is needed, etomidate is the induction agent of choice; the minimum alveolar concentration for all agents is reduced.

### *PCP (Phencyclidine)*

This causes effects similar to those of ketamine or schizophrenia, with hypertension, tachycardia, sweating, and fever. It may also cause hallucinations, ataxia, tremors, and convulsions. It potentiates narcotics and sympathomimetic agents. A cooling blanket may be needed because of the tendency toward hyperthermia. Anticholinergic drugs are not necessary.

Pain relief measures for labor and delivery may be similar to those for nonusers, except: The patient is susceptible to narcotic and sympathomimetic drugs, and reduced doses are called for. If the patient is hallucinating, general anesthesia is required. Cholinesterase inhibition depresses succinylcholine metabolism, so that drug is best avoided.

### *LSD, Mescal, Nutmeg, and Psilocybin*

These all produce euphoria, hallucinations, and sympathomimetic effects. Acutely intoxicated patients require treatment similar to that described for PCP. The effects of muscle-relaxant drugs may be prolonged.

## Stimulants

### *Amphetamines*

These produce stimulation of both the CNS and cardiovascular system (10). Paranoia and psychotic symptoms may develop, in addition to hypertension and loss of appetite. Overdose causes chest pain, convulsions, coma, and respiratory failure (11). The myocardium is sensitized to catecholamines, and arrhythmia is frequent (12).

Gastric absorption continues, and toxic symptoms may increase after the patient comes under anesthetic care.

To control agitated patients, neuroleptics or barbiturates may be needed. Epidural block is the analgesic method of choice for labor and/or delivery. This results in improved uterine blood flow. Fluid administration and direct-acting sympathomimetic agents are required for control of blood pressure.

### *Cocaine*

Table 38–1 lists the effects of cocaine toxicity. The reuptake of norepinephrine at nerve endings is inhibited. The excess of free norepinephrine in the blood has the usual effect of increasing blood pressure and vasomotor tone. Coronary artery spasm occurs, producing intravascular thrombosis, ischemia, arrhythmias, myocardial infarction, and sudden death (13–15). Cerebral effects include excitement, seizures, depression, and paranoia. Cerebral vascular accidents may occur.

In pregnant women, cocaine increases blood pressure, decreases uterine blood flow, increases uterine contractility, and stimulates labor and placental separation. Miscarriage, premature labor, and fetal damage all occur with greater frequency (16–18).

Both alpha and beta adrenergic stimulation may be manifested and require treatment. Nitroglycerin, nitroprusside, alpha- and beta-blockers, and calcium blockers may be needed. Cerebrovascular accidents, respiratory failure, and seizures may occur.

When anesthesia is required, the patient should be managed as though she has severe coronary artery disease, which many chronic abusers have. Labor and delivery may occur during episodes of acute intoxication. Little additional analgesia is required because that is provided by cocaine. Psychotic behavior may require administration of a neuroleptic drug such as haldol, droperidol, or thorazine.

Epidural and spinal anesthesia are useful to reduce uterine artery spasm, but blood pressure is labile, blood volume may be depleted, and response to vasopressor drugs is variable. Here again the technique of external pump delivery of small concentrations of local anesthetic or opioid combinations by the continuous technique with small incremental doses permits better control. The toxicities of cocaine and the local anesthetic for epidural are additive; convulsions may result. Spinal anesthesia is preferable because of the very much smaller dose of local anes-

**Table 38–1.** Effects of Cocaine Toxicity

| Behavioral | Neurologic | Cardiovascular | Causes of Death |
|---|---|---|---|
| Euphoria | Tremor | Tachycardia | Asphyxia during convulsion |
| Irritability | Hyperreflexia | Arrhythmia | Cerebral hemorrhage |
| Restlessness | Convusions | Hypertension | Myocardial infarction |
| Insomnia | Fever | Angina | Ventricular fibrillation |
| Paranoia | Dilated pupils | Shock | |
| Psychosis | Coma | | |
| Hallucinations | | | |
| Delirium | | | |
| Suicidal | | | |

thetic drug used. Blood pressure is supported with a vasopressor infusion.

When general anesthesia is required, drugs that increase myocardial irritability should be avoided, such as halothane. Drugs with sympathomimetic properties should be avoided, such as ketamine or nitrous oxide. Adequate depth of anesthesia must be provided during stimulating procedures, to avoid triggering an adrenergic surge.

If abruption of the placenta occurs, general anesthesia is usually required. The minimum alveolar concentration for anesthetic drugs often increases. In spite of careful induction, avoidance of sympathetic stimulation and treatment with sympathetic blocking drugs, arrhythmia, or myocardial infarction may occur.

## Tobacco

The harmful effects of smoking tobacco can be considered from the standpoints of local irritation, chemical absorption, and late stimulation of neoplastic activity. It also has an adverse effect on the fetus. Fetal growth retardation and increased mortality also occur.

The local irritation caused by inhaling tobacco smoke causes reactive airway disease, manifested by bronchospasm, mucosal edema, susceptibility to infection, thick mucus in the bronchioles, spasmodic coughing, irritable vocal cords, and tendency to bouts of acute laryngospasm and bronchospasm (19). The principal chemical absorbed, nicotine, stimulates both the CNS and autonomic ganglia, with release of epinephrin.

Carbon monoxide is inhaled along with nicotine. This combines with hemoglobin and interferes with its oxygen transport function. If smoking is stopped, both mother and fetus benefit by a greater availability of hemoglobin to carry oxygen.

Pain relief for labor and delivery is best accomplished by regional anesthesia. Bouts of wheezing and coughing may occur, but they are not dangerous. General anesthesia may be complicated by laryngeal spasm at induction and emergence, and by bronchospasm at any time. Atelectasis may complicate the recovery period.

## Food and Obesity

In the vast majority of cases, obesity is a result of self-abuse by excessive food intake. Many systemic diseases are worsened by the presence of obesity, including cardiac, vascular, and hepatic disease, and diabetes (20). The work of the heart increases. Metabolism increases to support the extra weight, and oxygen consumption and $CO_2$ production rise. To compensate, respiratory rate increases more than tidal volume. The weight of the chest wall and the abdominal mass decreases compliance and ventilatory capacity. Decreased functional residual capacity and increased closing volume lead to hypoxia and intolerance of the supine position. Pregnancy makes the problems worse, and the patient may be unable to lay flat (21,22).

The patient is said to have morbid obesity when actual weight approaches or exceeds twice the ideal weight. The patient is Pickwickian when fat cells increase within the muscle mass, pulmonary ventilation decompensates intermittently, and when there is right heart overload (23). Anesthetic concerns include the above, plus the increase in gastric contents (24,25). Obstetric complications are more frequent, as are emergency cesarean deliveries, and surgery takes longer. Moving the heavy patient and accommodating the equipment to her bulk, require extra help (Figure 38–1). The blood pressure cuff must be wider than the circumference of the arm, otherwise the readings are falsely elevated. Avoid placing the patient in full supine position.

It may be impossible to place a reliable intravenous line of adequate size to deal with transfusion needs. If a 16-gauge catheter cannot be placed percutaneously, a subclavian, internal jugular or surgical cutdown should be done before any emergency arises.

For vaginal delivery, mild analgesia with intravenous narcotics, followed by local anesthesia of the perineum, is the simplest and best choice. Nitrous oxide and oxygen may be used as a supplement.

For epidural and spinal, longer and heavier gauge needles should be available. Very thin needles bend excessively. Catheters should be inserted a greater distance than usual, as the shifting outer fat layers tend to pull the catheter out. Securing the catheter along the midline crease on the back minimizes the amount of displacement as the patient moves about. Extra slack should be left at the insertion site as the catheter is secured, and there should be a little extra padding to protect against kinking. It is advisable to insert the catheter early on while there is ample time because of anticipated greater difficulty in needle placement (26–28).

Continuous spinal is a more reliable technique than is

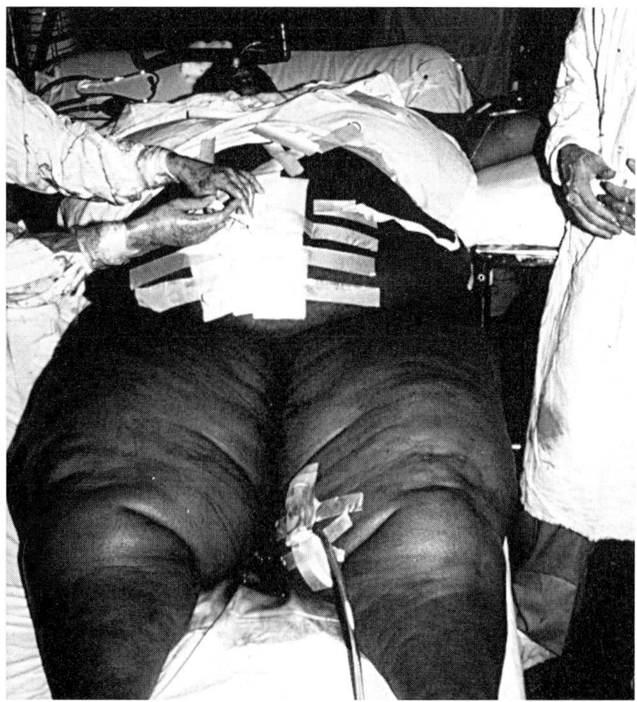

**Fig. 38–1.** This figure demonstrates the tremendous problem a patient with morbid obesity presents to the anesthesiologist.

epidural because of the positive endpoint (29). For control of labor pain, small increments of dilute local anesthetic provide analgesia without motor paralysis. Start with 3 ml Tetracaine or Marcaine 0.25 mg/ml (0.025%). For cesarean, use 5 ml Tetracaine or Marcaine 1 mg/ml (0.1%), with incremental additions of 2 ml until the level of anesthesia is satisfactory. For rapid onset, use 1 ml Lidocaine 50 mg/ml (5%) with incremental additions of 0.25 ml.

For general anesthesia, difficult intubation must be expected. Awake intubation under local anesthesia is the safest technique. Fiberoptic equipment may be needed. Sedation should be adequate to make intubation easier, but respiratory difficulty may occur even though the patient is still conscious. Sitting or semi-sitting position may be required until the endotracheal tube is in place so that control of respiration is readily established. The pediatrician should be alerted to the possibility of fetal depression. After the patient is intubated, a heavy duty respirator or a strong hand on the breathing bag is needed to maintain adequate pulmonary ventilation.

General anesthetic drugs should be titrated into the patient after endotracheal intubation has been accomplished. The mg/kg method is not a reliable way of determining dosage (30,31). Actual weight gives too large a number; ideal weight gives too small a number. As the procedure is ending, apply topical anesthesia to the pharynx, larynx, and trachea or administer intravenous lidocaine, so that the endotracheal tube is tolerated easily. Do not remove the endotracheal tube until consciousness, motor power, and spontaneous breathing have returned fully.

If regional anesthesia (spinal or epidural) cannot be established and if an endotracheal tube cannot be inserted while the patient is conscious and breathing spontaneously, there are two options: tracheotomy under local anesthesia followed by general anesthesia or delivery under local anesthesia. Either vaginal or cesarean delivery can be done using local infiltration of a dilute anesthetic solution, along with sedation that preserves consciousness and spontaneous breathing. The anesthesiologist should avoid being forced into administering general anesthesia before intubation is accomplished.

## TRAUMA

Trauma is the most common cause of death during the child-bearing years. (32,33). All other causes of maternal mortality account for only half as many deaths. Trauma may initiate obstetric complications, such as ruptured uterus and separation of the placenta. If the mother survives, abruption of the placenta is the most common cause of fetal death.

The principles of treatment of a trauma patient must be followed; if she is pregnant, these factors must be taken into account (34): Normal blood pressure is lower; systemic vascular resistance decreases. Blood loss is better tolerated because of the increased blood volume, but replacement needs are greater. Elevated blood pressure may be due to pregnancy-induced hypertension (PIH) or to catecholamine release related to the trauma. Impaired placental perfusion may occur and cause fetal hypoxia in spite of normal maternal blood pressure. Respiratory alkalosis from hyperventilation also decreases uterine perfusion. Alpha-adrenergic drugs should not be used; ephedrine and dobutamine preserve uterine perfusion. Fetal monitoring should be continuous.

Knife or gunshot wounds of the lower abdomen require exploration. Blunt trauma may also jeopardize both fetus and mother. Placental separation, ruptured uterus, direct injury of the fetus, or major bleeding from engorged vessels may necessitate removal of the fetus and/or the uterus.

If death of the mother is imminent in spite of vigorous resuscitation, immediate cesarean delivery should be considered. Not only can the fetus be saved, but some correctable injury of the mother may be found, making resuscitation more effective. The longer the delay of delivery, the poorer the prospect for fetal survival. Prompt, aggressive, and efficient treatment may save both. Do not delay surgery to place invasive monitors. The patients need: intubation, oxygen, and ventilation; vigorous fluid therapy; surgical intervention. Intubation having been previously accomplished, drugs recommended for anesthesia are ketamine in small doses, and Norcuron as needed. If the patient is in extremis, intubation can be done without anesthesia, with only Norcuron used to facilitate the surgery; anesthetic drugs may be entirely unnecessary or contraindicated.

## COMPLICATIONS OF PREGNANCY

### Miscarriage

Normally, this is not a critical emergency, but a D&C may be required. In the presence of emotional trauma and abdominal pain, the stomach retains its contents for many hours. Postponing the D&C to allow the stomach time to empty is neither effective nor appropriate. Delay cannot be relied upon to provide an empty stomach, so anesthesia must be carried out with suitable precautions to prevent aspiration, whenever it is done.

Unless there has been severe bleeding and shock, any acceptable method of anesthesia may be used. This may be general anesthesia with a rapid sequence induction or local/regional analgesia with paracervical block.

### Incompetent Cervix

Painless dilatation occurring in the second or early third trimester may be a cause of threatened abortion. Treatment consists of placing a circumferential heavy suture through the cervix and pulling it closed. The suture remains in place until its removal when delivery occurs.

The anesthetic consideration is whether any technique or drug is teratogenic, or prone to increase uterine activity and the risk of miscarriage. Although most anesthesiologists favor regional anesthesia for the circlage, there is no evidence that it is either better or worse than general anesthesia. No special recommendation is made for either type, except that it should be carried out with due diligence and skill (35–39).

## Ectopic Pregnancy

This may be manifested by irregular vaginal bleeding, without the patient knowing she is pregnant. A tender abdominal mass after missed periods may be enough to make the diagnosis. Sudden abdominal pain and faintness indicate that the ectopic pregnancy has ruptured, and there may be major intraperitoneal blood loss.

Anesthesia for such cases follows the standard practice for emergency abdominal surgery: a large IV access; fluid administration based on symptoms and signs; blood transfusion availability; secure the airway; titrate the anesthetic to avoid overdose.

## Trophoblastic Neoplasm

This includes hydatidiform mole, invasive mole, and choriocarcinoma. Symptoms include irregular vaginal bleeding and rapid enlargement of the uterus. The trophoblast normally is slightly invasive; in these conditions, it grows more rapidly and invades more deeply; it may become malignant and metastasize.

Anesthesia is required for treatment, which is immediate evacuation of the uterus, and/or chemotherapy. Severe bleeding and uterine perforation may occur at any time during or after a normal or abnormal pregnancy. Pregnancy-induced hypertension and coagulopathy may be additional complications.

Before regional anesthesia is decided upon, consider the possibility of coagulopathy and severe hemorrhage. General anesthesia, with suitable precautions to protect the airway and manage hemorrhage, is a better choice.

## Retained Placenta

After the fetus has been delivered, the placenta may be slow to separate. Massage of the fundus of the uterus to encourage contraction usually is successful in causing the placenta to separate and be expelled. This does not occur in about 1% of patients, and after a 30-minute wait, manual removal is usually attempted (40). It may be found that the cervix and lower uterine segment are tightly contracted, so that insertion of the hand is not possible. The anesthesiologist is called upon to assist, both to provide analgesia and to relax the uterus.

Spinal and epidural anesthesia do not cause uterine relaxation. Because of the possibility of major blood loss, both would be relatively contraindicated for analgesia. However, if there has been little blood loss, and a catheter is already present and the regional block can be activated with a small additional dose of drug, it is acceptable to do so.

Muscle relaxant drugs do not relax the uterus.

Uterine relaxation can be best obtained by administration of a potent inhalation agent, amyl nitrate, or nitroglycerin.

For use of a potent inhalation agent, full general anesthesia precautions must be taken, including tracheal intubation. Several minutes are required for induction and relaxation and for return of contractility after the inhalation agent is discontinued. During this period, severe bleeding may occur. This is not the method of choice.

Amyl nitrate may be administered by breaking an ampule and having the patient inhale the vapor. The dose is difficult to control or even estimate. Hypotension and headache are common (41). An explosion, though rare, may occur, especially in an oxygen-enriched environment (42).

Nitroglycerin is the drug of choice to relax the uterus. Given intravenously, a dose of 50 to 100 micrograms causes uterine relaxation in about 40 to 60 seconds. In some cases, 500 micrograms and 90 seconds may be required. The smaller doses cause no significant changes in blood pressure. A loading dose of crystalloid IV fluid is recommended before treatment, particularly if there has been significant blood loss. After relaxation develops, placental separation occurs spontaneously or can easily be accomplished manually. The uterus rapidly regains its tone.

Analgesia for the procedure can be obtained without producing unconsciousness or requiring general anesthesia precautions. For a person who has had no recent previous narcotic or sedative, give: Fentanyl 50 micrograms, ketamine 5 mg repeated every 2 or 3 minutes, and 50% nitrous oxide and oxygen. Consciousness, spontaneous respiration, and reflexes are retained (43–45).

## Placenta Accreta or Percreta

This is a condition of abnormally strong attachment or penetration of placental tissue into the uterus. It does not separate normally after delivery, and bleeding may be massive, resulting in complete exsanguination and death. Clamping of the aorta followed by hysterectomy may be required. There are several important points to make in regard to the anesthesiologist's and the obstetrician's reactions in regard to this diagnostic problem. One is that if there is evidence of a previous cesarean section there is a naturally increased risk of placenta accreta (46–48). This can be diagnosed in some instances by the obstetrician's application of detailed ultrasound diagnosis, in which he/she can determine that certain criterion, which are well-known and defined in the literature, would certainly be diagnostic of this syndrome. Therefore, it would seem axiomatic that in all cases of previous cesarean section, the obstetrician should alert the anesthesiologist of his/her intent to perform a complete ultrasound examination to rule out the possibility of placenta accreta. A second very important point to make in regard to this diagnosis is to recall that, according to Read and associates'(49) 1980 study, the incidence of placenta accreta has increased to 1:2,500 deliveries, with accreta 78% of the time, increta 17% of the time, and percreta 5% of the time. The 600 cases subsequently reviewed by Fox (50) revealed that there was only one reasonable method after delivery of the baby at the time of cesarean section, and that was hysterectomy, not manual removal of the placenta. Our reasoning follows Fox's case review, in which 25% of the women died when manual removal of the placenta occurred. Reflecting upon this for a moment, one can imagine the scenario in a small hospital, late at night, with a single anesthesiologist and nursing staff available together, an obstetrician who is surprised by a situation such as placenta accreta. In such a situation, because the obstetrician was not aware of placenta accreta, he/she may attempt a manual removal of the placenta, with massive amounts of blood loss occurring within the next several minutes, of which the single anesthesiologist cannot keep up with because he/she was not alerted, without benefit of prior warning. In these instances, the mother's bleeding is so rapid that there is often just not enough time to react to the massive losses of both volume of blood and its oxygen-carrying capacity. Third, in acute hypotensive crises, especially in obstetrics, the primary pressor agent in the past has always been ephedrine. However, there are many who believe today that small aliqouts of phenylephrine in 25 to 50 µmg can be used as an alpha agonist to support the maternal pressure, especially if the maternal heart rate is already elevated.

The situation is managed as are other hemorrhagic emergencies, with large-bore IV access, pumping fluids and blood, minimal general anesthesia, intubation, and ventilation. The most important aspect of management of a patient with placenta accreta or percreta is, first of all, recognition that the situation may be possible. In all instances in which a previous placenta accreta has occurred, and/or low-lying placenta has been diagnosed with subsequent cesarean section, the patient is suspect. In cases in which the patient is suspect and a cesarean section is planned, very careful attention must be given to monitoring. Large-bore IV needles should be placed in both arms. The possibility of placing a CVP with a swan introducer for large volume correction of hemorrhage may be lifesaving. It is also important to think about monitoring blood pressure during severe hypotensive episodes in such cases. To alleviate the worry from this latter concern, an arterial catheter may be placed prior to induction of the patient. This takes a very short period of time, is innocuous, and in a healthy young patient, can be vital in regard to management of the patient intraoperatively. The administration of the anesthesia may be done with primarily oxygen and narcotics with addition of some type of anxolytic, such as scopolamine for depressing memory during periods of minimal analgesia when the patient is hypotensive and/or in shock. In addition, it is very important for the obstetrician to have standing by or nearby someone who is able to help him/her with possible vascular clamps, management of major vascular correction intra-abdominally, if such diagnosis is made.

In summary, it can be said that management of this diagnostic problem is one of the major threats to the perinatal team. Certainly, there must be close communication and coordination among the various members of the perinatal team, including the obstetrician and the anesthesiologist, and certainly by the nursing staff, and support by the hematology lab. Certainly these five components are necessary to the survival of these patients: (1) a member of the obstetric team whose job it is to coordinate the amount of blood replacement and ensure the blood gets to the operating room so the anesthesiologist can administer it; (2) communication between the obstetrician and anesthesiologist regarding the coagulation status, and, if necessary, a member of the obstetric team again calling in a hematologist specialist in regard to the changing status of the coagulation during acute blood loss; (3) management of the patient during the massive transfusion time, as it requires volume administration with colloid and crystalloid agents before blood may be available—and this must be done with an extra set of hands that must provide help to the anesthesiologist, who is a single physician all by himself/herself; (4) certainly, a significant amount of whole blood should be made available, and, again, this is why a preemptive diagnosis is so important in these cases and also why obstetricians can be very helpful in regard to performing the ultrasound diagnostic work-up; and (5) as mentioned before, the baseline coagulation tests need to be done on a rapid time line during the massive period of blood loss, and there may be instances in which a hematologist should be at the elbow of the anesthesiologist, working with the anesthesiologist and obstetrician in determining the CBC, the platelet count, the fibrinogen, the prothrombin time (PT), and the partial prothrombin time (PTT) because fluxes and changes are so rapid as to be life-threatening.

## Inversion of the Uterus

Inversion (eversion) of the uterus is a rare complication, most often encountered immediately after vaginal delivery. During vigorous efforts to expel the placenta by fundal pressure, the corpus of the uterus is forced through the cervix, which then tightens and prevents replacement of the corpus. The condition has also been noted during cesarean section. The inverted tissue has sharply restricted blood flow, especially venous return, because the cervix acts like a tourniquet. As time goes by, the everted mass enlarges due to venous engorgement and edema formation. Forceful attempts to push the corpus back through the cervical ring are very painful, and the anesthesiologist is called to assist.

The need for haste reduces the desirability of epidural, so spinal anesthesia or general anesthesia with intubation is chosen. But neither of these relax the cervix. Relaxation may be obtained by administering ritodrine, terbutaline, nitroglycerin, or amyl nitrate by inhalation.

In one particular case, the following occurred: The patient had a vaginal delivery under saddle block anesthesia. The intern caused uterine inversion while removing the placenta. Repeated efforts to replace the uterine corpus were made by staff members of increasing rank and experience, without success. The patient complained of severe pain as the saddle block wore off. Decision was made to give general anesthesia with intubation. A small dose of thiopental was followed by 100 mg of succinylcholine. When fasciculations ceased, and before the endotracheal tube could be inserted, the obstetrician announced that he/she had just achieved success: the cervix had relaxed, and the fundus popped back in.

In a parturient with acute inversion of the uterus during cesarean section, Emmott and Bennett found no increase in hypotension or blood loss with epidural anesthesia (51). To the contrary, they theorize that an epidural may actually decrease hypotension by blocking a visceral afferent, autonomic reflex which can decrease blood pressure in this unusual event even in the absence of significant blood loss. If re-inversion is accumulated, toxic metabolic products can cause hemodynamic adversity when suddenly released into the systemic circulation. Uterine inversion is more common after vaginal delivery and may require uterine relaxation with terbutaline, ritodrine, IV nitroglycerin, or inhaled amyl nitrate for re-inversion.

## QUADRUPLET DELIVERY

In one series of deliveries of over 39,000, there were two sets of quadruplets recorded. Both of these cases presented with maternal and significant logistic delivery problems. Some of the maternal problems included greatly distended abdomen due to the pendulous uterus and extreme hypotension in the supine position. Exaggerated lordosis was also a problem. Toxemia of pregnancy was a threat, and finally the possibility of hemorrhage after delivery because of uterine atony was a consideration. Fetal problems were restricted primarily to prematurity because of the multiple fetuses and tendency to deliver early. Anesthesia for pain relief at the time of labor can certainly be lumbar epidural with minimal delivery of local anesthetic via the method mentioned multiple times in this textbook that consists of a small amount of local anesthetic mixed with opioid and epinephrine via a continuous delivery by a pump. This results in minimal or no sympathectomy, and minimal effect upon maternal blood pressure. Perhaps the most important aspect or consideration in regard to the mother with quadruplets is that she be kept on her side at all times during labor and perhaps even during labor, or at least moved to her back just prior to labor. For the second stage, or analgesia for delivery, an ideal anesthetic would be a caudal block that allows for analgesia of the S2, S3, S4 area and pain relief at the outlet, allowing the mother to deliver without sympathectomy above that area and certainly minimizing any effect upon the mother because of its use. (52). Other considerations include very careful placement of IV lines for treatment of uterine atony and/or replacement of blood volume in case of hemorrhage. In addition, consideration must be given to careful monitoring of the mother in that situation, including monitoring of the maternal saturation, heart rate, and blood pressure, done either on a semicontinuous basis in which a noninvasive blood pressure device or a cesarean section is considered because of the threat of uterine atony and hemorrhage, or it is possible that an arterial line could be considered. Certainly in lieu of any obstetric complications such as a history of previous bleeding and/or low lying placenta, this latter consideration should be entertained. With the advent of more effective noninvasive blood pressure monitors today, it is possible to detect blood pressures in the very low ranges and much more frequently than was possible in the past. Therefore, in many instances, noninvasive blood pressure monitor may be adequate.

## EXTREMES OF AGE

Very young women who become pregnant are likely to have nutritional deficiencies and receive poor prenatal care. Cephalopelvic disproportion is rarely a problem, and the need for cesarean section is not greater than average (53). There is a higher incidence of premature labor. Although below the legal age for voting, in most states any girl who becomes pregnant is considered to be an emancipated child, and legally capable of giving consent for medical treatment. It is advisable, however, to obtain consent as well from a husband, legal guardian, or parent.

Barring any specific disease condition, the choice of anesthesia for the young pregnant person is based on similar considerations as for mature women. Apprehension and fear are major concerns, and repeated reassurances are needed.

Older women who become pregnant often are obsessed with the health of the fetus (54). Professional career women, for example, often delay having children. And beyond age 35, congenital anomalies become more common. There is a higher incidence of maternal disease, pregnancy-induced hypertension, diabetes, cardiac disease, and thyroid problems. There is greater likelihood of prolonged labor, malpresentation, and placental abnormalities. There are more forceps deliveries and more cesareans than for younger women; blood loss is greater.

Most older mothers prefer regional anesthesia so they can experience the birth process fully; it may be their only chance, and it is a much desired baby. The anesthesiologist should comply with the request to use regional anesthesia, with minimal or no sedation.

## INFECTION AND FEVER

Body temperature is closely regulated by a center in the hypothalamus. The heat generated by metabolism is dissipated by convection, conduction, and evaporation. Fine tuning of the mechanism is accomplished by vasodilation or vasoconstriction of peripheral blood vessels, as well as panting for increased evaporation.

Changes in body temperature may result from infections, metabolic alterations, the effects of drugs, and environmental changes. The common infections during pregnancy are respiratory, urologic, and venereal. Chorioamnionitis rarely occurs until the membranes are ruptured and the pregnancy near termination. The metabolic factors most likely to cause fever are dehydration and thyrotoxicosis. Overdoses of stimulant drugs may cause fever; depressant drugs may allow body cooling sufficient to cause hypothermia. General anesthetics disturb the temperature regulating mechanism. In air conditioned operating rooms, hypothermia is common. Malignant hyperthermia is considered in Chapter 20 on Complications of General Anesthesia.

In pregnant women, fever causes increased secretion of oxytocin and increased plasma norepinephrine. Uterine blood flow is reduced while uterine activity is increased, leading to premature labor. The mother develops tachycardia, increased cardiac output, increased metabolic rate, and sometimes arrhythmias.

Whenever possible, administration of anesthesia should be delayed until the fever is brought under control. The cause of the fever should be identified, and treated with fluids, antibiotics, acetaminophen rather than aspirin, and perhaps a cooling blanket. Reducing the fever reduces oxygen consumption, cardiac work, and arrhythmia potential.

Infections of special concern to anesthesiologists include those with transmission potential, and those that affect the choice of anesthetic.

## Herpes Simplex

The incidence of genital herpes simplex is increasing (55,56). It causes painful ulcerations and enlarged lymph nodes, as well as fever, emesis, malaise, and photophobia, and signs of meningeal irritation. Mild caudal equina symptoms may develop, involving both motor and sensory fibers. The initial episode lasts almost 2 weeks, and there are recurrences.

The lesions shed virus particles that may infect the fetus during vaginal delivery. Genital herpes simplex is transmitted between genital partners. It is not normally transmitted to health care workers, but suitable protective measures should be used: gowns and gloves should be worn if active lesions are present or suspected (57).

Herpes genitalis remains in the genital region, usually. However, it may and does spread. The buttocks and thighs and other areas may be affected.

Because the possibility of transmission or spread is real, vaginal delivery is avoided by many obstetricians. Cesarean delivery is recommended unless there has been complete absence of lesions and symptoms for 2 weeks and negative cultures. General anesthesia is acceptable.

No evidence exists that epidural or spinal anesthesia acts to spread the infection to the nervous system (58,59). There is no uniformity of opinion among anesthesiologists as to what circumstances are acceptable and what constitutes a contraindication to regional anesthesia when the patient has had herpes genitalis. However, intraspinal narcotics should not be used.

The behavior of viruses and the reactivation of viral infections are not well understood. If a patient has had oral herpes and epidural narcotics are administered, the oral herpes may be reactivated (60). Recurrent oral herpes occurred in 10% of women who received epidural morphine, but in only 0.6% of those who did not. In another study, the proportions were 3.24% in those who had received epidural morphine, and 0.36% in those who did not. The trigeminal ganglion is a site of action of both epidural morphine and the herpes simplex virus. Therefore, it may be prudent to use a general analgesia, that is, nitrous oxide administration during vaginal delivery supplemented by IV medication for pain control, or the use of pudendal block for perineal pain relief and concommitant administration of $N_2O$ with analgesic levels for pain relief just during expulsion and delivery of the baby (61). Figure 38–2 lists the number and type of anesthetics administered to mothers with herpes simplex virus at the time of delivery.

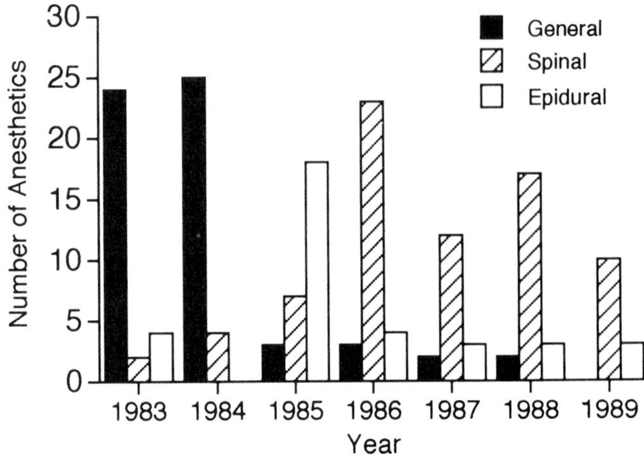


**Fig. 38–2.** Total number of anesthetics administered annually from January 1983 through September 1989. All patients carried a diagnosis of herpes simplex virus (HSV) at the time of delivery. The three categories of analgesia include general, spinal, and epidural. (Redrawn from Bader AM, Camann WR, Datta S: Anesthesia for cesarean delivery inpatients with herpes simplex virus type-2 infections. Reg. Anesth. 15:261, 1990.)

## Aids

Acquired immunodeficiency syndrome is also a viral disease. The virus invades the T cell lymphocytes and makes the patient vulnerable to opportunistic organisms; unusual infections develop, as well as malignancies. The antibody response indicates the presence of infection with the virus; it does not signify immunity. The development of antibodies requires from 2 weeks to 5 months, so a person may be infected although the blood test is still negative.

The most common sources of infection include transmission by sexual contact and by injection of blood from an infected person (62,63). This may occur by shared use of contaminated needles by IV drug users and by transfusion of infected blood products. Transmission from mother to fetus or newborn occurs in about two-thirds of pregnancies of infected women (64,65). It is not spread by casual contact, and an exceedingly small number of cases have ever been attributed to this, but not proven.

A person infected with the virus may have no signs or symptoms, or the illness may become progressively worse. Three stages are recognized: asymptomatic carrier state, ARC (AIDS related complex), with enlarged lymph nodes, and full-blown AIDS, with a variety of infections and malignancies.

Pregnant women have decreased immune mechanisms. They are, therefore, more vulnerable to acquiring the infection and of having a latent infection progress to a more active stage. Of 16 women who were in the asymptomatic carrier stage, seven developed AIDS related complex and five developed fulminate AIDS within 3 years (66).

The opportunistic infections associated with AIDS are both bacterial and viral (cytomegalovirus, herpes simplex, and progressive leukoencephalopathy). There are also infections by protozoa, worms, and fungi (histoplasmosis, candidiasis and aspergillosis)

Systemic manifestations of AIDS vary considerably and involve different physiologic systems, but may include the following:

CNS: encephalopathy, meningitis, dementia, paresis, ataxia, seizures.

Respiratory: pneumonia (pneumocystitis carinii), herpes, candidiasis, coccidiomycosis.
GI: colitis, proctitis, anorexia, malabsorption, dehydration (67).
Hematologic: anemia, leukopenia, thrombocytopenia.

Anesthetic considerations for the patient with AIDS include protection of other people: patients, nurses, doctors (68,69). Special attention should be given to isolation, disposal of contaminated linen, and handling of pointed or sharp objects.

Respiratory complications should be anticipated, both during and after parturition. Impaired oxygenation and respiratory failure may occur because of concurrent pulmonary infections. There may be fungal infections in the mouth and throat, making tissues edematous and friable. Gentle awake intubation may be required.

Cardiovascular problems arise because of dehydration, fever, and electrolyte abnormalities. Fluid therapy may be difficult to manage. Correction of coagulation defects may be required whether or not regional anesthesia is selected.

CNS involvement results in dementia and lack of cooperation. Neurologic defects occur in about one-third of AIDS patients, involving both spinal cord and brain.

The choice of anesthesia essentially involves judging what manifestations of the disease are least and most troublesome, and how the anesthetic will interact.

For vaginal delivery, systemic analgesia with intravenous narcotics, followed by local anesthesia of the perineum, is the best choice. The analgesia may be supplemented by an inhalation agent with increased oxygen concentration. However, it is imperative that the dose be limited to avoid the development of unconsciousness and the need for airway assistance. Small doses of ketamine may be useful during the actual delivery.

For cesarean section, local infiltration with a dilute local anesthetic drug is the safest, although not the most comfortable method. It may also be supplemented by narcotics, ketamine, or inhalation analgesia, avoiding the need for airway intervention. If the patient is not cooperative, and general anesthesia must be used, intubation under local anesthesia is the safest approach, but may not be practical. Rapid sequence induction may be required. In the anticipation that oral pathology may make intubation impossible due to swelling, friable and bleeding tissues, a standby team should be present, ready to do a tracheotomy.

The problems of regional anesthesia may include: lack of cooperation, dehydration, coagulation defect, and neurologic disease. If neurologic disease is not already present, it may develop soon after (perhaps facilitated by a breach of the blood- brain barrier); if it is present, it may become more advanced. If the patient has severe respiratory problems, regional anesthesia may well be the best choice, in spite of the potential complications.

In dealing with any complicated problem such as AIDS, one of the anesthesiologist's concerns is that he/she may be accused of having made matters worse, and become the subject of a malpractice suit. The best way to prevent this is to show that you have given careful attention to the matter: write a note in the hospital chart before you begin, stating what the potential problems are, what the possible choices are, what your selection is among those choices, and the reasoning for your selection. This should be supplemented by a thorough description of all the findings of this particular patient. You may later be said to have used poor judgment, but that is not negligence, and it does not constitute malpractice.

Although transmission of disease from patient to anesthesiologist is extremely unlikely, protective clothing, double gloving and eye shields are mandatory. Do not get secretions or blood on yourself, and do not get them on your equipment and papers. Use disposable equipment whenever possible. Use a nonrebreathing system for general anesthesia. Use a disposable pen and discard it after use because your gloved hand may have contaminated it. Whenever your gloves become contaminated, change to a clean pair. See Chapter 37 for an in-depth discussion of AIDS and precautions.

## Tuberculosis

The influx of immigrants from the orient and third world countries has resulted in an increase of the frequency of this disease. A tuberculin test, and chest x ray when indicated, should be used for people in high-risk groups. Treatment usually controls the disease, so that it does not pose an unusual problem for the recent anesthesiologist. The anesthetic used is guided by the clinical situation.

If the patient has a positive sputum or active disease, precautions must be taken to prevent the spread of the disease to personnel and other patients, with use of appropriate masks, gowns, and gloves. The anesthesiologist should use disposable equipment when possible. For general anesthesia, use a nonrebreathing system to avoid contamination of the anesthetic machine. All reused items should be disinfected.

## Pneumonia

Pneumonia may be caused by bacteria, viruses, or fungi. Fever, cough, excessive secretions, debility, and hypoxia may be present. Appropriate medical treatment is called for, including antibiotics, fluids, and oxygen as indicated by pulse oximetry.

If a blood stream infection is suspected, as in bacteremia or viremia, there is concern that regional anesthesia may breach the blood-brain barrier. Apparently, this concern is groundless, and spinal or epidural anesthesia may be used.

## Excessive Pulmonary Secretions

For all patients with excessive pulmonary secretions, management of anesthesia for labor and delivery is best done with a continuous regional technique, allowing the patient to cough at will, to clear the secretions. The use of narcotics with the regional technique must be tempered by concern that the patient may be vulnerable to respiratory depressant drugs. Limited exertion, supplemental oxygen, and continuous monitoring with a pulse oximeter are recommended. If general anesthesia is needed, frequent suctioning through the endotracheal tube should be carried out, attempting to clear the bronchi on both sides. This can be done by twisting the endotracheal tube 90° to the right and to the left alternatively, before inserting the suction catheter. Be sure to hyperventilate with oxygen before and after each suction effort.

## Cystic Fibrosis

Cystic fibrosis is a genetic disease, transmitted as a recessive trait. Impaired ciliary function, thick and tenacious secretions, and recurrent respiratory infections are characteristic. These may lead to bronchiectasis, hemoptysis, and pneumothorax. Chronic hypoxia may cause clubbed fingers. Dysfunction of other glands also occurs, with decreased pancreatic enzymes, cirrhosis of the liver, and portal hypertension. Dehydration and salt depletion may be present.

## Sarcoidosis

Sarcoidosis is a granulomatous disease of the lungs and other organs. It may require no treatment; it responds to steroid therapy, and there are remissions. Severe cases develop into restrictive-type lung disease, with hypoxia. Patients often improve when pregnant.

Any form of anesthesia, as appropriate, may be used. There may be granulomatous involvement of the vocal cords, and patients may develop laryngeal edema after extubation, being at risk for 2 days post-intubation. Steroid administration and prophylactic use of humidified air or oxygen may be needed, along with careful observation and pulse oximetry.

## Respiratory Failure

Respiratory failure may be the end result of a host of disease conditions, with two common denominators: inadequate ventilation of the lungs and inadequate gas exchange from alveoli to blood. Some of the blood passes through the lungs without unloading its $CO_2$ and without uptake of oxygen. In the case of the pregnant patient with carbon monoxide poisoning, the primary problem is inability for oxygen uptake due to CO-hemoglobin binding. The most expedient and efficacious method of reducing such a blockade is to expose the mother to the hyperbaric oxygen atmosphere. The short exposure of hyperoxia does not appear to have adverse fetal effects and is the treatment of choice for saving the mother and fetus (Figure 38–3 and Table 38–2) (70). Whatever the cause, the patient must be treated for the pulmonary condition rather than the pregnancy. Whatever is best for the mother is best for the fetus. If an obstetric emergency develops, the same principle applies. See Chapter 33 for more detailed information.

## Peripartum Cardiomyopathy

Peripartum cardiomyopathy (PPCM) often presents for the first time during cesarean under regional anesthesia or in the postpartum period because of the increased cardiac output demands and the augmentation of intravascular volume after delivery. Malinow, et al had a patient whose heart rate plummeted to 35 bpm after a spinal (T4 level) and a BP that decreased to 80/40 (71). She responded to 0.8 mg atropine and 15 mg ephedrine, but was intubated when she developed severe pulmonary edema ($PaO_2$ 42, pH 7.25). The systolic blood pressure dropped to 60 mm Hg two times subsequently, requiring CaCl IV and dopa-

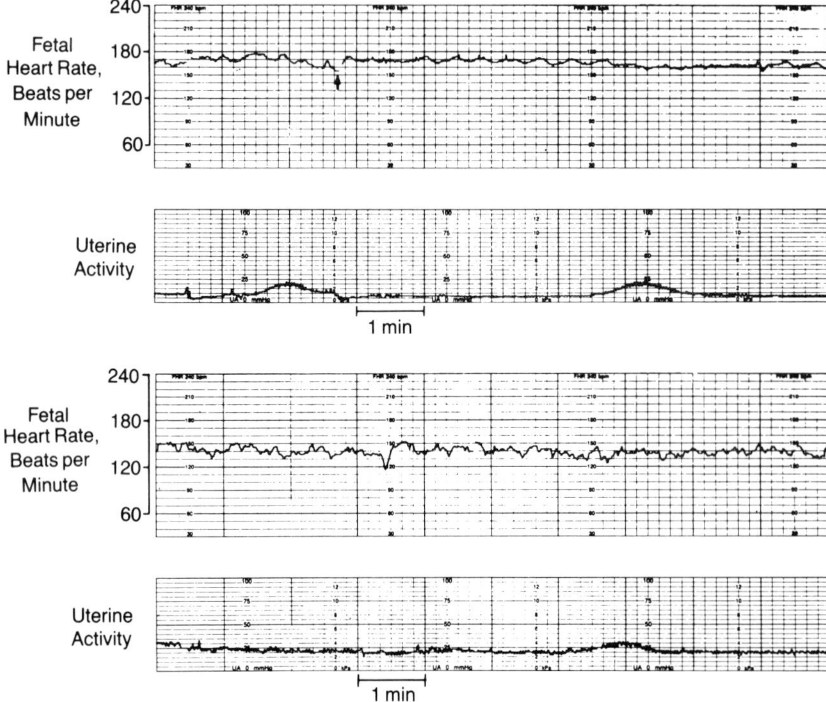


**Fig. 38–3.** The advantages of hyperbaric oxygen therapy. In this instance, prior to hyperbaric oxygen therapy there was an elevated baseline fetal heart rate at 170 beats per minute, with decreased beat-to-beat pattern, as shown in the top two tracings. After 90 minutes of hyperbaric oxygen therapy (100% at 2.4 atmospheres) the heart rate slowed to 140 beats per minute and beat-to-beat variability was normal, as shown in the lower two tracings. (From Van Hoesen KB, Camporesi EM, Moon RE, Hage ML, et al: Should hyperbaric oxygen be used to treat the pregnant patient for acute carbon monoxide poisoning? J.A.M.A. 261: 1039, 1989.)

**Table 38–2.** Carbon Monoxide Poisoning

| Author | Pregnant Subject | Oxygen Exposure† | Pregnancy Outcome |
|---|---|---|---|
| Opposing use* | | | |
| Ferm | Hamster | 3.6 ATA × 3 h<br>4.0 ATA × 2 h | Increased fetal anomaly rate |
| Fujikura | Rabbit | 1.2 ATA × 15 h | Increased retrolental fibroplasia and prematurity |
| Telford et al | Rat | 2.0 ATA × 6 h | Increased fetal resorption |
| Miller et al | Rat | 3.0 ATA × 6 h | Increased cardiovascular defects |
| Supporting use | | | |
| Ferm | Hamster | 3.0 ATA × 3 h | No malformations |
| Cho and Yun | Rat (exposed to CO prior to HBO) | 3.0 ATA × 20 min | Significant decrease in pregnancy resorption compared with untreated group |
| Gilman et al | Hamster | US Navy Table 6‡ | No significant differences between fetuses from treated group and control |
| Hollander et al | Human | 3.0 ATA × 46 min | Healthy newborn |
| Present case | Human | 2.4 ATA × 90 min | Healthy newborn |

* All pressures and/or duration of treatment in the opposing group exceed those recommended for therapeutic treatment of carbon monoxide (CO) intoxication in humans.
† ATA indicates atmosphere absolute.
‡ See text for details.
(From Van Hoesen KB, Camporesi EM, Moon RE, Hage ML, et : Should hyperbaric oxygen be used to treat the pregnant patient for acute carbon monoxide poisoning? JAMA 261:1039–1043, 1989.)

mine 5 g/Kg/min. A PA catheter was placed in the recovery room and CO measured 4.5 L/min with a pulmonary capillary wedge pressure (PCWP) of 28 mm Hg. Three days postpartum, the ejection fraction was 0.30 but increased to 0.70 3 days later and the patient was discharged. Overall mortality is as high as 30 to 60% in parturients with peripartum cardiomyopathy.

A primigravida with severe preeclampsia and aortic regurgitation developed heart failure late in her pregnancy (72). She was taking 250 mg of Methyldopa every six hours and 80 mg Lasix daily. An elective cesarean was planned and an epidural was dosed with a single bolus of 18 ml of 0.5% bupivacaine to a T4 level after a 1 liter fluid bolus. No central venous catheter was placed because "it would be difficult to interpret with aortic regurgitation." An automated BP cuff was used rather than an arterial catheter. The BP decreased from 158/98 to 70/50 but came up to 98/50 with a 500 ml fluid bolus. Because there was no sacral anesthesia, the patient was given a further 6 ml of 0.5% bupivacaine and placed sitting for caudal spread. BP dropped to 45/20 and then was too low to measure despite aggressive fluid boluses and 15 mg IV ephedrine. She was intubated as CPR was begun. Ventricular fibrillation was initially converted with epinephrine, lidocaine, calcium, and defibrillation and an infant with an Apgar of 1 at 1 minute was delivered (who did well). Soon the QRS widened once more and the mother could not be resuscitated again. The authors stated that the cardiac failure in this case might have been reversed with earlier elevation of the SVR with alpha agonists. They also suggest that epidural anesthesia may be contraindicated in "symptomatic aortic incompetence," but another possibility may have been the administration of the local anesthetic as a single bolus and then giving a further dose while the patient was sitting, which may have precipitated this catastrophe. As the authors mention in their discussion, Judge, et al have stated that lowering the SVR is beneficial in aortic regurgitation (73). They further relate how the proximate cause of the fatal arrythmia was probably ischemia due to hypoperfusion in an already abnormally perfused heart (coronary artery blood flow is mainly systolic in severe aortic regurgitation). Even with optimal anesthetic and obstetric management, some patients with advanced heart disease will succumb to the enormous hemodynamic demands of delivery, especially surgical delivery.

## Cardiomyopathy

There are abundant case reports detailing the successful management of labor epidurals in parturients with mitral stenosis (74), Eisenmenger's complex (75–77), pulmonary hypertension (78–80), status asthmaticus (81), paroxysmal ventricular achycardia (82), and idiopathic hypertrophic subaortic stenosis (IHSS) (83,84). Heytens and Alexander used a segmental epidural dosed with 8 ml of 0.125% bupivacaine in a patient with Eisenmenger's syndrome for labor without any significant hemodynamic changes or reversal of shunt (85). This patient did die on the fourth postpartum day from an embolic stroke. Boccio, et al state that regional anesthesia is relatively contraindicated in patients with idiopathic hypertrophic subaortic stenosis (86), but Minnich, et al (84) used an epidural for labor in their case study and found the decreased catecholeamine release to be a definite advantage in idiopathic hypertrophic subaortic stenosis. Their patient did not require a cesarean, but the authors say that they would have used the epidural for this procedure. Both groups of authors would use fluid as a first-line defense against hypotension but would use phenylephrine if necessary, despite the decreased uterine blood flow associated with its use. Phenylephrine is also named the vasopressor of choice in case reports from parturients with pulmonary hypertension (87) and preeclampsia associated with myocardial ischemia in a woman with severe coronary artery disease (88).

The amelioration of dangerous hemodynamic changes with labor can be seen in a case in which pulmonary artery pressure increased from 88/36 to 102/61 during labor in a patient with primary pulmonary hypertension, but decreased to 82/56 with epidural analgesia and 65/40 after delivery (87). Epidural technique has been avoided by many in this condition because of a fear of circulatory collapse with a decreased SVR and venous return. More recently, epidurals have been useful adjuncts to prevent malignant pulmonary hypertension and right heart failure, which can also rapidly lead to a circulatory collapse. Roessler and Lambert consider general anesthesia hazardous for cesarean with pulmonary hypertension and choose epidural (89).

In some patients who were judged not able to tolerate epidural analgesia for labor pain, intrathecal morphine (0.5 to 1.0 mg) has provided excellent analgesia with no adverse hemodynamic changes, although severe pruritus can complicate this method (90–93). Writer, et al found that epidural morphine alone did not compare favorably with bupivacaine for labor pain (94). Cohen reported better pain relief with a combination of dilute bupivacaine and fentanyl (95). Epidural fentanyl can also be used either alone or in combination with 6 to 10 ml of 0.125% bupivacaine during active labor with little or no hemodynamic change. If respiratory depression occurs, it can be reversed by 0.04 to 0.08 mg of IV naloxone followed by an infusion of 0.04 mg per hour (96).

Examination of the literature provides a convincing argument that epidural analgesia is appropriate for any patient, except one with uncorrected hypovolemia, sepsis, or a bleeding diathesis. It is unusual for congenital or acquired cardiac disease to be a contraindication to epidural anesthesia as long as it is well managed and appropriate monitoring and support are given.

## ORTHOPEDIC PROBLEMS

Pregnancy occurs in women with many varieties of orthopedic disease. It may precede the pregnancy, or develop in the pregnant woman as a result of accidents.

Orthopedic conditions of the extremities are essentially of no concern. Deformities of the spine are the major concern, as well as their effects on the contents of the thoracic cage. Other types of congenital abnormalities may be present.

### Rheumatic Disease

Rheumatic disease is a chronic disease that affects other areas of the body besides the joints (97–99). Granulomas may occur in the coronaries, the heart valves, the myocardium, and the cardiac conduction system; the lungs may have granulomas that become necrotic, and there may be pleurisy or pericarditis. Although most manifestations of rheumatic disease improve with pregnancy—in fact there are remissions—the respiratory effects become worse (100). Restricted activity of the costochondral joints causes decreased pulmonary function. Restrictive pulmonary disease becomes worse. The cricoarytenoid joints may limit vocal cord movement and cause obstruction; the neck may be unstable. Awake fiberoptic intubation may be needed. The choice of anesthesia should be based on the severity and nature of associated diseases. Regional anesthesia is preferred; it does not adversely effect the patient.

Pulmonary and cardiac granulomas cause problems related to their location. The coronary arteries, the heart valves, and the conduction system may be affected, and pericarditis may also be present. Laryngeal cartilage involvement limits vocal cord movement, causes edema, distorts the anatomy, and makes intubation difficult. The atlanto-occipital joint may be unstable, making neck extension very hazardous. Severe impairment of exposure may require the fiberoptic technique. Nasal intubation, with great care to prevent bleeding, may be the easiest route.

#### *Ankylosing Spondylitis*

Ankylosing spondylitis is a special form of rheumatic disease, in which many joints become fused (101,102). With this, the patient may turn to stone in the shape of a wheelchair, with head flexed, making tracheotomy impossible. In our experience, one such patient was successfully and easily anesthetized with a paramedian spinal, although the spinal column appeared to be solidly fused on x ray. A continuous technique would be ideal for obstetric delivery.

Ankylosing spondylitis may become more symptomatic during pregnancy (103). Abnormalities of the cervical spine may make oral intubation impossible.

The continuous catheter technique for either epidural or spinal anesthesia is usually the best choice for either type of delivery. Extra caution is required to avoid fluid overload. Depending on the nature of the visceral involvement, full invasive monitoring may be desirable.

General anesthesia should not be started until successful awake intubation has been accomplished. Awake intubation may be performed by use of the fiberoptic. Some of these patients may be so fixed with their chin—that basically opposes the sternum—that it is impossible to intubate them from behind. It may be necessary to approach the patient from the front, sit on the bed next to them with the fiberoptic and the tube in front of them, with the entire fiberoptic technique performed in the frontal position. Calcification of spinal ligaments may make spinal or epidural anesthesia impossible, unless a paramedian approach is used. The Taylor technique may be best: paramedian insertion of the needle and catheter through the junction of L5 and the sacrum.

### Spinal Abnormalities

#### *Backache*

Backache develops in pregnant women because the retaining ligaments are softened by hormones, such as relaxin. The spinal column develops lordosis, the pelvis rotates anteriorly, and the pubic symphysis and sacroiliac joints become unstable (104). Previous back trouble becomes worse. Epidural and spinal anesthesia do not cause these changes to become worse after delivery, and may be used in spite of severe backache. However, it is important that good communication exists between the anesthesiologist and the patient in such instances. For example, although it is pointed out to the patient that in the experience of the anesthesiologist, patients he or she has managed with such problems have not worsened with administration of a regional anesthetic, it is important for each individual patient to make a decision on her own whether or not she wants to have an epidural spinal administered in cases of backache and/or neurologic problems. In the final analysis, it is the patient—not the anesthesiologist—who is impacted by any problems. The patient therefore must give to the physician complete, informed consent and the patient must make the decision for a regional anesthetic, i.e, spinal or epidural in such instances.

### *Herniated Intervertebral Disc*

Herniated intervertebral disc is not a contraindication to spinal or epidural anesthesia. However, the onset of epidural anesthesia may be delayed, and distribution may be spotty and incomplete. Two catheters, one above and one below the herniation, are more certain to provide complete anesthesia (105). However, spinal anesthesia is not impaired, and is more reliable.

### *Scoliosis*

Scoliosis may develop in childhood or adolescence (106). Abnormalities of the vertebrae, the nervous system, and the muscles may be present. A variety of connective tissue disorders may also be present. Both heart and lungs may be affected, particularly with restriction of chest motion and lung function (107,108). Ventilation perfusion defects, compression of the lungs, inability to take deep breaths and cough well, lead to hypoxia, and pulmonary vascular resistance increases. Associated cardiovascular disease includes mitral prolapse, cyanotic heart disease, and coarctation of the aorta. Right heart failure and increased pulmonary vascular disease may be present (109).

The effect of pregnancy increases the cardiovascular and pulmonary deficiencies, especially if the chest deformity cannot accommodate to the increased abdominal size (110). Oxygen administration should begin early, and narcotics must be cautiously used because the respiratory system may be unable to accommodate to the requirements of labor and to the effects of the drugs (111).

Regional anesthesia is not contraindicated. It does not worsen the orthopedic condition. Pain relief reduces the demands on the cardiac and respiratory systems. One drawback of regional anesthesia is that patients may be unable to breathe adequately while supine, making a cesarean operation mechanically very difficult. General anesthesia with intubation and control of respiration is best for such a case.

Epidural anesthesia is commonly recommended, but may be impossible to accomplish (112). Location and verification of the epidural space may be time-consuming or even impossible. We recommend that continuous spinal be considered as the method of choice. A paramedian approach on the convex side of the spinal curve, where the bony aperture is larger, may be surprisingly easy. Once spinal fluid is obtained, the problems are almost over. Thread in a catheter, anchor it securely, and then administer small doses of very dilute local anesthetic solutions. Sensory analgesia without motor paralysis should be obtained using Marcaine or Tetracaine 0.25 mg/ml, starting with 3 ml and titrating to effect. Raising the concentration to 1 mg/ml produces motor paralysis if desired for cesarean section.

Scoliosis often causes chronic restrictive pulmonary disease, with respiratory acidosis and hypoxemia. Pulmonary vascular resistance is increased, and right heart failure results. Congenital heart disease and coarctation of the aorta may also be present. All of these are likely to become worse during pregnancy, particularly if the curvature is in the thoracic area. If the pelvis is normal, delivery from below can occur without difficulty. If the pelvis is deformed, cesarean section is required.

Technical problems occur with both anesthesia and cesarean delivery. With adequate regional anesthesia, the patient may be unable to lie flat because of cardiac or respiratory problems, and there may be additional impairment of respiration due to the block. The surgical approach for cesarean is very difficult or impossible if the patient must remain in a sitting position. It is also very difficult if the spinal deformity causes the rib cage and pubic bone to become closer together, decreasing the available abdominal exposure.

Because of the problems of difficult catheter insertion, adequacy of breathing, and intolerance of supine posture, general anesthesia is a better choice than regional. If neck and jaw mobility is normal, the usual rapid sequence induction is acceptable. If there is doubt about ability to expose the larynx, awake intubation should be done.

## Unstable Neck

This is a most important consideration. Extension, or even flexion in some cases, may cause spinal cord injury. The neck must be stabilized before intubation is done, so that its position does not change. A collar is not adequate for this purpose, and the patient must not be allowed to cough vigorously when the tube enters the trachea. Intubation should be accomplished under local anesthesia because it may be difficult and time consuming. The local anesthesia should be so thorough that the gag and cough reflexes are fully obtunded. An assistant should have medication prepared, attached to the IV line, ready for administration as soon as the intubation placement is verified. Fiberoptic visualization, here again, may be the best technique.

## Spinal Cord Injury

Severe injury resulting in paraplegia may cause miscarriage or premature labor. Otherwise, pregnancy can go to full term with painless vaginal delivery. Incomplete spinal cord damage allows varying degrees of sensation and/or pain.

Anesthesia concerns for severe spinal injury include especially autonomic instability and excess potassium release from damaged muscle tissue. Patients with injury above the T6 level may have autonomic hyperreflexia, with severe hypertensive episodes, and have also severe hypotension when spinal or epidural anesthesia is administered (113,114). If succinylcholine is used for general anesthesia, there may be a serious rise in the blood potassium level, so this drug is contraindicated.

For patients who have no pain in labor, but who have exhibited hyperreflexia, and for those who need pain relief, the best method of management is continuous spinal or epidural, with slow incremental doses and careful control of blood pressure. Spinal narcotics may be best to avoid both hypotension and hypertension, while providing adequate pain relief (115).

## Miscellaneous Skeletal Abnormalities

These may be of many varieties: traumatic, congenital, present at birth or appearing later. The congenital type may relate to closure of the neural tube, with spinal and neurologic abnormalities. There may be abnormal growth, ossification of bones, development of cartilage, fusion of sutures, softening or calcification of ligaments, fragility of bones, and distortion of the skeleton. In all cases, the anesthesia must be tailored to the particular problem.

Miscellaneous disorders of the skeleton and the neural tube are often associated with complications of the respiratory and cardiovascular systems, as well as coagulation defects. In addition, pathological fractures of bones and small pelvic outlets may be among these disorders. The anesthesiologist must weigh the relative problems of achieving endotracheal intubation against those of getting a needle into the spine. Our choice: Correct any coagulation defect and do a paramedian continuous spinal.

When all other approaches to the problems are too hazardous, remember the virtues and values of proceeding with local infiltration and intravenous sedation. Use very dilute solutions, so as a large volume can be employed. Maintain patient consciousness and spontaneous breathing. Assist if necessary, with a mask and high flow of oxygen and perhaps a trace of inhalation analgesic.

## *McArdle's Disease*

McArdle's disease was first described in 1951 and is a hereditary myopathy due to an enzyme deficiency. The condition is secondary to absence of muscle phospharylase that results in inability of glycogen conversion to lactate. This condition appears to be a single recessive autosomal gene, approximately three times more evident in males than females.

The primary consideration in regard to anesthesiology is the use of a muscle relaxant for induction and intubation. Ordinarily, succinycholine hydrochloride is used because of its rapid action. However, such a drug used in this disease process may cause serious problems. The primary reason to avoid use of a potent depolarizing muscle relaxant such as succinycholine hydrochloride is due to the risk of myoglobinaemia and the possibility of serious renal damage after the fact. Other methods of intubation may be used in this disease process such as awake intubation under local analgesic spray and the use of the fiberoptic instrument. In addition, substitution of the newer, effective muscle relaxants of a nondepolarizing nature such as vecuronium and atracurium for succinycholine hydrochloride can be used. Before using these latter muscle relaxants for induction, especially in a rapid sequence induction, careful attention should be given to the planning and sequencing of the rapid sequence induction and continuation of the cricoid pressure because of the necessity to avoid any possible regurgitation or aspiration (116).

## *Jervell, Lange-Nielson Syndrome*

The Jervell, Lange-Nielson syndrome, described in 1957, is a hereditary disease of autosomal recessive origin, and it is rather rare (1:300,000) in incidence (117). The primary markers of the disease process are syncopal problems combined with congenital deafness and a prolongation of the Q-T interval. In some instances, there may be a family history of sudden death, which most probably is related to syncopal attacks with associated Stokes-Adams attacks. The ultimate cause of death in the aforementioned cases are asystole or ventricular fibrillation due to an increasingly evident atrio-ventricular block. Patients with the Jervell, Lange-Nielson syndrome may also exhibit the most unusual Torsades des pointe phenomenon, which is described as a rapid ventricular tachycardia with consistently changing QRS configurations. It appears that recent developments in various blocking agents such as β-blocking drugs have improved survival in this class of patients. One case report in the literature of a patient with Jervell, Lange-Nielson syndrome who underwent a cesarean section revealed that the patient was treated with 20 mg propranolol twice a day until her cesarean section. The patient received a general anesthetic with a typical induction with thiopental and succinycholine hydrochloride for intubation of the trachea. Maintenance for the anesthetic was $N_2O$, oxygen, and halothane. The outcome of the pregnancy was good, with delivery of a healthy neonate, and the mother did well in the immediate postoperative period and throughout her postpartum course. This same patient was delivered 2 years subsequently and had a nearly identical induction and anesthetic maintenance as previously described. Again, she delivered a healthy neonate and recovered uneventfully. It would appear that the patient's maintenance on propranolol 20 mg twice per day was a successful therapeutic measure for her because she had not suffered any Stokes-Adams syncopal attacks since early childhood and subsequent to her placement on propranolol.

The pathology of this condition is confusing, but certainly involves the relationship between the cardiac sympathetic nerves and the sympathetic tone in relationship to depolarization and repolarization of the ventricles. The latter relationship is often imbalanced in favor of the sympathetic tone that may lead to a tendency toward fibrillation. Support for the latter theory comes from work done in the late 1970s in regard to the performance of stellate ganglion block to effect a sympathectomy per se. Patients who received these blocks showed clinical improvement with decreases also in the frequency of syncopal attacks and in the duration of the Q-T interval (117–119).

Propranolol certainly seems to be the treatment of choice in this syndrome. In addition, careful consideration of the anesthetic agent together with a general anesthesia to allay the anxiety that might be experienced by a patient should she be concerned about being awake during her surgery should be made. Otherwise, in a patient who prefers to be awake and who does not appear to have a high level of anxiety, regional anesthesia could be a consideration if a low T10 to T8 block would be used with supplementation with fentanyl 50 to 100 μmg as previously suggested in Chapter 30 on Cesarean Section. The problem with the use of a regional anesthetic is the concern for hypotension in lieu of a patient who is β-blocked. Therefore, the typical epidural with an anticipated level of T4 would certainly not be appropriate with these patients, and the authors favor the use of general anesthesia in patients who are suitable candidates for this technique and who are not absolutely determined to be awake for the delivery of their baby.

## ENDOCRINE DISEASE

### Adrenal

#### *Glucocorticoid Hormonal Excess*

This may be iatrogenic, or due to disease. These features constitute the Cushing's syndrome due to excess glucocorticoid hormone: buffalo hump, thick neck, obesity, moon-shaped face, abdominal striae, hirsutism, ecchymoses, diabetes, hypertension, osteoporosis, hypokalemia (120–122). Cushing's syndrome becomes worse with pregnancy, with increased susceptibility to infection. Anesthetists must give extra attention to strict sterility and to careful movement of patients to prevent fractures.

In spite of having excessive levels of glucocorticoids, the patients have inadequate response to stress, and may require additional steroid administration. The following is recommended: Hydrocortisone 100 mg IV before a cesarean, or every 8 hours during labor; taper to 1 dose each 12 hours on Days 2 and 3 and a single dose on Day 4

There is no contraindication to regional anesthesia, and this is the best choice, although the procedure may be difficult due to edema or vertebral fractures. For general anesthesia, a difficult intubation must be expected, due to the buffalo hump, thick neck, obesity, and vascular fragility. Awake intubation is recommended.

#### *Primary Hyperaldosteronism*

This causes potassium loss and sodium retention. Nephropathy may develop, with polyuria, and hypokalemia causing muscle weakness. Hypertension occurs and is confused with preeclampsia. The patient should be prepared before anesthesia with potassium supplements and spironolactone. Hypokalemia predisposes to cardiac arrhythmia and prolonged effect of muscle relaxants.

#### *Adrenal Insufficiency*

Also known as Addison's disease, this may be iatrogenic, and may occur spontaneously during pregnancy or as a result of hemorrhagic shock (Sheehan's syndrome). Sodium loss and potassium retention occur. Anemia, hypovolemia, hypoglycemia, and general debility develop.

Before anesthesia is begun, the patient should be given a large dose of hydrocortisone, 200 mg IV, a liter of 5% dextrose in saline, followed by 1 or 2 liters of normal saline, each containing 100 mg hydrocortisone. These patients are excessively susceptible to all anesthetic agents and are prone to severe hypotension. Regional or general anesthesia may be used, with lower doses of drugs and special attention to the need for additional fluid and steroid.

#### *Pheochromocytoma*

This produces epinephrin and norepinephrine. Most of those tumors occur in the adrenal medulla, but some are in other chromaffin tissue. Failure to diagnose and treat cause over 50% mortality for both mother and fetus. Hypertensive crisis and cardiac failure are the cause of death; after the tumor is removed, hypotension is the cause of death.

The condition is suspected because of a history of headaches, symptoms resembling those of hyperthyroidism, and hypertension, usually intermittent. Diagnosis is confirmed by measurement of catecholamines or vanillylmandelic acid in urine and blood. Treatment is started with α and β adrenergic blocking drugs, phenoxybenzamine and propranolol, or similar drugs. If diagnosed early in pregnancy, prompt surgical removal is recommended. If diagnosed late, the plan entails waiting until the fetus is viable, delivering by cesarean, and, immediately thereafter, removing the tumor.

The choice of anesthesia is based upon how best to control the effects of the tumor and its hormone secretions. There is no particular best choice of anesthesia, but whatever is used should be managed so as to avoid a surge in catecholamine output. Whatever is best for the mother is best for the fetus. This should be treated as an endocrine problem, not an obstetric problem (122–125).

If the patient is well controlled by medical treatment, she may be allowed to deliver normally. Any appropriate anesthesia may be used, with special attention to adequate fluid administration. Be prepared to treat sudden severe swings of blood pressure from one extreme to the other.

### Pituitary

The pregnant patient with a pituitary tumor that is symptomatic is treated for the tumor rather than the pregnancy. If the tumor is not symptomatic, the delivery is managed as appropriate, with regional anesthesia if possible to prevent straining during labor. Acromegalic features are likely to cause difficulty with airway and intubation; awake intubation should be considered if general anesthesia is needed.

#### *Hypopituitarism*

This condition may be caused by necrosis of the pituitary as a result of hemorrhagic shock. The signs leading to this diagnosis are those of failure of the other endocrine glands, especially the adrenal (Sheehan's syndrome).

## Thyroid

Pregnant women remain euthyroid, although there is an increase in metabolic rate. There are increases of laboratory values for T3 and T4 because thyroid-binding globulin increases. The free thyroid index remains normal (126).

### *Nontoxic Goiter*

This may increase in size during pregnancy. The anesthesia used for delivery may be managed without regard to the goiter, unless acute respiratory distress develops due to tracheal compression. In that case, under local anesthesia, an endotracheal tube is inserted far enough to overcome the obstruction to breathing, and left in until after the delivery, when the goiter may be removed surgically.

### *Thyrotoxicosis*

This may be masked by symptom changes normal with pregnancy (127). Exaggerated symptoms and a resting pulse rate of over 100 raise suspicions. Laboratory findings that confirm the diagnosis include: Serum T4 over 15 mg/dl and serum T3 over 250 ng per dl; normal T3 resin uptake and elevated free T4 or T3 index. TSH levels should be normal.

Medical management is best done with propylthiouracil to inhibit synthesis of thyroid hormone (128),it has the least placental transfer of available alternatives. Propranolol may be used in addition to propylthiouracil to control symptoms of increased catecholamine release. Surgical treatment is rarely needed before delivery. For the patient who has been made euthyroid by therapy, choice of anesthesia for delivery is whatever is appropriate without regard to the thyroid.

If anesthesia must be administered for an emergency to a patient who has not been treated for thyrotoxicosis, a method should be chosen that gives swift control without making matters worse. Use preliminary sedation with a barbiturate (pentobarbital) or versed to control apprehension, as well as a blocking drug (propranolol, esmolol) to reduce catecholamine effects. Spinal and epidural anesthesia diminish catecholamine release from the adrenals, and either is the preferred method of anesthesia for delivery. The patient should be closely monitored for signs of developing thyroid storm. Preparations should be made for treating thyroid storm, having available a cooling blanket and ice, steroids, morphine, propranolol, esmolol, iodine, antihypertensive drugs, and antithyroid drugs. Vigilance must continue through the postpartum period.

### *Hypothyroidism*

Reduced thyroid function may develop spontaneously or be a result of medical treatment. Besides the common symptoms, pregnant patients may have slow pulse, low voltage EKG, cardiomegaly, and congestive heart failure. A low level of serum T4 confirms the diagnosis.

Pitfalls to watch for in treating reduced thyroid function include: sensitivity to sedatives, narcotics and anesthetics, vulnerability to hypothermia and hypoglycemia, tolerance of blood loss but easy susceptibility to heart failure by fluid overload or stress.

Preferred anesthesia for delivery is continuous epidural or spinal, with slow raising of the level, and care to maintain blood pressure without a large fluid load. General anesthesia should be induced slowly and incrementally to allow for slow circulation of blood. Recovery is slower than normal.

## Parathyroid

### *Hyperparathyroidism*

This causes elevated serum calcium levels due to bone resorption and increased absorption of calcium from the GI tract (129). Symptoms are not alarming unless a hypercalcemic crisis occurs, with mental deterioration, coma, renal failure, cardiac arrhythmia, or congestive failure.

Preparation for anesthesia includes checking for electrolyte and fluid balance. The serum calcium level may be reduced by administering steroids and phosphate. Regional or general anesthesia may be given, as appropriate, for the obstetric condition. Responses to muscle relaxants may be abnormal (130).

### *Hyperaldosteronism*

Usually iatrogenic, this results in low serum ionized calcium and high serum phosphorus (131). Further decrease in ionized calcium is caused by fetal calcium removal and alkalosis, due to hyperventilation, citrated blood transfusions, or uremia. The patient develops neuromuscular irritability, exaggerated tendon reflexes, and tetany. Acute treatment and preparation for anesthesia are by administration of intravenous calcium gluconate or calcium chloride with EKG monitoring. During labor, hyperventilation should be prevented by adequate regional anesthesia. General anesthesia may be used for delivery as appropriate for the obstetric condition.

## Blood Sugar Control

The management of diabetes is fully discussed elsewhere.

Hypoglycemia may be a cause of refractory hypotension in women who have had regional anesthesia for delivery. After a prolonged period of being NPO and fluid load of salt solution without added glucose, a spinal or epidural anesthetic is administered. Adrenal catecholamine secretion and hepatic glycogenolysis are reduced under these conditions. Symptoms develop if the blood sugar level falls below 40 to 50 mg%: agitation, tremors, confusion, diaphoresis, hunger, tachycardia, hypotension, hypertension, seizures, and coma may also occur (132).

Treatment is intravenous administration of 50% dextrose, up to 50 ml. Refractory hypotension after regional anesthesia may respond favorably.

# HEMATOLOGIC PROBLEMS

Coagulation defect and/or prolonged bleeding time are contraindications to regional blocks, including spinal, epidural, and pudendal. Pain relief should be accomplished with narcotics, inhalation analgesia, and/or small doses of ketamine for delivery. For cesarean section, general anesthesia is used for cases in which regional is contraindicated, with special attention to avoid trauma and bleeding, especially a hematoma in the tissues of the airway. See Chapter 26 for more information.

### Lupus Erythematosus

Lupus erythematosus is a disorder of the immune system with multiple and varied presentations, with coagulation defects, low platelets, vasculitis, purpura, and disseminated thrombosis (133,134). It is exacerbated by pregnancy. It increases the risk of fetal loss by miscarriage or later hypertension and renal failure. It causes heart defects in the fetus. Treatment is with steroids and aspirin.

### Idiopathic Thrombocytic Purpura

Idiopathic thrombocytic purpura may affect mother and fetus (135–138). Pregnancy causes exacerbation of the disease. Easy bruising, petechiae, and bleeding from multiple sites may occur. Prednisone administration improves both mother and fetus. The patient who is seriously ill and fails to respond may require platelet transfusions, immunoglobulin, and/or splenectomy.

### Von Willebrand's Disease

Von Willebrand's disease is a hereditary coagulation defect involving factor VIII. Bleeding time is prolonged, and bleeding may occur in any area of the body. During pregnancy, the tendency to bleed is diminished, but there is increased risk of postpartum hemorrhage. Cryoprecipitate or fresh frozen plasma bring the factor VIII levels to near normal, and bleeding time becomes normal.

The complication of epidural or intrathecal or intrapelvic hemorrhage is so serious that it is not worth the risk to use a regional block. When in doubt, analgesia or general anesthesia is the method of choice. With modern techniques of general anesthesia and neonatal care, the risk to the fetus is not significantly greater.

### Anticoagulant Treatment

Anticoagulant treatment is given to patients who suffer from thromboembolic disease. Pregnancy increases the risk of this condition. Pulmonary embolism presents as both cardiac and pulmonary disturbances. Various emergency surgical interventions may be required, and the patient is treated for the embolism without specific regard to the pregnancy.

Anticoagulant therapy with heparin or other drugs is used to prevent recurrent emboli. The partial prothrombin time is maintained at twice the norm. Low, prophylactic doses of heparin do not affect the coagulation tests. Although the frequency of hemorrhage is low in those receiving mini doses of heparin, the consequences of such hemorrhage are severe. Regional anesthesia is contraindicated unless there is an even more severe contraindication to other forms of pain relief.

### Sickle Cell Disease

Sickle cell disease is an inherited condition that ranges in severity from asymptomatic sickle cell trait to fatal sickle cell anemia and crisis. It is mostly limited to black people, but white individuals of Mediterranean origin may be affected (138–140).

Hemoglobin S is deformed into sickle shape when deoxygenated because the hemoglobin precipitates in long crystals. These cells aggregate, causing circulatory stasis or vascular occlusion and infarction of affected tissue or organs. Sickling is induced by low oxygen pressure, low pH, low blood pressure, hypothermia, dehydration, or any other factor that slows blood flow, including venous obstruction and tourniquets. The anesthesiologist caring for a patient with sickle cell disease is often urged to give special attention to maintain good oxygenation, blood pressure, adequate fluid, etc. In fact, this is no more than we should do for every patient. Ideal treatment for every patient includes what is ideal for blacks with or without sickle cell disease.

## Bleeding Tendencies

Occasionally, an obstetric case arises in which there is a clear advantage to regional anesthesia, but a bleeding tendency will incur the risk of neurological compromise. Dr. Abouleish recounted such a situation in a parturient with Ehlers-Danlos syndrome (141). This disorder involves a defect in collagen synthesis in almost every system in the body and predisposes the victim to bleed from any open wound. While associated micrognathia and a higher risk for pneumothorax with positive pressure ventilation make regional anesthesia attractive, exaggerated lordosis, restrictive pulmonary disease, and a bleeding tendency can complicate the technique. In this particular case, it was felt that a continuous caudal technique would be less likely to disrupt epidural veins due to the angle at which the catheter enters the epidural space. As is typical for this condition, the blood coagulation tests were normal. Dr. Abouleish also described another patient with this syndrome for whom a subarachnoid anesthetic was chosen for cesarean section. In both patients, Dr. Abouleish believed that the risk of aspiration pneumonitis was greater than was the remote possibility of bleeding with a regional anesthetic.

Kotelko reported on a woman with May-Hegglin anomaly, characterized by thrombocytopenia, and in whom a platelet count of 24,000 was increased to 35,000 with six units of platelets prior to a spinal anesthetic for cesarean section (142). Kotelko had informed the patient of a reported incidence of epidural venous puncture of 1.0% with a spinal or epidural needle (143); knowing this risk, the woman preferred a regional anesthetic. Kotelko reviews the literature concerning May-Hegglin as reported by Owens, et al in 33 cases of spinal hematoma (six after spinal anesthesia and 27 following diagnostic lumbar puncture (LP); 26 had some evidence of a bleeding abnormality (13 had received anticoagulants and nine had thrombocytopenia) (144). Forty-five percent had partial or good neurologic recovery.

In a similar case, a woman with osteogenesis imperfecta

required cesarean section for breech presentation (145). These patients have a bleeding tendency due to decreased platelet adhesion and aggregation. In this case, the bleeding time was normal and she had reduced cervical spine movement and a receding mandible, so a continuous epidural anesthetic was chosen. Had there been an abnormal bleeding time, the authors state that awake intubation would have been indicated. Crosby and Elliott report a woman with a quintuplet gestation and a rapidly dropping platelet count who required a cesarean section (146). In her case, a general anesthetic was chosen. Her severe pulmonary edema and hypoxia required her to be anesthetized in the sitting position. For this reason, she probably would not have tolerated regional anesthesia even if her platelet count had been stable. Incidentally, the patient was aggressively diuresed with pulmonary artery catheter guidance prior to induction and was not extubated until the second postoperative day.

People with a lupus anticoagulant autoantibody often have a partial thromboplastin time (PTT) higher than the upper limit for regional anesthesia but who are clinically hypercoagulable. They are frequently on low-dose aspirin and steroids to prevent thrombosis. Malinow, et al used conduction analgesia for labor in such a patient with a partial thromboplastin time 50% over controls (147). Although the bleeding time was normal, the paper quotes a study that showed that a hemorrhagic diathesis is possible in people on aspirin with a normal bleeding time. In this case, Malinow, et al decided that the benefit of decreased catecholeamines (in the face of a decreased prostacyclin production by an infarcted placenta) outweighed the bleeding risk. They would have used general anesthesia for a cesarean because the airway was normal. Without antiplatelet therapy, less than one in six pregnancies will be successful in women with lupus anticoagulant.

Patients with known bleeding disorders such as Von Willebrand's disease receive epidural anesthesia for labor and cesarean section as long as the partial thromboplastin time and bleeding time are near normal (148,149). In fact, it is common for factor VIII levels to be higher in the third trimester of pregnancy. Fresh frozen plasma, cryoprecipitate, and desmopressin are frequently used if excessive bleeding occurs. Desmopressin can be used prophylactically before delivery, although it will result in minimal correction of laboratory abnormalities and lasts only a short time.

All of the case reports that the present authors have reviewed stress that a disease or history of bleeding are not enough to deny a patient an epidural anesthetic as long as coagulation tests are near normal and there is no evidence of unusual bleeding. Most authors will not do regional anesthesia with a platelet count of less than 50,000, or when the platelet count is rapidly falling, without transfusion of platelets prior to the block (150).

## RENAL INSUFFICIENCY OR FAILURE

Preexisting renal disease is worsened by pregnancy (151–153). Renal disease may develop as a result of complications of pregnancy. Renal disease affects the major systems of the body, including cardiovascular, respiratory, metabolic, endocrine, neurologic, and hematopoetic.

When the patient requires anesthesia, there may be a combination of problems present, some of which may be immediately improved by suitable intervention: hypertension, pericardial effusion, pleural effusion, acid-base and electrolyte disorders, blood volume abnormality, coagulopathy, and anemia. Treatment with insulin, steroids, antihypertensive medications, and renal dialysis, all may be necessary (154,155).

Anesthesia may worsen the renal condition by causing hypotension or by causing a rise in the serum fluoride level. With methoxyflurane no longer available, enflurane is the drug to avoid (156).

For pain relief during labor, fentanyl is the drug of choice because it is metabolized by the liver with only little renal excretion. It does not affect renal function. It does cross the placenta, but has minimal effect on the fetus. Small amounts of diazepam may be used in addition, but phenothiazines should be avoided because they may cause psychotic reactions. During vaginal delivery, nitrous oxide with 50% or more of oxygen provides additional analgesia, and local anesthesia of the perineum or pudendal blocks are satisfactory.

Continuous epidural or spinal anesthesia may be used, but there are special concerns about bleeding tendency and blood volume. Coagulopathy should be corrected before the block is performed. If coagulation status is borderline, the smaller needle and catheter of continuous spinal and lesser venous network within the thecal space make this technique preferable to continuous epidural. Adjusting the concentration and dose of local anesthetic drug makes the technique suitable for labor and delivery (157).

It is common practice to give a fluid load before administering spinal or epidural anesthesia. But the renal patient may be intolerant of any fluid load, and great caution must be exercised. Measuring CVP or PA pressures may be desirable. Usually, however, both fluid loading and hypotension may be avoided by slow titration of small doses of drug, so that onset of anesthesia is gradual, and blood pressure is supported with small doses of ephedrine.

If general anesthesia is required, hyperkalemia is the principal added concern. Along with the usual precautions for general anesthesia, avoid succinylcholine (158). Atracurium and vecuronium are cleared at an almost normal rate even in anephric subjects. Balanced anesthesia is satisfactory, and fluid administration must be sharply limited. Antihypertensive agents are preferable to halogenated anesthetics for control of elevated blood pressure, partly because of concern about renal damage, and partly to prevent causing a boggy relaxed uterus.

Blood transfusion to correct anemia or treat blood loss is no longer considered especially objectionable. Later renal transplant is not endangered by transfusions.

## NEUROLOGIC DISEASE

### Convulsions in the Labor Room

Seizures of a laboring patient may be due to idiopathic epilepsy, toxemia of pregnancy (eclampsia), or local anesthetic reaction. The differential diagnosis is usually not difficult to make: a history of epilepsy; signs and symptoms associated with preeclampsia; recent injection of a local anesthetic. Although eclampsia may occur de novo, without preliminary warning signs, that is quite unusual. Local anesthetic toxic reactions may occur immediately because of intravascular injection, or rapid absorption of the drug from tissues, or as long as 20 minutes after injection following slower absorption of the drug from tissues.

The emergency treatment of convulsions, whatever the cause, is to assure pulmonary ventilation with oxygen and then to control cardiovascular abnormalities. The muscles of the throat and jaw participate in the rigidity, so that the airway becomes obstructed. Spontaneous respiratory activity ceases because the muscles of chest and abdomen are involved as well.

Every labor room should be supplied with, or have readily available, a supply of oxygen and a bag and mask device for artificial respiration. Using these may be adequate to ventilate the lungs should the seizure cease spontaneously within a short time. Endotracheal equipment should also be readily available and should be used should more active treatment be required. The seizure is then terminated by administration of the most readily available drug: thiopental in 50 mg increments, diazepam in 2 mg increments, or midazolam in 2 mg increments. If there is a need to intubate, succinylcholine is administered and intubation is accomplished with cuff inflation. Maintaining pulmonary ventilation is the primary concern.

The patient may not have an intravenous infusion, and efforts to start one may be unsuccessful. Intubation cannot be done because of rigidity of the jaw and throat muscles. There are several options while you continue efforts to ventilate with the mask: (1) have someone do a tracheotomy or cricothyrotomy; (2) use a transtracheal needle or mini tracheotomy device; (3) give an intramuscular injection of succinylcholine—twice the usual dose, and massage the injection site to produce more rapid absorption. Within 3 minutes, there should be sufficient relaxation to intubate and ventilate.

If the cardiovascular system shows no great aberration, nothing more need be done. If the blood pressure is either too low or too high, or the pulse is too slow, appropriate medication is administered. For cardiac arrhythmia, lidocaine or bretylium may be adequate; cardioversion or defibrillation may be needed.

Having control of the basic life support needs, attention can turn to the cause. If there are indications of eclampsia, the obstetricians can administer their favorite treatments, including IV magnesium. If the likely cause is local anesthetic toxicity, the problem will abate without other treatment.

Fetal monitoring, which has been conducted throughout this episode, should show no particular detrimental effect if maternal respiration and circulation have been maintained. The fetus is more tolerant of local anesthetics than the mother, provided there has been no acidosis or asphyxia.

If the treatment efforts have not produced a stable, well-oxygenated patient and fetal distress is apparent, an emergency cesarean is indicated. This is particularly true if cardiac compression (CPR) is needed. CPR is more effective when the baby is out, so that a prompt cesarean may save both baby and mother.

Local anesthetic drugs may trigger a catastrophe (159,160) if injected directly into a blood vessel or if a large dose is deposited in a vascular area. The standard precautions of aspiration, incremental injection, low concentration of drug, and limited total dose should prevent such occurrences. Bupivacaine should be used only in very low concentrations because of its particular cardiotoxicity.

### *Von Recklinghausen's Disease (Neurofibromatosis)*

The lesions increase in size during pregnancy (161). There may be pelvic obstruction requiring a cesarean section (162). Lesions on the vocal cords may cause obstruction. Patients have a higher incidence than normal of hypertension, pheochromocytoma, and of brain tumors (meningioma, glioma, acoustic neuroma, and obstructed cerebral spinal fluid (CSF) flow).

Patients with Von Recklinghausen's disease have abnormal responses to the depolarizing relaxants and may develop contracture rather than relaxation after succinylcholine (163). They are also more sensitive to the nondepolarizing relaxants, requiring smaller doses that produce a duration of action longer than normal.

The choice of anesthesia depends upon the particular manifestations of the disease in the individual patient. The usual preference for regional anesthesia for labor and delivery applies, unless there is the contraindication of brain tumor, elevated cerebral spinal fluid pressure, or other neurologic manifestation. If general anesthesia is required, avoid succinylcholine, and use smaller doses of other relaxant drugs.

### *Spinal Cord Injury or Disease*

Spinal cord injury or disease may deprive the patient of painful sensation, as well as cause motor paralysis. Vaginal delivery may occur even if the patient is totally paralyzed and unable to push; low forceps may be needed. Whether any anesthesia or analgesia is required may be questioned.

If the spinal cord damage is at the level of T7 or above, autonomic hyperreflexia may be a serious problem for half the patients (164,165). Afferent stimuli from skin or viscera reach the spinal cord and cause a sympathetic response, without modulation from the higher centers. The blood pressure may rise suddenly to very high levels, and a vagal reflex slows the heart. Facial flushing and severe headache and sweating occur. There may be convulsions, coma, and intracranial bleeding.

Control of the excessive autonomic lability is best obtained by placing an intrathecal or epidural catheter (166). A local anesthetic or a narcotic or both may be used as for normal people. If general anesthesia is needed for any reason, avoid use of succinylcholine because the affected muscles respond with a surge of potassium output that elevates the blood level excessively.

### *Ruptured Cerebral Aneurysm or Arteriovenous Anomaly*

Ruptured cerebral aneurysm or arteriovenous anomaly may require repair during pregnancy because of intracranial bleeding (167,168). The anesthesia for the craniotomy is carried out with the same technique and with the same attention to detail as if the patient were not pregnant. The fetal heart should be monitored with a tracing. Beat-to-beat variability usually disappears, but the rate remains normal. Induced hypotension is usually employed for the mother. A maternal mean blood pressure of 50 mm Hg is tolerated by the fetus; below that, the fetal heart rate may drop. The best drug to induce hypotension is trimethaphan because its relatively high molecular weight limits placental transmission. Maternal hypotension induced by drugs is better tolerated by the fetus than that induced by hypovolemia, perhaps because the drugs cause vasodilation while hypovolemia causes vasoconstriction, reducing uterine blood flow.

There is no need to deliver the fetus immediately after the craniotomy (169,170). Most patients can go to term and deliver vaginally. Bearing down is a stress that may initiate an intracranial bleeding episode, so an assisted delivery under regional anesthesia is desirable.

## *Multiple Sclerosis*

Multiple sclerosis and pregnancy do not affect each other. The method of delivery is also not affected (171,172).

Multiple sclerosis is an intermittent and progressive disease. Its course apparently is not affected by any form of anesthesia, so general or regional anesthesia may be used (Figure 38–4) (173).

With the litigious attitude of many patients, an exacerbation of symptoms after regional anesthesia may be attributed to the anesthetic. Therefore, before a spinal or epidural is administered, a full discussion should be conducted with the patient and her family. They should state in writing that they understand the possibility of exacerbation of symptoms, but that they nevertheless prefer and wish to have the regional anesthetic (Figure 38–5) (174).

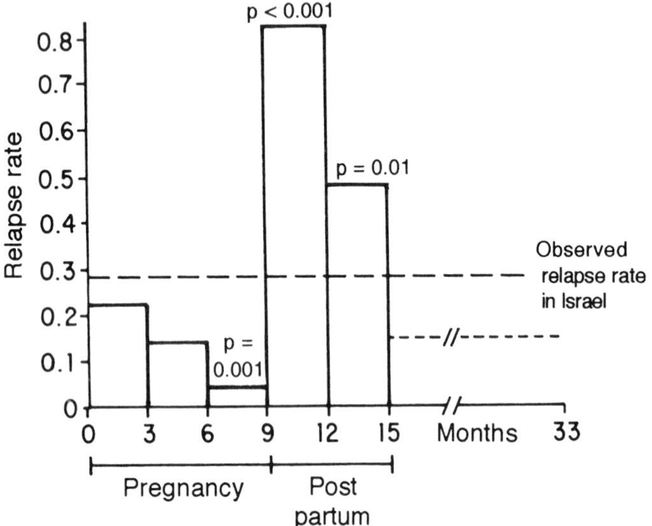


**Fig. 38–4.** Relapse rate for multiple sclerosis during two time periods. The pregnancy rate is shown in the first three bars (First, second, and third trimesters), and the postpartum rate is shown in the next two bars (first three months after delivery and next three months thereafter). This is contrasted against the overall observed relapse rate per person per year in Israel, which is just below 0.3 (see broken line). (Redrawn from Korn-Lubetzki I, Kahana E, Cooper G, Abramsky O: Activity of multiple sclerosis during pregnancy and puerperium. Ann. Neurol. 16:2229, 1984.)

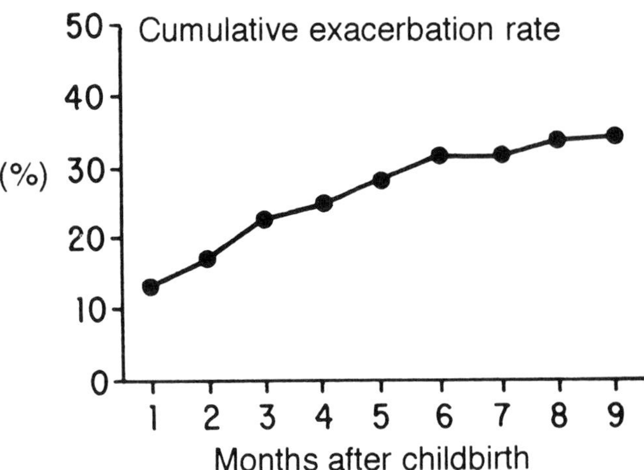


**Fig. 38–5.** Cumulative exacerbation rate of multiple sclerosis in a study group in the 9 months following delivery. (Redrawn from Nelson LM, Franklin GM, Jones MC: Multiple Sclerosis Study Group: Risk of multiple sclerosis exacerbation during pregnancy and breast-feeding. J.A.M.A. 259:3441, 1988.)

## *Brain Tumors*

Brain tumors may be diagnosed during a pregnancy, the tumor causing increasing symptoms because of enlargement (175). Steroids may be administered to reduce the cerebral edema. The decision of when to operate depends on the nature and symptomatology of the tumor. Brain surgery should be delayed if possible until the fetus is a good size—32 weeks gestation—and then delivery accomplished by cesarean under general anesthesia. If brain surgery is urgent before 32 weeks, the standard methods of anesthesia may be used—hyperventilation, hypothermia—without harm to the fetus, but mannitol should be avoided because it affects the fetus. Spinal and epidural anesthesia are contraindicated at any time because of complication possibilities due to increased intracranial pressure.

## *Benign Intracranial Hypertension*

Benign intracranial hypertension, "pseudotumor cerebri," occurs without a focal lesion (176,177). Spinal tap is said to be safe and therapeutic. It is safe because there is uniform brain swelling, and herniation does not occur when the pressure is lowered by a lumbar tap. It is therapeutic because a continuous leak occurs at the puncture site, acting as a safety valve to release the pressure. This is best left to the neurologist to treat.

## *Epilepsy*

Seizures may occur for the first time during a pregnancy, or a pregnant woman may have epilepsy since childhood (178,179). Epilepsy tends to become more severe during pregnancy because of emotional stress, water retention, and respiratory alkalosis. Vigorous treatment with anticonvulsants is required. Enzyme induction occurs. Status epilepticus is treated in the standard way.

Obstetric complications occur more frequently in epileptic women: toxemia, premature labor, growth retardation, fetal anomalies, elevated perinatal mortality. Fetal anomalies include heart disease, cleft lip and palate, spina bifida, and urinary tract abnormalities, probably due to teratogenic effects of the anticonvulsant drugs, which cross the placenta. The newborn may have vitamin K deficiency and may have drug withdrawal symptoms.

Anesthesia for epileptic patients may be conducted as for any other, except: High doses of local anesthetics should be avoided because of their seizure potential; spinal is preferred to epidural, and a continuous spinal can effectively be used for labor. With general anesthesia, avoid convulsion-inducing hyperventilation with enflurane, ketamine, methohexital, and althesin.

Awake intubation is not always easy in pregnant patients because the nasal mucosa is relatively vascular. Mokriski, et al describe a post-ictal eclamptic patient who could not be intubated orally because of a lacerated and edematous tongue (180). They used a solution of 0.125% phenylephrine and 3% lidocaine for vasoconstriction and local anesthesia of the nose and were able to nasally intubate (in a patient with platelets of 35,000) without hemorrhage or an exacerbation of her hypertension. Nasal cocaine may reduce placental blood flow, but at the same time increase maternal BP to an unacceptable extent.

## *Muscle Diseases*

Muscular dystrophy is characterized by weakness and loss of function (181–183). Myotonia causes rigidity and hypertrophy of striated muscle. Myotonia atrophica causes wasting of muscle, including cardiac and smooth muscle, as well as other organ and endocrine abnormalities. Fetal abnormalities are most likely to occur with myotonia atrophica. The patient's symptoms tend to be worsened during pregnancy, and labor may be prolonged.

Because of the varied presentation of muscular disease, anesthesia management must depend on the patient's condition (184–187). Pulmonary function tests, EKG, and blood chemistry tests should be done. Reduced respiratory function or reserve must be anticipated in all cases. All sedative and narcotic drugs may cause excessive respiratory depression. Local infiltration anesthesia may be used for any procedure. Before regional block, the patient should be informed that later exacerbation of symptoms are not to be attributed to the procedure.

Succinylcholine causes contractures in myotonic patients, and changes that may resemble malignant hyperthermia. Nondepolarizing relaxants may have increased effects, and reversal with neostigmine may precipitate a myotonic crisis. Atracurium is the best relaxant to use because of its breakdown by the Hoffman mechanism. In myotonic patients, contractures may be precipitated by shivering, so the patient and the OR should be kept warm. Nerve or muscle stimulation by electric current may cause contracture, so the usual nerve stimulation test for relaxant effect should not be used. Strong retraction of the abdominal wall may cause a contracture that can only be relieved by direct infiltration of a local anesthetic into the affected muscle. Generalized contractures and acute myotonic crisis may be treated with steroid administration (1 to 2 grams) or quinidine (up to 600 mg) or Dantrolene.

## *Myasthenia Gravis*

Myasthenia gravis occurs during the child-bearing age (188–192). Motor endplates and acetylcholine receptor sites are reduced in number and size, probably due to an autoimmune mechanism triggered by a viral infection of the thymus that normally causes the receptors to regenerate.

Well-controlled patients with myasthenia gravis may have a normal delivery (Table 38–3). Muscle weakness and respiratory insufficiency are the problems to be anticipated. They may be caused by inadequate treatment or over-treatment (cholinergic crisis). Many antibiotics have muscle-relaxant properties and should be avoided; among the safe ones are penicillin G, cephradine, and cephaloridine. Magnesium sulfate should also be avoided because it increases muscle weakness. The condition worsens during the immediate postpartum period, and without any emotional stress.

Elements of myotonia may also be present, and the patient should be fully evaluated for respiratory and cardiac function. Cardiac muscle may be affected. Hyperthyroidism may be present, as well as a thymoma.

The newborn infant may also have myasthenic symptoms and require respiratory support and drug therapy (193).

Narcotics and sedatives may have exaggerated effects. Regional anesthesia is satisfactory if the level is kept low enough (T8 to T10) to avoid affecting the intercostal muscles. A T8 level is adequate for cesarean section, and a dilute solution will provide sensory anesthesia without causing motor paralysis. Titrate the dose by the continuous catheter technique. Ester-type local anesthetics should only be used in small (spinal) doses because the anticholinesterase therapy of the patient interferes with their breakdown. Amide local anesthetics are a better choice. During labor, progressive muscle weakening may occur, and additional anticholinesterase medication may be required.

For general anesthesia, cricoid pressure and rapid intubation are required. Succinylcholine should not be used because of unpredictable effect and duration. Nondepolarizing relaxants have rapid onset, exaggerated effect, and normal excretion. Only a small amount is needed. Atracurium is the best choice because it is destroyed by the Hoffmann mechanism. After intubation, no additional muscle relaxant is required. Many patients require postoperative respiratory support.

Cardiomyopathy, myocarditis, and cardiomegaly may

**Table 38–3.** Myasthenia Gravis

| Case | Age/ Parity | Duration of Disease (y) | Thymectomy (Years Before Index Pregnancy) | Antepartum Complications | Mode and Timing of Delivery (wk/d) | Puerperal Course of Myasthenia Gravis | Infant Outcome |
|---|---|---|---|---|---|---|---|
| 1 | 34/1 | 6 | No | None | Spontaneous vertex at 40/2 | Unchanged | 4080 g, well, breast-fed |
| 2 | 31/0 | 10 | Yes (9) | None | Augmented vertex at 39 | Unchanged | 3090 g, well, formula-fed |
| 3 | 29/0 | 11 | No | Excalating generalized weakness at 38 wk | Oxytocin induction, lower-segment cesarean at 38/6 for failure to progress and fetal compromise | Improved | 3420 g, neonatal myasthenia gravis treated with neostigmine until day 16, formula-fed |
| 4 | 31/0 | 8 | No | None | Spontaneous vertex at 40/3 | Unchanged | 3860 g, well, breast-fed |
| 5 | 25/0 | 15 | Yes (15) | None | Spontaneous vertex at 40/5 | Unchanged | 3660 g, well, breast-fed |
| 6 | 32/4 | 8 | Yes (7) | Hospitalized from 34 wk to delivery for ptosis, dysphasia, and shortness of breath | Induced vertex at 39/3 | Improved | 3200 g, well, breast-fed |
| 7 | 35/0 | 16 | Yes (15) | None | Spontaneous compound at 41/3 | Unchanged | 3320 g, well, breast-fed |
| 8 | 27/2 | 2 | Yes (2) | Escalating blurred vision, ptosis, and fatigue at 36 wk | Induced vertex at 39/1 | Improved | 3000 g, well, breast-fed |
| 9 | 18/0 | 11 | Yes (4) | Periodic weakness of both skeletal and respiratory muscles | Induced vertex at 39 | Unchanged | 2820 g, well, formula-fed |
| 10 | 19/1 | 12 | Yes (5) | No prenatal care | Induced footling breech at 28 | Unchanged | 1554 g, stillbirth, nonimmune hydrops fetalis, multiple anomalies |
| 11 | 20/2 | 13 | Yes (6) | Respiratory failure at 30 wk requiring intubation and ventilation | Induced vertex at 35 for oligohydramnios | Unchanged | 2460 g, well, formula-fed |

(From Mitchell PJ, Bebbington M: Myasthenia gravis in pregnancy. Obstet. Gynecol. 80:178–181, 1992.)

also be present. Circulatory instability may occur during labor and the postpartum period.

## Klippel-Feil Syndrome

A woman with Klippel-Feil syndrome and congenital hydrocephalus was felt to be unsuitable for regional anesthesia because a dural puncture could cause neurologic deterioration and the volume of anesthetic in the epidural space could raise intracranial pressure (ICP) (194). On the other hand, a normal intubation was prohibited by fusion of the altlanto-occipital joint, a large posterior cranium, and a two-finger-breadth oral opening. There was a risk of intracranial hemorrhage with hypertension, and she was dyspneic at rest. An awake, nasal, fiberoptic intubation was chosen after topical nasal cocaine and 10% lidocaine (1 cc) over the larynx through the suction port of the fiberoptic scope. There was difficulty in passing the endotracheal tube over the bronchoscope because it kept hanging up on the epiglottis and arytenoids, so the procedure took 55 minutes. Clearly this would have been too long in a case of fetal or maternal distress.

## Severe Spinal Deformities

The next important consideration in this case was the possibility of a difficult airway in a patient with a deformity of the spine. Several case reports have described management in such cases. Quance reported a patient with arthrogryposis multiplex congenita who had kyphoscoliosis and extreme limitation of cervical movement (195). An epidural was attempted for cesarean section but it was totally unilateral. They proceeded with a rapid sequence induction during which they were only able to place a 6.0 endotracheal tube with great difficulty. Incidentally, the succinylcholine lasted 20 minutes in this patient.

One parturient with Noonan's syndrome was a dwarf with kyphoscoliosis, webbed neck, shield-shaped chest, flat face, small nasal passages, and high palatal arch (Figure 38–6) (196). Again an epidural was selected but could not be accomplished. A spinal was successful with a sensory level of T1. In the 30 to 50% of these patients who also have pulmonary stenosis, the authors recommend general anesthesia because the extra fluid required to prevent hypotension may not be tolerated. Quance, et al sug-

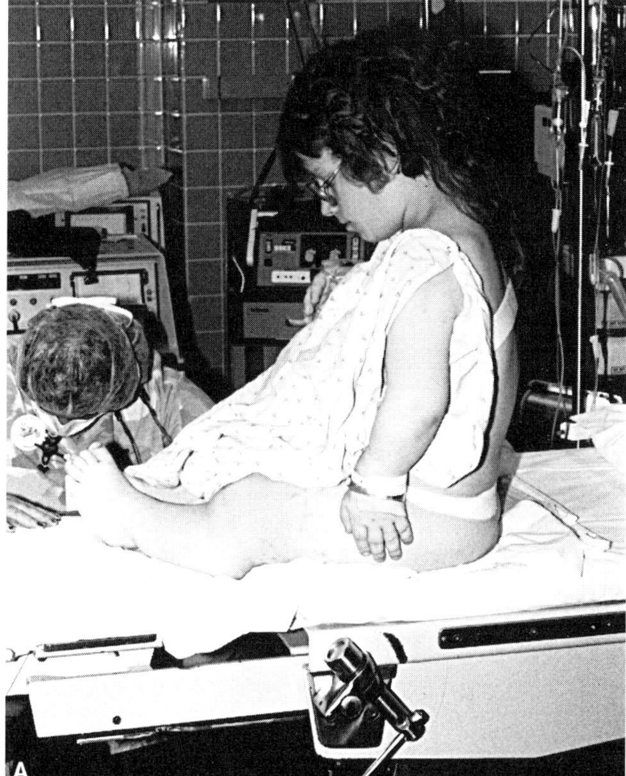

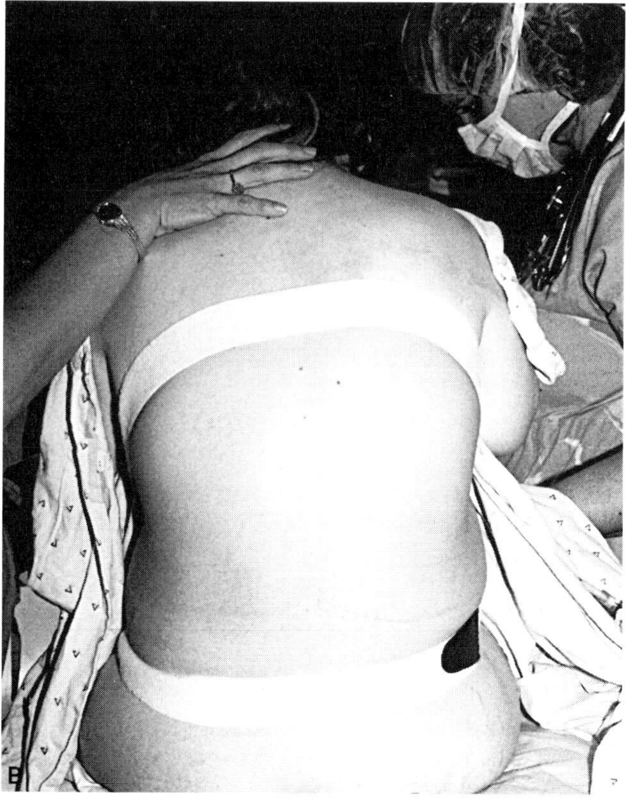

Fig. 38–6A & B. The management of these special people demands understanding of their altered physiology including skeletal, cardiovascular, pulmonary and nervous systems, and highlights the importance of individualized therapy.

**Table 38–4.** Diagnostic Criteria for Landry-Guillian-Barré Syndrome

1. Often begins one to three weeks after an infection that is usually respiratory;
2. Occurs in all ages and both sexes;
3. Onset of paralysis is usually preceded by dysesthesias of the feet or hands;
4. Symmetrical loss of muscle power but the degree of loss may be unequal;
5. Minimal and transient objective sensory loss;
6. Never severe or direct bladder involvement but there may be difficulty in voiding secondary to confinement in bed;
7. Tendon reflexes lost or at least diminished;
8. All cranial nerves except the optic and auditory nerves are often involved;
9. Cerebrospinal fluid protein elevated without a marked increase in the number of cells; albuminocytologic dissociation:
10. Complete functional recovery without residua in six months.

(From Nelson LH, McLean WT: Management of Landry-Guillain-Barré Syndrome in Pregnancy. Obstet Gynecol 65:25S, 1985.)

gest an oral, awake, fiberoptic intubation in the presence of an ear, nose, and throat (ENT) surgeon, and if all else fails, to mask ventilate with cricoid pressure.

Cunningham, et al warns us that patients with osteogenesis imperfecta can be difficult to intubate (195). Epidural is recommended, although kyphoscoliosis can make it technically difficult. Their patient had a normal bleeding time, which is important, as these patients have a mild bleeding tendency. An awake intubation is recommended for any general anesthetic.

## *Landry-Guillain-Barré Syndrome*

Landry first described a neurologic disorder of pregnancy in 1859 that was essentially a paralyzing disorder. A followup description occurred in 1916 with an article by Guillain, Barré, and Strohl. Over the intervening years,

**Table 38–5.** Polyneuritis in Pregnancy

| Name | Etiology | Laboratory Tests |
|---|---|---|
| Polyneuritis | Vitaqmin $B_{12}$ deficiency | Measure vitamin $B_{12}$ levels |
| Porphyria | | Blood porphyrobilinogen, urinary-coproporphyrins and uroprophyrins |
| Lead poisoning | Excess lead | Lead assay |
| Arsenic poisoning | Excess arsenic | Urine arsenic |
| Polyneuritis | Secondary to vaccination with a viral agent | None |
| Insecticide poisoning | Specific agent | Assay for specific agent if possible |
| Diptheria | *C. Diphtheriae* | Culture |

(From Nelson LM, Franklin GM, Jones MC, Multiple Sclerosis Study Group: Risk of multiple sclerosis exacerbation during pregnancy and breast-feeding. JAMA 259:3441–3443, 1988.)

**Table 38–6.** Case Review of Landry-Guillain-Barré Syndrome

| Case and Year | Onset of Symptoms | Delivery | Condition at Delivery vs Onset | Condition after Delivery (Total Time for Recovery) | Infant |
|---|---|---|---|---|---|
| (1) Spire, 1913 | 6 mo | 6 mo | Worse | Slow improvement (6 mo) | Premature, died |
| (2) Maisel and Woltman, 1934 | 34 wk | | Stable | Improvement | Unknown |
| (3) Biemond, 1937 | 6 wk | D&C for macerated fetus | Unchanged | Slow improvement (6 mo) | Macerated fetus described at D&C |
| (4) Ford and Walsh, 1943 | 4 mo | Term | Worse | Improvement PP | Unknown |
| (5) Zfass et al, 1954 | 3 mo | Term | No sequelae (responding to vitamin B complex over 4 wk) | Recovered before delivery | ? normal |
| (6) Feldman et al, 1955 | 5 mo minor, beginning muscular | 8 mo | Worse | Prolonged over 21 mo, papilledema with residual scotomata | Died from erythroblastosis |
| (7) Kalstone and Pearce 1959 | 36 wk | 38 wk | Worse | Slow improvement (4 mo) | Normal |
| (8) Betson and Golden, 1960 | 7 mo | 37 wk | Tracheostomy, improved | Burning of feet only (9 wk) | Normal |
| (9) Osler and Sidell, 1960 | Near term | Near term | Respirator, emergency cesarean delivery | Respiratory collapse, 2 grand-mal seizures, died 8 days after admission | ? normal |
| (10) Heller and Dejong, 1963 | 6.5 mo | Term | Normal | Full recovery | ? normal |
| (11) Gendre et al, 1963 | 11 mo | Term | Poorer | Improvement (6 mo) | Normal |
| (12) Rudolph et al, 1965 | 34 wk | 39 wk | Bulbar paralysis, worse, induced | Improvement | Normal |
| (13) Rudolph et al, 1965 | 34 wk | 35–36 wk | Worse, pneumonia respirator sp labor | Died PP day 3, icteric, bronchopneumonia, inf mono | Premature |
| (14) Pavlovic, 1965 | 5 mo | Term | Respirator, improved | Improvement | Normal |
| (15) Provvidenza, 1965 | 4 mo | Term | Stable | Normal (3 mo) | Normal |
| (16) Ravn, 1967 | 32 days | 45 days | Therapeutic D&C, began to improve 2 days later | Normal | |

PP = post partum: D&C = dilatation and curettage; inf mono. = infectious mononucleosis; sp labor = spontaneous labor; PROM = premature rupture of the membranes.
* Occured in three pregnancies, clearing at delivery. No history or dietary or toxic. Cranial nerves were normal .
(From Nelson LM, Jones MC, Multiple Sclerosis Study Group: Risk of multiple sclerosis exacerbation during pregnancy and breast-feeding. JAMA 259:3441–3443, 1988.)

the medical entity of acute polyradiculitis in pregnancy has been known by various names. The most accepted name by far today in the literature is Landry-Gillian-Barré syndrome. The criteria are identified as diagnostic for this syndrome, and are noted in Table 38–4 (198). Other differential diagnoses that should be considered are noted in Table 38–5. These alternative diagnoses should be considered because they concern neurologic disorders that are accompanied by paralysis. Over the past 70 years, some 29 cases have been reported in the literature and are reviewed in Table 38–6.

There is no question that the Landry-Guillain-Barré syndrome is a demyelinating neurologic disorder that may confound a physician in the obstetric practice because of the many complaints that patients often have during pregnancy, e.g, tingling in the extremities, malaise, and some respiratory discomfort. Nevertheless, a physician who encounters a patient who has the aforementioned complaints, when the predominant picture becomes a progressively increasing complaint over time, and when these complaints are also of apparent beginning motor weakness in the lower extremities, the Landry-Guillain-Barré syndrome must be considered immediately because of the importance in making an early diagnosis to prevent serious consequences to both the mother and fetus (199).

This disorder is relatively rare, occurring in an estimated less than 2 per 100,000 people. It is, however, currently the most common cause of weakness in patients under the age of 40. Poliomyelitis in the past had the distinction of being the most common disease process causing weakness in patients under 40 years of age (200). As mentioned, the disorder usually begins in a rather subacute fashion, but is noticeably progressive and eventually results in flaccid paralysis of the lower extremities with

| Case and Year | Onset of Symptoms | Delivery | Condition at Delivery vs Onset | Condition after Delivery (Total Time for Recovery) | Infant |
|---|---|---|---|---|---|
| (17) Ravn, 1967 | 13 days postconception | Term | Slight facial nerve impairment | Same | Normal |
| (18) Radman, 1967 | 32.5 wk | 37 wk | Slight facial muscle weakness | Normal (4 mo PP) | Normal |
| (19) Calderón-González et al, 1970* | Last trimester | Term | Quadraplegic, areflexic | Normal 2 mo PP | Normal |
| | Second trimester | Unknown | Quadraplegic, areflexic | | ? normal |
| | First trimester | Unknown | Quadraplegic, areflexic | Normal 4–6 mo PP | ? normal |
| | 2 mo after changing oral contraceptive type | | Stopped oral contraceptives and improved | | |
| (20) Notter and Gaja, 1970 | 2 mo before pregnancy | Term | Occasional exacerbation of paresthesias and motor deficit | Unknown | Normal |
| (21) Tse et al, 1971 | 30 wk | Unknown | Unknown | Unknown | Unknown |
| (22) Elstein et al, 1971 | 32 wk | 34 wk | Worse, respirator | 17 days died from second hemorrhage from tracheostomy | Premature |
| (23) Novak and Johnson, 1973 | 1967, 29 wk | 42 wk | Worse | Gradual improvement over 2 yr PP | Normal |
| | 1969, 18 wk | PROM, 36 wk | Worse | Gradual improvement deficit in lower extremities | Normal |
| (24, 25) Sudo and Weingold, 1975 | 30 wk | 32 wk | Worse | Normal | Premature |
| | 23.5 wk | 42 wk | Improved | Improvement | Normal |
| (26) Gronsky, 1975 | 38 wk | 39 wk | Worse | Worse, intubated for 19 days then improved | Normal |
| (27) Ahlberg and Ahlmark, 1978 | 32 wk | 34 wk | Worse | Worse, 10 wk PP off respirator | Premature, mono/vgotic male twins |
| (28) Barvo et al, 1982 | 29 wk | 39 wk | Improved, off respirator | Improvement referred for therapy | Normal |
| (29) Nelson and McLean (present case) | 18 wk | 40 wk | Improved, off respirator | Improvement, some decreased sensation on plantar surface of feet after 2 yr | Normal |

loss of medullary reflexes in that area also. The problem is that subsequent involvement moves upward and the respiratory musculature can be affected, resulting in significant embarrassment of respiratory function. If the patient tends to be in the third trimester, already with some respiratory embarrassment, it can be well understood that this type of problem can cause significant respiratory embarrassment or even death if not treated.

Unfortunately, the etiology of this syndrome is not well understood. There have been three cases reported in the literature of this syndrome being associated with serologic evidence of cytomegalic virus infection (201). The authors of that report confirm that the implication of cytomegalic virus as a causative agent for the Landry-Guillain-Barré syndrome must have serum samples before the onset of the patient's illnesses, which they did not have in their patients. Nevertheless, all three of the patients that they reported have positive IgM results, which they felt definitely supported the diagnosis of primary cytomegalovirus infection. The typical clinical signs of Guillain-Barré syndrome are noted in Table 38–7

Certainly, the successful treatment of Landry-Guillain-

**Table 38–7.** Typical Clinical Signs in Landry-Gillain-Barré Syndrome

| |
|---|
| *Motor* |
| Progressive skeletal muscle paralysis |
| Loss of deep tendon reflexes |
| Decreased pulmonary vital capacity |
| Peripheral facial weakness |
| Dysphagia |
| *Sensory* |
| Distal paresthesias |
| Decreased appreciation of vibration and proprioceptive senses |
| Distal glove-and-stocking anesthesia to pinprick (late manifestation implying axonal destruction) |
| *Autonomic* |
| Cardiac arrhythmias |
| Altered blood pressure (hypertension or hypotension) |

(From Koski CL, Khurana R, Mayer RF: Gullain-Barré syndrome. Am. Fam. Physician. 34(3):198–210, 1986.)

Barré syndrome associated with pregnancy demands a multidisciplinary team approach, including the obstetricians, the anesthesiologists who have expertise in respiratory management and intensive care management of respiratory disorders, an internist with a superb background in infectious diseases, and the involvement of the pediatrician early on. Fortunately, the progress of the disease process is usually limited and most of the time a complete recovery occurs. Subsequent to complete recovery, however, there may be relapses, and this is absolutely important to keep in mind because recurrences may occur months or even years after the initial onset of the illness. Treatment is truly based upon treatment of clinical symptoms and signs, including respiratory support and nutritional support. The use of steroids is controversial, and felt by some to be detrimental (202).

Plasmapheresis has been suggested as a therapy, and this is suggested for use early in the course, i.e., within 7 days of the onset of symptoms that appear to be rapidly progressive or in patients who may require assisted ventilation. Others are less impressed with plasmapheresis because of the concern and complications that plasmapheresis may cause during pregnancy (203).

Etiology of the syndrome is still unknown, although it is usually preceded by a viral, respiratory, or gastrointestinal illness. Some investigations have revealed cytomegalovirus antibodies in as much as 25% of cases (199). Certainly aggressive longitudinal care is necessary for both the mother and baby if maternal and perinatal morbidity and mortality are to be favorably affected.

Obstetric management is done by following the patient carefully with serial ultrasonographic studies and nonstress tests and other methods of detecting fetal threats such as growth retardation. Delivery often and usually is by the vaginal route, with second stage support by either forceps delivery or vacuum extraction.

Anesthetic management can be by an epidural in the first stage of labor with a continuous opioid anesthetic concentration of drug. Nitrous oxide supported with pudendal block by the obstetrician is used during the second stage of labor. For cesarean section, there has been a report of one case performed with an epidural with a fairly low level that provided satisfactory anesthesia for delivery. In regard to the latter, it is suggested that if regional anesthesia is used, certainly the dermatome levels should be kept low so as to provide no further respiratory embarrassment of the patient (204). Certainly, if necessary, a general anesthetic could also be performed with careful attention to details of general anesthesia, as mentioned in detail in Chapters 19, 20, and 30.

These patients must be followed carefully postoperatively and also carefully for several days and even weeks after delivery because of the possibility of recurrence. Therefore, it must be mentioned to the patient that at any signs of similar onset of disease processes as recorded earlier, the patient must contact her physician immediately. An example of some of the respiratory embarrassment that can occur during pregnancy is shown in Figure 38–7. Naturally, because some of these patients have severe respiratory embarrassment in the second and/or third trimester of pregnancy, it may necessitate placement

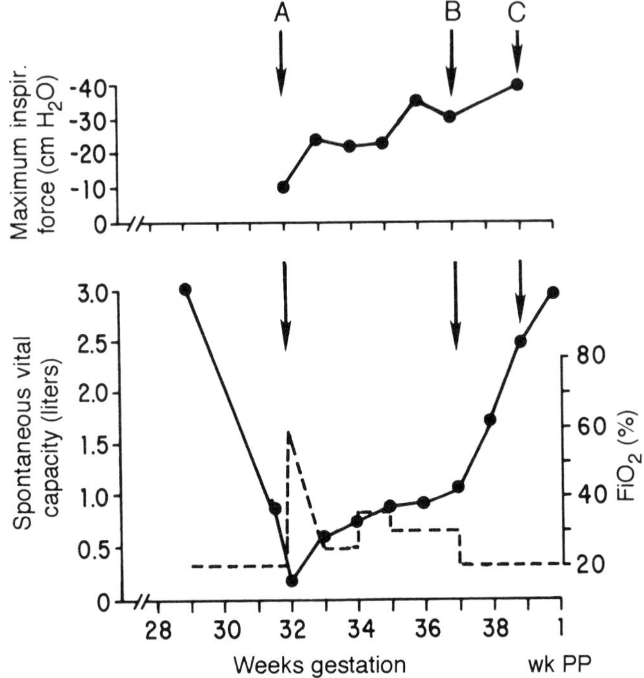


**Fig. 38–7.** Pulmonary mechanisms in a patient with Landry-Guillian-Barré syndrome. The top graph shows maximum inspiratory force, with changes denoted from 32 to 40 weeks of pregnancy. The bottom graph shows vital capacity during the same time period. Note that in both tracings, the mechanical ventilation was begun at point A, mechanical ventilation was closed at point B, and delivery was affected at point C. (Redrawn from Bravo RH, Katz M, Inturrisi M, Cohen NH: Obstetric management of Landry-Guillain-Barré syndrome: A case report. Am. J. Obstet. Gynecol. 142:714, 1982.)

of an endotracheal tube with ventilation and subsequent conversion to tracheostomy if long-term respiratory support is necessary. There have been two case reports of tracheal erosion from subsequent long-term ventilation, and, unfortunately, because of the anatomical relationships, often this erosion occurs in the area of the innominate artery, which can result in massive blood loss and death (Figure 38–8) (205). From the laboratory standpoint, there is a marked increase in the cerebrospinal fluid protein without an increase in the number of cerebrospinal cells, with the resultant so called "albiminalcytologic dissociation."

The maternal and perinatal mortality can be between 7 and 10%, which certainly makes it a major concern in regard to careful management and detection of the disease as early as possible. Management of such a patient during pregnancy focuses upon the advantage of the obstetrician having a close relationship with the anesthesiologist, as the latter is an expert in respiratory management. Because of the aforementioned maternal and perinatal mortality, certainly these patients should be delivered at a Level 4 center, which can respond to the intensity of management necessary by the team efforts of the obstetricians, anesthesiologists, and pediatricians.

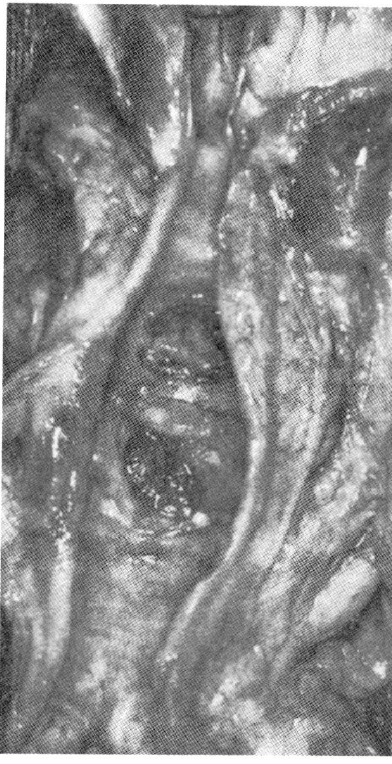

**Fig. 38–8.** The pathologic erosion of the trachea from the posterior view, demonstrating the erosion just below the tracheostomy site in the interior wall of the trachea. (From Elstein M, Legg NJ, Murphy M, Park DM, et al: Guillain-Barré syndrome in pregnancy. Respiratory paralysis complicated by a fatal tracheo-innominate artery fistula. Anaesthesia 26:216, 1971.)

## REFERENCES


1. Semlitz L, Gold MS: Adolescent drug abuse. Diagnosis, treatment and prevention. Psychiatr. Clin. North. Am.1986;9:455.
2. Keith LG, MacGregor S, Friedell S, Rosner M, et al: Substance abuse in pregnant women: recent experience at the perinatal center for chemical dependence of Northwestern Memorial Hospital. Obstet. Gynecol. 1989;73:715.
3. New JA, Dooley SL, Keith LG: The prevalence of substance abuse in patients with suspected preterm labor. Am. J. Obstet. Gynecol. 1990;162:1562.
4. Eridsson M, Larsson G, Zetterstrom R: Abuse of alcohol, drugs and tobacco during pregnancy: consequences for the child. Paediatrician. 1979;8:228.
5. Nakada T, Knight RT: Alcohol and the central nervous system. Med. Clin. North. Am. 1984;68:121.
6. Segel LD, Klausner SC, Harney Gnadt JT, Amsterdam EA: Alcohol and the heart. Med. Clin. North. Am. 1984;68:147.
7. El-Ganzouri AR, Ivankovich AD, Braverman B, McCarthy R: Monoamine oxidase inhibitors: should they be discontinued preoperatively? Anesth. Analg. 1985;64:592–6.
8. Fried PA, Watkinson B, Willan A: Marijuana use during pregnancy and decreased length of gestation. Am. J. Obstet. Gynecol. 1984;150:23.
9. Wu TC, Tashkin DP, Djahed B, Rose JE: Pulmonary hazards of smoking marijuana. N. Engl. J. Med. 1988;318:347.
10. New JA, Dooley SL, Keith LG: The prevalence of substance abuse in patients with suspected preterm labor. Am. J. Obstet. Gynecol. 1990;37:130.
11. Elliot RH, Rees GB: Amphetamine ingestion presenting as eclampsia. Can. J. Anaesth. 1990;37:130.
12. Eriksson M, Larsson G, Zetterstrom R: Amphetamine addiction and pregnancy. II: Pregnancy, delivery and the neonatal period. Sociomedical aspects. Acta. Obstet. Gynecol. Scand. 1981;60:253.
13. Howard RE, Hueter DC, Davis GJ: Acute myocardial infarction following cocaine abuse in a young woman with normal coronary arteries. JAMA. 1985;254:95.
14. Pasternack PF, Colvin SB, Baumann FG: Cocaine-induced angina pectoris and acute myocardial infarction in patients younger than 40 years. Am. J. Cardiol. 1985;55:847.
15. Nahas G: A calcium channel blocker as antidote to the cardiac effects of cocaine intoxication. N. Engl. J. Med. 1986;313:519.
16. Chasnoff IJ, Burns WJ, Schnoll SH, Burns KA: Cocaine use in pregnancy. N. Engl. J. Med. 1985;313:666.
17. Oro AS, Dixon SD: Perinatal cocaine and methamphetamine exposure. Maternal and neonatal correlates. Pediatrics. 1987;111:571.
18. Little BB, Snell LM, Palmore MK, Gilstrap LC: Cocaine use in pregnant women in a large public hospital. Am. J. Perinatol. 1988;5:206.
19. Pearce AC, Jones RM: Smoking and anesthesia: preoperative abstinence and perioperative morbidity. Anesthesiology. 1984;61:576.
20. Bray G: Complications of obesity. Ann. Intern. Med. 1985; 103:1052.
21. Eng M, Butler J, Bonica J: Respiratory function in pregnant obese women. Am. J. Obstet. Gynecol. 1975;123:241.
22. Johnson SR, Kolberg BH, Varner MW, Railsback LD: Maternal obesity and pregnancy. Surg. Gynecol. Obstet. 1987; 164:431.
23. Neuman GG, Baldwin CC, Petrini AJ, Wise L, et al: Perioperative management of a 430-kilogram (946 pound) patient with Pickwickian syndrome. Anesth. Analg. 1986;65:985.
24. Fisher A, Waterhouse TD, Adams AP: Obesity: its relation to anesthesia. Anesthesia. 1975;30:633.
25. Vaughn RW, Bauer S, Wise L: Volume and pH of gastric juice in obese patients. Anesthesiology. 1975;43:686.
26. Blass NH: Regional anesthesia in the morbidly obese. Reg. Anaesth. 1979;4:20.
27. Hodgkinson R, Husain F: Obesity and the cephalad spread of analgesia following epidural administration of bupivacaine for cesarean section. Anesth. Analg. 1980;59:89.28.
28. Hodgkinson R, Husain F: Obesity, gravity, and spread of epidural anesthesia. Anesth. Analg. 1981;60:421.
29. Jacobs L, Berger H, Fierro F: Obesity and continuous spinal anesthesia: A case report. Anesth. Analg. 1963;42:547.
30. Jung D, Mayersohn M, Perrier D, Calkins J, et al: Thiopental disposition in lean and obese patients undergoing surgery. Anesthesiology. 1982;56:269.
31. Bentley JB, Borel JD, Vaughan RW, Gandolfi AJ: Weight, pseudocholinesterase activity, and succinylcholine requirement. Anesthesiology. 1982;57:48.
32. Patterson RM: Trauma in pregnancy. Clin. Obstet. Gynecol. 1984;27:32.
33. Crosby WM: Traumatic injuries during pregnancy. Clin. Obstet. Gynecol. 1983;26: 902.
34. Haycock CE: Emergency care of the pregnant traumatized patient. Emerg. Med. Clin. North. Am. 1984;2:849.
35. Duncan PG, Pope WDB, Cohen MM, Greer N: Fetal risk of anesthesia and surgery during pregnancy. Anesthesiology. 1986;64:790.
36. Delaney AG: Anesthesia in the pregnant woman. Clin. Obstet. Gynecol. 1983;26:795.
37. Aldridge LM, Tunstall ME: Nitrous oxide and the fetus: a

review and the results of a retrospective study of 175 cases of anaesthesia for insertion of Shirodkhar suture. Br. J. Anaesth. 1986;58:1348.

38. Konieczko KM, Chapk JN, Nonh OF: Fitotoxic potential of general anesthesia in relation to pregnancy. Br. J. Anaesth. 1987;59:449.
39. Mazze RI, Kallen B: Reproductive outcome after anesthesia and operation during pregnancy: a registry study of 5405 cases. Am. J. Obstet. Gynecol. 1989;161:1178.
40. Biehl DR: Antepartum and postpartum hemorrhage. *In* Anesthesia for Obstetrics. Edited by S Shnider, G Levinson. Baltimore, Williams & Wilkins; 1987, p. 288.
41. Plummer MH: Bleeding problems. *In* Obstetric anesthesia: The Complicated Patient. Edited by F James, A Wheeler, D Dewan. Philadelphia, F. A. Davis, 1988, p. 321.
42. Reynolds JEF: Martindale's The Extra Pharmacopoeia. London: Pharmaceutical Press; 1989, p. 1492.
43. Peng ATC, Gorman RS, Shulman SM, Demarchis E, Nyunt K, Blancato L: Intravenous nitroglycerin for uterine relaxation in patients with retained placenta. Anesthesiology. 1989;71:172.
44. Kates RA: Antianginal drug therapy. *In* Cardiac Anesthesia, vol. 1. Edited by JA Kaplan. Orlando, Grune and Stratton, 1987, p. 451.
45. DeSimone CA, Norris MC, Leighton BC: Intravenous nitroglycerin aids manual extraction of a retained placenta. Anesthesiology. 1990;73:787.
46. Clark SL, Koonings PP, Phelan JP: Placenta previa/accreta and prior cesarean section. Obstet. Gynecol. 66:89–92, 1985.
47. Singh PM, Rodrigues C, Gupta AN: Placenta previa and previous cesarean section. Acta. Obstet. Gynecol. Scand. 60:367–368, 1981.
48. Clark SL, Yeh SY, Phelan JP, Bruce S, et al: Emergency hysterectomy for obstetric hemorrhage. Obstet. Gynecol. 64: 376–380, 1984.
49. Read JA, Cotton DB, Miller FC: Placenta accreta: changing clinical aspects and outcome. Obstet. Gynecol. 56:31, 1980.
50. Fox H: Placenta accreta, 1945–1969. Obstet. Gynecol. Surv. 27:475, 1972.
51. Emmott, RS, Bennett, A: Acute inversion of the uterus at cesarean section: Implications for the anaesthetist. Anaesthesia 43:118, 1988.
52. Abouleish, E: Caudal analgesia for quadruplet delivery. Anesthesia and Analgesia (Current Researches) 55(1):61–66, 1976.
53. Leppert PC, Namerow PB, Horowitz E: Cesarean section deliveries among adolescent mothers enrolled in a comprehensive prenatal care program. Am. J. Obstet. Gynecol. 1985;152:623.
54. Kirz DS, Dorchester W, Freeman RK: Advanced maternal age: the mature gravida. Am. J. Obstet. Gynecol. 1985; 152:7.
55. Jacob AJ, Epstein J, Madden DL, Sever JL: Genital herpes infection in pregnant women near term. Obstet. Gynecol. 1984;63:480.
56. Guinan ME, Wolinsky SM, Reichman RC: Epidemiology of genital herpes simplex virus infection. Epidemiol. Rev. 1985;7:127.
57. Brown ZA, Berry S, Vontver LA: Genital herpes simplex virus infections complicating pregnancy. Natural history and peripartum management. J. Reprod. Med. 1986;31: S420.
58. Ravindran RS, Gupta CD, Stoops CA: Epidural analgesia in the presence of herpes simplex virus (type 2) infection. Anesth. Analg. 1982;61:714.
59. Joyce TH, Marx GF: Regional anesthesia and herpes. Soc. Obstet. Anesth. Perinatology Newsletter. 1983;14:1.
60. Crone LA, Conly JM, Storgard C, Zbitnew A, et al: Herpes labialis in parturients receiving epidural morphine following cesarean section. South. Med. J. 1993;86(1):33–7.
61. Bader, AM, Camann, WR, Datta, S: Anesthesia for cesarean delivery in patients with herpes simplex virus type-2 infections. Reg. Anesth. 15:261–263, 1990.
62. Curran JW: The epidemiology and preventions of the acquired immunodeficiency syndrome. Ann. Intern. Med. 1985;103:657.
63. Marcus R: Surveillance of health care workers exposed to blood from patients infected with human immunodeficiency virus. N. Engl. J. Med. 1988;319:1118.
64. Centers for Disease Control: Recommendations for assisting in the prevention of perinatal transmission of human T-lymphotropic virus type III/lymphadenopathy-associated virus and acquired immunodeficiency syndrome. MMWR. 1985;34:721.
65. Cowan MJ, Hellman D, Chudwin D, Wara DW, Chang RS, et al: Maternal transmission of acquired immune deficiency syndrome. Pediatrics. 1984;73:382–6.
66. Scott GB, Fischl MA, Klimas N, Fletcher MA, et al: Mothers of infants with the acquired immunodeficiency syndrome. JAMA 1985;253:363.
67. Krilov LR, Rubin LG, Frogel M, Gloster E, et al: Disseminated adenovirus infection with hepatic necrosis in patients with human immunodeficiency virus infection and other immunodeficiency states. Rev. Infect. Dis. 1990;12: 303.
68. Lee KG, Soni N: AIDS and anaesthesia. Anaesthesia. 1986; 41:1011.
69. Cantineau JP: AIDS and implications for anesthesiologists. Cur. Opin. Anaesthesiol. 1989;2:349.
70. Van Hoesen, KB, Camporesi, EM, Moon, RE, Hage, ML, et al: Should hyperbaric oxygen be used to treat the pregnant patient for acute carbon monoxide poisoning? JAMA 261: 1039–1043, 1989.
71. Malinow AM, Butterworth JF, Johnson MD, Safon L, et al.: Peripartum cardiomyopathy presenting at cesarean delivery. Anesthesiology 63:545, 1985.
72. Alderson, JD: Cardiovascular collapse following epidural anaesthesia for cesarean section in a patient with aortic incompetence. Anaesthesia 42:643, 1987.
73. Judge TP, Kennedy JW, Bennett LJ, Wills RE, et al: Quantitative hemodynamic effects of heart rate in aortic regurgitation. Circulation 44:355–367, 1971.
74. Hemmings GT, Whalley DG, O'Connor PJ, Dunn C: Invasive monitoring and anaesthetic management of a parturient with mitral stenosis. Can. J. Anaesth. 34:182, 1987.
75. Pirlo, A, Herren, AL: Eisenmenger's Syndrome and pregnancy. A case report and review of the literature. Anesth. Review VI:9, 1979.
76. Heytens, L, Alexander, J: Maternal and neonatal death associated with Eisenmenger's Syndrome. Acta. Anaesth. Belgica. 37:45, 1986.
77. Camba Rodriguez, MA, Yanez Gonzalez, AM, Gonzalez Rviz, F: Epidural anesthesia for cesarean section in a patient with Eisenmenger's syndrome. Rev. Esp. Anestesiol. Reanim. (Spain) 36:45, 1989.
78. Robinson, DE, Leicht, CH: Epidural analgesia with low-dose bupivacaine and fentanyl for labor and delivery in a parturient with severe pulmonary hypertension. Anesthesiology 68:285, 1988.
79. Slomka, F, Salmeron, S, Zetlaoui, P, Cohen, H, et al: Primary pulmonary hypertension and pregnancy: anesthetic management for delivery. Anesthesiology 69:959, 1988.

80. Power, KJ, Avery, AF: Extradural analgesia in the intrapartum management of a patient with pulmonary hypertension. Br. J. Anaesth. 63:116, 1989.
81. Younker, D, Clark R, Tessem J, Joyce III TH, et al: Bupivacaine-fentanyl epidural analgesia for a parturient in status asthmaticus. Can J Anaesth 34:609, 1987.
82. Nakagawa, H, Yoda, K, Fujiwara, A, Miyazaki, M: Painless delivery under lumbar epidural anesthesia for a pregnant woman with syncope caused by paroxysmal ventricular tachycardia. Masui (Japan) 38:560, 1989.
83. Boccio, RV, Chung, JH, Harrison, DM: Anesthetic management of cesarean section in a patient with idiopathic hypertrophic subaortic stenosis. Anesthesiology 65:663, 1986.
84. Minnich, ME, Quirk, JG, Clark, RB: Epidural anesthesia for vaginal delivery in a patient with idiopathic hypertrophic subaortic stenosis. Anesthesiology 67:590, 1987.
85. Heytens, L, Alexander, J: Maternal and neonatal death associated with Eisenmenger's Syndrome. Acta. Anaesth. Belgica. 37:45, 1986.
86. Boccio, RV, Chung, JH, Harrison, DM: Anesthetic management of cesarean section on a patient with idiopathic hypertrophic subaortic stenosis. Anesthesiology 65:663, 1986.
87. Power, KJ, Avery, AF: Extradural analgesia in the intrapartum management of a patient with pulmonary hypertension. Br. J. Anaesth. 63:116, 1989.
88. Dawson PJ, Ross AW: Pre-eclampsia in a parturient with a history of myocardial infarction. A case report and literature review. Anaesthesia 43:659, 1988.
89. Roessler, P, Lambert, TF: Anesthesia for cesarean section in the presence of primary pulmonary hypertension. Anaesth Intensive Care 14:317, 1986.
90. Abboud, TK, Shnider, SM, Dailey, PA, Raya, JA, et al: Intrathecal administration of hyperbaric morphine for the relief of pain in labor. Br. J. Anaesth. 56:1351, 1984.
91. Copel, JA, Harrison, D, Whittemore, R, Hobbins, JC: Intrathecal morphine analgesia for vaginal delivery in a woman with a single ventricle. A case report. J. Reproductive Med. 31:274, 1986.
92. Hyde, NH, Harrison, DM: Intrathecal morphine in a parturient with cystic fibrosis. Anesth. Analg. 65:1357, 1986.
93. Abboud, TK, Novhihed, R, Daniel, J: Intrathecal morphine for relief of labor pain in a parturient with severe pulmonary hypertension. Anesthesiology 59:477, 1983.
94. Writer, WDR, James III, FM, Wheeler, AS: Double-blind comparison of morphine and bupivacaine for continuous epidural analgesia in labor. Anesthesiology 54:215, 1981.
95. Cohen, SE, Tan, S, Albright, GA, Halpern, J: Epidural fentanyl/bupivacaine combinations for labor analgesia: effect of varying dosages. Anesthesiology 65:368, 1986.
96. Joyce III TH, Palacios QT: Cardiac disease. *In* Obstetric Anesthesia: The Complicated Patient. 2nd Ed. Edited by FM James III, AS Wheeler, DM Dewan. Philadelphia, F.A. Davis Company, 1988, p. 168.
97. Thurnaau GR: Rheumatoid arthritis. Clin. Obstet. Gynecol. 1983;26:558.
98. Hollingsworth JW, Saykaly RJ: Systemic complications of rheumatoid arthritis. Med. Clin. North. Am. 1977;61:217.
99. Sachs BP, Lorell, BH, Mehrez, M, Damien, N: Constrictive pericarditis and pregnancy. Am. J. Obstet. Gynecol. 1986; 154:156.
100. Cecere FA, Persellin RH: The interaction of pregnancy and the rheumatic diseases. Clin. Rheum. Dis. 1981;7:747.
101. Pirlo AF, Herren AL: Ankylosing spondylitis. Case report and review of literature. Anesth. Rev. 1978;5:13.
102. Ostensen M, Romberg O, Husby G: Ankylosing spondylitis and motherhood. Arthritis Rheum. 1982;25:140.
103. Ostensen M, Husby G: A prospective clinical study of the effect of pregnancy on rheumatoid arthritis and ankylosing spondylitis. Arthritis Rheum. 1983;26:1155.
104. MacLennan AH, Nicolson, R, Green RC, Bath, M: Serum relaxin and pelvic pain of pregnancy. Lancet. 1986;2:243.
105. Schachner SM, Abram SE: Use of two epidural catheters to provide analgesia of unblocked segments in a patient with lumbar disc disease. Anesthesiology. 1982;56:150.
106. Gibbons PA, Lee IS: Scoliosis and anesthesia. Int. Anesthesiol. Clin. 1985;23:149.107.
107. Hirschfeld SS, Rudner C, Nash Jr CL, Nussbaum E, et al: Incidence of mitral valve prolapse in adolescent scoliosis and thoracic hypokyphosis. Pediatrics. 1982;70:451.
108. Turino GM, Goldring RM, Rishman AP: Corpulmonale in musculoskeletal abnormalities of the thorax. Bull. N.Y. Acad. Med. 1965;41:959.
109. Kafer ER: Respiratory and cardiovascular functions in scoliosis and the principles of anesthetic management. Anesthesiology. 1980;52:339.
110. Berman AT, Cohen DL, Schwentker EP: The effects of pregnancy on idiopathic scoliosis: A preliminary report on eight cases and a review of the literature. Spine. 1982; 7:76.
111. Sawicka EH, Spencer GT, Branthwaite MA: Management of respiratory failure complicating pregnancy in severe kyphoscoliosis: A new use for an old technique? Br. J. Dis. Chest. 1986;80:191.
112. Feldstein G, Ramanthan S: Obstetrical lumbar epidural anesthesia in patients with previous posterior spinal fusion for kyphoscoliosis. Anesth. Analg. 1985;64:83.
113. McGregor JA, Meeuwen J: Autonomic hyperreflexia: A mortal danger for spinal cord-damaged women in labor. Am. J. Obstet. Gynecol. 1985;151:330.
114. Stirt JA, Marco A, Conklin KA: Obstetric anesthesia for a quadriplegic patient with autonomic hyperreflexia. Anesthesiology. 1979;51:560.
115. Baraka A: Epidural meperidine for control of autonomic hyperreflexia in a paraplegic parturient. Anesthesiology. 1985;62:688.
116. Coleman P: McArdle's disease: Problems of anaesthetic management for caesarean section. Anaesthesia 39: 784–787, 1984.
117. Moss AJ, McDonald J: Unilateral cervicothoracic sympathetic ganglionectomy for the treatment of long Q-T interval syndrome. N. Engl. J. Med. 285:903, 1971.
118. Callaghan ML, Nichols AB, Sweet RB: Anesthetic management of prolonged Q-T interval syndrome. Anesthesiology 47:67, 1977.
119. Freshwater, JV: Anaesthesia for caesarean section and the Jervell, Lange-Nielson Syndrome (prolonged Q-T interval syndrome). Br. J. Anaesth. 56:655–57, 1984.
120. Koerten JM, Morales WJ, Washington III SR, Castaldo TW: Cushing's syndrome in pregnancy: A case report and literature review. Am. J. Obstet. Gynecol. 1986;154:626.
121. Glassford J, Eagle C, McMorland GH: Cesarean section in a patient with Cushing's syndrome. Can. Anaesth. Soc. J. 1984;31:447.
122. Mitchell SZ, Freilich JD, Brant, D, Flynn, M: Anesthetic management of pheochromocytoma resection during pregnancy. Anesth. Analg. 1987;66:478.
123. Pinaud M, Souron R, Le Neel J-C, Lopes P, et al: Bilateral phaeochromocytomas in pregnancy: Anesthetic management of combined cesarean section and tumor removal. Eur. J. Anaesth. 1985;2:395.

124. Desmonts JM, Marty J: Anaesthetic management of patients with phaeochromocytoma. Br. J. Anaesth. 1984;56:781.
125. Stonham J, Wakefield C: Phaeochromocytoma in pregnancy: Cesarean section under epidural analgesia. Anaesthesia. 1983;38:654.
126. Mestman JH: Thyroid disease in pregnancy. Clinics Perinatol. 1985;12:3.
127. Burrow GN: The management of thyrotoxicosis in pregnancy. N. Engl. J. Med. 1985;313:562.
128. Momotani N, Noh J, Oyanagi H, Ishikawa N, et al: Antithyroid drug therapy for Graves disease during pregnancy: optimal regimen for fetal thyroid status. N. Engl. J. Med. 1986;315:24.
129. Rossai RL, ReMine SG, Clerkin EP: Hyperparathyroidism. Surg. Clin. North. Am. 1985;65:187.
130. Al-Mohaya S, Naguib M, Abdelatif M: Abnormal responses to muscle relaxants in a patient with primary hyperparathyroidism. Anesthesiology. 1986;65:554.
131. Bolen JW: Hypoparathyroidism in pregnancy. Am. J. Obstet. Gynecol. 1973;117:178.
132. Fischer KF, Lees JA, Newman JH: Hypoglycemia in hospitalized patients. N. Engl. J. Med. 1986;315:1245.
133. Dombrowski RA: Autoimmune disease in pregnancy. Med. Clin. North. Am. 1989;73:605.
134. Malinow AM, Rickford WJK, Mokriski BLK, Saller DN, et al: Lupus anticoagulant: implications for obstetric anaesthetists. Anesthesia. 1987;42:1291.
135. Scott JR, Rote NS, Cruikshank DP: Antiplatelet antibodies and platelet counts in pregnancies complicated by autoimmune thrombocytopenic purpura. Am. J. Obstet. Gynecol. 1987;145:932.
136. Burrows RF, Kelton JG: Incidentally detected thrombocytopenia in healthy mothers and their infants. N. Engl. J. Med. 1988;319:142.
137. Samuels P, Bussel JB, Braitman LE, Tomaski A, et al: Estimation of the risk of thrombocytopenia in the offspring of pregnant women with presumed immune thrombocytopenic purpura. N. Engl. J. Med. 1990;323:229.
138. Charache S, Niebyl JR: Pregnancy in sickle cell disease. Clin. Haematol. 1985;14:729.
139. Martin JN, Morrison JC: Managing the parturient with sickle cell crisis. Clin. Obstet. Gynecol. 1984;27:39.
140. Morrison JC, Blake PG, Reed CD: Therapy for the pregnant patient with sickle hemoglobinopathies: a national focus. Am. J. Obstet. Gynecol. 1984;27:39.
141. Abouleish, E: Obstetric anaesthesia and Ehlers-Danlos Syndrome. Br. J. Anaesth. 52:1283, 1980.
142. Kotelko, DM: Anaesthesia for caesarean delivery in a patient with May-Hegglin anomaly. Can. J. Anaesth. 36:328, 1989.
143. Bromage, PR: Epidural Analgesia. Philadelphia, W.B. Saunders Company, 1978; pp. 659–60.
144. Owens EL, Kasten GW, Hessel EA: spinal subarachnoid hematoma after lumbar puncture and heparinization: a case report, review of the literature, and discussion of anesthetic implications. Anesth. Analg. 65:1201, 1986.
145. Cunningham AJ, Donnelly M, Comerford J: Osteogenesis imperfecta: anesthetic management of a patient for cesarean section: a case report. Anesthesiology 61(1):91–3, 1984.
146. Crosby, ET, Elliott, RD: Anaesthesia for caesarean section in a parturient with quintuplet gestation, pulmonary edema, and thrombocytopenia. Can. J. Anaesth. 35:417, 1988.
147. Malinow AM, Rickford WJK, Mokriski BLK, Saller DN, et al: Lupus anticoagulant: Implications for obstetric anaesthetists. Anesthesia. 1987;42:1291.
148. Cohen, S, Goldiner, PL: Epidural analgesia for labor and delivery in a patient with Von Willebrand's disease. Reg. Anesth. 14:95, 1989.
149. Chediak, J, Alban, G, Maxey, B: Von Willebrand's disease and pregnancy: management during delivery and outcome of offspring. Am. J. Obstet. Gynecol. 155:618, 1986.
150. Rolbin, SH, Abbott, D, Musclow, E, Papsin, F, et al: Epidural anesthesia in pregnant patients with low platelet counts. Obstet. Gynecol. 71:918, 1988.
151. Davison JM, Katz AI, Lindheimer MD: Kidney disease and pregnancy: Obstetric outcome and long-term renal prognosis. Clin. Perinatol. 1986;15:103.
152. Jungers P, Forget D, Henry-Amar M, Albouze G, et al: Chronic kidney disease and pregnancy. Adv. Nephrol. 1986;15:103.
153. Gabert HA, Miller JM Jr: Renal disease in pregnancy. Obstet. Gynecol. Surg. 1985;40:449.
154. Knuppel RA, Montenegro R, O'Brien WF: Acute renal failure in pregnancy. Clin. Obstet. Gynecol. 1985;28:288.
155. Oken DE: Hemodynamic basis for human acute renal failure (vasomotor nephropathy). Am. J. Med. 1984;76:702.
156. Maddern PJ: Anaesthesia for the patient with impaired renal function. Anesth Intens Care. 1983;11:321.
157. Orko R, Pitkanen M, Rosenberg PH: Subarachnoid anaesthesia with 0.75% bupivacaine in patients with chronic renal failure. Br. J. Anaesth. 1986;58:605.
158. Shanks CA: Muscle relaxants in renal failure patients. *In* Muscle Relaxants: Basic Clinical Aspects. Edited by RL Katz. New York: Grune & Stratton, 1985.
159. Lund PC, Covino BG: Distribution of local anesthetics in man following peridural anesthesia. J. Clin. Pharm. 1967; 7:324.
160. Norishima HO, Pederson H: Finster toxicity of lidocaine in the adult, newborn and fetal sheep. Anesthesiology. 1981;55:57.
161. Swapp GH, Main RA: Neurofibromatosis in pregnancy. Br. J. Dermatol. 1973;80:431.
162. Griffiths ML, Theron EJ: Obstructed labor from pelvic neurofibroma. S. Afr. Med. J. 1978;53:781.
163. Baraka A: Myasthenic response to muscle relaxants in von Recklinghausen's disease. Br. J. Anaesth. 1974;46:701.
164. Abouleish E: Hypertension in a paraplegic parturient. Anesthesiology. 1980;53:348.
165. Stirt JA, Marco A, Conklin KA: Obstetric anesthesia for a quadriplegic patient with autonomic hyperflexia. Anesthesiology. 1979;51:560.
166. Baraka A: Epidural meperidine for control of autonomic hyperreflexia in a paraplegic parturient. Anesthesiology. 1985;62:688.
167. Kofke WA, Wuest HP, McGinnis LA: Cesarean section following ruptured cerebral aneurysm and neuroresuscitation. Anesthesiology. 1984;60:242.
168. Minielly R, Yuzpe AA, Drake CG: Subarachnoid hemorrhage secondary to ruptured cerebral aneurysm in pregnancy. Obstet. Gynecol. 1979;53:64.
169. Conklin KA, Herr G, Fung D: Anesthesia for cesarean section and cerebral aneurysm clipping. Can. Anaesth. Soc. J. 1984;34:451.
170. Lennon RL, Sundt TM Jr, Gronert GA: Combined cesarean section and clipping of intracerebral aneurysm clipping. Can. Anaesth. Soc. J. 1984;60:240.
171. Bamford C, Sibley W, Laguna J: Anesthesia in multiple sclerosis. Can. J. Neurol. Sci. 1978;5:41.
172. Crawford JS, James III FM, Nolte H, Van Steenberge A, et al: Regional anesthesia for patients with chronic neurological disease and similar conditions. Anaesthesia. 1981;36:821.
173. Korn-Lubetzki, I, Kahana, E, Cooper, G, Abramsky, O: Activ-

ity of multiple sclerosis during pregnancy and puerperium. Ann. Neurol. 16:2229–231, 1984.

174. Nelson, LM, Franklin, GM, Jones, MC, Multiple Sclerosis Study Group: risk of multiple sclerosis exacerbation during pregnancy and breast-feeding. JAMA 259:3441–3443, 1988.
175. Haas JF, Janisch W, Stanczek W: Newly diagnosed primary intracranial neoplasms in pregnant women: a population-based assessment. J. Neurol. Neurosurg. Psychiatry. 1986; 49:874.
176. Ahlskog JE, O'Neill BP: Pseudotumor cerebri. Ann. Intern. Med. 1982;97:249.
177. Koontz WL, Herbert WNP, Cefalo RC: Pseudotumor cerebri in pregnancy. Obstet. Gynecol. 1983;62:324.
178. Evans DE: Anaesthesia and the epileptic patient: A review. Anaesthesia. 1975;30:34.
179. Robertson IG: Prescribing in pregnancy: Epilepsy in pregnancy. Clin. Obstet. Gynaecol. 1986;13:365.
180. Mokriski, BK, Malinow AM, Gray WC, McGuinn WJ: Topical nasopharyngeal anaesthesia with vasoconstriction in pre-eclampsia-eclampsia. Can. J. Anaesth. 35:641, 1988.
181. Smith CL, Bush GH: Anesthesia and progressive muscular dystrophy. Br. J. Anaesth. 1985;57:1113.
182. Sokoll MD, Gergis SD: Anesthesia and neuromuscular disease. Anesth. Rev. 1975;2:20.
183. Azar I: The response of patients with neuromuscular disorders to muscle relaxants: A review. Anesthesiology. 1984; 61:173.
184. Sarnat HB, O'Connor T, Byrne PA: Clinical effects of myotonic dystrophy on pregnancy and the neonate. Arch. Neurol. 1976;33:459.
185. Mitchell MM, Ali HH, Savarese JJ: Myotonia and neuromuscular blocking agents. Anesthesiology. 1978;49:44.
186. Hook R, Anderson EF, Note P: Anesthetic management of a parturient with myotonia atrophica. Anesthesiology. 1975; 43:689.
187. Cope DK, Miller JN: Local and spinal anesthesia for cesarean section in a patient with myotonic dystrophy. Anesth. Analg. 1986;65:687.
188. Rolbin SH, Levinson G, Shnider SM, Wright RG: Anesthetic considerations for myasthenia gravis and pregnancy. Anesth. Analg. 1978;57:441.
189. Drachman DB: Myasthenia gravis: Part 2. N. Engl. J. Med. 1978;298:186.
190. Fennel D, Ringel S: Myasthenia gravis and pregnancy. Obstet. Gynecol. Surv. 1987;41:414.
191. Luz-Tobias A, Ramilo N, Yu K, Rigor B: Anesthetic management of a parturient with myasthenia gravis. J. Kentucky Med. Assoc. 1987;Feb:78–80.
192. Mitchell PJ, Bebbington M: Myasthenia gravis in pregnancy. Obstet. Gynecol. 80:178–181, 1992.
193. Dunn JM: Neonatal myasthenia. Am. J. Obstet. Gynecol. 1976;125:265.
194. Burns AM, Dorje P, Lawes EG, Nielsen MS: Anesthetic management of cesarean section for a mother with preeclampsia, the Klippel-Feil syndrome and congenital hydrocephalus. Br. J. Anaesth. 61:350, 1988.
195. Quance DR: Anaesthetic management of an obstetrical patient with arthrogryposis multiplex congenita. Can. J. Anaesth. 35:612, 1988.
196. Dadabhoy ZP, Winnie AP: Regional anesthesia for cesarean section in a parturient with Noonan's Syndrome. Anesthesiology 68:636, 1988.
197. Cunningham AJ, Donnelly MB, Comerford J: Osteogenesis Imperfecta: anesthetic management of a patient for cesarean section: a case report. Anesthesiology 61:91, 1984.
198. Nelson LH, McLean Jr WT: Management of Landry-Guillain-Barré syndrome in pregnancy. Obstet. Gynecol. 65:25S-29S, 1985.
199. Laufenburg HF, Sirus SR: Guillain-Barr syndrome in pregnancy. AFP 39:147–150, 1989.
200. Miller RG: Guillain-Barré syndrome. Current methods of diagnosis and treatment. Postgrad. Med. 77:57–9, 62–4, 1985.
201. Hart IK, Kennedy PGE: Guillain-Barré syndrome associated with cytomegalovirus infection. Quart. J. Med. 67(253): 425–430, 1988.
202. Swick HM, McQuillen MP: The use of steroids in the treatment of idiopathic polyneuritis. Neurology 26:205–15, 1976.
203. Caudle MR, Scott JR: The potential role of immunosuppression, plasmapheresis, and desensitization as treatment modalities for Rh isoimmunization. Clin. Obstet. Gynecol. 25: 3131, 1982.
204. McGrady EM: Management of labour and delivery in a patient with Guillain-Barré syndrome. Anaesthesia (Letter) 42:899, 1987.
205. Elstein M, Legg NJ, Murphy M, Park DM, et al: Guillain-Barré syndrome in pregnancy. Respiratory paralysis complicated by a fatal tracheo-innominate artery fistula. Anaesthesia 26:216–224, 1971.

# Chapter 39

# SURGICAL DISEASES DURING PREGNANCY

MARK B. LANDON

Surgery other than cesarean section is a relatively uncommon event for the pregnant patient. Overall, less than 1% of women undergo some type of surgical procedure during pregnancy. As a rule, when surgical care is not emergent, it is best deferred until the second trimester or, more often, the postpartum period. The timing of many procedures is thus dictated by concerns regarding anesthesia and its potential risks to mother and fetus. These issues have been largely addressed elsewhere in this book. This chapter focuses on the pathophysiology, diagnosis, and treatment of certain specific surgical diseases during pregnancy. Wherever possible, specific anesthesia-related considerations are discussed. However, an understanding of the general approach to the pregnant surgical patient is essential for the obstetric anesthesiologist.

The diagnosis of many surgical conditions is hampered by pregnancy. Altered abdominal anatomy and physiologic changes can make certain diagnoses extremely difficult to establish. Diagnostic procedures such as radiography are often avoided in the pregnant woman, despite the need to establish a prompt diagnosis. Radiologic studies, when indicated for the health and well-being of the mother, should not be withheld. For example, a single chest radiograph delivers less than 1 rad to the first trimester fetus, which is far below the accepted potentially teratogenic dose of 5 to 10 rads.[1] Furthermore, the use of magnetic resonance imaging (MRI) is becoming increasingly popular as a diagnostic medium. It does not pose a threat to either the mother or fetus, and enables the physician to make a definitive diagnosis in most instances. Delay in providing acute surgical care when indicated is in part responsible for an increase in maternal mortality, and morbidity, and fetal loss when surgical diseases complicate pregnancy.

## PREGNANCY LOSS AND PRETERM LABOR

It is unlikely that a brief anesthetic exposure alone is associated with an increased risk of first trimester miscarriage. On the other hand, even minor surgery under local anesthesia may be associated with preterm labor and delivery. However, no single anesthetic agent or technique has been found to be associated with a higher or lower incidence of preterm labor. Abdominal procedures are clearly more likely to result in preterm labor, and uterine manipulation is believed to be a causative factor. In one study, 95 such operations were associated with preterm labor.[2] Excellent abdominal relaxation so as to minimize uterine handling can be helpful in these cases. The role of prophylactic tocolytic administration is poorly defined, yet many obstetricians employ these drugs during the postoperative period. The β-mimetic ritodrine and terbutaline are used as well as magnesium sulfate. Most recently, indomethacin has become a popular tocolytic agent for use in this setting because it is rarely associated with significant cardiovascular side effects.

### Anesthetic Concerns

As a general rule, pregnant patients are in excellent health, and are usually classified as physical status Class 1 patients, per the American Society of Anesthesiologists (ASA) classification (see Table 39–1). As a rule, the shortest exposure to the lowest concentration of anesthetic should be the goal of the obstetric anesthesiologist. There are few prospective data to support a teratogenic risk of most commonly employed anesthetic agents.[3] Shnider and Webster reviewed the records of 147 women who received anesthesia for surgery during pregnancy, including 47 during the first trimester. When compared to over 8000 women who delivered during this time period, the frequency of congenital anomalies was not significantly different in this group.[2] The authors also compared outcome data on 60 000 women from the National Collaborative Perinatal Study, with 50 women undergoing appendectomy during pregnancy, and noted no difference in malformation rates among the two groups.[2] It is generally appreciated that such theoretic risks are greatest during the period of organogenesis, at 4 to 12 weeks. Thus, nonemergent surgery should be postponed until after the first trimester. In cases where surgery is indicated during organ development, documentation of fetal age and viability by ultrasound may be critical in determining whether a procedure or anesthetic may have untoward effects on the fetus. All patients should understand that the background risk of malformations which exists in the general population is 2% to 3%.

It would appear that, as a blanket statement, neither general anesthesia nor regional anesthesia may be superior for surgery during pregnancy. During early pregnancy, regional techniques may minimize fetal drug exposure, especially for extremity surgery. With spinal anesthesia, fetal exposure to local anesthetics is much less than with other regional blocks. Local techniques for upper abdominal and thoracic surgery may cause great maternal stress, and are often avoided unless the anesthe-

**Table 39–1.** Classification of Physical Status Adopted by the American Society of Anesthesiologists (Modified for Parturients)

| | |
|---|---|
| Class 1. | Parturients who have no organic, physiologic, biochemical or psychiatric disturbances other than the normal changes of pregnancy. |
| Class 2. | Mild systemic disease or moderate obstetric pathology complicating the pregnancy and delivery. Examples: Patients with Class 1 or 2a heart disease, mild diabetes, mild hypertension, or anemia. |
| Class 3. | Moderate to severe systemic disease or severe obstetric pathology. Examples: Class 2b heart disease, severe diabetes with vascular complications, moderate to severe pulmonary, renal, or hepatic insufficiency, moderate to severe preeclampsia. |
| Class 4. | Patients with severe systemic disease that threatens the life of the gravida. Examples: Class 3 heart disease, eclampsia, hemorrhagic shock, or advanced pulmonary, renal, hepatic, or endocrine insufficiency. |
| Class 5. | A moribund patient who has little chance of survival but who is submitted to operation in desperation. Examples: Parturients with ruptured uterus and in profound shock, major cerebral trauma or ruptured aneurysm with rapidly increasing intracranial pressure. Such patients require resuscitative measures rather than an anesthetic. |
| Emergency (E). | All parturients except those who have a scheduled (elective) induction of labor or cesarean section should be considered emergency cases and the letter E placed beside the numerical classification. Thus a parturient who is otherwise normal but has a full stomach and requires an anesthetic should be classified 1E. One with mild heart disease should be classified 2E. The unprepared parturient with moderate to severe preeclampsia should be classified 3E, whereas one with eclampsia should be classified 4E. |

(From Bonica JJ, Kohn GC: Analgesia during normal labor. *In* Principles and Practice of Obstetric Analgesia and Anesthesia. Vol. 2. Edited by JJ Bonica. Philadelphia, FA Davis Company, 1967, p. 858.)

siologist is very skilled with these procedures. When employing regional anesthesia associated with significant sympathetic blockade, rapid infusion of isotonic crystalloid (approximately 1 liter) should be performed prior to drug infusion. Continuous epidural and spinal techniques have the advantage of allowing titration of the block, while avoiding extensive sympathectomy and hypotension.

In general, anesthesia induction and maintenance doses are similar to those given to patients in nonpregnant states. The lowest *effective dose* is preferred. The emphasis is on effective dose, since it is inappropriate and inhumane not to provide adequate anesthesia in operative procedures, regardless of whether the patient is pregnant or not. Either halothane or isoflurane can provide uterine relaxation if intrauterine manipulation is indicated. As always, careful attention to airway control and avoidance of aspiration are primary concerns, and are discussed elsewhere in this book, as detailed in Chapter 20.

After a patient has reached 20 weeks gestation, the strict supine position should be avoided. Aortocaval compression can usually be reduced by the left lateral tilt position. A wedge facilitates this rather well, particularly in late second and third trimester patients.

## SPECIFIC SURGICAL DISEASES

### Appendicitis

Acute appendicitis is the most common pathologic entity necessitating exploratory laparotomy during pregnancy. Babaknia, et al noted an average of 1 : 1500 deliveries in several series totaling over 500 000 pregnancies.[4] There is little evidence that this disease is more common during pregnancy, despite the concept that progesterone impairs intestinal motility. Appendicitis appears to complicate pregnancy more frequently during the second and third trimesters.[5]

Alterations of maternal physiology and anatomic upward displacement of the appendix may make the diagnosis of acute inflammation more difficult during gestation (Figure 39–1). Delay in diagnosis is thus not uncommon and may result in more advanced disease (perforation, etc.) than seen in nonpregnant individuals. Large appendicular mucoceles can present a challenge to the physi-

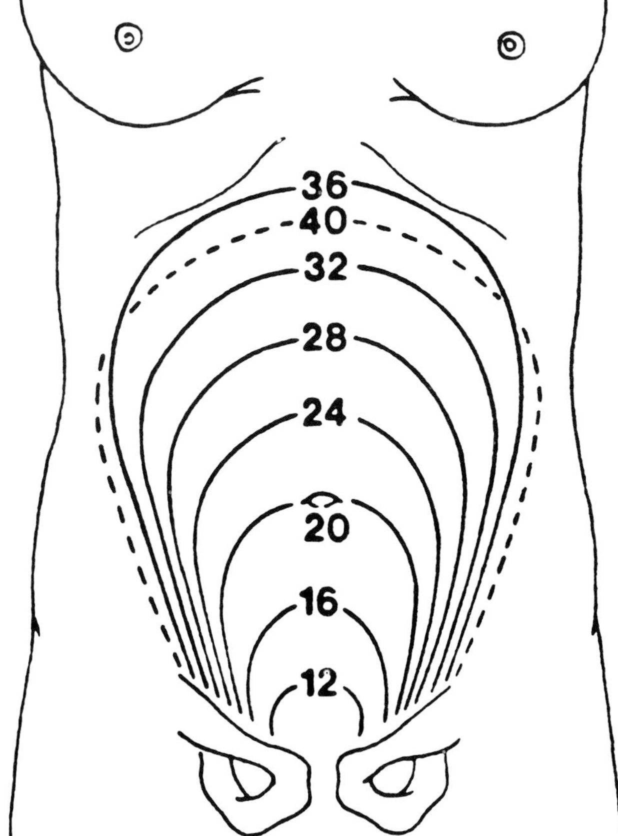


**Fig. 39–1.** Increasing fundal height according to week of gestation. At term, the fundus approaches the xiphoid process, which can obscure normal physical signs associated with intra-abdominal disease. (From Depp R: Cesarean delivery and other surgical procedures. *In* Obstetrics: Normal and Problem Pregnancies. 2nd Ed. Edited by SG Gabbe, JR Niebyl, JL Simpson. New York, Churchill Livingstone, 1991, p. 685.)

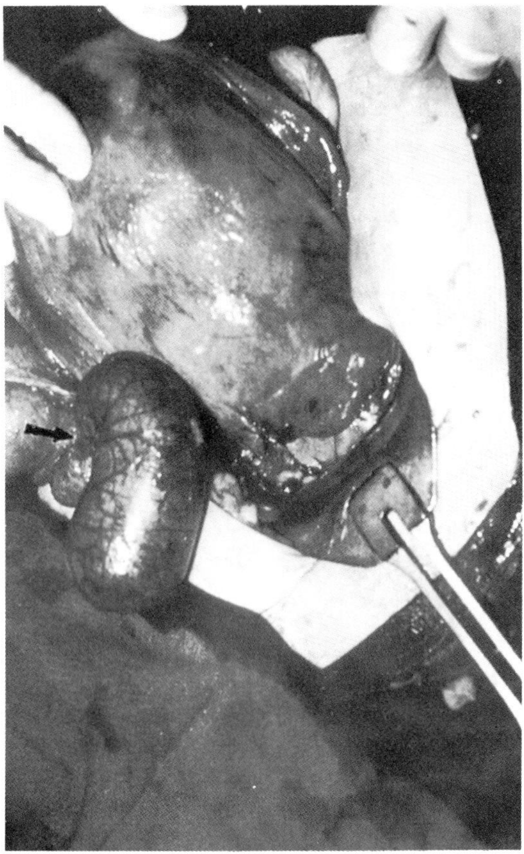

Fig. 39–2. An appendix mucocele immediately adjacent to a gravid uterus. (From Abu Zidan FM, Al-Hilaly MA, Al-Atrabi N: Torsion of a mucocele of the appendix in a pregnant woman. Acta. Obstet. Gynecol. Scand. 71:140, 1992.)

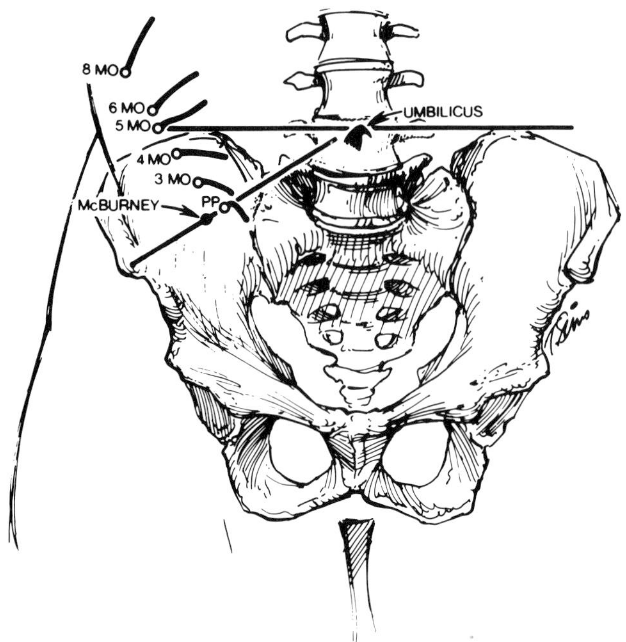


Fig. 39–3. Adaptation of Baer et al description of position of the appendix during normal pregnancy according to month of gestation. (MO = month; PP = postpartum). (From Baer JL, Reis RA, Arens RA: Appendicitis in pregnancy with changes in position and axis of the normal appendix in pregnancy. J.A.M.A. 98:1359, 1932; with permission from Cunningham FG, MacDonald PC, Gant NF (Eds): Williams Obstetrics. 18th Ed. Norwalk, Appleton & Lange, 1989, p. 833.)

cian in regard to diagnosis. One such case with torsion resulted in an acute abdomen in a third trimester gestation (Figure 39–2).[6]

In the nonpregnant patient, the appendix is located in the right lower quadrant or in the pelvis in 95% of cases. Retrocecal appendices account for the remaining 5%. Classic barium enema studies performed by Baer in 1932 demonstrated that by the mid-third trimester, over 90% of patients' appendices were above the iliac crest, and many approached the right subcostal area (Figure 39–3).[7] This should be kept in mind for the rate instance where regional anesthetic techniques might be used.

Right-sided abdominal pain is a constant feature in women presenting with acute appendicitis. Early in the process, obstruction of the appendiceal lumen may produce periumbilical pain. With perforation or gangrene, peritoneal irritation will produce a point of maximal tenderness. The pregnant uterus may limit contact of the appendix with the anterior abdominal wall, resulting in a more diffuse pain. Anorexia is seen in the majority of cases (67%), as is nausea and vomiting, which are common features of normal early gestation. Temperature elevation (over 38° C) is seen in roughly 50% of cases, with tachycardia being mild at best. Laboratory data are nonspecific, and usually reveal a mild leukocytosis or normal white blood cell (WBC) count with a shift. The differential diagnosis includes: ruptured corpus luteum; ectopic pregnancy; adnexal torsion; amnionitis; pyelonephritis; cholangitis; degenerating myoma; and preterm labor.

Appendicitis late in pregnancy is more likely to result in perforation. Delay in diagnosis should therefore be avoided. Perinatal mortality increases several-fold if perforation occurs. The surgeon who suspects the diagnosis of appendicitis should seek anesthetic consultation promptly. The planned incision should be discussed. During early pregnancy, a midline incision may be preferred because of the high frequency of false-positive diagnosis. Laparoscopy has been employed in uncertain cases as well. In later pregnancy, a muscle-splitting incision over the point of maximal tenderness is preferred. The patient is tilted slightly to the left side to enhance exposure, as well as to displace the uterus off the vena cava. Conduction anesthesia has been advocated as the method of choice for early pregnancy, where potential teratogenicity is a concern. In later pregnancy, general anesthesia is clearly preferred to allow maximal oxygenation, uterine relaxation, and avoidance of hypotension.

The surgical management of this condition is not altered during the first two trimesters. If generalized peritonitis is encountered, drainage is indicated. Antibiotics are generally reserved for cases of gangrene or perforation. In late pregnancy, cesarean section may be performed if there is perforation and peritonitis, as the risk of preterm labor, sepsis, and fetal distress are present. To prevent uterine abscess formation, cesarean hysterectomy should be considered in such cases as well.

It is important to be aware of the most important safety aspect in regard to fetal protection during surgical procedures. This is care in maintaining adequate uterine blood flow on the maternal side of the placenta, and in turn, maintaining adequate perfusion on the fetal side of the placenta. The latter is compromised if surgical traction reduces the umbilical blood flow by direct compression. To guard against this, one must use a fetal monitor to record a continuous fetal heart tracing during the procedure. It is a simple matter to ask the surgeon to change retractor tension or direction when a sudden bradycardia is encountered during the surgical procedure.

## *Gallbladder and Biliary Tract Disease*

### Liver Disease

Following acute appendicitis, diseases of the biliary tract are the most common surgical conditions complicating pregnancy. The diagnosis of biliary tract disease during pregnancy can be extremely difficult, as certain conditions unique to pregnancy can affect liver function, such as acute fatty liver, severe preeclampsia, and intrahepatic cholestanes. Marked changes in liver function during normal pregnancy must be appreciated as well. For example, alkaline phosphatase levels may double, whereas total protein and albumin fall during early pregnancy. In contrast, most globulins and carrier proteins increase in concentration. Biliary stasis or incomplete gallbladder emptying is a normal phenomenon during pregnancy.

The liver may be involved in up to 50% of cases of severe preeclampsia. Laboratory values for mild and severe preeclampsia are compared in Table 39–2. Elevation of liver transaminases and mild elevations of bilirubin are part of the syndrome of hemolysis, elevated liver enzymes, and low platelet count.[8] Laboratory values used to diagnose HELLP syndrome are listed in Table 39–3. Histologically, fibrin is deposited periportally with areas of hemorrhage present. If bleeding is significant, subcapsular hemorrhage may occur with the potential for rupture (Figure 39–4). Early in the disease process, these patients complain of right upper quadrant pain and, frequently, nausea and vomiting. Hypotension, shock, and tachycardia ensue. Disseminated intravascular coagulation may be present as well. Following emergency cesarean section, pressure should be applied by the obstetrician to the bleeding area on the liver. Cesarean section improves exposure for the vascular surgeon while facilitating venous return by evacuating the uterus. Postoperative complications, including renal failure and adult respiratory distress syndrome (ARDS), are common in such cases and warrant an intensive care setting for postoperative care.[9]

**Table 39–2.** Comparison of Laboratory Findings in Women with Mild Versus Severe Preeclampsia

| Laboratory Value | Mild[a] | Severe[a] |
|---|---|---|
| Hematocrit (%) | 34 ± 4 | 35.5 ± 4.2 |
| Fibrinogen (mg/dl) | 401 ± 80 | 404 ± 91.3 |
| Platelet count (× 10³/mm³) | 240 ± 90 | 230 ± 83 |
| Uric acid (mg/dl)[b] | 6 ± 1.6 | 6.5 ± 1.6 |
| Creatinine (mg/dl)[b] | 0.8 ± 0.2 | 0.9 ± 0.4 |
| Creatinine clearance (mg/dl)[b] | 86 ± 22 | 98 ± 36 |
| SGOT (IU/liter)[b] | 28 ± 66 | 37 ± 69 |
| Bilirubin (mg/dl)[b] | 0.7 ± 0.8 | 0.4 ± 0.3 |
| Albumin (g/dl) | 3.1 ± 0.3 | 2.9 ± 0.5 |

[a] Mean ± 1 SD.
[b] $p < 0.05$
(From Anderson GD, Sibai BM: Hypertension in pregnancy. *In* Obstetrics: Normal & Problem Pregnancies. Edited by SG Gabbe, JR Niebyl, JL Simpson. New York, Churchill Livingstone, 1986, p. 822)

**Table 39–3.** Laboratory Values Used to Diagnose HELLP Syndrome

Hemolysis
- Abnormal peripheral blood smear
- Increased bilirubin greater than or equal to 1.2 mg/dl
- Increased lactic dehydrogenase greater than 600 IU/L

Elevated liver enzymes
- Increased SGOT greater than 72 IU/L
- Increased lactic dehydrogenase as above

Low platelets
- Platelet count less than 100 × 10³/μl

HELLP = Hemolysis, elevated liver enzymes, and low platelets

(From Sibai BM, Anderson GD: Hypertension. *In* Obstetrics: Normal and Problem Pregnancies. 2nd Ed. Edited by SG Gabbe, JR Niebyl, JL Simpson. New York, Churchill Livingstone, 1991, p. 1006.)

Cirrhosis of the liver is uncommon during pregnancy, as is portal hypertension. Women with severe liver disease are often beyond childbearing age or experience infertility secondary to oligo-ovulation. The risk of spontaneous abortion may also be slightly increased in cirrhotic women.[10] Bleeding from esophageal varices is unpredictable during pregnancy. Plans should be made for this potential event involving the vascular surgeon, anesthesiologist, and obstetrician. Shunt surgery has been successfully performed during pregnancy. The timing of such elective procedures is debated, yet most women who have undergone splenorenal shunts deliver vaginally without complications.[11] The risk of hemorrhage is increased in such women, who may be deficient in factors V and VIII. Thus, epidural anesthesia may be contraindicated if a coagulopathy is present. Thrombocytopenia secondary to hypersplenism may add to this problem. Nonetheless, some form of analgesia should be provided to lessen bearing-down efforts, which may increase portal pressure. For this reason, prophylactic forceps have been advocated to shorten the second stage. Pudendal block with $N_2O/O_2$ inhalation analgesia may be used for second stage pain relief. This may be supplemental to or even supplanted with local injection perineal analgesia with $N_2O/O_2$ inhalation analgesia.

Liver transplantation has become successful over the past few years with several instances of subsequent pregnancies after transplantation noted in the literature (12–15). More remarkable is the feat of liver transplantation *during* pregnancy, which occurred twice in documented reports of 1990[16] and 1991.[17] Both cases were

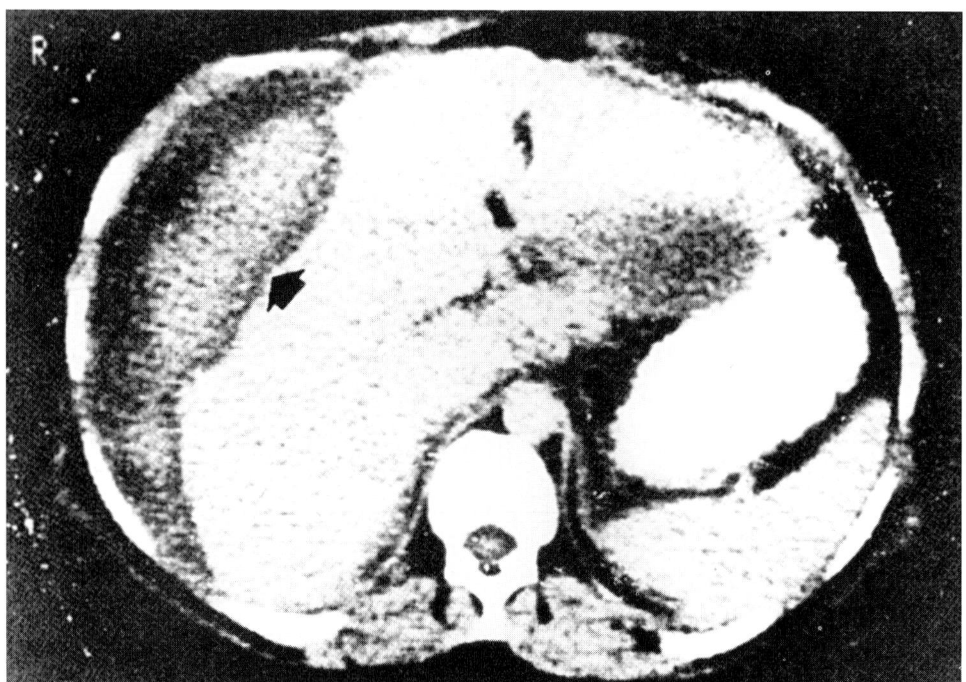


**Fig. 39–4.** Computed tomogram of the liver depicting a subscapular (arrow) hematoma along the right aspect of the liver in a woman with preeclampsia. (Produced with permission from Manas KJ, Welsh JD, Rankin RA, Miller DD: Hepatic hemorrhage without rupture in preeclampsia. N. Engl. J. Med. 312:424, 1985.)

instances of fulminant hepatic failure in pregnancy, but had successful outcomes in regard to their transplantation and eventual delivery status (Figure 39–5).

## *Cholecystitis*

Pregnancy does appear to increase the likelihood of gallstone formation, but not the risk of developing acute cholecystitis.[18,19] Cholecystectomy, however, accounts for more nonobstetrical/gynecologic surgery during pregnancy than any condition other than appendicitis. As mentioned previously, pregnancy markedly alters gallbladder function. Ultrasound studies in early pregnancy have demonstrated that the fasting gallbladder volume is twice the size of a normal gallbladder. The rate of gallbladder emptying is slower, and the percentage emptying is lower than in the nonpregnant female.[19]

In general, attacks of biliary colic should be treated symptomatically during gestation. Ultrasound is helpful in the evaluation of patients suspected of having gallbladder disease. During pregnancy, naturally, medical management is preferred whenever possible. A response to intravenous hydration, analgesia, nasogastric suction, and antibiotics is most often observed. In cases refractory to these standard measures, cholecystectomy may be performed after several days of conservative therapy. If ascending cholangitis develops, cholecystectomy should not be postponed. Cholecystectomy is also indicated if common bile duct obstruction is present or if severe pancreatitis develops. As with other surgical emergencies, temporizing can increase perinatal mortality and morbidity as well as maternal risks. When cholecystectomy is performed during the second or third trimester, fetal mortality is around 5% (Table 39–4).[20] However, if pancreatitis secondary to biliary tract stones remains untreated, fetal mortality exceeds 50%.[21] In the classic surgical approach to

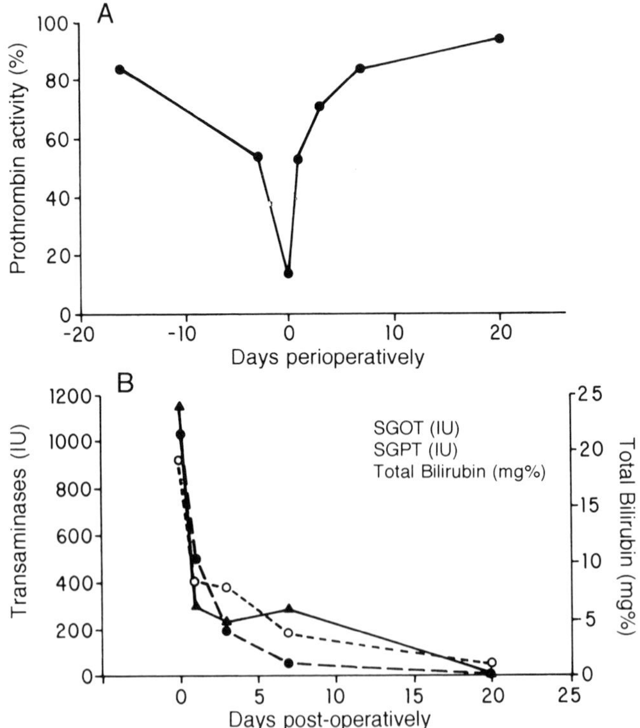


**Fig. 39–5.** **A,** perioperative prothrombin activity percentages. **B,** postoperative transaminases levels on the left and bilirubin levels on the right. (Redrawn from Moreno EG, García GI, Gómez SR, González-Pinto I, et al: Fulminant hepatic failure during pregnancy successfully treated by orthotopic liver transplantation. Transplantation 52:923, 1991.)

**Table 39–4.** Cholecystectomy During 1st, 2nd, and 3rd Trimesters, Related to Spontaneous Abortion and Premature Labor

| Trimester | Spontaneous Abortion, No. of Pts./Total | | | Premature Labor, No. of Pts./Total | | |
|---|---|---|---|---|---|---|
| | I | II | III | I | II | III |
| Greene et al. (2), 1963 | 2/10 | 2/5 | 0/2 | 0/10 | 0/5 | 0/2 |
| O'Neill (8), 1969 | 0/2 | 0/5 | 0/1 | 0/2 | 0/5 | 0/1 |
| Friley and Douglas (1), 1972 | 0/3 | 0/3 | 0/0 | 0/3 | 0/3 | 0/0 |
| Printen (9), 1978 | 0/2 | 0/4 | 0/0 | 0/2 | 0/4 | 0/0 |
| Landers et al. (5), 1987 | 1/3 | 0/3 | 0/3 | 0/3 | 0/3 | 2/3 |
| Dixon et al. (6), 1987 | 0/3 | 0/12 | 0/1 | 0/3 | 0/12 | 1/1 |
| McKellar | 0/2 | 0/4 | 0/3 | 0/2 | 1/4 | 1/3 |
| Total | 3/25 (12) | 2/36 (5.6) | 0/10 (–) | 0/25 (–) | 1/36 (–) | 4/10 (–) |

* Pregnancy not known preoperatively.
† Elective abortion chosen by patients and performed preoperatively.
‡ Outcome of two pregnancies not known, so results excluded.
Numbers in parentheses are percentages.
(Modified from McKellar DP, Anderson CT, Boynton CJ, Peoples JB: Cholecystectomy during pregnancy without fetal loss. Surg. Gynecol. Obstet. 174:465–468, 1992.)

cholecystectomy, the preferred anesthetic technique is general anesthesia with either intravenous analgesia and/or inhalation analgesia. Regional anesthesia is really not ideal for pregnant patients due to the fact that the sensory level may need to be at T2-T4 which may precipitate hypotension. To complicate matters, there may be inadequate analgesia which may need to be supplemental with intravenous analgesia. In the *laparoscopic cholecystectomy* technique, *general anesthesia* is a good choice.

## Breast Disease

Examination of the breast during early pregnancy is important, because as gestation proceeds, hypertrophy, engorgement, and increased vascularity make this evaluation considerably more difficult. Delay in the diagnosis of breast cancer during pregnancy has often been attributed to the physician's reluctance to properly evaluate complaints relating to the breast.[22] While bilateral serosanguinous discharge may normally accompany late pregnancy, masses with or without unilateral discharge require prompt and definitive evaluation.[23]

Because the hyperplastic breast of pregnancy is characterized by an increase in radiographic density, mammography is of limited value in evaluation of suspected masses. Fine-needle aspiration of a mass for cytologic study should be the primary diagnostic procedure during pregnancy. Equivocal cytologic diagnosis requires excision of the tumor under local anesthesia. This approach minimizes any risk to the fetus and, should a malignancy be detected, it permits discussion between patient and physician before planning definitive therapy. One cancer per four biopsies can be expected, a figure similar to that found in nonpregnant patients.[22]

Breast cancers found in pregnant women are histologically identical to neoplasms recovered from nonpregnant women of similar age. The 5-year and 10-year survivals of pregnant women with breast cancer are similar to those observed in nonpregnant women. The prognosis depends mainly on the stage of the disease at the time of diagnosis. The presence and degree of lymph node involvement clearly help predict the likelihood of recurrence after radical mastectomy. During pregnancy, 62% to 85% of women have positive axillary nodes at the time of diagnosis.[24,25] This increased proportion of patients with advanced disease may be due in part to delay in diagnosis, or hormonal and vascular changes that promote tumor growth and metastases.

Mastectomy appears to be the treatment of choice for patients with early disease, regardless of gestational age. A modified radical procedure with or without primary reconstruction is performed under general anesthesia. The risk of miscarriage is approximately 1%.[22] Patients who are candidates for wide local excision and axillary node sampling followed by radiation are most often advised to terminate pregnancy if this therapeutic option is elected. In such cases, the amount of radiation delivered to the fetus must be calculated and the patient counselled appropriately.

## Ovarian Disease

Ovarian pathology is uncommon in pregnancy, yet with the increasing utilization of ultrasound, it is likely that more adnexal masses will be detected. The frequency of adnexal pathology varies, but ovarian masses may be as common as 1 in 556 pregnancies (Figure 39–6 and Table 39–5).[26] The management of uncomplicated ovarian cysts represents a difficult clinical decision for the obstetrician. During the first trimester, simple thin-walled cysts are likely to represent corpus luteum cysts, which can be managed expectantly. Large cysts (over 78 cm) and smaller multilocular cysts or thick-walled semisolid cysts should be surgically removed. Conservative management in these later conditions may result in torsion, rupture, or spread of an undiagnosed malignancy. Emergency surgery or surgery in late pregnancy is more likely to be difficult and with increased uterine manipulation, prema-

**Table 39–5.** Pathology at Time of Surgery

| Trimester | Pathology | No. |
|---|---|---|
| 1st | Torsion of corpus luteum | 5 |
| 2nd | Dermoid | 5 |
| | Fibroid | 2 |
| | Endometrioma | 1 |
| 3rd | Dermoid | 3 |
| | Corpus luteum | 2 |
| | Luteoma | 2 |
| | Granulosa | 1 |
| | Thecoma | 1 |
| | Cystadenoma | 1 |
| Total | | 23 |

(From Hopkins MP, Duchon MA: Adnexel surgery in pregnancy. J Reprod Med. 31:1035, 1986.)

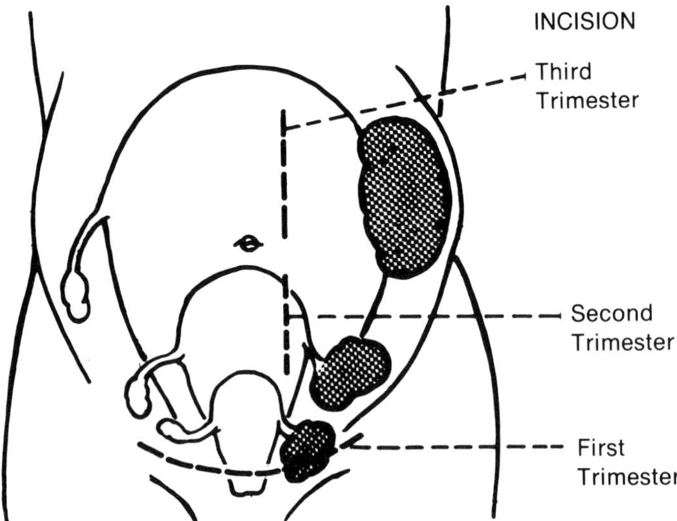


**Fig. 39–6.** Surgical incisions used in first, second, and third trimesters, including abdominal locations. The incision in the first trimester, the Pfannensteil incision, is the most popular. (Redrawn from Hopkins MP, Duchon MA: Adnexal surgery in pregnancy. J. Reprod. Med. 31:1035, 1986.)

ture labor may follow such cases. For this reason, adnexal surgery is preferably undertaken between 14 and 18 weeks gestation.

While the risk of malignancy is approximately 2% to 3% for ovarian tumors diagnosed during pregnancy, a midline incision is indicated to allow for adequate exposure and exploration of the upper abdomen if malignancy is encountered.[27] Benign cystic teratoma and mucinous cystadenoma are the most common tumors found in pregnancy. These benign neoplasms should be removed in the shortest period of time possible, thus minimizing the risk of uterine irritability and preterm labor.

Either regional techniques or general anesthesia may be employed for exploratory laparotomy for adnexal disease during pregnancy. If a malignant condition is found, however, prolonged surgery should be anticipated with upper abdominal biopsies and retroperitoneal lymph node sampling. Regardless of the pathology encountered, avoidance of the supine position in the second and third trimesters, as well as hypotension, remains an important principle in these cases. As discussed previously, the role of prophylactic tocolytic therapy has yet to be defined, though many obstetricians will administer such medications during the immediate postoperative period.

## *Endocrine Glands*

### *Thyroid*

Thyroid disorders are common in women of childbearing age and have been estimated to occur in 0.2% of all pregnancies. The thyroid gland appears to be functioning maximally during normal pregnancy. Basal metabolic rate, which in the past was employed as indirect measurement of thyroid function, is elevated in pregnant women. The size of the thyroid gland may be increased, although the incidence of goiter in pregnancy is likely to be related to the availability of iodine in the diet. Laboratory assessment of thyroid function is dramatically altered by the hormonal changes of pregnancy. These are reviewed elsewhere in this text.

Thyrotoxicosis is encountered in approximately 0.2% of pregnancies.[28] Most women with mild-to-moderate disease appear to tolerate pregnancy well. There is no clear evidence that pregnancy worsens the disease or makes it more difficult to treat. Uncontrolled disease, however, is associated with an increased incidence of neonatal morbidity resulting from preterm birth and low birth weight.[28,29] Graves' disease is the most common cause of hyperthyroidism in pregnancy. Medical therapy is generally preferred, employing thiourea compounds as they present less risk than surgery. The risks from thyroidectomy include anesthesia blood loss, recurrent laryngeal nerve paralysis, and hypoparathyroidism. An occasional patient may be allergic to thioureas or refractory to this therapy which may be attempted with concurrent β-blockade in difficult cases.[28,29] In general, surgery is planned for the second trimester. General anesthesia is the preferred method for these patients with either intravenous analgesia or inhalation analgesia as the mainstay for pain relief. Thyroid storm precipitated by the stress of surgery is a life-threatening complication of thyrotoxicosis which should be anticipated. Standard prophylactic measures include the administration of antithyroid drugs to block the synthesis of thyroid hormone, and iodine solution to block release of the hormone stored in the gland.

Thyroidectomy is a procedure which is well tolerated by pregnant women, with a mortality risk equivalent to the use of general anesthesia alone. Fetal loss, however, is more likely, although a 90% salvage rate is reported in the literature.[30] Surgical exploration of the thyroid for suspicious nodules where the mother is euthyroid is probably less hazardous, although such procedures are performed preferably in midpregnancy. Recurrence of a cyst after aspiration, suspicious cytology, and symptomatic compression remain indications for exploration. With upper airway obstruction, awake fiberoptic intubation would be the procedure of choice.

### Parathyroid

A discussion of normal parathyroid function and calcium metabolism during pregnancy is found in Chapter 32. The treatment for severe hypercalcemia secondary to hyperparathyroidism during pregnancy is surgical exploration. Hyperparathyroidism during pregnancy is associated with increased perinatal morbidity and mortality. Shangold's review of 159 pregnancies in 63 women revealed that 11 ended in intrauterine fetal death.[31] Four neonatal deaths followed episodes of tetany. During recent years, the incidence of stillbirths and neonatal deaths has fallen to 2%. Neonatal tetany is observed in 15% of cases, and often leads to the diagnosis of maternal disease.[31] Reduced serum calcium levels in the neonatal period are believed to result from chronic maternal hypercalcemia and resultant fetal hypercalcemia, which suppresses fetal parathyroid hormone synthesis. After delivery, the fetus is relatively hypoparathyroid.

Because of the high rate of perinatal complications, many authorities recommend prompt excision of the abnormal parathyroid tissue once the diagnosis is established. In Shangold's series, surgery was performed in 16 cases. Of these women, 14 were cured by the procedure and of these, 12 subsequently had a successful pregnancy. Surgical therapy is indicated in patients with severe disease, indicated by markedly elevated serum calcium levels and progressive symptoms, including bone disease and nephrocalcinosis. Hypercalcemic crisis should be treated medically with careful administration of isotonic saline along with furosemide, which inhibits tubular resorption of calcium. Mithramycin should not be used in the pregnant individual.

In patients with mild disease, particularly in late pregnancy, medical treatment of hyperparathyroidism may be attempted. Oral phosphate therapy has been employed successfully in a limited number of cases.[32] This therapy is reserved for women with mild disease and normal renal function, as phosphate retention may precipitate soft tissue calcification. General anesthesia is the preferred method for these patients, with either intravenous analgesia or inhalation analgesia as the mainstay for pain relief.

### Pheochromocytoma

Pheochromocytoma is a rare catecholamine-producing tumor uncommonly associated with pregnancy. The tumor arises from chromaffin cells of the adrenal medulla or sympathetic nervous tissue, including remnants of the organs of Zuckerkandl, neural crest tissue lying along the abdominal aorta. The tumor is located in the adrenal gland in 90% of cases.[33] The incidence of malignancy, diagnosed by metastases, is approximately 10%.

In pregnancy, pheochromocytoma may be present as hypertensive crisis marked by cerebral hemorrhage or severe congestive heart failure. Over one-third of cases may not be diagnosed until postmortem examination.[33] The outcome of pregnancy is largely determined by whether the diagnosis is established before labor and delivery. In one series, half of the mothers entering labor with undiagnosed pheochromocytoma died.[33] Similarly, fetal mortality is related to the timing of diagnosis. When diagnosed antepartum, half of fetuses died compared to two-thirds when the disease was undiagnosed prior to delivery.[33]

The signs and symptoms of pheochromocytomas may mimic those of severe pregnancy-induced hypertension. Headache, blurry vision, abdominal pain, and hypertension are common to both entities. The presence of paroxysmal hypertension, particularly prior to 20 weeks gestation, as well as orthostasis and absence of proteinuria should alert the clinician to this possible diagnosis. Thyrotoxicosis may also resemble this disease; however, significant hypertension is uncommon with Graves' disease.

The definitive diagnosis rests on laboratory measurements of catecholamines and their metabolites in urine and blood. Radiologic techniques including computerized tomography (CT) scanning are then employed to localize the tumor. Selective catheterization of the adrenals has been employed during pregnancy. It should be appreciated that such invasive techniques may provide a powerful stress to patients with pheochromocytoma, so that pharmacologic preparation and monitoring are essential.

Once the diagnosis is established, the patient should be prepared for removal of the tumor. Preferably, this is carried out prior to labor and delivery, when the risks are greatest. Before surgery, the patient should be stabilized on either oral doses of phenoxybenzamine or intravenous phentolamine in an effort to reduce the catecholamine-mediated effects.

Anesthesia is provided by the general technique with careful attention to preparation of the patient prior to surgery and detailed monitoring during surgery because of the labile blood pressure problems associated with this disease. Careful evaluation of fluid status with central monitoring is preferred when using those preparations. β-blockade is reserved for the treatment of tachyarrhythmias, and should not be instituted before α-blockade, as hypertensive crises may ensue. In the mid-trimester, the choice of treatment is resection of the tumor, after which the patient continues to term, with cesarean section only for obstetric indications. In the third trimester, once the patient is stabilized, laparotomy with cesarean section is the procedure of choice.

## Urinary Tract

During pregnancy, marked changes take place in renal physiology and anatomy of the urinary tract. The renal physiologic adjustments include an increase of 50% to 75% in renal plasma flow, and an average 50% increase in glomerular filtration.[34] The latter occurs by the end of the first trimester of pregnancy.

Morphologic changes of the urinary tract are most pronounced during the third trimester. Ureteral and caliceal dilatation are believed to result from hormonal factors such as progesterone-mediated smooth-muscle relaxation as well as uterine and pelvic vein compression of the ureters leading to stasis. Upper urinary tract dilatation is rare

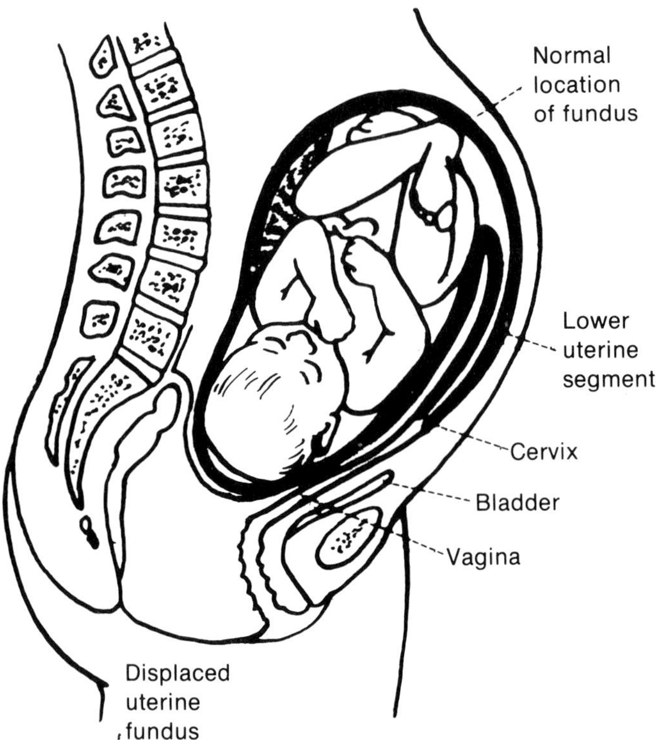


**Fig. 39–7.** Sagittal section (full fetal view) demonstrating the incarcerated retroverted gravid uterus. (Redrawn from Keating PJ, Walton SM, Maouris P: Incarceration of a bicornuate retroverted gravid uterus presenting with bilateral ureteric obstruction. Br. J. Obstet. Gynaecol. 99:345, 1992.)

in early pregnancy and usually develops after the twentieth week of gestation. The right side is dilated greater than the left in 86% of cases.[35] The kidney itself also increases approximately 1 cm in length during normal gestation. The increment in size is likely due to enhanced glomerular filtration rate and upper tract dilatation. One very remarkable case of gross hydronephrosis occurred in a patient who presented with bilateral uterine obstruction. This patient was delivered by cesarean section, at which time it was discovered that the patient also had incarceration of a bicornuate retroverted gravid uterus (Figure 39–7).[36]

The most common surgical entity of the urinary tract during pregnancy is calculus disease. The incidence of ureteral calculi found during pregnancy ranges from 0.05% to 0.35%.[37] Its presentation may be confused and overlap with those of acute cystitis and pyelonephritis. Failure to respond to appropriate antibiotic therapy in a pregnant woman with pyelonephritis should prompt consideration of calculus disease.

Nonobstructing stones may be unrecognized until they lodge within the ureter. Microhematuria may only be observed in 50% of these cases.[37] Flank pain, dysuria, urgency, nausea, and vomiting are common presenting symptoms. If a stone is suspected, a limited excretory urogram is performed. A flat plate followed by a 20-minute delay film will often suffice.

Management of calculi is generally not different from that in the nonpregnant population. The majority of stones will pass spontaneously, requiring narcotics and vigorous hydration. Conservative management is the rule, although unrelenting pain, obstruction, and unresponsive infection require active surgical intervention. A ureteral catheter may be passed or even a percutaneous nephrostomy performed if laparotomy is to be avoided. One such example of a Hippuran I 131 isotope study where percutaneous nephrostomy to relieve renal obstruction in the right kidney was used is shown in Figure 39–8.[38] This

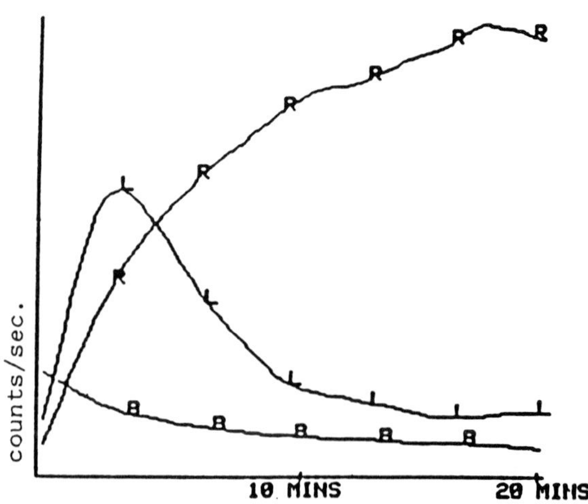


**Fig. 39–8.** Different $^{131}$I isotope excretion curves performed at 25 weeks gestation. (From Trewhella M, Reid B, Gillespie A, Jones D: Percutaneous nephrostomy to relieve renal tract obstruction in pregnancy. Br. J. Radiol. 64:471, 1991.)

1991 case was noted as being the first case report of percutaneous nephrotomy being performed during pregnancy. The 1991 case and a 1984 case by F.H. Renny[39] reported by Lewis in 1985[40] signify that this operative intervention during pregnancy is indeed rare yet effective. Open surgery or a new technique of ultrasonic stone destruction via a ureteral approach can be used safely throughout pregnancy without the presence of significant preterm labor.[37,41] General anesthesia has been employed in the majority of these cases due to positioning demands.

## *Traumatic Injury*

Trauma is the most frequent cause of death of women younger than age 35 in the United States.[42] Trauma is a leading nonobstetric cause of maternal mortality, accounting for approximately 20% of deaths during pregnancy. It has been suggested that the pregnant woman is at increased risk for trauma with the incidence of accidental injury being reported at 7%.[43] However, this was a 1963 study, and a recent 1992 study of a 5-year period of ICU admissions revealed no admissions were directly related to trauma (Table 39–6).[44] Alteration in habitus with impairment in balance increases the risk of trauma as pregnancy advances.[45]

Minor trauma is rarely associated with poor maternal or fetal outcome. In contrast, the severely injured gravida is at great risk and requires appropriate emergency medical care. A multidisciplinary team approach is required as the emergency room personnel rarely care for the gravid female, just as the perinatal team uncommonly treats the trauma victim. The obstetrician, emergency room physician, trauma surgeon, anesthesiologist, and neonatologist form the team required to render expert care in this setting. An organized approach to the pregnant trauma victim requires an understanding of maternal-fetal physiology and its alterations which may impact on the fetoplacental unit. The basic approach of the ABCs of trauma are applied to the gravid woman. Patency of the airway and adequate ventilation are primary considerations. Supplemental oxygen should be administered until a blood gas determination is performed. The unconscious patient should be evaluated for spontaneous respiration and, if absent, endotracheal intubation and mechanical ventilation should be accomplished. General anesthesia is preferred in all of the following trauma-associated problems due to the need for airway protection and control of ventilation. As a full stomach may at least functionally exist, antacid administration may reduce the risk of aspiration in these patients. Maintenance of blood pressure and blood volume is essential to both maternal and fetal well-being. Significantly greater blood and volume replacement may be required by the pregnant individual because of the expanded state associated with pregnancy. At a minimum, a single large-bore intravenous catheter is introduced. In unstable patients, a second large-bone line should be placed.

The massively bleeding patient requires prompt replacement of intravascular volume. Lactated Ringer's solution administered in volumes larger than the estimated blood loss may be successful in returning the fetal heart rate to normal. For hypotensive patients, fresh whole blood is ideal, as it has sufficient coagulation factors, platelets, and adequate levels of 2,3-diphosphoglycerate. Type-specific banked blood should be used in emergent situations where full crossmatching would be too time-consuming. If whole blood is unavailable, packed cells and plasma are an alternative. Packed cells and crystalloid or crystalloid alone are less effective at restoring volume.

The serious trauma victim should have several standard laboratory studies performed. These include: type and crossmatch, complete blood count with platelets, SMA-

**Table 39–6.** Admitting Diagnoses to the ICU

| | | Admitting Diagnoses | | |
|---|---|---|---|---|
| Primary Diagnoses | No. | Respiratory Failure | Hemodynamic Instability | Neurologic Dysfunction |
| Obstetric | 21 | | | |
| Preeclampsia | 7 | 1 | 3 | 3 |
| Sepsis/infection | 5 | 2 | 3 | |
| Hemorrhage | 4 | | 4 | |
| AFLP* | 3 | 1 | 1 | 1 |
| Pulmonary edema† | 2 | 2 | | |
| Nonobstetric | 11 | | | |
| Pneumonia | 3 | 3 | | |
| Asthma | 1 | 1 | | |
| Cardiac | 2 | | 2 | |
| Substance OD* | 2 | 1 | | 1 |
| Guillain-Barré syndrome | 1 | 1 | | |
| Myasthenia gravis | 1 | | | 1 |
| Sepsis | 1 | 1 | | |
| Totals | 32 | 13 (41%) | 13 (41%) | 6 (18%) |

* AFLP acute fatty liver of pregnancy; OD = overdose.
† Pulmonary edema was associated with obstetric events: one patient with triplets was receiving oral tocolytics and one patient had fetal surgery.
(From Kilpatrick SJ, Matthay MA: Obstetric patients requiring critical care.* A five-year review. Chest. 101:1407–12, 1992.)

**Table 39–7.** Approach to the Pregnant Trauma Patient

Management
1. Evaluate cardiopulmonary status—begin CPR if necessary.
2. Control hemorrhage and evaluate the need for surgery. Establish large-bore intravenous access.
3. Maintain lateral decubitus position.
4. Maintain maternal $pO_2 > 60$ mm Hg.
5. Volume replacement/Transfusion as necessary.
6. Fetal monitoring.
7. Foley catheter.

Evaluation
1. CBC, electrolytes.
2. Type and crossmatch.
3. Arterial blood gas.
4. Serum amylase.
5. Urinalysis.
6. Peritoneal lavage as appropriate.
7. Radiologic studies.

6, urinalysis, and coagulation panel, including fibrinogen levels and serum amylase. The baseline coagulation studies are particularly important in cases of abdominal trauma, where abruptio placentae is a known complication. As fibrinogen concentrations double in normal pregnancy, levels below 250 mg/dl are often indicative of a coagulopathy. An easy, rapid test to assess coagulation status is to determine clot formation time in a plain red top tube. Clot formation should occur within 5 to 7 minutes. While maternal stabilization is being accomplished, fetal monitoring should be instituted. Continuous fetal monitoring may be a useful adjunct in treatment. For example, late decelerations may respond to volume replacement and allow further stabilization of the mother. However, unresponsive fetal distress in a hemodynamically stable mother demands prompt delivery. Table 39–7 lists the management and evaluation steps to be taken in the approach to the pregnant trauma patient. The reader is referred to Chapter 43 for a detailed description of intensive care management.

## *Specific Injuries*

### Head and Chest Injury

Severe head or chest injury demand full attention as these types of trauma are often life-threatening. Patients in coma or those bleeding with increased pressure or brain trauma require prompt neurosurgical intervention. Fetal consideration often becomes secondary in these cases. Similarly, thoracic injury with open chest wounds must be managed expeditiously, as exsanguination of the mother will lead to fetal death as well. Antemortem cesarean section should be considered when maternal survival seems unlikely. This may be preferable to postmortem cesarean section which is generally carried out only if gestational age exceeds 28 weeks. Postmortem cesarean section requires anticipation of maternal death with continued resuscitation (ventilation and cardiac massage) accompanied by prompt delivery.

### Blunt Abdominal Injury

Mild abdominal trauma rarely results in fetal compromise.[46] Prolonged fetal monitoring is recommended following such events. Some have suggested routine performance of the Kleihauer-Betke test to determine if fetomaternal bleeding has occurred.

Automobile accidents are the most common cause of serious abdominal trauma in pregnancy.[44] In pregnant women involved in serious car accidents, the maternal mortality has been reported to be 7.2%.[47] Fetal mortality is nearly twice as likely. Uterine rupture can occur with blunt abdominal trauma. Crosby and coworkers have demonstrated marked increases in intrauterine pressure in primates subjected to acute deceleration injuries.[46] These authors specify that untoward fetal effects are only likely to be significant if uterine rupture or placental abruption follows blunt trauma.

Direct fetal injury is rare as the fetus is cushioned by amniotic fluid, the anterior abdominal wall, and uterus. In spite of this, skull and long-bone fetal fractures have been reported. Skull fractures are most likely to occur in late pregnancy accompanying maternal pelvic fracture. A maternal pelvic fracture, unless producing true bony obstruction, is not an indication for cesarean delivery.[48]

The potential for intraperitoneal bleeding must be considered in patients sustaining blunt abdominal trauma. Peritoneal lavage is advocated when there are: (1) multiple severe injuries including thoracic injury; (2) abdominal signs and symptoms of intraperitoneal hemorrhage; and (3) hypotensive shock. An open technique as opposed to blind paracentesis is suggested, particularly in late pregnancy.[49] A positive paracentesis consists of: (1) free-flowing blood; (2) lavage fluid in the Foley catheter; or (3) a red cell count more than 100 000/mm$^3$. If one of these criteria are met, laparotomy is indicated.

### Penetrating Abdominal Injury

Gunshot wounds and knife stabbings are the most common penetrating injuries found in pregnant women. The uterus is the most likely organ to be involved in such cases. When the uterus is involved, fetal injury occurs in 59% to 89% of cases, whereas fetal mortality varies from 41% to 71%.[50] Penetrating gunshot wounds always require exploratory laparotomy. Primary repair of bowel and urinary tract injuries is accomplished in cases where the uterus is intact. Incidental cesarean section offers little advantage in this situation. If uterine injury is encountered, and the fetus is beyond 32 weeks gestation, delivery is recommended. In the period between 28 to 32 weeks, the ease of uterine repair and presence of possible fetal injury will mandate whether delivery is undertaken.

The management of stab wounds is somewhat controversial. However, when the extent of injury is in doubt, laparotomy is indicated. Peritoneal lavage or fistulogram studies may reduce the need for exploration in certain cases. If intrathoracic or intraperitoneal penetration is suspected, exploration is necessary.

Uterine injury is common with stab wounds. A cesarean section should be performed if fetal injury is encountered in the third trimester. Fetal fractures and wounds have been reported to heal in utero.[44] Thus, in the previable fetus (less than 26 weeks), observation is undertaken in lieu of cesarean delivery. Small uterine injuries may be closed primarily, although a substantial risk for preterm labor and delivery does exist. If labor ensues, preterm vaginal delivery is preferable to cesarean section in such cases.

The pregnant woman requiring surgery represents a considerable challenge to both the anesthesiologist and obstetrician. Altered maternal anatomy and physiology may make the diagnosis of surgical complications more difficult. Delay in providing surgical care when indicated (eg, appendicitis, perforated viscus) is clearly responsible for increased maternal morbidity and perinatal mortality. However, when surgical care is not emergent, it is best deferred until the second trimester or during the puerperium. Anesthetic concerns center on the potential teratogenecity of anesthetic agents during the first trimester, appropriate oxygenation, and avoidance of spine hypotension. In most cases, surgical procedures are well tolerated by mother and fetus, making preterm delivery unnecessary.

## REFERENCES


1. Brent RL: The effects of embryonic and fetal exposure to X-ray, microwaves, and ultrasound. Clin. Perinatol. 13:615, 1986.
2. Shnider SM, Webster GM. Maternal and fetal hazards of surgery during pregnancy. Am. J. Obstet. Gynecol. 92:891, 1965.
3. Spence AA, Knill-Jones RP: Is there a health hazard in anesthetic practice? Br. J. Anaesth. 50:713, 1978.
4. Babaknia A, Parsa H, Woodruff JD: Appendicitis during pregnancy. Obstet. Gynecol. 50:40, 1977.
5. Cunningham FG, McDubbin JH: Appendicitis complicating pregnancy. Obstet. Gynecol. 45:415, 1975.
6. Abu Zidan FM, Al-Hilaly MA, Al-Atrabi N: Torsion of a mucocele of the appendix in a pregnant woman. Acta. Obstet. Gynecol. Scand. 71:140–142, 1992.
7. Baer JL, Reis RA, Arens RA: Appendicitis in pregnancy with changes in position and axis of the normal appendix in pregnancy. JAMA 98:1359, 1932.
8. Wernstein L: Syndrome of hemolysis, elevated liver enzymes, and low platelet count: A severe consequence of hypertension in pregnancy. Am. J. Obstet. Gynecol. 142: 159, 1982.
9. Sibai BM, Anderson GD: Hypertension. *In* Obstetrics: Normal & Problem Pregnancies. 2nd Ed. SG Gabbe, JR Niebyl, JL Simpson. New York, Churchill Livingstone, 1991, pp. 993–1055.
10. Cheng YS: Pregnancy in liver cirrhosis and/or portal hypertension. Am. J. Obstet. Gynecol. 110:1100, 1971.
11. Brown HJ: Splenorenal shunt during pregnancy. Am. J. Surg. 37:441, 1971.
12. Walcott WO, Derick DE, Jolley JJ, Snyder DL, et al: Successful pregnancy in a liver transplant patient. Am. J. Obstet. Gynecol. 132:340, 1978.
13. Myers RL, Schmid R, Newton JJ: Childbirth after liver transplantation. Transplantation. 29:432, 1980.
14. Newton ER, Tovksoy N, Kaplan M, Reinhold R: Pregnancy and liver transplantation. Obstet. Gynecol. 71:499, 1988.
15. Haagsma EB, Visser GH, Klompmaker IJ, Verwer R, et al: Successful pregnancy after orthotopic liver transplantation. Obstet. Gynecol. 74:442, 1989.
16. Fair J, Klein AS, Feng T, Merritt WT, et al: Intrapartum orthotopic liver transplantation with successful outcome of pregnancy. Transplantation 50:534–535, 1990.
17. Moreno EG, García GI, Gómez SR, González-Pinto I, et al: Fulminant hepatic failure during pregnancy successfully treated by orthotopic liver transplantation. Transplantation 52:923–926, 1991.
18. Kammerer WS: Nonobstetric surgery during pregnancy. Med. Clin. North Am. 63:1157, 1979.
19. Bennion LJ, Grundy SM: Risk factors for the development of cholelithiasis in man. N. Engl. J. Med. 229:1221, 1978.
20. McKellar DP, Anderson CT, Boynton CJ, Peoples JB: Cholecystectomy during pregnancy without fetal loss. Surg. Gynecol. Obstet. 174:465–468, 1992.
21. Printen KJ, Ott RA: Cholecystectomy during pregnancy. Am. Surg. 44:432, 1978.
22. Byrd BF, Bayer DS, Robertson JC: Treatment of breast tumors associated with pregnancy and lactation. Ann. Surg. 155:940, 1962.
23. Donnegan WL: Cancer and pregnancy. CA. 33:194, 1983.
24. White TT, White WC: Breast cancer and pregnancy: Report of 49 cases followed 5 years. Ann. Surg. 144:384, 1956.
25. Thomas DB: Do hormones cause breast cancer? Cancer 53: 595, 1984.
26. Hopkins MP, Duchon MA: Adnexal surgeon in pregnancy. J. Reprod. Med. 31:1035, 1986.
27. Hill LM, Johnson CE, Lee RA: Ovarian surgery in pregnancy. Am. J. Obstet. Gynecol. 122:565, 1975.
28. Niswander KR, Gordon M, Berendes HW: The Women and Their Pregnancies. Philadelphia, W.B. Saunders, 1972.
29. Mestman JH, Manning PR, Hodgman J: Hyperthyroidism and pregnancy. Arch. Intern. Med. 134:4334, 1974.
30. Bruner JP, Landon MB, Gabbe SG: Diabetes mellitus and Grave's disease in pregnancy. Obstet. Gynecol. 72:443, 1988.
31. Shangold MM, Doz N, Welt SI: Hyperparathyroidism and pregnancy: A review. Obstet. Gynecol. Surv. 37:217, 1982.
32. Montora MM, Collea JV, Mestman JH: Management of hyperparathyroidism in pregnancy with oral phosphate therapy. Obstet. Gynecol. 55:431, 1980.
33. Schenker JG, Chowers I: Pheochromocytoma and pregnancy. Review of 89 cases. Obstet. Gynecol. Surv. 26:1173, 1971.
34. Dunlop W: Serial changes in renal hemodynamics during normal human pregnancy. Br. J. Obstet. Gynecol. 88:1, 1981.
35. Fayad MM, Youssef AF, Zahran MC: The ureterocalyceal system in normal pregnancy. Acta. Obstet. Gynecol. Scand. 52: 69, 1973.
36. Keating PJ, Walton SM, Maouris P: Incarceration of a bicornuate retroverted gravid uterus presenting with bilateral ureteric obstruction. Br. J. Obstet. Gynaecol. 99:345–347, 1992.
37. Harris RE, Dunnihoo DR: The incidence and significance of urinary calculi in pregnancy. Am. J. Obstet. Gynecol. 99: 237, 1967.
38. Trewhella M, Reid B, Gillespie A, Jones D: Percutaneous nephrostomy to relieve renal tract obstruction in pregnancy. Br. J. Radiol. 64:471–472, 1991.
39. Renny RH: Percutaneous nephrostomy to relive renal tract obstruction in pregnancy. Br. J. Radiol. 64:976, 1991.
40. Lewis GJ, Chatterjee SP, Rowse AD: Acute renal failure in pregnancy secondary to idiopathic hydronephrosis. Br. Med. J. 290:1250, 1985.
41. Freed SZ, Herig N: Urology in pregnancy. Baltimore, Williams & Wilkins, 1982, p. 150.
42. National Safety Council: Accidental Facts. Chicago, 1975.
43. Peckham CH, King RW: A study of intercurrent conditions

observed during pregnancy. Am. J. Obstet. Gynecol. 87:609, 1963.

44. Kilpatrick SJ, Matthay MA: Obstetric patients requiring critical care.* A five-year review. Chest 101:1407–12, 1992.
45. Crosby WM: Trauma during pregnancy. Maternal and fetal injury. Obstet. Gynecol. Surv. 29:683, 1974.
46. Fort AJ, Harli RS: Pregnancy outcome after noncatastrophic maternal trauma during pregnancy. Obstet. Gynecol. 35: 912, 1970.
47. Crosby WM, Costiloe DJ: Safety of lap-belt restraint for pregnant victims of automobile collisions. N. Engl. J. Med. 284: 362, 1971.
48. Speer DP, Peltier LF: Pelvic fractures and pregnancy. J. Trauma. 12:474, 1972.
49. Rothenberger DA, Quattlebaum FW, Zabel J: Diagnostic peritoneal lavage for blunt trauma in pregnant women. Am. J. Obstet. Gynecol. 129:479, 1977.
50. Buchsbaum HJ: Penetrating Injury of the Abdomen. *In* Trauma in Pregnancy. Edited by HJ Buchsbaum: Philadelphia, W.B. Saunders, 1979.

Section I

# OBSTETRIC ANALGESIA AND ANESTHESIA FOR FETAL COMPLICATIONS

# Chapter 40

# ANTEPARTUM FETAL EVALUATION AND SURVEILLANCE

ROGER K. FREEMAN

Antepartum fetal evaluation and surveillance are the keystone elements in assuring the health and well-being of the growing fetus. These measures continue up to and include the intrapartum period, during which the greatest stresses to the fetus occur because of both the labor process and the delivery process. The oxygenation removal of $CO_2$ and the blood flow in the placenta maintain growth and development in the healthy fetus. The methods currently in use today, a correlation with outcome, a discussion of the use of sonography, the current status of intrapartum fetal monitoring, and a discussion of anesthetic considerations follow.

## ANTEPARTUM FETAL SURVEILLANCE FOR WELL-BEING

The primary aim of antepartum fetal surveillance is to detect evidence of uteroplacental insufficiency (UPI). Uteroplacental insufficiency is defined as a deficient function of the placenta in terms of oxygenation of, and carbon dioxide removal from the fetus. Current methods available for identification of fetal well-being are reviewed in Table 40–1.

### Auscultation

Listening for fetal heart tones is done during most prenatal visits. Unfortunately, unless one attempts to evaluate the presence of reactivity, which is hard to do by auscultation, this has very little value during the third trimester other than to document whether the fetus is alive or dead. During the first trimester, after the eighth to tenth week, it is possible to document fetal heart activity by Doppler; this may be very useful in evaluating a patient with a threatened abortion, or when there is a question of a missed abortion. Certainly, when there is a question of fetal well-being after the twenty-sixth week, simple auscultation is insufficient to answer any question other than to document life.

### *Assessment of Fetal Movement*

Long before electronic monitoring devices were available, clinicians recognized that a perceived decrease in fetal movement could be a sign of impending fetal death. In a prospectively randomized antepartum fetal surveillance study by Neldam,[1] 1000 patients followed by a fetal-movement-counting protocol had no antepartum fetal deaths, compared to 1000 patients followed with no fetal-movement-counting protocol with 8 fetal deaths. This certainly supports the value of this method as reasonable for use by all patients. In our experience, however, many patients who perceive a decrease in fetal movements subsequently have normally reactive nonstress tests (NSTs) with obvious fetal movement when tested. It has also been long recognized that the reliability of the patient as an observer of fetal movement is less than perfect. Inasmuch as this method of fetal surveillance costs nothing and, when done in a systematic fashion, may contribute significantly to the detection of otherwise unsuspected fetal jeopardy, its use is recommended, especially in low risk populations.

Sadovsky has been responsible for the systematization of an approach to the assessment of fetal well-being.[2] If there are more than three movements in 30 minutes, the fetus is considered to be in good condition, but fewer than three movements in 30 minutes indicates either a fetal sleep state, or that there may be reason for concern, and further counting should continue. At this point we instruct our patients to count for another 30 minutes, and if there are less than three movements in the second counting period, we ask the patient to come to the hospital for an NST. If the NST is nonreactive, subsequent management is according to antepartum fetal heart rate testing (AFHRT) protocols. If the NST is reactive (which is usually the case), the patient is reassured and asked to continue her counting schedule. At the time of the NST, we like to teach the patient more about counting movement, since the reason for her decreased movement count is often due not to lack of fetal movement, but rather to her lack of recognition of that movement. When simultaneous real-time ultrasound scanning has been done with patients who were asked to note the fetal movements, there have usually been more movements observed by ultrasound than perceived by the patient.[3] Most patients feel three movements in just a few minutes, so that this technique requires very little of the patient's time.

Sadovsky has shown that when the fetal movement count drops below 3 in 12 hours, or when movements cease for 12 hours, fetal death is imminent; he designates this ominous drop in movement count the movement alarm signal (MAS).[4,5,6] He has also ranked various ante-

**Table 40–1.** Fetal Surveillance Methods

1. Auscultation of fetal heart tones
2. Assessment of fetal movement
3. Measurement of uterine growth
4. Assessment of fetal heart rate
5. Sonography

partum tests according to the sequence with which they become abnormal in a fetus in jeopardy (Table 40–2).[2]

## *Assessment of Uterine Growth*

During the third trimester of pregnancy, the assessment of uterine growth should be done on all patients at the time of their routine prenatal visits. As a general rule, the fundal height in centimeters as measured with a tape measure will equal the number of weeks of gestation (Figure 40–1). Several factors could negate this relationship (Table 40–3) and, except for maternal obesity, which would already be obvious, the other causes are all things about which the clinician would want to know. Specifically, abnormalities in the amniotic fluid volume may lead to the diagnosis of a fetal malformation or intrauterine growth retardation (IUGR). Thus, abnormalities in the gross uterine size or abnormal growth rates of the fundal height should lead to further investigation with either sonography or fetal heart rate testing. Unfortunately, the accuracy of clinical assessment leaves something to be desired. In a recent study from our institution, the diagnosis of IUGR by clinical estimates had very poor correlation with outcome measurements.[7] Generally speaking, however, any time the uterine size is significantly larger or smaller than expected for gestational age, or there is a lack of uterine growth, or a decrease in the rate of growth, the patient should be evaluated by sonography. If the findings suggest uteroplacental insufficiency, AFHRT or biophysical profile testing (BPP) should be used.

## *Antepartum Fetal Heart Rate Testing*

In 1961, Hon observed *late deceleration* of the fetal heart rate following maternal exercise in patients with clinical UPI.[8] Late deceleration is typically a slowing of the fetal heart rate that begins after the peak of contraction. In the mid-1960s, others reported an association between late deceleration after oxytocin-induced uterine contractions prior to labor and other signs of UPI, including IUGR,

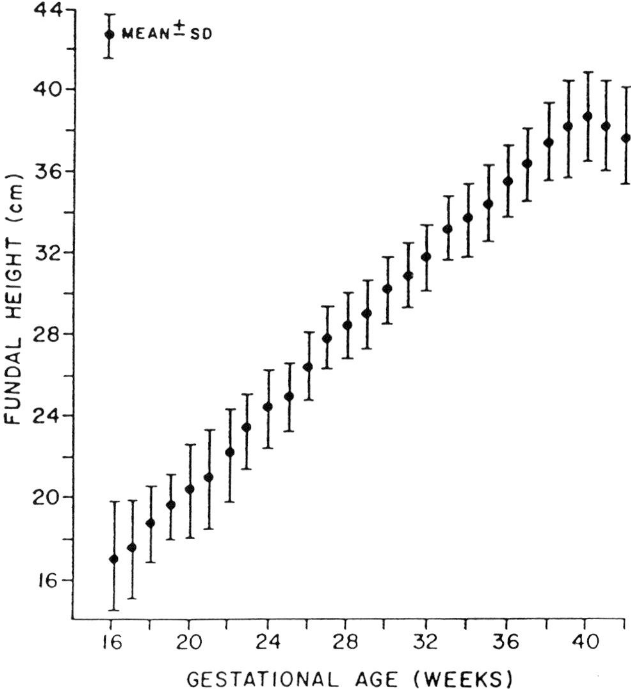


**Fig. 40–1.** Fundal height versus gestational age. (From Johnson TRB, Walker MA, Niebyl JR: Preconception and prenatal care. *In* Obstetrics: Normal and Problem Pregnancies. 2nd ed. Edited by SG Gabbe, JR Niebyl, JL Simpson. New York, Churchill Livingstone, 1991, p. 227.)

late deceleration and fetal acidosis during subsequent labor, and, in the extreme case, fetal death.[9–11]

In 1972, we reported on a group of high-risk patients studied systematically with the oxytocin challenge test (OCT) and found a relationship between a positive OCT and subsequent fetal death, but perhaps more importantly, the reassuring value of a negative OCT in predicting the absence of fetal death for the subsequent week.[12] Several subsequent studies have supported the value of the OCT, which is better referred to as the contraction stress test (CST).[13–15] The CST is time consuming and may be difficult to interpret; there are significant numbers of equivocal and false-positive tests.[16] Because of this, the nonstress test (NST) has gained popularity as people have realized that acceleration with fetal movement (reactivity) is a very good measure of fetal well-being at the time the test is done. Actually, the two methods are complementary

**Table 40–2.** Sadovsky's Sequence of Abnormal Tests Prior to Fetal Death

1. Contraction stress test
2. Nonstress test
3. Decreased fetal movement
4. Movement alarm signal
5. Severe changes on nonstress test

**Table 40–3.** Factors Which Negate Fundal Height = Weeks Gestation Relationship

1. Maternal obesity
2. Multiple gestation
3. Polyhydramnios
4. Abnormal fetal lie
5. Oligohydramnios
6. Fetal growth retardation

and, indeed, reactivity is an important part of the interpretation of a CST, and the fetal heart rate response to any spontaneously occurring uterine contractions is an important part of the interpretation of the NST. There does remain, however, a controversy as to the best method for primary surveillance. In addition, real-time ultrasound and the BPP are being utilized by many for surveillance of the fetus at risk for chronic UPI. The following sections will describe the methodology and interpretation for the CST, NST, and BPP.

## *The Contraction Stress Test*

### Methodology

The best equipment for performing antepartum testing today employs Doppler ultrasound with second- or third-generation logic systems using either short-term averaging or autocorrelation. The test should be done with a one-to-one nurse/patient ratio and should not be relegated to the labor-and-delivery area with a busy nurse who cannot be with the patient throughout the test. The conduction of the CST is done as follows in our unit:

1. The patient is placed in the semi-Fowler position, often in mild lateral tilt to prevent supine hypotension.
2. The fetal monitor is attached and a baseline fetal heart rate (FHR) and uterine contraction recording is made to determine the baseline rate, reactivity, and uterine contraction frequency, if any.
3. The mother's blood pressure is recorded before, then every 10 to 15 minutes during the test with special attention to any supine hypotension which may affect the test result.
4. If there are fewer than three uterine contractions per 10-minute period, uterine contractions are stimulated as follows.
   A. Nipple stimulation: The patient is asked to begin unilateral nipple massage through her clothing and to tug and roll the nipple for 5 minutes. If uterine activity does not begin, bilateral stimulation is used. There are many variations on the exact methodology and timing of stimulation, but most investigators indicate about 70% effectiveness with this method.
   B. Oxytocin stimulation: If the patient fails to respond to breast stimulation, an IV is started and an infusion of dilute oxytocin is begun at 0.5 to 1.0 mU per minute. This is increased every 15 to 20 minutes until uterine activity of three contractions per 10 minute interval is achieved. The oxytocin is then turned off and the fetal monitor tracing is observed until uterine activity returns to baseline levels.

### Interpretation

***Negative.*** A test is considered negative if there are no late decelerations with a contraction frequency of 3 in 10 minutes. With most negative tests, there is good fetal reactivity. Causes for reduced fetal reactivity with a negative CST include maternal sedation, congenital malformations and gestational age under 30 weeks. One must be sure that, if a test is nonreactive and negative, there are no very subtle late decelerations present that are being missed, especially if there is significant Doppler artifact on the FHR.

***Positive.*** If late decelerations are present with more than 50% of the uterine contractions, the test is positive (Figure 40–2). Once late decelerations are seen, the test should be continued to determine if they will be persistent. Late decelerations with absent fetal reactivity (a nonreactive positive test) may be very subtle.

***Equivocal.*** If late decelerations are present but intermittent, or if they do not persist, the test is only suspicious. Sometimes, late decelerations will occur with excessive uterine activity, or there may be prolonged or variable decelerations present, in which case the test would also be regarded as equivocal. Variable or prolonged decelerations may indicate oligohydramnios.

***Unsatisfactory.*** If the FHR cannot be clearly seen, or if the uterine activity does not reach a frequency of 3 in 10 minutes, the test is not satisfactory.

***Sinusoidal.*** A sinusoidal pattern (Figure 40–3) is considered ominous. It has been reported with severe erythroblastosis fetalis, fetal-maternal hemorrhage, and severe intrapartum asphyxia. It is always nonreactive and is present during the whole test, but may alternate with flat heart rate.

### Management

The CST, when negative, appears to be very reliable in predicting the absence of fetal death within 1 week.[17] Under certain circumstances, it is wise to shorten this testing interval, even if the last test was negative (Table 40–4). Equivocal tests should be repeated in 24 hours. They are not reassuring, but they do not usually herald rapid fetal deterioration. Reactions to equivocal tests should be tempered by consideration of the overall clinical situation.

Patients with positive CSTs are uncommon but demand careful management. With a reactive fetus, the chance is about 50% that the test is false-positive as measured by fetal distress in subsequent labor.[12] However, if the fetus is mature, intervention will almost always result in a fetus in good condition. A trial of labor, preferably with internal monitoring, is appropriate in these patients if the cervix is at all favorable. If a reactive positive CST occurs prior to fetal maturity, we follow the NST on a daily basis and

**Table 40–4.** Indications for Shortening Interval Between Contraction Stress Tests

A. Change in maternal status such as:
   1. Worsening hypertension or preeclampsia
   2. Deterioration of diabetic control
   3. Vaginal bleeding
B. Change in fetal status such as:
   1. Decreased or absent movement
   2. Falling estriol
   3. Discovery of meconium at the time of amniocentesis

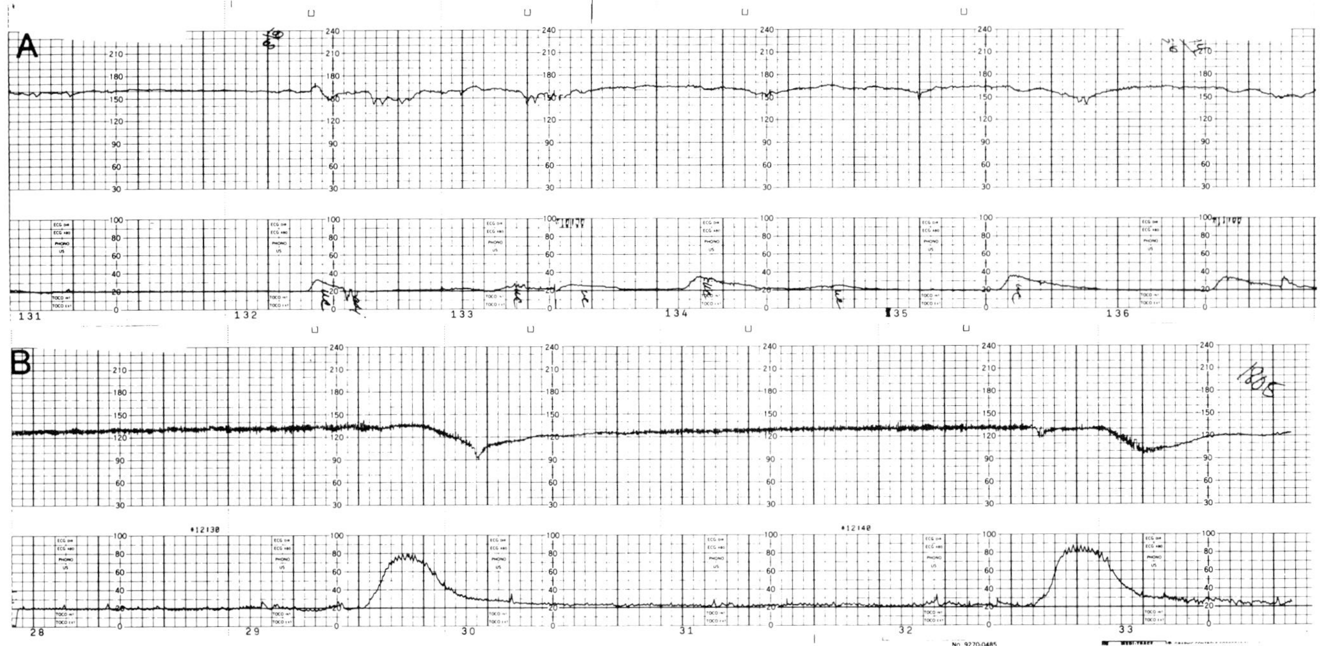

**Fig. 40–2.** Nonreactive positive contraction stress tests using oxytocin. **A,** Note that while some minimal longterm variability is present, there are no accelerations that meet the criteria for reactivity. **B,** Note that there is no longterm variability and there is complete absence of accelerations. The contraction frequency is less than 10 minutes, but with a tracing like this it is not necessary to stimulate further. (From Freeman RK, Garite J, Nageotte P: Fetal Heart Rate Monitoring. 2nd Ed. Baltimore, Williams & Wilkins, 1991.)

avoid intervention as long as reactivity is present and fetal maturity has not been demonstrated.

Patients with completely nonreactive positive CSTs do not tolerate labor in our experience,[18] and the likelihood of more benefit from continued intrauterine existence is doubtful; in fact, the risk of intrauterine death if not delivered is great. For this reason, if gestation is over 30 to 32 weeks, we recommend delivery by cesarean section even prior to demonstrated pulmonary maturity. If the patient is below 30 to 32 weeks, the absence of reactivity may be a function of prematurity rather than fetal jeopardy, and since intervention is much more risky for the fetus at this stage, we use daily BPP studies in such situations, and avoid intervention unless the BPP is significantly abnormal.

## *The Nonstress Test*

### Methodology

The fetal heart rate and uterine activity are recorded as noted under stress testing.

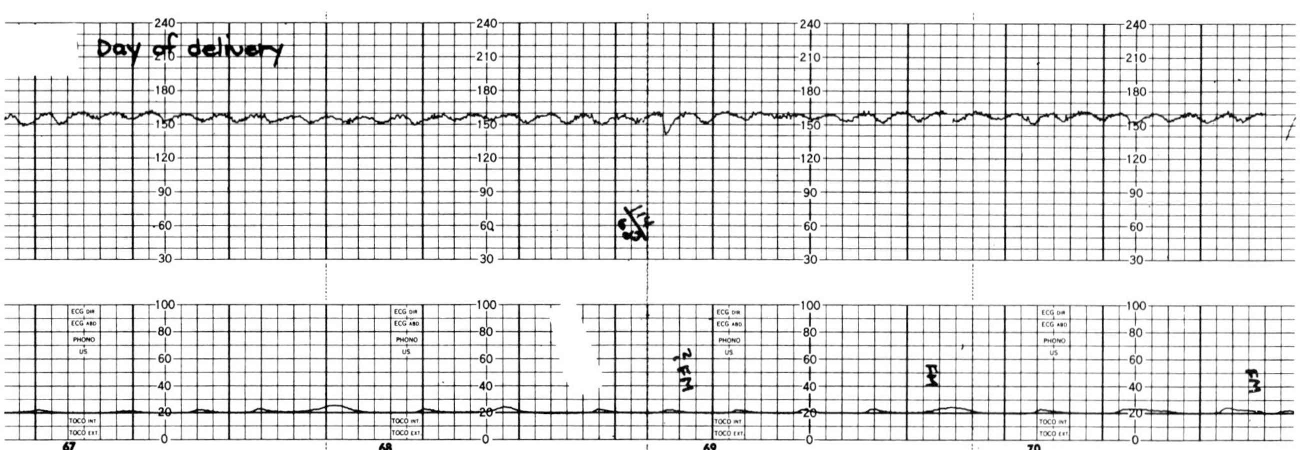


**Fig. 40–3.** Antepartum sinusoidal heart rate pattern. The sine wave, a longterm variability, may be seen to fluctuate above and below the baseline, is constant, and may be seen with late decelerations. This often represents severe fetal anemia or hypoxia. (From Freeman RK, Garite J, Nageotte P: Fetal Heart Rate Monitoring. 2nd ed. Baltimore, Williams & Wilkins, 1991.)

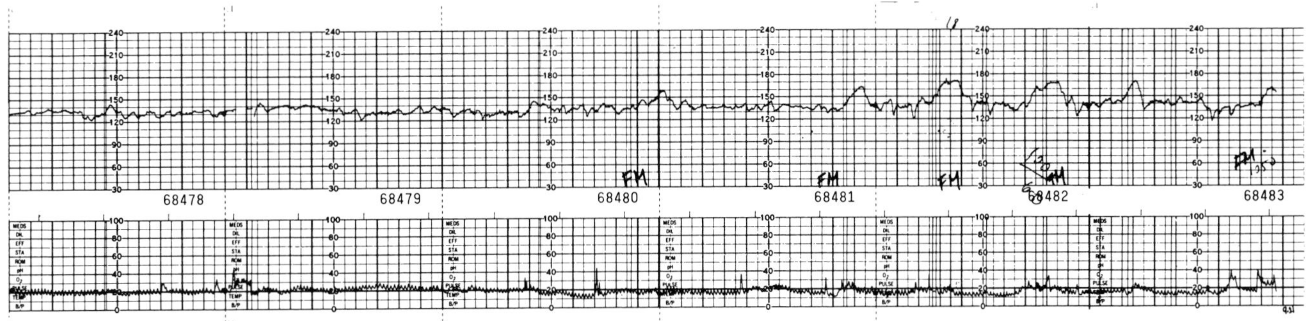


**Fig. 40–4.** Reactive nonstress test showing accelerations associated with fetal movement, marked by the notation "FM." (From Freeman RK, Garite J, Nageotte P: Fetal Heart Rate Monitoring. 2nd Ed. Baltimore, Williams & Wilkins, 1991.)

## Interpretation

The definition of what constitutes adequate fetal reactivity is not universally agreed upon. Most people use a definition of FHR acceleration of 15 beats per minute lasting 15 seconds from onset to offset, occurring twice in 20 minutes (Figure 40–4). It has been shown that when FHR accelerations occur, there are virtually always fetal movements present, but when fetal movement occurs, there is not always an accompanying acceleration of the FHR.[3] The definition of nonreactivity is anything that does not meet the criteria for reactivity. Most clinicians do not feel that the above criteria are applicable to very premature fetuses; often the magnitude of change is much less in fetuses under 30 weeks gestation. If spontaneously occurring uterine contractions elicit decelerations, the test should be interpreted as a CST and, indeed, it may become necessary to induce uterine contractions in such situations in order to determine the significance of these decelerations. Many clinicians feel that the presence of spontaneously occurring decelerations is more ominous than those elicited by induced contractions.[19]

## Management

Most clinicians use the NST on a weekly basis if it is reactive. However, recently some authors have recommended more frequent testing in postdate pregnancies,[20] and perhaps in diabetics. In addition, the recommendation has been made to combine the NST with real-time scanning in order to improve its predictive power. If the NST is nonreactive, it should be followed by an immediate CST or BPP. Many times the nonreactive fetus will become reactive during the CST.

## *The Biophysical Profile*

Manning and Platt[21] have developed a technique, called the biophysical profile (BPP), that utilizes real-time ultrasound to assess fetal well-being. With this technique, five parameters are studied and a score of 0 or 2 is assigned to each (Table 40–5). In their original study, Manning and Platt found no perinatal mortality if all parameters were normal (score = 10), and 60% mortality if all parameters were abnormal (score = 0). A subsequent study by Baskett, et al[22] in 2400 high risk pregnancies showed that only 1.2% of biophysical profiles were abnormal and 1.7% were equivocal. Their corrected perinatal mortality rate was 1:1000.

In our experience, when using the CST for primary surveillance, the BPP is useful in assessing the nonreactive fetus prior to 30 weeks gestation, where the lack of reactivity may be a function of immaturity rather than jeopardy. The role of this technique for primary surveillance is currently increasing. Data suggest that it is comparable to contraction stress testing with fewer equivocal tests.[22] A randomized prospective trial comparing the BPP to the CST for primary surveillance is clearly needed.

## *Correlation With Outcome*

On review of the literature, the incidence of a fetal death within 1 week of a negative CST is about 2:1000 patients tested, and many of those deaths were due to causes other than UPI.[17] A collaborative study involving over 7000 patients and over 18 000 tests compared patients followed with the CST for primary surveillance to a nonrandomized, but comparable, risk group of patients followed with the NST for primary surveillance.[23,24] The nonstress test group had a significantly higher perinatal mortality rate, and the corrected antepartum death rate was 8 times higher in the NST group than the CST group (3.2:1000 versus 0.4:1000). In postdate pregnancies, a study by Miyazaki showed no benefit of NST surveillance over no surveillance.[25] Another recent study comparing weekly NST surveillance in postdate pregnancies to weekly CST surveillance revealed that the former group had a perinatal mortality of 11:1000 compared to 0:1000

**Table 40–5.** Manning and Platt's Biophysical Profile

| | Score | |
|---|---|---|
| | **0** | **2** |
| 1. Nonstress test | nonreactive | reactive |
| 2. Fetal movement | decreased | present |
| 3. Fetal tone | decreased | normal |
| 4. Fetal breathing | absent | present |
| 5. Amniotic fluid volume | decreased | normal |

in the latter group.[20] In this same study, a small number of patients, followed with a biweekly NST and a weekly real-time scan, had a mortality rate comparable with that of the group followed with the CST.[20] Three randomized prospective studies comparing patients followed with NST surveillance to patients with no surveillance have failed to demonstrate any benefits to patients being followed with the NST.[26–28] A large study by Manning suggests that weekly BPP surveillance yields mortality rates comparable to CST surveillance, often with less time needed for testing.[29]

The clinician should use the method with which he feels most comfortable, and which is most logistically feasible. Whether there is any value to screening all patients is as yet unresolved; at present, we use fetal movement counting for low-risk patients.

### Sonography

For the purposes of this chapter, the discussion on sonography will be confined here to its use in studying fetal well-being in the third trimester, and in the next section, on its use in estimating gestational age and fetal maturity.

When sonography first became available for use in obstetrics, it was noted that the biparietal diameter (BPD) of the fetal head was a measurement that could usually be made with reasonable accuracy, and that it correlated with gestational age with decreasing accuracy as gestation progressed. In cases of severe IUGR, it was noted that the BPD exhibited a decreased rate of growth with serial examinations. More recently, it was recognized that the growth rate of the BPD is the least affected measurement in the fetus suffering from IUGR and that the abdominal circumference (AC) is much more sensitive. In addition, decreased amniotic fluid volume is often, but not always, associated with IUGR when the cause is UPI.

Gohari[30] first showed that total intrauterine volume (TIUV), as measured by a static scanner, could be used to predict a very high likelihood of IUGR if this volume was 1.5 standard deviations or more below the mean volume for gestational age. In patients with TIUV within 1 standard deviation of the mean, there were no instances of IUGR. A problem with this test is that a gray area exists between 1 and 1.5 standard deviation below the mean; in this range, there was a 67% false-positive rate.

The ultrasonic estimation of fetal weight has gone through a steady evolution, with each investigator proposing a somewhat modified formula and claiming it to be more accurate than its predecessor. Most methods utilize the real-time assessment of BPD and AC. Most authorities agree, however, that the 95% confidence limits for accuracy are about ± 10% of body weight, and that this probably decreases near term, and with very large macrosomic babies.

The measurement of the fetal femur length has been proposed by O'Brian et al[31] to estimate gestational age. It is useful in confirming or disputing the BPD, especially where there may be abnormalities in its shape. The ratio between the fetal femur length and the AC is also useful in assessing fetal growth symmetry. In addition, it is of value in detecting abnormalities of fetal limb growth, such as that seen in dwarfism.

In patients with medically complicated pregnancies, the most common sonographic application is in the investigation of abnormal growth. In the diabetic, the usual question is whether there is macrosomia. The difference in size between the biparietal diameter and the thorax or abdomen is a reliable predictor of a body configuration that correlates with the risk of shoulder dystocia. Some studies indicate that if the BPD exceeds the thoracic diameter by $<$ 1.5 cm, the risk of shoulder dystocia appears to be increased.[32,33] Recent work by Nageotte, et al,[34] however, is more supportive of an estimated fetal weight greater than 4500 g as a predictor of shoulder dystocia, and his data call into question the value of the head/chest ratio.

When IUGR is suspected, the BPD alone is insufficient to assess the fetus. It is very difficult to assess a pregnancy for IUGR if the dates are not known, especially if the IUGR is symmetrical. If the IUGR is symmetrical (NBD:AC ratio), one must be very suspicious of either a very early fetal insult or anomalies. Characteristically, the symmetrically growth-retarded fetus will have normal amniotic fluid volume (AFV). Once symmetrical growth retardation is suspected, a careful search for anomalies should be made, and the patient should be considered for an amniotic fluid karyotype. Since UPI can cause symmetric IUGR, in the absence of genetic anomalies, fetal surveillance by AFHRT or BPP should be used until delivery is decided upon.

With asymmetrical IUGR, the body is more affected than the BPD, with an increased BPD/AC ratio, and there is usually decreased amniotic fluid volume. This type of growth retardation is most commonly found where there is a maternal disease state associated with decreased uterine perfusion, such as hypertension, collagen vascular diseases, or diabetes with severe vascular involvement. Once IUGR is suspected, fetal surveillance by AFHRT or BPP is indicated.

Timing of delivery in patients with IUGR presents a dilemma. One school of thought recommends delivery as soon as the diagnosis is made by ultrasound and there is reasonable potential for fetal survival, reasoning that it is important to get the fetus out of its hostile intrauterine environment as soon as possible. Another school of thought would not intervene before 36 to 37 weeks, with amniotic fluid tests indicating maturity, so long as fetal surveillance by APFHRT or BPP is normal. They reason that there is a significant error in diagnosing IUGR even in the hands of the best ultrasonographer, and if there is no evidence of hypoxia by APFHRT, it is probably safe to follow the patient and allow the fetus to mature. Certainly in the absence of hypoxia, asymmetrically growth-retarded babies do fairly well.

## Fetal Maturity Determination

### Clinical Methods

Too often, a careful history is not taken, or an opportunity to evaluate a patient early in pregnancy is missed. This can result in problems in the third trimester, when

**Table 40–6.** Clinical Findings Which Help Date a Pregnancy

1. Early examination prior to the 10th week of gestation
2. Documentation of the first appearance of fetal heart tones (by stethoscope) prior to the 20th week
3. Documentation of conception by basal body temperature
4. Quickening reported by a reliable patient at 16 to 18 weeks

intervention decisions may be required and there are no reliable data for estimating gestational age. There are numerous clinical findings which can help date a pregnancy accurately (Table 40–6), and the importance of using one or more of them at the appropriate times cannot be overstated.

## Laboratory Methods

### Human Chorionic Gonadotropin Assays

Pregnancy tests are frequently done in settings other than the obstetrician's office, and it is worth asking the patient if she had one done earlier, and, if so, documenting the result. Human Chorionic Gonadotropin (HCG) is first detectable in serum by radioimmunoassay about 9 days after conception[35] and rises rapidly thereafter. Urine pregnancy tests usually don't become positive until about 4 weeks after conception. There are recent data to suggest that an early quantitative serum beta HCG determination is as accurate as early sonography in dating a pregnancy.[36]

### Amniotic Fluid Phospholipid Tests

The appeal of amniotic fluid analysis for the estimation of fetal maturity lies in the fact that it is based on the specific maturity of the fetal lung, which is the system that usually determines survivability in the premature neonate. We must caution, however, that other systems may not mature in parallel with the lung and, while the knowledge of fetal lung maturity is important, it is not the whole answer.

It has long been known that a mixture of substances, known as surfactant, appears to be necessary to reduce surface tension within the lung in order for it to remain expanded. Surfactant is primarily made up of phospholipids, and it appears that lecithin is the principle substance responsible for reducing surface tension in the lung. Neonates born prior to the adequate production of lecithin will suffer from respiratory distress syndrome (RDS) due to hyaline membrane disease (HMD). This was the basis for Gluck's original work on amniotic fluid phospholipids as a predictor of HMD.[37] In order to correct for dilutional problems, Gluck originally related the lecithin concentration to the sphingomyelin concentration, as determined by thin-layer chromatography, and called this the L/S ratio. Today, this remains the most commonly used method for determination of fetal lung maturity, although there have been many variations on this, some of which we will discuss.

A word of caution is in order. Many of the attempts to vary Gluck's method for determination of the L/S ratio have resulted in decreased accuracy. For example, when the L/S ratio is above 2.0, the likelihood of HMD is less than 2%, and the majority of babies with HMD who have had recent L/S ratios greater than 2.0 will have had acute asphyxia or will be diabetic.[38,39] However, probably no more than 50% of those fetuses with amniotic fluid L/S ratios less than 2.0 will get RDS if delivered soon after the test.[40]

Because of the problem with false predictions of lung maturity in diabetics, further work was done by Gluck and coworkers that demonstrated that the presence of phosphotidylglycerol (PG) in concentrations over 5% reliably predicts fetal lung maturity even in fetuses of diabetics.[39,41] In addition, PG is useful when specimens have been contaminated by blood, meconium, and vaginal secretions, and the L/S ratio might therefore be unreliable. Unfortunately, in nondiabetic pregnancies where the L/S is reliable, PG is usually not present prior to 35 or 36 weeks gestation, and one cannot rely on its absence to predict the likelihood of HMD. This false-negative problem is present with all methods used to predict fetal lung maturity from amniotic fluid.

Other amniotic fluid analyses that are available for the prediction of RDS include foam stability tests (shake[42] and foam shake index[43]), fluorescence polarization[44] (which gives a P-value), and the Amniostat-FLM slide agglutination test for phosphotidylglycerol.[45] Our experience has been that all of these tests are quite reliable as predictors of fetal lung maturity, but have a high error rate when predicting fetal lung immaturity. However, the value of these three tests is that they cost between 1/3 and 1/6 as much as the L/S or PG in our laboratory, and they also give much quicker results. For this reason, we have devised a "cascade system" where the tests are done in order of their simplicity and rapidity, and if any test indicates fetal lung maturity in the nondiabetic, we don't run the others. This has resulted in a major savings in both cost and time.[46]

## The Sonographic Estimation of Fetal Maturity

Ultrasound has added a great dimension to the estimation of fetal maturity, but one must be careful to understand the limitations of this technique. Like clinical and laboratory estimations of gestational age, the accuracy diminishes as pregnancy progresses. Four measurements that are of value in determining gestational age via sonography are listed in Table 40–7.

The gestational sac can be measured in three dimensions and its volume calculated and related to a nomogram in patients under 8 weeks gestation, with a resulting accu-

**Table 40–7.** Sonographic Measurements for Determination of Gestational Age

1. Gestational sac volume
2. Crown-rump length
3. Biparietal diameter
4. Fetal femur length

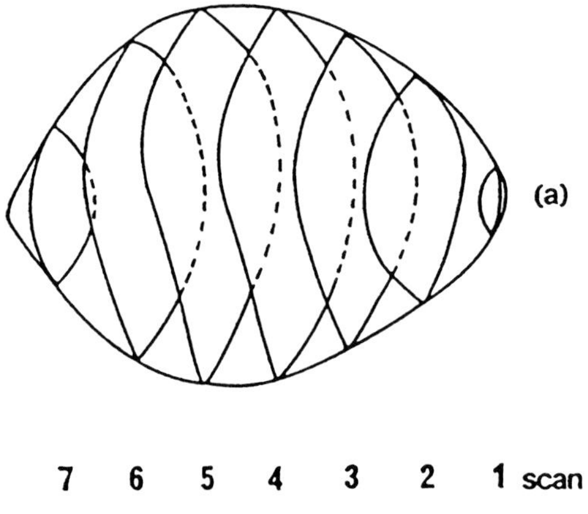


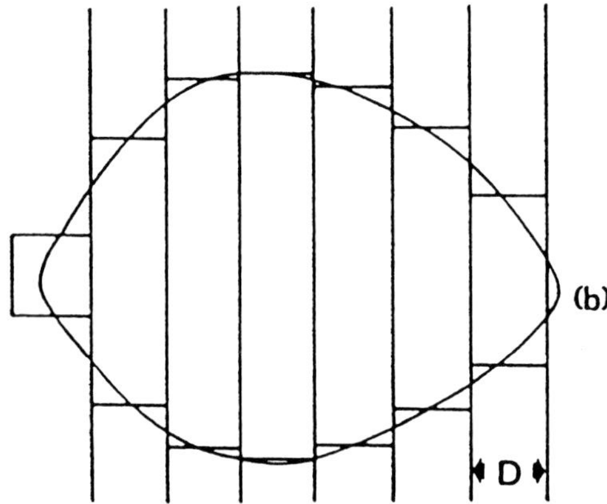


**Fig. 40–5.** A diagrammatic representation of the technique employed in the sonar estimation of "gestation sac" volume. The vertical lines correspond to serial parallel section scans taken at either 0.5-cm or 1-cm intervals **(D).** The sac volume is thereby divided into a series of flat, truncated cones. The upper part of the figure **(a)** demonstrates this subdivision in a two-dimensional form. The mathematical method used to estimate the volume of the gestation sac is illustrated in the lower part of the figure **(b).** The mean area of each adjoining pair of areas is calculated, and the resulting value is multiplied by the distance between them **(D),** thus giving an estimate for the volume of each "truncated cone." The overall volume of the gestation sac is then taken to be the sum of these volumes. (From Robinson H: Gestational sac: Volumes as determined by sonar in the first trimester of pregnancy. Br. J. Obstet. Gynaecol. 82:100, 1975.)

racy range of less than a week (Figure 40–5).[47] Certainly, if one has access to a patient this early in gestation, clinical and laboratory methods (quantitative HCG) ordinarily yield the same degree of accuracy. This method is helpful, however, in determining gestational age in circumstances where pelvic pathologies, such as fibroids or marked obesity, confuse the picture.

Probably the most accurate means of determining gestational age in early pregnancy by sonography is the *fetal crown-rump length.* This may be done between 6 and 12 weeks gestation and is said to have an accuracy range within just a few days.[48] The technique requires considerable skill and should be made on the largest of several measurements.

The most commonly used method to assess fetal gestational age by ultrasound is the BPD (Figure 40–6). The BPD cannot be measured accurately before 12 weeks, and is most accurate prior to 26 weeks gestation. In the third trimester, the accuracy of the BPD falls off rapidly; it may have a range as great as 8 weeks in late pregnancy. For this reason, attempts to assess maturity by BPD late in pregnancy are at best only gross, and intervention decisions should not be made on the basis of a third trimester BPD alone. Fetuses with misshapen heads following rupture of the membranes or during premature labor present special problems. In these situations, the occipito-frontal diameter as well as the BPD should be measured and the cephalic index calculated in an attempt to improve the accuracy of the measurement. Late in pregnancy, when the fetal head is deep in the pelvis, it may also be impossible to get an accurate BPD measurement.

The measurement of the fetal femur length has been suggested as a means of determining gestational age.[31] This serves as a correlative finding when a good BPD cannot be measured. Most investigators agree that multiple measurements of different parts of the anatomy on different occasions will give the most accurate measurement of gestational age by sonography, and may also uncover discrepancies that suggest other problems, such as IUGR, dwarfism, microcephalus or hydrocephalus.

In 1979, Grannum et al[49] suggested that the placenta could be graded for maturity (Figure 40–7). They noted no immature L/S ratios in 23 patients with grade III placentas, 12.5% immature L/S ratios in 28 patients with grade II placentas, and 32.3% low L/S ratios in patients with grade I placentas. A subsequent study by Harman[50] found 3.4% immature L/S ratios in 84 patients with grade III placentas. This suggests that placental grading should probably not be used as a substitute for amniotic fluid phospholipid determinations.

## Intrapartum Electronic Fetal Monitoring

Prospectively randomized studies of intrapartum electronic fetal heart rate monitoring have not indicated a clear advantage of this technique over intermittent auscultation every 15 minutes in the first stage of active labor and every 5 minutes in the second stage of labor.[51–56] Patients who are not monitored electronically during labor should have intermittent auscultation every 15 minutes during the first stage of active labor and every 5 minutes during the second stage. It is also prudent to listen frequently following activation of a major conduction anesthetic. For example, the most common complication of regional anesthesia is hypotension. Hypotension can reduce effective placental blood flow to the fetus and result in fetal compromise which may be detected by changes in the fetal heart rate. Close attention to monitoring in the 20 minutes or so after activation of regional anesthesia may pick up such changes. More specifically, such monitoring should include maternal blood pressure and fetal heart rate determination every 5 minutes.

Intrapartum electronic fetal heart rate monitoring

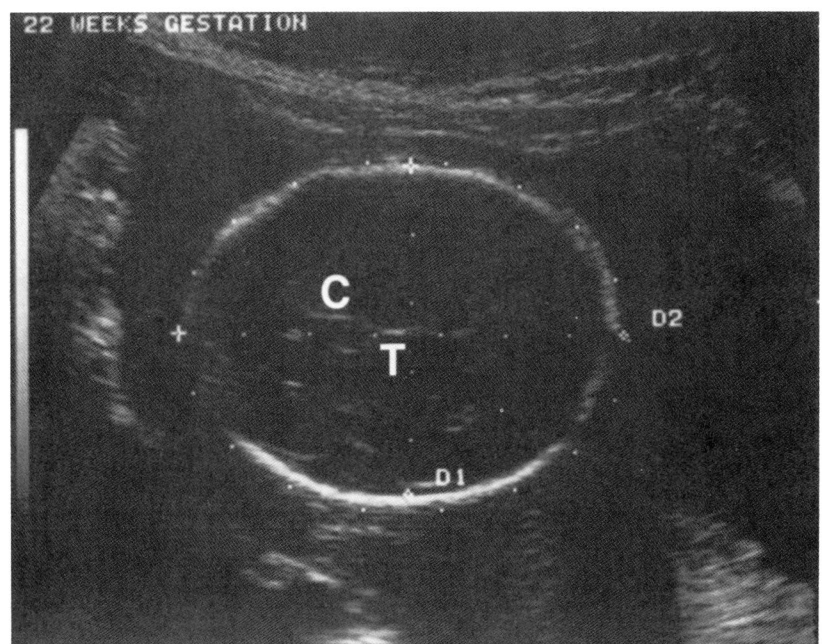


**Fig. 40–6.** A determination of the BPD at the level of thalami **(T)** and cavum septum pellucidum **(C).** The BPD measurement is made from the outer edge of the skull to the opposite inner edge **(D1)** and on a line perpendicular to the midline. The occipitofrontal diameter **(D2)** is also shown. The electronic calipers (dots) have been placed to obtain a measurement of the HC. (From Gabbe SG et al: Obstetrics: Normal and Problem Pregnancies. 2nd ed. New York, Churchill Livingstone, 1991.)

(EFM) gives information about baseline fetal heart rate, the variability of the baseline rate, and periodic fetal heart rate changes. Uterine contraction monitoring gives information about the frequency, duration and, if an intrauterine pressure catheter is used, amplitude of contractions. The relationship between uterine contractions and FHR changes may be helpful in diagnosing evidence of UPI, umbilical cord compression or fetal head compression.

## *Baseline FHR*

The baseline fetal heart rate usually resides between 120 and 160 BPM, but normal fetuses may have baseline rates outside of this usual range. Fetal tachycardia refers to an elevated baseline FHR and may be caused by a number of factors (Table 40–8). Following an episode of acute fetal hypoxia, there is frequently a rise in the baseline rate for a few minutes (Figure 40–8). Chronic fetal hypoxia is usually not associated with fetal tachycardia. Fetal tachycardia in the absence of the first 5 causes mentioned in Table 40–8, and in the absence of nonreassuring periodic FHR changes, is not an indication of fetal compromise.

Baseline variability of the FHR may be average, increased or decreased (Figure 40–9). The variability probably reflects the integrity of the CNS autonomic control of the FHR. With developing fetal hypoxia, one may see increased variability of the FHR that is believed to be due to chemoreceptor detection of decreased oxygen, resulting in reflex CNS sympathetic and parasympathetic discharge. After fetal hypoxia has become more severe, and fetal acidosis has developed, FHR variability tends to decrease, probably secondary to CNS depression. However, anything that causes fetal CNS depression will manifest itself in decreased variability (Table 40–9).

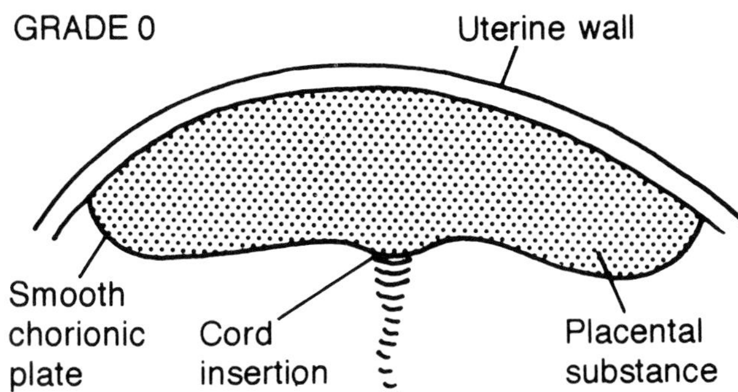


**Fig. 40–7.** Diagram showing the ultrasonic appearance of a Grade 0 placenta. (Redrawn from Granum P, Berkowitz R, Hobbins J: The ultrasonic changes in the maturing placenta and their relation to fetal pulmonic maturity. Am. J. Obstet. Gynecol. 133: 915, 1979.)

## *Periodic FHR Changes*

Acceleration of the FHR begins to occur in association with fetal movement at about 24 weeks gestation, and by 30 weeks more than 90% of normal fetuses have fetal heart rate acceleration that can be observed.[57] When periodic accelerations occur, simultaneous real-time sonography will show accompanying fetal movement.[3] It is a reas-

**Table 40–8.** Causes of Intrapartum Fetal Tachycardia

1. Maternal fever
2. Drugs (sympathomimetic or parasympatholytic)
3. Fetal arrhythmias (P.A.T. usually over 200 BPM)
4. Maternal hyperthyroidism in some cases
5. Acute fetal anemia
6. Fetal hypoxia (not consistent)

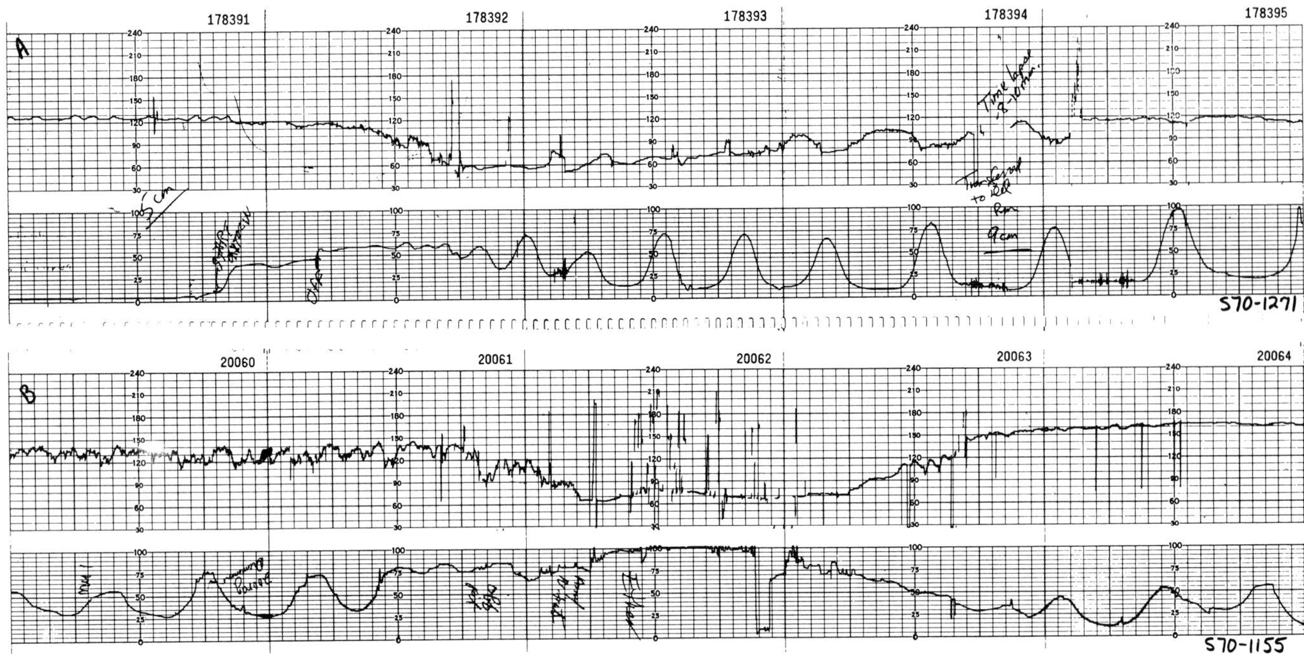

**Fig. 40–8.** A tetanic contraction with a severe prolonged FHR deceleration after IV Dramamine followed by fetal tachycardia. (From Freeman RK, Garite J, Nageotte P: Fetal Heart Rate Monitoring. 2nd Ed. Baltimore, Williams & Wilkins, 1991.)

suring sign and forms the basis of the NST. There is some evidence that accelerations, especially if associated with contractions, may represent umbilical venous compression and, in some instances, may develop into variable deceleration if the artery also becomes occluded.[58] The fetal scalp stimulation test can be used to assess fetal well-being in the face of nonreassuring periodic FHR changes. If fetal scalp stimulation is associated with an acceleration, there is very little likelihood that the fetus is acidotic; for this reason, stimulation has replaced fetal scalp blood sampling in many situations.[59]

Early deceleration is characterized by symmetrical FHR decelerations resembling a mirror image of the uterine contraction both in shape and timing (Figure 40–10). It is usually seen between 4 cm and 6 cm dilatation and is caused by fetal head compression, presumably as the edge of the cervix crosses the anterior fontanelle. It is a vagal reflex, and therefore can be blocked by the administration of atropine. It has no ominous connotation and its main importance is that it resembles late deceleration in configuration, but begins early in the contraction phase.

Variable deceleration occurs at any time in the contraction phase and is characterized by an abrupt fall in heart rate followed by an abrupt return (Figure 40–11), except when there is fetal hypoxemia. It is probably due to umbilical cord compression and occurs in over half of labors. When it is present before the onset of labor, it suggests oligohydramnios resulting in decreased umbilical cord protection. There are four factors which, if present, suggest that there may be some element of fetal hypoxia present (Table 40–10). Most patients with variable decelerations do not develop these changes, and therefore don't

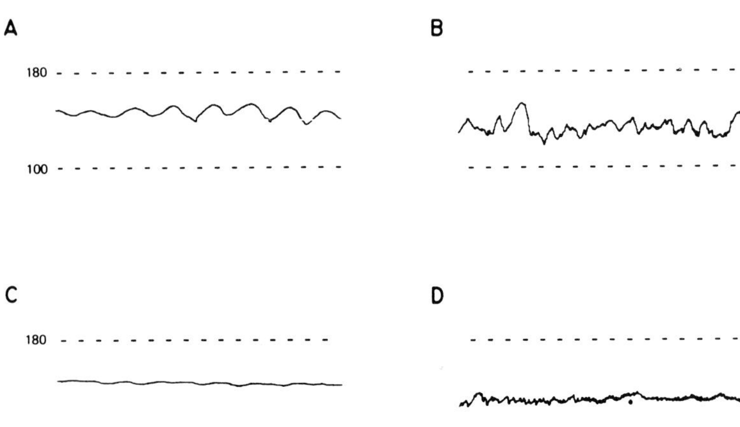


**Fig. 40–9.** Longterm variability (LTV) is demonstrated in **A** and **B** and is absent in **C** and **D.** Shortterm variability (STV) alone is shown in **D** and its concurrent presence with LTV is shown in **B.** Absence of both LTV and STV is seen in **C.** (From Zanini B, Paul RA, Huey JR: Fetal heart rate after tetanic contraction. Am. J. Obstet. Gynecol. 136:43, 1980.)

**Table 40–9.** Causes of Decreased Fetal Heart Rate Variability

1. Fetal CNS anomalies
2. Drugs (central depressants)
3. Fetal CNS infection
4. Prior fetal CNS damage
5. Ongoing fetal hypoxia if accompanied by nonreassuring periodic FHR changes

**Table 40–10.** Indicators of Fetal Hypoxia (When Accompanied by Variable Decelerations)

1. Increasing baseline FHR
2. Decreasing FHR variability
3. Slow return to the baseline
4. Variable deceleration exceeding 45 seconds on repetitive occasions

have any evidence of significant fetal hypoxia. When variable deceleration develops repeatedly, it is often easily relieved by maternal position change. Recently, intrauterine amnioinfusion via a transcervical catheter has been used to relieve variable deceleration in patients with decreased amniotic fluid volume following rupture of membranes during progressive labor.[60,61] If persistent variable deceleration with one or more of the above criteria occurs prior to the second stage of labor and cannot be corrected, expeditious delivery should be considered. At the very least, fetal scalp stimulation or blood sampling should be done, followed by expeditious delivery if results indicate a lack of acceleration or metabolic acidosis, respectively.

Late deceleration is characterized by symmetrical slowing of the FHR beginning at or after the peak of the contraction, and occurring with several contractions (Figure 40–12). It is believed to be due to UPI. Numerous techniques exist for correcting late decelerations (Table 40–11). As late deceleration evolves, it is first associated with increased or normal FHR variability, and fetal pH usually remains in the normal range. With the nonacidemic fetus, late deceleration appears to be primarily a vagal reflex. As hypoxemia becomes more significant, the FHR variability decreases, and there is an increasing incidence of metabolic acidosis. Late deceleration in the acidemic fetus cannot be blocked by atropine, and is believed to be due to myocardial depression.[62] If late deceleration with good FHR variability cannot be corrected and persists with most uterine contractions, consideration should be given to expeditious delivery, or fetal scalp stimulation or blood sampling, followed by expeditious delivery, if indicated. Late deceleration that is persistent, in association with decreased or absent FHR variability, is best managed by expeditious delivery.

## Anesthetic Considerations

When planning analgesia and anesthesia for a laboring patient, the FHR pattern preceding the procedure should

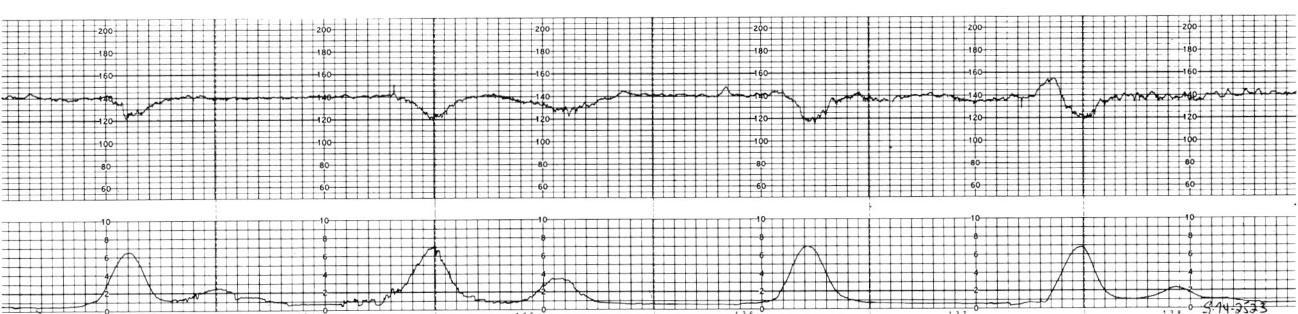

**Fig. 40–10.** Early decelerations are seen with each contraction on this panel. They are uniform, mirror the contractions, and decelerate only 10 to 20 BPM. (From Freeman RK, Garite J, Nageotte P: Fetal Heart Rate Monitoring. 2nd Ed. Baltimore, Williams & Wilkins, 1991.)

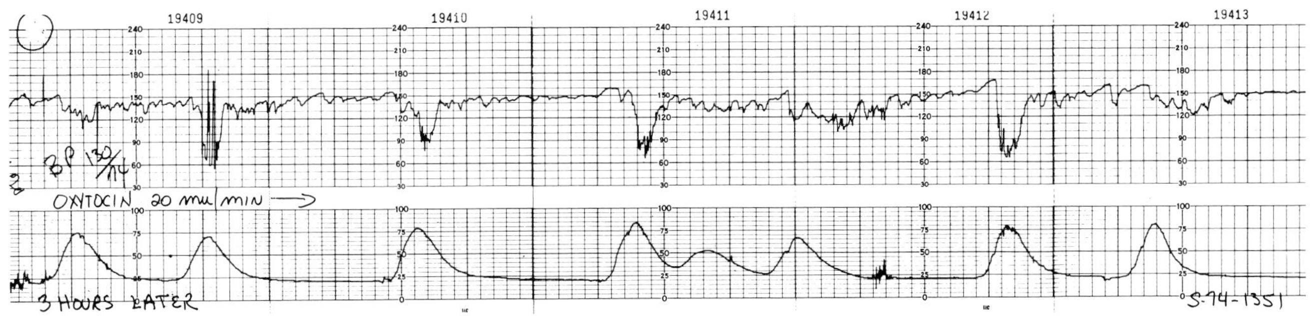


**Fig. 40–11.** Moderate variable decelerations are seen in this panel. Baseline heart rate and variability are normal. (From Freeman RK, Garite J, Nageotte P: Fetal Heart Rate Monitoring. 2nd Ed. Baltimore, Williams & Wilkins, 1991.)

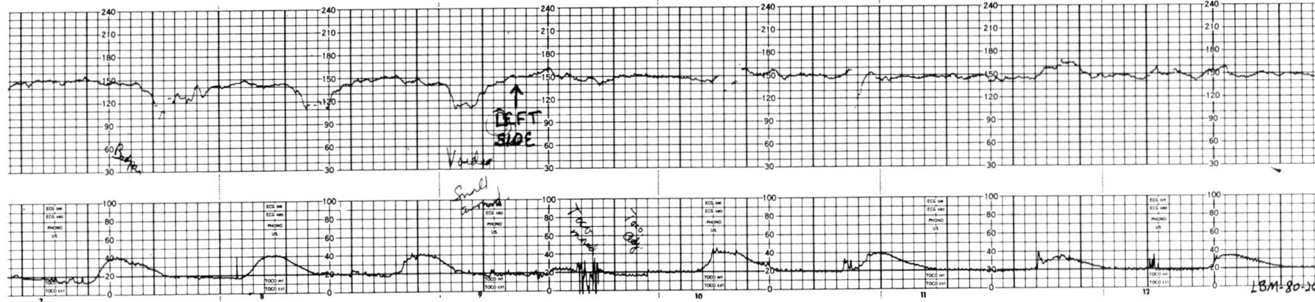

**Fig. 40–12.** Late deceleration corrected by turning patient on her side. (From Freeman RK, Garite J, Nageotte P: Fetal Heart Rate Monitoring. 2nd Ed. Baltimore, Williams & Wilkins, 1991.)

be taken into account. If there is evidence of UPI, the anesthesiologist and obstetrician should be aware of the increased risk to the fetus should a conduction anesthetic precipitate maternal hypotension. As mentioned many times in this text, the new 1990s technique of epidural analgesia for labor, eg, low dosage combination, that is, drug-continuous infusion technique, allows analgesia without the threat of hypotension. Perhaps this is one of the most remarkable advances made during the decade of 1980 to 1990. Delivery of small doses has been found to be adequate from the maternal standpoint, and at the same time it does not result in sympathectomy, and therefore does not precipitate hypotensive threats.

For first stage labor analgesia, one may consider use of the segmental epidural with continuous infusion of local anesthesia. For second stage, one may consider use of the caudal or subarachnoid block technique or pudendal block with or without nitrous oxide supplementation.

For nonemergent cesarean section, one may consider use of the epidural after careful attention to prehydration and maternal positioning (left uterine displacement with legs elevated), but even then it should be used only if the FHR is both stable and at a normal rate. In unstable FHR situations, general anesthesia is preferred unless there are maternal complicating factors, such as morbid obesity or a difficult airway; in such cases, a low spinal or local anesthesia is preferred. In emergency cesarean section, a general anesthetic is preferred, because less time is required for general anesthesia than for conduction anesthesia, and because of the need for preservation of maternal blood pressure in cases of fetal compromise. However, a recent innovation in this area is use of the continuous spinal catheter with administration of an opioid for first stage analgesia with conversion to 5% lidocaine for cesarean section. The latter provides rapid onset of block and the ability to keep the level low enough to avoid hypotension.

**Table 40–11.** Maneuvers for Relieving Late Decelerations

1. Positioning patient on her side
2. Administering oxygen via face mask
3. Discontinuing oxytocin
4. Correcting any hypotension
5. Increasing the IV infusion rate

## CONCLUSION

Over the past decade, there has been tremendous progress in our ability to determine antepartum and intrapartum fetal condition, but a great deal remains to be done before we can also treat the fetus, short of delivery, when the fetal condition is deteriorating. As such, it is critical for the clinician to be aware of the relationship between maternal disease and fetal condition, and to be able to employ fetal surveillance techniques to make intervention decisions appropriately.

## REFERENCES


1. Neldam S: Fetal movements as an indicator of fetal wellbeing. Lancet 1(8180):1222, June 7, 1980.
2. Sadovsky E: When prompt delivery is indicated. Contemp. Obstet. Gynecol. 16:109, 1980.
3. Rabinowitz R, Persitz E, Sadovsky E: The relation between fetal heart rate accelerations and fetal movements. Obstet. Gynecol. 61:16, 1983.
4. Sadovsky E, Polishuk W: Fetal movements in utero. Obstet. Gynecol. 50:49, 1977.
5. Sadovsky E, Yaffe H: Daily fetal movement recording and fetal prognosis. Obstet. Gynecol. 31:845, 1973.
6. Sadovsky E, Yaffe H, Polishuk W: Fetal movements monitoring in normal and pathological pregnancy. Int. J. Gynecol. Obstet. 12:75, 1974.
7. Freeman RK, Dorchester W, Anderson G, Garite TJ: The significance of a previous stillbirth. Am. J. Obstet. Gynecol. 151:7, 1985.
8. Hon EH, Wohlgemuth R: The electronic evaluation of fetal heart rate. IV. The effect of maternal exercise. Am. J. Obstet. Gynecol. 81:36, 1961.
9. Pose SV, Castilo JB, Mora-Rojas EO, Soto-Yances A, et al: Test of fetal tolerance to induced uterine contractions for the diagnosis of chronic distress. *In* Perinatal Factors Affecting Human Development. Pan Am Health Org. Pub. #185, 1969.
10. Kubil FW, Kaeser D, Kinselman M: Diagnostic management of chronic placental insufficiency. *In* The Foetal Placental Unit. Edited by A Pecile, E Finzi. Amsterdam, Excerpta Medical Foundation, 1969, p. 323.
11. Hammacher K: The clinical significance of cariotography. *In* Perinatal Medicine. Proceedings of the First European Congress, Berlin. Edited by PS Huntington, KA Hunter, E. Saling. New York, Academic Press, 1969, p. 80.
12. Ray M, Freeman R, Pine S, Hesselgesser R: Clinical experiences with the oxytocin challenge test. Am. J. Obstet. Gynecol. 114:1, 1972.

13. Schifrin BS, Lapidus M, Doctor GS, Leviton A: Contraction stress test for antepartum fetal evaluation. Obstet. Gynecol. 45:433, 1975.
14. Freeman RK: The use of oxytocin challenge test for antepartum clinical evaluation of uteroplacental respiratory function. Am. J. Obstet. Gynecol. 121:418, 1975.
15. Farahani G, Vasudeva K, Petrie R, Fenton AN: Oxytocin challenge test in high risk pregnancy. Obstet. Gynecol. 47:159, 1976.
16. Freeman RK, Goebelsman U, Nochimson D, Cetrulo C: An evaluation of the significance of a positive oxytocin challenge test. Obstet. Gynecol. 47:8, 1976.
17. Huddleston J, Freeman RK: The oxytocin challenge test. *In* Perinatal Medicine. Edited by S Corson, R Bolognese. Baltimore, Williams & Wilkins, 1977.
18. Braly P, Freeman RK: The significance of fetal heart rate activity with a positive oxytocin challenge test. Obstet. Gynecol. 5:689, 1977.
19. Visser GHA, Redman CWG, Huisjes HJ, Turnbull AC: Nonstressed antepartum heart rate monitoring: Implications of decelerations after spontaneous contractions. Am. J. Obstet. Gynecol. 138:429, 1980.
20. Eden RD, Gergely RZ, Schifrin BS, Wade ME: Comparison of antepartum fetal heart rate testing schemes in post date pregnancies. Am. J. Obstet. Gynecol. 144:683, 1982.
21. Manning F, Platt L, Sipos L: Antepartum fetal evaluation: Development of a fetal biophysical profile. Am. J. Obstet. Gynecol. 136:787, 1980.
22. Baskett TF, Gray JH, Prewett SJ, Young LM, et al.: Antepartum fetal assessment using a fetal biophysical profile score. Am. J. Obstet. Gynecol. 148:630, 1984.
23. Freeman RK, Anderson G, Dorchester W: A prospective multi-institutional study of antepartum fetal heart rate monitoring. I. Risk of perinatal mortality and morbidity according to antepartum fetal heart rate test results. Am. J. Obstet. Gynecol. 143:771, 1982.
24. Freeman RK, Anderson G, Dorchester W: A prospective multi-institutional study of antepartum fetal heart rate monitoring. II. Contraction stress test versus nonstress test for primary surveillance. Am. J. Obstet. Gynecol. 143:778, 1982.
25. Miyazaki FS, Miyazaki BA: False reactive nonstress test in postterm pregnancies. Am. J. Obstet. Gynecol. 140:269, 1981.
26. Lumley J, Lester A, Anderson I, Renou P, et al: A randomized trial of weekly cardiotocography in high-risk obstetric patients. Br. J. Obstet. Gynaecol. 90:1018, 1983.
27. Kidd LC, Patel NB, Smith R: Non-stress antenatal cardiotocography—A prospective randomized clinical trial. Br. J. Obstet. Gynaecol. 92:1156, 1985.
28. Brown VA, Sawers RS, Parsons RJ, Duncan SLB, et al: The value of antenatal cardiotocography in the management of high-risk pregnancy: A randomized controlled trial. Br. J. Obstet. Gynaecol. 89:716, 1982.
29. Manning FA: Determination of fetal health: Methods for antepartum and intrapartum fetal assessment. Current Problems in Obstetrics and Gynecology, Vol VII, No. 4, Dec 1983.
30. Gohari P, Berkowitz R, Hobbins J: Prediction of intrauterine growth retardation by determination of total intrauterine volume. Am. J. Obstet. Gynecol. 127:255, 1977.
31. O'Brian G, Queenan J, Campbell S: Assessment of gestational age in the second trimester by real-time ultrasound measurement of the femur length. Am. J. Obstet. Gynecol. 139: 540, 1981.
32. Modanlou HD, Komatsu G, Dorchester W, Freeman RK, et al: Large-for-gestational age neonates: Anthropometric reasons for shoulder dystocia. Obstet. Gynecol. 60:417, 1982.
33. Williams J, et al: Ultrasound predictions of shoulder dystocia. Presented at 5th Annual Society of Perinatal Obstetricians Meeting, Las Vegas, NV, February 1985.
34. Nageotte MP, et al: Antenatal decision of shoulder dystocia. Presented at 8th Annual Society of Perinatal Obstetricians Meeting, 1988.
35. Mishell D, Nakamura R, Barberia J: Initial detection of human chorionic gonadotropin in serum in normal gestation. Am. J. Obstet. Gynecol. 118:90, 1974.
36. Lagrew DC, Wilson EA, Jawad MJ: Determination of gestational age by serum concentration of human chorionic gonadotropin by progestational steroid. Am. J. Obstet. Gynecol. 138:708, 1980.
37. Gluck L, Kulovich MV, Borer RC Jr, Brenner PH, et al: Diagnosis of the respiratory distress syndrome by amniocentesis. Am. J. Obstet. Gynecol. 109:440, 1971.
38. Donald IR, Freeman RK, Goebelsmann U, Chan WH, et al: Clinical experience with the amniotic fluid lecithin sphingomyelin ratio. I. Antenatal prediction of pulmonary maturity. Am. J. Obstet. Gynecol. 115:547, 1973.
39. Gabbe SG, Lowensohn RI, Mestman JH, Freeman RK, et al: The lecithin sphingomyelin ratio in pregnancies complicated by diabetes mellitus. Am. J. Obstet. Gynecol. 128:757, 1977.
40. Bustos R, Kulovich MV, Gluck L, Gabbe SG, et al: Significance of phosphatidylglycerol in amniotic fluid in complicated pregnancies. Am. J. Obstet. Gynecol. 133:899, 1979.
41. Kulovich M, Gluck L: The lung profile, II: Complicated pregnancy. Am. J. Obstet. Gynecol. 135:64, 1979.
42. Clements JA, Platzker ACG, Tierney DF, Hobel CJ, et al: Assessment of the risk of the respiratory distress syndrome by a rapid test for surfactant in amniotic fluid. N. Engl. J. Med. 286:1077, 1972.
43. Sher G, Statland BE, Freer DE, Kraybill EN: Assessing fetal lung maturation by the foam stability index test. Obstet. Gynecol. 52:673, 1978.
44. Golde SH, Mosley GH: A blind comparison study of the lung phospholipid profile, fluorescence microviscosimetry, and the lecithin/sphingomyelin ratio. Am. J. Obstet. Gynecol. 136:222, 1980.
45. Garite TJ, Yabusaki KK, Moberg LJ, Symons JL, et al: A new rapid slide agglutination test for amniotic fluid phosphatidylglycerol: Laboratoy and clinical correlation. Am. J. Obstet. Gynecol. 147:681, 1983.
46. Garite TJ, Freeman RK, Nageotte MP: Fetal maturity cascade: A rapid and cost-effective method for fetal lung maturity testing. Obstet. Gynecol. 67:619, 1986.
47. Robinson H: Gestational sac: Volumes as determined by sonar in the first trimester of pregnancy. Br. J. Obstet. Gynaecol. 82:100, 1975.
48. Robinson H: Sonar measurement of fetal crown-rump length as a means of assessing maturity in the first trimester of pregnancy. Br. J. Obstet. Gynaecol. 4:28, 1973.
49. Granum P, Berkowitz R, Hobbins J: The ultrasonic changes in the maturing placenta and their relation to fetal pulmonic maturity. Am. J. Obstet. Gynecol. 133:915, 1979.
50. Harman CR, Manning FA, Stearns E, Morrison I: Placental maturity grade and L/S ratio: A prospective study of 314 consecutive patients. Am. J. Obstet. Gynecol. 143:941, 1982.
51. Neldam S, Osler M, Hansen PK, Nim J, et al: Intrapartum fetal heart rate monitoring in a combined low- and high-risk population: A controlled clinical trial. Eur. J. Obstet. Gynecol. Reprod. Biol. 23:1, 1986.
52. MacDonald D, Grant A, Sheridan-Pereira M, Boylan P, et al: The Dublin randomized controlled trial of intrapartum fetal heart rate monitoring. Am. J. Obstet. Gynecol. 152:524, 1985.

53. Haverkamp AD, Orleans M, Langendoerfer S, McFee J, et al: A controlled trial of the differential effects of intrapartum fetal monitoring. Am. J. Obstet. Gynecol. 134:399, 1979.
54. Renou P, Chang A, Anderson I, Wood C: Controlled trial of fetal intensive care. Am. J. Obstet. Gynecol. 126:170, 1976.
55. Haverkamp AD, Thompson HE, McFee JG, Cetrulo C: The evaluation of continuous fetal heart rate monitoring in high-risk pregnancy. Am. J. Obstet. Gynecol. 125:310, 1976.
56. Freeman R: Intrapartum fetal monitoring: a disappointing story. New Engl. J. Med. 322:624–626, 1990.
57. Druzin ML, Fox A, Kogut E, Carlson C: The relationship of the nonstress test to gestational age. Am. J. Obstet. Gynecol. 153:386, 1985.
58. James LS, Yeh MN, Morishima HO, Daniel SS, et al: Umbilical vein occlusion and transient acceleration of the fetal heart rate. Experimental observations in subhuman primates. Am. J. Obstet. Gynecol. 126:276, 1976.
59. Clark S, Gimovsky M, Miller F: The scalp stimulation test: A clinical alternative to fetal scalp blood sampling. Am. J. Obstet. Gynecol. 148:274, 1984.
60. Miyazaki FS, Nevarez F: Saline amnioinfusion for relief of repetitive variable decelerations: A prospective randomized study. Am. J. Obstet. Gynecol. 153:301, 1985.
61. Nageotte MP, Freeman RK, Garite TJ, Dorchester W: Prophylactic intrapartum amnioinfusion in patients with preterm premature rupture of membranes. Am. J. Obstet. Gynecol. 153:557, 1985.
62. Martin C, et al: Mechanisms of late decelerations in the fetal heart rate. A study with autonomic blocking agents in fetal lambs. Eur. J. Obstet. Gynecol. Reprod. Biol. 9:361, 1979.

Chapter 41

# FETAL CARE IN LABOR AND EMERGENCY DELIVERY FOR FETAL INDICATIONS

ROBIN J. WILLCOURT
RONALD E. MYERS
GABRIELLE DE COURTEN-MYERS
SARAH L. ARTMAN
RICHARD W. O'SHAUGHNESSY
JOHN S. McDONALD

As maternal mortality has been impressively reduced in this century due to improvement in care, attention has shifted to protecting the fetus. Evaluation of the fetus during labor and delivery is the responsibility of the obstetrician. For the obstetric anesthesiologist, understanding the methods of monitoring the fetus and the interpretation of the findings will improve the ability of the anesthesiologist to care for the mother.

## FETAL DISTRESS

The term *fetal distress* is commonly used to imply that there is a deficiency in fetal oxygenation to the extent that the fetus is somehow endangered. The term is often used very loosely in the day-to-day practice of obstetrics, producing an inconsistent approach to the management of the mother and fetus.

The diagnosis of fetal distress is difficult to make. In practice, the use of scalp blood sampling during labor is limited by the tediousness of the procedure, so that the diagnosis is usually based on the appearance of the fetal heart-rate patterns prior to delivery, and is therefore often erroneous.[1] Thus, a predelivery diagnosis of fetal distress may not be confirmed in the newborn once the Apgar scores and and the cord blood gases are obtained. This tends to confer an impression of vagueness and imprecision to the diagnosis of fetal distress, which is especially difficult for the anesthesiologist, who may have seen unexpectedly normal outcomes in the neonates who were diagnosed as having fetal distress while in utero. It is of great value for the anesthesiologist to understand the physiological mechanisms involved in the clinical entity we call fetal distress, so that the treatment of the condition is understood, and also to provide the anesthesiologist with information that will benefit the fetus if there is a need for his or her services.

Once the diagnosis of fetal distress is made, it is the role of the obstetrician and the anesthesiologist to maximize a favorable outcome for the fetus, while at the same time ensuring that the mother suffers no lasting ill effects from the proposed therapy. The treatment of the mother and fetus will depend to some extent on the underlying problem and to the degree of the perceived threat to the well-being of the fetus. Clearly, one transitory episode of fetal heart rate abnormality would not inevitably lead to an immediate operative delivery.

Fetal distress is preceded by a period of fetal stress which carries no long term morbidity, but which signals a warning that the fetus is in a potentially harmful environment. A persistent pattern of stress will turn to one of distress if the fetal environment is not altered favorably. This can only be achieved if adverse factors can be changed quickly, and if no other deleterious effects to the fetus are added. Since the end point of fetal distress is reached through different physiologic mechanisms, these will be discussed separately.

### Effects

Fetal heart rate late decelerations during labor may indicate the presence of fetal asphyxia, as experimental studies with monkeys have demonstrated.[2,3] Neuropathologic studies demonstrate that initially healthy, well-oxygenated fetuses can endure moderate or, indeed, even marked asphyxia lasting up to several hours without risking brain injury, until or unless several further, significant fetal physiologic changes take place.[4,5] Fetal asphyxia finally damages the brain: (1) when its severity is very marked; (2) when it is sustained sufficiently long (from 15 minutes to more than several hours) as to cause marked fetal acidosis; and (3) when the accompanying acidosis depresses fetal cardiovascular performance to such an extent as to reduce blood pressure or, ultimately, to cause cardiovascular collapse. When the fetal blood pressure declines, the fetal asphyxia is accompanied by cerebral ischemia. The marked fetal asphyxia combined with cerebral ischemia eventually provides the setting for cerebral anoxia. Animal experimental studies have demonstrated that it is specifically these circumstances accompanied by cerebral anoxia that risk permanent brain injury or fetal death.[4,6–8]

Fetal heart rate late decelerations may signify the presence of fetal asphyxia. The identification of late decelerations dictates that measures be taken to relieve any associated fetal asphyxia lest it persist, aggravate, and, with its prolongation, compromise the fetus and, eventually, cause brain injury or death. If fetuses develop late decelerations when oxytocic agents are being infused, these agents must be discontinued since they may cause fetal asphyxia or, if fetal asphyxia already exists, aggravate it. Failure to respond to the warning of fetal heart rate late decelerations by continuing the infusion of oxytocic agents risks asphyxia that may progress to the extent of damaging the fetus.

Other measures may reduce fetal asphyxia. These include changing the posture of the mother by placing her in a lateral rather than supine position to improve uterine blood flow, and administering oxygen to the mother by face mask. However, fetal recovery from short-term asphyxia may be possible when the inciting causes are removed.[4,9] Intrauterine recovery from asphyxia explains why fetuses may be born with satisfactory Apgar scores and yet develop an acute hypoxic/ischemic encephalopathy during the newborn period as a consequence of intrapartum or prepartum asphyxia.

A marked fetal asphyxia which lasts for hours depresses the fetal cardiovascular performance and risks fetal brain injury or demise. The combination of a fetal asphyxia and an ischemia of bodily organs caused by an associated depression of cardiovascular performance may adversely affect organs other than the brain, including the heart, kidneys, and gastrointestinal tract. However, the risk of brain damage remains paramount because it is brain injury that causes lifelong disabilities diminishing the quality of life and restricting an individual's developmental potential. Since the brain already loses the ability to generate new neurons by midgestation, neurons lost as a consequence of asphyxia as a part of damage to brain tissue are not replaced, and the associated functional deficits are permanent.

The brain also is among the organs most vulnerable to injury from asphyxia. In adult man, periods of asphyxia associated with brain anoxia as brief as 4 to 5 minutes may markedly damage the brain, while in the newborn, periods of asphyxia causing brain anoxia as short lived as 6 to 10 minutes may be required.[10–13] Other organs including the heart, kidneys, and gastrointestinal tract likewise may be affected by asphyxia.

Interpreting fetal well-being in labor is a topic about which entire texts are written for obstetricians. In this chapter we will review fetal physiology, discuss the methods of fetal heart-rate monitoring, and the basic interpretation of that monitoring. Obstetrical management in the course of abnormal fetal heart rate patterns and other obstetrical conditions is discussed, along with anesthetic considerations.

## Fetal Physiology and Mechanisms of Brain Injury

Fetuses exposed to intrapartum asphyxia may sustain brain damage (Figures 41–1, 41–2, 41–3, 41–4). However, in most cases of antepartum asphyxia, damage to the brain cannot be demonstrated. Animal experimental studies have demonstrated that, for asphyxia to damage the brain, the brain or some tissue component of the brain must experience a period of anoxia or near-anoxia.[6,7,8] (See Table 41–1.) For this to occur, the fetus itself must

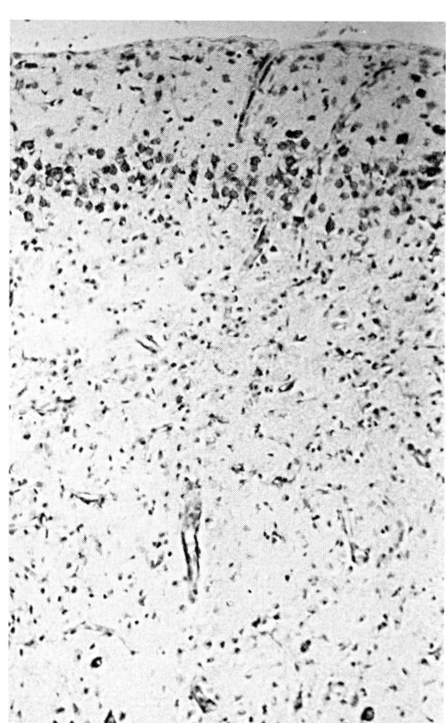

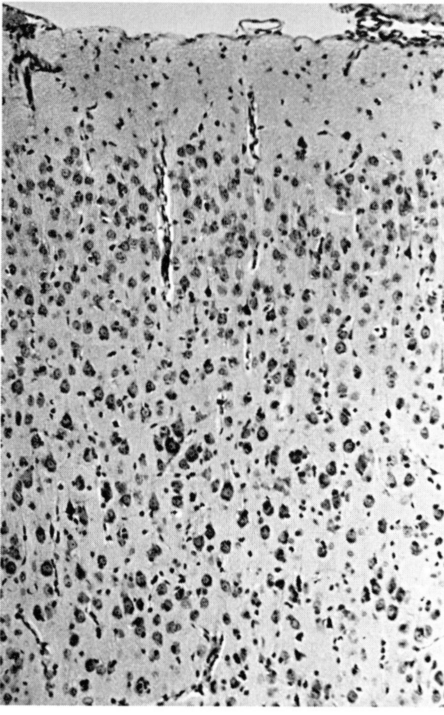

**Fig. 41–1.** Detrimental effect of hyperglycemia on anoxic brain injury. Micrographs of cerebral cortex from cats exposed to the same marked hypoxia and hypotension (leading to brain anoxia) illustrate extensive neuronal loss when hyperglycemic (left panel) but no injury when normoglycemic (right panel).

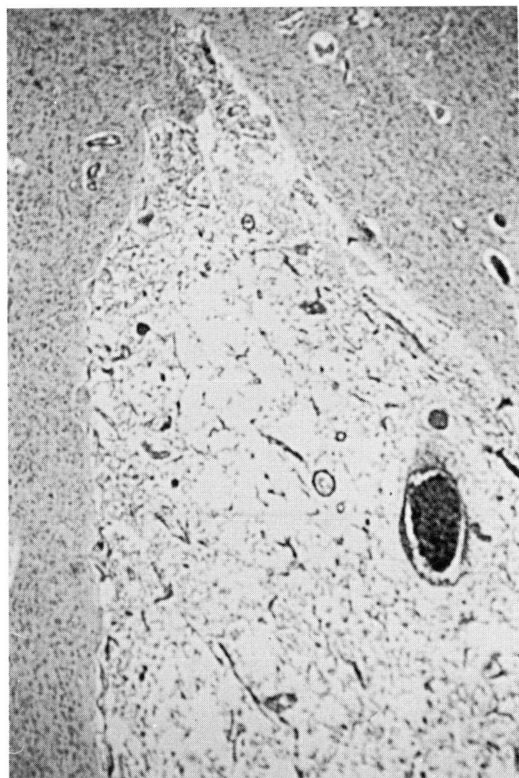

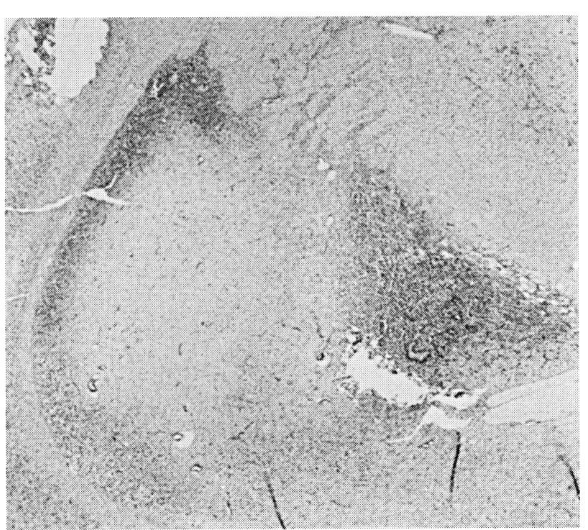

**Fig. 41–2.** Perinatal basal ganglia necrosis. Top, Loss of all brain cells except vessels (en bloc necrosis) in the putamen of an asphyxiated human newborn. Bottom, Similar damage to the putamen of a rhesus monkey fetus exposed to 12.5 minutes of umbilical cord clamping.

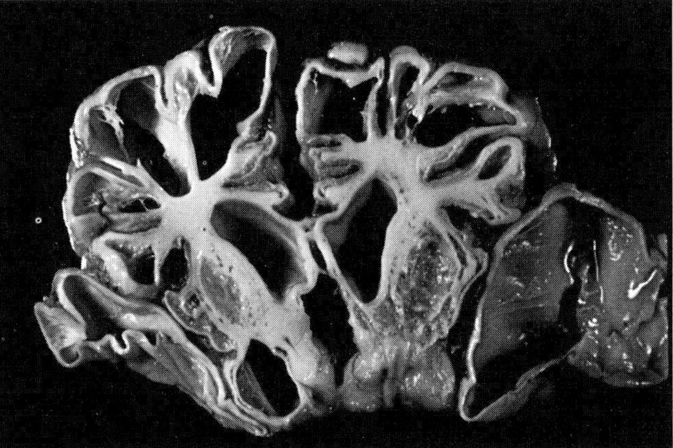

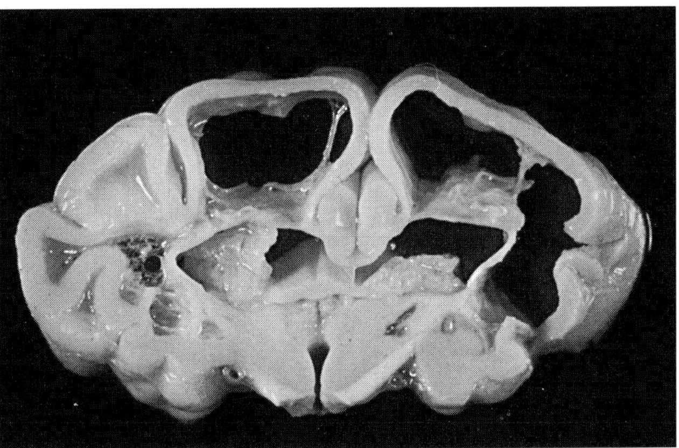

**Fig. 41–3.** Multicystic encephalomalacia. Top, Coronal brain section from a human newborn with survived perinatal asphyxia showing multiple grey and particularly white matter cysts. Bottom, Similar brain pathology produced in a sheep fetus exposed to 1 hour of marked asphyxia in utero delivered 3 weeks later.

experience an anoxia such that its arterial blood is fully deprived of oxygen, i.e., carries no oxygen, or alternatively, the fetus itself may experience only a marked hypoxia while the brain experiences an anoxia. However, for a marked systemic hypoxia to cause a cerebral anoxia, the hypoxia must be lengthy (>20 minutes to several hours) and, ultimately, depress fetal cardiovascular performance, leading to hypotension with or without a circulatory collapse.[4,7,8] The hypoxia-induced fall in blood pressure leads to a cerebral ischemia. Whether the fetus is totally asphyxiated or, rather, experiences an ischemia-induced cerebral anoxia, the failed oxygen delivery to the brain precipitates, for the first time, marked changes in brain chemistry that damage the brain. In contrast, when fetuses are exposed to marked asphyxia but maintain an adequate blood pressure, the presence of the marked systemic hypoxia fails to significantly alter brain energy metabolism and induces only minor changes in brain chemistry that are not brain destructive.[14] Fetuses exposed to marked hypoxia ultimately develop a noticeable metabolic and respiratory acidosis. Because this acidosis is progressive in nature, if it is sufficiently prolonged and intense, it will depress cardiovascular performance and cause a circulatory collapse. Thus, allowing a marked fetal asphyxia to induce will eventually precipitate a circulatory collapse, cause a brain anoxia, and risk damage to the brain and death.

The experimental findings that established these relations accord well with clinical experience. The Apgar scores at delivery are extremely low, reflecting a conspicuous depression of both nervous system function (reduced responsiveness to stimulation, reduced muscle tone, and absent or gasping respiration) and of cardiovas-

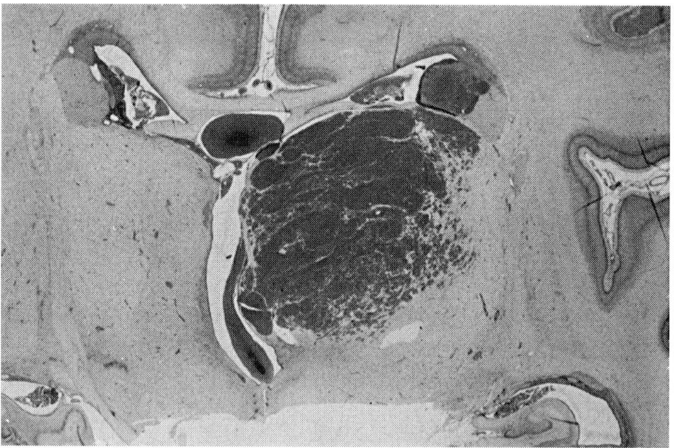

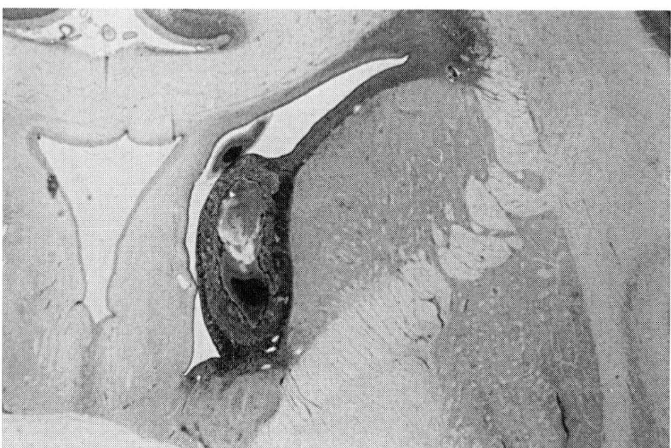

**Fig. 41–4.** Comparison of intraventricular hemorrhage (IVH) Grade II with Grade IV. Top, Grade IV IVH with extensive parenchymal hemorrhages in the thalamus and caudate nucleus with minor germinal matrix hemorrhage in a 32-week gestational newborn. Bottom, Typical Grade II IVH with germinal matrix hemorrhage restricted to the ganglionic eminence and rupture into the ventricle in a 30-week gestational premature newborn.

**Table 41–1.** Hypoxic Brain Injury Requires Hypotension in Fetuses, Newborns, and Adults

| Animal/Age | N | art$PO_2$/duration mmHg/minutes | Lowest MABP mmHg | Pathology |
|---|---|---|---|---|
| Cat/adult | 13 | 17/25 | >65 | all intact |
| Cat/adult | 13 | 17/25 | <45 | 12 damaged |
| Pig/newborn | 6 | 27/40 | 25 ± 1 | all intact |
| Pig/newborn | 3 | 27/40 | 12 ± 4 | all damaged |
| Sheep/fetus | 21 | 10/120 | 36 ± 2 | all intact |
| Sheep/fetus | 8 | 10/120 | 28 ± 2 | all damaged |

(From de Courten-Myers GM, Yamaguchi S-I, Wagner KR, Ting P, et al: Brain injury from marked hypoxia in cats: Role of hypotension and hyperglycemia. Stroke 16(6):1016–1021, 1985; de Courten-Myers GM, Fogelson HM, Kleinholz M, Myers RE: Hypoxic brain and heart injury thresholds in piglets. Biomed. Biochem. Acta. 48:143, 1989; and Ting P, Yamaguchi S, Bacher JD, Killens RH, et al: Hypoxic-ischemic cerebral necrosis in midgestational sheep fetuses: Physiopathologic correlations. Exper. Neurol. 80:227–245, 1983.)

cular function (reduced or absent heart beat and pallor). Very low Apgar scores generally signify a fetal circulatory collapse. That fetal cardiovascular function must be depressed to the point of collapse before brain damage develops explains why fetal death is about as common as brain-damaged survival following severe intrapartum asphyxia. However, a significantly depressed Apgar score at birth only increases the risk of death or brain injury; most infants with very low Apgar scores are resuscitated successfully and later show no evidence of brain damage.[15] Thus, extended asphyxia leading to hypotension or a circulatory collapse is necessary but, in most instances, not sufficient to cause brain injury.

What do we know about what constitutes the additional "sufficient conditions"? Fetuses exposed to marked asphyxia that yet maintain an adequate blood flow to the brain show only minor changes in brain energy metabolism.[16,17] Their brains show essentially unchanged concentrations of adenosinetriphosphate (ATP), glucose and glycogen, slight reductions of phosphocreatine (PCr) and slight-to-moderate increases in lactic acid concentration. However, when their cardiovascular function begins to decline even slightly, reducing their cerebral blood flow, their brain chemistry, for the first time, dramatically changes, showing noticeable reductions in phosphocreatine, ATP, glycogen and glucose, and marked increases in lactic acid concentrations. Exposure to anoxia or marked hypoxia combined with critical blood pressure lowering leading to brain anoxia alters brain chemistry primarily by stimulating glycolysis. The stimulation of glycolysis in the brain causes all available carbohydrate substrates—including brain glucose and glycogen—to break down.

Markedly reduced ATP and PCr, and increased lactic acid concentrations from asphyxia are strongly associated with brain injury. Episodes of asphyxia that cause lactic acid to accumulate in the brain to concentrations greater than 17 μmoles to 20 μmoles per gram damages the brain in all instances.[16,18,19,20] When brain anoxia develops and glycolysis is stimulated, it is the brain's stores of carbohydrate substrates in the form of glucose and glycogen that define the extent to which lactic acid accumulates. During glycolysis, 1 mol of glucose is converted to 2 mols of lactate and 2 mols of ATP. However, the hydrolysis of the 2 mols of ATP yields 2 mols of hydrogen ions, and it is the accumulation of the hydrogen rather than of the lactate ions that appears to damage the brain during asphyxia. Because brain glucose concentrations parallel those of blood throughout the normal ranges of glycemia, hyperglycemic animals exposed to anoxia develop high lactic acid concentrations throughout widespread regions of their brains, exceeding the threshold values for injury. Conversely, normoglycemic and, especially, slightly hypoglycemic animals that contain brain carbohydrate stores at or below normal that are exposed to anoxia, fail to develop lactic acid concentrations throughout most of their brain regions when exposed to anoxia. Thus, normoglycemia and slight hypoglycemia during anoxia is brain protective.

Both animal and human fetuses and newborns generally exhibit greater tolerances to asphyxia than do adults.[4] Their higher brain tolerances are understandable because both fetuses and newborns maintain serum glucose concentrations well below those of adults. Further, the brains of early fetuses generally show much lower glycogen concentrations than do the brains of near-term fetuses, newborns, or adults. Both the fetuses' lower serum glucose and their lower brain glycogen concentrations reduce the severity of brain tissue acidosis during brain exposure to anoxia. The fetuses' reduced brain tissue acidosis from exposure to anoxia produces a circumstance where most fetal brain areas fall short of reaching the threshold for injury. A similar brain protection against anoxia can be achieved in adults by inducing a slight hypoglycemia by food deprivation. Unfortunately, the stress of asphyxia itself generally produces a fetal hyperglycemia as a consequence of glucose release from hepatic glycogen stores due to catecholamine stimulation. These relations point out the importance of avoiding maternal and fetal hyperglycemia during labor, since the fetus' glycemia is influenced by that of the mother, and hyperglycemia is a risk factor for brain damage from asphyxia.

An infant born with a very low Apgar score as a consequence of asphyxia who nonetheless survives without brain injury averts injury through one of three mechanisms: (1) the fetus was hypoxic but never brain anoxic; (2) the fetus was exposed to a brief anoxia, the duration of which limited brain tissue lactic acid accumulation; and (3) the brain anoxia of the fetus was sufficiently long as to provoke a maximum lactic acid accumulation (4 to 8 minutes), but the resultant acidosis remained below the threshold for injury as a consequence of an insufficient supply of carbohydrate substrates (low glycemia). One or another of these mechanisms account for the fact that the great majority of asphyxiated fetuses escape brain injury.

It is sometimes mistakenly assumed that increasing the severity of fetal asphyxia increases the severity of brain damage that may be produced. Thus, according to this assumption, if a severe asphyxia is markedly damaging, then a slight asphyxia must be minimally damaging. The continuum of severity of clinical deficit which may be seen developmentally ranges from minor learning disability on the one hand, to a disabling cerebral palsy and mental handicap on the other. Slight learning disability then, according to this scheme, would be interpreted as reflecting exposure to a slight degree of birth asphyxia. This view of a relation between the continuum of severity of asphyxia a fetus may experience and the continuum of severity of clinical deficit and of brain damage produced is *not* supported by animal experimental studies. Rather, fetal exposure to intrapartum asphyxia either produces focally destructive lesions of the brain or fails to damage the brain at all. Furthermore, the experimental evidence would indicate that both slight and moderate degrees of asphyxia are well tolerated by fetuses without producing pathologic change in the brain.

In summary, intrapartum asphyxia damages the brain only if this organ experiences an episode of anoxia and if its available carbohydrate substrates as influenced by glycemia are sufficient to produce a marked brain tissue lactic acidosis. Prolonged intrapartum asphyxia produces a progressive systemic acidosis which ultimately imparts cardiovascular collapse. The very low fetal blood oxygen values induced by the asphyxia combined with significant reduction in cerebral blood flow produced as a consequence of the depressed cardiovascular performance eventually renders the brain anoxic and causes fetal brain injury or death (Table 41–1). Fetuses' physiologically low serum glucose concentrations protect the brain during anoxia and result in a brainstem/thalamic pattern of injury if anoxia brain injury occurs. Elevation of the fetal serum glucose concentration at the time cerebral anoxia takes place, on the other hand, significantly reduces the brain tolerance to anoxia and causes cerebral hemispheric patterns of brain injury. A prolonged steady hypotension without circulatory collapse caused by hypoxia, particularly as it occurs in earlier fetuses, selectively damages the white matter. In the majority of instances of intrapartum asphyxia, a fetal circulatory collapse caused by the asphyxia is a necessary condition for brain injury.

## Perspectives of Brain Injury

Intrapartum asphyxia damages the brain only if this organ experiences an episode of anoxia and if its available carbohydrate substrates as influenced by glycemia are sufficient to produce a marked brain tissue lactic acidosis. Prolonged intrapartum asphyxia produces a progressive systemic acidosis which ultimately impairs cardiovascular performance leading, first, to a systemic hypotension and, later, to a cardiovascular collapse. The very low fetal blood oxygen values induced by the asphyxia combined with significant reductions in cerebral blood flow produced as a consequence of the depressed cardiovascular performance eventually renders the brain anoxic and causes fetal brain injury or death. Fetuses' physiologically low serum glucose concentrations protect the brain during anoxia and result in a brainstem/thalamic pattern of injury if anoxia brain injury occurs. Elevation of the fetal serum glucose concentration at the time cerebral anoxia takes place, on the other hand, markedly reduces the brain tolerance to anoxia and causes cerebral hemispheric patterns of brain injury. A prolonged steady hypotension without circulatory collapse caused by hypoxia, particularly as it occurs in earlier fetuses, selectively damages the white matter. Grades 1 to 3 intraventricular hemorrhage bear little relation to hypoxic-ischemic events, while Grade 4 intraventricular hemorrhage, unrelated to Grades 1 to 3 intraventricular hemorrhage, arises as hemorrhages from areas of parenchymal necrosis caused by anoxia/ischemia. Only Grade 4 intraventricular hemorrhage risks marked neurologic impairment. In the majority of instances of intrapartum asphyxia, a fetal circulatory collapse caused by the asphyxia is a necessary condition for brain injury.

## *Evaluating Fetal Condition During Labor*

Continuous electronic fetal monitoring, first introduced by Hon in the 1950s, gained widespread use in the 1970s. Animal experimentation had indicated that fetal hypoxia and acidosis often produced abnormalities in the recorded fetal heart beat. The dramatic improvement in the precision with which fetal cardiac activity could be

**Table 41–2.** Guidelines for Minimum Frequency of Auscultation* of Fetal Heart Rate in Labor

| | Low Risk | With Risk Factors |
|---|---|---|
| Active phase of first stage | Every 30 minutes | Every 15 minutes |
| Second stage | Every 15 minutes | Every 5 minutes |

* Auscultation should occur after a contraction whenever possible.

observed and recorded was expected to provide an improvement in fetal outcome. Randomized prospective trials of continuous fetal monitoring have not, however, been able to demonstrate a significant reduction in mortality or an improvement in several measures of morbidity. Thus, while continuous monitoring may be more effective than intermittent auscultation of fetal heart rate in detecting intrapartum fetal compromise, the benefit of that detection in terms of a recognizable decrease in fetal morbidity and mortality has not yet been apparent (Table 41–2).

Reflecting this, the current American College of Obstetrics and Gynecology guidelines (September 1989) state that either intermittent auscultation or continuous monitoring may be used during labor to assess fetal status. The frequency of auscultation or evaluation of a continuous fetal heart rate tracing depends upon the presence of risk factors, and is increased during the second stage of labor or during changes in maternal hemodynamic status, such as during conduction anesthesia dosing. There has been much concern about the possibly unnecessary operative delivery of fetuses with fetal heart rate tracings interpreted as "asphyxia," "hypoxia," or "fetal distress" who show no evidence of compromise in the immediate or delayed neonatal period. Such operative deliveries would, of course, hinder clinical research attempts to demonstrate a measurable benefit of continuous electronic fetal monitoring. Recently, a move has been made to follow the American College of Obstetrics and Gynecology guidelines that the terms "asphyxia," "hypoxia," and "fetal distress" should be abandoned in descriptions of fetal monitoring, whether continuous or intermittent (Table 41–3). Rather, a fetal heart rate should be considered either reassuring or nonreassuring, or ominous. Any nonreassuring fetal heart rate pattern must be interpreted along with other clinical data (Table 41–3). The increasing availability of fetal scalp pH can assist in interpretation and management of a nonreassuring fetal heart rate. Recently, the technique of observing fetal heart rate response to scalp stimulation or acoustic stimulation has also been shown to correlate well with fetal well-being.

## *Monitoring Methods*

Intermittent auscultation of fetal heart rate may be done with a fetal stethoscope or a Doppler ultrasound monitor. The fetal heart should be auscultated for at least 30 seconds following a contraction at the frequency recommended in the American College of Obstetrics and Gynecology guidelines (Table 41–2). If continuous electronic fetal monitoring is used, then the same guidelines are used to determine the frequency of evaluation of the tracing. Continuous electronic fetal heart rate monitoring can be accomplished by external or internal devices. An external monitor device usually employs Doppler ultrasound to detect movement of a cardiac structure. The transducer is gently strapped to the maternal abdomen. Each movement of the structure aligned beneath the transducer is interpreted as a heart beat. The time between two beats is measured and the frequency of beats per minute instantly calculated and displayed. A continuous recording of the frequency is generated along the top portion of a standardized paper strip. Because the transducer may detect cardiac movement at slightly different points in the cardiac cycle, the beat-to-beat variations in frequency known as the short-term variability may be artificially depicted. Improvements in the capability of the ultrasound devices have improved the precision of external monitors in detecting short-term variability, but internal fetal heart rate monitoring provides an even more exact evaluation of the cardiac event. For example, unusual fetal heart rate patterns such as the rare sinusoidal type could not be detected by the periodic auscultation of the fetal heart (Figure 41–4). This method employs a spiral electrode attached through the open cervix to the fetal scalp after the membranes are ruptured, with the second contact immersed in the electrolyte-rich vaginal fluids. These are attached to a ground plate applied to the maternal leg. This allows precise detection of the electrocardiac event, and again, the frequency of events is instantly calculated and displayed. Because of the greater precision of this device, the beat-to-beat variability of rate can be reliably determined, which is an important prognosticator of fetal well-being.

Both internal and external methods are subject to error. The external monitor may either pick up a strong maternal pulse or have a very high fetal rate providing misleading information. The internal monitor may display maternal pulse if mistakenly applied to maternal tissue, or may

**Table 41–3.** Fetal Heart Rate Tracings

| | Rate (bpm) | Variability | Variable Decelerations | Late Decelerations |
|---|---|---|---|---|
| Reassuring | 120–160 | Present | Occasional, Mild | None |
| Nonreassuring | 100–180 | Present or Reduced | Moderate, Frequent | Occasional, Not Persistent |
| Ominous | $<100$ or $>180$ | Normal or Reduced | Severe | Persistent |

Note: Not all the described abnormalities need be present for a tracing to be considered nonreassuring or ominous.

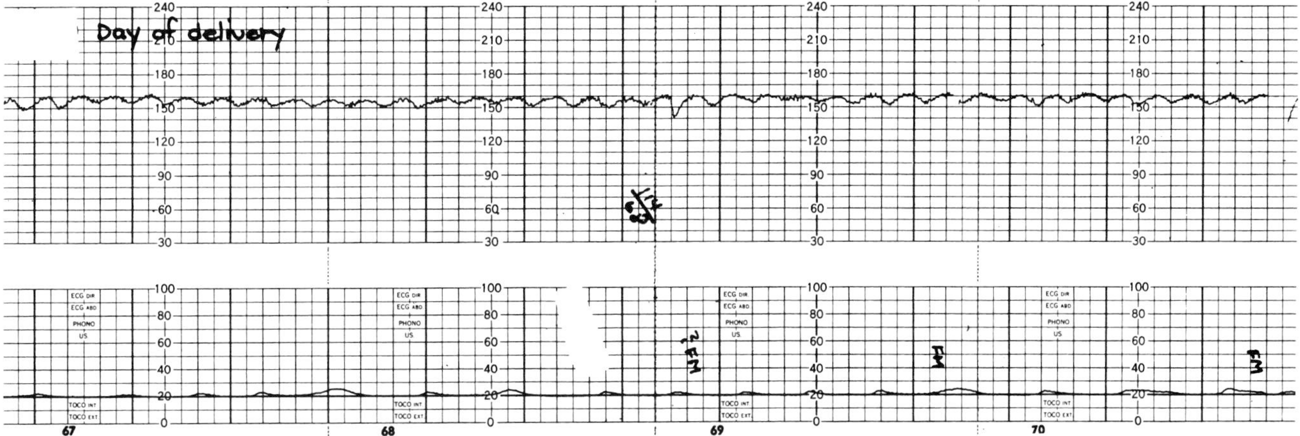


**Fig. 41–5.** Antepartum sinusoidal heart rate pattern. The sine wave, a longterm variability, may be seen to fluctuate above and below the baseline, is constant, and may be seen with late decelerations. This often represents severe fetal anemia or hypoxia. (From Freeman RK, Garite J, Nageotte P: Fetal Heart Rate Monitoring. 2nd ed. Baltimore, Williams & Wilkins, 1991.)

even detect maternal electrocardiogram activity transmitted through a dead fetus.

Uterine contraction activity may also be monitored, and the relationship of certain fetal heart rate patterns to uterine contractions is very important. External monitoring uses a tocodynamometer applied to the maternal abdomen over the uterus. The tocodynamometer detects pressure changes through the abdominal wall as the uterus contracts. The length and frequency of the contractions are recorded along the lower portion of the paper strip. The tocodynamometer cannot determine absolute intensity of contractions.

Internal intrauterine contraction monitoring employs a plastic catheter placed through the open cervix to rest within the uterine cavity. The catheter is filled with sterile water and internal pressure changes caused by contractions are transmitted to a strain transducer and converted to an electrical signal which is displayed. This intrauterine device can measure absolute intensity of contractions, as well as length and frequency of contractions.

## Advantages and Disadvantages

An obvious advantage of internal monitoring is more precise observation of fetal heart rate and uterine contractions. However, external monitoring can be used prior to rupture of membranes and cervical dilatation while internal monitoring cannot. Internal monitoring does carry a very low risk of fetal damage due to incorrect placement of the electrode, e.g., on an eye or a fontanelle. This can be prevented by careful application. The intrauterine pressure catheter has been implicated in uterine rupture, but again this is prevented by correct application. Studies have suggested that internal monitoring may increase the rate of postpartum endometritis, but this has not been confirmed by randomized trials.

## Fetal Scalp pH and Scalp Stimulation

Additional information on fetal welfare may be obtained by sampling fetal blood for pH determination.[21,22,23] The presence or absence of acidemia can then be helpful in management. To perform this sampling, the fetal membranes must be ruptured, the cervix must be dilated enough to allow visualization of the fetal scalp, and the vertex must be low enough in the pelvis to be reached. A cone with a 2 cm opening at its tip is placed against the scalp and the visible portion of scalp is wiped dry. A puncture is made with a 2 mm blade and the blood is drawn into a heparinized capillary tube. While the blood is being analyzed for pH, firm pressure must be applied to the puncture site for at least 2 contractions or 5 minutes to assure hemostasis. Prepackaged kits are available which include the items needed to obtain the sample, and the procedure has become common in many hospitals. However, the capability to measure pH on very small samples is not available in some small hospitals. Recently, attention has been directed towards scalp stimulation and acoustic stimulation response. The fetal scalp is vigorously stroked with the examiner's finger and any change in the fetal heart rate is observed closely. Acoustic stimulation through the maternal abdomen with an artificial larynx has also been employed to induce a response in the fetal heart rate. Prospective trials have shown that an acceleration in fetal heart rate in response to scalp or acoustic stimulation has a strong positive predictive value for a normal pH. Thus, a reassuring response to scalp stimulation may obviate the need for blood sampling.

## Fetal Monitoring Interpretation

A normal fetal heart rate is between 120 to 160 beats per minute. If intermittent auscultation is used, a fetal heart rate is considered reassuring if it falls within these limits. Occasionally, a rate between 100 to 119 beats per minute may be detected, though this does not usually indicate fetal compromise. Three instances of a nonreassuring fetal heart rate detected during intermittent auscultation are specified in American College of Obstetrics and Gynecology guidelines: (1) a baseline rate between contractions of less than 100 bpm; (2) a rate less than 100 bpm persisting more than 30 seconds beyond a contraction; and (3) baseline tachycardia over 160 bpm. When any of these instances occur, further investigation into fetal status should be made. Usually, this involves continuous electronic fetal monitoring, preferably internal monitoring. If continuous monitoring is not available and an auscultated nonreassuring heart rate persists, then immediate delivery may be indicated.

When continuous monitoring is employed, much more information about fetal status is available; for example, the unusual pattern such as sinusoidal as shown in Figure 41–5. As above, a normal fetal heart rate baseline is between 120 to 160 bpm, while a rate between 100 to 119 bpm may sometimes be seen, and usually does not indicate fetal compromise. Any rate below 100 which lasts for 3 minutes or longer is termed bradycardia.

Moderate bradycardia is a rate between 80 to 100 bpm and may be seen intermittently with head compression such as during the second stage of labor. Severe bradycardia is a rate less than 80 bpm and suggests fetal compromise. This may be seen in instances where blood supply to the fetus is acutely reduced, such as placental abruption, prolonged cord compression as in cord prolapse, hypertonus of the uterus during oxytocin stimulation, or maternal hypotension as may occur with epidural anesthesia or the supine position (Figures 41–6, 41–7). Prolonged bradycardia requires intervention to correct the underlying cause if possible, or immediate delivery may be warranted. In rare instances, bradycardia is due to congenital fetal heartblock which can be shown by fetal electrocardiogram and does not require immediate intervention. This uncommon condition would usually be detected during prenatal care and would not initially present in labor.

Tachycardia is defined as mild when the fetal heart rate is 161 to 180 bpm and severe when over 180 bpm. Fetal tachycardia is seen in maternal dehydration, in fetal or maternal infection (often even preceding development of maternal fever), in fetal anemia, in maternal hyperthyroidism, or after sympathomimetic drugs including caffeine, amphetamines, or cocaine. Hydration should be initiated along with detection and correction of underlying causes. Tachycardia does not usually suggest significant fetal compromise, although its presence does cause extra work for the fetus, and such fetal tracings should be closely watched for the development of other signs of fetal compromise. Like bradycardia, fetal tachycardia may also rarely be caused by a dysrhythmia. In these cases, the rate is usually over 200 bpm.

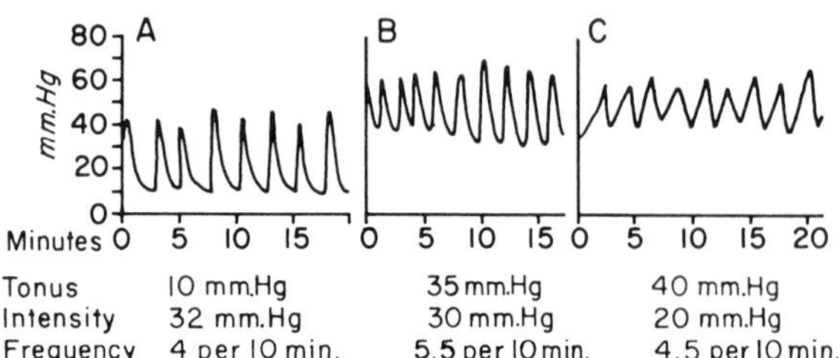


**Fig. 41–7.** Record of amniotic fluid pressure in a normal parturient **(A)** and in patients with abruptio placentae (B, C). Note the high resting tonus and low intensity of contractions in abruptio. (From Caldeyro-Barcia R, Alvarez H: Amniotic Fluid Pressure. J. Obstet. Gynaec. Brit. Emp. 59:655, 1952.)

Any significant change in the baseline fetal heart rate during the course of labor may be a sign of fetal compromise, even if the baseline rate remains within normal limits. Such fetal heart rates should be evaluated for the presence of other signs of compromise.

Following assessment of fetal heart rate, the baseline variability should be considered. Long-term variability is the difference in rate seen over 10 to 20 second intervals. This appears as an irregular flowing pattern of amplitude change in the fetal heart rate. Though internal monitoring provides the most precise information, long-term variability can sometimes be adequately appreciated by external

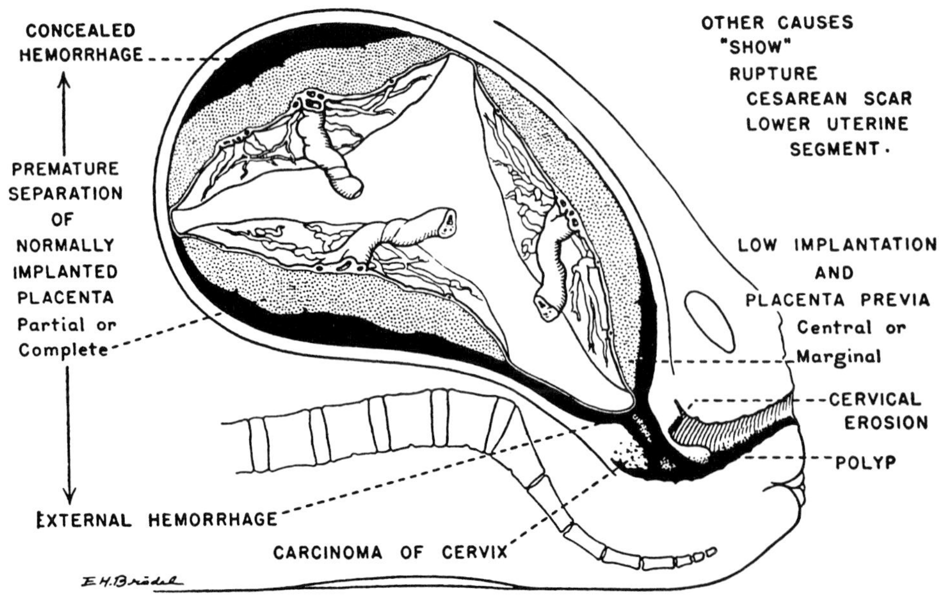


**Fig. 41–6.** Hemorrhage from premature placental separation. Extensive placental abruption (upper left) but with the periphery of the placenta and the membranes still adherent, resulting in completely concealed hemorrhage. Placental abruption (lower portion of figure) with the placenta detached peripherally and with the membranes between the placenta and cervical canal stripped from underlying decidua, allowing external hemorrhage. Partial placenta previa (right) with placental separation and external hemorrhage. (From Cunningham FG, MacDonald PC, Gant NF: Williams Obstetrics. 18th ed. East Norwalk, Appleton and Lange, 1989.)

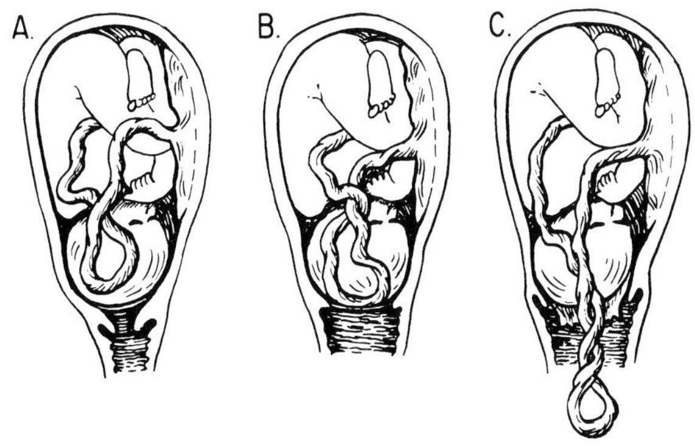


**Fig. 41–8.** Prolapse of the umbilical cord. **A,** Occult prolapse with intact membranes; little risk of pressure on the cord. **B,** Forelying cord; increasing risk of compression. **C,** Frank prolapse; high risk of compression. (From Greenhill JP: Obstetrics. 13th ed. Philadelphia, WB Saunders Co., 1965.)

monitoring. Long-term variability may be described as normal (more than 6 bpm), reduced (2 to 6 bpm), or absent (less than 2 bpm).

Short-term variability is the small but measurable difference in rate between each cardiac cycle and is a very important sign of fetal status. Generally, a healthy fetus exhibits a variability of 3 to 8 bpm in baseline heart rate, indicating an active autonomic nervous system. Absence of variability reflects a decrease in autonomic nervous system activity which could be due to many causes, including fetal compromise and acidosis. However, variability is also absent following administration of medications, including narcotics in doses commonly used in labor and during naturally occurring fetal sleep cycles which may last up to 40 minutes. Absence of variability is also seen in anencephalic fetuses and other congenital or induced fetal neurologic impairment. During labor, if a fetal heart rate tracing initially exhibits good variability which then disappears, and the absent variability cannot be attributed to a fetal sleep cycle or narcotic medication, close observation is required. If persistent, a need for further assessment of fetal status must be undertaken (Figure 41–8).

The next aspect of a fetal heart rate tracing that should be evaluated is the presence of periodic changes. These are changes in rate that occur either spontaneously or with a regular relationship to uterine contractions. The relationship of the fetal heart rate tracing to simultaneously recorded uterine contractions is an important component of elective fetal monitoring. During a contraction, intervillous space blood flow is reduced and maternal-fetal oxygen transport may be impaired. The response of the fetal heart rate to the stress of uterine contractions, therefore, must be carefully analyzed for characteristics which suggest fetal hypoxia.

## Accelerations of Fetal Heart Rate

Accelerations during antepartum testing are a reassuring finding and are thought to represent increased fetal sympathetic activity. When occurring with a contraction, they also probably represent sympathetic activity as a response to the contraction, perhaps as a compensation to mildly reduced uteroplacental blood flow due to the contraction. While generally not considered an ominous sign, neither are accelerations with contractions considered reassuring.

## Early Decelerations of Fetal Heart Rate

Decelerations that occur concomitantly with contractions and have a gradual beginning and ending are termed *early decelerations.* The deceleration must coincide completely with the contraction and cannot last longer than the contraction. They are generally mild, and have the appearance of a mirror image of the contraction, falling only 15 to 20 bpm below the baseline. They are theoretically due to a vagal response to fetal head compression, but this has not been thoroughly proven. Over time, it has been determined that these are benign patterns of interest, but of no alarm from the clinician's standpoint.

## Late Decelerations of Fetal Heart Rate

Late decelerations have the same shape as early decelerations, with a gradual slope to the amplitude changes and with the appearance of a mirror image of the contraction. However, late decelerations are delayed in both onset and conclusion by 10 to 20 seconds after onset and conclusion of the contraction. Late decelerations may have an amplitude ranging from 10 to over 45 bpm. While a larger drop in heart rate is seen in more severe decelerations, even mild (less than 20 bpm) late decelerations should be immediately evaluated.

Parer has described two types of late decelerations.[24] The first is termed *reflex late deceleration* and is a response of the previously well-oxygenated fetus to an acute fall in uterine blood flow during a contraction. Blood which has not been reoxygenated is returned from the placental bed to the fetus, where chemoreceptors respond by triggering vagal activity, resulting in the circulation time from the placenta to the chemoreceptors. There remains adequate uterine blood flow to oxygenation between contractions so variability, reflecting adequate cerebral oxygenation, is maintained.

The second type of late deceleration is that accompanied by absent variability, suggesting impaired autonomic nervous system oxygenation. This is thought to occur when the deoxygenated blood returning from the placenta not only triggers chemoreceptor response, but also directly suppresses the myocardial tissue function. The associated absent variability indicates the more ominous nature of this type of late deceleration.

Late decelerations occur as the result of intermittent decreases in the oxygen content of the fetal blood.[25] The fetal heart slows in response to a vagal stimulus in the early stages of fetal stress. Once the fetus has become profoundly acidotic, there is loss of central nervous system control and the late decelerations are produced by direct myocardial hypoxia.[26] The treatment for repetitive late decelerations is dependent, therefore, on the stage of the problem, inasmuch as stress requires less immediate action than distress.

In the early stages of a late deceleration pattern, the

fluctuations in the oxygen level produce a relative deficiency in the oxygen content of the fetal blood. During this period, the fetus is able to continue its normal metabolic functions, although some shunting of the blood supply will take place in order to maintain optimum perfusion to the heart and brain.[27] As the peripheral tissues continue to be underperfused, there will be a gradual accumulation of lactic acid which, if allowed to continue, will lead to a metabolic acidosis. Intervention at this point may prevent the acidosis and any potential harm from occurring.

In a study using a transcutaneous oxygen electrode placed on the fetal scalp, Willcourt, et al found that although the fetal oxygen level was not always elevated by placing the mother on her left side, in many cases positioning the mother on the right side could improve the fetal oxygen tension. They concluded that there is a *preferred* lateral position for each patient.[28] Therefore, one can position the mother on either side, using the usual parameters of fetal assessment to evaluate the efficacy of this approach (Figure 41–9).

Next, the mother should be given oxygen by face mask. If an open mask is used, the oxygen flow rate must be at 10 liters per minute, as flow rates less than this do not raise the fetal oxygen tension to its potential maximum.[29] The fetal $tcPO_2$ can be elevated by as much as 8 mmHg by keeping the $FIO_2$ as high as possible. This represents an increase in the oxygen-carrying capacity of the fetal blood of as much as 5 ml to 6 ml of oxygen per kg.[30–33] Any underlying maternal disease such as asthma, pneumonia, or pulmonary edema must be aggressively treated. The efficacy of maternal hyperoxygenation is dependent on the ability of the uteroplacental unit to transfer oxygen to the fetus, and if this is already impaired, the additional oxygen supplied to the fetus may not be sufficient to overcome the problem.

Thus, the blood flow to the uterus needs to be enhanced so that an adequate maternal blood flow through the intervillous space is maintained. A liter of intravenous electrolyte fluid is usually sufficient, along with the other components of the treatment, to begin the process of intrauterine resuscitation. Caution must always be taken, however, to monitor the patient's fluid intake and output to avoid excessive replacement. Similarly, the patient's blood pressure must be closely observed, as even mild maternal hypotension may reduce uterine blood flow enough to lead to a very worrisome fetal heart rate tracing. As discussed previously, ephedrine may occasionally be necessary to restore adequate uterine and fetal blood flow.

All of these steps are important in the process of in utero fetal resuscitation. However, the factor limiting the efficacy of this treatment is the microscopic anatomical structure of the placenta. If there is structural damage to the placenta from preexisting maternal disease such as diabetes mellitus or hypertension, for example, the above techniques will have only a limited effect, since exchange

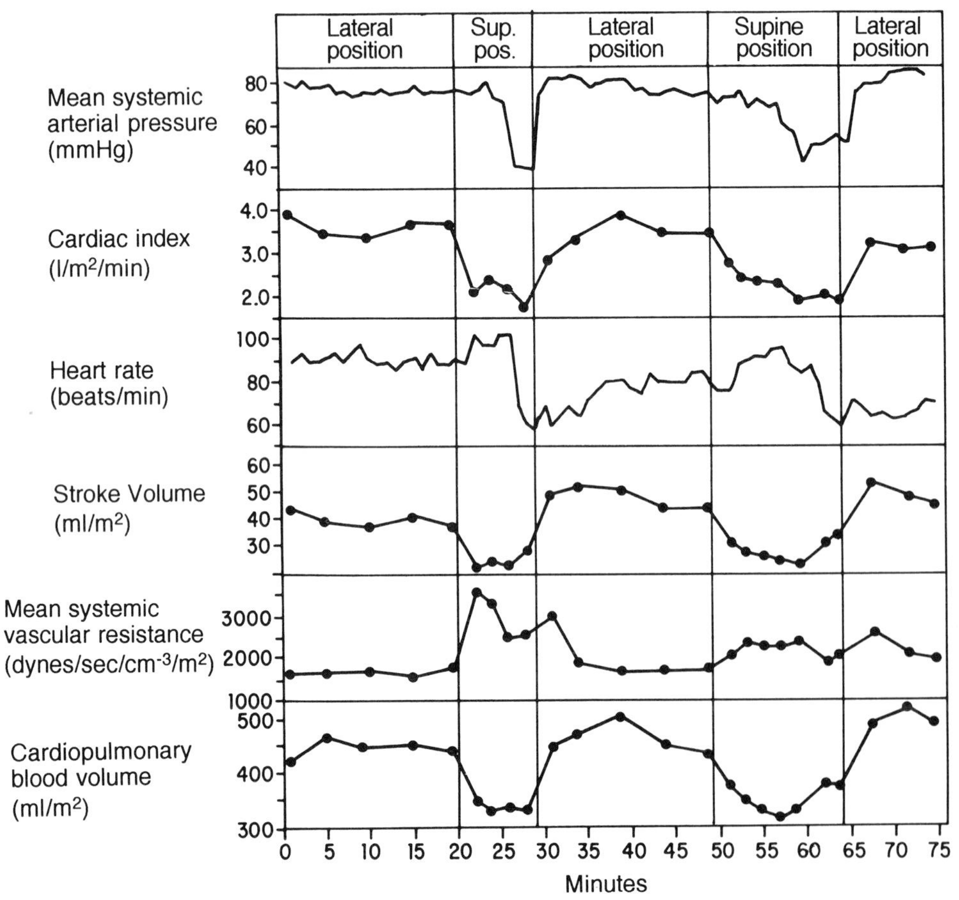


**Fig. 41–9.** Serial hemodynamic studies in a patient who exhibited supine hypotension. After the patient was lying supine for 6 minutes, a profound fall in arterial pressure and pulse rate was seen. (Redrawn from Kerr MG: Cardiovascular dynamics in pregnancy and labour. Br. Med. Bull. 24:19, 1968.)

across the intervillous space will continue to be impaired.[34]

Under these circumstances, cessation of the uterine contractions may improve the fetal environment. Tocolytic agents such as terbutaline can be given subcutaneously to the mother.[35] The fetal oxygen tension will rise once the contractions cease, allowing time to evaluate the fetal status before deciding whether to let the labor resume.

The betamimetics are the tocolytic drugs of choice for this purpose as they can be given quickly, which is an essential aspect of intrauterine resuscitation.[35] The fetal heart rate should indicate that there is an improvement in the fetal oxygen tensions within a few minutes of instituting treatment, though if one has had to resort to these techniques to resuscitate the fetus, there is a great likelihood that the labor will not be allowed to continue and the fetus will be delivered abdominally.

By maintaining the mother in the lateral position, using hyperoxygenation, expanding her blood volume, and possibly using a tocolytic drug, one should be able to alleviate the immediate fetal heart rate abnormalities and gain some time in which to plan a further course of action. This is the essence of fetal resuscitation as applied to a late deceleration pattern. If the pattern is allowed to persist, the oxygen deficit can lead to severe acidosis and central nervous system dysfunction in the fetus.

## *Variable Decelerations of Fetal Heart Rate*

Unlike early and late decelerations, variable decelerations may have any configuration and any temporal relationship to contractions. They generally have an abrupt beginning and ending, though the return to baseline may sometimes occur more gradually. The abrupt fall in fetal heart rate is caused by sudden vagal activity, which may be stimulated by several events (Table 41–4). Umbilical cord compression has been shown to directly cause variable decelerations, and head compression may also lead to variable decelerations. Generally, short term fetal heart rate variability is maintained, indicating adequate central oxygenation. Loss of variability, or severe (less than 60 bpm or a drop of more than 60 bpm from the baseline) variable decelerations may signal fetal compromise.

Variable decelerations occur frequently in the second stage of labor, probably due to head compression and, if variability is maintained, probably do not indicate fetal compromise. Variable decelerations are a manifestation of umbilical cord compression,[36] and are seen when the umbilical cord becomes entangled around the fetus, or when the uterus presses on the cord during a contraction. A similar situation is seen with oligohydramnios, where the normally protected floating cord may be compressed against the uterine wall.

**Table 41–4.** Ordinary Causes of Severe Decelerations

1. Overt cord problems
2. Occult cord problems
3. Abruptio placenta
4. Fetal bleed
5. Idiosyncratic drug reaction
6. Severe maternal hypotension

In these cases, the fetal systemic blood pressure may increase as the normal flow pattern confronts an impediment; this mechanism at the same time may elicit a vagally mediated baroreceptor reflex to slow the heart rate.[37] The blood flow from the placenta is impaired only for the duration of the cord compression, and once the obstruction is relieved, the flow returns to normal. It is during the period of impaired blood flow that the fetus experiences reduced delivery of oxygen to the peripheral tissues. At first, the blockage will slow the velocity of the blood returning to the placenta. This means that the blood that is already present in the periphery will remain there a little longer. This allows for greater extraction of oxygen and results in a higher level of carbon dioxide in the fetal blood. If this process is transient, with full recovery of the blood flow within a few seconds, there will not be any significant hypoxemia, and the fetal metabolic processes will continue normally. The initial effects of umbilical cord compression, therefore, include a lowered oxygen content and a higher level of carbon dioxide in the blood returning to the placenta. This is a respiratory acidosis. A severe respiratory acidosis exists when the fetal $PCO_2$ rises above 60 mmHg in the umbilical artery.[38] If the cord compression continues, the pH will fall and, by virtue of the fact that the fetal blood entering the intervillous space will not be able to unload all the carbon dioxide and fully exchange with oxygen, an oxygen debt will develop. Thus, a mixed respiratory and metabolic acidosis will occur.

## *Obstetric Management*

It is important to remember that electronic fetal heart rate monitoring is a sensitive but not specific test for fetal compromise. Electronic monitoring should be used primarily as a screening measure. An abnormal tracing is not in itself diagnostic of fetal compromise. Many normal women demonstrate some abnormalities in their fetal monitoring tracing, usually only intermittently, and it is important that the clinician not overreact to transient fetal heart rate abnormalities when the patient and her fetus appear otherwise. An abnormal fetal heart tracing should prompt the clinician to look closer at the clinical context to decide if the tracing is truly indicative of fetal compromise.

In evaluating and managing fetal well-being in labor, the underlying condition of both the mother and fetus must be considered. Any maternal disease may affect the fetal heart rate tracing and should be corrected immediately. In some cases, restraint is necessary to keep from delivering the fetus with a concerning tracing during a reversible state of maternal compromise. In diabetic ketoacidosis, for example, poor variability and late decelerations that may be seen will almost always resolve with correction of the maternal metabolic state. During a grand mal seizure of any etiology, fetal bradycardia may be seen which usually resolves as the post-ictal state resolves. The concerning fetal heart rate tracings seen during these reversible maternal states are managed differently from concerning tracings seen during labor.

In addition, the ability of a given fetus to withstand stresses must be considered. Prematurity, infection, and uteroplacental insufficiency of any etiology all place a fetus at greater risk of an abnormal fetal heart rate tracing and, ultimately, a poor outcome. In these situations, earlier evaluation and treatment of mild abnormal fetal heart rate tracings may be warranted.

Three specific conditions warrant further discussion: uterine hyperstimulation, maternal hypotension, and umbilical cord prolapse.

### Hyperstimulation

One of the most common causes of fetal distress is that caused by overzealous administration of oxytocin which elicits uterine hyperstimulation. This complication is simply due to the overshoot in intravenous dosage that results in the development of a uterine hypercontractile state. It may be manifest by an increase in frequency referred to as polystole, or as already alluded to, it may be manifest by hyperstimulation or a hypertonic uterus. Either of these have a negative total effect upon fetal blood flow due to interruption of normal placental intervillous blood exchange. The most common result is the development of fetal distress limited to the duration of the hyperstimulation. The healthy fetus will rebound immediately and without sequelae after the oxytocin is stopped. The pathophysiology behind this result is the reduction in exchange of oxygen and carbon dioxide at the intervillous level (Figure 41–1). The pathologic continuum consists of mild reductions in fetal $PaO_2$ slight elevations in $PaCO_2$ and mild respiratory acidosis in mild cases on the one hand to severe disturbance in exchange with hypoxia and even asphyxia with severe metabolic acidosis in severe cases on the other hand. Fortunately the biologic half-life of oxytocin is very short; therefore, the most important element in therapy is detection of the problem, followed by immediate cessation of the exogenous oxytocin. In rare instances, it may be necessary to administer a tocolytic such as magnesium sulfate or terbutaline to counteract the stimulatory effect of oxytocin. These tocolytic agents provide freedom from the continued contractions allowing a period of time wherein the fetus may be revitalized or resuscitated.

### Hypotension

This has been the most frequent complication of regional anesthesia in the past, but today, with the newer methods of minimal dosages along with adequate intravenous hydration anesthetics, this threat has nearly been eliminated. The reason for hypotension is simply that the most common effect of regional analgesia is its substantial reduction in peripheral vascular resistance. This results in a fall in pressure according to the level of reduction in vascular resistance. The pathologic continuum of this complication advances from very mild reductions in systemic pressure in mild cases on the one hand to the substantial reductions accompanied by near shock states in severe cases. Most of these hypotensive reactions can be managed with early detection and immediate action consisting of the following tenets used successfully in management of hypotension over many years:

1. elevation of the legs to a 90° angle; with
2. simultaneous left uterine displacement;
3. administration of 500 ml to 600 ml of intravenous fluid within 5 to 15 minutes; and
4. administration of 25 mg to 50 mg of ephedrine in 10 mg IV aliquots

Hypotension associated with regional anesthesia for cesarean section can still be a problem today, but even this has been managed somewhat by slow dosage regimens and thus reduction in sudden changes in peripheral vascular resistance. For instance, today, the patient may be given a 3 ml test dose, followed by 5 ml given at 5 minute periods with dermatome testing done before each injection. Usually, the dosage regimen would consist of four separate injections over a 20 minute period.

### Umbilical Cord Prolapse

Umbilical cord prolapse is a condition in which a loop of the cord has exited the cervix after rupture of the membranes. As presenting fetal part presses on the cervix, the cord is compressed. The fetal heart rate pattern in this condition will usually be bradycardia, or severe variable decelerations. In either situation, a vaginal exam should be immediately performed (Figure 41–10). If there is a cord prolapse, the presenting part can be elevated by the examiner's hand, and preparation for immediately delivery should be made.

### Other Obstetric Management

In the absence of the three specific conditions discussed above, after considering each of the described aspects of the fetal tracing and the maternal and fetal underlying status as described, the elements should be considered together. For example, mild-to-moderate variable decelerations with good variability are not as worrisome as late decelerations with absent variability. The more abnormalities and the more severe, the more concerning the tracing. Fetal heart rate tracings may be divided into three categories: reassuring, nonreassuring, and ominous (Table 41–3). In the case of a reassuring tracing, labor may be allowed to continue. If a tracing is nonreassuring, then in utero resuscitation and further evaluation as described below should be initiated. If a tracing is ominous, in utero resuscitation should be immediately begun while arrangements for prompt delivery are made.

Initial management of a tracing which is nonreassuring due to severe variable decelerations should involve a vaginal exam to rule out umbilical cord prolapse. Such a tracing could also reflect rapid descent of the fetal head. If neither of these is detected, then management should be directed at relieving possible intrauterine cord compression. Repositioning the mother allows the fetus to move within the uterus and may relieve the pressure on the umbilical cord, as well as improve uterine blood flow. If

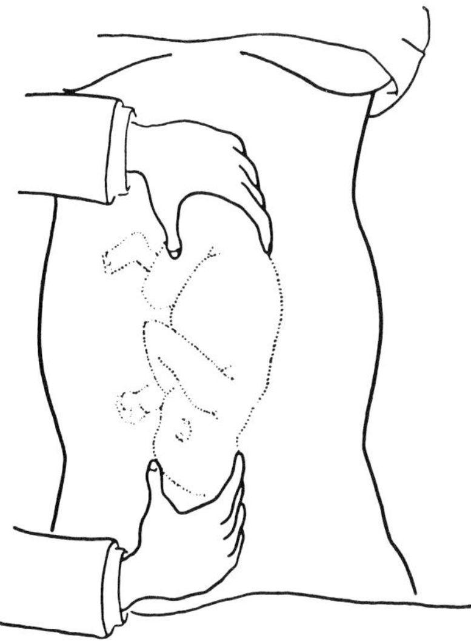

**Fig. 41–10.** Maneuver for the diagnosis of umbilical cord complications. After allowing at least 60 seconds for the fetal heart rate to stabilize following contraction (or following any procedure), the left hand is placed over the fundus of the uterus and firm pressure is applied along the long axis of the uterus for about 10 seconds. All manipulations are noted on the fetal ECG record. The presenting part of the fetus is then grasped firmly in the right hand and pushed upward toward the pelvic inlet for 20 to 50 seconds (depending on the response of the fetal heart). Following release, the fetal heart rate is observed for at least 30 to 40 seconds. The maneuver then is repeated with pressure on the presenting part applied in different directions. In this way, the entire pelvic rim is explored for possible malposition of the umbilical cord. (From Hon EH: Umbilical Cord Problems. Obstet. Gynecol. 14:154, 1959.)

an oxytocic drug is being used, stopping it will reduce the strength and frequency of the contractions and the variable decelerations may resolve. If no oxytocin is in use, a tocolytic drug may be used to abolish contractions and thus relieve variable decelerations. If these techniques do not relieve severe variable decelerations, and delivery is not imminent, then an amnioinfusion may be performed.

Amnioinfusion is gaining popularity as a technique to improve fetal heart rate tracing. Warmed saline is infused through an intrauterine contraction monitor catheter (Figure 41–11). This has been shown to dilute meconium, thereby improving fetal outcome in some cases. By adding to the volume of fluid bathing the umbilical cord, this technique may also reduce cord compression and improve the fetal heart rate tracing. Studies have reported the use of amnioinfusionwhen oligohydramnios has been suspected as a cause of cord compression (Table 41–5).[39,40] Oligohydramnios may occur under the following conditions: as a complication of a pregnancy with intrauterine growth retardation, with prolonged rupture of the membranes complicating a preterm labor in which tocolysis is used; or it may occur in a normal term pregnancy following spontaneous or artificial rupture of the membranes. The umbilical cord in each of these cases is vulnerable to cord compression. Amnioinfusion attempts

**Table 41–5.** Complete Relief of Repetitive Variable Decelerations

| | Infusion | | Noninfusion | | | |
|---|---|---|---|---|---|---|
| | No. | % | No. | % | $X^2y$* | p |
| Total group | 25/49 | 51 | 2/47 | 4.2 | 23.69 | 0.001 |
| Multiparous group | 7/22 | 31.8 | 2/26 | 7.6 | 3.11 | 0.078 |
| Nulliparous group | 18/27 | 66.7 | 0/21 | 0 | 19.65 | 0.001 |

* $x^2$ calculated with Yates correction

(From Miyazawa FS, Nevarez F: Saline amnioinfusion for relief of repetitive variable decelerations: A prospective randomized study. Am. J. Obstet. Gynecol. 153:301, 1985.)

to restore some of the lost amniotic fluid so that the cord may float freely in the uterine cavity again.

To perform this procedure, an intrauterine pressure catheter is inserted into the intrauterine cavity, if one has not been placed already (Figure 41–11). Then 300 ml to 500 ml of warm lactated Ringer's solution is infused over 15 to 30 minutes. A constant infusion of the same solution can be started by pumping at a rate of 100 ml to 200 ml per hour thereafter. One must be certain not to overdistend the capacity of the uterus as this may compress the intervillous space to such an extent that uteroplacental insufficiency develops.[41] In practice, this means infusing no more than 800 ml. The technique has been used with good results, i.e., significant relief of variable decelerations as shown in Table 41–5, and it seems likely to become a standard part of the procedures to deal with fetal distress from this particular cause.

Amnioinfusion may also be helpful in the management of persistent late decelerations. However, the first line of treatment of persistent late decelerations or absent variability is to increase oxygen delivery to the fetus by increasing uteroplacental perfusion. This is often accomplished by repositioning the patient. Maternal supine position in particular reduces uterine blood flow both by direct compression of the aortic and iliac arteries by the gravid uterus, and by decreased cardiac output due to compression of the vena cava. The supine position should thus be avoided at all times in the third trimester and especially in labor.

If the described maneuvers to improve oxygen delivery to the fetus do not lead to an improved fetal heart rate tracing, then more aggressive management is needed. If the tracing remains nonreassuring but not worrisome, then fetal scalp stimulation should be done. If an acceleration of at least 15 bpm for 15 seconds is seen, this is reassuring. However, the tracing must be closely observed and if improvement does not occur, then further assessment by scalp pH should be considered. A scalp pH should also be done if the scalp stimulation is not followed by an acceleration meeting criteria.

As referred to earlier, the interpretation of fetal scalp pH has undergone some debate, with some studies recently suggesting that the lower limit of normal may be much lower than previously thought.[38] It is well accepted that a scalp pH greater than 7.25 is normal. If a value above 7.25 is obtained, close observation should be continued

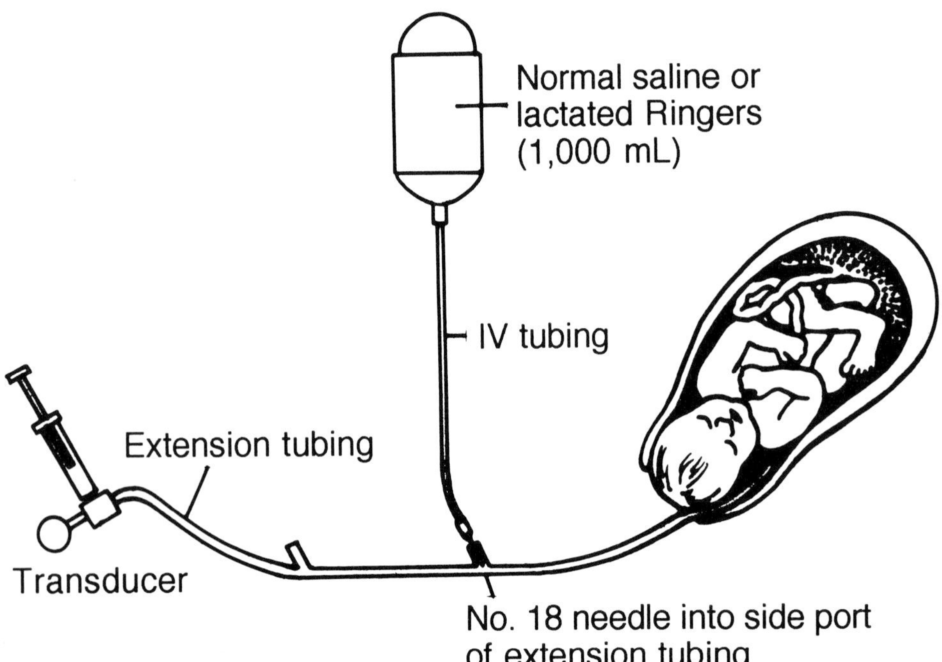


**Fig. 41–11.** Insertion of intrauterine pressure catheter. A setup of treating repetitive variable decelerations permits continuous internal monitoring of uterine contractions during amnioinfusion. (Redrawn from Miyazaki FS: Relieving variable decelerations. Cont. OB-Gyn, February, 1987.)

and scalp sampling repeated as indicated by the fetal heart rate tracing. Scalp pH between 7.20 and 7.25 is considered borderline and should be repeated in 15 to 30 minutes to evaluate for a possible decline in pH. A value below 7.20 is considered abnormal and necessitates intervention, and probably rapid delivery.

### *Emergency Delivery*

In addition to a fetal scalp pH $< 7.20$, an ominous fetal heart rate tracing is an indication for an immediate delivery. Immediate delivery may also be indicated in the presence of a nonreassuring tracing which is persistent despite in utero resuscitation techniques as previously described. Delivery must be accomplished either by a vaginal or abdominal route. Anesthetic considerations for emergency cesarean section are discussed elsewhere. Immediate vaginal delivery may be accomplished by the use of forceps or a vacuum extractor, or, in the case of breech presentation, by a vaginal breech extraction. For immediate vaginal delivery, the cervix must be fully dilated and adequate anesthesia is essential.

If the fetal head is on the perineum, then outlet forceps may be applied. Low outlet forceps usually can be performed with just a pudendal block. For the more extensive placements of the mid forceps or vacuum extraction from the mid-pelvis, or vaginal breech extraction, rotational maneuvers are sometimes necessary up to 90° on either side of the midline. In this situation, the preferred method of analgesia is conduction block, either caudal, epidural with sacral blockade, or a subarachnoid block with the saddle block configuration. If the block is spotty, the obstetrician and the anesthesiologist can cooperate in a joint maneuver to offer some extra analgesia to the patient with $N_2O$, and even small aliquots of ketamine (in 5 mg to 10 mg increments, up to a total of 25 mg to 35 mg over 5 minutes) during application and traction with the forceps. This is one of these close working situations where the obstetrician and the anesthesiologist must be able to communicate during the actual progress of the case. The obstetrician has a difficult job in that he or she must deliver a baby in a situation which is not certain, i.e., perhaps vaginal delivery may not be accomplishable and an emergent cesarean section may be necessary for ultimate delivery. Throughout the actual process, the two colleagues must work closely together and be reactive to each other's needs for the benefit of providing an optimum outcome for the mother and her baby. Intense motor and sensory block is found to be the best situation most of the time, and this allows freedom in attempting to deliver from below without the distress or negative efforts of the mother hindering the process.

If a vaginal delivery cannot be attempted, or is attempted but unsuccessful, then cesarean delivery is indicated. The safety of the mother must be maintained, however, despite the urgency of the situation. Careful consideration to maternal welfare must be given by both the obstetrician and the anesthesiologist.

## Summary

Intrapartum fetal heart rate monitoring has become an accepted standard of care in the hospitals of the United States. The techniques include intermittent auscultation and continuous electronic monitoring by external or internal devices. The information provided by these techniques must be interpreted along with careful consideration of the underlying maternal and fetal conditions. All of this information is used by health care providers in attempts to assure and, if indicated, improve fetal well-being. The inability of clinical trials to demonstrate a recognizable reduction in fetal morbidity and mortality when continuous monitoring is used has not led to a significant reduction in its use. In today's society, the saving of even a few lives, too few to be "significant" in a clinical trial, to say nothing of the presumed decrease in morbidity, is felt to justify the application of the technology to the majority of patients. In practice, many hospitals are currently suffering from a nursing shortage such that adequate personnel to perform intermittent auscultation are not available. Continuous electronic monitoring enables nurses to provide care for more than one patient simultaneously. This fact alone has made continuous electronic monitoring a necessity in many hospitals. In addition, in the current medico-legal environment, there may be a benefit to having an electronically generated record of fetal cardiac activity as compared to a handwritten notation of the auscultated rates.

## REFERENCES


1. Gillmer MDG, Combe B: Intrapartum fetal monitoring practice in the United Kingdom. Br. J. Obstet. Gynaecol. 86:753, 1979.
2. Adamsons K, Myers RH: Late decelerations and brain tolerance of the fetal monkey to intrapartum asphyxia. Am. J. Obstet. Gynecol. 128:893, 1977.
3. Huddleston JF, Perlis HW, Macy J Jr, Myers RE, et al: The prediction of fetal oxygenation by an on-line computer analysis of fetal monitor output. Am. J. Obstet. Gynecol. 128: 599, 1977.
4. Myers RE: Experimental models of perinatal brain damage: Relevance to human pathology. *In* Intrauterine Asphyxia and the Developing Brain. Edited by L Gluck. Chicago, Year Book Medical Publishers, Inc., 1977, pp. 37–97.
5. Myers RE, de Courten-Myers GM: Metabolic principles of patterns of perinatal brain injury. *In* Risks of Labour. Edited by JW Crawford. New York, John Wiley and Sons, 1985, pp 119–145.
6. de Courten-Myers GM, Yamaguchi S-I, Wagner KR, Ting P, et al: Brain injury from marked hypoxia in cats: Role of hypotension and hyperglycemia. Stroke 16(6):1016–1021, 1985.
7. de Courten-Myers GM, Fogelson HM, Kleinholz M, Myers RE: Hypoxic brain and heart injury thresholds in piglets. Biomed. Biochem. Acta. 48:143, 1989.
8. Ting P, Yamaguchi S, Bacher JD, Killens RH, et al: Hypoxic-ischemic cerebral necrosis in midgestational sheep fetuses: Physiopathologic correlations. Exper. Neurol. 80:227–245, 1983.
9. Myers RE: Threshold values of oxygen deficiency leading to cardiovascular and brain pathological changes in term monkey fetuses. *In* Oxygen Transport of Tissue: Instrumentation, Methods, and Physiology. Edited by DF Bruley, HI Bicker. New York, Plenum Press, 1973, pp. 1047–1054.
10. Brierley JB, Adams JH, Graham DI, Simpson JA: Neocortical death after cardiac arrest. A clinical, neurophysiological and neuropathological report of two cases. Lancet 11:560–565, 1971.
11. Brierley JB, Meldrum BS, Brown AW: The threshold and neuropathology of cerebral anoxic-ischemic cell change. Arch. Neurol. 29:367–374, 1973.
12. Cole SI, Corday E: Four-minute limit for cardiac resuscitation. JAMA 1454–1458, Aug 11, 1956.
13. Schneider M: Critical blood pressure in the cerebral circulation. *In* Selective Vulnerability of the Brain in Hypoxemia. Edited by JP Schade, WH McMenemy. Philadelphia, FA Davis Co., 1963, p. 17.
14. Myers RE, de Courten GM, Yamaguchi S, Ting et al: Failure of marked hypoxia with maintained blood pressure to produce brain injury. J. Neuropath. Exp. Neurol. 39:378, 1980.
15. Nelson KB, Ellenberg JH: Apgar scores as predictors of chronic neurologic disability. Pediatrics 68:36, 1981.
16. Myers RE, de Courten-Myers GM, Wagner KR: The effects of asphyxia on the fetal brain. *In* Fetal Physiology and Medicine. Edited by RW Beard, P Nathaniels. New York, Marcel Dekker, 1984, pp. 419–458.
17. Wagner KR, Myers RE: Metabolic basis for fetal brain tolerance to anoxia. Trans. Amer. Soc. Neurochem. 12:227, 1981.
18. Myers RE, Yamaguchi M: Tissue lactate accumulation (> 15 to 20 μmoles/g) as cause of cerebral edema. Soc. Neurosci. Abs. 2:730, 1976.
19. Myers RE: Lactic acid accumulation as cause of brain edema and cerebral necrosis resulting from oxygen deprivation. *In* Advances in Perinatal Neurology. Edited by R Korobkin, C Guilleminault. New York, Spectrum Publishers, 1979, pp. 85–114.
20. Myers RE, Wagner KR, de Courten-Myers GM: Brain metabolic and pathologic consequences of asphyxia: Role played by serum glucose concentration. *In* Advances in Perinatal Medicine. Edited by A Milunski, EA Friedman, L Gluck. New York, Plenum Medical Book Co., 1983, pp 67–115.
21. McDonald JS: Evaluation of fetal blood pH as a reflection of fetal well-being. Am. J. Obstet. Gynecol. 97:912–918, 1967.
22. Maclachlan NA, Spencer JA, Harding K, Arulkumaran S: TI Fetal acidaemia, the cardiotocograph and the T/QRS ratio of the fetal ECG in labour. Br. J. Obstet. Gynaecol. 99:26–31, 1992.
23. Endersheim TG, Hutson JM, Druzin ML, Kogut EA: Fetal heart rate response to vibratory acoustic stimulation predicts fetal pH in labor. Am. J. Obstet. Gynecol. 157: 1557–1560, 1987.
24. Parer JT, Livingston EG: What is fetal distress? Am. J. Obstet. Gynecol. 162(6):1421–1425, 1990.
25. Quilligan EJ, Katibak E, Hofschild J: Correlation of fetal heart rate patterns and blood gas values. II. Bradycardia. Am. J. Obstet. Gynecol. 91:1123, 1965.
26. Martin CB Jr, de Haan J, van der Wildt B, Jongsma HW, et al: Mechanisms of late decelerations in the fetal heart rate: A study with autonomic blocking agents in fetal lambs. Eur. J. Obstet. Gynecol. Reprod. Biol. 9:361, 1979.
27. Cohn HE, Sacks EJ, Heymann MA, Rudolph AM: Cardiovascular responses to hypoxemia and acidemia in fetal sheep. Am. J. Obstet. Gynecol. 120:817, 1974.
28. Willcourt RJ, Paust JC, Queenan JT: Changes in fetal $tcPO_2$ occurring during labour in association with lumbar extradural analgesia. Br. J. Anaesth. 54:635, 1982.
29. Kihlstrom I: Blood pressure in the fetal guinea pig. Acta. Physiol. Scand. 113:51, 1981.
30. Paulick RP, Meyers RL, Rudolph CD, Rudolph AM: Hemodynamic responses to alpha-adrenergic blockade during hypoxia in the fetal lamb. J. Dev. Physiol. 16:63, 1991.
31. Gudmundsson S, Linblad A, Marsal K: Cord blood gases and absence of end-diastolic blood velocities in the umbilical artery. Early Hum. Dev. 24:231, 1990.
32. Kokholm G: Simultaneous measurements of blood pH, $pCO_2$, $pO_2$ and concentrations of hemoglobin and its derivatives—a multicenter study. Scand. J. Clin. Lab. Invest. Suppl. 203:75, 1990.
33. Wilkening RB, Boyle DW, Meschia G: Fetal neuromuscular blockade: effect on oxygen demand and placental transport. Am. J. Physiol. 257:H734, 1989.
34. Las Heras J, Baskerville JC, Harding PG, Haust MD: Morpho-

metric studies of fetal placental stem arteries in hypertensive disorders of pregnancy. Placenta 6:217, 1985.

35. Patriarco MS, Viechnicki BM, Hutchinson TA, Klasko SK, et al: A study on intrauterine fetal resuscitation with terbutaline. Am. J. Obstet. Gynecol. 157:384, 1987.
36. Tejani N, Mann LI, Bhakthavathsalan A: Correlation of fetal heart rate patterns and fetal pH with neonatal outcome. Obstet. Gynecol. 48:460, 1976.
37. Itskovitz J, Rudolph AM: Denervation of arterial chemoreceptors and baroreceptors in fetal lambs in utero. Am. J. Physiol. 242:H916, 1982.
38. Lumley J, McKinnon L, Wood C: Lack of agreement and normal values for fetal scalp blood. J. Obstet. Gynaecol. Br. Commonw. 78:13, 1971.
39. Miyazawa FS, Nevarez F: Saline amnioinfusion for relief of repetitive variable decelerations: A prospective randomized study. Am. J. Obstet. Gynecol. 153:301, 1985.
40. Nageotte MP, Freeman RK, Garite TJ, Dorchester W: Prophylactic intrapartum amnioinfusion in patients with preterm premature rupture of the membranes. Am. J. Obstet. Gynecol. 153:557, 1985.
41. Tabor BL, Maier JA: Polyhydramnios and elevated intrauterine pressure during amnioinfusion. Am. J. Obstet. Gynecol. 156:130, 1987.

Chapter 42

# ANESTHESIA FOR FETAL INTERVENTION

JOHN W. SEEDS,
BARRY C. CORKE

---

The accurate diagnosis and subsequent treatment of fetal pathological conditions by medical or surgical means is a relatively recent development. Amniocentesis, fetoscopy, dynamic image ultrasound imaging of fetal anatomy, and percutaneous fetal blood sampling are the current methods of diagnosing fetal conditions that have evolved over the past 3 decades (Figure 42–1).[1,2,3,4,5,6] Since treatment follows diagnosis, consideration of fetal treatment followed the development of these techniques for the more accurate diagnosis of various fetal conditions.[7–18]

One of the highest visibility techniques has been intrauterine vascular transfer to benefit the fetus. Early attempts at this procedure were done blindly by using x-ray-guided grid transfer. Fortunately, today we have the ultrasound-guided percutaneous method. Table 42–1 summarizes some of the benefits of this technique.

Techniques of anesthesia can be of great assistance in these invasive methods of both diagnosis and treatment because they allow the physician to proceed with accuracy and assurance that sudden unexpected movements of either the mother or fetus will not disrupt their sensitive and specifically directed operative action. This chapter will review the historical perspective of the various methods used today and will discuss the human fetal therapeutic intervention methods and their anesthetic implications. It is acknowledged that many of the medical treatment methods available for fetal disease by administration of pharmacological agents to the mother do not require consideration of anesthetic therapy. Digitalis, for example, may be given to the mother for the treatment of fetal supraventricular tachycardia without consideration of anesthetic therapy. The direct surgical treatment of the fetus does, however, raise the issue of the need for anesthesia for both mother and fetus and will be the primary focus for this chapter.[19]

## HISTORICAL PERSPECTIVE

Animal models for fetal surgical intervention have been used for many years for laboratory investigation. Guinea pigs, lambs, and dogs have provided experimental models for fetal intestinal obstruction, coarctation of the aorta, and diaphragmatic hernia since the early 1920s.[20]

Surgical techniques for intervention in humans were researched and reported in 1963 by Liley, and focused upon the treatment of one of the great clinical challenges at that time, severe fetal hemolytic disease.[21] The original method as described involved localization of the fetus with fluoroscopy, followed by the placement of a needle percutaneously into the fetal peritoneal cavity. Tightly packed compatible red cells were then infused into the fetal peritoneal cavity. Absorption of these red cells via the thoracic duct provided effective transfusion therapy in the majority of cases. Just a few short years afterward, in 1966, Asensio reported the exteriorization of the lower limb of the human fetus through a laparotomy and hysterotomy, which allowed cannulation of the exposed femoral vessels and the luxury of complete exchange transfusion of a fetus suffering from severe hemolytic disease.[22] General anesthesia was used for this original unique operation and was described as a normal halothane anesthetic. There was no other description in the original paper beyond this, but presumably the usual induction in the endotracheal tube prior to general anesthesia was used as noted. Also, an oxygen/nitrous oxide environment of 50%, or perhaps a greater percentage of nitrous oxide, was made available.

Difficulty with maintenance of the pregnancy after exteriorization of the fetal limb through hysterotomy, and a low level of successful outcome compared to the relative success of the Liley method, soon resulted in abandonment of this approach. There was an interlude of several years before new methods became available to push onward in regard to fetal manipulative methods.

The first of these included an exciting new method of successful direct visualization of the fetus with sampling of pure fetal blood using a small fiberoptic endoscope. This method was described in 1974.[23] This revolutionary technique enabled aspiration of fetal blood, and later, direct transfusion of donor red cells through the same narrow-gauge needle used for the aspiration of the diagnostic sample.[24,25] In essence, it was the earlier method of Liley rejuvenated but now with the aid of visualization through the use of a small fiberoptic scope passed via a number 10-gauge needle. Naturally, a 10-gauge needle elicited considerable maternal pain upon penetration of the various maternal abdominal layers before reaching the fetus in utero. To offset this, heavy maternal sedation in the form of 2 cc to 3 cc midazolam and 1 cc to 2 cc fentanyl was used to ablate the painful maternal response. At the same time, these aforementioned drugs gained access to the fetal circulation and simultaneously minimized fetal

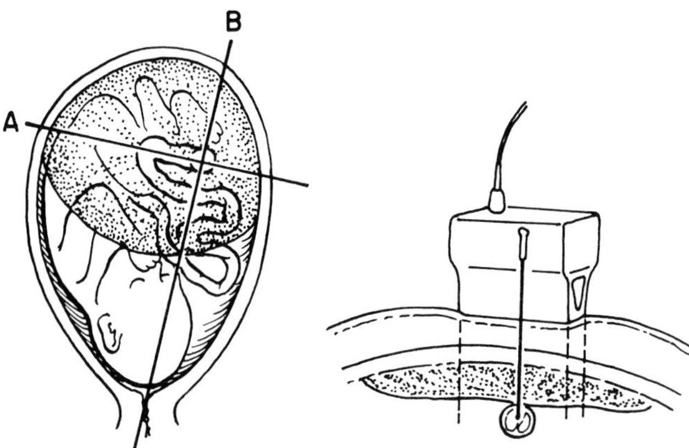


**Fig. 42–1.** Right image: Schematic demonstrating scanning planes A and B through the umbilical cord insertion on anterior placenta. Left image: Schematic demonstrating a sampling plane B through a cross section of the umbilical cord at right angles to plane A.

movement as well because of fetal cerebral depression. This method of fiberoptic visualization was introduced in and around the time the potent combination of a tranquilizer and a narcotic was popular and known as Sublimaze or Innovar. The two agents in this drug combination were droperidol and fentanyl, and were combined into one. If there was one criticism of this method, it was that the danger of producing a light plane of anesthesia without adequate protection of the maternal airway was unappreciated.

## Human Fetal Therapeutic Intervention

The commercial introduction of dynamic image (real-time) ultrasound visualization of fetal anatomy in 1977 marked the beginning of the modern era of prenatal diagnosis of fetal conditions.

Generally, fetal conditions that benefit from intervention involve malformations which result in the accumulation of fluids above an obstruction, with subsequent damage of vital organs (Figure 42–2). These malformations may also constitute a threat to the pregnancy itself by promoting preterm labor and delivery.[5,6,12,14,26–28]

Narrow-gauge needle aspiration of cerebrospinal fluid from the dilated ventricles of a human fetus with severe congenital hydrocephalus using ultrasound guidance was first reported in 1981.[29] Needle aspiration of fluid from the renal pelvis of a fetus with ureteropelvic junction obstruction was described in 1982.[12] Placement of continuous diversion catheters for both hydrocephalus and obstructive uropathies was accomplished in 1982,[18] and finally, percutaneous ultrasound-guided fine-needle aspiration of fetal blood, followed by transfusion in the case of hemolytic disease, was successfully performed by Bang and reported in 1982.[7] This technique has since gained wide popularity, both for diagnosis and treatment of fetal hemolytic disease.[1,2,3,4,8,9,10]

### *Hydrocephalus*

Isolated hydrocephalus due to aqueductal stenosis or atresia is a fetal malformation that was once considered a candidate for antenatal therapy (Figure 42–3).[18] Poor outcomes reported in cases of congenital hydrocephalus

**Table 42–1** Summary of Results of Intrauterine Vascular Transfer Using Ultrasound-Guided Percutaneous Method.

| | | | | | | Cord Blood Values | | | | | |
|---|---|---|---|---|---|---|---|---|---|---|---|
| Case # | Gestational Age (wk) | Delivery Mode | Interval Between Last Transfusion and Delivery (days) | Neonatal Weight (gm) | Birth Status | Hematocrit (%) | Bilirubin (mg/100 ml) | Adult Transfused Red Blood Cells (%) * | Total Exchange Transfusions (N) | Neonatal Hospital Stay (days) | Outcome |
| 1 | 34 | Cesarean (a) | 18 | 2300 | Good | 23 | 7.4 | 50 | 3 | 19 | Alive and well |
| 2A | 26.5 | Cesarean (b) | 1 | — | Stillborn (aa) | – | – | — | – | — | Stillborn (aaa) |
| 2B | 34.5 | Cesarean (b) | 22 | 2470 | Good | 19.0 | 10.5 | NA | 7 | 17 | Alive and well |
| 3 | 30 | Cesarean (c) | 1.5 | 1550 | Hydrops (bb) | 26.5 | 7.0 | 80 | 4 | 48 | Alive and well |
| 4 | 29.5 | Cesarean (d) | 0 | 1470 | Hydrops (cc) | 10.0 | 2.2 | — | 2 | 40 | Alive and well |
| 5 | 25.5 | Vaginal | 1 | 840 | Stillborn (aa) | 12.0 | NA | NA | — | — | Stillborn (bbb) |
| 6 | 34.5 | Cesarean (b) | 29 | 2600 | Good | 21 | 4.1 | 99 | 1 | 18 | Alive and well |
| 7 | 35 | Cesarean (e) | 24 | 2600 | Good | 16 | 4.2 | 85 | 1 | 17 | Alive and well |

NA, not available
* Kleihauer-Betke test
*Delivery Mode Abbreviations:*
(a) failed induction
(b) repeat
(c) preterm labor rupture of membranes, and fetal distress
(d) suspected cord trauma during intrauterine transfusion
(e) breech presentation
*Birth Status Abbreviations:*
(aa) hydrops
(bb) hyaline membrane disease grade II, ventral septal defect (VSD), patent ductus arteriosus (PDA)
(cc) evidence of cord or placental hematoma
*Outcome Abbreviations:*
(aaa) autopsy refused
(bbb) autopsy showed hydrops

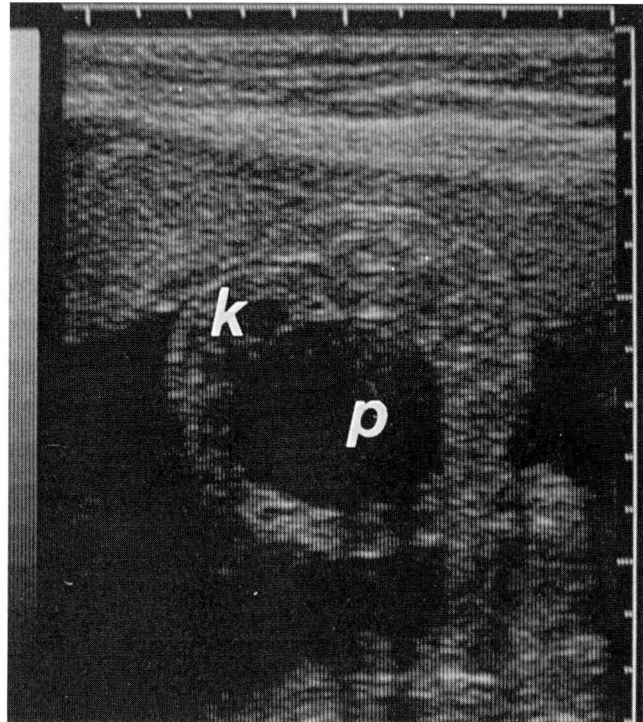


**Fig. 42–2.** This transverse midabdominal fetal sonogram shows a severely dilated fetal renal pelvis (p) and caliectasis of the affected kidney (k) in the case of a severe congenital uretero-pelvic junction obstruction. The accumulated urine appears black (anechoic) on the scan.

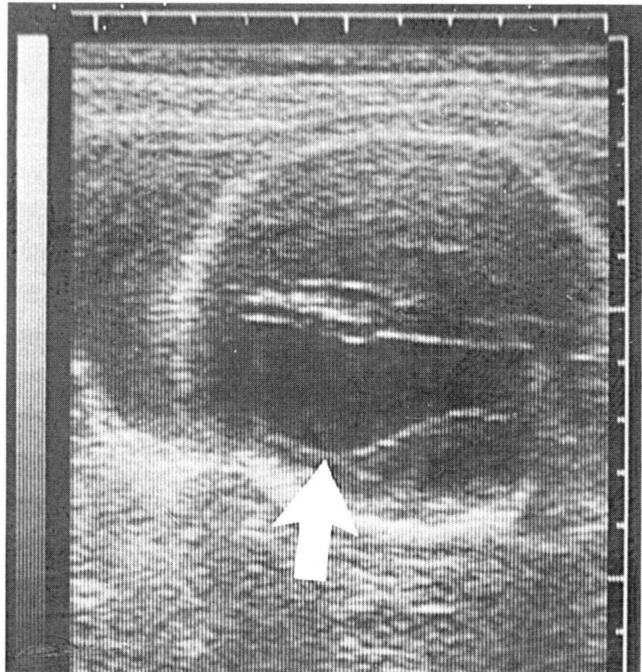

**Fig. 42–3.** This moderately dilated fetal lateral ventricle (arrow) is well shown on ultrasound. The cerebrospinal fluid filling the ventricle appears black (anechoic) as any homogeneous fluid does on ultrasound.

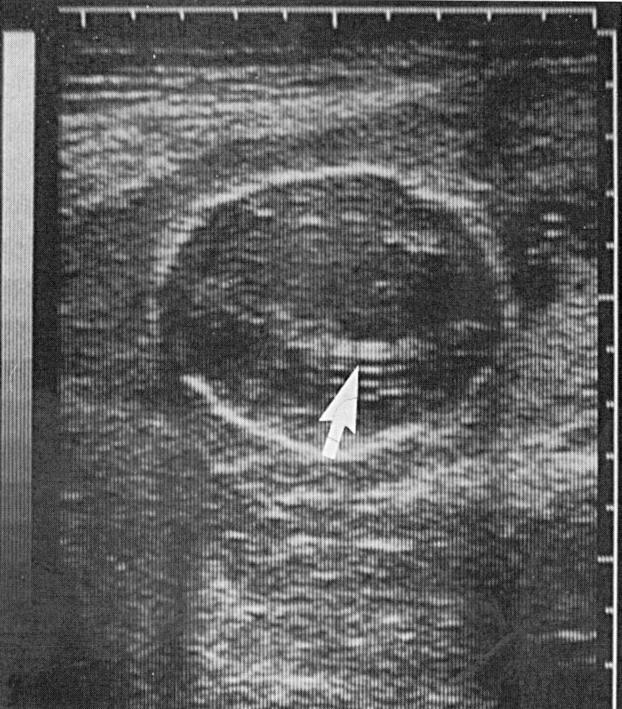

**Fig. 42–4.** This occipitofrontal scanplane of the cranium of a 26-week fetus after intervention shows the ventriculo-amniotic diversion shunt (arrow) within the ventricle.

that were overt at birth supported the thesis that prenatal treatment might improve outcome. However, prenatal treatment of severe fetal hydrocephalus was studied from 1981 to 1985 by many investigators with some technical success, but only limited clinical benefit (Figure 42–4).

Furthermore, significant improvement in the neurological status of these infants using conventional neonatal neurosurgical care has made antenatal intervention difficult to justify,[27,28] Therefore, since prenatal treatment of fetal hydrocephalus subjects the fetus to some considerable risks, and the benefits of such therapy remain unclear, this fetal procedure has largely come to a stop.

### *Obstructive Uropathies*

Ureteropelvic junction obstruction producing unilateral fetal hydronephrosis is, in the vast majority of cases, not an appropriate condition for antenatal intervention.[5,16,17,30] In most cases, expectant management with neonatal evaluation and treatment will result in a successful outcome of the pregnancy, and even survival of the affected kidney.[31] Complete obstruction, however, may result in a dilated fetal kidney of sufficient size to influence bowel function, leading to polyhydramnios and preterm labor (Figure 42–5).[14] Antenatal drainage or diversion may be of benefit in improving amniotic fluid volume equilibrium and diminishing the risk of premature delivery.[14] Each case must be evaluated individually as to the need for treatment. Anesthetic involvement in such cases includes:

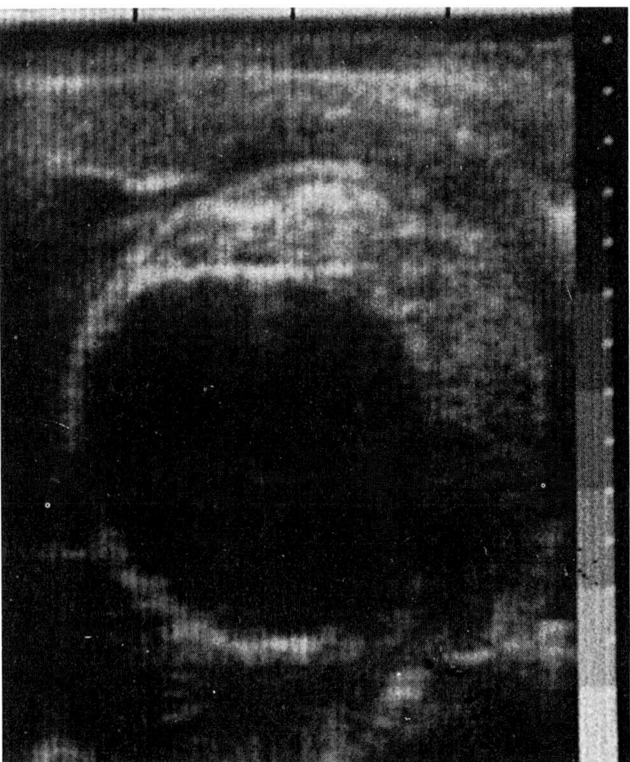

**Fig. 42–5.** Another transverse midabdominal scan of a fetus with severe ureteropelvic junction obstruction resulting in extreme dilatation of the renal pelvis that caused polyhydramnios and maternal renal failure.

1. anesthetic evaluation of the mother (Figure 42–6)
2. surgical needs—
   consideration for any special surgical needs, such as immobility of fetus during actual procedure;
3. monitoring needs—
   *maternal:* intra-anesthetic maternal monitoring includes but is not limited to inspired $O_2$, expired $O_2$, $SaO_2$, EKG, heart rate, blood pressure, uterine contractions;
   *fetal:* fetal heart rate; and
4. recovery needs—
   for the most part, the usual standard tenets of recovery are followed with the additional concern for any signs of uterine irritability which might predispose to premature labor. The usual treatments are then instituted for use in uterine relaxation.

## Fetal Bladder Obstruction

Fetal bladder outlet obstruction resulting in oligohydramnios and fetal hydronephrosis before 32 weeks gestation represents a fetal condition that may benefit from antenatal intervention (Figure 42–7).[13,17] Not every affected fetus, however, will benefit from diversion catheterization, and careful evaluation by a team of experienced clinicians is necessary to avoid treatment of infants with no hope of benefit.

Two somewhat similar methods of treatment for obstructive uropathy have been described. Both approaches result in the placement of a small diversion catheter between the obstructed fetal urinary tract and the sterile amniotic cavity. The Harrison Bladder Stent is a 5 Fr double-pigtail catheter loaded over a needle-trocar, which is then inserted percutaneously into the obstructed organ using ultrasound guidance. The needle is removed as the catheter is advanced by using a sliding pusher. Difficulty is often encountered from frictional resistance between both maternal and then fetal tissues and the advancing catheter. The alternative system uses a similar catheter but delivers it through the lumen of a thin-walled 13-gauge cannula placed into the obstructed organ also with ultrasound guidance. The placement of a catheter by either method is made more difficult by severe oligohydramnios secondary to fetal bladder obstruction. Warm sterile saline can be injected to expand the amniotic cavity, facilitating the placement of either catheter (Figure 42–8). Maternal analgesia consists of a sedative of 10 mg diazepam and an anesthetic injected for local area block. In addition, a continuous infusion of ritodrine is given for uterine relaxation.

In 1982, the exteriorization of a fetus with bladder obstruction and bilateral hydronephrosis for surgical creation of bilateral cutaneous nephrostomies was reported.[30] This was accomplished by laparotomy and hysterotomy, as was described for some earlier procedures for the treatment of fetal hemolytic disease by exchange transfusion. The exteriorization and nephrostomy procedure was technically successful, but the infant died of pulmonary hypoplasia after birth. The maternal anesthetic technique was general, similar to the previous exteriorization technique. Although it is remarkable that the pregnancy was sustained after such a significant uterine intrusion, the immediate surgical risks to the mother and the implications for subsequent obstetrical care, including the necessity for each subsequent pregnancy to be delivered by cesarean section because of the danger of uterine rupture during labor, are serious drawbacks to this technique. Furthermore, the availability of feasible and less radical methods of diverting urine, such as percutaneous catheterization, make exteriorization of the fetus for direct treatment less attractive.

## *Percutaneous Umbilical Vein Blood Sampling*

Bang, in 1982, first described the successful ultrasonic guidance of a narrow-gauge needle to the umbilical vein within the fetal liver for aspiration and transfusion.[7] Since that time, multiple investigators have reported the successful use of this technique for acquisition of fetal blood samples for a variety of indications.[1,2,3,4,8,9,10] The use of direct fetal blood transfusions has gained wide popularity, and in many centers has replaced the intraperitoneal approach (Figure 42–9).[9,10,15] As mentioned earlier, maternal anesthetic considerations here are limited to sedation, analgesia, and monitoring of the mother's cardiovascular and respiratory parameters and monitoring of the fetus' gross movements, respiratory efforts, and cardiovascular parameters.

THE OHIO STATE UNIVERSITY
THE OHIO STATE UNIVERSITY HOSPITALS
ARTHUR G. JAMES CANCER HOSPITAL AND RESEARCH INSTITUTE
COLUMBUS, OHIO

**Department of Anesthesiology**
**Anesthesiology Preoperative Form (#1)**

Date of Visit ____/____/____ Time of Visit ____________

Age ____. Status: Inpatient ____

**Outpatient** ____ **SDA** ____ **OB** ____
**N.P.O Status Date** ____/____/____ **Time** ____________

Operative Procedure ____________________ Wt. ________ Ht. ________

| **History: Cardic Eval:** | | | **Pulmonary Eval:** | | | **Misc:** | | | |
|---|---|---|---|---|---|---|---|---|---|
| M.I. | Y | N | Smoke | Y | N | Allergy | Y | N | |
| C.H.F. | Y | N | D.O.E. | Y | N | Antibiotics | Y | N | |
| Hyprtn | Y | N | Asthma | Y | N | Medication | Y | N | ________ |
| Angina | Y | N | | | | Other | Y | N | ________ |

| **Central Nervous System:** | | | **Anesthesia History:** | | | **Metabolic Problems:** | | | |
|---|---|---|---|---|---|---|---|---|---|
| Seizrs | Y | N | Past Anesth. | Y | N | Hepatic | Y | N | ________ |
| C.V.A. | Y | N | Problems | Y | N | Renal | Y | N | ________ |
| Syncope | Y | N | M.H. | Y | N | G.I. | Y | N | ________ |
| Paresis | Y | N | Family Deaths | Y | N | Diabetes | Y | N | |
| | | | | | | Bleeding | Y | N | |
| | | | | | | Others | Y | N | ________ |

Comments: ______________________________

**Lab:**

HB ____ HCT ____ Electrolytes NA ____ K ___.___ Other ________ Ekg Normal Y N Coags Normal Y N

**Physical:**

B.P. ____/____ Temp ______.___ Pulse ______ Resp. Rate ______

| **Head:** | | | **Central Nervous System:** | | | **Heart:** | | |
|---|---|---|---|---|---|---|---|---|
| Pupils | N | A | Orient | Yes | No | Murmurs | No | Yes |
| Oral opening | N | A | Sensory | N | A | Rhythm | N | A |
| Teeth | N | A | Motor | N | A | JVD | N | A |
| Mntm-Cric | N | A | | | | | | |
| Neck rom | N | A | | | | | | |

| **Lung:** | | |
|---|---|---|
| Clear: | Y | N |
| Rales | No | Yes |
| Rhonchi | No | Yes |
| Wheezes | No | Yes |

Comments: ______________________________

ASA PS ____

**Anes Plan:** General Regional L. Stdy

**Monitoring:** Std **Others:** A Line CVP Line PAC

**Recovery:** Std SICU

Signature: ____________________ MD/CRNA ____________________ Faculty

The Ohio State University
Form 10838

**Fig. 42–6.** Form used at The Ohio State University Hospitals for maternal anesthetic evaluation.

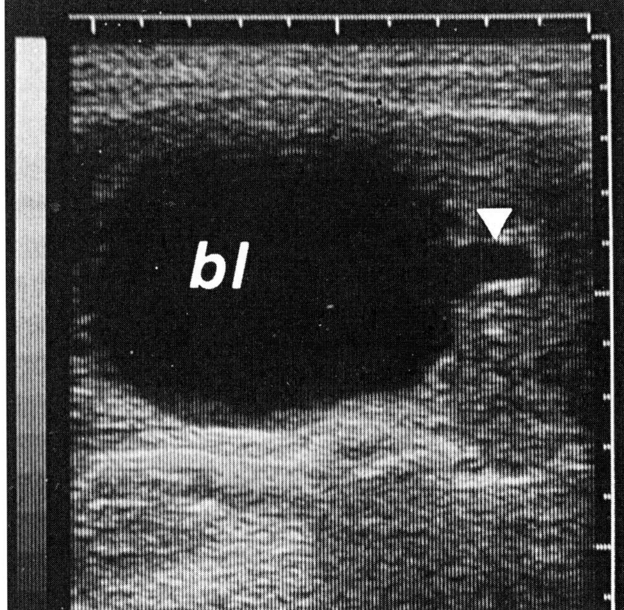


**Fig. 42–7.** Ureteral atresia in the fetus results in severe oligohydramnios and extreme dilatation of the fetal bladder (bl) as shown here. The closed triangle indicates the pelvic portion of the fetal bladder.

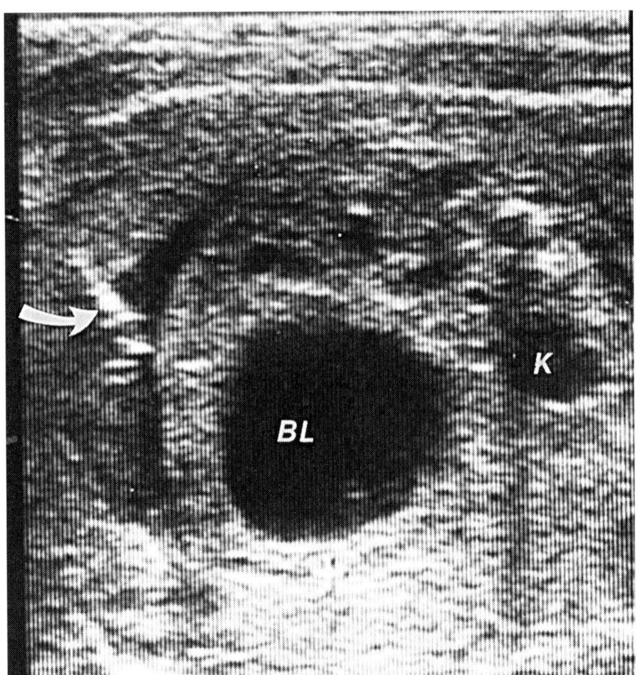


**Fig. 42–8.** This transverse fetal scan was done at the time of intervention. The dilated, obstructed bladder is seen (BL), as is one hydronephrotic kidney (K). The needle tip (arrow) is seen during the injection of saline to facilitate shunt placement.

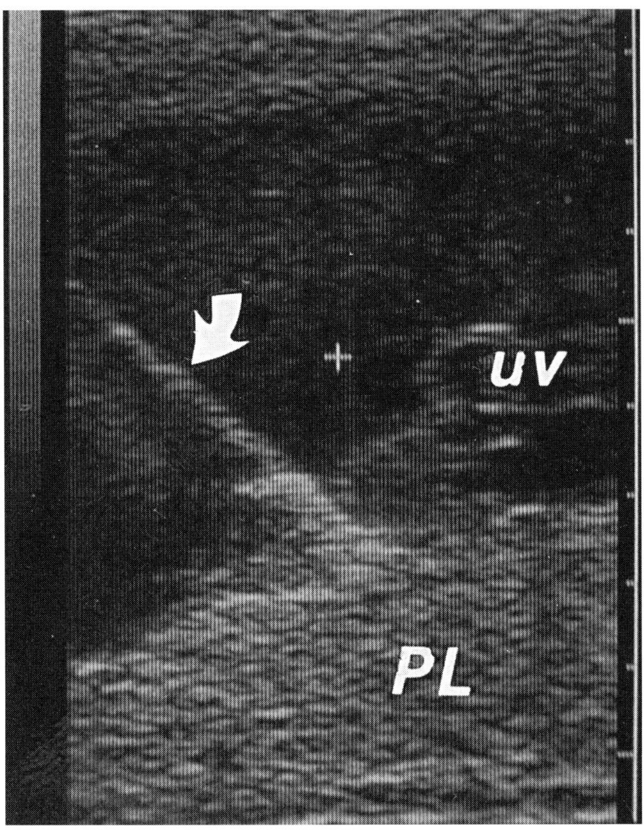


**Fig. 42–9.** Taken during an ultrasound-guided fetal blood sampling procedure, this sonogram illustrates the aspiration needle (curved arrow) crossing the amniotic cavity to puncture the umbilical vein (uv) at the cord insertion on the placenta (PL).

### *Other Possible Interventions*

The precise guidance of aspiration or biopsy needles to specific fetal organs enables a wide variety of both diagnostic and therapeutic procedures.[32] These include:

1. aspiration of fetal thoracic cysts;
2. aspiration of pleural effusions;
3. aspiration of ascites (Figure 42–10);
4. biopsy of fetal skin;
5. biopsy of fetal muscle; and
6. biopsy of fetal liver.

All of the above aspirations are usually performed using ultrasound as a guide and the biopsies are usually via the guided-needle technique.

## ANESTHETIC CONSIDERATIONS FOR FETAL INTERVENTION

In general, the use of anesthetic and neuromuscular blocking agents to facilitate fetal interventions are aimed at reduction of maternal pain and maternal anxiety, as well as reduction or elimination of fetal movement.[33–35] The added advantage of need for anesthetic intervention to reduce fetal pain remains generally controversial and the issue of whether the fetus needs "pain relief" is now

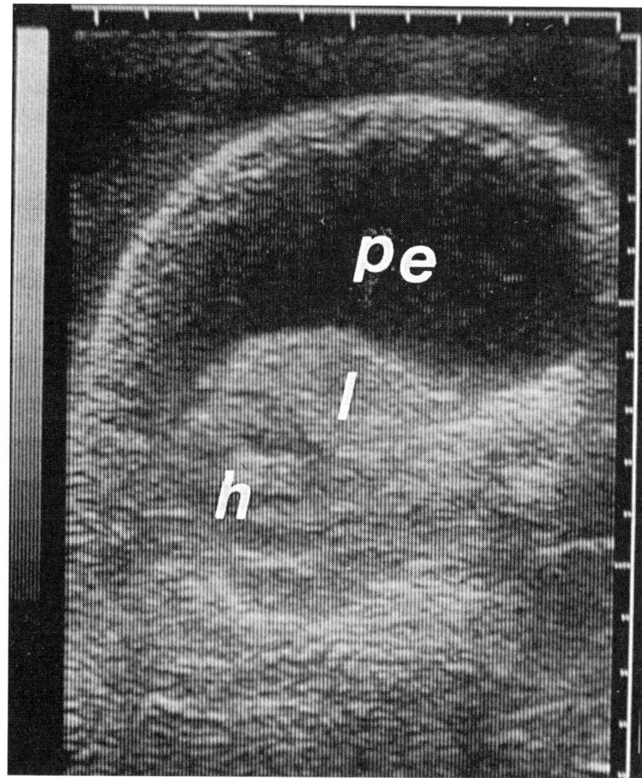


**Fig. 42–10.** Severe congenital pleural effusion or hydrothorax is another possible candidate for aspiration or diversion therapy. This transverse thoracic fetal sonogram shows a severe pleural effusion (pe). The fetal heart (h) and the right lung (l) may also be seen. The effusion appears black (anechoic) on scan.

being challenged. Some reported data appear to show that neonates benefit from anesthesia or analgesia while undergoing surgical procedures even as limited as circumcision.[19] Not only does the use of adequate medication avoid the difficult questions of pain awareness and pain memory in the case of the neonate, but the data appear to show improved surgical outcome.[19] Since these observations were made in premature infants as well as full term neonates, it may be assumed that perhaps the same considerations would apply to the fetus of a similar gestational age and neurological maturity.[19] There are obvious differences, including the presence of fetal circulation, but it should be assumed that some form of abatement of noxious stimuli to the fetus might be advantageous. In the majority of fetal procedures, the mother receives some form of medication that will cross the placenta and reach the fetal circulation. It has been assumed that in most cases, this transplacental analgesia and sedation is sufficient to ameliorate lasting effects of the noxious stimuli associated with fetal interventions. Maternal safety should be the major consideration, however, and anesthetic medication should be tailored to the requisites of the individual surgical procedure. Yet, anesthetic considerations must not end here, with the fetus assuming a secondary role. The fetus is, after all, the reason for the operative procedure, i.e., improved salvage of the fetus at risk of an intrauterine malady. Previously, consideration must have been for the mother, with lesser concern about the prime effect upon the fetus. Now, it is possible to consider the fetus as a separate entity within the mother with specific anesthetic requirements, for lack of movement, for example, provided by muscle relaxants injected directly into the fetus, not experienced solely as a side effect. Analgesia might similarly be considered and again administered directly to the fetus without maternal-to-fetal transport considerations. In this way, the anesthesiologist could develop a tailor-made anesthetic regimen for the fetus complete and separate from that of the mother.

Fetal movement can have significant impact on the success and safety of many fetal interventions.[10] Fetal movement during the placement of a catheter or during fetal blood sampling or transfusion could cause needle displacement, procedural failure, or significant fetal trauma.[10] It can do much to increase the frustration level for the surgeon and perhaps be the difference between success and failure. Most intervention protocols address the issue of reduction of fetal movement, either indirectly with heavy sedation or directly with fetal administration of neuromuscular blocking agents.[34,35]

## *Pain Relief for Major Surgical Intervention*

Laparotomy with hysterotomy may require the use of a major general anesthetic technique.[11] The reason for this is that with the one technique, adequate conditions for both the mother and the fetus may be forthcoming. Adequate anesthesia for laparotomy may be provided by general anesthesia using a balanced endotracheal approach. Regional anesthesia may also be satisfactory but may require supplementary drugs to provide adequate sedation and, occasionally, analgesia. In the context of major surgical intervention, spinal or epidural analgesia will be necessary to ensure a pain-free patient who will remain still during the procedure. The specific technique for lumbar or spinal will not be described in this chapter since they are discussed in detail in Chapters 13 (epidural) and 14 (spinal). In the general consideration of the technique best suited for the operative procedure, the various complications must be identified. The complications of regional techniques, particularly hypotension, are likely to be hazardous to the fetus as well as the mother, and every effort should be made to maintain maternal hemodynamic homeostasis throughout the procedure. The anesthesiologist and the obstetrician should confer before making a decision in regard to the specific technique to be used since the surgeon may have past experience dictating a preference for a certain technique, awareness of the demands of the operative procedure itself, or the wishes of the patient.

It must be admitted, therefore, that balanced endotracheal anesthetic with careful attention to the adequacy of narcotic analgesia is, in the majority of cases, the technique of choice by the authors of this chapter due to our past exposure and experience in cases where intrauterine intervention is undertaken with the intention of preservation of the pregnancy after the procedure. This conclusion does not preclude the use of other techniques on an individual basis when specific advantages are apparent.

General anesthesia can be safely used for laparotomy and hysterotomy procedures with little difficulty for the mother or fetus if certain protective tenets are adhered to. These will be described later in this paragraph. Induction of general anesthesia can be accomplished with use of the standard short-acting amnestic and muscle relaxant, thiopental and succinylcholine. Their use primarily assures rapid sequence induction and rapid tracheal cannulation. As noted in many other areas of this book, this rapid sequence induction with concomitant protection of the mother's airway is necessary in order to prevent aspiration of foreign materials into the lungs. Anesthesia maintenance can be by either $O_2$ 100%, plus low levels of isoflurane, endflurane or desflurane; or $O_2$ 50% with $N_2O$ 50%, plus low levels of the same three inhalation agents. Since these fetal interventions are performed in the second trimester or beyond, there is no concern in regard to $N_2O$ being considered as a possible cause of first trimester deformity. During the maintenance period of anesthesia, the use of an intermediate muscle relaxant for the mother assures easy control over ventilation, and this becomes important to the success of the operation during periods of surgical needle placement. At such times, the anesthesiologist can guarantee periods of apnea during which very accurate needle placements can be performed by the surgeon. There may also be instances where additional fetal injection of muscle relaxants are indicated to prevent any movement of the fetus during specific operative maneuvers. Some of the pertinent maternal safety tenets in regard to general anesthesia include:

1. use of the rapid sequence induction methods;
2. use of cricoid pressure;
3. no institution of positive-pressure breathing until after successful tracheal intubation; and
4. use of at least two of the three following maternal aspiration preventatives: (a) 30 ml of nonparticulate antacid, i.e., sodium citrate or bicitra; (b) $H_2$ antagonist, i.e., 50 mg IV ranitidine; (c) 10 mg IV of clopromide (metoclopramide).

Some of the pertinent fetal safety tenets in regard to general anesthesia include:

1. use of fetal monitoring during induction and the surgical procedure; and
2. careful attention to prevention of the supine hypotensive syndrome.

Adequate anesthesia for laparotomy may be provided by general anesthesia using a balanced endotracheal approach. Regional anesthesia may also be satisfactory. In the context of major surgical intervention, spinal or epidural analgesia will be necessary to ensure a pain-free patient who will remain still during the procedure. Adequate blocks of the above will provide good analgesia and muscular relaxation so that the same conditions found during general anesthesia should be present. The one complication of the regional technique, hypotension, could be hazardous to the fetus even though it may not be severe enough to be hazardous to the mother, thus every effort should be made to maintain maternal hemodynamic homeostasis. In situations where there is potential preexisting compromise to the fetus, this method should not be a consideration.

It appears, therefore, that balanced endotracheal anesthetic with careful attention to the adequacy of narcotic analgesia may be, in the majority of cases, the technique of choice if intrauterine intervention is undertaken with the intention of preservation of the pregnancy after the procedure. This conclusion does not preclude the use of other techniques on an individual basis when specific advantages are apparent.

### *Pain Relief for Minor Surgical Intervention*

Percutaneous placement of a large needle such as is necessary with the methods previously described can be and most often is associated with significant pain; the larger the needle, the greater the pain. It is possible to minimize, but not totally eliminate, such pain using local infiltration of the site and deeper tissues with an anesthetic.[33] A reasonable technique to consider for infiltration is use of a 26-gauge needle with 0.5 ml of 1% lidocaine to develop a skin wheal at the desired site. Subsequent use of the larger diagnostic/therapeutic needle can then be done with some significant reduction in pain. Nevertheless, sometimes the use of these larger-bore needles and instruments may necessitate an actual field block as described earlier. Often peritoneal and/or uterine mural pain associated with the procedure cannot be blocked. Experience has demonstrated, however, that the discomfort attributable to deeper tissues is not as great as that from the superficial tissues and, in the majority of cases, this pain is tolerable and does not require systemic analgesia.

### *Anxiety Relief*

Maternal anxiety associated with fetal surgery can itself significantly impact on outcome and arises both out of concern for the seriousness of the fetal condition and fear of pain and complications from the procedure. Such anxiety varies greatly in intensity and can complicate the procedure. Sudden unexpected maternal movements during the procedure can directly cause procedure failure. Often, only mild sedation is needed to provide adequate maternal relaxation. It is unnecessary and potentially dangerous to substitute heavy parenteral analgesia for light sedation—for example, *do not use 15 mg of morphine in a situation where 5 mg of valium would do.* It is vital, furthermore, to minimize the need for such sedation. Heavy medication can compromise maternal safety because of inadequate airway protection, increasing the possibility of aspiration of stomach contents, which remains a source of danger in the pregnant patient despite appropriate preoperative preparation. It is appropriate at this point to mention that there must be an appreciation of the difference between sedation, amnesia, and anesthesia. Sedation is usually referred to in those cases where just a small amount of a drug is used to elicit a sleepy, relaxed state. The drug usually used is benzodiazepam or another barbiturate. It does not necessarily include the state of analgesia that is a separate entity altogether, and refers to a loss of pain sensation in a given area or in a general sense if a systemic analgesic such as a narcotic is administered.

It is very important to emphasize the best method of preoperative anxiety reduction is patient education. Careful, informative preparation for the procedure by the responsible physician can minimize the need for pharmacological agents. Each step of the procedure should be reviewed and the operating area toured. A confident and informed relationship between the physician and the patient is the soundest and safest method of anxiety control. Often, but not always, the presence in the operating room of the husband or another personal support person is helpful in anxiety reduction. If adequate relaxation cannot be achieved with light analgesia, consideration should be given to general endotracheal anesthesia in order to preserve maximum airway protection, as well as optimal control over sudden maternal movement.

### *Complications of Fetal Movement*

Fetal movement during the course of antenatal intervention also poses a significant risk to the fetus. When placing a diversion catheter for obstructive uropathy, for example, fetal movement makes appropriate placement more difficult and increases the probability of technical error. Even after a successful catheter placement, fetal movement may cause displacement of a correctly placed device. During a real-time ultrasound examination of a fetus shortly after placement of a hydrocephalus diversion catheter at 26 weeks gestation, the fetus was seen to grasp the catheter with his hand and remove it, despite the fact that his mother was asleep from parenteral analgesia.

Fetal movement at the time of percutaneous umbilical vein blood sampling could result in difficulty gaining appropriate intravenous access or subsequent displacement of a properly placed needle. Such technical failure leads to undesirable multiple needle placements.

Fetal movement while a needle is present within an internal organ could also result in significant traumatic damage, including laceration of vital organs or vascular structures.

## Available Anesthetic Techniques

### *Maternal Sedation and Local Anesthesia*

Sedation combined with local infiltration is an inadequate technique for major surgical interventions, but would provide adequate pain relief in the case of percutaneous needle aspirations or catheter insertions. The method is inexpensive, and avoids most of the risks of major general anesthesia. The chief danger is that when sufficient sedation is administered to reduce fetal movement, a light plane of anesthesia may result in an unprotected airway. This leaves the patient at risk for both hypoxia and aspiration of gastric contents. When this method is selected, any of several sedative agents may be chosen, all of which cross the placenta and will be found in fetal plasma at near-maternal levels. The most commonly used drugs are the benzodiazepines, including diazepam and midazolam, and the narcotics, including morphine sulphate and fentanyl.

The problem of fetal movement remains, however, even with large doses of these drugs, and the temptation is to repeat doses at short intervals whenever fetal movements complicate the procedure. Whenever this technique is used, it is essential that the maternal airway be monitored by a responsible operator. This means that the patient must be placed in a monitored area after the procedure for up to 3 to 4 hours where her respirations, adequacy of ventilation and normalcy of cardiovascular parameters can be closely followed.

### *Local Anesthesia with Fetal Paralysis*

Since local anesthesia with minimal parenteral analgesia provides adequate pain relief for the mother in most cases, the greatest remaining problem is that of arresting fetal movement. Paralysis is a logical consideration. The intravenous injection of curare into the fetal circulation to transiently arrest fetal movement for the purpose of promoting the success of intrauterine transfusion was first reported by Ch de Crespigny in 1983.[8,34] He reported 16 transfusions in 4 fetuses, using ultrasound-guided percutaneous venipuncture of the umbilical vein within the fetal liver. He administered 3 mg of curare intravenously with great success and with no observed complications. Seeds, et al, in 1986, reported the use of fetal intramuscular pancuronium bromide (0.5 mg/kg) for the same purpose in six cases with no complications.[34] Other investigators since have confirmed the safe application of this technique for the temporary arrest of fetal movement during a variety of fetal interventions.[35]

Both curare and pancuronium bromide have been used with safety and effectiveness. Neither crosses the placenta and will not therefore, lead to maternal neuromuscular blockade. Both produce effective fetal paralysis for 2 to 4 hours. The dose of drug must be adjusted depending on whether the route of administration is intravenous or intramuscular. In general, the dosages consist of those in Table 42–2.

During percutaneous fetal umbilical vein blood sampling, if it is necessary for the aspiration needle to cross the amniotic cavity, the needle is at risk for displacement should fetal movement occur, and consideration of fetal paralysis is appropriate. The paralytic agent may be administered with either a separate needle injection intramuscularly into a thigh or shoulder, or the agent may be given as soon as the needle enters the umbilical vein. Although the intramuscular route requires a second needle passage, it offers the advantage of arrested movement before the

**Table 42–2** Dosages to Produce Effective Fetal Paralysis.

| Drug | Route of Administration: Intravenous | Route of Administration: Intramuscular |
|---|---|---|
| Pancuronium Bromide | 0.1 mg/kg | 0.5 mg/kg |
| Curare | * | 3.0 mg ** |

* Fetal intravenous curare has not been reported.
** Fetal intramuscular curare dose reported was not weight indexed.

aspiration needle is placed and becomes vulnerable. The intravenous injection offers the advantage of perhaps a reduction in the number of needle passes, but has the disadvantage that fetal movement prior to the paralysis could delay the acquisition of intravenous access, or cause dislodgement of the needle before adequate paralysis. The dosage used in early reports for third trimester reports was 3 mg of curare, and 0.4 mg to 0.6 mg of pancuronium bromide.[34,35]

Local anesthesia with fetal paralysis offers the advantages of maximum reduction of fetal movement with minimal risk to the maternal airway. Fetal paralysis may, however, require additional needle placements, and does not provide any fetal anesthesia or analgesia. The significance of this latter consideration remains controversial and difficult to evaluate in the case of the unborn, as mentioned above. Furthermore, if as a result of a complication of the procedure the fetus required delivery, the neonate will be paralyzed and require assisted ventilation until the paralysis is reversed. This is not a life-threatening problem for the infant since it should be anticipated, and appropriate resuscitation equipment and personnel can be provided.

## Regional Anesthesia

Regional anesthesia for use in these procedures can offer excellent analgesia for the mother and also good muscular relaxation of the abdominal area. If there are problems with fetal movement and if difficulties occur due to that movement, then one can add direct fetal injection of a muscle relaxant for the fetal effect only. The advantages of the regional anesthetic for the mother include being awake, aware, and alert during the operative procedure. In addition, this technique avoids the necessity for intubation and all the problems associated with it. The disadvantage is chiefly the possibility of hypotension as mentioned earlier. However, this need not be a major concern if early diagnosis and immediate treatment are effected so that there is no direct fetal compromise. Both lumbar epidural and spinal block techniques may be used to obtain regional analgesia. Both are perfectly acceptable and really have more to do with the personal preferences of the anesthesiologist who may feel more comfortable with one method over the other.

## General Anesthesia

General anesthesia provides certain advantages both for maternal and fetal pain relief, with reduction of both maternal and fetal movements during an antenatal intervention. Maternal analgesia and amnesia will be provided, and it is likely that, at the same time, the fetus will receive sufficient anesthetic agents through the placenta to minimize movement. The maternal airway will be adequately protected if an endotracheal tube is placed.

There remain the risks of anesthetic complications, including aspiration during induction. Balanced anesthesia, using a combination of inhalation agents, narcotics, and neuromuscular blockers will provide adequate maternal analgesia and amnesia. Induction of anesthesia is often associated with transient hypertension and significant catecholamine release, which could result in uterine irritability and adverse fetal effects. Maintenance with halogenated hydrocarbon agents, including isoflurane and halothane, are associated with hypotension and uterine relaxation. The use of general anesthesia requires the presence of a trained anesthesiologist and a full operating room setting, which will markedly increase the cost of such procedures.

## Procedure-Specific Anesthetic Choices

In the case of laparotomy with hysterotomy, general endotracheal anesthesia is the method used most often in our experience. The specific anesthetic agent chosen may remain a matter of individual choice for the anesthesiologist, but again in our experience in the majority of cases, a balanced technique with a minimum concentration of halogenated agent was optimal.

The placement of a fetal diversion catheter that requires passage of a relatively large diameter cannula or needle will most often be successfully completed using light maternal sedation, local anesthetic, and fetal paralysis. In our experience, this provides good pain and anxiety relief along with fetal movement control, while maintaining a high level of maternal safety.

Light or no sedation along with local anesthesia and fetal paralysis is also an appropriate method for percutaneous fetal umbilical vein blood sampling and intrauterine intravascular blood transfusion.

Fetal paralysis alone can also be used to optimize either magnetic resonance imaging or tomographic radiography.

A field block is the establishment of a wall of anesthesia around an operative field, without infiltrating the operative site itself. This is especially applicable when the nerve supply enters from one aspect of the area; field block of the proximal side renders the distal area numb. Field block is most valuable for plastic surgery, where it is undesirable to distort the operative site by distension of the tissues.

Field block differs from nerve block in that no specific nerve is targeted, but a wall of anesthetic solution affects the multiple small nerve branches entering the area. To be most effective, a field block should be done with a large volume of dilute solution, slightly distending each tissue layer.

For laparotomy, the injection is done just beneath the skin, beneath the fascia, and just above the peritoneum. Each layer may be injected, then incised; then the next layer is injected and incised. Little or no solution is needed in the fat. To obtain intraperitoneal analgesia, 25 ml of dilute local anesthetic solution should be sprayed into the peritoneal cavity and gently distributed over all surfaces. For cesarean section, an additional layer of solution should be injected just under the uterine peritoneal layer, along the line of incision.

The secret of success for field blocks is to use very dilute solutions and large volumes. Be sure that no area is left without its layer of solution. The use of concentrated solutions is counter-productive—only a small volume is available, some areas are missed, and painful impulses escape through the gap in the wall. Whatever drug is chosen should be used only up to its maximum safe dose. The addition of dilute epinephrine prolongs the duration of action and retards absorption, resulting in lower blood concentration, and greater safety. Inject gently as the needle is moving in and out, parallel to the surface. Aspiration is not necessary as long as the needle is in motion; do not inject without aspiration if the needle is motionless.

For cesarean section, the technique should be modified to inject along the linea alba and its adjacent tissue. The abdominal wall may be thin in the patient at term, so care must be exercised not to go through the peritoneum and pierce the uterus inadvertently. Please refer to Figure 42–11 for reference points for abdominal wall analgesia for a vertical incision. For Pfannensteil incision, see Figure 42–12, where the iliohypogastric and iliolingual nerves are blocked.

Dilute solutions of the long-acting local anesthetic drugs give the surgeon ample time to accomplish this task without haste. With these drugs, onset of anesthesia is rapid when used in this way, although the onset is delayed for nerve blocks. Marcaine or tetracaine may be used in 0.1% concentration (1 mg/ml); average dose up to 1 ml/lb, allows use of an ample volume of solution. Add 0.5 ml of 1:1000 epinephrine to 200 ml of solution unless the patient has heart disease or hypertension.

## Conclusion

Considerations of safety and the adequacy of a given technique must include effects on both the mother and the fetus. The use of heavy sedation is not only dangerous because of potential compromise of maternal airway but also because it does not ensure arrest of fetal movement. General anesthesia is indicated for the rare case of major operative intervention or unusual anxiety unrelieved by light sedation. Fetal paralysis by direct injection of small doses of muscle relaxants injected directly into the fetus and local analgesia by injection of local anesthetics into the maternal abdomen at the point of needle entry is an acceptable method.

## REFERENCES


1. Daffos F, Capella-Pavlovsky M, Forestier F: Fetal blood sampling via the umbilical cord using a needle guided by ultrasound. Prenat. Diagn. 3:271, 1983.
2. Hsieh F-J, Chang F-M, Ko T-M, Chen H-Y: Percutaneous ultrasound guided fetal blood sampling in the management of non-immune hydrops fetalis. Am. J. Obstet. Gynecol. 157: 44, 1987.
3. Hobbins JC, Grannum PA, Romero R, Reece EA, et al: Percutaneous umbilical blood sampling. Am. J. Obstet. Gynecol. 152:1, 1985.
4. Daffos F, Capella-Pavlovsky M, Forestier F: Fetal blood sampling during pregnancy with use of a needle guided by ultrasound: A study of 606 consecutive cases. Am. J. Obstet. Gynecol. 153:655, 1985.
5. Vintzileos AM, Campbell WA, Nochimson DJ, Weinbaum PJ: Antenatal evaluation and management of ultrasonically detected fetal anomalies. Obstet. Gynecol. 69:640, 1987.
6. Hadlock FP, Deter RL, Carpenter R, Gonzalez ET, et al: Review: Sonography of fetal urinary tract anomalies. Am. J. Roentgenol. 137:261, 1981.
7. Bang J, Bock JE, Trolle D: Ultrasound-guided fetal intravenous transfusion for severe rhesus haemolytic disease. Br. Med. J. 284:373, 1982.
8. Ch de Crespigny L, Robinson HP, Quinn M, Doyle L, et al: Ultrasound-guided fetal blood transfusion for severe rhesus isoimmunization. Obstet. Gynecol. 66:529, 1985.
9. Seeds JW, Bowes WA Jr: Ultrasound-guided fetal intravascular transfusion in severe rhesus immunization. Am. J. Obstet. Gynecol. 154:1105, 1986.
10. Berkowitz RL, Chitkara U, Goldberg JD, Wilkins I, et al: Intrauterine intravascular transfusions for severe red blood cell isoimmunization: Ultrasound-guided percutaneous approach. Am. J. Obstet. Gynecol. 155:574, 1986.
11. Harrison MR, Golbus MS, Filly RA, Callen PW, et al: Fetal surgery for congenital hydronephrosis. N. Engl. J. Med. 306: 591, 1982.
12. Kirkinen P, Jouppila P, Tuononen S: Repeated transabdominal renocenteses in a case of fetal hydronephrotic kidney. Am. J. Obstet. Gynecol. 142:1049, 1982.
13. Manning FA, Harman CR, Lange IR, Brown R, et al: Antepartum chronic fetal vesicoamniotic shunts for obstructive uropathy: A report of two cases. Am. J. Obstet. Gynecol. 145:819, 1983.
14. Seeds JW, Cefalo RC, Herbert WN, Bowes WA Jr: Hydramnios and maternal renal failure: Relief with fetal therapy. Obstet. Gynecol. 64:26S, 1984.
15. Grannum PA, Copel JA, Plaxe SC, Scioscia AL, et al: In utero exchange transfusion by direct intravascular injection in severe erythroblastosis fetalis. N. Engl. J. Med. 314:1431, 1986.
16. Berkowitz RL, Glickman MG, Smith GJW, Siegel NJ, et al: Fetal urinary tract obstruction: What is the role of surgical intervention in utero? Am. J. Obstet. Gynecol. 144:367, 1982.
17. Harrison MR, Filly RA, Parer JT, Faer MJ, et al: Management of the fetus with a urinary tract malformation. JAMA 246: 635, 1981.
18. Clewell WH, Johnson ML, Meier PR, Newkirk JB, et al: A surgical approach to the treatment of fetal hydrocephalus. N. Engl. J. Med. 306:1320, 1982.
19. Anand KJS, Hickey PR: Pain and its effects in the human neonate and fetus. N. Engl. J. Med. 317:1321, 1987.
20. Rosenkrantz JG, Simon RC, Carlisle JH: Fetal surgery in the pig with a review of other mammalian fetal techniques. J. Pediatr. Surg. 3:392–97, 1965.
21. Liley AW: Intrauterine transfusion of foetus in haemolytic disease. Br. Med. J. 2:1107, 1963.
22. Asensio SH, Figueroa-Longo JG, Pelegrina IA: Intrauterine exchange transfusion. Am. J. Obstet. Gynecol. 95:1129, 1966.
23. Hobbins JC, Mahoney MJ: In utero diagnosis of hemoglobinopathies: Technique for obtaining pure fetal blood. N. Engl. J. Med. 290:1065, 1974.
24. Rodeck CH, Kemp JR, Holman CA, Whitmore DN, et al: Direct intravascular fetal blood transfusion by fetoscopy in severe rhesus isoimmunization. Lancet 1:625, 1981.
25. Rodeck CH, Nicolaides KH, Warsof SL, Fysh WJ, et al: The management of severe rhesus isoimmunization by fetoscopic intravascular transfusions. Am. J. Obstet. Gynecol. 150:769, 1984.
26. Manning FA: International Fetal Surgery Registry, 59 Emily Street, Winnipeg, Canada, R3E 0W3, May 1986.
27. Manning FA, Harrison MR, Rodeck C: Catheter shunts for fetal hydronephrosis and hydrocephalus. Report of the International Fetal Surgery Registry. N. Engl. J. Med. 315:336, 1986.

28. Chervenak FA, Duncan C, Ment LR, Hobbins JC, et al: Outcome of fetal ventriculomegaly. Lancet 2(8396):179–181, 1984.
29. Birnholz JC, Frigoletto FD: Antenatal treatment by hydrocephalus. N. Engl. J. Med. 304:1021–23, 1981.
30. Golbus MS, Harrison MR, Filly RA, Callen PW, et al: In utero treatment of urinary tract obstruction. Am. J. Obstet. Gynecol. 142:383, 1982.
31. Mandell J, Kinard HW, Mittelstaedt CA, Seeds JW: Prenatal diagnosis of unilateral hydronephrosis with early postnatal reconstruction. J. Urol. 132:303, 1984.
32. Asher JB, Sabbagha RE, Tamura RK, Luck S, et al: Fetal pulmonary cyst: Intrauterine diagnosis and management. Am. J. Obstet. Gynecol 151:97, 1985.
33. Spielman FJ, Seeds JW, Corke BC: Anaesthesia for fetal surgery. Anaesthesia 39:756, 1984.
34. Seeds JW, Corke BC, Spielman FJ: Prevention of fetal movement during invasive procedures with pancuronium bromide. Am. J. Obstet. Gynecol. 155:818, 1986.
35. Moise KJ Jr, Carpenter RJ, Deter RL, Kirshon B, et al: The use of fetal neuromuscular blockade during intrauterine procedures. Am. J. Obstet. Gynecol. 157:874, 1987.

Chapter 43

# INTENSIVE CARE MANAGEMENT OF THE MOTHER

THOMAS M. FUHRMAN,
ROBERT R. KIRBY

The growing epidemics of trauma, illicit drug use, and violence have combined to make the pregnant patient no longer a rarity in the Intensive Care Unit (ICU). In addition, patients whose conditions are directly associated with pregnancy, such as severe pregnancy-induced hypertension and hemorrhage, can often benefit from the resuscitation and invasive monitoring available in the ICU. Finally, many patients have conditions that previously made pregnancy an unacceptable high risk. Now these problems frequently can be dealt with, but may, in the course of management, necessitate ICU care. Which patients are transferred to the intensive care unit depends on several considerations.

In general, admissions are based on the need for specialized care not available in a regular hospital setting. Invasive hemodynamic monitoring, intensive respiratory care and an increased level of nursing care are indications. The level of nursing care that can be provided outside of an intensive care unit is determined on an individual hospital basis. Logically, nursing for the parturient and fetus should be provided by those most versed in obstetrical care. Certainly many situations can be handled in the labor and delivery unit. The nurse-to-patient ratio usually is better here than in other areas of the hospital. Patients who need primarily intensive nursing effort can remain on that unit rather than be transferred to the ICU. When more than extra nursing care is required, however, transfer is indicated. Each obstetrical service must have its guidelines that dictate the specific circumstances requiring ICU admission.

The guiding tenet is that the fetus is best served by optimizing care for the compromised mother-to-be. Few obstetrical services routinely care for patients requiring invasive monitoring and mechanical ventilation. Fewer ICUs routinely care for patients during the peripartum period. The complexities of caring for an obstetrical intensive care unit patient truly requires the team approach. The obstetrician and the intensivist must combine forces and be co-primary care providers. Many other specialties may be needed as consultants. Coordination is essential.

## PATIENT POPULATION

Stephens reported the incidence of intensive care unit admissions in a large obstetrical hospital[1] (Table 43–1). From 1979 to 1989, 61,435 deliveries occurred. One hundred and twenty six patients (0.2%) were admitted to the ICU during the peripartum period. Others have reported 0.4% to 0.9% of deliveries resulting in the need for ICU admission.[2,3] The ICU was in a general hospital associated with the obstetrical hospital. Only those patients first admitted to the latter were included in this report. Direct admissions for trauma, therefore, were not included.

Hypertensive disease of pregnancy accounted for 30 admissions (24%). Twenty eight patients (22%) suffered excessive blood loss. Sixteen patients (13%) had complications associated with anesthesia. Eleven patients (9%) had preexisting disease (cardiac or musculoskeletal). Other reasons for admission included infection, pulmonary embolism, or morbid obesity. Noteworthy was the five-fold higher incidence of anesthetic complications with general as compared to regional anesthesia. Based upon this information, in a hospital in which general anesthesia predominates for obstetrical procedures, an increased number of complications and thus ICU admissions may be anticipated.

Another recent study reviewed a 5-year period in which 32 obstetric patients required admission to an ICU (Table 43–2).[2] Eight of these patients developed acute lung injury and required aggressive respiratory care and high levels of positive-end expiratory pressure. Figure 43–1 reveals an example of necessary aggressive respiratory care in a 17-year-old patient who had a prolonged period of mechanical ventilation and who eventually recovered.

### Trauma

Trauma caused by accidental injury has been estimated to occur in up to 7% of all pregnancies.[4] Over a 34-year period, it was the leading nonobstetrical cause of maternal mortality in Iowa.[5] Rottenberger, et al, reported that a large Minnesota trauma service admitted 103 pregnant women.[6] The majority of these injuries occurred during motor vehicle accidents (54%). Falls accounted for another 29% of the injuries and 17% were caused by physical assaults. The injuries were classified as major (20%), minor (17%), and insignificant (63%). Following major injuries, 61% of the women suffered fetal demise, whereas only one fourth of these women died as a result of their injuries. Of the women who had minor injuries, 27% suffered fetal demise, with no maternal deaths. None of the cases with insignificant injuries had fetal demise or maternal deaths.

**Table 43–1.** Obstetrical Intensive Care Unit Admissions (1979 To 1989)*

| | |
|---|---|
| Number Deliveries | 61,435 |
| Intensive Care Unit (ICU) Admissions | 126 |
| Reasons for Admission | |
| Pregnancy-induced hypertension | 30 |
| Excessive blood loss | 28 |
| Anesthetic complications | 16 |
| Preexisting disease | 11 |
| Miscellaneous (infection, pulmonary embolism, morbid obesity, etc.) | 41 |

(* Data from Stephens ID: ICU admissions from an obstetrical hospital. Canad. J. Anaesth. 38:677, 1991.)

Maternal demise is the leading cause of fetal demise. The second most common cause of fetal demise in trauma is placental abruption, which occurs in 1% to 5% of minor injuries, and up to 50% in cases of major maternal injury.[6,7] Uterine activity after trauma can help to predict placental abruption.[7,8] Frequent contractions, greater than 8 per hour, within the first few hours after a traumatic injury have been observed in almost all patients with this complication.

Fetal heart rate monitoring can be helpful to detect loss of variability or late decelerations. A 4-hour period of monitoring has been recommended after traumatic injury. Pregnant patients who have not developed complications with their pregnancies within 4 hours of injury can be expected to have normal outcomes.[7]

Another important aspect of trauma care is the potential for maternal-fetal hemorrhage. A prospective study of 205 cases of noncatastrophic trauma detected 18 occurrences of fetomaternal hemorrhage, or 8.78%.[8] A history of direct abdominal trauma did not increase the incidence of fetomaternal hemorrhage, except in incidences of motor vehicle accidents (MVA) (Table 43–3). However, all the hemorrhages greater than 0.1% (percent of fetal cells in maternal circulation) were found in patients with direct abdominal trauma. Should the mother be Rh negative, $Rh_o$ (D) immune globulin should be administered within 72 hours to prevent Rh isoimmunization.[7]

One other important aspect should be remembered. Not all pregnant patients will be obviously pregnant or able to communicate their status on admission to a trauma center. All female patients of childbearing age must have a pregnancy test at the time of admission.

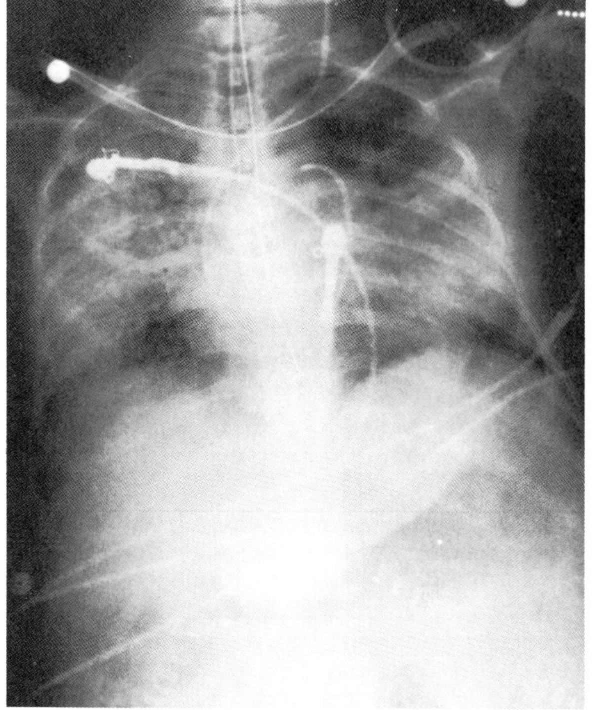

**Fig. 43–1.** Anteroposterior chest roentgenogram of a 17-year-old woman with acute lung injury associated with cryptogenic cirrhosis and Hemophilus influenza pneumonia. Note the presence of an endotracheal tube and a pulmonary arterial catheter. (From Kilpatrick SJ, Matthay MA: Obstetric patients requiring critical care. A five year review. Chest 101:1407, 1992.)

## Respiratory Care

Intensive respiratory care of the obstetrical patient should only be undertaken in the ICU. The specialized equipment and personnel required for intensive respiratory care are concentrated here.

**Table 43–2.** Antepartum and Postpartum ICU Admitting Diagnoses

| ICU Admitting Diagnosis | Antepartum | Ventilated | Postpartum | Ventilated |
|---|---|---|---|---|
| Respiratory failure | 7* | 5 | 6 | 5 |
| Hemodynamic instability | 2** | 0 | 11 | 5 |
| Neurologic dysfunction | 2 | 2 | 4 | 2 |
| Total | 11 | 7 (64%) | 21 | 12 (57%) |

* One patient in this group had a previable pregnancy at 20 weeks.
** Both patients had fetal death prior to transfer to ICU.
(From Kilpatrick SJ, Matthay MA: Obstetric patients requiring critical care. A 5-year review. Chest 101:1407–1412, 1992.)

**Table 43–3.** Incidence of Fetomaternal Hemorrhage From MVA and Trauma

| | Complications | | Fetomaternal Hemorrhage | |
|---|---|---|---|---|
| | No. | % | No. | % |
| Trauma | | | | |
| Motor vehicle accident | 4/56 | 7.1 | 10/56 | 17.9 |
| Fall | 6/87 | 6.9 | 5/87 | 5.7 |
| Assault | 7/41 | 17.1 | 2/41 | 4.9 |
| Other | 1/21 | 4.8 | 1/21 | 4.8 |
| Direct abdominal trauma | | | | |
| Yes | 15/125 | 12.0 | 12/175 | 6.9 |
| No | 3/80 | 3.8 | 6/80 | 7.5 |

(From Goodwin TM, Breen MT: Pregnancy outcome and fetomaternal hemorrhage after noncatastrophic trauma. *In* Current Concepts—Review Article. Edited by JF Desforges. Am. J. Obstet. Gynecol. 162:665, 1990.)

**Table 43–4.** Methods of Delivering Oxygen Therapy

| Method | Maximum $FIO_2$ |
|---|---|
| Nasal cannulae | 0.40 |
| Simple mask | 0.60 |
| Partial rebreathing mask | 0.80–0.9 |
| Nonrebreathing mask | 0.9–1.0 |
| Air entrainment (Venturi) mask | 0.24–0.50 |
| Continuous Positive Airway Pressure (CPAP) mask | 1.0 |
| Tracheal intubation | 1.0 |
| Spontaneous breathing | |
| Mechanical ventilation | |

The reasons for intubation and mechanical ventilation are similar for pregnant and nonpregnant patients. Intervention is required for failure of adequate oxygenation or ventilation.[9]

## *Oxygen Therapy*

A number of techniques are available to support oxygenation (Table 43–4). The minimal acceptable level of oxygenation is suggested to be a $PaO_2$ of 60 mmHg when the patient breathes a fraction of inspired oxygen ($FIO_2$) of 0.6. A $PaO_2$ of 60 mmHg normally represents an arterial oxyhemoglobin saturation ($SaO_2$) of 90% (Figure 43–2). A substantial increase in $PaO_2$ above 60 mmHg can only effect a maximal 10% increase in $SaO_2$. Conversely, a $PaO_2$ less than 60 mmHg produces a significant reduction in saturation.

The maximal $FIO_2$ generally achieved with nasal cannulae at an oxygen flowrate of 6 L/min is 0.40. Increasing flow to higher levels will not increase the $FIO_2$ at the trachea. The $FIO_2$ of 0.6 can usually be provided with a simple face mask. A $FIO_2$ greater than 0.6 requires a nonrebreather, a partial rebreather, or a continuous positive airway pressure (CPAP) mask.[10] However, a patient who requires a $FIO_2$ greater than 0.6 with a mask to achieve an $SaO_2$ of 90% is at constant risk of significant hypoxemia. Should the mask be removed for only a short period of time, an obstetrical patient with a pregnancy-induced reduction of functional residual capacity (FRC) will desaturate faster than a nonpregnant patient.[11,12] Fetal hypoxia, with possible catastrophic results, will quickly follow.

A failure of ventilation is defined by the development of a respiratory acidemia, as the partial pressure of arterial carbon dioxide ($PaCO_2$) rises and the pH decreases. However, the normal $PaCO_2$ in the pregnant patient is approximately 30 mmHg to 34 mmHg.[13] This respiratory alkalosis begins during the first trimester.[14] (Figure 43–3) Thus a seemingly normal $PaCO_2$ of 40 mmHg in a pregnant patient is really elevated and must be thoroughly assessed as a possible indicator of acute respiratory failure. Causes of acute respiratory failure during pregnancy include aspiration, pulmonary infection, asthma, beta adrenergic tocolytic therapy, air embolism, amniotic fluid embolism, and thromboembolism[15] (see Chapter 33).

Only a few therapeutic options are available for patients who require respiratory support beyond supplemental oxygen. CPAP delivered with a face mask may be sufficient in patients who can protect their own airway. Even patients who were tachypneic with respiratory acidosis have been successfully treated with mask CPAP.[16] Positive pressure helps to maintain the FRC and may decrease the work of breathing. If successful, it eliminates the need

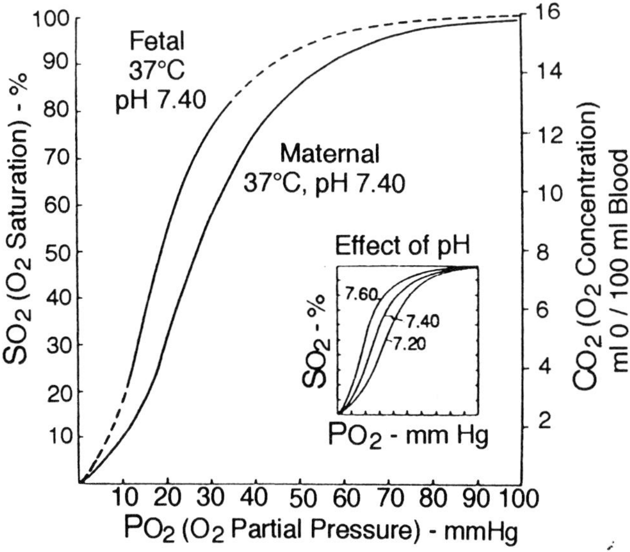


**Fig. 43–2.** Oxygen dissociation (equilibrium) curves of human fetal and maternal blood. The effect of pH on the position of the curve (Bohr effect) is shown on the insert. The oxygen capacity of 16 ml/100 ml blood on the right ordinate refers to maternal blood (Modified from Novy MJ, Edwards MJ: Respiratory problems in pregnancy. Am. J. Obstet. Gynecol. 99:1024, 1967.)

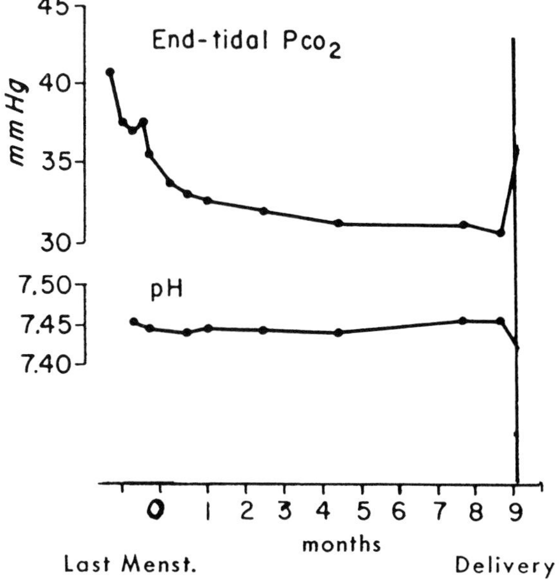


**Fig. 43–3.** The decrease in $PaCO_2$, noted here by decreased $PECO_2$, begins early in pregnancy. The pH reflects this respiratory effect and is alkalotic throughout the period. (Modified from Prowse CM, Gaensler EA: Anesthesiology 26:381, 1965.)

for tracheal intubation, a potentially traumatic event in obstetrical patients with airway edema.

If the patient cannot protect her airway or suffers from significant respiratory impairment, tracheal intubation and aggressive ventilatory support are indicated.

## *Tracheal Intubation*

A decision to intubate the trachea should not be taken lightly. Nasotracheal intubation is relatively contraindicated during pregnancy. The nasal mucosa is engorged, hyperemic, and friable. Bleeding is easily started and difficult to stop. Even if successful, the tube size that will pass the turbinates is often so small as to make spontaneous breathing difficult and may even compromise mechanical support.

Orotracheal intubation can be performed in an awake patient, but even in the best of circumstances is problematic. Mechanical difficulties, including manipulation of a standard laryngoscope handle between the patient's chin and enlarged breasts is tricky, and visualization of the larynx is rendered difficult by the frequent presence of oropharyngeal and supraglottic edema. The predisposition to vomiting (pregnancy and an invariably full stomach) increases the risk of pulmonary aspiration of gastric contents even in an awake individual. Fiberoptic bronchoscopy can be used successfully to aid tube placement but requires skill and experience.

In most cases, a rapid sequence induction with sodium thiopental and muscle relaxation with succinylcholine, together with cricoid pressure (Sellick maneuver) will be employed. Severe hypertension may result from laryngoscopy (in both awake and asleep intubation) and is particularly marked in patients with hypertensive disorders of pregnancy. Increased blood pressure, cerebral edema, and intracranial hemorrhage have been reported to occur under these circumstances in severely preeclamptic patients.[17]

As with nasotracheal intubation, a small-diameter tube may be needed because of laryngeal and tracheal edema. However, the work of breathing is increased significantly, and occult positive end-expiratory pressure (PEEP) may occur because of the increased expiratory resistance in a small-diameter tube. As large a tube as can be inserted atraumatically should be placed to offset these problems. In addition, endotracheal tube cuff design can also affect the pressure transmitted to the mucosa. Three different cuff designs are noted in Figure 43–4. These were then evaluated in laboratory models of high- and reduced-lung compliance (Figure 43–5). In the model of significantly reduced lung compliance analogous to acute lung injury, cuff pressures met or exceeded 25 mmHg in every instance except with the HI cuff, 8.0 ETT with a 10% leak in ventilation. This would indicate that some tracheal damage is likely in the worst case scenario, but that use of the largest endotracheal tube possible would minimize the possibility of injury. A larger tube size means that a smaller volume of air needs to be injected into the pilot tube to effect a cuff seal.[18] Hence, pressure necrosis is less likely to result from the cuff's approximation to the edematous tracheal mucosa.[19]

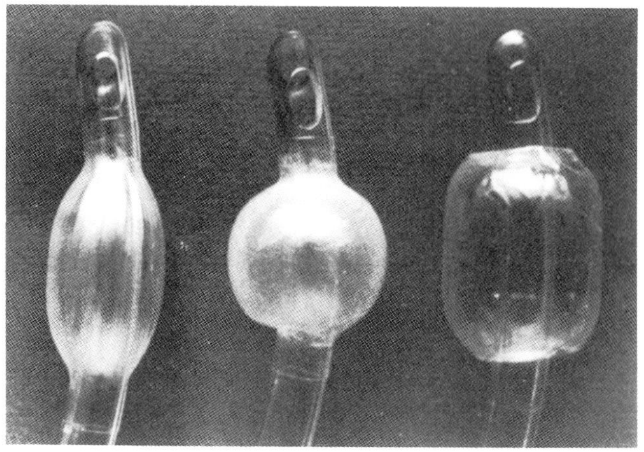

**Fig. 43–4.** Cuff designs: left, LO; center, MED; right, HI. (Modified from Guyton DC, Banner MJ, Kirby RR: High-volume, low-pressure cuffs: Are they always low pressure? Chest 100:1076, 1991.)

Once the tube is inserted, a CPAP system may be used if the patient's problem is primarily hypoxemia and not hypercarbia. Such an approach is relatively simple,[20] providing that central respiratory control mechanisms are intact and the work of breathing caused by the disease state and endotracheal tube is not excessive. Good results are reported with such therapy, but it is not tolerated in all cases, and some form of mechanical ventilatory support is often necessary.

## *Mechanical Ventilation*

A variety of support modes can be employed (Table 43–5). Controlled ventilation, assisted ventilation, and assist-control ventilation are traditional techniques that have been employed for decades but have become obsolete except in selected circumstances.[21] Intermittent mandatory ventilation (IMV) and synchronized intermittent mandatory ventilation (SIMV), both of which combine spontaneous breathing with mechanical ventilation were (and perhaps are) the most popular forms of support in the United States for both long-term ventilation and weaning.[22] The relative merits of these and other techniques for weaning have been discussed and challenged by Morganroth and Grum.[23] They note a small number of patients (<5% to 10%) are not easily weaned, regardless of the methodologies employed. Further studies on the monitoring of the work of breathing and on ventilatory modes specifically designed to decrease or selectively increase the work of breathing might provide a reduction in the number of difficult-to-wean patients. One example of a patient who developed problems secondary to weaning is shown in Figure 43–6. The patient does well for nearly 6 minutes, but slowly begins to accumulate $CO_2$ with an increase in respiratory rate and minute ventilation, as noted in the figure. These changes are difficult, if not impossible, to detect visually, and necessitate attention to careful laboratory monitoring techniques, eg, blood gases, respiratory rate, and minute ventilation pa-

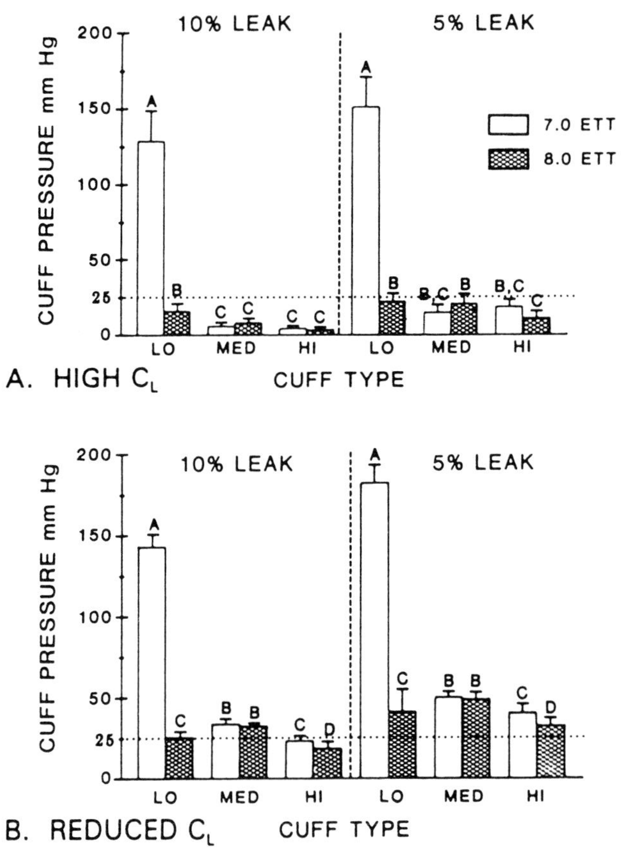


MEANS IN EACH GROUP ARE SIGNIFICANTLY DIFFERENT UNLESS THEY SHARE THE SAME LETTER (P=0.05)

**Fig. 43–5.** Baseline cuff inflation pressures for each cuff type under conditions of **(A)** high lung compliance (100 ml/cm $H_2O$) and **(B)** reduced lung compliance (15 ml/cm $H_2O$) with 10% and 5% leaks in delivered $V_T$. A reference line is drawn at 25 mmHg, indicating the maximum safe cuff pressure, ie, one that will not cause significant interference with tracheal wall blood flow. (Modified from Guyton DC, Banner MJ, Kirby RR: High-volume, low-pressure cuffs: Are they always low pressure? Chest. 100:1078, 1991.)

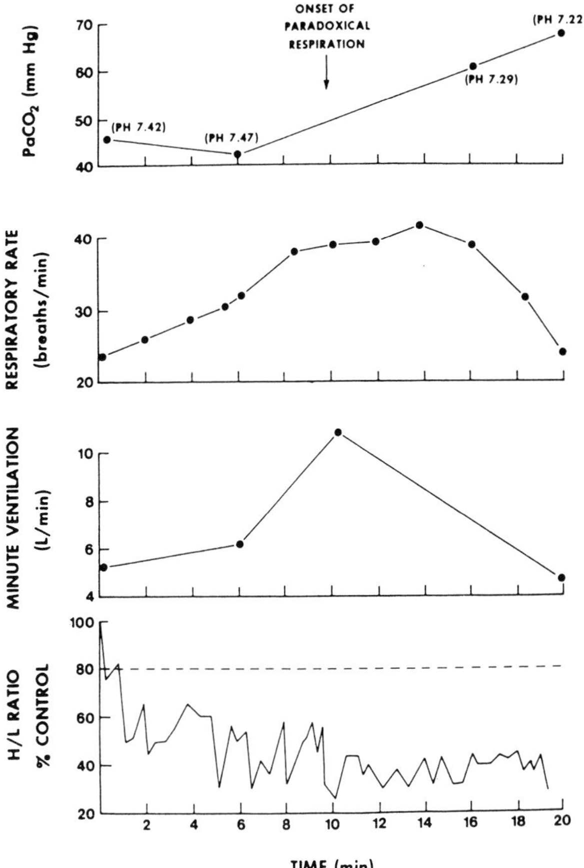


**Fig. 43–6.** Sequence of changes in $PaCO_2$, respiratory rate, minute ventilation, and high/low ratio of the diaphragm in a patient during a 20-minute attempt at discontinuation of ventilator support. (Modified from Cohen CA, Zagelbaum G, Gross D, et al: Clinical manifestations of inspiratory muscle fatigue. Am. J. Med. 73:308, 1982.)

**Table 43–5.** Techniques of Mechanical Ventilation

| | |
|---|---|
| Assisted (Patient-Triggered) | Initiated by patient who controls rate of cycling |
| Controlled | Ventilator rate set by physician/respiratory technician |
| Assist-Control | Initiated by patient but back-up control rate provided if spontaneous effort ceases or is inadequate |
| IMV/SIMV | Combination of spontaneous and controlled breaths; latter set by physician, former initiated by patient |
| Inverse-Ratio Ventilation (IRV) | Controlled ventilation with prolonged inspiratory time (so-called reverse I:E ratio); generally requires neuromuscular paralysis and/or heavy sedation |
| Pressure Support Ventilation (PSV) | Adjunct to IMV/SIMV or stand-alone mode; augments the patient's spontaneous breaths |

rameters. Two other ventilation methods will be discussed briefly which are, perhaps, less familiar to anesthesiologists and obstetricians caring for obstetrical patients.

## *Inverse-Ratio Ventilation*

Inverse-ratio ventilation (IRV)[24,25] extends the inspiratory time of a conventional mechanical tidal volume using: (1) volume-cycled or time-cycled ventilators with an inspiratory pause (Figure 43–7A); or (2) pressure-controlled ventilation with a decelerating inspiratory flow (Figure 43–7B).

Two effects are sought. First is a lowering of peak inspiratory pressure (PIP), and potentially a lesser incidence of barotrauma. Second is an improved distribution of inspired gas so that areas of the lungs with longer time constants (which require more time for filling because of increased airway resistance and decreased compliance) will fill more completely, thus improving the overall distribution of inspired gas and V/Q relationships. To date, no prospective randomized studies have demonstrated improvement in outcome with IRV compared to other tech-

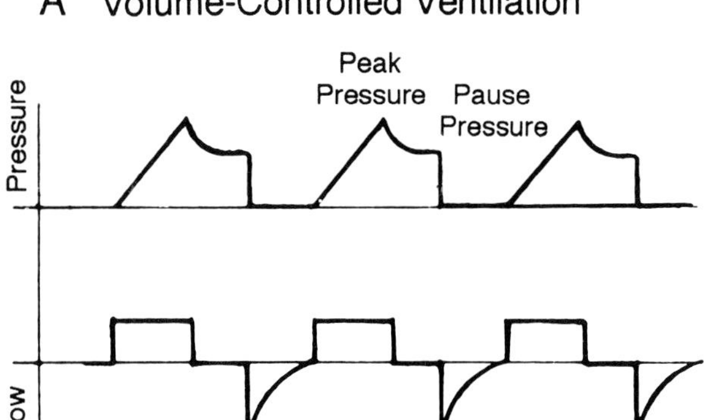


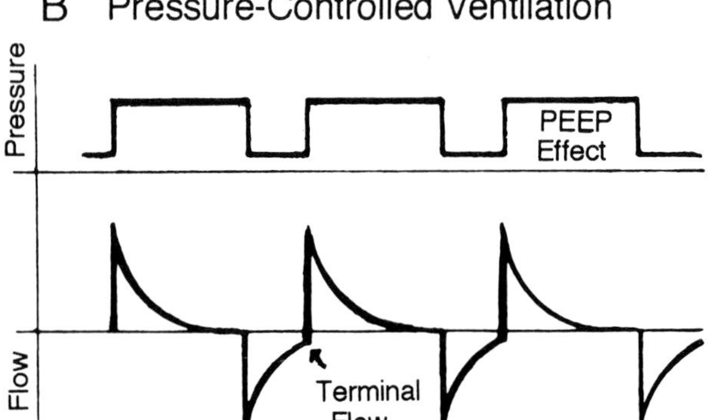


**Fig. 43–7.** Methods of increasing inspiratory/expiratory ratio. **A,** Volume-controlled; the use of an inspiratory pause. Note the pressure is held while no gas flow occurs. **B,** Pressure-controlled; the use of a decelerating inspiratory flow pattern. (Modified from Gurevitch MJ: Inverse ratio ventilation and the inspiratory/expiratory ratio. *In* Handbook of Mechanical Ventilatory Support. Edited by A. Perel. Baltimore, Williams & Wilkins, 1991.)

niques of mechanical ventilation and positive-end expiratory resistance.

Doubt has been expressed as to the efficacy and purported reduction in complications.[26] Of particular concern is the possibility that the prolonged inspiratory phase, hence decreased time for exhalation, will lead to gas trapping in the lungs and to occult or "auto" positive-end expiratory resistance, which is not detectable by conventional airway pressure monitoring. In addition, almost without exception, patients must be heavily sedated and frequently paralyzed so that they will tolerate this so-called reverse I:E ratio technique. Potentially adverse maternal and fetal effects of such medications must be considered before embarking upon IRV.

### *Pressure Support Ventilation*

Much less controversial, but also unproven, is pressure support ventilation (PSV).[27,28] Most forms of acute respiratory failure, particularly in obstetrical patients, are associated with increased work of breathing. Many ventilator circuits further increase this work because of high resistance.[20] Finally, the resistance of a small endotracheal

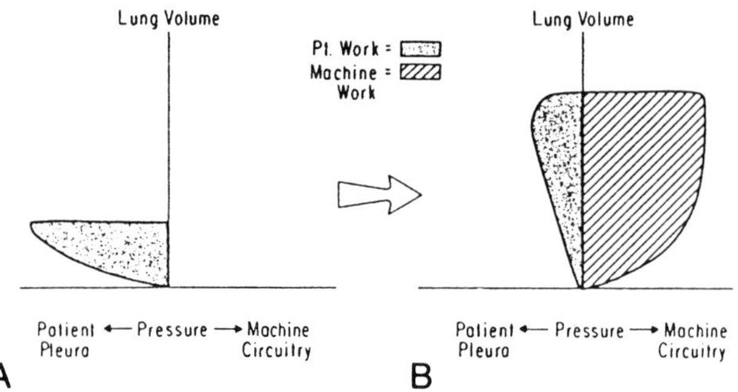


**Fig. 43–8.** Diagram depicting the pressure/volume work of a patient with reduced compliance in **A,** significant pressure work and resultant small volume achieved with an unassisted breath, versus **B,** reduced pressure work resulting in a significantly increased volume achieved in a pressure assisted breath. The shaded areas indicating patient work are approximately equal in both **A** and **B**. (From MacIntyre NR: Respiratory function during pressure support ventilation. Chest 89:677, 1986.)

tube and its associated work increment already have been mentioned.

Pressure support ventilation is used to decrease this intrinsic and extrinsic spontaneous work of breathing (IMV, SIMV, or as a stand-alone mode). When a spontaneous breath is initiated, the ventilator detects the reduction of airway pressure and responds by generating a high flow of gas into the circuit, increasing pressure up to a preselected maximum level (eg, 10 cm to 50 cm $H_2O$ above the baseline pressure of zero or some level of positive-end expiratory resistance). Gas flow continues and pressure is maintained so long as the spontaneous effort is maintained. Generally, when the flow is reduced to 25% of its peak level, the ventilator cycles off, allowing exhalation to commence. Weaning is achieved by a gradual reduction of the pressure level as the patient improves.

That PSV achieves a reduction of respiratory work is well established.[27-29] An example of modifying patient work of breathing during ventilatory support is by the use of PSV, whereby pressure/volume ratio may be reduced (Figure 43–8). Patients need to be more comfortable when it is in use, and thus the need for sedation can be reduced. Such considerations are of obvious importance to obstetrical patients in whom increased work of breathing and oxygen consumption have important maternal and fetal implications. As with most other popular forms of ventilator therapy, pressure support ventilation's final role awaits additional study.

## *Positive-End Expiratory Resistance/Continuous Positive Airway Pressure (PEEP/CPAP)*

Obstetrical patients have a naturally occurring reduction of FRC.[12,30] When this "physiologic" phenomenon is further compromised by an additional superimposed reduction of FRC in acute respiratory failure, profound increases in intrapulmonary shunting and reductions of $PaO_2$ will occur. Fetal compromise is a real possibility.

PEEP and CPAP are utilized to increase functional residual capacity, reduce shunting, and improve oxygenation.

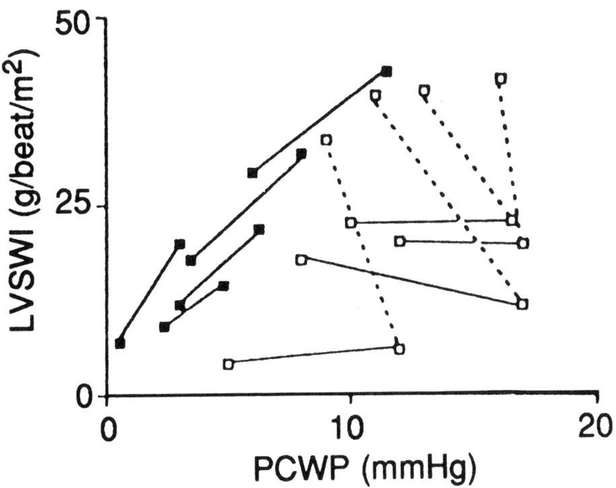


**Fig. 43–9.** The effect of therapy on left ventricular stroke work index (LVSWI) and pulmonary capillary wedge pressure (PCWP) in patients with the adult respiratory distress syndrome. Treatment with volume expansion (-----) resulted in an improved LVSWI in some patients (■). In other patients, volume expansion increased PCWP without an improvement in LVSWI (□). (Modified from Jardin F, et al: Pulmonary and systemic haemodynamic disorders in the adult respiratory distress syndrome. Intensive Care Med. 5:127, 1979.)

Such therapy in neonatal respiratory distress syndrome is efficacious, markedly improving survival. In adults, efficacy is more difficult to document, perhaps because respiratory problems are multifactorial in origin and frequently associated with multiorgan system failure.

These observations have led some investigations to question the use of positive-end expiratory resistance/continuous positive airway pressure.[31] This is a short-sighted view, however, at least until the benefits of allowing hypoxic patients to remain so are demonstrated. What level of pressure should be used has been debated for almost 20 years.[32–36] Clearly the potentially adverse effects of a reduction in cardiac output on uteroplacental circulation cannot be overlooked. This problem may result from a high level of mechanical ventilation and positive-end expiratory resistance. Conversely, failure to reverse hypoxemia is also detrimental. When maternal hyperventilation from inappropriate ventilator support is superimposed, adverse fetal effects may be profound.[37–39] What is needed is careful titration looking for both beneficial and adverse effects on both mother and fetus.[40,41] Management of patients with adult respiratory distress syndrome typifies the complexity in patient management, with decision-making necessarily including judgment regarding respiratory and cardiovascular parameters (Figure 43–9).

## Hemorrhage

Normal changes in the obstetrical patient's blood volume are summarized in Chapter 2. Red cell mass is increased, but less so than plasma volume. As a result, a fall in hemoglobin and hematocrit values is to be expected, but a hematocrit less than 33% is abnormal until proven otherwise.

**Table 43–6.** Maternal Hemorrhage

| Cause | Incidence (%) |
|---|---|
| Placental abruption | 0.5 to 1.0 |
| Placenta previa | 0.3 to 1.9 |
| Uterine rupture | 0.02 to 0.08 |
| Postpartum hemorrhage | 3.0 to 5.0 |

Four conditions are of special concern to the ICU management team (Table 43–6). All of these include major maternal hemorrhagic conditions.[42] Most often, the initial care will have been provided in the labor and delivery suite, but continued bleeding and resuscitation may well carry over to the ICU. In some cases, an underlying coagulopathy may be demonstrated. As an additional concern in eclampsia/preeclampsia, however, this is rare.

### Placental Abruption

Premature separation of the placenta occurs in 0.5% to 1% of deliveries and carries a mortality of 20% to 35%.[42,43] Its occurrence in traumatic injury was discussed previously.[6–8] Presenting signs and symptoms include vaginal bleeding, uterine tenderness, back pain, and fetal distress. Significant maternal or fetal distress requires an emergency cesarean section. Otherwise, vaginal delivery may be attempted with continuous fetal monitoring. Disseminated intravascular coagulation may occur. Clotting studies, and typing and crossmatching of packed red blood cells are essential to management.

### Placenta Previa

Implantation of the placenta in the lower uterine segment or cervical os is termed *placenta previa.* Four grades are described, ranging from full coverage of the os to a low-lying implantation in the lower uterine segment without encroachment of the os. The incidence of this condition ranges from 0.3% to 1.9%, and the associated fetal mortality is 8% to 24%.[42,44]

Vaginal bleeding in this condition usually is painless in contrast to placental abruption. Vaginal examination can induce life-threatening hemorrhage and should be performed only after ultrasound examination has excluded the problem, or in an operating room with immediate cesarean section capabilities.

Parturients who present prior to term are managed with transfusion and bed rest whenever possible until fetal maturity is demonstrated. Perinatal hypoxia is a real danger to both premature and mature infants.

Uterine bleeding at the time of surgery and in the postpartum period can be severe because of poor contractility, or if the placenta has grown into the myometrium and becomes abnormally adherent (placenta accreta). In severe cases with major blood loss, ICU management is essential.

### Uterine Rupture

This condition is rare (0.02% to 0.08%)[45] and usually occurs in patients in active labor. Bleeding into the peritoneal cavity may result in little vaginal appearance and may be painless. The sudden onset of fetal distress and an "unusual" abdominal mass are characteristic findings. Prompt operative intervention is necessary if maternal or fetal distress occurs, and a cesarean hysterectomy may be required.

### *Postpartum Hemorrhage*

Bleeding following delivery usually results from uterine atony, but may reflect trauma, coagulopathy, or retained products of conception. As mentioned in Table 43–6, this occurs in up to 3% to 5% of deliveries. Management entails uterine massage, oxygenation, and certain prostaglandins or ergot alkaloids (ergotrate, methylergonovine). If pharmacologic methods fail, surgical intervention is necessary. Inspection of the birth canal, curettage, uterine packing (controversial), uterine or hypogastric artery ligation, and even hysterectomy may be necessary.

### *Coagulopathy*

Coagulopathy-induced bleeding may occur with intrauterine fetal demise (though rare if the demise is less than 1 month's duration), following amniotic fluid embolism (see Chapter 41), and in association with sepsis.[42] Ventilatory and circulatory management in the ICU, transfusion and aggressive fluid therapy, and bleeding and clotting studies are indicated.

## Cardiovascular Disease

The incidence of cardiac disease in pregnancy ranges from 0.4% to 4% with an associated maternal mortality of 0.4% to 6.8%.[46,47] Rheumatic heart disease continues to predominate despite a declining incidence. Because of the associated cardiovascular changes in pregnancy, the parturient with heart disease is placed at particular risk during labor, delivery, and in the postpartum period. Improved management, however, allows many of these patients to give birth, whereas not too many years ago they would not have become pregnant or the pregnancy would have been terminated.

### *Mitral Stenosis*

Approximately 90% of rheumatic valvular lesions are mitral stenosis. The increased heart rate and blood volume in pregnancy predispose to pulmonary edema and atrial fibrillation. In moderate-to-severe mitral stenosis, labor and delivery should be monitored with an intraarterial catheter and central venous or pulmonary artery (PA) catheter. The pulmonary artery occlusion pressure (PAOP) may overestimate left ventricular end-diastolic pressure (LVEDP).

Whenever possible, tachycardia should be minimized, pulmonary artery pressure and central blood volume decreased, and systemic vascular resistance (SVR) increased. Epidural or intrathecal narcotics may be useful to reduce pain as they avoid the hemodynamic consequences of local anesthetics.[47]

### *Mitral Insufficiency and Prolapse*

Mitral insufficiency is the second most common valvular lesion in pregnancy and, when severe, is associated with left ventricular failure. In counterdistinction to mitral and aortic stenosis, a reduction of peripheral vascular resistance is preferred in order to increase forward flow and to decrease regurgitant blood flow. Decreased heart rate, atrial dysrhythmias, and myocardial depressants are poorly tolerated.[47] Mean pulmonary artery occlusion pressure measurements are frequently increased because of the large V wave associated with mitral regurgitation.

Mitral valve prolapse (MVP) occurs in 5% of the general population and up to 17% of young or child-bearing women.[48] Most patients are asymptomatic and tolerate pregnancy well. Tachycardia due to a reduction in ventricular volume can be expected to accentuate mitral valve prolapse and should therefore be minimized. In addition, patients with mitral valve prolapse should be treated with antibiotic prophylaxis.

### *Aortic Stenosis*

This lesion is rare in pregnancy but, when present, is a serious problem. A decrease of systemic vascular resistance is poorly tolerated, and because of the relatively fixed stroke volume, a reduction of heart rate and venous return should be avoided. As with mitral stenosis, severe aortic stenosis will benefit from invasive cardiovascular monitoring. However, major dysrhythmias may be associated with pulmonary artery catheter insertion. In addition, pulmonary artery occlusion pressure may underestimate the LVEDP depending upon ventricular compliance.[47] Thus the decision to employ such monitoring must be weighed carefully.

### *Aortic Insufficiency*

As with mitral insufficiency, aortic insufficiency is tolerated well during pregnancy. Increased systemic vascular resistance, decreased heart rate, and myocardial depressants are best avoided.

### *Peripartum Cardiomyopathy*

This disease is poorly understood but has a high mortality (up to 84%) in patients with cardiomegaly that persists beyond 6 months.[47] It seems to occur most commonly in women with twins, preeclamptics and eclamptics, blacks, and in patients with viral infections. Ventricular failure, pulmonary emboli, and myocardial infarction may be seen.

### *Myocardial Infarction*

Although rare, this problem may be increasing as parturients become older, and other risk factors such as cigarette smoking and cocaine use become increasingly prevalent. Maternal mortality has been noted to be as high as 35% at or within 2 weeks of the time of infarction.[49] Management is based upon the mother's condition prior to the stress of labor. Continual reassessment of the mother's condition is required and increasing the level of monitor-

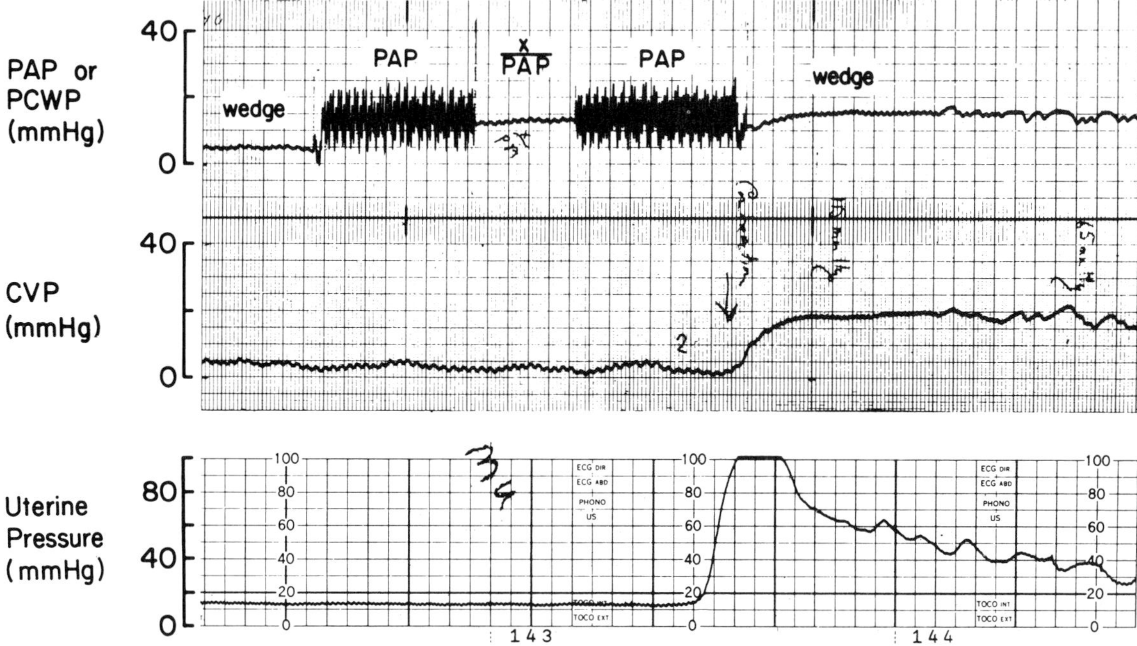


**Fig. 43–10.** Effect of a uterine contraction (change in uterine pressure) on maternal pulmonary capillary wedge and central venous pressures. PAP = pulmonary artery pressure; PCWP and wedge = pulmonary capillary wedge pressure; X/PAP = mean pulmonary artery pressures; CVP = central venous pressure. (From Hankins GDV, Wendel JR GD, Leveno KJ, Stoneham J: Myocardial infarction during pregnancy: A review. Obstet. Gynecol. 65:139, 1985.)

ing is warranted if her condition deteriorates. Invasive monitoring is recommended in the presence of unstable angina or heart failure. The effects of labor are noted in Figure 43–10. The pulmonary capillary wedge pressure rose from 5 mmHg to 15 mmHg, and the central venous pressure rose from 5 mmHg to 20 mmHg.

### *Hypertensive Disorders of Pregnancy*

These syndromes are discussed elsewhere but warrant some mention here (Table 43–7). Most important from an ICU management standpoint are preeclampsia and eclampsia. Severe preeclampsia is characterized by one or more of the following: (1) systolic blood pressure > 160 mmHg; (2) diastolic blood pressure > 110 mmHg; (3) proteinuria > 5 g/24 hours; (4) oliguria < 500 ml/24 hours; and (5) headaches, visual disturbances, epigastric pain, pulmonary edema, or cyanosis.[47,50] Eclampsia is present when the same complex of signs and symptoms occurs, plus seizures not caused by other underlying problems.

**Table 43–7.** Characteristics of Severe Preeclampsia/Eclampsia

| | |
|---|---|
| *Preeclampsia* | |
| Systolic BP | >160 mmHg |
| Diastolic BP | >110 mmHg |
| Proteinuria | > 5 g/24 hours |
| Oliguira | <500 ml/24 hours |
| Headaches | Common |
| Visual disturbances | Common |
| Epigastric pain | Common |
| Pulmonary edema | Common |
| Cyanosis | Common |
| *Eclampsia* | |
| All of the above plus seizure not caused by other conditions. | |

Blood volume is characteristically reduced and viscosity is increased. A decrease of renal blood flow and glomerular filtration rate is characteristic. Central nervous system irritability and hyperreflexia are present. Thrombocytopenia is common.

Definitive treatment is delivery of the fetus and placenta. Seizure control is achieved with magnesium sulfate, 2 g to 4 g as a slow intravenous bolus, followed by 1 g to 3 g/hour. Control of hypertension is best achieved by hydralazine or sodium nitroprusside (SNP). The latter is the most effective agent, although it must be used with caution prior to delivery to avoid fetal cyanide toxicity and an increase of maternal intracranial pressure (ICP) in those patients with central nervous system manifestations.

Severely preeclamptic patients may develop cardiac failure and pulmonary edema. Monitoring with a pulmonary artery catheter is advocated in such individuals, since central venous pressure measurements may be misleading.[41,51,52,72] A syndrome of hemolysis, elevated liver enzymes, and thrombocytopenia (HELLP) occurs in a subset of patients.[53] Increased maternal and fetal mortality occur, therefore expedient delivery is essential.

Following delivery, patient management in an ICU is indicated. The risk of pulmonary edema is increased in the postpartum period because of fluid shifts and centralization of blood volume.

**Table 43–8.** Hyponatremia and Water Intoxication Syndromes

| *Early Signs:* | Oliguria | *Late Signs:* | Nausea and vomiting |
|---|---|---|---|
| | Weakness | | Abdominal distention |
| | Lethargy | | Shock |
| | Disorientation | | Coma |
| | | | Death |

## Fluid and Electrolyte Therapy

Historically, few areas have been managed as poorly as fluid administration to the obstetrical patient. As late as the 1970s (and occasionally into the 80s), postpartum patients commonly received 2000 ml to 3000 ml or more of 5% dextrose in water ($D_5W$) on the day of delivery and the first postpartum day, with simultaneous infusions of an oxytocin compound containing significant amounts of vasopressin. The results were predictable, although seldom recognized until far advanced (Table 43–8): a reduction of urine output secondary to decreased glomerular filtration rate; fluid retention and hyponatremia; hypertension and tachycardia; and confusion, lethargy, stupor, convulsions, and sometimes death. The problem was water intoxication related to the administration of electrolyte-free fluid, increased endogenous antidiuretic hormones production as a result of pain, stress or narcotics, and the superimposed infusion of vasopressin.

The syndrome was well described by the 1950s, and even though antidiuretic hormones activity could not be directly assayed, the pathophysiology was reasonably well understood.[54–58] In 1951, Bristol[59] demonstrated that hyponatremia alone could significantly reduce glomerular filtration rate and urine output (Table 43–9). By the 1960s, fluid and electrolyte shifts in surgery, shock, and trauma were characterized,[60–63] and the rationale for the administration of balanced electrolyte solutions such as Ringer's lactate was established. Yet, even in the late 1980s, reports of severe water intoxication associated with excessive $D_5W$ infusion leading to death or permanent neurologic disability continued to appear.[64–66]

Why such events should occur, and why any obstetrician or obstetrical anesthesiologist should continue this basically irrational approach to fluid therapy is impossible to ascertain. No doubt the roots of such an approach germinated in the earlier work of Coller[67,68] and others who mistakenly ascribed postoperative oliguria to salt intolerance. They believed the stress of surgery somehow "stunned" the kidneys so that they were unable to excrete a salt-and-water load. Hence, the recommendation to minimize fluid administration, and to give no salt the day of surgery and 1 to 2 days thereafter became surgical doctrine until the aforementioned work of Shires in 1964.[62,63] Somehow, these later developments went unnoticed by the majority of obstetricians, and water intoxication continued to be a major clinical problem.

**Table 43–9.** Reduction in Ability to Excrete Water Load During Hyponatremia*

| Serum Sodium (mEq/L) | % Water Load Excreted |
|---|---|
| 140 | 71 |
| 135–139 | 60 |
| 130–134 | 48 |
| 125–129 | 43 |
| 120–124 | 43 |
| 110–119 | 30 |

(* Data from Bristol WR: Relations of sodium chloride depletion to urine excretion and $H_2O$ intoxication. Am. J. Med. Sciences 221:412, 1951.)

Obstetrical patients are perhaps least suited to the administration of large amounts of $D_5W$. They already have a total body water excess as a maternal consequence of pregnancy. In addition, for reasons that are not well understood, women have a higher incidence of severe and symptomatic hyponatremia postoperatively than do men, and a considerably higher incidence of major complications such as coma and death.[64]

Those individuals with preeclampsia, central nervous system manifestations, and an increase of intracranial pressure can be pushed into full blown eclampsia because of a sudden exacerbation of cerebral edema. The solution is to administer balanced electrolyte fluids rather than $D_5W$ intrapartum and immediately postpartum. Should hyponatremia develop, it may be handled by fluid restriction in mild cases, or by the judicious administration of hypertonic salt solutions, increasing serum sodium by no more than 2 mEq/L/hour in severe ones.[66,69] Once the sodium concentration reaches 125 mEq/L, such treatment should be stopped. Overly rapid correction has been suggested to predispose to central pontine myelinolysis (CPM), a lesion associated with progressive paraparesis, quadriparesis, dysphagia, and dysarthria.[70,71] However, the relationship between hyponatremia, rapid correction, and CPM is not clearly established.

## Monitoring

### *Maternal*

Invasive monitoring already has been discussed in other sections of this chapter. Of particular interest in recent years has been the use of pulmonary artery catheters to distinguish cardiogenic (high pressure) from noncardiogenic (permeability) pulmonary edema. Much attention has centered on preeclampsia because of its multiorgan system involvement and the delicate balance of fluid shifts.[41,47,72] Indications for such monitoring include severe hypertension unresponsive to conventional antihypertensive therapy, pulmonary edema, oliguria that does not respond to fluid challenges, and anesthetic management. Unfortunately, as is the case with essentially every other field in which pulmonary artery catheter monitoring is advocated, a documented improvement in outcome has yet to be demonstrated, although diagnostic capabilities appear to be increased. Pulmonary artery catheterization may be useful to monitor the progress of respiratory failure and its response to interventions such as positive-end expiratory resistance and continuous positive airway pressure.[32–36]

Of special concern with invasive monitoring is the association of catheter-related infections and sepsis. Some

50 000 cases of catheter sepsis are estimated to occur annually. Risk factors and catheter management recently were summarized and specific recommendations made.[73] Peripheral intravenous catheters from outside sources or the emergency department are considered to be contaminated and should be replaced aseptically. Arterial catheters do not have to be routinely changed. However, axillary artery catheter use should be restricted to less than 4 days' duration. Pulmonary artery catheters can be left in place so long as no evidence of catheter-related sepsis (unexplained fever more than 48 hours after insertion, positive blood cultures, infection at the insertion site) is present. Catheters may be changed once over a guidewire and the catheter tip cultured. Central venous pressure catheters may be used until there is an indication for change. In the absence of evidence for sepsis, they may be changed over a guidewire on multiple occasions.

### *Fetal*

Most critical care physicians have little first-hand knowledge concerning fetal monitoring and will rely on their obstetrician colleagues to assess fetal well-being. They must keep in mind that the techniques used were developed for obstetrics, not critical care.[74]

Fetal heart rate is considered to be the prime indication of well-being, and the normal values, variabilities, and abnormal patterns are discussed in detail elsewhere (Chapter 41). One thing should be considered when fetal monitoring is utilized so as not to jump to conclusions about "fetal distress." Maternal needs in the intensive care unit may dictate the use of narcotics, sedatives, tranquilizing drugs, and other agents which will secondarily alter fetal heart rate and variability. These changes do not indicate fetal difficulties, but rather a normal response to the drugs in question.

Caton has pointed out the inconsistencies of assuming that oxygen deprivation is the sole determinant of intrauterine distress.[74] He suggests that conditions such as severe hypoglycemia are equally devastating. In all other areas of medicine, complete batteries of tests are used to evaluate organ function. Only in obstetrics are 1 or 2 parameters (fetal heart rate, scalp pH) considered sufficient to evaluate the entire gamut of fetal physiologic activity. At best, this approach is provincial and shortsighted. This discussion would be largely philosophical were it not for the fact that maternal treatment decisions may be altered because of concern over a changing fetal heart rate and the presumption that hypoxia is present. The result is that neither mother or fetus is treated appropriately. Whenever decisions are to be made, maternal well-being must be the primary consideration.

## Cardiac Arrest in Pregnancy

Cardiac arrest in near-term pregnancy presents unique difficulties. Aortocaval compression with total inferior vena caval compression reduces the already compromised blood flow associated with closed-chest compres-

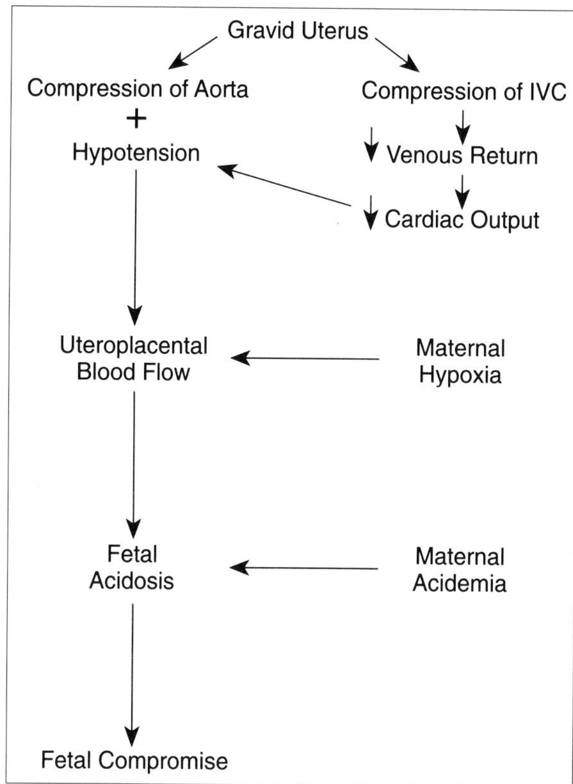


**Fig. 43–11.** Pathophysiology of cardiopulmonary arrest during pregnancy. IVC = inferior vena cava. (From Lee RV, Rodgers BD, White LM, Harvey RC: Cardiopulmonary resuscitation of pregnant women. Am. J. Med. 81:311, 1986.)

sion (Figure 43–11). As a result, an emergency cesarean section within 5 minutes of commencing cardiopulmonary resuscitation is recommended.[75–77] Other investigators have extended their allowable time period to as much as 15 minutes of continuous cardiopulmonary resuscitation in pregnancies of 32 weeks or greater.[78] In out-of-hospital cardiac arrests, a perimortem cesarean section should be performed immediately upon arrival at the hospital, regardless of the elapsed time.[79] In view of the difficulties in obtaining adequate cardiac output during cardiopulmonary resuscitation with the fetus in utero, and the reasonable maternal and fetal survival with prompt cesarean section, a delay beyond 5 minutes of resuscitative efforts seems unreasonable and should be discouraged. Thirty cases of successful postmortem cesarean deliveries were reported from 1971 to 1985.[75] Table 43-10 lists the causes of maternal death.

## Neurologic Problems

Central nervous system dysfunction following cardiac arrest or in severe preeclampsia and eclampsia are known to most clinicians and are important reasons for ICU admission. Less common conditions also may necessitate critical care intervention, and have been nicely summarized in a review article by Fox, et al.[80]

**Table 43–10.** Reported Cases of Postmortem Cesarean Deliveries with Surviving Infants

| Years | Causes of Maternal Death | Cases | % |
|---|---|---|---|
| 1971 to 1985 | Infection (meningitis) | 1 | 3.3 |
| | Trauma | 2 | 6.7 |
| | Anesthesia | 5 | 16.7 |
| | Cardiac | 1 | 3.3 |
| | Malignancy | 2 | 6.7 |
| | Cerebrovascular accident | 1 | 3.3 |
| | Embolism (pulmonary & amniotic fluid) | 3 | 10 |
| | Asthma | 1 | 3.3 |
| | Unspecified* | 14 | 46.7 |
| | Total | 30 | 100.0 |

(Modified from Katz VL, Dotters DJ, Droegemueller W: Perimortem cesarean delivery. Obstet. Gynecol. 68:571, 1986.)

## Pseudotumor Cerebri

Pseudotumor cerebri is characterized by an increase of intracranial pressure > 200 mm $H_2O$, without a structural intracranial cause. It results in papilledema, enlarged blind spots, and abducens palsies. Pseudotumor cerebri has an incidence of approximately 19 per 100,000 in young women.[81] It occurs less frequently during pregnancy,[82] and appears to have a shorter duration when it occurs during pregnancy than it has if the patient is not pregnant. Serious visual complications including permanent blindness in 5% to 10% of patients may result. The primary therapeutic goal, therefore, is to prevent blindness.[83] Lumbar tap, lumoperitoneal shunting,[84] and optic nerve decompression[85] have been utilized for this purpose. Diuretics may be of some benefit.

## Stroke

The risk of stroke during pregnancy is 13 times that of the nonpregnant, age-matched population occurring in 1 out of every 3000 pregnancies.[86]Arterial occlusion and cerebral venous occlusion are the leading causes. The latter is most common in the first postpartum month. Arthrosclerosis, the most common cause for strokes in the elderly, accounts for only 25% of strokes during pregnancy.[87]

## Subarachnoid Hemorrhage

Subarachnoid hemorrhage occurs in 1 of every 10,000 pregnant patients, a rate 5 times higher than in nonpregnant individuals. Approximately 2% of all subarachnoid hemorrhages occur during pregnancy.[88] It accounts for 5% to 10% of maternal deaths occurring during pregnancy.[89]

Management of the pregnant patient who has had a subarachnoid hemorrhage is complicated by the fetal presence. The use of diuretics may result in fetal dehydration. Barbiturates can depress fetal respiration. If delivery is imminent, the depressed fetal respiration can be managed by the neonatologist following delivery and should not play a major role in the decisions concerning maternal management.

## Epilepsy

Neurologic disorders affected by pregnancy include epilepsy. The incidence of unfavorable outcomes (fetal hypoxia, vaginal bleeding, placental abruption, toxemia, premature labor, small-for-date fetal size, and low I.Q.) is increased.[90] Some anticonvulsant medications (eg, valproic acid) are associated with teratogenicity.[91] A pregnant patient with a seizure disorder admitted to the ICU during the first trimester should have careful evaluation of her anticonvulsant therapy.

## Multiple Sclerosis and Myasthenia Gravis

Pregnancy does not seem to have a deleterious effect on the course of multiple sclerosis, although exacerbations do frequently occur during pregnancy.[92] There is evidence of a true increase in exacerbation during the postpartum period.[93]

Myasthenia gravis is often complicated with pregnancy[94] which has a definite but unpredictable effect:[95] one-third of women improve during pregnancy, one-third are unchanged, and one-third become worse. Premature labor may be increased, and during labor, the need for anticholinesterases increases. Neonatal myasthenia gravis occurs in 5% to 10% of the offspring of myasthenic mothers because of placental transfer of maternal acetylcholine receptor antibodies to the fetus; however, it is more often transient with a duration of less than 4 weeks.[96]

## Spinal Injuries

Paraplegics and quadriplegics can have normal conception and fetal development. However, they are at risk for several problems, including decubitus ulcers, urinary tract infections, deep venous thrombosis, and pulmonary complications.[97] A problem of particular concern is autonomic hyperreflexia in those patients with cord lesions above the T-6 level. Reflex sympathetic discharge ($T_4$-$L_2$) cannot be modulated by descending central inhibitory control. Episodes of bladder and bowel distention, cutaneous stimulation, and uterine contractions can elicit profound hypertension, anxiety, and severe headache. The onset of labor may be painless because of a lack of sensory input and can initiate the syndrome before the patient or physician is aware of the developing problem.

Treatment is directed toward lowering of the blood pressure with hydralazine, trimethophan, nitroglycerin or sodium nitroprusside. Prevention of seizures and stroke is a primary goal.[98] If labor cannot or should not be stopped, an epidural anesthetic can be used to prevent autonomic hyperreflexia or to control the blood pressure increase associated with it.[99] Most of these patients are managed successfully in labor and delivery suites. However, a few may be admitted to an intensive care unit for unrelated reasons. Medical and nursing personnel in the intensive care unit, therefore, should be aware of the possible development of the aforementioned problems and their relationship to unanticipated labor and delivery.

## Clinical Impact

During the peripartum period, the patient undergoes extreme changes in her physiology. As detailed in this book, many of these changes are part of the natural and wonderful process of childbirth. The proper delivery of analgesia and anesthesia is essential for this process. However, as detailed in this chapter, the obstetrical patient may have numerous physiological derangements. During this period these problems may threaten the lives of the mother-to-be and her fetus. Consider the example of the patient who has moderately severe pregnancy-induced hypertension. This patient might suffer significant hemorrhage during delivery. While this is certainly a serious problem, it could worsen with the development of coagulopathy and sepsis. The patient might next proceed into adult respiratory distress syndrome. Only a previously healthy young woman might survive such an insult, and her survival would depend on her care by the intensive care team. This team would consist of personnel well versed in the physiology of pregnancy and the peripartum period. This team must also be astute and knowledgeable about invasive monitoring, mechanical ventilation, and fluid therapy, particularly in those aspects that differ the obstetrical patient from other ICU patients.

The patient who suffers physiological derangements as noted above can only be cared for in an area dedicated strictly for that purpose. The equipment and monitors required for the intensive care of a patient are concentrated in this area for many reasons. In the same manner, the team caring for such a patient must be composed of experts in critical care and obstetrics. Only a few large centers will have people who are truly experts in both areas. Most hospitals must assemble a group of experts from several disciplines for this purpose. The true principles and practice of obstetric analgesia and anesthesia extend beyond the time of delivery. It seems only natural that anesthesiologists, as integral personnel in both the labor-and-delivery suite and the ICU, be at the forefront in delivering critical care to obstetrical patients and serve in an advisory capacity to our challenged obstetricians about what is and should be appropriate in critical care management.

## REFERENCES


1. Stephens ID: ICU admissions from an obstetrical hospital. Canad. J. Anaesth. 38:677, 1991.
2. Kilpatrick SJ, Matthay MA: Obstetric patients requiring critical care. A 5-year review. Chest 101:1407–1412, 1992.
3. Mabie WL, Sibai BM: Treatment in an obstetric intensive care unit. Am. J. Obstet. Gynecol. 162:104, 1990.
4. Patterson RM: Trauma in pregnancy. Clin. Obstet. Gynecol. 27:32, 1984.
5. Varner MW: Maternal mortality in Iowa from 1952 to 1986. Surg. Gynecol. Obstet. 168:555, 1989.
6. Rothenberger D, Quattlebaum FW, Perry JF Jr, Zabel J, et al: Blunt maternal trauma: A review of 103 cases. J. Trauma 18:173, 1978.
7. Pearlman MD, Tintinalli JE, Lorenz RP: Blunt trauma during pregnancy. N. Engl. J. Med. 323:1609, 1990.
8. Goodwin TM, Breen MT: Pregnancy outcome and fetomaternal hemorrhage after noncatastrophic trauma. *In* Current Concepts—Review Article. Edited by JF Desforges. Am. J. Obstet. Gynecol. 162:665, 1990.
9. Prater MR, Irwin RS: Respiratory failure I: An overview. *In* Intensive Care Medicine. Edited by JM Rippe, RS Irwin, JA Alpert, et al. Boston, Little, Brown, and Company, 1985, pp. 379–84.
10. Smith RA: Oxygen delivery systems. *In* Respiratory Care. Edited by RR Kirby, RW Taylor. Chicago, Year Book Medical Publishers, 1986, pp. 515–529.
11. Cugell DW, Frank NR, Gaensler EA, Badger TL: Pulmonary function in pregnancy: I. Serial observations in normal women. Amer. Rev. Tuberculosis 67:568, 1953.
12. Weinberger SE, Weiss ST, Cohen WR, Weiss JW, et al: State of the art—pregnancy and the lung. Am. Rev. Respir. Dis. 121:559, 1980.
13. Prowse CM, Gaensler EA: Respiratory and acid-base changes during pregnancy. Anesthesiology 26:381, 1965.
14. Skatrud JJB, Dempsey JA, Kaiser DG: Ventilatory response to medroxyprogesterone acetate in normal subjects. Time course and mechanism. J. Appl. Physiol.: Respir. Environ. Exercise. Physiol. 44:939, 1978.
15. Hollingsworth HM, Pratter MR, Irwin RS: Acute respiratory failure in pregnancy. J. Intens. Care Med. 4:11, 1989.
16. DeHaven CB, Fuhrman TM, Downs JB, Reilley TE: Treatment of hypercarbia and tachypnea with mask CPAP. Crit. Care Med. 17:S151, 1989.
17. Hodgkinson R, Husain FJ, Hayashi RH: Systemic and pulmonary blood pressure during cesarean section in parturients with gestational hypertension. Can. Anaesth. Soc. J. 27:389, 1980.
18. Guyton DC: Endotracheal and tracheotomy tube cuff design: Influence on tracheal damage. Crit. Care Update 1(3):1, 1990.
19. Guyton DC, Banner MJ, Kirby RR: High-volume, low-pressure cuffs: Are they always low pressure? Chest 100:1076, 1991.
20. Kirby RR: Positive airway pressure: System design and clinical application. *In* Critical Care: State of the Art. Edited by WC Shoemaker. Fullerton, CA, Society of Critical Care Medicine, 1985, pp. G1–G52.
21. Kirby RR: Modes of mechanical ventilation. *In* Current Respiratory Care. Edited by RM Kacmarek, JK Stoller. Toronto, BC Decker, Inc., 1988, pp. 128–131.
22. Venus B, Smith RA, Mathru M: National survey of methods and criteria used for weaning from mechanical ventilation. Crit. Care Med. 15:530, 1987.
23. Morganroth M, Grum C: Weaning from mechanical ventilation. J. Intens. Care Med. 3:109, 1988.
24. Perel A: Newer ventilation modes: Temptations and pitfalls. Crit. Care Med. 15:707, 1987.
25. Tharrat R, Allen R, Albertson T: Pressure controlled inverse-ratio ventilation in severe adult respiratory failure. Chest 94:755, 1988.
26. Kacmarek R, Hess D: Pressure-controlled inverse-ratio ventilation: Panacea or auto-PEEP? (Editorial) Respir. Care 33: 945, 1990.
27. MacIntyre NR: Respiratory function during pressure support ventilation. Chest 89:677, 1986.
28. Räsänen J, Downs JB: Modes of mechanical ventilatory support. *In* Clinical Applications of Ventilatory Support. Edited by RR Kirby, MJ Banner, JB Downs. New York, Churchill Livingstone, 1990, p. 173.
29. Banner MJ, Kirby RR, MacIntyre NR: Patient and ventilator work of breathing and ventilatory muscle loads at different levels of pressure support ventilation. Chest 100:531, 1991.
30. Caton D: Pregnancy: Essential physiologic concerns. *In* Critical Care. 2nd Ed. Edited by JM Civetta, RW Taylor, RR Kirby. Philadelphia, JB Lippincott Co, 1992.
31. Grum C, Morganroth M: Initiating mechanical ventilation. J. Intens. Care Med. 3:6, 1988.
32. Suter PM, Fairley B, Isenberg MD: Optimum end-expiratory

pressure in patients with acute pulmonary failure. N. Engl. J. Med. 292:284, 1975.

33. Gallagher TJ, Civetta JM, Kirby RR: Terminology update: Optimal PEEP. Crit Care Med. 6:323, 1978.
34. Shapiro BA, Cane RD, Harrison RA; Positive end-expiratory pressure therapy in adults with special reference to acute lung injury: A review of the literature and suggested clinical correlations. Crit. Care Med. 12:127, 1984.
35. Räsänen J, Downs JB, DeHaven B: Titration of continuous positive airway pressure by real-time dual oximetry. Chest 92:853, 1987.
36. Kirby RR, Downs JB, Civetta JM, Modell JH, et al: High level positive end-expiratory pressure (PEEP) in acute respiratory insufficiency. Chest 67:156, 1975.
37. Motoyama E, Acheson F, Rivard G: Adverse effect of maternal hyperventilation on the foetus. Lancet 1:286, 1966.
38. Morishma HO, Daniel SS, Adamson K Jr, James LS: Effects of positive pressure ventilation of the mother upon the acid-base status of the fetus. Am. J. Obstet. Gynecol. 93:269, 1965.
39. Levinson G, Shnider SM, de Lorimer AA, Steffenson JL: Effect of maternal hyperventilation on uterine blood flow and fetal oxygenation and acid-base status. Anesthesiology 40:340, 1974.
40. Broaddus VC, Berthiaume Y, Biondi JW, Matthay MA: Hemodynamic management of the adult respiratory distress syndrome. J. Intens. Care Med. 2:190, 1987.
41. Strauss RG, Keefer JR, Burke T, Civetta JM: Hemodynamic monitoring of cardiogenic pulmonary edema complicating toxemia of pregnancy. Obstet. Gynecol. 55:170, 1980.
42. Taylor CE: Hemorrhagic disorders in the obstetric patient. *In* Critical Care. 2nd Ed. Edited by JM Civetta, RW Taylor, RR Kirby. Philadelphia, JB Lippincott Co., 1992.
43. Hurd WW, Miodovnik M, Hertzberg D: Selective management of abruptio placentae: A prospective study. Obstet. Gynecol. 61:467, 1983.
44. Crenshaw C, Jones DED, Parker RT: Placenta previa: A survey of 20 years' experience with improved perinatal survival by expectant therapy and cesarean delivery. Obstet. Gynecol. Surv. 28:461, 1973.
45. Phelan JP: Uterine rupture. Clin. Obstet. Gynecol. 33:432, 1990.
46. Sullivan JM, Ramanathan KB: Management of medical problems in pregnancy—Severe cardiac disease. N. Engl. J. Med. 313:304, 1985.
47. James CF: Cardiac disease in the obstetrical patient. *In* Critical Care. 2nd Ed. Edited by JM Civetta, RW Taylor, RR Kirby. Philadelphia, JB Lippincott Co., 1992.
48. Nishimura RA, McGoon MD, Shub C, Miller FA, et al: Echocardiographically documented mitral-valve prolapse. Long-term followup of 237 patients. N. Engl. J. Med. 313:1305, 1985.
49. Hankins GDV, Wendel GD Jr, Leveno KJ, Stoneham J: Myocardial infarction during pregnancy: A review. Obstet. Gynecol. 65:139, 1985.
50. Hood DD: Hypertensive disorders: Preeclampsia and eclampsia. *In* Critical Care. 2nd Ed. Edited by JM Civetta, RW Taylor, RR Kirby. Philadelphia, JB Lippincott Co., 1992.
51. Benedetti TJ, Cotton DB, Read JC, Miller FC: Hemodynamic observations in severe preeclampsia with a flow-directed pulmonary artery catheter. Am. J. Obstet. Gynecol. 136:465, 1980.
52. Cotton DB, Gonik B, Dorman K, Harrist R: Cardiovascular alterations in severe pregnancy-induced hypertension: Relationship of central venous pressure to pulmonary capillary wedge pressure. Am. J. Obstet. Gynecol. 151:762–4, 1985.
53. Weinstein L: Syndrome of hemolysis, elevated liver enzymes, and low platelet count: A severe consequence of hypertension in pregnancy. Am. J. Obstet. Gynecol. 142: 159, 1982.
54. Ariel IM, Kremen AJ, Wangensteen OH: An expanded interstitial (thiocyanate) space in surgical patients. Surgery 27: 827, 1950.
55. Zimmerman B, Wangensteen OH: Observations on water intoxication in surgical patients. Surgery 31:654, 1952.
56. LeQuesne LP: Postoperative water retention—with a report of a case of water intoxication. Lancet 1:172, 1954.
57. Ariel IM: Effects of a water load administered to patients during the immediate postoperative period. Arch. Surg. 62: 303, 1951.
58. Kennedy JH, Sabga GA, Hopkins RW, Penn I, et al: Urine volume and osmolality. Arch. Surg. 88:155, 1964.
59. Bristol WR: Relations of sodium chloride depletion to urine excretion and $H_2O$ intoxication. Am. J. Med. Sciences 221: 412, 1951.
60. Williams J, Grable E, Frank HA, Fine J: Blood losses and plasma volume shifts during and following major surgical operations. Ann. Surg. 156:648, 1962.
61. Scott JC Jr, Welch JS, Berman IB: Water intoxication and sodium depletion in surgical patients. Obstet. Gynecol 26: 168, 1965.
62. Shires GT, Carrico CT, Cohn D: The role of extracellular fluid in shock. Int. Anaesth. Clin. 2:435, 1964.
63. Shires T, Coln D, Carrico J, Lightfoot S: Fluid therapy in hemorrhagic shock. Arch. Surg. 88:688, 1964.
64. Arieff AI: Hyponatremia, convulsions, respiratory arrest, and permanent brain damage after elective surgery in healthy women. N. Engl. J. Med. 314:1529, 1986.
65. Ayus JC, Krothapalli RK, Arieff AI: Treatment of symptomatic hyponatremia and its relation to brain damage. N. Engl. J. Med. 317:1190, 1987.
66. Layon AJ, Bernards WC, Kirby RR: Fluids and electrolytes in the critically ill. *In* Critical Care. 2nd Ed. Edited by JM Civetta, RW Taylor, RR Kirby. Philadelphia, JB Lippincott Co., 1992.
67. Coller FA, Campbell KN, Vaughan HH, Iob LV: Postoperative salt intolerance. Ann. Surg. 119:533, 1944.
68. Coller FA, Iob V, Vaughan HH, Kalder NB, et al: Translocation of fluid produced by the intravenous administration of isotonic salt solutions in man postoperatively. Ann. Surg. 122:663, 1945.
69. Sterns RH: Severe hyponatremia: the acre for conservative management. Crit. Care Med. 20:534–539, 1992.
70. Kleinschmidt-DeMasters BK, Norenberg MD: Rapid correction of hyponatremia causes demyelination: relation to central pontine myelinolysis. Science 211:1068:70, 1981.
71. Laureno R: Central pontine myelinolysis following rapid correction of hyponatremia. Ann. Neurol. 13:232, 1983.
72. Clark SL, Cotton DB: Clinical indications for pulmonary artery catheterization in the patient with severe preeclampsia. Am. J. Obstet. Gynecol. 158:453, 1988.
73. Norwood S, Ruby A, Civetta JM, Cortes V: Catheter-related infections and associated septicemia. Chest 99:968, 1991.
74. Caton D: Fetal monitoring concerns. *In* Critical Care. 2nd Ed. Edited by JM Civetta, RW Taylor, RR Kirby. Philadelphia, JB Lippincott Co., 1992.
75. Katz VL, Dotters DJ, Droegemueller W: Perimortem cesarean delivery. Obstet. Gynecol. 68:571, 1986.
76. Lindsay SL, Hanson GC: Cardiac arrest in near-term pregnancy. Anaesthesia 42:1074, 1987.
77. Oates S, Williams GL, Rees GAD: Cardiopulmonary resuscitation in late pregnancy. Brit. Med. J. 297:404, 1988.
78. Lee RV, Rodgers BD, White LM, Harvey RC: Cardiopulmo-

nary resuscitation of pregnant women. Am. J. Med. 81:311, 1986.
79. Zakowski MI, Ramanathan S: CPR in pregnancy. Curr. Rev. Clin. Anesth. 10:105, 1990.
80. Fox MW, Harms RW, Davis DH: Selected neurologic complications of pregnancy. Mayo Clin. Proc. 65:1595, 1990.
81. Durcan FJ, Corbett JJ, Wall M: The incidence of pseudotumor cerebri: population studies in Iowa and Louisiana. Arch. Neurol. 45:875–77, 1988.
82. Kassam SH, Hadi HA, Fadel HE, Sims W, et al: Benign intracranial hypertension in pregnancy: current diagnostic and therapeutic approach. Obstet. Gynecol. Surv. 38:314–21, 1983.
83. Rush JA: Pseudotumor cerebri: Clinical profile and visual outcome in 63 patients. Mayo Clin. Proc. 55:541, 1980.
84. Selman WR, Spetzler RF, Wilson CB, Grollmus JW: Percutaneous lumboperitoneal shunt: Review of 130 cases. Neurosurgery 6:255, 1980.
85. Brourman ND, Spoor TC, Ramocki JM: Optic nerve sheath decompression for pseudotumor cerebri. Arch. Opthalmol. 106:1378, 1988.
86. Wiebers DO: Ischemic cerebrovascular complications of pregnancy. Arch. Neurol. 42:1106–13, 1985.
87. Stern BJ: Cerebrovascular disease and pregnancy. *In* Neurologic Disorders of Pregnancy. Edited by PJ Goldstein. Mt. Kisco, NY, Futura Publishing Co., 1986, pp. 19–40.
88. Robinson JL, Hall CS, Sedzimir CB: Arteriovenous malformations, aneurysms, and pregnancy. J. Neurosurg. 41:63, 1974.
89. Wiebers DO: Subarachnoid hemorrhage in pregnancy. Semin. Neurol. 8:226–229, 1988.
90. Yerby M, Koepsell T, Daling J: Pregnancy complications and outcomes in a cohort of women with epilepsy. Epilepsia 26: 631–635, 1985.
91. Janz D: Antiepileptic drugs and pregnancy: Altered utilization patterns and teratogenesis. Epilepsia 23 (suppl 1):553, 1982.
92. Birk K, Rudick R: Pregnancy and multiple sclerosis. Arch. Neurol. 43:719–726, 1986.
93. Birk K, Smeltzer SC, Rudick R: Pregnancy and multiple sclerosis. Semin. Neurol. 8:205–213, 1988.
94. Fennel DF, Ringel SP: Myasthenia gravis and pregnancy. Obstet. Gynecol. Surv. 42:414–421, 1987.
95. Mitchell PJ, Bebbington M: Myasthenia gravis in pregnancy. Obstet. Gynecol. 80:178, 1992.
96. Parry GJ, Helman-Patterson TD: Pregnancy and autoimmune neuromuscular disease. Semin. Neurol. 8:197–204, 1988.
97. Young BK, Katz M, Klein SA: Pregnancy after spinal cord injury: Altered maternal and fetal responses to labor. Obstet. Gynecol. 62:59, 1983.
98. Lindan R, Joiner E, Freehaven AA, Hazel C: Incidence and clinical features of autonomic dysreflexia in patients with spinal cord injury. Paraplegia 18:285, 1980.
99. Cohen BS, Hilton EB: Spinal cord disorders and pregnancy. *In* Neurologic Disorders of Pregnancy. Edited by PJ Goldstein. Mt. Kisco, NY, Futura Publishing Co., 1986, pp. 139–152.

Chapter 44

# NEONATAL GENETIC CHALLENGES

ANNEMARIE SOMMER

Birth defects, many of them of genetic origin, present a special challenge to the practitioners of anesthesiology, as well as obstetricians and pediatricians caring for a neonate. Often the patient may have a well-known syndrome and management does not present a problem, but on occasion the patient may have a malformation not readily associated with a recognizable disorder, and in this case, guidelines for management may be important. Craniofacial malformations such as clefting or obstructive lesions may make intubation and resuscitation difficult, and an understanding of underlying associated conditions and malformations is important.

Some of the more common conditions are outlined in this chapter and it is hoped that the practitioners presented with the challenge of a malformed neonate will be able to use it in their practices.

## INCIDENCE

Although major progress has been made in the delineation and diagnosis of birth defects and genetic diseases, a significant number of these infants continue to be born and present a challenge to all personnel involved in their care. Even today, approximately 2% to 3% of infants born will have a major malformation, and many will have multiple malformations. It is important to evaluate such an infant immediately after birth and to institute appropriate measures of management. Congenital malformations account for approximately 10% of neonatal deaths, and within this group many infants may suffer from recognizable syndromes or genetic conditions with known etiologies.[1] This has a significant impact on the families as well as society, and proper neonatal management will be the most important aspect of the care of such a newborn in order to affect mortality as well as morbidity.

## CHROMOSOME DISORDERS

Chromosome abnormalities occurring in the newborn are frequently recognizable by specific phenotypic appearance, but any multiple malformation syndrome should probably have a chromosome analysis performed. It is estimated that about 5 of every 1000 liveborn infants have a chromosome abnormality, and although these figures may change with the increasing availability of prenatal diagnosis, one should still be familiar with the most common conditions.[1]

### Trisomy 21

The most common chromosome abnormality seen in liveborn infants is trisomy 21. It occurs with a frequency of approximately 1 in 700 live births. The trisomy is often associated with advanced maternal age, but recent findings suggest that about 6% are due to nondisjunction occurring in the father.[2] Of all the babies born with trisomy 21, 80% are born to mothers under 35 years of age, while 20% are born to women over 35. Trisomy 21 is a sporadic condition also called Down syndrome, and is not hereditary.

The most common clinical manifestations of Down syndrome at birth are severe hypotonia, poor Moro reflex, hyperflexible joints, a flat facial profile, upslanting palpebral fissures, and redundant skin at the back of the neck (Figure 44–1).

Frequently in the newborn, surgical intervention is indicated immediately, and anesthesia may present a challenge. Approximately 3% of infants with Down syndrome have duodenal atresia which needs an operation, another 40% to 60% of babies with trisomy 21 have congenital heart disease, and 1% have a neural tube defect. The problems which have to be considered are not only the surgical complications, but rather it has to be remembered also that 10% of children with Down syndrome have a significant neck instability at the C-1 to C-2 level. Individuals with trisomy 21 present a lifelong challenge since additional problems such as strabismus, dysplastic hips, and hormonal deficiencies such as hypothyroidism all occur with increased frequency. Another constant feature of Down syndrome is developmental delay. In all instances, trisomy 21 has to be recognized, the findings discussed with the family, and a proper course of intervention outlined so as to have the best outcome possible.

### Trisomy 18

The second most common autosomal trisomy is that for chromosome 18. The overall incidence ranges from 1 in 3500 to 1 in 8000 live births. Approximately three-fourths of the neonates with this condition are females. All are born either premature or postmature for dates, and all exhibit mild-to-severe intrauterine growth retardation.

The most common anomalies[3] observed at birth include a prominent occiput, small palpebral fissures, small pinched faces, microstomia, and low-set, malformed simple auricles. In addition, they have a short sternum, a small pelvis, limited hip abduction, hypoplastic labia majora,

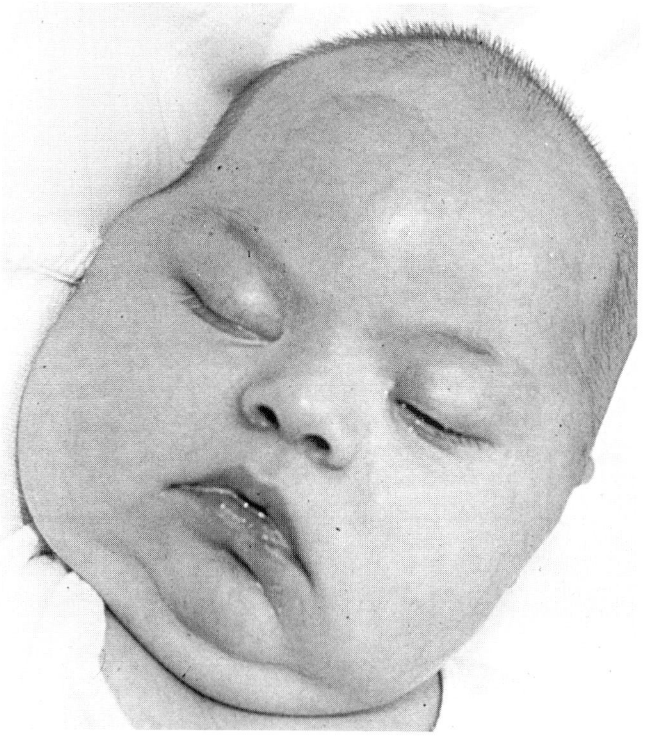

**Fig. 44–1.** Newborn with Down's syndrome.

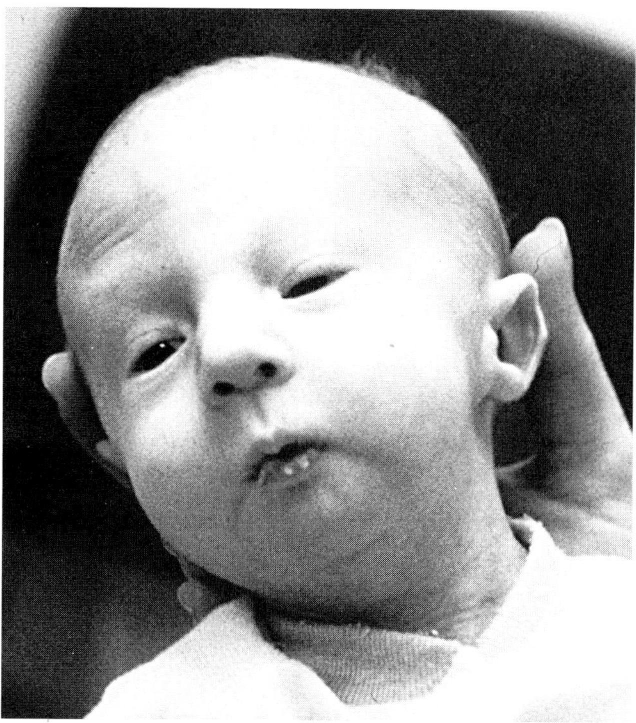

**Fig. 44–2.** Patient with trisomy 18.

prominent heels ("rocker bottom feet"), and proximally implanted dorsiflexed big toes. The hands are usually held in a position of clasped thumbs, with the second and fifth fingers overlapping the third and fourth ones (Figure 44–2).

Malformations which would indicate early intervention including surgical procedures include renal anomalies, a cleft lip/cleft palate complex, which occurs in 15% of these infants, and congenital heart disease, which is present in 99% of cases, and most commonly involves ventricular septal defects, patent ductus arteriosus and atrial septal defects. All infants with trisomy 18 have central nervous system malformations, most often a hypoplastic cerebellum. The natural history of trisomy 18 reveals that the mean survival time is 2.5 months, with 90% of all cases dying within a year.[4] Most infants with trisomy 18 will not require neonatal resuscitation unless clefting conditions or central nervous system malformations cause aspiration, but if it becomes necessary, it should be provided.

## Trisomy 13

Trisomy of chromosome 13 is also seen in the neonate with an estimated incidence of approximately 1 in 5000 live births.

These infants have multiple congenital anomalies, with the central nervous system being most severely affected. The anomalies include microcephaly with a sloping forehead which is the most common craniofacial manifestation of holoprosencephaly. These infants also have microphthalmia, iris colobomata and cleft lip/palate in 75% of cases. Other malformations include localized scalp defects, abnormal auricles, polydactyly, hyperconvex fingernails, thin ribs and cryptorchidism. Congenital heart disease occurs in 80% of patients with trisomy 13, most commonly ventricular septal defect, patent ductus arteriosus and atrial septal defect (Figure 44–3). The natural

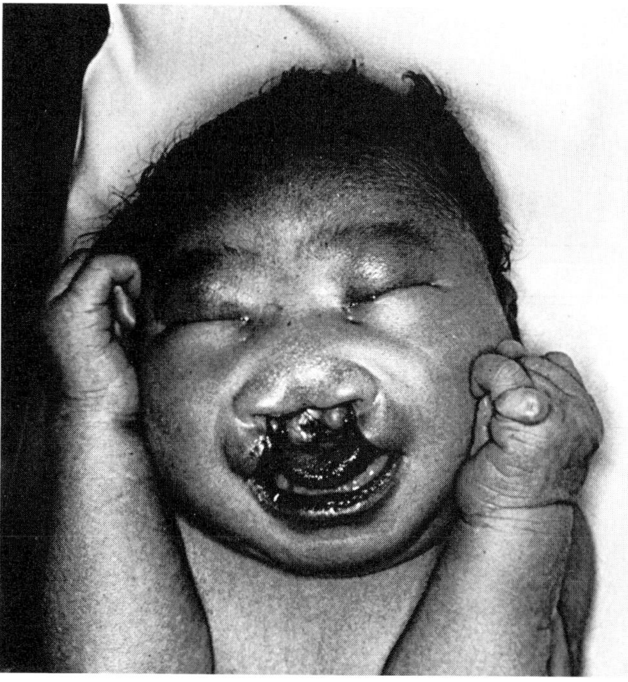

**Fig. 44–3.** Patient with trisomy 13.

history of trisomy 13 reveals a mean survival time of 3 months with 80% of all cases dying within a year of birth.[3] The high infant mortality is secondary to the severe brain defect which is invariably present and neonatal resuscitation may be complicated not only by the structural malformations making intubation difficult, but also by seizures and apnea as well. In most instances of trisomy 13, symptomatic care only seems indicated.

## Turner's Syndrome

One of the more common sex chromosome abnormalities is Turner's syndrome, with a karyotype of 45X. It is known that most XO conceptuses are early lethals and only about 1 in 95 of these are ever born.

The clinical manifestations include short stature, transient congenital lymphedema, a narrow palate, small mandible, ptosis, abnormal auricles, a webbed neck, and a low posterior hairline (Figure 44–4). All of them have ovarian dysgenesis and 60% have renal anomalies, the most common being a horseshoe kidney.[3] In addition, 35% of patients with Turner's syndrome will have cardiac defects such as coarctation of the aorta, a bicuspid aortic valve or valvular aortic stenosis. Turner's syndrome diagnosed in the neonate is compatible with a normal life expectancy.[5] Generalized lymphedema, which is frequently very evident in the extremities and the structures of the neck, may therefore present difficulties on neonatal resuscitation if that should become necessary, but because of a generally favorable prognosis, no effort should be spared to give any such neonate the optimal medical care.

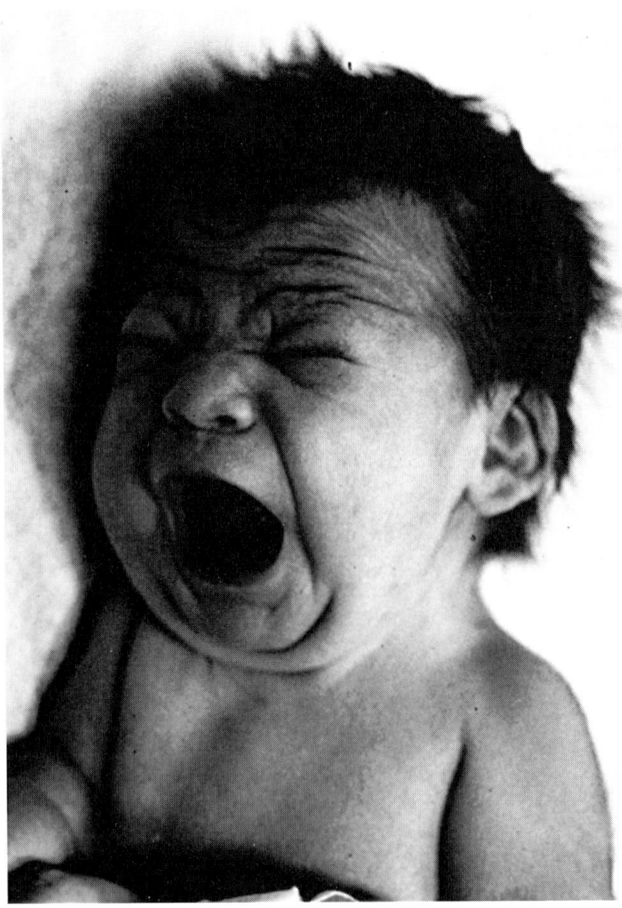

**Fig. 44–4.** Newborn with Turner's syndrome.

## *Chromosome Rearrangements*

At times, chromosomal rearrangements, especially unbalanced translocations, may be anticipated if a positive family history of previously malformed infants or increased fetal wastage is obtained. Often, one of the parents will be a balanced translocation carrier and phenotypically normal, but an offspring with an unbalanced rearrangement may well have multiple congenital anomalies.

Duplications and deletions may occur, and as a rule, duplications lead to less severe phenotype alterations than deletions. Large segment deletions may not allow for intrauterine survival and smaller deletions may lead to severe malformations.[6]

Some of the malformations seen more commonly in autosomal aberrations include cleft lip/palate, esophageal atresia, trachealesophageal fistula, omphalocele and other gastrointestinal malformations, renal anomalies, and congenital heart disease. Other frequent findings include absences or hypoplasia of the radial side of the arms, postaxial hexadactyly, and brain malformations, especially holoprosencephaly and agenesis of the corpus callosum.[6]

Neonatal resuscitation may be needed for many of these infants, and knowledge of individual malformations is necessary. It is uniformly anticipated that holoprosencephaly is a brain anomaly incompatible with long-term survival.

### Partial Trisomy 6q

An example of a partial trisomy 6q resulting from a balanced chromosomal rearrangement in the mother was reported. The mother had had two previous spontaneous abortions and now had a newborn with multiple anomalies. The findings included microcephaly, hypertelorism, a flat nasal bridge, a short thin philtrum, upper-lip notching, a high-arched palate, and micrognathia. The infant also had flexion contractures at the elbows, hips and knees, as well as camptodactyly of all fingers. He had cyanotic congenital heart disease, an absent left kidney, and growth and psychomotor retardation (Figure 44–5). Multiple complications including central nervous system emboli and frequent infections led to a limited survival of only 3 years.[7]

### 5p- Syndrome

One of the better known deletion syndromes is the partial deletion of the short arm of chromosome 5, also called the cri du chat syndrome.

All infants born with this deletion have a cat-like cry, microcephaly, slow growth, and mental deficiency. Other frequent findings are hypotonia, a rounded face, hypertelorism, epicanthic folds, and down-slanting palpebral fissures. Congenital heart disease is present in about 30% of cases and multiple other anomalies including facial clefts occur less frequently (Figure 44–6).

Most of these infants will not require neonatal resuscita-

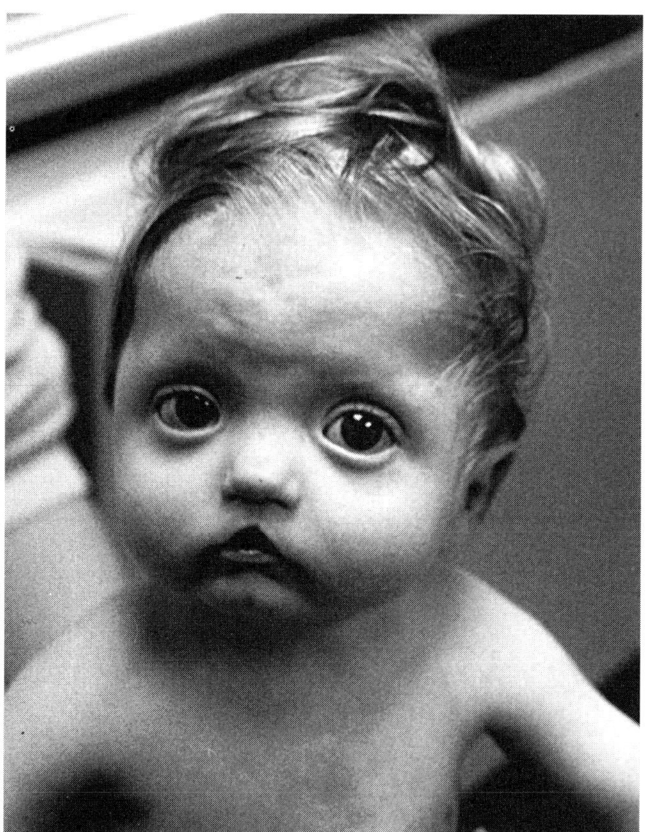

**Fig. 44–5.** Patient with partial trisomy 6q.

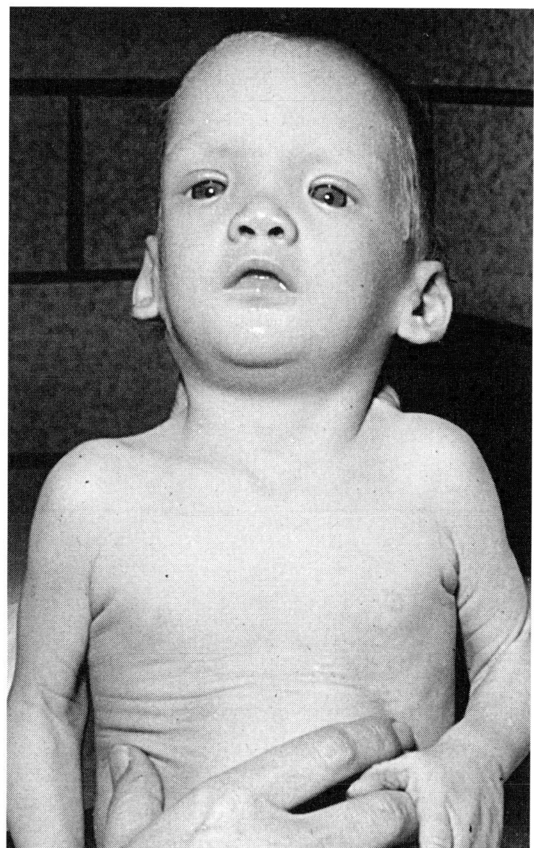

**Fig. 44–6.** Patient with cri-du-chat syndrome.

tion and most of them will enjoy a good life expectancy in spite of growth and psychomotor retardation.[5]

## Single Gene Disorders

Many single-gene disorders may result in malformation syndromes and often are recognizable in the newborn by specific anomalies. Recognition of known conditions is important since neonatal management must be based on this factor.

### *Autosomal Disorders*

In autosomal dominant inheritance, a single abnormal gene is expressed as an abnormality in the individual who has inherited it. The abnormal gene is then passed on to 50% of all the offspring of the affected parent. It is therefore important to have a good family history and to have seen the parents if a newborn shows anomalies. If the family history is negative and neither of the parents affected, a dominant condition might still be present and represent a fresh mutation.

#### Treacher Collins Syndrome

This autosomal dominant condition, also known as Franceschetti syndrome and mandibulo-facial dysostosis, has an incidence of 1 in 10 000 births.[8]

The disorder is characterized by most of the following anomalies: (1) down-slanting palpebral fissures; (2) lower lid coloboma; (3) absence of eyelashes medial to coloboma; (4) maxillary and mandibular hypoplasia; (5) ear anomalies; (6) ear tags; and (7) conductive hearing loss. Cleft palate may occur in 28% and incompetence of the soft palate in 32% of cases. A more common occurrence also includes choanal atresia. Most of the craniofacial anomalies may combine to form a very narrow upper airway and cause respiratory distress. Some of the patients may need a tracheostomy, but every support must be given since these patients usually have a normal life expectancy and normal development, and even the facial growth may be such as to improve the outward appearance with increasing age.

#### Achondroplasia

The prevalence of achondroplasia is about 1 in 10,000 to 1 in 25,000 births. Approximately 85% of all cases represent fresh mutations.[3]

Achondroplasia is a short-stature syndrome consisting most commonly of rhizomelic dwarfism, a large head with frontal bossing and a depressed nasal bridge. They also have short extremities, trident hands, lumbar lordosis, caudal narrowing of the spinal canal and a narrow foramen magnum (Figure 44–7). Occasionally, hydrocephalus may also be present and is thought to be secondary to raised intracranial venous pressure due to stenosis of the jugular foramen.[9] The foramen magnum is not only small

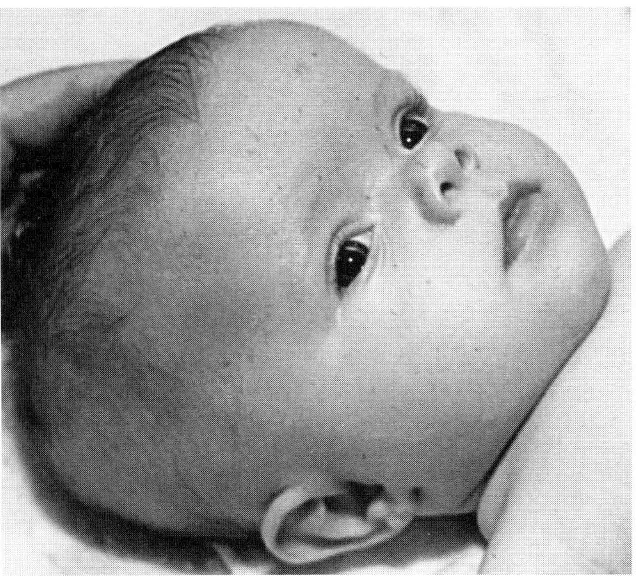

**Fig. 44–7.** Newborn with achondroplasia.

at birth, but has an impaired rate of growth during the first year of life.[10]

Infants with achondroplasia are at an increased risk for sudden infant death which may occur as a result of acute or chronic compression of the lower brain stem or cervical spinal cord.[11] Neonatal mortality and morbidity are also increased in achondroplasia because there is an increased risk for intracranial bleeds because of the large head, and uncontrolled neck movement may also cause problems because of impingement by structurally abnormal bony elements.

In addition, the adult female, if she becomes pregnant, presents her own problems at delivery. A cesarean section is universally necessary for the delivery of the baby, and not only will the mother have the already known narrowing of the caudal spinal canal, but she may indeed have to have surgery of her back and present a challenge to the anesthesiologist. Because of the complications of the vertebral skeletal problem in achondroplasia, some mothers may even be paraplegic prior to pregnancy.

Overall, the intelligence in achondroplasia is normal and prolonged survival is the rule, and utmost medical care is indicated.

### EEC Syndrome

Another example of an autosomal dominant condition is the ectrodactyly, ectodermal dysplasia, clefting (EEC) syndrome. Although not very common, it is well known. The most common clinical manifestations include: (1) ectrodactyly of the hands and feet; (2) sparse hair, eyebrows and eyelashes; (3) occasional hypodontia; and (4) lacrimal duct obstruction. Cleft lip and palate are also an integral part of the syndrome (Figure 44–8). Less frequent anomalies are genitourinary malformations.[12] and choanal atresia.[13]

The affected individuals usually have normal intelligence and life expectancy. Early aggressive management is indicated because clefting may cause upper airway complications, aspiration and failure to thrive. Most importantly, if choanal atresia is present in the newborn, respiratory distress will be evident almost immediately and an adequate airway needs to be provided.

## Autosomal Recessive Disorders

Autosomal recessive inheritance classically is characterized by having affected individuals in a single generation only. Therefore, only affected siblings may be found in the family history because for an autosomal recessive disorder to be expressed, both parents of the affected individual have to be carriers of the same recessive gene. If that is the case, then the risk for affected offspring from that mating is 25% for each pregnancy and is present in equal proportions in males and females.

### Ellis-van Creveld Syndrome

This autosomal recessive disorder is also called chondroectodermal dysplasia. Early reports include those of McKusick[14] in 1964 from an inbred Amish population, but the disorder has now been reported in other populations as well.

This disorder includes some of the following features: (1) short stature of prenatal onset resulting ultimately in dwarfism and an average adult height of 43 inches to 60 inches; and (2) abnormalities of the craniofacies consisting of oral webbing and a short upper lip bound by frenulae to the alveolar ridges (Figure 44–9). Later on, dental problems, including dysplastic teeth and delayed eruptions, have occurred. The affected individuals frequently have a narrow thorax with short ribs resulting in thoracic dystrophy and 50% will have congenital heart disease, most commonly an atrial septal defect. The skeletal manifestations include disproportionate irregularly short extremities, polydactyly, malformed carpal bones, fusion of capitate and hamate, and hypoplasia of the upper lateral tibiae. They also may have hypoplastic nails. The intelligence is usually normal. Cardiorespiratory problems secondary to thoracic dystrophy and/or congenital heart disease add to the high infant mortality in this disorder.[5]

### Werdnig-Hoffman Disease, SMA 1

The severe infantile form of spinal muscular atrophy (SMA) occurs in 1 in 10 000 to 1 in 25 000 newborns depending on the population surveyed.[1,15] It is an anterior horn-cell disease. Symptoms of hypotonia and weakness may be present at birth, and there may be a history of decreased or even absent fetal movement. The progressive loss of motor neurons results in progression of symptoms during the first few months of life.

Clinically, the tendon reflexes may be decreased or absent and there may be fasciculation of the tongue and fine tremors. Usually the lower extremities are first and most severely involved, but it is the progressive paralysis of respiratory muscles which leads to death during the first year of life, often with intercurrent infections. Paralysis of the diaphragm may also occur.[16] Although structural

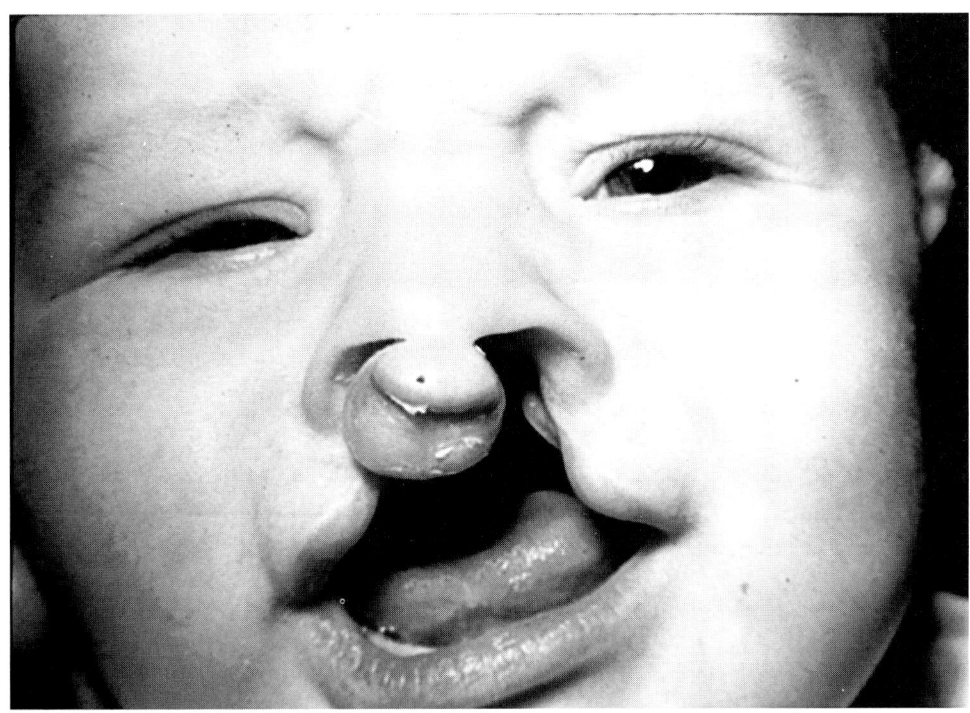

**Fig. 44–8.** Patient with EEC syndrome.

cardiac abnormalities usually are not found, an abnormal electrocardiogram is found in almost all cases of SMA 1.[17] The patients show regular and constant spikes on the isoelectric electrocardiographic line. The patients with spinal muscular atrophy have normal intelligence. No definite treatment for SMA 1 is available for these patients and death is inevitable during early infancy.

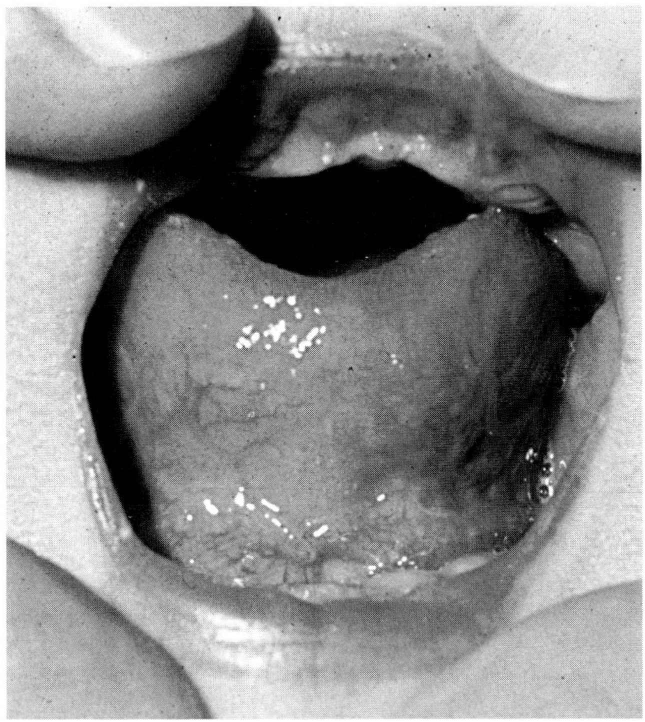

**Fig. 44–9.** Patient with Ellis-van Creveld syndrome, oral frenula.

### Glycogen Storage Diseases

Several forms of autosomal recessive glycogen storage diseases due to different enzyme deficiencies are known and some may lead to neonatal complications.

The infantile form of glycogen storage disease II (Pompe's) is an example of early onset manifestations.[18] The infants have a deficiency of the lysosomal enzyme acid alpha-1, 4-glucosidase (acid maltase) which results in severe prostration and hypotonia in those affected. The manifestations appear between birth and 6 months and, although the involvement is generalized, the infants usually will present with hypotonia and large hearts with congestive heart failure. The tongue may also be enlarged. Neonatal hydrops has also been reported with this disorder. Death occurs in the first year of life and no curative treatment has been found as yet.

Glycogen storage disease type Ia (von Gierke disease) may also lead to neonatal problems. The cause of the disorder is a glucose-6-phosphatase deficiency in liver and kidney, and the incidence has been estimated as 1 in 200 000 births. Hypoglycemia and acidosis occur during the first 6 months of life and may cause significant morbidity and mortality if left untreated. The infants also will have hepatomegaly.

The treatment consists of frequent feedings of carbohydrates, and cornstarch is often used as its source. If euglycemia is maintained, the outlook for normal development is excellent.[19]

## X-Linked Disorders

In X-linked disorders, the gene or genes responsible for causing clinical pathology are located on an X chromosome. The better known X-linked abnormalities are recessive. In these cases, the abnormal gene is carried by the mother in a single dose on one of her two X chromosomes and causes no disability. However, a male offspring who inherits the abnormal X from his mother will show signs and symptoms because males have one X chromosome only. Therefore, in an X-linked recessive disease, a carrier mother married to a normal male will have a 25% chance with each pregnancy of having an affected male child. All daughters will be normal, but half of them will be carriers of the abnormal gene.

### Hemophilia A (Factor VIII Deficiency)

One example of an X-linked recessive disorder is hemophilia A, also called "classical" hemophilia and Factor VIII deficiency. The incidence is estimated as 1 in 10 000 white male births.[1,3] The hereditary defect is the absence of antihemophilic globulin (Factor VIII) with the gene for the clotting factor mapped to Xq28.[20]

The level of Factor VIII coagulant activity will determine the severity of the clinical manifestations. All affected males have an increased tendency to bleed even from the most minimal trauma, and spontaneous bleeding into joint spaces may occur. This may lead to hemarthroses and severe joint limitations. Bleeding may also occur in any other area of the body.

Bleeding has been reported at the time of circumcision, although the presence of tissue thromboplastin may make this procedure a safe one even in hemophiliac boys. It should be noted that neonatal resuscitative procedures may cause bleeding in a hemophiliac male and early and correct diagnosis and proper treatment with Factor VIII are mandatory.

Greatly improved diagnostic and treatment modalities have resulted in a normal life expectancy for hemophiliacs. Normal intelligence and quality of life are routine. For known carrier females, prenatal diagnosis is available and a son with hemophilia should be identified and treated accordingly as a newborn.

### Ectodermal Dysplasia (Anhidrotic)

Anhidrotic ectodermal dysplasia is another example of an X-linked recessive disorder, with the gene having been mapped to Xq12.[3]

Affected males have hypotrichosis and absence or hypoplasia of teeth and sweat glands. Frequently there is absence of the mucous glands of the upper airway.

The clinical diagnosis in the newborn may be suggested by the absence of eyebrows and eyelashes. Because of the inability to sweat, control of body temperature is disturbed and most of the morbidity in ectodermal dysplasia is caused by hyperthermia. These boys also have an increased susceptibility to infections because of the defect in the mucous glands of the upper airway. In addition, the defective skin barrier also may result in skin infections such as monilia. Because of the decreased number and deformation of the teeth, the boys have to be watched for nutritional deficiency, since they may not be able to chew their food well and may not receive all necessary nutrients.

Although some boys with anhidrotic ectodermal dysplasia may exhibit developmental delay, early recognition of the condition and proper prospective management, especially of the hyperthermia, may result in near normal growth and development.

## Multifactorial Disorders

Many of the more common birth defects are inherited on a multifactorial basis. In multifactorial disorders, a trait is determined by the interaction of one or more genes and environmental factors. The risk of occurrence of such traits may vary with populations, and the risk of recurrence in families depends on the number of affected individuals and the degree of relationship.

Examples of disorders thought to be transmitted as multifactorial traits include cleft lip and palate, congenital heart disease, neural tube defects, congenital club foot, pyloric stenosis, and some allergic disorders.[3]

## *Craniofacial Anomalies*

Craniofacial anomalies may include malformations of the brain, the calvarium and the face. Facial anomalies in turn may involve various disorders of clefting and branchial arch syndromes. Anomalies in the fetal development of the brain may be reflected in the facial appearance, and defective induction of the prechordial plate may result in hypotelorism and cyclopia.[21] Abnormal development of the rhinencephalon can result in the malformation of the intermaxillary segment which may then be revealed as a median cleft lip, agenesis of the nasal septum and a single nasal fossa.[22]

### Isolated Clefts

Cleft lip and cleft palate are the results of defective closure of the primary and secondary palate and frequently are inherited as a multifactorial trait.[3] Syndromes as well as chromosome abnormalities and monogenic disorders may also be associated with cleft lip and palate, and teratogenic agents are known to cause clefting defects as well.

Because of differences in timing in embryological development, two multifactorial entities are usually distinguished: cleft lip with or without cleft palate; and isolated cleft palate.

Cleft lip with or without cleft palate is a relatively frequent condition and not associated with additional malformations. The overall incidence is thought to be 1 in 1000 births.[3] The recurrence risk in a given family will depend on the number of affected relatives. For first degree relatives of the affected patient, ie, for siblings and children, the risk is generally 4%, while the risk for uncles, aunts, nieces and nephews is approximately 0.7%.

Although a severe cleft lip and palate may cause neonatal respiratory problems because of aspiration, intubation may at times be difficult because of the structural anomalies (Figure 44–10). The overall life expectancy and quality of life for patients with the cleft lip/palate complex is normal.

Isolated cleft lip and palate may be seen with some

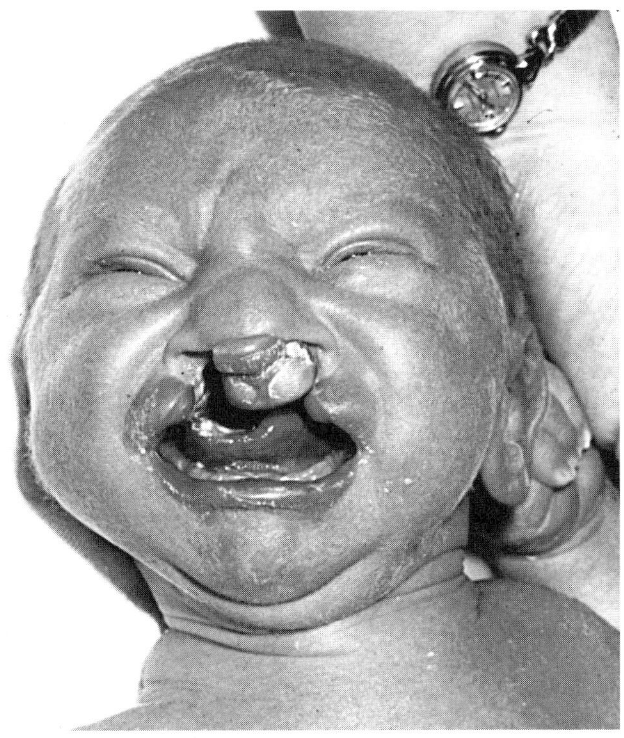

**Fig. 44–10.** Patient with cleft lip and palate malformation.

teratogens such as the antiepileptic drugs diphenylhydantoin, trimethadione, and valproic acid, but in most cases, associated anomalies will be present. The recurrence risk in these conditions becomes nonsignificant with the discontinuation of the use of the teratogen.

Facial clefting may also be the result of disruptive sequences such as early amnion rupture. Management of these cases will depend on associated disruptions and location of defects.

Cleft palate occurring as the only malformation is much rarer than cleft lip with or without cleft palate. It occurs with a frequency of 0.45 per 1000 births, and females are affected more often than males. For most families, multifactorial recurrence risks may be cited and normal survival is the rule.

## Clefts as Part of Associations and Malformation Syndromes

Craniofacial anomalies such as cleft lip and palate, hypotelorism, hypertelorism and other midline defects are frequent malformations in many conditions of various etiologies. Holoprosencephaly may be reflected in abnormal facial development as well.[21]

Chromosomal aberrations frequently associated with cleft lip and palate include trisomy 13, trisomy 18, the 4p-syndrome, dup 3q, and other chromosome rearrangements. The associated malformations may include holoprosencephaly, hypotelorism, congenital heart disease, skeletal malformations, intrauterine growth retardation, and developmental delay. A careful physical examination will suggest the diagnosis, and confirmation is provided by chromosome analysis.

Monogenic syndromes may also be characterized by clefts. Careful examination and family history will suggest the diagnosis.

One example of a severe clefting syndrome inherited as an autosomal dominant disorder is the ectrodactyly, ectodermal dysplasia, clefting syndrome discussed earlier. Newborns may appear to be severely malformed, but with appropriate management and surgical intervention, these individuals usually are of normal intelligence and have a normal life expectancy.

An autosomal recessive clefting syndrome is the Roberts-SC phocomelia syndrome. Affected individuals have various degrees of intrauterine growth retardation, microbrachycephaly, shallow orbits, cleft lip and palate, and other mid-facial defects.[5] In addition, there is hypomelia, more severe in the upper extremities and varying from phocomelia to lesser limb reduction defects. Many Roberts-SC phocomelia syndrome infants are stillborn or have died in early infancy, but long-term survivors have also been reported. Growth deficiency and mental deficiency have been seen in all of them.

The holoprosencephaly sequence is frequently associated with cleft lip and palate and hypotelorism.[21] The name holoprosencephaly denotes a severe central nervous system malformation which results in severe postnatal growth, and mental and endocrine dysfunction of the affected individual (Figure 44–11). Both lobar and alobar holoprosencephaly may be part of other syndromes, but also occur as isolated defects, frequently of unknown etiology.

The prognosis for individuals with facial clefting and associated holoprosencephaly is very poor and a severely

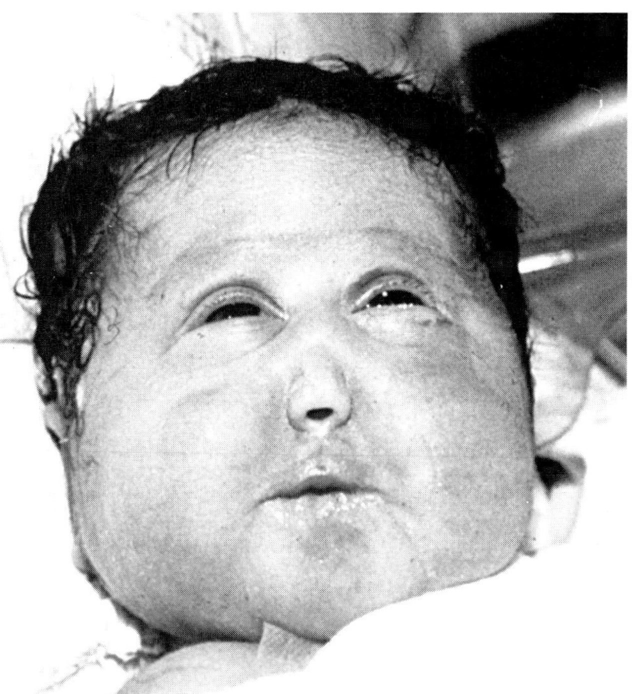

**Fig. 44–11.** Facial appearance of holoprosencephaly.

affected forebrain should guide the medical management since long-term survival is very low.

### Congenital Heart Disease

The incidence of congenital heart disease in liveborns is estimated as between 4.05 to 10.2 per 1000, and many of these infants may present with signs and symptoms during the neonatal period.[23]

Cyanosis may be present in some of the congenital heart lesions, such as D-transposition of the great arteries which accounts for 3.8% of all congenital heart disease. Other cyanotic newborns may have tricuspid atresia, tetralogy of Fallot, pulmonary artery atresia or total anomalous pulmonary venous return.

Most instances of congenital heart disease are best explained on a multifactorial base of inheritance, although the exact recurrence risk may vary slightly with the occurrence rate of a given defect.

Today, most forms of congenital heart disease are treatable, and therefore are consistent not only with a normal life expectancy, but also with reproduction. It appears that patients with congenital heart disease have an increased risk of transmitting it to some of their offspring, with the average risk still being multifactorial and in the 1% to 10% range.[23]

Congenital heart disease also occurs frequently in single gene as well as chromosome disorders. About 5% to 8% of patients with congenital heart lesions will have a chromosome abnormality such as trisomy 21, trisomy 18, trisomy 13, 5p- and others. Three percent will have disorders inherited on a Mendelian basis. Examples are Marfan syndrome. Ehlers-Danlos syndrome and other connective tissue disorders, Holt-Oram, Smith-Lemli-Opitz and thrombocytopenia-absent-radius (TAR) syndromes.

## Syndromes of Uncertain Etiology

Malformations occurring on a sporadic basis and those that may be due to as-yet poorly defined genetic mechanisms may still present as neonatal management problems and deserve the full attention of the physician.

### Amyoplasia Congenita

Amyoplasia congenita is also called the "classic arthrogryposis" and arthrogryposis multiplex congenita. It is a condition of unknown etiology, although viruses, maternal hypotension, and maternal multiple sclerosis have been implicated.[24,25] The "classical" presentation in the newborn includes contractures of all joints. Most commonly the arms will be extended with flexion at the hands and wrists, and the shoulders will be internally rotated. The lower extremities will have fixed hips and knees as well as equinovarus position of the feet in various degrees of severity. A rigid spine may also be present. There usually is decreased muscle mass of the extremities. Micrognathia is also a frequent neonatal presentation and some patients may have torticollis (Figure 44–12). Because of the contractures and abnormal positioning, infants with amyoplasia congenita may well have severe problems at the time of delivery and require the attention of the obstetric anesthesiologist. Neonatal airway compromise may also occur.

Most patients with amyoplasia congenita will have a normal life expectancy and normal intelligence, and neonatal resuscitation is a very critical aspect of their management. It was thought that malignant hyperthermia may be a risk in patients with amyoplasia congenita, but this has not been proven.[26]

### Beckwith-Wiedemann Syndrome

This condition described by Beckwith and Wiedemann is also known as the exomphalos-macroglossia-gigantism syndrome. The etiology is complex and still being delineated. Dominant mutations[27] as well as multifactorial causation and a chromosomal origin involving region 11p15.5 have all been proposed.

Infants present with multiple manifestations of over-

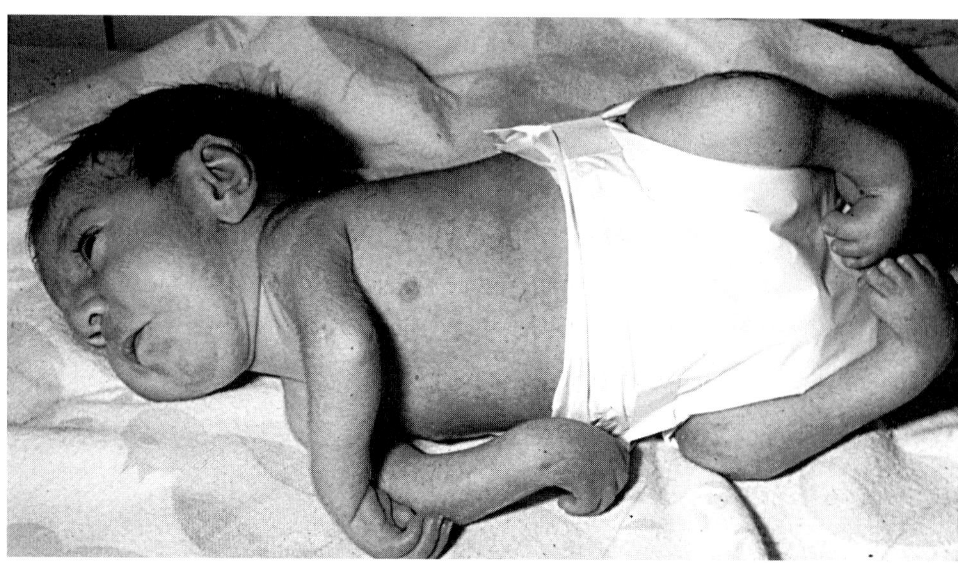

**Fig. 44–12.** Patient with arthrogryposis multiplex congenita.

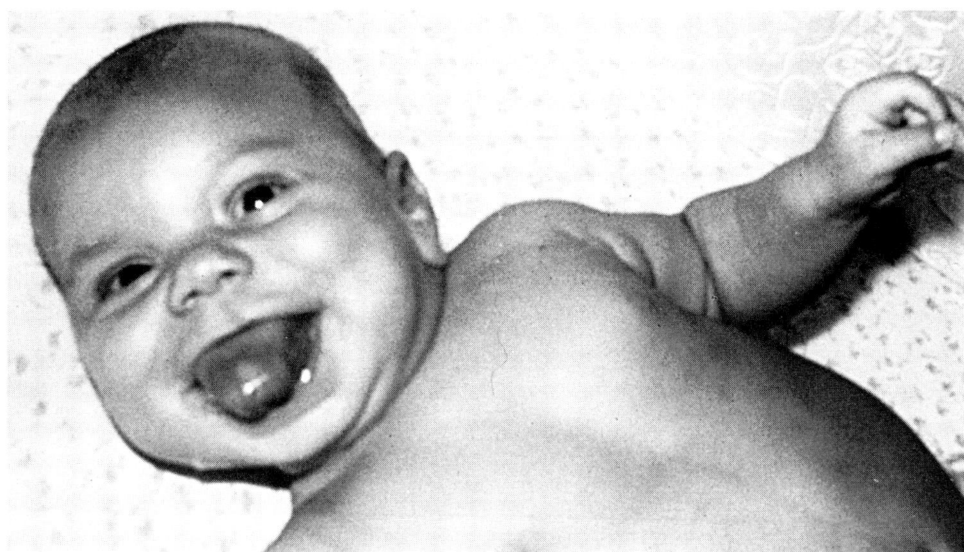

**Fig. 44–13.** Patient with Beckwith-Wiedemann syndrome: macroglossia.

growth. They are macrosomic and have macroglossia (Figure 44–13) as well as an omphalocele or other umbilical defect. Hyperplasias and dysplasias also occur in the form of large kidneys with medullary dysplasia, pancreatic hyperplasia and fetal adrenocortical cytomegaly. Neonatal polycythemia and severe hypoglycemia are common.

The craniofacial manifestations in addition to the macroglossia may include prominent eyes with relative infraorbital hypoplasia, capillary nevi over the eyelids and glabella, large fontanelles and a prominent occiput. Unusual earlobe creases and indentations on the posterior rim of the helix may also be seen. Neonatal management may be difficult because of airway compromise secondary to macroglossia, the need for surgical repair of the omphalocele, and the rather frequent neonatal hypoglycemia.

Although 43% of patients may develop growth hypertrophy and asymmetry, up to 11% may develop embryonal tumors such as Wilms' tumor, rhabdomyosarcoma, and hepatoblastoma.[28] The patients with Beckwith-Wiedemann syndrome have a normal life expectancy and most of them are of normal intelligence. The final height of these individuals is also within the range of normal despite early overgrowth. Patients with the Beckwith-Wiedemann syndrome are part of a population of newborns with omphalocele which occurs with a frequency of 1 in 6000 births and need to be properly diagnosed and treated.

## Environmental Agents

Some environmental agents may act as teratogens. A teratogen is defined as an agent that may produce physical or functional abnormalities in a developing human fetus and which is detected postnatally. Concerns about environmental changes have made the public aware of the potential damage caused by teratogens, but much more education is necessary to achieve the proper perspective. Teratogens, as a rule, have a specific action and cause a specific pattern of malformation. Before an agent is classified as a teratogen, it must be shown that specific criteria such as susceptible stages of development, genetic differences in susceptibility and dose-response relationships have all been evaluated to allow for the proper conclusion. It is also desirable to prove teratogenicity through animal models.[29]

### *Fetal Alcohol Syndrome*

Alcohol consumption at the time of conception and during pregnancy is common, and it is estimated that about 30% of all children of chronic alcoholic women have the full-blown fetal alcohol syndrome. An additional 1 in 300 babies may show some signs and symptoms and are best classified as showing a fetal alcohol effect.[3]

Fetal alcohol syndrome is characterized by prenatal and postnatal growth retardation, developmental delay and various abnormalities such as microcephaly, short palpebral fissures, epicanthic folds, a short nose, a smooth philtrum and a thin upper lip. Congenital heart disease also occurs. Neonatally, the infants are tremulous, and later on hyperactivity and distractibility are often seen. Although children with the fetal alcohol syndrome may "never catch up," the life expectancy is normal, and neonatal morbidity is most commonly related to heart disease or central nervous system malformations. Certainly, the fetal alcohol syndrome should be the most preventable congenital disorder.

### *Drugs*

A group of drugs which has been shown to cause congenital malformations are many of the antiepileptic agents. Refer to Chapter 36 for a more detailed discussion of these agents. Other drugs such as retinoic acid and illicit agents such as cocaine also are associated with fetal malformations.

#### Fetal Hydantoin Syndrome

The original antiepileptic agent implicated was hydantoin and led to the description of the fetal hydantoin syndrome.[30] The most common anomalies seen are mild intrauterine and postnatal growth retardation, craniofacial signs such as a large anterior fontanelle, hypertelorism, epicanthic folds, a short nose and cleft lip and palate. Hypoplasia of the distal phalanges with small nails also is a frequent finding. Occasionally 33% of the hydantoin-exposed fetuses may show some effect of the teratogen, but nontreatment of the mother is not an alternative. If anticonvulsants are needed, the mother has to be informed of the potential risks to the fetus, and the safest effective antiepileptic agent should be used as treatment.

### Fetal Valproate Effect

One of the more recent anticonvulsants to enter the market was valproic acid, and in 1984 the fetal valproate syndrome was fully delineated.[31]

The craniofacial changes include a narrow bifrontal diameter, a high forehead, epicanthic folds which connect with an infraorbital crease, telecanthus, a short nose with an upturned tip, a long philtrum and a relatively small mouth. Additional findings include congenital heart disease and neural tube defects such as myelomeningocele which may occur in 5% of exposed offspring (Figure 44–14).

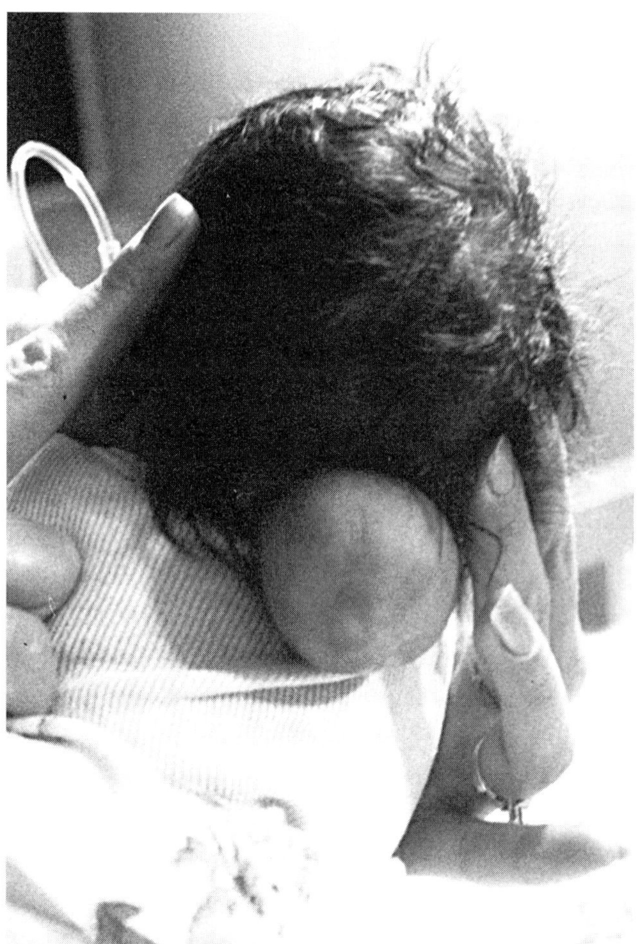

**Fig. 44–14.** Patient with fetal valproate effect.

### Retinoic Acid Embryopathy

In 1982, the drug isotretinoin (Accutane) was licensed for treatment of severe acne. This agent is an analog of vitamin A, and vitamin A was known to be teratogenic from animal studies. Accutane was found to cause malformations in humans as reported a year after the introduction of the drug.[32] Warnings had been issued not to use the drug during pregnancy, but women who had used Accutane before they knew they were pregnant had offspring with a spectrum of anomalies including the craniofacies, cardiac and central nervous systems. The most common craniofacial anomalies include microtia and anotia with stenosis of the external ear canal, a narrow sloping forehead, a U-shaped palatal cleft and micrognathia.

The cardiac defects are conotruncal malformations and aortic arch hypoplasia and others. The central nervous malformations have included hydrocephalus, microcephaly, errors in neuronal migration, as well as cerebellar hypoplasia and cerebellar microdysgenesis. Neonatal complications are related to the cardiac and central nervous system malformations.

Isotretinoin exposure also may result in spontaneous abortions with a risk as high as 40%, but there is virtually no evidence to suggest that isotretinoin prior to conception is teratogenic. Nevertheless, if Accutane is being used, the FDA recommends postponement of pregnancy "for an indefinite period of time."[33]

### Cocaine

Maternal cocaine abuse during pregnancy is on the rise and appears to be associated with an increased rate of spontaneous abortions, premature delivery, placental abruption and abnormal neonatal neurologic and behavioral assessment.[29] The unifying pathogenetic mechanisms are problems associated with vascular disruption. Negative outcomes of pregnancy relate most likely to two factors: (1) vasoconstriction of the uterine arteries may cause fetal hypoxia which then causes excessive release of fetal catecholamines; and (2) increased levels of circulating catecholamines in the mother due to blocking of the catecholamine reuptake receptors by cocaine are responsible for pharmacological effects such as hypertension and tachycardia.

Vascular disruption may cause a host of abnormalities such as intracranial hemorrhage with resulting porencephaly, limb defects, gastroschisis and intestinal atresias, and genitourinary anomalies. Neonates may suffer withdrawal, jitteriness and seizures. Long-term effects have not been well defined yet.

## Radiation

Very little evidence exists for a teratogenic effect of diagnostic radiation.[29] Only large doses of radiation exceeding 10 rads have been shown to cause increased fetal loss and increased rate of microcephaly and mental retardation. These large doses are never used other than in treatment for malignancies, or are an accidental exposure to atomic blasts or atomic plant accidents. Diagnostic X-rays result in millirad exposure only and are not considered teratogenic unless a cumulative dose of 5000 to 10 000 millirads is exceeded, which is not very likely at all.

## Clinical Impact and Conclusion

Since significant progress has been made in the management of the pregnant mother and her fetus, and outcomes of pregnancies complicated by maternal conditions such as diabetes and other chronic illnesses have been greatly improved, the incidence and complications resulting from birth defects and genetic disorders have not changed much.

We have certainly learned about genetic conditions by recognizing the impact of advanced maternal age on the incidence of chromosome abnormalities, by being aware that advanced paternal age is associated with some recognizable dominant mutations, and that mothers who have phenylketonuria must be treated during their entire lifetime to prevent offspring with microcephaly and mental retardation. These and other conditions can be ascertained by careful history taking, and genetic counseling should be provided.

Prenatal diagnosis is a part of any pregnancy at risk for birth defects and genetic diseases, and often special tests can guide the practitioner to specific diagnoses.

While alpha-fetoprotein measurements in the mother may help identify pregnancies at risk for neural tube defects or for chromosome abnormalities, additional studies such as ultrasound imaging and measurements, amniocentesis for fetal chromosome analysis, and metabolic tests may confirm certain congenital defects.

The prenatal diagnosis should then be carefully evaluated and discussed by a team consisting at least of the managing obstetrician and a genetic counselor before presenting the results to the family. The pregnant woman should also have the support of other family members and professionals providing psychosocial support. The ultimate outcome of the pregnancy should then be determined by all of them.

The difficult decision to terminate a pregnancy is most frequently made for known lethal conditions such as some chromosome abnormalities like trisomy 13 and triploidy or skeletal dysplasias such as achondrogenesis or thanatophoric dysplasia. However, not all birth defects and genetic conditions are diagnosed prenatally, and are therefore recognized only at birth. If a decision is made to terminate the pregnancy, this would be the appropriate time to have the obstetrician consult the anesthesiologist to make him or her aware of the situation and discuss anesthetic requirements for termination of the pregnancy, including analgesia to offset the pain associated with the procedure, and amnesia to offset the psychologic impact.

It is recommended that in cases where neonatal resuscitation becomes necessary, all such resuscitative measures should be applied, except for newborns with anencephaly. In the case of anencephaly, it may be prudent for the obstetrician, anesthesiologist, and mother to discuss the method of handling the neonate at delivery. For example, it may be that a mask will be placed over the baby's nose and mouth for passive administration of $O_2$. Active resuscitative methods, eg, positive pressure ventilation, may be avoided according to the wishes of the three aforementioned individuals. For the remaining patients, early consultations with a geneticist and other appropriate consultants will assist in further management decisions.

In addition to prematurity, genetic conditions and birth defects account for a large part of neonatal morbidity and mortality. Recognizing the most common newborn birth defects and the ability to make the proper decisions in management will have an impact on the entire life of the newborn.

## REFERENCES


1. Berini RY (exec ed), Kahn E (ed): Clinical Genetics Handbook. National Genetics Foundation Inc. Oradell, New Jersey, Medical Economics Books, 1987.
2. Sherman SL, Takaesu N, Freeman S, Phillips C, et al: Trisomy 21: Association between reduced recombination and nondisjunction. Am. J. Hum. Genet. 47:A97, 1990.
3. Nora JJ, Fraser FC: Medical Genetics. Principles and Practice, Ed. 3. Philadelphia, Lea and Febiger, 1989.
4. Mange AP, Mange EJ: Genetics: Human Aspects, Ed 2. Sunderland, Massachusetts, Sinauer Associates Inc, 1990.
5. Jones KL: Smith's Recognizable Patterns of Human Malformations, Ed 4. Philadelphia, WB Saunders Co, 1988.
6. Schinzel A: Catalogue of Unbalanced Chromosome Aberrations in Man. New York, Walter de Gruyter, 1984, p. 38.
7. Sommer A, Westman J, Stallard R: Partial trisomy 6q. Proc. Greenwood Genet. Center 3:22, 1984.
8. Argenta LC, Iacobucci JJ: Treacher-Collins syndrome: Present concepts of the disorder and their surgical correction. World J. Surg. 13:401, 1989.
9. Steinbok P, Hall J, Flodmark O: Hydrocephalus in achondroplasia: The possible role of intracranial venous hypertension. J. Neurosurg. 71:42, 1989.
10. Hecht JT, Horton WA, Reid CS, Pyeritz RE, et al: Growth of the foramen magnum in achondroplasia. Am. J. Med. Genet. 32:528, 1989.
11. Pauli RM, Scott CI, Wassman ER Jr, Gilbert EF, et al: Apnea and sudden unexpected death in infants with achondroplasia. J. Ped. 104:342, 1984.
12. Rollnick BR, Hoo JJ: Genitourinary anomalies are a component manifestation in the ectodermal dysplasia, ectrodactyly, cleft lip/palate (EEC) syndrome. Am. J. Med. Genet. 29: 131, 1988.
13. Christodoulou J, McDougall PM, Sheffield LJ: Choanal atresia as a feature of ectrodactyly-ectodermal dysplasia-clefting (EEC) syndrome. J. Med. Genet. 26:586, 1989.
14. McKusick VA, Egeland JA, Eldridge R, et al: Dwarfism in the Amish. I. The Ellis-van Crevel syndrome. Bull. Hopkins Hosp. 115:306, 1964.
15. Czeisel A, Hamula J: A Hungarian study on Werdnig-Hoffman disease. J. Med. Genet. 26:761, 1989.
16. Sivan Y, Galvis A: Early diaphragmatic paralysis in infants with genetic disorders. Clin. Pediatr. 29:169, (Philadelphia) 1990.
17. Coletta C, Carboni P, Carunchio A, Porro G, et al: Electrocardiographic abnormalities in childhood spinal muscular atrophy. Int. J. Cardiol. 24:283, 1989.
18. Emery AEH, Rimoin DL (eds): Principles and Practice of Medical Genetics. New York, Churchill Livingstone, 1983.
19. Levy HL: Nutritional therapy for selected inborn errors of metabolism. J. Am. Coll. Nutr. 8(suppl):54S, 1989.
20. Harper K, Pembrey ME, Davies KE, Winter RM, et al: A clini-

cally useful DNA probe closely linked to Haemophilia A. Lancet 2:6, 1984.
21. Cohen MM Jr: Selected clinical research involving the central nervous system. J. Craniofacial Genet. and Developm. Biol. 10:215, 1990.
22. Tuchman-Duplessis J, Auroux M, Haegel P: Illustrated Human Embryology, Vol. 3: Nervous System and Endocrine Glands. New York, Springer Verlag, 1975, p. 87.
23. Hoffman JIE: Congenital heart disease: Incidence and inheritance. Pediatr. Clin. N. Am. 37:25, 1990.
24. Schnabel R: Intrauterine coxsackie B infection in arthrogryposis multiplex congenita syndrome. Verh. Dtsch. Ges. Pathol. 65:311, 1981.
25. Livingstone JR, Sack GH Jr: Arthrogryposis multiplex congenita occurring with maternal multiple sclerosis. Arch. Neurol. 41:1216, 1984.
26. Baines DR, Douglas ID, Overton JH: Anaesthesia for patients with arthrogryposis multiplex congenita: What is the risk of malignant hyperthermia? Anaesthesia and Intensive Care 14:370, 1986.
27. Sommer A, Cutler EA, Cohen BL, Harper D, et al: Familial occurrence of the Wiedemann-Beckwith syndrome and persistent fontanel. Am. J. Med. Genet. 1:59, 1977.
28. Carlin ME, Escobar LF, Ward RL, Wielgus TY: Beckwith-Wiedemann syndrome (BWS) revisited. 11th Annual David W. Smith Workshop on Malformations and Morphogenesis. Lexington, Kentucky, 1990.
29. Hoyme HE; Teratogenically induced fetal anomalies. Clin. Perinatol. 17:547, 1990.
30. Monson RR, Rosenberg L, Hartz SC, Shapiro S, et al: Diphenylhydantoin and selected congenital malformations. N. Engl. J. Med. 289:1049, 1973.
31. DiLiberti JH, Farndon PA, Dennis NR, Curry JR: The fetal Valproate syndrome. Am. J. Med. Genet. 19:473, 1984.
32. Lammer EJ, Hayes AM, Schunior A, Holmes LB: Unusually high risk for adverse outcomes of pregnancy following fetal Isotretinoin exposure. Am. J. Hum. Genet. 43:A58, 1988.
33. Etretinate approved. FDA Drug Bulletin 16:16, 1986.

Chapter 45

# NEONATAL MANAGEMENT OF THE COMPLICATED OBSTETRIC LABOR AND DELIVERY

AVROY FANAROFF

The modern era of perinatal medicine has been characterized by rapid technologic advances and improved care of the mother, fetus, and newly born infant. The team concept remains central to providing optimal care for the patients and wise and judicious application of the tools available to the health care team is mandated by cost-conscious consumers and vigilant managed health-care supervisors. Communication among all the health care providers is essential to provide optimal care for the perinatal patients.[1] This chapter has been designed to complement specific sections addressing high risk pregnancy and intrapartum care, and will cover the following broad topics: Regionalization of perinatal care, Fetal evaluation, Selected maternal disorders—Effects on the fetus, Amniotic fluid disorders, Hematologic disorders, Problems in the delivery room, Selected respiratory disorders, and Infections.

## REGIONALIZATION OF PERINATAL CARE

The concept of regionalization implies uniform access to appropriate levels of care for all pregnant women and their offspring. Effective regionalization of perinatal care allows appropriate transfer of pregnant women and newborns at high risk to a regional center, whereas patients at low risk are cared for in community hospitals. Driven by a number of factors, including major financial considerations, regionalization in the United States has come under considerable attack. The term deregionalization has even crept into discussions on organization of perinatal care, and tne flow of patients is dictated in many instances by managed medicine.

It has been reassuring to observe that in Ontario, Canada the perinatal outcomes reaffirm the principles of regionalization. From 1982 to 1985, the transfer rate for labor or threatened labor prior to 37 weeks gestation, hypertension or toxemia increased, and there was a large increase (from 49% to 69%) of infants weighing 500 to 1500 grams delivering at the tertiary units. Infant death rates decreased throughout the region and the death rate among low-birth-weight infants was lowest among those born at the level III center.[2]

The data from the NICHD are similarly encouraging in that 80% of infants with birth weights below 1500 grams delivered at the tertiary centers.[3] (Figure 45–1 The importance of hospital of birth for low-birth-weight infants was highlighted in New York where preterm and low-birth-weight-infants were at a 24% higher risk of death if birth occurred at either a level I or II unit. Furthermore, infants below 1500 grams accounted for 70% of the perinatal deaths.[4]

Over the past 3 decades, the patterns of fetal deaths have changed markedly. The fetal death rate (per 1000 births) diminished from 11.5 in the 1960s to 5.1 in the 1980s, resulting from virtual elimination of fetal deaths due to intrapartum asphyxia and Rh isoimmunization, significant decreases in unexplained fetal deaths and those caused by fetal growth retardation. The continued toll is due to intrauterine infections, lethal malformations, growth retardation and abruptio placenta, which remains the largest identifiable cause of fetal death.[5]

Low birth weight (<2500 grams) accounts for 75% of poor perinatal outcomes. Strategies to improve the outcome of these babies has focused on antenatal prevention of conditions associated with low birth weight, together with intensive education, extensive intrapartum evaluation, and monitoring, along with sophisticated and aggressive care of the low-birth-weight fetus and infant.

Simple measures in antenatal care, such as elimination of cigarette smoking, improved nutrition, eradication of genitourinary tract infection, and increased awareness of the hazards of preterm birth have led to lower rates of prematurity in some centers.[6,7]

Regionalization was developed to provide uniform access to quality care for all pregnant women and their offspring. The principles remain noble and, above all, regionalization provides cost-effective care.

### Fetal Evaluation

#### *Alpha-Fetoprotein Screening*

Maternal serum alpha-fetoprotein (AFP) measurement has proven to be the most effective prenatal screening program yet devised (Table 45–1). The liver is the primary site of synthesis of alpha-fetoprotein, and by 15 to 20 weeks of pregnancy, AFP is a major serum component. The AFP in amniotic fluid at 15 to 20 weeks is mainly derived from fetal urination with a small contribution through the fetal skin. Any pregnancy complication or birth defect that causes fetal serum to leak or exude into the amniotic fluid will elevate amniotic fluid AFP and sub-

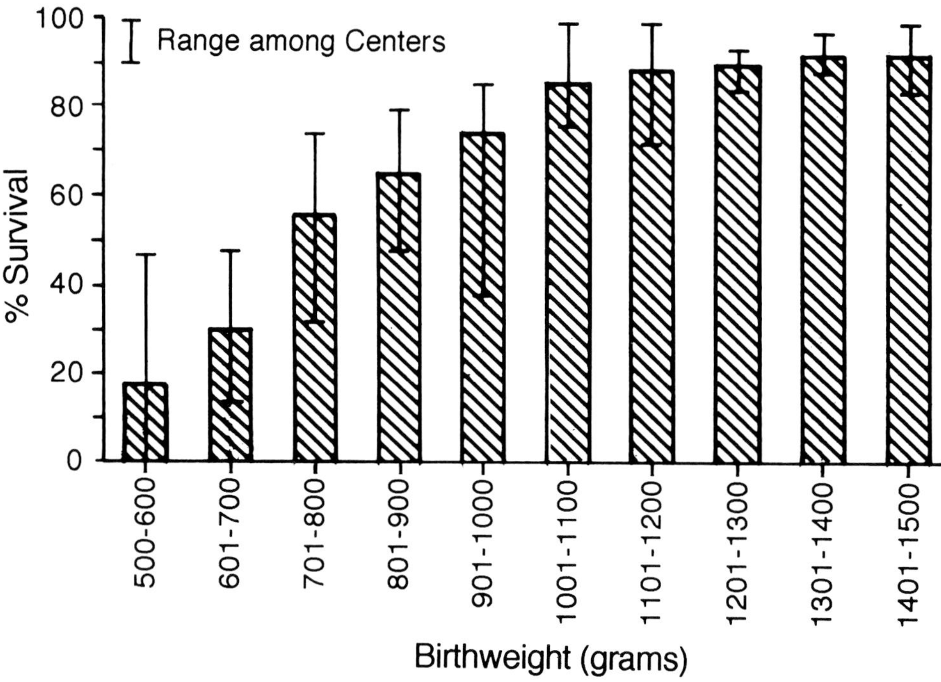


**Fig. 45–1.** Very low birth weight outcomes of the National Institute of Child Health and Human Development Neonatal Network. (Redrawn from Hack M, Horbar JD, Malloy MH, et al: Very low birth weight outcomes of the National Institute of Child Health and Human Development Neonatal Network. Pediatrics 87:587, 1991.)

sequently maternal serum AFP levels. Examples include anencephaly, open spina bifida, epidermolysis bullosa, gastroschisis, omphalocele and amniotic bands. Furthermore, abnormalities in the volume of amniotic fluid may be reflected by abnormal AFP values. Additionally, abnormalities in placental function may also alter maternal AFP (Table 45–2).

The maternal serum alpha-fetoprotein measurements have now replaced amniotic fluid measurements. Routine obstetric care includes screening for maternal serum alpha-fetoprotein between 15 and 18 weeks after the last menstrual period. If the levels are elevated in two samples after adjustment for weight and race, an ultrasound examination is performed. This may suggest an explanation such as incorrect estimation of gestational age, multiple gestation, fetal death or definite congenital anomaly. If doubt persists, an amniocentesis for measurement of the levels of alpha-fetoprotein and acetylcholinesterase, an enzyme found in fetal spinal fluid, in amniotic fluid is recommended to exclude anomalies possibly missed by sonography. With improved ultrasonographic techniques, most lesions can be confidently identified minimizing the need for the amniocentesis.[8]

**Table 45–1.** Assessment of the Fetus

| |
|---|
| Throughout Pregnancy |
| Gestational age: history, uterine growth, quickening, first heart sounds, ultrasound |
| Fetal growth |
| Serology, maternal antibodies |
| Amniotic fluid volume |
| Ultrasound: fetal number, growth, anomalies, fetal well-being |
| Risk assessment |
| First and Second Trimesters |
| Alpha-fetoprotein |
| Chorionic villus sampling |
| Amniocentesis |
| Cordocentesis |
| Third Trimester |
| Nonstress, stress tests |
| Formal fetal movement counting |
| Fetal biophysical profile |
| Estriol |
| Amniotic fluid phospholipids and bilirubin |
| Perinatal Period |
| Continuous FHR monitoring |
| Fetal scalp pH |
| Cord blood gases |

(From Klaus & Fanaroff, (Eds): Care of the High-Risk Neonate. 4th Edition. Philadelphia, WB Saunders, Co., 1993, with permission.)

### *Formal Fetal Movement Counting*

With a goal of decreasing the stillbirth rate near term, there has been an increased tendency to use fetal movements as an indicator of fetal well-being. The test is simple and can be administered frequently by a compliant and perceptive mother, preferably every night when the fetus is usually more active. The mother documents how long it takes to feel ten kicks and maintains accurate "kick sheets" for review by the medical staff. Fifty percent of women will feel ten kicks in less than 20 minutes, and if she does not feel ten kicks in 2 hours, she is instructed to come to the hospital for a nonstress test. The use of kick counts has been associated with a 50% increase in the number of nonstress tests and an increased rate of obstetric intervention for fetal compromise. In San Diego, the test reduced fetal mortality, as compared with historical controls,[9] but a larger prospective controlled trial from Europe failed to demonstrate that routine formal fetal counting achieved such an effect.[10] The test does merit further trial and is certainly worth instituting for selected high risk patients as they approach term.

### Fetal Benefits of Ultrasound

#### Detection of Fetal Anomalies

There is an ongoing debate as to the value of routine ultrasound in pregnancy (Table 45–3). In a prospective trial of ultrasound screening, perinatal mortality was decreased, and there was a reduced need for antenatal hospitalization and even clinic visits among the women assigned to the ultrasound group.[11] Somewhat ironically, the reduced perinatal mortality resulted from termination of pregnancies with major malformations. A retrospective study on the effectiveness of routine ultrasonography to detect structural abnormalities in a low-risk population revealed that most major malformations could be recognized by ultrasound in the second trimester.[12] (The onus is on the patient to report for care before this time.) The false-positive rate was exceptionally low and no fetus so identified came to harm, although the families were subjected to unnecessary anxiety. In view of the large number of patients examined, the many technicians and technical difficulties that can always be anticipated particularly with maternal obesity, multiple gestation, and abnormal fetal position, the results are extraordinarily good. It is apparent, however, that there are still great gaps in knowledge regarding the natural history of certain ultrasonographic findings, eg, choroidal cysts or dilated renal pelvis. Only when the natural history has been established will families be appropriately counseled.

#### Evaluation of Fetal Well-Being

In addition to determining fetal number, fetal size, and anatomy, the fetus is being bombarded by ultrasound and Doppler waves in efforts to determine its welfare. Doppler patterns from the placenta, the aorta, the umbilical artery, middle cerebral artery, the umbilical vein and the inferior vena cava are evaluated in conditions ranging from maternal hypertension through fetal hydrops. In some instances, they have predicted fetal and neonatal outcome; at other times the findings are inconclusive.[13] An elevated systolic/diastolic ratio was predictive of a greater incidence of growth retardation, meconium-stained amniotic fluid, fetal distress, and neonatal depression.[14–16]

#### Percutaneous Fetal Blood Sampling

Percutaneous Fetal Umbilical Blood sampling (PUBS) or cordocentesis provides direct access to the fetal circulation for both diagnostic and therapeutic purposes. The procedure is carried out under high resolution ultrasound guidance and has had a major impact on the evaluation and treatment of the residual patients with Rh isoimmunization and other hemolytic diseases in pregnancy. Other indications for PUBS include rapid karyotyping evaluation of fetal malformations detected later in pregnancy, and the evaluation of fetal acid-base status, fetal metabolic and infectious diseases—notably toxoplasmosis and other hematologic disorders including hemoglobinopathies, thrombocytopenia and twin-to-twin transfusions. The technique may also be used for directly transfusing or administering medications to the fetus.[17,18]

Ultrasound has become an indispensable and integral component of antenatal care. It is cost effective and in my opinion should be offered to all pregnant women.

## Selected Maternal Disorders—Effects on the Fetus

### Hypertension in Pregnancy

#### Background and Incidence

Hypertensive disorders with a host of different etiologies affect 10% to 20% of pregnant women. The term *pregnancy-induced hypertension* has replaced preeclampsia to denote the syndrome which occurs predominantly during the first pregnancy in 6% to 8% of pregnancies. The syndrome is characterized by the sequential development of facial and hand edema, hypertension, and proteinuria after the twentieth week of gestation. If seizures supervene, then the condition is known as eclampsia. Preeclampsia is a complex clinical syndrome with hypertension representing but one manifestation.[19,20]

#### Etiology

Events in the development of preeclampsia include incomplete trophoblastic invasion of the maternal spiral arteries, poor trophoblastic perfusion, endothelial cell injury with activation of coagulation, and altered endothelial permeability. The goal is to detect the onset of preeclampsia early and to intervene so that severe complications for the mother and fetus are prevented. Close supervision of all hypertensive pregnant women, with frequent evaluation of fetal growth and well-being are indicated. Preliminary reports have been encouraging with the use of newer therapies for preeclampsia, including low-dose aspirin therapy and calcium supplementation.

#### Definitions

Preeclampsia is defined by a blood pressure >140/90 mmHg and proteinuria >300 mg/liter in 24 hours I9 (WHO). The presence of proteinuria >5 grams/liter, a persistent diastolic pressure >110 mmHg, platelets <100 000, elevated liver enzymes or jaundice, oliguria <400 ml/24 hours and symptoms including epigastric pain, visual disturbance or severe headache identify the sickest women, the so called HELLP syndrome.[19,20]

#### Neonatal Problems

Neonatal problems include prematurity, intrauterine growth retardation, asphyxia, and hypoglycemia. Anemia and respiratory distress syndrome must be anticipated in preterm infants born after a placental abruption (see below). In pregnant women with mild hypertension without proteinuria, fetal growth is normal. However, pregnancy-induced hypertension associated with proteinuria is detrimental to fetal growth.[15]

**Table 45–2.** Risk of Fetal Death With Maternal Levels of Alpha-Fetoprotein at Least 2 Times the Median, According to Reported Cause of Death

| Reported Cause of Death | # of Deaths | # w/Alpha-Fetoprotein >2× Median | Odds Ratio | 95% Confidence Interval |
|---|---|---|---|---|
| Birth defects* | 35 | 2 | 1.3 | 0.3–5.5 |
| Hydrops fetalis | 10 | 1 | 2.4 | 0.3–18.9 |
| Maternal hypertension | 45 | 13 | 8.7 | 4.4–17.0 |
| Maternal or fetal infection | 23 | 1 | 1.0 | 0.1–7.3 |
| Placenta previa | 4 | 2 | 21.3 | 3.0–152.8 |
| Placental abruption | 54 | 7 | 3.2 | 1.4–7.2 |
| Placental infarction | 33 | 10 | 9.3 | 4.3–20.0 |
| Prolapsed cord | 6 | 2 | 10.7 | 1.9–58.9 |
| Other types of cord compression | 85 | 7 | 1.9 | 0.9–4.2 |
| Structural abnormality of the cord | 59 | 5 | 2.0 | 0.8–5.0 |
| Premature rupture of the membranes | 24 | 5 | 5.6 | 2.1–15.3 |
| Prematurity | 18 | 2 | 2.7 | 0.6–11.7 |
| Anoxia | 43 | 4 | 2.3 | 0.8–6.2 |
| Other** | 45 | 1 | 0.5 | 0.1–3.6 |
| Not specified | 128 | 16 | 3.1 | 1.8–5.4 |
| Total fetal deaths | 612 | 78 | 3.2 | 2.3–4.2 |
| Total live births | — | 112 | Referent | — |

* Alpha-fetoprotein-related birth defects are excluded

** Includes 9 deaths reported as resulting from maternal injury; 3 from unspecified maternal conditions; 10 from incompetent cervix; 4 from oligohydramnios; 1 each from unspecified complications of pregnancy, breech presentation, other complications of labor, fetal blood loss, and hemolytic diseases; 3 from intrauterine growth retardation; 9 from aspiration syndrome; and 2 from maternal complications of diabetes.

(From Waller K, Lusog LS, Cunningham GC, et al: N. Engl. J. Med. 325:6–10, 1991, with permission.)

## Hypertension Intrauterine Treatment of Growth Retardation

Intrauterine fetal growth retardation is an important cause of preterm birth and a major cause of neonatal morbidity. It is imperative that the growth regarded fetuses be identified. Maternal dates are always important, and abdominal circumference and estimated fetal weight are more reliable than head circumference in determination of growth retardation.[21] Vigilance throughout gestation combined with a comprehensive and reliable medical history, including dating of pregnancy, may prevent more growth-retarded fetuses slipping through the diagnostic nets before delivery. At present, almost 20% continue to declare themselves only after delivery.

Several studies suggest that low-dose aspirin administration may prevent fetal growth retardation in women at risk for this complication.[22–25] (Table 45–4) These conditions include previous delivery of growth-retarded infants, maternal lupus erythematosis or hypertension, and fetuses with abnormal umbilical artery flow velocity. Low-dose aspirin therapy appears to be safe for both mother and fetus. Whereas ingestion of large quantities of aspirin have been associated with premature closure of the ductus arteriosus, pulmonary hypertension, and bleeding disorders in the newborn, these complications are not observed with low-dose therapy.

**Table 45–3.** Indications for Ultrasound

Confirmation of pregnancy
Determination of:
- Gestational age
- Fetal number and presentation
- Placental location (vaginal bleeding)
- Fetal anatomy (previous malformations)

Assessment of:
- Size/date discrepancy
- Fetal well-being (biophysical profile—fetal tone, movements, and respiration)
- Volume of amniotic fluid (suspected oligohydramnios or polyhydramnios
- Fetal arrhythmias
- Fetal anatomy

Assist with procedures:
- Amniocentesis
- Intrauterine transfusion

(From Klaus & Fanaroff, (Eds): Care of the High-Risk Neonate. 4th Ed. Philadelphia, WB Saunders Co., 1993, with permission.)

### *The Diabetic Pregnancy*

The metabolic derangements are the major abnormality affecting individuals with diabetes mellitus. Pregnant women with diabetes should be managed by suitably trained individuals and teams who comprehensively monitor mother and fetus throughout pregnancy. Optimal care of women with diabetes must begin prior to conception to optimize the pregnancy outcome for herself and her offspring. Strict glucose control at this time reduces the frequency of congenital malformations and may also diminish other perinatal complications, including intrauterine demise, macrosomia, and neonatal disorders.[26–28] All pregnancies should be screened so that women with ges-

**Table 45–4.** Pregnancy Outcomes

| | Placebo Group | Aspirin Group | 95% CL (%)* | p |
|---|---|---|---|---|
| No. (%) with | | | | |
| Pregnancy-induced hypertension | 13 (25%) | 6 (13%) | −3 to 28 | NS** |
| Proteinuric hypertension | 10 (19%) | 1 (2%) | 7 to 27 | <0.02 |
| Onset of hypertension before 37 wk | 9 (17%) | 0 | 7 to 27 | <0.01 |
| Mean (SD) | | | | |
| Gestation at delivery (wk) | 38.7 (3.9) | 39.5 (2.1) | | NS |
| Birthweight (g) | 2954 (852) | 3068 (555) | | NS |
| No. (%) of infants | | | | |
| <2500 g | 13 (25%) | 7 (15%) | −5 to 25 | NS |
| <1500 g | 4 (8%) | 0 | 0 to 15 | NS |
| Below 5th centile | 7 (14%) | 7 (14%) | | NS |
| Mean (SD) blood loss at delivery | 358 (228) | 289 (188) | | NS |
| Perinatal deaths | 3 | 1 | | NS |

* 95% CL = 95% confidence limits for difference in proportions
** Abbreviation NS, not significant.
(From McParland P, Pearce JM, Chamberlain GVP: Lancet 335:1552–1555, 1990, with permission.)

tational diabetes can be identified and appropriately managed.

### *Management of Diabetics Prior to Conception*

The goal is to achieve a mean fasting glucose below 100 mg/dl and a 2-hour post-prandial level around 120 mg/dl. Glycosylated hemoglobin should be maintained within the normal range. The objective is to achieve glycemic control prior to conception, throughout embryogenesis, and then continue throughout gestation. In this way, major abnormalities may be averted. Outpatient management of the diabetic pregnancy has replaced the obligatory period of hospitalization. However, in the face of deteriorating glycemic control, maternal complications including hypertensive disorders, infection, preterm labor or evidence of fetal compromise, hospitalization is mandated. (Table 45–5)

The major problems encountered in the offspring of diabetic women include macrosomia, birth asphyxia, hypoglycemia, cardiorespiratory disorders, polycythemia, jaundice, and congenital malformations. Improved surveillance during pregnancy and labor has reduced the incidence of stillbirth and severe birth asphyxia as well as respiratory distress syndrome. (Table 45–6)

Macrosomia, however, remains a significant problem despite efforts at strict control of maternal glucose homeostasis. Marosomia, variously defined as birth weight greater than 4 kg, 4.5 kg, or 5 kg, is increasing in the United States.[29] Maternal diabetes was the strongest single risk for macrosomia. Male sex of the infant, increasing parity, and increasing duration of gestation are other important contributory factors associated with macrosomia. Maternal smoking, on the other hand, was associated with a marked decrease in the risk of macrosomia.[29] (Table 45–7)

Cesarean section is indicated if there is cephalopelvic disproportion associated with macrosomia, and every effort is expended to prevent birth trauma and asphyxia.

Hypoglycemia is still a common problem in infants of diabetic mothers. Infants may be asymptomatic or present

**Table 45–5.** Risks for CNS, Cardiovascular System and All Major Defects Among Infants of Diabetic Mothers, Atlanta Birth Defects Case-Control Study, 1988

| | Central Nervous System | | Cardiovascular System | | All Major Defects | |
|---|---|---|---|---|---|---|
| Diabetic Group | RR | R% | RR | R% | RR | R% |
| All insulin users (n = 47) | 7.4 (2.5,21.8) | 2.5 | 12.9 (4.8,34.6) | 6.1 | 5.2 (2.1,13.2) | 12.1 |
| Insulin-dependent | | | | | | |
| Diabetes mellitus (n = 28) | 15.5 (3.3,73.8) | 5.3 | 18.0 (3.9,82.5) | 8.5 | 7.9 (1.9,33.5) | 18.4 |
| Noninsulin-dependent | | | | | | |
| Diabetic insulin users-all (n = 19) | 2.1 (0.3,13.3) | 0.7 | 9.7 (2.7,35.3) | 3.3 | 3.4 (1.0,11.7) | 7.9 |
| Gestational diabetic | 3.0 (0.2,50.6) | 1.0 | 20.6 (2.5,168.5) | 9.7 | 6.5 (0.8,50.6) | 15.1 |
| Noninsulin users | | | | | | |
| All (n = 30) | 0.4 (0.1,3.4) | 0.1 | 1.8 (0.6,4.9) | 0.8 | 1.0 (0.5,2.0) | 2.3 |
| Gestational diabetic | 0 | 0 | 1.9 (0.5,6.8) | 0.9 | 0.8 (0.3,2.1) | 1.8 |

Abbreviations: RR, relative risk (compared with that of nondiabetic mothers); R% , absolute risk (per 100 live births).
Notes: Risks were adjusted for race, hospital, and year of birth, maternal education, maternal age, and maternal history of other chronic illnesses and alcohol intake during the first trimester of pregnancy. Results in parentheses are 95% confidence intervals.
(From Becerra JE, Khoury MJ, Cordero JF, et al: Pediatrics 85:1–9, 1990, with permission.)

**Table 45–6.** Pathophysiology of Morbidity and Mortality of IDM

| Problem | Pathophysiology |
|---|---|
| Fetal demise | Acute placental failure?<br>Hyperglycemia—lactic acidosis—hypoxia? |
| Macrosomia | Hyperinsulinism |
| RDS | Insulin antagonism of cortisol<br>Variant surfactant biochemical pathways |
| Wet lung syndrome | Cesarean delivery |
| Hypoglycemia | ↓ Glucose and fat mobilization |
| Polycythemia | Erythopoietic "macrosomia"?<br>Mild fetal hypoxia?<br>↓ $O_2$ delivery to fetus—HbA? |
| Hypocalcemia | ↓ Neonatal parathyroid hormone<br>↑ Calcitonin?<br>↓ Magnesium |
| Hyperbilirubinemia | ↑ Erythropoietic mass<br>↑ Bilirubin production<br>Immature hepatic conjugation?<br>Oxytocin induction |
| Congenital malformations (CNS, heart, skeletal) | Hyperglycemia?<br>Genetic linkage?<br>Insulin as teratogen?<br>Vascular accident? |
| Renal vein thrombosis | Polycythemia?<br>Dehydration? |
| Neonatal small left colon syndrome | Immature gastrointestinal motility? |
| Cardiomyopathy | Reversible septal hypertrophy<br>↑ Glycogen?<br>↑ Muscle? |
| Family psychologic stress | High-risk pregnancy<br>Fear of diabetes in infant |
| Subsequent development of insulin dependent diabetes | Genetic HLA markers; risk is greater for infant of diabetic father. |

From Klaus, Fanaroff A, (Eds): Care of the High-Risk Neonate, 4th Edition, Philadelphia, WB Saunders Co., 1993, with permission.)

with a constellation of symptoms including apathy, poor feeding, hypotonia, high-pithed cry, or even seizures. Close monitoring of the blood glucose at the bedside is mandatory. Efforts are made to maintain the blood glucose above 40 mg, with a combination of early oral feeding and intravenous supplementation if necessary. Infusing glucose at a rate of 8 mg/kg/min, increasing with 2 mg/kg/min increments will usually achieve normoglycemia.

The hypertrophic cardiomyopathy noted in infants of diabetic mothers is fortunately a transient phenomenon. Septal hypertrophy may be observed early in the second trimester, and the full-blown syndrome is more prevalent in pregnancies characterized by poor control. The converse does not hold true, and good glycemic control does not necessarily prevent the disorder, thereby implicating factors other than glucose in the etiology of the disorder.[30] Hormones such as insulin, epinephrine, and growth hormone and epidermal growth factor have been implicated but not necessarily incriminated in the etiology of the hypertrophy. Few infants are symptomatic; thus careful observation and monitoring are the treatments of choice.

### *The Effects of Drugs on the Fetus*

Drug use and abuse during pregnancy represents a major problem and hazard to both the mother and the fetus. The prevalence of drug abuse among pregnant women range between 0.4% and 27%.[31] A large prospective drug screening of newborns by meconium analysis documented 44% positive for cocaine, morphine, cannabinoid or combinations thereof.[32] (Table 45–8) Only 25% of these mothers admitted to illicit drug use.

The use of drugs during pregnancy is associated with a high incidence of stillbirths, maternal hemorrhage (abruptio placentae), premature rupture of the membranes, meconium-stained amniotic fluid, and fetal distress.[33,34]

For the newborn, there is increased morbidity and mortality. Complications which may be anticipated include birth asphyxia, prematurity, intrauterine growth retardation, cerebral infarction, and infection. There have been questions raised with regard to an increased incidence of congenital malformations, and the use of opiates is complicated by severe withdrawal syndromes. Data from the Atlanta birth defects case control study identified an increased risk of urinary tract defects with the maternal use of cocaine. No association was found between cocaine use and genital organ defects.[35] There are profound teratogenic effects of cocaine on the developing brain resulting in microcephaly, and defects in neuronal migration and differentiation.[36] (Table 45–9) Destructive lesions of the brain, including infarction and intraventricular hemorrhage, have been attributed to vasospasm and hypoxemia. The distribution of the lesions may relate to the developmental maturation of the brain at the time of exposure to cocaine.[36,37]

Long-term sequelae include delays in physical growth and mental development, sudden infant death syndrome and learning disabilities. There is evidence of diffuse brain involvement. Cocaine exposure only in the first trimester does not place the infant at risk for an adverse neonatal outcome compared with drug-free infants, but may place the infant at risk for neurobehavioral deficiencies that may have long term developmental implications.[31,36]

The identification of the drug-exposed neonate is difficult. The history is often unreliable and the effects of the drug on the fetus may not be apparent during the neonatal period. Screening of the infant's urine has severe limitations, and technical problems have rendered hair analysis impractical in the neonate. Meconium analysis has emerged as the most reliable method to detect intrauterine exposure of newborns to drugs.[32,38] The effect of cocaine use in pregnancy is of paramount importance because of the high prevalence of use and the devastating effects on the fetus. The long-term consequences are not yet known; however the constellation of prematurity, intrauterine growth retardation and microcephaly which characterize intrauterine cocaine exposure suggests that the neurodevelopmental future may be bleak for many of these infants.

## Disorders Associated with Alterations in Amniotic Fluid

The fetus is often compromised in the presence of disorders of amniotic fluid volume, leakage of amniotic fluid

**Table 45–7.** Clinical Status of Diabetes: Timing of Assessment

| Assessment | Non-Insulin Dependent | Insulin Dependent No Vasculopathy | Insulin Dependent, With Vasculopathy |
|---|---|---|---|
| *Maternal* | | | |
| History/physical examination | Preconceptual/initial visit | Preconceptual/initial visit | Preconceptual/initial visit |
| Opthamologic evaluation◇ | | | |
| No known abnormality | Preconceptual/initial visit | Preconceptual/early first trimester | Preconceptual/early first trimester |
| Known abnormality | Each trimester | Each trimester | Each trimester, as indicated |
| Electrocardiogram@ | NI | Preconceptual/initial visit@ | Preconceptual/initial visit@ |
| Prenatal screen panel and bacteriuria screen | Preconceptual/initial visit | Preconceptual/initial visit | Preconceptual/initial visit |
| Glycosylated proteins$ | NI | Initial visit/delivery$ | Initial visit/delivery$ |
| Thyroid panel screen | NI | Preconceptual/initial visit (repeat monthly until normal) | Preconceptual/initial visit (repeat monthly until normal) |
| Creatinine clearance | NI | Preconceptual/initial visit (if abnormal, each trimester) | Preconceptual/initial visit (if abnormal, each trimester) |
| Urine protein | | | |
| Dipstick | Serially | Serially | Serially |
| 24 h | NI | ≥1 + by dipstick | ≥1 + by dipstick |
| Lipid profile | NI | Preconceptual/initial visit | Preconceptual/initial visit |
| *Fetal (weeks gestation)* | | | |
| Alpha-fetoprotein (maternal serum) | 16–18 | 16–18 | 16–18 |
| Ultrasonography | | | |
| Dating/anomaly screen | 18–22 | 18–23 | 18–22 |
| Echocardiography | NI | 20–24 | 20–24 |
| Fetal growth/development | 37–39 | 30–32; 37–39 | 30–32; 37–39 |
| Fetal movement | 36 to intervention | 34 to intervention | 30 to intervention |
| CST/NST (biophysical profile; backup)! | NI | 32–34 to intervention | 32–34 to intervention |
| Lung maturity documentation | If intervention <38 wk | If intervention <39 wk | If intervention <39 wk |

* Not routinely indicated
◇ Implies pupillary dilation
@ Advised with diabetes >10 y duration or known cardiovascular disease or abnormal lipids profile.
$ More frequently if used as compliance evaluator.
! Earlier or more frequent assessment dependent on clinical status, eg, evidence of intrauterine growth retardation or multiple gestation.
(From Klaus, Fanaroff A, (eds): Care of the High-Risk Neonate 4th Edition, Philadelphia, WB Saunders Co., 1993, with permission.)

with superimposed infection, or the presence of meconium in the amniotic fluid. Refinements of ultrasonographic techniques have made recognition of these disorders more precise, in addition to often providing evidence of the underlying etiology of the disorder. Interventional therapy may thus be commenced prior to delivery. Hence, the amniotic fluid volume may be modified or direct therapy may be instituted with amnioinfusion. This section will consider polyhydramnios, oligohydramnios and meconium-stained amniotic fluid.

**Table 45–8.** Meconium Drug Screen of 3010 Neonates for the Metabolites of Cocaine, Morphine (Opiates) and Cannabinoid

| | |
|---|---|
| Total stools (meconium) analyzed | 3010 |
| Positive for drug metabolites (cocaine, morphine, or cannabinoid) | 1333 (44.3%)* |
| Positive for cocaine | 923 (30.7%) |
| Positive for morphine (opiate) | 617 (20.5%) |
| Positive for cannabinoid | 346 (11.5%) |
| Negative for any drug metabolite | 1677 (55.7%) |

* Drug exposure rate based on maternal self-report = 11.1%
(From Ostrea EM Jr, Brady M, Gause S, Raymundo AL, et al: Drug screening of newborns by meconium analysis: A large-scale prospective, epidemiology study. Pediatrics 39:107–113, 1992, with permission.)

## *Polyhydramnios*

Polyhydramnios is associated with a broad array of maternal and fetal disorders (Table 45–10). The overall incidence is less than 1% of all maternal and fetal disorders.[39,40] Despite increasingly sophisticated equipment and experienced obstetrical songraphers, the early diagnosis of polyhydramnios remains subjective. Later in ges-

**Table 45–9.** Selected Perinatal Outcomes, According to Whether or not the Mother Used Cocaine*

| Outcome | Cocaine Users (%) | Nonusers (%) | Adjusted Relative Risk |
|---|---|---|---|
| Birthweight <2500 g | 28 | 6 | 2.8 |
| Gestational age <37 wk | 29 | 9 | 2.4 |
| Small for Gestational age | 29 | 9 | 3.4 for smokers<br>2.1 for non-smokers |
| Decreased head circumference | 16 | 6 | 2.1 for smokers<br>1.1 for nonsmokers |
| Abruptio placentae | 4 | 1 | 4.5 |
| Perinatal death | 4 | 1 | 2.1 |

* Data are from Handler et al.
(From Volpe JJ: Effects of cocaine on the fetus. N. Engl. J. Med. 327: 399–407, 1992, with permission.)

**Table 45–10.** Natural History of Polyhydramnios

| | Mild (n = 92) | Moderate (n = 18) | Severe (n = 21) |
|---|---|---|---|
| *Anomalies* | 16 (17%) | 13 (72%) | 18 (87%) |
| *Resolution* | | | |
| Anomalies | 2/16 (13%) | 0 | 0 |
| No Anomalies | 69/76 (91%) | 4/5 (80%) | 0 |
| *Stillbirth* | | | |
| Anomaly | 0 | 1 | 1 |
| Multiple gestation | 0 | 3 | 2 |
| *Neonatal demise* | | | |
| Anomaly | 1 | 4 | 6 |
| Multiple gestation | 0 | 0 | 1 |

(From Hendricks SK, Conway L, Wang K, et al: Prenat. Diagn. 11: 649–654, 1991, with permission.)

tation, the ultrasonic determination of polyhydramnios is more reliable.[41] Current indicators of polyhydramnios include a single pocket of amniotic fluid of at least 8 cms[42] or an amniotic fluid index (AFI) of greater than 25 cms.[43] The AFI is determined by dividing the uterus into four quadrants, measuring the largest vertical pocket in each quadrant, and then summing the measurements. The AFI after 24 weeks gestation in the normal pregnancy is 16.2 cms ± 5.3 cms. The amniotic fluid volume reaches a maximum of approximately 1000 ml at 34 weeks gestation and then decreases progressively until delivery. Polyhydramnios is considered when the amniotic fluid volume exceeds 2000 ml. In the second half of pregnancy, fetal micturition, digestion and breathing are the major pathways for the formation and clearance of amniotic fluid.

### Conditions Associated with Polyhydramnios

In over one-third of cases there is no identifiable cause for polyhydramnios. There are many potential causes for the excessive fluid, hence the mother must be screened for diabetes, hypertension, lithium ingestion, multiple gestation, and erythroblastosis, and the fetus closely scrutinized for anomalies of the gastrointestinal tract, central nervous system, hydrops fetalis, renal, skeletal, and chromosomal abnormalities, in addition to TORCH infections. In some instances, no apparent cause for the polyhydramnios is established and vague disorders affecting the membranes have been implicated, with the mechanism yet to be determined. Resolution of hydramnios is associated with a good prognosis, whereas severe hydramnios carries a grave prognosis for the fetus.[39,40]

All pregnancies complicated by polyhydramnios should be closely monitored. Selected rather than universal fetal karyotyping can be justified by the ability to detect multiple anomalies and intrauterine growth retardation sonographically.

### Treatment of Polyhydramnios

No therapy is necessary in the asymptomatic patient with mild polyhydramnios. Therapy is indicated if there is evidence of maternal respiratory compromise or premature labor. Therapy is aimed at the underlying cause, hence tighter control of maternal diabetes, fetal transfusion in the case of erythroblastosis, and direct fetal therapy where polyhydramnios has been associated with fetal intra-abdominal masses. Amniocentesis under ultrasound guidance may be attempted, but this carries the risk of premature labor, amnionitis, or even abruptio placentae. It is necessary to remove 1500 to 2000 ml of fluid. More recently, the amniotic fluid volume has been reduced by maternal indomethacin therapy.[44]

### Assessment of the Newborn

Infants delivered following a pregnancy complicated by polyhydramnios should be carefully assessed for major malformations, including specific syndromes, and evaluated for evidence of toxoplasmosis, others, rubella, cytomegalovirus, Herpes (TORCH) infections or erythroblastosis fetalis. The incidence of malformations ranges from 9% to 50% with an average of 18% to 20%. The stomach should be aspirated and the aspirate carefully inspected and measured. This serves the dual purpose of establishing continuity of the esophagus and, if the gastric contents are of normal quantity and not bile-stained, helps rule out upper gastrointestinal obstruction. A careful neurologic assessment is mandatory, including measurement of the head circumference to rule out major anomalies of the central nervous system or neuromuscular disorders. Myopathies such as myotonia dystrophia will present with polyhydramnios, neonatal depression, and neonatal edema.

## Oligohydramnios—Pulmonary Hypoplasia

While total uterine volume increases linearly with gestational age, the amniotic fluid shows a steady increase until 25 weeks, then increases gradually until 30 weeks gestation and peaks at a volume of 900 ml to 100 ml. Fetal urine production is a major contributor to the amniotic fluid pool at urine flow increases from 3 ml to 4 ml/hour at 25 weeks gestation to >50 ml per hour at 38 weeks gestation.[45] Clearance of amniotic fluid relates to fetal swallowing.

Near term, there is a normal decline in amniotic fluid volume. The relationship between fetal urine production, fetal swallowing, and the fetal membranes in the development of oligohydramnios is complex. Trimmer and associates, after carefully measuring urine production ultrasonographically, concluded that the decreased urine production in the post-term infant with oligohydramnios was the result of, not the cause of, the oligohydramnios. Structural changes in the amniotic epithelial layer have been documented with oligohydramnios. The abnormal membranes thus become part of the vicious cycle as the amniotic fluid volume will not be reconstituted.

Oligohydramnios has been defined ultrasonographically by general descriptors which include an obvious lack of amniotic fluid, crowding of the fetal limbs, and a poor fetal-fluid interface. Objective criteria include the maximal vertical axis ranging from <1 cm to <3 cms, or the amniotic fluid index, as defined above, <5 cms. Oligohydramnios associated with intact fetal membranes has been associated with intrauterine growth retardation, asphyxia,

**Table 45–11.** Clinical Profile of Infants Born After Rupture of Membranes of 7 Days or More That Occurred Before 29 Weeks Gestation

| | No Pulmonary Hypoplasia (n = 74) | Pulmonary Hypoplasia (n = 14) |
|---|---|---|
| Gestational age at birth (wk)* | 28.2 ± 2.16 (24–34) | 26.2 ± 2.14 (24–31) |
| Birth weight (gm)* | 1191 ± 362 (640–2280) | 903 ± 278 (580–1590) |
| Gestational age at ROM (wk)* | 25.1 ± 2.68 (15–28) | 20.9 ± 3.17 (16–26) |
| ROM (days)* | 22.4 ± 18.5 (7–126) | 38.4 ± 20.9 (8–67) |
| Oligohydromnios | | |
| Severe | 26 (35%) | 7 (50%) |
| Moderate | 20 (27%) | 5 (36%) |
| Deformities | | |
| Severe | 0 (0%) | 5 (36%) |
| Moderate | 9 (12%) | 4 (29%) |
| Pneumothoraces | 11 (15%) | 9 (64%) |
| Persistent pulmonary hypertension of the newborn | 8 (11%) | 6 (43%) |
| Maternal amnionitis | 35 (47%) | 8 (57%) |
| Neonatal infection | 4 (5%) | 0 (0%) |
| Small for gestational age | 6 (8%) | 1 (7%) |
| Died | 8 (11%) | 10 (71%) |

* Values are mean ± standard deviation (range).
(From Rotschild A, Ling EW, Puterman ML, Farquharson D: Neonatal outcome after prolonged preterm rupture of membranes. Am. J. Obstet. Gynecol. 162:46–52, 1990, with permission.)

and increased perinatal morbidity and mortality.[46,47] Furthermore, the syndrome of post-maturity and meconium-stained fluid is more likely with oligohydramnios. Severe skeletal deformities and pulmonary hypoplasia can be anticipated if membranes rupture prior to 26 weeks gestation.[48] (Table 45–11)

Neonatal death caused by pulmonary hypoplasia may result from oligohydramnios because of premature and prolonged rupture of the membranes. Oligohydramnios may result in lung hypoplasia both as a direct result of fetal thoracic compression, and indirectly through inhibition of fetal breathing. Rotschild[48] concluded that the gestational age at the time of rupture of membranes was the single best predictor of pulmonary hypoplasia. The probability of pulmonary hypoplasia diminished from 50% if membranes ruptured at 19 weeks gestation, to 30% at 22 weeks, to less than 10% by 26 weeks gestation, and trivial thereafter (Figure 45–2). Roberts[49] noted that pulmonary hypoplasia was more common if membranes ruptured prior to 22 weeks gestation.

The absence of fetal breathing movements and reduced thoracic circumference have been suggested as useful markers in prenatal prediction of pulmonary hypoplasia. In normal pregnancies, there is a linear growth of internal thoracic circumference and lung area with gestational age. Fetuses with circumferences below the third percentile were more likely to have pulmonary hypoplasia, but this was not invariable.[50] Fetal lung length is an additional measurement that is computed in attempting to predict pulmonary hypoplasia. Measured by ultrasound from the tip of the apex to the base on the diaphragmatic dome, normative data has been generated which correctly identified 11 of 12 fetuses with pulmonary hypoplasia.[49] (Figure 45–3, 45–4) Kilbride reported that in pregnancies with Premature Rupture of Membranes (PROM) >2 weeks, prior to 28 weeks gestation, oligo-hydramnios (fluid < 1 cm) was a better predictor of pulmonary hypoplasia than fetal breathing or thoracic circumference.[51]

In terms of relating fetal breathing and lung hypoplasia, it all comes down to the definition. With Blott's strict definition of 60 seconds, there is a relationship between lack of fetal breathing and lung hypoplasia.[52] When a more liberal definition is utilized, a variable relationship is noted and the documentation of episodic fetal breathing is not necessarily reassuring.

In summary, there remains much to be learned about pulmonary hypoplasia. Pulmonary hypoplasia may be pro-

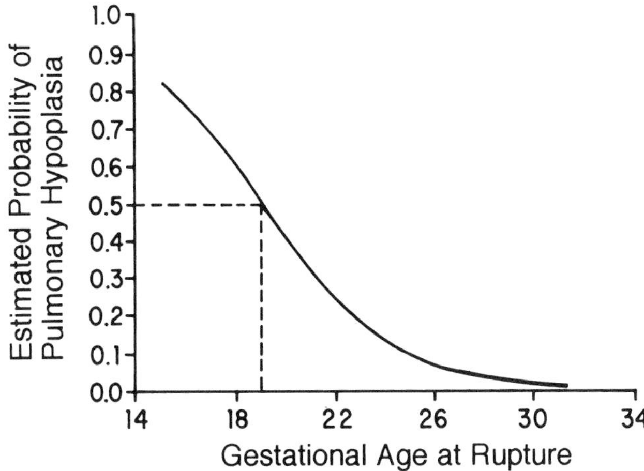


**Fig. 45–2.** Relationship between gestational age at rupture of membranes, duration of rupture, and pulmonary hypoplasia in 88 infants. (Redrawn from Rotschild A, Ling EW, Puterman ML, Farquharson D: Neonatal outcome after prolonged preterm rupture of membranes. Am. J. Obstet. Gynecol. 162:46, 1990.)

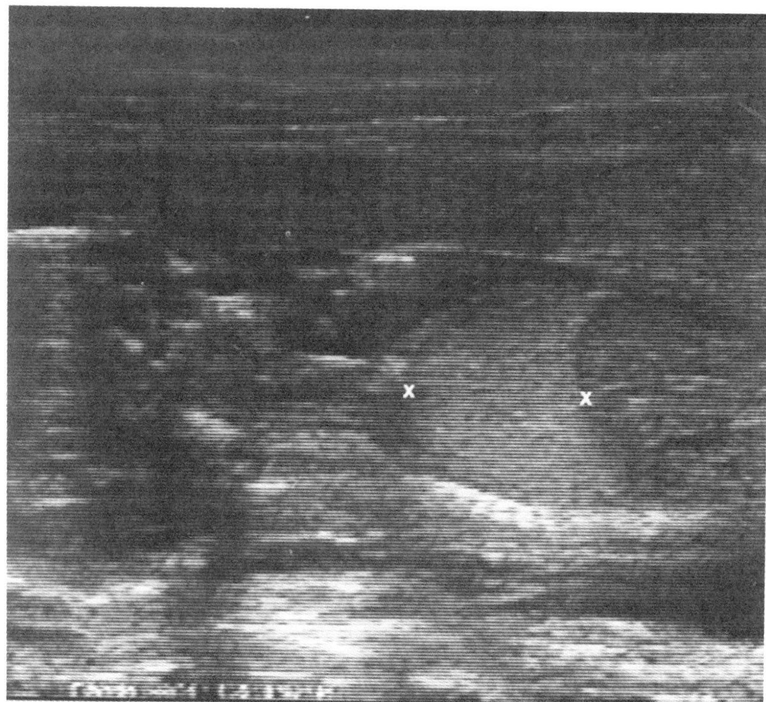

Fig. 45–3. Ultrasonogram of fetal lung in sagittal section with crosses indicating method of measurement from base of lung at dome of diaphragm to apex of lung adjacent to clavicle. (From Roberts AB, Mitchell JM: Direct ultrasonographic measurement of fetal lung length in normal pregnancies and pregnancies complicated by prolonged rupture of membranes. Am. J. Obstet. Gynecol. 163:1560, 1990, with permission.)

duced experimentally by draining the amniotic fluid, producing urinary tract obstruction, or creating a diaphragmatic hernia. Spinal cord injury may also be used to produce pulmonary hypoplasia in the absence of oligohydramnios. The precise contributions of thoracic compression, restriction of fetal respiration, or disturbance of pulmonary fluid dynamics in pulmonary hypoplasia remain to be clarified. With the advent of surfactant and improved survival of immature infants, malformations are responsible for an incremental number of perinatal deaths. Pulmonary hypoplasia predominates in association with congenital diaphragmatic hernia, renal dysplasia, thoracic dystrophies and prolonged rupture of the membranes.

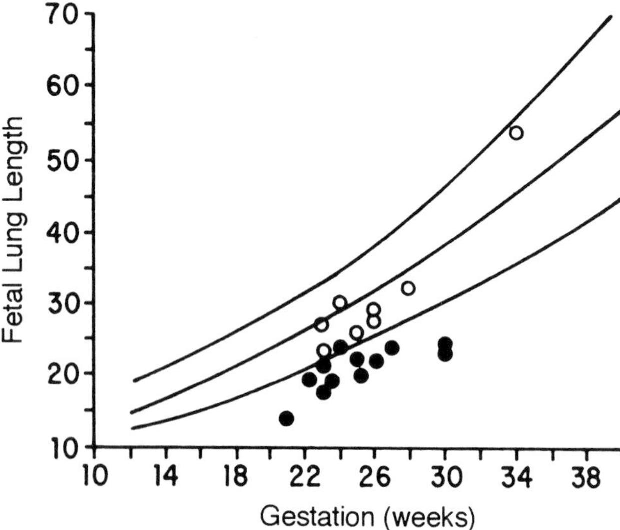


Fig. 45–4. Mean + 95% prediction intervals for normal fetal lung length plotted against gestational age. Superimposed circles represent lung length measurements in patients with ruptured membranes. Open circles represent patients with normally grown lungs; solid circles represent those with pulmonary hypoplasia. (Redrawn from Roberts AB, Mitchell JM: Direct ultrasonographic measurement of fetal lung length in normal pregnancies and pregnancies complicated by prolonged rupture of membranes. Am. J. Obstet. Gynecol. 163:1560, 1990.)

As with the evolution of many disorders, the ability to identify patients at risk for and with pulmonary hypoplasia exists. The next steps are to establish ways and means of reversing the process and reestablishing lung growth. Lung transplantation appears a hopeless alternative for those afflicted with this malady at birth.

In managing patients with PROM, it is first necessary to establish that membranes have ruptured (nitrazine paper and fern) and, with speculum examination, to culture the cervix. Accurate assessment of gestational age, amniotic fluid volume, together with thoracic volume, lung length, and pulmonary maturity follow. Fetal wellbeing is then closely monitored via biophysical profile with close attention to fetal breathing patterns.[53,54] The mother is closely observed for signs of chorioamnionitis. Amnioinfusion may be considered, but the use of tocolytics or steroids are controversial in cases of PROM associated with oligohydramnios.[55]

A skilled neonatal resuscitation team should be alerted for the delivery room as these infants will often be depressed and acidotic. Preparations for oxygenation, intubation, and mechanical ventilation, as well as circulatory support, will be necessary. A careful physical examination will be necessary to identify the classical features of Potter's syndrome or the contractures and deformations associated with oligohydramnios. The lungs are often extremely noncompliant, pneumothoraces are common, and severe pulmonary insufficiency with hypoxemia and hypercarbia must be anticipated. The role of surfactant therapy, steroids, and newer modes of mechanical ventilation in infants with hypoplastic lungs are still evolving.

## Meconium-Stained Amniotic Fluid

Since the mid-1970's, the combined obstetrical/pediatric approach to the prevention of meconium aspiration has been widely practiced.[56–58] The pharynx was suctioned with delivery of the head and the trachea intubated, regardless of the consistency of the meconium or the condition of the infant. The concept that meconium aspiration syndrome is entirely preventable has proven to be fallacious. Despite a combined aggressive perinatal approach as outlined above, severe complications of meconium aspiration are still encountered.[59–61] Meconium staining is noted in approximately 10% of deliveries and significant meconium aspiration syndrome will occur in approximately 3% of these deliveries, for an overall incidence of 3 in 1000 live births.[62] (Figure 45–5) The risk is greatest when the meconium is thick, ie, contains particulate matter, in combination with abnormal fetal monitor tracings.[63] These infants with severe meconium aspiration syndrome have evidence of severe pulmonary hypertension and the muscular hypertrophy in the intra-acinar pulmonary arteries strongly supports a long-standing intrauterine event.[64]

The additional benefits of tracheal intubation following pharyngeal suctioning have been challenged in those situations where the amniotic fluid is lightly stained and the infant is vigorous. Under these circumstances, fewer complications, ie, stridor, were encountered in the group of infants not intubated.[65] Although this was not a well-randomized trial, it has now become standard practice at many centers in North America not to intubate infants who have been suctioned on the perineum, if the meconium staining is light, and the infant is vigorous at birth.

If thick meconium is identified, then the fetal status should be closely monitored with a scalp electrode. The scalp pH should be measured if there is evidence of fetal distress, ie, tachycardia, decelerations, decreased long-term variability. Obstetric management is guided by the above findings and amnioinfusion may be considered (see below). At delivery, the oro- and nasopharynx should be well-suctioned by the obstetrician before delivery of the shoulders and the trachea visualized and suctioned by the pediatrician. This approach diminishes the chances for meconium aspiration syndrome. The prevailing theory is that meconium aspiration syndrome is predominantly an intrauterine event associated with fetal compromise, and the meconium in the airways is merely a marker of previous fetal hypoxia.[61]

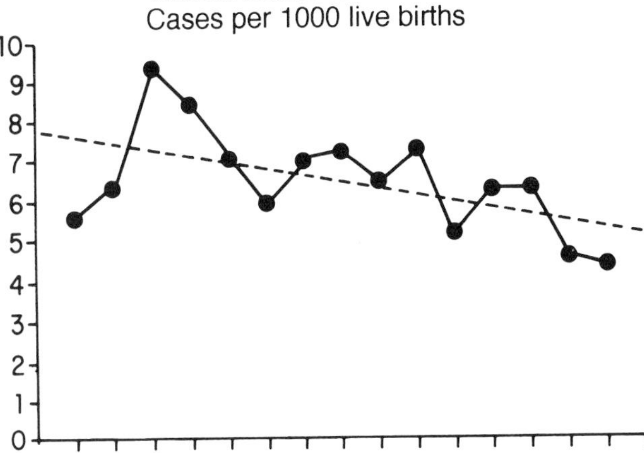


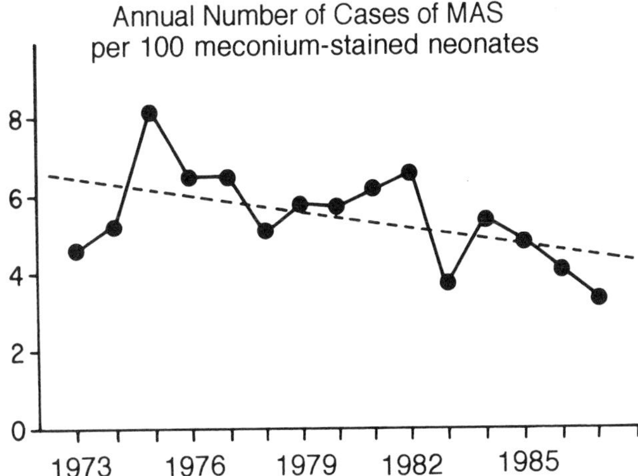


**Fig. 45–5.** Incidence of meconium aspiration syndrome (MAS) from 1973 through 1987. **A,** Annual incidence of MAS per 1000 live births. **B,** Annual number of cases of MAS per 100 meconium-stained neonates. (From Wiswell TE, Tuggle JM, Turner BS: Meconium aspiration syndrome: Have we made a difference? Pediatrics 85:715, 1990, with permission.)

## Amnioinfusion[66–71]

The fluid-filled amniotic sac serves a number of important functions for the fetus. This includes protection from trauma, bacteriostasis, intrauterine temperature homeostasis, nutrition, hemostasis, umbilical cord protection, and providing the correct milieu for normal development of limbs and lungs.

Amnioinfusion is used under a variety of circumstances including the prophylaxis and treatment of chorioamnionitis, umbilical cord compression, and meconium aspiration syndrome, or to improve imaging of the fetus in the presence of oligohydramnios. Amnioinfusion is designed to infuse a sterile solution into the amniotic sac for the purpose of expanding the amniotic fluid volume. (Table 45–12)

Antibiotics such as ampicillin, cephalosporins, and gentamicin have been infused into women with chorioamnionitis. There have been insufficient studies to establish the efficacy of such therapy, although there has been no evidence of major neonatal or maternal morbidity.

Severe variable or umbilical cord compression deceler-

**Table 45–12.** Characteristics of Delivery

| | Routine care (N = 44) | Amnio-infusion (N = 36) | Difference (P) |
|---|---|---|---|
| Fetal distress | | | |
| Present | 10 | 1 | |
| Absent | 34 | 35 | <.05 |
| Meconium below the cords | | | |
| Present | 16 | 2 | |
| Absent | 28 | 34 | <.01 |
| Meconium Aspiration Syndrome | | | |
| Present | 3 | 0 | |
| Absent | 41 | 36 | NS* |

* Not significant.
(From Wenstrom KD, Parsons MT: The prevention of meconium aspiration in labor using amnioinfusion. Obstet. Gynecol. 73:647–651, 1989, with permission.)

ations are defined as decelerations that last for >60 seconds in which the deceleration nadir is <70 beats per minute. The nadir heart rate of <70 bpm approximates the atrioventricular nodal rate and thereby implies maximal vagal stimulation and probable complete cord occlusion, ie, cessation of umbilical circulation. Complete cord occlusion will lead to metabolic acidosis. Severe variables are encountered with PROM, severe oligohydramnios, nuchal cord, true knot in the cord, and cord prolapse. Standard therapy for severe variable decelerations includes changing the maternal position, discontinuation of oxytocics, ruling out cord prolapse, and administration of 100% oxygen to the mother by face mask. Amnioinfusion has been suggested for variable decelerations not responding to standard therapy. Preliminary data indicate that amnioinfusion reduces the incidence of variable decelerations and improves fetal blood gas status. Amnioinfusion has also reduced the incidence of meconium staining and the need for operative intervention for fetal distress in women with oligohydramnios.[66–68] Thus, by restoring amniotic fluid during labor, the umbilical cord appears to be protected from compression. Additionally, in the presence of oligohydramnios, amnioinfusion may improve the ability to visualize the fetus ultrasonographically and permit better identification of the cause of the oligohydramnios.

Intrapartum amnioinfusion may be of benefit to patients with meconium-stained amniotic fluid. The incidence of thick meconium was reduced after amnioinfusion. There was also less fetal acidemia at birth, fewer cases with meconium below the cord, and reduced need for positive pressure ventilation in the amnioinfused group.[69] Others have reported the need for fewer operative deliveries for fetal distress and less meconium below the cord following amnioinfusion.[70] The amnioinfusion appears to correct oligohydramnios, reduce cord compression and thereby decrease the risk of acidemia and antepartum aspiration of meconium.

In summary, oligohydramnios, chorioamnionitis, and fetal deformation frequently complicate preterm, premature rupture of membranes. Amnioinfusion may be used to restore the amniotic fluid volume and prevent cord compression or deformation. Direct therapy may also prevent chorioamnionitis and meconium aspiration syndrome.

## Hematologic Problems

### *Anemia Book*[71,72]

Anemia may result from hemorrhage, hemolysis, or failure of red cell production. The presence of severe anemia at the time of delivery or on the first day of life is usually the result of hemorrhage or hemolysis due to isoimmunization. When the anemia is secondary to acute blood loss at the time of delivery, there may be evidence of circulatory insufficiency.

Obstetric accidents and malformations of the placenta and cord may result in hemorrhage which can be life threatening to both the mother and fetus. Hence, severe hemorrhage may be observed with placenta previa, abruptio placentae, or accidental incision of the placenta or umbilical cord during cesarean section. The infant may not receive the usual placental transfusion during the section, and clamping the cord with the infant elevated above the placenta may result in fetoplacental hemorrhage. Infants delivered with tight nuchal cords are also at risk for fetoplacental hemorrhage. The cord rarely ruptures but may during an attended precipitous delivery.

Signs of acute blood loss include pallor, tachycardia, tachypnea or gasping respiration, hypotension, and evidence of poor perfusion with slow capillary refill. The hemoglobin content may initially be normal but with restoration of circulating blood volume will drop precipitously. Remember that capillary values for both hematocrit and hemoglobin are consistently higher than venous or arterial measurements, and that the hematocrit rises 3% to 6% to peak between 3 and 12 hours of life in the normal newborn.

It is often extremely difficult to distinguish the infant with hypovolemic shock from the severely asphyxiated newborn. Both may be extremely pale with evidence of poor perfusion and hypotension and both conditions may be present in the same patient.

The fundamental approach to resuscitation with regard to the airway, oxygenation and support of the circulation are initiated, irrespective of the underlying cause. Thereafter, metabolic acidosis and circulating volume can be restored.

#### *Occult Hemorrhage Prior to Birth*

Fetomaternal hemorrhage may be precipitated by amniocentesis, external version, fundal pressure during the second stage of labor, the use of intravenous oxytocics, trauma, placenta previa, and abruptio placentae.[73] The clinical manifestations are dependent on the timing and acuity. Chronic bleeding results in a very pale but not necessarily distressed or hypotensive infant. The blood smear reveals microcytic hypochromic red cells with no features of hemolysis. Acute and massive bleeding (more than 150 ml of fetal blood) results in a pale, distressed, hypotensive, acidotic infant, with normocytic, normochromic red cells. Fetal cells can be detected in the maternal circulation by the Kleihauer-Betke acid elution test.

These infants need rapid restoration of circulating blood volume, whereas the chronic bleeds may only require iron supplementation.

Intrauterine twin-to-twin transfusions represent another form of occult hemorrhage in utero. Both twins are at risk. The donor twin is often pale and undergrown compared with the plethoric recipient.

### Neonatal Anemia

Because of the relatively large amounts of blood withdrawn from sick preterm infants and a refractory bone marrow, most such infants require blood transfusions. It is disquieting to note that neonates account for 15% of blood transfusions in the U.S.A., and that translated into 500 000 transfusions in 1988.[74] One can only speculate as to how many were absolutely indicated. In order to eliminate the need for transfusions, there are a number of studies underway evaluating the role of erythropoietin in the anemia of prematurity. The preliminary reports have included a small but growing number of premature infants. These have yielded encouraging but not startling results, and the associated neutropenia, for which no valid cause has been established, is disturbing.[75,76] Erythropoietin is only one of the factors needed to correct the anemia of prematurity, and though it may be dominant, needs a supporting cast of iron and other red cell constituents.[77] Reports to date have only included relatively well low-birth-weight infants. If the number of transfusions in ventilator-dependent infants who are having significant quantities of blood withdrawn can be significantly reduced, a powerful weapon will have been given to the neonatal team. The optimal dose of erythropoietin and the iron and other needs of the red cell need to be established.[75–77]

### Platelet Disorders

The etiology of neonatal thrombocytopenia may be decreased platelet production, increased peripheral platelet destruction, or a combination thereof. Accelerated platelet destruction is reflected by decreased platelet survival, increased mean platelet volume, normal numbers of megakaryocytes in the bone marrow, and an attenuated post-transfusion platelet increment after transfusion.[78]

#### Immune Thrombocytopenia

Syndromes of immune-mediated platelet destruction may occur during pregnancy, affecting the mother, the fetus or both. Antibodies directed against blood platelets may rapidly destroy them, resulting in thrombocytopenia with an attendant risk of hemorrhage. Better understanding of the mechanisms of platelet destruction has resulted in significant changes in the monitoring and management of immune thrombocytopenic states during pregnancy and in the neonatal period.

#### Neonatal Alloimmune Thrombocytopenia[79,80]

In neonatal alloimmune thrombocytopenic purpura alloantibodies, the result of alloantigenic differences between maternal and fetal platelets can cross the placenta and destroy the fetal platelets. This leads to severe thrombocytopenia, which in turn can lead to severe central nervous system hemorrhage, either in the fetus or in the newborn after delivery.

Alloimmune thrombocytopenia has been estimated to occur in 1 of every 5000 births despite the fact that 2% to 3% of women have PIAI-negative platelets and 85% of their offspring are PIAI positive. Platelet antigen incompatibility thus occurs once in every 50 pregnancies, yet alloimmunization only occurs in 1% of the incompatible situations. This has been attributed to linkage to particular immune-response genes. The infant may present with scattered petechiae and ecchymoses accompanied 10% to 20% of the time by varying grades of intracranial hemorrhage. Hence, careful neurologic examination and imaging of the brain by ultrasound or computerized tomography is indicated. The timing of bleeds in utero may be aided by the presence of hemosiderin which can be detected by magnetic resonance imaging. Platelet counts are often below 5000/mm$^3$.

The diagnosis may be established by allotyping platelets from the mother and infant or detecting platelet alloantibody in the maternal serum. It is often necessary to treat the neonate prior to establishing the diagnosis.

Treatment options include transfusion with maternal or other antigen negative platelets, exchange transfusion, steroids, or intravenous immunoglobulin. Intravenous immunoglobulin in a dose of 400 mg/kg/day for 5 days or 1 g/kg/day for 3 days, has become the most widely adopted therapy for infants with platelets <50 000/mm$^3$ at birth, rapidly declining platelet counts, or those with hemorrhage. The platelet count usually rises within a week. Maternal platelets, which should be washed to remove alloantibody before administration, will increase the platelet count immediately, and are reserved for infants with life-threatening hemorrhage.[79–81]

Although this is a rare entity, subsequent pregnancies in platelet AI negative women with an already affected infant carry an 85% risk of recurrence. A number of approaches have been adopted to prevent hemorrhage in the fetus. These include percutaneous umbilical blood sampling during the second trimester to identify the affected fetuses and direct intravascular transfusion of maternal platelets at term to allow safe delivery.[79] An alternate approach has been the weekly infusion of intravenous immunoglobulin ( 1 G/kg/weekly ) in addition to treatment with oral steroid.[80]

#### Idiopathic (Immune) Thrombocytopenic Purpura (ITP)

This syndrome results from the production of autoantibodies against platelet antigens. IgG autoantibodies, which may cross the placenta, are more frequent than IgM, so that the fetus is at risk for thrombocytopenia. The risk to the fetus, 10% to 50%, cannot be established from the maternal platelet count, nor have the platelet antibodies associated with greatest risk to the fetus been identified. In contrast with alloimmune thrombocytopenia, where hemorrhage may occur prior to delivery, the greatest risk for serious hemorrhage in ITP occurs during delivery. Platelet destruction may continue for the first 3 months of life, however, after labor and delivery thrombocytopenia is usually mild and well tolerated.

An approach to preventing intrapartum hemorrhage is to perform caesarean section for all fetuses with a platelet count below 50 000/mm$^3$ as determined from the fetal scalp or by umbilical sampling.

The major goal is to protect the mother from hemorrhage during pregnancy and then ensure an atraumatic delivery for the at-risk fetus. Intravenous immunoglobulin complemented by steroids has become the mainstay in therapy. In the newly born, intravenous immunoglobulin (400 mg/kg/5 days) is used when the platelet count is below 50 000/mm$^3$ and declining. Platelet transfusions are reserved for infants with active bleeding. Random donor platelets may survive only long enough to contribute to hemostasis if not to increase the platelet count.[78]

### Nonimmune Platelet Destruction

Nonimmune platelet destruction may occur with a variety of conditions and underlying circumstances. These include bacterial and viral infections, certain drugs administered to the mother or infant, following exchange transfusion, extracorporeal membrane oxygenation or cardiac surgery, as a component of disseminated intravascular coagulopathy, or as the result of platelet destruction within giant hemangiomas (Kasabach-Merritt syndrome). These disorders are usually easily distinguishable from the immune thrombocytopenia.

## Problems in the Delivery Room

### *Initial Steps in Resuscitation*[81–85]

In most instances, resuscitation is not required, and the infant's transition to extrauterine life may be assisted by a few simple steps.

### *Thermal Management*

Immediately after birth, the newborn infant should be placed under a preheated radiant warmer. In order to avoid evaporative heat loss, the infant should be thoroughly dried and the wet blankets promptly removed. Minimizing heat loss, particularly in premature infants, is important as heat loss is exaggerated by their lack of subcutaneous fat, and the increased surface area-to-weight ratio. Moreover, the preterm infant is poorly equipped to generate additional heat because of reduced stores of brown fat and glycogen. Hypothermia may precipitate a cascade of dangerous physiologic changes including hypoglycemia, metabolic acidosis, and a reversion to the fetal circulation pattern, with resulting hypoxemia. Placement of knitted cap on the infant's head in the delivery room is an important step that also decreases evaporative heat loss.

### *Respiratory Evaluation*

The next step in initial care should be to clear the pharynx and nose of fluid. This can be accomplished easily by using a bulb syringe to suction first the infant's mouth, then the nose. During the first minute of life, the infant's respirations, heart rate and color are evaluated. The mildly depressed infant may experience primary apnea at birth. This type of apnea is due to mild depression of the brain stem respiratory control area by hypoxia or reflex inhibition, and has been found to respond well to tactile stimulation and exposure to oxygen. Thus, if the infant is still apneic after initial drying and suctioning, tactile stimulation may be provided through flicking the soles of the feet or rubbing the infant's back.

### *Cardiovascular Assessment*

The next step in initial stabilization of an infant is evaluation of the heart rate. If the heart rate is above 100 bpm and perfusion is normal, the infant can be considered to be adapting normally to extrauterine life. If the heart rate is below 100 bpm, initiation of positive pressure ventilation may be necessary to restore a heart rate above 100 bpm.

Next, assess the color and determine core temperature, if there is peripheral cyanosis. If central cyanosis is present, free-flow 100% oxygen should be provided, and further evaluation to determine the cause of the cyanosis should be undertaken.

### *The Apgar Score*

These simple steps, usually completed before the end of the first minute of life, are sufficient for the initial delivery room care of the majority of healthy infants. The next step in an infant's evaluation is assignment of the Apgar score at 1 minute and 5 minutes of life. The Apgar score is a qualitative measure of the infant's success in adapting to the extrauterine environment. The score consists of two vital signs (respiratory effort and heart rate), color, and two neurologic responses (response to stimulation and general tone). Each of these components is given a score of 0 to 2, with 2 being the best score, and 0 indicating no response. Each component is evaluated at 1 minute and 5 minutes, and a total score is calculated. When the Apgar score is less than 6 at 5 minutes, it is recommended that a 10 minute and 15 minute score be determined. The Apgar score assigned at 10 minutes or 15 minutes may indicate the infant's risk of a later neurologic deficit.

Although the Apgar score is useful in the initial steps of evaluation, resuscitation of the infant should not be delayed until 1 minute. A low Apgar score, in premature infants $<$32 weeks gestation or $<$1500 grams at birth, can occur in the absence of asphyxia (Tooley, et al., 1977).

### *Care of the Depressed Newborn Infant*

Antenatal monitoring and anticipatory management of the mother-infant dyad have increasingly been utilized to decrease the possibility of antenatal or perinatal birth asphyxia. Nonetheless, severely depressed infants are still encountered who require advanced skill in resuscitations.

Hypoxic-ischemic injury in utero may lead to a form of severe central depression of respiration which is termed "secondary apnea." An infant with this form of apnea is unresponsive to stimulation, and mechanical ventilation with oxygen must be initiated at once if the infant fails to respond to the initial resuscitative steps outlined above. Ventilation should be promptly provided through positive pressure ventilation with a bag and mask. While positive pressure ventilation is being provided to the depressed infant, the heart rate should also be assessed. If the infant has suffered prolonged asphyxia, the heart rate may be depressed, and bag and mask ventilation may restore a normal heart rate over 100 bpm, accompanied by an improvement in cardiac output.

If after 15 to 30 seconds of positive pressure ventilation the infant's heart rate fails to rise above 80 bpm, chest compressions should be begun at 120 times per minute and continued so as to provide circulatory support, and minimize the effects of hypoperfusion. Furthermore, endotracheal intubation should be promptly performed if the infant is not responding to positive pressure ventilation, or if prolonged positive pressure ventilation is required to support respiration. Even in the moderately depressed infant, restoration of circulation and artificial ventilation will usually dramatically improve color and perfusion before 5 minutes of life, and prolonged cardiorespiratory support may not be necessary.

An ethical issue arises with the infant who appears lifeless at birth with an assigned Apgar score of 0. In a regional report, attempts at reanimation were restricted to those infants who demonstrated signs of life shortly prior to delivery.[86] These were few and far between, when one considers only 93 such resuscitative encounters over a period of 5 years. Only 36 of these survived until discharge and one-third of the long-term survivors were lost to follow-up. Although 61% of those followed appeared to be normal, most had only a brief period of follow-up. This retrospective case collection generated insufficient data to guide the resuscitation teams confronted by the apparently stillborn infant. Their data did suggest that if there was no response to resuscitation within 10 minutes, the prognosis for either life or normal development was hopeless. If the Apgar score is still zero at that point, despite ventilation, cardiac compression and medications, it is probably prudent to discontinue. We recommend that all institutions comply with the guidelines of the American Academy of Pediatrics and the American Heart Association so that each and every delivery is attended by two people skilled in resuscitation of the newborn, and with sole responsibility for the newborn. In this manner, at least there will never be a delay in instituting therapy.

### *Advanced Resuscitation and the Specific Problems of the Severely Depressed Newborn*

The use of medications to support circulation may be required in those rare infants who have a heart rate below 80 bpm despite adequate ventilation and chest compressions for a minimum of 30 seconds, or who have an undetectable heart rate. Epinephrine, volume expanders, and sodium bicarbonate are the medications for advanced newborn resuscitation that should be available in all delivery rooms.

Two routes are available for administration of such medications to a newborn in an emergency. Epinephrine may be given intratracheally, from which site rapid absorption into the circulation occurs. For administration of volume expanders or bicarbonate, placement of an umbilical venous line provides prompt and convenient access.

Epinephrine is the first drug to be considered during advanced resuscitation. Epinephrine increases the strength and rate of cardiac contractions, and may be given at a dose of 0.1–0.3 ml/kg (concentration 1:10 000) by the intravenously or intratracheal route, and repeated every 5 minutes if required. Usually within 15 to 30 seconds, an improvement in heart rate and perfusion occurs.

The severely depressed infant may present with circulatory shock at birth, due to such problems as asphyxia, hemorrhage, sepsis, pulmonary insufficiency or structural heart disease. The antenatal history may give valuable clues allowing anticipation of shock in the infant, eg, if the mother has abruptio placentae, or if severe fetal depression has been diagnosed prior to delivery. Clinical signs of hypovolemia in the infant include pallor, weak pulses, cold extremities, poor capillary refill, poor response to resuscitation, or low blood pressure. In the delivery room, the infant's blood pressure may be measured by the noninvasive dynamap technique, however this may underestimate hypotension in low-birth-weight infants. More accurate monitoring of blood pressure can be achieved by an indwelling umbilical arterial catheter. Tachypnea, poor urine output, metabolic acidosis, and central nervous system depression may also accompany the picture of shock in infants.

The management of shock depends on the underlying mechanism of the hypotension. Three mechanisms which may contribute to shock are decreased blood volume (usually due to perinatal blood loss or twin-to-twin transfusion), decreased cardiac contractility (asphyxia, congenital heart disease) or decreased peripheral vascular resistance (sepsis).

Volume expansion is the first line of treatment of the clinical picture of shock. This is effective for infants with reduced volume due to blood loss as well as septic vasodilated infants with effective reduction of blood volume. The four most commonly used volume expanders are normal saline, 5% albumin/saline, whole blood (cross-matched with mother), and Ringer's lactate. Volume expanders are given intravenously at a dose of 10 ml/kg over 5 to 10 minutes. Care should be taken, however, not to administer excessive fluids to the infant with asphyxia and myocardial dysfunction. In such infants, a combination of fluid administration at the dose indicated above, and use of inotropic agents such as dopamine, dobutamine and Isuprel may yield the best outcome. Within minutes of restoration of peripheral circulation, there may be a remarkable and rapid improvement in blood pressure, color, peripheral perfusion and neurologic state as function is restored to all organ systems.

During prolonged asphyxia, diminished oxygen delivery to the tissues may result in a buildup of lactic acid, with a resultant metabolic acidosis. When ventilation of the asphyxiated infant has been established and metabolic acidosis is documented or strongly suspected on clinical grounds, sodium bicarbonate may be administered intravenously at a dose of 2 mEq/kg of a 0.5 mEq/ml (4.2%)

solution. Resolution of the metabolic acidosis will reverse pulmonary vasoconstriction, and aid in establishment of normal aerobic metabolism. Bicarbonate should not be administered if ventilation has not been established because this will result in an accumulation of $CO_2$ in the blood, and superimpose a respiratory acidosis on a preexisting metabolic acidosis.

Hypoglycemia may accompany profound asphyxia. The provision of glucose is invaluable for the recovery of all tissues of the asphyxiated infant. Therefore, if asphyxia is suspected, the serum glucose level should be promptly assessed and intravenous glucose infusion provided so as to normalize glucose concentration in the blood.

## Birth Injuries

Birth injuries are not entirely avoidable and may follow the most skilled and careful obstetric care. The fetus may be injured during amniocentesis, cordocentesis, intrauterine transfusions, surgical procedures in utero, or even with the scalp electrode during labor.[18,54] Labor and delivery account for the bulk of birth injuries, which occur in 2 to 7 per 1000 live births. The infants at greatest risk are macrosomic, premature, or those with an abnormal presentation.[87] Gross prolonged labor, dystocia, and cephalopelvic disproportion predispose to injury as does instrumental intervention with forceps or vacuum extractor. Delivery by caesarean section is no guarantee against birth trauma. During a breech presentation the brachial plexus may be injured as a result of traction on the shoulder when delivery of the head is attempted.

In infants delivered in the breech position, there is a three-fold increase in perinatal mortality rate and admissions into neonatal intensive care units. There is a 12-fold increase in neonatal depression, as defined by a low Apgar score, in those infants delivered in the breech position.[88] In a prospective trial, external cephalic version reduced the frequency of breech position in labor and also the need for abdominal delivery. The versions were well tolerated by the mothers as well as the fetuses and by convention the procedure had a success rate of 83%. Even with the use of inexperienced personnel the procedure can be accomplished in less than 5 minutes. This represents a means of reducing operative deliveries and birth trauma.

Most cases of brachial palsy follow prolonged labor and difficult deliveries in which traction is exerted on the neck.[89] To quantitate the forces applied to the fetal head during delivery of the shoulders, engineers and obstetricians joined forces. The obstetrician was hot-wired with sensors on his fingers and the force determined by applying the same sensors against a precalibrated strain gauge load cell. Remarkably, two shoulder dystocias were encountered during a small series of 29 random births. (Shoulder dystocia complicates 0.15% to 2% of vaginal births, more frequently if there is fetal macrosomia, and lateral traction on the head and neck away from one of the shoulders may injure the nerves.)[87–91] A wide range of forces was applied to the fetus, with the force increasing as the deliveries increased in difficulty. Injury to the fetus was associated with a higher impulse and considerably higher peak force. Thus, the obstetrician must be trained in force perception, bearing in mind that the faster the force is applied the more vulnerable is the newborn to injury.[89]

Infants with Erb's palsy will hold the hand limply alongside the body with the forearm pronated. The affected limb does not move, the Moro reflex is asymmetric, and the tendon reflexes cannot be elicited; however, the grasp reflex remains intact. Treatment is expectant with physiotherapy and appropriate splinting. Recovery is usually complete within 3 to 6 months. If recovery is delayed, operative intervention is available.

Injuries and palsies may also occur in utero, in the absence of any external forces. These are often symmetric and bilateral, and multiple nerves are involved.

### Respiratory Disorders

The respiratory system plays a critical role in successful early adaptation to extrauterine life. Interruption of the fetal-placental circulation at birth requires the newborn infant to immediately achieve gas exchange and undergo major circulatory changes. This section will be confined to disorders in maturation of the developing lung, pulmonary hypoplasia, congenital diaphragmatic hernia, an anatomic disorder which must be recognized in the delivery room, and a brief consideration of primary pulmonary hypertension or persistence of the fetal circulation.

## Respiratory Distress Syndrome[92]

Respiratory disorders are the major cause of mortality and morbidity in the newborn period. Respiratory distress syndrome (RDS) is the most common disorder, although the lack of a precise clinical definition necessitates cautious interpretation of statistics regarding its incidence and associated outcome. The diagnosis can be established biochemically by documentation of surfactant deficiency in amniotic fluid, tracheal or gastric aspirate, but this is rarely done and a combination of clinical and radiological diagnosis is used.

Respiratory distress syndrome is encountered most commonly in immature infants, infants of diabetic mothers, and following perinatal asphyxia. Gestational age is the key determinant; hence, approximately 70% of infants less than 28 weeks gestation will manifest RDS.

Infants with RDS typically present with a combination of cyanosis, grunting, tachypnea, flaring, and retractions. These are not distinguishing features and may also be observed with hypothermia, hypoglycemia, anemia, polycythemia, and metabolic acidosis, together with a wide array of pulmonary parenchymal and nonpulmonary disorders. To avoid serious diagnostic errors, a broad and flexible approach to the infant presenting with these features is necessary. Review of the pregnancy history, delivery and neonatal transition is necessary in addition to careful observation and physical examination of the infant. The initial laboratory screen requires an arterial blood gas, complete blood count and differential, blood culture and blood sugar in addition to appropriate roentgenographic studies. In this manner, the underlying cause of the respiratory distress can easily be discerned. The typical roentgenographic features of surfactant deficiency consist of a diffuse reticulogranular pattern in both lung fields with superimposed air bronchograms. It is not possible to distinguish between surfactant deficiency and pneumonia, particularly due to group B streptococci; hence the widespread use of antibiotics in treating infants with respiratory disorders.[92]

Impaired or delayed surfactant synthesis is the key element in the pathogenesis of RDS. The resultant decrease in lung compliance leads to alveolar hypoventilation and ventilation perfusion imbalance. The resultant hypoxemia may cause a metabolic acidosis, and both may contribute to pulmonary vasoconstriction. Surfactant replacement therapy has become the cornerstone of therapy for infants with RDS.

The ability to replace surfactant has resulted in substantial improvements in survival rates and reduced the morbidity for infants with respiratory distress syndrome. All regimens of surfactant therapy appear to improve oxygenation of preterm infants, decrease the incidence of air leaks, and reduce mortality.[93–97] It is still debated whether prophylactic therapy, wherein many infants who would not require therapy are treated with surfactant, is superior to rescue therapy, ie, treating infants who meet specific criteria. Earlier therapy, however, may be beneficial in reducing bronchopulmonary dysplasia.[98] The incidence of patent ductus arteriosus and intraventricular hemorrhage appears unaltered by surfactant administration. Pulmonary hemorrhage appears to be increased in lower-birth-weight infants receiving surfactant. The use of surfactant therapy is also being investigated in term infants with meconium aspiration syndrome, pneumonia, and pulmonary hypertension.[99] (Table 45–13)

Assisted ventilation has also contributed considerably to improving the outcome of infants with respiratory failure. In neonates with RDS, the pulmonary mechanics are rapidly changing, and appropriate ventilatory changes are determined from the blood gases. Oxygenation is dependent upon the mean airway pressure and the matching of ventilation with perfusion. Carbon dioxide elimination is adjusted by altering rates and pressure.[100] New modes of assisted ventilation gradients (including high-frequency jet ventilation and high-frequency oscillation) deliver small volumes of gas at high frequencies and limit the development of high airway pressure which may contribute to lung injury. However, neither high frequency or jet ventilation have reduced the incidence of bronchopulmonary dysplasia or the mortality rate in controlled trials.[101,102]

In summary, surfactant replacement therapy represents a major advance in the care of infants with respiratory disorders. Maintenance of a neutral thermal environment, nutritional support, and a gentle approach to mechanical ventilation are other components which have led to the improved overall outcome for infants with respiratory disorders.

### *Pulmonary Hypoplasia*[48–52]

(See also Disorders of Amniotic Fluid—Oligohydramnios)

Pulmonary hypoplasia may be unilateral or bilateral and occurs as an isolated entity or secondary to disorders or anomalies which restrict lung growth. Bilateral pulmonary hypoplasia occurs most commonly in association with oligohydramnios secondary to renal disease in the fetus or premature and prolonged leakage of amniotic fluid. Accompanying clinical features include a characteristic appearance of the skull and face, limb deformities, and severe respiratory insufficiency often manifesting with air leaks.

Unilateral pulmonary hypoplasia is seen most often in infants with a diaphragmatic hernia. The clinical course is dependent upon the extent of the hernia and other accompanying malformations. The prognosis is worse if there has been polyhydramnios, other major malformations, or if the liver has herniated into the thorax.[103]

**Table 45–13.** Typical Odds Ratios and 95% Confidence Intervals (CI) For the Effects of Surfactants in Prophylaxis and Treatment Trials

| | N | Odds Ratio | 95% CI | N | Odds Ratio | 95% CI |
|---|---|---|---|---|---|---|
| *Prophylaxis* | Natural Surfactant | | Synthetic Surfactant | | | |
| Neonatal death | 9 | 0.55 | 0.38–0.80 | 7 | 0.65 | 0.50–0.86 |
| PTX | 9 | 0.31 | 0.22–0.44 | 3 | 0.62 | 0.40–0.96 |
| IVH | 7 | 0.90 | 0.62–1.30 | 2 | 0.87 | 0.60–1.27 |
| PDA | 8 | 1.17 | 0.88–1.57 | 4 | 1.33 | 1.01–1.75 |
| BPD | 6 | 0.59 | 0.40–0.86 | 6 | 0.99 | 0.75–1.31 |
| Death or BPD | 6 | 0.43 | 0.30–0.63 | 3 | 0.84 | 0.64–1.09 |
| *Treatment* | Natural Surfactant | | Synthetic Surfactant | | | |
| Neonatal death | 13 | 0.60 | 0.47–0.76 | 5 | 0.61 | 0.46–0.80 |
| PTX | 12 | 0.34 | 0.26–0.43 | 4 | 0.52 | 0.42–0.65 |
| IVH | 9 | 0.93 | 0.68–1.27 | 2 | 0.83 | 0.65–1.05 |
| PDA | 10 | 1.14 | 0.85–1.53 | 3 | 0.72 | 0.60–0.87 |
| Death or BPD | 9 | 0.61 | 0.45–0.84 | 3 | 0.56 | 0.45–0.72 |

N = number of trials; PTX = pneumothorax; IVH = intraventricular hemorrhage; PDA = patent ductus arteriosus; BPD = bronchopulmonary dysplasia.
(From Halliday HL: Yearbook, 1991, p. xiii, with permission.)

### *Congenital Diaphragmatic Hernia*[103–107]

Persistent cyanosis and a scaphoid abdomen in a cyanotic infant who has been intubated is the classical presentation of a congenital diaphragmatic hernia. Most commonly, hernias involve the left diaphragm, and the cardiac impulse and sounds are shifted to the right with the abdominal contents present in the thorax. When the hernia is on the right side, the diagnosis is more difficult because the clinical signs are not as striking. An x-ray is mandatory in any infant who does not respond to cardiopulmonary resuscitation. When a diaphragmatic hernia is confirmed, the infant should be intubated and mechanically ventilated. Bag-and-mask ventilation are contraindicated, as this will further distend the bowel and compromise ventilation. A nasogastric tube must be placed immediately to decompress the gastrointestinal tract.

The surgical approach to the infant with a congenital diaphragmatic hernia is being reevaluated. Until relatively recently congenital diaphragmatic hernia has been treated as a surgical emergency. However, the reduction of the viscera from the chest did not always improve oxygenation, hypercapnea persisted and thoracic compliance worsened following repair.[104] The mortality remained substantial. Delayed operative intervention was advocated and outcome was not adversely affected by delays of 4 to 24 hours.[105,106] An evaluation of delayed repair and preoperative extracorporeal membrane oxygenation versus immediate operation did not improve survival in 101 high risk congenital diaphragmatic hernias. There were however, fewer late deaths and pulmonary sequelae with the delayed repair.[107]

### *Primary Pulmonary Hypertension*

The syndrome of persistent fetal circulation or primary pulmonary hypertension is characterized by pulmonary hypertension with right-to-left shunting at either the foramen ovale, ductus arteriosus or both. Persistent fetal circulation is associated with perinatal asphyxia, meconium aspiration syndrome, pulmonary hypoplasia, neonatal sepsis, hyperviscosity secondary to polycythemia, and hypoglycemia. Echocardiographic assessment distinguishes pulmonary hypertension from structural congenital heart disease. The diagnosis of even the most complex congenital heart disease can be established by a constellation of noninvasive techniques including echocardiography with color flow sequencing and magnetic resonance imaging. Precise diagnosis is necessary, particularly if surgical intervention is needed. The surgical techniques continue to improve so that formerly lethal congenital cardiac malformations are being tackled with some degree of confidence.

Extracorporeal membrane oxygenation (ECMO) is an innovative technique that has dramatically changed the outcome for selective infants with intractable respiratory failure and pulmonary hypertension. Perfusion and gas exchange are maintained by means of veno-arterial or veno-venous cardiopulmonary bypass through a membrane lung. ECMO has rescued moribund infants with respiratory failure from a variety of causes. In the past decade, 83% of 3528 infants so treated have survived. These infants had a predicted mortality rate of >80%. The infants were placed on ECMO because of persistent hypoxemia (a-$AdO_2$ >600 for 6–8 hours, oxygenation index >40 for 4 hours), or acute deterioration despite maximal therapy including hyperventilation, pressors, tolazoline, etc. The survival rates on ECMO depended on the underlying cause of respiratory failure; hence, 93% of the infants with meconium aspiration survived, 84% with respiratory distress syndrome, 77% with sepsis, 83% with persistent pulmonary hypertension of the newborn with no clear etiology,[108] and 63% of infants with congenital diaphragmatic hernia (Table 45–14)

**Table 45–14.** ECMO Registry

| Aggregate Survival By Diagnosis | N | Survival | Survival % |
|---|---|---|---|
| Meconium Aspiration Syndrome | 1356 | 1262 | 93 |
| Hyaline Membrane Disease | 532 | 446 | 84 |
| Congenital Diphragmatic Hernia | 585 | 364 | 62 |
| Sepsis | 416 | 321 | 77 |
| Persistent Pulmonary Hypertension of the Newborn | 480 | 414 | 86 |
| Other | 156 | 120 | 77 |

(From Stolar CJH, Snedecor SM, Bartlett RH: Extracorporeal membrane oxygenation and neonatal respiratory failure: Experience from the extracorporeal life support organization. J. Peds. Surg. 26:563–571, 1991, with permission.)

## Infection

### *Overview*

The overall incidence of septicemia is 2 to 5 per 1000 live births. However, among infants with a birth weight under 1500 grams, the rate exceeds 10% and is inversely related to gestational age. A high index of suspicion has resulted in early diagnosis and vigorous intervention with supportive care and broad spectrum antibiotics. Nonetheless, sepsis contributes to the ongoing morbidity, and the mortality rates have decreased slowly in the past decade.[109] Despite the availability of effective and broad spectrum antibiotics, sepsis contributes in a major way to the morbidity and mortality of low-birth-weight infants who, as a result of improved survival rates, have prolonged hospital stays and multiple invasive procedures which render them vulnerable to nosocomial infections.[1,3] The mortality risk remains 20% to 30% for gram-negative sepsis and is far greater in the presence of hypotension or multiple organ dysfunction.

Defects in the immune system predispose the newborn to higher rates of infection. They include neutrophil-functional defects such as impaired chemotaxis, abnormal opsonic activity, reduced phagocytosis, and bactericidal activity and defects in the complement pathway.[110] The preterm infant is further handicapped by reduced levels of circulating immunoglobulins which traverse the placenta in the latter stages of the third trimester.

The amniotic fluid provides a sterile intrauterine environment supplemented by phagocytic activity. Premature rupture of the membranes breaches this environment and exposes the infant to organisms colonizing the birth canal. Pathogenic organisms may also reach the fetus via the blood stream. Maternal viral infections, for example, may spread to the fetus resulting in intrauterine infection with a broad range of sequelae. The rubella syndrome and cytomegalovirus infections are prime examples of this manner of transmission. Other viruses may first reach the fetus during the birthing process and subsequently result in acute or chronic changes. Herpes and hepatitis B fit into this category.

Group B streptococci remain the principal organisms responsible for neonatal septicemia and meningitis in the term newborn. The organism colonizes approximately 30% of pregnant women, yet the attack rate for the newborn remains <1%, perhaps due to passive acquisition of protective antibody. Early onset streptococcal disease is more common with maternal fever, prolonged rupture of membranes, prematurity, and multiple pregnancy. Symptoms of infection include lethargy, poor feeding, temperature instability-tachypnea, abdominal distension and hypoglycemia. Infants may present with apnea, respiratory distress, shock or even seizures. The complete blood count may reveal leucocytosis, neutropenia or a shift to the left with an elevated band count and thrombocytopenia. The early initiation of antibiotic therapy has improved the outcome for this illness.[110–112]

## Perinatal Human Immunodeficiency Virus Infection

The newborn with human immunodeficiency virus (HIV) infection is not currently identifiable in the nursery. All babies of HIV-infected women have antibodies to HIV. It is the rare baby that has clinical or laboratory findings diagnostic of infection in the newborn period. However, there are suggestive maternal behaviors which indicate that the infant may be at risk. Hence, infants of women with syphilis, herpes, or those who abuse drugs are at greatest risk.[113]

About 30% of the infants of HIV-infected women will be infected with the virus. The infants may also acquire the virus through breast feeding. An embryopathy with growth failure, microcephaly, and distinct facial features including a box-like appearance of the forehead, ocular hypertelorism, and a short nose with patulous lips was reported.[114] The features closely resemble the fetal alcohol syndrome and the embryopathy concept has been rejected. A cardiomyopathy has also been observed.[115] Other features to look for include resistant oral thrush, lymphadenopathy and pneumonitis. These tend to appear beyond the neonatal period.

Infants born of HIV-positive mothers are generally treated like other infants in the nursery. They are, however, closely followed to ascertain whether they have the disease, so that therapy can be instituted in a timely fashion.[116]

In summary, there is a high rate of transmission of virus from mother to infant but no single test which can confirm true infection in infants born to infected mothers.

## Immunoglobulin Therapy for Neonatal Sepsis

Whereas there is a sound rationale for the administration of intravenous immunoglobulin (IVIG) to immature infants, there have been major concerns about its infusion into septic neonates. This stems from neonatal animal studies wherein mortality has been increased by combining IVIG with antibiotics for septicemia. It has been postulated that high doses of IVIG could cause blockade of the Fc receptors of the reticulo-endothelial system. In the premature infant, already a compromised host with impaired defenses, this might delay the clearance of pathogenic organisms. Also, the immune complexes resulting from the rapid infusion of antibodies directed to an infecting organism could cause the release of inflammatory mediators, resulting in more serious illness, or could deposit in the tissues of the lung and kidney causing subsequent tissue damage. Nonetheless, there is animal data to show augmentation of the opsonic and bactericidal capability of neonatal sera with the addition of IVIG.

There have been few reports of IVIG therapy for fetuses with suspected infection or neonates with established bacterial sepsis. The reports may be criticized as they are not well-controlled randomized prospective studies. However, the primary outcome variable has been mortality, and the preliminary results support the hypothesis that the administration of IVIG to neonates with sepsis might result in a more rapid clearance of bacteria and a lower mortality rate. Consequently there may be a role for adjunctive immunoglobulin therapy particularly in septic preterm infants.

Sidiropoulos[117] administered immunoglobulin G (IgG) to mothers with chorioamnionitis who were at risk for preterm delivery and demonstrated that IgG traversed the placenta after 32 weeks gestation. Those infants delivered prior to 32 weeks showed no increment in their cord serum IgG levels. However, the infants beyond 32 weeks gestation had dose-dependent increments of all classes of IgG and the transplacental passage of specific antibodies could be proven. All babies delivered prior to 32 weeks gestation had clinical, laboratory or radiologic evidence of infection and required antibiotic therapy, irrespective of the treatment given the mother. None of the babies delivered after 32 weeks gestation in whom the mothers received high dose IVIG had evidence of infection.

The initial reports of the successful use of intravenous immunoglobulin therapy for neonates with bacterial sepsis can also be attributed to Sidiropoulos, who reported that by supplementing antibiotic therapy with daily IVIG (15 ml/day if birth weight <2500 grams and 30 ml/day if birth weight >2500 grams) for 6 days, a lower mortality was noted in the infants <2500 grams, 1/13 (compared with 4/9 if the infants received antibiotics along [P = *04]). Haque[118] reported on a series of 44 septic infants from Saudi Arabia randomized to receive Pentaglobulin (IgG with IgA and IgM). Four of the 17 placebo recipients died, compared with 1 of the 21 infants treated with Pentaglobulin (P >0.1). Thirty-nine of the infants were infected with gram negative organisms. This is very different from the prevailing nosocomial pathogens in the United States which are gram-positive cocci, mainly coagulase-negative staphylococci and streptococcal species.

Another small series involved the administration of 800 mg Sandoglobulin/kg/day for up to four doses, to 12 presumed septic neonates with neutropenia and positive latex agglutination for group B streptococci. Two (17%) of these infants died in contrast with 7 (58%) of the infants treated with supportive care and antibiotics alone. Although this is statistically significant (P <.05), the series is small, the controls were selected post hoc, and the data are supportive of the administration of IVIG to septic neonates with group B streptococcal septicemia with neutropenia.[119,120] This demonstrated a dramatic improvement in the neutrophil response and a marked shift to the left in presumed septic neutropenic neonates treated with intravenous immunoglobulin. Concerns about reticuloendothelial blockade if IVIG is administered to septic neonates have not materialized.

Weisman[121] randomized 753 neonates between 500 and 2000 grams to receive 500 mg/kg of Sandoglobulin (n = 372) or albumin (n = 381) before 12 hours of life. Thirty-one infants enrolled were septic at the time of the initial infusion. In the placebo group, death from sepsis was observed in 5 of the 17 infants (29%), whereas only 1 of the 14 IVIG recipients (7%) died. If the post-infusion serum IgG level was >800 mg (n = 11), no deaths occurred, whereas 7 out of 20 (35%) neonates with values <800 mg/dl (35%) died (P < −05). This series implies that there is a critical serum IgG level.

In summary, the administration of intravenous immunoglobulin to preterm septic neonates has been accomplished without obvious side effects and appears to improve outcome. Further trials are needed to establish whether adjunctive IVIG is efficacious and whether there is a critical serum IgG level necessary to reduce the mortality and morbidity from sepsis. There is insufficient data at present to establish the efficacy of the therapy.

## REFERENCES


1. Martin RJ, Fanaroff AA (eds): Neonatal-Perinatal Medicine: "Diseases of the Fetus and Infant, Ed 5. St. Louis, Mosby Year Book, 1992.
2. Campbell MK, Chance GW, Natale R, Dodman N, et al: Is perinatal care in southwestern Ontario regionalized? Can. Med. Assoc. J. 144:305–312, 1991.
3. Hack M, Horbar JD, Malloy MH, Tyson JE, et al: Very low birth weight outcomes of the NICHD Network. Pediatrics 87:587–597, 1991.
4. Paneth N, Kiely L, Wallenstein S, Susser M: The choice of place of delivery: Effect of hospital level on mortality in all singleton births in New York City. AJDC 141:60–64, 1987.
5. Fretts RC, Boyd ME, Usher RH, Usher HA: The changing pattern of fetal death, 1961–1988. Obstet. Gynecol. 79: 35–39, 1992.
6. Laurin J, Persson P-H: The effect of bedrest in hospital on fetal outcome in pregnancies complicated by intra-uterine growth retardation. Acta. Obstet. Gynecol. Scand. 66: 407–411, 1987.
7. Bouyer J, Papiernik E, Dreyfus J: Prevention of preterm birth and perinatal risk reduction. Isr. J. Med. Sci. 22: 313–317, 1986.
8. Milunsky A, Jick SS, Bruell CL, MacLaughlin DS, et al: Predictive values, relative risks and overall benefits of high and low maternal alpha fetoprotein screening in singleton pregnancies. New epidemiologic data. Am. J. Obstet. Gynecol. 161:291–297, 1989.
9. Moore TR, Piacquadio K: A prospective assessment of fetal movement screening to reduce fetal mortality. Am. J. Obstet. Gynecol. 160:1075, 1989.
10. Grant A, Elbourne D, Valentin L, Alexander S: Routine formal fetal movement counting and risk of antepartum late death in normally formed singletons. Lancet 2:345–349, 1989.
11. Saari-Kemppainen A, Karjalainen O, Ylostalo P, Heinonen OP: Ultrasound screening and perinatal mortality: Controlled trial of systematic one-stage screening in pregnancy (The Helsinki Ultrasound Trial). Lancet 336:387–391, 1990.
12. Waldenstrom U, Axelsson O, Nilsson S, Eklund G, et al: Effects of routine one-stage ultrasound screening in pregnancy: A randomized controlled trial. Lancet 2:585–588, 1988.
13. Brar HS, Platt LD, Paul RH: Fetal umbilical blood flow velocity waveforms using Doppler ultrasonography in patients with late decelerations. Obstet. Gynecol. 73: 363–366, 1989.
14. Brar HS, Medearis AL, DeVore GR, Platt LD: A comparative study of fetal umbilical velocimetry with continuous and pulsed-wave Doppler ultrasongraphy in high-risk pregnancies: Relationship to outcome. Am. J. Obstet. Gynecol. 160: 375–387, 1989.
15. Steel SA, Pearce JM, McParland P, Chamberlain GVP: Early doppler ultrasound screening in prediction of hypertensive disorders of pregnancy. Lancet 335:1548–1551, 1990.
16. Lombardi SJ, Rosemond R, Ball R, Entman SS, et al: Umbilical artery velocimetry as a predictor of adverse outcome in pregnancies complicated by oligohydramnios. Obstet. Gynecol. 74:338–341, 1989.
17. Daffos F, Capello-Pavlovsky M, Forestier F: Fetal blood sampling during pregnancy with use of needle guided by ultrasound: A study of 606 consecutive cases. Am. J. Obstet. Gynecol. 153:655, 1985.
18. Orlandi F, Damiani G, Jakil C, Lauricella S, et al: The risks of early cordocentesis (12–21 weeks): Analysis of 500 procedures. Prenat. Diag. 10:425–428, 1990.
19. Zuspan FP, Macgillivray I, Gant N, et al: (members of the Hypertension in Pregnancy Working Group): National High Blood Pressure in Pregnancy. Am. J. Obstet. Gynecol. 163:1689–1712, 1990.
20. Zuspan FP: The hypertensive disorders of pregnancy: Report of WHO study group. Technical report series 758. Geneva WHO, 1987.
21. Campbell S: Fetal growth. *In* Beard R, Nathanielsz P (eds): Fetal Physiology and Medicine: The Basis of Perinatology. Edited by R Beard, P Nathanielsz. Philadelphia, WB Saunders Co, 1976.
22. Barton JR, Sibai BM: Low dose aspirin therapy to improve perinatal outcome. Clin. Obstet. Gynecol. 34:251–261, 1991.
23. Sibai BM, Mirro R, Chesney CM: Low dose aspirin in pregnancy. Obstet. Gynecol. 74:551–557, 1989.
24. Uzan S, Beaufils M, Breart G, Bazin B, et al: Prevention of fetal growth retardation with low-dose aspirin: Finding of the EPREDA trial. Lancet 337:1427–1431, 1991.
25. Wallenberg HCS, Rotmans N: Prevention of recurrent fetal growth retardation. Lancet 1:939, 1988.
26. Jovanovic-Peterson L, Peterson CM, Reed GF, Metzger BE, et al: Maternal postprandial glucose levels and infant birth weight: The diabetes in early pregnancy study. Am. J. Obstet. Gynecol. 164:103–111, 1991.
27. Steel JM, Johnstone FD, Hepburn DA, Smith AF: Can pre-

pregnancy care of diabetic women reduce the risk of abnormal babies? Br. Med. J. 301:1070–1074, 1990.
28. Mills JL, Knapp RH, Simpson JL, Jovanovic-Peterson L, et al: Lack of relation of increased malformation rates in infants of diabetic mothers to glycemic control during organogenesis. N. Engl. J. Med. 318:671–676, 1988.
29. Brunskill AJ, Rossing MA, Connell FA, Daling J: Antecedents of macrosomia. Pediatr. Perinat. Epidem. 5:392–401, 1991.
30. Veille JC, Sivakoff M, Hanson R, Fanaroff A: Intraventricular septal thickness of fetuses of diabetic mothers. Am. J. Obstet. Gynecol. 79:51–4, 1992.
31. Chasnoff IJ: Drug use and women: Establishing a standard of care. Ann. NY Acad. Sci. 562:208–210, 1989.
32. Ostrea EM Jr, Brady M, Gause S, Raymundo AL, et al: Drug screening of newborns by meconium analysis: A large-scale prospective, epidemiologic study. Pediatrics 89:107–113, 1992.
33. Chasnoff IJ, Burns WJ, Schnoll SH, et al: Cocaine use in pregnancy. N. Engl. J. Med. 313:666–669, 1985.
34. Keith LG, MacGregor S, Friedell S, Rosner M, et al: Substance abuse in pregnant women: Recent experience at the Perinatal Center for Chemical Dependence of Northwestern Memorial Hospital. Obstet. Gynecol. 73:715–720, 1989.
35. Chavez GF, Mulinare J, Cordero JF: Maternal cocaine use during early pregnancy as a risk factor for congenital urogenital anomalies. JAMA 262:795–798, 1989.
36. Volpe JJ: Effects of cocaine on the fetus. N. Engl. J. Med. 327:339–407, 1992.
37. Ryan L, Ehrlich S, Finnegan L: Cocaine abuse in pregnancy: Effects on the fetus and newborn. Neurotoxicol. Teratol. 9:295–299, 1987.
38. Ostrea EM Jr, Brady MJ, Parks PM, Asensio DC, et al: Drug screening of meconium in infants of drug-dependent mothers: An alternative to urine testing. J. Pediatr. 115: 474–477, 1989.
39. Hill LM, Breckle R, Thomas ML: Polyhydramnios: Ultrasonically detected prevalence and neonatal outcome. Obstet. Gynecol. 69:21–25, 1987.
40. Hill LM: Resolving polyhydramnios: A sign of improved fetal status. Am. J. Perinatol. 5:61–63, 1988.
41. Alexander EX, Spintz HP, Clark RA: Sonography of polyhydramnios. Am. J. Roentgenol. 138:343, 1982.
42. Chamberlain PF, Manning F, Morrison I, et al: Ultrasound evidence of amniotic fluid volume: II. The relationship of increased amniotic fluid to perinatal outcome. Am. J. Obstet. Gynecol. 150:250–254, 1984.
43. Phelan JP, Smith CV, Broussard P, et al: Amniotic fluid assessment with four quadrant technique at 36–42 weeks gestation. J. Reprod. Med. 32:540–42, 1987.
44. Carlson D, Platt L, Mederis A, et al: Quantifiable polyhydramnios: Diagnosis and treatment. Obstet. Gynecol. 75: 989–993, 1990.
45. Trimmer KJ, Leveno KJ, Peters MT, Kelley MA: Observations on the Cause of Oligohydramnios in Prolonged Pregnancy. Am. J. Obstet. Gynecol. 163:1900–1903, 1990.
46. Batside A, Manning F, Harman C, et al: Ultrasound evaluation of amniotic fluid: Outcome of pregnancies with severe oligohydramnios. Am. J. Obstet. Gynecol. 154:895, 1986.
47. Chamberlain PF, Manning F, Morrison I, et al: Ultrasound evidence of amniotic fluid volume: I. The relationship of marginal and decreased amniotic fluid volumes to perinatal outcome. Am. J. Obstet. Gynecol. 150:245–250, 1984.
48. Rotschild A, Ling EW, Puterman ML, Farquharson D: Neonatal outcome after prolonged preterm rupture of membranes. Am. J. Obstet. Gynecol. 162:46–52, 1990.
49. Roberts AB, Mitchell JM: Direct ultrasonographic measurement of fetal lung length in normal pregnancies and pregnancies complicated by prolonged rupture of membranes. Am. J. Obstet. Gynecol. 163:1560–1566, 1990.
50. Nimrod C, Davies D, Iwanicki S, et al: Ultrasound prediction of pulmonary hypoplasia. Obstet. Gynecol. 68:495, 1986.
51. Kilbride HW, Yeast JD, Thibeault DW: Intrapartum and delivery room management of premature rupture of membranes complicated by oligohydramnios. Clinics in Perinatology 16:863–888, 1989.
52. Blott M, Greenough A, Nicolaides KH, Campbell S: The ultrasonographic assessment of the fetal thorax and fetal breathing movements in the prediction of pulmonary hypoplasia. Early Hum. Dev. 21:143–151, 1990.
53. Manning FA, Harman CR, Morrison I, Menticoglou S, et al: Fetal assessment based on fetal biophysical profile scoring. IV: An analysis of perinatal morbidity and mortality. Am. J. Obstet. Gynecol. 162:703–709, 1990.
54. Grant A: Monitoring the Fetus During Labour. *In* Effective Care in Pregnancy and Childbirth. Edited by I Chalmers, M Enkin, M Keirse. New York, Oxford University Press, 1990, p. 855.
55. Ohlsson A: Treatments of premature rupture of membranes: A meta-analysis. Am. J. Obstet. Gynecol. 160: 890–906, 1989.
56. Gregory G, Gooding CA, Phibbs RH, et al: Meconium aspiration in infants—a prospective study. J. Pediatr. 85:848, 1974.
57. Ting P, Brady J: Tracheal suction in meconium aspiration. Am. J. Obstet. Gynecol. 122:767, 1975.
58. Carson BS, Losey RW, Bowes WA Jr, et al: Combined pediatric and obstetric approach to prevent meconium aspiration syndrome. Am. J. Obstet. Gynecol. 126:712, 1976.
59. Davis RO, Philips JB, Harris BA Jr, et al: Fatal meconium aspiration syndrome occurring despite airway management considered appropriate. Am. J. Obstet. Gynecol. 151: 731, 1985.
60. Falciglia HS: Failure to prevent meconium aspiration syndrome. Obstet. Gynecol. 71:349, 1988.
61. Falciglia HS, Henderschott C, Potter P, Helmchen R: Does DeLee suction at the perineum prevent meconium aspiration syndrome. Am. J. Obstet. Gynecol. 167:1243–1249, 1992.
62. Wiswell TE, Tuggle JM, Turner BS: Meconium aspiration syndrome: Have we made a difference? Pediatrics 85: 715–721, 1990.
63. Rossi EM, Philipson EH, Williams TG, et al: Meconium aspiration syndrome: intrapartum and neonatal attributes. Am. J. Obstet. Gynecol. 161:1106, 1989.
64. Murphy JD, Vawter GF, Reid LM: Pulmonary vascular disease in fetal meconium aspiration. J. Pediatr. 104:758, 1984.
65. Linder N, Aranda JV, Tsur M, et al: Need for endotracheal intubation and suction in meconium-stained neonates. J. Pediatr. 112:613, 1988.
66. Miyazaki FS, Nevarez F: Saline amnioinfusion for relief of repetitive variable decelerations: A prospective randomized study. Am. J. Obstet. Gynecol. 153:301, 1985.
67. Nageotte MP, Freeman RK, Garite TJ, et al: Prophylactic intrapartum amnioinfusion in patients with premature rupture of membranes. Am. J. Obstet. Gynecol. 153:557, 1985.
68. Nageotte MP, Bertucci L, Towers CV, Lagrew DL, et al: Prophylactic amnioinfusion infusion in pregnancies complicated by oligohydramnios: A prospective study. Obstet. Gynecol. 77:677–680, 1991.
69. Sadovsky Y, Amon E, Bade ME, et al: Prophylactic amnioin-

fusion during labor complicated by meconium: A preliminary report. SPO #18, 1989.

70. Wenstrom KD, Parsons MT: The prevention of meconium aspiration in labor using amnioinfusion. Obstet. Gynecol. 73:647, 1989.

71. Fisk NM, Ronderos-Dumit D, Soliani A, Nicolini U, et al: Diagnostic and therapeutic transabdominal amniotransfusion in oligohydramnios. Obstet. Gynecol. 78:270–278, 1991.

72. Nathan DG, Oski FA, (eds): Hematology of Infancy and Childhood, Ed 2. Philadelphia, WB Saunders Co, 1981.

73. Moya ER, Perez A, Reece EA: Severe fetomaternal hemorrhage: A report of 4 cases. J. Reprod. Med. 32:243, 1987.

74. Wegman ME: Annual Summary of Vital Statistics—1991. Pediatrics 90:835–845, 1992.

75. Halperin DS: Use of recombinant erythropoietin in treatment of the anemia of prematurity. Am. Journal. Ped. Hem./Onc. 13:351–363, 1991.

76. Halperin DS, Wacker P, Lacourt G, Felix M, et al: Effects of recombinant human erythropoietin in infants with the anemia of prematurity: A pilot study. J. Pediatr. 116: 779–786, 1990.

77. Heese H de V, Smith S, Watermeyer S, Dempster WS, et al: Prevention of iron deficiency in preterm neonates during infancy. S. Afr. Med. J. 77:339–345, 1990.

78. Beardsley DS: Immune thrombocytopenia in the perinatal period. Seminars in Perinatology: Perinatal Hematology 14: 368–373, 1990.

79. Kaplan C, Daffos F, Forestier F, et al: Antenatal treatment of alloimmune thrombocytopenia: Antenatal diagnosis and in-utero transfusion of maternal platelets. Blood 70: 340–343, 1988.

80. Bussel J, Berkowitz R, McFarland J, et al: Antenatal treatment of neonatal alloimmune thrombocytopenia. N. Engl. J. Med. 319:1374–1378, 1988.

81. Andrew M, Castle V, Saigal S, Carter G, Kelton JG: Clinical impact of neonatal thrombocytopenia. J. Pediatr. 110: 457–464, 1987.

82. Hack M, Fanaroff AA: Changes in the delivery room of the extremely small infant (<750 gram): Effects on morbidity and outcome. N. Engl. J. Med. 314:660, 1986.

83. Standards for CPR and ECC, Part VII: Neonatal advanced life support. JAMA 268:2276, 1992.

84. Bloom RS, Cropley C: Textbook of Neonatal Resuscitation. American Heart Association/American Academy of Pediatrics. American Heart Association, 1987.

85. Freeman RK, Poland RL (eds): Antepartum and Intrapartum Care. *In* Guidelines for Perinatal Care, Ed 3. Elk Grove Village, American Academy of Pediatrics, 1992.

86. Jain L, Ferre C, Vidyasagar D, Nath S, et al: Cardiopulmonary resuscitation of apparently-stillborn infants: Survival and long-term outcome. J. Pediatr. 118:778–782, 1991.

87. Gross TL, Sokol RJ, Williams T, Thompson K: Shoulder dystocia: A fetal-physician risk. Am. J. Obstet. Gynecol. 156: 1408–1414, 1987.

88. Mohamed K, Seeras R, Coulson R: External cephalic version at term: A randomized controlled trial using tocolysis. Br. J. Obstet. Gynaecol. 98:8–13, 1991.

89. Allen R, Sorab J, Gonik B: Risk factors for shoulder dystocia: An engineering study of clinician-applied forces. Obstet. Gynecol. 77:352–355, 1991.

90. Gonik B, Hollyer VL, Allen R: Shoulder dystocia recognition: Differences in neonatal risk for injury. Am. J. Perinatol. 8:31–34, 1991.

91. Acker DB, Sachs BP, Friedman EA: Risk factors for shoulder dystocia in the average-weight infant. Obstet. Gynecol. 67: 614–618, 1986.

92. Martin RJ, Fanaroff AA (eds): The respiratory distress syndrome and its management. *In* Ed. 5, Neonatal—Perinatal Medicine—Diseases of the Fetus and Infant. St. Louis, Mosby Year Book, 1992.

93. Soll RF: 1. Prophylactic administration of synthetic surfactant. 2. Prophylactic administration of natural surfactant. 3. Synthetic surfactant treatment of RDS. 4. Natural surfactant treatment of RDS. *In* Chalmers I (ed): Oxford Database of Perinatal Trials. Edited by I Chalmers. Version 1.I Disk Issue 3, February 1990.

94. Soll RF, Hockstra RE, Fangman JJ, et al: Multi-center trial of single-dose modified bovine surfactant extract (Survanta) for prevention of respiratory distress syndrome. Pediatrics 85:1092–1102, 1990.

95. Fujiwara T, Konishi M, Chida S, et al: Surfactant replacement therapy with a single postventilatory dose of reconstituted bovine surfactant in preterm neonates with respiratory distress syndrome: Final analysis of a multi-center, double-blind, randomized trial and comparison with similar trials. Pediatrics 86:753–764, 1990.

96. Bose C, Corbet A, Bose G, et al: Improved outcome at 28 days of age for verty low birth weight infants treated with a single dose of synthetic surfactant. J. Pediatr. 117: 947–953, 1990.

97. Horbar JD, Soll RF, Schachinger H, et al: A European multicenter randomized controlled trial of single dose surfactant therapy for idiopathic respiratory distress syndrome. Eur. J. Pediatr. 149:416–423, 1990.

98. OSIRIS Collaborative Group: Early versus delayed neonatal administration of a synthetic surfactant—the judgment of OSIRIS. Lancet 340:1363–69, 1992.

99. Auten RL, Notter RH, Kendig JW, et al: Surfactant treatment of full-term newborns with respiratory failure. Pediatrics 87:101–107, 1991.

100. Carlo WA, Martin RJ: Principles of neonatal assisted ventilation. Pediatr. Clin. N. Am. 33:221, 1986.

101. Carlo WA, Siner B, Chatburn RL, Robertson S, et al: Early randomized intervention with high-frequency jet ventilation in respiratory distress syndrome. J. Pediatr. 117: 765–770, 1990.

102. HIFI Study Group: High-frequency oscillatory ventilation compared with conventional mechanical ventilation in the treatment of respiratory failure in preterm infants. N. Engl. J. Med. 320:88, 1989.

103. Adzick NS, Vacanti JP, Lillehei CW, O'Rourke P, et al: Fetal diaphragmatic hernia: Ultrasound diagnosis and clinical outcome in 38 cases. J. Pediatr. Surg. 24:654–658, 1989.

104. Sakai H, Tamura M, Bryan AC, et al: The effect of surgical repair on respiratory mechanics in congenital diaphragmatic hernia. J. Pediatr. 3:432–438, 1987.

105. Langer JC, ┌ıller RM, Bohn DJ, et al: Timing of surgery for congenital diaphragmatic hernia: Is emergency operation necessary? Pediatr. Surg. 23:731–734, 1988.

106. Hazebroek FWJ, Tibboel D, Bos AT, et al: Congenital diaphragmatic hernia: Impact of preoperative stabilization. A prospective pilot study in 13 patients. J. Pediatr. Surg. 23: 1139–1146, 1988.

107. Wilson JM, Lund DP, Lillehei CW, O'Rourke PP: Delayed repair and preoperative ECMO does not improve survival in high-risk congenital diaphragmatic hernia. J. Pediatr. Surg. 27:368–375, 1992.

108. Stolar CJH, Snedecor SM, Bartlett RH: Extracorporeal membrane oxygenation and neonatal respiratory failure: Experience from the extracorporeal life support organization. J. Peds. Surg. 26:563–571, 1991.

109. Vesikari T, Janas M, Gronroos P, Tuppurainen N, et al: Neonatal septicemia. Arch. Dis. Child. 60:542–546, 1985.

110. Wilson CB: Immunologic basis for increased susceptibility of the neonate to infection. J. Pediatrics 108:1–12, 1986.
111. Philip AGS: Neonatal sepsis: Problems of diagnosis and the need for prevention. *In* Preventions of infections and the role of immunoglobulins in the neonatal period. Edited by G Duc. London, Royal Society of Medicine Services, 1990.
112. Boyer KM, Gotoff SP: Prevention of early-onset neonatal group B streptococcal disease with selective intrapartum chemoprophylaxis. N. Engl. J. Med. 314:1655–9, 1986.
113. Pitt J: Perinatal human Immunodeficiency virus infection. Clinics in Perinatology. Vol. 18, No. 2, June 1991.
114. Marion R, Wiznia A, Hutcheon R, et al: Human T-cell lymphotropic virus Type III (HTLV-III) infection. A new dysmorphic syndrome associated with intrauterine HTLV-III infections. Am. J. Dis. Child. 140:638–674.
115. Lipschultz S, Chanock S, Sanders S, et al: Cardiovascular manifestations of human immunodeficiency virus infection in infants and children. Am. J. Cardiol. 63:1489–1497.
116. Centers for Disease Control: Recommendations for prevention of perinatal transmission of human T cell lymphotropic virus III/LAV and AIDS. MMWR 34:721–726, 1985.
117. Sidiropoulos D, Boehme U, Von Muralt G, Morrell A, et al: Immunoglobulin supplementation in prevention or treatment of neonatal sepsis. Pediatr. Inf. Dis. 5:S193–5194, 1986.
118. Haque KN, Zaidi MH: IgM-enriched intravenous immunoglobulin therapy in neonatal sepsis. Am. J. Dis. Child. 142: 1293–1296, 1988.
119. Friedman CA, Wender DF, Temple DM, Rawson JE: Intravenous gamma globulin as adjunct therapy for severe group B streptoccal disease in the newborn. Am. J. Perinatol. 6: 453–6, 1989.
120. Christensen RD, Hardman T, Thornton J, Hill HR: A randomized, double-blind, placebo-controlled investigation of the safety of immune globulin administration to preterm neonates. J. Perinatol. 9:126–130, 1988.
121. Weisman LE, Kueser TJ, Rubio TT, Frank G, et al: Intravenous immune globulin therapy for early-onset sepsis in premature neonates. J. Pediatrics 121:434–443, 1992.

Chapter 46

# MEDICOLEGAL ASPECTS

NIKOLAI TEHIN
JOHN R. FEEGEL
HAROLD J. HUNTER, JR.

This chapter deals with selected medico-legal aspects of obstetrical anesthesia and analgesia. Legal principles are presented to provide basic information on the nature of liability and negligence. Then selected topics which seem to provide the bases for malpractice suits are approached. The Standard of Care and the role of expert witnesses are briefly addressed, along with informed consent, staff privileges and credentialling, privacy and confidentiality, midwives and CRNAs, and selected federal issues including Medicare and Medicaid. Lastly, selected suggestions for avoidance of legal problems are offered. Obviously, this chapter cannot be used as a handbook for defending one's own lawsuit or contracting with other agencies or institutions. Only a competent lawyer can provide the required expertise for the practitioner of anesthesia who receives notice of an impending lawsuit. Usually, the defendant's lawyer is provided by the professional liability insurance carrier; however, it is not unreasonable for a defendant anesthesiologist or anesthetist to retain personal counsel in addition. A personal attorney provides a watchful eye on the insurance lawyer, even though both should have common interests in the defense of the claim. Consideration of coverage limits, applicability of the policy and problems of settlement at various stages of the lawsuit are often facilitated by a defendant talking to a personal lawyer.

Since all cases vary regardless of apparent similarity, none of the statements provided in this chapter should be relied on in lieu of competent legal advice.

## LIABILITY

It is accepted in our society that rational adults are responsible for the consequences of their own acts.[1] Under some circumstances, a person or corporation may also be liable for the acts of others, through the principle of *respondeat superior* or vicarious liability.[2] Thus, an employer may be required to pay for damage or injury caused by an employee ("servant") acting within the scope of employment. Application of these principles in the practice of obstetrical anesthesia may be obvious and, at times, obscure, though no less legally binding. A patient may directly contract with a person to administer anesthesia, and that person may be an agent of a professional group or an employee of a hospital. Alternatively, the hospital may supply the anesthesia professional to the patient without a direct contract between patient and professional. Here, the hospital may contend that the anesthesia professional is a "private contractor" for whose acts the hospital should not be held liable. Yet, a growing trend of cases hold the anesthesiologist (and other hospital-based physicians, such as emergency room doctors, pathologists, and radiologist) to be "apparent agents" of the hospital, depending on the absence of contractual contact with the patient, and the degree of control the hospital can exercise over the anesthesiologist.[3] Further application of liability to the hospital for acts of its "independent contractors" may be found in the emerging doctrine of *non-delegable duty,*[4] which may be imposed by statute or by case law, and under which a hospital is not permitted to delegate to a contractor its responsibility to the patient to provide reasonably safe anesthesia. Under the doctrine of *"borrowed servant,"* particularly in the operating room, a surgeon (or anesthesiologist) may be held responsible for the negligent acts of a nurse or technician whom he "borrows" from the hospital, by whom the nurse is actually employed, for a specific technical purpose, provided that he directly supervises the borrowed person and directs her to perform a task that is not simply administrative.[5] For example, the counting of surgical instruments by the nurse may be ministerial, causing the hospital-employer to remain liable for the negligent miscount and harm.

### Damages

Damages are the actual loss or harm to another which result from the negligent acts alluded to above. Such damages may be profound or relatively slight, yet be actionable under the law when shown to be closely and legally caused by the negligent act. Since, in obstetrics, the anesthesia professional works with mother and child, two lives and two nervous systems are at risk. Elements of damage may include past and future medical costs, loss of future earning capacity, pain and suffering, and loss of companionship for survivors. Life-long medical support for a patient rendered comatose by negligent administration of anesthesia or the death of a highly paid professional can obviously result in enormous, yet fair dollar amounts to compensate for the loss.

The elements of damage may vary from state to state.

## Negligence

A legal cause of action based on negligence requires the showing of a duty on the part of the actor to conform to a certain standard of conduct so as to protect others from unreasonable harm, a breach of that duty, and harm or damages closely resulting from that breach.[6] In the absence of any one of these necessary elements, there can be no negligence under the law. Duty and the standard of care may be demonstrated from statutes, published practice standards[7] of medical specialty societies,[8] authoritative textbooks, hospital policies, and more often by testimony of expert witnesses. The judge determines which of these the plaintiff may use to demonstrate these elements while the jury, if any, is allowed to give these sources whatever weight if deems proper.

## Res Ipsa Loquitur

*Res Ipsa Loquitur*[9] is a rule of evidence which under some circumstances lessens the plaintiff's burden of proving his case. To be applicable, a plaintiff must show that in the ordinary course of events, his injury would not have occurred but for negligence, and that the instrumentality causing the damage was solely under the control of the defendant, and that there was no way the plaintiff could have caused or contributed to the injury. The circumstances of obstetric anesthesia, where the patient is rendered helpless by the anesthetic and is injured by the negligence of the anesthesiologist may sufficiently satisfy these judgments. Cases arising from foreign bodies left in the patient at surgery may also involve a res ipsa approach. Here, the burden of proof is shifted to the defendant who must overcome the presumption of negligence.

## Medical Expert

The medical expert witness is essential to the review and prosecution of a medical negligence action against an anesthesiologist. The medical expert, in giving his medical opinion, may rely upon his own education, training, and experience as well as treatises, journals and other published material which is generally available to members of the specialty. The role of the medical expert is to review the medical record for the purposes of evaluating (1) the technical competence of the physician; (2) the reasonableness of the medical judgments made under the circumstances; (3) whether the physician's personal interaction with the patient, other physicians, nurses or family members materially and adversely impacted the patient's care; and (4) establishing within reasonable medical probabilities the nexus between the breach of the standard of care and the resulting injury.

The law recognizes that the physician whose care is being reviewed (the defendant) is also an expert qualified to render an opinion as to whether the standard of care was met, and whether any alleged breach of the standard was a substantial factor in causing an injury.

Because the obligations of the standard of care go beyond technical competence and extend into the area of reasonable medical judgment and personal interaction with other health care providers, one can reasonably expect there to be differences of opinion between well-trained and highly regarded physicians as to what is required. In temporary injuries and nondisabling permanent injuries, the physician is more apt to be judged as having met the standards of care. An analysis of reviewer inclinations indicates that if the outcome results in a significant permanent injury or death, the care is much more likely to be judged to be substandard by the reviewers.[10]

## Informed Consent

With the rise of self-determination and the health care provider's recognition of the respect due to the patient's autonomy, the need for clearly informed and fully voluntary consent to medical treatment has emerged as an essential part of professional practices.[11] Consent to anesthesia and invasive analgesia is no exception. Most hospitals provide a separate form on which to record the patient's consent to anesthesia. Hence, while a patient might fully consent to, say, a cesarian section, a separate document showing consent to anesthesia should be obtained and made part of the patient's chart.

The consent is not synonymous with the form which the patient signs, although hospital vocabulary may sound like it is. Consent implies the meeting of the minds of two or more persons, a reasonable understanding of what is to take place, and a submission of one of these persons to allow the other to perform the act. To be valid, consent must be noncoerced and freely given by a competent person who is rational.[12] To meet these requirements, the patient should not be influenced by medication, drugs or alcohol, should be of age and not mentally incompetent, and obviously fully understanding the thing to which she consents. *Informed consent* by most statutes also requires that the health care providers explain the reasonable risks of the procedure, the alternative procedures available and the risks of those as well. It is prudent, therefore, that the anesthesia professional obtain the consent personally, even though getting the signature on the hospital form as evidence of it is routinely delegated to a nurse or clerk. These ancillary personnel may not be capable of fully explaining the procedure, alternatives, and risks.[13] In obtaining the patient's consent, it is the physician's duty to disclose to the patient, whose knowledge of medical science is presumed less than that of the physician, all material information necessary to enable the patient to make an informed decision regarding the proposed treatment. In many states, the physician's duty to disclose is measured by a professional standard: either the customary disclosure practice of physicians in the community, or what a reasonable physician would disclose to the patient under similar circumstances.[14] In other jurisdictions, the trend has been to measure the duty from the perspective of the patient, requiring the physician to disclose the information necessary for the patient to make an intelligent, informed decision.[15]

The disclosure of all material information involves informing the patient of matters which the physician knows or should know would be regarded as significant by a reasonable person in the patient's position when deciding to accept or reject a recommended medical procedure.[16]

When a procedure inherently involves a known risk of death or serious injury, the physician must inform the patient of the possibility of such an outcome and must explain to the patient, in lay terms, the potential complications. To be material, a fact must also be one that is not commonly appreciated.[17] The duty involves, in addition to information about recommended treatment, advising a patient of the material risks of not consenting to a procedure such as a pap smear, and to matters involving the physician's personal interest.[18] However, in the words of the California Supreme Court, "the patient's interest in information does not extend to a lengthy polysyllabic disclosure on all possible complications. A mini-course in medical science is not required."[19] The patient's concern is with the risk of death or bodily harm and problems of recuperation. Also, there is no duty to discuss relatively minor risks inherent in common procedure when it is known that such risks are remote.

Recently, a court has held that a physician has a duty to a patient who specifically asks to be told the truth regarding his life expectancy. The patient with pancreatic cancer was not advised of the probability that his chances for survival, even with treatment, were extremely low and that his remaining time was short. The patient consented to fruitless treatment which had severe side effects, the patient and his wife did not alter their wills, and the family did not make appropriate plans for the patient's impending death, such as selling the family business and foregoing new business ventures.[20]

As a general rule, the responsibility for obtaining the patient's informed consent rests only on the physician performing the medical procedure. In the surgical setting, the question arises as to which physician—the surgeon or the anesthesiologist—must disclose to the patient the risks associated with anesthesia, as opposed to the risks of the operation itself. There are no clear legal guidelines on this point, although a recent Connecticut case held that the allocation of responsibility to disclose, among a surgeon and other specialists employed to assist the surgeon, was a question for expert testimony, to be determined by the standard of the professional community.[21] Clearly, the prudent anesthesiologist will fully inform the surgical patient of the risks associated with anesthesia and will obtain that patient's consent to all anticipated anesthetic procedures.

The properly signed form is, in some states, rebuttably presumed to be properly obtained in the absence of fraud.[22] The rule of informed consent may be overridden by impossibility, such as an emergency, by another obligation such as a strong claim for public health, by therapeutic privilege, where full disclosure would seriously harm the patient and sometimes by the physician's own conscientious objection.[23]

## Condition Precedent to Malpractice Action

A number of states require as a condition precedent to the pursuit of a malpractice suit, that notice of an impending action be given in advance to the health care provider, or require that the case be reviewed by a panel of physicians and attorneys to evaluate its relative merits. Typically, the panel will review the medical records, take testimony from the parties and hear expert medical opinion before rendering a judgment as to the merits of the case. The procedural requirements and the consequences of submission to a panel vary widely from state to state. In some instances the findings of the panel may be introduced into evidence at the trial of the action, and in others it is utilized as a mediation tool intended to influence settlement or dismissal of the claims.

These variable conditions should never be ignored by the defendant anesthesiologist or not fully met. To do so may fatally jeopardize the defense, and may lead to a withdrawal of coverage by the insurance carrier for failing to cooperate with the terms of the policy.

Similarly, a subpoena or a properly filed request for the production of documents should be considered as issued by the court and taken very seriously to avoid sanctions. Where compliance may work a significant hardship, one should bring the difficulty to the attention of the lawyer issuing the subpoena. When that approach fails, the problem can be presented to the judge along with the reasons why full and prompt compliance would not be reached. Under no circumstances should a subpoena be ignored simply because the defendant anesthesiologist doesn't like it.

## Alternative Dispute Resolutions

In many states, differing attempts have been made to remedy patients' complaints of medical care without resorting to trial. These measures, intended to reform health-related malpractice actions, have been fostered by medical societies and many medical specialty colleges as well as by federal and state administrations, past and present. Fears of run-away jury awards and the purported effects on health care costs have generated discussions often characterized by more heat than light. Examples of alternative resolution measures include binding and nonbinding arbitration (where a committee hears the case), mediation (where an acceptable person attempts to bridge the gap between demand and offer), screening committees (to determine if there are genuine issues in dispute), no-fault insurance plans (where negligence need not be proved in exchange for a predetermined payment or benefit), and on the federal level, delegation to a magistrate (in lieu of a judge). It is premature to identify any of these as a panacea, but short of denying citizens their constitutionally protected access to the court, efforts to improve the system must be encouraged and, where warranted, applauded.

## Personal Interaction

Even the most technically proficient physician exercising reasonable medical judgment may find himself in litigation due to a failure of communication. Lack of personal interaction with nurses, surgeons, attending physicians, obstetricians, or other anesthesiologists and family members can give rise to catastrophic consequences. It is generally accepted that a patient who has been treated courteously is less apt to sue the health care provider, despite a poor outcome. Conversely, an angry patient or survivor may try to sue even where there is an insufficient legal or medical basis. Danzon[24] has provided an in-depth study of the economic profile of medical malpractice actions and cites a California Medical Association Study which shows that roughly 1 in 126 patients admitted to hospital were injured due to negligent care, with only 1 in 10 of these filing a claim, and of these, only 40% resulting in any payment of the plaintiff. The reasons for not filing claims frequently remain unknown, but good physician-patient rapport probably helps.

## *Documentation—Record Keeping*

The best shield against claims of medical negligence are medical records that are conscientiously prepared for the purpose of assuring the quality and continuity of a patient's care, and which document information regarding the patient preoperatively, intraoperatively, and postoperatively. The Joint Commission on Accreditation of Hospitals provides the principal framework for the maintenance of appropriate medical records.[25] A physician conforming to the American Society of Anesthesiologists' guidelines for "appropriate care"[26] should document the pertinent medical findings, so that there is a clear and progressive picture of the anesthetic care delivered and the patient's response. Corrections, addenda and supplements to a record for purposes of clarity or explanation are permitted but should be clearly identified as such, and entered in the record in the appropriate chronological sequence. Interlineation, insertion, or obliteration of charted notes is to be avoided at all times.

Anesthesia records are characterized by technical symbols, abbreviations and often jargon that is mandated by the nature of the practice and the circumstances. Extra care therefore must be taken to be accurate, legible and complete.[27,28] The record should be thought of as the anesthesiologist's proof of adequate anesthesia care. Incomplete records will prove to be difficult to explain after a lawsuit is filed.[29]

## *Obstetric and Nonobstetric Malpractice Claims*

Using the American Society of Anesthesiologists' Closed Claims database, Chadwick and others,[30] found that the most common complications in obstetric claims were maternal death (22%), newborn brain damage (20%), and headache (12%). In nonobstetrical claims, the most common complications were death (39%), nerve damage (16%), and brain damage (13%). Complications due to aspirations and convulsions were more common in the obstetrical cases. The standard of care was met in 46% of the obstetrical cases and 39% of the nonobstetrical cases. Newborn brain injury was the leading cause of claims in the obstetrical cases, but only 50% of these were considered to be anesthesia related.[31]

An earlier study of anesthesia-related maternal mortality[32] identified anesthesia as the primary cause of death in 15 cases (6.9% of direct maternal death, or 0.82 per 100 000 births), and a contributing factor in 4 cases. The failure to provide a patent airway was the predominant cause of anesthesia-related deaths since 1980, although no anesthesia-related deaths were identified in the last 2 years of the study.[32] The patient was described as obese or morbidly obese in 10 of the 15 deaths in which anesthesia was the primary cause. In this same study, all but two were black, although 84.9% of the state's population was white.[32] Eleven of the 15 were cesarian sections, with 10 classified as emergencies.[32] Of the 15 cases, 10 were by general anesthesia, 4 by spinal and 1 by epidural.[32]

## Case Examples

A review of cases throughout the country involving anesthesia misadventures consistently reveal that laxity in preparation and lack of vigilance in monitoring combine to give rise to catastrophic results. The following are case examples illustrating common risk areas.

*CASE NO. 1. Patient, age 44, suffered renal failure and was a chronic hemodialysis patient. She was admitted to hospital, with fever, hypertension, confusion, right-sided weakness and aphasia. A full neurologic workup was essentially negative. Her blood pressure was treated with IV medications, and as her blood pressure stabilized, her neurologic symptoms resolved. Discharge was arranged but on the morning of planned discharge, the patient developed a warm fluctuant swelling in the lower aspect of her right arm. Hospital discharge was cancelled and the surgical consultant diagnosed a false aneurysm at the site of an abandoned and previously repaired dialysis shunt and ordered emergent surgery to repair the disrupted graft.*

*Surgery commenced under local anesthetic at 4:15 p.m. and concluded at 7:30 p.m. The patient was taken awake and alert to the recovery room. Two hours later at 9:29 p.m., she arrested. Resuscitation attempts were unsuccessful and she was pronounced dead at 10:20 p.m.*

*At the time of arrest, the serum potassium was measured at 8.5 mEq/L on two occasions. No order for serum potassium was given either preoperatively, intraoperatively or postoperatively. The arrest was precipitated by hyperkalemia.*

COMMENTS: This case illustrates the importance of the preoperative visit and the necessity of discussing the patient with the surgeon and personal physician, in this case a nephrologist. At the time of the surgery, the patient was presumed to be stable physiologically, but in fact her potassium levels were elevated, something that should have been considered in a patient who is a chronic hemodialysis patient and who had not been dialyzed for several days due to her admission. If she had her serum potassium measure preoperatively, intraoperatively, or even immediately postoperatively, the reasonable medical probabilities are that she would not have died.

*CASE NO. 2. Patient is sent to the community hospital by her midwife with third trimester bleeding. The patient arrives and an on-call obstetrician admits the patient to labor and delivery at 7:30 a.m. and immediately diagnoses fetal distress and probable placental abruption, and orders emergency cesarean section. The patient was immediately taken to the operating room and a full presurgical preparation undertaken. Anesthesiologist "A" is present in the operating room and in the initial stages of preparing another patient for an 8:00 a.m. elective surgery. His patient has not yet been anesthetized and he agrees to cover the cesarean in the absence of the on-call anesthesiologist. Anesthesiologist "A" took a history, positioned the patient, ascertained that her IV was patent, and is ready for delivery of the anesthetic agent that he had prepared for crash induction at 7:55 a.m. Within 1 minute of induction, the on-call anesthesiologist, "B", chief of the department, arrives and it is agreed that he shall replace "A." Anesthesiologist "B" then proceeds to duplicate the preparations accomplished by "A." The infant is delivered 3 minutes after induction at 8:10 a.m. At all times, a complete operating room team was available including assistant surgeon and pediatrician.*

COMMENTS: The case illustrates the need for strong personal interaction among members of the health care team. Although the emergency was declared at 7:30 a.m., with full operating room crew available and both an obstetrician and anesthesiologist present, there was no interaction on the emergency plan. A full surgical preparation of the patient was undertaken without objection from the anesthesiologist. At literally the last minute, anesthesiologist "A" stepped aside in favor of "B," causing further delay in an emergency situation.

*CASE NO. 3. The obstetrician for a 32-year-old patient admitted to labor and delivery performed a full rectal and vaginal examination despite his awareness that placenta previa was present. The patient suffered a massive hemorrhage requiring emergency cesarean section. Before the operation, the anesthesiologist failed to complete prompt intubation of the airway and was required to make three intubation attempts. After the second attempt, the patient had a massive regurgitation of stomach contents into the airway further complicating the third intubation. The child was born without residual problems but the mother died 7 hours after the delivery as a consequence of the hypoxic episode.*

COMMENTS: The most frequent critical incidents leading to patient death are related to management of the respiratory system. In the use of general anesthesia, the most common problems are difficult tracheal intubation, aspiration, and inadequate ventilation. Before an anesthetic drug is administered, all equipment that may be required to establish an airway and to deliver oxygen must be at hand and in place.

*CASE NO. 4. A 29-year-old patient was admitted for surgery for treatment of choledocholithiasis and right posterior lobe abscess of liver. Anesthesia was performed by a certified registered nurse anesthetist under the direction of a supervising anesthesiologist. During the course of the surgery, the patient suffered anoxic brain damage. The Positive End Expiratory Pressure valve (PEEP) was incorrectly placed into the anesthesia circuit by the nurse anesthetist, who had not performed an appropriate equipment check which would have disclosed the misplaced valve. The supervising anesthesiologist had not performed a preanesthetic check of the equipment, and had not required the PEEP valve to be present in the operating room, in the circuit, and tested prior to the patient's arrival, and had not reviewed the setup of the nurse anesthetist.*

COMMENTS: The anesthesiologist must always insist on a thorough equipment check before beginning anesthetic administration. Modern equipment is subject to unanticipated disconnection, one-way exhaust valves may be inadvertently shut tight, improper connection of the system may occur and alarms may malfunction. Equipment malfunction and improper assembly still continues to occur even though efforts are made to incorporate into the design systems which will avoid or minimize human error.

*CASE NO. 5. Patient, age 62, was admitted to the hospital for surgical repair of inguinal hernia. Following the surgery, the patient had an episode of shortness of breath and cyanosis requiring oxygen. The anesthesiologist did not monitor the patient in recovery and, in particular, had not reviewed blood gases which had been drawn in recovery. Patient suffered a severe brain injury.*

COMMENTS: The patient had not recovered from the anesthetic and the transition to self sufficiency from the supported environment of anesthesia had not been made. This transition in most instances is made without complication, but the consequences of not monitoring it and assuring that the patient is physiologically back to the preanesthetic state can be catastrophic.

## Staff Privileges, Contracts and Credentialing

Full discussion of the modern legal implications of a hospital granting privileges to a practitioner who is later shown in a malpractice suit to have been incompetent before appointment is well beyond the scope of this chapter, although it is a significant topic of interest for all physicians, anesthesiologists, and hospital administrators. However, the problems for the anesthesiologist or an independent CRNA, must be mentioned if only to sound an alert. Since hospitals are now held responsible for negligent appointment and retention of its medical staff,[33] and since the hospital's board of trustees is usually incapable of adequate assessment of applicant's credentials, these issues are submitted to a committee chosen from the medical staff, which logically, but dangerously, may include a staff member of the specialty involved. This may put the presently contracted anesthesiologist in judgement over the qualifications and appointment of a potential competitor. Unsubstantiated rejection may result in an antitrust lawsuit by the disappointed applicant, requiring a complex and expensive defense for the unwitting anesthesiologist or his group. Since these federal cases allow for treble damages, the demands may be enormous.

Couple these thorny issues with legal problems surrounding "exclusive contracts," and other restrictive contractual provisions, and one might conclude that the prudent anesthesiologist needs competent legal advice at almost every turn.[34] The anesthesiologist may also arrive in the difficult position of being one of the closest, knowledgeable witnesses in an obstetrical disaster that warrants cancellation of staff privileges or other disciplinary and malpractice actions against the surgeon or the hospital itself. Obviously, that anesthesiologist needs immediate and personal legal counsel, and should not fully rely on the hospital's attorney, who might not recognize his own conflicts of interest.

State and federal laws may confer full or limited immunity for some of the duties suggested above, but competent local legal advice is mandatory before the prudent anesthesiologist can rely on a personal understanding of these protections.[35]

## MEDICARE AND OTHER FEDERAL ISSUES

Federal prosecution for fraud and abuse under Medicare promises to be very active during the 1990s, if only for attempted cost containment. Payment for the service of a CRNA is authorized under certain conditions, but only on an assignment basis, to the anesthetist or to the hospital, physician, group practice, hospital or ambulatory care center as the employer or contractor.[36] Penalties for fraudulently billing for CRNA services are included. Somewhat complicated and often confusing Medicare regulations and penalties also apply to overcharges by physicians for services of a certified registered nurse anesthetist, and should be specifically consulted, with concurrent legal advice, by any anesthesiologist whose practice involves Medicare.[37] Similarly, the state and federal provisions of Medi*caid,* should be of interest to anesthesiologists, their hospital administrators and their attorneys, since the welfare program includes childbirth.[38]

The intended scope of this chapter does not permit an exhaustive presentation of the often arcane federal regulations and penalties applicable to obstetrical anesthesia. However, mere reference to sanctions under the above-cited programs as well as those found under Title XI of the Social Security Act[39] and applicable provisions of The Health Care Quality Improvement Act of 1986,[40] should serve as notice. Those engaged in administering obstetrical or other types of anesthesia also need to be aware of the stiff provisions prohibiting kickbacks, bribes, rebates, and the so called "Safe Harbors" whereby institutions may attempt to devise lawful or illegal cooperative business arrangements for professional services, equipment or office space and personnel.[41]

These areas of the law are very much in flux and anything said about them is *de facto* dated and subject to error, particularly in a changing administration. Forewarned can be forearmed, but vigilance is required.

### Privacy and Confidentiality

The right to privacy is overtly included in the Constitutions of some states and recognized, if not spelled out as part of The Constitution of the United States.[42] Violations of privacy are recognized nationwide as grounds for civil lawsuits. Invasions of privacy applicable to anesthesiology might include the presence of unwarranted persons in the operating room or delivery suites or photography during the procedure without permission. Noble motives such as medical education will not suffice to overcome these violations where permission has not been given by the patient. Sometimes teaching hospitals will anticipate these potential invasions and seek prior approval from the patient through use of a broadly worded form signed at admission. The prudent anesthesiologist will personally check the patient's record prior to becoming a party to these educational violations, particularly when the procedure is an emergency with less time to obtain routine blanket permissions.

Confidentiality is closely related.[43] The anesthesiologist as a co-equal on the surgical/obstetrical team is coresponsible in the respect due to the patient's confidentiality. The patient's awareness of communications to third parties without permission is not required for this violation. Publication of an identifiable patient's condition or discussion of the case without justification or permission may be sufficient grounds for a civil lawsuit and disciplinary action by the state medical regulatory board.

Under partial anesthesia, patients may disclose intimate facts to the anesthesiologist and others without rational intention to do so. These disclosures must be held in professional confidence by all personnel and not disclosed without permission regardless of how humorous or scandalous the inadvertent disclosure may have been. Indeed, a prudent anesthesiologist will carefully weigh the therapeutic benefit of including such remarks in the patient's medical record.

The degree to which a patient places her trust in the anesthesiologist is no less than that afforded to psychiatrists and clergy. Not every state recognizes physician-patient privilege to prevent disclosure, but all courts recognize breaches of confidentiality as actionable. This is particularly true where the disclosure may have profited the physician, such as in his research[44] or the publication of a book or journal article.

### Midwives, Nurse Anesthetists and Anesthesiologists

Cost reduction in providing medical care is a significant political issue for the 1990s. Participants in this tug-of-war include physicians with and without specialty certification, professional societies such as The American College of Obstetricians and Gynecologists (ACOG), The American Society of Anesthesiologists (ASA), The American Association of Nurse Anesthetists (AANA), The American College of Nurse-Midwives (ACNM), The Joint Commission on Accreditation of Health Care Organizations (JCAHO), The Health Care Finance Administration (HCFA), The Federal Trade Commission (FTC), The American Hospital Association (AHA), the various state professional licensure boards, and numerous health insurance organizations, to name a few. Some of these groups will see their goal as that of maintaining the highest professional standards and thus demand regulation by which only licensed or certified physicians can provide anesthesia for, or participate in, the delivery of babies. Others may champion the cause of nonphysician performance of these duties. Still others, concerned with cost reduction or the economic and legal effects of monopolies will concentrate on the financial or the restraint of trade aspects. Obviously, there is no single solution demonstrable here. Anesthesiologists must be aware of these evolving principles and regulations and be ready to conform where applicable. Similar advice is offered to the members of the other competing groups. Keen attention must be given to the forthcoming literature of each of these interested parties, as well as to the federal and state regulatory agencies. There is no doubt that such information will be plentiful.

The prudent anesthesiologist and nurse anesthetist will research as well their contractual and supervisory relationships to others who, by virtue of state or federal law or hospital policies and by-laws are also involved in obstetrical anesthesia and analgesia. These relationships will no doubt vary from state to state and hospital to hospital. In some, a nurse anesthetist may be an independent contractor of the hospital or patient, with or without direct supervision by an anesthesiologist or anesthesiology group, who in turn may be an independent contractor, employee, or agent of the hospital. Restrictive policies originally designed to prohibit direct professional association of physicians with nonphysicians in the practice of medicine, have often been abandoned as an alternative to an antitrust action by the FTC. Anesthesiology practices and institutional policies must therefore be kept very up-to-date to avoid these legal conflicts.

A joint survey by The Committee on Obstetric Anesthesia of The American Society of Anesthesiologists and The American College of Obstetricians and Gynecologists showed that anesthetic procedures were most often provided by the obstetricians or by CRNAs regardless of the size or volume of the birthing unit.[45] (Midwives were not surveyed in this study.) Among anesthesia respondents 73% believed obstetricians lack sufficient background in obstetric anesthesia, and 46% of obstetricians believed anesthesiologists and CRNAs lack sufficient training in obstetric anesthesia.[46] Obviously, this level of mutual distrust must have an impact on the medical-legal relationship between anesthesia and birthing personnel. While obstetric anesthesia is considered to be a high risk practice with increased medicolegal exposure for the anesthesiologist, Chadwick and others[47] showed that nonobstetric anesthesia malpractice claims were seven times more likely than obstetric-anesthesia claims.

From an anesthesia, and possibly from a surgical standpoint, labor and imminent childbirth should be viewed, in a real sense, as a potentially emergent situation. What may begin as a routine delivery can, without warning, change into a frantic battle to avoid death and severe injury. Emergency cesarean section is among the most common situations in which the anesthesiologist must marshal not only his technical and interpersonal skills but also his best medical judgment. If the patient is not doing well, confidence in one's abilities must not prevent an immediate review of technique and equipment. The change of circumstance must be immediately communicated to the obstetrical surgeon and corrective action must immediately be initiated to address the problem. Because of the unique role of being charged with the life and well-being of two patients, the anesthesiologist must be an active participant, willing and able to direct the response to the emergency.

The leading causes of anesthetic-related maternal mortality are complications arising from aspiration of gastric contents[48] or to failed endotracheal intubation.[49] Maternal death and complications related to the respiratory system are significantly more common in cases involving general anesthetics.[50]

## "Captain of the Ship"

Under this outdated doctrine,[51] the surgeon and obstetrician were considered fully in charge and therefore responsible for all other personnel in the operating room. The recognition of the expertise required to select and administer anesthesia has elevated the anesthesiologist to a co-equal member of the team, and thus, responsible for his own acts. The law now recognizes that the obstetrician is entitled to rely on the anesthesiologist and should not be held liable where only the anesthetic aspects are substandard.[52] However, many lawyers will consider it their duty to include the obstetrician as a co-equal defendant in a lawsuit where the actual responsibilities cannot be clearly determined. The discovery process may later more accurately define responsibility and wrong doing more precisely, with one or more of the OR personnel being dismissed from the lawsuit. Hence, initial inclusion in the lawsuit should not be considered a vindictive act by the plaintiff's lawyer nor evoke pessimism in the defendant anesthesiologist. Prompt legal consultation is warranted.

## Helpful Suggestions

The avoidance of a lawsuit is superior to winning. The following comments are aimed at prevention as well as contributing to a successful defense.

*1. **Rapport.*** There is no substitute for good rapport with the patient and her family. Even a patient who is seriously malpracticed may be reluctant to sue a kind and considerate friend. Conversely, the angry patient who is disappointed by the anesthesiologist's nasty and discourteous attitude may try to sue even if the procedure was not done negligently.

*2. **Examination.*** The anesthesiologist should examine his patient and explain the procedure along with the risks. This important step should not be delegated to an incompetent assistant or omitted because it is bothersome and time consuming. The obstetrician or the internist may not fully comprehend the proposed anesthesia and thereby falsely announce that the patient is "cleared."

*3. **Chart Review.*** A review of the medical record *before* anesthesia, rather than catching up during the procedure is mandated by prudent practice. The anesthesiologist who later finds a charted contraindication is poorly armed for the defense.

*4. **Visit.*** The patient and the baby should be visited postpartum and the visit meaningfully charted. This step demonstrates concern and negates a later charge that no one saw or cared about the postpartum anesthesia patient. A greeting from the door will not do, but a rapid and reasonable demonstration of limb movements, orientation and coordination will come closer to the ideal.

***5. Record Keeping.*** The anesthesiologist *must* produce accurate, legible, and complete records as contemporaneously as prudent practice allows. These must never be altered, although later additions or corrections are allowed by obvious measures and with preservation of the original.

***6. Literature.*** There is a professional obligation to stay up-to-date with the art and science of one's profession. When a complication arises because the anesthesiologist was out-of-date, his defense suffers greatly.

***7. Contact and Candor with the Defense Attorney.*** When a threat of suit arises, the matter must be promptly reported to the insurance carrier in writing, with a copy kept on reserve. When a defense attorney is identified, the defendant-anesthesiologist should treat her/him as a friend and a confidant. Nothing can ruin a defense more thoroughly than a defendant who misleads or lies to his own lawyer.

***8. Plaintiffs and Their Lawyers.*** The defendant-anesthesiologist should treat the one suing and his or her lawyer with courtesy and professionalism. The plaintiff's lawyer did not cause the problem, and, along with the defense attorney should be recognized as a problem solver. Animosity and rancor add nothing to the situation.

***9. Contracts.*** These legally binding documents are the specialty of only selected attorneys, since they frequently contain clauses of specific compliance, promises to not compete on dissolution, and areas involving state and federal regulations, about which lawyers engaged in general practice may not be fully aware. A good rule of thumb is that anesthesiologists do not approve contracts without counsel and lawyers do not administer anesthesia.

***10. Medicare, Medicaid, and Government Programs.*** The ever-changing regulations for Medicare, Medicaid, OBRA, Social Security, Federal Trade Commission (antitrust issues), HCFA (safe harbors and RBRVS payments) and others are legal minefields for the unwary obstetrical anesthesiologist and everyone else. Since these medically related regulations are recent progeny of even more complex social issues which evoked legislation, highly specialized legal advice should be sought.

***11. Confidentiality and Privacy.*** Just because a health professional learns or knows something about another person, there is no license to tell others. Indeed, there may be a stiff penalty for invasions of privacy and breaches of confidentiality, particularly where the vulnerability and intimacy of childbirth are involved. In this area, at least, the conspiracy of silence may be praiseworthy.

***12. Truthtelling.*** Common decency and professional bearing demand truthtelling under all circumstances, whether one is under oath or not. Truthtelling, either to the patient or to her family, is mandated whatever the circumstances. Untruths are not justified.[53]

***13. Visibility.*** Every anesthesiologist should remember that one is not alone or unseen in the operating room. Any conduct, comment, or demeanor may be recalled by other OR personnel when they are served with a subpoena and sworn to testify.

## REFERENCES


1. Wigmore: Responsibility for Tortious Acts: Its History. Harv. Law. Rev. 7:315, 1894.
2. Keeton WP, et al: Prosser and Keeton on the Law of Torts. 5th Ed. St. Paul, MN. West Pub. Co., (1984) 500 et seq.
3. Williams v St. Claire Medical Center, 657 SW 2d 590 (Ky App 1983) (Nurse anesthetist employed by professional corporation rather than hospital). Paintsville Hosp. Co. v Rose, 683 SW 2d 255 (Ky 1985) (Emergency room physician—apparent agency).
4. Jackson v Power, 743 P2d 1376 (Alaska 1987).
5. Buzan v Mercy Hosp. Inc., 203 So2d 11 (Fla 3 DCA 1967).
6. Keeton: op cit. p. 160 et seq.
7. Cheney FW, Posner K, Caplan RA, Ward RJ: Standard of Care and Anesthesia Liability. JAMA 261(11):1599, 1989.
8. Joint Commission on Accreditation of Health Care Organizations. Accreditation Manual for Hospital, 1992.
9. Ybarra v Spangard, 154 P2d 687 (Cal 1944).
10. Cheney FW, Posner K, Caplan RA, Ward RJ: Standard of Care and Anesthesia Liability. JAMA 261(11):1599, 1989.
11. Beauchamp TL, Childress JF: Principles of Biomedical Ethics. Ed. 3. New York, Oxford University Press, 1989.
12. Rozovsky FA: Consent to Treatment: A Personal Guide. Ed. 2. Boston, Little Brown & Company, 1990.
13. Southwick AR, Slee DA: The Law of Hospital and Health Care Administration. Ed. 2. Ann Arbor, Health Administration Press, 1988.
14. See, eg, Charley v Cameron, 528 P2d 1205 (Kan. 1974).
15. See, eg, Cobbs v Grant, 8 Cal3d 229, 243 (1972).
16. Sard v Hardy, 379 A2d 1014 (Md 1977). Wilkinson v Vesey, 295 A2d 676, (RI 1972). 69 ALR.3d 1202.
17. See: Moore v Regents University of California, 793 P2d 479 (Cal 1990). Truman v Thomas, 611 P2d 902 (Cal 1980).
18. Cobbs v Grant, 502 P2d 1 (Cal 1972).
19. Arato v Avedon, 839 P2d 983 (Cal 1992).
20. See: Mason v Walsh, 600 A2d 326 (Conn.App. 1991).
21. Mazzia VDB: Anesthesiology: Its Perils and Pitfalls. Trauma 33:88–96, 1991.
22. e.g, Fla.Stat. 766.103(4) (1991). Parr v Palmyra Hospital, 228 SE2d 596 (Ga Appl. 1976).
23. American College of Obstetricians and Gynecologists. Ethical Considerations of Informal Consent. ACOG Committee Opinion 108, Washington, DC, ACOG, 1992.
24. Danzon PM: Medical Malpractice. Theory, Evidence and Public Policy. Cambridge, Harvard University Press, 1985.
25. Joint Commission on Accreditation of Health Care Organizations. Accreditation Manual for Hospitals, 1991.
26. Cheney FW, Posner K, Caplan RA, Ward RJ: Standard of Care and Anesthesia Liability. JAMA 261(11):1599, 1989.
27. Collins VJ: Principles of Anesthesiology. Ed. 2. Philadelphia, Lea and Febiger, 1976.
28. Gion H: Charting and the Anesthetic Record. *In* Introduction to the Practice of Anesthesia. Ed. 2. Edited by M Lichtiger, F Moya. Hagerstown, Harper and Row, 1978.
29. Dillon JB: The Prevention of Claims for Malpractice. Anesthesiology 18:794, 1957.
30. Chadwick HS, Posner K, Caplan RA, Ward RJ, Cheney FW: A Comparison of Obstetric and Nonobstetric Anesthesia Malpractice Claims. Anesthesiology 74:242, 1991.
31. ibid.
32. Endler GC, Mariona FG, Sokol RJ, Stevenson LB: Anesthesia-related Maternal Mortality in Michigan, 1972–1984. Am. J. Obstet. Gynecol. 159(1):187, 1988.
33. See: Insigna v LaBella, 543 So2d 209 (Fla 1989).
34. Blum JD: Economic Credentialing. J. Legal Medicine 12(4):

427, 1991. (A review of the legal aspects of staff credentialing and contracts).

35. Health Care Quality Improvement Act of 1986: 42 U.S.C. 11101–11152 (1991) But see: Patrick v Burget, 486 US 94 (1988), and Austin v McNamarra, 731 F Supp. 934 (C.D. Cal 1990).
36. 42 U.S.C. 13951(1)(5)(B), Sec. 1833 (1)(5)(B) See also: Anesthesiologists Affiliated et al v Sullivan, 941 F2d 678 (8th Cir. 1991) (Claims for CRNA services not employed by the anesthesiologists and other issues.)
37. 42 U.S.C. 13951(1)(6), Sec. 1833 (1)(6).
38. See: Fossett JW, et al: Medicaid in The Inner City: The Case of Maternity Care in Chicago. Milbank Quarterly 68(1):111, 1990. Mitchell JB Schurman R: Access to Private Obstetric/Gynecology Services Under Medicaid. Medical Care 22(11): 1026, 1984.
39. eg, 42 U.S.C. 1320a-7a, Sec 4.08, 4.09
40. eg, 42 U.S.C. 11131, Sec. 421 (Failure to report medical malpractice payments)
41. eg 42 U.S.C. 1320a-7b, Sec. 1128(B)(b)(1) et seq. See also: Copeland Wm: Recruiting Physicians: Avoiding The Legal Minefield. Hospital and Health Services Administration 37(2):269, 1992. 56 Fed. Reg. 35,952 1992 (questionably final Safe Harbor definitions). Tedrick S: Legal Issues in Physician Self-Referral and Other Health Care Business Relationships. J. Legal. Medicine 13(4):521, 1992.
42. See: Roe v Wade 410 U.S. 113 (1973) (Women's Rights to abortion. Decision based on privacy).
43. Dellinger AM, Brannon JG: Medical Records: Refusal to Disclose or Improper Disclosure. *In* Healthcare Facilities Law. Edited by AM Dellinger. Boston, Little Brown, 1991, Sec. 8.12.
44. Moore v Regents of University of California, 793 P2d 479 (Cal 1990) (Patient's cells used for alleged profit-making research).
45. Gibbs CP, Krischer J, Peckhan BM, Sharp H, Kirschbaum TH: Obstetric Anesthesia: A National Survey. Anesthesiology 65(3):298–306, 1986.
46. ibid.
47. Chadwick HS, Posner K, Caplan RA, Ward RJ, Cheney FW: A Comparison of Obstetric and Nonobstetric Anesethesia Malpractice Claims. Anesthesiology 74:242–249, 1991.
48. Cheek TG, Gutsche BB: Pulmonary Aspiration of Gastric Contents. *In* Anesthesia for Obstetrics. Ed. 2. Edited by SM Shnider, G Levinson. Baltimore, Williams & Wilkins, 1987.
49. Endler GC, Mariona FG, Sokol RJ, Stevenson LB: Anesthesia-related Maternal Mortality in Michigan 1972–1984. Am. J. Obstet. Gynecol. 159(1):187, 1988.
50. Chadwick HS, op cit.
51. Foster v Englewood Hosp. Assn., 313 NE2d 255 (III App 1974). Sesselman v Muhlenberg Hosp., 306 A2d 474 (NJ Super 1973). Sparger v Worley Hosp. Inc., 547 SW2d 582 (Tex 197).
52. Dohr v Smith 104 So2d 29 (Fla 1958).
53. Bok S: Lying: Moral Choice in Public and Private Life. New York, Vintage, 1979.

# INDEX

Note: Page numbers in *italics* indicate figures; page numbers followed by t indicate tables.